SMITH'S
Anesthesia for Infants and Children

EIGHTH EDITION

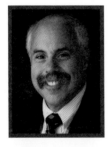

Peter J. Davis, MD, FAAP
Professor
Department of Anesthesiology
Department of Pediatrics
University of Pittsburgh School of Medicine;
Anesthesiologist-in-Chief
Children's Hospital of Pittsburgh of UPMC
Pittsburgh, Pennsylvania

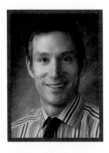

Franklyn P. Cladis, MD
Assistant Professor
Department of Anesthesiology
University of Pittsburgh School of Medicine
Children's Hospital of Pittsburgh of UPMC
Pittsburgh, Pennsylvania

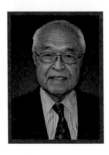

Etsuro K. Motoyama, MD, FAAP
Professor Emeritus
Department of Anesthesiology
Department of Pediatrics (Pulmonology)
University of Pittsburgh School of Medicine;
Former Director, Pediatric Pulmonology Laboratory
Children's Hospital of Pittsburgh of UPMC
Pittsburgh, Pennsylvania

ELSEVIER
MOSBY

ELSEVIER
MOSBY

1600 John F. Kennedy Blvd.
Ste 1800
Philadelphia, PA 19103-2899

SMITH'S ANESTHESIA FOR INFANTS AND CHILDREN   ISBN: 978-0-323-06612-9

Previous editions copyrighted 1959, 1963, 1968, 1980, 1990, 1996, 2006

International Standard Book Number 978-0-323-06612-9

Acquisitions Editor: Natasha Andjelkovic
Developmental Editor: Julie Mirra
Publishing Services Manager: Anne Altepeter
Team Manager: Radhika Pallamparthy
Senior Project Manager: Cheryl A. Abbott
Project Manager: Antony Prince
Design Direction: Steven Stave

Printed in the United States of America

Last digit is the print number: 9 8 7 6 5 4 3 2 1

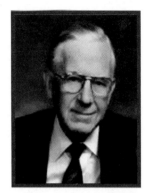

Dr. Robert Moors Smith

The eighth edition of *Smith's Anesthesia for Infants and Children* is dedicated to Dr. Robert Moors Smith, who died on November 25, 2009, 2 weeks before he would have been 97. The eulogy published by the Harvard Medical School's Office of Communications began with this statement: "The Harvard Medical School flag is at half-mast today in memory of Robert M. Smith, MD, Clinical Professor of Anesthesia, former Chief of Anesthesiology at Children's Hospital Boston and pioneer in clinical anesthesiology in children." This was an extraordinary tribute from an institution that has produced literally hundreds of world leaders in medicine.

Dr. Smith was one of the most distinguished pioneers of modern anesthesia for children in the world. In the United States he was considered the "Father of Pediatric Anesthesiology." During his tenure at Children's Hospital Boston, Dr. Smith was a superb and compassionate clinician and educator who continually advanced practices in pediatric anesthesia and kept abreast with the fast progress of increasingly complex surgery on smaller and younger patients. He was an early advocate of compassionate patient safety—more than 30 years before the term even existed.

Along with Dr. Margo Deming of Philadelphia, Dr. Smith was an early supporter of endotracheal intubation with sterile and child-appropriate–sized tubes to prevent aspiration and postintubation croup. He also encouraged the wrapping of small children to prevent heat loss. In the early 1950s when the monitoring of infants and children consisted of visual observation of the patient and intermittent palpation of the patient's radial pulse, Dr. Smith pioneered a new approach of continuous physiological monitoring. By using a stethoscope taped on the chest wall over the trachea and heart, Dr. Smith could assess ongoing changes in heart and breath sounds. Furthermore, Dr. Smith, together with Ms. Betty Lank, his chief nurse anesthetist, developed a homemade latex infant blood pressure cuff (referred to as the *Smith cuff*) and advocated its routine use for patient safety when inhaled anesthetics consisted of diethyl-ether and cyclopropane. These advancements were early steps in the development of elaborate physiological monitoring systems that are essential for safe anesthesia care today.

In 1959, Dr. Smith published the first comprehensive textbook for pediatric anesthesia, entitled *Anesthesia for Infants and Children*. It was well received among practitioners and trainees in pediatric anesthesia and soon became a classic, often referred to as the "Bible of Pediatric Anesthesia." For the ensuing 20 years until his retirement from Harvard in 1980, Dr. Smith revised and expanded the book through the fourth edition, as he kept abreast with the rapid progress in the practice and science of pediatric anesthesia and other pediatric surgical specialties. Shortly thereafter, Dr. Smith asked the current editors to assume the editorship. To continue his vision, the book was modified and expanded to a multi-authored volume and was renamed *Smith's Anesthesia for Infants and Children* in Dr. Smith's honor. The fifth through the seventh editions were published between 1990 and 2006. With this eighth edition, *Smith's Anesthesia for Infants and Children* has been in publication for more than half a century, making it the longest ongoing textbook of pediatric anesthesiology in the world. It has been a great honor and privilege for us to carry on Dr. Smith's legacy.

CONTRIBUTORS

Ann G. Bailey, MD
Professor, Anesthesiology and Pediatrics
University of North Carolina
Chapel Hill, North Carolina

David Barinholtz, MD
President and CEO, Mobile Anesthesiologists, LLC
Chicago, Illinois

Victor C. Baum, MD
Professor, Anesthesiology and Pediatrics
Executive Vice-Chair, Department of Anesthesiology
Director, Cardiac Anesthesia
University of Virginia
Charlottesville, Virginia

David S. Beebe, MD
Professor, Department of Anesthesiology
University of Minnesota
Minneapolis, Minnesota

Kumar G. Belani, MBBS, MS
Professor, Departments of Anesthesiology, Medicine,
    and Pediatrics
University of Minnesota
Minneapolis, Minnesota

Richard Berkowitz, MD
Chairman and Medical Director, Department of Anesthesiology
    and Pain Medicine
Community Hospital
Munster, Indiana;
Visiting Associate Professor, Department of Anesthesiology
    and Pediatrics
University of Illinois College of Medicine
Chicago, Illinois

Bruno Bissonnette, MD, FRCPC
Professor Emeritus of Anesthesia
University of Toronto
Toronto, Ontario;
Founder and President, Children of the World Anesthesia
    Foundation
Rimouski, Quebec

Adrian Bosenberg, MB ChB, FFA(SA)
Professor, University of Washington School
    of Medicine;
Director, Regional Anesthesia Services
Seattle Children's Hospital
Seattle, Washington

Barbara W. Brandom, MD
Professor, Department of Anesthesiology
University of Pittsburgh School of Medicine;
Attending Physician, Department of Anesthesiology
Children's Hospital of Pittsburgh of UPMC;
Director, North American Malignant Hyperthermia Registry
    of MHAUS
Pittsburgh, Pennsylvania

Claire Brett, MD
Professor, Clinical Anesthesia and Pediatrics
Department of Anesthesiology and Perioperative Care
University of California, San Francisco
San Francisco, California

Robert B. Bryskin, MD
Regional Anesthesia Coordinator
Nemours Children's Hospitals;
Assistant Professor, Anesthesiology
College of Medicine, Mayo Clinic
Jacksonville, Florida

Patrick Callahan, MD
Assistant Professor of Anesthesiology
University of Pittsburgh School of Medicine
Children's Hospital of Pittsburgh of UPMC
Pittsburgh, Pennsylvania

Franklyn P. Cladis, MD
Assistant Professor
Department of Anesthesiology
University of Pittsburgh School of Medicine
Children's Hospital of Pittsburgh of UPMC
Pittsburgh, Pennsylvania

David E. Cohen, MD
Associate Professor, Anesthesiology and Critical Care
   and Pediatrics
University of Pennsylvania;
Perioperative Medical Director, The Children's Hospital
   of Philadelphia
Philadelphia, Pennsylvania

Ira Todd Cohen, MD, MEd
Professor, Anesthesiology and Pediatrics
Director of Education, Department of Anesthesiology
   and Pain Medicine
Children's National Medical Center
Washington, DC

Andrew Davidson, MBBS, MD
Associate Professor, University of Melbourne;
Staff Anaesthetist, Royal Children's Hospital;
Head, Clinical Research Development
Murdoch Children's Research Institute
Melbourne, Victoria, Australia

Jessica Davis, BA, JD, LLM
Adjunct Professor, Widener University School of Law
Wilmington, Delaware

Peter J. Davis, MD, FAAP
Professor
Department of Anesthesiology
Department of Pediatrics
University of Pittsburgh School of Medicine;
Anesthesiologist-in-Chief
Children's Hospital of Pittsburgh of UPMC
Pittsburgh, Pennsylvania

Duncan de Souza, MD, FRCP(C)
Assistant Professor, Anesthesiology and Pediatrics
Department of Anesthesiology
University of Virginia
Charlottesville, Virginia

Nina Deutsch, MD
Assistant Professor, Anesthesiology and Pediatrics
Children's National Medical Center
Washington, DC

James A. DiNardo, MD, FAAP
Associate Professor of Anesthesia
Harvard Medical School;
Senior Associate in Cardiac Anesthesia
Program Director, Pediatric Cardiac Anesthesia Fellowship
Children's Hospital Boston
Boston, Massachusetts

Peter Ehrlich, MD, Msc, RCPS(C), FACS
Associate Professor of Surgery, Section of Pediatric Surgery
University of Michigan Medical School;
Medical Director, Pediatric Trauma
University of Michigan CS Mott Children's Hospital
Ann Arbor, Michigan

Demetrius Ellis, MD
Professor, Nephrology and Pediatrics
University of Pittsburgh School of Medicine;
Director, Pediatric Nephrology
Children's Hospital of Pittsburgh of UPMC
Pittsburgh, Pennsylvania

Jeffrey M. Feldman, MD, MSE
Division Chief, General Anesthesia
Children's Hospital of Philadelphia;
Associate Professor, Clinical Anesthesia
University of Pennsylvania School of Medicine
Philadelphia, Pennsylvania

Kathryn Felmet, MD
Assistant Professor, Critical Care Medicine and Pediatrics
University of Pittsburgh School of Medicine
Children's Hospital of Pittsburgh of UPMC
Pittsburgh, Pennsylvania

John E. Fiadjoe, MD
Assistant Professor, Anesthesia
Children's Hospital of Philadelphia
Philadelphia, Pennsylvania

Jonathan D. Finder, MD
Professor of Pediatrics
University of Pittsburgh School of Medicine
Clinical Director, Pulmonary Medicine
Children's Hospital of Pittsburgh of UPMC
Pittsburgh, Pennsylvania

Randall P. Flick, MD, MPH, FAAP
Associate Professor of Anesthesiology
Chair, Division of Pediatric Anesthesiology
Medical Director, Eugenio Litta Children's Hospital
Mayo Clinic
Rochester, Minnesota

Michelle Fortier, PhD
Licensed Psychologist
Center for the Advancement of Pediatric Health
University of California Irvine School of Medicine;
Department of Anesthesiology and Perioperative Care
Center for Pain Management
Orange, California

Salvatore R. Goodwin, MD
Associate Professor, Anesthesiology
Mayo Medical School
Rochester, Minnesota;
Chairman, Department of Anesthesia
Nemours Children's Clinic
Jacksonville, Florida

George A. Gregory, MD
Professor Emeritus of Anesthesia and Pediatrics
University of California, San Francisco
San Francisco, California

Lorelei Grunwaldt, MD
Assistant Professor of Surgery
University of Pittsburgh School of Medicine
Division of Pediatric Plastic Surgery
Children's Hospital of Pittsburgh of UPMC
Pittsburgh, Pennsylvania

Dawit T. Haile, MD
Instructor of Anesthesiology
Mayo Clinic
Rochester, Minnesota

Steven Hall, MD
Arthur C. King Professor of Pediatric Anesthesia
Feinberg School of Medicine
Northwestern University;
Anesthesiologist-in-Chief
Children's Memorial Hospital
Chicago, Illinois

Gregory Hammer, MD
Professor, Anesthesia and Pediatrics
Stanford University School of Medicine;
Associate Director, Pediatric ICU
Director, Pediatric Anesthesia Research
Lucile Packard Children's Hospital at Stanford
Stanford, California

Michael W. Hauser, MD
Staff Anesthesiologist
Cleveland Clinic
Cleveland, Ohio

Eugenie S. Heitmiller, MD
Associate Professor, Anesthesiology and Pediatrics
Department of Anesthesiology and Critical Care Medicine
The Johns Hopkins University School of Medicine;
Vice Chairman for Clinical Affairs
Department of Anesthesiology and Critical Care Medicine
The Johns Hopkins Hospital
Baltimore, Maryland

Andrew Herlich, DMD, MD
Professor of Anesthesia, Department of Anesthesiology
University of Pittsburgh School of Medicine;
Chief of Anesthesia, UPMC Mercy Hospital
Pittsburgh, Pennsylvania

Robert S. Holzman, MD, FAAP
Associate Professor of Anesthesia
Harvard Medical School;
Senior Associate, Perioperative Anesthesia
Children's Hospital Boston
Boston, Massachusetts

Elizabeth A. Hunt, MD, MPH, PhD
Assistant Professor, Department of Anesthesiology and Critical Care Medicine
The Johns Hopkins University School of Medicine;
Drs. David S. and Marilyn M. Zamierowski Director
The Johns Hopkins Medicine Simulation Center
Baltimore, Maryland

Nathalia Jimenez, MD, MPH
Assistant Professor, Department of Anesthesiology and Pain Medicine
University of Washington School of Medicine
Seattle Children's Hospital
Seattle, Washington

Lori T. Justice, MD, FAAP
Clinical Staff Pediatric Anesthesiologist
Children's Anesthesiologists, PC
East Tennessee Children's Hospital
Knoxville, Tennessee

Zeev N. Kain, MD, MBA
Professor, Anesthesiology and Pediatrics and Psychiatry and Human Behavior
Chair, Department of Anesthesiology and Perioperative Care
Associate Dean of Clinical Operations, School of Medicine
University of California, Irvine
Orange, California

Evan Kharasch, MD, PhD
Vice Chancellor for Research
Russell D. and Mary B. Shelden Professor of Anesthesiology
Director, Division of Clinical and Translational Research
Department of Anesthesiology;
Professor of Biochemistry and Molecular Biophysics
Washington University in St. Louis
St. Louis, Missouri

Sabine Kost-Byerly, MD, FAAP
Director, Pediatric Pain Management
Department of Anesthesiology and Critical Care Medicine
The Johns Hopkins Hospital;
Associate Professor of Anesthesiology
The Johns Hopkins University School of Medicine
Baltimore, Maryland

Elliot J. Krane, MD
Professor, Department of Anesthesia and Pediatrics
Stanford University School of Medicine
Stanford, California;
Director of Pain Management
Lucile Packard Children's Hospital at Stanford
Palo Alto, California

Barry D. Kussman, MBBCh, FFA (SA)
Assistant Professor of Anesthesia
Harvard Medical School;
Senior Associate in Cardiac Anesthesia
Children's Hospital Boston
Boston, Massachusetts

Ira S. Landsman, MD
Associate Professor, Department of Anesthesiology and Pediatrics;
Chief, Division of Pediatric Anesthesiology
Vanderbilt University Medical Center
Nashville, Tennessee

Ronald S. Litman, DO
Attending Anesthesiologist
The Children's Hospital of Philadelphia;
Professor, Anesthesiology and Pediatrics
University of Pennsylvania School of Medicine
Philadelphia, Pennsylvania

Joseph Losee, MD, FACS, FAAP
Professor of Surgery and Pediatrics
University of Pittsburgh School of Medicine
Chief, Division Pediatric Plastic Surgery
Children's Hospital of Pittsburgh of UPMC
Pittsburgh, Pennsylvania

Igor Luginbuehl, MD
Associate Professor of Anesthesia
Department of Anesthesia and Pain Medicine
The Hospital for Sick Children
Toronto, Ontario

Anne M. Lynn, MD
Professor, Department of Anesthesiology
   and Pain Medicine
Adjunct Professor, Pediatrics
University of Washington School of Medicine
Seattle Children's Hospital
Seattle, Washington

Thomas J. Mancuso, MD
Associate Professor of Anesthesia
Harvard Medical School;
Senior Associate in Anesthesia
Children's Hospital Boston
Boston, Massachusetts

Brian P. Martin, DMD
Clinical Assistant Professor
University of Pittsburgh School of Dental
   Medicine;
Chief, Division of Pediatric Dentistry
Children's Hospital of Pittsburgh of UPMC
Pittsburgh, Pennsylvania

Keira Mason, MD
Associate Professor of Anesthesia
Harvard Medical School;
Director, Department of Radiology, Anesthesia,
   and Sedation
Children's Hospital Boston
Boston, Massachusetts

William J. Mauermann, MD
Assistant Professor of Anesthesia
Mayo Clinic
Rochester, Minnesota

Lynne G. Maxwell, MD
Associate Professor of Anesthesiology and Critical Care
University of Pennsylvania
Senior Anesthesiologist
Children's Hospital of Philadelphia
Philadelphia, Pennsylvania

George M. McDaniel, MD, MS
Assistant Professor of Pediatrics and Internal
   Medicine
Director, Pediatric Electrophysiology
University of Virginia
Charlottesville, Virginia

Francis X. McGowan, Jr., MD
Professor of Anesthesia
Harvard Medical School;
Chief, Division of Cardiac Anesthesia
Director, Anesthesia and Critical Care
   Medicine
Research Laboratory
Children's Hospital Boston
Boston, Massachusetts

Constance L. Monitto, MD
Assistant Professor, Anesthesiology and Critical
   Care Medicine
The Johns Hopkins University School
   of Medicine
Baltimore, Maryland

Philip G. Morgan, MD
Professor, Department of Anesthesiology
University of Washington;
Seattle Children's Research Institute
Seattle, Washington

Etsuro K. Motoyama, MD, FAAP
Professor Emeritus
Department of Anesthesiology
Department of Pediatrics (Pulmonology)
University of Pittsburgh School of Medicine;
Former Director, Pediatric Pulmonology Laboratory
Children's Hospital of Pittsburgh of UPMC
Pittsburgh, Pennsylvania

Julie Niezgoda, MD
Pediatric Anesthesiology
Children's Hospital Cleveland Clinic
Cleveland Clinic
Cleveland, Ohio

David M. Polaner, MD, FAAP
Professor of Anesthesiology and Pediatrics
University of Colorado School of Medicine;
Attending Pediatric Anesthesiologist
Chief, Acute Pain Service
Anesthesia Informatics
The Children's Hospital, Denver
Aurora, Colorado

Paul Reynolds, MD
Uma and Sujit Pandit Professor and Chief of Pediatric
   Anesthesiology
Department of Anesthesiology
University of Michigan
Ann Arbor, Michigan

Mark A. Rockoff, MD
Professor of Anesthesia
Harvard Medical School;
Vice-Chairman, Department of Anesthesiology, Perioperative
    and Pain Medicine
Children's Hospital Boston
Boston, Massachusetts

Thomas Romanelli, MD, FAAP
Clinical Instructor, Harvard Medical School;
Consultant Anesthesiologist
Shriners Burns Hospital Boston;
Assistant in Anesthesia
Massachusetts General Hospital
Boston, Massachusetts

Allison Kinder Ross, MD
Associate Professor and Chief, Division of Pediatric Anesthesia
Duke University Medical Center
Durham, North Carolina

Joseph A. Scattoloni, MD
Clinical Lecturer, Department of Anesthesia
Section of Pediatric Anesthesia
University of Michigan Health System
Ann Arbor, Michigan

Jamie McElrath Schwartz, MD
Assistant Professor, Departments of Anesthesiology and
    Critical Care Medicine and Pediatrics
The Johns Hopkins University School of Medicine
Baltimore, Maryland

Robert J. Sclabassi, MD, PhD, DABNM, FASNM
Attending Neurophysiologist
Chief, Intraoperative Monitoring Service
West Penn Alleghany Health System
Pittsburgh, Pennsylvania

Victor L. Scott, II, BSc, MD
Professor of Anesthesiology, Department of Anesthesiology
University of Pittsburgh School of Medicine
Children's Hospital of Pittsburgh of UPMC
Pittsburgh, Pennsylvania

Donald H. Shaffner, MD
Associate Professor, Department of Anesthesiology
Critical Care Medicine and Pediatrics
The Johns Hopkins University School of Medicine
Baltimore, Maryland

Avinash C. Shukla, MBBS, FRCA
Associate in Cardiac Anesthesia
Children's Hospital Boston
Boston, Massachusetts

†Robert M. Smith, MD
Clinical Professor Emeritus of Anesthesia
Harvard Medical School and Children's Hospital Boston
Boston, Massachusetts

Kyle Soltys, MD
Assistant Professor of Surgery
University of Pittsburgh School of Medicine
Thomas E. Starzl Transplant Institute
Hillman Center For Pediatric Transplantation
Children's Hospital of Pittsburgh of UPMC
Pittsburgh, Pennsylvania

Sulpicio G. Soriano, MD
Children's Hospital Boston Endowed Chair in Pediatric
    Neuroanesthesia
Associate Professor of Anesthesia
Harvard Medical School;
Senior Associate, Department of Anesthesiology, Perioperative
    and Pain Medicine
Children's Hospital Boston
Boston, Massachusetts

Brian P. Struyk, MD
Assistant Professor, Clinical Anesthesiology
    and Critical Care
University of Pennsylvania School of Medicine;
Director, Radiology Anesthesia
Children's Hospital of Philadelphia
Philadelphia, Pennsylvania

Kevin J. Sullivan, MD
Assistant Professor of Anesthesiology
Rochester, Minnesota;
Clinical Associate Professor of Pediatrics
University of Florida Health Science Center
Jacksonville, Florida;
Staff Pediatric Anesthesiologist, Critical Care Physician,
    and Medical Director
Pediatric Intensive Care Unit
Wolfson Children's Hospital
Jacksonville, Florida

Jennifer Thomas, MBChB, FFA (SA), BSc (Ed)
Associate Professor, Department of Pediatric Anaesthesia
Red Cross War Memorial Children's Hospital
University of Cape Town
Cape Town, Western Cape, South Africa

Stevan P. Tofovic, MD, PhD, FAHA, FASN
Assistant Professor of Medicine
University of Pittsburgh School of Medicine
Pittsburgh, Pennsylvania

Kha Tran, MD
Assistant Professor of Anesthesia and Critical Care Medicine
University of Pennsylvania School of Medicine;
Attending Anesthesiologist and Clinical Director, Fetal
    Anesthesia Team
Children's Hospital of Philadelphia
Philadelphia, Pennsylvania

Donald C. Tyler, MD, MBA
Associate Professor of Anesthesiology and Critical Care
University of Pennsylvania
Department of Anesthesiology and Critical Care Medicine
The Hospital of the University of Pennsylvania
    and Children's Hospital of Philadelphia
Philadelphia, Pennsylvania

---

†Deceased.

Robert D. Valley, MD
Professor of Anesthesiology and Pediatrics
University of North Carolina School of Medicine
Chapel Hill, North Carolina

Monica S. Vavilala, MD
Associate Professor, Department of Anesthesiology and Pain
   Medicine and Pediatrics
Adjunct Associate Professor, Neurological Surgery
   and Radiology
University of Washington;
Associate Director, Harborview Injury Prevention
   and Research Center
Seattle, Washington

Lisa Vecchione, DMD, MDS
Director, Orthodontic Services
Cleft-Craniofacial Center
Children's Hospital of Pittsburgh of UPMC;
Assistant Clinical Professor of Surgery
University of Pittsburgh School of Medicine
Pittsburgh, Pennsylvania

Kerri M. Wahl, MD, FRCP(C)
Associate Professor, Department
   of Anesthesiology
Duke University Medical Center
Durham, North Carolina

Jay A. Werkhaven, MD
Associate Professor and Director, Pediatric Otolaryngology
Vanderbilt Bill Wilkerson Center for Otolaryngology
   and Communication Sciences
Vanderbilt University
Nashville, Tennessee

Susan Woelfel, MD
Associate Professor of Anesthesiology
University of Pittsburgh School of Medicine
Children's Hospital of Pittsburgh of UPMC
Pittsburgh, Pennsylvania

Myron Yaster, MD
Richard J. Traystman Professor
Departments of Anesthesiology, Critical Care Medicine,
   and Pediatrics
The Johns Hopkins University School of Medicine
Baltimore, Maryland

Aaron L. Zuckerberg, MD
Director, Pediatric Anesthesia and Critical Care Medicine
Director, Children's Diagnostic Center Department
   of Pediatrics and Anesthesia
Sinai Hospital;
Assistant Professor, Department of Pediatrics
University of Maryland Medical School;
Director of Pediatric Anesthesia, Department of Anesthesia,
   NAPA/MD
Baltimore, Maryland

CONTRIBUTORS TO THE SUPPLEMENTAL MATERIAL

Cuneyt M. Alper, MD
Professor of Otolaryngology
University of Pittsburgh School of Medicine
Division of Pediatric Otolaryngology
Children's Hospital of Pittsburgh of UPMC
Pittsburgh, Pennsylvania

Lawrence M. Borland, MD
Associate Professor
Departments of Anesthesiology and Pediatrics
University of Pittsburgh School of Medicine
Children's Hospital of Pittsburgh of UPMC
Pittsburgh, Pennsylvania

Robert B. Bryskin, MD
Regional Anesthesia Coordinator
Nemours Children's Hospitals;
Assistant Professor, Anesthesiology
College of Medicine, Mayo Clinic
Jacksonville, Florida

James G. Cain, MD
Visiting Associate Professor
Department of Anesthesiology
University of Pittsburgh School of Medicine
Pittsburgh, Pennsylvania

Franklyn P. Cladis, MD
Assistant Professor
Department of Anesthesiology
University of Pittsburgh School of Medicine
Children's Hospital of Pittsburgh of UPMC
Pittsburgh, Pennsylvania

Peter J. Davis, MD, FAAP
Professor
Department of Anesthesiology
Department of Pediatrics
University of Pittsburgh School of Medicine;
Anesthesiologist-in-Chief
Children's Hospital of Pittsburgh of UPMC
Pittsburgh, Pennsylvania

William A. Devine
Curator of the Frank E. Sherman, MD, and
   Cora C. Lenox, MD, Heart Museum
Department of Pathology
Children's Hospital of Pittsburgh of UPMC
Pittsburgh, Pennsylvania

Joseph E. Dohar, MD, MS, FAAP, FACS
Professor of Otolaryngology
University of Pittsburgh School of Medicine;
Clinical Director, Pediatric Voice, Resonance,
   and Swallowing Center
Department of Otolaryngology
Children's Hospital of Pittsburgh of UPMC
Pittsburgh, Pennsylvania

Christopher M. Grande, MD, MPH
Anesthesiologist and Intensivist
Executive Director, International Trauma Anesthesia
   and Critical Care Society (ITACCS)
Baltimore, Maryland

Gregory Hammer, MD
Professor, Departments of Anesthesia and Pediatrics
Stanford University School of Medicine;
Associate Director, Pediatric ICU
Director, Pediatric Anesthesia Research
Lucile Packard Children's Hospital at Stanford
Stanford, California

Timothy D. Kane, MD, FACS
Associate Professor of Surgery and Pediatrics
George Washington University School of Medicine
Children's National Medical Center and Sheikh
   Zayed Institute for Pediatric Surgical Innovation
Washington, DC

Lizabeth M. Lanford, MD
Clinical Assistant Professor of Pediatrics
University of Pittsburgh School of Medicine
Division of Pediatric Cardiology
Children's Hospital of Pittsburgh of UPMC
Pittsburgh, Pennsylvania

George V. Mazariegos, MD
Professor of Surgery and Critical Care
University of Pittsburgh School of Medicine;
Chief, Pediatric Transplantation
Children's Hospital of Pittsburgh of UPMC
Pittsburgh, Pennsylvania

Etsuro K. Motoyama, MD, FAAP
Professor Emeritus
Department of Anesthesiology
Department of Pediatrics (Pulmonology)
University of Pittsburgh School of Medicine;
Former Director, Pediatric Pulmonology Laboratory
Children's Hospital of Pittsburgh of UPMC
Pittsburgh, Pennsylvania

Douglas A. Potoka, MD
Assistant Professor of Surgery
University of Pittsburgh School of Medicine
Department of Pediatric General and Thoracic Surgery
Children's Hospital of Pittsburgh of UPMC
Pittsburgh, Pennsylvania

Paul Reynolds, MD
Uma and Sujit Pandit Professor and Chief of Pediatric
   Anesthesiology
Department of Anesthesiology
University of Michigan
Ann Arbor, Michigan

Allison Kinder Ross, MD
Associate Professor and Chief
Division of Pediatric Anesthesia
Duke University Medical Center
Durham, North Carolina

Kenneth P. Rothfield, MD
Chairman, Department of Anesthesiology
Saint Agnes Hospital
Baltimore, Maryland

Victor L. Scott, II, BSc, MD
Professor of Anesthesiology
Department of Anesthesiology
University of Pittsburgh School of Medicine
Children's Hospital of Pittsburgh of UPMC
Pittsburgh, Pennsylvania

Robert F. Yellon, MD, FACS
Professor, Department of Otolaryngology
University of Pittsburgh School of Medicine;
Director of Clinical Services
Department of Pediatric Otolaryngology
Children's Hospital of Pittsburgh of UPMC
Pittsburgh, Pennsylvania

Dr. Robert Moors Smith, a distinguished pioneer of modern pediatric anesthesia who was known as the "Father of Pediatric Anesthesia" in the United States, passed away on November 25, 2009, 2 weeks before he would have turned 97. In 1959, Dr. Smith wrote the first comprehensive textbook, *Anesthesia for Infants and Children,* specifically dedicated to the anesthetic management and care of children when pediatric anesthesia was in its infancy and the essentials of pediatric anesthesia practice were barely taking form.

During the following 2 decades as pediatric anesthesia expanded along with the rapid development and expansion of pediatric surgery, Dr. Smith published three additional revised and updated editions with few contributors. The book remained popular as the primary reference source of pediatric anesthesia practice and was often referred to as the "Bible" for practicing pediatric anesthesiologists.

After the fourth edition was published in 1980 and before his retirement from Children's Hospital Boston and Harvard Medical School, Dr. Smith transferred the honor and responsibility of continuing the legacy of his textbook to me, a former fellow and associate in the 1960s and one of the few contributors to the later editions.

From the 1980s and onward, we witnessed continual, if not exponential, expansions in pediatric anesthesia and related fields, with the expansion of pediatric surgical subspecialties and techniques, including the development of neonatal and pediatric intensive care units and intensive care medicine; improvements in anesthesia-related equipment, monitors, and newer anesthetic and adjuvant drugs; establishment of clinical practice standards; expansions in postgraduate anesthesiology training programs; and the development of clinical and basic research activities directly or indirectly related to anesthesiology, physiology, pharmacology, and cell and molecular biology. It became obvious that a single-author textbook in our subspecialty was no longer feasible or desirable.

I was extremely fortunate to have Dr. Peter J. Davis join me to face the new challenge. Our cordial and productive collaboration has lasted for more than 2 decades and still continues today. Peter and I changed the format of the book and expanded it to a multi-author textbook. We published the fifth edition in 1990 with the modified title *Smith's Anesthesia for Infants and Children* to honor Dr. Smith's legacy (against Dr. Smith's initial protest). In subsequent editions in 1996 (sixth edition) and 2006 (seventh edition), we added new chapters authored by experts in specific fields to keep up with the development and expansion of science and practice of pediatric anesthesia, including critical care medicine, psychology, regional anesthesia, pain medicine, and bariatric surgery.

Anesthesia for Infants and Children has surpassed half a century of continual publication since the first edition in 1959, and I have been extremely fortunate to have been closely associated with Bob Smith professionally as well as personally since my fellowship days in Boston in the 1960s. (Bob was particularly pleased to note the half-century mark of his publication when I visited him for the last time in the early summer of 2009 in his lifelong hometown of Winchester, Massachusetts.) With the passing of a giant in the field, it is also the time to pass the torch to Peter Davis as the principal editor, with Dr. Franklyn Cladis as a new member, for the eighth edition, which is dedicated to the memory of Dr. Robert Moors Smith and his glorious life as a family man, compassionate pediatric physician, and a kind mentor to former trainees.

Etsuro K. Motoyama, MD, FAAP

Dr. Robert Moors Smith's legacy is as a pioneer and a great educator in pediatric anesthesia. Long before the terminology became fashionable—before it even existed—Dr. Smith advocated patient monitoring and safety. In the 1950s, when pediatric anesthesia was still in its infancy, he made the use of the precordial stethoscope and the pediatric blood pressure cuff (Smith cuff) a standard of care. In 1959, he wrote a major comprehensive anesthesia textbook, *Anesthesia for Infants and Children,* which was specifically dedicated to the anesthetic management and care of children.

The first four editions of this book were written almost entirely by Dr. Smith himself. The scope of Dr. Smith's scholarship was reflected in the breadth of his firsthand clinical experience, his keen sense of observation, and his ability to apply scientific and technical developments in medicine and anesthesia to the field of pediatric anesthesia. In 1988, Dr. Smith became the first pediatric anesthesiologist to receive the Distinguished Service Award from the American Society of Anesthesiologists.

In 1980, with Dr. Smith's retirement from the Harvard Medical School faculty and the anesthesia directorship of Children's Hospital Boston, the task of updating this classic textbook was bestowed upon Drs. Motoyama and Davis. The fifth edition, published in 1990, was multi-authored and was reorganized to include new subjects of importance in the ever-expanding field of anesthesiology and pediatric anesthesiology in particular. In the fifth edition, the editors tried to maintain Dr. Smith's compassion, philosophy, and emphasis on the personal approach to patients. To honor his pioneering work and leadership (and against Dr. Smith's initial strong resistance), the title of the fifth edition of the textbook was modified to read *Smith's Anesthesia for Infants and Children.*

In 1996, the sixth edition of the textbook was published. New developments with inhaled anesthetic agents (sevoflurane and desflurane), intravenous agents (propofol), neuromuscular-blocking agents, and anesthetic adjuncts, coupled with changes in the approach to pediatric pain management and airway management, were highlights.

In 2006, the seventh edition further expanded those areas of development. The roles of airway management, regional anesthesia, new local anesthetic agents, and innovative regional anesthetic techniques had been further developed. Newer intravenous anesthetic agents and adjuncts were also included in this edition while maintaining Dr. Smith's principles regarding patient safety and compassion.

The eighth edition has been prepared with the same considerations as the previous seven editions: to give anesthesia care providers comprehensive coverage of the physiology, pharmacology, and clinical anesthetic management of infants and children of all ages. This edition remains organized into four sections. Part I, Basic Principles, has been updated with major revisions to the chapters Respiratory Physiology in Infants and Children, Cardiovascular Physiology, Regulation of Fluids and Electrolytes, Thermoregulation: Physiology and Perioperative Disturbances, and Pharmacology of Pediatric Anesthesia. A chapter on Behavioral Development has been added to this section to help the clinician to better understand the normal behavioral responses of children. Part II, General Approach to Pediatric Anesthesia, has had a number of changes in the authorship of the chapters. New chapters on Pain Managemant, Blood Conservation, Airway Management, and Regional Anesthesia have been added. In addition, real-time use of ultrasound has been incorporated into the website to further enhance the techniques of regional anesthesia. All other chapters in this section have been updated by the same group of contributors as in the seventh edition. Part III, Clinical Management of Specialized Surgical Problems, contains new material. In response to the increasing number of neonatal and fetal surgeries, a new chapter on Neonatology for Anesthesiologists has been added. This is a chapter designed to explore the physiology, development, and care of high-risk neonates. This chapter complements the chapters Anesthesia for Fetal Surgery and Anesthesia for General Surgery in the Neonate. In addition to Neonatology for Anesthesiologists, a chapter on Anesthesia for Conjoined Twins has been added. The chapters on congenital heart disease have been reorganized and written by new contributors. Other chapters with new contributors include Anesthesia for Plastic Surgery, Anesthesia for Neurosurgery, Anesthesia for Fetal Surgery, and Anesthesia for Burn Injuries. The remaining chapters in this section have been updated by the same group of contributors. Part IV, Associated Problems in Pediatric Anesthesia, contains updated and revised chapters on Cardiopulmonary Resuscitation, Medicolegal and Ethical Aspects, Malignant Hyperthermia, and Systemic Disorders. A new chapter on Critical Care Medicine has been added. Of note, the chapter History of Pediatric Anesthesia has been updated by Dr. Mark A. Rockoff, who had direct consultation with Dr. Robert M. Smith before Dr. Smith's death. The appendixes, which can be found online at www.expertconsult.com, include an updated list of drugs and their dosages, normal growth curves, normal values for pulmonary function tests in children, and an expanded list of common and uncommon syndromes of clinical importance for pediatric anesthesiologists.

In keeping with the advancement in technology, this edition is now in color and the text material is further supplemented by a website. Videos of airway techniques, single-lung isolation, regional anesthesia, the use of ultrasound, and anatomic disections of congenital heart lesions are accessible with just a click of the mouse. In addition, supplemental materials on organ transplantation, airway lesions, and pediatric syndromes are available.

In summary, considerable developments and progress in the practice of pediatric anesthesia over the past decade are reflected in this new edition. The emphasis on the safety and well-being of our young patients during the perianesthetic period remains unchanged.

Peter J. Davis, MD, FAAP
Franklyn P. Cladis, MD
Etsuro K. Motoyama, MD, FAAP

ACKNOWLEDGMENTS

The project of revising a classic medical textbook presents many opportunities and challenges. The chance to review the many new developments that have emerged in pediatric anesthesia since the publication of the last edition of *Smith's Anesthesia for Infants and Children* in 2006 and to evaluate their effects on clinical practice has indeed been exciting. As always, we are deeply indebted to the extraordinary work done and commitment made by Dr. Robert M. Smith. Beginning shortly after World War II, Dr. Smith pioneered pediatric anesthesia in the United States. Between 1959 and 1980, he published the first four editions of his book, *Anesthesia for Infants and Children*. His work made this textbook a classic, establishing a quality and record of longevity. The first through fourth editions were written almost exclusively by Dr. Smith, except for the chapter on respiratory physiology by E.K. Motoyama. Since the late 1980s when Dr. Smith passed the book to Drs. Motoyama and Davis, the subsequent fifth, sixth, and seventh editions have utilized the talents and expertise of many renowned pediatric anesthesiologists throughout North America. The seventh edition had been expanded by the addition of new chapters, new contributors, and an enclosed DVD. The eighth edition brings change to the book in both content and presentation. New chapters and new contributors have further advanced our knowledge base. The presentation of the material has been enhanced by the use of color and by providing access to a website to further supplement the book's written text material. In addition, the editorial components of the book have been changed and expanded. Franklyn Cladis has joined the book's lineage of editors.

Our ability to maintain this book's standard of excellence is not just a reflection of the many gifted contributors but is also a result of the level of support that we have received at work and at home. We wish to thank the staff members of the Department of Anesthesiology at Children's Hospital of Pittsburgh of UPMC and the University of Pittsburgh Medical Center for their support and tolerance.

Our special thanks go to Shannon Barnes, editorial assistant, as well as Susan Danfelt and Patty Klein, administrative assistants, of the Department of Anesthesiology, Children's Hospital of Pittsburgh of UPMC, for their many hours of diligent work on the book. We are also appreciative of Dr. Basil Zitelli, Professor of Pediatrics, University of Pittsburgh at Children's Hospital of Pittsburgh of UPMC, for his generosity in allowing us to use many of the photographs published in his own book, *Atlas of Pediatric Physical Diagnosis*.

Our special thanks also go to Elsevier's Natasha Andjelkovic, acquisitions editor; Julie Mirra, developmental editor; and Cheryl Abbott, senior project manager, for their editorial assistance.

Finally, as with the previous two editions, we are deeply indebted to our family members Katie, Evan, Julie, and Zara Davis; Yoko, Eugene, and Ray Motoyama; and Joseph Losee and Hudson Cladis Losee for remaining loyal, for being understanding, and for providing moral support throughout the lengthy and, at times, seemingly endless project.

Peter J. Davis, MD, FAAP
Franklyn P. Cladis, MD
Etsuro K. Motoyama, MD, FAAP

CONTENTS

PART IV: Associated Problems in Pediatric Anesthesia

Abbreviations

See inside back cover of this text.

Supplemental Material

To all of the children we care for and from whom we learn every day

Basic Principles

Special Characteristics of Pediatric Anesthesia

Peter J. Davis, Etsuro K. Motoyama, and Franklyn P. Cladis

CONTENTS

In the past few decades, new scientific knowledge of physiology and pharmacology in developing humans, as well as technologic advancements in equipment and monitoring, has markedly changed the practice of pediatric anesthesia. In addition, further emphasis on patient safety (e.g., correct side-site surgery, correct patient identification, correct procedure, appropriate prophylactic antibiotics) coupled with advances in minimally invasive pediatric surgery, have created a need for better pharmacologic approaches to infants and children, as well as improved skills in pediatric anesthetic management.

As a result of the advancements and emphasis on pediatric subspecialty training and practice, the American Board of Anesthesiology has now come to recognize the subspecialty of pediatric anesthesiology in its certification process.

PERIOPERATIVE MONITORING

In the 1940s and 1950s, the techniques of pediatric anesthesia, as well as the skills of those using and teaching them, evolved more as an art than as a science, as [†]Dr. Robert Smith vividly and eloquently recollects through his firsthand experiences in his chapter on the history of pediatric anesthesia (see Chapter 41, History of Pediatric Anesthesia, as updated by Mark Rockoff). The anesthetic agents and methods available were limited, as was the scientific knowledge of developmental differences in organ-system function and anesthetic effect in infants and children. Monitoring pediatric patients was limited to inspection of chest movement and occasional palpation of the pulse until the late 1940s, when Smith introduced the first physiologic monitoring to pediatric anesthesia by using the precordial stethoscope

for continuous auscultation of heartbeat and breath sounds (Smith, 1953; 1968). Until the mid-1960s, many anesthesiologists monitored only the heart rate in infants and small children during anesthesia and surgery. Electrocardiographic and blood-pressure measurements were either too difficult or too extravagant and were thought to provide little or no useful information. Measurements of central venous pressure were thought to be inaccurate and too invasive even in major surgical procedures. The insertion of an indwelling urinary (Foley) catheter in infants was considered invasive and was resisted by surgeons.

Smith also added an additional physiologic monitoring: soft, latex blood-pressure cuffs suitable for newborn and older infants, which encouraged the use of blood pressure monitoring in children (Smith, 1968). The "Smith cuff" (see Chapter 41, History of Pediatric Anesthesia, Fig. 41-4) remained the standard monitoring device in infants and children until the late 1970s, when it began to be replaced by automated blood pressure devices.

The introduction of pulse oximetry for routine clinical use in the early 1990s has been the single most important development in monitoring and patient safety, especially related to pediatric anesthesia, since the advent of the precordial stethoscope in the 1950s (see Chapters 10, Equipment; 11, Monitoring; and 40, Safety and Outcome) (Smith, 1956). Pulse oximetry is superior to clinical observation and other means of monitoring, such as capnography, for the detection of intraoperative hypoxemia (Coté et al., 1988, 1991). In addition, Spears and colleagues (1991) have indicated that experienced pediatric anesthesiologists may not have an "educated hand" or a "feel" adequate to detect changes in pulmonary compliance in infants. Pulse oximetry has revealed that postoperative hypoxemia occurs commonly among otherwise healthy infants and children undergoing simple surgical

---

[†]Deceased.

procedures, presumably as a result of significant reductions in functional residual capacity (FRC) and resultant airway closure and atelectasis (Motoyama and Glazener, 1986). Consequently, the use of supplemental oxygen in the postanesthesia care unit (PACU) has become a part of routine postanesthetic care (see Chapter 3, Respiratory Physiology).

Although pulse oximetry greatly improved patient monitoring, there were some limitations, namely motion artifact and inaccuracy in low-flow states, and in children with levels of low oxygen saturation (e.g., cyanotic congenital heart disease). Advances have been made in the new generation of pulse oximetry, most notably through the use of Masimo Signal Extraction Technology (SET). This device minimizes the effect of motion artifact, improves accuracy, and has been shown to have advantages over the existing system in low-flow states, mild hypothermia, and moving patients (Malviya et al., 2000; Hay et al., 2002; Irita et al., 2003).

Monitoring of cerebral function and blood flow, as well as infrared brain oximetry have advanced the anesthetic care and perioperative management of infants and children with congenital heart disease and traumatic brain injuries. Depth of anesthesia can be difficult to assess in children, and anesthetic overdose was a major cause of anesthesia-associated cardiac arrest and mortality. Depth-of-anesthesia monitors (bisectral index monitor [BIS], Patient State Index, Narcotrend) have been used in children and have been associated with the administration of less anesthetic agent and faster recovery from anesthesia. However, because these monitors use electroencephalography and a sophisticated algorithm to predict consciousness, the reliability of these monitors in children younger than 1 year old is limited.

In addition to advances in monitors for individual patients, hospital, patient, and outside-agency initiatives have focused on more global issues. Issues of patient safety, side-site markings, time outs, and proper patient identification together with the appropriate administration of prophylactic antibiotics have now become major priorities for health care systems. The World Health Organization (WHO) checklists have been positive initiatives that have ensured that the correct procedure is performed on the correct patient, as well as fostered better communication among health care workers. In anesthesia, patient safety continues to be a mantra for the specialty. Improved monitoring, better use of anesthetic agents, and the development of improved airway devices coupled with advancements in minimally invasive surgery, continue to advance the frontiers of pediatric anesthesia as a specialty medicine, as well as improve patient outcome and patient safety.

ANESTHETIC AGENTS

More than a decade after the release of isoflurane for clinical use, two volatile anesthetics, desflurane and sevoflurane, became available in the 1990s in most industrialized countries. Although these two agents are dissimilar in many ways, they share common physiochemical and pharmacologic characteristics: very low blood-gas partition coefficients (0.4 and 0.6, respectively), which are close to those of nitrous oxide and are only fractions of those of halothane and isoflurane; rapid induction of and emergence from surgical anesthesia; and hemodynamic stability (see Chapters 7, Pharmacology; 13, Induction Maintenance and recovery; and 34, Same-Day Surgical Procedures). In animal models, the use of inhaled anesthetic agents has been shown to attenuate the adverse effects of ischemia in the brain, heart, and kidneys.

Although these newer, less-soluble, inhaled agents allow for faster emergence from anesthesia, emergence excitation or delirium associated with their use has become a major concern to pediatric anesthesiologists (Davis et al., 1994; Sarner et al., 1995; Lerman et al., 1996; Welborn et al., 1996; Cravero et al., 2000; Kuratani and Oi, 2008). Adjuncts, such as opioids, analgesics, serotonin antagonists, and α_1-adrenergic agonists, have been found to decrease the incidence of emergence agitation (Aono et al., 1999; Davis et al., 1999; Galinkin et al., 2000; Cohen et al., 2001; Ko et al., 2001; Kulka et al., 2001; Voepel-Lewis et al., 2003; Lankinen et al., 2006; Aouad et al., 2007; Tazeroualti et al., 2007; Erdil et al., 2009; Bryan et al., 2009; Kim et al., 2009).

Propofol has increasingly been used in pediatric anesthesia as an induction agent, for intravenous sedation, or as the primary agent of a total intravenous technique (Martin et al., 1992). Propofol has the advantage of aiding rapid emergence and causes less nausea and vomiting during the postoperative period, particularly in children with a high risk of vomiting. When administered as a single dose (1 mg/kg) at the end of surgery, propofol has also been shown to decrease the incidence of sevoflurane-associated emergence agitation (Aouad et al., 2007).

Remifentanil, a μ-receptor agonist, is metabolized by nonspecific plasma and tissue esterases. The organ-independent elimination of remifentanil, coupled with its clearance rate (highest in neonates and infants compared with older children), makes its kinetic profile different from that of any other opioids (Davis et al., 1999; Ross et al., 2001). In addition, its ability to provide hemodynamic stability, coupled with its kinetic profile of rapid elimination and nonaccumulation, makes it an attractive anesthetic option for infants and children. Numerous clinical studies have described its use for pediatric anesthesia (Wee et al., 1999; Chiaretti et al., 2000; Davis et al., 2000, 2001; German et al., 2000; Dönmez et al., 2001; Galinkin et al., 2001; Keidan et al., 2001; Chambers et al., 2002; Friesen et al., 2003). When combined, intravenous hypnotic agents (remifentanil and propofol) have been shown to be as effective and of similar duration as propofol and succinylcholine for tracheal intubation.

The development of more predictable, shorter-acting anesthetic agents (see Chapter 7, Pharmacology) has increased the opportunities for pediatric anesthesiologists to provide safe and stable anesthesia with less dependence on the use of neuromuscular blocking agents.

AIRWAY DEVICES AND ADJUNCTS

Significant changes in pediatric airway management that have patient-safety implications have emerged over the past few years. The laryngeal mask airway (LMA), in addition to other supraglottic airway devices (e.g., the King LT-D, the Cobra pharyngeal airway), has become an integral part of pediatric airway management. Although the LMA is not a substitute for the endotracheal tube, LMAs can be safely used for routine anesthesia in both spontaneously ventilated patients and patients requiring pressure-controlled support. The LMA can also be used in the patient with a difficult airway to aid in ventilation and to act as a conduit to endotracheal intubation both with and without a fiber optic bronchoscope.

In addition to supraglottic devices, advances in technology for visualizing the airway have also improved patient safety. Since the larynx could be visualized, at least 50 devices intended for laryngoscopy have been invented. The newer airway-visualization devices have combined better visualizations, video capabilities, and high resolution.

The development and refinement of airway visualization equipment such as the Glidescope, Shikani Seeing Stylet, and the Bullard laryngoscope have added more options to the management of the pediatric airway and literally give the laryngoscopist the ability to see around corners (see Chapters 10, Equipment; and 12, Airway Management).

The variety of pediatric endotracheal tubes (ETTs) has focused on improved materials and designs. ETTs are sized according to the internal diameter; however, the outer diameter (the parameter most likely involved with airway complications) varies according to the manufacturer (Table 1-1). Tube tips are both flat and beveled, and a Murphy eye may or may not be present. The position of the cuff varies with the manufacturer. The use of cuffed endotracheal tubes in pediatrics continues to be controversial. In a multicenter, randomized prospective study of 2246 children from birth to 5 years of age undergoing general anesthesia, Weiss and colleagues (2009) noted that cuffed ETTs compared with uncuffed ETTs did not increase the risk of postextubation stridor (4.4% vs. 4.7%) but did reduce the need for ETT exchanges (2.1% vs. 30.8%). However, the role of cuffed ETTs in neonates and infants who require prolonged ventilation has yet to be determined.

INTRAOPERATIVE AND POSTOPERATIVE ANALGESIA IN NEONATES

It has long been thought that newborn infants do not feel pain the way older children and adults do and therefore do not require anesthetic or analgesic agents (Lippman et al., 1976). Thus, in the past, neonates undergoing surgery were often not afforded the benefits of anesthesia. Later studies, however, indicated that pain experienced by neonates can affect behavioral development (Dixon et al., 1984; Taddio et al., 1995, 2005). Rats exposed to chronic pain without the benefit of anesthesia or analgesia showed varying degrees of neuroapoptosis (Anand et al., 2007). However, to add further controversy to the issue of adequate anesthesia for infants, concerns regarding the neurotoxic effects of both intravenous and inhalational anesthetic agents (GABAminergic and NMDA antagonists) have been raised. Postoperative cognitive dysfunction (POCD) has been noted in adult surgical patients (Johnson et al., 2002; Monk et al., 2008). In adults, POCD may also be a marker for 1-year survival after surgery. Although POCD is an adult phenomenon, animal studies by multiple investigators have raised concerns about anesthetic agents being toxic to the developing brains of infants and small children (Jevtovic-Todorovic et al., 2003, 2008; Mellon et al., 2007; Wang and Slikker, 2008). Early work by Uemura and others (1985) noted that synaptic density was decreased in rats exposed to halothane in utero. Further work with rodents, by multiple investigators, has shown evidence of apoptosis in multiple areas of the central nervous system during the rapid synaptogenesis period. This window of vulnerability appears to be a function of time, dose, and duration of anesthetic exposure. In addition to the histochemical changes of apoptosis, the exposed animals also demonstrated learning and behavioral deficits later in life.

In addition to apoptotic changes that occurred in rodents, Slikker and colleagues have demonstrated neuroapoptotic changes in nonhuman primates (rhesus monkeys) exposed to ketamine (an NMDA antagonist). As with the rodents, ketamine exposure in monkeys resulted in long-lasting deficits in brain function (Dr. Merle Poule, personal communication on the Safety of Key Inhaled and Intravenous Drugs in Pediatric Anesthesia [SAFEKIDS] Scientific Workshop, November 2009, White Oaks Campus Symposium). How these animal studies relate to human findings is unclear to date. However, three clinical studies have been reported, and all three studies are retrospective. Wilder et al. (2009) studied a cohort group of children from Rochester, Minnesota, and noted that children exposed to two or more anesthetics in the first 4 years of life were more likely to have learning

TABLE 1-1. Measured Outer Diameters (OD) of Pediatric Cuffed Tracheal Tubes According to the Internal Diameter (ID) of Tracheal Tubes Supplied by Different Manufacturers

ID	Tracheal Tube Brand	2.5	3.0	3.5	4.0	4.5	5.0	5.5
OD (mm)	Sheridan Tracheal Tube Cuffed Murphy	NA	4.2	4.9	5.5	6.2	6.8	7.5
	Sheridan Tracheal Tube Cuffed Magill	NA	4.3	NA	5.5	NA	6.9	NA
	Mallinckrodt TT High-Contour Murphy	NA	4.4	4.9	5.7	6.3	7.0	7.6
	Mallinckrodt TT High-Contour Murphy P-Series	NA	4.3	5.0	5.7	6.4	6.7	7.7
	Mallinckrodt TT Lo-Contour Magill	NA	4.5	4.9	5.7	6.2	6.9	7.5
	Mallinckrodt TT Lo-Contour Murphy	NA	4.4	5.0	5.6	6.2	7.0	7.5
	Mallinckrodt TT Hi-Lo Murphy	NA	NA	NA	NA	NA	6.9	7.5
	Mallinckrodt TT Safety Flex	NA	5.2	5.5	6.2	6.7	7.2	7.9
	Portex TT-Profile Soft Seal Cuff, Murphy	NA	NA	NA	NA	NA	7.0	7.6
	Rüsch Ruschelit Super Safety Clear Magill	4.0	5.1	5.3	5.9	6.2	6.7	7.2
	Rüsch Ruschelit Super Safety Clear Murphy	NA	NA	NA	NA	NA	6.7	7.3

Modified from Weiss et al.: Shortcomings of cuffed paediatric tracheal tubes. *Brit J Anaesth* 92:78–88, 2004.

disabilities, compared with children exposed to one anesthetic or none at all. Kalkman and others (2009) studied a group of children undergoing urologic surgery before age 6 years and reported that there was a tendency for parents to report more behavioral disturbances than those operated on at a later age. However, in a twin cohort study from the Netherlands, Bartels and coworkers (2009) reported no causal relationship between anesthesia and learning deficits in 1,143 monozygotic twin pairs.

In an effort to determine the impact of anesthetic agents or neurocognitive development, a collaborative partnership between the U.S. Food and Drug Administration (FDA) and the International Anesthesia Research Society has formed Safety of Key Inhaled and Intravenous Drugs in Pediatric Anesthesia (SAFEKIDS), a program designed to fund and promote research in this area.

REGIONAL ANALGESIA IN INFANTS AND CHILDREN

Although conduction analgesia has been used in infants and children since the beginning of the twentieth century, the controversy about whether anesthetic agents can be neurotoxic has caused a resurgence of interest in regional anesthesia (Abajian et al., 1984; Williams et al., 2006).

As newer local anesthetic agents with less systemic toxicity become available, their role in the anesthetic/analgesic management of children is increasing. Studies of levobupivacaine and ropivacaine have demonstrated safety and efficacy in children that is greater than that of bupivacaine, the standard regional anesthetic used in the 1990s (Ivani et al., 1998, 2002, 2003; Hansen et al., 2000, 2001; Lönnqvist et al., 2000; McCann et al., 2001; Karmakar et al., 2002). A single dose of local anesthetics through the caudal and epidural spaces is most often used for a variety of surgical procedures as part of general anesthesia and for postoperative analgesia. Insertion of an epidural catheter for continuous or repeated bolus injections of local anesthetics (often with opioids and other adjunct drugs) for postoperative analgesia has become a common practice in pediatric anesthesia. The addition of adjunct drugs, such as midazolam, neostigmine, tramadol, ketamine, and clonidine, to prolong the neuroaxial blockade from local anesthetic agents has become more popular, even though the safety of these agents on the neuroaxis has not been determined (see Chapters 15, Pain Management; and 16, Regional Anesthesia) (Ansermino et al., 2003; de Beer and Thomas, 2003).

In addition to neuroaxial blockade, specific nerve blocks that are performed with or without ultrasound guidance have become an integral part of pediatric anesthesia (see Chapter 16, Regional Anesthesia). The use of ultrasound has allowed for the administration of smaller volumes of local anesthetic and for more accurate placement of the local anesthetic (Ganesh et al., 2009; Gurnaney et al., 2007; Willschke et al., 2006). The use of catheters in peripheral nerve blocks has also changed the perioperative management for a number of pediatric surgical patients. Continuous peripheral nerve catheters with infusions are being used by pediatric patients at home after they have been discharged from the hospital (Ganesh et al., 2007). The use of these at-home catheters has allowed for shorter hospital stays. In addition, the use of regional techniques with ultrasound guidance, coupled with the natural interest in pain management,

has allowed for pediatric anesthesiologists to spearhead pediatric acute and chronic pain management programs.

In addition to advances in anesthetic pharmacology and equipment, advances in the area of pediatric minimal invasive surgery have improved patient morbidity, shortened the length of hospital stays, and improved surgical outcomes (Fujimoto et al., 1999).

Although minimally invasive surgery (MIS) imposes physiologic challenges in the neonate and small infant, numerous neonatal surgical procedures can nevertheless be successfully approached with such methods, even in infants with single ventricle physiology (Georgeson, 2003; Ponsky and Rothenberg, 2008). The success of MIS has allowed for the evolution of robotic techniques, stealth surgery (scarless surgery), and Natural Orifice Transluminal Endoscopic Surgery (NOTES) (Dutta and Albanese, 2008; Dutta et al., 2008; Isaza et al., 2008).

FUNDAMENTAL DIFFERENCES IN INFANTS AND CHILDREN

Regardless of all the advances in equipment, monitoring, and patient safety initiatives, pediatric anesthesia still requires a special understanding of anatomic, psychological, and physiologic development. The reason for undertaking a special study of pediatric anesthesia is that children, especially infants younger than a few months, differ markedly from adolescents and adults. Many of the important differences, however are not the most obvious. Although the most apparent difference is size, it is the physiologic differences related to general metabolism and immature function of the various organ systems (including the heart, lungs, kidneys, liver, blood, muscles, and central nervous system) that are of major importance to the anesthesiologist.

Psychological Differences

For a child's normal psychological development, continuous support of a nurturing family is indispensable at all stages of development; serious social and emotional deprivation (including separation from the parents during hospitalization), especially during the first 2 years of development, may cause temporary or even lasting damage to psychosocial development (Forman et al., 1987). A young child who is hospitalized for surgery is forced to cope with separation from parents, to adapt to a new environment and strange people, and to experience the pain and discomfort associated with anesthesia and surgery (see Chapters 2, Behavioral Development; and 8, Psychological Aspects).

The most intense fear of an infant or a young child is created by separation from the parents, and it is often conceived as loss of love or abandonment. The sequence of reactions observed is often as follows: angry protest with panicky anxiety, depression and despair, and eventually apathy and detachment (Bowlby, 1973). Older children may be more concerned with painful procedures and the loss of self-control that is implicit with general anesthesia (Forman et al., 1987). Repeated hospitalizations for anesthesia and surgery may be associated with psychosocial disturbances in later childhood (Dombro, 1970). In children who are old enough to experience fear and apprehension during anesthesia and surgery, the emotional factor may be of greater concern than the physical condition; in fact, it may represent the greatest problem of the perioperative course (see Chapter 8, Psychological Aspects) (Smith, 1980).

All of these responses can and should be reduced or abolished through preventive measures to ease the child's adaptation to the hospitalization, anesthesia, and surgery. The anesthesiologist's role in this process, as well as having a basic understanding of neurobehavioral development, are important (Table 1-2).

TABLE 1-2. Aspects of Developmental Assessment and Common Developmental Milestones

Follows dangling object from midline through a range of 90°	1 mo
Follows dangling object from midline through a range of 180°	3 mo
Consistent conjugate gaze (binocular vision)	4 mo
Alerts or quiets to sound	0-2 mo
Head up 45°	2 mo
Head up 90°	3-4 mo
Weight on forearms	3-5 mo
Weight on hands with arms extended	5-6 mo
Complete head lag, back uniformly rounded	Newborn
Slight head lag	3 mo
Rolls front to back	4-5 mo
Rolls back to front	5-6 mo
Sits with no support	7 mo
Hands predominantly closed	1 mo
Hands predominantly open	3 mo
Foot play	5 mo
Transfers objects from hand to hand	6 mo
Index finger approach to small objects and finger-thumb opposition	10 mo
Plays pat-a-cake	9-10 mo
Pulls to stand	9 mo
Walks with one hand held	12 mo
Runs well	2 y
Social smile	1-2 mo
Smiles at image in mirror	5 mo
Separation anxiety/stranger awareness	6-12 mo
Interactive games: peek-a-boo and pat-a-cake	9-12 mo
Waves "bye-bye"	10 mo
Cooing	2-4 mo
Babbles with labial consonants ("ba, ma, ga")	5-8 mo
Imitates sounds made by others	9-12 mo
First words (≈4-6, including "mama," "dada")	9-12 mo
Understands one-step command (with gesture)	15 mo

Modified from Illingworth RS: *The development of the infant and young child: normal and abnormal*, New York, 1987, Churchill Livingstone; ages are averages based primarily on data from Arnold Gesell.

Differences in Response to Pharmacologic Agents

The extent of the differences among infants, children, and adults in response to the administration of drugs is not just a size conversion. During the first several months after birth, rapid development and growth of organ systems take place, altering the factors involved in uptake, distribution, metabolism, and elimination of anesthetics and related drugs. Interindividual variability of a response to a given drug may be determined by a variety of genetic factors. Genetic influences in biotransformation, metabolism, transport, and receptor site all affect an individual's response to a drug. These changes appear to be responsible for developmental differences in drug response and can be further modified by age-related and environmental-related factors. The pharmacology of anesthetics and adjuvant drugs and their different effects in neonates, infants, and children are discussed in detail in Chapter 7, Pharmacology.

Anatomic and Physiologic Differences

Body Size

As stated, the most striking difference between children and adults is size, but the degree of difference and the variation even within the pediatric age group are hard to appreciate. The contrast between an infant weighing 1 kg and an overgrown and obese adolescent weighing more than 100 kg who appear in succession in the same operating room is overwhelming. It makes considerable difference whether body weight, height, or body surface area is used as the basis for size comparison. As pointed out by Harris (1957), a normal newborn infant who weighs 3 kg is one third the size of an adult in length but $\frac{1}{9}$th the adult size in body surface area and $\frac{1}{21}$ of adult size in weight (Fig. 1-1). Of these body measurements, body surface area (BSA) is probably the most important, because it closely parallels variations in basal metabolic rate measured in kilocalories per hour per square meter. For this reason, BSA is believed to be a better criterion than age or weight in judging basal fluid and nutritional requirements. For clinical use, however, BSA proves somewhat difficult to determine, although a nomogram such as that of Talbot and associates (1952) facilitates the procedure considerably (Fig. 1-2). For the anesthesiologist who carries a pocket calculator, the following formulas may be useful to calculate BSA:

Formula of DuBois and DuBois (1916)

$$BSA(m^2) = 0.007184 \times Height^{0.725} \times Weight^{0.425}$$

Formula of Gehan and George (1970)

$$BSA(m^2) = 0.0235 \times Height^{0.42246} \times Weight^{0.51456}$$

At full-term birth, BSA averages 0.2 m², whereas in the adult it averages 1.75 m². A table of average height, weight, and BSA is given for reference in Table 1-3. A simpler, crude estimate of BSA for children of average height and weight is given in Table 1-4. The formula:

$$BSA(m^2) = (002 \times kg) + 0.40$$

is also reasonably accurate in children of normal physique weighing 21 to 40 kg (Vaughan and Litt, 1987).

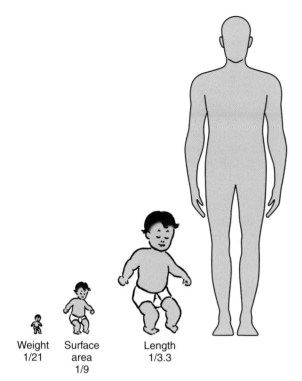

■ FIGURE 1-1. Proportions of newborn to adult with respect to weight, surface area, and length. *(From Crawford JD, Terry ME, Rourke GM: Simplification of drug dosage calculation by application of the surface area principle, Pediatrics 5:785, 1950.)*

The caloric need in relation to BSA of a full-term infant is about 30 kcal/m² per hour. It increases to about 50 kcal/m² per hour by 2 years of age and then decreases gradually to the adult level of 35 to 40 kcal/m² per hour.

Relative Size or Proportion

Less obvious than the difference in overall size is the difference in relative size of body structure in infants and children. This is particularly true with the head, which is large at birth (35 cm in circumference)—in fact, larger than chest circumference. Head circumference increases by 10 cm during the first year and an additional 2 to 3 cm during the second year, when it reaches three-fourths of the adult size (Box 1-1).

At full-term birth, the infant has a short neck and a chin that often meets the chest at the level of the second rib; these infants are prone to upper airway obstruction during sleep. In infants with tracheostomy, the orifice is often buried under the chin unless the head is extended with a roll under the neck. The chest is relatively small in relation to the abdomen, which is protuberant with weak abdominal muscles (Fig. 1-3). Furthermore, the rib cage is cartilaginous and the thorax is too compliant to resist inward recoil of the lungs. In the awake state, the chest wall is maintained relatively rigid with sustained inspiratory muscle tension, which maintains the end-expiratory lung volume functional residual capacity (FRC). Under general anesthesia, however, the muscle tension is abolished and FRC collapses, resulting in airway closure, atelectasis, and venous admixture unless continuous positive airway pressure (CPAP) or positive end-expiratory pressure (PEEP) is maintained.

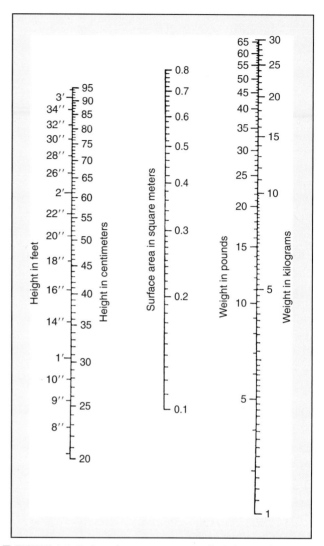

■ FIGURE 1-2. Body surface area nomogram for infants and young children. *(From Talbot NB, Sobel FH, McArthur JW, et al.: Functional endocrinology from birth through adolescence, Cambridge, 1952, Harvard University Press.)*

TABLE 1-3. Relation of Age, Height, and Weight to Body Surface Area (BSA)*

Age (y)	Height (cm)	Weight (kg)	BSA (m²)
Premature	40	1	0.1
Newborn	50	3	0.2
1	75	10	0.47
2	87	12	0.57
3	96	14	0.63
5	109	18	0.74
10	138	32	1.10
13	157	46	1.42
16 (Female)	163	50	1.59
16 (Male)	173	62	1.74

* Based on standard growth chart and the formula of DuBois and DuBois (1916): BSA (m²) = 0.007184 × Height$^{0.725}$ × Weight$^{0.425}$.

TABLE 1-4. Approximation of Body Surface Area (BSA) Based on Weight

Weight (kg)	Approximate BSA (m²)
1-5	$0.05 \times kg + 0.05$
6-10	$0.04 \times kg + 0.10$
11-20	$0.03 \times kg + 0.20$
21-40	$0.02 \times kg + 0.40$

Modified from Vaughan VC III, Litt IF: Assessment of growth and development. In Behrman RE, Vaughn VC III, editors: *Nelson's textbook of pediatrics,* ed 13, Philadelphia, 1987, WB Saunders.

Box 1-1 Typical Patterns of Physical Growth

WEIGHT
Birth weight (BW) is regained by the tenth to fourteenth day.
Average weight gain per day: 0-6 mo = 20 g; 6-12 mo = 15 g.
BW doubles at ≈4 mo, triples at ≈12 mo, quadruples at ≈24 mo.
During second year, average weight gain per month: ≈0.25 kg.
After age 2 years, average annual gain until adolescence: ≈2.3 kg.

LENGTH/HEIGHT
By end of first year, birth length increases by 50%.
Birth length doubles by age 4 years, triples by 13 years.
Average height gain during second year: ≈12 cm.
After age 2 years, average annual growth until adolescence: ≈5 cm.

HEAD CIRCUMFERENCE
Average head growth per week: 0-2 mo = ≈0.5 cm; 2-6 mo = ≈0.25 cm.
Average total head growth: 0-3 mo = ≈5 cm; 3-6 mo = ≈4 cm; 6-9 mo = ≈2 cm; 9-12 mo = ≈1 cm.

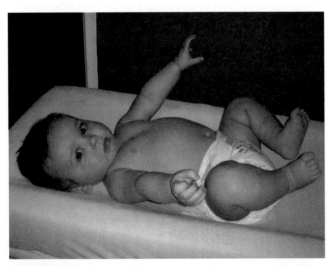

■ **FIGURE 1-3.** A normal infant has a large head, narrow shoulders and chest, and a large abdomen.

Central and Autonomic Nervous Systems

The brain of the neonate is relatively large, weighing about 1/10 of body weight compared with about 1/50 of body weight in the adult. The brain grows rapidly; its weight doubles by 6 months of age and triples by 1 year. By the third week of gestation, the neural plate appears, and by 5 weeks the three main subdivisions of the forebrain, midbrain, and hindbrain are evident. By the eighth week of gestation, neurons migrate to form the cortical layers, and migration is complete by the sixth month. Cell differentiation continues as neurons, astrocytes, aligodendrocytes, and glial cells form. Axons and synaptic connections continually form and remodel. At birth, about one fourth of the neuronal cells are present. The development of cells in the cortex and brain stem is nearly complete by 1 year of age. Myelinization and elaboration of dendritic processes continue well into the third year. Incomplete myelinization is associated with primitive reflexes, such as the Moro and grasp reflexes in the neonate; these are valuable in the assessment of neural development.

At birth the spinal cord extends to the third lumbar vertebra. By the time the infant is 1 year old, the cord has assumed its permanent position, ending at the first lumbar vertebra (Gray, 1973).

In contrast to the central nervous system, the autonomic nervous system is relatively well developed in the newborn. The parasympathetic components of the cardiovascular system are fully functional at birth. The sympathetic components, however, are not fully developed until 4 to 6 months of age (Friedman, 1973). Baroreflexes to maintain blood pressure and heart rate, which involve medullary vasomotor centers (pressor and depressor areas), are functional at birth in awake newborn infants (Moss et al., 1968; Gootman, 1983). In anesthetized newborn animals, however, both pressor and depressor reflexes are diminished (Wear et al., 1982; Gallagher et al., 1987).

The laryngeal reflex is activated by the stimulation of receptors on the face, nose, and upper airways of the newborn. Reflex apnea, bradycardia, or laryngospasm may occur. Various mechanical and chemical stimuli, including water, foreign bodies, and noxious gases, can trigger this response. This protective response is so potent that it can cause death in the newborn (see Chapters 3, Respiratory Physiology; and 4, Cardiovascular Physiology).

Respiratory System

At full-term birth, the lungs are still in the stage of active development. The formation of adult-type alveoli begins at 36 weeks post conception but represents only a fraction of the terminal air sacs with thick septa at full-term birth. It takes more than several years for functional and morphologic development to be completed, with a 10-fold increase in the number of terminal air sacs to 400 to 500 million by 18 months of age, along with the development of rich capillary networks surrounding the alveoli. Similarly, control of breathing during the first several weeks of extrauterine life differs notably from control in older children and adults. Of particular importance is the fact that hypoxemia depresses, rather than stimulates, respiration. Anatomic differences in the airway occur with growth and development. Recently, the concept of the child having a funnel-shaped airway with the cricoid as the narrowest portion of the airway has been challenged. Based on bronchoscopic images, Dalal and colleagues (2009) suggest for infants and children the glottis not the cricoid, may be the narrowest portion. The development of the respiratory system and its physiology are detailed in Chapter 3, Respiratory Physiology.

Cardiovascular System

During the first minutes after birth, the newborn infant must change his or her circulatory pattern dramatically from fetal to adult types of circulation to survive in the extrauterine environment. Even for several months after initial adaptation, the pulmonary vascular bed remains exceptionally reactive to hypoxia and acidosis. The heart remains extremely sensitive to volatile anesthetics during early infancy, whereas the central nervous system is relatively insensitive to these anesthetics. Cardiovascular physiology in infants and children is discussed in Chapter 4.

Fluid and Electrolyte Metabolism

Like the lungs, the kidneys are not fully mature at birth, although the formation of nephrons is complete by 36 weeks' gestation. Maturation continues for about 6 months after full-term birth. The glomerular filtration rate (GFR) is lower in the neonate because of the high renal vascular resistance associated with the relatively small surface area for filtration. Despite a low GFR and limited tubular function, the full-term newborn can conserve sodium. Premature infants, however, experience prolonged glomerulotubular imbalance, resulting in sodium wastage and hyponatremia (Spitzer, 1982). On the other hand, both full-term and premature infants are limited in their ability to handle excessive sodium loads. Even after water deprivation, concentrating ability is limited at birth, especially in premature infants. After several days, neonates can produce diluted urine; however, diluting capacity does not mature fully until after 3 to 5 weeks of life (Spitzer, 1978). The premature infant is prone to hyponatremia when sodium supplementation is inadequate or with overhydration. Furthermore, dehydration is detrimental to the neonate regardless of gestational age. The physiology of fluid and electrolyte balance is detailed in Chapter 5, Regulation of Fluids and Electrolytes.

Temperature Regulation

Temperature regulation is of particular interest and importance in pediatric anesthesia. There is a better understanding of the physiology of temperature regulation and the effect of anesthesia on the control mechanisms. General anesthesia is associated with mild to moderate hypothermia, resulting from environmental exposure, anesthesia-induced central thermoregulatory inhibition, redistribution of body heat, and up to 30% reduction in metabolic heat production (Bissonette, 1991). Small infants have disproportionately large BSAs, and heat loss is exaggerated during anesthesia, particularly during the induction of anesthesia, unless the heat loss is actively prevented. General anesthesia decreases but does not completely abolish thermoregulatory threshold temperature to hypothermia. Mild hypothermia can sometimes be beneficial intraoperatively, and profound hypothermia is effectively used during open heart surgery in infants to reduce oxygen consumption. Postoperative hypothermia, however, is detrimental because of marked increases in oxygen consumption, oxygen debt (dysoxia), and resultant metabolic acidosis. Regulation of body temperature is discussed in detail in Chapter 6, Thermoregulation.

SUMMARY

Pediatric anesthesia as a subspecialty has evolved, because the needs of infants and young children are fundamentally different from those of adults. The pediatric anesthesiologist should be aware of the child's cardiovascular, respiratory, renal, neuromuscular, and central nervous system responses to various drugs, as well as to physical and chemical stimuli, such as changes in blood oxygen and carbon dioxide tensions, pH, and body temperature. Their responses are different both qualitatively and quantitatively from those of adults and among different pediatric age groups. More importantly, the pediatric anesthesiologist should always consider the child's emotional needs and create an environment that minimizes or abolishes fear and distress.

There have been many advances in the practice of anesthesia to improve the comfort of young patients since the seventh edition of this book was published in 2006. These advances include a relaxation of preoperative fluid restriction, more focused attention to the child's psychological needs with more extensive use of preoperative sedation via the transmucosal route, the wide use of topical analgesia with a eutectic mixture of local anesthetic cream before intravenous catheterization, expanded use of regional anesthesia with improved accuracy and safety by means of ultrasound devices, and more generalized acceptance of parental presence during anesthetic induction and in the recovery room. Furthermore, a more diverse anesthetic approach has evolved through the combined use of regional analgesia, together with the advent of newer and less soluble volatile anesthetics, intravenous anesthetics, and shorter-acting synthetic opioids and muscle relaxants. Finally, the scope of pediatric anesthesia has significantly expanded with the recent development of organized pain services in most pediatric institutions. As a result, pediatric anesthesiologists have assumed the leading role as pain management specialists, thus further extending anesthesia services and influence beyond the boundary of the operating room.

REFERENCES

Complete references used in this text can be found online at www.expertconsult.com.

Behavioral Development

Julie Niezgoda

Assessment of growth and development of infants and children typically falls under the domain of the pediatrician or pediatric subspecialist. Delays or deviations from normal often dictate the need to conduct extensive diagnostic evaluations and management strategies. Familiarity with developmental stages may also benefit the pediatric anesthesiologist, allowing the practitioner to recognize the different coping mechanisms children use to respond to the anxiety and stresses throughout the perioperative period. Growth issues, especially failure to thrive, may indicate a serious underlying medical condition that could affect the management and anesthetic plan for children.

A variety of processes are encompassed in growth and development: the formation of tissue; an increase in physical size; the progressive increases in strength and ability to control large and small muscles (gross motor and fine motor development); and the advancement of complexities of thought, problem solving, learning, and verbal skills (cognitive and language development). There is a systematic approach for tracking neurologic development and physical growth in infants, because attainment of milestones is orderly and predictable. However, a wide range exists for normal achievement. The mastering of a particular skill often builds on the achievement of an earlier skill. Delays in one developmental domain may impair development in another (Gessel and Amatruda, 1951). For example, immobility caused by a neuromuscular disorder prevents an infant from exploration of the environment, thus impeding cognitive development. A deficit in one domain might interfere with the ability to assess progress in another area. For example, a child with cerebral palsy who is capable of conceptualizing matching geometric shapes but does not have the gross or fine motor skills necessary to perform the function could erroneously be labeled as developmentally delayed.

It is possible for the anesthesiologist to obtain a gestalt of a child's growth and development level while recording a preoperative history and during the physical examination. However, the anesthesiologist needs to realize that these assessments are usually done by pediatricians over time and are best performed when the child is physically well, familiar with the examiner, and under minimal stress. Therefore, a child who is developing normally could be assessed as delayed during a preoperative assessment.

The goal of this chapter is to review the developmental and behavioral issues faced in routine pediatric practice to help the anesthesiologist tailor an anesthetic plan that is geared to the appropriate age of the child with the goal of decreasing postoperative complications such as behavioral disturbances, emotional reactions, or escalation in medical care. The chapter is divided into sections addressing growth and developmental milestones, including gross motor skills, fine motor skills, cognition, and language, followed by a section of clinical scenarios illustrating the relevance of developmental issues in pediatric anesthesia. The last section contains several common developmental disorders and related anesthetic issues.

PRENATAL GROWTH

The most dramatic events in growth and development occur before birth. These changes are overwhelmingly somatic, with the transformation of a single cell into an infant. The first eight weeks of gestation are known as the embryonic period and encompasses the time when the rudiments of all of the major organs are developed. This period denotes a time that the fetus is highly sensitive to teratogens such as alcohol, tobacco, mercury, thalidomide, and antiepileptic drugs. The average embryo weighs 9 g and has a crown-to-rump length of 5 cm. The fetal stage (more than 9 weeks' gestation) consists of increases in cell number and size and structural remodeling of organ systems (Moore, 1972).

During the third trimester, weight triples and length doubles as body stores of protein, calcium, and fat increase. Low birth weight can result from prematurity, intrauterine growth retardation (small for gestational age, SGA) or both. Large-for-gestational-age (LGA) infants are those whose weight is above the 90th percentile at any gestational age. Deviations from the normal relationship of infant weight gain with increasing gestational age can be multifactorial. Potential causes include maternal diseases (e.g., diabetes, pregnancy-induced hypertension, and seizure disorders), prenatal exposure to toxins (e.g., alcohol, drugs, and tobacco), fetal toxoplasmosis-rubella-cytomegalovirus-herpes simplex-syphilis (TORCHES) infections, genetic abnormalities (e.g., trisomies 13, 18, and 21), fetal congenital malformations (e.g., cardiopulmonary or renal malformations), and maternal malnutrition or placental insufficiency (Kinney and Kumar, 1988).

POSTNATAL GROWTH

Postnatal growth is measured by changes in weight, length, and head circumference plotted chronologically on growth charts. This is an essential component of pediatric health surveillance, because almost any problem involving physiologic, interpersonal, or social domains can adversely affect growth.

Growth milestones are the most predictable, taking into context each child's specific genetic and ethnic influences (Johnson and Blasco, 1997). It is essential to plot the child's growth on gender- and age-appropriate percentile charts. Charts are now available for certain ethnic groups and genetic syndromes such as Trisomy 21 and Turner's syndrome. Deviation from growth over time across percentiles is of greater significance for a child than a single weight measurement. For example, an infant at the fifth percentile of weight for age may be growing normally, may be failing to grow, or may be recovering from growth failure, depending on the trajectory of the growth curve.

Of the three parameters, weight is the most sensitive measurement of well-being and is the first to show deviance as an indication of an underlying problem. Causes of weight loss and failure to thrive include congestive heart failure, metabolic or endocrine disorders, malignancy, infections, and malabsorption problems. Inadequate increases in height over time occur secondary to significant weight loss, and decreased head circumference is the last parameter to change, signifying severe malnutrition. Pathologies such as hydrocephalus or increased intracranial pressure may appear on growth charts as head-circumference measurements that are rapidly increasing and crossing percentiles. Small head size can be associated with craniosynostosis or a syndromic feature. Significant changes in head-circumference measurements in children should alert the anesthesiologist to the potential of underlying neurologic problems.

Because significant weight fluctuation is a potential red flag for serious underlying medical conditions, anesthesiologists should be familiar with the normal weight gain expected for children. It is not unusual for a newborn's weight to decrease by 10% in the first week of life because of the excretion of excess extravascular fluid or possibly poor oral intake. Infants should regain or exceed birth weight by 2 weeks of age and continue to gain approximately 30 g/day, with a gradual decrease to 12 g/day by the first year. Healthy, full-term infants typically double their birth weight at 6 months and triple it by 1 year of age. Many complex formulas are available to estimate the average weight for normal infants and children. A relatively simple calculation to recall is the "rule of tens"; e.g., the weight of a child increases by about 10 pounds per year until approximately 12 to 13 years of age for females and age 16 to 17 years for males. Therefore, one could expect weight gain of 20 pounds by age 2 years, 30 pounds by 3 years, 40 pounds by 4 years, and so on. The weight in pounds can be converted to kilograms by dividing it by 2.2. Length in centimeters is estimated by the following formula: (age in years × 6) + 77.

DEVELOPMENTAL ASSESSMENT

Developmental assessment serves different purposes, depending on the age of the child. In the neonatal period, behavioral assessment can detect a wide range of neurologic impairments. During infancy, assessment serves to reassure parents and to identify sensory, motor, cognitive, and emotional problems early, when they are most amenable to treatment. Middle-childhood and adolescence assessments often help with addressing academic and social problems.

Milestones are useful indicators of mental and physical development and possible deviations from normal. It should be emphasized that milestones represent the average for children to attain and that there can be variable rates of mastery that fall into the normal range. An acceptable developmental screening test must be highly sensitive (detect nearly all children with problems); specific (not identify too many children without problems); have content validity, test-retest, and interrater reliability; and be relatively quick and inexpensive to administer. The most widely used developmental screening test is the Denver Developmental Screening Test (DDST), which provides a pass/fail rating in four domains of developmental milestones: gross motor, fine motor, language, and personal-social. The original DDST was criticized for underidentification of children with developmental disabilities, particularity in the area of language. The reissued DDST-II is a better assessment for language delays, which is important because of the strong link between language and overall cognitive development. Table 2-1 lists the prevalence of some common developmental disabilities (Levy and Hyman, 1993).

TABLE 2-1. Prevalence of Developmental Disabilities

Condition	Prevalence per 1000
Cerebral palsy	2-3
Visual impairment	0.3-0.6
Hearing impairment	0.8-2
Mental retardation	25
Learning disability	75
Attention deficit hyperactivity disorder	150
Behavioral disorders	60-130
Autism	9-10

MOTOR DEVELOPMENT

Primitive Reflexes

The earliest motor neuromaturational markers are primitive reflexes that development during uterine life and generally disappear between the third and sixth months after birth. Newborn movements are largely uncontrolled, with the exception of eye gaze, head turning, and sucking. Development of the infant's central nervous system involves strengthening of the higher cortical center that gradually takes over function of the primitive reflexes. Postural reflexes replace primitive reflexes between three and six months of age as a result of this development (Schott and Rossor, 2003). These reactions allow children to maintain a stable posture even if they are rapidly moved or jolted (Box 2-1).

The asymmetric tonic neck reflex (ATNR) or "fencing posture" is an example of a primitive reflex that is not immediately present at birth because of the high flexor tone of the newborn infant. When the neonate's head is turned to one side, there is increased extensor tone of the upper extremity on the same side and increased flexor tone on the occipital side. The ATNR is a precursor to hand-eye coordination, preparing the infant for gazing along the upper arm and voluntary reaching. The

disappearances of this reflex at 4 to 6 months allows the infant mobility to roll over and begin to examine and manipulate objects in the midline with both hands.

The palmar grasp reflex is present at birth and persists until 4 to 6 months of age. When an object is placed in the infant's hand, the fingers close and tightly grasp the object. The grip is strong but unpredictable. The waning of the early grasp reflex allows infants to hold objects in both hands and ultimately to voluntarily let them go.

The Moro reflex is probably the most well-known primitive reflex and is present at birth. It is likely to occur as a startle to a loud noise or sudden changes in head position. The legs and head extend while the arms jerk up and out, followed by adduction of the arms and tightly clenched fists. Bilateral absence of the reflex may mean damage to the infant's central nervous system. Unilateral absence could indicate birth trauma such as a fractured clavicle or brachial plexus injury.

Postural reflexes support control of balance, posture, and movement in a gravity-based environment. The protective equilibrium response can be elicited in a sitting infant by abruptly pushing the infant laterally. The infant will extend the arm on the contralateral side and flex the trunk toward the side of the force to regain the center of gravity (Fig. 2-1). The parachute response develops around 9 months and is a response to a free-fall motion, where the infant extends the extremities in an outward motion to distribute weight over a broader area. Postural reactions are markedly slow in appearance in the infant who has central nervous system damage. Children who fail to gain postural control continue to display traces of primitive reflexes. They also have difficulty with control of movement affecting coordination, fine and gross motor development, and other associated aspects of learning, including reading and writing. Table 2-2 is a list of the average times of appearance and disappearance of the more common primitive reflexes.

Box 2-1 Definitions of Primitive Reflexes

Automatic stepping reflex: Although the infant cannot support his or her weight when a flat surface is presented to the sole of the foot, he or she makes a stepping motion by bringing one foot in front of the other.

Crossed extension reflex: When an extremity is acutely stimulated to withdraw, the flexor muscles in the withdrawing limb contract completely, whereas the extensor muscles relax. The opposite occurs (full extension, with relaxation of contracting muscles) in the opposite limb.

Galant reflex: An infant has the one side of the back stroked moves or swings in that direction.

Moro reflex: When the infant is startled with a loud noise or when the head is lowered suddenly, the head and legs extend and the arms raise up and out. Then the arms are brought in and the fingers close to make fists.

Palmar reflex: When an object is placed into the infant's hand or when the palm of the infant's hand is stroked with an object, the hand closes around the object.

Asymmetric tonic neck reflex ("fencing"): When the infant's head is rotated to one side, the arm on that side straightens and the opposite arm flexes.

Landau reflex: When the infant is held in a horizontal position, he or she raises the head and bring the legs up into a horizontal position. If the head is forced down (flexed) the legs also lower into a vertical position.

Derotational righting reflex: When the infant turns the head one direction, the body leans in the same direction to maintain balance.

Protective equilibrium reflex: When a lateral force is applied to the infant, he or she responds by leaning into the force and extending the contralateral arm.

Parachute reflex: When the infant is facing down and lowered suddenly, the arms extend out in a protective maneuver.

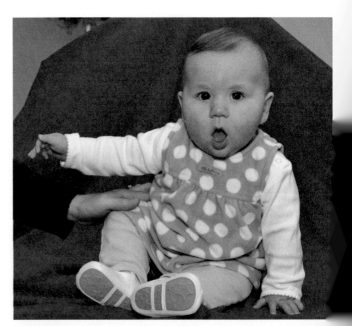

■ **FIGURE 2-1.** The protective equilibrium response is demonstrated in an infant being pushed laterally. Note the extended contralateral arm.

TABLE 2-2. Primitive Reflexes

Reflex	Present by (Months)	Gone by (Months)
Automatic stepping	Birth	2
Crossed extension	Birth	2
Galant	Birth	2
Moro	Birth	3-6
Palmar	Birth	4-6
Asymmetric tonic neck ("fencing")	1	4-6
Landau	3	12-24
Derotational head righting	4	Persists
Protective equilibrium	4-6	Persists
Parachute	8-9	Persists

Gross Motor Skills

One principle in neuromaturational development during infancy is that it proceeds from cephalad to caudad and proximal to distal. Thus, arm movement comes before leg movement (Feldman, 2007). The upper extremity attains increasing accuracy in reaching, grasping, transferring, and manipulating objects. Gross motor development in the prone position begins with the infant tightly flexing the upper and lower extremities and evolves to hip extension while lifting the head and shoulders from a table surface around 4 to 6 months of age. When pulled to a sitting position, the newborn has significant head lag, whereas the 6-month-old baby, because of development of muscle tone in the neck, raises the head in anticipation of being pulled up.

Rolling movements start from front to back at approximately 4 months of age as the muscles of the lower extremities strengthen. An infant begins to roll from back to front at about 5 months. The abilities to sit unsupported (about 6 months old) and to pivot while sitting (around 9 to 10 month of age) provide increasing opportunities to manipulate several objects at a time (Needleman, 1996). Once thoracolumbar control is achieved and the sitting position mastered, the child focuses motor development on ambulation and more complex skills. Locomotion begins with commando-style crawling, advances to creeping on hands and knees, and eventually reaches pulling to stand around 9 months of age, with further advancement to cruising around furniture or toys. Standing alone and walking independently occur around the first birthday. Advanced motor achievements correlate with increasing myelinization and cerebellum growth. Walking several steps alone has one of the widest ranges for mastery of all of the gross motor milestones and occurs between 9 and 17 months of age. Milestones of gross motor development are presented in Table 2-3 and Figure 2-2. The accomplishment of locomotion not only expands the infant's exploratory range and offers new opportunities for cognitive and motor growth, but it also increases the potential for physical dangers (Vaughan, 1992).

Most children walk with a mature gait, run steadily, and balance on one foot for 1 second by 3½ years of age. The sequence for additional gross motor development is as follows: running, jumping on two feet, balancing on one foot, hopping, and skipping. Finally, more complex activities such as throwing, catching, and kicking balls, riding bicycles, and climbing on playground equipment are mastered. Development beyond walking incorporates improved balance and coordination and progressive narrowing of additional physical support. Complex motor skills also incorporate advanced cognitive and emotional development that is necessary for interactive play with other children. Figure 2-3 shows the red flags to watch for in the abnormal physical development of the infant.

TABLE 2-3. Cognitive and Language Communication Skills Development

Average Age of Attainment (Months)	Cognitive	Language Communication
2	Stares briefly at area when object is removed	Smiles in response to face or voice
4	Stares at own hand	Monosyllabic babble
8	Object permanence—uncovers toy after seeing it covered	Inhibits to "no" Follows one-step command *with* gesture (wave to "come here")
10	Separation anxiety from familiar people	Follows one-step command without gesture ("give it to me")
12	Egocentric play (pretends to drink from cup)	Speaks first real word
18	Cause and effect relationships no longer need to be demonstrated to understand (pushes car to move, winds toy on own) Distraction techniques may no longer succeed	Speaks 20 to 50 words
24	Mental activity is independent of sensory processing or motor manipulation (sees a child in a book with a mask on face and can later reenact event)	Speaks in two-word sentences
36	Capable of symbolic thinking	Speaks in three-word sentences
48	Immature logic is replaced Conventional logic and wisdom	Speaks in four-word sentences Follows three-step commands

1 Month
Prone, lies tightly
flexed with pelvis
high. Head lags
after shoulders
when pulled to sit

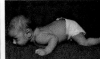
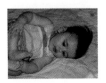

12 Months
Walks alone

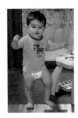

3 Months
Prone, rests on forearms.
Partial head lag when
pulled to sit

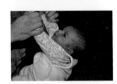

18 Months
Runs

5 Months
Rolls back to front

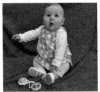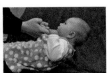

24 Months
Jumps in place,
throws overhand,
walks down stairs
holding rail

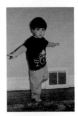

6 Months
Sit without support.
Lifts head before
shoulders when
pulled to sit

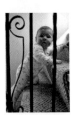

36 Months
Balance on one foot
for one second

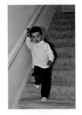

7 Months
Commando crawl

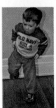

48 Months
Hopes on one foot

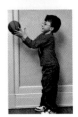

8 Months
Four point kneeling,
reaches with one
hand. Aquires sitting
position without
support

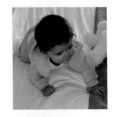

60 Months
Catches a ball

10 Months
Cruises
around
furniture

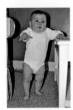

■ **FIGURE 2-2.** Gross motor skills development chart.

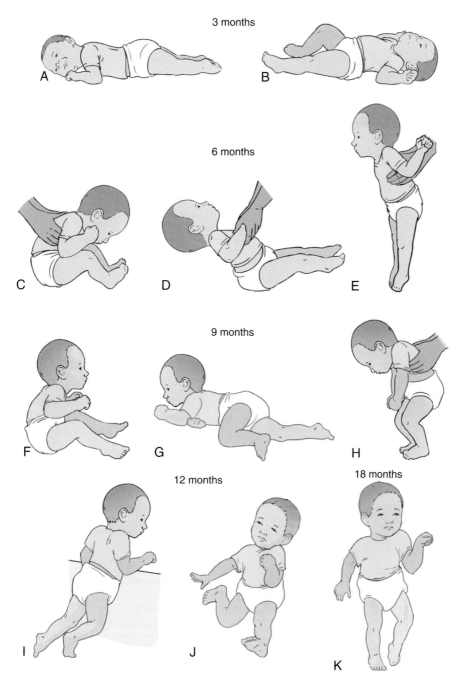

FIGURE 2-3. Abnormal developmental findings. **A,** Difficulty lifting head and stiff legs with little or no movement. **B,** Pushing back with head, keeping hands fisted, and lacking arm movement. **C,** Rounded back, inability to lift head up, and poor head control. **D,** Difficulty bringing arms forward to reach out, arching back, and stiffening legs. **E,** Arms held back and stiff legs. **F,** Using one hand predominantly; rounded back and poor use of arms when sitting. **G,** Difficulty crawling and using only one side of the body to move. **H,** Inability to straighten back and cannot bear weight on legs. **I,** Difficulty getting to standing position because of stiff legs and pointed toes; only using arms to pull up to standing. **J,** Sitting with weight to one side and strongly flexed or stiffly extended arms; using hand to maintain seated position. **K,** Inability to take steps independently, poor standing balance, many falls, and walking on toes. *(Redrawn from* What Every Parent Should Know *[pamphlet], 2006, Pathways Awareness Foundation.)*

Fine Motor Development

At birth, the neonate's fingers and thumbs are typically tightly flexed. Normal development moves from the primitive grasp reflex, where the infant reflexively grabs an object but is unable to release it to a voluntary grasp and release of the object. By 2 to 3 months of age the hands are no longer tightly fisted, and the infant begins to bring them toward the mouth, sucking on the digits for self comfort. Objects can be held in either hand by age 3 months and transferred back and forth by 6 months.

1 Month
Hands tightly fisted

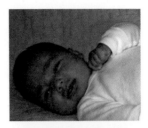

2 Months
Grasps rattle

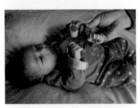

3 Months
Hands unfisted most
of the time

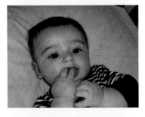

4 Months
Reaches for and retains
rattle, uses both hands

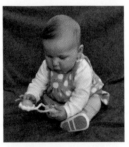

6 Months
Transfers objects hand
to hand, immature
hand rake of pellat

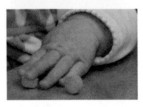

10 Months
Pincer grasp between
thumb and index finger

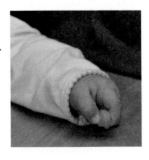

12 Months
Pincer grasp
between finger tips

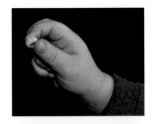

18 Months
Tower of four cubes,
scribbles spontaneously

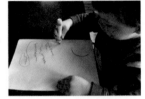

24 Months
Tower of six cubes,
turns pages of books
one at a time, imitate
vertical stroke

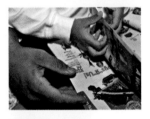

36 Months
Copies circle,
cuts with
small scissors

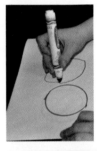

48 Months
Copies cross,
draws a person
with three parts

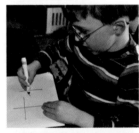

60 Months
Copies triangle

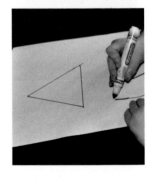

■ **FIGURE 2-4.** Fine motor skills development chart.

In early development, the upper extremities assist with balance and mobility. As the sitting position is mastered with improved balance, the hands become more available for manipulation and exploration. The evolution of the pincer grasp is the highlight of fine motor development during the first year. The infant advances from "raking" small objects into the palm to the finer pincer grasp, allowing opposition of the thumb and the index finger, whereby small items are picked up with precision. Children younger than 18 months of age generally use both hands equally well, and true "handedness" is not established until 36 months (Levine et al., 1999). Advancements in fine motor skills continue throughout the preschool years, when the child develops better eye-hand coordination with which to stack objects or reproduce drawings (e.g., crosses, circles, and triangles). Figure 2-4 lists and demonstrates the chronologic order of fine motor development.

LANGUAGE DEVELOPMENT

Delays in language development are more common than delays in any other developmental domain (Glascoe, 2000). Language includes receptive and expressive skills. Receptive skills are the ability to understand the language, and expressive skills include the ability to make thoughts, ideas, and desires known to others. Because receptive language precedes expressive language, infants respond to several simple statements such as "no," "bye-bye," and "give me" before they are capable of speaking intelligible words. In addition to speech, expression of language can take the forms of gestures, signing, typing, and "body language." Thus, speech and language are not synonymous. The hearing-impaired child or child with cerebral palsy may have normal receptive language skills and intellect to understand dialogue but needs other forms of expressive language to vocalize responses. Conversely, children may talk but fail to communicate; for example, a child with autism may vocalize by using "parrot talk" or echolalia that has no meaningful content and does not represent language.

Language development can be divided into the three stages of pre-speech, naming, and word combination. Pre-speech is characterized by cooing or babbling until around 8 to 10 months of age, when babbling becomes more complex with multiple syllables. Eventually random vocalization ("da-da") is interpreted and reinforced by the parents as a real word, and the child begins to repeat it. The naming period (ages 10 to 18 months) is when the infant realizes that people have names and objects have labels. Once the infant's vocalizations are reinforced as people or things, the infant begins to use them appropriately. At around 12 months of age some infants understand as many as 100 words and can respond to simple commands that are accompanied by gestures. Early into the second year a command without a gesture is understood. Expressive language is slower, and an 18-month-old child has a limited vocabulary of around 25 words. After the realization that words can stand for things, the child's vocabulary expands at a rapid pace. Preschool language development begins with word combination at 18 to 24 months and is the foundation for later success in school. Vocabulary increases from 50 to 100 words to more than 2000 words during this time. Sentence structure advances from two- and three-word phrases to sentences incorporating all of the major grammatic rules. A simple correlate is that a child should increase the number of words in a sentence with advancing age; e.g., two-word sentences by 2 years of age, three-word sentences by age 3 years (Table 2-3).

Language is a critical barometer of both cognitive and emotional development (Coplan, 1995). Mental retardation may first surface as a concern with delayed speech and language development around 2 years of age; however, the average age of diagnosis is 3 to 4 years. All children whose language development is delayed should undergo audiologic testing. If a child's expressive skills are advanced compared with his or her receptive skills (e.g., child speaks five-word sentences but does not understand simple commands), a pervasive development disorder could be the cause.

COGNITIVE DEVELOPMENT

The concept of a developmental line implies that a child passes through successive stages. The psychoanalytic theories of Sigmund Freud and Erik Erikson and the cognitive theory of Jean Piaget describe stages in the development of cognition and emotion that are as qualitatively different as the milestones attained in gross motor development.

At the core of Freudian theory is the idea of biologically determined drives. The core drive is sexual, broadly defined to include sensations that include excitation or tension and satisfaction or release (Freud, 1952). There are discrete stages: oral, anal, oedipal, latent, and genital. During these stages the focus of the sexual drive shifts with maturation and is at first influenced primarily by the parents and subsequently by an enlarging circle of social contacts. Defense mechanisms in early childhood can develop pathologically to disguise the presence of conflict. The emotional health of the child and adult depends on the resolution of the conflicts that arise throughout these stages.

Erikson's chief contribution was to recast Freud's stages in terms of the emerging personality (Erikson, 1963). For example, basic trust, the first of Erickson's psychosocial stages, develops as infants learn that their urgent needs are met regularly. The consistent availability of a trusted adult creates the conditions for secure attachment. The next stage establishes the child's internal sense of either autonomy vs. shame and doubt and corresponds to Freud's anal stage. A sense of either identity or role confusion corresponds to the crisis experienced in Freud's genital stage (puberty) (Table 2-4).

Piaget's name is synonymous with the study of cognitive development. A central tenet of his theory is that cognition is qualitatively different at different stages of development (Hobson, 1985). During the sensorimotor stage, children learn basic things about their relationship with their environment. Thoughts about the nature of objects and their relationships are acted out and tied immediately to sensations and manipulation. With the arrival of language the nature of thinking changes dramatically, and symbols increasingly take the place of things and actions. Stages of preoperational thinking, concrete operations, and formal operations correspond to the different ages of preschool, school age, and adolescence, respectively. At all stages, children are not passive recipients of knowledge but actively seek out experience (assimilation) and use them to build on how things work.

Cognitive development and neuromaturational development are closely related, and it is sometimes difficult to distinguish between the two in the infant and child. Early in the neonatal period, cognitive development begins when the infant responds to visual and auditory stimuli by interacting with surroundings

TABLE 2-4. Classic Stage Theories of the Development of Emotion and Cognition

Theory	0-1 Years (Infancy)	2-3 Years (Toddler)	3-6 Years (Preschool)	6-12 Years (School Age)	12-20 Years (Adolescents)
Freud: psychosexual	Oral	Anal	Oedipal phallic	Latency	Puberty and genital
Erikson: psychosocial	Basic trust	Autonomy vs. shame and doubt	Initiative vs. guilt	Industry vs. inferiority	Identity vs. role confusion
Piaget: cognitive	Sensorimotor (stages I-IV)	Sensorimotor (stages V and VI) Egocentric thought	Preoperational	Concrete operational	Formal operational

to gain information. Activities such as mouthing, shaking, and banging objects provide information to the infant beyond the visual features. Infant exploration begins with the body, with activities such as staring intently at a hand and touching other body parts. These explorations represent an early discovery of "cause and effect," as the infant learns that voluntary movements generate predictable tactile and visual sensations (e.g., kicking the side of the bed moves a mobile). Signs of abnormal cognitive development are outlined in Box 2-2.

A communication system develops between the infant and mother or primary caregiver. Accordingly, the infant begins to display anxiety at the end of this developmental period if the person most familiar to the child is not available. The ability to maintain an image of a person develops before that of an object, and therefore the infant may display separation anxiety when a loved one leaves the room. Object permanence, a major milestone, develops around 9 months when the infant understands that objects continue to exist even if they are covered up and not seen. With locomotion the child explores greater areas and develops a substantial sense of social self, as well as an early appreciation of the behavior standards expected by adults. Interactive and pretend play begins at 30 months, and playing in pairs occurs around 24 to 36 months.

Childhood cognitive development and the effect it has on the child's perception of the hospitalization and surgery are important for the pediatric anesthesiologist to understand in order to help the child deal with the stresses during this time. One out of four children will be hospitalized by age 5 years. Although extreme emotional reactions are rare, at least 60% of children demonstrate signs of stress-related anxiety during the perioperative period. Children between the ages of 1 and 3 years, previously hospitalized children, and children who have undergone turbulent anesthetic inductions are at increased risk for exhibiting adverse postoperative behavioral reactions.

Box 2-2 Abnormal Cognitive Signs

1 month: Failure to be alert to environmental stimuli. May indicate sensory impairment

5 months: Failure to reach for objects. May indicate motor, visual, and/or cognitive deficit

6 months: Absent babbling. May indicate hearing deficit

7 months: Absent stranger anxiety. May be due to multiple care providers (eg, neonatal intensive care unit)

11 months: Inability to localize sound. May indicate unilateral hearing loss

(Modified from Seid M et al.: Perioperative psychosocial interventions for autistic children undergoing ENT surgery, *Int J Ped Otorhinolaryngology*, 40:107, 1997.)

Stress and anxiety can be manifested by behavioral problems such as nightmares, phobias, agitation, avoidance of caregivers, emotional distress, and regressive behaviors (e.g., temper tantrums, bedwetting, and loss of previously acquired developmental milestones). Allowing adequate preoperative evaluation and psychological preparation for both the parent and child based on specific needs relative to the child's developmental stage is a method the anesthesiologist can invoke to reduce the emotional trauma of anesthesia.

Erikson (1963) describes the infants' motivations as dependent on the satisfaction of basic human needs (e.g., food, shelter, and love). According to Freud, the child directs all of his or her energies to the mother and fears her loss because her absence may jeopardize the child's satisfaction creating tension and anxiety. This dependence is the essence of separation anxiety. Before this stage infants are able to accept surrogates and respond favorably to anyone holding them. Once stranger anxiety develops, active participation of the parents during the hospitalization should be encouraged to maintain a sense of security for the child and promote bonding (Thompson and Standford, 1981).

Toddlers have developed ambulation skills that allow exploration, but they are well bonded to their parents and much less willing to be separated, especially when they are stressed. They are too young to understand detailed explanations so procedures should be told in simple, nonthreatening language. Comprehension of conversation is more advanced than verbal expression. The receptive and expressive language discordance often results in frustration on the child's behalf, putting toddlers at increased risk for stormy inductions and postoperative emotional and behavioral reactions. Toddlers also fear pain and bodily harm. Whenever possible, a parent or trusted caregiver should be present for potentially painful or threatening procedures. Children at this age are comforted by a familiar toy or treasured object and respond to magical thinking or stories.

The preschooler's view of the world is egocentric or self-centered. The child is unable to understand or conceptualize another individual's point of view, does not comprehend when people do not understand him or her, and has no appreciation for others' feelings. These children have concerns with bodily integrity and demonstrate the need for reassurances. Anxiety can be allayed by giving the child a sense of mastery and participation, such as allowing him or her to "hold" the mask for induction. Their preoperational thinking is very literal, and it is important to use caution when using similes or metaphors, e.g., if a provider states that the child will be given a "stick" (intravenous line or shot), the child may wait to be handed a tree branch. At this stage, any explanation appears to be more important than the actual content of the explanation. Children given explanations, whether accurate or not, were found to have fewer postoperative behavioral changes than those who were not given explanations (Bothe and Gladston, 1972). Although the preschooler's vocabulary is improving, cognitively the child may have difficulty remembering a sequence of events or establishing causality, leading to misconceptions about procedures.

School-age children, during the "concrete operations" stage, are more independent. Their activities become goal-oriented, and their language skills develop rapidly. They have a sense of conscience and can appreciate feelings of others. Children are able to draw on previous experience and knowledge to formulate predictions about related issues. They have an increased need for explanation and participation. Rather than giving children choices in the operating room (e.g., intravenous injection vs. mask for going to sleep), details about the procedure and options available for the child should be discussed preoperatively in a nonthreatening environment (McGraw, 1994).

Adolescents are caught in a difficult period between childhood and adulthood. Physically, they are maturing and may feel self-conscious about their bodies. Psychologically, they are striving to know who they are. Adolescents have developed the ability to recognize and exhibit mature defense mechanisms (e.g., the adolescent whose appendicitis "at least gets me out of my math test"). They are more likely to cooperate with a physician perceived to be attentive and nonjudgmental. Concerns regarding coping, pain, losing control, waking up prematurely, not waking up, and dying are very real for teenagers. Clear explanations and assurances should be provided regarding these issues. The need for independence and privacy is important and should be respected.

CLINICAL RELEVANCE OF GROWTH AND DEVELOPMENT IN PEDIATRIC ANESTHESIA

An overview of basic growth and development can be obtained in a preoperative consultation by reviewing the history and observing for gross and fine motor milestones during the physical examination. A 1-month-old infant displaying well-developed extensor tone when suspended in a ventral position might be interpreted by the parent as having advanced motor development when, in reality, issues of an upper motor neuron lesion should be considered. Other signs of spasticity are early rolling, pulling to a direct stand at 4 months of age, and walking on the toes. Persistent closing of fists beyond 3 months of age could be the earliest indication of neuromotor dysfunction. An afebrile 2-month-old baby with tachypnea, rales, audible murmur, and failure to gain weight should raise concerns about a significant cardiac lesion and the need for a cardiac consultation. A 7-month-old infant with poor head control who is unable to sit without support or to lift his or her chest off the table in the prone position may indicate hypotonia and a possible neuromuscular disorder. Spontaneous postures, such as "frog legging" when prone or scissoring may provide visual physical clues of hypotonia or spasticity, respectively. At 9 months of age, the child should stand erect on a parent's lap or cruise around office furniture, and the 12-month-old child will want to get down and walk. Weakness in the 3- or 4-year-old child may be best discovered by observing the quality of stationary posture and transition movements. Gower's sign (arising from sitting on the floor to standing using the hands to "walk up" the legs) is a classic example of pelvic girdle and quadriceps muscular weakness. Fine motor evaluation can be easily evaluated

by handing the infant a tongue depressor or toy. The newborn infant should grasp it reflexively; by 4 months of age, the infant should reach and retain the object, and by the age of 6 months, the child can transfer an object from hand to hand. The development of fine pincer grasp by 12 months of age allows the child to pick up small objects with precision, and increases the risk for foreign body aspiration. The observation of a child who constantly uses one hand while neglecting the other should prompt the clinician to examine the contralateral upper extremity for weakness associated with hemiparesis.

Abnormal head size, significant weight gain or loss, and short-stature issues may be indicative of genetic issues. The presence of three or more dysmorphic features should raise concerns of a syndromic feature with possible difficult airway issues. Almost 75% of superficial dysmorphic features can be found by examining the head, hands, and skin.

Down's Syndrome

Down's syndrome is the most common genetic abnormality worldwide, with an estimated prevalence of 1 out of 800 children (Sherman et al., 2007). Although this syndrome was described centuries earlier, Dr. John Langon Down first reported its clinical description in 1866 (Megarbane et al., 2009). Down's syndrome is the most recognizable and best known chromosomal disorder. The extra copy in chromosome 21 affects several organs and results in a wide spectrum of phenotypical changes (Hartway, 2009). Down's syndrome is usually identified soon after birth by a characteristic pattern of dysmorphic features (Fig. 2-5) (Ranweiler, 2009). The diagnosis is confirmed by karyotype analysis with trisomy 21 present in 95% of persons with this syndrome (Gardiner and Davisson, 2000).

Perioperative responsibility is shared between the anesthesiologist and the surgeon. The anesthesiologist is responsible for preoperative risk evaluation, perioperative management, and subsequent patient optimization (Hartley et al., 1998). The preoperative evaluation provides the best opportunity to stratify the potential risks, because children with Down's syndrome often have multiple congenital anomalies, each of which has anesthetic implications (Fig. 2-5) (Santamaria et al., 2007). Important considerations in the operative management of these patients include assessment of their behavioral development, atlantoaxial instability, airway narrowing, and respiratory and cardiac malformations; these are critical issues that require special attention when considering anesthesia (Bhattarai et al., 2008). Wherever possible, preoperative therapeutic interventions must be initiated to reduce the risks associated with these concurrent diseases (Borland et al., 2004). For the anesthesiologist, a system-based approach to the patient with Down's syndrome may be most useful. For a complete discussion of the anesthetic concerns related to Down's Syndrome, see Chapter 36, Systemic Disorders.

Behavioral Considerations

Down's syndrome is the most common cause of mental retardation, which is characterized by developmental delays, language and memory deficits, and other cognitive abnormalities (Roizen and Patterson, 2003). The child's cognitive state and psychological status often allow the anesthesia provider to ascertain the appropriate technique based on the child's needs.

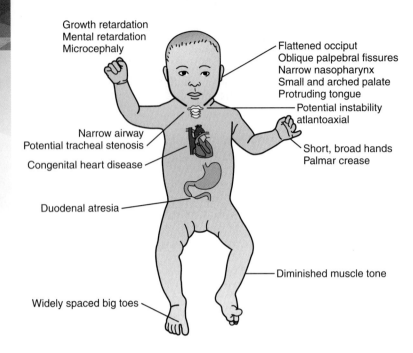

Growth retardation
Mental retardation
Microcephaly

Flattened occiput
Oblique palpebral fissures
Narrow nasopharynx
Small and arched palate
Protruding tongue

Potential instability
atlantoaxial

Narrow airway
Potential tracheal stenosis

Congenital heart disease

Short, broad hands
Palmar crease

Duodenal atresia

Diminished muscle tone

Widely spaced big toes

■ **FIGURE 2-5.** The congenital anomalies of Down's syndrome. *(Modified from Ranweiler R: Assessment and care of the newborn with Down syndrome,* Adv Neonatal Care *9:17, 2009; and Santamaria LB, Di Paola C, Mafrica F, et al: Preanesthetic evaluation and assessment of children with Down's syndrome,* The Scientific World Journal *7:242, 2007.)*

Older children and young adults with Down's syndrome have a higher prevalence of early Alzheimer's disease, further impairing cognitive function (Nieuwenhuis-Mark, 2009). Interestingly, children up to 6 years of age show age-related gains in adaptive function, but older children show no correlation between age and adaptive function (Dykens et al., 2006). In addition, the incidence of seizure disorders in those with Down's syndrome is 5% to 10% (Stafstrom et al., 1991).

Attention Deficit Hyperactivity Disorder

Attention deficit hyperactivity disorder (ADHD) is a disorder of inattention, hyperactivity, and impulsivity that affects 8% to 12% of children worldwide, with boys overrepresented by a ratio of about 3:1 (Biederman and Faraone, 2005). During child and adolescent development, ADHD is associated with greater risks for low academic achievement, poor school performance, retention in grade level, school suspensions and expulsions, poor peer and family relations, anxiety and depression, aggression, conduct problems, and delinquency (Barkley, 1997). The means of inheritance acquisition is probably multifactorial, but family, twin, and adoption studies have documented a strong genetic basis for ADHD (Thapar et al., 1999). The cellular theory suggests the frontosubcortical cerebellar regions of the brain have inadequate dopamine and noradrenaline to effectively provide inhibitory regulation (Biederman and Faraone, 2005).

Both the American Academy of Pediatrics (AAP) and the American Academy of Child and Adolescent Psychiatry (AACA) recommend psychoactive medications for children, adolescents, and adults with ADHD. These medications are classified as stimulants or nonstimulants. Perioperative consequences of these medications include resistance to premedication, cardiovascular instability, altered anesthesia requirements (monitored anesthesia care), lower seizure thresholds, and increased postoperative nausea and vomiting (Forsyth et al., 2006).

As an example of medication interaction, one patient required large doses of midazolam while receiving methylphenidate (Ririe et al., 1997). ADHD drugs are associated with increased blood pressure as a result of increased catecholamine levels, but the chronic use of stimulants can deplete these stores or downregulate catecholamine receptors. Prolonged hypotension has been reported in older patients with ADHD, and cardiac arrest (requiring cardiopulmonary resuscitation) during anesthetic induction was reported in a teenager (Bohringer et al., 2000; Perruchoud and Chollett-Rivier, 2008).

Medications such as buproprion are associated with seizures in a dose-related manner. The seizure threshold can be lowered by concomitant administration of drugs such as antipsychotics, antidepressants, systemic steroids, tramadol, and sedating antihistamines. In addition, bupropion inhibits the enzyme responsible for converting tramadol to morphine, thereby reducing the analgesic effect of tramadol (Corner et al., 2002).

These cases highlight the potential difficulties of the drug–drug interactions while a patient is undergoing general anesthesia. Based on these observations, the anesthesiologist should request more details about the medications a patient is taking for ADHD, particularly if they are stimulants or nonstimulants and the length of time the patient has been taking the medications. As in cardiac arrest, the implications and ramifications of anesthesia can be quite significant (Tables 2-5 and 2-6 (Perruchoud and Chollett-Rivier, 2008).

Autism

Autism affects 5 to 7 in 10,000 births, is found in all racial, ethnic, and social backgrounds, and is four times more common in males than females (Rudolph and Rudolph, 2003). Current data suggest that the actual rate is 40 out of 10, 000 births and that one out of every 150 children in the United States is affected (Rutter, 2005). Autism is now recognized a psychiatric childhood disorder, and is listed in the Diagnostic and Statistic Manual of Mental Disorders (DSM-IV) under the section Pervasive Developmental Disorders (PDD). The diagnostic criteria for autistic disorders include qualitative impairments social interactions, impairment in verbal and nonverbal communications, restricted range of interests, and resistance

TABLE 2-5. The Mechanisms of Action of Commonly Used ADHD Medications

Commonly Used Drug	Mechanism of Action
Methylphenidate (Ritalin)	Blocks the reuptake of norepinephrine and dopamine Stimulates the cerebral cortex similarly to amphetamines
Dexamphetamine (Dexedrin)	Promotes the release of catecholamines through sympathomimetic amines, primarily dopamine and norepinephrine Competitively inhibits catecholamine reuptake by the presynaptic nerve terminal
Buproprion (Wellbutrin)	Inhibits the neuronal uptake of norepinephrine and dopamine
Atomoxetine, 25 mg (Strattera)	Selectively inhibits norepinephrine reuptake by the presynaptic nerve terminal

From Forsyth I et al.: Attention deficit hyperactivity disorder and anesthesia, *Paediatric anaesthesia*, 16:371, 2006.

change (APA, 2000). These children exhibit hyperactivity and patterns of behavior, activity, and interests that are restrictive, repetitive, and stereotyped.

The etiology is unknown in the vast majority of the cases. However, there is a small minority of patients with notable coexisting medical diseases, including macrocephaly (15% to 35%), seizure disorders (30%), fragile X syndrome (2% to 8%), and tuberous sclerosis (1% to 3%) (Box 2-2) (Bailey and Rutter, 1991; Williams et al., 2008).

TABLE 2-6. Possible Drug–Drug Interactions with ADHD

Potential Side Effects	Medications
Sympathomimetic drugs that may produce exaggerated cardiovascular effects	Ephedrine, tramadol, SSRIs, MAOIs, tricyclics, herbal remedies, and dietary supplements (e.g., ephedra, St. John's wort)
Stimulants with potential to increase anesthetic requirements	Methylphenidate, dexamphetamine
Stimulants with potential to exacerbate seizure activity	Tramadol, detropropoxyphene, SSRIs, tricyclics

From Forsyth I et al.: Attention deficit hyperactivity disorder and anesthesia, *Paediatric anaesthesia*, 16:371, 2006.
SSRI, Selective serotonin reuptake inhibitor; *MAOI*, monoamine oxidase inhibitor.

Children with autism can present perioperative challenges to a pediatric anesthesia team (van der Walt and Moran, 2001). They are less able to understand the need for the procedures involved in surgery and have difficulty adjusting to the new routine of the hospital visit. Their perioperative anxiety level can be very high, and it may be difficult for them to interact with strangers, even caring and attentive perioperative staff. They are more sensitive to the visual and auditory stimuli of the hospital, particularly in the operating room, and even simple tactile stimuli such as the face mask may overwhelm their senses. Overall, these children are at high risk for severe distress and anxiety; consequently, morbidity and cost may be increased, and patient and parental satisfaction may be decreased.

Premedication varies depending on the requirements of each child, as well as the preferences of the individual anesthesiologist, who might generally use oral, intramuscular, or intravenous medications. Most institutions employ oral midazolam 0.5 mg/kg; however, the side effects are unpredictable and may not allow optimal anesthetic induction (Rainey and van der Walt, 1998). Ketamine is also an effective preoperative sedative, available in intravenous, intramuscular, and oral dosing. Oral ketamine has a 17% bioavailability, compared with 93% when given intramuscularly or intravenously (Clements et al., 1982). An effective transmucosal dosing combines ketamine 3 mg/kg mixed with midazolam 0.5 mg/kg (Funk et al., 2000).

If possible, the patient should undergo conditioning to become familiar with the hospital and the upcoming procedure (Nelson and Amplo, 2009). Diminished waiting time in the preoperative area can lessen fear and stress. Short, clear commands, with empathic positive and negative reinforcements, can help guide the patient through this difficult ordeal. Anesthesia management can be optimized by judicial use of premedication and parental presence during induction. The actual administration of an adequate dose of premedication can be the biggest challenge for the anesthesiologist working with an uncooperative or frightened child with delayed cognitive abilities. A balanced approach can help minimize the use of force, which is sometimes necessary, but nonetheless upsetting to the patient, the family, and the perioperative team. A discussion regarding the potential use of restraints during the perioperative period is imperative to clearly define the caregiver's expectations regarding this treatment modality. In summary, children with autism can present perioperative challenges, but thoughtful psychosocial and medical interventions can improve patient and parent satisfaction.

For questions and answers on topics in this chapter, go to "Chapter Questions" at www.expertconsult.com.

REFERENCES

Complete references used in this text can be found online at www.expertconsult.com.

CHAPTER 3

Respiratory Physiology in Infants and Children

Etsuro K. Motoyama and Jonathan D. Finder

CONTENTS

A mong many physiologic adaptations for the survival of humans at birth, cardiorespiratory adaptation is by far the most crucial. The respiratory and circulatory systems must be developed sufficiently in utero for the newborn infant to withstand drastic changes at birth—from the fetal circulatory pattern with liquid-filled lungs to air breathing with transitional circulatory adaptation in a matter of a few minutes. The newborn infant must exercise an effective neuronal drive and respiratory muscles to displace the liquid filling the airway system and to introduce sufficient air against the surface for[ce] in order to establish sufficient alveolar surface for gas exchang[e]. At the same time, pulmonary blood vessels must dilate rapid[ly] to increase pulmonary blood flow and to establish adequa[te] regional alveolar ventilation/pulmonary perfusion ($\dot{V}_A/\dot{Q}$) for sufficient pulmonary gas exchange. The neonatal adapta[tion] of lung mechanics and respiratory control takes seve[ral] weeks to complete. Beyond this immediate neonatal period, t[he] infant's lungs continue to mature at a rapid pace, and postna[tal] development of the lungs and the thorax surrounding the lungs continues well beyond the first year of life. Respiratory function in infants and toddlers, especially during the first several months of life, as with cardiovascular system and hepatic function, is both qualitatively and quantitatively different from that in older children and adults, and so is their responses to pharmacologic agents, especially anesthetics.

This chapter reviews clinically relevant aspects of the development of the respiratory system and function in infants and children and their application to pediatric anesthesia. Such knowledge is indispensable for the proper care of infants and children before, during, and after general anesthesia and surgery, as well as for the care of those with respiratory insufficiency.

The respiratory system consists of the respiratory centers in the brainstem; the central and peripheral chemoreceptors; the phrenic, intercostal, hypoglossal (efferent), and vagal (afferent) nerves; the thorax (including the thoracic cage; the muscles of the chest, abdomen, and diaphragm); the upper (extrathoracic) and lower (intrathoracic) airways; the lungs; and the pulmonary vascular system. The principal function of the respiratory system is to maintain the oxygen and carbon dioxide (CO_2) equilibrium in the body. The lungs also make an important contribution to the regulation of acid-base (pH) balance. The maintenance of body temperature (via loss of water through the lungs) is an additional but secondary function of the lungs. The lungs are also an important organ of metabolism.

DEVELOPMENT OF THE RESPIRATORY SYSTEM

Prenatal Development of the Lungs

The morphologic development of the human lung is seen as early as several weeks into the embryonic period and continues well into the first decade of postnatal life and beyond

(Fig. 3-1). The fetal lungs begin to form within the first several weeks of the embryonic period, when the fetus is merely 3 mm in length. A groove appears in the ventral aspect of the foregut, creating a small pouch. The outgrowth of the endodermal cavity, with a mass of surrounding mesenchymal tissue, projects into the pleuroperitoneal cavity and forms lung buds. The future alveolar membranes and mucous glands are derived from the endoderm, whereas the cartilage, muscle, elastic tissue, and lymph vessels originate from the mesenchymal elements surrounding the lung buds (Emery, 1969).

During the pseudoglandular period, which extends until 17 weeks' gestation, the budding of the bronchi and lung growth rapidly take place, forming a loose mass of connective tissue. The morphologic development of the human lung is illustrated in Figure 3-2. By 16 weeks' gestation, preacinar branching of the airways (down to the terminal bronchioli) is complete (Reid, 1967). A disturbance of the free expansion of the developing lung during this stage, as occurs with diaphragmatic hernia, results in hypoplasia of the airways and lung tissue (Areechon and Reid, 1963). During the canalicular period, in midgestation, the future respiratory bronchioli develop as the relative amount of connective tissue diminishes. Capillaries grow adjacent to the respiratory bronchioli, and the whole lung becomes more vascular (Emery, 1969).

At about 24 weeks' gestation, the lung enters the terminal sac period, which is characterized by the appearance of clusters of terminal air sacs, termed *saccules,* with flattened epithelium (Hislop and Reid, 1974). These saccules are large and irregular with thick septa and have few capillaries in comparison with the adult alveoli (Boyden, 1969). At about 26 to 28 weeks' gestation, proliferation of the capillary network surrounding the terminal air spaces becomes sufficient for pulmonary gas exchange (Potter, 1961). These morphologic developments may occur earlier in some premature infants (born at 24 to 25 weeks' gestation) who have survived through neonatal intensive care. Starting at 28 weeks' gestation, air space wall

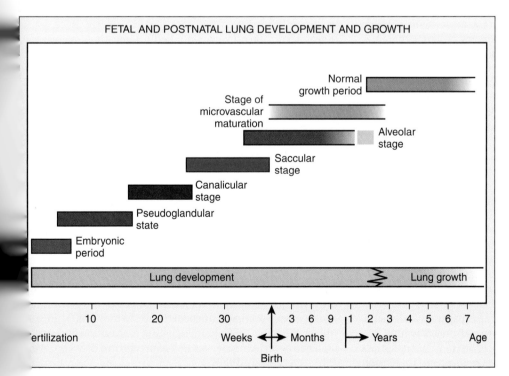

FETAL AND POSTNATAL LUNG DEVELOPMENT AND GROWTH

Normal growth period

Stage of microvascular maturation

Alveolar stage

Saccular stage

Canalicular stage

Pseudoglandular state

Embryonic period

Lung development   Lung growth

10   20   30   3 6 9   1 2 3 4 5 6 7

Fertilization   Weeks ←→ Months   Years   Age

Birth

■ **FIGURE 3-1.** Stages of human lung development and their timing. Note the overlap between stages, particularly between the alveolar stage and the stage of microvascular maturation. Open-ended bars indicate uncertainty as to exact timing. *(From Zeltner TB, Burri PH: The postnatal development and growth of the human lung. II. morphology, Respir Physiol 67:269, 1987.)*

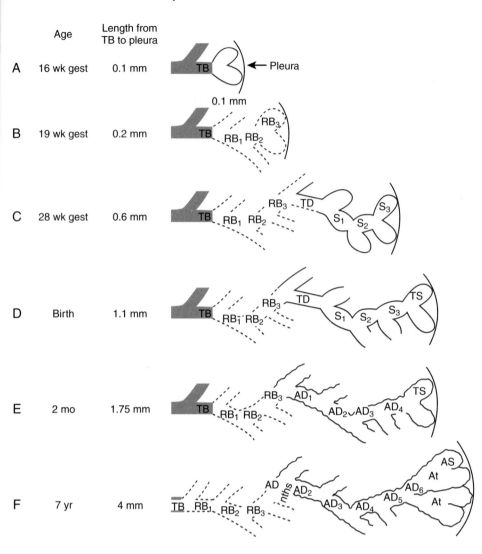

■ **FIGURE 3-2.** Development of the acinus in human lungs at various ages. *TB,* Terminal bronchiole; *RB,* respiratory bronchiole; *TD,* transitional duct; *S,* saccule; *TS,* terminal saccule; *AD,* alveolar duct; *At,* atrium; *AS,* alveolar sac, *(From Hislop A, Reid L: Development of the acinus in the human lung,* Thorax 29:90, 1974.)

thickness decreases rapidly. From this period onward toward term, there is further lengthening of saccules with possible growth of additional generations of air spaces. Some mammalian species, such as the rat, have no mature alveoli at birth (Burri, 1974). In contrast, alveolar development from saccules begins in some human fetuses as early as 32 weeks' gestation, but alveoli are not uniformly present until 36 weeks' gestation (Langston et al., 1984). Most alveolar formation in humans takes place postnatally during the first 12 to 18 months of postnatal life, and development of respiratory bronchioles by transformation of preexisting terminal airways does not take place until after birth (Langston et al., 1984).

The fetal lung produces a large quantity of liquid, which expands the airways while the larynx is closed. This expansion produces the growth factor, such as human bombesin, and helps to stimulate lung growth and development (Sunday et al., 1988). The lung fluid is periodically expelled into the uterine cavity and contributes about one third of the total amniotic fluid. Prenatal ligation or occlusion of the trachea was tried in the 1990s with some success for the treatment of the fetus with congenital diaphragmatic hernia (Harrison et al., 1993). This treatment causes the expansion of the fetal airways and results in an accelerated growth of the otherwise hypoplastic lung.

The type II pneumocytes, which produce pulmonary surfactant that forms the alveolar lining layer, reduces surface tension and stabilizes air spaces after air breathing, appear at about 24 to 26 weeks' gestation but occasionally as early as 20 weeks (Spear et al., 1969; Lauweryns, 1970). Idiopathic (or infantile) respiratory distress syndrome (IRDS), also known as hyaline membrane disease (HMD), which occurs in premature infants, is caused by the immaturity of the lungs with their insufficient pulmonary surfactant production and their inactivation by plasma proteins exuding onto the alveolar surface (see Surface Activity and Pulmonary Surfactant).

Experimental evidence from animals indicates that certain pharmacologic agents such as cortisol and thyroxin administered to the mother or directly to the fetus accelerate the maturation of the lungs, resulting in the early appearance of type II pneumocytes and surfactant (deLemos et al., 1970; Motoyama et al., 1971; Wu et al., 1973; Smith and Bogue, 1982; Rooney, 1985). Liggins and Howie (1972) reported accelerated maturation of human fetal lungs after the administration of corticosteroids to mothers 24 to 48 hours before the delivery of premature babies. Despite initial concern that steroids might potentially be toxic to other organs of the fetus, particularly to the development of the central nervous system, prenatal glucocorticoid therapy has been used widely since the 1980s to induce lung maturation and surfactant synthesis in mothers at risk of premature delivery (Avery, 1984; Avery et al., 1986).

NEONATAL RESPIRATORY ADAPTATION

Respiratory rhythmogenesis occurs in the fetus long before partition. The clamping of the umbilical cord and increasing arterial oxygen tensions and relative hyperoxia with air breathing (but not transient hypoxia) initiate and maintain rhythmic breathing at birth.

To introduce air into the fluid-filled lungs at birth, the newborn infant must overcome large surface force with the first few breaths. Usually a negative pressure of 30 cm H_2O is necessary to introduce air into the fluid-filled lungs. In some normal full-term infants, even with sufficient surfactant, a force of as much as –70 cm H_2O or more must be exerted to overcome the surface force (Fig. 3-3) (Karlberg et al., 1962). Usually fluid is rapidly expelled via the upper airways. The residual fluid leaves the lungs through the pulmonary capillaries and lymphatic channels over the first few days of life, and changes in compliance parallel this time course. All changes are delayed in the premature infant.

As the lungs expand with air, pulmonary vascular resistance decreases dramatically and pulmonary blood flow increases markedly, thus allowing gas exchange between alveolar air and pulmonary capillaries to occur. Changes in Po_2, Pco_2 *(P stands for partial pressure)*, and pH are largely responsible for the dramatic decrease in pulmonary vascular resistance (Cook et al., 1963). The resultant large increases in pulmonary blood flow and the increase in left atrial pressure with a decrease in right atrial pressure reverse the pressure gradient across the atria and close (initially functionally and eventually anatomically) the foramen ovale, a right-to-left one-way valve. With these adjustments, the cardiopulmonary system approaches adult levels of ventilation/perfusion ($\dot{V}A/\dot{Q}$ balance within a few days (Nelson et al., 1962, 1963). The process of expansion of the lungs during the first few hours of life and the resultant circulatory adaptation for establishing pulmonary gas exchange are greatly influenced by the adequacy of pulmonary surfactant. It should be remembered that these changes are delayed in immature newborns.

Postnatal Development of the Lungs and Thorax

The development and growth of the lungs and surrounding thorax continue with amazing speed during the first year of life. Although the formation of the airway system all the way to the terminal bronchioles is complete by 16 weeks' gestation, alveolar formation begins only at about 36 weeks' gestation. At birth, the number of terminal air sacs (most of which are saccules) is between 20 and 50 million, only one tenth that of fully grown lungs of the child. Most postnatal development of alveoli from primitive saccules occurs during the first year and is essentially completed by 18 months of age (Langston et al., 1984). The morphologic and physiologic development of the lungs, however, continues throughout the first decade of life (Mansell et al., 1972).

During the early postnatal period, the lung volume of infants is disproportionately small in relation to body size. In addition, because of higher metabolic rates in infants (oxygen consumption per unit body weight is twice as high as that of adults), the ventilatory requirement per unit of lung volume in infants is markedly increased. Infants, therefore, have much less reserve of lung volume and surface area for gas exchange. This is the primary reason why infants and young children become rapidly desaturated with hypoventilation or apnea of relatively short duration.

In the neonate, static (elastic) recoil pressure of the lungs is very low (i.e., compliance, normalized for volume, is unusually high), which is not dissimilar to that of geriatric or emphysematous lungs, because the elastic fibers do not develop until the postnatal period (whereas elastic fibers in geriatric lungs are brittle and not functional) (Mansel et al., 1972; Fagan, 1976; Bryan and Wohl, 1986). In addition, the elastic recoil pressure of the infant's thorax (chest wall) is extremely low because of its compliant cartilaginous rib cage with poorly developed thoracic muscle mass, which does not add rigidity. These unique characteristics make infants more prone to lung collapse, especially under general anesthesia when inspiratory muscles are markedly relaxed (see maintenance of FRC below). Throughout

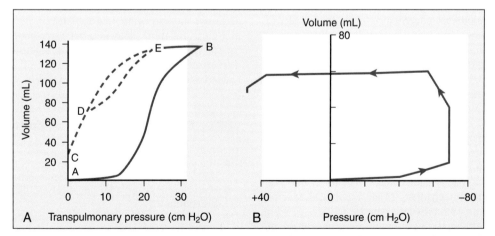

FIGURE 3-3. A, Typical pressure-volume curve of expansion of a gas-free lung. *A-B,* initial expansion. In the example, approximately 30 cm H_2O pressure will be necessary to overcome surface forces. *C,* Deflation to zero pressure with gas trapping. *D-E,* Subsequent breaths with a further increase in FRC (from C to D). **B,** Pressure-volume relationships during the first breath of a newborn weighing 4.3 kg. Here, 60 to 70 cm H_2O negative pressure was necessary to overcome the surface forces. *(From Karlberg P et al.: Respiratory studies in newborn infants. II. Pulmonary ventilation and mechanics of breathing in the first minutes of life, including the onset of respiration, Acta Paediatr Scand 51:121, 1962.)*

infancy and childhood, static recoil pressure of the lungs and thorax steadily increases (compliance, normalized for volume, decreases) toward normal values for young adults (Zapletal et al., 1971; Motoyama, 1977).

The actual size of the airway from the larynx to the bronchioles in infants and children, of course, is much smaller than in adolescents and adults, and flow resistance in absolute terms is extremely high. When normalized for lung volume or body size, however, infants' airway size is relatively much larger; airway resistance is much lower than in adults (Polgar, 1967; Motoyama, 1977; Stocks and Godfrey, 1977). Infants and toddlers, however, are more prone to severe obstruction of the upper and lower airways because their absolute (not relative) airway diameters are much smaller than those in adults. As a consequence, relatively mild airway inflammation, edema, or secretions can lead to far greater degrees of airway obstruction than in adults (e.g., as with subglottic croup [laryngotracheo-bronchitis] or acute supraglottitis [epiglottitis]).

Further description on the development of the lungs and thorax and their effects on lung function, especially under general anesthesia, are described later in the chapter. Perinatal and postnatal adaptations of respiratory control are included in the following section on the control of breathing.

Prenatal Development of Breathing

Respiratory rhythmogenesis occurs long before parturition. Dawes and others (1970) were the first to demonstrate "breathing" activities with rhythmic diaphragmatic contractions in the fetal lamb. They found it to be episodic and highly variable in frequency. Boddy and Robinson (1971) recorded movement of the human fetal thorax with an ultrasound device and interpreted this as evidence of fetal breathing. Later studies have shown that during the last 10 weeks of pregnancy, fetal breathing is present approximately 30% of the time (Patrick et al., 1980). The breathing rate in the fetus at 30 to 31 weeks' gestation is higher (58 breaths/min) than that in the near-term fetus (47 breaths/min). A significant increase in fetal breathing movements occurs 2 to 3 hours after a maternal meal and is correlated with the increase in the maternal blood sugar level (Patrick et al., 1980).

Spontaneous breathing movements in the fetus occur only during active, or rapid eye movement (REM), sleep and with low-voltage electrocortical activity, and they appear to be independent of the usual chemical and nonchemical stimuli of postnatal breathing (Dawes et al., 1972; Jansen and Chernick, 1983). Later studies, however, have clearly shown that the fetus can respond to chemical stimuli known to modify breathing patterns postnatally (Dawes et al., 1982; Jansen et al., 1982; Rigatto et al., 1988, 1992). In contrast, hypoxemia in the fetus abolishes, rather than stimulates, breathing movements. This may be related to the fact that hypoxemia diminishes the incidence of REM sleep (Boddy et al., 1974). It appears that normally low arterial oxygen tension, or Pao_2 (19 to 23 mm Hg), in the fetus is a normal mechanism inhibiting breathing activities in utero (Rigatto, 1992). Severe hypoxia induces gasping, which is independent of the peripheral chemoreceptors and apparently independent of rhythmic fetal breathing (Jansen and Chernick, 1974).

The near-term fetus is relatively insensitive to $Paco_2$ changes. Extreme hypercapnia ($Paco_2$ greater than 60 mm Hg) in the fetal lamb, however, can induce rhythmic breathing movement that is preceded by a sudden activation of inspiratory muscle tone with expansion of the thorax and inward movement (inspiration) of amniotic fluid, as much as 30 to 40 mL/kg (an apparent increase in functional residual capacity [FRC]) (Motoyama, unpublished observation). When Pao_2 was reduced, breathing activities ceased, and there was a reversal of the sequence of events noted above (i.e., relaxation of the thorax, decreased FRC as evidenced by outward flow of amniotic fluid) (Motoyama, 2001).

The Hering-Breuer (inflation) reflex is present in the fetus. Distention of the lungs by saline infusion slows the frequency of breathing (Dawes et al., 1982). Transection of the vagi, however, does not change the breathing pattern (Dawes, 1974).

Maternal ingestion of alcoholic beverages abolishes human fetal breathing for up to 1 hour. Fetal breathing movement is also abolished by maternal cigarette smoking. These effects may be related to fetal hypoxemia resulting from changes in placental circulation Jansen and Chernick, 1983). It is not clear why the fetus must "breathe" in utero, when gas exchange is handled by the placental circulation. Dawes (1974) suggested that fetal breathing might represent "prenatal practice" to ensure that the respiratory system is well developed and ready at the moment of birth. Another reason may be that the stretching of the airways and lung parenchyma is an important stimulus for lung development; bilateral phrenic nerve sectioning in the fetal lamb results in hypoplasia of the lungs (Alcorn et al., 1980).

Perinatal Adaptation of Breathing

During normal labor and vaginal delivery, the human fetus goes through a period of transient hypoxia, hypercapnia, and acidemia. The traditional view of the mechanism of the onset of breathing at birth until the 1980s was that the transient fetal asphyxia stimulates the chemoreceptors and produces gasping, which is followed by rhythmic breathing at birth that is aided by thermal, tactile, and other sensory stimuli. Subsequent studies have challenged this concept (Chernick et al., 1975; Baier et al., 1990; Rigatto, 1992). The current concept regarding the mechanism of continuous neonatal breathing is summarized in Box 3-1.

Once the newborn has begun rhythmic breathing, ventilation is adjusted to achieve a lower $Paco_2$ than is found in older children and adults (Table 3-1). The reason for this difference is not clear but most likely is related to a poor buffering capacity in the neonate and a ventilatory compensation for metabolic acidosis. The Pao_2 of the infant approximates the adult level within a few weeks of birth (Nelson, 1976).

Box 3-1 Mechanism of Continuous Neonatal Breathing

- The onset of breathing activities occurs not at birth but in utero, as a part of normal fetal development.
- The clamping of the umbilical cord initiates rhythmic breathing.
- Relative hyperoxia with air breathing, compared with low fetal Pao_2, augments and maintains continuous and rhythmic breathing.
- Continuous breathing is independent of the level of $Paco_2$.
- Breathing is unaffected by carotid denervation.
- Hypoxia depresses or abolishes continuous breathing.

TABLE 3-1. Normal Blood-Gas Values

	Pao$_2$ (mm Hg)	Sao$_2$ (%)	Paco$_2$ (mm Hg)	pH
Pregnant woman at term	88*	96	32	7.40
Umbilical vein	31	72*	42	7.35
Umbilical artery	19	38*	51	7.29
1 hour of life (artery)	62	95	28	7.36
24 hours of life (artery)	68	94	29	7.37
Child and adult (artery)	99	97	41	7.40

*Estimated values.

Control of breathing in the neonate evolves gradually during the first month of extrauterine life and beyond and is different from that in older children and adults, especially in the response to hypoxemia and hyperoxia. The neonates' breathing patterns and responses to chemical stimuli are detailed after a general overview of the control of breathing.

CONTROL OF BREATHING

The mechanism that regulates and maintains pulmonary gas exchange is remarkably efficient. In a normal person, the level of Paco$_2$ is maintained within a very narrow range, whereas oxygen demand and carbon dioxide production vary greatly during rest and exercise. This control is achieved by a precise matching of the level of ventilation to the output of carbon dioxide. Breathing is produced by the coordinated action of a number of inspiratory and expiratory muscles. Inspiration is produced principally by the contraction of the diaphragm, which creates negative intrathoracic pressure that draws air into the lungs. Expiration, on the other hand, is normally produced passively by the elastic recoil of the lungs and thorax. It may be increased actively by the contraction of abdominal and thoracic expiratory muscles during exercise. During the early phase of expiration, sustained contraction of the diaphragm with decreasing intensity (braking action) and the upper airway muscles' activities and narrowing of the glottic aperture impede and smoothen the rate of expiratory flow.

Rhythmic contraction of the respiratory muscles is governed by the respiratory centers in the brainstem and tightly regulated by feedback systems so as to match the level of ventilation to metabolic needs (Fig. 3-4) (Cherniack and Pack, 1988). These feedback mechanisms include central and peripheral chemoreceptors, stretch receptors in the airways and lung parenchyma via the vagal afferent nerves, and segmental reflexes in the spinal cord provided by muscle spindles (Cherniack and Pack, 1988). The control of breathing comprises neural and chemical controls that are closely interrelated.

Neural Control of Breathing

Respiratory neurons in the medulla have inherent rhythmicity even when they are separated from the higher levels of the

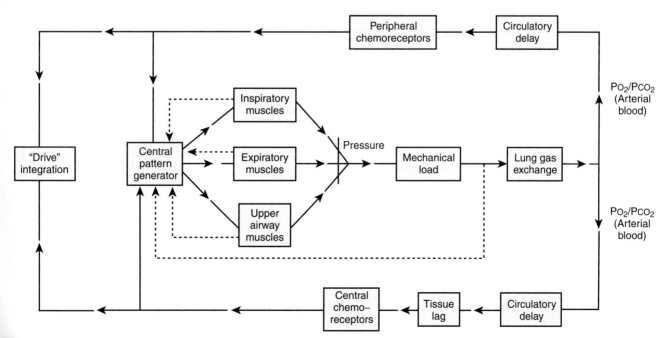

FIGURE 3-4. Block diagram of multi-input, multi-output system that controls ventilation.

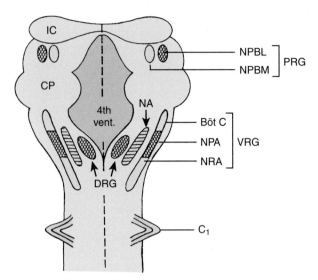

■ FIGURE 3-5. Schematic representation of the respiratory neurons on the dorsal surface of the brainstem. Cross-hatched areas contain predominantly inspiratory neurons, blank areas contain predominantly expiratory neurons, and dashed areas contain both inspiratory and expiratory neurons. *Böt C,* Bötzinger complex; *C,* first cervical spinal nerve; *CP,* cerebellar peduncle; *DRG,* dorsal respiratory group; *4th Vent,* fourth ventricle; *IC,* inferior colliculus; *NA,* nucleus ambiguus; *NPA,* nucleus paraambigualis; *NPBL,* nucleus parabrachialis lateralis; *NPBM,* nucleus parabrachialis medialis; *NRA,* nucleus retroambigualis; *PRG,* pontine respiratory group; *VRG,* ventral respiratory group. *(From Tabatabai M, Behnia R: Neurochemical regulation of respiration. In Collins VJ, editor: Physiological and pharmacological basis of anesthesia, Philadelphia, 1995, Williams & Wilkins.)*

brainstem. In the cat, respiratory neurons are concentrated in two bilaterally symmetric areas in the medulla near the level of the obex. The dorsal respiratory group of neurons (DRG) is located in the dorsomedial medulla just ventrolateral to the nucleus tractus solitarius and contains predominantly inspiratory neurons. The ventral respiratory group of neurons (VRG), located in the ventrolateral medulla, consists of both inspiratory and expiratory neurons (Fig. 3-5) (von Euler, 1986; Tabatabai and Behnia, 1995; Berger, 2000).

Dorsal Respiratory Group of Neurons

The DRG is spatially associated with the tractus solitarius, which is the principal tract for the ninth and tenth cranial (glossopharyngeal and vagus) nerves. These nerves carry afferent fibers from the airways and lungs, heart, and peripheral arterial chemoreceptors. The DRG may constitute the initial intracranial site for processing some of these visceral sensory afferent inputs into a respiratory motor response (Berger, 2000).

On the basis of lung inflation, three types of neurons have been recognized in the DRG: type Iα *(I stands for inspiratory),* type Iβ, and pump (P) cells. Type Iα is inhibited by lung inflation (Cohen, 1981a). The axons of these neurons project to both the phrenic and the external (inspiratory) intercostal motoneurons of the spinal cord. Some type Iα neurons have medullary collaterals that terminate among the inspiratory and expiratory neurons of the ipsilateral VRG (Merrill, 1970).

The second type, Iβ, is excited by lung inflation and receives synaptic inputs from pulmonary stretch receptors. There is

controversy as to whether Iβ axons project into the spinal cord respiratory neurons; the possible functional significance of such spinal projections is unknown. Both Iα and Iβ neurons receive excitatory inputs from the central pattern generator (or central inspiratory activity) for breathing, so that when lung inflation is terminated or the vagi in the neck are cut, the rhythmic firing activity of these neurons continues (Cohen, 1981a, 1981b; Feldman and Speck, 1983).

The third type of neurons in the DRG receives no input from the central pattern generator. The impulse of these neurons, the P cells, closely follows lung inflation during either spontaneous or controlled ventilation (Berger, 1977). The P cells are assumed to be relay neurons for visceral afferent inputs (Berger, 2000).

The excitation of Iβ neurons by lung inflation is associated with the shortening of inspiratory duration. The Iβ neurons appear to promote inspiration-to-expiration phase-switching by inhibiting Iα neurons. This network seems to be responsible for the Hering-Breuer reflex inhibition of inspiration by lung inflation (Cohen, 1981a, 1981b; von Euler, 1986, 1991).

The DRG thus functions as an important primary and possibly secondary relay site for visceral sensory inputs via glossopharyngeal and vagal afferent fibers. Because many of the inspiratory neurons in the DRG project to the contralateral spinal cord and make excitatory connections with phrenic motoneurons, the DRG serves as a source of inspiratory drive to phrenic and possibly to external intercostal motoneurons (Berger, 2000).

Ventral Respiratory Group of Neurons

The VRG extends from the rostral to the caudal end of the medulla and has three subdivisions (Fig. 3-5). The Bötzinger complex, located in the most rostral part of the medulla in the vicinity of the retrofacial nucleus, contains mostly expiratory neurons (Lipski and Merrill, 1980; Merrill et al., 1983). These neurons send inhibitory signals to DRG and VRG neurons and project into the phrenic motoneurons of the spinal cord, causing its inhibition (Bianchi and Barillot, 1982; Merrill et al., 1983). The physiologic significance of these connections may be to ensure inspiratory neuronal silence during expiration (reciprocal inhibition) and to contribute to the "inspiratory off-switch" mechanism.

The nucleus ambiguus (NA) and nucleus paraambigualis (NPA), lying side by side, occupy the middle portion of the VRG. Axons of the respiratory motoneurons originating from the NA project along with other vagal efferent fibers and innervate the laryngeal abductor (inspiratory) and adductor (expiratory) muscles via the recurrent laryngeal nerve (Barillot and Bianchi, 1971; Bastel and Lines, 1975). The NPA contains mainly inspiratory (Iγ) neurons, which respond to lung inflation in a manner similar to that of Iα neurons. The axons of these neurons project both to phrenic and external (inspiratory) intercostal motoneuron pools in the spinal cord. The nucleus retroambigualis (NRA) occupies the caudal part of the VRG and contains expiratory neurons whose axons project into the spinal motoneuron pools for the internal (expiratory) intercostal and abdominal muscles (Merrill, 1970; Miller et al., 1985).

The inspiratory neurons of the DRG send collateral fibers to the inspiratory neurons of the NPA in the VRG. These connections may provide the means for ipsilateral synchronization of the inspiratory activity between the neurons in the DRG and those in the VRG (Merrill, 1979, 1983). Furthermore, axon collaterals of the inspiratory neurons of the NPA on one side project to the inspiratory neurons of the contralateral NPA, and vice versa. These connections may be responsible for the bilateral synchronization of the medullary inspiratory motoneuron output, as evidenced by synchronous bilateral phrenic nerve activity (Merrill, 1979, 1983).

Pontine Respiratory Group of Neurons

In the dorsolateral portion of the rostral pons, both inspiratory and expiratory neurons have been found. Inspiratory neuronal activity is concentrated ventrolaterally in the region of the nucleus parabrachialis lateralis (NPBL). The expiratory activity is centered more medially in the vicinity of the nucleus parabrachialis medialis (NPBM) (Fig. 3-5) (Cohen, 1979; Mitchell and Berger, 1981). The respiratory neurons of these nuclei are referred to as the pontine respiratory group (PRG), which was, and sometimes still is, called the pneumotaxic center, although the term is generally considered obsolete (Feldman, 1986). There are reciprocal projections between the PRG neurons and the DRG and VRG neurons in the medulla. Electrical stimulation of the PRG produces rapid breathing with premature switching of respiratory phases, whereas transaction of the brainstem at a level caudal to the PRG prolongs inspiratory time (Cohen, 1971; Feldman and Gautier, 1976). Bilateral cervical vagotomies produce a similar pattern of slow breathing with prolonged inspiratory time; a combination of PRG lesions and bilateral vagotomy in the cat results in apneusis (apnea with sustained inspiration) or apneustic breathing (slow rhythmic respiration with marked increase end inspiratory hold) (Feldman and Gaultier, 1976; Feldman, 1986). The PRG probably plays a secondary role in modifying the inspiratory off-switch mechanism (Gautier and Bertrand, 1975; von Euler and Trippenbach, 1975).

Respiratory Rhythm Generation

Rhythmic breathing in mammals can occur in the absence of feedback from peripheral receptors. Because transection of the brain rostral to the pons or high spinal transection has little effect on the respiratory pattern, respiratory rhythmogenesis apparently takes place in the brainstem. The PRG, DRG, and VRG have all been considered as possible sites of the central pattern generator, although its exact location is still unknown (Cohen, 1981b; von Euler, 1983, 1986). A study with an in vitro brainstem preparation of neonatal rats has indicated that respiratory rhythm is generated in the small area in the ventrolateral medulla just rostral to the Bötzinger complex (pre-Bötzinger complex), which contains pacemaker neurons (Smith et al., 1991).

The pre-Bötzinger complex contains a group of neurons that is responsible for respiratory rhythmogenesis (Smith et al., 1991; Pierrefiche et al., 1998; Rekling and Feldman, 1998). Although the specific cellular mechanism responsible for rhythmogenesis is not known, two possible mechanisms have been proposed (Funk and Feldman, 1995; Ramirez and Richter, 1996). One hypothesis is that the pacemaker neurons possess intrinsic properties associated with various voltage- and time-dependent ion channels that are responsible for rhythm generation. Rhythmic activity in these neurons may depend on the presence of an input system that may be necessary to maintain the neuron's membrane potential in a range in which the voltage-dependent properties of the cell's ion channels result in rhythmic behavior. The network hypothesis is the alternative model in which the interaction between the neurons produces respiratory rhythmicity, such as reciprocal inhibition between inhibitory and excitatory neurons and recurrent excitation within any population of neurons (Berger, 2000). The output of this central pattern generator is influenced by various inputs from chemoreceptors (central and peripheral), mechanoreceptors (e.g., pulmonary receptors and muscle and joint receptors), thermoreceptors (central and peripheral), nociceptors, and higher central structures (such as the PRG). The function of these inputs is to modify the breathing pattern to meet and adjust to ever-changing metabolic and behavioral needs (Smith et al., 1991).

Airway and Pulmonary Receptors

The upper airways, trachea and bronchi, lungs, and chest wall have a number of sensory receptors sensitive to mechanical and chemical stimulation. These receptors affect ventilation as well as circulatory and other nonrespiratory functions.

Upper Airway Receptors

Stimulation of receptors in the nose can produce sneezing, apnea, changes in bronchomotor tone, and the diving reflex, which involves both the respiratory and the cardiovascular systems. Stimulation of the epipharynx causes the sniffing reflex, a short, strong inspiration to bring material (mucus, foreign body) in the epipharynx into the pharynx to be swallowed or expelled. The major role of receptors in the pharynx is associated with swallowing. It involves the inhibition of breathing, closure of the larynx, and coordinated contractions of pharyngeal muscles (Widdicombe, 1985; Nishino, 1993; Sant'Ambrogio et al., 1995).

The larynx has a rich innervation of receptors. The activation of these receptors can cause apnea, coughing, and changes in the ventilatory pattern (Widdicombe, 1981, 1985). These reflexes, which influence both the patency of the upper airway and the breathing pattern, are related to transmural pressure and air flow. Based on single-fiber action-potential recordings from the superior laryngeal nerve in the spontaneously breathing dog preparation in which the upper airway is isolated from the lower airways, three types of receptors have been identified: pressure receptors (most common, about 65%), "drive" (or irritant) receptors (stimulated by upper airway muscle activities), and flow or cold receptors (Sant'Ambrogio et al., 1983; Fisher et al., 1985). The laryngeal flow receptors show inspiratory modulation with room air breathing but become silent when inspired air temperature is raised to body temperature and 100% humidity or saturation (Sant'Ambrogio et al., 1985). The activity of pressure receptors increases markedly with upper airway obstruction (Sant'Ambrogio et al., 1983).

Tracheobronchial and Pulmonary Receptors

Three major types of tracheobronchial and pulmonary receptors have been recognized: slowly adapting (pulmonary stretch) receptors and rapidly adapting (irritant or deflation) receptors, both of which lead to myelinated vagal afferent fibers and unmyelinated C-fiber endings (J-receptors). Excellent reviews on pulmonary receptors have been published (Pack, 1981; Widdicombe, 1981; Sant'Ambrogio, 1982; Coleridge and Coleridge, 1984).

Slowly adapting (pulmonary stretch) receptors. Slowly adapting (pulmonary stretch) receptors (SARs) are mechanoreceptors that lie within the submucosal smooth muscles in the membranous posterior wall of the trachea and central airways (Bartlett et al., 1976). A small proportion of the receptors are located in the extrathoracic upper trachea (Berger, 2000). SARs are activated by the distention of the airways during lung inflation and inhibit inspiratory activity (Hering-Breuer inflation reflex), whereas they show little response to steady levels of lung inflation. The Hering-Breuer reflex also produces dilation of the upper airways from the larynx to the bronchi. Although SARs are predominantly mechanoreceptors, hypocapnia stimulates their discharge, and hypercapnia inhibits it (Pack, 1981). In addition, SARs are thought to be responsible for the accelerated heart rate and systemic vasoconstriction observed with moderate lung inflation (Widdicombe, 1974). These effects are abolished by bilateral vagotomy.

Studies by Clark and von Euler (1972) have demonstrated the importance of the inflation reflex in adjusting the pattern of ventilation in the cat and the human. In cats anesthetized with pentobarbital, inspiratory time decreases as tidal volume increases with hypercapnia, indicating the presence of the inflation reflex in the normal tidal volume range. Clark and von Euler demonstrated an inverse hyperbolic relationship between the tidal volume and inspiratory time. In the adult human, inspiratory time is independent of tidal volume until the latter increases to about twice the normal tidal volume, when the inflation reflex appears (Fig. 3-6). In the newborn, particularly the premature newborn, the inflation reflex is present in the eupneic range for a few months (Olinsky et al., 1974).

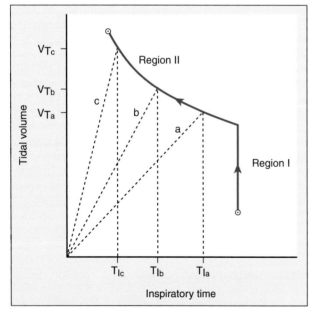

■ **FIGURE 3-6.** Relationship between tidal volume (V_T) and inspiratory time (T_I) as ventilation is increased in response to respiratory stimuli. Note that in region I, Vt increases without changes in T_I. Also shown as dashed lines are the V_T trajectories for three different tidal volumes in region II. *(From Berger AJ: Control of breathing. In Murray JF, Nadel JA: Textbook of respiratory medicine, Philadelphia, 1994, WB Saunders.)*

Apnea, commonly observed in adult patients at the end of surgery and anesthesia with the endotracheal tube cuff still inflated, may be related to the inflation reflex, because the trachea has a high concentration of stretch receptors (Bartlett et al., 1976; Sant'Ambrogio, 1982). Deflation of the cuff promptly restores rhythmic spontaneous ventilation.

Rapidly adapting (irritant) receptors. Rapidly adapting (irritant) receptors (RARs) are located superficially within the airway epithelial cells, mostly in the region of the carina and the large bronchi (Pack, 1981; Sant'Ambrogio, 1982). RARs respond to both mechanical and chemical stimuli. In contrast to SARs, RARs adapt rapidly to large lung inflation, distortion, or deflation, thus possessing marked dynamic sensitivity (Pack, 1981). RARs are stimulated by cigarette smoke, ammonia, and other irritant gases including inhaled anesthetics, with significant interindividual variability (Sampson and Vidruk, 1975). RARs are stimulated more consistently by histamine and prostaglandins, suggesting their role in response to pathologic states (Coleridge et al., 1976; Sampson and Vidruk, 1977; Vidruk et al., 1977; Berger, 2000). The activation of RARs in the large airways may be responsible for various reflexes, including coughing, bronchoconstriction, and mucus secretion. Stimulation of RARs in the periphery of the lungs may produce hyperpnea. Because RARs are stimulated by deflation of the lungs to produce hyperpnea in animals, they are considered to play an important role in the Hering-Breuer deflation reflex (Sellick and Widdicombe, 1970). This reflex, if it exists in humans, may partly account for increased respiratory drive when the lung volume is abnormally decreased, as in premature infants with IRDS and in pneumothorax.

When vagal conduction is partially blocked by cold, inflation of the lung produces prolonged contraction of the diaphragm and deep inspiration instead of inspiratory inhibition. This reflex, the paradoxical reflex of Head, is most likely mediated by RARs. It may be related to the complementary cycle of respiration, or the sigh mechanism, that functions to reinflate and reaerate parts of the lungs that have collapsed because of increased surface force during quiet, shallow breathing (Mead and Collier, 1959). In the newborn, inflation of the lungs initiates gasping. This mechanism, which was considered to be analogous to the paradoxical reflex of Head, may help to inflate unaerated portions of the newborn lung (Cross et al., 1960).

C-Fiber endings. Most afferent axons arising from the lungs, heart, and other abdominal viscera are slow conducting (slower than 2.5 m/sec), unmyelinated vagal fibers (C-fibers). Extensive studies by Paintal (1973) have suggested the presence of receptors supposedly located near the pulmonary or capillary wall (juxtapulmonary capillary or J-receptors) innervated by such C-fibers. C-fiber endings are stimulated by pulmonary congestion, pulmonary edema, pulmonary microemboli, and irritant gases such as anesthetics. Such stimulation causes apnea followed by rapid, shallow breathing, hypotension, and bradycardia. Stimulation of J-receptors also produces bronchoconstriction and increases mucus secretion. All these responses are abolished by bilateral vagotomy. In addition, stimulation of C-fiber endings can provoke severe reflex contraction of the laryngeal muscles, which may be partly responsible for the laryngospasm observed during induction of anesthesia with isoflurane or halothane.

In addition to receptors within the lung parenchyma (pulmonary C-fiber endings), there appear to be similar nonmyelinated nerve endings in the bronchial wall (bronchial C-fiber endings) (Coleridge and Coleridge, 1984). Both chemical and, to a lesser degree, mechanical stimuli excite these bronchial C-fiber endings. They are also stimulated by endogenous mediators of inflammation, including histamine, prostaglandins, serotonin, and bradykinin. Such stimulation may be a mechanism of C-fiber involvement in disease states such as pulmonary edema, pulmonary embolism, and asthma (Coleridge and Coleridge, 1984).

The inhalation of irritant gases or particles causes a sensation of tightness or distress in the chest, probably caused by its activation of pulmonary receptors. The pulmonary receptors may contribute to the sensation of dyspnea in lung congestion, atelectasis, and pulmonary edema. Bilateral vagal blockade in patients with lung disease abolished dyspneic sensation and increased breath-holding time (Noble et al., 1970).

Chest-Wall Receptors

The chest-wall muscles, including the diaphragm and the intercostal muscles, contain various types of receptors that can produce respiratory reflexes. This subject has been reviewed extensively (Newsom-Davis, 1974; Duron, 1981). The two types of receptors that have been most extensively studied are muscle spindles, which lie parallel to the extrafusal muscle fibers, and the Golgi tendon organs, which lie in series with the muscle fibers (Berger, 2000).

Muscle spindles are a type of slowly adapting mechanoreceptors that detect muscle stretch. As in other skeletal muscles, the muscle spindles of respiratory muscles are innervated by γ-motoneurons that excite intrafusal fibers of the spindle.

Intercostal muscles have a density of muscle spindles comparable with those of other skeletal muscles. The arrangement of muscle spindles is appropriate for the respiratory muscle load-compensation mechanism (Berger, 2000). By comparison with the intercostal muscles, the diaphragm has a very low density of muscle spindles and is poorly innervated by the γ-motoneurons. Reflex excitation of the diaphragm, however, can be achieved via proprioceptive excitation within the intercostal system (Decima and von Euler, 1969).

Golgi tendon organs are located at the point of insertion of the muscle fiber into its tendon and, like muscle spindles, are a slowly adapting mechanoreceptor. Activation of the Golgi tendon organs inhibits the homonymous motoneurons, possibly preventing the muscle from being overloaded (Berger, 2000). In the intercostal muscles, fewer Golgi tendon organs are present than muscle spindles, whereas the ratio is reversed in the diaphragm.

Chemical Control of Breathing

Regulation of alveolar ventilation and maintenance of normal arterial Pco_2, pH, and Po_2 are the principal functions of the medullary and peripheral chemoreceptors (Leusen, 1972).

Central Chemoreceptors

The medullary, or central, chemoreceptors, located near the surface of the ventrolateral medulla, are anatomically separated from the medullary respiratory center (Fig. 3-7). They respond to changes in hydrogen ion concentration in the adjacent

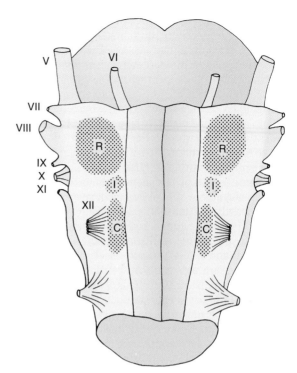

■ **FIGURE 3-7.** View of the ventral surface of the medulla shows the chemosensitive zones. The rostral *(R)* and caudal *(C)* zones are chemosensitive. The intermediate *(I)* zone is not chemosensitive but may have a function in the overall central chemosensory response. The roman numerals indicate the cranial nerves. *(From Berger AJ, Hornbein TF: Control of respiration. In Patton HD et al., editors:* Textbook of physiology, *ed 21, Philadelphia, 1989, WB Saunders.)*

cerebrospinal fluid rather than to changes in arterial Pco_2 or pH (Pappenheimer et al., 1965). Since CO_2 rapidly passes through the blood-brain barrier into the cerebrospinal fluid, which has poor buffering capacity, the medullary chemoreceptors are readily stimulated by respiratory acidemia. In contrast, ventilatory responses of the medullary chemoreceptors to acute metabolic acidemia and alkalemia are limited because changes in the hydrogen ion concentration in arterial blood are not rapidly transmitted to the cerebrospinal fluid. In chronic acid-base disturbances, the pH of cerebrospinal fluid (and presumably that of interstitial fluid) surrounding the medullary chemoreceptors is generally maintained close to the normal value of about 7.3 regardless of arterial pH (Mitchell et al., 1965). Under these circumstances, ventilation becomes more dependent on the hypoxic response of peripheral chemoreceptors.

Peripheral Chemoreceptors

The carotid bodies, located near the bifurcation of the common carotid artery, react rapidly to changes in Pao_2 and pH. Their contribution to the respiratory drive amounts to about 15% of resting ventilation (Severinghaus, 1972). The carotid body has three types of neural components: type I (glomus) cells, presumably the primary site of chemotransduction; type II (sheath) cells; and sensory nerve fibers (McDonald, 1981). Sensory nerve fibers originate from terminals in apposition to the glomus cells, travel via the carotid sinus nerve to join the glossopharyngeal nerve, and then enter the brainstem. The sheath cells envelop both the glomus cells and the sensory nerve terminals.

A variety of neurochemicals have been found in the carotid body, including acetylcholine, dopamine, substance P, enkephalins, and vasoactive intestinal peptide. The exact functions of these cell types and the mechanisms of chemotransduction and the specific roles of these neurochemicals have not been well established (Berger, 2000).

The carotid bodies are perfused with extremely high levels of blood flow and respond rapidly to an oscillating Pao_2 rather than a constant Pao_2 at the same mean values (Dutton et al., 1964; Fenner et al., 1968). This mechanism may be partly responsible for hyperventilation during exercise.

The primary role of peripheral chemoreceptors is their response to changes in arterial Po_2. Moderate to severe hypoxemia (Pao_2 less than 60 mm Hg) results in a significant increase in ventilation in all age groups except for newborn, particularly premature, infants, whose ventilation is decreased by hypoxemia (Dripps and Comroe, 1947; Rigatto et al., 1975b). Peripheral chemoreceptors are also partly responsible for hyperventilation in hypotensive patients. Respiratory stimulation is absent in certain states of tissue hypoxia, such as moderate to severe anemia and carbon monoxide poisoning; despite a decrease in oxygen content, Pao_2 in the carotid bodies is maintained near normal levels, so that the chemoreceptors are not stimulated.

In acute hypoxemia, the ventilatory response via the peripheral chemoreceptors is partially opposed by hypocapnia, which depresses the medullary chemoreceptors. When a hypoxemic environment persists for a few days, for example, during an ascent to high altitude, ventilation increases further as cerebrospinal fluid bicarbonate decreases and pH returns toward normal (Severinghaus et al., 1963). However, later studies demonstrated that the return of cerebrospinal fluid pH toward normal is incomplete, and a secondary increase in ventilation precedes the decrease in pH, indicating that some other mechanisms are involved (Bureau and Bouverot, 1975; Foster et al., 1975). In chronic hypoxemia that lasts for a number of years, the carotid bodies initially exhibit some adaptation to hypoxemia and then gradually lose their hypoxic response. In people native to high altitudes, the blunted response of carotid chemoreceptors to hypoxemia takes 10 to 15 years to develop and is sustained thereafter (Sorensen and Severinghaus, 1968; Lahiri et al., 1978). In cyanotic heart diseases, the hypoxic response is lost much sooner but returns after surgical correction of the right-to-left shunts (Edelman et al., 1970).

In patients who have chronic respiratory insufficiency with hypercapnia, hypoxemic stimulation of the peripheral chemoreceptors provides the primary impulse to the respiratory center. If these patients are given excessive levels of oxygen, the stimulus of hypoxemia is removed, and ventilation decreases or ceases. Pco_2 further increases, patients become comatose (CO_2 narcosis), and death may follow unless ventilation is supported. Rather than oxygen therapy, such patients need their effective ventilation increased artificially with or without added inspired oxygen.

Response to Carbon Dioxide

The graphic demonstration of relations between the alveolar or arterial Pco_2 and the minute ventilation ($\dot{V}E/Pco_2$) is commonly known as the CO_2 response curve (Fig. 3-8). This curve normally reflects the response of the chemoreceptors and respiratory center to CO_2. The CO_2 response curve is a useful means for evaluation of the chemical control of breathing, provided that

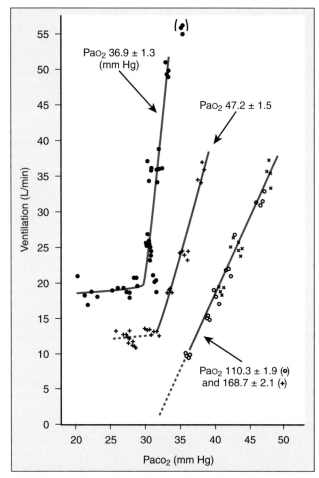

■ FIGURE 3-8. Effect of acute hypoxemia on the ventilatory response to steady-state Pao_2 in one subject. Inspired oxygen was adjusted in each experiment to keep Pao_2 constant at the level as indicated. *(From Nielsen M, Smith H: Studies on the regulation of respiration in acute hypoxia,* Acta Physiol Scand *24:293, 1951.)*

the mechanical properties of the respiratory system, including the neuromuscular transmission, respiratory muscles, thorax, and lungs, are intact. In normal persons, ventilation increases more or less linearly as the inspired concentration of carbon dioxide increases up to 9% to 10%, above which ventilation starts to decrease (Dripps and Comroe, 1947). Under hypoxemic conditions the CO_2 response is potentiated, primarily via carotid body stimulation, resulting in a shift to the left of the CO_2 response curve (Fig. 3-8) (Nielsen and Smith, 1951). On the other hand, anesthetics, opioids, and barbiturates in general depress the medullary chemoreceptors and, by decreasing the slope, shift the CO_2 response curve progressively to the right as the anesthetic concentration increases (Fig. 3-9) (Munson et al., 1966).

A shift to the right of the CO_2 response curve in an awake human may be caused by decreased chemoreceptor sensitivity to CO_2, as seen in patients whose carotid bodies had been destroyed (Wade et al., 1970). It may also be caused by lung disease and resultant mechanical failure to increase ventilation despite intact neuronal response to carbon dioxide. In patients with various central nervous system dysfunctions, the CO_2 response may be partially or completely lost (Ondine's curse) (Severinghaus and Mitchell, 1962). In the awake state

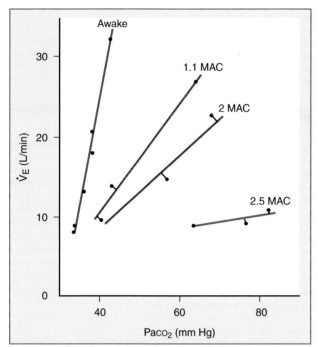

FIGURE 3-9. CO_2 response curve with halothane. Family of steady-state CO_2 response curves in one subject awake and at three levels of halothane anesthesia. Note progressive decrease in ventilatory response to Pao_2 with increasing anesthetic depth (MAC; ventilatory response in awake state was measured in response to end-tidal Pco_2). *(Courtesy Dr. Edwin S. Munson; data from Munson ES, et al.: The effects of halothane, fluroxene, and cyclopropane on ventilation: a comparative study in man,* Anesthesiology *27:716, 1966.)*

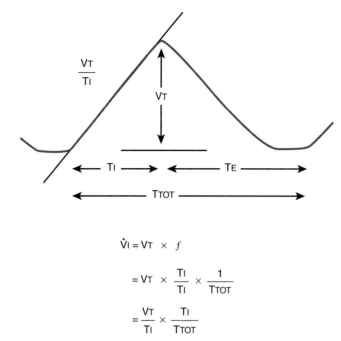

FIGURE 3-10. Schematic drawing of tidal volume and timing components on time-volume axes. V_T, Tidal volume; T_I, inspiratory time; T_E, expiratory time; T_{TOT}, total time for respiratory cycle; f, respiratory frequency; V_T/T_I, mean inspiratory flow rate; T_I/T_{TOT}, respiratory duty cycle.

these patients have chronic hypoventilation but can breathe on command. During sleep, they further hypoventilate or become apneic to the point of CO_2 narcosis and death unless mechanically ventilated or implanted with a phrenic pacemaker (Glenn et al., 1973).

It has been difficult to separate the neuronal component from the mechanical failure of the lungs and thorax, because the two factors often coexist in patients with chronic lung diseases (Guz et al., 1970). Whitelaw and others (1975) demonstrated that occlusion pressure at 0.1 second ($P_{0.1}$, or the negative mouth pressure generated by inspiratory effort against airway occlusion at FRC) correlates well with neuronal (phrenic) discharges but is uninfluenced by mechanical properties of the lungs and thorax. The occlusion pressure is a useful means for the clinical evaluation of the ventilatory drive.

As mentioned previously, hypoxemia potentiates the chemical drive and increases the slope of the CO_2 response curve ($\dot{V}_E/Pco_2$). Such a change has been interpreted as "a synergistic (or multiplicative) effect" of the stimulus, whereas a parallel shift of the curve has been considered as "an additive effect." This analysis may be useful for descriptive purposes, but it is misleading. Because ventilation is the product of tidal volume and frequency ($\dot{V}_E = V_T \times f$), an additive effect on its components could result in a change in the slope of the CO_2 response curve. Obviously, the responses of tidal volume and frequency to CO_2 should be examined separately to understand the effect of various respiratory stimulants and depressants.

Milic-Emili and Grunstein (1975) proposed that ventilatory response to CO_2 be analyzed in terms of the mean inspiratory flow (V_T/T_I, where V_T is tidal volume and T_I is the inspiratory time) and in terms of the ratio of inspiratory time to total ventilatory cycle duration or respiratory duty cycle (T_I/T_{TOT}) (Fig. 3-10). Because the tidal volume is equal to $V_T/T_I \times T_I$ and respiratory frequency (f) is $1/T_{TOT}$, ventilation can be expressed as follows:

$$\dot{V}_E = V_T \times f = V_T / T_I \times T_I / T_{TOT}$$

The advantage of analyzing the ventilatory response in this fashion is that V_T/T_I is an index of inspiratory drive, which is independent of the timing element. The tidal volume, on the other hand, is time dependent, because it is $(V_T/T_I) \times T_I$. The second parameter, T_I/T_{TOT}, is a dimensionless index of effective respiratory timing (respiratory duty cycle) that is determined by the vagal afferent or central inspiratory off-switch mechanism or by both (Bradley et al., 1975). From this equation, it is apparent that in respiratory disease or under anesthesia, changes in pulmonary ventilation may result from a change in V_T/T_I, T_I/T_{TOT}, or both. A reduction in T_I/T_{TOT} indicates that the relative duration of inspiration decreased or that expiration increased. Such a reduction in the T_I/T_{TOT} ratio may result from changes in central or peripheral mechanisms. In contrast, a reduction in V_T/T_I may indicate a decrease in the medullary inspiratory drive or neuromuscular transmission or an increase in inspiratory impedance (i.e., increased flow resistance, decreased compliance, or both). By relating the mouth occlusion pressure to V_T/T_I, it becomes clinically possible to determine whether changes in the mechanics of the respiratory system contribute to the reduction in V_T/T_I (Milic-Emili, 1977).

Analysis of inspiratory and expiratory durations provides useful information on the mechanism of anesthetic effects

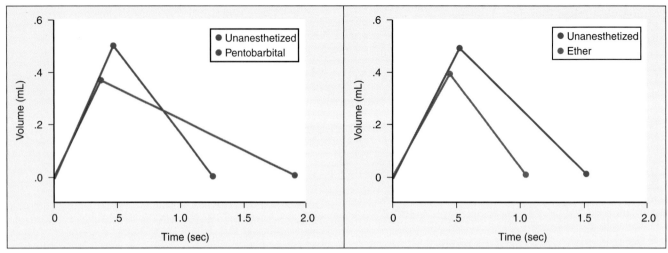

■ **FIGURE 3-11.** Schematic summary of changes in the average respiratory cycle in a group of newborn rabbits before and after sodium pentobarbital anesthesia *(left)* and before and during ether anesthesia *(right).* Measurements obtained during spontaneous room air breathing. Zero on the time axis indicates onset of inspiration. Mean inspiratory flow is represented by the slope of the ascending limb of the spirograms. *(Modified from Milic-Emili J: Recent advances in the evaluation of respiratory drive,* Int Anesthesiol Clin *15:75, 1977.)*

on ventilation. Figure 3-11 illustrates the effect of pentobarbital, which depresses minute ventilation, and diethyl ether, which "stimulates" ventilation in newborn rabbits. With both anesthetics the mean inspiratory flow (V_T/T_I) did not change, but V_T decreased because T_I was shortened. With pentobarbital, however, T_E was prolonged disproportionately, and T_I/T_{TOT} and frequency decreased; consequently, minute ventilation was decreased. With ether, on the other hand, ventilation increased as the result of disproportionate decrease in Te and consequent increases in T_I/T_{TOT} and frequency (Milic-Emili, 1977).

Control of Breathing in Neonates and Infants

Response to Hypoxemia in Infants

During the first 2 to 3 weeks of age, both full-term and premature infants in a warm environment respond to hypoxemia (15% oxygen) with a transient increase in ventilation followed by sustained ventilatory depression (Brady and Ceruti, 1966; Rigatto and Brady, 1972a, 1972b; Rigatto et al., 1975a) (Fig. 3-12). In infants born at 32 to 37 weeks' gestation, the initial period of transient hyperpnea is abolished in a cool environment, indicating the importance of maintaining a neutral thermal environment (Cross and Oppe, 1952; Ceruti, 1966; Perlstein et al., 1970). When 100% oxygen is given, a transient decrease in ventilation is followed by sustained hyperventilation. This ventilatory response to oxygen is similar to that of the fetus and is different from that of the adult, in whom a sustained decrease in ventilation is followed by little or no increase in ventilation (Dripps and Comroe, 1947). By 3 weeks after birth, hypoxemia induces sustained hyperventilation, as it does in older children and adults.

The biphasic depression in ventilation has been attributed to central depression rather than to depression of peripheral chemoreceptors (Albersheim et al., 1976). In newborn monkeys, however, tracheal occlusion pressure, an index of central neural drive, and diaphragmatic electromyographic output were increased above the control level during both the

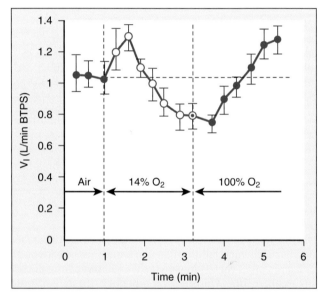

■ **FIGURE 3-12.** Effect on ventilation of 14% oxygen (hypoxia) from room air and then to 100% oxygen (hyperoxia) in three newborn infants. Ventilation (mean ± SEM) is plotted against time. During acute hypoxia there was a transient increase in ventilation followed by depression. Hyperoxia increased ventilation. *(Modified from Lahiri S, et al.: Regulation of breathing in newborns,* J Appl Physiol *44:673, 1978.)*

hyperpneic and the hypopneic phases in response to hypoxic gas mixture (LaFramboise et al., 1981; LaFramboise and Woodrum, 1985). These findings imply that the biphasic ventilatory response to hypoxemia results from changes in the mechanics of the respiratory system (thoracic stiffness or airway obstruction), rather than from neuronal depression, as has been assumed (Jansen and Chernick, 1983). Premature infants continue to show a biphasic response to hypoxemia even at 25 days after birth (Rigatto, 1986). Thus, in terms of a proper response to hypoxemic challenge, maturation of the respiratory system may be related to postconceptional rather than postnatal age.

Response to Carbon Dioxide in Infants

Newborn infants respond to hypercapnia by increasing ventilation but less so than do older infants. The slope of the CO_2 response curve increases appreciably with gestational age as well as with postnatal age, independent of postconceptional age (Rigatto et al., 1975a, 1975b, 1982; Frantz et al., 1976). This increase in slope may represent an increase in chemosensitivity, but it may also result from more effective mechanics of the respiratory system. In adults the CO_2 response curve both increases in slope and shifts to the left with the severity of hypoxemia (Fig. 3-8). In contrast, in newborn infants breathing 15% oxygen, the CO_2 response curve decreases in slope and shifts to the right (Fig. 3-13). Inversely, hyperoxemia increases the slope and shifts the curve to the left (Rigatto et al., 1975a).

Upper Airway Receptor Responses in the Neonatal Period

Newborn animals are particularly sensitive to the stimulation of the superior laryngeal nerve either directly or through the receptors (such as water in the larynx), which results in ventilatory depression or apnea. In anesthetized newborn puppies and kittens, negative pressure or air flow through the larynx isolated from the lower airways produced apnea or significant prolongation of inspiratory and expiratory time and a decrease in tidal volume, whereas similar stimulation caused little or no effect in 4- to 5-week-old puppies or in adult dogs and cats (Al-Shway and Mortola, 1982; Fisher et al., 1985).

In a similar preparation using puppies anesthetized with pentobarbital, water in the laryngeal lumen produced apnea, whereas phosphate buffer with sodium chloride and neutral pH did not. The principal stimulus for the apneic reflex was the absence or reduced concentrations of chloride ion (Boggs and

Bartlett, 1982). In awake newborn piglets, direct electric stimulation of the superior laryngeal nerve caused periodic breathing and apnea associated with marked decreases in respiratory frequency, hypoxemia, and hypercapnia with minimal cardiovascular effects. Breathing during superior laryngeal nerve stimulation was sustained by an arousal system (Donnelly and Haddad, 1986). The strong inhibitory responses elicited in newborn animals by various upper airway receptor stimulations have been attributed to the immaturity of the central nervous system (Lucier et al., 1979; Boggs and Bartlett, 1982).

Active Vs. Quiet Sleep

During the early postnatal period, full-term infants spend 50% of their sleep time in active or REM sleep compared with 20% REM sleep in adults (Stern et al., 1969; Rigatto et al., 1982). Wakefulness rarely occurs in neonates. Premature neonates stay in REM sleep most of the time, and quiet (non-REM) sleep is difficult to define before 32 weeks' postconception (Rigatto, 1992). Neonates, particularly prematurely born neonates, therefore breathe irregularly.

Neurologic and chemical control of breathing in infants is related to the state of sleep (Scher et al., 1992). During quiet sleep, breathing is regulated primarily by the medullary respiratory centers and breathing is regular with respect to timing as well as amplitude and is tightly linked to chemoreceptor input (Bryan and Wohl, 1986). During REM sleep, however, breathing is controlled primarily by the behavioral system and is irregular with respect to timing and amplitude (Phillipson, 1994).

Periodic Breathing and Apnea

Periodic Breathing

Periodic breathing, in which breathing is interposed with repetitive short apneic spells lasting 5 to 10 seconds with minimal hemoglobin desaturation or cyanosis, occurs normally even in healthy neonates and young infants during wakefulness, REM sleep, and non-REM sleep (Rigatto et al., 1982). Periodic breathing tends to be more regular in quiet sleep than in active sleep and has been observed more often during active sleep (Rigatto et al., 1982) or during quiet sleep (Kelly et al., 1985). Minute ventilation increases during REM sleep due to increases in respiratory frequency with little change in tidal volume (Kalapezi et al., 1981; Rigatto et al., 1982).

An addition of 2% to 4% CO_2 to the inspired gas mixture abolishes periodic breathing, probably by causing respiratory stimulation (Chernick et al., 1964). Nevertheless, the ventilatory response to hypercapnia seems to be diminished during periodic breathing (Rigatto and Brady, 1972a). The decreased hypercapnic response appears to result from changes in respiratory mechanics rather than from a reduction in chemosensitivity, because respiratory center output as determined by airway occlusion pressure is greater during REM sleep than during non-REM sleep.

The incidence of periodic breathing was reported to be 78% in full-term neonates, whereas the incidence was much higher (93%) in preterm infants (mean postconceptional age of 37.5 weeks) (Kelly et al., 1985; Glotzbach et al., 1989). The incidence of periodic breathing diminishes with increasing postconceptual age and decreases to 29% by 10 to 12 months of age (Fenner et al., 1973; Kelly et al., 1985).

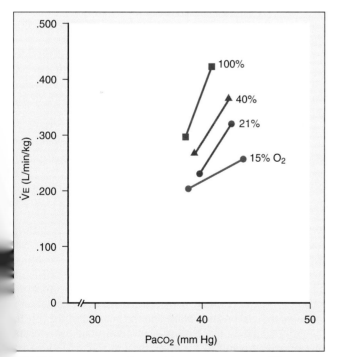

FIGURE 3-13. Mean steady-state CO_2 response curves at different inspired oxygen concentrations in eight preterm infants. The slope of the CO_2 response decreases with decreasing oxygen. *(From Rigatto H et al.: Effects of O_2 on the ventilatory response, J Appl Physiol 39:896, 1975.)*

Apnea of Prematurity and Hypoxia

Central apnea of infancy is defined as cessation of breathing for 15 seconds or longer or a shorter respiratory pause associated with bradycardia (heart rate less than 100 beats/min, cyanosis, or pallor (Brooks, 1982). Apnea is common in preterm infants and may be related to an immature respiratory control mechanism (Jansen and Chernick, 1983). Most preterm infants with a birth weight of less than 2 kg have apneic spells at some time (Spitzer and Fox, 1984). Glotzbach and others (1989) reported a 55% incidence of central apnea in preterm infants, whereas it was rarely found in full-term infants (Kelly et al., 1985). These studies, however, were based on a relatively small number of infants admitted to a single institution.

The report by the Collaborative Home Infant Monitoring Evaluation (CHIME) Study Group has shed a new light on the understanding of the incidence and extent of apnea in infancy (Hunt et al., 1999; Ramanathan et al., 2001). The CHIME study was based on the recordings of respiratory inductive plethysmography, electrocardiography (ECG), and pulse oximetry in normal infants and those with increased risk of sudden infant death syndrome (SIDS), and it involved a total of 1079 infants during the first 6 months after birth (Hunt et al., 1999; Ramanathan et al., 2001). This report has revealed evidence that the control of breathing and oxygenation during sleep in healthy term infants are not as precise as have been assumed. Normal infants, up to 2% to 3%, commonly have prolonged central, obstructive, or mixed apnea lasting up to 30 seconds, which is associated with oxygen desaturation (Ramanathan et al., 2001). With a simple upper respiratory infection, prolonged obstructive sleep apneas were recorded in a few normal full-term infants but were present in 15% to 30% of preterm infants. The risk of having such episodes was 20 to 30 times higher among preterm infants than in full-term infants before 43 weeks' postconception (Hunt et al., 1999). Healthy term infants had an average baseline SpO_2 of 98% throughout the recorded period. However, hypoxemia (SpO_2 less than 90%, occasionally in the 70% to 80% range) occurred in 59% of these normal term infants in 0.6% of recorded cases (Hunt et al., 1999). Thus, levels of hypoxemia or hypoxia previously considered pathologic are relatively common occurrences among normal infants.

Apparent life-threatening events (ALTE) are characterized by an episode of sudden onset characterized by color change (cyanosis or pallor), tone change (limpness or rarely stiffness), and apnea, which requires immediate resuscitation to revive the infant and restore normal breathing (National Heart, Lung, and Blood Consensus Development Conference, National Institutes of Health, 1987). The incidence of ALTE is as high as 3% and may occur in previously healthy infants. Overnight polysomnography (PSG) is particularly useful in the evaluation of infants with a history of unexplained apnea. Treatable pathologic conditions, however, were found only in about 30% of infants, and thus normal PSG results are not necessarily diagnostic for the purpose of ruling out ALTE (Ramanathan et al., 2001).

Postoperative Apnea

Life-threatening apnea has been reported postoperatively in prematurely born infants earlier than 41 weeks' postconception, particularly in those with a history of apneic spells after simple surgical procedures, such as inguinal herniorrhaphy, and can occur up to 12 hours postoperatively (Steward, 1982;

Liu et al., 1983). These reports resulted in a general consensus among the pediatric anesthesiologists that infants younger than 44 weeks' postconception be admitted for overnight observation after inguinal hernia repair for safety. In a subsequent report, including various surgical procedures, apnea was reported in 4 of 18 prematurely born infants who were 49 to 55 weeks' postconceptional age (Kurth et al., 1987). The authors of this report proposed that premature infants younger than 60 weeks' postconception should be admitted for overnight observation, which raised a controversy as to what postconceptional age is safe and appropriate for the same-day discharge from the hospital for the prematurely born infant (Kurth et al., 1987). Malviya and others (1993) analyzed the relationship between the incidence of postoperative apnea and maturation. They reported a high incidence of postoperative apnea (26%) in infants younger than 44 weeks' postconception, whereas the incidence of apnea in those older than 44 weeks was only 3%.

Subsequently, Coté and others (1995) performed a meta-analysis of the data from previously published studies of postoperative apnea in expremature infants after inguinal hernia repairs. They concluded that postoperative apnea was strongly and inversely correlated to both gestational age as well as postconceptual age and was associated with a previous history of apnea. The probability of postoperative apnea in those older than 44 weeks postconceptual age decreases significantly (to 5%) but still exists. Another important finding of this classic paper was that postoperative hypoxemia, hypothermia, and (most importantly) anemia (hematocrit value of less than 30) are significant risk factors regardless of gestational or postconceptual age (see Chapter 13, Induction, Maintenance, and Recovery). Most of these studies occurred in the period when infants were predominantly anesthetized with halothane and without regional (caudal) block to maintain a lighter level of anesthesia with spontaneous breathing during surgery. Postoperative apnea still exists with newer anesthetic agents (e.g., sevoflurane or desflurane), but appears to occur much less often.

Both theophylline and caffeine have been effective in reducing apneic spells in preterm infants (Aranda and Trumen, 1979). Caffeine is especially useful for premature infants during the postanesthetic period (Welborn et al., 1988). Xanthine derivatives are known to prevent muscle fatigue, and their respiratory stimulation in the premature infant may occur via both central and peripheral mechanisms (Aubier et al., 1981).

Maintenance of the Upper Airway and Airway Protective Reflexes

Pharyngeal Airway

The pharyngeal airway, unlike the laryngeal airway, is not supported by a rigid bony or cartilaginous structure. Its wall consists of soft tissues and is surrounded by muscles for breathing and for swallowing and is contained in a fixed bony structure (i.e., the maxilla, mandible, and spine) (Isono, 2006). Anatomic imbalance between the bony structure (the container—micrognathia, facial anomalies) and the amount of the soft tissues (the content—macroglossia, adenotonsillar hypertrophy, obesity) would result in the pharyngeal airway narrowing and obstruction (Fig. 3-14) (Isono, 2006).

Even the normal pharyngeal airway is easily obstructed by the relaxation of the velopharynx (soft palate), posterior displacement of the mandible (and the base of the tongue) in the

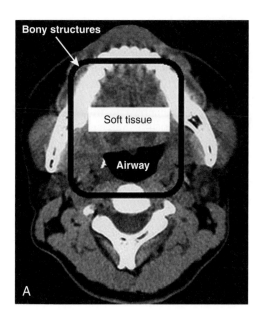

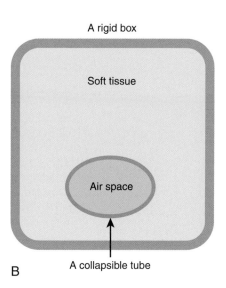

■ **FIGURE 3-14.** A mechanical model of the pharyngeal airway *(right)* is produced based on structures surrounding the pharyngeal airway on a CT scan *(left). (From Isono S: Developmental changes of pharyngeal airway patency: implications for pediatric anesthesia,* Pediatr Anesth *16:109, 2006.)*

supine position during sleep, flexion of the neck, or external compression over the hyoid bone. The pharyngeal airway also is easily collapsed by negative pressure within the pharyngeal lumen created by inspiratory effort, especially when airway-maintaining muscles are depressed or paralyzed (Issa and Sullivan, 1984; Reed et al., 1985; Roberts et al., 1985). In neonates, with a relatively hypoplastic mandible, the oropharynx and the entrance to the larynx at the level of the aryepiglottic folds are the areas most easily collapsed (Reed et al., 1985).

Mechanical support to sustain the patency of the pharynx against the collapsing force of luminal negative pressure during inspiration is given by both the sustained muscle tension and cyclic contraction of the pharyngeal dilator muscles, acting synchronously with the contraction of the diaphragm. These include the genioglossus, geniohyoid, sternohyoid, sternothyroid, and thyrohyoid muscles (Fig. 3-15) (Bartlett et al., 1973; Pack et al., 1988; Thach, 1992). Similar phasic activities have been recorded in the scalene and sternomastoid muscles in humans (Onal et al., 1981; Drummond, 1987).

A neural balance model of pharyngeal airway maintenance proposed by Remmers et al. (1978) and Brouillette and Thach (1979) and further modified by Isono (2006) is shown in Figure 3-16. In this model, the suction (collapsing) force created in the pharyngeal lumen by the inspiratory pump muscles (primarily the diaphragm) must be well balanced by the activities of pharyngeal airway dilator muscles to maintain upper airway patency. Increased nasal and pharyngeal airway resistance (partial obstruction) exaggerates the suction force. In addition, once pharyngeal closure occurs, the mucosal adhesion force of the collapsed pharyngeal wall becomes an added force acting against the opening of pharyngeal air passages (Reed et al., 1985).

Several reflex mechanisms are present to maintain the balance between the dilating and collapsing forces in the pharynx. Chemoreceptor stimuli such as hypercapnia and hypoxemia stimulate the airway dilators preferentially over the stimulation of the diaphragm so as to maintain airway patency (Brouillette and Thach, 1980; Onal et al., 1981, 1982). Negative pressure in the nose, pharynx, or larynx activates the pharyngeal dilator muscles and simultaneously decreases the diaphragmatic activity (Fig. 3-17) (Mathew et al., 1982a, 1982b; Hwang et al., 1984; Thach, 1992). Such an airway pressure reflex is especially prominent in infants younger than 1 year of age (Thach et al., 1989). Upper airway mechanoreceptors are located superficially in the airway mucosa and are easily blocked by topical anesthesia (Mathew et al., 1982a, 1982b). Sleep, sedatives, and anesthesia depress upper airway muscles more than they do the diaphragm (Sauerland and Harper, 1976; Ochiai et al., 1989, 1992). The arousal from sleep shifts the balance toward pharyngeal dilation (Thach, 1992).

Laryngeal Airway

The larynx is composed of a group of cartilage, connecting ligaments, and muscles. It maintains the airway, and the glottis functions as a valve to occlude and protect the lower airways from the alimentary tract. It is also an organ for phonation (Proctor, 1977a, 1977b, 1986; Fink and Demarest, 1978). With

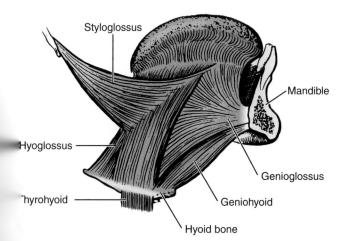

FIGURE 3-15. Lateral view of the musculature of the tongue and relationship with a mandible and hyoid bone. *(From Kuna ST, Remmers JE: Pathophysiology and mechanisms of sleep apnea. In Fletcher EC, editor:* Abnormalities of respiration during sleep, *Orlando, 1986, Grune & Stratton.)*

Pharyngeal airway (PA) size

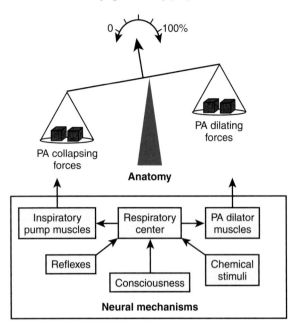

■ **FIGURE 3-16.** A neural and anatomic balance model of the pharyngeal airway *(PA)* maintenance by Remmers et al. (1978) in adults and Brouillette and Thach (1979) in infants illustrating the balance of opposing forces that affect PA size. Airway collapsing forces (suction force created by inspiratory pump muscles) and dilating forces (pharyngeal dilator muscles) are shown on either side of the fulcrum, and neural mechanisms controlling this balance are in the box below the balance. *(Redrawn from Isono S: Developmental changes of pharyngeal airway patency: implications for pediatric anesthesia,* Pediatr Anesth *16:109, 2006.)*

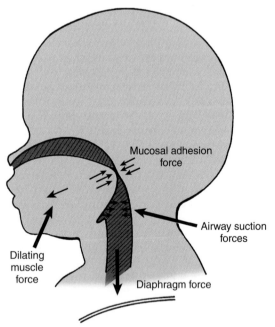

■ **FIGURE 3-17.** Schematic illustration of sequence of events showing one of the ways in which the upper airway pressure reflex operates to preserve pharyngeal airway patency. *(From Thach BT: Neuromuscular control of the upper airway. In Beckerman RC et al., editors:* Respiratory control disorders in infants and children, *Baltimore, 1992, Williams & Wilkins.)*

the exception of the anterior nasal passages, the larynx at the subglottis is the narrowest portion of the entire airway system in all ages (Eckenhoff, 1951). The cricoid cartilage forms a complete ring, protecting the upper airway from compression.

For over half a century, the shape of pediatric larynx was thought to be "funnel shaped," with the narrowest point at the laryngeal exit (cricoid ring), in contrast to the adult larynx, which is "cylindrical" in shape. This belief was based on the well-referenced classic paper by Eckenhoff in 1951; Eckenhoff quoted the work of Bayeux in 1897, more than half a century before his time, whose description was based on moulages (plaster casting) made from cadaveric larynx from 15 children between the ages of 4 months and 14 years. Indeed, Eckenhoff's original paper cautioned that "the measurements so derived may not be completely applicable to the living" (Eckenhoff, 1951; Motoyama, 2009). More recently, however, both Litman and colleagues (2003) and Dalal and colleagues (2009) using two entirely different methodologies in living infants and children under general anesthesia, found that the dimensions of the larynx in infants and children are more cylindrical than funnel-shaped, as in adults, and the cylindrical shape does not change significantly with growth. In addition, both Litman and Dalal's papers confirmed that the cricoid opening is the narrowest point of the larynx; however, in paralyzed children the opening at the vocal cords (lima glottidis) may be narrower than the opening of the cricoid cartilage, but it is expandable beyond the opening of the cricoid ring (Eckenhoff, 1951; Dalal et al., 2009). Perhaps more important clinically, both groups found with statistical significance that the cricoid opening is not circular but mildly elliptic with a smaller transverse diameter. This means that a tight-fitting, uncuffed endotracheal tube or even a "best-fitted" tube in young children with acceptable pressure leak (i.e., 20 cm H$_2$O) would exert more compression, if not ischemia, on the transverse mucosa of the cricoid ring (Motoyama, 2009). This finding provides theoretic evidence and further supports the recent trend of favoring cuffed endotracheal tubes over uncuffed endotracheal tubes in infants and children for their safety.

The glottis widens slightly during tidal inspiration and narrows during expiration, thus increasing laryngeal air flow resistance (Bartlett et al., 1973). Laryngeal resistance is finely regulated in neonates and young infants to dynamically maintain end expiratory lung volume (FRC) well above the small lung volume determined by the opposing elastic recoil forces of the thorax and the lungs, as is discussed in a later part of this chapter (Harding, 1984; England and Stogren, 1986). In infants with IRDS, expiration is often associated with "grunting" caused by narrowing of the glottic aperture. This grunting apparently maintains intrinsic positive end-expiratory pressure (PEEP), also known as *PEEP$_i$* or *autoPEEP,* during the expiratory phase and presumably prevent or reduce premature closure of airways and air spaces. In infants with IRDS, when grunting is eliminated by endotracheal intubation, respiratory gas exchange deteriorates rapidly and critically to the point of cardiorespiratory arrest unless continuous positive airway pressure (CPAP) is applied (Gregory et al., 1971).

Airway Protective Reflexes

Upper airway protective mechanisms involve both the pharynx and larynx and include sneezing, swallowing, coughing, and pharyngeal or laryngeal closure. Laryngospasm is a sustained tight closure of the vocal cords caused by the stimulation of the superior laryngeal nerve, a branch of the vagus, and contraction of the adductor muscles that persists beyond the removal of the stimulus. In puppies, it is elicited by repetitive stimulation of the superior laryngeal nerve with typical adductor after-discharge activity. This response is not evoked by the stimulation of the recurrent laryngeal nerve (Suzuki and Sasaki, 1977). Hyperventilation and hypocapnia, as well as light anesthesia, increase the activity of adductor neurons, reduce the mean threshold of the adductor reflex, or increase upper airway resistance (Suzuki and Sasaki, 1977; Nishino et al., 1981). Hyperthermia and decreased lung volume also facilitate laryngospasm produced by stimulation of the superior laryngeal nerve (Sasaki, 1979; Haraguchi et al., 1983). Contrarily, hypoventilation and hypercapnia, positive intrathoracic pressure, and deep anesthesia depress excitatory adductor after-discharge activity and increase the threshold of the reflex that precipitates laryngospasm (Suzuki and Sasaki, 1977; Ikari and Sasaki, 1980; Nishino et al., 1981). Hypoxia below an arterial Po_2 of 50 mm Hg also increases the threshold for laryngospasm (Ikari and Sasaki, 1980).

These findings are clinically relevant, suggesting a fail-safe mechanism by which asphyxia (hypoxia and hypercapnia) tends to prevent sustained laryngospasm. In healthy, awake adults, laryngospasm by itself is self-limited and not a threat to life. On the other hand, in the presence of cardiopulmonary compromise, such as may occur during anesthesia (particularly in infants), laryngospasm may indeed become life threatening (Ikari and Sasaki, 1980). Increased depth of anesthesia increases the reflex threshold and diminishes excitatory adductor after discharge in puppies (Suzuki and Sasaki, 1977). This finding is in accord with the clinical experience that laryngospasm occurs most readily under light anesthesia and that it can be broken by deepening anesthesia or awakening the patient. In puppies, positive intrathoracic pressure inhibits the glottic closure reflex and laryngospasm. This supports the clinical observation that during the emergence from anesthesia in infants and young children, maintenance of PEEP and inflation of the lungs at the time of extubation seem to reduce both the incidence and severity of laryngospasm (Motoyama, unpublished observation).

Infants are particularly vulnerable to laryngospasm. Animal studies suggest that during a discrete interval after birth and before complete neurologic maturation, there is a period of transient laryngeal hyperexcitability. This may relate to the transient reduction in central latency and a reduction in central inhibition of the vagal afferent nerve. If these observations in puppies are applicable to human infants, they may explain the susceptibility of infants and young children to laryngospasm and have some causal relation in unexpected infant death such as SIDS (Sasaki, 1979).

Infants, particularly premature neonates, exhibit clinically important airway protective responses to fluid at the entrance to the larynx (Davies et al., 1988; Pickens et al., 1989). This response seems to trigger prolonged apnea in neonates and breath-holding during inhalation induction of anesthesia in children. When a small quantity (less than 1 mL) of warm saline solution is dripped into the nasopharynx in a sleeping infant, it pools in the piriform fossa and then overflows into the interarytenoid space at the entrance to the larynx. This area is densely populated with various nerve endings, including a structure resembling a taste bud. The most common response to fluid accumulation is swallowing. The infant also develops central apnea with either the glottis open or closed; coughing

is rare (Pickens et al., 1989). Apneic responses are more prominent with water than with saline solution (Davies et al., 1988).

These findings appear clinically important in pediatric anesthesia. During inhalation induction, pharyngeal reflexes (swallowing) are abolished, whereas laryngeal reflexes remain intact, as Guedel (1937) originally described for ether anesthesia. Secretions would accumulate in the hypopharynx without swallowing and cause breath-holding, resulting from central apnea, a closure of the glottis, or both. Positive pressure ventilation using a mask and bag instead of suctioning the pharynx would push secretions farther down into the larynx, stimulate the superior laryngeal nerve, and trigger real laryngospasm.

Anesthetic Effects on Control of Breathing

Effects of Anesthetic on Upper Airway Receptors

Inhalation induction of anesthesia is often associated with reflex responses such as coughing, breath-holding, and laryngospasm. Volatile anesthetics stimulate upper airway receptors directly and affect ventilation. In dogs spontaneously breathing through tracheostomy under urethane-chloralose anesthesia, an exposure of isolated upper airways to halothane caused depression of respiratory-modulated mechanoreceptors or pressure receptors, whereas irritant receptors and flow (cold) receptors were consistently stimulated in a dose-dependent manner (Nishino et al., 1993). Responses to isoflurane and enflurane were less consistent. Laryngeal respiratory-modulated mechanoreceptors may be a part of a feedback mechanism that maintains the patency of upper airways; the depression of this feedback mechanism may play an important role in the collapse of upper airways during the induction of anesthesia. Furthermore, activation of irritant receptors by halothane and other volatile anesthetics may be responsible for laryngeal reflexes such as coughing, apnea, laryngospasm, and bronchoconstriction seen during inhalation induction of anesthesia (Nishino et al., 1993).

The same group of investigators showed that in young puppies (younger than 2 weeks old), exposure of isolated upper airways to halothane (and to a lesser extent to isoflurane) resulted in a marked depression of ventilation (less than 40% of control) associated with decreases in both tidal volume and respiratory frequency (Sant'Ambrogio et al., 1993). Ventilatory effects caused by the exposure of isolated upper airways to volatile anesthetics were present but only mildly in 4-week-old puppies, whereas adult dogs were not affected. The superior laryngeal nerve section and topical anesthesia of the nasal cavity completely abolished the effects of halothane and isoflurane in the isolated upper airways of puppies (Sant'Ambrogio et al., 1993). Laryngeal receptor output in response to volatile anesthetics was not measured in this study. These findings in puppies appear to be clinically relevant because infants and young children often develop manifestations of upper airway reflexes during inhalation induction.

Effects of Anesthetics on Upper Airway Muscles

The genioglossus, geniohyoid, and other pharyngeal and laryngeal abductor muscles have phasic inspiratory activity synchronous with diaphragmatic contraction, in addition to their tonic activities that maintain upper airway patency in both animals and human neonates (Bartlett et al., 1973; Brouillette

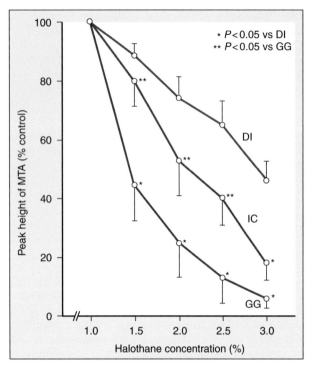

■ FIGURE 3-18. Decrease in phasic inspiratory muscle activity, expressed as peak height of moving time average *(MTA)*, in percent change from control (1% halothane), during halothane anesthesia in adult cats. Values are mean ± SEM. *P < 0.05 compared with the diaphragm *(DI)*; **P < 0.05 compared with the genioglossus muscle *(GG)*. *(From Ochiai R et al.: Effects of varying concentrations of halothane on the activity of the genioglossus, intercostals, and diaphragm in cats: an electromyographic study,* Anesthesiology *70:812, 1989.)*

and Thach, 1979). The genioglossus and geniohyoid muscles increase the caliber of the pharynx by displacing the hyoid bone and the tongue anteriorly and are the most important muscles for the maintenance of oropharynx patency (Fig. 3-15). They have both phasic inspiratory activity and tonic activity throughout the respiratory cycle in awake humans (Onal et al., 1981). These activities of the genioglossus muscle and presumably other pharyngeal and laryngeal abductor muscles are easily depressed by alcohol ingestion, sleep, and general anesthesia; their depression would result in upper airway obstruction (Remmers et al., 1978; Brouillette and Thach, 1979; Nishino et al., 1984, 1985; Bartlett et al., 1990).

Sensitivity to anesthetics differs among various inspiratory muscles and their neurons. In studies in cats with the use of electromyography, Ochiai et al. (1989) demonstrated that the phasic inspiratory activity of the genioglossus muscle was most sensitive to the depressant effect of halothane at a given concentration, whereas the diaphragm was most resistant; the sensitivity of inspiratory intercostal muscles was intermediate (Fig. 3-18). In addition, phasic genioglossus activity was more readily depressed in kittens than in adult cats. Phasic genioglossus activity was completely abolished with 1.5% halothane or more in all kittens studied, whereas the activity was diminished but present in most adult cats even at 2.5% (Ochiai et al., 1992).

Early depression of the genioglossus muscle and other pharyngeal dilator muscles appears to be responsible for upper airway obstruction in infants and young children, especially during the induction of inhalation anesthesia. Because of the higher sensitivity to anesthetic depression, the upper airway muscles failed to increase the intensity of contraction to keep the pharynx patent while the diaphragm continues to contract vigorously and the negative feedback mechanism to attenuate its contraction may be diminished or lost (Brouillette and Thach, 1979; Ochiai et al., 1989; Isono et al., 2002). Partial upper airway obstruction may occur more often in infants and young children than is clinically apparent during anesthesia by mask without an oral airway. Keidan et al. (2000) found in infants and children breathing spontaneously under halothane anesthesia that the work of breathing (as an index of the degree of upper airway obstruction) significantly increased when breathing by mask without an oral airway than with an oral airway in place, even when partial upper airway obstruction was not clinically apparent. An addition of CPAP (5 to 6 cm H_2O) further improved airway patency as evidenced by significant decreases in the work of breathing (Keidan et al., 2000).

Effects of Anesthetic on Neural Control of Breathing

Most general anesthetics, opioids, and sedatives depress ventilation. They variably affect minute ventilation ($\dot{V}E$), its components (V_T, f, V_T/T_I), and respiratory duty cycle (T_I/T_{TOT}). All inhaled anesthetics significantly depress ventilation in a dose-dependent fashion (Fig. 3-9). This subject has been extensively reviewed; information in human infants and children, however, remains limited (Hickey and Severinghaus, 1981; Pavlin and Hornbein, 1986).

Studies in adult human volunteers using the occlusion technique and the timing component analysis have indicated that the reduction in tidal volume with anesthetics results primarily from a reduction in the neural drive of ventilation (Milic-Emili and Grunstein, 1975; Whitelaw et al., 1975; Derenne et al., 1976; Wahba, 1980). Inspiratory time tends to decrease, but the respiratory duty cycle is relatively unaffected. In several studies in children 2 to 5 years of age, breathing was relatively well maintained at a light level of halothane (0.5 minimum alveolar concentration [MAC]) (Murat et al., 1985; Lindahl et al., 1987; Benameur et al., 1993). In deeper, surgical levels of anesthesia (1.0 to 1.5 MAC), breathing was depressed in a dose-dependent manner and hypercapnia resulted. Decreased $\dot{V}E$ was associated with reduced V_T and increased respiratory frequency. The neural respiratory drive was depressed as evidenced by reduced V_T/T_I, whereas the duty cycle (T_I/T_{TOT}) either tended to increase without changes in T_I or decreased slightly (Murat et al., 1985; Lindahl et al., 1987; Benameur et al., 1993). In infants younger than 12 months of age, ventilatory depression was more pronounced and the duty cycle did not increase, partly because of high chest-wall compliance and pronounced thoracic deformity (thoracoabdominal asynchrony) compared with older children (Benameur et al., 1993).

When an external load was imposed on the airway system of an awake individual, ventilation was maintained by increased inspiratory effort (Whitelaw et al., 1975). This response was greatly diminished or abolished by the effect of general anesthetics, opioids, and barbiturates (Nunn and Ezi-Ashi, 1966; Isaza et al., 1976; Kryger et al., 1976b; Savoy et al., 1982). In children under light halothane anesthesia (0.5 MAC), an addition of a resistive load initially decreased tidal volume. However, tidal volume returned to baseline within 5 minutes (Lindahl et al., 1987).

Effects of Anesthetic on Chemical Control of Breathing

In the dog, inhaled anesthetics diminish or abolish the ventilatory response to hypoxemia in a dose-dependent manner (Weiskopf et al., 1974; Hirshman et al., 1977). In human adult volunteers, the hypoxic ventilatory response was disproportionately depressed in light halothane anesthesia compared with the response to hypercapnia (Knill and Gelb, 1978). At 1.1 MAC of halothane, the hypoxic ventilatory response was completely abolished, whereas the hypercapnic response was about 40% of control in the awake state. Even at a subanesthetic or trace level (0.05 to 0.1 MAC), halothane, isoflurane, and enflurane attenuated the hypoxic ventilatory response to about 30% of the control group, whereas hypercapnic response was essentially intact (Knill and Gelb, 1978; Knill and Clement, 1984). The site of the anesthetics' action appears to be at the peripheral (carotid) chemoreceptors, because of the rapid response in humans as well as the direct measurement of neuronal chemoreceptor output in the cat (Davies et al., 1982; Knill and Clement, 1984).

Subsequently, Temp and others (1992, 1994) challenged these findings by demonstrating that 0.1 MAC of isoflurane had no demonstrable ventilatory effect on hypoxia. On the other hand, Dahan and others (1994) confirmed the original findings by Knill and Gelb (1978). The reason for the conflicting results appeared to be related to the contribution of visual and auditory inputs (Robotham, 1994). The study by Temp and others (1994) was conducted while the volunteers were watching television (open-eyed), whereas the volunteers in the study by Dahan and others (1994) were listening to soothing music with their eyes closed (but not asleep).

Pandit (2004) conducted a meta-analysis of 37 studies in 21 publications and analyzed the conflicting response to hypoxia under trace levels of anesthetics. Pandit's analysis supported the prediction by Robotham (1994) that the study condition has a major impact on the outcome of the study. Bandit concluded that the main factor for the difference in hypoxic response was the anesthetic agent used ($p < 0.002$). Additional factors included subject stimulation ($p < 0.014$) and agent-stimulation interaction ($p < 0.04$), whereas the rate of induction of hypoxia or the level of Pco_2 had no effect (Pandit, 2000).

The effect of subanesthetic concentrations of inhaled anesthetics on ventilation in infants and children has not been studied. However, high incidences of postoperative hypoxemia in otherwise healthy infants and children without an apparent hypoxic ventilatory response in the postanesthetic period suggest that the hypoxic ventilatory drive in infants and children may be blunted with the presence of residual, subanesthetic levels of inhaled anesthetics (Motoyama and Glazener, 1986).

Summary

The understanding of the control of breathing during the perinatal and early postnatal periods has increased significantly. In general, neural and chemical controls of breathing in older infants and children are similar to those in adolescents and adults. A major exception to this general statement is found in neonates and young infants, especially prematurely born infants younger than 40 to 44 weeks' postconception. In these infants, hypoxemia is a potent respiratory depressant, rather than a stimulant, either centrally or because of changes in respiratory mechanics. These infants often develop periodic breathing without apparent hypoxemia, and occasionally they experience central apnea with possible serious consequences, most likely because of immature respiratory control mechanisms.

LUNG VOLUMES

Postnatal Development of the Lungs

In the human fetus, alveolar formation does not begin until about 4 weeks before birth, although development of the airways, including the terminal bronchioles, are completed by 16 weeks' gestation (Reid, 1967; Langston et al., 1984). The full-term newborn infant has 20 to 50 million terminal airspaces, mostly primitive saccules from which alveoli later develop (Thurlbeck, 1975; Langston et al., 1984). During the early postnatal years, development and growth of the lungs continue at a rapid pace, particularly with respect to the development of new alveoli. By 12 to 18 months of age, the number of alveoli reaches the adult level of 400 million or more; subsequent lung development and growth are associated with increases in alveolar size as well as further structural development (see Development of the Respiratory System) (Dunnill, 1962; Langston et al., 1984).

During the early period of postnatal lung development, the lung volume of infants is disproportionately small in relation to body size. Furthermore, because the infant's metabolic rate in relation to body weight is nearly twice that of the adult, the ventilatory requirement per unit of lung volume in infants is greatly increased. Infants seem to have far less reserve in lung surface area for gas exchange. Furthermore, general anesthesia markedly reduces the end expiratory lung volume (FRC, or relaxation volume, Vr), especially in young infants, reducing their oxygen reserve severely. Normal values for lung volumes and function in persons of various ages are compiled in Table 3-2.

Total lung capacity (TLC) is the maximum lung volume allowed by the strength of the inspiratory muscles stretching the thorax and lungs. Subdivisions of TLC are shown schematically in Figure 3-19. Residual volume (RV) is the amount of air remaining in the lungs after maximum expiration and is approximately 25% of TLC in healthy children. FRC is determined by the balance between the outward stretch of the thorax and the inward recoil of the lungs and is normally roughly 50% of TLC in the upright posture in healthy children and young adults; it is about 40% when they are in the supine position (Fig. 3-20). The two opposing forces create an average negative average pleural pressure of approximately –5 cm H_2O in older children and adults. In the neonate the pleural pressure is only slightly negative or nearly atmospheric.

Functional Residual Capacity and Its Determinants

In infants, outward recoil of the thorax is exceedingly low, and inward recoil of the lungs is only slightly lower than that of adults (Agostoni, 1959; Bryan and Wohl, 1986). Consequently, the FRC (or, more appropriately, Vr) of young infants at static conditions (e.g., apnea, under general anesthesia, or paralysis) decreases to 10% to 15% of TLC, a level incompatible with normal gas exchange because of airway closure, atelectasis, and V/Q imbalance (Fig. 3-21) (Agostoni, 1959). In awake infants and young children, however, FRC is dynamically maintained by a number of mechanisms for preventing the collapse of the

TABLE 3-2. Normal Values for Lung Functions in Persons of Various Ages

					Age		Male 15 yr	Male 21 yr	Female 21 yr
	1 wk	1 yr	3 yr	5 yr	8 yr	12 yr			
Height (cm)	48	75	96	109	130	150	170	174	162
Weight (kg)	3.3	10	15	18	26	39	57	73	57
FRC (mL)	75*	(263)	(532)	660	1174	1855	2800	3030	2350
FRC/weight (mL/kg)	(25)	(26)	(37)	(36)	(46)	(48)	(49)	(42)	(41)
VC (mL)	100†	(475)	(910)	1100	1855	2830	4300	4620	3380
V_E (mL/min)	550	(1775)	(2460)	(2600)	(3240)	(4150)	5030	6000	5030
V_T (mL)	17	(78)	(112)	(130)	(180)	(260)	360	500	420
f (frequency)	30	(24)	(22)	(20)	(18)	16	14	12	12
V_A (mL/min)	385	(1245)	(1760)	(1800)	(2195)	(2790)	3070	4140	3530
V_D (mL)	75	21	37	49	75	105	141	150	126
C_l (mL/cm H_2O)	5	(16)	(32)	44	71	91	130	163	130
Peak flow rates (L/min)	10			136	231	325	437	457	365
R (cm H_2O/L/sec)	29‡	(13)	(10)	8	6	5	3	2	2
DLco (mL/mm Hg/min)§				11	15	20	27	28	24
Cardiac output (L/min)	(0.9)	1.9	2.7	3.2	4.4	5.7	(7.0)	(7.6)	(7.2)
Lung weight (g)	49	120	166	211	290	470	640	730	

Data from Bucci G, Cook CD, Barrie H: Studies of respiratory physiology in children. V. Total lung diffusion, diffusing capacity of pulmonary membrane, and pulmonary capillary blood volume in normal subjects from 7 to 40 years of age. *J Pediatr* 58:820, 1961; Comroe JH Jr et al.: *The lung,* Chicago, 1962, Year Book; Cook CD et al.: Studies of respiratory physiology in the newborn infant. I. Observations on the normal premature and full-term infants, *J Clin Invest* 34:975, 1955; Cook CD et al.: Studies of respiratory physiology in the newborn infant. VI. Measurements of mechanics of respiration, *J Clin Invest* 36:440, 1957; Cook CD, Hamann JF: Relation of lung volumes to height in healthy persons between the ages of 5 and 38 years, *J Pediatr* 59:710, 1961; Koch G: Alveolar ventilation, diffusing capacity and the A-a PO_2 difference in the newborn infant, *Respir Physiol* 4:168, 1968; Long EC, Hull WE: Respiratory volume-flow in the crying newborn infant, *Pediatrics* 27:373, 1961; and Murray AB, Cook CD: Measurement of peak expiratory flow rates in 220 normal children from 4.5 to 18.5 years of age, *J Pediatr* 62:186, 1963.

*Supine.
†Crying vital capacity.
‡Nose breathing.
§Single-breath technique.
Parentheses, Interpolated values.

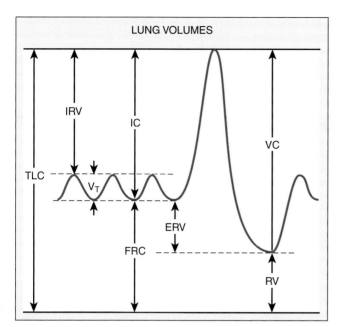

■ FIGURE 3-19. TLC and lung volume subdivisions. *ERV,* Expiratory reserve volume; *FRC,* functional residual capacity; *IC,* inspiratory capacity; *IRV,* inspiratory reserve volume; *RV,* residual volume; *TLC,* total lung capacity; *VC,* vital capacity; *VT,* tidal volume. *(From Motoyama EK: Airway function tests in infants and children,* Int Anesthesiol Clin *26:6, 1988.)*

lungs, tincluding a sustained inspiratory muscle tension to make the thorax stiffer (Box 3-2) (see Elastic Properties). FRC in young infants is therefore dynamically determined; there is no fixed level of FRC.

In normal children and adolescents, lung volumes are related to body size, especially height. In most instances, the relative size of the lung compartment appears to be approximately constant from school-aged children to young adults (see Table 3-2). A study in anesthetized and paralyzed infants and children indicates that TLC, as measured with a tracer gas washout technique, is relatively small in infants (60 mL/kg) when the lungs are inflated with relatively low inflation pressure (20 to 25 cm H_2O; the recruitment of previously collapsed air space with this

pressure might not have been complete) (Thorsteinsson et al., 1994). TLC in children older than 1.5 years of age (determined with inflation pressures of 35 to 40 cm H_2O) increases with growth until about 5 years of age (body weight, 20 kg), when it reaches that of older children and adolescents (90 mL/kg).

Negative pressure surrounding the lungs is the same, with respect to lung expansion, as positive pressure within the airways; thus, the net transpulmonary pressure represents the force expanding or contracting the lungs. In contrast, negative intrathoracic pressure has quite a different effect from positive airway pressure with respect to pulmonary circulation and the ventilation/pulmonary perfusion relationship.

Anesthesia, surgery, abdominal distention, and disease may all alter lung volumes. The patient in the prone or supine position has a smaller FRC than the patient standing or sitting, because the abdominal contents shift. FRC is further decreased under general anesthesia with or without muscle relaxants (Westbrook et al., 1973). (see Effect of General Anesthesia on FRC)

The importance of the air remaining in the lungs at the end of normal expiration is often overlooked. This gas volume (FRC) serves as a buffer to minimize cyclic changes in Pco_2 and Po_2 of the blood during each breath. In addition, the fact that air normally remains in the lungs throughout the respiratory cycle means that relatively few alveoli collapse. Although alveolar collapse does not occur during normal breathing in healthy, awake infants and children, unusually high pressures are needed to expand the lungs when they are liquid filled at birth, collapsed after open-chest surgery, or during general anesthesia without the maintenance of PEEP, especially in young infants (von Ungern-Sternbery, 2006). Transpulmonary pressure of 30 to 40 cm H_2O (and occasionally even more) is needed to reexpand the collapsed lungs. Thereafter, 5 to 7 cm H_2O of PEEP appears adequate to prevent airway closure and to maintain FRC.

Mechanics of Breathing

To ventilate the lungs, the respiratory muscles must overcome certain opposing forces within the lungs themselves. These forces have both elastic and resistive properties. Although respiratory mechanics in adults have been studied extensively

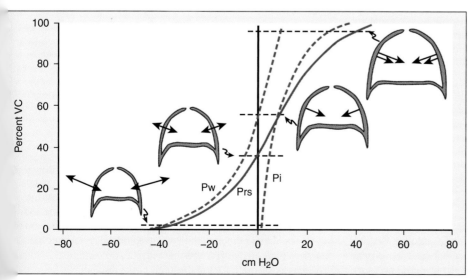

■ FIGURE 3-20. Static volume-pressure curves of the lung *(Pi),* chest wall *(Pw),* and respiratory system *(Prs)* during relaxation in the sitting position. The static forces of the lung and chest wall are pictured by the arrows in the side drawings. The dimensions of the arrows are not to scale; the volume corresponding to each drawing is indicated by the horizontal broken lines. *(From Agostoni E, Mead J: Statics of the respiratory system. In Fenn WO, Rahn H, editors:* Handbook of physiology: section 3, respiration, vol 1, Washington, DC, 1986, American Physiological Society.)

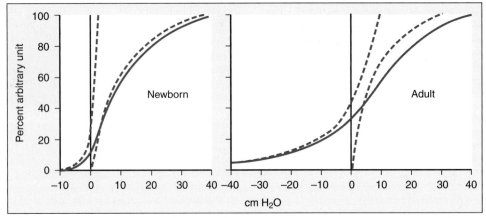

■ **FIGURE 3-21.** Static pressure-volume curve of lung *(right dashed line)*, chest wall *(left dashed line)*, and total respiratory system *(solid line)* in the newborn and adult. *(From Agostoni E: Volume-pressure relationships of the thorax,* J Appl Physiol *14:909, 1959.)*

Box 3-2 Maintenance of Functional Residual Capacity in Young Infants

- Sustained tonic activities of inspiratory muscles throughout the respiratory cycle.
- Breaking of expiration with continual but diminishing diaphragmatic activity.
- Narrowing of the glottis during expiration.
- Inspiration starting in midexpiration.*
- High respiratory rate in relation to expiratory time constant.*

All mechanisms of sustaining FRC are lost with anesthesia or muscle relaxant.

*Create $PEEP_i$ or autoPEEP.

over the past five decades, most available information on infants and young children has emerged relatively recently (Bryan and Wohl, 1986; ATS/ERS Joint Committee, 1993).

Elastic Properties

Compliance of the Lungs and Thorax

When the lungs are expanded by the contraction of inspiratory muscles or by positive pressure applied to the airways, elastic recoil of the lungs and thoracic structures surrounding the lungs counterreacts to reduce lung volume. This elastic force is fairly constant over the range of normal tidal volumes, but it increases at the extremes of deflation or inflation (Fig. 3-22). The elastic properties of the lungs and respiratory system (lungs and thorax) are measured and expressed as lung compliance (C_L) or respiratory system compliance (Crs) in units of volume change per unit of pressure change. The following equation is derived:

$$C_L = \Delta V / \Delta P$$

where ΔV is usually the tidal volume and ΔP is the change in transpulmonary pressure (the difference between the airway and pleural pressures [$\Delta P = Pao- Ppl$]) for C_L, and for Crs, ΔP is transrespiratory pressure (the difference between the airway pressure at end-inspiratory occlusion and atmospheric pressure

[$\Delta P = Pao - P_B$]) necessary to produce the tidal volume. These measurements are made at points of no flow, that is, at the extremes of tidal volume when there is no flow-resistive component (static compliance). Lung compliance may vary with changes in the midposition of tidal ventilation with no inherent alteration in the elastic characteristics of the lungs (Fig. 3-22). The elastic properties of the lungs are described more accurately by measuring pressure-volume relationships over the entire range of TLC.

In normal persons, lung compliance measured during the respiratory cycle (i.e., the dynamic compliance during quiet breathing) is approximately the same as the static compliance. When there is airway obstruction, however, the ventilation of some lung units may be functionally decreased, resulting in decreased dynamic compliance, whereas the static compliance is relatively unaffected. This difference between static and

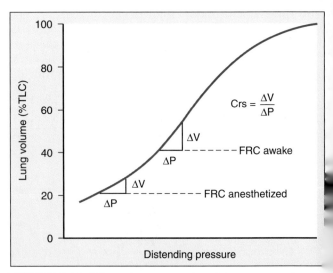

■ **FIGURE 3-22.** Schematic representation of the pressure-volume (P-V) curve and compliance of the respiratory system (Crs). At the midpoint of the P-V curve (indicated as FRC awake), the slope and compliance (Crs = $\Delta P/\Delta V$) are the highest. When FRC is decreased to the lower, flatter portion of the P-V curve under general anesthesia or paralysis (indicated as FRC anesthetized), Crs decreases even without changes in the mechanics of the lungs or the respiratory system.

dynamic compliance increases with increasing respiratory frequency (frequency dependence of compliance) and is a sign of airway obstruction (Woolcock et al., 1969).

Quiet, normal expiration occurs passively, resulting from the elastic recoil of the lungs and chest wall and involves little or no additional work. The situation in the infant or in the anesthetized and spontaneously breathing patient may be somewhat different, because expiration may have an active phase (Munson et al., 1966). To consider volume-pressure relationships from another point of view, a normal tidal volume may be obtained using transpulmonary pressures of approximately 4 to 6 cm H_2O in persons of all sizes, provided that the lungs are normal, they are normally expanded initially, and the airways are patent. The total transthoracopulmonary pressure needed to ventilate the lungs with positive pressure in a closed chest is, in the adult, approximately twice the required transpulmonary pressure during spontaneous breathing, because the thoracic structures must also be expanded. The chest wall in the newborn is extremely compliant and therefore requires almost no force for expansion (Fig. 3-21). The combined compliance of the chest wall and lungs, or the compliance of the total respiratory system (Crs), is expressed as follows:

$$1/Crs = 1/C_L + 1/Cw$$

where C_L is lung compliance and Cw is chest-wall compliance. The equation can be expressed in terms of elastance (E), an inverse of compliance (E = 1/C):

$$Ers = E_L + Ew$$

where Ers is the elastance of the total respiratory system, E_l is lung elastance, and Ew is chest wall elastance. Lung compliance in normal humans of different sizes is generally directly proportional to lung size (see Table 3-2). The compliance is expressed per unit of lung volume (e.g., per FRC, vital capacity [VC], or TLC) for comparison (termed *specific compliance*).

Developmental Changes in the Compliance of the Lungs and Thorax

After the initial period of neonatal adaptation, the compliance of the infant's lungs is extremely high (elastic recoil is low), probably because of absent or poorly developed elastic fibers (Fig. 3-23) (Fagan, 1976, 1977; Motoyama, 1977). Oddly enough, their functional characteristics resemble those of geriatric, emphysematous lungs with pathologically high compliance caused by the loss of functioning elastic fibers (Fig. 3-24). Thus, both extremes of human life, the lungs are prone to premature airway closure (Mansell et al., 1972). Elastic recoil pressure the lungs at 60% TLC increases from about 1 cm H_2O in the newborn to 5 cm H_2O at 7 years of age and 9 cm H_2O at 16 years age (Fagan, 1976, 1977; Zapletal et al., 1987).

In infants the outward recoil of the chest wall is exceedingly small, because the rib cage is cartilaginous and horizontal, and the respiratory muscles are not well developed, whereas the inward recoil of the lungs is only moderately decreased compared with that in adults (Agostoni, 1959; Gerhardt and Bancalari, 1980). Consequently, the static balance of these opposing forces would decrease FRC to a very low level (Fig. 3-22). Such a reduction in FRC would make parenchymal airways unstable and subject them to collapse. In reality, however,

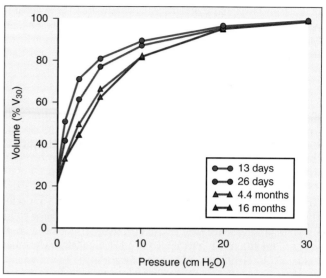

■ FIGURE 3-23. Pressure-volume curves obtained from excised lungs at autopsy. Data are grouped by postnatal ages, as shown by symbols. It is evident that elastic recoil pressure (horizontal distance between nil distending pressure and the curve at a given distending volume) increases with postnatal development of the lungs. *(Data from Fagan DG: Post-mortem studies of the semistatic volume-pressure characteristics of infants' lungs, Thorax 31:534, 1976; Fagan DG: Shape changes in static V-P loops for children's lungs related to growth, Thorax 32:193, 1977.)*

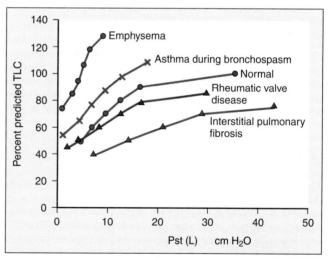

■ FIGURE 3-24. Static pressure-volume curves (deflation limbs) of the lungs in various conditions as indicated. *(From Bates DV, editor: Respiratory function in disease, ed 3, Philadelphia, 1989, WB Saunders.)*

dynamic FRC in spontaneously breathing infants is maintained at around 40% TLC, a value similar to that in adults in the supine position, because of a number of possible mechanisms or their combinations (Bryan and Wohl, 1986).

Maintenance of Functional Residual Capacity in Infants

Infants terminate the expiratory phase of the breathing cycle before lung volume reaches the relaxation volume, or true FRC, determined by the balance of opposing chest wall and lung elastic recoil (Kosch and Stark, 1979). This "premature" cessation of the expiratory phase, which PEEP$_i$ with higher FRC, probably results partly from the relatively long time constant of the respiratory system in infants in relation to their high respiratory rate (Olinsky et al., 1974). Additional mechanisms may also help maintain dynamic FRC above the relaxation volume. Glottic closure, or laryngeal braking, during the expiratory phase of the breathing cycle is an important mechanism for the establishment of sufficient air space in the lungs during the early postnatal period (Fisher et al., 1982). Diaphragmatic braking, the diminishing diaphragmatic activity extending to the expiratory phase of breathing, is another important mechanism that extends expiratory time and maintains FRC (Box 3-2).

Among all mechanisms that maintain FRC, tonic contractions of both the diaphragm and the intercostal muscles throughout the respiratory cycle in awake infants appear to be most important. This mechanism effectively stiffens the chest wall and maintains a higher end expiratory lung volume (Muller et al., 1979). Henderson-Smart and Read (1979) have shown a 30% decrease in thoracic gas volume in sleeping infants changing from non-REM to REM sleep. This large reduction in dynamic FRC may result from loss of tonic activity of the respiratory muscles, loss of laryngeal braking, diaphragmatic braking, or all of these factors. All of these important mechanisms for maintaining FRC in infants (and to a lesser extent in older children) are lost with general anesthesia or muscle relaxants, causing marked reductions in FRC, airway closure and atelectasis (Serafini et al., 1999).

When is the FRC no longer determined dynamically but determined by the balance between the recoils of the thorax and the lungs to the opposing direction, as in adults? Colin and others (1989) have shown that, in infants and children during quiet, natural sleep, the transition from dynamically determined to relaxed end expiratory volume or FRC takes place between 6 and 12 months of age. By 1 year of age the breathing pattern is predominantly that of relaxed end-expiratory volume, just as in older children and adults. These findings coincide with the upright posture and development of thoracic tissue and muscle strength in infants.

The breathing pattern of infants younger than 6 months of age is predominantly abdominal (diaphragmatic) and the contribution of the rib cage (external intercostal muscles) to tidal volume is relatively small (20 to 40%), reflecting instability of the thorax or weakness of the intercostal muscles. After 9 months of age, the rib cage component of tidal volume increases to a level (50%) similar to that of older children and adolescents, reflecting the maturation of the thoracic structures (Hershenson et al., 1990). Furthermore, a study by Papastamelos and others (1995) has shown that the stiffening of the chest wall continues throughout infancy and early childhood. By 12 months of age, however, chest wall compliance (which is extremely high in neonates) decreases and nearly equals lung compliance. The chest wall becomes more stable and can resist the inward recoil of the lungs and maintain FRC passively. These relatively recent findings support the notion that the stability of the respiratory system is achieved by 1 year of age.

Effects of General Anesthesia on Functional Residual Capacity

General anesthesia with or without muscle relaxation results in a significant reduction of FRC in adult patients in the supine position soon after the induction of anesthesia, whereas FRC is unchanged during anesthesia in the sitting position (Rehder et al., 1971, 1972b, 1974; Westbrook et al., 1973). A decrease in FRC is associated with reductions in both lung and thoracic compliance, but the mechanism responsible for the reduction in FRC and the sequence of events that changes respiratory mechanics were not understood for many years.

In an excellent study, deTroyer and Bastenier-Geens (1979) showed that when a healthy volunteer was partially paralyzed with pancuronium, the outward recoil of the thorax decreased, whereas lung recoil (compliance) did not. This change altered the balance between the elastic recoil of the lung and thorax in opposite directions, and consequently FRC diminished. The compliance of the lungs decreased shortly thereafter, resulting from the reduced FRC and resultant airway closure. Based on their findings, deTroyer and Bastenier-Geens postulated that, in the awake state, inspiratory muscles have intrinsic tone that maintains the outward recoil and rigidity of the thorax. Anesthesia or paralysis would abolish this muscle tone, reducing thoracic compliance followed by a reduction in FRC, and eventually lung compliance in rapid succession (in a matter of a few minutes).

In healthy young adults, a reduction of FRC during general anesthesia is limited to between 9% and 25% from the awake control levels (Laws, 1968; Rehder et al., 1972; Westbrook et al., 1973; Hewlett et al., 1974; Juno et al., 1978). In older individuals, the average reduction in FRC is more (30%), probably because of lower elastic recoil pressure, increased closing capacity and further airway closure, and eventual atelectasis (Bergman, 1963).

With the more compliant thoraces of infants and young children, general anesthesia and muscle relaxation would be expected to produce more profound reductions in FRC than in adolescents and adults. Henderson-Smart and Read (1979) have shown a 30% reduction in thoracic gas volume (FRC) in infants, changing the sleep pattern from non-REM to REM sleep with increased muscle flaccidity. In children 6 to 18 years of age under general anesthesia and paralysis, Dobbinson and others (1973) found marked reductions in FRC (average reduction, 35%) from their own awake control values, as measured with a helium dilution technique. The average decrease in FRC among those younger than 12 years of age was 46%. Fletcher and others (1990) demonstrated that compliance of the respiratory system (Crs) in infants and children under general anesthesia decreased about 35%, a value comparable with the reduction reported in adults under similar conditions (Westbrook et al., 1973; Rehder and Marsh, 1986). This reduction in Crs occurred both during spontaneous breathing and during manual ventilation with low tidal volume after muscle relaxants were given. When tidal volume was doubled, however, Crs returned to preanesthetic control levels.

These findings are in accord with previous findings in adults and support the notion that anesthesia reduces FRC (deTroyer and Bastenier-Geens, 1979; Hedenstierna and McCarthy, 198_). The finding that a larger tidal volume increases Crs toward control values also indicates that FRC decreases to the lower, flatter portion of the pressure-volume curve, which would lead to airway closure (Fig. 3-22). Motoyama and others (1982a) reported moderate decreases in FRC (−46%) in children as measured with helium dilution and a marked decrease (−71%) in infants under halothane anesthesia and muscle paralysis, approaching the relaxation volume in the newborn infant reported by Agostoni (1959).

Until recently, the possible differential effect on FRC of general anesthesia without muscle paralysis vs. general anesthesia with muscle paralysis was not critically compared. Westbrook et al. (1973) reported a 25% reduction in FRC in healthy young adults in the supine position after anesthesia with intravenous sodium thiopental. They did not find a statistically significant difference in the extent of reductions in FRC with thiopental alone vs. those with an addition of muscle relaxant (d-tubocurarine), although the mean reduction in FRC was somewhat more with the relaxant. A more recent study in anesthetized infants and toddlers clearly demonstrated that addition of muscle paralysis in anesthetized children results in additional marked reductions in FRC (on top of the reduction by the effect of general anesthesia) (von Ungern-Sternberg et al., 2006). Furthermore, the reduction in FRC in infants less than 6 months of age was extreme (FRC, 21.3 to 12.2 mL/kg or −43%) as compared with reductions in toddlers (25.6 to 23.0 mL/kg or −10%) (von Ungern-Sternberg et al., 2006). This marked loss of FRC in infants represents the collapse of their extremely compliant thorax with inspiratory muscle paralysis and massive airway closure that would eventually result in atelectasis, uneven distribution of ventilation, V/Q imbalance, and hypoxemia unless the lungs are reexpanded and supported with PEEP.

Effect of Positive End-Expiratory Pressure Under General Anesthesia

Thorsteinsson and others (1994) reported that the lung volume at FRC (or relaxation volume, Vr) was at a lower, flatter portion of the pressure-volume (P-V) curve in all anesthetized infants and children studied. To restore FRC to the normal or steepest portion of the P-V curve of the respiratory system seen in the awake state (with the highest compliance), a PEEP of 5 to 6 cm H_2O had to be added to infants younger than 6 months of age and more than 12 cm H_2O in older children (Thorsteinsson et al., 1994). A more recent study in children (aged 2 to 6 years) also showed that PEEP as high as 17 cm H_2O is needed to raise the lung volume to the steepest portion (highest compliance) of the P-V curve (Kaditis et al., 2008).

Shortly after the induction of anesthesia and muscle relaxation in adult patients, increased density appearing on computed tomography (CT) scans in the dependent portion of the lung has been described in the literature. This increased density could be reduced or eliminated by adding PEEP (Brismar et al., 1985). Serafini and others (1999) were the first to report evidence of airway closure and atelectasis in young children (aged . to 3 years; mean age of 1.8 years) on a CT scan in the dependent portion of the lungs shortly after the inhalation induction of anesthesia and intubation. These patients were given three deep inflations of the lungs (sighs) with 40% oxygen in nitrous oxide and ventilated with 10 mL/kg of tidal volume. Atelectasis-increased density (airway closure or atelectasis) appeared n the CT scan almost immediately when patients were ventilated without PEEP (Fig. 3-25, A). When the patients were entilated for 5 minutes with an addition of PEEP (5 cm H_2O) ith the same ventilator settings and end tidal P_{CO_2}, the density disappeared from the repeated CT scans in all 10 children udied, indicating the recruitment of atelectic lung segments ig. 3-25, B) (Serafini et al., 1999).

Because the stability of the thorax increases during the first ar of life, it is likely that the thorax would resist the airway lapse and atelectasis with increasing age (Papastamelos

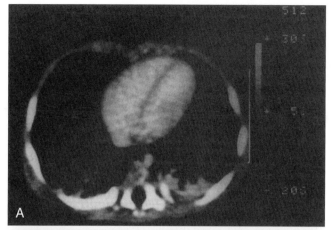

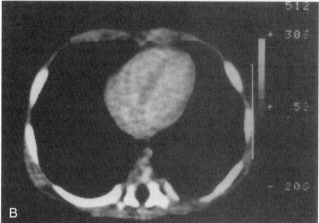

■ **FIGURE 3-25.** Computed tomography (CT) scan of the thorax during general endotracheal anesthesia. **A,** Transverse CT scan of the thorax 5 minutes after the induction of anesthesia without PEEP. Note the appearance of atelectasis (density) in the dependent regions of both lungs. **B,** Transverse CT scan of the thorax during anesthesia with a PEEP of 5 cm H_2O, showing the complete disappearance of atelectasis in the dependent regions of both lungs. *(From Serafini G et al.: Pulmonary atelectasis during paediatric anaesthesia: CT scan evaluation and effects of positive end-expiratory pressure (PEEP),* Paediatr Anaesth *9:225, 1999.)*

et al., 1995). Motoyama (1996) examined this possibility by measuring respiratory system compliance in infants and young children under 6 years of age who were undergoing halothane-nitrous oxide endotracheal anesthesia. These patients were ventilated either with or without PEEP (6 cm H_2O) for 15 minutes preceded by deep sighs. After a period of ventilation with PEEP, respiratory system compliance was consistently higher after PEEP than without PEEP. There were significant age-related differences in the degree of increase in compliance after PEEP (6 cm H_2O) vs. no PEEP (Fig. 3-26). The average increase of respiratory system compliance with PEEP was greatest in infants younger than 8 months of age (75% higher with PEEP vs. without PEEP). In contrast, in older infants and toddlers (aged 9 months to 2.5 years), an average increase in compliance with PEEP was 22%; in children (aged 2.5 and 5.5 years), the increase was 9%, the level one would expect in adults. These results reflect greater reductions in FRC (or increases in airway closure and atelectasis) in the younger age groups (Motoyama, 1996).

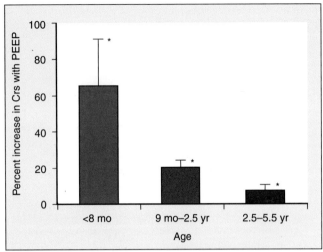

■ **FIGURE 3-26.** Compliance of the respiratory system (Crs) under general anesthesia in infants and children and the effect of PEEP. An addition of PEEP (5 to 6 cm H$_2$O) improves (restores) Crs significantly in all age groups studied. The beneficial effect of PEEP was most dramatic in infants younger than 8 months (see text). *(From Motoyama EK: Effects of positive end-expiratory pressure (PEEP) on respiratory mechanics and oxygen saturation (SpO$_2$) in infants and children under general anesthesia, Anesthesiology 85:A1099, 1996.)*

Persistent airway closure during general anesthesia would result in resorption atelectasis because alveolar gas (mostly oxygen and nitrous oxide) trapped below the occluded airways would be rapidly absorbed. Resultant pulmonary V/Q imbalance and right-to-left shunting of blood in the lung may reduce arterial Po$_2$ in the postanesthetic recovery room. Such an effect would be expected to be more profound in infants. Motoyama and Glazener (1986) studied arterial oxygen saturation (SpO$_2$) with a pulse oximeter in otherwise healthy infants and children before and after general anesthesia for simple, relatively short, surgical procedures (e.g., inguinal hernia repair or myringotomy tube insertions). On arrival at the postanesthetic care unit (PACU), the mean SpO$_2$ was 93% (estimated Pao$_2$, 66 mm Hg), significantly reduced from the preoperative value of 97%. In some children, SpO$_2$ decreased to the low 70s (estimated Pao$_2$ of less than 40 mm Hg). These patients showed no sign of hypoxic ventilatory stimulation with normal cutaneous Pco$_2$ (Motoyama and Glazener, 1986).

A large percentage (20% to 40%) of otherwise healthy infants and children develop oxygen desaturation (SpO$_2$ of less than or equal to 94%) during transport and on arrival at the PACU (Motoyama and Glazener, 1986; Pullertis et al., 1987; Patel et al., 1988). A later study of postoperative hypoxemia involving 1152 patients ranging from infants to adults has demonstrated that hemoglobin desaturation occurs sooner, is more pronounced, and lasts longer in infants than in children and longer in children than in adults (Xue et al., 1996). All children, therefore, should be given oxygen by mask during the transport from the operating room and on arrival at the PACU until they can maintain satisfactory oxygen saturation by pulse oximeter without supplemental oxygen (see Chapter 11, Monitoring).

Closing Volume and Closing Capacity

Beside the lungs and chest wall, the air passages themselves have a compliance that may be important. With deep inspiration,

the airway caliber increases in size (interdependent of airways and lung volume), whereas the airway caliber decreases during passive expiration, with an even bigger increase during forced expiration with dynamic compression. Closing volume (CV) is the lung volume above RV at which air flow during expiration ceases from dependent lung zones (i.e., lower lung segments in the upright position), presumably because of the closure or collapse of small airways. Closing capacity (CC) is the sum of CV above RV plus RV.

$$CC = CV + RV$$

Whether this closure is anatomic or merely the result of dynamic compression and reduction in flow (see Dynamic Properties) is controversial (Hughes et al., 1970; Hyatt et al., 1973). Because the patency of small airways depends in part on the elastic recoil of the lungs, CC as a percentage of TLC is relatively high in young children and would be even higher, at least theoretically, in infants (Mansell et al., 1972). CC increases with aging as well as with small airway disease, such as chronic bronchitis caused by smoking and emphysema in adults.

Lung compliance is reduced in most situations in which lung volume is decreased (e.g., the removal of lung tissue, atelectasis, and intrapulmonary tumors), although it is normal when corrected for lung volumes. Compliance is also decreased when surface forces are increased, as it is in IRDS with increased surface force (or decreased surfactant), or when elastic recoil is abnormally increased (e.g., in interstitial pulmonary fibrosis).

Emphysema is associated with a loss of elastic recoil and therefore an abnormal increase in compliance. Chest-wall compliance decreases with conditions such as scleroderma, kyphoscoliosis, and ankylosing spondylitis involving the thoracic structures.

Dynamic Properties

Breathing involves cyclic contractions of respiratory muscles and the generation of force, which must overcome resistive and elastic properties of the lung and chest wall. The resistive properties of the respiratory system include the resistance to air flow within the airways, the tissue viscoelastic resistance or the resistance of the lung and thoracic tissues themselves to deformation, and inertial resistance (inertance) resulting from the movement of gas molecules within the airways, especially at high velocities. In contrast to compliance (or elastance), which is measured at points of no flow, flow resistance is present only when the lung is in motion.

Airway Resistance

The pressure required to overcome frictional resistance and produce flow between the alveoli (Palv) and the airway opening (Pao) is proportional to flow rate. Airway resistance (Raw) expressed as pressure gradient across the airways (P = Pao − Palv) per unit flow ($\dot{V}$):

$$Raw = \frac{P}{\dot{V}(cmH_2O/L/sec)}$$

If the respiratory system is assumed to have a single compartment with a constant elastance or compliance (E = 1/C) and a constant resistance (R), the equation of forces acting on the respiratory system can be expressed as follows:

$$P = E\dot{V} + R\dot{V} + I\dot{V}$$

In tidal breathing, inertance (I) is very small and can be ignored. During normal tidal breathing, approximately 90% of the pressure gradient required is needed to overcome the elastic forces, and the remaining 10% of the pressure is expended to counter the flow resistance (Sly and Hayden, 1998).

Flow resistance is related to the length (l), radius of the tube (r), and the viscosity of the gas (η) as follows:

$$R = \frac{8l\eta}{\pi r^4}$$

Assuming a laminar flow (as seen in small or peripheral airways), it is apparent from this equation (Poiseuille's law) that the most important factor affecting flow resistance is the change in the radius of the tube (airways), because resistance is inversely proportional to the fourth power of the radius. (When the flow is turbulent, as occurs in large airways, the flow resistance increases approximately with r^5.) Therefore, airway resistance in infants with smaller airway diameters is much higher, in absolute terms, than airway resistance in older children and adults. It might also be expected that inflammation or secretions in the airway system would result in exaggerated degrees of obstruction in infants compared with older children and adults (Fig. 3-27). One such example may be the severe and often life-threatening obstruction of upper airways seen only in infants and young children with acute supraglottitis (epiglottitis) and subglottic croup (laryngotracheobronchitis). However, in relation to body size, the caliber of airways in general is wider, and airway resistance is lower in infants and children compared with adults (Motoyama, 1977; Stocks and Godfrey, 1977).

In absolute terms, airway resistance in the newborn is very high (19 to 28 cm H_2O/L per second). It decreases to less than 2 cm H_2O/L per second in the adolescent and the adult. In relative terms (as expressed per unit of lung volume, usually FRC or specific resistance), specific airway resistance is relatively low, or conductance (Gaw, the reciprocal of resistance; G = 1/R) is very high in the newborn. The specific conductance (sGaw = Gaw/FRC) decreases rapidly during the first year of life, indicating a rapid increase in lung volume (alveolar formation) in relation to airway size (Stocks and Godfrey, 1977, 1978). Between 6 and 18 years of age, Gaw increases linearly with increases in height; However, sGaw stays fairly constant throughout this period at about 0.2 L/sec per cm H_2O (Zapletal et al., 1969, 1976, 1987).

Distribution of Airway Resistance

Rohrer's earlier work (1915) led to the belief that peripheral airways of small caliber were the major contributors to total airway resistance. However, the elegant morphometric studies of Weibel (1963) with airway castings in inflated lungs proved that the total cross-sectional area of each generation of airways increases dramatically toward the periphery, like a cross section of a trumpet, on the cross-sectional area vs. airway-generation plot (Fig. 3-28). Indeed, about two thirds of the total airway resistance exists between the airway opening and the trachea, and most of the remaining resistance is in the large central airways. The airways smaller than a few millimeters in diameter (peripheral airways) contribute only about 10% of total resistance (Macklem and Mead, 1967).

These findings have important clinical implications. If the peripheral airways contribute little to the total airway resistance, disease processes involving small airways—such as emphysema in adults, cystic fibrosis (CF) in children, and bronchopulmonary dysplasia (BPD) in infants—will not be detectable by measurement of the total airway resistance. For instance, complete obstruction of half of the peripheral airways would increase the total airway resistance by only 5% to 6 %, an increase within the usual variation in measurements. For this reason, the peripheral airways used to be called the "quiet zone" of the lung (Mead, 1970). Apparently, the measurement of total airway resistance is not a sensitive clinical test for detecting small airway obstruction.

The airway system extends from the airway opening at the nares or the mouth to the alveolar duct at the periphery of the lung. Functionally, the airway system can be subdivided into the upper (extrathoracic) and lower (intrathoracic) airways. The upper airway begin at the airway opening (the mouth or the nose—normally the mouth in quiet breathing) and include the nasal or oral cavity, the pharynx, the larynx, and the uppermost segment of the trachea before it enters into the thorax. The lower airway begins with the thoracic inlet of the trachea, the trachea, bronchi, bronchioli, and alveolar ducts entering the alveoli (Box 3-3).

Upper Airway Resistance

During quiet breathing, air-flow resistance through the nasal passages accounts for approximately 65% of total airway resistance in adults (Ferris et al., 1964). This is more than twice the resistance during mouth breathing. For air warming, humidification, and particle filtration, it is important that one preferentially or instinctively breathe through the nose despite its higher resistance (Proctor, 1977a, 1977b). Stocks and Godfrey (1978) found nasal resistance comprised approximately 49% of the total airway resistance in European infants, whereas it was significantly less in infants of African origin (31%). Overall, upper airway resistance is approximately two thirds of the total airway resistance.

Except when crying, newborn infants are obligatory nose breathers. The cephalad position of the epiglottis and close approximation of the soft palate to the tongue and epiglottis in neonates may be a reason why mouth breathing is more

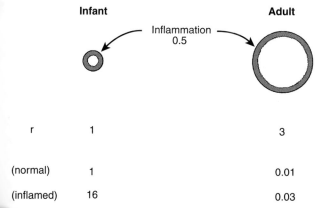

	Infant	Adult
		Inflammation 0.5
r	1	3
(normal)	1	0.01
(inflamed)	16	0.03

FIGURE 3-27. Effect of inflammation on airway resistance in infants and adults. *R*, Flow resistance; *r*, radius of an air passage.

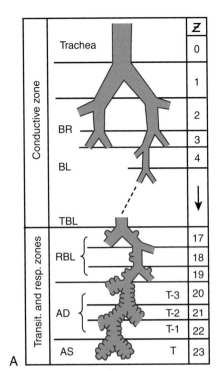

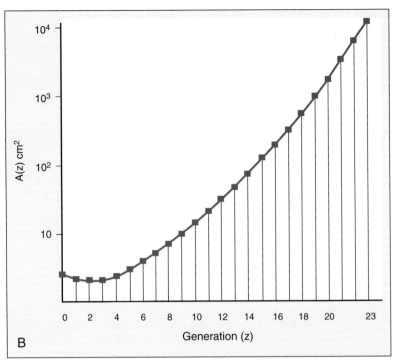

■ **FIGURE 3-28. A,** Diagrammatic representation of the sequence of elements in the conductive, transitory, and respiratory zones of the airways. **B,** Total airway cross-sectional area, *AD,* alveolar ducts; *AS,* alveolar sacs; *z,* order of generation of branching; *A(z),* in each generation, *z. BR,* Bronchi; *BL,* bronchioles; *RBL,* respiratory bronchioles; *T,* terminal generation; *TBL,* terminal bronchioles. *(From Weibel ER:* Morphometry of the human lung, *New York, 1963, Academic Press.)*

Box 3-3 Airway System and Resistance

UPPER AIRWAYS: EXTRATHORACIC
Mouth/nose, pharynx, larynx (the narrowest segment)
Upper airway resistance: 65% of total Raw

LOWER AIRWAYS: INTRATHORACIC
Lower airway resistance: 35% of total Raw
Central (large) airways: trachea, large bronchi
Peripheral (small) airways: small bronchi, bronchioli
Central airways: 90% of lower Raw (30%)
Peripheral airways: 10% of lower Raw (<5%)

---

cross-sectional area of the airway segments increases dramatically toward the periphery, although the diameter of successive single airways decreases. This is because the number of airways increases markedly and, consequently, the flow resistance of airways decreases toward the periphery (Weibel, 1963) (Fig. 3-28). Using a retrograde catheter technique, Macklem and Mead (1967) demonstrated that the peripheral airways, less than about 1 mm in diameter (around 14th generation), contribute less than 10% of the lower airway resistance (or 3% of the total airway resistance).

Tissue Viscoelastic Resistance

It has been assumed that airway (frictional) resistance represents the majority of total respiratory system resistance during breathing, and the pressure needed to overcome tissue viscous resistance during inspiration was estimated to be about 35% in adults and 28% in children (Bryan and Wohl, 1986). However, studies since the 1980s in both anesthetized animals and humans on mechanical ventilation have indicated that viscoelastic resistance, or the energy required to counter the hysteresis or viscoelasticity of the lungs and thoracic tissues, contributes a significantly greater proportion of the total resistance than previously assumed (Milic-Emili et al., 199). Furthermore, both airway resistance (Raw) and viscoelastic resistance (Rvis or ΔR) have been found to be flow and volume dependent (i.e., both Raw and Rvis change with volume and/or flow changes) and to the opposite directions. Airway resistance (Raw) increases with increasing flow as a result of higher turbulence, whereas Raw decreases with increasing lung volume, because airway caliber also increases w

difficult than nose breathing (Moss, 1965; Sasaki et al., 1977a). When the nasal airway is occluded, some infants, especially during REM sleep, do not respond sufficiently to initiate adequate mouth breathing and obstructive apnea ensues. In infants, the insertion of a nasogastric tube significantly increases total resistance by as much as 50% and may compromise breathing (Stocks, 1980).

Lower Airway Resistance

Between the trachea and the alveolar duct are an average of 23 (mean of 17 to 27) airway generations or branchings (Fig. 3-28) (Weibel, 1963). As gas molecules move from the trachea toward the terminal airways during inspiration, the radius of the successive generations of airways becomes smaller and the flow resistance is expected to increase. In reality, however, the total

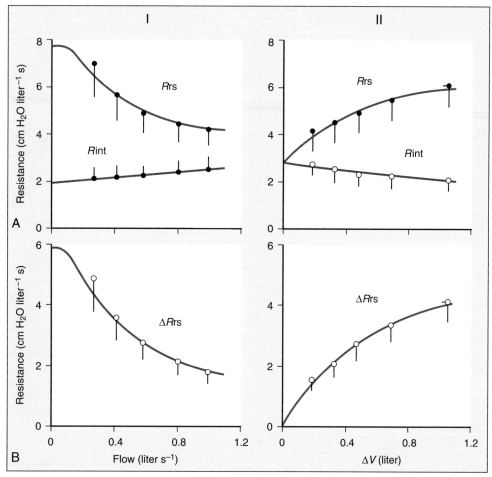

■ **FIGURE 3-29.** Flow and volume dependence of respiratory system resistance (Rrs) and its subdivisions, resistive component (Rint, mostly airway resistance, Raw) and viscoelastic component (ΔRrs or Rvisc) (Rrs = Rint + ΔRrs). **A,** *I,* Average relationship of Rrs and Rint with increasing inspiratory flow on X-axis at a constant inspiratory volume (0.47 L) in 16 anesthetized and paralyzed adult subjects. **B,** *I,* Similar relationship between ΔRrs with variable inspiratory flow. **A,** *II,* Average relationship of Rrs and Rint with variable inspiratory volume on X-axis at a constant inspiratory flow (0.56L/sec) in the same subjects as **A,** *I,* **B,** *II,* Similar relationship in terms of ΔRrs. *Bars,* 1SD. *(Modified from D'Angelo E et al.: Respiratory mechanics in anesthetized paralyzed humans,* J Appl Physiol *67:2556, 1989.)*

volume. The traditional view had been that the total resistance followed the same direction of flow resistance because it was thought to be the majority of total respiratory system resistance. Paradoxically, Rvis decreases with increasing flow, when the volume is kept constant, and when the flow rate is kept constant Rvis increases with increasing lung volume (Fig. 3-29) (D'Angelo et al., 1989). Furthermore, the direction of changes in total resistance followed that of Rvis rather than that of Raw. Studies in children who have been anesthetized and ventilated have shown a similar flow and volume dependence of RV exist in adults; that is, opposite of the direction of changes in Raw, although the total resistance did not necessarily follow the changes in Rvis that occurred in adults (Fig. 3-30) (Kaditis et al., 2008).

This evidence and new understanding on the behavior of viscoelastic resistance have important clinical implications. Traditionally, the patient with airway obstruction has been treated with large tidal volumes and a slow respiratory rate to allow complete exhalation to avoid intrinsic PEEP$_i$ and air trapping. With the new understanding, it makes more sense to have patients breathe with a smaller tidal volume and higher respiratory rate in order to minimize total respiratory system resistance and decrease work of breathing (Kaditis et al., 1999b, 2008).

Time Constant of the Respiratory System

When the lung is allowed to empty passively from end inspiration to FRC, the speed of lung deflation is determined by the product of respiratory system resistance and compliance (R × C or R/E), which is a unit of time (time constant, τ). If the respiratory system is considered as a single compartment with a constant resistance and compliance within the tidal volume range of breathing (which is a reasonable assumption in healthy individuals), then τ = R × C.

Under these conditions, the volume-time profile can be represented by an exponential decay and at 1 time constant (1τ), tidal volume is reduced by 63%. It requires 3 × τ to nearly complete exhalation to FRC. In healthy children and adults, τ is 0.4 to 0.5 seconds; it is slightly shorter in neonates (0.2 to 0.3 seconds) (Bryan and Wohl, 1986). In patients with obstructive lung disease, such as bronchial asthma, τ is increased because of an

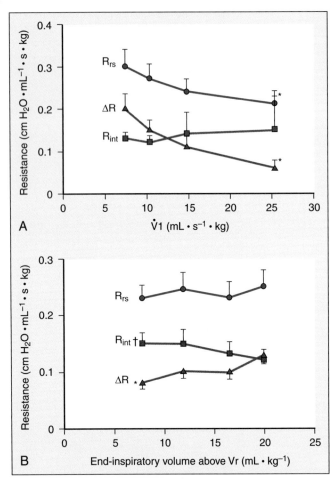

A

B

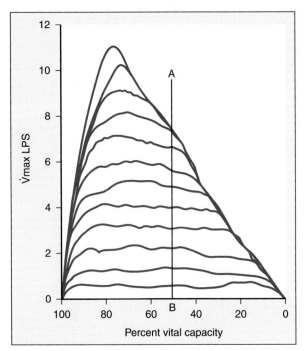

A

B

■ FIGURE 3-31. Flow-volume curves obtained when a subject performs a series of vital capacity expirations of graded effort, varying from a very slow breath out to one of maximal speed and effort. *(From Bates DV et al., editors:* Respiratory function in disease: an introduction to the integrated study of the lung, *Philadelphia, 1971, WB Saunders.)*

■ FIGURE 3-30. Flow and volume dependence of respiratory system resistance (Rrs) and its subdivisions, flow-resistive component (Rint or Raw) and viscoelastic component (ΔR or Rvis) (Rrs = Rint + ΔR), in eight healthy children aged 2.3 to 6.5 years under general endotracheal anesthesia. **A,** Average relationship of Rrs, Rint, and ΔR with increasing inspiratory flow on X-axis at a constant end-inspiratory volume (VT, 12 mL/kg). ΔR and Rrs decreased significantly with increasing flow as in adults (see Fig. 3-29). **B,** Average relationship of Rrs, Rint, and ΔR with increasing volume on x-axis while flow was kept constant (15 mL/sec per kg) in the same subjects as in **A.** Rint decreases with increasing volume as expected, whereas ΔR increased with increasing volume. Unlike in adults, there was no volume dependence of Rrs; *Bars,* 1 SEM; $\dot{V}_1$ inspiratory flow; *Vr,* relaxation volume or end expiratory volume. *(From Kaditis AG et al.: Effect of lung expansion and PEEP on respiratory mechanics in anesthetized children,* Pediatr Anesth *106:775, 2008.)*

increase in airway resistance; it is also increased markedly in patients breathing through an endotracheal tube under general anesthesia.

The Concept of Flow Limitation and Maximum Expiratory Flow-Volume Curves

During quiet breathing, pleural pressure remains subatmospheric, whereas during forced expiration, pleural pressure increases considerably above atmospheric pressure and in turn increases alveolar pressure. The resultant pressure gradient between the alveoli and the airway opening (atmospheric)

produces the expiratory flow. In the periphery of the lungs this pressure within the airways is even higher than the increased pleural pressure by effort because of the additional elastic recoil pressure of the lung. In comparison, in major intrathoracic airways the pressure within the lumen is near atmospheric and lower than the surrounding pleural pressure. At some point along the airways the pressure within the airway lumen should equal the pleural pressure surrounding the airway (equal pressure point [EPP]) (Mead et al., 1967). During forced expiration, the airway between EPP and the trachea is dynamically compressed, and the flow rates consequently become independent of effort (i.e., additional expiratory effort or pressure does not increase flow) (Fig. 3-31). Under these circumstances (dynamic flow limitation), the maximum expiratory flow rate (Vmax or MEF) is determined by the flow resistance of the upstream segment (Rus) between the alveoli and the EPP and the elastic recoil pressure of the lung (Pstl), as follows (Mead et al., 1967):

$$\dot{V}max = \frac{Pstl}{Rus}$$

According to the wave-speed theory of expiratory flow limitation, compliance or collapsibility of lower airways around the EPP (choke point) is an additional determinant of MEF rate (Dawson and Elliott, 1977; Hyatt, 1986).

The maximum expiratory flow volume (MEFV) curve obtained during forced expiration from TLC to residual volume relates instantaneous MEFs to corresponding lung volume (Fig. 3-32). Clinically, the measurement of MEF rate is an extremely sensitive test for the detection of obstruction of the lower airways toward the periphery (quiet zone) of the lung because it eliminates the component of upper airway resistance

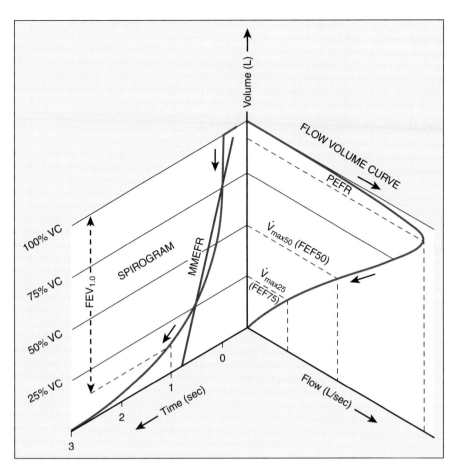

■ **FIGURE 3-32.** MEFV curve on volume-flow axis on the right is contrasted with spirometric tracing (spirogram) on volume-time axis on the left during a single forced vital capacity (VC) maneuver. *FEV$_{1.0}$,* Forced expiratory volume in 1 second; *PEFR,* peak expiratory flow rate; *MEF$_{50}$, MEF$_{25}$,* MEF at 50% and 25%, respectively, of forced VC. *(From Motoyama EK: Airway function tests in infants and children,* Int Anesthesiol Clin *26:6, 1988.)*

between the mouth and EPP and is independent of the degree of effort or cooperation by the patient (Zapletal et al., 1971) (see Measurements of Pulmonary Function).

Distribution of Flow Resistance

On the basis of physiologic measurements in lungs obtained at autopsy, Hogg and others (1970) reported that airway conductance of the peripheral airways in children younger than 6 years of age was disproportionately low (i.e., resistance was high). They postulated that the diameter of small airways of the same generation was disproportionately smaller in infants than in older children and adults. Although this theory is consistent with the high incidence of severe lower airway disease in infants, it conflicts with later physiologic data obtained from healthy infants. Studies of MEFV curves in anesthetized infants and children, and more recently in sedated infants, showed that at low lung volumes, the MEF normalizes for lung volume and that the conductance of the upstream segment is disproportionately high in infants and decreases with age, indicating that lower airway resistance toward the periphery of the lung parenchyma is relatively lower, rather than higher, in the early postnatal years (Fig. 3-33) (Motoyama, 1977; Lambert et al., 2004).

Summary

Compliance of the respiratory system has both lung and chestwall components. During artificial ventilation of a healthy adult, about one half of the inspiratory pressure is required to expand

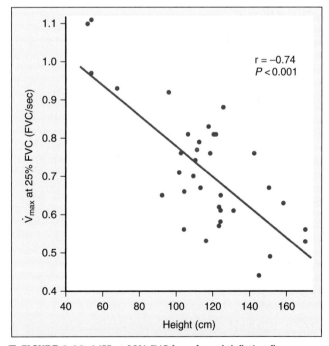

■ **FIGURE 3-33.** MEF at 25% FVC from forced deflation flow-volume curves vs. height in anesthetized boys and girls. MEF$_{25}$ is expressed in FVC units per second to normalize for lung size. FVC-adjusted MEF$_{25}$ is disproportionately higher in infants than in older children. *(From Motoyama EK: Pulmonary mechanics during early postnatal years,* Pediatr Res *11:220, 1977.)*

the lungs and one half is needed to expand the chest wall. In infants, the chest wall is extremely compliant and requires little pressure to expand. Accordingly, airway pressure during artificial ventilation should be reduced. In absolute terms, lung compliance increases with body or lung size. In relative terms, however, lung compliance is relatively high in infants and decreases with age, as elastic recoil pressure of the lungs increases. Most of the flow resistive force against breathing is exerted within the upper and large central airways; the small airways contribute only a fraction of total flow resistance. Flow resistance in absolute terms is largest when air passages are smallest; thus, infants are more prone to airway obstruction of the upper and lower airways. When lung volumes are taken into account, however, total airway resistance is relatively low during the newborn period and increases rapidly during the first year, as lung volume increases with alveolar formation. Resistance of smaller (parenchymal) airways appears to be relatively low at birth and increases with age. The contribution of viscoelastic resistance from the lungs and thoracic tissue hysteresis has been found to be much larger than had been recognized in the past. Both flow-resistive and tissue viscoelastic resistance change with increasing flow and volume, but the directions of changes are opposite to each other. Forming a complex mechanism, the tonic activities of the pharyngeal and laryngeal dilator muscles protect the pharyngeal airway from collapse. During spontaneous breathing, the genioglossus and other upper airway muscles contract synchronously with the diaphragm and increase upper airway caliber. These muscles are easily depressed by sleep and anesthesia, causing upper airway obstruction both at the velopharynx and, to a lesser extent, at the base of the tongue, resulting in upper airway obstruction during anesthesia.

VENTILATION

Ventilation involves the movement of air in and out of the lungs. The diaphragm is the most important muscle for normal inspiration, although the intercostal and accessory respiratory muscles aid in a maximal inspiratory effort. Quiet expiration results from the elastic recoil of the lungs and chest wall and the relaxation of the diaphragm. The expiration of a newborn, even when resting or asleep, appears active rather than passive, as it appears in the older child and adult. A similar active expiration has been observed in anesthetized patients, but the mechanism is unknown (Freund et al., 1964). Forced expiration is accomplished with the aid of the spinal flexors, the intercostal muscles, and especially the abdominal muscles.

Tidal volume (VT) is the amount of air moved into or out of the lungs with each breath. Minute volume ($\dot{V}E$) is the amount of air breathed in or out in a minute, or as follows:

$$\dot{V}E = VT \times f$$

The frequency (f) of quiet breathing decreases with increasing age. The exact basis for this change is unknown but may be related to the work of breathing. Humans seem to adjust their respiratory rate and tidal volume so that ventilatory needs are accomplished with a minimum of work (McIlroy et al., 1954). The relatively high rate in newborns (average, 34 breaths/min) as compared with adults (10 to 12 breaths/min) is consistent with this minimum work concept (Fig. 3-34) (Cook et al., 1957). Mead (1960), however, has presented data indicating that in the

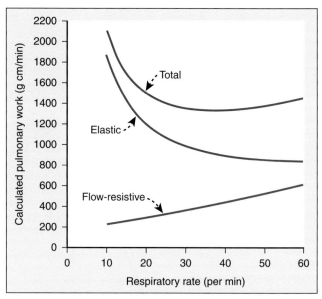

■ **FIGURE 3-34.** Calculated pulmonary work in newborns vs. respiratory rate. The theoretical minimum work of respiration occurs at a rate of 37 breaths/min. Observed resting respiratory rates were 38 breaths/min. *(From Cook CD et al.: Studies of respiratory physiology in the newborn infant. VI. measurements of mechanics of respiration,* J Clin Invest 36:440, 1957.)

normal resting state, respiration is adjusted to require a minimum average force of the respiratory muscles. Mead postulated that the principal site of the sensory end of the control mechanism is in the lungs. In certain situations, the minimum work of breathing and minimum average force required would occur at the same frequency of respiration, but this would not invariably be true.

Dead Space and Alveolar Ventilation

Only part of the minute volume is effective in gas exchange—the alveolar ventilation ($\dot{V}A$). The remainder merely ventilates the respiratory dead space. If the minute noneffective ventilation ($\dot{V}E–\dot{V}A$) is divided by the frequency, the physiologic respiratory dead space is calculated. In the normal person, the physiologic and anatomic dead spaces are approximately equal because alveolar dead space is negligible. Because the air passages are compliant structures, the size of the dead space correlates closely with the degree of lung expansion. When airway obstruction and emphysema are present, dead space increases. However, physiologic dead space is influenced more by the evenness of gas distribution within the lungs and by the perfusion of the alveoli. Thus, when ventilation of the lungs is uneven (as in asthma or CF) or the blood supply to various areas of the lungs decreases (as with pulmonary emboli), the physiologic dead space increases.

Although the anatomic dead space represents an inefficient part of the respiratory tract with respect to gas exchange, it does have two important functions: warming and humidifying gas on inspiration. These functions are compromised by endotracheal intubation or tracheostomy.

In a healthy person, dead space can be estimated as 1 ml pound of body weight (Radford et al., 1954). In children and young adults, a more exact estimate may be obtained from the relation of dead space to body height (Hart et al., 1963).

The dead space to tidal volume (V_D/V_T) ratio in normal lungs is approximately constant (0.3) from infancy to adulthood (Table 3-2). An absolute increase in dead space, however, whether caused by respiratory abnormalities or external apparatus, is much more critical to the infant than to the adult because of the infant's small tidal volume and the relatively larger volume of dead space added.

Alveolar ventilation, or the minute effective ventilation, may be expressed in terms of the carbon dioxide in the peripheral arterial blood. Thus, the following equation is applicable:

$$\dot{V}_A = \frac{(P_B - 47) \times \dot{V}CO_2}{Paco_2}$$

where CO_2 is the carbon dioxide production per minute, $Paco_2$ is the arterial carbon dioxide tension, and $PB - 47$ is the barometric pressure minus water vapor tension at 37° C.

The difference between minute volume and alveolar ventilation ($\dot{V}_E - \dot{V}_A$) is the wasted ventilation caused by physiologic dead space. The concept of alveolar ventilation may be easier to understand if it is considered similar in some way to the renal clearance of a substance; in the lungs, CO_2 is the substance being cleared. If CO_2 remains constant when alveolar ventilation is halved, $Paco_2$ doubles. Measurement of alveolar ventilation provides a far better index of the efficacy of ventilation than measurement of minute volume. Minute volume may be very large, but if it is composed mostly of dead space or ineffective ventilation, it may be inadequate and $Paco_2$ may start to increase.

Physiologic dead space is calculated from the CO_2 tensions between arterial blood and mixed expired gas ($Petco_2$) and is often expressed as a fraction of the tidal volume:

$$V_D / V_T = \frac{Paco_2 - Petco_2}{Paco_2}$$

Alveolar ventilation is considerably higher per unit of lung volume in the healthy infant than in the adult. This is expected because the oxygen consumption is also higher per unit of lung volume or body weight in the infant (Cook et al., 1955).

Distribution of Ventilation

The distribution of ventilation is affected by a number of factors. At end expiration with the mouth open and the larynx relaxed, alveolar pressure is zero, or atmospheric. The interpleural pressure is negative, and there is a vertical pressure gradient. The pressure surrounding the apex of the lung is more negative than that at the base. Accordingly, the transmural or distending pressure at the apex is greater and the regional FRC is larger than that at the base (Fig. 3-35, A). At the end of tidal inspiration, a greater proportion of the inspired air is distributed to the base because the regional FRC is at the steepest portion of the pressure-volume curve at the base. In a lateral decubitus position, the lower part of the lung receives a larger tidal volume than the upper part (Kaneko et al., 1966). In adults with unilateral lung disease, pulmonary gas exchange can be improved by positioning with the healthy lung down, or dependent (Remolina et al., 1981).

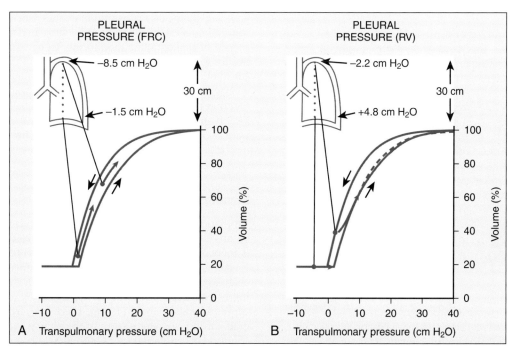

FIGURE 3-35. Effect of vertical gradient of pleural surface pressure on distribution of tidal ventilation. **A,** At the beginning of lung inflation ⸺m functional residual capacity (FRC), lower regions are operating on a steeper part of the compliance curve of lungs than upper regions. ⸺cordingly, during slow inspiration from FRC, ventilation is greater in lower lung regions *(arrows)*. **B,** At RV, pleural surface pressure at lung ⸺se is positive (+4.8 cm H_2O) and lower airways are closed. Consequently, at the beginning of slow inspiration from RV, lower lung regions ⸺ not ventilated and the uppermost part of the lung is preferentially ventilated *(arrows)*. *(From Milic-Emili J: Pulmonary statics. In Widdicomb JG,* ⸺tor: *Respiratory physiology, MTP international review of science, Series I, vol 2, Borough Green, Kent, 1974, Butterworth.)*

In infants with unilateral lung disease, however, the opposite seems to be the case. In the lateral decubitus position, oxygenation improves when the healthy lung is uppermost (Heaf et al., 1983; Davies et al., 1985). Furthermore, Heaf and others (1983) have shown by means of a krypton-81m ventilation scan that in infants and children up to 27 months of age, with or without radiologic evidence of lung disease, ventilation is preferentially increased in the uppermost part of the lung and diminished in the dependent lung (Fig. 3-36). This paradoxical distribution of ventilation in young children may be explained by premature airway closure (Davies et al., 1985). Because the infant's chest wall is extremely compliant, the pleural pressure is near atmospheric. The condition resembles that of adults breathing at extremely low lung volumes (or near RV) (Fig. 3-35, *B*). Under these circumstances, airway closure occurs and, in the lateral decubitus position, ventilation preferentially shifts to the uppermost part of the lung (Milic-Emili et al., 1966). In paralyzed, mechanically ventilated adults, tidal ventilation is preferentially shifted to the uppermost part of the lung, presumably by a similar mechanism (i.e., reduction of FRC and airway closure) (Rehder et al., 1972).

Distortion of regional mechanical properties in the lungs results in far greater variations in the distribution of ventilation than is produced by gravitational forces. The product of regional flow resistance (R, expressed as pressure/flow in cm H_2O/mL per second) and compliance (C, expressed as volume/pressure in mL/cm H_2O) determines the regional ventilation in the lungs. The product of resistance and compliance (R × C) is a unit of time, termed the time constant (τ), as previously discussed. In diseased lungs, such as with asthma, BPD, and CF, the regional time constant becomes abnormal in affected areas, resulting in an uneven distribution of ventilation. The distribution of ventilation may be studied by measuring a nitrogen wash-out curve. The subject breathes 100% oxygen, and the decay of the alveolar nitrogen concentration is measured in successive expirations. Both in normal children and adults, nitrogen concentration is less than 2.5% after 7 minutes of oxygen breathing. This value is increased in patients with an uneven distribution of ventilation because the elimination of nitrogen from poorly ventilated areas is prolonged. In addition, radioactive xenon ventilation scans have been used to demonstrate macroscopic ventilatory abnormalities to aid in the interpretation of perfusion lung scans.

Clinical Implications

The anesthesiologist often controls a patient's ventilation manually or mechanically during general anesthesia, because most anesthetic techniques cause spontaneous ventilation to decrease or cease. This is because most anesthetics are potent respiratory depressants, and because the endotracheal tube and the anesthesia circuit add elastic and resistive loads to breathing. Because anesthesia generally causes a decrease in FRC, the uneven distribution of ventilation, and an increase in physiologic dead space, the tidal volume must be increased. The mechanical dead space and internal compliance of anesthetic equipment also must be taken into account for the proper estimation of a patient's ventilatory requirement. Physiologic dead space is further increased in patients with preexistent lung dysfunction. For these reasons, it is practical to start with a tidal volume of 10 to 15 mL/kg, or roughly 1.5 to 2.0 times that required in awake individuals.

The inspiratory-to-expiratory (I/E) ratio is set to 1:2, a duty cycle (TI/TTOT) of 0.33. Respiratory frequency should be 10 to 14 breaths/min in adolescents, 14 to 20 breaths/min in children, and 20 to 30 breaths/min in infants. Once the mechanical ventilation is established, it can be decreased and refined with the aid of capnographic monitoring. In patients with obstructive lung disease who have a prolonged respiratory system time constant, expiratory time is increased to allow sufficient time for passive lung deflation. Passive expiration is an exponential function and takes three times the time constant to return to FRC (Lamb, 2000). The addition of a low level of PEEP (5 to 7 cm H_2O) restores the volume (FRC) lost from the relaxation of inspiratory muscles and helps prevent airway closure.

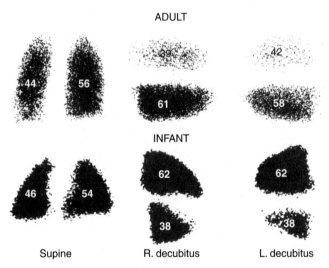

ADULT

INFANT

Supine   R. decubitus   L. decubitus

■ **FIGURE 3-36.** Posterior krypton 81m ventilation lung scan in a healthy 31-year-old man and in a 2-month-old girl. In the adult, ventilation is preferentially distributed to the dependent lung; in the infant, the reverse is seen, with ventilation greater in the uppermost lung. For all scans, the distribution of ventilation to each lung is expressed as a percentage of the total to both lungs. *(From Heaf DP et al.: Postural effects on gas exchange in infants,* N Engl J Med *308:1505, 1983.)*

Summary

Ventilation comprises effective (alveolar) and dead space ventilation. In healthy subjects, ventilation in relation to body size is increased in early infancy and then remains fairly constant throughout childhood and adolescence. Changes in Pao_2 reflect changes in alveolar ventilation; thus, capnographic monitoring of end tidal Pco_2 is useful for adjusting and maintaining appropriate alveolar ventilation. There is a vertical, hydrostatic gradient in negative pressure in the pleural space. Uneven distribution of ventilation exists both in health and in disease. The regional resting volume (FRC) is highest in the uppermost part of the lung, whereas the regional tidal volume is largest in the lowermost region of the lung in a spontaneously breathing subject. The opposite relationship exists in spontaneously breathing infants as well as in patients under anesthesia who are mechanically ventilated. In diseased lungs, uneven distribution of regional compliance (C), resistance (R), and a time constant (R × C) cause maldistribution of ventilation and increased physiologic dead space.

GAS DIFFUSION

The ultimate purpose of pulmonary ventilation is to allow the diffusion of oxygen through the alveolar epithelial lining, basement membrane, and capillary endothelial wall into the plasma and red cells and diffusion of CO_2 in the opposite direction. The distance for gases to diffuse between the alveolar space and the capillary lumen is extremely small, about 0.3 mcm in humans (Weibel, 1973). Because these processes apparently follow the physical laws of diffusion, without any active participation by the lung tissue, pressure gradients must exist or gas exchange will not occur. On the other hand, if the gradient is increased by changes in gas tension either within the alveoli or in the blood, gas exchange is more rapid. Furthermore, because the blood Po_2 affects the blood Pco_2, changes in one moiety alter diffusion of the other. CO_2 diffuses approximately 20 times faster than oxygen in a gas-liquid environment. Therefore impairment of CO_2 diffusion does not become apparent in clinical situations until extremely severe disease is present.

The diffusing capacity of the lungs may be measured with a foreign gas, carbon monoxide (CO), used in small concentrations (less than or equal to 0.3%), or with various concentrations of inspired oxygen (Forster, 1957). The subjects of diffusion and diffusing capacity have been reviewed.

The diffusing capacity of carbon monoxide (D_{LCO}) can be measured with a single breath technique by adding an inert gas to the inhaled gas mixture with a single alveolar gas sample (Ogilve et al., 1957). The D_{LCO} test is not exactly a measure of diffusing capacity, because *diffusing* implies that the uptake of CO is attributable to diffusion alone and *capacity* implies it is a maximal limit (Crapo et al., 2001). Indeed, the term *transfer factor* (T_{LCO}) has become a standard term in most countries outside of North America (Forster, 1983; Cotes et al., 1993). The role of D_{LCO} measurement in lung function testing is to provide information on the transport of gas from alveolar air to hemoglobin in pulmonary capillaries. More specifically, D_{LCO} measures the uptake of CO from the lungs per minute per unit of CO driving pressure, as follows:

$$D_{LCO} = \frac{\dot{V}_{CO}}{P_{ACO} - P_{CCO}}$$

where *CO* is uptake of $\dot{V}CO$ (mL/min), *PACO* is alveolar partial pressure of CO, and *Pcco* is average pulmonary capillary partial pressure of CO. Because the basic equation is flow/pressure change ($\dot{V}/\Delta P$), D_{LCO} is a measure of conductance (G = 1/R).

Although the diffusion of gases within the lungs is necessary for survival, comparatively few conditions occurring in children affect diffusion per se. Diffusing capacity is decreased in the "alveolar capillary block syndrome" (Bates, 1962). This decrease was considered to result primarily from increased thickness of the alveolocapillary membranes; but it is now believed that uneven distribution of ventilation with a resulting V/Q imbalance is the more important cause of arterial oxygen desaturation (Finley et al., 1962). Diffusing capacity changes with hemoglobin concentrations; it increases as hemoglobin concentration increases. A correction factor has to be used according to the recommendation of American Thoracic Society guidelines (1995). Anemia,

on the other hand, is associated with a decrease in diffusing capacity. This is partially explained by the decreased ability of blood to carry the inspired gases. Patients with congenital heart disease and left-to-right shunts often have an increased D_{LCO} caused by increased blood volume and flow in the lungs (Bucci and Cook, 1961). Conversely, diffusing capacity may be reduced when the pulmonary blood flow is markedly decreased, as in pulmonic stenosis.

PULMONARY CIRCULATION

Perinatal and Postnatal Adaptation

In prenatal life, pulmonary vascular resistance is high and most of the right ventricular output runs parallel to the left ventricular output, bypassing the lungs and flowing into the descending aorta through the ductus arteriosus. With the onset of ventilation at birth, the pulmonary vascular resistance suddenly decreases and blood flow through the lungs increases, enabling the organism to exchange oxygen and CO_2 and sustain independent existence. The principal factors that control this vital adjustment in vascular resistance are chemical changes (i.e., changes in Po_2 and Pco_2 or pH) in the environment of the pulmonary vessels (Cook et al., 1963). An increase in Po_2 also produces constriction and subsequent closure of the ductus arteriosus. The pulmonary arterial pressure, which is slightly higher than the pressure in the ascending aorta in the fetus, suddenly decreases at birth and then continues to decrease, with a gradual decline in pulmonary vascular smooth muscle mass approaching the adult level within the first year of life (Assali and Morris, 1964; Rudolph, 1970). If the lungs do not expand adequately (as in IRDS of the neonate) and Po_2 remains low, the pulmonary vascular resistance and pressure may remain high, and there may be prolonged patency of the ductus arteriosus and persistent right-to-left shunting of blood (Strang and MacLeish, 1961) (see Chapter 4, Cardiovascular Physiology).

Under normal postnatal conditions, the systemic and pulmonary vascular beds are connected in series to form a continuous circuit. Although the systemic circulation has a high vascular resistance with a large pressure gradient between the arteries and veins, the pulmonary circulation presents a low resistance to flow.

Both hypoxemia and hypercapnia constrict the pulmonary vascular bed and increase resistance to flow. Chronic hypoxemia is associated with a pulmonary hypertension that returns to or toward normal when the hypoxemia is corrected (Goldring et al., 1964). Pulmonary hypertension that persists for months or years results in right-sided heart failure (cor pulmonale), which then further complicates the existing pulmonary insufficiency.

Under normal circumstances, the arterial blood from the left ventricle contains up to 5% unsaturated blood (venous admixture). This comes mainly from the bronchial circulation but also in part from blood in the pulmonary circulation bypassing the alveoli and from blood flowing through the thebesian veins. This physiologic venous admixture depresses the arterial Po_2 from approximately 102 to 97 mm Hg. In certain conditions, such as V/Q imbalance (including decreased diffusing capacity), the amount of the venous admixture through the lungs increases sufficiently to cause significant arterial hypoxemia. Venous admixture also occurs because of intrapulmonary shunting as the result of atelectasis, pulmonary arteriovenous fistula, pulmonary hemangiomas, and increased collateral (bronchial) circulation, as in bronchiectasis. In addition, shunting may occur at the cardiac level when there is congenital heart disease with right-to-left shunting.

Nitric Oxide and Postnatal Adaptation

The vascular endothelial cells release various vasoactive factors that affect vascular tone. Nitric oxide (NO) is a unique endogenous regulatory molecule involved in a wide variety of biological activities, including systemic and pulmonary vasodilation, neurotransmission, and immunomodulation (Welch and Loscalzo, 1994). Under physiologic conditions, NO is produced from the amino acid L-arginine catalyzed by constitutive NO synthase (cNOS) with a number of cofactors (nicotinamide adenine dinucleotide phosphate [NADPH], flavoproteins, tetrahydrobiopterin, reduced glutathione, and heme complex) and with the presence of ionized calcium and calmodulin. NO in the vascular endothelial cells diffuses into the adjacent vascular smooth muscle cells, stimulates guanylate cyclase activity, and increases cyclic guanylate monophosphate (cGMP), resulting in controlled smooth muscle relaxation and vasodilation (Furchgott and Vanhoutte, 1989; Moncada et al., 1989). In normal lungs, basal release of endothelium-derived NO contributes to the maintenance of low pulmonary vascular resistance (Celemajer et al., 1994; Stamler et al., 1994).

Certain cytokines and bacterial endotoxins induce a NO synthase isoform (inducible NOS [iNOS]) in macrophages, neutrophils, vascular and airway smooth muscles, and other cell types that normally do not produce cNOS. A massive release of NO by iNOS via activated macrophages and other cell types appears to be the primary cause of profound vasodilation and systemic hypotension in septic shock (Cohen, 1995).

Distribution of Pulmonary Perfusion

As with regional ventilation, gravity results in a nonuniform distribution of pulmonary blood flow in normal lungs. West (1965) divided the characteristics of upright lung perfusion into three zones, which were later modified to four zones, of flow distribution (Fig. 3-37) (Hughes et al., 1968). Perfusion of lung tissue depends on the interrelation among three pressures: alveolar pressure (PA), pulmonary arterial pressure (Pa), and pulmonary venous pressure (Pv). Because pulmonary circulation normally is a low-pressure circuit, the pulmonary perfusion pressure varies from the top to the bottom of the lung, barely overcoming the hydrostatic pressure to reach the apex of the tall upright adult lung. Both pulmonary perfusion pressure and flow are relatively increased at the lung base (West, 1994).

In zone I, the apical-most part, alveolar pressure is higher than both pulmonary arterial and venous pressures. Alveolar capillary blood flow is absent in this zone or is only intermittently occurring with peak pulsatile pressure and flow. Ventilation in zone I is mostly wasted. Excessive PEEP increases zone I, thus increasing alveolar dead space, whereas increased pulmonary perfusion pressure, as occurs in exercise or hypoxemia, decreases or abolishes zone I.

In zone II (the waterfall zone), as the vertical distance above the heart decreases (with alveolar pressure uniform throughout the lung), arterial pressure becomes higher than surrounding

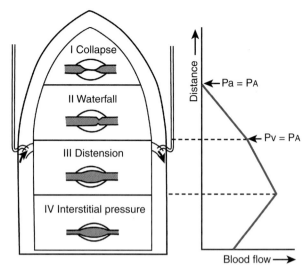

■ **FIGURE 3-37.** Four zones of lung perfusion. Zone I has no flow because alveolar pressure exceeds pulmonary arterial pressure, thereby collapsing alveolar vessels. Zone II is present when pulmonary arterial pressure exceeds alveolar pressure and both are greater than pulmonary venous pressure. This is termed the *vascular waterfall,* because flow is unaffected by downstream (pulmonary venous) pressure. Zone III is characterized by a constant driving force, the difference between pulmonary arterial and venous pressure. Both are greater than alveolar pressure. Flow increases throughout zone III, even though driving pressure is constant because the absolute pressures lower in the lung distend the vessels to a greater extent, thereby lowering resistance. Zone IV has less flow per unit lung volume, probably because of the increased parenchymal pressure surrounding pulmonary vessels. *(From Hughes JMB et al.: Effect of lung volume on the distribution of pulmonary blood flow in man,* Respir Physiol *4:58, 1968.)*

alveolar pressure while venous pressure remains lower than alveolar pressure. The driving pressure in this zone is the difference between arterial and alveolar pressures (Pa – PA), which determines blood flow regardless of venous or downstream pressure (waterfall phenomenon). The blood flow increases linearly as the driving pressure increases toward the base of the lung until pulmonary venous pressure equals alveolar pressure.

In zone III, both arterial and venous pressures are higher than alveolar pressure. The driving pressure for blood flow becomes the difference between arterial and venous pressures (Pa – Pv) throughout this zone. Although the pressure gradient is the same throughout zone III, blood flow is greater toward the base, presumably because both arterial and venous pressures are greater and the pulmonary vascular bed is more distended. The relationships among arterial, venous, and alveolar pressures in zones I to III are summarized as follows:

Zone I: PA > Pa > Pv
Zone II: Pa > PA > Pv
Zone III: Pa > Pv > PA

In zone IV, blood flow is progressively decreased toward the base of the lung, presumably because of increased interstitial pressure surrounding the extraalveolar vessels. This zone increases in size with reduction in the lung volume toward R (Hughes et al., 1968; West, 1994).

The vertical distance between the top and the bottom of the lung is decreased in the supine position, resulting in the disappearance of zone I. Zone II also decreases as pulmonary venous pressure becomes higher throughout the lung in the supine position. The effect of gravity in infants and small children, particularly in the supine position, would be small, although it has not been documented.

Ventilation/Perfusion Relationships

To achieve normal gas exchange in the lung the regional distribution of ventilation and pulmonary perfusion must be balanced. Without this balance, pulmonary gas exchange is impaired, even when the overall levels of ventilation and perfusion are adequate. The normal value for the ventilation/perfusion ($\dot{V}_A/\dot{V}_P$, $\dot{V}_A/\dot{Q}$, or simply V/Q) ratio is about 0.8. Studies with radioactive gases have shown that the elastic and resistive properties of various parts of the lung, as well as the pulmonary blood flow, are influenced by gravity. Both components of the V/Q ratio are affected by changes in a patient's position (West, 1965).

When the patient is in the upright position, blood flow and ventilation are both less in the apex than in the base of the lungs. Because the difference in blood flow between the apex and the base is relatively greater than that in ventilation, the V/Q ratio increases from the bottom to the top of the lungs, as shown in Figures 3-38 and 3-39. The apical regions (high V/Q) have higher alveolar P_{O_2} and lower P_{CO_2} and partial pressure of nitrogen (P_{N_2}), whereas the basal areas (low V/Q) have lower P_{O_2} and higher P_{CO_2} and P_{N_2}. Gravity has a greater effect on the V/Q ratio in hypotensive and hypovolemic patients and may be exaggerated with positive-pressure ventilation. In the supine position, similar differences exist between the anterior and posterior parts of the lung, but they are smaller. During exercise, pulmonary arterial pressure and blood flow, as well as ventilation, are increased and more evenly distributed. In infants and children the distribution of pulmonary blood flow is more uniform than in adults because the pulmonary arterial pressure is relatively high, and the gravity effect in the lungs is less.

In diseased lungs, changes in the V/Q ratio occur as the result of uneven ventilation, uneven perfusion, or both; for example,

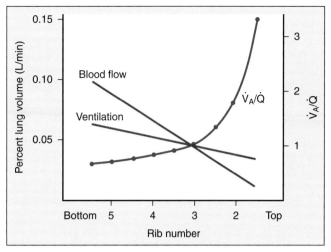

■ **FIGURE 3-39.** Effect of vertical height (expressed as the level of the anterior ends of the ribs) on ventilation and pulmonary blood flow *(left ordinate)* and the V/Q ratio *(right ordinate). (From West JB:* Ventilation/blood flow and gas exchange, *ed 2, Oxford, 1970, Blackwell Scientific Publications.)*

compression or occlusion of pulmonary vessels, reduced pulmonary vascular bed, or intrapulmonary-anatomic right-to-left shunting may contribute to nonuniform perfusion. In congenital heart diseases with increased pulmonary blood flow caused by left-to-right shunting, the V/Q ratio is decreased. When perfusion is diminished, as in tricuspid atresia or pulmonic stenosis with tetralogy of Fallot, V/Q is increased.

The lungs appear to have an intrinsic regulatory mechanism that, to a limited extent, preserves a normal V/Q ratio. In areas with a high V/Q ratio, a low P_{CO_2} tends to constrict airways and dilate pulmonary vessels, and the opposite occurs in areas with a low V/Q ratio. In the latter case, in addition to the effect of P_{CO_2}, hypoxic pulmonary vasoconstriction (HPV) decreases regional blood flow and helps to increase V/Q ratios toward normal. The administration of drugs such as isoproterenol, nitroglycerin,

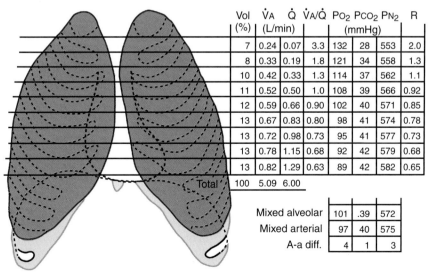

Vol (%)	$\dot{V}_A$ (L/min)	$\dot{Q}$	$\dot{V}_A/\dot{Q}$	P_{O_2}	P_{CO_2} (mmHg)	P_{N_2}	R
7	0.24	0.07	3.3	132	28	553	2.0
8	0.33	0.19	1.8	121	34	558	1.3
10	0.42	0.33	1.3	114	37	562	1.1
11	0.52	0.50	1.0	108	39	566	0.92
12	0.59	0.66	0.90	102	40	571	0.85
13	0.67	0.83	0.80	98	41	574	0.78
13	0.72	0.98	0.73	95	41	577	0.73
13	0.78	1.15	0.68	92	42	579	0.68
13	0.82	1.29	0.63	89	42	582	0.65
Total 100	5.09	6.00					

Mixed alveolar	101	.39	572
Mixed arterial	97	40	575
A-a diff.	4	1	3

FIGURE 3-38. Effect of distribution of ventilation and perfusion on regional gas tensions in erect man. The lung is divided into nine horizontal slices, and the position of each slice is shown by its anterior rib markings. *Vol,* Relative lung volume; *$\dot{V}_A$,* regional alveolar ventilation; *$\dot{Q}$,* regional perfusion; *$\dot{V}_A/\dot{Q}$,* V/Q ratio; *R,* respiratory exchange ratio. *(From West JB: Regional differences in gas exchange in the lung of erect man,* Appl Physiol *17:893, 1962.)*

theophylline, and sodium nitroprusside diminishes or abolishes HPV and increases intrapulmonary shunting (Goldzimer et al., 1974; Colley et al., 1979; Hill et al., 1979; Benumof, 1994). All inhaled anesthetics depress HPV in vitro, contributing to an increase in venous admixture during general anesthesia (Sykes et al., 1972; Bjertnaes, 1978). The effect of inhaled anesthetics on HPV, however, has not been conclusive in vivo (Marshall and Marshall, 1980, 1985; Pavlin and Su, 1994).

Wagner and others (1974) have developed a quantitative method of studying the continuous spectrum of V/Q mismatch. The technique is based on the pattern of elimination of multiple inert gases infused intravenously. At steady state after intravenous infusion of test gases dissolved in saline solution, arterial, mixed-venous, and expired gas samples are obtained, and minute ventilation and cardiac output are measured. The ratio of arterial to mixed venous concentration (retention) and the ratio of expired to mixed venous concentration (excretion) are computed for each gas, and retention-solubility and excretion-solubility curves are drawn by the computer. The ratio of the two curves represents the distribution of perfusion and ventilation on the spectrum of V/Q ratios (Fig. 3-40) (West, 1974, 1994; Benumof, 1994).

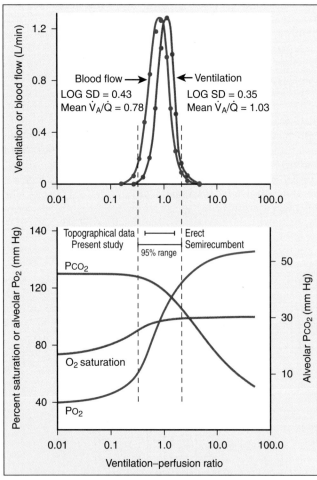

■ **FIGURE 3-40.** Upper graph shows the average distribution of V/Q ratios in young semirecumbent normal subjects. The 95% range covers V/Q from 0.3 to 2.1. The corresponding variations of Po_2, Pco_2, and oxygen saturation in the end-capillary blood can be seen in the lower panel. *(From West JB: Blood flow to the lung and gas exchange,* Anesthesiology 41:124, 1974.)*

Low Ventilation/Perfusion Ratio and Lung Collapse While Breathing Oxygen

In a lung unit with a low regional V/Q ratio while breathing oxygen, collapse of the lung unit occurs, leading to atelectasis. As alveolar ventilation to the lung unit ($\dot{V}A$) decreases, regional expiratory volume (VE) decreases progressively in comparison with regional inspiratory volume (VI) as it approaches the amount of oxygen taken up by regional pulmonary blood flow. A point is reached at which the expired alveolar volume falls to zero (West, 1974). This situation occurs at the "critical" inspired V/Q. With inspired ratios less than the critical V/Q value, the lung unit becomes unstable; oxygen may enter rather than leave the lung unit during the expiratory phase or the unit may gradually collapse (Figure 3-41) (West, 1975). Figure 3-42 shows the calculated relationship between the critical inspired V/Q and the concentration of inspired oxygen (assuming mixed venous Po_2 of 40 mm Hg and Pco_2 of 45 mm Hg and no nitrogen exchange occurring across the whole lung). From Figure 3-42, it can be seen that lung units with V/Q of less than 0.01 become vulnerable when Fio_2 is increased above 0.5, whereas lung units with inspiratory $\dot{V}AI/\dot{Q}$ of 0.1 are not at risk even with 100% oxygen (West, 1975). Although a V/Q of less than 0.1 is uncommon in normal awake children, lung units with a V/Q of less than 0.1 may occur in the diseased lung as well as in the normal lung under general anesthesia.

OXYGEN TRANSPORT

For normal metabolism, oxygen must be transported continuously to all body tissues. Changes in oxygen demand are met by the integrated response of three major functional components of the oxygen transport system: pulmonary ventilation, cardiac output, and blood hemoglobin concentration and characteristics. With acute oxygen demand, such as with extreme exercise, high fever, or acute hypoxemia (less than 60 mm Hg), oxygen transport is increased mainly by increased cardiac output, whereas alveolar ventilation is increased to maintain proper levels of alveolar Po_2 and Pco_2. Chronic hypoxemia increases erythropoietin production, thereby increasing erythrocyte

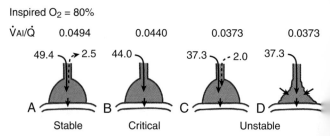

■ **FIGURE 3-41.** Schematic drawings to explain the development of shunts in lung units with low inspiratory $\dot{V}A/\dot{Q}P$ ($\dot{V}AI/\dot{Q}$) caused by breathing high concentrations of oxygen. **A,** Stable; there is a small expired alveolar ventilation ($\dot{V}A$) and the unit is stable. **B,** Critical; inspired $\dot{V}A$ is decreased slightly from A and expired $\dot{V}A$ falls to zero. **C,** Unstable; inspired $\dot{V}A$ is further reduced and gas enters into the lung unit during the expiratory phase. **D,** Unstable; reverse inspiration during expiratory phase is prevented and the unit gradually collapses. *(From West JB: New advances in pulmonary gas exchange,* Anesth Analg 54:409, 1975.)*

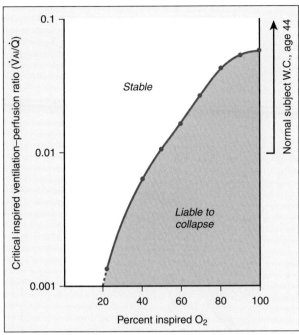

■ FIGURE 3-42. Relationship between inspired oxygen concentration and critical inspiratory $\dot{V}_{AI}/\dot{Q}$, the value at which the expired ventilation of a given lung unit falls to zero. Lung units whose $\dot{V}_A/\dot{Q}$ is less than the critical value may be unstable and easily collapse. *(From West JB: New advances in pulmonary gas exchange, Anesth Analg 54:409, 1975.)*

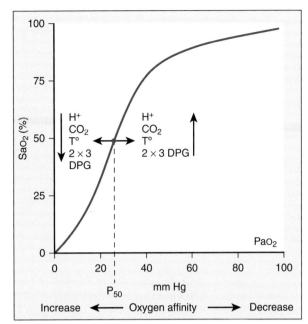

■ FIGURE 3-43. Schematic representation of oxygen dissociation curve and factors that affect blood oxygen affinity. Oxygen partial pressure at 50% oxygen saturation (P_{50}) is a convenient index of oxygen affinity. P_{50} of adult blood (at 37° C; pH, 7.40; P_{CO_2}, 40 mm Hg) is roughly 27 mm Hg and is influenced by a number of factors. H^+, hydrogen ion concentration; Pao_2, arterial oxygen tension; Sao_2, Arterial oxygen saturation; *T8*, blood temperature; *2,3 DPG*, 2,3-diphosphoglycerate.

production from the normal daily rate of approximately 1% of circulating red cell mass to about 2%. Thus, increasing red cell mass in response to chronic hypoxemia is a slow process (Finch and Lenfant, 1972). Hemoglobin concentrations greater than the normal level (15 g/dL) raise viscosity and increase blood flow resistance until the plasma volume is also increased (Thorling and Erslev, 1968).

The amount of oxygen carried by the plasma depends on its solubility and is small (0.31 mL/dL per 100 mm Hg). Most oxygen molecules in blood combine reversibly with hemoglobin to form oxyhemoglobin. Each molecule of hemoglobin combines with four molecules of oxygen; 1 g of oxyhemoglobin combines with 1.34 mL of oxygen.

Oxygen Affinity of Hemoglobin and P_{50}

The oxygen-hemoglobin dissociation curve reflects the affinity of hemoglobin for oxygen (Fig. 3-43). As blood circulates through the normal lungs, oxygen tension increases from the mixed-venous P_{O_2} of around 40 mm Hg to pulmonary capillary P_{O_2} of above 105 mm Hg, and hemoglobin is saturated to about 97% in arterial blood. (Unfortunately, most pulse oximeters commercially available today are artificially modified to read 100% saturation in healthy subjects breathing room air rather than 97%; see later discussion.) The shape of the dissociation curve is such that further increases in P_{O_2} result in a very small increase in oxygen saturation (S_{O_2}) of hemoglobin.

The blood of normal adults has S_{O_2} of 50% when P_{O_2} is 27 mm Hg at 37° C and a pH of 7.4. The P_{50}, which is the P_{O_2} of whole blood at 50% S_{O_2}, indicates the affinity of hemoglobin for oxygen. An increase in blood pH increases the oxygen affinity

of hemoglobin (Bohr effect) and shifts the oxygen-hemoglobin (O_2-Hb) dissociation curve to the left. Similarly, a decrease in temperature also increases oxygen affinity and shifts the O_2-Hb dissociation curve to the left; a decrease in pH or an increase in temperature has the opposite effect and the O_2-Hb curve shifts to the right (Comroe, 1974) (Fig. 3-43).

Benesch and Benesch (1967) and Chanutin and Curnish (1967) demonstrated that the oxygen affinity of a hemoglobin solution decreases by the addition of organic phosphates, in particular 2,3-diphosphoglycerate (2,3-DPG) and adenosine triphosphate (ATP), which bind to deoxyhemoglobin but not to oxyhemoglobin. Human erythrocytes contain an extremely high concentration of 2,3-DPG, averaging about 4.5 mol/mL, compared with ATP (1 mol/mL) and other organic phosphates (Oski and Delivoria-Papadopoulos, 1970). Thus, an increase in red cell 2,3-DPG decreases the oxygen affinity of hemoglobin, increases P_{50} (shifts the dissociation curve to the right), and increases the unloading of oxygen at the tissue level. Increases in 2,3-DPG and P_{50} have been found in chronic hypoxemia.

In the newborn, blood oxygen affinity is extremely high and P_{50} is low (18 to 19 mm Hg), because 2,3-DPG is low and fetal hemoglobin (HbF) reacts poorly with 2,3-DPG (Fig. 3-44). Oxygen delivery at the tissue level is low despite high red blood cell mass and hemoglobin level. After birth, the total hemoglobin level decreases rapidly as the proportion of HbF diminishes, reaching its lowest level by 2 to 3 months of age (physiologic anemia of infancy) (Fig. 3-45). During the same early postnatal period, P_{50} increases rapidly; it exceeds the normal adult value by 4 to 6 months of age and reaches the highest value ($P_{50} = 30$) by 10 months and remains high during the first decade of life

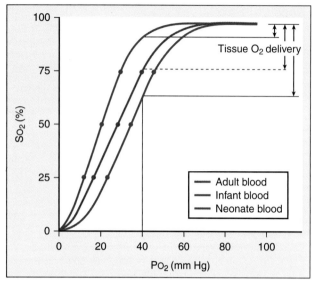

■ **FIGURE 3-44.** Schematic representation of oxygen-hemoglobin dissociation curves with different oxygen affinities. In infants older than 3 months with high P_{50} (30 mm Hg vs. 27 mm Hg in adults), tissue oxygen delivery per gram of hemoglobin is increased. In neonates with a lower P_{50} (20 mm Hg) and a higher blood oxygen affinity, tissue oxygen unloading at the same tissue P_{O_2} is reduced.

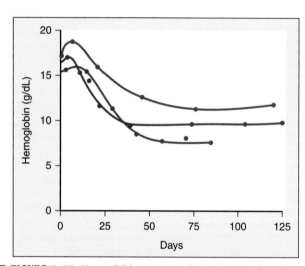

■ **FIGURE 3-45.** Hemoglobin concentration in infants of varying degrees of maturation at birth. *Blue,* Full-term infants; *brown,* premature infants with birth weights of 1200 to 2350 g; *purple,* premature infants with birth weights less than 1200 g. *(From Nathan DG, Oski FA: Hematology of infancy and childhood, ed 3, Philadelphia, 1987, WB Saunders.)*

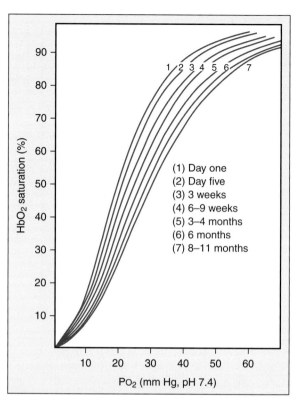

■ **FIGURE 3-46.** Oxyhemoglobin equilibrium curve of blood from normal term infants at different postnatal ages. The P_{50} on day 1 is 19.4 ± 1.8 mm Hg and has shifted to 30.3 ± 0.7 at age 11 months (normal adults = 27.0 ± 1.1 mm Hg). *(From Oski FA: The unique fetal red cell and its function, Pediatrics 51:494, 1973b.)*

TABLE 3-3. Oxygen Unloading Changes with Age

Age	P_{50} (mm Hg)	Percent Saturation at Venous Oxygen Tension of 40 mm Hg	Hemoglobin (g/100 mL)	Oxygen Unloaded* (mL/100 mL)
1 day	19.4	87	17.2	1.84
3 wk	22.7	80	13.0	2.61
6-9 wk	24.4	77	11.0	2.65
3-4 mo	26.5	73	10.5	3.10
6 mo	27.8	69	11.3	3.94
8-11 mo	30.0	65	11.8	4.74
5-8 yr	29.0	67	12.6	4.73
9-12 yr	27.9	69	13.4	4.67
Adult	27.0	71	15.0	4.92

Data from Oski FA: Designation of anemia on a functional basis, *J Pediatr* 83:353, 1973a.
*Assumes arterial oxygen saturation of 95%.

(Fig. 3-46) (Oski and Delivoria-Papadopoulos, 1970; Oski, 1973a, 1973b). This high P_{50} is associated with a relatively low hemoglobin level (10 to 11 g/dL) and an increased level of 2,3-DPG, probably related to the process of general growth and development and high plasma levels of inorganic phosphate (Card and Brain, 1973). These observations engendered a hypothesis to explain why hemoglobin levels are relatively lower in children than in adults (physiologic "anemia" of childhood) (Card and Brain, 1973). Because children have a lower oxygen affinity for hemoglobin, oxygen unloading at the tissue level is increased.

Thus, a lower level of hemoglobin in infants and children is just as efficient, in terms of tissue oxygen delivery, as a higher hemoglobin level in adults (Oski, 1973a) (Table 3-3). Table 3-4 compares the hemoglobin concentrations at different ages in terms of equal tissue oxygen unloading (Motoyama et al., 1974).

TABLE 3-4. Hemoglobin Requirements for Equivalent Tissue Oxygen Delivery

	P_{50} (mm Hg)	Hemoglobin for Equivalent O_2 Delivery (g/dL)						
Adult	27	7	8	9	10	11	12	13
Infant >6 mo	30	5.7	6.5	7.3	8.2	9.0	9.8	10.6
Neonate <2 mo	24	10.3	11.7	13.2	14.7	16.1	17.6	19.1

Data calculated from Motoyama EK et al.: Functional basis of childhood anemia [abstract], *Am Soc Anesthesiology* 283, 1974.

Acceptable Hemoglobin Levels

These findings have important clinical implications for anesthesiologists. Until the 1980s it was assumed that children with a hemoglobin level of less than 10 g/dL were not acceptable for general anesthesia and surgery. This level of hemoglobin has been used arbitrarily without the knowledge of different oxygen affinity and tissue oxygen unloading at different ages. It appears from Table 3-4 that if a hemoglobin level of 10 g/dL is acceptable for an adult with a P_{50} of 27 mm Hg, 8.2 g/dL should theoretically be adequate for an infant older than 8 months of age with an average P_{50} of 30 mm Hg (without considering the high level of metabolism and oxygen consumption). In contrast, for a 2-month-old premature infant with a P_{50} of 24 mm Hg, a hemoglobin level of 10 g/dL is equivalent to only 6.8 g/dL in adults, and this may be inadequate to provide sufficient tissue oxygenation in patients with limited cardiac output or oxygen desaturation.

With the advent of human immunodeficiency virus (HIV) and acquired immunodeficiency syndrome (AIDS) and the resultant anxiety among the medical community and the lay public about homologous blood transfusion, the criteria for transfusion have changed significantly since the 1980s. At the consensus-developing conference by the National Institutes of Health and the Food and Drug Administration on Perioperative Red Blood Cell Transfusion, it was agreed that the available evidence does not support the "10/30" rule (that is, hemoglobin, 10 g/dL, or hematocrit, 30%), although the literature is remarkable for its lack of carefully controlled, randomized studies that would provide definitive conclusions (Consensus Conference, 1988). Other data suggest that cardiac output does not increase dramatically in healthy adult humans until the hemoglobin value decreases to approximately 7 g/dL.

At the Consensus Conference (1988) it was also agreed that the decision to transfuse red blood cells in a specific patient should take into consideration the many factors that comprise clinical judgment. These factors include the duration of anemia, the intravascular volume, the extent of surgery, the probability of massive blood loss, and the presence of coexisting conditions such as impaired cardiopulmonary function and inadequate cardiac output. A general consensus on the acceptable perioperative levels of hemoglobin and hematocrit in infants and young children has not emerged, and the lowest safe limit of hemoglobin for infants less than 2 months of age has not been determined, although in sick infants it is desirable to maintain a hemoglobin level of 12 to 13 g/dL or a hematocrit of 40% (equivalent to 8 g/dL in adults) (see Chapter 14, Blood Conservation).

There has been controversy about what constitutes abnormally low oxygen saturation in infants and children postoperatively and what is considered clinically unsafe. Mok and others (1986) reported that during the first week of life, oxygen saturation as monitored with pulse oximetry (SpO_2) was noticeably decreased, especially during REM sleep (mean SpO_2, 92%) and during feeding (SpO_2, 91%). After 4 weeks of age, however, SpO_2 was more stable and was maintained at or above 94% during sleep. Thus, an SpO_2 of less than 94% can be considered as physiologically abnormal in infants beyond the first week of age. A study in preterm infants (mean gestational age, 33 weeks; postconceptional age, 37 weeks) has shown that median SpO_2 at the time of discharge was 99.5% and increased to 100% at follow-up 6 weeks later. The preterm infants had higher baseline saturation and no more incidence of desaturation than full-term infants of equivalent postconceptional ages (Poets et al., 1992). It is generally agreed that SpO_2 less than 95% in otherwise healthy infants and children is abnormal and that these patients require oxygen supplementation.

The routine use of pulse oximetry has dramatically improved the anesthesiologist's ability to monitor and properly maintain proper oxygenation (Coté et al., 1988, 1991). This is especially true for premature infants, who are susceptible to oxygen toxicity and retinopathy of prematurity, even when breathing room air (Wilson-Mikity syndrome). In premature infants weighing less than 1300 g, the incidence of retinopathy of prematurity increases markedly with exposure to 12 or more hours of PaO_2 exceeding 80 mm Hg (Flynn et al., 1992). Arterial oxygen saturation (SaO_2) must be adjusted properly so as to maintain PaO_2 in the normal neonatal range of 60 to 80 mm Hg (Orzalesi et al., 1967). As mentioned, oxygen affinity to hemoglobin is very high in the neonate and decreases rapidly during the first 3 to 6 months of life (Oski, 1973a, 1973b, 1981). Estimated PaO_2 should be adjusted according to age, as shown in Table 3-5. In the newborn, whose P_{50} is 18 to 20 mm Hg, the range of SaO_2 to maintain adequate PaO_2 (60 to 80 mm Hg) is 97% to 98% (assuming no transfusion with adult blood has been given), whereas in the adult (P_{50}, 27), it is 91% to 96%. In the neonate, SaO_2 of 91% corresponds to PaO_2 of 41 mm Hg. Although the values in Table 3-5, based on Severinghaus's nomogram for the Bohr effect, are only estimates, published data comparing arterial PO_2 and oxygen saturation seem to agree well with values in the nomogram (Severinghaus, 1966; Ramanathan et al., 1987; Bucher et al., 1989).

Unfortunately, another factor compounding the confusion (and clinically too important to ignore) is that the most commonly used pulse oximeters in the United States are artificially set to read 2% to 3% higher at the 90% to 95% range than actual arterial oxygen hemoglobin saturation (as measured by means of cooximetry), and that the pulse oximeters most commonly used in Europe tend to read somewhat lower than actual arterial oxygen saturation (Jennis and Peabody, 1987; Bucher et al., 1989). Unfortunately, a newer and technologically advanced pulse oximeter with less motion artifact, which has increasingly been used in the United States and elsewhere, also has artificially increased readings; it also reads 2% to 3% higher, matching the reading of the more traditionally used pulse oximeter (M. Patterson, 1995, personal communications). In view of these findings, the range of SpO_2 of 93% to 95%, corresponding to an estimated PaO_2 of 66 to 74 mm Hg in adults (but only 40 to 50 mm Hg in neonates), often recommended as desirable maintenance levels for neonates and premature infants intraoperatively or in the intensive care settings, appears much too low

TABLE 3-5. Estimated PO₂ at Different P₅₀ Values of Hemoglobin*

SO₂ (%)	Age				
	1 day	2 wk	6-9 wk	6 mo-6 yr	Adult
P₅₀ (mm Hg)†	19	22	24	29	27
	Estimated PO₂ (mm Hg) at Neutral pH (7.40)				
99	108	130	143	171	156
98	77	92	101	122	111
97	64	77	84	101	92
96	56	68	74	89	82
95	52	62	68	82	74
94	48	58	63	76	69
93	45	55	60	72	66
92	43	52	57	68	62
91	41	50	55	66	60
90	40	48	53	63	58
88	37	45	49	59	54
86	35	42	47	56	51
84	34	40	44	53	49
82	32	39	42	51	47
80	31	37	41	49	45
78	30	36	39	47	43
76	29	34	38	45	41
74	28	33	36	44	40
72	27	32	35	42	39
70	26	31	34	41	37

Data calculated from Severinghaus JW: Blood gas calculator, *J Appl Physiol* 21:1108, 1966.

*Data are calculated with the assumption that the shift in oxygen dissociation curve of hemoglobin because of changes in its oxygen affinity at neutral pH (7.40) is the same as the shift caused by the Bohr effect.

†PO₂ at which oxygen saturation of hemoglobin (SO₂) is 50%.

for adequate tissue oxygenation. Furthermore, respiratory alkalosis, which may result from assisted or controlled ventilation, would shift the oxygen hemoglobin dissociation curve further to the left (P₅₀, even lower than it already is) and decrease PaO₂ and tissue oxygen delivery even further at this range of oxygen saturation (Fig. 3-43). Therefore, in clinical practice, SpO₂ levels of 95% to 97% (corresponding PaO₂ of 50 to 70 mm Hg in neonates and 60 to 80 mm Hg in infants 1 to 2 months old) but not higher, should be considered.

Some anesthetics affect the oxygen affinity of hemoglobin. The presence of cyclopropane (although it has not been used since the 1970s) significantly decreases oxygen affinity and increases P₅₀ by 3 mm Hg without changes in the 2,3-DPG levels, whereas halothane has minimal effects (Orzalesi et al., 1971). Exposure to 50% nitrous oxide, on the other hand, has been reported to produce a marked reversible increase in oxygen affinity; P₅₀ decreased from 26 to 18 mm Hg, a level similar to that of HbF (Fournier and Major, 1984). This finding contrasts with a report based on one patient by Prime (1951), who found no effect with 70% nitrous oxide, and with a study by

Smith and others (1970) who reported a 3 mm Hg rightward shift of P₅₀ with an unspecified concentration of nitrous oxide. The finding of Fournier and Major above may be of considerable clinical importance. Although less often used of late, nitrous oxide anesthesia combined with hyperventilation would markedly increase the oxygen affinity of hemoglobin and decrease oxygen unloading at the tissue level. This effect could be hazardous in neonates whose P₅₀ is unusually low even without respiratory alkalosis or nitrous oxide.

Surface Activity and Pulmonary Surfactant

The alveolar surfaces of human lungs are lined with surface-active materials with unique properties that are responsible for the stability of air spaces. These materials, which contain specific phospholipids and proteins (discussed later), are collectively called pulmonary surfactant.

The relationship among pressure (P), surface tension (T), and radius (r) of a sphere, such as a soap bubble, is expressed by the Laplace equation as follows:

$$P = 2T / r$$

It can be seen from this equation that if surface tension is constant, in a number of connected spheres the smallest sphere has the highest pressure. Thus, the smaller spheres would empty their gas contents into the larger ones. If this concept applied to lung units, the lungs would be unstable, with most units collapsing into several large ones, as seen in the lung of an infant with IRDS. Fortunately, such instability does not exist in normal lungs. As Clements and others (1958) first demonstrated, saline extract of normal lungs exhibits extremely low surface tensions (0 to 5 dynes/cm) with dynamic compression of the surface area increasing surface tension (up to 30 to 50 dynes/cm) during expansion of the surface area. In comparison, pure water has a fixed surface tension of about 72 dynes/cm in room temperature and soap bubbles exhibit relatively low (20+ dynes/cm) but fixed surface tension. These findings by Clements et al. indicate that, in normal lungs, the surface tension decreases as the alveolar radius decreases during exhalation and vice versa; the stability of the air spaces is maintained regardless of the size of each alveolus or lung unit (Fig. 3-47).

The alveolar lining layer obtained from lung lavage contains approximately 10% lipoprotein and 90% phospholipid. Of the phospholipid fraction of surfactant, phosphatidylcholine constitutes about 70%, of which about 60% (about 40% of total phospholipid fraction) is surface active "disaturated" dipalmitoylphosphatidylcholine with saturated palmitate (C-16) in both R₁ and R₂ positions of the three carbon skeleton of phospholipid, whereas other phosphatidylcholines contain unsaturated fatty acids in the R₂ position and are not surface active (Figs. 3-48 and 3-49). Phosphatidylglycerol, another surface active phospholipid, was subsequently identified in the lung extract and comprises about 10% of surfactant fraction (Rooney et al. 1974). Phosphatidylglycerol appears late during the development; its appearance or reappearance coincide with the recovery from IRDS and acute respiratory distress syndrome (ARDS in adults and with the loss of surfactant (Lewis and Jobe, 1993). Other phospholipids include sphingomyelin (also surface active), phosphatidylethanolamine and phosphatidylinositol which are not surface active (Rooney, 1985). The production of phosphatidylcholine increases towards term, whereas that c

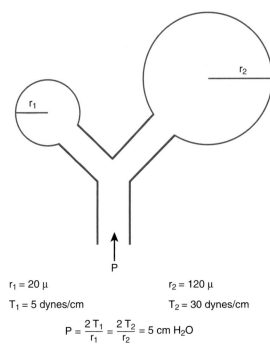

$r_1 = 20\ \mu$ $r_2 = 120\ \mu$

$T_1 = 5$ dynes/cm $T_2 = 30$ dynes/cm

$$P = \frac{2\,T_1}{r_1} = \frac{2\,T_2}{r_2} = 5\ \text{cm H}_2\text{O}$$

■ **FIGURE 3-47.** Schematic drawing of stable alveoli of different sizes.

Phospholipids

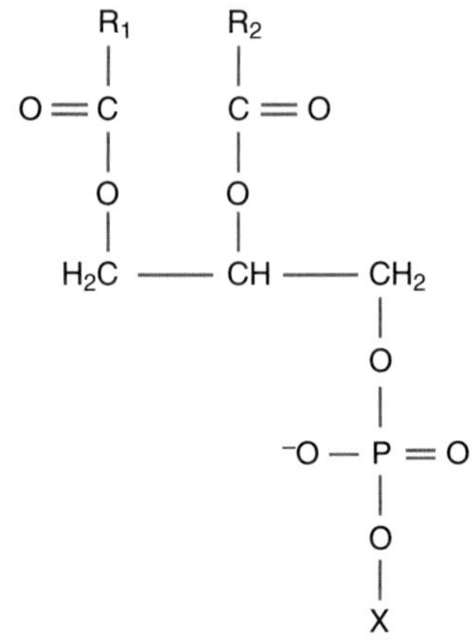

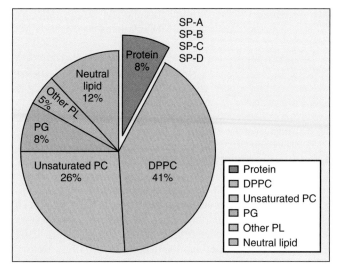

■ **FIGURE 3-49.** Composition of surfactant. *DPPC,* Dipalmitoylphosphatidylcholine; *PC,* phosphatidylcholine; *PG,* phosphatidylglyrerol; *PL,* phospholipids.

Phospholipid classes

Phosphatidylcholine:	X = CH$_2$ – CH$_2$ – $^+$N(CH$_3$)$_3$
Phosphatidylethanolamine:	X = CH$_2$ – CH$_2$ – $^+$NH$_3$
Phosphatidylglycerol:	X = CH$_2$ – CHOH – CH$_2$OH
Phosphatidylinositol:	X = C$_6$H$_6$(OH)$_5$
Phosphatidylserine:	X = CH$_2$ – CH(COO$^-$) – $^+$NH$_3$

■ **FIGURE 3-48.** Molecular structure of glycerophospholipids. Glycerophospholipids have two fatty acyl chains (R$_1$ and R$_2$) attached by ester linkages to a three-carbon glycerol backbone. A polar head group, which determines the phospholipid class, is also attached to the glycerol backbone. The classes shown are *PC,* phosphatidylcholine or lecithin; *PE,* phosphatidylethanolamine; *PG,* phosphatidylglycerol; *PI,* phosphatidylinositol; and *PS,* phosphatidylserine. Only the disaturated PC (DPPC) with saturated 16 carbon fatty acid chains (palmitates) on both R$_1$ and R$_2$ positions and PG are surface active and constitutes major fractions of surfactant phospholipids. *(From Notter RH: Lung surfactants: basic science and clinical applications, New York, 2000, Marcel Dekker.)*

sphingomyelin decreases. The ratio of these phospholipids (L/S ratio) in the amniotic fluid has been used as an index of fetal lung maturity (Kulovich et al., 1979).

Inadequacy or deficiency of the surfactant system is important in several clinical conditions. Historically, Avery and Mead (1959) showed that the minimum surface tension of lung extracts from premature infants dying of IRDS was unusually high when measured on the Wilhelmy balance. Surface-active phosphatidylcholine is markedly decreased or even absent in the alveolar linings in these lungs (Boughton et al., 1970). These findings partially explain the atelectasis and low compliance in the lungs of infants with this syndrome.

There are four surfactant proteins (SP) that have been identified (SP-A, SP-B, SP-C, and SP-D), which comprise about 10% of surfactant on the mature alveolar surface (see Fig. 3-49). Of these, SP-B and SP-C are intimately linked to the stability of surface active monolayer at the alveolar surface. They are both predominantly expressed in type II alveolar epithelial cells (pneumocytes) and Clara cells in the bronchioles. SP-B is essential for myelin formation of the lamellar inclusions in type II cells and promotes surface adsorption of dipalmitoylphosphatidylcholine in the lipid mixtures and an addition of the mixture of surface active phospholipids, and SP-B restores the normal pressure-volume curves of the lungs in the animal model of IRDS (Suzuki et al., 1989; Rider et al., 1993).

Surfactant proteins SP-A and SP-D are similar in structure, containing proline-rich collagen domain in addition to carbohydrate domain (called collectins). In mature lungs, SP-A is predominantly expressed in type II pneumocytes and Clara cells, whereas SP-D is widely expressed in various epithelial surfaces in the body (Hull et al., 2000). SP-A and SP-D seems to function primarily as innate host defense molecules in the airways and alveoli (Jobe and Weaver, 2002). SP-A increases production of NO by macrophages and promotes killing of pathogens. SP-A also down-regulates general inflammatory responses of the lung by decreasing the generation of TNF-alpha and other inflammatory cytokines and granulocyte recruitment and activation (Jobe and Weaver, 2002). A decrease in SP-A is probably common in patients with severe lung injury. Infants born with decreased SP-A/dipalmitoylphosphatidylcholine ratio are at increased risk of developing BPD and dying (Hallman et al., 1991).

Surfactant phospholipids and proteins are produced within the type II pneumocytes, stored in the osmiophilic lamellar inclusions within these cells, and excreted into the alveolar surface, forming tubular myelins and subsequently spreading to form surface-active alveolar lining layers (Figs. 3-50, 3-51, and 3-52) (Kikkawa et al., 1965).

Fujiwara and others first reported, with impressive results, the instillation in the trachea of bovine surfactant in premature infants born with surfactant deficiency (Fujiwara et al., 1980). Surfactant replacement therapy using human, bovine, or synthetic surfactant in premature infants with IRDS has been established as an important and essential form of therapy, reducing morbidity and mortality (Merritt et al., 1986; Lang et al., 1990; Hoekstra et al., 1991; Long et al., 1991; Holms, 1993). Surfactant replacement therapy has been extended to cover other clinical conditions with surfactant deficiency or inactivation not only in premature infants but also in full-term infants, children, and adults. These conditions include neonates with persistent pulmonary hypertension (PPHN) in whom surfactant production by type II pneumocytes is depressed because of severe pulmonary hypoperfusion and hypoxia; neonates with severe congenital diaphragmatic hernia (CDH) whose immature lungs are damaged by ventilator-induced lung injury and surfactant inactivation by plasma protein leak on the alveolar surface; meconium aspiration syndrome caused by pulmonary

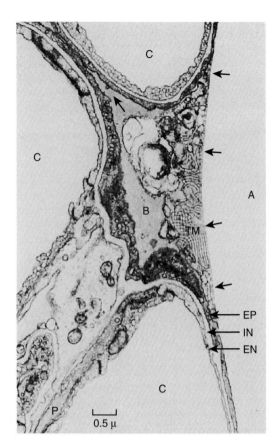

■ **FIGURE 3-51.** Perfusion-fixed rat lung showing three capillaries *(C)* and the extracellular lining layer toward the alveolus *(A)* composed of a base layer *(B)* and an osmophilic lining layer *(short arrows).* Base layer contains tubular myelin figures *(TM)* and extends into a cleft between capillaries closely opposed because of septal folding *(long arrows).* EP, Alveolar epithelial cell (type I); EN, capillary endothelial cell; IN, interstitium; P, pericyte (×23,000). *(From Weibel ER: Morphological basis of alveolar-capillary gas exchange,* Physiol Rev *53:419, 1973.)*

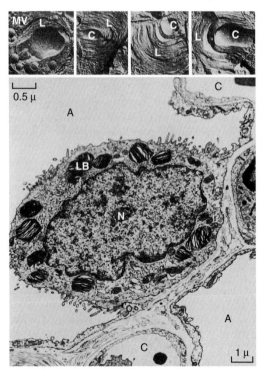

■ **FIGURE 3-50.** Granular pneumocyte (type II). Cytoplasm around the nucleus *(N)* contains many organelles, particularly osmophilic lamellar bodies *(LB).* Insets show lamellar bodies in freeze-etched preparation revealing form and existence of central core *(C)* around which lamellae *(L)* are stacked. (×22,400). A; Alveolar space; C, capillary space. *(From Weibel ER: Morphological basis of alveolar-capillary gas exchange,* Physiol Rev *53:419, 1973.)*

hypoperfusion, inflammation, and inactivation of surfactant by protein leak; and ARDS in children and adults (Jobe, 1993; Pramanik et al., 1993).

CILIARY ACTIVITY

The tracheal and bronchial walls are lined with pseudostratified epithelium that consists of ciliated cells, nonciliated serous and brush cells, and abundant mucus-secreting goblet cells. The submucosal area contains numerous serous and mucous cell glands, which are major contributors of the mucus in the respiratory tract. Under normal circumstances both goblet cells and mucus-secreting glands diminish in number toward the periphery of the airway system. The mucosal surface is covered by a serous fluid layer, in which the cilia beat. Above this periciliary layer of serous fluid lie discontinuous flakes of mucus (rather than the continuous mucous blanket assumed previously), which are moved cephalad by the cilia (Fig. 3-53) (Jeffery and Reid, 1977).

The cilia in the respiratory tract play an important role in the removal of mucoid secretions, foreign particles, and ce

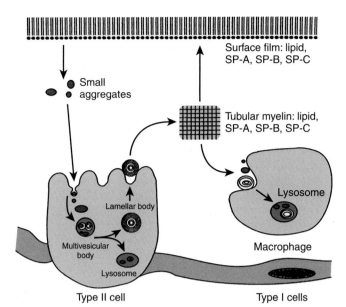

■ **FIGURE 3-52.** Life cycle of pulmonary surfactant. SP-A, SP-B, SP-C, and phospholipids are packaged in lamellar inclusion bodies and secreted by type II alveolar epithelial cells (pneumocytes) into the air space. Lamellar bodies unfold into tubular myelin, which gives rise to the phospholipid-surfactant protein film at the air-liquid interface. Used surfactant phospholipids are released from the film as small vesicles, which are taken up and recycled or degraded by type II cells. Alveolar macrophages also take up surfactant and degrade it. *SP-A, SP-B, SP-C,* Surfactant proteins A, B, and C.

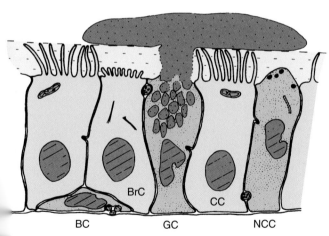

FIGURE 3-53. The ultrastructure of airway epithelium represented diagrammatically. Cilia beat in a fluid layer of low viscosity above which move flakes of mucus. Ciliated cells *(CC)*, goblet cells *(GC)*, nonciliated "serous" cells *(NCC)*, brush cells *(BrC)*, and basal cells *(BC)* are shown, as are nerves penetrating the epithelium. *(From Jeffery PK, Reid LM: The respiratory mucous membrane. In Brain JD et al., editors:* Respiratory defense mechanisms, *New York, 1977, Marcel Dekker.)*

bris and are an essential defense mechanism of the airway system. These cilia move in a synchronous, whip-like fashion a rate of 600 to 1300 times per minute. They can move particles toward the mouth at the rate of about 1.5 to 2 cm/min (Lichtiger et al., 1975).

Ciliary function is influenced by the thickness of the mucous layer and other factors that can occur with dehydration or infection. In tissue culture, some viral infections reduce ciliary motion as much as 50%, and repeated infections in vivo can destroy the cilia completely (Kilburn and Salzano, 1966). Inhalation of warm air with 50% humidity maintains normal ciliary activity, whereas breathing dry air for 3 hours results in a complete cessation of mucus movement. Ciliary activity can be restored by breathing warm, saturated air (Forbes, 1974; Hirsch et al., 1975). Breathing 100% oxygen and controlled positive-pressure ventilation also affect ciliary function (Wolfe et al., 1972; Forbes, 1976; Forbes and Gamsu, 1979).

Inhaled anesthetics seem to decrease ciliary function in both animals and humans. Forbes and Horrigan (1977) observed a dose-related depression of ciliary activity during halothane and enflurane anesthesia. The same group of investigators found delayed mucus clearance during and 6 hours after discontinuation of halothane or diethyl ether anesthesia (Forbes and Gamsu, 1979). These findings suggest that inhaled anesthesia has adverse effects on mucociliary clearance, especially in patients with pulmonary disease. The effect of anesthetics on mucociliary clearance in infants and children has not been reported.

MEASUREMENTS OF PULMONARY FUNCTION IN INFANTS AND CHILDREN

Airway obstruction is often difficult to assess clinically, particularly in young infants. For instance, what appears to be stridor may not indicate obstruction of the upper or extrathoracic airways. Similarly, although wheezing commonly represents disorders of relatively large intrathoracic airways (such as bronchial asthma), other airway dysfunction, from the upper airways (such as stridors) to the lower airways (such as rhonchi from secretions) can be mistaken for wheezing.

Another cause of abnormal breath sounds is an airway abnormality as narrowing of the airway lumen by mucosal edema, compression, secretions, foreign objects, or hyperreactive airway smooth muscles. Stridor and wheezing may also be caused by increased collapsibility of the airways, as seen in laryngotracheomalacia that involves both the upper and lower (large central) airways. A careful evaluation of the medical history and physical examination are obviously essential and helpful but may be inadequate to determine the exact nature of the disorder.

Pulmonary function tests (PFTs) are most effective in evaluating the respiratory status of infants and children and in documenting the site(s), nature, and extent of airway dysfunction. In addition, pulmonary function tests allow objective and quantitative assessment of airway reactivity such as occurs with bronchial asthma and BPD and the response of airway reactivity to bronchodilator therapy. For a detailed account of various measurements of pulmonary function in children and adolescents, the publications by Polgar and Promadhat (1971) and Bates (1989) should be consulted.

Until recently, PFTs relied almost entirely on the understanding and cooperation of children who could respond to the commands of pulmonary technicians to perform various test maneuvers. PFTs, therefore, have been effective only for intelligent and cooperative children older than 5 or 6 (sometimes as young as 3) years of age. More recently, new techniques have been developed to perform modified PFTs in anesthetized, paralyzed, and intubated infants and children using a forced deflation or in infants and toddlers under heavy sedation with chest compression (also known as a "squeeze technique") (Motoyama et al., 1987; Frey et al., 2000; Weiner et al., 2003). Both of these techniques produce MEFV curves for analysis.

The most common types of pulmonary disability may be classified under the general headings of restrictive diseases and obstructive diseases, although there is considerable overlap between the two groups. Restrictive disorders, whether intrapulmonary or extrapulmonary in origin, result in reduced lung volumes. Relatively common restrictive disorders in infants and children, from the anesthesiologist's point of view, include persistent PPHN and CDH in the newborn period, congestive (also obstructive) heart failure, pulmonary fibrosis, kyphoscoliosis, obesity, and abdominal distention in older children.

In patients after surgery, especially those given muscle relaxants, the VC is a practical guide to muscle strength. A VC of at least twice the tidal volume (15 mL/kg; normal range, 60 to 70 mL/kg) appears necessary to maintain adequate spontaneous ventilation. The measurement of peak inspiratory and expiratory pressures against airway occlusion at FRC provides additional information. A minimum of 30 cm H_2O is needed for effective coughing and adequate spontaneous breathing.

Obstructive pulmonary disorders may be classified into upper and lower airway diseases. Most of the severe upper airway diseases, such as acute epiglottitis and subglottic croup, occur in infancy and early childhood. Occasionally, however, upper airway obstruction can be seen in children with obstructive sleep apnea syndrome (OSAS) with chronic adenotonsillar hypertrophy, as well as in children with subglottic stenosis associated with prolonged intubation or tracheostomy. Vascular ring and vascular sling are rare but are associated with severe tracheobronchial (large central airway) obstruction.

The lower airway disorders commonly seen among children include BPD, CF, bronchial asthma, reactive airways disease associated with gastroesophageal reflux, and heart disease with left-to-right shunting and pulmonary hypertension.

Standard Tests of Pulmonary Function

As mentioned above, Standard PFTs are largely limited to children older than 5 years who can understand and cooperate with the test procedures. In newborns, some physiologic indicators of pulmonary function can be measured using modifications of standard tests. The relatively recent introduction of tests that are applicable in infants and young children has considerably broadened the ability to assess their pulmonary dysfunction (Weiner et al., 2003). Zapletal and others (1987) compiled pulmonary function indices in children from the data he and his coworkers accumulated over the last two decades. Some of these normal values are reproduced in Appendix C (see www.expertconsult.com).

Measurement of Lung Volumes

TLC and its subdivisions (see Fig. 3-19 and the discussion of lung volumes) are measured either with spirometry and the gas dilution technique or with body plethysmography. FRC is commonly measured by the gas dilution technique with rebreathing of a known concentration of helium (10% He in O_2). TLC is obtained by adding inspiratory capacity (IC) and FRC. RV is

the difference between TLC and VC, the maximum amount of air one can breathe out from TLC. Forced vital capacity (FVC) is the VC obtained during maximum expiratory effort. Normally, FVC and VC in the same healthy person are nearly identical, but in patients with obstructive airway disease, airway closure worsens with effort and FVC may become considerably smaller than VC. VC per se is not a useful indicator for differential diagnosis, because it decreases in both obstructive and restrictive lung disorders such as atelectasis and pulmonary fibrosis. TLC, on the other hand, is decreased in restrictive disease but is increased by air trapping in obstructive disorders.

Gas dilution techniques underestimate TLC in obstructive lung disease, because the test gas molecules (helium) do not sufficiently penetrate into trapped gas compartments. Under these circumstances, body plethysmography should be used to measure FRC more accurately. Measurement of FRC (or thoracic gas volume [TGV]) with body plethysmography is accomplished with a panting (or short, rapid breathing) maneuver against mouth occlusion. TGV is derived from simultaneous changes in lung volume (V) and airway pressure (P) using Boyle's law ($P \times V = k$). When body plethysmography is not available, addition of a low level of end-expiratory positive airway pressure (EPAP) during helium rebreathing increases gas mixing, probably by preventing airway closure or by keeping the collateral channels open. The difference in calculated FRC with and without EPAP correlates well with the degree of air trapping in the lung (Motoyama et al., 1982b). In obstructive lung disease, FRC and in particular RV, in relation to TLC (FRC/TLC, RV/TLC), are markedly increased.

Flow Function with Spirometry

In clinical pulmonary function laboratories, airway obstruction is usually assessed by the analysis of maximal forced expiration using a spirometer. The resultant volume change in relation to time is displayed on a kymograph (Fig. 3-54). Peak expiratory flow rate (PEFR) is by far the simplest of all expiratory flow

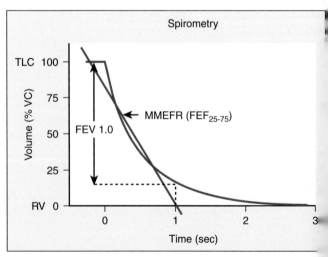

■ FIGURE 3-54. A spirometric tracing of forced vital capacity (FVC; $FEV_{1.0}$, forced expiratory volume in 1 second; MMEFR, maximum mid expiratory flow rate, or FEF_{25-75}; RV, residual volume; TLC, total lung capacity. (From Motoyama EK: Physiologic alterations in tracheostomy. In Myers EN et al., editors: Tracheotomy, New York, 1985, Churchill Livingstone.)

measurements. PEFR is decreased most drastically by obstruction of the upper or large lower (central) airways, even when other indices of airway function are within normal limits. It is also decreased in patients with typical asthma, which primarily involves central airways, with severe peripheral airway disease such as CF, and with neuromuscular disorders. The measurement of PEFR is not a sensitive test for discriminating among various types of lung disease. Another major disadvantage of PEFR is that it varies with the degree of effort and cooperation, particularly in young children.

For many decades, the forced expiratory volume in 1 second ($FEV_{1.0}$) and maximum mid-expiratory flow rate (MMEFR or FEF_{25-75}) have been used extensively to evaluate airway function. These parameters are obtained from spirographic tracings made during an FVC maneuver from maximal inspiration (TLC) down to RV (see Fig. 3-54).

A reduction in $FEV_{1.0}$ correlates well with the clinical severity of lung disease, both in adults and in children. $FEV_{1.0}$ is expressed both in absolute terms and as a percentage of the value predicted on the basis of gender, age, and height. It is also expressed in relation to FVC ($FEV_{1.0}/FVC$). In obstructive lung disease, $FEV_{1.0}$ is decreased both in absolute terms and in relation to FVC because of prolonged expiration. On the other hand, in restrictive lung disease such as pulmonary fibrosis, in which airways are wide open, $FEV_{1.0}$ is decreased but $FEV_{1.0}/FVC$ may be normal or even increased. The FEF_{25-75} is the average flow rate between 25% and 75% of FVC. Compared with $FEV_{1.0}$, FEF_{25-75} is a more sensitive index of airway disease involving smaller airways.

The major limitations of these indices of airway function are that they are variable depending on the patient's effort; they are also inadequate for identifying the site of obstruction (e.g., the upper vs. lower airways or the central vs. peripheral airways).

Measurement of Airway Resistance

The standard technique for evaluating airway obstruction has been the measurement of airway resistance (Raw) and forced expiratory flow. Airway resistance is the most direct index of airway obstruction. It is, however, rarely used in clinical settings for several reasons: it requires a body plethysmograph, which is too costly, needs a trained pulmonology technician to perform it, and is too complicated for routine use. Furthermore, airway resistance is not a sensitive indicator of disease involving the lower airways, particularly small, peripheral airways, because the latter contribute only a fraction of total airway resistance, and abnormally high airway resistance does not indicate the site or location of airway disease.

Airway resistance is influenced by the degree of lung inflation. As the lung volume increases, the airways expand and airway resistance falls. The airway conductance (G_{aw}), the reciprocal of resistance, changes linearly with lung volume in children (Zapletal et al., 1969).

Maximum Expiratory Flow-Volume Curves

Unlike other conventional indices of airway function that express volume change per unit of time (i.e., flow rates), MEFV curves relate MEF rates to corresponding lung volumes during FVC maneuver (see Fig. 3-32). As mentioned previously, the intrathoracic airways downstream (toward the mouth) from the

EPP are subjected to dynamic compression during forced exhalation. As a result, the MEF rate at low lung volumes (i.e., less than 50% FVC) becomes independent of effort and is determined by the flow resistance of the upstream segment of airways between the alveoli and EPP (Rus) and by the static recoil pressure of the lung (Pstl):

$$\dot{V}max = Pstl / Rus$$

The measurement of MEF rate is a very sensitive test of lower airway obstruction, because it eliminates the component of the upper and lower central airway resistance between the mouth and EPP, which may amount to as much as 80% to 90% of the total airway resistance. Another advantage of MEFV curve analysis over conventional spirometry is that it is independent of effort put forth in determining the MEF rate, particularly in young children, whose effort may be submaximal or inconsistent. The normal values of MEF rate in children are shown in Appendix C (see www.expertconsult.com).

Figure 3-55 is a schematic representation of MEFV curves from a patient with CF whose flow function is only mildly affected with a classic spirometry. PEFR is within normal limits, whereas values of MEF rate at 50% and 25% of FVC (FEF_{50} and FEF_{75}, respectively) are markedly reduced. With MEFV curves, lower airway disease can be further divided into central vs. peripheral airway disorders by repeating MEFV curves with air (21% oxygen in nitrogen) vs. a 20% oxygen–80% helium mixture.

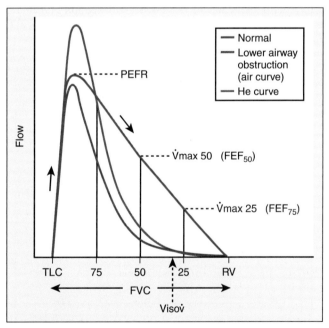

■ **FIGURE 3-55.** MEFV curve of a 13-year-old boy with CF *(brown line)* compared with predicted MEFV curve *(blue line)* breathing air. Note that PEFR is within normal limits, whereas MEFs at 50% (MEF_{50}) and at 25% (MEF_{25} or MEF_{25}) are markedly reduced, indicating lower airway obstruction. The second MEFV curve *(purple line)* was obtained while he was breathing an 80% helium/20% oxygen mixture *(He curve)*. The He curve crosses the air curve at 30% FVC ($\dot{V}iso/\dot{V}$), indicating peripheral airway disease. *TLC,* Total lung capacity; *RV,* residual volume; *FVC,* forced vital capacity. *(From Motoyama EK: Physiologic alterations in tracheostomy. In Myers EN et al., editors:* Tracheotomy, *New York, 1985, Churchill Livingstone.)*

In healthy persons, the flow-limiting segment (EPP) is located in the central airways, usually within the first five generations of the tracheobronchial tree (Zapletal et al., 1969). Because the flow pattern is turbulent and dependent on density, air, with an average molecular weight of 29, has a lower flow rate than does the helium-oxygen mixture, with a much lighter average molecular weight of 9.6. In the case of peripheral airway obstruction, EPP moves upstream (peripherally) toward the area of obstruction, where the flow pattern is laminar and therefore dependent on viscosity. The viscosity of helium is higher than that of nitrogen, so flow rates in helium MEFV curves (He curve) at lower lung volumes become less than those in MEFV curves with air (air curve). In Figure 3-55, the He curve crosses the air curve at 30% of FVC (volume of isoflow). Volume of isoflow of more than 20% of FVC is considered evidence of peripheral airway obstruction (Hutcheon et al., 1974). In children with mild to moderate asthma, both PEFR, an indicator of large airway function, and MEF_{25} (or FEF_{75}), an indicator of lower airway function, are decreased because asthma involves constriction of both large and medium or even smaller airways (Fig. 3-56).

In contrast, in a typical case of mild CF with primary peripheral airway disease, MEF_{25} is markedly reduced but PEFR is within normal limits (Fig. 3-55). Figures 3-56 and 3-57 illustrate changes in flow and volume function in a 9-year-old boy with bronchial asthma. The control or baseline MEFV curve (curve 1 in Fig. 3-56) is markedly reduced from the predicted curve (curve 3). His FVC is decreased because of air trapping and increases in RV. After an inhalation of nebulized bronchodilator, there is a marked increase in overall expiratory flow rates with decreased air trapping and a resultant increase in FVC (curve 2). TLC is increased toward the predicted value.

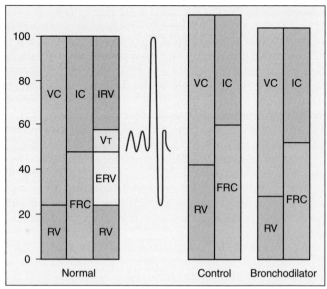

■ FIGURE 3-57. Bar graphs representing changes in TLC and its subdivisions in a 9-year-old boy with bronchial asthma before (control) and after bronchodilator use in relation to predicted values. Note the increase in TLC and RV and the reduction in VC in the control period caused by air trapping. The RV/TLC and FRC/TLC ratios are abnormally increased. Bronchodilator use nearly abolished air trapping and restored VC. Compare these values with his flow function in Figure 3-56. *IRV,* Inspiratory reserve volume; *ERV,* expiratory reserve volume; *VT,* tidal volume; *IC,* inspiratory capacity. *(From Motoyama EK: Airway function tests in infants and children,* Int Anesthesiol Clin *26:6, 1988.)*

Evaluation of Upper Airway Function

Upper airway obstruction is not uncommon in infants and young children because of anatomic factors such as a relatively large heads, short necks, and small mandibles in relation to tongue size. Also, the caliber of the upper airways is smaller in absolute terms than in older children and adults. Common causes of upper airway obstruction include, in descending order, obstructive sleep apnea (pharyngeal obstruction), laryngomalacia, vocal cord paralysis and dysfunction, laryngeal papillomas, and subglottic stenosis of various causes. In addition, in older children, severe inspiratory obstruction may occur as the result of conversion reaction (Appelblatt and Baker, 1981). This condition may be mistakenly diagnosed as severe bronchial asthma. In some patients with bronchial asthma, the primary site of airway obstruction is in the upper airways, with the clinical manifestation of coughing (Christopher et al., 1983).

The conventional pulmonary function tests already described are used primarily to detect impairment of lower, intrathoracic airway function and are inadequate for the evaluation of upper airway obstruction.

The intrathoracic airways narrow during forced expiration because of dynamic compression, whereas during forced inspiration they expand because of increases in surrounding negative pleural pressure. By contrast, the caliber of the extrathoracic trachea and larynx expands during forced expiration and narrows during forced inspiration, particularly when there is obstruction.

Functionally, obstructive airway lesions in the upper airways and large intrathoracic (central) airways can be clas-

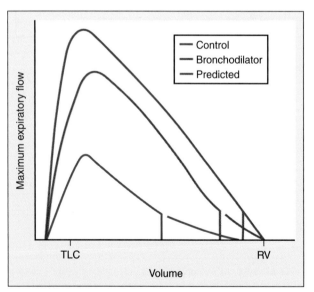

■ FIGURE 3-56. MEFV curves of a 9-year-old boy with bronchial asthma before (1) and after (2) inhalation of nebulized bronchodilator compared with a predicted MEFV curve (3). The volume between TLC and the vertical line for each MEFV curve is the forced expiratory volume in 1 sec ($FEV_{1.0}$). Note that PEFR, $FEV_{1.0}$, and MEFs at same volumes are all markedly diminished in the control curve. The bronchodilator produced a marked improvement in all flow parameters. *(From Motoyama EK: Airway function tests in infants and children,* Int Anesthesiol Clin *26:6, 1988.)*

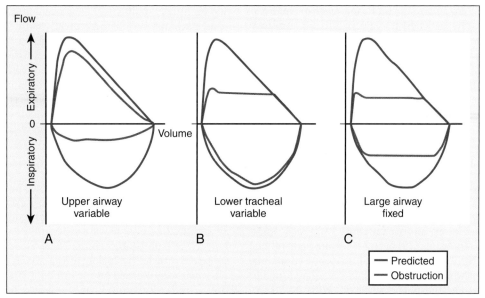

■ FIGURE 3-58. Schematic tracing of maximum expiratory-inspiratory flow-volume curves. **A,** Variable upper airway obstruction caused by papillomatosis of the larynx. **B,** Variable central (intrathoracic) airway obstruction caused by tracheomalacia. **C,** Fixed-type obstruction due to tracheal stenosis. *(From Motoyama EK: Physiologic alterations in tracheostomy. In Myers et al., editors:* Tracheotomy, *New York, 1985, Churchill Livingstone.)*

fied into "variable" and "fixed" types of obstruction, based on the ability of the obstructed segment of the airways to alter its caliber in response to changes in transmural pressure. In variable extrathoracic airway obstruction, inspiratory flow is markedly reduced because of pharyngeal collapse during inspiration, whereas expiratory flow is relatively unchanged (Fig. 3-58, *A*). The opposite is true with variable intrathoracic large airway obstruction (Fig. 3-58, *B*). Large-airway obstruction of a fixed type limits both inspiratory and expiratory flows nearly equally, because the changes in transmural pressure do not affect airway caliber (Fig. 3-58, *C*). The measurement of maximum expiratory-inspiratory–flow-volume curves is useful in diagnosing the location (extrathoracic vs. intrathoracic) and the nature (variable vs. fixed) of large airway obstruction (Kryger et al., 1976a; Frenkiel et al., 1980). Figure 3-58, *A* shows the maximum expiratory-inspiratory–flow-volume curve of a 7-year-old girl with laryngeal papillomatosis, who, because of her "wheezing" (in reality, it was stridor) had previously been thought to have bronchial asthma. She had nearly normal MEFV curves with severe reductions in inspiratory flow. She did not respond to bronchodilators.

Airway Reactivity

Because wheezing is often a manifestation of airway reactivity or airway hyperresponsiveness, it is important to examine positive response to bronchodilators (hyperresponsiveness) or to stimuli that provoke bronchoconstriction (airway reactivity). The most commonly used pulmonary function test for this purpose is the measurement of flow rates during forced expiration. Traditionally, $FEV_{1.0}$ and FEF_{25-75} have been used. More recently, however, measurements of MEF on MEFV curves at 50% and 25% of FVC (MEF_{50}, MEF_{75}) have shown to be most sensitive (Zapletal et al., 1971). Some healthy children (up to 5% of the general population) may respond to a bronchomotor

challenge, but the degree of response is relatively small, usually less than 5% of the control value in $FEV_{1.0}$ and not more than 20% of the control value in FEF_{25-75} and MEFs. When the response is beyond these ranges, airway hyperreactivity or bronchial asthma is suspected. In children, inhalation of aerosolized β_2-adrenergic agonists, such as albuterol (salbutamol) and metaproterenol, is used for bronchodilation. To provoke bronchoconstriction, exercise challenge has been used widely in children. The inhalation of bronchoconstrictors such as methacholine and histamine, although a more definitive test, is used less often because of its discomfort in patients whose cooperation is less than optimal (Chatham et al., 1982).

It has been recognized that exercise-induced bronchoconstriction results not from exercise per se but from reduction in tracheobronchial mucosal temperature caused by vigorous mouth breathing of dry air and resultant evaporative heat loss (McFadden et al., 1982). The exercise challenge test, therefore, has been replaced by cold air challenge with normocapnic hyperpnea with added CO_2, which gives more consistent results (Deal et al., 1980). When MEFV curves are used to evaluate bronchial reactivity, MEF must be compared at the same lung volume before and after the challenge, which could change RV and, therefore, FVC. Because the absolute lung volume often is not available in clinical settings, MEF (at 50% or 25% FVC) should be compared at the same volume below TLC, rather than at the volume above RV. The rationale for this practice is that TLC is altered relatively little (although affected by severe air trapping or its release) by comparison with large changes in RV.

Pulmonary Function Tests in Infants

Advances in neonatal intensive care and improved survival of premature infants with varying degrees of chronic lung disease of prematurity since the 1980s prompted the focused interest and development of innovative techniques for pulmonary function testing in neonates, infants, and young children. A position paper was published by the International Committee on Infant Lung Mechanics based on critical evaluation of these techniques (American Thoracic Society/European Respiratory Society [ATS/ERS] Joint Committee, 1993). Guidelines for laboratory conditions, preparation of infants, sedation, and patient safety have also been published by the same group and by others (Gaultier et al., 1995; Quanjer et al., 1995; Frey et al., 2000; Weiner et al., 2003).

Measurements of Dynamic Respiratory Mechanics

Maximum or Partial Expiratory Flow-Volume Curves

Two techniques have been developed to produce flow-volume curves to evaluate lower airway function (ATS/ERS Joint Committee, 1993). Motoyama (1977) and Motoyama and others (1987) produced MEFV curves by "forced deflation" in infants and young children who were intubated and ventilated under sedation or general anesthesia and paralysis. With this technique, a moderate negative pressure is applied to the endotracheal tube at maximal inflation of the lung (TLC). While the lungs are rapidly deflated (within a few seconds), instantaneous expiratory flow and integrated volume signals produce an MEFV curve. MEF is obtained at 25% and 10% of FEV. This forced deflation technique was found to be safe and reproducible and extremely sensitive for the evaluation of smaller airway function. The average normal value for FEF_{75} in full-term infants was 49 mL/kg per second and MEF_{75}/FVC, an index of upstream conductance (or the caliber of airways toward the periphery), was 1.12, whereas in preterm infants without apparent lung disease MEF_{75} was 95 mL/kg per second and the MEF_{75}/FVC was 1.67. This indicates that in preterm infants, airway caliber in relation to lung volume is much larger than in full-term infants (Nakayama et al., 1991; ATS/ERS Joint Committee, 1993). A major drawback of this technique, however, is that its application is limited to the infants already intubated under general anesthesia or being cared for in the intensive care unit setting.

Another technique is the infant "squeeze" or "hugging" (thoracoabdominal compression) technique, originally reported by Adler and Wohl (1978) and later improved by Taussig and others (1982). In this technique a double-layer inflatable "jacket" is wrapped around the thorax and abdomen of a sedated infant. The inner compression bag is attached to a reservoir of compressed air, and the jacket is inflated rapidly at the end of spontaneous tidal inspiration. A partial flow-volume curve is produced, and MEF at the end tidal volume (MEF_{FRC}) is measured. Although the reproducibility of this test is somewhat limited, it has an advantage over the deflation technique in that it can be applied to infants who are not intubated. One major problem with this technique is that although it seems to work in infants with lower airway obstruction by producing flow limitation, the pressure and flow developed by external thoracoabdominal compression are insufficient to produce dynamic compression of the intrathoracic airways in healthy infants; no predicted normal values could be obtained (ATS/ERS Joint Committee, 1993).

After the discussion at the mentioned ATS/ERS Joint Committee meetings, a modification of the "infant hugging" technique was developed. This technique, a raised volume thoracoabdominal compression technique, is accomplished by increasing the end-inspiratory volume initially to 20 cm H_2O and eventually to 30 cm H_2O by occluding the expiratory valve and "stacking" several tidal breaths while inspiratory flow is maintained (Feher et al., 1996; Goldstein et al., 2001; Weiner et al., 2003). With this modified squeeze technique, expiratory flow limitation was achieved even in healthy infants (Lambert et al., 2004). The advantage of this technique over the forced deflation technique is that infants can be studied with sedation alone, rather than under general endotracheal anesthesia or under sedation with muscle relaxation in ICU settings.

Measurements of Passive Respiratory Mechanics

The total respiratory system compliance (dynamic compliance) can be measured during the respiratory cycle by measuring the tidal volume and peak inspiratory pressure. In patients with airway dysfunction, however, dynamic compliance does not reflect the true (static) compliance. This problem is circumvented by a brief occlusion of the airway at end inspiration. This approach is based on the principle that the active Hering-Breuer reflex in young infants causes a brief period of apnea during occlusion of the airway at lung volumes above FRC. The passive mechanical properties of the respiratory system can then be determined during this brief moment of respiratory muscle relaxation by removing the upper airway occlusion and allowing the lungs to deflate passively to FRC or relaxation volume (Mortola et al., 1982; Zin et al., 1982). The static compliance of the total respiratory system (Crs) is obtained by dividing the tidal volume by the relaxation pressure at the mouth during the occlusion and relaxation of the respiratory muscles, which reflects the elastic recoil of the respiratory system (LeSouef et al., 1984). In addition, by extrapolation from the plot of a flow-volume loop during passive deflation from airway occlusion, the resistance of the total respiratory system and the time constant can be obtained (LeSouef et al., 1984). This technique can also be applied in intubated patients under general anesthesia or in intensive-care–unit settings, although the resistance of the endotracheal tube per se would be a major component of measured resistance.

According to published data compiled by the ATS/ERS Joint Committee (1993) dynamic lung compliance values for infants and both term and preterm infants range from 1.1 to 2.0 mL/kg per cm H_2O, whereas static compliance values range from 1.0 to 1.6 mL/kg per cm H_2O. Quasistatic compliance of the thorax (Cw) in preterm infants (6.4) exceeds that of term infants (4.2) (ATS/ERS Joint Committee, 1993). Compliance of the total respiratory system (Crs) between 1 and 12 months of age can be expressed as follows:

$$Crs = 0.87 + 26.3 \times Height^3 \text{ (Masters et al., 1987) or}$$
$$Crs = 0.88 \times Weight \text{ in } kg^{1.09} \text{ (Marchal and Crance, 1987)}$$

Values for airway resistance (Raw) have been reported as:

$$Raw = 0.047 - 0.036 \times Height^3 \text{ (Masters et al., 1987) or}$$
$$Raw = 5.36 \times Weight \text{ in } kg^{-0.75} \text{ (Marchal et al., 1988)}$$

FRC is low in infants. As measured with the gas (helium) dilution method in infants sedated with chloral hydrate, the mean FRC was reported as 20.2 ± 4.7 mL/kg (SD; range, 2 to 24 mL/kg) up to 18 months of age, whereas FRC or TG obtained by means of body plethysmography was highe 23.8 ± 5.3 mL/kg (range, 29 to 34 mL/kg) (ATS/ERS Joi Committee, 1993; McCoy et al., 1995). The reason for th discrepancy between the two methods is unknown, but th

TABLE 3-6. Predicted Values of Respiratory Rate and Tidal Volume in Infants*

Age (mo)	Birth	3	6	9	12
Respiratory rate (breaths/min)	47	38	33	29	26
Tidal volume (mL/kg)	7.4	9	9	9	9

Modified from ATS Assembly on Pediatrics and the ERS Paediatrics Assembly: ATS statement. Respiratory mechanics in infants: physiologic evaluation in health and disease, *Am Rev Respir Dis* 147:474, 1993.
*Weighted mean from published data.

magnitude of difference in FRC measured with gas dilution versus body plethysmograph (15% to 23%) was similar (ATS/ERS Joint Committee, 1993; Gappa et al., 1993; McCoy et al., 1995). The values for boys and girls are similar in most studies. Table 3-6 shows the average values of respiratory rate and tidal volume in infants between birth and 12 months of age based on published data (ATS/ERS Joint Committee, 1993). The average respiratory rate is high at birth (47 breaths/min) and decreases rapidly with growth (26 breaths/min at 12 months). In contrast, average tidal volume is larger in infants (9 mL/kg) than in older children and adults (7 mL/kg) but is remarkably consistent between 3 and 12 months of age, whereas the respiratory rate changes markedly.

Indications for and Interpretation of Pulmonary Function Tests

Although pulmonary function tests usually do not help in diagnosing the exact location of a pathophysiologic process (e.g., left vs. right lung), they do provide qualitative and quantitative assessments of the general type of disability (e.g., restrictive vs. obstructive, upper vs. lower airway, or central vs. peripheral airway), the extent of impairment, and the efficacy of various treatments, either medical or surgical.

Various indices of pulmonary function, as already described, are expressed in absolute terms as well as in percentage of the predicted normal values. Normal values are based usually on gender and height, because height is better correlated with lung volumes and other ventilatory parameters than is body weight or age. More complicated multiple regression formulas include all these parameters. Ideally, each pulmonary function laboratory should establish normal values based on its own sample population, using the same instruments and techniques that are used to evaluate patients with pulmonary dysfunction as recommended by the ATS/ERS Joint Committee (1993). In reality, however, laboratories usually choose values from published data. Polgar and Promadhat (1971) compiled and compared all of the predicting formulas of pulmonary function in children published by 1969. Their data are still valid and useful today. Once the "normal" values are chosen, it is important to test a sample population of healthy children to make sure that the results fall within the predicted range of values.

For most pulmonary function indices, the normal range (mean ± 2 SDs) is within 20% to 25% of the predicted values, with the exception MEF values on MEFV curves, which go up to 40% of the mean. This does not necessarily indicate that patients with some pulmonary function indices outside of this range have lung disease. Serial pulmonary function tests in these patients are invaluable for a better understanding of the presence or absence of disease and its progression with time.

What particular test or combination of tests is most useful? In a child who "wheezes," it is essential to investigate lower airway function, because wheezing is most often caused by airway hyperreactivity (e.g., bronchial asthma or BPD). Wheezing is usually caused by the narrowing of relatively large intrathoracic (lower) airways (i.e., tracheal and large bronchi) and occurs during expiration. It should be kept in mind that both stridors (mostly inspiratory), coming from narrowing of the extrathoracic (laryngopharyngeal) airways, and rhonchi (both inspiratory and expiratory), usually caused by rattling of secretions in the trachea or large bronchi, are often mistaken as wheezing.

If there is considerable lower airway dysfunction, lung volume should be measured to determine the extent of dysfunction and air trapping. Evaluation of bronchial hyperresponsiveness with a bronchodilator must also be done in these patients and, if it is present, the extent of reversibility should be evaluated. Upper airway function should be examined in patients with stridor and in those in whom lower airway dysfunction is absent or mild in relation to overall respiratory symptoms.

Which children should have pulmonary function tests and pulmonology consultations preoperatively? All children with a history of severe neonatal respiratory disease, such as BPD, meconium aspiration, severe bronchiolitis, and those who wheeze (asthma) should have a consultation with a pulmonologist and have a baseline pulmonary function test performed to establish the nature of the lung dysfunction. These children often have lower airway obstruction and abnormal gas exchange with reactive airways whether or not they wheeze; infants with BPD do not wheeze, because the primary site of airway reactivity and narrowing is in relatively small airways and does not cause wheezing (Motoyama, 1988). At the minimum, oxygen saturation should be measured in room air with a pulse oximeter preoperatively as a guide for postoperative management. In addition, children with history of asthma, CF, or gastroesophageal reflux often have moderate to severe lung dysfunction, and they should be evaluated by a pulmonologist. Another condition requiring pulmonary-function testing before surgical repair is scoliosis. Adolescents with scoliosis may have a moderate to severe restrictive defect, especially those with Duchenne's muscular dystrophy (DMD) and other forms of muscular dystrophy; some of these patients cannot generate sufficient airway pressure for effective coughing or lung expansion postoperatively. These patients, as well as surgeons, should know what to expect postoperatively, and the anesthesiologist should make sure that an intensive care unit bed is reserved for postoperative care (Finder et al., 2004; Birnkrant et al., 2007; Finder, 2010).

With advanced knowledge and new technology, the ability of a pulmonary-function laboratory to evaluate and document pulmonary dysfunction has improved considerably. Standard pulmonary-function testing is effective in identifying the site, nature, and extent of airway dysfunction, as well as changes in volume function in children. With new developments in the various noninvasive test methods, it is now possible in an increasing number of pediatric medical centers to evaluate lung function and the presence of reversible (reactive) airways disease in infants, even those experiencing respiratory failure. Pulmonary-function test results are helpful for planning the anesthetic approach and postoperative management of infants and children with known pulmonary dysfunction.

SPECIAL CONSIDERATIONS FOR PEDIATRIC LUNG DISEASE

The pathophysiology of the child with lung disease can complicate perioperative management of these children by the anesthesiologist (see Chapter 36, Systemic Disorders). Careful preoperative history taking and baseline assessment of the patient with lung disease is essential for patient safety for the perioperative and postoperative periods. Depending on the age and condition of the patient, this assessment may include, beyond the basic H&P, pulse oximetry, capnography, chest radiography, pulmonary function testing, and consultation with a pulmonologist.

Asthma

Asthma (bronchial asthma) is the most common respiratory disease of childhood and can affect up to 10% of pediatric patients. Asthma is a chronic inflammatory disease of the airways in which many cell types, but in particular, mast cells, eosinophils, neutrophils, and T lymphocytes play important roles. In susceptible individuals, the inflammation causes recurrent episodes of widespread airway constriction and obstruction with symptoms of wheezing, breathlessness, chest tightness, and cough—particularly at night or in the early morning—with or without oxygen desaturation. The airway obstruction is partly reversible either spontaneously or with pharmacologic treatments. The inflammation also causes an associated increase in airway reactivity to a variety of stimuli. The most common trigger for asthma in all age groups is respiratory viral infections, especially respiratory syncytial virus infection in infants. Other factors that can influence asthma control include environmental allergies, environmental tobacco smoke exposure, and (often unrecognized) gastroesophageal reflux. Cold, dry air can exacerbate asthma or trigger bronchospasm in susceptible individuals.

Pediatric asthma can be difficult to define in children younger than 6, but in general can be diagnosed in the setting of recurrent bronchospasm that is responsive to bronchodilators or systemic steroids. The hallmark of asthma is episodic airway obstruction that is caused by a combination of bronchospasm (increased smooth muscle tone), epithelial edema, and increased secretions in the airways. Asthma in childhood has at least two subtypes that largely fall into groups defined by the age at onset (Martinez et al., 1995). Early-onset asthma (before the third birthday) tends to be nonallergic and triggered predominantly by respiratory viral infections. The term *reactive airways disease* is often invoked, but there is no physiologic differentiation from this purported disease and childhood asthma. As a result, the term *reactive airways disease* has recently been discarded by many (Fahy et al., 1995). There is evidence that patients with early-onset asthma have reduced lung function at birth (Martinez et al. 1995). Later onset (after age 3 years) is more likely to be associated with an allergic phenotype (with positive allergy tests and most often a positive family history for allergy). Although treatment is similar, the earlier onset group is more likely to be free of asthma symptoms by the sixth birthday.

Treatment of asthma depends on severity and persistence of symptoms. The most recent guidelines document from the National Heart, Lung, and Blood Institute of the National Institutes of Health (Expert Panel Report 3) (National Asthma Education and Prevention Program, 2007) uses a stepwise approach to asthma control by defining patients as having intermittent, mild persistent, moderate persistent, and severe persistent asthma. The "controller" therapies for these differing patient groups include low, medium, and high-dose inhaled corticosteroids, long-acting β-agonists (in conjunction with an inhaled glucocorticoid), leukotriene modifiers, mast-cell stabilizers, theophylline, and oral corticosteroids. Additional add-on therapies for poorly controlled, severe persistent asthma include a monoclonal antibody to IgE (omalizumab) in patients with documented allergies.

Management of acute exacerbations of asthma (bronchoconstriction or bronchospasm) is also managed in a step-wise approach (see Chapter 36, Systemic Disorders). β-adrenergic agonists are the mainstay of therapy, especially inhaled albuterol. Inhaled therapy can range from intermittent use of metered-dose inhaler treatments to continuous nebulized albuterol in a monitored setting in the emergency department or intensive care unit. Intravenous β-adrenergic agonists (terbutaline and others) are used in the intensive care setting. Intravenous magnesium sulfate and helium-oxygen mixture (Heliox) are also given in the intensive care setting for refractory bronchoconstriction. Anticholinergic medications have been recommended in the emergency care setting but not the hospital setting in the most recent NIH asthma guidelines.

Careful preoperative assessment for asthma control can reduce risk of intraoperative or postoperative complications from bronchoconstriction and secretions. In children aged 6 and older it is useful to have pulmonary-function testing performed before the procedure requiring general anesthesia. Normal function does not preclude the possibility of intraoperative bronchospastic episodes, but it does reduce the likelihood. Abnormal spirometry showing an obstructive pattern primarily affecting relatively large lower airways, especially with baseline responsiveness to albuterol, suggests poorly controlled asthma and therefore increased perioperative risks (Figs. 3-59 and 3-60). How the anesthesiologist deals with this information depends on the urgency of the procedure; elective procedures may have to be delayed until the child has been seen by pulmonology or allergy consultants and the asthma control has improved. Intraoperative systemic corticosteroids and inhaled bronchodilators may lessen the likelihood of perioperative bronchospasm. V/Qs imbalance may be manifest in the operating room as an increasing inspired oxygen concentration to avoid oxygen desaturation. It is important to bear in mind that with increased Fio_2 during general anesthesia, significant V/Q imbalance could be masked and be revealed soon after the child is extubated and brought to a lower Fio_2 environment in the postoperative care unit.

Bronchopulmonary Dysplasia (BPD)

BPD, or "chronic lung disease of infancy" remains a common problem in the 21st century despite significant advances in neonatology and neonatal intensive care. The term *BPD* was coined by Northway in 1967 to describe the lung disease seen in premature infants who survived the early days of positive pressure ventilatory support (with a primitive respirator by today's standards) and with inadvertent high inspired oxygen concentration in the neonatal period (Northway et al., 1967). They described radiographic and pathologic changes seen in this patient population. Although BPD is associated with prematurity, it c

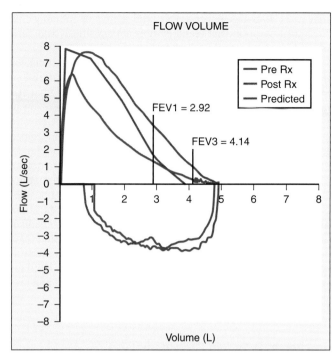

■ **FIGURE 3-59.** Spirometry (MEFV curves) of a 15-year-old boy with mild asthma. Baseline (before treatment) flow-volume curve *(blue)* shows moderate flattening (decreased expiratory flows) of the entire flow-volume curve. FEF$_{25\ to\ 75}$, 41% pred. FVC >100%. After treatment with a bronchodilator *(brown)*, there is a marked increased in MEF rates throughout the expiratory phase.

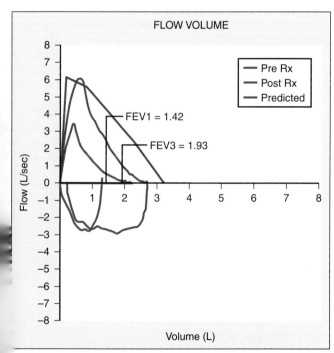

◀ **FIGURE 3-60.** Spirometry of a 15-year-old girl with asthma with marked air trapping. Baseline (before treatment) flow-volume curve *(blue)* shows marked decreases in both expiratory flows and volume. After treatment with a bronchodilator *(brown)*, both FVC and FEF$_{25\ to\ 75}$ increased markedly. FVC (Pre Rx), 68%, (Post Rx), 83% pred.; FEF$_{25\ to\ 75}$ (Pre Rx), 19%, (Post Rx), 51% pred. SpO$_2$ (Pre Rx), 96%, (Post Rx), 98%. *VC,* Forced vital capacity; *FEF$_{25\ to\ 75}$,* maximum midexpiratory flow rate.

occur in full-term infants who receive prolonged intubation and ventilator-induced lung injury (VILI) in the neonatal period.

The lung injury originally described resulted from a combination of volutrauma and shear stress trauma from positive pressure ventilation, inadequate PEEP, and oxygen toxicity. The early descriptions of BPD included necrotizing bronchiolitis, alveolar septal fibrosis, inflammation, and increased airway smooth muscle (O'Brodovich and Mellins, 1985). Patients with this disorder as originally described had complex pathophysiology, with a combination of noncompliant, collapsed areas side by side with compliant and overly distended areas of lung parenchyma, a combination of fixed and reversible obstructive airway disease, with resultant maldistribution of ventilation, and decreased vascular surface area with increased pulmonary vascular resistance.

The original and simplest definition of BPD was the need for oxygen at 28 days of age with characteristic chest radiographic findings. Others have recommended a definition of oxygen requirement after 36 weeks postconceptional age (Shennan et al., 1988).

Recently a differentiation between "old" and "new" BPD has been made, reflecting the changes in management of these patients: New strategies include antenatal glucocorticoids, instillation into the airway of exogenous surfactant, lower ventilator pressures with PEEP, permissive hypercapnia, and accepting lower oxygen levels or "lung protective ventilatory strategy" to minimize VILI, which predominated early BPD. These treatment strategies have resulted in a different pathology in the "new" BPD, in which the primary abnormality is a simplified alveolar architecture (fewer and larger alveoli), abnormal and reduced capillary beds, and evidence of interstitial fibrosis (Jobe, 1999; Merritt et al., 2009). The overall result appears to be an arrest in lung development, with less inflammation and fibrosis. This results in what is predominantly a restrictive rather than obstructive lung disease with a large component of vascular insufficiency (decreased vascular surface area). Modern clinical variability in lung disease seen in premature infants has prompted many clinicians to adopt the term *chronic lung disease of infancy,* because it can incorporate both the "old" and "new" forms of BPD, as well as related diseases like Wilson-Mikity syndrome.

Hypoxemia in BPD, which is one of the defining features of the disease, has numerous pathophysiologic etiologies. These include bronchobronchiolar hyperreactivity, maldistribution of ventilation and V/Q imbalance, hypoventilation (both because of respiratory insufficiency and potentially from abnormal control of breathing), and right-to-left shunting through the foramen ovale, resulting in sudden oxygen desaturation. Pulmonary artery hypertension is common in severe cases of BPD. V/Q imbalance is very common in this population, as is a baseline oxygen requirement. Hypoxia can contribute to increased pulmonary vascular resistance in an already limited vascular bed. Bronchospasm involving relatively small airways without audible wheezing is common even in the first few months of life; increased smooth muscle in the airway has been demonstrated even in very young infants (Motoyama et al. 1987; Margraf et al., 1991).

Inadequate cartilaginous support of the central airways (e.g., tracheomalacia or bronchomalacia) is also common, and it can lead to episodic complete airway obstruction with Valsalva maneuvers. Alveolar hypoxia increases pulmonary vascular resistance and can induce sudden right-to-left shunting through the foramen ovale, resulting in profound systemic hypoxia. Anesthetic management can therefore be complicated by many factors, including bronchospasm, PA hypertension, central airway malacia, and V/Q imbalance. PEEP can be useful and essential in overcoming both large central airway collapsibility and preventing parencymal airway closure caused by anesthesia-induced loss of inspiratory muscle tone and resultant reductions in end expiratory lung volume (FRC). Close monitoring of ventilation and end tidal CO_2 in this patient population is essential to avoid hypoventilation and hypoxemia/hypercarbia, which lead to worsened pulmonary artery hypertension, as well as to control peak inspiratory pressure (less than 20 cm H_2O) to avoid further damage to the fragile lung. Electrolyte abnormalities in patients receiving diuretic therapy for lung disease are common and therefore should be assessed before induction of anesthesia (Ramanathan, 2008).

Chronic Aspiration

Chronic aspiration is a common clinical problem in pediatric medicine. Aspiration can be viewed as falling into the categories of anterograde ("from above," or to the result of a dysfunctional swallow) and retrograde ("from below," or from gastroesophageal reflux disease). Patients can have both varieties simultaneously, especially in the setting of neurocognitive disabilities. Evaluation of the respiratory tract for aspiration is a common reason for bronchoscopy.

Airway protective mechanisms that occur during swallowing include cessation of breathing, adduction of the vocal cords, elevation of the soft palate and larynx in synchrony (closure of the supraglottic larynx), and a rise in intratracheal pressure during swallowing. Foreign materials are also kept out of the airway by very sensitive laryngeal and tracheal irritant receptors, which can induce cough and laryngospasm. The upper and lower esophageal sphincters also protect from reflux and penetration of gastric contents into the respiratory tract. The presence of a tracheostomy tube does not protect the airways and can reduce airway protection by anchoring the larynx and preventing rise in the larynx that helps to close the supraglottic structures during swallowing (Sasaki et al., 1977b). Thus, patients with tracheostomy tubes are at increased risk for aspiration (Finder et al., 2001). General anesthesia also reduces or abolishes airway protective reflexes.

Patients with swallowing disorders, particularly those with significant neurocognitive impairment (cerebral palsy with mental retardation) are at very high risk for airway disease and thereby perioperative anesthetic complications. Quite often children with swallowing disorders are identified early in the course of their disease as requiring gastrostomy to allow for a safe means of feeding. They are usually identified through study of their swallowing as having aspiration with thin liquids. Although the nutrition now bypasses the mouth, there remains another thin liquid—saliva in the mouth—that can be aspirated and lead to significant airway disease. Chronic aspiration of saliva leads to airway inflammation, airway hyperreactivity, airway obstruction, and eventually chronic bacterial bronchitis and bronchiectasis. This leads to a fixed airway obstruction and worsening V/Q imbalance. An important clue to V/Q mismatch in this population is low or borderline oxyhemoglobin saturation on pulse oximetry at baseline assessment in room air. Although in the setting of a hospital a saturation of 94%

may meet discharge criteria, this finding may be the only clue to silent aspiration that could complicate anesthesia and perioperative management.

In this setting, careful preoperative assessment is crucial for avoiding perioperative complications. Limiting the volume of saliva penetrating the lower airways can be achieved pharmacologically (systemic anticholinergics), surgically (excision of the submandibular salivary glands and ligation of the parotid glands), and also minimally invasively with ultrasound-guided injections of botulism toxin into the four main saliva glands. Treatment for acquired airway reactivity (asthma) with inhaled glucocorticoids can also minimize airway inflammation, thereby reducing the likelihood of intraoperative and postoperative atelectasis, bronchospasm with hypoxemia, aspiration, and pneumonia. Children with impaired coughing mechanism and especially those whose surgery may impair coughing (e.g., scoliosis repair or major laparotomy) benefit from mechanically assisted cough therapy (CoughAssist device, Phillips Respironics; Murrysville, PA) to avoid mucus plugging and prevent postoperative pneumonia (Finder, 2010).

Tracheomalacia and Bronchomalacia

Chondromalacia of the trachea or bronchus is fairly common, occurring at an estimated 1:2100 children (Boogaard et al., 2005). The most common presentation is persistent respiratory congestion in the first 6 months of life. Airway malacia can be differentiated from more distal lower airway diseases (such as bronchial asthma or bronchiolitis) by the absence of hypoxemia and the lack of other signs of lung disease (e.g., hyperinflation, subcostal retractions, and increased work of breathing). Indeed, these patients are given the title of "happy wheezers" to describe the "wheeze"(noisy inspiratory breathing, rather than true expiratory wheeze) that occurs in the absence of distress. In general these patients do not experience airway obstruction when intubated, as the positive pressure would "stent" the collapsible central airways open.

Spirometry typically shows fixed MEF caused by large airway collapse, whereas maximum inspiratory flow is unaffected (Fig. 3-58, B). Primary tracheomalacia and bronchomalacia do not lead to V/Q imbalance and therefore are not associated with hypoxemia. Removal of the distending pressure after extubation may result in increased central-airway noises, which are perceived as a central, monophonic wheeze in the postoperative recovery room. Because β-agonists act by relaxing smooth muscle, they do not lead to improvement in wheezing from large airway malacia, and they possibly exacerbate the symptoms. Ipratropium bromide appears to be the most efficacious therapy for symptomatic relief in children with tracheomalacia and bronchomalacia (Finder, 1997).

Cystic Fibrosis (CF)

Cystic fibrosis is a primary disease of impaired mucociliar clearance caused by a mutation in the gene encoding th CF transmembrane conductance regulator (CFTR) prote (Davis, 2006). CFTR functions as a chloride channel and influences the activity of other channels, including the epitheli sodium channel. As a result, the airway surface liquid, whic bathes the epithelial cells and in which the cilia function, reduced in volume. Ciliary beating is thereby impaired, reducing mucociliary transport, and leading to stasis of secretions, chronic infection, chronic airway inflammation, and destruction of airway elastin. This eventually leads to increasingly worsening fixed airway obstruction and to premature death from respiratory failure.

Survival in CF patients has improved dramatically since the disease was first described in 1938 and continues to increase (Davis, 2006). This can be ascribed to improved nutrition (the addition of supplemental pancreatic enzymes, vitamins, and dietary supplements), improved antibiotics (oral, intravenous, and inhaled), other inhaled therapies (nebulized recombinant human deoxyribonuclease [Dnase] or nebulized hypertonic saline), and improved attention to airway clearance (Davis, 2006). High-frequency chest-wall compression ("vest" therapy) is thought to work by rapidly and repetitively compressing the intrathoracic airways, producing "minicoughs," which help shear airway secretions from the airway wall and aid in their clearance. This therapy has gained widespread acceptance, and it is likely responsible for the continuing rise in survival. The predicted mean survival reported by the Cystic Fibrosis Foundation was 37.4 years in 2008, which compares with 32 years in 2000 (see www.cff.org/AboutCF; Cystic Fibrosis Foundation).

CF can be viewed as a multisystem exocrinopathy that affects the sweat ducts, liver, pancreas, intestines, reproductive tract, and respiratory tract (both upper and lower airways). Indications for anesthesia and surgery are therefore diverse, ranging from vascular access (implantable ports), bronchoscopy, nasal polypectomy, and sinus surgery to lung and liver transplantations.

Because general anesthesia impedes mucociliary clearance, it is expected that even brief periods of general anesthesia in mildly affected patients can lead to accumulation of lower airway secretions, mucus plugging, airway closure, and hypoxemia (Forbes and Gamsu, 1979). It is therefore important for the anesthesiologist to get a sense of the baseline lung function in patients with CF before planning general anesthesia. If the patient is old enough to perform pulmonary-function testing (generally 6 years and older), spirometry is a useful tool to identify those at increased risk because there are varying degrees of lower airway obstruction involving primarily smaller airways and air trapping (Fig. 3-61). Bronchiectasis is also common in CF and is associated with fixed lower airways obstruction and increased volume of bronchial secretions. This may be evident on plain chest radiographs, but it may require computed tomography (CT) for identification. The finding of bronchiectasis predicts increased bronchial secretions and a need for thorough intraoperative airway clearance (tracheal suctioning). Response to bronchodilator varies; most patients with CF do not have coexisting asthma and airway reactivity, although positive responses to bronchodilators have been documented at times in these patients—apparently to the result of acute infection and increased airway reactivity (Motoyama, personal observations).

Because of the increased risk of perioperative mucus plugging, airway closure, and atelectasis with resultant hypoxemia, elective surgery in individuals with CF should always follow a period of intensified airway clearance therapy (including antibiotic therapy when appropriate) in the intensive care settings as dictated by the pulmonologist and intensivist managing the CF lung disease for those with advanced airway obstruction and bronchiectasis. Postoperative hypoventilation and atelectasis should be anticipated and treated. Adequate pain control is key to maximizing cough clearance.

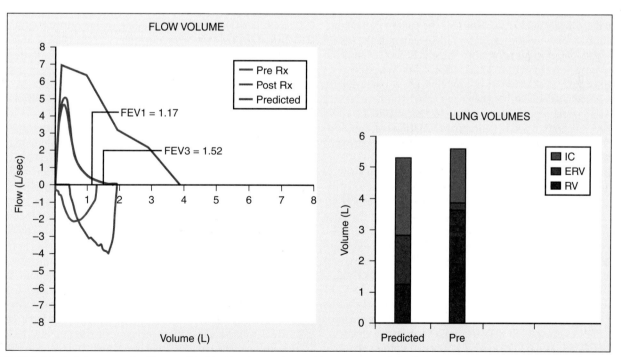

FIGURE 3-61. A, Spirometry of a 19-year-old girl with advanced cystic fibrosis. FVC is markedly decreased. Maximum expiratory flow rates are ~erely decreased with increasing concavity toward the volume axis as she exhales toward RV, indicating severe lower airway obstruction primarily ~cting the smaller airways. There is no difference before *(green)* and after *(red)* treatment with a bronchodilator. FVC, 47% pred.; FEF$_{25\text{ to }75}$, ~% pred. **B,** Lung volume measurement shows severe air trapping with a marked increase in RV. SpO$_2$, 95%. *FVC,* Forced vital capacity; *FEF*$_{25\text{ to }75}$, ~ximum midexpiratory flow rate; *IC,* inspiratory capacity; *ERV,* expiratory reserve volume; *RV,* residual volume.

Duchenne's Muscular Dystrophy (DMD) and Other Congenital Disorders of Neuromuscular Weakness

DMD is caused by a mutation in the gene coding for the protein dystrophin, which acts as a "shock absorber" for the muscle cell, connecting the cytoskeleton of the muscle cell to the membrane and extracellular matrix (Bushby et al., 2010a, 2010b). It is a critical part of a complex of proteins (referred to as the dystroglycan complex) at the cell membrane that connect the actin-myosin filament to the cell membrane. Absence of dystrophin, which is a rodlike protein, leads to a secondary loss of the rest of the dystroglycan complex. This leads to fragility of the muscle-cell membrane. Repeated injury to the muscle-cell membrane with contraction of the actin-myosin apparatus causes leak of cytosol into the plasma, inflammation, and eventual fibrosis. Skeletal muscle is most affected by this disease, but cardiac muscle is also affected quite commonly in this disease.

DMD is X-linked and therefore is almost exclusively a disease of boys. The incidence of DMD is 1:3500 boys. The muscle weakness is progressive in nature, and it may not be recognized until early childhood. Delayed walking is common, as is calf pseudohypertrophy. Increased falling in middle childhood can also lead to suspicion of this disease. The classic physical finding of proximal lower extremity weakness (Gower's sign), in which the patient uses his upper extremities to push his torso upright, is strongly suggestive of this diagnosis. Patients with DMD often have elevated levels of transaminases, which are mistaken as a sign of liver dysfunction, when the enzymes are leaking from the skeletal muscle. The usual screening test is the creatine kinase enzyme assay from peripheral blood, which can be extremely elevated. Diagnosis is most often confirmed by genetic testing, although muscle biopsy is occasionally performed.

Eventual involvement of the respiratory tract in DMD is the rule. This involvement does not occur until after the muscle disease has progressed to the point that the patient can no longer ambulate. The earliest respiratory involvement is the loss of an adequate cough. This is because there is loss of strength in the abdominal musculature. Weak diaphragm and glottis can also contribute to loss of an adequate cough (Finder, 2010). Patients may not realize that they have lost this function until they develop pneumonia. This stage of respiratory involvement, however, can be predicted by pulmonary-function testing (Bach et al., 1997). Management of inadequate cough includes manual and mechanically assisted coughing (Finder, 2010).

The next stage of respiratory involvement after loss of adequate cough is the development of insufficient ventilation during sleep, especially during REM sleep (Suresh et al., 2005). Signs and symptoms of this stage can be subtle, such as increasing nocturnal awakenings, morning headache (from CO_2 retention), and decreasing school performance. Current management of this stage is the institution of noninvasive ventilation (often bilevel pressure support via a nasal or face mask) (Finder et al., 2004).

When the patient with DMD begins to develop respiratory failure when awake, hypoventilation leads to hypercapnia and eventually to hemoglobin desaturation. Noninvasive measurement of CO_2 (end tidal CO_2) can be performed in the outpatient setting, along with pulse oximetry and venous measurement of blood gases—obviating the need for arterial puncture in the outpatient. Noninvasive ventilation (generally, with a ventilator attached to an angled mouthpiece for delivered breaths that are assisted and controlled) is also becoming increasingly common for management of respiratory failure in this population (Gomez-Merino and Bach, 2002). Other management of DMD includes special attention to stretching to reduce contractures and the use of corticosteroids to slow the progression of the muscle disease (Moxley et al., 2005; Bushby et al., 2010b). Scoliosis is common in this population and often requires surgical correction. Another common surgery in the DMD population is placement of gastrostomy tubes when patients can no longer adequately chew and swallow.

Patients with DMD and other muscular dystrophies are at increased risk for life-threatening intraoperative hyperkalemia with or without hyperthermia when inhaled anesthetics or a depolarizing muscle relaxant (succinylcholine) are administered, although they are distinct from malignant hyperthermia (see Chapter 37: Malignant Hyperthermia). Although this is widely recognized, this population is also at increased risk for hypoventilation, upper airway obstruction, and impaired cough clearance. Glossomegaly is also common in boys with DMD and can obstruct the upper airway during induction of anesthesia and in the postoperative period; weakened upper airway dilator muscles contribute to airway obstruction. Limited mobility of the mandible and cervical spine limit maneuvers like a jaw thrust and may pose difficulty in visualization of the larynx and can complicate intubation.

Hypoventilation is common in patients with neuromuscular weakness, although it may not be apparent in the immediate preoperative assessment (which is largely limited to measurement of oxyhemoglobin saturation). Preoperative measurement of end tidal CO_2 is recommended, because it may reveal CO_2 retention and therefore increased risk of hypoventilation during the postoperative period. In addition, it is not uncommon for individuals with DMD to have cardiomyopathy with impaired cardiac output. This impairment is often unrecognized and untested because involved patients are nonambulatory and require relatively little cardiac output for normal activities of daily living. This impairment can be worsened by perioperative psychological and physical stresses with general anesthesia, as well as with hypoxemia and hypercapnia. It is therefore critical that any elective surgery in a patient with neuromuscular weakness be preceded by a careful assessment of both respiratory and cardiac function.

Pulmonary function testing usually shows decreased maximum inspiratory and expiratory pressures, decreased peak flows, and decreased VC (restrictive defect) caused by muscle weakness resulting in both incomplete inspiration and expiration (Fig. 3-62). Measurements of peak cough flow and of maximum inspiratory and expiratory pressures are also helpful in assessing risk for poor cough clearance postoperatively. Outpatient measurement of end tidal CO_2 (or venous blood gas during clinical visits is useful for identifying patients at risk for hypoventilation and who might benefit from postoperative noninvasive support of ventilation. Although hemoglobin saturation may be within normal limits, the anesthesiologist should not presume that the pulmonary function is normal. An elevation in the RV/TLC ratio is not uncommon, even in those with normal minute ventilation, because of the inability to exhale forcefully to the true RV. Impaired cough clearance in the neuromuscularly weak patient should be expected.

Active postoperative involvement of the respiratory therapists and pulmonologists is essential to avoid postoperative complications of atelectasis and pneumonia. Assisted or artificial coughing using a mechanical insufflation-exsufflat

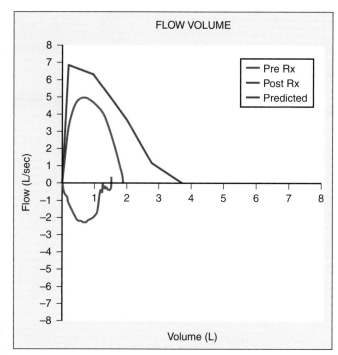

FLOW VOLUME

— Pre Rx
— Post Rx
— Predicted

■ FIGURE 3-62. Spirometry of a 14-year-old boy with DMD with progressive muscle weakness. FVC is decreased because of both decreased inspiratory capacity (IC) and a weak or decreased expiratory force and incomplete exhalation and resultant increases in RV. FVC, 50% pred. SpO_2, 96%, *FVC*, Forced vital capacity; *RV,* residual volume.

device as part of a coordinated care program along with meticulous pain control is very useful in managing these individuals in the postoperative period. The reader is referred to an excellent review of this topic (Birnkrant et al., 2007).

SUMMARY

It is apparent that the respiration of pediatric patients, especially neonates and young infants, is considerably different from that of older children and adults. Respiratory control mechanisms are not fully developed in young infants until at least 42 to 44 weeks' postconception, especially in terms of their response to hypoxia.

The lungs are immature at birth, even in full-term infants. Most alveolar formation and elastogenesis occur postnatally during the first year of life. Thoracic structure is insufficient to support the negative pleural pressure generated during the respiratory cycle, at least until the infant develops the muscle strength for upright posture toward the end of the first year. Weakness of the thoracic structure is in part compensated by

Box 3-4 Infants Are Prone to Perioperative Hypoxemia

● Immature respiratory control and irregular breathing; hypoxia does not stimulate, but rather depresses, ventilation. Trace anesthetics abolish hypoxic ventilatory response.
● Infants have small FRC and high oxygen demand.
● Anesthesia reduces FRC; airway closure and atelectasis result
● Prone to hypoxemia (SpO_2 < 94%) in PACU without O_2.
● Infants are prone to upper airway obstruction.
● High oxygen affinity (low oxygen unloading) of fetal hemoglobin.

tonic contractions of the intercostal and accessory muscles. Anesthesia diminishes or abolishes this compensatory mechanism and the end expiratory lung volume decreases to the point of airway closure, resulting in widespread alveolar collapse and atelectasis. An addition of muscle relaxants in anesthetized infants significantly decreases FRC further and collapses the thorax even more, resulting in further V/Q imbalance and hypoxemia. Infants are prone to upper airway obstruction because of anatomic and physiologic differences, as discussed in this chapter. Anesthesia preferentially depresses tonic and phasic activities of the pharyngeal and other neck muscles, which normally resist the collapsing forces in the pharynx.

Fetal hemoglobin has high oxygen affinity and limits oxygen unloading at the tissue level. These factors, unique to infants younger than 3 months of age, result in decreases in oxygen delivery to the tissues that have much higher oxygen demands than those of adults. Thus, infants and young children are prone to perioperative hypoxemia and tissue hypoxia (Box 3-4).

Pulmonary surfactant, which normally maintains the surface tension on the alveolar lining extremely low and variable during the breathing cycle, is lacking or inhibited in premature neonates and in those with IRDS, which causes alveolar collapse and atelactasis.

Lung function can be evaluated with pulmonary-function testing, even in infants, for preoperative assessment with the recent development of new technologies in certain pediatric centers. Finally, common and not so common pediatric lung diseases, which would affect anesthetic and perioperative managements, have been discussed.

For questions and answers on topics in this chapter, go to "Chapter Questions" at www.expertconsult.com.

REFERENCES

Complete references used in this text can be found online at www.expertconsult.com.

CHAPTER

4

Cardiovascular Physiology

**Duncan de Souza, George M. McDaniel,
and Victor C. Baum**

CONTENTS

Pediatric anesthesiologists are notorious for remarking that their patients are not simply small adults. This is only partially correct, because the healthy adolescent really is a small adult. At the other end of the spectrum, the statement rings most true for neonates and infants whose cardiovascular systems are profoundly different from that of an adult. All organ systems undergo a maturation process that exists as a continuum from fetal life through childhood. The immaturity of the cardiovascular system is obvious; one need only look at the heart rate and blood pressure to see that what is normal for a healthy newborn is very abnormal for an adult. Understanding the limitations of the developing cardiovascular system is one of the central challenges of pediatric anesthesia.

This chapter reviews pediatric cardiovascular physiology and begins with a thorough study of the unique anatomy and physiology of fetal circulation, as well as the remarkable changes that occur at birth. The changes at birth, termed *transitional circulation*, take on added importance in states of prematurity, congenital heart disease, or critical illness. The basic determinants of myocardial performance are the same for patients of any age, but there are important differences between the neonatal and adult hearts. Reviews of electrophysiologic development and of the maturation of the neurohumoral control of circulation comprise the first part of this chapter. With this solid foundation of knowledge, the effects of anesthetics on the developing cardiovascular system can be understood. Integrating the basic physiology with the response to anesthetic agents allows care to be provided safely for pediatric patients across the entire spectrum of age and disease.

FETAL CIRCULATION

Current knowledge of fetal anatomy and physiology owes a great debt to the pioneering work of Rudolph and colleagues in fetal and neonatal sheep (Rudolph et al., 2001). The advent of fetal echocardiography has provided greater insight into the developing cardiovascular system. Knowledge of cardiac function and its regulation still relies on animal studies with extrapolation to the human fetus and neonate. A problem is that animals that are routinely studied are born at very differing stages of cardiovascular development. The human infant is somewhere in the middle of this developmental spectrum, with rats and rabbits less mature, and guinea pigs and sheep more mature at birth. Despite these limitations, the large body of knowledge gained from animal study has been confirmed by clinical observation in humans.

Anatomy

The organ of prenatal respiration is the placenta. It is a large, low-resistance circuit that has an enormous influence on the pattern of fetal blood flow. The lungs are almost completely excluded from fetal circulation, and three special shunts (the ductus venosus, the foramen ovale, and the ductus arteriosus) allow the most oxygenated blood to perfuse the heart and brain (Fig. 4-1). Two umbilical arteries originate from the internal iliac arteries and deliver fetal blood to the placenta. One umbilical vein carries oxygenated blood from the placenta to the fetus. When umbilical venous blood approaches the liver, it can take two pathways. It is estimated that 50% to 50% of umbilical venous blood bypasses the liver via the ductus venosus, while the remainder perfuses the left lobe of the liver. Blood flow to the right lobe of the liver is predominantly from the portal circulation. The right and left hepatic veins, along with the ductus venosus, merge into the suprahepatic inferior vena cava (IVC) (Fig. 4-2). Bypassing the high-resistance hepatic microcirculation, umbilical venous blood in the ductus venosus remains not only more oxygenated, but it also ows at a higher velocity. Within the suprahepatic IVC there re now two streams of blood. The stream of blood with higher elocity is derived from the ductus venosus and drainage from ne left hepatic vein. The stream of blood with slower velocity onsists of drainage from the right hepatic vein mixed with nous return from the abdominal IVC. Upon entering the ght atrium, these two streams of blood diverge. The blood th higher velocity is primarily directed across the foramen ale to the left atrium. This right-to-left shunt is possible cause left atrial pressure is low due to minimal pulmonary nous return. The Eustachian valve is a flap of tissue at the nction of the IVC and the right atrium. It functions to help ect the higher-velocity stream of blood across the foramen ale and into the left atrium (Fig. 4-3). The lower-velocity eam of blood crosses the tricuspid valve and is ejected by right ventricle. This anatomic arrangement allows the st oxygenated blood from the umbilical vein to bypass the r and the right side of heart.

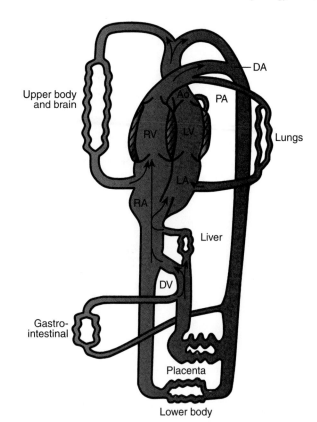

■ FIGURE 4-1. Fetal circulation. *Ao*, Aorta; *DA*, ductus arteriosus; *DV*, ductus venosus; *LA*, left atrium; *LV*, left ventricle; *PA*, pulmonary artery; *RA*, right atrium; *RV*, right ventricle. *(From Rudolph AM: The fetal circulation and postnatal adaptation. In Rudolph AM, editor:* Congenital diseases of the heart, *ed 2, Armonk, NY, 2001, Futura.)*

The majority of blood in the left atrium originates from the higher-velocity stream that crosses the foramen ovale. In the left atrium it mixes with a small amount of pulmonary venous return. The purpose of the ductus venosus and foramen ovale is to allow the most oxygenated blood from the umbilical vein to reach the left ventricle with the least drop in oxygen saturation possible. Oxygen saturation in the umbilical vein is approximately 80%. Inevitable mixing with more deoxygenated blood from the liver, IVC, and superior vena cava (SVC) results in the left ventricle ejecting blood with a saturation of 65% to 70% when the mother is breathing room air. The left ventricle pumps blood primarily to the heart and brain through the ascending aorta and great vessels of the aortic arch. SVC blood enters the right atrium and crosses the tricuspid valve into the right ventricle. Only a small amount of SVC blood and poorly oxygenated IVC blood enters the left atrium via the foramen ovale. High pulmonary vascular resistance (PVR) forces almost all of the right ventricular output to enter the systemic circulation via the ductus arteriosus. The ductus arteriosus is the continuation of the main pulmonary artery and inserts into the aorta at a point immediately distal to the origin of the left subclavian artery. The blood in the descending aorta is a mixture of left and right ventricular outputs with the right ventricle predominating. Consequently, the gut, kidneys, and lower extremities are perfused with blood that has an oxygen saturation of approximately 55%. Two umbilical arteries, branches from the internal iliac arteries, return blood to the placenta.

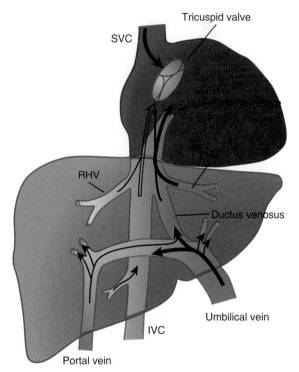

■ FIGURE 4-2. The course of umbilical venous blood as it reaches the liver. The left lobe of the liver is supplied mainly by the umbilical vein, and the right lobe of the liver is supplied by the portal circulation. *IVC,* Inferior vena cava; *SVC,* superior vena cava; *LHV,* left hepatic vein; *RHV,* right hepatic vein. *(Modified from Rudolph AM: The fetal circulation and postnatal adaptation. In Rudolph AM, editor: Congenital diseases of the heart, ed 2, Armonk, NY, 2001, Futura.)*

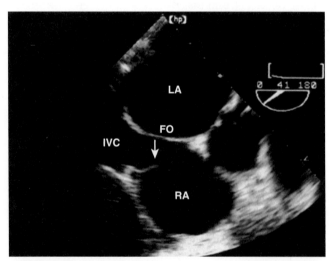

■ FIGURE 4-3. Transesophageal echocardiogram of an adult patient with a prominent Eustachian valve remnant *(arrow).* The Eustachian valve directs blood from the inferior vena cava across the foramen ovale into the left atrium. The thinnest part of the atrial septum is where the foramen ovale is during fetal life. *IVC,* Inferior vena cava; *RA,* right atrium; *LA,* left atrium; *FO,* foramen ovale. *(From Sawhney N, Palakodeti V, Raisinghani A et al.: Eustachian valve endocarditis: a case series and analysis of the literature,* J Am Soc Echocardiogr *14:11, 2001.)*

The key features of fetal circulation are shown in Figure 4-4 and listed below:

1. Low systemic vascular resistance (SVR) secondary to the low-resistance placenta
2. High PVR secondary to fluid-filled lungs and a hypoxic environment
3. Minimal pulmonary blood flow and low left atrial pressure
4. High pulmonary artery pressure
5. The most oxygenated blood from the umbilical vein perfuses the brain and heart, bypassing the liver via the ductus venosus and bypassing the right ventricle via the foramen ovale.
6. High PVR forces most right ventricular output across the ductus arteriosus into the descending aorta, allowing deoxygenated blood to return to the placenta.

Fetal Cardiac Output

The three important fetal shunts create a circulation that is parallel rather than the more efficient postnatal series circulation. Furthermore, the shunts do not function perfectly, which increases the work of the heart. Some of the oxygenated umbilical venous blood enters the right ventricle, crosses the ductus arteriosus, and flows into the descending aorta. Delivering this highly oxygenated blood back to the placenta is the equivalent of a left-to-right shunt, which increases the myocardial work. Additionally, some deoxygenated blood from the SVC and IVC flows across the foramen ovale and is ejected by the left ventricle. This is an effective right-to-left shunt, which decreases the oxygen saturation of the blood ejected by the left ventricle. The fetus and most critically, its very metabolically active heart and brain, grow and develop in a cyanotic environment.

In the fetus, right and left ventricular outputs are not equal. The ventricles, acting in parallel, pump different amounts of blood, and organs receive blood flow from both ventricles. Thus, it is customary to refer to the combined ventricular output (CVO) of fetal circulation. The fetal CVO is estimated at 400 mL/kg per minute, a value that is similar to that of the neonate but almost threefold higher than it is in adults. The ratio of right ventricular to left ventricular output is approximately 1.3:1 (Kenny et al., 1986). The volume load borne by the right ventricle combined with the high fetal PVR results in significant hypertrophy. After birth, the right ventricle remodels over time under the influence of a series circulation and lowered PVR (Fig. 4-5). The demands of a parallel circulation result in increased myocardial work superimposed on the demand of a fetus having to grow and develop in a cyanotic milieu. Nevertheless, the fetal circulation is an efficient arrangement with adequate physiologic reserve. This is demonstrated by the full spectrum of congenital heart lesions that are well tolerated *in utero.*

Oxygen Delivery

The transfer of oxygen across the placental bed is inefficient when compared with the transfer of oxygen in the lungs. The normal alveolar-arterial gradient for oxygen is minimal for a patient with healthy lungs breathing room air. This is in contrast to the fetal state, in which maternal arterial oxygen tension (Pao_2) is close to 100 mm Hg, and the partial pressure

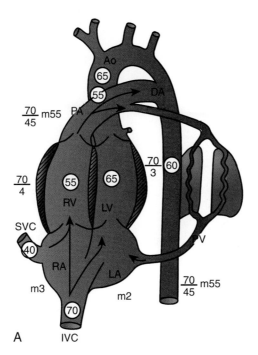

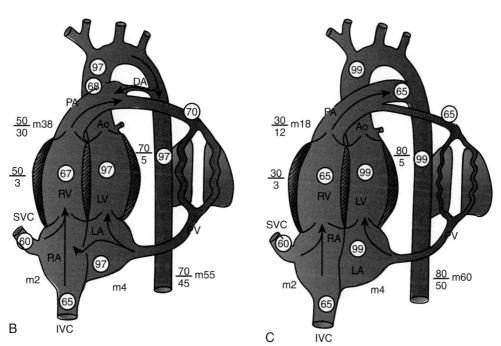

FIGURE 4-4. Fetal and neonatal circulation. Circled values are oxygen saturation, with values for pressure (systolic, diastolic, and mean) appearing beside their respective chamber or vessel. **A,** Fetal circulation near term. **B,** Transitional circulation at younger than 1 day old. **C,** Neonatal circulation at several days old. *Ao,* Aorta; *DA,* ductus arteriosus; *IVC,* inferior vena cava; *LA,* left atrium; *LV,* left ventricle; *PA,* pulmonary artery; *PV,* pulmonary veins; *RA,* right atrium; *RV,* right ventricle; *SVC,* superior vena cava. *(From Rudolph AM: The fetal circulation and Rudolph AM: Changes in the circulation after birth. In Rudolph AM, editor:* Congenital diseases of the heart, *Chicago, 1974, Mosby.)*

f oxygen (Po₂) in the umbilical vein is no more than 30 to 5 mm Hg. It should be recalled that after umbilical venous ood is diluted with more poorly oxygenated blood, the Po₂ the blood ejected by the left ventricle is about 25 to 30 m Hg when the mother is breathing room air. With such a w fetal oxygen tension, any reductions in maternal oxygen-ion could severely impact the fetus. The large gradient for ygen across the placenta means that when the mother is eathing 100% oxygen, maternal Pao₂ can be as high as 400

to 500 mm Hg, but the Po₂ in the umbilical vein rises to no higher than 40 mm Hg. In cases of suspected uteroplacental compromise, this small increase in umbilical vein Po₂ may be critical and justifies administering supplemental oxygen to the mother. The modest rise in umbilical vein Po₂ that occurs when the mother is breathing 100% oxygen can result in a large increase in fetal oxygen saturation. This occurs because fetal hemoglobin has a different oxygen-hemoglobin dissocia-tion curve than adult hemoglobin.

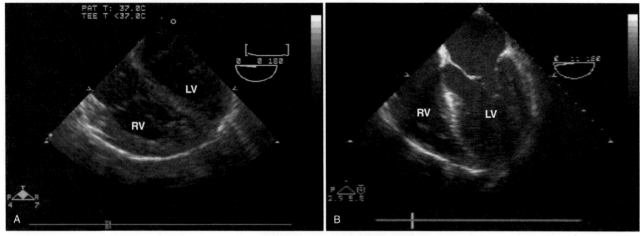

■ **FIGURE 4-5.** Transesophageal echocardiogram four-chamber view of a healthy newborn, **A,** and adult **B.** The ventricles are equal in the newborn heart. Growth of the left ventricle and remodeling of the right ventricle create the usual adult appearance.

Oxygen transport must be achieved in a relatively hypoxic environment (Lister et al., 1979). How does the fetus ensure adequate oxygen delivery? Fetal hemoglobin (HbF) has unique properties that allow the fetus to transport oxygen despite a low Po_2. Approximately 80% of fetal hemoglobin is HbF compared with an adult who has over 90% adult hemoglobin (HbA). The Pao_2 at which Hb is 50% saturated is called the P_{50}. Fetal hemoglobin (HbF P_{50}:19 mm Hg) is shifted to the left in comparison with adult hemoglobin (HbA P_{50}:26 mm Hg). A low level of 2,3-diphosphoglycerate (2,3-DPG) and the decreased affinity of HbF for 2,3-DPG cause the leftward shift of HbF. *In vitro,* HbF has a sigmoidal oxygen dissociation curve similar to that of HbA. The result is that for any given Po_2, the oxygen saturation is higher for HbF than for HbA.

Assuming a Pao_2 of 30 mm Hg in the blood ejected by the left ventricle, this value falls in the steepest part of the oxygen-hemoglobin dissociation curve. At a Pao_2 of 30 mm Hg, fetal hemoglobin would be approximately 70% saturated, and adult hemoglobin would only be 50% saturated (Fig. 4-6). Using the equation for oxygen content of the blood (Cao_2) demonstrates how the fetus can achieve levels of oxygen transport that are near those of an adult. Oxygen content of blood is defined by the following equation, Sao_2 is the arterial oxygen saturation of hemoglobin, and Hb is the hemoglobin concentration in g/dL:

$$Cao_2(mL\ O_2/dL) = [Sao_2/100 \times Hb \times 1.34\ mL\ O_2\ Hb] + Pao_2 \times 0.003\ mL\ O_2/mm\ Hg$$

At normal levels of Pao_2, when an adult is breathing room air, the amount of oxygen dissolved in blood is negligible, because it is only 0.003 mL O_2/mm Hg. Therefore, the Cao_2 is typically calculated by determining the amount of oxygen that is carried bound to hemoglobin. For example, an adult with a Sao_2 of 100% and a Hb of 11 g/dL would have the following Cao_2:

$$Cao_2 = 1.0 \times 11 \times 1.34 = 14.7\ mL\ O_2/dL\ of\ blood$$

The fetus maintains Cao_2 through two mechanisms. In addition to the leftward shift of HbF, the fetus is erythrocytotic compared with the adult. Using the equation for Cao_2 for a fetus with a Hb of 17 g/dL and an oxygen saturation of 65% yields the following:

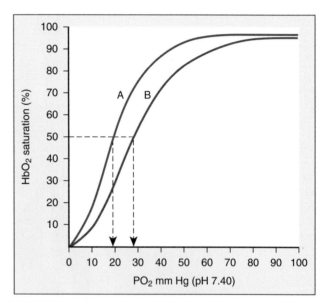

■ **FIGURE 4-6.** Oxygen-hemoglobin dissociation curves for fetal *(A)* and adult *(B)* hemoglobin. The dashed lines represent the P_{50} for fetal and adult hemoglobin, respectively. For any given Po_2, fetal hemoglobin has a higher oxygen saturation than adult hemoglobin. *(From Delivoria-Papadopoulos M, McGowan JE: Oxygen transport and delivery. In Polin RA, Fox WW, Abman SH, editors: Fetal and neonatal physiology, ed 3, Philadelphia, 2004, Saunders.)*

$$Cao_2 = 0.65 \times 17 \times 1.34 = 14.8\ mL\ O_2/dL\ of\ blood$$

Fetal hemoglobin's greater affinity for oxygen improve oxygen uptake at the placenta. A greater affinity for oxygen i an advantage for uptake at the placenta but a drawback for th unloading of oxygen at the tissue level. Given that the purpos of hemoglobin is to deliver oxygen to the tissues, this pose a problem. The fetus copes with this problem with anothe modification to its internal milieu. Oxygen release, or righ ward shifting of the oxygen-hemoglobin curve, is increase by acidosis. Fetal pH (normal values 7.25–7.35) is lower tha it is in adults, facilitating oxygen release at the tissue lev It is important to realize that the preceding discussion h involved only oxygen content of the blood. Oxygen delive which is the goal, can only be achieved when an adequate capacity to carry oxygen is matched with a cardiac output that is sufficient to meet metabolic needs.

TRANSITIONAL CIRCULATION

At birth, the fetus must make a transition to an adult circulatory system. The fact that the vast majority of newborns make this transition smoothly does not mean that the changes required are inconsequential. On the contrary, the events precipitating the transition from fetal to adult circulation are profound and immediate, requiring the fetus to make dramatic changes to ensure survival. The primary events that occur at birth are the clamping of the umbilical cord and initiation of breathing, with inflation of the lungs with air. These changes markedly alter the resistances in the cardiovascular system, changing the pattern of blood flow through the three vital shunts that characterize the fetal circulation. The fetus moves from a circulation that functions in parallel to one that is in a series. The lungs must now become the organs of oxygen supply and ventilation. Lung inflation and increased oxygen tension lower PVR dramatically, causing increased pulmonary blood flow and increased blood return to the left atrium. Cord clamping removes the low-resistance placenta from the circulation system and raises SVR. Left atrial pressure now exceeds right atrial pressure, closing the flap of tissue covering the foramen ovale. Normal intracardiac pressures keep the tissue flap over the foramen ovale closed, and over weeks it will completely seal. However, permanent occlusion does not occur in up to 25% of adults who retain a small defect or probe patency of the patent foramen ovale (PFO) (Hagen et al., 1984). Left atrial pressure rises for two reasons. First, left atrial volume increases significantly because of the increase in pulmonary blood flow. Second, left-sided pressures in the heart rise because of the increase in SVR. With the increase in systemic blood pressure and fall in PVR, flow through the ductus arteriosus becomes initially bidirectional and then very quickly evolves into a left-to-right shunt. Within the first hours of life the ductus arteriosus begins to close under the influence of the increased oxygen tension, loss of placental prostaglandins, and the more alkalotic environment of the newborn. Permanent closure of the ductus arteriosus takes weeks to occur.

Cardiac output *in utero* is considered to be the combined output of both ventricles and has been estimated at 400 mL/kg per minute. The right ventricle does more of this work, resulting in its hypertrophied state at birth. After birth, right ventricular work decreases because the volume load is reduced and PVR falls. In a series circulation, the cardiac output is the equal volume of blood ejected by each ventricle. Newborn cardiac output is the same as that *in utero* but by convention is calculated as 200 mL/kg per minute, which is the output of each ventricle (Lister et al., 1979). In the transition to postnatal life, it is the left ventricle that must cope with increased demands. Left ventricular output increases two- to threefold. This is accomplished by an increase in the left ventricular preload and stroke volume and heart rate. The volume load increase and rise in SVR represent a significant increase from the fetal state (Anderson, 1996). Additionally, as a result of the high beta stimulation associated with labor and delivery, heart rate increases and is near maximum. The newborn must maintain a high cardiac output because its metabolic rate ($\dot{V}O_2$:6-7 mL O_2/kg per

minute) is double that of an adult (Anderson, 1990). With a large surface-to-mass ratio, the newborn is at a significant disadvantage for maintaining temperature. Its compensation is to use its high metabolic rate to generate heat for temperature homeostasis (Hill and Rahimtulla, 1965). The remainder of the increased $\dot{V}O_2$ is devoted to growth and the oxygen requirement of the brain, which is proportionally much larger in newborns.

After umbilical cord clamping, flow through the ductus venosus ceases, causing it to involute. With no possibility of any flow, the ductus venosus does not play a role in problems during the state of transitional circulation. However, the foramen ovale and the ductus arteriosus have the ability to maintain fetal circulatory flow patterns under certain circumstances. The ductus arteriosus remains patent *in utero* as a result of hypoxemia, mild acidosis, and placental prostaglandins. Removal of these factors after delivery causes vasoconstriction of the ductus arteriosus. This functional closure of the ductus arteriosus is reversible until fibrosis leads to anatomic closure, which does not occur for weeks. Newborns with significant lung disease can have persistence of fetal circulation, which is defined as fetal shunting that occurs beyond the usual transition period in the absence of structural heart disease.

Persistence of fetal circulation most commonly occurs in instances of severe prematurity with respiratory distress syndrome (RDS). Hypoxemia is a potent stimulus, maintaining a patent ductus arteriosus (PDA). Flow through the ductus arteriosus remains possible as long as it is patent. The direction of that flow depends solely on the relative resistances between the systemic and pulmonary circulations. Flow through the PDA is usually left to right, adding an additional volume burden to the lung that is already coping with RDS. Significant RDS can be accompanied by elevations in PVR that are high enough to cause bidirectional or even right-to-left shunting at the PDA. The elevated PVR also raises right heart pressures, causing the same phenomenon to occur at the foramen ovale. A patent foramen ovale (PFO) provides an opportunity for intracardiac right-to-left shunting. Any other type of lung disease (e.g., meconium aspiration or pneumonia) that is severe enough can also cause persistence of the fetal circulation. Nonsteroidal antiinflammatory drugs, via their antiprostaglandin action, can be used to induce closure of a PDA. Indomethacin is the preferred agent (Giroud and Jacobs, 2007).

Reversion to fetal circulation can occur in some infants who have made a smooth transition from fetal circulation. The usual scenario is a previously healthy infant who has developed a critical illness. The cause is most often sepsis, although certain newborn surgical emergencies (such as necrotizing enterocolitis) may also be precipitants. Hypothermia, hypercarbia, acidosis, and hypoxemia can all accompany sepsis and may cause a reversion to fetal circulation. During the period before anatomic closure of the ductus arteriosus and foramen ovale, marked physiologic stresses can cause the newborn to revert to fetal circulation. This reversion is characterized by increased pulmonary vascular reactivity, raised PVR, and shunting at the PFO and PDA. The direction of shunting depends on the balance between SVR and PVR. In this scenario, vigorous resuscitation of the infant is required, and nonsteroidal antiinflammatory drugs to close the PDA do not have a role.

Pulmonary Blood Flow and Pulmonary Vascular Resistance

It is clear that the most fundamental and critical transition necessary for postnatal life is the establishment of breathing, accompanied by a fall in PVR. Therapeutic attempts to manipulate PVR occur in certain newborns with congenital heart disease. Deleterious changes in PVR also accompany critical neonatal disease states. Therefore, a brief discussion of pulmonary circulatory physiology is warranted.

At midgestation, PVR is estimated to be tenfold higher than it is 24 hours after an uncomplicated birth. During the last trimester, PVR decreases slightly to levels seven- to eightfold greater than it is 24 hours after delivery (Rudolph, 1979). This reduction results from the physical growth of the pulmonary vasculature that increases the cross-sectional area by more than the corresponding increase in blood flow. Yet, PVR still remains high immediately prior to birth and must fall dramatically in the first postnatal minutes to ensure survival. Pulmonary blood flow increases by an amount corresponding to the decrease in PVR, and pulmonary blood pressure falls by 50% (Fig. 4-7). Thus, the pulmonary vasculature presents a puzzle that flies in the face of the normal principles of cardiovascular embryology. The guiding principle of cardiac and vascular development is that once normal structures form, the correct pathway for blood flow is established. Once flow is established, normal growth ensues. The pulmonary vasculature must grow normally despite greatly reduced flow. The elevated PVR necessary for fetal existence cannot be solely the result of anatomic hypoplasia. If this were the case, the transition to postnatal life would be rocky indeed. Rather, the pulmonary vessels must be of normal size but retain the ability to markedly vasoconstrict. Even more remarkable is that the ductus arteriosus is an outgrowth of the pulmonary arterial system, yet it responds in a completely opposite fashion to the pulmonary vasculature. The very stimuli that raise PVR *in utero* cause dilation of the ductus arteriosus. The factors that govern pulmonary vasoreactivity have still not been fully elucidated, but our understanding has grown considerably in the last 20 years (Martin et al., 2006).

The primary force driving high fetal PVR is hypoxemia. The estimated Po_2 in the pulmonary arteries is less than 20 mm Hg. This phenomenon of hypoxemia-induced pulmonary vasoconstriction (HPV) persists into adulthood, where it is vital in maintaining oxygen saturation during one-lung anesthesia. *In utero*, the mechanism of HPV is not fully understood. Oxygen is a potent stimulator of endothelial-derived vasodilating substances such as nitric oxide and prostacyclin. Nitric oxide activates soluble guanylate cyclase, which increases guanylate 3'-5'-cyclic monophosphate (cGMP). Prostacyclin stimulates adenylate cyclase to

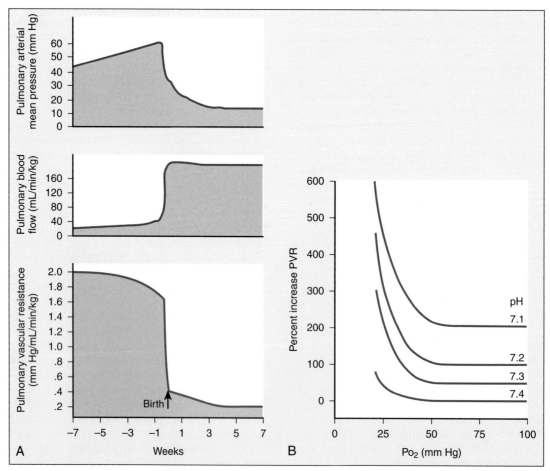

■ **FIGURE 4-7. A,** The changes in pulmonary arterial pressure, blood flow, and PVR from late gestation through the neonatal period in lambs and other species. **B,** The effect of oxygen tension and acid–base balance on PVR in newborn calves. A low Po_2 results in minimal increase in PVR if pH is maintained at 7.4. Conversely, dramatic rises in PVR occur when acidosis is combined with a low Po_2. *(From Rudolph AM: Prenatal and postnatal pulmonary circulation. In Rudolph AM, editor: Congenital diseases of the heart, ed 2, Armonk, 2001, Futura.)*

increase adenylate or adenosine 3′-5′-cyclic monophosphate (cAMP). Both cGMP and cAMP initiate vasodilation in pulmonary vessels. Under conditions of low oxygen tension, the release of nitric oxide and prostacyclin is presumably attenuated, tipping the balance in favor of vasoconstriction. The specific substances inducing pulmonary vasoconstriction are not well understood. Attention is focused on arachidonic acid and its metabolites and the potent vasoconstrictor endothelin (Tod and Cassin, 1984; Hickey et al., 1985a; Ivy et al., 1996).

At delivery, mechanical and biochemical factors lead to the abrupt fall in PVR (Teitel et al., 1990). Aeration of the previously fluid-filled lungs removes the external compressive force on the pulmonary vasculature. Responding to the sudden rise in oxygen tension, the endothelium secretes potent vasodilators, nitric oxide and prostacyclin. Luminal diameter increases as endothelial and smooth muscle cells become thinner. The increase in blood flow further recruits small lumen vessels, leading to an overall increase in the cross-sectional area of the pulmonary vascular bed. Smooth muscle relaxation occurs in the larger pulmonary vessels. This first, rapid phase of pulmonary vasodilation is followed by a period of remodeling that lasts for months. During this time there is maturation of vascular smooth muscles with continuing modest declines in PVR. PVR approximates adult values by about 2 months of age, and the remodeling process is usually complete by 6 months of age. During the first few years of life, new vessels develop to supply the growing lung parenchyma (Fig. 4-8). It is important to understand that in the early postnatal period, PVR is markedly affected by hypoxia and acidosis (Rudolph and Yuan, 1966). More recently, pain has also been associated with increasing PVR.

MYOCARDIAL PERFORMANCE

At which point the newborn heart does mature is a very important issue. In this context one must distinguish between functional maturity of the heart and the state of the cardiovascular system. The histologic and physiologic changes that translate into important clinical limitations are believed to be complete by about 6 months of age and certainly by the end of the first year of life. After this age, a child is expected to respond to changes in preload, afterload, contractility, heart rate, and calcium in a manner similar to the adult. However, the cardiovascular system is still driven by the demands of growth and will not reach adult values for blood pressure and heart rate until adolescence.

Ohm's law mathematically describes the relationship between voltage, current, and resistance in electrical circuits. The well-known adaptation of Ohm's law to the cardiovascular system states the following:

$$Blood\ Pressure = Cardiac\ Output \times SVR$$

Cardiac output is the product of stroke volume and heart rate. Heart rate is easily measured. Stroke volume, on the other hand, is not easily measured in most clinical settings. The clinician must know the factors affecting stroke volume and how they can be manipulated to optimize cardiac function. The physiologic parameters underlying myocardial performance are no different in the newborn and the adult. These parameters are preload, afterload, and contractility. Additionally, newborns and infants have an altered ability to transport calcium, which affects both diastolic relaxation and systolic contraction. Within the important areas of preload, afterload, contractility, and heart rate, pediatric patients have unique limitations. The younger the patient, the more the limitation. This section attempts to explain the key differences between the immature and adult heart.

Cardiac cells are known as myocytes. Hyperplasia, which is an increase in cell number, is responsible for growth of the myocardium during fetal life. Hyperplasia continues into the early newborn period, after which increased demands on the heart can only be met by hypertrophy (increase in myocyte size). The functional unit of each myocyte is the myofibril. Myofibrils consist of contractile proteins arranged in repeating units called sarcomeres. The immature myocyte shape is rounded compared with the rodlike appearance of the adult

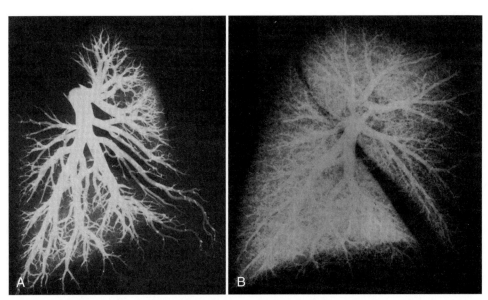

FIGURE 4-8. Pulmonary angiograms at birth **(A)** and from an 18-month-old infant **(B).** Growth of existing vessels and development of ra-acinar arteries create the prominent hazy background appearance. *(From Haworth SG: Pulmonary vascular development. In Long WA, editor: al and neonatal cardiology, Philadelphia, 1990, Saunders.)*

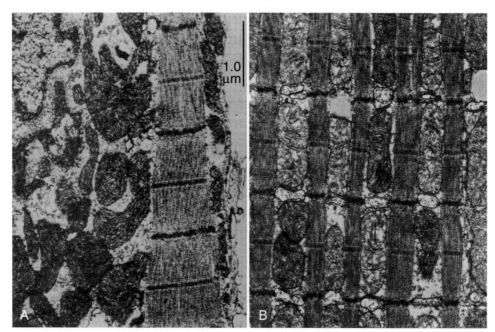

■ **FIGURE 4-9.** Electron micrographs of a rabbit myocyte at aged 3 weeks **(A)** and fully mature **(B)**. The infant myocyte has one myofibril. The adult myocyte has organized, repeating rows of myofibrils separated by mitochondria. *(From Anderson PAW: Myocardial development. In Long WA, editor:* Fetal and neonatal cardiology, *Philadelphia, 1990, Saunders.)*

myocyte. Immature myocytes also have a much larger surface-area to volume ratio. Adult myocytes contain multiple repeating rows of longitudinally arranged myofibrils. The newborn myocyte has fewer myofibrils in a more chaotic and scattered intracellular arrangement (Fig. 4-9). Sarcomere volume is only 30% of the newborn myocyte compared with 60% in the adult (Baum and Palmisano, 1997). The T-tubule system is a series of invaginations of the sarcolemma, or cell membrane, bringing it in close contact with the myofibrils. In this way, the action potential can rapidly disperse itself throughout the myocyte. Both the sarcolemma and T-tubule system are relatively well developed in the human newborn. The sarcoplasmic reticulum (SR) is a tubular network regulating the uptake, storage, and release of intracellular calcium. The adult heart relies on the SR to fully regulate calcium transport. Contrastingly, the newborn heart has an underdeveloped sarcoplasmic reticulum. There is more reliance on the sarcolemma and T-tubule system for the appropriate movement of calcium necessary for contraction and relaxation. The newborn has decreased contractile reserve on the basis of reduced sarcomere number and an immature system of calcium transport. The reduction in sarcomeres also reduces the compliance of the immature heart.

Preload

In 1895, the German physiologist Otto Frank published his observations on the relationship of diastolic filling of the heart and the pressure the heart was able to generate during systole (Frank, 1895). Ernest Starling, an English physiologist, conducted the classic experiment in the early 1900s that defined the length-tension relationship for cardiac muscle (Fig. 4-10). Understanding his experiment is important, because in the laboratory he was able to isolate that which is impossible to isolate

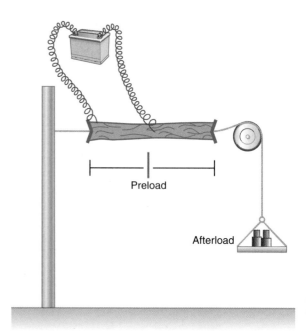

■ **FIGURE 4-10.** A schematic diagram of the classic Starling experiment. The suspended weight (afterload) is held constant, allowing the tension developed to be measured at different lengths (preload) of the muscle strip. *(From Epstein D, Wetzel RC: Cardiovascular physiology and shock. In Nichols DG, Ungerleider RM, Spevak PS, et al., editors:* Critical heart disease in infants and children, *ed 2, Philadelphia, 2006, Mosby.)*

in vivo. Using a fixed weight to keep afterload constant, he w[...] able to prove that the tension developed was proportional [...] the length of the muscle strip prior to stimulation. The grea[...] the length of the muscle strip, the greater the tension it w[...] able to develop. The Frank-Starling mechanism, or Starlin[...]

Law of the Heart, is taken from a famous lecture by Dr. Starling himself, in which he stated, "the energy of contraction, however measured, is a function of the length of the muscle fiber" (Starling, 1918).

The clinical correlates of length and tension are left ventricular end-diastolic volume (LVEDV) and stroke volume, respectively. In the laboratory, the length of a muscle strip is easily determined because both ends can be fixed. This is very different from the intact heart, where the ventricle is a three-dimensional structure with complex geometry that defies the simple concept of length. Nevertheless, it is clinically appropriate to regard length as LVEDV. The LVEDV represents the loading of the ventricle. It is present before contraction, and therefore has come to be called *preload*. The force of ventricular contraction increases with increasing preload until a point is reached where the ventricle is over stretched and the force of contraction decreases. This point is the apex of the well-known Starling curve. Force of contraction is not synonymous with contractility, and for all points along a Starling curve, contractility is equal. Changes in the force of contraction, however, occur when preload changes (Fig. 4-11). Laboratory evidence has shown that resting sarcomere distance is 1.6 microns, with optimal conditions occurring at 2.2 microns. Excessive stretch, causing decreased force of contraction, does not occur until sarcomere length reaches 3.5 microns (Sonnenblick, 1974). In the laboratory the force of contraction increases until the sarcomere is stretched to over twice its resting length. If this translated fully to the intact heart, any increase in preload would result in increased force of contraction, because physiologically achieving a doubling of resting sarcomere length is almost impossible. However, well before a doubling of resting sarcomere length is reached,

the patient falls on to the descending limb of the Starling curve. The reason is the relationship between volume and pressure, which is known as compliance.

The Starling curve describes the relationship between LVEDV and stroke volume. The problem is that measuring LVEDV in a way that is simple, accurate, and available in real time is not possible. Echocardiography is the best method to quantify LVEDV. However, the two-dimensional images seen echocardiographically may not faithfully represent the volume contained in a three-dimensional ventricle with its elliptical shape. The equations used to objectively measure volume are not practical in most clinical situations and certainly not in the dynamic environment of the operating room. Subjective assessments of LVEDV using echocardiography depend on the skill of the operator and will detect only the extremes of preload conditions. Given the problems in measuring volume, the clinician is forced to use a surrogate measure of LVEDV. A catheter placed in a central vein and connected to a transducer measures pressures simply, accurately and continuously. Using pressure as a guide to volume requires understanding the relationship between the two variables, defined as compliance and described by the following equation:

$$\text{Compliance} = \frac{\Delta \text{ Volume}}{\Delta \text{ Pressure}}$$

The change in pressure resulting from a change in volume is compliance. Volume is in the numerator of the equation meaning that if a large increase in volume is met by a relatively small rise in pressure, compliance is high. As a completely empty ventricle is filled, the initial rise in LVEDP is small. In this situation the ventricle is said to be compliant. When the ventricle is full, a small increase in volume results in a large increase in pressure. The ventricle is now poorly compliant or "stiff." As with the Starling curve, it is important to note that moving to different points on the compliance curve does not mean that the intrinsic compliance of the ventricle has changed. A true intrinsic change in compliance will be reflected in a new compliance curve (Fig. 4-12). In adult cardiac medicine it is readily

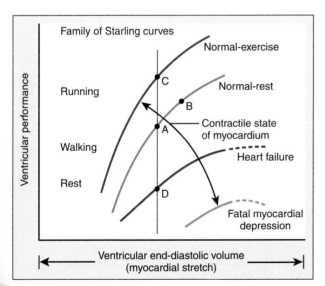

◀ **FIGURE 4-11.** Starling's Law of the Heart. Contractility is the same for each curve. Moving from point *A* to point *B* requires an increase in LVEDV. Moving to point *C* or point *D* can only occur if there is a change in contractility. For the same LVEDV, the stroke volume falls progressively with impaired contractility. The figure demonstrates that the failing ventricle is dependent on preload. (*Modified from Opie LH, Perlroth MG: Ventricular function. In Opie LH, editor: The heart: physiology from cell to circulation. Philadelphia, 1998, Lippincott-Raven.*)

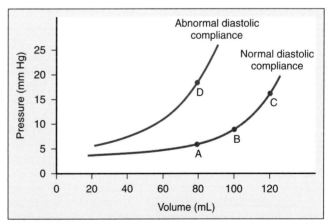

■ **FIGURE 4-12.** Diastolic-compliance curves. Each curve represents a different intrinsic compliance. Movement between points *A, B,* and *C* reflects a change in preload with no change in compliance. Movement from point *A* to point *D* can only occur when the ventricle becomes less compliant. (*From Mark JB: Atlas of cardiovascular monitoring, New York, 1998, Churchill Livingstone.*)

appreciated that ischemia, infarction, or hypertrophy result in a stiffer, or less compliant, ventricle. However, no ventricle, regardless of its intrinsic compliance, has an infinite ability to accept volume. Eventually the inflection point on the curve will be reached and pressure will climb rapidly for any given increase in volume. It is this sharp increase in pressure beyond the inflection point that is responsible for the descending limb of the Staring curve.

Decreases in the force of contraction represented by the descending limb of the Starling curve are due to the result of pressure and not volume or "overstretch." The reason is that the rise in pressure causes an imbalance in the myocardial oxygen supply/demand ratio that results in decreased force of contraction. The left ventricle is perfused according to the following equation:

$$\text{Coronary perfusion pressure} = \text{Diastolic blood pressure} - \text{LVEDP}$$

When the maximum increase in blood pressure achieved by volume loading has been reached, further volume only serves to increase LVEDP at the expense of coronary perfusion pressure. Thus, myocardial oxygen supply decreases. A key determinant of myocardial oxygen demand is wall stress defined by the modified Law of Laplace:

$$\text{Wall stress} = \frac{\text{Pressure} \times \text{radius}}{\text{Ventricular wall thickness} \times 2}$$

Wall stress is usually, but erroneously, thought of as similar to afterload, because the value for pressure in the numerator is assumed to be systolic blood pressure. In fact, blood pressure is a key component of wall stress, but they are clearly not the same. Oxygen consumption increases with increasing wall stress, and wall stress has both systolic and diastolic components. During systole the value for pressure in the wall stress equation is the systolic blood pressure. In the diastole the value for pressure is LVEDP. A patient with a value on the steep part of the compliance curve has sharp increases in LVEDP disproportionate to the increase in volume. Concomitantly, the ventricular cavity is fully distended from the volume load. Thus, excessively high LVEDP combined with an enlarged ventricular radius simultaneously causes an increase in myocardial oxygen demand and a decrease in myocardial oxygen supply. This situation, if unchecked, leads to ischemia and a decrease in the force of contraction.

The response of the newborn heart to volume loading (relative insensitivity) has been the source of great confusion (Rudolph, 1974). This confusion stems from experimental work done in the 1970s and is the logical extension of the known structural differences in the newborn heart (Romero and Friedman, 1979; Gilbert, 1980). The response to preload was investigated in fetal sheep for the left and right ventricles. For either ventricle, isolated output rose only slightly with increases in filling pressures. Using a microsphere technique in fetal sheep, alterations in combined cardiac output were measured as blood volume was modulated (Gilbert, 1980). With a decrease of 10% in circulating volume, there was a significant drop in right atrial pressure, as well as in cardiac output. In contrast, cardiac output did not significantly change despite a significant change in right atrial pressure with a 10% increase in circulating blood volume from baseline. These data lead the author to conclude that the fetus operates at the upper end of the Starling curve and possesses limited cardiac reserve.

With only half the amount of sarcomere volume that is in an adult, connective tissue comprises a much greater percentage of the newborn heart. The myofibrils are fewer in number with a disorderly arrangement in the myocyte. There is much more stiff connective tissue. The sum total of these changes makes it plausible that the relatively noncompliant newborn heart does function at the upper end of its Starling curve, where the response to volume loading is blunted. In fact, the original experiments failed to account for an inevitable consequence of increases in preload. An increase in the preload leads to greater stroke volume, and if heart rate is unchanged, cardiac output must increase as well. Blood pressure must now rise unless there is a corresponding drop in SVR. Therefore, an increase in preload leads to an increase in afterload, which then acts to reduce stroke volume. This created the impression that the newborn heart could not increase stroke volume in response to volume loading. Other work, controlling for arterial pressure, shows that the newborn heart is indeed responsive to volume *within the limitations of its decreased compliance* (Fig. 4-13) (Kirkpatrick et al.; 1976, Hawkins et al., 1989). This has been shown in the laboratory with a sheep model and though echocardiography in the human fetus. The newborn can be likened to the hypertensive adult with diastolic dysfunction. This is not to suggest that the otherwise healthy newborn has diastolic dysfunction, because the newborn heart is not dysfunctional but normal for its stage of development. Rather, the lesson of diastolic dysfunction is that the ventricle is preload dependent. At the low end of the Starling curve, reduced preload is poorly tolerated. The upper end of the Starling curve is flattened, reflecting its reduced compliance. Between these two points is the steepest part of the curve, where increases in LVEDV result in significantly greater stroke volume. Clinical experience observing the response to volume infusion confirms this property of the newborn heart.

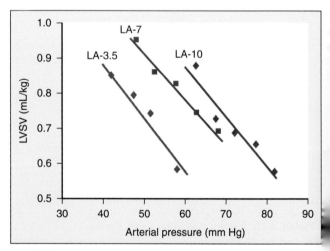

■ **FIGURE 4-13.** The response of the immature heart to changes in preload and afterload. When afterload is held constant, left ventricular stroke volume (LVSV) increases linearly with increased left atrial (LA) pressure. Increasing afterload creates an inverse linear relationship with LVSV when LA pressure is constant. *(From Hawkins J, Van Hare GF, Schmid KG, et al.: Effects of increasing afterload on left ventricular output in fetal lambs,* Circ Res 65:127, 1989.)

Afterload

In addition to preload, there is another loading force that influences myocardial performance. The force that resists the ejection of blood is known as afterload. In isolated muscle strip experiments, the afterload is represented by the weight against which the muscle contracts or shortens. The stretch applied to the isolated muscle strip before contraction is fixed, allowing the experiment to be conducted at a constant length, or preload. Plotting the velocity of myocardial shortening against progressively increasing afterload reveals an inverse relationship. The shape of the curve is exponential with the points of maximal and zero shortening both occurring at physiologically impossible limits. The greatest shortening velocity occurs at zero load. When the load is so great that no muscle fiber shortening can occur, isometric contraction occurs. Between these two extremes, it is intuitive that increasing afterload results in reduced velocity of muscle fiber shortening. Transferring this straightforward laboratory concept to the intact circulation is difficult (Martin et al., 2006). The force generated by the shortening of an isolated muscle strip is directed in only one plane. This is very different from the three-dimensional contraction of the left ventricle with its asymmetric geometry. Additionally, in the laboratory the force that resists the shortening of the muscle is the weight applied to the muscle strip. Physiologically, the force that resists the ejection of blood is a complex interplay between blood pressure, vascular impedance, walls stress, and inertia. Finally, blood pressure and SVR are commonly used measures of afterload, but neither is fully accurate.

In most situations, the systemic blood pressure does provide an appropriate surrogate for afterload. One common exception is in conditions in which there is obstruction to left ventricular outflow. In adults, the most common cause is aortic stenosis, but pediatric patients may also have congenital lesions that cause obstruction at the subvalvular level in the left ventricular outflow tract (LVOT) in addition to aortic valve disease. The left ventricle must generate enough pressure to overcome both the systolic blood pressure and the gradient across the valve or the LVOT obstruction. Assuming that the ventricle must only overcome the systolic blood pressure leads to a significant under estimation of afterload. The use of SVR to approximate afterload is also problematic. The concept of SVR describes resistance, which is defined as the pressure drop across a system divided by the flow across that same system. This is reflected in the equation for SVR:

$$SVR = \frac{\text{Mean arterial pressure} - CVP}{\text{Cardiac output}} \times 80$$

Multiplication by 80 converts SVR from mm Hg/L/min/m into SI units (dynes•s•cm^{-5}). The calculated SVR may be similar for patients with very different cardiovascular performance. Consider these two patients:

Patient 1: Blood pressure, 120/80; central venous pressure, 10; cardiac output, 5 L/min. The calculated SVR is 1328 dynes•s•cm^5.

Patient 2: Blood pressure, 110/70; central venous pressure, 15; cardiac output, 4 L/min. The calculated SVR is 1360 dynes•s•cm^5.

These two hypothetical patients are very different, yet the SVR similar. The first patient has normal cardiovascular function and the second patient's cardiovascular function is compromised. reduction in contractility has caused a fall in cardiac output despite the attempts of the ventricle to compensate with a higher diastolic filling pressure. This example demonstrates how SVR in isolation does not necessarily reflect large changes in loading conditions and cardiac output. The modified Law of Laplace describes a better approximation of afterload (see Preload section p. 91). As discussed in the section on preload, wall stress was demonstrated to be a key component of myocardial oxygen demand. During left ventricular ejection, the value for pressure is the systolic blood pressure. By including the radius and accounting for the compensatory mechanism of left ventricular hypertrophy the modified Law of Laplace provides a more comprehensive view of the forces that resist ventricular ejection. Importantly, it demonstrates the concept that the dilated ventricle with an increased radius must eject blood under increased afterload conditions. Given the inability to easily measure ventricular radius and thickness, the modified Law of Laplace is not a clinical parameter to guide management. It is presented here to help the reader conceptualize afterload. It still cannot describe all the variables that account for afterload in the intact cardiovascular system.

Studies of the intact heart that assess the effect of changes in afterload on cardiac output are difficult to interpret without controlling for the other variables. The most important additional variable is preload. Preload and afterload are linked. For instance, pharmacologically increasing afterload decreases stroke volume. As the heart ejects less blood with each contraction, the end-diastolic volume must increase if venous return is held constant. With an increase in LVEDV the Starling curve dictates an enhanced ventricular force of contraction, which acts to return stroke volume to its previous level. The general inverse relationship between afterload and stroke volume holds across the spectrum from fetal life to adulthood (Friedman, 1972). The question is whether the immature myocardium is excessively sensitive to increases in afterload. In the laboratory, afterload can be assessed while strictly controlling for preload. These studies have revealed that the fetal myocardium is indeed more sensitive to increases in afterload than the adult myocardium (Friedman, 1972). Animal experiments with an intact circulation also show a decrease in ventricular output under conditions of increasing afterload (Fig. 4-13) (Gilbert, 1982; Thornburg and Morton, 1986). Van Hare and colleagues (1990) used a balloon occluder in the aortas of fetal sheep to modulate afterload while keeping preload constant. Combined ventricular output was measured by transducing aortic flow. They noted that at physiologic mean atrial pressures, there was an inverse linear relationship between mean arterial pressure and stroke volume. This exists for both right and left ventricles. Despite this, a fetus normally makes a smooth transition to postnatal life when the low-resistance placenta is removed. At birth, pulmonary blood flow dramatically increases, raising left-ventricular preload. Stroke volume increases, which leads to an increase in systemic blood pressure. Despite the rise in blood pressure and the loss of the low-resistance placenta, cardiac performance in the newborn is not compromised. The explanation is that much of the rise in afterload is secondary to increased preload. In clinical practice with newborns and young children, it is rare to encounter conditions of purely increased afterload. A more likely situation is significant hypovolemia that results in hypotension. Despite the low afterload state, overall cardiac performance is impaired, because the decrease in afterload is caused by decreased preload. The correct therapy is to restore intravascular volume.

Blood pressure improves, and the increased afterload is well tolerated. This example illustrates the interrelationship between these two variables of cardiac output.

It has been shown that when preload is held relatively constant, cardiac output moves inversely within the physiologic range of afterload. The relevance of afterload in the newborn stage might be questioned, because systemic hypertension is so rare. The right ventricle develops in an environment of raised PVR, yet after birth it is more sensitive to increases in afterload. Although there is limited ability of the systemic circulation to become hypertensive, the pulmonary circulation, under appropriately provocative conditions, can revert to its fetal state. Postnatally, the right ventricle begins to remodel in response to decreasing pulmonary artery pressures. Sustained elevations in pulmonary artery pressures decrease right ventricular output and reduce left-ventricular preload (Thornburg and Morton, 1983). Because both ventricles share the septum, the strain on the right ventricle impairs left-ventricular filling and contraction (Rein et al., 1987). Reductions in left-sided preload and contractile force demonstrate how the inability of the right ventricle to cope with increased afterload can lead to decreases in systemic cardiac output. In the newborn stage, the potential for pulmonary hypertension far exceeds that of systemic hypertension. This is the most common scenario for a significant rise in afterload while preload remains relatively unchanged. The strain on the right side of the heart and ventricular interdependence may lead to biventricular failure.

Contractility

The third parameter of myocardial performance is contractility. Seemingly intuitive, contractility is often confused with changes in stroke volume brought about by alterations in loading conditions. Contractility, synonymous with inotropy, is the intrinsic ability of the myocardium to contract *when loading conditions are held constant*. The Starling curve is the first source of confusion. As discussed in the section on preload, every point on an individual patient's Starling curve represents the same inotropic state. Movement along the curve is solely because of changing conditions of preload. In the same way, the demonstration in the laboratory of decreased myocardial shortening velocity in response to increased weight (afterload) is not evidence of a fall in contractility. Contractility has remained constant, but the force of contraction is reduced. Contractility and force of contraction are clearly not the same. The force of contraction, related to loading conditions, can vary widely. Contractility is relatively fixed. It can be increased pharmacologically but is usually either normal or reduced. Further demonstrating misconceptions about contractility, a hypertrophied ventricle is often assumed to have increased contractility. Hypertrophy is a response to increased afterload, but contractility, once corrected for the greater cross-sectional area of the ventricular muscle mass, is normal. Any disease process that injures the myocardium decreases global contractility. In adults, this most commonly occurs secondary to ischemia or infarction. In addition to these causes, pediatric patients may suffer decreased contractility on the basis of genetic disorders, infiltrative diseases, infections, or nutritional deficiencies.

The immature myocardium has a reduced sarcomere concentration combined with a transport system for calcium that is not fully developed. The myofibrillar arrangement is also more disorganized in the infant heart when compared with the adult heart. Mitochondria, the energy powerhouse of the myocyte, are reduced in number in the immature heart (Barth et al., 1992). Based on the above differences, a reduction in contractility is expected. Contractility is measured by the tension developed in the isolated muscle strip. This expected reduction in contractility of the immature myocardium is confirmed in laboratory experiments where preload and afterload are controlled. Across the entire range of loading conditions, fetal cardiac muscle generates less tension than adult myocardium (Fig. 4-14) (Friedman, 1972; Romero et al., 1972). In an intact heart it is not possible to fully separate the influences of different loading conditions. Nevertheless, fractional area shortening of the ventricle measured echocardiographically is used as a measure of contractility. Decreased fractional area shortening has been observed in the fetal heart (St. John Sutton et al., 1984). Effecting a true increase in contractility requires either a greater number of contractile elements or more vigorous action by the contractile elements already present. Increasing the number of contractile elements (hyperplasia and hypertrophy) occurs as a normal part of development. Improving the action of the contractile elements already present requires an understanding of the singular role of calcium. Therapy to improve inotropy exerts its action at the myocyte level by affecting the levels of intracellular calcium.

Calcium and Diastolic Function

A comprehensive understanding of the excitation-contraction coupling mechanism of contraction and relaxation is important for the safe practice of pediatric anesthesia. The relevant points are included here. The formation of actin-myosin cross-bridges

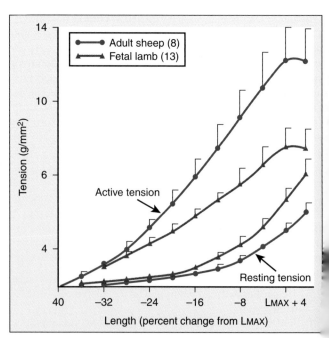

■ FIGURE 4-14. Length-tension relationships in adult sheep compared with fetal lambs. The fetal myocardium has greater resting tension but is able to generate less active tension. This represents a state of decreased compliance or a "stiffer" ventricle combined with decreased contractility. (*From Friedman WF: The intrinsic properties of the developing heart,* Prog Cardiovasc Dis *15:87, 1972.*)

occurs under the influence of calcium. Tropomyosin and troponin are inhibitory proteins that prevent the formation of actin-myosin cross-bridges. Calcium induces conformational changes in tropomyosin and troponin that remove their inhibition to actin-myosin cross-bridge formation. This is the basis of contraction and requires major changes to intracellular calcium content. It is estimated that the difference between diastolic and systolic calcium levels is 100-fold (10^{-7} M to 10^{-5} M) (Shah et al., 1994). Responsibility for these large changes in intracellular calcium concentration lies with the integrated function of the sarcolemma, the T-tubule system, and the SR. Breaking the actin-myosin cross-bridges and returning the ventricle to its baseline state is an energy-consuming process that requires adenosine triphosphate (ATP) and calcium reuptake. This is primarily accomplished by the removal of calcium into the SR and the sarcolemmal Na^+–Ca^{2+} exchanger (Mahony, 2007). Ryanodine is an inhibitor of SR function. In the presence of ryanodine, fetal and newborn hearts are minimally affected, whereas adult hearts suffer a significant decline in contractility (Penefsky, 1974).

Experimental modulation of calcium handling has been shown to alter ventricular mechanics. In a study with mice that overexpressed the Ca^{2+} ATPase, the rate of myocardial relaxation was directly correlated with the rate of calcium uptake by the SR (He et al., 1997). In guinea pigs, ryanodine blockade of SR function caused impaired relaxation (Kaufman et al., 1990). Additionally, there were age-dependent changes in the relaxation response. In adult hearts, ryanodine blockade produced a greater impairment of relaxation compared with immature hearts. Concomitantly, there was greater density of Ca^{2+} pumps, greater calcium-dependent ATPase activity, and greater uptake of calcium in isolated SR vesicles from adult hearts as compared with those isolated from immature hearts. With decreased SR function in the immature heart, the extrusion of calcium across the cell membrane assumes greater importance. The Na^+–Ca^{2+} exchanger provides the primary mechanism for this. The exchanger is sensitive to membrane potential as it exchanges three sodium ions for one calcium ion. Developmental changes in the exchanger function have been demonstrated, and there are differences among species in relative function (Nakanishi and Jarmakani, 1981; Artman, 1992; Boerth et al., 1994). In the rabbit, with its poorly developed SR exchanger, mRNA is significantly elevated in the neonate versus the adult (Artman, 1992). The relative contribution of calcium sequestration between the SR and the exchanger in the human is similar to that of the rabbit (Mahony, 2007). In addition to reduced calcium handling, there may be developmental changes in troponin interactions that effect calcium binding. There is differential expression of cardiac and slow skeletal-muscle isoforms. In fetal hearts, the predominant form is the slow-skeletal form. Shifts to the cardiac isoform are completed in the first year of life. This is significant in that the cardiac isoform has a decreased affinity for calcium when phosphorylated, potentially aiding the removal of calcium from troponin C.

The sum total of these events is to demonstrate that across all age ranges the intracellular handling of calcium is critical for systolic function and even more important for diastolic function. The diastolic characteristics of the immature myocardium have been studied. The immature myocardium has been described as "stiffer" when compared with the adult myocardium. Ventricular compliance increases with maturation (Friedman, 1972; Romero et al., 1972; Kaufman et al.,

1990). Measurements of rates of pressure change demonstrate decreased relaxation capabilities in neonatal hearts when compared with adult hearts (Palmisano et al., 1994). There are a number of potential factors involved. Structural and contractile protein changes, extra-cardiac structures, and maturing organelle function have been studied. The diastolic relaxation properties of the ventricle are a key determinant of the ventricle's compliance. Reductions in calcium reuptake lead to expected decreases in diastolic relaxation (Kaufman et al., 1990). Echocardiographic studies on human fetuses with normal hearts have demonstrated age-related changes in early diastolic flow that are consistent with improved relaxation (Kenny et al., 1986; Harada et al., 1997). Consequently, intracellular calcium homeostasis in the newborn is more dependent on a normal serum ionized calcium level, and the newborn tolerates hypocalcemia poorly. Immaturity of calcium transport leads to a decrease in systolic-force generation and a decrease in diastolic relaxation. The manifestation of impaired diastolic relaxation is a reduction in compliance. Clinically, these issues must be appreciated when interpreting assessments of volume based on pressure readings such as the central venous pressure (CVP).

Heart Rate

As mentioned in the section on preload, it has long been considered that the newborn's heart rate is dependent on and relatively insensitive to changes in end-diastolic volume. Assuming the maintenance of sinus rhythm, heart rate is believed to determine cardiac performance through its influence on preload and myocardial oxygen supply and demand. At very high heart rates, hypotension ensues, because diastolic filling time is severely restricted and preload markedly falls. Coronary perfusion to the left ventricle occurs during diastole, and systolic ejection time is fixed. Thus, tachycardia shortens the time for perfusion of the left ventricle and results in an increased oxygen demand combined with a decreased oxygen supply. The absence of coronary artery disease in newborns offers them some protection in accepting imbalances in myocardial oxygen supply and demand. However, extremes of heart rate are poorly tolerated by adults and newborns alike.

The question is whether the newborn who has a heart rate within normal range is fundamentally different than the adult. When corrected for weight, stroke volume is similar across all ages. The high cardiac output of newborns and infants can only be achieved with a heart rate that is significantly higher than in adults. This has created the idea that the newborn is dependent on heart rate. Here it becomes difficult to sort out the isolated effect of heart rate from its effects on loading conditions and contractility. It is not intuitive as to why changes in heart rate alter contractility. The mechanism is known as the force-frequency relationship. Experiments using atrial pacing, while controlling loading conditions, demonstrate an increase in stroke volume with an increase in heart rate (Anderson et al., 1982). With constant loading conditions, the only explanation for increased stroke volume is that contractility has increased. Thus, an increased heart rate improves contractility. The basis for the force-frequency relationship is that an increase in heart rate is accompanied by enhanced release of intracellular calcium (Parilak et al., 2009). There is a suggestion that the force-frequency relationship has minimal effect in newborns but is present during infancy (Wiegerinck et al., 2008). Spontaneous increases in heart rate also improve cardiac output. In this scenario, the increase in heart rate is the result of a neurohumoral stimulus with an effect that cannot be isolated to producing tachycardia. Both preload and contractility can be expected to increase, as long as the increase in heart rate does not lead to deleterious changes in preload or myocardial oxygen supply and demand. The combination of these factors allows the newborn and infant to use heart rate to significantly augment cardiac output.

Integrating Preload, Afterload, and Contractility

The determinants of myocardial performance, while discussed in isolation, are actually intricately linked. Diagrammatically, the determinants of myocardial performance can be represented by ventricular pressure-volume loops (Suga et al., 1973). The loop shows the pressure and ventricular volume changes that occur during one cardiac cycle. Increases in preload while afterload is held constant result in greater stroke volume (Fig. 4-15). This simple curve does not provide any information about contractility. The end systolic pressure-volume relationship (ESPVR) is a family of curves that is generated by rapidly altering preload or afterload. The curves create a series of points that are connected to become the ESPVR line. The slope of this line represents contractility (Fig. 4-16). The pressure-volume loop illustrates the concept that movement along the ESPVR line reflects changes in loading conditions while contractility remains constant. In Figure 4-16, the increases in afterload result in a series of points that are connected to become the ESPVR line. The slope of the ESPVR line represents contractility. The two figures of ventricular pressure-volume loops represent an idealized situation where preload and afterload can be manipulated independent of each other. In the intact organism, preload and afterload are linked. The interdependence of preload and afterload is shown in a new ventricular pressure-volume loop (Fig. 4-17).

In states of decreased contractility, the ventricular pressure-volume loop displays the limitations of the failing heart. Analysis of the ventricular pressure-volume loop shows that the failing ventricle is sensitive to changes in loading conditions (Fig. 4-18). The ESPVR line has shifted down and to the right. With preload held constant, stroke volume is reduced.

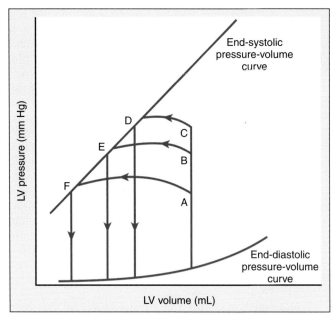

■ **FIGURE 4-16.** Ventricular pressure-volume loop. As afterload is increased, stroke volume falls when preload is held constant. The slope of the line connecting points D, E, and F is the end-systolic pressure-volume relationship and represents contractility. Only alterations in the slope of the line represent changes in contractility. The contractility at points D, E, and F is identical. (*Modified from Braunwald E, Ross J, Sonnenblick EH: Mechanisms of contraction of the normal and failing heart, Boston, 1976, Little, Brown.*)

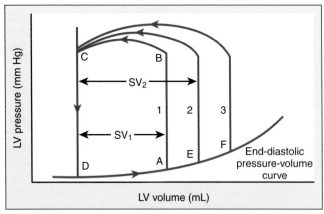

■ **FIGURE 4-15.** Ventricular pressure-volume loop. As preload increases from point A to points E and F, the end-diastolic pressure-volume curve represents compliance. The increased preload results in greater stroke volume (SV) when afterload is held constant. (*Modified from Braunwald E, Ross J, Sonnenblick EH: Mechanisms of contraction of the normal and failing heart, Boston, 1976, Little, Brown.*)

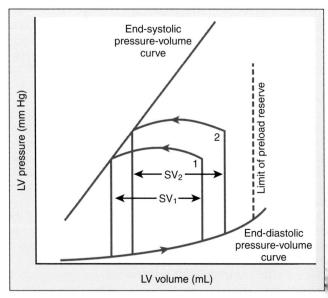

■ **FIGURE 4-17.** Ventricular pressure-volume loop. The interdependence of preload and afterload is demonstrated. The increase in preload from point 1 to point 2 results in a rise in stroke volume (SV₁ to SV₂) that is less than anticipated because the increase in preload causes a corresponding increase in afterload. (*Modified from Strobeck JE, Sonnenblick EH: Myocardial contractile properties and ventricular performance. In Fozzard HA, Haber E, Jennings RB, et al., editors: The heart and cardiovascular system, New York, 1986, Raven.*)

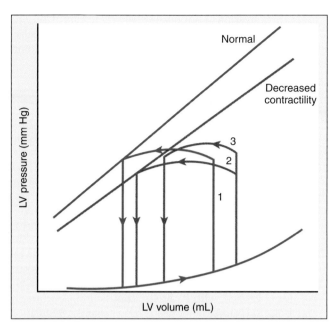

FIGURE 4-18. Ventricular-pressure volume loop with decreased contractility. The line representing contractility is shifted down and to the right. *Curve 1* is the stroke volume with normal contractility. *Curve 2* shows that when contractility is reduced, stroke volume can be maintained through increased preload. *Curve 3* demonstrates a significant reduction in stroke volume when afterload is increased in the presence of decreased contractility. *(Modified from Braunwald E, Ross J, Sonnenblick EH: Mechanisms of contraction of the normal and failing heart, Boston, 1976, Little, Brown.)*

The body's response to this situation is to increase LVEDV in an attempt to preserve stroke volume. Stroke volume has improved at the expense of a higher end-diastolic pressure. The ventricular pressure-volume loop demonstrates why afterload reduction is the cornerstone of medical therapy for the failing heart. Any increases in afterload come at the expense of stroke volume, with a limited ability for compensatory changes in preload.

The reflex of the trainee when confronted with a patient with significantly decreased contractility is to withhold or restrict fluids in a well-meaning attempt to avoid pulmonary edema. The ventricular pressure-volume loop for the patient with heart failure shows the fallacy and danger of this approach. Positive pressure ventilation is associated with decreases in preload. Venous tone is decreased by most anesthetic agents. The combination of these two events means that while the patient's global volume status is unchanged, he or she has become relatively hypovolemic. He or she is below the optimum LVEDV for his or her failing heart. Far from being on the verge of pulmonary edema, this patient now requires intravascular volume to compensate for the effects of anesthesia and positive pressure ventilation. Although maintaining LVEDV is critical for patients, there are currently limited means to accurately assess preload. Central venous pressure must be interpreted in light of the altered ventricular compliance of the failing heart. Lastly, while the failing heart requires adequate preload, its ability to accept volume rapidly is limited. Cautious infusion of volume with frequent reassessment is necessary lest a rapid bolus of fluid results in pulmonary edema, which is exactly the outcome the trainee sought to avoid by restricting volume in the first place.

DEVELOPMENTAL ASPECTS OF CARDIOMYOCYTE STRUCTURE AND FUNCTION

Ultrastructural maturation of several aspects of the cardiomyocyte as it relates to calcium homeostasis has been addressed previously. This section addresses these aspects in greater detail, as well as the maturation of additional subcellular components. Most of the knowledge of ultrastructural maturation derives from animal studies, and the timing in humans is often not yet defined.

Subcellular Structures

Sarcolemmal Ion Channels

Numerous voltage-dependent and ligand-gated ion channels reside in the sarcolemma, and a full discussion far exceeds the space available in this chapter. Although developmental changes in the inward sodium current have been noted in several species, there appear to be few developmental changes in the human atrium (Sakakibara et al., 1992). A variety of inward and outward potassium channels exists. Although developmental changes have been documented, methodologic differences and differences among species do not allow application to human development (Sanchez-Chapula et al., 1994; Xie et al., 1997; Morrissey et al., 2005). Na^+,K^+ ATPase maintains the sodium gradient across the cell and is inhibited by the cardiac glycosides, such as digitalis. There are developmental changes in the isoform distribution of the enzyme subunits, and this enzyme has less activity in immature myocardium. Calcium handling is crucial to myocardial contraction. Calcium channel (I_{ca}) density increases two to threefold in the developing rabbit, although the voltage sensitive activation is similar to that of humans (Osaka, 1991; Huynh et al., 1992; Wetzel et al., 1993). In one study of human atrial myocytes (presumably from ill children), younger hearts had decreased calcium channel density, and in another study, more rapid inactivation of calcium current was evident (Hatem et al., 1995; Roca et al., 1996). However, in the realm of human myocardial development, many of these hearts were fairly mature when studied. The Na^+–Ca^+ exchanger, which can serve to bring calcium either into or out of the cell, has higher activity in immature myocardium in a variety of species (Artman et al., 1995). This is a purported source of additional calcium entry into the contractile apparatus in immature myocardial cells that have relatively deficient sarcoplasmic reticulum. There is increased activity of the Na^+–H^+ exchanger in immature myocardium, and this has been implicated as a factor in the greater resistance of immature myocardium to acidosis (Downing et al., 1966; Haworth et al., 1997).

Transverse Tubules

Transverse tubules, or *T-tubules,* invaginations of the sarcolemma in ventricular, but not atrial, myocardial cells have been mentioned in the discussion of myocardial performance. They allow transmission of the action potential, with its attendant ion shifts, to all parts of the cell, which allows rapid activation of the entire cell. T-tubules are thus a required component of larger cells (Gotoh, 1983). Maturation of T-tubules is associated with the increased size of mature myocardial cells, with the sarcolemmal calcium channels further from the contractile apparatus. Species that have a relatively mature myocardium at birth have well-developed T-tubules at birth, whereas animals with immature myocardium at birth do not. T-tubules first appear at about 30 weeks gestation in humans (Kim et al., 1992).

Mitochondria

Mitochondria increase in size, relative volume, and internal compactness and complexity during myocardial development, and their growth may continue into the postnatal period (Barth et al., 1992). In some species, maturation is postnatal. Maturation of mitochondria mirrors the shift from a primary carbohydrate energy source of immature myocardium to the primary long-chain free fatty-acid energy source of mature myocardium (Fisher et al., 1980, 1981).

Cytoskeleton

An intracellular construction of microtubules and microfilaments links the contractile elements, T-tubules, sarcolemma, mitochondria, and nucleus. This scaffolding organizes the subcellular components that participate in cell signaling and allows transmission of the force of contraction to be applied to the myocyte. Mutations in several of these can be responsible for several familial cardiomyopathic conditions. The cytoskeleton not only undergoes modification with myocardial development, but microfilaments also play a role in the adaptive response to mechanical loading of the heart (Small et al., 1992; van der Loop et al., 1995; Schroder et al., 2002). One of the most important roles of the cytoskeleton is to link the thick filaments. Titin, the largest protein in the human, extends from the Z-disc to the M-line of the sarcomere. It both aligns the thick filament and has a spring-like function that determines passive tension. Titin isoforms are under developmental regulation, with fetal myocardium having the more compliant N2BA isoform, which is then replaced with the stiffer isoforms. The conversion of isoforms is species dependent, but it correlates with the shift from the more compliant fetal myocardial cells (when studied removed from the surrounding matrix) to the less compliant cells of the adult.

Sarcoplasmic Reticulum

The tubular network of SR regulates intracytosolic calcium concentration. The ryanodine receptor is located in the SR, as are a variety of proteins and channels that regulate calcium. Calcium regulation by the SR is critically important for the release of calcium (contraction) and its re-uptake (diastole). In the mature cardiac myocyte, the SR is the primary source of calcium to the cell. The amount of SR is significantly reduced in immature myocardium, as are indices of SR function, in a variety of species (Maylie, 1982; Nakanishi et al., 1987; Nassar et al., 1987).

Contractile Proteins

These proteins compose the thin filaments of the I-band (actin, the troponin complex and tropomyosin) and the thick filaments (myosin and titin) are composed of contractile proteins. All of these proteins have developmentally regulated changes in isoform expression. Additionally, their expression is specific to cell type (e.g., cardiac vs. noncardiac or atrial vs. ventricular) and is regulated by physiologic signaling, such as thyroid hormone or diabetes (Baum et al., 1989).

Myosin

Myosin is the most abundant contractile protein and is responsible for transducing chemical energy (ATP) into mechanical energy. It is composed of two heavy and two light chains. Different heavy-chain myosin isoforms have different ATPase activity, conferring different calcium sensitivity. Developmental changes in myosin are species specific. In humans, the V3 isoform is most common in the fetus (90% at 30 weeks, gestation), decreases in the neonate, and reaccumulates beginning in the second month of life to become predominant in the adult. The V3 isoform, consisting of two β heavy chains, has the lowest ATPase activity of the various myosin types and consumes less ATP for the same amount of force generation (Cummins et al., 1980). Atrial myosin, with its briefer contraction, is primarily the V1 isoform (consisting of two α heavy chains). Regulation of the myosin heavy chain is at the transcriptional level and appears to account, at least in part, for the rapid conditioning of a ventricle after the placement of a pulmonary artery band (Lompre et al., 1984). The myosin light chain, located near the head of the heavy chain, has a variety of subunits that regulate myosin ATPase activity and that are also under developmental regulation.

Actin

The thin filament consists of two intertwined bands of actin monomers. Both skeletal and cardiac forms of actin are present during human cardiac development. In the early embryonic heart the skeletal form predominates (more than 80%). The cardiac form is present in the early stages of heart tube development and gradually increases. The onset of rhythmic contraction coincides with the disappearance of the skeletal isoform. In humans, cardiac actin increases to approximately 50% in the first decade, but the physiologic implication of this shift is not known (Boheler et al., 1991). Skeletal actin rapidly increases after the imposition of an acute pressure load to the ventricle before declining slowly.

Tropomyosin

Tropomyosin lies in the groove between the two actin bands and, depending on its deformation by troponin, either permits or prevents the interaction of actin and myosin. There are two isomers, and the isomer distribution depends on the intrinsic heart rate (and therefore the species). In humans, the amount of β isoform increases from 5% in the fetal ventricle to 10% in the adult, but the physiologic implication of this shift is not known (Humphreys and Cummins, 1984).

Troponins

The three distinct but functionally coupled proteins of the troponin complex (troponins T, C, and I) confer calcium sensitivity to actin-myosin cross-bridge formation, and each has multiple developmental and species specificity (Anderson et al., 1991). Troponin T binds the complex to tropomyosin troponin C binds calcium; and troponin I regulates the interaction of the complex with tropomyosin, binding to troponin C during systole and to actin during diastole. Four forms of cardiac troponin T are present in the human as the result of alternative splicing of a single gene, and their expression is developmentally regulated (Anderson et al., 1991). All isoforms are expressed in the fetal heart, but only one (cTnT3) is expressed in the adult. In failing human hearts, including those of children, cTnT1 and cTnT4 are upregulated (Saba et al., 1996). These isoform shifts likely affect contractility, as they modify the calcium sensitivity of the contractile apparatus. Troponin I has both cardiac and slow skeletal forms. Both are found in fetal hearts. Approximately 70% of troponin I is the skeletal form, but the isoform shift to the adult form of troponin I (all cardiac) is complete in the human by 9 months of age (Sasse et al., 1993). Phosphorylation of the cardiac isoform, but not the skeletal isoform, decreases the sensitivity of troponin C and the myofilament for calcium, as well as the affinity of troponin I for troponin C, with both decreases altering contractile performance. The slow skeletal form of troponin I in neonates may contribute to the resistance of the neonatal myofilament to deactivation at acid pH, perhaps contributing to the greater recovery of neonatal myocardium from an acidotic insult (Solaro et al., 1986). Although there are several isoforms of troponin C, only the cardiac isoform is expressed in cardiac muscle.

Myocardial Energy

Newborn sheep have a higher myocardial oxygen consumption than adult sheep. These metabolic demands of the developing heart are met by a capillary network of higher density than that found in adults (Fisher et al., 1982).

The immature myocardium uses lactate as a primary energy source. This is in contrast to the mature myocardium, where fatty acids are the primary energy source. To be metabolized, fatty acids must first be transported into the mitochondria. This is accomplished by carnitine palmitoyl-CoA transferase. Activity of this enzyme is reduced in the immature myocardium, suggesting the necessity of carbohydrate as the primary energy source (Fisher et al., 1980, 1981).

Electrophysiology

The sinus node can initially be identified as a horseshoe-shaped structure at the lateral junction of the superior vena cava and the right atrium. As the heart develops, it assumes the elongated spindle shape that is seen in the mature heart. Using voltage-sensitive dyes, spontaneous cellular depolarization has been observed prior to the development of contractile function. Although spontaneous depolarization is also seen in the developing atrium and bulboventricular portion, cells that are destined to form the sinus node have a higher intrinsic rate of depolarization (Pickoff, 2007).

Discrete connections between the sinus node and the atrioventricular (AV) node are a matter for debate. The lack of an identified cell type insulated from the surrounding atrial myocardium has been considered evidence of a lack of specialized internodal conducting pathways (Anderson et al., 1981). Preferential conduction along bands of atrial myo-

cytes in the anterior septum may be to the result of a more organized cellular alignment (Racker, 1989). More recent evidence from studies of developing human hearts has demonstrated three internodal pathways identified by antibody staining (Blom et al., 1999).

Functional changes in the electrophysiologic properties of the atrium have been described. Action potential duration in human neonates is shorter than in adults. This is relevant in that it may explain the highest incidence in childhood of atrial arrhythmias in the fetus and neonate (Pickoff, 2007). Once these dysrhythmias are terminated in the newborn, there is a low incidence of recurrence.

Delay in contraction between the atrium and ventricle is seen before the development of the AV node. Action-potential recordings from the AV canal area of the developing chicken heart demonstrate characteristics that are to be expected of slowing areas of conduction—namely, a slow rate of rise and a prolonged duration. These characteristics are further linked to differential expression of acetylcholinesterase. Expression is higher in the AV canal region compared with expression in the free wall of the atrium or ventricle (Mikawa and Hurtado, 2007; Pickoff, 2007).

AV nodal cells are distinct from the other embryonic myocardial cells. They have differential expression of calcium-regulatory proteins and membrane channels (Mikawa and Hurtado, 2007). Formation of the AV node is an incompletely understood complex series of events that likely involve modulation by the gene *NKx2-5* (Mikawa and Hurtado, 2007; Briggs et al., 2008).

Formation of the Purkinje system is an area of active investigation. Purkinje-like function is seen after cardiac looping (Pickoff, 2007). However, the network is still developing in the fetal heart. Studies suggest a paracrine interaction between the fetal myocardium and the cardiac endothelial cells. Purkinje fiber development is seen primarily in two sites, periarterially and subendocardially. Phenotypical recruitment of a beating myocyte to a conduction fiber is thought to be modulated by endothelin-1 (ET-1). The ET-1–induced expression of conduction-tissue markers in myocytes is dependent on dosage and inhibited by ET-1 antagonists (Mikawa and Hurtado, 2007). Exposure of myocytes to ET-1 is also associated with downward regulation of markers found primarily on muscle cells.

In chicken embryos, conduction velocities increase with age and are related to the emergence of fast-conducting sodium channels (Shigenobu and Sperelakis, 1971; Pickoff, 2007). Findings have been similar in mammalian systems (Rosen et al., 1981; Pickoff, 2007). Of note is the maintenance of conduction slowing from atrium to ventricle seen in the primitive heart. In a canine model, measurement of AV-nodal conduction demonstrated that conduction was faster in immature hearts, but the AV node, not the ventricular myocardium, remained the site of conduction slowing with differential atrial pacing (McCormack et al., 1988).

Through fetal magnetocardiography, conduction times have been noted to increase with gestational age (Kahler et al., 2002; Stinstra et al., 2002; van Leeuwen et al., 2004). This is thought to be related to myocardial growth (van Leeuwen et al., 2004). Intracardiac conduction times have been measured in children and compared with those in adults. There were no age-related differences in atrial, AV-nodal, or His Purkinje-conduction times (Gillette et al., 1975).

Central Nervous System Regulation of Cardiovascular Function

The regulation of cardiac output and blood flow is controlled by neural and circulation mechanisms. Neural regulation is accomplished by modulating the output through the sympathetic and parasympathetic nervous systems in response to input from receptors in the heart and vasculature. Hormonal regulation occurs by receptor stimulation by circulating molecules.

The autonomic nervous system is developed in the human by about 27 weeks' gestation. Parasympathetic innervation precedes sympathetic innervation (Fig. 4-19). In sheep, at least, the postnatal increase in contractile function with adrenergic stimulation is a consequence of higher resting adrenergic tone rather than a maturation of the myocardium (Teitel et al., 1985). The β-adrenergic/adenylate cyclase system develops during fetal life. The density of the β-adrenergic receptor density peaks at term and declines postnatally, mirroring the maturation of cardiac sympathetic innervation. Calcium channels in neonatal myocardium do, however, respond less to β-adrenergic stimulation than they do in the adult, and isoproterenol stimulation of adenyl cyclase is blunted in the late fetus and neonate (Osaka and Joyner, 1992). In the late term fetus and the neonate, coupling of the β-receptor and adenylate cyclase may be decreased, because differential β-adrenergic response to isoproterenol and forskolin, a direct activator of adenylate cyclase, has been observed (Schumacher et al., 1982; Tanaka and Shigenobu, 1990). This finding may help explain the decreased response of calcium channels to β-adrenergic stimulation in the neonatal myocardium (Baum and Palmisano, 1997).

The sinoatrial node is sensitive to β-adrenergic stimulation in the fetus before the development of ventricular sensitivity, and this sensitivity tends to parallel the development of autonomic innervation to these regions of the heart.

Vagal myelination in humans continues through the fetal period and reaches adult levels by about 50 weeks postconceptual age (Sachis et al., 1982). In humans, parasympathetic input to the heart is from the superior, inferior, and thoracic branches of the vagus nerve (Hildreth et al., 2009). The relative balance of sympathetic and parasympathetic stimulation is reflected in the decreasing mean heart rate as a child reaches adolescence.

The aortic arch and carotid bodies have baroreceptors that provide the afferent limb of the feedback circuit. Stimulation of these receptors sends impulses to the cardioinhibitory and vasomotor centers of the medulla. In turn, the efferent signals result in decreased blood pressure, vasodilation, and slowing of the heart rate. Arterial baroreflexes are present and operational in healthy and critically ill human neonates; human neonates, even preterm neonates, have well-developed vagally mediated cardiac responses to hypoxemia and other stimuli, although the course of maturation is unclear (Thoresen et al., 1991; Buckner et al., 1993). Decreasing sensitivity in studies of awake animals suggests a decreasing role for heart rate in the control of blood pressure in aging animals (Palmisano et al., 1990).

Stretch receptors in the myocardium also provide afferent signals to the central nervous system. Within the atrium there are two types of stretch receptors. Type A receptors are sensitive to pressure and are activated by atrial systole. Type B receptors are sensitive to volume and fire during ventricular systole. They have opposing effects on the sympathetic nervous system, with Type A receptors stimulating sympathetic activity. Secretion of vasopressin is inhibited by stimulation of stretch receptors. Stretch receptors are also found in the ventricular myocardium and when activated cause hypotension and bradycardia (Teitel et al., 2007).

Pulmonary Vascular Development

The pulmonary vasculature is a unique low-flow, high-pressure system *in utero* that must convert to a high-flow, low-pressure system after birth. In the absence of shunts, the right and left sides of the heart are connected through the pulmonary vasculature, which becomes the major determinant of right-ventricular afterload and left-ventricular preload. Effective cardiopulmonary interactions are crucial for a smooth transition to postnatal life. Primary lung problems, such as severe meconium aspiration or respiratory distress syndrome, through their effects on the pulmonary vasculature, can severely stress the heart. Congenital heart disease causes abnormalities of pulmonary blood flow, which can profoundly influence the pulmonary vasculature in its transition to postnatal life. This section begins with a review of normal pulmonary vascular development and concludes with a discussion of the changes present in pulmonary arterial hypertension.

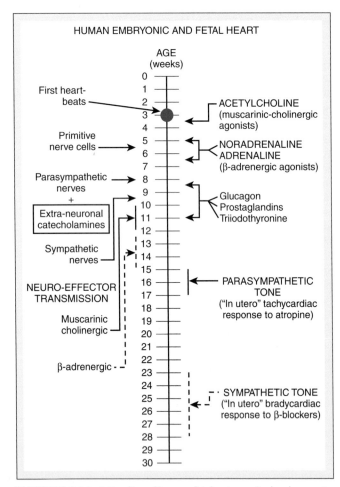

■ **FIGURE 4-19.** A timeline of human fetal autonomic development. *(From Papp JG: Autonomic responses and neurohumeral control in the early antenatal heart,* Basic Res Cardiol *83:2, 1988.)*

Pulmonary vessels are described by their relation to the bronchioles. Terminal bronchioles are the smallest purely conductive airways. Beyond them lie respiratory bronchioles, with dual conductive and gas-exchange functions, and then more distally, the alveolar units. Resistance in the pulmonary vasculature is at the level of the small pulmonary arteries (approximately fifth to sixth generation), which are defined as preacinar if they are proximal to the terminal bronchioles and intraacinar if they course parallel to the respiratory bronchioles and alveolar units. Conductive airways and preacinar arteries are fully present by 16 weeks' gestation (Hislop and Reid, 1973). There is a thickened muscular layer in the medial wall of preacinar vessels, most prominent at the fifth and sixth generation arteries (Hlastala et al., 1998). Beyond the preacinar arteries there is a transition zone of vessels at the level of the respiratory bronchioles with incomplete muscularization in the medial layer. The medial layer of these incompletely muscularized vessels contains pericytes (mesenchymal cells capable of differentiation) and precursor smooth muscle cells. Compared with a complete muscular layer, partial muscularization is believed necessary to aid the gas exchange function of respiratory bronchioles because alveolar development at birth is very immature. Arteries associated with immature alveoli are completely free of a muscular medial layer at birth.

The developing pulmonary vasculature must be of a caliber that can accommodate the enormous increase in postnatal blood flow without a damaging rise in pressure. In a setting of low blood flow, the pulmonary vasculature grows normally but retains a high resistance because of increased vascular tone. The increased vascular tone is primarily modulated by hypoxemia. Expansion of the lungs and a rise in alveolar oxygen tension after birth leads to the marked vasodilation of small arteries required to accept the increase in blood flow. Normal volume, low pressure pulmonary blood flow in the newborn period begins a process of regression of the muscular medial layer of the small arteries. Morphologically recognizable alveoli develop over the first 2 months of postnatal life with continued development until 18 months of age. After this, growth of existing alveoli continues until late childhood. The sparse numbers of alveoli at birth are associated with nonmuscularized intraacinar arteries. The rapid period of alveolar development is matched by growth of new intraacinar arteries. Both existing and new intraacinar arteries develop a thin, muscular medial layer. Thus, the process of normal pulmonary vascular development involves both the regression of muscularity in preacinar existing vessels and the growth of new intraacinar vessels that acquire a thin muscular layer. Disturbances of flow or pressure during this time can have profound consequences.

Diseases that affect normal pulmonary blood flow patterns have far-reaching consequences. In fetuses with abnormal restriction of pulmonary blood flow, there is often hypoplasia of the pulmonary arterial system. The degree of hypoplasia can be mild to fulminant, with atresia of all or parts of the pulmonary arterial system. For example, with tetralogy of Fallot, the level of pulmonary outflow obstruction is typically in the infundibulum of the right ventricular outflow tract. The resulting decrease in pulmonary blood flow affects the main and branch pulmonary arteries, which can be variably hypoplastic. Despite being hypoplastic, the vasculature has the ability to remodel and grow with improved blood flow. In patients who receive an early modified Blalock-Taussig shunt that provides augmentation of pulmonary blood flow, growth of the pulmonary arteries

is seen. Also, in patients with hypoplastic pulmonary arteries, patch augmentation can result in reversal of pulmonary artery hypoplasia (Agnoletti et al., 2004).

Disruption of normal pulmonary vasculature has also been observed when the perturbation to pulmonary flow is on the venous side. In hypoplastic left heart syndrome, blood returning to the left atrium must cross over to the right atrium via the foramen ovale. If the foramen ovale is widely patent, blood returning via the pulmonary veins to the left atrium is shunted across to the right atrium. Right-sided structures are often enlarged to accommodate the flow. However, if the patent foramen ovale is restrictive, pulmonary venous pressure rises and development of the pulmonary arterial vasculature is compromised. There is pressure rather than volume stress on the pulmonary vasculature. At birth, the increase in pulmonary blood flow with lung expansion leads quickly to left-atrial hypertension, compromising pulmonary blood flow and resulting in severe hypoxemia. Even if the emergent situation is optimally treated, surgical mortality remains high. At autopsy, the pulmonary veins of these infants are thickened and "arterialized" (Rychik et al., 1999). In juxtaposition to the pulmonary hypoplasia seen in patients with reduced pulmonary blood flow, patients with increased pulmonary blood flow may develop enlarged pulmonary arteries. In an uncommon variant of tetralogy of Fallot, the pulmonary valve is absent, resulting in free pulmonary insufficiency. This increased volume of blood flowing back and forth through the main and branch pulmonary arteries leads to massive dilation.

PVR decreases to near adult levels over the first 2 months of life. During these early months of life the concepts of pulmonary resistance and pulmonary reactivity are well demonstrated. Compared with the in utero state, resistance in young infants is low, though not quite yet at adult levels. However, the pulmonary reactivity is high, because the muscular pulmonary vasculature retains an impressive ability to increase vascular tone. By age 4 to 6 months, if the pulmonary vasculature has developed normally, both resistance and reactivity are low. The appropriate regression of the muscular layer of small pulmonary arteries leaves a healthy older infant unable to mount significant pulmonary hypertension. The contrast with the neonate is striking. Stressed by surgery that involves cardiopulmonary bypass or by pulmonary insults (such as respiratory distress syndrome or meconium aspiration) the neonate's reactive pulmonary vasculature is primed for a dangerous pulmonary hypertensive crisis.

The most common scenario of altered postnatal pulmonary blood flow occurs in patients with left-to-right shunts. Despite the increased pulmonary blood flow in the first few months of life, PVR continues to fall, leading to even greater pulmonary blood flow. The consequence of increased flow through the same cross-sectional vascular area is pulmonary hypertension. Because resistance is defined as pressure divided by flow, the diagnosis of pulmonary hypertension is not synonymous with increased PVR. The pulmonary vasculature accepts the increased blood flow at the expense of a rise in pressure. Resistance only increases when pressure remains high and pulmonary blood flow falls. Untreated, the natural result of this situation is a condition of pulmonary hypertension, elevated PVR, and fixed, irreversible pulmonary vascular disease. This is known as Eisenmenger's syndrome. In 1897, Dr. Eisenmenger described a 32-year-old male with cyanosis and exercise intolerance who died from massive hemoptysis (Eisenmenger, 1897).

The autopsy revealed a large ventricular septal defect (VSD) and overriding aorta. It was the first demonstration of congenital heart disease causing pulmonary vascular changes.

The normal process of pulmonary vascular remodeling consists of a reduction in the thickness of the muscular layer in preacinar small pulmonary arteries. Simultaneously, there is development of new intraacinar arteries and growth of existing intraacinar arteries that acquire a thin, muscular layer. The overall cross-sectional area of the pulmonary vasculature increases in concert with alveolar growth and development. Persistent high pulmonary blood flow from left-to-right shunting profoundly alters this process. The thickened muscular medial layer of small pulmonary arteries persists instead of involuting. In the transition zone of the respiratory bronchioles, precursor cells transform into vascular smooth muscle. Increased blood flow induces a shear stress in the pulmonary bed. Although felt to be a protective mechanism, this induces a reactive process that stimulates the muscularization of the pulmonary arteries and reduces the capacity for vasodilation. Development of new acinar arteries is impaired. Pulmonary artery pressure remains elevated. With persistent pulmonary hypertension, there are progressive changes in the pulmonary arteries that have been histologically characterized.

Heath and Edwards (1958) first described the following histologic changes in the pulmonary vasculature that are created by excessive blood flow and pressure:

- Stage I: Medial hypertrophy (reversible)
- Stage II: Cellular intimal hyperplasia in an abnormally muscular artery (reversible)
- Stage III: Lumen occlusion from intimal hyperplasia of fibroelastic tissue (partially reversible)
- Stage IV: Arteriolar dilation and medial thinning (irreversible)
- Stage V: Plexiform lesion, an angiomatoid formation (terminal and irreversible)
- Stage VI: Fibrinoid/necrotizing arteritis (terminal and irreversible)

Abnormal pulmonary vascular remodeling begins at birth if there is excessive pulmonary blood flow (Hall and Haworth, 1992). The Heath and Edwards scale is prognostic but limited, because pathologic stages are not correlated with clinical parameters. Rabinovitch overcame this problem by correlating pathologic severity with the hemodynamic state and assigning a simple three-stage grading system (Rabinovitch, 1999):

- Grade A: Extension of muscle into normally nonmuscularized vessels. This occurs because precursor cells in distal small pulmonary arteries differentiate into vascular smooth muscle. Pulmonary blood flow is increased but pulmonary artery pressure is not.
- Grade B: Medial hypertrophy of proximal muscular arteries. There are hyperplasia and hypertrophy of vascular smooth muscle. The mean pulmonary-artery pressure is elevated. Grade B made be further classified as mild or severe, depending on the thickness of the medial wall.
- Grade C: Reduction in the number of distal vessels. The vasculature is unable to keep up with the growth of alveolar units. There may also be loss of distal vessels due to luminal occlusion.

Grade A or mild grade B changes are histologically equivalent to Heath-Edwards Stage I. Grade C changes are associated with Heath-Edwards stage II or III and the possibility of irreversible changes in the pulmonary vasculature. Severe grade B or grade C disease is predictive of postoperative pulmonary hypertensive problems after surgery to repair the defect (Rabinovitch et al., 1984).

Any discussion of the pulmonary vasculature would be incomplete without exploring the role of the endothelium. Far from being a passive structure, modern understanding of the endothelium has evolved to recognize its singular place in the regulation of vascular tone (Rabinovitch, 1999). Exposure to high flow has multiple negative effects. Endothelial barrier function is compromised, which leads to the release of growth factors that increase vascular smooth muscle and deposition of subendothelial matrix proteins. Luminal diameter eventually decreases with superimposed increased vascular reactivity. Normally antithrombogenic, damaged endothelium reacts abnormally with marginating platelets, resulting in activation of the coagulation system. The endothelium is a key source of the endogenous vasodilators prostacyclin and nitric oxide. When subjected to high flow and shear stress, the release of the endogenous vasodilators is increased, but it may not be enough of an increase to counteract the increased vascular reactivity when pulmonary blood flow is high.

ASSESSMENT OF THE CARDIOVASCULAR SYSTEM

The evaluation of a pediatric patient for anesthesia requires knowledge of age-appropriate history, physical findings, and laboratory data. Age correction is implicit in all facets of the cardiovascular examination. A heart rate of 110 beats per minute in a 6-month-old infant, for example, is normal, not "sinus tachycardia, normal for age," as one often sees when cardiovascular data are reported by adult cardiologists. This section relates to the examination of the child with a nominally healthy and normal cardiovascular system (see Chapter 36, Systemic Disorders; issues of the child with congenital heart disease are discussed in Chapter 20, Anesthesia for Congenital Heart Surgery).

History

One of the most basic indicators of adequate cardiac function is age-appropriate exercise tolerance. In infants, heart failure is marked by a history of tachypnea and diaphoresis, particularly with feeding. A history of cyanosis may be abnormal or may be a normal finding. Many healthy infants develop acrocyanosis or perioral cyanosis with crying or cold.

Physical Examination

"Failure to thrive" is determined by plotting patient data on weight, height, and head circumference growth charts. Specific growth charts are available, for example, for children with Down syndrome, where normal growth may not mirror that of the population at large (Cronk et al., 1988). More important than the current position on growth charts is the child's trajectory. The tenth percentile may be adequate for an individual patient. However, it becomes worrisome if the child's growth had previously been recorded at the fiftieth percentile. In general, me conditions causing failure to thrive will result first in loss of weight, followed by loss of height, preserving head circumference if at all possible. Certain metabolic disorders, however, show a preferential loss in height first.

Vital signs need to be corrected for age, as indicated above. Normal values for heart rate, respiratory rate, and blood pressure are shown in Tables 4-1 and 4-2 and Figures 4-20 and 4-21. Blood pressure cuffs need to be appropriately sized to avoid artifact. Although it was originally taught that the cuff width should be approximately two-thirds the length of the humerus, the current recommendation is now similar to that for adults. The width of the cuff should be approximately 40% to 50% of the circumference (approximately 125% to 155% of the diameter) of the limb where the pressure is being measured and long enough to approximately encircle it. The cardiovascular physical examination begins with inspection, and proceeds to palpation and then auscultation.

Inspection

Is the chest symmetric? Is there jugular venous distention? Jugular venous distention is unlikely be observed in infants with short, fat necks. Is there cyanosis? Is there clubbing of the fingers?

TABLE 4-1. Normal Respiratory Rates in Children

Age	Respiratory Rate (min⁻¹)
Birth-6 weeks	45-60
6 weeks-2 years	40
2-6 years	30
6-10 years	25
> 10 years	20

TABLE 4-2. Acceptable Ranges of Heart Rates (Beats/Min)

	Awake	Asleep	Exercise/Fever
Newborn	100-180	80-160	<220
1 week-3 months	100-220	80-200	<220
3 months-2 years	80-150	70-120	<200
2-10 years	70-110	60-90	<200
> 10 years	55-90	50-90	<200

Data from Adams FH, Emmanouilides GC, editors: *Moss' heart disease in infants, children, and adolescents*, ed 3, Baltimore, 1983, Williams and Wilkins.

Palpation

Is the precordium quiet? Is there a palpable thrill? Are the arterial pulses symmetric without radial-femoral delay (suggesting coarctation of the aorta)? Where is the liver palpated? The liver is normally palpable 1 to 2 cm below the right costal margin in the midclavicular line in infants, and is a window to the central venous pressure. As central venous pressure increases, the liver edge descends reliably.

Auscultation

Are the lungs clear without wheezing or rales, both of which could result from cardiac dysfunction? Are there any murmurs? Murmurs are almost universally heard in all children at some point, as heart sounds readily transmit through the thinner pediatric thorax. The differentiation between functional (innocent) murmurs and pathologic murmurs is often easy, but it can at times be challenging. A further discussion of murmurs is included in Chapter 36, Systemic Disorders. Figure 4-22 summarizes the changes in heart rate, cardiac output (CO), and stroke volume (SV) that occur in childhood.

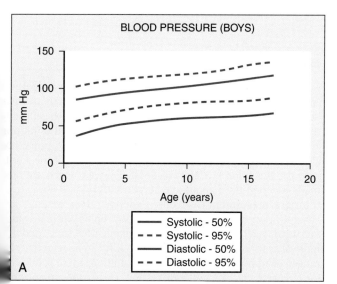
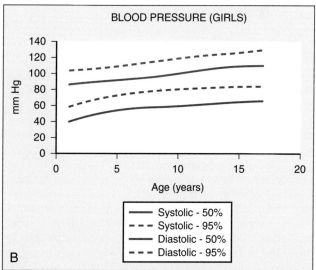

FIGURE 4-20. Normal resting blood pressures in boys **(A)** and girls **(B)** aged 1 to 17 years. Pressures reflect those in children at the fiftieth percentile for height. Blood pressure varies slightly in children who are significantly taller (several mm Hg higher) or shorter (several mm Hg lower). Blood pressures also do not reflect normal values obtained when children are under anesthesia. *(Data from National High Blood Pressure Education Program Working Group on High Blood Pressure in Children and Adolescents:* The fourth report on the diagnosis, evaluation, and treatment of high blood pressure in children and adolescents. *Available at www.nhlbi.nih.gov/guidelines/hypertension/child_tbl.htm.)*

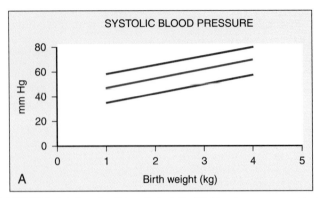
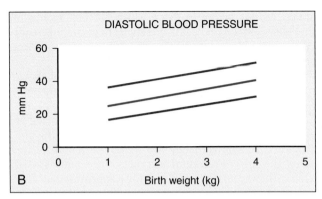

■ **FIGURE 4-21.** Systolic **(A)** and diastolic **(B)** blood pressures on the first day of life. Data are shown as the regression line and 95% confidence limits. *(Data from Versmold HT, et al.: Aortic blood pressure during the first 12 hours of life in infants with birth weight 610 to 4,220 grams.* Pediatrics, *67:607, 1981.)*

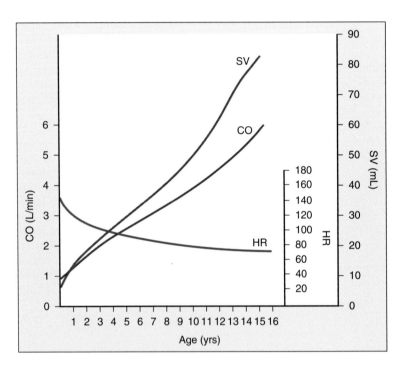

■ **FIGURE 4-22.** Changes in cardiac output *(CO)*, stroke volume *(SV)*, and heart rate *(HR)* with age. *(From Rudolph AM, editor:* Congenital diseases of the heart, *Chicago, 1974, Mosby.)*

Chest Radiograph

Evidence of heart disease on the routine chest radiograph includes cardiomegaly (heart failure or large left-to-right shunts), decreased pulmonary blood flow (right-to-left shunts), abnormal cardiac silhouette (small pulmonary artery segment with tetralogy of Fallot), widened angle at the carina (large left atrium), pruning (decreased peripheral pulmonary arteries, as in pulmonary arterial hypertension), and rib notching (in children over about age 5 years with coarctation). Artifacts are more commonly seen in children. Given the inability of young children to cooperate, films taken during exhalation are more common in children, and the cardiac silhouette may appear artifactually large (Fig. 4-23). Although the lungs may appear abnormally small in an expiratory film, a more sensitive finding on a film taken in exhalation is buckling of the trachea. The shadow of a normal large thymus in infants can overlay the heart shadow, tempting a diagnosis of cardiomegaly. Sometimes a "sail sign" can be seen at the inferolateral border of the thymus, where it separates from the cardiac shadow, clearly identifying it as the thymus and not the heart (Fig. 4-24).

Electrocardiogram

Normal values of the electrocardiogram are dependent on age and heart rate. With development and growth, neonatal right-ventricular predominance is replaced with left ventricular predominance, the heart rate slows, and all durations and intervals lengthen. Between the ages of 3 and 8 years, the electrocardiogram of a child looks similar to that of the adult with the exception of right precordial T waves, which are normally inverted until about age 10 years. Upright T waves over the right precordium in children younger than 10 years are an indication of right ventricular hypertrophy. Normal values for heart rate, QRS width, frontal-plane QRS axis, and P interval are shown in Tables 4-3 and 4-4. It can be seen that the ranges of normal are fairly wide. In addition, these values are for children who are awake or resting. Heart rates in anesthetized children are likely to be somewhat lower. The QT interval (QTc), corrected by Bazett's formula (QTc = QT/$\sqrt{\text{R - R interval}}$) has an upper limit of normal of 0.44 seconds in infants and children 6 months of age and older. The upper limit of normal is 0. seconds in the first week of life and 0.45 in the first 6 months.

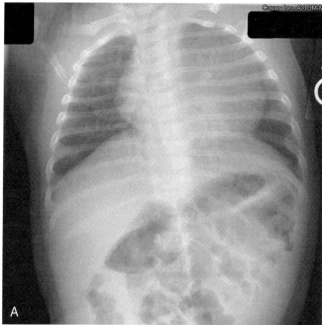

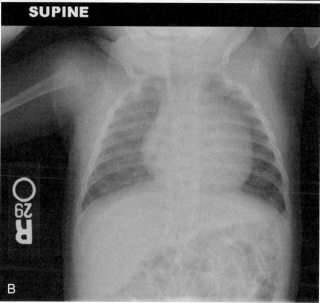

FIGURE 4-23. A, Apparent cardiomegaly that is really an artifact of an expiratory film (and a large thymus). **B,** A repeat film taken shortly thereafter shows a normal cardiac size.

Cardiac Catheterization

A cardiac catheterization includes one or more of the following:

Anatomic diagnosis: This is done with a combination of hemodynamic data and angiographic evaluation. Radiographic contrast is injected through a catheter with its tip near the region of interest.

Hemodynamic data: Measures are made of oxygen saturation and pressure in the various cardiac chambers and great vessels. From these, indicators of cardiovascular function can be derived (see below).

Response to vasodilators: Hemodynamic measures are repeated in the absence and presence of a vasodilator, typically a pulmonary vasodilator such as nitric oxide or

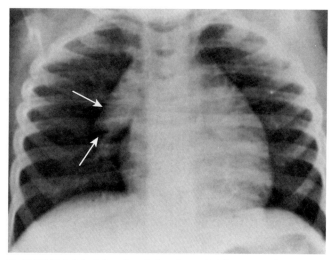

FIGURE 4-24. A thymic sail sign *(arrows)*. When seen, this can aid in differentiation of true cardiomegaly from a large thymic shadow. *(From Keats TE, Anderson MW: Atlas of Roentgen variants that may simulate disease, Philadelphia, 2007, Mosby.)*

oxygen, to evaluate the responsiveness of the pulmonary vasculature and to determine whether the patient is a surgical candidate.

Evaluation of arrhythmias: Several electrode catheters are placed in or near the right- and possibly left-sided chambers to map the locus and pathway of aberrant tracts (for example, Wolff-Parkinson-White syndrome or the site of an ectopic focus of an atrial or ventricular tachyarrhythmia). Attempts may be made to provoke the arrhythmia with electrical stimulation (a series of premature extrasystoles) or with drugs (isoproterenol).

Although major advances have been made in deriving physiologic measures of cardiac function by means of echocardiography and magnetic resonance imaging (MRI), cardiac catheterization remains the gold standard for many of these, in addition to providing images of radiologic anatomy and

TABLE 4-3. Normal Electrocardiogram Variables in Children

	Rate/min	QRS axis	QRS Duration (sec)
0-1 day	122 (94-155)	135 (59-189)	0.05 (0.02-0.07)
1-3 days	122 (91-158)	134 (64-197)	0.05 (0.02-0.07)
3-7 days	128 (90-166)	133 (76-191)	0.05 (0.02-0.07)
7-30 days	149 (106-182)	109 (70-160)	0.05 (0.02-0.08)
1-3 mo	149 (120-179)	75 (30-115)	0.05 (0.02-0.08)
3-6 mo	141 (105-185)	60 (7-105)	0.05 (0.02-0.08)
6-12 mo	131 (108-169)	55 (6-98)	0.05 (0.03-0.08)
1-3 yr	119 (89-152)	55 (7-102)	0.06 (0.03-0.08)
3-5 yr	109 (73-137)	56 (6-104)	0.06 (0.03-0.07)
5-8 yr	100 (65-133)	65 (10-139)	0.06 (0.03-0.08)
8-12 yr	91 (62-130)	60 (6-116)	0.06 (0.04-0.09)
12-16 yr	80 (60-120)	59 (9-128)	0.07 (0.04-0.09)

Data from Davignon A, Rautaharju P, Boisselle E, et al.: Normal ECG standards for infants and children, *Pediatr Cardiol* 1:123–131, 1979.

TABLE 4-4. Upper Limits of Normal for PR Interval (Sec)

Rate (min-1)	0-1 mo	1-6 mo	6-12 mo	1-3 yr	3-8 yr	8-12 yr	12-16 yr	Adult
<60						0.18	0.19	0.17
60-80					0.17	0.17	0.18	0.21
80-100	0.12				0.14	0.15	0.15	0.15
100-120	0.12			0.15	0.16	0.15	0.16	0.19
120-140	0.11	0.14	0.14	0.14	0.15	0.15		0.18
140-160	0.11	0.13	0.13	0.14	0.14			0.17
160-180	0.11	0.12	0.12	0.12				
>180	0.09	0.11	0.11					

Modified from Park MK, Guneroth WG: *How to read pediatric ECGs,* ed 4, Philadelphia, 2006, Mosby; original data from Davignon A, Rautaharju P, Boisselle E, et al.: Normal ECE standards for infants and children, *Pediatr Cardiol* 1:123–131, 1979.

function (Odegard et al., 2004). In addition, the number of interventional procedures performed or proposed is expanding, while the patient population is increasingly complex. New procedures, including stenting of a variety of vessels, closure of atrial and ventricular septal defects, percutaneous placement of prosthetic valves, and hybrid repairs of defects jointly in the catheterization laboratory by both cardiac surgeon and an interventional cardiologist have expanded therapeutic options for patients (Kapoor et al., 2006; Galantowicz et al., 2008; Lurz et al., 2008). Transvascular replacement of pulmonary and aortic valves is also on the near horizon. These increasingly complex procedures require the attendance of an anesthesiologist, and the care rendered transcends beyond keeping the child from moving. The physiologic state of children undergoing such procedures can be tenuous, and the anesthetic care is provided in an environment that is foreign to many anesthesiologists (Cua et al., 2007) (See Chapter 21, Anesthesia for Children with Congenital Heart Disease Undergoing Non-Cardiac Surgery, Closed Cardiac Procedures, and Cardiac Catheterization). The environment may become increasingly foreign, because there are proposals to develop MRI suites for cardiac catheterization procedures in order to lower the radiation exposure to patients. More and more complex electrophysiologic procedures are also being done, some of which can take many hours to complete. All of these factors have contributed to a general shift from sedation toward general anesthesia in the pediatric cardiac catheterization laboratory. Additionally, transesophageal echocardiography guidance is required for many of the procedures, which requires endotracheal intubation.

Over the years, cardiac catheterization has become safer despite the increasing complexity of the procedures. Beyond routine potential anesthetic complications, complications include cardiac perforation and arrhythmias from catheter manipulation, embolization of closure devices, hypothermia (readily addressed with forced-air warming mattresses) and brachial-plexus injury from positioning (cardiologists try to extend the arms over the head to remove the upper arms from the field of the lateral x-ray tube), and vascular complications. Femoral venous injury is marked by a bluish color to the leg, whereas femoral arterial insufficiency is marked by a cold, white leg. However, these are almost always transient.

Vitiello and colleagues (1998) studied pediatric cardiac catheterization laboratory complications in a consecutive series of almost 5000 patients. One or more complications occurred in 8.8% of children. Vascular complications were most common (in 3.8%) and death occurred in 0.14%, most commonly in infants. With the large introducer sheaths needed for many newer interventional procedures, one might expect the incidence of vascular complications to increase.

Hemodynamic Assessment

A complete cardiac catheterization includes measures of oxygen saturation and pressures in all the cardiac chambers and great vessels. From these, additional hemodynamic measures such as vascular resistance and cardiac index can be derived.

Pressure

Normal intracardiac pressures are shown in Tables 4-5 and 4-6. The difference between pressures obtained on both sides of a valve, referred to as the gradient, is obtained with two separate catheters, or more commonly by withdrawing a single catheter

TABLE 4-5. Normal Values of Intracardiac Cardiac and Vascular Pressures (in mm Hg)

Location	Term Newborns	Infants and Children
Right atrium	m = 0-4	a = 5-10 v = 4-8 m = 2-6
Right ventricle	35-50/1-5	15-25/2-5
Pulmonary artery	35-80/20-50 m = 25-60	15-25/8-12 10-6
Pulmonary wedge	m = 3-6	a = 6-12 v = 8-15 m = 5-10
Left atrium	m = 3-6	a = 6-12 v = 8-15 m = 5-10
Left ventricle		80-130/5-10
Systemic artery	65-80/45-60 m = 60-65	90-130/60-80 m = 70-95

Data from Rudolph AM: *Congenital Disease of the Heart,* Chicago, 1974, Mosby. *a,* A wave; *m,* mean; *v,* v wave.

TABLE 4-6. Normal Hemodynamic Variables Beyond Infancy

Location	Average	Range
Mean right atrial pressure (CVP) (mm Hg)	3	1-5
Right ventricle pressure (mm Hg)		
Systolic	25	17-32
Diastolic	5	1-7
Pulmonary artery pressure (mm Hg)		
Systolic	25	9-19
Diastolic	10	17-32
Mean	15	4-13
Mean pulmonary wedge pressure (mm Hg)	9	6-12
Mean left atrial pressure (mm Hg)	8	2-12
Cardiac index (L/min/m²)	3.5	2.5-4.2
Stroke volume index (mL/m²)	45	
Oxygen consumption (mL/min/m²)	150	110-150
Vascular resistance index		
Pulmonary (Wood units/m²)		1-3
Pulmonary (dynes•sec•cm⁻⁵•m²)		80-240
Systemic (Wood units/m²)		10-20
Systemic (dynes•sec•cm⁻⁵•m²)		800-1600

Data from Rudolph AM: *Congenital disease of the heart*, Chicago, 1974, Mosby.
Pressures are in mm Hg.

across the valve. Unlike valve area that is fixed (and can be measured by echocardiography or derived from hemodynamic data), the gradient varies depending on the cardiac output—the higher the output, the higher the gradient for a specific valve area. Similarly, the gradient for a fixed lesion can decrease in the face of falling cardiac output.

Oxygen Content and Saturation

Oxygen capacity refers to the maximum amount of oxygen that can be bound to hemoglobin. Oxygen content, the amount of oxygen transported in blood, is calculated as

$$[(1.34 \times \text{oxygen saturation} \times \text{patient's hemoglobin}) + (0.003 \times \text{Po}_2)]$$

where $(0.003 \times \text{Po}_2)$ reflects the amount of oxygen dissolved in plasma. This is the oxygen content in milliliters of oxygen per 100 mL of blood. Sometimes the content is referenced in milliliters per liter, in which case everything is multiplied by 10. Because the contribution of oxygen in plasma is small, this component is typically neglected in calculations done at physiologic Po_2. Oxygen saturation, the fraction of hemoglobin that is bound to oxygen, is readily measured in samples of blood from each cardiac chamber or vessel by oximetry.

Oxygen Consumption

Oxygen consumption is required to derive cardiac output by the Fick equation. Historically, oxygen consumption was measured by comparing the volume of oxygen in a timed sample of expiratory gas collected in a large (Douglas) bag with that inspired

over the same time (Rudolph, 2001). This is cumbersome and was replaced by a simpler method that uses a mouthpiece or a head hood, making it usable even in infants (Lister et al., 1974). In most centers, however, oxygen consumption ($\dot{V}O_2$) is simply derived from a nomogram that uses age, gender, and heart rate (LaFarge and Miettinen, 1970). In any event, after the immediate newborn period, oxygen consumption in the resting child is approximately 150 mL/min/m²; during the first 3 weeks of life, it is approximately 120-130 mL/min/m² (Rudolph, 2001). When a child is under general anesthesia, oxygen consumption reliably decreases (Table 4-7).

Cardiac Output

Cardiac output increases with increased size. Pediatric cardiologists, however, always normalize for body surface area (converting to cardiac index). Beyond the first week of life, cardiac index remains fairly constant at about 4 L/min/m². Older children and adults can have cardiac output that is readily measured in the catheterization laboratory by means of a pulmonary artery thermodilution catheter. However, small size and the presence of intracardiac shunts make this technique of less utility in pediatric cardiology. Other indicator dilution techniques, which historically preceded thermodilution, are generally obsolete and no longer used.

The method routinely used to measure cardiac output is the Fick principle, or the Fick equation. This states that in a state of equilibrium, blood flow through an organ is proportional to the amount of indicator taken up or added. In this specific modification of the indicator dilution technique, oxygen acts as the indicator. In the case of pulmonary blood flow, oxygen is added, and in the case of the systemic blood flow, oxygen is withdrawn. In a normal healthy person these must be equal, because the amount of oxygen consumed by the body must equal the amount delivered to the blood during its passage through the pulmonary circulation.

Cardiac output is derived from the Fick principle as follows:

$$\dot{Q} = \frac{I}{(C_{I_1} - C_{I_2})}$$

where $\dot{Q}$ is the flow rate, I is the amount of indicator added and CI_1 and CI_2 are the concentrations of indicator before and after the addition (or subtraction) of indicator I. Using oxygen extraction in the systemic circulation as the indicator:

$$\dot{Q} = \frac{\dot{V}O_2}{(CaO_2 - CmvO_2)}$$

where $\dot{V}O_2$ is oxygen consumption, CaO_2 is the content of oxygen in the systemic arteries and $Cmvo_2$ is the mixed venous oxygen content. $\dot{Q}$ now represents cardiac output. The units of $\dot{Q}$ are L/min, and the units of CaO_2 and $Cmvo_2$ are mL oxygen/L blood. However, in children, $\dot{V}O_2$ is typically expressed as mL/min/m², so that the resulting number represents cardiac index rather than cardiac output. Because pulmonary flow and systemic flow are almost identical in normal individuals, oxygen uptake across the pulmonary circulation provides identical results as oxygen consumption across the systemic circulation. When the components of oxygen content are substituted, the equation becomes:

$$\dot{Q} = \frac{\dot{V}O_2}{[(1.34 \times Hb \times sat_a) + (0.003 \times PaO_2) - (1.34 \times Hb \times sat_{mv}) + (0.003 \times PmvO_2)]}$$

TABLE 4-7. Oxygen Consumption Table (mL/min/m²)

Age	| Heart Rate (beats/min) 50	60	70	80	90	100	110	120	130	140	150	160	170
Male patients													
3				155	159	163	167	171	175	178	182	186	190
4		149		152	156	160	163	168	171	175	179	182	186
6		141	144	148	151	155	159	162	167	171	174	178	181
8		136	141	145	148	152	156	159	163	167	171	175	178
10	130	134	139	142	146	149	153	157	160	165	169	172	176
12	128	132	136	140	144	147	151	155	158	162	167	170	174
14	127	130	134	137	142	146	149	153	157	160	165	169	172
16	125	129	132	136	141	144	148	152	155	159	162	167	
18	124	127	131	135	139	143	147	150	154	157	161	166	
20	123	126	130	134	137	142	145	149	153	156	160	165	
25	120	124	127	131	135	139	143	147	150	154	157		
30	118	122	125	129	133	136	141	145	148	152	155		
35	116	120	124	127	131	135	139	143	147	150			
40	115	119	122	126	130	133	137	141	145	149			
Female patients													
3				150	153	157	161	165	169	172	176	180	183
4			141	145	149	152	156	159	163	168	171	175	179
6		130	134	137	142	146	149	153	156	160	165	168	172
8		125	129	133	136	141	144	148	152	155	159	163	167
10	118	122	125	129	133	136	141	144	148	152	155	159	163
12	115	119	122	126	130	133	137	141	145	149	152	156	160
14	112	116	120	123	127	131	134	133	143	146	150	153	157
16	109	114	118	121	125	128	132	136	140	144	148	151	
18	107	111	116	119	123	127	130	134	137	142	146	149	
20	106	109	114	118	121	125	128	132	136	140	144	148	
25	102	106	109	114	118	121	125	128	132	136	140		
30	99	103	106	110	115	118	122	125	129	133	136		
35	97	100	104	107	111	116	119	123	127	130			
50	94	98	102	105	109	112	117	121	124	128			

Data From LaFarge CG, Miettinen OS: The estimation of oxygen consumption, *Cardiovas Res* 4:23, 1970.

Hb is the hemoglobin concentration in g/dL, sat_a is the systemic arterial saturation, PaO_2 is the partial pressure of oxygen in the systemic arteries sat_{mv} is the mixed venous arterial saturation, and $PmvO_2$ is the partial pressure of oxygen in mixed venous blood. Since the amount of oxygen carried dissolved in the blood is so relatively low, this equation can be simplified to:

$$\dot{Q} = \frac{\dot{V}O_2}{[(1.34 \times Hb) \times (sat_a - sat_{mv})]}$$

Pulmonary and arterial blood flows are not similar in instances of left-to-right or right-to-left shunting, in which case both pulmonary (Q_p) and systemic flows (Q_s) need to be calculated independently. In these cases:

$$\dot{Q}_p = \frac{\dot{V}O_2}{[(1.34 \times Hb) \times (sat_{pv} - sat_{pa})]}$$

In the above equation, sat_{pv} is the pulmonary venous oxygen saturation, and sat_{pa} is pulmonary arterial oxygen saturation.

Shunts

Left-to-right shunting results in an increase or step up in oxygen saturation at some level of the right side of the heart. An atrial septal defect, for example, results in a step up from the systemic veins to the right ventricle and a ventricular septal defect results in a step up from the right atrium to the pulmonary artery. Streaming patterns allow a certain amount of normal variability, and a step up may take a distance to become apparent, based on the position of the sampling catheter relative to the shunt. For example, the saturation in the inferior vena cava is typically higher than that of the superior vena cava. Thus, there can be up to a 9 mm Hg step up in Po_2 from the superior vena cava to the right atrium, which can be a normal finding. The step up from an atrial-septal defect may not be fully recognized from a sample drawn from the right atrium, because the tip of the catheter may be outside the stream of the shunt. The step up will not be fully recognized until a sample is drawn from the right ventricle. Similarly, a catheter tip could be directly within the streaming shunted blood before full mixing, allowing for an overestimation of the degree of shunt. Right-to-left shunts result in a step down at some level on the left side of the circulation, with the same provisos for potential artifact as for left-to-right shunts. As a general rule, samples should be obtained from the most distal chamber possible (excluding an additional level of shunt) to allow maximal mixing. The following example shows how to determine the degree of shunt (the pulmonary:systemic flow ratio, or $\dot{Q}_p : \dot{Q}_s$). This becomes somewhat more complex in the case of multiple levels of shunt or bidirectional shunting. Dividing equation 4.5 by equation 4.4 results in the pulmonary:systemic flow ratio:

$$\dot{Q}_p / \dot{Q}_s = \frac{\dot{V}O_2(1.34 \times Hb) \times (sat_{pv} - sat_{pa})}{\dot{V}O_2(1.34 \times Hb) \times (sat_a - 4.6\, sat_{mv})}$$

Rearranging and canceling simplifies this to:

$$\dot{Q}_p : \dot{Q}_s = \frac{sat_a - sat_{mv}}{sat_{pv} - sat_{pa}}$$

This has the fortunate effect of having the term for $\dot{V}O_2$ cancel. Thus, if only an estimation of $\dot{Q}_p : \dot{Q}_s$ is of interest, $\dot{V}O_2$ has to be neither measured nor assumed. As an example, presume a ventricular septal defect with a left-to-right shunt. The mixed venous (right atrial) saturation is 70%, the pulmonary arterial saturation is 85%, and the pulmonary venous and systemic arterial saturations are 100%. Substituting into equation 4.7 shows that the $\dot{Q}_p : \dot{Q}_s$ is: (100-70)/(100-85), or 30/15, or 2:1. There is twice as much pulmonary blood flow as systemic.

Vascular Resistance

Measurement of the resistance across a vascular bed relates to Ohm's law. In hemodynamic terms, I = E/R can be seen as I = flow, E = the pressure drop across the vascular bed, and R = resistance. Solving for R yields R = E/I. Thus:

$$SVR = \frac{map - cvp}{\dot{Q}_s}$$

SVR = systemic vascular resistance, map = mean systemic arterial pressure, and cvp = central venous pressure.

By analogy:

$$PVR = \frac{pap - pvp}{\dot{Q}_p}$$

PVR = pulmonary vascular resistance, pap = mean pulmonary arterial pressure, and pvp = pulmonary venous pressure

(pulmonary arterial wedge pressure, mean left atrial pressure, or left ventricular end-diastolic pressure can be substituted for pvp).

Again, oxygen consumption must be calculated or assumed in order to calculate $\dot{Q}_p$ and $\dot{Q}_s$. In general, pulmonary capillary wedge, left atrial, or left ventricular end-diastolic pressures can be substituted for pulmonary venous pressure, assuming the absence of obstructions to pulmonary venous or left atrial drainage. Pediatric cardiologists have historically expressed vascular resistance in terms of Wood units. Wood units are derived when the units are pressure in mm Hg and blood flow in L/min (or, more typically, L/min/m²) to give a resistance index. Multiplying Wood units by approximately 80 converts to SI units (dyne•cm^{-5}/sec). Normal values (Wood units) in children are systemic vascular resistance index of 20, with a range of 15 to 30 (10 to 15 in neonates, with adult levels by 12 to 18 months of age), and pulmonary vascular resistance of 1 to 3 in infants older than 6 to 8 weeks of age, after the normal postnatal fall.

Echocardiography

For many infants and children, echocardiography has supplanted the need for cardiac catheterization, and many children now have cardiac surgery based on the results of echocardiography rather than catheterization. For some problems, such as AV valve anatomy, echocardiography is distinctly superior to catheterization (see www.expertconsult.com for further discussion). The thin chests and lack of hyperinflated lungs in children mean that echocardiographic views in children are often superior to those in adults. In common parlance, echocardiography also includes the use of Doppler to assess blood flow and to infer intracardiac pressures, shunts, and pressure gradients (see Doppler Echocardiography Basics, p. 110).

Modern echocardiography is derived from sonar used on ships. A brief electrical impulse is sent to a transducer, which converts (transduces) it and emits it as high frequency sound. As the sound wave encounters a change in density, such as a cardiac structure, some of the sound energy continues on and some is reflected. The echo transducer acts as a receiver and converts the transmitted sound to electrical energy, which is sent to an image processor and displayed on a screen. Because the speed of sound through the body is both known and constant, the distance of the structure from the transducer is easily calculated. This process occurs many times each second. The original format was A-mode echocardiography, where A stood for amplitude. The intensity of the reflected wave was shown as the height or amplitude, like a series of mountain peaks. The first clinical use was echoencephalography, where a beam was directed across the skull looking for shifts of midline structures. The next modification was B-mode echocardiography, where the intensity of the reflected wave was shown as the brightness of a dot. If the reflected waves were recorded on a rolling piece of paper, the series of dots would meld into a series of moving lines, with each line representing a separate cardiac structure with its own distinctive movement pattern. This was the M-mode echocardiograph. M-mode echocardiography was particularly useful for measuring vessel and chamber size and thickness. Although it showed only a one-dimensional representation of the heart (an "ice pick view"), ventricular function could be estimated by ventricular end-systolic and end-diastolic dimensions or by measuring systolic time intervals. The next major advance was two-dimensional echocardiography. Several (32, then 64) separate B-mode ultrasound emitting transducers were mounted together such that a fan-shaped series of lines of light and dark was created. These were repeated rapidly and formed a real-time image of the moving heart. This was exactly analogous to a black-and-white television set, where there is not really a picture but rather a series of rapidly refreshed lines of bright dots that the eyes and brain integrate into a picture. Quality improved with the development of phased array transducers, which generated multiple B-mode lines electronically. These transducers were miniaturized so that they could be mounted onto a gastroscope, resulting in transesophageal echocardiography. Current pediatric transesophageal probes are useful down to infants who weigh approximately 3 kg. Finally, electronic manipulation has allowed the representation of three-dimensional views of the heart. This is currently available on transesophageal probes, although as of this writing, it is not available on pediatric transesophageal probes. Intraoperative transesophageal echocardiography has been shown in several studies to improve intraoperative surgical repairs in a cost-effective manner and is routine in centers with the capability (Sutherland et al., 1989; Muhiudeen et al., 1992; Bettex et al., 2005). This technique is not totally without risk, however. In addition to the risks of local pharyngeal and esophageal injury, which attend its use in both children and adults, introduction or manipulation of the probe can cause acute and massive obstruction of the easily compressible aorta or large bronchi in infants.

Cardiac shunts, particularly right-to-left shunts, can be qualitatively visualized through contrast echocardiography with extraordinary sensitivity in terms of both the presence of the shunt and the site of the shunt. A milliliter or two of air is drawn up into a syringe of saline or other fluid and vigorously agitated. The gross air is expelled and the aerated fluid rapidly injected into a systemic vein. The numerous tiny bubbles (microcavitations) appear somewhat like the snow in an agitated snow globe. Normally these transverse the right side of the heart to be eliminated via the pulmonary capillaries into the alveoli, leaving the left atrium, left ventricle, and aorta without any contrast. If there is a right-to-left shunt, these bubbles pass to the left atrium (atrial level shunt), ventricle (ventricular level shunt), or descending aorta (ductal level shunt). This technique is not helpful in determining whether there are multiple levels of shunts (unlike catheterization), and it is not particularly qualitative, also unlike catheterization.

A variety of advanced measurement techniques, such as automated (endocardial) border detection and tissue velocity measurement are available, but they are not generally used in routine intraoperative clinical management. They are useful to more fully quantitate myocardial mechanics.

Evaluation of Cardiac Function by Echocardiography

Preload

In the intact heart, pressure is easily measured and used as a surrogate for volume. The end-diastolic volume can be assessed using pulmonary arterial wedge pressure, left atrial pressure, or central venous pressure. However, given the different diastolic compliances of individual ventricles, pressure provides a crude estimate of volume—the parameter that is actually sought. Echocardiography provides the best estimate of preload. This is readily measured either as end-diastolic dimension (M-mode), end-diastolic area (two-dimensional echocardiography), or end-diastolic volume (derived from two-dimensional echocardiography).

Afterload

Clinical measures of wall stress are difficult, leaving SVR as the typical clinical indicator. Recall the following equation.

$$SVR = \frac{map - cvp}{\dot{Q}_s}$$

In normal circumstances, systemic blood flow = cardiac output (or index). Arterial and central venous pressures are obtained from indwelling catheters. Cardiac output can be derived from Doppler measures of blood flow and echo measures of valve or aortic area.

Contractility

Ejection fraction is the most common surrogate for contractility, although it suffers from being load dependent. Ejection fraction (EF), is shown in the following equation:

$$EF = \frac{(\text{End-diastolic volume}) - (\text{End-systolic volume})}{(\text{End-diastolic volume})}$$

EF is normally 65% to 80% and does not change appreciably with age. Shortening fraction (SF) is the equivalent measure in the common setting when only the ventricular diameters are known.

$$SF = \frac{(\text{End-diastolic diameter}) - (\text{End-systolic diameter})}{(\text{End-diastolic diameter})}$$

The normal value for SF is >0.28, with a range of 0.28 to 0.44 (Gutgesell et al., 1977). The concept of SF was developed when the only echocardiographic modality available was M-mode, which utilizes an echo representation in only one dimension. A variety of mathematical manipulations were derived to convert a one-dimensional measurement into three-dimensions, which would allow for expression of contractility as the already recognized concept of ejection fraction. This was particularly useful to adult cardiologists, who routinely used EF derived from other methods. However, this conversion also resulted in a cubing of any inherent error in the measurement and made these formulae somewhat less than adequate. Advances in two-dimensional echocardiography have improved the ability to generate a realistic measure of ejection fraction (three-dimensional from echocardiography (two-dimensional); however, SF remains in common use, particularly among pediatric cardiologists. Velocity of circumferential fiber shortening (Vcf) is a somewhat outdated measure of contractility, and also suffers from being dependent on afterload. In circumferences/sec, it is:

$$Vcf = \frac{(\text{End-diastolic diameter}) - (\text{End-systolic diameter})}{(\text{End-diastolic diameter}) \times \text{Ejection time}}$$

The general increase in afterload with aging in childhood and with certain diseases limits the absolute usefulness of these measures as a pure indicator of ventricular function.

Additional measures of left-ventricular contractility can be derived from echocardiographic measures in conjunction with hemodynamic measures. These include the end-systolic pressure-volume relationship popularized by Suga and colleagues (1973). However, this is not done routinely because it requires measures of hemodynamic data and ventricular volume data at multiple levels of ventricular volume to derive the slope of the line connecting the end-systolic pressure volume points. Unlike the other measures of ventricular function, it is load independent.

Doppler Echocardiography Basics

This technique utilizes the Doppler phenomenon, the frequency shift well-known to anyone who has heard a train whistle approach with increasing frequency and then depart with decreasing frequency. In general, this technique involves insonating the heart with a high-frequency sound wave. Using fast Fourier transformation and filtering to prevent measuring the velocity of other structures, such as heart and vascular components, the velocity (and direction) of moving blood can be determined. There are three modes of Doppler in routine use. Continuous mode shows the fastest velocity along the Doppler beam, but cannot resolve distance. Pulse wave mode can resolve distance from the transducer. Thus, it can be "aimed" from the real-time two-dimensional echocardiograph image so that specific areas of the heart can be interrogated. Finally, color-flow mapping allows the color coding of specific pixels on the two-dimensional echocardiograph in essentially real time to allow superposition of blood flow and cardiac anatomy.

Data obtained from Doppler interrogation can be used to derive a wide variety of physiologic information. For example, cardiac output (or output across a specific valve or area) can be determined as follows:

$$Flow = CSA \times Vm$$

CSA = cross-sectional area, and Vm = mean flow velocity. Vm is the integral of the flow under the spectral Doppler velocity display, also known as time-velocity integral (TVI). Thus, with each beat:

$$Stroke\ volume = CSA \times TVI$$

and

$$Cardiac\ output = Stroke\ volume \times Heart\ rate$$

If flow is measured across both the aortic and pulmonary valves, the presence and degree of an intracardiac shunt can be determined.

Valve area can also be determined by Doppler examination by using the principle of continuity. This states that in the absence of shunts that either add or subtract volume, the stroke volume at any two points in the heart must be equal. The continuity principle leads to the continuity equation, where $CSA_1 \times TVI_1 = CSA_2 \times TVI_2$. Knowing three of the values in the equation allows one to rearrange the equation and solve for the fourth.

$$CSA_2 = \frac{(CSA_1 \times TVI_1)}{TVI_2}$$

Consider the example of aortic stenosis. CSA_2 is aortic valve area, CSA_1 and TVI_1 are measured in the left ventricular outflow tract, and TVI_2 is a high-velocity jet across the stenotic valve.

The continuous-wave function of Doppler echocardiography allows the calculation of pressure gradients. If the flow between the two points occurs across a narrow orifice, for example in aortic stenosis, blood-flow velocity increases. Measuring the peak velocity allows the calculation of a pressure gradient. This technique is widely used in echocardiography but has certain limitations. The angle of interrogation of the Doppler beam must be accurately aligned with the direction of blood flow. The more poorly aligned the direction of blood flow is with the Doppler beam, the greater the underestimation of the true velocity of blood flow. Mathematically, the degree of underestimation is described by the cosine of the angle theta (θ) between the direction of blood flow and the Doppler beam, the angle of incidence. The cosine function is nonlinear between 0 degrees (cosine 0 = 1) and 90 degrees (cosine 90 = 0). For example, if θ is 30 degrees, cosine 30 = 0.87. Therefore, at an angle of 30 degrees, the measured velocity is only 87% of the true blood velocity. The software of the echocardiography works on the assumption that the direction of blood flow and the Doppler beam are in perfect alignment.

The equation that relates peak velocity to pressure is known as the modified Bernoulli equation, where V is velocity in meters/sec:

$$\Delta\ Pressure\ (mm\ Hg) = 4V^2$$

Readers are referred to textbooks of echocardiography for a complete derivation of the modified Bernoulli equation. Assuming good alignment of the Doppler beam and the direction of blood flow, peak velocity is now easily converted into the pressure gradient across the lesion (Fig 4-25).

CARDIAC MAGNETIC RESONANCE IMAGING

The 1990s and early 2000s saw explosive growth in the use of cardiac MRI. The images produced truly bring the anatomy of the cardiovascular system to life. The use of MRI was extended to cardiac imaging when "gating" technology was developed. The beating of the heart posed a problem for MRI because it created movement artifact. Gating refers to imaging the heart in conjunction with its cardiac cycle in order to minimize artifact. It is usually linked to the electrocardiograph, but can be paired with pulse-wave plethysmography or any other modality that reflects the cardiac cycle. As a first line of investigation, MRI is generally not recommended. Echocardiography remains the initial modality for almost all pediatric patients with heart disease because of its speed and portability, as well as the information that can be obtained about cardiac anatomy and function. Nevertheless, echocardiography does have limits. Poor acoustic windows, especially in older children, may limit its usefulness. Even with good quality echocardiographic images, the major thoracic vessels, both arterial and venous, are not well visualized because of the surrounding air-filled lungs. Before the advent of MRI, the thoracic vessels could only be seen well with cardiac catheterization. MRI now provides a noninvasive method for imaging the thoracic vasculature. However, to limit the use of MRI to diagnosing abnormalities of the thoracic vessels is to underestimate its power. When it comes to imaging the cardiovascular system, MRI is only limited by the skill and expertise of the cardiologist or radiologist who is directing and interpreting the scan.

MRI has proven safe in pediatric patients. There are no known harmful effects from exposure to the magnetic field. Implanted devices containing metal can make MRI unsafe. The dangers of implanted metal exposed to a magnetic field are threefold. First,

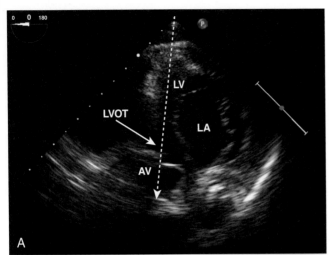

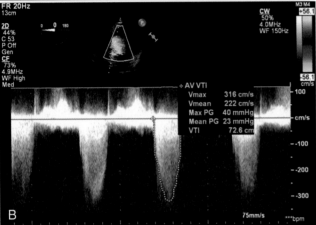

■ FIGURE 4-25. Transesophageal echocardiogram in aortic stenosis. **A,** Deep transgastric view with very good alignment of the Doppler beam *(dashed arrow)* with the left-ventricular outflow tract and aortic valve. *AV,* aortic valve, *LA,* left atrium, *LV,* left ventricle, *LVOT,* left-ventricular outflow tract. **B,** Spectral Doppler tracing of the velocity of blood as it accelerates across the stenotic aortic valve. Velocity *(y axis)* is plotted versus time *(x axis)*. The peak velocity is 3.16 m/sec, which translates into a peak gradient of 40 mm Hg using the modified Bernoulli equation.

preoperative questioning should delay the scan while advice is sought from the manufacturer and MRI personnel. MRI demands a still patient who is confined in a small tube. Children who have not reached adolescence require some form of sedation that covers the spectrum from "light" sedation to general anesthesia, with or without the airway being secured. The reader is referred to Chapter 33, Anesthesia and Sedation for Pediatric Procedures Outside the Operating Room, for a more complete discussion on the challenges of anesthesia and sedation in remote locations such as the MRI suite.

MRI concepts of imaging are often difficult to understand and made more so by terminology that is unfamiliar. By way of simple explanation, MRI images are created by placing a patient in a strong magnetic field that aligns the protons on hydrogen atoms. A directed pulse of radiofrequency wave is directed at the area of interest, and the hydrogen protons emit their own radiofrequency wave. These emitted radiofrequency waves are constructed into the MR image. Terms often seen on MRI reports are T1 and T2 weighting. T1 refers to the longitudinal relaxation time and is a measure of time it takes for a substance to become magnetized. T2 is transverse relaxation time and refers to how long protons remain "in phase" after the radiofrequency pulse. Depending on the molecular structure (e.g., water content, blood, soft tissue, or bone) in the anatomic area of interest, T1 and T2 images are different. These differences become important, because the pathologic abnormality being sought may be better seen on either T1 or T2 weighted images.

The lesions most commonly sought by MRI are coarctation, vascular rings, aortic arch abnormalities, and branch pulmonary artery stenosis. The common feature of these lesions is that they usually all lie beyond the reach of the echocardiography probe. The original cardiovascular imaging technique was a technique called *spin echo*, which has been improved and may now be called *fast* or *turbo-spin echo*. Flowing blood appeared black, resulting in the term "black blood imaging." The technique was good for imaging structural abnormalities of the heart and vascular system, but it only provided still images that could not display cardiac function. After the diagnosis of a lesion on two-dimensional imaging, a three-dimensional reconstruction can display the lesion in astounding detail and clarity (Fig. 4-26). Intravenous contrast (gadolinium) can be injected rapidly to create magnetic resonance angiography and better demonstrate the pathology (Fig. 4-27). The obvious drawback to MRI for stenotic vascular lesions is that no information about the pressure gradient can be obtained. Sometimes, on visualization, the stenosis appears so severe that it demands repair. However, in cases in which even more information is needed, cardiac catheterization remains the benchmark for visualization and measurement of pressure gradients. The ability of MRI to accurately diagnose lesions of the thoracic vasculature is obvious, but a more exciting application of cardiac MRI testing is in the quantitative and qualitative assessments of cardiac function. In contrast to "black blood imaging," gradient echo MR produces bright blood images and is done at high speed, which allows the creation of a cine loop that displays the entire cardiac cycle in real time (Fig. 4-28). Freezing the image at end-diastole and end-systole allows the calculation of ventricular volume. The ventricle is divided into "slices," and the blood volume of each slice is calculated by multiplying its cross-sectional area and thickness. Knowing precisely end-diastolic and end-systolic volumes allows the calculation of stroke volume, ejection fraction, and cardiac output. Very good correlation has been made

the implanted metallic devices may heat up. Second, under the influence of a magnetic field, implanted metal devices may move, causing tissue damage in the area of implantation. This is relevant to the pediatric cardiac population because patients often have various stents, coils, sternal wires, pacemakers, and other foreign material. Manufacturers attempt to make their devices "MRI compatible" but there are no hard and fast rules. The presence of a pacemaker generally contraindicates MRI imaging, although most other foreign material is safe. Foreign material implanted in pediatric cardiac patients is usually weakly ferromagnetic, which results in little heat being generated. The caveat is that the implanted device may move in the presence of a strong magnetic field. Manufacturers and clinicians often wait 4 to 6 weeks after implantation to use MRI. During this time it is believed that the device becomes fixed by surrounding fibrosis and cannot move in response to a magnetic field. The 4-to-6-week recommendation is arbitrary and not based on good data. Finally, implanted devices may pose negligible risk to the patient, but they can cause image artifacts. The discovery of possible dangerous foreign material on

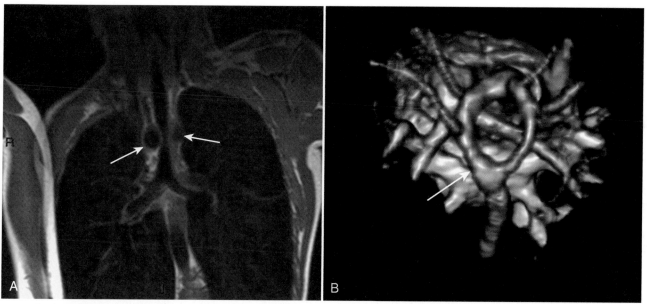

■ FIGURE 4-26. Double aortic arch. **A,** Coronal MRI of the chest showing lateral tracheal compression from right and left secondary to a double aortic arch *(white arrows).* **B,** Three-dimensional reconstruction of the double aortic arch *(white arrow)* as viewed from above. The double arch encircles both the trachea and esophagus, which are not seen in this three-dimensional image.

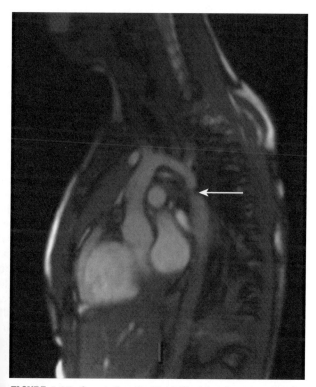

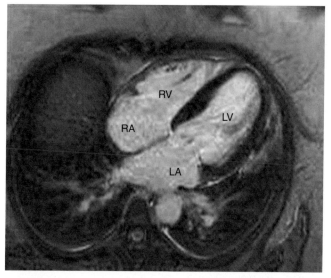

■ FIGURE 4-28. Cardiac MRI. The four-chamber view clearly shows the four cardiac chambers. A high-speed cine loop displays the four-chamber image in a real-time image, giving important information about ventricular function and valvular regurgitation. *LA,* Left atrium; *LV,* left ventricle; *RA,* right atrium; *RV,* right ventricle.

FIGURE 4-27. Coarctation. Sagittal MRI of the chest showing the coarctation *(white arrow)* beyond the origin of the left subclavian artery.

with other methods of calculating cardiac output (Bellenger et al., 2000; Ioannidis et al., 2002). In fact, the ability of MRI to detect small changes in ventricular volume (10 mL) exceeds that of echocardiography.

In addition to static measurements of ventricular volume, MRI can also measure blood-flow velocity, which allows the calculation of blood flow. Blood flowing through a magnetic field produces a phase shift proportional to its velocity. Plotting blood-flow velocity versus time (one cardiac cycle) creates a curve. The integration of the area under the curve is stroke volume. Calculation of cardiac output by MRI compares favorably with the Fick and thermodilution methods (Hundley et al., 1995). Measuring stroke volume in the aorta and pulmonary artery simultaneously allows the measurement of pulmonary to systemic ($\dot{Q}_p : \dot{Q}_s$) ratio. For pediatric patients with septal defects or intracardiac mixing and single ventricle physiology, accurate noninvasive measurements of $\dot{Q}_p : \dot{Q}_s$ ratios can now be made. The agreement with oximetry-based calculations obtained in the cardiac catheterization laboratory is very good (Beerbaum et al., 2001).

Although less relevant to pediatric patients, MRI can also be used to assess wall motion, diagnose ischemic heart disease, and evaluate myocardial viability. Wall motion can be assessed qualitatively by analyzing a real-time image of ventricular contraction. For these purposes, the left ventricle is divided into the same anatomic regions recommended for echocardiographic assessment (Shanewise et al., 1999). Function is graded as normal, variably hypokinetic, akinetic, or dyskinetic. Quantification of regional wall motion can be done by measuring myocardial thickening throughout the cardiac cycle, but this is time consuming. Dobutamine-stress MRI operates under the same principles as other noninvasive stress tests. Regional wall-motion abnormalities that result from coronary stenoses are unmasked by increasing the inotropic and chronotropic state of the heart. The regional wall-motion defects are assessed qualitatively. Lastly, akinetic areas of myocardium may consist of fixed scar (nonviable myocardium) or hibernating (viable myocardium) tissue, which take up and release intravenous contrast differently. Myocardial delayed enhancement is a technique that allows the differentiation of viable, chronically ischemic myocardium from that which is permanently damaged (Fig. 4-29).

EFFECTS OF ANESTHESIA ON THE CARDIOVASCULAR SYSTEM

Any use of anesthetics in young children needs to take into account the variable effects of anesthetics on the immature myocardium, recognize the time frame of myocardial development, and consider the clinical appropriateness of various anesthetic regimens for specific surgical procedures. Cardiopulmonary interactions also need to be considered, given the numerous and potentially potent effects of some anesthetics on the respiratory system. Unfortunately, many if not most, studies have been done in children, not infants, in whom myocardial maturation is essentially complete, leaving less information about the cardiac effects of anesthetics in young and premature infants. In addition, many earlier studies have not been repeated with sevoflurane or desflurane, leaving much of the available information centered on halothane and isoflurane.

Anesthetic Effects on Ion Currents

Both volatile anesthetics and several intravenous anesthetics can affect many of the voltage-dependent myocardial ion currents, although studies in immature myocardium are limited. Halothane, for example, can inhibit $I_{Ca,L}$ the L-type calcium current in fetal as well as adult myocardium (Fig. 4-30). Baum and Klitzner (1991) have shown that both halothane and isoflurane

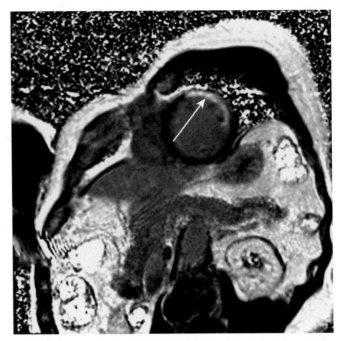

■ FIGURE 4-29. Cardiac MRI. The short-axis view of the left ventricle demonstrates a scarred and akinetic segment of myocardium (*white arrow*). The area has delayed uptake of gadolinium contrast.

can decrease the height of the action potential in neonatal right-ventricular papillary muscle, consistent with an effect on trans-sarcolemmal calcium entry. A variety of anesthetics are known to shift the activation and inactivation kinetics of $I_{Ca,L}$. These include halothane and ketamine (Baum et al., 1994). These might decrease calcium entry via $I_{Ca,L}$ in cells with more negative resting potential, such as immature myocardial cells.

BAY K8644, a calcium-channel agonist, can only partially prevent or reverse halothane- or isoflurane-induced depression in right-ventricular papillary muscles of neonatal rabbits (Baum and Klitzner, 1993). This is consistent with the view that mechanisms other than decreased trans-sarcolemmal calcium entry contribute to anesthetic-induced myocardial depression. Halothane, even in clinically appropriate doses, reversibly inhibits Na^+-Ca^{2+} exchange in neonatal ventricular myocytes. This provides for an additional mechanism for the more pronounced volatile anesthetic-induced depression of immature myocardium, with its increased reliance on Na^+-Ca^{2+} exchange relative to adult myocardium (Baum et al., 1994).

A variety of volatile and intravenous anesthetics can affect the various K^+ channels, with implications for arrhythmia generation and anesthetic-induced myocardial preconditioning (Baum, 1993; Buljubasic et al., 1996; Stadnicka et al., 1997; Stadnicka et al., 2000; Fujimoto et al., 2002; Suzuki et al., 2003). However, there is no information on the effects in the young or

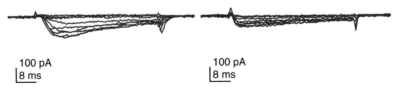

100 pA
8 ms

100 pA
8 ms

■ FIGURE 4-30. Calcium current ($I_{Ca,L}$) measured from a single ventricular myocyte isolated from a 28-day-old rabbit fetus (term = 31 days). Control to the left, 0.125% halothane to the right. The axes are picoamps (pA) and milliseconds (ms). (*From Baum VC, Palmisano BW: The immature heart and anesthesia*, Anesthesiology *87:1529, 1997.*)

immature heart, and the phenomenon of anesthesia-induced preconditioning, mediated at least in part by potassium current, has not been fully evaluated in immature myocardium.

Anesthetic Effects on the Conduction System

In vitro, infant rabbit hearts are more resistant than adult rabbit hearts to the direct sinus-node pacemaker depression of halothane and isoflurane (Palmisano et al., 1994). Maximal depression of the sinus node is about 10%, suggesting that indirect effects rather than direct effects are primarily responsible for the bradycardia seen during clinical anesthesia. It is likely that cholinergic effects play a major role, as baseline cholinergic tone is present in neonates and infants, and under halothane and nitrous-oxide anesthesia there is a dose-related increase in heart rate with atropine (Palmisano et al., 1991b).

For both infant and adult hearts, the sinus rate is more resistant to the effects of halothane and isoflurane than are other measurements of cardiac function (Palmisano et al., 1994). These anesthetics decrease spontaneous pacemaker discharge by decreasing the rate of diastolic depolarization and increasing the action potential duration (Bosnjak and Kampine, 1983). In the adult heart, where it has been studied, halothane decreases the rate of diastolic depolarization and moves the maximal diastolic depolarization (V_m) closer to threshold potential. These two effects counterbalance with little effect on sinus rate (Hauswirth and Schaer, 1967).

Halothane prolongs AV conduction time more than isoflurane, and the effect in infants is greater than it is in adults (Palmisano et al., 1994). The age difference for isoflurane is much less marked than for halothane. There has been little information evaluating the effects of the newer inhalational agents on sinus-node function in healthy children. Sevoflurane and isoflurane have little effects on sinus node function or AV conduction in children with pre-excitation conditions such as Wolff-Parkinson-White syndrome, suggesting they have little if any effects on normal tissue (Chang et al., 1996; Sharpe et al., 1999). In a study of *in vitro* rabbit hearts, propofol had no effects on atrial or AV conduction, although it did prolong AV conduction in adult hearts of rabbits (Wu et al., 1997).

Anesthetic Effects on Myocardial Metabolism

Reactivity of the coronary vasculature to a variety of physiologic and pharmacologic stimuli has been shown to be present in newborn animals of a variety of species (Toma et al., 1985; Downing and Chen, 1986; Buss et al., 1987; Hickey et al., 1988; Muscuitto et al., 1992). In infant rabbit and *in vitro* fetal lamb hearts, both halothane and isoflurane vasodilate coronary arteries and result in increased coronary flow, and these effects are similar to those in adult hearts of those animals (Palmisano et al., 1994; Davis et al., 1995). Isoflurane decreases oxygen consumption, which coupled with increased coronary flow, results in relative overperfusion (Hickey et al., 1988; Stowe et al., 1991; Palmisano et al., 1994). Because isoflurane causes a greater increase in heart rate in adults, the decrement in oxygen consumption is more pronounced in adult hearts than in neonatal hearts (Palmisano et al., 1994). However, when heart rates are kept similar, there are no age differences. In the hypoxic, stressed, neonatal lamb, neither halothane nor isoflurane alter

redistribution of blood flow to vital organs, including the heart (Cameron et al., 1985; Brett et al., 1989).

Myocardial flow in the neonatal lamb decreases at 1 MAC isoflurane (from 250 to 88 mL/100g per minute), but this fall is in exact proportion to the decrease in myocardial oxygen consumption, resulting in unchanged myocardial oxygen extraction and endocardial-to-epicardial flow ratios (Brett et al., 1987). Consistent with this, 1.5% halothane was not found to affect steady state levels of myocardial high energy phosphates or intracellular pH in neonatal myocardium, despite a decrement in myocardial performance (McAuliffe and Hickey, 1987). This indicates that uncoupling of oxidative phosphorylation does not account for volatile anesthetics' depressant effect on myocardial function.

Anesthetic Effects on Systolic Function

Young hearts show an increased susceptibility to myocardial depression from the volatile anesthetics (Cook et al., 1981). Although it has been suggested that the apparent increased hemodynamic depression in the young human heart may be the result of differences in anesthetic uptake and distribution, several studies have indicated that the increased hemodynamic effects of the volatile anesthetics are a result of increased direct action on the myocardium in the immature heart (Barash et al., 1978; Boudreaux et al., 1984; Schieber et al., 1986; Murray et al., 1992).

A major effect on myocardial contractility is via limitation of calcium availability to the contractile apparatus. Transsarcolemmal and sarcoplasmic reticular calcium flux are altered with the net effect of depleting intracellular stores (Nakao et al., 1989; Wilde et al., 1991; Frazer and Lynch, 1992; Schmidt et al., 1993; Wilde et al., 1993). Halothane depresses contractility more than isoflurane does (Lynch, 1986; Krane and Su, 1987; Baum and Klitzner, 1991; Palmisano et al., 1994). Halothane decreases peak intracellular calcium concentration more than isoflurane does and is a more potent depressant of contractile function *in vitro* in both neonatal and adult hearts (Komai and Rusy, 1987; Krane and Su, 1989; Lynch, 1990; Bosnjak et al., 1992; Pan and Potter, 1992; Palmisano et al., 1994). Although there were no age effects of isoflurane, halothane was more depressant to neonatal hearts than adult hearts. However, there may be some dependence on species, because a study in isolated rat atrium did not find that the depression was dependent on age (Rao et al., 1986).

Studies in neonatal lambs have shown that both halothane and isoflurane decrease cardiac output to the same degree that they decrease myocardial oxygen consumption (Cameron et al., 1985; Brett et al., 1987; Brett et al., 1989). Isoflurane at 1 MAC decreased blood pressure primarily by decreasing cardiac output rather than by affecting vascular resistance (Brett et al., 1987). Results in human neonates, infants, and children are more variable, probably because of differing techniques and the confounders of changes in heart rate and afterload. Nicodemus, in an early study, showed increased hypotension in neonates and less hypotension in older children (Nicodemus et al., 1969).

Murray et al. (1992), using echocardiographic indexes of cardiac function, could show no difference between halothane and isoflurane at equipotent concentrations. Sevoflurane has been shown to cause less myocardial depression in young children than halothane, although very young infants were not studied (Holzman et al., 1996).

Anesthetic Effects on Diastolic Function

Anesthetic effects of calcium flux that might impair systolic function could also affect diastolic function, which requires temporary reuptake of released calcium into stores. Indexes of diastolic relaxation show a more depressant effect of halothane than isoflurane, and the effects are greater in infant rabbit hearts than in adult rabbit hearts (Palmisano et al., 1994). There was no age effect seen with isoflurane. This prominent effect of halothane may be a reflection of immature myocardium's limited capacity to remove calcium from the contractile proteins. The principle mechanism for relaxation in adult myocardium is sequestration of calcium in the sarcoplasmic reticulum, and this is relatively undeveloped in immature myocardium; thus, these hearts may depend more on removal via Na^+-Ca^{2+} exchange (Hoerter et al., 1981; Bers and Bridge, 1989; Fisher and Tate, 1992). It is possible that developmental changes in the actin-regulatory proteins could also affect anesthetic mediation of relaxation.

Anesthetic Effects on Autonomic Control

Halothane, isoflurane, fentanyl, sevoflurane, and nitrous oxide all depress baroreceptor control of heart rate through the central nervous system, autonomic ganglia, and the heart (Biscoe and Millar, 1966; Duke et al., 1977; Duncan et al., 1981; Seagard et al., 1982; Seagard et al., 1983; Kotrly et al., 1984; Murat et al., 1988; Murat et al., 1989). The effect of halothane is more pronounced in younger animals when animals are made pharmacologically hypertensive, but there does not seem to be an age effect when animals are made pharmacologically hypotensive (Wear et al., 1982; Dise et al., 1991; Palmisano et al., 1991a). In (anesthetized) infants undergoing ligation of a patent ductus arteriosus, a heart rate change is typically not seen with acute alterations in blood pressure (Gregory, 1982). Constant showed that while halothane preserves cardiac vagal activity in children, it does not preserve baroreceptor activity any better than sevoflurane (Constant et al., 1999; Constant et al., 2004). Murat showed that isoflurane-mediated tachycardia may be less pronounced in neonates (Murat et al., 1989). Although acute increases in the inspiratory concentration of desflurane or isoflurane can cause an abrupt increase in heart rate and systemic blood pressure from stimulation of the tracheobronchial tree, this effect is not seen with acute increases in sevoflurane concentration (Ebert et al., 1995).

Hemodynamic Effects of Specific Agents

Preanesthetic Medications

Appropriate preanesthetic management of pediatric patients has been an area of much interest for quite a few years. Preoperative education, parental presence, and pharmacologic agents have all been used and all have a place in providing a smoother and safer induction. These are considered in Chapter 9 (Preoperative Preparation) and only cardiac effects of pharmacologic agents will be considered here. Although numerous oral, intramuscular, and intranasal drugs have been proposed as pediatric premedicants, the current most popular agent is oral midazolam. Intravenous midazolam can decrease cardiac output when it is combined with intravenous morphine (Shekerdemian et al., 1997). Midazolam in routine oral doses of 0.5 to 1.0 mg/kg is well tolerated hemodynamically, even in children with cardiac disease. In a study by Masue and colleagues (2003), larger doses of 1.5 mg/kg did not cause any overall decrease in blood pressure, heart rate, or oxygen saturation, although a small number of patients did have a decrease in blood pressure or saturation (6% and 4%, respectively). This was likely related to baseline agitation or underlying cyanotic heart disease confounding the measurements (Masue et al., 2003). If used for sedation in the intensive care unit, abrupt cessation after several days of use can result in cardiovascular withdrawal phenomena. Audenaert et al. (1995) used Doppler echocardiography to compare three premedication regimens in children. They compared oral premedication (meperidine, 3 mg/kg + pentobarbital 4 mg/kg), nasal premedication (ketamine, 5 mg/kg + midazolam, 0.2 mg/kg), and rectal premedication (methohexital, 30 mg/kg). All had relatively modest effects if any. Meperidine + pentobarbital decreased heart rate, mean arterial pressure, and cardiac index. Ketamine + midazolam had no significant cardiovascular effects, and methohexital increased heart rate with a consequent decrease in stroke volume, but without additional effects.

Inhalational Anesthetics

To some extent, all the currently used volatile anesthetics are myocardial depressants. Many studies in humans suffer from studying relatively older children, where differences in myocardial function from adults would be expected to be limited if at all. In general, halothane decreases blood pressure by decreasing myocardial contractility without a compensatory rise in heart rate. Thus, cardiac output decreases. Isoflurane, desflurane, and sevoflurane decrease blood pressure by decreasing left-ventricular afterload. Cardiac output is also maintained by these three agents because they preserve autonomic function and baroreceptor-mediated tachycardia. Children older than age 3 years will have an increase in heart rate with sevoflurane but no change in cardiac output, whereas halothane results in a lower blood pressure and no change in heart rate (Piat et al., 1994; Sarner et al., 1995; Kern et al., 1997). The greatest decrease in blood pressure and the least increase in heart rate with sevoflurane occur in infants younger than 6 months of age (Lerman et al., 1994). The myocardial effects of volatile anesthetics may be more pronounced in the myopathic heart, which mirrors clinical experience (Hettrick et al., 1997).

Ejection fraction and cardiac index are decreased at 1.25 MAC by both isoflurane and halothane (Murray et al., 1987). Halothane has a more pronounced effect on contractility than isoflurane or sevoflurane. In a group of children (not neonates) with congenital heart disease, sevoflurane and isoflurane maintained cardiac output with minimal effect on contractility. Sevoflurane decreased contractility less than halothane. Isoflurane, as it did in other studies, increased heart rate and lowered systemic vascular resistance. Halothane depressed contractility, cardiac output, mean arterial pressure, and systemic vascular resistance (Rivenes et al., 2001). The addition of nitrous oxide to halothane or isoflurane at 1.0 MAC does not seem to change contractility, although it may decrease heart rate, blood pressure, and cardiac index (Murray et al., 1988). Cardiac output has been shown to improve, particularly with halothane, with the administration of atropine in several studies (Miller and Friesen, 1988; Murray et al., 1989). The effect of atropine on cardiac output was because of its effect on heart rate.

Sevoflurane has gained widespread acceptance in the practice of pediatric anesthesia. It produces less tachycardia than isoflurane, as well as less myocardial depression and fewer arrhythmias than halothane (Lerman et al., 1990; Frink et al., 1992; Holzman et al., 1996; Paris et al., 1997; Wodey et al., 1997). Sevoflurane does not cause heart rate or cardiac output to change appreciably; however; it does lower systemic vascular resistance and blood pressure compared with those values of awake patients.

Desflurane has been shown to either decrease or increase heart rate before an incision is made (Taylor and Lerman, 1991; Zwass et al., 1992).

Nitrous oxide is a direct myocardial depressant; however, this is likely offset by an increase in sympathetic tone (Ebert and Kampine, 1989). In the intact animal, it is a very mild cardiac depressant, and its effects are similar to its effects in infants and adults. Its use in infants does not result in an increase in pulmonary vascular resistance (Hickey et al., 1986). The effects of sympathetic stimulation that can be seen with nitrous oxide in adults are absent in young children (Murray et al., 1988).

Xenon has significant potential as a general anesthetic, and it has been shown to not have significant cardiac affects *in vitro*, however both clinical and pediatric uses are very limited (Stowe et al., 2000).

Opioids

Opioids have long been used in the field of pediatric cardiac anesthesia for their cardiovascular stability, and even a high dose of an opioid has minimal or no effect on heart rate, cardiac output, PVR, mean arterial pressure, and SVR (Robinson and Gregory, 1981; Hickey et al., 1985c; Hansen and Hickey, 1986). As when they are used in adults, opioids used in pediatric patients can blunt the increases in PVR that are associated with tracheal suctioning. The effects of high-dose sufentanil are qualitatively similar to those of high-dose fentanyl (Hickey and Hansen, 1984; Davis et al., 1987). Other opioids have not been studied as intensively in infants and young children. However, given their similar effects in adults, similar findings can be expected in children.

Propofol

Propofol can cause decrease in blood pressure and heart rate, even in healthy children (Short and Aun, 1991). Hannallah and coworkers, however, noted no significant hemodynamic differences when induction/maintenance was done with propofol/propofol infusion, propofol/halothane, thiopentone/halothane, or halothane/halothane (1994). Intracardiac hemodynamic values, including shunts, measured in the catheterization laboratory tend to remain unchanged with propofol (Gozal et al., 2001).

Ketamine

Ketamine has long history of use in the arena of pediatric anesthesia. It can be given orally or intramuscularly as a premedication, in can be given intravenously to induce or maintain anesthesia. Ketamine's benefits particularly concern its hemodynamic stability. Although it is a direct myocardial depressant, possibly related to its effects on $I_{Ca,L}$ (Baum et al., 1991b; Baum et al., 1994), its actions a sympathomimetic preserve myocardial function. However, hearts that are depleted of catecholamine or beta-blocked, one would expect to see a more prominent depressant effect. In the pediatric cardiac catheterization laboratory, ketamine has been shown to have little hemodynamic effects if given as a 2 mg/kg bolus or as an infusion of 50 to 75 mcg/kg per minute (Morray et al., 1984; Oklu et al., 2003). Compared with an infusion of propofol, ketamine causes an increase in systemic arterial pressure and has fewer effects on shunting, because PVR and SVR were unchanged. After cardiac surgery, ketamine at a dose of 2 mg/kg has also been shown to cause no change in heart rate, cardiac output, PVR, or SVR (Hickey et al., 1985b). This statement, however, presumes adequate ventilation. That said, a study in children with pulmonary hypertension showed that even with sevoflurane and spontaneous ventilation, ketamine did not change pulmonary arterial pressure or PVR (Williams et al., 2007). Two studies in children have evaluated the effects of ketamine at altitude (Denver and Albuquerque) and found significant increases in pulmonary vascular resistance with ketamine (Berman et al., 1990; Wolfe et al., 1991).

Regional Anesthetics

Regional anesthesia is discussed more fully in Chapter 16 (Regional Anesthesia). Both spinal and epidural anesthesia with local anesthetics in children have minimal hemodynamic effects compared with the vasodilation noted in adults. Routine prophylactic fluid loading is not required in pediatric practice. A caudal and thoracic epidural block with local anesthetic and fentanyl had no effect unless epinephrine (5 mcg/mL) was added, when it was associated with increased cardiac output accompanied by decreased arterial blood pressure and SVR (Raux et al., 2004). There are no hemodynamic differences noted between spinal or epidural anesthesia (combined with general anesthesia) when used for pediatric cardiac anesthesia (Hammer et al., 2000). Regional anesthesia has such a negligible hemodynamic effect in children that high or even total spinal anesthesia has in fact been suggested by some groups for use in pediatric cardiac anesthesia (Finkel et al., 2003).

SUMMARY

The developmental stage of myocardium at the time of birth is dependent on species, and much of the knowledge of myocardial development derives from animal studies, leaving the specifics in humans unclear. For most purposes, human myocardium can certainly be considered mature by 12 months of age and to a good extent by 6 months of age. Developmental changes in myocardial maturation are apparent in numerous extracellular and intracellular components of heart muscle, and many have to do with calcium handling and excitation-con traction coupling. Current clinically useful anesthetics have multiple sites of interaction with the myocardium and its neural regulation, but are generally safe. Noninvasive evaluation of the heart by echo-Doppler and MRI have supplanted many of the indications for cardiac catheterization in evaluating both cardiac anatomy and cardiac physiology.

For questions and answers on topics in this chapter, go to "Chapter Questions" at www.expertconsult.com.

REFERENCES

Complete references used in this text can be found online at www.expertconsult.com.

Regulation of Fluids and Electrolytes

Demetrius Ellis

CONTENTS

Concentrations of minerals and electrolytes in extracellular fluid (ECF) are maintained nearly constant, despite large day-to-day variations in the dietary intake of salt and water. Such homeostasis is governed primarily by the kidneys through an array of intricate processes that may be influenced by intrarenal and extrarenal vasoactive substances and hormones. Although the basic tenants governing nephron function and homeostasis of body fluid composition have changed little over the past decade, major advances stemming from genetic research have greatly elucidated the structure and function of many renal tubular electrolyte transporters during both health and disease. A major objective of this chapter is to enhance the understanding of electrolyte (and fluid) pathophysiology based on newer information.

OVERVIEW OF ANATOMY AND PHYSIOLOGY

Anatomy

The kidneys are retroperitoneal paired organs located on each side of the vertebral column. A normal adult kidney measures 11 to 12 cm in length, 5 to 7.5 cm in width, and 2.5 to 3.0 cm in thickness. In the adult male, it weighs 125 to 170 g, and in the adult female, it weighs 115 to 155 g. Beneath its fibrous capsule lies the cortex, which contains the glomeruli, the convoluted proximal tubules, the distal tubules, and the early portions of the collecting tubules. The remainder of the tissue, the medulla, contains the pars recta, the loop of Henle, and the middle and distal portions of the collecting duct. The inner medulla borders the renal pelvis, where urine is received from the collecting ducts. The ducts and loops are arranged into cone-shaped bundles called *pyramids,* which have tips that project into the renal pelvis and form papillae. The pelvis drains into the ureter, which in the adult human descend a distance of 28 to 34 cm open into the fundus of the bladder. The walls of the pelvis and ureters contain smooth muscles that contract in a peristaltic manner to propel urine to the bladder.

Renal Blood Flow

Despite accounting for only 0.5% of body weight, the kidneys receive about 25% of the cardiac output, with a blood flow of approximately 4 mL/min per gram of kidney tissue. Renal plasma flow (RPF) in women is slightly lower than it is in men, even when normalized for body surface area, averaging 592 ± 153 mL/min per 1.73 m² and 654 ± 163 mL/min per 1.73 m², respectively (Smith, 1943). In children between the ages of 6 months and 1 year, normalized RPF is half that of adults but increases progressively to reach adult levels at about 3 years of age (McCrory, 1972). After the age of 30 years, renal blood flow (RBF) decreases progressively; by the age of 90 years, it is approximately half of the value present at 20 years (Davies and Shock, 1950). This generous supply provides not only for the basal metabolic needs of the kidneys but also for the high demands of ultrafiltration.

The basic arterial supply of the kidneys is a single renal artery that divides into large anterior and posterior branches and subsequently into segmental or interlobar arteries. The latter form the arcuate and interlobular arteries. These blood vessels are end-arteries and therefore predisposed to tissue infarction in the presence of emboli. The arcuate arteries are short, large-caliber vessels that supply blood to the afferent arterioles of the glomeruli at a mean pressure of 45 mm Hg, which is higher than that found in most capillary beds. This high hydraulic pressure and large endothelial pore size lead to enhanced glomerular filtration (Brenner and Beeuwkes, 1978).

Glomerular capillaries have many anastomoses but recombine to form the efferent arteriole. The latter subdivide into an extensive peritubular capillary network. This arrangement allows solute and water to move between the tubular lumen and blood. These networks rejoin to form the venous channels, through which blood exits the kidneys.

Ninety percent of RBF goes to the cortex, which accounts for 75% of the renal weight, whereas the medulla and the rest of the kidneys receive 25% of the RBF. Although cortical blood flow is 5 to 6 mL/g per minute, outer medullary blood flow decreases to 1.3 to 2.3 mL/g per minute, and the flow to the papilla is as low as 0.22 to 0.42 mL/g per minute (Dorkin and Brenner, 1991). The unevenness in the distribution of RBF between the cortex and the medulla is necessary to develop and maintain the medullary gradient of osmotically active solutes that drive the countercurrent exchange/multiplier, which is essential for the elaboration of concentrated urine. Outer medullary blood flow may preferentially supply the loop of Henle, thereby accounting for the striking influence of loop diuretics in that region. Furthermore, papillary blood flow is far greater than the metabolic needs of the renal parenchyma and is well adapted to the countercurrent concentrating mechanism characteristic of this region.

RBF remains almost constant over a range of systolic blood pressures from 80 to 180 mm Hg, a phenomenon known as autoregulation. Consequently, glomerular filtration is also constant over this range of pressures as a result of adaptations in the renal vascular resistance (Selkurt et al., 1949, Gertz et al., 1966). Because the changes in resistance that accompany graded reductions in renal perfusion pressure occur in both denervated and isolated perfused kidneys, autoregulation appears not to depend on extrinsic neural or hormonal factors (Thurau, 1964). According to the "myogenic hypothesis" first proposed by Bayliss (1902), the stimulus for vascular smooth muscle contraction in response to increasing intraluminal pressure is either the transmural pressure itself or the increase in the tension of the vascular wall. An increase in perfusion pressure, which initially tends the vascular wall, is followed by a contraction of the resistance vessels and a return of blood flow to basal levels.

There are only a few studies of autoregulation of RBF in developing animals. Aortic constriction in adult animals reduces renal perfusion by 30% but has minimal effects on RBF and glomerular filtration rate, compared with the significant changes observed in 4- to 5-week-old rats (Yared and Yoshioka, 1989). Furthermore, it has been demonstrated that autoregulation of RBF in young rats occurs at renal perfusion pressures between 70 and 100 mm Hg, compared with pressures of 100 to 130 mm Hg in adult rats (Chevalier and Kaiser, 1985). A similar increase in the pressure set point for autoregulation has been found in dogs (Jose et al., 1975). It appears that autoregulation of RBF occurs in the very young and is sufficient to maintain blood flow constant over a wide range of perfusion pressures that are physiologically adequate for the age. No such human studies are available.

Several substances have been proposed to participate in the autoregulation of RBF, including vasoconstrictor and vasodilator prostaglandins, kinins, adenosine, vasopressin, the renin-angiotensin-aldosterone system, endothelin, and endopeptidases (Herbacznska-Cedro and Vane, 1973, Osswald et al., 1978, Maier et al., 1981, Schnermann et al., 1984). Nitric oxide (NO), previously known as endothelium-derived relaxing factor (EDRF), has also been shown to play an important role in regulating renal vascular tone through its vasodilatory action. Bradykinin, thrombin, histamine, serotonin, and acetylcholine act on endothelial receptors to activate phospholipase C, which in turn results in the formation of inositol triphosphate and diacylglycerol, resulting in the release of intracellular calcium (Marsden and Brenner, 1991, Luscher et al., 1992). This in turn stimulates the synthesis of NO from L-arginine. Other factors that stimulate the formation of NO include hypoxia, calcium ionophores, and mechanical stimuli to the endothelium. NO increases RBF by decreasing efferent arteriolar vascular resistance, while glomerular filtration remains unchanged (Marsden and Brenner, 1991).

Because in mature kidneys, autoregulation is lost at arterial pressures less than 80 mm Hg, the lower physiologic pressures prevailing in the newborn period may be expected to limit this important control mechanism. There is evidence both to support and to refute this conclusion (Kleinman and Lubbe, 1972, Jose et al., 1975).

Renal Physiology

The glomerulus is a specialized capillary cluster arranged in loops that functions as a filtering unit. The capillary walls may be viewed as a basement membrane lined by a single layer of cells on either side. In contact with blood are endothelial cells, which contain many fenestrations; podocytes, with their foot processes, line the other side of the basement membrane.

The route by which water and other solutes are filtered from the blood is not fully understood, but it appears that plasma ultrafiltrate traverses the large fenestrations of the glomerular capillary endothelium and penetrates the basement membrane and the slit pores located between the podocyte foot processes. Filtration of large molecules is greatly influenced by the size and charge of the specific molecule, as well as by the integrity and charge of the glomerular basement membrane. Abnormalities in various structural proteins of the slit-pore diaphragm such as nephrin, podocin, and α-actinin may be responsible for several proteinuric disorders (Mundel and Shankland,

2002). In general, the endothelium and the *lamina rara interna* of the glomerular basement membrane slow the filtration of circulating polyanions such as albumin (Ryan and Karnovsky, 1976). The *lamina rara externa* and the slit pores slow the filtration of cationic macromoleculess such as lactoperoxidase (Graham and Kellermeyer, 1968). Neutral polymers such as ferritin are not filtered because of their large molecular size and shape (Farauhar et al., 1961). Molecules with a radius of 4.2 nm or more are excluded from the glomerular filtrate. In practical terms, red cells, white cells, platelets, and most proteins are restricted to the circulation.

Glomerular Filtration

Among the main functions performed by the kidneys is the process of glomerular filtration. The glomerulus is primarily responsible for the filtration of plasma. The glomerular filtration rate (GFR) is the product of the filtration rate in a single nephron and the number of such nephrons, which range from 0.7 to 1.4 million in each kidney (Keller et al., 2003). Clearance, which is defined as the volume of plasma cleared of a substance within a given time, provides only an estimate or approximation of GFR.

Although tubular reabsorption and tubular secretion may influence the blood level of numerous medications and endogenously-produced substances such as urea, creatinine, and uric acid, the degree of elimination of such substances depends largely on GFR. Hence, in individuals with renal impairment, estimation or measurement of GFR is crucial in determining the dosage adjustment and choice of medications needed to achieve effectiveness while avoiding toxicity. GFR is also a major factor that affects electrolyte composition and volume of body fluids, as well as acid-base homeostasis.

Glomerular filtration is driven by hydrostatic pressure, which forces water and small solutes across the filtration barrier. In healthy individuals, changes in hydrostatic pressure rarely affect single-nephron GFR because autoregulatory mechanisms sustain or maintain a constant glomerular capillary pressure over a large range of systemic blood pressure (Robertson et al., 1972). Hydrostatic pressure is opposed by the oncotic pressure produced by plasma proteins and the hydrostatic pressure within Bowman's capsule. Mathematically, this relation can be expressed by the following equation:

$$SNGFR = K_f \times (P - p) = K_f \times P_{UF}$$

SNGFR is the single-nephron glomerular filtration rate; K_f is the glomerular ultrafiltration coefficient; P and p are the average hydraulic and osmotic pressure differences, respectively; and P_{UF} is the net ultrafiltration pressure. As plasma water is filtered, the proteins within the capillaries become more concentrated, so oncotic pressure increases at the distal end of the glomerular capillary loop and the rate of filtration ceases at the efferent capillary (Blantz, 1977). Under normal conditions, about 20% of the plasma water that enters the glomerular capillary bed is filtered; this quantity is referred to as the filtration fraction

RBF has the greatest influence on GFR. Renal parenchymal disorders interfere with autoregulation of RBF, such that GFR may fall, even with low-normal mean arterial blood pressure (MABP). Still more pronounced changes in GFR may occur with hypotension or hypertension, which may accelerate

ischemic or hypertensive injury. Clearance of a molecule may serve as an indicator of GFR only if the assayed molecule is biologically inert and freely permeable across the glomerular capillary, if it remains unchanged after filtration, and if it is neither reabsorbed nor secreted by the tubule. The exogenous-filtration marker inulin (a fructose polymer) has all of these attributes and is the ideal standard for measuring GFR. However, inulin-clearance measurement is rarely used clinically because it is an expensive and cumbersome method. Instead, measurement of an endogenous small molecule such as serum creatinine (molecular weight, 0.113 kDa), which is derived from muscle metabolism at a relatively constant rate and is freely filtered at the glomerulus, is a practical, rapid, and inexpensive means for estimating GFR, thereby aiding clinical decisions. Thus, in the steady state, creatinine production and urinary creatinine excretion are equal even when GFR is reduced.

Serum-creatinine concentrations vary by age and gender. In 1-year-old girls values are 0.35 ± 0.05 mg/dL (mean ± SD) and rise gradually to 0.7 ± 0.02 mg/dL (mean ± SD) by 17 years of age; boys have corresponding mean values that are 0.05 mg/dL higher until 15 years of age and 0.1 mg/dL higher subsequently (Schwartz et al., 1987). Expected creatinine-excretion rates in 24-hour urine collections are often used to validate such collections. Values range from 8 to 14 mg/kg per day in neonates and in infants younger than 1 year of age, with an increase to about 22 ± 7 mg/kg per day (mean ± SD) in preadolescent children of either gender (Hellerstein et al., 2001). Subsequently, creatinine excretion in boys is 27 ± 3.4 mg/kg per day.

In healthy children with proportional height and weight, GFR can be estimated by creatinine clearance (CrCl) as calculated by Schwartz's formula, which does not rely on measurement of urinary creatinine or timed urine collections:

$$CrCl\ (mL/min\ per\ 1.73\ m^2) = (Height/P_{CR}) \times k,$$

where height is in centimeters, P_{CR} is the plasma-creatinine concentration in mg/dL, and k is a constant proportion to muscle mass. The value of k is 0.45 in full-term newborns and until 1 year of age, 0.55 in children 2 years of age and older and in adolescent girls, and 0.70 in adolescent boys (Schwartz et al., 1987). Normal CrCl ranges from 90 to 143 mL/min per 1.73 m², with a mean of 120 mL/min per 1.73 m²

Although more cumbersome, calculation of CrCl based on values obtained in 12- or 24-hour urine collections provide a better estimate of GFR. Once the completeness of such collections is validated based on expected creatinine excretion, CrCl is calculated using the following formula:

$$CrCl\ (mL/min/1.73\ m^2) = \frac{U \times V \times SA\ m^2}{min \times P_{CR} \times 1.73\ m^2}$$

U is the urinary concentration of creatinine in mg/dL, V is the total urine volume in mL, min is the time of collection in minutes, and P_{CR} is the serum concentration of creatinine in mg/dL. To standardize the clearance of children of different sizes, the calculated result is multiplied by 1.73 m² (surface area of a standard man in meters squared) and divided by the surface area of the child in meters squared

In children with impaired renal function, GFR estimated based on creatinine methods may grossly overestimate the true GFR, because tubular and gastrointestinal secretion of creatinine increases disproportionately. Hence, serum creatinine concentrations are less reflective of filtration at the glomerulus

For example, Schwartz's formulas overestimate GFR by 10% ± 3% when GFR is greater than 50 mL/min per 1.73 m² but by 90% ± 15% when GFR is less than 50 mL/min per 1.73 m². Other limitations of creatinine-based GFR determinations stem from variations of analytical assays, reference values ranging from 0.1 to 0.6 mg/dL in children younger than 9 years of age, diurnal variation in serum creatinine levels resulting from high intake of cooked meat or intense exercise, influence of body mass index, and inaccurate urine collections—all of which make comparisons of GFR difficult over time, especially in growing children (Levey et al., 1988). Using cimetidine to block tubular secretion of creatinine before measuring CrCl in urine collections may improve such measurements (Hellerstein et al., 1998).

Measurement of cystatin-C, a 13-kDa serine proteinase produced at a constant rate by all nucleated cells, is purported to be a superior endogenous marker of filtration, because cystatin-C is less susceptible to variation than is plasma creatinine. A meta-analysis compared the correlation between GFR measured by inulin clearance, radiolabeled methods, nonlabeled iothalamate or iohexol, and either plasma creatinine or cystatin-C concentrations measured nephelometrically (Dharnidharka et al., 2002).The correlation between GFR and cystatin-C was significantly higher compared with plasma creatinine (0.846 versus 0.742, P < 0.001). Thus, cystatin-C measurements are becoming increasingly popular in clinical practice, and reference ranges have been generated in children up to 16 years of age (Table 5-1) (Bokenkamp et al., 1998; Finney et al., 2000; Harmoinen et al., 2000).

Studies in renal transplant donors and in individuals with various renal disorders have shown that plasma-creatinine concentration changes minimally as GFR falls to about 50 mL/min per 1.73 m² (Fig. 5-1) (Shemesh, 1985). This compensation is largely the result of hypertrophy and hyperfiltration of the remaining nephrons. When more than 50% of the nephrons cease to function and "renal reserve" is outstripped, serum creatinine may rise rapidly in a parabolic fashion (Fig. 5-1). Thus, when a more accurate clinical assessment of GFR is desirable for research purposes, radiolabeled methods with an identity exceeding 97% give a better approximation of GFR relative to inulin clearance and may be more useful in aiding clinical decisions. In multicenter investigations conducted in the United States using a uniform method for GFR measurement, ¹²⁵I-iothalamate is often used because this isotope has low radiation exposure and long isotope half-life and can be assayed

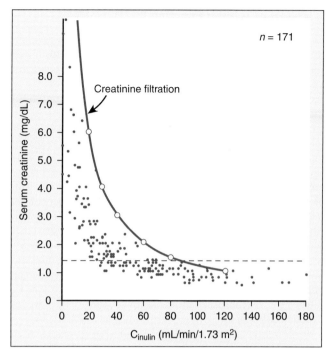

■ **FIGURE 5-1.** Relationship of serum creatinine to GFR. *(From Shemesh O, Golbetz H, Kriss JP, et al.: Limitation of creatinine as a filtration marker in glomerulopathic patients, Kidney Int 28:830, 1985.)*

at a central laboratory (Bajaj et al., 1996). Otherwise, ⁹⁹ᵐTc-diethylenetriaminepenta-acetic acid (Tc-DTPA) is commonly used to estimate GFR for routine clinical purposes. In other countries, ⁵¹Cr-ethylenediaminetetra-acetic acid (Cr-EDTA), which delivers a greater radiation dosage, is also popular, as are nonlabeled iothalamate and iohexol methods.

Although GFR may fluctuate, the kidneys retain the ability to regulate the rate of solute and water excretion according to changes in intake. This regulation is achieved by changes in tubular reabsorption rates—a phenomenon known as glomerular-tubular balance (Tucker and Blantz, 1977). The end result is preservation of ECF volume and chemical composition. Glomerular-tubular balance can be disturbed by several factors, including volume expansion, loop diuretics, and inappropriate secretion of antidiuretic hormone (ADH).

TABLE 5-1. Nonparametric 95% Reference Intervals for Cystatin C in Different Age Groups

Age Group	n	Reference Interval	90% Confidence Limits		P*
			Lower Limit	Upper Limit	
Preterm infants	58	1.34-2.57	1.07-1.42	2.47-2.86	0.000
Full-term infants	50	1.36-2.23	1.24-1.44	2.03-2.32	0.000
>8 days to 1 yr	65	0.75-1.87	0.71-0.86	1.78-1.91	0.000
>1 to 3 yr	72	0.68-1.60	0.65-0.79	1.39-1.67	0.011
>3 to 16 yr	162	0.51-1.31	0.48-0.68	1.26-1.35	—

Modified from Harmoinen A, Ylinen E, Ala-Houhala M, et al.: Reference intervals for cystatin C in pre- and full-term infants and children, *Pediatr Nephrol* 15:105–108, 2000, 107, Table 1. (With permission of Springer Science and Business Media.)
*Statistical significance versus the oldest group (including Bonferroni's correction factor 5).

Overview of Tubular Function

The proximal tubule is the site of reabsorption of large quantities of solute and filtered fluid (Fig. 5-2). Many transporters subserving tubular electrolyte transport have been characterized at the genetic level, and various pathologic disorders have been elucidated (Epstein, 1999). Under physiologic conditions, the proximal convoluted tubule isotonically reabsorbs 50% to 60% of the glomerular filtrate (Berry and Rector, 1991). The initial portion of the proximal convoluted tubule reabsorbs most of the filtered glucose, amino acids, and bicarbonate. Glucose and amino acids are absorbed actively, whereby they are transported against their electrochemical gradient, coupled to sodium (Na^+). Active Na^+ transport at the peritubular membrane provides the driving force that ultimately is responsible for other transport processes. The system is driven by sodium, Na^+, K^+, (activated) adenosine triphosphatase (Na^+-, K^+-ATPase), or the Na^+ "pump," which requires the presence of K^+ in the peritubular fluid and is inhibited by ouabain. Micropuncture studies show that around 50% to 70% of the filtered Na^+ is reabsorbed in this segment, mostly by a process of active cotransport.

The major fraction of filtered bicarbonate (HCO_3^-) is absorbed early in the proximal convoluted tubule. Hydrogen (H^+) gains access to luminal fluid via an Na^+/H^+ electroneutral exchange mechanism and forms carbonic acid. The latter is dehydrated to H_2O and CO_2 under the influence of carbonic anhydrase. CO_2 diffuses into the cell, and HCO_3^- is re-formed and ultimately absorbed into the bloodstream. In general, the concentration of HCO_3^- is maintained at 26 mmol/L, which is slightly below the renal threshold of approximately 28 mmol/L (Pitts and Lotspeich, 1946).

The renal clearance of glucose is exceedingly low, even after complete maturation of glomerular filtration. The amount filtered increases linearly as plasma glucose increases. Initially, all filtered glucose is reabsorbed until the renal threshold has been exceeded (at around 180 mg/dL), at which point filtered glucose appears in the urine. However, maximal tubular glucose (T_{mG}) reabsorption is attained at a filtrate glucose concentration of about 350 mg/mL (Pitts, 1974). The reabsorption of glucose in the proximal tubule occurs via a carrier-mediated, $Na^+/glucose$ cotransport process across the apical membrane, followed by passive facilitated diffusion and active Na^+ extrusion across the basolateral membrane.

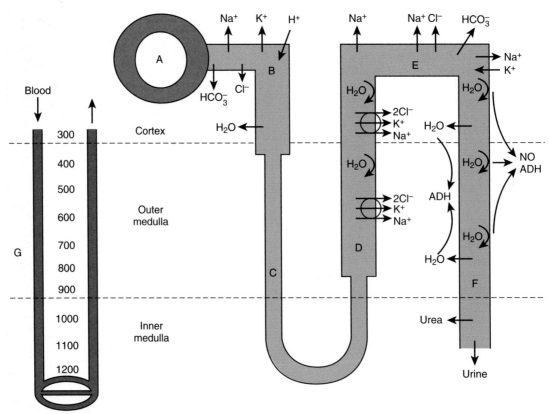

■ **FIGURE 5-2.** Sodium and water handling by the nephron. *A,* Glomerulus. *B,* Proximal tubule, the major site for the reabsorption of Na^+ (70%), Cl^-, K^+ (80%), HCO_3^- (80% to 90%), and water. The reabsorptive process is isomotic, regardless of whether the kidneys are concentrating or diluting urine. *C,* Thin descending loop of Henle. *D,* Thick ascending loop of Henle. It is always impermeable to water. The medullary portion is important for the generation of free water. There is active Na^+, K^+, and Cl^- (20% to 25%) reabsorption, which is responsible for driving the countercurrent multiplier and creating increased medullary tonicity. The cortical thick ascending limb and the early distal tubule *(E)* are responsible for the reabsorption of the remaining HCO_3^-, to as well as 5% of the filtered Na^+ and Cl^-. These segments are impermeable to water and are unaffected by ADH. In the late distal tubule and the cortical collecting duct *(F),* aldosterone action controls Na^+ and K^+ reabsorption and excretion. The medullary portion of the collecting duct is the major site for ADH-dependent water reabsorption. This segment is permeable to water in the presence of ADH. The *vasa recta (G)* is important in maintaining a concentrated medullary interstitium.

Apart from Na^+, other solutes reabsorbed in the proximal tubule include K^+, Ca^{2+}, P^{2-}, Mg^{2+}, and amino acids. These are discussed in detail in other sections of this chapter.

The loop of Henle makes the formation of concentrated urine possible and contributes to the formation of dilute urine (Kokko, 1979). This dual function is achieved through the unique membrane properties of the loop, the postglomerular capillaries, and the hypertonicity of the interstitium. The proximity of the descending and ascending portions of loop allows it to function as a countercurrent multiplier, whereas the capillaries serve as countercurrent exchangers (Fig. 5-2). The descending loop of Henle abstracts water from tubular fluid, increasing the intraluminal concentrations of NaCl and other solutes. However, the intraluminal osmolality remains in equilibrium with the interstitium, where 50% of the osmolality results from urea. In the thin ascending limb of the loop of Henle, there is passive efflux of NaCl and urea into the interstitium. The thick ascending limb of the loop of Henle, by being impermeable to water, contributes to the formation of dilute urine.

The final creation of hypotonic or hypertonic urine depends on the distal tubules and collecting ducts and their interaction with ADH. In the distal convoluted tubule, Na^+ reabsorption occurs against a steep gradient, largely under the influence of aldosterone. K^+ is secreted by the distal tubule in association with Na^+ reabsorption and H^+ secretion. Moreover, this segment of the nephron acidifies the urine and is the only site of new bicarbonate formation. At the end of the collecting duct, about 1% of the filtered water and about 0.5% of the filtered Na^+ appear in the final urine.

The Kidneys and Antidiuretic Hormone

ADH plays a pivotal role in water homeostasis by acting on the most distal portion of the nephron. ADH is a cyclic octapeptide that, along with its carrier protein, neurophysin, is synthesized in the supraoptic and paraventricular nuclei of the hypothalamus (Zimmerman and Defendini, 1977). The prohormone migrates along the nerve axons to the posterior pituitary gland, where it is stored as arginine vasopressin. It is released through exocytosis (Douglas, 1973).

Several variables affect ADH secretion. Physiologically, the most important factor is plasma osmolality. A very small rise in plasma osmolality is sufficient to trigger a response from the sensitive osmoreceptors located in and around the hypothalamic nuclei, leading to ADH secretion. Conversely, plasma ADH concentrations are less than 1 pg/mL at a physiologic plasma osmolality of less than 280 mOsm/kg water. The antidiuretic activity of ADH is maximal at plasma osmolality of greater than 295 mOsm/kg water, when plasma ADH exceeds 5 pg/mL (Robertson, 2001). Once plasma osmolality exceeds this limit—thus surpassing the capacity of the ADH system to affect maximal fluid retention—the organism depends on thirst to defend against dehydration. Intracerebral synthesis of angiotensin II largely mediates this thirst response and the oropharyngeal reflex. Atrial natriuretic peptide (ANP) opposes the release of ADH and of angiotensin II. In summary, plasma osmolality and Na^+ are maintained within a narrow range. The upper limit of this range is determined by the sensitivity of the thirst mechanism located in the hypothalamus, whereas its lower range is affected by ADH release.

Nonosmolar factors also influence ADH secretion and may be the key stimuli of ADH secretion in pathologic disorders, leading to hypovolemia and hypotension. These changes are mediated by low-pressure (located in the left atrium) and high-pressure (located in the carotid sinus) baroreceptors. Experimental studies suggest that this nonosmotic pathway of ADH release is less sensitive than the osmotic pathway and is triggered by a 5% to 10% fall in blood volume, whereas a 1% to 2% increase in ECF osmolality can trigger ADH release.

Nonhypovolemic conditions that stimulate ADH release often result in diminished urine volume, hyponatremia, fractional excretion of uric acid greater than 10%, low serum uric acid level (<4 mg/dL), and urinary sodium greater than 20 mEq/L (Albanese et al., 2001). These conditions result in hyponatremia. Conversely, inhibitors of ADH release or primary or acquired nephropathies may result in the inability to respond to ADH or to conserve water, and these inhibitors are often accompanied by polyuria with Uosm of less than 150 mOsm/kg, dehydration, and hypernatremia.

ADH has a major effect on the medullary thick ascending limb and thereby influences the countercurrent multiplier mechanism and urinary concentration. More directly, ADH binds to V_2 receptors in the basolateral membrane of the collecting duct, causing the activation of adenylate cyclase and the formation of cyclic 3',5'-adenosine monophosphate (cAMP) (Dorisa and Valtin, 1976; Schwartz et al., 1974). This results in insertion of aquaporin-2 water channels in apical membranes and in the activation of apical Na^+ channels, which causes water conservation (Andreoli, 2001). These effects are counterbalanced by prostaglandin E_2 (PGE_2) and the calcium-sensing receptor in cells of the medullary thick ascending limb that mediate saluresis and diuresis.

Polyuric syndromes can be separated on the basis of urine osmolality and generally consist of water diuresis, solute diuresis, or a mixed water-solute diuresis with typical Uosm of less than 150 mOsm/kg, 300 to 500 mOsm/kg, and 150 to 300 mOsm/kg, respectively (Oster et al., 1997). The etiology of polyuria may be facilitated by obtaining a urinalysis; a measurement of urine pH; and measurements of electrolytes, creatinine, osmolality, glucose, urea nitrogen, and bicarbonate, preferably in a timed urine collection together with the corresponding serum values. Such assessment may serve to prevent dehydration, acid-base disturbances, hypokalemia, or hypernatremia, which often accompany such polyuric disorders (Table 5-2) (Oster et al., 1997). Proper correction of acute hypernatremia is needed to prevent brain demyelination. Normal saline infusion may be the agent of choice in polyuric conditions associated with solute diuresis, whereas ADH and electrolyte-free fluid administration may be appropriate in cases of "pure" water diuresis. The recommended rate of correction of hypernatremia is about 10 mEq/L per 24 hours, amounting to a fall in plasma osmolality of about 20 mOsm/kg H_2O per day (Adrogue and Madias, 2000b).

Renin-Angiotensin-Aldosterone System

The renin-angiotensin-aldosterone axis plays a key role in control of vascular tone, Na^+ and K^+ homeostasis, and, ultimately, circulatory volume and cardiovascular and renal function. Renin is an enzyme with a molecular weight of 40 kDa that is synthesized and stored in the juxtaglomerular apparatus

TABLE 5-2. Studies Used in the Evaluation of Polyuria

Abbreviation (Term)	Definition	Formula*	Comment
C_{osm} (osmolal clearance)	Urine flow (volume/unit time) necessary to excrete the urinary solution isotonically (i.e., at osmolality of the plasma)	$\dfrac{(U_{osm})V}{P_{osm}}$	Classic clearance formula applied to solute
$C_{osm(E)}$ (electrolyte osmolal clearance)	Urine flow (volume/unit time) necessary to excrete urinary electrolytes at concentration of plasma Na	$\dfrac{(U_{[Na]} + U_{[K]})V}{P_{[Na]}}$	Assumes that contribution of $P_{[K]}$ is negligible compared with $P_{[Na]}$
$C_{osm(NE)}$ (nonelectrolyte osmolal clearance)	Urine flow (volume/unit time) necessary to excrete urinary nonelectrolytes isotonically (i.e., at osmolality of plasma)	$C_{osm} - C_{osm(E)}$	—
Ch_2o (free water clearance)	Volume of urinary solute–free water excreted per unit time	$V - C_{osm}$	—
$Ch_2o(e)$ (electrolyte–free water clearance	Volume of urinary electrolyte–free water excreted per unit time	$V - C_{osm(E)}$	$Ch_2o(e)$, rather than Ch_2o, influences $S_{[Na]}$
U_{TS} (urine total solute)	Measured total amount of urinary solute in 24 hr	$(U_{osm})(TV)$	—
U_E (urine electrolyte solute)	Estimated total amount of urinary solute in 24 hr accounted for by electrolytes	$(2)(U_{[Na]} + U_{[K]})(TV)^†$	—
U_{NE} (urine nonelectrolyte solute)	Estimated total amount of urinary solute in 24 hr not accounted for by electrolytes	$U_{TS} - U_E$	—
UAG (urinary anion gap)	Difference (in mEq/L) between sum of urinary concentrations of Na and K, and that of Cl	$U_{[Na]} + U_{[K]} - U_{[Cl]}$	A large (positive) value usually implies a large concentration of anions other than Cl
PS (principal solute)	Principal urinary solute in millimoles per 24 hr	—	If PS is a monovalent ion such as Na^+ or Cl^-, PS is calculated as twice its total excretion
PS% (percent principal solute)	Contribution of principal solute to total solute excretion	$\dfrac{(100)(PS)}{(U_{osm})(TV)}$	The solute with the highest osmolal concentration in a 24-hr urine collection, expressed as a percentage of total solute excretion

Modified from Oster JR, Singer I, Thatte L, et al.: The polyuria of solute diuresis, *Arch Intern Med* 157:721–729, 1997.
*$P_{[Na]}$, Plasma sodium concentration; P_{osm}, plasma osmolality; *TV*, total 24-hr urinary volume; $U_{[Cl]}$, urine chloride concentration; $U_{[K]}$, urine potassium concentration; $U_{[Na]}$, urine sodium concentration; U_{osm}, urine osmolality; and *V*, urine volume/unit time.
†U_E calculations assume that the corresponding anions are monovalent.

surrounding the afferent arterioles of the glomeruli (Davis and Freeman, 1976). The primary stimuli for renal renin release are reductions in renal-perfusion pressure, Na^+ restriction, and Na^+ loss as detected by the specialized *macula densa* cells located in the distal tubule. Mechanical (stretch of the afferent glomerular arterioles), neural (sympathetic nervous system), and hormonal (PGE_2 and prostacyclin) stimuli act in an integrated fashion to regulate the rate of renin secretion (Fig. 5-3).

Once released into the circulation, renin cleaves the leucine-valine bond of angiotensinogen, forming angiotensin I. Angiotensin-converting enzyme that is present in the lungs, as well as in the kidneys, large caliber vessels, and other tissues, cleaves the carboxyl terminal (histidine-leucine dipeptide) from angiotensin I to form the biologically active angiotensin II (Ng and Vane, 1967).

Angiotensin II has numerous important hemodynamic functions that are mediated largely by binding to angiotensin-II T1-receptors in endothelial cells, tubular epithelial cells, and smooth muscle (Box 5-1) (Burnier and Brunner, 2000). It plays a key role in regulating blood volume and long-term blood pressure through stimulation of several tubular transporters of Na^+-conversation that are mainly located in the proximal tubule, as well as through its effects in enhancing aldosterone secretion

and Na^+ reabsorption in the distal tubule. As a potent direct smooth-muscle vasoconstrictor and as an enhancer of ADH and sympathetic nervous system activity, angiotensin II also participates in short-term blood-pressure regulation in disorders associated with volume depletion or circulatory depression. Research has uncovered multiple nonhemodynamic functions that are primarily mediated by binding to T1 receptors of angiotensin II, which are particularly important in the pathophysiology of progressive renal injury (Hall et al., 1999).

A rise in plasma aldosterone concentration stimulates urinary K^+ secretion, thus allowing maintenance of K^+ balance. Aldosterone also increases the excretion of ammonium (NH_4^+) and magnesium (Mg^{2+}) and increases the absorption of Na^+ in the distal tubule, both by increasing the permeability of the apical membrane and by increasing the activity of Na^+, K^+ adenosine triphosphatase (ATPase) (Marver and Kokko, 1983). The net effect is to generate more negative potential in the lumen, a driving force for increased K^+ secretion. In addition, aldosterone enhances reabsorption of sodium in the cortical collecting duct through activation of the epithelial sodium-specific channel, ENaC (Greger, 2000). In performing these functions, aldosterone plays a key role in regulating fluid and electrolyte balance. Long-term aldosterone administration

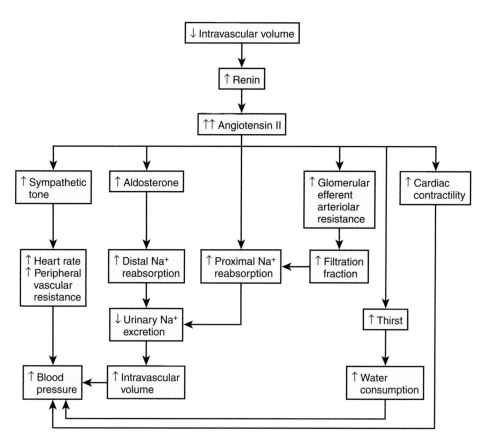

■ **FIGURE 5-3.** Effects of decreased intravascular volume on the renin-angiotensin-aldosterone system.

Box 5-1 Effects of Angiotensin II Mediated via AT₁ and AT₂ Receptor Stimulation

AT₁ RECEPTOR STIMULATION
Vasoconstriction (preferentially coronary, renal, cerebral)
Sodium retention (angiotensin, aldosterone production)
Water retention (vasopressin release)
Renin suppression (negative feedback)
Myocyte and smooth muscle cell hypertrophy
Stimulation of vascular and myocardial fibrosis
Inotropic/contractile (cardiomyocytes)
Chronotropic/arrhythmogenic (cardiomyocytes)
Stimulation of plasminogen activator inhibitor-1
Stimulation of superoxide formation
Activation of sympathetic nervous system
Increased endothelin secretion

AT₂ RECEPTOR STIMULATION
Antiproliferation/inhibition of cell growth
Cell differentiation
Tissue repair
Apoptosis
Possible vasodilation
Kidney and urinary-tract development

Modified from Burnier M, Brunner HR: Angiotensin II receptor antagonists, *Lancet* 355:637, 2000.

...ealthy volunteers increases the ECF volume. Clinical edema ...oes not occur, however, because after several days the kidneys ...escape" from the Na⁺-retaining effect while maintaining the ...⁺-secretory effect (August et al., 1958).

The Kidneys and Atrial Natriuretic Peptide

ANP is secreted by atrial monocytes in response to local stretching of the atrial wall in cases of hypervolemia (e.g., congestive heart failure or renal failure) and ultimately results in the reduction of intravascular volume and systemic blood pressure (Brenner et al., 1990). In the kidneys, ANP acts in the medullary collecting duct to inhibit sodium reabsorption during ECF expansion. ANP induces hyperfiltration, natriuresis, and suppression of renin release, and it inhibits receptor-mediated aldosterone biosynthesis (Greger, 2000). In the cardiovascular system, it diminishes cardiac output and stroke volume and reduces peripheral vascular resistance. Some of these effects are mediated through the influence of ANP on vagal and sympathetic nerve activity.

Body Fluid Compartments

The internal environment of the body consists of fluids contained within compartments. Water accounts for 50% to 80% of the human body by weight. The variation in water content depends on tissue type: adipose tissue contains only 10% water, whereas muscle contains 75% water. Total body water (TBW) decreases with age, mainly as a result of loss of water in ECF. For clinical purposes, TBW is estimated at 60% of body weight in infants older than age 6 months, as well as in children and adolescents. This value is very inaccurate for low–birth-weight premature infants in whom TBW comprises as much as 80% of total body weight (Friis-Hensen, 1971; Kagan et al., 1972). In term infants younger than 6 months of age, TBW may be approximated as 75% of total body weight (Hill, 1990). Newer formulas that consider the height (cm) and weight (kg), but

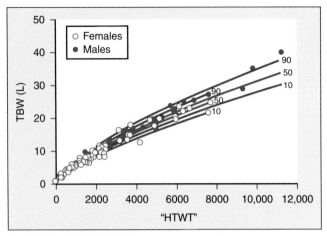

■ **FIGURE 5-4.** Total body water (TBW) plotted against the parameter (Ht × Wt) for children from 3 months to 13 years of age. The 10th, 50th, and 90th percentile curves, generated from the equations in the text, are shown. The curves for both males and females are presented. *(From Morgenstern BZ, Mahoney DW, Warady BA: Estimating total body water in children on the basis of height and weight: a reevaluation of the formulas of Mellits and Cheek,* J Am Soc Nephrol *13:1884-1888, 2002.)*

not the degree of adiposity or the child's surface area, have improved the estimation of TBW, particularly in healthy children between 3 months and 13 years of age (Fig. 5-4) (Mellits and Cheek, 1970; Morgenstern, 2002). TBW can be determined as follows:

$$0 \text{ to } 3 \text{ Months: TBW} = 0.887 \times (Wt)^{0.83}$$

$$\text{Children 4 to 13 years: TBW} = 0.0846 \times 0.95^{[if \text{ female}]} \times$$
$$(Ht \times Wt)^{0.65}$$

$$\text{Children over 13 years: TBW} = 0.0758 \times 0.84^{[if \text{ female}]} \times$$
$$(Ht = \times Wt)^{0.69}$$

Intracellular Fluid

Intracellular fluid (ICF) represents about two thirds of the TBW, which is equivalent to 30% to 40% of total body weight. However, the proportion of ECF is much greater than that of ICF in preterm infants and reaches 60% of TBW at term. The membranes retaining this fluid allow the passive diffusion of water, whereas active transport mechanisms maintain an internal solute milieu different from that found outside the cells. K^+, P^{2-}, and Mg^{2+} are intracellular ions, and Na^+ and Cl^- are predominantly extracellular.

Extracellular Fluid

ECF accounts for about one third of TBW and is made up of two compartments: plasma and interstitial fluid. Plasma water represents 4% to 5% of body weight and 10% of TBW. It is the milieu in which blood cells, platelets, and proteins are suspended. Blood volume is usually estimated as a changing proportion with respect to body weight. When expressed as milliliters per kilogram of body weight, it decreases with age from 80 mL/kg at birth to 60 mL/kg in adulthood.

Interstitial Fluid

Interstital fluid accounts for 16% of body weight and has a solute composition almost identical to that of intravascular fluid, except for a lower protein concentration. In general, the bulk distribution of ions and fluids between these two compartments is determined by the Donnan effect and Starling forces.

Transcellular Fluid

The transcellular fluid compartment (1% to 3% of body weight) is a specialized subdivision of the ECF compartment. Separated from blood by endothelium and epithelium, it represents fluid collections such as cerebrospinal fluid, aqueous and vitreous humors of the eyes, synovial fluid, pleural fluid, and peritoneal fluid.

MATURATION OF RENAL FUNCTION

Although all nephrons of the mature kidneys are formed by 36 weeks' gestation during healthy intrauterine life, hyperplasia continues until the sixth postnatal month; thereafter, cell hypertrophy is responsible for increases in renal size. Growth in the size of the kidney tends to be directly proportional to increase in height (Schultz et al., 1962).

While the fetal kidney receives 3% to 7% of cardiac output, RBF increases gradually after birth (Rudolph et al., 1971). RBF, as measured by paraaminohippuric acid (PAH) clearance (C_{PAH}), correlates with gestational age. For example, C_{PAH} is 10 mL/min per square meter at 28 weeks of gestation and 35 mL/min per square meter at 35 weeks of gestation (Fawer et al., 1979). C_{PAH} corrected for body surface area doubles by 2 weeks of age and reaches adult levels at 2 years. Furthermore, changes in RBF are associated with considerable increases in the relative RBF to the outer cortex, where most glomeruli are located (Olbing et al., 1973).

Selected renal functions measured at different ages are summarized in Table 5-3. The GFR in the full-term newborn infant averages 40.6 ± 14.8 mL/min per 1.73 m^2 and increases to 65.8 ± 24.8 mL/min per 1.73 m^2 by the end of the second postnatal week (Schwartz et al., 1987). GFR reaches adult levels after 2 years of age. Premature newborns have a lower GFR that increases more slowly than that in full-term infants. The low GFR at birth is attributed to the low systemic arterial blood pressure, high renal-vascular resistance, and low ultrafiltration pressure, together with decreased capillary surface area for filtration.

Despite a low GFR, full-term infants are able to conserve Na^+ (Spitzer, 1982). This is explained by the existence of glomerulotubular balance, such that as GFR and the filtered load of Na^+ increase, so does the ability of the proximal tubule to reabsorb Na^+. In contrast, preterm infants have a prolonged glomerulotubular imbalance, so that GFR is high relative to tubular capacity to reabsorb Na^+. The glomerulotubular imbalance is caused by structural immaturity of the proximal convoluted tubule and the incomplete development of the transport system responsible for conserving Na^+. This, together with poor response of the distal tubule to mineralocorticoids in preterm infants, results in Na^+ wastage and susceptibility to hyponatremia.

TABLE 5-3. Maturation of Renal Function with Age

Measurement	Premature Newborn	Full-term Newborn	1 to 2 weeks	6 Months to 1 Year	1 to 3 Years	Adult
GFR (mL/min /1.73 m²)*	14 ± 3	40.6 ± 14.8	65.8 ± 24.8	77 ± 14	96 ± 22	Male: 125 ± 15 Female: 110 ± 15
RBF (mL/min /1.73 m²)	40 ± 6	88 ± 4	220 ± 40	352 ± 73	540 ± 118	620 ± 92
Tm_{PAH} (mg/min/ 1.73 m²)	10 ± 2	16 ± 5	38 ± 8	51 ± 20	66 ± 19	79 ± 12
Maximal concentration ability (mOsm/kg)	480	700	900	1200	1400	1400
Serum creatinine (mg/dL)	1.3	1.1	0.4	0.2	0.4	0.8-1.5
Tm_P/GFR (mg/dL)	—	7.39 ± 0.37	—	5.58 ± 0.28	5.71 ± 0.28	3.55 ± 19
Fractional excretion of sodium (%)	2% to 6%	<1	<1	<1	<1	<1
Tm_G (mg/min /1.73 m²)	—	—	71 ± 20	—	—	339 ± 51

*GFR, Glomerular filtration rate; RBF, renal blood flow; Tm_{PAH}, tubular maximum for para-aminohippuric acid; Tm_P, tubular maximum for phosphorus; Tm_G, tubular maximum for reabsorption of glucose.

The tubular mechanisms involved in the excretion of organic acids are poorly developed in neonates. The tubular transport of PAH, which is a weak acid, is around 16 ± 5 mg/min per 1.73 m² in full-term infants and about half this value in premature babies. It increases with age and reaches adult rates, ranging from 55 to 104 mg/min per 1.73 m² by 12 to 18 months (Spitzer, 1978). PAH excretion is limited by a number of factors, including low GFR, immaturity of the systems providing energy for transport, and a low number of transporter molecules. This is further accentuated by a low extraction ratio for PAH and other organic acids caused by the predominance of juxtamedullary circulation in the immature kidney, a phenomenon that allows increased shunting of blood through the *vasa recta* and exclusion of postglomerular blood from the proximal tubular excretory surface (Calcagno and Rubin, 1963).

The kidneys' ability to concentrate urine is lower at birth, especially in premature infants. After water deprivation in the full-term newborn, urine concentrates to only 600 to 700 mOsm/kg, or 50% to 60% of maximum adult levels. Healthy children ranging from 6 months to 3 years of age who were given 20 mcg of desmopressin intranasally demonstrated a gradual rise in urinary concentration, starting from a mean value of 525 mOsmol/kg to reach a mean maximum plateau of 825 mOsm/kg (Marild et al., 1992). The major cause for the reduced concentration of urine in the neonate is the hypotonicity of the renal medulla (Aperia and Zetterstrom, 1982). Several mechanisms that contribute to interstitial hypertonicity are not well developed, including urea accumulation in the medulla, length of the loop of Henle and the collecting ducts within the medulla, and Na⁺ reabsorption in the ascending, water-impermeable loop (Trimble, 1970; Horster, 1978; Edwards, 1981). In addition, the collecting duct cells in immature kidneys may be less sensitive to ADH than those of mature nephrons (Schlondorff et al., 1978).

A water-loaded infant can excrete diluted urine with osmolity as low as 50 mOsm/kg. In the first 24 hours of life, however, the infant may be unable to increase water excretion to approximate water intake (Aperia and Zetterstrom, 1982). The diluting capacity becomes mature by 3 to 5 weeks of postnatal life.

FLUID AND ELECTROLYTE NEEDS IN HEALTHY INFANTS AND CHILDREN

The normal need for fluids varies markedly in low–birth-weight and full-term neonates, as well as during infancy and later childhood. This variability in fluid needs is caused by differences in the rate of caloric expenditure and growth, the ratio of evaporative surface area to body weight, the degree of renal functional maturation and reserve, and the amount of TBW at different ages. For instance, compared with older children and adults, infants have greater fluid needs because of higher rates of metabolism and growth; a surface area-to-weight ratio that is about three times greater, resulting in higher insensible fluid loss; and greater urinary excretion of solutes combined with lower tubular concentrating ability, which increases obligatory fluid loss. On the other hand, as previously noted, low–birth-weight and full-term neonates have a greater percentage of TBW compared with older children and adults (Friis-Hensen, 1971; Kagan et al., 1972). This increase in TBW results mainly from expansion of the ECF compartment, which at birth may comprise as much as 50% of the TBW. During the first 3 postnatal days, when this "extra fluid" is eliminated by the kidneys, full-term neonates require less fluid intake (Silverman, 1961; Oh, 1980; Winters, 1982).

The needs of low–birth-weight infants are more variable and may be markedly altered by relatively minor changes in ambient temperature or by phototherapy (Table 5-4) (Fanaroff et al., 1972; Oh and Karecki, 1972; Wu and Hodgman, 1974). In contrast to more mature infants, the immature skin in very low–birth-weight infants (<1500 g) allows disproportionate evaporative heat loss relative to basal metabolic rate (Levine et al., 1929; Levinson et al., 1966). This greater evaporative heat loss, together with a large body surface area, accounts for the much greater insensible fluid needs in infants with very low birth weight.

Parenteral and Oral Fluids and Electrolytes

Except for the first 3 postnatal days when full-term neonates require only 40 to 60 mL/kg fluid per day, in general, 100 mL

TABLE 5-4. Average Fluid Needs of Low–Birth-Weight Infants (mL/kg per 24 hr) During First Week of Life*

Age (days)	Component	Body Weight (g)			
		751 to 1000	1001 to 1250	1251 to 1500	1501 to 2000
1	IWL[†]	65	55	40	30
	Urine[‡]	20	20	30	30
	Stool	0	0	0	0
	Total	85	75	70	60
2 to 3	IWL	65	55	40	30
	Urine	40	40	40	40
	Stool	0	0	0	5
	Total	105	95	80	75
4 to 7	IWL	65	55	40	30
	Urine	60	60	60	60
	Stool	5	5	5	5
	Total	130	120	105	95

From Oh W: Fluid and electrolyte therapy in low birth weight infants, *Pediatr Rev* 1:313, 1980.

*Allowances for increased metabolic rate (cold stress, increased activity) are not included; these infants are in an incubator and naked.

[†]Insensible water loss.

[‡]Volume required to achieve a urine osmolarity of 250 mOsm/kg of renal solute load during the first day (no sodium and protein added), 10 mOsm/kg per day on the second and third days, and 15 mOsm/kg per day on the fourth to seventh days.

TABLE 5-5. Normal Losses and Maintenance Requirements for Fluid, Electrolytes, and Dextrose in Infants and Children

H_2O = 100 to 125 mL/100 kcal Expended

Components:	Insensible loss (mL)	45
	Sweat (mL)	0 to 25
	Urine (mL)	50 to 75
	Stool (mL)	5 to 10
	Food oxidation (mL)	12

Na^+ = 2.5 mmol/100 kcal Expended

Components:	Body growth	
	Sweat	Variable
	Urine	Variable
	Stool	Variable

K^+ = 2.5 mmol/100 kcal Expended

Components:	As for Na^+

Cl^- = 5 mmol/100 kcal Expended

Components:	As for Na^+

Dextrose = 25 g/100 kcal Expended

Components:	Basal metabolic rate
	Growth and tissue repair
	Physical activity

Maintenance Solution (per liter of water)

Dextrose (g)	50
Na^+ (mmol)	25
K^+ (mmol)	25
Cl^- (mmol)	50

Adapted from Winters RW: *Principles of pediatric fluid therapy*, ed 2. Boston, 1982, Little, Brown.

TABLE 5-6. Method to Predict Metabolic Rates During Critical Illness

Average Hospital Energy Requirements		Increases in Energy Expenditure with Stress	
Body Weight(kg)	kcal/kg/day		
0 to 10	100	Fever	12% per °C
10 to 20	1000 + 50/kg	Cardiac failure	>37° C
>20	1500 + 20/kg	Major surgery	15% to 25%
		Burns	20% to 30%
		Severe sepsis	Up to 100%
			40% to 50%

Modified from Holliday MA: Fluid and nutrition support. In Holliday MA, Barratt TM, Avner ED, editors: *Pediatric nephrology*, ed 3, Williams and Wilkins, 1994, Baltimore.

of water is needed for each 100 kcal expended. Notably, an additional 15 mL of water is generated endogenously for each 100 kcal used (water of oxidation), which is also available for body functions. In preterm infants, fluid intake may be gradually increased to 150 mL/kg per day, whereas 100 to 125 mL/kg per day generally suffices for infants weighing less than 10 kg. The fluid requirement decreases to 50 mL/kg per day for those weighing 11 to 20 kg and to 20 mL/kg per day for those with body weights above 20 kg. These fluid volumes are sufficient to allow excretion of dietary solute load, as well as to replace insensible fluid loss through the skin, lungs, and intestines (Table 5-5) (Winters, 1982). It should be noted that energy expenditure and, therefore, fluid intake may be significantly increased with stress (Table 5-6) (Holliday et al., 1994).

The high fractional excretion of Na^+ (FE_{Na+}) in premature infants can lead to negative Na^+ balance, hyponatremia, neurologic disturbances, and poor growth unless an Na^+ intake of 3 to 5 mmol/kg per day is given; in full-term infants and older children, 2 to 3 mmol/kg per day is sufficient (Drukker et al., 1980). Premature infants have a lower renal threshold for bicarbonate. In addition, several functional and anatomic factors combine to limit tubular excretion of weak organic acids (Avner et al., 1990). Consequently, premature infants may need small supplements of base. Sodium bicarbonate at 1 to 2 mmol/kg per day is generally recommended for the very small premature infant. Clinically important disturbances in acid-base status are unusual in full-term neonates unless they consume excessive amounts of protein.

DEHYDRATION IN INFANTS AND CHILDREN

Because premature infants and mature neonates have a great TBW-to-body weight ratio than older infants and children, th tolerate a greater degree of dehydration before manifestin clinical symptoms. A 10% fluid deficit in such patients may produce symptoms consistent with moderate dehydration, whereas a similar deficit in adults produces severe symptoms. However, dehydration can occur very quickly in infants because disorders such as vomiting or diarrhea very rapidly produce deficits of 50 to 100 mL/kg. Dehydration can also develop in healthy premature infants if insensible water losses are underestimated and are not adequately replaced. This situation may result from use of an open radiant warmer without appropriate plastic shields; forced convection in nonhumidified incubators; skin immaturity, resulting in greater transcutaneous evaporative fluid loss; use of phototherapy, causing insensible fluid loss; hyperthermia; or tachypnea. In older infants and children, gastrointestinal disorders are the major causes of dehydration.

Assessment of Dehydration

Assessment of the extent and type of dehydration is important for formulating a therapeutic strategy. Table 5-7 provides guidelines for the clinical assessment of the severity of dehydration in children (Ellis and Avner, 1985). Laboratory measurements should include hematocrit, blood gases, glucose, calcium, blood urea nitrogen, and albumin, as well as serum and urinary creatinine, osmolality, and electrolytes. A urinalysis should be done to detect cellular elements and to measure specific gravity. Urinary osmolality and specific gravity are of minimal value in assessing dehydration in premature infants with tubular immaturity and in infants with reduced urinary concentrating ability

caused by low protein intake. In general, however, such data, together with a careful medical history, physical examination, and assessment of fluid input and loss, aid in the diagnosis of dehydration and guide adjustment of the amount and composition of fluid administration during various phases of therapy.

Treatment of Dehydration

Severely dehydrated infants and children should be cared for in the intensive care unit with constant monitoring of central venous pressure and serial measurements of the initial laboratory studies. Box 5-2 shows a stepwise approach to the treatment of isotonic, hypotonic, and hypertonic dehydration (Ellis and Avner, 1985). Particular attention should be given to hypernatremic dehydration and brain injury. The initial measures for fluid resuscitation are to stabilize the vital signs by administering crystalloid or colloid solutions and to correct severe acid-base imbalance, hypoglycemia, and other metabolic disturbances. The objective of subsequent measures is to assess further the kind of dehydration and to plan a time course for administration of the appropriate fluid volume and chemical composition needed to correct previous deficits and to replace ongoing losses.

The composition of select parenteral and oral rehydration solutions are shown in Tables 5-8 and 5-9. In most infants and children receiving parenteral solutions for brief periods, the normal fluid and electrolyte needs can be easily satisfied. The caloric needs, however, are not readily met. It is customary

TABLE 5-7. Clinical and Laboratory Assessments of the Severity of Dehydration in Children*

Signs and Symptoms	Mild Dehydration	Moderate Dehydration	Severe Dehydration
Weight loss (%)	5	10	15
Fluid deficit (mL/kg)	50	100	150
Vital Signs			
Pulse	Normal	Increased; weak	Greatly increased; feeble
Blood pressure	Normal	Normal to low	Reduced and orthostatic
Respiration	Normal	Deep	Deep and rapid
General Appearance			
Infants	Thirsty, restless, alert	Thirsty, restless, or lethargic, but arousable	Drowsy to comatose; limp, cold, sweaty; gray color
Older children	Thirsty, restless, alert	Thirsty, alert, postural hypotension	Usually comatose; apprehensive, cyanotic, cold
Skin turgor†	Normal	Decreased	Greatly decreased
Anterior fontanel	Normal	Sunken	Markedly depressed
Eyes	Normal	Sunken	Markedly sunken
Mucous membranes	Moist	Dry	Very dry
Urine			
Flow (mL/kg/hr)	<2	<1	<0.5
Specific gravity	1.020	1.020-1.030	>1.030

*When hypernatremia is present, the severity of dehydration may be clinically underestimated because of the relative preservation of extracellular fluid volume (ECFV) at the expense of intracellular fluid volume (ICFV). In such states, neurologic symptoms (lethargy alternating with hyperexcitability, progressing to focal or generalized seizures) may predominate.
†With hypernatremia, the skin may have a thick, "doughy" consistency or a soft, velvety texture.

Box 5-2 Stepwise Approach to Fluid Therapy in Infants and Young Children with Moderate (100 mL/kg) to Severe (150 mL/kg) Dehydration*

PHASE I (0 TO 4 HOURS)

1. Assess vital signs and body weight, approximate fluid deficit, and begin fluid balance sheet.
2. Obtain blood for immediate chemical and acid-base analysis, and if possible, obtain a urine sample for chemical and microscopic determinations.
3. Regardless of the type of dehydration (see p ***), begin immediately with 0.9% NaCl at 20 to 30 mL/kg given over 1 hr or faster, depending on the severity of circulatory compromise. If the major cause of dehydration is diarrhea, a mixture of 0.45% NaCl and 0.45% NaHCO$_3$ is preferred as the initial hydrating solution. If shock is present, administer 5% salt-poor albumin (10 mL/kg).
4. Stabilize vital signs by repeating Step 3 if needed, and continue fluid administration at 10 mL/kg per hour until urine output is established.
5. On the basis of serum electrolyte values, determine the type of dehydration. Also, make a more precise assessment of the total fluid deficit and proceed to phase II.

PHASE II (4 HOURS TO 2 DAYS)

1. Repeat Phase I, Steps 1 and 2.
2. Isotonic dehydration (serum [Na$^+$] = 130 to 150 mmol/L).
   a. Replace 60% to 70% of the remaining fluid deficit over the next 24 hours using a solution containing 0.45% NaCl with 20 mmol/L KCl and 50 g/L dextrose; add 20 mmol NaHCO$_3$/L if serum pH is <7.25. Replace maintenance fluid plus continued fluid loss using the same solution.
   b. Replace remainder of fluid deficit over the subsequent 24 hours, in addition to maintenance fluid and ongoing fluid loss, with solution containing 0.2% NaCl with 20 mmol KCl and 50 g/L dextrose.
   c. Additional dextrose, K$^+$, or HCO$_3{}_-$ may be needed and may be added according to serial serum measurements.
3. Hypotonic dehydration (serum [Na$^+$] < 130 mmol/L).
   a. Estimate Na$^+$ deficit as follows: [Na$^+$] deficit (mmol) = (135 – Serum [Na$^+$]) × Total body water (L). Replace 60%

of fluid deficit over the next 24 hours using a similar choice of solution as in Phase I, Step 3, plus 5% to 10% dextrose. If serum [Na$^+$] is <120 mmol/L or symptoms of water intoxication are present, give 12 mL/kg of 3% saline solution over 1 hour. During this time, replace maintenance fluid and ongoing fluid loss with the solution noted in Phase II, Step 2b.
   b. Same as for Phase II, Step 2b.
   c. Same as for Phase II, Step 2c.
4. Hypertonic dehydration (serum (Na$^+$) > 150 mmol/L).
   a. Add fluid deficit, 48 hours of maintenance water, and estimate of continued fluid loss to determine total volume of fluid to be administered initially at a constant rate over 48 hours.
   b. Use a solution containing 0.2% NaCl with 40 mmol KCl/L and 25 g/L dextrose.
   c. Add 20 mmol lactate or acetate if plasma pH is <7.25. (Do not use NaHCO$_3$, because calcium may need to be added to the fluid.)
   d. If serum calcium level is <8.5 mg/dL, add 1 g calcium gluconate to every 500 mL of administered fluid. Additional calcium is administered as required by serial serum values or clinical symptoms of hypocalcemia. Discontinue when serum calcium level equals 9.0 mg/dL.
   e. If serum [Na$^+$] is decreasing at 0.50 mmol/L per hour, decrease rate of administration by 30% to 50%. If serum [Na$^+$] is decreasing at <0.25 mmol/L per hour, increase rate of fluid administration by 30% to 50%.

PHASE III (3 TO 6 DAYS)

1. Same as for Phase I, Steps 1 and 2.
2. Replace any residual fluid or solute deficits over the next 2 to 4 days using the solution described in Phase II, Step 2b.
3. For severe hypertonic dehydration (serum [Na$^+$] > 175 mmol/L), Phase II therapy is continued for 3 to 4 days and subsequently may be switched to Phase III therapy, Step 2, when serum [Na$^+$] is <145 mmol/L.

*For mild dehydration (50 mL/kg) that requires parenteral fluid therapy, start therapy with phase II.

TABLE 5-8. Composition of Frequently Used Parenteral Fluids

Liquid	CHO	Prot.*	Cal/L	Na$^+$	K$^+$	Cl$^-$	HCO$_3^{-\dagger}$	Ca^{2+}	P‡
	(g/100 mL)				(mEq/L)			(mg/dL)	
D$_5$W	5	—	170	—	—	—	—	—	—
D$_{10}$W	10	—	340	—	—	—	—	—	—
Normal saline (0.9% NaCl)	—	—	—	154	—	154	—	—	—
½ Normal saline (0.45% NaCl)	—	—	—	77	—	77	—	—	—
D$_5$ (0.2% NaCl)	5	—	170	34	—	34	—	—	—
3% Saline	—	—	—	513	—	513	—	—	—
8.4% Sodium bicarbonate (1 mEq/mL)	—	—	—	1000	—	—	1000	—	—
Ringer's solution	0 to 10	—	0 to 340	147	4	155.5	—	4.5	—
Ringer's lactate	0 to 10	—	0 to 340	130	4	109	28	3	—
Amino acid 8.5% (Travasol)	—	8.5	340	3	—	34	52	—	—

TABLE 5-8. Composition of Frequently Used Parenteral Fluids—cont'd

Liquid	CHO	Prot.*	Cal/L	Na+	K+	Cl-	HCO₃⁻ †	Ca²⁺	P‡
	(g/100 mL)					(mEq/L)		(mg/dL)	
Plasmanate	—	5	200	110	2	50	29	—	—
Albumin 25% (Salt poor)	—	25	1000	150 to 160	—	<120	—	—	—
Intralipid	2.25	—	1100	2.5	0.5	4.0	—	—	0.8

Modified from DeYoung L, Patterson J, Johns Hopkins Hospital, Children's Medical and Surgical Center: *The Harriet Lane handbook: a manual for pediatric house officers,* ed 14, Mosby.
*Protein or amino acid equivalent.
†Bicarbonate or equivalent (citrate, acetate, lactate)
‡Approximate values; actual values may vary somewhat in various localities depending on electrolyte composition of water supply used to reconstitute solution. Values may vary from lot to lot.

TABLE 5-9. Comparison of Oral Rehydration Solutions (ORS) and "Clear Fluids"

Product	Na⁺*	K⁺	Cl⁻	Base	CHO, g/L	Glucose/Na⁺ Ratio	Osmolality
World Health Organization Oral Rehydration Therapy (ORT)	90	20	80	30	20	1.2	310
Pedialyte	45	20	35	30	25	3.1	250
Rehydralyte	75	20	65	30	25	1.6	305
Infalyte	50	25	45	10	30	—	200
Cereal-based ORT	90	20	80	30	50	—	175
Gatorade	23	3	17	3	46	11.1	330
Cola	2	2	0.1	13	120	—	750
Ginger ale	3	3	1	4	90	—	540
Apple juice	3	3	28	0	120	—	730
Chicken broth	250	8	250	0	0	—	450
Tea	0	5	0	0	0	—	5

Modified from Meyers A: Fluid and electrolyte therapy for children, *Curr Opin Pediatr* 6:303–309, 1994.
*Na⁺, K⁺, Cl⁻, and base levels are measured in mmol/L.

to provide 5% dextrose in parenteral solutions. Although this concentration provides only a fraction of the optimal number of calories (20% of total kilocalories needed by infants younger than 1 year of age), it is sufficient to prevent ketosis. In less mature neonates, higher infusion rates of 5% dextrose generally suffice to maintain blood glucose concentrations between 50 to 90 mg/dL (Roy and Sinclair, 1975; Winters, 1982).

Provided that infants and children are less than 10% dehydrated and have minimal electrolyte abnormalities, a good level of consciousness, adequate bowel sounds, and absence of signs of hypovolemia, oral rehydration may be used to replace deficits and maintain fluid volume. Commercially available preparations, such as Pedialyte RS (Ross) with a Na⁺ content of 45 mmol/L may be used. In children with diarrhea in developing countries, the World Health Organization (WHO) has recommended the use of an inexpensive and effective oral rehydration solution consisting of 90 mmol/L Na⁺ and 111 mmol/L of glucose (total osmolarity, 311 mOsmol/L). However, glucose-based solutions with a lower osmolality may further optimize fluid and glucose-sodium coupled absorption in the small intestine (Hahn et al., 2001).

PERIOPERATIVE PARENTERAL GUIDELINES OF FLUIDS AND ELECTROLYTES

The optimal perioperative fluid volume and composition requirements in infants and children have not been adequately investigated. The formulas provided by Berry in Table 5-10 are widely used to determine the hourly rates of intraoperative fluid volume administration, which consists of four major components (1986):

1. Maintenance fluid established by Holliday and Segar based on calorie expenditure at different ages (1957).
2. Estimated volume deficit incurred during preoperative fasting or gastrointestinal or by other fluid deficits. One third of such deficits may be replaced during the first hour of surgery, while the remaining volume may be spread over the duration of the surgery.
3. Severity of surgical and nonsurgical trauma. This may comprise the largest volume of fluid loss or fluid redistribution, which derives largely from the ECF compartment.

TABLE 5-10. Guidelines for Fluids for Newborn and Children during the Perioperative Period*

Age (yr)	Hydrating Solution During First Hour (mL/kg)	Hydrating Solution During Following Hours
Neonates		Maintenance fluid: 4 mL/kg /hr 5% to 10% dextrose in 0.75 normal saline plus 20 mEq sodium bicarbonate/L Trauma: 6 to 10 mL/kg/ hr for intra-abdominal or 4 to 7 mL/kg/hr for intrathoracic surgery replaced with Ringer's lactate
<3	25	Maintenance fluid: 4 mL/kg /hr 5% Dextrose in normal saline
3 to 4	20	Maintenance and trauma: basic hourly fluid 4 mL/kg 5% Dextrose in normal saline + If mild trauma 2 mL/kg = 6 mL/kg/hr
>4	15	+ If moderate trauma 4 mL/kg = 8 mL/kg/hr + If maximal trauma 6 mL/kg = 10 mL/kg/hr

Modified from Berry FA: Practical aspects of fluid and electrolyte therapy. In Berry FA, editor: *Anesthetic management of difficult and routine pediatric patients,* New York, 1986, Churchill Livingstone.
*Plus blood replacement with blood or 3:1 volume replacement with crystalloid. Replace blood loss in excess of 20 mL/kg with equal volume of packed red blood cells.

4. Blood losses and fluids needed to support systemic blood pressure.

A key goal of perioperative fluid management is to maintain an adequate intravascular volume without the development of hyponatremia. Perioperative patients are at risk for developing hyponatremia because of multiple factors, including prehydration with hypotonic fluid, and nausea, pain, and stress associated with surgery that may result in nonhypovolemic stimulation of ADH release during and after surgery (that is, the inappropriate secretion of ADH) (Burrows et al., 1983; Arieff, 1998). The limited ability of such individuals to excrete a large water load may be influenced by any preexisting edema-forming disorder, obstructive uropathy, or the use of thiazide diuretics or other drugs such as narcotics and antiemetics. However, hypotonic fluid infusion is the most important cause of acute hyponatremia developing in the intraoperative period. Acute hyponatremia results in increased water content in neurons (brain edema) without a change in solute content. This may cause subclinical symptoms such as headache, nausea, vomiting, or muscle weakness in any age group. Younger children are more susceptible to more severe hyponatremic encephalopathy because of their larger brain-to-skull ratio (Moritz and Ayus, 2002). Unless there is a free water deficit, isotonic fluid infusion is recommended during the perioperative period. The need for potassium, calcium, chloride, and bicarbonate (or lactate or citrate, which may be converted to bicarbonate in individuals without hepatic failure) is more controversial. Such components are contained in lactated Ringer's solution, which is nearly isonatremic (Na^+ = 130 mEq/L) and isotonic but also

contains K^+ (4 mEq/L), Ca^{2+} (0.9 mmol/L), Cl^- (109 mEq/L), and lactate (27.7 mmol/L).

The amount of dextrose commonly used is 5% (equals 5000 mg/dL or 278 mmol/L). Although this is more than 50 times more concentrated than normal plasma glucose concentration (90 to 100 mg/dL or ≈5 mmol/L), the energy delivery based on the volume of fluid given to an infant weighing 10 kg amounts to 50 kcal for the first hour of surgery. Such energy supply is particularly important in preventing hypoglycemia in premature and full-term neonates, who have greater energy requirements than older children, but it may lead to hyperglycemia in 0.5% to 2% of pediatric patients. This disorder may be less common in children receiving regional anesthesia, which reduces the hyperglycemic effects of surgery. Although such transient hyperglycemia is purported to have various potential deleterious consequences, these have not been well substantiated. A review suggests that a solution of lactated Ringer's solution with 1% dextrose is sufficient to prevent both hypoglycemia and hyperglycemia in most children, excluding premature and full-term neonates (Berleur et al., 2003). This practice, however, is not yet widely used.

Perioperative Fluid Management of Premature and Full-Term Neonates

Guidelines for the intraoperative fluid and electrolyte management of premature and full-term neonates are largely based on available knowledge of renal physiology rather than on data obtained from clinical investigations. The physiology of the healthy neonate is influenced by the short tubular length and is characterized by immature reabsorption mechanisms, an activated renin-angiotensin-aldosterone system, and low circulating ADH concentrations (Avner et al., 1990; El-Dahr and Chevalier, 1990). Thus, healthy preterm neonates weighing less than 1300 g, or of fewer than 32 weeks' gestation, have FE_{Na+} rates that range from 8.2% to 2.1% between 28 and 32 weeks' gestation, with further gradual decrease to less than 1% at term; such rates may increase to 15% with stress (Arant, 1978; Delgado et al., 2003). The high FE_{Na+} in preterm infants is ascribed to decreased Na^+ reabsorption in the proximal tubule, together with hyporesponsiveness of the distal tubule to aldosterone (Sulyok et al., 1979). When combined with a negative Na^+ balance that results from inadequate Na^+ supplementation as well as decreased sensitivity of the collecting duct to ADH, up to one third of such infants develop significant hyponatremia (Na^+ < 130 mEq/L), often manifesting with neurologic disturbances during the first 6 weeks of life (Roy and Sinclair, 1975).

Both premature and term neonates have a limited capacity to excrete K^+, possibly because of distal tubular insensitivity to aldosterone. Hence, baseline reference plasma K^+ concentrations range from 3.9 to 5.9 mEq/L. Moreover, both preterm and term neonates are capable of producing maximally diluted urine while concentrating capacity is limited. Yet, hyponatremia may develop after administration of large volumes of hypotonic fluids, because fluid excretion may be limited mainly because of low GFR. Stress may cause profound reduction in GFR in premature and term neonates through release of various extrarenal vasoactive and hormonal substances that modify the response of "immature kidneys," thereby further disturbing fluid and electrolyte homeostasis. The higher body content of water and the higher metabolic rate, as well as a propensity to metabolic acidosis and hypocalcemia in premature newborns, are other important factors in deciding the volume and composition of intraoperative fluids.

Such considerations support the avoidance of boluses of hypotonic fluids while keeping in mind the lower age- and size-appropriate circulatory pressures that may serve as the goal of fluid management. In the absence of the expected physiologic fluid loss, which may range from 5% to 15% of body weight during the first 3 days of postnatal life, fluid volume during this time period may be limited to 60 mL/kg per day, whereas blood pressure support may be sustained with small infusions (5 mL/kg) of 5% albumin or other blood products as needed. Beyond 3 days of life, maintenance fluid volume is gradually increased to 150 mL/kg per day. Deficits beyond the expected physiologic losses and ongoing losses and allowance for surgical trauma may be replaced by a similar fluid composition, but the volume replacement may be more gradual or less rapid than outlined for older infants and children (Table 5-10). Na^+ bicarbonate and calcium may be supplemented, while K^+ should be limited. Also, a higher glucose concentration is generally desirable in premature infants. A recommended fluid composition is 0.75 normal saline with 20 mEq sodium bicarbonate/L (total Na^+ = 135 mmol/L) in 5% to 10% dextrose, as well as 20 mEq/L KCl if plasma K^+ falls below 3.5 mEq/L. Close attention to change in body weight and urine output and serial measurements of plasma electrolytes are essential in guiding the perioperative fluid management of the sick premature and full-term neonate.

Fluid Management of Children Undergoing Renal Transplantation

The key goal of intraoperative management is to expand the circulatory volume and to maintain systemic blood pressure between the 90th and 95th percentiles for age, gender, and height percentile, so as to allow for adequate perfusion of the renal allograft (Update on the 1987 Task Force Report on High Blood Pressure in Children and Adolescents, 1996). An adult kidney may sequester up to 250 mL of blood, and in infants nearly 50% of the cardiac output may be directed toward perfusion of the allograft. To ensure adequate perfusion of the allograft, the anesthesiologist actually needs to maximize the circulatory volume of the recipient, mainly with crystalloid or packed cytomegalovirus-safe, leukocyte-poor red blood cells if hemoglobin is below 9 g/dL, while closely monitoring the central venous pressure (CVP) and systemic MABP during vessel anastomosis. Near the completion of the vascular anastomoses, 20% mannitol (0.5 to 1.0 g/kg) and intravenous furosemide, 1 mg/kg, may be given before the cross-clamps are released. Before cross-clamp release, CVP should be maintained at 8 to 12 cm H_2O, and the systolic blood pressure and MABP should be kept above 120 mm and 70 mm Hg, respectively. If the MABP is inadequate to achieve good renal perfusion of the adult kidneys, a constant dopamine infusion of up to 5 mcg/kg per minute may be started. Intraoperative blood gases may be monitored frequently, because clamping of the aorta and accumulation of lactic acid can result in metabolic acidosis and vasoconstriction. The critical goal is to obtain immediate allograft function; hypotension after cross-clamp release in an infant with inadequate circulatory volume and an underperfused allograft is a potential catastrophe.

Intravenous furosemide (1 to 2 mg/kg per dose), 25% salt-poor albumin (0.5 g/kg per dose), 20% mannitol (0.3 to 0.5 g/kg per dose), or 0.9 normal saline solution (10 mL/kg bolus) may be given to help promote urine output in the immediate postoperative period.

The volume and composition of intravenous fluid administered during the first 48 postoperative hours are essential to ensure continued renal function. The urine output often exceeds 5 mL/kg per hour. Thus, insensible losses are quantitatively less important. In children with such high urine output, the concentration of dextrose to 1% is routinely reduced to prevent hyperglycemia, which may compound osmotic diuresis because of high preoperative blood urea nitrogen concentrations. Urine output is replaced on a milliliter-for-milliliter basis. In infants and children with body weight below 30 kg, the CVP should be maintained in the range of 5 to 10 cm H_2O, and the MABP should be at greater than 70 mm Hg. One fluid solution that may be used during the first 24 to 48 hours consists of 1% dextrose, 0.45 mEq/L NaCl solution, and 10 to 20 mEq sodium bicarbonate per liter. During the first 24 to 36 hours, additional fluid boluses of 10 mL/kg of normal saline or a 5% albumin solution may be given if CVP falls below 5 cm H_2O, with the goal of maintaining a urine output above certain arbitrary limits (5, 4, and 3 mL/kg per hour for body weight <10 kg, <20 kg, and <30 kg, respectively). In conjunction with such fluid boluses, intravenous furosemide (1 mg/kg) is also administered because renal allografts tend to be dependent on diuretics in the early perioperative setting.

Serum electrolytes (Na^+, K^+, Cl^-, HCO_3^-, Ca^{2+}, P^{2-}, Mg^{2+}) may be monitored at 8- to 12-hour intervals during the first 2 postoperative days. Potassium chloride is given separately as needed when the plasma K^+ falls below 3.5 mEq/L. In infants and young children, close monitoring of fluid balance and cardiovascular examination are essential to prevent electrolyte imbalance and fluid overload, which may result in severe hypertension or pulmonary edema, or, in reduction of intravascular volume and acute tubular necrosis (ATN). A bladder catheter inserted intraoperatively is necessary for accurate measurement of urine volume. Unless there are specific urologic indications, the catheter is removed after 4 to 5 days.

Immediate measures must be undertaken to improve postoperative oliguria. Beside the most easily correctable causes of oliguria, such as hypovolemia or a malfunctioning catheter, other potential causes include vascular bleeding or occlusion, ATN caused by prolonged cold ischemia storage, hyperacute rejection, or urinary extravasation or obstruction. In patients with oxalosis, precipitation of calcium oxalate crystals in the graft may cause acute allograft failure. Children with delayed graft function, congestive heart failure, or marked electrolyte abnormalities may require removal of fluid by hemodialysis or peritoneal dialysis. Fluid removal should be performed cautiously to avoid allograft hypoperfusion.

DISORDERS OF SODIUM METABOLISM

Among the many kidney functions, sodium homeostasis via multiple or redundant systems is paramount (Greger, 2000). About 75% of the filtered Na^+ is reabsorbed in the proximal tubule by the luminal Na^+/H^+ exchanger and by the basolateral Na^+, K^+-ATPase. Such reabsorption is increased by the action of angiotensin II, which preferentially constricts the efferent arteriole, thereby increasing filtration fraction and limiting fluid reentry into the peritubular capillaries. Dopamine has an opposing effect in this tubule segment, causing natriuresis. About 20% of NaCl reabsorption occurs in the ascending loop of Henle via the electroneutral $Na^+/K^+/2Cl^-$ transporter (NKCC2), causing the formation of dilute urine. Vasopressin and loop diuretics inhibit such reabsorption. In the distal tubule, Na^+ is reabsorbed by a thiazide-sensitive Na^+/Cl^- cotransporter. In the connecting tubule and in the cortical collecting duct, Na^+ is reabsorbed by the sodium-specific amiloride-sensitive ENaC. The ENaC is activated by aldosterone. In the medullary collecting duct, Na^+ reabsorption is under the influence of ANP.

Much experimental evidence suggests that regulation of ECF volume and maintenance of systemic blood pressure prevail over Na^+ homeostasis; plasma Na^+ concentration and plasma osmolality are secondary regulators (Bricker, 1982; Rees et al., 1984; Gennari, 1998a; Kumar and Berl, 1998; Scheinman et al., 1999). Thus, virtually all of the conditions associated with hyponatremia are primarily disorders of ADH excess with an impaired ability to excrete free water. Disturbances in serum Na^+ concentration may be associated with hypervolemia, normovolemia, or hypovolemia.

Hyponatremia (Plasma NA⁺ <135 mmol/L)

In infants and children, hyponatremia occurs much more often than hypernatremia. Although premature and full-term infants are capable of producing hypotonic urine, large, hypotonic fluid loads cannot be excreted, especially during the first 6 weeks of postnatal life. This is most evident during the first week of life, when only 10% to 50%, rather than 80%, of an intravenous challenge of 5% dextrose in water is excreted within 4 hours. The major factor limiting the response to a fluid challenge, especially in preterm infants during the first 5 weeks of postnatal life, is the physiologically low GFR and low urinary flow rate (Svenningsen and Aronson, 1974; Leake et al., 1976). Moreover, high urinary Na^+ excretion and negative Na^+ balance may contribute to the hyponatremia found in about one third of low–birth-weight premature infants (Engelke et al., 1978). This Na^+ wasting has been attributed to deficient proximal and distal tubular reabsorption of Na^+ in such infants (Sulyok et al., 1979).

A positive water balance, rather than Na^+ wasting, has also been implicated in the hyponatremia of healthy premature infants (Rees et al., 1984; Sulyok et al., 1985). Low serum albumin concentrations and reduced plasma oncotic pressure may also bring about fluid retention and "late hyponatremia" in preterm infants (Menon et al., 1986). Thus, independent of the specific pathologic process, preterm infants are at high risk of developing hyponatremia. Therefore, electrolytes should be monitored frequently during the first 4 to 6 weeks of life, especially in infants of fewer than 34 weeks' gestation. Other causes of hyponatremia in neonates are shown in Table 5-11. In older infants and children, hyponatremia may occur with dehydration, edema-forming states, and syndrome of inappropriate secretion of antidiuretic hormone (SIADH). Such conditions may be differentiated clinically at the bedside. In addition, the simple laboratory studies described in the section on dehydration may reveal urinary hypotonicity, suggesting water intoxication or the dilutional hyponatremia associated with renal failure.

TABLE 5-11. Causes of Hyponatremia

Neonates	Infants and Children
Drugs	
Prolonged use of diuretics in mother or infant	Diuretics (thiazides, osmotic diuretics)
Oxytocin for labor	Arginine vasopressin
Dopamine >5 mcg/kg/min	Carbamazepine
Prostaglandin infusion	Vincristine
Excessive administration of electrolyte-free solutions	Theophylline
	Cyclophosphamide
	Morphine
	Estrogen
	Barbiturates
	Nonsteroidal antiinflammatory agents
	Mannitol
	Hypotonic 1.5% glycine irrigant
	Ecstasy
	Selective serotonin reuptake inhibitors
	All conditions listed for neonates
Endocrine Disorders	
Pseudohypoaldosteronism	Hyperglycemia
Adrenogenital syndrome	Myxedema
Adrenal insufficiency problems	Glucocorticoid deficiency
Hypothyroidism	Decreased atrial natriuretic peptide
SIADH caused by asphyxia	Diabetes/ketonuria
	All conditions listed for neonates
Renal Disorders	
Dysplasia	Nephrotic syndrome
Multicystic kidneys	Acute or chronic renal failure
Obstructive uropathy	Medullary cystic kidneys
Polycystic kidney disease	Nephronophthisis
Renal tubular acidosis	Chronic pyelonephritis
Acute or chronic renal failure	Drug-induced tubulointerstitial nephritis
	Hypokalemic nephropathy
	Metabolic alkalosis
	Bicarbonaturia
	Postobstructive diuresis
	All conditions listed for neonates
Gastrointestinal Disorders	
Dilute formulas	Pancreatitis
	Cirrhosis
	Vomiting
	Diarrhea
	Ileus
	Bowel edema
	Protein-losing enteropathy
	Colonoscopy
Central Nervous System Disorders	
	SIADH
	Cerebral salt wasting
	Reset osmostat

TABLE 5-11. Causes of Hyponatremia—cont'd

Neonates	Infants and Children
Miscellaneous	
Negative Na⁺ balance caused by high FE_{Na^+} in infants ≤34 weeks gestation	Congestive heart failure
Hypoalbuminemia and decreased oncotic pressure	"Third-space" from burns, peritonitis, or severe muscle injury
Osmotic diuresis caused by hyperalimentation and low TmG	Water intoxication (psychogenic polydipsia, dilute formulas)
Ketonuria	Physical and emotional stress
Congestive heart failure	Cystic fibrosis
Hydrops fetalis	Pain
Congenital nephrotic syndrome	Postoperative
Surgery	Porphyria
Infection	Rickettsial disease
Pulmonary disorders	Fresh-water drowning Pseudohyponatremia in patients with hypoproteinemia, hyperglycemia, or hyperlipidemia Prolonged exercise

FE_{Na^+}, Excreted fraction of filtered sodium; *SIADH*, syndrome of inappropriate antidiuretic hormone; *TmG*, tubular maximum for glucose reabsorption.

Surgery and anesthesia stimulate ADH release. This may persist for 2 or more days and may result in acute hypotonic hyponatremia, particularly when hypotonic fluids are also administered. Even isotonic fluid administration may not prevent hyponatremia caused by ADH release, because such individuals often excrete urine with sodium and potassium concentrations higher than plasma. This is partly because of high ANP concentrations that may coexist in this setting. The syndrome of SIADH is discussed in a later section of this chapter.

Several causes of hyponatremia require special emphasis. Pseudohyponatremia is associated with normal plasma osmolality and occurs in the setting of severe hyperlipidemia, hyperproteinemia, or disorders in which solutes other than sodium such as glucose, mannitol, or sorbitol result in high plasma osmolality. Administration of thiazide diuretics to individuals with cardiac failure may impair distal tubular dilution of urine and the ability to excrete a water load. Finally, large amounts of hypotonic fluid intake during prolonged exercise can cause acute symptomatic hyponatremia and noncardiogenic pulmonary edema, particularly under high ambient temperatures when sweat sodium and chloride are high or when nonsteroidal antiinflammatory agents are administered.

In hyponatremic patients who require parenteral fluids, the decision to correct the plasma Na⁺ level may be based both on clinical symptoms and signs and on the rapidity with which the disorder developed. Children are especially prone to neurologic symptoms (Laureno and Karp, 1997; Lauriat and Berl, 1997, Albanese et al., 2001). In clinical practice, the most important prophylactic measure for preventing hyponatremia is to avoid the infusion of hypotonic fluids. Common symptoms and signs of hyponatremia include headache, fatigue,

nausea, and vomiting; seizures and respiratory arrest are more severe and sometimes delayed manifestations. Guidelines for replacing such sodium deficits may be based on the following formula:

$$Na^+ \text{ Deficit (mmol)} = TBW \times (Desired - Actual \text{ plasma } Na^+)$$

For example, the amount of 3% saline solution needed to raise the plasma Na⁺ to 125 mmol/L in a 10-kg infant with a plasma Na⁺ concentration of 115 mmol/L (assuming that TBW is 65% of body weight) may be calculated as follows:

$$TBW = 0.65\,TBW \times 10\,kg = 6.5\,L$$

$$Na^+ \text{Deficit} = 6.5\,L(125\,mmol/L - 115\,mmol/L) = 65\,mmol$$

In asymptomatic children, the Na⁺ deficit of 65 mmol may be replaced by 422 mL of normal saline (154 mmol/L) given over 24 hours; symptomatic children may receive 127 mL of 3% saline solution (513 mmol/L) given at a rate of about 5 mL/kg per hour, that is, 2.5 mmol/kg per hour

With chronic hyponatremia (over 48 hours in duration), adaptive increases in neuronal osmolytes (glutamine, taurine, phosphocreatinine, myoinositol) diminish cellular uptake of water, thereby preventing brain edema (Gullans and Verbalis, 1993). Thus, in contrast to acute hyponatremia, in which brain edema combined with noncardiogenic pulmonary edema and hypoxia can disrupt neuronal function, such events are uncommon with chronic hyponatremia. Edema-forming disorders such as nephrosis, liver failure, or congestive heart failure are commonly associated with chronic hyponatremia in children. Although physiologic mechanisms stimulate both sodium and fluid retention aimed at preventing hypovolemia, hypovolemic stimuli for ADH release result in free-fluid retention and hyponatremia. Treatment includes the possible correction of the primary disorder, the elimination of diuretics and other offending agents, and limitation of electrolyte-free water intake. Because most individuals with chronic hyponatremia are asymptomatic, and because slow recovery of brain osmolytes coupled with iatrogenic correction of chronic hyponatremia can result in fatal or serious pontine and extrapontine myelinolysis, the rate of correction of serum sodium should be slow (about 0.3 mEq/L per hour) (Ayus et al., 1987; Adrogue and Madias, 2000a).

Syndrome of Inappropriate Secretion of Antidiuretic Hormone

SIADH is a diagnosis by exclusion. It is a hypo-osmolar, saline-resistant form of hyponatremia that occurs in the absence of dehydration, hypoadrenalism, renal failure, hypothyroidism, or myxedema. The nonhypovolemic and nonhypotonic release of ADH impairs the ability of the kidneys to excrete free water.

The main causes of SIADH in infants and children are shown in Box 5-3. Hyponatremia attributable to SIADH is uncommon in premature and full-term infants younger than 4 to 6 weeks old because of factors that limit the urinary concentrating ability to values below 600 mOsm/kg. These factors include a low dietary-solute intake, low circulating levels of ADH, and tubular hyporesponsiveness to endogenous ADH (Svenningsen and Aronson, 1974; Godard et al., 1979). Because of these circumstances, it is indeed difficult to establish the diagnosis of SIADH in such infants. In children with bacterial meningitis,

Box 5-3   Disorders Associated with Syndrome of Inappropriate Secretion of Antidiuretic Hormone

CENTRAL NERVOUS SYSTEM DISORDERS

Asphyxia in newborns: Intraventricular hemorrhage in neonates, mask ventilation
Encephalitis
Meningitis (viral, bacterial, tuberculous)
Cerebrovascular accident (stroke)
Postpituitary surgery
Brain tumors
Brain abscesses
Hydrocephalus
Head trauma
Guillain-Barré syndrome
Lupus cerebritis

PULMONARY DISORDERS

Atelectasis or pneumothorax in newborns
Positive pressure ventilation
Pneumothorax
Hyaline membrane disease
Pneumonia (viral, bacterial)
Abscess
Tuberculosis
Aspergillosis
Positive-airway pressure breathing
Ligation of patent ductus arteriosus

MEDICATIONS

Vincristine
Cyclophosphamide
Carbamazepine
Selected serotonin reuptake inhibitors

ADH may be directly released through leaky, inflamed vessels, with secondary alterations in the blood-brain barrier. Despite the hyponatremia, mean plasma ADH levels are relatively high rather than suppressed in such children (3.3 U/mL versus 1 U/mL), and SIADH develops in about 50% of them (Kaplan and Feigin, 1978).

The diagnosis of SIADH should be suspected in any child who has or has had asphyxia, meningitis, a brain tumor, trauma, surgery, or pulmonary disease, as well as in any child who does not appear dehydrated but has hyponatremia, hypochloremia, persistent natriuresis, decreased plasma osmolality (<270 mOsm/kg), and urine that is not maximally dilute (>100 mOsm/kg). The blood urea nitrogen (BUN) and plasma uric acid levels are often reduced.

Na^+ excretion in SIADH may vary according to the extent of ECF expansion, which may raise the GFR and suppress aldosterone release. In addition, intravascular volume expansion stimulates the secretion of ANP, which enhances the renal excretion of Na^+. Moreover, Na^+ excretion matches or exceeds Na^+ intake.

The initial treatment of children with SIADH who have few or no symptoms may consist of restricting fluid intake to between one half and two thirds of the maintenance rate, or 800 to 1000 mL/m²/day. For severely symptomatic children, 3% saline may be given at a rate of 2.5 mmol/kg per hour, or 5 mL/kg per hour to maintain serum Na^+ concentrations at or above 125 mmol/L. In patients with urinary osmolality greater than 500 mOsm/kg, an alternative method for faster correction of severe hyponatremia is to use loop diuretics to inhibit reabsorption of free water while replacing measured urinary Na^+ losses. In young children, such treatment must be monitored especially closely to prevent volume contraction, hypokalemia, or acid-base imbalance. Furosemide at a dose of 1 mg/kg may be given intravenously one or two times daily. Other therapies used to manage adults with SIADH, such as osmotically active agents, dimethyl chlortetracycline, and lithium carbonate, are generally not used in children with this condition. V_{1a} and V_2 receptor blockers are newer agents that may soon become available and may be more effective in managing this disorder (Palm et al., 2001).

Hypernatremia (Plasma NA⁺ >145 mmol/L)

The causes of hypernatremia in infants and children are listed in Box 5-4. Hypernatremia commonly results from excessive water loss and inadequate water intake and occurs most often in individuals who are unable to communicate or satisfy their own thirst by accessing water. Thus, infants and debilitated individuals of any age are particularly susceptible to this disorder. A primary lack of thirst sensation is a rare cause of this disorder in children. The condition has been caused by improper mixing of formulas and is also increasingly reported with inadequate breastfeeding (Manganaro et al., 2001; Oddie et al., 2001). It is also increasingly recognized as a complication in hospitalized individuals who are very ill and have edema in association with renal failure, heart failure, hypotension, or liver failure, resulting in impaired sodium excretion and sodium overload (Kahn, 1999; Adrogue and Madias, 2000b). Administration of isotonic saline to maintain systemic blood pressure, together with associated hyperglycemia, may promote hypernatremia in these settings. Also, the deliberate use of hypertonic saline for the treatment of brain edema has occasionally resulted in severe hypernatremia (Peterson et al., 2000).

Premature infants and full-term neonates are also prone to hypernatremia because, in addition to an inability to excrete a water load, they are unable to excrete a large solute load (Aperia et al., 1975a, 1975b, 1977). The renal response to an Na^+ load improves gradually, so that by the end of the first year of life, Na^+ excretion reaches maximal levels of 16 mmol/hr per 1.73 m² (Aperia et al., 1975b). The limited ability to excrete an Na^+ load appears to result from a reduced GFR and tubular inability to significantly increase the FE_{Na^+} because of the effect of aldosterone in increasing distal tubular Na^+ reabsorption.

Signs and symptoms associated with hypernatremia in infants include muscle weakness, hyperpnea, apnea, bradycardia, restlessness, a high-pitched cry, lethargy, insomnia or coma, and muscular hypertonicity (Finberg and Harrison, 1955). Older children may exhibit thirst, lethargy, confusion, muscle irritability, rhabdomyolysis, respiratory arrest, seizures, or coma. Tachycardia and hypotension are symptoms of hypovolemia, which is an ominous sign suggestive of extreme dehydration. Because of hypertonicity, fluid shift from the intracellular compartment may result in brain shrinkage, subarachnoid hemorrhage, and permanent brain injury when chronic adaptive solute gain fails to maintain cell volume. Even with such correction, the ensuing neuronal hyperosmolality may predispose a patient to cerebral edema and serious neurologic consequences when rehydration with hypotonic fluid is used aggressively.

Box 5-4 Causes of Hypernatremia

HYPERNATREMIA CAUSED BY PURE WATER LOSS

Inadequate water replacement of mucocutaneous fluid losses, especially in low–birth-weight infants or young children with fever and lack of access to water; phototherapy; or use of radiant warmers.

Central diabetes insipidus: Low plasma ADH concentration
Congenital thalamic/pituitary disorders
Acquired: Trauma or tumor involving the thalamic/pituitary areas

Nephrogenic diabetes insipidus with failure of thirst response: High plasma ADH concentration
Congenital distal tubular and collecting duct unresponsiveness to ADH
Biochemical: Hypercalcemia, hypokalemia
Dietary: Severe protein malnutrition or marked restriction in NaCl intake
Drug-induced: Lithium carbonate, demeclocycline, amphotericin B
Anesthetic-induced: Methoxyflurane
Hyperventilation

HYPERNATREMIA CAUSED BY WATER LOSS IN EXCESS OF SODIUM LOSS

Lactation failure: Breastfeeding
Overdressing of neonates and infants

Neonates receiving phototherapy or kept in incubators without normothermal control
Diarrhea or colitis
Vomiting
Profuse sweating
Hyperosmolar nonketotic coma
Hypertonic dialysis
Renal disorders with partial diabetes insipidus or limited concentrating ability, including chronic renal failure, polycystic kidney disease, medullary cystic disease, pyelonephritis, obstructive uropathy, amyloidosis, and sickle-cell nephropathy
High protein intake with high urea appearance rate
Diuretics: Mannitol, furosemide

HYPERNATREMIA CAUSED BY SODIUM EXCESS

Excess NaCl intake secondary to improper preparation of oral formulas or electrolyte solutions
Excessive administration of $NaHCO_3$
Ingestion of NaCl tablets, sea water, or near-drowning in sea water
Inadequate free fluid relative to NaCl intake because of defective thirst mechanism or unconsciousness
Cushing's syndrome or excessive administration of glucocorticoids
Hyperaldosteronism or excessive administration of mineralocorticoids

---

The initial laboratory investigation of hypernatremia is similar to that noted in the section on dehydration. In the absence of dehydration, the treatment of hypernatremia depends largely on the underlying disorder. The judicious administration of insulin and avoidance of colloids may be needed in patients with hyperosmolar nonketotic hyperglycemic coma. On the other hand, the administration of free water, together with appropriate replacement of arginine vasopressin, is useful for the treatment of central diabetes insipidus. Surgery may be used to treat several endocrinopathic conditions, whereas thiazides and a diet low in osmotic activity may be of benefit in nephrogenic diabetes insipidus.

In children with acute hypernatremia resulting from pure water loss, such as those with nephrogenic diabetes insipidus, a hypotonic fluid may be given at a rate that decreases plasma osmolality by no more than 2 mOsmol/kg per hour. The rate can be calculated using the following formula:

$$\text{Current TBW} = 65\% \text{ of body weight (kg)}$$

$$\text{Former TBW} = \frac{\text{Current Na}^+ \times \text{Current TBW}}{\text{Desired Na}^+}$$

$$\text{Water deficit (L)} = \text{Former TBW} - \text{Current TBW}$$

For example, to calculate the water deficit in a 10-kg infant with diabetes insipidus, a current serum-Na^+ concentration of 160 mmol/L, and a desired plasma-Na^+ concentration of 140 mmol/L, the following applies:

$$\text{Current TBW} = 0.65 \times 10 \text{ kg} = 6.5 \text{ L}$$

$$\text{Former TBW} = \frac{160 \text{ mmol/L} \times 6.5 \text{L}}{140 \text{ mmol/L}} = 7.43 \text{ L}$$

$$\text{Water deficit} = 7.43 \text{ L} - 6.5 \text{ L} = 0.93 \text{ L}$$

In children with hypotonic sodium loss, this fluid deficit, together with ongoing fluid losses that occurring during replacement of such a deficit, may be infused as ⅛ or ¼ saline with 1% to 2% dextrose

With chronic hypernatremia, correction of plasma osmolality may occur at a rate of less than 1 mOsmol/kg per hour, or a reduction in serum sodium of less than 0.5 mEq/L. Hypotonic fluids given at a low rate are the most suitable for this purpose. In individuals with accidental sodium loading, furosemide combined with adequate replacement of urine volume with 5% dextrose in water, is usually effective unless renal failure is present, in which case dialysis may be of benefit.

Hypernatremic Dehydration

This disorder is relatively common in premature infants of fewer than 27 weeks' gestation (Baumgart, 1982; Baumgart et al., 1982). Its typical presentation, however, is in infants younger than 12 months of age, with diarrhea being the usual predisposing cause. Such infants have inadequate access to free water, increased insensible water loss, proportionally greater water loss than Na^+ loss from the gastrointestinal tract, and at times, a positive solute balance from the improper use of electrolyte solutions used to manage the diarrhea (Paneth, 1980). Patients with hypertonic dehydration often do not have dehydration of the interstitial fluid compartment and thus may not manifest the poor skin turgor, dryness of mucous membranes, and postural changes in pulse and blood pressure that are often associated with isotonic or hypotonic dehydration. Muscular hypertonicity may result in nuchal rigidity. Other potential complications include brain hemorrhage and edema after rehydration because of fluid shifting into the brain. Because of impaired insulin secretion, initial serum glucose concentrations often exceed 130 mg/dL in 50% and 200 mg/dL in 25% of children with hypernatremia. Hence, the amount of dextrose administered to such individuals may be limited, or insulin may be given to prevent further hyperglycemia, osmotic diuresis, and hypernatremia. Hypocalcemia also occurs in 10% to 20% of patients with hypertonic dehydration. The management of this disorder is outlined in Box 5-2.

DISORDERS OF POTASSIUM METABOLISM

Potassium (K^+) is the principal cation in the ICF, ranging in concentration from 140 to 160 mmol/L; the normal K^+ concentration in ECF varies between 3.5 and 5.5 mmol/L (same as 3.5 and 5.5 mEq/L). The low proportion of ECF K^+ to ICF K^+ is necessary to maintain transmembrane electrical potential, which is essential for proper functioning of muscle and neural tissue (Suki, 1976).

Potassium Homeostasis

Total body K^+ content correlates with body weight and height and depends on muscle mass (Pierson et al., 1974; Patrick, 1977). In a healthy 20-year-old adult, total body K^+ approximates 58 mmol/kg, a value that decreases progressively with age as muscle mass decreases and body fat increases. In children, the total body K^+ is 38 mmol/kg or less (Pierson et al., 1974). More than 90% of body K^+ is intracellular, and most of that is in muscle tissue. Of the extracellular K^+, only 1.4% is contained within the ECF, whereas the remaining 8.6% is contained in the bone matrix.

The daily need for K^+ is about 2 mmol/100 kcal of expended energy. The daily intake from a standard Western diet is estimated to be 0.75 to 1.5 mmol/kg of body weight. Typically, approximately 90% of the K^+ ingested each day is eliminated in the urine. Less than 15% is eliminated in the stool, while a negligible amount is lost through the skin. The amount of K^+ eliminated in stool increases, however, with a significant degree of renal failure, reaching 34% of dietary intake at a GFR of less than 5 mL/min per 1.73 m² (Hayes et al., 1967).

The renal tubular mechanisms involved in K^+ homeostasis have been extensively reviewed (Halperin and Kamel, 1998). Nearly 85% of the filtered K^+ is reabsorbed in the proximal tubule and the ascending thick limb of the loop of Henle. The amount of K^+ in the final urine depends on the amount of intake and on the tubular secretion of K^+.

Two key hormones lower ECF K^+ acutely through redistribution in various tissues. Insulin causes Na^+ to enter and H^+ to exit cells through the electroneutral Na^+/H^+ exchanger, and epinephrine (and β_2-adrenergic agonists) activates the Na^+, K^+-ATPase, which exports three Na^+ ions for each two K^+ ions that enter the cell. Although epinephrine possesses both α- and β-adrenergic properties, it first causes a hyperkalemic response (during the first 1 to 3 minutes) and then a sustained decrease in plasma K^+ concentration through trapping of K^+ in cells by maintenance of an intracellular net negative charge that is essential in determining the electronegative resting membrane potential. By contrast, α-adrenergic agonists raise plasma K^+ concentration by modifying muscle K^+ uptake (Rosa et al., 1980).

Chronic K^+ homeostasis is largely regulated by secretion of K^+ by principal cells that predominate in the renal cortical collecting duct and are located in smaller numbers in the connecting tubule. The main mechanisms of K^+ secretion are depicted in Figure 5-5. Secretion is aided by the following factors:

1. The plasma aldosterone level that is stimulated by angiotensin II and by high plasma K^+ concentrations. Aldosterone activates the ENaC. This results in Na^+ reabsorption and the development of an electronegative lumen voltage that favors K^+ secretion. An ATP-sensitive ROMK channel aids the efflux of K^+ into the tubular lumen. Many primary adrenal disorders or renal disorders associated with high circulating levels of renin and angiotensin II may lead to secondary stimulation of aldosterone and result in hypokalemia.
2. The peritubular-fluid K^+ concentration directly stimulates Na^+/K^+-ATPase and may be the most important mediator of K^+ secretion.
3. High urinary flow rates.
4. Hypomagnesemia, possibly through inactivation of the Na^+/K^+-ATPase pump.
5. Higher pH in the lumen of the cortical collecting duct.
6. Reabsorption of bicarbonate and Na^+ that influences the electronegativity in the lumen of the cortical collecting duct.

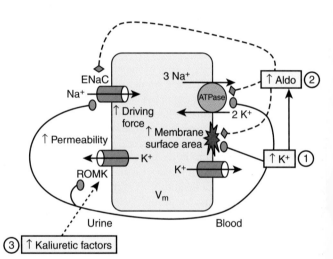

■ **FIGURE 5-5.** Major factors that regulate K^+ secretion in principal cells. Sodium is reabsorbed across the luminal membrane through ENaC Na^+ channels, with the resultant cellular depolarization increasing the electrical driving force for K^+ secretion through ROMK K^+ channels. *1,* Elevation of peritubular [K^+] *(oval arrowheads)* increases the density of luminal ENaC and ROMK channels, which promote both K^+ secretion by increasing the electrical driving force and K^+ permeability, respectively. Increases in peritubular [K^+] also activate the Na^+,K^+-ATPase pump in the basolateral membrane and stimulate aldosterone release. *2,* Aldosterone *(diamond arrowheads)* increases the density of ENaC (but not ROMK) channels and activates the Na^+,K^+-ATPase pump, both of which increase the driving force for K^+ secretion. The surface area of the BLM containing the Na^+, K^+-ATPase pump undergoes amplification during prolonged exposure to either increased peritubular [K^+] or aldosterone. *3,* Kaliuretic factors, including K^+ itself, have been proposed to somehow directly increase K^+ secretion. For example, high luminal [K^+] may directly increase the activity of ROMK channels. *(From Gennari FJ, Segal AS: Hyperkalemia: An adaptive response in chronic renal insufficiency,* Kidney Int *62:1-9, 2002.)*

Understanding such mechanisms provides physiologic explanations for plasma K+ alterations and for therapeutic rationale. An example is the individual with hypovolemia and hyperkalemia. The kidneys guard against extracellular volume contraction by raising angiotensin II levels. The latter increases bicarbonate reabsorption in the proximal and distal tubules such that the cortical collecting duct lumen becomes less electronegative and favors NaCl retention but reduced K+ secretion despite elevated aldosterone levels. In this clinical setting, low urinary flow rate also contributes to hyperkalemia. This is in contrast to individuals with euvolemia or hypervolemia, in whom a high plasma K+ concentration inhibits proximal tubular bicarbonate reabsorption while it directly stimulates aldosterone release, thereby promoting K+ secretion (along with Cl^- and HCO_3^-) in the cortical collecting duct. In this setting Na^+ is reabsorbed through the important effect of aldosterone in activating the specific ENaC at the apical membrane of principal cells (Halperin and Kamel, 1998). When ENaC is blocked by trimethoprim, amiloride, or triamterene, kaliuresis is inhibited.

Hypokalemia (Plasma K+ <3.5 mmol/L or <3.5 mEq/L)

Although hypokalemia usually implies total body K+ depletion, it can also be caused by transcellular shifts of K+ without extrarenal losses. Several classifications of hypokalemia have been devised according to whether the condition is acute or chronic, with or without K+ shift, renal or extrarenal. One classification is shown in Box 5-5. Because the etiology of renal K+ wasting is extensive, it may be facilitated by further subclassification on the basis of systemic blood pressure (Box 5-6).

Hypokalemia without Potassium Depletion

Pseudohypokalemia can result from increased uptake of K+ when large numbers of leukemic cells (white blood cell count of 100,000 to 250,000 mm³) are allowed to stand at room temperature (Adams et al., 1981). This confounding effect is eliminated by rapid separation of plasma or by cold storage of blood samples at 4°C.

Hypokalemia caused by intracellular shift of K+ is particularly common in metabolic or respiratory alkalosis, and approximates a 0.6-mmol/L fall for every 0.1-unit increase in blood pH (Kim and Brown, 1968; Adrogue and Madias, 1981). Endogenous or exogenous β-adrenergic agonists such as albuterol, dopamine, dobutamine, and theophylline mediate transcellular shifts of K+. Barium poisoning or toluene intoxication resulting from the inhalation of paint or glue vapors can produce hypokalemia by trapping K+ within the cells (Roza and Berman, 1971; Streicher et al., 1981). Insulin administration activates the Na^+, K^+-ATPase, resulting in active K+ uptake and hypokalemia. This is commonly encountered during the treatment of diabetic ketoacidosis.

Hypokalemic periodic paralysis is a rare autosomal dominant disorder characterized by recurrent episodes of flaccid paralysis of the trunk and limbs that lasts 6 to 24 hours. Paralysis may be accompanied by cardiac arrhythmias, which may be provoked by high carbohydrate intake, exertion, and a

---

Box 5-5 Causes of Hypokalemia

HYPOKALEMIA WITHOUT POTASSIUM DEPLETION
Spurious
High white blood cell count

Transcellular Shifts
Metabolic alkalosis
Insulin excess
β-Adrenergic agonists
Barium intoxication
Toluene intoxication
Hypokalemic periodic paralysis
Delirium tremens

HYPOKALEMIA WITH POTASSIUM DEPLETION
Nutritional
Inadequate nutritional intake
Chloride-deficient infant formula

Extrarenal Causes
Copious perspiration: cystic fibrosis
Gastrointestinal losses/malabsorption
Chronic diarrhea
Vomiting
Gastrointestinal fistulas
Ostomy/short gut syndrome
Ureterosigmoidostomy
Rectal villous adenoma
Geophagia
Laxative abuse
Full-thickness burns

Renal Causes
Renal tubular acidosis (types I and II)
Fanconi's syndrome
Carbonic anhydrase inhibitors
Correction phase of metabolic alkalosis

Chloride Depletion
Vomiting/gastric drainage with metabolic alkalosis
Congenital chloride diarrhea
Cystic fibrosis
Diuretics (thiazide, loop, osmotic)
Cisplatin

Potassium Wasting
Bartter's syndrome
Gitelman's syndrome
Liddle's syndrome
Renal artery stenosis: high renin and aldosterone release
Mineralocorticoid excess: Cushing's syndrome, hyperaldosteronism, prolonged use of glucocorticoids, licorice ingestion, 17α- or 11β-hydroxylase deficiency
Pyelonephritis and other interstitial nephritides
Magnesium depletion
Postobstructive diuresis
Diuretic phase of acute tubular necrosis
Antibiotics: carbenicillin, penicillins, amphotericin B, aminoglycosides, cidofovir

Box 5-6 Renal Wasting of Potassium in Relation to Systemic Blood Pressure

RENAL WASTING OF K⁺ ASSOCIATED WITH NORMAL BLOOD PRESSURE

High Renin, High Aldosterone

Renal tubular acidosis
Bartter's syndrome
Gitelman's syndrome
Magnesium-losing tubulopathy
Calcium-losing tubulopathy
Osmotic diuresis: Hyperglycemia
Covert diuretic abuse
Prolonged emesis or nasogastric suction
Drugs: Penicillins, amphotericin B, aminoglycosides, cisplatin, ifosfamide

RENAL WASTING OF K⁺ ASSOCIATED WITH HYPERTENSION

Low Renin, High Aldosterone

Aldosterone-producing adenoma
Idiopathic hyperaldosteronism
Dexamethasone-suppressible hyperaldosteronism
Adrenocortical carcinoma

Low Renin, Low Aldosterone

17α-Hydroxylase deficiency
11β-Hydroxylase deficiency
11β-Hydroxysteroid dehydrogenase deficiency, licorice ingestion
Liddle's syndrome

High Renin, High Aldosterone

Malignant hypertension
Renal artery stenosis
Renin-secreting tumor (Wilms, nephroblastomatosis)
Chronic renal disease

Gill JR, Santos F, Chan JCM: Disorders of potassium metabolism. In Chan JCM, Gill JR, editors: *Kidney electrolyte disorders,* New York, 1990, Churchill Livingstone.

---

high Na⁺ diet (Griggs et al., 1970). This condition is more common in the Asian population and is characterized by low urinary K⁺ excretion, low transtubular potassium gradient (TTKG), and no acid-base disturbances (Lin et al., 2001). Dietary restriction of salt and carbohydrates together with spironolactone may help prevent such attacks. Intravenous K⁺ infusion should be avoided, because rebound hyperkalemia can occur. Potassium-sparing diuretics and the ingestion of foods rich in K⁺ are of limited benefit in treating or in preventing the disorder. Notably, affected individuals are susceptible to malignant hyperthermia with administration of general anesthesia.

Potassium Depletion

K⁺ depletion accounts for most cases of hypokalemia. Three basic disturbances can affect total body K⁺ balance and result in cellular depletion: poor nutritional intake, extrarenal loss of K⁺, and renal loss of K⁺.

Nutritional Causes

A deficient diet alone is seldom the only cause of symptomatic hypokalemia, because K⁺ is ubiquitous in foodstuffs. In adults, a reduction in K⁺ intake to less than 10 mmol/day for 7 to 10 days does cause a relative total body K⁺ deficit of 250 to 300 mmol, or a decrement of 7% to 8% (Wormersley and Darragh, 1955). Occasionally K⁺ depletion occurs in hospitalized patients maintained on K⁺-free intravenous fluids. In these instances, the kidney responds by appropriately decreasing K⁺ excretion, although it cannot produce K⁺-free urine.

Extrarenal Causes

Diarrhea, vomiting, and abuse of laxatives result in hypokalemia via a complex process. In addition to K⁺ loss (through vomit and stool), these conditions cause intravascular volume contraction, secondary hyperaldosteronism, and enhanced urinary excretion of K⁺. In children, diarrhea is often accompanied by hyperchloremic metabolic acidosis, whereas laxative abuse is associated with normal acid-base status or mild metabolic alkalosis (Welfare et al., 2002).

Copious perspiration from intense physical exertion in a hot environment causes K⁺ depletion (Knochel et al., 1972). This condition is characterized by normal plasma K⁺ concentration with total body K⁺ depletion and a high rate of urinary K⁺ excretion. Loss of K⁺ via sweat and secondary hyperaldosteronism explains the depletion state and the urinary loss; the sustained normal plasma K⁺ level, however, is not adequately explained. The human colon responds to aldosterone in a similar fashion, resulting in an increase in the renal collecting duct transepithelial potential difference followed by an increase in Na⁺, K⁺-ATPase activity (Thompson and Edmonds, 1971). Glucocorticoids are kaliuretic, and evidence suggests that their effect is independent of any action on the mineralocorticoid receptor (Bia et al., 1982). Furthermore, glucocorticoids appear to cause an increase in K⁺ and a decrease in Na⁺ stool concentration that can be associated with increased Na⁺, K⁺-ATPase activity (Charney et al., 1975).

Renal Causes

Renal wastage of K⁺ occurs by several different but interrelated mechanisms. First, an increased Na⁺/K⁺ exchange may occur in the distal tubule in conditions associated with increased circulating mineralocorticoid or glucocorticoid concentrations, resulting in circulatory volume expansion and suppression of plasma renin and aldosterone levels. Hypokalemia often occurs in Conn's syndrome (Ganguly and Donohue, 1983). It also occurs in 30% of patients with adrenal hyperplasia (Cushing's syndrome) (Prunty et al., 1963). The ingestion of certain food and the use of glucocorticoids or other drugs that possess mineralocorticoid activity can also result in hypokalemia. Licorice, for example, contains large amounts of glycyrrhizic acid, which impairs adrenal 11β-hydroxysteroid dehydrogenase action. This impairs the degradation of endogenous glucocorticoids, resulting in a mineralocorticoid-like response (Brem, 2001).

Second, increased delivery of Na⁺ to the distal tubule, which occurs in various proximal tubulopathic conditions (including proximal renal tubular acidosis and Fanconi's syndrome) may enhance K⁺ secretion. Similarly, thiazides and loop diuretics increase the delivery of Na⁺ to the distal nephron, thus promoting K⁺ excretion (Kassirer and Harrington, 1977). This effect by diuretics is augmented by concomitant Cl⁻ depletion and by contraction alkalosis (Seldin and Rector, 1972; Kassirer and Harrington, 1977).

Third, large concentrations of nonabsorbable anions in the distal tubules, such as penicillins, increase the electronegativity of tubular fluid and induce kaliuresis and hydrogen ion secretion (Lipner et al., 1975). Carbenicillin is particularly notorious for causing hypokalemia, because it is secreted actively in the proximal tubule, and high concentrations of the anion are delivered to the distal nephron (Stapleton et al., 1976).

Fourth, kaliuresis may occur secondary to direct damage to the renal epithelium. Conditions such as pyelonephritis and other interstitial nephritides may be associated with hypokalemia. Similarly, antibiotics such as amphotericin B, polymyxin, and outdated tetracycline can lead to K^+ depletion through their direct toxic effects on the renal tubules (Chesney, 1976). Aminoglycosides result in magnesium and K^+ wasting, probably because of a change in the permeability of the renal epithelium to these cations (Humes et al., 1982). Experimentally, hypokalemia tends to occur within the first 7 days of aminoglycoside administration and often occurs in the absence of overt acute tubular necrosis and renal failure. This tubular defect and the risk of hypokalemia usually resolve within 1 to 2 weeks after discontinuation of the drug.

Fifth, several genetic disorders are known to cause K^+ depletion. Box 5-6 characterizes such disorders of hypokalemia based on the presence or absence of hypertension. Hypertensive disorders may be associated with high peripheral renin activity (renovascular disorders comprise the majority of such causes in children) or low renin states that are then associated with either increased plasma mineralocorticoid or glucocorticoid levels, or with more direct activation of the principal cell amiloride-sensitive ENaC in the cortical collecting duct. The result may be salt retention, chronic volume expansion, renin and aldosterone suppression (hence "pseudoaldosteronism"), and hypertension as exemplified in Liddle's syndrome. In Liddle's syndrome, treatment that consists of blocking the mineralocorticoid receptor with spironolactone, or blocking the aldosterone receptor with amiloride, is less effective than the combination of triamterene and a low-salt diet.

Manifestations of Potassium Depletion

Hypokalemia results in multiple biochemical and neurophysiologic disturbances (Box 5-7) (Weiner and Wingo, 1997). Chronic hypokalemia and moderate degrees of acute K^+ depletion (5% to 10% of total body K^+) are generally well tolerated. More profound deficits result in clinical manifestations that are independent of the underlying cause of hypokalemia.

Biochemical consequences of hypokalemia include impairment in insulin release and insulin end-organ sensitivity, thereby increasing the risk of hyperglycemia or precipitation of frank diabetes mellitus (Rowe et al., 1980). Metabolic alkalosis results from direct stimulation of proximal tubular bicarbonate reabsorption and ammonia genesis by increased proton secretion via H^+, K^+-ATPase located in the collecting duct and by decreasing citrate excretion. Inadequate ADH response and increased synthesis of angiotensin II in the central nervous system may cause polyuria. Hypokalemia may raise plasma ammonia levels in patients with reduced hepatic function. Also, chronic renal K^+ wasting may predispose to formation of renal cysts and interstitial fibrosis (Torres et al., 1990).

Many of the symptoms of acute hypokalemia relate to disturbed neuromuscular functions. Skeletal muscle weakness caused by cell hyperpolarization is the earliest manifestation of K^+ depletion. Plasma K^+ concentrations below 3.0 mEq/L lower the resting cell membrane potential and thereby increase the voltage needed to reach the threshold and initiate an action potential (Fig. 5-6). The symptoms include restless legs syndrome, fatigue, muscle cramps, paralysis, and rhabdomyolysis. Frank muscle necrosis may occur with serum K^+ concentrations below 2.0 mEq/L (Knochel, 1982). Cardiac manifestations of hypokalemia include abnormalities in rhythm as a result of slowed repolarization (Helfant, 1986). The presence of electrocardiographic changes helps to exclude spurious hypokalemia and may aid the decision to manage the hypokalemia urgently (see Fig. 5-6). Abnormalities include depression of the ST segment, lower T-wave voltage, and appearance of U waves. Patients receiving cardiac glycosides are especially at risk of developing such abnormalities. Hypokalemia also impairs the cardiovascular responses to norepinephrine and angiotensin II.

K^+ depletion may lead to several functional and structural abnormalities in the kidneys, including reduced RBF and GFR, renal hypertrophy, tubuloepithelial dilation, vacuolization, and sclerosis (Relman and Schwartz, 1956). Functionally, patients develop urinary acidification and concentration defects and polyuria.

Box 5-7 Pathophysiologic Consequences of Hypokalemia

NEUROMUSCULAR
Peripheral nerves: Paresthesias
Skeletal muscle: Fatigue, weakness, cramps, flaccid paralysis, rhabdomyolysis, myoglobinuria
Smooth muscle: Paralytic ileus, increased vascular pressor resistance

RENAL
Concentration defect: Polyuria, nocturia
Sodium retention
Increased ammonia production, enhanced bicarbonate reabsorption
Reduced renal blood flow, decreased GFR
Predisposition to urinary tract infection
Interstitial fibrosis
Cyst formation

METABOLIC
Metabolic alkalosis
Impaired hepatic glycogen storage
Impaired protein metabolism
Insulin resistance
Increased plasma ammonia
Growth retardation

HORMONAL
Impaired growth hormone release
Impaired insulin secretion
Decreased aldosterone secretion
Increased renin release
Increased synthesis of prostaglandins

Gill JR, Santos F, Chan JCM: Disorders of potassium metabolism. In Chan JCM, Gill JR, editors: *Kidney electrolyte disorders,* New York, 1990, Churchill Livingstone.

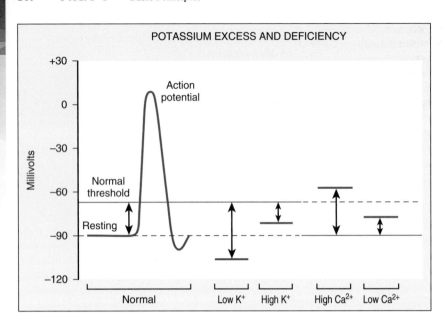

POTASSIUM EXCESS AND DEFICIENCY

■ **FIGURE 5-6.** Typical action potential profile. Normal threshold is influenced by Ca^{2+} concentrations, whereas K^+ concentrations affect the resting potential. *(From Leaf A, Cotran RS: Renal pathophysiology, ed 2, New York, 1980, Oxford University Press.)*

Diagnosis of Hypokalemia

When hypokalemia is diagnosed, the underlying pathophysiologic cause may not be apparent. Measurement of urinary K^+ levels may be helpful. A urinary concentration of less than 10 mEq/L suggests nearly maximal conservation and usually implies extrarenal loss of K^+. Urinary K^+ concentrations exceeding 30 mEq/L suggest the kidneys are a likely route for the depletion. In patients maintained on diuretics, the caveat is that within hours of discontinuation of these agents, the kidneys respond by conserving K^+.

Treatment of Hypokalemia

The treatment of hypokalemia requires extreme caution, as the magnitude of loss is difficult to measure clinically. In the absence of cellular shifts, the percent of total body K^+ deficit may be grossly estimated from the plasma concentration and intracellular K^+ content ($0.40 \times$ body weight $\times$ 145 mEq/L) as follows:

$$Plasma\ K^+\ 2.6\ to\ 3.5\ mEq/L\ =\ 5\%\ to\ 10\%$$
$$Plasma\ K^+\ 1.8\ to\ 2.5\ mEq/L\ =\ 10\%\ to\ 20\%$$
$$Plasma\ K^+ < 1.8\ mEq/L\ \ \ =\ >20\%$$

The concurrence of hypokalemia and metabolic acidosis suggests an even greater K^+ depletion. In such children the correction of the acidosis should follow, rather than precede, the correction of hypokalemia. Guidelines for potassium supplementation in dietary or medication forms are available for adults but not for children (Cohn et al., 2000). Such supplements should be given with close monitoring of blood levels, particularly when combined with potassium-sparing diuretics such as amiloride and spironolactone. Providing details of managing children with specific disorders associated with chronic hypokalemia is beyond the scope of this chapter. Supplemental K^+ at a dosage of 3 to 5 mEq/kg per day (plus maintenance amounts) may be given orally as the chloride salt, because most disorders are associated with chloride depletion. Several liquid and salt preparations are available. Microencapsulated

salt preparations are associated with a lower rate of gastrointestinal bleeding and hemorrhage. In patients with combined K^+ and phosphate depletion, the phosphate salt is recommended. Magnesium correction may help improve the hypokalemia, especially in refractory states such as appears in Gitelman's syndrome (Whang et al., 1992). High K^+-containing foods are useful in individuals whose conditions are managed with laxatives and diuretics

Intravenous K^+ repletion is often desirable for the management of acute hyperkalemia, particularly when neuromuscular or electrocardiographic alterations are clinically evident. Concentrations as high as 40 mEq/L may be given peripherally. Higher concentrations should be administered in large veins to prevent phlebitis. Concentrations exceeding 60 mEq/L generally are not recommended. In special clinical situations, higher K^+ concentrations may be delivered in limited fluid volumes by diluting 20 mEq of KCl in 100 mL in a Soluset with a microdrip and infusing it at a rate not to exceed 0.5 mEq/kg per hour (maximum, 30 to 40 mEq/hr). Such higher infusion rates, although reserved for life-threatening situations, can be given perioperatively in hypokalemic children with close cardiac monitoring and frequent measurement of plasma K^+ concentrations.

Hyperkalemia (Plasma K^+ >5.5 mEq/L in Infants and Children, or >6 mmol/L in Neonates)

Conditions causing hyperkalemia are listed in Box 5-. Hyperkalemia may result from a surprisingly small increa in total body K^+ or may result rapidly from transcellular shi Normally, the kidneys provide the crucial defense against slig elevations in serum K^+ level. Thus, with a few exceptior hyperkalemia commonly occurs in conditions characterized decreased urine flow rates or marked reduction in GFR. In t absence of renal insufficiency, drugs are responsible for m cases of hyperkalemia. Several agents may cause hyperkalen by increasing the K^+ load, by facilitating transcellular K^+ effl or by impairing renal excretion of K^+ (Table 5-12) (Peraze 2000).

Box 5-8 Causes of Hyperkalemia

PSEUDOHYPERKALEMIA
Ischemic blood drawing
Hemolysis
Thrombocytosis (>1,000,000/mm³)
Leukocytosis (>500,000/mm³)
Familial "leaky red blood cell"
Infectious mononucleosis

TRANSCELLULAR SHIFTS
Metabolic acidosis
Hyperglycemia with insulin insufficiency
Extracellular hypertonicity
Tissue damage: Trauma, exercise, burns, rhabdomyolysis,
    asphyxia, catabolic states, sepsis, rejection of transplanted
    organs (such as liver, kidney)
Drugs (see Table 5-12)
Familial hyperkalemic periodic paralysis

INCREASED POTASSIUM LOAD
Dietary excess, oral or intravenous K^+ supplementation
Use of aged bank blood/hemolysis
Geophagia
High doses of K^+-containing medications (such as potassium
    penicillin)

DECREASED RENAL EXCRETION OF POTASSIUM
Acute renal failure
Chronic renal failure
Low–birth-weight infants
Spitzer-Weinstein syndrome
Drugs (see Table 5-12)
Hyporeninemic hypoaldosteronism
Type I and type II pseudohypoaldosteronism
Addison's disease (hypoaldosteronism)
Obstructive uropathy
Impaired steroidogenesis: Congenital adrenal hyperplasia,
    mitochondrial disorders, Smith-Lemli-Opitz syndrome

TABLE 5-12. Medications That Can Cause Hyperkalemia and Their Mechanisms of Action

Medication	Mechanism
Increased Potassium Input	
Potassium supplements and salt substitutes	Potassium ingestion
Nutritional and herbal supplements	Potassium ingestion
Stored packed red blood cells	Potassium infusion
Penicillin G potassium	Potassium ingestion
Transcellular Potassium Shifts	
β-Blockers	Decrease β-driven potassium uptake
Intravenous amino acids (lysine, arginine, and ε-aminocaproic acid)	Release of potassium from cells
Succinylcholine	Depolarize cell membranes
Digoxin intoxication	Decrease Na^+, K^+-ATPase activity
Impaired Renal Excretion	
Potassium-sparing diuretics	
Spironolactone	Aldosterone antagonism
Triamterene	Block Na^+ channels in principal cells
Amiloride	Block Na^+ channels in principal cells
Nonsteroidal antiinflammatory drugs	Decrease aldosterone synthesis Decrease renal blood flow and glomerular filtration rate
ACE Inhibitors and Angiotensin II Receptor Blockers	
	Decrease aldosterone synthesis
	Decrease renal blood flow and glomerular filtration rate
Trimethoprim and pentamidine	Block Na^+ channels in principal cells
Cyclosporine and tacrolimus	Decrease aldosterone synthesis Decrease Na^+, K^+-ATPase activity Decrease K^+ channel activity
Heparin	Decrease aldosterone synthesis

Modified from Perazella MA: Drug-induced hyperkalemia: old culprits and new offenders, *Am J Med* 109:307–314, 2000.
ACE, Angiotensin-converting enzyme.

Transcellular Shift

Among the conditions associated with altered K^+ distribution across cell membranes is poorly controlled insulin-dependent diabetes mellitus. The mechanism is twofold: hyperglycemia causes hypertonicity with resultant extrusion of K^+ from cells, whereas insulin deficiency does not promote K^+ entry into the cells (Ammon et al., 1978). These effects are independent of aldosterone response and level of renal function.

Cellular damage from rhabdomyolysis, burns, tissue necrosis, or fulminant rejection of a grafted organ may release large quantities of K^+ into the extracellular space. In patients with normal renal function, most of the excess K^+ is easily excreted. In those with large tumor lysis after induction of chemotherapy or those with renal impairment, however, hyperkalemia may occur (Araseneau et al., 1973).

During metabolic acidosis, part of the H^+ load is buffered within cells in exchange for K^+. It has been noted that for every 0.1-U decrease in blood pH, serum K^+ changes by $0.6 \, mEq/L$. Changes in plasma HCO_3^- concentration may influence K^+ concentration independent of changes in pH. Clinically, serum K^+ can be decreased with bicarbonate administration in the absence of metabolic acidosis (Fraley and Adler, 1977).

Pseudohyperkalemia

Ischemic blood drawing is a very common cause of pseudohyperkalemia, especially in infants and young children who undergo blood sampling by lancing and squeezing the finger or heel, or because of hemolysis from prolonged application of tourniquets. Several conditions cause false elevations in plasma K^+ concentrations, including thrombocytosis, leukocytosis, hemolysis, and sampling of ischemic blood (Chumbley, 1970; Ingram and Seki, 1962). In general, immediate determination of K^+ in plasma instead of in serum minimizes the release of K^+ from the cellular components and avoids the development of pseudohyperkalemia.

High Potassium Intake

An oral intake of as little as 50 mmol of K^+ (<2% of normal body K^+ content) by an adult can cause a transient increase in plasma K^+ of 0.5 to 1.0 mmol/L. From 70% to 90% of this load is sequestered intracellularly within 15 to 30 minutes and ultimately excreted in the urine. Thus, when renal function is normal, large amounts of K^+ may be ingested without adverse sequelae. However, the intravenous administration of K+ at a rate higher than 0.5 mmol/kg per hour may result in life-threatening hyperkalemia. In patients with renal insufficiency, hyperkalemia may occur because of increased excretory burden associated with large doses of potassium penicillin (10^6 units contain 1.7 mEq K^+), juices with high K^+ content, overuse of salt substitutes (1 g contains 10 to 13 mEq of K^+), and the administration of banked stored blood (1 L contains 15 to 20 mEq of K^+) (Bostic and Duvernoy, 1972).

Decreased Potassium Excretory Capacity

Regardless of the underlying cause, impaired renal function predisposes a patient to K^+ retention and hyperkalemia. However, hyperkalemia is uncommon even in advanced renal failure unless endogenous or exogenous loads are excessive. Nonoliguric individuals with impaired GFR can excrete ordinary dietary intakes of K^+ until GFR decreases to as low as 5 mL/min per 1.73 m^2 (Gonick et al., 1971). An increase in K^+ secretion per nephron, as well as increased colonic secretion, helps to prevent hyperkalemia in severe renal failure (van Ypersele de Strihou, 1977). If hyperkalemia occurs with a GFR above 10% of normal, other causes should be sought, such as worsening metabolic acidosis, increased catabolism, cell injury, hemorrhage, or use of potassium-sparing diuretics.

The most common clinical setting in which hyperkalemia occurs is acute oliguric renal failure of any etiology. In addition to the decreased excretory capacity, an increased K^+ burden is imposed by an increased catabolic rate. The daily increase in K^+ concentration averages 0.3 to 0.5 mmol/L in oliguric acute renal failure under optimal conditions of nutrition, whereas the increase exceeds 0.7 mmol/L in patients with trauma, a high rate of catabolism, or both (Schrier, 1979).

Hyporeninemic hypoaldosteronism accounts for more than 50% of adults or older children with unexplained hyperkalemia accompanying adequate, albeit decreased, GFR (Schambelan et al., 1980). Most such patients have a component of chronic interstitial renal disease, and more than half have diabetes mellitus.

Obstructive uropathy may be associated with a defect in K^+ excretion associated with a mild hyperchloremic acidosis, decreased fractional excretion of K^+, and mild hyperkalemia (Battle et al., 1981) because of end-organ resistance to the action of aldosterone or because of hypoaldosteronism by itself.

Many drugs or drug combinations can cause hyperkalemia, particularly when KCl supplements are coadministered (Table 5-12) (Perazella, 2000). For example, a potassium-sparing diuretic and an angiotensin-converting enzyme inhibitor can result in life-threatening hyperkalemia-induced arrhythmia, especially in diabetic patients with renal insufficiency or other high-risk groups. The mechanisms may involve one or more of the following:

- Direct suppression of renin release by β-blockers or by prostaglandin synthetase inhibitors leading to secondary hypoaldosteronism
- Lowered aldosterone synthesis caused by angiotensin-converting enzyme inhibitors
- Inhibition of Na^+, K^+-ATPase and other transporters in principal cells by digitalis, trimethoprim, cyclosporine, or tacrolimus. Succinylcholine increases plasma K^+ concentration by increasing the permeability of muscle membranes during depolarization (Gronert and Theye, 1975).

Adrenal destruction brought on by hemorrhage, tumor, infection, autoimmune polyglandular syndrome, or adrenoleukodystrophy can cause an Addison-like presentation with fatigue, muscle weakness, hypotension, and hyponatremia. Congenital disorders associated with reduced steroidogenesis may have a similar clinical presentation (Ten et al., 2001; Bonny and Rossier, 2002). Hereditary disorders that exhibit similar sodium wasting and hyperkalemia, but that show increased, rather than low, plasma renin and aldosterone levels, include the autosomal dominant (self-limited) and autosomal recessive (permanent) forms of pseudohypoaldosteronism I. In these disorders, a defective mineralocorticoid receptor is responsible for hyponatremia, hyperkalemia, and metabolic acidosis (Ten et al., 2001; Bonny and Rossier, 2002). In contrast, pseudohypoaldosteronism Type II (Gordon's syndrome) is a sporadic or autosomal dominant condition associated with hypertension, suppressed plasma renin activity, normal plasma aldosterone concentration, and mild hyperchloremic acidosis that respond well to thiazide diuretics (Milford, 1999).

Manifestations of Hyperkalemia

The clinical manifestations of hyperkalemia relate to interference with the electrophysiologic activities of muscle. Under the influence of hyperkalemia, the ratio of intracellular to extracellular K^+ is decreased, resulting in delayed depolarization, hastened repolarization, and slow conduction velocity (Knochel, 1982). The most important effect involves the heart. Diagnostic electrocardiographic alterations include tenting or symmetric peaking of the T wave in the precordial leads and depression of the ST wave (Fig. 5-7). In severe hyperkalemia, there is widening of the QRS complex, lengthening of the PR interval, first-degree or second-degree heart block, disappearance of the P wave, and, finally, atrial standstill. Ventricular fibrillation or asystole follows the development of a sinusoid wave. Although the magnitudes of hyperkalemia and of cardiotoxicity correlate well, arrhythmias may develop with even mild hyperkalemia when other metabolic abnormalities such as hyponatremia, acidosis, or calcium disorders coexist.

Hyperkalemia affects electrical activities in noncardiac muscle as well. Such manifestations as paresthesias, weakness, and flaccid paralysis that spare the head and trunk are not rare.

Clinical Evaluation of Dyskalemia

The initial step involves a clinical assessment of circulatory volume (Halperin and Kamel, 1998; Rodriguez-Soriano et al., 1990). Assuming that Na^+ and fluid conservation mechanisms are intact, the next step is to determine whether the excretion of K^+ is appropriate relative to expected values in healthy children (Rodriguez-Soriano et al., 1990). If K^+ excretion is abnormal, urinary flow rate and K^+ excretion rate are measured separately. The flow rate in the terminal portion of the cortical collecting duct (CCD) is proportional to the osmolar particles in urine

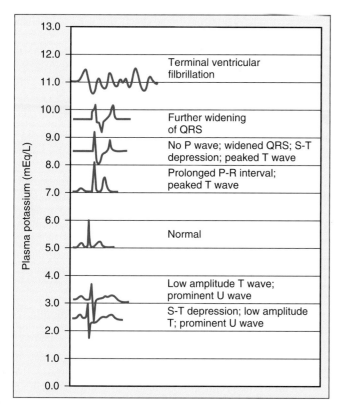

FIGURE 5-7. The relationship between plasma potassium concentration and electrocardiographic changes. *(From Winters RW: The body fluids in pediatrics, Boston, 1973, Little, Brown.)*

which consist primarily of urea derived from protein metabolism, with Na^+ and Cl^- contributing to a lesser extent. This is derived as follows:

$$\text{Flow rate in CCD} = (U_{osm} \times U_{vol})\, P_{osm}$$

where U refers to urine and P refers to plasma. Under the influence of ADH, a minimum flow rate in the CCD is 1 L for each 300 mOsmol excreted, which is approximately the osmolality of plasma. Thus, a lesser osmolality in the CCD would result in a lower flow rate and reduced net K^+ secretion

If the flow rate in the CCD is adequate, then the ability of principal cells to secrete K^+ depends largely on the appropriate activity and secretion of K^+ by ENaC and ROMK channels (see Fig. 5-5). This is assessed by measurement of urinary chloride excretion and by estimation of the transtubular $[K^+]$ gradient, or, TTKG:

$$\text{TTKG} = ([K^+]_U) \div (U_{osm} / P_{osm}) \div [K^+]_P$$

This equation provides an estimate of the K^+ concentration in the CCD relative to plasma K^+ concentration after correcting for further water reabsorption past the CCD, in the medullary collecting duct, under the influence of ADH. TTKG values under 4.9 in infants or under 4.1 in children indicate a reduced ability to secrete K^+ as a result of hypoaldosteronism or pseudohypoaldosteronism, and the situation requires further investigation of renal and adrenal disorders (Rodriguez-Soriano, 1990). Such evaluation may consist of venous blood gas measurements; electrolyte measurement of gastric fluids,

urinary nitrogen, plasma renin, aldosterone, and cortisol and corticosterone concentrations; and, possibly, identification of mutated genes.

Treatment of Hyperkalemia

The strategy of managing hyperkalemia depends on the plasma K^+ concentration, renal function, and cardiac manifestations (Box 5-9). Mild to moderate hyperkalemia without major electrocardiographic changes responds to a simultaneous decrease in K^+ intake and increase in Na^+ intake. In certain instances, loop diuretics may be used to increase K^+ excretion.

The fastest means of reversing cardiotoxicity is to antagonize the membrane effects of high plasma K^+ concentration. Calcium decreases the threshold potential of excitable tissue, thus restoring the normal differences between threshold and transmembrane potentials (see Fig. 5-6).

Calcium gluconate, infused intravenously at 100 to 200 mg/kg per dose, is an effective initial measure even in the absence of hypocalcemia.

If the clinical setting permits administration of a high fluid volume rate, a solution consisting of glucose and insulin added to 0.9 N NaCl is the most effective means for lowering plasma K^+ concentration (10% glucose solution, with insulin added at a ratio of 1 unit per 4 or 5 g of glucose). In children with metabolic acidosis, K^+ can be driven intracellularly by intravenous $NaHCO_3$ given at 1 to 2 mEq/kg per dose. Both treatment measures decrease plasma K^+ levels within minutes and are effective regardless of acid-base or insulin status. Hyperventilation (with resultant hypocapnia and respiratory alkalosis) abruptly increases the urinary excretion of K^+. Its effect, however, is not sustained beyond 24 hours (Gennari and Segal, 2002).

Sodium polystyrene sulfonate (Kayexalate), a cation-exchange resin, can be administered at a dose of 1 g/kg, in

---

Box 5-9 Treatment of Hyperkalemia

TREATMENT OF MILD HYPERKALEMIA
Decrease dietary K^+ burden
Discontinue K^+-containing medications or K^+-sparing diuretics
Eliminate conditions that favor hyperkalemia: Acidosis, sodium restriction

TREATMENT OF MODERATE TO SEVERE HYPERKALEMIA
To Reverse Membrane Effects
Calcium gluconate, 100 to 200 mg/kg per dose

To Produce Transcellular Shifts
Sodium bicarbonate, 1 to 2 mmol/kg per dose
Glucose, 0.3 to 0.5 g/kg as 10% glucose solution with insulin, 1 unit per 4 to 5 g glucose IV
Albuterol by nebulizer
Hyperventilation

To Remove Potassium
Kayexalate, 1 g/kg per dose PO or enema
Furosemide, 1 mg/kg per dose IV
Dialysis (hemodialysis or peritoneal dialysis)
Hemofiltration (continuous arteriovenous hemofiltration or continuous venovenous hemofiltration with or without dialysis)

sorbitol for oral use, or in mineral oil for rectal instillation. This dosage may be repeated every 2 to 4 hours. Typically, plasma K⁺ concentration decreases by 1 mEq/L per dose. The onset of action for the oral route is 1 to 4 hours, whereas an enema removes K⁺ within 30 to 60 minutes. In patients with renal failure, repeated administration of sodium polystyrene sulfonate may impose a high Na⁺ load with resultant hypertension and edema.

Dialysis may be useful in the treatment of hyperkalemia, especially in patients with renal failure. Hemodialysis can remove 1 mEq K⁺/kg per hour. The duration of this effect depends on the rate of ongoing endogenous release of K⁺. Peritoneal dialysis is less efficient than hemodialysis, but it can be performed more safely in small infants and children.

DIURETIC THERAPY

Pharmacologic agents that promote diuresis represent a major advance in the treatment of edema and hypertension. The principal therapeutic purpose of these agents is to induce a negative Na⁺ and fluid balance. The increase in urine output merely reflects the linkage of salt and water transport in the kidneys: solute reabsorption limits the osmotic reabsorption of water, and diuresis ensues.

Classification of Diuretics and Site of Action

In this section diuretics are classified according to the site of action in the nephron. This system is oversimplified, because several agents have pharmacologic effects that are not localized to a single tubular site (Table 5-13).

Proximal Tubule Diuretics

Mannitol

This is a nonmetabolizable sugar that is osmotically active. Mannitol is freely filtered at the glomerulus, but it is poorly reabsorbed and therefore obligates the renal excretion of water (Warren and Blantz, 1981). It limits water reabsorption in segments of the nephron that are freely permeable to water, namely, the proximal tubule, the descending limb of Henle's loop, and the collecting tubule. This results in a decreased gradient for NaCl reabsorption in the late proximal and distal tubule, which, together with a mannitol-induced washout of the hypertonic medullary interstitium brought about by increased blood flow, potentiates natriuresis. The magnitude of the natriuresis depends on the pretreatment intravascular volume status and on RBF.

Mannitol has limited use when GFR is severely compromised and may aggravate congestive heart failure or other conditions in which intravascular volume is often increased.

In nonedematous oliguric conditions, mannitol may be used to increase water excretion rather than natriuresis. It is also useful in the prophylaxis of acute renal failure because of its ability to expand the extracellular volume, increase tubular-fluid flow, redistribute blood to hypoxic inner cortical and outer medullary regions, and scavenge free radicals (Warren and Blantz, 1981). The rationale for using mannitol in oliguric acute renal failure is to convert the condition into a nonoliguric

TABLE 5-13. Site, Mechanism, Duration of Action, and Dose of Diuretics

Site of Action	Diuretic	Mechanism of Action*	Onset	Peak	Duration	Dose (mg/kg/day)	Potency
Proximal tubule	Acetazolamide (Diamox)	Carbonic anhydrase inhibitor	1-2	2	4-6	5-7	Mild
	Mannitol	Osmotic diuretic	1-2	2	Variable	0.5-1.0 g/kg per dose	Moderate
Ascending loop of Henle	Furosemide (Lasix)	Inhibition of chloride reabsorption	0.5-1	2-4	6-8	2-6 (oral), 1-6 (IV)	Very potent
	Bumetanide (Bumex)		0.25-0.5	0.45	5-8	0.08-0.6 (oral), 0.04-0.4 (IV)	Very potent
	Ethacrynic acid (Edecrin)		0.5-1	2-4	6-8	1-2	Very potent
Distal convoluted tubule (early)	Hydrochlorothiazide (HydroDiuril)	Inhibition of sodium reabsorption	1-2	4-6	12-24	2-3.5	Moderate
	Chlorothiazide (Diuril)		1-2	4-6	12-24	20-40	Moderate
	Metolazone† (Zaroxolyn)		2	6	24-6	0.5-5.0 mg/day	Moderate to potent
Distal convoluted tubule (late) and collecting duct	Spironolactone (Aldactone)	Competitive inhibitor of aldosterone	8-24	24-48	48-72	1-2	Mild
	Triamterene (Dyrenium)	Direct effect by reducing electrical potential between cell and lumen	2-4	6-8	19-24	3	Mild

*See text for details of mechanisms of action.
†Metolazone acts at the proximal tubule (as a carbonic anhydrase inhibitor) and unlike the other thiazides, can be used in patients with renal failure. It is only available in oral form.

one, thereby permitting easier management of fluids, nutritional support, and electrolytes. In addition, mannitol has been reported to decrease the incidence of acute renal failure in cardiopulmonary bypass surgery, myoglobinuria, transfusion of mismatched blood, and contrast nephropathy (in patients with chronic renal failure) (Byme, 1966; Eneas et al., 1979; Anto et al., 1981, Rigden et al., 1984). The usual dose is 0.5 g/kg given intravenously as a 12.5% solution. A good response is usually observed within 2 hours and consists of a urine output of at least three times the volume injected (10 to 12 mL/kg). In oliguric conditions, however, loop diuretics may be used initially because these may be effective without risking further intravascular volume expansion.

Because osmotic diuretics such as mannitol reduce TBW and intracellular volume, they help to decrease intracranial pressure in neurosurgical conditions associated with brain edema and to decrease intraocular pressure in ophthalmologic procedures. They also ameliorate symptoms associated with dialysis-related disequilibrium syndrome (Arieff, 1982).

Acetazolamide

This carbonic anhydrase inhibitor causes sodium bicarbonate diuresis and a reduction in total body bicarbonate stores. Its effectiveness is limited by the development of hyperchloremic metabolic acidosis. The bicarbonaturia induces phosphaturia, whereas the metabolic acidosis increases calcium excretion (Lemman et al., 1967; Beck and Goldberg, 1973). Both factors are responsible for renal stone formation and nephrocalcinosis during prolonged use of acetazolamide. It can cause severe K^+ wasting, especially during the acute bicarbonaturic phase.

Therapeutically, acetazolamide may be effective in the chronic treatment of glaucoma, in alkalinization of the urine, in the treatment of acute mountain sickness, to stimulate ventilation in central sleep apnea, to reduce endolymph formation in Meniere's disease, and in the treatment of refractory hydrocephalus (Conger and Falk, 1977; Vogh, 1980; Greene et al., 1981; Brookes et al., 1982; White et al., 1982; Maren, 1987).

Loop Diuretics

These agents are rapidly absorbed from the gastrointestinal tract and are excreted by glomerular filtration and by tubular secretion (Rane et al., 1978). Diuretic response is usually very rapid after intravenous administration and greatly exceeds that produced by most other diuretic agents.

Loop diuretics inhibit the NKCC2 electroneutral cotransport system in the luminal membrane of both the medullary and the cortical segments of the ascending limb of the loop of Henle, where 20% of the filtered Na^+ and Cl^- are reabsorbed (Burg et al., 1973). They also inhibit NaCl transport at the level of the proximal and distal tubules and are known to possess weak carbonic anhydrase inhibitory properties (Radtke et al., 1972; Imbs et al., 1987). Loop diuretics tend to increase RBF without increasing GFR, especially after intravenous administration. Increased RBF is associated with a redistribution of blood flow from the medulla to the cortex and within the cortex (Higashio et al., 1978). The hemodynamic effects appear to involve the renin-angiotensin system and vasodilatory prostaglandins (Gerger, 1983). These hemodynamic effects have not been linked to the diuretic response, however, and tend to be short-lived.

By markedly increasing the movement of solute in the distal segments of the nephron, loop diuretics induce potent diuresis and natriuresis. The large Na^+ load presented to the distal tubule is associated with increased K^+ and H^+ ion secretion. Thus, hypokalemia and metabolic alkalosis may ensue. The hypercalciuric action of loop diuretics makes them suitable agents for treatment of hypercalcemia, but their use in newborns with chronic respiratory disorders has been implicated in the development of nephrocalcinosis (Dirks, 1979; Schell-Feith et al., 2000).

In addition to inducing rapid diuresis, loop diuretics appear to improve cardiac function before the onset of diuresis by increasing venous capacitance (Dikshit et al., 1973). These drugs are also effective in the treatment of refractory edema as long as interstitial fluid can be mobilized without compromising intravascular volume. Because furosemide, ethacrynic acid, and bumetanide are effective with GFR as low as 10 mL/min per 1.73 m^2, they are useful for the management of edema in patients with chronic renal failure. Despite the obvious benefits of high-dose furosemide in certain experimental models of acute renal failure (deTorrente et al., 1978), its use in humans for conversion of oliguric acute renal failure to a nonoliguric state is controversial (Brown et al., 1981). All loop diuretics are ototoxic when given in large dosages to patients with severe renal failure (Gallagher and Jones, 1979). Unique to the loop diuretics, ototoxicity has been ascribed to drug-induced changes in the electrolyte composition of endolymph.

Finally, furosemide must be used cautiously in infants with hyperbilirubinemia because it is highly protein bound (Prandota and Pruitt, 1975) and thus capable of displacing bilirubin from albumin (Wenneberg et al., 1977). This phenomenon usually occurs with repeated dosages exceeding 1 mg/kg (Aranda et al., 1978).

Distal Convoluted Tubule Diuretics

The diuretic action of thiazides depends on the direct inhibition of the Na^+/Cl^- cotransporter in the distal convoluted tubule, which is accompanied by enhanced excretion of K^+ and hypokalemia (Kunau et al., 1975). By increasing Na^+ delivery to the cortical collecting duct, thiazides induce a kaliuresis that rivals that of loop diuretics, whereas the natriuresis of furosemide is 5 to 10 times greater than that produced by thiazides.

Apart from their use in managing edema and hypertension, thiazides have also been used successfully for treatment of hypercalciuria because they augment the reabsorption of calcium in the distal tubule (Sutton, 1986). Thiazides can also reduce polyuria and polydipsia in nephrogenic diabetes insipidus (Shirley et al., 1982). Such beneficial effect probably results from plasma volume depletion with an attendant decrease in GFR, which promotes NaCl and obligatory fluid reabsorption in the proximal tubule. This effect of thiazides is augmented by dietary salt restriction. Finally, thiazides are useful in the treatment of proximal renal tubular acidosis, characterized by marked bicarbonaturia. Depletion of intravascular volume is necessary to increase proximal bicarbonate reabsorption, an effect that is also promoted by restricting dietary Na^+ (Donckerwolke et al., 1970).

Combined therapy with thiazides and loop diuretics can be used to manage refractory edema that is caused by cirrhosis, nephrotic syndrome, or severe cardiac dysfunction. Synergy occurs when these classes of diuretics are administered together. NaCl delivery out of the proximal tubule is increased, whereas Na^+ reabsorption is inhibited in the loop of Henle and distal tubule. Thus, the resulting diuretic action is greater than that achieved with either agent alone (Ghose and Gupta, 1981). Similarly, metolazone, a thiazide-like diuretic, is particularly useful in the management of edema that accompanies congestive heart failure, renal disorders such nephrotic syndrome, and states of decreased renal function. While other thiazides lose their diuretic effectiveness at a CrCl of about 30 to 40 mL/min, metolazone retains its effectiveness, especially when used in conjunction with loop diuretics. This is attributed to its action on the proximal tubule in addition to its action on the distal diluting tubular segments. A limiting factor to the use of metolazone is its availability in tablet form, which may preclude its use in patients whose gastrointestinal tract cannot be used. In such instances, chlorothiazide may be used intravenously in conjunction with loop diuretics.

Adverse effects of thiazides include hypokalemia, metabolic alkalosis, carbohydrate intolerance, hyperuricemia, hyponatremia in the presence of severe restriction of dietary Na^+, and hypercalcemia (Manuel and Steele, 1974; Popovtzer et al., 1975; Hoskins and Jackson, 1978). In general, the hypercalcemia resolves within a few days.

Late Distal Tubule Diuretic

These diuretics are primarily K^+-sparing diuretics. Because of their distal site of action, they are not potent when they are used alone. Their major use is as adjuncts to thiazide or loop diuretics. Spironolactone competitively antagonizes aldosterone, whereas triamterene and amiloride inhibit the ENaC in the cortical collecting duct and thereby limit kaliuresis (Stoner et al., 1974; Corvol et al., 1981). In addition, triamterene may depress the GFR through its effect on urinary prostaglandin E_2 excretion (Favre et al., 1982). In general, these agents should be used cautiously in children with renal failure because of the danger of hyperkalemia. Furthermore, concurrent use of K^+-sparing diuretics and K^+ supplements is hazardous.

ANESTHETIC AGENTS AND THE KIDNEYS

Inhalational and intravenous anesthetics and many intravenous and oral analgesics and sedatives may influence renal function through their hemodynamic, cardiovascular, autonomic, and neuroendocrine effects. The trauma of surgery and possible accompanying dehydration are more likely, however, to result in renal dysfunction through elevations in plasma renin, aldosterone, and ADH that accompany surgery. These perturbations are reduced by morphine or halothane anesthesia (Philbin and Coggins, 1978). Prolonged release of ADH associated with surgical stress and use of anesthetics, combined with high infusions of hypotonic fluids, may result in hyponatremia. Moreover, well-hydrated patients may not experience reductions in glomerular filtration and may actually experience increases in RBF with subsequent increases in urine output and sodium excretion (Bastron et al., 1981; Philbin et al., 1981).

More direct nephrotoxic acute renal failure was common before discontinued use of the fluorinated anesthetic methoxyflurane (Pezzi et al., 1966; Halpren et al., 1973). Inhaled anesthetics in current use, such as sevoflurane and halothane,

result in fewer metabolic byproducts composed of inorganic fluoride, as well as oxalic acid; hence renal dysfunction is rare with these agents. Fluoride, in particular, may decrease ATP availability and thereby impair the action of the Na^+, K^+-ATPase in the loop of Henle and in the collecting duct. This may result in a salt-losing, vasopressin-resistant high–urine-output renal dysfunction (Whitford and Taves, 1973). Conversely, a preexisting reduction in GFR may prolong the pharmacologic half-life of many agents that have significant renal elimination, such as morphine, and thereby exacerbate their hemodynamic and other systemic adverse effects. Moreover, because of short tubular length and enzymatically immature secretory mechanisms, proximal tubular secretion of propofol metabolites and of other substances may be limited in infants under 6 months of age. Awareness of the previously discussed developmental differences in GFR and tubular function in preterm and term neonates and early infancy is essential in determineing the choice and dosage modification of many such agents.

DISORDERS OF DIVALENT ION METABOLISM

Calcium

Calcium plays many vital physiologic roles, not the least of which is to maintain the health of bones. It is essential for the stability of cellular membranes and regular neuromuscular excitation-contraction coupling, blood coagulation, and transport and secretory functions of the cell. Furthermore, Ca^{2+} acts as a "second messenger" in the signal transduction of extracellular hormones and other substances that affect numerous cellular functions.

Calcium Homeostasis

A typical adult diet contains about 800 mg of elemental Ca^{2+}, of which only 20%, or about 4 mmol (160 mg), is absorbed principally in the duodenum and jejunum. This net Ca^{2+} absorption is closely matched by renal excretion such that all but 4 mmol of the 270 mmol of Ca^{2+} filtered by the kidneys is excreted in the urine. This contrasts with a net Ca^{2+} absorption of 40% to 45% in infants and a rate as high as 80% in low–birth-weight infants and breastfed babies (Liu et al., 1989; Matkovic and Heaney, 1992). Normal daily bone turnover in adults accounts for 14 mmol of Ca^{2+} and comprises only a small proportion of the bone reservoir consisting of about 20 mmol, or 800 g.

Plasma Ca^{2+} is maintained at a concentration of 9 to 10.5 mg/dL (2.2 to 2.4 mmol/L) as total calcium, with approximately 40% of this value comprising the protein-bound nonfiltratable fraction, and 10% is chelated. Ionized calcium accounts for 47% the total circulating Ca^{2+} and ranges from 4 to 5 mg/dL (1.0 1.25 mmol/L) (Moore, 1970).

The extent of protein binding per deciliter of plasma approximately 0.8 mg of Ca^{2+} for every 1 g of albumin a 0.16 mg for each 1 g of globulin. Furthermore, a threefold increase in serum phosphate or sulfate concentration resu in a 10% decrease in serum Ca^{2+} concentration. In additio the binding of Ca^{2+} to albumin is pH-dependent between 7 and 9. An acute increase or decrease in the pH by 0.1 ur results in an increase or a decrease, respectively, of prote bound Ca^{2+} of 0.2 mg/dL (0.05 mmol/L). Thus, infusion of bl products, rapid correction of metabolic acidosis by infusion of sodium bicarbonate, or acute alkalosis caused by hyperventilation in the presence of hypocalcemia may all precipitate tetany and/or seizures because of increased binding of Ca²⁺ to albumin. Calcium homeostasis is complex and occurs at three main levels, often involving similar calcitropic hormones, receptors, and transporters.

In the small intestine, Ca²⁺ is absorbed via two mechanisms: a nonsaturable passive paracellular pathway such that a high Ca²⁺ intake results in higher Ca²⁺ absorption, and an active energy-dependent intracellular pathway that predominates when calcium intake is low. This latter mechanism is highly influenced by 1,25-dihydroxyvitamin D₃ [1,25(OH)₂D₃ or calcitriol], which stimulates the synthesis and/or activity of enterocyte apical Ca²⁺ transporters known as CaT1 and ECaC. Calcium crosses the cytoplasm bound to calbindin-D₉ₖ and then is extruded against an electrochemical gradient at the basolateral side by plasma membrane Ca²⁺-ATPase (PMCA). Disorders leading to hypersensitivity or increased synthesis of 1,25(OH)₂D₃ can result in increased intestinal absorption and hypercalciuria. Lactose stimulates calcium absorption even in the absence of vitamin D via an effect that may involve 25-hydroxylase (Lester et al., 1982). This may explain the higher plasma Ca²⁺ levels seen in infants. The efficiency of intestinal Ca²⁺ absorption depends on needs, age, gender, dietary intake, pregnancy, and vitamin D status.

The kidneys play a major role in Ca²⁺ homeostasis. The mechanisms of renal transport have been reviewed extensively by Suki and Rouse (1991), Bushinsky (2001), and Frick and Bushinsky (2003) and are reviewed here briefly. Only the fraction of Ca²⁺ not bound to protein is filtered, accounting for 60% of the plasma concentration. About 70% of the filtered Ca²⁺ is reabsorbed in the proximal convoluted tubule through a paracellular pathway involving solvent drag of salt and water (convection). It is then returned to the circulation from the interstitium. About 20% of the filtered Ca²⁺ is reabsorbed in the thick ascending limb of the loop of Henle via both paracellular and transcellular processes. Paracellin is the major protein component of the paracellular tight junction. Similar to the pathway of magnesium reabsorption, the Ca²⁺-sensing receptor (CaSR) detects small changes in interstitial Ca²⁺ concentrations and regulates the apical ROMK channel, thereby producing a lumen-positive voltage that drives Ca²⁺ through the tight junctions (Fig. 5-8, A and B). In this tubular segment mutations in paracellin, NKCC2 transporter, ROMK, CaSR, or inhibition of the NKCC2 transporter by loop diuretics can result in significant hypercalciuria, nephrocalcinosis, and osteopenia. The distal convoluted tubule reabsorbs 8% of the filtered calcium mainly via an active transcellular transport. This mechanism is similar to that found in enterocytes, except that intracellular calcium transport occurs through binding to calbindin-D₂₈ₖ and extrusion takes place mainly through a Na⁺/Ca²⁺ exchanger and less by PMCA. This mechanism is influenced by parathyroid hormone (PTH) and perhaps by other calcitropic hormones.

Bone reabsorption and formation also contribute to calcium homeostasis. The mechanisms by which osteoclasts and osteoblasts affect these processes are less well understood, but several hormonal regulators and transport processes are thought to resemble those found in the intestine and kidneys.

PTH is a major regulator of serum Ca²⁺ homeostasis. PTH acts via cAMP to increase proximal tubular Ca²⁺ excretion while it increases reabsorption in the distal and collecting ducts, so that the net effect is conservation of Ca²⁺ (Suki and Rouse, 1991). PTH also resorbs Ca²⁺ from the vast skeletal reservoir

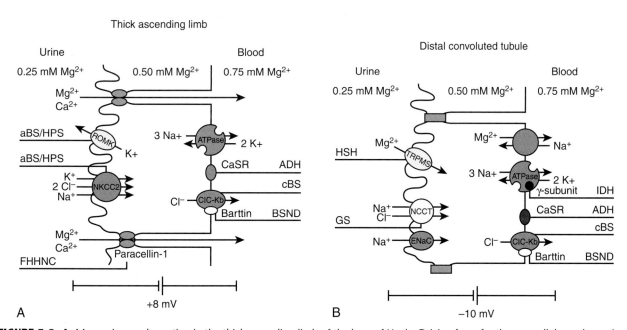

FIGURE 5-8. A, Magnesium reabsorption in the thick ascending limb of the loop of Henle. Driving force for the paracellular reabsorption of magnesium and calcium is the lumen-positive electrochemical gradient generated by the transcellular reabsorption of NaCl. **B,** Magnesium reabsorption in the distal convoluted tubule. In this segment, magnesium is reabsorbed by an active transcellular pathway involving an apical entry step probably via a magnesium permeable ion channel and a basolateral exchange mechanism, presumably an Na⁺/Mg²⁺ exchanger. The molecular identity of this exchanger is still unknown. See text for details. *ADH,* Autosomal dominant hypocalcemia. *(From Konrad M, Weber S: Recent advances in molecular genetics of hereditary magnesium-losing disorders,* J Am Soc Nephrol *14:249-260, 2003.)*

of Ca^{2+} and increases intestinal Ca^{2+} absorption by stimulating 1α-hydroxylase and calcitriol synthesis by proximal tubular epithelium, thereby guarding against hypocalcemia. High plasma phosphorus concentrations directly stimulate PTH release. This causes phosphaturia and raises serum Ca^{2+} concentration by the body's tendency to maintain a constant $Ca^{2+} \times P^{2-}$ product. Conversely, preterm infants who are fed diets low in phosphorus develop hypophosphatemia and are susceptible to hypercalcemia through direct stimulation of calcitriol synthesis.

Calcitriol is another major independent homeostatic factor. It increases intestinal absorption of Ca^{2+}, and in concert with PTH, it stimulates osteoclast-mediated resorption of bone. High serum calcium concentrations, on the other hand, interact with the parathyroid cell Ca^{2+}-sensing receptors to inhibit PTH secretion. High calcitriol levels also exert a negative feedback role on PTH secretion.

Other endogenous or exogenous substances play a lesser role in Ca^{2+} homeostasis. A hypercalcemic substance produced in several malignant or paraneoplastic syndromes is known as PTH-related peptide (PTHrP). The N-terminal of PTHrP functions like PTH and often contributes to humoral or tumoral hypercalcemia. Increased synthesis of other hypercalcemic cytokines, such as interleukins-1,-6, and -11, as well as tumor necrosis factor-α and prostaglandins, may also be released in various malignancies (Mundy and Guise, 1997). Macrophages may be an important source of such factors that act synergistically to produce significant osteolysis. Glucocorticoids lower calcium levels by reducing its intestinal absorption. Excessive thyroid hormone accelerates bone turnover, and calcitonin lowers serum calcium by increasing its excretion at the medullary portion of the thick ascending limb of the loop of Henle while inhibiting bone turnover. Immobilization may raise serum calcium levels by lowering the inflow of calcium into bone hydroxyapatite. Hypervitaminosis D, or a combination of vitamin A administration and decreased vitamin A catabolism in individuals with reduced renal function, may cause hypercalcemia by stimulating intestinal absorption.

Hypocalcemia (Plasma Ionized Calcium <1.0 mmol/L, or Total Calcium <7.0, 8.0, and 8.8 mg/dL, or <1.7, 2.0, and 2.2 mmol/L in Preterm, Term Newborns, and Children, Respectively)

The causes of hypocalcemia in neonates and children are listed in Box 5-10, and the biochemical features of these disorders are shown in Table 5-14 (Umpaichitra et al., 2001). "Early neonatal hypocalcemia" develops within the first 48 hours after birth in about 33% of infants of fewer than 37 weeks' gestation, in 50% of infants of insulin-dependent diabetic mothers, and in 30% of infants with neonatal asphyxia. In this disorder, there appears to be a significant correlation between gestational age and serum calcium levels. Plasma PTH concentrations are usually normal. Hence, the mechanism for the hypocalcemia may involve decreased calcium intake associated with increased P^{2-} loading and possibly resistance to the action of PTH (Linarelli et al., 1972; Tsang et al., 1973). Elevated calcitonin levels have been recently suggested as a cause of early hypocalcemia, particularly in neonatal asphyxia (Venkataraman et al., 1987).

In term infants, hypocalcemia may occur 5 to 7 days after birth and is often associated with the ingestion of cow's milk

Box 5-10 Causes of Hypocalcemia* in Neonates and Children

EARLY NEONATAL HYPOCALCEMIA
Preterm: Related to decreased PTH secretion
Neonates with asphyxia: Limitation of calcium intake
Infants of mothers with diabetes: Related to maternal urinary magnesium loss because of glycosuria, which results in hypomagnesemia

LATE NEONATAL HYPOCALCEMIA (END OF THE FIRST WEEK OF LIFE)
Dietary phosphate loading
Hypoparathyroidism
Hypomagnesemia

CHILDHOOD HYPOCALCEMIA
Vitamin D-related: Vitamin D-deficient rickets, vitamin D-dependent rickets type I (1β-hydroxylase deficiency), and type II (end-organ resistance to calcitriol)
Parathyroid hormone-related: Hypoparathyroidism, pseudohypoparathyroidism type I and type II
Calcium/phosphorus-related: Malabsorption, hyperphosphatemia
Organ-related: Hepatic rickets, acute pancreatitis, renal osteodystrophy
Miscellaneous: Drugs, such as calcitonin, phosphate, and bisphosphonates; magnesium deficiency; calcium-sensing receptor defect

Modified from Umpaichitra V, Bastian W, Castells S: Hypocalcemia in children: pathogenesis and management, *Clin Pediatr* 40:305-312, 2001.
*Causes, at different ages at onset, can overlap.

(Root and Harrison, 1976). Maternal vitamin D status may also play an important role in late neonatal hypocalcemia (Cockburn et al., 1980). Nutritional deficiency of vitamin D, inadequate photoconversion of vitamin D, and decreased calcium intake are currently uncommon causes of hypocalcemia and rickets in infants. In neonates with micrognathia, hypertelorism, fishmouth, low-set posteriorly rotated ears, cardiac disease, branchial dysembryogenesis, or DiGeorge's anomaly, must be considered. In this disorder, there is aplasia or hypoplasia of the parathyroid glands in association with diverse genetic deletions that can be detected by fluorescent in situ hybridization (FISH) DNA probes (Hong, 1998).

In children, autoimmune disorders that are either isolated or associated with other polyglandular syndromes comprise the majority of causes of acquired hypoparathyroidism and are often diagnosed by detection of specific autoantibodies directed against various endocrine tissues. Pseudohypoparathyroidism is associated with mutations in the PTH receptor, which is a G protein-coupled receptor. Circulating PTH levels are high, but there is PTH resistance in bone and the kidneys or in the kidneys alone (Farfel et al., 1999). In the first subtype (Ia), the phenotype consists of hereditary osteodystrophy (Albright dystrophy), short fingers, short stature, mental retardation, and subcutaneous calcifications, whereas in subtype Ib, the phenotype is normal. Pseudohypoparathyroidism type II is caused by disturbances in the pathway past the PTH receptor. Plasma PTH levels are also increased in this disorder.

Hypocalcemia is a common complication of hypomagnesemia. Three mechanisms have been suggested: resistance to the action of PTH; subnormal secretion of PTH; and defective

TABLE 5-14. Causes of Hypocalcemia and Their Biochemical Profile Clues

Causes of Hypocalcemia	Serum						Urine	
	Ca	P	PTH	Alk Phos	250D₃	1,25(OH) 2D₃	Mg	Ca
Vitamin D-deficient rickets	↓, ↔	↔, ↓	↑	↑	↓	*	↔	↓
Vitamin D-dependent rickets type I	↓	↓, ↔	↑	↑	↔	↓	↔	↓
Vitamin D-dependent rickets type II	↓	↓, ↔	↑	↑	↔	↑	↔	↓
Hypoparathyroidism	↓	↑	↓	↔	↔	↔, ↓	↔	↓
Pseudohypoparathyroidism	↓	↑	↑	↔	↔	↔, ↓	↔	↓
Rickets of prematurity	↔, ↓	↔, ↓	↑	↑	↔	↔, ↓	↔	?
Renal osteodystrophy	↓	↑	↑	↑	↔	↓	↔, ↑	↓
Calcium-sensing receptor defect	↓	↔	**	↔	↔	↔, ↓	↔	↑
Mg deficiency	↓	↔	**	↔	↔	↓	↓	↑

Modified from Umpaichitra V, Bastian W, Castells S: Hypocalcemia in children: pathogenesis and management, *Clin Pediatr* 40:305–312, 2001.
Ca, Calcium; *P*, phosphorus; *PTH*, parathyroid hormone; *Alk Phos*, alkaline phosphatase; *Mg*, magnesium; ↔, normal; ↓, decrease; ↑,increase; ?, difficult to interpret owing to different degree of renal immaturity in preterm infants; *, decrease or normal or increase; **, decrease or normal or slight increase (relatively low for degree of hypocalcemia).

Ca^{2+}/Mg^{2+} exchange in bone (Estep et al., 1969; Suh et al., 1973; Chase and Slatopolsky, 1974). Correction of hypomagnesemia has been shown to restore calcium homeostasis.

Hepatic disorders that interfere with vitamin D and other fat-soluble vitamin absorption and conversion to 25-vitamin D_3, or calcidiol, can cause hypocalcemia, particularly in debilitated or immobilized individuals. In children with renal failure resulting from a variety of chronic renal disorders, impaired conversion of calcitriol by proximal tubular α-hydroxylase to the active calcitriol form, along with phosphate retention, impaired intestinal absorption of Ca^{2+}, and high circulating PTH concentrations that impair osteoclastic activity all combine to cause hypocalcemia (Slatopolski and Delmez, 1992). Mutations in 1α-hydroxylase lead to vitamin D-resistant rickets, an autosomal dominant disorder that appears at 4 to 12 months of age with low serum Ca^{2+} but normal 25-vitamin D_3 levels. If calcitriol levels are normal, hypocalcemia can be the result of mutations in the vitamin (calcitriol) D receptor (VDR), which is also an autosomal dominant, vitamin D-resistant condition that appears at 3 to 12 months with rickets and alopecia (Levine and Carpenter, 1999).

Manifestations of Hypocalcemia

Many of the symptoms associated with hypocalcemia are attributed to increased neuromuscular excitability. These symptoms include numbness and tingling of the hands, toes, and lips; irritability, anxiety, and depression; a prolonged QT interval; cardiac arrhythmias; and congestive heart failure. In the neonatal period, jitteriness, twitching, and seizures are more common. The seizures may be generalized or focal and usually are short-lived but repetitive, with very little postictal depression. Chvostek's and Trousseau's signs and a high-pitched cry are useful indications, especially in the older infant and child. Infants may have cyanosis, vomiting, or feeding intolerance, whereas older children may experience laryngospasm. With prolonged hypocalcemia, cataracts can develop because of the increased intake of Na^+ and water by the lens (Ireland et al., 1968).

Treatment of Hypocalcemia

If hypocalcemia is not life threatening, it is preferable to administer a calcium-containing solution amounting to 15 mg of elemental calcium/kg body weight infused over a period of 4 to 6 hours. For clinical emergencies (seizures, tetany), 10% calcium gluconate is infused, preferably in a large vein or central venous catheter, to provide an elemental Ca^{2+} dosage of 2 to 4 mg/kg body weight in newborns and 2 to 3 mg/kg body weight in children, given over 5 to 10 minutes under constant electrocardiographic monitoring. Subsequently, 25 to 50 mg of intravenous elemental Ca^{2+}/kg per day may be used until hypocalcemia resolves. If hypomagnesemia is also present, 50% magnesium sulfate (48 mg elemental Mg^{2+}/mL) at a dosage of 6 mg of elemental Mg^{2+}/kg body weight may be infused over 1 hour.

Hypoparathyroidism requires the use of calcitriol at an initial dosage of 0.01 mcg/kg body weight daily to maintain plasma Ca^{2+} concentrations between 8.5 and 9.0 mg/dL. Monitoring of plasma levels and urinary Ca^{2+} excretion may limit the risk of hypercalcemia, hypercalciuria, and nephrocalcinosis (evident on renal ultrasound). In vitamin D-dependent rickets type I, the dose of calcitriol is 10 to 15 ng/kg per day combined with elemental calcium of 500 to 1000 mg/day. Children with vitamin D-deficient rickets may receive vitamin D (ergocalciferol, 8000 units/mL = 0.2 mg/mL) at 2000 to 10,000 IU/day orally for 4 to 8 weeks, or a single oral megadose of 200,000 to 600,000 IU (Strosstherapy), which is safe and more effective, particularly when compliance is in question. Oral or intravenous calcitriol may be used in pseudohypoparathyroidism or in children with chronic renal failure to increase intestinal absorption Ca^{2+} and suppress PTH secretion.

Hypercalcemia (Plasma Ionized Calcium >1.35 mmol/L or >5.4 mg/dL, or Total Calcium >10.5 mg/dL, or 2.6 mmol/L)

It is important to exclude pseudohypercalcemia as a cause of hypercalcemia in individuals with essential thrombocytosis after clotting of phlebotomized blood. The causes of

Box 5-11 Causes of Hypercalcemia

NEONATES
Iatrogenic (calcium salts)
Idiopathic infantile hypercalcemia
Williams' syndrome

Vitamin D
Vitamin D intoxication
Subcutaneous fat necrosis

Parathyroid related
Hyperparathyroidism
Neonatal severe hyperparathyroidism
Secondary hyperparathyroidism
Familial hypocalciuric hypercalcemia
PTHrP (humoral hypercalcemia) tumor related
PTH receptor mutation: Jansen's disease (metaphyseal chondrodysplasia)

Miscellaneous
Hypophosphatasia
Hypophosphatemia
Vitamin A intoxication
Blue diaper syndrome
Thiazide diuretics

CHILDREN
Primary hyperparathyroidism
Tertiary hyperparathyroidism
Ectopic secretion of PTH by tumors
Neoplasms (bony metastases)
Neoplastic production of 1,25(OH)$_2$D$_3$
Phosphate depletion with hypophosphatemia
Sarcoidosis, tuberculosis, and other granulomatous disorders
Immobilization
Milk-alkali syndrome
Medications: Thiazide diuretics, theophylline, lithium, salicylate intoxication, vitamin D or vitamin A intoxication
Thyrotoxicosis
Exsiccosis
Acquired immunodeficiency syndrome (AIDS)
Multiple fractures
Acute renal failure
PTH, PTHrP

Box 5-12 Evaluation of Infants with Persistent Hypercalcemia

Blood-total and ionized calcium, pH, phosphorus, alkaline phosphatase, creatinine, intact PTH, 25-hydroxyvitamin D, 1,25-dihydroxyvitamin D
Urine-calcium/creatinine ratio, tubular reabsorption of phosphate
Renal ultrasonography
Other tests that can be performed if the above do not yield a diagnosis:
  PTHrP
  Vitamin A
  Parents' serum calcium and urine calcium
  Long bone X-rays

From Rodd C, Goodyer P: Hypercalcemia of the newborn: etiology, evaluation, and management, *Pediatr Nephrol* 13:542-547, 1999.

Diagnostic Studies

Diagnostic studies to consider in newborns and in children with hypocalcemia or hypercalcemia are shown in Box 5-12 (Rodd and Goodyer, 1999). In general, PTHrP and calcitrophic cytokines need not be measured unless plasma PTH levels are normal or suppressed and the cause of hypercalcemia is cryptic. If PTHrP is measured, the blood tube should contain a proteinase inhibitor.

Manifestations of Hypercalcemia

Newborns and infants with hypercalcemia have nonspecific symptoms, such as failure to thrive because of anorexia and vomiting. Irritability, lethargy, hypotonia, and seizures are common with more severe hypercalcemia. Bradycardia, a short OT interval, and hypertension are other findings. In older children, nausea, vomiting, constipation, and vague central nervous system symptoms of headaches and fatigue may be apparent. Renal function may be markedly decreased because of diminished RBF caused by hypercalcemia-induced vasoconstriction and by circulatory volume depletion resulting from acquired nephrogenic diabetes insipidus. Nephrocalcinosis, nephrolithiasis, hematuria, and sterile pyuria may occur secondary to hypercalciuria. An inability to concentrate the urine because of resistance to the action of ADH may result in polyuria, polydipsia, and dehydration. Hypokalemia may occur secondary to diuresis. The development of rapid and severe hypercalcemia (>17 mg/dL) can result in dehydration, azotemia, coma, and death.

Management of Hypercalcemia

The first step in the management of acute hypercalcemia is to discontinue all of the sources of calcium and vitamin D. In neonates, a formula with low calcium and vitamin D content may be used, as well as immediate provision of hydration consisting of normal saline at 20 mL/kg per hour for 4 hours. Excretion of calcium may be further promoted by intravenous furosemide at a dosage of 0.5 to 1.0 mg/kg body weight given every 6 hours with frequent monitoring of plasma ionized Ca^{2+}, Na$^+$, K$^+$, Cl and Mg^{2+} concentrations. Supplementation with such ions is essential. Thiazides are anticalciuric and are contraindicated. Calcitonin given at 4 to 8 IU/kg body weight subcutaneous

hypercalcemia vary by age (Box 5-11) (Rodd and Goodyer, 1999; Ziegler, 2001). Although hypercalcemia is uncommon in newborns, the most common cause is iatrogenic, resulting from excessive administration of calcium salts. Other causes in this age group include idiopathic infantile hypercalcemia, which is usually mild; more severe hypercalcemia occurs in Williams' syndrome. Primary neonatal hyperparathyroidism is a rare disorder caused by homozygous inheritance of mutations in the Ca^{2+}-sensing receptor that result in familial hypocalciuric hypercalcemia (FHH). Although these patients' heterozygous parents are often asymptomatic, the condition may be life threatening in the offspring because of plasma calcium 15 to 30 mg/dL, unexplained anemia, hepatosplenomegaly, and nephrocalcinosis. Primary hyperparathyroidism is extremely rare in childhood but may occur in the multiple endocrine adenoma syndrome, in which hypercalcemia, hypercalciuria, and nephrolithiasis relate to elevated levels of 1,25(OH)$_2$D$_3$ (Broadus et al., 1980).

every 6 hours is particularly useful if there is concurrent renal insufficiency. Methylprednisolone at 1 mg/kg per 24 hours may be useful in this setting. Biphosphonates inhibit macrophage and osteoclast activity and are increasingly used to treat hypercalcemia but also to prevent osteoporosis, osteopathy, or calcinosis. Pamidronate at a single dose of 0.5 mg/kg intravenously (may be repeated daily as needed for 3 days) is the agent of choice in tumoral hypercalcemia, vitamin D intoxication, resistant hypercalcemia, or in newborns with subcutaneous fat necrosis and elevated plasma $1,25(OH)_2D_3$ concentrations. Etidronate at an oral dosage of 5 mg/kg given twice daily along with sodium supplementation at 3 mmol/kg per day is also effective for managing chronic disorders. In severe hypercalcemia or when oliguria or renal insufficiency is present, dialysis with a low calcium dialysate concentration (1.25 mmol/L) is recommended. In cases of severe neonatal hyperparathyroidism resulting from homozygous FHH or other forms of primary hyperparathyroidism, expeditious parathyroidectomy may be lifesaving.

Magnesium

Magnesium is the fourth most abundant cation in the body, and it is largely located intracellularly. Its principal role is to stabilize electrically excitable membranes. Magnesium is also an important co-factor of numerous important enzymes, including Na^+, K^+-ATPase, alkaline phosphatase, and adenylate cyclase (Gums, 1987). It is essential in oxidative phosphorylation, protein synthesis, and DNA metabolism.

Magnesium Homeostasis

Normal plasma magnesium levels range from 1.7 to 2.5 mg/dL or 0.7 to 1.0 mmol/L. In general, plasma levels of Mg^{2+} correlate well with tissue levels; such correlation is poor, however, in circumstances such as renal failure or hepatic cirrhosis (Cohen and Kitzes, 1982).

Despite being very abundant in the body, defense against hypomagnesemia is limited by the following factors:

- An inappropriately low parathyroid secretion when plasma levels are below 1.0 mg/dL
- PTH resistance at the skeletal level, and
- Decreased calcitriol levels predisposing to combined hypocalcemia (Agus, 1999)

Hypomagnesemia is common in hospitalized individuals, particularly when nutritional intake is low for 3 or more days.

An average Western diet provides 400 mg of Mg^{2+} (16 mmol) per day, of which 30% to 50% is absorbed in the jejunum and ileum (Brannan et al., 1976). Intestinal absorption can increase to 80% in the presence of mild hypomagnesemia (plasma Mg^{2+} 1.2 mg/dL, <1.0 mEq/L, or <0.5 mmol/L). In the blood, 30% of Mg^{2+} is bound to proteins and is not filtered at the glomerulus. Of the filtered Mg^{2+}, about 3% is excreted in the urine.

Once filtered, Mg^{2+} is reabsorbed in the proximal tubule (5% to 20%), in the thick ascending limb of the loop of Henle (5% to 76%), and in the distal convoluted tubule (5% to 10%). As with Ca^{2+}, the bulk of Mg^{2+} reabsorption occurs in the thick ascending limb of the loop of Henle via a passive paracellular mechanism. This mechanism is facilitated by the positive transepithelial voltage that is generated by apical Na^+ entry and by diffusion of K^+ into the lumen that is generated by the interplay of the apical NKCC2 cotransporter, the basolateral Na^+-K^+-ATPase, and the return of K^+ into the tubular lumen via the action of ROMK(Fig. 5-8, A) (Konrad and Weber, 2003). The resultant change in luminal charge affects the configuration of structural proteins, especially that of paracellin-1 (also known as *claudin 16*) present in tight junctions. Mutations in paracellin-1 become manifest in early childhood and are often accompanied by familial hypomagnesemia, hypercalciuria, hematuria, and nephrocalcinosis, and they can cause polyuria and progressive decline in GFR, such that one third of these children develop renal failure by age 15 years (Weber et al., 2001).

Interference with NKCC2 cotransport by loop diuretics diminishes the luminal voltage and leads to Mg^{2+} wasting, hypomagnesemia, and hypocalcemia. Metabolic acidosis, K^+ depletion, and hypophosphatemia may cause magnesuria by affecting the transepithelial voltage. In contrast, Mg^{2+} transport in the distal convoluted tubule is active and transcellular (Fig. 5-8, B). Specific, but not well-characterized, Mg^{2+} channels transport Mg^{2+} in and out of the cells in this region and are influenced by multiple agents, including the Mg^{2+}-sparing diuretics amiloride and chlorothiazide (Cole and Quamme, 2000, Konrad and Weber, 2003). Mutations in these channels or in the Ca^{2+}/Mg^{2+}-sensing receptor (CaSR), which inhibits Na^+, Ca^{2+}, and Mg^{2+} absorption at the basolateral membrane, are responsible for several inherited disorders that are often present in infancy and childhood with symptoms related to hypomagnesemia (Box 5-13) (DiStefano et al., 1997).

Box 5-13 Inherited Disorders of Renal Magnesium Handling

PRIMARY INHERITED DISORDERS OF RENAL MAGNESIUM HANDLING
Hypomagnesemia with secondary hypocalcemia (HSH)
Infantile isolated hypomagnesemia with autosomal dominant inheritance (IDH)
Infantile primary hypomagnesemia with autosomal recessive inheritance

Other Inherited Disorders
Idiopathic hypermagnesuria
Congenital hypomagnesemia not yet classified

HYPOMAGNESEMIA ASSOCIATED WITH HYPERCALCIURIA AND NEPHROCALCINOSIS
Familial hypomagnesemia with hypercalciuria and nephrocalcinosis (FHHNC)

Inherited Disorders Associated With Abnormal Extracellular Mg^{2+}/Ca^{2+} Sensing
Autosomal dominant hypoparathyroidism
Familial hypocalciuric hypercalcemia and neonatal severe hyperparathyroidism (FHH)

HYPOMAGNESEMIA ASSOCIATED WITH ABNORMAL RENAL NACL TRANSPORT
Gitelman's syndrome
Bartter's syndrome
Classic form (cBS)
Antenatal form with hyperprostaglandin E (aBS/HPS)
With sensorineural hearing loss (BSND)

Cole D, Quamme GA: Inherited disorders of renal magnesium handling. *J Am Soc Nephrol* 11:1937-1947, 2000, p 1940, Table 2. (With permission of Springer Science and Business Media.)

Etiology and Manifestations of Dysmagnesemia

Hypomagnesemia (Plasma Concentration <1.7 mg/dL, or <0.7 mmol/L)

Hypomagnesemia is far more common and more clinically relevant than hypermagnesemia (>2.5 mg/dL, or >1.0 mmol/L). Genetic disorders resulting in renal Mg^{2+} wasting are highlighted in Box 5-13, and noninheritable or acquired causes of hypomagnesemia and its clinical manifestations are shown in Boxes 5-14 and 5-15 (Elin, 1988). Pediatric transplant recipients maintained on cyclosporine or tacrolimus are particularly susceptible to hypomagnesemia. This disorder is associated with an increase in the fractional excretion of Mg^{2+} (Barton et al., 1987). Experimental studies demonstrate that cyclosporine leads to a decrease in the serum magnesium concentration that is associated with renal Mg^{2+} wasting and Mg^{2+} shift into tissue compartments with no effect on intestinal absorption of Mg^{2+} (Barton et al., 1989).

Because of the type of clinical conditions that cause hypomagnesemia and because hypomagnesemia itself may contribute to refractory hypokalemia and hypocalcemia, it is common to find concurrent hypokalemia, hypocalcemia, and metabolic alkalosis. Symptoms may be exclusively attributed to hypomagnesemia only after excluding these other electrolyte disturbances. Patients with renal wasting of magnesium have nephrocalcinosis, nephrolithiasis, and decreased GFR. Neurologic symptoms resemble those of hypocalcemia and may include personality changes, tremors, seizures, and carpopedal spasm.

Hypermagnesemia

Hypermagnesemia often occurs in individuals with acute renal failure who also consume a high level of dietary Mg^{2+} or who experience cellular efflux in association with acute ketoacidosis or pheochromocytoma crisis. Although individuals with plasma Mg^{2+} concentrations below 10 mg/dL are usually asymptomatic,

---

Box 5-14 Causes of Hypomagnesemia

GASTROINTESTINAL
Chronic diarrhea
Bowel bypass or resection
Congenital inflammatory bowel disease
Malabsorption syndromes
Tropical sprue
Gluten enteropathy
Laxative abuse
Pancreatitis
Specific magnesium malabsorption
Prolonged nasogastric suctioning
Caloric malnutrition

RENAL EXCRETION
Gitelman's syndrome
Acute renal failure
Renal tubular acidosis
Chronic pyelonephritis
Postobstructive diuresis
Primary renal tubular magnesium wasting
Drugs
    Acetazolamide
    Alcohol
    Aminoglycosides
    Amphotericin B
    Bumetanide
    Capreomycin
    Carbenicillin
    Chlorthalidone
    Cisplatin
    Cyclosporine
    Digoxin
    Ethacrynic acid
    Furosemide
    Mannitol
    Methotrexate
    Osmotic agents
    Pentamidine
    Tacrolimus

    Theophylline
    Thiazides
    Torsemide
    Viomycin

NUTRITIONAL DEFICIENCIES
Malnutrition or eating disorders
Magnesium-free parenteral feedings
Long-term alcohol abuse

ENDOCRINE DISORDERS
Hyperaldosteronism
Hypocalcemia
Hyperparathyroidism
Hyperthyroidism
Diabetes mellitus
Ketoacidosis
Diabetic
Alcoholic
Hypoparathyroidism
SIADH
Excessive lactation

REDISTRIBUTION
Insulin treatment for diabetic ketoacidosis
High-catecholamine states
Major trauma or stress
Hungry-bone syndrome

MULTIPLE MECHANISMS
Chronic alcoholism
Alcohol withdrawal
Major burns
Liquid-protein diet
Acute porphyria

NEONATES
Gestational diabetes
Gestational hyperparathyroidism
Gestational hypoparathyroidism
Exchange transfusion (citrate)

Modified from Elin RJ: Magnesium metabolism in health and disease, *Dis Mon* 34:161-218, 1988.

Box 5-15 Clinical and Laboratory Manifestations of Hypomagnesemia

NEUROMUSCULAR
Weakness
Tremors
Muscle fasciculation
Positive Chvostek's sign
Positive Trousseau's sign
Dysphagia

CARDIAC
Arrhythmias (torsades de pointes)
ECG changes

CENTRAL NERVOUS SYSTEM
Personality change
Depression
Agitation
Psychosis
Nystagmus
Seizure

METABOLIC
Hypokalemia
Hypocalcemia

Modified from Elin RJ: Magnesium metabolism in health and disease, *Dis Mon* 34:161-218, 1988.

hypermagnesemia may cause central nervous system depression, decreased deep-tendon reflexes, muscle weakness, respiratory muscle paralysis, hypotension, bradycardia, heart block, and other arrhythmias.

Etiology and Management of Dysmagnesemia

Diagnosis of Dysmagnesemia

In individuals with normal renal function and absence of renal Mg^{2+} wasting, a fractional excretion of Mg^{2+} (FE_{Mg2+}) below 0.5% indicates low dietary intake or gastrointestinal losses of Mg^{2+}, whereas an FE_{Mg2+} over 2% suggests renal Mg^{2+} wasting.

$$FE_{Mg}^{2+} = \frac{U_{Mg}^{2+} \times Pcr}{(0.7 \times P_{Mg2+}) \times Ucr} \times 100$$

U_{Mg2+} and P_{Mg2+} and Ucr and Pcr are the urinary and plasma concentrations of Mg^{2+} and creatinine, respectively. In this equation, plasma Mg^{2+} concentration is multiplied by 0.7 because only 70% of plasma Mg^{2+} is free. This implies that administration of albumin or blood products may further lower the ionized form of Mg^{2+} and precipitate symptoms. In individuals with low normal plasma Mg^{2+} concentrations, total body Mg^{2+} depletion may be confirmed by an Mg^{2+} excretion in a 24-hour urine collection amounting to less than 70% after an intravenous or intramuscular load of 2.4 mg/kg of lean body mass (this may be administered over 4 hours as the chloride or the sulfate solution in 5% dextrose in water or normal saline) (Gullestad et al., 1994)

Management of Dysmagnesemia

The first steps in the management of dysmagnesemia are to discontinue offending medications and to attempt to correct the primary cause of hypomagnesemia (Box 5-16). In individuals with tetany or cardiac arrhythmias, intravenous Mg^{2+} may be infused slowly to avoid hypotension. The usual dosage is 0.2 mEq/kg (0.1 mmol/kg or 2.4 mg/kg) every 4 to 6 hours until blood levels exceed 1.0 mg/dL (0.4 mmol/L or 0.8 mEq/L). The intravenous or intramuscular administration of 25 to 50 mg/kg body weight of magnesium sulfate solution, or 0.2 to 0.4 mEq/kg body weight of elemental Mg^{2+}, is also preferred in symptomatic individuals with normomagnesemia who exhibit refractory hypokalemia or hypocalcemia. Amiloride may be used to reduce renal Mg^{2+} wasting by stimulating reabsorption in the cortical collecting duct. Because Mg^{2+} has a low renal tubular threshold (1.3 to 1.7 mEq/L), intravenous infusions or large single oral loads of Mg^{2+} are quickly excreted in the urine. Thus, smaller, more frequent doses or use of oral sustained-release preparations are more effective. Symptomatic hypermagnesemia may be acutely managed by dialysis using a dialysate Mg^{2+} concentration of 0.2 mmol/L, as well as calcium infusion or anticholinesterase administration.

Phosphorus

Most total body P^{2-} exists in the form of the inorganic phosphate, but it also exists in an organic intracellular form, where it is the major anion. Phosphorus is an integral component of intracellular nucleic acids and cell membrane phospholipids and it is involved in phosphorylation of proteins and lipids. Severe hypophosphatemia (<1 mg/mL) may have profound effects on all body functions by limiting 2,3-diphosphoglycerate and oxygen dissociation from hemoglobin and by reducing phosphate available for synthesis of high-energy bonds in the form of ATP, which is involved in virtually all energy-requiring processes (Knochel, 1977). Phosphorus, along with Ca^{2+}, is a major constituent of bone.

Phosphorus Homeostasis

Approximately 85% of the total body P^{2-} is in bone (hydroxyapatite, octacalcium phosphate, and amorphous calcium phosphate) and teeth, whereas 15% is a constituent of carbohydrate, lipid, and protein in soft tissues, and 0.1% is in the ECF (Raisz, 1977).

Serum P^{2-} concentration is maintained between 3.0 and 8.5 mg/dL, depending on age (Parfitt and Kleerekoper, 1980). It is highest in infants (4.5 to 8.5 mg/dL) and relatively high in children (3.7 to 5.9 mg/dL), presumably because of increased concentrations of growth hormone and reduced levels of gonadal hormones until the completion of adolescence.

About 50% to 60% of dietary P^{2-} is absorbed in the small intestine, especially in the duodenum and jejunum, through an active vitamin D-dependent process that is also dependent on Na^+, and by passive diffusional flux through paracellular pathways (Harrison and Harrison, 1961). The absorption of P^{2-} depends on the availability of adequate glucose, Na^+, P^{2-}, and Ca^{2+}. Absorption is decreased by the ingestion of antacids such as aluminum hydroxide, which binds phosphorus in the gut and thereby inhibits gastrointestinal absorption.

Box 5-16 Treatment of Magnesium Depletion

The following guidelines are suggested for the treatment of magnesium deficiency regardless of etiology:

1. It is important to know that the kidneys are producing urine and that the blood urea nitrogen (BUN) and/or creatinine is normal. Magnesium may be needed and may be administered even in an instance of renal insufficiency, but the treatment must be monitored by frequent serum or plasma level assays.
2. On the first day of therapy, at least 1 mEq mg/kg per day should be given parenterally. Subsequently, at least 0.5 mEq mg/kg per day should be given for 3 to 5 days. If parenteral fluid therapy continues, at least 0.2 mEq/kg per day should be given.
3. Give the above in intravenous infusions if such infusions are being given anyway; otherwise, intramuscular administration is satisfactory.
4. The following schedule for an average adult is safe and effective.
   a. Intramuscular route: [ampules of 1 g $MgSO_4(H_2O)_7$, 50% solution = 8.13 mEq Mg^{2+}]. Day 1: 2.0 g (16.3 mEq) every 4 hours for six doses. Days 2-5: 1.0 g (9.1 mEq) every 6 hours.
   b. Intravenous route (same ampules) Day 1: 6 g (41 mEq) in each liter of fluid and at least 2 L of 83 mEq. Days 2 to 5: A total of 6 g (49 mEq) distributed equally in total fluids of the day.

   If the patient's condition requires continued intravenous infusions, 2 g of $MgSO_4$ should be given daily in the infusion as long as infusions are necessary. When a patient who has a reason to have magnesium deficiency is convulsing, 2.0 g of $MgSO_4$ solution may be administered intravenously in a 10-minute period. For infants and children with symptoms, such doses may be 0.025 g $MgSO_4$/kg, or 0.2-0.3 mEq/kg per dose of elemental mg^{2+}, in 10 minutes.

5. Oral preparations

Magnesium oxide	(Uro-Mg) 50 mEq magnesium per g of salt
	(Mag-Ox) 50 mEq magnesium per g of salt
Magnesium chloride	(Slo-Mag) 9.75 mEq magnesium per g of salt
Magnesium lactate	(MagTab) 7.6 mEq magnesium per g of salt

- Note: 50% solution of $MgSO_4$ = 500 mg/mL (1 g/2 mL), or 49.3 mg elemental Mg^{2+}/mL, or 98.6 mg elemental Mg^{2+}/2 mL. Given an atomic gram weight of 24.3 and a valence of 2 for Mg^{2+}, 98.6 mg = 4.058 mmol or 8.13 mEq elemental Mg^{2+}/g salt.
- Example: A 10-kg infant with seizures, hypomagnesemia, and an adequate serum calcium level may receive 2.0 mEq elemental Mg^{2+} (0.2 mEq/kg • 10 kg). This may be accomplished by diluting 0.5 mL of the 50% $MgSO_4$ in 9.5 mL of dextrose and infusing over 2 to 10 minutes.

Adapted from Flink EB, et al.: Magnesium deficiency and magnesium toxicity in man. In Prasad AS, Oberleas D, editors: *Trace elements in human health and disease.* New York, 1976, Academic Press, p 13.

At least 90% of plasma P^{2-} appears in the glomerular ultrafiltrate. Most of the filtered P^{2-} is reabsorbed in the proximal tubule. The process is active and Na^+ dependent, and it occurs against an electrochemical gradient (Suki and Rouse, 1991). The amount of P^{2-} in the urine closely parallels the amount absorbed by the intestine. Normally the kidney excretes 10% to 20% of the filtered P^{2-}, suggesting that the maximal capacity of the tubules to reabsorb P^{2-} is met or exceeded. Saline expansion causes phosphaturia, which can be blocked by total parathyroidectomy. In the absence of PTH, the reabsorption of P^{2-} by the *pars recta* and the distal nephron is complete and accounts for the hyperphosphatemia in hypoparathyroidism (Knox et al., 1977).

The urinary excretion of P^{2-} depends on the oral intake of P^{2-} (high intake causes increased excretion), the oral intake of Ca^{2+} (high intake causes hypophosphaturia), the presence of catabolism (high catabolic rates cause hyperphosphatemia and hyperphosphaturia), acid-base status (chronic metabolic acidosis decreases the tubular reabsorption of P^{2-} by decreasing the Vmax of Na^+/P^{2-} cotransport in the brush border membrane of the proximal tubule), and the levels of PTH and calcitriol (Kempson, 1982). Severe respiratory alkalosis stimulates glycolysis and carbohydrate phosphorylation, resulting in secondary intracellular shift of phosphate. Untreated diabetes causes hypophosphatemia through volume expansion, osmotic diuresis, or ketonuria, and also through extracellular shift after insulin administration.

Phosphate transport at the proximal tubule is the main means for regulating total body phosphate balance. The latter process is largely mediated by a type IIa Na^+/P^{2-} electrogenic cotransporter (NPT2a) in the proximal tubule (Murer et al., 2000; Kronenberg, 2002; Tenenhouse and Murer, 2003). An increase or a decrease in the number of NPT2a in the brush border cell membrane is associated with either an increase or a decrease in P^{2-} reabsorption. Modulators of NPT2a endocytosis, internalization, recycling, and lysosomal degradation include PTH, fibroblast growth factor 23 (FGF-23), and several proteins that interact with this phosphate transporter. High levels of PTH or FGF-23 increase NPT2a endocytosis and breakdown and cause phosphaturia. Reduction in dietary phosphate lowers PTH levels while concurrently promoting insertion of NPT2a at the apical membrane, thereby promoting phosphate reabsorption (Fig. 5-9).

Human disorders of phosphate transport may relate to aberrations in these phosphate-regulating genes. Certain tumors can cause oncogenic hypophosphatemic osteomalacia (OHO) by stimulating mRNA encoding for FGF-23, whereas activating mutations of FGF-23 can cause autosomal dominant hypophosphatemic rickets (ADHR). Another phosphate-regulating gene is named the *phosphate-regulating gene with homology to endopeptidases on the X chromosome (PHEX)*. Many mutations in this gene that are largely expressed in osteoblasts, osteoclasts, and odontoblasts, lead to decreased degradation of FGF-23, which may be the key defect in X-linked hypophosphatemic rickets (XLH). However, the mechanism by which PHEX dysfunction leads to renal phosphate wasting is unclear (Kronenberg, 2002).

Regulation of phosphate shifts in and out of bone is principally mediated by PTH and calcitriol that is synthesized mainly by proximal tubular epithelial cells. Several plasma proteins prevent precipitation of calcium phosphate in vessels and soft tissues, whereas alkaline phosphatase aids deposition of such minerals in bone. Other hormones that may affect the renal handling of P^{2-} include vasopressin, thyroxin, glucagon, insu

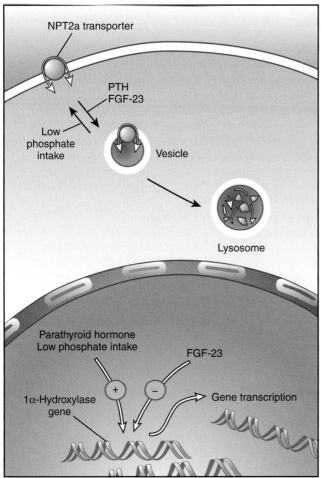

■ FIGURE 5-9. Regulation of the NPT2a sodium-phosphate cotransporter and synthesis of 1,25-dihydroxyvitamin D$_3$ in the renal proximal tubule. PTH and fibroblast growth factor 23 (FGF-23) both lead to rapid internalization and subsequent lysosomal destruction of NPT2a. A low-phosphate diet causes the insertion of NPT2a into the plasma membrane. PTH and a low-phosphate diet both stimulate production of 25-hydroxyvitamin D 1α-hydroxylase messenger RNA (mRNA), whereas FGF-23 lowers mRNA levels. *(From Kronenberg HM: NPT2a-The key to phosphate homeostasis, N Engl J Med 347:1022-1024, 2002.)*

lin, and glucocorticoids (Ritz et al., 1980). The antiphosphaturic action of growth hormone is believed to occur via mechanisms involving increased reabsorption of Na$^+$, release of insulin, or increased synthesis of $1,25(OH)_2D_3$.

Hypophosphatemia stimulates calcitriol synthesis. The adaptive increases in plasma calcitriol concentrations on bone and intestine raise serum phosphate levels and cause hypercalciuria. This is evident in hereditary hypophosphatemic rickets (HHPR) but not in the disorders involving excessive amounts or activating mutations of FGF-23 (XLH, ADHR, or OHO), in which calcitriol expression is suppressed. The transporter abnormality in HHPR remains elusive.

Hypophosphatemia (Plasma Concentration <2.5 mg/dL)

The etiologies of hypophosphatemia are summarized in Box 5-17. Because it is found in most foods, particularly in dairy

products, and because intestinal absorption is efficient and minimally regulated, phosphorus depletion is rare except in patients with hyperparathyroidism. Hypophosphatemia usually coexists with total body P^{2-} depletion, which is defined precisely as P^{2-} content in lean muscle below 0.28 mol/g dry weight. One may occur without the other, however, particularly when the decrease in serum P^{2-} results from intracellular shifts (Popovtzer and Knochel, 1986).

Clinical manifestations of hypophosphatemia are quite diverse and may be attributable to the underlying disorder (for example, pseudofractures and osteopenia in chronic hypoparathyroidism) or because of hypoxic effects on any and all body processes resulting in hemolysis, rhabdomyolysis, respiratory muscle paralysis, myocardial failure, encephalopathy, or neuropsychiatric symptoms and in secondary disturbances in renal tubular bicarbonate, magnesium, calcium, and glucose reabsorption. Plasma Ca^{2+} concentration may increase as a result of stimulation of calcitriol and from mobilization of bone Ca^{2+} caused by reduction in the blood Ca$^{2+} \times$ P^{2-} product. Glucose intolerance may occur with severe P^{2-} depletion (Marshall et al., 1978). Osteomalacia, rickets, hypercalcemia, hypercalciuria, and distal tubular acidification

---

Box 5-17 Causes of Hypophosphatemia

EXCESSIVE RENAL LOSSES AS PRIMARY CAUSE
Drugs: Cyclosporine, tacrolimus, diuretics, salicylates, carbonic anhydrase inhibitors
Primary hypophosphatemic rickets
Hereditary hypophosphatemic rickets with hypercalciuria
Postobstructive diuresis
Renal tubular acidosis
Postrenal transplantation
Fanconi's syndrome
Recovery from acute tubular necrosis
Potassium deficiency
Oncogenic osteomalacia or rickets
Vitamin D deficiency and dependency (also related to decreased intestinal absorption)
Volume expansion or osmotic diuresis (hyperglycemia)

NEGATIVE INTESTINAL BALANCE AS PRIMARY CAUSE
Breastfed premature infants
Term infants fed with low phosphate source
Use of phosphate-binding antacids
Decreased dietary intake (rare) especially with dialysis and phosphate binders
Vomiting or gastric suction
Glucocorticoids

ACUTE FLUX OF PLASMA PHOSPHATE TO INTRACELLULAR AND SKELETAL POOLS*
Nutritional recovery, usually TPN associated
Therapy of diabetic ketoacidosis
Salicylate intoxication
Alkalosis (especially respiratory)
Androgen therapy
Burn therapy
Hungry-bone phenomenon
Increased tumor burden (uptake by tumor cells)

*The serum phosphate is maintained but total body pools are depressed. In many of these conditions, recovery results in restoration of intracellular phosphate, precipitating acute hypophosphatemia.

defects are known to occur in chronic hypophosphatemia of any cause (Kurtz and Hsu, 1978). Chronic administration of antacids (such as calcium carbonate or aluminum hydroxide) combined with inadequate P^{2-} intake may result in severe hypophosphatemia. In addition to acting as P^{2-} binders, antacids can induce net P^{2-} secretion in the gut and create a negative P^{2-} balance.

Many genetic disorders causing hypophosphatemia are characterized by an abnormal response to PTH, alteration in the structure and function of renal tubular transporters, or defective regulatory proteins within the proximal tubular epithelium. Several of these disorders are inherited and are associated with other metabolic disturbances such as aminoaciduria, glucosuria, hypocalcemia, rickets, and growth failure.

Hypophosphatemia is commonly seen after successful renal transplantation. Contributory factors include the persistence of preexisting parathyroid hyperplasia, volume expansion and osmotic diuresis in the immediate postoperative period, glucocorticoid administration (which increases the renal excretion of P^{2-} and inhibits the gastrointestinal absorption of this ion), ingestion of antacids (which also function as phosphate binders), and an inherent renal tubular defect for P^{2-} reabsorption that is independent of all other hormonal and metabolic factors (Parfitt et al., 1986).

Moderate hypophosphatemia (plasma concentrations of 1.0 to 2.5 mg/dL) generally results in few symptoms and can be managed with oral rather than intravenous phosphate salts. Whenever possible, this may be accomplished through dietary supplements. One quart of milk provides about 1 g of elemental phosphorus (≈ 32 mmol). The dosage of oral salt supplements ranges from 1.0 to 3.0 mmol/kg per day, with the larger dosages given to infants. Children with hypophosphatemia after renal transplantation may temporarily require phosphate replacement with calcitriol supplements. This drug combination is also effective in the management of children with hypophosphatemic rickets.

Children who show symptoms, those with profound hypophosphatemia (plasma concentration <1.0 mg/dL), or children requiring parenteral nutrition may be treated with intravenous phosphate at about 50% of the oral dosage. The choice of the preparation, including sodium phosphate or potassium phosphate, of either oral or intravenous phosphate preparations (Table 5-12), depends on plasma K^+ concentrations and level of renal function.

Hyperphosphatemia

The pathogenesis of hyperphosphatemia is related to the redistribution of P^{2-} from the intracellular compartment, P^{2-} overdose, or decreased renal clearance of P^{2-} (Box 5-18). Symptoms result from the reciprocal decrease in serum calcium. Convulsions, cardiac arrhythmias, laryngospasm, and tetany may reflect hypocalcemia. Also, hyperphosphatemia can produce, contribute to, or be associated with acute renal failure. Conditions such as crush injury, tumor lysis syndrome, rhabdomyolysis, and hemolysis are often associated with oliguria and acute renal failure. The most serious side effect of

---

Box 5-18 Causes of Hyperphosphatemia

DECREASED GLOMERULAR FILTRATION RATE
Acute and chronic renal failure

INCREASED TUBULAR REABSORPTION OF PHOSPHATE
Parathyroid Dysfunction
Hypoparathyroidism (transient hypoparathyroidism of infancy, pseudohypoparathyroidism; transient parathyroid resistance of infancy)

Other Endocrine Causes
Hyperthyroidism, tumoral calcinosis, growth hormone excess; juvenile hypogonadism
High ambient temperature

INCREASED PHOSPHATE LOADS
Exogenous Loads
Enemas and laxatives; vitamin D intoxication; parenteral phosphate; blood transfusions; white phosphorus burns; phosphorus-rich cow's milk

Endogenous Loads
Cellular shift in diabetic ketoacidosis; lactic acidosis; tissue hypoxia; rhabdomyolysis; cytotoxic therapy of neoplasms; hemolysis; malignant hyperthermia

Miscellaneous
Familial intermittent hyperphosphatemia

---

hyperphosphatemia relates to calcium-phosphorus precipitation in the form of hydroxyapatite crystals in nonosseous tissue, including the cornea, lungs, kidneys, pancreas, blood vessels, and brain.

SUMMARY

Elucidation of nephron transporters and their interacting substrates has greatly enhanced our understanding of fluid and electrolyte regulation in children and in adults. However, unlike in adults, anatomic, metabolic, and physiologic differences stemming from the evolving aspects of development (ranging from prematurity to adolescence) result in a spectrum of responses of the nephron to perturbations in fluid and electrolyte balance. This treatise provides the guidelines for fluid and electrolyte management based on an understanding of renal function and tubular transporter physiology in health and disease and during various periods of childhood.

For questions and answers on topics in this chapter, go to "Chapter Questions" at www.expertconsult.com.

REFERENCES

Complete references used in this text can be found online at www.expertconsult.com.

Thermoregulation: Physiology and Perioperative Disturbances

Igor Luginbuehl, Bruno Bissonnette, and Peter J. Davis

CHAPTER

6

One of the many physiologic adaptations required for the survival of homeothermic species is the ability to maintain constant core body temperature within narrow limits. The significance of thermal regulation for neonates was first appreciated by two French obstetricians, Tarnier and later Budin, who in 1907 published the finding of significantly higher survival rates in normothermic versus hypothermic neonates (Budin, 1907). Several other investigators later confirmed the importance of thermal stability in the adaptive process and further elucidated the mechanisms by which neonates, infants, and children are able to behave as homeotherms (Silverman and Blanc, 1957; Cross et al., 1958; Silverman et al., 1958; Bruck, 1961). A homeothermic organism is characterized by its ability to maintain constant core (or central) body temperature despite changes in the ambient temperature. Not many physiologic parameters are as vigorously and effectively controlled as the core temperature. In humans, the central body temperature refers to the temperature of the vessel-rich group organs (i.e., brain, heart, lungs, liver, and kidneys) and is normally maintained within ±0.2° C of its set point of 37.0° C. This so-called interthreshold range defines the limits within which no thermoregulatory effector responses are triggered and the human organism behaves poikilothermically. The musculoskeletal system makes up the major part of the peripheral compartment, which is considered to be a dynamic buffer in the thermoregulatory system. The skin, representing the shell compartment, acts as a barrier to the environment.

Temperature control is subjected to circadian rhythms, some of which begin in the first days of life. The circadian rhythm of body temperature is generally age dependent (less pronounced at very young and very old ages) and generally closely associated with the sleep-wake cycle. In fertile women, a monthly rhythm in body temperature exists because of a higher set-point temperature in the luteal phase of the menstrual cycle (Hardy, 1961). Despite the fluctuations of body temperature within these rhythms, temperature control is tight and is accomplished by a sophisticated system that balances heat production and heat loss.

However, despite this effective regulatory system, the body's ability to dissipate or generate heat by means of skin–blood-flow regulation, sweat production, changes in minute ventilation, and metabolism, it can easily be overwhelmed by external factors.

Anesthesia and surgery have a powerful effect on thermoregulation, and otherwise minor changes in body temperature may result in cellular and tissue dysfunction, thus explaining the need not only for tight temperature regulation within narrow limits, but also for perioperative temperature monitoring.

Accidental hypothermia occurs commonly in patients of any age who are undergoing anesthesia and surgery, and it has often been accepted as an unfortunate but unavoidable consequence of the surgical procedure. This high rate of hypothermia led Pickering to his famous statement, "The practical difficulty in cooling men is to break through the defenses of the body; the most effective means is to give an anesthetic…" (Pickering, 1958).

This chapter discusses the relative merits of different anatomic sites of temperature monitoring; the principles and physiology of thermoregulation in adults and children of all ages; and reviews the influence of anesthetic agents on thermoregulation, the physiologic consequences of hypothermia and hyperthermia, and the techniques used to prevent perioperative hypothermia.

TEMPERATURE MONITORING

Temperature is one of the seven base quantities as defined in the International System of Units (Système Internationale, SI). The unit is Kelvin (K; not "degrees Kelvin"), where 0 K = −273.15° C. Most countries measure temperature in degrees Celsius (°C), whereas a few use degrees Fahrenheit (°F). Normal body temperature is 37.0° C, 98.6° F, or 310.15 K. The following formulas can be used to easily convert from one unit into the other:

$$°\text{Celsius} = [(°\text{Fahrenheit} - 32) \times 5] \div 9$$

$$°\text{Fahrenheit} = (9 \times °\text{Celsius} \div 5) \times 32$$

$$\text{Kelvin} = °\text{C} + 273.15$$

Perioperative detection of changes in body temperature requires appropriate monitoring and monitoring sites. Most national anesthetic societies now have guidelines that require that one method for measuring body temperature during anesthesia be available (La Société Française d'Anesthésie et de Réanimation, 1994; American Society of Anesthesiologists, 2005; Australian and New Zealand College of Anaesthetists, 2006; Canadian Anesthesiologists' Society, 2007).

Although mercury-in-glass thermometers were standard for decades, the most common thermometers used in the perioperative setting are thermocouples and thermistors.

A thermocouple consists of two different metals, often copper and constantan (an alloy of copper, nickel, manganese, and iron). At the junction of any two different metals from the thermoelectric series, a small current is produced. The voltage magnitude of the current depends on the temperature and can therefore be used to measure the temperature. This principle is named *Seebeck's effect* after the physicist, Thomas Johann Seebeck, who discovered it.

The fact that electrical resistance changes exponentially with different temperatures forms the basis of the thermistor type of thermometer, which consists of a semiconductor resistor made of a tiny piece of metal (copper, nickel, manganese, or cobalt). The change in resistance is analyzed to measure temperature. Both thermocouple and thermistor probes are inexpensive and considered sufficiently accurate for clinical purposes.

Infrared thermometers (thermopiles) are quite popular in postanesthesia care units and on hospital wards; however, for continuous temperature monitoring during anesthesia they are not suitable. Despite a fast response time, their accuracy in clinical practice has not been confirmed (particularly when they are not used properly) (Craig et al., 2002; Heusch and McCarthy, 2005; Leon et al., 2005; Dodd et al., 2006).

Temperature-sensitive liquid crystals have been used to measure skin temperature. Although these devices are easy and convenient to handle, they generally do not meet the accuracy criteria required for clinical use. Their readouts can easily be affected by changes that are related not only to body temperature but also to skin blood flow (Leon et al., 1990; MacKenzie and Asbury, 1994). The suggestion of simply adding a constant correcting value (e.g., 2.2° C) to an arbitrary skin temperature to estimate central temperature has been shown to be unreliable (Burgess et al., 1978; Leon et al., 1990).

Body temperature varies widely within the body. Because of their high perfusion rates, core tissues tend to maintain a constant temperature, whereas peripheral tissues usually have significantly lower and less uniform temperatures that may differ by several degrees within a short distance from each other (Colin et al., 1971).

It has been suggested that hypothalamic temperature reflects core temperature, although there is no physiologic evidence that hypothalamic temperature precisely represents central temperature (Benzinger, 1969). Core-temperature measuring sites recommended for clinical use are the tympanic membrane, nasopharynx, distal esophagus, pulmonary artery, and, with some limitations, bladder and rectum. These sites usually provide equal readings in humans who are awake and in those who are anesthetized and undergoing noncardiac surgery (Cork et al., 1983). However, different temperatures may be measured at different monitoring sites and under certain clinical conditions, and the physiologic and clinical significance of these differences may vary.

The precision and accuracy of measurements at different body sites have been studied, and each site has its advantages and disadvantages (Cork et al., 1983; Bissonnette et al., 1989b). Ideally, the temperature-monitoring site reflects core temperature and is associated with only minimal or no morbidity.

Skin temperature measurements offer little as a reflection of core temperature (Lacoumenta and Hall, 1984; Bissonnette et al., 1989b). Because there is a wide variation in skin temperature, depending on the site of monitoring, several investigators have suggested monitoring between 4 and 15 sites, using different formulas to accurately describe the mean skin temperature (Shanks, 1975; Puhakka et al., 1994; Ram et al. 2002). For skin temperature to be of clinical value, it must closely reflect central temperature in the perioperative setting so that mild hypothermia and early signs of malignant hyperthermia (MH) can be detected. Beside the fact that increased body temperature is a late sign of MH, it is unlikely that skin temperature correlates well with central temperature during the early stages of MH, because circulating catecholamine concentrations may be up to 20 times higher than normal and result in significant changes of skin perfusion (Sessler, 1986; Sessler and Moayeri, 1990).

Tympanic-membrane temperature has been suggested as the most ideal temperature-monitoring site. Although it is not necessary for the temperature probe to be in direct contact with the tympanic membrane to accurately reflect tympanic temperature, the external auditory canal needs to be sealed by the probe to allow the air column trapped between the probe and the tympanic membrane to reach a steady-state temperature. During the initial postoperative period after infants and children have had cardiac reconstructive surgery, tympanic temperature does not correlate well with brain temperature and therefore does not provide a reliable estimate of central body temperature (Muma et al., 1991; Bissonnette et al., 2000). Because of difficulties associated with obtaining appropriate-sized thermistors and reports of tympanic membrane perforation, the clinical use of continuous intraoperative temperature measurement has been discouraged.

For a nasopharyngeal temperature probe to accurately reflect core temperature, its tip needs to be placed in the posterior nasopharynx close to the soft palate. This should provide a good estimate of the core temperature. However, using the probe with an uncuffed endotracheal tube that has a moderate to large air leak may lead to falsely low readings. Slight and self-limited bleeding from the nose may occur (especially in children with large adenoids), and its impracticability with mask anesthesia has limited its routine use. Nevertheless, because of the ease of its application and its reliability, this mode of temperature monitoring has been widely accepted in clinical practice.

In contrast, oral temperature is generally considered less adequate and is therefore not recommended as an accurate site for intraoperative temperature-monitoring (Cork et al., 1983).

Esophageal temperature probes are often combined with an esophageal stethoscope, which makes this site particularly attractive for the pediatric population. In infants and children, and in patients who are cachetic, the thermal insulation between the tracheobronchial tree and the esophagus is minimal. Therefore, the respiratory gas flow may result in erroneous temperature readings, particularly when the fresh gas flow is high and its temperature differs significantly from body temperature (Bissonnette et al., 1989b). Furthermore, central temperature is measured only if the tip of the probe is placed in the distal third of the esophagus at the point where the heart sounds are the loudest (Bissonnette et al., 1989b; Stoen and Sessler, 1990). In patients with endotracheal tubes, monitoring of esophageal temperature is more reliable than rectal temperature and more practical than tympanic temperature.

Axillary temperature is not only the most commonly used method of measuring temperature, but it is also the most convenient site for temperature monitoring. It has been reported to be as accurate in measuring central temperature as tympanic membrane, esophageal, and rectal temperature sites. However, this accuracy is only achieved when the tip of the thermometer is carefully placed over the axillary artery and the arm is closely adducted (Bissonnette et al., 1989b). Unfortunately, malpositioning of the probe may result in unreliable estimates of core temperature. Infusion of cool solutions at high flow rates in small children on the ipsilateral side of the thermometer probe may result in falsely low temperature readings.

Rectal temperature monitoring can provide a central temperature reading; it is associated with minimal morbidity and its ease of insertion confers major advantages (Bissonnette et al., 1989b). Problems to be considered with its use pertain to the probe's insulation by feces, its exposure to cooler blood

returning from the legs, the influence of an open abdominal cavity during laparotomy, or irrigations of the bladder or the abdomen with either cold or warm solutions. Relative contraindications for rectal temperature probe insertion are inflammatory bowel disease, neutropenia and/or thrombocytopenia, and the need to irrigate the bowel or bladder.

Bladder-temperature monitoring is considered to be one of the most accurate methods of measuring core temperature. Its precision has been demonstrated to be identical to pulmonary-artery–temperature monitoring as long as urinary output is high; however, when urinary output is normal or less than normal, this site may become inaccurate in reflecting central temperature (Horrow and Rosenberg, 1988; Brauer et al., 2000).

A pulmonary artery catheter with a distal-tip thermistor represents the gold standard for core temperature measurement in noncardiac surgery. Because of its invasive nature, its use—particularly in the pediatric population—has been limited to special situations, such as in critically ill children.

The site or sites for temperature monitoring are often guided by the surgical procedure. For patients undergoing cardiac surgery, in whom temperatures from different body sites convey useful information, temperature is usually measured in at least two sites (e.g., the rectum, bladder, esophagus, nasopharynx, or tympanic membrane).

For pediatric patients undergoing a short surgical procedure that does not require endotracheal intubation, either rectal or axillary temperature monitoring can be used safely. If the child is intubated, an additional option includes the use of a distal esophageal temperature probe.

PHYSIOLOGY OF THERMAL REGULATION

Survival from body temperatures as low as 13.7° C has been reported, whereas death resulting from protein denaturation occurs within 7° C above normality at approximately 44° C (Gilbert et al., 2000). This illustrates a tolerance for cold that is more than three times higher than that for heat, which explains why the system for heat dissipation needs to be much more effective than the system for defense against cold.

The thermoregulatory system is similar to other physiologic control systems in the sense that the brain uses negative feedback mechanisms to keep temperature variations from normal values minimal. The principal site of temperature regulation is the hypothalamus, which integrates afferent signals from temperature-sensitive cells found in most tissues, including other parts of the brain, spinal cord, central core tissues, respiratory tract, gastrointestinal tract, and the skin's surface. The processing and regulation of thermoregulatory information occurs in three stages: afferent thermal sensing, central regulation, and efferent response (Fig. 6-1).

Afferent Thermal Sensing

Anatomically distinct warm and cold receptors in the body periphery sense the ambient temperature. The skin contains about 10 times more cold receptors than warm receptors, acknowledging the important function of the skin in the detection of cold (Poulos, 1981). Thermosensitive receptors are also located in close proximity to the great vessels, the viscera, and the abdominal wall, as well as in the brain and in the spinal

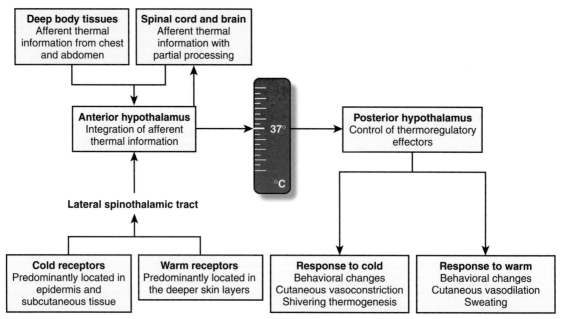

■ **FIGURE 6-1.** Illustration of the thermoregulatory pathways with afferent thermal information from various body parts being integrated in the anterior hypothalamus and triggering efferent responses in the posterior hypothalamus.

cord. Each receptor type transmits its information through an afferent-nerve–conduction pathway. Although information originates from anatomically different nerve fibers, the speed of transmission is mainly influenced by the intensity of the stimulus rather than the type of nerve fiber. It is well established that the rate of change in skin temperature alters the apparent importance of the change. Rapid changes contribute up to five times as much to the central regulatory system as slower changes with comparable intensity (Wyss et al., 1975). However, other than in patients undergoing cardiopulmonary bypass surgery (where rapid temperature changes are common), the rate of change in core temperature does not appear to substantially influence the magnitude of the provoked regulatory responses.

The thermal information from cold-sensitive receptors, which have their maximal discharge rate of impulses at a temperature between 25° and 30° C, is transmitted to the preoptic area of the hypothalamus by A-delta fibers.

Thermal information gathered from peripheral warm receptors, whose maximal discharge rate is between 45° and 50° C, is carried by unmyelinated C fibers. These C fibers also convey pain sensations, which explains why intense heat cannot be distinguished from severe pain (Pierau and Wurster, 1981; Poulos, 1981). Although most ascending thermal information travels along the spinothalamic tracts in the anterolateral spinal cord, no single spinal tract is solely responsible for conveying thermal information (Hellon, 1981).

Central Regulation

Integration of afferent thermal information takes place in the anterior hypothalamus, whereas the posterior hypothalamus controls the descending pathways to the effectors. Thermal inputs from the skin's surface, spinal cord, and deep body tissues are integrated in the preoptic area of the anterior hypothalamus and compared with the threshold temperatures, triggering heat gain or loss. Once the threshold has been reached, the

hypothalamus then carefully orchestrates the mechanisms for heat generation and dissipation in order to maintain body temperature within the narrow limits of its set point (interthreshold range).

The preoptic area of the hypothalamus contains cold- and heat-sensitive neurons, with the latter predominating by a ratio of 4:1 (Boulant and Bignall, 1973). However, the vast majority of the neurons in this area are insensitive to temperature (Nakayama et al., 1963). This area also receives and processes nonthermic afferent information, which seems to be important in controlling the adaptive mechanisms and the behavior of the organism (Hori and Katafuchi, 1998).

Direct heat stimulation of this area results in increased discharge rates from the heat-sensitive neurons and activation of heat-loss mechanisms. Conversely, hypothalamic cold-sensitive neurons respond with increased discharge rates to direct cooling of the preoptic area of the hypothalamus (Boulant, 1974; Boulant and Demieville, 1977). Other centers involved in thermoregulation include the dorsomedial hypothalamus, periaqueductal gray matter, the *nucleus raphe pallidus* in the medulla oblongata, and the spinal cord, although their functions are not yet fully elucidated (Guieu and Hardy, 1970; Simon, 1974; Cabanac, 1975; Dickenson, 1977).

The contribution of the central thermoreceptors to thermal regulation under normal conditions is limited by the marked predominance of thermal input from peripheral receptors (Downey et al., 1964). These central receptors take over thermoregulation if the sensory input from peripheral sensors is disrupted (e.g., through central neuraxial anesthesia or spinal cord transection), but they are less efficient when compared with peripheral thermoreceptors (Downey et al., 1967).

The threshold temperature defines the central temperature at which a particular regulatory effector is activated (Box 6-1). When the integrated input from all sources is signaling that the interthreshold range is exceeded on either side, efferent responses are initiated from the hypothalamus to maintain normal body temperature.

Box 6-1 Definition of Temperature Regulation Terms

Threshold temperature: Central temperature that elicits a regulating effect to maintain normothermia, e.g., vasoconstriction, vasodilation, shivering, sweating, or nonshivering thermogenesis

Interthreshold range: Temperature range over which no regulatory response occurs

Gain: Intensity of regulatory response

Mean body temperature: Physiologically weighted average temperature from various tissues

Nonshivering heat production: Metabolic thermogenesis above basal metabolism not associated with muscle activity

Shivering: Heat production through voluntary muscle activity

Dietary thermogenesis: Heat production through metabolism of nutrients

---

The slope of the response intensity plotted against the difference between the thermal input temperature and the threshold temperature is called the *gain* of that response (i.e., the intensity of the response).

The difference between the lowest temperature at which warm responses are triggered and the highest temperature at which cold responses are triggered indicates the thermal sensitivity of the system. As previously stated, the interthreshold range defines the temperature range over which no regulatory responses occur (although the brain presumably detects these temperature changes). This range changes from approximately 0.4° C in the awake state to approximately 3.5° C during general anesthesia. Compared with normal body temperature (37.0° ± 0.2° C), the interthreshold range during general anesthesia expands further into the hypothermic than into the hyperthermic range. This physiologic system acts as an "all-or-none" phenomenon. The mechanism by which the body determines the absolute threshold temperatures is not known, but it appears that the thresholds are influenced by multiple factors, including plasma concentrations of sodium, calcium, thyroid hormones, tryptophan, general anesthetics, and other drugs; circadian rhythm; exercise; pyrogens; food intake; and adaptation to cold and warm environments. Central regulation is already fully functional in neonates, but it may be impaired in the premature, elderly, or critically ill patient. It is now known that regulatory responses are based on mean body temperature.

Efferent Response

Mean body temperature (MBT) is a physiologically weighted average temperature that reflects the thermoregulatory importance of various tissues, but in particular that of the central compartment. In unanesthetized humans, the MBT can be calculated as follows:

$$MBT = 0.85 \times (Central\ T) + 0.15 \times (Skin\ T)$$

where T denotes the temperature measured in °C. Other formulas do exist (Ramanathan, 1964; Colin et al., 1971; Shanks, 1975; Puhakka et al., 1994). See the following example:

$$MBT = 0.66 \ \times (Rectal\ T + 0.34\ MSK)$$

where MSK reflects the mean skin temperature (in °C), which then equals:

$$MSK = 0.3 \times (Chest\ T + Arm\ T) + 0.2 \times (Thigh\ T + Calf\ T)$$

From that it follows:

$$MBT = 0.66 \times Rectal\ T + 0.34 \times$$
$$(0.3 \times [Chest\ T + Forearm\ T] +$$
$$0.2 \times [Thigh\ T + Calf\ T])$$

Skin temperature is the most important parameter in triggering behavioral changes; however, in terms of impact on the thermoregulatory autonomic response, the thermal input from the skin contributes only about 20% (Cheung and Mekjavic, 1995; Lenhardt et al., 1999). The main part of this autonomic response depends on afferent information from the central core, which includes the brain (parts other than the hypothalamus), the spinal cord, and deep abdominal and thoracic tissues, with each of them contributing about 20% to the central thermoregulatory control (Jessen and Mayer, 1971; Simon, 1974; Mercer and Jessen, 1978; Jessen et al., 1984).

The thermal steady state is actively defended by the hypothalamus responding to thermal changes, that is, temperatures exceeding the interthreshold range to either side. Thus, thermal deviations from the threshold temperature initiate efferent responses that either increase metabolic heat production (shivering or nonshivering thermogenesis) and decrease environmental heat loss (active vasoconstriction and behavioral changes) or increase heat loss (active vasodilation, sweating, and behavioral maneuvers).

Efferent responses (behavioral changes, cutaneous vasoconstriction or vasodilation, nonshivering thermogenesis, shivering, and sweating) appear to be mediated according to the central interpretation of the afferent input.

The most commonly described thermoregulatory model is a set-point system in which hypothalamic integration of thermal information indicates a body temperature above or below a predetermined threshold and then triggers warm or cold defenses. This set-point model, borrowed from engineering models, provides an easy way to explain how the thermoregulatory system functions and how temperature is regulated. In this model, the body compares its actual central temperature against a set reference temperature and then balances heat loss and heat-generating mechanisms to keep the temperature at this set reference point. However, while convenient, this model may not be accurate. More recent research suggests that peripheral and central thermoreceptors are connected through several other neurons to a thermoregulatory effector cell to form a thermoeffector loop (Kobayashi, 1989). In this set-up, once the temperature reaches the range for which the particular thermosensitive neuron has its highest sensitivity, its firing rate increases significantly and—independent of a central nervous system controller—triggers a response in the thermoregulatory effector. Central body temperature in this model is then the averaged result of all the thermoeffector loop actions combined, basically making a central controller (i.e., the hypothalamus) redundant (Kobayashi, 1989; Romanovsky, 2004). Although this more recent model has received a fair amount of attention, it has not been widely accepted in clinical practice.

Regardless of the actual model used, if an effective thermoregulatory system is in place, behavioral responses (e.g., heating the home, looking for shelter, or putting on a jacket) to environmental temperatures outside the thermoneutral range (approximately 28° C for an unclothed adult) remain the quantitatively most important thermoregulatory effectors in humans and are far more efficient than all of the autonomic responses combined. Cutaneous vasoconstriction is the first and most consistent thermoregulatory response to hypothermia. Total digital skin blood flow can be divided into nutritional (capillaries) and thermoregulatory (arteriovenous shunts) components. Cold-mediated decreases in cutaneous blood flow are most pronounced (down to 1% of the normal blood flow seen in a thermoneutral environment) in arteriovenous shunts of the hands, feet, ears, lips, and nose (Grant and Bland, 1931; Hillman et al., 1982). These shunts are typically 100 μm in diameter, which means that one can divert 10,000 times as much blood as a capillary with a 10 μm diameter under otherwise unchanged conditions (i.e., same length and pressure gradient) (Hales, 1985).

Neuronal regulation of blood flow in cutaneous arteriovenous shunts is different in glabrous (nonhairy) and nonglabrous (hairy) skin. In glabrous skin, blood flow is controlled by norepinephrine, whereas nonglabrous arteriovenous shunt flow is controlled by the opposing actions of noradrenergic vasoconstriction and cholinergic vasodilation.

Flow changes not only in the arteriovenous shunts, but also in the far more numerous capillaries (Coffman and Cohen, 1971). The impressive decrease in cutaneous perfusion secondary to thermoregulatory vasoconstriction results in a heat-loss reduction of 50% from the hands and feet, but only of 17% from the trunk, resulting in an overall heat-loss reduction of only 25% (Sessler et al., 1991).

Voluntary muscle activity, nonshivering thermogenesis, and shivering are the efferent mechanisms that lead to heat generation.

In contrast, exposure to warmth initially results in sweating, which triggers massive precapillary vasodilation with marked increase in skin blood flow. This allows for huge amounts of heat to be transported to the skin, from where it then dissipates to the environment, mainly by evaporation because of the preconditioning by sweat.

THERMAL REGULATION IN THE NEWBORN

Premature infants, infants who are small for gestational age, and even full-term neonates have an exceptionally large skin surface area compared with their body mass (assuming a normal ratio for a full-term neonate of 1, then the ratio for an adult is approximately 0.40). Heat loss is further increased because there is only a thin layer of subcutaneous fat and reduced keratin content of the infant's skin, which results in increased thermal conductance and increased evaporative heat loss. (Therefore, when compared with adults, neonates lose proportionately more heat through their skin in similar environments). In contrast to adults, the capabilities and the functional range of the neonate's thermoregulatory system are significantly limited and easily overwhelmed by environmental factors. The lower ambient temperature limit of thermal regulation in adults is

0° C, whereas that in newborns is 22° C. The combination of increased heat loss and a diminished efficacy of the thermoregulatory response with a reduced ability to generate heat puts these infants at high risk for hypothermia. The same anatomic properties that are responsible for the increased risk of hypothermia also allow for rewarming that is three to four times faster in infants and children compared with adults (Szmuk et al., 2001).

The neutral temperature (or the thermoneutral zone) is defined as the ambient temperature range, at which the oxygen demand (as a reflection of metabolic heat production) is minimal and temperature regulation is achieved through nonevaporative physical processes only (i.e., vasoconstriction or vasodilation). The upper limit of this range is called the *upper critical temperature* and marks the ambient temperature at which evaporative heat losses are triggered. Similarly, the lower critical temperature defines the ambient temperature below which metabolic heat generation is activated (nonshivering and/or shivering thermogenesis). Depending on the neonate's weight, this neutral temperature zone is in the range of 32° to 35° C (unclothed in a draft-free environment with uniform temperature and moderate humidity), whereas for an unclothed adult it is approximately 28° C (Hey, 1975). In a thermoneutral environment, the cutaneous arteriovenous shunts are open and skin blood flow is maximal.

Maintaining core temperature in a cool environment results in increased oxygen consumption and potentially metabolic acidosis. It was demonstrated long ago that oxygen consumption does not correlate with rectal temperature in full-term neonates, but rather it increases directly with the skin surface-to-environment temperature gradient (Adamson et al., 1965). Oxygen consumption is minimal at gradients of 2° to 4° C. Thus, at environmental temperatures of 32° to 34° C and an abdominal skin temperature of 36° C, the resting newborn infant is in a state of minimal oxygen consumption (i.e., in a neutral thermal state). Normal rectal temperature, therefore, does not necessarily imply a state of minimal oxygen consumption in this age group, because the baby could activate all its physiologic defense mechanisms to maintain normal rectal temperature (Fig. 6-2).

Of particular concern in view of thermoregulation in the newborn is the head, which comprises up to 20% of the skin's total surface area and shows the highest regional heat flux ability (Anttonen et al., 1995). In neonates and infants, the head may account for up to 85% of body-heat losses, which can be explained by the thin skull bones and the usually sparse scalp hair in combination with the close proximity to the highly perfused brain (core temperature) (Fleming et al., 1992). Facial cooling may increase oxygen requirements in the term and preterm infant by up to 23% and 36%, respectively, thereby further demonstrating the effectiveness of protecting the infant from heat loss by covering the head (Sinclair, 1972).

Thermoregulatory vasoconstriction and vasodilation are already present during the first day of life in both the premature and the full-term infant (Bruck, 1961; Lyons et al., 1996). With vasoconstriction, cutaneous blood flow decreases and the effect of tissue insulation increases, which results in an overall reduction in conductive and convective heat losses.

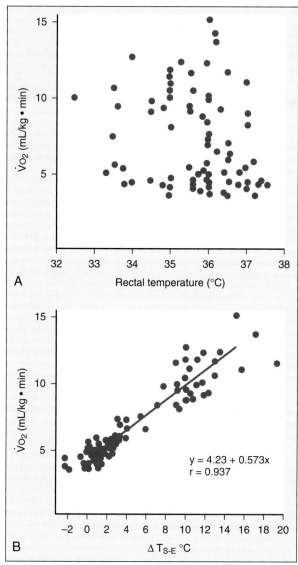

■ FIGURE 6-2. A, Relation of oxygen consumption (Vo$_2$) to rectal temperature. Note complete lack of correlation. **B,** Relationship between oxygen consumption and temperature gradient between skin temperature and environment (ΔT_{S-E}) in full-term human newborns with varying deep body and skin temperatures. *(From Adamson KJ, Jr, Gandy GM, James LS: The influence of thermal factors upon oxygen consumption of the newborn human infant. J Pediatr 66:495, 1965.)*

Heat loss for the premature infant or the infant who is small for gestational age represents the extreme of thermal regulation. The small size and decreased subcutaneous insulation tissue result in increased thermal transfer coefficients, thereby challenging the thermoregulatory capacity of these infants. The anatomic disadvantages further narrow the temperature range for thermoregulatory stability. In small-for-gestational-age infants, a slightly lower skin surface area-to-volume ratio and an increased motor tone offer some (although minor) protection, compared with the premature infant with regard to heat loss or transfer. In addition to the physical limitations of heat conservation in infants and children, surgery can further increase heat loss and fluid requirements by exposing the visceral surfaces of the abdomen and thorax, thereby exacerbating evaporative heat and water losses.

HEAT LOSS MECHANISMS

The abilities to produce and dissipate heat are fundamental for a homeothermic organism. Controlled heat loss in homeotherms is accomplished in two stages, both governed by the physical laws of conduction, radiation, convection, and evaporation (Box 6-2) (Swyer, 1973). The second law of thermodynamics states that heat can be transferred from a warmer to a cooler object but never from a cooler to a warmer object. What this means is that the warmer object (in the operating room setting, this is almost exclusively the patient) is used to warm up the surrounding cooler objects (e.g., the operating room walls, tables, and instruments). Although most anesthesiologists consider heat loss to be a nuisance, without any heat loss to the environment (i.e., perfect insulation), the body of an awake adult at rest (assuming a metabolic rate of 75 W) would warm up by at least 1° C per hour. (Keep in mind that during exercise, metabolic heat generation can increase up to tenfold.) This can be calculated with the following formula:

$$HSR = mk \, dT_B / dt$$

where HSR is the heat storage rate (W), m is the body mass (kg), k is the specific heat coefficient of the human body ($3.5 \bullet 10^3$ J/°C), dT$_B$ is the change in body temperature (°C), and dt is the time interval (sec) (Burton, 1935).

The first stage of heat loss during anesthesia occurs with the transfer of heat from the body core (central compartment) to the periphery and the skin's surface, which is referred to as the concept of internal redistribution of heat. In the second stage, heat is dissipated from the skin's surface to the environment (see "Anesthesia and Hypothermia," p. 168). Physiologic manipulations of regional blood flow and changes in the thermal conductance properties of the insulation tissue can influence both gradients. Most studies of thermal regulation in infants and children have quantified the relative contributions of radiation, convection, evaporation, and conduction to heat loss. A study in newborns in a thermoneutral environment found radiation, convection, evaporation, and conduction to account for 39%, 34%, 24%, and 3%, respectively, of total heat loss (Hey, 1973). However, the conditions in the operating room rarely meet the criteria for thermoneutrality and the relative contributions of each of these four physical components to total heat loss can vary significantly. Figure 6-3 gives an overview of the heat loss mechanisms involved in the operating room setting.

Conduction

Conduction describes heat transfer between two surfaces in direct contact. The amount of heat transferred (C) depends on the temperature difference between the two objects in contact (T$_1$ – T$_2$), the surface area of the objects in contact (A), and the

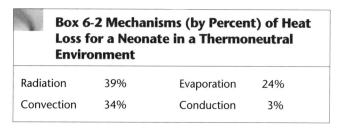

Box 6-2 Mechanisms (by Percent) of Heat Loss for a Neonate in a Thermoneutral Environment			
Radiation	39%	Evaporation	24%
Convection	34%	Conduction	3%

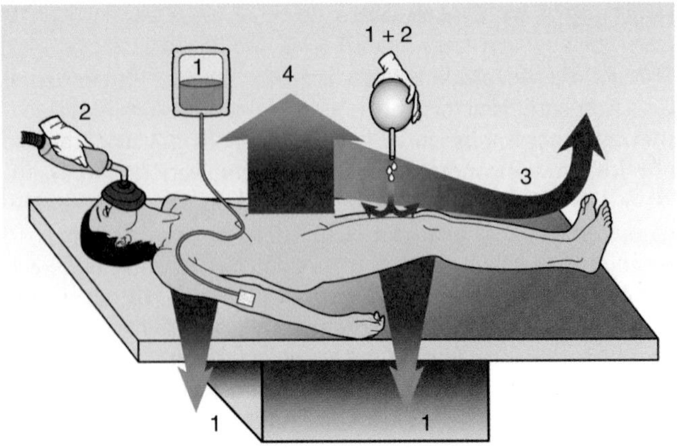

FIGURE 6-3. Schematic illustration of the four mechanisms contributing to perioperative hypothermia: *(1)* conduction, *(2)* evaporation, *(3)* convection, and *(4)* radiation. *(Modified from Gurtner C, Paul O, Bissonnette B: Temperature regulation: physiology and pharmacology. In Bissonnette B, Dalens B, editors:* Pediatric anesthesia: principles and practice, *New York, 2002, McGraw-Hill.)*

conductive heat transfer coefficient (h_k) of the materials and can be calculated as follows:

$$C = h_k \, A(T_1 - T_2)$$

The coefficient h_k is a property of the material or interface between the two objects that determines the rate of heat transfer per unit area per unit temperature difference (W/m² • °C). During surgery, relatively little heat should be lost to the environment via conduction, because the patient is supposed to be well insulated from surrounding objects (Allen, 1987). However, conduction is also responsible for heat loss created by warming up cool intravenous fluids and irrigation solutions, which have the potential to significantly and quickly reduce body temperature. Attention should also be paid to ensure that the patient's skin is not in contact with any metallic surfaces, because metals have a high thermal conductivity, thereby facilitating heat transfer. (In addition, contact with metallic surfaces during surgery must be avoided to prevent skin burns from electrocautery.) The physiologic factors controlling conductive heat loss are cutaneous blood flow and the thickness of the subcutaneous tissue (insulation).

Radiation

Radiant heat loss refers to transfer of heat between two objects of different temperatures that are not in contact with each other (e.g., radiation is the mechanism by which the sun warms the earth). The emitted radiation carries the energy from the warmer object to the cooler object, thereby causing the warmer object to cool and the cooler object to warm. This heat transfer occurs in the infrared light spectrum. Heat exchange by radiation depends on the difference of the fourth power of the absolute temperatures of the two objects:

$$R = e \, s \, A \, (T_{sk}^4 - T_r^4)$$

where R is heat transfer by radiation (W), e is the emissivity (a material property with a value between 0 and 1), s is the Stefan Boltzmann constant ($5.67 • 10^{-8}$ J/sec • m² • K⁴), A denotes the surface area of the object (m²), T_{sk} is the skin temperature, and T_r is the temperature of the second object (both temperature values in K).

Because the temperature differences for clinical purposes are rather small, it is acceptable to use a first-power relationship for T_{sk} and T_r, which then allows the calculation of radiation heat exchange as follows:

$$R = h_r A(T_{sk} - T_r)$$

where h_r denotes the radiation coefficient, an integration of emissivity and the Stefan Boltzmann constant. Heat transfer by radiation principally depends on the temperatures of the two surfaces concerned and is unaffected by air movement or the distance between the surfaces, and it can take place even across a vacuum (Allen, 1987).

As previously stated, newborns and infants have a large surface area-to-mass ratio, thus radiant heat loss is proportionally greater the smaller the infant. In both the infant who is awake and the infant who is anesthetized, radiation is the major factor for heat loss under normal conditions. The human body is an excellent emitter of energy at wavelengths relevant to heat transfer, and the probability of photon reflection in the standard operating room is almost zero. Radiant heat loss in the operating room is therefore a function of the temperature difference between the patient's body and the room (i.e., the floor, walls, and ceiling) and all the objects in it. Warming up the operating room (and its contents) reduces not only the temperature gradient between the patient and the environment but also radiant heat losses. However, as long as a temperature gradient exists, the patient continues to warm up the surrounding environment. At a room temperature of 22° C, about 70% of the total heat loss is a result of radiation (Hardy et al., 1941). A simple single-layer covering of the body dramatically reduces the heat loss by convection and radiation; thus, a thin shirt (e.g., a silk blouse, although it provides only negligible insulation) already results in considerably increased thermal comfort.

Convection

Convective heat loss describes the transfer of heat to moving molecules, such as air or liquids. The thin layer of air directly adjacent to the skin is warmed by conduction from the body, from which heat is then lost by convection. Changes in body posture and minute ventilation may also affect convective heat loss. In the case of an unclothed individual who is exposed to air, the rate and direction of convective heat exchange depend on airflow velocity ("wind speed") and the temperature difference between air and the skin's surface. The situation is more complex for a clothed individual. Convective heat transfer may be calculated as follows:

$$Q = h_c A \, (T_{sk} - T_a)$$

where Q is the heat exchange by convection (W), A is the surface area (m²), h_q is the convective heat transfer coefficient (W/m² • °C), T_{sk} is the mean skin temperature (°C), and T_a is the ambient temperature (°C). The convective heat exchange coefficient h_c is not a constant and depends on the rate of air movement (or fluid current), the shape of the body, and the surrounding medium (i.e., gas or liquid). Thus, convective heat loss increases in proportion to the temperature difference between the body surface and the surrounding gas (or liquid) and the square root of the flow velocity of the gas (or liquid) in contact with the patient. Convective loss is best experienced outdoors in the form of the wind chill factor.

Evaporation

Evaporative heat loss occurs through the skin and the respiratory system. Under conditions of thermal neutrality, evaporation accounts for 10% to 25% of heat loss. Physical factors governing evaporative heat loss include relative humidity of the ambient air, velocity of airflow, and lung minute ventilation. The driving force behind evaporation is the vapor pressure difference between the body surface and the environment. Evaporative losses include mainly three components: sweat (sensible water loss); insensible water loss from the skin, respiratory tract, and open surgical wounds; and evaporation of liquids applied to the skin, such as antibacterial solutions. The evaporation of water from a surface is dependent on energy that is absorbed from the surface during the transition from a liquid to a gaseous state. This energy is called the *latent heat of vaporization,* and in the case of sweat, it has a value of 2.5 $\times 10^6$ J/kg. This figure emphasizes the extraordinary power of the human sweating mechanism as a means of dissipating heat, especially considering that an adult in excellent physical condition can produce up to 2 or 3 liters of sweat per hour (Armstrong et al., 1986; Godek et al., 2008). In an environment where the air temperature is equal to or higher than the skin temperature, sweating is the only mechanism available for dissipation of heat that originates from metabolic production. In this situation, anything that limits evaporation, such as high ambient humidity or impermeable clothing, may easily lead to heat storage and a potentially fatal rise in body temperature. Evaporative heat loss can be calculated as follows:

$$E = h_e A_{wet}(P_{sk} - P_a)$$

where E is the evaporative heat loss (W); h_e is the evaporative heat transfer coefficient (W/m² • kPa); P_{sk} is the water vapor pressure at the skin's surface; and P_a is the ambient water vapor pressure (both pressure values in kPa). The coefficient for evaporative heat exchange (h_e) incorporates the latent heat of vaporization of water and the paramount effect of air movement on evaporation. For practical purposes, h_e may be calculated from the following formula:

$$h_e = 124V^{0.5}(W/m^2 \bullet kPa)$$

where V is the airflow velocity (m/sec). The important point to note is that evaporation is determined by the vapor pressure gradient between the exposed body surface and the ambient air and the rate of airflow across the surface (Allen, 1987).

Physiologic factors affecting evaporative losses relate to an infant's ability to sweat and to increase the minute ventilation. Although the physical characteristics of the newborn predispose him or her to heat loss, it has been demonstrated that neonates are capable of sweating in a warm environment (Bruck, 1961). Full-term neonates begin to sweat when rectal temperature reaches 37.5° to 37.9° C and ambient temperature exceeds 35° C. Although the onset of sweat production in infants who are small for gestational age is slower than it is in full-term infants, the maximum rates of sweat production are comparable (Sulyok et al., 1973). However, premature infants with a gesta-

tional age below 30 weeks show no sweating response because the lumen of their sweat glands are not yet fully developed.

Only a small amount of heat is lost when dry, inspired respiratory gases are humidified by water evaporating from the tracheobronchial epithelium. In adults, respiratory losses account for only 5% to 10% of total heat loss during anesthesia and surgery, and total insensible losses account for approximately 25% of the total heat dissipated (Bickler and Sessler, 1990). Minute ventilation on a per-kilogram basis in infants and children is significantly higher than in adults; thus, respiratory heat loss represents about one third of the total heat loss. Obviously, respiratory heat loss increases if the patient breathes cool, dry air as opposed to warm, moisturized air (Bissonnette et al., 1989a, 1989b).

Evaporative heat loss from a large surgical incision may equal all other sources of intraoperative heat loss combined (Roe, 1971). Because of increased evaporative heat loss, hypothermia is also more likely to occur if the skin of the patient is wet or comes in contact with wet drapes.

HEAT GENERATION

The ability to produce heat by increasing the metabolic rate and oxygen consumption is the other prerequisite of thermal regulation for a homeothermic organism (Hull and Smales, 1978). Beside the fact that three of the physical mechanisms leading to heat loss (i.e., conduction, radiation, and convection) can theoretically also be used to passively warm up a patient, the body has the ability to actively produce heat. Heat generation can be achieved through four mechanisms:

1. Voluntary muscle activity
2. Nonshivering thermogenesis
3. Involuntary muscle activity (shivering)
4. Dietary thermogenesis

The behavioral aspect of heat production (voluntary muscle activity) is usually not functional in the perioperative period and therefore its role in heat production will not be discussed further here. Of the three remaining mechanisms for heat production, nonshivering thermogenesis is the major component in the newborn, whereas shivering thermogenesis is the main mechanism for heat production in older children and adults. The contribution of nonshivering thermogenesis in adults is debatable (Jessen, 1980a).

Although both the time course and the relationship between nonshivering and shivering thermogenesis in infants have been described, the exact time sequence and factors involved in the developmental aspects of switching on shivering thermogenesis and nonshivering thermogenesis off remain to be elucidated (Hull and Smales, 1978). The importance of nonshivering thermogenesis seems to decrease rapidly after the first year of life, while at the same time shivering thermogenesis is becoming more and more effective (Fig. 6-4B). Under normal conditions, dietary thermogenesis will not contribute significantly to thermogenesis during anesthesia. It only affects temperature if the patient is given food with a high protein or fructose content before or during anesthesia, which is normally not the case.

Nonshivering Thermogenesis

Nonshivering thermogenesis is defined as an increase in metabolic heat production (above the basal metabolism) that is not associated with muscle activity. It occurs mainly through

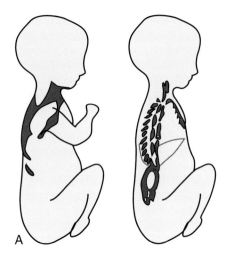

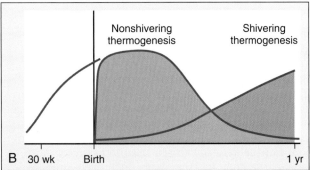

■ **FIGURE 6-4. A,** Brown adipose tissue in superficial *(left)* and deep *(right)* sites in the newborn. **B,** Relation of shivering thermogenesis to nonshivering thermogenesis as it appears in certain newborn animals. The time scale represents human development. *(A, From Aherne W, Hull D: The site of heat production in the newborn infant. Proc R Soc Med 57:1172, 1964. B, From Hull D, Smales ORC: Heat production in the newborn. In Sinclair JC, editor: Temperature regulation and energy metabolism in the newborn, New York, 1978, Grune and Stratton.)*

metabolism in brown fat and to a lesser degree also in skeletal muscle, liver, brain, and white fat.

Brown fat differentiates in the human fetus between 20 and 30 weeks of gestational age (Lean et al., 1986a). It comprises only 2% to 6% of the infant's total body weight and is found in six main locations: between the scapulae, in small masses around blood vessels of the neck, in large deposits in the axillae, in medium-size masses in the mediastinum, around the internal mammary vessels, and around the adrenal glands or kidneys (Fig. 6-4A).

Brown fat is a highly specialized tissue; the brown color is secondary to the abundant content of mitochondria in the cytoplasm of its multinucleated cells. These mitochondria are densely packed with cristae and have an increased content of respiratory-chain components (Himms-Hagen, 1976). They are unique in their ability to uncouple oxidative phosphorylation, resulting in heat production instead of generating adenosine triphosphate. This uncoupling process is mediated by the presence of the uncoupling protein 1 (UCP-1, or thermogenin) that is located on the inner mitochondrial membrane (Himms-Hagen, 1976; Ricquier and Kader, 1976).

Brown fat is highly vascularized and has a rich sympathetic innervation, which appears to be primarily β-sympathetic in

origin and responsible for the uncoupling of oxidative phosphorylation (Karlberg et al., 1962, 1965). In respect to nonshivering thermogenesis, mature brown fat cells mainly rely on activation by β_3-receptors. Cold stress increases sympathetic nervous system activity and norepinephrine release, which causes increased lipase activity in the brown fat tissue (Schiff et al., 1966). As a consequence, hydroxylation of triglycerides and release of free fatty acids occur. These free fatty acids act on UCP-1 and thereby increase the protein conductance across the mitochondrial membrane. In addition to norepinephrine, glucocorticoids and thyroxin have been implicated as factors that trigger nonshivering thermogenesis (Gale, 1973; Jessen, 1980b, 1980c). The heat produced by nonshivering thermogenesis is mainly a by-product of fatty acid metabolism, but to a minor degree it can also result from glucose metabolism. The activation of brown fat metabolism results in an increased proportion of the cardiac output being diverted through the brown fat. This proportion may reach as much as 25% of the cardiac output, which facilitates the direct warming of the blood.

Pharmacologic inhibition of nonshivering thermogenesis can be achieved with ganglionic and β-receptor blockade, inhalational anesthetics, and surgically by sympathectomy (Silverman et al., 1964; Stern et al., 1965; Ohlson et al., 1994). Inhibition of nonshivering thermogenesis by inhalational anesthetics starts as early as 5 minutes after turning on the vapor and starts to wean off within approximately 15 minutes after discontinuation of the inhalational anesthetic (Ohlson et al., 1994). Nonshivering thermogenesis is also inhibited in infants who have been anesthetized with fentanyl and propofol (Plattner et al., 1997).

In general, nonshivering thermogenesis seems to be quite variable in adults, but most often it does not appear to be functional or relevant (Ohlson et al., 1994; van Marken Lichtenbelt and Daanen, 2003). This assumption is supported by the fact that oxygen consumption does not increase significantly when patients exhibit thermoregulatory vasoconstriction (Mestyan et al., 1964; Dawkins and Scopes, 1965). However, it seems that adults have the potential to regenerate brown fat tissue under certain pathologic conditions, such as pheochromocytoma (secondary to high and sustained sympathetic stimulation), Chagas' disease, hibernoma (a benign brown-fat tissue tumor), or marked cold acclimatization (Garruti and Ricquier, 1992; Lean et al., 1986b; Vybiral et al., 2000).

In contrast, premature and full-term neonates, as well as infants, are able to double their metabolic heat production during cold exposure (Mestyan et al., 1964; Dawkins and Scopes, 1965; Hey and Katz, 1969). Clinically significant nonshivering thermogenesis is possible within hours after birth and may persist up to the age of 2 years (Fig. 6-4, B) (Oya et al., 1997). Despite the fact that nonshivering thermogenesis is the main source of thermoregulatory heat production in infants, it should be kept in mind that its effect and sustainability are limited and do not compensate for the decreased ability of newborns and infants to effectively reduce heat loss through cutaneous vasoconstriction or the lack of heat production through shivering.

Core hypothermia or exposure to cold during general anesthesia with propofol and fentanyl do not trigger nonshivering thermogenesis in children; therefore, nonshivering thermogenesis seems to be nonfunctional (Plattner et al., 1997). Halothane anesthesia has been shown to block nonshivering thermogenesis in children (Ohlson et al., 1994; Dicker et al., 1995). It has been demonstrated in animal studies that pharmacologic inhibition of nonshivering thermogenesis by β-blockade also affects shivering thermogenesis (Bruck and Wunnenberg, 1965). In the animals studied, shivering did not fully compensate for the lack of heat produced by nonshivering thermogenesis. The magnitude of nonshivering thermogenesis in animals varies among species, but it appears that in newborn versus adult animals and in cold-adapted versus warm-adapted animals, the contribution of nonshivering thermogenesis to heat generation is significant (Himms-Hagen, 1976).

Shivering Thermogenesis

The precise mechanisms and factors that govern the onset of shivering and the decline of nonshivering thermogenesis are unclear. With increasing age, shivering thermogenesis takes over a more prominent role in thermoregulation. It has been shown that shivering is triggered only after all the other cold defense mechanisms, such as behavioral responses, nonshivering thermogenesis (both ineffective under anesthesia), and maximal thermoregulatory vasoconstriction, have failed to maintain body temperature within the interthreshold range (Hemingway, 1963; Hemingway and Price, 1968). Until recently, newborns and infants were considered to be unable to shiver, presumably because of the general immaturity of the musculoskeletal system on the one hand and the limited muscle mass on the other hand, which would render muscle activity ineffective in defense against cold. However, a few reports exist about shivering in neonates occurring at rectal temperatures of 35.0° to 35.3°C (Brück, 1992; Petrikovsky et al., 1997). It is debatable whether this shivering was indeed thermoregulatory in origin or whether drugs and other factors (all mothers received an intrapartum amnioinfusion) were to blame. For clinical purposes, it is probably reasonable to say that neonates do not shiver, and if they do, it is of no (or only minor) significance for thermoregulation.

For a short time and only in an otherwise healthy and young person, shivering can result in an up to a sixfold increase in metabolic heat production and oxygen consumption, but only a twofold increase is sustainable (Horvath et al., 1956; Benzinger, 1969; Ciofolo et al., 1989; Just et al., 1992; Giesbrecht et al., 1994). Oxygen consumption in elderly patients (usually the age group with the highest risk for adverse cardiac events) increases on average by approximately 130% during shivering (Bay et al., 1968).

Shivering is characterized by involuntary, irregular muscular activity usually beginning in the muscles of the upper body (commonly the masseter). Overt shivering is preceded by a generalized increase in muscle tone, and only once this muscle tone reaches a certain threshold will shivering be detectable (Guyton, 2000). The intensity of shivering is higher in central muscles than it is in peripheral muscles (Bell et al., 1992).

Shivering occurs in two different electromyographic patterns: a basal, continuous shivering with low intensity at a rate of 4 to 8 Hz and superimposed bursts of high intensity at a rate of 0.1 to 0.2 Hz. The former is associated with type 1 and the latter with type 2 muscle fibers, with the bursts creating the typical "waxing and waning" pattern in the electromyogram (Stuart et al., 1966; Haman et al., 2004).

Impulses from cold receptors impinge at the motor center for shivering in the dorsomedial part of the posterior hypothalamus, adjacent to the wall of the third ventricle. In warm conditions, this center is inhibited by impulses from the heat-sensitive area in the preoptic region of the anterior hypothalamus. However, predominantly cold impulses from the skin and the spinal cord activate the shivering center, resulting in stimulation of anterior motor neurons of the spinal cord. Initially, this leads to the described generalized increase in skeletal muscle tone throughout the body, but it does not cause the actual shivering.

In healthy patients, this rise in oxygen consumption is easily met by increased cardiac output without any signs of cardiopulmonary compromise. In patients with already limited hemodynamic, coronary, or pulmonary reserves, this increase in oxygen demand can lead to decreased mixed venous oxygen content and eventually to decreased arterial oxygen content and tissue hypoxia. An inverse correlation has been shown between intraoperative temperature and postoperative oxygen demand, as well as between different anesthetics (see "Thermoregulation and General Anesthesia," p. 172) (Roe et al., 1966). Shivering is not only an unpleasant experience for the patient in the postoperative period; it has also been implicated in increased intracranial and intraocular pressure, wound dehiscence, and dental damage (Mahajan et al., 1987; Rosa et al., 1995; Alfonsi, 2001).

Although the incidence of postoperative shivering is inversely related to the core temperature, shivering was also found in patients who were kept strictly normothermic during isoflurane or desflurane anesthesia, indicating that a substantial fraction of shivering is nonthermoregulatory, with pain being one potential trigger (Horn et al., 1998, 1999). Inhibition of shivering with meperidine in awake, actively cooled volunteers resulted in a more than threefold higher and more than four-times prolonged core temperature afterdrop with a rewarming rate decreased by 37% when compared with the shivering control group (Giesbrecht et al., 1997).

Dietary Thermogenesis

Stimulation of energy expenditure and thermogenesis by certain nutrients (i.e., proteins and amino acids) is a well-known phenomenon (Lindahl, 2006). Despite muscle paralysis and decreased metabolism during general anesthesia, the infusion of small amounts of amino acids resulted in up to a fivefold increase in heat generation during anesthesia compared with that in adults who were awake (Sellden et al., 1994). Using pre- and intraoperative amino-acid infusions, the same researchers were able to use this advantage clinically to achieve a core temperature of 36.5° ± 0.1° C at the end of surgery, whereas the temperature dropped to 35.7° ± 0.1° C in the control group (Sellden and Lindahl, 1999). Similar findings have been reported for preoperative amino-acid infusion in patients undergoing spinal anesthesia (Kasai et al., 2003). Although effective, the exact mechanism behind this form of thermogenesis has not yet been fully elucidated. It seems that stimulation of cellular amino-acid oxidation is crucial. Furthermore, protein synthesis and breakdown in extrasplanchnic tissues that require extra synthesis of ATP, could be a contributing factor as well. Approximately half of the heat generated in association with amino-acid infusions is splanchnic in origin. Blood flow in extrasplanchnic (but not splanchnic) tissues increases

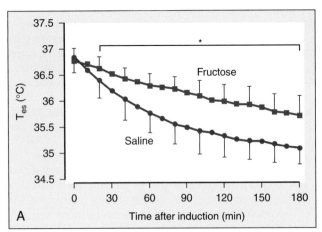
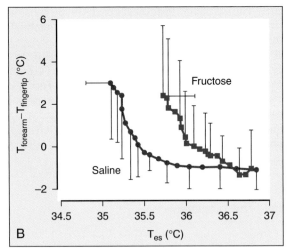

■ **FIGURE 6-5. A,** Core temperature measured at the distal esophagus (T$_{es}$) during surgery. Patients receiving the fructose infusion had significantly greater core temperatures than those receiving saline (*P = 0.001). **B,** Relationship between the forearm-minus-fingertip temperature gradient (T$_{forearm}$ – T$_{fingertip}$) and distal esophageal (core) temperature (T$_{es}$). Patients assigned to fructose infusion experienced vasoconstriction (increased in the gradient) at a significantly higher core temperature than did those receiving saline infusion (P < 0.001). *(From Mizobe T, et al.: Fructose administration increases intraoperative core temperature by augmenting both metabolic rate and the vasoconstriction threshold.* Anesthesiology *104:1124-1130, 2006.)*

significantly, reflected by a raise in cardiac output of almost 20% (Brundin and Wahren, 1994). Except for a different time course, the average whole-body thermic effect of intravenous amino-acid administration is not different from the one seen with oral protein ingestion. Fructose administration has also been shown to increase the metabolic rate by 20% in anesthetized adult surgical patients. In a study of 20 patients, Mizobe et al. (2006) noted that intravenous fructose increased the intraoperative core temperature, oxygen consumption, and the vasoconstrictive threshold (Fig. 6-5). Dietary thermogenesis has the potential to cause hyperthermia not only during general anesthesia with attenuated thermoregulation, but also in the patient who is awake (Sellden, 2002).

EFFECT OF ANESTHESIA ON THERMOREGULATION

Anesthesia and Hypothermia

There is no generally accepted definition for hypothermia, but the distinction between mild (core temperature 34.0° to 35.9° C), moderate (32.0° to 33.9° C), and severe hypothermia (below 32.0° C) appears useful and reasonable for clinical purposes (Brux et al., 2005). General anesthesia reduces the threshold at which the body initiates a thermoregulatory response to cold stress (Boxes 6-3 and 6-4). Mild intraoperative hypothermia (1° to 3° C below normal) is common and results from a combination of the following events:

1. A reduction of approximately 30% in metabolic heat generation during anesthesia (Brismar et al., 1982).
2. Increased environmental exposure.
3. Anesthetic-induced central inhibition of thermoregulation (Sessler and Ponte, 1982; Sessler, 1991).
4. Redistribution of heat within the body (Hynson et al., 1991a).

Box 6-3 General Effects of Anesthetics on Thermoregulation

1. Lowering of the threshold temperature for cold defense
2. Increasing the threshold temperature for heat defense
3. Tenfold widening of the interthreshold range to approximately 2° to 4° C
4. Generally no effect on the gain of the thermoregulatory response (except for desflurane)

Box 6-4 Specific Effects of Anesthetics on Thermoregulation

1. Opioids reduce threshold temperature for vasoconstriction and shivering as a linear function of dose.
2. Propofol reduces threshold temperature for vasoconstriction and shivering as a linear function of dose.
3. Volatile anesthetics produce a nonlinear inhibition of the thermoregulatory defense mechanisms, with the inhibition being proportionally greater at higher end-tidal concentrations.
4. Volatile anesthetics at comparable minimum alveolar concentrations produce similar degrees of thermoregulatory inhibition.
5. N$_2$O decreases vasoconstriction threshold less than halogenated volatile agents.

Hypothermia during general anesthesia has a typical profile and usually develops in three phases (Fig. 6-6):

1. Internal redistribution of heat.
2. Thermal imbalance.
3. Thermal steady state (plateau or rewarming).

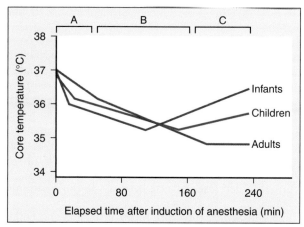

■ FIGURE 6-6. This graph illustrates the three phases typical for the course of intraoperative hypothermia during general anesthesia. *A* represents the internal redistribution of heat; *B* is the thermal imbalance phase with ongoing net loss of heat to the environment; and *C* is the thermal steady state, which in children and infants is a rewarming phase. *(Modified from Bissonnette B: Thermoregulation and paediatric anaesthesia. Curr Opin Anaesthesia 6:537, 1993.)*

Internal Redistribution

In order to understand the concept of internal redistribution, it is helpful to use the previously described division of the human body into three thermal compartments, the central, peripheral, and skin (or "shell") compartments. The core temperature represents the central compartment temperature, which contains the vessel-rich group organs receiving approximately 75% of the cardiac output and representing about 10% of the body weight in adults and up to 22% in neonates. In an awake adult at rest, the entire central compartment accounts for approximately 66% of the body mass and extends to about 71% during general anesthesia (Deakin, 1998).

The peripheral compartment comprises the remaining part of the body mass (mainly muscles) and acts as a dynamic buffer to accommodate any changes in core temperature by thermoregulatory vasodilation or vasoconstriction. Its estimated buffer capacity of over 600 kJ allows the body to maintain core temperature constant with a minimal amount of energy expenditure for thermoregulation despite absorption or dissipation of significant amounts of heat.

The skin compartment is almost virtual and represents the barrier between the previous two compartments and the environment. After induction of anesthesia, peripheral vasodilation causes an increase in the size of the central compartment, forcing it to redistribute its heat within a larger volume. In addition, the anesthesia-induced reduction in metabolic heat generation decreases the amount of energy available to compensate for the enlargement of this compartment. The concept of internal redistribution of heat, therefore, consists primarily not of heat loss to the environment, but of a measurable decrease in core temperature and an increase in the peripheral and skin compartment temperatures because of redistribution of heat.

With induction of anesthesia, the central core temperature starts to decrease rapidly by approximately 0.5° to 1.5° C during the first 30 to 45 minutes of anesthesia (Fig. 6-7). Although this process results in reduced core temperature, the total body-heat content decreases only slightly. Heat—as the name implies—is mainly redistributed and not dissipated. This redistribution of heat accounts for 81% of the core temperature

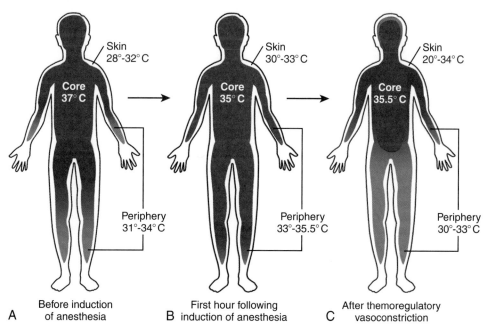

■ FIGURE 6-7. The dynamic changes within the three temperature compartments of a child before induction of anesthesia, during the first hour of anesthesia, and after thermoregulatory vasoconstriction. In the awake human, temperature and size of the compartments are considered normal **(A)**. After the first hour of anesthesia, the internal redistribution of heat results in a rapid decrease in core temperature and an increase in peripheral temperature, together causing enlargement of the central compartment and shrinkage of the peripheral compartment **(B)**. The drop in central temperature is mainly caused by the distribution of its heat to a larger volume, and actual heat loss is minimal at this stage. **C,** Once thermoregulatory vasoconstriction has been initiated (after about 3 hours of anesthesia), the central compartment is shrinking in favor of the peripheral compartment. The rise in central temperature is now due to the fact that generated heat is contained in a smaller volume.

decrease in the first hour of anesthesia, whereas the remainder is the result of the anesthesia-induced reduction in metabolism and increased heat loss. For the subsequent 2 hours of anesthesia, the impact of redistribution on total heat loss decreases to approximately 43% (Matsukawa et al., 1995b). Accordingly, administration of a vasoconstrictor, such as phenylephrine, can limit the drop in core temperature caused by redistribution (Ikeda et al., 1999a).

Internal redistribution results in shrinkage of the peripheral compartment and enlargement of the central compartment, which explains not only the decreased core temperature, but also the increased temperature in the peripheral and skin compartments (Fig. 6-7). This is reflected by a more than fourfold increase in the perfusion of the forearms and particularly the legs after induction of anesthesia, and a forearm-fingertip or calf-toe temperature gradient that may exceed 8° C (Matsukawa et al., 1995b).

Thermal Imbalance

The second phase, which is the result of reduced heat production combined with increased heat loss to the environment, lasts about 2 to 3 hours (see Fig. 6-6). This heat loss leads to an approximately linear decrease in mean body temperature (typically 0.5° to 1.0° C/hr). Decreased heat production during anesthesia is caused by limited or absent muscle activity, work of breathing, and the reduced metabolic rate (Stoen and Sessler, 1990; Washington et al., 1992). Heat loss to the environment is a function of the temperature difference between body surface and ambient structures (concept of patient warming up the environment), and therefore decreases passively as the patient becomes more hypothermic. As mentioned earlier, radiation, convection, evaporation, and conduction all contribute to heat loss from the patient to the environment during anesthesia and surgery.

Thermal Steady State (Plateau or Rewarming Phase)

The third stage of the hypothermic response to anesthesia consists of a thermal steady state, in which metabolic heat production equals heat dissipation to the environment, and the core temperature therefore remains constant (see Fig. 6-6). This plateau normally occurs between a core temperature of 34.5° to 35.5° C. This is only possible if the patient increases the heat production, decreases the heat loss, or both to prevent further hypothermia.

A study of adults who were anesthetized with isoflurane showed that the effect of thermoregulatory vasoconstriction reduces heat loss by a maximum of 25%, which is relatively small compared with the fall in metabolic rate and the increase in evaporative heat loss from the surgical incision (Sessler et al., 1992). Heat loss to the environment is determined mainly by the capillary blood flow in large areas of the skin that cover the limbs and the trunk. These capillaries markedly outnumber the arteriovenous shunts, but they cannot constrict as effectively as the shunts. It is possible that vasoconstriction contributes to the thermal plateau by reestablishing the temperature gradient between the central and the peripheral compartments and thereby preventing metabolic heat from being transported to the periphery, from which it would dissipate (see Fig. 6-7). The metabolic heat produced in the body core is once again confined to a smaller central compartment, allowing the core temperature to remain constant.

To reinforce this theory of compartment size, it should be noted that the use of a limb tourniquet during surgical procedures can influence the thermoregulatory response in children and adults (Bloch et al., 1992; Estebe et al., 1996). The tourniquet may induce hyperthermia, which is most likely the result of decreased effective heat loss from distal skin areas, as well as from metabolic heat constraint to the central thermal compartment. Upon release of the tourniquets, the core temperature drops quickly to levels similar to those in patients who were part of a control group without a tourniquet (Estebe et al., 1996; Sanders et al., 1996; Akata et al., 1998). Despite having a constant core temperature, total body-heat content continues to decrease, because heat loss to the environment continues.

Unlike in adults, this third phase in infants and children is a rewarming rather than a plateau (see Fig. 6-6). As mentioned, general anesthesia decreases heat production by inhibiting muscular activity and nonshivering thermogenesis and by reducing the metabolic rate. Thus, the only possible explanation for this rewarming phase must be the occurrence of marked vasoconstriction within the peripheral and central compartments that results in shrinkage of the central compartment. The amount of metabolic heat produced is then distributed within a smaller central compartment volume and results in a higher core temperature. This is associated with a simultaneous increase in oxygen consumption, carbon dioxide production, and systemic norepinephrine levels, an effect that has been observed in infants who were anesthetized with isoflurane and paralyzed with vecuronium (Bissonnette, personal observation).

In contrast to adult responses, intraoperative thermoregulatory responses in infants are effective enough to significantly increase the core temperature despite a constant ambient temperature. A clinical study in anesthetized children found a twofold increase in oxygen consumption during mild hypothermia (Ryan, 1982). Both active and passive rewarming imposes significant physiologic stress on the infant. Passive surface rewarming (with the use of warm blankets, bundling, or other measures) turns off the skin's cold receptors. If normal core temperature is not reached or maintained with passive surface rewarming, hypothermia may result in hypoventilation or even apnea, relative anesthetic overdose (reduced minimum alveolar concentration [MAC] at lower temperatures), and metabolic acidosis. The increased oxygen demand to maintain normal core temperature in the anesthetized infant may create or exacerbate a preexisting cardiopulmonary insufficiency. The release of norepinephrine to trigger vasoconstriction may contribute to the development of acidosis and hypoxia, thereby facilitating right-to-left pulmonary shunting. Sustained pulmonary artery hypertension and right-to-left pulmonary shunting may begin a vicious cycle of hypothermia (Fig. 6-8).

In infants, a correlation between intraoperative hypothermia and an early increase in postoperative oxygen consumption has been demonstrated (Roe et al., 1966).

Anesthesia and Hyperthermia

Similar to hypothermia, hyperthermia triggers important physiologic thermoregulatory responses by using threshold and gains. Similar to hypothermia, the threshold temperature

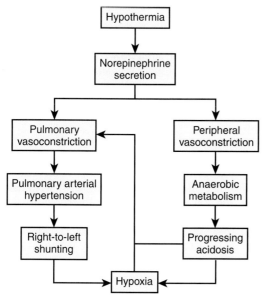

■ FIGURE 6-8. The vicious cycle of hypothermia in neonates and infants. *(Modified from Klaus M, Faranoff A: Care of the high-risk neonate, Philadelphia, 1986, WB Saunders.)*

represents the central temperature for which a particular regulatory effector becomes active, whereas the gain quantifies the intensity of the response (Fig. 6-9). The effector mechanisms during hyperthermia are well preserved during anesthesia (Lopez et al., 1993). The efferent-response thresholds are shifted to higher temperatures with an expansion of the interthreshold range, which corresponds to the difference between the normal central temperature and the first efferent response triggered by the hypothalamus. An interesting observation with regard to the interthreshold range resides in the difference between the shift observed for hypothermia and the shift seen for hyperthermia.

The poikilothermic range to the hypothermic side in the anesthetized patient may be expanded by up to 3.5° C. In contrast, clinical studies in human volunteers have demonstrated that the threshold for active vasodilation and sweating is only 1.0° to 1.4° C higher in anesthetized patients than in those who are awake (Lopez et al., 1993). This observation suggests that the human physiology responds more aggressively to the threats from hyperthermia than from hypothermia. Thus, hyperthermia seems to be a far more dangerous threat to the body than a comparable degree of hypothermia (Lopez et al., 1993).

The efferent responses during hyperthermic stress are limited to two mechanisms: active thermoregulatory vasodilation and sweating. Vasodilation triggered in response to warm stress is not simply the absence of vasoconstriction, but rather an active process mediated by sympathetic cholinergic impulses and release of vasoactive substances (e.g., vasoactive intestinal peptide [VIP], histamine) that results in increased dissipation of heat (Detry et al., 1972; Rübsamen and Hales, 1984; Kellogg et al., 1998; Bennett et al., 2003; Wilkins et al., 2004). It has been demonstrated that the effect of hyperthermia on the peripheral vasculature results in a significant increase in blood flow (Tankersley et al., 1991; Matsukawa et al., 1995b). The observation of active cutaneous vasodilation in infants under anesthesia, although difficult to quantify (skin flushing), suggests that this thermoregulatory response to hyperthermia is preserved.

Sweating represents an increase in evaporative cutaneous heat loss during episodes of heat stress. The relatively high heat of vaporization of sweat (2.5×10^6 J/kg) makes sweating an extremely effective process. This allows for up to a fivefold increase in heat loss to the environment, making it proportionally more effective than all the cold-defense mechanisms combined (Fusi et al., 1989).

A study in adult volunteers showed that sweating remains functional during isoflurane anesthesia (Sessler, 1991b).

The benefits provided by induced hyperthermia (vasodilation) may be desirable during peripheral microvascular surgery, where an increase in regional blood flow is important. One of the clinical limitations of induced hyperthermia to increase cutaneous blood flow is the efficiency of the sweating mechanism. Despite active transfer of approximately 50 W of heat across the patient's skin via convection and radiation, it was possible to demonstrate that the central temperature remains relatively constant or even decreases for exactly this reason (Sessler, 1993). Although shivering can easily double the heat production, sweating can result in the dissipation of more than 10 times the amount of normal basal heat production (Guyton, 2000).

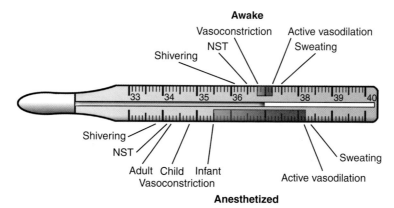

FIGURE 6-9. Thermoregulatory thresholds and gains in awake and anesthetized adults, children, and infants. The vertical height/depth of each [lin]e indicating the threshold temperature represents the maximal intensity of each effector response, whereas the slope of the lines represents the gain [of] the response. The temperature scale corresponds to the core temperature. The sensitivity of the thermoregulatory system is the range between the [firs]t cold response *(vasoconstriction)* and the first warm response *(sweating)* and is called *interthreshold range,* which is significantly expanded during [an]esthesia. *NST,* Nonshivering thermogenesis.

Thermoregulation and General Anesthesia

Both intravenous and inhalational anesthetics can interfere with thermal regulation at peripheral and central receptor sites. In adults, general anesthesia has been shown to lower the thermoregulatory threshold temperature, triggering an average response to hypothermia by approximately 2.5° C, while the increases in the threshold temperature initiating a response to hyperthermia is less pronounced (approximately 1.3° C) (see Fig. 6-9) (Sessler et al., 1988a; 1988b). This anesthesia-induced expansion of the interthreshold range results in a wider temperature range over which active thermoregulatory responses are absent. Within this range, humans behave poikilothermically, with the body temperature changing passively in proportion to the difference between metabolic heat production and heat loss to the environment. Vasoconstriction and nonshivering thermogenesis are the only thermoregulatory responses available to anesthetized, paralyzed, hypothermic infants and children. Patients with mild hypothermia during surgery (e.g., a central body temperature of about 34.5° C) demonstrate profound peripheral vasoconstriction, which can easily be verified using the skin's surface temperature gradients (e.g., forearm versus fingertip skin temperature), volume plethysmography, a laser Doppler flowmeter, or other techniques (Stuart et al., 1966; Sessler et al., 1988a, 1988b).

Thermoregulation and Inhalational Anesthetics

The maximum intensity of peripheral thermoregulatory vasoconstriction during anesthesia is similar to that in volunteers who are awake, indicating that the gain of the response is preserved, but that it is triggered at a markedly lower threshold temperature. The only exception seems to be desflurane, which lowers not only the threshold temperature for vasoconstriction but also its gain (Kurz et al., 1995b). The temperature at which vasoconstriction and nonshivering thermogenesis are triggered identifies the corresponding lower thermoregulatory threshold for the anesthetic agent at any given concentration or dose.

Halothane administration in a concentration of 1.0% in oxygen to healthy adults undergoing donor nephrectomy reduced the threshold temperature for thermoregulatory vasoconstriction to 34.4° ± 0.2° C (Sessler et al., 1988a). In infants and children who were anesthetized with 0.6% halothane combined with a caudal epidural block with bupivacaine, the threshold temperature for vasoconstriction was 35.7° C (Bissonnette and Sessler, 1992). Of note, in children with a body weight of over 30 kg, the central temperature continued to drop even after the vasoconstriction threshold temperature had been reached, whereas children and infants with a body weight below 30 kg were able to maintain or even slightly increase their central temperature. This shows that thermoregulatory defense in infants and younger children is more effective than in older children and adults.

The administration of subanesthetic concentrations of nitrous oxide (10% to 25% in a normoxic mixture) to healthy adult volunteers resulted in a significant but dose-independent reduction of shivering thermogenesis (Cheung and Mekjavic, 1995).

In a concentration of 0.6 (63%) MAC, administration of nitrous oxide resulted in a calculated reduction of the vasoconstriction threshold to 35.7° ± 0.6° C (Goto et al., 1999). Overall, nitrous oxide decreased the thermoregulatory vasoconstriction threshold less than equally potent concentrations of sevoflurane and isoflurane.

In a small study of adults anesthetized with isoflurane, the decrease in the threshold temperature for thermoregulatory vasoconstriction was found to be inversely correlated to the isoflurane concentration, with the threshold temperature decreasing by approximately 3° C per 1% increase in end-tidal isoflurane concentration (Stoen and Sessler, 1990). In a more recent study, the same group found that this dependence on dose was not linear, with isoflurane reducing the threshold temperature disproportionately at higher anesthetic concentrations (Xiong et al., 1996). In adults anesthetized with 0.7% isoflurane, the shivering-temperature threshold decreased, as did the maximum intensity of shivering. The gain of shivering increased significantly and was associated with a pattern of clonic muscular activity that was not a component of regular shivering (Ikeda et al., 1998a).

The thermoregulatory vasoconstriction-threshold temperature in infants and children anesthetized with isoflurane differs only slightly from that in adults (Bissonnette and Sessler, 1990). In pediatric patients anesthetized with 1 MAC halothane in 70% nitrous oxide, this same threshold temperature is higher (35.8° ± 0.5° C) than reported for adults (34.4° C) (Bissonnette and Sessler, 1990; Sessler et al., 1988a). In the adult study, the patients were anesthetized without nitrous oxide and the administered halothane concentration (1.3 MAC) was significantly higher than the one used in the pediatric study (1.0 MAC). In a separate study, a similar thermoregulatory threshold (35.8° ± 0.3° C) was found in pediatric patients who were anesthetized with 1 MAC of halothane in oxygen combined with a caudal epidural block with bupivacaine (Nebbia et al., 1996).

Thermoregulatory inhibition during general anesthesia with equally potent concentrations of halothane is therefore likely to affect adults and children similarly. The high surface area-to-mass ratio in infants, which allows for a rapid loss of heat to the environment, is largely offset by the high intrinsic metabolic rate. Heat loss is further reduced by the well-developed thermoregulatory vasoconstriction mechanism (Bissonnette and Sessler, 1990). Although a trend toward increased threshold temperatures was noted in smaller infants and children anesthetized with similar (age-corrected) concentrations of isoflurane, differences between groups were not statistically significant and spanned only about 0.3° C. This indicates that inhibition of thermoregulatory vasoconstriction is similar in anesthetized infants and children and relatively independent of body weight (Bissonnette and Sessler, 1990). This relatively constant degree of thermoregulatory inhibition in infants and children of different ages is in marked contrast to the age-related changes in the MAC of isoflurane. In infants 1 to 6 months of age, the MAC for isoflurane is approximately 1.5 times higher than the MAC for adults.

With regard to decreasing the threshold temperature for thermoregulatory vasoconstriction, sevoflurane was found to be similar to, although slower than, isoflurane, (Ozaki et al., 1997; Saito, 1997).

Desflurane increases the sweating threshold temperature in a concentration-dependent, linear way. The threshold temperatures for vasoconstriction and shivering at 0.8 MAC are comparable with the other volatile anesthetics, however, at 0 MAC, the drop in vasoconstriction threshold temperature was less pronounced. Thus, for desflurane there may be a nonlinear concentration-response relationship for cold-defense mechanisms (Annadata et al., 1995b). Desflurane also reduces the gain of thermoregulatory vasoconstriction (Kurz et al., 1995).

Enflurane is a peculiar inhalational agent with respect to its thermoregulatory effects. In healthy adult volunteers anesthetized with 1.3% enflurane (equivalent to approximately 0.77 MAC), the threshold temperature for thermoregulatory vasoconstriction was $35.1° \pm 0.6°$ C without any patient stimulation and $35.5° \pm 0.8°$ C during painful electrical stimulation. This result demonstrated a slight, although clinically insignificant, effect of nociception in offsetting the anesthesia-induced thermoregulatory inhibition (Washington et al., 1992). Combination with caudal or lumbar epidural blockade eliminates this effect during abdominal and peripheral surgical procedures. Thermoregulatory studies with enflurane in the pediatric population are hampered by the lack of enflurane MAC studies for this age group. In pediatric patients aged 1 to 12 years, 1.67% enflurane (equal to 1 MAC in adults, which is estimated to be equivalent to 0.75 to 1.0 MAC for the age group studied) combined with caudal bupivacaine caused a profound drop in the threshold temperature for thermoregulatory vasoconstriction (Nebbia et al., 1996). Most patients in this study failed to achieve thermoregulatory vasoconstriction despite reaching a mean core temperature of $33.9° \pm 0.9°$ C. It was therefore concluded that the risk of hypothermia with enflurane is significantly higher when compared with the risk for isoflurane or halothane.

The effects of different inhalational anesthetics on the threshold temperature for thermoregulatory vasoconstriction are summarized in Figure 6-10. In addition, hypothermia can affect the physical characteristics of inhalational anesthet-

ics, as well as the pharmacokinetics and pharmacodynamics of intravenous anesthetic drugs. Hypothermia reduces the MAC of inhalational agents (for isoflurane there is a linear MAC decrease of 5.1% per °C drop in core temperature) and increases their tissue solubility (Vitez et al., 1974; Eger and Johnson, 1987; Antognini, 1993; Antognini et al., 1994; Liu et al., 2001). Thus, for any inspired concentration of an inhalational anesthetic agent in a hypothermic patient, an increased amount of the agent is delivered to the tissues, when in fact the anesthetic requirements are decreased. Hypothermia also affects the pharmacokinetics of barbiturates and narcotics (Kadar et al., 1982; Koren et al., 1987).

Thermoregulation and Intravenous Agents

The effect of opioids on thermoregulation remained unclear until a few years ago. Alfentanil has been shown to significantly reduce the threshold temperature for thermoregulatory vasoconstriction. This reduction appears to be linear and in proportion to the plasma drug concentration (Kurz et al., 1995a). Meperidine and sufentanil linearly reduce the shivering threshold temperature (Alfonsi et al., 1998). Meperidine reduces the threshold temperature for shivering twice as much as it does the temperature for vasoconstriction, a side effect that is clinically used to treat postoperative shivering (Ikeda et al., 1997). Neither meperidine nor alfentanil reduce the gain and the maximum shivering intensity (Ikeda et al., 1998b). Tramadol slightly decreases the threshold temperature for sweating, whereas the threshold temperatures for vasoconstriction and shivering decrease linearly with the tramadol plasma concentration. In adult surgical patients, Mohta et al. (2009) have shown that tramadol is an effective prophylactic drug for reducing the incidence of postanesthetic shivering. Overall, with a doubling only of the interthreshold range, its effects on thermoregulation can be considered mild (De Witte et al., 1998).

A comparison between the temperature effects in children anesthetized with either ketamine or halothane showed that halothane decreases rectal temperature more than ketamine. Regardless of the agent used, children with the highest surface area-to-body weight ratio (i.e., the smallest children) had the greatest decrease in body temperature (Engelman and Lockhart, 1972). Core hypothermia in adults who are induced with ketamine is less pronounced when compared with the effect when they are induced with propofol. This finding was preserved during maintenance of anesthesia with sevoflurane in nitrous oxide/oxygen (Ikeda et al., 2001).

In the case of propofol, a small study of adult volunteers showed a significant and linear decrease in the threshold temperatures for vasoconstriction and shivering, whereas in another study the sweating threshold temperature increased only slightly (Leslie et al., 1994; Matsukawa et al., 1995c). Furthermore, induction of anesthesia with a single bolus dose of propofol (2.5 mg/kg) in adults and maintenance of anesthesia with sevoflurane in 60% nitrous oxide/oxygen resulted in lower core temperatures ($35.5° \pm 0.3°$ C) when compared with patients who only received sevoflurane in nitrous oxide/oxygen for induction and maintenance of anesthesia ($36.2° \pm 0.2°$ C) (Ikeda et al., 1999b). This led to the suggestion that brief propofol-induced vasodilation is sufficient enough to facilitate the core-to-peripheral redistribution of body heat, resulting in nonrecoverable heat loss to the environment.

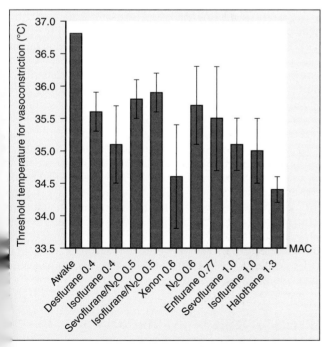

FIGURE 6-10. Threshold temperature (in °C) for thermoregulatory vasoconstriction in adults for different concentrations of inhalational anesthetics either alone or in combination with nitrous oxide. The x-axis denotes the MAC equivalents of the different inhalational anesthetics. *(Data compiled from Sessler and Ponte, 1982; Washington et al., 1992; Annadata et al., 1995; Kurz et al., 1995b; Ozaki et al., 1995; Goto et al., 1999.)*

Midazolam slightly reduces the threshold temperature for sweating, whereas the decrease in the threshold temperature for vasoconstriction is more profound, resulting in a threefold expansion of the interthreshold range, which is comparable with the results found for central neuraxial nerve blockade (Kurz et al., 1995c). These results contrast with the findings for inhalational anesthetics, propofol or opioids, which can expand the interthreshold range by a factor of 10 to 15 (Kurz et al., 1995c).

A bolus dose of clonidine followed by an infusion results in a dose-independent increase in the threshold temperature for sweating, but its gain remains unchanged (Delaunay et al., 1996). The use of clonidine for premedication neither affects redistribution hypothermia nor does it worsen hypothermia during general anesthesia (Bernard et al., 1998).

Dexmedetomidine given to healthy adult volunteers does not affect the threshold temperature for sweating, but reduces the threshold temperatures for vasoconstriction and shivering in a dose-dependent way (Talke et al., 1997). Easley et al. (2007) have reported that dexmedetomidine (0.5 mcg/kg) was effective in the treatment of shivering within 5 minutes.

Atropine blocks sympathetic cholinergic-mediated sweating and increases the threshold temperature for sweating and therefore may lead to hyperthermia (Fraser, 1978).

Thermoregulation and Regional Anesthesia

During regional anesthesia, central thermoregulation remains functional, as does metabolic heat generation, thereby providing some protection against hypothermia (Hynson et al., 1991). Regional anesthesia interferes with regional thermal sensation (afferent and efferent pathways) and inhibition of thermoregulatory vasoconstriction and shivering in the anesthetized area. Increased internal redistribution of body heat followed by increased heat loss to the environment may contribute to intraoperative hypothermia. In many aspects, the factors responsible for intraoperative hypothermia during neuraxial blockade are similar to those for patients under general anesthesia: redistribution of body heat from the core to the peripheral compartment accounts for 89% of the initial drop (i.e., in the first hour) in core temperature. In the following 2 hours, redistribution contributes to 62% of the core temperature decrease (Matsukawa et al., 1995a; 1995b). The extent of this redistribution, and thus the decrease in core temperature, depend on inhibition of peripheral vasoconstriction rather than on centrally mediated effects. Neuraxial anesthesia usually affects a major part of the body mass and the decrease in core temperature can be quite pronounced. However, heat production during regional anesthesia is only minimally decreased (Hynson et al., 1991).

In contrast to patients undergoing general anesthesia, patients under central neuraxial anesthesia may fail to reach a steady state in which heat loss and heat generation are equal, because peripheral vasoconstriction is completely abolished in the area affected by neuraxial blockade. In addition, extensive regional anesthesia may alter or even block the thermal input to the hypothalamus from the anesthetized body part, with the number of dermatomes blocked being directly proportional to the inhibition of central thermoregulation (Ozaki et al., 1994; Leslie and Sessler, 1996; Frank et al., 2000). Heat loss may therefore be an ongoing issue until

sympathetic function and consequently the ability for vasoconstriction have been restored. Under these circumstances, hypothermia during regional anesthesia may become even more profound than during general anesthesia. In an attempt at compensation, peripheral vessels not affected by regional anesthesia are maximally vasoconstricted, although this is often not sufficient to prevent a further drop in core temperature, particularly when the body mass affected by regional anesthesia is approximately the same or even larger than the unblocked mass.

Shivering is initiated once the patient's core temperature reaches the shivering threshold; however, neuraxial blockade reduces the gain of shivering by more than 60%, mainly because the upper body muscles fail to compensate for lower body paralysis (Kim et al., 1998). It seems unlikely that systemic absorption of local anesthetics contributes to the thermoregulatory changes seen under regional anesthesia, because a study generating equal plasma drug concentrations without regional anesthesia failed to reproduce these thermoregulatory disturbances (Glosten et al., 1991).

Compared with general anesthesia, the use of regional anesthesia reduces the risk of hypothermia, especially during surgery with small incisions where the patient can be kept well insulated. In contrast, regional anesthesia for large surgical incisions predisposes a patient to more profound hypothermia than with general anesthesia, and recovery to normal body temperature may be prolonged (Cattaneo et al., 2000).

In adults, the changes in threshold temperatures for sweating, vasoconstriction, and shivering during spinal anesthesia and epidural anesthesia seem to be comparable and result in a twofold expansion of the interthreshold range (Ozaki et al., 1994). In adults, the combination of general anesthesia with thoracic epidural anesthesia further reduced the threshold temperature for thermoregulatory vasoconstriction and thus significantly aggravated hypothermia compared with general anesthesia alone (Joris et al., 1994). Interestingly enough, diabetic patients with autonomic neuropathy showed lower core temperatures and delayed thermoregulatory vasoconstriction during general anesthesia than diabetic patients without autonomic dysfunction (Kitamura et al., 2000).

Unlike the thermoregulatory effects of regional anesthesia in adults, the institution of a caudal block in children anesthetized with halothane does not significantly alter the threshold temperature for thermoregulatory vasoconstriction in children (35.7° C without versus 35.9° C with caudal block) (Bissonnette and Sessler, 1992). Nevertheless, temperatures during regional anesthesia should be monitored in adult and pediatric patients, because significant hypothermia is common and remains otherwise undetected and therefore also untreated. However, a survey revealed that only a third of clinicians monitors body temperature during regional anesthesia in adults (Frank et al., 1999).

ADVERSE EFFECTS OF HYPOTHERMIA

Heat loss in children undergoing surgery can occur for a variety of reasons. Exposure of body cavities to low environment temperatures and humidity, infusion of cold fluids, and ventilation with cold and dry gases, in combination with the infant physical characteristics of the large body surface area-to-mass ratio and the minimal insulating tissue layer, the potential f an infant or a child to become hypothermic during anesthesia is significantly increased. Nevertheless, hypothermia must not be viewed as an inevitable consequence of surgery. Although hypothermia may be protective for a small subgroup of patients with certain ischemic conditions, in the majority of patients the adverse effects outweigh the benefits, and inadvertent core hypothermia must be avoided (Illievich et al., 1994). In a review of temperature monitoring and perioperative thermoregulation, Sessler (2008) noted that hypothermia-related complications include increased morbidity, surgical wound infections, coagulopathies, increased allogenic transfusions, negative nitrogen balance, delayed wound healing, delayed postoperative anesthetic recovery, prolonged hospitalization, shivering, and patient discomfort.

A study of 200 adult patients scheduled for colorectal surgery showed that patients who were allowed to become hypothermic (core temperature 34.7° ± 0.6° C) during the procedure suffered from a more than threefold higher rate of surgical wound infections than the group who was actively warmed and kept normothermic (36.6° ± 0.5° C) (Kurz et al., 1996). Furthermore, the times until suture removal and discharge from hospital in the hypothermia group were prolonged by 1 and 2.6 days, respectively. It has been suggested by these and other researchers that the vasoconstriction triggered by hypothermia may result in a decreased tissue partial pressure of oxygen, which leads to increased wound infection and finally delayed wound healing, even in the absence of an infection (Fig. 6-11) (Jonsson et al., 1991). A shorter

hospital stay (2.7 fewer days) for normothermic versus hypothermic patients has also been reported by others (Sellden and Lindahl, 1999). In addition, hypothermia itself has been shown to reduce chemotaxis and phagocytosis of granulocytes, natural killer cell cytotoxicity, migration of macrophages, and synthesis of immunoglobulins, thereby directly affecting the immune response (Leijh et al., 1979; van Oss et al., 1980; Wenisch et al., 1996; Beilin et al., 1998).

Hypothermia significantly delays the reactions in the coagulation cascade (most likely because of a direct effect on the activity of the coagulation factors) with prolongation of prothrombin time and partial thromboplastin time (Rohrer and Natale, 1992). Inhibition of platelet function with prolonged bleeding time was found during hypothermia, secondary to inhibited up-regulation of platelet surface protein GMP-140 and down-regulation of the glycoprotein GP Ib-IX complex, reduced platelet aggregation, and thromboxane B_2 generation (the stable metabolite of thromboxane A_2) (Michelson et al., 1994). This platelet dysfunction is fully reversible with rewarming. Thromboelastography confirms these findings with a prolongation of the reaction and coagulation times, as well as a reduction in the clot formation rate (Douning et al., 1995). It is therefore not surprising that blood loss in patients undergoing hip arthroplasty was found to be significantly higher in the hypothermia group (core temperature, 35° ± 0.5° C) than in the normothermia group (core temperature, 36.6° ± 0.4° C) (Schmied et al., 1996). Similar results have been confirmed by other researchers (Bock et al., 1998; Rajagopalan et al., 2008).

Notably greater incidences of myocardial ischemia and PaO_2 values below 80 mm Hg have been reported in hypothermic patients (defined by sublingual temperature measured on arrival to the recovery room) when compared with normothermic patients in the first 24 hours after lower extremity vascular surgery with either epidural or general anesthesia (Frank et al., 1993). Although these findings are most likely not relevant to most pediatric patients because of the lack of coronary heart disease, they nevertheless demonstrate the widespread and potential impact of hypothermia on the body in surgical patients.

Hypothermia results in diminished metabolism of drugs and prolongs their action. Although intraoperative hypothermia in adults resulted in delayed recovery from anesthesia when compared with normothermic patients, no such differences could be demonstrated in children (Bissonnette and Sessler, 1993; Lenhardt et al., 1997).

Studies on the effects of hypothermia and muscle relaxants have demonstrated that hypothermia decreases the requirements for nondepolarizing muscle relaxants because there is an increased sensitivity of the neuromuscular junction, as well as diminished biliary (indicating a reduced affinity for the drug substrate to microsomal enzymes) and renal elimination of the drug (Ham et al., 1978; Miller et al., 1978). Similar findings have been confirmed for other medications (McAllister and Tan, 1980).

Although similar studies are lacking for the pediatric population, there are no reasons to believe that the results would be significantly different from those in adults. Avoiding hypothermia in the infant and child is therefore as crucial as in adults and requires not only an understanding of thermal physiology, but also meticulous attention to detail in anesthetic care.

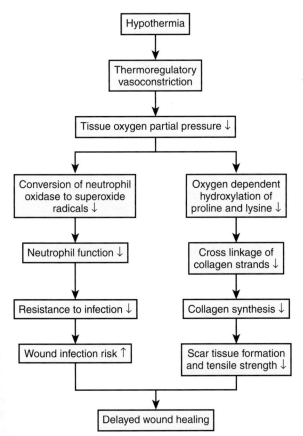

FIGURE 6-11. Hypothermia and its adverse effects on immune function and wound healing (↓ represents a decrease; ↑ indicates an increase in the corresponding response).

PREVENTION OF HYPOTHERMIA

Operating Room Temperature

Keeping the operating room temperature at an optimal level is crucial in the prevention of hypothermia. The major source of heat loss in the anesthetized patient is caused by radiation. As mentioned previously, radiant heat loss is a function of the temperature difference between the patient and the environment. The effectiveness of controlling ambient operating room temperature in controlling the temperature of newborns during surgery has been confirmed (Bennett et al., 1977). In adults, 21° C is reported as the critical ambient temperature for maintaining normal nasopharyngeal or esophageal temperatures (36° to 37.5° C) (Morris and Wilkey, 1970; Morris, 1971a, 1971b). Operating room temperatures of 27° and 29° C are recommended for full-term and premature newborns, respectively. It is essential that every operating room be equipped with an individual thermistor control unit so that the temperature in each operating room can be controlled independently to meet the needs of each patient.

Convective heat loss in the operating room is due to the constant air draft caused by the air conditioning system. Keeping the patient covered provides the best protection against this form of heat loss.

Evaporative heat loss from the respiratory tract accounts for only 5% to 10% of total heat loss during anesthesia. However, more important are the evaporative heat losses from open body cavities during surgery. In order to reduce this form of heat loss, the relative humidity of the operating room should be kept in the range of 40% to 60%.

Radiant Heaters

Radiant heaters are mainly used during induction of anesthesia and insertion of catheters, until the patient is prepared and draped. Prolonged use of radiant heaters may result in increased insensible water losses. The minimal manufacturer-recommended distance of the radiant heater from the skin must be respected at all times in order to avoid skin burns.

Reflecting Blankets

The use of reflective blankets in adults has produced conflicting results, and data on their use in infants and children are sparse. In adults, it has been reported that intraoperative normothermia can be maintained when the reflective blanket covers 60% or more of the patient's body surface area (Bourke et al., 1984). One drawback of reflective blankets is the potential build-up of condensation on the inner side, which can result in wet clothes or skin, putting the patient at high risk for evaporative heat loss. With regard to heat conservation, it seems not that important what material the cover is made of; instead, it is important to cover as much of the body surface as possible (Sessler et al., 1991). The practice of covering the head with a plastic bag provides an easy, inexpensive way to significantly reduce radiant, convective, and evaporative heat losses (Fig. 6-12).

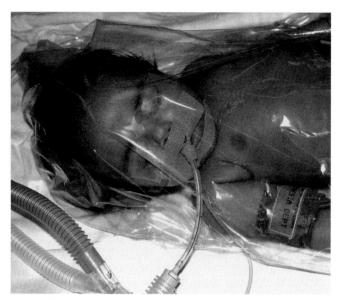

■ **FIGURE 6-12.** The head of an infant constitutes a large fraction of its body size; therefore, covering the infant's head and as much as possible of the remaining body surface with plastic wrap can significantly reduce evaporative and convective heat loss.

Skin-Surface–Warming Devices

The use of skin-surface–warming devices in adults before the induction of anesthesia reduces the magnitude of hypothermia that results from internal redistribution of heat (Glosten et al., 1993). Aggressive skin-surface warming induces peripheral vasodilation and favorably increases the temperature of the peripheral compartment to values approaching those of the central compartment. The net result is an increased mean body temperature, and the skin-surface warming reduces the amount of energy transferred from the central to the peripheral compartment after induction of anesthesia. A variety of passive and active skin-surface warmers are available, including circulating hot-water blankets, infrared radiant heaters, and convective forced-air heaters, which blow warm air through a disposable blanket to raise the effective ambient temperature immediately surrounding the patient (Stephen et al., 1960; Vale and Lunn, 1969; Morris, 1971b; Goldblat and Miller, 1972; Sessler and Moayeri, 1990; Steele et al., 1996). A newer system that simulates water immersion using a special garment and feedback algorithms analyzed by computer to achieve a preset body temperature is available, seems to perform well, and is also safe in children (Nesher et al., 2001a, 2001b; Nesher et al., 2002). Of all these devices, convective forced-air warmers are by far the most effective, not only from a thermoregulatory perspective, but also from a cost and convenience point of view. Not only can they maintain normal body temperature, but they can also rewarm a hypothermic patient (Sessler and Moayeri, 1990; Kurz et al., 1993; Ciufo et al., 1995; Karayan et al., 1996). In patients with decreased peripheral perfusion (e.g., because of high doses of vasoconstrictors, aortic cross clamping for coarctation or abdominal aortic aneurysm repair, or severe peripheral arterial occlusive disease) the device should be used with great caution only and not for extended lengths of time to avoid skin burns, particularly in infants and neonates (Azzam and Krock, 1995; True et al., 2000; Siddik-Sayyid et al., 2008).

Warming Mattresses

The use of warming mattresses reduces conductive heat loss. Warming mattresses set at 40° C and covered with two layers of cotton blankets have been demonstrated to effectively conserve heat (Goudsouzian et al., 1973). This measure is mainly efficient for infants with a body surface area of less than 0.5 m². In older children and adults, only a small proportion of the skin's surface area is in direct contact with the heating mattress, which makes these devices generally less effective to maintain normothermia.

Warming of Intravenous Fluids

Rapid infusion of chilled intravenous fluids (1° to 6° C) can be used effectively to induce hypothermia. The administration of 1 L of an ice-cold infusion in an adult is expected to decrease the core temperature by approximately 1.7° C, but values of up to 3° C are possible (Baumgardner et al., 1999; Rajek et al., 2000). Thus, intravenous fluids and blood products should be warmed before administration. It is particularly important to warm fluids in instances of rapid or massive fluid administration. In addition, attention should be paid to the length and the type of the infusion tubing, because significant heat loss of the infusion during transit from the warming device to the intravenous cannula may occur (Faries et al., 1991; Bissonnette and Paut, 2002). Even when warming the infusion to 37° C, a flow rate of more than 750 mL/hr is required to keep its temperature above 32° C at a distance of 25 cm away from the warmer when the infusion tubing is exposed to ambient air (20° C) (Faries et al., 1991). Because this flow rate is usually beyond the needs of regular pediatric cases, the length of the infusion tubing distal to the warmer should be kept as short as possible. Although a study demonstrated that conservative fluid management (1 mL/kg per hour of crystalloids warmed to 37° C) in patients aged 1 to 3 years resulted in less core hypothermia when compared with the control group who received a more aggressive fluid replacement (10 mL/kg per hour) (Ezri et al., 2003), this should not preclude pediatric patients from receiving appropriate intraoperative fluid resuscitation.

Because both the peritoneal and thoracic cavities are large heat-exchanging areas, solutions for intraoperative irrigation should always be warmed to body temperature. Although desirable from a thermoregulatory point of view, antimicrobial solutions for surgical skin preparation should not be warmed, because heat can cause chemical breakdown of the iodine solution and thereby inactivate its antimicrobial properties.

Humidified and Heated Gases

When breathing spontaneously (without an endotracheal tube or laryngeal mask airway in place), the tracheobronchial epithelium heats and moistens the inspired air, an energy-dependent process (evaporation and convection). Intubation significantly reduces the epithelial surface area that is available for warming and humidification of inspired gases. In order to minimize convective and evaporative heat losses from the respiratory tract and to minimize adverse effects on the tracheobronchial epithelium, inspiratory gases should be heated and humidified. Airway humidification in intubated patients prevents tracheal damage caused by dry inspired gases, increases tracheal mucus flow, and minimizes respiratory heat losses (Berry et al., 1973; Forbes 1974; Mercke 1975; Chalon et al., 1979b; Tollofsrud et al., 1984). Heat and humidity can be added to inspired gases either actively by evaporative or ultrasonic heated humidifiers or passively by heat and moisture exchanging filters ("artificial noses") (Newton, 1975; Chalon et al., 1979a, 1984; Bissonnette et al., 1989a). Furthermore, there is considerable evidence that a relative humidity level of at least 50% is required to maintain normal ciliary function in the respiratory tract and to help prevent bronchospasm (Forbes, 1974; Mercke, 1975; Chalon et al., 1979a; Chan et al., 1980). More recent research, however, suggests an even higher humidity level of 75% to 100% to effectively maintain mucociliary function (Kilgour et al., 2004). Humidification to 50% (but not to 75% to 100%) is easily obtained with heat and moisture exchanging filters and should be standard for long procedures (Forbes, 1974; Mercke, 1975; Chalon et al., 1979a). In adults, heating and humidification of gases to 37° C and 100% relative humidity not only effectively helps maintain normothermia, but it also helps reverse hypothermia during general surgery (Pflug et al., 1978; Stone et al., 1981).

Because of the higher minute ventilation per kilogram of body weight in pediatric patients, airway humidification for infants is even more important and effective in helping to maintain normothermia than it is for adults (Bissonnette and Sessler, 1989a; Bissonnette et al., 1989). In newborns, heat loss during general anesthesia is significantly reduced when gases are heated and when humidified gases are used instead of dry anesthetic gases (Fonkalsrud et al., 1980). Although high-temperature humidification devices can decrease intraoperative evaporative heat loss, they may cause tracheal burns. Because there may be a large temperature gradient between the humidifier and the endotracheal tube, it is important to measure airway temperature as close to the patient as possible. This has the advantage of preventing heated gases from accidentally burning the trachea while providing the warmest possible inspiratory gas. In addition, intraoperative heat loss can be minimized. If these devices are used, it is recommended to heat inspiratory gases to normal body temperature only. Although heat and moisture exchanging filters are less effective than active humidifiers (especially in the first hour after induction of anesthesia), they seem to provide a reasonable, convenient, and cost-effective alternative (Bissonnette et al., 1989a).

Additional advantages of heat and moisture exchangers in small infants include the lack of risk for airway burns and over-humidification with the consequences of overhydration, and the reduced risk for breathing-circuit disconnection (Smith and Allen, 1986; Shroff and Skerman, 1988). Heat and moisture may falsely increase the esophageal temperature by about 0.35° C when compared with tympanic or mean body temperature (Bissonnette et al., 1989b).

All heat and moisture exchangers increase the dead space of the anesthesia tubing; however, the smallest ones have a dead space of less than 2 mL. At a fresh gas flow of 30 to 60 L/min, the increase in airway resistance is minimal, typically creating a pressure gradient of less than 2 cm H_2O. Most heat and moisture exchangers now commonly have an in-built filter for bacteria, viruses, and latex particles (Barbara et al., 2001). Copious secretions from the tracheobronchial tree may result in partial or complete obstruction of the filter and thereby severely affect ventilation (Prasad and

Chen, 1990; Barnes and Normoyle, 1996; Stacey et al., 1996). The in vitro specifications of the heat and moisture exchangers given by the manufacturers do not always match the actual in vivo performance (Lemmens and Brock-Utne, 2004).

Transportation

Care in the transportation of an infant with regard to temperature management cannot be overemphasized. One short transport (e.g., to the critical care unit) can be enough to render all successful intraoperative efforts to maintain normothermia ineffective. It is therefore essential that the incubator (if available) be fully warmed before transport both to and from the operating room. Older infants and children should at least be covered with a warmed blanket for transport, and if the patient is hypothermic despite all the measures taken in the operating room, it is helpful to bring the forced-air warming blanket with the patient to the critical-care or the post-anesthesia care unit, so that the rewarming process can be continued there.

SUMMARY

Because of the small size with increased body surface area-to-body weight ratio and increased thermal conductance, infants and young children are at significant risk for thermal instability. This risk is even higher for premature infants and infants who are small for gestational age. Although awake infants are able to maintain normothermia, they can do so only within a narrow range of ambient temperatures and only for a limited amount of time. The exposure to the operating room with its normally low ambient temperature combined with the high airflow from the air-conditioning system during anesthesia and surgery, and the use of cold infusions and dry anesthetic gases can easily overwhelm the thermal homeostatic mechanisms and, in certain instances, result in potentially serious complications. A sound understanding of the physiology and the limitations of the thermoregulatory system during anesthesia has improved the recognition, prevention, and management of these perioperative disturbances. The knowledge of the different effects of each anesthetic agent on the thermoregulatory mechanism undoubtedly proves useful in providing safe anesthesia.

For questions and answers on topics in this chapter, go to "Chapter Questions" at www.expertconsult.com.

REFERENCES

Complete references used in this text can be found online at www.expertconsult.com.

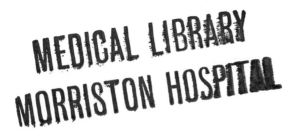

Pharmacology of Pediatric Anesthesia

Peter J. Davis, Adrian Bosenberg, Andrew Davidson, Nathalia Jimenez, Evan Kharasch, Anne M. Lynn, Stevan P. Tofovic, and Susan Woelfel

CONTENTS

DEVELOPMENTAL PHARMACOLOGY

Developmental changes profoundly affect the clinical response to medicines. Dr. Abraham Jacobi, a founder of American pediatrics, recognized more than a century ago that children are not "miniature men and women, with reduced doses and the same class of disease in smaller bodies," that pediatrics "has its own independent range and horizon," and that age-appropriate pharmacotherapy was important (Kearns et al., 2003). More recently, as the immaturity of renal and metabolic systems has been recognized, the pharmacologic uniqueness of babies and infants has been specifically recognized (Anderson and Holford, 2008). Physical growth, development, organ maturation, physiologic changes, and coexisting disease that occur throughout the spectrum of development—from preterm newborn to adolescence and adulthood—profoundly influence drug pharmacokinetics and pharmacodynamics, and ultimately the panoply of both desirable and undesirable clinical responses. This chapter presents the basic pharmacologic principles relevant to understanding basic pediatric pharmacology in general, and that of pediatric anesthetic pharmacology in particular.

Medications that are commonly used in children are not regularly tested in children, and drug labeling often consists exclusively of adult data. Of the 140 new molecular entities of potential use in pediatrics, only 38% were labeled for use in children when they were initially approved (Tod et al., 2008). Much use of drugs in pediatrics, particularly in newborns and infants, is off-label use. About one third of drugs prescribed in office-based pediatric practice, two thirds of those prescribed in hospitals, and 90% of drugs used in pediatric intensive care units are used for indications other than those for which they have been approved (Tod et al., 2008). When data were submitted to the

U.S. Food and Drug Administration (FDA) to support labeling changes intended to guide pediatric drug use, on average, only 2.2 pediatric studies were represented (Abdel-Rahman et al., 2007). A considerable amount of pediatric drug use is based on "extrapolation" (or worse) from adult dosing and use guidelines. A major address of pediatric pharmacology research in the past decade has focused on the challenge of characterizing developmental changes in pharmacokinetics and pharmacodynamics, as well as determining proper pediatric dosing guidelines, particularly the downward scaling of adult doses to children.

Physiology and Development

Growth and maturation are seminal features of pediatric development, and it is important to understand that they vary independently (Anderson and Holford, 2008; Rhodin et al., 2009; Sumpter and Anderson, 2009). Growth is an increase in size, often characterized by changes in weight. Maturation is a time-dependent phenomenon, often characterized by age. Traditionally, the common metric of maturation was postnatal age (PNA), the time since birth. With the superiority of neonatal intensive care and the survival of neonates as small as 500 g and 24 weeks' gestation, who have clearly immature and widely variant degrees of development at birth, it is now well established that PNA is an inadequate metric of organ maturation, which actually begins before birth. Postconceptual age (PCA), the sum of gestational age (the period between conception and birth) and PNA, is a superior metric. Because of the inexactitude in determining the date of conception, the alternate metric of postmenstrual age (PMA) is often used instead. Particularly for infants and very small children, use of PCA or PMA rather than PNA is important in pediatric pharmacology and therapeutics.

Body composition changes dramatically during growth and development (Anderson and Holford, 2008). Simply stated, compared with adults, infants have big heads, large torsos, and short, stumpy legs. Figure 7-1 depicts developmental changes in pediatric physiology that can affect drug disposition. Table 7-1 describes the changes in organ weight that occur during growth. The most significant changes with age are in total body water, the intracellular vs. extracellular distribution of body water, and muscle and fat mass (Tables 7-2 and 7-3). Total body water content constitutes 75% of body weight in the full-term newborn and 80% to 85% of body weight in the preterm neonate. This decreases to about 60% at 5 months and remains relatively constant until puberty. Extracellular water redistributes intracellularly during the first year of life. Extracellular fluid is 45% to 50% of body weight in premature and newborn infants, decreasing to 26% at 1 year and 18% in adults. In contrast, body fat increases with age, from 3% in premature neonates and 12% in full-term newborns, to 30% at 1 year of age. "Baby fat" is shed when toddlers start walking and drops to adult levels of about 18%, concomitant with an increase in muscle mass. A major consequence of body-composition changes may be differences in drug volume of distribution, with neonates and infants having larger volumes of water-soluble drugs, as described below.

The relative lack of dosing data for many drugs used in pediatrics has necessitated the use of extrapolations from adult dosing. Considerable effort has been expended to provide a scientific basis for such extrapolations, such as of volumes of distribution, clearance, renal function, and dose. Basic models for predicting physiologic function and drug dose based on size include the linear per-kilogram model, the surface-area model, and the allometric model. It is now increasingly evident and accepted that allometric scaling provides the most accurate information. Throughout nature, many body-size relationships are of the form:

$$Y = a \bullet W^b$$

where Y is the biological characteristic, W is the body mass, and a and b are empirically derived constants. For physiologic functions such as cardiac output, metabolic rate, oxygen consumption, glomerular filtration rate (GFR), and pharmacologic functions such as drug clearance, the power exponent b is 0.75. For physiologic volumes such as blood volume, lung volume, tidal volume, and stroke volume, and pharmacologic volumes such as the volume of distribution, the power exponent is 1. For time-based physiologic functions such as circulation time, heart rate, and respiratory rate, and pharmacologic functions such as drug elimination half-life, the exponent is 0.25 (Johnson and Thomson, 2008). This allometric model may then be used to scale metabolic processes across size:

$$Y_i = Y_{std} \bullet \left(\frac{W_i}{W_{std}} \right)^{power}$$

where W_i is the weight of any individual and W_{std} is the weight of a standardized individual (such as a mythical 70-kg adult). The applicability of scaling will subsequently become apparent.

Pharmacokinetic Parameters

Pharmacokinetics refers to the time course of drug disposition in the body and the processes that affect it. These processes include absorption, distribution, metabolism and transport, and excretion. Conceptually, pharmacokinetics is characterized by the fundamental primary parameters of volume of distribution and clearance and by the secondary parameter of half-life (which is proportional to volume of distribution and inversely proportional to clearance).

Volume of Distribution

Volume of distribution (V_d) is a theoretic concept that relates the amount of drug in the body (dose) to the concentration (C) of drug that is measured (in blood, plasma, and unbound in tissue water). Volume of distribution is the volume of fluid "apparently" required to contain the total-body amount of drug homogeneously at a concentration equal to that in plasma (or blood) (Fig. 7-2):

$$C_0 = \frac{dose(X)}{V_d} \text{ or } V_d = \frac{dose(X)}{C_0}$$

The volume of distribution does not necessarily correspond to any specific physiologic volume or space. Drugs such as highly water-soluble compounds, which are confined intravascularly, have a small volume of distribution (approximately equal to intravascular volume), whereas lipophilic drugs that distribute to tissues have a large volume of distribution (that may be so large as to exceed total body water). For example, in adults the volume of distribution of gentamicin is 0.2 to 0.3 L/kg, whereas that of digoxin is 8 to 10 L/kg. Plasma protein binding of drugs decreases the apparent volume of distribution

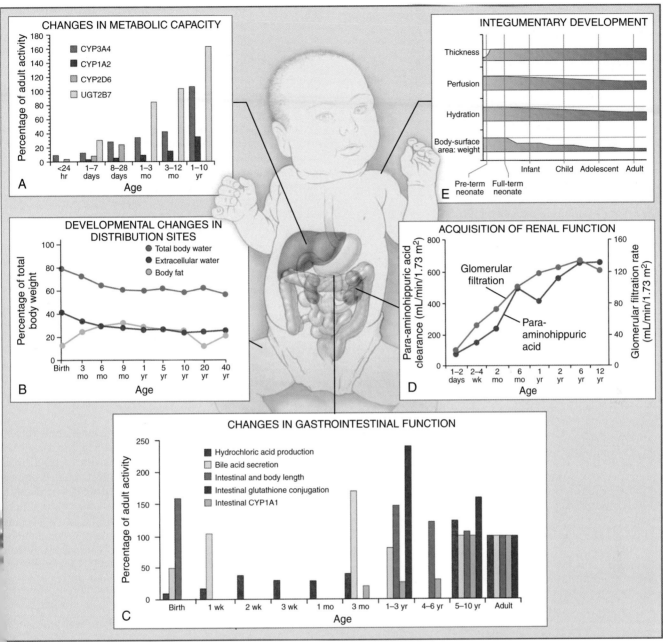

FIGURE 7-1. Developmental changes in physiologic factors that influence drug disposition in infants, children, and adolescents. **A,** Activity of many cytochrome P450 (CYP) isoforms and a specific UGT isoform is markedly diminished during the first two months of life. Increases to adult activity over time are enzyme- and isoform-specific. **B,** Age-dependent changes in body composition, which influence the apparent volume of distribution for drugs. Infants in the first 6 months of life have markedly expanded total body water and extracellular water as compared with older infants and adults. This is expressed as a percentage of total body weight. **C,** Age-dependent changes in both the structure and function of the gastrointestinal tract. As with hepatic drug-metabolizing enzymes **(A),** the activity of cytochrome CYP1A1 in the intestine is low during early life. **D,** Effect of postnatal development on the processes of active tubular secretion—represented by the clearance of para-aminohippuric acid and the GFR, both of which approximate adult activity by 6 to 12 months of age. **E,** Age dependence in the thickness, extent of perfusion, and extent of hydration of the skin and the relative size of the skin surface area (reflected by the ratio of body surface area to body weight). Although skin thickness is similar in infants and adults, the extent of perfusion and hydration diminishes from infancy to adulthood. *(From Kearns GL et al: Developmental pharmacology: drug disposition, action, and therapy in infants and children,* N Engl J Med *349:1157, 2003.)*

and tissue binding increases the apparent volume of distribution. The major practical value of volume of distribution lies in the calculation of initial drug dosing (loading):

$$dose(X) = C_0 \bullet V_d$$

A major consequence of growth and maturational changes in body composition may be differences in volume of distribution. In general, neonates and infants have larger distribution volumes for water-soluble drugs and smaller volumes for lipophilic drugs. For example, the volume of distribution of gentamicin is

TABLE 7-1. Changes in Organ Weights with Age (Percentage of Body Weight)

Organ System	Fetus	Full-Term Newborn	Adult
Skeletal muscle	25.0	25.0	40.0
Skin	13.0	4.0	6.0
Skeleton	22.0	18.0	14.0
Heart	0.6	0.5	0.4
Liver	4.0	5.0	2.0
Kidneys	0.7	1.0	0.5
Brain	13.0	12.0	2.0

From Widdowson EM: *Scientific foundations of pediatrics*, ed 2, Baltimore, 1982, University Park Press.

TABLE 7-2. Body Composition during Growth

Body Compartment	Premature Infant (1.5 kg)	Full-Term Infant (3.5 kg)	Adult (70 kg)
Total body water (% body weight)	83	73	60
Extracellular fluid (% body weight)	62	44	20
Blood volume (mL/kg)	60	85-105	70
Intracellular water (% body weight)	25	33	40
Muscle mass (% body weight)	15	20	50
Fat (% body weight)	3	12	18

From Cook DR, Marcy JH: *Neonatal anesthesia*, Pasadena, Calif, 1988, Appleton Davies.

TABLE 7-3. Age-Related Estimates of Gas and Tissue Volumes and Blood Flow

Tissue Volume	Gas and Tissue Volume (mL/kg) Adult	Gas and Tissue Volume (mL/kg) Infant	Tissue Blood Flow (% CO) Adult	Tissue Blood Flow (% CO) Infant
Tidal volume (V_T)	7	7	—	—
Functional residual capacity (FRC)	40	25	—	—
Blood volume	70	90	—	—
Brain	21	90	14.3	34
Heart	4	4.5	4.3	3
Abdominal viscera	57	70	28.6	25
Kidneys	6	10	25.7	18
Muscle	425	180	11.4	10
Fat	150	100	5.7	5
Poorly perfused tissue	270	270	10.0	5

From Cook DR, Marcy JH: *Neonatal anesthesia*, Pasadena, Calif, 1988, Appleton Davies.

0.5 to 1.2 L/kg in neonates and infants compared with 0.2 to 0.3 L/kg in adults (Echeverrisa).

Clearance

Clearance is the fundamental parameter describing the ability to eliminate a drug. Clearance may refer to elimination from the body (systemic or total clearance) or by a specific organ (renal or hepatic clearance). Clearance is not the amount of drug actually eliminated, but rather represents the theoretic amount of biologic fluid (blood or plasma) from which the drug is completely removed per unit time (mL/min, L/hr). Systemic clearance represents the sum of hepatic clearance; renal clearance; and for some drugs, other routes of clearance (e.g., pulmonary elimination of volatile anesthetics, hydrolysis in blood, or dialysis).

$$CL_{total} = CL_{renal} + CL_{hepatic} + CL_{other}$$

where *CL* indicates clearance. Clearance is achieved through the processes of metabolism and excretion. A major practical value of understanding clearance is that at steady-state, total clearance is a primary determinant of dose and dosing interval (dose rate) when the desired steady-state plasma concentration (C_{ss}) is known:

$$Dose\ rate = C_{ss} \bullet CL_{total}$$

Renal Clearance

The kidney is the most important organ for elimination of water-soluble drugs and metabolites. This is particularly true for infants and small children, in whom hepatic metabolism is underdeveloped, and in whom age-dependent renal clearance is a major determinant of age-appropriate drug dosing (Kearns et al., 2003). Maturation of renal function, which occurs independently of PNA, is a dynamic process. Nephrogenesis begins between about weeks 5 and 9 of gestation and is complete by week 36, after which there are changes in renal blood flow (Kearns et al., 2003; Rhodin et al., 2009). GFR is approximately 5 mL/min in full-term neonates, but about one fifth that in preterm neonates. GFR increases with PMA, at a rate described as a maturation function (MF), based on the sigmoidal hyperbolic Hill equation, where $PMA_{50}{}^{\gamma}$ is the maturation half-time, and γ is the Hill coefficient:

$$MF = \frac{PMA^{\gamma}}{PMA_{50}{}^{\gamma} + PMA^{\gamma}}$$

The rate of GFR maturation is nonlinear and maximum at about 48 weeks' PMA. It varies with prematurity, with preterm neonates (33 to 34 weeks' PMA) having a slower increase (14 mL/min per 1.73 m² per week PMA) in the first few weeks of life than full-term neonates (39 to 41 weeks' PMA; 94 mL/min per 1.73 m² per week PMA). In general, healthy newborns' GFR is about 30% of adult GFR and reaches adult values at about 8 to 12 months of age. Renal tubular function matures more slowly, reaching adult levels at about 12 to 18 months of age. For example, the dosing interval for tobramycin, which is eliminated renally, is 24 hours in full-term newborns but 36 to 48 hours in preterm newborns (Kearns et al., 2003).

Renal drug clearance depends on glomerular filtration, active tubular secretion, and active and passive tubular reabsorption. In addition to both the growth and the maturation

Dose 50 mg

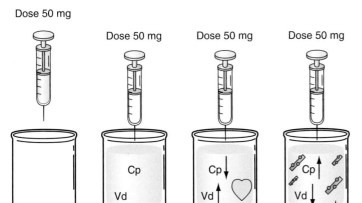

FIGURE 7-2. Apparent volume of distribution. The real volume of the beaker is 5 L (V_d = 50 mg/10 mcg/mL = 5 L). However, based on measured concentrations in fluid and calculated according to the equation for V_d on p. 180, the volume of distribution may vary (thus *apparent volume*). It depends on significant tissue or plasma protein binding. Significant tissue binding (i.e., significant digoxin binding to myocardial Na^+, K^+-ATPase) increases volume of distribution (V_d = 10 L; see the text for explanation). Because routinely measured fluid concentration includes both free unbound and plasma protein bound drug, the increased protein binding reduces volume of distribution (V_d = 2.5 L).

aspects of renal function, disease and concomitant drug administration (either directly or by altering rates of renal maturation) can also affect renal function.

Hepatic Clearance

For many drugs, including several used in anesthesia (e.g., sedative hypnotics, benzodiazepines, opioids, and neuromuscular blockers), hepatic clearance (CL_H in the following formulas) is a major route of elimination (Wilkinson, 1987). Hepatic clearance is the product of liver blood flow (Q_H) and the hepatic extraction ratio (E_H) of a drug.

$$CL_H = Q_H \cdot E_H$$

E_H is defined as the fraction of drug entering the liver that is eliminated in one pass through the liver.

$$E_H = \frac{C_{in} - C_{out}}{C_{in}}$$

E_H depends on liver blood flow and the intrinsic clearance of the drug (CL_{int}), defined as the total capacity of the liver to eliminate drug in the absence of limitations from blood flow.

$$E_H = \left(\frac{CL_{int}}{Q_H + CL_{int}} \right)$$

CL_{int} functionally represents drug biotransformation (the total activity of enzymes and transporters involved in metabolism and biliary secretion). Thus, combining the previous equation with the equation for hepatic clearance:

$$CL_H = Q_H \cdot \left(\frac{CL_{int}}{Q_H + CL_{int}} \right)$$

Since only an unbound drug is considered diffusible into liver cells (although in reality a simplification), E_H also depends on the fraction of unbound drug in the blood (f_u) (Baker and Barton, 2007). Therefore the three theoretic primary determinants of hepatic drug clearance are liver blood flow, intrinsic clearance (biotransformation), and plasma protein binding.

$$CL_H = Q_H \cdot E_H = Q_H \cdot \left(\frac{CL_{int} \cdot f_u}{Q_H + CL_{int} \cdot f_u} \right)$$

In reality, the important determinants of hepatic clearance are liver blood flow and the extraction ratio (Fig. 7-3). For drugs with a high extraction ratio (e.g., lidocaine, fentanyl, sufentanil, and propofol), hepatic clearance depends primarily on hepatic blood flow (because intrinsic clearance is so efficient, drug delivery to the liver becomes rate limiting). For low-extraction drugs (e.g., methadone, diazepam, and alfentanil), hepatic clearance is independent of hepatic blood flow and depends primarily on intrinsic clearance (metabolism).

Absorption

Although the predominant route of drug administration in pediatric anesthesiology is intravenous, the oral route is the

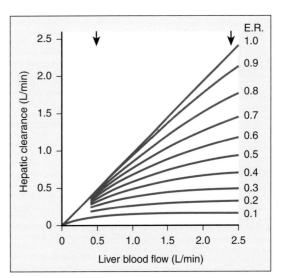

FIGURE 7-3. Effect of increasing liver blood flow on the hepatic clearance of drugs with varying extraction ratios. Each curve represents a drug whose extraction ratio at 1.5 L/min is shown above that flow. For drugs with a low extraction ratio, an increase in liver blood flow within the physiologic range *(arrow)* produces very little change in hepatic clearance. For a drug with a high extraction ratio, however, increases in liver blood flow produce an almost proportional increase in hepatic clearance. *(From Wilkinson GR, Shank DG: Commentary: a physiological approach to hepatic drug clearance,* Clin Pharmacol Ther *18:377, 1975.)*

most commonly used in children. Changes in physiologic processes that accompany normal growth and development can affect drug absorption (Kearns et al., 2003; Abdel-Rahman et al., 2007). In general, neonates and small children absorb drugs more slowly than older children and adults, resulting in delayed and lower peak drug concentrations. Neonatal gastric pH is relatively high (greater than 4) compared with older children and adults, thus acid-labile drugs (such as penicillin G) are more efficiently absorbed and have greater bioavailability. Conversely, weak acids (such as phenobarbital) may require larger doses because of reduced bioavailability. In the first few months of life, gastric emptying, intestinal motility, and intestinal drug transport increase.

Parenteral drug absorption may also be affected by development. Transdermal bioavailability is increased in infants because there is a thinner strateum corneum in preterm neonates, better skin hydration and perfusion in small children, and a larger surface area-to-volume ratio. Intramuscular bioavailability is greater in neonates and infants than in older children because of a higher density of skeletal muscle capillaries. Rectal-drug bioavailability in drugs undergoing extensive first-pass metabolism is higher in neonates and infants, because hepatic metabolism is immature. Conversely, rectal formulations may be expelled more quickly in young children because of more frequent high-amplitude pulsatile contractions.

Distribution

The age-dependent changes in body composition described above can result in developmental differences in drug distribution. For hydrophilic drugs with relatively small volumes of distribution, greater total body water and larger extracellular fluid spaces result in larger volume of distribution, and hence lower intravascular drug concentrations. Lipophilic drugs with relatively large volumes of distribution are not similarly affected.

Plasma protein binding can exhibit developmental differences, although the clinical significance of protein binding in pharmacokinetics and pharmacodynamics remains unresolved (Benet and Hoener, 2002; Trainor, 2007). The primary binding proteins are albumin (for acidic drugs) and α_1-acid glycoprotein (for basic drugs). Decreased plasma albumin and α_1-acid glycoprotein concentrations in neonates may result in increased unbound (free) drug concentrations and hence pharmacologic effect.

Metabolism

Metabolism of a drug can result in bioactivation of an inactive prodrug, formation of an active or inactive metabolite, or occasionally a toxic metabolite. The liver is the primary site of drug metabolism, although the intestine can metabolize oral drugs before they reach the systemic circulation and extrahepatic metabolism (e.g., renal, blood, and other tissues) may be important for certain drugs (i.e., remifentanil and propofol). Phase I reactions (oxidation, reduction, and hydrolysis) chemically modify the drug structure to add, form, or uncover a functional group and render the molecule more water soluble. Phase II reactions (glucuronidation, sulphation, and glutathione conjugation) add an endogenous molecule to the drug or metabolite to render it even more water soluble for elimination. Typical pathways of drug metabolism are provided in Table 7-4.

TABLE 7-4. Pathways in Drug Metabolism

Reaction	Examples
Phase I	
Oxidation reactions	Thiopental, methohexital
Aliphatic hydroxylation	Pentazocine, meperidine, glutethimide, doxapram, ketamine, chlorpromazine, fentanyl, propranolol
Aromatic	Lidocaine, bupivacaine, mepivacaine
Expoxidation	Phenytoin
O-Dealkylation	Pancuronium, vecuronium, codeine, phenacetin, methoxyflurane
N-Dealkylation	Morphine, meperidine, fentanyl, diazepam, amide local anesthetics, ketamine, codeine, atropine, methadone
N-Oxidation	Meperidine, normeperidine, morphine, tetracaine
S-Oxidation	Chlorpromazine
Oxidative deamination	Amphetamine, epinephrine
Desulfuration	Thiopental
Dehalogenation	Halogenated anesthetics
Dehydrogenation	Ethanol
Reduction Reactions	
Axo reduction	Fazadinium
Nitroreduction	Nitrazepam, dantrolene
Carbonyl reduction	Prednisolone
Alcohol dehydrogenation	Ethanol, chloral hydrate
Hydrolysis Reactions	
Ester hydrolysis	Ester local anesthetics, succinylcholine, acetylsalicyclic acid, propanidid amide local anesthetics
Phase II: Conjugation Reactions	
Glucuronamide	Oxazepam, lorazepam, morphine, nalorphine, codeine, fentanyl, naloxone
Sulfate	Acetaminophen, morphine, isoproterenol, cimetidine
Methylation	Norepinephrine
Acetylation	Procainamide
Amino acid	Salicyclic acid
Mercapturic acid	Sulfobromophthalein
Glutathione	Acetaminophen

Modified from Tucker GT: Drug metabolism, *Br J Anaesth* 51:603, 1979.

Comprehensive reviews of human drug metabolism are available, but a generalized overview is instructive for understanding developmental changes in biotransformation (Kramer and Testa, 2008; Pelkonen et al., 2008; Zanger et al., 2008). Cytochrome P450 (CYP) is the main oxidative (phase I) metabolizing enzyme system, and more than 50 human P450s have been identified, although only a small fraction are responsible for the majority of drug metabolism (Fig. 7-4) (Paine et al., 2006; Zanger et al., 2008). Individual CYPs are classified by their sequence evolution and amino-acid similarities (Ingelman-Sundberg et al., 2007; Zanger et al., 2008). Those with great

PERCENT OF TOTAL HEPATIC P450

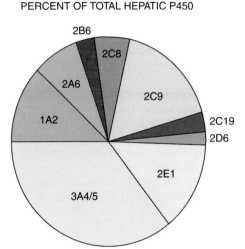

PERCENT OF TOTAL INTESTINAL P450

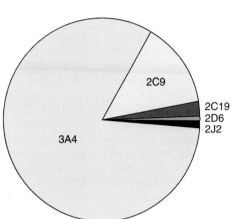

■ **FIGURE 7-4.** Cytochrome P450 isoform content in human liver and intestine. *(Data from Rowland-Yeo K et al.: Abundance of cytochromes P450 in human liver: a metaanalysis, Br J Clin Pharmacol 57:687, 2004; Paine et al.: The human intestinal cytochrome P450 "pie," Drug Metab Dispos 34:880, 2006.)*

than 40% sequence homology are grouped in a family (designated by an Arabic number, e.g., *CYP3*); those with more than 55% homology are in a subfamily (designated by a letter, e.g., *CYP3A*), and individual CYPs are identified by a third number (e.g., *CYP3A4*). The majority of drugs in humans are metabolized by CYPs 1, 2, and 3 (particularly CYPs 1A2, 2B6, 2C8, 2C9, 2C19, 2D6 and 3A4, 3A5, and 3A7). CYPs can have numerous genetic variants, and there are several highly polymorphic CYPs. Allelic CYP variants are designated by an asterisk and number (e.g., *CYP3A5*3*, where the "wild-type" is always *1) (Ingelman-Sundberg et al., 2007; Zanger et al., 2008). CYPs can have varying degrees of substrate specificity, and some are very accommodating, like CYP3A, which metabolizes approximately one third to one half of all therapeutically used drugs.

The developmental pattern of biotransformation activity generally follows a hyperbolic curve with age that begins in fetal development, with hepatic drug metabolism and very low clearance before and during the first month. It reaches near adult levels at approximately 1 year, becomes maximum before puberty, and declines slightly into adulthood

(Johnson and Thomson, 2008). There are, however, enzyme and isoform-specific patterns of developmental maturation of drug-metabolizing enzymes (Blake et al., 2005; Hines, 2008). Several pertinent examples are in the following paragraphs.

The CYP3A family is the most important drug-metabolizing enzyme. The important isoforms are CYP3A4 (the major CYP present in the adult liver and the intestine), CYP3A5 (which metabolizes very many of the CYP3A4 substrates with equal or diminished activity and is polymorphically expressed), and CYP3A7 (a fetal form that is usually less active than 3A4 or 3A5). CYP3A undergoes a "developmental switch" with CYP3A7, the predominant CYP3A expressed in fetal liver (Stevens, 2006; Hines, 2008). Indeed it is the most abundant of any CYP and is thought to be important in fetal steroid metabolism and homeostasis (Fig. 7-5, *A*). CYP3A7 expression decreases during gestation, declines further after birth, and is typically undetectable after the first year. CYP3A4 expression is low during development and then increases after the first 6 months of age. CYP3A metabolizes many drugs of importance in anesthesiology, including all of the fentanyl series opioids (except remifentanil), most benzodiazepines, and local

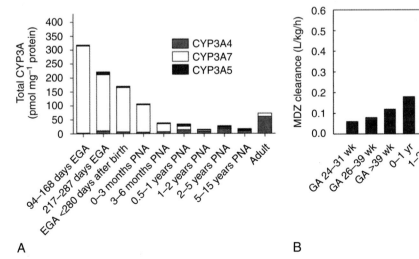

FIGURE 7-5. Developmental aspects of hepatic CYP3A expression and activity. **A,** Content of hepatic CYP3A4, CYP3A5, and CYP3A7 proteins as a function of age. **B,** Clearance of the CYP3A substrate midazolam. *EGA,* Estimated gestational age; *PNA,* postnatal age. (**A** *From Stevens JC: New perspectives on the impact of cytochrome P450 3A expression for pediatric pharmacology,* Drug Discov Today *11:440, 2006;* **B,** *redrawn from de Wildt SN et al.: Cytochrome P450 3A: ontogeny and drug disposition,* Clin Pharmacokinet *37:485, 1999.)*

anesthetics. Although high in abundance, CYP3A7 has low activity toward many drugs (1% to 3% of the activity of CYP3A4 towards midazolam and alfentanil) (Björkman, 2006). Therefore, CYP3A-catalyzed drug metabolism and clearance increases with age. For example, the hepatic extraction of midazolam is only 0.04 in neonates, compared with 0.38 in adults (Björkman, 2006). Midazolam clearance is similarly very low in neonates, particularly in preterm infants. The age-dependent maturation of midazolam clearance is shown in Figure 7-5, B.

Other hepatic CYP isoforms also demonstrate maturation of expression. CYPs 1A2, 2C9, 2C19, 2D6, and 2E1 are expressed minimally or not at all in the fetus, but substantial increases occur after birth. CYP2D6 metabolizes about one fourth of all drugs, including antidepressants, antipsychotics, β-blockers, and numerous orally administered opioids, most notably catalyzing bioactivation of the inactive prodrugs codeine and tramadol (to the pharmacologically active metabolites morphine and O-desmethyltramadol, respectively) (Ingelman-Sundberg et al., 2007; Madadi and Koren, 2008). Isoform-dependent maturation of CYP enzymes in infants is exemplified by the development of tramadol metabolism and disposition, which shows that CYP2D6-catalyzed O-demethylation matures faster than CYP3A-catalyzed N-demethylation (Fig. 7-6). CYP1A2 metabolizes caffeine and theophylline, two methylxanthines that are commonly used in pediatrics. CYP1A2 is essentially absent in fetal liver and minimally active in neonates, such that 85% of caffeine is eliminated unchanged renally in neonates (Cazeneuve et al., 1994). CYP1A2 activity matures rapidly thereafter, reaching adult values by age 6 months, and caffeine clearance in these children reflects primarily hepatic demethylation (Kearns et al., 2003).

Compared with hepatic CYP enzymes, the ontogeny of CYPs in the intestine is far less understood. CYPs 3A4, 3A5, and 2C9 are the predominant intestinal isoforms, accounting for approximately 80% (3As) and 15% (2C9) of the total, respectively, with the remainder comprising CYPs 1A1, 1A2, 2C19, 2J2, and 2D6 (Paine et al., 2006). CYP3A expression declines from the proximal to distal intestine, with 75% occurring in the duodenum and jejunum (Paine et al., 1997). In the intestine, like in the liver, CYP3A4 is the predominant CYP3A isoform, and CYP3A5 is polymorphically expressed in 20% to 70% of adults (Paine et al., 1997). In otherwise histologically normal duodenal biopsies from a population of 74 children, CYP3A4 protein expression increased steadily with age (Fig. 7-7) (Johnson and Thomson, 2008). In fetal duodenum it was essentially absent, and in neonates it was expressed at about half the level seen in mature children. Intestinal CYP3A enzyme activity followed the same pattern as enzyme expression (Johnson and Thomson, 2008).

Other phase I enzymes are important in drug metabolism. Ester hydrolysis is a ubiquitous reaction catalyzed by a diverse array of esterases in blood and tissue. Esterase activity is important in the hydrolysis of remifentanil to an inactive metabolite, resulting in termination of clinical effect. Remifentanil is hydrolyzed by nonspecific esterases in plasma and (more so) tissue, but not by plasma cholinesterase (Manullang and Egan, 1999). In contrast, and unlike most ester drugs, red-cell rather than plasma esterases metabolize esmolol. Whereas CYPs mostly mature in the first months to year of life, esterase activity in neonates is already at levels nearly equivalent to those in adults (Allegaert et al., 2008). For example, remifentanil clearance in children from the ages of 1 month to 9 years old resembles that in adults (Sumpter and Anderson, 2009).

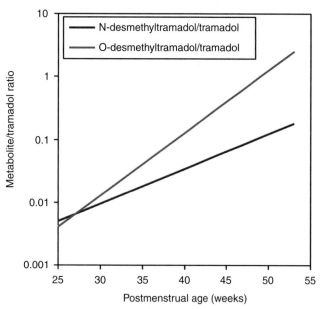

■ **FIGURE 7-6.** Age-dependent and cytochrome P450 (CYP) isoform-dependent development of tramadol metabolism and disposition. Tramadol is a relatively inactive prodrug. Tramadol undergoes CYP2D6-catalyzed O-demethylation to the active analgesic metabolite O-desmethyltramadol, and CYP3A4-catalyzed N-demethylation to the inactive metabolite N-desmethyltramadol. The O-desmethyltramadol/tramadol concentration ratio represents a bioactivation pathway and reflects CYP2D6 activity. The N-desmethyltramadol/tramadol concentration ratio represents an inactivation pathway, and reflects CYP3A4 activity. The figure shows the influence of age on metabolite/tramadol concentration ratios in 24-hour urine collections in neonates and infants after administration of intravenous tramadol. Maturation of CYP2D6 activity is faster than that of CYP3A4. *(Redrawn from Allegaert K et al.: Determinants of drug metabolism in early neonatal life, Curr Clin Pharmacol 2:23, 2007.)*

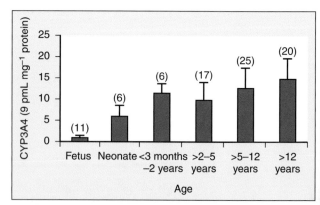

■ **FIGURE 7-7.** Developmental aspects of duodenal CYP3A4 expression and activity (mean ± SD). The number of patients in each group is given in brackets. CYP3A protein expression was measured by Western blotting. Statistically significant differences were observed between the fetus group and all of the other groups and between neonates and children older than 5 years (p < 0.05). The age-related pattern of duodenal CYP3A activity was similar to that of CYP3A protein expression (not shown). *(From Johnson TN et al.: Enterocytic CYP3A4 in a paediatric population: developmental changes and the effect of coeliac disease and cystic fibrosis, Br J Clin Pharmacol 51:451, 2001.)*

Phase II drug-metabolizing enzymes include glucuronosyltransferases (UGTs), sulfotransferases (SULTs), acetyltransferases, and glutathione transferases, all catalyzing conjugation reactions with multiple isoforms of each enzyme, often with isoform-dependent ontogeny (Blake et al., 2005; Hines, 2008). The two main UGT families are UGT1 and UGT2. UGT1A1, the major enzyme responsible for bilirubin conjugation, is not detectable in fetal liver, increases immediately after birth, and reaches adult levels by 3 to 6 months of age. UGT2B7 is of particular interest, because it conjugates morphine. UGT2B7 activity in fetal liver is present at 10% to 20% of adult values and increases in neonates to reach adult values by 2 to 3 months after birth. Morphine clearance is very low in premature infants and increases substantially over the first year of life. SULT ontogeny is isoform-specific, with SULT1E1 activity highest in the fetus and declining thereafter, SULT2A1 activity is barely detectable in neonates and increases in neonates, whereas SULT1A1 activity is constant from fetal age to adulthood.

Elimination

Elimination refers to all processes that remove a drug from the body, including drug metabolism (biotransformation) and excretion. Returning to the concept of drug elimination in general, it is now appreciated that several elements affect the development of drug elimination from fetus to adult, including patient size, organ maturation, organ function, and coexisting disease. Developmental patterns of drug clearance are shown for several drugs in Figure 7-8. For drugs in which renal elimination largely determines systemic clearance, the age-dependence of such clearance approximates that of GFR. In contrast, when hepatic metabolism predominates, the pattern differs.

The complexity of developmental pharmacokinetics can be appreciated using a drug such as propacetamol. Propacetamol is an N, N-diethylglycine ester prodrug of acetaminophen (paracetamol), which is hydrolyzed by plasma esterases after intravenous administration to the active metabolite acetaminophen. Acetaminophen in turn undergoes both phase I, and more so phase II metabolism, to glucuronic acid, sulfate, cysteine, and glutathione conjugates. Figure 7-9 shows the developmental aspects of propacetamol pharmacokinetics (Anderson et al., 2005). Consistent with the relative age invariance of esterase expression, ester hydrolysis to the active metabolite, acetaminophen, was also age invariant. The central compartment volume of distribution was also age invariant, whereas the peripheral compartment volume was somewhat decreased in neonates. Clearance increased markedly with age in the first year, from 12% of adult values at 27 weeks' PCA to 84% of its mature value by 1 year. Importantly, PCA was more important than PNA, as described above.

Scaling Pediatric Dosing

Ideal clinical practice would be informed by age-specific clinical pharmacokinetic data for every drug used in children. As this remains an unattained ideal, considerable effort has been expended to establish pharmacokinetic models to predict age-dependent dosing based on adult data (Anderson and Holford, 2008; Johnson, 2008; Tod et al., 2008; Sumpter and Anderson, 2009). Several principles are now apparent, some of which have been described previously in this chapter. Loading doses depend on concentration and central volume of distribution. For central volumes, allometric modeling (p. 195) suggests that the volume of distribution scales with a power of 1, such that

$$V_{child} = V_{std} \cdot \left(\frac{W_i}{70} \right)$$

where W_i is the weight of any individual and V_{std} is the volume of a standardized 70-kg adult. Because maintenance dosing equals the product of concentration and clearance, the fidelity of clearance models is important. Historically, the linear per-kilogram model, the body-surface area model, and the allometric three-fourths power model have been used. There is a nonlinear relationship between clearance and size. The linear per-kilogram model, although widely used, is the most inaccurate of the three models, because clearance (per kg) is larger in children than in adults. It leads to underprediction by more than 10% at body weights less than 47 kg, and approaches 50% for a 3.5-kg newborn. The body-surface area model, which assumes that adults and children are geometrically similar (although they in fact are not), over-predicts clearance by more than 10% at body weights below 20 kg. The allometric model, which is based on physiologic principles and has been well-validated clinically, is the most accurate.

$$CL_{child} = CL_{adult} \cdot \left(\frac{W_{child}}{70} \right)^{0.75}$$

Figure 7-10 compares the accuracy of the linear per-kilogram, the body-surface area, and the allometric three-fourths power models.

Clearance, however, depends on not just growth (size), but also on maturation of organ clearance processes (i.e., PCA). It is also influenced by concomitant diseases and potentially by drug interactions, which can influence organ function. While allometry alone provides reasonable estimates of clearance in older children using adult data, it alone is insufficient to

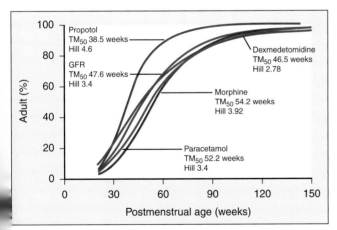

FIGURE 7-8. Clearance maturation, expressed as a percentage of mature clearance. Maturation profiles for acetaminophen, morphine, and dexmedetomidine, in which glucuronidation and renal excretion play a major role, resemble that for renal function (GFR). For propofol, cytochrome P450 enzymes also contribute to biotransformation and elimination, thus causing faster maturation than that predicted from renal excretion alone. The maturation half-time (TM_{50}) and Hill coefficient are shown for each drug. (From Sumpter A, Anderson BJ: Pediatric pharmacology in the first year of life, Curr Opin Anaesthesiol 22:469, 2009.)

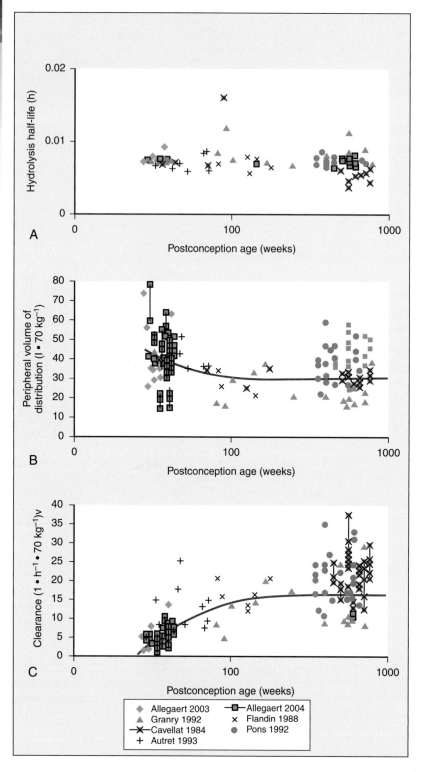

■ **FIGURE 7-9.** Developmental aspects of intravenous propacetamol disposition. **A,** Lack of effect of age on the half-life of propacetamol hydrolysis to acetaminophen. **B,** Influence of age on the peripheral compartment volume of distribution (V_3) of acetaminophen, standardized to a 70-kg person. The solid line represents the nonlinear relation between V_3 and age. Peripheral volume of distribution decreased from 27 weeks' postconceptional age to reach 110% of the value in older children by 6 months. The central volume of distribution did not change with age. **C,** Influence of age on acetaminophen's apparent systemic clearance, standardized to a 70-kg person. The solid line represents the nonlinear relation between clearance and age. Clearance increased from 27 weeks' postconceptional age to reach 84% of the value in older children by 1 year. Data are from a meta-analysis, with different symbols representing different individual studies. *(From Anderson BJ et al.: Pediatric intravenous paracetamol (propacetamol) pharmacokinetics: a population analysis,* Pediatr Anesth *15:282, 2005.)*

predict clearance in infants and young children (Sumpter and Anderson, 2009). Therefore, the most parsimonious model for prediction drug clearance is as follows:

$$CL_{child} = CL_{adult} \bullet \left(\frac{W_{child}}{70} \right)^{0.75} \bullet MF \bullet OF$$

where *MF* is the maturation function (with a value from 0 to 1), and *OF* is organ function (also with a value from 0 to 1). The only major exception to this rule is in neonates, where organ maturation is relatively uninitiated, and the practical relationship is best approximated by the linear per-kilogram model.

For practical purposes, size models have been simplified for clinical use. This is also influenced by regulatory considerations, which sort children into the categories of neonates (younger than 1 month), infants (1 month to 2 years), children (2 to 12 years), and adolescents (12 to 18 years). Table 7-5 presents age-specific dose adjustments. An even simpler method suggest

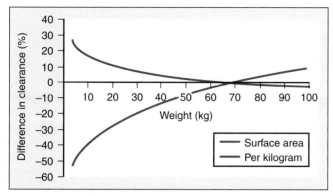

■ **FIGURE 7-10.** Relative differences in clearance determined by the dose per surface area and the dose per kilogram of weight models when compared with the allometric ¾-power weight model. *(From Anderson BJ, Holford NH: Mechanism-based concepts of size and maturity in pharmacokinetics,* Ann Rev Pharmacol Toxicol *48:303, 2008.)*

1 month, 1 year, 7 years, and 12 years, respectively for doses that are one eighth, one fourth, one half, and three fourths of the adult doses (Anderson and Holford, 2008). It is important to remember that these dose adjustments are for drug disposition only, and they do not take into account any age-dependent differences in pharmacodynamic response.

Pharmacodynamics

Pharmacodynamics refers to the biological effect of a drug, specifically the concentration (usually plasma)-effect relationship (or more precisely, the effect site concentration-effect relationship, although the effect-site concentration is rarely actually measured). Far less is known about the developmental aspects of pharmacodynamics than of pharmacokinetics. The concentration-effect relationship defining drug pharmacodynamics is characterized by potency and efficacy. Potency (drug concentration, or less correctly drug dose, that produces a specific effect) is characterized by the ED_{50}, defined as the concentration producing half-maximal effect in a graded dose-response (from zero to maximal response) curve in a single experiment, cell, animal, or individual. Potency can also be characterized by the ED_{50}, or as the concentration producing an all-or-nothing (quantal) response in a quantal dose-response curve in 50% of a population of cells, animals, or individuals. Efficacy is the maximum possible response at the highest possible drug concentration. The developmental aspects of drug pharmacodynamics are therefore best described by age-dependent changes in potency and efficacy. Often, however, the only information available is age dependence of clinical drug response, which may reflect both pharmacokinetic and pharmacodynamic changes.

True age-related pharmacodynamic changes may be qualitative or quantitative, and they may apply to both therapeutic and adverse effects (Stephenson, 2005). One example of quantitative differences in therapeutic response is the effect of warfarin in prepubertal, pubertal, and adult patients. Despite equivalent plasma drug concentrations, warfarin effects on prothrombin fragments 1 and 2 and on the international normalized ratio (INR) were higher in prepubertal patients than in adults. Similarly, augmented response was observed with cyclosporine, in which peripheral blood monocytes from infants had twofold lower proliferation and sevenfold lower interleukin-2 expression compared with older subjects. Examples of age-dependent adverse effects occurring only in children include chloramphenicol toxicity ("gray baby syndrome"), limb deformation from thalidomide during embryogenesis, tetracycline staining of dental enamel, and valproic acid hepatotoxicity, which is increased in young children. Generalized factors leading to age-dependent drug responses include physiology, pathology,

TABLE 7-5. Pediatric Maintenance Doses of Drugs Expressed as a Percentage of Adult Dose Using an Allometric ¾ Power Model*

Approximate Age	Weight (kg)	Percentage of Adult Dose	Fraction of Adult Dose
Birth	3.2	5	1/20
2 months	4.5	13	1/8
4 months	6.5	17	
12 months	10	23	1/4
18 months	11	25	
5 years	18	36	
7 years	23	43.5	
10 years	30	53	1/2
11 years	36	61	
12 years	40	66	
14 years	45	72	3/4
16 years	54	82	
Adult	70	100	1

Modified from Holford NH, Anderson BJ: Paediatric dosages. In: *New ethical catalogue,* Auckland, New Zealand, 1997, Adis International; with permission from Anderson et al: *Eur J Pediatr* 165:819, 2006.
* The neonatal estimate based on size is reduced further by 50% to account for age-related maturational changes of clearance.

host response to disease, and adverse drug reactions, as well as pharmacodynamics (Stephenson, 2005).

For drugs used in anesthesia, the best information on developmental pharmacodynamics has been obtained for inhaled anesthetics, and to a lesser extent, certain intravenous anesthetics. The potency of inhaled anesthetics is significantly affected by developmental age. The principal metric of inhaled anesthetic potency (the median effective concentration, or EC_{50}), has been called the *minimum alveolar concentration (MAC)* and defined as the "minimum alveolar concentration of anesthetic at 1 atmosphere that produces immobility in 50% of those patients or animals exposed to a noxious stimulus," where the stimulus is usually an incision (Mapleson, 1996). Other endpoints have been analogously defined, such as MAC_{AWAKE} endpoint, which defines loss (or return) of consciousness. The quantal EC_{50} of all inhaled anesthetics is similarly influenced by age, with a common log-linear negative slope (for age older than 1 year) (Mapleson, 1996). For decreasing ages younger than 40 years, EC_{50} (MAC) increases 6% per decade. Thus, the MAC for sevoflurane is conceptually 20% greater at age 10 and 27% greater at age 1 (i.e., 2.16% and 2.29% at ages 10 and 1, respectively, for a MAC of 1.8% at age 40 (Mapleson, 1996). A clinical study found the MAC of sevoflurane to be 2.5% in children between 1 and 12 years old and 3.2% in infants 6 to 12 months old, compared with 2% at age 40 (Lerman et al., 1994; Mapleson, 1996). The MAC_{AWAKE} endpoint for sevoflurane was 0.43%, 0.45%, and 0.66% in children 8 to 12 years old, 5 to younger than 8 years, and 2 to younger than 5 years, respectively (Davidson et al., 2008c). The ratio between the MAC_{AWAKE} endpoint and MAC did not differ with age.

Measures of the age-dependent change in apparent anesthetic potency may be influenced by the clinical drug effect used as the index of response. For example, various electroencephalogram (EEG)-derived parameters (e.g., spectral edge frequency, bispectrum, and bispectral index [BIS]) have been used to measure volatile anesthetic effects in children (Wodey et al., 2005; Tirel et al., 2006; Davidson et al., 2008b). Although there were age-dependent effects of volatile anesthetics on various EEG parameters, the EEG itself was found to be highly age-dependent. Specifically, EEG was fundamentally different in infants between 0 and 6 months old, and caution was suggested in the use of BIS to determine volatile anesthetic pharmacodynamics in children (Wodey et al., 2005; Davidson et al., 2008b). Similar results were obtained when EEG-derived parameters were used to evaluate age and propofol effects, and EEG results in children younger than 1 year old were considered inaccurate (Jeleazcov et al., 2007).

Compared with inhaled anesthetics, much less is known about developmental aspects of intravenous drug pharmacodynamics. In part, this reflects the ease, lack of expense, ubiquity, and real-time availability of measuring end-tidal inhaled anesthetic concentrations, compared with measuring plasma concentrations of intravenous anesthetics. Limited data are available for propofol, which suggests slightly lower sensitivity (diminished potency) in children. Plasma propofol concentration-effect (BIS) curves analyzed in children (mean age of 10 years, range of 6 to 13 years) and adults (mean age of 18 years, range of 14 to 32 years) found graded EC_{50} means values of 4 vs. 3.3 mcg/mL, respectively. When propofol infusions were targeted to maintain a steady-state BIS of 50, measured mean plasma concentrations were 4.3 ± 1.1 and 3.4 ± 1.2 mcg/mL, respectively (Rigouzzo et al., 2008). Somewhat lower propofol

potency was also reported by others (Jeleazcov et al., 2008). In contrast, one study found no difference in propofol EC_{50} in adults and children, however, predicted rather than measured plasma concentrations were used in the analysis, which is a limitation of such studies (Munoz et al., 2006). Increased propofol EC_{50} in children is consistent with diminished EC_{50} in older adults (Schnider et al., 1999). No data are available regarding propofol pharmacodynamics in neonates.

In summary, available data suggest some developmental age-dependence of inhaled and intravenous anesthetic pharmacodynamics, with somewhat lower potency in young children. Nonetheless, developmental changes in drug pharmacodynamics, in general, appear to be much smaller and of less clinical significance than developmental changes in drug pharmacokinetics.

Nonlinear Pharmacokinetics

For some drugs, an increase in dose is not followed by proportional increases in plasma C_{ss} and area-under-the-plasma-concentration curve (AUC). Instead, the C_{ss} and AUC increase more than expected. The explanation for this nonlinear pharmacokinetics is that the enzymes responsible for metabolism and elimination of the drug may be saturated. The nonlinear pharmacokinetics, also called *Michaelis-Menten kinetics*, occur when the maximum rate of metabolism (V_{max}) for the drug is approached. Michaelis-Menten pharmacokinetics describes the rate of production of molecules (drug metabolites) produced by enzymatic chemical reactions. Enzymes can perform up to several million catalytic reactions per second. To determine the maximum rate of an enzymatic reaction, the substrate (plasma drug) concentration should be increased until a constant rate of product (drug metabolite) formation is achieved. This is the maximum velocity (V_{max}) of the enzyme. At this point, the active sites of the enzymes are saturated with drug, and a constant amount of drug begins to be eliminated per unit of time ("zero-order" kinetics). Because the substrate (drug plasma) concentration at V_{max} cannot be measured exactly, the metabolism of drug can be characterized by Michaelis-Menten constant (K_m), or the drug plasma concentration at which the rate of metabolism is half of its maximum ($K_m = V_{max}/2$). For practical purposes, the K_m is the plasma concentration at which, when the dose is increased, the nonproportional increase in C_{ss} and AUC start to occur.

For most of drugs that are metabolized by hepatic enzymes and eliminated by the liver, the K_m is above the required therapeutic range and the drugs follow linear kinetics. However, when the therapeutic range is above the K_m, nonlinear kinetics occurs. For example, the average K_m and therapeutic range for phenytoin are 4 mg/L and 10 to 20 mg/L, respectively, and many patients on phenytoin experience nonlinear pharmacokinetics.

The nonlinear pharmacokinetics may also be seen in low clearance drugs for which elimination is significantly influenced by the binding of the drug to plasma proteins. In this scenario, after increasing the dose of the drug, a less-than-expected increase in C_{ss} and AUC occurs. This would suggest that the plasma protein-binding sites have been saturated and that the free fraction of low-clearance drug has increased. The latter would result with increased clearance and a less-than-expected increase C_{ss} occurs. However, if measured, the free fraction of the low-clearance drug increases proportional

Both valproic acid and disopyramide follow this type of nonlinear pharmacokinetics (Bowdle et al., 1980; Lima et al., 1991).

Compartment Models

For many drugs, after intravenous administration, the process of distribution throughout plasma and tissues occurs rapidly and simultaneously, and the whole body could be thought of as a single compartment. In this single-compartment model, after bolus intravenous administration of the drug, there is a monoexponential decrease in plasma concentration. The latter is the result of the elimination process that allows a constant portion of the drug (not amount) in the body to be eliminated per unit of time. In this case, the drug follows the first-order kinetic. The first order elimination of a drug from the body or plasma (C_p) is defined as follows:

$$A_B \times A_B^{\,0} \times e^{-Kdt}, \text{ or } C_p \times C_p^{\,0} \times e^{-Kdt}$$

$A_B^{\,0}$ is the initial amount in the body and $C_p^{\,0}$ is plasma concentration immediately after the bolus; t is the time since bolus, and K_d is the rate constant of elimination. The e^{-Kdt} represents the fraction of the $A_B^{\,0}$ remaining at time t. The K_d is an index of the body's capacity to remove the drug. The elimination rate constant K_d is the fraction of the total amount of drug in the body that is removed per unit of time. It is a function of clearance and volume of distribution:

$$K_d = CL / V_d$$

The elimination rate constant (K_d) can be also thought of as the fraction of the volume of distribution that is effectively cleared of drug per unit of time. Because the drug plasma concentration diminishes monoexponentially, a graph plot of the logarithm of the plasma concentrations vs. time yields a straight line. The elimination rate constant defines the slope of this curve, and two plasma concentrations measured during the decay or elimination phase can be used to calculate the K_d (Fig. 7-11):

$$K_d = \ln C_{p1} - \ln C_{p2} / (t_2 - t_1)$$

The K_d is often expressed in terms of a time required for one half of the total amount of drug in the body to be eliminated, or the plasma concentrations to decrease by one half, that is, by the half-life of the drug $(t_{1/2})$. If plasma concentrations decrease by 50% and $C_{p1} = 2C_{p2}$, then in the previous equation, $t_2 - t_1 = t_{1/2}$ and:

$$K_d = \ln 2 / t_{1/2}$$

$$t_{1/2} = 0.693 / K_d$$

The half-life, like K_d, is dependent on volume of distribution and clearance, and this relationship is shown in the next equation:

$$t_{1/2} = (0.693 \times V_d) / CL$$

The half-life is a variable that determines the following factors:

1. The time needed $(5 \times t_{1/2})$ to reach plasma C_{ss} of the drug after initiation of an infusion;
2. The time needed to reach new C_{ss}'s after increasing or decreasing the infusion rate;
3. The time needed for the drug to disappear from plasma after the infusion is stopped; and
4. The time it takes for all the drug from the body to be eliminated after cessation of the drug infusion (Fig. 7-12).

The short half-life is an obvious advantage for drugs given by intravenous infusion. It allows for drug effects to be easily and dynamically titrated; it requires a relatively shorter time for C_{ss}'s to be achieved; and if toxicity occurs, it is easier to handle. For drugs administered intermittently (oral or parenteral) a short half-life is a disadvantage because multiple doses are needed, it is difficult to keep the plasma concentration within the therapeutic window, and a missed dose could drop plasma concentrations below the minimal therapeutic level. It should be emphasized that volume of distribution and clearance may change independently of one another and alter the half-life in the same or opposite directions. For the given clearance, drugs with smaller volume of distribution have a shorter half-life and a faster recovery after the infusion of an anesthetic agent. Reduced clearance, with no changes in volume of distribution, increases the half-life and recovery time after intravenous infusion.

Most of the drugs used in anesthesia do not follow the simple, one-compartment pharmacokinetics but rather behave like a two- or even three-compartment model. Distribution of anesthetic drugs into and out of peripheral tissues determines the pharmacokinetic profile and the time course of the anesthetic drug's effect. For the two-compartment model, the central compartment includes the blood and organs or tissues that have high blood flow and can be thought of as a rapidly equilibrating volume. The second compartment has a volume (V_t) that equilibrates at a much slower pace. After bolus administration of a drug that follows the two-compartment model, the two distinct phases of distribution and terminal elimination can be distinguished, and the decay of plasma concentration over time is defined by the biexponential equation (Fig. 7-13). Changes in plasma and the site-of-action concentrations would depend on drug elimination and on the equilibrium between central and peripheral tissue compartments.

For many anesthetic drugs, three phases can be distinguished after intravenous bolus administration. This three-compartment model is composed of the central compartment

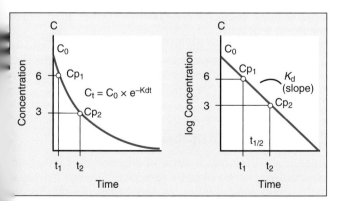

FIGURE 7-11. Single-compartment model. The initial plasma (body) drug concentration $(C_p^{\,0})$ produced by single loading dose diminishes monoexponentially (left). The semilogarithmic graph of concentration vs. time yields a straight line (right).

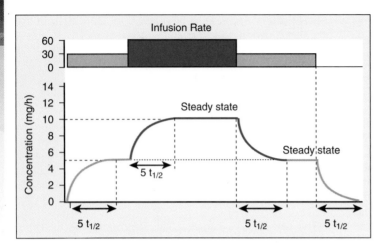

■ **FIGURE 7-12.** Changes in plasma concentration and steady-state level after intravenous infusion are in the function of half-life.

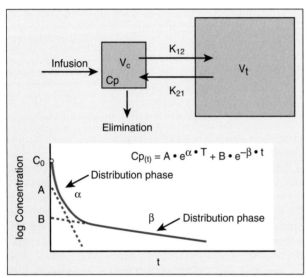

■ **FIGURE 7-13.** Two-compartment model. For many drugs, after an intravenous bolus, there is no "instantaneous" and even distribution of the drug throughout the body (as in the one-compartment model). Drugs distribute with different paces between the initial or central (V_c) compartment (i.e., circulation and well-perfused organs, including the brain) and the tissue or peripheral compartment (V_t). The changes in plasma concentrations follow the biexponential decay.

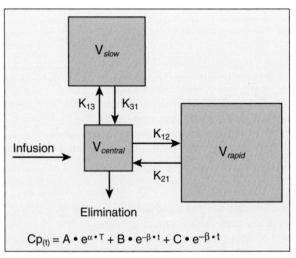

■ **FIGURE 7-14.** Three-compartment model. For many anesthetic drugs, three phases in distribution can be distinguished after intravenous administration. After immediate distribution into the central compartment (i.e., bloodstream and highly perfused organs), there is redistribution of drugs (i.e., from the brain) back into circulation (K_{21}) and to peripheral tissue with rapid equilibrium (K_{12}). The drug also diffuses at a very slow pace into and out from the poorly perfused tissues (K_{13}, K_{31}). The triexponential decay describes the changes in plasma concentrations.

and two additional compartments that include the respective rapid and slow equilibrating tissues and organs (Fig. 7-14). Likewise, the three-compartment model is characterized by the triexponential plasma concentration equation, three volumes of distribution, and five rate constants of distribution and terminal elimination $(K_{12}, K_{21}, K_{13}, K_{31},$ and $K_{10})$.

After an intravenous bolus, the anesthetic or hypnotic drug dilutes almost immediately, within the single circulation time, into the central compartment (i.e., in the bloodstream and in the highly perfused organs such as the brain and spinal cord). The central volume of distribution can be used to calculate the loading dose. Subsequently, there is a redistribution of drug out from the CNS back into the blood and to the peripheral compartments with rapid equilibrium (muscles viscera; V_{drapid}). Finally, the drug diffuses into poorly perfused tissues (fat) that slowly equilibrate with the central compartment. The initial redistribution, rather than metabolic clearance, determines the termination of the

effect of single boluses of parenteral anesthetics. If prolonged anesthesia is required, the maintenance infusion rate should compensate not only for the drug clearance but initially also for the transient loss of anesthetic by redistribution to the peripheral compartments that are governed by "intercompartmental clearance" and elimination rate constants $(K_{12}, K_{21}, K_{13},$ and $K_{31})$.

Context-Sensitive Half-Time

Traditionally, clearance, volume of distribution, and half-life are standard pharmacokinetic parameters used to characterize the drug's offset of action. As discussed previously, they are derived from one- and two-compartment models or, through the use of computer simulation programs, from multicompartment models. These pharmacokinetic parameters can be relatively easy to apply to calculate the infusion rate and predict the offset of action of water-soluble drugs with small volumes of distribution and relatively simple patterns of disposition (i.e., muscle relaxants).

For the anesthesiologist, pharmacokinetic factors are often used for the routine selection and use of various intravenous anesthetic agents. Drugs with short elimination half-lives are commonly selected for brief procedures, whereas drugs with longer half-lives are selected for lengthier procedures. Drugs with small volumes of distribution tend to decrease the time required for recovery after intravenous infusion, and agents with decreased plasma clearances may increase the time for recovery. In general, formulas for the calculation of continuous infusions incorporate knowledge of these pharmacokinetics. For bolus administration of drug, the volume of distribution and the desired plasma concentration are needed. Table 7-6 lists plasma concentrations in adults for some of the opioids. The bolus dose is calculated as the product of the volume of distribution and the desired plasma concentration (C_p):

$$\text{Bolus dose} = V_d \times C_p$$

The maintenance infusion rate (MIR) is calculated as the product of the desired plasma concentration and the clearance:

$$\text{MIR} = CL \times C_p$$

Although these formulas work well, Shafer and Varvel (1991) and Hughes et al. (1992) have demonstrated the complex interactions that occur with prolonged infusions, especially in drugs that are lipid soluble.

The offset of drug effect depends on reduction of the plasma concentrations and the withdrawal of drug from the site of action; that is, for anesthetic from the receptor site in the CNS. If steady state is achieved and all compartments are saturated, then the half-life of elimination phase, which is a function of the first-order processes of elimination, correlates with a decrease in the site-of-action drug concentrations and with the offset of drug action. However, after infusion of a highly lipophilic anesthetic agent, when steady state is not achieved and not all compartments are saturated, the decline in concentrations (i.e., the offset of action and recovery from anesthesia) depends on complex interactions between the duration of the infusion and initial distribution, redistribution, and metabolic and elimination first-order processes. The classic descriptors of a drug's pharmacokinetics and offset of action (terminal half-time) are of little help to anesthesiologists in predicting the offset of action and recovery from anesthesia for the intravenous anesthetic drugs. Fortunately, with the help of pharmacokinetic and pharmacodynamic simulation models, new predictors of offset of drug effects have evolved (Shafer and Varvel, 1991; Hughes et al., 1992; Youngs and Shafer, 1994).

Using pharmacokinetic and pharmacodynamic models and basic pharmacokinetic profiles of commonly used synthetic opioid analogs, Shafer and Varvel (1991) were the first to construct the offset of action (recovery) curves as a function of the duration of infusion for fentanyl, alfentanil, and sufentanil (Fig. 7-15). Hughes et al. (1992) introduced the term *context-sensitive half-time* (context refers to the duration of infusion) as a time required for a drug concentration to decrease to half of its value after drug infusion of a given duration. Of importance is that for any given drug, its context-sensitive half-time varies with the duration of the drug infusion. Because for most intravenous anesthetic drugs the 50% fall in concentration is not sufficient for recovery from anesthesia, other decrement times have been introduced (Youngs and Shafer, 1994), for example, 80% and 90% decrements.

After a short intravenous infusion (0 to 15 minutes), fentanyl and other synthetic opioid analogs have similar context-sensitive half-times (Fig. 7-15). However, after prolonged infusion (longer than 1 hour), there is a marked difference among four synthetic opioid analogs (fentanyl, sufentanil, alfentanil, and remifentanil), and these differences do not correlate with their classic pharmacokinetic parameters (Table 7-7). In contrast to its older congeners, remifentanil has a short and steady context-sensitive half-life of 3 minutes, which does not change with the increasing duration of infusion (Egan et al., 1996). This contrasts with alfentanil, which has a context-sensitive half-time that increases to 1 hour after a 4-hour infusion (Ebling et al., 1990; Scholz et al., 1996). This difference is because of the unique pharmacokinetic profile of remifentanil. It is a highly liposoluble (volume of distribution at steady state [V_{dss}] of 30 L) opioid analog that undergoes widespread metabolism (deesterification), including metabolism in the circulation. Unlike other opioids, the termination of action of remifentanil does

TABLE 7-6. Opioid Concentrations that Ablate Responsiveness to Intraoperative Noxious Stimuli and Permit Adequate Ventilation on Emergence*

	Fentanyl	Alfentanil	Sufentanil
Induction and Intubation			
Thiopental	3 to 5	250 to 400	0.4 to 0.6
O_2/N_2O only	8 to 10	400 to 750	0.8 to 1.2
Maintenance			
N_2O/potent vapor	1.5 to 4	100 to 300	0.25 to 0.5
O_2/N_2O only	1.5 to 10	100 to 750	0.25 to 1.0
O_2 only	15 to 60	1000 to 4000	10 to 60
Adequate ventilation	1.5	125	0.25 on emergence

* Opioid concentrations given in ng/mL.

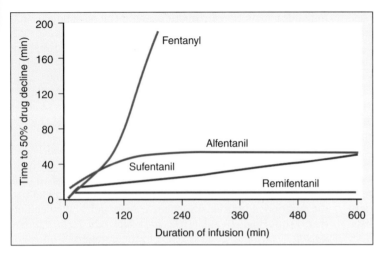

■ **FIGURE 7-15.** Context-sensitive half-time: the time required for drug concentration to decrease by half of its value (*Y axis*) after cessation of infusion of given duration (*X axis*) for fentanyl and its congeners, sufentanil, alfentanil, and remifentanil (see the text for explanation). *(Modified from Shafer SL, Varvel MD: Pharmacokinetics, pharmacodynamics, and rational opioid selection,* Anesthesiology *74:53, 1991;* Egan TD: Clin Pharmacokinet *29:80, 1995.)*

TABLE 7-7. Pharmacokinetic Parameters of Synthetic Opioids after Single Intravenous Bolus Administration

	Volume of Distribution ($V_d$ss; L/kg)	Elimination Half-Life ($t_{1/2}\alpha$ min)	Distribution Half-Life ($t_{1/2}\beta$ min)	Total Body Clearance (mL/min/kg)	Context-Sensitive Half-Time (3-hr Infusion)
Fentanyl	4	2 to 3	220 to 300	10 to 20	100
Sufentanil	1.7	1.4	160	10 to 15	30
Alfentanil	0.75	0.6 to 12	90 to 120	8	50
Remifentanil	0.3 to 0.4	1 to 1.5	6 to 14	50	3

Data from Egan TD et al.: Remifentanil versus alfentanil: comparative pharmacokinetics and pharmacodynamics in healthy adult male volunteers, *Anesthesiology* 84:821, 1996; Ebling WF et al.: Understanding pharmacokinetics and pharmacodynamics through computer simulation I: the comparative clinical profiles of fentanyl and alfentanil, *Anesthesiology* 72:650, 1990; Scholz J et al.: Clinical pharmacokinetics of alfentanil, fentanyl and sufentanil, an update, *Clin Pharmacokinet* 31:275, 1996.

not depend on redistribution but rather on extremely rapid metabolic clearance. Kapila et al. (1995) demonstrated that the context-sensitive half-times of remifentanil (3 minutes) and alfentanil (50 to 55 minutes) derived from computer modeling are similar to measured context-sensitive half-times (3.2 and 47 minutes for remifentanil and alfentanil, respectively), and both correlate with measured pharmacodynamic offset (recovery of minute ventilation). The latter confirms the value and clinical applicability of this new pharmacokinetic-pharmacodynamic parameter in predicting the offset of anesthetic drugs.

The context-sensitive half-time curves provide a better, clinically more relevant comparison of the pharmacokinetic profiles of anesthetic drugs than the traditional pharmacokinetic parameters (Fig. 7-16). After a single intravenous dose, commonly used anesthetic and hypnotic drugs have a short duration of action. However, after prolonged infusions the context-sensitive half-times and duration of action increase. For some drugs (e.g., propofol and ketamine), this increase is modest, whereas for others (e.g., diazepam and thiopental), it is quite dramatic. In the case of midazolam, the rapid increase in its context-sensitive half-time with prolonged duration of infusion occurs in the presence of a relatively short elimination half-life ($t_{1/2}\beta$), and this is most likely because of the low clearance of midazolam.

The data regarding the context-sensitive half-times and other decrement times of anesthetic agents in the pediatric population are limited, at best. In children aged 3 to 11 years, longer context-sensitive half-times than in adults were reported for propofol. After a 1-hour infusion in children and

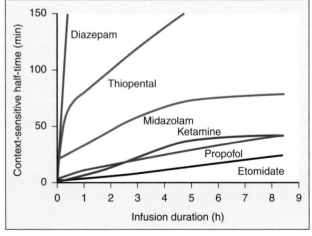

■ **FIGURE 7-16.** Context-sensitive half-time for commonly used general anesthetics. *(From Reves JG et al.: Nonbarbiturate intravenous anesthetics. In Miller RD, editor:* Anesthesia, *ed 5, New York, 2000, Churchill Livingstone.)*

adults, the context-sensitive half-times for propofol are 10.4 and 6.6 minutes, respectively, and after a 4-hour infusion they are 19.6 and 9.5 minutes, respectively (McFarlan et al. 1999). This is probably due to the altered compartment volumes and may lead to slower recovery from a propofol infusion in children than in adults (Short et al., 1994). In contrast the shorter context-sensitive half-time of fentanyl was determined in pediatric population (2 to 11 years old) compared with published data in adults (Ginsberg et al., 1996).

Population Pharmacokinetics

Pharmacokinetics and pharmacodynamics of drugs in the pediatric population and in adults are different. Furthermore, neonates, infants, children, and adolescents have distinct differences in physiologic development, and the pediatric population is quite heterogeneous with regard to pharmacokinetics and pharmacodynamics of drugs across different age groups. These differences justify studying pharmacokinetics and pharmacodynamics in children of various ages. However, the testing of medications in children presents a dilemma: while society wants to spare children from the potential risk involved in research, children may be harmed if they are given medications that have been inadequately studied (Steinbrook, 2002).

Classical nontherapeutic pharmacokinetics studies involve administering either single or multiple doses of a drug to a relatively small group of subjects and require multiple sampling to characterize the concentration and time profile of the drug. Conducting standard nontherapeutic pharmacokinetic studies with frequent sampling in children imposes many ethical and practical issues, and an alternative and preferable approach in many pediatric situations is the population pharmacokinetics (PPK) approach. This approach, in addition to dense data and frequent sampling, deal with sparse data and infrequent sampling of blood from a larger population, and it allows many obstacles related to classical nontherapeutic pharmacokinetic studies in children to be overcome.

PPK is an area of clinical pharmacology that studies the sources and the correlates of variability in drug-plasma concentration parameters among individuals in the target population of patients who are receiving clinically effective doses of a drug (Shen and Lu, 2007). PPK is focused on the quantitative assessment of the typical pharmacokinetic parameters, as well as the within- and between-individual and residual variability in drug absorption, distribution, metabolism, and excretion (Steiner, 1992; Ette and Williams, 2004). The population approaches use mathematic and statistic modeling to investigate the dose-concentration-effect relationship and to quantitatively and qualitatively assess factors that may explain interindividual variability (Sheiner et al., 1979). In the early 1980s, Sheiner and Beal introduced the new PPK data analysis approach (i.e., the population approach) and demonstrated that estimates of PPK parameters could be obtained even if only two or three samples are collected per patient (Sheiner and Beal, 1980, 1981, 1982). They also introduced a new software program (the Nonlinear Mixed Effects Model, or NONMEM) that was capable of performing the new type of analysis, and this is now the most commonly used population modeling program (Sheiner and Beal, 1980; Sheiner et al., 1979).

The PPK approach allows not only major contributions to variability of key pharmacokinetic parameters to be established, but it also goes one step further and allows the relative contributions of different factors to be determined. In this regard, size, age, and renal function are major contributors to vancomycin clearance variability in neonates. Using the PPK and NONMEM modeling, Anderson and colleagues (2002a) have shown that size explains 49.8%, age accounts for 18.2%, and renal function explains 14.1% of clearance variability of vancomycin in neonates. The small unexplained percentage (18%) is residual variability in clearance and suggests that target concentration intervention is unnecessary if size, age, and renal function are used to predict the dose (Anderson et al., 2002a).

Body Size and Maturation Adjustments

Two major features of children that are not seen in adults are growth and development, and these unique characteristics of the pediatric population can be studied by using size and age as covariates. PPK studies in children cover a population with much wider range in body size than similar studies in adults, and body weight can vary in the pediatric population up to 200-fold (i.e., 0.5 to 100 kg). Even when only one particular age group is studied, it is not uncommon that tenfold differences in body weight are reported. Both primary pharmacokinetic parameters, clearance, and volume of distribution are functions of body size. Therefore, to identify the potential effects of other covariates in predicting pharmacokinetic parameters, it is necessary to use size as a primary covariate and standardized clearance and volume of distribution to appropriate body size.

In adults, to account for impact of body size, pharmacokinetic parameters are traditionally adjusted to body weight or body surface area. However, these empirical approaches, although appropriate when adjusting for dose, clearance, or volume of distribution in adults, may be inappropriate for scaling small children to adults (Holford, 1996). The body-weight adjustments may underpredict clearance, whereas the body surface area model may overpredict clearance in children (and the error increases with decreasing weight) (Mitchell et al., 1971; Holford, 1996; Anderson et al., 2006). Measurement of body surface area, which can be calculated from height and weight by DuBois formula:

$$BSA = \left(W^{0.425} \times H^{0.725} \right) \times 0.007184$$

where *BSA* represents body surface area, *W* is weight, and *H* is height. It may also be calculated by using several very similar formulas; however, all formulas may be inaccurate, especially in younger pediatric patients (Holford, 1996; Anderson et al., 2006). Infants are not morphologically similar to adults (they have short legs, relatively big heads, and large body trunks), and direct photometric measurement has been suggested to be an inaccurate prediction of body surface area in children younger than 12 years old, or BSA greater than 1.3 m^2 (Mitchell et al., 1971).

A method for body-size adjustment that has begun to be used regularly in PPK studies in children is allometric size adjustment. Allometry is a methodology used to relate morphology and body function to the size of an organism. This methodology had found wide application in drug development to predict pharmacokinetic parameters in humans based on data from different animal species. Gillooly and colleagues (2001) have shown that in almost all species, including humans, when the log of the basal metabolic rate is plotted against the log of body weight, a straight line with a slope of 0.75 is produced (Fig. 7-17).

In the allometric size adjustment model, pharmacokinetic parameters are studied by body weight of an individual by power model:

$$F_{size} = (W / W_{adult})^{PWR}$$

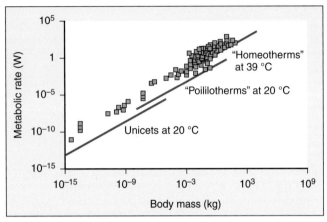

■ **FIGURE 7-17.** A comparison of the temperature-standardized relation for whole-organism metabolic rate *(W)* as a function of the body mass *(kg)*. Data points represent unicells, plants, ectotherms, and endotherms, all standardized to 20° C. The three lines indicate that the "allometric 0.75 power model" fits for unicells, poikilotherms and homeotherms. *(From Gillooly JF et al.: Effects of size and temperature on metabolic rate,* Science *293:2248, 2001.)*

where F_{size} is a factor for size, W is a body weight of an individual, W_{adult} is body weight of an adult of standard 70-kg size, and *PWR* is allometric power exponent.

The allometric "0.25 power" model can be used to predict the pharmacokinetic estimates in children with PWRs of 0.75, 0.25, and 1 for clearance, half-life, and volume of distribution, respectively (West et al., 1997, 1999; Anderson et al., 2006). Using the fixed power exponent allows investigators to delineate secondary covariate effects from the effects of size. The allometric scaling also allows direct comparison of pediatric and adult pharmacokinetic estimates and can be used to predict the pediatric dose based on the adult dose (Table 7-5).

Age is used as a covariate to describe the maturation process in the pediatric population. Several quantitative models that describe the maturation of clearance have been developed, and they vary depending on age group studied (Allegaert et al., 2006; Anderson et al., 2000). Rhodin and colleagues (2009) have studied the effects of size and maturation on GFR in 923 individuals from eight studies, from 22 weeks' PMA to 31 years of age. They demonstrated that PMA is a better descriptor of maturation changes than PNA and that a sigmoid hyperbolic model describes the nonlinear relationship between GFR and PMA. Half of the adult values are reached at 48 weeks PMA, and at 1 year PNA the predicted GFR is 90% of the adult GFR (Rhodin et al., 2009).

Data Modeling

There are three main approaches to modeling data collected from a group of subjects: naïve pooled data, the standard two-stage approach, and mixed-effects models. In the naïve pooled-data approach, time-concentration data pooled together from different subjects are treated as if all doses and all observations pertain to a single subject. This approach does not allow information about the magnitude and the causes of between-subject variability to be collected, and it is adequate only if data are extensive for each subject and if there is only minor between-subject variability. In the standard two-stage approach,

individual time-concentration profiles are analyzed, and the individual parameters (i.e., volume of distribution and clearance) are estimated in the first stage by separately fitting each subject's data. In the second stage, individual estimates are used as variables and combined to obtain summary measures. If data are sparse, misrepresentation may occur easily.

In contrast to the naïve pooled-data and the two-stage approaches that use dense data from a small group of subjects, the mixed-effects models study the variability in drug response in the population of interest, using sparse data (often only two or three samples) from a large number of subjects. The mixed-effects modeling approach, similar to the naïve pooled-data approach, analyzes the data of all individuals at once, but it takes into consideration the interindividual effects. The modeling is "mixed" because it describes the data using a mixture of fixed effects (parameters' differences predicted by covariates) and random effects (between subject and residual or unexplained variability). In their seminal work in the early 1980s, by using phenytoin data collected from therapeutic monitoring in epileptic patients, Sheiner and Beal showed not only how estimates of PPK could be obtained from few samples per patient, but they also demonstrated that the naïve pooled-data and the two-stage approaches may both result in biased parameter estimates. The advantages of this approach are that in addition to sparse data, it can handle the imbalance in data per individual and it can estimate the between-observation variability. Obviously, the use of sparse data and imbalanced data allows many ethical concerns and practical problems related to frequent sampling to be overcome. The disadvantage is that this approach needs advanced training for the use of specialized software such as NONMEM, and fitting complicated models can be time consuming.

NEUROTOXICITY

One of the most active areas of investigation in the past several years involves the potentially toxic effects of sedative and anesthetic agents on the developing nervous system. Newborn animal model studies have reported apoptosis in multiple areas in the CNS during the period of rapid synaptogenesis, when exposure to agents that work via *N*-methyl-D-aspartate (NMDA) antagonists or γ-aminobutyric acid (GABA) agonist pathways occurs (Ikonomidu, 1999; Jevtovic-Todorovic et al., 2003; Mellon et al., 2007). Although this effect was originally shown in newborn rodent models, recent work has demonstrated the same histologic changes in nonhuman primates (Wang and Slikker, 2008). Ketamine, isoflurane, and sevoflurane have all been shown to produce apoptosis in the brains of developing rodents in a dose-dependent manner (Ikonomidu et al., 1999; Jevtovic-Todorovic et al., 2003; Fredriksson et al., 2007; Loepke et al., 2009; Satomoto et al., 2009; Stratmann et al., 2009). Apoptosis has also been demonstrated in the spinal cord (Sanders et al., 2008). The period of vulnerability is thought to coincide with the period of synaptogenesis, which is at about day 7 in rats and from late pregnancy through early toddlerhood in humans. Concern and interest increased with the demonstration of long-term learning deficits at early maturity in rats when they were exposed to an "anesthetic cocktail" of midazolam, nitrous oxide and isoflurane for 6 hours on postnatal day 7 (Jevtovic-Todorovic et al., 2003). Combinations of nitrous oxide, midazolam, and isoflurane may cause more apoptosis than single agent (Jevtovic-Todorovic et al., 2003; Fredriksson et al., 2007). I monkeys, ketamine produced apoptosis when given for 24 hours in late gestation or to 5-day-old monkeys but not to 30-day-old monkeys (Slikker et al., 2007). Also a shorter administration period of ketamine did not produce apoptosis in 5-day-old monkeys. There is mixed evidence for long-term measurable changes in cognitive function or behavior in rodents exposed to anesthesia in the neonatal period (Jevtovic-Todorovic et al., 2003; Fredriksson et al., 2007; Loepke et al., 2009; Stratmann et al., 2009). No data have been presented that examine long-term effects in primates. The application of these findings to human neonates and infants has many unknown elements, including the window of vulnerability, the duration of exposure, and the dose of agent necessary to affect long-term neurodevelopment. The mechanism that triggers apoptosis is not clear, but there is some evidence that apoptosis may be triggered as a result of decreased release of trophic factors from the axon (Head et al., 2009). The possibility that GABA receptors may be involved is complicated by the observation that the morphology of GABA receptors changes during this period, as do their downstream actions, and that the addition of a GABA agonist does not completely reverse the apoptotic effect of GABA antagonists. In addition to apoptosis, there is also increasing evidence that anesthetics can cause a change in dendritic morphology. This may also be to the result of anesthesia causing relative inactivity of neurons and a decrease in relevant trophic factors. A series of articles in *Anesthesia & Analgesia* in June 2008 presented the data and controversies well. Editorials in *Anesthesiology* in November 2008 through January 2009 presented several approaches to investigating the presence and extent of such a neurotoxic effect in human infants and young children who are exposed to anesthetic agents (Cattano et al., 2008; Davidson et al., 2008a; Jevtovic-Todorovic et al., 2008; Loepke et al., 2008; Loepke and Soriano, 2008; McGowen and Davis, 2008; Sanders et al., 2008; Sun et al., 2008, Wang and Slikker, 2008; Hansen and Flick, 2009). Great efforts will be ongoing in the near future to further delineate the mechanisms, to investigate the extent of the problem in humans, and to study possible therapeutic options to minimize such toxicity. An FDA advisory panel held in April 2007 concluded "there was no scientific basis to recommend changes in clinical practice" with the current data (the meeting transcript can be found at *www.fda.gov/ohrms/dockets/ac/2007-4285t1.pdf*).

INTRAVENOUS AGENTS

Sedative Hypnotics and Barbiturates

A variety of sedative-hypnotic agents can be used for premedication or induction of anesthesia. These agents are administered intravenously, but for premedication oral, sublingual, intranasal, rectal, or less commonly, intramuscular routes are used.

On a milligram-per-kilogram basis, barbiturates are more lethal to newborns than to more mature animals (Carmichael, 1947; Weatherall, 1960; Goldenthal, 1971). The sleeping times of newborn animals are markedly prolonged at sublethal doses given on an equal milligram-per-kilogram basis (Weatherall, 1960). Greater penetration of the blood-brain barrier by barbiturates has been found in neonates compared with older animals (Domek et al., 1960).

Neonates have a decreased ability to metabolize barbiturates (Mirkin, 1975). The longer-acting barbiturates, which are in part excreted unmetabolized in the urine, would be expected to have prolonged or elevated blood levels (Knauer et al., 1973; Boreus et al., 1975). Glucuronic acid conjugation of barbiturates develops rapidly and increases 30-fold during the first 3 weeks of life (Brown et al., 1958).

Short-acting barbiturates (e.g., methohexital, thiamylal, and thiopental) can be used to induce anesthesia in infants and children. These agents produce rapid induction of hypnosis with minimal relaxation or analgesia. The pharmacokinetics of short-acting barbiturates in infants, children, and adults were studied extensively by Brodie (1952), Dundee and Barron (1962), Mark (1963), Saidman and Eger (1966), and Lindsay and Shepherd (1969). Because of the child's proportionately greater amount of vessel-rich tissue, the uptake of short-acting barbiturates should be more rapid; the effect more quickly achieved; and metabolism, excretion, and recovery more prompt unless retarded by supplementary agents (Eger, 1974). These agents are used less commonly now than in the past in many centers where other short-acting sedatives have supplanted the short-acting barbiturates.

Thiopental

Thiopental is an ultra short-acting barbiturate used as an intravenous induction agent in anesthesia. It has been also used in critical care settings as a continuous infusion for the treatment of intracranial hypertension and status epilepticus. Hiccoughs, sneezing, and other respiratory irregularities are rarely seen on induction, and there is no excitement or extrapyramidal activity associated with its use. It decreases cerebrospinal fluid pressure, making it useful for diagnostic and operative neurologic procedures (Dawson et al., 1971). Intraocular pressure also is decreased. Awakening is quiet, occasionally interrupted by shivering, and associated with a low incidence of nausea (Smith et al., 1955). Porphyria, seldom encountered in the United States, is a specific contraindication to barbiturates (Dundee and Barron, 1962). Thiopental requirements for induction of anesthesia reveal an inverse relation with age. Jonmarker et al. (1987) reported that the ED_{50} of thiopental in infants is significantly greater (7 mg/kg) than that in adults (4 mg/kg) (Fig. 7-18). Westrin et al. (1989) determined the dose of thiopental needed for satisfactory induction of 10 healthy, unpremedicated neonates who were 0 to 14 days old and 20

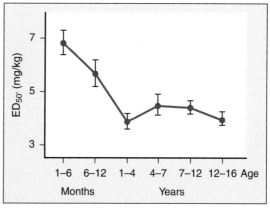

■ **FIGURE 7-18.** Estimated ED_{50} ± SD for thiopental in the various age groups. *(From Jonmarker C et al.: Thiopental requirements for induction of anesthesia in children, Anesthesiology 67:104, 1987.)*

infants who were between 1 and 6 months old. In this study, the ED_{50} for thiopental induction was 3.4 ± 0.2 mg/kg in neonates and 6.3 ± 0.7 mg/kg in infants aged 1 to 6 months. In an in-vitro study in which the free fraction of thiopental was measured in the serum of neonates and adult volunteers, Kingston et al. (1990) noted that neonates had a free drug fraction that was 1.5 to two times greater than that of adults. The increased free fraction of thiopental may explain the decreased induction dose required by the neonate. Sorbo et al. (1984) studied the pharmacokinetics of thiopental in 24 surgical patients aged 5 months to 13 years. The volume of distribution of the central compartment ranged from 0.3 to 0.4 L/kg. The steady-state volume of distribution was approximately 2 L/kg and did not differ statistically from values previously measured in adults. The elimination half-time and clearance of thiopental in these infants and children were 6.1 ± 3.3 hours and 6.6 ± 2.2 mL/kg per minute, respectively. These values were significantly different from the values of 12 ± 6 hours and 3.1 ± 0.5 mL/kg per minute, respectively, observed in adults. After a single intravenous dose, clinical effect is mainly terminated by redistribution. When repetitive or larger doses are used, redistribution becomes less effective and metabolism plays a more important role, explaining the shorter recovery times in children when compared with adults.

Methohexital

Methohexital, a methylated oxybarbiturate, is more potent than thiopental by a ratio of about 3:1, is more rapidly eliminated, and produces more undesirable side effects (Clarke et al., 1968). Greater speed of recovery provides its principal indication, especially for outpatient care or for situations where very brief effect is wanted, such as for cardioversion or electroconvulsive therapy. The incidence of involuntary muscular movement, hiccoughs, and respiratory irregularity during induction is definitely greater with methohexital than with thiopental. Although methohexital has been used via the intramuscular or rectal route without tissue damage, some studies suggest that the high concentration of rectal methohexital can cause mucosal damage (Miller et al., 1961). Administration of 10% methohexital to rats via the rectal route produces minor, self-limited lesions in the rectal mucosa (Hinkle and Weinlander,

1989). The recommended dose for intravenous use is 1 to 2 mg/kg, and in children younger than 5 years, 25 to 30 mg/kg can be administered rectally.

In a study of 85 children, Khalil et al. (1990) compared 25 mg/kg of rectal methohexital in a 10% and a 1% concentration. In this study, 1% was associated with a better success rate, faster onset time, high plasma concentration, and longer recovery time than the 10% concentration. In addition, they noted that the length of the rectal catheter had no effect on the pharmacodynamics of the drug. A 10% solution of methohexital at a dose of 25 mg/kg usually produced sleep in 6 to 10 minutes, which coincided with peak serum levels (Goresky and Steward, 1979; Letty et al., 1985).

Forbes et al. (1989a) reported on the plasma concentrations of 60 children after doses of 15, 20, 25, or 30 mg/kg of rectal methohexital (Fig. 7-19). The dose of 30 mg/kg resulted in significantly higher plasma concentrations for up to 20 minutes. In addition, in a separate study of 12 patients who were premedicated with 25 mg/kg of 2% rectal methohexital, Forbes et al. (1989b), using pulsed Doppler and two-dimensional echocardiography, noted a significant increase in heart rate but no change in cardiac index, stroke volume, ejection fraction, or blood pressure.

Audenaert et al. (1995) prospectively reviewed the effects of rectal methohexital in 648 patients. They noted that after a 30 mg/kg dose of 10% methohexital, children fell asleep 85% of the time. Sleep usually occurred in 6 minutes. Sleep was less likely to occur in patients with myelomeningocele or in patients receiving phenobarbital or phenytoin therapy. Side effects of defecation after administration occurred in 10% of patients, and hiccoughs occurred in 13% (Audenaert et al., 1995). The intravenous dose for induction using methohexital dissolved in a lipid emulsion was determined by Westrin (1992), who noted that the dose (adjusted by body weight) needed for induction in infants younger than 5 months was almost twice that for older children (Fig. 7-20).

Beskow et al. (1995) compared intravenous induction of methohexital (3 mg/kg) and thiopental (7.3 mg/kg) in 41 infants aged 1 month to 1 year. In this study of short surgical procedures, recovery as measured by spontaneous eye opening after methohexital was significantly shorter than it was for thiopental.

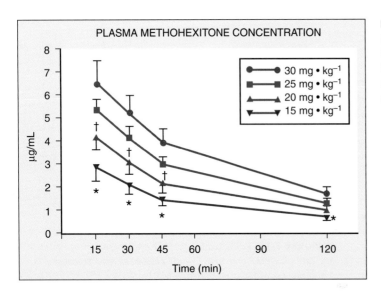

■ FIGURE 7-19. Plasma methohexitone concentrations after rectal administration of methohexitone 15 mg/kg, 20 mg/kg, 25 mg/kg, or 30 mg/kg. Mean ± SEM. *P < 0.05, 15 mg/kg vs. 30 mg/kg; †P < 0.05, 20 mg/kg vs. 30 mg/kg. *(From Forbes RB et al.: Pharmacokinetics of two percent rectal methohexitone in children, Can J Anaesth 36:160, 1989a.)*

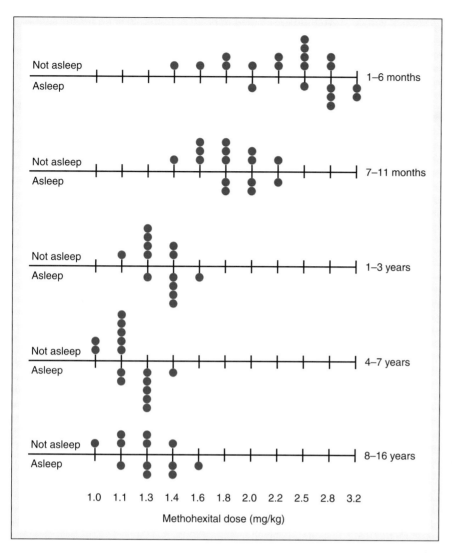

■ **FIGURE 7-20.** Results of injection of different doses of methohexital. Each filled circle represents one patient. The position of the circle below or above the line indicates whether induction was classified as satisfactory or not satisfactory. *(From Westrin P: Methohexital dissolved in lipid emulsion for intravenous induction of anesthesia in infants and children, Anesthesiology 76:917, 1992.)*

Benzodiazepines and Antagonists

Diazepam

Diazepam produces relatively pleasant sedation or hypnosis with few side effects and prompt recovery. Its action is caused by depression of the amygdala of the limbic system and spinal internuncial neurons. It is a specific treatment of seizure disorders in children (Lombroso, 1966; Carter and Gold, 1977). Intravenous administration of 0.2 to 0.3 mg/kg usually induces hypnosis, but the requirement varies widely. Diazepam appears to cause less cardiac depression than do barbiturates (Muenster et al., 1967; Abel and Reis, 1971).

Diazepam is metabolized by the CYP-linked monooxygenase system. In adults, the metabolite, desmethyldiazepam, is eliminated more slowly ($t_{1/2}$ = 150 hours) than the parent compound ($t_{1/2}$ = 20 to 30 hours) (Meberg et al., 1978).

The plasma half-life of diazepam and the nature of the diazepam metabolites formed vary with maturity (Morselli et al., 1974). The premature infant and the mature infant at term eliminate diazepam at a slower rate than older infants, children, and adults. In premature infants, a demethylated derivative of diazepam, N-desmethyldiazepam, could not be measured in plasma until 4 hours after injection, in comparison with older infants and children, in whom N-desmethyldiazepam was

measured in the plasma by 1 hour and had peaked by 24 hours. In adults, 71% of diazepam or its metabolites was excreted in the urine, and about 10% was excreted in the feces. As an oral premedicant or intravenous induction agent, the recommended dose of diazepam is 0.1 to 0.2 mg/kg. The local pain on injection intravenously has decreased its current use, along with the availability of other short-acting benzodiazepines (e.g., midazolam).

Midazolam

Midazolam is a water-soluble, short-acting benzodiazepine. Its chemical configuration confers a pH-dependent ring phenomenon. At pH 4, the diazepine ring opens, and a highly stable water-soluble compound results. At physiologic pH values, the ring closes and thereby increases the drug lipophilic activity. Cardiovascular stability, transient mild respiratory depression, minimal venous irritation, amnesia, and short duration of action are reasons why midazolam has replaced diazepam.

Midazolam is metabolized in the liver; less than 1% is excreted unchanged in the urine. Midazolam undergoes extensive metabolism (involving CYP3A4, CYP3A5, and CYP3A7) to a major hydroxylated form, 1-OH-midazolam. The protein binding of midazolam is extensive, with a free fraction of only 3% to 6%. Midazolam has an intermediate rate of absorption (0.5 to 1.5

hours) and a bioavailability of 30% to 50%. The terminal elimination phase ranges from 1 to 4 hours (Smith et al., 1981).

In children, the pharmacokinetics of midazolam have been reported. Payne et al. (1989) noted that in healthy children, midazolam administered at 0.15 mg/kg intravenously, the volume of distribution at steady state, the elimination half-life, and the clearance were 1.29 L/kg, 70 minutes, and 9.1 mL/kg per minute, respectively. Jones et al. (1993) have also reported on the kinetics of intravenous midazolam (0.5 mg/kg) in 12 healthy children and noted that the kinetics were consistent with a three-compartment model with a volume of distribution of 1.9 L/kg, $t_{1/2}\beta$ of 107 minutes, and a clearance of 15.4 mL/kg per minute. However, because the drug exhibits dose-related changes in clearance, comparisons between studies become difficult (Salonen et al., 1987). The kinetics of midazolam have also been determined after intramuscular, rectal, and oral administration. Payne et al. (1989) noted that times for peak serum concentrations after intramuscular, rectal, and oral administration were 15, 30, and 53 minutes, respectively, whereas the drug clearance and bioavailability via these three different routes were 10.4, 50.8, and 33.4 mL/kg per minute and 87%, 18%, and 27%, respectively. The lower bioavailability after oral or rectal administration is consistent with the commonly used oral dose of 0.5 mg/kg, which is almost five times higher than intravenous dosing.

In a study involving pediatric patients aged 6 months to 16 years, Reed et al. (2001) characterized the pharmacokinetic profile of both oral and intravenous midazolam using noncompartmental models. After oral administration, midazolam absorption was rapid, with adolescents absorbing the drug at half the rate seen in children younger than 12 years old. In young children, the volumes of distribution were larger; the largest volume of distribution was observed in children, whereas adolescents had a slower clearance and longer half-life after intravenous administration. There was great variability between patients in oral bioavailability, which averaged 36% (with a range of 9% to 71%) and in metabolism. An oral dose of 0.2 to 0.3 mg/kg was suggested as adequate in most children for sedation. The authors emphasized the importance of titrating intravenous dosing in the individual patient (Reed et al., 2001).

The pharmacokinetics of rectally administered midazolam in children were reported by Saint-Maurice and colleagues (1986). In this study of 16 children who were administered midazolam at 0.3 mg/kg, the terminal half-life and clearance were 106 minutes and 42.5 mL/kg per minute, respectively. Differences in the plasma clearance rates between pharmacokinetic studies involving rectal, oral, and intramuscular forms of administration were probably related to changes in drug bioavailability. Decreases in bioavailability increase the apparent drug clearance.

Commercially prepared solutions for oral midazolam are available. Literature on the pharmacokinetics and pharmacodynamics of oral midazolam has been hindered by the fact that studies have used different vehicles for administering the drug. Different vehicles affect drug absorption and, consequently, onset time and drug bioavailability (Brosius and Bannister, 2003). In addition, concurrent antacid use and grapefruit juice may increase the onset time and drug bioavailability of midazolam (Goho, 2001; Lammers et al., 2002).

Population studies involving the pharmacokinetics of midazolam in neonates have been reported. Using NONMEM and a two-compartment model, 531 midazolam concentrations from 187 infants were analyzed. The clearance and the central

volume were noted to be 70 ± 13 mL/kg per hour (or 1.02 mL/kg per minute) and 591 ± 65 mL/kg, respectively. Of interest was that the clearance was 1.6 times higher in full-term neonates with a gestational age of more than 39 weeks than in neonates of fewer than 39 weeks' gestation (Burtin et al., 1994).

The pharmacokinetics of midazolam in premature infants after both oral and intravenous administration were described by de Wildt and colleagues (2001, 2002). In premature infants with 24 to 34 weeks' gestational age and at 3 to 11 days of life, de Wildt et al. noted the apparent volume of distribution, clearance, and half-life were 1.1 L/kg, 1.8 mL/kg per minute, and 6.3 hours, respectively, after a single 0.1-mg/kg bolus dose. In addition, the metabolite 1-OH midazolam was markedly reduced compared with reports in older children. Also of note was that in those infants exposed to indomethacin, midazolam clearance was increased (Fig. 7-21) (de Wildt et al., 2001).

In a separate study of preterm infants who were administered oral midazolam, de Wildt et al. (2002) noted that midazolam clearance was markedly decreased and that the bioavailability was 0.4. The decrease in clearance was thought to mirror the pattern of CYP3A4 intestinal and hepatic activity (de Wildt et al., 2002). The kinetics of midazolam are affected by the use of extracorporeal membrane oxygenation (ECMO); Mulla et al. (2003) noted that the volume of distribution and half-life of midazolam are significantly increased in neonates requiring ECMO.

The cardiovascular and respiratory effects of midazolam have been reported in adults. Midazolam decreases systolic and diastolic blood pressures by 5% to 10%, decreases systemic vascular resistance by 15% to 30%, and increases heart rate by 20%. Right- and left-sided filling pressures are usually unaffected. Reeves et al. (1979) observed that 0.2 mg/kg midazolam was a safe agent for induction of anesthesia in patients with compromised myocardial function. In healthy patients, no significant difference was found in the hemodynamic effects of induction doses of 0.25 mg/kg midazolam and 4 mg/kg thiopental (Lebowitz et al., 1982).

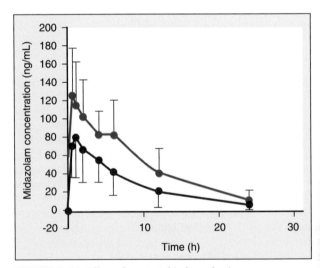

■ **FIGURE 7-21.** Effect of postnatal indomethacin exposure on midazolam disposition in preterm infants. Midazolam concentration vs. time curve after a single intravenous dose (0.1 mg/kg) to preterm infants with (n = 11, open circles) and without (n = 13, solid circles) postnatal indomethacin exposure. Each dot represents mean ± SD concentration at each time point. *(Redrawn from de Wildt SN et al.: Pharmacokinetics and metabolism of intravenous medazolam in preterm infants, Clin Pharmacol Ther 70:525-531, 2001.)*

Respiratory depression is commonly associated with midazolam administration, and this respiratory depression is poorly related to dose, not reversed by naloxone, and independent of the rate of administration of the drug (Forster et al., 1983; Alexander and Gross, 1988; Alexander et al., 1992).

As an intravenous induction agent in children, midazolam in doses as high as 0.6 mg/kg was not as reliable as thiopental (Salonen et al., 1987). The most common pediatric use for intravenous midazolam other than as an anesthetic adjunct has been its use as a sedative for intensive care patients. Rosen and Rosen (1991) demonstrated the usefulness of continuous midazolam in critically ill pediatric patients. In their retrospective report of patients sedated for 4 to 72 hours who received a slow intravenous bolus (0.25 mg/kg) followed by a continuous infusion at 0.4 to 4 mg/kg per hour, they noted that all of their patients were adequately sedated, their patients' oxygen consumption was significantly reduced, and enteral feedings were successful in all of those in whom it was attempted. However, others have noted reversible neurologic abnormalities associated with prolonged intravenous midazolam infusions (Engstrom and Cohen, 1989; Sury et al., 1989; Bergman et al., 1991).

Even with the extensive experience of intravenous midazolam in adult patients and volunteers, most of the pediatric experience with midazolam is derived from its use as a preanesthetic medication delivered via the intramuscular, oral, rectal, intranasal, and sublingual routes of administration. More than 85% of anesthesiologists responding to a survey of premedication practices indicated that they prescribe midazolam (Kain et al., 1997). In children, midazolam has been shown to produce tranquil and calm sedation, reduce separation anxiety, facilitate induction of anesthesia, and enhance antegrade amnesia (Twersky et al., 1993). Kain et al. (2000) have shown that 0.5 mg/kg of oral midazolam can produce significant anterograde amnesia at 10 and 20 minutes and anxiolysis as early as 15 minutes after administration. Numerous studies have documented the efficacy of orally administered midazolam (Feld et al., 1990; Weldon et al., 1992; Levine et al., 1993b). The appropriate dose appears to range between 0.5 and 1 mg/kg. Its time of onset ranges from 15 to 30 minutes. Oral midazolam can also be safely administered to children with cyanotic heart disease without affecting oxygen saturation (Levine et al., 1993a). Serious side effects of midazolam are uncommon. However, several postoperative behavioral problems (fearfulness, nightmares, food rejection) were observed in children premedicated with oral midazolam (0.5 mg/kg) (McGraw, 1993). Postoperative dysphoria and crying can be very difficult for families when it occurs; a duration of 15 to 20 minutes sounds short but may seem very long for those caring for such a child. In addition, McMillan et al. (1992) have noted loss of balance, dysphoria, and blurred vision in some patients receiving 0.75 and 1 mg/kg orally. Hiccups have been associated with midazolam administration via the rectal, nasal, and oral routes (Marhofer et al., 1999). One major disadvantage of oral midazolam is its bitter taste. It should be administered in a flavored syrup or drink; however, a commercially available liquid preparation is now available. Almenrader et al. (2007) reported that 14% of children refused oral midazolam in a study comparing oral clonidine with oral midazolam premedication. They also reported a trend toward an increased incidence of emergence agitation in the midazolam group, with parental satisfaction favoring clonidine. Alternatively, Ko et al. (2001) in a study of 88 children having outpatient surgery, reported a lower incidence of emergence agitation after a sevoflurane/N$_2$O/O$_2$ anesthetic when oral midazolam 0.2 mg/kg was given.

Oral midazolam has been associated with prolonged recovery times in some studies, but others, using BIS and measured end-tidal gases, did not find this problem (Viitanen et al., 1999; Brosius and Bannister 2001, 2002).

In a multicenter study involving 455 children, Coté et al. (2002) reported on the effectiveness of commercially prepared midazolam syrup. In this study, oral midazolam was effective for sedation and anxiolysis at a dose as low as 0.25 mg/kg. Doses as high as 1 mg/kg had minimal effects on respiration and oxygen saturation (Fig. 7-22).

Rectal administration of midazolam has also been successfully used to sedate patients. Saint-Maurice et al. (1986) have shown that after a dose of 0.3 mg/kg, a maximum plasma concentration of 100 ng/mL was achieved with levels of sedation as judged by mask acceptance, with patient cooperation being satisfactory in all 16 patients. Coventry et al. (1991), in a double-blind study of pediatric patients requiring sedation for computed tomography evaluations, noted that 0.3 and 0.6 mg/kg of rectal midazolam was ineffective in providing satisfactory sedation. Spear et al. (1991) noted that the optimum dose of rectal midazolam was 1 mg/kg and that doses of 0.3 mg/kg resulted in patient struggling during anesthesia induction.

Nasal and sublingual transmucosal routes of administration have also been used for midazolam preanesthesia medications. Wilton et al. (1988) and Davis et al. (1995) demonstrated the usefulness of preanesthetic sedation of preschool children with 0.2 to 0.3 mg/kg of intranasal midazolam. Walbergh et al. (1991) determined plasma concentrations after administration of 0.1 mg/kg of intranasal midazolam. In these patients, peak plasma concentrations of midazolam occurred within 10 minutes after its administration, with peak plasma concentrations ranging from 43 to 106 ng/mL. In this study, plasma midazolam concentrations exceeded threshold sedation values for adults (40 ng/mL) as early as 3 minutes after its nasal administration

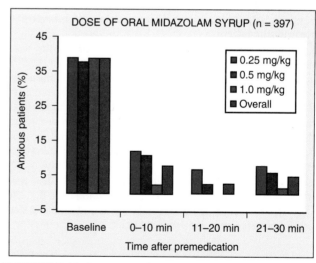

■ **FIGURE 7-22.** Percentage of patients exhibiting anxiety from baseline to time elapsed after administration of oral midazolam. There was a positive association between dose and onset of anxiolysis (P = 0.01); a larger proportion of children achieved satisfactory anxiolysis within 10 minutes at the higher doses. *(From Coté CJ et al.: A comparison of three doses of a commercially prepared oral midazolam syrup in children,* Anesth Analg *94:37, 2002.)*

and exceeded this level for as long as 30 minutes. Because intranasal midazolam can irritate the nasal mucosa, its use is limited by the volume of drug to be administered. The sublingual mucosa has a rich vascular supply and drugs are absorbed systemically, thereby eliminating hepatic first-pass metabolism. Karl et al. (1993), in a comparative study of intranasal and sublingual midazolam administration, demonstrated the two routes to be equally effective but that the sublingual route of administration had better patient acceptance.

Pandit et al. (2001) demonstrated that when aliquots of midazolam dissolved in strawberry syrup were placed on the anterosuperior aspect of the child's tongue, 0.2 mg of midazolam was effective in 95% of patients for parental separation. When midazolam was administered sublingually, Khalil et al. (1998) noted that in children aged 12 to 129 months who received either placebo or 1 of 3 doses of midazolam (with none of these children receiving placebo), 28% of those receiving 0.25 mg/kg, 52% of those receiving 0.5 mg/kg, and 64% of those receiving 0.75 mg/kg of midazolam showed satisfactory sedation (drowsy) 15 minutes after drug administration. Children receiving the two higher doses of midazolam (0.5 and 0.75 mg/kg) accepted mask induction willingly, whereas the group receiving 0.25 mg/kg resembled the placebo group.

Flumazenil

Flumazenil blocks the effects of benzodiazepines on the GABAergic inhibition pathway in the CNS. Flumazenil does not have significant agonist activity of its own and does not appear to reverse the effects of opioids. Flumazenil has a short duration of action. Its plasma half-life is between 0.7 and 1.3 hours. It is metabolized and cleared by the liver and excreted in the urine (Rocari et al., 1986). Adverse effects of flumazenil include nausea, vomiting, blurred vision, sweating, anxiety, and emotional lability. Serious adverse effects include seizures and cardiac dysrhythmias; these events have been associated with patients physically dependent on benzodiazepines, patients with epilepsy, and patients having taken multiple drug ingestions or overdoses. Clinical trials in adults suggest a use of flumazenil in reversing the effects of conscious sedation, general anesthesia in benzodiazepine overdose, and hepatic encephalopathy.

Use of flumazenil in pediatric patients has been related to clinical situations requiring benzodiazepine reversal in anesthesia and for the treatment of benzodiazepine overdose (Roald and Dohl, 1989; Jones et al., 1991). Doses of flumazenil varied between 0.005 and 0.1 mg/kg, with 0.01 mg/kg being the most commonly used dose. In a study of 107 children undergoing procedural sedation, Shannon et al. (1997) noted that a mean dose of 0.017 mg/kg of flumazenil was used to reverse a mean midazolam dose of 0.18 mg/kg. Because of its short half-life relative to the half-life of most benzodiazepines, resedation is a common finding after flumazenil use. Consequently, repeat administrations and careful patient observations are necessary (Jones et al., 1993).

Other Sedative Agents

Etomidate

Etomidate is a potent, short-acting, nonbarbiturate sedative-hypnotic agent without analgesic properties. After a single intravenous bolus injection, it has a rapid onset (5 to 15 seconds) with a peak effect at 60 seconds and a short duration of action (3 to 5 minutes) that is terminated by redistribution. It produces a central depressant effect through GABA mimetic action. Administered intravenously, it has been used for induction and maintenance of anesthesia; use for prolonged sedation in critically ill patients has become very uncommon because of steroid-synthesis effects. Little information is available about the use of etomidate in infants and small children.

Etomidate is metabolized in the liver. Only 2% of the drug appears unchanged in the urine. Etomidate causes little change in cardiovascular function in either healthy or compromised patients (Guldner et al., 2003). In a study of children with atrial septal defects (ASDs) undergoing cardiac catheterization, Sarkar et al. (2005) noted that induction doses of intravenous etomidate had no significant effect on the hemodynamics or on the shunt fraction. Myoclonic movements that are not associated with epileptiform electroencephalographic activity occur in 30% to 75% of patients after induction with etomidate (Ghonheim and Yamanda, 1977). Pain at the injection site is a common side effect. A new formulation of etomidate dissolved in a fat emulsion of medium and long-chain triglycerides is available. A study in children using this formulation reported a low incidence (5%) of pain at injection; however, a higher incidence of myoclonic movements (85%) is reported as well (Nyman et al., 2006).

Etomidate has both anticonvulsant and proconvulsant qualities. In patients with known seizure disorders, etomidate can produce epileptiform activity (Ebrahim et al., 1986; Modica et al., 1990). A major side effect limiting etomidate use is its suppression of adrenal steroid synthesis and reports of increased mortality after its use (Ledingham and Watt, 1983). Etomidate blocks adrenal steroid synthesis through inhibition of two mitochondrial enzymes dependent on CYP: cholesterol side-chain cleavage enzyme and 11β-hydroxylase (Wagner et al., 1984). The inhibition of steroid synthesis occurs with both prolonged continuous infusions and with single induction doses (Longnecker, 1984; Wagner and White, 1984). Dönmez et al. (1998) noted in a randomized prospective study of 30 children undergoing cardiopulmonary bypass that when etomidate (0.3 mg/kg) was used as an induction agent, it significantly suppressed the increased cortisol levels associated with the stress responses of surgery and cardiopulmonary bypass. In critically ill children a single bolus dose has shown impaired adrenal function associated with increased mortality (den Brinker et al., 2008). In adult trauma patients, single-dose etomidate administration for rapid-sequence intubation was associated with chemical evidence of adrenal suppression, increased length of stay in the intensive care unit (ICU), and an increased number of days using a ventilator (Hildreth et al., 2008). However, other studies of adults suggest that for ICU patients receiving etomidate for induction their clinical outcome and therapy were no different from patients induced with other sedative hypnotic agents (Ray and McKeown, 2007). For induction of anesthesia, the recommended intravenous dose is 0.3 to 0.4 mg/kg. Recent studies by Cotton et al. (2009) with an etomidate analog suggests that the analog undergoes ultra rapid metabolism, maintains the drug's sedative properties, and has no adrenal suppression. It is probably best to avoid etomidate use in patients with adrenally suppressed states.

Propofol

Propofol is an alkylphenol that is formulated in 10% soybean oil, 2.25% glycerol, and 12% purified egg phosphatide. This form of reconstitution is used because of anaphylactic reactions that occurred when propofol was reconstituted with polyethoxylated castor oil (Cremophor-EL). The rapid redistribution and metabolism of propofol result in a short duration of action and allow for the drug to be administered via repeated injections or continuous infusions with minimal accumulation. Kinetic studies in both adults and children reveal a drug with a large steady-state volume of distribution, a slow elimination half-life, and a rapid clearance. Glucuronidation of propofol is a major route of elimination. Uridine 5-diphosphate-glucuronosyltransferases (UGTs) are the drug metabolizing enzymes for phase II. Extrahepatic metabolism of propofol occurs, and at these extrahepatic sites, conjugation is governed by different exons than in the liver (Takahashi, 2008). Mutations in these locations can markedly affect glucuronidation. In radiolabeled isotope studies, 88% of the radioactivity is excreted in the urine, 2% is excreted in the feces, and the remainder is excreted as 1- and 4-glucuronides and 4-sulfate conjugates. In patients with hepatic and renal impairments, no statistically significant alterations occur in the pharmacokinetics. Because the clearance of the drug exceeds the capacity of the liver blood supply, extrahepatic sites of metabolism appear to be involved with the clearance of propofol. These extrahepatic sites of metabolism were suggested in studies of patients undergoing liver transplantation where metabolic products of propofol metabolism were produced when propofol was administered only during the anhepatic phase of the operation. The effect of fentanyl on propofol clearance is not clear. In studies by Cockshott et al. (1987), fentanyl decreased propofol clearance, whereas in other studies, no effect was noted (Saint-Maurice et al., 1989; Gill et al., 1990).

Another important aspect of propofol pharmacokinetics is that the drug can limit its own clearance. Propofol is eliminated by hepatic conjugation to inactive metabolites, which are excreted by the kidneys. A 2-mg/kg bolus dose of propofol for the induction of anesthesia can reduce blood flow to the liver by 14%. Bolus doses of propofol may cause a small but persistent change in blood flow to the liver, resulting in decreased clearance and higher-than-predicted plasma concentrations.

The pharmacokinetics of propofol in children have been described by numerous investigators (Saint-Maurice et al., 1989; Jones et al., 1990; Marsh et al., 1991; Kataria et al., 1994; Knibbe et al., 2002; Zuppa et al., 2003). In computer-controlled infusions of propofol in children younger than 10 years, Marsh et al. (1991) noted the volume of the central compartment to be 0.34 L/kg and the clearance of the drug to be 34.3 mL/kg per minute. Kataria et al. (1994) using three different pharmacokinetic modeling approaches, analyzed the kinetics of single-bolus and continuous infusions of propofol in children. In all three models, the pharmacokinetics were well described by a three-compartment model with a central compartment of 0.52 L/kg and a clearance of 34 mL/kg per minute.

The pharmacokinetics of propofol were studied in a small number of children after cardiac surgery. When propofol was used to provide sedation for 6 hours, Knibbe et al. (2002), using population kinetics, reported propofol to fit a two-compartment model with a clearance of 35 mL/kg per minute and a central compartment of 0.78 L/kg. In addition, the authors suggested that children may have a lower pharmacodynamic sensitivity to propofol in that higher plasma concentrations were needed to maintain sedation than those reported in adults.

The pharmacodynamics of propofol have been well described and reviewed (Shafer, 1993). Because of the pharmacokinetic properties of propofol, infusions allow for more rapid decreases

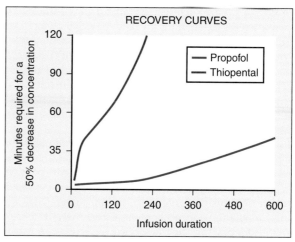

■ FIGURE 7-23. Curves showing time required for 50% decreases in propofol and thiopental concentrations after discontinuation of a continuous infusion. *(From Shafer SL: Advances in propofol pharmacokinetics and pharmacodynamics,* J Clin Anesth *5:14S, 1993.)*

in plasma concentrations and faster patient recoveries from anesthesia (Fig. 7-23) (Mirakhur, 1988; Borgeat et al., 1990; Watcha et al., 1991; Larsson et al., 1992; Lebovic et al., 1992; Nightingale and Lewis, 1992; Reimer et al., 1993; Shafer, 1993). One of the newer pharmacokinetic terms is *context-sensitive half-life,* used to describe the time to decrease drug concentration by 50% after variable infusion durations. Such values can show how long a drug's effects may persists after discontinuing infusions, based on how long it has been infused. McFarlan et al. (1999) reported a propofol infusion simulation to keep blood concentration of propofol at 3 mcg/mL in children aged 3 to 11 years. After a bolus of 2.5 mg/kg, infusions rates were 250 mcg/kg per minute for 15 minutes, then 216 mcg/kg per minute for 15 minutes, 183 mcg/kg per minute for 30 minutes, 166 mcg/kg per minute for 1 hour, and 150 mcg/kg per minute for the second and fourth hours. The predicted context-sensitive half-life in children was 10.4 minutes (for a 1-hour infusion) to 19.6 minutes (4-hour infusion), compared with values of 6.7 to 9.5 minutes in adults. Engelhardt et al. (2008) prospectively used this changing infusion schema to reach predicted propofol concentrations in 17 healthy children between 1 and 6 years of age. They found concentrations were higher than predicted in the first 30 minutes (7.1 mcg/mL vs. 6.6 mcg/mL) but the differences at 30, 50, and 70 minutes were not significant and no child needed rescue doses of propofol.

In general, with induction doses of propofol, blood pressure decreases, as does systemic vascular resistance. Changes in heart rate are variable, and cardiac output decreases slightly. In studies evaluating propofol requirements for induction of anesthesia in children, Manschot et al. (1992) noted that in children aged 3 to 15 years receiving 5 mcg/kg of alfentanil to reduce the pain of propofol injection, age-related differences in propofol requirements were demonstrated. In children aged 10 to 15 years, 1.5 mg/kg of propofol was sufficient to induce sleep, whereas in children aged 3 to 9 years, a dose of 2.5 mg/kg was needed. In a study by Hannallah et al. (1991) in which alfentanil was not administered, the ED_{50} and ED_{95} for loss of eyelash reflex were 1.3 and 2 mg/kg, whereas the ED_{50} and ED_{95} for induction of anesthesia were 1.5 and 2.3 mg/kg, respectively. Westrin (1991), in a study of infants aged 1 to 6 months and children aged 10 to 16 years, noted that the ED_{50} of propofol was 3 mg/kg for infants and 2.4 mg/kg for the older children. In all three of these studies, propofol was administered over 10 to 30 seconds. However, as with most hypnotic agents, propofol also demonstrates a rate-dependent induction. Stokes and Hutton (1991) demonstrated that with the use of slower infusion rates, induction time for anesthesia increases but smaller doses could be used.

Peeters et al., (2006) studied propofol pharmacokinetics and pharmacodynamics in unventilated infants after craniofacial surgery. Twenty-two infants, aged 1 month to 2 years, received propofol at 33 to 66 mcg/kg per minute in the ICU, based on Comfort-B scores and bispectral index (BIS) monitoring. Population kinetic analysis using NONMEM showed propofol kinetics was best described by a two-compartment model. Body weight was a significant covariate (i.e., use of body weight made the model fit the measured concentrations more closely). Clearance was 0.169 L/min (or 77 mL/min per kilogram), steady-state volume of distribution 144 L (or 16.1 L/kg) and central volume 20.3 L (or 2.3 L/kg). These values are much higher than those reported in children receiving ventilation. The importance of dose titration was emphasized by the great interpatient variability in propofol effect on Comfort-B scores or BIS readings.

In patients with congenital heart disease, Gozal et al. (2001) demonstrated that despite lower systemic and pulmonary pressures, propofol did not modify the characteristics of the patient's underlying intracardiac shunts.

In normal children aged 1 to 6 years, Karsli et al. (2002), using transcranial Doppler, noted that propofol decreases cerebral blood flow velocity and that there is a relationship between cerebral blood flow velocity and propofol dosing. In addition, Wilson-Smith et al. (2003) noted that in healthy children who were given propofol for their elective surgery, the effects of nitrous oxide on cerebral blood flow velocity were preserved.

In addition to its anesthetic action, propofol appears to have antiemetic properties. In adult patients, Borgeat et al. (1992) demonstrated that 10 mg of propofol administered in the recovery room was effective in reducing the incidence of nausea and vomiting. Watcha et al. (1991) noted that in pediatric patients undergoing strabismus surgery, propofol alone effectively decreased the incidence of postoperative emesis (23%) compared with a similar group of patients anesthetized with halothane and nitrous oxide and supplemented with prophylactic droperidol (50%). However, in patients who received propofol and nitrous oxide, Watcha et al. (1991) noted that the incidence of emesis increased significantly (60%). Weil et al. (1993) also noted the antiemetic effect in pediatric patients with strabismus who were anesthetized with propofol and nitrous oxide compared with patients anesthetized with halothane and nitrous oxide. This antiemetic effect of propofol was even more pronounced in patients who received no opioids. Reimer et al. (1993) noted no difference in the incidence of emesis between pediatric patients undergoing strabismus repair who were anesthetized with halothane and nitrous oxide and those receiving propofol in oxygen or propofol with nitrous oxide. Differences between studies with regard to the antiemetic effect of propofol may be a function of the basic design of each study. Variations in premedications, opioid administration, and postoperative fluid intake may be factors that make comparisons of the studies difficult.

The antiemetic effects of propofol have also been demonstrated in pediatric patients undergoing short ear, nose, and throat surgical procedures and ambulatory surgical procedures (Borgeat et al., 1990; Martin et al., 1993).

In patients undergoing radiofrequency ablation, a procedure that is associated with an incidence of emesis as high as 60%, Erb et al. (2002) noted that propofol-based anesthesia was associated with a markedly decreased incidence of nausea (21%) and emesis (6%) compared with rates of nausea and vomiting of 63% and 55%, respectively, in children anesthetized with isoflurane.

Side effects from propofol include tolerance to the drug, pain on injection, spontaneous excitatory movements, and anaphylactic reactions. Tolerance has been reported in a pediatric patient undergoing numerous exposures for radiation therapy (Deer and Rich, 1992). Pain from injection is a common problem with propofol administration and may be related to the size of the vein in which it is administered. Westrin (1991) noted that pain during the injection occurred more often in the infants (50%) than in the older children (18%). The addition of 5 to 15 mcg/kg of alfentanil, 1% lidocaine (1 mg), or 0.1 mg/kg lidocaine can markedly attenuate the pain on injection (Valtonen et al., 1989; Manschot et al., 1992; Kwak et al., 2009). The addition of thiopental and the use of inhaled nitrous oxide also have been shown to attenuate the pain on injection (Beh et al., 2002; Cox, 2002).

Involuntary motor movements have been associated with propofol, and these spontaneous movement disorders appear to occur in the absence of epileptic form activity on electroencephalography (Borgeat et al., 1993; Reynolds and Koh, 1993). Anaphylactic reactions have also been reported. Initial studies with propofol using 10% polyethoxylated castor oil as a solubilizing agent had reported instances of anaphylactic reactions (Briggs et al., 1982). Laxenaire et al. (1992) have reported on 14 patients with life-threatening reactions within minutes after receiving propofol in its current preparation. In some patients, these anaphylactic reactions occurred during the patient's first exposure to propofol.

Because of its lipid base, propofol has been associated with bacterial growth and patient infection if strict aseptic techniques during handling are not observed. Because of patient safety concerns, 0.005% ethylenediaminetetraacetate (EDTA) or metabisulfite was added to the formulation by different manufacturers. In a study comparing propofol with and without EDTA, Cohen et al. (2001) noted no differences in clinical profiles between the two drugs and noted that both formulations lower ionized calcium without any apparent clinical effect.

A major concern with propofol administration is the development of the propofol infusion syndrome (PRIS). PRIS has been defined as arrhythmias during the infusion plus one or more of the following: lipemic plasma, hepatomegaly, metabolic acidosis with or without an increase in serum lactate, or rhabdomyolysis with myoglobinuria. The occurrence of death in infants, children, and adults has raised concerns regarding the safety of propofol infusions for ICU-patient sedations. The pathogenesis of PRIS is unclear. Proposed mechanisms include enzyme block steps in mitochondrial fatty acid oxidation and inhibition of β-adrenergic receptors and calcium channel function. The rare occurrence of PRIS suggests a genetic susceptibility. PRIS is associated with concomitant catecholamine and steroid administration and high-dose infusion. Although monitoring of biochemical markers has been proposed to detect the development of PRIS, it may result in a false sense of security (Veldhoen et al., 2009).

Ketamine

Ketamine is a racemic, nonbarbiturate cyclohexamine derivative that produces dissociation of the cerebral cortex from the limbic system. Ketamine appears to block afferent impulses in the diencephalon and associated pathways of the cortex, sparing the reticular formation of the brain stem. This may be the mechanism of its action. It may also act on the brain stem (Domino et al., 1965). There is often electroencephalographic seizure activity, particularly in the limbic system and cortex, without clinical manifestations (Schwartz et al., 1974). Clinically, a ketamine anesthetic produces effective sedation and analgesia, but patients may keep their eyes open. Many reflexes are preserved. Preservation of gag reflex, laryngeal irritability, and continued muscle tension occur. Intravenous doses of 2 mg/kg produce a highly predictable response in children. On a milligram-per-kilogram basis, the amount of ketamine required to prevent gross movements is four times greater in infants younger than 6 months than in 6-year-old children (Lockhart and Nelson, 1974).

White et al. (1980) compared both the l- and d-isomers of ketamine in adult surgical patients with respect to the efficacy and side effects of these isomers. In this study, they noted that the d-isomer produced the most satisfactory anesthetic state and the lowest incidence of negative emergence reactions, whereas the l-isomer produced the least satisfactory anesthesia and the highest incidence of emergence reactions.

The pharmacokinetics of ketamine in patients of different ages were determined (Table 7-8). In infants younger than 3 months old, the volume of distribution was similar to that in older infants but the elimination half-life was prolonged. Clearance was reduced in the younger infants; reduced metabolism and renal excretion in the young infant are the likely causes. Ketamine is metabolized in the liver, and its major metabolite is norketamine. Norketamine has about 30% of the clinical activity of ketamine.

In the anesthetic state associated with ketamine, respiration and blood pressure are usually well maintained. The use of ketamine in infants, particularly at the high doses required for lack of movement, has been associated with respiratory depression and apnea (Eng et al., 1975). Generalized extensor spasm with opisthotonos also has been seen in infants (Radney and Badola, 1973). In addition, acute increases in pulmonary artery pressure have occasionally occurred in infants with congenital heart disease during ketamine anesthesia for cardiac catheterization. Studies suggest that pulmonary vascular resistance is not changed by ketamine in infants with either normal or elevated pulmonary vascular resistance, as long as the airway and ventilation are maintained (Hickey et al., 1984; Morray et al., 1984). In a study of 60 children with congenital heart disease randomized to receive propofol infusion or propofol with ketamine 0.5 mg/kg during cardiac catheterization, Akin et al. (2005) reported that hypotension and bradycardia were higher in the group that received propofol alone. Williams et al. (2007) studied ketamine 2 mg/kg bolus over 5 minutes followed by infusion at 10 mcg/kg per minute in 15 children with pulmonary hypertension having cardiac catheterization with sevoflurane (1 MAC decreased to 0.5 MAC after ketamine) and spontaneous ventilation. No changes in pulmonary artery pressure or resistance index were found.

The mechanism of cardiorespiratory stimulation has not been entirely clarified. Dowdy and Kaya (1968), Traber et al. (1970), and other groups have shown that there is a direct negative inotropic action on the denervated heart. In the presence of intact sympathetic and autonomic nervous systems, however, a pressor effect causes increased blood pressure, heart rate, and cardiac output, a response present in all ages. This serves as a most valuable adjunct in the management of poor-risk patients but is a contraindication in the presence of hypertension or tachycardia. In their investigation of ketamine, Dowdy and Kaya (1968) also found evidence of antiarrhythmic activity.

Ketamine increases cerebrospinal fluid pressure significantly for 5 to 15 minutes, but as shown by Dawson et al. (1971), the increase may be held within acceptable limits by pretreatment with thiopental (Gardner et al., 1971; Lockhart and Jenkins, 1972). Elevation of intraocular pressure also occurs after ketamine administration. In a group of 15 children, Yoshikawa and Murai (1971) noted an average increase of 30% that was maximum within 15 minutes after administration of ketamine and evident for approximately 30 minutes. In addition to the elevation of intraocular pressure, nystagmus limits its usefulness in eye surgery.

Ketamine had the advantage of a clean record with no known toxic effects on the liver, kidneys, or other organ systems. However, it has been the most thoroughly studied anesthetic/sedative agent implicated in causing neuronal apoptosis after exposure in newborn animal model studies.

A major drawback to ketamine administration in older children is the high incidence of hallucinations and bad dreams. In adults, this occurs in 30% to 50% of patients, and in prepubescent children, the incidence is noted at 5% to 10%. Hallucinations were uncommon in children, but the awakening phase may entail considerable excitement (Wilson et al., 1970).

Ketamine can be administered orally, and part of its effect is secondary to its metabolite norketamine. Gutstein and colleagues (1992) compared oral premedication with ketamine at either 3 or 6 mg/kg. With 3 mg/kg, 73% of the children were sedated within 30 minutes. At the 6 mg/kg dose, 100% of the patients were sedated, and 67% tolerated intravenous cannulation. Onset times for the 3- and 6-mg/kg dose groups were 19.6 and 11.2 minutes, respectively (Gutstein et al., 1992).

Use of low-dose ketamine as an analgesic adjunct has emerged in select populations in recent work. Aouad et al. (2008) conducted a prospective randomized double-blind comparison of propofol alone (1 mg/kg) to propofol and ketamine (0.5 mg/kg of each) in 63 children undergoing anesthesia for oncologic procedures. The combination group had fewer patients needing rescue propofol (83% vs. 100%) or fentanyl (43% vs. 75%) and showed more stable hemodynamics. However, 40% of the

TABLE 7-8. Pharmacokinetics of Ketamine: Effect of Age

Age	$t_{1/2}\beta$ (min)	$V_d$ss (L/kg)	CL (mL/min per kg)
<3 Months	184.7	3.46	12.9
4-12 Months	65.1	3.03	35.0
4 Years	31.6	1.18	25.1
Adult	107.3	0.75	20.0

Modified from Lake CL: *Pediatric anesthesia*, East Norwalk, CT, 1988, Appleton & Lange.

$t_{1/2}\beta$ Elimination half-life; $V_d$ss, volume of distribution at steady state; CL, clearance.

combination group had agitation during recovery (vs. 6% with propofol alone). Slavik and Zed (2007) reviewed studies of ketamine and propofol for procedural sedation and anesthesia using MEDLINE, EMBASE, and the Cochrane databases and found eight clinical trials to include. They found that the ideal ratio of ketamine to propofol was unclear; better clinical efficacy of the combination over propofol alone was not shown; better hemodynamic and respiratory status was demonstrated in some studies; and at higher ketamine doses, greater adverse effects were apparent (Slavik and Zed, 2007).

Several investigators have studied low dose-ketamine given intravenously or into the tonsillar bed in children undergoing tonsillectomy with conflicting results (O'Flaherty et al., 2003; Conceicao et al., 2006; Batra et al., 2007; Dal et al., 2007; Erk et al., 2007; Abu-Shahwan, 2008; Honarmand et al., 2008). Most studies involved 60 to 100 children and compared the perioperative course looking at pain scores, rescue analgesics, and side effects compared with patients in a control group (receiving saline). Ketamine at doses less than 0.25 mg/kg were ineffective, and at 0.5 mg/kg results were positive in some studies and negative in others. The addition of low-dose ketamine infusions in 11 children with advanced cancer and pain that was inadequately treated with high doses of opiates (0.1 to 0.2 mg/kg per hour titrated up to 0.5 mg/kg per hour in 3 of 11 patients) improved pain control and allowed decreases in opiate pain medications in 8 (Finkel et al., 2007).

Clonidine

Clonidine is an α_2-adrenergic agonist that has been used as a premedication, anesthetic adjunct, extender for postoperative analgesic duration, and to prolong the analgesia associated with regional anesthetic blocks. In one prospective, randomized, blinded study, 60 children (aged 5 to 11 years) received placebo, 2 mcg/kg or 4 mcg/kg oral clonidine 100 minutes before inhalation induction of anesthesia with halothane/N_2O/O_2 (Nishina et al., 1996). Sedation, separation from family, and tolerance to mask application were better in the 4 mcg/kg clonidine group. Halothane was titrated to maintain blood pressure and heart rate within 20% of baseline, and the 4-mcg/kg group used 45% less halothane. No delay in transfer to ward postoperatively was found (15 to 17 minutes). Heart rates were slower in the group receiving 4 mcg/kg, but bradycardia did not occur, although all children received atropine 30 mcg/kg with the premedication.

Bergendahl et al., (2006) reviewed clonidine use in pediatric anesthesia both as premedication and for intraoperative use. Rectal absorption is rapid, and clonidine shows high bioavailability. Some studies included in this review found improved postoperative analgesia with oral clonidine, decreased vomiting, and shivering. Postoperative confusion and agitation in young children receiving clonidine compared with children receiving placebo or midazolam was reported by some. Persistence of postoperative sedation (or calmness) is a desirable feature to some assessors.

Addition of clonidine to local anesthetics for caudal blocks has been successful in extending duration of analgesia in most studies, although some increases in side effects have occurred in some studies. Two case reports of caudal blocks with clonidine in formerly premature infants with the appearance of postoperative apnea have limited its use in this population.

Atropine use is often recommended to minimize heart rate decreases, and this extra step may be a partial explanation for the lack of more extensive use of this agent.

Potts et al. (2007) recently reported a population analysis of clonidine in children using NONMEM and reporting their results using allometric scaling (to a standard of 70 kg). Published data from four studies (two intravenous, one rectal, and one epidural clonidine) were combined with an open-label group of children who received clonidine 1 to 2 mcg/kg after cardiac surgery (380 observations). The mean age was 4 years, and the mean weight was 17.8 kg. Clearance was 14.6 L/hr per 70 kg, central volume was 62.5 L/70 kg, and peripheral volume was 119 L/70 kg with the distribution half-life of 12 minutes and elimination half-life of 9 hours. At birth, clearance was low at 3.8 L/hr per 70 kg, reaching 82% of adult values by age 1 year. Absorption was slower from epidural sites than the rectum (Fig. 7-24; Table 7-9). Simulations showed context-sensitive half-lives increased with infusion duration (1, 3, 6, and 10 hours) and decreased with increasing age (Table 7-10). The relatively long elimination half-life and importance of intact renal function for clearance may be features explaining the current preference for the newer α_2-agonist dexmedetomidine.

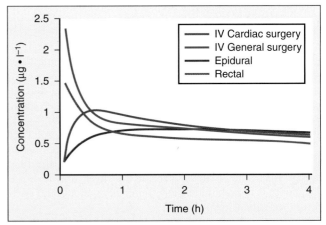

■ **FIGURE 7-24.** Typical time-concentration profiles for a 5-year-old child (20 kg) given intravenous, epidural, and rectal clonidine (2.5 mcg/kg^{-1}). *(From Potts AL et al.: Clonidine disposition in children: a population analysis,* Pediatr Anesth *17:924, 2007.)*

TABLE 7-9. Age-Related Clonidine Clearances Described Using Both the Allometric "¾ Power" Model (70 kg^{-1}) and the Linear per Kilogram Models (kg^{-1})*

Age	Weight (kg)	CL$_{std}$ (L/h^{-1}/70 kg^{-1})	CL (L/h^{-1}/kg^{-1})
0	3.5	3.83	0.116
1 Month	4.5	4.93	0.140
3 Months	6	6.80	0.180
6 Months	7.5	8.96	0.224
1 Year	10	12.0	0.278
2 Years	12	13.9	0.310
4 Years	16	14.6	0.273
10 Years	30	14.6	0.258

From Potts AL et al.: Clonidine disposition in children: a population analysis, *Pediatr Anesth* 17:924, 2007.

*Residual errors were similar between data from children undergoing cardiac surgery (additive error 0.02 mcg/L^{-1}, proportional error 0.09%) and those undergoing general surgery (additive error 0.03 mcg/L^{-1}, proportional error 0.11%).

TABLE 7-10. Changes in Context-Sensitive Half-Life with Age after an Infusion of 0.3 mcg/kg^{-1}/h^{-1}

	1 Hour	3 Hours	6 Hours	10 Hours
Neonate	8	10.75	11.5	11.75
3 Months	5.5	8	8.25	8.5
6 Months	4.25	6.5	7	7.25
1 Year	3.3	5.25	6	6.25
5 Years	2.8	5.25	6	6.25
10 Years	2.75	5.75	6.25	6.75
Adult	2.5	6.5	7.5	8.25

From Potts AL et al.: Clonidine disposition in children: a population analysis, *Pediatr Anesth* 17:924, 2007.

Dexmedetomidine

One of the newer additions to the list of intravenous sedative and anesthetic drugs is dexmedetomidine. It is a selective α_2-agonist with sedative and analgesic properties. Dexmedetomidine is more selective for the α_2-adrenoreceptor with a reported ratio of α_2 to α_1 of 1600:1, which is seven to eight times higher than that reported for clonidine. Its sedative effect is attributed to hyperpolarization of noradrenergic neurons in the locus coeruleus (Carollo et al., 2008). This suppression of locus coeruleus neurons is similar to normal sleep. It provides respiratory stability, with no ventilatory depression accompanying its sedative, anxiolytic, and analgesic effects in adults. Mahmoud et al. (2009) have shown dexmedetomidine to be a useful anesthetic agent for magnetic resonance imaging (MRI) evaluations of airways in children with obstructive sleep apnea (OSA). Although hemodynamic effects of hypotension or bradycardia are less commonly seen than with clonidine, they have been reported. Dexmedetomidine has also been suggested as a novel treatment for atrial and junctional tachyarrhythmias (Chrysostomou et al., 2008). Tobias and Berkenbosch (2004) reported early experience with dexmedetomidine infusions in 30 ventilated infants and children, comparing it with midazolam. Decreases in morphine use were found in the high-dose dexmedetomidine group (0.5 mcg/kg per hour) compared with those receiving midazolam (0.1 mg/kg per hour). Heart rates were slower in the dexmedetomidine group, but hypotension was not seen. In pediatric cardiac surgical patients, Chrysostomou et al. (2009) suggest that higher doses may be needed in the younger patients.

In neurosurgeries requiring an intraoperative "awake" period to assess patient responses during deep brain stimulation for Parkinson's disease, or in surgeries near speech areas, or in surgery for epilepsy, dexmedetomidine has proved very useful to allow anesthesia without intubation (Mack et al., 2004).

Koroguli et al. (2005) noted that in children aged 1 to 7 years undergoing MRI that dexmedetomidine was superior to midazolam. However, in a separate study, Koroguli et al. (2006), also noted that dexmedetomidine has slower recovery and discharge compared with propofol. The slower recovery times with dexmedetomidine compared with propofol have also been observed by Heard and others (2008).

Hammer and colleagues (2008) reported dexmedetomidine effects on cardiac electrophysiology in 12 children (aged 5 to 17 years). One mcg/kg administered over 10 minutes and then 0.7 mcg/kg per hour for 10 minutes led to decreased heart rates, increased blood pressure, and depressed sinus and atrioventricular (AV) node function. Respiratory rate and end-tidal CO_2 during spontaneous ventilation were unchanged (Hammer et al., 2008). Caution in dexmedetomidine use for patients who are poorly tolerant of bradycardia or at risk for AV nodal block was emphasized. Jooste and others (2010) demonstrated in post-cardiac transplant patients that a rapid IV bolus dose had a transient increase in systemic and pulmonary pressures, as well as a decrease in heart rate. These transient changes were more pronounced in the systemic system as opposed to the pulmonary circulation.

Because dexmedetomidine has pharmacolytic properties that simulate normal sleep, Mahmoud et al. (2009) have demonstrated its usefulness in patients with sleep apnea.

Pharmacokinetics for dexmedetomidine in adults demonstrate desirable characteristics for use as titrated intravenous infusions for sedation and anxiolysis. Its elimination half-life is 2 hours (8 hour for clonidine), and its distribution half-life is 6 minutes (Carollo et al., 2008). Several groups have reported pharmacokinetics in children of dexmedetomidine. Petroz et al. (2006) studied 36 children, 18 from Canada and 18 from South Africa, in an open-label study. Blood was sampled for 24 hours after 10-minute infusions of 2, 4, or 6 mcg/kg per hour and analyzed by NONMEM. Concentrations were below detection after 6 hours; a two-compartment model central volume of distribution of 0.8 L/kg was constructed with a systemic clearance of 0.013 L/kg per minute and an elimination half-life of 110 minutes. Table 7-11 lists the pharmacokinetic values from this and other studies; a puzzling finding was dexmedetomidine concentrations that were consistently 30% higher in Canadian

TABLE 7-11. Dexmedetomidine Pharmacokinetic Studies

Author	N	Age	Analysis	CL mL/min/kg	V$_d$ L/kg	t$_{1/2}$β (min)	Protein Binding
Petroz	36	2-12 yr	Population	13	1	110	92.6% (n=11)
Vilo	8	<2 yr	Traditional	17.4	3.8 1.2	139	
	8	2-11 yr		17.3		96	
Potts	45	4d-14 yr	Population	7.8-13.6	0.97		
Diaz	10	4 mo-7.9 yr	Traditional	9.5	1.53	159	

Data from Petroz GC, Sikich N, James M et al.: A phase 1, two-center study of the pharmacokinetics and pharmacodynamics of dexmedetomidine in children, *Anesthesiol* 105:1098, 2006; Vilo S, Rautiainen P, Kaisti K et al.: Pharmacokinetics of intravenous dexmedetomidine in children under 11 years of age, *Br J Anaesth* 100:697, 2008; Potts L, Warman GR, Anderson BJ: Dexmedetomidine disposition in children: a population analysis, *Pediatr Anesth* 18:722, 2008; Diaz SM, Rodarte A, Foley J: Pharamacokinetics of dexmedetomidine in postsurgical pediatric intensive care patients: preliminary study, *Ped Crit Care Med* 8:419-24, 2007.

children, which was thought to have occurred because of a handling problem with specimens. Context-sensitive decrement times did not increase after 90- to 120-minute infusions with the context-sensitive half-life, plateauing at about 70 minutes and the 80% decrement time at about 220 minutes. Heart rate and blood pressure decreased over the hour after the infusion and decreased with higher infusion doses, whereas respiration and oximetry were stable. Sedation lasted less than 1 hour. Vilo et al. (2008) studied eight children (aged 2 to 11 years) and eight infants (aged 1 to 23 months) after receiving dexmedetomidine at 1 mcg/kg. Analysis of blood samples used noncompartmental methods. Data are summarized in Table 7-11. Clearance was similar in the two age groups, but volume of distribution (steady state) was larger in the younger group, making the half-life longer. Interindividual variation was large, especially in the infants. All were sedated by the dexmedetomidine but easily aroused, and five of the eight children needed extra sedation during MRIs. Based on the volume at steady state, younger children would be predicted to need larger initial dexmedetomidine doses with similar maintenance rates to older children or adults.

Potts et al. (2008) looked at population pharmacokinetics in 45 children after cardiac surgery aged 4 days to 14 years (mean age of 3.4 years). Population parameter estimates for a two-compartment model using NONMEM were reported using allometric scaling to 70 kg. In Table 7-11 the results are corrected for comparison with others' work. Clearance increased from 15.5 L/hour per 70 kg at birth to reach 72% adult values at 6 months and 87% by 1 year (Table 7-12). Clearance in children at 39.2 L/hour per 70 kg is slightly less than adult values of 44.8 to 52.5 L/hour per 70 kg. Volumes of distribution were 103.5 to 126 L/70 kg, and half-lives were 12 minutes (α, distribution) and 2.3 hours (β, elimination), similar to adult reports. Context-sensitive half-lives after infusions of 1, 3, and 10 hours were longer in neonates (1.24 for 1 hour to 2.07 for 10 hours) than at age 1 year (0.49 to 1.09 hours) or in adults (0.49 to 1.45 hours). Large intersubject variability was attributed to age and size differences (Fig. 7-25).

In addition to intravenous administration, dexmedetomidine can also be administered intramuscularly and intranasally. Dyck et al. (1993) demonstrated a 73% bioavailability after intramuscular

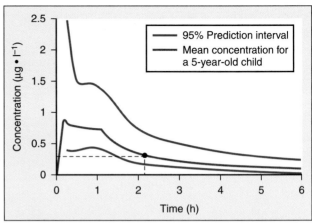

■ **FIGURE 7-25.** Simulated dexmedetomidine concentration-time profile after a dosage regimen of 1 mcg/kg^{-1} for 10 minutes and a maintenance infusion of 0.7 mcg/kg^{-1} per hour^{-1} for 50 minutes in a 5-year-old child (20 kg), with 95% prediction interval simulated using 1000 children with an age range of 2.4 to 14.5 years. Pharmacokinetic parameters for the simulation are those determined from this study. A concentration of 0.304 mcg/L^{-1} is associated with recovery from sedation (return to baseline alertness) and is represented by the dashed line. *(From Potts AL et al.: Dexmedetomidine disposition in children: a population analysis, Pediatr Anesth 18:722, 2008.)*

administration in adult volunteers and that intramuscular injection did not result in the biphasic hemodynamic response observed with intravenous administration. Intranasal doses of 1 to 2 mcg/kg have been shown to induce sedation in children (Yuen et al., 2007, 2008; Talon et al., 2009). Transmucosal dexmedetomidine has a bioavailability of 80% (Anttila et al., 2003).

In addition to its use as a sedative agent, dexmedetomidine has been demonstrated to decrease the incidence of postoperative emergence agitation and effectively treat postemergence shivering. Ibacache et al. (2004) noted that a single dose of dexmedetomidine (0.3 mcg/kg) markedly attenuated the incidence of sevoflurane-associated emergence agitation, while Easley et al. (2007) reported that 0.5 mcg/kg of dexmedetomidine effectively stopped postoperative shivering in children within 5 minutes.

OPIOIDS

To avoid the major adverse hemodynamic effects caused by potent inhalation anesthetic agents, the use of narcotic anesthesia has reemerged. Relative potencies of the various narcotics are listed in Table 7-13. Initially, meperidine (0.5 to 1 mg/kg

TABLE 7-12. Age-Related Dexmedetomidine Clearances Described Using Both the Allometric "¾ Power" Model (per 70 kg) and the Linear per Kilogram Model (per kg)

Age (years)	Weight (kg)	CL_{std} (L/h^{-1}/70 kg^{-1})	CL (L/h^{-1}/kg^{-1})
0	3.5	15.56	0.47
1 Months	4.5	18.10	0.51
3 Months	6	22.62	0.60
6 Months	7.5	28.45	0.71
1 Year	10	34.09	0.79
2 Years	12	37.58	0.83
3 Years	14	38.49	0.82
4 Years	16	38.83	0.80
8 Years	25	39.13	0.72
12 Years	38	39.18	0.65

From Potts AL et al.: Dexmedetomidine disposition in children: a population analysis, *Pediatr Anesth* 18:722, 2008.

TABLE 7-13. Comparative Opioid Potencies

Drug	Potency
Morphine	1
Methadone	1
Meperidine	0.1
Alfentanil	40
Fentanyl	150
Sufentanil	1500

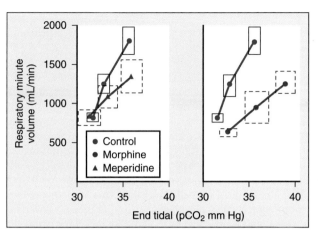

■ **FIGURE 7-26.** CO_2 response curves in infants after intramuscular injection of morphine or meperidine. *(From Way et al.: Respiratory sensitivity of the newborn infant to meperidine and morphine, Clin Pharmacol Ther 6:454, 1965.)*

and morphine (0.05 to 0.1 mg/kg) were used to reinforce nitrous oxide anesthesia in the neonate. However, concerns regarding the toxicity and increased sensitivity of neonates to narcotics were raised. Way et al. (1965) demonstrated that morphine depresses newborn respiration more than meperidine and that these decreases in ventilatory response to increased CO_2 concentrations occur at a dose one third (on a milligram-per-kilogram basis) of that administered to adults (Fig. 7-26). In laboratory animals, narcotics are more toxic to newborn animals than to older animals (Goldenthal, 1971). For morphine and dihydromorphine, the blood-brain barrier is more permeable in newborn animals than in older animals. The brain concentration of morphine several hours after injection was two to four times greater in brains of younger rats despite equal blood concentration (Fig. 7-27). This finding may be related to greater perfusion, to greater permeability, or to both in the

newborn. Whereas increased permeability of the blood-brain barrier (BBB) to morphine occurs in neonatal nonhuman primates (1 to 3 days after birth), the adult BBB permeability is achieved by two months of age (Lynn et al., 1991). Such developmentally increased permeability is not seen with meperidine; this is not surprising because the lipid solubility of meperidine is quite high (Kupferberg and Way, 1963).

Studies involving opiate receptor-binding sites in rats have suggested that changes in receptor ontogeny also may be responsible for the respiratory depressant and analgesic effects observed in newborns. Zhang and Pasternak (1981) have shown that both low-affinity and high-affinity opiate receptors are present in rats. Low-affinity receptors are associated with respiratory depression, whereas high-affinity receptors are associated with analgesia. In the rat model, low-affinity receptors are present in large numbers at birth, and the number remains constant through 18 days of life. By contrast, high-affinity receptors are scarce at birth and do not reach significant proportions (50% of the adult value) until 15 days of life. Respiratory depression in infants may be a function not only of the lipophilicity of opioids but also of the maturational changes in the opiate receptor pool. In addition to age-related changes in opioid receptor pools, genetic factors may affect the μ-opioid receptor (OPRM1). Single nucleotide polymorphisms (SNPs) resulting in a single amino-acid change can have effects on opioid side effects and analgesia. Individuals homozygous for the G allele of the 118 A > G polymorphism seem to require higher doses of intravenous and oral morphine to achieve adequate levels of analgesia (Matthes et al., 1996; Klepstad et al., 2004; Romberg et al., 2004, 2005; Chou et al., 2006).

Clinical studies on opioid sensitivity have been conflicting. Early reports by Kupferberg and Way (1963) suggested neonates had more respiratory depression after opioid administration than did adults. However, Lynn et al. (1993) evaluated the respiratory depressant effects of intravenous morphine infusions in 30 postoperative patients aged 2 to 570 days and noted no evidence of a relationship of any given morphine concentration

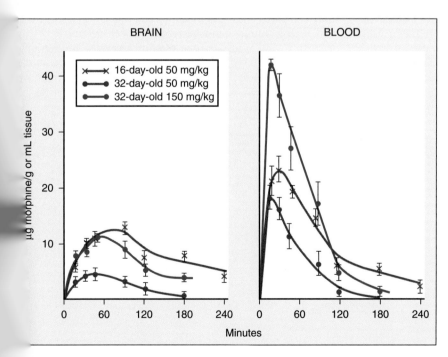

■ **FIGURE 7-27.** Brain and blood levels of morphine in young and older rats. Note that in young rats, brain concentrations of lower dose (50 mg/kg) were equivalent to brain concentrations of a higher dose of 150 mg/kg in older animals, even though the plasma concentrations were lower in the younger animals. *(From Kupferberg HI, Way EL: Pharmacologic basis for the increased sensitivity of the newborn rat to morphine, J Pharmacol Exp Ther 109:141, 1963.)*

with respiratory depression and age. Infants who had a morphine C_{ss} over 20 ng/mL, 67% of subjects, had elevated levels of arterial P_{CO_2} during spontaneous ventilation (six of nine infants), perhaps showing evidence of a threshold concentration.

Nichols et al. (1993) studied the extent and duration of respiratory depression after intrathecal administration of 0.02 mg/kg of morphine to 10 patients aged 4 months to 15 years. Although intrathecal morphine depresses ventilation for at least 18 hours, there was no relationship of age and ventilatory depression.

Age-related sensitivities have also been studied after intravenous fentanyl administration. Hertzka et al. (1989) determined that fentanyl-induced ventilatory depression as assessed by skin surface P_{CO_2} and ventilatory patterns was not greater in infants (older than 3 months) than in children or adults. In addition to age sensitivities, Zhou et al. (1993) demonstrated ethnic differences in the disposition and effects of morphine. In a study in Chinese and Caucasian adult volunteers, they found that Chinese subjects had an increased morphine clearance with decreased respiratory and hemodynamic depressant effects. Interestingly, the decreased respiratory and hemodynamic susceptibility did not correlate with the gastrointestinal effects, with Chinese subjects experiencing more nausea and vomiting than Caucasians. The complexities of opioid actions, both related to analgesia and to side-effect profiles, are still incompletely studied for "old" agents like morphine, as well as newer ones like the fentanyl derivatives.

Morphine

The pharmacology of morphine has been studied in both adults and children. In adults, morphine is 30% to 35% protein bound, whereas in neonates, it is 18% to 22% bound (Bhat et al., 1990, McRorie et al., 1992). Morphine is a drug with a high hepatic extraction coefficient; consequently, morphine clearance is determined by hepatic blood flow. Increases in hepatic blood flow can further increase morphine clearance, whereas decreases in hepatic blood flow can lower drug clearance. Morphine is inactivated by N-demethylation and glucuronidation. The two major metabolic products are morphine 6-glucuronide and morphine 3-glucuronide, which are mainly excreted by the kidneys. In adults, sulfate metabolism accounts for 5% to 10% of the drug's metabolism. In neonates the enzymes for glucuronide metabolism are immature, and the role of sulfation in morphine metabolism may be more pronounced. McRorie et al. (1992) demonstrated that in the neonate, sulfation contribution to morphine metabolism is proportionately higher, because glucuronidation is deficient. This effect diminishes by 4 to 6 months of age as glucuronidation reaches adult values.

As with other drugs, morphine appears to undergo age-related changes in its pharmacokinetic profile (Table 7-14). The presence of age-related changes in the neonatal period appears somewhat controversial. Bhat et al. (1990) studied the pharmacokinetics in 20 newborn infants younger than 5 days of age after a single bolus administration of intravenous morphine. In this study, they concluded that with increasing gestational age, drug clearance increases by 0.9 mL/kg per minute per week of gestation and that with increasing gestational age, both distribution and elimination half-life also decreased. Compared with term infants, Bhat et al. noted that in infants with fewer than 30 weeks' gestation, morphine had a longer elimination half-life (10 ± 3.7 h) and slower clearances (3.4 vs. 15 mL/kg per minute). However, Chay et al. (1992) reported no difference in the pharmacokinetics of continuous morphine infusions in preterm and term infants. There was no reported correlation of gestational age or conceptual age with drug clearance or elimination half-life. In addition, these investigators noted that a plasma concentration of 125 ng/mL was necessary to provide adequate sedation in 50% of the neonates. These values are quite high compared with the analgesic values of 12 ng/mL needed after cardiac surgery (Lynn et al., 1984). How much of this difference is related to the desired effect (sedation during mechanical ventilation vs. postoperative analgesia) is not clear.

Most studies of morphine pharmacokinetics in infants and children have reported large interindividual variability, as shown in Fig. 7-28. This makes predicting effect and duration of action in an individual problematic. The same variability has been seen with meperidine and even with fentanyl (Pokela et al.,1992).

Bouwmeester et al. (2004) using an allometric model standardized to a 70-kg person, described a total-body clearance for morphine of 80% of that of adults at 6 months of age and 96% of that predicted in adults by 1 year of age; these findings correlate with the ones previously described by McRorie et al. (1992) (Table 7-15). It was also estimated that the formation of M3G in 1-year old infants accounts for 86% of morphine elimination, compared with 55% in adults, and that the morphine volume of distribution increased exponentially from 83 L per 70 kg at birth to 136 L per 70 kg at 6 months of age. Interestingly, Anand et al. (2008), using the same allometric model, found higher volumes of distribution (190 L per 70 kg) in preterm neonates (23 to 32 weeks' gestation) than the ones described by Bouwmeester et al. (2004).

TABLE 7-14. Morphine Age-Related Pharmacokinetics

Reference	Age	No. of Patients	V_d (L/kg)	CL (mL/kg/min)	$t_{1/2}\beta$ (min)
Dahlstrom et al. (1979)	1-7 yr	8	1.13	6.17	183
Dahlstrom et al. (1979)	7-15 yr	8	1.36	6.71	202
Lynn and Slattery (1987)	2 to 4 d	7	3.3	6.3	408
Lynn and Slattery (1987)	17-65 d	4	5.15	23.8	234
Barret et al. (1991)	1-37 d	26	2.7	3.6	534

Data from Dahlstrom B, Bolme P, Feyching H, et al: Morphine kinetics in children, *Clin Pharmacol Ther* 26: 354-65, 1979; Lynn AM, Slattery JT: Morphine pharmacokinetic in early infancy, *Anesthesiology* 66:136-39, 1987; Barret DA, Elias-Jones AC, Rutter N et al: Morphine kinetics after diamorphine infusion in premature neonates, *Br. J Pharmacol* 32: 31-37, 1991.
CL, Clearance; $t_{1/2}\beta$, elimination half-life; V_d, Volume of distribution.

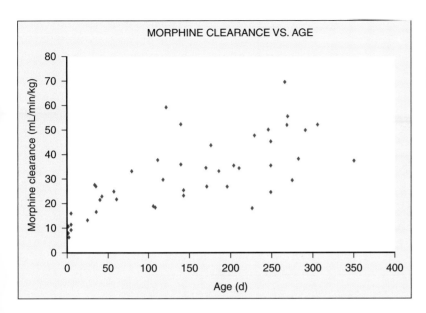

MORPHINE CLEARANCE VS. AGE

■ **FIGURE 7-28.** Morphine clearance (mL/min⁻¹ per kg⁻¹) vs. age (days) in infants receiving morphine. *(From Lynn AM et al.: Intravenous morphine in postoperative infants: intermittent bolus dosing versus targeted continuous infusions,* Pain *88[1]:89, 2000.)*

TABLE 7-15. Morphine Sulphate Clearance Changes with Postnatal Age in Term Neonates

Age (days)	Weight* (kg)	Clearance (mL/min⁻¹/kg⁻¹)	CLTstd (L/hr⁻¹/70 kg)	Weight (kg)	Clearance (mL/min⁻¹/kg⁻¹)	CLTstd (L/hr⁻¹/70 kg)
0-7	3	9.8	18.7 (12.0-30.6)	3.2	5.5	10.6 (6.2-16.3)
8-30	4	13.3	27.3	3.9	7.4	15.1 (6.9-38.4)
31-90	5.6	23.9	53.4 (37.3-74.4)	4.3	10.5	22.0 (20.5-42.0)
91-180	7.5	32.3	77.6 (44.5-125.2)	5.1	13.9	30.3 (18.2-52.6)
181-365	8.5	38.1	94.5 (44.6-172.1)	7.2	21.7	51.6 (13.7-68.0)
Adult	70	22	92.4 (CV% 38)			

Data from Bouwmeester NJ et al.: Developmental pharmacokinetics of morphine and its metabolites in neonates, infants, and young children, *Br J Anaesth* 92:208, 2004; Lynn AM, Nespeca MK, Bratton SL et al: Intravenous morphine in postoperative infants: intermittent bolus dosing versus targeted continuous infusions, *Pain* 88(1):89, 2000; McRorie TI, Lynn AM, Nespeca MK et al: The maturation of morphine clearance and metabolism, *Am J Dis Child* 146(8):972, 1992; adult data from Kart T, Christup LL, Ramussen M: Recommended use of morphine in neonates, infants and children based on a literature review: Part 1—pharmacokinetics, *Pediatr Anesth* 7:5-11, 1997. *Weights are estimates only.

In addition to age, morphine pharmacokinetics can be influenced by disease. Patients with renal failure were reported to be sensitive to narcotic intoxication after morphine administration. Chauvin et al. (1987b) studied the pharmacokinetics of morphine in adult patients with renal insufficiency. For morphine, they found that morphine in patients with chronic renal failure has similar rates of clearance and half-lives but significantly smaller steady-state volumes of distribution compared with morphine in age- and weight-matched control patients. Although chronic renal failure did not alter the elimination of unchanged morphine, metabolites of morphine accumulated at higher plasma levels for longer periods of time in the patients with chronic renal failure. In studies of patients with renal failure, Osbourne et al. (1993) noted that morphine metabolism is impaired and that the metabolites of morphine (morphine glucuronide and morphine 6-glucuronide) accumulate in the plasma (Fig. 7-29). Hanna et al. (1993) have also demonstrated abnormal kinetics of morphine metabolites in patients with renal failure. Patients with renal failure had a prolonged elimination half-life and decreased clearance in the pharmacokinetic profile of morphine 6-glucuronide. In patients with renal impairment, the increased opioid sensitivity may be a function

of decreased morphine metabolism coupled with impaired clearance of the metabolites, which have analgesic and respiratory activity.

In patients with liver disease, the effects of disease can be unpredictable. Patwardhan et al. (1981) described the effects of liver disease on morphine kinetics in adult patients with cirrhosis and in healthy adult volunteers. Compared with healthy subjects, patients with moderate-to-severe cirrhosis had a normal elimination and disposition of morphine but a prolonged elimination half-life and decreased clearance of indocyanine. (Indocyanine is taken up and excreted solely by the hepatocytes, making it a reliable indicator of liver disease). Because morphine is a highly extracted drug and its clearance depends on hepatic blood flow, the investigators postulated that morphine has extrahepatic sites of metabolism in the gastrointestinal tract and kidneys.

In a limited study of 21 children aged 6 months to 10 years who underwent cardiopulmonary bypass for repair of their underlying heart defects, Dagan et al. (1993) noted that in the postbypass period, for patients requiring inotropic support, morphine clearance was 50% less than that reported for other children. Similarly Lynn et al. (1998) reported increased

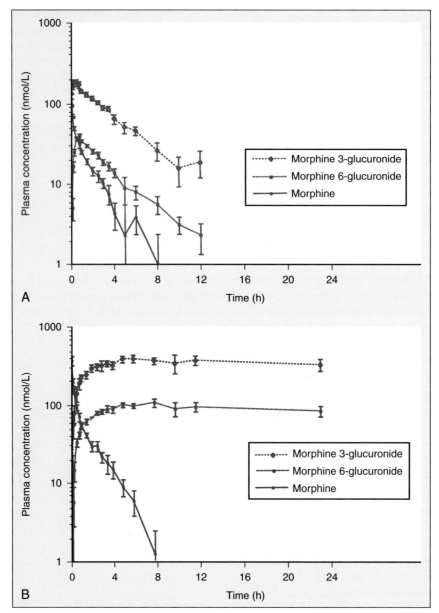

■ FIGURE 7-29. A, Morphine and metabolite levels in normal volunteers (mean ± SEM; data correction to 10 mg/70 kg). **B,** Pharmacokinetic of morphine and morphine glucuronides in patients with kidney failure. *(From Osborne R et al.: The pharmacokinetics of morphine and morphine glucuronides in kidney failure,* Clin Pharmacol Ther *54:158, 1993.)*

morphine clearance in infants after noncardiac surgery than in age-matched infants receiving morphine after cardiac procedures.

Geiduschek et al. (1997) described a morphine clearance of 11.7 ± 9.3 mL/kg/min in neonates supported by ECMO. Peters et al. (2005), using an allometric model, described an initial reduced morphine clearance at the start of ECMO (2.2 L/hr per 70 kg) that rapidly normalizes after 2 weeks of therapy.

In addition to intravenous infusions, intraspinal axis administration of opioids has been studied. Nordberg et al. (1984) noted that in adults, after 0.5 mg of intrathecally administered morphine (L2-4), the cerebrospinal fluid kinetics revealed a terminal half-life of 175 minutes, a volume of cerebrospinal fluid distribution of 0.88 mL/kg, and a clearance of 2.8 mL/kg per minute. In pediatric patients undergoing craniofacial surgical repairs, Nichols et al. (1993) noted that the cerebrospinal

fluid concentrations at 6, 12, and 18 hours after 0.02 mg/k of intrathecal administration were 2860, 640, and 220 n mL, respectively. These children had good analgesia, but were mechanically ventilated, so respiratory effects were n assessed.

In children, Attia et al. (1986) demonstrated that t pharmacokinetics of epidural morphine were similar to v ues reported in adults. After a 50-mcg/kg epidural bolus, t volume of distribution was 7.9 L/kg, the elimination half-l was 74 minutes, and the clearance was 28 mL/kg per m ute. In addition to morphine pharmacokinetics, Attia et (1986) noted that the onset and duration of analgesia w 30 minutes and 19 hours, respectively, and that respirat depression as evidenced by changes in the slope of the vent tory response to CO_2 was impaired for 22 hours after epidu administration.

Intranasal use of morphine has been reported in adults. Fitzgibbon et al. (2003) after an intranasal dose of 40 mg of morphine in adults receiving opioids (i.e., not naïve to opioid effects) found an absolute bioavailability of 22% and a relative (to oral) bioavailability of 226%, with a C_{max} of 62 ± 22.8 ng/mL and a $t_{\frac{1}{2}}$ of 2 ± 0.7 hours. In a clinical trial, Stoker et al. (2007) found that reduced intranasal morphine doses (7.5 mg and 15 mg) are effective for moderate to severe pain as well. There are no reported studies in children.

Meperidine

Meperidine, like morphine, is an agonist at the μ-opioid receptor that shows great interindividual variability. In infants and neonates, the pharmacokinetics varied greatly between subjects, with a $t_{\frac{1}{2}}\beta$ of 10.7 hours (range of 3.3 to 59.4 hours), median clearance of 8 mL/kg per minute (range of 1.8 to 34.9 mL/kg per minute), and a median steady-state volume of distribution of 7.2 L/kg (range of 3.3 to 11) (Pokela et al.,1992). Normeperidine, its active metabolite, has a half-life that is dependent on renal function and can accumulate with high doses or in patients with decreased renal function; normeperidine may precipitate tremors or seizures (Saneto et al., 1996; Kussman and Sethna, 1998). Meperidine also has local anesthetic activity because of its interactions with sodium ion channels. It has been used as a local anesthetic after tonsillectomy and adenoidectomy procedures in children with mixed results (Elhakim et al., 1997; Nikandish et al., 2008). Its routine use in many pediatric centers has become very uncommon because of the undesirable effects of accumulating normeperidine and because there are a host of other agents available. However, meperidine in small doses can be used to treat postoperative shivering.

Fentanyl

Fentanyl is a synthetic opiate with a clinical potency 50 to 100 times that of morphine. It is metabolized by dealkylation, hydroxylation, and amide hydrolysis to inactive metabolites. It has a high hepatic extraction coefficient and a high pulmonary uptake (Roerig et al., 1987). Heberer noted that cirrhosis in adults had no effect on fentanyl kinetics. Fentanyl has relatively minimal hemodynamic effects and is used both as an adjunct to nitrous oxide anesthesia and as a sole anesthetic agent. Bradycardia and chest-wall rigidity are potential problematic features of high-dose fentanyl anesthesia. The cardiovascular effects of fentanyl at doses of 30 to 75 mcg/kg fentanyl (with pancuronium) are minimal (Hickey et al., 1984). Modest increases in mean arterial pressure and systemic vascular resistance index were noted by Hickey and colleagues (1985).

In neonates, Murat et al. (1988) have shown that although baroreceptor control of heart rate is present, fentanyl anesthesia (10 mcg/kg) can significantly depress the baroreceptor response to both hypotension and hypertension. In comparative studies of opioid-induced respiratory depression with sufentanil and fentanyl administration in adults, Bailey et al. (1990) noted that ventilatory depression (both magnitude and duration) was less after sufentanil administration. In addition, although the two drugs have similar half-lives, analgesia lasted longer after sufentanil administration. The dose of fentanyl needed to ensure satisfactory anesthesia for infants varies with the surgical stress

and disease comorbidity. Hickey and Retzack (1993) have shown that in a pediatric patient with reactive pulmonary vasculature, 25 mcg/kg of fentanyl was needed to prevent an acute episode of right ventricular failure secondary to pulmonary hypertension in the patient who was undergoing upper airway instrumentation and manipulation. Ellis and Steward (1990) have shown that in children undergoing hypothermic cardiopulmonary bypass or profound hypothermia with circulatory arrest who were anesthetized with fentanyl, a dose of at least 50 mcg/kg of fentanyl was needed to blunt the hyperglycemic response to hypothermia and circulatory arrest. Yaster (1987) noted that in neonates anesthetized with fentanyl, metocurine, and oxygen who were undergoing a wide variety of surgical procedures, fentanyl (10 to 12.5 mcg/kg) provided reliable hemodynamic stability for 75 minutes.

In a study of children aged 6 months to 6 years undergoing cardiac surgery with cardiopulmonary bypass, Pirat et al. (2002) compared three groups of patients. One group received intravenous fentanyl, the second group received intrathecal fentanyl, and the third group received both intravenous and intrathecal fentanyl. In this study, intrathecal fentanyl offered no advantage over intravenous fentanyl with regard to hemodynamic stability or suppression of the biochemical stress response. However, the combination of intrathecal and intravenous fentanyl was associated with better hemodynamic stability in the prebypass period compared with either group alone.

Duncan et al. (2000) reported a dose-ranging study of 40 pediatric patients undergoing cardiac surgery using one of five intravenous fentanyl doses: 2, 25, 50, 100, and 150 mcg/kg. In this study, patients in the 2 mcg/kg group had significant rises in prebypass glucose, prebypass and postbypass cortisol, and prebypass and postbypass norepinephrine. No significant rises occurred in glucose, cortisol, and catecholamines in any of the higher dosage groups. Patients in the group receiving 2 mcg/kg had significantly higher mean systolic blood pressures and heart rates. Higher doses of fentanyl (100 and 150 mcg/kg) offered little advantage over 50 mcg/kg in controlling these neuroendocrine stress responses.

Age-related differences in the kinetics and sensitivity to fentanyl and changes in kinetics associated with pathophysiologic conditions and types of surgery create variability and make generalizations difficult (Johnson et al., 1984; Koren et al., 1984; Collins et al., 1985; Koehntop et al., 1986; Singleton et al., 1987). In the neonate, fentanyl clearance seems comparable with that of the older child or adult, whereas in the premature infant, fentanyl clearance is markedly reduced. In premature infants, fentanyl half-life was reported as 6 to 32 hours (Collins et al., 1985). In infants and children, fentanyl plasma concentrations were less than those in adults after similarly administered intravenous doses (milligrams per kilogram) (Fig. 7-30) (Singleton et al., 1987). These marked variations in kinetics reflect age differences and perhaps differences in anesthetics, surgeries, or duration of sampling.

Fentanyl pharmacokinetics after continuous infusions for fewer than 24 hours in critically ill children have demonstrated increased steady-state volume of distribution (15.2 L/kg), prolonged terminal elimination half-life (24 hours), and normal clearances (Katz and Kelly, 1993). The pharmacokinetics after 48 hours of continuous fentanyl infusion in newborns were reported for 12 neonates. In these infants (mean gestational age, 32 weeks; mean weight, 1.88 kg; mean PNA, 6 ± 9 days), the volume of distribution was noted as 17 ± 9 L/kg, total body

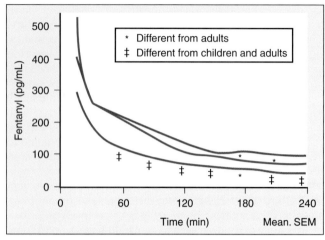

■ FIGURE 7-30. Fentanyl concentration-vs-time curves for adults *(top curve),* children *(middle curve),* and infants *(bottom curve).* *(From Singleton MA et al.: Plasma concentrations of fentanyl in infants, children, and adults,* Can Anaesth Soc J *34:152, 1987.)*

clearance was 1154 mL/kg per hour, and the half-life was 9.5 ± 2.6 hours (Santeiro et al., 1997). In addition, the relatively high total body clearance was noted to correlate with PNA, suggesting that hepatic blood flow increases with age. Gauntlett et al. (1988) found that fentanyl clearance increased with PNA, with most of the increase occurring by 2 weeks of age.

In a study of neonates who were not undergoing surgery, Saarenmaa et al. (2000) studied the fentanyl clearance in the first few days of life of 38 infants who were at 26 to 42 weeks' gestation and had birth weights of 835 to 3550 g. This study reported a correlation of fentanyl clearances with gestational age and birth weight (Fig. 7-31).

Prolonged fentanyl infusions, however, were associated with tolerance. In this context, tolerance is defined as the need to increase drug doses to maintain a stable drug effect (e.g., an increased dose of fentanyl to achieve pain relief on day 7 vs. day 1 of use). In neonates sedated with fentanyl via continuous infusion while undergoing ECMO, Arnold et al. (1991) noted that the daily infusion rates and plasma concentrations required to keep the infant sedated increased over time. Although prolonged continuous infusions of fentanyl may increase the volume of distribution, prolong the elimination half-life of the drug, and consequently prolong recovery on discontinuation, the development of tolerance may minimize this pharmacologic consequence.

In addition to intravenous administration, fentanyl has been administered transmucosally as a means of providing sedation to children. The pharmacokinetics and bioavailability of oral transmucosal fentanyl citrate (OTFC) were studied by Streisand et al. (1991) using adult volunteers studied on three separate occasions (Fig. 7-32). Plasma levels of fentanyl were determined after intravenous, transmucosal, or gastrointestinal (oral) administration. Regardless of the mode of administration, the terminal elimination half-life was similar in all three groups (425 to 469 minutes). Compared with the oral group, peak plasma concentrations of fentanyl occurred earlier (22 vs.101 minutes) and were higher (30 vs. 1.6 ng/mL) in the OTFC groups. The bioavailability of OTFC was 50%, compared with 30% in the oral group. This difference in the bioavailability probably relates to the first-pass (hepatic

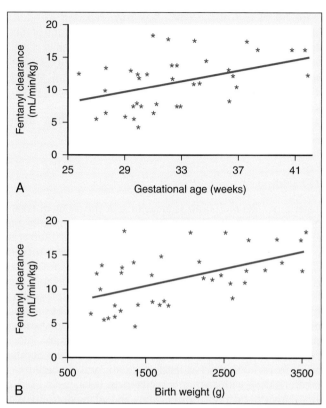

■ FIGURE 7-31. Plasma clearance of fentanyl correlates with gestational age and birth weight. *(From Saarenmaa E et al.: Gestational age and birth weight effects on plasma clearance of fentanyl in newborn infants,* J Pediatr *136:767, 2000.)*

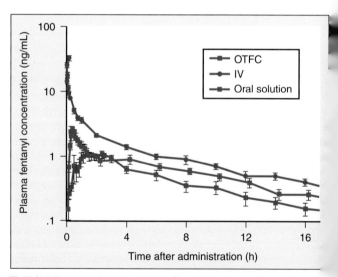

■ FIGURE 7-32. Plasma concentrations of fentanyl after oral transmucosal, intravenous, and oral administration. *(From Streisand JB et al.: Absorption and bioavailability of oral transmucosal fentanyl citrate,* Anesthesiology *75:226, 1991.)*

extraction) effect observed with orally administered dru... (Streisand et al., 1991). In children, Dsida et al. (1998) a... Wheeler et al. (2002) found less bioavailability of OTFC, w... levels similar to the ones achieved by adults after oral adm... istration (33% and 36% ± 1%). In a subsequent study co... paring pharmacokinetic parameters of oral administration...

the intravenous formulation of fentanyl and OTFC, Wheeler et al. (2004) found similar pharmacokinetic parameters. However, there was a high interpatient variability, especially in the early hours after oral administration of intravenous fentanyl; the pharmacokinetic variables for the orally administered intravenous formulation were peak plasma concentrations (C_{max}: 1.83 ng/mL, standard deviation [SD] 1.19 ng/mL), time to C_{max} (1.74 hours, SD 1.54 hours), apparent volume of distribution at steady state (17.5 L/kg, SD 7.20 L/kg), and apparent oral fentanyl clearance (3.33 L/kg, SD 2.25 L/kg^{-1} per hour^{-1}). Therefore, as stated by the authors, this method of administration should be used with caution until further data are available.

Intranasal administration of fentanyl has also been used to provide postoperative analgesia for pediatric patients (Galinkin et al., 2000; Manjushree et al., 2002). After 2 mcg/kg of intranasal fentanyl, Galinkin et al. (2000) noted the mean fentanyl concentrations at 10 and 34 minutes were 0.8 and 0.6 ng/mL, respectively. In a study comparing intranasal fentanyl with intravenous fentanyl, Manjushree et al. (2002) noted that onset time to analgesia after 1 mcg/kg of fentanyl was slower (13 minutes) for the intranasal route than for the intravenous route of administration (8 minutes).

Darwish and collaborators (2007), using a fentanyl buccal tablet of 400 mcg in healthy adult volunteers, have found predictable pharmacokinetics after single- and multiple-dose administration. In 2008, the FDA posted a safety alert for this formulation. This formulation is intended only for management of breakthrough pain in adult patients with cancer who are tolerant to opioid therapy. In pediatrics, the applicability for this formulation is unlikely given its high dose.

Sufentanil

With the hypothesis that increase in potency is associated with increased opiate effects and decreased nonspecific cardiovascular effects, other fentanyl congeners have been developed. Sufentanil, a potent synthetic opioid, is an N-4 substituted derivative of fentanyl. It is a highly lipophilic compound that is distributed rapidly and extensively to all tissues. Sufentanil is approximately five to 10 times more potent than fentanyl and has an extremely high margin of safety. The major pathways for sufentanil metabolism involve O-demethylation and N-dealkylation; minimal amounts are excreted unchanged in urine. Desmethyl sufentanil, the major metabolite of sufentanil, possesses about 10% the activity of the parent compound.

Pharmacokinetic and pharmacodynamic studies of sufentanil were conducted in infants, children, and adults. In adults, compared with fentanyl, the smaller volume of distribution (2.48 L/kg) and high clearance rate (11.3 mL/kg per minute) of sufentanil contribute to its short terminal elimination half-life (149 minutes). Meuldermans et al. (1982) demonstrated that sufentanil is more protein bound (92%) than fentanyl (84%), and that pH affects protein binding. Decreasing pH from 7.4 to increased protein binding by 28%; conversely, increasing pH from 7.4 to 7.8 decreased protein binding by 28%.

Clinical studies assessing the hemodynamic and endocrine stress response of sufentanil have been done in adults undergoing cardiopulmonary bypass (deLange et al., 1982; Sebel and Bovill, 1982). Sufentanil appears to block some of the stress responses to cardiac surgery. Stress-induced increases

in antidiuretic hormone and growth hormone appear to be blocked before, during, and after cardiopulmonary bypass, whereas the catecholamines (norepinephrine, epinephrine, and dopamine) show a large surge during the bypass and postbypass periods (deLange et al., 1982; Bovill et al., 1983). In a double-blind study, Rosow et al. (1984) found the drugs fentanyl and sufentanil to be comparable with regard to hemodynamic stability.

The pharmacokinetic and pharmacodynamic effects of sufentanil in children have been studied. Hickey et al. (1984) compared the hemodynamic response of 5 and 10 mcg/kg of sufentanil to 50 to 75 mcg/kg of fentanyl in patients with complex congenital heart disease. Although heart rate and blood pressure changed slightly, they noted marked improvement in the patient's oxygenation with both fentanyl and sufentanil. They concluded that both sufentanil and fentanyl were safe anesthetics in high doses, and that both agents favorably decreased pulmonary vascular resistance and thereby increased pulmonary blood flow and systemic oxygenation in patients with cyanotic heart disease. Davis et al. (1987) examined both the pharmacodynamics and pharmacokinetics of high-dose sufentanil (15 mcg/kg) and oxygen in infants and children undergoing cardiac surgery. Sufentanil provided marked hemodynamic stability after an infusion and during the stress periods of incision and sternotomy (Table 7-16). The hemodynamic responses to sufentanil were similar to those noted by Hickey et al. (1984) but differed from the increases in blood pressure and heart rate occurring after intubation, sternotomy, and incision observed in older children undergoing repair of their congenital heart defect (Moore et al., 1985).

Greeley et al. (1987) investigated age-related changes in the pharmacokinetics of sufentanil in pediatric patients undergoing cardiothoracic surgery. They noted that sufentanil best fit a three-compartment model and that neonates had significantly smaller clearance rates, larger volumes of distribution at steady state, and longer elimination half-lives than infants, children, and adolescents (Table 7-17). The developmental pharmacokinetic changes of improved clearance and elimination for sufentanil were further substantiated in another report in which infants were studied within the first 8 days of life and then again at 3 to 4 weeks of age (Greeley and de Bruijn, 1988).

TABLE 7-16. Hemodynamics during Sufentanil Anesthesia in Infants and Children Undergoing Open-Heart Surgery

Variable	Baseline	1 min	5 min	Incision	Sternotomy
Heart rate	140 ± 14	129 ± 25	118 ± 23*	116 ± 20*	123 ± 32
Systolic blood pressure	101 ± 9	86 ± 15*	74 ± 11*	99 ± 15	106 ± 13
Diastolic blood pressure	65 ± 10	48 ± 9*	46 ± 12*	65 ± 14	67 ± 13

From Davis PJ et al.: Pharmacodynamics and pharmacokinetics of high-dose sufentanil in infants and children undergoing cardiac surgery, *Anesth Analg* 66:203, 1987.
Values are mean ± SD.
*P<0.01 compared with baseline.

TABLE 7-17. Age-Related Pharmacokinetic Values for Sufentanil

Age	N	$t_{1/2}\alpha$ (min)	$t_{1/2}\beta$ (min)	CL (mL/kg/min)	$V_d$ss (L/kg)
Neonates (0 to 8 days)	3	20.5	635	4.2	2.7
Neonates (20 to 28 days)	3	8.8	217	17.3	3.4
0 to 1 mo	9	23.4	737	6.7	4.15
1 mo to 2 yr	7	15.8	214	18.1	3.09
2 to 12 yr	7	19.6	140	16.9	2.73
12 to 16 yr	5	20.4	209	13.1	2.75

From Greeley WJ, de Bruijn NP: Sufentanil pharmacokinetics in pediatric cardiovascular patients, *Anesth Analg* 67:86, 1988.
$t_{1/2}\alpha$, Distribution phase half-life; $t_{1/2}\beta$, elimination phase half-life; *CL*, clearance; V_d*ss*, volume of distribution at steady state.

Guay et al. (1992) studied the pharmacokinetics of sufentanil in 20 healthy pediatric patients aged 2 to 8 years. After intravenous administration of 1 to 3 mcg/kg of sufentanil, the elimination half-life was 97 ± 42 minutes, the volume of distribution at steady state was 2.9 ± 0.6 L/kg, and the plasma clearance was 30.5 ± 8.8 mL/kg^{-1} per minute^{-1}. It is unclear whether the doubling of the plasma clearance value in healthy children was a function of the study design or the patient's underlying disease. A similar effect was noted for morphine in infants with and without cardiac disease (Lynn et al., 1998).

In addition to its use as an anesthetic agent, sufentanil has been used as a preanesthetic medication in children. Pharmacokinetic studies in adults after intravenous and intranasal administration show that the area under the curve from 0 to 120 minutes after intranasal dosing was 78% of that after intravenous injection (Helmers et al., 1989). By 30 minutes after drug administration, plasma sufentanil concentrations were identical for the two routes of administration.

The role of the kidneys in sufentanil elimination and metabolism has not been well defined. The effects of renal failure in sufentanil kinetics were assessed in adolescent patients with chronic renal failure (Davis et al., 1988). There was no statistical difference in apparent volume of distribution, elimination, and clearance between patients with renal failure and patients in a control group. However, there was a large amount of variability in both groups of patients. In patients with renal failure, sufentanil must be administered carefully on the basis of responses elicited in individual patients.

The pharmacodynamics of sufentanil were also evaluated in neurosurgical patients. The effects of opioids on intracranial pressure (ICP) and cerebral perfusion pressure have been controversial. In intubated patients with severe head injuries (less than 8 on the Glasgow Coma Scale), sufentanil administration was associated with an increase in ICP, a decrease in mean arterial blood pressure, and a decrease in cerebral perfusion pressure (Albanese et al., 1993). The effects of sufentanil in the EEGs of premature infants were reported by Nguyen and colleagues (2003). Bolus injection and continuous infusion increased EEG discontinuity, decreased burst suppression, and increased interburst intervals.

In adult patients undergoing nonintracranial neurosurgical procedures, Trindle et al. (1993) noted that cerebral blood flow velocity (as assessed by transcranial Doppler) increased after sufentanil infusion. This increase in velocity was similar for equipotent doses of fentanyl (Trindle et al., 1993).

In a study of adult patients with head trauma, Scholz et al. (1994) noted that sufentanil bolus (2 mcg/kg), combined with a sufentanil continuous infusion (150 mcg/hr) and midazolam continuous infusion (9 mg/hr), resulted in decreases in both ICP and mean arterial pressure. Perfusion pressure was noted to be stable.

Alfentanil

Alfentanil, a potent, short-acting analog of fentanyl, is rapidly distributed to the brain and central organs and then rapidly redistributed to more remote sites. It is about one fourth as potent as fentanyl and has one third the duration of action. After a single bolus injection, the drug's decreased volume of distribution results in a significantly shorter elimination half-life. Its low lipid solubility allows less penetration of the blood-brain barrier. The concentration in brain tissue is markedly less than that in plasma. The duration of narcotic effect appears to be governed by redistribution and elimination. The redistribution principle is most important after a small single-dose infusion, whereas elimination determines the effect of a large single bolus, multiple small-bolus infusions, or a continuous infusion. Alfentanil is metabolized in the liver by oxidative N-dealkylation and O-demethylation in the CYP3A4 system (Yun et al., 1992). The pharmacologically inactive metabolites are excreted in the urine, with the major metabolite being noralfentanil (Camu et al., 1982). Alfentanil metabolism is catalyzed by CYP3A3/4 and CYP3A5 (Klees et al., 2005). Interindividual differences in the expression of this cytochrome and its susceptibility to inducers and inhibitors may account for the clinical variability in alfentanil kinetics and dynamics (Kharasch and Thummel, 1993). Although gender differences in CYP activity can affect drug metabolism, Kharasch et al. (1997a), in a study of young women, could find no differences in alfentanil clearance on different days of the menstrual cycle. Differences in CYP activity can markedly influence the pharmacokinetics of alfentanil, specifically its context-sensitive half-time. Using normal, low, and high CYP3A4 activity, Kharasch et al. (1997b) have postulated through computer simulations that alfentanil can behave similarly to remifentanil (high CYP3A4 activity) or fentanyl (low CYP3A4 activity) (Fig. 7-33).

Protein binding has a significant influence on the pharmacokinetics of alfentanil. Alfentanil is 88% to 95% protein bound in the plasma and is independent of concentration and blood pH. The plasma protein most responsible for binding of alfentanil is α_1-acid glycoprotein. In adults, changes in the binding and in the pharmacokinetics of alfentanil occur during and after cardiopulmonary bypass (Hug, 1984). Disease states, including end-stage kidney or liver failure, can alter protein binding of opioids in children. Davis et al. (1989b) studied the effects of liver disease and kidney disease on the binding characteristics of alfentanil. Compared with healthy children, patients with kidney disease had a significant decrease in protein binding (89.2% ± 5.4% vs. 93.1% ± 3.2%), an increase in α_1-acid glycoprotein concentration (108.8 ± 44.3 vs. 71.8 ± 30.7 mg/dL), and no change in albumin concentration (3910 ± 754 vs. 4555 ± 524 mg/dL), where

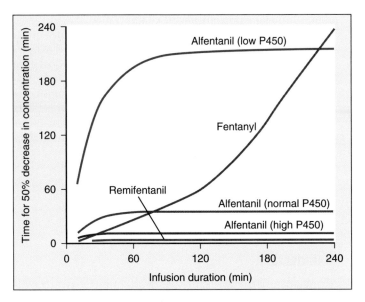

FIGURE 7-33. Effect of P450 3A4 activity on the time required for a 50% decrease in alfentanil venous plasma concentration after targeted infusions of variable durations. Half-times for fentanyl and remifentanil in normal participants were calculated using reported kinetic parameters. *(From Kharasch E et al.: The role of cytochrome P450 3A4 in alfentanil clearance: implications for interindividual variability in disposition and perioperative drug interactions, Anesthesiology 87:36, 1997.)*

patients with liver disease had a significant decrease in protein binding (85.9% ± 6.2% vs. 93.1% ± 3.2%), no change in a 1-acid glycoprotein concentration (65.8 ± 31.8 vs. 71.8 ± 30.7 mg/dL), and a decrease in albumin concentration (3045 ± 1255 vs. 4555 ± 524 mg/dL). Alfentanil binding has been studied in adult burn patients and noted to be increased from 90% to 94% protein bound (Macfie et al., 1992). Because alfentanil is highly protein bound, even small changes in the drug's free fraction could have marked pharmacodynamic effects in patients with kidney or liver failure.

The pharmacokinetics of alfentanil have been studied in both adults and children, but limited information is available for children of different ages. The limited, age-related, developmental pharmacokinetic data for alfentanil are presented in Table 7-18. In a study by Meistelman et al. (1987), children aged 5 (± 1.1 years) had significantly smaller volumes of distri-

bution and shorter elimination half-lives but similar clearance values compared with those young adult patients aged 31 (± 4 years). Goreskey et al. (1987) noted no differences in volume of distribution, elimination half-life, or clearance in infants aged 3 to 12 months compared with children aged 1 to 14 years. On the other hand, Roure et al. (1987) noted that children aged 33 (± 18) months had faster clearance rates and elimination half-lives but similar volumes of distribution compared with those of adults. As Maitre et al. (1987) noted in population studies of alfentanil pharmacokinetics in adults, differences in the pharmacokinetic profiles among the pediatric studies may be related to the large interpatient variability of alfentanil. Davis et al. (1989a) have studied the pharmacokinetics of a single bolus of alfentanil in newborn premature infants and older children. In their study, newborn premature infants had considerably longer elimination half-lives (525 ± 305 vs. 60 ± 11 minutes), slower clearance rates (2.2 ± 2.4 vs. 5.6 ± 2.4 mL/kg per minute), and larger volumes of distribution (1 ± 0.39 vs. 0.48 ± 0.19 L/kg) than those observed in the older children (Fig. 7-34).

In a report on the influence of gestational age on the pharmacokinetics of alfentanil in neonates, Killian et al. (1990) noted no changes in alfentanil kinetics between preterm and term infants. Wiest et al. (1991) studied the kinetics of alfentanil in neonates after a loading dose and variable continuous infusion route. Noncompartmental analysis revealed a clearance rate of 3.24 mL/kg per minute, a volume of distribution of 0.54 L/kg, and an elimination half-life of 4.1 hours. However, they noted an effect of alfentanil plasma concentration on plasma clearance, suggesting dose-dependent pharmacokinetics in these ill neonates.

The effects of renal failure and cirrhosis on alfentanil kinetics were studied in adult and in pediatric patients. Chauvin et al. (1987a) have studied the pharmacokinetics of alfentanil in adult patients with chronic renal failure. The clearance and half-life values for alfentanil were similar in patients with renal failure and in control patients, but the steady-state volumes of distribution of alfentanil were significantly greater in patients with renal disease than in control patients. However, when the kinetic values for alfentanil were corrected

TABLE 7-18. Alfentanil Age-Related Pharmacokinetics

Reference	Age	No. of Patients	V_d (L/kg)	CL (mL/min per kg)	$T_{1/2}\beta$ (min)
Meistelman et al. (1987)	4 to 8 yr	8	0.163	4.7	40
Meistelman et al. (1987)	25 to 40 yr	5	0.457	4.2	97
Goresky et al. (1987)	4 to 12 mo	5	0.500	8.3	76
Goresky et al. (1987)	1 to 14 yr	8	0.416	7.7	84
Davis et al. (1989a)	1 to 3 days (premature, 26 to 35 wk)	5	0.840	1.35	455
Killian et al. (1990)	1 to 3 days (term)	5	0.820	1.7	328

$_d$, Volume of distribution; *CL*, clearance; $t_{1/2}\beta$, elimination half-life.

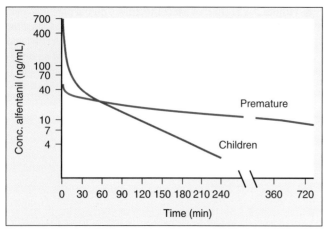

■ **FIGURE 7-34.** Alfentanil concentration-vs.-time curves in newborn premature infants and older children. Both groups received 25 mcg/kg of alfentanil. *(From Davis PJ et al.: Pharmacokinetics of alfentanil in newly born premature infants and older children, Dev Pharmacol Ther 13:21, 1989.)*

for protein binding, the steady-state volumes of distribution and rates of clearance of unbound drug were similar in both groups of patients.

The effects of cirrhosis on alfentanil pharmacokinetics in adults were demonstrated by Ferrier et al. in 1985. Patients with cirrhosis have lower total plasma clearance (1.60 vs. 3.06 mL/kg per minute) and prolonged terminal elimination half-life (219 vs. 97 minutes) but a similar volume of distribution (0.390 vs. 0.355 L/kg) as those values of patients in a control group.

In contrast to the studies in adults, the pharmacokinetics of alfentanil in children with cholestatic hepatitis or end-stage kidney disease who are about to undergo either liver or kidney transplantation appear to be unaffected by the disease process (Davis et al., 1989b). Whether this difference is related to age or to the underlying pathophysiology of the disease states remains unanswered.

As do other opiates, alfentanil produces a shift to the right in the ventilatory response curve. Although this shift is dose dependent, the ventilatory depressant effects dissipate by 30 to 50 minutes after the dose is given (Kay and Pleuvry, 1980; Kay and Stephenson, 1980).

Goldberg et al. (1992) noted that in healthy adult patients, prolonged alfentanil administration sometimes resulted in arterial oxygen desaturation and depression of the hypercapneic respiratory drive even though the patients were easily arousable. Muscle rigidity can occur with rapid-acting opiates such as fentanyl, sufentanil, and alfentanil. Pokela et al. (1992) have reported that rigidity, which requires changes in ventilator settings, occurs in neonates after alfentanil administration.

The cardiovascular effects of alfentanil were assessed during both low- and high-dose infusions (Kay and Pleuvry, 1980; Kay and Stephenson, 1980). At doses of 150 mcg/kg, heart rate, mean arterial pressure, and systemic vascular resistance were noted to decrease. Pulmonary capillary wedge pressure, pulmonary vascular resistance, right atrial pressure, and pulmonary artery pressure increased slightly (Kramer et al., 1983).

The neuroendocrine stress response with alfentanil has been studied in adults. Alfentanil incompletely suppresses the stress response. High-dose alfentanil can blunt the growth hormone, antidiuretic hormone, and cortisol responses to bypass.

Epinephrine and norepinephrine concentrations are increased with the onset of bypass (deLange et al., 1982; Stanley et al., 1983).

Meretoja and Rautiainen (1990) noted that in children aged 1 month to 2 years, oral flunitrazepam premedication and alfentanil bolus of 20 mcg/kg followed by a continuous infusion of 0.5 mcg/kg per minute provided adequate sedation for patients spontaneously breathing room air who were undergoing cardiac catheterization. In these patients, hemodynamic variables changed less than 11%.

In adults, Ausems et al. (1986) have defined the Cp50 values of alfentanil for various surgical and anesthetic stimulations (Fig. 7-35). Using these adult Cp50 plasma values, initial bolus and infusion rates can be estimated for children.

Remifentanil

Remifentanil is the hydrochloride salt of 3-[4-methoxycarbonyl]-4-[(1-oxopropyl)phenylamino]-1-piperidine] propanoic acid methyl ester. Because of its ester linkage, remifentanil is susceptible to metabolism by blood and tissue esterases. Its primary metabolic pathway is through de-esterification to form a carboxylic acid metabolite, which is only one 300th to one 1000th the potency of the parent compound. In adult studies, the pharmacokinetic profile of remifentanil is best described by a biexponential decay curve, with a small volume of distribution (0.39 L/kg), a rapid distribution phase (0.94 minute), and an extremely short elimination half-life (10 minutes) (Egan et al., 1993; Glass et al., 1993; Westmoreland et al., 1993).

In addition, computer simulations show that the duration of remifentanil infusion has no effect on the time to decrease the plasma or effect site concentration by 50%. The half-time for achieving an equilibration constant between plasma and the effect compartment ($t_{1/2}K_{eo}$) is 1.3 minutes. Thus, the context-sensitive half-time is a flat line.

For opioids, which undergo organ elimination, the neonatal profile of opioids demonstrates prolonged clearances, large volumes of distribution, and markedly prolonged half-lives. However, in neonates remifentanil has a rapid clearance, a large volume of distribution, and a half-life that does not change with age. In an

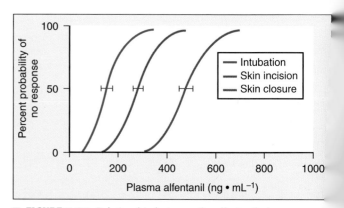

■ **FIGURE 7-35.** Relationship between the alfentanil plasma concentrations (with 66% nitrous oxide) and their effects for three specific events of short duration (intubation, skin incision, and skin closure). *(From Ausems ME et al.: Plasma concentrations of alfentanil required to supplement nitrous oxide anesthesia for general surgery, Anesthesiology 65:362, 1986.)*

age-related study of remifentanil pharmacokinetics, Ross et al. (2001) noted that the volume of distribution was largest in the infants younger than 2 months (mean value of 452 mL/kg) and decreased to mean values of 223 to 308 mL/kg in the older patients. There was a more rapid clearance in the infants younger than 2 months (90 mL/kg per minute) and infants aged 2 months to 2 years (92 mL/kg per minute) than in the other groups (mean of 46 to 76 mL/kg per minute). The half-life was similar in all age groups, with mean values of 3.4 to 5.7 minutes. Because the redistribution phase and elimination half-life are so rapid, a bolus injection before a continuous infusion of remifentanil is usually unnecessary.

Another unique feature of remifentanil kinetics in children is that its pharmacokinetic profile is unchanged by cardiopulmonary bypass. For opioids, which undergo organ elimination, cardiopulmonary bypass prolongs drug clearance, increases volume of distribution, and increases half-life. The pharmacokinetic profile of remifentanil appears to be unaffected by cardiopulmonary bypass (Fig. 7-36) (Davis et al., 1999).

The pharmacodynamics of remifentanil were studied in children and infants. Multiple case reports of remifentanil use in neonates and infants suggest its usefulness (Wee and Stokes, 1999; Chiaretti et al., 2000; German et al., 2000; Dönmez et al., 2001; Foubert et al., 2002). In a multicenter trial of infants younger than 2 months who were undergoing pyloromyotomy, Galinkin et al. (2001) and Davis et al. (2001) noted that remifentanil provides stable hemodynamic conditions and that new onset of postoperative apnea, as detected by pneumograms, did not occur with remifentanil.

Pharmacodynamic studies suggest that the short duration of remifentanil in older children can be used to promote faster emergence times (Davis et al., 1997, 2000). As with other opioids, the issue of tolerance is a concern with remifentanil. In a systematic review of randomized controlled trials comparing remifentanil with other opioids in adult patients, Komatsu et al. (2007) found a 40% additional need for postoperative analgesics (RR 1.36, 95%; CI 1.21-1.53); confirming earlier studies by Guignard et al. (2000) and Vinik and Kissin (1998). In pediatrics Crawford et al. (2006) demonstrated increased cumulative morphine consumption during the first 24 hours after spine instrumentation, in patients who had remifentanil infusion when compared with patients who received morphine intraoperatively. In a study done on cultured rat dorsal horn neurons exposed to different levels of remifentanil comparable with the ones used in clinical practice, Zhao and Joo (2008) found an increase in NMDA responses that is consistent with remifentanil-induced hyperalgesia and tolerance.

The incidence of postoperative nausea and vomiting appears to be similar to the incidence seen with other opioids (Eltzschig et al., 2002; Komatusu et al., 2007). A higher incidence of postoperative shivering is described in patients receiving remifentanil (RR 2.15, 95%; CI 1.73-2.69) when compared with alfentanil, fentanyl, and sulfentanil (Komatsu et al., 2007).

The short context-sensitive half-life of remifentanil and the issue of rapid appearance of tolerance make it mandatory to have a plan for ongoing analgesia if postoperative pain is anticipated before stopping remifentanil infusions.

Methadone

Methadone is a synthetic opioid analgesic. It is a racemic mixture with the l-isomer that is 10 to 50 times more potent than the d-isomer. Methadone has an oral bioavailability of 80% with a range of 41% to 99%. It is 60% to 90% protein bound, and α_1-acid glycoprotein is the main determinant of the free fraction of methadone. After an intravenous dose in adults, the pharmacokinetic profile fits a two-compartment model with a distribution half-life of 6 minutes and an elimination half-life of 35 hours (Gourlay et al., 1982). Findings of the pharmacokinetics of methadone in children suggest that it has a large volume of distribution (7.1 L/kg), a high plasma clearance (5.4 mL/kg per minute), and a long half-life (19.2 hours) (Berde et al., 1991).

Methadone metabolism clearance and disposition have been thought to be governed by hepatic CYP3A4 activity. However, Kharasch et al. (2009), in a set of studies with adult volunteers, have shown that methadone disposition and clearance are unchanged despite profound inhibition of the CYP3A4 and that oral absorption and bioavailability are not affected by glycoprotein transporter activity. Little information is available with respect to methadone's pharmacokinetic profile in end-stage liver or kidney failure. Urinary pH is another important determinant of the elimination half-life of methadone. Acidifying the urine markedly decreases the half-life of methadone and increases its renal clearance (Bellward et al., 1977).

Although methadone has become a cornerstone therapy for opiate dependence and the management of chronic neuropathic and cancer pain, clinical use in children is somewhat limited. In a randomized, double-blind study of morphine and methadone, Berde et al. (1991) noted that the children receiving methadone perioperatively had significantly less opioid requirements in the immediate postoperative period and better pain scores in the entire postoperative period than did children receiving equipotent doses of morphine. However, no differences in opioid requirements were found after the immediate postoperative period. Also, no differences in sedation scores were described; however, the maximum time of methadone administration was 48 hours. Recommended doses of perioperative methadone include a loading dose of 0.1 to 0.2 mg/kg with 0.05 mg/kg

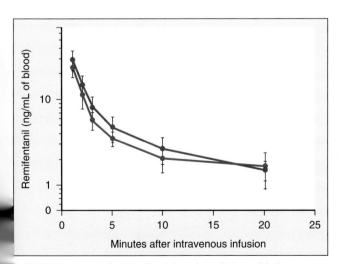

FIGURE 7-36. Prebypass (*brown*) and postbypass (*blue*) pharmacokinetic decay curves of remifentanil were constructed from the average concentrations of the 12 patients.
From Davis PJ et al.: The effects of cardiopulmonary bypass on remifentanil kinetics in children undergoing atrial septal defect repair, Anesth Analg 89:904, 1999.)

supplemental dose every 4 to 12 hours for a maximum of 2 to 3 days to avoid the possibility of excessive sedation secondary to drug accumulation as a result of the prolonged elimination half-life of methadone.

Among opioid analgesics, methadone is unique as a potent blocker of the delayed rectifier potassium ion channel. This results in QT prolongation and can produce torsade de pointes ventricular tachycardia in susceptible individuals and may explain the sudden death associated with its use (Andrews et al., 2009). The effects of methadone on the QT interval may be enhanced by hypokalemia, drugs that increase the QT interval such as erythromycin and ondansetron, or by CYP 3A4 inhibitors such as fluoxetine, fluconazole, valproate, and clarithromycin (Ehret et al., 2006).

Tramadol

Tramadol is a centrally acting agent with two distinct mechanisms of action: opioid and nonopioid. Tramadol acts as an opioid agonist. Tramadol also acts on monoamine systems to inhibit the reuptake of norepinephrine and serotonin. Tramadol is structurally related to codeine. It is metabolized by liver CYP2D6; about 0.8% of the white population is deficient in this enzyme. Its metabolite, O-demethyl metabolic intermediate, has some analgesic effect. Tramadol is a stereoisomer. The pharmacokinetic profile of the stereoisomer was reported by Bressolle et al. in 2009. The (+)-stereoisomer form provides similar analgesia as the racemic form. The bioavailability of tramadol in adults is 68%, and it is 20% protein bound. Tramadol is metabolized by the 2D6, 2B6, and 3A4 P450 cytochromes. It has an active metabolite with more affinity for the μ receptor than the parent compound. In 14 children aged 1 to 12 years, the intravenous tramadol pharmacokinetic profile demonstrated a volume of distribution, clearance, and half-life of 3.1 L/kg, 6.1 mL/kg per minute, and 6.4 hours, respectively. In the same study, the kinetics of tramadol after caudal administration revealed a volume of distribution, clearance, and half-life of 2.06 L/kg, 6.6 mL/kg per minute, and 3.7 hours, respectively. Of note was that the ratio of caudal and intravenous AUC was 0.83, suggesting there is extensive systemic absorption of caudal tramadol (Murthy et al., 2000) (Fig. 7-37).

The clinical efficacy of tramadol has been reviewed in adults and children by Scott and Perry (2000); in summary, the overall efficacy of tramadol is comparable with equianalgesic doses of parenteral opioids. In children, tramadol has been administered

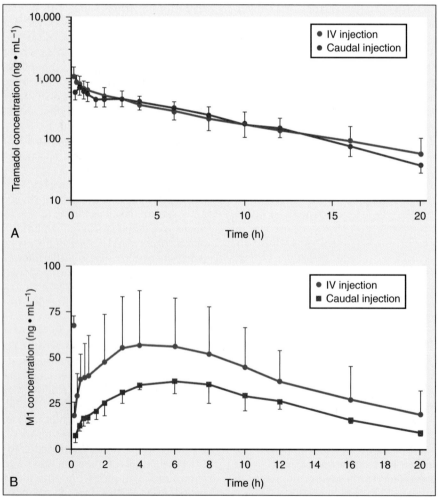

■ **FIGURE 7-37. A,** Mean (SD) serum concentrations of total tramadol after intravenous or caudal injection of tramadol 2 mg/kg. **B,** Mean (SD) serum concentrations of O-dimethyl tramadol *(M1)* after intravenous or caudal injection of tramadol 2 mg/kg. *(From Murthy BVS et al.: Pharmacokinetics of tramadol in children after IV or caudal epidural administration, Br J Anaesth 84:346, 2000.)*

Box 7-1 Tramadol: Recommended Dosages for Children

ROUTE: FORM
    DOSAGE (REPEATED DOSES × 4-6 PER DAY)
Oral, drops
    2-3 mg/kg^{-1}
Oral, tablets
    1-2 mg/kg^{-1}
Rectal, suppositories
    1.5 to 3 mg/kg^{-1}
IV, bolus
    2 to 2.5 mg/kg^{-1}
IV, continuous infusion
    0.1 to 0.25 mg/kg^{1}/hr^{-1}

From Bozkurt P: Use of tramadol in children, *Paediatr Anaesth* 15:1041, 2005. *IV*, Intravenous.

---

orally, intravenously, intramuscularly, and caudally. Its major advantage is its lack of respiratory depression after its administration (Scott and Perry, 2000; Ozcengiz et al., 2001; Viitanen and Annila, 2001; Finkel et al., 2002; Engelhardt et al., 2003; Rose et al., 2003). Doses are presented in Box 7-1.

Hydrocodone

Hydrocodone is a synthetic opiate, available in oral preparations, usually in combination with acetaminophen. It is most commonly used in transitioning from intravenous to oral opiate pain medications or as an oral treatment for acute pain. Oral bioavailability is reported to be 60%, with onset of effect 10 to 20 minutes after dosing and a duration of 3 to 6 hours. Pediatric dosing is suggested as 0.05 to 0.1 mg/kg. Since hydrocodone is combined with acetaminophen, in an elixir form with 2.5 mg hydrocodone and 167 mg acetaminophen in 5 mL, dosing must account for all sources of acetaminophen in order to avoid toxicity related to doses of the acetaminophen that are higher than desired.

In a report comparing oxycodone with hydrocodone in 67 patients older than 12 years of age, with a mean age of 35 years, who were treated in an emergency department after acute fractures, oxycodone 5 mg and hydrocodone 5 mg both combined with acetaminophen gave equivalent pain relief at 30 and 60 minutes after medication. Side effects were similar, except the hydrocodone group showed a higher incidence of constipation (Marco et al., 2005). Litkowski (2005) compared analgesia from oxycodone with ibuprofen, oxycodone with acetaminophen, and hydrocodone with acetaminophen with placebo after third molar extraction in a multicenter trial. There were 249 patients with a mean age of 19 years, and pain relief was equivalent in the acetaminophen groups but less than in the group that received oxycodone with ibuprofen. Onset of pain relief was also faster in the group that received oxycodone with ibuprofen.

The only study of hydrocodone use in children found in several online searches compared 60 children (of a planned 94) receiving either rofecoxib or hydrocodone with acetaminophen dosed for 0.2 mg/kg hydrocodone every 6 hours) after elective tonsillectomy. Pain was assessed at 6-hour intervals initially by recovery staff and then by parents. Pain at rest was similar between the two groups (3 to 5 on a 10-point scale), but with swallowing, the group that received rofecoxib had scores that

were lower (2 to 4 vs. 4 to 6 in hydrocodone group). Side effects were not compared, because the number of patients was insufficient when the study was stopped early because of a recall of rofecoxib (Bean-Lijewski et al., 2007).

Hydrocodone has been used in the past in cough-suppressant medications because of its strong antitussive effects, but now it is rarely used, partially because reports about adverse effects, including death, have been published (Morrow and Faris, 1987).

Oxycodone

Oxycodone is a semisynthetic opioid analgesic (6-deoxy-7, 8-dihydro-14-hydroxy-3-O-methyl-6-oxomorphine) that was introduced into clinical practice in 1917. It is well absorbed after oral administration, and its bioavailability ranges between 60% to 80%, three times higher than morphine (with an oral bioavailability of 20%). N-demethylation to noroxycodone is the major metabolic pathway. A smaller fraction is metabolized by O-demethylation to oxymorphone. A fraction of both noroxycodone and oxymorphone are further metabolized to noroxymorphone (Kalso, 2005).

Metabolites show variable pharmacologic activity. Oxymorphone is an active metabolite with higher μ-opioid affinity than the parent compound. However, its low plasma concentration suggests a minor role in the analgesic response to oxycodone. Both noroxycodone and noroxymorphone are inactive metabolites. Excretion is mainly by renal elimination. Ten percent is eliminated as unchanged oxycodone; 50% is eliminated as noroxycodone and oxymorphone; and 18% is eliminated as noroxymorphone (Olkkola and Hagelberg, 2009).

In adults, after intravenous administration, the maximum concentration is reached after 25 minutes with a $t_{1/2}$ of 2 to 3 hours and clearance values between 15 and 18 mL/min^{-1} per kg^{-1} (Pöhyiä et al., 1991). In children aged 2 to 10 years, mean clearance is similar to adult values at 15.2 (with a range of 8.5 to 21.2) mL/min^{-1} per kg^{-1} (Olkkola et al., 1994). For infants younger than 1 week of age, clearance values are lower, with a median value of 9.9 (and a range of 2.3 to 17.2) mL/min^{-1} per kg^{-1}. Clearance increases with age, reaching adult values by age 2 to 6 months (Pokela et al., 2005). However, high interindividual variability in clearance is described.

Other forms of administration have been used in children. Kokki et al. (2004) studied the pharmacokinetic parameters of 0.1 mg kg^{-1} oxycodone administered intramuscularly, orally, and transmucosally and compared them with the intravenous form of administration. The mean (SD) $t_{1/2}\beta$ were similar between groups: 163 (26) min for IV administration, 150 (39) min for IM, 150 (44) min for mucosal and 147 (61) for oral administration. Oral and mucosal administration showed greater interindividual variability (Kokki et al., 2004). In a subsequent study, Kokki et al. (2006) used a higher dose of 0.2 mg/kg that was given transmucosally and reported better bioavailability than previously described. However, the median noroxycodone-to-oxycodone AUC ratio reported was 0.78, showing significant hepatic metabolism and suggesting that children probably swallowed some of the oxycodone at the time of administration (Kokki et al., 2006). The recommended dose for intravenous, oral, and intramuscular administration in children is 0.1 mg kg^{-1} (Kokki et al., 2004). For transmucosal administration a dose of 0.2 mg kg^{-1} is suggested, but it is still not clear if part of the increase in availability is because of oral absorption.

Controlled-release (CR) oxycodone is recommended for chronic pain treatment in adults. There are no pharmacokinetic studies on CR oxycodone in children. From adult studies it is known that CR oxycodone is absorbed in a biexponential way with a rapid phase that has a mean half-life of 37 minutes and a slow phase with a mean half-life of 6.2 hours (Mandema et al., 1996). The most significant difference from the normal-release form is the time for maximum concentration, which is reported as 3.2 (SD 2.2) hours for the CR form and 1.4 (SD 0.7) hours for the normal-release form (Reder et al., 1996; Benzinger et al., 1997). Czarnecki and colleagues (2004) studied the use of CR oxycodone for postoperative pain treatment after spinal fusion in children 10 to 19 years of age. In this study, the mean initial dose used was 1.24 mg/kg^{-1} per day^{-1} and the average use 13.3 days. Even though the authors did not report any adverse events and suggested that CR oxycodone is a plausible analgesic choice, there are no studies in children and it is not recommended (per manufacturer) for use in pediatrics. Additionally, there is increasing concern about the abuse of CR oxycodone, especially in adolescents (Cicero et al., 2005; Rogers and Copley, 2009).

Oxycodone is a μ-opioid receptor agonist with equianalgesic potency to intravenous morphine, despite the fact that its affinity to the μ-opioid receptor is over 20 times less than morphine. It has been suggested that oxycodone's potency is explained by higher CNS concentration caused by active transport across the BBB (Boström et al., 2006). In adult studies oxycodone showed a similar analgesic profile and incidence of side effects when compared with morphine, except for smaller changes in blood pressure and less sedation (Kalso et al., 1991; Silvasti et al., 1998). Also, in adults it has been shown that side effects are caused by the parent compound and not to metabolites (Lalovic et al., 2006). There is only one study in children that looks at the ventilatory effects of intravenous oxycodone. In this study Olkkola et al. (1994) suggested that oxycodone produced greater ventilatory depression than morphine. Other authors believe it has the same ventilatory effects as morphine in this population (Kalso, 1995).

In patients with renal and hepatic dysfunction, some extra considerations should be taken. Patients with severe hepatic dysfunction show impaired oxycodone elimination with 75% decreased plasma clearance, 50% increased volume of distribution, and an increased elimination half-life of from 3 to 14 hours (Tallgren, 1997). Patients with renal dysfunction show an increased volume of distribution and a prolonged elimination half-life as a result of reduced clearance (Kirvelä et al., 1996).

Codeine

Codeine (7,8-didehydro-4,5-epoxy-3-methoxy-17-methyl-morphinan-6 alpha-ol phosphate) is considered a weak opioid according to the World Health Organization's three-step analgesic ladder and is recommended for the treatment of mild to moderate pain. In children, codeine has been administered by oral, rectal, and intramuscular routes. It is not used in the intravenous form because of reported cases of severe hypotension (Parke et al., 1992). The recommended dose is 1 mg/kg to a maximum dose of 3 mg/kg per day. It is often used in combination with other analgesics such as acetaminophen, aspirin, and nonsteroidal antiinflammatory drugs.

Despite the widespread use of codeine in children, there are very few studies related to codeine pharmacokinetics in this age population. In adults, after oral administration codeine peak plasma concentration is reached after 60 minutes, compared with only 30 minutes after intramuscular administration. Terminal half-life is 3 to 3.5 hours, the volume of distribution is 3.6 l kg^{-1}, and the clearance rate 0.85 L/min^{-1} (Williams et al., 2001). In healthy adult volunteers, rectal and oral administration show good systemic bioavailability with reported values of 90% (Moolenaar et al., 1983). However, when administered in the postoperative period, values after rectal administration are less predictable, with systemic availability reported between 12% and 84% (Persson et al., 1992).

McEwan (2000) studied children between 3 months and 12 years of age and reported peak plasma values at 30 minutes after intramuscular and oral administration of codeine. Additionally, higher peak levels are described after intramuscular administration, which seem to correlate with better analgesia at 30 minutes. However, this effect is not persistent, and both routes showed similar performances after 1 hour. Codeine is metabolized in the liver by three different pathways: glucuronidation to codeine 6-glucuronide (the principal route), N-demethylation to norcodeine (10% to 20%) and O-demethylation to morphine (5% to 15%). Five to 15% of codeine is excreted unchanged in urine (Williams et al., 2001).

In a study of infants (0 to 10 months of age) and young children (3 to 4 years of age), Quiding et al. (1992) found that after administration of rectal codeine, the terminal half-life of codeine and morphine is 2.5 hours in infants; in children, the half-lives are 2.5 hours for codeine and 1.6 hours for morphine. Additionally, they found that AUC of morphine as a percentage of AUC of codeine ranged from 0% to 0.3%, similar to those previously described in adults; the authors concluded that infants at 6 months of age already have O-demethylation activity similar to that of adults (Quiding et al., 1986).

It is generally accepted that codeine's analgesic efficacy is explained by its conversion to morphine (Desmeules et al., 1991; Poulsen et al., 1996). O-demethylation to morphine is dependent on the enzyme cytochrome P450 (CYP2D6). The CYP2D6 gene is highly polymorphic, explaining wide levels of enzyme activity between individuals. There are four described phenotype levels of activity: poor metabolizers (PMs), intermediate metabolizers (IMs), extensive metabolizers (EMs), and ultrarapid metabolizers (UMs). The clinical implication of this variability is the unpredictability of analgesia and side effects of this medication. PMs show no analgesic effect, whereas UMs can show profound levels of analgesia with marked and potentially dangerous side effects (Poulsen et al., 1996; Ciszkowski et al., 2009). An example of this is found in a report by Voronov and colleagues (2007) on apnea and subsequent brain injury after administration of oral codeine in a child (of African origin) who was subsequently found to be an UM. The estimated incidence of UMs varies among racial and ethnic groups. It can be as low as 1% in the European, Caucasian, and Chinese populations, or up to 29% in Ethiopian (DeLeon, 2008, Stamer and Stuber, 2008).

Additionally, reports of randomized clinical trials in children evidenced lower analgesic efficacy of codeine when compared with oxycodone and higher failure rates when combined with acetaminophen and compared with ibuprofen (Charney et al., 2008; Drendel et al., 2009). There are two systematic reviews in adults that show only a small benefit of adding codeine acetaminophen (de Craen et al., 1996; Moore et al., 1997). These reports, plus the potential development of severe side effects in UMs, question the use of codeine when more predictable medications are available.

Opioid Agonist-Antagonists

Under this category are opioids that have a high affinity but poor efficacy at the μ-opioid receptor. Because of poor efficacy they act as μ-opioid receptor antagonists. Pentazocine, nalbuphine, and butorphanol belong to this class.

Nalbuphine

Nalbuphine is a phenanthrene opioid derivative, structurally similar to oxymorphone and naloxone. It has an analgesic potency equivalent to morphine with a respiratory depressant and analgesic ceiling effect between 150 and 300 mcg/kg (Beaver and Feise, 1978; Romagnoli and Keats., 1980; Gal and DiFazio, 1982; Julien, 1982). After intravenous administration in adults, it has an elimination half-life of 135.5 ± 55.4 minutes with a clearance of 217.6 mL/min (Sears et al., 1987). After intramuscular and subcutaneous administration, bioavailability is high, with mean values of 83% and 79%, respectively. Absorption is rapid with a C_{max} of 59.96 ± 9.52 ng/mL and 56.14 ± 14.48 ng/mL after intramuscular and subcutaneous injection of 20 mg in adults (Lo et al., 1987). After oral administration the bioavailability is low at 11.8% because of the high clearance rate (Aitkenhead et al., 1988). In children the distribution is similar to adults, but the elimination half-life is shorter (57 ± 14 minutes) (Jaillon et al., 1989). In a study in children receiving 0.3 mg/kg of nalbuphine rectally, the maximum plasma concentration achieved was 24 ± 15 ng/mL in a mean time of 25 ± 11 minutes with an elimination half-life of 162 ± 42 minutes (Bessard et al., 1997).

Nalbuphine has been used for treatment of opioid-induced pruritus. In adults, studies show similar effects to naloxone (Penning et al., 1988; Kendrick et al., 1996). However, one study in pediatrics did not have a similar finding, suggesting that nalbuphine may not be as effective in treating opioid-induced pruritus in children (Nakatsuka et al., 2006). Nalbuphine has also been used to decrease the incidence of emergence delirium after general anesthesia with sevoflurane as the sole agent for nonpainful procedures in children. Dalens et al. (2006) report that administration of a single dose of 0.1 mg/kg of nalbuphine before extubation decreases by 30% the development of emergence delirium without prolonging the postanesthesia recovery time when compared with placebo. The use of nalbuphine as a sole agent for postoperative pain treatment is scarce. There are two studies describing its use with positive reports after tonsillectomy and adenoidectomy procedures (Habre and McLeod, 1997; Van den Berg et al., 1999). However, the ceiling analgesic effect makes its use difficult for moderate to severe pain treatment.

Opioid Antagonists

Naloxone and naltrexone are competitive opioid antagonists at the μ-, k-, and d-receptors. At the μ-receptor, both have high affinity but total lack of efficacy, making them act as competitive inhibitors of exogenous and endogenous opiates. Both have central and peripheral actions but different pharmacokinetic profiles. Naltrexone is orally effective and has a long duration of action, making it excellent for detoxification in opiate-addicted patients. However, when it is used in patients receiving opiates for ongoing pain, acute withdrawal symptoms may be precipitated.

Naloxone has poor bioavailability after oral administration but a very fast onset of action after intravenous administration, making it the most common opioid antagonist used in anesthesia. It is structurally related to morphine and oxymorphone. After intravenous administration in adults, it has a peak effect at 1 to 2 minutes and a half-life of 64 ± 12 minutes (Ngai, 1976). Pharmacokinetic studies in newborns have been conflicting. Early reports in full-term newborns found an increased half-life (233 ± 140 minutes) after intraumbilical administration of 35 mcg of naloxone (Moreland et al., 1980). However, Stile et al. (1987) reported a shorter half-life of 70 ± 35.6 minutes in premature newborns (26 to 34 weeks' gestation). The discrepancies between the two neonatal studies may be explained by differences in the route of administration. Intramuscular naloxone has a bioavailability of 35% in adults with detectable blood levels up to 4 hours after administration (Dowling et al., 2008). In neonates blood levels after intramuscular administration are similar to the ones achieved after intravenous administration, with duration of action up to 24 hours (Moreland et al., 1980). For opioid reversal after anesthesia, doses of 0.01 mg/kg repeated every 2 to 3 minutes are recommended. Lower doses are used to treat opioid side effects, either in bolus or continuous infusion (Gan et al., 1997; Cepeda et al., 2004). Maxwell et al. (2005) described a significant reduction in the incidence of pruritus (50%) and nausea (40%) after morphine as patient-controlled analgesia with the use of a continuous low-dose naloxone infusion (0.25 mcg/kg^{-1} per hour^{-1}) in children, confirming previous studies in adults. A new peripherally acting μ-opioid receptor antagonist, methylnaltrexone, has been recently approved by the FDA for treatment of opioid-induced constipation in adults (Thomas et al., 2008). There are no studies of this agent in children.

INHALED ANESTHETIC AGENTS

Inhalation anesthesia remains the most common anesthetic technique in children. For people of all ages, the ideal agent would include properties such as rapid change in effect with change in delivery, low toxicity, minimal effects on cardiovascular and respiratory systems, and low cost. An inhalational agent that has a nonpungent odor and low airway irritability would be highly favored, particularly for children in whom inhalational induction is common. For these reasons, and also because of its relatively more favorable cardiovascular profile, sevoflurane is probably the most widely used agent for induction of anesthesia in children. Sevoflurane, isoflurane, and desflurane are all routinely used for maintenance of anesthesia. The use of halothane is now largely limited to countries where the cost of other agents is prohibitive. Although xenon has many potentially favorable properties, experience in children is limited and its high cost may be prohibitive. Nitrous oxide is still widely used as an adjunct to other agents during induction and maintenance of anesthesia. Nitrous oxide is also used by itself for procedural sedation.

Physical Properties

At atmospheric pressure and room temperatures, nitrous oxide and xenon are gases, whereas the other agents are all liquids. Desflurane's boiling point is close to room temperature, so a heated pressurized vaporizer is used to provide a reliable delivery of the agent independent of ambient temperature. Halothane is a polyhalogenated alkane, and sevoflurane, isoflurane, and desflurane are polyhalogenated ethers. Xenon is a naturally occurring element that exists as 0.05 ppm in the atmosphere. It is produced as a byproduct in the fractional distillation of air. Properties of the anesthetic agents are summarized in Table 7-19.

Nitrous Oxide

The physical properties of nitrous oxide may produce some particular clinical considerations. Nitrous oxide reduces the anesthetic requirements for the more potent inhalational agents, speeds the uptake of the more potent agents, and serves to dilute the inspired oxygen content. Inhaling high concentrations of nitrous oxide causes air-filled body cavities to expand. This is because nitrous oxide is considerably more soluble in blood than is nitrogen (partition coefficients of 0.47 for nitrous oxide and 0.014 for nitrogen), and therefore the volume of nitrous oxide diffusing into the cavity exceeds the volume of nitrogen that can diffuse out (Eger, 1974). Assuming a trivial quantity of nitrogen diffuses out of the space while ventilating the lungs with nitrous oxide, then the maximum multiple expansion of the original space that can occur is as follows (Eger, 1974):

$$\text{Multiple} = 100 / (100 - \% \text{ nitrous oxide})$$

Using this equation, if 75% nitrous oxide is inspired, then the space volume may expand up to threefold. The rate at which the space expands varies with the site; a pneumothorax may double in size in 12 minutes, whereas a small bowel obstruction may double in 120 minutes (Eger, 1974). This 10-fold difference in the rate of expansion is determined in part by the reduction in (mural) blood flow to the bowel as the gas volume within the lumen expands. The same limitation of blood flow does not occur with a pneumothorax. Other cavities that may expand in the presence of nitrous oxide include the middle ear, gas within the ocular globe, and CNS air from a pneumoencephalogram. In situations where oxygenation (either inspired oxygen concentration or tissue oxygenation) must be maximized, the use of nitrous oxide, particularly in concentrations in excess of 50%, must be judiciously reviewed. The potency of nitrous oxide is affected by barometric pressure, being less effective at high altitude than at sea level or below.

Once believed to be entirely nontoxic, nitrous oxide has aroused increasing suspicion of cellular and atmospheric toxicity on several counts. Lymphocyte depression, miscarriage (first trimester), cancer, defects in spermatogenesis, and apoptosis have raised concerns about health risks after prolonged exposure (Brodsky et al., 1984; Rowland et al., 1995; Jevtovic-Todorovic et al., 2003). The half-life of nitrous oxide, an oxygen-free radical scavenger, in the troposphere is approximately 150 years, compared with the half-lives of the polyhalogenated inhalational anesthetics, which have tropospheric half-lives of 5 to 10 years. Although less than 5% of the nitrous oxide released into the atmosphere originates from medical sources, limiting the waste of nitrous oxide through the use of low fresh gas flows and smoke stack scrubbers curbs the depletion of the ozone layer. In infants the expansion of bowel can make abdominal surgery technically difficult. Many surgeons prefer nitrous oxide to be avoided in laparoscopic and laparotomy procedures. Nitrous oxide should be discontinued if bowel expansion becomes problematic or is likely to be problematic (Orhan-Sungur et al., 2005).

Nitrous oxide and xenon are odorless, whereas the halogenated agents all have distinct odors. Desflurane and isoflurane are significantly more pungent than halothane or sevoflurane. Therefore, inhalational induction in a child is considerably more acceptable with sevoflurane or halothane.

TABLE 7-19. The Pharmacology and Solubility of Inhalational Anesthetics

	Halothane	Isoflurane	Sevoflurane	Desflurane	Nitrous Oxide	Xenon
Molecular weight	197.4	184.5	200.1	168	44	131
Boiling point (°C)	50.2	48.5	58.6	23.5	−88.5	−108.1
Vapor pressure (mm hg)	244	240	185	664	—	—
Metabolized (%)	15-25	0.2	5	0.02	—	—
Solubility						
Blood: gas partitian coefficient	2.4	1.4	0.66	0.42	0.47	0.115
Fat: blood partitian coefficient	51	45	48	27	2.3	Not known
MAC						
MAC in adults (%)	0.75	1.2	2.05	7.0	104	71
MAC in a 2 year old (%)	0.97	1.60	2.6	8.73	Not known	Not known

Pharmacokinetics

Many principles of pharmacokinetics are common between the inhalation and intravenous anesthetics, but there are some subtle differences. With inhalation agents, differences in partial pressure drive the agent across tissues rather concentration gradients. For intravenous agents, central compartment (blood) concentrations can change directly as more drug is delivered. Changing inspired partial pressure with inhalation anesthetics has a more indirect effect on the central compartment because of the differences between inspired and alveolar partial pressures. Similarly, the elimination of inhalational agent through the lung also adds a layer of complexity. In spite of these differences, multicompartmental modeling and the concept of effect-site concentration can be applied to both inhalational and intravenous agents.

Wash-in is the uptake and wash-out is the elimination of inhalation anesthetics through the lung. Wash-in is often summarized as the increase over time in the alveolar fraction (F_A) over inspired fraction (F_I) of the agent (F_A/F_I). The F_A is important, because it approximates partial pressure in the blood and because it is measured clinically as the end-tidal concentration.

Wash-In

The F_I is determined largely by the inspired concentration, the circuit characteristics such as the degree of mixing between fresh and exhaled gas, the total fresh gas flow, and the dead space in the circuit. The rate of rise of F_A/F_I is determined by the ratio of alveolar ventilation compared with functional residual capacity, the solubility of the agent in blood, the cardiac output (total perfusion of the lungs), and the gradient of partial pressure of inhalation agent between the alveolus and the pulmonary arterial blood. More soluble agents have a slower wash-in, and lower ventilation itself also results in a slower wash-in (Fig. 7-38). Wash-in of the more soluble agents is also affected to a greater degree by ventilation than is wash-in of less soluble anesthetics (Figs. 7-39 and 7-40). For example, changing ventilation has little effect on wash-in of highly blood-insoluble agents such as nitrous oxide but a substantial effect on wash-in of more blood-soluble agents such as halothane (Eger, 1974). As cardiac output increases, wash-in decreases as the agent is removed more rapidly from the alveolus. Once again the effect changes with solubility, with a greater effect seen in more soluble agents (Eger, 1974). Lastly, wash-in is faster with a lower gradient of partial pressure between alveolus and mixed venous blood (pulmonary arterial blood). In other words, if mixed venous partial pressures are very low and alveolar pressures are high, then wash-in is slower.

The pulmonary arterial partial pressure of the inhalation agent is determined by the redistribution of the agent into the body tissues. This redistribution can be modeled like any other pharmacokinetic system, with the blood being the central compartment and any number of additional peripheral compartments that correlate to organ groups that rich, moderate, and poor with vessels. In the classic model of compartments grouped by vascular richness, the rate of redistribution to peripheral compartments is determined by the blood flow, tissue and blood solubility, and volume of the compartments. The effect-site partial pressure can also be modeled along with the K_{eo}.

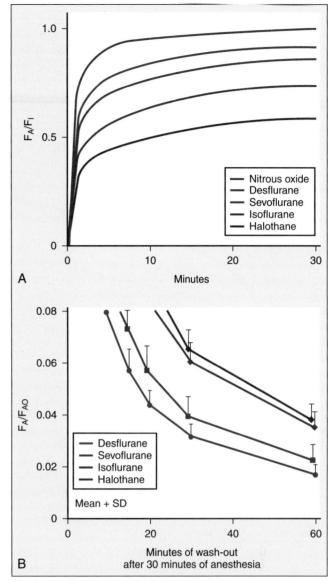

■ FIGURE 7-38. A, In unstimulated human volunteers, the increase in the alveolar concentration (F_A) toward the inspired concentration (F_I) is more rapid with the least soluble potent inhaled anesthetic (desflurane) and slowest with the most soluble potent inhaled anesthetic (halothane). Only nitrous oxide has a more rapid increase in F_A/F_I than desflurane. Nitrous oxide has a still more rapid increase because of its low solubility in blood and tissues and because of the employment of a greater inspired concentration (i.e., its rise is influenced by the concentration effect). **B,** Elimination, as defined by the decrease in alveolar concentration relative to the last alveolar concentration found during anesthesia (F_{AO}), is most rapid with desflurane, less rapid with sevoflurane, and slowest with isoflurane and halothane. Despite its greater solubility, the decrease with halothane is as rapid as the decrease with isoflurane, because halothane is metabolized and thus is cleared from the body by both the lungs and liver, whereas isoflurane is cleared only by the lungs.

Right to-left shunting of blood influences the relationship between wash-in and the systemic arterial partial pressure of the inhalational anesthetic. Again, the influence of shunt varies with blood-gas solubility. Right-to-left shunting has a greater influence with a less soluble agent than with a more soluble

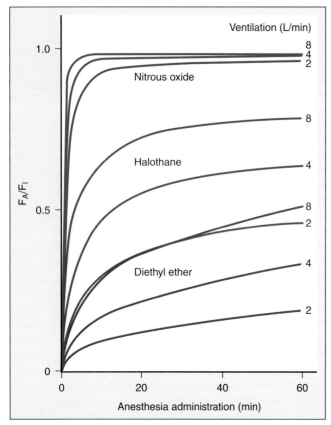

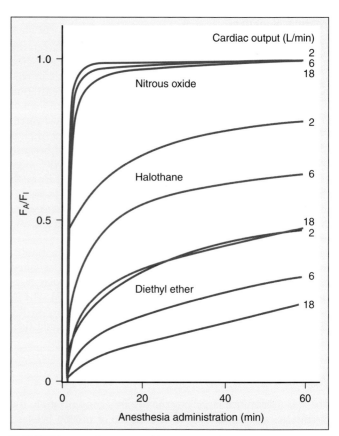

■ **FIGURE 7-39.** The alveolar concentration of anesthetic/concentration of inspired anesthetic (F_A/F_I ratio) rises more rapidly if ventilation is increased. Solubility modifies this impact of ventilation; the effect on the anesthetizing partial pressure is greatest with the most soluble anesthetic (ether) and least with the least soluble anesthetic (nitrous oxide). *(Modified from Eger EI II: Ventilation, circulation, and uptake. In Eger EI II, editor: Anesthetic uptake and action, Baltimore, 1974, Williams & Wilkins.)*

■ **FIGURE 7-40.** If unopposed by a concomitant increase in ventilation, an increase in cardiac output decreases alveolar anesthetic concentration by augmenting uptake. The resulting alveolar anesthetic change is greatest with the most soluble anesthetic. F_A/F_I is the ration of alveolar concentration of anesthetic to the concentration of inspired anesthetic. *(Modified from Eger EI II: Ventilation, circulation, and uptake. In Eger EI II, editor: Anesthetic uptake and action, Baltimore, 1974, Williams & Wilkins.)*

agent (Fig. 7-41). Thus, in principle for sevoflurane, presence of congenital cyanotic heart disease would slow the onset of anesthesia, whereas if halothane were used the effect of the shunt would be less. Although in theory such shunts may indeed slow wash-in, this is of questionable clinical relevance because the children with shunts may have many factors that can influence induction technique and choice of anesthetic.

Wash-in changes with age. Wash-in is faster in infants than in adults and older children (Fig. 7-42) (Salanitre and Rackow, 1969; Steward and Creighton, 1978; Brandom et al., 1983a; Gallagher and Black, 1985). All reasons for these changes are not completely understood, but the following explanations are included:

● Infants have greater ventilation relative to functional residual capacity (5:1 in neonates and 1.5:1 in adults).
● Agents in neonatal blood have less solubility than in adult blood (Lerman et al., 1984).
● There are different cardiac output and different redistribution of agents from the central compartment in neonates (movement of agent blood into peripheral tissues). Even though neonates have relatively large cardiac output, relatively more is initially distributed to tissues with

less agent solubility and consequently less initial uptake of agent peripherally, leading to greater pulmonary arterial partial pressures and thereby increasing wash-in.
● Total tissue solubility is generally less in infants (Lerman et al., 1986). This leads to a faster rise in pulmonary arterial pressures, as previously described. This change with age may be the result of greater water content in neonates and less protein and lipid. This difference in solubility is the most apparent for halothane.

The effect of age on wash-in varies between inhalational anesthetics. The influence of age is least for less soluble agents such as sevoflurane and desflurane.

Although there are good data describing the faster wash-in in infants, there are fewer data describing in detail how fast concentrations rise in the brain compared with the blood. For halothane, modeling has predicated faster rises in brain and myocardium for infants compared with adults (Fig. 7-43) (Brandom et al., 1983a). This modeling uses the classic model of pharmacokinetics. The time constant (τ) for equilibrium between blood and brain can be roughly estimated from the brain volume, brain-blood solubility, and blood flow. If blood flow to the brain is 50 mL/min per 100 g, and the brain-blood

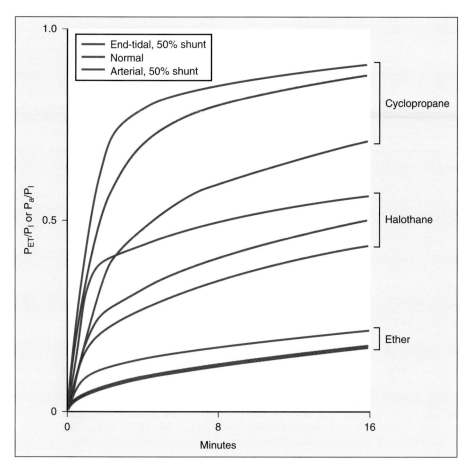

■ **FIGURE 7-41.** When no ventilation-perfusion abnormalities exist, the alveolar (P_A or P_{ET}) and arterial (*a*) anesthetic partial pressures rise together (*brown lines*) toward the inspired partial pressure (P_a). When 50% of the cardiac output is shunted through the lungs, the rate of rise of the end-tidal partial pressure (*blue lines*) is accelerated, whereas the rate of rise of the arterial partial pressure (*purple lines*) is retarded. The greatest retardation is found with the least soluble anesthetic, cyclopropane. *(From Eger El II, editor:* Anesthetic uptake and action, *Baltimore, 1974, Williams & Wilkins.)*

Legend in figure:
— End-tidal, 50% shunt
— Normal
— Arterial, 50% shunt

Cyclopropane
Halothane
Ether

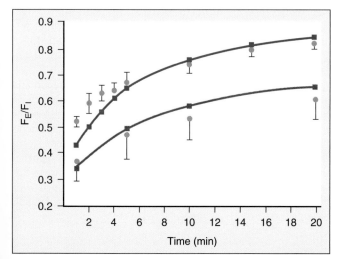

■ **FIGURE 7-42.** The observed ratio of expired to inspired halothane (F_E/F_I) in infants demonstrates their more rapid uptake of halothane compared with adults. *Blue circles,* Infant observed (mean ± SD); *blue line,* infant predicted; *brown circles,* adult observed (mean ± SD); *brown line,* adult predicted. Predicted curves generated from a computerized model. *(Data from Sechzer PH et al.:* Anesthesiology *24:779, 1963; Eger El II et al.:* Anesthesiology *35:365, 1971a; International Anesthesia Research Society; Brandom BW et al.: Uptake and distribution of halothane in infants: in vivo measurements and computer simulations,* Anesth Analg *62[4]:404, 1983.)*

solubility is 2, then τ equals 4 minutes. Given that three time constants achieve 95% equilibrium, the total time to achieve equilibrium equals 12 minutes. If in neonates the solubility is only 1, then τ = 2 minutes and 95% equilibrium occurs in 6 minutes. It may be important to note that in such classic models there is an assumption that there is no delay between brain concentration and anesthetic effect. This assumption may not always be valid, because an anesthetic effect such as loss of consciousness involves complex neural networks that may themselves have some time constants.

There are few data describing the $t_{1/2}K_{eo}$ constants for inhalational anesthetics. In one study, Fuentes et al. (2008) describe a decreased $t_{1/2}K_{eo}$ for sevoflurane in children compared with that in adults. This fits with the predicted results in the modeling mentioned previously. There are no data yet for the $t_{1/2}K_{eo}$ in children who are younger than 3 years of age. This lack of information is important, because anesthesiologists monitor F_A with end-tidal gas analysis but have no direct way of monitoring effect-site concentration, so any age-dependent difference in $t_{1/2}K_{eo}$ would influence the lag between observed end-tidal concentration and targeted clinical effect.

In summary, small children have a faster induction because of both faster wash-in and shorter $t_{1/2}K_{eo}$. Clinically, a rapid inhalational induction is also facilitated by using a high F_I (overpressure). The maximum concentration that can be delivered varies between agents depending on the maximum incorporated into the design of the vaporizer. Halothane can be administered at up

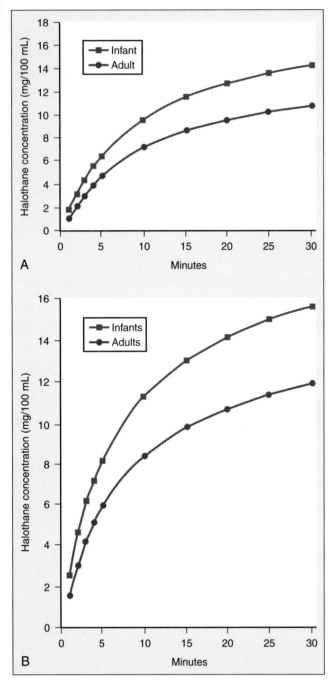

■ FIGURE 7-43. A, Predicted concentration of halothane in the brain. Values were derived from a computerized model of anesthetic uptake and distribution. **B,** Predicted concentration of halothane in the heart. *(From Brandom BW et al.: Uptake and distribution of halothane in infants: in vivo measurements and computer simulations, Anesth Analg 62[4]:404, 1983.)*

to 5%, whereas sevoflurane can be given at up to 8% (although some vaporizers restrict the maximum sevoflurane concentration to 5% to 7%). Halothane, however, is more than three times as potent as sevoflurane; therefore, halothane vaporizers can deliver more multiples of MAC. Even though sevoflurane may have a faster wash-in than halothane, if 5% halothane is delivered, it will have faster clinical effect than 8% sevoflurane. Because halothane has significant toxic cardiac effects, 5% halothane may quickly lead to cardiovascular collapse.

Wash-Out

When the inhalation anesthetic is discontinued, wash-out represents the decrease over time in F_A/F_I. Factors influencing wash-out are similar to those affecting wash-in (e.g., blood solubility, tissue solubility, and ventilation). In general, wash-out increases as blood solubility decreases. Wash-out may also be influenced by duration of anesthetic, reflecting redistribution from peripheral compartments. This influence is less for less-soluble agents. Comparing context sensitive half-times, there is little difference between sevoflurane, isoflurane, and desflurane after short anesthesia, whereas substantial changes occur after prolonged anesthesia. After 6 hours, decrement time is least for desflurane, followed by sevoflurane and then isoflurane (Bailey, 1997). The wash-out and decrement characteristics of halothane are more complex in that a substantial quantity of halothane is metabolized. Although the context-sensitive half-time for halothane may be higher than for other less soluble agents after short anesthesia, because a substantial amount of halothane is metabolized, its context-sensitive half-time does not rise substantially with time, so that after anesthesia of some hours' duration it is less than sevoflurane.

As many of the factors influencing wash-out are similar to those determining wash-in, it would be expected that age-related effects would be similar, with wash-out being faster in infants. However, no clinical studies have been performed to confirm this expectation. The effect of age on time to recovery from anesthesia may also be influenced by maturational changes in the neurophysiology of arousal and awakening.

Metabolism and Toxicity

Xenon, an inert element, is not metabolized. Nitrous oxide is also not metabolized to any appreciable degree by human tissue; however, in the presence of vitamin B_{12}, intestinal bacteria may reduce nitrous oxide to nitrogen. Amongst the halogenated inhalational anesthetics, desflurane is the least metabolized (0.02%), followed by isoflurane (0.2%), sevoflurane (5%), and halothane (25%) (Kharasch, 1995). The metabolism of isoflurane and desflurane is of no clinical significance (Box 7-2).

Sevoflurane is oxidized *in vivo* to inorganic fluoride ion and hexafluoroisopropanol. This is mainly through the CYP2E1 enzyme system (Kharasch, 1995). The activity of CYP2E1 is low at birth and then gradually increases during childhood (Vieira et al., 1996). Hexafluoroisopropanol is in turn conjugated to form glucuronide and excreted. No renal toxicity has been reported after sevoflurane anesthesia in spite of measured plasma fluoride levels greater than 50 mcm/L, the level associated with methoxyflurane and nephrotoxicity (Ebert et al., 1998a, 1998b).

Box 7-2 *In Vivo* Metabolism of Inhalational Anesthetics

INHALATIONAL AGENT; PERCENT METABOLIZED
Methoxyflurane; 50
Halothane; 20
Sevoflurane; 5
Enflurane; 2.4
Isoflurane; 0.2
Desflurane; 0.02

The lack of toxicity compared with methoxyflurane may be to the result of differences in where the metabolism occurs. With methoxyflurane, intrarenal metabolism is substantial, leading to high local concentrations of fluoride, whereas most metabolism of sevoflurane occurs in the liver rather than the kidneys, so intrarenal levels of fluorides are not as great.

Sevoflurane is absorbed by and degraded by alkaline hydrolysis in the presence of soda lime or baralyme into five compounds (A through E) (Hanaki et al., 1987; Morio et al., 1992). Only compound A is produced in significant concentrations, with levels of 20 to 40 ppm after several hours of 2.5% sevoflurane and a low fresh gas flow (Liu et al., 1991; Bito and Ikeda, 1994; Frink et al., 1996). Alkaline hydrolysis is enhanced by increased temperatures, low water content, high concentration of sevoflurane, the use of baralyme rather than soda lime, or the use of new soda lime. Although 100 ppm of compound A has been found to cause renal damage in rats, no evidence for injury has been seen in humans. The production of compound A is less with newer CO_2 absorbents (Kharasch et al., 2002). In spite of the lack of human evidence, some authorities suggest that if sevoflurane is used in a closed circuit system with baralyme or soda lime, then the fresh gas flow should not be less than 2 liters/min.

Carbon monoxide (CO) can also be produced by sevoflurane, isoflurane, or desflurane in the presence of desiccated soda lime or baralyme, although only in minute and clinically inconsequential concentrations. The magnitude of CO production is desflurane > isoflurane > halothane and sevoflurane. Newer CO_2 absorbents that do not have the strong bases such as KOH or NaOH produce effectively no CO (Kharasch et al., 2002).

Potency

The potency of inhaled agents is defined in terms of MAC. The MAC at which 50% of patients do not move on skin incision is termed *1 MAC*. MAC varies between inhalation anesthetics and is generally inversely related to lipid solubility. Another general rule is that MAC is additive; i.e., 0.5 MAC of sevoflurane delivered with 0.5 MAC of isoflurane is equivalent to 1 MAC of isoflurane. In children there are exceptions to the rule; notably, MAC for nitrous oxide and halothane are additive, but MAC is less than additive for both nitrous oxide with sevoflurane and nitrous oxide with desflurane (Fisher and Zwass, 1992; Lerman et al., 1994).

MAC has also been determined in terms of the concentration at which 50% of subjects respond to other forms of stimuli, such as endotracheal intubation (MAC_{INT}), laryngeal mask airway insertion (MAC_{LMA}), and endotracheal extubation (MAC_{EXT}) and in terms of concentration at which 50% of subjects have other types of responses for defined stimuli, such as hemodynamic response to pain (MAC_{BAR}) or awakening (MAC_{AWAKE}). MAC_{INT} is usually 50% higher than MAC, whereas MAC_{LMA} is similar to MAC (Inomata et al., 1994; Kihara et al., 2003). MAC_{BAR} is approximately 30% greater than MAC. MAC_{EXT} is approximately 25% less than MAC, whereas MAC_{AWAKE} for most inhalational anesthetics is about 30% of MAC (Cranfield and Bromley, 1997; Inomata et al., 1998; Kihara et al., 2000). These relationships are often agent dependent; e.g., MAC_{AWAKE} for halothane and nitrous oxide is relatively high at 0.5 MAC (Stoelting et al., 1970; Gaumann et al., 1992). MAC and MAC_{BAR} may be significantly reduced by the addition of antinociceptive agents such as opioids (Katoh et al., 1999). In contrast, MAC_{AWAKE} is less affected by these agents (Katoh et al., 1993a, 1993b).

In clinical practice, anesthesia is given to guarantee that nearly all patients do not respond, so indeed we are far more interested in MAC at which 95% or 99% of subjects do not respond. In spite of this most MAC studies define MAC at 50% response. MAC is also determined for a short skin incision. A typical surgery involves a wide variety of stimuli; some are greater than that used to determine MAC, and many are smaller. Finally, when considering MAC studies it is important to consider the certainty (standard error or 95% confidence interval) around the estimates of MAC. The degree of uncertainty in MAC at 50% and the uncertainty in how to relate MAC at 50% to MAC at 95% make clinical interpretation of MAC data very difficult. This is particularly relevant to children, for whom studies are relatively few.

MAC changes with age (Fig. 7-44 and Table 7-20) (Lerman et al., 1983; Cameron et al., 1984; LeDez and Lerman, 1987; Murray et al., 1991; Taylor and Lerman, 1991; Katoh and Ikeda, 1992; Mapleson, 1996; Nickalls and Mapleson, 2003). In general, MAC rises during the neonatal period to peak in infancy and then declines throughout life, reaching the lowest values in old age. The MAC for sevoflurane is somewhat different. With sevoflurane the MAC the peak occurs in neonates and is therefore not less than it is infants (Lerman et al., 1994). It is not known exactly why MAC changes with age. The MAC for xenon and nitrous oxide has not been determined in children.

Although studies are few, MAC_{INT}, MAC_{LMA}, MAC_{EXT}, MAC_{BAR}, and MAC_{AWAKE} have a similar relationship to MAC in children (Katoh et al., 1993a, 1993b; Inomata et al., 1994, 1998; Cranfield and Bromley, 1997; Kihara et al., 2003). There is some evidence that MAC_{AWAKE} in children is relatively less in small children (Davidson et al., 2008a). Although this is consistent with animal data, these studies need to be interpreted with caution given the difficulty of measuring wakefulness in small children.

Effects on Systems and Side Effects

Cardiovascular System

Inhalational anesthetics affect the cardiovascular system through many different and often linked mechanisms. They may have direct effects on myocardial contractility, cardiac conduction, or vascular smooth muscle, or there may be indirect activity via autonomic, neurohumoral, or cardiovascular reflex systems. The responses in children may differ from those in adults because of differences in maturation and differences in patterns of coexisting pathology. The contractility of neonatal myocardium is more sensitive to inhalational anesthetics in comparison with adult myocardium, resulting in a greater decrease in contractility (Rao et al., 1986; Krane and Su, 1987; Murat et al., 1990). This effect may be related to a reduced amount of contractile elements in the neonatal myocardium or to differences in the functional maturity of the sarcoplasmic reticulum and calcium channel function.

In children, halothane, isoflurane, desflurane, and sevoflurane all decrease systemic blood pressure in a dose-dependent way. The percentage of decrease in blood pressure compared with blood pressure in the nonanesthetized state is greater in infants than it is in older children. One MAC of sevoflurane results in about a 20% to 30% reduction in systolic blood pressure in neonates and infants, compared with a reduction of about a 10%

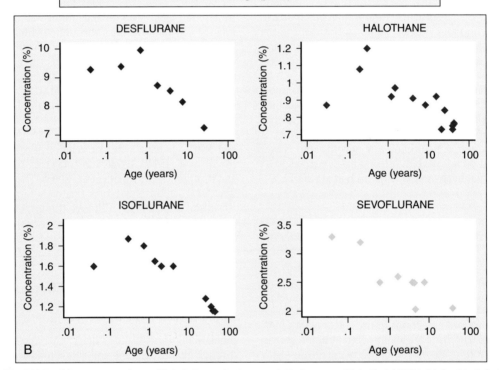

■ **FIGURE 7-44.** The MACs of four commonly used inhaled anesthetics are plotted vs. age. Note that MAC is highest in infants 3 to 6 months of age. The reasons for this are not clear. *(From Coté CJ: Pediatric anesthesia. In: Miller RD, Eriksson LI, Fleisher LA, et al: Miller's anesthesia, ed 7, Philadelphia, 2010, Churchill Livingstone.)*

reduction in older children. Similarly, 1 MAC of desflurane results in about a 30% reduction in blood pressure in neonates and infants but only about a 20% reduction in older children (Taylor and Lerman, 1991; Lerman et al., 1994). Halothane has a substantially greater effect on myocardial contractility, whereas the other agents decrease blood pressure mainly by decreasing systemic vascular resistance (Wolf et al., 1986). Halothane also results in a dose-dependent decrease in heart rate, but the other agents cause a dose-dependent increase in heart rate. The effect of halothane on atrioventricular conduction is greater in infants than it is in adults and older children (Palmisano et al., 1994). Halothane also sensitizes the myocardium to catecholamines, increasing the risk of arrhythmias particularly during hypercarbia (Karl et al., 1983). Sevoflurane has no effect on atrioventricular conduction and does not change the sensitivity

of myocardium to catecholamines (Navarro et al., 1994). The cardiovascular effects of nitrous oxide have been incompletely studied in children. Xenon has minimal cardiovascular effects in adults but has not been studied specifically for its cardiovascular effects in children.

Respiratory System

Halothane, isoflurane, sevoflurane, and desflurane all depress ventilatory drive and response to CO_2 resulting in a dose-dependent decrease in alveolar ventilation occurring mainly through reduced tidal volume (Murat et al., 1985, 1987; Brown et al., 1998). Respiratory rate tends to increase up to 1 MAC and then decreases at concentrations greater than 1 MAC. There is some evidence that halothane causes less depression o

TABLE 7-20. Minimum Alveolar Concentrations (MAC) of Volatile Anesthetics in Children

Parameter	MAC Anesthetic Concentration
Halothane	
Neonates	0.87
1-6 mo	1.20
15 ± 7 mo	0.94
Isoflurane	
Preterm <32 weeks' gestation	1.28
Preterm 32-37 weeks' gestation	1.41
7-30 mo	1.69
4-10 yr	1.69
Sevoflurane	
Neonates	3.3
1-6 mo	3.2
6-12 mo	2.5
1-3 yr	2.6
2-12 yr	2.3-2.5
Desflurane	
Neonates	9.16
1-6 mo	9.42
6-12 mo	9.92
1-3 yr	8.72
3-5 yr	8.62
5-12 yr	7.98

From Mazoit JX: Pharmacokinetic/pharmacodynamic modeling of anesthetics in children: therapeutic implications, *Paediatr Drugs* 8(3):139, 2006.

respiratory drive than sevoflurane (Brown et al., 1998). Similarly all agents depress the tone of airway musculature, causing an increased risk of airway obstruction and there is some suggestion that halothane may once again cause less depression.

Halothane, isoflurane, and sevoflurane are all bronchodilators (Rooke and Su, 1993). Whereas sevoflurane improves airway and respiratory mechanics in children with airway sensitivity, desflurane causes worsening mechanics (von Ungern-Sternberg et al., 2008). Sevoflurane and halothane are minimally irritating to the airways, but isoflurane, and particularly desflurane, are more irritating and pungent. Induction with desflurane is associated with a substantial risk of airway complications; however, extubation after desflurane anesthesia is not associated with a high rate of complications (Taylor and Lerman, 1991, 1992; Fisher and Zwass, 1992; Zwass et al., 1992; Cranfield and Bromley, 1997). Even though sevoflurane is a minimal irritant, in some measures of airway irritability it is still more irritating than propofol anesthesia (Oberer et al., 2005).

Xenon is odorless and nonirritating to the airways, but it has density of 5.9 g/L compared with 1.5 g/L for nitrous oxide and g/L for air. The greater density can result in increased work of breathing. This may be clinically significant in neonates.

Central Nervous System

In children, the influence of inhalational anesthetics on the cerebral vasculature is complex and incompletely studied (Szabo et al., 2009). All inhalational agents depress the CNS and reduce cerebral metabolic rate as measured by the cerebral metabolic rate for oxygen (CMR_{O_2}). Agents may also have direct effects on the cerebral vascular tone both directly and indirectly through alterations to autoregulation and responsiveness to CO_2. During inhalation, cerebral blood flow (CBF) during anesthesia and hence cerebral blood volume and intracranial pressure, are thus determined by the direct effect on cerebral vascular tone, the CMR_{O_2}, the capacity for autoregulation, and the cerebral perfusion pressure. All of these can be influenced by inhalational anesthetics to differing degrees, and hence the action of inhalational anesthetics on CBF is varied and difficult to predict. In general, an ideal agent would reduce CMR_{O_2} with a matched decrease in CBF and minimal effect on autoregulation or responsiveness to CO_2.

All volatile agents are direct cerebral vasodilators, with halothane and desflurane being the most potent and sevoflurane the least potent (Matta et al., 1999; Bedforth et al., 2000; Fairgrieve et al., 2003; Luginbuehl et al., 2003; Sponheim et al., 2003; Barlow et al., 2004). Children may have an increased sensitivity to the vasodilation of inhalational anesthetics (Luginbuehl et al., 2003). Most inhalational anesthetics agents decrease CMR_{O_2}. The decrease in CMR_{O_2} is greatest with isoflurane and sevoflurane, and least with halothane (Oshima et al., 2003). Considering the effect of the agent on CMR_{O_2} and direct effects on the vasculature, the total CBF is greatest with halothane, followed by desflurane, isoflurane, and then sevoflurane. The effect is dose-dependent. With isoflurane and sevoflurane there is minimal change in CBF at less than 1 MAC, and any small rise that occurs can be overcome with very mild hyperventilation (Leon and Bissonnette, 1991). Similarly, at less than 1 MAC, isoflurane and sevoflurane have minimal effects on autoregulation and responsiveness to CO_2 (Fairgrieve et al., 2003; Vavilala et al., 2003; McCulloch et al., 2005; Wong et al., 2006).

Nitrous oxide increases CBF and CMR_{O_2} and impairs autoregulation. It is therefore generally avoided in children at risk of impaired cerebral perfusion (Bedforth et al., 1999; Girling et al., 1999; Rowney et al., 2004). The effect of xenon on cerebral vasculature has been incompletely studied in adults, and there are no studies in children. There is some evidence to suggest xenon has a similar effect as other inhalational anesthetics (Laitio et al., 2009).

Inhalational anesthetics produce reproducible and dose-dependent changes in the EEG. Low concentrations result in an increase in power, especially in the higher frequencies. Increasing concentrations result in a gradual shift of power to the lower frequencies and a decrease in total power. High doses result in burst suppression and an isoelectic EEG. The shifts in frequencies and power differ between agents, with halothane and nitrous oxide rarely exhibiting burst suppression. In older children the EEG patterns are similar to those of adults, but in infants there are significant differences. Infants have substantially lower total power, less obvious shifts in frequency with dose, and greater variability in the time domain (Davidson et al., 2008a).

There are several commercially available processed EEG devices that use the EEG to measure anesthesia depth. Several studies have shown that in older children the indices derived by these devices correlate with the doses of sevoflurane and isoflurane, and they have some capacity to differentiate conscious states (Davidson, 2006). The indices derived from these devices do not correlate well to concentration of nitrous oxide and xenon, and at 1 MAC they show different values for halothane than for isoflurane or sevoflurane (Davidson and Czarnecki, 2004). In infants the performance of these EEG-derived depth monitors is significantly worse, and they are not recommended for use in infants (Davidson et al., 2005). Although EEG-derived anesthesia depth monitor indices correlate with the dose of anesthesia, there are only a few studies investigating their usefulness in clinical practice in children. These studies have generally found that BIS-guided anesthesia results in slightly lower agent consumption, shorter awakening times, and slightly faster recovery (Bannister et al., 2001; Messieha et al., 2004, 2005). Similar modest differences have been demonstrated for propofol anesthesia (Weber et al., 2005a, 2005b). They have not been shown to reduce awareness in children.

There is great controversy surrounding epileptiform activity and sevoflurane in children. Spiking has been reported by several authors during induction with sevoflurane (Yli-Hankala et al., 1999; Vakkuri et al., 2001; Sonkajärvi et al., 2009). The phenomenon is poorly understood and may be associated with clinical signs of seizures such as myoclonic activity (Voss et al., 2008). There is no evidence to suggest a link between these EEG findings and any adverse postanesthesia outcome, so the clinical significance of unusual or spiking activity during sevoflurane anesthesia is unknown. To limit epileptiform activity, some recommend limiting the inspired concentration of sevoflurane to less than 6%. Note that limiting inspired sevoflurane concentration in this way may only have an indirect effect on limiting cortical concentration caused by wash-in and the time taken to achieve equilibrium with effect site. Similarly, any limitation in inspired sevoflurane concentration and overpressure should be accompanied by increased care that time is taken to achieve equilibrium to avoid the complications of inadequate anesthesia. Although sevoflurane does increase spiking in patients with epilepsy, there is no evidence that sevoflurane increases the risk of adverse outcome in children with epilepsy, and opinion is divided as to whether or not sevoflurane should be avoided in children with epilepsy (Kurita et al., 2005).

Other Side Effects

Malignant Hyperthermia

Halothane, isoflurane, sevoflurane, and desflurane may all trigger malignant hyperthermia in susceptible individuals, including children. Xenon and nitrous oxide are thought not to trigger malignant hypothermia (see Chapter 37, Malignant Hyperthermia).

Nitrous Oxide Toxicity

Nitrous oxide can oxidize vitamin B_{12} and hence inhibit its coenzyme function. This may reduce the activity of methionine synthase, which produces methionine from homocysteine, which in turn may impair DNA synthesis. The clinical relevance of this toxicity is unlikely to be relevant after only brief exposure.

Hepatotoxcity

Halothane, isoflurane, sevoflurane, and desflurane have all been associated with transient hepatic dysfunction and raised transaminase enzymes in adults, although the evidence for a causal link is particularly poor for sevoflurane and desflurane. The mechanism of hepatic failure or "halothane hepatitis" is unclear, but it may be the result of an immunologic response to a metabolite. This metabolite is not a product of the other inhalation anesthetics. Although controversial, there is evidence to suggest "halothane hepatitis" can occur in children (Kenna et al., 1987).

Properties of Specific Inhaled Agents

Sevoflurane

Sevoflurane is a polyfluorinated methyl isopropyl ether anesthetic that is the first ether anesthetic to be widely used for the induction of anesthesia in children. Its low blood solubility, half that of isoflurane, speeds the equilibration of alveolar and inspired anesthetic partial pressures (Fig. 7-38). However, the tissue and blood solubilities of sevoflurane and isoflurane in the vessel-rich group (brain, heart, liver, kidneys, and endocrine glands), muscle, and fat groups are indistinguishable. Because the wash-in of inhalational anesthetics is increased by use of the overpressure technique, these physicochemical differences affect the wash-in of the anesthetics to a lesser extent than they do the rate of wash-out and the rate of emergence from anesthesia. In terms of the pharmacokinetics of inhaled anesthetics, changes in alveolar ventilation and cardiac output affect the wash-in of more soluble anesthetics (halothane and methoxyflurane) more than that of the less soluble anesthetic agents (sevoflurane and desflurane) (Eger, 1974). In contrast, increases in the right-to-left shunt (as in an intrapulmonary or intracardiac shunt) affect the wash-in of the less soluble anesthetics (sevoflurane) compared with the more soluble anesthetics (halothane and methoxyflurane) (Lerman, 2002). Because of the low blood and tissue solubilities of sevoflurane, its elimination in infants and children is rapid.

Sevoflurane is a far less potent anesthetic than isoflurane and halothane, as reflected by the MAC of sevoflurane. The MAC of sevoflurane is twice that of isoflurane and three times that of halothane (Lerman et al., 1994). The relationship between age (in the pediatric range) and the MAC of sevoflurane differs from the relationships for isoflurane and halothane in two respects. First, the MAC of sevoflurane does not increase steadily as age decreases, and second, the contribution of nitrous oxide to the MAC of sevoflurane in children is less than it is for halothane. MAC of sevoflurane in neonates and infants younger than 6 months (3.2%) and in infants older than 6 months and children up to 12 years (2.5%) is constant. Why the MAC of sevoflurane does not increase as age decreases as it does with the other inhalational anesthetics is unclear. Although nitrous oxide reduces the MAC of inhalational anesthetics in proportion to its concentration, the same does not hold true for sevoflurane in children. In the case of sevoflurane in children aged 1 to 3 years, nitrous oxide (inspired concentration, 60%) decreases the MAC of sevoflurane by only 25%. The explanation for the blunted effect of nitrous oxide on the MAC of sevoflurane in children also remains unclear.

Sevoflurane is unique among the currently used ether anesthetics in that in unpremedicated children, it is well tolerated when administered for induction of anesthesia, even without nitrous oxide. The incidences of breath holding, coughing, laryngospasm, and desaturation during induction of anesthesia with sevoflurane and halothane are few and similar with the two anesthetics (Black, 1996; Lerman et al., 1996). However, induction of anesthesia with sevoflurane is not always uneventful. Although exceedingly rare, EEG and epileptiform activities were reported during inhalational inductions with sevoflurane in children (Komatsu et al., 1994; Vakkuri et al., 2001; Jaaskelainen et al., 2003). Investigations failed to identify a cause for these episodes (Constant et al., 1999). Rare instances of twitching of the face or limb usually dissipate rapidly as the depth of anesthesia is increased. If the inspired concentration of sevoflurane is increased slowly (i.e., in 0.5% to 1% increments every few breaths), a protracted excitement phase may ensue during the induction. This can be obviated by increasing the inspired concentration of sevoflurane very quickly, without inducing airway reflex responses. Administering 60% to 70% nitrous oxide for approximately 1 minute and then adding 8% (inspired concentration) sevoflurane to the nitrous oxide makes the induction rapid and smooth. Recall of the odor of sevoflurane is rare, and excitement during the induction of anesthesia is minimal. Other techniques for rapid induction of anesthesia in children with sevoflurane have included a single-breath (vital capacity) induction with 8% sevoflurane, which is 40% more rapid than a single-breath induction with 5% halothane (Agnor et al., 1998). Whichever technique is used to induce anesthesia, clinicians continue to be surprised by anesthetized children who withdrew on attempted cannulation of a vein. This results not from a flaw in the anesthetic, sevoflurane, but rather in the combination of its pharmacology and delivery. Compared with halothane, the modestly increased maximum vaporizer concentration of sevoflurane is overshadowed by the 250% greater MAC. This limits the alveolar concentration that can be achieved in the first few minutes of anesthesia. This may reduce the probability of circulatory depression during induction of anesthesia with sevoflurane, but it also prevents clinicians from inducing a deep level of anesthesia quickly and thereby preventing a response to stimulation.

Like halothane, sevoflurane is a potent respiratory depressant. At concentrations greater than 1.5 MAC, sevoflurane is a more potent respiratory depressant than halothane. Indeed, apnea may occur in the unstimulated child breathing 8% inspired sevoflurane. Premedication with midazolam or other medications may potentiate the respiratory depression with sevoflurane. After an inhalational induction with sevoflurane, spontaneous ventilation usually resumes after a brief period of apnea or manual ventilation of the lungs and a reduction in the inspired concentration of sevoflurane. Sevoflurane maintains cardiovascular homeostasis in infants and children. At 1 MAC for sevoflurane, heart rate is usually maintained in infants and children even when they are not pretreated with atropine, although rare instances of a slowing of the heart rate have been reported, particularly at concentrations exceeding 1 MAC (Lerman et al., 1994). Systolic pressure is usually reduced 20% to 25% from awake values. These responses to 1 MAC sevoflurane are similar to those after other inhalational anesthetics. Arrhythmias during sevoflurane anesthesia are uncommon; the incidence of arrhythmias during sevoflurane anesthesia after exogenous epinephrine is similar to that during isoflurane

anesthesia. In infants and children with congenital heart disease undergoing cardiac surgery, hypotension and desaturation in cyanotic children after sevoflurane anesthesia occurred less often than they did after halothane anesthesia (Russell et al., 2001). In parallel with the rapid elimination of sevoflurane, the recovery profile for sevoflurane is rapid compared with that for halothane. Transient agitation and involuntary movements during emergence from anesthesia have been reported. Emergence agitation occurs primarily in preschool-aged children, lasts 10 to 20 minutes, and is often self-limited. Although agitation has been attributed to pain, pain as the sole explanation was dispelled when agitation was noted in children after lower abdominal surgery with a working caudal block in situ and after sevoflurane for MRI procedures, where no pain occurs (Aono et al., 1997; Cravero et al., 2000). One of the most difficult problems has been defining emergence agitation, which could not previously be assessed with any scale or measurement (Sikich and Lerman, 2004). It is important to note that emergence agitation is not unique to sevoflurane; it also occurs after other anesthetic agents, including isoflurane and desflurane.

Sevoflurane is degraded both *in vivo* (to inorganic fluoride and hexafluoroisopropanol) and *in vitro* (via alkaline hydrolysis in the presence of soda lime or baralyme to five compounds (A through E) (Hanaki et al., 1987; Morio et al., 1992). *In vivo*, sevoflurane is metabolized by microsomal CYP IIE1 isozyme in both the liver and kidneys (Kharasch et al., 1995a, 1995b). The peak plasma concentration of inorganic fluoride is proportional to the duration of exposure to sevoflurane in children. However, there have been no instances of sevoflurane-induced nephrotoxicity after several million anesthetic procedures. Two plausible explanations for the absence of nephrotoxicity are the rapid elimination of sevoflurane and the small extent of intrarenal metabolism of sevoflurane, the putative source of inorganic fluoride-induced nephrotoxicity (Kharasch et al., 1995a). *In vitro*, sevoflurane is both absorbed and degraded in the presence of soda lime and baralyme, yielding only compound A in significant concentrations; up to 20 to 40 ppm in closed circuits in humans (Liu et al., 1991). Alkaline hydrolysis of sevoflurane is enhanced by high temperatures, decreased water content in the absorbent, increased inspired concentration of sevoflurane, and new absorbent. In infants and children, compound A concentrations during sevoflurane anesthesia in a closed circuit increase in parallel with increasing in age (Frink et al., 1996). In concentrations up to 100 ppm for 3 hours, compound A causes histopathologic changes in the kidneys of rats, although no evidence of histopathologic or pathophysiologic renal changes have been reported in humans (Gonsowski et al., 1994a, 1994b). In the presence of desiccated soda lime and baralyme, sevoflurane is degraded to only an extremely small extent to CO (Fang et al., 1995; Wissing et al., 2001). When both potassium hydroxide and sodium hydroxide are eliminated from the absorbent, sevoflurane produces only minute concentrations of CO (Murray et al., 1999; Versichelen et al., 2001). The combination of high-dose sevoflurane with desiccated baralyme has resulted in instances of extreme heat and fire within the absorbent canister (Previte et al., 2004; Wu et al., 2004; Dunning et al., 2007).

Desflurane

Desflurane is a potent polyfluorinated methyl ethyl ether anesthetic available for use in infants and children. The single substitution of a fluorine atom for a chlorine atom on the carbon atom of isoflurane dramatically changes the physicochemical properties of this anesthetic (Table 7-19). Blood-gas and tissue-blood solubilities are only fractions of those of halothane and isoflurane (Yasuda et al., 1989). As a result, the wash-in of desflurane is the fastest of all of the available potent inhalational anesthetics (Fig. 7-38). As in the case of sevoflurane, changes in alveolar ventilation and cardiac output exert small effects on the pharmacokinetics of this anesthetic, whereas changes in right-to-left shunting exert a large effect (Eger, 1974; Lerman, 2002). Just as the wash-in of desflurane is extremely fast, the wash-out of desflurane is extremely rapid. Of the potent inhalational anesthetics, the elimination of desflurane is most rapid (Fig. 7-38) (Yasuda et al., 1991).

The MAC of desflurane in infants and children is least in neonates, increasing throughout infancy and reaching a zenith of 9.9% in infants aged 6 to 12 months. MAC decreases thereafter with increasing age through adolescence (Taylor and Lerman, 1991). Nitrous oxide (60%) decreases the MAC of desflurane by only 26% in children, an effect similar to that of sevoflurane (Fisher and Zwass, 1992).

Inhalational inductions with desflurane are not recommended because upper airway reflexes are often triggered (50% incidence of breath holding, 40% incidence of laryngospasm) (Taylor and Lerman, 1992; Zwass et al., 1992). If anesthesia is induced by either the intravenous or inhalational route, desflurane may be used to maintain anesthesia (Taylor and Lerman, 1992; Zwass et al., 1992). Like sevoflurane, desflurane maintains cardiovascular homeostasis at 1 MAC (Taylor and Lerman, 1991). At this concentration, heart rate and systolic blood pressure are depressed 20% to 25% compared with awake values (Taylor and Lerman, 1991). Arrhythmias and bradycardia are uncommon with this anesthetic.

The rate of recovery after desflurane anesthesia parallels the extremely rapid wash-out of this anesthetic (Taylor and Lerman, 1992; Davis et al., 1994). Early experience with the rapid recovery after discontinuation of desflurane resulted in the precipitous onset of excruciating surgical pain. A strategy to prevent pain on emergence must be considered and the intervention instituted before discontinuation of this anesthetic.

Desflurane resists metabolism both *in vivo* (0.02%) and *in vitro* (in the presence of soda lime and baralyme) (Smiley et al., 1991). *In vivo*, insignificant blood concentrations of inorganic fluoride are produced after desflurane anesthesia. However, *in vitro* degradation of desflurane may be problematic. If the CO_2 absorbent becomes desiccated and is incubated with desflurane, then desflurane may react with the constituents to release CO_2 into the inspired limb of the breathing circuit (Fang et al., 1995; Wissing et al., 2001). Other ether anesthetics, including isoflurane and enflurane, and all difluoromethyl ethyl ether anesthetics (including desflurane), undergo a similar path of degradation to CO in the presence of desiccated absorbent, albeit to a lesser extent than desflurane (Baxter et al., 1998). Absorbent becomes desiccated by circulating fresh gas through an absorbent canister for a prolonged period of time without a reservoir bag in place. In some anesthetic machines, this continuous fresh gas flow desiccates the absorbent by flowing retrograde through the canister, exiting where the reservoir bag usually is attached. Without the ability to detect CO in the breathing circuit, contamination of the breathing circuit with CO might present a serious risk to patients, particularly those anesthetized after the anesthetic machine has not been used for a prolonged period (i.e., Monday mornings). To preclude

this complication, the fresh gas flow should be discontinued when the anesthetic machine is not in use, the reservoir bag should never be removed from the canister, and most importantly, the anesthetic machine should be turned off when it is not in use. If there is a suspicion that the absorbent has been desiccated, the absorbent must be replaced before any anesthetic is administered. There are no guidelines for rehumidifying desiccated absorbents. Not all absorbents produce CO when they are exposed to the desflurane. Those absorbents that lack both potassium hydroxide and sodium hydroxide do not produce CO.

With a boiling point close to room temperature, a heated, pressurized vaporizer was developed to deliver a predictable concentration of desflurane. This vaporizer requires electrical current to maintain a predictable temperature and pressure that are independent of ambient conditions.

Isoflurane

The pharmacology of isoflurane is very similar to that of desflurane with a few exceptions. As mentioned, the chemical structure of isoflurane is identical to that of desflurane except that isoflurane has a chlorine atom instead of a fluoride atom on the carbon atom (Table 7-19). Because isoflurane is more soluble in blood and tissues than desflurane, the wash-in and wash-out of isoflurane are slower than those of desflurane (Fig. 7-38) (Yasuda et al., 1991). The MAC of isoflurane is between those of halothane and sevoflurane (Table 7-19) (Cameron et al., 1984).

Like desflurane, isoflurane triggers airway reflex responses during inhalational inductions and is not suited for this purpose. Although numerous attempts were made to ameliorate the airway responses to an inhalational induction, clinicians abandoned the notion of using it for this purpose. Isoflurane is used similarly to desflurane for the maintenance phase of anesthesia.

Once anesthesia is induced, whether the airway is instrumented or not, children and adults breathe isoflurane without difficulty. Similarly, they emerge from isoflurane anesthesia without difficulty.

Isoflurane, like desflurane, does not depress the circulation in children. In fact heart rate often increases during isoflurane anesthesia, and blood pressure is well maintained. Unlike in the adult, rapid increases in the inspired concentration of isoflurane do not trigger a central sympathetic (tachycardia and hypertension) response that requires intervention with an opioid or other agent.

The *in vivo* metabolism of isoflurane, 0.2%, yields small concentrations of inorganic fluoride in the blood without significant intrarenal production. Nephrotoxicity after isoflurane anesthesia is not a substantive risk. However, in the presence of desiccated soda lime and baralyme, isoflurane can produce CO

Halothane

Halothane was the standard of practice with which all other inhalational anesthetics were compared until the introduction of sevoflurane. Halothane is the only nonether anesthetic that is used today, being an alkane in structure. The wash-in of halothane is the slowest of the currently used anesthetic agents because it is the most soluble (see Table 7-19). This means that the time to equilibration of inspired and alveolar (or brain) partial pressures of halothane is the greatest of the anesthetic

Although this may be viewed as a safety factor, the potency of halothane is the strongest of the anesthetic agents. These two factors, together with the ability to deliver a maximum inspired concentration of 5% halothane with all vaporizers, resulted in numerous episodes of cardiorespiratory instability that included hypotension and bradycardia or arrhythmias. In particular, concern was expressed in the 1980s about the ability of neonates to tolerate halothane anesthesia because of the hemodynamic consequences. Based on the current understanding of the pharmacology of halothane, several conclusions may be made about the past experience with this anesthetic in pediatric anesthesia:

- The MAC for halothane in neonates is less than that in older infants.
- Halothane depresses both the circulation and respiration in infants and children.
- With the design of the vaporizer and given the potency of halothane, it is easier to overdose children with halothane than with other anesthetic agents.

Halothane is metabolized approximately 15% to 20% in humans. Immunologic responses, including hepatitis, have been documented after repeated halothane anesthesia, even in children (Kenna et al., 1987). With the declining use of this agent in clinical practice, it is unlikely to pose a serious threat to children.

LOCAL ANESTHETIC AGENTS

All local anesthetic agents in clinical use consist essentially of three parts tertiary amine and an aromatic ring linked by an intermediate chain. The tertiary amine is a weak base and is positively charged at physiologic pH. The intermediate chain contains either an ester or an amide. The substituted aromatic ring is lipophilic, whereas the positively charged tertiary-amine end is relatively hydrophilic (Fig. 7-45).

Local anesthetics are thus classified as either amino-esters (e.g., cocaine, tetracaine, chloroprocaine, and procaine) or amino-amides (e.g., lidocaine, bupivacaine, ropivacaine, and

levobupivacaine). Amino-amides are more commonly used in pediatric practice, and the pharmacology of these agents in pediatrics has been reviewed by Mazoit and Dalens (2004).

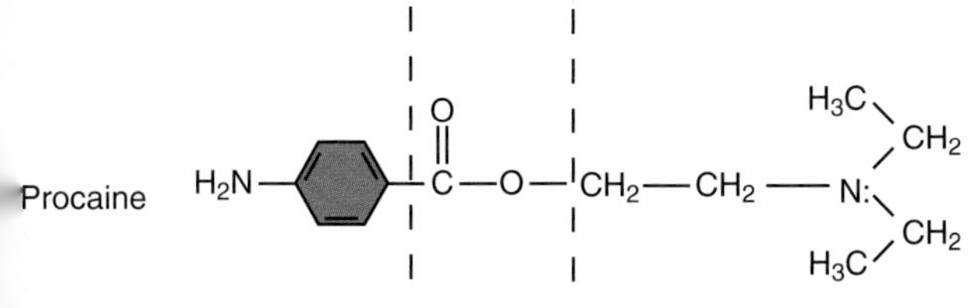

Physiochemical Properties

The potency and duration of action of local anesthetic agents are dependent on the lipophilicity of the local anesthetic molecule, the degree of ionization (pK_a), the pH of the preparation and of the tissue, the degree of protein binding, the intrinsic vasoconstrictor properties of the drug, and temperature (Heavner, 2007). Lipophilicity determines the affinity of the molecule for lipid membranes and increases the potency and the duration of action. Lipophilicity is increased by increasing the size of the alkyl substitution on the aromatic ring or on or near the tertiary amine (Heavner, 2007).

The pKa of a drug is the hydrogen ion concentration (pH) at which 50% of the drug exists in its ionized hydrophilic form (i.e., in equilibrium with its un-ionized lipophilic form). All local anesthetic agents are weak bases. At physiologic pH, the lower the pKa the greater the lipophilicity. The pH of the site where the local anesthetic is placed determines the degree of ionization and thus the activity of the drug. Sodium bicarbonate has been used clinically to increase the speed of onset by raising the pH of a local anesthetic solution by increasing the un-ionized fraction (lipophilicity).

Bupivacaine, mepivacaine, and ropivacaine—but not lidocaine—have an asymmetric carbon atom that allows these drugs to exist as different isomers or S– and R+ enantiomers. A racemic mixture contains equal amounts of the S– and R+ enantiomers. Bupivacaine is a racemic mixture of equiosmolar amounts of R+ bupivacaine and S– bupivacaine (Leone et al., 2008).

The pharmacokinetic properties of enantiomers are essentially the same, but their stereospecificity influences the protein binding and pharmacodynamics (Burm, 1994, 1997; Kremer et al., 1988). Ropivacaine and levobupivacaine are pure S– enantiomers that have less cardiac toxicity and a greater sensory motor differential (Bardsley et al., 1998; Mazoit et al., 2000; Leone et al., 2008). This differential effect is poorly understood but may be related to the length of spread along the nerve, to selective inhibition of the Na^+ and K^+ channels that are present in different proportions in different nerve types, or to preferential blockade of the tetrodotoxin-resistant sodium channels (Oda et al., 2000; Berde, 2004).

The intrinsic vasoconstrictor properties of a local anesthetic drug influence the initial rate of uptake from the site of injection into the central circulation (T_{max}) and the duration of action. It may also influence the peak plasma concentration (C_{max}). Some local anesthetic agents have a biphasic effect on the blood vessels, for example, ropivacaine at low concentrations vasoconstricts, but at higher concentration it has vasodilator effects.

Finally, the duration of action of local anesthetic agents is shorter in neonates and infants despite the use of larger weight-scaled doses for both central and peripheral nerve blockade (Berde, 2004). This may be because of age-related differences in the pharmacodynamic responses, the degree of myelination of the nerves that increases with age, spacing of the nodes of Ranvier, the length of nerve exposed, tissue barriers, and other factors including pharmacogenetic variation.

FIGURE 7-45. Structures of two local anesthetics, the aminoamide ~~l~~ocaine and the aminoester procaine. In both drugs a hydrophobic ~~ar~~omatic group is joined to a more hydrophilic base, the tertiary ~~am~~ine, by an intermediate amide or ester bond. *(From Coté CJ: ~~Pe~~diatric anesthesia. In: Miller RD, Eriksson LI, Fleisher LA, et al: Miller's ~~An~~esthesia, ed 7, Philadelphia, 2010, Churchill Livingstone.)*

Mechanisms of Action

Local anesthetics are potent reversible sodium channel blockers with marked stereospecificity that influences their action. They interfere with nerve cell membrane excitation and subsequent conduction of action potentials in excitable tissue. They bind to the inner vestibule of the voltage-gated sodium channel after passing through the cell membrane. Various subtypes of sodium channel exist that are tetrodotoxin sensitive or resistant in different nerve fibers (Baker and Wood, 2001; Heavner, 2007). Nerve fibers vary in their sensitivity to local anesthetic agents. Small myelinated axons, Aγ motor and Aδ sensory axons, are the most sensitive, followed by the large myelinated Aα and Aβ fibers. The least susceptible are the slow conducting fibers, the small unmyelinated C fibers.

The local anesthetic agents enter the sodium channels in the "active" or "open" state and render them "inactive" or "closed." The membrane is thus stabilized, and propagation of a depolarizing wave is prevented. The affinity of the local anesthetic drug to the sodium channel varies with the gating state of the channel. Their affinity is high when the sodium channel is open and activated (during sensory transmission, motor activity, or tachydysrhythmias of the myocardium), and the affinity is low at slow excitation rates or when the sodium channel is inactivated or closed (Heavner, 2007). Neonates have a higher heart rate than adults and may thus be more prone to myocardial toxicity. Hypoxia, acidosis, hypothermia, and electrolyte disorders increase the risk of toxicity (Freysz et al, 1989, 1993; Timour et al., 1990).

Local anesthetic agents also inhibit the K2P channel, blocking repolarization and delaying recovery after depolarization. This effectively prolongs the action potential and adds to risk of toxicity (i.e., convulsions or dysrhythmias) (Kindler and Yost, 2005). The distribution of Na+ and K+ ions in the channel varies from one nerve type to another and may explain the differential blockade of sensory and motor nerves by individual local anesthetic agents (Kindler and Yost, 2005).

Local anesthetic agents may also have beneficial systemic actions on inflammatory cells and in chronic pain by interaction with G-protein receptors (Hollman et al., 2004).

Systemic Absorption

When local anesthetics are used to perform a nerve block they are injected into a specific space (e.g., spinal, caudal, or epidural) or location (e.g., peripheral nerve block, skin infiltration, topical). The speed of absorption is a function of the site of injection, the speed of injection, the amount and concentration of the local anesthetic injected, the intrinsic vasoconstrictor properties of the drug, the blood supply to the site, lipid solubility, absorption into the surrounding tissue, and the pH of the tissue.

Local diffusion into the nerve at the site of injection produces regional anesthesia. Diffusion into the bloodstream produces blood concentrations that can be measured. After a single shot injection, the rate of absorption and the volume of distribution determine the rate at which peak plasma levels are reached. Clearance has little impact, but on the other hand clearance is the major factor that impacts steady-state plasma concentrations during continuous infusions.

Highly vascular areas are more prone to rapid local anesthetic uptake and consequently, toxicity. The rate of absorption is greatest from the intercostal space and trachea; intermediate from the caudal and epidural spaces and lowest following skin infiltration. The order of site absorption from highest to lowest is intercostal, intratracheal, caudal, epidural, brachial plexus, and subcutaneous.

Absorption from the epidural space is considered biphasic (McCann et al., 2001). The buffering properties of the epidural space are important, and the epidural fat acts as a store where the injected drug can accumulate. The slow release is responsible for a longer terminal half-life. Epidural fat in neonates and infants is less abundant, and the peak plasma concentration occurs earlier in this age group (Eyres et al., 1978).

The systemic effects of local anesthetics are a function of dose, rapidity of injection, site of injection, and ultimately the rate of rise and the plasma concentration reached. Toxic effects involving either the CNS or the heart are directly related to the free (unbound) drug concentration. In general, CNS toxicity occurs at lower plasma concentrations than cardiac toxicity in infants and young children.

Cardiac output also has an influence. A higher cardiac output increases the uptake, producing higher initial plasma concentrations and decreasing the duration of action. Ropivacaine is considered a better agent than bupivacaine for epidural infusions because the vasoconstrictor properties of ropivacaine slow the absorption of the drug into the blood, decreasing the peak plasma levels. Karmakar et al. (2002) have shown that after 2 mg/kg of either caudal ropivacaine or bupivacaine, ropivacaine undergoes slower systemic absorption from the caudal space, but the peak venous plasma concentrations are comparable.

Vasoconstrictors may also be used to reduce the absorption of local anesthetic into the systemic circulation. The efficacy of epinephrine varies with the patient's age but is also dependent on the vascularity at the site of injection. Epinephrine prolongs the duration of bupivacaine and ropivacaine by approximately 50% in neonates, 25% in infants younger than 4 years old, and 10% in older children (Warner et al., 1987; Hansen et al., 2001). Epinephrine is usually diluted to various concentrations. Box 7-3 is a quick reference guide for converting concentrations to mcg/mL.

Distribution

The volume of distribution is difficult to evaluate and is largely unknown in children. Pharmacokinetic analysis after extravascular injection is difficult. In conventional pharmacokinetic modeling it is assumed that elimination is longer than absorption and that the terminal phase occurs when absorption is almost totally completed (Mazoit and Dalens, 2004). If absorption is longer than elimination, such as when local anesthetic agents are injected extravascularly, the terminal half-life represents the comple

---

Box 7-3 Epinephrine Dilution and Conversion to mcg/mL

Epinephrine Dilution	mcg/mL
1:100,000	10
1:200,000	5
1:400,000	2.5
1:800,000	1.25

absorption process as well as elimination. It is thus impossible to accurately calculate the volume of distribution, but the total body clearance can be calculated accurately if sampling is long enough. A further confounding factor is that clearance also varies with time (Mazoit and Dalens, 2004).

Tissue binding is another important factor, because the local anesthetic agents are widely distributed outside the blood. Furthermore, the extracellular fluid volume in newborns and young infants is almost twice that of an adult. Theoretically, volume of distribution should be much larger in neonates and infants.

Protein binding and volume of distribution influence the Cmax of a drug. The peak plasma Cmax of ropivacaine is delayed in infants and children when compared with adults. The time to Cmax decreases from 90 to 120 minutes in infants younger than 6 months of age to 30 minutes in adults and children older than 8 years of age.

In infants and children, the pharmacokinetics of ropivacaine has been reported after caudal, epidural, and ilioinguinal blocks (Hansen et al., 2000a, 2000b, 2001a; Lonnqvist et al., 2000; Wulf et al., 2000). Hansen et al. (2001a) showed that infants between the ages of 0 and 3 months have higher free ropivacaine concentrations than infants who are 3 to 12 months of age, and for both these groups of infants the free drug concentrations were within the concentrations reported for adults. However, Wulf et al. (2000) noted that infants had higher peak plasma concentrations than toddlers aged 1 to 5 years, with the peak concentration occurring at 60 minutes in both groups. In a dosing study of children 4 to 12 years of age, Bosenberg et al. (2001) noted that single-shot caudals in doses of 1 to 3 mg/kg resulted in peak plasma levels of free ropivacaine that increased proportionately with increasing doses.

The lungs may also influence the plasma levels. The lungs slow the rate of rise and influence the peak plasma concentration. The lung extraction ratio for amide local anesthetic agents is high (approximately 0.8), resulting in a difference between mixed venous and arterial concentrations. Infants with right-to-left cardiac shunts may therefore be at greater risk of toxicity. Bokesch et al. (1987) demonstrated higher plasma lidocaine levels in the systemic circulation in animals with right-to-left shunts.

Protein Binding

Amide local anesthetics are weak bases and are bound to serum proteins albumen and α_1-acid glycoprotein (AAG). Protein binding ranges from 65% (lidocaine) to more than 95% (bupivacaine and ropivacaine). The binding properties of these proteins are very different. Albumen has a low affinity but greater capacity for local anesthetics than AAG, which has a high affinity but low capacity. Protein binding is pH dependent; metabolic or respiratory acidosis increases the free fraction, thereby increasing the risk of toxicity. Bilirubin also competes with amide drugs for albumen binding sites (Meunier et al., 2001).

Neonates and infants have lower AAG levels (approximately 0.2 to 0.3g/L) compared with children older than 1 year and adults (about 0.7 to 1 g/L). The free fraction of local anesthetics is therefore increased in neonates. In the first 24 to 48 hours after surgery or other inflammatory processes, however, the plasma level of AAG, an acute phase protein, rapidly increases (Kremer et al., 1988; Bosenberg et al., 2005). This effectively lowers the free fraction, theoretically providing some protective effect. This effect may abate at approximately 48 hours.

Amide local anesthetics are also linearly bound to red cells (blood-plasma concentration ratio of about 0.60 to 0.85) (Tucker et al., 1970; Meunier et al., 2001). Although this only accounts for less than 20% to 30% of the total amount in blood, it may be relevant in term neonates, especially those with intrauterine growth retardation where the hematocrit may exceed 45% to 60% (Lonnqvist and Herngren, 1995).

Metabolism

The rate and route of metabolism vary with age. Amide local anesthetics are metabolized in the liver by the cytochrome P450 (CYP) enzyme system. The main CYP isoforms involved are CYP3A4 for lidocaine and bupivacaine and CYP1A2 for ropivacaine. These systems are immature at birth. CYP3A4 is partly replaced by CYP3A7 at birth and matures by 9 months. The intrinsic clearance of bupivacaine is only one third that of adults at 1 month of age, and two thirds at 6 months. The major metabolites are 2,6-pipecoloxylidide (PPX) for both bupivacaine and ropivacaine, with the addition of 3-hydroxy-ropivacaine for ropivacaine.

Ropivacaine metabolism also varies with age. Even though CYP1A2 is only fully mature at 3 years, the majority of ropivacaine (70%) is excreted as PPX, whereas 24% of ropivacaine is excreted unchanged by the kidneys at birth (Larsson et al., 1997). In early infancy, only 4% is excreted as 3-hydroxy-ropivacaine, the major metabolite in adults (Bosenberg et al., 2005).

With regard to the ester compounds, those derived from para-aminobenzoic acid (PABA; e.g., procaine, chloroprocaine, and tetracaine) undergo hydrolysis by esterases in the blood (plasma cholinesterase) or tissues. PABA undergoes hepatic biotransformation and clearance. PABA metabolites are thought to be responsible for the allergic reactions seen with this group of drugs. Because of its extremely short duration of action, chloroprocaine has been used primarily for continuous epidural techniques in infants and neonates. The use of tetracaine has generally been limited to spinal and topical anesthesia.

Clearance

Lidocaine has a high hepatic extraction ratio, and its clearance is dependent on hepatic blood flow (Tucker, 1986). In addition, the product of lidocaine metabolism monoethylglycine xylidine (MEGX) may inhibit the intrinsic enzyme involved with its degradation (Bax et al., 1985). MEGX is an active metabolite slightly less potent than lidocaine (Bax et al., 1985). Lidocaine has a longer elimination half-life and larger volume of distribution in children than in adults after either intratracheal or caudal anesthesia (Eyres et al., 1978; Ecoffey et al., 1984). Bupivacaine and ropivacaine have a relatively low hepatic extraction ratio. Protein binding and CYP enzyme activity affect drug clearance, which is low at birth, increasing throughout the first year of life (Mazoit, 1988; Lonnqvist et al., 2000; Hansen et al., 2001a, 2001b; Meunier et al., 2001).

Pharmacokinetic studies have demonstrated age-related differences in clearance between infants and children (Eyres et al., 1983; Ecoffey et al., 1985; Desparmet et al., 1987; Mazoit, 1988; Mazoit and Dalens, 2004). Clearance of bound and unbound ropivacaine is lower in neonates (33 to 60 mL/min^{-1} per kg^{-1}, compared with that of infants (160 to 220 mL/min^{-1} per kg^{-1} (Hansen, 2000a, 2000b; Lonnqvist et al., 2000; Rapp et al., 2004b; Bosenberg et al., 2005).

All studies of prolonged administration in children have assumed that clearance is unchanged during the whole period of the continuous infusion. In theory, after several hours the clearance of bupivacaine and ropivacaine decreases; this decrease is probably related to the decrease in free fraction, which is related to the increase in AAG plasma levels. The plasma concentration of total bupivacaine tends to increase after 48 hours, especially in infants younger than 4 months old, when the AAG is said to fall. Based on this premise, some authors recommend terminating continuous infusions of bupivacaine after 48 hours in infants under 6 months.

However, there was no decrease observed in AAG levels after 72 hours in the only study to date that has measured AAG levels beyond 48 hours (Bosenberg et al., 2005). In this study, both total and unbound ropivacaine levels were similar at 48 and 72 hours.

Extrapolation of pharmacokinetic data after single-bolus bupivacaine administration for infants and children suggests that for continuous caudal and epidural infusions, rates of 0.2 to 0.4 mg/kg per hour for infants and 0.2 to 0.75 mg/kg per hour for children would provide efficacious and safe plasma concentrations (McCloskey et al., 1992).

Lidocaine

The amide local anesthetics are bound to serum proteins. AAG is the major binding protein. The free drug fraction for lidocaine ranges from 30% to 40%, and for both ropivacaine and bupivacaine it ranges from 4% to 7%. Metabolism of amides is by the liver's cytochrome P450 system. CYP3A4 metabolizes bupivacaine, and CYP1A2 is mostly involved with ropivacaine's metabolism. Lidocaine has a high hepatic-extraction ratio, and its clearance is dependent on hepatic blood flow. In addition, the metabolic product of lidocaine metabolism (MEGX) may inhibit the intrinsic enzyme involved with its degradation. Lidocaine has a longer elimination half-life and a larger volume of distribution in children than in adults after either intratracheal or caudal anesthesia (Eyres et al., 1978; Ecoffey et al., 1984). Bokesch and others (1987) demonstrated higher plasma lidocaine levels in the systemic circulation in animals with right-to-left shunts.

Bupivacaine

Bupivacaine and ropivacaine have a low hepatic-extraction ratio. Thus, protein binding and CYP enzyme activity effect drug clearance (Lonnqvist et al., 2000). Bupivacaine is a racemic mixture of equiosmolar amounts of R$^+$ bupivacaine and S$^-$ bupivacaine. Drug clearance is low at birth and increases throughout the first year of life. Pharmacokinetic studies have demonstrated age-related differences between infants and children (Eyres et al., 1983; Ecoffey et al., 1985; Desparmet et al., 1987; Mazoit et al., 1988; Mazoit and Dalens, 2004). Extrapolation of pharmacokinetic data after single-bolus bupivacaine administration for infants and children suggests that for continuous caudal and epidural infusions, rates of 0.2 to 0.4 mg/kg per hour for infants and 0.2 to 0.75 mg/kg per hour for children would provide efficacious and safe plasma concentrations (McCloskey et al., 1992).

Ropivacaine

Ropivacaine is a long-acting amide, local anesthetic agent with fewer cardiac and CNS toxicities. It is thought to provide a greater separation of sensory and motor effects. Karmakar and others (2002) have shown that after 2 mg/kg of either caudal ropivacaine or bupivacaine, ropivacaine undergoes slower systemic absorption from the caudal space but with comparable peak venous plasma concentrations. In comparative studies of caudal blocks with ropivacaine and bupivacaine, Khalil and others (1999) and Ivani and others (1998) noted that for children the quality and duration of postoperative pain relief, motor and sensory effects, and time to first micturition were similar.

In infants and children, the pharmacokinetics of ropivacaine have been reported after caudal, epidural, and ilioinguinal blocks (Hansen, 2000a, 2000b, 2001a; Lonnqvist et al., 2000; Wulf et al., 2000; Dalens et al., 2001). Hansen and others (2001) have shown that infants who are 0 to 3 months of age have higher to medium maximum free ropivacaine concentrations than infants who are 3 to 12 months of age, and for both these groups of infants the free drug concentrations are within the concentrations reported for adults. However, Wulf and others (2000) noted that in infants less than one year of age and toddlers 1 to 5 years of age, infants had higher peak plasma concentrations than toddlers, with the peak concentration occurring at 60 minutes in both groups. In a dosing study of children 4 to 12 years of age, Bosenberg and others (2001) noted that single shot caudals in doses of 1 to 3 mg/kg resulted in peak plasma levels of free ropivacaine that increased proportionately to the increase in dose.

McCann and others (2001) reported on the pharmacokinetics of epidural ropivacaine (1.7 mg/kg) in infants and young children. In this study, researchers noted that ropivacaine has a biphasic absorption. As with bupivacaine, ropivacaine shows age-related clearance changes with infants having slower clearance than children, but in both groups the peak plasma concentrations were well below the maximum tolerated venous concentration (2100 mcg/mL for adults). In children receiving 24- to 72-hour epidural infusions of ropivacaine, Berde et al. (2008) noted stable concentrations of unbound ropivacaine with no age dependency or sign of systemic toxicity.

The pharmacodynamics of ropivacaine after caudal blocks have been shown to be similar to bupivacaine with regard to onset time, efficacy, duration of analgesia, and incidence of motor block. In children receiving caudal blocks with 1 MAC of sevoflurane, Ingelmo et al. (2009) noted that the potencies (ED$_{50}$ and ED$_{95}$) for ropivacaine and levobupivacaine were similar. Local anesthetic supplements can also affect their duration of action. Ropivacaine's duration of action can be prolonged with neostigmine, clonidine, or ketamine supplementation (Da Conceicao and Coelho, 1998; Ivani et al., 1998, 1999, 2000; Khalil et al., 1999; Morton, 2000; Turan et al., 2003).

Levobupivacaine

Levobupivacaine is one of the enantiomers of bupivacaine. There is less information regarding its use in children than for the other local anesthetics (Gunter et al., 1999; Ivani et al., 2003, 2005; Chalkiadis et al., 2004; DeNegri et al., 2004; Kokki et al., 2004a; Locatelli et al., 2005).

In studies of children 1 to 7 years of age, Ivani and others (2002) noted that caudal bupivacaine, levobupivacaine, and ropivacaine were thought to be clinically comparable. Locatelli and others (2005) reported that caudal bupivacaine was associated with more motor block and longer analgesic block. However, in a study of over 300 children aged 1 month to 10 years, Frawley et al. (2006) noted that onset time, motor block, and analgesia of levobupivacaine was comparable with bupivacaine. In addition, 0.21% levobupivacaine appears to have equivalent potency to racemic bupivacaine. In pediatric patients with continuous infusions of epidurals, DeNegri and others (2004) noted that ropivacaine and levobupivacaine were associated with less motor block than bupivacaine. Cortinez et al. (2008) reported on the pharmacokinetics of levobupivacaine (2.5 mg/kg) after caudal administration in 10 patients 1 to 36 months of age and found that the median range of levobupivacaine's C_{max} and T_{max} were $1.48^{(0.62\ to\ 2.40)}$ mcg/mL and $37^{(10\ to\ 60)}$ minutes, respectively. No patient had a toxic level.

In a dose-response study by Ivani et al. (2003) of children undergoing caudal block for subumbilical surgical procedures, three concentrations (0.125%, 0.20%, and 0.25%) of levobupivacaine were compared. A dose-response relationship was observed, and they noted the optimal concentration to be 0.2% (Ivani et al., 2003). More information on local anesthetics is given in Chapter 14, Regional Anesthesia.

NEUROMUSCULAR BLOCKING AGENTS

Neuromuscular blocking agents (NMBAs) are used to facilitate intubation, provide surgical relaxation, and control ventilation in the operating room and ICU. NMBAs have no sedative, hypnotic, or analgesic side effects, but they may indirectly decrease metabolic demand, prevent shivering, decrease nonsynchronous ventilation and compliance of the respiratory system, and decrease ICP. The purposes of this section are to review the growth and development of the neuromuscular junction and muscle, the age-related pharmacologic characteristics of NMBA and their antagonists, and the monitoring equipment available for evaluating neuromuscular function.

Neuromuscular Junction and Neuromuscular Transmission

The general anatomy, age-related physiology, and pharmacology of the neuromuscular junction have been well defined (Bowman, 1980; Meakin et al., 1992; Wareham et al., 1994; Calakos and Scheller, 1996; Prince and Since, 1998; Sanes and Lichtman, 1999; Naguib et al., 2002). The neuromuscular system is incompletely developed at birth. The conduction velocity of motor nerves increases throughout gestation as nerve fibers are myelinated. The myotubules connect to mature muscle fibers in the latter part of intrauterine life and in the first several weeks after birth (Table 7-21). Some slow-contracting muscle (e.g., intrinsic muscles of the hand) is progressively converted to fast-contracting muscle, with a concomitant change in the force-velocity relationship. However, both the diaphragm and the intercostal muscles increase their percentage of slow muscle fibers in the first months of life. Synaptic transmission is slow at birth, and the rate at which acetylcholine (ACh) is released during repeated nerve stimulation is limited in the infant.

TABLE 7-21. Development of Skeletal Muscle Fibers

Age	Development
4 wk	Mesenchyumal cells become syncytial; myoblasts become myotube
5 wk	Syncytial myotube grows in length; primitive muscle fibers with myofilaments appear
9 wk	More myofilaments appear, grow in length; nuclei centralized
5 mo	Muscle fibers become thicker, longer; myofilaments multiply; myofilaments differentiate into actin and myosin; nuclei move more peripherally
Birth	Myofilaments aggregate into bundles, form myofibrils; muscle fibers grow still thicker, longer; nuclei have shifted peripherally
Adult	Muscle fibers thick and mature; alternating actin and myosin myofilaments aggregate into longitudinal bundles

Box 7-4 Characteristics of the Neonatal Neuromuscular Junction

Acetylcholine receptors change in function and distribution.
Slow twitch fibers (type I increase several-fold in first 6 months).
Infants younger than 2 months have lower TOF ratio.
Infants younger than 2 months have increased fade.
Differences are more pronounced in premature infants than in term infants.

Age-related changes in the ACh receptor may also contribute to the reduced margin of safety of neurotransmission in infants compared with adults (Box 7-4).

Acetylcholine Receptors

Prejunctional, postjunctional, and extrajunctional ACh receptors are involved with neuromuscular transmission. The postjunctional, adult ACh receptor consists of five units, that form a rosette with a central pit at the mouth of the ion channel (Fig. 7-46). Each rosette is made up of two α_1 units and β_1, ε, and δ units. These subunits are arranged in a specific order (counterclockwise α^*-ε-α-δ-β) The α^* subunit has a binding site with higher affinity for d-tubocurarine. The two binding sites for ACh are at α and δ (Blount and Merlie, 1989; Gu et al., 1990; Pederson and Cohen, 1990). Both sites must interact with the ACh in order for the channel to open and allow the flow of ions (Na^+, K^+, Ca^{2+}). If a competitive nondepolarizing NMBA prevents the interaction of ACh with one or two of the subunits α and α^*, the channel cannot open. The immature or fetal ACh receptor subtypes differ in the structure of one subunit from the adult subtype (i.e., a γ subunit which is present in the fetal ACh receptor instead of the ε subunit, which is present in the adult ACh receptor). Neonates have a mix of both adult and fetal receptors, but at term the adult subtypes are more common (Table 7-22; Fig. 7-47). A limited number of extrajunctional ACh receptors are also incorporated in the muscle membrane of older infants, children, and adults. Nerve activity inhibits the biosynthesis of ACh receptors at extrajunctional sites.

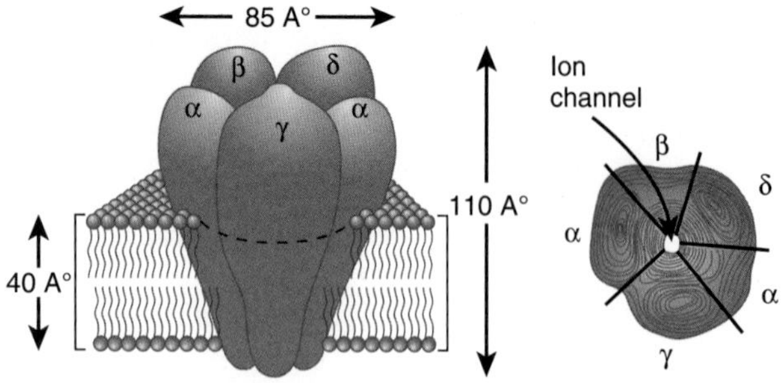

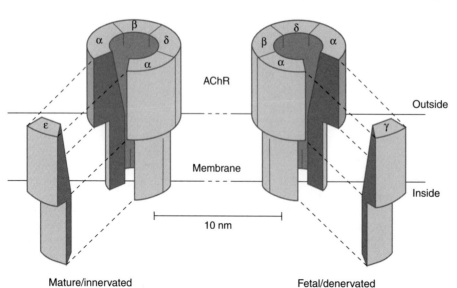

■ FIGURE 7-46. Structure of the fetal nicotinic ACh receptor and a description of the requirements to activate and competitively antagonize receptor function. The five subunits (two αs, β, ε, and δ with apparent molecular masses of 40, 50, 60, and 65 kDa, respectively), which are partly homologous in sequence, are arranged to form the perimeter of an internal cavity, which is believed to be the ion channel. Each of the subunits has an extracellular and a cytoplasmic exposure, with the bulk of the peptide chain existing on the extracellular side. The α subunits each carry a recognition site for agonists and competitive antagonists *(From Taylor P: Are neuromuscular blocking agents more efficacious in pairs? Anesthesiology 63:1, 1985.)*

Neuromuscular Transmission in the Neonate

The issues of ACh transfer, release, or reformation in the nerve terminal have been well reviewed (Lee, 1987; Naguib et al., 2002). Mobilization of ACh during tetanic stimulation may be limited in the neonate and particularly in the premature infant. Unanesthetized newborns appear to have less neuromuscular reserve during tetanic stimulation than do adults. In neonates, there is no fade of twitch height with repeated stimulation at rates of 1 to 2 Hz; however, there is significant fade at 20 Hz. Premature infants may show post-tetanic exhaustion that lasts for 15 to 20 minutes. Goudsouzian (1980) noted slower contraction times of the thumb after slow and rapid rates of stimulation in full-term infants (aged 1 to 10 days, anesthetized with halothane) than in older children. The percentage of fade at 20, 50, or 100 Hz did not differ between the infants and the older children, but the tetanic stimulus was applied for only 5 seconds. The train-of-four (TOF) ratio, the degree of post-

TABLE 7-22. Distinguishing Features of Mature and Fetal Receptors

Mature Receptors	Fetal Receptors*
ε Subunit	γ Subunit
Localized to end-plate region	Junctional and extrajunctional sites
Metabolically stable (half-life = 2 wk)	Metabolically unstable (half-life = 24 hr)
Larger single-channel conductance	Smaller single-channel conductance
Shorter mean open time	Twofold to 10-fold longer mean open time
Agonists depolarize less easily	Agonists depolarize more easily
Competitive agents block more easily	Competitive agents block less easily†

Data from Martyn JA et al.: Up-and-down regulation of skeletal muscle acetylcholine receptors, *Anesthesiology* 76:822, 1992.
*Immature junctional receptors have the same characteristics as upregulated extrajunctional receptors.
†Recent data conflict with this statement: Paul M et al.: The potency of new muscle relaxants on recombinant muscle-type acetylcholine receptors, *Anesth Analg* 94:597, 2002.
Fetal receptors are more sensitive to pancuronium, vecuronium, mivacurium, and rocuronium but not to d-tubocurarine or gallamine.

tetanic facilitation, and the tetanus/twitch ratio increase with age. Crumrine and Yodlowski (1981) noted a decrease in the amplitude of the frequency sweep electromyogram (FS-EMG) at frequencies of 50 to 100 Hz in infants younger than 12 weeks who had been given methohexital (Fig. 7-48). The FS-EMG is a recording of the action potential from an electrical stimulus rate that increases exponentially from one pulse per second to 100 Hz during a stimulation period of 10 seconds. The exponential increase in frequency allows assessment of neuromuscular transmission at tetanic rates without inducing fatigue. Older infants and children responded like adults. The addition of 70% nitrous oxide depressed the FS-EMG 11% to 38% in the group of infants younger than 12 weeks old, and this correlated with failure to sustain tetanus.

■ FIGURE 7-47. ACh receptor channels with the subunits (α, β, ε, and δ or α, β, γ, and δ) arranged around the central cation channel. Binding of acetylcholine to the two α subunits induces the conformational change that converts the channel from closed to open, although the mean channel open times differ between the two types of ACh receptors depicted here *(From Martyn JAJ et al.: Up-and-down regulation of skeletal muscle acetylcholine receptors, Anesthesiology 76:822, 1992.)*

Mature/innervated   Fetal/denervated

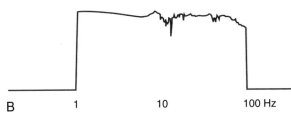

■ FIGURE 7-48. Tracings of the FS-EMG responses from the tibialis anterior muscles of a 1-day-old infant **(A)** and a 4-month-old infant **(B)** premedicated with methohexital. *(From Crumrine RS, Yodlowski EH: Assessment of neuromuscular function in infants,* Anesthesiology *54:29, 1981.)*

Mechanism of Action of Depolarizing and Nondepolarizing Neuromuscular Blocking Agents

Succinylcholine, the only depolarizing relaxant used clinically, produces two different types of blockade: phase I and phase II (Fig. 7-49). During phase I, succinylcholine binds to ACh receptors, causing ion channels to open or depolarize in the same fashion as does ACh. The molecules remain bound to the receptor for an extended period and cause the membrane to remain depolarized and unable to trigger any further muscle action potentials. This initial depolarization and movement of the individual muscle bundles may be seen clinically as fasciculations.

With an infusion or an increased amount of accumulated drug (dose of 4 to 6 mg/kg), a succinylcholine-induced block begins to assume the characteristics of a nondepolarizing block, which is referred to as *phase II block, desensitization,* or *dual blockade* (Lee and Katz, 1980; Sutherland et al., 1980; Donati and Bevan, 1983; Goudsouzian and Liu, 1984; Lee, 1986). Post-tetanic facilitation occurs, as well as fade with tetanus and TOF ratio of less than 0.4. These clinical characteristics of a phase II block are identical to those that occur with a nondepolarizing agent. Because a phase II block is functionally a nondepolarizing blockade, anticholinesterase drugs (reversal drugs) are effective, but only when four twitches are present and the plasma concentration of succinylcholine is low. On the other hand, nondepolarizing agents competitively bind one or two α units of the ACh receptor; this prevents both units from binding with ACh to open the ion channel. The drug may also physically block the ion channel in the motor end-plate, this is described as channel blockade. The NMBAs are classified either according to chemical structure or duration of action and are listed in on p. 250 (Table 7-34).

Basic Definitions

ED$_{95}$ and Intubating Dose

ED$_{95}$ is the dose of neuromuscular blocking agent that is expected to produce 95% block at the adductor pollicis. Several multiples of the ED$_{95}$ (e.g., two to three times ED95) are usually administered to ensure adequate neuromuscular blockade for intubation and to minimize the time to maximum block, which is also called the *onset time* (Kopman et al., 2001). The ED$_{95}$'s (relative potencies), onset, and duration of effect of various neuromuscular blocking agents in infants and children are illustrated in Tables 7-23, 7-24, and 7-25. ED$_{95}$ values tend to be higher in children than in infants or adults for most nondepolarizing neuromuscular blocking agents, with the exception of atracurium.

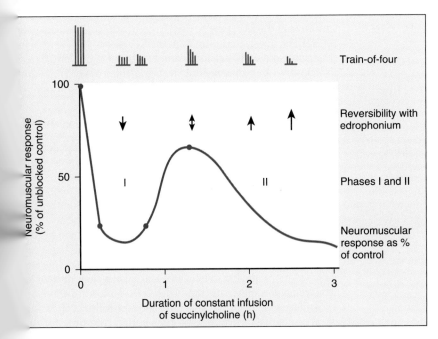

■ FIGURE 7-49. During continuous infusion of succinylcholine, a phase I block characterized by reduced neuromuscular response, little fade of TOF, and increased blockade with edrophonium is seen initially. During phase II, there is a fade of TOF, and increasing reversibility of the block by edrophonium, and accumulation of the slowly recovering residual block.

TABLE 7-23. Potency (ED$_{95}$) of Nondepolarizing NMBAs in Infants, Children, and Adults (mcg/kg)*

Drug	Anesthetic	Infant	Child	Adult
Mivacurium	Halothane	85	89	67
Cisatracurium	Narcotic	43	47	40
Vecuronium	Halothane	25	47-60	33
	Narcotic	47-60	81-100	43
Rocuronium	Halothane		300	
	Narcotic	255	402	350
Pancuronium	Halothane	45-50	61-70	67
	Narcotic	66	93	70

Data from Blinn A et al: Pancuronium dose-response revisited, *Paediatr Anesth* 2:153, 1992; de Ruiter J, Crawford MW: Dose-response relationship and infusion requirement of cisatracurium besylate in infants and children during nitrous oxide-narcotic anesthesia, *Anesthesiology* 94:790, 2001; Kalli I, Meretoja OA: Duration of action of vecuronium in infnats and children anaesthetized without potent inhalation agents, *Acta Anaesthesiol Scand* 33:29; 1989; Meretoja OA: 1988: Meretoja OA, Luosto T: Dose-response characteristics of pancuronium in neonates, infants and children, *Anaesth Intensive Care* 18:455, 1990, 1994; Meretoja OA, Taivainen T, Erkola O, et al: Dose-response and time-course of effect of rocuronium bromide in paediatric patients, *Eur J Anaesthesiol* 11(Suppl):19, 1995a; Meretoja OA, Taivainen T, Wirtavuori K: Pharmacodynamic effects of 51 W89, an isomer of atracurium, in children during halothane anaesthesia, *Br J Anaesth* 74:6, 1995b, 1995; Taivainen T, Meretoja OA: The neuromuscular blocking effects of vecuronium during sevoflurane, halothane, and balanced anaesthesia in children, *Anaesthesia* 50:1046, 1995; Woelfel SK et al.: Clinical pharmacology of mivacurium in pediatric patients less than two years old during nitrous oxide-halothane anesthesia, *Anesth Analg* 77:713, 1993; Taivainen T, Meretoja OA, Erkola O, et al: Rocuronium in infant, children and adults during balanced anaesthesia, *Paediatr Anaesth* 6:271, 1996.

*Determined according to anesthetic background. Intubation dose is usually 2 to 3 times the ED$_{95}$. Values are means.

TABLE 7-24. Time to Onset of Maximum Block and Recovery During Inhalational Anesthesia in Infants*

Drug	Dose (mg/kg)	Maximum Block (%)	Onset Time (min)	Time to T$_{25}$ Recovery (min)	Time to T$_{90}$ Recovery (min) (mean ± SD)
Succinylcholine	1.6	90	0.9	4	
Mivacurium	0.15	90	1.1	10.3	
Cisatracurium	0.1	100	1.2	55	
Vecuronium	0.07	MAX	1.5	NA	73 ± 27
Rocuronium	0.6	90	0.6	41.9	
Pancuronium	0.07	90	1.3	70	

Data from Fisher DM, Miller RD: Neuromuscular effects of vecuronium (ORG NC45) in infants and children during N$_2$O-halothane anesthesia, *Anesthesiology* 58:519, 1983b; Kalli I, Meretoja OA: Duration of action of vecuronium in infants and children anaesthetized without potent inhalation agents. *Acta Anaesthesiol Scand* 33:29; 1989; Soltész S et al.: Neuromuscular blockade with cisatracurium in infants and children: its course under sevoflurane anesthesia. *Anaesthesist* 51:374, 2002; Taivainen T et al.: The safety and efficacy of cisatracurium 0.15 mg/kg^{-1} during nitrous oxide-opioid anaesthesia in infants and children. *Anaesthesia* 55:1047, 2000. Woelfel SK et al.: Neuromuscular effects of 600 mcg/kg^{-1} of rocuronium in infants during nitrous oxide-halothane anaesthesia. *Paediatr Anaesth* 4:173, 1994; Woelfel SK, Brandom BW, McGowan FX et al.: Clinical pharmacology of mivacurium in pediatric patients less than two years old during nitrous oxide-halothane anesthesia, *Anesth Analg* 77:713, 1993.

*Values are means.

TABLE 7-25. Time to Onset of Maximum Block and Recovery During Inhalational Anesthesia in Children*

Drug	Dose (mg/kg)	Block (%)	Time to Onset (min)	Time to T$_{25}$ (min)	Time to T$_{90}$ (min) (mean ± SD)
Succinylcholine	2	90	0.5	4	
Mivacurium	0.3	90	1.5	10.6	
Cisatracurium	0.15	100	2.2	34	
Vecuronium	0.07	MAX	2.4	25.5	35
	0.1	100	1.3	24	
Rocuronium	0.6		1.3	26	
Pancuronium	0.1	100	2.5	45–60	>120
	0.4	100	0.7	75	

Data from Brandom, 1995; Fisher, 1983; Kalli I, Meretoja OA: Duration of action of vecuronium in infants and children anaesthetized without potent inhalation agents, *Acta Anaesthesiol Scand* 33:29; 1989; Soltész S et al.: Neuromuscular blockade with cisatracurium in infants and children: its course under sevoflurane anesthesia, *Anaesthesist* 51:374, 2002; Taivainen T et al.: The safety and efficacy of cisatracurium 0.15 mg/kg^{-1} during nitrous oxide-opioid anaesthesia in infants and children, *Anaesthesia* 55:1047, 2000. Woelfel SK et al: Neuromuscular effects of 600 mcg/kg^{-1} of rocuronium in infants during nitrous oxide-halothane anaesthesia, *Paediatr Anaesth* 4:173, 1994; Gronert BJ, Brandom BW: Neuromuscular blocking drugs in infants and children, *Pediatr Clin North Am* 41:73, 1994.

*Values are means.

Dose-Response Curves

Dose-response studies in children and then infants are undertaken after adult clinical trials for safety and efficacy have been performed. Three or four doses expected to produce a measurable or less than maximum effect are administered during a standardized anesthetic with standard monitoring conditions (e.g., these TOF every 10 seconds). The ED$_{50}$ and ED$_{95}$ are determined from data (Fig. 7-50). ED$_{50}$ is determined from the middle of the dose-response curve where there is less variability resulting in a more robust measure. The intubating dose as a multiple of the ED$_{50}$ may be used to compare onset and duration of NMBAs; however, multiples of the ED$_{95}$ are routinely used for this comparison. Onset times and lengths of action of different NMBAs may be compared only if equivalent doses or equal multiples of the ED$_{95}$ are administered.

Onset and Duration of Block, Maintenance Doses, Recovery Index

By current convention, onset is the time to maximum effect, and duration is the time for return of neuromuscular transmission to 25% of baseline, or T$_{25}$ (Bedford, 1995). In general, the dose of a specific nondepolarizing agent required to produce a particular degree of relaxation is similar in neonates (younger than 1 month), infants (aged 1 to 12 months), and adolescents (older than 13 years). However, in children (aged 3 to 10 years) the dose (ED$_{95}$) tends to be greater and the onset of block tends to be more rapid than in adults. In addition, the maximal effect (onset) is reached more quickly in neonates and infants than in the older children and adolescents (see Tables 7-23, 7-24, and 7-25).

Differences in onset and duration are influenced by age-related changes in volume of distribution, the time for dr

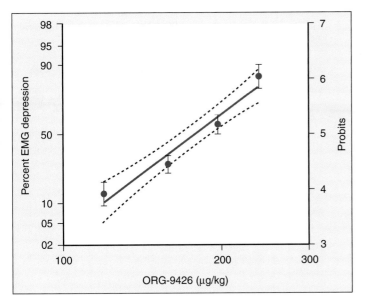

■ **FIGURE 7-50.** Dose-response curve (n = 61) for rocuronium in children during nitrous oxide-halothane anesthesia. *Filled circles,* Group mean values ± SEM; *dashed lines,* the 95% confidence limits. *(From Woelfel SK et al.: Effects of bolus administration of ORG-9426 in children during nitrous oxide-halothane anesthesia,* Anesthesiology *76:940, 1992.)*

to reach the effected site (muscle tissue and the neuromuscular junction), as well as clearance. The effect of a bolus of a specific NMBA depends on tissue sensitivity (Cp_{ss}), the pharmacokinetics (plasma concentration of drug, volume of distribution, clearance, and elimination half-life), and the pharmacodynamic parameter K_{eo} for the resultant effect or block. Unfortunately, it is difficult to measure the concentration at the neuromuscular junction, because there is a lag time between concentration in the plasma and the neuromuscular junction. Therefore the pharmacodynamic parameters, Cp_{ss} and K_{eo}, are measured using a model to determine concentration at the neuromuscular junction.

Duration of block in infants. A prolonged duration of action occurs for both vecuronium and recuronium in neonates and infants (younger than 6 mo) compared with children and adults. Age does not have this effect on the duration of atracurium

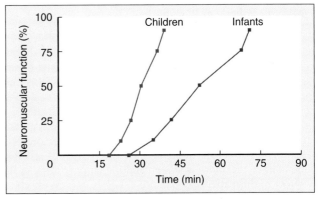

■ **FIGURE 7-51.** Recovery of T_1 after 600 mcg/kg rocuronium in infants and children during halothane. *(Data from Woelfel SK et al.: Effects of bolus administration of ORG-9426 in children during nitrous oxide-halothane anesthesia,* Anesthesiology *76:940, 1992.)*

or cisatracurium (Table 7-26 and Fig. 7-51) (Meretoja, 1990; Driessen et al., 2000; Rapp, 2004a).

When neuromuscular transmission has recovered to T_{25}, four twitches using TOF stimuli are usually present. The clinical importance of T_{25} is that maintenance doses of the neuromuscular blocking drug should be administered at this point if muscle relaxation is required for the surgical procedure. Maintenance doses are 0.25 to 0.3 times the intubation dose (Table 7-27). In addition, T_{25} recovery is the earliest time that the pharmacologic reversal agents should be administered for a rapid and full recovery to 100% of baseline neuromuscular transmission.

A recovery index (i.e., RI_{25-75}) is the difference in time to recovery from 25% to 75% of the final baseline (T_{25} to T_{75}). Published indices of recovery provide an expected duration of effect, but monitoring of neuromuscular transmission is preferable. Common recovery indices are from 5% to 25%, 25% to 75%, or 5% to 95% recovery and are another means of comparing NMBAs.

TABLE 7-26. Duration of Action of Rocuronium in Infants Under 1 Year of Age*

Dose of Rocuronium (mg/kg)	Age (mo)	T_{75} (min)	TOF > 0.7 (min)
0.45	0-1	56.4 ± 16[†]	62.3 ± 18
	2-4	62.7 ± 32	64.1 ± 27
	5-12	45.8 ± 18	43.7 ± 12
0.6	0-1	100.8 ± 35[†]	94.8 ± 31
	2-4	70.6 ± 19	63.8 ± 14
	5-12	63.4 ± 21	67.5 ± 18

Modified from Rapp HJ et al.: Neuromuscular recovery following rocuronium bromide single dose in infants, *Paediatr Anaesth* 14:329, 2004c.
*Data are from 61 infants and children under isoflurane anesthesia. Values are means.
†Age group "0-1 mo" is significantly different from age group "5-12 mo" for both doses of rocuronium at p ≤ 0.05.

TABLE 7-27. Intubation and Maintenance Doses (mg/kg) of NMBAs in Infants and Children

	Intubation Dose*	Maintenance
Succinylcholine	1-2	—
Cisatracurium	0.1-0.2	0.02-0.05
Vecuronium	0.05-0.1	0.02
Rocuronium	0.3-1.0[†]	0.1
Pancuronium	0.08-0.1	0.02

Adapted from Rapp HJ, Altenmueller CA, Waschke C: Neuromuscular recovery following rocuronium bromide single dose in infants, *Paediatr Anaesth* 14:329, 2004a.
*The recommended dose range for intubation in infants and children is two to three times ED_{95}. Increasing the dose speeds the onset of neuromuscular block.
[†]0.6-1.0 mg/kg of rocuronium in the infant may have a prolonged duration of action with up to 100 min for recovery to T_{75}. Maintenance dose is one fourth to one third of the intubation dose.

TABLE 7-28. Continuous Infusion Dose Range (mcg/kg/min) Required to Maintain $T_1 < 5\%-10\%$*

Drug	Type	Infant	Child	Adult
Cisatracurium	ICU	2.8 (0.6-4.9)	3.9±1.3	1.0-2.6
	Opioid Anesthesia	1.3-2.5	1.3-2.9	N/A
Vecuronium	ICU	1.1 (0.9-2.9)	1.5-2.6	0.9
	Opioid Anesthesia	0.8-1	1.6-2.5	0.8-1.6
Rocuronium	Inhaled Anesthesia	N/A	13.1-16.7	5.9-6.1
	Opioid Anesthesia	N/A	8.4	9.8

Data from Burmester M, Mok Q: Randomised controlled trial comparing cisatracurium and vecuronium infusions in a paediatric intensive care unit, *Intensive Care Med* 31:686, 2005; Hodges UM: Vecuronium infusion requirements in paediatric patients in intensive care units: the use of acceleromyography, *Br J Anaesth* 76:23, 1996; Prielipp RC et al: *Crit Care Trauma* 81:3, 1995; Odetola FO, Bhatt-Mehta V, Zahraa J et al: Cisatracurium infusion for neuromuscular blockade in the pediatric intensive care unit: a dose-fiding study, *Pediatr Crit Care Med* 3(3):250-254, 2002; Reich DL et al.: Comparison of cisatracurium and vecuronium by infusion in neonates and small infants after congenital heart surgery, *Anesthesiology* 101:112, 2004; Woloszczuk-Gebicka B et al.: The influence of halothane, isoflurane, and sevoflurane on rocuronium infusion in children, *Acta Anaesthesiol Scand* 45:73, 2001.
*Values are means (range).

Pharmacologic Differences in Infants and Children: Sensitivity, Volume of Distribution, Clearance

The drug concentration in plasma that produces 50% to 90% twitch suppression at steady-state conditions (C_p or C_p), such as with an infusion, provides a means of comparing drug potencies. Neonates and infants are more sensitive to all NMBAs than children and adults. D-tubocurarine has been well studied in all age groups, and the concentration at the effect site (C_{ss}) for neonates is one half to one third of that for children and adults. However, initial dosing of d-tubocurarine for the neonate should not be decreased, because the volume of distribution is larger, clearance is slower, and the elimination half-life is longer in this patient population.

Different patterns emerge between atracurium and cisatracurium vs. vecuronium and rocuronium in infants. For cisatracurium, the ED_{95} values are similar for infants, children, and adults at 43, 47, and 40 mcg/kg, respectively (see Table 7-23). The volume of distribution of cisatracurium is increased, and the clearance is more rapid in infants than in children and adults. Thus, the same multiple of ED_{95} dose has a similar and predictable duration in infants, children, and adults. Mean infusion rates to maintain block at 95% are also similar in infants, children, and adults during the same anesthetic exposure (Table 7-28).

On the other hand, ED_{95} values for vecuronium in infants and children are 47 and 81 mcg/kg, respectively, with narcotic anesthesia and 25 and 45 mcg/kg with halothane anesthesia. Onset is more rapid in the infant (0.6 to 0.8 times that of the child), and duration is increased with the RI at 1.7 to 2.9 times that of a child. Infants have both increased volume of distribution and mean residence time, but clearance is basically unchanged or slightly less in the infant (5.6 mL/kg per minute) compared with children (5.9 mL/kg minute) (Table 7-29). The Cp_{ss50} is lower in the infant. After a single dose of relaxant, recovery depends on both distribution and elimination. The combination of a longer mean residence time and a lower sensitivity for vecuronium explains the prolongation of neuromuscular block in infants. Vecuronium should be considered a long-acting NMBA in neonates and infants.

TABLE 7-29. Pharmacokinetics and Pharmacodynamics of Vecuronium*

Age Group	$t_{1/2}\beta$ (min)	CL (mL/kg/min)	Vd_{ss} (mL/kg)	Cp_{ss50} (ng/mL)
Infants	64.7 ± 30.2	5.6 ± 1.0	357 ± 70	57.3 ± 17.7
Children	41.0 ± 15.1	5.9 ± 2.4	204 ± 116	109.8 ± 28.1
Adults	70.7 ± 20.4	5.2 ± 0.7	269 ± 42	93.7 ± 33.5

From Cook DR, Marcy JH: *Neonatal anesthesia*, Pasadena, CA, 1988, Appleton Davies.
*Values are means ± SD.
$t_{1/2}\beta$, Elimination half-life; *CL*, clearance; *Vd_{ss}*, volume of distribution at steady state; *Cp_{ss50}*, steady-state plasma concentration associated with 50% neuromuscular blockade.

Similarly, rocuronium acts as a long-acting NMBA in infants. It has the most rapid onset of action in all age groups because of its low potency (ED_{95} of 255 to 400 mcg/kg) compared with the other commonly used NMBAs (which have higher potency, with ED_{95} values between 40 to 90 mcg/kg for mivacurium, cisatracurium, vecuronium, and pancuronium). The most rapid onset occurs in infants when rocuronium is compared with all the other age groups. Here, both the volume of distribution and mean residence time are greater in infants (aged 3 to 12 months) than children (aged 4 to years), but for rocuronium, the clearance is slower for the infant but more rapid in the child than the adult. The effect site concentration that produces 50% block is also less in the infant (Table 7-30) (Wierda et al., 1997; Saldein et al., 200). These factors contribute to the prolonged length of action of rocuronium in infants.

TABLE 7-30. Pharmacodynamic Data for Rocuronium in Infants, Children, and Adults*

	Infants	Children	Adults
EC_{50} ng/kg	652 ± 215	1200 ± 295	954 ± 276
EC_{90} ng/kg	1705	2230	2035

Data from Saldien V et al.: Target-controlled infusion of rocuronium in infants, children, and adults: a comparison of the pharmacokinetic and pharmacodynamic relationship, *Anesth Analg* 97:44, 2003; Wierda JM et al.: Pharmacokinetics and pharmacokinetic-dynamic modelling of rocuronium in infants and children, *Br J Anaesth* 78:690, 1997.
*Effect site concentration of rocuronium to produce 50% and 90% neuromuscular block in infants, children, and adults. Note that these concentrations are decreased for the infant, whereas those of children and adults are similar.

Monitoring Neuromuscular Block

Types of Monitoring: Peripheral Nerve Stimulation and Acceleromyography

Restoration of complete skeletal muscle strength is essential to ensure that patients are able to sustain adequate ventilation, cough, and maintain a patent airway after administration of relaxants. Peripheral nerve stimulation (PNS) is routinely used, resulting in a visual or tactile subjective observation of response to an electrical stimulation, single twitch stimulus or TOF. However, expert researchers in the field of neuromuscular study cannot reliably detect fade when the TOF ratio is greater than 0.4 but less than 0.9, either visually or tactilely (Viby-Mogensen et al., 1985, 2007; Kopman, 2009). The TOF-Watch objectively measures acceleration of the thumb using a piezoelectric transducer placed on the tip of the thumb. Acceleromyography (AMG) is based on Newton's Second Law: Force = Mass × Acceleration. When TOF stimulation is used, the percentage of TOF ratio is displayed on a digital screen, so fade is quantified without a subjective interpretation (Fig. 7-52).

Neuromuscular Block Effects at Different Muscles

The adductor pollicis is commonly monitored; however, the diaphragm, larynx, flexor hallucis brevis, and orbicularis oculi are also observed clinically. The onset, depth, and duration of action of NMBAs differ at different muscle sites. In adults, block develops faster, is less profound, and recovers more quickly in the centrally located muscles such as the larynx, the masseter (jaw), and the diaphragm than in more peripherally located muscles (such as the adductor pollicis) (Fig. 7-53). In children aged 18 months to 9 years), complete block occurs earlier in the orbicularis oculi than at the adductor pollicis (0.7 minutes on average), but observation of complete block at either muscle leads to excellent intubation conditions (Plaud et al., 1997). Also, in children (aged 2 to 18 years), onset and recovery are both slower at the flexor hallucis brevis than at the adductor pollicis during inhalational anesthesia. In addition, the ED_{90} for the diaphragm is 1.6 times the ED_{90} of the adductor pollicis in infants and children. Doses of pancuronium for 90% relaxation of the adductor pollicis and diaphragm are 42 vs. 70 mcg/kg (0 to 1 year), 47 vs. 81 mcg/kg (1 to 3 years), and 62 vs. 101 mcg/kg (3 to

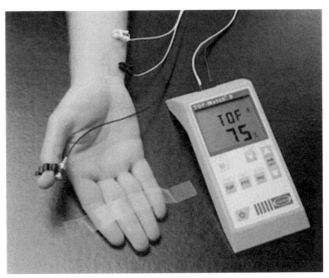

FIGURE 7-52. TOF-Watch (Organon Ltd., Dublin, Ireland). This neuromuscular transmission monitor is based on measurement of acceleration using a piezoelectric transducer. Note the transducer fastened to the thumb and the stimulating electrodes. On the display of the TOF-Watch, the TOF ratio is given in percentage. *(From Viby-Mogensen J: Neuromuscular monitoring. In Miller ED, Eriksson LI, Fleisher LA, et al: Miller's anesthesia, ed 7, Philadelphia, 2010, Churchill Livingstone.)*

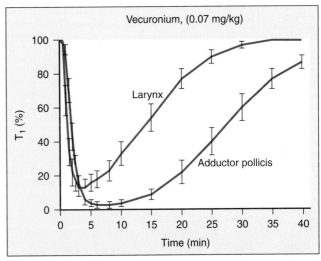

FIGURE 7-53. First twitch height (T_1) against time for vocal cords and adductor pollicis, after vecuronium 0.07 mg/kg. Bars indicate SEM. *(From Donati F, Meistelman C, Plaud B: Vecuronium neuromuscular blockaded at the adductor muscles of the larynx and adductor pollicis, Anesthesiology 74:833-837, 1991.)*

10 years), respectively. Therefore, when there is a 90% block of the adductor pollicis, there is much less block of the diaphragm in infants and children (Laycock et al., 1988). Intubation and supplemental doses of NMBAs are listed in Table 7-27.

Types of Stimuli

Peripheral nerve stimulation can be delivered at different frequencies to assess the depth of neuromuscular block (e.g., TOF, post-tetanic count [PTC], and double burst stimulation [DBS])

and is often used instead of tests of ventilation and grip strength in pediatric patients. TOF stimulation is the most common pattern of stimulation for clinical monitoring of neuromuscular blockade in the operating room, because the response can be elicited without an established baseline, and the peripheral nerve stimulator may be placed at any time during the surgical procedure. This stimulation mode allows for convenient visual and tactile evaluation of moderate degrees of nondepolarizing blockade without the undue discomfort that accompanies tetanic bursts (i.e., 50 to 100 Hz for 5 seconds) (Brull et al., 1990).

In adults, at a TOF ratio of greater than 0.9, vital capacity returns to normal (more than 15 to 20 mL/kg), pharyngeal muscle strengthens to allow recovery of swallowing, diplopia disappears, and maximum inspiratory and expiratory forces are only slightly depressed (−50 cm H_2O) (Kopman and Yee, 1997). No similar data are available for infants and children, but recovery to TOF ratio of greater than 0.9 is recommended (Table 7-31).

Post-tetanic stimulation. PTC is 20 single-twitch stimuli after a tetanic stimulation. This monitoring mode is usually used intraoperatively when there is no response to TOF stimuli. The time to return of TOF can be predicted when PTC is 5 to 10 counts, and this recovery time is more rapid in children than in adults. For example, in children (aged 2 to 5 yrs) who have been given rocuronium (1 mg/kg), when PTC of 1 occurs, the TOF returns in 7 minutes, whereas in adults (aged 18 to 60 years) TOF returns in 16 minutes, and in those aged 65 to 80 years, 22.3 minutes are required (Bakayra et al., 2002, 2003).

Children receiving an atracurium infusion who have a PTC of less than 10 show only one response to TOF stimuli, although a PTC of 15 correlates with 3 to 4 responses to TOF, which is a stage where pharmacologic reversal may be administered (Ridley and Hatch, 1988).

In contrast, children with vecuronium infusions who have a PTC of 5 to 15 have adequate surgical relaxation, and pharmacologic reversal of block can be administered in 6 to 18 minutes (Ridley and Braude, 1988).

In addition to predicting the amount of time for a TOF ratio of three to four twitches to return and therefore when block can be reversed, PTC is useful in the timing of NMBA administration

so that the diaphragm is relaxed in children. When the PTC is zero at the AP, it is likely that the diaphragm is also relaxed. In children, the diaphragm recovers from relaxants more rapidly than the adductor pollicis (Laycock et al., 1988).

Double burst stimulation. Because it is difficult to estimate the TOF ratio with sufficient certainty to exclude residual paralysis, DBS was developed (Viby-Mogensen et al., 1985; Ueda et al., 1988; Drenck et al., 1989; Engbaek et al., 1989). DBS consists of two short tetanic bursts of 50 Hz separated by 750 milliseconds, and the ratio of the second to the first response is evaluated. DBS is more sensitive than TOF in children (aged 3 to 10 years) as well as adults when manually detecting residual neuromuscular block. Fade could not be detected manually with TOF greater than 0.44 and with DBS greater than 0.67 (Saddler et al., 1990). Therefore, absence of fade in response to DBS excludes severe residual neuromuscular block but does not indicate adequate clinical recovery of TOF ratio to greater than 0.9 (Fig. 7-54) (Fruergaard et al., 1998; Gätke et al., 2002).

Monitoring Recovery

Complete recovery from neuromuscular block requires a TOF of greater than 0.9 (Kopman et al., 1997, 2009). A large body of evidence in adults exists that depressed pharyngeal and upper esophageal function, decreased chemoreceptor sensitivity to hypoxia, impaired ability to maintain the airway, and increased risk for the development of postoperative pulmonary complications are all consequences of postoperative residual neuromuscular block (Berg et al., 1997; Eriksson et al., 1997).

Residual paralysis (TOF of less than 0.7 to 0.9) in the recovery room occurs in 19% to 54% of patients when long-acting, intermediate-acting, or a single intubating dose of NMBA are used in adults (Debaene et al., 2003). In one study evaluating this effect,

TABLE 7-31. Clinical Signs and Symptoms in Awake Adult Volunteers When the TOF Ratio is Between 0.7 and 0.9

TOF Ratio	Signs and Symptoms*
0.7-0.75	Double vision Decreased hand grip strength Inability to oppose incisors Unable to clench tongue depressor with teeth Facial weakness Overall weakness Lethargy
0.85-0.90	Double vision Generalized fatigue Able to clench tongue depressor with teeth

From Kopman AF et al.: Relationship of the train-of-four fade ratio to clinical signs and symptoms of residual paralysis in awake volunteers, *Anesthesiology* 86:765, 1997.

*Awake volunteers recovering from mivacurium infusion had these clinical signs before full neuromuscular recovery.

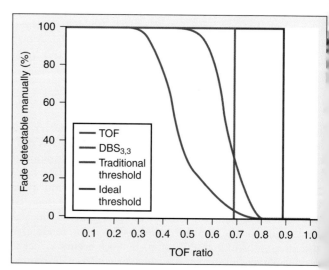

FIGURE 7-54. Fade detected by touch in the response to TOF and DBS in relation to the true TOF ratio, as measured mechanically. The axis indicates the percentage of instances in which fade can be felt at a given TOF ratio. It is not possible to exclude residual neuromuscular block by TOF or DBS with certainty, whether a TOF ratio of 0.7 or 0.9 is taken to reflect adequate recovery of neuromuscular function. *(From Viby-Mogensen J: Neuromuscular monitoring. In Miller ED, editor: Miller's anesthesia, ed 6, Philadelphia, Elsevier Churchill Livingstone.)*

no similar residual block was found in children (older than 2 years); however, children always recover faster than adults from NMBA. The block was monitored carefully intraoperatively, and all children received pharmacologic reversal drugs when three or four twitches were present (Baxter et al., 1991). It is appropriate to ensure full recovery in all pediatric patients and especially in infants, because they have a narrow margin of safety.

Timing of Antagonists

Neurotransmission returns promptly if few receptors are blocked at the time of reversal (e.g., T_{25} or when three or four twitches of TOF are present). At this stage, 70% to 75% of receptors may still be occupied (Waud, 1971). Neostigmine (50 mcg/kg) is the recommended dose in infants (Fisher et al., 1983). There is no clinical advantage in attempting to antagonize intense neuromuscular block (fewer than three or four twitches) in children or in administering increased doses of neostigmine or edrophonium (Gwinnutt et al., 1991; Kopman and Eikerman, 2009). Data for this phenomena in children are shown in Figure 7-55 (Meistelman et al., 1988; Donati et al., 1989; Gwinnutt et al., 1991; Bevan et al., 1999). The plasma level of the NMBA should be low enough that the competitive effect of the anticholinesterases allow enough muscle strength to ensure TOF of 0.9 to 1 (Kopman et al., 1997). In addition, certain antibiotics, hypothermia, acidosis, hypocalcemia, and especially inhalational agents can prolong or potentiate neuromuscular block from nondepolarizing relaxants.

The present use of primarily short- and intermediate-acting relaxants may change the rule to "always reverse blockade" with ACHs to "always document return of full neuromuscular function (TOF of greater than 0.9)" at the end of the case with either spontaneous or pharmacologically induced (anticholinesterases

or sugammadex) recovery. Clearly, the margin of safety of relaxants is increased by using objective rather than subjective criteria to judge the adequacy of neuromuscular transmission. Experts in neuromuscular studies have documented the difficulty with subjective (visual and tactile) assessment of TOF and DBS in determining complete recovery (Drenck, 1989; Fruergaard, 1998). For these reasons, an objective monitor (see Fig. 7-52), such as the accelerometer (AMG) is highly recommended. In addition, when objective monitoring is used, anticholinesterases can be administered at T25 (when 3 to 4 twitches are present) so that the drugs can have a complete response.

Potency or Dose of Neuromuscular Blocking Agent

Intubation doses (two to three times the ED_{95}) for depolarizing and nondepolarizing neuromuscular relaxants for infants and children are shown in Table 7-27. The length of action of recovery to T_{25} is also available (see Tables 7-24 and 7-25). Both age and inhalational anesthetic have an effect on potency. The speed of onset is inversely proportional to the potency of the nondepolarizing agents. With the exception of atracurium, molar potency is highly predictive of a drug's rate of onset of effect. Rocuronium has a more rapid onset than cisatracurium or vecuronium (Kopman, 2009).

Types of Neuromuscular Blocking Agents

Depolarizing Neuromuscular Relaxant: Succinylcholine

Succinylcholine, a rapid-acting and usually short-duration depolarizing muscle relaxant, is useful for rapid-sequence induction and endotracheal intubation. The onset time for 2 mg/kg is 30 ± 7 seconds in children (aged 2 to 10 years) with a T_{25} of 5.2 ± 1.9 min (Woolf et al., 1997). Succinylcholine is metabolized by butyrylcholinesterase, which effects both the onset and duration of action. Prolonged neuromuscular blockade can result from abnormally low or atypical enzyme concentrations. The former ranges from 9 to 23 minutes, whereas the latter genetic variations may last from 4 to 8 hours (Viby-Mogensen and Hanel, 1978; Viby-Mogensen, 1980). This enzyme activity is reduced in neonates, but there is little change in butyrylcholinesterase activity between 3 months and 12 years of age. Clinically, this reduction in neonates has no effect.

Dose, Onset, and Duration in Infants and Children

Neonates and infants require about twice as much succinylcholine (mcg/kg) as older children or adults (Table 7-32). Neonates and infants (younger than 2 years old) have an ED_{95} of 625 and 729 mcg/kg, respectively, for succinylcholine; they also have a faster clearance, larger volume of distribution and have a shorter onset time than children older than 2 years of age, with an ED_{95} of 523 mcg/kg, and adults, with ED_{95} of 290 mcg/kg.

In infants, 1 to 2 mg/kg of succinylcholine produces a block equal to that produced by 0.5 to 1 mg/kg in children aged 6 to 8 years (Cook and Fischer, 1975; Meakin et al., 1990). At equipotent doses, there is no statistically significant difference between the times to recover to 50% and 90% neuromuscular transmission in the two groups. Complete neuromuscular block develops in children given 1 mg/kg of succinylcholine. Because of marked variability in block produced by small

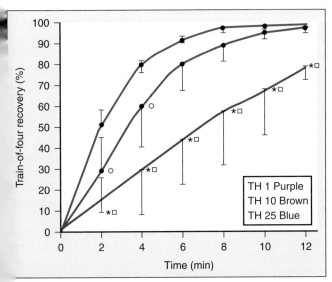

FIGURE 7-55. Recovery characteristics of vecuronium TOF after administration of neostigmine (30 mcg/kg) and atropine (10 mcg/kg) three predetermined twitch height values during nitrous oxide halothane anesthesia in children: TH 1 vs. TH 10, * P < 0.01; TH 1 vs. TH 25, □ P < 0.01; TH 10 vs. TH 25, ○ P < 0.01. *TH*, Twitch height. *Modified from Meistelman C et al.: Importance of the level of paralysis recovery for a rapid antagonism of vecuronium with neostigmine in children during halothane anesthesia,* Anesthesiology 69:98, 1988.)

TABLE 7-32. Calculated ED$_{50}$ and ED$_{95}$ for Succinylcholine as a Function of Age

Age	ED$_{50}$ (mcg/kg)	ED$_{95}$ (mcg/kg)	ED$_{50}$ (mcg/m²)	ED$_{95}$ Group (mcg/m²)
Neonates	250	625	3952	9881
Infants	317	729	6277	14,436
Children	184	423	4416	10,154
Adults	—	290	—	11,940

Data from Meakin G et al.: Dose-response curves for suxamethonium in neonates, infants, and children, *Br J Anaesth* 62:655, 1989.

doses of succinylcholine, it is recommended to select doses at the upper end of the range for children undergoing rapid-sequence induction. Succinylcholine (1 mg/kg) in adults reaches complete block in 60 seconds and lasts 6 to 8 minutes; for infants, 3 to 4 mg/kg is necessary, and for children 2 mg/kg is required to achieve the same duration (Meakin et al., 1989). It should be noted that treatment of laryngospasm does not require the full intubating dose of succinylcholine, and a minimal dose such as 0.2 mg/kg allows positive pressure ventilation in children.

Side Effects

Side effects of succinylcholine are well described and include dysrhythmias, increased intraocular pressure, prolonged apnea, injured muscle membranes with associated hyperkalemia, association with masseter spasm and malignant hyperthermia, and death.

Cardiac Arrest

Intractable, unexpected cardiac arrest (ventricular fibrillation or asystole) associated with a 40% to 50% mortality, was reported after the use of succinylcholine in children with undiagnosed Duchenne's muscular dystrophy (Larach et al., 1997). This series of case reports resulted in the FDA issuing a "black box" warning against the elective use of succinylcholine in children. Succinylcholine can also cause rhabdomyolysis and massive hyperkalemia (Tang et al., 1992; Hopkins, 1995; Gronert, 2001, 2002; Holak et al., 2007; Piotrowski and Fendler, 2007; Al-Takrouri et al., 2004). A survey (in 221 patients undergoing 444 anesthetics) in families identified with Duchenne's muscular dystrophy and Becker's muscular dystrophy revealed only six cardiac arrests, all in children who were not suspected of having the myopathy; in addition, they were all successfully resuscitated. Patients in whom myopathies were suspected had no cardiac arrests because succinylcholine was avoided (Breucking et al., 2000).

Life-threatening anaphylactic or anaphylactoid reactions have been reported, and drug-specific immunoglobulin-E antibodies to succinylcholine have been demonstrated (Naguib and Magboul, 1998).

Dysrhythmias. In the infant and small child, profound sustained sinus bradycardia (rates of 50 to 60 beats/min) is often observed; asystole occurs rarely. Nodal rhythm and ventricular ectopic beats are seen in about 80% of children given a single intravenous injection of succinylcholine; however, such dysrhythmias are rarely seen after an intramuscular injection of succinylcho-line. The incidence of bradycardia and other dysrhythmias is increased after a second dose of succinylcholine. Atropine appears to offer adequate protection against these bradyarrhythmias in all age groups. In infants, vagolytic doses of 0.02 to 0.03 mg/kg are required for protection; in older children, adequate protection is provided by doses of 0.005 mg/kg of atropine.

Intragastric pressure. Succinylcholine may increase intragastric pressure caused by the intensity of muscle fasciculations that have been recorded as high as 40 cm H_2O in adults, making them at risk for regurgitation and aspiration. Because of limited muscle mass, the infant or small child seldom has strong fasciculations; only a 4 cm H_2O increase or a decrease in intragastric pressure in infants was observed (Salem et al., 1972).

Intraocular pressure. Intravenous or intramuscular administration of succinylcholine increases intraocular pressure in infants and adults. Dilation of choroidal vessels and contraction of extraocular muscles may be the mechanism. A patient undergoing an enucleation with all extraocular muscles released showed an increase of intraocular pressure with succinylcholine. Typically, the intraocular pressure increases in 60 seconds, peaks at 2 to 3 minutes, and then returns to control levels 5 to 7 minutes after injection. The increase in intraocular pressure can be controlled by pretreatment with a nondepolarizing NMBA. This transient increase in intraocular pressure may be misinterpreted and lead to unnecessary surgery in a patient with glaucoma if tonometry is performed within 5 to 7 minutes of the injection of succinylcholine (see Chapter 27 Anesthesia for Ophthalmic Surgery).

Increased intracranial pressure. Increases in ICP after the administration of succinylcholine are produced by cerebral metabolic stimulation and increases in cerebral blood flow (Lanier et al., 1986, 1989; Minton et al., 1986). These effects are attenuated by prior administration of a nondepolarizing agent, by treatment with thiopental or lidocaine, and by hyperventilation.

Hyperkalemia, myoglobinemia, and increase in creatine phosphokinase. In normal adult patients, succinylcholine increases plasma levels of potassium by 0.3 to 0.5 mEq/L. Alarming levels of potassium, as high as 11 mEq/L, along with cardiovascular collapse, were often reported with succinylcholine in a variety of conditions, including burns, massive trauma, stroke, spinal cord injury, and muscle diseases (Delphin et al., 1987; Rosenberg and Gronert, 1992; Schow et al., 2002). The common denominator is existence of extrajunctional ACh receptors that occurs with massive tissue destruction or CNS injury with muscle wasting. Strong fasciculations are not necessary to produce hyperkalemia in susceptible patients. There are no data to suggest that the infant is any less vulnerable than the adult to massive potassium flux from the listed conditions (Henning and Bush, 1982; Dierdorf et al., 1984).

A high incidence of myoglobinemia occurs after succinylcholine use (1 mg/kg) in prepubertal patients, especially those anesthetized with halothane. Increased muscle fasciculations and myoglobin levels are seen in children younger than 4 years old compared with children between the ages of 4 and 9 years who received succinylcholine (Blanc et al., 1986). Others, however, report no change in fasciculations or myoglobin with age (infant to midteens) (Sekino et al., 1990). Pretreatment with "self-taming" succinylcholine (0.1 mg/kg) did not reduce the fasciculations or the change in myoglobin. Pretreatment with pancuronium and d-tubocurarine decreases the fasciculations but does not obliterate the release of myoglobin.

Plasma levels of creatine phosphokinase, an indicator of muscle injury, increase significantly after succinylcholine administration in children. Children (aged 3 to 15 years) undergoing emergency surgical procedures and who have been pretreated with mivacurium, gallamine, or normal saline before the administration of succinylcholine showed no differences in fasciculations or reported myalgias. However, pretreatment with mivacurium showed decreases in the rise of myoglobin, potassium, and creatine phosphokinase (CPK) levels. A significant association was observed between fasciculations and the release of both myoglobin and CPK (Theroux et al., 2001). The tendency of muscle in children to release myoglobin after depolarization with succinylcholine is not readily explained. Such changes seem to be rare in infants.

Masseter spasm and malignant hyperthermia. Masseter spasm is a marked increase in tension of the masseter muscle that prevents opening of the mouth after succinylcholine has produced neuromuscular block. Resting tension or stiffness in the masseter muscle increases in a dose-related manner as succinylcholine blocks neuromuscular function (DeCook and Goudsouzian, 1980; Van Der Spek et al., 1988, 1989; Plumley et al., 1990; Sadler et al., 1990). Masseter spasm is probably the extreme end of the normal dose-related increase in resting tension seen with succinylcholine. Of 500 children who had halothane and nitrous-oxide anesthetic with 2 mg/kg of succinylcholine, 4.4% had incomplete relaxation and one patient had masseter spasm (Hannallah and Kaplan, 1994). Masseter rigidity alone is not diagnostic of malignant hyperthermia, and this is not currently an indication to change to a nontriggering anesthetic (see Chapter 37, Malignant Hyperthermia).

Present Status of Succinylcholine Use in Infants and Children

Routine use of succinylcholine in infants and children should be avoided because of risk for cardiac arrest, hyperkalemia, and rhabdomyolysis in patients with unsuspected Duchenne's muscular dystrophy. Succinylcholine is only recommended for emergency control of the airways in infants and children.

The introduction of the new ultra-short–, short-, and intermediate-acting relaxants and other strategies to increase the speed of onset of NMBAs has reduced the need for succinylcholine in children. A large intubating dose (four to five times ED_{95}) can be used to accelerate the onset of block with the necessary result of effectively converting the intermediate-acting drugs, cisatracurium, rocuronium, and vecuronium to long-acting relaxants, especially in infants. Rocuronium (1.2 mg/kg, four times ED_{95}) produces good intubating conditions (90% depression of twitch height) in 33 ± 5 seconds in children (aged 2 to 10 years) with the resulting T_{25} of 41 ± 13 minutes (Woolf et al., 1997). Priming is rarely used in children because onset time is already more rapid in children than that in adults. In addition, intubation is routinely performed in pediatric patients without neuromuscular blocking drugs for nonemergent (not rapid-sequence or full-stomach precautions) intubations with a combination of inhalational agents, opioids, propofol, and sedatives. In fact, for rapid sequence in infants and children, remifentanil 3 mcg/kg and propofol mg/kg produce good to excellent intubating conditions compared with propofol and succinylcholine (2 mg/kg) (Crawford al., 2005; Simon et al., 2002).

Contraindications to Succinylcholine: Absolute and Relative

The absolute contraindications to succinylcholine include patient or immediate family history of malignant hyperthermia, suspected myopathy, and hyperkalemia.

Relative contraindications include patients with plasma cholinesterase deficiency, hypercarbia, moderate hyperkalemia, increased extrajunctional ACh receptors because of trauma, stroke, immobility, burns, sepsis, or when the other side effects are undesirable.

Nondepolarizing Neuromuscular Relaxants

Selection of Nondepolarizing Relaxant: Dose, Onset, Duration, Side Effects, and Metabolism

At appropriate doses, all nondepolarizing relaxants produce neuromuscular blockade; at equipotent doses, each relaxant produces the same degree of relaxation as any other. Increasing the dose speeds the onset of block. Onset time is more rapid with relaxants that have high ED_{95} values (and therefore low potency; e.g., rocuronium). Potent inhaled anesthetic agents speed the onset of block, but they also lengthen the duration of block in a concentration-dependent manner (Jalkanen and Meretoja, 1997). Factors in selecting one relaxant over another include the onset time, duration of effect, side effects, and routes of elimination (renal or hepatic). In addition, age (neonate, infant, child, adolescent, or adult) and the disease state of the patient are important.

The side effects of the nondepolarizing relaxants are primarily cardiovascular and relate to the amount of histamine release, ganglionic blockade, and vagolysis and are age-related. In infants and children, minimal cardiovascular effects are seen after administration of atracurium or vecuronium at several multiples of the ED_{95} (Brandom et al., 1983b, 1984; Fisher and Miller, 1983; Goudsouzian et al., 1983a, 1983b). At two times ED_{95}, increases in heart rate are seen with pancuronium and rocuronium in children; in contrast, both have minimal effects on heart rate in infants. Because the infant responds with bradycardia to a variety of stimuli (e.g., hypoxia and tracheal intubation), the "potential" vagolytic effects of pancuronium or rocuronium may be a desirable effect.

In adults, atracurium (three times ED_{95}) causes histamine release, whereas vecuronium (at any multiple of ED_{95}) is not associated with histamine release (Tullock et al., 1990). Infants and children appear to be less susceptible than adults to histamine release after administration of relaxants. In a small series of infants, five times ED_{95} of atracurium did not elicit flushing or alter heart rate or blood pressure (Brandom et al., 1984; Goudsouzian et al., 1985). However, local signs of histamine release after direct intravenous injection of atracurium in infants and children have been described; rarely, flushing with or without mild hypotension is seen at high multiples of the ED_{95} (Nightingale and Bush, 1983). At high doses, d-tubocurarine may cause hypotension and histamine release in children. The different pattern of tryptase release by the various types of relaxants suggests different mechanisms of mast-cell activation (Koppert et al., 2001). Bronchospasm may be related to histamine release or release of leukotrienes. Some relaxants may block prejunctional muscarinic receptors in the airway.

Another area of importance with neuromuscular blocking agents is the risk of anaphylaxis. A 12-year survey at a French pediatric center showed 60.8% of the IgE-mediated anaphylaxis reported with neuromuscular blocking agents, and vecuronium caused the largest number of reactions (Karila et al., 2005). The second most common agent to produce this reaction is latex. As in adults, NMBAs are responsible for most anaphylactic reactions occurring during anesthesia. Succinylcholine and rocuronium can also have this reaction.

Routes of Elimination of Nondepolarizing Agents

Nondepolarizing NMBAs are eliminated by renal excretion, hepatic uptake and excretion, and biotransformation, including Hofmann elimination (Table 7-33). These drugs filter freely through the glomerulus, and the renal clearance does not exceed the GFR (1 to 2 mL/kg per minute). The degree of metabolism of NMBA varies widely. Hofmann elimination and ester hydrolysis are largely responsible for the breakdown of atracurium and cisatracurium; butyrylcholinesterase is primarily associated with the metabolism of mivacurium. Gantacurium appears to be degraded by two chemical mechanisms, neither which is enzymatic: rapid formation of an inactive cysteine product, and a slower hydrolysis of the ester bond to inactive products.

Hepatic biodegradation has been demonstrated for steroidal relaxants (Savage et al., 1980; Bencini et al., 1983). Rocuronium is primarily eliminated by the liver with no metabolites, and with only a small fraction (10%) eliminated in urine. Only a small fraction (20% to 30%) of pancuronium undergoes metabolism. In contrast, the hepatic metabolism of vecuronium is significant (Savage et al., 1980; Marshall et al., 1983). Spontaneous deacetylation occurs in the liver, and the by-products are 3-hydroxy and 17-hydroxy derivatives. In addition, the 3-hydroxy metabolite is a potent (approximately 80% of vecuronium) neuromuscular blocking agent, and because it has a slower plasma clearance this contributes to the prolonged duration of action, especially in pediatric ICU patients on infusions of vecuronium (Caldwell et al., 1994). The 17-hydroxy and 3, 17-hydroxy metabolites however are far less active (Marshall et al., 1983).

Classification of Nondepolarizing Blocking Drugs

All but one nondepolarizing NMBA fall into the two groups of either aminosteroids (e.g., pancuronium, vecuronium, rocuronium, and rapacuronium) or benzylisoquinolinium (e.g., d-tubocurarine, atracurium, cisatracurium, and mivacurium) compounds. Gantacurium is an asymmetric mixed-onium chlorofumarate compound.

Nondepolarizing NMBA can also be categorized by the time to maximum blockade (i.e., onset time) and by the clinical duration of effect (i.e., T_{25}) (Table 7-34). Long-acting (duration of greater than 50 minutes) agents include pancuronium, and intermediate-acting (duration of 20 to 50 minutes) agents are vecuronium, rocuronium, and cisatracurium, but the only short-acting (duration of 10 to 20 minutes) agent of mivacurium is no longer available in the United States. It is still used in Europe. An ultra-short–acting agent (duration of fewer than 10 minutes), gantacurium, is in development. Sugammadex, a drug that irreversibly encapsulates rocuronium molecules and restores neuromuscular function, if approved by the FDA, may transform some intermediate-acting NMBAs (e.g., rocuronium and vecuronium) into agents with an effective short or ultra-short duration.

Long-acting relaxants (e.g., pancuronium) are generally reserved for surgical procedures such as cardiac operations, which last longer than 3 or 4 hours and where an increase in heart rate is desirable in infants and children and postoperative ventilation is planned. Intermediate-acting agents are also commonly chosen for surgical procedures for which postoperative ventilation is anticipated, and NMBAs are titrated

TABLE 7-34. Classification of NMBAs by Chemical Structure and Duration of Action*

	Benzylisoquinolinium Compound	Aminosteroidal Compound
Short-acting (10-20 min)	Mivacurium	Rapacuronium
Intermediate-acting (20-50 min)	Atracurium, cisatracurium	Vecuronium, rocuronium
Long-acting (>50 min)	D-tubocurarine	Pancuronium

Modified from Bedford RF: The FDA protects the public by regulating the manufacture of anesthetic agents and the production devices used in anesthetic practice, *Anesthesiology* 82:33A, 1995.
*The ultra-short acting (<10 min) agent, gantacurium, an asymmetric mixed-onoim chlorofumarate, is in development.

TABLE 7-33. Metabolism and Elimination of NMBAs

		Elimination		
Drug	Metabolism (%)	Kidney	Liver	Metabolites
Succinylcholine	Butyrylcholinesterase (98%-99%)	<2%	None	Monoester
Mivacurium	Butyrylcholinesterase (95%-98%)	<5%	None	Inactive monoester and quaternary alcohol
Cisatracurium	Hoffman elimination (77%)	16%		Laudanosine and acrylates; no clinical effect
Vecuronium	Liver (30%-40%)	40%-50%	50%-60%	3-OH metabolite accumulates in renal failure and is active (80% potency of vecuronium)
Rocuronium	None	10%-25%	>70%	None
Pancuronium	Liver (10%-20%)	85%	15%	3-OH metabolite (66% potency of pancuronium)

Modified from Naguib M, Lien CA: Pharmacology of muscle relaxants and their antagonists. In Miller RD, Eriksson LI, Fleisher LA, et al., editors: *Miller's anesthesia*, ed 7, Philadelphia, 2010, Churchill Livingstone.

with infusions. Intravenous infusions or intermittant bolus of vecuronium, rocuronium, or cisatracurium are the most common neuromuscular drugs that are presently used in the operating room for pediatric patients in the United States (Table 7-27).

Interactions with Inhaled Anesthetics

Inhaled anesthetics both decrease the dose of NMBA needed for intubation and prolong the duration of action and recovery. The duration of anesthesia, concentration of agent and specific inhaled agent all have an effect. The order of potentiation from greatest to least is desflurane, sevoflurane, isoflurane, halothane, and nitrous-oxide-opioid or propofol anesthesia. The proposed pharmacodynamic mechanism is a central effect on motor neurons, inhibition of the ACh receptor, and an increased affinity for the NMBA at the receptor site (Fig. 7-56) (Stanski et al., 1979; Dickinson et al., 1995; Péréon et al., 1999; Paul et al., 2002a).

Ultra-Short–Acting Agents

Gantacurium

Gantacurium, an ultra-short–acting nondepolarizing NMBA in development, may be an alternative to succinylcholine. The chemical structure is a bis-tetrahydroisoquinolinium chloro-fumarate, with a wide margin of safety. A study of adult volunteers determined the ED_{95} to be 0.19 mg/kg; with time to onset of 90% block from 1.3 to 2.1 minutes (dose-dependent). Duration is 4.7 to 10.1 minutes and increases with increasing dose. Recovery rates from T_5 to T_{95} and from T_{25} to T_{75} are 7 and 3 min, respectively, and they are independent of the dose administered. Transient cardiovascular side effects observed (with doses beginning at three times ED_{95}) are suggestive of histamine release. Significant histamine release at four times ED_{95} was exhibited. No pediatric studies are available (Belmont et al., 2004; Lien et al., 2005).

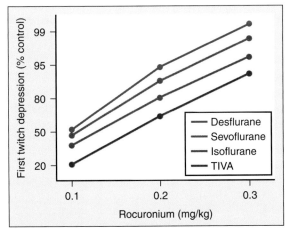

FIGURE 7-56. Cumulative dose-response curves for rocuronium-induced neuromuscular blockade during 1.5 MAC anesthesia with desflurane, sevoflurane, isoflurane, and total intravenous anesthesia. *From Wulf H et al.: Neuromuscular blocking effect of rocuronium during desflurane, isoflurane, and sevoflurane anaesthesia,* Can J Anaesth *45:526, 1998.)*

Short-Acting Agents

Mivacurium

Mivacurium was discontinued in the United States market in June 2006; however, it is still available in Europe. Mivacurium is metabolized by butyrylcholinesterase more slowly than succinylcholine, and this influences the duration of action (Beaufort et al., 1998; Ostergaard et al., 2000; Gatke et al., 2001). The chemical structure is a bis-benzylisoquinolinium compound, a mixture of three optical isomers. The two active isomers of mivacurium (trans-trans and cis-trans) have a short half-life and rapid clearance because of rapid enzymatic hydrolysis. The cis-cis isomer has minimal neuromuscular blocking effects but is slowly hydrolyzed (Cook et al., 1992a, 1992b; Head-Rapson et al., 1994; Lien et al., 1994). The ED_{95} of mivacurium during halothane anesthesia in infants and children is 85 and 89 mcg/kg, respectively, compared with an ED_{95} of 45 to 81 mcg/kg in adults (Woelfel et al., 1993; Meretoja et al., 1994). In infants, mivacurium produces complete neuromuscular blockade as quickly as succinylcholine, but the intubating conditions are less desirable after mivacurium (i.e., a higher incidence of coughing and diaphragmatic movement) (Cook et al., 1995). In children, mivacurium produces complete neuromuscular blockade more slowly than does succinylcholine. During halothane anesthesia, increasing the dose of mivacurium from 0.2 to 0.3 mg/kg (two to three times ED_{95}) does not shorten the time to complete paralysis (1.5 minutes) or produce hypotension or cutaneous flushing (Gronert and Brandom, 1994). Mivacurium can induce histamine release when large bolus doses (e.g., 0.4 mg/kg) are administered rapidly. The most common manifestation of histamine release is transient cutaneous flushing and mild decreases in blood pressure. Recovery to T_{25} was faster in infants (6.3 minutes) compared with children (10 minutes). Increasing the dose of mivacurium given to children from 0.2 to 0.3 mg/kg did not significantly prolong the time to spontaneous recovery of neuromuscular function to 25% of baseline (Cook et al., 1995). Mivacurium (0.3 mg/kg) has little or no effect on lung mechanics as measured with flow-volume loops (Fine et al., 2002).

The infusion rate of mivacurium to maintain constant neuromuscular block at approximately 95% twitch depression is about twice as great in infants and children as in adults (Markakis et al., 1998). An advantage of mivacurium is that it can be given via infusion for hours without accumulation or prolongation of recovery once the infusion is stopped (Brandom et al., 1990; Goudsouzian et al., 1994).

Rapacuronium

Rapacuronium is a short-acting aminosteroid with low potency and rapid onset of action. In spite of appropriate studies in infants and children prior to FDA release in 1999, it was withdrawn from the market in 2001 due to the high incidence of respiratory complications, especially bronchospasm (Meakin, 2001; Fine et al., 2002). The affinity of rapacuronium to block M_2 receptors is 15 times higher than its affinity to block M_3 receptors, which would explain the high incidence of severe bronchospasm (Fig. 7-57) (Jooste et al., 2003). The doses that produce good to excellent intubating conditions at 60 seconds in infants and children with nitrous oxide-oxygen and alfentanil (12.5 to 50 mcg/kg) are 1.5 and 2 mg/kg, respectively (Meakin et al., 2000). Rapacuronium

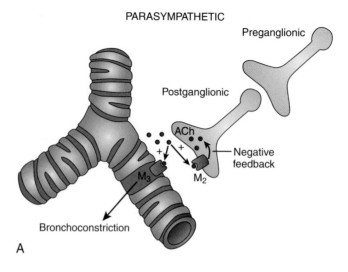

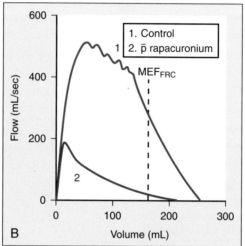

■ **FIGURE 7-57. A,** Muscarinic (M_3) receptors are located postsynaptically on airway smooth muscle. ACh stimulates M_3 receptors to cause contraction. M_2 muscarinic receptors are located presynaptically at the postganglionic parasympathetic nerve endings, and they function in a negative feedback mechanism to limit the release of acetylcholine. **B,** A typical example of the effect of rapacuronium on partial expiratory flow-volume curves, as obtained by the forced deflation technique, from a 3-year-old child under total intravenous anesthesia (propofol/ remifentanil). *1,* The baseline flow-volume curve; *2,* a flow-volume curve, executed under the same volume and pressure settings as *1,* but obtained after a single-dose infusion of rapacuronium. There is a severe decrease in peak expiratory flow, a flattening of the forced expiratory flow-volume curve, and a decreased forced expiratory volume. The severe decrease in maximal expiratory flow at functional residual capacity (MEF_{FRC}) from the baseline value together with the concavity of the curve toward the volume axis indicate the involvement of relatively small airways. (**A,** *From Naguib M, Lien CA: Pharmacology of muscle relaxants and their antagonists. In Miller RD, Eriksson LI, Fleisher LA, et al.: Miller's anesthesia, ed 7, Philadelphia, 2010, Churchill Livingstone.* **B,** *From Fine GF, Motoyama EK, Brandom BW et al.: The effect on lung mechanics in anesthetized children with rapacuroinium: a comparative study with mivacurium, Anesth Analg 95(1):56-61, 2002.)*

produces block earlier than mivacurium, and recovery is dose related and slower than that from mivacurium during halothane anesthesia (Brandom et al., 2000).

Intermediate-Acting Agents

Atracurium

Atracurium has been replaced in the United States by its metabolite, cisatracurium, because of the histamine-releasing side effect, which is more common in adults than in children (Goudsouzian et al., 1986; Shorten et al., 1993). Atracurium is primarily metabolized by nonspecific esters (ester hydrolysis) and is spontaneously decomposed by Hofmann degradation. Both processes are sensitive to pH and temperature. Deficient

or abnormal butyryl cholinesterases have no effect on atracurium degradation.

The effect of potent inhaled anesthetics on the dose-response relationships of atracurium in infants, children, and adolescents have been studied extensively (Brandom et al., 1985a; Goudsouzian et al., 1983a, 1985; Stiller et al., 1985a, 1985b; Meretoja et al., 1994).

The ED_{95} for atracurium is similar in infants aged 1 to 6 months (150 mcg/kg) and in adolescents, whereas it is greater (280 mcg/kg) in children with both halothane and isoflurane anesthesia. For anesthesia with nitrous oxide and fentanyl neonates and infants (younger than 1 year old) have an ED_{9} of 226 mcg/kg and children (older than 1 year) have an ED_{95} o 316 mcg/kg (Meretoja and Wirtavuori, 1988). In addition, infu sion requirements for children ages 2 to 10 years are decrease with both halothane and isoflurane (6.3 mcg/kg per minute) compared with balanced anesthesia with fentanyl (9.3 mcg/kg per minute). Neonates, up to 1 month old, have an infusion requirement of atracurium of 0.40 ± 0.02 mg/kg per hour that is 25% less than that of infants and children (0.52 ± 0.02 mg/kg per hour) (Kalli and Meretoja, 1988).

At equipotent doses (ED_{95}), the duration of effect (time from injection to 95% recovery) is 23 minutes in infants and 29 minutes in both children and adolescents, compared with 44 minutes in adults. The T_{25} recovery (minimum time when pharmacologic reversal can be administered) is 10 minutes in infants, 15 minutes in children and adolescents, and 16 minutes in adults. At higher multiples of the ED_{95}, the duration of effect is longer, but the times from T_5 to T_{25} recovery (recovery index) are the same. The shorter duration of effect in the infant results from a difference in pharmacokinetics compared with those of both children and adults. In infants (1 to 8 months), the volume of distribution is larger, clearance is more rapid, and the elimination half-life is shorter than in children (aged 2 to 10 years) or adults. The ED_{95} of atracurium is comparable for neonates and infants (226 mcg/kg).

Cisatracurium

Cisatracurium is a metabolite of atracurium, a mixture of 10 optical and geometric isomers (Welch et al., 1995). The R-R[1] optical isomer in the cis-cis configuration, cisatracurium, is about 1.5 times more potent than atracurium and does not liberate histamine even at very high doses (five times the ED_{95}) (Soukup et al., 1997). Cisatracurium is primarily degraded by Hofmann degradation to laudanosine and a monoquaternary acrylate, which is hydrolyzed by plasma esterases. The by-products of metabolism have no neuromuscular blocking effect, and they are excreted by the liver and the kidneys (Neill et al., 1983).

Cisatracurium is equipotent in infants, children, and adults (Table 7-23). During nitrous oxide-narcotic thiopentone administration, the ED_{50} and ED_{95} values for infants (29 ± 3 mcg/kg and 43 ± 9 mcg/kg, respectively) were similar for children (29 ± 2 mcg/kg and 47 ± 7 mcg/kg) (DeRuiter and Crawford, 2001).

With halothane anesthesia in children, the rate of recovery after a dose of one to two times the ED_{95} was rapid, with a recovery index from T_{25} to T_{75} of 9 to 11 minutes and a recovery index from T_5 to T_{95} 25 to 30 minutes (Meretoja et al., 1996). In a separate study of infants and children anesthetized with nitrous oxide and opioids, 0.15 mg/kg (three times the ED_{95}) of cisatracurium had a mean onset time of maximum blockade in infants of 2 ± 0.8 minutes, whereas that in children was less rapid at 3 ± 1.2 minutes. The clinical duration of action of cisatracurium to T_{25} was significantly longer in infants (43.3 ± 6.2 minutes) than in children (36 ± 5.4 minutes); however, once neuromuscular function started to recover, the rate of recovery was similar in both age groups (Taivainen et al., 2000). Another study with 0.1 mg/kg (two times ED_{95}) of cisatracurium in 15 infants and 15 children with remifentanil and sevoflurane anesthesia (2% end-tidal) also reported a significantly faster onset (74 vs. 98 seconds), longer clinical duration to T_{25} (55 vs. 41 minutes), and longer recovery to TOF greater than 0.9, 73 (range 56 to 95) minutes vs. 59 (range 43 to 72) minutes in the infants than in children. Here, the inhalational agent accelerated the onset and prolonged the recovery to T_{25} in spite of a smaller dose of cisatracurium. Again, the recovery index was comparable in

both infants and children at 21 vs. 16 minutes (Soltész et al., 2002). One of the benefits of cisatracurium is that once recovery begins, full recovery is rapid and predictable in both infants and children. Also of note is that there were negligible changes in heart rate or blood pressure for both age groups at the larger dose (Brandom, 1998; Taivainen et al., 2000; Meakin et al., 2007).

Cisatracurium infusions have a place in the ICU for postoperative care, especially in patients with organ failure. Postoperative cardiac patients (younger than age 2 years) receiving cisatracurium infusions had a high clearance, low duration of residual block, and a mean return to TOF of greater than 0.9 of 30 minutes (Reich et al., 2004). Another ICU study in children (aged 3 months to 16 years) had an average cisatracurium infusion rate of 3.9 ±1.3 mcg/kg per minute with a median time to recovery significantly shorter with cisatracurium (52 minutes, with a range of 35 to 73 minutes) compared with vecuronium (123 minutes, with a range of 80 to 480 minutes) (Burmester and Mok, 2005). Steady-state volume of distribution (207 ± 31 mL/kg) and total body clearance (6.8 ± 0.7 mL/min per kg) for cisatracurium are significantly larger in children than those published for adults. Both renal failure and liver disease have minimal effects on the pharmacodynamics of cisatracurium (Table 7-35) (Prielipp et al., 1995; DeWolf et al., 1996).

Vecuronium

Vecuronium has an intermediate duration of action in children and adults; however, the neuromuscular block lasts longer in infants. The ED_{95} of vecuronium in infants and adults is 43 to 47 mcg/kg, whereas in children it is 81 mcg/kg (D'Hollander et al., 1982a; Fisher and Miller, 1983; Meretoja et al., 1988). Onset in the infant (68 seconds) is 0.6 to 0.8 times more rapid than that in the child after 0.1 mg/kg of vecuronium; however, the multiple of the ED_{95} is greater for the infant (two times vs. 1.2 times) (Kalli and Meretoja, 1989). Onset to maximum block from 0.07 mg/kg in the infant with halothane anesthesia occurs in 1.5 ± 0.6 minutes.

ED_{95}, onset and duration in children. The ED_{95} for vecuronium for children with halothane is 45 mcg/kg and with a narcotic is 81 mcg/kg, which is greater than that of adults at 33 mcg/kg

TABLE 7-35. Pharmacokinetic Data for Cistracurium in Children and Adults*

Variable	Children	Adults
$t_{1/2}\alpha$ (min)	3.5 ± 0.9	
$t_{1/2}\beta$ (min)	22.9 ± 4.5	23 ± 2.7
V_d (mL/kg)	207 ± 31	144 ± 34
CL (mL/kg/min)	6.8 ± 0.7	5.3 ± 1.2

From Kisor DF et al: Importance of the organ-independent elimination of cisatracurium, *Anesth Analg* 83:901, 1996; data for CL values from Imbeault K et al: Pharmacokinetics and pharmacodynamics of a 0.1 mg/kg dose of cisatracurium besylate in children during N_2O/O_2/propofol anesthesia, *Anesth Analg* 102:738, 2006.

*Values are mean ± SEM.

$t_{1/2}\alpha$, Half-life of the distribution phase; $t_{1/2}\beta$, elimination half-life; V_d, volume of distribution, *CL*, clearance.

for halothane and 43 mcg/kg for narcotic anesthesia. The time to onset of maximum block after 0.07 mg/kg of vecuronium is 2.4 ± 1.4 minutes in the child under halothane anesthesia with time to recovery of T_{90} of 35 ± 6 minutes, whereas that for adults is 2.9 ± 0.2 minutes for onset and T_{90} of 53 ± 21 minutes (Table 7-25).

Duration of block in the infant and child. At equal doses (0.07 mg/kg) of vecuronium with halothane anesthesia, the duration to T_{90} is longest in infants (73 ± 27 minutes) compared with that in children (35 ± 6 minutes) and adults (53 ± 21 minutes). Vecuronium is a long-acting NMBA in infants.

Recovery to 10% of initial twitch height from 0.1 mg/kg of vecuronium (two times ED_{95}) is also prolonged, at 42 minutes, in the infant (younger than 1 year of age) with nitrous-oxide-fentanyl anesthesia. Time to T_{10} and the recovery index (time from 25% to 75% recovery) were 1.7 to 2.9 times longer in the infant, than in the child (aged 1 to 14 years). Time to full recovery to 100% of T_1 from the start of recovery occurred in 55 minutes for the infant but took only 20 to 24 minutes for the child. Interestingly, TOF was observed to recover more rapidly in younger children. The clinical implication of this observation is not known (Kalli and Meretoja, 1989). In addition, a 100 and 150 mcg/kg initial bolus of vecuronium (two to three times ED_{95}) produced a block of greater than 90% from 59 to 110 minutes respectively, in the neonate and infant group, but only from 18 to 37 minutes for children and from 37 to 68 minutes in adolescents (Meretoja, 1989a). Vecuronium should be regarded as a long-acting NMBA in infants (younger than 1 year old).

Volume of distribution and clearance. Fisher et al. (1983) determined the pharmacodynamics and pharmacokinetics of vecuronium in infants and children. The volume of distribution and the mean residence time are greater in infants than in children. Clearance is similar in the two groups; the Cp_{ss50} was lower in infants than in children. The combination of a large volume of distribution in infants and fixed clearance results in a longer mean residence time. After a single dose of relaxant, recovery of neuromuscular transmission depends on both distribution and elimination. The combination of a longer mean residence time and a greater sensitivity for vecuronium explains the prolongation of neuromuscular blockade in infants. Little or no 3-hydroxy vecuronium is formed after a single dose of vecuronium (0.1 to 0.2 mg/kg). Decreased clearance of vecuronium and the accumulation of 3-hydroxy vecuronium may contribute to prolonged spontaneous recovery times after infusions in ICU (Reich et al., 2004).

Infants vs. children. In a similar fashion, infusions of vecuronium in infants also act as long-acting rather than intermediate-acting agents. The clearance of vecuronium is low in infants (younger than aged 2 years), significant amounts of the metabolite 3-hydroxy vecuronium are found, and return to full neuromuscular transmission of TOF greater than 0.9 is quite slow (180 minutes) compared with a cisatracurium infusion, which takes only 30 minutes to attain the same level of neuromuscular transmission (Reich et al., 2004). A 45% decrease of vecuronium mean infusion rate of 54.7 ± 4.23 mcg/kg per hour is required in infants (aged 2 to 5 months) compared with that of the older children (aged 2 to 10 years) at 98.7 ± 7.07 mcg/kg per hour to keep block at 1 twitch. Recovery to TOF of greater than 0.7 is more rapid at 45 minutes for infants than 65 minutes for children. This faster recovery may be related to the decreased

total amount of vecuronium infused in the infants (Hodges, 1996). In the operating room with fentanyl and nitrous-oxide anesthesia, neonates (younger than 1 month) and infants (aged 1 to 12 months) require 40% less vecuronium at 62 ± 15 mcg/kg per hour compared with children (aged 3 to 10 years) at 154 ± 49 mcg/kg per hour and adolescents (older than age 13 years) and adults at 89 ± 13 mcg/kg per hour. Interindividual variation is quite large (Meretoja, 1989a, 1989b). These data correlate with the pharmacokinetic/pharmacodynamic studies in infants that reveal the increased volume of distribution, longer mean residence time and smaller Cp_{ss50}. Since the clearance is no different in infants than in children, the factors just mentioned explain the prolonged action of vecuronium in infants. Therefore, great interindividual variation makes routine monitoring of neuromuscular block in both the ICU and operating room essential; AMG is one convenient and reliable method in neonates and infants (Hodges, 1996).

Children vs. adults. An infusion rate of 144 mcg/kg per hour (2.4 mcg/kg per minute) vecuronium is required to maintain approximately 95% neuromuscular blockade in children during narcotic and nitrous-oxide anesthesia. These infusion rates are several times higher than those in adults (aged 18 to 85 years) (D'Hollander et al., 1982b). Young adults required 54 mcg/kg per hour (0.9 mcg/kg per minute) to maintain 95% neuromuscular blockade. This suggests that clearance is more rapid in children than in adults, and children do recover more rapidly from vecuronium infusions than do adults (Table 7-29). Several groups have described long-term vecuronium infusion requirements in adults with multiple organ failure in the ICU (Segredo et al., 1992). Infusion rates of about 1.6 mcg/kg per minute were required, and the degree of block gradually increased, a sign of accumulation. Increasing vecuronium infusion requirements, by contrast, may be seen during very prolonged infusions (i.e., lasting 3 to 14 days). These increased requirements could not be clearly associated with various pathophysiologic states, concurrent drug administration, or biochemical abnormalities. Proliferation of extrajunctional cholinergic receptors resulting from prolonged nondepolarizing blockade has also been offered as an explanation (Hogue et al., 1992; Martyn et al., 1992).

Patients with organ failure. Adults with liver failure have a decreased clearance (50%) of vecuronium and time to recovery to T_{50} is twice (130 minutes) and the RI (25% to 75%) is three times (68 minutes) that of normal patients in spite of the Cp_{ss50} being equal (Lebrault et al., 1985). The similarity of Cp_{ss50} suggests that patients with cirrhosis have normal sensitivity to vecuronium. Despite the prolonged duration of action of vecuronium in patients cirrhosis, it was still shorter than that of pancuronium in patients free of liver disease. No studies are available in pediatric patients with liver failure.

Vecuronium is only slightly dependent on renal elimination (10% to 30%), and it is minimally affected by renal failure. Some adult studies demonstrated a longer duration of neuromuscular block in this patient population (Lynam et al., 1988). The increased duration is related to both a decreased plasma clearance and a prolonged elimination half-life of vecuronium in the renal failure group. Similarly, Bencini et al. (1983) found a 50% decrease in clearance, an increase in volume of distribution, and a 50% increase in elimination half-life. The duration of action was not reported. Metabolites of vecuronium were not measured in these adult studies.

Chronic phenytoin therapy reduces the effect of vecuronium by mechanisms that include both increased vecuronium metabolism and reduced sensitivity of the patient to circulating concentrations of vecuronium (Wright et al., 2004).

Rocuronium

ED$_{95}$, onset, intubating conditions, and recovery. Rocuronium (ORG 9426), an aminosteroid, with no metabolites, has a chemical structure similar to vecuronium (with active metabolites). Rocuronium has one eighth to one tenth the potency of vecuronium. The lesser potency of rocuronium produces a more rapid onset of block in comparison with equipotent doses of other drugs (i.e., equal multiples of the ED$_{95}$) (Kopman, 1989). Table 7-23 shows the ED$_{95}$ for infants and children for rocuronium. Bolus administration of 0.6 mg/kg of rocuronium at two times ED$_{95}$ is associated with a transient increase in heart rate of about 15 beats/min and produces complete neuromuscular blockade (at the adductor pollicis) in infants and children in 50 and 80 seconds, respectively (Woelfel et al., 1992; O'Kelly et al., 1994). Increasing the dose to 0.8 mg/kg in children shortens this time to an average of 30 seconds (O'Kelly et al., 1994). Low-dose rocuronium for tracheal intubation in children during inhalational induction is 0.3 mg/kg (ED$_{95}$) and allows acceptable intubating conditions in 95% of children (aged 2 to 7 years) with sevoflurane anesthesia within 2 minutes, or in children (aged 1 to 3 years) of age in 60 seconds (Eikermann et al., 2002). Another study shows that children (aged 4 to 6 years) have good intubation conditions in 90 seconds, 80% of the time (Hung et al., 2005). Recovery to TOF of greater than 0.8 occurs in 24 ± 8 minutes with a low dose of rocuronium (0.3 mg/kg) (Eikermann et al., 2002). Rocuronium 0.3 mg/kg with halothane anesthesia in children (older than 1 year of age) shows a slower onset than the larger dose, but does not cause a prolonged block (Driessen et al., 2002).

Recovery in infants. There is significant variability in time to recovery with 0.6 mg/kg of rocuronium in infants compared with children; and time to T$_{25}$ is almost twice as long at 41.9 minutes in infants (older than 10 months) compared with children (aged 1 to 5 years) at 26.7 minutes (Woelfel et al., 1994; Driessen et al., 2005). Prolonged recovery to T$_{75}$ and TOF of greater than 0.7 with both 0.45 mg/kg and 0.6 mg/kg of rocuronium in infants 0 to 1 months, 2 to 4 months, and 5 to 12 months under isoflurane anesthesia can be seen in Table 7-26 (Rapp et al., 2004a). Even the low dose of 0.3 mg/kg of rocuronium with halothane nitrous-oxide anesthesia has a prolonged recovery to T$_{25}$, T$_{75}$, RI, and TOF of greater than 0.7 in the 0 to 6-month age group compared with those children older than 2 years of age (Driessen et al., 2000). This age-related difference is similar to that observed with vecuronium (Meretoja, 1989a). Both of these drugs are long-acting NMBAs instead of an intermediate-acting agent in the infant (Fig. 7-51). This is true for infants with balanced anesthesia (Taivainen et al., 1996).

Recovery in children vs. adults. Time to appearance of the fourth twitch after 1 mg/kg rocuronium is more rapid in children than adults, with ranges from 27 to 62 minutes in children (younger than 5 years of age) vs. 37 to 94 minutes in adults. In addition, once PTC is detected, recovery to one twitch in the TOF is also more rapid in children, at 7 minutes compared with 16 minutes in the adults (Baykara et al., 2002). No data on PTC in infants are presently available. Steady-state target-controlled infusions

of rocuronium in infants, children, and adults revealed infants had the lowest infusion rates of rocuronium and children had the greatest (Saldien et al., 2003). The data are shown in Table 7-28.

Rapid onset of action with minimal tachycardia and intermediate duration of action in children (older than age 2 years) makes rocuronium an attractive neuromuscular blocking drug. However, in infants rocuronium functions as a long-acting nondepolarizing agent and the recovery time is quite variable. The monitoring device AMG has been shown to be practical even in the neonate and small infant and should be used (Driessen et al., 2005).

Infusions of rocuronium in ICU patients are variable, with rates reported from 0.3 to 2.2 mg/kg per hour (5 to 36.6 mcg/kg per minute), so use of neuromuscular monitoring equipment is highly recommended. In the operating room, infusion rates in children are influenced by inhalational anesthetics. Values range when using nitrous oxide from 16.7 ± 2.3 mcg/kg per minute for fentanyl anesthesia, 13.6 ± 3.7 mcg/kg per minute for halothane, 13.1 ± 5.1 mcg/kg per minute for isoflurane, and 8.49 ± 1.6 mcg/kg per minute for sevoflurane. The rocuronium infusion rate required to maintain stable 90% to 99% T$_1$ depression is reduced 20% with halothane and isoflurane, and by 50% with sevoflurane. No data are available for rocuronium infusions in children with desflurane. However, adult studies show no differences between isoflurane, sevoflurane, and desflurane with respect to potency (121 to 136 mcg/kg), infusion rate (6.1 to 6.3 mcg/kg per minute) or recovery (26 to 28 minutes) from rocuronium (Bock et al., 2000).

Intramuscular rocuronium. A multicenter study evaluated the intubating conditions, onset, and duration of intramuscular rocuronium in infants (1 mg/kg) and children (1.8 mg/kg) under halothane anesthesia. Conditions were not satisfactory in a consistent manner in this patient population. Rocuronium delivered intramuscularly is not an adequate alternative to intramuscular succinylcholine when rapid intubation is necessary (Kaplan et al., 1999).

Organ failure. A single bolus dose of rocuronium 0.3 mg/kg in children (older than 1 year of age) with renal failure does not cause a prolonged block, but it has a slower onset, 139 ± 71 vs. 87 ± 43 seconds, than in healthy children (Driessen et al., 2002).

No change in clearance is found in adults with renal disease or cirrhosis for patients receiving 0.6 to 0.8 mg/kg of rocuronium.

Long-Acting Agents

Pancuronium

Pancuronium, a steroidal bis-quaternary muscle relaxant, is still used for infants and children because of its predictable neuromuscular blocking action and associated cardiovascular stimulating properties. Older children require a larger dose than do infants and small children (Table 7-36) (Goudsouzian, 1974; Meretoja, 1990; Blinn et al., 1992).

Sixty-seven percent of pancuronium is recovered within 24 hours in the urine (Duvaldestin, 1982). About 25% of pancuronium appears in the urine in the form of the 3-hydroxy metabolite, and less than 5% each appeared in the form of the 17-hydroxy and 3,17-dehydroxy metabolites. Approximately 11% of the pancuronium was excreted in the bile.

TABLE 7-36. Cumulative Dose-Response Relationship of Pancuronium

Age	ED$_{50}$ (mg/kg)	ED$_{95}$ (mg/kg)
3 to 6 mo	24 ± 7	45 ± 7
7 to 12 mo	30 ± 5	52 ± 9
1 to 3 yr	34 ± 9*	62 ± 18*
4 to 6 yr	29 ± 8	62 ± 13*

Data from Blinn A et al: Pancuronium dose-response revisited, *Paediatr Anesth* 2:153, 1992.
*Statistically significant difference from the 3- to 6-month age group (analysis of variance).

Antagonists for Neuromuscular Blocking Agents: Anticholinesterases and Sugammadex

Doses of Anticholinesterase Drugs in Infants and Children

Three anticholinesterases are available to antagonize neuromuscular blockade: neostigmine, edrophonium, and pyridostigmine. Reviews by Bevan et al. (1992) and Aquilonius and Hartvig (1986) are available on the mechanisms of action of these drugs. When the enzyme acetylcholinesterase, which breaks down ACh, is inhibited, the concentration of ACh increases at the motor end plate and competes with the nondepolarizing NMBA. In addition, anticholinesterases may also increase the release of ACh from the presynaptic nerve terminals, block neural potassium channels, and have a direct agonist effect (Bevan et al., 1992).

Fisher et al. (1983, 1984) examined the dose of neostigmine and edrophonium required in infants, children, and adults to reverse a 90% blockade from a continuous d-tubocurarine infusion. In infants and children, 15 mcg/kg of neostigmine produced a 50% antagonism of the d-tubocurarine blockade; in adults, 23 mcg/kg was required. The duration of antagonism was equal in all three age groups, although the elimination half-life was clearly shorter in infants. A larger dose would give a higher sustained blood concentration. The dissociation between the elimination half-life and the duration of antagonism may result from the carbamylation of cholinesterase by neostigmine.

In infants, 145 mcg/kg of edrophonium produced a 50% antagonism of the d-tubocurarine blockade; for children and adults, 233 mcg/kg and 128 mcg/kg, respectively, were required. The volume of distribution of edrophonium is similar in all age groups. The elimination half-life of edrophonium is shorter in infants than in children or adults; hence, clearance is more rapid in infants.

Meakin et al. (1983) compared the rate of recovery from pancuronium-induced neuromuscular blockade after various doses of neostigmine (0.036 or 0.07 mg/kg) or edrophonium (0.7 or 1.43 mg/kg) in infants, children and adults. In the first 5 minutes, recovery of neuromuscular transmission was more rapid after edrophonium than after neostigmine in all age groups; recovery was more rapid in infants and children than in adults. By 10 minutes, there was no difference in neuromuscular transmission achieved in infants and children with either reversal agent (at either dose); adults had lower neuromuscular transmission at the lower dose (0.036 mg/kg) of neostigmine. If speed of initial recovery is a critical issue, edrophonium is better than neostigmine, and a high dose of neostigmine is better than a low dose. At 30 minutes after injection of either reversal agent (at any dose), there was no difference between neuromuscular transmission among age groups. Another study shows no advantage in increasing the neostigmine dose more than 20 mcg/kg to antagonize a rocuronium block (at only 10% recovery of the first twitch at which three or four twitches are present), and reaffirms that recovery is more rapid in children than adults (Abdulatif et al., 1996). Debaene et al. (1989) document that recovery with neostigmine 30 mcg/kg for infants and children and 40 mcg/kg for the adults under halothane from vecuronium also produces a more rapid response in children.

Edrophonium (0.5 to 1 mg/kg) has a more rapid effect than neostigmine (50 to 70 mcg/kg) when the block has recovered to three or four twitches, but it is not as effective for a profound block (only one twitch present). Pyridostigmine (350 mcg/kg) is rarely used clinically.

Side Effects of Anticholinesterases

Cardiovascular effects. The muscarinic effects of the anticholinesterases are blocked by administration of either atropine (7 to 10 mcg/kg) or glycopyrrolate (5 mcg/kg). An increase in heart rate should be observed from glycopyrrolate before administration of edrophonium because of its rapid onset; atropine can be administered at the same time as edrophonium.

Nausea and vomiting. Conflicting reports are available on the incidence of postoperative nausea and vomiting (PONV) related to anticholinesterase administration. Some evidence suggests that this incidence is dose dependent, with the lower dose of neostigmine 1.5 mg in adults having a lower incidence of PONV. The well-known risk of residual neuromuscular block far outweighs the concern for nausea and vomiting, especially in infants and children.

Sugammadex

Sugammadex appears to be a novel reversal agent that rapidly and effectively reverses rocuronium-induced neuromuscular blockade in less than 5 minutes, similar to that of anticholinesterases when administered at appropriate times. Sugammadex, a γ-cyclodextrin, is highly water soluble with a hydrophobic cavity that encapsulates steroidal neuromuscular blocking drugs, rocuronium at a rate greater than that for vecuronium, which has a greater rate than pancuronium (Figs. 7-58 and 7-59). Efficacy and safety have been demonstrated for sugammadex in infants (28 days to 23 months old), children (aged 2 to 11 years), adolescents (aged 12 to 17 years), and adults (aged 18 to 65 years) as a method for eliminating rocuronium (0.6 mg/kg). Sugammadex (0.5, 1, 2, or 4 mg/kg) was compared with placebo at reappearance of the second twitch of TOF with AMG monitor. Time to TOF of greater than 0.9 was 21, 19, 23.4, and 28.5 minutes in infants, children, adolescents, and adults, respectively, after placebo administration. With sugammadex (2 mg/kg), the TOF of greater than 0.9 was attained in 0.6, 1.2, 1.1, and 1.1 minutes, respectively, with no adverse events. The sugammadex plasma concentrations were similar for children, adolescents, and adults across the dose range. The drug was well tolerated and no recurrence of blockade, inadequate reversal, significant

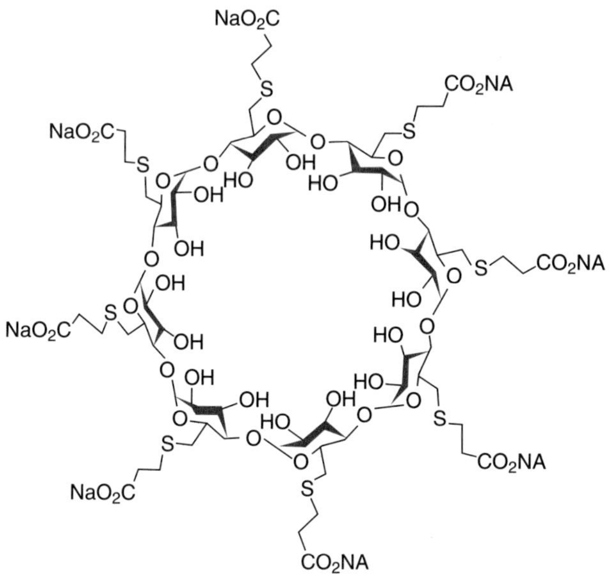

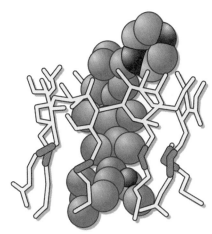

■ FIGURE 7-58. Structure of the synthetic γ-cyclodextrin sugammadex (ORG 25969). *(From Naguib M, Lien CA: Pharmacology of muscle relaxants and their antagonists. In Miller ED, Eriksson LI, Fleisher LA, et al: Miller's anesthesia, ed 7, Philadelphia, 2010, Churchill Livingstone.)*

■ FIGURE 7-59. The sugammadex-rocuronium complex. *(From Bom A et al.: A novel concept of reversing neuromuscular block: chemical encapsulation of rocuronium bromide by a cyclodextrin-based synthetic host, Angew Chem 41:266, 2002.)*

QT prolongation, or other abnormalities were observed (Plaud et al., 2009). The encapsulated aminosteroid is excreted in urine; studies of adult patients in end-stage renal failure conclude that sugammadex appears to be safe in this patient population (Staals et al., 2008). Studies are ongoing at this time. Sugammadex also has a high affinity for vecuronium.

A 2009 review recommends the dose of 2 mg/kg sugammadex for shallow block, and 4 mg/kg for deep block in adults. A larger dose of 16 mg/kg may be administered 3 minutes after 1 to 1.2 mg/kg of rocuronium is administered (deep block), and recovery is rapid. No recurrence of block has been reported, the safety profile is unremarkable, no change in dose requirement has been found as a result of age or type of volatile anesthetic (Mirakhur, 2009). Another review recommends sugammadex to antagonize both deep and moderate rocuronium and

vecuronium block in adults and moderate block in children (aged 2 to 17 years). The drug is approved in Australia, Iceland, New Zealand, and Norway (Yang and Keam, 2009).

COMMONLY ADMINISTERED ANESTHETIC ADJUNCTS

Anticholinergic Agents

Atropine

Strong cholinergic stimulation, such as that which occurs from halothane and succinylcholine, can produce profound bradycardia and reduce cardiac output in infants. The primary purpose of atropine in pediatric anesthesia is to protect against cholinergic stimulation; its secondary purpose is to inhibit the production of secretions.

If atropine is administered intravenously in incremental doses, more atropine (on a weight basis) is needed to accelerate the heart rate in children younger than 2 years; however, acceleration uniformly occurs with 14.3 mcg/kg (Dauchot and Gravenstein, 1971). Infants need higher doses of atropine to increase heart rate compared with adults (Palmisano et al., 1991). The onset of the chronotropic effects of atropine appears to be related to the underlying heart rate at the time of administration of atropine. Children with slower heart rates have longer onset times than do children with faster heart rates (Zimmerman and Steward, 1986). Although atropine can increase heart rate and cardiac output, it does not appear to change the neuromuscular blocking onset time of atracurium (Simhi et al., 1997). A dose of 30 mg/kg appears to be vagolytic in infants, children, and adults. This dose provides adequate protection against a cholinergic challenge. In a study of 20 healthy children aged 1 to 36 months undergoing elective surgery, McAuliffe et al. (1997) noted that 20 mcg/kg intravenously caused a variable increase in heart rate and cardiac output in anesthetized children. In 40 children ranging from 2 to 6 years in age, intratracheal atropine (20 mcg/kg) produced only a modest increase in heart rate after 5 minutes (Jorgensen and Ostergaard, 1997). However, 50 mcg/kg increased heart rate rapidly (Howard and Bingham, 1990). The site of injection has a role in the onset time of atropine effect. In a randomized study of children 1 to 10 years of age who were anesthetized with nitrous oxide, oxygen, and halothane, Sullivan et al. (1997) noted that a subglossal injection resulted in a faster onset time than either a deltoid or vastus lateralis intramuscular injection.

In all age groups, 5 to 10 mcg/kg atropine minimally decreases salivation (Gaviotaki and Smith, 1962). Children with Down syndrome may have an increased sensitivity to atropine; the pupils dilate in response to atropine, and large increases in heart rate occur after repeated doses of atropine (Berg et al., 1960; Priest, 1960; Harris and Goodman, 1968). In a retrospective study by Kobel et al. (1982), however, patients with Down syndrome were no more sensitive to intravenous atropine than were other patients.

Glycopyrrolate is another anticholinergic agent. It is a quaternary amine that penetrates the CNS less than atropine. It inhibits the muscarinic action of ACh at postganglionic parasympathetic neuroeffector sites in smooth muscle secretory glands and in the CNS. Adverse reactions include tachycardia; palpitations; restlessness; delirium; dry, hot skin; myostasis;

xerostomia; and urinary retention. The intravenous dose is usually 0.005 to 0.01 mg/kg.

Scopolamine is a nonselective muscarinic antagonist, which has both peripheral antimuscarinic properties as well as central sedative, antiemetic, and amnestic effects. The pharmacokinetics and dynamics of scopolamine for clinical use have been reviewed by Renner and colleagues (2005). It has been used clinically as a premedication and as an antiemetic. Scopolamine has a short half-life—approximately 70 minutes after intravenous administration—and has dose-dependent adverse effects. The transdermal delivery system was developed to minimize the drug's adverse effects. The drug is also well absorbed after intranasal and ocular administration. The dose of scopolamine for intravenous, intramuscular, and subcutaneous administration is 6 to 10 mcg/kg.

Analgesic Agents

Ketorolac

Ketorolac is a nonsteroidal antiinflammatory drug. The analgesic properties of nonsteroidal antiinflammatory drugs are thought to be related to their ability to attenuate the hyperalgesic state caused by prostaglandins as opposed to producing analgesia directly. Ketorolac may act both peripherally and centrally. Ketorolac is an enantiomeric compound. The pharmacokinetics of ketorolac were described after single and continuous infusion (Olkkola and Maunuksela, 1991; Gillis et al., 1997; Hamunen et al., 1999; Kauffman et al., 1999; Dsida et al., 2002; Kokki et al., 2002; Zuppa et al., 2009). Ketorolac has also been administered intranasally to adults (Brown et al., 2009).

In a study of 43 pediatric surgical patients, Dsida et al. (2002) noted no age-related differences in the pharmacokinetics, and the kinetic profile was similar to that reported for adults. In a pharmacokinetic study of the stereoisomers of ketorolac in children, Kauffman et al. (1999) noted that concentrations of the S– enantiomer were lower than those of the R++ enantiomer and that the S– enantiomer had a shorter half-life, greater clearance, and larger volume of distribution. Similar findings were noted by Lynn and colleagues (2007). These differences in the enantiomer kinetic profile appear to be similar for children, adolescents, and adults (Fig. 7-60) (Hamunen et al., 1999). In addition to its analgesic properties, ketorolac may have antiemetic properties (Munro et al., 1994). In children undergoing ureteral reimplantation procedures, ketorolac can decrease the incidence and severity of postoperative bladder spasms, and in children undergoing low-risk cardiac surgery, ketorolac did not affect serum creatinine values differently than the control group of children who did not receive ketorolac (Park et al., 2000; Inoue et al., 2009). A major determinant to the use of ketorolac has been the potential that nonsteroidal agents affect bone healing. In a study of 349 adolescent patients undergoing posterior spinal fusions, Sucato et al. (2009) noted that the incidence of pseudoorthosis was the same in adolescents given ketorolac to those who did not receive nonsteroidal antiinflammatory drugs.

Acetaminophen (Paracetamol)

Acetaminophen (paracetamol in European countries and the United Kingdom), N-acetyl-p-aminophenol, was first used widely in 1949 and has been available in the United States without prescription since 1955. Its analgesic and antipyretic action may be related to its inhibition of prostaglandin synthesis in the CNS. Adult absorption from the gastrointestinal tract is rapid, with maximum levels at 30 to 60 minutes and a half-life of 2 hours. Acetaminophen is metabolized in the liver primarily by conjugation. Large doses result in the formation of hepatotoxic metabolites generated by the cytochrome P450 CYP2E1 system. Although the immaturity of the P450 system appears to increase the margin of safety for acetaminophen use in infancy, there have been reports of hepatotoxicity in infants (Greene et al., 1983). For accidental overdosing of a single dose, use of the Rumack-Matthew nomogram has become standard in deciding whether N-acetyl cysteine is appropriate. Dosing above 140 mg/kg per day for several days has been suggested to carry significant risk of liver damage (Cranswick and Coghlan, 2000).

It has been reported that therapeutic concentrations of acetaminophen for antipyresis are 10 to 20 mg/L to achieve 50% of maximal fever reduction (Rumack, 1978). Information of the ideal analgesic concentrations for acetaminophen is incomplete. Anderson and Holford (1999) modeled acetaminophen pharmacodynamics for analgesia after tonsillectomy. The population-based model in 120 children, with a mean age of 8 years and a mean weight of 34 kg, suggested that a mean pain score of 3.6 of 10 would be found with an acetaminophen concentration of 10 mg/L (Anderson et al., 2001). A subsequent study by the same authors reported that an acetaminophen concentration of 10 mg/L was associated with a pain score reduction of 2.6 out of 10 in children after tonsillectomy (Anderson et al., 2001). Using a different paradigm, Korpela et al. (1999) reported that children's pain scores in the postoperative recovery unit were significantly lower with rectal acetaminophen doses of 40 or 60 mg/kg compared with scores for children who received placebo or 20 mg/kg. Rescue morphine use was related to acetaminophen doses, with reduction in the number of children needing rescue medication reaching significance at the 40 and 60 mg/kg dose groups. Most surgeries were herniorrhaphies or orchiectomies. These authors suggest that concentrations with doses of 40 mg/kg rectal acetaminophen would be expected to be in the range of 13 to 17 mg/L.

Acetaminophen is the most widely used analgesic in pediatric anesthesia. An intravenous formulation (propacetamol) has been in use in Europe for over 10 years and for a somewhat shorter time in the United Kingdom, while in the United States only the oral and rectal formulations have been available. Acetaminophen's pharmacokinetics has been studied in children, infants, and neonates. Reports from multiple investigators of rectal acetaminophen dosing establish that higher doses are needed to achieve concentrations in the 10 to 20 mg/L range. Rectal absorption is also erratic, with longer onset times for analgesia compared with those for oral administration (Anderson; Montgomery et al., 1995; Birmingham et al., 1997; Cormack et al., 2006).

Arana et al. (2001) reviewed the use of paracetamol in infants. Metabolism by conjugation is the most important pathway, with sulfation most important in neonates because glucuronidation is deficient for several weeks. Oxidation via the cytochrome P450 system is a minor pathway, but it can generate N-acetyl-p-benzoquinone imine, which is hepatotoxic. Most reports suggest infants generate less of this compound, perhaps explaining the wider margin of safety for acetaminophen in infants. Elimination half-life averages 3.5 hour, compared

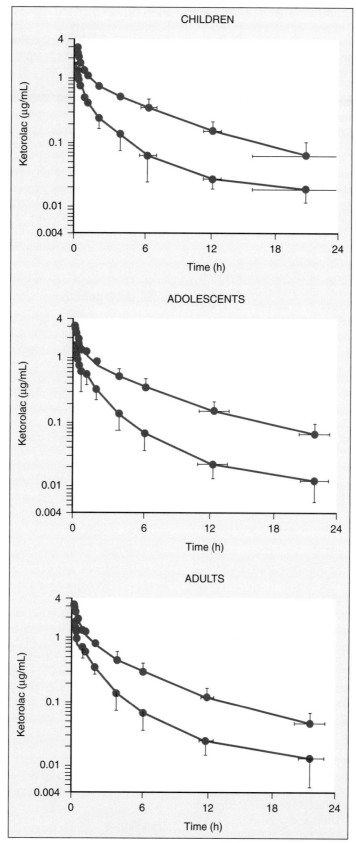

FIGURE 7-60. Concentrations (mean ± SD) of S– ketorolac *(brown circles)* and R– ketorolac *(blue circles)* in plasma after intravenous administration of 0.5 mg/kg of racemic ketorolac tromethamine to 18 children, 28 adolescents, and 18 adults. *(From Hamunen K et al.: Stereoselective pharmacokinetics of ketorolac in children, adolescents, and adults,* Acta Anaesthesiol Scand *43:1041, 1999.)*

with 1.9 to 2.2 hours in adults. Premature infants showed even longer half-lives of 11 hours in infants with 28 to 30 weeks' gestation and 4.8 hours in infants with 32 to 36 weeks' gestation. Clearance is reduced in neonates, so dosing intervals may need to be longer (8 to 12 hours rather than 4 to 6 hours). The intravenous prodrug, propacetamol, which is hydrolyzed to acetaminophen, shows measurable amounts of acetaminophen immediately after intravenous injection in neonates, infants, and children, suggesting the plasma esterases are active even in newborns. Maximum increases in pain thresholds were found 2 hours after maximum plasma concentrations but correlating with peak cerebrospinal fluid concentrations, implying a CNS site of action. This review also reports several studies that suggest higher rectal dosing at 30 to 40 mg/kg are needed to get concentrations in the 10 to 20 mg/L range. Only premature infants at 28 to 32 weeks' gestation achieved these levels from rectal doses of 20 mg/kg.

Anderson et al. (2002b) gathered pooled data of acetaminophen concentrations from six studies of premature infants, neonates, term infants, and children who received acetaminophen orally or rectally. Of the 283 children included, 124 were younger than 6 months of age. A NONMEM analysis using a one-compartment model and a "one fourth power" model found a volume of distribution of 66.6 L and a clearance of 12.5 L/hr per 70-kg person. Weight and age were the covariates most important to account for the pharmacokinetic variability. The volume of distribution decreased from 109.7 L/70 kg at 28 weeks postconception to 72.9 L/70 kg at 60 weeks postconception. Clearance increased from 0.74 L/hr per 70 kg at 28 weeks postconception to 10.8 L/hr per 70 kg at 60 weeks postconception. Using these parameters to achieve a mean C_{ss} above 10 mg/L at its trough, the authors suggest oral dosing of 25 mg/kg per day at 30 weeks postconception, 45 mg/kg per day at 34 weeks postconception, 60 mg/kg per day at 60 weeks postconception, and 90 mg/kg per day at 6 months of age. Especially for the higher dose recommendations, Anderson and colleagues caution that the effect of these dose levels on the formation of hepatotoxic metabolites from the CYP2E1 pathway are unknown, and that the dose schedule should be limited to fewer than 3 days.

In the United States, clinical trials of an intravenous formulation of acetaminophen that would have advantages for use in the perioperative period are currently underway. One gram of propacetamol generates 0.5 grams of acetaminophen. Since similar formulas have been available for several years in Europe and the United Kingdom, some information for children and infants is available to guide dosing. Allegaert et al. (2004) used a population analysis of 48 neonates; 30 infants were studied after a single dose of 20 or 40 mg/kg propacetamol, and 18 received multiple doses with a 30 mg/kg load and then 20 mg/kg at 6-hour intervals (for 36 weeks postconception or older), 8-hour intervals (for 32 to 36 weeks postconception), or 12-hour intervals (for younger than 32 weeks postconception). The volume of distribution was 70.4 L/70 kg, and clearance increased from 2.85L/h per 70 kg at 27 weeks postconception to 7.05 L/h per 70 kg at 42 weeks postconception. Tables of model predictions to keep acetaminophen concentration above 10 mg/L suggest loading with 40 mg/kg propacetamol with maintenance doses of 10 to 15 mg/kg at 4-hour intervals for infants past 30 weeks postconception (6-hour intervals in 28-week prematures).

Recently Anderson and colleagues (2005) did NONMEM population-based modeling of propacetamol in 144 children (aged 27 weeks postconception to 14 years) based on pooled data from seven studies. Size was used as the primary covariate. The data fit a three-compartment (depot, central, and peripheral) linear model best. Central volume was 24 L/70 kg, and peripheral volume was 30 L/70 kg, with clearance of 16 L/hr per 70 kg. Clearance increased from 1.87 L/hr per 70 kg at 27 weeks postconception to 84% of mature values (16.3 L/hr per 70 kg) by age 1 year. Peripheral volume of distribution decreased from 45 L/70 kg at 27 weeks postconception to mature values (30.4 L/70 kg) by 6 months of age. They also confirmed that the relative bioavailability of propacetamol was 0.5 compared with oral acetaminophen elixir. A mean acetaminophen concentration of 10 mg/L can be achieved in children aged 2 to 15 years with doses of 30 mg/kg propacetamol every 6 hours. In young infants, maintenance doses should be decreased according to postconceptual age because of lower clearance to 9 mg/kg (28 weeks), 11 mg/kg (30 weeks), 14 mg/kg (34 weeks), 18 mg/kg (40 weeks), 23 mg/kg (3 months), and 27 mg/kg (6 months).

5-HT$_3$ Antagonists

Ondansetron

Ondansetron is a serotonin 5-hydroxytryptamine$_3$ (5-HT$_3$)-receptor antagonist. The mechanism of action, although not totally elucidated, appears to block the effects of serotonin on 5-HT$_3$ receptors on vagal afferents. Ondansetron is well absorbed orally and has an oral bioavailability of 60%. Ondansetron is metabolized in the liver by CYPIA2, CYP2D6, and CYP3A4 (Sweetland et al., 1992; Gregory et al., 1998). After oral administration, peak plasma levels occur in 1 to 2 hours. In adults, after oral, intramuscular, or intravenous administration, the volume of distribution and half-life are 140 L/kg and 3.5 hours. In children, the half-life ranged from 2.5 to 3 hours, the volume of distribution ranged from 1.9 to 2.4 L/kg, and the clearance ranged from 6.6 to 15.6 mL/kg per minute (Bryson et al., 1991; Spahr-Schopfer et al., 1995). The major clinical use in anesthesia has been for prophylaxis and treatment of postoperative nausea and vomiting. Both large-scale studies and meta-analyses noted ondansetron to be a superior prophylactic drug compared with placebo, droperidol, and metoclopramide (Patel et al., 1997; Domino et al., 1999; Lim et al., 1999). The addition of dexamethasone to prophylactic ondansetron further increases the antiemetic efficacy of the drugs (Splinter et al., 1998). When used for treatment of postoperative nausea and vomiting, ondansetron (0.1 mg/kg, maximum 4 mg) appears to be superior to placebo (Khalil et al., 1996; Culy et al., 2001).

Granisetron

Granisetron, with an elimination half-life of 9 to 12 hours, has been reported to be effective at a dose of 40 mcg/kg when administered either orally or intravenously (Fujii et al., 1998, 1999a, 1999b, 2001; Fujii and Tanaka, 1999, 2001, 2002).

Tropisetron

Tropisetron is another 5-HT$_3$-receptor antagonist whose half-life is two to three times longer than that of ondansetron. In studies of children, doses ranging from 0.1 to 0.2 mg/kg were found to be effective for postoperative nausea and vomiting (Ang et al., 1998; Holt et al., 2000; Jensen et al., 2000).

Dolasetron

Dolasetron, a highly potent and selective 5-HT$_3$-receptor antagonist, appears to provide prophylactic antiemetic efficiency similar to that of ondansetron (Sukhani et al., 2002; Olutoye et al., 2003). Dolasetron appears to have an active metabolite that has a half-life of about 8 hours. In a pharmacokinetic study of 30 children, the kinetics of the metabolite were similar after both intravenous and oral administration. The volume of distribution, clearance, and half-life were 5.2 L/kg, 22.1 mL/kg per minute, and 5.7 hours, respectively. Bioavailability has been estimated at 59% (Lerman et al., 1996).

SUMMARY

The pediatric anesthesiologist should have an appreciation of the pathophysiology of the child's disease and a firm understanding of how developmental changes affect the pharmacology of anesthetic agents. In contrast to inhalational anesthetics, the effects of intravenous agents are in part delivered by pharmacokinetic parameters; that is, volume of distribution and clearance. Consequently, drug dosages are often age-dependent and need to be individualized. The anesthetic management of the infant and child requires a careful approach; both knowledge of pharmacologic and physiologic development and monitoring of neuromuscular function are essential.

The authors are indebted to Dr. Jerrold Lerman and Dr. D. Ryan Cook for their previous contribution to this chapter in the seventh edition of *Smith's Anesthesia for Infants and Children*.

For questions and answers on topics in this chapter, go to "Chapter Questions" at www.expertconsult.com.

REFERENCES

Complete references used in this text can be found online at www.expertconsult.com.

General Approach to Pediatric Anesthesia

Psychological Aspects of Pediatric Anesthesia

Zeev N. Kain and Michelle Fortier

CONTENTS

Surgery and anesthesia are causes for considerable emotional stress in both parents and children. Because the consequences of this stress occur in the immediate postoperative period and may remain long after the hospital experience has passed, one of the main tasks of the pediatric anesthesiologist is to ensure the psychological, as well as the physiologic, well-being of patients (Chapman et al., 1956; Kain and Mayes, 1996; Kotiniemi et al., 1997a, 1997b; Holm-Knudsen et al., 1998; Aono et al., 1999; Kain et al., 1999a, 1999b, 2006a). To minimize the emotional stress of anesthesia and surgery, the anesthesiologist must understand the psychological developmental milestones of childhood and anticipate situations that a child may find threatening. The latter can often be accomplished with preoperative education, a careful and thoughtful preoperative visit, and the administration of preoperative sedation when other measures are inadequate. During the preoperative visit with the patient, the anesthesiologist can optimally evaluate the levels of anxiety of both the parent(s) and the child, while assessing the child's medical condition. Of interest is that anesthesiologists are best at predicting which child in the preoperative holding area will be most anxious during induction of anesthesia (MacLaren et al., 2009). In this chapter, the psychological facets of hospitalization and surgery for children and the psychological and medical preparation of pediatric patients for anesthesia and surgery are discussed. A summary of premedications used for children undergoing anesthesia is included.

PSYCHOLOGICAL PREPARATION FOR ANESTHESIA AND SURGERY

More than 4 million children undergo surgery in the United States each year, and it is estimated that 50% to 75% of these children experience significant fear and anxiety before their operations (Corman et al., 1958; Vernon et al., 1965; Melamed and Siegel, 1975; Beeby and Hughes, 1980; Kain et al., 1996c). Based on behavioral and physiologic measures of anxiety, induction of anesthesia in children has been identified as the most stressful point during the entire preoperative period (Kain and Mayes, 1996). Appropriate understanding and management of fear and anxiety before surgery are important, because if not managed well, they can lead to both psychological and physiologic adverse outcomes, including postoperative maladaptive behavioral changes and increased postoperative pain and analgesic requirements. As an indicator of the importance of preoperative anxiety, a panel of 72 anesthesiologists ranked various clinical outcomes with low anesthesia morbidity according to importance and frequency (Macario et al., 1999). The three clinical outcomes with the highest combined scores were incisional pain, nausea and vomiting, and preoperative anxiety. Thus, it is important to understand the psychological issues involved when a child undergoes surgery.

Incidence and Definition

Although the exact prevalence of preoperative anxiety in children is difficult to assess because of issues related to measurement and developmental variations, it is estimated that up to 75% of children are reported to exhibit significant psychological or physiologic manifestations of anxiety during the preoperative period (Corman et al., 1958; Vernon et al., 1965; Melamed and Siegel, 1975; Beeby and Hughes, 1980; Kain et al., 1996c). That is, every year up to 3 million children in the United States exhibit significant fear and anxiety before undergoing surgery.

Preoperative anxiety is operationally defined as a subjective feeling of tension, apprehension, nervousness, worry, and vigilance that is associated with increased autonomic nervous system activity (Burton, 1984; Kain and Mayes, 1996). Children are threatened by anticipated parental separation, pain or discomfort, loss of control, uncertainty about "going to sleep," and masked strangers working in a technical, sterile, non–child-focused environment. Younger children tend to be concerned about separation from parents, and older children are more anxious about the anesthetic and surgical processes. The stress and anxiety experienced by children during induction of anesthesia represent an interaction between child-related factors and environmental conditions in the operating room. Child-related factors include age and developmental maturity, previous experience with medical procedures and illness, individual capacity for affect regulation and trait anxiety, and parental trait anxiety (Lumley et al., 1990, 1993; Kain et al., 1996c; Davidson et al., 2006).

Environmental factors related to the operating room include factors such as interactions with the medical staff, intensity of lights, level of noise produced by the staff and instrument preparation, and the number of medical personnel who interact with the child. Children may appear frightened or agitated, breathe deeply, tremble, stop talking or playing, or start to cry. Other children may become nauseated, wet themselves, have increased motor tone, or attempt to escape from the operating room personnel (Burton, 1984; Kain and Mayes, 1996). These behaviors, which are likely to prolong the induction of anesthesia, give children a sense of control over the situation and therefore diminish the sense of helplessness.

Identification of Children at Risk

The first step in psychologically preparing children to undergo surgery is to identify those children who are at a particularly high risk to develop extreme anxiety and fear before surgery. This is particularly important in an environment that is sensitive to hospital and operating room costs. To date, studies looking into risk factors that affect the behavioral responses of children during the preoperative period have identified several categories, including age, temperament and developmental stage of the child, trait (baseline) and state (situational) anxiety of the parent, various demographic characteristics of the child and parent, and quality of previous experience of the child with medical procedures.

Young children, between the ages of 1 and 5 years old, are reported to be at the highest risk for developing significant anxiety before anesthesia and surgery (Brophy and Erickson, 1990; Lumley et al., 1993; Vetter, 1993; Kain et al., 1996a, 1996c). At this age, children are particularly vulnerable because they are young enough to be dependent on their parents, yet old enough to recognize parental absence. Additional factors that enhance the vulnerability of this age group include the degree of inexperience in social contact, ability to communicate and benefit from psychological preparation, and ability to relieve anxiety through play (Hyson, 1983). Although the younger child may not have the cognitive ability to anticipate potential dangers or painful situations during induction of anesthesia, the older child (older than age 6 years) may anticipate pain and fear "going to sleep" (Sparrow et al., 1984). Older children may also rely on a number of coping strategies, including verbal questioning and cognitive mastery (e.g., learning about heart monitors or about what surgeons do) to mediate their anxiety.

Children who have high trait anxiety and who have experienced poor-quality medical encounters in the past are at a particularly high risk to develop high anxiety during the preoperative period (Kain et al., 1996a, 1996c; Davidson et al., 2006). Interestingly, a child who must undergo repeated surgical procedures may respond with either higher-than-expected preoperative anxiety levels or lower-than-expected preoperative anxiety levels. Based on a conditioned learning model, the preoperative situation presents unconditioned fear stimuli that occur repeatedly over short intervals. Thus, children's previous surgical and medical histories may either exacerbate or attenuate their fear conditioning, and the quality of the previous medical experience (e.g., how distressing it was to the child) is more crucial than its occurrence (Box 8-1).

Several investigations indicate that children who have a shy and inhibited temperament show higher levels of fear and anxiety on the day of surgery compared with other children (Melamed and Ridley-Johnson, 1988; Kain et al., 2001). Conversely, children who have a more socially adaptive temperament are less anxious in the perioperative settings (Kain et al., 2001). Temperament in a child refers to individual patterns of behavior and has been compared with personality traits in adults (Buss et al., 1973; Buss and Plomin, 1975). Kagan et al. (1987) reported that temperament characteristics can be used to predict how a child responds emotionally in a stressful situation; for example, children who are "shy" or "inhibited" tend to become more anxious in novel settings, as suggested by the adrenocortical response and elevated heart rate.

A child's anxiety before surgery is strongly affected by the state and trait anxiety of the parent (Kain et al., 1996c, 2001). Parental anxiety mediates the child's response to stressful situations through two pathways (Kain and Mayes, 1996). First, whereas some parents may act as stress reducers for their children, parents who are anxious themselves are typically less available to respond to their children's needs. Indeed, in these cases the child's distress may further compound parental anxiety, thus diminishing the parent's ability to respond effectively. The second pathway of the effect of parental anxiety on a child's response reflects the genetics of parental disposition and anxiety.

Box 8-1 Risk Factors for Preoperative Anxiety

CHILD RELATED
Young age (1 to 5 years of age)
Poor previous experience with medical procedures and illness
Shy and inhibited temperament
Lack of developmental maturity and social adaptability
High cognitive levels
Not enrolled in daycare

PARENT RELATED
High trait and state anxiety
Divorced parents
Multiple surgical procedures for parents

ENVIRONMENT RELATED
Sensory overload
Conflicting messages
Operating

Previous research has illustrated that mothers who were more anxious in the surgical setting had children who were also more anxious and that these mothers were less able to respond to their children's anxiety (Kagan et al., 1987).

Divorced parents, parents with lower educational levels, and parents of children who were not enrolled in a daycare setting rate themselves as significantly more anxious preoperatively (Kain et al., 1996a, 1996c). Finally, parents of children who are younger than 1 year old, parents who themselves underwent multiple hospitalizations, and parents of children who underwent multiple admissions all report being more anxious (Litman et al., 1996; Shirley et al., 1998). Preoperative anxiety in young children undergoing surgery can be managed with behavioral or pharmacologic (preoperative sedative medication) interventions, or both (Fig. 8-1).

Psychological Preparation Programs

The concept of psychological preparation of children and parents who undergo surgery was introduced almost 50 years ago (Mellish, 1969; Robinson and Kobayashi, 1991). Earlier programs provided the child with information regarding the surgical and anesthetic procedures and sought to develop a rapport between the medical staff and the child (Melamed and Siegel, 1975; Melamed et al., 1976, 1978). In the 1970s, modeling preparation programs were introduced to multiple hospitals in the United States. These modeling programs included the use of illustrated books, video programs, and puppet shows (Melamed and Siegel, 1975; Melamed et al., 1976, 1978). The theory behind these programs was that children would be prepared for the surgical experience by observing other children who underwent similar procedures. During the 1990s, the idea of family-centered care was introduced to medicine in general and to the area of preoperative preparation in particular (Melamed, 1993). Coupled with the development of the child-life discipline and the teaching of coping skills, this concept dominates the preparation programs in current use. Child-life specialists are individuals who facilitate the child's coping and the perioperative adjustment of children and parents by providing play experiences using modeling techniques (AAP statement, 1993). Child-life specialists incorporate descriptions of the perioperative

sensations children experience and provide opportunities to examine, rehearse, and play with perioperative equipment to be used in their care. Child-life specialists also aim to establish supportive relationships with children and parents and to teach relaxation skills, as well as present information to the child and parent about the anesthetic and surgical procedures (AAP statement, 1993).

The regularity with which preparation programs aimed at children undergoing surgery are being used has changed over the past decades. Although these programs were scarce in the 1970s and 1980s, they became quite popular in the 1990s. In fact, in 1996 about 80% of all major acute care children's hospitals in the United States offered such programs to children and their parents (O'Byrne et al., 1997). Unfortunately, the number of comprehensive preparation programs has been reported as decreasing over the past few years; this new trend is likely the result of new economical constraints in the perioperative environment.

O'Byrne et al. (1997) state that he type of preparation program used varies significantly among different children's hospitals in the United States. About 89% of children's hospitals are reported to provide narrative preparation, 87% provide operating-room tours, 86% provide play therapy, and 84% provide printed material. More comprehensive preparation, such as child-life preparation is provided at about 50% of children's hospitals, and relaxation is taught at about 40% of the hospitals. Interestingly, a panel of experts indicated their consensus regarding the effectiveness of psychological preparation programs before surgery. On a scale of 1 (least effective) to 9 (most effective), child-life preparation was ranked the most effective, followed by play therapy, an operating-room tour, and printed material (O'Byrne et al., 1997).

Although the effectiveness of preparation programs in reduction of anxiety in the holding area is well established, their effectiveness for reducing anxiety during the induction process is questionable (Kain et al., 1996a, 1998a). Methodologic flaws, such as the absence of an appropriate outcome instrument and small sample size, hinder many of the studies that report reduced anxiety in children. In fact, a study that included a validated outcome measure has clearly documented that although a comprehensive psychological preparation program (i.e., child life) is effective in reduction of anxiety in the holding area, it is

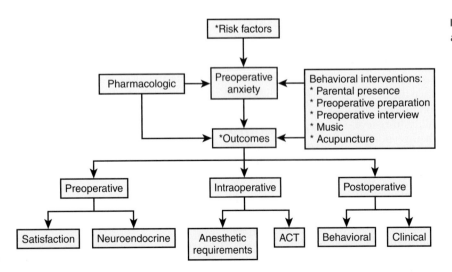

■ **FIGURE 8-1.** Operational view of preoperative anxiety in children. *ACT,* Anesthesia control time.

not effective during the induction of anesthesia or in the recovery room (Kain et al., 1998a). It is likely that the extreme anxiety experienced during induction of anesthesia inhibits children's abilities to process and implement of the content of the preoperative-preparation program.

Considerations in Choosing a Preparation Program

It is vital to realize that psychological preparation programs have to be tailored based on the individual needs of each child. That is, a preparation program that is appropriate for a 3-year-old child is not appropriate for a 12-year-old child. Thus, once the type of the preparation has been chosen (e.g., child-life vs. a tour of the operating room), the preparation has to be individualized based on developmental considerations of the child.

Timing of the preparation in relation to the day of surgery is a significant factor. That is, children aged 6 years and older benefit most if they participate in the program more than 5 to 7 days before surgery and benefit the least if the program is given 1 day before surgery (Melamed et al., 1976; Robinson and Kobayashi, 1991; Kain et al., 1996a). This extended interval between the preparation and the surgery is needed for older children to have adequate time to process new information provided to them during the preparation process (Melamed et al., 1983; Kain et al., 1996a, 1998a). Typically, older children prepared 1 week ahead of surgery show an immediate increase in the anxiety during the preparation period, with a gradual decrease until the time of surgery (Melamed et al., 1983). Interestingly, there may be a negative effect of a preparation program on younger children. This may be a result of the inability of children younger than age 3 years to separate fantasy from reality (Melamed et al., 1976; Robinson and Kobayashi, 1991). From ages 3 to 6 years, children experience increased ability to separate fantasy from reality, and by the age of 6 years, this distinction of fantasy vs. reality is typically completed (Piaget, 1955).

It is particularly challenging to design a preparation program for children who have been previously hospitalized. Information about what occurs on the day of surgery does not provide new information for these children. Studies have documented that simple modeling and play programs are not beneficial for these children and may actually sensitize these children (Melamed et al., 1983; Faust and Melamed, 1984). Alternative psychological programs, such as teaching extensive, individualized coping skills combined with actual practice, are more helpful for these children (Melamed et al., 1983; Kain et al., 1996a). These alternative programs should be based on the particular experiences the child had during previous surgeries.

Parental Issues

Clearly, preoperative preparation should be directed to parents as well as to children. Multiple studies have reported that parents typically become very anxious when their child undergoes surgery, and parental anxiety was identified as a significant risk factor for increased preoperative anxiety in children (Pinto and Hollandsworth, 1989; Kain et al., 1996a, 1996c; Litman et al., 1996; Shirley et al., 1998; Cassady et al., 1999). Parents experience preoperative anxiety for reasons such as fear of separation and bodily harm to their children, guilt, and financial stress (Cassady et al., 1999). Indeed many parents are more anxious about their children's health than their own (Kain et al., 1997d). Mothers are more prone to preoperative anxiety than are fathers, particularly when a child is younger than 1 year old or when they are coping with a child's first surgical experience (Litman et al., 1996; Shirley et al., 1998). Previous research has also documented that women are significantly more concerned with risks and side effects in general, although men specifically articulate a fear of death twice as often as women.

Parents who undergo a preoperative preparation program or who have viewed a preoperative videotape featuring factual information about anesthesia show reduced preoperative anxiety on the day of surgery, but this reduction in anxiety is transient and does not extend to the anesthetic induction, the recovery room, or 2 weeks postoperatively (Table 8-1) (Pinto and Hollandsworth, 1989; Kain et al., 1996a; 1998a; Cassady et al., 1999). Nonetheless, the use of videotapes has received increased attention as a supplementary educational modality for parents, because the tapes are informative, perhaps anxiolytic, and cost effective in certain settings (Pinto and Hollandsworth, 1989; Karl et al., 1990; Cassady et al., 1999; Cassady and Kain, 2000).

Future of Preparation Programs

Most surgeries in the United States are currently conducted on an outpatient basis, and as a result, many children receive preparation for surgery on the morning of the procedure. A major

TABLE 8-1. Use of Preoperative Videos for Increased Parental Education and Decreased Parental Anxiety

| Measure | Experimental Group[†] | | Control Group | | |
	Prevideo	Postvideo	Prevideo	Postvideo	P Value
SALT (% Correct)	75.2 ± 1.8*	84.9 ± 2.3	73.4 ± 1.4	75.4 ± 1.9	<.0220
STAI State Anxiety	40.5 ± 1.7	36.0 ± 1.4	39.2 ± 1.5	37.7 ± 1.2	<.0310
APAIS Total	22.0 ± 1.2	17.0 ± 0.9	22.0 ± 0.8	21.6 ± 0.7	<.0001
APAIS Anxiety	12.7 ± 0.8	9.0 ± 0.6	12.6 ± 0.6	12.2 ± 0.5	<.0001
APAIS Need for Information	9.3 ± 0.7	8.0 ± 0.3	9.4 ± 0.6	9.3 ± 0.6	<.0001

From Cassady et al.: Use of a preanesthetic video for facilitation of parental education and anxiolysis before pediatric ambulatory surgery, *Anesth Analg* 88:246, 1999.
Values are given as mean ± SEM.
Group x time interaction obtained by repeated-measures analyses of variance.
SALT, Standard Anesthesia Learning Test; *STAI State Anxiety*, State-Trait Anxiety Inventory (State Anxiety); *APAIS*, Amsterdam Preoperative Anxiety and Information Scale.

issue with this approach is that because of production pressure, health care providers rarely spend more than a few minutes with the child before surgery (Kain et al., 2009a). As such, a different approach is needed.

The absence of cost-sensitive preoperative preparation programs will inevitably be filled by technological advancements. The future will be characterized by the development and implementation of computerized multimedia displays and interactive technology. The latter offers particular appeal, because its multimodal capability can provide specific interventions for individuals with a wide range of medical problems and coping styles. The capacity, programmability, and rapid response of current interactive technology are suitable for such tasks, but the cost remains high. In the future, it is the hope that all children and their parents will be able to realize the benefits of specialized, technologically advanced, tailored educational systems programmed to meet their individual and cultural needs and coping styles.

Parental Presence

Parental presence during the induction of anesthesia has been suggested as an alternative to sedative premedication. Although there is general agreement about the desirability of parents visiting during their child's hospitalization, their presence during invasive medical procedures, such as induction of anesthesia, remains very controversial (Lerman, 2000; Kain, 2001). Potential benefits from parental presence include reducing the need for preoperative sedatives and reducing the child's anxiety and distress on separation to the operating room. Increased child compliance and reduced child anxiety during induction of anesthesia have been suggested to be benefits as well. Common objections to this practice include delays in operating-room schedules, crowded operating rooms, and a possible adverse reaction of the parent during the induction process.

A large-scale, nationwide survey indicated that there is a large variability in hospital policy in the United States toward parental presence in operating rooms. Thirty-two percent of the hospitals allow parental presence; 11% encourage parental presence; 23% have no formal hospital policy; and 26% do not allow it (Kain et al., 2004c).

The same survey reported that only 10% of anesthesiologists have parents present during induction of anesthesia in more than 75% of cases, and that 27% of anesthesiologists have parents present during induction in less than 25% of cases. About 50% of all anesthesiologists never have parents present during induction (Kain et al., 2004c). The reported prevalence of parental presence varies widely among the different geographic locations in the United States.

The survey showed that parental presence during induction of anesthesia was practiced most often in the northeast region and least often in the south-central region of the United States (Fig. 8-2). Interestingly, the findings in this survey are very much different from the findings in a nationwide survey conducted in 1995 (Kain et al., 1997c, 2004c) (Fig. 8-3). Overall, there was an increase in the rate of parental presence from 1995 to 2002, and the number of anesthesiologists who never allow parental presence dropped in every geographic region (Kain et al., 1997c, 2004c). These findings may represent a new trend in this practice in the United States.

Parental Perspectives

A number of surveys have indicated that most parents prefer to be present during the induction of anesthesia regardless of the child's age (Braude et al., 1990; Ryder and Spargo, 1991). Furthermore, a majority of parents believe that they are of some help to their child and to the anesthesiologist during the induction process (Ryder and Spargo, 1991). A study indicates that over 80% of parents chose to be present in the operating room when returning for a second operation regardless of whether they were present in the operating room in the first operation

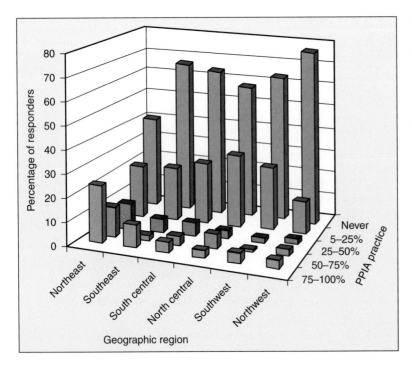

■ **FIGURE 8-2.** Practice of parental presence during induction of anesthesia as a function of geographic areas in the United States as of 1995. *PPIA,* Parental presence during induction of anesthesia. *(From Kain ZN et al.: Trends in the practice of parental presence during induction of anesthesia and the use of preoperative sedative premedication in the United States 1995–2002: results of a follow-up national survey,* Anesth Analg *98:1252–1259, 2004c.)*

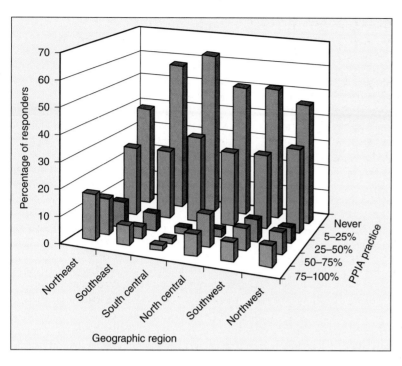

■ **FIGURE 8-3.** Practice of parental presence during induction of anesthesia as a function of geographic areas in the United States as of 2002. *PPIA,* Parental presence during induction of anesthesia. *(From Kain ZN et al.: Trends in the practice of parental presence during inductions of anesthesia and the use of preoperative sedative premedication in the United States 1995–2002,* Anesth Analg *98:1252–1259, 2004c.)*

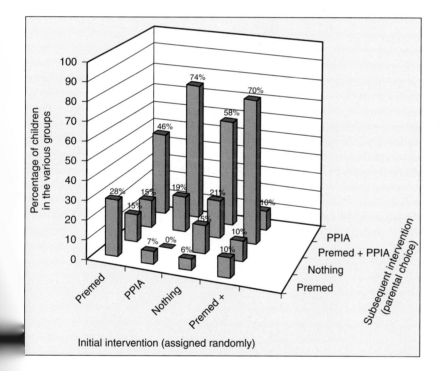

■ **FIGURE 8-4.** Data regarding the parental intervention choice in the subsequent surgery as a function of the initial surgery. For example, 28% of the parents who were assigned to the premedication group in the initial intervention chose to be in the premedication group in the subsequent surgery. *PPIA,* Parental presence during induction of anesthesia. *(From Kain ZN et al.: Parental intervention choices for children undergoing repeated surgeries,* Anesth Analg *96:970, 2003b.)*

(Kain et al., 2003b). This preference for parental presence during induction shown by parents who had experience with other interventions, including preoperative midazolam, is similar to the preference for parental presence shown by parents of children undergoing surgery for the first time (Kain et al., 2003b) (Fig. 8-4). It is no surprise, therefore, that parental presence during the induction of anesthesia is associated with increased parental satisfaction regarding not only the separation process from their child but also with the overall functioning of the hospital (Kain et al., 2000).

Many parents report increased anxiety when they are present during induction of anesthesia (Vessey et al., 1994). An investigation found, however, that anxiety after induction of anesthesia among parents who were present during induction did not differ significantly from anxiety among parents who were not present during the induction process (Kain et al., 2003a). This finding is in agreement with previous randomized controlled trials that have examined this issue (Bevan et al., 1990; Kain et al., 1996b, 1998b, 2000).

Parental physiologic responses during induction of anesthesia have been examined as well (Kain et al., 2003a). It was found that parental heart rate and skin conductance levels significantly increase as the parents walk to the operating room. Interestingly, once the induction begins, parental heart rate

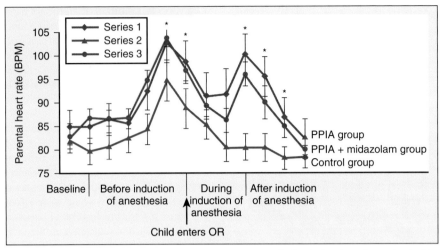

■ **FIGURE 8-5.** Changes in parental heart rate *(HR)* from baseline measurement until after induction of anesthesia. Data are reported as mean *(SE)*. ***, Time points at which differences between groups are statistically significant (P < .05); *OR*, Operating room; *PPIA*, Parental presence during induction of anesthesia. *(From Kain ZN et al.: Parental intervention choices for children undergoing repeated surgeries, Anesth Analg 96:970, 2003b.)*

decreases, only to peak again once the parents have to leave the operating room. This second peak in heart rate is in agreement with previous data indicating that the most upsetting factors are seeing the child go limp during induction and then having to leave the child (Vessey et al., 1994). Parental blood pressure after induction of anesthesia was not elevated, and examination of parental data from a Holter monitor revealed no rhythmic abnormalities and no electrocardiographic changes indicative of ischemia (Fig. 8-5) (Kain et al., 2003a).

There have been isolated reports of parental presence resulting in disruptive behavior and even a report of the removal of a child from the operating room by a grandmother (Schofield and White, 1989; Bowie, 1993). In contrast, a 4-year experience with 3086 children in a free-standing ambulatory surgery center found that no parent needed to be escorted from the operating room (Gauderer et al., 1989).

Experimental Studies Involving Parental Presence

Early studies involving parental presence during induction of anesthesia indicated that the presence of a parent might lower the anxiety of the child (Schulman et al., 1967; Hannallah and Rosales, 1983). These studies, however, were nonrandomized, did not control for confounding variables, and lacked appropriate outcome measurement tools. It is important to note that measurement of a child's anxiety during induction of anesthesia is a complex issue that necessitates the use of a validated and reliable instrument of a child's anxiety. Such an instrument, the Yale Preoperative Anxiety Scale, was developed and validated a number of years ago (Kain et al., 1995, 1997b). Later studies that used appropriate sample size, eliminated confounding variables, and used appropriate end points and assessment instruments concluded that parental presence does not result in decreased anxiety on the part of the child during the induction process (Hickmott et al., 1989; Bevan et al., 1990; Kain et al., 1996b, 1998b, 2000; Kain, 2001). Further, parental presence during induction of anesthesia was also compared with the use of oral midazolam (0.5 mg/kg) administered 30 minutes before surgery (Kain et al., 1998b). The investigations concluded that the use of oral midazolam is significantly more

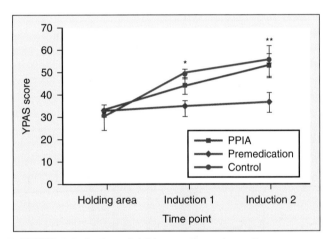

■ **FIGURE 8-6.** Anxiety of child across the perioperative period. *Induction 1*, Entrance to the operating room; *Induction 2*, Introduction of the anesthesia mask to the child. Premedication group was significantly less anxious compared with the parental presence and control groups at Induction 1 *(*)* and induction 2 *(**)*. *PPIA*, Parental presence during induction of anesthesia; *YPAS*, Yale Preoperative Anxiety Scale. *(From Kain ZN, Mayes LC, Caramico LA, et al.: Postoperative behavioral outcomes in children: effects of sedative premedication, Anesthesiology 90:758–765, 1999b.)*

effective than parental presence in terms of both reducing a child's anxiety and increasing a child's compliance (Fig. 8-6) (Kain et al., 1998b).

However, it is clear that research related to the basic concepts underlying parental presence during induction of anesthesia has not changed during the past 2 decades and that the present body of research simply deals with the question of whether parents should be present during induction of anesthesia. Research interests should shift toward an emphasis on what parents actually do during induction of anesthesia rather than simply on their presence. A preliminary publication reports the development of an intervention that consists of an informational and modeling video, instructed graduated exposure and shaping exercises, coached distraction technique supportive telephone coaching, and adherence checks (Kain et al., 2002b). This informative modeling intervention is directed at parents of children undergoing surgery and is quite extensive. Results show that children and parents who underwent the extensive parental-preparation program were significantly less anxious than were children whose parents were present during induction of anesthesia and who did not receive the preparation program. More data regarding this preparation program are needed.

Moreover, more recent studies have also attempted to illustrate which children may benefit most from parental presence. In a large-scale prospective cohort study of over 400 children, Kain and colleagues (2006c) demonstrated that children who were older, had lower levels of temperamental activity, and had less anxious parents who valued preparation and coping skills for medical situations benefitted from parental presence at anesthesia induction in terms of anxiety levels and cooperation ratings. In addition, calm parents were found to benefit anxious children during induction of anesthesia, whereas there were no benefits of parental presence when parents were highly anxious (Kain et al., 2006a). In fact, in this large cohort study, calm children who had overly anxious parents present at anesthesia induction were significantly more anxious than calm children who had no parental presence. Finally, it should be noted that the number of parents who are allowed into the operating rooms does not impact the anxiety of the child (Kain et al., 2009b). That is, a child's anxiety during induction is not higher or lower based on the presence of only one parent as opposed to both parents.

Satisfaction Issues

Previously, the medical community held the view that the only "real" outcomes are those that have an immediate and direct impact on patient morbidity and mortality. This view has changed dramatically, and issues such as patient satisfaction and quality of life are considered by many as equally important as morbidity (Ford et al., 1997). This new development is echoed in review articles in the anesthesia literature suggesting that patient satisfaction should serve as an important end point and indicator of overall quality of anesthesia care (Fung and Cohen, 1998).

Typically, parents are not aware of the events that take place inside an operating room. To parents, the most important thing is their child's safety. However, with anesthetic mortality rates approaching 1:100,000, safety is expected. In contrast, parents evaluate an anesthesiologist, in part, based on the separation experience with their child. That is, if their child is taken to the operating room upset and crying, their satisfaction and impression of the anesthesiologist and the surgery center may be poor.

A study evaluated parental presence during induction of anesthesia as a contributing factor to their satisfaction. The study also evaluated the effectiveness of parental presence when used in conjunction with oral midazolam (0.5 mg/kg) (Kain et al., 2000). The study has demonstrated that while parental presence did not provide added value in terms of reducing child's anxiety or increasing a child's compliance, it did improve parental satisfaction with both the separation process and the entire perioperative process (Kain et al., 2000). Thus, although experimental studies fail to demonstrate the effectiveness of parental presence with regard to anxiety reduction or increased compliance,

parental satisfaction seems to improve if the parents are present during the induction of anesthesia.

Medicolegal Issues

The practicing anesthesiologist should also be aware of legal issues associated with parental presence during induction of anesthesia—that is, the additional risks the anesthesiologist incurs because of the presence of a parent in the operating room. The legal literature is not clear with this issue. Of note, however, is a decision made by the Illinois Supreme Court with regard to parental presence during an invasive procedure. In its verdict, the Illinois Supreme Court stated that a hospital that allows a nonpatient to accompany a patient during treatment does not have a duty to protect the nonpatient from fainting (Lewyn, 1993). If medical personnel invite the nonpatient to be present during the treatment, however, the hospital has a legal responsibility toward the nonpatient. Thus, there is an important distinction between allowing parental presence and inviting parental presence. As a response to such possible litigation, a number of hospitals require parents to sign a separate consent form when they express the wish to be present during induction of anesthesia. In a nationwide survey, Kain et al. (2004c) reported that only 5% of all hospitals in the United States indicate that they routinely obtain a separate written consent for parental presence during induction of anesthesia.

Behavioral Interventions

Family-Centered Preparation

In the contexts of increased attention to family-centered care in the past decade and of the relationship between a parent and a child's anxiety, Kain and colleagues recently developed a multicomponent, behavioral preoperative-preparation program targeting the family as a whole, rather than the individual child (Kain et al., 2007). Termed ADVANCE (*A*nxiety-reduction, *D*istraction, *V*ideo modeling and education, *A*dding parents, *N*o excessive reassurance, *C*oaching, and *E*xposure/shaping), this program consists of psychological techniques of shaping, exposure, and modeling with coaching in combination with empirically supported distraction techniques. A randomized controlled trial comparing ADVANCE with standard of care (no premedication or parental presence), standard of care plus parental presence at induction of anesthesia, or standard of care plus midazolam indicated that parents and children in the ADVANCE group exhibited significantly lower levels of preoperative anxiety in the holding area compared with all other groups and lower anxiety during anesthesia induction when compared with the standard-of-care and parental-presence groups (Kain et al., 2007). Moreover, children in the ADVANCE groups had a lower incidence of emergence delirium, required fewer analgesics in recovery, and had a shorter length of stay in recovery as compared with children in the other three groups.

Music

Music has well-established psychological effects, including the induction and modification of moods and emotions (Baeck, 2002; Kain et al., 2002a; Lipe, 2002). Kane, in 1914, is reported to have been one of the first individuals to provide intraoperative music to distract patients from "the horror of surgery." It was not until about 1960, however, that a group of dentists reported that 65% to 90% of their patients needed little or no anesthesia for dental extractions with the routine use of music during dental surgery (Gardner and Licklider, 1959; Gardner et al., 1960). Music has gained popularity as a part of complementary medicine directed at patients undergoing medical and surgical procedures (Wang et al., 2002a, 2002b, 2003).

The role of music as a therapeutic modality for the treatment of preoperative anxiety in adult patients has been evaluated in several studies. Although a number of studies conducted in this area were hindered by multiple methodologic flaws, the anxiolytic effects of perioperative music are well documented in adults (Standley, 1986; Thompson and Kam, 1995; Miluck-Kolasa et al., 1996; Wang et al., 2002a). As indicated earlier, the anxiety experienced by a child during the induction period is related to personality factors, as well as to operating room factors such as bright lights and high noise levels. Several studies that have assessed noise levels in the operating room concluded that while overall sound levels are not excessive, loud intermittent noises up to 108 dB are present intermittently (Hodge and Thompson, 1990; Nott and West, 2003). Cohen (1970) classified noises as just audible (10 dB), very quiet (50 dB, comparable with light traffic at 30 miles/hr), moderately loud (70 dB, comparable with a dishwasher), very loud (90 dB, comparable with a food blender), and uncomfortably loud (130 dB, comparable with a rock-and-roll band). Interestingly, a sudden noise with a level as little as 30 dB above the background noise (e.g., an SpO_2 alarm) might cause an immediate startle response, which is associated with an activation of the sympathetic system, and an anxiolytic response (Falk and Woods, 1973). A study introduced an intervention that consisted of dimmed operating room lights (200 lux) and soft background music (Bach's "Air on a G String" at 50 to 60 dB), and only the attending anesthesiologist was allowed to interact with the child during induction (Fig. 8-7) (Kain et al., 2002b). The number of medical personnel interacting with the child is of particular importance, as it is not uncommon that the surgeon, the circulating nurse, the anesthesia resident, and the anesthesiologist attending all try to help the child through the induction process. This may result in conflicting messages and increased anxiety on the part of the child. This study found that this combination of music, dim light, and only the attending anesthesiologist interacting with the child was effective and that the children who received this intervention exhibited significantly less anxiety during induction of anesthesia (Kain et al., 2002b).

To date, most reported studies of music therapy in the medical literature describe interventions that consist of patients passively listening to music. Studies that examined live-participation music therapy with children undergoing surgery concluded that this type of music therapy resulted in reduced anxiety in children undergoing surgery (Chetta, 1981; Robb et al., 1995). These studies, however, were limited because of a small sample size and a lack of reliable and valid outcome measures. A more recent trial that used an appropriate sample size and a reliable instrument for measuring outcome indicated some complexities related to this issue (Kain et al., 2004b). The study found that both at separation from parents and on entrance to the operating room, only children who received music therapy from one of the therapists involved in the study were significantly less anxious than the control group. This anxiolytic effect was present only in the holding area and

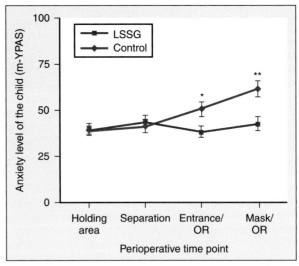

■ **FIGURE 8-7.** Levels of anxiety manifested by children during the perioperative period. Anxiety was assessed by the modified Yale Preoperative Anxiety Scale (m-PAS). Observed anxiety differed significantly between the two groups (F[1,67] = 6.3, P = .014). *LSSG,* Low sensory stimulation group; *OR,* Operating room. *, P = .03; **, P = .003. *(From Kain ZN, Wang SM, Mayes LC, et al.: Sensory stimuli and anxiety in children undergoing surgery: a randomized controlled trial, Anesth Analg 92:897–903, 2001.)*

at separation but not during induction of anesthesia. Thus, it can be concluded that the provision of live-participation music therapy is quite expensive, and considering the results of the more recent study, it is doubtful as to whether this modality should be routinely used to reduce preoperative anxiety in all children undergoing surgery.

Acupuncture

Acupuncture originated in China between the years 2000 and 100 BCE (Hsu, 1996). Despite the slow progression of scientific evidence, acupuncture and related techniques have become very popular in the western medical culture over the last few decades.

Several studies have examined whether acupuncture is an effective treatment modality for preoperative anxiety. Wang and Kain (2001a, 2001b) found that both healthy volunteers and adult patients undergoing routine outpatient surgery report lower levels of state anxiety after auricular acupuncture provided in specific points. This effect started as early as 30 minutes after insertion of the acupuncture needles. The use of acupuncture as a treatment for parental anxiety was examined as well. Wang and Kain randomized mothers of children who were scheduled for surgery to an acupuncture intervention group or a sham acupuncture control group (Fig. 8-8). The intervention was performed at least 30 minutes before the child's induction of anesthesia and all mothers were present during induction of anesthesia (Wang et al., 2004).

The investigators found that after induction, maternal anxiety in the acupuncture group was significantly lower, and children whose mothers received the acupuncture intervention were significantly less anxious on entrance to the operating room (Wang et al., 2004). Thus, auricular acupuncture may have various uses in the pediatric perioperative environment.

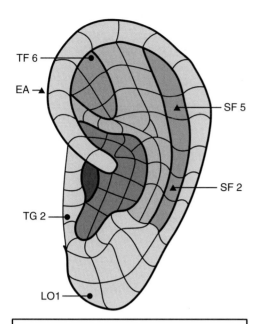

FIGURE 8-8. Auricular acupuncture points that are used to treat parental anxiety. *(From Wang S, Maranets I, Weinberg M, et al.: Parental auricular acupuncture as an adjunct for parental presence during induction of anesthesia, Anesthesiology 100(6):1399–1404, 2004.)*

In addition to acupuncture, Wang and colleagues (2005) have also examined parental acupressure as an intervention for preoperative anxiety and found that acupressure at the Yintang point significantly reduced parental self-reported anxiety in the preoperative holding area.

Preoperative Interview

Anesthesiologists undoubtedly have the ability to increase or decrease the anxiety levels of patients; therefore, one should consider the preoperative interview as a psychological intervention that is administered routinely to parents and children (Egbert et al., 1963; Kain et al., 2002a). The anxiety-moderating effect of anesthesiologists is dependent on multiple variables, such as environmental stimuli and the coping style of the parent. That is, patients undergoing surgery generally ask for all relevant information to be provided to them, although some patients and parents have a coping style that is information-seeking, whereas others have a coping style that is information-avoiding (Miller, 1995; Kain et al., 1997a, 1997d). The challenge for the anesthesiologist is to identify the individual coping style of a parent without the benefit of using structured psychological instruments during the preoperative visit.

The impact of information given in the preoperative setting on the anxiety of patients was examined by Miller and Mangan (1983). They found that adult patients who were given extensive information preoperatively were more anxious and uncomfortable. In contrast, no increase in preoperative anxiety was

demonstrated in a study that involved English and Scottish men undergoing elective herniorrhaphy who were presented with detailed risk information (Kerrigan et al., 1993). Similarly, a study that involved parents of children undergoing surgery found that the provision of detailed anesthetic information in the setting of a randomized controlled trial did not increase the anxiety of the parents (Kain et al., 1997d). In terms of information desired by children, Fortier and colleagues (2009) recently demonstrated that the majority of children report a strong desire for comprehensive preoperative information, particularly information about pain; however, the impact of providing such information on perioperative outcomes, including anxiety, is not known. Thus, the practicing anesthesiologist should be aware of these data and provide information in the perioperative settings as dictated by the settings and the needs of the parents and the children.

BEHAVIORAL OUTCOMES OF PREOPERATIVE ANXIETY IN CHILDREN

Postoperative Behavioral Changes

Epidemiology

In 1945, Levy described 25 cases of children who developed significant fear of physicians after tonsillectomy. Vernon et al. (1966) developed a structured parental instrument (Posthospitalization Behavior Questionnaire [PHBQ]) that addressed the issue of postoperative behavioral changes in children. Earlier studies that used the PHBQ reported that up to 88% of all children undergoing anesthesia and surgery develop new behavioral changes postoperatively (Vernon et al., 1966; Peterson and Shigetomi, 1982; Thompson and Vernon, 1993). More recent studies conducted in the United States and Europe documented that up to 54% of young children undergoing outpatient surgery experience general anxiety, nighttime crying, enuresis, separation anxiety, and temper tantrums 2 weeks postoperatively (Fig. 8-9) (Kain et al., 1996c; Kotiniemi et al., 1996, 1997a; Kain, 2000). Nearly one-fifth of children continue to demonstrate maladaptive behavior changes 6 months postoperatively, and in 6% of children these behaviors persist at 1 year (Kain et al., 1996c).

Nightmares and waking up crying are particularly common problems after surgery in children, and the incidence of these behaviors is as high as 20% 2 weeks postoperatively (Kain et al., 1996c). The effect of outpatient surgery on postoperative sleep patterns was also addressed in a study that used actigraphy, which is an objective measure that aims to quantify sleep (Kain et al., 2002c). The study found that 47% of all children developed postoperative sleeping problems as assessed by either actigraphy or the PHBQ (Kain et al., 2002c). Fourteen percent of children experienced a decrease of at least 1 standard deviation in percentage sleep as assessed by actigraphy (Fig. 8-10) (Kain et al., 2002d).

Considering the dramatic changes that have occurred with health care delivery, this relatively high incidence of postoperative behavioral changes is surprising (Kain, 2000). That is, considering that these were studies that were conducted with outpatients, a lower incidence would be expected. It is important to appreciate, however, that because of economic issues, outpatient surgery for children is being performed with high levels of medical acuity. Children with similar issues underwent

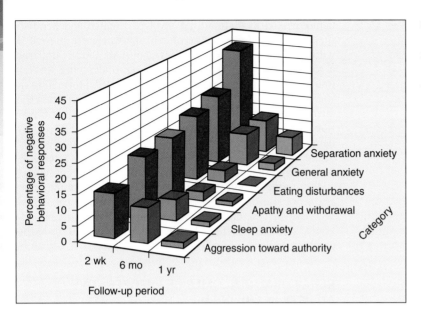

■ **FIGURE 8-9.** The incidence of postoperative behavioral changes as a function of time after surgery. *(From Kain ZN, Mayes LC, O'Connor T, et al.: Preoperative anxiety in children: predictors and outcomes,* Arch Pediatr Adolesc Med *150:1238–1245, 1996c.)*

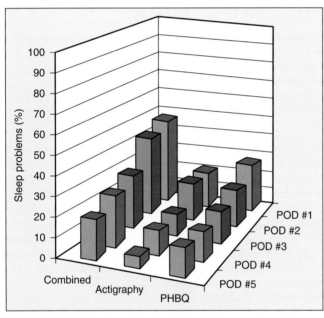

■ **FIGURE 8-10.** Postoperative sleeping disturbances during the first five postoperative nights, as determined either by actigraphy or the PHBQ. *(From Kain ZN, Mayes LC, Alexander GM, et al.: Sleeping characteristics of children undergoing outpatient elective surgery,* Anesthesiology *97:1093–1101, 2002.)*

inpatient surgery just a few years ago; it may be that efforts to improve the psychological climate of hospitals have been neutralized by other variables.

Predictors

Several studies report that young age is a significant risk factor for the development of postoperative behavioral changes. In 1945, Levy noted a marked reduction in the emotional reaction after surgery in children older than age of 3 years, when the incidence of the new-onset behaviors dropped from 50% to 10%. More recent investigations confirm this observation and report that these postoperative behavioral changes are most common

between the ages of 1 and 4 years (Vernon et al., 1965; Kain et al., 1996c). At these ages, children are particularly vulnerable because of issues such as separation anxiety, social inexperience, limited ability to communicate and benefit from psychological preparation, and limited ability to relieve anxiety through play (Kain, 2000).

Increased anxiety of the child and of the parent in the holding area and during induction of anesthesia are both good predictors for later emergence of maladaptive postoperative behaviors (Eckenhoff, 1958; Kain et al., 1996c, 1999a, 2004a, 2006a; Lumley et al., 1993). Meyers and Muravchick (1977) compared postoperative behavioral responses in a group of children who underwent a "steal induction" with a group of children who underwent an "awake" induction. One month after the children were discharged from the hospital, the investigators reported that the rate of behavioral changes was 88% in the awake group and 58% in the steal group. Kain et al. (1999a) confirmed these previous findings and observed that extreme anxiety during induction of anesthesia and forcing the child to the table is associated with a significantly increased occurrence of negative postoperative behavioral changes. Several reports indicate that these behavioral changes are significantly more common among children undergoing tonsillectomy and genitourinary surgery (Manley, 1982; Kain et al., 1996c). Finally, positive behavioral changes have also been reported after surgery, particularly in children with chronic conditions (e.g., recurrent otitis media) that have been improved by the surgery (Kain et al., 1996c; Kotiniemi et al., 1996).

The issue of anesthetic techniques (intravenous vs. mask) has not been demonstrated to be a significant predictor of the incidence of postoperative maladaptive behavioral changes (Kotiniemi and Ryhanen, 1996). In addition, the type of anesthetic used (sevoflurane vs. halothane) has not been shown to predict the incidence of postoperative negative behavioral changes (Kain et al., 2005). Although a history of previous surgery predicted increased incidence of postoperative maladaptive behavior in one study, other studies did not confirm this finding (Lumley et al., 1993; Kain et al., 1996c; Kotiniemi et al., 1997b). It is likely that the quality of surgical experiences is a important predictor, not simply the history of surgery. Quality of past medical experience as a predictor of future anxiety of the child has been reported in studies exploring the issue of preoperative anxiety (Kain et al., 1996c).

Interventions

Preparation Programs

The impact of preparation programs on the incidence of postoperative behavioral changes is not clear. Vernon and Thompson (1993) completed a meta-analysis of published studies that evaluated the effects of preoperative behavioral preparation programs on postoperative behavior. The meta-analysis concluded that on the average, children who received preoperative interventions tended to have less postoperative maladaptive behavioral changes than did control subjects. In contrast, Kain et al. (1998a) compared several types of preoperative preparation programs in children and found no effect of preoperative preparation on the incidence of postoperative behavioral changes.

Parental Presence

The impact of parental presence during induction of anesthesia on the incidence of postoperative behavioral changes was evaluated (Kain et al., 1996b). To date, all studies concluded that the presence of a parent during induction does not have an impact on the issue of postoperative behavioral changes (Kain et al., 1996b; Kain, 2000).

Sedatives

Investigations that looked into the association between preoperative sedative premedication and postoperative behavioral changes report contradictory findings. Two investigations report some beneficial effects of premedication on postoperative behavior, but others report no effect (Padfield et al., 1986; Parnis et al., 1992; Payne et al., 1992). Furthermore, an investigation found a higher incidence of negative postoperative behavioral changes in children who were premedicated (McGraw and

Kendrick, 1998). These contradictory results may be explained by the methodologic complexity of this issue. Confounding variables such as the age of the child, surgical procedure, postoperative pain, and recent stressful major life events must be considered. An investigation by Kain and others (1999b) addressed all of these methodologic issues and screened all children for recent stressful life events. The investigators found that a significantly smaller number of children who were premedicated with oral midazolam before surgery demonstrated negative behavioral changes on postoperative days 1 through 7 (Fig. 8-11). Postoperative behaviors that were most improved included apathy and withdrawal, separation anxiety, and eating disturbances. At the second postoperative week, however, there were no significant differences between the placebo and midazolam groups. Thus, it can be concluded that in addition to its significant beneficial preoperative effects, sedative premedication improves immediate postoperative behavioral outcomes in young children undergoing general anesthesia and outpatient surgery.

Clinical Outcomes

Five decades ago, Janis (1958) proposed that moderate levels of preoperative anxiety in adult patients were associated with good postoperative behavioral recovery and that low and high levels of preoperative anxiety were associated with poor behavioral recovery. Although Janis' theory is intriguing, his studies were based on descriptive data from nonrandom, limited samples and retrospective reports of questionable validity. Subsequent studies have been critical of Janis' methodology and have reported a linear rather than a curvilinear relationship between anxiety level and postoperative behavioral recovery (Johnson et al., 1971; Johnston, 1980; Johnston and Carpenter, 1980; Newman, 1984; Pick et al., 1994). That is, low levels of preoperative anxiety are associated with good postoperative behavioral recovery, whereas high levels of preoperative anxiety are associated with poor postoperative behavioral recovery. To date, the literature on adults indicates that intensity of pain, analgesic requirements, postsurgical complications, length of hospital stay,

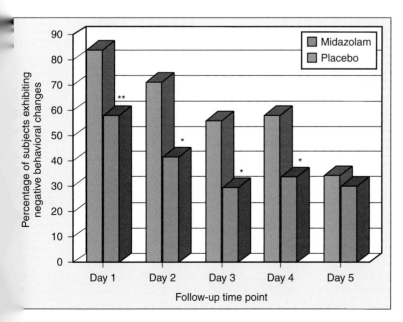

■ **FIGURE 8-11.** The effect of oral midazolam on the incidence of postoperative behavioral outcomes. *(From Kain ZN, Mayes LC, Caramico LA: Postoperative behavioral outcomes in children: effects of sedative premedication,* Anesthesiology *90:758–765, 1999b.)*

poor patient satisfaction, and blood cortisol levels have all been reported to be associated with high levels of preoperative anxiety (Devine, 1992; Johnston and Vogele, 1993; Contrada et al., 1994; Kiecolt-Glaser et al., 1998).

Many reviews of this research have appeared that, although critical of the methodology of a large number of studies, concluded that high preoperative anxiety is associated with impaired postoperative recovery (Mumford et al., 1982; Mathews and Ridgeway, 1984; Rogers and Reich, 1986; Anderson, 1987; Suls and Wan, 1989; Johnston and Wallace, 1990; Kincey and Saltmore, 1990; Devine, 1992; Johnston and Vogele, 1993; Contrada et al., 1994; Kiecolt-Glaser et al., 1998).

The fact that low preoperative anxiety is predictive of good postoperative outcome underlies many interventions in which the aim is to reduce preoperative anxiety. As with the cohort studies described earlier, preparation studies have used diverse postoperative outcome measures, including pain, analgesic requirements, length of hospital stays, patient satisfaction, cortisol levels, blood pressure, heart rate, and behavioral indices of recovery (Mumford et al., 1982; Andersen and Masur, 1983; Mathews and Ridgeway, 1984; Anderson, 1987; Johnston and Vogele, 1993). Reviews of this research concluded that psychologically prepared adult patients have improved postoperative recovery results (Mumford et al., 1982; Suls and Wan, 1989; Johnston and Wallace, 1990; Devine, 1992; Johnston and Vogele, 1993; Contrada et al., 1994; Kiecolt-Glaser et al., 1998).

In contrast to the adult literature, there is a paucity of peer-reviewed, published-outcome data regarding the question of whether heightened preoperative anxiety impairs postoperative recovery in children undergoing surgery. A large-scale study assessed this question with convergent clinical, neuroendocrinologic, and behavioral measures and found that increased preoperative anxiety in children is associated with impaired postoperative behavioral and clinical recovery. Analysis of the data indicated that children who were more anxious preoperatively showed poorer immediate clinical recovery (Kain et al., 2002c). The study also found a significant relationship between preoperative anxiety and postoperative pain and postoperative behavioral recovery. That is, children who were more anxious preoperatively were in more pain postoperatively and had a higher incidence of postoperative behavioral changes. More recently, Kain and colleagues (2004a, 2006a) demonstrated that preoperative anxiety was a predictor of emergence delirium, postoperative anxiety and sleep problems, and new behavioral problems after surgery.

SUMMARY

The perioperative period may be very stressful for the young child undergoing surgery. The fear and anxiety during this period are associated not only with immediate hardship to parents and children but also with outcomes such as parental satisfaction, as well as postoperative behavioral and clinical recovery. In this chapter, a variety of behavioral interventions have been described that can and should be used for the management of anxiety during this perioperative period. Although some interventions, such as preparation programs, are well established, others, such as parental presence, music, and acupuncture, are still under development. The individual clinician should have the knowledge of the risk factors, management, and outcome of this important clinical phenomenon.

REFERENCES

Complete references used in this text can be found online at www.expertconsult.com.

Preoperative Preparation

Elliot J. Krane, Peter J. Davis, and Zeev N. Kain

CHAPTER

9

CONTENTS

In addition to having a sound understanding of a child's medical disease and anticipated surgical procedure, the anesthesiologist must also appreciate the emotional stresses that affect both the child and parent. The preoperative meeting with the patient and his or her parents is not only a responsibility of the anesthesiologist but also an important opportunity to learn facts that could otherwise be missed. It is a chance to win the confidence of the patient and the parents, if they are present (Fig. 9-1).

A careful preoperative examination of the child and the child's medical record enables the anesthesiologist to assess the child's general state of health and to identify the presence of chronic, acute, or intercurrent diseases, as well as to recognize previous anesthetic problems (Black, 1999). From this knowledge, appropriate subspecialty consultation can be sought, the operative medical condition can be optimized for the surgery, and the anesthetic plans can be made. In addition to monitoring practices and anesthetic techniques, anesthetic plans should include provisions for the patient's postoperative care, particularly an analgesic plan. It is the general goal of the preanesthetic visit to anticipate potential complications before they occur, to avert them when possible, and, in so doing, to minimize the risks to the health of the child. The risk of anesthesia is assessed during the preoperative visit, and the child's parents should be informed of the plans for anesthesia and monitoring, and they should be apprised of the anticipated risk.

PREANESTHETIC VISIT

The preanesthetic visit should begin with a careful review of the medical record; particular attention should be paid to previous anesthetic agents and problems encountered, the successful and unsuccessful techniques used in the past for airway management, and any history of cardiorespiratory diseases or airway anomalies. A history of medical or environmental allergies should be elicited, and it should include questions specifically directed toward evaluating the presence of allergy to latex in children at risk, notably those with meningomyelocele or urogenital anomalies, those who undergo bladder self-catheterization, or those whose medical histories indicate a significant amount of latex exposure in the past (Holzman 1997; Porri et al., 1997; Hollnberger et al., 2002; Pires et al., 2002; Eustachio et al., 2003; Dehlink et al., 2009; Rendeli et al., 2006; Bostancy et al., 2007; Dieguez et al., 2007; Garcia 2007; Baker and Hourihane, 2008; De Queiroz et al., 2009). Results of laboratory tests should be reviewed, focusing on hematologic evaluations, renal function, and electrolyte profiles, as well as blood gas analysis and pulmonary function tests when appropriate.

The anesthesiologist must be aware of the child's current drug therapy and how it may interact with the anesthetic. The perioperative administration of bronchodilators, cancer chemotherapeutic agents, or anticholinesterases has significant implications for anesthesia (Schein and Winoker, 1975; Selvin,

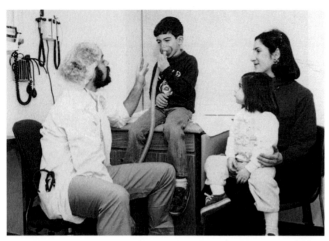

■ **FIGURE 9-1.** An instructive approach to the anesthesia induction can be taken during the preoperative visit, enabling the anesthesiologist to gain the child's trust and confidence.

1981; Drummond, 1984). Corticosteroid administration is traditionally recommended for patients who receive chronic corticosteroid therapy and for patients who have received steroids in the past, although evidence for the necessity of doing so is lacking (see Chapter 36, Systemic Disorders). Current drug therapy must also include questions regarding the use of herbal medications. Potential complications in the perioperative period have been attributed to the use of complementary medicines. Table 9-1 summarizes the most commonly used herbal remedies (Ang-lee et al., 2001).

Many unusual syndromes occur in childhood, and they often have multisystem involvement; consequently, they have an important impact on anesthetic management. An important caveat in pediatric medicine is that when one congenital anomaly exists, there is a significant likelihood of anomalies involving other organs. For example, infants with tracheoesophageal fistulas have an increased incidence of congenital heart disease, and some forms of radial dysplasia are associated with thrombocytopenia or atrial septal defects. The topic of congenital anomalies was extensively discussed in a review by Lynn (1985). The remainder of this section is a review of pediatric diseases that may be important to the anesthesiologist. Information regarding these problems may be forthcoming from the child's medical history, the physical examination, or both.

PHYSICAL EXAMINATION

The extent of the physical examination that the anesthesiologist performs depends on the circumstances. If a small infant scheduled for a minor operation has been crying and has finally dropped off to sleep, one can observe from the bedside the child's general nutritional state, skin color, character of respiration, and presence or absence of nasal discharge. Although the surgeon's or pediatrician's notes are helpful, they should not be a substitute for the anesthesiologist's independent examination.

Certain general principles are applied to the preoperative evaluation. When examining a child, the anesthesiologist should look for somewhat different signs than when examining an adult. Between the ages of 4 and 8 years, children must be examined for loose primary teeth. Finding an empty dental socket after an operation is not disturbing if one knows that the child lost the tooth before admission. There is always the danger of the recent onset of an upper respiratory tract infection with cough, rhinitis, and pharyngitis. If an infant or child has rhinitis, it may be challenging to determine whether it is because of an infection, seasonal allergies, or simply the result of crying. Enlarged cervical nodes and otitis media occur in association

TABLE 9-1. Pharmacologic Effects and Potential Perioperative Complications of Eight Commonly Used Herbal Remedies

Name of Herb	Common Uses	Potential Perioperative Complications
Echinacea, purple cone flower root	Prophylaxis and treatment of viral, bacterial, and fungal infections	Reduced effectiveness of immunosuppressants; potential for wound infection; may cause hepatotoxicity when used with other hepatotoxic drugs
Ephedra, ma-huang	Diet aid	Dose-dependent increase in heart rate and blood pressure; arrhythmias with halothane; tachyphylaxis with intraoperative ephedrine
Garlic, ajo	Antihypertensive, lipid-lowering agent, anti-thrombus forming	May potentiate other platelet inhibitors; perioperative bleeding
Ginkgo, maidenhair; fossil tree	Circulatory stimulant; Alzheimer's disease, peripheral vascular disease, and erectile dysfunction	May potentiate other platelet inhibitors; perioperative bleeding
Ginseng	To protect the body against stress and restore homeostasis	Perioperative bleeding; potential for hypoglycemia
Kavakava, pepper	Anxiolytic	Potentiates sedative effects of anesthetic agents; possible withdrawal syndrome after sudden abstinence; kavakava-induced hepatotoxicity
St. John's wort, goatweek, amber, hardhay	Treatment for depression and anxiety	Decreased effectiveness of cyclosporine, alfentanil, midazolam, lidocaine, calcium channel blockers, and digoxin
Valerian, vandal root, all heal	Anxiolytic and sleep aid	Potentiates sedative effects of anesthetic agents; withdrawal-type syndrome with sudden abstinence

From Skinner CM, Rangasami J: Preoperative use of herbal medicines: a patient survey, *Br J Anaesth* 89:792-795, 2002.

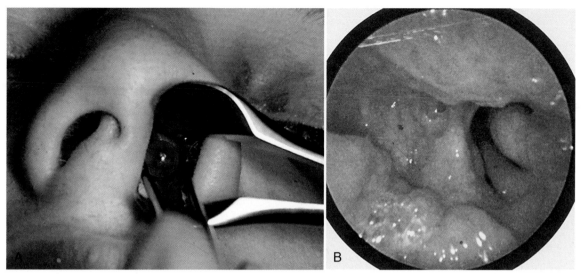

■ **FIGURE 9-2.** Unilateral nasal discharge can be from a foreign body like a bead (**A**), or a unilateral choanal atresia (**B**). *(From Yellon RF, McBride TP, Davis HW: Otolaryngology. In Zitelli J and Davis HW, editors:* Atlas of pediatric physical diagnosis, *ed 5, St Louis, 2007, Mosby.)*

with respiratory tract infections; clear, colorless rhinitis suggests crying or an allergic etiology.

Partial airway obstruction may result from infection, anatomic anomalies, or tumors. When possible, a diagnosis should be made before anesthesia is begun. Unilateral nasal discharge is unusual and suggests a foreign body (or, less often, choanal atresia) (Fig. 9-2).

Whenever possible the anesthesiologist should personally observe or palpate the location and size of the lesion, such as a laceration, tumor, or nevus, that may be the reason for surgery. A tumor may be the size of a pea or a melon, and a nevus may be a spot on a child's elbow or cover half a limb. The anesthesia cannot be planned intelligently without knowledge of these points.

Review of Body Systems (Table 9-2)

Central Nervous System

Disorders of the neuromuscular system only rarely escape notice during the history and review of systems; the purpose of the central nervous system (CNS) examination is primarily to assess the severity of the abnormality and the implications for anesthetic care.

Trauma is the most common cause of death in children, and most fatal trauma involves injury to the CNS. Head injuries often result in an altered level of consciousness, cerebral edema, and elevated intracranial pressure. Tumors of the brain

TABLE 9-2. Medical History and Review of Systems: Anesthetic Implications

System	History	Potential Anesthetic Implication
Central nervous and neuromuscular systems	Seizure	Medications: drug interactions, inadequate anticonvulsant therapy, drug-induced hepatopathology
	Head trauma	Elevated intracranial pressure
		Anemia
	Hydrocephalus	Elevated intracranial pressure
	Central nervous system tumor	Elevated intracranial pressure
		Chemotherapeutic drug interactions
		History of steroid use
	Developmental delay	Bulbar dysfunction
		Risk of aspiration
	Neuromuscular disease	Altered response to relaxants
	Muscle disease	Risk of malignant hyperthermia
		Risk of rhabdomyolysis and hyperkalemia
Cardiovascular system	Heart murmur	Risk of right-to-left air embolism of intravenous air bubbles
		Need for SBE prophylaxis
	Cyanotic heart defect	Right-to-left cardiac shunt
		Risk of right-to-left air embolism of intravenous air bubbles
		Hemoconcentration
		Need for SBE prophylaxis
	History of squatting	Teratology of Fallot
	Diaphoresis with feeding or crying	Congestive heart failure
	Hypertension	Coarctation of the aorta, renal disease, or pheochromacytoma

Continued

TABLE 9-2. Medical History and Review of Systems: Anesthetic Implications—cont'd

System	History	Potential Anesthetic Implication
Respiratory system	Prematurity	Increased risk of postoperative apnea
	Bronchopulmonary dysplasia	Lower airway obstruction
		Reactive airways disease
		Subglottic stenosis
		Pulmonary hypertension
	Respiratory infection, cough	Reactive airways and bronchospasm
	Croup	Medication history
	Snoring	Subglottic stenosis or anomaly
		Obstructive sleep apnea
		Perioperative airway obstruction
	Asthma	β-Agonist or theophylline therapy
		History of steroid use
	Cystic fibrosis	Drug interactions
		Pulmonary toilet
		Pulmonary dysfunction and VQ mismatch
		Reactive airways disease
Gastrointestinal/hepatic systems	Vomiting, diarrhea	Electrolyte abnormality, especially hypokalemia
		Dehydration
		Risk of aspiration
	Growth failure	Low glycogen reserves/risk of hypoglycemia
		Anemia
	Gastroesophageal reflux	Risk of aspiration
		Reactive airways disease
		Anemia
	Jaundice	Altered drug metabolism
		Risk of hypoglycemia
		Coagulopathy
	Liver transplant recipient	Altered drug metabolism
		Immunosuppression
		Coagulopathy
Renal system	Frequency, nocturia	Occult diabetes mellitus
		Electrolyte disturbance
		Urinary sepsis
	Renal failure/dialysis	Electrolyte disturbance
		Hypervolemia or hypovolemia
		Anemia
		Medication history
	Kidney transplant recipient	Immunosuppression
		Poor toleration of hypotension
		Hypertension
Endocrine system	Diabetes	Insulin requirement
		Intraoperative hyperglycemia or hypoglycemia
	Steroid therapy	Adrenocorticoid suppression
Genitourinary system	Pregnancy	Teratogenic effects
		Risk of spontaneous abortion
Hematologic system	Anemia	Transfusion requirement
		Occult hemoglobinopathy
	Bruising, history of bleeding	Coagulopathy
	Sickle cell disease	Anemia
		Need for hydration
		Limb tourniquet use
	Human immunodeficiency virus infection	Susceptibility to infection
		Infectious risk to medical personnel
Dental system	Loose primary teeth	Risk of aspiration if tooth avulsed

Modified from Coté CJ, Todres ID, Ryan JF: Preoperative evaluation of pediatric patients. In Ryan JF, Todres ID, Coté CJ, et al., editors: *A practice of anesthesia for infants and children,* New York, 1986, Grune & Stratton. (With permission from Elsevier.)
SBE, Subacute bacterial endocarditis; *VQ,* ventilation perfusion.

are the most common solid tumors of childhood and usually occur in the posterior fossa. They generally increase intracranial pressure as a mass effect but also often obstruct cerebrospinal fluid pathways, resulting in hydrocephalus. The anesthetic care of children with elevated intracranial pressure is discussed in Chapter 22, Anesthesia for Neurosurgery.

To ensure both therapeutic levels and the absence of toxic levels, serum levels of certain anticonvulsant drugs should be measured or should have been measured before elective surgery in children with chronic seizure disorders. Most anticonvulsants have a long plasma half-life; therefore, missing one dose in the perioperative period does not significantly diminish the serum level and efficacy. Of the commonly used anticonvulsants, only phenobarbital, phenytoin, or valproate may be given intravenously in the perioperative period. Other commonly administered anticonvulsants, however, such as gabapentin, pregabalin, levatiracetam, or lamotrigene, are available only as oral medications. If a prolonged period without oral intake is anticipated (such as after abdominal surgery), a neurologist should be consulted about possible alternative parenteral drug therapy.

Conditions such as developmental delay and spastic cerebral palsy have important implications for anesthesia. In such children, the response to opioids and anesthetic agents is less predictable than that with healthy children. Many patients with cerebral palsy or intellectual impairment have difficulty managing oral secretions, and gastroesophageal reflux is particularly common in these children. They are at a greater risk of aspirating oral or gastric contents during induction. Cerebral palsy in older children often produces restrictive lung disease as a result of deformities of the spine and thoracic cage and from uncoordinated respiratory muscle function.

Neuromuscular diseases, such as congenital myotonia, muscular dystrophy, and the various forms of myositis, contraindicate the use of succinylcholine even in emergency airway management, although it is rarely used in current pediatric anesthetic practice (see Chapter 36, Systemic Disorders). In myotonia, succinylcholine produces a sustained contracture of skeletal muscle that may impede the ability to maintain a patent airway and ventilate the lungs. In other myopathies, such as clinically active dermatomyositis, succinylcholine produces life-threatening hyperkalemia. Some forms of muscular dystrophy (central core disease) are statistically associated with malignant hyperthermia, whereas others may result in a malignant hyperthermia-like syndrome that is equally life threatening (Guis et al., 2004; Rosenberg et al., 2007; Driessen and Snoeck, 2008; Hayes et al., 2008; Puel et al., 2008; Takagi and Nakase, 2008; Schwartz and Raghunathan, 2009). Although not all children with Duchenne's or other muscular dystrophies are genetically susceptible, Rosenberg and Heiman-Patterson (1983), as well as Takagi and Nakase (2008), recommend that precautions against malignant hyperthermia be taken in patients with this disorder because of rhabdomyolysis and hypermetabolism that may occur in myopathic children after exposure to triggering agents. For further discussion please refer to Chapter 37, Malignant Hyperthermia.

Cardiovascular System

Evaluation of the cardiovascular system is critical to the delivery of safe anesthesia. The physical examination seldom reveals an unexpected CNS lesion, but a careful history and auscultation of the child's chest often reveal a congenital cardiac lesion that may be unknown to the parents or the child's surgeon.

The history-and-systems review yields information regarding known cardiac anomalies of an acquired disease, cyanotic defects, or the presence of congestive heart failure. Symptoms of congestive heart failure may be insidious. In an infant, whose level of activity is not high, the symptoms of congestive heart failure or cyanosis are most likely limited to a few times of physical exertion, such as feeding and crying, and the only symptoms of congestive heart failure may be pallor and diaphoresis, which are subtle findings. Parents should be asked about diaphoresis during nursing or sucking. Resting

tachypnea and failure to thrive are also consequences of more advanced degrees of congestive heart failure, which may be the result of ventricular volume overload (most commonly, a ventricular septal defect, patent ductus arteriosus, or anomalous pulmonary venous return), either right- or left-sided outflow obstruction, or pulmonary hypertension.

Preoperative evaluation of a patient with a known or suspected heart defect that is physiologically significant should include a thorough history and physical examination; an electrocardiogram (ECG) and echocardiogram; determination of hematocrit value, a baseline oxygen saturation value (SpO_2); a chest radiograph; and a definitive understanding of the type of cardiac lesion, its degree of severity, and its physiologic effect on cardiac efficiency and oxygen delivery. Such patients should be examined meticulously and should not be accepted for anesthesia until they are in the best possible physical condition. For children with compromising lesions or those requiring cardiac medication, it is advisable to consult the cardiologist shortly before surgery.

The presence of polycythemia is uncommon in modern clinical practice but still should be ruled out in children with cyanotic heart disease; a hematocrit value of greater than 65% may be reduced by red blood cell pheresis or isovolemic hemodilution. Dehydration must be avoided, preferably through the use of controlled intravenous hydration beginning the night before surgery or by following the *nil per os* (NPO) guidelines and ensuring adequate oral intake of clear liquids up until 2 hours before surgery.

Particular care must be taken to rule out the existence of any infection, especially in the throat, ears, skin, or genitourinary tract. Bacteremia and infections of the teeth or gums should be controlled with appropriate antibiotics. The preoperative occurrence of fever or rhinitis or a significant preoperative exposure to a source of infection should be considered a possible indication for postponement of the operation.

Asymptomatic cardiac murmurs occasionally have implications for anesthesia. If they represent small ventricular septal defects or mild valvular disease, prophylaxis against bacterial endocarditis is indicated for procedures that may result in bacteremia, such as dental surgery, gastrointestinal or urogenital endoscopy, and nasotracheal intubation (Wilson et al., 2007). Atrial septal defects contraindicate the use of the sitting position for suboccipital craniotomies in order to minimize the risk of paradoxical air embolism (Fischler, 1992). The defects may also make intraoperative transesophageal echocardiography desirable in certain cases that have been associated with venous air embolism (e.g., posterior spine fusions or liver transplantation), so the movement of air from the pulmonary to the systemic circulation may be detected. If the anesthesiologist detects a previously undescribed murmur in these circumstances, a consultation with the cardiologist is indicated to further delineate the nature of the lesion (Fig. 9-3). Many congenital anomalies and syndromes are associated with cardiac defects or other cardiovascular problems; Box 9-1 provides an outline of these conditions.

Respiratory System

Chapter 3, Respiratory Physiology in Infants and Children, describes the anatomic and physiologic differences between the pediatric and adult respiratory systems. The differences in dimension and function predispose the child to perioperative airway

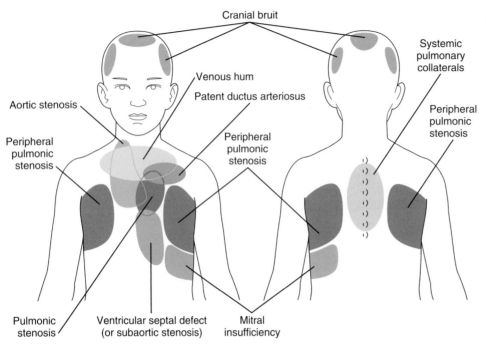

■ **FIGURE 9-3.** Sites for auscultation where murmurs are heard best. *(From Beerman LB, Kreutzer J, Park SC: Cardiology. In Zitelli J, Davis HW, editors: Atlas of pediatric physical diagnosis, ed 5, St Louis, 2007, Mosby.)*

Box 9-1 Pediatric Syndromes Associated with Cardiac Conditions

SYNDROMES ASSOCIATED WITH CONGENITAL HEART DISEASE
Apert's syndrome
Asplenia syndrome (Ivemark's syndrome)
Conradi's syndrome
DiGeorge's syndrome
Down syndrome (trisomy 21)
Edwards' syndrome (trisomy 18)
Ellis-van Creveld syndrome
Goldenhar's syndrome
Holt-Oram syndrome
I-cell disease
Laurence-Moon-Biedl syndrome
LEOPARD syndrome (multiple lentigines syndrome)
Marfan syndrome
Meckel's syndrome
Noonan's syndrome
Patau's syndrome (trisomy 13)
Polysplenia
Rubinstein's syndrome
Sebaceous nevi syndrome
TAR syndrome (thrombocytopenia-absent radius syndrome)
VACTERL (vertebral, anal, cardiac, tracheal, esophageal, renal, and limb) association
VATER (vertebral defects, imperforate anus, tracheoesophageal fistula, radial and renal dysplasia) association
Williams syndrome

SYNDROMES ASSOCIATED WITH CARDIOMYOPATHY
Cretinism
Duchenne's muscular dystrophy

Farber's disease
Friedreich's ataxia
Hunter's syndrome
Hurler's syndrome
Maroteaux-Lamy syndrome
Myotonic dystrophy
McArdle's disease
Pompe's disease
Stevens-Johnson syndrome

SYNDROMES ASSOCIATED WITH AUTONOMIC DYSFUNCTION OR ARRHYTHMIAS
Albright's osteodystrophy
Guillain-Barré syndrome
Jervell and Lange-Nielsen syndrome
Riley-Day syndrome
Shy-Drager syndrome
Short QT syndrome
Sipple's syndrome
Wolff-Parkinson-White syndrome

SYNDROMES ASSOCIATED WITH THROMBOSES OR ISCHEMIC HEART DISEASE
Ehlers-Danlos syndrome
Fabry's disease
Grönblad-Strandberg syndrome
Homocystinuria
Progeria
Tangier disease
Werner's syndrome

obstruction, which mandates a critical preoperative evaluation of the airway. The upper airway of the child may be further compromised by many entities, including: tonsillar or adenoidal hypertrophy or both; craniofacial anomalies such as Crouzon's disease, Apert's syndrome, hemifacial microsomia, Goldenhar's syndrome, Treacher Collins syndrome (or Pierre Robin syndrome); lingular hypertrophy (common in trisomy 21); Beckwith's syndrome and the various forms of mucopolysaccharidosis (Hurler's syndrome and Hunter's syndrome being the most common); isolated airway anomalies, such as cleft palate, laryngeal web cleft, laryngomalacia, or subglottic stenosis; or tumors, such as hemangiomas and lymphangiomas, which may occur anywhere along the airway. Cutaneous cervicofacial hemangiomas along a beard distribution are suggestive of an association with upper airway or subglottic hemangiomas (Orlo et al., 1997).

Acute upper respiratory tract infections provide a common dilemma for the anesthesiologist. The mere volume of publications that evaluate the risk of adverse events of anesthesia in children with upper airway infections speaks to the ongoing controversy (Tait and Malviya, 2005). In the best of all worlds, no child would be anesthetized electively during an acute respiratory illness. Although not all studies have identified acute respiratory illness as a cause of perioperative complications in children, there is compelling evidence that the occurrence of both intraoperative and postoperative hypoxemia and other airway complications are increased in children with upper respiratory tract infections (DeSoto et al., 1988; Cohen and Cameron, 1991; Kinouchi et al., 1992; Levy et al., 1992; Rolf and Coté, 1992; Parnis et al., 2001; Bordet et al., 2002; Elwood et al., 2003; Tait, 2005). There is also evidence that the incidence of bronchospasm is increased in the presence of upper respiratory infections in children who are intubated (Rolf and Coté, 1992; Rachel Homer et al., 2007; von Ungern-Sternberg et al., 2007). In a prospective study, Tait and colleagues (2001) noted that endotracheal intubation, a history of prematurity, reactive airways disease, parental smoking, airway surgery, and nasal congestion are all risk factors associated with respiratory complications in infants and children who have upper respiratory infections and who are undergoing anesthesia. Furthermore, the child with an acute respiratory disease exposes other patients and health care workers to their contagion, which may not be a trivial concern when these individuals are immunocompromised.

Other considerations, however, must be taken into account before making the decision to postpone surgery. For example, the relatively small risk to the child must be weighed against the expense and effort the family has made to come to the hospital, often from a distant locale and at the cost of lost income. Some children, particularly those seen for otolaryngologic surgery, appear to never be free from respiratory infections during much of the year. Postponement of surgery may not be practical in these circumstances. Indeed, one study indicates that myringotomy is therapeutic in these children and is not associated with an increased incidence of postoperative pulmonary complications (Tait and Knight, 1987).

The presence of acute disease of the lower airways, however, should generally delay elective surgery. The presence of fever, cough, and an abnormal auscultatory examination is reason for radiographic evaluation and possibly cancellation of scheduled surgery. Patients with a viral lower respiratory tract infection such as influenza may develop airway hyperreactivity that is indistinguishable from bronchial asthma and can last as long as 6 or 7 weeks from onset.

Chronic diseases of the lower respiratory tract occur in both children and adults. Asthma and cystic fibrosis are the most common chronic pulmonary diseases of childhood. A careful history and physical examination usually suffice in the preoperative evaluation of these diseases. If preoperative impairment is severe, however, or if the planned surgery is extensive, formal pulmonology consultation and pulmonary function testing may provide the anesthesiologist with information that can be used to provide optimal postoperative care. Children with asthma are commonly medicated with β_2-adrenergic agents

and inhaled corticosteroids. Other first-line drugs include cromolyn sodium and leukotriene receptor antagonists; rarely are theophylline preparations administered at this time. However, when theophylline is a part of the patient's treatment, serum concentration of theophylline should be measured preoperatively to ensure blood levels in a therapeutic range (10-20 mcg/mL), and the anesthesiologist should be aware of potential interactions among theophylline, β_2-adrenergic drugs, and halothane (although it is not often used). Asthmatic children who receive corticosteroids should also be considered for perioperative therapy with stress doses of corticosteroids if steroid therapy has been recent, although as previously stated, the evidence to support this convention is lacking. For those children who have required systemic steroids in the past, a short course of steroids beginning 1 to 2 days before the day of surgery may be beneficial (see Chapter 36, Systemic Disorders).

Severe kyphoscoliosis typically leads to significant restrictive lung disease. This is particularly true in cases of kyphoscoliosis that occur before the teenage years. Particularly in this age group, the cause of the kyphoscoliosis should be assessed, because it typically results from neuromuscular diseases such as cerebral palsy or muscular dystrophy or from anatomic anomalies such as hemivertebrae, which may be part of a syndrome that is associated with other congenital anomalies of importance to the anesthesiologist (e.g., VATER association). Preoperative testing of pulmonary function may be useful in predicting which children will require admission to an intensive care unit with or without mechanical ventilation postoperatively, but usually the decision to mechanically ventilate patients after spinal surgery is based on general preoperative condition, duration and difficulty of surgery, blood loss, and other surgical factors, rather than on the test of pulmonary function itself (see Chapter 26, Anesthesia for Orthopedic Surgery).

An infant who was born prematurely is often left with a residual chronic obstructive pulmonary disease called *bronchopulmonary dysplasia,* the consequence of both oxygen toxicity and ventilator-induced lung injury to immature lungs. The incidence and severity of this disabling condition have been dramatically reduced by the use of surfactant in neonatal intensive care units. Children with bronchopulmonary dysplasia exhibit a combination of fibrotic and cystic changes in the lung parenchyma with reactive small airways disease, with or without wheezing and air trapping. These children may respond to steroids and bronchodilators in varying degrees. More advanced bronchopulmonary dysplasia is associated with chronic hypoxia, carbon dioxide retention, pulmonary hypertension, and ultimately *cor pulmonale* (Berman et al., 1982).

As in the adult with chronic pulmonary disease, elective surgery is best delayed until preoperative cardiopulmonary function has been optimized. Children with severe bronchopulmonary dysplasia are usually treated with diuretics to reduce extravascular lung water; consequently, abnormal serum electrolyte levels are common preoperatively (e.g., hypokalemia, hypochloremia, or metabolic alkalosis). Arterial saturation should be maximized at all times to reduce pulmonary hypertension, and perioperative bronchodilator therapy should be considered. Alterations in anesthetic care include: judicious, if any, use of nitrous oxide to avoid exacerbation of pulmonary gas trapping and pulmonary vascular resistance; very conservative fluid therapy and restriction of sodium; and continuation of bronchodilator therapy. Postoperative mechanical ventilation may be required in this population.

Life-threatening apnea and bradycardia may occur after general anesthesia, most commonly in the preterm infant who is still younger than 45 weeks' or as old as 60 weeks' postconceptional age (the sum of gestational age and postnatal age) (Liu et al., 1980; Kurth et al., 1986; Wellborn et al., 1986). Hospital admission and respiratory monitoring are necessary for infants at risk, even after brief general anesthesia. Risk factors for postoperative apnea in preterm infants include: a history of mechanical ventilation, history of apnea and bradycardia, and anemia at the time of surgery (Kurth and LeBard, 1991; Wellborn et al., 1991; Spear, 1992; Malviya et al., 1993; Coté et al., 1995). In a meta-analysis of eight studies, Coté et al. (1995) reported that the postconceptual age required to reduce the risk of postoperative apnea to 1% was 54 weeks for infants born at 35 weeks' gestation and 56 weeks for infants born before 32 weeks' gestation. For further information, see Chapter 17, Neonatology for Anesthesiologists, Figure 17-10.

Congenital diseases of the lungs are usually recognized and surgically corrected in the newborn period. These conditions and their anesthetic management are discussed in Chapters 18 and 23, Anesthesia for General Surgery in the Neonate, and Anesthesia for General Abdominal, Thoracic, Urologic, and Bariatric Surgery.

Gastrointestinal System

The primary concern of the anesthesiologist is to assess the integrity of the gastroesophageal sphincter, the emptiness of the stomach, and, hence, the risk of aspiration on induction of or emergence from anesthesia. Gastroesophageal reflux occurs as an isolated entity in some otherwise healthy infants. Parents describe regular spitting up after meals, and there may be a history of recurrent lower respiratory tract infections, small airways disease, wheezing, or esophagitis that points to the diagnosis. Gastroesophageal reflux is very common in the child with developmental delays. After repair of tracheoesophageal fistulas, abnormalities of esophageal motility and decreased competence of the gastroesophageal sphincter are often present, increasing the risks of vomiting and aspiration on induction of anesthesia. Children who fall into these categories should be considered to have a "full stomach."

Renal System

Renal failure is uncommon in childhood. Chronic renal failure is typically managed with either peritoneal dialysis or, in the older child, hemodialysis. The evaluation of the child with preoperative renal disease includes serial measurements of blood pressure to assess the adequacy of antihypertensive therapy; careful determination of vascular volume; and measurement of serum levels of electrolytes, urea nitrogen, creatinine, phosphate, calcium, and magnesium, as well as hematocrit value. Electrolyte levels should be within a reasonably normal range; if significant derangement exists, additional electrolyte therapy or dialysis should be performed before elective surgery. The acceptable lower limit of hematocrit is generally considered to be about 20% with chronic renal failure. Such an assumption of adaptation, however, is controversial because the blood levels of 2,3-diphosphoglycerate in these children are not necessarily increased, depending on the chronicity of anemia or recent history of dialysis.

Milder degrees of renal dysfunction may also affect anesthetic care. In small children with mild or moderate underlying renal disease, clinically significant hypervolemia may occur without compensation by augmented urine output, and an excessive sodium or free-water load further deranges the serum electrolyte level. Particular caution is important in the management of fluids in children, and central venous pressure monitoring is required during major surgery in which significant blood loss or fluid shifts are anticipated (see Chapter 5, Regulation of Fluids and Electrolytes).

Hematologic System

Underlying disorders of the hematologic system are not common. The systems review should include an inquiry into unusual bleeding in the family's or child's medical history to explore possible genetic coagulopathies. A report of excessive bleeding from a circumcision or tonsillectomy should raise the possibility of thrombocytopenia, von Willebrand's disease, or one of the inherited factor deficiencies and is a reason to measure platelet count, bleeding time, and coagulation time (see Chapter 36, Systemic Disorders).

Sickle cell disease typically produces no symptoms in early childhood, so a systems review is unlikely to detect its presence. For this reason, children of African heritage should be screened for sickle cell disease before surgery. A positive result should be followed by a hemoglobin electrophoresis to confirm the diagnosis or to define other hemoglobinopathies. The anesthetic plan may then be altered to ensure preoperative and postoperative hydration and to provide a high concentration of inspired oxygen. To prevent ischemia and subsequent sickling in the operated limb, the use of a tourniquet during orthopedic surgery is contraindicated when sickle cell disease or trait is present. This has become controversial, however.

In a report by the Preoperative Transfusion in Sickle Cell Disease Study Group, aggressive treatment (transfusion to a hemoglobin S level of less than 30%) was compared with a more conservative management regimen (hemoglobin maintained at 10 g/dL). The conservative approach was equally as effective as the aggressive approach in preventing serious complications but was associated with half the number of transfusion-associated complications (Vichinsky et al., 1995). A hematologic consultation should be sought or institutional protocols be developed for children with hemoglobinopathies who are undergoing anesthesia (see Chapter 36, Systemic Disorders).

THE CHILD WITH PHYSICAL OR MENTAL DISABILITIES

One of the most important principles in dealing with all types of physically and/or mentally disabled children is to be considerate. In any situation involving the care of patients with disabilities, it is appropriate to show appreciation for the position of the families and the dedication they show and deprivation they endure, usually with remarkably little complaint. It is often inspiring to learn about their abilities to cope with misfortune.

Brain Damage

Children who survive severe hypoxic or traumatic brain damage and children with postinfectious encephalopathy may need to undergo various surgical procedures. Preoperative evaluation should include determination of the type and degree of the original neurologic lesion and the patient's present neurologic status. Patients with severe neurologic lesions may depend on implanted ventriculoperitoneal shunts, and shunt patency should be ensured before the administration of anesthesia. Signs and symptoms of a blocked shunt include an abnormally low or high heart rate or blood pressure, headache, vomiting, irritability, and drowsiness. At some point in the child's past, pulmonary management may have required a tracheostomy, which, if still present, may simplify the induction of anesthesia. However, if the patient was decannulated in the past, the upper airway may have been rendered stenotic.

Because they may have difficulty swallowing, these patients often aspirate secretions, and atelectasis or pneumonia may develop. Consequently, a chest radiograph may be indicated to determine the presence and degree of ventilatory compromise. The same patients commonly have gastrostomy tubes for feeding, which should be identified, drained before the induction of anesthesia, and then left open throughout the operative period to prevent gastric distension.

Old injuries, strictures, flexions, deformities, and scars should be noted, with careful descriptions made of signs of recent injuries, pressure sores, or self-inflicted scratches and marks that might otherwise be attributed to anesthetic care. During anesthesia, added care is taken to protect all parts of the body from abnormal pressure and positioning.

Cerebral Palsy

Special consideration is needed when caring for patients with the diagnosis of cerebral palsy, spastic diplegia, or quadriplegia (Nolan et al., 2000). Inexperienced personnel commonly make the serious mistake of assuming that patients with spastic diplegia or quadriplegia also suffer from cognitive impairment, which may not be true. *Cerebral palsy* is a general term applied to several different forms of neuromuscular disability, arising from various anatomic lesions of the brain and not always involving intellectual impairment (Stiles, 1981). The treatment of patients with cerebral palsy should include careful assessment of their level of intelligence. When in doubt, as with all patients who have difficulty communicating, one should assume that they can both hear and understand what is said.

Developmental Delay, Cognitive Dysfunction, and Psychological Disorders

The term *mental retardation* is one of the broadest in medicine, encompassing many different forms, and it is pejorative in its tone. The anesthesiologist is encouraged to use more sensitive terminology, such as *cognitive dysfunction, developmental delay,* or *intellectual impairment,* to name a few more acceptable terms. Trisomy 21 (or other trisomies), autism, and phenylketonuria are well-known forms of this affliction; information on more obscure forms may be found in special texts, such as that of Katz and Steward (1993). Developmental delays that are genetic bear no specific outward stigmata or congenital anomalies, and anesthesia is adapted to the child's level of consciousness and cooperation. Trisomy 21 and other chromosomal forms of intellectual impairment are often associated with congenital heart defects, as well as other congenital organ defects. Trisomy 21 is

also commonly associated with blunting of the styloid process of the second cervical vertebra, which combined with the ligamental laxity of the syndrome allows atlanto-occipital subluxation, or dislocation on marked flexion of the head and neck, resulting in spinal cord injury (Moore et al., 1987; Williams et al., 1987) For more on this subject, see Chapter 36, Systemic Disorders.

Children with autism are difficult to deal with and are sometimes wildly resistant to any intervention. These patients may appear to be remarkably alert, but they also appear to be locked within themselves. The management of the autistic child must be individualized to the dynamics particular to each child's circumstances (Rainey et al., 1998; van der Walt and Moran, 2001). As for other intellectually impaired children, the presence of a parent at induction often has a soothing effect. Premedication with oral midazolam or clonidine is often effective for sedating these children and improving cooperation.

Hyperactivity and Lack of Cooperation

Hyperactive, aggressive, resistant, and uncooperative children offer challenging situations to the anesthesiologist. Such attitudes are seen in pure behavioral syndromes without developmental handicaps, as well as in various forms of neurologic disease or posthypoxic encephalopathy.

The history is carefully reviewed to determine the extent of the hyperactivity and factors that affect the behavior. Parents or attendants are questioned as to which approaches have succeeded in the past and which have not. Trial-and-error methods are not advisable. Oral premedication with midazolam, clonidine, or ketamine may be helpful. Intramuscular ketamine (2 to 4 mg/kg) may be used as a last resort (Hannallah and Patel, 1989).

DRUG ABUSE IN THE CHILD AND ADOLESCENT

Abuse of illicit drugs is unfortunately not limited to adults. Drugs such as cocaine, marijuana, and lysergic acid diethylamide (LSD) are of social and medical concerns. In 1993, about 1 in 3 high school seniors in the United States (35.5%) had used marijuana in their lifetime (Fig. 9-4) (Johnston et al., 1994). A survey of schoolchildren in Great Britain showed that 15.8% of boys have been offered the drug Ecstasy and that 5.7% have

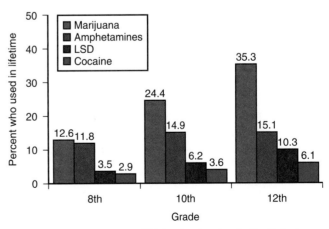

■ **FIGURE 9-4.** Percentage of high school seniors in the United States who have used marijuana and other illegal substances in their lifetime.

taken it (Milroy, 1999). A survey among college students in Great Britain indicated that the most commonly used drugs are marijuana (59%), amphetamines (19%), cocaine (18%), and LSD (18%) (Christophersen, 2000). Because drug abuse may result in increased morbidity and mortality, a thorough understanding of the consequences of drug abuse is essential for the practicing anesthesiologist.

Cocaine

Cocaine is an alkaloid derived from the leaves of the South American shrub, *Erythroxylum coca*. Cocaine can be abused via every possible route, including oral, nasal, intravenous, and rectal. The hydrochloride form can be chemically altered to the base form, which is then concentrated by extraction in ether or baking soda (Perez-Reyes et al., 1982; Fleming et al., 1990). The residue from this method is a form of cocaine base commonly called *crack* (based on the cracking sounds it makes when heated) (Fleming et al., 1990; Julien, 1994). High levels of cocaine may persist in a person for 6 hours after nasal administration (Inaba et al., 1978). The metabolism of cocaine occurs primarily through plasma and hepatic cholinesterase, and patients with pseudocholinesterase deficiency are at increased risk for cocaine toxicity. Less than 5% of ingested cocaine is excreted unchanged in the urine (Inaba et al., 1978). Ecgonine methyl ester and benzoylecgonine constitute over 80% of cocaine metabolites and are detected in the urine for 14 to 60 hours after cocaine use.

Medical Complications

Myocardial ischemia and infarction have been described among young cocaine users with no other known cardiac risk factors (Box 9-2) (Mittleman et al., 1999; Feldman et al., 2000). The pathophysiologic basis for cocaine-related cardiac effects is not clear, and multiple mechanisms have been postulated, including increases in myocardial oxygen demand, accelerated atherosclerosis, thrombus formation, coronary vasospasm and vasoconstriction, and abnormally enhanced platelet aggregation (Pitts et al., 1997). Endothelin-1, a potent vasoconstrictor, is released by cocaine and may play a significant role in vasospastic angina, acute myocardial infarction, and sudden cardiac death (Wilbert-Lampen et al., 1998). Cocaine abuse has also been associated with ventricular hypertrophy, myocardial depression, and cardiomyopathy (Ghuran and Nolan, 2000). Dysrhythmias associated with cocaine use include sinus tachycardia, ventricular premature contractions, ventricular tachycardia or fibrillation, and asystole (Mouhaffel et al., 1995). Dilated cardiomyopathy, myocarditis, and congestive heart failure have also been reported secondary to cocaine use (Kloner et al., 1992; Mouhaffel et al., 1995). In addition, there is an increased incidence of hemorrhagic cerebrovascular accidents in patients who abuse cocaine (Brust, 1993). The smoking of crack cocaine produces alteration in pulmonary function, as would be expected.

Anesthetic Management

Identification of the cocaine user during the preoperative assessment presents a special challenge to the anesthesiologist, because self-reporting of drug abuse is notoriously unreliable. The nasal mucosa may show signs of ulceration. Extremities should be examined for sclerosis of peripheral veins and needle

Box 9-2 Medical Complications of Cocaine Abuse

Cardiac
Myocardial ischemia/infarction
Arrhythmias
Cardiomyopathy
Myocardial depression
Neurologic complications
Seizures
Cerebral infarctions
Subarachnoid hemorrhage
Intracerebral bleed
Obstetric complications
Preterm labor
Premature rupture of membranes
Abruptio placentae
Precipitate delivery
Sudden infant death syndrome
Pediatric complications
Prematurity
Congenital anomalies
Neurobehavioral abnormalities
Partial ankyloglossia
Necrotizing enterocolitis
Pulmonary complications
Cocaine-induced asthma
Hypersensitivity pneumonitis
Chronic cough
Pulmonary edema
Pneumothorax
Pulmonary hemorrhage

marks from intravenous injections. Auscultation over the lungs is important to exclude cocaine-induced asthma, and a careful cardiovascular and neurologic examination is necessary (Fleming et al., 1990; Kain and Rosenbaum, 1994).

When cocaine use is suspected or confirmed, preoperative laboratory tests include: complete blood cell count with a platelet count to rule out thrombocytopenia; ECG to identify signs of rhythm disturbance or myocardial ischemia; chest radiography to rule out any pulmonary or cardiac involvement; and abdominal radiography—cocaine and heroin addicts may experience pseudo-obstruction.

Induction and Maintenance of Anesthesia

Of concern is that ketamine should be used with extreme caution in these patients because it can markedly potentiate the cardiovascular toxicity of cocaine. Because both cocaine and succinylcholine undergo metabolism by plasma cholinesterase, the use of succinylcholine may result in prolonged paralysis, an increased anesthetic requirement for volatile anesthetics may be present in the acutely intoxicated patient, and the temperature rise and sympathomimetic effects associated with cocaine can mimic malignant hyperthermia (MH), so it may be difficult to differentiate between the MH and the influence of cocaine.

Acutely Intoxicated Patient

General stabilization and hemodynamic control should precede induction of anesthesia. Propranolol was used successfully in the past to treat the β-adrenergic cardiac effects of cocaine

(Fleming et al., 1990). Propranolol may worsen coronary vasoconstriction and should not be used if the patient is experiencing chest pain. Intravenous nitroglycerin, which has been shown to reverse both cocaine-induced hypertension and coronary vasoconstriction, may be the preferable drug. Furthermore, Brogan et al. (1991) reported that sublingual nitroglycerin, in a dose sufficient to reduce the mean arterial pressure by 10% to 15%, reverses cocaine-induced coronary artery vasoconstriction. Labetalol, hydralazine, and esmolol have been documented to adequately control cocaine-induced hypertension (Hollander, 1995).

Clinical experience and experimental evidence support the use of benzodiazepines as a first-line treatment for cocaine-intoxicated patients (Hollander, 1995). In addition to anxiolytic effects, benzodiazepines may lower blood pressure and heart rate, thereby decreasing myocardial oxygen consumption. Benzodiazepines are recommended for patients who are experiencing cocaine-associated chest pain and cardiac ischemic changes, as well as for patients who are having convulsions. In addition, although no clinical data exist to support the use of acetylsalicylic acid (aspirin) in patients with cocaine-associated ischemia, some experimental evidence supports the use of aspirin (Rezkalla et al., 1993).

Amphetamine-Related Designer Drugs

The term *designer drugs* includes compounds that have been chemically altered from federally controlled substances to produce special effects and to bypass legal regulation. The largest group consists of the methylenedioxy derivatives of amphetamine and methamphetamine. Amphetamine designer drugs produce indirect sympathetic activation by releasing norepinephrine, dopamine, and serotonin from terminals in the central and autonomic central nervous system (Albertson et al., 1999; Christophersen, 2000). The best known and most widely used designer drug is 3,4-methylenedioxymethamphetamine (MDMA, or Ecstasy), which chemically resembles a combination of amphetamine and mescaline (Milroy, 1999). The drug can be ingested orally, injected, smoked, or snorted. The onset of action is directly related to the route of administration, and for an oral dose, onset usually occurs in 20 to 45 minutes and lasts up to 6 hours (Milroy, 1999). Ecstasy is metabolized by the liver and excreted by the kidneys.

Most people who use Ecstasy experience no complications, but a number of deaths have occurred as a result of hyperthermia or idiosyncratic reactions to the drug. The most commonly seen reaction to severe or toxic ingestion of Ecstasy is a syndrome of altered mental status, tachycardia, tachypnea, profuse sweating, and hyperthermia (Henry, 2000). This constellation of symptoms closely resembles that caused by acute amphetamine overdose, which is not surprising given the chemical similarity of MDMA. Reported severe complications from ingestion of Ecstasy include hyperthermia, rhabdomyolysis, renal failure, cardiovascular collapse, disseminated intravascular coagulation, hepatic failure, hyponatremia, urinary retention, cerebral infarct, and cerebral hemorrhage (Hall, 1997a; Milroy, 1999; Ghuran and Nolan, 2000; Henry, 2000; Reneman et al., 2000). Liver damage was recognized among the first deaths in the United Kingdom and seems to be a function of hyperthermia and the resulting shock and disseminated intravascular coagulopathy (Henry, 2000).

The usual presentation in cases of acute toxicity includes hyperthermia, muscle rigidity, and a rise in creatinine kinase (CK) (Hall, 1997b). These patients may deteriorate toward multiple-organ failure, requiring intensive cardiovascular and respiratory support. These patients should be treated with active cooling and dantrolene given over 72 hours (Dar and McBrien, 1996). MDMA-induced hyperthermia results from augmentation of central serotonin function by stimulation of neuronal serotonin release (Dar and McBrien, 1996). Interestingly, Rittoo and Rittoo (1992) suggest that serum MDMA concentrations be measured in the admission blood sample of young adults who develop hyperthermia during general anesthesia. They also raise the question of whether patients who develop hyperthermia after Ecstasy use are at higher risk for the development of severe hyperthermia after general anesthesia.

Management is aimed at controlling symptoms. Benzodiazepines are suggested for agitation or seizures, and dopamine or norepinephrine is recommended for hypotension unresponsive to fluid challenges. Also suggested are phentolamine or nitroprusside for hypertension, lidocaine for ventricular dysrhythmias, and aggressive cooling and possibly the use of dantrolene (Milroy, 1999; Ghuran and Nolan, 2000; Henry, 2000). Additionally, the use of bicarbonate for rhabdomyolysis and correction of electrolyte abnormalities may be needed in the management of these patients.

Marijuana

Marijuana is the most commonly used illegal drug. The hemp plant *Cannabis sativa*, from which marijuana grows throughout the world, flourishes in most temperate and tropical regions. Marijuana is commonly ingested by smoking, which increases the bioavailability of the primary psychoactive constituent, tetrahydrocannabinol (THC) (Musty et al., 1995; Hall and Solowij, 1998). Inhalation of marijuana smoke produces euphoria, signs of increased sympathetic nervous system activity, and decreased parasympathetic nervous system activity (Schwartz, 1987). At high doses, however, sympathetic activity is inhibited and parasympathetic activity is increased, leading to bradycardia and hypotension. Reversible ECG abnormalities have been reported, as have increases in supraventricular and ventricular ectopic activity (Ghuran and Nolan, 2000). The clinical relevance of this finding is unclear.

Pharmacologic effects of inhaled marijuana occur within minutes but rarely persist longer than 2 to 3 hours. The likelihood that an acutely intoxicated patient would come to the operating room is small. Severe tachycardia should be controlled preoperatively with labetalol or esmolol. Animal studies have demonstrated decreased dose requirements for volatile anesthetics, barbiturates, and ketamine after the intravenous injection of THC. Possible intraoperative complications include bronchospasm secondary to airway irritability by the marijuana smoke, although marijuana is a bronchodilator.

Phencyclidine and Lysergic Acid Diethylamide Abuse

Phencyclidine (PCP) was developed in 1956, and it was briefly used as an anesthetic in humans before being abandoned because of the high incidence of bizarre and serious psychiatric reactions, including agitation, excitement, delirium, disorientation, and hallucinatory phenomena (Abraham et al., 1996). If taken orally, the effects of PCP develop in 1 to 2 hours and last from 8 to 12 hours. The mechanisms of action of both PCP and LSD are quite complex and include agonist, partial agonist, and antagonist effects at various serotonin, dopaminergic, and adrenergic receptors (Abraham et al., 1996). No data exist that examine PCP and its effect on patients undergoing general anesthesia, but anesthesiologists should be familiar with the management of issues related to PCP, because this product is a structural analogue of ketamine (Jansen, 1993).

The CNS effects of LSD begin approximately 15 to 30 minutes after intake and last about 6 to 12 hours (Abraham et al., 1996). The psychological effects related to LSD are intense and include alterations in mood and emotion, euphoria, dysphoria, and visual hallucinations (Abraham and Aldridge, 1993). LSD abuse is associated with only a mild sympathetic discharge that does not resemble those of cocaine, Ecstasy, or amphetamines (Ghuran and Nolan, 2000). These patients may also experience severe attacks of anxiety and panic. Anesthesia and surgery may precipitate these uncontrollable panic responses; diazepam or midazolam may be useful for the management of such responses. Postoperative hallucinations in patients undergoing general anesthesia have been reported as well (Morris and Magee, 1995).

PREOPERATIVE PREGNANCY TESTING

Although the pregnancy rates for teenagers fell to record lows for the United States in 2002, teen pregnancy rates have since risen, and teen pregnancy remains a significant public health concern and poses a dilemma for pediatric anesthesiologists. The birth rate for the youngest teenagers is about 0.7 birth per 1000 females aged 10 to 14 years and about 44 per 1000 for girls aged 15 to 19 years (Martin et al., 2003). At least 5% of girls are or have been pregnant by the time they reach their nineteenth birthday, and a substantial percentage of girls who are screened for elective or emergency surgery in their teen years have unsuspected or unrecognized pregnancies. General anesthesia and surgery in this population place the patient at risk for spontaneous abortion and the fetus at risk of exposure to known teratogenic substances during both anesthesia and the perioperative period, when the patient is no longer under the control of the anesthesiologist. It is this knowledge that leads many anesthesiology departments to have a policy of routinely screening postmenarchal girls for pregnancy.

On the other hand, routine pregnancy screening opens a Pandora's box of legal, ethical, and practical concerns. Some of the issues are discussed in the following paragraphs.

If an unsuspected (and, chances are, unwanted) pregnancy is discovered, the disclosure of this information to the patient and her family is a challenging task best done by a physician who is well acquainted with the family. The likelihood is that the anesthesiologist, and often the surgeon, have little personal knowledge of the patient and the family. How to best disclose test results and then ensure appropriate high-risk obstetric care must be prospectively determined before embarking on a testing program.

Complicating test result disclosure further is the fact that in the United States, the Health Insurance Portability and Accountability Act (HIPAA) restricts the disclosure of confidential medical information to a third party (parent) without the

consent of the patient (pregnant child). This creates a challenging logistical problem for the anesthesiologist.

The fact that there is a teenage pregnancy may imply a previous criminal offense against the child, such as rape or incest. Because of mandatory reporting requirements when child abuse is suspected, there may be criminal legal overtones to a positive pregnancy test that the anesthesiologist must address.

Finally, although the recognition of an unsuspected teen pregnancy may be a theoretically advantageous accomplishment before elective anesthesia, the fact is that within a hospital there are many more potentially injurious events that can occur to a fetus, including exposure to ionizing radiation, teratogenic antibiotics, and antineoplastic agents. A pregnancy screening program makes more sense if instituted on a hospital-wide basis rather than strictly within a preoperative screening program. Hospital-wide institution of such a program relieves the anesthesiologist of the burden of test-result disclosure and institution of appropriate social services.

PREOPERATIVE ORDERS

After the medical history and physical examination have been completed, preoperative orders are written.

For preoperative fasting, the anesthesiologist must consider the patient's age, size, and general medical condition, as well as the scheduled time of surgery if it is known (Table 9-3). The younger the child, the smaller the glycogen stores; therefore, the occurrence of hypoglycemia with prolonged intervals of fasting is more likely. For this reason, fasting time is reduced in the infant and young child. In general, solid food and milk products are prohibited within 8 and 6 hours, respectively, before surgery (generally after midnight); breast milk is prohibited within 4 hours of surgery; and clear liquids are prohibited within 2 hours of surgery. Liquids such as apple or grape juice, flat cola, and sugar water may be encouraged up to 2 hours before the induction of anesthesia. Ample experience has shown that shortened fasting times are safe, diminish preoperative anxiety and agitation, and may reduce the volume of gastric contents (Coté, 1990; Miller et al., 1990; Schreiner et al., 1990; Emerson et al., 1998; American Society of Anesthesiologist Task Force on Preoperative Fasting, 1999; Ferrari et al., 1999). When surgery is to be delayed beyond the anticipated time, it is important that small infants, generally those younger than 12 to 18 months old, are offered clear fluids or given intravenous fluids to prevent dehydration or hypovolemia.

TABLE 9-3. Fasting (NPO) Guidelines for Elective Surgery in Infants and Children

Substance	Minimum Hours of Fasting
Solid food	8
Commercial formula	6
Milk or milk products	6
Citrus juices	6
Breast milk	4
Clear liquids	2

Regardless of how long the patient fasts, there remains a defined population of children who are at an increased risk for regurgitation and aspiration of stomach contents. This group of children includes patients who have not fasted the requisite length of time and have sustained a severe injury during this period and children with esophageal dysmotility, incompetent gastroesophageal sphincters (gastroesophageal reflux diseases), delayed gastric emptying times, and abdominal conditions that are associated with ileus, vomiting, and electrolyte disorders. In addition, children with medical disorders that are associated with fluid and electrolyte abnormalities (such as diabetic ketoacidosis) are at risk for regurgitation and aspiration secondary to delayed gastric emptying.

In children at risk for aspiration, appropriate medical evaluation is important and preanesthetic medication with a nonparticulate antacid such as sodium citrate/citric acid (0.5 mL/kg), metoclopramide (0.1 mg/kg), and/or H_2-blocking agents (e.g., ranitidine 2.5 mg/kg) may be considered.

Two issues related to the NPO guidelines that commonly arise involve the safety of clear-liquid fasting in overweight and/or obese children for the recommended 2 hours before surgery and gastric fluid volume in children who have been chewing gum before the induction of anesthesia. Cook-Sather and colleagues (2009) noted in a study of ambulatory surgical patients, in which 27% of the patients were overweight or obese, that weight and obesity did not change the ratio of the patients' gastric fluid volume to their ideal body weights. Thus, the 2-hour fasting interval is appropriate in overweight and obese patients.

Chewing gum has the potential to increase gastric fluid volume and acidity. In adults who chewed sugared or sugarless gum before surgery, gastric fluid volume and pH did not change (Dubin et al., 1994). However, Schoenfelder et al. (2006) noted that children who chewed gum had larger gastric volumes than those children who did not. The significance of these findings remains unclear in that the incidence of aspiration is still exceedingly low.

PREANESTHETIC MEDICATIONS

Preoperative anxiety not only is an unpleasant experience for the patient but also makes the induction and recovery from anesthesia more complicated (Holm-Knudsen et al., 1998; Aono et al., 1999; Kain et al., 1999; Zuwala and Barber, 2001; Wollin et al., 2003). Indeed, inadequate preoperative premedication not only results in stormier anesthetic inductions, but also greater postoperative pain and behavioral abnormalities in children that persist long after surgical recovery occurs (Kain et al., 2006). In addition to allaying the anxieties of surgery, separation, pain, and body disfigurement, premedication should therefore allow a smoother and safer induction of anesthesia. The issue of which child should be premedicated and what agent should be used, and whether a parent may be present during induction of anesthesia must be considered according to the specific needs of each child and within the context of the anesthetic practice and clinical setting (Coté, 1999; McCann and Kain, 2001; Leelanukrom et al., 2002; Caldwell-Andrews et al., 2005; Kain et al., 2007a; 2007b).

Which is the best agent to use for premedication? The sheer volume of articles on the subject attests to the lack of an ideal agent or combination of agents as premedication for children.

Most preoperative medication is dictated by tradition. As Beecher remarked more than 50 years ago, "Empirical procedures firmly entrenched in habits of good doctors seem to have a vigor and life, not to say an immortality of their own" (1959).

The remainder of this chapter offers a discussion on the various premedications according to their drug classification. In selecting premedication, three important factors must be remembered:

1. A child's major fear concerning hospitalization is pain from needles and injections. Often hospitalization is synonymous with needles. Many children remember the premedication injection more than they do the pain associated with the operative procedure. Thus in selecting a premedication agent, most any route of administration is preferable to intramuscular injection.
2. Children who undergo regular hospitalizations need as much, or more, preoperative medication than patients undergoing anesthesia for the first time. Previous hospital experiences have formed the basis of their fears, so questions directed at determining their past experiences are invaluable. The previous anesthetic record should be reviewed, with careful attention given to the premedication agent and its effect.
3. The effects of premedications in children vary significantly. Some children may be sedated, others may be excited and restless after drug administration. In addition, to obtain a given level of sedation, some children may need half a recommended dose, and others may need twice the recommended dose. Therefore the dosages in Table 9-4 are intended to serve only as useful guidelines.

Anticholinergic Agents

Anticholinergic agents are mentioned in this chapter only for historical reference; in years past they were routinely administered to prevent unwanted autonomic vagal reflexes or bradycardia associated with airway instrumentation, nasopharyngeal stimulation, and anesthetic drugs (particularly halothane and morphine). Before that use, these compounds were administered to block the excessive secretions that were caused by the administration of diethyl ether at induction of anesthesia. At present they are uncommonly used and have few indications; fewer still are the indications that cannot wait until the patient has had anesthesia induced and intravenous access established, allowing intravenous administration of an anticholinergic. As with all pharmacologic agents, the use of anticholinergic agents—whether as an antisialagogue premedication

TABLE 9-4. Guidelines for Commonly Used Preanesthesia Medications in Children

Medication	Oral	Intravenous	Transmucosal
		Route of Administration	
Midazolam (mg/kg)	0.5-1	0.1	0.2-0.3 (nasal)
Morphine (mg/kg)		0.05-0.1	
Fentanyl (mcg/kg)		0.5-1	10 (oral transmucosal)
Ketamine (mg/kg)	5-10	1-2	5-10
Clonidine (mcg/kg)	2.5-5	1-2	

or as a vagolytic agent during surgery—should be governed by specific considerations of the potential side effects (temperature elevation, flushing, dry mouth, tachycardia, and CNS irritability) that can be significant.

Although atropine is the most commonly used agent, scopolamine and glycopyrrolate may also be used to premedicate children. Atropine, in doses of 0.02 mg/kg (0.03 mg/kg in infants), is an extremely effective vagolytic agent.

Oral atropine has been shown to be effective in preventing the adverse cardiovascular changes during induction of anesthesia (Miller and Friesen, 1987). Although injection is avoided with the use of oral atropine, the timing of its use relative to the operative procedure must still be anticipated.

Glycopyrrolate is a quaternary ammonium complex that does not cross the blood-brain barrier. As a result, it has a minimal CNS effect. It causes less tachycardia than atropine, but it is as effective as atropine at half the dose (0.01 mg/kg) as a vagolytic and antisialagogue. Studies in children have shown that glycopyrrolate reduced gastric fluid volume and altered its pH (Brock-Utne et al., 1978; Stoelting, 1978).

Opioids

Opioid premedication, once routinely administered as an intramuscular morphine injection in children, is nearly as uncommon and unnecessary as anticholinergic premedication. Opioid premedication can result in unpleasant dysphoria and an increased incidence of preoperative and postoperative vomiting. When given, opioids can be administered via the oral, rectal, intravenous, intramuscular, or transmucosal route. Interest in the use of opioids as preanesthetic medications has focused on the intranasal and oral transmucosal forms of administration (Leiman et al., 1987; Henderson et al., 1988; Nelson et al., 1989). The advantage of the latter technique is that the dose of premedication can be titrated to effect. Oral transmucosal fentanyl (OTFC) appears to have a relatively short onset time without adversely increasing gastric pH, but it does slightly increase gastric volume and delays the time that children need to tolerate postoperative fluids (Stanley et al., 1989; Ashburn et al., 1990).

Pharmacokinetic studies have demonstrated that OTFC is absorbed well through the buccal mucosa (Streisand et al., 1991). In volunteers administered an oral drink of both fentanyl and OTFC, OTFC produced higher and earlier peak plasma concentrations, as well as increased bioavailability (50% versus 30%), compared with swallowed fentanyl. In blinded studies of children in which OTFC (15 to 20 mcg/kg) was compared with placebo, OTFC is superior to placebo in allowing children to separate from parents and undergo inhalation induction of anesthesia (Moore et al., 2000; Tamura, et al., 2003). However, it was associated with considerable untoward side effects, including nausea and vomiting, oversedation, and oxygen desaturation (Nelson et al., 1989; Streisand et al., 1989, 1991; Ashburn et al., 1990; Goldstein-Dresner et al., 1991; Moore et al., 2000). The postoperative nausea and vomiting are not attenuated by intraoperative intravenous droperidol (50 mcg/kg) (Freisen and Lockhart, 1992). Because of the high incidence of reported side effects, as well as the need for continuous pulse oximetry while and after this drug is administered, OTFC as a preoperative sedative in children has not gained widespread use or popularity.

Hypnotics

Midazolam is a water-soluble benzodiazepine with a more rapid onset time and a shorter duration of action than diazepam. Its water solubility allows better absorption after intramuscular injection and eliminates the venous irritant properties associated with diazepam (Ghoneim and Korttila, 1977). Midazolam's peak plasma concentration occurs 45 minutes after intramuscular injection, but its anxiolytic effects occur in as little as 5 minutes. Its duration of action is usually 2 hours, with a range of 1 to 6 hours (Reves et al., 1985).

Now approved as a premedication for children and marketed as an oral preparation, midazolam has become the most commonly administered premedication before routine surgery in virtually every pediatric center; it is now the gold standard with which other premedications are compared. A national survey of over 5000 anesthesiologists has indicated that midazolam is the preoperative sedative of choice in more than 90% of all routine cases in children (Kain et al., 1997; Brosius and Bannister, 2002). The experience with midazolam is extensive and demonstrates the drug to be highly effective in alleviating anxiety, increasing cooperation, and diminishing antegrade recall without affecting retrograde memory (Payne et al., 1991a; Parnis et al., 1992; Twersky et al., 1993; Gillerman et al., 1996; McCann and Kain, 2001; Millar et al., 2007). Premedication with midazolam is safe and free of side effects, and it does not prolong recovery times (Payne et al., 1991b; Sievers et al., 1991; McMillan et al., 1992; Weldon et al., 1992; Davis et al., 1995; Viitanen et al., 1999; Brosius and Bannister, 2002). Finally, midazolam premedication smoothes the postoperative recovery of children and diminishes the incidence of delirium (Ko et al., 2001).

Nasal midazolam has also been reported to be highly effective in reducing anxiety in children within 10 to 12 minutes of administration (Griffith et al., 1998; Gautam et al., 2007). Furthermore, Davis et al. (1995) demonstrated that nasal midazolam (0.2-0.3 mg/kg) administered to patients undergoing myringotomies led to reduced preoperative anxiety and did not prolong recovery time and hospital discharge time. A drawback of nasal midazolam, however, is that more than 50% of children cry at administration because it irritates the nasal passages. The only rationale for administration of nasal midazolam is if a child without intravenous access cannot or will not swallow the oral preparation. Occasionally, younger children who refuse to take oral or nasal midazolam are more inclined to accept the midazolam rectally (McCann and Kain, 2001). Midazolam administered rectally in doses of 0.5 to 1 mg/kg effectively reduces the anxiety of children before induction of anesthesia.

Other benzodiazepines have not gained the popularity of midazolam nor have shown any advantage over the use of midazolam. Studies of flunitrazepam in children are limited, but it appears to be an effective pediatric premedication (Richardson and Manford, 1979). As with other benzodiazepines, flunitrazepam can be administered as a rectal premedication. In a double-blind, placebo-controlled study, 0.04 mg/kg of rectal flunitrazepam provided better sedation and mask-acceptance scores without prolonging recovery from anesthesia (Esteve and Saint-Maurice, 1990). Triazolam has been used as a preanesthetic medication in adults (Yamakage et al., 2002) but its use in children has not been evaluated, nor has it been compared with conventional agents.

Ketamine

In high doses (4 to 12 mg/kg), intramuscular ketamine has often been used to induce and maintain anesthesia in children (Wyant, 1971). Hannallah and Patel (1989) demonstrated that at low doses (2 mg/kg), intramuscular ketamine can facilitate inhalation induction of anesthesia. In this study of uncooperative children undergoing tympanostomy tube insertion, low-dose intramuscular ketamine was very effective in completing a mask induction with halothane in a shorter time than in cooperative children who did not need premedication. Although the induction time was shorter in the group receiving ketamine, ketamine did prolong the hospital discharge times.

As an alternative to intramuscular administration, rectal, nasal transmucosal, and oral routes of ketamine administration have been described. Rectal administration of ketamine has been reported in children undergoing a wide variety of surgical procedures. Van der Bijl and colleagues (1991) compared rectal administration of midazolam (0.3 mg/kg) with rectal administration of ketamine (5 mg/kg). Thirty minutes after the administration of either drug, good anxiolysis, cooperation, and sedation were achieved. In doses of 8 to 10 mg/kg, Saint-Maurice et al. (1979) noted that the interval from rectal administration to loss of verbal contact and acceptance of the facemask was 7 and 9 minutes, respectively.

Nasal transmucosal ketamine is an effective means of premedicating children. Weksler and colleagues demonstrated that 6 mg/kg of nasal ketamine administered 20 to 40 minutes before surgery achieved satisfactory sedation in 78% of the patients, whereas smaller doses of 5 mg/kg produced comparable sedation and ease of separation from parents as nasal midazolam (Weksler et al., 1993; Gautam et al., 2007).

Oral ketamine, of course the most acceptable route in most situations, has been used for nearly 20 years as a preoperative anesthetic medication in healthy children who are undergoing routine surgical procedures and in children undergoing corrective surgery for congenital heart defects (Stewart et al., 1990). Gutstein et al. (1992), in a double-blind, prospective study, evaluated placebo and oral ketamine at both 3 and 6 mg/kg doses as a preanesthetic medication in children. At some time during the study, 100% of the children administered 6 mg/kg were sedated as opposed to 73% of the children administered 3 mg/kg. In both groups of children who received ketamine, the onset of sedation occurred in 12 minutes, and in the 6 mg/kg group, 67% of patients were sufficiently sedated to have an intravenous cannula inserted. Similarly, the combination of oral midazolam and oral ketamine has a very high success rate of satisfactory anxiolysis compared with a somewhat lower success rate for either drug alone (Funk et al., 2000; Ghai et al., 2005). Postanesthesia care-unit discharge time of children who received orally administered ketamine is reported not to be prolonged compared with orally administered midazolam, provided that the duration of surgery is longer than 30 minutes (Funk et al., 2000). Oral ketamine has also been found to be an effective premedication in alleviating the distress of invasive procedures in pediatric oncology patients (Tobias et al., 1992). An oral transmucosal lozenge containing ketamine was under development for some time as a surgical premedication, and was found to be equally effective as oral midazolam; the present status of this drug development project is unknown at the time of this writing (Horiuchi et al., 2005).

Alpha-2-Adrenoreceptor Agonists

The role of α_2-adrenoreceptor agonists for both premedication of children before surgery and as analgesics during and after surgery is continuing to evolve. In adults, α_2-adrenoreceptor agonists have been shown to provide perioperative sedation, postoperative analgesia, improved perioperative hemodynamic stability, and reduced anesthetic requirements (Ghignone et al., 1987; Wright et al., 1990; Carabine et al., 1991). The MAC-sparing effect of premedication with 1 to 10 mcg/kg of oral clonidine has been demonstrated (Nishina et al., 1996; 1997; Inomata et al., 2002).

Clonidine

In a double-blind, randomized study, Mikawa and colleagues demonstrated that in children, oral clonidine produces sedation in a dose-dependent manner, and that at a dose of 4 mcg/kg, clonidine provides satisfactory sedation, a better quality of child/parent separation, and better mask acceptance than does standard oral diazepam premedication (0.4 mg/kg) (1993). Fazi and colleagues (2001) showed that oral clonidine was generally inferior to oral midazolam; however, clonidine 4 mcg/kg was associated with faster awakening than midazolam 0.5 mg/kg. These authors found that after clonidine premedication, children were more distressed and agitated during inhalation induction and had higher pain scores and greater analgesic requirements in the postoperative period. Yet few other citations in the literature have found similar results. Virtually all other authors have shown that oral clonidine in doses of 4 to 5 mcg/kg is comparable in efficacy with oral midazolam 0.5 mg/kg; whereas the onset of sedation tends to be less after the use of clonidine, the degree of sedation tends to be greater (Inomata et al., 2002; Bergendahl et al., 2004; Almenrader et al., 2007a; 2007b). Clonidine may be a useful premedication in children who have previously experienced delirium, agitation, or paradoxical reactions to midazolam or other benzodiazepines in the past (Stella and Bailey, 2008).

Importantly, clonidine premedication has beneficial effects that go beyond the preoperative period. It has become clear both from clinical experience and from clinical research that the analgesic effect of clonidine persists well into the postoperative period, reducing measures of surgical pain in children (Schmidt et al., 2007). This may be closely related to why the incidence of emergence delirium is reduced following clonidine premedication (Ko et al., 2001; Bock et al., 2002; Malviya et al., 2006) and is not after midazolam premedication (Breschan et al., 2007), and why the neuroendocrine stress response to surgery is attenuated in those children who were premedicated with clonidine (Kain et al., 2000).

Clonidine, therefore, is emerging as a premedication that is equal in sedative efficacy to midazolam, but that possesses salutory effects over and above midazolam. Its role in pediatric anesthesia will continue to evolve and be better defined in the future.

Dexmedetomidine

Dexmedetomidine is another α_2-agonist that has an α_2 selectivity that is seven to eight times greater than clonidine. Although approved to be used as an infusion for sedation of adult intensive care unit (ICU) patients, dexmedetomidine has also been used as a premedication, an anesthetic adjuvant, a procedural sedation agent, and a treatment for postoperative shivering and agitation resulting from an emergency situation. In addition, when applied to intra-articular surfaces after orthoscopic surgery, dexmedetomidine enhances postoperative analgesia and decreases the need for postoperative analgesic agents (Ibacache 2004; Easley et al., 2007; Yuen et al., 2007, 2008; Mason et al., 2006, 2008; Al-Metwalli et al., 2008; Heard et al., 2008; Mahmoud et al., 2009; Talon et al., 2009). As a premedication, Yuen and colleagues (2007, 2008) have shown that 1.7 mcg/kg of dexmedetomidine intranasally can provide sedation in children but has an onset time and peak effect of 45 minutes and 90 to 150 minutes, respectively. In burn patients, Talon et al. (2009) suggested that 2 mcg/kg of dexmedetomidine was comparable with 0.5 mg oral midazolam with respect to preoperative sedation, conditions at induction, and emergence from anesthesia. The bioavailabilities of dexmedetomidine after oral and buccal administration were 16% and 82%, respectively (Anttila et al., 2003). Dyck et al. (1993) have reported that after intramuscular administration, peak concentrations of dexmedetomidine occur at 12 minutes and that the bioavailability is 73%.

SUMMARY

The pediatric anesthesiologist must recognize developmental differences in anatomy and physiology and also must understand and deal effectively with the emotional reactions and needs of children of various ages and developmental stages. Although premedication agents often alleviate the anxieties of anesthesia and surgery, these pharmacologic adjuncts cannot substitute for a thorough and thoughtful preoperative visit and discussion with the patient and family.

For questions and answers on topics in this chapter, go to "Chapter Questions" at www.expertconsult.com.

REFERENCES

Complete references used in this text can be found online at www.expertconsult.com.

Equipment

John E. Fiadjoe, Jeffrey M. Feldman,
and David E. Cohen

CHAPTER

10

CONTENTS

T he pediatric anesthesiologist is charged with caring for a diverse patient population. Anesthetizing a 500-g newborn can be immediately followed by the care of a 100-kg adolescent. This broad range of patient sizes requires an equally diverse and unique spectrum of equipment. This chapter focuses on the types of equipment that are used in pediatric anesthesia and highlights unique adaptations of equipment for pediatric use.

HUMIDIFIERS

During normal breathing, the nasal mucosa and upper airway serve as a reservoir for condensed water. This water is evaporated during breathing and reduces the heat expended by the body in warming and humidifying inhaled gases. In typical atmospheric conditions, air in the pulmonary periphery contains 44 mg of water per liter at 37° C (100% relative humidity). Breathing ambient air at a temperature of 22° C, water content of 10 mg/dL would require the addition of 34 mg/L of evaporated water. This evaporation results in a loss of energy with the resultant cooling of the respiratory mucosa. The caloric expenditure of humidification consumes approximately five times the energy required to heat the inspired gases; this may amount to 20% of the basal metabolic rate of an infant (Rashad and Benson, 1967). Nasopharyngeal humidification is bypassed with the placement of common airway devices such as tracheal tubes, tracheostomy tubes, and laryngeal masks. Benefits of heating and humidifying anesthetic gases include prevention of intraoperative hypothermia, decreased atelectasis, and improved mucociliary clearance. Consequences of overhumidification include impaired mucociliary clearance related to reduced mucus viscosity, atelectasis, accumulation of secretions, infection, thermal injury, and surfactant inactivation (Schiffmann, 2006). Partial humidification of gas in the anesthesia breathing circuit

takes place within the carbon-dioxide absorber, which uses an exothermic reaction that may raise the water vapor content to as much as 29 mg/L. Further humidification is accomplished by reducing the amount of fresh-gas flow, thereby increasing rebreathing of humidified gases and using a heat and moisture exchanger (HME, or "artificial nose"). The HME uses a fine mesh to cause condensation of exhaled water vapor. The HME may increase the resistance to breathing or the dead space for some infants and children, although these changes are usually tolerable. Low fresh-gas flow alone is often inadequate at maintaining humidity and temperature in infants and neonates, therefore active or passive humidification devices should always be incorporated when ventilating this population (Hunter et al., 2005). HMEs increase airway humidification and preserve temperature in anesthetized children at a lower cost than active humidification systems (Bissonnette and Sessler, 1989) and they require 80 minutes to achieve optimal saturation of the membrane, during which time they are less efficient. HMEs come in a variety of sizes, enabling selection based on size of the patient, so that dead space or resistance can be minimized. Specially designed HMEs filter out infectious pathogens and minimize the risk of cross-infection between patients (Wilkes et al., 2000).

Active humidification is the most efficient means by which to heat and humidify inspired gases (Bissonnette and Sessler, 1989). A servocontrolled, shielded heated wire in the fresh gas line helps to prevent cooling and condensation of the water as it passes through the inspiratory limb. The temperature should be regulated by a probe near the patient connection, because overheating of the inspired gases can produce injury to the airway (Klein and Graves, 1974). Active humidifiers may also increase the compression volume of the breathing circuit; thus, compensatory increases in the tidal volume during controlled ventilation may be necessary except in ventilators with compliance compensation (Coté et al., 1983).

ANESTHESIA BREATHING SYSTEMS

Since Philip Ayre's (1937) landmark article began the modern era of breathing systems for pediatric anesthesia, this has been a topic of controversy. Using Magill's technique of tracheal intubation for the repair of cleft lip and palate in infants, Ayre noted adverse results. Breathing through a "closed" high-resistance system, these infants often developed "rapid, 'sighing' respirations" and "ashy pallor and sweating." They exhibited a "dark, congested oozing at the site of operation." Postoperatively, the infants were "in varying degrees of shock: some...for days" (Ayre, 1937). The contribution of hypotension or hypovolemia to this picture remains unknown, because blood pressure was not measured, and blood loss was difficult to quantify by Ayre's account.

Ayre noted dramatic clinical improvement when he adopted an open T-piece breathing system. The T piece, an extremely simple device, consists of an inspiratory limb, a connection to the patient, and an expiratory limb. It has no unidirectional or overflow valves, and there is no breathing bag. The expiratory limb serves as a reservoir for fresh gas, a means of monitoring the infant's respirations, and if the distal end is intermittently occluded, a means of providing positive pressure ventilation. If the volume of the expiratory limb is one third of the tidal volume, rebreathing can be virtually eliminated during spontaneous ventilation with a fresh-gas flow that is twice the minute ventilation (Ayre, 1956). Ayre attributed the salutary effect of the T piece to marked reductions in resistance to gas flow and rebreathing.

Nonrebreathing and Partial Rebreathing Systems

Despite its apparent benefits, the T piece is far from ideal. The major flaws are its release of anesthetic gases into the operating room and its inability to provide assisted or controlled ventilation. A series of modifications occurred. Rees (1950) first proposed the addition of a breathing bag to the expiratory limb. Another system, the Magill attachment, which predated Ayre's publication, introduced fresh gas distal to a breathing bag and an overflow valve near the patient connection. These and other variations were brought together under a single classification scheme proposed by Mapleson (1954), in which each system was distinguished on the basis of the location of its fresh gas inflow and overflow valves relative to the patient connection.

These Mapleson circuits share the benefit of reduced resistance to breathing by virtue of the absence of unidirectional valves and canisters; the elimination of these components results in varying degrees of rebreathing that depend on the fresh-gas flow (Fig. 10-1, A). Rebreathing is not necessarily bad because it serves to conserve heat, humidity, and anesthetic gases. Yet in the absence of a mechanism by which to monitor the accumulation of carbon dioxide, the consequences of hypercarbia and respiratory acidosis probably outweigh these benefits.

Each circuit has different rebreathing characteristics depending on the locations of the fresh gas inflow, the overflow valves, and the fresh-gas flow rate; the respiratory rate (i.e., expiratory time) and tidal volume, carbon dioxide production, and the mode of ventilation (i.e., spontaneous or controlled) also contribute to the degree of rebreathing. The following sections describe the Mapleson A (Magill attachment) and D systems. The B and C systems are rarely used today. The Mapleson E system is the T piece described in the previous section of this chapter.

Mapleson A System

The Mapleson A system results in no rebreathing during spontaneous ventilation when the fresh-gas flow is more than 75% of the minute ventilation; it requires a larger fresh-gas flow to eliminate rebreathing during controlled ventilation (Fig. 10-1, B) (Waters and Mapleson, 1961; Kain and Nunn, 1967). This design is impractical in the operating room, because the proximal location of the overflow valve makes it cumbersome for scavenging waste gases, difficult to adjust during head-and-neck surgery, and potentially dangerous, because the heavy valve could dislodge a small tracheal tube.

Mapleson D System

The Mapleson D system is characterized by a proximal fresh-gas inflow and a distal overflow valve. It is a modification of the T piece, in which a breathing bag and an overflow valve have been added to the distal expiratory limb. Although it requires slightly more fresh-gas flow to eliminate rebreathing during spontaneous ventilation than the Mapleson A system, it is the most economical during controlled ventilation (Waters and Mapleson, 1961). On balance, considering both spontaneous and controlled ventilation, the Mapleson D requires the lowest fresh-gas flow rates among all Mapleson circuits. This system has become the most widely used of the Mapleson circuits for pediatric anesthesia.

The precise flow dynamics in the Mapleson D system have been a subject of discussion that has resulted in a variety of complex recommendations (Mapleson, 1954; Waters and Mapleson, 1961, Nightingale et al., 1965; Bain and Spoerel, 1973; Rose et al., 1978; Spoerel et al., 1978; Rose and Froese, 1979). To eliminate rebreathing, higher fresh-gas flows are needed during spontaneous ventilation than during controlled ventilation. With spontaneous ventilation, rebreathing is eliminated by provision of fresh-gas flow equal to the mean inspiratory flow rate (Mapleson, 1954; Rose et al., 1978). If an inspiratory/expiratory ratio is 1:1 or 1:2, the mean inspiratory flow rate is 2 to 3 times the minute ventilation. Although Spoerel and others (Bain, 1979) have demonstrated that a normal arterial carbon dioxide tension ($Paco_2$) can be maintained during spontaneous ventilation at fresh-gas flows as low as 100 mL/kg per minute, an increased minute ventilation (and hence more respiratory work) is required to compensate for rebreathed carbon dioxide.

The recommendations for fresh-gas flow during controlled ventilation are complex and varied (Waters and Mapleson, 1961; Nightingale et al., 1965; Bain and Spoerel, 1973). This reflects the importance of several factors that were summarized by Rose and Froese (1979) (Fig. 10-2). When a high fresh-gas flow (greater than 100 mL/kg per minute) is used, the $Paco_2$ is governed by minute ventilation (ventilation limited). At low fresh-gas flow (less than 90 mL/kg per minute), $Paco_2$ is independent of minute ventilation, varying instead as a function of the amount of rebreathing, which is governed by the fresh-gas-flow rate (flow limited).

Additional important factors that govern the magnitude of rebreathing include carbon dioxide production, respiratory rate, and respiratory waveform characteristics (e.g., inspiratory flow, inspiratory and expiratory times, and expiratory

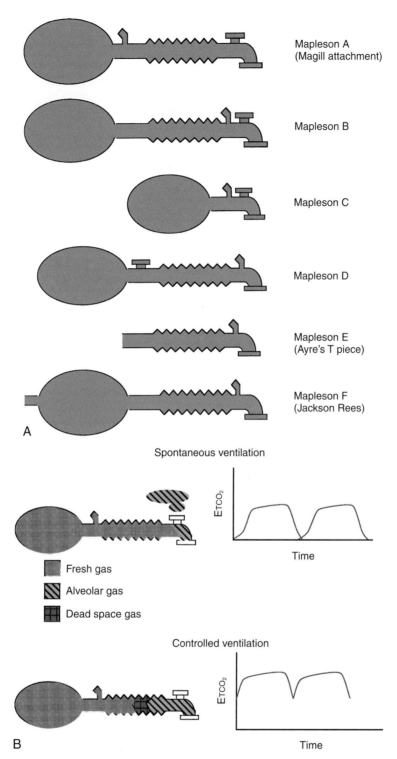

Mapleson A
(Magill attachment)

Mapleson B

Mapleson C

Mapleson D

Mapleson E
(Ayre's T piece)

Mapleson F
(Jackson Rees)

A

Spontaneous ventilation

E_{TCO_2}

Time

Fresh gas

Alveolar gas

Dead space gas

Controlled ventilation

E_{TCO_2}

B   Time

FIGURE 10-1. A, The Mapleson circuits. Each circuit is classified on the basis of the relative positions of the fresh-gas inlet, overflow valve, corrugated tubing, and reservoir bag in relation to the patient connection. **B,** Mapleson A system during spontaneous and controlled ventilation. *(Adapted from Mapleson WW: The elimination of rebreathing in various semiclosed anesthetic systems, Br J Anaesth 26:323, 1954.)*

pause) (Rose and Froese, 1979). Adjustments to the ventilatory pattern that allow the fresh-gas flow to constitute a larger proportion of the inspired gas (e.g., slow inspiratory time or low inspiratory flow) or that enable exhaled gases to be more completely washed out (e.g., long expiratory pause or slow rate) reduce the amount of rebreathing. With a Mapleson D circuit that has controlled ventilation and low fresh-gas flow

(flow limited), an attempt to reduce the $Paco_2$ by increasing the respiratory rate would reduce the expiratory pause and thus promote rebreathing (Fig. 10-3). In this situation, the increased ventilation is offset by increased fraction of inspired oxygen ($Fico_2$), resulting in no net change in $Paco_2$. To wash out the exhaled gas at this higher respiratory rate and take advantage of the increased minute ventilation, the fresh-gas

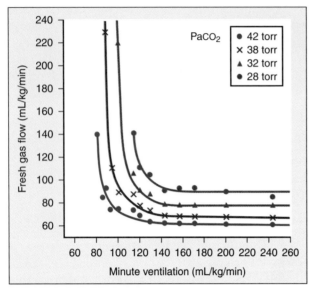

■ **FIGURE 10-2.** Fresh-gas flow as it relates to minute ventilation in the Mapleson D system.

flow must be increased. These fresh-gas flow and ventilatory recommendations are predicated for a normal metabolic rate and hence normal carbon dioxide production (Bain and Spoerel, 1977; Nightingale and Lambert, 1978). Conditions that increase carbon dioxide production (e.g., fever, catabolic state, or malignant hyperthermia) must be met with a proportional increase in fresh-gas flow or ventilation.

Bain Modification of Mapleson D

The Bain modification of the Mapleson D circuit incorporates the fresh-gas supply within the expiratory limb in a coaxial arrangement (Fig. 10-4) (Bain and Spoerel, 1972). This circuit is light and streamlined with only a single hose to the patient. It also provides some countercurrent warming of the inspired gases and effective scavenging of expired gases. Its major disadvantage lies in the inability to directly inspect the integrity of the inspiratory limb. Pethick (1975) described an indirect test of the Bain inspiratory-limb integrity in which the oxygen flush is passed through the circuit for several seconds. If the inspiratory limb is intact, the rapid flow of gas through it exerts a Venturi effect on the expiratory limb, resulting in a slight negative pressure and collapse of the breathing bag. With a leak from the inspiratory limb into the expiratory limb, the pressure in the latter rises, tending to inflate the reservoir bag. The rebreathing characteristics of the Bain circuit are identical to those of any other Mapleson D. The major reasons that proponents have advocated the use of these Bain circuits for pediatric anesthesia are their relatively lower resistance to breathing offered by an open system, the countercurrent warming of gases, and the low profile of a single hose attached to the patient.

The primary sources of resistance in an anesthesia delivery system are the tracheal tube, the valves, and the carbon dioxide absorber. With modern equipment, the tracheal tube represents a major source of resistance in the neonate (Cave and Fletcher, 1968; Brown and Hustead, 1969). Light-weight, large-diameter, modern disc valves exert resistance in two ways. There is a minimum, flow-independent resistance necessary to displace the valve, usually much less than 1 cm H_2O (Hunt, 1955). A much higher resistance

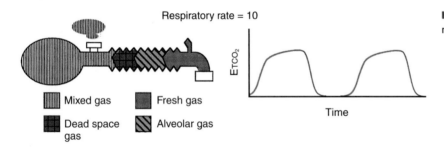

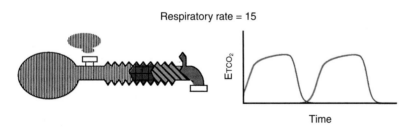

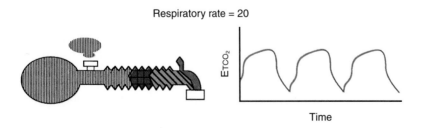

■ **FIGURE 10-3.** Influence of respiratory rate on rebreathing in the Mapleson D system.

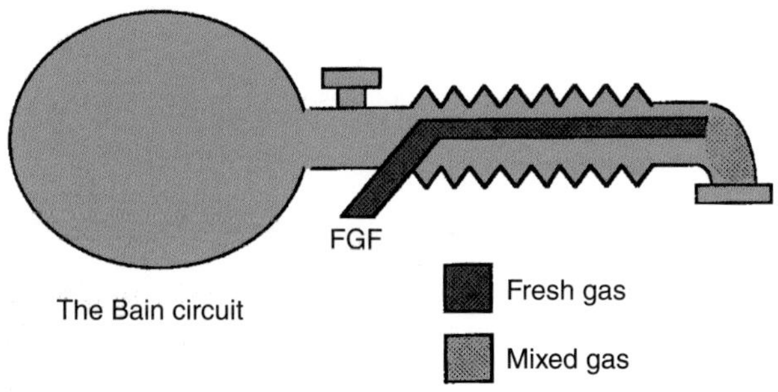

FGF

The Bain circuit

■ Fresh gas

▨ Mixed gas

■ **FIGURE 10-4.** The Bain modifications of the Mapleson D circuit provide a low-profile circuit and allow simple connections to the patient's airway.

may be required when the expiratory valve is wet. At high gas flows (more than 30 L/min), the valves also become a source of turbulent resistance proportional to the flow through them. Carbon dioxide canisters are also a source of turbulence. Their resistance is inversely proportional to the length of the path the gas must take through the resistor. Modern absorbers are short and wide to minimize this path of resistance.

Approximately a half century after Ayre introduced the T piece, the extent to which his work applies remains unclear. Perhaps the infants Ayre studied were subjected to the significant resistance imposed by the valves of that era. Although the neonate has a lower proportion of fatigue-resistant fibers in the diaphragm, infants as young as 2 weeks old have been shown to compensate for increases in resistance of 200% without changes in blood gases, at least for relatively short lengths of time (Muller et al., 1979). The benefits of the Mapleson systems must be weighed against their inherent problems on an individual basis. If a practitioner seldom uses Mapleson circuits and is unfamiliar with their characteristics, or if a practitioner has to make substantial alterations to an anesthesia machine to accommodate them, the additional risks of the situation must be considered. Even if a circle system is used for most children, it is important to understand the flow requirements of these circuits, as they continue to be used for resuscitation outside of the operating room and for transporting critically ill patients.

Circle Systems

The circle system is standard equipment on anesthesia machines that have been designed to meet the standards specified in ASTM 1850-00 (2005). When functioning properly, it enables lower fresh-gas flows than the Mapleson D circuit; a circle system conserves heat, humidity, and anesthetic agent. It also minimizes environmental pollution. Compared with the resistance of an endotracheal tube, the additional resistance imposed by the addition of unidirectional valves and a carbon-dioxide canister is trivial. Because the ratio of the patient's tidal volume to the volume of the inspiratory limb is small in young children, changes in the anesthetic concentration can take some time to reach equilibrium unless higher fresh-gas flows are used. It is important to be vigilant for the manifestations of stuck (resistance) or floating (rebreathing) unidirectional valves, because both have harmful consequences in small children.

Special circle-breathing systems have been designed for infants and children that incorporate the same components as the standard adult circuits but have been modified to minimize

dead space and resistance to breathing. Most incorporate short, narrow-caliber hoses and Y connections to minimize the weight and compliance of the circuit. These smaller hoses, along with smaller carbon dioxide absorbers, are also used to reduce the time needed to effect a change in the concentration of vapor or gases in the circuit.

ANESTHESIA MACHINES

Anesthesia machines serve two basic functions. The first function is to enable the anesthesia provider to control the concentrations of gases and anesthetic vapors delivered to the patient. The second function is to support both spontaneous and mechanical ventilation. There are no anesthesia machines specifically designed for pediatric applications, and for the most part, the available machines function as they do for adult care. There are, however, certain characteristics that should be sought in an anesthesia machine that is to be used for pediatric patients.

Gas and Anesthetic Vapor Delivery

Oxygen

All modern anesthesia machines are designed to ensure continuous oxygen delivery from either pipeline or cylinder supplies and to notify the user if the oxygen-supply pressure fails. Because pressure in the oxygen supply does not guarantee that oxygen is indeed flowing through the pipes, an oxygen analyzer located in the inspiratory limb of the anesthesia circuit is an essential safety monitor for every anesthetic (Dorsch and Dorsch, 2007). Indeed, an inspired oxygen-concentration monitor is considered to be the standard of care for every anesthetic according to the American Society of Anesthesiologists (2005) (Box 10-1).

The oxygen analyzer is also important when caring for the anesthetized pediatric patient, because certain clinical conditions mandate precise control of the delivered oxygen concentration, and the oxygen analyzer serves to confirm delivery of the desired oxygen concentration.

The inspired oxygen concentration (Fio_2) is typically controlled by mixing oxygen with either air or nitrous oxide to achieve the desired result. When mixing oxygen and nitrous oxide, it is relatively easy to predict the resulting concentration of oxygen, because the ratio of the flows determines the percentage of inspired oxygen (1:1 oxygen/nitrous oxide is 50% oxygen, and a 1:3 ratio is 25% oxygen). When mixing air and oxygen, it is not as intuitive to predict the resulting oxygen concentration, because the air supply contains 21% oxygen. Furthermore, it can be difficult to minimize the oxygen concentration and use a low-flow technique. For example, if 200 mL/min of oxygen is delivered (minimum mandatory flow on some anesthesia machines), air flowing at 4 L/min results in a 25% concentration of oxygen. A table of flow ratios and resulting oxygen concentrations can be useful to guide flow settings, but the oxygen analyzer is an ideal tool to document the delivered oxygen concentration. When caring for pediatric patients, it is useful to have an anesthesia machine capable of delivering air only (no minimum oxygen flow), so that low concentrations of oxygen can be delivered without using excessive gas flows. Nitrous oxide and air are most commonly mixed with oxygen to control Fio_2, but there are conditions in which helium or carbon dioxide are used.

Box 10-1 Standards for Basic Anesthetic Monitoring Committee of Origin: Standards and Practice Parameters

(Approved by the ASA House of Delegates on October 21, 1986, and Last Amended on October 25, 2005)

These standards apply to all anesthesia care although, in emergency circumstances, appropriate life support measures take precedence. These standards may be exceeded at any time based on the judgment of the responsible anesthesiologist. They are intended to encourage quality patient care, but observing them cannot guarantee any specific patient outcome. They are subject to revision from time to time, as warranted by the evolution of technology and practice. They apply to all general anesthetics, regional anesthetics and monitored anesthesia care. This set of standards addresses only the issue of basic anesthetic monitoring, which is one component of anesthesia care. In certain rare or unusual circumstances, 1) some of these methods of monitoring may be clinically impractical, and 2) appropriate use of the described monitoring methods may fail to detect untoward clinical developments. Brief interruptions of continual† monitoring may be unavoidable. These standards are not intended for application to the care of the obstetrical patient in labor or in the conduct of pain management.

STANDARD I

Qualified anesthesia personnel shall be present in the room throughout the conduct of all general anesthetics, regional anesthetics and monitored anesthesia care.

Objective

Because of the rapid changes in patient status during anesthesia, qualified anesthesia personnel shall be continuously present to monitor the patient and provide anesthesia care. In the event there is a direct known hazard, e.g., radiation, to the anesthesia personnel which might require intermittent remote observation of the patient, some provision for monitoring the patient must be made. In the event that an emergency requires the temporary absence of the person primarily responsible for the anesthetic, the best judgment of the anesthesiologist will be exercised in comparing the emergency with the anesthetized patient's condition and in the selection of the person left responsible for the anesthetic during the temporary absence.

STANDARD II

During all anesthetics, the patient's oxygenation, ventilation, circulation and temperature shall be continually evaluated.

Oxygenation
Objective

To ensure adequate oxygen concentration in the inspired gas and the blood during all anesthetics.

Methods

1. Inspired gas: During every administration of general anesthesia using an anesthesia machine, the concentration of oxygen in the patient breathing system shall be measured by an oxygen analyzer with a low oxygen concentration limit alarm in use.*
2. Blood oxygenation: During all anesthetics, a quantitative method of assessing oxygenation such as pulse oximetry shall be employed.* When the pulse oximeter is utilized, the variable pitch pulse tone and the low threshold alarm shall be audible to the anesthesiologist or the anesthesia care team personnel.* Adequate illumination and exposure of the patient are necessary to assess color.*

Ventilation
Objective

To ensure adequate ventilation of the patient during all anesthetics.

Methods

1. Every patient receiving general anesthesia shall have the adequacy of ventilation continually evaluated. Qualitative clinical signs such as chest excursion, observation of the reservoir breathing bag and auscultation of breath sounds are useful. Continual monitoring for the presence of expired carbon dioxide shall be performed unless invalidated by the nature of the patient, procedure or equipment. Quantitative monitoring of the volume of expired gas is strongly encouraged.*
2. When an endotracheal tube or laryngeal mask is inserted, its correct positioning must be verified by clinical assessment and by identification of carbon dioxide in the expired gas. Continual end-tidal carbon dioxide analysis, in use from the time of endotracheal tube/laryngeal mask placement, until extubation/removal or initiating transfer to a postoperative care location, shall be performed using a quantitative method such as capnography, capnometry or mass spectroscopy.* When capnography or capnometry is utilized, the end tidal CO_2 alarm shall be audible to the anesthesiologist or the anesthesia care team personnel.*
3. When ventilation is controlled by a mechanical ventilator, there shall be in continuous use a device that is capable of detecting disconnection of components of the breathing system. The device must give an audible signal when its alarm threshold is exceeded.
4. During regional anesthesia and monitored anesthesia care, the adequacy of ventilation shall be evaluated by continual observation of qualitative clinical signs and/or monitoring for the presence of exhaled carbon dioxide.

Circulation
Objective

To ensure the adequacy of the patient's circulatory function during all anesthetics.

Methods

1. Every patient receiving anesthesia shall have the electrocardiogram continuously displayed from the beginning of anesthesia until preparing to leave the anesthetizing location.*
2. Every patient receiving anesthesia shall have arterial blood pressure and heart rate determined and evaluated at least every five minutes.*
3. Every patient receiving general anesthesia shall have, in addition to the above, circulatory function continually evaluated by at least one of the following: palpation of a pulse, auscultation of heart sounds, monitoring of a tracing of intra-arterial pressure, ultrasound peripheral pulse monitoring, or pulse plethysmography or oximetry.

Body Temperature
Objective

To aid in the maintenance of appropriate body temperature during all anesthetics.

Methods

Every patient receiving anesthesia shall have temperature monitored when clinically significant changes in body temperature are intended, anticipated or suspected.

---

*Under extenuating circumstances, the responsible anesthesiologist may waive the requirements marked with an asterisk (*); it is recommended that when this is done, it should be so stated (including the reasons) in a note in the patient's medical record.

†Note that "continual" is defined as "repeated regularly and frequently in steady rapid succession," whereas "continuous" means "prolonged without any interruption at any time."

Indications for Careful Control of Fio$_2$

Studies have implicated arterial oxygen tension as one of several variables linked to retinopathy of prematurity (ROP) in preterm infants (weighing less than 1300 g) whose retinas are immature (Flynn et al., 1992). The contribution of brief episodes of intraoperative hyperoxemia to the development of ROP remains unknown, and oxygen concentrations greater than necessary should be avoided in this vulnerable population. It is not known whether there is any real impact on outcome dependent on whether air or nitrous oxide is used as the balance gas in these patients. Given the potential for nitrous oxide to interfere with deoxyribonucleic acid (DNA) synthesis, it may be prudent to avoid this gas in the developing neonate, although there are no definitive data indicating that nitrous oxide is dangerous for these patients.

During airway laser surgery it is desirable to reduce the inspired oxygen concentration to less than 30% to minimize the risk of igniting the tracheal tube or any other combustible materials. Because nitrous oxide also supports combustion, it should not be used in these cases. Air can be used alone or with small amounts of additional oxygen. Helium is also a useful balance gas in these cases, because it does not support combustion and can improve the flow of inspired gases beyond any obstructions in the airway (Pashayan et al., 1988). Specially adapted anesthesia machines capable of delivering inspired carbon dioxide to achieve hypercarbia or increased inspired nitrogen to produce hypoxia may be indicated in the care of the neonate with specific types of congenital heart disease (Tabbutt et al., 2001). The important aspect of caring for these patients is to maintain the balance of pulmonary and systemic blood flow by controlling pulmonary vascular resistance. Both hypoxic oxygen concentrations and carbon dioxide can be used toward this end.

In addition to the inspired oxygen analyzer, the pulse oximeter is also a mandatory patient monitor and facilitates reducing the Fio$_2$ comfortably. As the Fio$_2$ is reduced, the pulse oximeter becomes a better indicator of problems with oxygenation. Because the pulse oximeter only measures the saturation of hemoglobin, it is not useful for assessing the alveolar-to-arterial oxygen gradient when an enriched oxygen concentration is being delivered. If an inspired oxygen concentration of 25% or less is used, the pulse oximeter can rapidly indicate a problem with oxygen delivery to the blood by measuring the reduced oxygen saturation. As the Fio$_2$ is increased, the pulse oximeter becomes a delayed indicator of an oxygenation problem.

Anesthetic Vapor Delivery

All modern anesthesia machines deliver anesthetic vapor by vaporizing a controlled amount of liquid anesthetic and mixing it with the fresh gas entering the anesthesia circuit. The only exception is the Zeus anesthesia machine (Draeger Medical; Lubeck, Germany), which injects liquid anesthetic directly into the anesthesia circuit under closed-loop control. There are excellent sources of information on the details of vaporizer design; however, they are beyond the scope of this chapter (Dorsch and Dorsch, 2007).

The limitation of using fresh-gas flow to vaporize liquid anesthetic is that the rate of change of anesthetic vapor concentration delivered to the patient depends primarily on the total fresh-gas flow. This becomes important for the pediatric patient because inhaled inductions are commonly used. In this case, a rapid and sustained increase in anesthetic vapor concentration is desired, and a high fresh-gas flow must be used. Typical settings are 3 L/min of oxygen and 7 L/min of nitrous oxide. These flows are wasteful in that most of the gas ultimately ends up in the scavenging system, but high flows are required to maintain the high inspired-agent concentration during induction. Once the desired concentration of anesthetic vapor is established in the breathing circuit, the fresh-gas flow can be reduced to the minimum rate necessary, a "low-flow" anesthesia technique. When attempting to minimize fresh-gas flows, both the inspired-oxygen monitor and the agent-concentration monitor should be used. The oxygen monitor confirms that adequate oxygen flow is being delivered. Measuring the exhaled-agent concentration helps assure proper depth of anesthesia. If the fresh-gas flow entering the circuit is reduced too early in the induction process, ongoing anesthetic uptake from the lungs may exceed the delivery of anesthetic vapor in the inspired gas and the concentration in the alveolus will fall.

Anesthesia Machine Ventilators

The most important advances in modern anesthesia machines germane to pediatric patients are improvements in anesthesia ventilators. For many years, anesthesia ventilators were not capable of delivering small tidal volumes precisely, did not function well at the higher respiratory rates required by children, and offered few if any modes of ventilation other than a volume-controlled mode. As a result, pediatric patients who were difficult to ventilate required an intensive-care–unit (ICU) ventilator in the operating room. Pressure-controlled ventilation has been an available mode of ventilation on many anesthesia machines for some time and has made it easier to ventilate a wider range of pediatric patients. The most modern anesthesia machines now incorporate ventilation capabilities that approach those of ICU ventilators. Not only are these modern anesthesia ventilators capable of accurately delivering small tidal volumes at high respiratory rates, but they offer a variety of ventilation modes and settings. Furthermore, the modern anesthesia ventilators are paired with flow sensors that are capable of monitoring delivered volumes precisely, even for small infants. In the past, setting the ventilator for small patients necessitated observing the chest for adequate expansion. Although there is no electronic or mechanical substitute for observing the patient, newer anesthesia ventilators are quite capable of ventilating even the smallest patients.

The standard ventilators used in pediatric intensive care units can be used in the operating room, but intravenous anesthesia techniques are typically required because anesthetic vapor delivery is either inefficient or simply not possible. Because anesthesia providers may not be familiar with the available ICU ventilators, it is best to have a respiratory therapist in attendance or immediately available if an ICU ventilator is brought to the operating room. Depending on the capabilities of the anesthesia machine, the added cost and complexity of using an ICU ventilator in the operating room, as well as the inability to administer a volatile anesthetic with the ICU ventilator, may be avoided. For those practitioners who care for small children routinely in the operating room, especially children with significant medical problems, a modern anesthesia machine with a capable ventilator becomes important.

Patients requiring nitric oxide need special adaptation of the breathing circuit. There are no anesthesia machines designed specifically to facilitate nitric oxide delivery, and common practice is to introduce nitric oxide into the breathing circuit through an adapter. This special arrangement is therefore needed for patients receiving nitric oxide and for patients with significant pulmonary hypertension who may require nitric oxide for intraoperative management.

Controlled Ventilation

Controlled ventilation in the operating room can take the form of pressure- or volume-controlled ventilation (VCV). In either case, the goal is to provide all of the patient's ventilation needs with mechanical ventilation—no spontaneous ventilation efforts are expected. Controlled ventilation is commonly used for pediatric patients, especially very small patients, because the work of breathing imposed by the breathing circuit and small endotracheal tube makes effective spontaneous ventilation impossible.

Pressure-controlled ventilation (PCV) is commonly used for pediatric patients and has become the standard approach to pediatric ventilation in many centers. PCV has become popular because it compensates for some of the limitations of the circle anesthesia system for ventilating small patients. Traditionally, it has been difficult to deliver small tidal volumes reliably when using a circle system. Using VCV where the desired tidal volume is delivered by the ventilator is likely to result in hypoventilation because the compliance of the breathing system (i.e., the ventilator components, internal piping, and the breathing circuit itself) can reduce the delivered tidal volume significantly. When using PCV, the ventilator delivers whatever volume is required to achieve the set inspiratory pressure. The resulting tidal volume will depend entirely on the patient's lung compliance, independent of the breathing circuit. The impact of compliance on delivered tidal volume may not be completely apparent when using PCV, because the flow sensor is typically mounted on the expiratory valve and therefore measures both exhaled gas, as well as the gas that was compressed during inspiration in the breathing circuit and never delivered to the patient. Delivered tidal volume is also influenced by adjustments to the fresh-gas flow when using VCV with an older anesthesia machine. PCV obviates the need to be concerned about changing fresh-gas flow, because the ventilator's target is to deliver the set inspiratory pressure. At higher fresh-gas flows the ventilator can deliver less gas to achieve the desired pressure and vice versa. When using PCV, as long as the inspiratory pressure is set so that the desired tidal volume is achieved, the patient is ventilated effectively. The primary disadvantage of PCV is that the delivered tidal volume is not guaranteed. Any change in lung compliance is associated with a change in tidal volume, and inspiratory pressure needs to be adjusted if tidal volume is to be maintained.

The most important change to date in modern anesthesia machines is the ability to precisely deliver small tidal volumes accurately by compensating for breathing-circuit compliance and changes in fresh-gas flow. Newer anesthesia machines have ventilators that can precisely deliver small volumes at high rates (Stayer et al., 2000). Delivering small tidal volumes requires not only an accurate ventilator, but a means for compensating for the compliance of the breathing system and the interaction between fresh-gas flow and inspired tidal volume. Breathing-system compliance exists in any ventilator-circuit combination and results from the compression of gas within the breathing circuit as pressure builds in the circuit, as well as the elastic expansion of the breathing-circuit tubing. Breathing-system compliance is expressed as milliliters of volume that are taken up per centimeter of water pressure, and it is determined by the internal volume of the breathing system and circuit, as well as the elastic properties of the circuit. Longer breathing circuits have an increased compliance primarily because of the greater internal volume. To better understand the impact of breathing-circuit compliance on delivered tidal volume, consider a case where the compliance value is 1 mL/cm H_2O and the inspiratory pressure is 20 cm H_2O. In that case, 20 mL of tidal volume delivered by the ventilator will not reach the patient. If the desired tidal volume is small, for example 100 mL or less, the fraction that does not reach the patient because of circuit compliance becomes a significant fraction of the desired tidal volume.

To compensate for the compliance of the breathing system, the preuse checkout must be performed to allow the ventilator to measure the compliance of the breathing system and then compensate for that compliance factor during VCV. To use these ventilators effectively, it is essential that the preuse checkout procedures be followed with the breathing-circuit configuration that is to be used during the procedure (Fig. 10-5, *A*) (Bachiller et al., 2008). Different anesthesia-machine vendors have different approaches to eliminate the interaction between fresh-gas flow and tidal volume. Some anesthesia machines (e.g., Draeger Medical; Lubeck, Germany) use a decoupling valve between the ventilator and the fresh-gas inflow so that the valve closes during inspiration. Other anesthesia machine designs (e.g., General Electric; Madison, Wisconsin) compensate for the fresh-gas flow by using closed-loop feedback between the inspiratory flow sensor and the ventilator.

Because modern anesthesia machines can now deliver and monitor small tidal volumes effectively, it is possible to use VCV routinely for pediatric patients. When using VCV, by definition, tidal volume is constant and pressure varies with changes in lung compliance. To protect the patient from high pressures caused by sudden changes in effective lung compliance (e.g., coughing or external pressure on the chest), a pressure limit can be set when using VCV. This limit should be set above the inspiratory pressure required to deliver the set tidal volume; otherwise, the desired volume will not be delivered.

Assisted Spontaneous Ventilation

Another advantage of modern anesthesia ventilators for pediatric patients is the advent of pressure-supported modes of ventilation. These modes are specifically designed to allow for spontaneous ventilation when an endotracheal tube or supralaryngeal airway is in place and the associated work of breathing would be an impediment to effective spontaneous ventilation. In pediatric patients the work of breathing is a major problem because small endotracheal tubes impose a significant resistance to inspiration, the ventilator circuits and valves add to the work of breathing, and the anesthetized patients have reduced inspiratory force. In general, long periods of unassisted spontaneous ventilation during anesthesia are undesirable and can result in progressive atelectasis. Supported ventilation is an excellent method for allowing a patient to breathe spontaneously, and it has been demonstrated to improve gas exchange during anesthesia (von Goedecke et al., 2005).

Depending on the manufacturer of the anesthesia machine, assisted spontaneous-ventilation modes can have different names; however, the basic controls and implementations for the

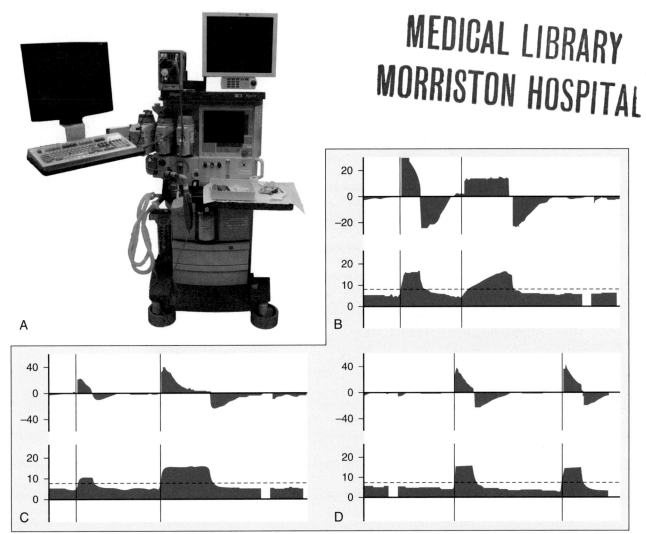

■ **FIGURE 10-5. A,** Modern anesthesia ventilator (Draeger Apollo Workstation) capable of pressure support ventilation and circuit compliance compensation. **B,** Typical flow (L/min) *(top)* and pressure (cm H$_2$O) *(bottom)* waveforms indicating mixed VCV and PSV. The vertical black spike indicates that a breath has been triggered by the patient. The mandatory volume breath is indicated by the constant inspiratory flow and ascending pressure waveforms and, in this case, was synchronized with the patient's inspiration. The pressure support breath is indicated by the constant inspiratory pressure and decelerating flow waveforms. **C,** Typical flow (L/min) *(top)* and pressure (cm H$_2$O) *(bottom)* waveforms indicating mixed PCV and PSV. The synchronized PCV breath can be distinguished from the pressure support breath by the magnitude and duration of the pressure waveform. **D,** Typical flow *(top)* and pressure *(bottom)* waveforms indicating PSV.

assisted part of the ventilation mode are similar. The common settings for the degree of ventilator assistance are the inspiratory flow needed to trigger a supported breath, the inspiratory pressure that will be provided when the patient initiates a breath, and any positive end-expiratory pressure (PEEP) that will be provided. The tidal volume that results from a supported breath depends on the inspiratory pressure provided by the ventilator and the amount of patient effort. Typical inspiratory support settings are between 5 and 15 cm H$_2$O above PEEP. The duration of a supported breath is typically determined by the patient. Once the inspiratory pressure is triggered, the ventilator supplies gas to maintain that pressure until the inspiratory flow falls to a predetermined fraction of the peak inspiratory flow (25% is common).

The most important ventilator control when using assisted spontaneous ventilation is the inspiratory flow that is needed to trigger an assisted breath. The trigger setting tells the ventilator how much inspiratory flow the patient must generate to cause the ventilator to assist the spontaneous effort. Pediatric patients may require lower trigger settings than adult patients, which increases the chance of autotriggering. Supported breaths are usually flow-triggered, whereby support is initiated when inspiratory flow exceeds a preset threshold. If the threshold is very low (0.5 to 1 L/min), it is possible that a breath may be triggered by a practitioner leaning on the patient's chest or simply by small movements of gas in the breathing circuit. Monitoring the pressure waveform as well as the rate and regularity of triggered breaths can help identify when autotriggering is occurring. If there is a concern that autotriggering is occurring, the trigger threshold can be gradually increased until triggering stops. At that point the patient, as well as the pressure and flow waveforms, can be inspected to see if there are any underlying spontaneous breathing efforts. The goal would be to determine whether there are sufficient spontaneous efforts to warrant using an assisted rather than a controlled mode of ventilation. If not, a mode of ventilation should be chosen with enough mandatory support to achieve the ventilation goals.

Three typical options for assisted spontaneous ventilation are listed as follows:

VCV plus pressure support: When using this mode, the user selects a volume to be delivered, the respiratory rate, the inspiratory/expiratory ratio, or the inspiratory time and PEEP as indicated. In addition, the user selects the inspiratory pressure for assisted breaths and the trigger threshold. The set respiratory rate and tidal volume determine the minimum mandatory ventilation the patient receives. If the patient initiates a breath within the window of a mandatory breath, the effort triggers a synchronized breath at the set tidal volume. If spontaneous efforts occur at a greater rate than the set mandatory rate, assisted breaths are triggered and provided at the set level of inspiratory-pressure support above PEEP. Observation of the pressure waveform allows the anesthetist to distinguish synchronized mandatory breaths from triggered pressure support breaths. The synchronized volume breath appears as a gradually ascending pressure waveform, whereas the pressure support breath appears as a square wave (Fig. 10-5, B).

PCV plus pressure support: When using this mode, the user selects an inspiratory pressure to be delivered, the respiratory rate, the inspiratory/expiratory ratio, or the inspiratory time and PEEP as indicated. In addition, the user selects the inspiratory pressure for assisted breaths and the trigger threshold. The set respiratory rate and inspiratory pressure determine the minimum mandatory ventilation the patient receives. If the patient initiates a breath within the window of a mandatory breath, the effort triggers a synchronized breath at the set inspiratory pressure. If spontaneous efforts occur at a greater rate than the set mandatory rate, assisted breaths are triggered and provided at the set level of inspiratory pressure support above PEEP. Observation of the pressure waveform allow one to distinguish synchronized mandatory breaths from triggered pressure support breaths. The synchronized pressure breath appears as a square wave at the set inspiratory pressure. The pressure support breath also appears as a square wave but typically at a lower maximum pressure and often a shorter inspiratory time (Fig. 10-5, C).

Pressure Support Ventilation (PSV): When this mode is selected, all of the breaths are supported at the set inspiratory pressure above PEEP. In that case, the minute ventilation that results is completely dependent on the inspiratory pressure setting, the patient's effort, and the patient's respiratory rate. Most of these modes allow for a minimum backup ventilation rate, whereby the ventilator delivers a breath if the patient does not trigger breaths at a rate that exceeds the backup rate. Untriggered breaths delivered by the backup setting alone may not result in an acceptable minute ventilation, because there is no patient effort to augment the delivered tidal volume. If a patient does not exceed the backup setting and trigger breaths when using PSV, it may be prudent to use a mandatory mode (VCV or PCV) with pressure support to ensure adequate minute ventilation (Fig. 10-5, D).

Warming Devices

Heat conservation is critical in the care of the newborn infant. A decrease of 2° C in the environmental temperature is sufficient to double the oxygen consumption of a full-term infant (Hill and Rahimtulla, 1965). To meet this increase in oxygen consumption, the neonate must double its minute ventilation. For a critically ill premature infant who is unable to mount this increase in ventilation, an oxygen debt and progressive lactic acidosis ensue (see Chapter 6, Thermoregulation: Physiology and Perioperative Disturbances). The rate of heat loss in newborn infants is four times that in adults because of a higher surface area-to-body weight ratio, increased curvature of body surfaces, and decreased insulation from skin and subcutaneous fat (Adamson and Towell, 1965). Special efforts must be made to maintain body temperature during anesthesia, especially in small infants undergoing operative procedures accompanied by large insensible heat losses.

Forced Warm-Air Device

The flow of warm air across a child's skin produced by a forced-air warming blanket prevents heat loss to the environment and may even effectively warm patients via radiant shielding and convection. Of all devices, this is one of the most effective and should be used in all cases where hypothermia is a possibility (Sessler et al., 1991; Camus et al., 1993; Kurz et al., 1993). Forced-air systems inject warm air through a connecting hose into a quiltlike blanket that has small holes on one surface. Warm air escaping through these holes provides conductive and convective warming to the patient. Different sizes of blankets permit maximum coverage of specific body areas over a range of patient sizes. The most effective units direct flow toward areas with major blood vessels, like the chest, axillae, abdomen, and groin, where convective heating is most effective (Giesbrecht et al., 1994). Like overhead radiant warmers and circulating-water blankets, forced-air systems can produce burns and overheating when used inappropriately (Truell et al., 2000). Maximum air temperatures on these devices are designed to minimize the risk of burns. Ensuring that the tube carrying the warm air to the blanket does not touch the patient also decreases the likelihood of thermal injury. Furthermore, directing warm air from the hose without the blanket ("free-hosing") has been associated with patient burns. Patients with compromised circulations are at a higher risk of burns even when the blanket is used correctly; the temperature should not be set to the highest setting in these patients, especially during prolonged surgery (Siddik-Sayyid et al., 2008). Blankets that are wet are ineffective at maintaining temperature and should be replaced (Lin et al., 2008).

Wrapping and Draping with Plastic Sheets

Because of their large surface area, infants have significant evaporative and radiant heat loss. Wrapping and draping the patient with special blankets is also effective in decreasing heat loss during prolonged surgery, especially when forced-air devices are impractical. Radiant heat loss can be decreased with the use of Webril cotton wrapping (Kendall Corporation; Boston, Massachusetts) covered with plastic bags over exposed extremities. For small infants with relatively large heads, cranial heat loss can be decreased up to 73% by wrapping the head in insulated hat or plastic bag. This is significant for neonates, because their brains are responsible for 44% of their total heat production (Rowe et al., 1983). The use of reflective blankets, made from the material used in outdoor survival apparel (e.g., space blankets), is also effective in reducing heat loss (Bourke, et al., 1984). Cutaneous heat loss is proportional to the surface area of the patient, making the percentage of skin surface covered far more important than the region of the body covered or the type of material used for passive insulation (Sessler et al., 1991).

Humidification of Inspired Gases

Humidification of inspired gases, as noted previously, is an important technique for conserving heat in anesthetized patients. Because 12% to 14% of body heat is lost through the respiratory tract, the use of warm, humidified gases decreases the potential heat drain in addition to preventing damage to the ciliated cells of the tracheobronchial tree caused by dry gases (Clarke et al., 1954). The humidifier should be servocontrolled, with a temperature sensor close to the patient to automatically shut off the heater when the preset temperature equals the patient's airway temperature, minimizing the risk of airway burns. Maximum temperature limits, causing automatic shut-off, should also be an integral aspect of the humidifier. Special anesthesia circuits with a heated wire in the expiratory limb minimizes condensation that can occur with humidifiers. HMEs (e.g., Humid-Vent) can provide 80% inspired humidity when 80 minutes of use is allowed to saturate the hygroscopic membrane (Bissonnette et al., 1989a, 1989b). Many HMEs are incorporated into breathing-system filters. These serve to minimize the passage of infectious materials to the breathing circuit and provide warmth and humidification of inhaled gases. The efficacy of various HME brands to perform these functions is variable. The internal volumes of these devices can range from 10 to 60 mL, and small volume filters are preferred in the neonatal population. HME filters may increase the work of breathing and dead space and should be accounted for when ventilating small children. Filtration efficacy is assessed by the penetrance of sodium chloride particles (0.1 to 0.3 mcm); tests in pediatric HME filters show that their filtration ability is less than in adult filters. Based on these findings the Centers for Disease Control (CDC) recommend changing the breathing circuit for each new case. Berry and Nolte (1991) examined the efficacy of the Pall HME filter in preventing bacterial contamination of the circle-breathing system in a laboratory model and found it to be an effective microbial barrier between the patient and the circle system. They concluded that when using the Pall HME filter the components beyond the filter may be reused. However the reuse of single-use equipment is not recommended and use borne by the individual practitioner or institution. To date there has not been a reported case of infection transmission between patients related to anesthesia-breathing systems with filters in place.

Face Masks

The most appropriate anesthesia face mask for a child spans vertically from the bridge of the nose to just below the lower lip, without compressing the nasal passages. It should contain the least volume (i.e., dead space) possible. The pediatric face mask should be constructed with a clear (nonlatex) plastic that

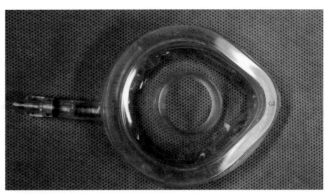

■ FIGURE 10-6. Plastic disposable face mask with pneumatic cushion.

allows recognition of cyanosis, the condensation of exhaled gas, and the presence of excess secretions or vomitus. A constant challenge in pediatric anesthesia, especially for small infants, is to find a face mask that conforms to the shape of an infant's face without a significant leak. During positive pressure ventilation the anesthesiologist often must twist or torque a face mask without applying undue pressure against a child's face to reduce the amount of air that escapes from within the mask. To achieve these purposes, a variety of face masks have been used in the pediatric population.

The most common anesthesia face mask in use today is the plastic disposable type that contains an adjustable pneumatic cushion, which when inflated or deflated with air can be altered to conform to the shape of a child's face. A variety of different manufacturers produce this type of face mask (Fig. 10-6). An alternative variety for use in pediatric patients is the Rendell-Baker-Soucek mask, which remains in use in many centers (Fig. 10-7). This mask is available in malleable rubber or non-latex silicone and allows an effective seal on a child's face while minimizing internal dead space. It was originally designed on the basis of anatomic molds taken from a large number of children (Rendell-Baker and Soucek, 1962).

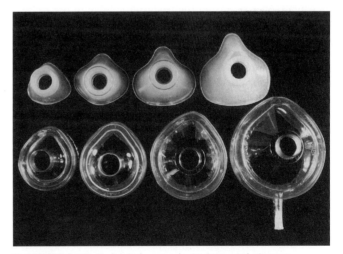

■ FIGURE 10-7. Pediatric face masks. Various mask sizes are available for the wide range of pediatric patients. *Top row,* Four different Rendell-Baker-Soucek masks (From Willy Rusch, Kernen, Germany); *Bottom row,* Disposable bubble masks (From Vital Signs, Totowa, New Jersey).

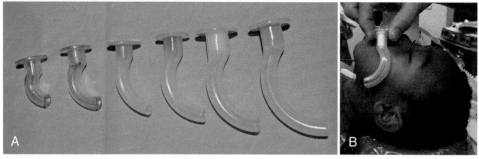

■ **FIGURE 10-8. A,** Oral airway devices for the spectrum of pediatric patients. **B,** The appropriately-sized oral airway device is chosen by placing it adjacent to the face to approximate its position in the oral cavity.

Oral and Nasal Airway Devices

Oral and nasal pharyngeal airway devices are used in pediatric anesthesia to improve patency of the upper airway and to facilitate delivery of oxygen or anesthetic gases to the lungs. Minimum requirements for these devices are noted in ANSI/ISO5364-08 (ANSI/ISO, 2008). The Guedel-type oral airway device is probably most commonly used in pediatric patients. It contains a central lumen for the passage of airflow and for suctioning of the posterior pharynx (Fig. 10-8, A). The oral airway device is primarily used to alleviate upper airway obstruction caused by tonsillar or adenoidal hypertrophy, or normal pharyngeal tissue obstruction, as often occurs in small infants (see Chapter 3, Respiratory Physiology).

Oral airway devices are usually manufactured from plastic or polyethylene and are latex-free. They are sized according to the total length of the device (50 to 80 mm, flange to tip, for most children) or based on an arbitrary scale designated by the manufacturer. The appropriate size is determined by placing the airway device adjacent to the child's face to approximate its position in the oral cavity. The appropriately-sized oropharyngeal airway device should extend from the corner of the mouth to the angle of the mandible (Fig. 10-8, B). When appropriately placed, its distal end snugly curves around the base of the tongue, without the proximal end protruding out of the mouth. Too small a device pushes the posterior portion of the tongue against the posterior pharyngeal wall, and too large a device may cause upper airway obstruction at the laryngeal inlet by compressing or distorting the epiglottis.

The oral airway device should be inserted in its normal orientation with the aid of a tongue depressor. In older children, insertion may be accomplished with the distal tip oriented cephalad and then turned 180 degrees when the tip has reached the posterior aspect of the palate. In younger children, this maneuver may push the tongue posteriorly and exacerbate airway obstruction.

Complications of using oral airway devices in children are not uncommon and usually occur during emergence. Lip or tooth damage is possible; a loose tooth may become dislodged and lost in the oral cavity, where it may accidentally travel into the bronchopulmonary tree. Compression of oral structures by the oral airway device may result in transient postoperative numbness and a sore throat.

The nasal airway device is made from soft, latex-free rubber to allow easy insertion through the nasal passage and into the nasal or oropharynx. It can be bathed in warm or cold water to decrease or increase its stiffness, respectively. Some nasal airway devices contain an enlarged flange at the proximal end to prevent unintentional advancement into the nasal cavity. Others contain an adjustable ring that can be secured against the outside of the nasal opening. Nasal airways are available in sizes 12 to 36F (outer diameter, or OD) (Fig. 10-9). If required, a stiffer nasal airway can be fashioned out of a standard tracheal tube by cutting it off at the appropriate length. An anesthesia breathing circuit can be connected to any type of nasal airway device using an appropriately sized tracheal tube adaptor (Fig. 10-10). This technique may facilitate intubation in patients with difficult airways by allowing the administration of anesthesia and oxygen during airway manipulation via a modified nasal airway connected to the anesthesia breathing circuit (Holm-Knudsen et al., 2005). The use of an adaptor also permits delivery of continuous positive airway pressure (CPAP).

To avoid trauma and bleeding of the delicate nasal mucosa, the nasal airway device should be lubricated and gently inserted in a posterocaudad direction along the floor of the nasal cavity. A topical vasoconstrictor, such as 0.05% oxymetazoline, can be applied to the nasal mucosa before inserting the nasal airway device to shrink nasal mucosal tissue and reduce bleeding.

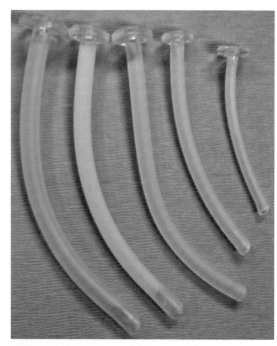

■ **FIGURE 10-9.** Nasopharyngeal airway devices.

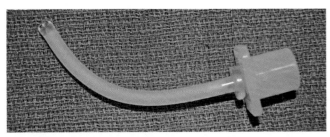

■ FIGURE 10-10. Nasopharyngeal airway device modified with 15-mm tracheal-tube adapter.

Vasoconstrictors should be used in recommended doses, particularly because topical phenylephrine use has been associated with cardiac arrest and death in children. The circumstances of these arrests usually involve the topical administration of an unmeasured dose of phenylephrine with resultant hypertension. The anesthesiologists in these cases administered a β-blocking or calcium-channel blocking agent in response to the hypertension, with the consequence of pulmonary edema and cardiac arrest (Groudine et al., 2000). Hypertension secondary to α-agonists should be treated with a α-antagonists and direct vasodilating agents. In children weighing up to 25 kg, the initial dose of phenylephrine should not exceed 20 mcg/kg (Groudine et al., 2000). Oxymetazoline can also cause hypertension, tachycardia, and peripheral vasoconstriction by stimulation of peripheral α_2-receptors; some patients exhibit hypotension, bradycardia, and neurologic and respiratory depression related to stimulation of central α_2-receptors. Current dosing guidelines recommend oxymetazoline use in children at 6 years of age, although it is safely utilized in children of all ages. A 0.025% solution is recommended for ophthalmic use (1 to 2 drops to affected eye every 6 hours) and a 0.05% solution for nasal use (2 to 3 sprays in each nostril twice a day). The proper diameter of the nasal airway device is determined by approximating the circular diameter of the nasal opening. The proper length of the nasal airway device is estimated by measuring the distance from the nares to the tragus of the ear. When appropriately placed, its distal tip should lie at the level of the angle of the mandible, between the posterior aspect of the tongue and above the tip of the epiglottis.

The most common complication resulting from inserting a nasal airway device is trauma to the nasal or pharyngeal mucosa that results in minor bleeding. Adenoidal tissue may be disrupted and may bleed into the oropharynx. Occasionally, a variable vessel is encountered in the nasal mucosa and bleeding brisk. Sequential dilation of the nasal passage with nasal airway devices of increasing size is sometimes used in an attempt to minimize trauma during nasal intubation. Adamson et al. (1988) investigated the influence of dilation vs. no dilation on bleeding and found an increased incidence of hemorrhage with dilation and no difference in resistance to passage of the tracheal tube. There are two pathways that devices can take when placed into the nasal passage: a lower pathway below the inferior turbinate and an upper pathway between the middle and inferior turbinates. The middle turbinate is attached anteriorly to the cribriform plate and posteriorly to the ethmoid bone by thin lamella, making it vulnerable to trauma and avulsion when an airway device is forcibly passed through the upper pathway. The lower pathway is therefore preferred, and airway devices should be inserted perpendicular to the patient's nare

and directed caudally to increase the likelihood of passage into the lower pathway (Hall and Shutt, 2003; Ahmed-Nusrath et al., 2008). Nasal airways should not be inserted in children with a coagulopathy, neutropenia, or suspicion of a traumatic basilar skull fracture.

Tracheal Tubes

The most commonly used tracheal tubes are made of nonreactive polyvinylchloride (PVC). Tracheal tubes should bear a designation that they comply with ANSI/ISO Standard 5361 (1999), which confirms that they are inert, as well as meet dimension, material, and product-marking standards. Biologically inert materials reduce the risk of airway inflammatory reactions.

PVC tubes are flammable and cannot be used in laser surgery performed on airways. A tube that is either nonflammable (e.g., metal) or laser-resistant (e.g., red rubber tube wrapped with aluminum foil or manufactured with special surface treatments) must be substituted (see Chapter 24, Anesthesia for Pediatric Otorhinolaryngologic Surgery). These special tubes should have a label indicating that they are intended for use in laser surgery. Patients with difficult airways or tracheal abnormalities often require a spiral wire-embedded silicone, or "anode," tube (Fig. 10-11). This tube has the flexibility to assume virtually any position, while the wire coil embedded in its wall preserves the lumen. Extreme caution must be taken with anode tubes, because their flexibility makes accidental extubation more likely.

In evaluating tracheal tubes for use in infants and children, their influence on dead space, resistance to breathing, and tracheal or laryngeal injury must be considered. Tracheal intubation reduces the dead space of the natural extrathoracic airway but can have a dramatic negative impact on the resistance to breathing (Glauser et al., 1961). Resistance to laminar flow through a tube is governed by the Hagen-Poiseuille Law, which dictates that resistance is proportional to the length of the tube and inversely proportional to the fourth power of the radius. Thus, small changes in the lumen of a tube can dramatically increase the resistance to flow through it. Assuming that flow is laminar and that all other variables are constant, one can predict that a reduction in internal diameter (ID) from 7.5 to 7.0 mm increases resistance 24%, whereas a reduction from 3.5 to 3.0 mm increases resistance by nearly 50%. Because luminal

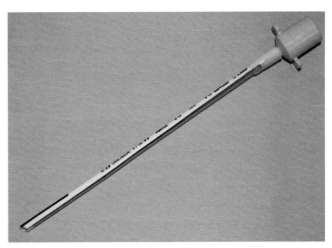

■ FIGURE 10-11. Wire reinforced anode tube.

changes between the tracheal tube and the adapter promote turbulent flow, measured differences are even more exaggerated. The resistance to breathing through the natural airway of a neonate is greater than that through a 3.5-mm ID tracheal tube but significantly less than that through a 2.5-mm ID tracheal tube (Polgar and Kong, 1965). A small amount of secretions or debris can increase resistance substantially, yet these accumulations are difficult to avoid in small-lumen tubes. The use of 2.5-mm ID tracheal tubes should be restricted to situations in which no other tube fits.

Resistance to breathing is governed by the ID of a tube, but the potential for laryngeal or tracheal mucosal injury is related to the OD. Mild trauma to the airway, producing as little as 1-mm mucosal edema, can result in significant narrowing of the infant's airway. As little as 25 mm Hg pressure on the lateral wall of the trachea causes local ischemia and mucosal injury in adults and presumably in children as well (Nordin et al., 1977; Seegobin and van Hasselt, 1984).

Historically, uncuffed tracheal tubes have been used for children under 8 years. Based on the interpretation of statements by Eckenhoff (1951), the child's larynx was thought to be conical with a circular cricoid ring at its most narrow dimension and only assumed a more cylindrical shape as the child matured into an adult (Motoyama, 2009). A circular, uncuffed tracheal tube would then conform well to this narrow, circular portion of the airway. More recent data suggest that the cricoid is slightly elliptical with the rima glottidis (the vocal cords) as the narrowest point in the pediatric airway (Litman et al., 2003; Dalal et al., 2009). A snug-fitting tracheal tube would exert more pressure on the lateral mucosa of the trachea than in the anterior-posterior direction. (Motoyama, 2009). This conclusion might suggest the use of smaller, uncuffed tracheal tubes. However, smaller tracheal tubes would increase resistance to spontaneous breathing, make controlled ventilation more difficult caused by a larger leak around the tube, increase environmental pollution, and possibly risk increased rates of pulmonary aspiration.

Yet with the reduction in tube size necessary to pass the glottic opening and the fear of laryngeal and tracheal damage, cuffed tracheal tubes have not been recommended in young children in the past. With the regular use of mechanical ventilation and the advent of pressure-support anesthesia ventilators, increased tracheal tube resistance may be less of an issue for most children undergoing anesthesia. Tissue damage may be the result of overinflated cuffs or prolonged intubation in intensive care settings (Nordin, 1977; Holski, 1997). Several series, however, have demonstrated that cuffed, tracheal tubes perform as well or better than uncuffed tubes in children undergoing anesthesia with muscle relaxant, noting fewer required intubation attempts and no difference in the incidence of postoperative croup (Khine et al., 1997; Murat, 2001; Weiss et al., 2009).

The development of a new, microcuff tracheal tube (Kimberly-Clark Worldwide; Roswell, Georgia) may add additional advantages to management of the pediatric airway (Weiss and Dullenkopf, 2007). These tubes have an anatomically-based intubation depth mark for placement at the level of the cords, providing a margin of safety for tube-tip displacement with head flexion and extension (Weiss et al., 2006). Additionally, these tubes have a distally placed cuff with a smooth, thin membrane that allows the cuff to avoid the cricoid and larynx and facilitates lower inflation pressures to seal the trachea (Fig. 10-12, A).

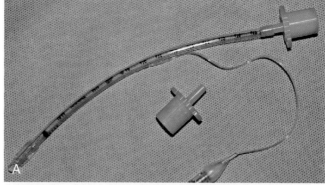

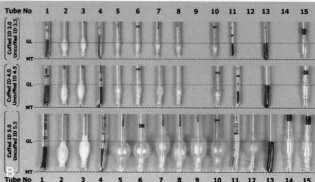

■ **FIGURE 10-12. A,** Microcuff tube. **B,** 3.0-, 4.0-, and 5.0-mm ID cuffed tracheal tubes and age-related corresponding (ID + 0.5 mm) uncuffed tracheal tubes are shown for each of the 15 tube brands. Age-related mid-tracheal placement of the tube tip according to the depth marking of the uncuffed tracheal tube results in laryngeal or even glottic level position of the cuff for all the cuffed tracheal tubes, *(From Weiss M et al.: Shortcomings of cuffed paediatric tracheal tubes, Br J Anaesth 92(1):78, 2004.)*

Whether cuffed tracheal tubes should replace uncuffed tubes in pediatrics is unclear. In a large, randomized, controlled, multicenter trial comparing cuffed with uncuffed endotracheal tubes, Weiss and others (2009) reported that in children from birth to 5 years of age undergoing general anesthesia, the incidence of postextubation stridor was similar for the cuffed tube group (4.4%) vs. the uncuffed group (4.7%). However, the rate of tube exchange was significantly greater in the uncuffed group (30.8%) compared with the cuffed group (2.1%). Unfortunately, some of the major shortcomings of cuffed tracheal tubes are the relative inconsistency of the distance of the distal tube tip to the lower and upper borders of the cuff, the ODs of the tubes, and the maximal cross-sectional area of the inflated cuff and depth markers for positioning of the tube at the appropriate depth of the trachea (Fig. 10-12, *B*; see Chapter 1, Special Characteristics of Pediatric Anesthesia, Table 1-1) (Weiss et al., 2004a).

A variety of tracheal tubes are available for special needs. A Ring, Adaire, Elwyn (RAE) tube has a preformed contour that facilitates access to the surgical field (Fig. 10-13, *A*). Oral RAE tubes were initially developed for cleft-palate surgery. The proximal end of the oral RAE tube rests over the middle of the mandible, whereas the proximal end of a nasal RAE tube rests on the forehead (Fig. 10-13, *B*; see Chapter 25, Anesthesia for Plastic Surgery, Fig. 25-12). These preformed tracheal tubes can be used for any type of head or neck surgery in which the operating room table is turned away from the anesthesiologist.

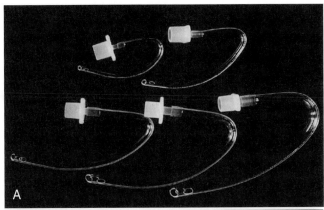

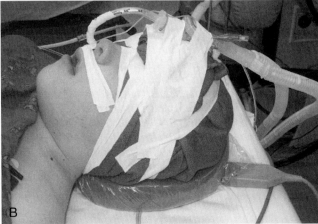

■ **FIGURE 10-13. A,** Oral RAE tubes. Preformed oral RAE tubes are made in a variety of sizes. They are especially useful in facial surgery. **B,** The nasal RAE tube is preformed to sit on the forehead for procedures in the oral cavity or neck. *(From Litman RS: Pediatric airway management. In Litman RS, editor:* Pediatric anesthesia: the requisites, *St. Louis, 2004, Mosby.)*

and the head is maintained in a neutral position. The greatest disadvantage of preformed tubes is that the flexion point is fixed. The length may be inappropriate, especially in patients whose cricoid diameter is unusually large or small, increasing the risk of endobronchial intubation or accidental extubation, respectively. Similarly, in a patient with a laryngeal or proximal tracheal stenosis, a standard tracheal tube of a caliber small enough to be admitted to the airway may be too short. Tubes of small caliber with extra length are commercially available for this purpose.

Double-Lumen Tracheal Tubes

A double-lumen tracheal tube is commonly used to attain lung separation in adults. Its advantages include rapid and easy separation of the lungs, access to both lungs to facilitate suctioning, the ability to rapidly switch to two-lung ventilation if needed, and the ability to administer CPAP or oxygen insufflation to the operative lung, when necessary. The smallest commercially available double-lumen tracheal tube is size 26F, which precludes its placement in children weighing less than 30 to 35 kg or younger than 8 to 10 years old (Table 10-1; see Chapter 23, Anesthesia for General Abdominal, Thoracic, Urologic, and Bariatric Surgery, Table 23-9). With this small,

TABLE 10-1. Comparative Diameters of Single-Lumen and Double-Lumen Tubes

Fresh Size (fr)	Double Lumen Tubes (Teleflex Medical-Rusch, Durham, NC)			Comparable Single Lumen Tubes (Coviden-Nellcor, Boulder, CO)	
	External Diameter (mm)*	Bronchial Lumen Internal Diameter (mm)	FOB Size (mm)†	Internal Dameter (mm)	External Diameter (mm)
26	8.3	3.4	2.4	6.0	8.2
28	8.9	3.8	2.4	6.5	8.9
35	11.1	4.2	>3.5	8.0	10.8
37	11.8	4.5	>3.5	9.0	12.1
39	12.4	4.8	>3.5	9.5	12.8
41	13.1	5.0	>3.5	10.0	13.5

*The approximate external metric diameter of the double lumen tube.
†The maximum diameter of FOB that will pass through lumen of given double lumen tube.
FOB, Fiberoptic tube.

double-lumen tracheal tube, bronchoscopic confirmation of its appropriate location within the trachea and bronchus requires use of an ultrathin flexible bronchoscope (Wood, 1985).

Tracheal Tubes for One-Lung Ventilation

Because of mechanical difficulties of one-lung ventilation in small children, pediatric surgeons historically have used retractors and surgical packs to improve surgical exposure during thoracic surgery. With the increasing popularity of thoracoscopic surgical techniques in children, there is an increasing need to provide one-lung ventilation to facilitate surgical exposure (Rowe et al., 1994; Tobias, 1999; Hammer, 2001). The pediatric anesthesiologist has a number of choices for the provision of one-lung ventilation.

Univent Tracheal Tubes. The Univent Tracheal Tube (Fuji Systems Corporation; Tokyo, Japan) is a single-lumen tracheal tube with a moveable bronchial blocker built into its side wall (Fig. 10-14) (Kamaya and Krishna, 1985; Hammer et al., 1998; MacGillivray, 1988). The bronchial blocker contains a low-pressure high-volume cuff and has a central channel used to suction the blocked lung and to insufflate oxygen. The Univent Tracheal Tube is inserted into the trachea like a standard tracheal tube with the bronchial blocker withdrawn into the main tube. The bronchial blocker can then be advanced into the main-stem bronchus of the operative lung under bronchoscopic guidance. Rotation of the tracheal tube determines the direction that the blocker takes as it is advanced. Inflation of the endobronchial cuff on the balloon-tip catheter enables isolation of the operative lung. At the end of the procedure, the blocker tube can be withdrawn into the main tube, permitting postoperative ventilation without the need to change to a separate single-lumen tube.

Advantages of the Univent Tracheal Tube include ease of placement and the ability to easily change from one-lung ventilation to two-lung ventilation. In addition, unlike the standard double-lumen tracheal tube, the bronchial blocker can be pulled back into its channel with the Univent tube left in place

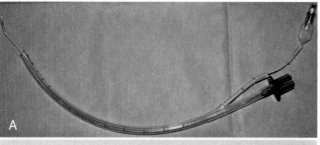

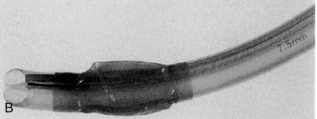

■ **FIGURE 10-14. A,** Univent tube. The bronchial blocker is incorporated into the tracheal tube to allow for isolation of one of the lungs during the anesthesia. The blocker can be withdrawn from the tube, and ventilation can be continued in the postoperative period without the need to exchange to a single-lumen tube. **B,** The blocker in the retracted state.

for postoperative ventilation. The Univent Tracheal Tube is available in sizes 3.5- (uncuffed), 4.5-, 6.0-, 6.5-, 7.5-, 8.0-, 8.5-, and 9.0-mm ID. The OD is larger than that of a conventional tracheal tube of the same ID. The IDs of the 3.5- and 4.0-mm ID Univent Tracheal Tubes limit the passage of a standard pediatric bronchoscope with an OD of 3.5 mm or greater, thereby requiring an ultrathin pediatric bronchoscope to visualize the bronchial blocker.

Selective Endobronchial Intubation

In infants and young children whose small size precludes placement of a double-lumen tracheal tube or a Univent tube, there are two additional options for one-lung ventilation: selective endobronchial intubation with a standard tracheal tube or placement of a separate "bronchial-blocker" device.

Endobronchial Intubation with a Standard Tracheal Tube. A tracheal tube can be inserted into either main bronchus with the use of bronchoscopic guidance or fluoroscopic guidance. In small neonates, an uncuffed tracheal tube can provide adequate isolation of the lungs. In older infants and children, a cuffed tracheal tube maintains an effective seal of the lungs while maintaining the tube in a proximal position within the main bronchus. A tube with a distally placed cuff facilitates this placement. The major disadvantage of selective endobronchial intubation is that it is not possible to quickly change from one-lung ventilation to two-lung ventilation because it requires repositioning the tracheal tube from the bronchus into the trachea and vice versa. Furthermore, with unintentional movement of the tracheal tube and minimal cephalad displacement, selective intubation may be lost because of bronchial extubation, a phenomenon that occasionally happens with surgery around the hilum of the lung.

Bronchial-Blocker Devices. A bronchial-blocker device consists of a small balloon that is purposefully inflated within the proximal portion of the main bronchus to isolate one of the lungs under bronchoscopic guidance. Several different devices can be used as bronchial blockers, including a Fogarty embolectomy catheter and the Arndt endobronchial blocker (Cook Critical Care; Bloomington, Indiana) (Fig. 10-15). The latter device contains a central channel that allows suctioning (for lung deflation) and the application of oxygen and CPAP. It is too large for use in neonates and infants.

A Fogarty embolectomy catheter contains a balloon at its distal end that can be placed within the proximal main bronchus to isolate the lung either with bronchoscopic or fluoroscopic guidance. A disadvantage of the embolectomy catheter is that the distal tip can be displaced proximally during the course of a surgical procedure, especially if the patient's position changes. Total airway obstruction can result if the inflated balloon slips back into the trachea. Suctioning or application of CPAP is not possible because of the lack of an inner channel. The catheter is usually placed outside of the tracheal tube in small infants, so that the small lumen of the tube is not further compromised.

The Arndt endobronchial blocker is a bronchial blocker with an inflatable cuff and a central lumen, through which a wire with a looped end has been passed (Arndt et al., 1999; Hammer, 2002). The bronchial blocker is passed through a specialized adapter that is placed at the proximal end of the tracheal tube. This adapter contains the following four ports:

1. A connection to the tracheal tube,
2. A standard 15-mm adaptor for the anesthesia circuit,
3. A port for the bronchial blocker with a self-sealing diaphragm that can be tightened around the bronchial blocker to hold it in place, and
4. A port for the flexible bronchoscope.

The bronchial blocker is passed through its port and placed at the entrance of the tracheal tube. The bronchoscope is passed through its port and then through the wire loop at the end of the bronchial blocker. The bronchoscope and bronchial blocker are then passed under direct vision as a single unit into the main bronchus of the operative side. The bronchoscope is withdrawn into the trachea, and the balloon is inflated under direct visualization. When correct placement has been confirmed, the wire loop is removed from the central channel. Once the wire guide is removed from the channel, it cannot be replaced. The Arndt endobronchial blocker is currently available in three sizes (5F, 7F, and 9F), with the 9F recommended for tracheal tubes of 7.5 mm and above, 7F for tracheal tubes of 6.0 to 7.0 mm, and 5F for tracheal tubes of 4.5 to 5.5 mm.

Tracheostomy Tubes

The three most common indications for tracheostomy in children are the need for prolonged mechanical ventilation (more than 50% of cases), upper airway obstruction (40%), and pulmonary toilet (10%) (Wetmore et al., 1999). Within each category are congenital, traumatic, metabolic, infectious, and neoplastic conditions that require tracheostomy. Although the underlying medical conditions may be numerous, the most common diagnoses in pediatric tracheostomy patients are bronchopulmonary dysplasia and neurologic disorders.

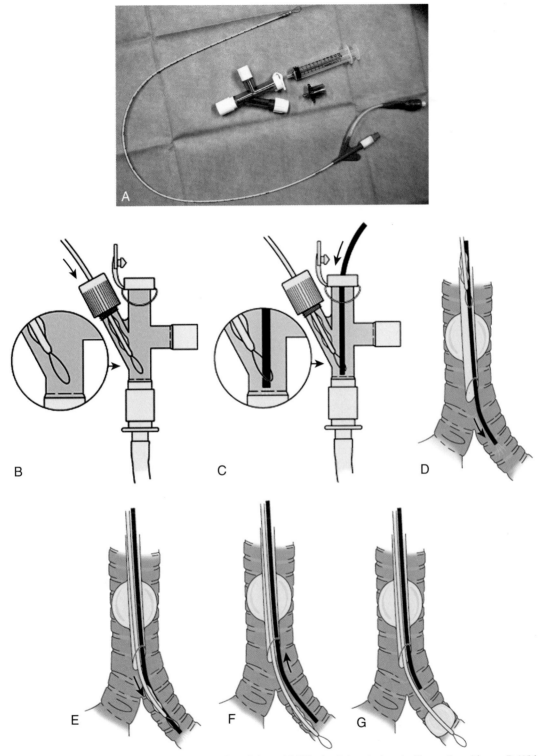

FIGURE 10-15. A, Arndt endobronchial blocker kit. The Arndt endobronchial blocker is inserted under fiberoptic guidance. **B,** With a special ultiport adapter that is attached to the tracheal tube, the blocker is inserted through a side port into the main body of the connector. Ventilation ith 100% oxygen is enabled through a second side port. **C,** A flexible bronchoscope is inserted through the remaining port, engaging the wire op at the end of the bronchial blocker. **D,** The bronchoscope is advanced into the bronchus to be isolated. **E,** The blocker is advanced into the onchus, sliding down the bronchoscope. **F,** The bronchoscope is withdrawn, leaving the blocker in place. **G,** The blocker's balloon is inflated, and acement is verified using the bronchoscope before it is withdrawn completely. *(B-G Courtesy of Cook, Inc., Bloomington, Ind.)*

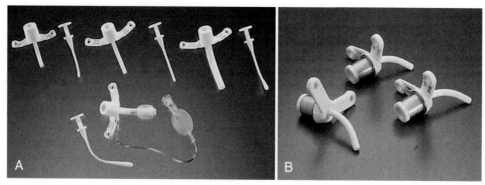

■ **FIGURE 10-16.** Representative models of pediatric tracheostomy tubes include the Shiley **(A)** and the Bivona **(B)**.

The ideal tracheostomy tube should be made of a material that causes minimal tissue reactivity, can be easily cleaned and maintained, and is available in a variety of shapes, diameters, and lengths (Fig. 10-16). The tube needs to be rigid enough to prevent kinking or collapse, yet soft enough to be comfortable for the patient. Early tracheostomy tubes were made of stainless steel or silver (Downes and Schreiner, 1985). These tubes had the advantages of causing minimal tissue reaction and averting tracheal collapse. Their rigidity caused significant discomfort to the patient because of injury to the tracheal mucosa. Most manufacturers use silicone tubes that have minimal tissue reactivity and conform to the structure of the airway. The ideal tube also contains an inner cannula that can be removed and cleaned. Modern tracheostomy tubes have a 15-mm male connector for the attachment of standard respiratory equipment. To improve the patient's comfort and ease of care, a low-profile swivel is commonly added to the tracheostomy tube. This allows unrestricted neck movement and easy care through a suction port. Tracheostomy tubes for infants are uncuffed; in larger children and adolescents, cuffed tracheostomy tubes are preferred. Attachments are available to promote verbal communication.

The appropriate tracheostomy tube is selected on the basis of ID, OD, and length (Table 10-2). The OD determines the size of the tube that may be inserted, whereas the ID determines the actual airway size. The diameter of the tube should be large enough to allow adequate air exchange, easy suctioning, and clearance of secretions. If the indication for tracheostomy is assisted ventilation, the size of the tube should be adjusted to prevent excessive air leak. Predictors of the appropriate tube size include the child's age and the size of a preexisting tracheal tube. A tube that is too large compromises the capillary blood flow in the tracheal wall, which may result in mucosal ischemia, ulceration, and development of fibrous stenosis. Overinflation of a cuffed tracheostomy tube for a prolonged period of time may produce similar injuries. This complication may be avoided by selecting the proper size of tracheostomy tube and adjusting the cuff pressure to less than 20 cm H_2O (Table 10-2). The choice of the tube size is also influenced by visualization of the size of the tracheal lumen.

The length of the tube is important, especially in neonates and infants. A tube that is too short may result in accidental decannulation or the development of a false passage. If a tube is too long, the tip may abrade the carina or become situated in the right main bronchus. Some plastic tubes may be cut to the desired length as necessary. Extra-long, custom-made tubes may be helpful in unusual situations, such as tracheomalacia or tracheal stenosis, to span the diseased area.

Supralaryngeal Airways

Laryngeal Masks

Since the invention of the original laryngeal mask, the Laryngeal Mask Airway (LMA; LMA North America; San Diego, California) (Brain, 1983), several manufacturers have developed laryngeal masks of various designs for use in children (Fig. 10-17, Table 10-3). Examples include the Ambu AuraOnce (Ambu A/S; Ballerup, Denmark), air-Q (Cookgas; St. Louis, Missouri), and the Portex Soft Seal Laryngeal Mask (SS-LM; Portex; Kent, United Kingdom) (Fig. 10-18). Most of these masks share common features, such as a bowl-shaped inflatable cuff attached to an airway tube and a detachable or fixed 15-mm adaptor at the proximal end of the airway tube. Some designs have curved airway tubes, whereas others maintain the original straight configuration. Some of the new designs incorporate a separate gastric access channel to facilitate correct placement and to allow gastric decompression; however, only the Proseal LMA is available in all pediatric sizes (Fig. 10-19). Despite variations in design, one simple principle applies to the use of these devices in children. The incidence of problems with positioning laryngeal masks is inversely proportional to the age of the child; consequently, the use of laryngeal masks in infants and neonates requires an experienced provider with a high level of vigilance. Fiberoptic bronchoscopy and magnetic resonance imaging (MRI) studies in pediatric patients demonstrate high incidence of malpositioning of the LMA in children (Keidan et al., 2000; Monclus et al., 2007). When placed properly, the distal cuff overlies the laryngeal inlet, and the aperture bars, when present, prevent the epiglottis from obstructing the lumen (Fig. 10-20). Once inflated through a pilot tube, the cuff creates a seal in the pharynx that permits both spontaneous and controlled ventilation without large gas leak, provided the peak pressure is below 15 cm H_2O (Epstein and Halmi, 1994; Lardner et al., 2008). A variety of methods of LMA placement in children is possible. The original "Brain" (1990) technique requires that the mask

TABLE 10-2. Tracheostomy Tube Dimensions

Model	Inner Diameter (mm)	Outer Diameter (mm)	Overall Length (mm)	Model	Inner Diameter (mm)	Outer Diameter (mm)	Overall Length (mm)
Shiley*				*Standard Pediatric Uncuffed*			
				60P025	2.5	4.0	38
Shiley Neonatal				60P030	3.0	4.7	39
				60P035	3.5	5.3	40
3.0	3.0	4.5	30	60P040	4.0	6.0	41
3.5	3.5	5.2	32	60P045	4.5	6.7	42
4.0	4.0	5.9	34	60P050	5.0	7.3	44
4.5	4.5	6.5	36	60P055	5.5	8.0	46
Shiley Pediatric				*Standard Pediatric FlexTend Plus‡*			
				60PFS25	2.5	4.0	38
3.0	3.0	4.5	39	60PFS30	3.0	4.7	39
3.5	3.5	5.2	40	60PFS35	3.5	5.3	40
4.0	4.0	5.9	41	60PFS40	4.0	6.0	41
4.5	4.5	6.5	42	60PFS45	4.5	6.7	42
5.0	5.0	7.1	44	60PFS50	5.0	7.3	44
5.5	5.5	7.7	46	60PFS55	5.5	8.0	46
Shiley Pediatric Long				*Extra Long Pediatric FlexTend Plus‡*			
5.0	5.0	7.1	50	60PFS35	3.5	5.3	40
5.5	5.5	7.7	52	60PFS40	4.0	6.0	44
6.0	6.0	8.3	54	60PFS45	4.5	6.7	48
6.5	6.5	9.0	56	60PFS50	5.0	7.3	50
				60PFS55	5.5	8.0	52
Shiley Cuffed Pediatric				*Neonatal Cuffed§*			
4.0	4.0	5.9	41	N025	2.5	4.0	30
4.5	4.5	6.5	42	N030	3.0	4.7	32
5.0	5.0	7.1	44	N035	3.5	5.3	34
5.5	5.5	7.7	46	N040	4.0	6.0	36
Shiley Cuffed Pediatric Long				*Pediatric Cuffed§*			
5.0	5.0	7.1	50	P025	2.5	4.0	38
5.5	5.5	7.7	52	P030	3.0	4.7	39
6.0	6.0	8.3	54	P035	3.5	5.3	40
6.5	6.5	9.0	56	P040	4.0	6.0	41
Bivona†				P045	4.5	6.7	42
				P050	5.0	7.3	44
Standard Neonatal Uncuffed				P055	5.5	8.0	46
60N025	2.5	4.0	30	*Adjustable and Extra Length¶*			
60N030	3.0	4.7	32				
60N035	3.5	5.3	34	60HA25	2.5	4.0	55
60N040	4.0	6.0	36	60HA30	3.0	4.7	60
60N045	4.5	6.5	36	60HA35	3.5	5.3	65
				60HA40	4.0	6.0	70
Neonatal FlexTend Plus‡				60HA45	4.5	6.7	75
				60HA50	5.0	7.3	80
60NFP25	2.5	4.0	30	60HA55	5.5	8.0	85
60NFP30	3.0	4.7	32	550050	5.0	7.7	50
60NFP35	3.5	5.3	34	550055	5.5	8.3	52
60NFP40	4.0	6.0	36	550060	6.0	8.3	55

*Shiley is manufactured by Mallinckrodt Inc., St. Louis, Missouri.

†Bivona is manufactured by Portex, Keene, New Hampshire.

‡FlexTend tubes feature a flexible, kink-resistant proximal extension that allows easier access and enables distal connections away from the infant's chin, neck, and chest.

§Bivona cuffed tubes are available in three different models: Fome-Cuf tubes (85 series) include a SidePort AutoControl Adapter that synchronizes cuff and ventilator pressure. A complete seal is possible for patients with high PEEP or high inspiratory pressure needs. Aire-Cuf tubes (65 series) feature a traditional air-filled cuff. TTS cuffs (67 series) feature an uncuffed tube profile when the cuff is deflated but provide the protection of a cuff when it is inflated.

¶Adjustable Hyperflex (HA series) is an instantly customizable, soft, flexible, kink-resistant, silicone tube with an adjustable neck flange. The flexible shaft adapts to the unique contours of each patient's anatomy. The Adjustable Hyperflex tube is primarily used as a measuring device and temporizing measure until the child can receive a permanent tube with a fixed neck flange. The 550 series is made of PVC that softens at body temperature. It features a long tube shaft and a traditional anatomic curve.

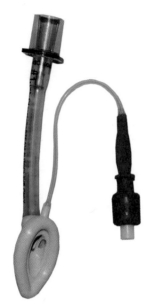

■ **FIGURE 10-17.** Classic LMA.

TABLE 10-3. Laryngeal Mask Sizes

	Weight (kg)	Maximum Endotracheal Tube Accepted*
Air-Q Size		
1	<7	5.0 Cuffed
1.5	7-15	6.0 Cuffed
2.0	15-30	6.0 Cuffed
2.5	20-50	6.5 Cuffed
3.5	50-70	7.5 Cuffed
4.5	70-100	8.5 Cuffed
Ambu AuraOnce Size		
1	<5	3.5 Uncuffed
1.5	5-10	4.5 Uncuffed
2	10-20	4.5 Cuffed
2.5	20-30	5.0 Cuffed
3	30-50	6.0 Cuffed
4	50-70	6.0 Cuffed
5	70-100	7.0 Cuffed
6	>100	7.0 Cuffed
LMA Classic		
1	<5	3.5 Uncuffed
1.5	5-10	4.0 Uncuffed
2	10-20	4.5 Uncuffed
2.5	20-30	5.0 Uncuffed
3	30-50	6.0 Cuffed
4	50-70	6.0 Cuffed
5	70-100	7.0 Cuffed
6	>100	7.0 Cuffed
LMA Proseal		
1	<5	
1.5	5-10	4.5 Uncuffed
2	10-20	4.5 Uncuffed
2.5	20-30	4.5 Uncuffed
3	30-50	5.0 Uncuffed
4	50-70	5.0 Uncuffed
5	70-100	6.0 Uncuffed

*Based on Mallinckrodt tracheal tubes.

advanced across the hard palate with the cuff fully deflated, the distal aperture facing anteriorly, and the head in the classic "sniffing" position. The index finger of the right hand helps guide the LMA over the surface of the tongue while pressing the mask against the palate, thereby simulating the action of the tongue on a bolus of food. A water-based lubricant applied to the posterior surface of the LMA helps to decrease the resistance to insertion. On meeting the characteristic resistance of the upper esophageal sphincter, the cuff is inflated through the pilot tube. With cuff inflation, the tube usually moves outward a short distance as the tube centers itself over the laryngeal inlet. Inflation of the cuff to recommended maximum volumes and the use of clinical endpoints such as outward movement of the LMA may result in cuff pressures that are higher than the maximum recommended pressure of 60 cm H_2O (Maino et al., 2006). High cuff pressures are associated with increased incidence of leak around the LMA, excess mucosal pressures, and an increased incidence of sore throat (Wong et al., 2009). Only a fraction of the recommended volume is required to obtain an effective seal, and using a manometer to guide inflation has been shown to decrease leakage around the LMA by promoting more effective molding of the device to the airway (Licina et al., 2008).

The LMA can also be inserted with the cuff partially inflated or with the aperture facing posteriorly and then turned 180 degrees once it is in the larynx (Chow et al., 1991; O'Neill et al., 1994; Nakayama et al., 2002). Clinical evaluations of the different insertion techniques suggest that the rotational technique is an acceptable alternative to the standard approach and may improve placement success in children (Tsujimura, 2001; Nakayama et al., 2002; Ghai et al., 2008).

Additional maneuvers that may facilitate ease of insertion include increasing head extension, performing a jaw-thrust maneuver, inserting the LMA slightly laterally in the pharynx to avoid the uvula, or using a laryngoscope to lift the tongue anteriorly (Brain, 1989; van Heerden and Kirrage, 1989; Cass, 1991). Nevertheless, in some children, insertion is difficult and associated with pharyngeal bleeding (Marjot, 1991). The LMA is usually placed in an anesthetized child; insertion in a conscious or sedated neonate is occasionally necessary in situations in which traditional mask ventilation and endoscopy is problematic (Denny et al., 1990; Markakis et al., 1992; Stricker et al., 2008). The LMA can be placed successfully in the prone pediatric patient in the case of accidental extubation and allows for rapid airway control without having to reposition the patient supine. (Dingeman et al., 2005).

Diagnostic and interventional flexible bronchoscopy is facilitated with LMA use. After LMA placement, the airway is anesthetized with topical lidocaine, and the patient is allowed to breathe spontaneously. Adequate anesthetic depth is maintained with volatile or intravenous anesthetic (Nussbaum and Zagnoev, 2001; Yazbeck-Karam et al., 2003).

Laryngeal masks are critical tools in the management of the airways in children. They have been used successfully to rescue ventilation in patients who have difficult airways and can serve as conduits to intubation (Yang and Son, 2003; Batra, et al., 2006). Attaching a swivel connector (Swivel Connector, Ref. 60-60.305; VBM; Sulz, Germany) to the 15-mm end of an LMA facilitates ventilation during fiberoptic intubation through the LMA and subsequent LMA removal (Weiss et al., 2004b). The use of this adaptor significantly shortens apnea time and allows uninterrupted ventilation of the patient during tracheal tube placement and LMA removal. Despite its many benefits, the LMA has several limitations in children. Cuffed tracheal tubes do not pass through small LMAs, because the pilot balloon becomes lodged in the airway tube (Weiss and Goldmann, 2004). In order to place a cuffed tracheal tube, an uncuffed tube is first inserted and the LMA is removed; a tube exchange is then performed, leaving a cuffed tube. This added step can cause additional morbidity or mortality if the exchange should fail.

Standard tracheal tubes are similar in length to their corresponding LMA sizes. This similarity results in the tracheal tube disappearing into the airway tube before a significant length of tube can be slid over a fiberoptic scope into the trachea. This presents challenges with advancing the tube into the trachea and removing the LMA. Several techniques have been described to address this problem, including using a second tracheal tube or laryngeal forceps as a stabilizer, cutting the airway tube of the LMA to shorten its length, using an extra-long tracheal tube, or leaving the LMA in place after intubation (Benumof, 1992; Yamashita, 1997; Selim et al., 1999; Muraika et al., 2003; Osborn and Soper, 2003; Yang and Son, 2003; Machotta and Hoeve, 2008).

The air-Q is uniquely designed to facilitate tracheal tube placement in children of all ages (Fig. 10-18, *B*). This laryngeal mask is a curved device with a uniquely designed airway tube. The airway tube readily accommodates the pilot balloon of cuffed tracheal tubes in all its sizes, and the length is shortened, thereby ensuring that the tracheal tube is in the trachea when the proximal end disappears into the device (Table 10-3).

A limitation of the classic LMA is its inability to protect the airway against regurgitation of gastric contents into the trachea. In a 1992 study by Barker et al., in adults without significant risk for reflux or aspiration there was a 25% incidence of regurgitation of methylene blue into the laryngeal mask, though no tracheal soiling was noted. Pulmonary aspiration during LMA use remains an uncommon event, with the incidence reported to be approximately 2 in 10,000 (Brimacombe and Berry, 1995; Keller et al., 2004a).

In general, the smaller size of the LMA, the higher the incidence of malpositioning, usually with the epiglottis contained within the grill of the LMA (Rowbottom et al., 1991; Mizushima et al., 1992; Dubreuil et al., 1993). Even in the presence of this type of malpositioning, ventilation is not usually impaired, although ventilation is more likely to become

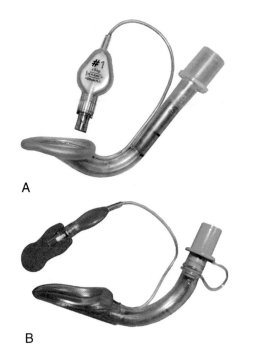

■ **FIGURE 10-18. A,** Ambu AuraOnce. **B,** Air-Q airway.

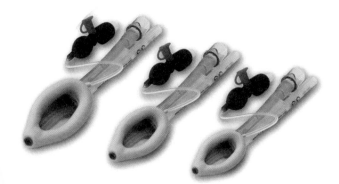

■ **FIGURE 10-19.** The pediatric Proseal LMA.

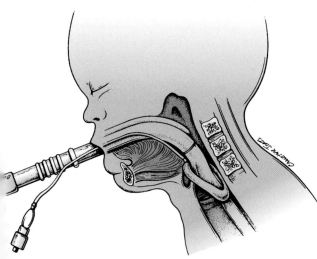

FIGURE 10-20. When properly inserted, the distal outlet of the ⅃MA is situated over the laryngeal inlet.

problematic with small movements of the child or LMA when the initial position is not optimal. (Mason and Bingham, 1990; Rowbottom et al., 1991).

The Proseal LMA is designed to separate the alimentary and respiratory tracts. It integrates a drain tube placed lateral to the airway tube of the LMA and ending at the tip of the mask (Fig. 10-19) (Brain et al., 2000). When the Proseal LMA is placed correctly, the second tube is contiguous with the alimentary tract and is sealed against the upper esophageal sphincter, allowing the passage of a nasogastric tube and confirmation of adequate positioning of the device. The Proseal LMA forms a more effective airway seal and is associated with higher oropharyngeal leak pressures (11 to 18 cm H_2O higher) and less gastric insufflation than the classic LMA in children (Goldmann and Jakob, 2005; Lopez-Gil and Brimacombe, 2005; Wheeler, 2006; Lardner et al., 2008). The first-attempt success rate of placement is reported to be about 90% in children (Wheeler, 2006). The Proseal LMA may effectively separate the gastrointestinal system from the airway; however, much of the evidence for this comes from case reports and requires the assumption that the device position does not change after it has been assessed to be correctly placed (Keller et al., 2004b).

The Proseal LMA is available for use in all infants. The incidence of complications with the Proseal LMA is highest in the youngest patients (size 1.5), most of these relating to poor positioning of the LMA, obstruction, or laryngospasm (Bagshaw, 2002).

The choice of which laryngeal mask to use depends on the clinical application, cost, personal preference, and experience. The practitioner needs to examine these variables when selecting the mask to use in the surgical environment.

Cobra Perilaryngeal Airway

The Cobra Perilaryngeal Airway (Cobra PLA; Engineered Medical Systems, Indianapolis, Indiana) is another supraglottic device that aids in airway management. The Cobra PLA consists of a softened distal tip that has slotted openings for ventilation and is designed to be positioned in the hypopharynx overlying the laryngeal inlet (Fig. 10-21). It is secured in place by a more proximal cuff and has a proximal 15-mm connector that attaches to the anesthesia breathing circuit. The Cobra PLA is available in eight different sizes, five of which are suitable for pediatric age and weight ranges (Table 10-4). It is suitable for use during spontaneous or controlled ventilation, and the larger sizes can accommodate an appropriately sized fiberoptic bronchoscope and tracheal tube for difficult intubations.

The Cobra PLA is inserted in a similar manner to the LMA. A preliminary study in adults demonstrated that the Cobra PLA often requires readjustment up or down to affect adequate ventilation once inserted (Agro et al., 2003). A comparison examining the anatomic positions of the LMA Unique, Softseal LMA, and the Cobra PLA found that herniation of the arytenoids through the mask aperture bars was more common with the Cobra PLA than with the other devices (van Zundert et al., 2006). Polaner et al. (2006) assessed the orientation of the Cobra PLA using flexible bronchoscopy in infants and children. They found the airway to be acceptable in all children; however, the laryngeal view was nearly or completely obstructed in 76.9% of the patients who weighed 10 kg or less. A comparison of the Cobra PLA to the LMA Unique in children revealed higher seal pressures for the

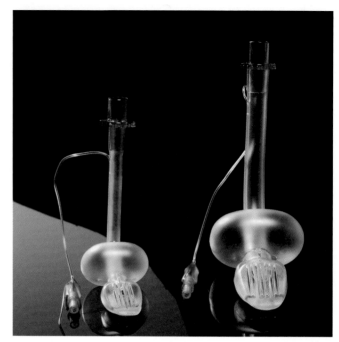

■ **FIGURE 10-21.** The Cobra PLA consists of a distal softened tip that contains slotted openings for ventilation, a more proximal cuff to secure the airway, and a proximal 15-mm connector that attaches to the anesthesia breathing circuit. *(Courtesy of Engineered Medical Systems, Inc., Indianapolis, Ind.)*

TABLE 10-4. Classification of the Cobra Perilaryngeal Airway

Perilaryngeal Airway Size	Perilaryngeal Airway Characteristics			
	Patient Size	Weight (kg)	Internal Diameter (mm)	Cuff Volume (mL)
0.5	Neonatal	>2.5	5	<8
1	Infant	>5	6	<10
1.5	Child	>10	6	<25
2	Child	>15	10.5	<40
3	Child/small adult	>35	10.5	<65
4	Adult	>70	12.5	<70
5	Large adult	>100	12.5	<85
6	Large adult	>130	12.5	<85

From Engineered Medical Systems, Inc., Indianapolis, Ind.

Cobra PLA, with similar insertion ease and times and less gastric insufflation. The fiberoptic view was found to be better based on the comparison of fiberoptic views immediately after induction to views before emergence (Szmuk et al., 2008). Airway obstruction secondary to epiglottic incarceration into the aperture bars has been reported and may be more likely if the device moves upward from the hypopharynx after insertion (Yamaguchi et al., 2006).

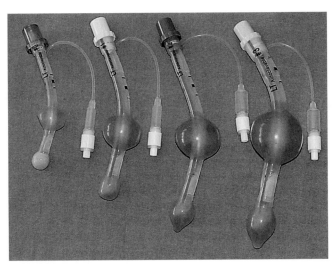

■ **FIGURE 10-22.** The laryngeal tube consists of an oval ventilation aperture placed between two distal low-pressure cuffs. The distal (esophageal) balloon is designed to seal the airway distally and protect against regurgitation. *(Courtesy of VBM Medical Inc., Noblesville, Ind.)*

Laryngeal Tube

The Laryngeal Tube (LT; VBM Medical; Noblesville, Indiana) is a single-lumen tube consisting of an oval ventilation aperture placed between two distal low-pressure cuffs and is inserted in a similar manner as the LMA (Fig. 10-22). The distal (esophageal) balloon is designed to seal the airway distally and protect against regurgitation. The proximal (oropharyngeal) balloon is designed to seal off the pharynx above the ventilation port. The two balloons are inflated sequentially via a unique connector at a pressure of 60 cm H_2O by using a manometer. There are seven sizes that encompass all age ranges. The LT is available in four designs: the standard LT reusable version, a disposable LT-D version, a reusable version with a gastric access channel (LTS-II), and the LTS-D, a disposable single use version with a gastric access channel (Table 10-5). Like the LMA and Cobra PLA, the LT is designed as an alternative to the anesthesia face mask and as a potential tool for providing ventilation in patients with difficult airways. It can be used during spontaneous or controlled ventilation. In adult studies, the rate of successful placement exceeds 90% (Cook et al., 2003). A prospective comparison of the LT with the LMA in children demonstrated similar insertion success rates

and higher airway leak pressures with the LT (Genzwuerker et al., 2006). The LT allows higher positive inspiratory pressure than the classic LMA; like other supralaryngeal airway devices it is associated with more ventilation failures in children who weigh less than 10 kg (Genzwuerker et al., 2005). Removal of the LT in an anesthetized state reduces cough, hypersalivation, hypoxia, and tube displacement (Lee et al., 2007).

Flexible Fiberoptic Bronchoscopy

Fiberoptic intubation remains the gold standard for the management of difficult pediatric intubation. Miniaturization of fiberoptic and digital image technology has allowed the design of ultrathin bronchoscopes that facilitate intubation with tracheal tube sizes down to 2.5 mm ID (Fan et al., 1986; de Blic et al., 1991; Roth et al., 1994). In addition, the optical aspects of the equipment have improved with these smaller fiberscopes to allow better screen resolution. With the child sedated or anesthetized and breathing spontaneously, a fiberoptic bronchoscope that has been passed through a tracheal tube is inserted through the mouth or nose to visualize the larynx. The tracheal tube is advanced off the bronchoscope after its entrance into the trachea.

Some ultrathin bronchoscopes contain a working channel, but it is often too narrow to allow effective suctioning of secretions, so secretions and blood are more likely to obscure the view in smaller children. Furthermore, oxygen insufflation should be judiciously applied through this channel in small children because of the possibilities of generating dangerously high intrabronchial pressures and development of a tension pneumothorax (Iannoli and Litman, 2002).

Ventilation can be accomplished during bronchoscopy by the use of a special endoscopy mask (VBM Medical, Noblesville, Indiana) that incorporates a conduit for passage of the bronchoscope or by placement of a modified nasal trumpet in the nare.

Lighted Stylets

The lighted stylet ("light wand") consists of a semirigid stylet with a bright light at the distal-most end (Fiberoptic Intubation Stylet, Anesthesia Medical Specialties; Santa Fe Springs, California; and Trachlight, Laerdal Medical, Armonk, New Jersey) (Fig. 10-23). The lighted stylet is prepared by inserting it inside a standard tracheal tube, the tip is then bent at a 60- to 120-degree angle, depending on the anatomy of the patient. The length of the bend may influence intubation success with the lighted stylet and should ideally be approximately equal to the distance from the thyroid prominence to the mandibular angle (Chen et al., 2003). After dimming of the operating room lights, a jaw thrust is performed with the nondominant hand, and the lighted stylet is placed in the midline of the pharynx and advanced slowly. A characteristic glow is noted with transillumination at the cricothyroid membrane, and the tracheal tube is advanced off the stylet into the trachea. Difficulty with placement of the lighted stylet may be caused by entrapment in the vallecula or a nonmidline insertion. In this event, the stylet should be withdrawn and reoriented in the midline to reduce the risk of airway trauma before subsequent insertion attempts (Fisher and Tunkel, 1997). A transient disappearance of the transilluminated light, followed by a reappearance more distally suggests passage behind the larynx into the esophagus.

TABLE 10-5. Laryngeal Tube Sizing

Size	Patient	Weight/Height
0	Newborn	<5 kg
1	Baby	5-12 kg
2	Child	12-25 kg
2.5	Adult	125-150 cm
3	Adult	<155 cm
4	Adult	155-180 cm
5	Adult	>180 cm

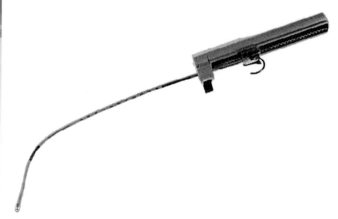

■ **FIGURE 10-23.** Using a lighted stylet, the endotracheal tube can be guided into the trachea with the use of the surface anatomy of the child and projection of the lighted stylet tip. *(From Litman RS: Pediatric airway management. In Litman RS, editor:* Pediatric anesthesia: the requisites, *St. Louis, 2004, Mosby.)*

The lighted stylet is useful when a child has an anatomically normal larynx that is difficult to visualize with direct methods. This may occur with micrognathia, temporomandibular joint disorders (or any condition that limits mandibular mobility), cervical spine instability, or facial trauma (Krucylak and Schreiner, 1992). It is particularly suited to children with limited neck and mandible mobility, but it is not useful in cases of fixed upper or lower airway obstructive pathology or in the presence of a foreign body.

Commercially made lighted stylets can be used in tracheal tubes as small as 4.5 mm ID. For small infants and neonates, a standard tracheal tube stylet can be combined with a 20-gauge fiberoptic illuminating light pipe (Storz Ophthalmics Inc., St. Louis, Missouri) attached to any standard fiberoptic light source (Davis et al., 2000). Few complications have been reported with lighted stylet use. However, arytenoid dislocation and dislodgement of the lighted stylet bulb have been described. The latter complication is less likely with newer stylet designs, and potential for arytenoid dislocation may be decreased by avoiding rotation of the stylet in the pharynx when it slides off the midline. The skill required for lighted-stylet guided intubation is easily acquired, and it remains a very useful adjunct in the management of children who present with difficult intubation.

Optical Stylets

The Shikani Optical Stylet (SOS) is a modification of the lighted stylet, which has a fiberoptic core that allows transmission of the image from the distal tip to an eyepiece (Fig. 10-24). It integrates a battery-operated light source and is manufactured in pediatric and adult versions. The pediatric version can accommodate tubes down to 2.5 mm ID. The SOS has an integrated oxygen insufflation port that allows the insufflation of oxygen. Similar to the lighted stylet, a jaw thrust with the nondominant hand facilitates the elevation of the epiglottis off the posterior pharyngeal wall and allows the SOS to be placed in the midline along the tongue base until the epiglottis and glottic opening are visualized. The device can be placed just past the vocal cords, and the tube can then be advanced into the trachea.

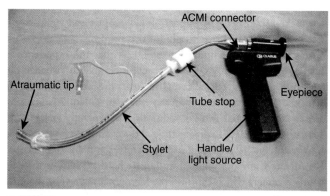

■ **FIGURE 10-24.** The Shikani Optical Stylet with a fiberoptic case that allows transmission of the image from the distal tip to an eyepiece.

The SOS combines the benefits of fiberoptics with a light wand and has been used successfully in patients who are difficult to intubate (Shukry et al., 2005). The SOS is limited by blood, secretions, and fogging, although fogging can be reduced by the application of an antifog solution or warming the device before use.

Bonfils Retromolar Scope

With mechanics of use similar to the SOS, The Bonfils Retromolar Scope is a rigid J-shaped optical stylet with a fixed anterior curve of 40 degrees. The manufacturer suggests a retromolar approach to the glottic opening to shorten the distance travelled to the glottis. Limited by blood, secretions, and fogging, the first-attempt success rate is reported to be about 70% in children (Bein et al., 2008).

Laryngoscopes

A variety of pediatric-sized laryngoscope blades are available (Table 10-6). The laryngoscope has three basic parts: a handle, a blade, and a light. The blade consists of a spatula, a flange, and a tip. Blades differ in length, width, and curvature. Laryngoscopes can be purchased with incandescent or fiberoptic light sources. Those with fiberoptic light sources provide extremely bright, highly focused light that occasionally can be obscured by the

TABLE 10-6. Laryngoscope Blade Types and Sizes

Age	Blade Type and Size		
	Miller	Wis-Hippel	MacIntosh
Premature neonate	0	—	—
Term neonate	0 to 1	—	—
1 to 12 mo	1	1	—
1 to 2 yr	1	1.5	2
2 to 6 yr	2	—	2
6 to 12 yr	2	—	3

Modified from Coté CJ: *A practice of anesthesia for infants and children,* Philadelphia, 2001, WB Saunders.

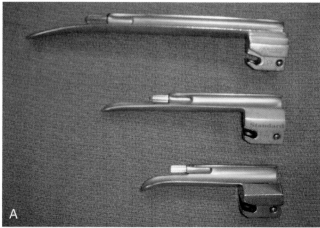

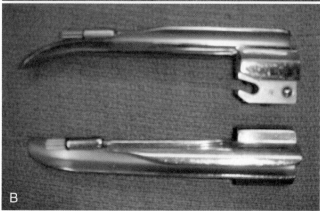

■ **FIGURE 10-25. A**, Miller blades and **B**, Phillips blades.

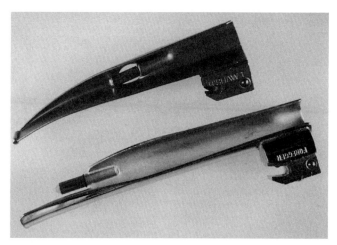

■ **FIGURE 10-26.** Robertshaw blade *(top)* and Flagg blade *(bottom)*.

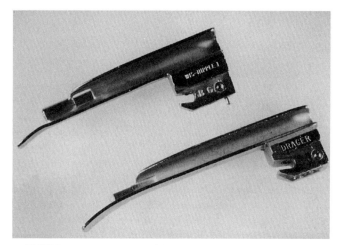

■ **FIGURE 10-27.** Two sizes of the Wis-Hipple blade are available.

tongue and soft tissue. Selection of a particular laryngoscope is usually based on personal preference and experience, the size of the child, and the peculiarities of a specific airway problem.

Generally, the straight Miller or Phillips blade is used in children (Fig. 10-25). This blade allows the cephalad aspect of the larynx to be exposed more easily, because the base of the tongue can be lifted out of the line of sight, and the protruding epiglottis can be retracted with the tip. Wide blades and large-flange blades, like the Robertshaw, the Flagg, and the Wis-Hipple blades, allow the wide tongue of the small child to be flattened during laryngoscopy (Fig. 10-26) (Robertshaw, 1962). The length of a 1.5 Wis-Hipple blade is especially useful in toddlers (Fig. 10-27). For older children and young adults, longer straight blades (e.g., the Miller 2) or curved blades (e.g., the MacIntosh) allow the anesthesiologist to achieve good exposure and avoid prominent dentition (Fig. 10-28).

During laryngoscopy, neonates may rapidly develop hypoxemia secondary to apnea, decreased functional residual capacity, and increased oxygen consumption. The Oxyscope is a modified Miller blade that allows insufflation of oxygen into the pharynx and decreases the rapidity with which hypoxemia occurs during laryngoscopy (Fig. 10-29) (Todres and Crone, 1981).

Video Laryngoscopes

Video laryngoscopes of various designs are being manufactured for use in children. Much of the data regarding the efficacy of these devices comes from case reports and case series with very few data from prospective trials. The Bullard laryngoscope represents one of the early designs of an optically enhanced laryngoscope for pediatric use (Fig. 10-30). It incorporates fiberoptics and mirrors to provide an indirect glottic view and has been used successfully in children of all ages (Borland and Casselbrant, 1990). Video laryngoscopes can play an important role in the successful management of the child who is difficult to intubate by direct laryngoscopy. One issue that seems to apply to many of these devices is that even with full view of the glottic opening, guiding the tracheal tube into the trachea may sometimes be difficult.

Glidescope

The Glidescope (Verathon Medical, Bothwell, Washington, U.S.) is a plastic laryngoscope with a MacIntosh-style curved blade. The blade has an integrated digital video camera that transmits the image from the tip to a portable video monitor. The Glidescope Cobalt consists of a video baton with a disposable plastic blade; the camera is positioned at the inflection point of the blade, providing a wide-angled view on the monitor (Fig. 10-31) (Cooper et al., 2005). After sweeping the tongue to the

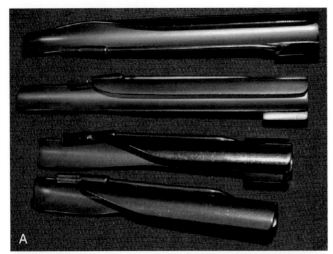

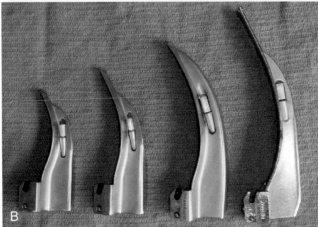

■ **FIGURE 10-28. A,** Miller blades. The top two blades compared with Wis-Hippel blades. Note that different manufacturers of the Miller blades have created slightly different nuances to the blade (i.e., the position of the bulb on the blade and the distance of the blade tip to the bulb). **B,** The four different sizes of the MacIntosh blade.

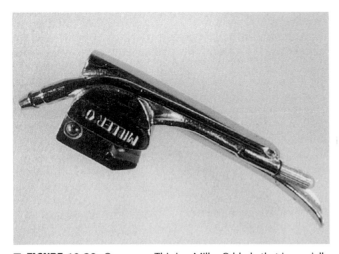

■ **FIGURE 10-29.** Oxyscope. This is a Miller O blade that is specially fitted; 2 to 3 L/min of oxygen is connected to the cannula on the left side of the blade, as shown. The oxygen is then directed by the lumen of this cannula into the trachea.

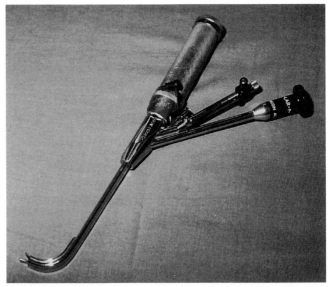

■ **FIGURE 10-30.** The Bullard laryngoscope allows a view of the larynx in children with limited ability to open their mouths and in cases where the larynx is positioned relatively anterior (cephalad).

left, the Glidescope is placed in the midline of the pharynx or slightly to the left to create space for the passage of the tracheal tube. Because the view of the larynx is not directly in the line of sight as in conventional laryngoscopy, a styleted tracheal tube with similar angulation as the blade or a hockey stick configuration is required for intubation and should be prepared before laryngoscopy. The manufacturer also provides a preformed rigid stylet (Gliderite Rigid Stylet) to facilitate intubation with the Glidescope. During passage of the tracheal tube, the laryngoscopist's attention should be directed to the passage of the styleted tube to minimize pharyngeal injury caused by blind advancement (Leong et al., 2008).

Storz Video Laryngoscope

The Storz Video Laryngoscope consists of a camera system that couples to several video blades. A Miller-type video blade is available for intubation in neonates and infants and has been used successfully after failed laryngoscopy in children (Hackell et al., 2009). A study in an infant mannequin compared the grade of view of the Miller-1 video blade to the standard Miller blade and demonstrated a one-grade improvement in view with the video blade (Wald et al., 2008; Xue et al., 2008; Fiadjoe et al., 2009). Because of the similarity in design of the Storz Video blades to standard blades, they allow documentation of the traditional direct laryngoscopy view while providing the option for visualization with video if the direct view is poor.

The Airtraq (Prodol Meditec SA; Vizcaya, Spain) is an indirect laryngoscope that uses a series of mirrors and prisms to provide a wide-angled view of the airway during intubation. The image is transmitted from a lens at the tip to a proximal viewfinder. The Airtraq incorporates a channel to house the tracheal tube during laryngoscopy (Fig. 10-32). The device is placed in the midline of the oropharynx, and the tip is advanced to the vallecula; the epiglottis may need to be elevated to obtain optimal exposure. Once adequate positioning has been obtained, the incorporated tracheal tube is advanced into the trachea. The Airtraq is currently manufactured in 4 sizes. The Airtraq

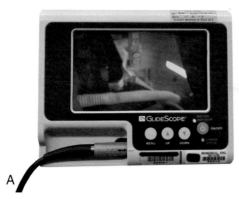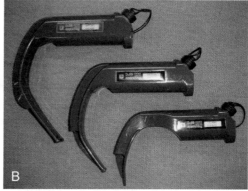

■ **FIGURE 10-31.** Glidescope video component **(A)** and blades **(B).** Three of the four blades are shown. From smallest to longest, the blade lengths (tip to handle) are 47, 82, and 102 mm. The widths of the camera, from the smallest to largest blade are 18, 20, and 27 mm.

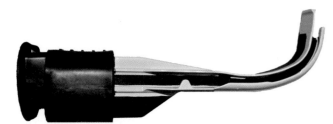

■ **FIGURE 10-32.** The Airtraq, manufactured in four sizes, incorporates a channel to house the endotracheal tube during laryngoscopy.

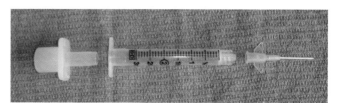

■ **FIGURE 10-33.** A makeshift cricothyrotomy airway. Note the catheter is attached to the barrel of a 3-mL syringe. A 7.0-mm endotracheal-tube adapter is firmly placed in the barrel of the syringe. This can then be attached to an anesthesia circuit or jet ventilator.

has been reported to facilitate difficult intubation in a child; however, further study in a large cohort of pediatric patients is warranted to evaluate its efficacy (Lejus et al., 2009).

Cricothyrotomy

The need for a surgical airway is imperative if intubation fails and ventilation becomes impossible. For the anesthesiologist, cricothyrotomy is an approach to creating an airway with a percutaneous needle and a catheter. The technique involves the following five steps:

1. Skin preparation and neck extension
2. Palpation of the cricothyroid membrane
3. Needle puncture of the membrane with an intravenous catheter attached to a syringe
4. Aspiration of air, advancement of catheter, and aspiration of catheter for air
5. Attach catheter to a 3-mL syringe barrel and a 7-mm ID endotracheal-tube adapter (Fig. 10-33).

Numerous kits for cricothyrotomy are on the market (Coté and Hartwick, 2009). In truth, the usefulness of these devices in infants and small children is questionable.

Intravenous Equipment

Catheters

Intravenous catheters appropriate for the smallest premature infant and the largest adolescent patient are made by a wide variety of companies. The appropriate catheter is usually dictated

by the patient's size, expected fluid requirements, and the operator's preference. In general, a 22- or 24-gauge catheter suffices in the small infant. Patients with significant fluid requirements, such as neonates undergoing gastroschisis repair, may need two or three intravenous catheters. In older children, a 22- or 20-gauge catheter usually suffices. Butterfly needles inserted into tiny veins are not adequate for infusions during surgery because they are easily dislodged, but they are convenient for performing rapid intravenous induction in a young child or an anxious adolescent. Pain from butterfly insertion can be minimized when using a 25- or 27-gauge butterfly needle.

In accordance with Poiseuille's relationship, the resistance to flow through an intravenous catheter is related to the radius of the lumen, length of the catheter, and the viscosity of the fluid (Table 10-7). Although small differences exist between comparable catheters of various manufacturers, major flow reductions occur when they are lengthened to enable central venous cannulation (Hodge et al., 1986; Rosen and Rosen, 1986). Viscosity of the infused fluid (e.g., blood vs. crystalloid) imposes significant resistance changes only when small (smaller than 20-gauge) or long (more than 3 inches) catheters are used (Hodge and Fleisher, 1985; Rothen et al., 1992). For example, an 18-gauge catheter lengthened to 8 inches to enable central venous placement exhibits the flow characteristics of a short 24-gauge catheter.

Central venous catheters are manufactured in various sizes lengths and materials for pediatric use. Catheters are constructed from Silicone, PVC, polyethylene or polyurethane. Each of these materials has unique advantages and disadvantages; however, the most common adverse events related to catheter use are infection and thrombosis. Polyurethane catheters have been shown to have greater pressure tolerance than

TABLE 10-7. Catheter Sizes and Their Flow Rates

Catheter Size (Gauge)	Length (Inches)	Mean Flow Rate Range (mL/min)		
		Crystalloid (Gravity)	Crystalloid (Pressure)	Blood (Pressure)
24	0.75	14 to 15	42 to 47	20 to 30
22	1	24 to 26	65 to 77	44 to 50
20	1.25 to 2	38 to 42	103 to 126	69 to 81
18	1.25 to 2	55 to 62	164 to 214	150 to 164
16	2	75 to 81	248 to 280	216 to 286
14	2	92 to 93	301 to 319	334 to 410
20	8	5	16	3
18	8	13	51	22
16	8	31	97	35

Data from Hodge D III, Fleisher G: Pediatric catheter flow rates, *Am J Emerg Med* 3:403, 1985.

silicone catheters in experimental models and are less likely to rupture (Smirk et al., 2009). Polyurethane and polyethylene catheters may increase the risk of vessel perforation as compared with silicone and PVC catheters. Silicone catheters are soft and pliable and may be more difficult to insert percutaneously; PVC catheters are stiff on insertion and soften after insertion, making them easier to place (Welch et al., 1997; Macdonald and Ramasethu, 2007). Peripherally inserted central catheters (PICCs) catheters are typically single lumen, made from silicone or polyurethane, and available in sizes as small as 1.2 French for neonatal use. Central venous catheters are available in sizes as small as 2.5 French and are typically single or double lumen for neonatal use—triple-lumen catheters are available for older children (Macdonald and Ramasethu, 2007). Central venous access can be obtained in children using several vessels; they can be peripherally inserted into central veins (PICC lines) or can be inserted using the femoral, subclavian, or jugular veins. The central circulation can also be accessed in neonates through the umbilical vessels. The risk of complications with subclavian access is increased when compared with cannulation of the internal jugular vein. Internal jugular access is associated with less pneumothorax, less accidental arterial puncture, and fewer attempts to puncture the vein (Iovino et al., 2001). Ultrasound facilitates catheter placement in children and lessens the number of attempts for successful cannulation even in experienced operators (Verghese et al., 1999). In young children, the combination of Valsalva's maneuver, liver compression, and Trendelenburg's position produces the largest increase in jugular venous size, with Valsalva's maneuver being the most effective single maneuver to achieve this increase. The optimal positioning of central venous catheters remains a subject of debate; however, avoiding intracardiac placement decreases the risk of cardiac perforation and tamponade. Central venous placement is not without risks, including pleural effusion, pneumothorax and hydrothorax, pneumomediastinum, and hemothorax. A risk factor for perforation is catheter stiffness; the more perpendicular the catheter is with the vessel wall the higher the chance of perforation, particularly in catheters placed on the left side of the head and neck. Ideally, the catheter tip should be placed at the superior vena

cava-right atrial (SVC-RA) junction outside of the heart, and the catheter axis should parallel the axis of the vein into which it is inserted (Fletcher and Bodenham, 2000). Central catheters should be placed 1 cm outside the cardiac silhouette in premature infants and 2 cm away in full-term infants, and x-ray technology should be routinely used to diagnose catheter migration into the heart (Nowlen et al., 2002). The carina may provide an estimate of the SVC-RA junction in older children, but this may not be the case in neonates and small children (Yoon et al., 2005; Inagawa et al., 2007).

Intraosseous Access

Intraosseous access should be considered in children who need acute resuscitation and have challenging peripheral or central vascular access (ILCOR, 2005) (see Chapter 30, Anesthesia for the Pediatric Trauma Patient). The intraosseous route provides noncollapsible access to the central venous circulation, making it an ideal route to administer drugs and fluid to patients with cardiovascular compromise or shock. Onset times of drugs administered via this route are similar to those given intravenously. The preferred access site in children and infants is the anteromedial surface of the tibia, approximately 1 to 2 cm below the tibial tuberosity. Other sites that have been successfully used include the sternum, the iliac crest, the distal radius, and several others. Several companies manufacture intraosseous needles; however, access may be obtained with any styleted needle. Spinal needles of 18 or 20 gauge have been successfully used for access. After sterile preparation of the chosen site, the needle is inserted perpendicular to the skin and advanced using a rotating motion until a loss of resistance is felt. Once seated, the stylet may be removed, and successful positioning is confirmed with aspiration of marrow and the ability to flush without extravasation. Risks of intraosseous access placement include infection, extravasation of fluid and medication, injury to the growth plate, and fracture (Tobias and Ross, 2010).

A number of studies have determined that needleless intravenous catheters reduce the rate of needlestick injuries by up to 60% (Orenstein et al., 1995; Needlestick, 2000). In 2001, the U.S. Occupational Safety and Health Administration (OSHA) authored the Needlestick Safety and Prevention Act (HR 5178), which provides a legislative mandate that health-care facility employers provide employees with safety-engineered sharp devices (Federal Register on January 18, 2001).

Infusion Sets

Intravenous infusion sets must also be tailored to the patient and the planned surgical procedure. Microdrip infusion sets (60 drops/mL) allow the anesthesiologist to more accurately deliver small volumes of infusate to the small child compared with the standard 15 drops/mL infusion set. For an older child (older than approximately 10 years), the standard adult infusion set is adequate. The addition of extension tubes to all pediatric infusion sets permits the intravenous catheter to be placed in any available extremity and allows a small child to be moved down on the operating table for better surgical access. Insertion of multiple stopcocks in the infusion tubing allows precise volumes of blood or colloid to be administered and minimizes the need to use needles to access the infusion. The blood set is attached to the stopcock closest to the patient, and a syringe is placed in the stopcock farthest from the patient. The stopcocks are opened to allow blood to flow into the syringe and then adjusted to allow an accurate volume of blood to be infused from the syringe into the patient. Before their use, all infusion sets should be "de-bubbled" to prevent air entrainment into the circulation, a task especially important in a premature infant, who is likely to have a patent foramen ovale or patent ductus arteriosus, or in a child with a known intracardiac defect or persistent patent foramen ovale. To decrease the incidence of accidental needlestick injuries, all manufacturers now offer injection ports throughout the length of the tubing that are accessible with standard syringes or specialized blunt adaptors. When these ports are accessed, care must be taken to avoid trapped air that often accumulates in these ports.

In the face of significant hypovolemia that results from brisk blood loss or other causes of severe intravascular volume depletion, the rapid infusion of blood or crystalloid may prevent an impending disaster. The speed of infusion is directly related to the driving pressure of the infusate and the resistance of the infusion. Unless small-bore infusion tubing is used to minimize infusion dead space, resistance of the infusion circuit is mainly related to the length and diameter of the intravenous catheter. Short catheters with large, IDs have less resistance than longer catheters with smaller diameters, irrespective of peripheral or central placement (Hodge and Fleisher, 1985). The driving pressure of the intravenous solution depends on the height of the fluid bag, gravity, or the mechanical force used to push the solution. A simple method to increase the fluid administration rate in neonates and small children uses the push-pull technique, as noted above. By drawing blood or fluid into a syringe, the fluid can be "pushed" into the patient with significant speed, especially in children weighing less than 40 kg (Stoner et al., 2007). Drawbacks of this technique include the need to manually perform the task and risk of infection that may increase as the same syringe is used repeatedly. Advantages include the ability to accurately deliver fluid at a brisk rate while manually sensing changes in system resistance that may indicate an intravenous catheter infiltration.

Pressurizing or mechanically pumping an intravenous solution or blood also dramatically increases the rate of infusion. By placing an inflatable sleeve over the infusion solution bag, the driving pressure of the solution can be markedly increased. By using a hand pump (C-Fusor, Smith Medical North America, Dublin; Ohio; Infu-Surg, Cardinal Health; Dublin, Ohio), the sleeve can be inflated incrementally to 300 mm Hg to drive blood or intravenous solution into the patient. Disadvantages with this system include the need to hand-inflate the pressurization device, the inability to accurately deliver small volumes of infusate, infiltration of infusate outside of the vein, and the risk of unintended infusion of air causing an air embolism (Linden et al., 1997). Special attention to removing residual air from the blood or infusion bags before spiking the bag is necessary. Before using a rapid-infuser system, the intravenous line should be checked for free flow and patency of the vein. Accuracy of infusion volumes can be increased by using the pressure system to fill a push-pull syringe that has been set up instead of having to manually fill the syringe. Any residual air can be removed using the syringe system. Automated pressure infusers (Level 1 H-1200, Smith Medical North America, Dublin, Ohio; Ranger A1400, Arizant Healthcare; Prairie, Minnesota) eliminate the need for manual inflation through the use of high pressure air or electrical power to create the driving pressure. These devices have fluid warmers and air detectors as integral parts or as accessories and can deliver large volumes of warmed fluids rapidly through special, disposable infusion sets. Roller pump technology has also been used to rapidly infuse blood or intravenous solution. Integrated with an electromagnetic heater, air detector, and electronic flow control, high volumes of warmed fluids can be accurately delivered using this technology (Belmont Rapid Infuser; Billerica, Massachusetts). Because the risk of air is greater with high-pressure infusers, it is crucial that any automated apparatus used stops delivery of fluid if air is detected in the line. Hemolysis and hyperkalemia may also be a concern if rapid infusers are used to deliver blood through 24-gauge intravenous catheters (Miller and Schlueter, 2004).

SUMMARY

Advances in medical technology have resulted in the design and production of a plethora of new equipment for the care of the child. This proliferation comes with many challenges. Careful organization and supervision of anesthesia supply rooms are essential to prevent the presence of expired supplies or nonfunctional equipment, as well as ensure that supplies are not out of stock. Equally as important is the need to standardize certain types of supplies or equipment, from both cost and knowledge perspectives. Having multiple pieces of equipment or supplies that perform the same or nearly the same function is costly to buy and stock. Even more critical is the need to maintain the clinical competency of each anesthesia provider in the use of the variety of specialized equipment, and this is something that is exceedingly difficult as the variety of equipment and supplies expand. Recurrent educational opportunities may be needed, particularly for devices that are rarely used. Lack of familiarity caused by small differences in a particular piece of equipment may impede function, especially in an urgent or emergent situation. Simplifying equipment and supply lists as much as possible is warranted, although safe and effective clinical care demands an extensive selection for the pediatric anesthesiologist.

REFERENCES

Complete references used in this text can be found online at www.expertconsult.com.

Monitoring

Ronald S. Litman, David E. Cohen, Robert J. Sclabassi, Patrick Callahan, Franklyn P. Cladis, and Etsuro K. Motoyama

MONITORING

Most studies that have determined the rate of cardiac arrests resulting from anesthesia have found a threefold to fivefold greater risk among children than adults (Graff et al., 1964; Keenan and Boyan, 1985). In children younger than 1 year, the incidence increases to 9.2 to 17 per 10,000 anesthesias, or 10 times the adult incidence (Olsson and Hallen, 1988; Cohen et al., 1990). Factors contributing to cardiac arrests in anesthetized children are likely to be related to the cardiovascular or respiratory system (Salem et al., 1975). Flick and others (2007) have reviewed cardiac arrest data at the Mayo Clinic. The incidences of cardiac arrest and mortality during noncardiac procedures were 2.9:10,000 and 1.6:10,000, respectively. However, the incidence of cardiac arrest in children undergoing cardiac operations was 127:10,000. The incidence of other serious complications is also greater for infants than for adults in the operating room (Tiret et al., 1988) and in the postanesthesia care unit (PACU) (Cohen et al., 1990). These data indicate that children are a high-risk population and should be monitored with particular attention to cardiovascular and respiratory variables.

Guidelines for the intraoperative monitoring of patients under anesthesia have been published by the American Society of Anesthesiologists (ASA) (2005) (see Box 10-1). These standards mandate the continuous presence of an anesthesiologist or a nurse anesthetist throughout the conduct of anesthesia and require continuous monitoring of oxygenation, electrocardiographic status, and adequacy of ventilation and circulation. The minimum standard for monitoring oxygenation includes an oxygen analyzer in the anesthesia breathing circuit, sufficient illumination to evaluate the patient's color, and a quantitative method such as pulse oximetry, except under extenuating circumstances. Tracheal intubation must be verified by physical examination and the qualitative detection of carbon dioxide in the exhaled gas. Regardless of whether endotracheal intubation has been performed, continuous capnography is required unless it is invalidated by the nature of the patient, procedure, or equipment. Furthermore, quantitative monitoring of the volume of expired gas is strongly encouraged. The ASA also recommends monitoring of ventilation using observation of chest excursion and the reservoir breathing bag, as well as auscultation of breath sounds. When ventilation is controlled by a mechanical ventilator, there should be in continuous use a device that is capable of detecting disconnection of components of the breathing system, and the device must give an audible signal when its alarm threshold is exceeded.

ASA monitoring standards for circulation mandate that every patient receiving anesthesia have continuous electrocardiography (ECG), and determination of arterial blood pressure and heart rate at least every 5 minutes. In addition, every patient's circulatory function should be evaluated continually, using at least one of the following methods: palpation of a pulse, auscultation of heart sounds, monitoring of an intraarterial pressure tracing, ultrasound peripheral pulse monitoring, and pulse plethysmography or oximetry. Finally, a method by which temperature can be measured should be readily available, and the patient's temperature should be monitored when clinically significant changes in body temperature are intended, anticipated, or suspected.

Many of these provisions have been extended to the PACU. In standards adopted by the ASA in 1988 and updated in 2009, PACU monitoring should emphasize oxygenation, ventilation, circulation, and temperature assessment, with specific capability for quantitative determination of systemic oxygenation by pulse oximetry or its equivalent. Equipment should be readily available to enable the practitioner to meet these standards in all pediatric patients. The anesthesiologist is the ultimate monitor.

Physical Examination

Observation

The anesthesiologist can gain a tremendous amount of information from observation alone. Anesthetic depth can be inferred from the rate and pattern of respiration, and airway obstruction can be detected by chest wall retractions or "see-saw" paradoxical motion. The skin and mucous membranes should be continually assessed to confirm adequate oxygenation, because a pulse oximeter reading can significantly lag behind other indices of hypoxemia when placed on an extremity (Reynolds et al., 1993), or it may not detect a pulse at all during intense vasoconstriction. In rare circumstances, pulse oximetry falsely indicates normal saturations during hypoxic conditions (Costarino et al., 1987).

Capillary refill can provide valuable information about the intravascular volume and cardiac output of a euthermic patient. A child with cool, mottled, poorly perfused extremities should be examined closely for additional evidence of hypovolemia or reduced cardiac output even if the systemic arterial pressure remains normal. Progression of this mottled appearance onto the trunk indicates the extreme vasoconstriction that may herald imminent cardiovascular collapse.

Auscultation

Continuous auscultation of heart and lung sounds by means of a precordial stethoscope is useful during all phases of general anesthesia, as well as during transport of the child between hospital locations. A precordial stethoscope allows the anesthesiologist to immediately detect changes in the rate and character of heart and breath sounds, and it often gives the first warning of a physiologic alteration (e.g., right main bronchial intubation, wheezing). Crisp heart tones are produced by the flow of blood through a briskly contracting heart. Myocardial depression initially results in a muffled and then in a distant quality to the heart tones. Careful auscultation may reveal arrhythmias or murmurs such as the mill-wheel murmur that results from a venous air embolus.

When selecting and placing a precordial or an esophageal stethoscope, one should consider the nature of the planned surgery, the proposed anesthetic, and any underlying patient condition that may affect auscultation. Breath sounds and heart tones are best heard when a precordial stethoscope is positioned near the left sternal border between the second and fourth interspaces (above the nipple line). An esophageal stethoscope is reserved for patients whose anesthetic management includes endotracheal intubation and in whom a precordial stethoscope either provides inadequate information or violates the surgical field. The proper method for accurate placement of the esophageal stethoscope is to listen while simultaneously advancing the device and placing it at the level where the heart and lung sounds are maximal. In small infants, unintentional placement of the esophageal stethoscope into the stomach can easily occur.

Esophageal stethoscopes are contraindicated in patients with esophageal atresia or in those who have a disease process involving the proximal portion of the esophagus. They confer a rigid feel to the esophagus, which might be mistaken for the trachea (Schwartz and Downes, 1977). As a result, the esophageal stethoscope is relatively contraindicated in neck dissections where the trachea is a critical landmark, such as a tracheostomy.

Electrocardiography

In pediatric anesthesia, ECG is most useful for tracking the heart rate and diagnosing intraoperative rate-related arrhythmias, of which the two most common are bradycardia and supraventricular tachycardia. ECG is much less prone to movement-related artifact than the original pulse oximeter, although new pulse oximeter devices have eliminated most motion artifacts. In small infants, hypoxemia-related bradycardia may occur before the pulse oximeter reveals oxyhemoglobin desaturation. Conversely, resolution of hypoxemia is heralded by the transition from bradycardia to normal sinus rhythm. Premature ventricular contractions are commonly observed when halothane is used as the general anesthetic agent, especially during periods of hypercapnia or catecholamine release. The precordial stethoscope as a single monitor provides a much better indication of cardiac contractility and thus the overall hemodynamic status.

Electrolyte abnormalities may also be uncovered through the use of ECG. Hyperkalemia produces the characteristically prominent T waves. Hypocalcemia, which may occur during rapid administration of citrated blood products, prolongs the QT interval. Because ischemic changes in normal pediatric patients are rare, and because lead II provides a good view of atrial activity for arrhythmia diagnosis, the latter is recommended for the routine intraoperative electrocardiographic monitoring of pediatric patients.

In children, the normal heart rate varies with age (Table 11-1). The normal heart rate of the newborn ranges from 120 to 160 beats per minute, although lower rates (e.g., 70) are frequently observed during sleep, and higher rates (>200) are common during anxiety or pain. Heart rates tend to decrease with age and in parallel with decreases in oxygen consumption. In addition, many children have a noticeable variation in heart rate with respiration (i.e., sinus arrhythmia).

Systemic Arterial Pressure

Noninvasive Measurement

Blood pressure is easily measured noninvasively in children and small infants using oscillotonometry. In children, oscillometric measurements of systolic arterial pressure (Bruner et al., 1981;

TABLE 11-1. Normal Resting Heart Rates of Infants and Children

Age	Heart Rate (beats/min)	
	Mean	Range (±2 SD)
0 to 24 hr	119	94 to 145
1 to 7 days	133	100 to 175
8 to 30 days	163	115 to 190
1 to 3 mo	152	124 to 190
3 to 12 mo	140	111 to 179
1 to 3 yr	126	98 to 163
3 to 5 yr	98	65 to 132
5 to 8 yr	96	70 to 115
8 to 16 yr	77	55 to 105

Modified from Liebman J, Plonsey R, Gillette PC, editors: *Pediatric electrocardiography*, Baltimore, Md, 1982, Williams & Wilkins.

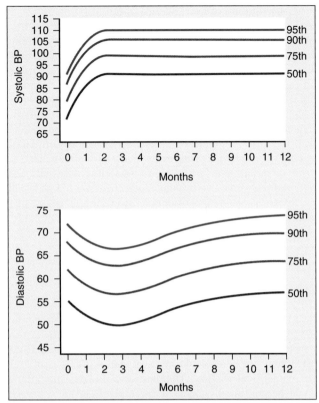

■ **FIGURE 11-1.** Age-specific percentiles of blood pressure measurements in boys, from birth to 12 months of age. Values for girls are slightly lower. *(From National Heart, Lung, and Blood Institute: Report of the Second Task Force on Blood Pressure Control in Children, Bethesda, Md, 1987, The Institute. Reproduced by permission of Pediatrics 79:1, copyright 1987.)*

Friesen and Lichtor, 1981) and mean arterial pressure (Kimble et al., 1981) usually correlate well with the Riva Rocci mercury column method, as well as with direct arterial pressure measurement, but oscillometric measurements tend to underestimate the diastolic component. During routine uncomplicated cases, measurement of blood pressure should be performed every 3 to 5 minutes while the child is anesthetized—determinations that are too frequent can result in limb ischemia. The blood pressure cuff is most commonly placed on the upper arm but can be placed on the forearm, thigh, or calf. There is inconsistent correlation of measurements obtained between the upper and lower limbs.

The width of the blood pressure cuff should cover approximately two thirds of the total length of the upper arm (or other extremity portion to which it is applied). A cuff that is too small or too narrow incompletely occludes the artery, resulting in the premature return of detectable flow and hence falsely increasing the pressure measurement (Park et al., 1976; Kimble et al., 1981). The error can be as great as 30 mm Hg. A cuff that is too wide can dampen the arterial wave and result in a falsely low pressure, but the magnitude of this error is small (Kimble et al., 1981). Blood pressure increases gradually throughout childhood (Figs. 11-1 and 11-2) and depends on the height of the child: taller children demonstrate a higher blood pressure (Table 11-2). Blood pressure ranges in premature infants have been defined (Table 11-3) and vary depending on the health status of the infant and mother.

Direct Measurement

Direct measurement of blood pressure via an arterial catheter is indicated when there is a need for precise beat-to-beat blood pressure monitoring or for frequent determination of arterial blood gas values. This patient population may include children who are expected to develop unstable hemodynamics or those undergoing a surgical procedure that could result in profound hemodynamic alterations related to blood loss (i.e., total loss >50% estimated blood volume [EBV], or acute loss >10% EBV), fluid shifts (i.e., third space losses >50% EBV), deliberate

hypotension, or nonpulsatile blood flow (e.g., cardiopulmonary bypass [CPB]). The respiratory indications for direct arterial monitoring include significant abnormalities in gas exchange caused by either preexisting disease or the procedure (e.g., thoracotomy). Rarely, direct arterial monitoring is necessary because of the inability to measure systemic arterial pressure by any indirect technique.

There are no absolute contraindications to placing an arterial catheter, but a risk-benefit analysis should be performed in patients with a hypercoagulable state or bleeding disorder. The radial artery is a favored site for arterial cannulation because the vessel is superficial and easily accessible. Other anatomic sites frequently used are the ulnar, dorsalis pedis, posterior tibial, and femoral arteries. The axillary artery has gained favor because of increased collateral blood flow compared with the brachial or femoral artery (Lawless and Orr, 1989; Cantwell et al., 1990; Greenwald et al., 1990; Piotrowski and Kawczynski, 1995). In general, the brachial artery should be avoided because of the risk for median nerve damage and poor collateral flow around the elbow. Umbilical vessels are an alternative site for cannulating the aorta and inferior vena cava in neonates. In determining a site, one needs to consider the history of that vessel (i.e., whether it has been cannulated before), its collateral flow, the experience of the person inserting the catheter, and special physiologic issues (e.g., whether it arises on an aortic root proximal to the ductus arteriosus) or surgical issues

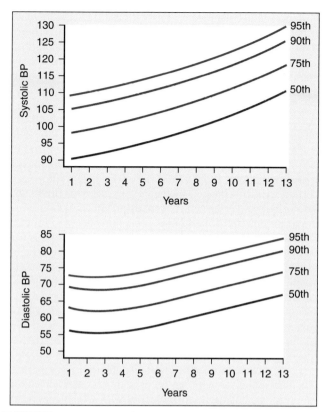

■ **FIGURE 11-2.** Age-specific percentiles for blood pressure measurements in boys, 1 to 13 years of age. Values for girls are slightly lower. *(From National Heart, Lung, and Blood Institute: Report of the Second Task Force on Blood Pressure Control in Children, Bethesda, Md, 1987, The Institute. Reproduced by permission of* Pediatrics *79:1, copyright 1987.)*

TABLE 11-3. Blood Pressure Ranges in Healthy Premature Infants*

Age (days)	Systolic Blood Pressure[†] (mm Hg)		Diastolic Blood Pressure[†] (mm Hg)	
	Minimum	**Maximum**	**Minimum**	**Maximum**
1	48 ± 9	63 ± 12	25 ± 7	35 ± 10
2	54 ± 10	63 ± 10	30 ± 0	39 ± 8
3	53 ± 9	67 ± 10	31 ± 8	43 ± 8
4	57 ± 10	71 ± 11	32 ± 8	45 ± 10
5	56 ± 9	72 ± 14	33 ± 9	47 ± 12
6	57 ± 9	71 ± 11	32 ± 7	47 ± 10

From Hegyi T, Anwar M, Carbone MT et al: Blood pressure ranges in premature infants: II. The first week of life, *Pediatrics* 97:336, 1996.
*Birth weight between 501 and 2000 g.
†Values are mean ± standard deviation.

(e.g., whether it arises from a vessel likely to be clamped or sacrificed during the procedure). Cannulation of vessels with good collateral flow, such as the arch vessels of the wrist or foot, may reduce the risk for ischemic tissue damage distal to the catheter.

As the largest superficial vessel, the femoral artery can be cannulated most predictably in situations when intense peripheral vasoconstriction may accompany low cardiac output and blood pressure. In less dire circumstances, the selection of a vessel may reflect a variety of anatomic and physiologic characteristics exhibited by certain vessels. The pedal vessels exhibit pressure wave amplification that results in pressure determinations exceeding aortic values by as much as 30% (Park et al., 1983).

After palpation and localization of the artery with the nondominant hand, one can cannulate the selected artery either by inserting the catheter directly into the artery using a catheter-over-needle device or by using the Seldinger technique. The Seldinger technique involves entering the vessel with a needle, placing a guidewire through the needle after the vessel is entered, removing the needle, and then placing the catheter over the wire into the vessel. A 22-gauge catheter is appropriate for peripheral artery cannulation in infants and children younger than 5 years, whereas a 20-gauge catheter may be substituted in older children. Aseptic technique should always be followed when placing an arterial line. When cannulating a peripheral artery, it is helpful to immobilize the extremity with a board.

A Doppler flow transducer is occasionally useful to locate an artery that is difficult to palpate. Surgical cutdown may be the preferred option when percutaneous placement is likely to be difficult or has failed. Indwelling arterial catheters are associated with several possible complications. Proximal emboli, distal ischemia, arterial thrombosis, and infection are common to all sites. Thrombosis of the radial artery is generally temporary, although it is more likely to persist after a cutdown (Miyasaka et al., 1976). Although small flush volumes (0.3 mL) in radial arterial catheters can be detected in the aortic arch vessels, cerebral infarcts have not been reported (Edmonds et al., 1980). The tip of an umbilical artery catheter should be placed in either a high (above the diaphragm) or a low (below L3) position to

TABLE 11-2. Systemic Arterial Pressure

Weight or Age	Systolic Pressure (±95% confidence limits) (mm Hg)	Diastolic Pressure (±95% confidence limits) (mm Hg)	Mean Pressure (±95% confidence limits) (mm Hg)
Newborn (kg)*			
1	47 (9)	27 (10)	35 (7)
2	54 (9)	32 (10)	40 (7)
3	62 (9)	37 (10)	45 (7)
4	69 (9)	42 (10)	50 (7)
6 wk to 9 yr[†]			
Boys	93 (9)	59 (9)	
Girls	96 (12)	62 (11)	
10 to 19 yr[†]			
Boys	108 (10)	67 (9)	
Girls	105 (10)	64 (11)	

*Adapted from Versmold HT, Kitterman JA, Phibbs RH et al: Aortic blood pressure during the first 12 hours of life in infants with birth weight 610 to 4,220 grams, *Pediatrics* 67:607, 1981.
†Adapted from Adams FH, Landaw EM: What are healthy blood pressures for children? *Pediatrics* 68:268, 1981.

avoid direct flushing into the renal arteries. Despite these precautions, as many as 10% of neonates exhibit hypertension as a late complication attributed to umbilical artery catheterization (Bauer et al., 1975; Plumer et al., 1976; Horgan et al., 1987). Minor complications of umbilical artery monitoring include vasospasm of the lower extremity vessels, which are more common with low tip placement. Major complications (e.g., necrotizing enterocolitis, renal artery thrombosis) occur independent of location (Mokrohisky et al., 1978; Umbilical Artery Catheter Trial Study Group, 1992). The rarity of clinical complications is remarkable given that the incidence of aortic thrombosis on removal of umbilical artery catheters approaches 95% in some series (Neal et al., 1972), although most series define the incidence at 12% to 31% of neonates (Symansky and Fox, 1972; Horgan et al., 1987; Seibert et al., 1987).

Systolic Pressure Variation

Systolic pressure variation is a noninvasive way to determine volume status and fluid responsiveness. It is defined as the difference between the maximal and minimal values of systolic blood pressure during a positive pressure breath. Initially during a positive pressure breath, there is a transient increase in systolic blood pressure (delta up) followed within four or five beats by a decrease in systolic blood pressure (delta down). Increases in intrathoracic pressure during positive pressure ventilation cause a decrease in systolic blood pressure because of decreased preload to the right ventricle, increased afterload to the right ventricle, and decreased afterload to the left ventricle. This decrease is greater during hypovolemia. Systolic pressure changes in response to respiratory variation have been used to determine hypovolemia (Greilich and Johnston, 2007).

The difference between the maximal systolic blood pressure and minimal systolic blood pressure during a respiratory cycle can help predict volume status. In fact, when this value is divided by the mean of the two systolic pressure values, it provides a percentage of respiratory change in arterial pulse pressure. The equation for this calculation is as follows:

$$\Delta PP\% = 100 \times (\text{maximum systolic pressure} -$$
$$\text{minimum systolic pressure}) \div$$
$$([\text{maximum systolic pressure} + \text{minimum systolic pressure}]/2)$$

where $\Delta PP\%$ is respiratory change in pulse pressure (mm Hg).

Michard and others (1999) demonstrated a strong relationship in adult ventilated patients between pulse pressure changes and cardiac output. Patients with pulse pressure changes (ΔPP) that are greater than 10% may be fluid responsive and benefit from the administration of intravenous fluids.

Changes in the pulse oximetry waveform (plethysmographic waveform amplitude) have been shown to predict fluid responsiveness (Pizov et al., 2010). Bedside use of this variable is challenging. The "pleth variability index" (Masimo Corp., Irvine, CA) automatically calculates the waveform amplitude variation and may predict fluid responsiveness noninvasively (Cannesson et al., 2008a, 2008b).

Central Venous Pressure

There are four relative indications for central venous catheterization: inadequate peripheral venous access, central venous pressure monitoring, infusion of hyperosmolar or sclerosing substances, and a planned operative procedure with a high risk for hemodynamically significant venous air embolism. There is no absolute indication for central venous pressure monitoring in pediatrics. Unlike direct systemic arterial pressures, central venous pressure itself rarely provides the sole basis for therapeutic action. It does, however, provide useful information that, taken together with other data, help to form a management plan. The procedures for which this monitoring deserves consideration include large estimated blood loss or fluid shifts (>50% EBV), deliberate hypotension, cardiac surgery with CPB, situations in which the usual signs of hypovolemia are likely to be misleading (e.g., renal failure, congestive heart failure), and procedures with expected moderate blood loss or fluid shifts. The normal values for central venous pressure in children are similar to those in adults (mean, 2 to 6 mm Hg).

Every insertion site that has been used in adults can be used in children. Access to the central circulation can be achieved from the internal and external jugular, subclavian, basilar, umbilical, and femoral veins. The site selected depends on the experience of the operator and the indication for the catheter. If venous access is the only requirement, one might elect to use visible veins (e.g., basilar, external jugular) or those with a lower risk for complications (e.g., femoral). Situations that require true intrathoracic central venous placement also require placement of the catheter into the internal jugular vein or subclavian vein. The umbilical vein can be used in neonates for volume resuscitation, but the high frequency with which these catheters enter the branch portal veins introduces a significant risk for permanent liver injury if sclerosing or hyperosmolar solutions are infused. Because a catheter tip can erode through the wall of the right atrium, care must be taken to avoid intracardiac tip placement. The catheter should be advanced only until the orifice lies in the intrathoracic great vessels, and its position should be confirmed radiographically.

Catheters of various sizes (2.5 to 10 French), lengths, and composition are available for pediatric applications (Cook Critical Care, Bloomington, IN, and other companies). Selection is based on the size of the patient (Andropoulos et al., 2001) and the purpose of the catheter. The composition of the catheter depends on its intended use. Teflon is fairly resistant to thrombus formation, but concerns about perforation by catheters have prompted the development of softer catheter materials, especially for long-term use (e.g., Silastic and polyurethane). The catheters are generally inserted via the Seldinger technique, using landmarks that are similar to those used in adults.

There are no absolute contraindications to placing a central venous catheter, but each site has potential risks. All sites share the common complications of infection (site cellulitis, bacteremia), venous thrombosis with potential emboli, air embolism, catheter malfunction (occlusion, dislodgment, or fractures), dysrhythmias (when the catheter tip is in the heart), and bleeding. Universal precautions and sterile technique should be used when placing a central venous catheter. The risks involved in cannulating the internal jugular vein include carotid artery puncture, Horner's syndrome, pneumothorax, and injury to the thoracic duct when the left internal jugular vein is cannulated. The high approach to the internal jugular vein, at the midpoint of the sternocleidomastoid muscle, results in comparable success with fewer complications than lower approaches (Coté et al., 1979). Two-dimensional ultrasound scanning improves localization of the internal jugular vein and increases the success rate of central venous cannulation in adults and children

(Verghese et al., 2002; Hind et al., 2003). Using this device, Alderson and others (1993) reported an 18% prevalence of anatomic variations in children younger than 6 years that would preclude or significantly hinder the successful cannulation of the internal jugular vein using anatomic landmarks alone. In addition, Hong and colleagues (2010) reported that rotating the head away from the neutral position increases the degree of carotid artery and internal jugular vein overlap, and decreases the incidence of lateral positioning of the internal jugular vein to the carotid artery.

Mixed Venous Oxygenation and Monitoring

Mixed venous oxygenation is defined as the oxygenation saturation or content of venous blood from the pulmonary artery. The collection of a mixed venous sample requires a pulmonary artery catheter. The Fick equation for mixed venous oxygen saturation (Svo_2) depends on four variables: oxygen consumption ($\dot{V}o_2$), cardiac output, hemoglobin, and arterial oxygen saturation.

Normal values for mixed venous saturation range from 65% to 75%. A decrease in Svo_2 occurs because of increased oxygen consumption (stress, pain, hyperthermia, shivering) or decreased oxygen delivery (anemia, decreased cardiac output, decreased Pao_2, decreased Sao_2). An increase in Svo_2 occurs because of a decrease in $\dot{V}o_2$ (hypothermia, anesthesia) or an increase in oxygen delivery (increased hemoglobin, increased cardiac output, increased Pao_2, increased Sao_2). Mixed venous oxygenation is used to assess the balance between oxygen delivery and oxygen consumption for patients in the operating room and intensive care unit. It is a global index of tissue oxygenation.

A significant limitation of mixed venous saturation is that it requires the collection of blood from the pulmonary artery. This is a particular limitation in the smaller pediatric patients. Blood from the superior vena cava (central venous saturation [$Scvo_2$]) and right atrium have been investigated as possible surrogate markers for mixed venous oxygen saturation, with mixed results.

Dueck and coworkers (2005) found a significant variation between central venous saturations and mixed venous saturations in the same patient, so individual values of $Scvo_2$ cannot be substituted for Svo_2 values. However, although the absolute values do not correlate, there is a correlation between the trends in $Scvo_2$ values and in Svo_2 values. Perez and colleagues (2009), in a retrospective pediatric study, identified a correlation between right atrial and mixed venous oxygen saturations. $Scvo_2$ is used clinically in pediatric patients. Continuous monitoring of $Scvo_2$ can be performed in neonates, infants, and children.

In infants, continuous monitoring of $Scvo_2$ can be achieved with a fiberoptic probe. One type of fiberoptic probe is designed as a percutaneous catheter from CeVOX (Pulsion Medical Systems AG, Munich, Germany). This 2-F probe is 31 cm in length and measures central venous oxygen saturations using spectrophotometry. Muller and coworkers (2007) described placing the catheter percutaneously through a 16-gauge single-lumen catheter in the femoral or subclavian vein. There were only three patients in this study, so accurate correlation with central venous blood samples cannot be determined.

The Pediasat system (Edwards Life Sciences) has been described in infants and children having orthopedic, craniofacial, and cardiac surgery. It comes in four sizes (4.5 F, 5 cm; 4.5 F, 8 cm; 5.5 F, 8 cm; and 5.5 F, 15 cm) and provides continuous readings of central venous oxygen saturation. Liakapolous and colleagues (2007) and Ranucci and colleagues (2008) demonstrated good correlation between $Scvo_2$ values from the Pediasat system when compared with co-oximetry values obtained from blood samples drawn from the distal port.

Artifact may limit the clinical usefulness of $Scvo_2$ catheters for intraoperative care. Manipulation of the catheter by the surgeon when the chest is open or direct light from the surgeon's headlight may alter the readings of the catheter.

Pulmonary Artery Catheters

Since its introduction in 1970, indications for the use of the flow-directed balloon-tipped pulmonary artery (Swan-Ganz) catheter in pediatric patients have been slow to evolve. Although the validity and value of the data that these catheters generate remain controversial in pediatrics, the technical difficulties and complications associated with their use are significant. Pulmonary artery pressure measurement can help guide therapy in children with elevated or volatile pulmonary vascular resistance, but the interpretation of the flow data they generate is hindered by several factors. First, the desired cardiac output varies according to age, disease state, and other elements of management that alter metabolic demand in complex ways, thereby introducing significant uncertainty in assigning a target value. Second, the prevalence of intracardiac communications that permit shunting of blood causes discrepancies in pulmonary and systemic blood flow that may vary continuously and are difficult to quantify. Finally, despite several studies demonstrating reasonable accuracy when thermodilution is compared with other methods of flow determination, such as the Fick equation (Freed and Keane, 1978) and dye dilution (Colgan and Stewart, 1977), the precision of these determinations in small infants is low and has a 25% intersample variability. In patients with congenital heart malformations, for example, measurement errors are introduced by shunting and complex anatomy, and the risks of improper placement of the flow-directed pulmonary artery catheter are increased. Alternatively, directly placed pulmonary artery catheters can provide the necessary information regarding pulmonary vascular resistance and residual left-to-right shunts, and left atrial catheters reflect filling and diastolic function of the left ventricle after cardiac surgery.

In some situations, pulmonary artery catheters provide useful information. In children who have severe coexisting pulmonary and circulatory failure, pulmonary artery catheters can help to quantify the hemodynamic impact of extreme respiratory support measures and guide complex fluid and pharmacologic regimens. They may also be useful in patients with underlying pulmonary hypertension or poorly compensated left ventricular dysfunction who undergo acute surgical stress (e.g., arteriovenous malformation clipping or aortic cross-clamping). Given the uncertainty about optimal systemic flow in a given child, mixed venous oxygen saturation may serve as a better indication of global perfusion. In the absence of left-to-right shunts, this sample is best obtained from the pulmonary artery.

Pulmonary artery catheters can be difficult to insert, especially in infants or in children with low cardiac output. They may be placed in any vein used for access to the central venous system, but the most reliable veins are the right internal jugular and the femoral. In infants and children smaller than 15 kg, it is technically difficult to place an introducer sheath in the neck vessels; the femoral veins are preferable. Multilumen catheters capable of thermodilution are available in two sizes, 5 and 7 F, with four options for the right atrium–to–pulmonary artery interluminal distance. Catheter recommendations are based on age (Table 11-4). The proper placement of these catheters can take a long time, and thus the assistance of fluoroscopy is recommended for infants and children less than 30 kg and for larger children who have a low cardiac output.

The risks of balloon-tipped pulmonary artery catheters are numerous and include the risks of central venous catheter placement discussed previously, as well as the complications seen in adult patients with pulmonary artery catheters: infection, air emboli, thrombus, pulmonary artery rupture, acute right bundle branch block, and intracardiac knots. Other complications are more common with children: misleading information, paradoxical systemic emboli, disruption of an intracardiac repair, and high-grade right ventricular outflow tract obstruction because of the relatively large balloon diameter. The presence of intracardiac and extracardiac malformations may result in an aberrant catheter course, leading to incorrect data and an increased risk for systemic emboli.

Cardiac output can be estimated in children through indicator dilution (e.g., thermodilution or dye dilution) and noninvasive techniques. Doppler determinations of aortic blood velocity can be used to quantify systemic flow if the angle of the incident ultrasound beam and the cross-sectional area of the aorta are reliably determined (Alverson et al., 1982). Transthoracic and transesophageal evaluations of Doppler cardiac output in children have proved to be less promising (Notterman et al., 1989; Muhiudeen et al., 1991). Thoracic bioimpedance, a method that estimates stroke volume on the basis of changes in thoracic impedance, has been applied to children as small as 3.6 kg. Although some correlation exists between bioimpedance and indicator dilution methods, reproducibility is poor (O'Connell et al., 1991). Further details and the complexities encountered in the measurement of cardiac output in children are beyond the scope of this chapter but have been reviewed previously (Tibby and Murdoch, 2002).

A noninvasive cardiac output monitor has been developed that determines cardiac output via the Fick principle for rebreathed CO_2 (Respironics; Novametrix Medical Systems Inc., Wallingford, CT) (Capek and Roy, 1988). The noninvasive cardiac output monitor has been clinically validated in adults and is approved by the U.S. Food and Drug Administration (FDA) for use, but it requires tidal volumes of 200 mL or greater (Guzzi et al., 2003; Watt et al., 2004).

Transesophageal Echocardiography

The value of transesophageal echocardiography (TEE) for monitoring hemodynamics and to evaluate preoperative and postoperative cardiac anatomy has been appreciated from the time of its introduction to the operating room. In the infancy of TEE in the late 1970s, an M-mode transducer was passed into the esophagus, plotting the distance of structures from the transducer on the y-axis and time on the x-axis (Frazin et al., 1976). Although they provided valuable information, M-mode images were too limited alone. In 1982, Schlüter and colleagues (1982) described their experience using a transducer capable of two-dimensional images mounted on a gastroscope. The usefulness of the images obtained was readily apparent, and since that time technology has catapulted the field of TEE to the forefront of cardiovascular monitoring. Now, multiple companies (Phillips, Acuson/Siemens, General Electric) manufacture advanced TEE-specific probes capable of two- and three-dimensional imaging on top of the original M-mode. Doppler has also been incorporated, providing the examiner the ability to extrapolate vast amounts of information from their patients.

The probes use ultrasound waves generated by the vibration of piezoelectric crystals in the tip of the transducer. Theses waves have frequencies between 2.5 and 7.5 MHz. The wave's ability to travel through tissues depends on the specific density of the tissues. Differences in impedance cause some of the energy generated by the crystals to be reflected and allow some to continue on to the next tissue plane until all the energy has dissipated. If the impedance is too great, as is the case with bone, all of the energy will be reflected. Images are then generated on the basis of the time from the impulse and the remaining energy found in the waves as they return to the transducer.

The quality of the image depends on a number of factors. The closer structures are to the transducer, the greater is the intensity of the image. Transducers with higher frequencies have less penetration than lower-frequency transducers; thus, if one is trying to visualize structures far away, a lower frequency provides better imaging. Images can also be adjusted with gain, so that unwanted echoes in the near field may be dampened and echoes in the far field enhanced.

Doppler technology uses low-intensity ultrasound reflected from moving columns of blood. The frequency of the returning echo is analyzed and estimations of direction and velocity are made. Accuracy of the estimation depends on the direction of flow relative to the direction of the beam. Parallel orientation provides the most accurate values, and increases in the angle of measurement falsely lower the predicted velocities. Measurements taken at angles greater than 20 degrees have a significant amount of error. Both pulsed-wave Doppler, if one is interested in determining velocity at a specific location, and continuous wave, to identify the highest velocity across an entire line of sight, are available for use during a TEE examination.

A modification of the Bernoulli equation allows an examiner to estimate pressure gradients using the measured velocities. Simplified, the change in pressure between two points is equal to four times the maximum velocity squared (Holen et al., 1977; Hatle et al., 1978). Using this principle, the stenosis of valves

TABLE 11-4. Guidelines for Multilumen Pulmonary Artery Catheters for Infants and Children

Age (yr)	Catheter Size (F)	CVP to Pulmonary Artery Port Distance (cm)
Newborn to 3	5	10
3 to 8	5	15
8 to 14	7	20
>14	7	30

severity of aortic coarctation, obstruction caused by muscle bundles or membranes, and a multitude of other clinical questions can be answered.

TEE has played a vital role in improving outcomes in pediatric patients with congenital heart disease. Typically, examinations are performed preoperatively to confirm anatomy, and postoperatively to assess repairs and evaluate function. One study looking at 865 consecutive examinations demonstrated alterations to surgical plans based on preoperative TEE examinations in 2% of patients. The same study found that 12% of patients had post-bypass examinations that led to surgical interventions. Many of these interventions saved patients from unnecessary revision operations and their associated morbidity. In addition to surgical interventions, medical management with drugs and fluids was affected in 20% of the examined patients (Bettex et al., 2003).

An earlier report found that pediatric patients leaving the operating room without residual defects seen on the echocardiographic examination had a risk for reoperation of 3%, versus 42% for those who were found to have residual defects (Ungerleider et al., 1989). This ability to detect problems early provides a significantly improved outcome and subsequently reduces costs, as the need for repeat operations is reduced (Randolph et al., 2002).

As evidence supporting the value of TEE in cardiac surgery has increased, recommendations for proper performance of the examination have matured. The American Society of Echocardiographers and the Society of Cardiovascular Anesthesiologists have developed guidelines for adult intraoperative TEE examinations to encourage complete examinations with standardized views and nomenclature so as to improve communication between various care providers (Shanewise et al., 1999). Discussion of the complete examinations is beyond the scope of this chapter, but some of the probe locations and angles are useful for obtaining basic information regarding a patient's condition (Table 11-5). Similar guidelines have also been published to assist clinicians with the pediatric examination (Lai et al., 2006).

Although the benefits have been demonstrated, providers must also be aware of the complications associated with the TEE examination. Problems that may be encountered include damage to the oral cavity, esophagus, or stomach; compromised ventilation; inadvertent extubation; right main stem advancement; vascular compression; and arrhythmias. In light of these serious but rare events, caution should precede placement of the transesophageal probe (Stevenson, 1999). Contraindications to the TEE examination include an unrepaired tracheoesophageal fistula, esophageal web, and recent esophageal or gastric surgery. Failure to ascertain a history of such events may lead to significant damage or even perforation of the esophagus.

Another issue encountered in the pediatric population is the size of the patient. Adult-sized probes are generally appropriate for patients older than 8 years or heavier than 20 kg. Pediatric probes are available for patients less than 20 kg. Most clinicians refrain from placing transesophageal probes in patients weighing less than 3 kg. If echocardiographic images are important to a particular surgery and TEE is contraindicated or impossible, an epicardial probe can be passed to the operative field via a sterile sleeve to obtain necessary imaging.

Temperature

Temperature monitoring is vital during pediatric anesthesia, as children may exhibit hypothermia or hyperthermia, both of which can have profound physiologic consequences (see Chapter 6, Thermoregulation).

Urine Output

Urine output often reflects intravascular volume status and cardiac output. Proper assessment of urine output requires recognition of the physiologic mechanisms that exert an affect on urine flow in children. During the first week of life, the glomerular filtration rate and renal plasma flow are only 25% of normal adult values (Arant, 1978). The neonatal kidney is limited in its ability to concentrate the urine (Simpson and Stephenson, 1993). By the end of the first week of life, the kidneys begin to reach absorption thresholds for sodium and glucose that approach adult levels.

Normal newborns produce between 0.5 and 4 mL urine/ kg per hour in the first 3 hours of life (Strauss et al., 1981). Urine flow, which initially ranges from 15 to 60 mL/kg per day, reaches as much as 120 mL/kg per day by the end of the first week of life, with 90% of neonates producing 0.5 to 5 mL/kg per hour (Douglas, 1972; Guignard, 1982). In the neonate who is less than 1 week old, urine flow alone is not a sensitive index of changes in cardiac output or intravascular volume. The limited capacity of the neonatal kidneys to compensate for diminished or excessive intravascular volume demands more precise management of blood and fluid replacement in these infants. Beyond the neonatal period, a urine flow of 0.5 to 1 mL/kg per hour usually indicates adequate renal perfusion and function.

Intraoperative monitoring of urine output is indicated in procedures in which large shifts in fluid, blood, or hemodynamics are anticipated, including blood loss greater than 20% of the EBV, third-space replacement exceeding 50% of the

TABLE 11-5. Transesophageal Echocardiography Cross Sections

Location	Angle (degrees)	Structures Visualized
Transgastric	0-20	Left and right ventricles, and both atrioventricular valves
	80-100	Two-chamber view of left side
	90-120	Long axis of left side, including left ventricular outflow tract
Midesophageal	0-20	Standard four-chamber view
	30-60	Aortic valve on short axis, coronary arteries
	60-90	Right ventricular inflow and outflow tracts
	80-110	Bicaval view
	120-160	Long-axis view of aortic valve and left ventricular outflow tract
Upper esophageal	0	Aortic arch on long axis
	90	Aortic arch on short axis

Modified from Shanewise JS, Cheung AT, Aronson S et al: ASE/SCA guidelines for performing a comprehensive intraoperative multiplane transesophageal echocardiography examination: recommendations of the American Society of Echocardiography Council for Intraoperative Echocardiography and the Society of Cardiovascular Anesthesiologists Task Force for Certification in Perioperative Transesophageal Echocardiography, *J Am Soc Echocardiogr* 12:884, 1999.

EBV, CPB, neurosurgery, deliberate hypotension, planned use of diuretics, or planned hemodilution. Silastic Foley catheters are available in sizes small enough (6 F) for full-term neonates. Alternatively, a small feeding tube can be used in premature infants and in those with a small urethra. In infants, urinary bladder catheters should be connected to a urinometer capable of measuring small volumes, or to a vented 10- to 20-mL syringe.

Noninvasive Respiratory Gas Monitoring

Carbon Dioxide

Capnometry is the instantaneous measurement of CO_2 in the breathing circuit; it depicts this information in a continuous graphic display in which both the quality and the quantity of ventilation can be evaluated (Figs. 11-3 to 11-6).

Before 1998, capnography was considered a standard monitor by the ASA for confirming the initial placement and continuous presence of an endotracheal tube. This section of the ASA monitoring standards was updated in 1998 and states that capnography should be used to confirm adequate ventilation during general anesthesia with or without an endotracheal tube (during laryngeal mask airway, face mask, or natural-airway anesthesia). Specifically, these guidelines state, "Continual monitoring for the presence of expired carbon dioxide shall be performed unless invalidated by the nature of the patient, procedure or equipment…. Continual end-tidal carbon dioxide analysis, in use from the time of endotracheal tube/laryngeal mask placement, until extubation/removal or initiating transfer to a

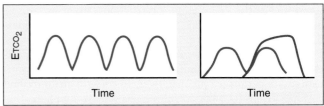

■ **FIGURE 11-4.** Common capnographic diagnoses: poor sampling. *Left:* Poor sampling as evidenced by absence of a plateau phase. This diagnosis could not be made with a capnometer that was incapable of real-time graphics. This is typical of small neonates whose small exhaled volumes are washed out by fresh gas flow. *Right:* The speckled curve projects the full exhaled breath that would be seen if fresh gas flow was diverted. Note that the plateau would be higher than the actual curve by an unpredictable amount. The digital information derived from a curve like the one on the left is useless.

postoperative care location, shall be performed using a quantitative method such as capnography, capnometry or mass spectroscopy" (ASA, 2003).

Most capnometers use the principle of infrared light absorption by sampling circuit gas in either a mainstream or a sidestream fashion. Sidestream analyzers aspirate a sample from the circuit and transport it via a long, narrow-bore tube to a distant analyzing chamber. Advantages include a lightweight airway adapter and the remote location of the delicate components of the analyzing chamber. Disadvantages of sidestream systems include potential occlusion of the sampling tube, distortion or dilution of the exhaled gas wave during aspiration and transport to the analyzing chamber, and the delay necessary to transport

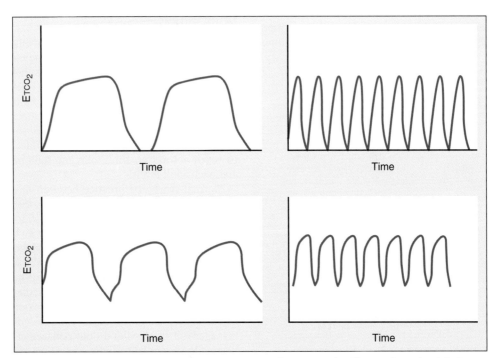

■ **FIGURE 11-3.** Common capnographic diagnoses: rebreathing. *Top:* Normal capnographs. The graph on the right is compressed over a longer time. Note the plateau, suggesting valid end-tidal CO_2 data and the return to baseline between breaths; there is no rebreathing. *Bottom:* Rebreathing, as there is no return to baseline. This can occur with inadequate fresh gas flow or floating unidirectional valves. The small initial deflection before exhalation (the preexhalation hump) can occasionally be seen. It represents the inhalation late in the inspiratory phase of more concentrated exhaled gas from the previous exhalation.

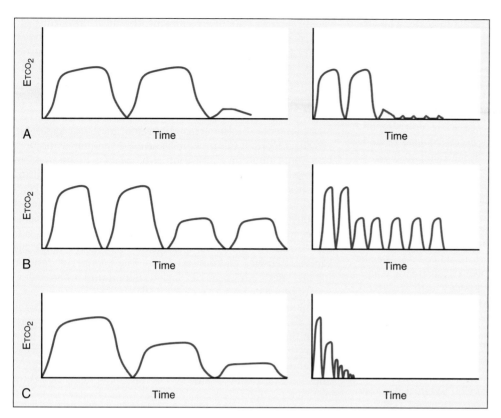

■ **FIGURE 11-5.** Common capnographic diagnoses: reduction in end-tidal carbon dioxide tension ($PETCO_2$). There are many reasons for sudden reduction in $PETCO_2$, some of which result in characteristic capnographic patterns. **A,** Abrupt reduction to zero (or nearly zero) typically indicates mechanical disruption, disconnection, accidental extubation, or plugged sampling line. **B,** Sudden reduction to a lower $PETCO_2$ while preserving plateau and characteristics of a good trace indicate sudden increase in dead space ventilation as occurs with a pulmonary embolus (either thrombus or air). **C,** Exponential reduction to zero (CO_2 washout curve) is characteristic of no pulmonary blood flow and thus either massive embolus or cardiac arrest.

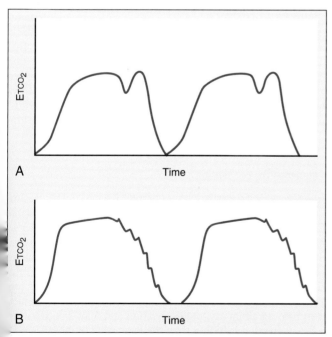

■ **FIGURE 11-6.** Common capnographic diagnoses: irregular tracings. Irregularities in the curve are common, especially at the end of exhalation when exhaled gas flow is lowest. **A,** Diaphragmatic activity indicating spontaneous respiratory effort, usually the result of dissipating neuromuscular blockade. **B,** Cardiac oscillations: fluctuations in intrathoracic gas volume as a result of cardiac activity, usually a benign finding.

and analyze the sample. Innovations in capnography technology have allowed a sampling rate as low as 30 mL/min (i.e., microstream technology).

Mainstream analyzers use a sample chamber placed directly into the circuit. They have the advantage of providing virtually instantaneous analysis by avoiding transport of the sample. Such a system necessitates the addition of a delicate and bulky sensor to the proximal airway connection, where it might easily serve as a fixation point to dislodge a small tracheal tube. Solid-state innovations have dramatically reduced the weight of the mainstream sensors, but they remain significantly more hazardous when added to the circuits of neonates and small infants. Although early mainstream sample chambers added as much as 17 mL of dead space to the circuit, currently available models reduce this volume to 2 mL or less.

Capnography in pediatric anesthesia is used to confirm placement of an endotracheal tube in the correct tracheal position and to continuously assess the adequacy of ventilation. Capnography also provides information about the respiratory rate, breathing pattern, endotracheal tube patency, and, indirectly, degree of neuromuscular blockade. Capnography can assist with the diagnosis of metabolic and cardiovascular events and can provide an early warning of a faulty anesthesia delivery system. In pediatric patients, an abnormal increase in end-tidal carbon dioxide tension ($PETCO_2$) most commonly signifies hypoventilation, but, rarely, it also indicates the presence of increased CO_2 production, as occurs with temperature elevation or as an early sign of malignant hyperthermia. On the other hand, an abnormally low $PETCO_2$ may indicate an increase in dead space or suggest a state of low pulmonary perfusion.

Sudden absence of the capnographic tracing indicates a breathing circuit disconnection, and the abnormal presence of inspired CO_2 signifies the presence of a faulty unidirectional valve, an exhausted CO_2 absorber, or, when a semiopen circuit is being used, rebreathing secondary to an insufficient fresh gas flow.

The capnographic tracing of small infants is often characterized by the lack of an apparent alveolar plateau. This is usually a result of a higher respiratory rate, an excessively high sampling flow for the volume of CO_2 produced, excessive dead space in the breathing circuit, or an excessive leak around an uncuffed endotracheal tube.

The degree to which P_{ETCO_2} reflects Pa_{CO_2} is subject to many variables, some technical and others physiologic. The technical issues of primary importance in the accurate measurement of mean alveolar CO_2 tension include the volume and flow rate of exhaled gas, the aspirating flow rate (for sidestream analyzers), the fresh gas flow rate, the type of breathing circuit, and the circuit location of the sampling chamber (mainstream analyzers) or lumen of the aspirating tubing (sidestream analyzers). These variables are of particular importance in the small neonate whose small exhaled volumes at low flow rates are often diluted by high fresh gas flows or aspirating gas flows (Badgwell et al., 1987, 1993; Rich et al., 1990; Spahr-Schopfer et al., 1993). Badgwell and others (1987) demonstrated exponential increases in the discrepancy between P_{ETCO_2} and Pa_{CO_2} values with progressive reduction in patients who weighed less than 12 kg (Fig. 11-7). The coaxial distal sampling tube that they advocated dramatically improved the correlation.

The physiologic variable that introduces the most significant error in P_{ETCO_2} is dead space ventilation (Swedlow, 1986). Apart from children with severe pulmonary pathology or acute

events such as pulmonary embolus, the most prevalent pediatric population in whom substantial dead space ventilation occurs are those with cyanotic congenital heart disease, particularly right-to-left shunts (Burrows, 1989; Fletcher, 1991).

Other Gases

Measurements of other respiratory and anesthetic gases can provide important information about cardiopulmonary physiology. Confirming the elimination of nitrogen is useful in determining adequate preoxygenation, whereas its presence during anesthesia may reveal a leak in the delivery system or, in combination with a sudden decrease in end-tidal CO_2, a venous air embolism. The measurement of anesthetic gases and vapors serves to illustrate the uptake and elimination of these agents and to confirm the purity and the accuracy of the tanks and vaporizers used to administer them. The quantity of residual inhaled anesthetic agent has obvious importance in the evaluation of prolonged emergence from anesthesia.

The techniques enabling multigas analysis that have found clinical application are based on properties such as ionized mass separation (mass spectrometry), ultraviolet and infrared light absorption, and absorption into lipophilic substances. A variety of manufacturers produce devices that quantify respiratory and anesthetic gases in the same unit as the capnograph; their complete description is beyond the scope of this chapter.

Monitoring Oxygen and Carbon Dioxide

Because of high oxygen consumption and small functional residual capacity of infants and small children, they are more likely to become hypoxemic during general anesthesia than adults. Careful tracking of arterial oxygenation is vitally important. Noninvasive monitors of oxygenation are ubiquitous in the perioperative setting because of technological advances that have improved their reliability and because of standards that require their application not only in the operating room but also in the PACU and sedation room. These devices are of two basic types: those that measure cutaneous (transcutaneous) oxygen tension, and others that evaluate arterial oxygen saturation (pulse oximeters).

Cutaneous Oxygen Tension

In 1972, a miniature Clark polarographic oxygen electrode, similar to those used in in vitro blood gas analysis, became available for application to the skin. When a probe heats the skin to 42° to 44° C, the cutaneous oxygen tension (Ps_{O_2}) approaches arterial oxygen tension because the skin blood flow and permeability to oxygen are increased (Barker and Tremper, 1985). The correlation may be better in neonates because their epidermis is less keratinized and their cutaneous capillary bed is denser. In fact, skin heating alters oxygen dissociation and may even result in a Ps_{O_2} value that is higher than the Pa_{O_2} value (Lubbers, 1981). In older children and adults, as the keratinized layer thickens, the diffusion gradient for oxygen becomes more significant. In practice, transcutaneous gas monitors are subject to the effect of these and myriad other nonlinear variables that influence skin perfusion, such as hypotension, hypothermia, and pharmacologic agents. They are the only noninvasive monitors that can provide information regarding significant hyperoxem

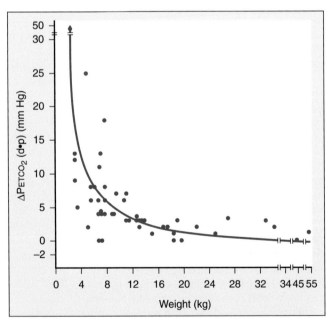

FIGURE 11-7. Gradient between end-tidal carbon dioxide (E_{TCO_2}) determinations made in the proximal and distal ends of a tracheal tube. Exponential increases in the gradient suggest substantial potential inaccuracy in proximal E_{TCO_2} determinations for children weighing less than 12 kg. (From Badgwell JM, McLeod ME, Lerman J, et al: End-tidal Pco2 measurements sampled at the distal and proximal ends of the endotracheal tube in infants and children, Anesth Analg 66:959, 1987.)

(Monaco et al., 1982; Rafferty et al., 1982; Barker and Tremper, 1985). The correlation, especially outside the physiologic range of Pao_2, is variable and depends on the individual conditions, and the data produced may differ from those provided by the Pso_2 by a substantial yet unpredictable amount (American Academy of Pediatrics, 1989). Such results led Barker and Tremper (1985) to propose a more reasonable role for this monitor in determining peripheral tissue oxygen delivery (perfusion) rather than arterial oxygenation.

From a practical standpoint, the monitor is cumbersome. It requires calibration, a warm-up time of 10 to 20 minutes, and meticulous skin preparation and probe placement. It is sensitive to electrosurgical interference and mechanical manipulation. The technical demands of this monitor have limited its current use to special applications, such as detection of hyperoxemia in premature infants. A frequent side effect of transcutaneous monitoring is the occurrence of first- and second-degree burns.

Cutaneous Carbon Dioxide Tension

Cutaneous carbon dioxide tension ($Psco_2$) measurement using a variant of the Severinghaus electrode is also available (Nosovitch et al., 2002). Although $Psco_2$ is always higher than $Paco_2$ as a result of tissue carbon dioxide production and the increased metabolism caused by a heating sensor, these monitors accurately follow trends in arterial carbon dioxide tension. The predictable gradient from arterial to cutaneous CO_2 tensions enables the monitors to calculate the gradient and display a "corrected" value. These devices are less altered by changes in skin temperature and perfusion than are cutaneous oxygen analyzers. The reasonably good correlation of end-tidal and arterial CO_2 tensions in all but extremely small subjects has limited the interest in cutaneous CO_2 tension monitoring in the operating room to very rare situations.

Pulse Oximetry

Pulse oximetry, invented by Takuo Aoyagi in 1974 and developed as a clinical monitor a decade later, has markedly improved patient safety, especially during the perioperative period (Yelderman and New, 1983; Aoyagi, 2003; Severinghaus, 2007). It provides an estimate of the oxyhemoglobin saturation in arterial blood with a probe on a fingertip (New, 1985). The pulse oximeter uses plethysmography to determine the systolic portion of the cardiac cycle. During systole, there is a greater volume of blood in a pulsatile arterial vascular bed. This vascular bed is positioned between a sensor that contains a two-wavelength (red and infrared, 660 and 940 nm) light-emitting diode and a photodiode receptor (the wavelength varies depending on the manufacturer). Less light is transmitted in systole than in diastole because of the increased volume of the arterial bed. Sophisticated algorithms based on the amount of light absorbed differentiate systole from diastole. Oxygenated and deoxygenated blood absorb different quantities of light, proportional to their concentrations or the percentage of saturation according to the Beer-Lambert law. Once systole is identified through plethysmography, the arterial saturation during this period is determined by using the ratio of light absorption at the two different wavelengths through this vascular bed. The ratio is matched to data acquired over a range of experimentally determined saturations and ratios of light absorption stored in the instrument's memory to determine the arterial saturation. Using the ratio of light absorption at two wavelengths makes unnecessary the calibration and zeroing to adjust to the size of the patient or to skin pigment (Aoyagi, 2003). In the 80% to 100% saturation range, arterial saturation values determined by this method correlated well with in vitro measurements (New, 1985). Based on the algorithm used to determine systole and the time-averaging process used over several cardiac cycles, different pulse oximeters have slightly different responses to a variety of clinical situations. Because the device must identify the pulse-added absorption, it may confuse motion of the extremity to which the sensor is attached with pulsating motion and abort the display of saturation data or, worse, display inaccurate data (see later).

Pulse oximetry was introduced into pediatric practice in the United States in the late 1980s (Salyer, 2003). It serves as an early warning signal of impending or actual hypoxemia, often before the onset of cyanosis, frequently reminding anesthesiologists of the alarming rapidity with which infants develop hypoxemia as compared with toddlers and older children (Xue et al., 1996). Continuous-use pulse oximetry is included in the basic monitoring standards of the ASA (2003). Anesthesiologist-blinded studies have demonstrated that the use of pulse oximetry facilitates earlier recognition and fewer episodes of hypoxemia (Coté et al., 1988, 1991). Pulse oximetry has rapidly evolved into a standard monitor during pediatric anesthesia and, as a result, has never been subjected to rigorous outcome studies with a true control group (an anesthetic without a pulse oximeter) (Cohen et al., 1988). There are no outcome studies that demonstrate proven benefit from the use of pulse oximetry (Moller et al., 1993a, 1993b; Pedersen et al., 2001).

A number of well-described limitations of pulse oximetry affect the accuracy of commercially available pulse oximeters. Among other factors, ambient lighting conditions, motion, peripheral circulation to the extremity, body temperature, and abnormal hemoglobins can interfere with accuracy and consistency of pulse oximeter performance (Schramm et al., 1997; Trivedi et al., 1997). Of all these factors, motion artifact is clinically the most common problem, resulting in inaccurate readings, data loss, missed alarms, and false alarms. Patient motion (e.g., shivering and seizures in adults and children, as well as kicking, stretching, and crying in infants) causes movement of venous blood, as well as other normally nonpulsatile body fluid components (e.g., tissue fluid in edematous patients), along with the arterial blood. The pulsatile components of the body fluids other than arterial blood may lead to falsely low saturation readings. If motion is combined with low perfusion at the sensor site, then the venous blood makes a more significant contribution to the pulsatile component and drives the Sao_2 as measured with a pulse oximeter (or SpO_2) even lower. Various algorithm-based motion rejection methods used by manufacturers to minimize the impact of motion artifact and reduce false alarms include averaging saturation data over longer periods of time, freezing values until uncorrupted signals are present, and implementing alarm delays (Petterson et al., 2007). Other technologies use parallel processing of multiple sophisticated algorithms to isolate the biological signal in the presence of noise. When compared with conventional and other motion-tolerant pulse oximeters, Signal Extraction Technology (Masimo Corp., Irvine, Calif) has been reported to have a better performance in a variety of pediatric clinical settings, including newborn and pediatric intensive care units, the PACU, and the pediatric sleep lab (Ahlborn et al., 2000; Bohnhorst et al., 2000; Malviya et al., 2000; Barker, 2002; Brouillette et al., 2002; Trang et al., 2004; Workie et al., 2005).

Although the pulse oximeter is a continuous monitor, it does not instantaneously reflect the arterial saturation or the degree of desaturation. Most commercially available pulse oximeters display the average SpO_2 numbers of the most recent 5 to 15 pulses, depending on models and manufacturers, causing a delay in detecting desaturation. When the patient is breathing high concentrations of oxygen and the blood is fully saturated, a substantial decrease in PaO_2 can occur without a change in SaO_2. Reynolds and associates (1993) detected desaturation in children 30 seconds earlier in probes placed centrally (forehead) than in those placed on a finger. By the time the value indicated by a peripheral sensor had decreased 5%, the value indicated on a central sensor was 30% to 40% lower (Agashe et al., 2006). The precise mechanism for this discrepancy remains unknown, although Severinghaus and Naifeh (1987) postulated that it reflects peripheral blood transit, capillary composition, and oxygen utilization. Centrally placed reflective forehead pulse oximeter sensors are reported to respond faster and to be less likely to be compromised by vasoconstriction than transmittance finger probes (Choi et al., 2010).

Pulse oximeters are designed to warn practitioners when the arterial saturation decreases to below normal, not to serve as quantitative devices in hypoxemic patients. Compared with measured arterial saturation in children with cyanotic congenital heart disease, most pulse oximeters exhibit a progressively positive bias, typically reaching 5% to 15% at an SaO_2 of 60%, in addition to a significant reduction in precision ($\pm 8\%$ to 10%) (Gidding, 1992; Schmitt et al., 1993) (Fig. 11-8). More recently, a pulse oximetry sensor designed specifically for patients who are chronically hypoxemic, such as children with congenital heart disease, has become available. This specialized sensor, called the Blue sensor, has reported precision of less than $\pm 4\%$ between saturations of 60% and 80%. When compared with a standard pulse oximetry sensor on postoperative palliative cardiac surgery patients, the Blue sensor had a bias of 0.21 and

an accuracy root-mean-square (RMS) error of 3.6% compared with SaO_2 values, whereas the standard sensor had a bias of 0.86 and an accuracy RMS error of 6.4% compared with SaO_2 values (Cannesson et al., 2008c). The Blue sensor demonstrates considerable improvement in the accuracy of pulse oximetry monitoring of cyanotic children.

Interference with the expected spectrophotometric absorption pattern also causes errors in measurement. Low hemoglobin (<5 g/dL) and abnormal hemoglobin species (e.g., methemoglobin, carboxyhemoglobin) cause inaccurate saturation estimates by pulse oximeters, which become progressively inaccurate as SaO_2 decreases (New, 1985; Barker and Tremper, 1987; Barker et al., 1989; Watcha et al., 1989). In contrast, unusual or abnormal hemoglobin molecules, such as fetal hemoglobin and sickle cell hemoglobin, apparently have little effect on the saturation measurement (Jennis and Peabody, 1987; Ortiz et al., 1999). Intravenous dyes such as methylene blue and indocyanine green, affect the expected light absorption and produce spurious information (Ralston et al., 1991). Aberrant radiation (e.g., electromagnetic energy from the electrocautery, infrared heat lamps, operating room lights) and infrared light pulses from lasers and neuronavigation systems also cause incorrect saturation determinations (Brooks et al., 1984; Costarino et al., 1987; Hanowell et al., 1987; Mathes et al., 2008; Zhang et al., 2009).

Multiple-Wavelength Pulse Oximetry

Pulse oximeters that use two wavelengths of light are subject to interference from other hemoglobin species that absorb light across similar spectra. Dyshemoglobins such as carboxyhemoglobin and methemoglobin cannot be detected by pulse oximetry, but their presence in arterial blood can bias the oximeter's estimate of SaO_2. Multiple-wavelength pulse oximetry (Pulse CO-Oximetry; Masimo Corp., Irvine, CA) has been developed to detect and measure both carboxyhemoglobin and methemoglobin levels noninvasively and continuously, although the accuracy of SaO_2 estimations from these devices is still compromised (Barker et al., 2006). Pulse CO-Oximetry devices that measure carboxyhemoglobin have been shown to be useful in the emergency room for detection of occult carbon monoxide poisoning, and for monitoring and guiding emergency treatment of CO exposure (Suner et al., 2008; Bledsoe et al., 2009; Piatkowski et al., 2009). Methemoglobinemia can be caused by a wide variety of oxidizing drugs and their metabolites and by exposure to industrial chemicals such as aniline dyes, chlorates, and bromates. The clinical usefulness of noninvasive methemoglobin detection and monitoring by Pulse CO-Oximetry has been demonstrated for the diagnosis and treatment of severe methemoglobinemia in the hospital setting (Annabi and Barker, 2009).

Plethysmographic Waveform Analysis

For many years, clinicians have used the shape and amplitude of the plethysmographic waveform from pulse oximetry as a crude and imprecise method to assess blood volume and cardiac output (Partridge, 1987). Respiratory variations in pulse oximetry plethysmographic waveform amplitude can predict fluid responsiveness noninvasively in mechanically ventilated patients, but this method of assessment is technically challenging—neither automated nor continuous, and not available in clinical practice

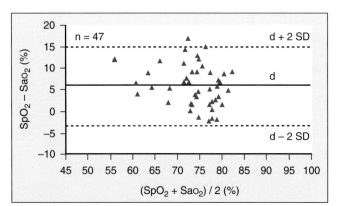

■ **FIGURE 11-8.** Accuracy and precision of pulse oximetry (Nellcor N-100) in chronically hypoxemic children with congenital heart malformations. Data comparing pulse oximetry (SpO_2) with CO-Oximetry (SaO_2) reflect a 5.8% mean positive bias for SpO_2, with wide discrepancies between the two techniques (± 2 SD = –3.8% to +15.4%). *(From Schmitt HJ, Schuetz WH, Proeschel PA, et al: Accuracy of pulse oximetry in children with cyanotic congenital heart disease, J Cardiothorac Vasc Anesth 7:61, 1993.)*

(Cannesson et al., 2007). An index that provides an automatic and continuous calculation of the respiratory variations in the waveform amplitude is now available with some pulse oximeters. The pleth variability index has been shown to predict fluid responsiveness during cardiac surgery (Cannesson et al., 2008b) and to predict changes in cardiac index with changes in positive end-expiratory pressure after cardiac surgery in mechanically ventilated, sedated patients (Desebbe et al. 2010). This index may allow the optimization of fluid loading noninvasively during and after surgery, but further validation is required before these results can be extrapolated to the general population.

Near-Infrared Spectroscopy

Near-infrared spectroscopy (NIRS) is another tool available to the anesthesiologist that provides information regarding tissue oxygenation. Its applications range from cerebral oximetry during circulatory arrest, to monitoring for compartment syndrome in the setting of trauma (Tobias and Hoernschemeyer, 2007; Bernal et al., 2010). Although NIRS continues to be studied for its impact on patient outcomes, it is increasing popular as a noninvasive monitor of vital data.

NIRS relies on principles similar to those of pulse oximetry, exploiting the variable absorption of light by color-containing compounds in the body. Infrared light emitted by the device enters the skin and scatters through the tissues beneath, some energy being absorbed and some reflected. The portion of the light that returns to the skin is analyzed and conclusions are drawn about the content of the tissues it passed through (Cohn, 2007).

The basis for analysis of the reflected light is found in the Beer-Lambert law. According to this law, reduction in the intensity of light passing through a substance depends on the absorbance of the substance and its thickness. These principles are used to quantify concentrations of oxygenated hemoglobin, which absorbs light at 805 nm, and deoxygenated hemoglobin, which absorbs at 730 nm, and to determine the regional oxygen saturation (rSo_2) of the tissue examined (Tobias, 2006).

Unlike pulse oximetry, NIRS does not require pulsatile flow, because it looks at all the blood in a given tissue including arterial, venous, and capillary blood. This means that NIRS is particularly valuable when pulsatility is lost (e.g., in CPB or circulatory arrest).

NIRS technology is commercially available from only a few companies. The INVOS Cerebral/Somatic Oximeter (Somanetics Corp., Troy, MI), which has been on the market for a long time, provides real-time monitoring capability for the rSo_2 of blood in tissues beneath the probe. To target specific tissues such as the brain or kidneys and not the skin and soft tissues between the probe and these organs, the device has been designed to eliminate data from the superficial tissues. The probe incorporates a light-emitting diode and two sensors located at fixed distances from the light. Infrared light passing through the superficial tissue is picked up by the closest sensor, and infrared light passing through the deeper tissues is picked up by the further sensor. Information from the superficial tissues is subtracted from the data returning from deeper tissues to provide accurate estimates of the deep tissue oxygenation (Tobias, 2006).

The Fore-Sight (Cass Medical Systems, Branford, CT) uses laser light at four wavelengths. Based on the same principles as the Sonametics device, it also accounts for the spurious information collected from the superficial tissues to focus

on the deeper areas of interest (Chakravarti et al., 2008). Both devices have approved uses in pediatrics, and probes of different sizes fit this population.

Clinicians presented with data on tissue oxygenation must know how to respond to it, and much has been written about the clinical usefulness of NIRS. Cerebral oximetry has been the most widely studied use of NIRS, and here NIRS has proved to be both a sensitive and specific indicator of cerebral tissue oxygenation (Al-Rawi et al., 2001). Kurth and coworkers (2002) noted thresholds for normal and abnormal values in a piglet model. They found baseline cerebral rSo_2 values of 68%, and they found that lactate began rising when the rSo_2 dropped to 44%, electroencephalographic changes started at around 42%, and ATP loss occurred at 33%. This information, along with corroborating findings in adult studies, has led to a weak consensus that an rSo_2 reduction of 20% from baseline, or an absolute value of 50%, serves as an indication of potential hypoxic injury and warrants intervention.

To establish the value of cerebral oximetry in the pediatric population, Hoffman and colleagues (2008) studied patients treated for hypoplastic left heart syndrome, and they demonstrated improved neurologic scores at age 4 to 5 years in patients who were monitored with cerebral oximetry at the time of their surgery and treated for abnormal values ($rSo_2 < 55\%$). This is encouraging, but most agree that there is still insufficient evidence to support clinical decisions based on NIRS values alone (Hirsch et al., 2009).

NIRS has generated interest in additional applications, including shock, compartment syndrome, plastics, and regional perfusion. Adult literature demonstrates NIRS ability to detect compartment syndrome as well as improvement in tissue oxygenation after fasciotomy (Giannotti et al., 2000). Studies of free flaps found that NIRS identified early evidence of flap failure prior to routine clinical evidence (Holzle et al., 2006).

NIRS provides information regarding tissue oxygenation for a broad spectrum of clinical scenarios. As studies continue, clinicians will better understand how to interpret and respond to the data so as to improve the outcomes of their patients.

Bispectral Index

In 1996, the FDA approved the use of the bispectral index (BIS) monitor (Aspect Medical Systems, Nattick, MA), a device based on electroencephalography (EEG) and used to predict the relative level of hypnosis, or unconsciousness, in anesthetized patients (Rosow and Manberg, 1998). Using a patch affixed to the patient's forehead, the BIS monitor integrates various EEG descriptors into a single, dimensionless, empirically calibrated number ranging from 0 to 100, where 0 represents electrical silence and 100 represents full wakefulness. A state of unconsciousness consistent with BIS values less than 60 usually ensures a lack of intraoperative recall (Glass et al., 1997). In adults, titration of anesthetics to a targeted BIS value between 40 and 60 results in the administration of relatively lower doses of anesthetics and earlier awakening (Gan et al., 1997). Studies in adults suggest that routine BIS monitoring is associated with reduced intraoperative awareness during high-risk surgical procedures (e.g., microlaryngeal surgery, cesarean section, cardiac bypass) (Myles et al., 2003).

In anesthetized children on mechanical ventilation, as well as in those spontaneously breathing through a face mask, BIS values are inversely proportional to the end-tidal concentration of halothane, sevoflurane, and desflurane (Denman et al., 2000; Davidson et al., 2001; Degoute et al., 2001; Tirel et al., 2006; Kern et al., 2007). Similar relationships between the depth of anesthesia (minimum alveolar concentration [MAC], plasma concentration) and BIS values have been studied during total intravenous anesthesia (TIVA), with or without additional opioids, in children with target-controlled infusion of propofol (Jeleazcov et al., 2007; Tirel et al., 2008; Rigouzzo et al., 2008; Malherbe et al., 2010). BIS values during sevoflurane anesthesia appear to be proportionately less in children with quadriplegic cerebral palsy and those who are mentally compromised (Choudhry and Brenn, 2002; Valkenburg et al., 2009).

In children, at a given depth of anesthesia (i.e., MAC), there are significant nonlinear inverse correlations between BIS values and age: BIS values are higher in toddlers than in older children in all studies, including TIVA with propofol. Furthermore, in addition to age-related variations in BIS values, interindividual variabilities in BIS index are much higher in infants and children than in adults (Tirel et al.; 2006, Kern et al., 2007; Rigouzzo et al., 2008). These characteristics of BIS in children may be associated with age-related differences in brain maturation and synapse formation throughout childhood (Watcha, 2001). The reliability of the BIS index is further diminished in infants younger than 1 year (Tirel et al., 2006; Jeleazcov et al., 2007; Kern et al., 2007; Rigouzzo et al., 2008).

The clinical benefits of measuring BIS and maintaining appropriate levels of anesthesia, such as reduced risk for intraoperative awareness and improved recovery time, may still be valid in pediatric patients, with the realization of certain characteristics of and differences in children. In adolescents undergoing scoliosis surgery, BIS can predict voluntary patient movement in response to commands during the intraoperative wake-up test (McCann et al., 2002). BIS monitoring was also used successfully for the intraoperative wake-up test in a neonate undergoing neurosurgery for the repair of myelomeningocele (Govindarajan et al., 2006). BIS monitoring in children aged 3 to 18 years who are undergoing tonsillectomy and adenoidectomy is associated with reduced recovery times (Bannister et al., 2001). However, in the same study, BIS monitoring did not affect recovery times in children younger than 3 years who were undergoing hernia repair.

More recently, interest in the efficacy of BIS in monitoring the depth of sedation has increased in other specialties, including critical care, emergency medicine, dentistry, and general pediatrics (Kerssens and Sebel, 2006; Malviya et al., 2006, 2007; Sadhasivam et al., 2006; Froom et al., 2008; Baygin et al., 2010). Also, BIS monitoring has been used in documenting positive sedative effects of regional and spinal blockade with local anesthetics in children, with or without general anesthesia (Davidson et al., 2006; Hermanns et al., 2006). Future studies are expected to further delineate the use of BIS in the pediatric population.

Neurophysiologic Monitoring

It has long been appreciated that the patient's physiologic status is dynamic, and that rapid and life-threatening changes may occur during surgery. The comparative abilities to evaluate the functional status of the nervous system by clinical means and by commonly used physiologic monitoring tools that are available to anesthesiologists is limited. Routine anesthesia monitoring may reflect stress on the central nervous system (CNS). For example, changes in heart rate related to both brainstem and vagal stimulation provide invaluable information when correlated with surgical activity. However, intraoperative neurophysiologic monitoring (IOM) adds yet another dimension, as well as specificity, to assessment of the status of the patient during surgery and anesthesia.

Neurophysiologic techniques provide important and reliable alternative tools for assessment of function of the pediatric CNS (Sclabassi and Krieger, 1995). These techniques provide objective measures of the functioning of the CNS and can serve to localize, warn of, and document deterioration in neuronal function. Intraoperatively, continuous monitoring of the area of the CNS that is at risk from surgical and anesthetic manipulation provides immediate insight into the effects of these manipulations. Rather than waiting to evaluate the neurologic examination of a child in the postoperative period, continuous IOM provides an immediate view of the integrity of the CNS, permitting changes in operative and anesthetic technique to minimize or correct the deleterious effects of intraoperative manipulations. Advantages of these methods are that the results are objective and quantifiable, the site of the lesion can be identified, and clinically latent and evolving lesions can frequently be demonstrated. These techniques have roles to play both in the diagnostic investigation of pediatric CNS function and in the field of intraoperative assessment of CNS function.

The measures used must be both specific to the neural tissue being manipulated and sensitive to changes in the functioning of the neural tissue produced by the surgical manipulations. Monitoring of the electrical activity dependent on the functioning of the brainstem (brainstem auditory evoked potential [BAEP] and brainstem somatosensory evoked potential [BSEP]), the cortex (EEG, somatosensory evoked potential [SEP], and visual evoked potential [VEP]), the spinal cord (SEP, motor evoked potential [MEP], and electromyogram [EMG]), the various cranial nerves (EMG), and peripheral nerves (compound action potential [CAP] and EMG) provides a multidimensional assessment of the integrity of the neural structures at risk. In addition, many of these measures provide information not only about function itself but also about variables that directly or indirectly affect function, such as blood flow, hypoxia, and hypotension. The goal of IOM is to provide information to the surgeon and anesthesiologist that allows them to modify their operative strategy before inducing additional deficits in the functioning of the CNS.

Perioperative Assessment and Communication

An important aspect of successful IOM is close communication among all members of the surgical team in the planning and execution of surgical procedures. The monitoring team need to be informed of the nature of the patient's disease process and of the planned operation. Preoperative studies are most useful in defining the effects of the pathology on the neurophysiologic measures to be used during the procedure, and in clarifying the maturational nature of these measures. The neurophysiologist should maintain close communication with members of the surgical team, including surgeons, anesthesiologists, and radiologists, before and during the procedure. This ensures that the monitoring approach is appropriately planned, that appropriate neurophysiologic measures are used during the procedure that the anesthesiologist can provide appropriate anesthesia to support the monitoring needed, and that the significance of observed changes is appreciated by all members of the team. The surgeon needs to understand the level of information that the neurophysiologist can provide as the operative procedure is evolving, and the anesthesiologist needs to understand the effects of the pharmacologic manipulations on the monitoring tools available to the neurophysiologist.

Technical Methodology

The recording of high-quality neurophysiologic data depends on the appropriate use of technology—the electrodes, amplifiers, stimulators, and other equipment used to acquire and display the data.

The bioelectrical activity at the scalp and the surface of the body is sensed using metal electrodes, and it is transferred through conducting leads to recording amplifiers. Subdermal needle electrodes are used in the operating room and may be used as stimulating electrodes as well as recording electrodes. The positions of the recording electrodes should be chosen in relation to the expected distribution of the responses to be recorded. Many laboratories place scalp electrodes at sites determined by the international 10-20 system (Jasper, 1958). This system, originally devised for EEG recordings, specifies the position of 21 evenly spaced locations on the scalp. Recording electrodes are placed symmetrically to provide control recordings from the side contralateral to the surgery, even when electrodes may not be positioned in the standard recording sites. Electrodes that are not in the operative field but are on the scalp and not accessible during surgery are either sutured or stapled in place. Electrodes on the face, which are placed to record electromyographic activity, are taped in place. Electrodes in the operative field are placed by the surgeons using sterile technique, usually early in the procedure.

Neurophysiologic signals are amplified using differential amplifiers (Goff, 1974), in which two input channels to the amplifier are differenced. This differencing has the effect of eliminating identical (in-phase) signal components that might be present at each recording electrode (presumably noise), and retaining the signals that are different (out of phase) and presumably produced by physiologic generators. The effectiveness with which a differential amplifier rejects in-phase signals compared with its ability to amplify out-of-phase signals is called the common mode rejection ratio (CMRR). Differential amplifiers typically have CMRRs of greater than 10,000:1 (80 dB). For efficient rejection of in-phase signals, it is extremely important that the impedances of each electrode in a pair be not only as low as possible but as similar as possible, because any inequality in electrode impedance will produce amplitude differences in the in-phase activity that will be amplified along with the desired signal.

In evoked potential recording, the observed neuroelectrical activity, either from the scalp or propagating activity from the cord, is assumed to consist of a signal component representative of underlying activity evoked by the stimulus and random noise consisting of both physiologic signals not relevant to the study and environmental noise generated by ubiquitous sources of electrical signals. Evoked potentials are typically a fraction of the size of the spontaneous brain activity appearing in the background EEG, and about one thousandth the size of the other physiologic and extraneous potentials with which they are intermixed. The aim of evoked potential recording is to acquire a large, clear response with the least possible noise contamination (i.e., the best signal-to-noise ratio possible); thus, the elimination of unwanted signal components is essential. This elimination is accomplished with analog and digital filtering techniques and signal averaging.

After signal amplification, the most effective method for extracting a signal of interest from background noise is signal averaging. Signal averaging is in effect a cross-correlation between a point-process defined by the occurrence of the stimuli and the recorded evoked activity (i.e., an optimal filter) (Lee, 1960). In averaging, the signal component at each point is coherent and adds directly, whereas the background and noise components tend to be statistically independent and summate in a more or less root-mean-square fashion.

Stimulators

SEP and MEP values are produced by electrical stimulators that produce a shock through the skin with electrodes positioned over a peripheral nerve or transcranially over an area of the cerebral cortex. Electroencephalographic scalp electrodes or electrode plates placed adjacent to the scalp or hard palate can be used to stimulate the cortex. Auditory stimulation is obtained using one of several techniques, depending on, among other things, the surgical procedure involved and whether the auricle is retracted. Options include miniature open-air high-fidelity earphones (commonly used with personal tape players or radios) that rest in the concha of the ear, and a tubal insert earphone. The tubal insert is attractive because it distances the transducer from the recording electrode (producing reduced stimulus artifact) and is easily supported. For stimulation of the visual system, a fiberoptic system, which is positioned directly under the eye but not on the globe, is designed to be mounted on the flash stimulator driven by a photic stimulator. With any of the stimulators, precise synchronization with the monitoring and averaging process must occur.

ANESTHETIC TECHNIQUES

The type of anesthesia as well as the patient's blood pressure, cerebral blood flow, body temperature, hematocrit, and blood gas tensions all affect the functioning of the patient's CNS and thus intraoperatively observed neurophysiologic measures (Grundy et al., 1981; Grundy, 1983; McPherson, 1994; Sloan, 1998). The neurophysiologist must discuss the anesthetic plan with the anesthesiologist before the start of the procedure to ensure that no conflicts exist over the required anesthetic and neurophysiologic monitoring. Both the neurophysiologist and anesthesiologist must understand one another's needs and develop a plan for monitoring and anesthesia that allows both individuals to provide appropriate care for each patient. The halogenated hydrocarbon inhalation agents tend to reduce the amplitude of somatosensory evoked responses (Salzman et al., 1986), and to suppress alpha motor neuron activity that interferes with obtaining MEPs. The best SEPs are often recorded when a narcotic relaxant technique (consisting of an opioid, nitrous oxide (<65%), and a muscle relaxant) is used, whereas the best MEPs are often recorded with TIVA. Thus, when both types of responses are needed, a balancing act with regard to anesthesia is required. Boluses of medications produce more disruption of signals than constant infusions. Regardless of how medications are delivered, the anesthesiologist must inform the neurophysiologist of medication administration, changes in patient temperature or blood pressure, and any change in the patient's condition.

In many situations, the use of halogenated hydrocarbon inhalation agents is desired to help control blood pressure. Once baseline responses have been obtained and compared with preoperative responses, many children can maintain their responses to an isoflurane level of approximately 0.3 MAC, whereas many adults can maintain their responses to 0.5 MAC or higher. This is highly variable, and it strongly depends on the individual patient's reaction to the inhalation agent. A slow increase in isoflurane until either the blood pressure is controlled or the responses significantly deteriorate usually leads to satisfactory results; however, a small number of patients cannot maintain their SEPs with any inhalation agent on board. Propofol, etomidate, and ketamine also appear to maintain SEPs at anesthetic concentrations and may be particularly useful when signals are expected to be difficult to obtain (Schubert et al., 1990; Kalkman et al., 1991; Taniguchi et al., 1992; McPherson, 1994). Close cooperation between the anesthesiologist and neurophysiologist is important, because some patients, particularly those with immature nervous systems, exhibit sensitivity to anesthetic agents (Sloan, 1998).

Neurophysiologic Measures

Neurophysiologic measures that are routinely used provide a functional map of much of the entire neuroaxis. These include the EEG, an unstimulated measure of cortical function suitable for providing the following information:

1. The degree of cortical activation related either to metabolic process (e.g., hypoxia) or to pharmacologic manipulation (e.g., pentobarbital-induced burst suppression to protect the patient's cortical function) (Niedermeyer and Lopes da Silva, 1993)
2. SEPs and VEPs, which provide additional measures of cortical function specific to certain pathways and vasculature

3. BAEPs and BSEPs, which provide information about the functioning of the brainstem, again specific to certain pathways (Regan, 1989)
4. EMGs, produced either by muscles innervated by the various cranial nerves (providing information about both the cranial nerves themselves and their underlying brainstem nuclei [Kamura, 1983]), or by somatic muscles (providing information about spinal cord or peripheral nerve function)

Maturational Effects

The functional assessment of the pediatric CNS presents difficult and unique problems. The pediatric CNS differs from the adult CNS in that it is maturing over the first several years of life; that is, the neural tissue, the myelin coating of the axonal processes, and the vascular supply to the CNS all show significant changes. These developmental anatomic changes are reflected in maturational functional changes as measured by ascending SEP and by descending MEP activity, VEPs, and BAEPs (Starr et al., 1977; Cracco et al., 1979; Guthkelch et al., 1982). A number of factors contribute to the maturational changes of evoked potentials, and the use of age- and size-matched normal controls is essential. For intraoperative monitoring purposes, infants act as their own controls. Central and peripheral myelination is believed to be completed by 5 years of age, and from then until maturity, the dominant factor affecting SEP latency is height (Yakovlev and Lecours, 1967; Gilmore et al., 1985) (Fig. 11-9).

GENERAL MONITORING PROCEDURES

Neurophysiologic recording during pediatric operations can rapidly become quite complex. It is not unusual to monitor several different neurophysiologic variables simultaneously, such as EEGs, BAEPs, BSEPs, SEPs, MEPs, and EMGs relating to multiple spinal and cranial nerves. This requires a well-organized and theoretically parsimonious approach to monitoring. Baseline responses are obtained before draping the patient and compared with the preoperative evaluation. Significant differences

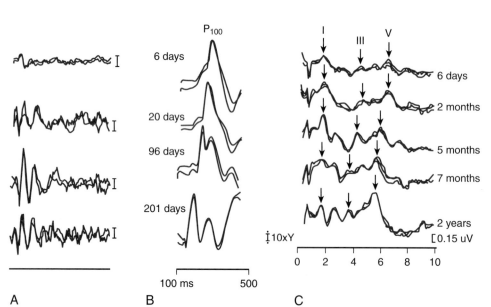

■ **FIGURE 11-9.** Maturational changes in cortical somatosensory median nerve evoked potentials (MSPs) **(A)**, flash visual evoked potentials (VEPs) **(B)**, and brainstem auditory evoked potentials (BAEPs) **(C)**, in early infancy. Note the decreasing latency (the time measured from the initiation of the stimulus to the point of maximum amplitude of the evoked potential) and enhancing morphology for the identified waves in all three modalities.

must be accounted for, because signal deterioration caused by the effects of inadequate patient positioning can produce functional deficits even before the start of the operation.

Electroencephalography

The functioning of the cerebral cortex is extremely sensitive to changes in arterial oxygenation and insufficient cerebral blood flow or an inadequate partial pressure of oxygen; this sensitivity is rapidly reflected in the EEG (Meyer and Marx, 1972). Oxidative metabolism supplies the energy for maintenance of the membrane potential of nerve cells, and the EEG depends directly on the transmembrane potentials of neurons, reflecting disturbances of cerebral metabolism such as hypoxia. Some factors that may contribute to ischemic events in surgical patients are decreased oxygen-carrying capacity resulting from hypovolemia, and decreased cerebral perfusion pressure resulting from factors associated with decreased systemic arterial pressure, increased intracranial pressure, and mechanical obstruction of cerebral vessels (Freye, 1990). It is thought that having two channels of continuous EEG monitoring is adequate, because the problems are related more to global or hemispheric effects than to precise focality. The EEG can be observed both as the ongoing unprocessed signal and in a Fourier-transformed representation. The electroencephalographic appearances of any ischemic or hypoxic events are similar, and differentiation between the various putative causative factors is made by being particularly attentive to the clinical situation. For example, blood pressure, ECG, oxygen saturation, administered drugs, and surgical manipulations may all have an observable effect. Other concurrent factors that may alter the EEG are changes in the depth of anesthesia, temperature changes, and changes in CO_2 content. These factors can be recognized by their relatively slow onset, lasting for several minutes, in contrast to the changes of ischemia, which generally occur within seconds. In some situations, the EEG may be acutely depressed on injection of an anesthetic that rapidly passes the blood-brain barrier. Such situations may be found with the use of high-dosage opioid anesthesia, in which fentanyl induces an immediate and marked reduction in fast-frequency activity in the EEG, with an increase in low-frequency, high-amplitude activity in the delta range (Freye, 1990).

A simplified but useful summary of possible changes includes the following:

1. Decreased frequency with increased amplitude (Van der Drift, 1972) implies an ischemic event to the cortex.
2. Widespread frequency slowing and decreased amplitude usually imply brainstem ischemia (Roger et al., 1954).
3. Ischemic events affecting the thalamus and the internal capsule produce unremarkable changes in the EEG (Van der Drift, 1972) but possibly significant changes in the SEPs.

Somatosensory and Motor Evoked Potentials

The neurophysiologic measures of value in assessing the spinal cord consist of SEPs, produced by stimulating various peripheral nerves, and MEPs, which may be observed as either compound muscle or nerve action potentials and which may be produced by either transcranial or spinal cord stimulation. It is advantageous to think of the SEPs as characterizing the ascending activity in the spinal cord and the MEPs as characterizing the descending activity in the spinal cord. This distinction, although not particularly important with respect to the sensory activity, is potentially extremely important with respect to the descending activity, because important questions remain as to what pathways are being stimulated (Rose, 1994), these distinctions are not as absolute as we would like to think.

Somatosensory Evoked Potentials (Ascending Activity)

SEPs depend on the stimulation of the large afferent fibers of peripheral nerves. After stimulation of peripheral nerves in the arms or the legs, SEPs can be reproducibly recorded over the spine and scalp. In the spinal cord, the SEPs are conducted primarily through the dorsal columns.

SEPs are a sequence of potentials generated in the peripheral nerves, dorsal horn nuclei, dorsal column pathways, and dorsal column nuclei of the spinal cord; the medial lemniscal pathways of the brainstem; and the thalamus and thalamocortical and parietal regions of the brain after the application of a transient electrical stimulus to a peripheral nerve (Sclabassi et al., 1993b). When recorded from electrodes on the surface of the body, the potentials of interest are very small, ranging in size from 2 to 5 mcV, and occur in approximately the first 100 msec after the application of a stimulus (often referred to as early and middle latency potentials). Evoked potentials are described in terms of latency and amplitude. Latency is the time measured from the application of a stimulus to the point of maximum amplitude of the evoked potential. Some types of SEP have more than one peak, and the time between peaks is the interpeak latency. The amplitude is the voltage difference between two peaks of opposite polarity, or a reference potential. Measurements of latencies, amplitudes, and interpeak latencies characterize SEP recordings. Changes in these measurements during a surgical procedure may represent injury to the neural tissue between the stimulus generator and the recording electrode.

In all cases, the stimuli are electrical impulses applied transcutaneously, at a rate of 0.7 to 5.3 Hz, depending on the robustness of the response, which is typically a function of the patient's age and pathology. Typically, responses to 128 stimuli are averaged; in many cases, as few as 12 responses may be averaged, providing near real-time updating of the responses.

All types of SEPs are used for intraoperative monitoring, primarily during spinal, cortical, and posterior fossa surgery. Potentials can be recorded after stimulation of the median nerve at the wrist, the common peroneal nerve, the posterior tibial nerve, and the dorsal nerve of the penis and the clitoris. Multiple types of responses from different stimuli and different sources are often simultaneously recorded, allowing the entire neuroaxis to be monitored. Monitoring multiple upper and lower extremity responses simultaneously during spinal surgery allows cord injury to be distinguished from global problems.

Median and Ulnar Nerve Evoked Potentials

The median (MSPs) and ulnar (USPs) nerve evoked potentials are all useful in assessing the brachial plexus, upper spinal cord, brainstem, and telencephalon. One important distinction is that the USPs provide information rostral to T1, whereas the MSPs provide information rostral to C6 (Fig. 11-10). At Erb's

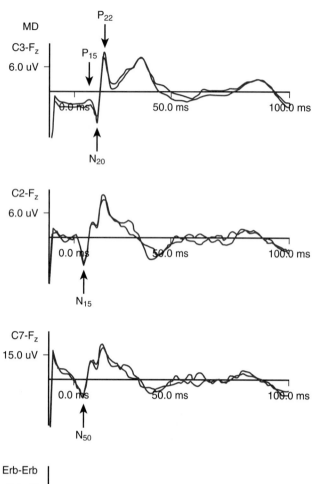

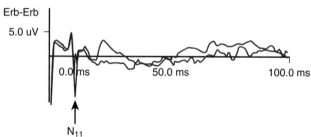

FIGURE 11-10. Median nerve evoked potentials (MSPs) produced by right median nerve stimulation (MD) stimulation. Data are recorded from Erb's point on the right referenced to Erb's point on the left *(bottom trace)*; cervical C7, cervical C2 and C3 (left parietal cortex), all referenced to F_z. Note the increase in latency of the large negative wave first identified as N11 at Erb's point, as the activity projects afferently.

point, the response consists of an apparently triphasic (positive-negative-positive) nerve action potential, reflecting the passage of the mixed nerve volley through the brachial plexus. This component is usually labeled N11 for the large negative-going component. At the cervical C7 recording site, the main component is a negative peak occurring at 14-msec latency, N14, with an associated complex structure. It has been postulated that these waves are generated in the dorsal roots, dorsal horn, posterior columns, and structures of the lower brainstem. During spinal fusions, monitoring of the brachial plexus may also alert the surgeon and anesthesiologist to compressive positioning of the arms.

Common Peroneal and Posterior Tibial Nerve Evoked Potentials

In the lower limb, nerves used to elicit cortical SEPs include the tibial, peroneal, and femoral. Spinal potentials are most consistently obtained through stimulation of the tibial nerve at the medial malleolus or peroneal nerve in the popliteal fossa.

SEPs recorded over the spine reflect the afferent volley traversing the dorsal columns. These responses can be recorded from electrodes attached to the skin over the spine, and they progressively increase in latency at more rostral recording locations. Spinal SEPs are relatively easy to obtain in children, with the amplitude and definition of the waves decreasing with increasing age, so that by the mid-teenage years, these responses are more difficult to obtain, as is the case with adults. More rostral recording locations reflect potentials arising in multiple ascending pathways, including the dorsal and dorsolateral columns, which lie primarily ipsilateral to the side of stimulation.

In our experience, SEPs are extremely sensitive and specific to spinal cord injury, whether it occurs in the dorsal or the ventral pathway. This is confirmed in the literature (Nuwer et al., 1995), where a false-negative rate of 0.063% was found for 51,263 spinal cases in which SEPs were the only potentials monitored. Furthermore, the negative predictive value (i.e., the likelihood of normal spinal cord function in the presence of stable SEPs) was 99.93%. This is a significant improvement over the 0.72% to 1.4% incidence of spinal cord injury reported for unmonitored cases (MacEwen et al., 1975).

Dermatomal Evoked Potentials

A disadvantage of SEPs produced by stimulation of large nerve trunks is that input to the spinal cord usually occurs over more than one level. This problem can be addressed by delivering the stimulus to a small cutaneous nerve that is believed to derive from a single dorsal root, or to the signature area of a particular dermatome. Significant disagreement exists concerning the cutaneous distributions of dermatomes, and care should be taken to stimulate the commonly accepted receptive fields of a root.

Pudendal nerve responses, a special type of dermatomal response, are particularly useful, especially in patients with spina bifida. The pudendal nerve carries sensory fibers from the penis, urethra, anus, and pelvic floor muscles and supplies motor innervation to the bulbocavernosus and pelvic floor muscles, the external urethral sphincter, and the external anal sphincter. Cortical responses to electrical stimulation of the dorsal nerve of the penis, the urethra, and the urinary bladder have all been described (Badr et al., 1982; Haldeman et al., 1982). Pudendal nerve responses are of similar morphology to the tibial nerve SEP (TSP) and are best recorded from the same area of the scalp (Fig. 11-11).

Motor Evoked Potentials (Descending Activity)

Because SEPs reflect function in the dorsal columns of the spinal cord, they do not directly assess the integrity of descending spinal motor tracts. It is possible to have focal damage to the motor areas in the spinal cord in which the SEPs remain normal. Accordingly, misleading results have occasionally been obtained when using SEPs alone for intraoperative monitoring and diagnosis (Lesser et al., 1986), b

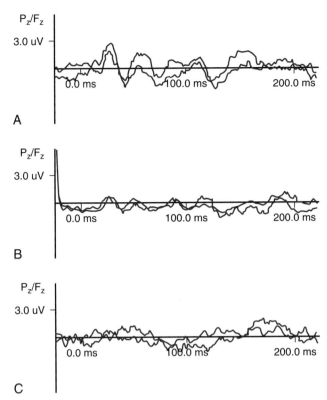

FIGURE 11-11. Pudendal nerve responses obtained from a male patient with tethered cord and symptoms referable to the pudendal nerve. All responses are recorded from P_z referenced to F_z. **A,** Responses obtained by stimulating the right branch of the dorsal nerve of the penis. **B,** Responses obtained by stimulating the left branch. Note the significant reduction in amplitude in response to the left-sided stimulation. **C,** Control data recorded during every procedure.

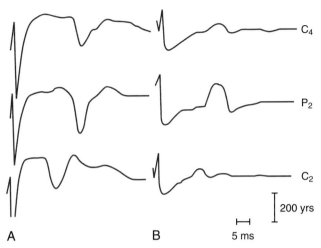

FIGURE 11-12. A, Compound muscle action potentials (CMAPs). **B,** Compound nerve action potentials (CNAPs). Both muscle and nerve action potentials were produced by transcranial magnetic stimulation at scalp positions C_4, P_z, and C_2. The CMAPs were recorded from the abductor pollicis brevis muscle, and the CNAPs were recorded from the left median nerve at the wrist.

MEPs are response threshold, onset latency, central conduction time, and response size (Fig. 11-13).

Combined Ascending and Descending Activity

Intraoperative monitoring of MEPS, CNAPs, and posterior TSPs are used to provide a simultaneous measure of the ascending and descending activities in the spinal cord. Through this approach, sequential stimulation is performed of the left tibial nerve, the right tibial nerve, and the spinal cord through the spinous processes. Recording electrodes positioned on the scalp record the bilateral SEPs from the tibial nerve stimuli as well as the afferent activity induced in the spinal area via direct spinal stimulation. Recording electrodes in the popliteal fossa allow the afferent stimulus compound action potentials to be observed, and then the descending compound action potentials produced by the spinal cord stimulation. This combined technique aids in localizing spinal cord dysfunction during surgery by continuously evaluating the adequacy of both the sensory and the motor components of spinal cord neural activity. Many times, both cannot be done because of technical difficulties relating to amplifier saturation and patient movement. In that case, MEPs and SEPs must be obtained separately.

Brainstem Auditory Evoked Potentials

Monitoring of the function of cranial nerve VIII through the use of BAEPs assists in preserving hearing, locating cranial nerve VIII, or determining whether the overall function of the brainstem is altered. BAEPs are also sensitive to retraction on the frontal poles, most likely because of force transmission to the brainstem.

The classic BAEP consists of a minimum of five and a maximum of seven peaks. All occur with 10 msec of a brief click or tone presentation. Wave I is generated in the auditory portion of nerve VIII. Wave II is generated bilaterally at or in the proximity of the cochlear nucleus. Wave III is generated bilaterally

this is rare (Nuwer et al., 1995). MEPs, which may be either evoked EMGs or compound action potentials, can be used to test the integrity of the motor pathways through either electrical or magnetic stimulation (Merton and Morton, 1980; Barker et al., 1985). MEPs can be obtained via stimulation of the motor areas of the brain or spinal cord through the intact skin, direct stimulation of exposed neuronal tissue, or direct root stimulation (e.g., during the release of a tethered cord), and recording of a stimulus-related response either as a compound muscle action potential (CMAP) or as an efferent compound nerve action potential (CNAP) (Fig. 11-12).

Transcranial electrical stimulation may be used to elicit motor responses. There is no general consensus about the location of recording electrodes, outside of specific muscle groups for evoked CMAPs or over the obvious peripheral nerves for evoked CNAPs, nor is there a general consensus concerning which class of these activities is more advantageous to record. CNAPs allow the patient to receive neuromuscular blockade agents. One of the most important stimulation parameters for eliciting reliable MEPs is the interstimulus interval (ISI) of a burst of stimuli (Taylor et al., 1993). It has been found that a burst of stimuli with ISIs between 2 and 5 msec (500 to 200 Hz) produce a maximal response by overcoming the depressed effect of general anesthesia (mentioned earlier) (Kalkman et al., 1995). The significant parameters and morphologic features of

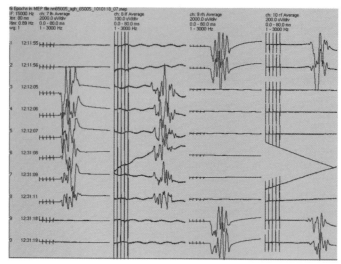

■ **FIGURE 11-13.** Motor evoked potentials (MEPs) obtained by transcranial electrical stimulation by needle electrode at C_3 and C_4 during stabilization of a cervical fracture. Channels 7 and 8 (columns 1 and 2) are recorded from the left abductor pollicis brevis and gastrocnemius muscles from stimulation of the right brain (anode at C_4), while channels 9 and 10 (columns 3 and 4) are recorded from the same muscle groups on the right side when the left brain is stimulated (anode at C_3). In many younger infants, both sides of the brain can be stimulated simultaneously. Note the 250-Hz burst of stimulus activity at the beginning of each trace.

from the lower pons near the superior olive and trapezoid body. Waves IV and V are probably generated in the upper pons or lower midbrain, near the lateral lemniscus or possibly near the inferior colliculus.

Waves I through V are relatively resistant to sedative medication and general anesthetics, but this places no constraints on the anesthesiologist. These waves are sensitive to temperature changes, with absolute and interpeak latencies increasing by approximately 0.20 msec. The latency of wave V is the primary concern in intraoperative monitoring of the BAEPs, because this is the most robust and easily identifiable of the waves in this response.

Visual System

VEPs are used to aid in determining the functional integrity of the visual system, primarily in the region of the optic nerves, chiasm, and optic radiations (Albright and Sclabassi, 1985). The recorded activity is generated either at the retina (electroretinogram) or at the cortex.

Stimulation of the visual system using a bright flash is not recommended for diagnostic purposes because of intersubject variability (Ciganek, 1961), except in select situations. In the operating room, this is a very helpful and effective technique (Fig. 11-14).

Electromyography

The EMG is electrical activity produced in muscle fibers below the skin; it has a frequency content ranging from 15 to 150 Hz. Three types of electrodes are used to record the EMGs: fine wire electrodes, which have the highest impedance and the narrowest field of view; subdermal needles, which have an intermediate impedance and a larger field of view; and disk surface electrodes, which have the lowest impedance and the largest field of view (field of view means the integrated level of electrical activity).

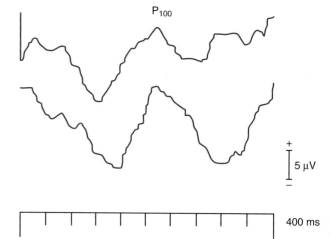

■ **FIGURE 11-14.** Intraoperative flash visual evoked potentials (VEPs), obtained between midline occipital (O_z) and vertex (C_z) electrodes. Data were from a 10-month-old girl who was operated on for a chiasmal glioma, which was 90% removed. *Top*: Response before resection. *Bottom*: Response after resection. The responses were obtained continuously during the procedure, were abnormal, and were highly variable from response to response, but they were unchanged during the procedure. *(From Albright AL, Sclabassi RJ: Cavitron ultrasonic surgical aspirator and visual evoked potential monitoring for chiasmal gliomas in children,* J Neurosurg 63:138, 1985.*)*

The recording techniques are essentially the same for all cranial nerves and all muscle groups. Subdermal platinum needle electrodes are used in bipolar recording configurations; that is, recordings are made between a pair of electrodes inserted into the same muscle group. Bipolar recordings are used to minimize confusion regarding which cranial nerve or branch of cranial nerve is producing the observed EMG. The electrodes are normally placed before the start of the procedure; occasionally, electrodes are placed in a sterile field by the surgeons.

These signals are listened to continuously for evaluation of nerve function both by the neurophysiologists and by the surgeons. Four categories of EMG activity are observed:

1. No activity, which in an intact nerve is the best situation but which may also be the case in a nerve that has been sharply dissected
2. Irritation activity, which sounds like soft intermittent flutter and is consistent with working near the nerve
3. Injury activity, which sounds like a continuous, nonaccelerating tapping and which can be an indicator of permanent injury to the cranial nerve
4. A "killed-end" response, which sounds like an accelerating firing pattern and is an unequivocal indicator of nerve injury

It is important to note that a sharply cut nerve may produce only a brief burst of activity; monitoring cannot be expected to replace extreme caution when working near the cranial nerves.

EMG is either spontaneous (e.g., anal sphincter activity produced by irritation of S3 to S5 roots during an untethering procedure involving the lower portion of the cauda equina) or evoked, of the type produced in selective rhyzotomy for the treatment of spasticity, for placement of pedicle screws, or for ongoing evaluation of the spinal cord. Evoked EMGs have a considerably larger amplitude (>1 mV) than sensory evoked potentials (<0.5 mcV) and therefore do not require averaging to extract them from the background noise.

Cranial Nerve Function

Cranial nerve function is monitored continuously during surgery for two reasons: first, to establish the location and orientation of the cranial nerves in the operative field, and second, to preserve functioning in the cranial nerves and their related brainstem nuclei (Sclabassi et al., 1993a). The major observed variables are the EMGs from the appropriate muscle group innervated by the cranial nerves of interest. In general, the cranial nerves ipsilateral to the operative side are monitored; when appropriate, bilateral activity is monitored.

In addition to monitoring the ongoing EMG activity related to the various cranial nerves, these cranial nerves may also be electrically stimulated. This is usually done to determine the location of the nerve in the operative field (because often the nerve is enveloped by tumor and may not be directly observable), or to determine the functional integrity of the nerve (Daube and Harper, 1989). The most common example of this procedure is the direct stimulation of nerve VII. The return path for the stimulating current is provided by a metal electrode inserted into the adjacent muscle mass. In some situations, when very precise localization of the nerve is required, bipolar stimulating electrodes are used. Most of the time, the question being asked is, Is the nerve there? These techniques are very useful when monitoring during surgery for posterior fossa tumors that extend to the floor of the fourth ventricle.

SUMMARY

The principal goal of intraoperative monitoring is to prevent morbidity, but a more fundamental goal is to provide the operative team with information that allows the operative objective to be accomplished with the best anesthetic and surgical strategy possible, with a clear view of any morbidity being induced along the way. This is particularly important when the degree of difficulty is high and morbidity is likely to be impossible to prevent.

Stringent time constraints exist in the intraoperative monitoring of neurophysiologic function, and damage to the CNS may occur rapidly, over seconds. This constraint has inspired the development of methods for extracting and analyzing evoked potential, EMG, and EEG waveforms rapidly and efficiently. A corollary of the increased sensitivity required to decrease the monitoring time is a higher rate of false-positive results.

False-positive results are also seen in baseline values acquired at the beginning of the procedure and from the preoperative studies. These are usually rapidly identified as such and produce no disruption in the flow of the case. Intraoperative monitoring requires rapid interpretations to be made of complex data, recorded under less-than-optimal conditions. It does no good to inform the surgeon 10 minutes after the fact that a significant change has occurred. Successful intraoperative monitoring of the pediatric CNS requires the acquisition of as many appropriate neurophysiologic variables as possible, and simultaneously. The correct interpretation of these responses is greatly aided by the ability to display the history of all of the acquired data in such a way as to facilitate a comparison of all of the data.

The anesthesiologist caring for infants and children has a wide array of equipment and monitors available. Their configuration depends primarily on the patient's illness, the experience of the anesthesiologist, and the proposed surgery. With the increasing complexity of anesthesia equipment and monitors, the anesthesiologist needs to understand thoroughly the operation and limitations of each device. Last, the anesthesiologist should never rely too heavily on the monitoring equipment and abandon the direct, close, personal surveillance of each patient during anesthesia and surgery.

REFERENCES

Complete references used in this text can be found online at www.expertconsult.com.

Airway Management

Robert S. Holzman

Airway management is the most important skill of the pediatric anesthesiologist, but what exactly *is* the pediatric airway? Examined through a broad lens, the pediatric airway is a composite of the anatomic development of the head, face, aerodigestive tract, and neck, structures contiguous as well as integral to the airway. It includes the differentiation of the primitive foregut into the trachea and esophagus and the subsequent development and differentiation of the upper and lower airways. It begins where air enters, normally at the nose and mouth, and is continuous through the upper (extrathoracic) and lower (intrathoracic) conducting airways. The dividing line between the upper and lower airways, the thoracic inlet, is bordered by T1 posteriorly, the first pair of ribs laterally, and the superior border of the manubrium anteriorly. Moreover, consideration of the pediatric airway would be incomplete without including its neurophysiology and gas-flow physics. Beyond that, the very practical details of the equipment needed to care for the pediatric airway are critical for the practitioner. In addition, medical conditions with specific airway challenges beget primary as well as secondary effects that must be accounted for as part of the anesthetic plan. Finally, an exit strategy must be established for patients with normal, and in particular, abnormal airways. The anesthesiologist, in collaboration with the surgeon and perioperative physicians and staff, is a critical stakeholder in that plan. Without elaborating on specific procedures covered elsewhere in this text and others, this chapter explores the developmental perspective on the anatomy and physiology of the upper airways and discusses gas-flow characteristics that change with age and abnormal airway conditions.

DEVELOPMENTAL ANATOMY*

The Upper Airway

Formation of the Cranial Vault and Base

The skull is a critical factor in the development of the face and therefore the upper airway. The skull develops from a membranous and cartilaginous neurocranium (Fig. 12-1). The membranous neurocranium gives rise to the flat bones of the cranial vault, and the cartilaginous neurocranium (chondrocranium) forms the skull base. The flat bones of the neurocranium, which form sutures from edge to edge, also form fontanels where more than two bones meet. The base of the skull is formed from the cartilaginous neurocranium, which then becomes the base of the occipital bone, the sphenoid, the ethmoid and petrous bones, and portions of the temporal bone.

The cranial base provides a floor for the calvarium and a roof for the face. The shaping of the skull base and contiguous structures is a dynamic process involving reciprocal influences between the cranial base, the pharynx, the face, and the primary and secondary palates. During fetal life and early childhood, neural influences predominate because of the rapid growth of the brain. During postnatal development of the airway, nasal influences play a major role, and because of speech and nutritional requirements, the pharynx also influences the development of the skull base. The anterior portion of the skull base is the ro

_____

*Information in this section is from Holzman, 1998.

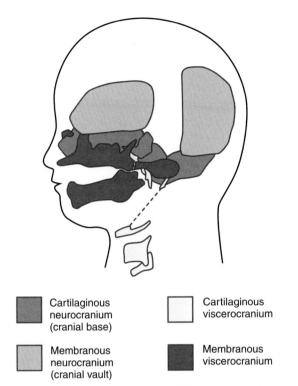

Cartilaginous
neurocranium
(cranial base)

Cartilaginous
viscerocranium

Membranous
neurocranium
(cranial vault)

Membranous
viscerocranium

■ **FIGURE 12-1.** Development of the skull from neurocranium and viscerocranium contributions at 20 weeks' gestation (lateral view). The skull base, the occipital bone, the body of the sphenoid, and the ethmoid are formed from cartilaginous neurocranium. Cell-signaling as well as geometric influences contribute to further growth of cranial and anterior facial structures.

of the nasomaxillary complex, whereas the posterior portion of the cranial base is the roof of the nasopharynx. During development, the depth of the nasopharynx increases as a result of remodeling of the palate, as well as changes in the angulation of the skull base, providing an enlarged nasal airway for the adult.

Clinical Correlation

The craniosynostoses were thought to occur because of premature fusion of cranial sutures. Coronal synostosis does consistently occur in Apert's syndrome; however, the craniosynostoses are much more complex in their pathoembryology. Current thought strongly suggests that malpositioning of the skull's basal points of dural attachment is the main initiating anomaly in craniosynostosis; this malpositioning theoretically results in the transmission of abnormal tensile forces upward through the dura to produce synostosis of the overlying suture. Growth reciprocity may also play a role; there is some evidence that cranial base malformations are partly caused by calvarial synostosis. Deformity of the skull base is recognizable in almost all patients, as are thinning and irregularity of the calvaria. Additional findings include sphenoid ridge abnormalities, thickening of the bone around the frontozygomatic suture, foreshortened anteroposterior length of the anterior cranial fossa, shallow orbits, anterior and superior displacement of the sphenoid bones, and anterior displacement of the petrous bones. The proptosis typically seen in the craniosynostoses, which can be the result of many factors, may include arrested maxillary growth, a shortened anterior cranial base,

sphenoidal hypoplasia, and forward displacement of the greater wing of the sphenoid bone. Ventricular dilation is consistent as well, although this may not represent hydrocephalus but rather distortion ventriculomegaly. Brain anomalies are also common, and optic nerve atrophy can occur because of the hypoplastic skull base. In addition, hypoplasia of the skull base foramina may result in cranial neuropathies. Hypoplastic, chronically congested sinuses and a challenging mask fit with a hypoplastic midface characterize the airway challenge. The larynx is seldom difficult to visualize with direct laryngoscopy, however, because branchial arch development is usually normal.

Craniovertebral Development

The paraxial mesoderm, a column of tissue on either side of the midline of the embryo, becomes divided into blocks of tissue (somites) at about the fourth week of development. Whereas most of the muscles of the head are derived from mesenchyme of the branchial arches, the cervical somites form the vertebrae of the neck that, under normal circumstances, undergo segmentation (Fig. 12-2). Failure of such segmentation can result in fusion and shortening with severely limited neck movement.

Clinical Correlation

Klippel-Feil syndrome is the result of varying combinations of fusions of the cervical vertebrae, such that the head appears to sit on the shoulders. The normal development of separate cervical vertebrae may be impaired, and fusion of adjacent vertebral bodies may occur. The degree of severity is variable; type I patients have a single-level fusion; type II patients have multiple, noncontiguous fused segments; and type III patients have multiple, contiguous fused segments (Samartzis et al., 2006). Klippel-Feil syndrome can occur with fetal alcohol syndrome, hemifacial microsomia (Goldenhar's syndrome), and anomalies of the extremities. The neck is short, and the hairline is low. In addition, the neck can be webbed. There may be atlanto-occipital fusion. Laryngoscopy and intubation can be extremely difficult, although laryngeal mask airways (LMAs) have been used successfully (Naguib et al., 1986; Nargozian, 2004).

The Face

Just as the neurocranium forms the cranial vault and base, the viscerocranium forms the face and is derived mainly from cartilage of the first two branchial arches (Fig. 12-3). Ectodermally-derived neural crest cells of the developing 3- to 4-week-old embryo migrate to branchial arch mesoderm, and the face develops as a result of these massive cell migrations and their interactions. Those cells forming the frontonasal process are derived from the forebrain fold and migrate a relatively short distance as they pass into the nasal region. Those cells that form the mesenchyme of the maxillary and mandibular processes have a considerably longer distance to migrate, because they must move into the branchial arches. At 28 days postconception, the face barely shows its eventual relation to the five primordia from which it is derived: the frontonasal prominence, which is the cranial boundary of the primitive mouth (stomodeum); the paired maxillary prominences (the first branchial arch); and the paired mandibular prominences (also the first branchial arch).

The paranasal sinuses begin developing at approximately 40 weeks of gestational age. The completion of turbinate development

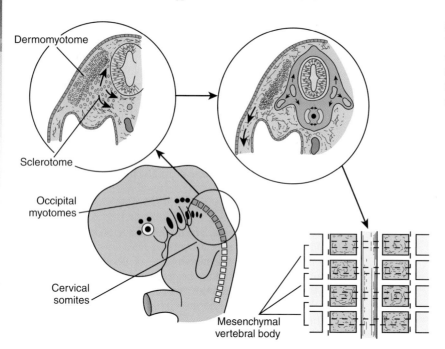

■ **FIGURE 12-2.** Craniovertebral development. Three pairs of occipital myotomes advance ventrally to form the muscles of the tongue, along with the hypoglossal nerve, as well as the facial muscles, which are innervated by the facial nerve.

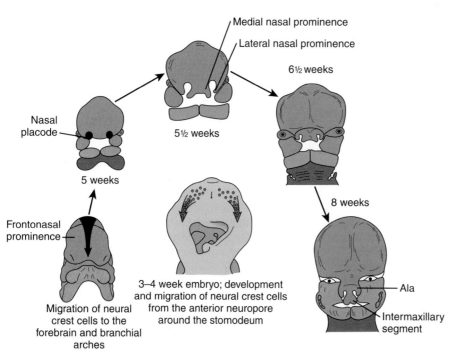

■ **FIGURE 12-3.** Development of the face. Neural crest cells form around the anterior neuropore and migrate to give rise to a variety of connective and nervous tissues of the skull, face, and branchial arches. With the frontonasal prominence developing for a shorter distance than the maxillary processes, there is a longer time for clefting of the lip and palate to occur. Severe rhinencephalic malformations may be accompanied by central nervous system abnormalities as well.

signals the beginning of sinus development, which continues until early adult life (Fig. 12-4). Although the exact function of the paranasal sinuses is not well understood, inflammatory, infectious, and neoplastic diseases of the sinuses are of major significance to the anesthesiologist, particularly if there is functional impairment before anesthesia and surgery. Sinus disorders are often comorbidities of asthma, immunoglobulin deficiencies, cystic fibrosis, or Kartagener's syndrome.

The oral cavity—a structure without structures—where much of the anesthesiologist's attention and skills are focused has a complex developmental heritage. The mouth (stomodeum) appears as a slight depression in the surface ectoderm, separated from the oral cavity by the oropharyngeal membrane. This membrane ruptures at about 24 to 26 days' gestation and the primitive foregut then communicates with the amniotic cavity. The involved germ layers are the endoderm internally and the

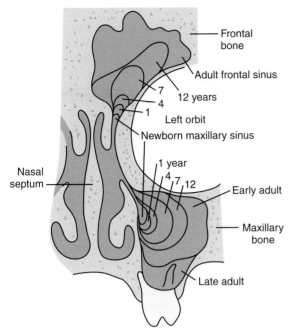

■ FIGURE 12-4. The paranasal sinuses begin their development at the end of fetal life from the mesenchyme of the lateral wall of the nasal cavity, developing into the turbinates. The completion of turbinate development signals the beginning of sinus development, which continues until early adult life.

ectoderm externally. The tongue surface arises primarily from first arch mesenchyme, with significant contributions from the third and fourth arches, hence its complex innervation by the facial nerve in the anterior two thirds and the hypoglossal nerve in the posterior one third (Fig. 12-5). The muscle bulk of the tongue

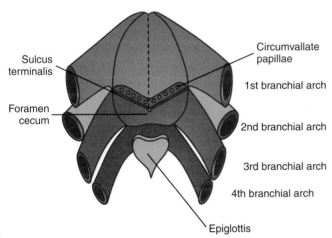

■ FIGURE 12-5. The tongue is a complex structure, derived as it is from elements of the first four branchial arches. This results in the first branchial arch contributing to the anterior two thirds of the tongue (lingual nerve, a branch of the mandibular division of the fifth cranial nerve), as well as the chorda tympani from the seventh cranial nerve. The third branchial arch contributes to the posterior third of the tongue, resulting in its innervation by the ninth cranial nerve. Tongue muscles, derived from the occipital myotomes in the region of the developing hindbrain, are innervated by the twelfth cranial nerve. The foramen cecum is the pharyngeal floor diverticulum in continuity with the developing thyroid.

arises primarily from occipital somites, explaining the hypoglossal nerve (XII) innervation and its susceptibility to injury from errant placement of dental rolls and pressure injury from overinflated LMA cuffs. The upper lip is formed by the merging of the maxillary prominences with the medial nasal prominences, with the lateral basal prominences forming the alae. The intermaxillary segment in the central portion of the upper lip area consists of a labial component (forming the philtrum), a maxillary component (associated with the four incisor teeth), and a palatal component (which becomes the primary palate).

The palate divides the nasomaxillary complex from the oral cavity (Fig. 12-6). The palatal processes advance in a medial direction from the maxillary processes of the first branchial arch, fusing in the midline in an anterior-to-posterior sequence and uniting with the premaxilla and the developing nasal septum. The soft palate forms from continued growth of the posterior edges of these palatal processes, ending with the formation and fusion of the two halves of the uvula.

Clinical Correlation

Cleft lip and palate are among the most common of congenital anomalies. They may occur alone, as part of a syndrome (there are over 300 syndromes associated with facial clefting), or as a component of a sequence, (e.g., as with Pierre-Robin syndrome). Clefts of the palate may occur by the same mechanism as cleft lip or be secondary to an anatomic obstruction preventing the medial fusion of the maxillary processes. For example, the cleft palate associated with Pierre-Robin syndrome occurs when the tongue, being displaced superiorly and posteriorly as a result of mandibular hypoplasia, interferes with palatal fusion.

Closure of the cleft palate may result in insufficient tissue for development of normal length or function of the soft palate and require a posterior pharyngeal flap. Velopharyngeal insufficiency is the cause of the hypernasal speech, nasal emission, and nasal turbulence (Sidman and Muntz, 2000).

The nose originates in the cranial ectoderm, which subsequently develops into the frontonasal prominence. The superior portion of the nose is formed from the lateral nasal processes, whereas the inferior portion of the nasal cavity is incomplete until the paired maxillary processes of the first branchial arch

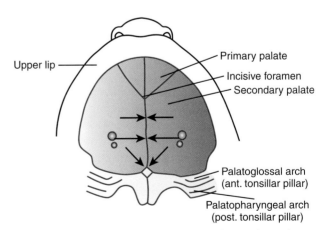

■ FIGURE 12-6. Formation of the primary and secondary palates, ultimately forming the floor of the nose and the roof of the mouth. The process of midline fusion occurs from posterior to anterior; clefting of the primary or secondary palate may occur in various combinations.

grow anteriorly and medially to fuse with the median nasal processes. The nasal cavities extend posteriorly during development, influenced by the posteriorly directed fusion of the palatal processes, thinning out the membrane that separates them from the oral cavity. By the thirty-eighth day of development, the two-layer membrane consisting of nasal and oral epithelia ruptures and forms the choanae (posterior nares). Failure of such rupture results in choanal atresia, although these choanae are not in the same location as the definitive choanae, which will eventually be located more posteriorly. Because the normal nasomaxillary complex grows both downward and forward, however, it does explain the unexpectedly anterior location in choanal atresia given the eventual normal development of the choanae.

Clinical Correlation

Choanal stenosis is not a blockage but rather a narrowing of less than 6 mm. Choanal atresia is also associated with various syndromes in up to 70% of patients, of which *c*olobomas, *h*eart disease, *a*tresia of the choanae, *r*etarded growth, *g*enital anomalies, *e*ar anomalies (the CHARGE association) is the major one. Repair of this form of choanal atresia may be more complicated, requiring a tracheostomy in infancy as an initial stage and more definitive repair later.

Bilateral choanal atresia is apparent immediately in the neonatal period because infants are obligate nasal breathers. These infants have respiratory distress, paradoxical cyanosis (crying relieves the cyanosis), and failure to thrive. The natural position of the tongue promotes obstruction that is relieved by an oral airway or a McGovern nipple (a standard nipple with an enlarged hole). Unilateral atresia often appears later (2 to 5 years of age) with rhinorrhea and chronic mucoid discharge and is often misdiagnosed. Because the intraoral airway is foreshortened as a result of the abnormally anterior choanal aperture, upper airway obstruction while breathing is common, and visualization of the laryngeal structures may be more difficult. Long-standing choanal atresia may also lead to obstructive sleep apnea.

The face, specifically the maxilla and mandible, grows in a dynamic fashion throughout childhood under the influence of bony deposition and resorption, soft-tissue contouring, and hormonal influences. In a reciprocal fashion, the skull base or neurocranium influences midfacial development via the growth of the sinuses, which in turn influence the skull base. Displacement of these structures of the nasomaxillary complex occurs in horizontal, vertical, and anteroposterior axes. These changes ultimately affect the proportions of the face and the morphology of all of the facial structures, including the upper airway.

The Branchial Apparatus

Branchial Arches

The branchial apparatus consists of four branchial arches visible on the surface of the embryo, as well as fifth and sixth arches that cannot be seen on the surface. Branchial pouches and clefts are likewise numbered craniocaudally (Fig. 12-7). The first branchial arch (Meckel's) cartilage is the position of the future mandible, as well as the eventual malleus and incus. The second branchial arch cartilage produces the stapes, the styloid process, the stylohyoid ligament, and the superior portion of the body of the hyoid. The other branchial arch cartilages contribute to the inferior portion of the hyoid as well as the thyroid cartilage.

Striated muscles are also formed in the respective branchial arch mesenchyme. Myoblasts differentiate and migrate to various parts of the head and neck, where they form the muscles of mastication and facial expression, each retaining their original nerve supply. Although muscular actions in the head and neck are thought of as far removed from the origin and course of the cranial nerves, fetal nerves that supply the branchial arch derivatives only have a short distance to travel from the brain. The trigeminal (V) nerve supplies the skin covering the parts of the face derived from the first branchial arch maxillary and

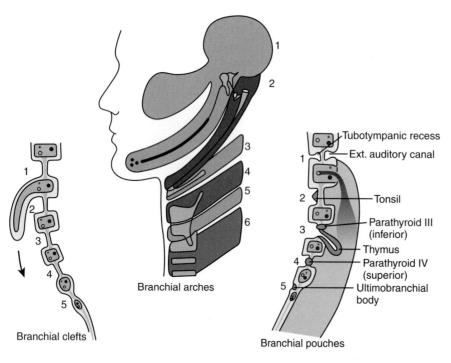

■ **FIGURE 12-7.** The branchial arches, pouches, and clefts. The musculature of each arch is supplied by the (cranial) nerve of its origin; the first arch by the mandibular division of the fifth cranial nerve, as well as the chorda tympani division of the seventh cranial nerve. The seventh cranial nerve supplies the second arch, the ninth cranial nerve the third arch, and the tenth and eleventh cranial nerves the remaining arches. Branchial clefts, when they fail to obliterate during normal development, may result in sinuses or cysts that communicate with the oropharynx through various pathways in the neck.

mandibular divisions (the ophthalmic division does not make a contribution). The facial (VII) nerve supplies the muscles derived from the first arch. The nerve of the third branchial arch is the glossopharyngeal (IX) nerve. Two branches of the vagus (X) nerve supply the remaining branchial arches. The superior laryngeal nerve innervates derivatives of the sixth branchial arch.

Branchial Pouches

The first branchial pouch develops into the tubotympanic recess, becoming the auditory tube and the middle ear cavity (Fig. 12-8). The cavity of the second branchial pouch is largely obliterated as the palatine tonsil develops, but part of it remains as the tonsillar fossa. The endoderm of the second branchial pouch becomes the surface epithelium of the tonsil and the lining of its crypts, with the mesenchyme around the pouch differentiating into lymphoid tissue. The endoderm of the dorsal part of the third branchial pouches differentiates into the inferior parathyroids, and the ventral parts unite to become the thymus. The paired parathyroid glands develop from separate pouches, with one pair derived from the third and the other from the fourth branchial pouch. At the seventh week of development, the parathyroid glands migrate caudally from their respective branchial pouches, with the third pouch parathyroids moving more caudally than the parathyroids of the fourth pouch. Accessory parathyroid tissue may be left along the line of migration. The endoderm of the fourth branchial pouches differentiates into the superior parathyroid glands, and the ventral parts develop into the ultimobranchial bodies, the calcitonin-secreting portion of the thyroid.

Branchial Clefts

Between the first and second arches, the first branchial cleft forms the external ear, which is the only normal structure to arise from a branchial cleft. However, if the second arch does not grow caudally over the third and fourth arches, as it normally should, then the second, third, and fourth clefts can remain as branchial fistulas, in contact with the skin surface between the clavicle and the mandible. Incomplete or arrested development of the branchial clefts may result in residual cysts, sinuses, and fistulas that may eventually become infected and require excision. The clinical significance of the specific embryology is that characteristic locations are of important surgical significance.

Clinical Correlation

The second branchial arch may occasionally fail to bury the second, third, and fourth branchial clefts completely, resulting in a cervical sinus communicating with the surface of the skin, and forming a branchial sinus, which may also contain a branchial cyst. These sinuses may be accompanied by a draining infection along the anterior border of the sternocleidomastoid muscle, requiring complete surgical dissection and removal. It is easy to understand embryologically how these tracts can open into the pharynx just posterior to the tonsils and may even pass between the external and internal carotid arteries.

The thyroid begins as a thickening of the endoderm of the floor of the pharynx, in the midline between the first and second pouches, at the foramen cecum. A thin connection, the thyroglossal duct, remains attached to the oral cavity, and its point of attachment marks the origin of the thyroid gland. The thyroid descends along the thyroglossal duct and reaches the level of the first tracheal ring at about the seventh week of gestation (Fig. 12-9). The thyroglossal duct is then normally obliterated. Accessory thyroid tissue may be deposited anywhere along this path; on the other hand, failure of the thyroid to descend may result in a lingual thyroid.

Anomalies associated with abnormal development of the branchial arches are varied, with a range of complexity and airway implications. Whereas too much variation among anomalies exists, an appreciation of the developmental anatomy explains (and helps the anesthesiologist anticipate) the following situations:

1. Unilateral or bilateral hypoplasia of upper airway structures, which may result in a small and hypomobile mandible, choanal stenosis or atresia, and hypoplastic or nonexistent sinuses.
2. Fusions or other abnormalities of various cervical vertebrae.
3. Cleft palate may be the result of failure to fuse, or it may be associated with hypoplastic mandibles and glossoptosis

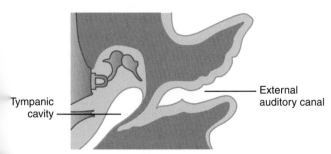

■ **FIGURE 12-8.** The tympanic cavity develops from the ubotympanic recess, an outgrowth of the first pharyngeal pouch, which extends laterally, contiguous with the external auditory canal having formed from the first pharyngeal cleft.

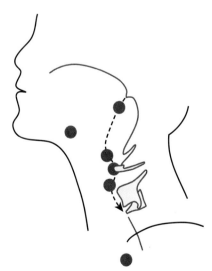

■ **FIGURE 12-9.** Descent of the thyroid along the thyroglossal duct. A lingual thyroid is the most common form of incomplete descent and is found inferior to the foramen cecum, where it may interfere with swallowing as well as breathing, particularly during anesthetic induction in infants.

(Pierre-Robin syndrome) or hemifacial microsomia (Goldenhar's syndrome).

4. Obstructive sleep apnea, which may result from chronic upper airway obstruction as a result of decreased available cross-sectional diameter of the airway with a relatively large volume occupied by the tongue and pharyngeal musculature, as well as an abnormally positioned palate.

The Larynx

Development of the larynx begins at approximately 3 weeks of gestational age with the formation of the laryngotracheal tube from the ventral wall of the foregut. The laryngotracheal tube then grows caudally into the splanchnic mesoderm on the ventral surface of the foregut, dividing into the right and left lung buds. The epiglottis begins to form from the hypobranchial eminence of the third and fourth arches at approximately 30 to 32 days' gestation. The aryepiglottic folds develop from the lateral boundaries of the fourth arch along a line from the hypobranchial eminence (epiglottis) to the arytenoid eminence of the sixth arch. Incomplete development at this stage may produce varying degrees of persistent laryngeal cleft (Fig. 12-10). A definite larynx may be seen by 41 days' gestation. (Fig. 12-11).

The cricoid and thyroid cartilages begin to develop before the arytenoid cartilages, with chondrification starting at about 7 weeks of gestation. As the thyroid cartilage develops, the glottis deepens, and the true vocal cords align within the thyroid laminae. Failure of the true vocal cords to split to form the primitive glottis at 10 weeks of gestation results in congenital atresia of the larynx or more often, a complete or partial congenital laryngeal web. Although webs may be supraglottic or subglottic, most occur at the level of the glottis. Congenital cysts of the supraglottic region are possibly remnants of the third branchial pouch and lie superior to the derivatives of the fourth arch. By the tenth to eleventh weeks of gestation, the major structures of the larynx have developed and the cartilages are

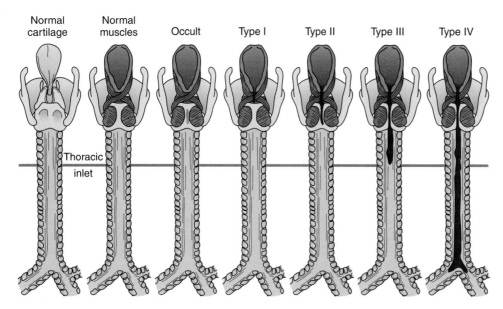

■ **FIGURE 12-10.** Laryngeal cleft, in various grades, results from a persistent communication between the trachea and esophagus, most commonly at the cranial end. Type I lesions are localized to the interarytenoid space superior to the vocal cords; type II lesions involve a partial cricoid cleft. Types III and IV lesions traverse the cricoid completely.

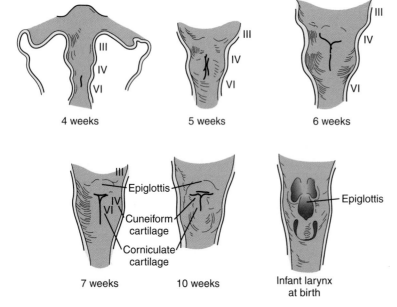

■ **FIGURE 12-11.** Development of the larynx. The epiglottis begins to form from elements of the third and fourth branchial arches at approximately 30 to 32 days of gestation, and early arytenoids cartilages can be identified on both sides of the laryngeal slit at this time as well. Incomplete development at this early stage may produce variable degrees of laryngeal cleft.

chondrifying. If the separation of the esophagus and trachea is slightly delayed and the margins of the laryngotracheal groove fail to fuse adequately, the rapidly growing trachea separates the proximal and distal esophagus, resulting in the most common form of proximal esophageal atresia and distal tracheoesophageal fistula.

Eckenhoff's (1951) review of the anatomy of the pediatric larynx has influenced more than a generation of pediatric anesthesiologists with regard to the selection of endotracheal tube size based on the concept of the narrowest (fixed) portion of the upper airway being the level of the cricoid cartilage, or the "funnel-morphing-into-cylinder" concept. Litman et al. (2003) examined laryngeal shape in sedated children undergoing MRI and determined that under sedated conditions with tonic maintenance of laryngeal shape, it is more cylindric than funnel-shaped, as it is in adults, and that the narrowest portion of the airway is at the level of the vocal cords. Furthermore, they concluded that there is no change in this relationship from childhood to adulthood. This finding has been confirmed by video-bronchoscopic imaging in anesthetized and paralyzed children as well and provides an intriguing challenge to traditional teaching (see Chapter 3, Respiratory Physiology) (Dalal et al., 2008, 2009). The adjudication of these disparate concepts, as well as the confirmation in both reports that the cricoid opening is elliptic rather than circular in shape, with the narrowest transverse diameter, help support the transition over the last 10 to 15 years to the common use of cuffed endotracheal tubes with a smaller diameter rather than tightly (or "appropriately") fitted, uncuffed endotracheal tubes. Moreover, advances in materials and design have allowed the development of thin-walled tubes with shorter, polyurethane cuffs, which provide an equivalent seal at a lower mucosal pressure (Dullenkopf et al., 2005). At this point, the increasingly routine use of cuffed endotracheal tubes, with appropriate care, appears to result in fewer repeated laryngoscopies and reintubations, less postintubation croup and less contamination in the operating room, and lower total fresh-gas flows.

DEVELOPMENTAL PHYSIOLOGY

The Upper Airway

It is almost axiomatic in pediatric training to be told that the infant is an obligate nasal breather, and the reasons are best understood by developmental anatomy. The epiglottis is located in a more cephalad position relative to the other mobile soft-tissue components of the oral cavity, the tongue and soft palate, and their close approximation even during normal respiration may impair transoral breathing. Nasal resistance may provide up to 50% of total airway resistance and varies depending on alar orientation, the pyriform aperture, the nasal cavity, and the choanae. This is of practical importance to the pediatric anesthesiologist particularly when anatomic or even therapeutic (e.g., nasogastric tube) obstructions are present, because airway resistance is significantly increased and therefore respiration may be compromised.

The tongue, palate, pharynx, epiglottis, and larynx all have to work together to accomplish feeding and breathing. With postnatal growth, the mandible enlarges, descends, and protrudes, and the oral cavity enlarges vertically. The tongue occupies a more anterior position as the oral cavity and pharynx grow, and

the larynx descends from its C2 position in the neck to C4 after one year of age. The clinical usefulness of the high-lying larynx is that it places the epiglottis into contact with the soft palate, allowing the infant to be a nasal breather while sucking and swallowing. With the growth of the oral cavity and the rearrangement of intraoral architecture during the first few months of life, infants convert from obligate nasal breathing to nasal and oral breathing.

Isono (2006) has reviewed the physiology of airway maintenance at the pharyngeal level and described the pharynx as a collapsible air-filled tube surrounded by soft tissues enclosed in a rigid box of bony structures, the mandible and vertebrae, with the lumen of the tube determined by the balance of the soft-tissue mass and the size of the surrounding rigid box. This simple approach explains the success of routine clinical airway maneuvers—continuous positive airway pressure (CPAP) serving as a pneumatic stent for the collapsed air-filled tube and surrounding soft tissue, and anterior displacement of the jaw serving to enlarge the rigid box. An oral airway displaces the base of the tongue anteriorly, thereby increasing the transpharyngeal luminal space and moving the base of the tongue away from the prevertebral bodies. Anesthetics, of course, depress the integrity of pharyngeal muscle tone through a variety of mechanisms, including the attenuation of neural input caused by the loss of consciousness and the decrease in tone of the diaphragm and intercostal musculature. The tongue and its muscular attachments such as the genioglossus, geniohyoid, sternohyoid, sternothyroid, and thyrohyoid are affected as well. All of this conspires to narrow the pharyngeal airway, more so in infants and small children than adults, especially during the first year of life (Isono et al., 2000). Adults are more equipped than children to defend against these effects, because they possess a more competent negative pressure reflex serving to augment pharyngeal tone, although the negative pressure reflex has been shown in infants younger than 1 year old as well (Thach et al., 1989; Horner et al., 1991). In addition, the progressive increase in pharyngeal cross-sectional area during the first year of life is positively influenced by the growth of the mandible and maxilla.

Pharyngeal airway obstruction has long been recognized as a significant component of the clinical entity called *laryngospasm*, and the application of CPAP, whether applied transnasally or transorally, depresses pharyngeal muscle tension and provides a mechanical pneumatic stent for the upper airway (Fink, 1956; Alex et al., 1987). This is a subtle component of the routine technique used by experienced pediatric anesthesiologists in applying gentle amounts of positive pressure during the induction phase, especially with infants and small children.

The fetus is an experienced swallower, well practiced from the age of 10 to 11 weeks' gestation, with suckling following at 18 to 24 weeks' gestation. This is fortunate, because coordination of this highly complex task is dependent on practice in utero and learning in pre- and postnatal life. However, breathing, even in utero, is a relatively late event, occurring at about 32 to 37 weeks' gestational age, and premature infants show their lack of experience with significant discoordination between swallowing and breathing, as do children who are neurologically impaired (Goldson, 1987; Arvedson et al., 1994).

Protective airway reflexes are initiated via adduction of the true and false vocal cords, closing the laryngeal vestibule. The epiglottis deflects posteriorly to cover the laryngeal inlet, diverting food into the pyriform sinuses. Finally, the larynx elevates through the effort of the suprahyoid musculature, contracting prior to the entrance of the food bolus into the hypopharynx, which aids in opening the cricopharyngeal sphincter. Moreover, activation of sensory receptors in the pharynx and anterior tonsillar pillars inhibits respiration during swallowing. Finally, the esophageal phase, from the upper esophageal sphincter to the lower esophageal sphincter (LES), is mediated by contractions that occur throughout the length of the esophagus via a coordinated peristaltic wave. The cricopharyngeal sphincter returns to a tonic state (+5 mm Hg) from its relaxed state (−15 mm Hg), as do the diaphragmatic crura, the angle of the gastroesophageal junction, and the diaphragm, thereby preventing reflux into the hypopharynx. Reflex protection of the airway occurs via two pathways: anterograde protection accomplished during normal swallowing, and retrograde protection accomplished by antireflux mechanisms. Laryngeal and nasopharyngeal closure occur via the influence of the superior laryngeal nerve on laryngeal mucosal receptors. Clinically, the adverse effects of laryngeal secretions manifest themselves as reflex closure of the larynx and sustained apnea (Perkett and Vaughan, 1982; Bartlett, 1985). With maturity, coughing replaces apnea as a protective mechanism (Miller et al., 1952; Leith, 1985). As far as gastrointestinal reflux is concerned, increasing attention has been devoted to its contribution to recurrent pneumonia, reactive airways disease, apnea, and respiratory failure. The upper and lower esophageal sphincters maintain a resting tone of 10 to 30 mm Hg over intragastric pressure, and in combination with crural support and the acute gastroesophageal angle, act to prevent regurgitation of stomach contents. However, premature infants have a lower LES pressure and a less acute gastroesophageal angle; central nervous system (CNS) immaturity is related to abnormalities of the LES relaxation pattern (Hillemeier, 1996).

DEVELOPMENTAL AIRWAY PHYSICS

Because of the variable diameter and length of the trachea, as well as the common (mainly in toddlers) problems of foreign body aspiration and anatomic or functional airway obstruction, understanding the physics of gas flow is even more crucial in pediatric anesthesia than in any other anesthesiology subspecialty. Noisy breathing is often an ominous sign in infants and small children. Stridor is noisy breathing coupled with increased inspiratory efforts, such as nasal and rib-cage flaring and suprasternal and sternal retraction. Severe airway obstruction may result in cyanosis, respiratory distress and fatigue, pneumothorax, pneumomediastinum, and death. Purely inspiratory stridor usually indicates lesions in the upper part of the airway. Lesions distal to the vocal cords usually produce expiratory stridor. Biphasic stridor is most characteristic of obstruction at the level of the subglottic space. Physical laws not only help explain the basis of these signs but provide guidance about effective clinical intervention (see Chapter 3, Respiratory Physiology in Infants and Children).

Laminar and Turbulent Flow

Laminar flow of a fluid (whether the fluid is a liquid or a relatively slowly-moving gas) through a tube is proportional to the pressure gradient (total pressure drop/length of tube), the fourth power of the radius of the tube and inversely proportional

to the viscosity of the fluid. This relationship is expressed mathematically in the Hagen-Poiseuille Law:

$$\dot{V} = \frac{P\pi r^4}{8\eta l}$$

where $\dot{V}$ equals the flow of the gas, P equals the total pressure drop, r equals the radius of the tube, η equals viscosity, and l equals length.

The most important implication of the Hagen-Poiseuille Law is that halving the radius, for example, decreases flow rate by the fourth power, or 16-fold. Likewise, doubling the radius increases the flow rate 16-fold; this is critically important, especially for infants and small children, and it explains the improvement in respiratory distress with appropriate treatment for conditions such as croup. In normal lungs, laminar flow occurs only in the periphery of the lung (small peripheral bronchi and bronchioli) where the flow is relatively slow in relation to the diameter of the airways. For the rest of the airway system, the flow pattern is predominantly turbulent because of uneven airway diameters and an average of 24 (19 to 27) airway branchings.

For turbulent conditions, the change in the expression from flow rate to the square of the flow rate illustrates that a much greater driving pressure is required to maintain gas flow. Fanning's equation expresses this relationship mathematically, where the radius of the tube to the fifth power now determines that flow.

$$\dot{V}^2 = \frac{P4\pi^2 r^5}{l\mu f}$$

where $\dot{V}$ equals the flow of the gas, P equals the total pressure drop, r equals the radius of the tube, μ equals density, l equals length, and f equals Fanning's friction factor.

Upper and lower conducting-airway air flow is turbulent, whereas the peripheral airways are characterized by laminar air flow, enhancing alveolar ventilation. The conducting airways bifurcate progressively (but not symmetrically). Cartilaginous support is characteristic of the main, lobar, and segmental bronchi, and more distal conducting airways have bronchial muscle forming a geodesic network. The total cross-sectional area of the respiratory tract is minimal at the third generation (Fig. 12-12). Small bronchi extend through about seven generations, and the total cross-sectional area increases by about sevenfold by generation 11. After the eleventh generation, cartilage

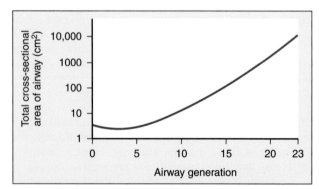

■ **FIGURE 12-12.** Cross-sectional area of the respiratory tract in relation to airway generations. With growth of the airways, compliance increases and resistance to gas flow falls according to the Hagen-Poiseuille Law, where resistance falls according to the fourth power of the radius. *(From Weibel ER: Morphometry of the human lung, New York, 1963, Academic Press.)*

disappears from the airway wall. With these noncartilaginous walls embedded within the lung parenchyma, contiguous elastic tissue serves to hold the airways open, and therefore lung volume plays a substantial role in the maintenance of conducting airway patency. In the terminal bronchioles, the total cross-sectional area is about 30 times the area at the level of the large bronchi. Flow resistance in these small airways is about 10% of lower airway resistance (Macklem and Mead, 1967).

Flow in laminar profiles enhances diffusivity, because flow at the center of the shear increases the rate of spread in that direction (Fig. 12-13). Fluids or gas molecules moving through a tube under constant pressure separate into a gradient of velocity profiles, with the fastest component in the center and the slowest components near the wall. When the cross-sectional area is reduced, the velocity must increase (and the pressure decrease) in order to maintain the same volume flow rate; resulting gas flow is much more turbulent. With abrupt narrowing, complete separation of the stream profiles occurs, the center stream constricts to a minimum value, and laminar flow may not be able to resume because of the turbulence. Pragmatically, when difficulty with positive pressure ventilation occurs, the natural response of the anesthesiologist is to apply more pressure to the rebreathing bag. For the patient whose airway is compromised, this results in more turbulence in the upper airways and less effective air flow downstream. Passive exhalation may also be impaired, and air trapping may result. However, if the pressure gradient (ΔP) across the obstruction is reduced (e.g., changing to spontaneous breathing from controlled ventilation in order to reduce the high pressure proximal to the obstruction), then air flow may be enhanced distally. This applies to airway narrowing, regardless of intrinsic or extrinsic causes.

Clinical Correlation

Causes of stridor include congenital, inflammatory, traumatic, and foreign bodies; a congenital cause is found in 85% of children younger than 2.5 years of age (Holzman, 2000). Severe airway obstruction may result in cyanosis, respiratory distress and fatigue, pneumothorax, pneumomediastinum, and death.

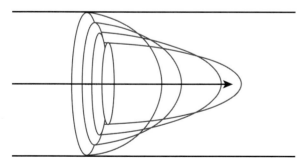

■ **FIGURE 12-13.** Taylor dispersion: fluids (or gases) moving through a tube under constant pressure separate into a gradient of velocity profiles with the fastest component in the center and the slowest components near the wall. With a reduction in cross-sectional area, the velocity must increase (and the pressure decrease) in order to maintain the same volume-flow rate. Turbulence results. Clinically, when resistance to air flow occurs, the natural response is to apply more pressure to the breathing bag; this will result in more turbulence in the upper airways and less effective air flow downstream.

Bubble Stability and Breathing: Laplace's Law

The pressure inside a vessel is always higher than the surrounding gas pressure, because the surface of the vessel is in a state of tension. In this respect, alveoli resemble bubbles, or spherical vessels. Laplace's Law describes the relationship between the radius of a vessel and the wall tension required to withstand a given internal fluid pressure. This is different for cylinders and spheres; a sphere has half the wall tension of a cylinder. Wall tension increases as the sphere becomes larger, and the radius of curvature decreases in order to balance the downward component of tension. A rough analogy is hanging heavy clothing on a clothesline; in order for the clothesline to sag less, its tension must be increased. The exact amount of pressure inside the sphere depends on the surface tension of the liquid and the radius of curvature. Laplace's equation expresses this mathematically:

$$P = 2T/R$$

where P equals pressure within the sphere, T equals surface tension of the liquid, and R equals the radius of the sphere. In addition to the amazing ability of pulmonary surfactant to dramatically reduce the surface tension at the alveolar surface (gas-liquid interface), the surfactant stabilizes the airspace by its ability to change the surface tension as the surface expands and contracts during the respiratory cycle; it decreases surface tension as the surface expands and increases the surface tension as the surface expands, affecting Laplace's Law so as to maintain and stabilize air space pressure during the respiratory cycle and prevent alveolar collapse (see Chapter 3, Respiratory Physiology in Infants and Children).

Understanding this relationship also helps explain the improvement in ventilation/perfusion matching with spontaneous breathing when there are two functional lung units of unequal compliance and resistance; an unusually high surface tension, along with interstitial fluid accumulation (edema) and fibrosis, would decrease compliance of the segment. Two functional units (e.g., lungs) of equal compliance and resistance increase their volumes equally when mouth pressure is increased to a constant level; the time course of wash-in is identical for both units. If the compliances of the two units are identical but the resistance of one is twice that of the other, however, the time constant is also twice normal and the unit with the higher resistance fills more slowly, although the volume increase in both units is the same if inflation is prolonged indefinitely. If inspiration ceases after 2 seconds, the pressure is higher in the unit with the lower resistance. Although it is true that paralysis and artificial ventilation do not greatly alter gas exchange ventilation/perfusion (V/Q) matching, dead space to tidal volume ratio (V_D/V_T), and shunt in young, healthy patients in comparison with spontaneous ventilation. This is not true for patients with inequalities in the distribution of ventilation because of asymmetric resistances between lung units (Fig. 12-14). Slow or sustained inflation permits increased distribution of gas to slow alveoli and so tends to distribute gas in accordance with the compliance of the different functional units. Such a situation is the principle underlying frequency-dependent compliance.

Clinical Correlation

Infantile (or idiopathic) respiratory distress syndrome (IRDS), or hyaline membrane disease, is a major cause of respiratory distress in preterm infants because of surfactant deficiency, as

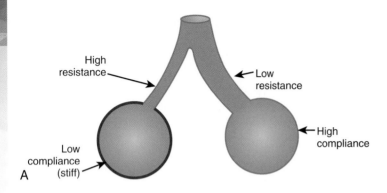

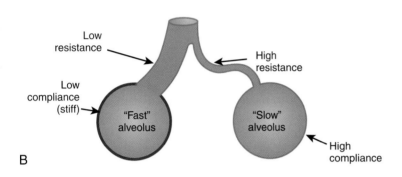

■ **FIGURE 12-14. A,** An idealized state showing the reciprocal relationship between resistance and compliance; gas flow is preferentially delivered to the most compliant regions, regardless of the rate of inflation. Static and dynamic compliance are equal. **B,** A typical state of respiratory disease, where alveoli exist in fast and slow groups. The relationship between compliance and resistance results in preferential delivery of inspired gas to the stiff alveoli if the rate of inflation is rapid; an end-inspiratory pause serves to redistribute gas from the fast alveoli to the slow alveoli.

well as ongoing respiratory embarrassment in bronchopulmonary dysplasia. Surfactant is a complex mixture of lipids and proteins secreted in type II respiratory epithelial cells that lowers alveolar surface tension and therefore decreases the pressure needed to keep alveoli open and inflated. Surfactant deficiency and the consequent alteration in the ability of alveoli to remain optimally inflated results in reduced compliance, reduced functional residual capacity, unevenly increased airway resistance, and decreased alveolar ventilation. These anatomic changes therefore result in an increased physiologic dead space, ventilation/perfusion imbalance, hypoxemia, hypercarbia, and mixed respiratory and metabolic acidosis. In addition, for children with peripheral airways obstruction who require assisted ventilation, the work of breathing during spontaneous breaths is decreased by the application of positive end-expiratory pressure (Graham et al., 2007).

Bernoulli's Principle and Venturi's Effect

In 1738, Bernoulli demonstrated that the pressure of a fluid is least where its speed is greatest. This decrease in pressure when a fluid passes through a region of constriction is the basis of Venturi's effect, demonstrated almost 60 years later when Venturi showed that as a liquid passes beyond a constriction to a wider part of a tube, its speed gradually decreases, accompanied by a gradual increase in pressure. Furthermore, Venturi showed that in order for a streaming fluid to regain a pressure much higher than that at the constriction, the tube immediately distal to the constriction has to open out very gradually, usually not more than a cone angle of about 15 degrees. This is really a conservation of energy principle; in a steady flow the sum of all forms of mechanical energy is the same at all points (i.e., the sum of the kinetic and potential energies are constant).

Clinical Correlation

In Venturi jet ventilation, actually based on Bernoulli's principle and initially described by Sanders in 1967 for clinical use, a jet replaces the constriction of a tube and the oropharynx or trachea acts as the diffuser. An activating toggle switch attached to an oxygen source at 50 psig via a variable pressure-reducing valve controls the stream of gas aimed at the trachea. This technique is often used for laser surgery of the vocal cords. Because the pressure is subatmospheric at the distal end of the jet, air is entrained to swell the stream of gas. This principle is also used during supplemental oxygen therapy (the "Venturi" mask with a variable-orifice air-entrainment port); it is also the principle behind the function of an atomizer.

AIRWAY EQUIPMENT

Routine Pediatric Airway Equipment

Face Masks

Because the cushion-seal face masks used for anesthetizing children have dead spaces from 50 to 80 mL, they add substantially to rebreathing. For this reason, Rendell-Baker and Soucek (1962) introduced a molded, low–dead-space face mask specifically for use with spontaneously breathing infants and children at a time when the administration of halothane anesthesia by mask was popular. However, it is easier to seal to the patient's face with a cushioned face mask than a Rendell-Baker model, and a good mask seal is particularly useful for the application of CPAP during the induction or emergence from general anesthesia.

The use of the proper technique by a clinician when employing a face mask is more important than the type of mask selected.

The clinician's fingers must not depress the submental soft tissues of small children, because the tongue will be forced against the hard and soft palates and an upper airway obstruction may result. Children who have craniofacial anomalies may present a special challenge when attempting to obtain a good mask seal. This includes children with midfacial dysmorphism such as occurs in Apert's syndrome, Crouzon's disease, choanal atresia, or more severe forms of frontonasal dysplasia. Obtaining an adequate mask fit in patients with craniofacial anomalies may be considerably more difficult than the laryngoscopy or tracheal intubation. A useful technique for the ventilation of the lungs of children with midface hypoplasia is to support their cheeks with dental rolls that are placed between the gingiva and buccal mucosa; this often results in a better mask fit.

Airway Adjuncts

Oropharyngeal airway devices should be available in the full range of sizes at each anesthetizing location. The required airway size can be estimated by a careful external examination of the child and by measuring the distance from the teeth to the base of the tongue. An oropharyngeal airway device that is too small can displace the base of the patient's tongue inferiorly toward the pharynx, thereby increasing the degree of obstruction, which may worsen with the application of CPAP in an effort to improve the airway obstruction. An airway that is too large may reach the laryngeal inlet and result in trauma or laryngeal hyperactivity and laryngospasm. It is common practice by some clinicians to insert an oropharyngeal airway device upside down, or convex to the natural curvature of the tongue and then to rotate the airway 180 degrees. However, this maneuver may abrade the hard palate and it is therefore not recommended. A less traumatic technique for the insertion of an oropharyngeal airway device is to use a tongue depressor to displace the tongue to the floor of the mouth and to insert the device concave to the tongue's surface.

Oropharyngeal airway devices are often used as "bite blocks" after a patient's trachea has been intubated, in order to prevent the clenching of the teeth on the endotracheal tube. This maneuver may, however, be hazardous in children between 5 and 10 years of age with loose deciduous teeth. Oropharyngeal airway devices are responsible for up to 55% of anesthesia-related dental complications (Clokie et al., 1989). Furthermore, when an oropharyngeal airway device is used as a bite block during long cases, it may cause necrosis of the tongue, uvular edema, or lip damage (Moore and Rauscher, 1977; Shulman, 1981). A gauze pad that has been rolled up and placed between the patient's upper and lower molar teeth is a better method of preventing the teeth from clenching on an endotracheal tube and minimizing dental trauma. Caution must be exercised, however, that the roll not slip and place undue pressure on the lateral aspect of the tongue (paraglossal sulcus), where the hypoglossal nerve runs.

Nasopharyngeal airway devices are generally constructed from red rubber or polyvinyl chloride and are available in various sizes. A nasal airway should be lubricated and gently inserted transnasally. Nasopharyngeal airway devices may traumatize the turbinates or adenoids of young children. Moreover, care must be exercised when using a nasopharyngeal airway device in children who have a bleeding diathesis or a congenital abnormality of the midface such as choanal atresia or frontonasal dysplasia. The proper length for the nasopharyngeal airway may be estimated by measuring the distance between the patient's auditory meatus and the tip of the nose. The insertion of a nasopharyngeal airway device that is too long may cause laryngospasm. Furthermore, if the airway is too short, the upper airway obstruction may not be relieved.

The LMA is used successfully for routine pediatric anesthetics and even for adenotonsillectomies (Webster et al., 1993; Williams and Bailey, 1993). LMAs are currently manufactured in several sizes, for patients ranging from neonates to large adults. With minimal inflation of the mask's cushion and thorough lubrication of the nonlaryngeal surface, an LMA should be seated at the laryngeal inlet and cause minimal discomfort to the patient postoperatively. Following its blind passage through the oral cavity, the proper seating of an LMA is generally heralded by a slight rise of the device when the mask's cushion is inflated with air. Care should be taken to use the minimal effective inflation pressure for the cuff, typically up to 60 cm H_2O. The routine use of a manometer is advocated. In some patients, the cushion of the LMA overrides the proximal portion of the esophagus, thereby exposing the patient to the risk of the aspiration of gastric contents, with the LMA serving as a conduit to the lungs (Nanji and Maltby, 1992). Nevertheless, although ideal positioning of an LMA appears to be achieved in only 50% of cases, the vast majority of patients fare very well (Rowbottom et al., 1991; Goudsouzian et al., 1992; Mizushima et al., 1992).

Although it was originally thought that pediatric-sized LMAs might not function adequately because of differences in airway anatomy, this fear proved to be unfounded. The #1 LMA, a miniature version of the adult LMA, was designed to fit infants who weigh less than 6.5 kg. It has worked satisfactorily even in premature infants as small as 1 kg, in newborn resuscitation, and in airway maintenance for infants with upper-airway congenital anomalies (e.g., Pierre-Robin, Goldenhar's, Treacher-Collins, and Schwartz-Jampel syndromes). In difficult intubating conditions, it has been used throughout the whole procedure or as a conduit for endotracheal intubation. The endotracheal tube can often be easily directed through an LMA without fiberoptic laryngoscopy.

Flexible LMAs in sizes 2, 2.5, and 3 are also available for pediatric use. The cuff is similar to a standard LMA, but the airway tube is wire-reinforced, longer, and more flexible, allowing it to be positioned away from the surgical field. Although the flexibility of the tube is advantageous for positioning, it is more difficult to insert, it may dislodge more easily, and biting can occlude it. Moreover, the flexibility of this LMA does not allow the rotation technique for insertion. Adenoidectomy or even tonsillectomy can be performed with the flexible LMA, because the cuff prevents soiling of the glottis and the trachea by blood and secretions from the surgical site. If tracheal intubation is planned via LMA, a standard LMA is a more logical choice in children, because it is shorter and has a larger diameter; in adolescents or adults, the intubating LMA (Fastrach) can be used.

The more cephalad and anterior position of the larynx of a child as compared with an adult has prompted the use of an alternate insertion technique in children. In this case, the LMA is inserted with its cushion placed against the hard palate. The device is then rotated through 180 degrees until the cushion is seated at the laryngeal inlet (McNicol, 1991). This method for the insertion of an LMA appears to be especially useful in preschool and young school-age children.

Endotracheal Tubes

The most definitive method for airway management in children remains intubation of the trachea. Polyvinylchloride is still the most popular material employed for the production of endotracheal tubes, although other materials continue to be used and newer technologies are evolving. For example, Weiss and Dullenkof (2007) have the reexamined design requirements of pediatric endotracheal tubes, including cuff placement below the cricoid cartilage, which requires a smaller, more distally placed cuff. Among other features, with polyurethane replacing the polyvinylchloride cuff, the sealing pressures for children are in the range of 6 to 14 cm H_2O (Weiss and Dullenkof, 2007). Recommended performance specifications, as well as detailed standards, for endotracheal tubes have been published (Carroll et al., 1973; Shupak and Deas, 1981).

Table 12-1 lists estimated values for the appropriate endotracheal tube sizes and lengths as well as those for pediatric LMAs (Cole, 1957; Penlington, 1974; Morgan and Steward, 1982; Steven and Cohen, 1990). In general, the size of the tube is more related to the age rather than size of the patient. When selecting an endotracheal tube for a child, it is important to remember that the presence of a deflated cuff adds about 0.5 mm to the tube's external diameter. However, the external diameters of endotracheal tubes differ widely among the manufacturers of the tubes. Cuffs also differ in their shapes and positions along the endotracheal tube. In addition, because nitrous oxide diffuses into the closed airspace of an endotracheal tube's cuff when the inflation valve is closed, this valve should be rendered incompetent during long procedures. Otherwise, the intracuff pressure should be monitored and maintained at a level below 25 cm H_2O (18.4 mm Hg). A variety of endotracheal tubes are available for special needs, including preformed oral or nasotracheal tubes (Ring-Adair-Elwyn [RAE] tubes) for oral or dental surgery and wire-reinforced (anode) endotracheal tubes for head and neck surgery or laryngotracheal reconstruction, when the tube may be inserted through the tracheal stoma and sutured to the anterior chest wall. The special precautions that must be taken with endotracheal tubes during laser surgery of the aerodigestive tract have been described (Sosis 1989, 1992; Sosis and Dillon, 1990, 1991, 1993). The majority of laser airway surgery in pediatrics is for the treatment of juvenile laryngeal papillomatosis or other laryngeal anomalies, and these are cases that lend themselves well to Venturi jet ventilation of the lungs. However, wrapped endotracheal tubes may be required for pediatric laser airway surgery when the laryngeal inlet is too narrow to permit a sufficient entrainment of pharyngeal gas for the Venturi technique (Holzman, 1991, 1992).

Since the seminal report by Koka et al. (1977), an air leak around an endotracheal tube has been strongly advocated for the prevention of postintubation croup in infants and children younger than 10 years of age. Surprisingly, a great deal of variability exists in the ability of a clinician to recognize an air leak around an uncuffed endotracheal tube (Schwartz et al., 1993). However, cuffed endotracheal tubes are advantageous for certain abdominal or thoracic procedures. Also, patients with pulmonary pathologic conditions with poor lung compliance may require high peak inspiratory pressures to assure adequate ventilation of the lungs, and a cuffed endotracheal tube may be necessary for these cases. Because of an increasingly sophisticated understanding of developing laryngeal anatomy and vastly improved materials science in the manufacture of endotracheal tubes, there is a currently a greatly expanded use of cuffed endotracheal tubes in all ages (see The Larynx, p. 350) Accordingly, the use of a cuffed endotracheal tube should be individualized (Table 12-2). Likewise, children who are susceptible to croup during a viral illness of the respiratory tract may benefit from tracheal intubation with a smaller endotracheal tube than is normally used, with or without a cuff, as long as the lungs can be ventilated adequately. A throat pack may help make a seal when an uncuffed endotracheal tube is employed.

Endotracheal tubes are available with or without a special opening known as a *Murphy eye* in the wall opposite the tube's distal bevel. Endotracheal tubes fabricated without the Murphy

TABLE 12-1. Airway Device Details

Age	Preterm	Full-Term Birth	6 mos	1 yr	2 yr	3 yr	4 yr	5 yr	6 yr	8 yr	10 yr	12 yr	14 yr	Adult
Average weight (kg)		3.5	7	10	12	14	16	18	20	25	30	40	50	70
Approx. BSA (m²)		0.25	0.38	0.49	0.55	0.64	0.74	0.76	0.82	0.95	1.18	1.34	1.5	1.73
ETT size (age + 16)/4	2.5-3	3-3.5	3.5-4	4	4.5	4.5	5	5	5.5	6	6.5	7	7	7.5-8
Teeth to midtrachea (cm)	7-8	9	11	12	13	14	14	15	15	16	17	18	20	20
Nare to midtrachea (cm)	8-9	10	12	14	15	16	17	18	19	20	21	22	23	24
Laryngeal mask airway		1	1.5	1.5	2	2	2	2	2.5	2.5	2.5	3	3	4

Calculations for estimating the internal diameter (ID) of an endotracheal tube:
(16 + age in years)/4
(Age in years/4) + 4
The diameter of the fifth finger
Calculations for estimating the length required for an orotracheal tube:
Height (in cm)/10 + 5
Weight (in kg)/5 + 12
Advance the endotracheal tube:
30 times the ID from the alveolar ridge
(Age in years/2) + 12
Insert the endotracheal tube to the first or second black line marked on the tube.
Advance the endotracheal tube into a bronchus, then withdraw it, 2 cm.
BSA, Body surface area; *ETT*, endotracheal tube.

TABLE 12-2. Advantages of Cuffed vs. Uncuffed Endotracheal Tubes

	Cuffed	Uncuffed
Advantages	Not important for subglottic stenosis	Larger tube, therefore less resistance for spontaneous breathing and mechanical ventilation
	Fewer repeat laryngoscopies and reintubations	Lower risk of occlusion
	Less contamination	No cuff = no ridges
	Lower fresh-gas flow	No concern about tip-to-cuff border distance
	Better protection against aspiration	No requirement for pressure monitoring
Indications	High risk of aspiration	Minus the concerns on the left, most likely does not matter much
	Preexisting or impending impaired pulmonary compliance Patient with poor lung compliance undergoing minimally invasive abdominal or chest surgery Cardiopulmonary bypass Requirement for precisely controlled mechanical ventilation	

eye are known as *Magill tubes*, whereas those that have this opening are called *Murphy tubes*. The Murphy eye was designed to provide an alternate pathway for the flow of ventilatory gases if the distal opening of the endotracheal tube was occluded—a common situation, especially in infants (Murphy, 1941). However, there are potential disadvantages to the presence of a Murphy eye on an endotracheal tube, including a tendency for accumulation of secretions and the possibility that a stylet, catheter, or bronchoscope may get stuck, requiring the removal of the entire assembly. Cuffed endotracheal tubes manufactured without a Murphy eye can have the cuff located closer to the tube's tip. Nevertheless, pediatric anesthesiologists generally favor the use of an endotracheal tube that is equipped with a Murphy eye because of the obstruction risk. Recently, Weiss and Dullenkof (2007) have reexamined the design requirements of a more anatomically suitable pediatric endotracheal tube, including cuff placement below the cricoid cartilage, thus requiring a smaller, more distally placed cuff and removal of the Murphy eye. Among other features, with a polyurethane as opposed to a polyvinylchloride cuff, the sealing pressures for children are in the range of 6 to 14 cm H_2O, well under the 20 to 25 cm H_2O for the leak test.

Stylets are often inserted into endotracheal tubes used for children to provide rigidity and bend the tube to a desired shape. However, the increased rigidity provided by a stylet can result in greater trauma. Moreover, because of metal fatigue, old wire stylets may break during their removal from an endotracheal tube, placing the patient at risk for the aspiration of a foreign body. Stylets should be of the proper size for the endotracheal tube, and they should be well lubricated so they can be removed easily. The tip of the stylet should be

properly recessed (1 to 2 cm) from the tip of the endotracheal tube to avoid its extrusion from the tube and direct trauma to the mucosa. Each stylet should be carefully inspected for any potential weak points.

The concerns about anatomic differences between children and adults were typically partisan enough that while an emerging acceptance of endotracheal intubation was obvious beginning in the 1950s and 1960s, it remained a relatively rare technique in pediatric anesthesia. Clinicians were warned about the narrowest part of the pediatric airway located at the cricoid cartilage. Outcome studies began to suggest the safety and efficacy of endotracheal intubation in infants and children, and pediatric anesthesia clinicians were becoming more vocal in defense of this emerging technique. See related video online at www.expertconsult.com.

Laryngoscopes

The ability to use standard straight and curved laryngoscope blades is mandatory in pediatric anesthesia. The laryngeal structures of infants are encountered at a more cephalad and anterior position, approximately the level of C2 to C3, depending on age, until the child reaches school age, when the laryngeal structures descend to a level opposite the body of C4. It is common practice to use a straight laryngoscope blade such as the Miller 0 or 1, or the Wis-Hippel 1.5, to intubate the trachea of an infant or a child up to school age. A curved laryngoscope blade with a wider spatula, such as the Macintosh blade may be advantageous to control the tongue of an older child. Whether to use the straight or the curved laryngoscope blades can be determined according to this approximate age distribution; however, the individual preferences of the clinician may vary, as can individual circumstances. The larger tongue of a patient with Down's syndrome, at any age, for example, may be easier to manipulate with the wider spatula of a Macintosh blade. A short laryngoscope handle is most useful for the intubation of the trachea of an infant, a small child, or an obese patient.

Equipment for the Management of a Difficult Airway in a Child

Line-of-sight devices have been the mainstay of direct laryngoscopy techniques, yet difficulties with laryngoscopy and intubation are not rare. Although it is typically acknowledged as a rare event, there is emerging literature that difficulty with laryngoscopy may be encountered in 5% to 20% of adult patients; although this may be substantially less of an issue in children and it may be age dependent (0.57% in newborns and toddlers, 0.12% in preschool, and 0.05% in school-age patients) (Rose and Cohen, 1994, 1996; Ezri et al., 2003; Schmidt and Koch, 2008).

Anterior commissure laryngoscopes, because of their tubular construction, are particularly useful with a difficult-to-visualize "anterior" (cephalad) larynx in the patient with a small oral cavity. They require a fiberoptic external light source. In addition, long bronchoscopy forceps must be available. The 15-mm connector is removed from the endotracheal tube, and the laryngoscope is inserted. With the epiglottis lifted directly from the laryngeal surface, the tip of the laryngoscope should be placed at the glottic opening. The endotracheal tube is inserted through the tubular laryngoscope blade. Although direct visualization of the glottis is usually lost at this point, correct positioning

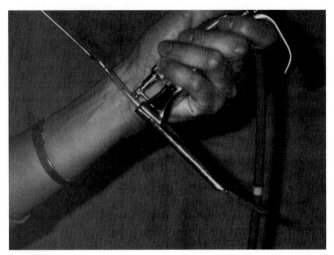

■ **FIGURE 12-15.** Use of an anterior commissure laryngoscope for endotracheal intubation; when an endotracheal tube with its 15-mm connector removed is inserted through the tubular blade after the epiglottis is lifted from the laryngeal surface and the tip of the blade is placed at the glottic opening, the bronchoscopy forceps can grasp the proximal end of the tube while the laryngoscope is removed over the tube and forceps.

and the tubular structure of the blade guide the tube into the trachea. Using the forceps, the tube is held in place while the laryngoscope is removed over the tube and forceps (Fig. 12-15). The endotracheal tube connector is then replaced, and the tube position is verified.

Newer technologies, such as fiberoptic bronchoscopy and the availability of video machines, are making it much easier to develop ways of viewing the larynx that are not directly line-of-sight dependent. The skills required for effective use of these devices are different, and although pediatric anesthesiologists must keep abreast of new technologic skills, conventional rigid laryngoscopy is used the majority of the time.

With fiberoptic and video modifications, flexible, malleable, and rigid devices have been developed that have added to the laryngoscopy tool shed in recent years. Optical stylets may be rigid, flexible, or malleable; resemble a conventional laryngoscope; or be more like a flexible fiberoptic bronchoscope (Liem et al., 2003). The basic design consists of a fiberoptic rod with an eyepiece at the user end that allows the anesthesiologist to view the advancement of the endotracheal tube, which is threaded over the device. Examples of these devices include the Bonfils Retromolar Intubation Fiberscope (Karl Storz Endoscopy; Culver City, California), the Shikani Optic Stylet (Clarus Medical LLC; Minneapolis, Minnesota), the StyletScope (Nihon Kohden Corp.; Tokyo, Japan), the Video Optical Intubation Stylet (VOIS, Acutronic Medical Systems, AG; Baar, Switzerland), and the Levitan FPS Scope (Clarus Medical LLC; Minneapolis, Minnesota) (see Chapter 10, Equipment, Fig. 10-24). The Bonfils laryngoscope is a nonmalleable scope, whereas the Shikani laryngoscope has a distally malleable stylet. It can accommodate a size 2.5 endotracheal tube in its pediatric version. All of these stylets can be used alone or in conjunction with rigid direct laryngoscopy. In the absence of direct laryngoscopy, a jaw lift or jaw thrust should be used to increase the anteroposterior distance of the hypopharyngeal space and move the base of the tongue away from the laryngeal inlet.

Rigid fiberoptic laryngoscopes have a fiberoptic bundle encased in a closed structure. They serve the same function as conventional rigid laryngoscopes, in that they are intended for viewing the larynx and confirming the insertion of the endotracheal tube. They cannot view the subglottic space or be inserted by any route other than transorally. Examples include the Bullard laryngoscope, UpsherScope, and WuScope. Only the Bullard laryngoscope is available in pediatric versions (see Chapter 10, Equipment, Fig. 10-30). The Acutronic Video Intubating laryngoscope (Acutronic Medical Systems, AG; Baar, Switzerland) was developed by Weiss and resembles a conventional laryngoscope and blade with a fiberoptic bundle that can be coupled to a video camera.

Rigid video laryngoscopes allow the image to be displayed to an eyepiece or a video screen. The video camera may be located within the handle, mounted on the handle, or displayed remotely. Other rigid video laryngoscopes include the Glidescope (Verathon, Inc.; Bothell, Washington) (see Chapter 10, Equipment, Fig. 10-31; see related video online at www.expertconsult.com). It is available in pediatric and neonatal versions. Because the larynx is not in the line of sight, the Glidescope should be used with a stylet. Exposure of the vocal cords on the image does not necessarily occur from exposure of the larynx. Antifogging solutions are not required, because a charge-coupled video chip covered by a heated glass window is incorporated into the blade, making it fog resistant.

The flexible fiberoptic laryngoscopes that are used for children are generally smaller than adult scopes, and not all small fiberscopes are designed with a channel for suctioning or oxygen insufflation. Also, pediatric fiberscopes may be limited in the extent of their tip excursion in comparison with larger fiberoptic laryngoscopes. A pediatric fiberoptic laryngoscope is often used to intubate the trachea of a child who is breathing spontaneously with a volatile anesthetic. In such cases, an airway intubation (Frei) mask or one with a similar design, which incorporates a grommet through which a fiberscope may be passed, is very useful (Frei, 1995) (see related video online at www.expertconsult.com).

It may seem counterintuitive to advocate blind intubation techniques amidst these advances in technology; however, in skilled and thoughtful hands, these methods are worthy of consideration because they have stood the test of time, and simply put, they work! Devices for blind intubation include the gum elastic bougie (e.g., Eschmann Stylet, Portex Limited; Hythe, United Kingdom) and the light wand (e.g., Trachlight, Laerdal Medical; Wappingers Falls, New York). In one study, children whose tracheas were found to be extremely difficult to intubate by conventional means were intubated without difficulty with the use of a light wand (Holzman et al., 1988). Finally, tactile intubation can be accomplished by using the index and middle fingers of the nondominant hand intraorally to palpate the epiglottis while the endotracheal tube or stylet is advanced along the palmar surface of the index finger to the larynx, laryngeal inlet, and intratracheally.

It is important to emphasize that these newer and developing technologies, as well as the older ones, require familiarization on the part of the anesthesiologist; no one can be expected to use these devices or techniques in the heat of battle with a difficult airway. Preparation and practice under controlled circumstances are the best preparation for emergency situations, and as always, chance favors the prepared mind. A well-stocked cart for use with difficult airways should be immediately available in every operating room suite.

Breathing Systems

The valved-circle anesthesia system or variations of Ayre's valveless T piece are the most common breathing circuits for pediatric patients (Mapleson, 1954). For years, the T piece was recommended for children weighing less than 10 kg because of the decreased resistance to spontaneous breathing, the better "feel" of the rebreathing bag in the hand of the anesthetist, and the faster anesthesia induction and emergence times using higher nonrebreathing fresh-gas flows. Improvements in machine components have resulted in low-resistance valves, reduced dead space at connections, improved CO_2-absorbent canister design, and the availability of capnography, as well as changes in philosophy that favor controlled pulmonary ventilation in small children; such improvements have rendered these arguments less durable. Likewise, modern, less-soluble inhalation agents make the influence of the breathing circuit less of an issue.

The compression volume of the breathing circuit is an important influence on alveolar ventilation in children, because their tidal volumes are so much smaller. Breathing circuits with large compression volumes can be "ventilated" far in excess of the volume delivered to the patient. Many circle systems modified for pediatric use are not only shorter, but they also have a smaller radius of curvature of the tubing, which according to Laplace's Law renders them less distensible and thus further decreases compression volume. Compliance of the tubing can also be decreased with fine wire or reinforced plastic.

Another important consideration for small children is the dead space of the breathing system. Dead space only exists when fresh and exhaled gases are mixed (i.e., at the Y piece); dead space no longer exists when fresh and exhaled gases are completely separated. Accordingly, the dead space of the Y piece in a circle system can be decreased by the addition of a median septum. Similarly, the dead space of an elbow in a Mapleson D system can be decreased by the addition of a fresh gas delivery port within the elbow (the Norman elbow).

CLINICAL AIRWAY CARE

Expert airway care is the most important skill in pediatric anesthesiology, and skill in understanding and controlling anesthetic depth is arguably the most important aspect of providing safe and expert airway care. It is critical to the success of spontaneous breathing techniques for diagnostic examination of the native airway, dynamic changes such as extrinsic compression or tracheomalacia, and for interventions such as the removal of a foreign body from the airway (see videoclip of infant bronchoscopy online at www.expertconsult.com). Aside from the assessment of heart rate, blood pressure, and patient movement, depth of anesthesia can also be evaluated by continuous monitoring of the heart sounds, the "classic" eye signs, and repeated examination of muscle tone. The arms and legs should feel completely relaxed, and the abdominal muscles should be soft and easily compressible, like bread dough, distinct from the boardlike rigidity of the excitement phase or the mild to moderate muscle tone of the awake or sedated state. Disconjugate gaze and pupillary dilation shortly after inhalation induction support the assessment of light anesthesia, whereas midsize pupils in midposition, along with other physical findings of acceptable anesthetic depth, add to the clinician's assessment. All signs together should be used to form a composite, so that

ideally the anesthesiologist should be able to ensure lack of patient movement in response to stimulation. Facility in determining anesthetic depth is also important for successful "deep" extubations—that is, the removal of the endotracheal tube while the patient is deeply anesthetized and breathing spontaneously. The presumption is that the patient will have less coughing, bucking, and airway irritability during the emergence process because of the lack of an endotracheal tube. In experienced hands, this technique is at least as safe as the more typical "awake" extubation (Patel et al., 1991; Pounder et al., 1991; Karam et al., 1995).

Profound surface analgesia of the oropharynx and laryngeal apparatus can be achieved by a combination of topical anesthesia of the tongue and posterior pharyngeal wall, glossopharyngeal nerve block, and superior laryngeal nerve block, as well as a transtracheal injection of local anesthetic (Cooper and Watson, 1975). Because most children will not tolerate this strategy well when they are awake, it is usually accomplished with sedation.

- Nebulized or gargled lidocaine can be used in older (i.e., school age) children to obtain surface analgesia of the tongue and pharyngeal surfaces.
- Local spray anesthesia can be used regardless of age by using age-appropriate concentrations of lidocaine (1% for infants, 2% for young school-age children, and up to 4% for older children and adolescents). Cooperative patients can gargle and swallow the accumulated spray; spray and suctioning sequences may have to be used for more deeply sedated patients.
- The internal branch of the superior laryngeal nerves can be blocked bilaterally as they pierce the thyrohyoid membrane just superior to the greater cornua of the thyroid cartilage (Fig. 12-16). Only a small amount of local

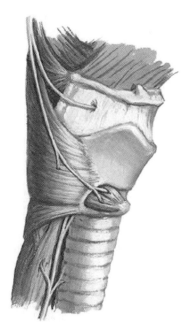

■ **FIGURE 12-16.** The internal branch of the superior laryngeal nerve pierces the thyrohyoid membrane at a vertical midpoint between the thyroid and hyoid cartilage, just superior to the greater cornua of the thyroid. It is here that the nerve can be percutaneously accessed to block sensation to the mucous membranes of the pharynx and supraglottic larynx.

anesthetic (e.g., lidocaine 1%) is required; after a sterile preparation of the skin, a fine needle is entered perpendicular to the skin at a point above the greater cornua of the thyroid cartilage, midway vertically between the thyroid and hyoid cartilages; the thyrohyoid membrane is pierced, and local anesthetic is deposited after careful aspiration just below. Then the needle is withdrawn slightly, just above the membrane. The onset of this block takes a few minutes, so it should be done before the glossopharyngeal nerve block.

● The glossopharyngeal nerves can be blocked bilaterally throughout their submucosal course in the posterior tonsillar (palatopharyngeal) pillar with the use of a tonsil block needle (Fig. 12-17). Only a small amount of local anesthetic volume of lidocaine 1% is required; careful aspiration before injection is a must. Typical injection locations are at the 2-, 4-, 8-, and 10-o'clock positions as the anesthesiologist faces the patient directly. The block is established quickly.

● A transtracheal block to anesthetize the recurrent laryngeal nerve can be accomplished with the use of a fine needle or small IV catheter piercing the cricothyroid membrane after the above blocks, using an age-appropriate concentration of lidocaine 1% to 4%. Accurate intratracheal location of the needle or catheter is confirmed by aspiration of air before injection, which is often accompanied by vigorous coughing; therefore, the needle or catheter should be withdrawn as soon as possible (Fig. 12-18).

Laryngospasm occurs more often in conjunction with airway-related procedures, and multiple strategies for the prevention and treatment of laryngospasm have been sought. CPAP is routinely used in preventing or treating laryngospasm and soft tissue upper airway obstruction. Usually, pressure at 5 to 10 cm H_2O as measured on the breathing circuit pressure gauge is effective; higher pressures are occasionally required. Care should be exercised, because opening pressure of the lower esophageal sphincter may be as low as 10 to 12 cm H_2O, and

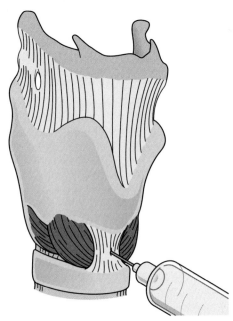

■ **FIGURE 12-18.** Transtracheal approach to the subglottic space, providing sensory blockade to the mucosa of the infraglottic trachea via the recurrent laryngeal nerve.

therefore the risk of gastric insufflation exists. Also, while CPAP is effective for soft-tissue obstruction, it is not necessarily effective for tumors of the airway or scar tissue.

CARE OF THE CHILD WITH A DIFFICULT AIRWAY

General Issues

The care of a child with a difficult airway must begin with an assessment of resources; the most important part of that assessment is a self-assessment. Questions to ask include:

1. Do I routinely take care of children? If not, then the pediatric airway may, for me, be relatively unique.
2. Do I routinely take care of children younger than 2 years of age? This population has consistently different anatomic and physiologic characteristics from those of older children, such as a much higher oxygen consumption and CO_2 production, a smaller functional residual capacity, and a greater reduction in intrathoracic volume when supine, anesthetized, and relaxed; therefore, this age range has substantially less oxygen reserve during airway misadventures.
3. Do I routinely take care of the subset of children with difficult airways? If not, then the pediatric difficult airway is definitely a special instance.

There is some evidence that the toll of providing care for children, especially resuscitation, may occasionally impose a substantially larger psychological burden on the pediatric specialist. For this reason, a color-coded resuscitation aid such as the Broselow-Luten system may decrease practitioner anxiety and afford more time for critical thinking during crises (Luten and Broselow, 1999, Luten et al., 2002). Although the evaluation of difficult airway anatomy in a child is, in principle, very similar to that of an adult, children often do not cooperate. With

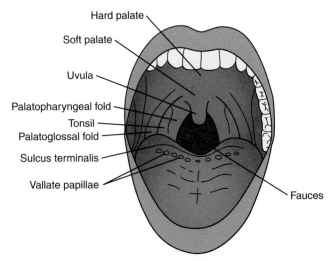

■ **FIGURE 12-17.** Intraoral approach to the glossopharyngeal nerve as it runs submucosally posterior to the posterior tonsillar pillar (palatopharyngeal fold). Blocking the nerve as it courses through the palatopharyngeal fold provides sensory analgesia to the mucosa over the palatine tonsil, the adjacent soft palate, the pharynx, and the posterior third of the tongue.

regard to the difficult airway, patients with a difficult airway as a "syndrome" are not usually the challenge; they have been previously identified, are often well categorized, and may even have a tracheostomy; the challenge is the patient who may look somewhat challenging to the less experienced evaluator but indeed has a difficult airway.

Specific Issues Unique to Children with Difficult Airways

Traditional clinical teaching is that the sniffing position is the optimal position for aligning the axes of the trachea, pharynx, and oral cavity. Because the anteroposterior dimension of the head in children is so much larger than that of the chest, a pillow or ring under the head may not be necessary to achieve this sniffing position; it may simply involve placing the patient on the flat mattress pad of the operating-room table, or even placing a small roll under the shoulders. This presumes normal mobility of adjacent structures of the larynx. With poor mobility of laryngeal structures, such as in the anteriorly placed larynx, direct laryngoscopy in the extended head position actually swings the larynx anteriorly as the anesthesiologist lifts the laryngoscope blade, making visualization more difficult. It is often better to flex the head onto the chest, as the glottic aperture then moves posteriorly and may be visualized directly. Indirect visualization may now be accomplished with many available devices, as described above. In order to develop comfort and expertise and retain familiarity, these devices must be used routinely.

Decision algorithms about the difficult airway are available, and most of the issues that are specific to the anticipated difficult pediatric airway are not that different from those for adults, including a broad range of appropriate equipment, occasional imaging studies, and preparation with sedation and topical local-anesthetic techniques (Fig. 12-19). If a spontaneous-breathing anesthetic technique is chosen, pediatric anesthesiologists are already comfortable with the assessment of anesthetic depth in children. Patient cooperation is a key crucial difference in the recognized difficult airway and in children is influenced by the chronologic, developmental, emotional, and intellectual components of the preoperative assessment. Surgical airway access, whether by needle cricothyroidotomy, open cricothyrotomy, or tracheostomy, is hazardous, especially in inexperienced hands, yet it may be the only option available. If this is a possible part of the airway plan, collaboration with a surgeon is essential.

The unexpected difficult pediatric airway patient is a different matter. Wheeler proposed a very reasonable modification to the well-accepted adult difficult airway algorithm (Fig. 12-20) (Wheeler, 1998). The key to this, or any other, algorithm is that it presents a reasoned and organized approach to a high-risk situation.

Care of the Patient with a Surgical or Reconstructed Airway

Tracheostomy

The need for pediatric tracheostomy is divided between the relief of airway obstruction (approximately 40%) and the need for prolonged ventilation of the lungs and pulmonary toilet (approximately 50%). Most patients remain with the basic underlying problem that resulted in the tracheostomy—typically severe subglottic stenosis—and a prolonged need for mechanical ventilation because of underlying lung disease or difficulty with maintaining an adequate translaryngeal airway caused by poor secretion control. Accidental decannulation and a tracheostomy tube plug are common perioperative events. Because a tracheostomy bypasses the natural sphincteric and glottic closure mechanisms responsible for warming and humidifying air and maintaining a functional residual capacity, children with a tracheostomy require airway humidification. Suctioning is usually required to clear accumulated secretions. The underlying disorders for which tracheostomy is performed are often chronic but potentially life threatening, especially after any surgical intervention; therefore, apnea with cardiac and respiratory monitoring including pulse oximetry, are routine whether the patient is in the intensive care unit (ICU) or another unit. Follow-up examinations for evaluating residual granulomas and evaluation for decannulation are common. Often, patients have mask aversion and posttraumatic stress disorder because of prolonged ICU care and life-threatening illness.

Pharyngeal Flap Surgery

Following cleft-palate repair, pharyngeal flap and oronasal fistula repair may be needed for velopharyngeal insufficiency. Different types of palatoplasties are performed to alleviate the hypernasality, depending on the cause and dynamics of the insufficiency. The length and width of the flap are tailored to the degree of velopharyngeal incompetence, and it is important for the anesthesiologist to know which kind of repair was done, especially if for subsequent surgery a nasal endotracheal tube or nasogastric tube will be placed, both of which are more problematic if a patient has had a superiorly based flap (Fig. 12-21). Direct vision with a fiberoptic laryngoscope is often the best technique to minimize trauma to the reconstructed area.

External Distraction Devices

Distraction osteogenesis for unilateral or bilateral advancement of maxillary or mandibular structures has become the major technique in craniofacial surgery. The use of distraction allows the surgeon better control in positioning the bony segments after the osteotomy, enables the segments to be moved a greater distance, and eliminates the need for bone grafts. However, the device may contribute to trismus and also decrease jaw opening. Its presence may interfere with routine airway techniques, and therefore advanced airway-management skills may be needed (Fig. 12-22). Midface advancement using a halo distractor or rigid external distraction (RED) device is favored by some surgeons, whereas others may use an internal midface distractor. Both types have drawbacks. For the anesthesiologist, the initial placement is not as much of a problem as the subsequent procedures to remove them. Limited ability to open the mouth may occur once the distraction is finished. This may be the result of the new position of the maxilla in relation to the mandible, or it may be caused from pain and swelling of the muscles through which the devices pass. The anesthesiologist must therefore be prepared for a more difficult intubation after the initial procedure.

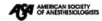

DIFFICULT AIRWAY ALGORITHM

1. Assess the likelihood and clinical impact of basic management problems:

    A. Difficult ventilation
    B. Difficult intubation
    C. Difficulty with patient cooperation or consent
    D. Difficult tracheostomy

2. Actively pursue opportunities to deliver supplemental oxygen throughout the process of difficult airway management

3. Consider the relative merits and feasibility of basic management choices:

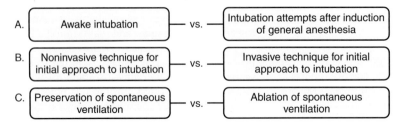

A.	Awake intubation	vs.	Intubation attempts after induction of general anesthesia
B.	Noninvasive technique for initial approach to intubation	vs.	Invasive technique for initial approach to intubation
C.	Preservation of spontaneous ventilation	vs.	Ablation of spontaneous ventilation

4. Develop primary and alternative strategies:

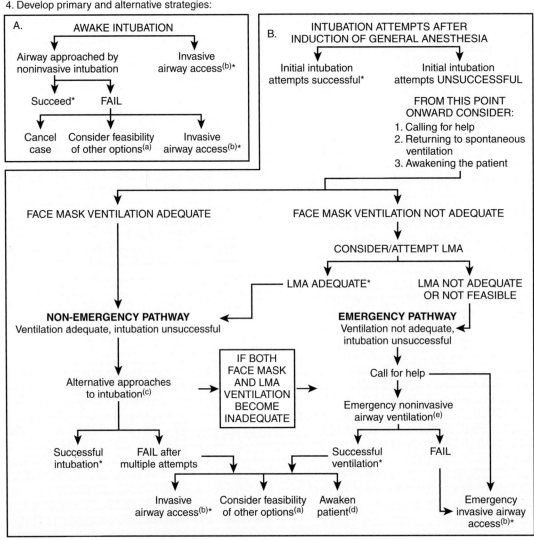

* Confirm ventilation, tracheal intubation, or LMA placement with exhaled CO_2

a. Other options include (but are not limited to): surgery utilizing face mask or LMA anesthesia, local anesthesia infiltration or regional nerve blockade. Pursuit of these options usually implies that mask ventilation will not be problematic. Therefore, these options may be of limited value if this step in the algorithm has been reached via the emergency pathway.

b. Invasive airway access includes surgical or percutaneous tracheostomy or cricothyrotomy.

c. Alternative non-invasive approaches to difficult intubation include (but are not limited to): use of different laryngoscope blades. LMA as an intubation conduit (with or without fiberoptic guidance), fiberoptic intubation, intubating stylet or tube changer, light wand, retrograde intubation, and blind oral or nasal intubation.

d. Consider re-preparation of the patient for awake intubation or canceling surgery.

e. Options for emergency non-invasive airway ventilation include (but are not limited to): rigid bronchoscope, esophageal-tracheal combitube ventilation, or transtracheal jet ventilation.

■ **FIGURE 12-19.** Difficult airway algorithm. *(Courtesy of the American Society of Anesthesiologists.)*

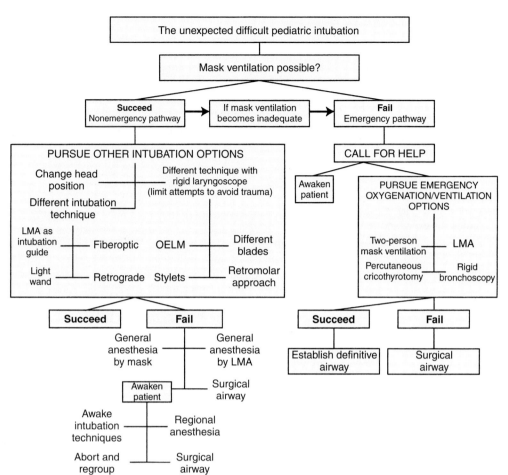

The unexpected difficult pediatric intubation

Mask ventilation possible?

Succeed
Nonemergency pathway → If mask ventilation becomes inadequate → **Fail**
Emergency pathway

PURSUE OTHER INTUBATION OPTIONS

Change head position — Different technique with rigid laryngoscope (limit attempts to avoid trauma)

Different intubation technique

LMA as intubation guide — Fiberoptic   OELM — Different blades

Light wand — Retrograde   Stylets — Retromolar approach

Succeed   **Fail**

General anesthesia by mask — General anesthesia by LMA

Awaken patient — Surgical airway

Awake intubation techniques — Regional anesthesia

Abort and regroup — Surgical airway

CALL FOR HELP

Awaken patient

PURSUE EMERGENCY OXYGENATION/VENTILATION OPTIONS

Two-person mask ventilation — LMA

Percutaneous cricothyrotomy — Rigid bronchoscopy

Succeed   **Fail**

Establish definitive airway   Surgical airway

■ **FIGURE 12-20.** A decision pathway for the difficult pediatric airway.

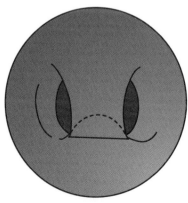

◀ **FIGURE 12-21.** Superiorly-based pharyngeal flap for velopharyngeal insufficiency. Pharyngeal flaps may be superiorly or inferiorly based, but the superiorly based repair has fewer complications. There are sphincter pharyngoplasty approaches as well. By decreasing the cross-sectional area of the airway, a previously adequate airway may be changed to a partially or totally obstructed airway; returning to the operating room to take down the flap may be lifesaving.

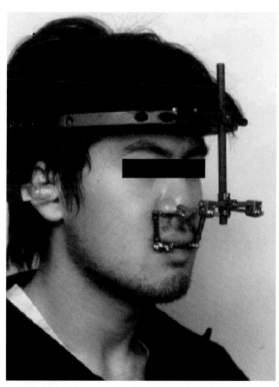

■ **FIGURE 12-22.** External maxillary distraction device. Distraction osteogenesis is a major technique in craniofacial surgery, and its use allows improved bone positioning after osteotomy, greater segmental movement, and elimination of bone grafts. The challenge for the anesthesiologist is the limitation in mouth movement, airway access, and planning for repeat procedures.

Restoring the Natural Airway

Airway Device Removal

The literature does not provide an extubation strategy for the difficult airway; however, it should probably be closely related to the intubation strategy. Awake extubation vs. extubation before the return of consciousness is a principal consideration, as are general clinical factors that may produce an adverse impact on ventilation after the patient has been extubated. Backup plans for airway management if the patient is not able to maintain adequate ventilation after extubation are a must, as is availability of a device that can serve as a guide for expedited reintubation such as a bougie or exchange catheter (Mort, 2007). Occasionally, a difficult extubation because of patient anxiety is facilitated by a sedation strategy (Arpino et al., 2008).

Decannulation of Tracheostomies

Decannulation should not usually be considered until the underlying disease that necessitated the tracheostomy has been resolved. A careful evaluation must be made of the effectiveness of the patient's own ventilatory efforts, efficiency of oxygenation, and ability to handle secretions. Decannulation evaluation is typically accomplished by endoscopic examination, with particular attention to edema, stenosis, or granuloma formation, with a sequencing of tracheal tube downsizing and capping, and followed by removal and closure of the tracheal stoma. Downsizing may be a more difficult strategy in smaller patients, for whom tracheostomy-tube removal and observation may be a better choice given their smaller airways and therefore greater relative resistance to breathing during the downsizing process. Finally, the anesthetic technique for decannulation is a matter of preference and experience; some prefer sedation, whereas many prefer a general anesthetic with a small endotracheal tube after the endoscopic examination.

SUMMARY

The airway is a composite of the anatomic development of the head, face, aerodigestive tract, and neck—structures contiguous as well as integral to the airway. This chapter considers the developmental anatomy, physiology, and air flow physics crucial to an informed plan for managing the pediatric airway. Airway equipment for routine and difficult airway applications is then considered, and a discussion of clinical care in these circumstances is included. Finally, restoration of the natural airway is addressed.

For questions and answers on topics in this chapter, go to "Chapter Questions" at www.expertconsult.com.

REFERENCES

Complete references used in this text can be found online at www.expertconsult.com.

Induction, Maintenance, and Recovery

Ira Todd Cohen, Nina Deutsch, and Etsuro K. Motoyama

CHAPTER

13

CONTENTS

Anesthetic induction, maintenance, and recovery pose unique challenges and considerations in infants and children. The anesthetic plan should be designed as a continuous process that cares for the patient from admission to discharge, anticipating the patient's preoperative anxiety, intraoperative requirements, and postoperative recovery. Each step in the continuum is interrelated and interdependent. All factors, including the patient's age, medical history, surgical procedure, and discharge disposition must be considered in selecting drugs and techniques to ensure safe induction, a stable intraoperative course, and a comfortable, rapid recovery.

The induction of general anesthesia in infants and children requires sensitivity, flexibility, and finesse, as well as specialized knowledge and skills. Eliciting concerns, perceiving fears, and predicting the degree of cooperation from patients and their families, in addition to obtaining the history of medical conditions, previous anesthetics, medication use, allergies, familial disorders, recent illnesses, loose teeth, and *nil per os* (NPO) status during the preoperative interview are all essential in formulating a plan for the anesthetic induction. The pediatric anesthesiologist must determine whether preinduction medications, topical anesthetics, or parental presence are indicated and whether an inhalation or intravenous technique is to be used. The setting, monitoring, and method of obtaining intravenous access and securing the airway also need to be determined in advance to ensure the smoothest course possible.

Once anesthesia is induced, the anesthesiologist is responsible for maintaining a state of analgesia, amnesia, adequate muscle relaxation, and autonomic nervous system stability while providing optimum surgical conditions. To achieve this goal, the anesthesiologist should choose appropriate anesthetic and adjuvant medications and continuously monitor anesthetic depth, oxygenation, ventilation, cardiovascular function, fluid balance, body temperature, and if indicated, glucose and electrolyte levels. For critically ill patients or for patients undergoing major or prolonged procedures, more extensive and invasive monitoring may be required. The pediatric anesthesiologist must ensure appropriate positioning and protective measures to avoid soft tissue injury in this at-risk population. Management of all factors, from the choice of pharmacologic agents, to the use of regional anesthetic adjuncts, to the adjustment of ambient temperature, is the role of the pediatric anesthesiologist.

Postoperatively, the pediatric anesthesiologist should plan a relatively swift awakening to ensure adequate airway maintenance, protective reflexes, and hemodynamic stability while avoiding pain, emergence agitation, nausea, and vomiting. A rapid return to the preoperative level of consciousness, although ideal for ambulatory and short-stay patients, may be frightening and disorienting to a child who is not prepared to awaken in a new and unfamiliar environment among strangers. Pain, however slight, magnifies these responses dramatically. Nonambulatory and critically ill patients may not need a rapid emergence and can benefit from an extended period of sedation and analgesia. If they are being transferred directly to an intensive care unit (ICU), continuous monitoring is indicated. Once the patient is in the postanesthesia care unit (PACU) or ICU, the anesthesiologist must assess airway patency, cardiovascular status, body temperature, and level of discomfort. Pain, nausea, and vomiting should be evaluated and treated appropriately.

INDUCTION OF GENERAL ANESTHESIA

The induction of general anesthesia can be the most critical yet rewarding interaction that a pediatric anesthesiologist has with young patients and their families. Minimizing anxiety, psychological trauma, and crying during induction has many advantages, including reduced occurrence of airway complications, emergence agitation, postoperative pain, short- and long-term behavioral changes, patient and family dissatisfaction, and difficult inductions with subsequent anesthetics (Laycock and McNicol, 1988; Kotiniemi et al., 1997; Kain et al., 1999; Przybylo et al., 2005; Kain et al., 2006). With the increased focus on family-centered care, including parents' concerns and priorities in the decision-making process being the norm, it is essential that all parties are prepared as well as possible regarding information, preferences, and expectations. If premedications or topical anesthetics are indicated, adequate time should be allotted to ensure maximal benefit. Smooth separation of child and family, be it before or after induction, should be facilitated by clearly stated instructions and participation of perioperative personnel.

Psychological Considerations

During the preoperative period, it is extremely important to identify the children and families who are likely to develop pronounced fear and anxiety before and during the induction of anesthesia. Because the level of stress and underlying temperament that predispose individuals to extreme anxiety may not be overtly apparent, it is essential that the pediatric anesthesiologist carefully evaluate each patient. Indicative behaviors, beyond the obvious crying and uncooperative child, include the absence of social interaction, vocalization, emotional expression, and age-appropriate independence from parents (Kain et al., 1997). It is also helpful to assess family members' levels of anxiety and coping styles. Premedication with anxiolytics has been shown to be the most consistently effective intervention for facilitating induction and reducing postoperative complications in anxious patients (Bergendahl et al., 2004; Almenrader et al., 2007; Schmidt et al., 2007).

Medical Considerations

Most children and infants scheduled for elective surgical procedures are in good health, but common disorders such as upper respiratory tract infection (URI), reactive airways disease, gastroesophageal reflux, obesity, and hemodynamically stable congenital heart lesions can pose diagnostic and management challenges for the pediatric anesthesiologist.

Patients with known medical problems should be carefully interviewed and examined, and if general anesthesia is to be induced, appropriate precautions and interventions should be taken. These issues are explored in detail elsewhere in this text (see Chapters 9, Preoperative Preparation, and 36, Systemic Disorders). An overview of some basic considerations is discussed below.

Upper Respiratory Tract Infections

URI is by far the most common problem the pediatric anesthesiologist encounters, especially in the ambulatory surgery setting. URI and the accompanying inflammation increase upper and lower airway irritability and secretions, and they may increase the incidence of laryngospasm, bronchospasm, and perioperative hypoxemia (see Chapter 36, Systemic Disorders) (DeSoto et al., 1988; Cohen and Cameron, 1991; Coté, 2001; Bordet et al., 2002; Elwood et al., 2003). Risk factors for associated complications include nasal congestion, copious secretions, reactive airways disease, history of prematurity, passive smoking, airway surgery, endotracheal intubation, and laryngeal mask airway insertion (Tait et al., 2001; von Ungern-Sternberg et al., 2007). Even in patients without a history of asthma, airway reactivity can develop with URI or lower respiratory tract infection and last as long as 6 to 8 weeks (Empey et al., 1976; de Kluijver et al., 2002). The decision to postpone the procedure depends on the urgency of the surgery, the severity of symptoms, and the need to instrument the airway (Tait and Malviya, 2005). In these patients, prophylactic bronchodilator treatment should be considered before the induction of anesthesia and before the emergence from anesthesia and extubation.

Reactive Airways Disease

In children with reactive airways disease (RAD), a detailed past medical history must be obtained to determine the severity of the disease and the effectiveness of current medical treatment. Recurrent emergency visits and hospital admissions, especially those to critical care units and/or involving the use of steroids, are red flags for poor control of symptoms. Mild asthma that is poorly controlled may improve with more aggressive treatment, whereas well-controlled severe RAD may require sustained optimized therapy. In a patient with active or recent bronchospasms, elective surgery should be postponed for 4 to 6 weeks. If surgery is required, preinduction treatment with a β_2-agonist is recommended to minimize respiratory complications (Scalfaro et al., 2001). Recent steroid use may require perioperative stress-dose steroid coverage (see Chapter 36, Systemic Disorders).

Congenital Heart Disease

Children with congenital heart disease (CHD) may require antibiotic prophylaxis preoperatively for the prevention of bacterial endocarditis. Recommendations by the American Heart Association (AHA) were updated by Wilson et al. in 2007. The recommendations can also be downloaded from the AHA website at *http://www.americanheart.org*. The guidelines for the AHA subacute bacterial endocarditis (SBE) prophylaxis, which were formulated by an AHA writing group with input from national and international experts, have been significantly modified. CHD conditions associated with the highest risk for SBE are listed as follows:

1. Unrepaired cyanotic lesions,
2. Repaired CHD with prosthetic material within 6 months of the procedure, and
3. Repaired CHD with residual defects at the site or adjacent to the site of a prosthetic patch or prosthetic device (which inhibit endothelialization).

Prophylaxis is only recommended for "dental procedures that involve manipulation of gingival tissue or the periapical region of teeth or perforation of the oral mucosa" and "invasive procedure of the respiratory tract that involves incision or biopsy of the respiratory mucosa, such as tonsillectomy and adenoidectomy" (Wilson et al., 2007). Standard antibiotic recommendations include amoxicillin PO or ampicillin IV 50 mg/kg (maximum dose 2 g) 30 to 60 minutes before the procedure. Alternative antibiotics for those patients allergic to penicillin or ampicillin include clindamycin, cefazolin, ceftriaxone, azithromycin, or clarithromycin.

Animal studies indicate that if the preoperative SBE dose is missed, the effective prophylaxis can be given within 2 hours (but not after 4 hours) after the procedure (Berney and Francioli, 1990; Dajani et al., 1997).

Preoperative Fasting

Preoperative fasting times allow for gastric emptying and reduction of aspiration risk. Evidence of rapid gastric emptying in infants and children and efforts to improve the perioperative experience of young patients and their families have resulted in liberalization of pediatric fasting guidelines. Based on clinical observation and studies of residual gastric volumes, international recommendations for NPO times before anesthetic induction in healthy children are 2 hours for clear liquids, 3 to 4 hours for breast milk, 4 hours for infant formula (in infants younger than 3 months), 6 hours for infant formula (in infants older than 6 months), 6 hours for light meals, and 8 hours for heavy meals (Schreiner et al., 1990; Litman et al., 1994; Cook-Sather et al., 2003; Søreide et al., 2005; Murat and Dubois, 2008). This growing consensus has given rise to the 2-4-6 rule. Although these fasting times do not apply to children with gastrointestinal or systemic disorders that may interfere with or slow gastric emptying, Cook-Sather and colleagues (2009) have reported that even in overweight and obese children undergoing elective surgery, the 2-hour minimum preoperative clear-liquid fasting guideline is adequate.

Allowing infants and children to have oral intake closer to the time of surgery can help reduce patient irritability, parental stress, and risk of dehydration. Conversely, the short and multiple fasting times can lead to confusion and NPO violations. It is extremely important that those giving and receiving instruction on preoperative food and fluid intake clearly understand the terminology (i.e., what constitutes a clear liquid), timing, and need for adherence to the guidelines (Schoenfelder et al., 2006). A clear liquid is a solution (as opposed to a suspension) that contains no particulate matter. Examples of clear liquids include water, Pedialyte, carbonated beverages, clear tea, plain gelatin, and fruit juices without pulp (American Society of Anesthesiologists, 1999; Ferrari et al., 1999).

Preanesthetic Preparations

The preoperative interview, which is essential for obtaining pertinent positive and negative findings in the patient's history and physical condition, may be the only opportunity for the anesthesiologist to assess child-family anxiety and establish a relationship of trust and confidence. Successful interaction with children requires skill and experience, but more importantly it requires honesty and playfulness. Most centers have presurgical tours and/or short movies to prepare children and families for the perioperative experience. Children are typically encouraged to bring a familiar object or favorite toy, and most pediatric waiting areas are designed as playrooms that are supplied with everything from busy boxes to video games. The anesthesiologist should take advantage of these preoperative tools during the preoperative interview. They should sit at the child's eye level and initiate communication based on the child's present activity. If the child offers an opening, such as asking to see their stethoscope, they should follow their lead. The anesthesiologist should express genuine interest or play with the child. This may help gain the child's confidence and divert or reduce fear and anxiety. Tone of voice and facial expression should be calm and friendly for all age groups. Infants can be engaged with varying facial expressions and games of "peek-a-boo." Good humor and empathy will go a long way in alleviating patient and family stress and anxiety.

Most children can be well managed in this friendly environment. An anesthesia mask may be given to the child to play with in the waiting area before induction (Fig. 13-1). Allowing children to choose a flavor (e.g., bubble gum, cherry, or grape) can provide them with a sense of control. The additional support of pacifiers, toys, and music boxes is often helpful.

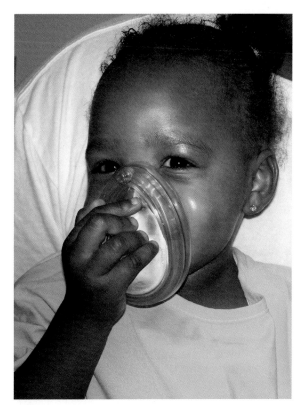

■ **FIGURE 13-1.** An anesthesia mask may be given to the child to play with in the waiting area before induction.

Children should keep the objects brought from home, particularly security blankets or other transitional objects, during the induction of anesthesia. Clowns have also been used for the prevention of preoperative anxiety in children (Vagnoli et al., 2005; Golan et al., 2009).

Family responses, questions, and interactions with the child are important to note. It is essential for the pediatric anesthesiologist to include patients and families in decisions regarding anesthetic induction and care. Together they should agree on the needs for premedication, parental presence, and the type of induction technique (inhalation vs. intravenous) to ensure the smoothest and safest induction possible. Unfortunately, even the best of plans can fail, and back-up measures such as another premedicant, induction room, or means of induction, must be readily at hand. For older, combative children scheduled for elective procedure, postponing the procedure until the child is properly prepared should be considered. Inhalation induction by force should be a measure of last resort.

Premedication

As stated above, the use of premedication is the most reliably effective intervention for reducing preinduction anxiety and stress for young patients and their parents. Preoperative medications are described in detail in Chapter 9, Preoperative Preparation, and are discussed only briefly here. Historically, premedication referred to long-acting sedatives and anticholinergic agents that were often given intramuscularly (IM) or rectally (PR) to prepare children in inpatients' units for their trip to the operating room. Contemporary administration of sedatives, typically by mouth, is administered just before induction to facilitate child-parent separation, anesthetic mask acceptance, and/or patient cooperation. IM administration is almost now solely reserved for extremely agitated, uncontrollable children.

Benzodiazepines

Midazolam, a water-soluble benzodiazepine, is the most commonly used preinduction medication (Kain et al., 1997). Given orally at 0.5 mg/kg mixed with fruit-flavored syrup, midazolam will create a calm, euphoric, or drowsy state in most children within 15 to 30 minutes. To potentiate its effect, children should be kept in a nonstimulating environment, and ambulatory children who may become unsteady should be held carefully on the parent's lap or placed in bed. Coté et al. (2002) showed that a wider range of doses can be effective, adjusting for time of onset, and that respiratory compromise does not occur in otherwise healthy, unmedicated children. Paradoxical reactions, including restlessness, agitation, and disinhibition, occur in approximately 1% to 3% of patients (McMillan et al., 1992; Golparvar et al., 2004). The bitter taste of midazolam, which is difficult to conceal, may reduce acceptance. Midazolam can also be administered via nasal mucosal delivery at 0.2 mg/kg with a more rapid onset but has the disadvantage of an unpleasant burning sensation (Zedie et al., 1996). Prolonged recovery times are not seen with the use of midazolam premedication (Davis et al., 1995b; Bevan et al., 1997). Acetaminophen (20 mg/kg), in fruit-flavored syrup, can also be mixed with midazolam as part of premedication for postoperative analgesia, especially for short ear cases, such as myringotomies (Watcha et al., 1992).

Opioids

The use of opioids for premedication is uncommon in healthy children who are undergoing elective procedures. Even with noninvasive delivery systems such as oral transmucosal fentanyl citrate (OTFC), the advantage of relatively rapid onset is offset by the disadvantages of dysphoria, pruritus, nausea, and vomiting (Goldstein-Dressner, 1991; Ashburn et al., 1993; Epstein et al., 1996). Opioid premedication is best reserved for children experiencing pain, in which analgesia and sedation can be synergistic. The risk of respiratory depression, especially in infants younger than 6 months of age, should always be taken into account.

Ketamine

Ketamine can be given via the oral, nasal, rectal, or IM route (Stewart et al., 1990; Gutstein et al., 1992; Weksler et al., 1993; Tanaka et al., 2000). Ketamine is an effective sedative, but it can also cause increased secretions, nausea, vomiting, psychological disturbances, and prolonged recovery. IM injection of ketamine, 2 to 3 mg/kg (undiluted) may be useful in uncooperative, combative children as the last resort to avoid inhalation induction by force, which increases the risk of physical and psychological trauma to patients (Hannallah and Patel, 1989).

Alpha 2-Adrenergic Receptor Agonists

Oral (4 mcg/kg) and rectal (5 mcg/kg) clonidine can produce excellent perioperative sedation and anxiolysis while reducing the anesthetic requirement, emergence agitation, and postoperative pain, shivering, nausea, and vomiting (Bergendahl et al., 2004; Schmidt et al., 2007; Tazeroualti et al., 2007). The prolonged postoperative sedation seen with clonidine premedication may be advantageous after major surgical procedures but can delay discharge for same-day surgery patients. Similar findings have been described with transmucosal dexmedetomidine 0.5 to 1 mcg/kg (Schmidt et al., 2007; Yuen et al., 2008).

Topical Anesthesia

For children who require or prefer an intravenous (IV) induction, there are multiple approaches to achieving topical anesthesia. Local anesthetics can be delivered without needles through the skin's protective stratum corneum into the innervated dermal layers via eutectic (EMLA) and liposomal (EL-MAX) creams or driven by mechanisms such as heat, iontophoresis, laser-assistance, or pressurized helium (Hung et al., 1997; Baron et al., 2003; Zempsky et al., 2004; 2008; Sawyer et al., 2009). These techniques, each with limitations, are capable of providing analgesia within 1 to 60 minutes of application. Reported satisfactory anesthesia varies with technique and patient age. Children younger than 6 or 7 years of age tend to report pain secondary to fear and anticipation of needlesticks, even with apparent anesthesia (Arts et al., 1994; Kleiber et al., 2002).

Parental Presence During Induction

Parental presence during induction of anesthesia (PPIA), in the operating room or a separate area such as an induction room, has increased significantly in the United States over the last decade

(Kain et al., 2004). Although the practice avoids separating children from their parents, it has not been shown to decrease patient anxiety or increase cooperation during induction (Kain et al., 1998; Arai et al., 2007). One benefit, which is important in terms of family-centered care, is an increase in parental satisfaction scores. Kain and colleagues, in 2006, confirmed the previous findings of Bevan et al. from 1990 that PPIA had a measurable benefit when a calm parent accompanied an anxious child, and a worsening effect when an anxious parent accompanied a calm child. There was no measurable benefit when both parent and child were calm. Subsequently, they have determined that parental preparation to reduce anxiety (e.g., learning distraction techniques, and avoiding reassuring behavior) can significantly improve the outcome of PPIA (Kain et al., 2007).

The logistical disadvantages of PPIA in the operating room include limited space, noise, unfamiliar equipment, and the need for parents to wear gowns and masks. Induction rooms can help anesthesiologists avoid some of these problems, but in both settings the parents must be prepared for the changes that can occur during induction, especially rapid loss of consciousness, uncoordinated movements, increased respiratory rate, and signs of upper airway obstruction. The anesthesiologist should be prepared to reassure the parent and respond quickly, especially if something goes wrong during induction. Parents need to be escorted to the waiting room as soon as their child loses consciousness.

Preparation for Induction

In the operating room or an induction room, anesthetic and monitoring equipment and supplies must be complete, confirmed, and readily available. The preinduction checklist for equipment should include a checked anesthesia machine, the gas pressures of accessory oxygen and nitrous oxide cylinders, an air-tight breathing circuit, the availability of a self-inflating bag, working suction, size-appropriate airway supplies (larger, smaller, and predicted, and including face masks, oral and nasal airways, laryngoscope blades and endotracheal tubes), and medications for induction and maintenance of anesthesia, as well as emergency medications. With the exception of patients suffering from malignant hyperthermia, emergency drugs for all pediatric inductions are atropine and succinylcholine, which should always be drawn into syringes of an appropriate size for the patient's age and weight and clearly labeled in case of severe laryngospasm. Supplies for starting and securing IV access should be prepared. Additional ancillary equipment such as tongue depressors, adhesive tape, and soft suction catheters should also be at hand. If laryngeal mask airway (LMA) use is planned, appropriate size LMAs should be included in the set up. Monitoring devices, such as an in-flow oxygen analyzer, a pulse oximeter, a capnograph, an electrocardiograph (ECG), and an automated blood pressure cuff, should all be checked and ready. The temperature of the operating room should be properly adjusted and warming devices (e.g., Bair Hugger and other warming blanket or a radiant heat lamp) should be used.

Monitoring During Induction

At a minimum, monitoring during induction should include pulse oximetry and capnography. The precordial stethoscope, once the *sine qua non* of pediatric anesthesia, has apparently been displaced by more accurate and adaptable monitors (Watson and Visram, 2001). However, the precordial stethoscope is still an essential and more sensitive and continuous monitor for changes in breath sounds and the quality of heart beat, especially in infants and young children. Vital signs can vary markedly during the induction of anesthesia and should be observed continuously with a precordial stethoscope and in accordance with the ASA standards for patient safety (1986). If the child is anxious, it is probably best to place additional monitors like ECG pads and a blood pressure cuff after induction instead of losing the opportunity for a calm induction. However, medical condition and early infancy may necessitate full monitoring before and during induction. If this is the case, the baseline measurements should be obtained before the patient is exposed to any anesthetic agent.

Methods of Induction

There are many approaches for safely inducing general anesthesia in children. The particular technique chosen depends on the patient's age; surgical procedure; underlying illness; discharge disposition; and in part, the preference of the anesthesiologist, the patient, and their family. The induction methods include: inhalational, IV, IM, and various combinations of these techniques.

Inhalation Induction

Whether sedated or awake, accompanied or alone, lying down or sitting up, a child breathing sevoflurane with or without nitrous oxide through a mask and circuit will become anesthetized. It is this simple fact that has made inhalation induction the most commonly used technique in pediatric anesthesia in the United States. In this manner, the induction of anesthesia is achieved with relative ease, speed, and safety, while avoiding the fear and pain of intravenous catheter insertion. Successfully selecting the approach, guiding the child and family through the process, and smoothly adapting to their needs is the challenge and reward of pediatric anesthesia induction.

When transitioning a child from the preoperative area to the site of induction, it is paramount that the well-sedated or asleep child is minimally stimulated or disturbed and that the awake or lightly sedated child is kept occupied and distracted by an anesthesiologist or family member. One person, either the anesthesiologist or a family member, should do all the talking, which should be reassuring and continuous. Giving patients and families the choice to have the child carried, walked, or wheeled to the induction location is another way to encourage participation and give them a sense of control. Perioperative staff need to remain quiet immediately before and during the induction, or they should be asked to step away. Regardless of location, age of the patient, or intended procedure, induction of anesthesia should be completely focused on the child and uninterrupted by other activities or last-minute preparations.

Once in the operating or induction room, the child may be given the choice to lie down or sit up. If sitting is elected and parents are present, the child can be offered the option to sit in a parent's lap or next to them (Fig. 13-2). The anesthetic mask, either one introduced in the waiting area or one detached from

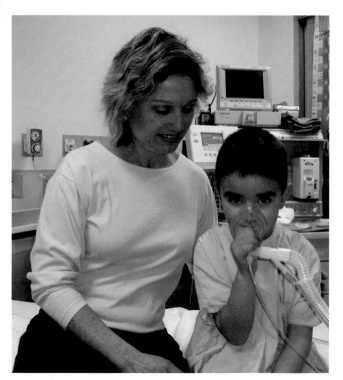

■ **FIGURE 13-2.** Sitting up during induction of anesthesia is an option. If parents are present, the child can sit in a parent's lap or next to a parent.

the anesthesia circuit, should be shown (again) to the child. Putting artificial fruit or candy flavors in the mask may help disguise the odor of the anesthetic. One should never place the mask on the child's face without warning. Even with preparation, some children, especially those with previous experience with inhalation inductions, may strongly reject the anesthesia mask (Przybylo et al., 2005). The mask may become more acceptable if a family or staff member initially tries it on, or if the anesthesiologist applies it to one of the child's toys or random body parts before placing it near his or her face. Other methods to introduce the mask include having the child watch the insufflation of the anesthetic bag or hold the mask him or herself as he or she begins to breathe into the circuit. Making a game out of this activity is far better than getting into battle of wills. Distraction techniques such as storytelling, singing, counting, or just talking nonsense are strongly encouraged. If the child still emphatically objects to the mask, other approaches such as supplemental sedation or an IV induction should be considered.

One way to initiate inhalation induction and avoid a negative reaction to the smell of the inhalation agent is to begin with a high flow of nitrous oxide and oxygen at a 2:1 ratio. The mask should be loosely applied to the child's face until sedation is evident. The full sedative effect of nitrous oxide will occur within 2 minutes and be observable as the respiratory rate slows. Sevoflurane can then be added and increased rapidly to 6% to 8%. Except in young infants, short exposure to high concentrations of sevoflurane does not cause significant hemodynamic changes. Timing of the introduction of sevoflurane, the rapidity of increase, and the distraction techniques employed should vary with the child and family's mood, level of anxiety, and degree of cooperation. Hyperventilation should be discouraged to avoid apnea

during the induction. If the child objects to the smell of the inhaled anesthetic, breathing through the mouth to reduce the smell can be suggested.

DuBois et al. (1999) compared three induction techniques of conventional tidal-volume breathing of sevoflurane: incremental increasing concentrations (2% to 6% to 8%) in 100% oxygen, 8% in 100% oxygen, and 8% in a 1:1 mixture of nitrous oxide and oxygen. There were minimal differences among the three approaches. Lejus and colleagues (2006) compared the two different breathing techniques of conventional tidal volume and single-breath vital capacity of 7% sevoflurane in children older than 5 years of age. Eyelash-reflex loss was more rapid in the vital-capacity group compared with the tidal-volume group, but the time to deep anesthesia, bispectral index values 60 and 40, and the incidences of side effects were similar in both groups. Of note, the vital-capacity technique was preferred over the tidal-volume technique by the children. The authors propose that the decreased exposure to the smell of sevoflurane and decreased awareness of losing consciousness explained the higher preference scores in the vital-capacity group.

If a child has fallen asleep or is well sedated in a parent's arms or on a stretcher, anesthesia can be induced by the "steal technique," as originally described by Guedel in 1921 (Calverley, 1986). While avoiding moving or awakening the child, 70% nitrous oxide at high flows via an anesthesia mask is held closely over the child's face. At first the mask should not touch the skin, but as sedation deepens it is placed gently on the face while incrementally increasing the concentration of sevoflurane. Monitoring devices should be attached as soon as possible. Once adequately anesthetized, the child can be transferred to a stretcher or operating-room bed if needed.

Once the patient has accepted the mask and is breathing the inhalation agent, it is extremely important to closely follow the progress of induction. The first sign is usually nystagmus, especially if nitrous oxide is being used. The eyes then usually close; the limbs and head may relax; and respiration becomes slower, regular, and deeper—then shallower and more rapid. Often children will have uncoordinated movements during the hyperreflexic phase of anesthesia and develop "snoring" or noisy breathing as the anesthetic depth deepens and as the patient develops partial upper airway obstruction. Although prepared for this preoperatively, parents should be reminded and reassured that this is normal during the induction of anesthesia. Until the eyelash reflex is gone, nothing should be done to move or stimulate the patient, unless airway obstruction or a similar need arises. Nurses and surgeons should not touch the patient without getting permission from the anesthesiologist. As soon as anesthesia is induced and the patient can tolerate moderately painful stimuli, an IV catheter can be started.

Unless excessive fluid or blood loss is anticipated, a 20-gauge catheter for children and a 22- or 24-gauge catheter for infants and small children fulfill the need for routine elective procedures. It is an error to use small-gauge catheters in infants and children merely because of their size. If adequate percutaneous sites are not available, use of a central venous catheter or surgical cut-downs may be indicated. Conversely, in children undergoing relatively minor procedures where major fluid shifts or blood loss are not anticipated, it is much better to have a working 22-gauge IV rather than a nonfunctioning 20-gauge catheter or multiple infiltrated IVs in an attempt to get larger venous access. If a scalp vein is used, caution is advised. Inadvertent subcutaneous injection of certain drugs, such as calcium, can cause tissue destruction and sloughing of the scalp.

Maintenance of the Upper-Airway Patency

Upper airway obstruction can arise during induction of anesthesia (even in healthy infants and children) for several reasons, including tongue displacement, excess soft tissue, velopharyngeal collapse, and laryngospasm. Applying pressure to the soft tissue between the rami of the mandible when holding a mask on a patient's face can push the tongue against the hard and soft palate or displace it posteriorly, leading to occlusion of the oral pharynx or its outlet, respectively. Even minimal relaxation of the pharyngeal and laryngeal muscles during induction can significantly reduce oral and nasal passages already compromised by enlarged or increased amounts of lymphoid tissue. Relaxation of the pharyngeal and laryngeal muscles, accompanied by a marked increase in respiratory effort and excessive generation of negative pressure, which can occur in response to pain and other stimulation, may result in collapse of the velopharynx. To prevent upper airway obstruction from these causes, the pediatric anesthesiologist must learn to hold the anesthesia mask snugly to the patient's face and perform the triple airway maneuver—neck extension, jaw thrust, and mouth opening—without applying pressure to the soft tissue or causing pain (Fig. 13-3). In addition, a moderate amount of continuous positive airway pressure (CPAP; 10 to 15 cm H_2O) can counteract the collapsing force on the relaxed airway (Motoyama, 1997; Hammer et al., 2001). Careful and

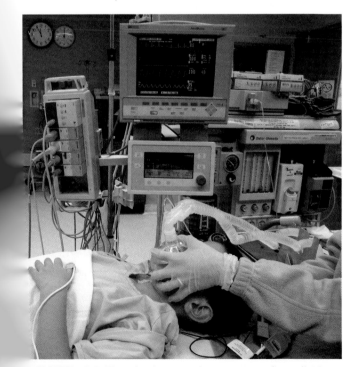

FIGURE 13-3. To maintain upper airway patency, the pediatric anesthesiologist holds the anesthesia mask snugly to the patient's face and performs the triple airway maneuver—neck extension, jaw thrust, and mouth opening—without applying pressure to the soft tissue or causing pain.

continuous monitoring of breath sounds via a precordial stethoscope is essential to guide and maximize the effectiveness of upper-airway maintenance by hand.

When the patient is sufficiently anesthetized, an oropharyngeal airway may be inserted to further aid in maintaining a patent airway. Insertion of an oral airway in an inadequately anesthetized patient risks triggering laryngospasm. The proper length of an oral airway, with the tip behind the base of the tongue, can be estimated by holding the airway over the side of the child's face extending from the ear to the angle of the mandible. A preferred method for inserting an oral airway is to slide it gently forward and downward over the tongue while the tongue is pulled outward by a tongue depressor. The technique of inserting the airway upside down and then correcting the orientation in the posterior pharynx should be avoided in children. It tends to push the tongue posteriorly and obstruct the oral pharynx, particularly in infants (Smith, 1980). A nasopharyngeal airway is better tolerated when the anesthesia is too light for insertion of an oropharyngeal airway. This type of airway should be well lubricated and inserted very gently to prevent mucosal injury and bleeding.

If the obstruction is not relieved by airway maneuvers, the patient may have laryngospasm, which can result from laryngeal mucosal irritation and is often initiated by the aspiration of saliva. Vigorous positive pressure ventilation may push the secretions down into the larynx, which intensifies the spasm and further inflates the stomach, compromising pulmonary gas exchange. The risk of regurgitation and aspiration of gastric contents also increases. A healthy child can tolerate a few moments of laryngospasm. A more successful approach is to maintain moderate continuous positive pressure and synchronous ventilation with the "expiratory" phase of laryngospasm, which is when the vocal cords momentarily relax. By using 100% oxygen and intermittent positive pressure, one can ventilate enough gas through the glottis to avoid serious hypoxemia. If rapid oxygen desaturation and bradycardia ensue, IV succinylcholine (2 mg/kg) and atropine (0.02 mg/kg) or 5 mg/kg of IM succinylcholine should be administered without delay (Liu et al., 1981; Hannallah et al., 1986). Airway patency needs to be reestablished with or without tracheal intubation.

Intravenous Induction

In children and adults, induction via the IV route has the advantage of speed and avoids the unpleasant odors and sensations of an inhalation induction. The major disadvantage involves the difficulty and fear associated with venipuncture in young children. Topical anesthetic, as discussed previously, can significantly reduce pain associated with catheter insertion if it is used appropriately and enough time is allowed. Children younger than 6 or 7 years of age have shown less overall benefit from the use of topical anesthetics than older children, probably because the fact that young children, although numb, continue to associate needles with pain. Children who are 8 to 10 years of age and older may prefer an IV induction to a mask, often because they have unpleasant memories from a previous experience. Dorsal hand, radial, and if needed, antecubital veins are typically most visible, accessible, and acceptable sites for IV catheter insertion. Wrist, foot, and saphenous veins are other possibilities, but they are difficult to access unless the extremity is immobilized and the skin is anesthetized.

The anesthesiologist should always be honest with children, explaining each step of the procedure without frightening them. Using distraction techniques during the placement of the catheter is superior for reducing pain and agitation, compared with using encouragement and complements on good behavior or courage. Before the delivery of any medications, the anesthesiologist should ensure that the IV catheter is easily flushed to avoid inadvertent subcutaneous infusions. Securing the IV insertion site is particularly important in children, because they often emerge in an uncooperative and agitated state. The extremity in which the catheter is inserted should be taped to a cushioned board with a loop of IV tubing to prevent accidental pull and removal of the catheter.

Propofol

An induction dose of propofol is 2.5 to 3.0 mg/kg in healthy unpremedicated children between the ages of 3 and 12 years (Manschot et al., 1992). In induction studies, children younger than 2 years of age required a significantly larger dose (2.6 to 3.4 mg/kg), whereas older children needed less (Aun et al., 1992; Manschot et al., 1992). Induction with propofol in children can cause significant decreases in blood pressure and inotropy, similar to those observed after thiopental (Mirakhur, 1988; Hannallah et al., 1991; Manschot et al., 1992).

A major drawback to propofol is the pain it causes on injection. In a quantitative systematic review, Picard and Tramèr (2000) determined that the only approach that had a reliably low number of needed-to-be-treated (NNT) patients was the lidocaine-tourniquet technique (similar to a Bier block; see Chapter 16, Regional Anesthesia) and that preinjection of local lidocaine and analgesics, temperature of medication, speed of infusion, and vein size had no significant effect. Yew et al. (2005) and Rochette et al. (2008) have shown that the addition of medium-chain triglyceride to propofol preparation also decreases pain on injection. Propofol offers the advantage of having antiemetic properties (Borgeat et al., 1990).

Thiopental

The induction dose of thiopental in healthy children is 5 to 6 mg/kg (Coté et al., 1981). In infants between 1 and 6 months of age, the median effective dose (ED50) is reported to be 6.8 mg/kg; in infants younger than 2 weeks of age, it is 3.4 mg/kg (Jonmarker et al., 1987). The dose for induction in infants younger than 5 months was almost twice that for older children (see Chapter 7, Pharmacology of Pediatric Anesthesia, Fig. 7-18). Like propofol, thiopental is a cardiac depressant and vasodilator, and it should be used with care in patients suspected to have hypovolemia or decreased cardiac function.

Etomidate

The induction dose of etomidate in healthy children is 0.3 mg/kg, and it is often recommended in patients who have limited hemodynamic reserve. Sarkar and colleagues (2005) confirmed that in children there are no significant changes in right atrial, aortic, or pulmonary artery pressure, or systemic or pulmonary vascular resistance after bolus dosing. Side effects include pain on injection and myoclonic movements.

Ketamine

Ketamine is a dissociative anesthetic, and a dose of 2 mg/kg produces a catatonic-like state in children within 1 to 2 minutes. Its ability to stimulate the release of endogenous catecholamine and subsequently elevate heart rate and blood pressure and dilate bronchial airways supports its use in patients who may benefit from these properties. Ketamine increases oral and airway secretions and is associated with psychological and behavioral sequelae in children. To minimize these side effects, antisialagogues (glycopyrrolate, 0.1 mg/kg) and benzodiazepines (0.5 mg/kg) are recommended, respectively.

MAINTENANCE OF ANESTHESIA

After induction, the anesthesiologist is responsible for maintaining patient analgesia, amnesia, and immobility, as well as maintaining autonomic and hemodynamic stability to allow for optimum working conditions for surgical procedures. Today, a balanced anesthetic technique that is tailored toward each patient and accounts for his or her medical conditions, as well as the surgical procedure and planned postoperative management, is preferred. To do this, the anesthesiologist has several options with respect to anesthetic drugs, including inhalational versus intravenous agents. Adjuvant drugs for pain control, muscle relaxation, and prevention of postoperative nausea and vomiting are also used. Furthermore, in certain patients, regional anesthesia allows for improved pain control with a reduction in the use of opioids that can have significant side effects.

During the maintenance phase, the anesthesiologist must always be vigilant, with careful and continual monitoring of anesthetic depth, oxygenation, ventilation, cardiovascular function, fluid balance, body temperature, and glucose and electrolyte levels. In more critically ill patients, the anesthesiologist may need to place more invasive monitors for more accurate observation of the patient's status. Ultimately, the anesthesiologist is the patient's advocate in the operating room, communicating with the surgeons and allowing for a safe, comfortable, and successful outcome in the perioperative period.

Pharmacologic Agents

Inhaled Anesthetics

Inhaled anesthetics are the most commonly used agents in the administration of general anesthesia in pediatric patients. Although halothane was a staple in pediatric anesthesia for years, the development of newer agents with better safety profiles has made halothane nearly obsolete (Lerman, 2004). With discontinuation of the production of halothane in the United States, sevoflurane, desflurane, and isoflurane are now the most commonly used inhalation agents. Nitrous oxide is also commonly used as an adjunct, although there remains some controversy regarding its use.

Introduced in 1995, sevoflurane became the agent of choice for inhalation inductions. In addition to its rapid and smooth induction of anesthesia, sevoflurane causes few arrhythmias, less cardiovascular depression, and minimal renal or hepatic toxicities, all of which are improvements over halothane

TABLE 13-1. Characteristics of Volatile Anesthetics

	Molecular Weight (Da)	Boiling Point (°C)	Vapor Pressure at 20° C (mm Hg)	Blood Gas Partition Coefficent	MAC (%) Infant (1-6 mo)	Child (3-10 yr)
Isoflurane	184.5	48.5	239	1.4	1.7	1.6
Desflurane	168.0	23.5	664	0.4	9.4	8.0
Sevoflurane	200.1	58.5	160	0.6	3.3	2.5

(Lerman, 2004). Isoflurane and desflurane also have more stable cardiovascular profiles and less associated toxicity compared with halothane. However, each agent has limitations that warrant consideration in certain patients and clinical situations. Table 13-1 summarizes the characteristics of the commonly used volatile anesthetics.

Nitrous Oxide

Nitrous oxide is the oldest and has been the most widely used anesthetic in both adults and children. It has an inoffensive odor and a very low solubility (blood-gas partition coefficient of 0.47) that results in rapid uptake and distribution. Because it has a minimum alveolar concentration of 104% for general anesthesia, nitrous oxide cannot be used as a sole anesthetic at normal atmospheric pressures. Therefore, it is generally used as an adjunct to reduce the minimum alveolar concentration of a primary inhalation agent, increasing the rate of induction of general anesthesia, as well as providing or augmenting the analgesic aspect of general anesthesia (Emmanouil and Quock, 2007).

Nitrous oxide has mechanisms of action that continue to be discovered. It appears that the anesthetic effect occurs through inhibition of N-methyl-d-aspartate (NMDA) glutamate receptors in the central nervous system. Analgesia occurs through release of endogenous opioids that then stimulate opioid receptors and spinal level γ-aminobutyric acid (GABA) receptors. Anxiolysis occurs through activation of GABA$_A$, although this pathway is still being investigated (Emmanouil and Quock, 2007).

Although nitrous oxide is widely used, there are certain patients and clinical situations in which its use is not recommended and even contraindicated. In adults with pulmonary hypertension, nitrous oxide increases pulmonary artery and pulmonary wedge pressures (Schulte-Sasse et al., 1982). However, in healthy infants, Hickey and colleagues (1986) observed mild decreases in heart rate, blood pressure, and cardiac index with no increase in pulmonary artery pressure or vascular resistance.

Nitrous oxide accumulates in closed, gas-containing spaces and should be avoided in patients at risk of toxicity caused by this expansion. This includes patients with obstructed loops of bowel, pneumothorax, pneumocephalus, and middle-ear surgery. Nitrous oxide also has been shown to increase middle cerebral-artery blood-flow velocity and may increase intracranial pressure (ICP), making its use in children with increased ICP contraindicated (Wilson-Smith et al., 2003). Furthermore, in situations in which maximal oxygen delivery is needed, such as shock, massive blood loss, severe anemia, and compromised cerebrospinal blood flow, nitrous oxide should be avoided. Children with abnormal vitamin B$_{12}$ and B$_{12}$-related metabolism may also be at risk of neurologic injury after exposure to nitrous oxide during a routine anesthetic procedure (Sanders et al., 2008).

The role of nitrous oxide in postoperative nausea and vomiting (PONV) has been examined extensively. Although the incidence was increased when used with propofol, no difference was seen in the incidence of PONV with or without nitrous oxide when used with sevoflurane or desflurane in children (Watcha et al., 1991; Kuhn et al., 1999; Bortone et al., 2002). Nitrous oxide supports combustion. Thus, its use in patients undergoing oral or facial procedures should be reevaluated with regard to the possibility of an airway fire.

Sevoflurane

Since its introduction in the mid 1990s, sevoflurane has replaced halothane as the agent of choice for inhalation inductions in pediatric patients. It is a fluorinated methyl isopropyl ether with a blood-gas partition coefficient of 0.68, allowing for rapid induction and recovery. With a nonpungent odor and minimal airway irritation, up to 8% sevoflurane can be delivered without significant breath holding, coughing, or laryngospasm. The minimum alveolar concentration (MAC) of sevoflurane decreases from 3.3% in neonates and infants younger than 6 months old to 2.5% in children between 6 months and 5 years old and to 2.0% in adults (Hatch, 1999). Lerman and colleagues (1994) found that the MAC-sparing effect of nitrous oxide was significantly less for sevoflurane.

Sevoflurane causes minimal cardiovascular side effects in children. Compared with desflurane, sevoflurane produces less hypotension. There is also less tachycardia than isoflurane and less myocardial depression than halothane (Frink et al., 1992b; Holzman et al., 1996). Using echocardiography, Wodey et al. (1997) found that sevoflurane did not affect heart rate, cardiac index, or myocardial contractility. Furthermore, it does not sensitize the myocardium to epinephrine (Hayashi et al., 1987). Arrhythmias are uncommon with sevoflurane compared with other agents (Hatch, 1999).

Sevoflurane affects respiratory function, with some studies suggesting it does so to a greater extent than other agents (Doi et al., 1994; Yamakage et al., 1994). Brown and colleagues (1998) found that compared with halothane, minute ventilation and respiratory frequency were lower in infants on 1 MAC of sevoflurane, but that there were only moderately increased end-tidal carbon dioxide (CO$_2$) levels. Sevoflurane is, however, an effective bronchodilator (May et al., 1996). Neurologically, sevoflurane has been associated with cortical epileptiform electroencephalograms, although no lasting clinical sequelae (such as seizures) have been attributed to sevoflurane alone. Further studies are necessary to determine which patients are at risk and what can be done to decrease the incidence of these EEG changes (Constant et al., 2005).

As much as 5% of sevoflurane is metabolized, with defluorination producing an inorganic fluoride that is then excreted in the urine. Peak fluoride concentrations, although higher in sevoflurane than in isoflurane, are still well below the accepted nephrotoxic level of 50 mmol/L. There is rapid elimination, and these levels remain below toxic levels even with prolonged anesthetics (Levine et al., 1996; Hatch, 1999). In addition, the metabolism of sevoflurane by the $P_{450}E_1$ system is mostly in the liver and not the kidneys. Thus, the concern of nephrogenic diabetes insipidus (DI) by elevated fluoride levels does not appear to be an issue.

Sevoflurane reacts with soda lime in the anesthesia circuit, resulting in the production of compound A. Compound A increases more when Baralyme brand (Allied Healthcare Products Inc., St. Louis, Mo) is used, when dry rather than wet absorbents are used, and when lower fresh gas flows (0.5 to 1 L) are used, resulting in increased canister temperatures (Frink et al., 1992a). Ebert and colleagues did not find evidence of renal injury after sevoflurane was administered in high concentrations (3% end-tidal) for 8 hours (1998). Kharasch and colleagues (1997) also found no significant renal dysfunction in patients with low-flow sevoflurane (1 L/min) when compound A was detected. Other studies have also documented no worsening of renal function after sevoflurane, even in patients with preexisting renal impairment (Conzen et al., 1995). New generation CO_2 absorbers, including DragerSorb Free and Amsorb Plus, have been shown to provide adequate CO_2 absorption while reducing the production of compound A, even at fresh gas flows as low as 500 mL/min (Marini et al., 2007).

Spontaneous ignition, fire, and explosion resulting from an exothermic reaction of sevoflurane with desiccated CO_2 absorbers have also been reported (Castro et al., 2004; Wu et al., 2004). With high fresh gas flow, the increasing dryness of the absorbent increases degradation of sevoflurane. Dunning et al. (2007) demonstrated that up to 3 mol of hydrogen were produced in the reaction of sevoflurane with heated, desiccated absorbent. The authors postulate that this hydrogen is the most likely fuel in anesthesia machine fires. Special attention should be paid to situations in which absorbent desiccation may be greater, such as in seldom-used anesthesia machines and in operating rooms where high fresh-gas flows relative to body size are used (Wu et al., 2004). The use of newer absorbents or Mapleson D circuits can also help avoid this problem (Woehlck, 2004).

While the question of sevoflurane-related hepatitis has been raised in case reports, metabolism of sevoflurane does not result in the trifluoroacetylated liver proteins that trigger the immune-mediated hepatitis seen with halothane, and immune-based hepatitis after sevoflurane has not been reported (Kharasch, 1995; 2008). Malignant hyperthermia has been reported with sevoflurane use (Otsuka et al., 1991).

Both postanesthetic emergence time and the time when discharge criteria are met are significantly lower in patients given sevoflurane compared with those receiving halothane; however, patients receiving sevoflurane had significantly higher pain scores that required analgesics to be administered earlier (Naito et al., 1991; Sarner et al., 1995). In a meta-analysis of randomized controlled trials, Kuratani and Oi (2008) demonstrated that sevoflurane had a higher probability of emergence agitation compared with halothane (Fig. 13-4). Treatment or pretreatment with either dexmedetomidine, fentanyl, or propofol can mitigate emergence agitation after sevoflurane anesthesia.

Desflurane

Desflurane is a fluorinated methyl ethyl ether with a blood:gas solubility coefficient of 0.42, which is close to nitrous oxide and lower than any other agent. With lower potency, the MAC in newborns is 9.2%, in infants it is 8% to 9.9%, and in older children and adults it is 6% (Hatch, 1999). Because of its lower boiling point (22.8° C), desflurane requires a heated pressurized vaporizer. It is also resistant to degradation and biotransformation.

Desflurane is highly irritating to the upper airway. Zwass and colleagues (1992) found that it caused moderate to severe laryngospasm in 49% of unpremedicated patients and moderate to severe coughing in 58%. These parameters did not improve with premedication. The authors concluded that desflurane, although safe for maintenance of anesthesia, was limited in its use for inhalation inductions. Recent changes in the package insert suggest that desflurane is not recommended for use in patients undergoing bag-and-mask ventilation or in patients with an LMA in place.

Studies in both adults and children have demonstrated a dose-related effect of desflurane on ventilation, with a decrease in tidal volume, minute ventilation, and the ventilatory response to CO_2. Respiratory rate was shown to increase (Lockhart et al., 1991; Behforouz et al., 1998). At 1 MAC, desflurane exhibits bronchodilator effects. However, with increasing concentration to 2 MAC, desflurane increased airway resistance as opposed to other inhalation agents that continued to produce bronchodilation (Dikmen et al., 2003). In children with known airway susceptibility, desflurane caused significant elevations in airway resistance and increased airway narrowing (von Ungern-Sternberg et al., 2008).

Desflurane has been shown to provide cardiovascular stability. Systemic vascular resistance decreases, which results in a decrease in systemic blood pressure without changes in cardiac output. Taylor and Lerman (1992) showed a mean percentage decrease in systolic arterial pressure of 29 + 13% from preanesthetic values in children, with the incidence of hypotension greatest in infants and least in children 5 to 12 years of age. These pressure differences, however, did not require intervention. Heart rate increases in a dose-dependent manner, and arrhythmias are uncommon. Sympathetic tone increases, but there does not appear to be increased sensitization of the myocardium to epinephrine as is seen with halothane (Hatch, 1999).

Because of its low blood:gas partition coefficient, desflurane allows for rapid emergence and recovery, which has been demonstrated in several studies of children (Taylor and Lerman, 1992; Welborn et al., 1996; Wolf et al., 1996). However, Welborn et al. (1996) found that recovery from desflurane was associated with a significantly greater incidence of agitation and excitement and that there was no difference in the time to meet discharge criteria as compared with other inhaled anesthetics. Wolf and colleagues (1996) found that desflurane, unlike isoflurane, was not associated with postoperative apnea and suggested that it may be useful in ex-premature infants. More recently, however, Sale et al. (2006) showed that although there was a faster time to awakening with desflurane, apnea did occur with desflurane and there was no difference between desflurane and sevoflurane

SEVOFLURANE AND EMERGENCE AGITATION

Study (ref. #)	Sevo n/N	Halo n/N	OR (95% CI)	Weight (%)	OR	(95% CI)
Cravero (16)	5/15	0/17		0.29	18.33	(0.92–366.2)
Villani (23)	3/32	0/32		0.42	7.71	(0.38–155.64)
Sury (20)	1/20	0/20		0.44	3.15	(0.12–82.16)
Rieger (25	21/22	17/19		0.78	2.47	(0.21–29.63)
Bebawy (26)	2/40	1/40		0.89	2.05	(0.18–23.59)
Hsieh (27)	8/20	2/20		1.13	6.00	(1.08–33.27)
Naito (28)	9/15	3/15		1.13	6.00	(1.17–30.72)
Weldon (14)	9/34	2/34		1.38	5.76	(1.14–29.08)
Johannesson (12)	14/22	4/18		1.50	6.13	(1.49–25.10)
Chiu (24)	3/20	2/20		1.60	1.59	(0.24–10.70)
Hallén (5)	3/30	2/30		1.69	1.56	(0.24–10.05)
Lerman (1)	19/250	2/125		2.31	5.06	(1.16–22.07)
Cravero (11)	12/21	6/22		2.36	3.56	(0.99–12.73)
Beskow (3)	12/31	7/31		4.03	2.17	(0.71–6.57)
Welborn (22)	1/20	5/20		4.46	0.16	(0.02–1.50)
Aono (2)	15/56	7/56		4.81	2.56	(0.95–6.88)
Galinkin (17)	17/133	7/127		5.86	2.51	(1.00–6.28)
Viitanen (21)	22/40	15/40		6.34	2.04	(0.83–4.98)
Lapin (18)	27/52	15/48		7.04	2.38	(1.05–5.38)
Murray (13)	31/64	20/66		9.53	2.16	(1.05–4.43)
Moore (19)	42/163	15/159		10.58	3.33	(1.76–6.30)
Kain (15)	25/52	26/52		12.67	0.93	(0.43–2.00)
Davis (4)	26/100	27/100		18.76	0.95	(0.51–1.78)
TOTAL	**327/1252**	**185/1111**		**100.00**	**2.21**	**(1.77–2.77)**

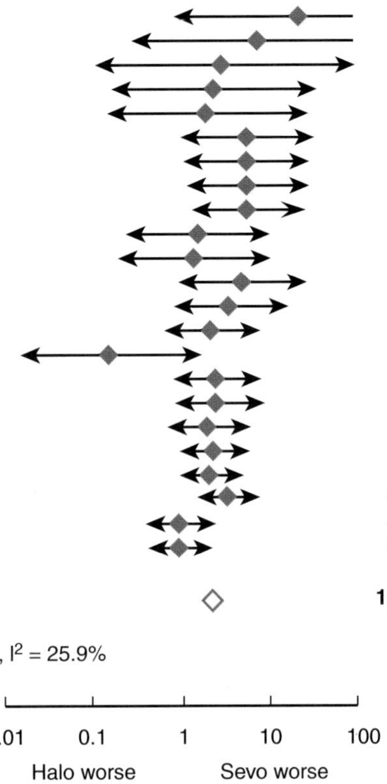

Test for heterogeneity: $x^2 = 29.69$, df = 22 (p = 0.13), $I^2 = 25.9\%$
Test for overall effect: z = 6.95 (p <0.00001)

0.01   0.1   1   10   100

Halo worse   Sevo worse

■ **FIGURE 13-4.** Meta-analysis of emergence agitation caused by sevoflurane *(Sevo)* versus halothane *(Halo)*. The center of each purple diamond is the odds ratio *(OR)* for individual trials, and the corresponding horizontal line is the 95% confidence interval *(CI)*. The open diamond is the pooled result. *(From Kuratani N, Oi Y: Greater incidence of emergence agitation in children after sevoflurane anesthesia as compared with halothane: a meta-analysis of randomized controlled trials,* Anesthesiology *109:229, 2008.)*

in the incidence of postoperative apnea in the ex-premature infant undergoing hernia repair (Kuratani et al., 2008).

Isoflurane

Isoflurane is a stable liquid that has a blood:gas partition coefficient of 1.4, which is much higher than both sevoflurane and desflurane. Like the other inhalation agents, the MAC of isoflurane is age-dependent, ranging from 1.3% in preterm infants to 1.7% in infants 6 to 12 months of age and decreasing to 1.6% in children 1 to 5 years old, compared with 1.2% in adults (Cameron et al., 1984; LeDez and Lerman, 1987). Because of its pungent odor, isoflurane causes coughing and laryngospasm, which precludes its use for inhalation inductions. Isoflurane is resistant to biodegradation, making the incidence of hepatotoxicity and nephrotoxicity minimal (Eger, 1984). The emergence profile is similar to that of halothane.

Like the other inhalation agents, isoflurane produces a dose-dependent respiratory depression, with an increase in respiratory rate and smaller tidal volumes that produce an increase in arterial CO_2 pressure. Isoflurane depresses ventilation to a greater extent than halothane, and isoflurane anesthesia requires mechanical ventilation (Eger, 1984). It is also a bronchodilator, with continued effects at higher concentrations (Dikmen et al., 2003).

Isoflurane, in a dose-dependent manner, decreases systemic vascular resistance, resulting in a subsequent drop in the systemic arterial pressure and increase in heart rate, all while maintaining cardiac output (Wolf et al., 1986). Tachycardia is particularly seen in younger patients (Eger, 1984). However, there is no reported increase in the incidence of arrhythmia, and it does not appear to sensitize the myocardium to epinephrine.

Isoflurane produces muscle relaxation and potentiates the intensity and duration of action of pancuronium and to a lesser extent vecuronium and atracurium. This results in the need to adjust dosing of these neuromuscular blockers accordingly.

Intravenous Agents

With more information available about IV agents and their pharmacokinetic and pharmacodynamic profiles in infants and children, their use has increased in these populations. Hypnotic and sedative agents, as well as the short-acting opioids, have been found to be both safe and effective in the pediatric population. In certain populations, including children who are susceptible to malignant hyperthermia, the use of total intravenous anesthesia (TIVA) has become essential.

The use of TIVA has both advantages and disadvantages. While TIVA allows for rapid recovery and does not require the sophisticated equipment needed to administer inhaled anesthetics, it can be associated with increased intraoperative awareness, prolonged recovery after long infusions, and the need for supplemental analgesia. In addition to this, newborns and young infants with immature hepatic enzyme systems and renal clearance can have significant accumulation of certain intravenous drugs. In the pediatric population, an inhalation induction for placement of an intravenous catheter often is done and negates some of the advantages of TIVA. All of these factors need to be considered when determining if TIVA is the ideal anesthetic for a particular patient.

Propofol

Propofol is a short-acting intravenous agent that is used for both induction and maintenance of anesthesia. With its fast onset, smooth maintenance, clear headed emergence, and decreased incidence of nausea and vomiting, it has many properties that make it ideal for TIVA. It is commonly used for procedures and sedation outside of the operating room, often as the sole agent in locations such as magnetic resonance imaging (MRI) and the endoscopy suite. Although propofol has no direct analgesic properties, patients receiving it seem to have lower analgesic requirements. At lower doses, it may not produce amnesia (Marik, 2004).

Propofol is highly lipid-soluble and rapidly cleared and redistributed into the peripheral tissues, with a short, context-sensitive half time (see Chapter 7, Pharmacology of Pediatric Anesthesia, Fig. 7-16). Relative to adults, children have a larger central compartment, and they have a higher clearance that can be twice that of adults, resulting in higher dosing requirements. Hannallah and colleagues (1994) showed that with a background of 60% nitrous oxide, pediatric patients required a dose of 250 to 300 mcg/kg per minute to prevent movement with surgical stimulation. A dose of 150 to 200 mcg/kg per minute stabilized the hemodynamic indices of those who received muscle relaxants. Moderate hypotension and bradycardia are associated with propofol administration, with a decrease in mean arterial pressure (MAP) of approximately 10% on induction and another 10% during the early maintenance phase. The arterial pressure subsequently returns to baseline (Passenbacher et al., 2002). The use of adjuncts such as opioids can accentuate these responses, while coadministration of ketamine has been shown to preserve hemodynamic stability, albeit with more postoperative agitation (Aouad et al., 2008).

Pain during injection is an issue with propofol. However, preadministering or mixing it with lidocaine appears to attenuate this somewhat. Often, an inhalation induction followed by the administration of propofol for maintenance also avoids this issue in children. Propofol is associated with a shorter recovery time and a shorter time until discharge. It is also associated with significantly decreased incidence of postoperative nausea and vomiting when compared with halothane (Marsh et al., 1991; Watcha et al., 1991; Hannallah et al., 1994). Cohen et al. (2004) found in patients aged 2 to 36 months that propofol at 200 mcg/kg with analgesic supplementation had the same hemodynamic, recovery, and antiemetic profile as sevoflurane. Emergence delirium does not appear to be an issue with propofol.

Although many properties of propofol make it ideal for sedation, it has been associated with several adverse effects in children and adults undergoing prolonged infusions (greater than 48 hours) at high doses of greater that 4 mg/kg per hour (Vasile et al., 2003). This propofol infusion syndrome (PRIS) is characterized by bradycardia, hypotension, lipemic plasma, fatty liver enlargement, significant lactic acidosis, rhabdomyolysis, and myoglobinuria. Usually, PRIS leads to fatal renal, cardiac, and circulatory failure (Fudickar and Bein, 2009).

PRIS is caused by propofol's impairment of oxygen utilization and inhibition of mitochondrial electron transport, leading to cytolysis of both skeletal and cardiac muscle cells (Kam and Cardone, 2007). Children appear to be more prone to PRIS because of low glycogen storage and high dependence on fat metabolism (Fudickar and Bein, 2009). Current therapy involves immediate stoppage of the propofol infusion, cardiorespiratory support, and hemodialysis or hemofiltration to eliminate the propofol and its toxic metabolites. Carbohydrate supplementation is also recommended (Fudickar and Bein, 2009).

Dexmedetomidine

Dexmedetomidine is a highly selective α_2-adrenoreceptor agonist with both sedative and analgesic properties. Its elimination half-life is 2 hours, with a rapid distribution half-life of only 6 minutes (Dyck and Shafer, 1993), making it ideal for IV infusion. U.S. Food and Drug Administration (USFDA)-approved for sedation in the intensive care unit in adult patients who are mechanically ventilated, dexmedetomidine has now been used in the pediatric ICU setting, as well as for sedation in noninvasive and invasive procedures (Chrysostomou et al., 2006; 2009). It has minimal effects on respiration, which may be beneficial in pediatric patients with upper airway obstruction, and it allows for agitation-free emergence (Mahmoud et al., 2010).

Several studies have reported efficacy of dexmedetomidine for sedation in noninvasive radiologic imaging. Compared with midazolam, dexmedetomidine provided better quality of sedation and less need for rescue sedation (Koroglu et al., 2005). In another study by Koroglu and colleagues (2006), patients randomly received either dexmedetomidine or propofol. Both agents demonstrated equally effective sedation, but propofol had shorter induction, recovery, and discharge times; however, hypotension and oxygen desaturation were more common with propofol. Mason and colleagues (2006) found that the effective mean loading dose of dexmedetomidine for children during radiologic imaging was 2.2 mcg/kg, followed by a continuous infusion of 1 mcg/kg per hour. There was no change in end-tidal CO_2 and no oxygen desaturation while these children were breathing room air.

For invasive procedures, use of dexmedetomidine as the sole agent for sedation has produced mixed results. For cardiac catheterization, Munro et al. (2007) used an average maintenance infusion rate of 1.15 + 0.29 mcg/kg per hour with a range of 0.[?] to 2 mcg/kg per hour. Hammer and colleagues (2008) noted that dexmedetomidine significantly depressed sinus and AV nodal function with sinus cycle length and sinus node recovery time increasing. Sixty percent of patients needed a propofol bolus for movement, for an increasing bispectral index (BIS) number, or in anticipation of stimulus. Because of dexmedetomidine's limited analgesic effects, use of ketamine or inhalational agents as an adjunct to dexmedetomidine has been shown to be effective in several studies (Ard et al., 2003; Tosun et al., 2006).

In adults, hypotension and bradycardia are reported, especially when propofol is given as a large and rapid bolus dose or with other agents that are negative chronotropes. There appears to be a biphasic response, with an initial increase in systolic blood pressure and a reflex decrease in heart rate, followed by stabilization of both parameters below baseline values (Bloor et al., 1992). In pediatric patients, Hammer and colleagues (2008) demonstrated an increase in MAP and a decrease in heart rate from baseline values after a 10-minute loading dose of dexmedetomidine 1 mcg/kg. These effects did not continue once an infusion of 0.7 mcg/kg per hour was administered. Respiratory rate and end-tidal CO_2 did not change. It also appears that concurrent use of medications that affect cardiac conduction, such as digoxin, enhance the risk of bradycardia. Mukhtar et al. (2006) demonstrated a sympatholytic effect of dexmedetomidine in pediatric patients undergoing cardiopulmonary bypass. Dexmedetomidine, through its centrally acting α_2-adrenergic agonist effect, also can reduce the shivering threshold in children and be used to reduce postoperative shivering (Blaine et al., 2007).

Adjuvant Agents

Today, there are numerous adjuvant agents available for use during the maintenance phase of anesthesia that allow for better intraoperative and postoperative management. Improved pain control, smoother emergence, and a more comfortable immediate postoperative period are all goals that are hopefully achieved through a balanced anesthetic technique. Furthermore, by decreasing the amount of the more noxious agents used, one reduces the undesirable side effects that can be associated with them. Opioids, nonsteroidal antiinflammatory drugs, hypnotics, antiemetics, and muscle relaxants all are commonly used in the pediatric population to improve quality of perioperative care.

Opioids

Opioids and their synthetic analogs are widely used in infants and children as adjuncts during maintenance of anesthesia, as well as to provide for better postoperative pain management. Whereas morphine and fentanyl have historically been the opioids of choice, newer agents such as remifentanil have become an important part of pediatric anesthesia. The agent chosen, as well as the dosage used, depends on the overall goal and the plan for postoperative management (spontaneous vs. mechanical ventilation). Opioids and other analgesics are discussed in greater detail in Chapter 7, Pharmacology of Pediatric Anesthesia. The intravenous dosages of opioids for children are listed in Table 13-2.

Morphine is a long-acting hydrophilic analgesic that is commonly used for management of both intraoperative and postoperative pain. There is a prolonged duration of action in very young infants because of its lower clearance and longer elimination half-life, which requires lower doses and a longer dosing interval in the newborn period (Lynn and Slattery, 1987). However, total body morphine clearance is 80% that of adults by 6 months of age (Bouwmeester et al., 2004). There does not appear to be an age-related difference in the respiratory depression that occurs (Lynn et al., 1993). Morphine can cause hypotension as a result of histamine release, and urticaria and bronchospasm can be seen. Postoperative nausea and vomiting can also occur.

Hydromorphone is a hydrogenated ketone derivative of morphine that is 7 to 10 times more potent. When compared with morphine, hydromorphone is more lipophilic and has a shorter time to onset and duration of action. It produces less sedation, nausea, and vomiting, but it can still produce significant respiratory depression. Both morphine and hydromorphone are widely used in patient-controlled and epidural analgesia.

Fentanyl is a lipophilic synthetic opioid that is approximately 100 times as potent as morphine but has a relatively short duration of action of 1 to 2 hours. Fentanyl is safely used as a primary anesthetic agent and as a supplemental analgesic during an inhalational anesthetic. Pharmacokinetic studies in neonates, infants, and children have demonstrated a highly variable volume of distribution, rate of clearance, and half-life (Koehntop et al. 1986; Singleton et al. 1987). Because the effect is less predictable in neonates and premature infants, postoperative ventilatory support should be considered.

In addition to the known side effects of the other opioid analgesics, fentanyl can cause chest wall rigidity and bradycardia. Chest wall rigidity may compromise the ability to bag-mask ventilate a patient and can necessitate the use of muscle relaxants to improve ventilation. Bradycardia, although beneficial in adults, can compromise cardiac output in small infants and may require treatment with vagolytic agents or muscle relaxants that cause tachycardia.

Fentanyl is ideal for patients who need short-term anesthesia and analgesia in which a quick return to baseline respiratory function is desired. It is widely used in outpatient procedures as well as in neurosurgical cases. In cardiac surgery patients, higher doses (upward of 50 mcg/kg) have been found to provide patients with hemodynamic stability. For longer procedures, it can also be administered as a continuous infusion. However, its context sensitive half-time profile changes dramatically after 2 hours of the infusion (see Chapter 7, Pharmacology of Pediatric Anesthesia, Fig. 7-15).

TABLE 13-2. Intravenous Dosages of Opioids in Children

Drug	As Major Anesthetic	As Adjunct	As Postoperative Analgesic
Morphine	0.2-2 mg/kg	0.05-0.1 mg/kg/hr	0.05-0.1 mg/kg
Fentanyl	50-100 mcg/kg	1-3 mcg/kg/hr	1-2 mcg/kg
Sufentanil	10-15 mcg/kg	0.1-0.3 mcg/kg/hr	—
Alfentanil	150-200 mcg/kg	1-3 mcg/kg/min	—
Remifentanil	0.2-1 mcg/kg/min	0.1-0.4 mcg/kg/min	—
Hydromorphone	5-10 mcg/kg	3-5 mcg/kg/hour	3-5 mcg/kg

Sufentanil is approximately 1000 times as potent as morphine, with an elimination half-life about half that of fentanyl but a similar neonatal pharmacokinetic profile (Davis et al., 1987a, 1987b). It is often administered as a continuous infusion.

Alfentanil is approximately 25 to 100 times as potent as morphine. It has a small volume of distribution and an elimination half-life one third that of fentanyl. In neonates, it has a prolonged elimination time and increased volume of distribution (Davis et al. 1989). It also has great patient-to-patient variability, making its effects more difficult to predict. Like other opioids, alfentanil has a high incidence of PONV.

Remifentanil is an ultrashort-acting opioid with potency similar to fentanyl. It undergoes esterase cleavage to inactive metabolites, making its clearance independent of hepatic or renal clearance. Ross et al. (2001) found a consistent pharmacokinetic profile, with neonates and infants younger than 2 years of age having the largest volume of distribution and most rapid clearance. It has a constant context-sensitive half-life of 3.4 to 5.7 minutes in all age groups despite the duration of administration and the dose infused. With a mean rate of 0.55 mcg/kg per minute, Davis et al. (2001) demonstrated that remifentanil was safe and provided stable intraoperative and postoperative conditions in premature and full-term infants undergoing pyloromyotomy. It allowed for rapid emergence without postoperative apnea. For tonsillectomy and adenoidectomy, remifentanil provided faster extubation times compared with fentanyl. However, these patients had higher pain discomfort scores postoperatively, indicating that supplemental analgesia for the postoperative period is necessary (Davis et al., 2000).

Methadone is a long-acting synthetic opioid with an elimination half-life of about 35 hours. It is equally as potent as morphine when administered intravenously. It is administered when protracted postoperative pain relief is anticipated.

Meperidine is one tenth as potent as morphine and does not have the increased narcotic effect in the newborn. In older infants and children, it offers the same advantages as morphine. Histamine release is associated with its use. Doses of meperidine that are less than 0.5 mg/kg reliably treat postanesthetic shivering (Macintyre et al., 1987).

Nonsteroidal Antiinflammatory Drugs

Nonsteroidal antiinflammatory drugs (NSAIDs) are often used intraoperatively to help decrease postoperative pain. Ketorolac has been shown to improve postoperative analgesia with a decrease in nausea and vomiting (Watcha et al., 1992; Cohen et al., 1993). There is continued controversy, however, as to whether the effects on platelet function should limit its use in the perioperative setting. Splinter and colleagues (1996) found that ketorolac increased bleeding in tonsillectomy patients. However, other studies have shown that ketorolac improved postoperative analgesia without increasing the incidence of bleeding after tonsillectomy and cardiac surgery (Romsing et al., 1998; Moffett et al., 2006). It has also been shown to be effective and safe in neonates and premature infants, and its kinetics have been described in children 6 to 18 months of age (Papacci et al., 2004; Lynn et al., 2007). It should be avoided in patients with compromised renal and hepatic function.

Acetaminophen is often given per rectum intraoperatively to supplement opioid analgesia. Korpela et al. (1999) found that there was a dose-related reduction in the number of children requiring a postoperative rescue opioid when given acetaminophen 40 or 60 mg/kg rectally after induction of anesthesia. There was also a decrease in PONV. Doses higher than 40 mg/kg, however, are at or near toxic levels, and higher dosing warrants further safety studies. Subsequent doses should be modified.

Intravenous acetaminophen provides effective analgesia, with 100% bioavailability, a rapid onset of action within 5 minutes of administration, and peak analgesic efficacy at 1 hour after administration (Wilson-Smith and Morton, 2009). Prins and colleagues (2008) compared IV with rectal acetaminophen in children younger than 2 years old who were undergoing craniofacial surgery. They found that the IV form was more effective, producing analgesia more rapidly and with less interpatient variability compared with the rectal administration. In the United States, ongoing studies are looking at the efficacy and safety of IV acetaminophen in the pediatric population for future approval by the Food and Drug Administration.

Hypnotics and Sedatives

Benzodiazepines, although most commonly used for premedication, can be used intraoperatively to ensure amnesia as part of a balanced anesthetic and to prevent emergence delirium. The shorter half-life of midazolam makes it well-suited for intraoperative use. In a meta-analysis, midazolam premedication was not found to cause a significant delay in either time to emergence or time to discharge from the PACU (Cox et al., 2006).

Ketamine

Ketamine, an NMDA-receptor antagonist, has long been used in pediatric anesthesia because of its analgesic properties and its ability to produce a dissociative state. Blood pressure is well maintained with spontaneous ventilation and preservation of laryngeal reflexes. However, it can produce psychodysmorphic symptoms that require supplementation with a benzodiazepine. To produce satisfactory conditions for diagnostic or therapeutic procedures, ketamine can be administered as intermittent bolus doses of 0.2 to 1 mg/kg along with glycopyrrolate to reduce oral secretions, or as an infusion of 1 to 2 mg/kg per hour after a loading dose (Morton, 1998). Ketamine at subanesthetic infusion doses of 0.1 to 0.25 mg/kg per hour has been shown to improve pain control and have an opioid-sparing effect (Finkel et al., 2007). Further studies to determine ketamine's antihyperalgesic properties in the pediatric population are needed.

The question of whether ketamine affects central nervous system development in newborns has been raised. In humans, organogenesis of the central nervous system begins in utero and continues for several years after birth. Ketamine is associated with neuronal apoptosis in animal models during organogenesis. However, no long-term learning or behavioral disturbance has ever been noted in children after ketamine administration for anesthesia (Lois and De Kock, 2008).

Antiemetics

Prevention of PONV is an important aspect of any anesthetic. Prophylactic use of serotonin receptor (5-HT$_3$) antagonists such as ondansetron and granisetron has decreased the incidence of PONV with minimal side effects and a decreased length of stay when compared with droperidol (Davis et al., 1995a; Fuj et al., 1996; Patel et al., 1997; Khalil et al., 2005). The half-life of ondansetron in infants and children younger than 2 years of age is 50% greater than in adults, making repeat dosing in the PACU unnecessary.

Metoclopramide (0.15 mg/kg) has antiemetic effects via antagonism of central dopaminergic receptors, as well as prokinetic effects caused by increased gastric emptying. Other agents with demonstrated effectiveness include dimenhydrinate at 0.5 mg/kg and perphenazine at 70 mcg/kg (Splinter and Rhine, 1998; Kranke et al., 2003).

Dexamethasone has been shown to be effective in reducing the incidence of PONV in children after tonsillectomy and after strabismus surgery (Splinter and Roberts, 1996; Madan et al., 2005). Kim et al. (2007) have shown no dose escalation response to dexamethasone in children having tonsillectomy or adenoidectomy. A dose of 0.0625 mcg/kg was as effective as 1.0 mcg/kg. There is also improved pain control in tonsillectomy patients (Elhakim et al., 2003). Several studies have shown that the best available treatment for patients at increased risk of PONV was a combination of a 5-HT$_3$ antagonist and dexamethasone (Henzi et al., 2000; Gombar et al., 2007).

Muscle Relaxants

Muscle relaxants are discussed in greater detail in Chapter 7, Pharmacology. The following overview briefly discusses the advantages and disadvantages of the different agents currently available.

Succinylcholine is a depolarizing muscle relaxant with a fast onset (able to produce intubating conditions within 1 minute) and short duration of action. It can be given IV (2 mg/kg in infants and small children or 1 mg/kg in older children) or IM (3 to 4 mg/kg with an onset of 3 to 4 minutes) (Liu et al., 1981). Because of the incidence of bradycardia and possible asystole, atropine (0.02 mg/kg) is administered before succinylcholine. Although its use in children is warranted in emergency situations, caution should be used because of the serious complications that can be associated with it. Succinylcholine can cause significant hyperkalemia in patients with neuromuscular disorders and burns, dysrhythmias, muscle rigidity, masseter spasm, and postoperative myalgias. In susceptible individuals, it can also trigger malignant hyperthermia.

Vecuronium is an intermediate-acting steroidal nondepolarizing muscle relaxant. Vecuronium does not produce the vagolytic response that one sees with pancuronium. In children, it has a higher ED$_{95}$ than in infants and adults (Meretoja et al., 1988). The duration of its effect is more prolonged in infants (73 minutes) compared with children (35 minutes) and adults (53 minutes) (Meretoja, 1988).

Rocuronium is an intermediate-acting steroidal nondepolarizing neuromuscular blocker that is similar in structure to vecuronium but one tenth as potent. It produces the most rapid onset of paralysis of the nondepolarizing agents and is used for rapid sequence inductions as an alternative to succinylcholine. At a dose of 0.6 mg/kg, the onset of maximal block is 1.3 + 2 minutes in children between 1 and 5 years old, and the time to recovery is 26.7 + 1.9 minutes (Woelfel et al., 1992). It can produce tachycardia and causes pain on injection in lightly anesthetized patients. Interaction of rocuronium with volatile anesthetic agents augments the intensity of neuromuscular blockade without effects on duration of or recovery from the block (Wulf et al., 1998).

Cisatracurium is an intermediate nondepolarizing agent that is a 1R-isomer of atracurium. At a dose of 0.15 mg/kg, the onset of maximal block is 2 + 0.8 minutes in infants and 3 + 1.2 minutes in children. Time to recovery was longer in infants (43.3 + 6.2 minutes) than in older children (36 + 5.4 minutes) (Taivainen et al., 2000). Cisatracurium undergoes hydrolysis at body temperature and physiologic pH (Hoffman elimination). It maintains hemodynamic stability and does not cause the release of histamine.

Pancuronium is a long-acting steroidal nondepolarizing muscle relaxant. It causes tachycardia by blocking vagal activity at the ganglionic level and through the release of norepinephrine. This tachycardia can be beneficial in young infants that depend on increased heart rate to improve cardiac output. Partially metabolized in the liver, the rest is then excreted by the kidneys, making its action prolonged in patients with hepatic or renal failure.

Regional Anesthesia

Regional anesthesia has become an important part of the anesthetic management of pediatric patients in the perioperative period. Regional techniques can decrease the intraoperative requirement of inhaled and intravenous agents and allow for a more rapid emergence with effective postoperative analgesia and minimal sedation (Markakis, 2000). Although caudal anesthesia remains the most popular regional technique in this population, epidural anesthesia, field blocks, ultrasound-guided peripheral nerve blocks, and neuroaxial opioids have also been used to a greater extent. The various regional analgesia techniques, as well as the choices and dosages of local anesthetics and opioids for regional analgesia are detailed in Chapter 16, Regional Anesthesia.

Caudal Anesthesia

Caudal blocks continue to be the most commonly used regional technique in infants and children. As an adjunct to general anesthesia, caudal blockade provides both intraoperative and postoperative analgesia for procedures in the lower abdomen, pelvis, or lower extremities. This block is easily performed with few associated complications, such as dural puncture and intravascular injection (Dalens and Hasnaoui, 1989). Anatomic features that contribute to these occurrences are the caudal position of the dural sac in infants at S3, the increased vascularity of the area, and the development of the sacral fat pad in school-aged children. Awareness of these factors should decrease the risk of complications.

Because infants and children do not cooperate and remain still while they are awake, caudal blocks are typically performed under general anesthesia. Once the airway is secured, the patient is placed in the lateral decubitus position and the sacral hiatus is identified and cleaned. Although several needle types and sizes have been investigated, short, beveled (22-gauge) needles have a lower incidence of intravascular injection compared with standard needles (Dalens and Hasnaoui, 1989). The needle is inserted through the sacrococcygeal ligament and advanced into the caudal space. Aspiration to confirm that there is no blood or cerebrospinal fluid (CSF), which would indicate inadvertent intravascular or intrathecal puncture, is performed before injection of the drug. Because the patient is under general anesthesia, the response to a standard test dose of epinephrine may be masked with minimal heart rate or blood pressure change seen. However, an increase of 25% or more in the T-wave amplitude appears to be a more reliable positive predictor of intravascular injection and was seen consistently with an epinephrine dose of 0.25 to 0.5 mcg/kg (Tanaka and Nishikawa, 1999; Kozek-Langenecker et al., 2000).

Bupivacaine is a local anesthetic that has long been used due to its relative safety and longer duration of action. It has a maximal safe dose of 2.5 mg/kg. Yaster and Maxwell (1989) recommend caudal dosing of bupivacaine 0.25% at 1 mL/kg, which should block approximately 10 spinal segments, with a maximal volume of 20 mL. For procedures longer than 3 hours, the caudal procedure can be repeated with a more dilute concentration of 0.125% or 0.175% to minimize the risk of toxicity as well as motor blockade. Levo-bupivacaine is the (S)-(-)-enantiomer of racemic bupivacaine, with similar local-anesthetic properties and potency. However, it is less toxic to the central nervous system and is less likely to cause myocardial depression and fatal arrhythmias than racemic bupivacaine (Tsui and Berde, 2005). Levo-bupivacaine 0.25% at a dose of 0.8 mL/kg provides adequate analgesia for penile or groin surgery (Taylor et al., 2003).

Ropivacaine is an S-enantiomer of bupivacaine with less cardiovascular and central nervous system toxicity than racemic bupivacaine. It produces significantly less motor blockade and stronger vasoconstriction at low concentrations (Zink and Graf, 2004). Several studies have shown comparable analgesic efficacy between ropivacaine, levo-bupivacaine, and bupivacaine (Ivani et al., 2002; Breschan et al., 2005; Locatelli et al., 2005). With lower systemic absorption and lower toxicity, ropivacaine is the drug of choice for prolonged use in neonates or patients with abnormal metabolism (Hansen et al., 2001). Hong and colleagues have shown that a high volume–low concentration of ropivacaine provides a higher level of block and longer duration of analgesia than a high concentration–low volume of ropivacaine (Hong et al., 2009), where the total drug amount is the same.

Other medications with analgesic properties, injected into the caudal space with and without local anesthetics, have been shown to be efficacious. Opioids, clonidine, and ketamine have been used with varying success and are discussed in greater detail in Chapter 16, Regional Anesthesia.

Contraindications to caudal anesthesia include active sepsis, local infection of the skin at the injection site, coagulopathy, sacral anomalies (including previous meningomyelocele), and uncorrected hypovolemia (Markakis, 2000). After caudal blockade, urinary retention occurs in approximately 10% of patients but is usually short-lived (Yaster and Maxwell, 1989).

Epidural Anesthesia

Placement of an epidural catheter through the caudal, lumbar, or thoracic route allows for continuous epidural delivery of local anesthesia both intraoperatively and postoperatively at the appropriate segmental level. Many have found success with catheters that were introduced caudally then threaded to the lumbar or thoracic level (Bosenberg et al., 1988). However, in 2002, Valairucha and colleagues found only 67% of catheter tips were in optimal position when threaded from below, and Blanco et al. (1996) could only advance 22% of catheters threaded from between L4 and L5 to predicted thoracic levels.

Direct placement at the lumbar and thoracic levels can be technically more challenging and present an increased risk of complications. However, weighing risks and benefits, anesthesiologists with experience in their placement and use have found that they provide successful analgesia for upper abdominal and thoracic procedures when specifically indicated. Rapp et al. (2005) demonstrated that ultrasound guidance allows for identification of the epidural space, ligamentum flavum, and dural structures, as well as the depth at which loss of resistance occurs. Willschke et al. (2006c) had a faster catheter placement, less bone contact, and direct visualization of epidural local anesthetic spread when ultrasound guidance was used instead of the standard loss-of-resistance technique. Further studies to evaluate whether there is a reduction in the complication rate in pediatric epidural anesthesia when using ultrasound for placement are ongoing.

Epidural analgesia can be provided through bolus dosing or continuous infusion of local anesthetics. Bupivacaine (0.125% to 0.25%) or ropivacaine (0.2%) can both be used. A continuous infusion through a lumbar catheter at a rate of 0.3 mL/kg per hour maintains an analgesic level between T10 and L1.

Epidural opioids can also provide effective analgesia without sympathetic, sensory, or motor blockade (Shapiro et al., 1984; Rosen and Rosen, 1989). Respiratory depression is a major complication that requires careful dosing and observation. Pruritus, nausea, vomiting, and urinary retention can also occur but can be minimized with smaller doses of opioids or a small dose of naloxone (0.5 to 1 mcg/kg). Preservative-free morphine (30 to 70 mcg/kg caudally or 50 mcg/kg epidurally) is hydrophilic, which allows for a delayed onset, decreased systemic uptake, and prolonged duration of action (15 to 20 hours) (Attia et al., 1986; Rash et al., 1990). Fentanyl and hydromorphone are lipophilic, with a more rapid onset, greater systemic absorption, and shorter duration of action, making them more appropriate as adjuncts for continuous infusions (Dalens et al., 1986).

Subarachnoid Opioids

Subarachnoid injection of morphine has been found to have a similar efficacy and side effect profile to epidurally placed morphine. The recommended dose is 10 to 20 mcg/kg (Krechel and Helikson, 1993). Delayed respiratory depression may occur and is typically more severe than when given in the epidural space (Nichols et al., 1993). Careful monitoring and delayed further dosing of opioids are necessary.

Peripheral Nerve Blocks and Field Blocks

With advances in technology, peripheral nerve blocks are increasingly being used in the pediatric population as adjuncts to general anesthesia and to manage postoperative pain. These blocks can supply analgesia for the upper and lower extremities and allow for one-sided blockade as opposed to the central regional techniques. Axillary, interscalene, sciatic, and femoral nerve blocks have all been described. The more recent use of ultrasound allows for real-time imaging of the anatomy and direct visualization of the needle in anesthetized patients who cannot indicate discomfort or pain caused by direct nerve injection. As a result, ultrasonography is gaining in popularity over landmark-based techniques and neurostimulation (Marhofer and Frickey, 2006; Roberts, 2006). It also decreases the volume of local anesthetic per block by 30% to 50%, which allows the anesthesiologist to stay within maximum dosing guidelines and still achieve success (Ecoffey, 2007). Toxicity can further be avoided by using diluted solutions and solutions that contain epinephrine (Berde, 1989). Disposable pumps that can deliver continuous peripheral nerve block infusions of local anesthesia can be used for continued postoperative pain control at the patient's home (Ganesh et al., 2007). Ludot and colleagues (2008) demonstrated successful analgesia and overall satisfaction with this technique in children who had a suitable family environment and proper parental instruction on the catheter's management.

Field blocks are also an important aspect of pediatric anesthesia and allow for improved postoperative pain control while decreasing the incidence of side effects associated with opioids. Compared with caudal anesthesia, ilioinguinal-iliohypogastric nerve block, wound infiltration, local anesthesia "splash," dorsal-penile nerve block, and subcutaneous ring block have all been shown to be effective for the chosen surgical procedure (Cross and Barrett, 1987; Hannallah et al., 1987; Fell et al., 1988; Casey et al., 1990). The use of ultrasound has also caused a revision in the technique of these blocks. The unpredictable depth of the posterior rectus sheath in children is more defined with ultrasound, allowing for improved analgesia. Furthermore, use of ultrasound for ilioinguinal-iliohypogastric nerve blocks reduced the volume of local anesthetic used to 0.075 mL/kg (Willschke et al., 2006a).

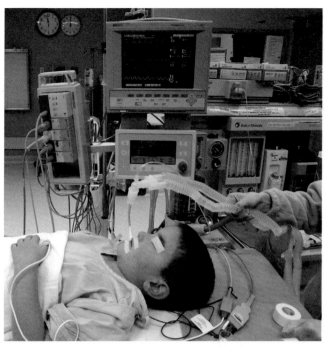

■ **FIGURE 13-5.** In addition to observation, standard monitoring devices in the operating room include a pulse oximeter, capnograph device, ECG machine, automated blood pressure measuring device, temperature probe, and precordial stethoscope.

Monitoring

In children, meticulous attention to the patient through both clinical observation and the use of monitors during the maintenance phase of anesthesia is of the utmost importance. Physiologic changes can be subtle and occur without warning, requiring a constant vigilance on the part of the anesthesiologist. Monitoring devices alone are not adequate to care for these patients. Through careful observation of changes in chest movement, breath sounds, and heart tones with a precordial stethoscope; skin color; and capillary refill, variations in children's ventilation and circulation can be found by the anesthesiologist long before a monitor indicates them.

In addition to observation, standard monitoring devices include a pulse oximeter, capnography, ECG, an automated blood pressure measuring device, a temperature probe, and a precordial stethoscope (Fig. 13-5). For longer surgical procedures or when there are anticipated fluid shifts, a Foley catheter to monitor urinary output as an indication of IV volume is also recommended. Invasive monitoring of arterial blood pressure or central venous pressure is also indicated in certain clinical situations.

Standards of Intraoperative Monitoring

In the tradition of safety that has been a hallmark of anesthesia care and practice, standards for basic anesthetic monitoring were initially proposed in 1986 by the Harvard University teaching hospitals (Eichhorn et al., 1986). These were then adopted and amended by the American Society of Anesthesiologists (ASA), with the last iteration approved in 2005. As stated in the document, these standards apply to all general anesthetics, regional anesthetics, and monitored anesthesia care. Although some rare

clinical situations may preclude use of all of the recommended monitors, it is expected that these standards are technologically attainable and should be used by all practitioners.

Standard I states that "qualified anesthesia personnel shall be present in the room throughout the conduct of all general anesthetics, regional anesthetics, and monitored anesthesia care" (ASA, 2005). It stipulates that this continuous care is "without any interruption at any time" because of the rapidly changing status of patients under anesthesia. Standard II stipulates that oxygenation, ventilation, circulation, and temperature be continually evaluated. "Continually" is defined as "repeated regularly and frequently in steady rapid succession" (ASA, 2005). For each component, specific objectives and methods are outlined. A combination of clinical observation and technical methods is recommended. Whereas there are no mandates for specific instrumentation, quantitative measurements are "strongly encouraged" over qualitative measures alone. Standard monitoring and supplemental measures recommended in pediatric anesthesia are shown in Box 13-1.

Pulse oximetry, introduced in the 1980s, has become a mandatory instrument in the perioperative care of pediatric patients. The pulse oximeter accurately reflects saturation in all age groups with various hematocrit values, including premature infants with fetal hemoglobin over the range of 60% to 100% Sao_2 (Deckardt and Steward, 1984). Recent advances in pulse oximetry include newer designs that claim to improve performance during low-perfusion states and patient motion, often a consideration in newborns and infants. Signal extraction technology (SET) uses algorithms that filter out interference, resulting in a 90% lower false-alarm rate (Miyasaka, 2002). Other devices provide continuous noninvasive measurement of total hemoglobin concentration and allow for differentiation between different hemoglobin types (Noiri et al.,

Box 13-1 Standard Monitors and Supplementary Measurements in Pediatric Anesthesia

STANDARD MONITORS
Physiology
Clinical observation by qualified anesthesiologist
Oxygenation: Pulse oximeter
Ventilation: Stethoscope, capnograph, gas flow meter
Circulation: Stethoscope, blood pressure cuff
ECG
Temperature probe: Rectal, esophageal, or axillary
Anesthetic depth: BIS monitor

Safety
Oxygen analyzer with low concentration alarm
Ventilator with low pressure and disconnect alarm

SUPPLEMENTAL MEASUREMENTS
Continual
Fluids given
Urine output (catheterization and urinometer)
Blood loss
Direct arterial pressure
Central venous pressure
Pulmonary arterial pressure and wedge pressure
Cardiac output (noninvasive or invasive)
EEG
Somatosensory-evoked potentials

Intermittent
Train-of-four twitch response on nerve stimulator
Arterial blood gas tensions, pH, hematocrit
Serum levels of Na^+, K^+, Ca^{2+}, glucose
Colloid oncotic pressure
Coagulation profile

2005; McMorrow and Mythen, 2006). The reliability of these new technologies continues to be investigated. Further information on monitoring devices, their mechanisms of action and clinical uses is presented in Chapter 11, Monitoring.

In addition to the information obtained through standard monitors, continuous clinical observation is imperative in the care of pediatric patients. It is often the first indication of an impending change in a patient's respiratory status. Through both visual observation and the use of a regular or precordial stethoscope, the anesthesiologist can determine the rate and depth of ventilation, as well as determine whether an endotracheal tube is one sided or if a patient is hypoxic. Stridor is indicative of extrathoracic airway narrowing and obstruction. Furthermore, periodic manual ventilation of the patient, with the anesthesiologist's hand on the bag, allows the anesthesiologist to detect changes in the patient's dynamic compliance and respiratory resistance that may be caused by air leaks in the anesthesia circuit, airway obstruction, or movement of the diaphragm.

Normal cardiovascular function is indicated by suitable heart tone and rate, rhythm, pulse volume, capillary refill, and skin color. Blood loss can be quantified by visual estimation of bleeding in the surgical field, pulse rate and volume, counting and

weighing of blood-soaked sponges, and measuring the volume of blood in suction bottles. Temperature, although monitored directly, can also be sensed by touch to confirm readings and avoid initiation of treatment for false hypothermia or hyperthermia. Through clinical observation, the anesthesiologist obtains a significant amount of information beyond that which monitors alone can offer.

Invasive Monitoring

Invasive arterial and central venous monitoring is technically more difficult in infants and children and not without risk. Even though there are definite indications for each, the anesthesiologist must weigh the risks and benefits to determine whether their use is appropriate.

Indications for direct arterial pressure monitoring are beat-to-beat monitoring of blood pressure when hemodynamic fluctuations are expected or pharmacologic manipulation can occur; an inability to measure blood pressure noninvasively; the need to frequently measure arterial blood gas samples; or other laboratory analyses to aid in management of the patient (Barbeito and Mark, 2006). Arterial catheters are typically placed percutaneously in the wrist (radial or ulnar), groin (femoral), or foot (posterior tibial or pedal). They should not be placed anywhere where there is evidence of vascular compromise or lack of collateral circulation. A noninvasive blood pressure monitor should always be available to verify the readings of the direct monitor.

Indications for a central venous catheter in the perioperative period include the need to measure central venous pressure to help quantify fluid balance; the need to infuse intravenous drugs for which peripheral access is inappropriate (i.e., vasoactive drugs, phlebitis-causing agents, hypertonic solutions); frequent blood draws; the need for prolonged access; difficult or impossible peripheral access; and the need for larger access for fluid administration than is achievable through peripheral catheter.

The risks of central catheter placement include vascular injury, unintentional arterial puncture, and pneumothorax, just to name a few. However, Verghese and colleagues (1999) showed that real-time ultrasound guidance for placement of an internal jugular catheter was superior to the landmark technique, with a high success rate and fewer carotid punctures. Another study demonstrated advantages of this technique in children older than 1 year of age or heavier than 10 kg (Leyvi et al., 2005).

Bispectral Index

The bispectral algorithm uses a statistical process to analyze EEG signals and compute a number between 0 and 100 that represents the degree of awareness. The variables analyzed include the frequency and power spectrum of the EEG, the amount of burst suppression, and the degree of synchronization of the EEG (Bowdle, 2006). In infants and children, studies have validated the bispectral index (BIS) and demonstrated that more accurate titration of general anesthesia is achieved with its use, resulting in shorter recovery times (Denman et al., 2000; Bannister et al., 2001; McCann et al. 2002; Powers et al., 2005). However, several studies have demonstrated low BIS values in young infants (younger than 1 year old) before awakening and poor correlations between anesthetic concentration and BIS (Davidson et al., 2005; Klockars et al., 2006; Malviya et al., 2007). Newer indices to measure anesthesia depth continue to be developed, including the Narcotrend index, the A-line ARX index, and the cerebral-state index. All of these are currently being studied for validation in children and with regard to BIS.

Anesthesia Record

The anesthesia record is extremely important as a data sheet during anesthesia, as a source of information for later anesthetics, and as a legal document. It should contain all of the pertinent preoperative information, including the patient's medical history, significant laboratory values, time of last food or liquid intake, vital signs, and a record of a focused physical examination. It should be signed by the trainee as well as the attending anesthesiologist, who is the legally responsible party.

After induction, a brief description of induction and intubation should be recorded, noting the drugs given, the size of the endotracheal tube, whether it is cuffed or uncuffed, and verification of proper air leak around the tube. Gas flow rates, maintenance concentrations, doses of anesthetic and adjuvant drugs, blood pressure, pulse, respiratory rate, temperature, oxygen saturation readings, and end-tidal CO_2 should be entered at regular intervals.

With advances in technology, automated anesthetic record systems have become more widely used (Egger Halbeis et al., 2008). Sanborn et al. (1996) found that electronic scanning recorded a higher incidence of intraoperative incidents than those reported voluntarily. Others have reported improvements in patient safety and care with automated systems (Junger et al., 2001; Merry et al., 2001). As automated records become more user friendly, affordable, and integrated with the care process, they eventually could be the standard method of recording information in the operating room.

Fluids and Electrolytes

Fluid therapy in the perioperative period needs to account for several different fluid requirements: fluid deficits, maintenance fluid, and the volume of fluid necessary to maintain adequate tissue perfusion. Fluid deficits come from numerous sources, including preoperative fasting, gastrointestinal and renal losses, hemorrhage and third space losses (see Chapter 5, Regulation of Fluids and Electrolytes).

Historically, maintenance fluid requirements were based on the recommendations of Holliday and Segar (1957), which state that the basal caloric needs of infants and children dictate their fluid requirements. They proposed that an infant needs 100 mL of water per 100 kcal of caloric expenditure. On the basis of 1 mL of fluid per 1 kcal of caloric requirement, the fluid requirements in infants and children were approximated by the following formulas:

$$0 \text{ to } 10 \text{ kg: } 4 \text{ mL/kg per hr}$$

$$10 \text{ to } 20 \text{ kg: } 40 \text{ mL} + 2 \text{ mL/kg per hr above } 10 \text{ kg}$$

$$>20 \text{ kg: } 60 \text{ mL} + 1 \text{ mL/kg per hr above } 20 \text{ kg}$$

For every 100 calories of energy expenditure or 100 mL of water, a child needs 3 mmol of sodium, 2 mmol of potassium,

5 mmol of chloride, and 5 g of dextrose. While 5% dextrose in 0.2% or 0.45% NaCl meets these requirements for maintenance fluids, several recent articles describing clinically significant hyponatremia caused by perioperative fluids have raised some concerns (Arieff, 1998; Halberthal et al., 2001). Practitioners are tending to reduce the average fluid maintenance volume to half or two thirds of the classic recommendations proposed by Holliday and Segar (1957) based on these findings or are using isotonic saline solutions (Paut and Lacroix, 2006; Bailey et al., 2010). Further studies are necessary to evaluate what the most appropriate maintenance fluids are; however, one must individualize fluid therapy and monitor blood sodium levels in patients who are receiving prolonged infusions.

Pediatric patients are typically kept fasting for 2 hours from clear fluids and 4 to 8 hours (sometimes longer) from breast milk and solid food before induction for elective surgery. To determine the fasting deficit, one multiplies the hourly maintenance fluid requirement by the number of hours of restriction. Half of the fluid deficit plus the hourly maintenance fluid requirement should be given during the first hour of anesthesia. One quarter of the fluid deficit plus the hourly maintenance fluid is infused during the second and third hours, along with the replacement of any third-space fluid loss (Furman et al., 1975). These deficits should be replaced with a balanced salt solution such as normal saline or Lactated Ringer's solution that does not contain glucose.

Glucose requirements in pediatric patients need to account for the hazards of both hyperglycemia and hypoglycemia. Hyperglycemia produces an osmotic diuresis that leads to dehydration and electrolyte abnormalities. It also appears to worsen neurologic outcome in cerebral ischemia and should be avoided (Lanier et al., 1987). On the other hand, hypoglycemia is known to cause cerebral ischemia and brain damage, especially in newborns. Infants and some children who have fasted for a prolonged period without glucose supplementation can become hypoglycemic during anesthesia yet show no overt clinical symptoms (Welborn et al., 1986). Intraoperative monitoring of blood glucose levels in these patients is recommended. However, preoperative hypoglycemia occurs rarely in normal, healthy infants and children (1% to 2%), making it less likely that the majority of patients need glucose administered in the perioperative period (Murat and Dubois, 2008).

Recommendations on the appropriate glucose-containing solution to administer, if IV glucose is to be given, have changed over the years (Bailey et al., 2010). Whereas a 5% dextrose solution consistently causes hyperglycemia, 2.5% dextrose in Lactated Ringer's solution maintains normal blood glucose levels (Welborn et al., 1987). Dubois et al. (1992) also investigated the use of lower dextrose solutions (1 or 0.9%) and found normal blood glucose concentrations without hypoglycemia.

A urethral catheter allows continual monitoring of urine output and the state of hydration and blood volume during major surgical procedures or when there is significant loss of blood and fluids. Urethral catheterization is recommended in surgeries lasting for 4 hours or longer. Urine output of more than 0.5 mg/kg per hour should be maintained to avoid damage to the renal tubules.

Ventilation

To maintain alveolar ventilation in infants and small children under general anesthesia, partial rebreathing or nonrebreathing Mapleson D- or F-type circuits (such as the Bain or Jackson-Reese) are commonly used. With their light weight and low flow resistance, they have desirable qualities for the pediatric population, although the lack of scavenging is a drawback. Today, adult circle systems with smaller pediatric circuits are safely used in children. However, in small infants, one must account for the potential for increased airway resistance and increased circuit compliance that diminishes the accuracy of measured tidal volume. For a more detailed discussion of pediatric anesthesia circuits and ventilators, refer to Chapter 10, Equipment.

For controlled ventilation in infants and children without major respiratory dysfunction, the ventilator can be set initially at a tidal volume of 10 mL/kg or peak pressure of 16 to 18 cm H_2O. Respiratory rates between 20/min for infants and 12/min for older children are sufficient, although higher respiratory rates are recommended for young infants (Peters et al., 1998). A positive end-expiratory pressure (PEEP) of at least 5 cm H_2O prevents airway closure and atelectasis in anesthetized infants and young children (Motoyama, 1996). Once the steady state of ventilation is established, tidal volume and respiratory rate can be adjusted to maintain an end-tidal CO_2 between 35 and 40 mm Hg (see Chapter 3, Respiratory Physiology in Infants and Children).

Temperature Maintenance

Infants and small children are at particular risk of hypothermia because of their relative lack of adipose tissue and their increased body surface area relative to their body weight, which increases the difference between heat loss and heat production. Under general anesthesia, core temperature control is impaired and regulatory defenses, including nonshivering thermogenesis, are not triggered (Sessler, 2008). Furthermore, vasodilation, exposure to the cold operating room environment, insensible heat loss, and infusion of cold intravenous fluids all contribute to the development of hypothermia. The mechanisms of thermoregulation are further discussed in Chapter 6, Thermoregulation: Physiology and Perioperative Disturbances.

Accurate monitoring of body temperature is imperative to maintaining normothermia as well as detecting malignant hyperthermia. Core temperature monitoring is the best indicator of thermal status and can be easily measured with an esophageal probe (Sessler, 2008). Because this is not always a possibility, near-core sites including the mouth, axillae, bladder, rectum, and skin surface are other possibilities, although they each have limitations. The safe range for a child's core temperature is between 35.5° and 37.5° C. To prevent complications caused by hypothermia, anesthesiologists need to be proactive and begin warming the patient as soon as or before the temperature deviates from this range.

There are several means by which body temperature can be maintained. Forced-air warmers preserve intraoperative normothermia better than circulating-water mattresses (Kurz et al., 1993). Humidifiers in the anesthesia circuit also help prevent evaporative heat loss, damage to the ciliated airway epithelia, and

postoperative pulmonary complications (Chalon et al., 1979). Additionally, increasing room temperature, using radiant warming lamps, wrapping the child's head and other exposed areas with plastic, and using warmed intravenous fluids help to conserve heat. Careful monitoring, however, is necessary to prevent hyperthermia that can sometimes occur when all of these measures are combined.

Blood Loss and Blood Component Therapy

Accurate and continuous monitoring of blood loss and its timely replacement are critical in pediatric patients. Relatively small losses in infants can produce significant changes in hemoglobin concentration and hemodynamic stability, making careful determination of acceptable blood loss mandatory. Estimated blood loss needs to account for the contents of suction bottles as well as a visual estimate of blood lost on the surgical drapes and the weight of blood-soaked sponges. Allowable blood loss is determined by the patient's estimated blood volume, preoperative and intraoperative hematocrit values, cardiopulmonary and general medical conditions to provide adequate oxygen transport, and risk versus benefit of the transfusion. Estimated blood volumes in pediatric patients are age dependent and are listed in Table 13-3.

Once the estimated blood volume (EBV) is known, one can determine the maximum allowable blood loss (MABL). This should be done for each patient before the induction of anesthesia and is achieved with the use of a simple mathematical calculation as follows (Barcelona et al., 2005):

$$MABL = \frac{EBV \times (\text{Starting HcT} - \text{Target HcT})}{\text{Starting HcT}}$$

For example, an 11-month-old infant weighing 10 kg with an initial hematocrit value of 35 would have an EBV of 750 mL (75 mL/kg). Assuming the minimum acceptable or target hematocrit value of 25, the MABL would be:

$$MABL = \frac{750 \times (35 - 25)}{35} = 214 \text{ mL}$$

The use of a trigger value alone to determine the need for transfusion is no longer recommended in most guidelines, because hemoglobin and hematocrit values may not accurately reflect blood volume or oxygen carrying capacity (Weldon, 2005). In actively bleeding patients without volume replacement, hematocrit values alone can be misleading (Hume and Limoges, 2002). However, the hematocrit value along with good clinical judgment can serve as a guideline for

TABLE 13-3. Estimates of Circulating Blood Volume

Age of Patient	Blood Volume (mL/kg)
Premature newborn	90-100
Full-term newborn	80-90
3 mo-1 yr	75-80
3-6 yr	70-75
>6 yr	65-70

when to consider transfusion (National Institutes of Health Consensus Conference, 1988).

Debate continues as to whether a crystalloid or colloid solution should be used to replace blood volume as the hematocrit is allowed to decrease (Bailey et al., 2010). The SAFE Study (2004) randomized adult ICU patients to receive either 4% albumin or normal saline for fluid resuscitation with the primary outcome being death from any cause. In 6997 patients, they found no difference in death rate or in number of days in either the ICU or the hospital between the groups. This was in contrast to a meta-analysis by the Cochrane Injuries Group Albumin Reviewers (1998), which suggested that the administration of albumin resulted in a 6% increase in the absolute risk of death when compared with the administration of crystalloid. If a colloid solution (e.g., albumen, hetastarch) is used, blood loss is replaced milliliter for milliliter. If a crystalloid solution is used, 2 to 3 times the volume of the blood loss is replaced. Although colloid may be more physiologic, it is more expensive and has not been shown definitively to be superior to crystalloid replacement. In otherwise healthy patients, the use of crystalloid is safe and effective to replace the MABL.

The minimum recommended hemoglobin concentration allowable has changed over the years. With the exception of patients who are in the early neonatal period (with high oxygen affinity of fetal hemoglobin and decreased oxygen unloading at tissue levels) and those with cyanotic cardiopulmonary disease, the previously recommended 10 g/dL is no longer a prerequisite hemoglobin concentration. Several studies have demonstrated cardiovascular stability with significant anemia (hemoglobin of 6 to 7 g/dL) in both animals and children who underwent acute normovolemic hemodilution (Stehling and Zauder, 1991; Fontana et al., 1995). Lacroix and colleagues (2007) found no difference in outcomes in children randomized to either a restrictive-strategy group (transfusion threshold of 7 g/dL) or a liberal-strategy group (transfusion threshold of 9.5 g/dL). However, a randomized, controlled trial comparing two hemodilution protocols (to a hematocrit value of 21.5% versus 27.8%) in children during hypothermic cardiopulmonary bypass found that a lower hematocrit value was associated with a poorer performance on psychomotor development tests at 1 year of age (Jonas et al., 2003).

The best recommendations to date appear to be those of the National Institutes of Health Consensus Conference on Perioperative Red Cell Transfusion (1988): healthy patients with hemoglobin values of 10 g/dL or greater rarely require transfusion, whereas those with values less than 7 g/dL often require transfusion. Thus, to keep operative hemorrhage and blood volume under control in a situation of continued blood loss, hemoglobin may be decreased temporarily to as low as (but not below) 7 g/dL (hematocrit 20%), with proper monitoring of blood pressure, arterial and mixed venous P_{O_2}. The hemoglobin level should be increased postoperatively (i.e., to 8 g/dL with a hematocrit of >25%) when the patient needs more oxygen uptake for increased metabolic needs.

Once the MABL is exceeded, transfusion is necessary, usually in the form of packed red blood cells (PRBCs). The hematocrit of PRBCs varies between 60% and 80% and can be adjusted according to the need of the physician administering the blood. The volume of PRBCs needed to replace the blood loss beyond MABL can be calculated as follows:

$$PRBCs\ (mL) = \frac{Blood\ loss\ MABL \times Desired\ HcT}{HcT\ of\ PRBCs}$$

Once the blood loss exceeds one blood volume (massive blood loss), a coagulopathy can develop because of both a reduction in platelets (dilutional thrombocytopenia) and a reduction in labile clotting factors. In patients with clinical signs of nonsurgical bleeding, the administration of other blood components, including platelets, fresh frozen plasma, and cryoprecipitate becomes necessary. The management of blood component therapy and massive blood loss is detailed in Chapter 14, Blood Conservation.

EMERGENCE AND EXTUBATION

Emergence

Prompt and safe emergence from general anesthesia begins with predicting the conclusion of surgery and assessment of the patient. The tapering or discontinuing of anesthetic agents must take into account the diverse pharmacokinetics and pharmacodynamics of inhaled anesthetics, intravenous anesthetics, muscle relaxants, and/or regional nerve blocks. The patient's age and medical condition must also be considered. For example, in infants the longer elimination half-lives for many agents may require earlier termination of agents than in children or adults. The patient's response to the pain, disorientation, or sudden awareness needs to be anticipated to ensure a gentle awakening. Judicious use of opioids for analgesia and hypnotics for sedation can help reduce agitation on emergence. With careful and appropriate planning, all anesthetized patients should emerge smoothly and on time.

As the anesthetics are curtailed, the respiratory rate and pattern should be observed. A rapid respiratory rate may be seen in cases of inadequate analgesia or stage 2 of anesthesia. Titrating subtherapeutic doses of an opioid can reduce pain experience on emergence. Increasing the fresh gas flow and moderately increasing the rate of controlled or assisted ventilation can facilitate the elimination of residual inhaled anesthetic. The criteria for adequate emergence from stage 2 of general anesthesia in pre- or nonverbal children include:

- Grimacing, using eyebrows and/or forehead,
- Spontaneous eye opening, and
- Purposeful movement, such as reaching for the endotracheal tube.

Paradoxical movement of the thorax and abdomen may indicate incomplete recovery from general anesthesia, residual paralysis, or upper airway obstruction, and they each need to be investigated and their causes addressed.

If neuromuscular blockers were used, recovery should be monitored using peripheral nerve stimulation and clinical assessment. Kopman et al. (1997) observed that recovery of a train-of-four (TOF) ratio over 0.90 is needed to assure adequate neuromuscular function, especially in the ambulatory setting. Neuromuscular blockade is reversed with intravenous atropine (0.02 mg/kg) followed by neostigmine (0.06 mg/kg). In infants, a higher dose of atropine (0.03 mg/kg) is recommended. Glycopyrrolate (0.01 mg/kg) is as effective as atropine and may produce a more stable heart rate (Warran et al., 1981).

Sugammadex, a new rapid-acting reversal agent, which has been approved for use in Europe, Australia, and New Zealand, encapsulates rocuronium and vecuronium, preventing binding to neuromuscular junction receptors. Studies in adults have shown recovery from weak blockade to a train-of-four ratio of 0.9 occurs in approximately 2 minutes with doses of 2 mg/kg or higher (Sorgenfrei et al., 2006; Suy et al., 2007; Vanacker et al. 2007). Plaud and colleagues (2009) demonstrated that in recovery from neuromuscular blockade from 0.6 mg/kg rocuronium, a train-of-four of 0.9 was attained in 0.6, 1.2, and 1.1 minutes in infants, children, and adolescents, respectively, with 2 mg/kg of sugammadex.

The clinical criteria for adequate recovery from nondepolarizing neuromuscular blockade in preverbal and uncooperative children include:

- Maintaining adequate, nonparadoxical breathing;
- Generating a negative inspiratory pressure greater than 30 cm H_2O;
- Sustaining tetanic contraction at 50 Hz;
- Sustaining hip flexion with leg elevation for 10 seconds; and,
- Lifting the head and/or coughing forcefully.

At the conclusion of surgery, while the child is still under general anesthesia, a lubricated suction catheter should be gently passed into the stomach to remove any gastric contents and gases that may have accumulated. This practice reduces the risk of vomiting and aspiration during emergence and decreases intra-abdominal pressure, allowing for greater expansion of the lungs. Gastric suctioning is especially important in patients thought to have a full stomach or an increased risk for gastroesophageal reflux. For all patients, mucosal injury and bleeding from suctioning should be avoided.

Extubation of the Trachea

The endotracheal tube can be removed from a patient who is well anesthetized (deep extubation) or from one who has successfully emerged from general anesthesia (awake extubation). Deep extubations should be performed in patients whose airway was well maintained by mask ventilation during induction of anesthesia and who are still receiving intravenous or inhalation agents at levels that will prevent coughing and laryngospasm. Before extubation, an oropharyngeal airway should be placed to avoid upper airway obstruction. Depth of anesthesia should be confirmed by the absence of any response to suctioning of the oral pharynx and deflation of the endotracheal tube cuff, if one is present. If airway patency was satisfactory before intubation, the return to spontaneous breathing is not a prerequisite for extubation. Deep extubation can be performed safely when using sevoflurane or desflurane to allow expedient awakening after extubation (Valley et al., 2003). This technique is especially useful for patients with a history of reactive airways disease.

Awake extubations, with protective laryngeal reflexes intact, should be performed in the child with difficult airways and full stomach risks. Before an awake extubation, infants and young children may respond to laryngeal stimulation by breath holding, bronchospasm, chest-wall rigidity, marked cyanosis, and oxygen desaturation. This phenomenon is impressive and may resemble the cyanotic spells seen in infants with tetralogy of Fallot. Fortunately, these episodes are self-limited, provided

that alveolar ventilation is maintained. Older children show less of a tendency toward sudden desaturation, but they are at a greater risk of forceful coughing against the endotracheal tube (bucking) when extubation is delayed. This may lead to a greater incidence of postintubation croup (Koka et al., 1977). Thus, older children should be extubated as soon as protective reflexes return.

Until recently, it was a widely accepted practice to ventilate the patient with high flows of 100% oxygen for several minutes before extubation in order to wash out residual anesthetics and replace them with pure oxygen. Recent studies, however, have demonstrated that this practice of "preoxygenation" should be modified and that patients should be ventilated with a mixture of oxygen and air (1:1 to 2:1 ratios of oxygen and air provide about 60% to 70% oxygen), instead of 100% oxygen, to minimize airway closure and atelectasis, which almost always develop during general anesthesia, especially in infants and children (see Chapter 3, Respiratory Physiology). To eliminate atelectasis, before extubation the lungs must be reinflated with several "vital capacity maneuvers" (sustained positive airway pressure of 35 to 40 cm H_2O for several seconds) with air-oxygen mixtures and then maintain PEEP/CPAP (5 to 7 cm H_2O) (Benoit et al., 2002; Lindahl and Mure, 2002; Tusman et al., 2003).

Technique of Extubation

The removal of the endotracheal tube should be performed with as much attention to detail as when it was inserted. Placement of an oral airway or a bite block before awakening can greatly reduce the risk of complete occlusion by the teeth on the endotracheal tube and compromise of the airways. Severe or complete occlusion of the tube or the upper airways associated with marked inspiratory effort, and intrathoracic negative pressure can result in postobstructive pulmonary edema (Galvis et al., 1980; Sofer et al., 1984). Oropharyngeal airways are preferred in patients whose airway patency was less than satisfactory during anesthetic induction. Soft bite blocks made of rolled gauze and tape can reduce the incidence of soft-tissue damage to the gums, palate, and lips associated with plastic airways. After reinflation of the lungs with high pressures to eliminate atelectasis, the lungs are inflated again with oxygen-air mixture synchronously with the child's inspiration by gently squeezing the anesthesia bag. The bag is then held momentarily at end-inspiration with a positive pressure of 15 to 20 cm H_2O to maintain a high lung volume as the endotracheal tube is gently pulled out. This last maneuver serves the following three functions:

1. It inflates the lungs with an oxygen-rich gas mixture, providing an increased oxygen reservoir that may be needed if breath holding or laryngospasm occurs (Motoyama et al., 1987).
2. Positive pressure (or stretching the airway walls) decreases the incidence and intensity of laryngospasm (Suzuki and Sasaki, 1977; Sasaki, 1979).
3. The patient's first response after extubation will be a cough-like forceful exhalation or coughing, expelling any secretions trapped between the ET tube and the laryngeal wall, thus minimizing the laryngeal reflex to secretions and laryngospasm.

The initial moments after extubation are critical; oxygen saturation, heart rate, and heart rhythm must be continuously monitored with a pulse oximeter, precordial stethoscope and ECG. The oral pharynx is suctioned quickly to remove any secretions, and a face mask is applied to reestablish the breathing circuit and application of CPAP. The patency of the airway is maintained by lifting the mandible forward into the jaw-thrust position. If spontaneous ventilation does not resume laryngospasm, often the results of secretions triggering laryngeal reflexes should be considered. Under these circumstances the pharynx and larynx must be cleared of secretions swiftly, even during laryngospasm, to prevent further irritation of the airway.

Once alveolar ventilation is reestablished, the patient is carefully examined for gastric distention and for signs of aspiration and pneumothorax. Even if the stomach was suctioned previously, the child may still retch and vomit. If vomiting occurs, it is often sufficient to turn the child's head to the side to allow secretions to fall into the cheek for removal or to roll the child on to the side.

Transport to the Postanesthetic Care Unit

When breathing is satisfactory, the patient is transported to the PACU in the lateral position with supplemental oxygen via a mask, keeping the airway clear of the tongue and secretions and protecting against aspiration (Smith, 1959; Isono et al., 2002). By holding the chin up and extending the neck, the anesthesiologist can further ensure a patent airway and feel the warm breaths, indicating gas exchange. During transport to the PACU, the guardrails should be up and the safety straps should be securely fastened to prevent injury. Patients should be covered with warmed blankets to reduce heat loss during transport. Monitoring during transport should include clinical observation of chest movement, color, and gas exchange in awake and active patients and heart and breath sounds with a precordial stethoscope in sleeping patients.

More extensive monitoring, including continuous pulse oximetry, electrocardiography, and invasive blood pressure measurements, should be maintained for compromised or critically ill patients. These patients, whether intubated or not, must have a self-inflating resuscitation bag or a Mapleson D circuit connected to an oxygen cylinder with a flow rate set to maintain adequate alveolar ventilation and oxygenation. Appropriately sized endotracheal tubes, a laryngoscope, and medications for intubation and resuscitation should be available in the PACU.

POSTANESTHETIC RECOVERY

The postanesthetic recovery period is a time of high risk for pediatric patients. A large percentage of otherwise healthy infants and children (20% to 40%) develop oxygen desaturation (SpO_2 = 94%) during transport and on arrival at the PACU (Patel et al., 1988). Oxygen desaturation occurs sooner, is more pronounced, and has a longer duration in infants than in children and a longer duration in children than in adults (Xue et al., 1996). Postoperative hypoxemia is most likely caused by atelectasis, but upper airway problems such as obstruction, croup, and laryngospasm, are more likely in children (4% to 5%) than adults (Cohen et al., 1990). All children, therefore, should be administered oxygen supplementation during their transport from the operating room and on arrival at the PACU, until they can maintain satisfactory oxygen saturation in room air or at their baseline Fio_2. Nausea,

vomiting, temperature instability, and postoperative pain also require prompt and effective treatment to ensure patient comfort and efficient discharge timing.

Recovery in the Postanesthetic Care Unit

The PACU should be situated adjacent to the operating rooms to facilitate rapid and safe patient transport and to allow the anesthesiologist ready access in case of an emergency. Each bed space should have an oxygen supply with humidification, a self-inflating resuscitation bag, a suction apparatus, a pulse oximeter, an ECG monitor, and an automated blood pressure apparatus. Other supplies and commonly used medications should be readily available. In addition, the PACU should be equipped to handle any emergency that may arise when caring for infants and children. Additional features needed for the PACU are an isolation room for either infectious or immunosuppressed patients and the ability to function as a critical care unit with additional mechanical ventilatory and invasive monitoring capabilities.

Initial Care

On arrival at the PACU, the anesthesiologist confirms the patency of the patient's airway, assesses the adequacy of ventilation, and ensures the supply of humidified oxygen. The anesthesiologist records the heart rate, respiratory rate, blood pressure, SpO_2, and temperature, which are reported to the nurse. The anesthesiologist then gives a report to the nurse concerning the child's condition, special problems related to any underlying illnesses, the events of the surgery, the anesthetic technique used, and medications given. The anesthesiologist should remain at the bedside until the child is reasonably stable and well attended. PACU staff must be competent in recognizing and initiating the treatment of commonly encountered problems, including inadequate ventilation, agitation, pain, vomiting, temperature instability, and delayed awakening. Before leaving the PACU, the anesthesiologist writes a summary note and postoperative orders.

Awakening Responses

With most currently used general anesthetic techniques, awakening occurs within a few minutes of the conclusion of surgery. Unfortunately, no one technique guarantees a smooth emergence, and agitation may occur in the early recovery period. Agitation may be caused by numerous factors, including emergence delirium caused by anesthetic agents, pain, metabolic disturbances (e.g., hypothermia, hyperthermia, hypoglycemia, hyponatremia), neurologic disturbances, a behavioral response to sudden awakening in a strange environment; separation anxiety, airway obstruction with resultant hypoventilation and hypoxia, and combinations of these factors. As discussed at the beginning of this chapter, a pediatric anesthesiologist should plan the general anesthetic approach to minimize or avoid many of these factors. The incidence of emergence delirium can be reduced with an opioid or hypnotic. Pain can be prevented in these patients by judicious use of analgesics or regional techniques intraoperatively. Any metabolic disturbances should be quickly recognized and treated swiftly and appropriately.

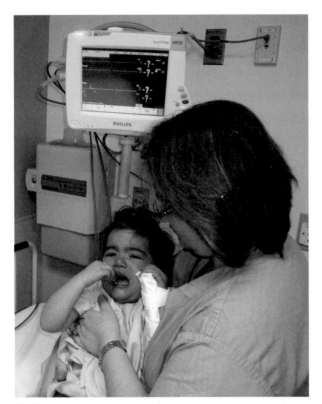

■ **FIGURE 13-6.** As pediatric patients awaken from anesthesia, they often need reassurance or the comfort of being touched or held to alleviate anxiety.

Measures other than the use of pharmacologic agents can often be effective in calming the awakening pediatric patient. Some patients simply need reassurance or the comfort of being touched or held to alleviate anxiety (Fig. 13-6). Parental presence has been shown to reduce the incidence of fear, crying, anger, and clinging during hospitalization (Fiorentini, 1993; Fina et al., 1997; Kamerling et al., 2008). Both parents and PACU staff have reported beneficial results from parental involvement. Once the infant or child has documented stable vital signs, a parent should be present.

Last but not least, the importance of detecting airway obstruction, inadequate ventilation, hypercarbia, and/or hypoxemia as causes of agitation cannot be overemphasized. Misdiagnosis can lead to inappropriate use of opioids and sedatives. Delayed and erroneous treatment of these problems can have serious consequences, including respiratory and cardiac arrests.

Common Problems in the Postanesthetic Care Unit

Apnea of Prematurity

Apnea may be central (no respiratory effort), obstructive (respiratory effort without gas flow), or mixed (both central and obstructive). Apnea is defined as cessation of breathing for longer than 15 seconds or for less than 15 seconds associated with bradycardia, cyanosis, or pallor (Nelson et al., 1978; Thatch, 1985). Repetitive pauses of breathing, lasting 5 to 10 seconds and not associated with other changes in infants, are termed periodic breathing. These abnormal respiratory patterns, which are observed commonly in neonates and preterm infants, can

appear or worsen in preterm infants after exposure to anesthetic agents (Rigatto, 1986). This is particularly true for prematurely born infants with a previous history of apnea (Liu et al., 1983).

In a combined analysis of eight studies from the halothane era, Coté et al. (1995) found that postoperative apnea was:

- Strongly and inversely correlated to both gestational age and postconceptual age (PCA)
- Associated with a previous history of apnea
- Not associated with being small-for-gestational age
- Associated with anemia (hematocrit <30) regardless of gestational age or PCA

They concluded that the risk of apnea in infants without a history of apnea or anemia is greater than 5% (95% CI) until PCA of 48 weeks with a gestational age of 35 weeks, and the risk remains greater than 1% until PCA of 54 to 56 weeks with gestational age of 32 weeks. They further concluded that older infants with apnea in the PACU and those with anemia should be admitted and monitored overnight. Because of these findings, it is generally recommended that preterm infants of fewer than 44 to 46 weeks PCA be admitted for monitoring after general anesthesia (Gregory et al., 1983; Coté et al., 1995). Regional anesthesia and subarachnoid blocks without sedation have been shown to decrease the risk of postoperative apnea (Williams et al., 2001). Sale et al. (2006) in a prospective comparison study, found no increase in respiratory events with the use of sevoflurane and desflurane. Welborn et al. (1998) found caffeine (10 mg/kg) to be effective in treating apnea in premature infants undergoing elective surgery. These patients, however, are still routinely admitted for observation and treatment.

Airway Obstruction

Although patients should be able to maintain airway patency before leaving the operating room, it is not uncommon for an infant or a child to have an obstruction after the stimulation of extubation and transportation has subsided. The anesthesiologist must be acutely aware of any changes in the breathing pattern at this time, because hypoventilation can lead to a reaccumulation of volatile agents in the alveoli that can further blunt the respiratory drive. Hypercarbia may result in dysrhythmias and hypertension, and hypoxemia in infants may lead to further suppression of breathing (Knill and Clement, 1984; Motoyama and Glazener, 1986). Neck extension, mouth opening, and jaw thrust alone or together may be enough to correct the problem. Nasopharyngeal airways, if necessary, are better tolerated than oropharyngeal airways in this setting. If obstruction continues, reassessment of anesthetic and neuromuscular blockade reversal should be conducted and possible reintubation may be considered.

Other causes of respiratory distress may be present in a way similar to upper airway obstruction. Pneumothorax, silent aspiration, and pulmonary edema should be considered and investigated if the patient continues to exhibit respiratory compromise.

Obstructive Sleep Apnea

Patients with obstructive sleep apnea syndrome (OSA) are predisposed to postoperative apnea (see Chapter 24, Anesthesia for Pediatric Otorhinolaryngologic Surgery). OSA is characterized by prolonged partial and/or intermittent complete upper airway obstruction that disrupts normal breathing and sleeping patterns (American Thoracic Society, 1996). Although OSA in adults is commonly associated with obesity, in children it more often arises from enlarged tonsils and adenoids (Young et al., 1993). Surgical removal of enlarged adenoids and tonsils often markedly improves upper airway patency (Schechter et al., 2002). OSA also occurs in infants and young children with a narrowing of upper airways secondary to craniofacial abnormalities, neuromuscular disorders, and Trisomy 21, which may worsen during the postoperative period (Marcus, 2001; Au and Li, 2009). Children with OSA have an increased sensitivity to opioids (Brown et al., 2004) (Fig. 13-7).

Postobstructive Pulmonary Edema

Pulmonary edema developing shortly after the relief of upper airway obstruction is known as postobstructive pulmonary edema (POPE) and negative pressure pulmonary edema (NPPE). It was first noted after difficult intubation in children and subsequently described after relief of laryngospasm both in infants and children (Travis et al., 1977; Galvis et al., 1980; Sofer et al., 1984). The first signs, which include rales, wheezing, desaturation, and copious production of pink, frothy respiratory secretions, may occur immediately after the relief of the obstruction. The cause of this type of pulmonary edema is attributed to the marked negative intrathoracic pressure generated by forced inspiration against a closed glottis (Mueller's maneuver), which leads to increased interstitial negative pressure, increased right-side cardiac preload, increased pulmonary vascular resistance, acute hypoxia, and increased capillary permeability (Thiagarajan and Laussen, 2007).

A high index of suspicion, as well as early recognition and intervention are essential to preventing complications secondary to postobstructive pulmonary edema. Once upper airway obstruction is relieved, patients should receive CPAP by mask (5 to 10 cm H_2O) with a high concentration of oxygen. Diuretics, along with intravenous fluid restriction, should be considered. If hypoxemia (SpO_2 <95%) persists, the patient may require endotracheal intubation and ventilation with a moderate PEEP (10 cm H_2O) until pulmonary edema is dissolved. Most cases are self-limited and usually resolve within 24 to 48 hours, but life-threatening complications are not unusual.

Postintubation Croup

The incidence of postintubation croup was reported to be about 1% (Koka et al., 1977). The most common cause is a tight-fitting endotracheal tube without an air leak at 30 to 40 cm H_2O with positive airway pressure (Koka et al.,

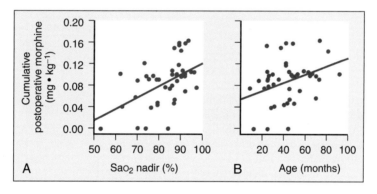

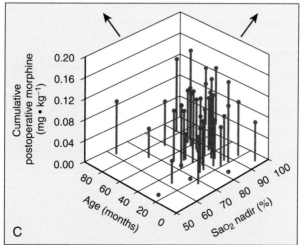

■ **FIGURE 13-7.** Age (in months) and preoperative arterial oxygen saturation (Sao_2) nadir (%) are significantly correlated with the cumulative postoperative morphine dose (mg/kg) required for analgesia after adenotonsillectomy. The correlation of each variable with the cumulative postoperative morphine dose is shown in the two-dimensional plots (**A** and **B**), and the correlation of the combined variables with the cumulative postoperative morphine dose is shown in a three-dimensional scatter plot (**C**). Estimates for each child are depicted with a filled circle. The magnitude of the cumulative postoperative morphine dose in the three-dimensional scatter plot is depicted by the height of the stem supporting each circle. *(From Brown KA, Laferriere A, Moss IR: Recurrent hypoxemia in young children with obstructive sleep apnea is associated with reduced opioid requirement for analgesia,* Anesthesiology *100:806–810, 2004.)*

1977). Other factors associated with postintubation croup may include traumatic or repeated intubation, "bucking" or coughing with the ET tube in place, changing the head position, the duration of surgery, and neck surgery. The incidence of postintubation croup seems to have decreased since this initial report. This may be secondary to the better quality of implant-tested sterile endotracheal tubes and the increased use of smaller-sized cuffed endotracheal tubes and corticosteroids.

The croup scoring system by Downs and Raphaely (1975) objectively quantifies the severity of the condition and its use can be helpful in treatment decisions (Table 13-4). Cool, humidified mist administered after extubation may be helpful in mild cases of croup. Racemic epinephrine (0.5 mL of 2.25% solution), diluted in 3 to 5 mL of normal saline solution and administered by nebulizer for 5 to 10 minutes, assists patients with progressively worsening symptoms and stridor by producing mucosal vasoconstriction, resulting in a shrinking of swollen airway mucosa. The "rebound effect" and recurrence of symptoms are well described and necessitate observing the patient for up to 4 hours after treatment. Anene et al. (1996), in a prospective, double-blind, placebo-controlled study, found that dexamethasone is effective in reducing the incidence of postintubation croup in children who have been intubated for longer than 48 hours.

Cardiovascular Instability

Cardiac rhythm disturbances and blood pressure fluctuations are rare in infants and children recovering from general anesthesia in comparison with adults (Hines et al., 1992; Murat et al., 2004). Bradycardia is typically a response to medications such as neuromuscular-blockade reversing agents or fentanyl, or it can be a normal variant that should be treated only if it is associated with hypotension. Hypoxia is also an important cause of bradycardia, especially in neonates and young infants. Tachycardia may be secondary to hypovolemia, inadequately treated pain, or anticholinergic medications. Careful assessment and appropriate therapy should be instituted to correct volume deficit or the need for analgesia. Hypertension may also reflect inadequate analgesia, an anticholinergic effect, or excessive hydration, or it may be an artifact caused by the use of an inappropriately small blood-pressure cuff. Hypotension is more unusual and is most often caused by hypovolemia secondary to inadequate fluid replacement or ongoing blood loss. Appropriate fluid resuscitation should be instituted.

Nausea and Vomiting

Postoperative vomiting (POV) is the most common complication of anesthesia in infants and children and a major cause of delayed PACU discharge and unscheduled admission for ambulatory patients (Patel and Hannallah, 1988; Murat et al., 2004). Nausea, also a common postoperative complication, is rarely included in pediatric studies because of the challenges of accurate assessment in infants and young children. Factors that increase the risk of POV include surgeries such as strabismus repair, adenotonsillectomy, and orchiopexy; age; gender; history of motion sickness; and intraoperative opioids. Eberhart noted four independent predictors of pediatric POV, including a duration of surgery equal to 30 minutes, an age of 3 years, strabismus surgery, and a positive history of POV in the patient's parent or sibling. When present, these risk factors increased the likelihood of POV (Fig. 13-8) (Gan et al., 2007). Early ambulation and clear liquids, in an attempt to meet the discharge criteria in the short-stay surgery settings, may precipitate vomiting, particularly in susceptible patients (Schreiner et al., 1992). Although rarely life threatening in the PACU, vomiting has the potential for causing aspiration, hypovolemia, and/or hypernatremia.

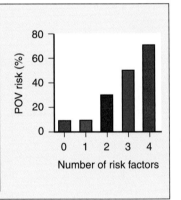

Risk factors	Points
Surgery ≥ 30 min	1
Age ≥ 3 years	1
Strabismus surgery	1
History of POV or PONV in relatives	1
Sum =	0-4

■ **FIGURE 13-8.** Simplified risk score from Eberhart and colleagues to predict the risk for POV in children. When 0, 1, 2, 3, or 4 of the depicted independent predictors are present, the corresponding risk for PONV is approximately 10%, 10%, 30%, 55%, or 70%, respectively. *(From Eberhart LH, Geldner G, Kranke P, et al.: The development and validation of a risk score to predict the probability of postoperative vomiting in pediatric patients,* Anesth Analg *99:1630, 2004.)*

TABLE 13-4. Clinical Croup Score

Criteria	Score 0	1	2
Inspiratory breathing sounds	Normal	Harsh with rhonchi	Delayed
Stridor	None	Inspiratory	Inspiratory and expiratory
Cough	None	Hoarse cry	Bark
Retraction and flaring	None	Suprasternal, (+) flaring	Suprasternal, subcostal, intercostal, (+) flaring
Cyanosis (sat <90%)	None	In room air	In 40% oxygen

From Downes JJ, Raphaely RC: Pediatric intensive care, *Anesthesiology* 43:238-250, 1975.

For prophylaxis against POV, intravenous serotonin (5-HT$_3$) receptor antagonists, such as ondansetron (0.1 to 0.15 mg/kg) and granisetron (0.04 mg/kg) given intraoperatively, have been shown to be highly effective with rare side effects (Patel et al., 1997; Fujii et al., 2002). Dexamethasone (0.2 to 0.5 mg/kg) given intraoperatively is effective in decreasing the incidence of both nausea and vomiting (Aouad et al., 2001). In combination these medications are synergistic (Davis et al., 2008). Gan and colleagues (2003) published guidelines for preventing and treating POV and recommended prophylaxis only in patients with moderate to high risk. In pretreated patients who develop POV in the PACU, a dose of an alternative 5-HT$_3$ blocker or an antiemetic from another family of medications (antihistamine, antidopaminergic) should be considered.

Temperature Instability

Even with the most careful attention to maintaining normothermia, patients often arrive in the PACU with lowered body temperature. Usually covering the patient with warmed blankets is sufficient, but radiant warming lamps and conductive warming blankets should be used in extreme cases. Hyperthermia that develops in the PACU may indicate the onset of an infectious process and should be watched closely. Malignant hyperthermia may be seen initially during the postanesthetic period. If malignant hyperthermia is suspected, appropriate investigation and therapy should be instituted without delay.

Emergence Delirium

Emergence delirium (ED) is a significant problem for children (Vlajkovic and Sindjelic, 2007). ED in children appears to be a dissociated state of consciousness characterized by inconsolability, thrashing, and incoherence (Fig. 13-9). Having all but disappeared with the discontinued use of older anesthetic agents, ED reemerged as a problem in children with the introduction of desflurane and sevoflurane (Davis et al., 1994; Aono et al., 1997; Grundmann et al., 1998). Theoretic explanations for this occurrence include rapid awakening in a strange environment, variable recovery of central nervous system function,

precipitous withdrawal from GABA receptors, and a yet-to-be-defined psychomotor side effect. Inadequately treated pain has also been proposed as a major contributor to this phenomenon, but studies have demonstrated a high incidence of ED in pain-free patients (Wells et al., 1999; Uezono et al., 2000). Risk factors include an age younger than 5 years old, otolaryngologic and ophthalmologic procedures, use of isoflurane, rapid emergence, the need for intraoperative opioids, anxious parents, poor socialization, and low adaptability scores (Voepel-Lewis et al., 2003; Kain et al., 2006). In this state, children pose a danger to themselves and care providers with complications arising in the forms of increased bleeding, pain, medication use, and need for staff. Other complications include patients pulling at surgical drains, loss of intravenous catheters and tubing, and longer PACU stays.

Several instruments and therapies have been proposed and studied to evaluate and prevent ED. The Pediatric Anesthesia Emergence Delirium Scale (PAEDS), using five criteria (eye contact, purposeful movement, awareness of environment, restlessness, inconsolability), has been demonstrated to be valid and reliable (Box 13-2) (Sikich and Lerman, 2004). A single intravenous prophylactic treatment of fentanyl 2.5 mcg/kg, clonidine 2 mcg/kg, ketamine 0.25 mg/kg, nalbuphine 0.1 mg/kg, or dexmedetomidine 0.15 mcg/kg has been shown to decrease incidence of ED (Cohen et al., 2001; Kulka et al., 2002; Dalens et al., 2006; Ibacache et al., 2004). Other routes of administration such as intranasal fentanyl 1 mcg/kg and oral clonidine 4 mg/kg are also effective (Finkel et al., 2001; Tazeroualti et al., 2007). Aouad and colleagues (2007) found that 1 mg/kg propofol after discontinuation of sevoflurane at the end of surgery decreases the incidence of ED without prolonging recovery.

Pain and Discomfort

All pediatric patients, including neonates and premature infants, experience pain if it is untreated. Differentiating between pain, anxiety, and other causes of stress in this age group is an ongoing challenge. Each age group and each patient has a different behavioral manifestation and communication ability regarding pain. The selection of the appropriate pain-assessment tool,

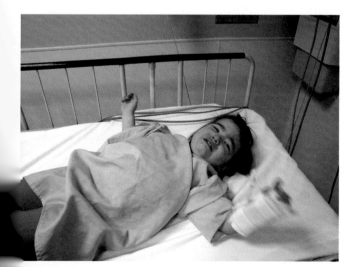

FIGURE 13-9. Emergence delirium in children appears to be a dissociated state of consciousness characterized by inconsolability, thrashing, and incoherence.

Box 13-2 The Pediatric Anesthesia Emergence Delirium Scale (PAEDS)

1. The child makes eye contact with the caregiver.
2. The child's actions are purposeful.
3. The child is aware of his or her surroundings.
4. The child is restless.
5. The child is inconsolable.

Items 1, 2, and 3 are scored on a scale of 0-4 as follows: 4 = not at all; 3 = just a little; 2 = quite a bit; 1 = very much; 0 = extremely. Items 4 and 5 are scored in reverse, as follows: 0 = not at all; 1 = just a little; 2 = quite a bit; 3 = very much; 4 = extremely. The scores of each item are added to obtain a total PAEDS score. The degree of emergence delirium increases directly with the total score.

(From Sikich N, Lerman J: Development and psychometric evaluation of the pediatric anesthesia emergence delirium scale, *Anesthesiology* 100(5):1142, 2004.)

from the multitude available, is crucial. Many of these tools are not designed for patients recovering from surgery and general anesthesia. Disorientation, fear, and regression may alter communication and behavior and cause misinterpretation. Some pain scales have a limited application in the clinical setting. As with pain assessment, selection of a pain management technique must be individualized for the patient, the surgical procedure, and the hospital setting. Selection must also be made with a good understanding of each technique's advantages and shortcomings. For these techniques to be successful, conscientious postoperative care must be given.

Pain Measurement and Assessment

Most techniques measure the intensity of pain by assigning incremental values. The most common technique, self-reporting, depends on verbal, cognitive, and developmental skills. Adapting adult patient surveying tools such as the McGill Pain Questionnaire, researchers have developed scales using verbal description and graphic rating (Melzack, 1975). Such tools are modified for age, culture, and cognitive ability (McGrath et al., 1985; Varni et al., 1987). Word lists and questioning techniques have been developed (Abu-Saad et al., 1990; Wilkie et al., 1990). Graphic or symbolic representations of pain intensity also require modification. The visual analog pain scale, initially developed for adult pain measurement, is typically a 10-cm horizontal line defined by "no pain" on the left end and "severe pain" on the right. In older children and adolescents, this instrument has been used with success (Abu-Saad, 1984; McGrath et al., 1985). In younger children, replacing the definers with different words, such as "no hurt" and "most hurt," numbers, or happy and sad faces has also been tested (Broadman et al., 1988; Savedra and Tesler, 1989). For younger children with preoperational reasoning, less abstract quantitative measurements, including counting poker chips, selecting color scales, and marking graduated thermometers, are more easily understood and used (Eland and Anderson, 1977; Hester, 1979; Jeans and Johnston, 1985). A further variation involves a progression of happy to crying faces; the faces are either illustrated, as in McGrath's Facial Affective Scale and the Wong-Baker FACES Pain Rating Scale, or photographed, as in Beyer's Oucher Scale (McGrath et al., 1985; Beyer and Aradine, 1988; Wong and Baker, 1988). Numeric values are assigned in each of these methods for progressive levels of pain intensity.

In infants and nonverbal children, observational pain scales must be implemented. For the evaluation of postoperative pain, the Children's Hospital of Eastern Ontario Pain Scale (CHEOPS) and the Objective Pain Scale grade behavioral manifestations of pain (McGrath et al., 1985; Hannallah et al., 1987). The CHEOPS assesses six categories—cry, facial expression, verbal response, torso position, leg activity, and arm movement—in relationship to the surgical wound. The Objective Pain Scale contains physiologic and behavioral changes associated with pain. These scales were designed for research purposes and are specific for age. The Facial Expression-Leg Movement-Activity-Cry-Consolability (FLACC) Scale has be shown to be valid and reliable in children who were preverbal, cognitively impaired, recovering from surgery, or undergoing painful procedures (Merkel et al., 1997; Voepel-Lewis et al., 2002; Manworren and Hynan, 2003; Nilsson et al., 2008). The Multidimensional Assessment of Pain Scale (MAP) has also shown promise of wide applicability (Ramelet et al., 2007). Neonatal and premature infant pain scales have been created and verified; these include the Neonatal Infant Pain Scale (NIPS), the Crying-Requires Oxygen-Increased Vital Signs-Expression-Sleep (CRIES) Scale, and the Premature Infant Pain Profile.

Observational pain assessment techniques are also fraught with variability. Studies have demonstrated that scoring by parents, nurses, and physicians can be unreliable when assessing pain by cry, behavior, and constructed pain scales (Wasz-Hocket et al., 1985; Beyer et al., 1990; Favaloro and Touzel, 1990; Watt-Watson et al., 1990). As with older children, previous experience, emotional and medical status, and clinician interaction can affect the response.

Because no single technique or approach is ideal, medical personnel assessing pain in children must be well versed and flexible. Verbal, graphic, behavioral, and physiologic measures have been examined and tested, but further work on psychology and emotional interplay is needed. Although cognitive development is well understood, a hospitalized child often regresses, and expected and previously observed abilities may be lost. Much progress has been made in acknowledging that infants and children experience pain, but a great deal of work is still needed to fully reveal the degree and manner of their experience.

Pain Management

The intraoperative use of opioids and regional anesthesia for preventing postoperative pain has been discussed. Even with the best planning, patients may still experience pain in the PACU. Although most pain and discomfort originate from surgical incision and tissue irritation, other causes, including tight bandages or casts, distended bladders, and corneal abrasions, should not be overlooked. Each of these problems requires immediate attention from the appropriate medical personnel. Foley catheters and nasogastric tubes may also be causes for distress. Preoperatively, patients should be prepared to expect these catheters, which will reduce anxiety during recovery. Treatment of pain in the PACU depends on the patient's medical condition, the surgical procedure, and discharge disposition. Oral acetaminophen (10 to 15 mg/kg) is useful in patients without intravenous access who have had minor surgical procedures. Rectal acetaminophen (30 to 40 mg/kg) may take up to 2 hours to achieve a therapeutic level and so is not effective for treating acute pain in the PACU. NSAIDs can play an important role in pain management for patients with compromised airways and respiratory function and can serve as adjuncts to opioid techniques, including neuroaxial and patient controlled analgesia use. Ketorolac should be avoided in patients with an increased risk for bleeding and those who underwent bone-grafting procedures.

Morphine (0.025 to 0.05 mg/kg) or fentanyl (0.5 to 1.0 mcg/kg), given in incremental doses, can be used to achieve an analgesic state in patients recovering from a general anesthetic. If hospital admission overnight or longer is planned, then morphine use is preferable because of its longer duration of action. For patients undergoing extensive surgical procedures with moderate to severe pain anticipated, continuous infusion of an opioid should be considered. Hendrickson et al. (1990) demonstrated better analgesia and greater patient satisfaction with continuous infusion compared with intermittent dosing. Continuous infusion can create consistent analgesic blood levels of morphine and remove the need for children to communicate their pain

(Berde, 1989; Esmail et al., 1999). Patient-controlled analgesia allows the patient to self-administer small incremental doses of a local anesthetic and an opioid. Patient-controlled analgesia has been extensively studied in children, and studies support its efficacy and safety (Gaukroger et al., 1989; Lawrie et al., 1990; Tyler, 1990; Berde et al., 1991). In younger children and infants, nurse-assisted patient-controlled analgesia is a useful alternative (Monitto et al., 2000; Anghelescu et al., 2005). However, there are risks associated with its use (Voepel-Lewis et al., 2008). It is most effective if patients are selected, evaluated, and instructed before surgery. Side effects of opioid use, including nausea, vomiting, pruritus, and urinary retention, should be anticipated and treated when they occur. Placement of indwelling catheters in the epidural space, body cavities, and nerve sheaths allows for continued use of local anesthetics and opioids for several days after surgery. In older children, patient-controlled epidural anesthesia (PCEA) has been shown to be safe and effective (Birmingham et al., 2003). Careful dosing and monitoring for side effects, including oversedation, respiratory arrest, and toxicity of local anesthetics, are essential. The advantages, limitations, and possible dangers of these techniques are discussed in Chapter 15, Pain Management.

Discharge from the Postanesthetic Care Unit

With more rapid recovery from general anesthesia and a greater variety of surgical cases being scheduled on an outpatient basis, strict time criteria for discharge from the PACU are becoming less useful. The Modified Aldrete Score examines the criteria of motor activity, respiration, blood pressure, consciousness, and color (Table 13-5). The Simplified Postanesthetic Recovery Score assesses consciousness, airway, and movement (Steward, 1975). Both scores can be helpful as guidelines in determining when a patient is ready for discharge. Inclusion of oxygen saturation by pulse oximetry is indicated. Before a child can be safely discharged from the PACU, a careful examination should

---

Box 13-3 PACU Discharge

1. The child is fully awake or easily aroused when called.
2. The airway is maintained and protective reflexes are present.
3. Oxygen saturation is maintained above 95% on room air or stable at the preoperative level with or without oxygen.
4. Hypothermia is absent, and hyperthermia is controlled.
5. Pain and nausea and vomiting are controlled.
6. There is no active bleeding.
7. Vital signs are stable.

---

be conducted to ensure safety on the patient floor, with its reduced nursing care and observation (Box 13-3).

From the PACU, patients can be admitted to a short-stay recovery unit or to a hospital ward. Regardless of the patient's disposition, the anesthesiologist is responsible for the follow-up, to ensure that no anesthetic complications occur, and to continue treatment for those patients receiving special pain management techniques. For ambulatory patients, a single visit is usually all that is needed. For patients with complicated medical conditions and/or extensive surgery, visits should continue until the patient is stable. Postanesthetic notes should be written in the patient's chart to communicate any findings or suggestions that may assist in the patient's recovery.

Short-Stay Recovery Unit

Patients undergoing outpatient procedures continue to recover in an ambulatory or a short-stay recovery unit (SSRU). Complications seen in the PACU can also occur here. The most common causes for unplanned hospital admission from the SSRU are vomiting, croup, fever, and family request (Patel and Hannallah, 1988). Criteria for discharge have been established (Box 13-4).

When discharged to home, the patient's family should be instructed concerning fluid intake, pain control, nausea and vomiting, and any special directives concerning the surgical procedure. In addition, a telephone number where someone will be available 24 hours a day should be supplied.

TABLE 13-5. Modified Aldrete Score

Criteria	Characteristics	Points
Activity	Voluntary movement of all limbs to command	2
	Voluntary movement of two extremities to command	1
	Unable to move	0
Respiration	Breathe deeply and cough	2
	Dyspnea, hypoventilation	1
	Apneic	0
Circulation	BP +/− 20 mm Hg of preanesthesia level	2
	BP >20-50 mm Hg of preanesthesia level	1
	BP >50 mm Hg of preanesthesia level	0
Consciousness	Fully awake	2
	Arousable	1
	Unresponsive	0
Color	Pink	2
	Pale, blotches	1
	Cyanotic	0

From Aldrete JA: The postanesthesia recovery score revisited, *J Clin Anesth* 7:89-91, 1995.

Box 13-4 Criteria for Discharge to Home

1. Vital signs are stable.
2. Intact gag reflex, swallowing, and cough, allowing for oral intake.
3. Ambulation or movements are appropriate for developmental level. (Patients who received regional analgesia must demonstrate returning motor function.)
4. Nausea and vomiting should be minimal, allowing for retention of ingested fluids.
5. No signs of respiratory distress, such as stridor retractions, nasal flaring, "barking" cough, wheezing, cyanosis, or dyspnea.
6. Patient is oriented to person, place, and time as appropriate for age.

Voiding is not necessary, but if present, it is helpful to assess fluid status and residual regional anesthesia.

(From Patel RI, Rice LJ: Special considerations in the recovery room of children from anesthesia, *Int Anesthesiol Clin* 29:55, 1991.)

SUMMARY

Maintenance of anesthesia, emergence, and postoperative care are parts of the continuous perioperative care of a patient. With improved technology in intraoperative monitoring under the guidelines for standards of monitoring and vigilance, anesthetic management of infants and children has become much safer in recent years. Yet the understanding of the young patient's special needs in terms of equipment, fluid requirement, airway management, and altered pharmacokinetics is essential. Newer anesthetic agents and adjuvant drugs, together with progress in regional analgesic techniques in infants and children, allow pediatric anesthesiologists to combine conduction analgesia with various general anesthetics for prompt and smooth emergence with appropriate postoperative analgesia. The great variety in patient age, size, and physiology necessitates planning and execution of postoperative management to be patient specific.

For questions and answers on topics in this chapter, go to "Chapter Questions" at www.expertconsult.com.

REFERENCES

Complete references used in this text can be found online at www.expertconsult.com.

CHAPTER

14

Blood Conservation

**William J. Mauermann, Dawit T. Haile, and
Randall P. Flick**

The year 1492 is often recalled as the year in which "Columbus sailed the ocean blue." Few recall that in that same year the first recorded attempt at therapeutic transfusion occurred in Rome. After having an apoplectic stroke, Pope Innocent VIII lapsed into a coma. His physician ordered that the blood of three of the Pope's young sons (he is said to have had many) be transfused in an attempt to revive him. Not surprisingly, the attempt failed, because the route of transfusion was *per os,* and led to the death of the Pope and to the deaths of his three sons, each of whom had been promised a ducat as payment.

Jean-Baptiste Denis is thought to be the first to attempt an intravenous transfusion of whole blood. He was a Parisian physician and astrologer who, in 1667, gave a teenage boy the blood of either a lamb or a dog in an attempt to restore him after he had been bled multiple times for fever. Denis was later tried for murder when another of his patients died. He was exonerated, but transfusion was subsequently banned throughout Europe for more than 100 years (Moore, 2003).

More than 300 years after the death of Pope Innocent VIII, the first successful human transfusion was performed in Philadelphia and credited to the University of Edinburgh-trained

"Father of American Surgery," Philip Syng Physick (Fig. 14-1). He did not publish any writings about his accomplishment and few details exist of the circumstances or outcome (Jepson, 1974).

The deaths of the Pope's three children are a reminder that the blood of a child is precious and should be conserved whenever possible. This chapter describes the techniques available to the pediatric anesthesiologist for conserving the blood of pediatric patients and provides insight into hemoglobin function, anemia, blood banking, and transfusion practices.

HEMOGLOBIN STRUCTURE AND FUNCTION IN THE NEONATE, INFANT, AND CHILD

Hemoglobin, the primary oxygen-carrying pigment, is a large complex tetrameric protein consisting of iron-containing heme groups (protoporphyrin IX ring with attached ferrous iron atom) and the globin protein moiety (Fig. 14-2). The paired arrangement of polypeptide globin chains each interacting with an attached heme group provides the complex reversible interactions that allow for the transport of oxygen.

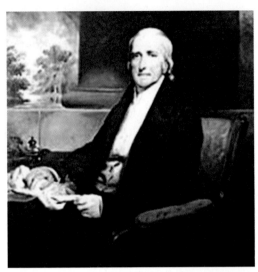

■ **FIGURE 14-1.** Philip Syng Physick. This portrait is by Robert Reynolds (circa 1840), who copied an earlier portrait (circa 1836) by Henry Inman (1801-1846). *(Adapted from Rutkow IM: Moments in surgical history: Philip Syng Physick [1768-1837],* Arch Surg *136[8]:968, 2001.)*

Because each heme moiety has the capacity to bind a single oxygen molecule, a molecule of hemoglobin can transport as many as four oxygen molecules; remarkably, this process is accomplished without the input of energy.

In the healthy child and adult the tetrameric structure of hemoglobin consists of two polypeptide alpha (α) chains and two beta (β) chains and is designated *hemoglobin A.* The chains differ in the number and sequence of amino acids and in the chromosomes on which their structure is coded. The gene for the α chain is located on chromosome 16, whereas the genes for the β chain and for the embryonic and fetal chains (gamma [γ], epsilon [ε], and zeta [ζ]) are closely linked on chromosome 11.

Hemoglobin structure during the embryologic period is characterized by three hemoglobin species, which include Gower-1($\zeta_2\varepsilon_2$), Gower-2 ($\alpha_2\varepsilon_2$), and Portland ($\zeta_2\gamma_2$) (Fig. 14-3). By the tenth week of gestation, these embryonic hemoglobin species are nearly completely replaced by fetal hemoglobin ($\alpha_2\gamma_2$), which is also called *hemoglobin F.* At 10 to 12 weeks of gestation, the distribution of hemoglobin is about 80% to 90% fetal hemoglobin and 10% hemoglobin A. Synthesis of fetal hemoglobin ceases at approximately 38 weeks of gestation; at birth, the percentage of fetal hemoglobin has decreased to about 70% to 80% and, under normal circumstances, continues to decrease thereafter. By 6 months of age, fetal hemoglobin levels typically have decreased to less than 5% and by 1 year of age, to 2%, which is a level similar to that in adults.

The primary physiologic function of hemoglobin is to carry oxygen acquired in the capillary beds of the pulmonary alveoli (or, in fetal life, the chorionic villi of the maternal placenta) and release it in the reduced-oxygen environment of the tissues. Hemoglobin also is important as a biological buffer and in the transport of both carbon dioxide (the Bohr effect) and nitric oxide (Fig. 14-4). In its primary role as an oxygen carrier, hemoglobin functions by altering its affinity for oxygen through changes in the quaternary structure of the protein moiety. This relationship can be usefully illustrated by examining the appearance of the oxyhemoglobin dissociation curve

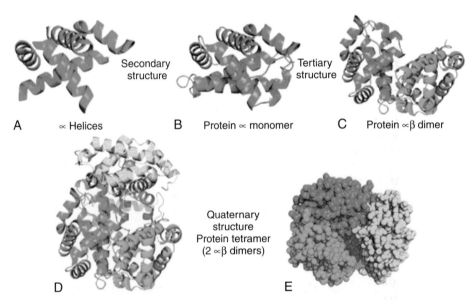

■ **FIGURE 14-2.** Hemoglobin. The structure of hemoglobin, made up of two α-globin chains and two β-globin chains, is used to illustrate the hierarchical nature of protein folding. **A,** Globin chains are composed almost entirely of α helices. **B,** The organization of secondary structural elements within a domain or protein defines the fold or tertiary structure, as is illustrated for the α helices *(green ribbon)* of an α-globin chain of deoxyhemoglobin. The spatial relationship of subunits in the assembled protein defines the protein's quaternary structure. **C,** To form a hemoglobin molecule, an α-globin chain and a β-globin chain *(green and blue,* respectively) assemble to form a dimer. **D,** Two αβ dimers assemble to form the hemoglobin tetramer (α chains, *green and magenta;* β chains, *blue and yellow*). **E,** A space-filling model of the hemoglobin tetramer in which the atoms are represented by spheres with radii proportional to their van der Waals radii is shown for the hemoglobin tetramer, colored as described. *(Modified from Rigby AC, Furie B, Furie BC: Protein architecture: relationship of form and function. In Hoffman R et al, editors:* Hematology: basic principles and practice, *ed 5, Philadelphia, 2009, Churchill Livingstone Elsevier.)*

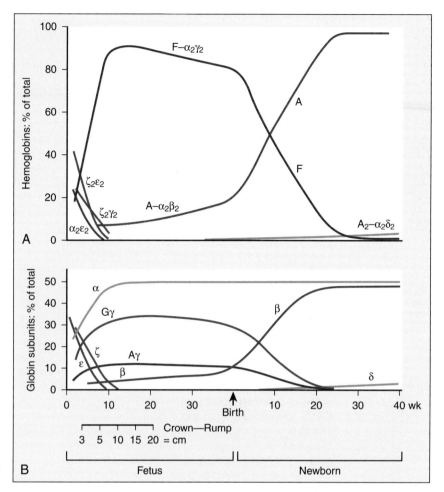

■ **FIGURE 14-3.** Hemoglobin structure during human development from embryo to early infancy. **A,** Hemoglobin tetramers. **B,** Globin subunits. *A* and *A₂,* Adult hemoglobin; *F,* fetal hemoglobin. *(Modified from Polin RA, Fox WW: Fetal and neonatal physiology, ed 2, Philadelphia, 1998, Saunders.)*

(Fig. 14-5). The sigmoidal shape of the curve, which describes the relationship of hemoglobin saturation at various levels of oxygen tension, results from the four globin chains individually interacting with oxygen and collectively affecting the affinity of the other chains for oxygen. This complex interaction results in an affinity curve that demonstrates hemoglobin's low affinity (flat portion of the lower curve) for oxygen in hypoxic environments and a rapidly increasing affinity (steep portion) as oxygenation of each heme group occurs until the molecule becomes saturated (flat portion of upper curve). The classic shape of the curve is described for hemoglobin A and reflects the physiologic requirement to load and unload oxygen within a narrow range of oxygen tensions. Other hemoglobin species and mixtures of species have different affinities for oxygen and therefore produce different dissociation curves that in turn reflect embryonic or fetal needs.

The dissociation curve for fetal hemoglobin reflects its function as an acceptor of oxygen carried by maternal hemoglobin A. Therefore, fetal hemoglobin must have a greater affinity for oxygen than maternal hemoglobin (hemoglobin A) to accept oxygen carried to the uterine villi. The increased affinity of fetal hemoglobin for oxygen can be traced to its lower capacity to interact with 2,3-diphosphoglycerate (2,3-DPG), because the binding site for 2,3-DPG is on the β chain, which is absent in fetal hemoglobin (Jepson, 1974). Although one would expect that the increased affinity for oxygen characteristic of fetal hemoglobin would be essential for adequate oxygen delivery in the fetus, that appears not to be the case, as illustrated by the lack of deleterious effects on the fetus when hemoglobin A is transfused in utero (Mathers et al., 1970). Furthermore, infants born to mothers with hemoglobinopathies characterized by an increased affinity for oxygen show no apparent effects (Moore et al., 1967). By extension, it can be presumed that in the neonate, transfusion with blood containing hemoglobin A is not harmful and may in fact have clear advantages, especially in critical illness (Oski, 1973).

As previously discussed, the characteristic sigmoidal shape of the oxyhemoglobin dissociation curve of hemoglobin A is a reflection of its structure, whereas its position with respect to oxygen saturation and oxygen tension is a function of various factors. Under normal circumstances, the oxygen tension at which hemoglobin A is 50% saturated (P_{50}) is 27 mm Hg. Temperature, pH, P_{CO_2}, and 2,3-DPG levels all have profound effects on oxygen affinity and therefore on P_{50}, resulting in a leftward or rightward shift in the position of the curve. Because the appearance of the oxyhemoglobin dissociation curve for the neonate is identical to that of the adult at a pH of 7.6, environmental differences are potentially more important to hemoglobin's functional affinity than are fundamental differences in the hemoglobin molecule itself (Nelson et al., 1964). Under normal circumstances, the P_{50} increases from about 19 mm Hg at 1 day of age to the adult level of 27 mm Hg at age 4 to 6 months (Fig. 14-6). At the end of the first year, the P_{50} actually exceeds that of the adult at a level slightly greater than 30 mm Hg (Oski, 1973). For further reading, see Chapter 3, Respiratory Physiology in Infants and Children.

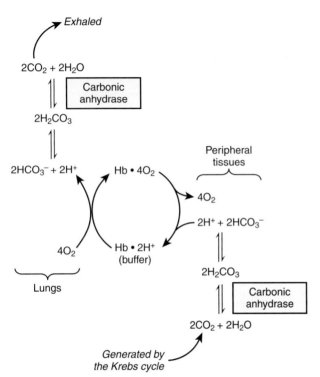

FIGURE 14-4. The Bohr effect. Carbon dioxide *(CO₂)* generated in peripheral tissues combines with water *(H₂O)* to form carbonic acid *(H₂CO₃),* which dissociates into protons *(H⁺)* and bicarbonate ions *(HCO₃⁻).* Deoxyhemoglobin acts as a buffer by binding protons and delivering them to the lungs. In the lungs, the uptake of oxygen *(O₂)* by hemoglobin *(Hb)* releases protons that combine with bicarbonate ion, forming carbonic acid, which, when dehydrated by carbonic anhydrase, becomes CO₂, which then is exhaled. *(Modified from Polin RA, Fox WW: Fetal and neonatal physiology, ed 2, Philadelphia, 1998, Saunders.)*

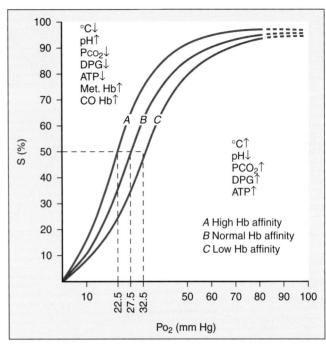

FIGURE 14-5. Oxyhemoglobin dissociation curve. Curve *B* is from a normal adult at 38° C, pH 7.40, and PCO₂ 35.0 mm Hg. Curves *A* (newborn) and *C* illustrate the effect on the affinity for oxygen of variations in temperature (°C), pH, PCO₂, 2,3-diphosphoglycerate (DPG), adenosine triphosphate (ATP), methemoglobin (Met Hb), and carboxyhemoglobin (CO Hb). *Hb,* Hemoglobin; *S,* Saturation. *(Modified from Duc G: Assessment of hypoxia in the newborn: suggestions for a practical approach,* Pediatrics 48[3]:469, 1971.)

The red blood cell (RBC) is of great importance to the function of hemoglobin. Loss of nuclear constituents during normal erythropoiesis imposes on the RBC a finite existence in the circulation. The absence of a nucleus allows it to function more effectively in oxygen transport but limits its ability to repair defects in the cell membrane, because it lacks the ability to synthesize the necessary proteins. The mature RBC maintains approximately 40 enzymes capable of various functions, such as electrolyte homeostasis, energy metabolism through anaerobic glycolysis, maintenance of cell membrane shape and integrity, maintenance of heme iron in the ferrous state, and maintenance of appropriate levels of 2,3-DPG. Free hemoglobin is rapidly removed and cannibalized, whereas hemoglobin maintained within the RBC membrane has a life span of up to 120 days. Fetal RBCs have a life span of only 60 to 90 days. With increasing prematurity, the life span of the RBC is progressively shorter, contributing to the frequency of transfusions required among the most premature patients. RBC senescence results from the loss of enzyme function necessary for maintenance of the membrane integrity. Ultimately, progressive loss of membrane results in the loss of the characteristic biconcave shape of the RBC, a shape that is less deformable and more fragile, and in sequestration and destruction of the RBC in the sluggish circulation of the spleen.

PHYSIOLOGIC ANEMIA AND THE ANEMIA OF PREMATURITY

At term, the neonate has a hemoglobin concentration of approximately 17 g/dL. As hemoglobin F is replaced with hemoglobin A over the ensuing months, the hemoglobin level decreases to a low of 10 g/dL, and the oxyhemoglobin dissociation curve shifts rightward. This shift is the result of the combination of increasing levels of hemoglobin A and increased levels of 2,3-DPG as described by Oski (1973). An increase in the levels of either one alone is insufficient. The importance of this is apparent in infants who have respiratory distress syndrome with abnormally low levels of 2,3-DPG and who show improved oxygen unloading at the tissue level after transfusion with fresh adult blood. The transition from a P₅₀ of 19 mm Hg in the term neonate to 27 mm Hg (as in the adult) typically occurs over 4 to 6 months. However, in the premature patient this transition may be delayed to as late as age 12 months.

As the conversion from hemoglobin F to hemoglobin A occurs, the hemoglobin concentration decreases from 17 to 18 g/dL at birth to a nadir of 10 to 11 g/dL at 8 to 12 weeks of age. This is termed the *physiologic anemia of infancy,* a condition that persists until the hemoglobin concentration increases to levels typical of the older child and adult over the second half of the first year. The anemia in the healthy

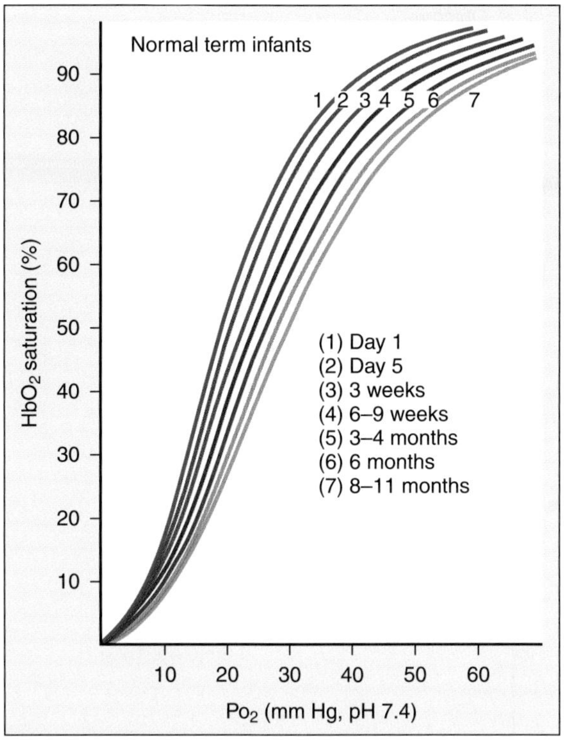
Normal term infants
1 2 3 4 5 6 7
(1) Day 1
(2) Day 5
(3) 3 weeks
(4) 6–9 weeks
(5) 3–4 months
(6) 6 months
(7) 8–11 months
HbO2 saturation (%)
Po2 (mm Hg, pH 7.4)

■ **FIGURE 14-6.** Oxygen equilibrium curve of blood at different postnatal ages. The mean ±SD oxygen tension at which hemoglobin A is 50% saturated shifts from 19.4 ±1.8 mm Hg on the first day of life to 30.3 ±0.7 mm Hg at age 11 months (normal in adults is 27.0 ±1.1 mm Hg). HbO_2, Oxyhemoglobin. *(Modified from Oski FA: The unique fetal red cell and its function: E. Mead Johnson Award address,* Pediatrics *51[3]:494, 1973.)*

neonate is asymptomatic and is therefore not a true anemia; thus, *physiologic* is used to differentiate the normal decrease in hemoglobin in the full-term neonate from that in the premature neonate. In the premature infant, this anemia occurs earlier, persists longer, and is symptomatic, with hemoglobin levels often decreasing to as low as 8.0 g/dL as early as the fourth week after birth.

The origin of physiologic anemia (and to a lesser extent, the anemia of prematurity) can be traced to a dramatic decrease in levels of erythropoietin. Erythropoietin, a glycoprotein of 34,000 Da, is synthesized in the fetal liver and thereafter in the kidneys and is the primary growth factor for erythroid progenitors. Its activity is primarily regulated by oxygen tension; as oxygen tension decreases, expression of the erythropoietin gene increases. In the fetus, erythropoietin gene expression is high, because oxygen tensions are low. The leftward position of the oxyhemoglobin dissociation curve necessitates that hemoglobin concentration be maintained at levels that will deliver sufficient oxygen to fetal tissues despite the high oxygen affinity of fetal hemoglobin.

At birth, oxygen tensions increase quickly, effectively halting erythropoietin synthesis, and consequently, erythropoiesis. In the full-term neonate, erythropoietin and, consequently, hemoglobin levels begin increasing around the age of 4 months, resulting in the correction of physiologic anemia, which is often called the *physiologic nadir* to emphasize the physiologic or nonpathologic nature of the decrease in hemoglobin. In premature infants, the phenomenon is more complex and is complicated by the need for repeated blood sampling in hospitalized premature infants. Often, the blood sampling requirements equal or exceed half of the total blood volume in infants weighing less than 1 kg (Stockman, 1986). The need for phlebotomy results in a need for the transfusion of adult banked blood—blood containing hemoglobin A with its characteristic lower affinity for oxygen. The resulting increase in tissue-oxygen tension further decreases erythropoietin synthesis and prolongs the duration of anemia for a period that is dependent on factors such as weight, gestational age, and the ongoing need for transfusion.

The *anemia of prematurity* is a true anemia that produces clinical signs and symptoms such as tachycardia, bradycardia, apnea, delayed growth, and poor weight gain. Treatment is directed at these consequences and consists of either transfusion, or more recently, the use of recombinant erythropoietin. Studies examining the potential benefit of booster transfusions targeted to keep hemoglobin levels greater than 10 g/dL in premature infants have been mixed; some have shown improvements in weight gain, and others have failed to demonstrate benefit (Blank et al., 1984; Stockman et al., 1984; Keyes et al., 1989).

The use of recombinant erythropoietin has also been studied extensively in the treatment of anemia of prematurity. A Cochrane Review described the results of 23 studies involving 2074 infants (Fig. 14-7) (Ohlsson and Aher, 2006). The end point of the majority of the studies was a reduction in the need for transfusion and donor exposure after enrollment. In the majority of studies, the need for transfusion was reduced; however, the reduction is of limited clinical significance. Several studies also found an increased incidence of retinopathy of prematurity among those treated with erythropoietin. The lack of clinically relevant benefit and the potential to increase the occurrence of retinopathy of prematurity prompted the recommendation against the use of erythropoietin as a means of reducing the need for transfusion in premature infants. Transfusion practices and indications in this group are discussed later in this chapter.

PERIOPERATIVE STRATEGIES FOR BLOOD CONSERVATION

This section discusses the following techniques and drugs that have been studied to limit allogenic blood transfusion in the pediatric population: erythropoietin, iron supplementation, hemostatic drugs, preoperative autologous blood donation, preoperative hemodilution, and deliberate hypotension. Not all these methods of blood conservation are ideal for every patient or surgical procedure, but each method has a place in the perioperative management of blood conservation in the pediatric patient.

Erythropoietin

As discussed in the previous section, erythropoietin is an inducible glycoprotein produced in the kidneys and extrarenal tissues. It regulates erythropoiesis in response to tissue hypoxia. Acute anemia is associated with exponential increases in erythropoietin in the plasma. However, in the critically ill, erythropoietin induction is blunted, as has also been observed

Analysis 01.03. Comparison 01 Erythropoietin vs. placebo or no treatment, Outcome 03, Use of one or more
red blood cell transfusions (low dose EPO)

Review: Early erythropoietin for preventing red blood cell transfusion in preterm and/or low–birth-weight infants
Comparison: 01 erythropoietin vs. placebo or no treatment
Outcome: 03 use of one or more RBC transfusions (low dose EPO)

Study	Treatment n/N	Control n/N	Relative risk (fixed) 95% CI	Weight (%)	Relative risk (fixed) 95% CI
01 High dose iron					
Chang 1999	0/15	0/15		0.0	Not estimable
Subtotal (95% CI)	15	15		0.0	Not estimable

Total events: 0 (Treatment), 0 (Control)
Test for heterogeneity: not applicable
Test for overall effect: not applicable

02 Low dose iron					
Otladen 1991	23/43	34/50		67.3	0.96 [0.72, 1.29]
Scubasi 1995	7/33	16/36		32.7	0.49 [0.22, 1.01]
Subtotal (95% CI)	76	86		100.0	0.80 [0.60, 1.07]

Total events 35 (Treatment), 50 (Control)
Test for heterogeneity chi-square = 3.29 df = I p = 0.07 I² = 69.69%
Test for overall effect z = 1.53 p = 0.1

| Total (95% CI) | 91 | 101 | | 100.0 | 0.80 [0.60, 1.07] |

Total events: 35 (Treatment), 50 (Control)
Test for heterogeneity chi-square = 129 df = I p = 0.07 I² = 69.69%
Test for overall effect z = 1.53 p = 0.1

0.2   0.5   1   2   5

Favors EPO   Favors control

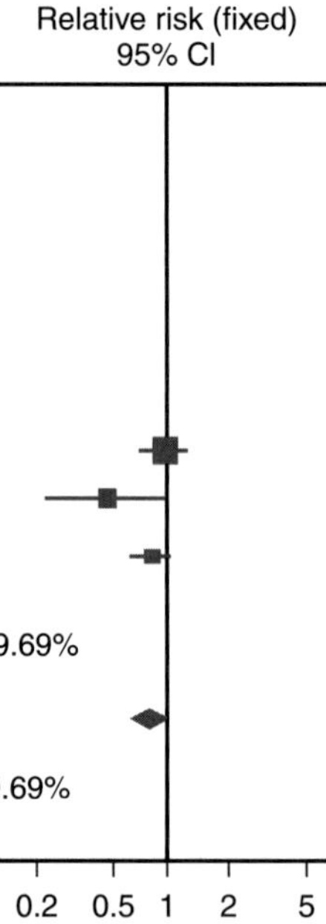

■ FIGURE 14-7. Erythropoietin and the need for transfusion among preterm and low–birth-weight infants: erythropoietin versus placebo or no treatment. Although the various outcomes of studies using erythropoietin *(EPO)* to decrease the need for transfusion among premature infants tend to favor its use, the effect sizes are small and may not be clinically relevant. *CI,* Confidence interval. *(Modified from Ohlsson A, Aher SM: Early erythropoietin for preventing red blood cell transfusion in preterm and/or low birth weight infants,* Cochrane Database Syst Rev, *19[3]:CD004863, 2006.)*

in various chronic illnesses in childhood. The exact mechanism of the inhibition observed in both critical illness and chronic illness has not been described (Krafte-Jacobs et al., 1994). Regardless of the mechanism, both situations often lead to the need for blood transfusion. The use of recombinant erythropoietin has been investigated as a means of reducing the need for transfusion or the frequency of transfusion in chronic or critical illness.

Adult studies have shown mixed results in the efficacy of recombinant human erythropoietin to avoid or limit blood transfusion. Several randomized controlled studies, including a study reported by Silver et al. (2006), have shown that at least 1 unit of blood was saved in patients in an adult intensive care unit (Corwin et al., 2002). More recently, however, Corwin and colleagues (2007) reported that in a large, prospective, randomized controlled trial involving more than 1400 adult patients, the group receiving erythropoietin had a 10% decrease in the need for transfusion compared with the control group. However, that study and others found an increase in the instances of thrombotic events among patients receiving erythropoietin.

A benefit, albeit small, was found in studies that examined the use of perioperative erythropoietin for reducing the need for transfusion during and after procedures in which transfusion is normally required. Laupacis and Fergusson (1998), in a meta-analysis involving adults undergoing either orthopedic or cardiac surgery, found a significant reduction in allogenic RBC transfusion in both groups of patients (Fig. 14-8). In a study of children undergoing craniofacial repair, Helfaer et al. (1998) found that

children receiving preoperative erythropoietin required transfusion significantly less often than controls (64% vs. 100%). Other small studies (183) and case reports have concluded that erythropoietin is efficacious in reducing the need for RBC transfusion in children, but in the absence of data from large, well-designed prospective trials, its use cannot be recommended.

Iron Supplementation

The main cause of iron-deficiency anemia in the developed world is blood loss, primarily from gastrointestinal tract bleeding, menstruation, numerous blood draws, or surgical blood loss. The development of iron deficiency is dependent on the individual's iron reserve, which in turn is dependent on the age, sex, rate of growth, and rate of absorption of iron.

The incidence of iron deficiency anemia is approximately 9% among children 1 to 2 years old in the United States (Looker et al., 1997). For adult patients with normal iron storage, there is conflicting evidence as to whether iron supplementation perioperatively improves the hemoglobin level. Several randomized control trials have failed to show that oral iron supplementation increases hemoglobin levels perioperatively (Crosby et al., 1994; Sutton et al., 2004; Mundy et al., 2005). However, two clinical trials (one randomized and one nonrandomized) with colorectal surgical patients have shown that treatment with oral iron supplementation for two weeks significantly increased hemoglobin levels and decreased blood transfusion rates (Okuyama et al.

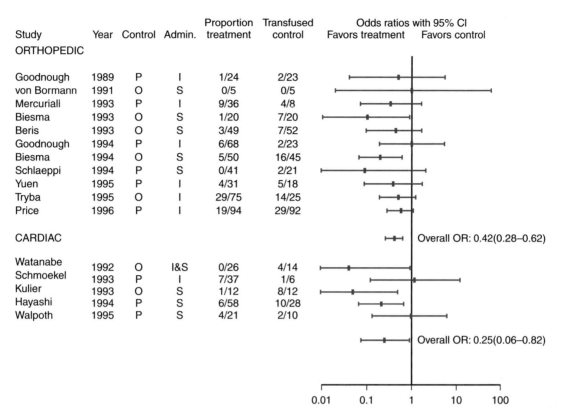

Study	Year	Control	Admin.	Proportion treatment	Transfused control	Odds ratios with 95% CI
ORTHOPEDIC						
Goodnough	1989	P	I	1/24	2/23	
von Bormann	1991	O	S	0/5	0/5	
Mercuriali	1993	P	I	9/36	4/8	
Biesma	1993	O	S	1/20	7/20	
Beris	1993	O	S	3/49	7/52	
Goodnough	1994	P	I	6/68	2/23	
Biesma	1994	O	S	5/50	16/45	
Schlaeppi	1994	P	S	0/41	2/21	
Yuen	1995	P	I	4/31	5/18	
Tryba	1995	O	I	29/75	14/25	
Price	1996	P	I	19/94	29/92	
CARDIAC						Overall OR: 0.42(0.28–0.62)
Watanabe	1992	O	I&S	0/26	4/14	
Schmoekel	1993	P	I	7/37	1/6	
Kulier	1993	O	S	1/12	8/12	
Hayashi	1994	P	S	6/58	10/28	
Walpoth	1995	P	S	4/21	2/10	
						Overall OR: 0.25(0.06–0.82)

■ **FIGURE 14-8.**   Proportion of patients receiving transfusions in studies of erythropoietin. *Admin,* Route of administration; *CI,* confidence interval; *I,* intravenous; *O,* open label control; *OR,* odds ratio; *P,* placebo; *S,* subcutaneous. *(Modified from Laupacis A, Fergusson D: Erythropoietin to minimize perioperative blood transfusion: a systematic review of randomized trials,* Transfus Med *8[4]:309, 1998.)*

2005; Lidder et al., 2007). The conclusion of a review by Beris et al. (2008) for the Network for Advancement of Transfusion Alternatives was that there is insufficient evidence to recommend the use of intravenous iron as a means of reducing the need for perioperative transfusion in adults. As with the use of erythropoietin, few data for children are available.

Hemostatic Drugs

Three currently available hemostatic drugs have been well investigated and extensively used to limit blood loss perioperatively. Two of the drugs, aminocaproic acid (EACA) and tranexamic acid (TA), are lysine amino-acid synthetic derivatives; the third, aprotinin, is a naturally occurring antifibrinolytic and proteinase inhibitor (Fig. 14-9). These drugs have been extensively used in adults and, more recently, in children.

Fibrinolysis, the lysis of formed fibrin clot, results from the enzymatic conversion of the proenzyme plasminogen to plasmin, a process that is mediated by tissue plasminogen activator, urokinase, factors XIa and XIIa, and kallikrein. Fibrinolysis results in the cleavage of polymerized fibrin strands at multiple sites and releases fibrin degradation products such as D dimer (Kolev and Machovich, 2003). EACA and TA exert their antifibrinolytic activity by reversibly blocking the lysine binding site on plasminogen, preventing binding to fibrin and conversion to active plasmin. As an inhibitor of fibrinolysis, TA is 10 times more potent than EACA. TA may also improve hemostasis by preventing plasmin-induced platelet activation, and both EACA and TA have antiinflammatory properties, but they are less than those of aprotinin (Eaton, 2008).

Antifibrinolytics have been used in children primarily for spine surgery and cardiac surgery, although they have been used for other procedures, including craniofacial reconstruction and repair of congenital diaphragmatic hernia during extracorporeal membrane oxygenation (ECMO). Sethna et al. (2005) reported on a randomized study of 44 pediatric patients undergoing elective spine surgery who received either TA (100 mg/kg loading dose followed by 10 mg/kg per hour) or saline placebo during the procedure; the treatment group had a 41% reduction in blood loss (Fig. 14-10). In a subsequent study involving children with Duchenne's muscular dystrophy, the same authors found a similar reduction in the transfusion requirement (Shapiro et al., 2007).

For adult cardiac surgery, the use of antifibrinolytics is well established. For children, although the efficacy data are less available and of lower quality, they support the use of TA and EACA primarily in children undergoing repair of cyanotic congenital heart disease. Bulutcu et al. (2005), in a series of studies involving 750 cyanotic patients, found that both TA and EACA were beneficial in reducing transfusion requirements by up to 50%, reducing blood loss by 44%, and significantly reducing times for sternal closure and rate of reexploration.

Few complications have been associated with the use of TA and EACA, although concerns have been related to thrombosis in patients, such as those undergoing ECMO or a Fontan procedure requiring the use of a baffle fenestration. Although case reports suggest the potential for concern, studies involving 71 patients undergoing a Fontan procedure and 431 patients undergoing ECMO have failed to demonstrate an increased risk of thrombosis (Hocker and Saving, 1995; Gruber et al., 2000; Downard et al., 2003).

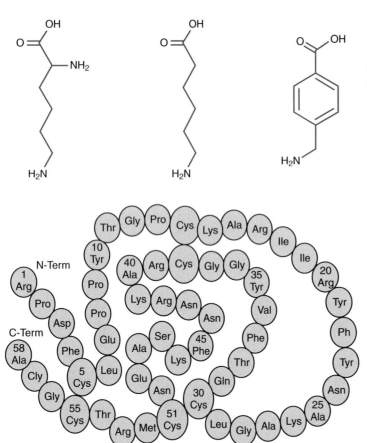

■ **FIGURE 14-9.** Molecular structures of three hemostatic drugs. Aminocaproic acid *(upper center)* and tranexamic acid *(upper right)* are synthetic derivatives of lysine *(upper left)*. Aprotinin *(lower)* is a proteinase inhibitor. *Term,* Terminal. *(Modified from Eaton MP: Antifibrinolytic therapy in surgery for congenital heart disease,* Anesth Analg *106[4]:1087, 2008.)*

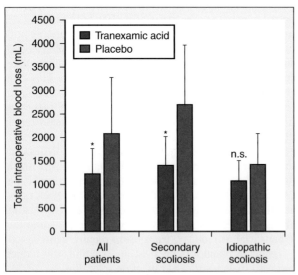

■ **FIGURE 14-10.** Mean intraoperative total blood loss in patients undergoing spinal surgery for scoliosis. Patients received either tranexamic acid or placebo. Blood loss was less in the tranexamic-acid group among patients with secondary scoliosis (*P* less than .01) and for all patients (*P* less than .01). *Asterisks,* Statistical significance; *error bars,* standard deviation; *N.S.,* not significant. *(Modified from Sethna NF, Zurakowski D, Brustowicz RM, et al.: Tranexamic acid reduces intraoperative blood loss in pediatric patients undergoing scoliosis surgery,* Anesthesiology *102[4]:727, 2005.)*

Aprotinin is a nonspecific serine protease inhibitor derived from bovine lung that inhibits proteases with active serine residues, especially plasmin. The resulting effects are an attenuation of inflammatory responses and antifibrinolysis. Aprotinin and the lysine analogues have very different modes and scopes of action, but ultimately both function by inhibiting fibrinolysis through the inhibition of plasmin. Additionally, aprotinin is thought to restore the adhesive properties of platelets independently of its effect on the inhibition of fibrinolysis (Bradfield and Bode, 2003). The efficacy of aprotinin is somewhat less clear than that of either EACA or TA. Eaton (2008), in a comprehensive review published in 2008, described in detail the available data on the efficacy of aprotinin use in pediatric cardiac surgery, in which it is most often used. Of the 14 randomized controlled trials, 11 showed a reduction in at least one parameter of blood loss or replacement. Three studies by Boldt et al. (1994, 1993a, 1993b) showed no benefit, whereas the majority of observational studies described in Eaton's review did show benefit. The difficulty in evaluating the extensive literature on the use of aprotinin in pediatric cardiac surgery lies in the differences in end points (e.g. transfusion requirement, or chest tube output), dosing regimens (i.e., high dose vs. low dose), surgical procedures (e.g. Fontan procedure or ventricular septal defect), cardiopulmonary bypass management, and patients (e.g., infants, neonates or reoperation). The relatively small numbers evaluated within each study and the virtually endless potential permutations of the resulting data make drawing conclusions about efficac difficult, although the weight of the existing evidence in adults and children suggests a benefit similar to that obtained with the lysine derivatives TA and EACA.

The use of aprotinin has raised concerns about the potential for complications, including thrombosis, anaphylaxis, and, most importantly, renal failure. In 2006 the Multicenter Study of Perioperative Ischemia Research Group reported on the largest observational prospective study of antifibrinolytic therapy (Mangano et al., 2006). The study tracked 4374 patients undergoing coronary artery bypass grafting and compared the use of aprotinin (1295 patients), EACA (883 patients), and TA (822 patients) with placebo (1374 patients). Aprotinin was associated with higher risks of death, cardiovascular event, cerebrovascular event, and renal failure. EACA and TA were not associated with increases in renal, cardiac, or neurologic complications. All three agents decreased blood loss to essentially the same degree.

In 1993, the Food and Drug Administration (FDA) approved aprotinin for patients at high risk of bleeding who were undergoing coronary artery bypass grafting with cardiopulmonary bypass (Ray and Stein, 2008). After the publication of the Blood Conservation Using Antifibrinolytics in a Randomized Trial (BART) study (Fergusson et al., 2008), Bayer Pharmaceuticals notified the FDA of its intent to withdraw aprotinin from the market. In that study of 2331 high-risk adult cardiac surgery patients, the investigators sought to determine whether aprotinin was superior to either TA or EACA in decreasing significant postoperative bleeding. The trial was terminated early because of an excess of deaths in the aprotinin group (6%) compared with the TA group (3.9%) and the EACA group (4.0%) (Fig. 14-11).

Preoperative Autologous Blood Donation

Since the 1980s, preoperative autologous donation (PAD) of blood 2 to 3 weeks before the operation has been used for adult cardiac and noncardiac surgical procedures in which blood loss and the need for blood transfusion are expected. The primary goal is to decrease the amount of allogenic blood transfused (Nath and Pogrel, 2005; Schved, 2005; Ferraris et al., 2007).

Numerous studies have documented the safety and benefit of this practice for adults in various settings. The main benefit is that it decreases the exposure to allogenic blood. A concern, though, is the amount of blood transfused (both allogenic and autologous) in patients who undergo PAD (Henry et al., 2002). The increased rate of transfusion is thought to lead to an increased risk of administrative errors with the increased number of units transfused (Schved, 2005). Vega et al. (2008) reported statistically higher complication rates among patients having reconstructive breast surgery who had PAD compared with patients in a control group who did not preoperatively donate their own blood.

Published studies of children and PAD are limited mostly to patients undergoing orthopedic or cardiac surgery. No large pediatric randomized controlled trials of this technique have been performed. Many of the case series involve a combination of PAD and other techniques, such as acute normovolemic hemodilution, erythropoietin, and controlled hypotension, making the evaluation of PAD alone difficult.

Masuda et al. (2000) studied children weighing less than 20 kg. The children were not given erythropoietin, and each child predonated a mean (with standard deviation indicated as SD) of 48 (SD = 17) mL/kg of blood over an average of 50 (SD = 16) days. No child in the study group received allogenic blood transfusion, but 80% of children in the control group did. Sonzogni et al. (2001) pretreated children in a PAD group with subcutaneous erythropoietin 3 times a week for 3 weeks preceding cardiac surgery and once intravenously on the day of the operation. The controls were 39 consecutive age-matched patients from the previous year. Children predonated 9 mL/kg of blood on two separate occasions if the hematocrit was greater than 33%. Three of the 39 children in the study group required transfusion with allogenic blood, compared with 24 of the 39 in the control group.

Most studies of PAD in orthopedics involve scoliosis surgery. Murray et al. (1997) studied 243 consecutive pediatric patients undergoing spinal fusion and found that 90% of the children who predonated did not require allogenic blood during surgery. Moran et al. (1995) reported similar results in their study of children undergoing spinal fusion. In that study, the proportion of patients who needed allogenic blood (11%) was nearly identical to that found by Murray and colleagues. In both studies, at

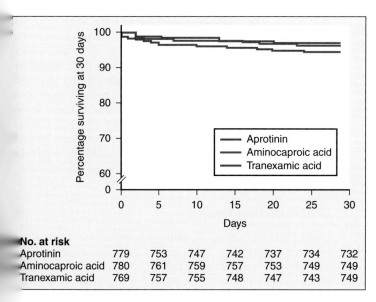

■ **FIGURE 14-11.** Kaplan-Meier curves showing survival at 30 days. Among the 2328 patients who were included in the analysis of death at 30 days after surgery, patients in the aprotinin group had a reduced rate of survival as compared with those in the tranexamic acid group ($P = 0.05$) and the aminocaproic acid group ($P = 0.06$). *(Modified from Fergusson DA, Hebert PC, Mazer CD, et al.: A comparison of aprotinin and lysine analogues in high-risk cardiac surgery, N Engl J Med 358[22]:2319, 2008.)*

No. at risk

Aprotinin	779	753	747	742	737	734	732
Aminocaproic acid	780	761	759	757	753	749	749
Tranexamic acid	769	757	755	748	747	743	749

least 70% of the children were able to complete the donation process. Concern about the ability of children, especially young children, to complete the donation program is often cited as an obstacle to PAD. However, in both of these studies, children younger than 10 years successfully completed the donation process. Clearly, the ability of infants, toddlers, and young school-aged children to tolerate the donation process is uncertain at best. The use of sedation or general anesthesia to facilitate this process would seem to be somewhat unreasonable and excessive, although it has been reported (Velardi et al., 1998). A contraindication for PAD includes predonation anemia.

Compared with acute normovolemic hemodilution (ANH), PAD has important disadvantages. The risk of transfusion errors (e.g., wrong unit or wrong patient) is not less with PAD than with the use of allogenic blood; the cost of obtaining, storing, and processing the predonated blood is not less with PAD; and the likelihood of contamination of the unit is not less with PAD. It is often unclear from the existing literature how the collection process occurs. For example, it is not clear whether these children require sedation before blood collection. Each of the problems is eliminated or nearly eliminated with ANH. ANH also has the advantage of returning fresh whole blood to the patient in contrast to PAD, which provides only the RBC component. Therefore, PAD should be reserved for older children, and the indications for the use of the predonated blood should be identical to those for allogenic units.

Acute Normovolemic Hemodilution

ANH is a technique designed to decrease the need for allogenic blood transfusion by the preoperative withdrawal of the patient's own blood to be reinfused as needed during the subsequent procedure. The withdrawn blood is collected in standard blood-collection bags containing anticoagulant. The circulating volume is restored with either colloid (1:1) or crystalloid (3:1), thereby reducing the hematocrit and the potential for loss of RBC mass as bleeding occurs during the procedure (Helm et al., 1996; Ferraris et al., 2007). Children weighing less than 35 kg typically do not fill an entire collection bag. As bags typically contain approximately 63 mL citrate-phosphate-dextrose (CPD) and hold 450 mL blood, the volume of the anticoagulant needs to be reduced if the volume of collected blood is less than 450 mL. Studies of adults have examined the potential benefits of various replacement fluids, including hetastarch, albumin, and Lactated Ringer's solution. All appear to be acceptable in adults, but few data exist to guide practice in children. Given that phlebotomy takes place just before the procedure and the withdrawn blood never leaves the patient's operating room, the potential for error in transfusing the wrong blood to the wrong patient is greatly reduced. The withdrawn fresh whole blood, which contains the non-RBC components not found in banked blood, is reinfused at the end of the procedure.

The volume of blood to be removed can be calculated with the following formula:

$$V = EBV \times Hi - Hf / Hav$$

where V is volume to be removed; EBV is estimated blood volume; Hi is initial or starting hematocrit value; Hf is the final or desired hematocrit value; and Hav is the average hematocrit value. The final or desired hematocrit is unclear and is dependent on various factors, including age, procedure, coexisting disease, and expected blood loss. Some have suggested that young infants are not appropriate candidates for ANH, because they have a limited capacity to increase cardiac output in response to anemia and the presence of fetal hemoglobin may limit oxygen unloading (Weldon, 2005). Supporting data, however, are lacking. In studies of older children and adolescents, hematocrit values have been allowed to decrease to as low as 9% without the development of lactic acidosis or other evidence of hypoperfusion (Fontana et al., 1995). The lowest appropriate or safe level of the desired hematocrit value is a function of the *critical hemoglobin*, which is the hemoglobin or hematocrit value below which oxygen consumption becomes delivery dependent and the ability to increase cardiac output is exceeded as lactic acidosis develops, reflecting insufficient oxygen delivery to the tissues. The critical hemoglobin concentration for humans is unknown, although studies in young healthy volunteers have failed to produce evidence of insufficient oxygen delivery at hemoglobin concentrations as low as 4.8 g/dL despite pharmacologic maneuvers that limited oxygen delivery to 7.3 mL/kg per minute (Lieberman et al., 2000). With the absence of cardiovascular disease in children, the ability to tolerate hematocrits of this level can be reasonably assumed; however, no large body of data exists to support the safety of the practice in children. Safety concerns must be balanced against the evidence for benefit usually determined by a reduction in total allogenic blood transfused or the reduction in exposure to units of allogenic blood. Linderkamp et al. (1992) calculated the following minimally acceptable hemoglobin concentrations: 6 g/dL for children and adults, 12 g/dL for preterm infants at birth, and 11 g/dL for full-term neonates at birth. These critical values were determined from oxygen transport parameters and oxygen consumptions (Linderkamp et al., 1992). Of course, the size of the preterm infant and the full-term neonate would preclude them from ANH; sufficient blood could not be drawn without risking a suboptimal hemoglobin concentration.

Several prospective randomized studies in adults show a modest decrease in the need for allogenic blood transfusion in both cardiac and noncardiac surgery (Goodnough et al., 1994; Moran et al., 1995; Kumar et al., 2002). In a 1998 meta-analysis, Bryson et al. did not demonstrate clear benefit with regard to a reduction in exposure to allogenic blood. According to the Society of Thoracic Surgeons Practice Guidelines, in the adult population the usefulness of ANH is not well established but may have benefit when used in conjunction with other blood conservation strategies (Masuda et al., 2000; Ferraris et al., 2007). A small series of adult patients of the Jehovah's Witness faith who underwent live donor hepatic transplants demonstrated a clear benefit when their results were compared with those of historical controls (Jabbour et al., 2005). The patients in this series not only underwent ANH but also were treated preoperatively with erythropoietin to increase the preoperative level of hemoglobin. The potential benefits of ANH or a combined approach to blood conservation remain unclear and can be addressed only by well-designed studies of sufficient size to provide clinicians with reassurance that the benefit outweighs any potential risk.

Deliberate Hypotension

Controlled, deliberate, or induced hypotension is a method of blood-conservation strategy first described by Cushing in 1917. Since then, the technique has been applied to numerous procedures in various settings, with a multitude of differe pharmacologic agents, and with patients of all ages. In a literature review, Tobias (2002) specifically looked at agents and techniques that can be used in infants and children.

Deliberate hypotension is defined as mean arterial pressure of 50 to 65 mm Hg, or 30% below baseline, which decreases bleeding in the surgical field and may be indicated for any procedure in which a relatively bloodless operating field is needed or whenever blood loss can be expected to require transfusion (Degoute, 2007). The ideal pharmacologic agent to induce controlled hypotension has the following characteristics: short onset, easily reversible and titratable, minimal toxic metabolites, minimal effects on vital organs, and predictable dose-dependent effect (Degoute, 2007). Numerous agents have been used successfully in both adults and children. A comprehensive review of agents useful in pediatrics was prepared by Degoute (2007). A summary of drugs is shown in Table 14-1.

The efficacy of deliberate hypotension to reduce the need for transfusion and improve the quality of the surgical field has been studied extensively for more than 30 years, although no large well-designed study or meta-analysis has demonstrated its efficacy in children. Still, the technique is widely accepted and used in children and infants. Most recent studies have focused on techniques and agents that may be used to achieve hypotension rather than on safety or efficacy. Shear and Tobias (2005), however, published a small study of cerebral oxygenation during controlled hypotension to 55 to 65 mm Hg using near infrared spectroscopy. They found that even with mean pressures of less than 54 mm Hg, oximetry values never decreased to less than 20% below baseline. They concluded that deliberate hypotension within the limits of 55 to 65 mm Hg was safe with regard to cerebral oxygenation.

Techniques for achieving deliberate hypotension are primarily pharmacologic, although positioning and regional techniques are occasionally used. The pharmacologic agents are derived from several different classes, including ganglionic blockers (e.g., trimethaphan), vasodilators (e.g., nitroglycerin and nitroprusside), β-blocking agents (e.g., esmolol), calcium channel blockers (most often nicardipine), and the volatile

TABLE 14-1. Drugs Used in Controlled Hypotension During Surgery

Drug	Site of Action	Predominant Action	Major Inconvenience
Anesthetics			
Bupivacaine (spinal anesthesia), ropivacaine (epidural anesthesia)	Medulla	Blockade of the sympathetic nervous system	On/off; need vasoconstrictor (ephedrine)
Inhalation anesthetics: Isoflurane, sevoflurane	Vessels: Vasodilation	Blockade of α-adrenoceptors	Resistance; need high concentrations or adjuvants
Opioids: Remifentanil	Heart: Bradycardia	Blockade of the sympathetic nervous system	None
Vasodilators			
Sodium nitroprusside	Resistance/capacitance vessels: Vasodilation	Direct acting	Cyanide toxicity; heavy monitoring
Nitroglycerin	Capacitance vessels: Vasodilation	Direct acting	Resistance; adequate monitoring
Adenosine	Resistance vessels: Vasodilation	Direct acting	Cost; histamine release
Alprostadil	Resistance vessels: Vasodilation Heart: ↓ Chronotropic effect	Direct acting	Cost
Calcium channel antagonists: Nicardipine, diltiazem	Resistance vessels: Vasodilation Heart: ↓ Inotropic effect	Direct acting	None
Fenoldopam	Resistance vessels: Vasodilation	Dopamine DA$_1$-receptor agonist	None; cost?
Autonomic Nervous System Inhibitors			
Trimethaphan	Vessels: Vasodilation heart: ↓ Contractility	Blockade of the ganglia of the autonomic nervous system	Histamine release; resistance
Clonidine	CNS	Presynaptic α-adrenoceptor agonist	Unpredictable effect
Urapidil, phentolamine	Vessels: Vasodilation	Postsynaptic α-adrenoceptor antagonist	Unpredictable effect
Labetalol	Heart: ↓ Contractility vessels: Vasodilation	α/β-Adrenoceptor antagonist	Slow-onset cardiac failure if used to treat profound arterial vasoconstriction
Esmolol	Heart: Bradycardia, ↓ contractility	β-Adrenoceptor antagonist	Resistance; cardiac failure
ACE Inhibitors			
Captopril, enalapril	Vessels: Vasodilation	Angiotensin II inhibitors	Long duration of action

Modified from Degoute Controlled hyptotension: a guide to drug choice, *Drugs* 67(7):1053, 2007.
ACE, Angiotensin-converting enzyme; *CNS*, central nervous system; ↓, decrease.

agents (presumably sevoflurane, with its greater titratability). The review by Tobias (2002) provides an extensive discussion of various agents. Often a combination of agents is required to provide adequate control of blood pressure, especially in young, healthy adolescents. The use of vasodilators such as nitroprusside or a volatile agent often results in reflex tachycardia that limits hypotension. Most practitioners find that satisfactory hypotension can be achieved only when heart rate is controlled, typically with a β-blocker (e.g., esmolol) or with a combination agent that blocks both α and β receptors (e.g., labetalol). Other agents that may be helpful in controlling heart rate, include clonidine (an α-receptor agonist) or a narcotic (especially remifentanil), as was shown in endoscopic sinus surgery and middle ear procedures (Degoute et al., 2003; Eberhart et al., 2003).

Dexmedetomidine has gained acceptance in various settings, but its use in this setting would appear to be limited. Nonetheless, it has been compared with remifentanil in two studies (one adult and one pediatric). In neither study was dexmedetomidine found to be superior (Tobias, 2002; Richa et al., 2008). A third article described only one patient for whom dexmedetomidine was used successfully to induce hypotension for spine instrumentation (Tobias and Berkenbosch, 2002). In the absence of additional data from larger prospective studies, the use of dexmedetomidine for controlled hypotension cannot be recommended.

Although the use of deliberate hypotension is widely accepted, the practitioner must be attentive to safety concerns, primarily those related to focal ischemia to such vital areas as the retina, spinal cord, and brain. Deliberate hypotension is contraindicated in patients with compromised circulation involving any critical vascular bed, elevated intracranial pressure, profound anemia or polycythemia, or sensitivity to any of the proposed hypotensive agents. The hematocrit concentration should be maintained at an adequate level. Despite the suggestion by some that deliberate hypotension and extreme ANH may be safely combined, deliberate hypotension should never be combined with ANH because of the risk of end organ ischemia (Schaller et al., 1983). The anesthesiologist must have experience with the technique and with the agents used to achieve hypotension. Adequate monitoring is essential, including invasive arterial blood pressure in all cases and central venous pressure monitoring in many or most cases. Patients placed in the reverse Trendelenburg position or in any position in which the head is higher than the heart must have the arterial pressure monitored and zeroed to reflect cerebral perfusion pressure. Arterial blood gases should be monitored frequently to ensure that a metabolic acidosis is not present, suggesting poor tissue perfusion or cyanide toxicity, when using sodium nitroprusside. Owing to its potential for toxicity, sodium nitroprusside deserves additional mention.

Sodium nitroprusside is 44% cyanide by weight. It interacts with oxyhemoglobin and spontaneously dissociates into methemoglobin, cyanide, and nitric oxide (Fig. 14-12). Its vasodilatory action is mediated principally through the action of nitric oxide. Although it is a highly efficacious vasodilator, when used in high doses for protracted periods, sodium nitroprusside may produce intoxication with its by-product, cyanide. Free cyanide radicals generated by the metabolism or breakdown of sodium nitroprusside are metabolized by one of the following four potential mechanisms:

1. Cyanide may bind and inactivate mitochondrial cytochrome oxidase and prevent oxidative phosphorylation, leaving anaerobic metabolism as the only path to energy production, leading to lactic acidosis.
2. Cyanide may be converted to thiocyanate by the enzyme rhodanase. Treatment with thiosulfate promotes metabolism of cyanide to thiocyanate, which may be excreted by the kidney.
3. Vitamin B_{12} converts cyanide to cyanocobalamin (this is a relatively minor pathway).
4. Free cyanide may be consumed by reversibly combining with methemoglobin into cyanomethemoglobin, a nontoxic compound.

The primary deleterious effect of cyanide intoxication is the poisoning of aerobic metabolism at the level of the mitochondria. Cyanide directly inhibits the functioning of the electron transport chain through its effects on cytochrome oxidase. When sodium nitroprusside infusion exceeds the capacity of thiocyanate to eliminate it, signs and symptoms become manifest. In addition, methemoglobinemia may develop if sodium nitroprusside is infused at doses exceeding 10 mcg/kg per minute for more than 10 to 12 hours.

Signs and symptoms of thiocyanate toxicity include nausea, disorientation, confusion, psychosis, weakness, muscle spasm, hyperreflexia, and convulsions. Cyanide toxicity has been known to result in "unexplained cardiac arrest," coma, encephalopathy,

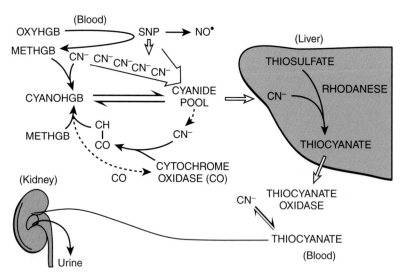

■ **FIGURE 14-12.** Primary pathways of sodium nitroprusside metabolism. *CN,* Cyanide; *CO,* cytochrome oxidase; *CYANOHGB,* cyanomethemoglobin; *METHGB,* methemoglobin; *NO,* nitric oxide; *OXYHGB,* oxyhemoglobin; *SNP,* sodium nitroprusside. *(Modified from Friederich JA, Butterworth JF: Sodium nitroprusside: twenty years and counting, Anesth Analg 81[1]:152, 1995.*

convulsions, and irreversible focal neurologic abnormalities. Regardless of the amount infused, any patient who receives sodium nitroprusside and who subsequently has neurologic abnormalities, cardiovascular instability, and increasing metabolic acidosis should be assessed for cyanide toxicity. The current method of monitoring for cyanide toxicity, particularly under general anesthesia, is insensitive. The value of measuring blood levels of cyanide is limited by the delay in obtaining results, which may not be available for several hours or days. Blood levels of cyanide exceeding 40 μmoL/dL are typically associated with toxicity; levels exceeding 70 to 80 μmoL/dL are potentially lethal. In otherwise healthy patients (such as those undergoing spinal fusion and a hypotensive technique), the presence and severity of metabolic acidosis correlates well with cyanide toxicity. However, among critically ill patients, ascertainment of cyanide toxicity may be confounded if the patient has acidosis from another cause. In children, the need for rapidly increasing doses or excessively large doses (greater than 10 mcg/kg per minute) of sodium nitroprusside within the first 60 minutes of initiation to maintain the desired clinical effect should alert the clinician of the potential for impending cyanide intoxication.

Prevention of cyanide toxicity can best be accomplished by limiting the dose and duration of the infusion and by close monitoring for signs and symptoms consistent with intoxication, especially metabolic acidosis. Infusions greater than 5 mcg/kg per minute should be avoided, and evidence for resistance or tachyphylaxis should be sought, especially early in the infusion. Patients with reduced renal function are at particular risk for the accumulation of thiocyanate and consequent intoxication.

Treatment, when required, usually consists of immediate discontinuation of the infusion, administration of oxygen, and correction of acidosis followed by the initiation of a thiosulfate infusion (at a dose of 60 mg/kg per hour after an initial bolus of 30 mg/kg infused over 20 to 30 minutes). Alternatively, dialysis may be beneficial to remove thiocyanate; hydroxocobalamin (50 mg/kg bolus followed by 100 mg/kg per hour) may assist by binding with cyanide to form nontoxic cyanocobalamin; or sodium thiosulfate (150 to 200 mg/kg slowly) with sodium nitrite (4 to 6 mg/kg, slowly) assists in converting hemoglobin to methemoglobin, which competes with cytochrome oxidase for cyanide (Friederich and Butterworth, 1995). Deliberate hypotension has become a useful and widely accepted technique in adults and children as experience has accumulated with its use over more than a generation. Still, the clinician must weigh the potential benefits against the risks associated with hypotensive anesthetic techniques.

Miscellaneous Techniques for Reducing Intraoperative Blood Loss

Vasoconstriction, positioning, and tourniquets are used to reduce operative blood loss and to optimize the surgical field. Tissue infiltration with epinephrine 1:200,000 as a vasoconstrictor for blood conservation has had positive outcomes in adult breast surgeries, but there are no reports from the pediatric population (Brantner and Peterson, 1985; Courtiss, 1987). Animal studies suggest that blood loss is limited for the duration of the epinephrine's effect, but delayed bleeding may occur (Rey et al., 1996). Karl et al. (1983) evaluated the safety of subcutaneous epinephrine infiltration under halothane anesthesia and reported that epinephrine, 10 mcg/kg, was safe in the pediatric population and that children tolerate a higher dose than adults.

The reverse Trendelenburg position, or head-up tilt position, is often used in head and neck surgery to minimize blood loss and to ensure a dry surgical field. Orthostatic stress experiments on healthy, awake, adult subjects have shown a decrease in cardiac output of up to 25% while maintaining mean arterial blood pressure. However, blood pressure is maintained by a baroreceptor reflex, and volatile anesthetics decrease the sensitivity of this reflex (Muzi and Ebert, 1995; Cooper and Hainsworth, 2001). Quantitative data are not available for the graded change in circulatory responses to various degrees of the reverse Trendelenburg position and the loss of compensatory baroreceptor reflex during general anesthesia in adults or children.

The use of pneumatic tourniquets after exsanguination of the upper or lower extremities significantly improves the operative conditions, particularly for cementing of bone (Abdel-Salam and Eyres, 1995; Wakankar et al., 1999). However, although tourniquet use as a blood conservation strategy is widely accepted in adults and children, there are potential risks, including nerve injury, increased infection, vascular injury, and cardiac and pulmonary injury (Estebe and Malledant, 1996; Kaabachi et al., 2005). In pediatric orthopedic surgery, the use of a tourniquet was identified by Kaabachi et al. (2005) as a risk factor for postoperative wound infection. The use of wide contour cuffs may reduce the likelihood of injury by decreasing mean tourniquet cuff pressure without compromising the quality of the surgical field (Reilly et al., 2009). In children with sickle cell disease (SCD) who require an extremity procedure, tourniquets have been used safely, provided that moderate hyperventilation with pH 7.40 to 7.45 and excellent oxygenation are maintained throughout the procedure (Adu-Gyamfi et al., 1993).

TRANSFUSION TRIGGERS

In 2005, approximately 29 million units of RBC and non-RBC blood components were transfused. Specific data are not available for the pediatric population, but at least one study indicates that approximately 1% of transfusions are administered to patients younger than 18 years (Sullivan et al., 2002). Although the present blood supply is safer than ever in terms of preventing transfusion-mediated infection, complications from blood component transfusions are not uncommon. Therefore, decisions about transfusion for any patient should weigh the potential benefits of transfusion against the risks, the occurrence of which may be unknown. Expert guidelines published for adult and pediatric patients all call for clinical judgments by the practitioner. As a result, transfusion practices vary considerably (Blanchette et al., 1991; Stehling et al., 1994; American Society of Anesthesiologists Task Force on Blood Component Therapy, 1996; Roseff et al., 2002; Desmet and Lacroix, 2004). The following sections summarize the existing guidelines and literature related to pediatric patients.

Transfusion of Fresh Whole Blood or Reconstituted Whole Blood

The transfusion of fresh whole blood (less than 5 days old) would appear to be the obvious choice for resuscitation of a bleeding child, because it replaces all the lost components. However, the storage of whole blood is problematic. In particular, factors

V and VIII are especially labile and tend to be rapidly depleted (Brecher, 2002). Also, refrigerated platelets lose their discoid shape, resulting in decreased survival (Murphy and Gardner, 1969). These factors, combined with the desire to optimize the number of usable components from only one donor and to treat patient-specific needs, have led to special requests for fresh whole blood, if available, in most centers (Roseff et al., 2002).

If fresh whole blood is not available but desired, stored RBCs can be reconstituted with fresh frozen plasma (FFP) (Roseff et al., 2002). This method of administering whole blood, however, provides no platelets and exposes the patient to twice as many donors. Few clinical scenarios require whole blood (Box 14-1). For massive transfusion, it can probably be used without further justification (Blanchette et al., 1991). However, for acute but controllable blood loss, particularly in the larger child, replacement with RBCs, crystalloid fluids, and colloid fluids are probably sufficient unless the clotting factors become excessively diluted (greater than 1 blood volume of replacement in adults). If that happens, plasma or platelets (or both) may be administered as needed.

TRANSFUSION OF RED BLOOD CELLS

There are only two accepted indications for the transfusion of RBCs: to increase oxygen-carrying capacity or avoid an impending inadequate oxygen-carrying state; and to suppress the production or dilute the amount of endogenous hemoglobin in selected patients with thalassemia or sickle cell disease (Hume and Limoges, 2002). Because neonates, particularly premature low–birth-weight patients, differ from infants and older children in terms of blood volume and physiology, they are discussed separately.

Transfusion in Patients Younger than 4 Months

Beside having a smaller absolute blood volume than older patients, children younger than 4 months have different physiologic processes than older patients. Examples include the premature infant's limited erythropoietin response to decreased oxygen delivery, as previously discussed, and the newborn's inefficient humoral system that precludes formation of antibodies to allogenic RBCs (Stockman et al., 1984; DePalma and Luban, 1990).

These young patients perhaps receive the most transfusions of all patient groups; infants receiving multiple transfusions are exposed to blood from approximately 10 different donors (Sacher et al., 1989; Strauss, 1991). Recent work has focused both on delineating guidelines for transfusion and on limiting the number of donors needed for these young patients.

Replacement of iatrogenic blood losses caused by blood draws for laboratory testing has historically accounted for approximately 90% of the transfusions in neonates (Kaabachi et al., 2005). Older guidelines and expert opinions have advocated replacing blood losses resulting from phlebotomy when losses exceed 5% to 10% of the total blood volume (Blanchette et al., 1991; Wakankar et al., 1999). These guidelines note that the decision to transfuse should not be made solely on the amount of blood lost but should include factors such as the clinical status of the patient, the patient's hemoglobin level, and the length of time over which the losses occurred (Blanchette et al., 1991). Currently transfusion simply to replace phlebotomy losses is much less common (Ramasethu, 1999; Simon et al., 1998; Shannon et al., 1995).

Maintenance of hematocrit levels greater than 35% (hemoglobin greater than 13 g/dL) for neonates with severe respiratory disease continues to be common practice without the support of evidence (Roseff et al., 2002). In a study of 10 oxygen-dependent infants with bronchopulmonary dysplasia, small-volume transfusions increased oxygen transport and decreased oxygen extraction. However, hemoglobin levels alone were not predictive of which children would benefit from transfusion (Alverson et al., 1988).

Transfusion in Patients Older than 4 Months

The transfusion practice guidelines of the American Society of Anesthesiologists Task Force on Blood Component Therapy (1996) are largely applicable to pediatric patients without cardiopulmonary disease. The points about RBC transfusions are summarized as follows:

1. Transfusion is rarely indicated when the hemoglobin concentration is greater than 10 g/dL.
2. Transfusion is almost always indicated when the hemoglobin concentration is less than 6 g/dL, especially if the anemia is acute.
3. The determination of whether intermediate hemoglobin concentrations (6.0 to 10 g/dL) justify transfusion should be based on the patient's risk of complications from inadequate oxygenation.
4. The use of a single hemoglobin trigger for all patients is not recommended.

Other guidelines have also been published specifically for pediatric patients older than 4 months (Roseff et al., 2002; Stehling et al., 1994) (Box 14-2).

Although numerous studies have been performed to delineate optimal hemoglobin levels in critically ill adults, few studies have been performed involving children. Traditionally, a hemoglobin level greater than 10 g/dL has been advocated for critically ill patients. In a landmark article by Hebert et al. (1999), a trial randomly assigned patients to receive RBC transfusions according to a liberal strategy (transfusion for hemoglobin less than 10 g/dL) or a restrictive strategy (transfusion for hemoglobin less than 7 g/dL). Although there was a higher

Box 14-1 Guidelines for Transfusion of Whole Blood

Exchange transfusion for the following:

Hemolytic disease of the newborn

Hyperbilirubinemia with risk of kernicterus

After cardiopulmonary bypass

Extracorporeal membrane oxygenation

Massive transfusion (i.e., transfusion of >1 blood volume in 24 hours)

Modified from Roseff SD, Luban NL, Manno CS.: Guidelines for assessing appropriateness of pediatric transfusion, *Transfusion* 42(11):1398-1413, 2002.

Box 14-2 Guidelines for Transfusion of Red Blood Cells in Patients Older Than 4 Months

Emergency surgical procedure in patient with clinically significant preoperative anemia

Preoperative anemia when other corrective therapy is not available

Intraoperative blood loss ≥15% of total blood volume

Hematocrit <24%

   In perioperative period, with signs and symptoms of anemia

   While receiving chemotherapy or radiotherapy

   With chronic congenital or acquired symptomatic anemia

Acute blood loss with hypovolemia not responsive to other therapy

Hematocrit <40%

   With severe pulmonary disease

   With extracorporeal membrane oxygenation

Sickle cell disease and any of the following:

   Cerebrovascular accident

   Acute chest syndrome

   Splenic sequestration

   Recurrent priapism

   Preoperatively when general anesthesia is planned, to increase hemoglobin to 10 g/dL

Chronic transfusion programs for disorders of RBC production (such as thalassemia major and Diamond-Blackfan syndrome unresponsive to therapy)

Modified from Roseff SD, Luban NL, Manno CS: Guidelines for assessing appropriateness of pediatric transfusion, *Transfusion* 42(11):1398-1413, 2002.

---

in-hospital mortality rate in the liberally transfused group, there was no difference between the groups in the 30-day mortality rate. The liberal strategy group also tended to have higher estimates of severity of multiple organ dysfunction and nosocomial infections.

The Hebert article spawned an interest in performing a similar study in children. The Transfusion Requirements in the Pediatric Intensive Care Unit (TRIPICU) trial was published in 2007 (Lacroix et al., 2007). In this trial, 637 infants and children in the intensive care unit were randomly assigned to a liberal strategy (transfusion for hemoglobin less than 9.5 g/dL) or a restrictive strategy (transfusion for hemoglobin less than 7 g/dL). There was no difference between the groups in the percentage of patients with new or progressive multiple organ dysfunction syndrome (the primary outcome) or death. However, patients in the restrictive strategy group received 44% fewer transfusions than did those in the liberal strategy group. This study suggests that in stable, critically ill children, a transfusion threshold of 7 g/dL decreases transfusion requirements without increasing adverse outcomes.

Clinicians should remember that the goal of RBC transfusion is to ensure adequate oxygen delivery to the tissues. The clinical picture of the patient is at least as important as the hemoglobin level in determining whether RBC transfusion is required or justified. At the minimum, findings of tachycardia or tachypnea, decreased urine output, or cool vasoconstricted extremities may indicate the need for increased oxygen-carrying capacity. Alternatively, acid-base balance or blood lactate levels can be monitored. More recently, central venous catheters that continually report mixed venous oxygen saturation have been developed in sizes appropriate for children. In addition, noninvasive cerebral oximetry measurements correlate well with measured mixed venous oxygenation in some patients (Cua et al., 2004; Tortoriello et al., 2005). In the future, these and other monitors under development may allow clinicians to better individualize treatment and predict which patients will benefit from RBC transfusion.

When the decision has been made to transfuse RBCs into a child, the appropriate volume must then be determined. Babies in the intensive care unit often receive "top-up" transfusions for slowly progressive anemia caused by phlebotomy. Typically, the dose is 10 to 15 mL/kg administered over 2 to 3 hours. For the larger child in the operating room, an estimate of allowable blood losses may be calculated before any procedure during which blood loss is expected. This can be accomplished with the patient's estimated blood volume (EBV), weight, initial hematocrit (Hi), and lowest allowable hematocrit (Hp) (Table 14-2). For example, the maximal allowable blood loss in a 5-kg infant with an Hi of 40% and in whom a hematocrit value of 24% is determined safe would be calculated as follows:

$$EBV = 5 \text{ kg} \times 80 \text{ mL/kg} = 400 \text{ mL blood}$$

$$\text{At hematocrit of 40\%, estimated RBC mass} = \\ 400 \text{ mL blood} \times 40\% = 160 \text{ mL of RBCs}$$

$$\text{At hematocrit of 24\%, estimated RBC mass} = \\ 400 \text{ mL blood} \times 24\% = 96 \text{ mL of RBCs}$$

$$\text{At hematocrit of 24\%, RBC loss} = 160 \text{ mL} - 96 \text{ mL} = 64 \text{ mL}$$

$$\text{Allowable blood loss} = 3 \times 64 \text{ mL} = \\ 192 \text{ mL (where 3 is a conversion factor for Hgb to HCT)}$$

A simpler method of calculating allowable blood loss uses the Hi, the Hp, and the average of the two hematocrits (Hav) as follows (Desmet and Lacroix, 2004):

$$\text{Allowable blood loss} = EBV \times (Hi - Hp) / Hav$$

$$\text{Allowable blood loss} = 400 \text{ mL} \times (40 - 24) / 32 = 200 \text{ mL}$$

Because blood loss is difficult to calculate in the operating suite, particularly with small patients and small wounds,

TABLE 14-2. Estimated Blood Volume

Age Group	Estimated Blood Volume (mL/kg)
Premature infants	90-100
Term newborns	80-90
Infants younger than 1 yr	75-80
Older children	70-75

these calculations should serve only as estimates and should be accompanied by laboratory measurements whenever possible before the decision to transfuse is made.

The effect that a volume of transfused RBCs will have on a child's hemoglobin level can also be estimated. In general, 10 mL/kg of RBCs will increase the hemoglobin by 1 to 2 g/dL. However, after a child has been exposed to a unit of blood, the child may be given as much of the unit as tolerated (avoiding polycythemia or volume overload) to avoid exposure to blood from other donors owing to ongoing postoperative blood loss or phlebotomy.

RBC Transfusion for Uncorrected Cyanotic Congenital Heart Disease

Children with uncorrected cyanotic congenital heart disease deserve special mention. Intuitively, cyanotic patients require a higher oxygen-carrying capacity to maintain adequate oxygen delivery in the presence of mixing lesions. Indeed, in the absence of phlebotomy in these children, polycythemia develops because of increased erythropoietin in response to poor tissue-oxygen tension. The usual recommendation for these children is to use transfusion to maintain hemoglobin concentrations of 13 to 18 g/dL, although support for this practice is lacking (Meliones et al., 1995; Stehling et al., 1994; Paridon, 1998; Lacroix et al., 2007). Anecdotal evidence from patients of the Jehovah's Witness faith who underwent operations to repair congenital heart disease suggests that lower hemoglobin levels may be tolerated in cyanotic patients (Kawaguchi et al., 1984; Henling et al., 1985).

Transfusion in patients with cyanotic heart disease may have effects beyond increasing oxygen-carrying capacity. Beekman and Tuuri (1985) studied seven children with right-to-left shunts in the catheterization laboratory. Partial exchange transfusions were used to increase the mean (shown with SD) baseline hemoglobin of 13.7 (0.5) g/dL to 16.4 (0.4) g/dL. This intervention not only increased the arterial oxygen saturation; it also decreased the degree of shunting by 59%. Presumably the decrease in shunting resulted from an increase in systemic vascular resistance as a result of an increase in blood viscosity.

RBC Transfusion for Sickle Cell Disease

Patients with SCD often have perioperative complications or a crisis. Early reports cited perioperative mortality rates of 10% and an incidence of postoperative complications of up to 50% (Vichinsky et al., 1995). The two indications for RBC transfusion in a patient with SCD are correction of a preexisting anemia and dilution of hemoglobin S concentration. Some experts advise a preoperative dilution of hemoglobin S levels to less than 30% (Bhattacharyya et al., 1993). However, this practice has never been shown to be of clear benefit.

To more completely address this controversy, Vichinsky and colleagues (1995) performed a multicenter, randomized trial that compared a conservative transfusion strategy (transfusion to increase the hemoglobin level to 10 g/dL) with an aggressive transfusion strategy (transfusion to decrease hemoglobin S to less than 30%). The patients underwent a total of 604 operations. The groups were well matched, and the mean preoperative hemoglobin levels were 10.6 g/dL in the conservative group and 11.0 g/dL in the aggressive group. When transfusion-associated complications were excluded, there was no difference in the incidence of major complications (e.g., acute chest syndrome, painful crisis, neurologic event, or death) even though the conservatively treated group had a higher concentration of hemoglobin S (59% vs. 31%). However, the incidence of transfusion-related complications was twice as high in the aggressively treated group (14% vs. 7%). These authors concluded that a transfusion protocol aimed at correcting anemia to a hemoglobin of 10 g/dL was as effective as a protocol designed to decrease the hemoglobin S concentration to less than 30% and resulted in half as many transfusion-related complications.

There seems to be no clear benefit to diluting hemoglobin S to a particular level. It then becomes necessary to determine which patients should receive prophylactic transfusion to attain an arbitrary hemoglobin level (usually a goal of 10 g/dL). Unfortunately, the clinical heterogeneity among patients with SCD makes the formation of uniform guidelines nearly impossible. However, some patient and operative characteristics allow the clinician to estimate the potential benefit of transfusion against the known risks.

The incidence of complications in patients with SCD varies widely with the type of operation. In a review by Koshy et al. (1995) of 1,079 procedures, the rates of perioperative complications were 0% for tonsillectomy and adenoidectomy, 2.9% for hip surgery, 3.9% for myringotomy, 7.8% for abdominal surgery, 16.9% for cesarean section and hysterectomy, and 18.6% for dilation and curettage. Patient characteristics that appear to be associated with increased postoperative complications include increased age, incidence of recent complications, inpatient hospital status, pregnancy, and preexisting infection (Firth and Head, 2004).

The clinician must use the above information to help decide whether the potential benefits of transfusion to reach a hemoglobin level of more than 10 g/dL outweigh the risks of transfusion in the patient with SCD who needs to have an operation. For example, a relatively asymptomatic child presenting for tonsillectomy is unlikely to benefit from transfusion for mild anemia. Conversely, it would seem that an adult female who is experiencing many symptoms because of her SCD and is going to undergo a cesarean section and hysterectomy (a procedure associated with a high incidence of perioperative complications) *may* benefit from correction of her anemia to a hemoglobin level greater than 10 g/dL.

TRANSFUSION OF FRESH FROZEN PLASMA

Indications for the transfusion of FFP in pediatric patients are essentially the same as the American Society of Anesthesiologists guidelines for adult patients (1996). FFP transfusion is indicated for the following conditions:

- Emergency reversal of the effects of warfarin
- Correction of coagulopathic bleeding with an increased prothrombin time (international normalized ratio greater than 1.5) or an increased partial thromboplastin time
- Correction of coagulopathic bleeding with massive transfusion (i.e., transfusion of more than 1 blood volume when coagulation profiles are not easily obtained

FFP is no longer indicated for volume replacement (Consensus conference, 1985; Northern Neonatal Nursing Initiative Trial Group, 1996). If colloid therapy is thought to be more beneficial than crystalloid therapy for volume replacement, albumin or a starch-based product such as hetastarch (≤20 mL/kg) may be used. In addition, nearly all congenital bleeding disorders can now be treated with factor-specific therapies and should not be treated with FFP or cryoprecipitate unless these targeted therapies are unavailable. The typical dose of FFP in the pediatric patient is 10 to 20 mL/kg (American Society of Anesthesiologists Task Force on Blood Component Therapy, 1996; Hume and Limoges, 2002; Roseff et al., 2002).

TRANSFUSION OF PLATELETS

Guidelines for the infusion of platelets in pediatric patients resemble those for adults (American Society of Anesthesiologists Task Force on Blood Component Therapy, 1996). If the rest of the coagulation system is normal, platelet counts greater than 50×10^9/L are probably sufficient for invasive procedures (McVay and Toy, 1991). If patients undergoing invasive procedures have platelet counts between 50×10^9/L and 100×10^9/L, platelets should be readily available for transfusion if needed. For massive transfusion with microvascular bleeding, platelet counts should be obtained before transfusion if possible. However, platelets may be given during a massive transfusion if a platelet count is not readily obtainable and there is evidence of microvascular bleeding. Platelet transfusions are probably not indicated when thrombocytopenia is caused by increased platelet destruction (idiopathic thrombocytopenic purpura) (American Society of Anesthesiologists Task Force on Blood Component Therapy, 1996).

Preterm infants who are critically ill are of great concern, because they are at high risk of intracranial hemorrhage. These patients have an underdeveloped subependymal matrix that is predisposed to rupture (Sacher et al., 1989; Strauss, 1991). Some experts recommend platelet transfusion for sick preterm babies when the platelet count is less than 100×10^9/L and for healthy preterm babies when the platelet count is less than 50×10^9/L. Andrew and colleagues (1993) randomly assigned 152 preterm thrombocytopenic babies to receive platelet transfusions to maintain a platelet count greater than 150×10^9/L (treatment group) or greater than 50×10^9/L (conventional group). The authors found no difference in the incidence of intracranial hemorrhage between the two groups (28% in the treatment group vs. 26% in the conventional group). They concluded that early infusion of platelet concentrates in thrombocytopenic premature infants did not alter the incidence of intracranial hemorrhage.

Platelets can be recovered from donors in two ways. One method is to remove whole blood from the donor and use centrifugal forces to separate its constituents. This results in the recovery of approximately 5.5×10^{10} platelets in 50 mL of plasma per 450 mL of whole blood removed from the donor. Typically, these platelet concentrates are then pooled with those recovered from other donors in groups of 6 to 8 for transfusion. Alternatively, apheresis can be used. This method draws blood into a circuit, separates the components with centrifugation or filtration, collects the desired blood component, and returns the remaining components to the donor. A single apheresis unit results in a similar number of platelets as 6 to 8 pooled platelet concentrates from whole blood, with the obvious advantage of exposure to only one donor (Fasano and Luban, 2008).

When dosing platelets for children, one can expect that one platelet concentrate per 10 kg of body weight will increase the platelet count by approximately 50×10^9/L. If platelets obtained by apheresis are used, an equivalent dose would be approximately 5 mL/kg body weight.

TRANSFUSION-ASSOCIATED COMPLICATIONS

Viral Infections

The current blood supply is safer than ever from the risks of transmitting viral infections. The estimated risk of transmission for some of the major viruses is shown in Table 14-3. The incidence of viral transmission is now too low to measure, so mathematical models are used to estimate risk (Goodnough et al., 1999a). Improvement in the safety of the blood supply has been multifactorial. After early descriptions of human immunodeficiency virus (HIV) transmission through blood transfusion in 1982 and 1983, the U.S. Public Health Service recommended that persons at increased risk of HIV not donate blood (Ammann et al., 1983). In addition, blood banks began asking donors about high-risk behaviors and giving donors the opportunity to specify that their blood should not be used (Hebert et al., 1999; Tortoriello et al., 2005). These simple interventions alone resulted in significant decreases in the incidence of transfusion-related HIV infection (Busch et al., 1991). With current donor-screening techniques and modern testing of donated blood, which includes antibody screening and nucleic acid testing, patients can generally be assured that the risk of acquiring a major viral infection is quite low. However, new infectious risks, such as exposure to West Nile virus, continue to emerge and will require ongoing surveillance to ensure the safety of the blood supply (Dodd, 2003a; 2003b).

TABLE 14-3. Risk of Transfusion-Transmitted Diseases

Disease	Incidence with Transfusion	Comments
Hepatitis B virus	1 in 137,000	Decreasing because of vaccination of health care professionals and school-aged children.
Hepatitis C virus	<1 in 1,000,000	Antibody screening began in 1990; NAT testing was added in 1999.
Human immunodeficiency virus	<1 in 1,900,000	First blood test was available in 1985; NAT testing was universal in 1999.
Human T lymphotropic virus types I and II	1 in 250,000 to 1 in 2,000,000	Viruses cause blood or nervous system disease in few infected patients.

Data from Goodnough LT et al.: Transfusion medicine: blood transfusion, parts 1 and 2, *N Engl J Med*, 340(6, 7):438,525, 1999, and AABB Buyers' Guide: *Transfusion-transmitted diseases* (website): http://www.aabb.org/Content/About_Blood/Facts_About_Blood_and_Blood_Banking/fabloodtrans.htm. Accessed April 2007.
NAT, Nucleic amplification testing.

Bacterial Infections

There has been an increasing focus on the bacteriologic safety of the blood supply. Between 1985 and 1999 in the United States, 694 transfusion-related deaths were reported to the FDA. Of these, 11.1% were attributed to bacterial contamination (Dodd, 2003a). The most likely bacterial contaminant of stored RBCs is *Yersinia enterocolitica*, but other gram-negative bacteria are possible as well (CDC, 1997). The risk of contamination is directly related to the duration of storage (Goodnough et al., 1999a; 1999b). In the United States, the risk of bacterial infection from the transfusion of RBCs is less than 1 in 1 million, but the mortality rate from infection is high: 12 of 20 patients who received RBCs infected with *Yersinia* died from 1987 to 1996 (Goodnough et al., 1999a; Dodd, 2003a). Symptoms of infection usually begin during the transfusion, and patients who die usually die within the next 24 hours.

The risk of sepsis from platelets is higher than from stored RBCs because platelets are stored warm. For this reason, the shelf life of platelets stored at 20° C to 24° C is only 5 days. The reported incidence of sepsis after platelet transfusion is 10 to 138 cases per million transfusions, and risk of death from platelet-associated infection is 2 to 18 per million transfusions (Kuehnert et al., 2001; Ness et al., 2001). There is evidence that the risk of infection is higher when pooled donors are used than when an apheresed unit is transfused from only one donor. The most common bacteria causing death after platelet transfusion are *Staphylococcus aureus*, *Klebsiella pneumoniae*, *Serratia marcescens*, and *Staphylococcus epidermidis* (Beekman and Tuuri, 1985). The clinical course for platelet-related bacterial infection is more variable than that associated with RBCs. Symptoms range from mild fever to florid sepsis with hypotension and death. The reported mortality rate is 26% (Goldman and Blajchman, 1991).

Hyperkalemia

There have been several reports of transfusion-associated hyperkalemic cardiac arrest in pediatric patients (Hall et al., 1993; Ivens and Camu, 1996; Buntain and Pabari, 1999; Chen et al., 1999; Smith et al., 2008). The RBC membrane is poorly permeable to potassium and relies on energy-dependent mechanisms to move potassium in and out of the cell. As RBCs age during storage, adenosine triphosphate synthesis and potassium pumping decrease, and potassium leaks into the supernatant (Ronquist and Waldenstrom, 2003). Indeed, among units stored for prolonged periods, the potassium concentration in the supernatant may exceed 60 mEq/L (Hall et al., 1993). In an analysis of 74 units of banked blood at the Mayo Clinic, Smith and colleagues (2008) found a range of potassium concentrations, from 7.3 to 77.2 mEq/L. In the first week of storage, the average (with SD) measured potassium was 19.0 (7.8) mEq/L; during the second week, 31.5 (14.1) mEq/L; and between 15 and 28 days of storage, 39.9 (10.3) mEq/L. Intraoperative washing of packed RBCs through autotransfusion and use of blood salvage devices may be effective at decreasing the potassium burden (Knichwitz et al., 2002). Alternatively, if notified in advance, blood banks can provide reduced-potassium blood. However, the emergent nature of many massive transfusions often precludes these interventions.

Hyperkalemic arrest seems to be more common among children than adults (Smith et al., 2008). This difference is likely because of smaller circulating volumes, immature renal function, and differences in autonomic tone. In most published reports, some degree of acidosis, hyperglycemia, or hypothermia was present before the arrest. Therefore, it is difficult to sort out the roles of these factors in augmenting the toxicity of potassium associated with the transfusion. Regardless, the combination of all these factors results in extremely high mortality for patients with transfusion-associated hyperkalemic arrest (87.5% mortality in one series [Smith et al., 2008]).

Immunomodulation

Allogenic blood transfusions seem to lead to modulation of the immune system. Indeed, targeted transfusions were initially used in the 1970s for immunosuppression after renal transplants, but the effect of transfusions on long-term outcome is still not understood (Opelz et al., 1973). More than 100 studies have been published on perioperative transfusion and postoperative infection (Mauermann and Nemergut, 2006). Although many of the conclusions were limited by the biases of small cohorts and retrospective studies, several prospective series showed that perioperative transfusion increased the infection rate in various settings, including cardiac surgery, orthopedic surgery, trauma, and colorectal surgery (Ammann et al., 1983; Busch et al., 1991; Goodnough et al., 1999a; Dodd, 2003). However, the transfusion literature remains divided on the subject of transfusion-associated infections; for every study with positive results, a study with negative results can also be found. The situation is similar for the risk of cancer recurrence after a presumed curative operation. In a 1996 article, Landers et al. (1996) reviewed the available studies, which included various surgical patients. The authors concluded that the burden of evidence pointed toward an association between transfusion and cancer recurrence. Other experts continue to argue that this is simply an association and not a causal relation (Vamvakas and Blajchman, 2001).

Most of the discussion surrounding immunosuppression and transfusion focuses on the effects of donor leukocytes (Kuehnert et al., 2001). Leukoreduction is thought to help reduce transfusion-associated nosocomial infections. Hebert and colleagues (2003) retrospectively reviewed the effects of a universal leukoreduction program in 23 Canadian centers. The patients were undergoing cardiac, orthopedic, or trauma surgery. Although leukoreduction appeared to decrease mortality and the incidence of antibiotic use, the overall rate of serious nosocomial infections was not affected. Fergusson et al. (2004) performed a meta-analysis of all available trials that used leukoreduction and found no difference in the infection rate. Although most of the trials studying this issue have been performed with adult patients, at least one analysis of patients in a pediatric intensive care unit suggested that increased numbers of RBC transfusions were independently associated with an increased incidence of bloodstream infections in critically ill children (Elward and Fraser, 2006).

Transfusion-Associated Graft-Versus-Host Disease

Not only can transfusions depress immune function, they also may activate it in adverse ways, as in the case of transfusion-associated graft-versus-host disease (TA-GVHD), a preventable disease associated with high mortality. Typically, adults with TA-GVHD show symptoms 10 days after transfusion and neonates with TA-GVHD experience symptoms 28 days after transfusion (Parshuram et al., 2002). The clinical features include fever, rash, diarrhea, hepatitis, and pancytopenia, with death occurring approximately 50 days after transfusion (Ohto and Anderson, 1996). Treatments include corticosteroids, azathioprine, methotrexate, cyclosporine, and bone marrow transplants. However, even with aggressive treatment, the mortality rate in children is nearly 100% (Leitman and Holland, 1985).

The pathophysiology of TA-GVHD has been described (Parshuram et al., 2002). Circulating donor leukocytes persist in transfusion recipients for up to 18 months (Lee et al., 1999). Normally these cells are recognized as foreign and are eliminated, but if they are not, donor leukocyte engraftment may occur, with proliferation of CD4 and CD8 T cells (Nishimura et al., 1997). The clinical effects are mediated by donor T-cell cytotoxicity and by recipient cytokines, including tumor necrosis factor α and interleukin 1 (Vogelsang and Hess, 1994).

The factors that may predispose patients to the development of TA-GVHD are all related to inadequate detection or removal of donor leukocytes. Immunocompromise potentially leads to both inadequate recognition and inactivation of leukocytes. Younger patients, including preterm and full-term infants and children, seem to be at higher risk, perhaps because their immune systems are immature. Congenital immunodeficiencies, including severe combined immunodeficiency syndrome, DiGeorge's syndrome, and Wiskott-Aldrich syndrome, have been associated with TA-GVHD. In addition, many children with congenital heart disease have associated immunodeficiency syndromes that may predispose them to TA-GVHD. Finally, the degree of similarity of human leukocyte antigens (HLAs) between donor and recipients is an important consideration. When donor lymphocytes are homozygous and a recipient is heterozygous for a particular haplotype, recognition of foreign leukocytes may not occur. On an individual level, this has significant implications for children receiving donor-directed platelet transfusions from family members. From an epidemiologic standpoint, the relatively high incidence of TA-GVHD in Japan may relate to a lack of HLA diversity.

Because TA-GVHD is mediated by donor leukocytes, it is preventable by removal of the same. Washing of donor RBCs and use of leukoreduction filters decrease the donor leukocyte burden but do not eliminate all the leukocytes. These methods may be effective at reducing the incidence of TA-GVHD, but they do not eliminate its occurrence (Ronquist and Waldenström, 2003; Smith et al., 2008). Gamma irradiation of 2,500 cGy is the only accepted and widely available method of preventing TA-GVHD. This degree of irradiation decreases the recovery of RBCs, so that the FDA recommends a shelf life of 28 days for irradiated RBCs compared with 42 days for nonirradiated packed RBCs (Davey et al., 1992). Potassium and free hemoglobin levels increase after irradiation and increase further with the duration of storage. Thus, it is preferable to irradiate blood products shortly before administration, particularly in small children, who may not tolerate a potassium load.

Transfusion-Related Acute Lung Injury

Transfusion-related acute lung injury (TRALI) is the leading cause of transfusion-related death in the United States (Kleinman et al., 2004). Although underreporting surely exists, the estimated risk of TRALI is one in 5000 transfusions, with FFP being the most commonly associated product (Goodnough et al., 1999a). This complication and its fatal consequences have been described in pediatric patients (Ririe et al., 2005). The originally proposed mechanism of TRALI is an interaction between antibodies from the donor and leukocyte antigens from the recipient (Opelz et al., 1973). Donor lipids and cytokines have also been implicated. Regardless of the mechanism, the end result is activation of recipient neutrophils in the pulmonary vascular bed. Neutrophil and complement activation culminates in increased pulmonary capillary permeability and pulmonary edema. Interestingly, the most commonly implicated donors are multiparous females, presumably as a result of an increase in human leukocyte antibodies to paternal antigens during pregnancy (Densmore et al., 1999).

The clinical features of TRALI are similar to those of acute respiratory distress syndrome and include dyspnea, hypoxia, and radiographic evidence of pulmonary edema without increased pulmonary capillary wedge pressure. Onset of symptoms usually occurs within 4 to 6 hours after transfusion. Treatment is supportive, because there is no evidence that corticosteroids or other specific therapy is helpful. It is estimated that 90% of patients with TRALI recover (Hebert et al., 1999). The majority of reported cases and studies of TRALI involve adults, but children are certainly at risk (Ririe et al., 2005; Church et al., 2006).

MASSIVE TRANSFUSION

Massive transfusion is typically defined as the need to transfuse more than 1 blood volume in a 24-hour period and, in the case of trauma, portends a poor prognosis (Vaslef et al., 2002; Como et al., 2004). Several potential complications of massive transfusion are listed in Table 14-4. The cause of coagulopathy during massive blood loss and resuscitation continues to be debated and is probably different for relatively controlled losses in the operating suite than for uncontrolled acute losses caused by trauma (Ketchum, 2006). The dilution and consumptive loss of coagulation factors (especially platelets) appear to vary widely. However, after losing 2 blood volumes, most adult patients have platelet counts less than 50×10^9/L, and many require correction of symptomatic thrombocytopenia before the platelet count decreases to that level (Hiippala et al., 1995). In otherwise healthy adults, the intraoperative loss of about 1.5 blood volumes requires replacement of coagulation factors with FFP. This is in contrast to trauma patients who appear to benefit from FFP administration early in the course of resuscitation (Ketchum, 2006; Shaz et al., 2009).

TABLE 14-4. Complications of Massive Transfusion

Complication	Mechanism
Acidosis	Poor oxygen delivery, lactate accumulation
Alkalosis	Citrate metabolism to bicarbonate by the liver
Hypocalcemia	Citrate binding of calcium
Hyperglycemia	Dextrose preservative in packed red blood cells
Hypothermia	Transfusion of cold blood products
Hyperkalemia	Multifactorial

Data from Smith HM et al.: Cardiac arrests associated with hyperkalemia during red blood cell transfusion: a case series, *Anesth Analg* 106(4):1062-1069, 2008.

It is difficult to conduct quality studies with patients experiencing major intraoperative blood loss, because measurements of blood loss, assumptions of intravascular volume status, and subjective observations of hemostasis are potential sources of error and bias. However, at least one observational study has attempted to identify the source of coagulopathy in pediatric patients undergoing a major operation. Murray and colleagues (1995) studied 32 patients (mean [SD] age, 15.6 [2.3] years) who lost more than 50% of their blood volume while undergoing major spine surgery and were resuscitated with packed RBCs and crystalloid solutions. In 17 of these 32 patients, coagulopathy developed, and it was felt that treatment with FFP was required. Patients with increased clinical bleeding had more blood loss and blood volume loss than the patients who did not have increased clinical bleeding. Although 30 of the 32 patients had increased prothrombin times and activated partial thromboplastin times, only 17 of these patients had excessive clinical bleeding. After loss of 1 blood volume, platelet counts estimated by regression analysis were 195,000/mL. In 14 of the 17 patients with excessive bleeding, FFP alone was adequate to achieve hemostasis. Two patients received platelets as well. The authors concluded that in pediatric patients

undergoing spinal fusion, coagulation factor dilution rather than thrombocytopenia is the major cause of coagulopathy and in the majority of cases FFP is the only blood component needed to correct the coagulopathy.

Whenever possible, the use of platelet and FFP transfusions should be guided by laboratory values, but even in an efficient hospital, prothrombin time results may not be available for 45 to 60 minutes, making laboratory guidance for blood component therapy difficult. For controlled blood loss in the operating room, therefore, the clinician must anticipate the need for blood products and evaluate coagulation status at regular intervals. As point-of-care testing becomes more widely available, values for prothrombin time and partial thromboplastin time may be accessible more quickly. Recently, thromboelastography has become an increasingly popular measure of dynamic clotting parameters (Fig. 14-13). Thromboelastography assesses the viscoelastic properties of blood under low shear conditions (Ganter and Hofer, 2008). Devices from different manufacturers use different technologies. However, the premise is similar. A pin is immersed in a blood sample. The blood sample or pin is then rotated through a specific cycle. As clot begins to form in the blood sample, torque is applied to the immersed pin.

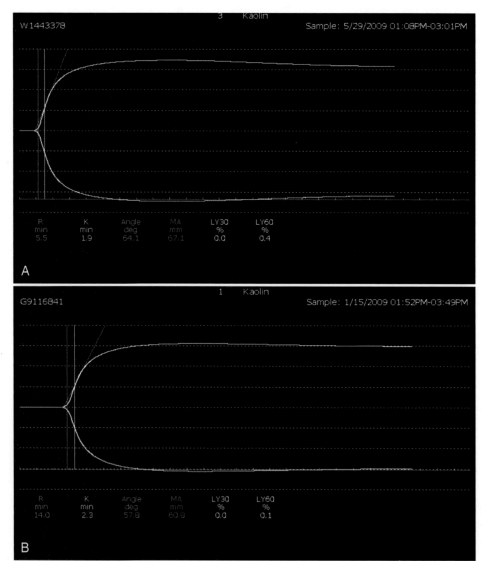

■ **FIGURE 14-13.** Thromboelastograms. **A,** Tracing shows normal clot formation. **B,** Prolonged reaction time *(R)* is shown for a child with an activated partial thromboplastin time of 56 seconds after cardiopulmonary bypass.

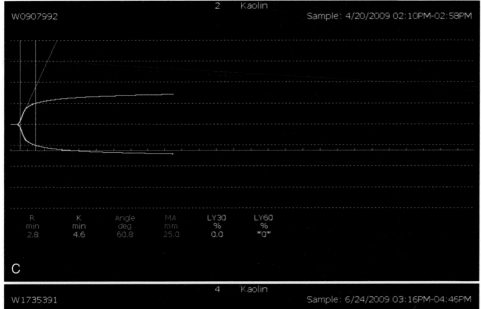

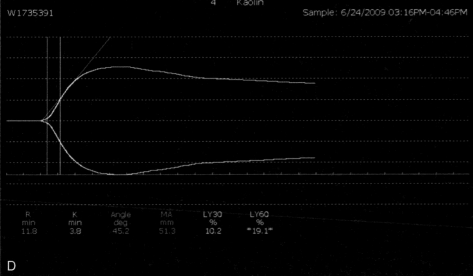

■ **FIGURE 14–13—cont'd.**
C, Tracing shows a low maximum amplitude *(MA)* in a child after cardiac surgery. The platelet count was 150 ×10⁹/L, indicating that the platelets were likely dysfunctional after cardiopulmonary bypass.
D, Tracing shows relatively normal initial clot formation but excessive fibrinolysis in a child in the intensive care unit after cardiac surgery. *Angle,* Kinetics of fibrin formation and clot development; *K,* coagulation time; *LY30,* percentage lysis at 30 minutes after maximum amplitude; *LY60,* percentage lysis at 60 minutes after maximum amplitude. *(All tracings were obtained using the TEG system, Courtesy of Haemoscope Corp, Niles, Ill.)*

The changes in torque are transmitted to a recording device. The devices record changes in viscoelasticity at all stages of clot formation. The terminology varies between devices, but the important measurements and the corresponding stages of clot formation for the TEG system (Haemoscope Corp, Niles, Illinois) are shown in Table 14-5 as an example (Ganter and Hofer, 2008).

Massive transfusion, particularly in trauma patients, predisposes the patient to hypothermia, a condition that worsens coagulopathy and blood loss. Monitoring for core body temperature is essential, and all fluids and blood products should be warmed. For small children, blood should be passed through the warmer into size-appropriate syringes for administration.

Citrate preservatives used for blood component storage must be considered in massive transfusions, because citrate binds serum calcium. Citrate metabolism is performed primarily by the liver, and patients with normal hepatic function usually do not have myocardial dysfunction as a result of citrate overload unless the transfusions are very rapid (greater than 1 unit of RBCs every 5 minutes in adults). Regardless, calcium levels should be monitored, and this can be quickly accomplished with point-of-care testing. Acidosis may occur with massive blood loss because of inadequate oxygen delivery and the accumulation of lactate. However, with adequate resuscitation, metabolic alkalosis is common, because the liver metabolizes citrate to bicarbonate.

TABLE 14-5. Measurements and Corresponding Stages of Clot Formation for the TEG System*

Output	Stage of Clot Formation	Potential Causes of Abnormal Results
Reaction time	Initial fibrin formation	Factor deficiency, heparin
Alpha angle	Kinetics of fibrin formation and clot development	Fibrinogen deficiency
Maximum amplitude	Ultimate strength and stability of clot	Platelet deficiency or dysfunction
Clot lysis	Clot lysis	Fibrinolysis

* Haemoscope Corp, Niles, Ill.

INTRAOPERATIVE BLOOD RECOVERY

Cell salvage devices are made by several manufacturers, but they all operate under the same general principles: centrifugal and hydrostatic forces are used to differentiate between blood constituents on the basis of their different densities (Waters, 2005). Suction is used to transfer blood from the surgical field to a collection reservoir. In the reservoir, the blood must be anticoagulated with either a heparin or a citrate-based anticoagulant. When a sufficient amount of blood has been captured for processing, a cycle is activated and the blood is drained into a centrifuge bowl. Blood enters the bowl while the centrifuge is spinning. Centrifugal forces separate the various blood components, with the larger, heavier RBCs forming sediment against the walls and the lighter particles (plasma) forming sediment closer to the center of the bowl. Hydrostatic forces then draw the plasma out through the center of the bowl. After separation of the RBCs, they are washed with a balanced salt solution to remove debris. Typically, the wash volume is at least three times the bowl volume. After washing, the RBCs are transferred to a collection bag for infusion into the patient (Waters, 2005).

The average hematocrit level of a properly processed salvaged unit is approximately 60%, and the survival of salvaged RBCs is reportedly similar to that of allogenic RBCs (Williamson and Taswell, 1991). The efficacy of intraoperative cell salvage depends largely on the efficiency of capturing the patient's shed blood. High suction pressures lead to turbulence that may ultimately destroy the RBCs, so the lowest suction pressure that is effective at clearing the surgical field should be used. Suction tips with larger orifices further decrease turbulence on the RBCs. Because sponges may contain a considerable amount of shed blood, they should be rinsed and wrung out into a basin; the rinse solution is then drawn into the collection reservoir (Waters, 2005).

Studies evaluating the efficacy of intraoperative cell salvage in pediatric patients have had mixed results. One potential obstacle is the use of a large, adult-sized collection system for small children (Weldon, 2005). Although infants may lose a large portion of their blood volume during an operation, this loss is likely not of sufficient volume to allow processing. An exception is the use of an adult cell-salvage device to recover RBCs from the cardiopulmonary circuit after cardiac surgery. When a smaller, 125-mL bowl is used, the results have been more encouraging. One retrospective study found that cell salvage using a 125-mL collection bowl decreased the need for banked RBCs from 100% to 67% during craniosynostosis surgery (Jimenez and Barone, 1995). A second study, using an even smaller system that required only 35 mL of shed blood for processing, also showed a reduction in the exposure to donor RBCs (Dahmani et al., 2000). Not all cell salvage devices are equal. In a study by Booke and colleagues (1999), three cell-salvage devices were compared. Of the three devices, the Continuous Autotransfusion System (CATSplus) was the most efficient, providing the highest hematocrit and the largest volume of salvaged blood. The cost-benefit ratio of cell salvage is directly proportional to the number of units processed (Waters, 2005). Thus, with small patients, a large financial savings is unlikely to be realized. Regardless of cost, fewer donor exposures appears to have clear benefits.

Intraoperative cell salvage is not without risk. Transfer of blood directly from the holding bag carries the potential for air embolism, requiring that blood be transferred from the holding bag to a transfusion bag with the air removed except in extreme emergencies when time does not allow. The wash solution must be a balanced salt solution, because the inadvertent substitution of sterile water would cause massive cell lysis and the readministration of lysed cells could result in potentially fatal hyperkalemia. Given that washing does not completely remove bacteria from the captured blood, gross bacterial contamination of the surgical field is a relative contraindication to the use of cell salvage (Hebert et al., 2003). Other relative contraindications include the presence of malignant cells or contaminants such as ascitic fluid, amniotic fluid, and thrombin gel.

BLOOD SUBSTITUTES

An oxygen-carrying substance that may be used as an alternative to donated RBCs for patients requiring transfusion has many potential advantages. This substance would likely have a longer shelf life, require less testing, be stored at room temperature, undergo viral inactivation, be universally biocompatible, and be easily supplied to areas where banked RBCs cannot be reliably obtained. Indeed, research has been ongoing in this area for at least 60 years. Two different substances have been studied: hemoglobin-based oxygen carriers (HBOCs) and perfluorocarbon (PFC) emulsions.

PFCs are inert substances that do not bind gases but act as solvents that can carry numerous gases, including oxygen. PFCs are insoluble in water and must be emulsified before administration. They are ultimately broken down by the reticuloendothelial system and exhaled as vapor; consequently they have a relatively short half-life (Tremper et al., 1982). Repeated administration results in hepatosplenomegaly in animals, and there appears to be a dose-dependent decrease in platelet count associated with administration (Leese et al., 2000). Because PFCs do not bind oxygen, their oxygen-carrying capacity is dependent on the partial pressure of oxygen. Patients must therefore receive high concentrations of inspired oxygen to have any meaningful oxygen delivery, and these high concentrations may carry the risk of pulmonary toxicity. In addition, unloading of oxygen at the tissue level is completely dependent on the oxygen gradients, and delivery tends to be poor. There are currently no FDA-approved PFCs, although third-generation PFCs are in preclinical development (Chang, 2000).

HBOCs were first studied in 1934 when Amberson purified bovine hemoglobin and administered it to animals (Jahr et al., 2007). These products consist of hemoglobin solutions that are polymerized or cross-linked (or both). When hemoglobin molecules are not contained by RBCs they rapidly scavenge nitric oxide, resulting in systemic (especially pulmonary) vasoconstriction, a release of proinflammatory mediators, and a loss of platelet inactivation (Wahr, 2003; Natanson et al., 2008). Cross-linking and polymerization of hemoglobin molecules has been proposed to increase the half-life of the molecules (free hemoglobin is rapidly scavenged by the reticuloendothelial system) and reduce nitric oxide-associated complications.

A meta-analysis of 16 trials that used five different HBOCs included a total of 3711 adult patients in various situations (Natanson et al., 2008). This analysis showed a significant increase in the risk of death (relative risk [RR], 1.30; 95% confidence interval [CI], 10.05 to 1.61) for patients treated with HBOCs. There was also a 2.7-fold increase in the risk of myocardial infarction for treatment patients (RR, 2.71; 95% CI, 1.67-4.40).

At present, there are no clinically viable alternatives to the transfusion of donor RBCs for the treatment of symptomatic anemia. As technology improves, more substances will be studied. However, with the poor track record of these substitutes thus far, rigorous study in animal models and adults will be required before substitutes are used in pediatric patients.

SUMMARY

In this chapter, we have attempted to provide the reader with the information required to understand hemoglobin function, techniques for RBC conservation, triggers that should prompt the clinician to consider blood product transfusion, and some of the safety and technical concerns related to the transfusion of various blood products. Ultimately, nothing can substitute for the sound clinical judgment of an experienced, well-informed pediatric anesthesiologist in the operating room or at the bedside. The recognition of the need for transfusion in any child, although grounded in science, must ultimately rest with the judgment of the clinician. Likewise, the timing and choice of blood product are determined by myriad factors, some of which have been mentioned in this chapter. As with all aspects of pediatric anesthesia care, thoughtful application of the information derived from this chapter and text can provide the science. It is up to each clinician to provide the art that is fundamental to the safety of the children for whose care we are entrusted.

For questions and answers on topics in this chapter, go to "Chapter Questions" at www.expertconsult.com.

REFERENCES

Complete references used in this text can be found online at www.expertconsult.com.

Pain Management

Constance L. Monitto, Sabine Kost-Byerly, and Myron Yaster

CONTENTS

"We must all die. But that I can save (a person) from days of torture, that is what I feel as my great and ever new privilege. Pain is a more terrible lord of mankind than even death itself" (Albert Schweitzer). The treatment and alleviation of pain is a basic human right that exists regardless of age (Yaster et al., 1997; Schechter et al., 2003). The old "wisdom" that young children neither respond to, nor remember, painful experiences to the same degree that adults do is simply untrue (Taddio and Katz, 2005). Many, if not all, of the nerve pathways essential for the transmission and perception of pain are present and functioning by 24 weeks' gestation (Lee et al., 2005; Lowery et al., 2007). Furthermore, recent research in newborn animals has revealed that the failure to provide analgesia for pain results in "rewiring" the nerve pathways responsible for pain transmission in the dorsal horn of the spinal cord and results in increased pain perception with future painful insults (Fitzgerald and Beggs,

2001; Pattinson and Fitzgerald, 2004). This confirms human newborn research in which the failure to provide anesthesia or analgesia for newborn circumcision resulted not only in short-term physiologic perturbations but also in longer term behavioral changes, particularly during immunization (Taddio et al., 1995; Maxwell et al., 1987; Taddio and Katz, 2005; Anand et al., 2006).

Providing effective analgesia to infants, preverbal children, adolescents, and the mentally and physically disabled poses unique challenges to those who practice pediatric medicine and surgery. In the past, several studies documented that physicians, nurses, and parents underestimate the amount of pain experienced by children and that they overestimate the risks inherent in the drugs used in the treatment of pain (Schechter et al., 1986; Finley et al., 1996; McGrath and Finley, 1996). This is not at all surprising; the guiding principle of medica practice is to do no harm, *primum non nocere*. Physicians are taught throughout their training that opioids, the analgesics most commonly prescribed in moderate to severe pain, cause respiratory depression, cardiovascular collapse, depressed levels of consciousness, constipation, nausea, vomiting, and, with repeated use, tolerance and addiction. Less potent analgesics, such as nonsteroidal antiinflammatory drugs (NSAIDs), can also cause problems such as bleeding, liver dysfunction, coagulopathies, and impaired wound and bone healing. Thus, physicians at times prescribe insufficiently potent analgesics, recommend inadequate doses, or use pharmacologically irrational dosing regimens because of their overriding concern that children may be harmed by the use of these drugs. The resulting conundrum often results in inadequate treatment for pain and for painful procedures. On the other hand, the adverse effects of pain and the failure to treat it are rarely discussed. In addition to its impact on neurodevelopment, it is known that unrelieved pain interferes with sleep, leads to fatigue and a sense of helplessness, enhances the stress and inflammatory response, and may result in increased morbidity or mortality (Anand et al., 1987).

Nurses may be wary of physicians' orders (and patients' requests) as well. The most common prescription order for potent analgesics is "to give as needed" (*pro re nata*, or PRN). Thus, the patient must know or remember to ask for pain medication, or the nurse must identify when a patient is in pain. These requirements may not always be met by children in pain. Children younger than 3 years of age may be unable to adequately verbalize when or where they hurt. Alternatively, they may be afraid to report their pain. Many children withdraw or deny their pain if pain relief involves yet another terrifying and painful experience—the intramuscular injection or "shot." Finally, several studies have documented the inability of nurses, physicians, and parents to correctly identify and treat pain, even in postoperative pediatric patients (McGrath and Finley, 1996; Romsing et al., 1996; Fortier et al., 2009).

Societal fears of opioid addiction and lack of advocacy are also causal factors in the under treatment of pediatric pain. Unlike adult patients, pain management in children is often dependent on the ability of parents to recognize and assess pain and on their decision to treat or not treat it (Romsing and Walther-Larsen, 1996; Sutters and Miaskowski, 1997). Even in hospitalized patients, most of the pain that children experience is managed by the patient's parents (Greenberg et al., 1999; Krane, 2008). Parental misconceptions concerning pain assessment and pain management may therefore result in inadequate pain treatment (Romsing and Walther-Larsen, 1996; Fortier et al., 2009). This is particularly true in patients who are too young or too developmentally handicapped to report their pain themselves. Parents may fail to report pain, either because they are unable to assess it or they are afraid of the consequences of pain therapy. False beliefs about addiction and the proper use of acetaminophen and other analgesics resulted in the failure to provide analgesia to children (Forward et al., 1996; Fortier et al., 2009). In another study, the belief that pain was useful or that repeated doses of analgesics lead to medication not working well resulted in the failure of the parents to provide or ask for prescribed analgesics to treat their children's pain (Finley et al., 1996). Parental education is therefore essential if children are to be adequately treated for pain. Unfortunately, the ability to educate parents properly about this issue is often limited by insufficient resources, time, and personnel (Greenberg et al., 1999).

Fortunately, the past 25 years have seen an increase in research and interest in pediatric pain management and in the development of pediatric pain services, primarily under the direction of pediatric anesthesiologists (Shapiro et al., 1991; Nelson et al., 2009). Pediatric-pain service teams provide pain management for acute, postoperative, terminal, neuropathic, and chronic pain. This chapter reviews the recent advances in opioid and local anesthetic pharmacology, as well as the various modalities that are useful in the treatment of acute childhood pain.

PAIN ASSESSMENT

The International Association for the Study of Pain (IASP) defines pain as "an unpleasant sensory and emotional experience associated with actual or potential tissue damage, or described in terms of such damage" (Merskey et al., 1979). Pain is a subjective experience; operationally it can be defined as "what the patient says hurts" and exists "when the patient says it does hurt." Infants, preverbal children, and children between the ages of 2 and 7 (Piaget's Preoperational Thought stage) may be unable to describe their pain or their subjective experiences. This has led many to conclude incorrectly that these children don't experience pain in the same way as adults. Clearly, children do not have to know (or be able to express) the meaning of an experience in order to have the experience (Anand and Craig, 1996). On the other hand, because pain is essentially a subjective experience, focusing on the child's perspective of pain is an indispensable facet of pediatric pain management and an essential element in the specialized study of childhood pain. Indeed, pain assessment and management are interdependent and one is essentially useless without the other. The goal of pain assessment is to provide accurate data about the location and intensity of pain, as well as the effectiveness of measures used to alleviate or abolish it.

Multiple validated instruments currently exist to measure and assess pain in children of all ages (von Baeyer and Spagrud, 2007; Crellin et al., 2007; Franck et al., 2000). The sensitivity and specificity of these instruments have been widely debated and have resulted in a plethora of studies to validate their reliability and validity. The most commonly used instruments that measure the quality and intensity of pain are "self-report measures." In older children and adults, the most commonly used self-report instruments are visual analogue scales (VASs) and numerical rating scales (0 = no pain; 10 = worst pain). However, pain intensity or severity can also be measured in children as young as 3 years of age by using pictures or word descriptors to describe pain. Two common examples include the Oucher Scale (developed by Dr. Judy Beyer), a two-part scale with a vertical numerical scale (0–100) on one side and six photographs of a young child on the other, or the Six-Face Pain Scale, first developed by Dr. Donna Wong and later modified by Bieri et al. (Fig. 15-1) (Beyer and Wells, 1989; Wong and Baker, 1988; Beyer et al., 1990). Because of its simplicity, the Six-Face Pain Scale-Revised is commonly used (Hicks et al., 2001; Bieri et al., 1990). Alternatively, color, word-graphic rating scales, and poker chips have been used to assess the intensity of pain in children. One obvious limitation of all of these self-report measures is their inability to be used in cognitively impaired children or in intubated, sedated, and paralyzed patients.

In infants, newborns, and the cognitively impaired, pain has been assessed by measuring physiologic responses to nociceptive

WBFPS

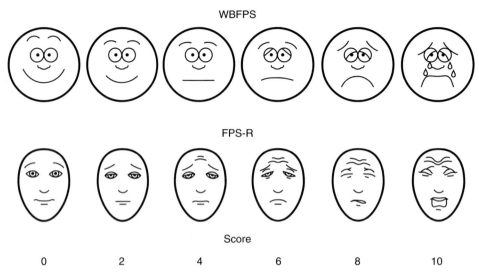

FPS-R

Score

0   2   4   6   8   10

■ **FIGURE 15-1.** Six-Face Pain Scale *(Top).* Original scale developed by Wong et al. *Lower,* Modified scale by Bieri et al. *(From Bieri D et al.: The Faces Pain Scale for the self-assessment of the severity of pain experienced by children: development, initial validation, and preliminary investigation for ratio scale properties,* Pain *41:139, 1990; Beyer JE et al.: Discordance between self-report and behavioral pain measures in children aged 3-7 years after surgery,* J Pain Symptom Manage *5:350, 1990.)*

stimuli, such as blood pressure and heart rate changes (observational pain scales, OPSs), or by measuring levels of adrenal stress hormones (Krechel and Bildner, 1995). Alternatively, behavioral approaches have used facial expression, body movements, and the intensity and quality of crying as indices of response to nociceptive stimuli. The most appropriate are the Crying, Requires oxygen, Increased vital signs, Expression, and Sleepless (CRIES) score for newborns and the revised Face, Legs, Activity, Cry, and Consolability (FLACC) pain tool for children who have difficulty verbalizing pain (Tables 15-1 and 15-2) (Grunau et al., 1990; Hadjistavropoulos et al., 1994; Voepel-Lewis et al., 2002). Another commonly used pain and sedation tool that uses both behaviors and physiologic parameters is the COMFORT scale, which relies on the measurement of five behavioral variables (alertness, facial tension, muscle tone, agitation, and movement) and three physiologic variables (heart rate, respiration, and blood pressure) (Table 15-3) (Ambuel et al., 1992; Bear and Ward-Smith, 2006). Each is assigned a score ranging

from 1 to 5, to give a total score ranging from 8 (deep sedation) to 40 (alert and agitated). A modified COMFORT scale that eliminates physiologic parameters has also been developed (Ista et al., 2005). It is also important to define accurately the location of pain. This is readily accomplished by using either dolls or action figures or by using drawings of body outlines, both front and back. Finally, in the research laboratory, sophisticated new tools such as functional magnetic resonance imaging (MRI) are being used to objectively assess and map pain and its pathways through the central nervous system (CNS) (Tracey and Mantyh, 2007).

NEUROPHYSIOLOGY OF PAIN

Pain is more than simply the physiologic transmission of nociceptive input from a site of injury to the brain and its modulation within the CNS. Rather, it is a complex sensation that is integrated and given value at higher, conscious brain centers. No two people experience it the same way. It is similar to symphonic music; despite the fact that the physiology of sound transmission is the same in everyone, symphonic music to some is simply awful and to others it is glorious. As individuals integrate neural transmissions, they give them personal, subjective value based on age, culture, genes, previous experience and education, values, and state of mind. The same is true for pain.

Many if not all of the nerve pathways essential for the transmission, perception, and modulation of pain are present and functioning by 24 weeks of gestation (Fig. 15-2) (Lowry et al., 2007; Lee et al., 2005). Although neural transmission in peripheral nerves is slower in neonates because myelination is incomplete at birth, the major nociceptive neurons in neonates as well as in adults are either unmyelinated C fibers or thinly myelinated Aδ fibers. After an acute injury such as surgical or accidental trauma, inflammatory mediators are released; they lower the pain threshold at the site of injury (primary hyperalgesia) and in the surrounding uninjured tissue (secondary

TABLE 15-1. CRIES Neonatal Pain Assessment Scale

Indicator	Score		
	0	1	2
Crying	No	High pitch but consolable	Inconsolable
Requires oxygen for Sat >95%	No	$Fio_2 < 30\%$	$Fio_2 > 30\%$
Increased vital signs	No	HR or BP increased <20%	HR or BP increased >20%
Expression	No	Grimace	Grimace and grunt
Sleepless	No	Wakes often	Constantly awake

Score <4: Initiate nonpharmacologic measures.
Score >4: Initiate pharmacologic and nonpharmacologic measures.
BP, Blood pressure; *HR,* heart rate.

TABLE 15-2. Revised FLACC for Pain Assessment in the Cognitively Impaired*

	0	1	2
Face	No particular expression or smile	Occasional grimace/frown; withdrawn or disinterested (appears sad or worried)	Consistent grimace or frown; frequent/constant quivering chin, clenched jaw (distressed-looking face; expression of fright or panic)
Legs	Normal position or relaxed	Uneasy, restless, tense (occasional tremors)	Kicking, or legs drawn up (marked increase in spasticity, constant tremors, or jerking)
Activity	Lying quietly, normal position, moves easily	Squirming, shifting back and forth, tense (mildly agitated [e.g., head back and forth, aggression]; shallow, splinting respirations, intermittent sighs)	Arched, rigid, or jerking (severe agitation, head banging; shivering [not rigors]; breath-holding, gasping or sharp intake of breath; severe splinting)
Cry	No cry (awake or asleep)	Moans or whimpers, occasional complaint (occasional verbal outburst or grunt)	Crying steadily, screams or sobs, frequent complaints (repeated outbursts, constant grunting)
Consolability	Content, relaxed	Reassured by occasional touching, hugging or talking; distractible	Difficult to console or comfort (pushing away caregiver, resisting care or comfort measures)

*Revised descriptors for children with disabilities shown in parentheses.
0 = Relaxed/comfortable; 1-3 = mild discomfort; 4-6 = moderate pain; 7-10 = severe pain.

TABLE 15-3. Comfort Scale

	1	2	3	4	5
Alertness	Deeply asleep	Lightly asleep	Drowsy	Fully awake and alert	Hyper-alert
Calmness or agitation	Calm	Slightly anxious	Anxious	Very anxious	Panicky
Respiratory response	No coughing and no spontaneous respirations	Spontaneous reparation with little or no response to ventilation	Occasional cough or resistance to ventilator	Actively breathes against ventilator or coughs regularly	Fights ventilator; coughing or choking
Physical movement	No movement	Occasional, slight movement	Slight movement often	Vigorous movement limited to extremities	Vigorous movement including torso and head
Blood pressure	Less than baseline	Consistently at baseline	Occasional increases of 15% or more (1-3 episodes during observation period)	Multiple increases of 15% or more (>3 episodes)	Sustained increase >15%
Muscle tone	Muscles totally relaxed; no muscle tone	Reduced muscle tone	Normal muscle tone	Increased muscle tone and flexion of fingers and toes	Extreme muscle rigidity and flexion of fingers and toes
Facial tension	Facial muscles totally relaxed	Facial muscle tone normal; no facial muscle tension evident	Tension evident in some facial muscles	Tension evident throughout facial muscles	Facial muscles contorted and grimacing

hyperalgesia). These inflammatory mediators, which include hydrogen and potassium ions, histamine, leukotrienes, prostaglandins, cytokines, serotonin (5-HT), bradykinins, and nerve-growth factors make a "sensitizing soup," which together with repeated stimuli of the nociceptive fibers cause decreased excitatory thresholds and result in peripheral sensitization. They are also targets of therapeutic intervention (Fig. 15-3). Secondary effects of peripheral sensitization include hyperalgesia, the increased response to a noxious stimulus and allodynia, whereby non-nociceptive fibers transmit noxious stimuli resulting in the sensation of pain from non-noxious stimuli.

Sensory afferent neurons have a unipolar cell body located in the dorsal root ganglion and are classified by fiber size into three major groups (A, B, C) (Table 15-4). Group A is further subclassified into four subgroups. Sensory fibers that respond to noxious stimulation include small caliber myelinated (Aδ) or fine unmyelinated C fibers. These fibers originate as free nerve endings that can be characterized by their response to specific stimuli such as pressure, heat, and chemical irritants and arise from epidermal and internal receptive fields, including the periosteum, joints, and viscera. The Aδ nociceptors transmit "first pain," which is well localized, sharp, and lasts as only as long as the original stimulus. The C-fiber, polymodal nociceptors display a slow conduction velocity and respond to mechanothermal and chemical stimuli. This "second pain" is diffuse, persistent, burning, slow to be perceived, and lasts well beyond the termination of the stimulus.

As the primary afferent neurons enter the spinal cord they segregate and occupy a lateral position in the dorsal horn (Fig. 15-4). The Aδ fibers terminate in laminae I, II (substantia

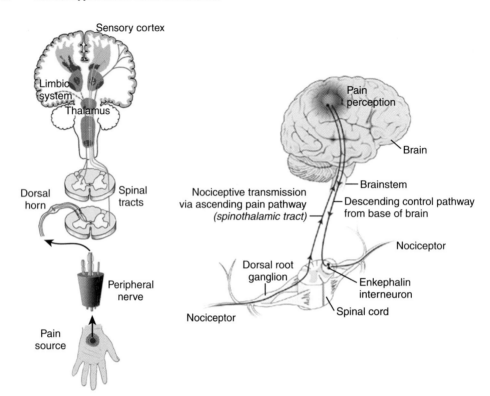

■ **FIGURE 15-2.** Nociceptive nerve pathways essential for the transmission, perception, and modulation of pain are depicted. *Left:* After an injury, nociceptive fibers carried in peripheral nerves enter the spinal cord via the dorsal horn. They are then transmitted via ascending spinothalamic, spinoreticular, and spinomesencephalic tracts to the thalamus, limbic system, and sensory cortex. *Right:* From the sensory cortex descending control pathways modulate pain in the spinal cord and in the periphery.

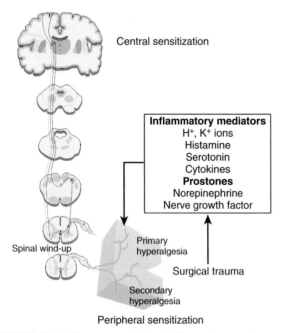

■ **FIGURE 15-3.** After an acute injury, inflammatory mediators are released. They lower the pain threshold at the site of injury (primary hyperalgesia) and in the surrounding uninjured tissue (secondary hyperalgesia). Repetitive stimulation of nociceptors and continuous neuronal discharge (peripheral sensitization) leads to central sensitization or windup. The combination of peripheral and central sensitization is responsible for a decrease in the pain threshold, both at the site of injury (primary hyperalgesia) and in the surrounding uninjured tissue (secondary hyperalgesia).

TABLE 15-4. Classification of Peripheral Nerve Fibers

Fiber Group	Innervation	Mean Diameter (mm)	Mean Conduction Velocity (mm/sec)
Aα (M)	Primary muscle spindle, motor to skeletal muscle	15	100
Aβ (M)	Cutaneous touch and pressure afferents	8	50
Aγ (M)	Motor to muscle spindles	6	20
Aδ (M)	Mechanoreceptors and nociceptors	< 3	15
B (M)	Sympathetic preganglionic	3	7
C (UM)	Mechanoreceptors, nociceptors, and sympathetic preganglionic fibers	1	1

M, Myelinated; *UM,* unmyelinated.

gelatinosa), V (nucleus proprius), and X (central canal). The C fibers terminate in laminae I, II, and V, and some enter the dorsal horn through the ventral root. These afferent neurons release one or more excitatory amino acids (e.g., glutamate and aspartate) or peptide neurotransmitters (e.g., substance P, neurokinin A, calcitonin gene-related peptide [CGRP], cholecystokinin,

THE DORSAL HORN

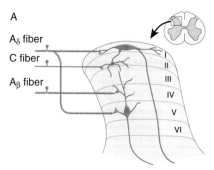

■ **FIGURE 15-4.** Primary afferent neurons enter the spinal cord, segregate, and occupy a lateral position in the dorsal horn. Their termination in distinct zones, or laminae, is depicted.

and somatostatin). Second-order neurons that receive these chemical signals integrate the afferent input with facilitatory and inhibitory influences of interneurons and descending neuronal projections. It is this convergence within the dorsal horn that is responsible for much of the processing, amplification, and modulation of pain. Furthermore, the ability to simultaneously process noxious and innocuous stimuli underlies the gate-control theory of pain described by Melzack and Wall (Melzack and Wall, 1965; DeLeo, 2006).

Second-order neurons are of two types: nociceptive specific neurons, which respond exclusively to nociceptive impulses from Aδ and C fibers, and wide dynamic range (WDR) neurons, which respond to both noxious and nonpainful stimuli. At a given dermatomal level, WDR neurons receive afferent input from the skin, muscle, and visceral nociceptors. Low-frequency stimulation of C fibers leads to a gradual increase in WDR neuronal discharge until it reaches a state of near continuous discharge called *central sensitization* or *wind-up*. Occupancy of the N-methyl-D-aspartic acid (NMDA) receptor by glutamate in the presence of glycine and the removal of the calcium channel's magnesium plug are crucial in the development of wind-up. In combination with peripheral sensitization, these two processes contribute to the postinjury hypersensitivity state that is responsible for a decrease in the pain threshold, both at the site of injury (primary hyperalgesia) and in the surrounding uninjured tissue (secondary hyperalgesia). It is largely as a result of this mechanism that pain may be prolonged beyond the duration normally expected after an acute insult. Prolonged central sensitization has the capacity to lead to permanent alterations in the CNS, including the death of inhibitory neurons, replacement with new afferent excitatory neurons, and the establishment of aberrant excitatory synaptic connections. These alterations can lead to a prolonged state of sensitization, resulting in intractable postoperative pain that is unresponsive to many analgesics.

Nociceptive activity in the spinal cord and the ascending spinothalamic, spinoreticular, and spinomesencephalic tracts carry messages to supraspinal centers (e.g., periaqueductal gray, locus coeruleus, hypothalamus, thalamus, and cerebral cortex) where they are modulated and integrated with autonomic, homeostatic, and arousal processes. This modulation, particularly by the endogenous opioids, γ-aminobutyric acid (GABA), and norepinephrine (NE), can either facilitate

pain transmission or inhibit it. Modulating pain at peripheral, spinal, and supraspinal sites helps achieve better pain management than targeting only one site and is the underlying principle of treating pain in a multimodal fashion (Fig. 15-3).

Although pain pathways are present at birth, they are often immature (Lee et al., 2005; Lowery et al., 2007). As a result, there are considerable differences in how an infant responds to injury compared with the way an adult does. Within the developing nervous system, inhibitory mechanisms in the dorsal horn of the spinal cord are immature, and inhibition of nociceptive input in the dorsal horn of the spinal cord is less than in the adult. Furthermore, dorsal horn neurons in the newborn have wider receptive fields and lower excitatory thresholds than those in older children (Torsney and Fitzgerald, 2003; Bremner and Fitzgerald, 2008; Fitzgerald and Walker, 2009). Thus, compared with adults, young infants have exaggerated reflex responses to pain. Furthermore, recent research in newborn animals has revealed that the failure to provide analgesia for pain results in "rewiring" the nerve pathways responsible for pain transmission in the dorsal horn of the spinal cord and results in increased pain perception for future painful insults (Fitzgerald and Beggs, 2001; Pattinson and Fitzgerald, 2004). This confirms human newborn research in which the failure to provide anesthesia or analgesia for newborn circumcision resulted not only in short-term physiologic perturbations but also in longer term behavioral changes, particularly during immunization (Maxwell et al., 1987; Taddio et al., 1995; Taddio and Katz, 2005).

Preemptive Analgesia, Preventive Analgesia, and Multimodal Analgesia

The possibility that pain after surgery might be preemptively prevented or ameliorated by the use of opioids or local anesthetics given preoperatively has been a concept under review (Katz and McCartney, 2002; Moiniche et al., 2002; Oong et al., 2005). Over the past few years the concept of preemptive analgesia has expanded and evolved to include the reduction of nociceptive inputs during and after surgery. This expanded conceptual framework, which includes preoperative, intraoperative, and postoperative analgesia, targets multiple sites along the pain pathway and is referred to as *preventive* or *multimodal* analgesia (Ballantyne, 2001; Katz and McCartney, 2002). Indeed, acute pediatric (and adult) pain management is increasingly characterized by a multimodal or "balanced" approach in which smaller doses of opioid and nonopioid analgesics, such NSAIDs, local anesthetics, NMDA antagonists, and α₂-adrenergic agonists, are combined to maximize pain control and minimize drug-induced adverse side effects (Fig. 15-5) (DeLeo, 2006). Additionally, a multimodal approach also uses nonpharmacologic complementary and alternative medicine therapies. These alternative medical therapies include distraction, guided imagery, hypnosis, relaxation techniques, biofeedback, transcutaneous nerve stimulation, and acupuncture (Rusy and Weisman, 2000). Taking this approach, activation of peripheral nociceptors can be attenuated with the use of NSAIDs, antihistamines, 5-HT antagonists, and local anesthetics (Fig. 15-5). Within the dorsal horn, nociceptive transmission and processing can be further affected by the administration of local anesthetics, neuraxial opioids, α₂-adrenergic agonists (e.g., clonidine and dexmedetomidine),

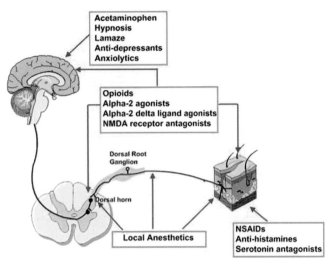

■ **FIGURE 15-5.** Supraspinal, spinal, and peripheral targets of multimodal pain therapy are depicted. Peripheral nociceptors are targets of NSAIDs, antihistamines, 5-HT antagonists, opioids, and local anesthetics. Within the dorsal horn, nociceptive transmission and processing can be affected by the administration of local anesthetics, opioids, α_2-adrenergic agonists and NMDA-receptor antagonists. Within the CNS, pain can be ameliorated by opioids, α_2-agonists, α_2-δ ligand agonists, and pharmacologic and nonpharmacologic therapies that reduce anxiety and induce rest and sleep.

and NMDA receptor antagonists (e.g., ketamine and methadone). Within the CNS, pain can be ameliorated by systemic opioids, α_2-agonists, anticonvulsants (e.g., gabapentin and pregabalin), pharmacologic therapies (e.g., benzodiazepines, α_2-agonists), and nonpharmacologic therapies (e.g., hypnosis, Lamaze, and acupuncture) that reduce anxiety and induce rest and sleep.

PHARMACOLOGIC MANAGEMENT OF PAIN: THE CONUNDRUM OF "OFF-LABEL" DRUG USE

Unfortunately, very few studies have evaluated the pharmacokinetic and pharmacodynamic properties of drugs in children (Conroy and Peden, 2001; Katz and Kelly, 1993). Most pharmacokinetic studies are performed using healthy adult volunteers, adult patients who are only minimally ill, or adult patients in a stable phase of a chronic disease. These data are then extrapolated to infants, children, and adolescents, and the medications are prescribed "off-label." So little pharmacokinetic and pharmacodynamic testing has been performed in children that they are often considered "therapeutic orphans" (Blumer, 1999). In addition, drug formulations designed for adults are often manipulated and altered by practitioners for use in children (e.g., tablets are dissolved to make a liquid formulation, or suppositories are cut in half). The U.S. Congress has enacted the Best Pharmaceuticals for Children Act, the Pediatric Research Equity Act, and the Food and Drug Administration (FDA) Amendments Act to promote standards and requirements for the use and labeling of pediatric drugs (BPCA, 2002; PREA, 2003; FDAAA, 2007).

PHARMACOLOGIC MANAGEMENT OF PAIN

Nonopioid Analgesics (or Weaker Analgesics with Antipyretic Activity)

The weaker or milder analgesics with antipyretic activity, of which acetaminophen (paracetamol), salicylate (aspirin), ibuprofen, naproxen, ketoprofen, and diclofenac are common examples, comprise a heterogenous group of NSAIDs and nonopioid analgesics (Table 15-5) (Agency for Health Care Policy and Research, 1992; Yaster, 1997; Tobias, 2000b; Kokki, 2003). They produce their analgesic, antiinflammatory, antiplatelet, and antipyretic effects primarily by blocking peripheral and central prostaglandin and thromboxane production by inhibiting cyclooxygenase (COX) types 1, 2, and 3 (Fig. 15-6). These metabolites of cyclooxygenase sensitize peripheral nerve endings and vasodilate the blood vessels causing pain, erythema, and inflammation.

These analgesic agents are administered enterally via the oral or, on occasion, the rectal route and are particularly useful for inflammatory, bony, or rheumatic pain. Parenterally administered agents, such as ketorolac and acetaminophen, are available for use in children in whom the oral or rectal routes of administration are not possible (Murat et al., 2005). Unfortunately, regardless of dose, the nonopioid analgesics are limited by a "ceiling effect" above which pain cannot be relieved by these drugs alone. Because of this, these weaker analgesics are often administered in oral combination forms with opioids such as codeine, oxycodone, or hydrocodone.

Only a few trials have compared the efficacy of these drugs in head to head competition, and in general these studies have shown that there are no major differences in their analgesic effects when appropriate doses of each drug are used. The commonly used NSAIDs, such as ketorolac, diclofenac, ibuprofen, and ketoprofen, have reversible antiplatelet adhesion and aggregation effects that are attributable to the inhibition of thromboxane synthesis (Niemi et al., 1997; Munsterhjelm et al., 2006). As a result, bleeding times are usually slightly increased, but in most instances they remain within normal limits in children with normal coagulation systems. Nevertheless this side effect is of such great concern, particularly in surgical procedures in which even a small amount of bleeding can be catastrophic (e.g., tonsillectomy and neurosurgery), that few clinicians prescribe them even though the evidence supporting increased bleeding is equivocal at best (Moiniche et al., 2003; Cardwell et al., 2005). Finally, many orthopedic surgeons are also concerned about the negative influence of all NSAIDs, both selective and nonselective COX inhibitors, on bone growth and healing (Simon et al., 2002; Einhorn, 2003; Dahners and Mullis, 2004). Thus, most pediatric orthopedic surgeons have recommended that these drugs not be used in their patients in the postoperative period.

The discovery of at least three COX isoenzymes (COX-1, COX-2, and COX-3) has enhanced our knowledge of NSAIDs (Cashman, 1996; Vane and Botting, 1998). The COX isoenzymes share structural and enzymatic similarities, but they are specifically regulated at the molecular level and may be distinguished by their functions. Protective prostaglandins, which preserve the integrity of the stomach lining and maintain normal renal function in a compromised kidney, are synthesized by COX-1 (Vane and Botting, 1998; Moiniche et al., 2003; Levesque et al.

TABLE 15-5. Dosage Guidelines for Commonly Used Nonsteroidal Antiinflammatory Drugs

Generic Name	Brand Name	Dose (mg/kg) Frequency	Maximum Adult Daily Dose (mg)	Comments
Acetaminophen (paracetamol)	Many brand names, e.g., Tylenol, Aspirin-Free Pain Relief, Panadol, Tempra	10-15 PO q 4 h 20-40 PR q 6-8 h	4000 60 mg/kg/d preterm 70 mg/kg/d term 90 mg/kg/d older	Lacks antiinflammatory activity No platelet effects Hepatic failure with overdose IV form available in Europe
Acetylsalicylic acid (aspirin)	Many brand names, e.g., Bayer, Bufferin, Anacin, Alka-Seltzer	10-15 PO/PR q 4 h	4000	Inhibits platelet aggregation GI irritability Reye's syndrome
Choline magnesium trisalicylate	Trilisate	7.5-15 PO q 6-12 h	4000	Aspirin compound that does not affect platelets
Ibuprofen	Many brand names, e.g., Motrin, Advil	4-10 PO q 6-8 h	2400	Available as an oral suspension Renal dysfunction Gastrointestinal irritability Inhibits platelet aggregation
Indomethacin	Indocin	0.3-1.0 PO q 6 h	150	Commonly used IV to close PDA (See Ibuprofen)
Naproxen	Naprosyn	5-10 PO q 12 h	1500	(See Ibuprofen)
Ketorolac	Toradol	IV or IM Load 0.5 Maint 0.2-0.5 q 6 h PO 0.25	120	May be given orally Maximum dose 30 mg Causes gastrointestinal upset and ulcer, discontinue after 5 days Expensive (See Ibuprofen)

PO, Orally; *PR*, rectally; *PDA*, patent ductus arteriosus; *IV*, intravenously; *IM*, intramuscularly.

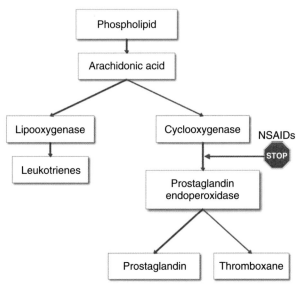

◄ FIGURE 15-6. The peripheral and central prostaglandin and thromboxane production inhibition by cyclooxygenase is depicted. Note that the inhibition of cyclooxygenase leads to increased production of leukotrienes.

005). The COX-2 isoenzyme is inducible by proinflammatory cytokines and growth factors, implying a role for COX-2 in both inflammation and control of cell growth. In addition to the induction of COX-2 in inflammatory lesions, it is expressed constitutively in the brain and spinal cord, where it may be involved in nerve transmission, particularly for pain and fever. Prostaglandins made by COX-2 are also important in ovulation and in the birth process (Vane and Botting, 1998; Moiniche et al., 2003; Levesque et al., 2005). The discovery of COX-2 has made possible the design of drugs that reduce inflammation without removing the protective prostaglandins in the stomach and kidneys made by COX-1. In fact, developing a more specific COX-2 inhibitor was a "holy grail" of drug research, because this class of drug was postulated to have all of the desired antiinflammatory and analgesic properties with none of the gastrointestinal and antiplatelet side effects. Unfortunately, the controversy regarding the potential adverse cardiovascular risks of prolonged use of COX-2 inhibitors has dampened much of the enthusiasm for these drugs and has led to the removal of rofecoxib from the market by its manufacturer (Johnsen et al., 2005; Levesque et al., 2005).

Aspirin

Aspirin, one of the oldest and most effective nonopioid analgesics, has been largely abandoned in pediatric practice because of its possible role in Reye's syndrome, its effects on platelet function, and its gastric irritant properties. Despite these problems, a "sister" compound, choline-magnesium trisalicylate is still prescribed, particularly in the management of postoperative pain and in the child with cancer. Choline-magnesium trisalicylate is a unique aspirin-like compound that does not bind to platelets and therefore has minimal, if any, effects on platelet function

(Yaster, 1997). As a result, it can be prescribed to patients with low platelet counts (cancer patients), dysfunctional platelets (uremia), and in the postoperative period. It is a convenient drug to give to children because it is available in both a liquid and tablet form and is administered either twice a day or every 6 hours. However, the association of salicylates with Reye's syndrome limits its use, even though the risk of developing this syndrome postoperatively is extremely unlikely.

Acetaminophen

The most commonly used nonopioid analgesic in pediatric practice remains acetaminophen, although its analgesic effectiveness in the neonate is unclear (Shah et al., 1998; Anderson, 2008). Unlike aspirin and other NSAIDs, acetaminophen produces analgesia centrally as a COX-3 inhibitor and via activation of descending serotonergic pathways (Graham and Scott, 2005; Anderson, 2008). It is also thought to produce analgesia as a cannabinoid agonist and by antagonizing NMDA and substance P in the spinal cord (Bertolini et al., 2006). Acetaminophen is an antipyretic analgesic with minimal, if any, antiinflammatory and antiplatelet activity and takes about 30 minutes to provide effective analgesia. When administered orally in standard doses, 10 to 15 mg/kg acetaminophen is extremely safe, effective, and has few serious side effects. When administered rectally, higher doses of 25 to 40 mg/kg are required (Rusy et al., 1995; Birmingham et al., 1997). Because of its known association with fulminant hepatic necrosis, the daily maximum acetaminophen dosages, regardless of formulation or route of delivery, in the preterm infant, full-term infant, and older child are 60, 80, and 90 mg/kg respectively (Table 15-5). Thus, when administering acetaminophen rectally it should be given every 8 hours rather than every 4 hours. Finally, an intravenous formulation of acetaminophen is now available in Europe and can be used in patients in whom the enteral route is unavailable. This formulation has been associated with better analgesia than oral acetaminophen in clinical trials in adult patients and is equally effective and less painful than the prodrug formulation of the drug in children (Murat et al., 2005).

Opioids

Overview

Over the past 30 years, multiple opioid receptors and subtypes have been identified and classified. There are 3 primary opioid receptor types, designated mu (μ) (for morphine), kappa (κ), and delta (δ). These receptors are primarily located in the brain and spinal cord, but they also exist peripherally on peripheral nerve cells, immune cells, and other cells (e.g., oocytes) (Sabbe and Yaksh, 1990; Snyder and Pasternak, 2003; Stein and Rosow, 2004). The μ-receptor is further subdivided into several subtypes such as the $\mu1$ (supraspinal analgesia), $\mu2$ (respiratory depression, inhibition of gastrointestinal motility), and $\mu3$ (antiinflammation, leukocytes), which affects the pharmacologic profiles of different opioids (Pasternak, 2001a, 2001b, 2005; Bonnet et al., 2008). Both endogenous and exogenous agonists and antagonists bind to various opioid receptors.

The differentiation of agonists and antagonists is fundamental to pharmacology. A neurotransmitter is defined as having agonist activity, whereas a drug that blocks the action of a neurotransmitter is an antagonist. By definition, receptor recognition of an agonist is "translated" into other cellular alterations (i.e., the agonist initiates a pharmacologic effect), whereas an antagonist occupies the receptor without initiating a transduction step (i.e., it has no intrinsic activity or efficacy). The intrinsic activity of a drug defines the ability of the drug-receptor complex to initiate a pharmacologic effect. Drugs that produce less than a maximal response have a lowered intrinsic activity and are called *partial agonists*. Partial agonists also have antagonistic properties, because by binding the receptor site, they block access of full agonists to the site. Morphine and related opioids are μ-agonists, whereas drugs that block the effects of opioids at the μ-receptor, such as naloxone, are designated antagonists. The opioids most commonly used in anesthetic practice and in the management of pain are μ-agonists. These include morphine, meperidine (pethidine), methadone, and the various fentanyls. Mixed agonist-antagonist drugs act as agonists or partial agonists at one receptor and antagonists at another receptor. Mixed (opioid) agonist-antagonist drugs include pentazocine, butorphanol, buprenorphine, nalorphine, and nalbuphine. Most of these drugs are agonists or partial agonists at the κ- and σ-receptors and antagonists at the μ-receptor. Naloxone and its oral equivalent, naltrexone, are nonspecific opioid antagonists.

Opioid receptors, which are found anchored to the plasma membrane both presynaptically and postsynaptically, decrease the release of excitatory neurotransmitters from terminals carrying nociceptive stimuli. These receptors belong to the steroid superfamily of G protein–coupled receptors. Their protein structure contains seven transmembrane regions with extracellular loops that confer subtype specificity and intracellular loops that mediate subreceptor phenomena (Stein and Rosow, 2004). These receptors are coupled to guanine nucleotide (GTP)-binding regulatory proteins (G proteins) and regulate transmembrane signaling by regulating adenylate cyclase (and therefore cyclic adenosine monophosphate [cAMP]), various ion channels (K^+, Ca^{++}, Na^+) and transport proteins, neuronal nitric oxide synthetase, and phospholipase C and A2 (Fig. 15-7) (Standifer and Pasternak, 1997; Maxwell et al., 2005; Pasternak, 2005). Signal transduction from opioid receptors occurs via bonding to inhibitory G proteins (Gi and Go). Analgesic effects are mediated by decreased neuronal excitability from an inwardly rectifying K^+ current, which hyperpolarizes the neuronal membrane, decreases cAMP production, increases nitric oxide synthesis, and increases the production of 12-lipoxygenase metabolites. Indeed, synergism between opioids and NSAIDs occurs as a result of the greater availability of arachidonic acid for metabolism by the 12-lipooxygenase pathway, after blockade of prostaglandin production by NSAIDs (Vaughan et al., 1997). Some of the unwanted side effects of opioids, such as pruritus, may be the result of opioid binding to stimulatory G proteins (Gs) and may be antagonized by low dose infusions of naloxone (Fig. 15-7) (Crain and Shen, 1998, 1996; Maxwell et al., 2005).

Pharmacokinetics

For opioids to effectively relieve or prevent most pain, the agonist must reach the receptor in the CNS. There are essentially two ways that this occurs, either via the bloodstream (after intravenous, intramuscular, oral, nasal, transdermal, or mucosal administration) or by direct application into the cerebrospinal fluid (intrathecal or epidural). Agonists administered via the bloodstream must cross the blood-brain barrier, a lipid membrane interface between the endothelial cells of the brain

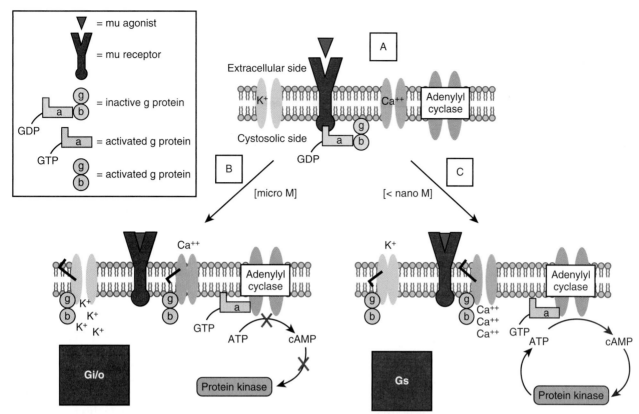

■ **FIGURE 15-7.** Opioid receptors are coupled to GTP binding regulatory proteins (G proteins) and regulate transmembrane signaling by regulating adenylate cyclase (cyclic AMP), various ion channels (K⁺, Ca⁺⁺, Na⁺) and transport proteins, neuronal nitric oxide synthetase, and phospholipase C and A2. **A,** Under basal conditions, G proteins exist in cell membranes as heterotrimers composed of single alpha (a), beta (b), and gamma (g) subunits. The α subunits are bound by GDP, and the G protein heterotrimer is anchored to the plasma membrane by the γ subunit. **B and C,** After the opioid receptor (Y) is activated by a μ-agonist ligand (▼) (e.g., morphine), it physically associates with the α subunit, causing the latter to release GDP and bind GTP. The GTP binding causes the dissociation of the α subunit from the β-γ subunit and from the receptor. Free α and β-γ subunits are functionally active and directly regulate a number of effector proteins, such as ion channels, adenylyl cyclase, and phospholipase C. **B,** Classically, the opioid receptor is thought to be a $G_{i/o}$ coupled receptor. Adenylyl cyclase is inhibited, the potassium channel is open, and the calcium channel is closed. **C,** At picomolar or nanomolar concentrations, opioid receptors are coupled to G_s proteins. Adenylyl cyclase is activated, the calcium channel is open, and the potassium channel is closed. *(From Maxwell LG et al: The effects of a small-dose naloxone infusion on opioid-induced side effects and analgesia in children and adolescents treated with intravenous patient-controlled analgesia: a double-blind, prospective, randomized, controlled study,* Anesth Analg *100:953, 2005.)*

vasculature and the extracellular fluid of the brain, to reach the receptor. Normally, highly lipid-soluble agonists, such as fentanyl, rapidly diffuse across the blood-brain barrier, whereas agonists with limited lipid solubility, such as morphine, have limited brain uptake. This rule, however, does not hold true for patients of all ages. The blood-brain barrier may be immature at birth and is known to be more permeable in neonates to morphine. Indeed, Kupferberg and Way (1963) demonstrated in a classic paper that morphine concentrations were two to four times greater in the brains of younger rats than older rats despite equal blood concentrations. Spinal administration, either intrathecally (subarachnoid) or epidurally, bypasses the blood and directly places an agonist into the cerebrospinal fluid, which bathes the receptor sites in the spinal cord (substantia gelatinosa) and brain. This "back door" to the receptor significantly reduces the amount of agonist needed to relieve pain and to induce opioid side effects such as pruritus, urinary retention, and respiratory depression (Cousins and Mather, 1984; Sabbe and Yaksh, 1990). After spinal administration, opi-

oids are absorbed by the epidural veins and redistributed to the systemic circulation, where they are metabolized and excreted. Hydrophilic agents such as morphine cross the dura more slowly than more lipid-soluble agents such as fentanyl or meperidine. This physical chemical property is responsible for the more prolonged duration of action of spinal morphine and its very slow onset of action after epidural administration (Sabbe and Yaksh, 1990).

Biotransformation

Effects of Age and Disease

Morphine, meperidine, methadone, codeine, and fentanyl are biotransformed in the liver before excretion by the kidneys. Many of these reactions are catalyzed in the liver by glucuronidation or microsomal mixed-function oxidases that require the cytochrome P450 system, nicotinamide adenine dinucleotide phosphate (NADPH), and oxygen. The cytochrome P450 system is immature at birth and does not reach adult levels of activity until the first month or two of life. The immaturity of this hepatic enzyme system may explain the prolonged clearance or elimination of some opioids in the first few days to weeks of life (Anderson and Lynn, 2009). On the other hand, the P450 system can be induced by various drugs (such as phenobarbital) and substrates, and once the infant is born, it matures regardless of gestational age. Thus, it is the age from birth and not the duration of gestation that determines how premature and full-term infants metabolize drugs.

Morphine is primarily glucuronidated into two forms: an inactive form, morphine-3-glucuronide, and an active form, morphine-6-glucuronide. Both glucuronides are excreted by the kidney. In patients with renal failure, morphine-6-glucuronide can accumulate and cause toxic side effects including respiratory depression (Murtagh et al., 2007; Lotsch, 2005). This is important to consider not only when prescribing morphine but when administering other opioids that are metabolized into morphine, such as codeine.

The pharmacokinetics of opioids in patients with liver disease and in critically ill patients requires special attention. Many disease states common in the critically ill may alter the metabolism and elimination of morphine (and other drugs). Severe cirrhosis, septic shock, and renal failure decrease the clearance of morphine and its metabolites, resulting in increased accumulation, prolonged duration of action, and possible toxicity. Oxidation of opioids is reduced in patients with hepatic cirrhosis, resulting in decreased drug clearance (e.g., meperidine, dextropropoxyphene, pentazocine, tramadol, and alfentanil) and increased oral bioavailability caused by a reduced first-pass metabolism (e.g., meperidine, pentazocine, and dihydrocodeine). Although glucuronidation is thought to be less affected by cirrhosis, the clearance of morphine is decreased and oral bioavailability is increased. The consequence of reduced drug metabolism is the risk of accumulation in the body, especially with repeated administration. Lower doses or longer administration intervals should be used to minimize this risk. Meperidine poses a special concern, because it is metabolized into normeperidine, a toxic metabolite that causes seizures and accumulates in liver disease. On the other hand, drugs that are inactive (prodrugs) but are metabolized in the liver into active forms (such as codeine) may be ineffective in patients with severe liver disease. Finally, the disposition of a few opioids, such as fentanyl, sufentanil, and remifentanil, appears to be unaffected in liver disease and are the drugs preferentially used in managing pain in patients with liver disease.

Distribution and Clearance

The pharmacokinetics of morphine have been extensively studied in adults, older children, and in premature and full-term newborns (Lynn et al., 1991, 1993). After an intravenous bolus, 30% of morphine is protein-bound in the adult vs. only 20% in the newborn. This increase in unbound ("free") morphine allows a greater proportion of active drug to penetrate the brain. This may in part explain the observation of Way et al. (1965) of increased brain levels of morphine in the newborn and its more profound respiratory depressant effects. The elimination half-life of morphine in adults and older children is 3 to 4 hours and is consistent with its duration of analgesic action. The half-life of elimination ($t_{\frac{1}{2}}\beta$) is more than twice as long in newborns younger than 1 week of age than in older children and adults

and is even longer in premature infants (Lynn and Slattery, 1987). Clearance is similarly decreased in the newborn compared with the older child and adult. Thus, infants younger than 1 month of age attain higher serum levels that decline more slowly than older children and adults. This may also account for the increased respiratory depression associated with morphine in this age group. Interestingly, the $t_{\frac{1}{2}}\beta$ and clearance of morphine in children older than 2 months of age are similar to adult values; thus, the hesitancy in prescribing and administering morphine in children younger than 1 year of age may not always be warranted. On the other hand, the use of any opioids in children who were born prematurely (fewer than 37 weeks' gestation) and are less than 52 to 60 weeks' postconceptional age or who were born at term and are younger than 2 months of age must be restricted to a monitored setting.

Based on its relatively short half-life (3 to 4 hours), one would expect older children and adults to require morphine supplementation every 2 to 3 hours when being treated for pain, particularly if the morphine is administered intravenously. This has led to the use of continuous infusion regimens of morphine and patient-controlled analgesia (see related section) or, alternatively, administration of longer-acting agonists such as methadone. When administered by continuous infusion, the duration of action of opioids that are rapidly redistributed (such as fentanyl, sufentanil, and alfentanil) and are thought to be short-acting may be longer than would be predicted simply by their pharmacokinetics (see Chapter 7, Pharmacology of Pediatric Anesthesia). An exception to this is remifentanil, a μ-opioid receptor agonist with unique pharmacokinetic properties (Burkle et al., 1996).

The pharmacokinetics of remifentanil are characterized by a small volume of distribution, rapid clearances, and low interpatient variability, compared with other intravenous anesthetic and analgesic agents. The drug has a rapid onset of action (the half-time for equilibration between blood and the effect compartment is 1.3 minutes) and a short context-sensitive half-life (3 to 5 minutes) (Bailey, 2002; Welzing and Roth, 2006). This latter property is attributable to hydrolytic metabolism of the compound by nonspecific tissue and plasma esterases. Virtually all (99.8%) of an administered remifentanil dose is eliminated during the half-life of redistribution $t_{\frac{1}{2}}\alpha$ (0.9 minutes) and the $t_{\frac{1}{2}}\beta$ (6.3 minutes). The pharmacokinetics of remifentanil suggest that within 10 minutes of starting an infusion, remifentanil blood levels will have nearly reached steady state. Thus, changing the infusion rate of remifentanil produces rapid changes in drug effect. The rapid metabolism of remifentanil and its small volume of distribution mean that remifentanil does not accumulate. Discontinuing the drug rapidly terminates its effect and has significant intraoperative implications. When remifentanil is administered intraoperatively as part of a balanced or primary opioid general anesthetic, some patients have reportedly awakened in severe pain. This can be because of inadequate loading of a longer-acting opioid, as well as "opioid-induced hyperalgesia," a paradoxical process by which opioid administration, even for short periods of time, increases the sensitivity to pain and worsens pain when the opioid is discontinued (Crawford et al., 1992; Chu et al., 2008). Finally, remifentanil may be a reasonable alternative to inhaled general anesthetic in newborn infants undergoing surgery, because it only briefly interferes with the control of breathing and because this effect is terminated shortly after discontinuing the drug (Davis et al., 2001; Galinkin et al., 2001).

Commonly Used Oral Opioids

Codeine, oxycodone (the opioid in Tylox and Percocet), and hydrocodone (the opioid in Vicodin and Lortab) are opioids that are commonly used to treat pain in children and adults, and are quite useful when making the transition from parenteral to enteral analgesia (Table 15-6). Methadone and sustained release formulations of morphine, oxycodone, oxymorphone, and hydromorphone are commonly used to treat chronic medical pain (e.g., cancer) and in postoperative surgical or trauma patients with long recuperative times (e.g., pectus excavatum or posterior spine surgery). Codeine, oxycodone, and hydrocodone are most commonly administered in the oral form, often in combination with acetaminophen. Although the combination drugs are convenient, and acetaminophen potentiates the analgesia produced by codeine—allowing the practitioner

TABLE 15-6. Commonly Used μ-Agonist Drugs

Agonist	Equipotent IV Dose (mg/kg)	Equipotent PO Dose (mg/kg)	Duration (hr)	Bioavailability (%)	Comments
Morphine	0.1	0.3	3-4	20-40	"Gold standard," very inexpensive Seizures in newborns Histamine release, vasodilation, avoid in circulatory compromise Poor oral bioavailability; give 3-5 times the IV dose Liquid morphine available in concentrations 2-20 mg/mL Renally cleared active metabolite, morphine 6-glucuronide
Meperidine (Demerol)	1.0	N/A	3-4	40-60	Catastrophic interactions with MAO inhibitors Tachycardia; negative inotrope Metabolite normeperidine produces seizures 0.25 mg/kg effectively treats shivering Not recommended for routine use
Hydromorphone (Dilaudid)	0.015	0.05	3-4	50-70	Commonly used when morphine produces too many undesirable systemic side effects No active metabolites
Fentanyl (Sublimaze)	0.001	N/A	0.5-1		Very effective for short painful procedures Vagotonic and can cause bradycardia Minimal hemodynamic alterations Chest wall rigidity/glottic closure (>5 mcg/kg rapid IV bolus); Rx naloxone or succinylcholine or pancuronium Oral transmucosal dose 10-15 mcg/kg Transdermal patch available for chronic pain
Methadone	0.1	0.1-0.2	4-24	70-100	Liquid preparation available Long duration of action makes it ideal for cancer pain, weaning dependent patients, etc. Useful for neuropathic pain (NMDA blockade) Because of incomplete cross tolerance, when used in opioid tolerant patients, conversion to morphine may be as low as 0.01 mg/kg

Codeine
Solution (codeine + acetaminophen)
  12 mg + 120 mg/5 mL
Tablets (codeine-acetaminophen)
  #2 15 mg + 300 mg
  #3 30 mg + 300 mg
	N/A	1.2	3-4	40-70	PO only
					Prodrug must be converted to morphine
					Often combined with acetaminophen

Hydrocodone
Elixir (Lortab) (hydrocodone + acetaminophen)
  7.5 mg + 500 mg/15 mL
Tablets (Vicodin or Lortab)
  Hydrocodone 2.5, 5, 7.5, or 10 mg
  + 325 or 500 mg acetaminophen
Oxycodone
Solution
  1 or 20 mg/mL
Tablets (oxycodone + acetaminophen)
  Percocet 5 mg + 325 mg
  Tylox 5 mg + 500 mg
	N/A	0.1	3-4	60-80	PO only
					Usually prescribed with acetaminophen
					Less nausea than codeine

Continued

TABLE 15-6. Commonly Used μ-Agonist Drugs—cont'd

Agonist	Equipotent IV Dose (mg/kg)	Equipotent PO Dose (mg/kg)	Duration (hr)	Bioavailability (%)	Comments
Oxycodone Tylox (5 mg/500 mg acetaminophen) (Percocet 5mg/325 mg acetaminophen) Roxicet solution (5 mL = 5 mg/325 mg acetaminophen)	N/A	0.1	3-4	60-80	PO only Sustained release tablet available that cannot be crushed or chewed. High abuse potential Usually prescribed with acetaminophen Less nausea than codeine

PO, Orally; *IV,* intravenously.

to use less opioid to achieve satisfactory analgesia—the combination of drugs significantly increases the risk of acetaminophen toxicity. Acetaminophen toxicity may result from a single toxic dose, from repeated ingestion of large doses of acetaminophen (e.g., in adults 7.5 to 10 g/day for 1 to 2 days, in children 60 to 420 mg/kg per day for 1 to 42 days), or from chronic ingestion. However, hepatotoxicity can also occur inadvertently when patients with poorly controlled pain increase the number of combination tablets they need to control their pain or when they are receiving more than one source of acetaminophen (Heubi et al., 1998). The latter occurs because so many prescription and over-the-counter drug products contain acetaminophen (e.g., cold remedies). Because of this risk, the preferred method is to prescribe opioids and acetaminophen (or ibuprofen) separately.

In equipotent doses, oral analgesics have similar effects and side effects including analgesia, sedation, cough suppression, pruritus, nausea, vomiting, constipation and respiratory depression (Table 15-6). Yet the responses of patients to individual opioids can vary markedly, even among these μ-opioid agonists (Pasternak, 2001a, 2005). Understanding this variability greatly enhances the ability to treat patients appropriately. Codeine is a case in point; although readily available, it is very nauseating, and many patients claim they are allergic to it because it so commonly induces vomiting. On the other hand, some differences may be more based on folklore rather than reality. Many physicians falsely believe that meperidine has less of an effect on the sphincter of Oddi than other opioids and therefore prescribe it for patients with gallbladder disease. In fact, meperidine offers no advantage over other opioids and has a serious disadvantage, namely catastrophic interactions with monoamine oxidase (MAO) inhibitors.

Codeine, hydrocodone, and oxycodone have an oral bioavailability of approximately 60%. They achieve their analgesic effects as early as 20 minutes after ingestion and have a $t_{1/2}\beta$ of 2.5 to 4 hours. Unlike oxycodone and hydrocodone, codeine is a prodrug. It has no intrinsic analgesic properties and must be metabolized into morphine by the liver's cytochrome P450 (CYP) 2D6 isoenzyme to become active. In patients with normal CYP 2D6, approximately 10% of codeine is metabolized into morphine. Unfortunately, approximately 7% of the American population has a complete or partial enzymatic deficiency of 2D6 making it impossible for them to metabolize codeine into morphine. Those patients with poor metabolizing ability get little if any analgesia from codeine. More ominously, approximately 3% to 5% of the U.S. population are rapid metabolizers, and in these patients, "normal" codeine doses may be toxic

because too much is converted into morphine. There is no way to predict who is a poor or rapid metabolizer.

Morphine is also effective when given orally, but only about 20% to 30% of an oral dose reaches the systemic circulation. Therefore, when converting a patient's intravenous morphine dose to oral maintenance therapy, one must multiply the intravenous dose by a factor of 3 to 4 to provide comparable analgesic efficacy. Hydrocodone is prescribed in a dose of 0.05 to 0.1 mg/kg. The elixir is available as 2.5 mg/5 mL combined with acetaminophen 167 mg/5 mL. As a tablet, it is available in hydrocodone doses between 2.5 to 10 mg, combined with 500 to 650 mg acetaminophen. Oxycodone is prescribed in a dose of 0.05 to 0.1 mg/kg. Unfortunately, oxycodone is not available in many countries outside of the United States, and even in the United States it is not available in most pharmacies. When it is available, it is usually in concentrations of 1 mg/mL or 20 mg/mL, which could lead to potentially catastrophic dispensing errors. In tablet form, oxycodone is commonly available as Tylox (500 mg acetaminophen and 5.0 mg oxycodone) and as Percocet (325 mg acetaminophen and 5 mg oxycodone). As mentioned previously, in all "combination preparations," there is a real possibility of inadvertently administering a hepatotoxic dose of acetaminophen in patients with uncontrolled pain.

Oxycodone is also available without acetaminophen in a sustained-release tablet (Oxycontin) for use in chronic pain. These pills must be swallowed whole and cannot be administered through a gastric tube or to children who cannot swallow pills, because when ground, crushed, or chewed, tremendous amounts of oxycodone become rapidly available and may result in catastrophic respiratory and cardiovascular collapse. Unfortunately, this property has also led to its diversion and abuse. Sustained-release opioids should only be prescribed to opioid-tolerant patients with chronic pain; they should not be used in routine postoperative pain management. In addition, in patients with rapid gastrointestinal transit, sustained-release preparations may not be absorbed at all; liquid methadone may be an alternative in these patients.

Oral morphine is available as a liquid in various concentrations (as much as 20 mg/mL), a tablet (morphine sulfate immediate release [MSIR]) that is available in 15- and 30-mg tablets, and as a sustained-release preparation (MSContin and Oramorph tablets or Kadian "sprinkle capsules"). Because it is so concentrated, morphine elixir is particularly easy to administer to children and severely debilitated patients. Indeed, in patients with terminal illness who cannot swallow, liquid morphine provides analgesia when it is simply dropped into the patient's mouth (buccal absorption).

Patient-Controlled Analgesia

Historically, pain medications have been administered on a demand or PRN basis (Krane, 2008). When drugs are given PRN, the patient or caregiver must recognize that pain exists, summon a nurse and await the preparation and administration of the analgesic. Even in the best of circumstances, there is a delay between the patient's request and the provider's response (Krane, 2008). Around-the-clock administration of analgesics at intervals based on population pharmacokinetics (e.g., every 4 hours) is not always effective because there are enormous individual variations in pain perception and opioid metabolism. Knowledge of opioid pharmacokinetics suggests that intravenous boluses of intermediate-acting opioids such as morphine may be needed as often as every 1 to 2 hours in order to avoid marked fluctuations in plasma drug levels, but generally they are ordered no more frequently than every 4 hours. One way to achieve this goal is via continuous intravenous opioid infusions. This approach provides steady analgesic levels and has been used with great safety and efficacy in children; however, because neither the perception nor the intensity of pain is constant, continuous opioid infusions do not adequately treat pain in all patients (Lynn et al., 2000). For example, a postoperative patient may be very comfortable resting in bed and may require little adjustment in opioid dosing. This same patient may experience excruciating pain when coughing, voiding, or getting out of bed. Receiving the same dose of opioid in both instances may result in either oversedation or under treatment. Thus, rational pain management requires some form of titration to effect whenever any opioid is administered. In order to give patients some measure of control over their pain therapy, analgesia on demand or patient-controlled analgesia (PCA) devices were developed (Berde et al., 1991; Yaster et al., 1997). These are microprocessor driven pumps that the patient controls to self-administer intermittent, predetermined, small doses of opioid whenever a need for more pain relief is felt. The opioid, usually morphine, hydromorphone, or fentanyl is administered either intravenously or subcutaneously (Table 15-7). The dosage of opioid, number of demand doses ("boluses") per hour, and the time interval between boluses (the "lock-out period") are programmed into the equipment by the pain-service physician to allow maximum patient flexibility and sense of control with minimal risk of overdosage. Generally, because older patients know that if they have severe pain they can obtain relief immediately, many prefer dosing regimens that result in mild to moderate pain in exchange for fewer side effects such as nausea or pruritus. Morphine is the most commonly prescribed opioid. Typically it is prescribed at a bolus dose of 20 mcg/kg, at a rate of up to 5 boluses/hour, and with a lock-out interval between each bolus of 6 to 8 minutes (Table 15-7). Variations include larger boluses (30 to 50 mcg/kg) and shorter time intervals (5 minutes).

The PCA pump computer stores within its memory how many boluses the patient has received, as well as how many attempts the patient has made at receiving boluses. This allows the provider to evaluate how well the patient understands the use of the pump and provides information to program the pump more efficiently. In addition, most PCA units allow low, continuous "background" infusions (e.g., morphine, 20 to 30 mcg/kg per hour, hydromorphone 3 to 4 mcg/kg per hour or fentanyl 0.5 mcg/kg per hour) in addition to self-administered boluses. Continuous background infusions can facilitate more restful sleep by preventing the patient from awakening in pain (Doyle et al., 1993). Although in adults a background infusion increases the potential for overdosage without significantly improving analgesia, this has not been the experience in pediatrics and in adult cancer patients (Fleming and Coombs, 1992). In these patients, a continuous infusion improves analgesia and makes the life easier for the health care provider, because with better analgesia there are fewer phone calls to rewrite orders or to change therapy (Monitto et al., 1998; Yildiz et al., 2003; Nelson et al., 2009). Contraindications to the use of PCA include inability to push the bolus button (because of weakness or arm restraints), inability to understand how to use the machine, and a patient's desire not to assume responsibility for personal care. Difficulties with PCA include increased costs; patient age limitations; and the need for physician, nursing, pharmacy protocols, education; and storage arrangements that must be instituted before its implementation. These policies, procedures, and protocols are essential for the safe use of opioids regardless of the method of administration. Essential features include age-appropriate parameters for monitoring respiratory status (e.g., respiratory rate and oxygen saturation), patient alertness, and pain assessment, as well as weight-based dosing. Additionally, because accurate prescribing requires a correct weight, proper conversion of pounds to kilograms, and the choice of an appropriate medication preparation

TABLE 15-7. IV Patient-Controlled Analgesia Dosing Guidelines

Drug (and Concentrations)	Continuous Basal Infusion* mcg/kg/hr (range, mcg/kg/hr)	Demand Dose mcg/kg (range, mcg/kg)	Lockout Interval Minutes (range)	Number of Demand Doses/Hour (range)	4-Hour Limit (mcg/kg)
Morphine (standard, 1 mg/mL; younger patients, 0.2 mg/mL; tolerant or high-need patients, 10 mg/mL)	20 (10-30)	20 (10-30)	8 (6-15)	5 (1-10)	250-400
Fentanyl (>30 kg, 0.02 mg/mL; 10-29 kg, 0.01 mg/mL; <10 kg, 0.005 mg/mL; tolerant or high-need patients, 0.05 mg/mL)	0.5 (0.2-1)	0.5 (0.2-1)	15 (6-15)	4 (1-10)	7-10
Hydromorphone (standard, 0.2 mg/mL; tolerant or high-need patients, 1 or 5 mg/mL)	4 (2-6)	4 (2-6)	8 (6-15)	5 (1-10)	50-80

*A basal infusion is not always used. It may increase the risk of respiratory depression and excessive sedation.

THE JOHNS HOPKINS HOSPITAL

PEDIATRIC PAIN SERVICE
INTRAVENOUS PCA ORDERS
HYDROMORPHONE

PAGE 1 OF 3

Last: Smith
First: John
number: 123-45-67
birthdate: 8/22/1997

floor: CMSC 9

addressograph plate

PAGE: _____

DATE	TIME	SIGN EACH ENTRY INCLUDE ID NUMBER	NOTED BY	COMPLETED BY		
				DATE	TIME	INITIALS
28-Jan	9:42	1 WEIGHT: **45** Kg.				
		2 ALLERGIES: NKDA				
		3 **DISCONTINUE ALL PREVIOUS OPIOID ORDERS.**				
		4 **INITIATE INTRAVENOUS PCA PROTOCOL**				
		5 Hydromorphone **0.2** mg/mL **20** mg in **100** mL 0.9% SALINE				
		6 UNITS: SET PUMP IN MILLIGRAMS (mg)				
		7 SET PUMP CONCENTRATION AT : **0.2** mg/ml				
		8 CONTINUOUS RATE: **0.18** mg/hr **4** mcg/Kg/hr				
		(FOR HYDROMORPHONE SUGGEST 3-5 mcg/kg/hr)				
		RANGE: **0** to **0.27** mg/hr				
		0 to 6 mcg/Kg/hr				
		9 DEMAND DOSE: **0.18** mg **4** mcg/Kg				
		(FOR HYDROMORPHONE SUGGEST START AT 4 mcg/Kg/Dose)				
		RANGE: **0** to **0.27** mg				
		0 to 6 mcg/Kg/Dose				
		10 DEMAND LOCKOUT: **8** MINS				
		(SUGGEST 7-15)				
		11 MAXIMUM DOSE(S): **5** PER HR:				
		(SUGGEST 0-5)				
		12 CLINICIAN BOLUS: **0.90** mg **0.02** mg/kg				
28-Jan	9:42	(PAIN SERVICE or PEDIATRIC RECOVERY ROOM NURSES ONLY!!)				

for pharmacy use only
Drug from floor stock

JHH 04-758-0094
JHH 15-193060 (04-775-08) 10/96

Dr. Myron Yaster   M.D.   A515(

ATTENDING PAIN SERVICE BEEPER: 283-2060

THE JOHNS HOPKINS HOSPITAL

PEDIATRIC PAIN SERVICE
INTRAVENOUS PCA ORDERS

Last: Smith
First: John
number: 123-45-67
birthdate: 8/22/1997

floor: CMSC 9

addressograph plate

PAGE: 2 of 3

DATE	TIME	SIGN EACH ENTRY INCLUDE ID NUMBER	NOTED BY	COMPLETED BY		
				DATE	TIME	INITIALS
28-Jan	10:15	1 WEIGHT **45** Kg.				
		2 FOR OXYGEN SATURATION < **94** %				
		BEGIN OXYGEN BY NASAL CANNULA AND TITRATE				
		TO OXYGEN SATURATION ≥ 95%				
		3 IF RESPIRATORY RATE < **12** AND Patient is UNAROUSABLE: Start the ABCs				
		Then, NALOXONE **0.04** mg IV/IM **1** mcg/Kg				
		TURN OFF the IVPCA pump				
		NOTIFY PAIN SERVICE, COVERING PHYSICIAN, and PICU				
		TRANSFER TO PICU, ONCE STABLE				
		4 IF NALOXONE IS NOT EFFECTIVE WITHIN 1 MINUTE: GIVE				
		NALOXONE **0.08** mg IV/IM **2** mcg/Kg				
		IF naloxone is ineffective; repeat dose in ONE MINUTE				
		FOR NAUSEA/ VOMITING/ PRURITUS:				
		5 DIPHENYDRAMINE **45** mg IV/PO q 4 hr PRN				
		(SUGGEST 0.5-1.0 mg) 1.00 mg/Kg				
		6 (butorphanol) **---** mg IV q 4hr PRN				
		(SUGGEST 0.03-0.05 mg/Kg) 0 mg/Kg				
		FOR NAUSEA/ VOMITING:				
		7 ONDANSETRON **4** mg IV Q4 PRN nausea/vomiting				
		0.1 mg/Kg, maximum dose 4 mg				
		FOR MUSCLE OR BLADDER SPASM				
		8 (diazepam) **---** mg IV/PO Q4 hours prn				
		(SUGGEST 0.1 mg/Kg) 0 mg/kg				
		Only with confirmation from Pediatric Pain Service:				
		9 HYDROMORPHONE **0.9** mg IV **0.02** mg/kg Q1hours PRN pain				
		Additional medications:				
		10 SENOKOT **1-2** tabs po once daily when tolerating PO				
		adult dose				
		11 ACETAMINOPHEN **650** mg q4HRS ATC PO when toleratec				
		(SUGGEST 120,240,325,650 MG, 10 TO 15 mg/Kg/dose) 14.4 mg/Kg				
		12 (ibuprofen) **---** mg PO q6HRS ATC				
		(SUGGEST 6-10 mg/Dose) mg/Kg				
		13 (ketorolac) **---** mg IV q6HRS ATC for 72 hrs				
28-Jan	10:15	(SUGGEST 0.5 mg/Kg; MAX 30 mg) mg/Kg				

ATTENDING PAIN SERVICE BEEPER: 283-2060

JHH 04-758-009

Dr. Myron Yaster   A5158   M.D.

JHH 15-193060 (04-775-22) 10/96

FIGURE 15-8. An electronic, computerized PCA provider order set is depicted. It provides clear, legible, weight-based (kg), calculated dosing using best prescription practice (e.g., no trailing zero after a decimal point). Additionally, it provides instructions to the pharmacist on the volume of drug to be dispensed and how the drug is to be prepared. Finally, it also provides the bedside nurse with monitoring guidelines and antidotes for opioid-induced complications.

and concentration, the computerization of analgesic medication prescribing is an important patient safety strategy (Wrona et al., 2007; Lee et al., 2008). Figure 15-8 is an example of an electronic, computerized PCA provider order set used in the Children's Center of the Johns Hopkins Hospital that incorporates many of these features.

Parent- and Nurse-Controlled Analgesia (Surrogate PCA or PCA by Proxy)

Independent use of PCA requires a patient with sufficient understanding, manual dexterity, and strength to initiate a demand dose. Thus, it was initially limited to adolescents and teenagers, but over time the lower age limit of patients has fallen. In general, many have found that any child able to play a video game can successfully operate a PCA pump independently. However, in very young children or children with developmental or physical handicaps, a similar but alternate mode of therapy is parent- or nurse-controlled analgesia (PNCA), sometimes referred to as *PCA by proxy* or *surrogate PCA* (Monitto et al., 2000). When using this technique, the child receives a basal opioid infusion when PCA bolus doses are initiated by a designated surrogate, generally a parent or nurse, when they perceive that the child appears to be in pain (Monitto et al., 2000; Nelson et al., 2009).

Allowing parents or nurses to initiate a PCA bolus is controversial. In 2004, the Joint Commission on Accreditation of Healthcare Organizations (JCAHO) issued a sentinel event alert warning that serious adverse events can result when surrogates become involved in administering analgesia by proxy (Joint Commission on Accreditation of Healthcare Organizations 2004). Of note, the JCAHO based this warning on a series of adverse events in adults who for the most part developed complications as a result of the preemptive use of the PCA bolus by spouses, children, or nurses when the patient was asleep. Although this alert was not meant to address cases in which caregivers were authorized to administer PCA boluses, it nevertheless raised serious concerns in the pediatric pain management community and changed the practice at some hospitals. Published studies have reported that up to 1% to 3% of patients receiving intravenous PCA by proxy may receive naloxone to treat cardiopulmonary complications (Monitto et al., 2000; Anghelescu et al., 2005; Voepel-Lewis et al., 2008). Interestingly, in a study comparing pediatric intravenous PCA and intravenous PCA by proxy, complication rates were similar between the two modes of therapy, but the use of naloxone was higher in the younger patients. However, it was unclear whether providers had a lower threshold for treating these children with naloxone given their younger age and an associated increased incidence of comorbidities (Voepel-Lewis et al., 2008). Because respirato depression does occur, safe institution of PCA by proxy as well as PCA requires close patient monitoring, established nursing protocols, and an understanding by surrogates of the appropriate use of the bolus dose.

Transdermal and Transmucosal Fentanyl

Because fentanyl is extremely lipophilic, it can be readily absorbed across any biological membrane, including the skin. Thus, fentanyl can be administered painlessly by nonintravenous routes, including transmucosal (nose and mouth) and transdermal routes. The transmucosal route of fentanyl administration is extremely effective for acute pain relief. When given intranasally (2 mcg/kg), it produces rapid analgesia that is equivalent to intravenously administered fentanyl (Galinkin et al., 2000). For transoral absorption, fentanyl is also available in a candy matrix (Actiq) attached to a plastic applicator device that looks like a lollipop. As the patient sucks on the lollipop, fentanyl is absorbed across the buccal mucosa and is rapidly absorbed (10 to 20 minutes) into the systemic circulation (Goldstein-Dresner et al., 1991; Streisand et al., 1989, 1991; Ashburn et al., 1993; Schechter et al., 1995). If excessive sedation occurs, the fentanyl is removed from the patient's mouth by the applicator. Transmucosal absorption is more efficient than ordinary oral-gastric intestinal administration because it bypasses the efficient first-pass hepatic metabolism of fentanyl that occurs after enteral absorption into the portal circulation. The candy matrix of fentanyl has been approved by the FDA for use in children for premedication before surgery and for procedure-related pain (e.g., lumbar puncture or bone marrow aspiration) (Dsida et al., 1998). It is also useful in the treatment of cancer pain and as a supplement to transdermal fentanyl (Portenoy et al., 1999). When administered transmucosally, a fentanyl dose of 10 to 15 mcg/kg is effective within 20 minutes and lasts approximately 2 hours. Because approximately 25% to 33% of the given dose is absorbed, blood levels equivalent to 3 to 5 mcg/kg intravenous fentanyl are achieved with this dose. The major side effect of treatment is nausea and vomiting, which occurs in approximately 20% to 33% of patients who receive it (Epstein et al., 1996). Finally, a new, rapidly dissolving, effervescent fentanyl buccal tablet, Fentora, has become available for breakthrough pain in patients who are already receiving opioids for persistent pain and who are tolerant to opioid therapy (Messina et al., 2008; Weinstein et al., 2009). These tablets come in various doses (100, 200, 400, 600, and 800 mcg). In adults, fentanyl buccal tablets have an absolute bioavailability of 65%; approximately 50% of the total administered dose is absorbed transmucosally, and the remaining half is swallowed and undergoes slow absorption from the gastrointestinal tract. There is little published pediatric experience with this drug.

The transdermal route is commonly used to administer many drugs, including scopolamine, clonidine, and nitroglycerin. Many factors, including body site, skin temperature, skin damage, ethnicity, and age affect the absorption of transdermally administered drugs. The transdermal fentanyl patch has revolutionized adult and pediatric cancer pain management (Zernikow et al., 2007; Finkel et al., 2005). Placed in a selective semipermeable membrane patch, which is attached to the skin by a contact adhesive, a reservoir of fentanyl provides slow, steady-state absorption of drug across the skin. As fentanyl is painlessly absorbed across the skin, a substantial amount is stored in the upper skin layers, which then act as a secondary reservoir. The presence of this "skin depot" has several implications:

1. It dampens the fluctuations of fentanyl effects.
2. It needs to be reasonably filled before significant vascular absorption occurs.
3. It contributes to a prolonged residual fentanyl plasma concentration after patch removal.

Indeed, the amount of fentanyl remaining within the system and skin depot after removal of the patch is substantial. At the end of a 24-hour period, a fentanyl patch releasing drug at the rate of 100 mcg/hr, 1.07 ± 0.43 mg fentanyl (approximately 30% of the total delivered dose from the patch) remains in the skin depot. Thus, even after removal of the patch, fentanyl continues to be absorbed from the subcutaneous fat reservoir for almost 24 hours (Grond et al., 2000).

Because of its long onset time, inability to rapidly adjust drug delivery, and long $t\frac{1}{2}\beta$, transdermal fentanyl is contraindicated for acute pain management. In fact, the use of this drug delivery system to treat acute pain has resulted in the death of an otherwise healthy patient. Transdermal fentanyl is appropriate only for patients who have developed opioid tolerance and for those with chronic pain (e.g., cancer) (Zernikow et al., 2007; Finkel et al., 2005). Even when transdermal fentanyl is appropriate, the vehicle imposes its own constraints; the patch with the lowest dose delivers 12.5 mcg of fentanyl per hour; others deliver 25, 50, 75, and 100 mcg of fentanyl per hour. The patches cannot be physically cut in smaller pieces to deliver less fentanyl.

Methadone

Primarily thought of as a drug to treat or wean patients who are addicted to or dependent on opioid, methadone is increasingly being used in the management of acute and chronic intractable pain. Unique among the opioids, methadone exists as a racemic mixture of two active isomers; one isomer binds as an agonist to the μ-receptor and the other as an antagonist at the NMDA receptor. It is this latter property that makes methadone unique among opioids. The NMDA system is involved in wind-up and the maintenance of chronic pain as well as opioid-induced hyperalgesia and the development of tolerance (Ebert et al., 1998; Gagnon and Bruera, 1999; Gorman et al., 1997). Thus, blockade of NMDA receptors can act to acutely enhance opioid-induced antinociception, impair the development of tolerance, and prevent the development of chronic pain (Raffa, 1996).

In addition, methadone is noted for its slow $t_{\frac{1}{2}}\beta$, very long duration of effective analgesia, high oral bioavailability, and inactive metabolites. The $t_{\frac{1}{2}}\beta$ of methadone averages 19 hours, and clearance averages 5.4 mL/kg per minute in children 1 to 18 years of age (Berde et al., 1991). Methadone has the longest $t_{\frac{1}{2}}\beta$ of any of the commonly available opiates and can provide up to 12 to 36 hours of analgesia after a single intravenous or oral dose (Gourlay et al., 1986, 1982, 1984; Berde 1989; Shannon and Berde, 1989). Pharmacokinetically, children are indistinguishable from young adults. Because a single dose of methadone can achieve and sustain a high drug-plasma level, it is a convenient way to provide prolonged analgesia without requiring an intramuscular injection or a continuous infusion. Berde et al. (1989) recommend methadone as a "poor man's PCA" and suggest loading patients with an initial dose of intravenous methadone (0.1 to 0.2 mg/kg) and then titrating in 0.05-mg/kg increments every 10 to 15 minutes until analgesia is achieved. Supplemental methadone can be administered in 0.05- to 0.1-mg/kg increments administered by slow intravenous infusion every 4 to 12 hours as needed. Shannon and Berde (1989) have also reported the use of small incremental doses administered by sliding scale. "Small increments of methadone are administered intravenously over 20 minutes every 4 hours via a 'sliding' scale on a 'reverse prn' (the nurse asks the patient) basis: 0.07 to 0.08 mg/kg for severe pain; 0.05 to 0.06 mg/kg for moderate pain; 0.03 mg/kg for little or no pain, if the patient is alert; and no drug if the patient has little pain and is somnolent" (Berde 1989; Shannon and Berde, 1989).

In addition, both methadone and sustained relief morphine can be used to wean patients who have become physically dependent on opioids after prolonged analgesic therapy (Yaster et al., 1996; Suresh and Anand, 1998; Tobias, 2000a). Finally, because methadone is extremely well absorbed from the gastrointestinal tract and has a bioavailability of 80% to 90%, it is extremely easy to convert intravenous dosing regimens to oral ones. Recently, however, the conversion dose of morphine to methadone has been challenged. Traditionally, it has been thought that the ratio of morphine to methadone was approximately 1:1; it now appears that when tolerance develops and morphine doses are "high," it is closer to 1:0.25 or even 1:0.1 (Lawlor et al., 1998; Ripamonti et al., 1998a, 1998b; Gagnon and Bruera, 1999). Tolerance to morphine and other opioids such as fentanyl is a significant problem in patients being treated for pain chronically or acutely in the intensive care unit setting. When this occurs, substituting methadone for morphine or fentanyl at the lower doses discussed in the previous section can rapidly reestablish analgesia even though all of these opioids work at the same μ-opioid receptor. This occurs because of "incomplete cross tolerance," which may be because methadone's antagonist actions at the NMDA receptor or because of multiple μ-receptor subtypes (Gorman et al., 1997; Ebert et al., 1998; Trujillo and Akil, 1991; Pasternak, 2001a).

Among opioid analgesics, methadone is unique as a potent blocker of the delayed rectifier potassium ion channel. This results in QT prolongation, can produce torsade de pointes ventricular tachycardia in susceptible individuals, and may explain the sudden death associated with its use (Andrews et al., 2009). The effects of methadone on the QT interval may be enhanced by hypokalemia, drugs that increase the QT interval such as erythromycin and ondansetron, or by CYP 3A4 inhibitors such as fluoxetine, fluconazole, valproate, and clarithromycin (Ehret et al., 2006). An updated list of medications causing torsade de pointes ventricular tachycardia can be found at www.azcert.org. Indeed, this is such a serious consequence of therapy that some have recommended that all patients treated with methadone have routine screening ECGs before or during their treatment.

Tramadol

Tramadol, a synthetic 4-phenylpiperidine analogue of codeine, is a centrally acting synthetic analgesic that has been used for 30 years in Europe and was approved by the FDA for adult use in the United States in 1995 (Raffa 1996; Minto and Power, 1997). It is a racemic mixture of two enantiomers: + tramadol and ⁻tramadol (Berde, 1989; Glare and Lickiss, 1992). The

+enantiomer has a moderate affinity for the μ-opioid receptor that is greater than that of the ⁻enantiomer (Raffa, 1993). In addition, the +enantiomer inhibits 5-HT uptake and the ⁻enantiomer blocks the reuptake of NE, complementary properties that result in a synergistic antinociceptive interaction between the two enantiomers. Tramadol may also produce analgesia as an α_2-agonist (Desmeules et al., 1996). A metabolite (O-desmethyltramadol) binds to opioid receptors with a greater affinity than the parent compound and could contribute to tramadol's analgesic effects as well. However, in most animal tests and human clinical trials, the analgesic effect of tramadol is only partially blocked by the opioid antagonist naloxone, suggesting an important nonopioid mechanism. Thus, tramadol provides analgesia synergistically by opioid (direct binding to the μ-opioid receptor by the parent compound and its metabolite) and nonopioid mechanisms (an increase in central neuronal synaptic levels of 5-HT and NE). Finally, animal and human studies have suggested that tramadol may have a selective spinal and local anesthetic action on peripheral nerves. Tramadol has been shown to provide effective, long-lasting analgesia after extradural administration in both adults and children and prolongs the duration of action of local anesthetics when used for brachial plexus and epidural blockade (Kapral et al., 1999; Prosser et al., 1997).

Tramadol's intravenous analgesic effect has been reported to be 10 to 15 times less than that of morphine and is roughly equianalgesic with NSAIDs (Raffa, 1996; Naguib et al., 1998). Unlike NSAIDs and opioid mixed agonist/antagonists, the therapeutic use of tramadol has not been associated with the clinically important side effects such as respiratory depression, constipation, or sedation. In addition, analgesic tolerance has not been a serious problem during repeated administration, and neither psychological dependence nor euphoric effects are observed in long-term clinical trials. Thus, tramadol may offer significant advantages in the management of pain in children by virtue of its dual mechanism of action, its lack of a ceiling effect, and its minimal respiratory depression.

Tramadol may be administered orally, rectally, intravenously, or epidurally (Gunes et al., 2004; Bozkurt, 2005). Oral and intravenous tramadol is administered in doses of 1 to 2 mg/kg; the higher dose provides a longer duration of action without increasing side effects (Finkel et al., 2002; Rose, 2003; Bozkurt, 2005).

COMPLICATIONS OF OPIOID THERAPY

Regardless of the method of administration, all opioids commonly produce unwanted side effects such as pruritus, nausea and vomiting, constipation, urinary retention, cognitive impairment, tolerance, and dependence (Yaster et al., 2003). Many patients suffer needlessly from pain in order to avoid these debilitating induced side effects (Watcha and White, 1992). Additionally, physicians are often reluctant to prescribe opioids because of these side effects and because of their fear of other, less common but more serious side effects such as respiratory depression. Several clinical and laboratory studies have demonstrated that low-dose naloxone infusions (0.25 to 1 mcg/kg per hour) can treat or prevent opioid-induced side effects without affecting the quality of analgesia or opioid requirements in adults, children, and adolescents (Maxwell et al., 2005; Gan et al., 1997).

Opioid-Induced Bowel Dysfunction

Opioid-induced bowel dysfunction (OBD), often described as constipation, is a constellation of symptoms that includes delayed gastric emptying, slow bowel motility, incomplete evacuation, bloating, abdominal distention, and gastric reflux. OBD occurs whether opioids are administered acutely or chronically, is found in 90% of patients treated with opioids, and is a significant problem in 50% to 60% of adult patients with advanced cancer (Glare and Lickiss, 1992; Fallon and Hanks, 1999). OBD is not really a side effect of opioid therapy; rather the effects of opioids on gastric emptying, peristalsis, and bowel motility are intrinsic opioid actions. Indeed, opium has been used in the treatment of dysentery for thousands of years. However, unlike the analgesic effects of opioids, the gastrointestinal ones are not accompanied by the development of tolerance.

In the postoperative surgical patient, OBD impacts how pain is managed because the return of bowel function and the ability to take nutrients and medicines orally are often the limiting factors in hospital length of stay. Surgeons often view opioids as the primary cause of bowel dysfunction, nausea, vomiting, and delayed hospital discharge. As a result, prescription and administration of opioids can become a balancing act between the need to provide appropriate analgesia and the need to facilitate bowel recovery and hospital discharge.

Therefore, patients treated with opioids, regardless of drug, route, or method of delivery, should be considered for a prophylactic bowel regimen of stool softeners and bulking agents (e.g., senna and lubiprostone) as soon as the patient can eat or drink. Indeed, there may be value in starting these agents preoperatively. Alternatively, several new peripherally-acting opioid antagonists, methylnaltrexone and alvimopan, have recently been approved by the FDA and may be of great utility (Moss and Rosow, 2008). These medications offer promise in the treatment of OBD in patients with late-stage advanced illness (methylnaltrexone), as well as postoperative ileus in adult patients (alvimopan). However, neither of these medications has been studied or approved for use in children. If these conservative measures fail, then stimulant laxatives (e.g., polyethylene glycol 3550) and enemas should be added to this regimen.

Opioid-Induced Pruritus

Opioid-induced pruritus (OIP) is one of the most common adverse side effects associated with opioid use. The incidence of OIP varies between 20% and 100% when opioids are administered neuroaxially (intrathecally or epidurally) and between 20% to 60% when administered intravenously (Ganesh and Maxwell, 2007). Surprisingly, the pathophysiology of clinical itch remains unclear. Over 300 years ago, the German physician Samuel Hafenreffer described itch as an "unpleasant sensation that elicits the desire to scratch," and this definition is still valid today. Much of the current research on itch focuses on identifying the neuronal mechanisms and the mediators responsible for itch in dermatological and systemic disease. OIP is primarily mediated by binding of μ-agonists with central μ-opioid receptors in the brain and spinal cord and can be blocked with centrally acting μ-receptor antagonists (Ko and Naughton, 2000). Binding of the dopamine D2 receptor and the release of prostaglandin E1 and E2 have also been implicated in the development of OIP. Blockade of the D2 receptor by antagonists such as droperidol or by inhibiting prostaglandin production with NSAIDs significantly reduces OIP (Horta et al., 1996). Whereas histamine is a potent pruritic agent, opioid-induced histamine release from mast cells plays almost no part in OIP.

A wide variety of drugs with different mechanisms of action have been used to treat or prevent OIP. Antihistamines, such as diphenhydramine or hydroxyzine are the most common and perhaps least effective drugs used to treat established OIP. They primarily interrupt the itch-scratch cycle by providing needed sleep but are not really effective at reducing the severity of itch. A more effective approach is to prophylactically administer a low-dose intravenous infusion of the opioid antagonist naloxone (0.25 to 1 mcg/kg per hour) or the partial agonist/antagonist nalbuphine (50 mcg/kg, maximum 5 mg/dose) (Kendrick et al., 1996; Maxwell and Yaster, 2003; Nakatsuka et al., 2006). Other strategies involve rotating opioids, reducing opioid dose, or switching to the oral route of administration.

Opioid-Induced Nausea and Vomiting

Nausea and vomiting occur in more than 50% of patients treated with opioids for acute pain. The pathophysiology of nausea and vomiting are well established. Nausea, a subjective unpleasant sensation in which the patient is aware of the urge to vomit but does not necessarily do so, is mediated by several neural pathways. Vomiting, the forceful expulsion of gastric contents, is coordinated by the vomiting center and chemoreceptor trigger zone (CTZ). The CTZ is rich in 5-HT type-3 (5-HT$_3$), histamine type-1 (H$_1$), muscarinic cholinergic type-1 (M$_1$), dopamine type-2 (D$_2$), neurokinin type-1 (NK$_1$), and μ-opioid receptors. Stimulation of these chemoreceptor triggers activates the vomiting center. In addition, stimulation of H$_1$ and/or M$_1$ receptors in the vestibular labyrinth can, via the CTZ, also activate the vomiting center. Finally, peripheral input via gastrointestinal vagal nerve fibers stimulates the brainstem vomiting center by activation of 5-HT$_3$, NK$_1$, or D$_2$ receptors. Most antiemetic drugs exert their effects by blocking one or more of these receptors.

A wide variety of drugs with different mechanism of actions have been used to treat or prevent opioid-induced nausea and vomiting (Watcha and White, 1992). The most commonly used antiemetics are antihistamines (diphenhydramine), phenothiazines (prochlorperazine and promethazine), butyrophenones (haloperidol and droperidol), benzamides (metoclopramide), 5-HT$_3$-receptor antagonists (ondansetron, dolasetron, granisetron), and dexamethasone. A low-dose intravenous naloxone infusion (1 mcg/kg per hour) has also been shown to be effective (Maxwell and Yaster, 2003). Many of the agents listed above work synergistically. Although it does not make sense to combine two drugs that act via the same mechanism (e.g., two antihistamines such as diphenhydramine and hydroxyzine), combinations of drugs that act via different mechanisms (e.g., ondansetron, a selective inhibitor of 5-HT$_3$ receptors and the steroid dexamethasone) can be effective (McKenzie et al., 1994). Finally, if these measures fail, opioid dose reduction, with or without the addition of NSAIDs, or opioid rotation may be effective.

Opioid-Induced Sedation

The sedating effects of opioids in opioid-naive patients are well known and can be thought of as either a desired effect or an adverse side effect. Although tolerance to sedation and drowsiness often develop, in some patients sedation and mental clouding are so debilitating that it leads to a reduced quality of life. Treatment is often dose reduction, opioid rotation, or the use of psychostimulants. Methylphenidate is the most commonly used stimulant to improve drowsiness, but others include dextroamphetamine, caffeine, and modafinil (Rozans et al., 2002; Prommer, 2006).

Tolerance, Dependence, and Withdrawal

Tolerance is the development of a need to increase the dose of an opioid (or benzodiazepine) agonist to achieve the same analgesic (or sedative) effect previously achieved with a lower dose (Nutt, 1996; Wise, 1996). Whereas tolerance to the sedative and analgesic effects of opioids usually develops after 5 to 21 days of morphine administration, tolerance to the constipating effects of opioids rarely occur. Additionally, cross-tolerance develops between all μ-opioid receptor agonists. However, because this cross tolerance is rarely complete, opioid rotation, that is, changing from one opioid (morphine, fentanyl, or hydromorphone) to another (usually methadone) can be helpful in preventing a continuous escalation in analgesic dosing. When it is necessary to switch, careful consideration must be given to the choice of opioid, dose, and expected degree of cross-tolerance. For example, when switching from high-dose morphine to methadone in patients who are tolerant of opioid, the equianalgesic dose is decreased by a factor of four- to fivefold. Even with this reduction, the calculated dose of methadone may be so high that it warrants a stepwise conversion while the patient remains in a high-surveillance care unit.

Physical dependence, sometimes referred to as *neuroadaptation,* is caused by repeated administration of an opioid that necessitates the continued administration of the drug to prevent the development of a withdrawal or abstinence syndrome characteristic for that particular drug (O'Brien, 1996). Physical dependence usually occurs after 2 to 3 weeks of morphine administration, but when high doses of opioid are administered it may occur after only a few days of therapy. Very young infants treated with high-dose fentanyl infusions after surgical repair of congenital heart disease and those who require extracorporeal membrane oxygenation (ECMO) have been identified to be at particular risk of developing dependence and withdrawal on discontinuation of therapy (Arnold et al., 1991, 1990; Kauffman 1991; Lane et al., 1991).

Physical dependence must be differentiated from addiction (O'Brien, 1996). *Addiction* is a term used to connote a severe degree of drug abuse and dependence that is an extreme of behavior in which drug use pervades the total life activity of the user and of the range of circumstances in which drug use controls the user's behavior. Patients who are addicted to opioids often spend large amounts of time acquiring or using the drug, abandon social or occupational activities because of drug use, and continue to use the drug despite adverse psychological or physical effects. In a sense, addiction is a subset of physical dependence. Anyone who is addicted to an opioid is physically dependent; however, not everyone who is physically dependent is addicted. Patients appropriately treated with opioid agonists for pain can become tolerant and physically dependent. They rarely become psychologically dependent or addicted (Porter and Jick, 1980).

When physical dependence has been established, sudden discontinuation of an opioid or benzodiazepine agonist produces a withdrawal syndrome within 24 hours of drug cessation. Symptoms reach their peak within 72 hours and include abdominal cramping, vomiting, diarrhea, tachycardia, hypertension, diaphoresis, restlessness, insomnia, movement disorders, reversible neurologic abnormalities, and seizures (O'Brien, 1996; Anand and Arnold, 1994; Katz et al., 1994; Nestler 1994, 1996; Norton 1988).

Clinical and experimental data suggest that the duration of opioid receptor occupancy is an important factor in the development of tolerance and dependence. Thus, continuous infusions may produce tolerance more rapidly than intermittent therapy (Katz et al., 1994; Anand and Arnold, 1994). This is particularly true for highly lipid-soluble opioids such as fentanyl. Tolerance and dependence predictably develops after only 5 to 10 days (2.5 mg/kg total fentanyl dose) of continuous fentanyl infusions (Arnold et al., 1991, 1990; Anand and Arnold, 1994; Katz et al., 1994). Nevertheless, prolonged therapy in excess of 10 days, even by intermittent bolus administration, should be expected to produce opioid dependence. As a result, tolerance and physical dependence to both opioid and benzodiazepines is a common phenomenon in the intensive care unit (Suresh and Anand, 1998; Anand and Arnold, 1994; O'Brien, 1996; Yaster et al., 1996; Koob and Nestler, 1997; Tobias, 2000a).

Withdrawal Scales and Weaning Strategies

Hospitalization and admission to the pediatric intensive care unit (PICU) are frightening and at times painful experiences to children and their families. In many critically ill patients, pharmacologically induced sedation verging on general anesthesia is often required to facilitate respiratory care and induce protective immobility that may last for days to weeks. These infants, children, and adolescents often require prodigious, constantly escalating, and on occasion, incomprehensibly high doses of analgesics and sedatives. How to wean these children and prevent withdrawal when they recover is a common problem facing pediatric pain specialists and intensivists. In the PICU, opioid and benzodiazepine withdrawal are common iatrogenic complications of the necessary analgesic and sedative strategies used to facilitate the care of critically ill children. Just as judicious monitoring and administration of these agents correlate with improved care, appropriate assessment tools to recognize withdrawal symptoms, as well as strategies to effectively wean patients at risk for withdrawal must be used when these medications are no longer necessary.

Withdrawal and Abstinence Scales for Infants and Children

In the neonatal intensive care unit (NICU), withdrawal scores were originally developed to care for infants born to drug addicted mothers. As in adults, neonatal opioid withdrawal is a disorder characterized by generalized irritability, respiratory and gastrointestinal distress, autonomic hyperactivity and, at times, seizures. Similar symptoms and degree of severity are seen in iatrogenic abstinence from opioids. Although less well described, comparable difficulties are also attributable to withdrawal from other sedatives and analgesics like benzodiazepines.

The most widely used tool to assess neonatal abstinence the Finnegan scale (Table 15-8). This tool is also among the most commonly used withdrawal scales in older infants and children, even though it has never been validated for this use. The Finnegan scale is a complicated assessment measure that

TABLE 15-8. The Finnegan Neonatal Abstinence Score

Sign/Symptoms	Score
Cry	
Excessive	2
Continuous	3
Sleep (# hours after feeding)	
<1 Hour	3
<2 Hours	2
<3 Hours	1
Moro Reflex	
Hyperactive	2
Markedly hyperactive	3
Tremors	
Mild	1
Moderate-severe	2
Moderate-severe when undisturbed	3
Increased tone	2
Frequent yawning	2
Sneezing	1
Nasal congestion	1
Nasal flaring	2
Respiratory Rate	
>60 Breaths per minute	1
>60 Breaths per minute with retractions	2
Excoriation	1
Seizures	5
Sweating	1
Fever	
100-101°F	1
>101°F	
Mottling	1
Excessive sucking	1
Poor feeding	2
Regurgitation	2
Projectile vomiting	3
Stooling	
Loose	2
Watery	3

Scoring: 0-7, Mild symptoms of withdrawal; 8-11, moderate withdrawal; 12-15, severe withdrawal.

ses a weighted scoring of 31 items that requires training and when used clinically, some assessment of interrater reliability. As a result, it may be too complicated for routine use. An alternative, the Lipsitz scale, offers the advantage of being a relatively simple numerical system, with a reported 77% sensi-

tivity using a value greater than 4 as an indication of significant signs of withdrawal (Table 15-9) (Lipsitz, 1975). The Lipsitz scale and the need for a scoring system to guide therapy was recommended by the American Academy of Pediatrics (AAP) in a 1998 consensus statement (AAP Committee on Drugs, 1998).

When pharmacologic treatment is needed to treat withdrawal, the AAP recommends dilute tincture of opium for neonatal opiate withdrawal. For sedative-hypnotic withdrawal, phenobarbital is the agent of choice. Agthe and others (2009) demonstrated that when tincture of opium is supplemented with oral clonidine (1 mcg/kg) every 4 hours, the duration of pharmacotherapy for neonatal abstinence syndrome is dramatically reduced. However, despite clear, evidence-based recommendations from the AAP, the management of the newborn with psychomotor behavior consistent with withdrawal varies widely. In a recently published survey of neonatal withdrawal treatment, Sarkar and Donn (2006) found inconsistent policies, scale utilization, and treatment regimens between institutions and individual physicians. These results reflect similar findings of earlier studies and reemphasize the disparity between the published evidence and recommendations supporting the use of withdrawal scoring and current clinical practice for neonatal withdrawal treatment.

Franck et al. (2004) investigated the use of an adapted neonatal assessment tool to older children. This 21-item checklist was initially used for opioid weaning and modified for the evaluation of opioid and benzodiazepine withdrawal symptoms (Franck et al., 2004). Their small study demonstrated good interrater reliability and content validity of the tool, as well as applicability to a wide range of ages (6 to 28 months). Thus, this withdrawal scale, named the *Opioid and Benzodiazepine Withdrawal Score (OBWS),* has a wide range of applicability. Adult withdrawal assessment tools often involve personal reporting of symptoms by the patient. Recently, a clinician-administered tool (the Clinical Opiate Withdrawal Scale [COWS]) was developed to provide a simplified 11-question score to assess withdrawal symptoms and to review its applicability in iatrogenic and abuse-related opioid withdrawal scenarios (Wesson and Ling, 2003). Although simplistic and promising, its applicability to other agents (such as benzodiazepines) and to the pediatric age group is unknown.

Weaning Strategies in Infants and Children

As previously discussed, tolerance and physical dependence develop as a result of the drug, dose, method of delivery, and duration of therapy. When the risk of withdrawal is high, weaning patients should be slow (Yaster et al., 1997, 1996). Unfortunately, abrupt withdrawal of opioids and sedatives to facilitate extubation and transfer of patients out of the PICU is commonplace. If sedative or opioid use has been of short duration (i.e., less than 72 hours), acute discontinuation is reasonable. If a patient has required infusions or repeated administration of an agent for more than 5 days, then an agent-specific weaning strategy should be employed.

One approach to the weaning process is to convert all of the patient's analgesic and sedative medications to intermittent parenteral therapy whenever possible. All forms of the drugs being used therapeutically must be counted in this conversion, including PRN medications. Furthermore, because it is quite common for patients to receive multiple opioids and sedatives, all of the opioids should be converted to morphine equivalents and the

TABLE 15-9. Lipsitz Abstinence Withdrawal Scale

Signs	0	1	2	3
			Score	
Tremors (muscle activity of limbs)	Normal	Minimally increased when hungry or disturbed	Moderate or marked increase when undisturbed; subside when fed or held snugly	Marked increase or continuous even when undisturbed, going onto seizure-like movements
Irritability (excessive crying)	None	Slightly increased	Moderate to severe when disturbed or hungry	Marked even when undisturbed
Reflexes	Normal	Increased	Markedly increased	
Stools	Normal	Explosive, but normal frequency	Explosive, more than 8 days	
Muscle tone	Normal	Increased	Rigidity	
Skin abrasions	No	Redness of knees and elbows	Breaking of the skin	
Respiratory rate/minute	< 55	55-75	76-95	
Repetitive sneezing	No	Yes		
Repetitive yawning	No	Yes		
Vomiting	No	Yes		
Fever	No	Yes		

Scoring: 0, No withdrawal symptoms; 1-2, mild withdrawal; 2-3, moderate withdrawal; >4, severe withdrawal.

benzodiazepines to diazepam equivalents (Yaster et al., 1996). How to proceed with weaning beyond this first step is not always clear, and there are no published evidence-based studies.

Initially, because of incomplete cross tolerance and because of the astronomic doses of medication that these patients are often receiving, one approach is to allow for a 24- to 48-hour transition period in which no attempt at weaning is made. During this time, opioids (e.g., methadone or morphine) and sedatives (e.g., diazepam) are administered every 6 to 8 hours around the clock and supplemental doses are allowed if symptoms of withdrawal occur. Once this transition period is completed, the patient's drug regimen is incrementally decreased. The speed of weaning is dictated by the chronicity of drug administration, the half-life of the opioid and benzodiazepine being used, the patient's sensitivity to the wean, and physician's experience and preference. Each medication is decreased by 10% to 20% of the original total dose daily. When the lowest doses are reached, usually in 5 to 7 days, the interval of drug dosing is increased from every 6 hours to every 8 or 12 hours, to once a day. Therapy is then stopped completely. If symptoms of withdrawal develop, they are treated symptomatically with clonidine 2 to 4 mcg/kg every 8 hours. Alternatively, another approach is to wean much more slowly, particularly in patients who have had a longer exposure to medication or are more physiologically fragile. In these patients, 10% of the original dose is reduced every 2 to 7 days, particularly if methadone is being used, because of its extremely long half-life. In addition, clonidine is prescribed prophylactically (in the doses previously described). If symptoms of withdrawal develop, breakthrough opioid or benzodiazepine dosing is provided as needed or the previous, higher, dose is restarted, and the weaning process is suspended for 1 to 2 days.

The α_2-adrenergic agents help prevent or mitigate the occurrence of drug withdrawal regardless of the drug causing addiction or dependence. Agthe and others (2009) have reported the use of clonidine in treating infants born to drug-addicted mothers as well as in patients who have become opioid and sedative dependent as a result of pain or sedation therapy. If tolerated hemodynamically, coadministered oral or transdermal clonidine (6 to 12 mcg/kg per day) can be used to ameliorate the signs and symptoms of withdrawal during the weaning process. In this instance, the clonidine is subsequently weaned. In addition, the use of dexmedetomidine has been reported to prevent withdrawal symptoms in patients dependent on opioids and sedatives (Finkel and Elrefai, 2004; Multz, 2003).

ANALGESIC ADJUVANTS

Adjuvant pain medications are drugs with a primary function that is not to treat pain, but that may have analgesic properties in specific circumstances. Many of the drugs that are discussed in the following section were initially used to treat neuropathic and chronic pain but are now increasingly being used to treat acute pain as a part of a multimodal therapeutic regimen (Fig. 15-3).

Antidepressants

Because 5-HT and NE mediate descending inhibition of ascending pain pathways in the brain and spinal cord (Figs. 15-2 and 15-3), 5-HT and NE reuptake inhibitor antidepressant medications may have efficacy in relieving pain (Saarto and Wiffen, 2007). Antidepressants that enhance NE action are more effective analgesics than those that predominantly enhance 5-HT action, such as with many of the newer antidepressants (Saarto and Wiffen, 2007). Older antidepressants, particularly the tricyclic antidepressants (TCAs) such as amitriptyline, doxepin, and nortriptyline have been the most thoroughly studied and are thought to cause analgesia by NE and 5-HT reuptake inhibition

(Wiffen et al., 2005). They also have other pharmacologic properties that may contribute to analgesia, such as reducing sympathetic activity, NMDA-receptor antagonism, anticholinergic activity, and sodium-channel blockade. Although generally administered orally, Collins et al. (1995) report using intravenous amitriptyline in eight children who could not tolerate oral medications. Newer non-TCAs seem to be less efficacious analgesics. Ironically, this may be in part because of their "cleaner" pharmacodynamic profiles. Of the newer antidepressants, duloxetine, a dual inhibitor of 5-HT and NE, has been shown to be effective in several randomized controlled trials in adult patients with fibromyalgia and other chronic pain conditions even in the absence of major depressive disorders (Arnold et al., 2009).

When using antidepressants in the management of neuropathic and other pain states, the response to therapy is at times remarkably fast. Unlike depression, in which response to these drugs may take or month or more, analgesia can be produced in as little as 1 to 2 weeks. However, side effects can limit the use of some of these drugs. Children bothered by anticholinergic side effects of TCAs, such as sedation, blurry vision, and dry mouth can be treated with nortriptyline or duloxetine. In addition, all TCAs have a quinidine-like effect on cardiac conduction. This calls for baseline and surveillance electrocardiograms in children who receive this therapy. Recent experience suggests that children, especially between 6 and 12 years of age, benefit from dividing the TCA dose to twice daily, to avoid cholinergic rebound symptoms in the afternoon when a single bedtime dose is used.

Antiepileptic Agents

Like the TCAs, antiepileptic adjuvant analgesics suffer an unfortunate name. Most families (and physicians who are unaware of their analgesic properties) question the use of an antiepileptic drug in a child who does not have seizures. Conceptually, these agents work by preventing "peripheral seizures" in the form of pathologic peripheral nerve discharge (Tanelian and Brose, 1991; Kingery, 1997; Rizzo, 1997). Carbamazepine is the most widely studied antiepileptic in the management of neuropathic pain, particularly in the treatment of lancinating neuropathic pain (such as pain caused by nerve-root compression or injury to a discrete peripheral nerve). Antiepileptic drugs can also help painful "glove and stocking" neuropathic conditions, disagreeable paresthesias, and intense sensitivity to innocuous stimuli (as seen in some human immunodeficiency virus [HIV] neuropathies and chemotherapeutic nerve injuries). Especially in oncology patients, carbamazepine's propensity for drug-drug interactions and risk of blood dyscrasias are of concern. As a result, these drugs have largely been replaced by gabapentin and pregabalin, an interesting class of weak anticonvulsant drugs that bind at voltage-gated–calcium-channel α_2-δ (Ca_v-α_2-δ) proteins (Taylor, 2009). Interestingly, despite their names, these drugs are not GABAergic and produce analgesia by reducing the presynaptic release of pain-inducing neurotransmitters such as glutamate, NE, substance P, and CGRP in the spinal cord and CNS.

Gabapentin and pregabalin have been most widely studied and used for the treatment of chronic pain conditions such as postherpetic neuralgia, diabetic neuropathy, complex regional pain syndromes, malignant pain, HIV-related neuropathy, and headaches. Increasingly, they are being used in the perioperative period as a component of multimodal pain therapy (see Fig. 15-3) (Joshi, 2005; Ho et al., 2006; Kong and Irwin, 2007; White, 2008). Adult studies have demonstrated their effectiveness (1200 mg gabapentin, 300 mg pregabalin orally) at enhancing postoperative analgesia and preoperative anxiolysis, preventing chronic postsurgical pain, attenuating the hemodynamic responses to laryngoscopy and intubation, and reducing postoperative delirium (Ho et al., 2006). The main side effect of both drugs is somnolence.

Alpha₂-Adrenergic Agonists: Clonidine, Tizanidine, and Dexmedetomidine

NE is involved in the control of pain by modulating pain-related responses through various pathways (Fig. 15-3). α_2-Adrenergic agonists, such as clonidine, tizanidine, and dexmedetomidine, have well-established analgesic and sedative profiles and wide application in perioperative multimodal pain management. Clonidine is the prototype and most widely studied of this class of drugs. It can be administered via the epidural, oral, and transdermal routes. Clonidine is traditionally used as an antihypertensive and to minimize the symptoms of opioid withdrawal (Agthe, 2009). However, when administered orally, intravenously, or transdermally, clonidine may reduce opioid requirements and improve analgesia. Similarly, the addition of clonidine to local anesthetic solutions for neuraxial or peripheral nerve blocks may enhance and prolong analgesia. However, the analgesic benefits of clonidine remain controversial. Finally, clonidine can be a useful antineuropathic agent, especially in children who cannot tolerate oral medications or who have coexisting problems like steroid-induced hypertension (Kingery, 1997). Clonidine is empirically started at 1 to 2 mcg/kg per dose, every 8 hours, and increased incrementally over days to doses up to 4 mcg/kg per dose. Alternatively, a transdermal patch can be applied in order to administer 6 to 12 mcg/kg per day. Clonidine use is limited by its side effects, which include bradycardia, hypotension, and excessive sedation (Joshi, 2005; White, 2008).

Compared with clonidine, dexmedetomidine is more selective, has a shorter duration of action, and has opioid-sparing and analgesic effects. Because dexmedetomidine does not cause respiratory depression, despite its potent sedative effects it is increasingly being used for deep procedural sedation, as a general anesthetic adjuvant, and for sedation in intubated patients in the intensive care unit.

N-Methyl-D-Aspartate Receptor Antagonists

NMDA receptor antagonists, such as ketamine and methadone, are important modulators of chronic pain and have been shown in some studies to be useful in preventive analgesia by reducing acute postoperative pain, analgesic consumption, or both when they are added to more conventional means of providing analgesia, such as opioids and NSAIDs, in the perioperative period (Fig. 15-3) (McCartney et al., 2004). NMDA receptor antagonists may reduce pain by two nonmutually exclusive mechanisms: a reduction in central hypersensitivity and a reduction of opioid tolerance. Nevertheless, the effectiveness of NMDA receptor antagonists in preventive analgesia has been equivocal at best (McCartney et al., 2004; Pogatzki-Zahn and Zahn, 2006). Ketamine is well known as a dissociative general anesthetic and may be an effective adjuvant in pain management when used in low doses (0.05 to 0.2 mg/kg per hour) (Tsui et al., 2007; Sveticic et al., 2008).

REGIONAL ANESTHESIA AND ANALGESIA

Overview

Since the late twentieth century, the use of local anesthetics and regional anesthetic techniques in pediatric practice has increased dramatically. Unlike most drugs used in medical practice, local anesthetics must be physically deposited at their sites of action by direct application and require patient cooperation and the use of specialized needles. Because of this, for decades children were considered poor candidates for regional anesthetic techniques. However, once it was recognized that regional anesthesia could be used as an adjunct and not a replacement for general anesthesia, its use increased dramatically. Regional anesthesia offers the anesthesiologist and pain specialist many benefits. It modifies the neuroendocrine stress response, provides profound postoperative pain relief, insures a more rapid recovery, and may shorten hospital stay with fewer opioid-induced side effects. Furthermore, because catheters placed in the epidural, pleural, femoral, sciatic, brachial plexus, and other spaces can be used for days or months, local anesthetics are increasingly being used not only for postoperative pain relief, but also for medical, neuropathic, and terminal pain (Dalens, 1989; Yaster and Maxwell, 1989; Giaufre et al., 1996; Golianu et al., 2000; Ross et al., 2000; Capdevila et al., 2003; Dadure et al., 2003). Peripheral nerve blocks provide

significant pain relief after many common pediatric procedures. Techniques range from simple infiltration of local anesthetics to neuraxial blocks like spinal and epidural analgesia. To be used safely, a working knowledge of the differences in how local anesthetics are metabolized in infants and children is necessary (Table 15-10) (Dalens, 1989, 1995; Yaster et al., 1993).

Effects of Age on Metabolism of Local Anesthetics

All local anesthetics in current use are either amino amides or amino esters and achieve their intended effect by blocking gated sodium channels. The ester local anesthetics are metabolized by plasma cholinesterase. Neonates and infants up to 6 months of age have less than half of the adult levels of this plasma enzyme. Theoretically, clearance may be reduced and the effects of ester local anesthetics prolonged. In reality this is never the case. Amides, on the other hand, are metabolized in the liver and bound by plasma proteins. Neonates and young infants (younger than 3 months of age) have reduced liver-blood flow and immature metabolic degradation pathways. Thus, larger fractions of local anesthetics are not metabolized and remain active in the plasma compared with adults. More local anesthetic is excreted in the urine unchanged. Furthermore, neonates and infants may be at increased risk for the toxic effects of amide local anesthetics because of lower levels of albumin and α_1-acid glycoproteins, which are proteins essential for drug binding (Lerman et al., 1989). This decreased binding leads to increased concentrations of free drug and potential toxicity, particularly with bupivacaine. On the other hand, the larger volume of distribution at steady state seen in the neonate for these (and other) drugs may confer some clinical protection by lowering plasma drug levels (see Chapter 7, Pharmacology of Pediatric Anesthesia).

TABLE 15-10. Suggested Maximal Doses of Local Anesthetics (mg/kg)*

Drug (Concentration) and Technique	Spinal	Caudal/Lumbar Epidural	Peripheral[†]	Subcutaneous[†]
Esters				
Chloroprocaine (1% infiltration) (2%-3% epidural)	NR	8-10[§]	8-10[§]	8-10[§]
Procaine	NR	NR	8-10[§]	8-10[§]
Tetracaine (0.5%-1%)	0.2-0.6[‡]	NR	NR	NR
Amides				
Lidocaine (0.5%-2%) (0.5%-1% infiltration) (1%-2% peripheral, epidural, subcutaneous) (5% spinal)	1-2.5	5-7[§]	5-7[§]	5-7[§]
Bupivacaine (0.0625%-0.5%) (0.125%-0.5% infiltration) (0.25%-0.5% peripheral, epidural, subcutaneous)	0.3-0.5	2-3[§]	2-3[§]	2-3[§]
Ropivacaine (0.125%-0.5% infiltration) (0.2%-0.5% peripheral, epidural)		2-3[§]	2-3[§]	
Etidocaine (0.5%-1%)	NR	3-4[§]	3-4[§]	3-4[§]
Prilocaine (0.5%-1% infiltration) (1%-1.5% peripheral) (2%-3% epidural)	NR	5-7[§¶]	5-7[§¶]	5-7[§¶]

*These are suggested safe upper limits when drug is administered at recommended location. Direct intraarterial or intravenous injection of even a fraction of these doses may result in systemic toxicity or death.

[†]Epinephrine should never be added to local anesthetic solution administered in area of an end artery (e.g., penile nerve block).

[‡]The minimal effective dose in children <10 kg is 1.5-2 mg.

[§]The higher dose is recommended only with the concomitant use of epinephrine 1:200,000.

[¶]Total adult dose should not exceed 600 mg.

NR, Not recommended. Concentrations are in mg percent. For example, a 1% solution contains 10 mg/mL.

Box 15-1 Intralipid Rescue for Local Anesthetic Toxicity

- Call for help and start CPR
- 20% Intralipid solution
- 1 to 2 mL/kg Bolus (adult dose, 150 mL)
- Once circulation is reestablished, start continuous infusion 0.5 mL/kg/minute

The metabolism of the amide local anesthetic prilocaine is unique in that it results in the production of oxidants that can lead to the development of methemoglobinemia. This occurs in adults with doses of prilocaine greater than 600 mg. Because premature and full-term infants have decreased levels of methemoglobin reductase, they are more susceptible to developing methemoglobinemia. An additional factor rendering newborns more susceptible to methemoglobinemia is the relative ease by which fetal hemoglobin is oxidized compared with adult hemoglobin. Because of this, prilocaine cannot be recommended for routine use in neonates.

Local Anesthetic Toxicity

Cardiovascular and CNS toxicity after local anesthetic administration in children is rare (Berde, 1992; McCloskey et al., 1992). Local anesthetic toxicity can be limited by careful attention to dose, route of administration, fractionating the dose, and rapidity of absorption of local anesthetic into the systemic circulation (Berde, 2004). Cardiovascular toxicity caused by bupivacaine is the most feared complication of local anesthetic administration, whether it is administered acutely (intermittent dosing) or continuously, because it presents as ventricular dysrhythmias that may be refractory to treatment. Neonates may be at increased risk for bupivacaine toxicity for reasons discussed earlier. Because of this, it is increasingly being replaced with either ropivacaine or levobupivacaine, which may have a greater therapeutic index and margin of safety (Dony et al., 2000; Groban et al., 2001). Patients who develop "lethal" cardiovascular collapse may be rescued with a 20% lipid solution bolus, 1 to 2 mL/kg or 150 mL for adults (Dalgleish and Katawaroo, 2005; Weinberg et al., 2006). This dose may be repeated while resuscitation continues. Once circulation is reestablished, a continuous lipid infusion of 0.5 mL/kg per minute is initiated, and the patient is transferred to an intensive care unit for further monitoring (Box 15-1). Other therapies include prolonged resuscitation efforts, extracorporeal membrane oxygenation, or another temporary circulatory-assistance device.

Topical Local Anesthetics EMLA and ELA-Max

There are several methods for providing topical anesthesia to minimize procedural pain (e.g., venipuncture, lumbar puncture, chest-tube insertion). These include injection of local anesthetic at the procedure site, application of topical anesthetic creams and ointments, iontophoresis, and laser-assisted delivery of anesthetics. An eutectic mixture of local anesthetics (EMLA) in the form of cream is a topical emulsion composed of 2.5% prilocaine and 2.5% lidocaine and produces complete anesthesia of intact skin after application. Unfortunately, for best effect, EMLA cream must be applied and covered with an occlusive dressing for 60 minutes before performing a procedure. This limits its use in the emergency room or office to situations in which the site can be prepared well in advance of anticipated use. Furthermore, if the procedure is a venipuncture, multiple sites must be prepared, in case the initial attempt is unsuccessful (a common problem in pediatric practice in general and more so when EMLA is applied, because it causes cutaneous blanching). Finally, as stated previously, the prilocaine component of EMLA can cause methemoglobinemia. Unfortunately, this has limited the use of EMLA in the newborn. Nevertheless, a single dose is safe and has been shown to be effective in the management of newborn circumcision (Taddio et al., 1997; Lehr and Taddio, 2007). Alternatives that do not contain prilocaine are readily available. Lidocane 4% (ELA-Max) is as effective as EMLA and requires only 30 minutes to become effective (Koh et al., 2004).

Interestingly, the effectiveness of topical local anesthetics at reducing pain is dependent on who makes the assessment. Soliman et al. (1988) studied the efficacy of EMLA cream compared with injected lidocaine at reducing the pain associated with venipuncture. Both an observer and a physician performing the procedure judged pain relief to be virtually complete in both groups. However, the children involved in the study were not so sanguine and were equally dissatisfied with both methods, particularly if the needle used for venipuncture was visible to them. Thus, despite the fact that two observers felt that the child was pain free, the child's cooperation with venipuncture did not improve. Therefore, it is not clear whether the delay that is involved in the use of EMLA (60-minute wait for effect) is always justified. On the other hand, topical local anesthetics may be more effective in children accustomed to numerous medical procedures (e.g., oncology patients) or for procedures in which the child cannot see the needle, such as lumbar puncture or bone marrow aspiration (although there is little evidence to support the effectiveness of EMLA even in these situations).

Local Infiltration

Infiltration of wound edges with local anesthetics (field block) or by directly instilling local anesthetic into a wound (splash) effectively provides intraoperative and postoperative analgesia for many minor (e.g., inguinal herniorrhaphy, laceration repair, or tonsillectomy) and some major surgical procedures (e.g., craniotomy) (Wong et al., 1995; Casey et al., 1990). Many studies have demonstrated the effectiveness of tetracaine-adrenaline [epinephrine]-cocaine (TAC), lidocaine-epinephrine-tetracaine (LET) and bupivacaine-norepinephrine (BN) in the management of lacerations in children (Schilling et al., 1995; Ernst et al., 1996). Unfortunately, cocaine, a key ingredient in making the TAC drug combination effective, is toxic. Indeed, toxicity has been reported even when TAC has been applied appropriately and according to recommended guidelines.

The most commonly used local anesthetics for local infiltration are lidocaine, mepivacaine, bupivacaine, ropivacaine, and levobupivacaine. As mentioned previously, local anesthetic toxicity is primarily related to how rapidly and how much local anesthetic is absorbed (or deposited) in the blood. Toxicity can be limited by careful attention to dose, route of administration, and by limiting the rate of rise of local anesthetic into the systemic circulation (Table 15-11). No more than 2 to 2.5 mg/kg of

TABLE 15-11. Local Anesthetic Maximum Dosing Guideline by Weight

Local Anesthetic	Bolus Dose (mg/kg)		Infusion (mg/kg/hour)	
	Infants <6 Months	Child	Infants <6 Months	Child
Bupivacaine	1.5	2.5	0.2	0.4
Ropivacaine	2	2.5	0.2	0.5
Chloroprocaine	10	10	15	15
Lidocaine	3	5	0.8	2

bupivacaine or 5 to 7 mg/kg of lidocaine should be used. Dilute solutions of the local anesthetics can be used to provide adequate spread of the anesthetic solution without exceeding the maximum dose. Epinephrine can also be added to the solution in vascular areas to slow the uptake of the anesthetic and to prolong its action. However, in order to avoid ischemic injury, epinephrine must never be used in procedures involving end-arteries, such as the penis or distal extremities. Finally, other adjuvants, particularly clonidine, can be added to the local anesthetic solution to improve the quality and duration of neural blockade (Cucchiaro and Ganesh, 2007). When performing nerve blocks, the pain of local anesthetic administration can be minimized by using small-gauge needles (25 to 30) and warm, buffered anesthetic solutions, and by injecting slowly. Adding bicarbonate to local anesthetic solutions shortens the onset time (faster block) and reduces the pain of injection (Christoph et al., 1988; Orlinsky et al., 1992). This is best accomplished by adding 1 mL (1 mEq) of 8.4% sodium bicarbonate to 9 mL lidocaine or by adding 1 mL (1 mEq) of 8.4% sodium bicarbonate to 29 mL bupivacaine (Yaster et al., 1993, 1994b).

Neural Blockade

The anatomy of peripheral nerves and the techniques of nerve blockade are basically the same for children and adults. The use of nerve stimulators, ultrasonography, and a description of the most common nerve blocks used in pediatric practice are discussed in Chapter 16, Regional Anesthesia. In the next sections the administration of analgesics through these catheters is discussed.

Continuous Epidural Analgesia

Continuous or intermittent epidural analgesia uses local anesthetics administered either alone or in combination with opioids, α_2-adrenergic agonists (clonidine) or NMDA receptor antagonists (ketamine) in order to block nociceptive impulses from entering the CNS and provide profound analgesia without systemic sedation (Dalens and Hasnaoui, 1989; Yaster and Maxwell, 1989; Llewellyn and Moriarty, 2007). Epidural analgesia has become the most commonly performed regional anesthetic technique for the intraoperative and postoperative management of patients with urologic, orthopedic, and general surgical procedures below the T4 dermatomal level in children. It has been used to provide continuous sympathetic blockade in

children with vascular insufficiency secondary to intense vasoconstriction (e.g., purpura fulminans), in patients with cancer unresponsive to parenteral and enteral opioids, and in the management of patients who have sickle cell trait with vasoocclusive crisis (Yaster et al., 1994a). How long an indwelling caudal or lumbar epidural catheter can be left in place without risking local or systemic infection is unknown; however, serious systemic infections after short-term (3 to 5 days) continuous lumbar and caudal epidural analgesia are extremely rare (Strafford et al., 1995; Kost-Byerly et al., 1998).

Epidural catheters can be inserted at the caudal, lumbar, or thoracic level. The closer the tip of the catheter lies to the dermatome to be blocked, the smaller the amount of drug required to produce neural blockade. Because local anesthetic toxicity is directly related to the total amount of drug infused, catheter placement plays a very important role in the overall safety of this technique. Epidural placement via the caudal and lumbar approach is most common, although even thoracic placement is advocated by some (Bosenberg et al., 1998). Of note, because the epidural space of young children is filled with loosely packed fat and blood vessels (compared with adults), it is possible to thread a caudally (or lumbar) placed catheter as far as the thorax. Bosenberg et al. (1998) first reported the use of the caudal approach for thoracic placement of an epidural catheter in children younger than 2 years of age. Gunter and Eng (1992) extended this observation to older children as well. In children under 5 years of age, caudal insertion and threading 8 to 10 cm of catheter is the preferred epidural technique for most surgery below T4. The key to success is to use short (5-cm), 18-gauge needles, through which 19- to 20-gauge, styletted catheters are inserted. The large-bore catheter offers many advantages over smaller bore (21- to 24-gauge) catheters that were initially used in pediatric epidural analgesia. These large-bore catheters allow for less resistance to flow, less likelihood of occlusion (kinking), and less back-leakage at the site of insertion.

Continuous infusions of local anesthetics either administered alone or with adjuvants (e.g., opioids or clonidine) provide pain relief during the entire period of infusion. This makes it very attractive for postoperative pain management and pain management where conventional therapy has proven ineffective (e.g., cancer or sickle cell crisis). Initially, high doses of local anesthetics, similar to those used intraoperatively, were used postoperatively, resulting in local anesthetic toxicity. Dilute concentrations given at much lower doses have been shown to provide sensory and autonomic blockade without risking local anesthetic toxicity. As an added benefit, lower concentrations of local anesthetics do not produce motor blockade, a side effect of local anesthetic administration that is disliked by patients, parents, and surgeons alike. Very dilute concentrations of local anesthetics (0.625 to 1.25 mg/mL bupivacaine or ropivacaine, 1 to 5 mg/mL lidocaine) are generally effective when combined with opioids and/or clonidine.

In North America, the most commonly used local anesthetics in continuous epidural blockade are bupivacaine and ropivacaine. Bupivacaine and ropivacaine are administered in concentrations ranging from 0.625 mg/mL (1/16th% solution) to as high as 2.5 mg/mL (0.25% solution). Concentrations above 1.25 mg/mL (1/8% solution) are rarely required for postoperative or medical analgesia and significantly increase the risks of toxicity and unwanted side effects (e.g., sensory, motor, autonomic dysfunction, urinary retention, and inability to walk). Berde, in the editorial accompanying McCloskey's report of bupivacaine toxicit in children, recommended that bupivacaine infusions be kept below 0.4 mg/kg per hour in children and 0.2 mg/kg per hour in neonates (Berde, 1992; McCloskey et al., 1992). Although this has not been formally studied, these recommended doses have become dosing guidelines. The most commonly used (and easiest) epidural concentration of bupivacaine or ropivacaine is 0.1% (1 mg/mL). Because in concentrations of 1 mg/mL, bupivacaine and ropivacaine do not always produce reliable analgesia, opioids such as fentanyl (2 to 2.5 mcg/mL), hydromorphone (10 mcg/mL), or morphine (20 to 30 mcg/mL) are almost always added to this dilute epidural solution. Which opioid to use is based on the site of the surgical procedure. For surgical procedures performed above the umbilicus (e.g., Nissen fundoplication or thoracotomy), many practitioners prefer hydromorphone or morphine, because they are less lipophilic than fentanyl and may have better rostral spread. For pain below the umbilicus, the initial starting infusion is 0.2 mL/kg per hour (0.2 mg/kg per hour bupivacaine or ropivacaine; 0.4 to 0.5 mcg/kg per hour fentanyl, or 2 mcg/kg per hour hydromorphone, or morphine 6 mcg/kg per hour); for pain above the umbilicus, the initial starting epidural infusion is 0.3 mL/kg per hour (0.3 mg/kg per hour bupivacaine or ropivacaine; 0.6 to 0.75 mcg/kg per hour fentanyl or 3 mcg/kg per hour hydromorphone, or morphine 9 mcg/kg per hour). Generally, infusion rates do not exceed 14 to 16 mL/hour.

If bupivacaine or ropivacaine is used in older children for epidural PCA, the basal infusion is generally administered at a rate that provides 0.2 mg/kg per hour of local anesthetic, while half of the basal rate is given as a bolus (Birmingham et al., 2003). A maximum of two boluses are allowed per hour with a lockout period of 15 minutes. This approach provides a maximum of 0.4 mg/kg per hour bupivacaine or ropivacaine.

As discussed previously, cardiovascular toxicity caused by bupivacaine is the most feared complication of local anesthetic administration, regardless of the method of administration. The newborn is particularly vulnerable. Because of this, bupivacaine has increasingly been replaced by either ropivacaine or levobupivacaine, which may have a greater therapeutic index and margin of safety. However, they are also significantly more expensive. Because lidocaine can be easily measured in most hospital clinical laboratories, is less cardiotoxic than bupivacaine, and is cheaper than ropivacaine, lidocaine can be used for continuous local anesthetic infusions in neonates. In neonates, lidocaine in 1 mg/mL concentrations can be administered at a rate of 0.8 mg/kg per hour. Blood levels are measured every 12 hours, and the infusion is titrated downward if the lidocaine blood levels are greater than 4 mg/L. In children older than 2 months of age, lidocaine can be administered in doses of 1.5 mg/kg per hour (lidocaine concentrations of 3 to 5 mg/mL).

Continuous Peripheral Nerve Blockade

Local anesthetics can be infused in continuous peripheral nerve blockade using either disposable elastomeric pumps or standard electronic PCA pumps. The most commonly used solution consists of 0.125% bupivacaine, 0.15% ropivacaine, or 0.1% ropivacaine at rates of 0.1 to 0.15 mL/kg per hour (maximum rate of 12 mL/h). The choice of local anesthetic is based on the anesthesiologist's preference and the need to prevent a motor blockade. Disposable elastomeric pumps have a rate selection of 2 to 14 mL/h (even numbers only) with a reservoir that can be filled with up to 400 mL of local anesthetic solution. They are not refillable but may be replaced to provide multiple days of peripheral neural blockade. In general, these catheters/pumps result in an opioid sparing effect as well as a low incidence of self-limited complications (Ganesh et al., 2007).

CHRONIC PAIN

For most pediatric anesthesiologists, the management of acute pain is an extension of their operating room experience, but this is not so with chronic pain. Although acute injury or disease may precede chronic or recurrent pain, once it becomes self-sustaining, chronic pain becomes its own condition independent of the original pathology that initiated it. Chronic pain in children is not unusual and can be incapacitating. Affected individuals become physically inactive and dependent on others for many of the tasks of daily living. As it progresses, it interferes with peer and family relationships and often results in the inability to go to school, which is the childhood equivalent of being unable to work. Thus, the management of chronic pain, in the absence of a treatable cause, is to restore function. This is often best accomplished through interdisciplinary cognitive-behavioral and physical rehabilitative programs that help return the child to physical activity even before pain reduction occurs. In the next sections the management of three archetypical chronic pain conditions in children and adolescents are discussed, namely complex regional pain syndromes (CRPSs), abdominal pain, and headaches.

Complex Regional Pain Syndromes

CRPS as a term was first proposed by Stanton-Hicks to describe a varied and dynamic presentation of symptoms including intense, almost incapacitating, regional pain and sensory, neurovascular, motor, and pseudomotor abnormalities (Stanton-Hicks et al., 1995; Stanton-Hicks, 2003; Berde and Lebel, 2005). Although the precise pathophysiology remains unclear, multiple abnormalities have been described in the peripheral nervous system and the CNS. Sympathetic nervous system involvement has been found in many but not all patients, as demonstrated by relief of pain by sympathetic blockade of the affected extremity or an abnormal hemodynamic response to tilt-table testing (Meier et al., 2006). The diagnosis of the syndrome continues to be based primarily on the patient's history and physical examination. Presentations without identifiable trauma to nervous system structures are classified as CRPS type I, or reflex sympathetic dystrophy (RSD) in older taxonomy. In cases in which a definable peripheral nerve lesion exists, the diagnosis is CRPS type II, or causalgia. The signs and symptoms for CRPS types I and II are clinically indistinguishable.

CRPS type I has been described in children as young as 5 years of age, and type II has been observed in children as young as 3 years old (Tan et al., 2008). Although uncommon, CRPS is not rare and is increasingly being recognized and diagnosed (Sherry et al., 1999; Lee et al., 2002). Unlike in adults, in children and adolescents CRPS is predominately a disease of females (female/male ratio 5:1) and most commonly affects a lower extremity. Furthermore, if a preceding injury is described, it is usually minor. In addition, psychosocial factors are thought to play a greater role than in adults. Finally, noninvasive, cognitive, behavioral, and physical therapies are more effective in the pediatric population than in adults (Sherry et al., 1999; Lee et al., 2002; Stanton-Hicks, 2003). However, in a minority of patients, persistent pain and a high degree of disability exist despite multimodal therapy including interventional therapy (Wilder et al., 1992).

Diagnosis

The diagnosis of CRPS is based primarily on the patient's history and physical examination rather than on laboratory testing. Examination or history often show that the affected child has sensory abnormalities such as intense, burning pain; allodynia; and hyperalgesia in the distal aspects of a single extremity. Even in CRPS type II, pain does not follow any sensory dermatomes but is present in a glove or stocking distribution. Whereas children may have all the symptoms generally associated with the syndrome, in adults there are several distinct differences: the temperature of the affected limb is often cooler in relation to the symmetric extremity, edema is less common, and atrophic changes are rare except for decreases in skeletal muscle mass (Tan et al., 2008). Just as in adults, spread of symptoms to other parts of the body, either in a continuous or in a discontinuous fashion, has been observed.

CRPS is primarily a clinical diagnosis. It is not an autoimmune, infectious, or a rheumatologic disorder. It is not associated with elevated erythrocyte sedimentation rates, and there are no elevations of any specific antigen or antibody titer. There is no fever or leukocytosis, which helps differentiate it from an infectious disease. Response to sympathetic blockade is not useful in diagnosis, because response can be seen with any form of sympathetically mediated pain.

The most common laboratory evaluations in CRPS involve nuclear medicine, quantitative sensory testing, and most recently, functional MRI (Intenzo et al., 2005; Lebel et al., 2008). Although a patient's nuclear medicine report often states that findings after bone scintigraphy are, or are not, consistent with CRPS, no particular pattern of hypofixation or hyperfixation on scintigraphic studies has been found to be diagnostic. Patients with a history and clinical presentation consistent with CRPS may have a decreased, increased, or normal uptake of tracer on a bone scan. Scintigraphy is more sensitive than plain x-rays and can be useful in supporting or confirming the diagnosis by helping to exclude other diagnoses such as arthritis, benign or malignant bony lesions, or metabolic bone diseases (Intenzo et al., 2005). Hypoperfusion corresponding to osteopenia on a plain radiograph may be used as a cautionary sign for conducting physical therapy sessions to avoid pathologic fractures.

Nerve-conduction studies (NCS) and electromyography (EMG) should be reserved for the occasional patient. These are painful tests and may not be well tolerated in highly sensitive patients. NCS and EMG are indicated when initially diffuse symptoms become more localized as therapy progresses, or when pain follows a distinct dermatomal pattern, because this may be indicative of a peripheral nerve entrapment. Quantitative sensory testing (QST) is primarily a research tool. Sethna et al. (2007) performed standardized neurologic examinations and QST in a group of 42 pediatric patients and found that cold allodynia was the most common abnormality. More than half of their patients also had mechanical, dynamic, and static allodynia and allodynia to punctuate temporal summation. The authors

suggested that these abnormal hyperexcitable sensory patterns may be consistent with a central sensitization pattern.

Finally, the importance of psychological disturbances both in the diagnosis and management of CRPS have been hotly debated. At one point, CRPS was thought to be an entirely psychosomatic disorder. Although this view is no longer tenable, the importance of psychological dysfunction and multiple stressors in affected children is clear and an important target of therapeutic intervention (Sherry et al., 1999; Tan et al., 2008). Indeed, Sherry et al. (1999) emphasize the importance of individual and family psychological issues in the perpetuation of this condition.

Treatment

There are currently no therapeutic modalities that predictably lead to resolution of CRPS. All treatment is directed at aggressive mobilization of the affected limb early in the process to prevent disability, refractoriness, and treatment failure and must include the family as well as the patient (Lee et al., 2002). Unquestionably, the key to therapy is physical reconditioning and mobilization of the affected limb by exercise, ambulation, and range of motion exercises (Lee et al., 2002). With reconditioning, affect, endurance, and pain improve. Medication may help alleviate pain, improve sleep, and facilitate physical therapy. Many drug classes, including opioids, NSAIDs, TCAs, and anticonvulsants are prescribed, but none has been subjected to the rigors of randomized controlled trials in the treatment of these patients. Finally, cognitive behavioral therapy is as important as physical therapy and medication, because it promotes positive coping skills and eliminates reinforcement of maladaptive behaviors.

Occasionally more aggressive intervention therapy, such as sympathetic nerve blocks, are used when pain is not well controlled by these more conservative measures, when allodynia is so severe that physical therapy is impossible, or when there is no improvement or even further loss of function despite adequate therapy. Sympathetic nerve blocks are not required for diagnosis and no association between the use of blocks and long-term outcome has been made. There are multiple case series and reports on the use of continuous infusions of local anesthetic with or without adjuvants such as opioids, clonidine, or ziconitide administered via peripheral nerve, lumbar sympathetic, epidural, and intrathecal catheters in these disorders (Dadure et al., 2005; Farid et al., 2007; Meier et al., 2009). Most infusions were limited to a few days, although some catheters remained in place for several months. Meier et al. (2009) demonstrated variable effectiveness of lumbar sympathetic blockade in lower extremity CRPS in the first randomized controlled crossover trial ever conducted in adolescent patients with this disease. However, no association between the response to sympathetic nerve blockade and long-term outcome has been shown. On the other hand, Sherry et al. (1999) believe that nerve blocks and medication are unnecessary and may be counterproductive because they reinforce the patient taking a passive, rather than active, role in recovery.

If blocks are considered, the practitioner along with the patient and the patient's family must weigh the risks of the procedure against their potential benefit. Which block to use is based not only on anatomy and physiology but also on local resources and availability and on the practitioner's skills with ultrasound or fluoroscopy for catheter guidance and placement.

When individual patients achieve a therapeutic response to sympathetic block, repeat blocks may be warranted, particularly if this allows the patient to more actively participate in physical therapy. The question of how often and when blocks should be repeated remains unanswered, and improvement in function is a guiding factor.

Finally, the use of neuromodulation (spinal-cord stimulators) in the management of pediatric CRPS is unclear. Spinal-cord stimulators are increasingly being used in adults with CRPS whose conservative treatment has failed, who are psychologically stable, and who can achieve functional status sufficient to participate in exercise after the procedure (Nelson and Stacey, 2006). However, their effectiveness is unclear. Initial favorable reports in adults were followed by less encouraging functional results in the same population 2 to 5 years later (Kemler et al., 2000, 2004, 2008). A case series of seven adolescent girls reported that at least some of the patients who received spinal-cord stimulators entered remission and no longer required the device at a long-term follow-up session, suggesting this modality has potential therapeutic use in pediatric CRPS (Olsson et al., 2008). However, much larger randomized controlled trials are required before this therapy can be recommended in young patients.

Functional Gastrointestinal Disorder

Functional gastrointestinal disorder (FGID) encompasses a group of conditions characterized by chronic or recurrent symptoms that are not explained by biochemical, anatomic, or structural abnormalities (Saps and Di, 2009; Yacob and Di, 2009). Normal gastrointestinal functions include transport, digestion, and absorption of nutrients, and removal of waste products. The gut is also an important immune barrier. Patients with FGIDs experience a constellation of symptoms consistent with abnormalities in these gastrointestinal functions. These include dysmotility, secretory dysfunction, malabsorption, diarrhea or constipation, and allergic enteritis. However, significant weight loss, growth failure, unexplained fever, pain far from the umbilicus, bloody diarrhea, and repeated emesis are rarely associated with FGIDs. Presence of these signs or symptoms should result in a search for an organic process, such as a tumor, mechanical obstruction, infection, or inflammatory bowel disease.

FGIDs are among the most common conditions in childhood and lead to numerous school absences and loss of work by parents. The FGIDs include functional abdominal pain (previously called recurrent abdominal pain), functional dyspepsia, irritable bowel syndrome, and abdominal migraine. Functional or recurrent abdominal pain is a description and not a diagnosis. It is commonly defined by at least three bouts of abdominal pain severe enough to affect the school-aged child's activities over a period of at least 3 months and is not feigned (malingering). The pain is often described as aching, cramping, and persistent and is commonly associated with headaches, recurrent limb pains, pallor, and vomiting. Additionally, there is no, or only an occasional, relationship of the pain with physiologic events such as eating or menses. The etiology is unclear. A diagnosis of abdominal migraine requires at least three or more episodes within 12 months. It is a paroxysmal, intense, acute, midline abdominal pain lasting 2 hours to several days with intervening symptom-free intervals lasting weeks to months. Associated with this abdominal pain are two of the following features:

headache or photophobia during the episode, family history of migraine, headache on one side only, and an aura or warning period. Finally, the patient with irritable bowel syndrome has abdominal discomfort and pain for at least 12 weeks, although not necessarily consecutive weeks over a 1-year span. The pain is relieved by defecation and is associated with a change in stooling form or frequency. To make this diagnosis, structural or metabolic abnormalities that might explain the symptoms must be ruled out.

Treatment

Therapy for FGIDs is largely supportive and has to address contributing psychosocial factors. There are no magic pills, and there is limited evidence to justify the use of drugs or herbal preparations outside of clinical trials (AAP, 2005; Huertas-Ceballos et al., 2008, 2009; Saps and Di, 2009; Yacob and Di, 2009). Pharmacologic therapy is focused on the control of symptoms with prokinetic, antispasmotic, secretory, and coating agents. Anxiolytics and antidepressants are used because of their ability to modulate pain transmission and perception, as well as their potential to address psychological comorbidities. However, if using drugs as a therapeutic trial, clinicians should be aware that these are fluctuating conditions and any response may reflect the natural history of the condition or a placebo effect rather than drug efficacy (Huertas-Ceballos et al., 2008). Indeed, this was confirmed in a large multicenter, randomized, placebo-controlled study of amitriptyline in 83 children with functional abdominal pain that found no statistical difference between amitriptyline and placebo therapy (Saps et al., 2009).

Chronic Abdominal Wall Pain

Although chronic abdominal pain arising from a visceral source is the most common type of abdominal pain, it must be differentiated from pain originating in the abdominal wall. Abdominal wall pain is localized, not diffuse, and on physical examination is exquisitely tender with abdominal wall tensing (Carnett's sign). The abdominal wall is innervated by the seventh to twelfth intercostal nerves. Entrapment of these nerves at the level of the anterior cutaneous branch, as well as in the rectus sheath, has been described in children (Skinner and Lauder, 2007). Successful treatment with rectus sheath blocks has been described and should be made easier with ultrasound guidance (Willschke et al., 2006; Skinner and Lauder, 2007).

Headache

Headaches are a universal feature of the human experience. Studies of Swedish schoolchildren have indicated that 40% of children experience a headache by age 7, 75% experience a headache by age 15, and migraine (one of the most common causes of headache in childhood) occurs in 1% of children by age 7 and 5% of children by age 15 (Bille, 1962). Headaches have a significant impact on the lives of children by causing school absences, poor school performance, and decreased extracurricular activities. Although the majority of patients have benign causes of headaches that can usually be diagnosed by a careful history and physical examination, radiologic evaluation using computed tomography (CT), MRI, or both may be necessary in select cases. Proper diagnosis, treatment, and close monitoring of these patients are extremely important to ensure that serious etiologies are not overlooked.

Pathophysiology

The brain and most of the overlying meninges have no pain receptors and are therefore insensitive to pain. Pain referred to the head arises from intracranial or extracranial arteries, large veins or venous sinuses, cranial and cervical muscles, the basal meninges, and extracranial structures, such as the teeth and sinuses. Thus, traction on vascular structures within the head, dilation or inflammation of cranial vascular structures, displacement of intracranial contents by tumor, abscess, increased intracranial pressure (ICP), and direct pressure on cranial nerves may result in headache. Also, sustained contraction of the head and neck muscles and pathologic processes outside of the head, such as diseases of the paranasal sinuses, eyes, teeth, and bones of the head and face also may result in pain referred to the head.

Pain arising from the cranial circulation and supratentorial structures travels in the trigeminal nerve. This pain is referred to the front of the head. Pain arising from the posterior fossa travels in the first three cervical nerves and is referred to the back of the head and neck and, occasionally, the forehead. Because the posterior fossa is also innervated by the glossopharyngeal and vagus nerves, pain arising from the posterior fossa also may be referred to the ears and throat.

The pathophysiology of a migraine headache requires a more detailed discussion. Migraine is the most common cause of chronic intermittent headaches in children and is associated with cortical hyperexcitability and vasomotor tone changes. During migraine attacks, cerebral blood flow is increased in the upper brainstem, which has a crucial role in initiating the attack. Complex neurochemical changes are associated with migraine; nitric oxide has a key role in the initiation and maintenance of migraine headache. Migraines may or may not be preceded by an aura (a focal neurologic sign). Auras are caused by "cortical spreading depression." This depolarization wave propagates across the brain cortex at 2 to 3 mm/min and is associated with transient depression of spontaneous and evoked neuronal activity. Activation of the trigeminovascular system is pivotal. Afferent fibers, arising from the trigeminal nerve and the upper cervical spinal cord segments, innervate the proximal parts of the large cerebral vessels and dura mater. These sensory fibers terminate within the lower brainstem and upper cervical cord. Nociceptive information is then relayed to the thalamus and cortical pain areas. Depolarization of the trigeminal ganglion or its perivascular nerve terminals activates the trigeminovascular system, giving rise to central transmission of nociceptive information and retrograde perivascular release of powerful vasoactive neuropeptides. Release of CGRP, neurokinin A, and substance P is associated with dural vasodilation and dural plasma extravasation. 5-HT plays an important role in migraine headaches, and 5-HT agonists and antagonists play important roles in therapy. Between attacks, 5-HT plasma levels are low and increase during attacks. These findings suggest selective stimulation of 5-HT_1 receptors to control attacks. Complex genetic factors are involved in migraine, increasing its risk up to fourfold.

Diagnosis

Standardized criteria have been developed to diagnose headache and divides headache into primary and secondary etiologies (Headache Classification Committee of the International Headache Society, 1988). Primary headaches are those that are directly attributed to a neurologic basis and include migraine, tension-type headaches, cluster headaches, and trigeminal autonomic cephalalgias. Secondary headaches are headaches directly attributed to another medical condition, such as headaches associated with space-occupying lesions, inflammation, sinusitis, and abnormalities of intracranial pressure (both high and low pressure) such as pseudotumor cerebri, Arnold-Chiari malformation, or hydrocephalus. Headaches that are associated with focal neurologic signs or symptoms, or that progressively worsen in severity or frequency are suggestive of intracranial pathology, and require neuroimaging by MRI or CT scan as appropriate and subsequent focused therapy. On physical examination, the clinician should look carefully for changes in consciousness, attention, language or memory, cranial nerve asymmetry or papilledema, nuchal rigidity, abnormal tone, gait ataxia, or any new neurologic abnormality.

Migraines and tension type headaches are the most common primary headaches of childhood. Approximately 10% of school-aged children suffer from migraine (Diamond et al., 2007; Silberstein et al., 2007). Migraine duration is generally between 1 to 48 hours. Migraine quality can be unilateral or bilateral, pulsating, moderate to severe in intensity, and aggravated by routine activity. The headache may be accompanied by nausea and vomiting or by photophobia and phonophobia (Headache Classification Committee of the International Headache Society, 1988). About 14% to 30% of children with migraine also experience a migraine aura, indicating focal cortical or brainstem dysfunction. Typical auras include spots, colors, images distortions, and visual scotoma. Interestingly, in adult patients a high prevalence of right-to-left shunting has been described in patients with migraine, especially migraine with aura, and symptoms have improved in some patients after closure of a patent foramen ovale (Nahas et al., 2009).

Migraine variants are headaches that are accompanied or manifested by transient neurologic symptoms. For example, hemiplegic migraine is characterized by the abrupt onset of hemiparesis that is usually followed by a headache. Basilar artery migraine is characterized by dizziness, weakness, ataxia, and severe occipital headache, and opthalmoplegic migraine is associated with orbital or periorbital pain and third, fourth, or sixth cranial nerve involvement. Cyclic vomiting and recurrent abdominal pain, in the absence of primary gastrointestinal disease, are also considered migraine variants. Status migraine is defined as a severely painful, continuous unremitting headache of more than 72 hours' duration (Olesen and Lipton, 2004).

Therapy

Treatment of migraine headaches often involves both pharmacologic and nonpharmacologic therapies. Lifestyle changes can be made to eliminate identifiable headache precipitants. Although these vary from patient to patient, they can include stress, fatigue or lack of sleep, hunger, food additives (e.g. nitrates, glutamate, caffeine, tyramine, and salt), and medications (e.g., oral contraceptives or indomethacin). Prophylacti therapy can be provided if headaches are recurrent or severe enough to interfere with the patient's life, or if they are resistant to acute therapy. The goal of prophylactic therapy is to reduce the frequency, duration, or severity of attacks. In general, these drugs can take as long as 6 to 8 weeks to show improvement in the patient's symptoms. When considering prophylactic therapy, consideration of the risks of long-term drug use as well as the side-effect profile of individual drugs must occur. Multiple classes of drugs have been used as prophylactic therapies, but few controlled studies in children are available.

Mechanisms of migraine prevention are not completely understood. In general, therapies have been focused on the three major theories proposed to explain migraine pathophysiology. The vascular theory attributes migraine pain to vasodilation. The second hypothesis focuses on cortical spreading depression, a neuronal depolarization wave followed by a suppression of bioelectric activity. The third theory postulates that migraine is related to the release of inflammatory neuropeptides from the trigeminal system, which subsequently dilate meningeal blood vessels (Galletti et al., 2009). Interestingly, mutations in voltage-gated calcium and sodium channels have been described in some patients with familial hemiplegic migraine, but whether similar pathologies occur in more standard cases of migraine is unknown (Pietrobon, 2005, 2007).

Prophylactic therapies include β-blockers (e.g., nadolol, propanolol), antidepressants (e.g., amitriptylline), cyproheptadine (periactin—an antihistaminergic, antiserotonergic drug), anticonvulsants (valproic acid, topiramate, gabapentin), and calcium channel blockers (flunarizine, verapamil). Emerging treatments in adults include angiotensin converting enzyme inhibitors, angiotensin II type 1 receptor blockers, and botulinum toxin. These classes of drugs can target multiple cortical and subcortical structures and also modulate peripheral neurogenic inflammation (Galletti et al., 2009).

β-Blockade with propranolol (1 to 3 mg/kg per day divided in 2 or 3 doses), calcium channel blockade with flurarizine, and topiramate treatment have been shown to be effective in ameliorating pediatric migraine (Victor and Ryan, 2003; Cruz et al., 2009). β-Blockade may decrease the frequency and intensity of migraines by increasing arterial tone and hampering vasodilation, or by reducing sympathetic tone. In addition, β-blockade reduces firing of some central noradrenergic neurons, and it may also interact with the serotonergic system, which plays an important role in migraine. Calcium channel blockers such as verapamil (4 to 8 mg/kg per day in three divided doses) may prevent migraine headaches by impairing the activation of neurogenic inflammation, a calcium-dependent process, or by increasing pain thresholds. Anticonvulsants can limit neuronal hyperexcitability through effects on voltage-gated sodium channels. In addition, antidepressants, anticonvulsants, and calcium channel blockers can also influence the serotonergic and dopaminergic systems, which play an important role in migraine pathophysiology.

Once a headache develops, the goals of therapy are to abort an attack and suppress pain, nausea, and vomiting. Often inducing or promoting sleep in a dark and quiet room is helpful in diminishing symptoms. Relaxation techniques, biofeedback, behavioral techniques, and acupuncture may also be helpful. Pharmacologic treatments to interrupt or abort the headache include a number of different classes of drugs. Mild analgesics such as acetaminophen and NSAIDs are often effective in chil-

dren (Hamalainen et al., 1997a; Hamalainen, 2006). Sumatriptan and other members of the triptan family are approved by the FDA for the treatment of adult migraine. Although commonly used in children, none has FDA approval for this indication. These medications are 5-HT$_1$ receptor agonists. Sumatriptan is available as an oral form (25 mg in adolescents), an injectable form (subcutaneous, 3 to 6 mg), and a nasal spray (5 to 20 mg). Nasal sumatriptan has been shown to be effective in pediatric migraine, whereas unlike in adults, the oral form of the drug has not (Hamalainen et al., 1997; Ueberall and Wenzel, 1999; Ahonen et al., 2004). Adverse effects associated with the use of triptans include tingling, dizziness, warm sensations, chest pain, and cardiac arrhythmias. Isometheptene and ergotamines have also been reported to be effective, especially when administered at the onset of the aura or start of the headache (Hamalainen, 2006). However, Hamalainen et al. (1997b) did not see an improvement in headaches after oral dihydroergotamine as compared with placebo in children with therapy-resistant migraines. In those children whose conservative therapy fails and who come to the hospital with status migraine, treatment with multiple doses of intravenous dihydroergotamine has been shown to be effective, although there is a significant incidence of adverse side effects, especially anxiety, nausea, and vomiting (Kabbouche et al., 2009). It should be noted that all abortive medications carry the risk of causing a headache from overuse of secondary medication, defined as a headache on more than 15 days of a month with overuse of acute treatment drugs for more than 3 months and headache that has developed or worsened during the period of medication overuse (Silberstein et al., 2005). When medication overuse headache occurs, a need for multisystem treatment approach may be beneficial (Pakalnis et al., 2007).

Sickle Cell Disease

Sickle cell disease (SCD) is an autosomal-recessive chronic hemolytic anemia characterized by the production of abnormal hemoglobin. A point mutation in the sickle cell β-globin gene results in the substitution of the hydrophobic amino acid valine for a glutamic acid at position 6 in the globin chain. When hemoglobin S tetramers become deoxygenated, valine is able to interact with other hydrophobic residues on neighboring globin chains to form insoluble globin polymers. Whereas polymerization rapidly reverts to normal once hemoglobin is reoxygenated, cells can become irreversibly sickled as a result of oxidative damage to the cell membrane after repeated cycles of sickling and unsickling. Sickle cells display abnormal adhesion to endothelial cells and initiate microvascular occlusion (Vijay et al., 1998; Kaul et al., 1989). Resultant hypoxia causes further sickling, tissue infarction, and the release of inflammatory cytokines. Repeated vasoocclusive crises (VOC) predispose to multiorgan dysfunction and shorten survival (Platt et al., 1991, 1994). In addition, patients with SCD are susceptible to bacterial infections caused by splenic autoinfarction as well as abnormal cell-mediated immunity. Other consequences of SCD include gallstone disease as a result of chronic hemolysis, priapisim, and stroke. Acute chest syndrome, caused by infection or embolic phenomena, is the leading cause of death (Vichinsky, 1991) (see Chapter 36, Systemic Disorders).

VOC are often characterized by excruciating and at times incapacitating pain. It is the most common and debilitating problem encountered by patients with SCD. Many factors have been associated with the onset of acute pain crises, including cold, dehydration, alcohol intake, stress, and intercurrent infection. However, over one half of episodes have no identifiable precipitant. Acute sickle cell pain is primarily the result of tissue ischemia and occlusion of the microcirculation, whereas acute bone pain appears to be the result of avascular necrosis of the bone marrow (Shapiro, 1989; Stinson and Naser, 2003). Painful episodes can begin as early as 6 months of age. Younger children often suffer from finger, toe, and limb pain, whereas in adolescents back and abdominal pain may be the most prominent symptoms. Acute painful episodes include a prodromal period followed by an infarctive phase. Subsequently, a postinfarctive phase characterized by signs of inflammation and persistent severe pain develops and is then followed by a resolving phase during which the pain gradually remits.

Although there is no intervention that completely abolishes sickle cell pain, provision of analgesics is the cornerstone of management, and their use is titrated to the individual patient by taking into account age, developmental status, and emotional state. Painful crises are often managed at home with hydration and oral analgesics. Treatment of mild-to-moderate pain generally includes NSAIDs or acetaminophen. However, because patients with SCD may have hepatic or renal impairment, care must be taken in prescribing these drugs to avoid systemic toxicity. If pain persists, an oral opioid is added to this regimen.

Patients coming to the hospital with sickle cell pain have commonly failed home therapy or may be unable to tolerate oral analgesics because of nausea and vomiting. Sickle cell crisis pain can be excruciating and is the leading cause of emergency room visits and hospital admissions in these patients. When studied, average VAS scores of 9.5 + 0.63 out of 10 have been reported (Ballas, 1997). In that setting, the use of parenteral opioids is common. Once pain has been appropriately assessed, medication is titrated to provide pain relief (Benjamin et al., 1999). Initial doses of opioid are based on a history of what has provided adequate analgesia in the past. Although historically, meperidine was the most commonly prescribed opioid for treatment of SCD pain, it is no longer a first line treatment of acute pain because of the CNS toxicity of its metabolite, normeperidine (Latta et al., 2002). In general, titration schemes involve administration of a loading dose of opioid (e.g., morphine 0.1 to 0.2 mg/kg or hydromorphone 0.01 to 0.04 mg/kg) followed by additional smaller bolus doses (generally one fourth or one half of the loading dose) or initiation of PCA (National Heart, Lung, and Blood Institute, 2002). A prospective controlled trial of morphine PCA showed that PCA was as effective as intermittent nurse-administered intravenous doses of morphine, with 80% of patients describing the PCA analgesic regimen as good to excellent (Shapiro et al., 1993). Once pain has stabilized and the patient can tolerate oral intake, analgesics can be transitioned to an equianalgesic sustained-release oral opioid, in conjunction with rescue analgesia, to treat breakthrough pain.

Unfortunately, even with aggressive, proactive pain management, pain in SCD is often difficult to treat, resulting in therapeutic failure and frustration for both patients and their health care providers. Patients with acute sickle cell crisis pain often report higher pain scores than postoperative patients until they enter the resolving phase of their crisis. They often report 10 out of 10 on a pain scale, even when they appear to their physicians and nurses to be comfortable. This disconnect between subjective and objective assessments can result in a therapeutic dilemma in which patients request more and more opioids and their physicians prescribe less and less. This lack of trust is in part caused by race and a fear of producing drug addiction (Geller and O'Connor, 2008). SCD is a disease primarily of African Americans and it is clear from other studies that African Americans are less likely than Caucasian and Hispanic Americans to be prescribed opioids for even common conditions in the emergency department, such as migraine headaches and fractures (Tamayo-Sarver et al., 2004, 2003).

Although patients with SCD do develop tolerance, as well as physical dependence and at times hyperalgesia, to opioids if they are administered for prolonged periods of time, they do not develop drug addiction at a higher rate than patients with other conditions (Waldrop and Mandry, 1995). Nevertheless, the failure to provide adequate analgesia often results in pseudoaddiction (Elander et al., 2003). Pseudoaddiction arises when a patient's pain is inadequately managed, and the response to this undertreatment is used as evidence for the diagnosis of drug addiction. Pseudoaddiction is postulated to progress through three phases. The cycle begins with "as-needed" dosing of inadequate analgesics for the treatment of continuous or recurrent pain. Initially, the patient merely requests more pain medication. When these requests are overlooked or ignored, the patient then tries to convince the physician of pain by moaning, grimacing, or crying. The physician interprets this behavior as aberrant and again refuses the requested dose escalation. Finally, the crisis phase occurs when the patient increases the level of bizarre, drug-seeking behavior. The cycle continues, with the patient persistently trying to acquire the drug and the physician consistently refusing to treat the pain, resulting in a lack of trust between the two parties and ultimately in the patient being viewed as a drug addict (Weissman and Haddox, 1989).

Opioids, even at high doses, often have limited efficacy in ameliorating sickle cell pain and often produce unwanted side effects such as sedation, constipation, nausea, and vomiting. Thus, other treatments have been used in place of or in conjunction with opioids in an attempt to diminish these side effects. Whereas single doses of an NSAID do not appear to significantly impact on opioid use, multidose parenteral NSAID infusions do seem to result in a significant opioid-sparing effect. Thus, ketorolac is often added to parenteral opioids in an attempt to improve analgesia and diminish opioid consumption. However, because of its impact on renal function, it is recommended that it not be given for more than 5 days in a given month (Feldman et al., 1997). Studies of parenteral corticosteroids also suggest that pain and length of hospital stay can be shortened by their use without producing short-term adverse effects (Dunlop and Bennett, 2006). However, concerns regarding increases in recurrent pain episodes, as well as the side effects of chronic steroids, have limited their clinical use in this setting (Couillard et al., 2007). Although not routinely employed, epidural analgesia with local anesthetic and opioid has also been shown to be effective in treating sickle cell pain and improving respiratory status in patients whose conventional therapy has failed (Yaster et al., 1994a). However, this modality is only effective if pain is localized to areas of the body that can be effectively blocked by epidural analgesia (e.g., chest, abdomen, and lower extremities). In addition, the impact of repeated epidural placements for the treatment of pain in patients with repeated pain crises is unknown. Finally, self-hypnosis, biofeedback, relaxation, and acupuncture have all been reported to be effective in reducing pain in some patients (Zeltzer et al., 1979; Sodipo, 1993).

In addition to recurrent, acute pain, patients with SCD are also at risk of developing chronic pain that can be physically and psychologically debilitating. Causes of chronic pain include arthritis, arthropathy, avascular necrosis, skin ulcers, and vertebral body collapse (National Heart, Lung, and Blood Institute, 2002). Although there are no studies addressing the management of chronic pain in patients with sickle cell disease, sustained-release opioids, such as MS-Contin or methadone, are at times prescribed to provide consistent analgesia (Dunlop and Bennett, 2006). Adjuvant drugs can be prescribed as well.

Ultimately, the best method of sickle cell pain control may involve therapies that decrease the likelihood of VOC by preventing sickling. Hydroxyurea was approved by the FDA for treatment of adults with sickle cell anemia in 1998, and in 2002 the National Heart, Lung, and Blood Institute issued recommendations for its use in children with SCD (National Heart, Lung, and Blood Institute, 2002; Strouse et al., 2008). Hydroxyurea acts in part by inducing the induction of fetal hemoglobin production, which inhibits hemoglobin polymerization and sickling. It also decreases hemolysis and reduces the expression of cell-adhesion molecules that contribute to vasoocclusion (Benkerrou et al., 2002). Studies in children have shown an increase in fetal hemoglobin concentration, a decline in the yearly rate of hospitalizations, and a reduction in pain crises, but long-term effects of hydroxyurea treatment in SCD are still unknown (Strouse et al., 2008).

PALLIATIVE CARE

Despite dramatic advances in the diagnosis and treatment of many pediatric diseases, death during childhood remains a persistent reality, and caring for children during their final days remains a compelling clinical responsibility for pediatric health care providers (Kang et al., 2007). The past decade has seen an enormous shift in the attitudes, beliefs, and practices of pediatric palliative medicine. Palliative care is increasingly being recommended for a variety of pediatric illnesses, including those for which a cure remains possible or even likely (Field and Behrman, 2009; Goldman et al., 2009). The most obvious are those life-threatening diseases for which curative treatment is possible but might fail, such as cancer. Less intuitive, are conditions with long periods of treatment devoted to prolonging life, but without cure, such as Duchenne's muscular dystrophy or children with severe neurologic disabilities (Wusthoff et al., 2007).

The goal of palliative care is to achieve the best quality of life possible for patients and their families. Control of pain, other physical symptoms, and psychological, social, and spiritual problems are vital components of this care. Pediatric palliative care focuses on three prominent aspects of care (Kang et al., 2007; Field and Behrman, 2009; Goldman et al., 2009). First, and arguably most important, is communication. Understanding how disease processes and a person's innate abilities and liabilities affect that communication is essential to building a foundation of collaboration and a sense of teamwork with the patient and family. Second, psychosocial aspects of pediatric palliative care are important to the present and future well-being of the child, the family, and the practitioner. Acknowledging and facil-

itating a family's spiritual needs and involvement in religious traditions that are comforting to them often helps provide meaning to this distressing experience (McSherry et al., 2007). For many families and health care providers the incorporation of religion and spirituality into the medical care of their child and patient can be an integral part of providing comprehensive high-quality palliative care (McSherry et al., 2007). Focusing on these and other issues that affect the children's, families', and practitioners' physical and mental health must be central when caring for dying children. Finally, the aspect that is most easily translated into clinical practice is caring for the specific physical needs of the child being treated. In the ensuing discussion, strategies are provided for managing common symptoms, including pain, dyspnea, agitation, gastrointestinal complaints, and seizures (Lin et al., 2009).

Pain Management

Assessing a child's and family's beliefs about the experience of pain and what it means, as well as the meaning of changes in pain medication, is an important part of pain interventions in palliative care. Pharmacologic management of pain is only one component of treatment and should always be accompanied by behavioral pain management strategies that pay attention to the beliefs that children and family have about the role of pain in the dying process. Communication within the multidisciplinary team is crucial in integrating information from all sources to provide the most accurate and complete assessment. In addition, addressing the family's concerns, as well as those of professional colleagues, openly and with clarity, is extremely important. This form of communication should happen regularly, with enough time for family members to express their concerns and for team members to address them.

No parent or health care provider wishes any child to suffer pain unnecessarily, particularly if they are dying. Indeed, watching a child die in pain is often a caregiver's greatest fear. And yet, there is often reluctance on the parts of parents and health care providers to manage pain aggressively. For many parents, the words *morphine* or *methadone* conjure up a fear of giving up. They also worry that their child will become addicted, that the drugs are too strong, or that the child's quality of life will be impaired by opioid-induced side effects, particularly excessive sedation. Health care providers share many of these beliefs and they may also worry that opioids will shorten their patient's life by inducing respiratory depression. Additionally, there is a fear that escalating opioid doses will induce tolerance and make pain control more difficult as the underlying disease progresses. Thus, there can be a concern about starting analgesics too soon.

Previously in this chapter the principles of pain assessment and the multimodal approach to pain management were discussed. In palliative care, the choice of appropriate analgesics often depends on both the nature of the patient's pain and on a medicine's formulation and route of administration. Thus, it is important to know whether the child is able to swallow liquid, sprinkles, or pills, or if medication can be administered via gastrostomy tube, rectally, or intravenously. For example, extended-release opioid preparations can be applied topically (transdermal fentanyl) or swallowed intact; however, the latter cannot be safely crushed for administration. Sprinkle formulations of morphine are very useful but clog feeding tubes and stick to bottles or cups. When oral administration is not an option, opioids can be given rectally if necessary, but it is preferable to use the intravenous route when available. Because of its unique long $t_{1/2}\beta$ and its NMDA-antagonist effects, methadone is increasingly a favored opioid to use in this patient population. It is equally effective orally and intravenously, can be administered 2 or 3 times a day, and it is particularly useful in managing opioid tolerance and neuropathic pain.

When prescribing opioids for palliative care (or chronic pain) it is essential for the prescriber to ascertain if the patient's local pharmacy has the drug and if the pharmacy will dispense it with subsequent refills. Furthermore, to avoid licensing authority investigation and error, prescribers must use best-prescribing practice (i.e., the prescriptions must be dated, signed, and clearly state that the opioid is being prescribed for a legitimate purpose [palliative care or chronic pain]) (Lee et al., 2008). Unfortunately, even when complying with these regulations, many pharmacies do not fill prescriptions for oral or parenteral methadone or sustained-release oxycodone. Furthermore, individuals who write these prescriptions are at risk of punitive investigations by their licensing authorities and the Drug Enforcement Agency (Jung and Reidenberg, 2006). Indeed, a practice with a large percentage of its patients who are patients with chronic pain and treated with opioids may be a trigger for an investigation.

Gastrointestinal Symptoms

The management of gastrointestinal symptoms, such as nausea, vomiting, constipation, diarrhea, anorexia (loss of appetite), and cachexia (involuntary weight loss and wasting) is fundamental in palliative care (Stanton-Hicks et al., 1995; American Academy of Pediatrics Subcommittee on Chronic Abdominal Pain, 2005). Although opioids are a common cause of these complaints, other causes must be suspected and ruled out. These include increased intracranial pressure, other medications (e.g., chemotherapeutics and antibiotics), metabolic abnormalities (e.g., uremia or hepatic failure), intestinal obstruction (e.g., gastric outlet or bowel), and mucositis. The management of opioid-induced nausea, vomiting, and constipation has been discussed previously, and the treatment strategies are the same in patients receiving palliative care.

Weight loss and malnutrition are often unavoidable symptoms experienced by patients at the end of life and are commonly associated with poor clinical outcome and increased morbidity and mortality (Stanton-Hicks et al., 1995; American Academy of Pediatrics Subcommittee on Chronic Abdominal Pain, 2005). Furthermore, eating and food can hold important meaning for patients and families; thus, anorexia and cachexia can have a negative impact on quality of life far in excess of their clinical impact. Mealtime commonly holds cultural, emotional, and religious significance, and the inability to enjoy food can affect the entire family. Families may believe that providing nutrition may stave off or reverse wasting; however, for children with certain malignant tumors or advanced disease, weight loss may be largely irreversible. Even so, several drugs have shown some benefit in palliating the cachexia associated with advanced cancer and disease. Appetite stimulants such as progestational drugs, corticosteroids, and cannabinoids can offer some improvement in appetite and weight gain, albeit primarily in adipose and not skeletal muscle tissue (Stanton-Hicks, 2003;

Tan et al., 2008). In addition, megestrol acetate and medroxyprogesterone, synthetic progestins, tend to increase a sense of well-being in addition to stimulating appetite (Stanton-Hicks, 2003; Tan et al., 2008).

Neurologic Symptoms

Many children who require end-of-life care may experience seizures, agitation, and somnolence or loss of consciousness as a result of a primary neurologic illness, an overwhelming systemic illness (chronic or acute), a metabolic derangement (e.g., hyponatremia, hypernatremia, or hypoglycemia), or disease progression (e.g., cerebral metastases) (Sherry et al., 1999). Although it is beyond the scope of this chapter to discuss the etiologies and management of these problems in great detail, a general overview of management is provided.

Seizures are paroxysmal discharges of neurons in the brain resulting in alteration of function or behavior. They are an indication of CNS irritability or disease and typically cause significant stress and distress to patients and families. Parents who have witnessed a child seizing commonly state that they believed their child was dying and that they never want to see their child have another seizure. Patients are more likely to express the fear of future mental handicap and embarrassment about losing control of consciousness, bladder, and/or bowel function in front of friends and family. Many seizures are provoked by fever, infection, and electrolyte abnormalities (e.g., hypoglycemia, hyponatremia, hypocalcemia, hypomagnesemia, or hypooxia). If no precipitating cause is found and the events witnessed are real seizures (some conditions, such as syncope, cardiac arrhythmias, and migraines, mimic seizures), the next step in management is to determine the type of seizure that is occurring, because most antiepileptic drugs are prescribed based on seizure type (Sherry et al., 1999).

The most common types of seizures are generalized and partial-onset seizures. Generalized seizures have no apparent focal onset, whereas partial-onset seizures have a focal onset and may remain focal or secondarily generalize. Table 15-12 lists the most common anticonvulsants and their routes of administration. Like opioids, which anticonvulsant to use depends in part on the anticonvulsant's formulation and the route of administration. For children who have recurrent seizures, physicians and caregivers must also plan for the possibility of status epilepticus. Status epilepticus is a single continuous seizure or repetitive seizures lasting more than 30 minutes without recovery of consciousness. Enabling caregivers to initiate treatment of prolonged or repetitive seizures can improve outcome, decrease anxiety, and prevent visits to an emergency department. Several abortive therapies are available. When intravenous access is not available, the most widely used anticonvulsant is rectal diazepam gel (0.2 to 0.5 mg/kg), although intranasal and buccal midazolam are effective alternatives (Farid and Heiner, 2007; Dadure et al., 2009; Rochette et al., 2009). The risk for respiratory compromise is lower with rectal diazepam than with intravenous formulations of the same medication, because absorption is slower and peak concentrations remain lower. When intravenous access is available, status epilepticus is best treated with lorazepam (0.05 to 0.1 mg/kg, at a rate of 2 mg/min) or with a slow infusion of fosphenytoin (20 mg/kg administered at a rate of 3 mg/min).

Agitation is an unpleasant state of increased arousal. It may present as loud or angry speech, crying, increased muscl

TABLE 15-12. Anticonvulsants

Drug	Dose	Therapeutic Plasma Levels (Toxic Levels)	Advantages	Disadvantages
Carbamazepine (Tegretol)	5-10 mg/kg two or three doses/day; Max dose: 35 mg/kg/day up to 1000 mg	8-12 mg/L	Sustained release formulation available Easily obtained blood levels	Bone marrow suppression, idiosyncratic leukopenia, aplastic anemia No IV formulation May sedate initially Hepatic enzyme inducer
Clonazepam (Klonopin)	Initial dose 0.005-0.015 mg/kg two or three doses/day; Max dose: 0.05 mg/kg/day	20-80 ng/mL (>80 ng/mL)	Oral rapid dissolving tablet Anxiolytic	Sedation
Lamotrigine (Lamictal)	Children >16 yr; Initial dose: 50 mg/day	0.25-0.29 mcg/mL	Not sedating BID dosing	No IV formulation Slow titration
Levetiracetam (Keppra)	Initial dose: PO/IV, 2.5-5 mg/kg two doses/day	6-20 mg/mL	Not sedating BID dosing IV formulation No drug interactions	Renal dosing required May exacerbate behavioral problems
Phenobarbital	Initial dose: PO/IV 2.5-4 mg/kg one or two doses/day	10-40 mg/L	Can quickly load via bolus dosing IV formulation Long half-life Readily available blood levels	Sedation Hepatic enzyme inducer Hyperactivity in younger children

IV, Intravenous; *PO,* oral; *BID,* twice daily.

tension, increased autonomic arousal (such as diaphoresis and tachycardia), or irritable affect. It can and often does evolve into delirium with sleep disturbance, confusion, and impaired attention. There are many treatable causes of agitation including pain, dyspnea, muscle spasm, bowel dysmotility, and bladder distention. In addition, acute withdrawal from several drugs, including opioids, benzodiazepines, corticosteroids, and some anticonvulsants can also cause agitation. The initial management of agitation is intuitive and nonpharmacologic. Familiar objects from home, a gentle touch, or a soothing voice are always the first steps. If these fail, and they often do, pharmacologic intervention may be warranted with either benzodiazepines, antipsychotics, or barbiturates (Truog et al., 1992; Sherry et al., 1999; Intenzo et al., 2005).

Dyspnea

Dyspnea, or a feeling of breathlessness, occurs when the respiratory system is unable to meet the body's need for oxygen uptake or carbon dioxide elimination. It commonly occurs in terminal illness either because of an increased oxygen demand (e.g., sepsis or organ system failure) or an inability to excrete carbon dioxide (e.g., muscle fatigue, pneumonia, interstitial lung disease, cystic fibrosis, or neoplasm) (Meier et al., 2009; Lin et al., 2009). There are several ways that dyspnea can be treated, namely positive pressure mechanical ventilation, noninvasive promotion of gas exchange (continuous positive airway pressure [CPAP] or supplemental oxygen), or pharmacologic measures to decrease or suppress the sensation of dyspnea. Positive pressure ventilation and CPAP may improve the physiologic disturbances causing dyspnea, but because they cannot reverse the underlying process, they are generally inappropriate in end-of-life situations. However, supplemental oxygen is not. Although

supplemental oxygen can often ameliorate the symptoms of hypoxemia and dyspnea, oxygen may also reverse the hypoxic drive to breathe and precipitate apnea.

Opioids are the drugs of choice in the treatment of dyspnea (McGrath et al., 2008; Meier et al., 2009; Saps and Di, 2009). All opioids raise the apneic threshold and shift the carbon dioxide response curve to the right; thus, there is no particular opioid that is superior to another for dyspnea. In a patient already receiving opioids, an increase of 25% in baseline dose effectively treats dyspnea. The use of nebulized morphine is controversial but has its advocates (McGrath et al., 2008; Meier et al., 2009; Saps and Di, 2009). It is hypothesized that the receptors in the lungs involved in the sensation of dyspnea are J-type stretch receptors and that the output from these receptors is attenuated by topically applied inhaled opioids (Sethna et al., 2005). Finally, dyspnea can cause anxiety, which can further worsen the sense of dyspnea. When this occurs, benzodiazepines are useful therapeutic adjuncts.

CONCLUSION

The past 30 years have seen a significant increase in research and interest in pediatric pain management. In this brief review the most commonly used agents and techniques in current practice have been consolidated in a comprehensive manner.

For questions and answers on topics in this chapter, go to "Chapter Questions" at www.expertconsult.com.

REFERENCES

Complete references used in this text can be found online at www.expertconsult.com.

Regional Anesthesia

Allison Kinder Ross and Robert B. Bryskin

CONTENTS

R egional anesthesia in infants and children has witnessed an increasing popularity over the years that has taken it from a practice of spinal and caudal procedures, to peripheral and truncal nerve blocks taking advantage of sonographic technology (Rochette et al., 2007). The advances that increased its popularity have presumably also improved the safety of blocks in children, which will ultimately encourage further use of this important practice in intraoperative and postoperative pain management. Despite the advances, it is still important to understand the basics of the practice: the pharmacokinetics and toxicities of local anesthetics and their additives, the anatomy of children at different ages, and the indications and complications of specific regional blocks.

LOCAL ANESTHESIA IN CHILDREN

The pharmacokinetics and pharmacodynamics of local anesthetics differ with the age of the child being treated. Amides, one class of local anesthetics, undergo enzymatic degradation in the liver and should be used carefully, particularly in neonates, infants, and children, because they lack the ability to distribute and metabolize these agents effectively. Ester anesthetic agents are metabolized by plasma cholinesterase and have fewer age-related metabolic differences.

Amides include lidocaine, etidocaine, prilocaine, mepivacaine, bupivacaine, ropivacaine, and levobupivacaine. Although all of these agents have been used for regional anesthesia in adults, etidocaine, mepivacaine, and prilocaine are rarely used in children. The choice of local anesthetic depends not only on the desired onset time and duration of action of the regional block, which will be discussed later, but also on the safety of the agent.

Amide anesthetics are primarily protein bound in the plasma. Bupivacaine, ropivacaine, and levobupivacaine are more than 90% bound to two plasma proteins: α1-acid glycoprotein (high affinity for local anesthetics) and albumin (high volume and relatively low affinity for local anesthetics). It is the free or unbound fraction of the local anesthetic that is physiologically active and is responsible for its effect on the cardiovascular system and the central nervous system (CNS). Infants less than 6 months of age have decreased levels of plasma proteins, resulting in a larger free fraction of local anesthetic, which consequently places this age group at a greater risk for toxicity from these agents (Lerman et al., 1989; Berde, 1992). As an infant matures, the level of plasma proteins increases, and the plasma free-fraction of the drug decreases. Adult levels of protein binding are reached near 1 year of age (Fig. 16-1). Of interest is that α1-acid glycoprotein levels increase in response to surgical stress, and the increased α1-acid glycoprotein ultimately decreases the free fraction of local anesthetic agent. This phenomenon occurs even when total plasma concentration appears to be near toxic levels (Tucker, 1994, 1996; Booker et al., 1996). The liver's cytochrome P450 system is responsible for the metabolism of amide local anesthetics. These enzymes reach adult activity by the first year of life. The immaturity of liver enzymes in neonates and infants contributes to the decreased clearance of amide local anesthetics seen in this time period.

Ester anesthetics such as chloroprocaine and tetracaine depend on plasma esterases for their elimination. The decreased levels of plasma proteins in neonates and infants are reflected in decreased levels of plasma esterases (Zsigmond and Downs, 1971). However, this has not been shown to be of clinical significance, and tetracaine is commonly used for spinal anesthetics in premature infants for inguinal hernia repairs. Chloroprocaine, although not a commonly used pediatric local anesthetic, has been used for caudal anesthesia. It is thought to afford a greater level of safety than amide anesthetics because of its rapid metabolism (Henderson et al., 1993; Tobias et al., 1996).

Safety Issues

Although numerous safety issues need to be considered when taking care of any patient for regional block, the specific issues in children that must be addressed include the age-related risks of local anesthetic toxicity, the placement of regional blocks in anesthetized children, direct nerve toxicity, risk for infection, and the risk for compartment syndrome. Other safety issues will be discussed in their respective sections as they pertain to specific blocks.

Local Anesthetic Toxicity

Children may be at increased risk for toxicity of local anesthetics because of their relatively increased cardiac output and increased systemic uptake of the agent. This increased systemic uptake may result either in direct CNS toxicity by increasing the amount of local anesthetic available to cross the blood-brain barrier, or in direct cardiac toxicity. Lidocaine at plasma levels of 2 to 4 mcg/mL acts as an anticonvulsant, but at 10 mcg/mL it produces convulsions (Dalens, 1995). Neonates, for example, will manifest symptoms of neurotoxicity such as depressed Apgar scores from lidocaine at umbilical venous blood concentrations of 2.5 mcg/mL, significantly lower than the 5 mcg/mL that is associated with neurotoxicity in adults (Foldes et al., 1960; Shnider and Way, 1968; Ralston and Shnider, 1978; Tucker, 1986).

In unmedicated patients, initial symptoms of neurotoxicity include headache, somnolence, vertigo, and perioral or lingual paresthesia. These symptoms and any objective signs of neurotoxicity such as tremors, twitching, shivering, or even convulsions may not be detected in infants and children under general anesthesia. Diagnosis of local anesthetic toxicity in the child under general anesthesia can be made with indirect signs such as muscular rigidity, hypoxemia without other causes, unexplained tachycardia, dysrhythmias, or cardiovascular collapse. General anesthetics are protective from the CNS effects, but general anesthetics are not protective against cardiac toxicity and may even further contribute to the toxicity (Badgwell et al., 1990). In fact, one study found that in anesthetized ewes, blood concentrations of local anesthetics were doubled because of decreased whole-body distribution and clearance (Copeland et al., 2008a). Net uptake of the local anesthetics in both the heart and brain were greater, with slower efflux, under general anesthesia. Although general anesthesia contributed to local anesthetic–induced cardiovascular depression and changed the overall pharmacokinetics, cardiovascular fatalities occurred only in conscious ewes—there were no fatalities in anesthetized ewes that received intravenous local anesthetics (Copeland et al., 2008b).

The original model that existed was that cardiac toxicity occurs because the local anesthetic prevents the fast inward sodium channels in the myocardium from opening. However, the action leading to toxicity is not at only one specific site, and there is evidence that potassium channels are involved with neuronal excitability and nerve conduction (Kindler and Yost, 2005). Manifestations of toxicity from bupivacaine consist of dysrhythmias with evidence of a high degree of conduction block, widening of the QRS, torsades de pointes, ventricular tachycardia related to reentry phenomena, and major cardiovascular collapse with decreased myocardial contractility (deLaCoussaye et al., 1992). Bupivacaine may produce cardiac

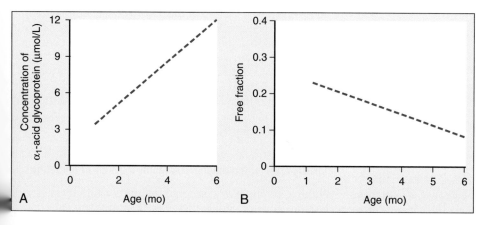

■ **FIGURE 16-1. A,** Age-related changes in plasma concentration of α₁-acid glycoprotein. **B,** Age-related changes in plasma free-fraction of bupivacaine. *(From Mazoit JX, Denson DD, Samii K: Pharmacokinetics of bupivacaine following caudal anesthesia in infants,* Anesthesiology *68:387, 1988.)*

and CNS toxicity at serum concentrations of 2 mcg/mL (Tucker, 1986; Dalens and Mazoit, 1998). Although 4 mcg/mL is considered the toxic threshold for bupivacaine in adults, the true toxic concentration of unbound bupivacaine is unknown in humans, particularly children (Knudsen et al., 1997; Luz et al., 1998; Meunier et al., 2001).

Bupivacaine. Bupivacaine is a racemic mixture of equimolar amounts of the enantiomers R(+) bupivacaine and S(–) bupivacaine. For many years, racemic bupivacaine was the only amide local anesthetic with long duration and therefore the most commonly used amide local anesthetic in children. Pharmacokinetic studies of a single dose of racemic bupivacaine (2.5 mg/kg) injected in the caudal space have demonstrated differences between infants and children (Ecoffey et al., 1985; Desparmet et al., 1987; Mazoit et al., 1988). Infants have a greater volume of distribution (3.9 L/kg versus 2.7 L/kg), an increased elimination half-life (7.7 versus 4.6 hours), and decreased clearance (7.1 versus 10.0 mL/kg per minute) compared with older children (Table 16-1). Although side effects from bupivacaine are rare, they can be serious, ranging from CNS excitation to cardiovascular collapse from direct cardiotoxicity. A series of case reports of possible toxicity of racemic bupivacaine secondary to continuous infusions of bupivacaine were reported in the early 1990s (Agarwal et al., 1992; McCloskey et al., 1992). In the report of McCloskey and coworkers, children had continuous caudal infusions of 0.25% bupivacaine at dosages between 1.67 and 2.5 mg/kg per hour. One neonate sustained bradycardia and hypotension, and two older children developed seizures. Bupivacaine serum concentrations at the time of the event ranged between 5.6 and 20.3 mcg/mL. In the cases reported by Agarwal and associates (1992), one child who developed a seizure had an intrapleural catheter with a bupivacaine infusion rate of 0.5 mg/kg per hour. The seizure occurred with a plasma bupivacaine level of 5.6 mcg/mL. The other child in this report had a continuous bupivacaine epidural infusion at 1.25 mg/kg per hour, and seizures occurred with a plasma bupivacaine level of 5.4 mcg/mL. Thus, all children in the reports from the McCloskey and Agarwal groups had plasma bupivacaine levels that exceeded bupivacaine's toxic threshold of 4 mcg/mL.

These early cases of toxicity prompted an editorial by Berde (1992), who addressed the false generalization that children were more resistant to local anesthetic toxicity than adults. Although earlier studies involving children noted no evidence of toxicity in patients with plasma concentrations of bupivacaine from 1 to 7 mcg/mL, the use of benzodiazepines in those children may have been protective (McIlvaine et al., 1988). Badgwell and coworkers (1990) reported greater resistance to toxicity in 2-day-old piglets compared with older piglets. However, the direct application of this study to neonates is difficult, because neonates have lower plasma protein concentrations and lower bupivacaine clearance. Berde (1992) recommended that maximal allowable dosages of local anesthetics should not be exceeded (Table 16-2), that infusion rates should be reduced in children with risk factors for seizures, and that the maximal allowable dosages should be reduced by at least 30% for infants less than 6 months of age.

Ropivacaine. Ropivacaine has become a commonly used local anesthetic in pediatric patients, with onset times similar to bupivacaine, and durations of actions that are similar or perhaps slightly longer than bupivacaine (Ivani et al., 1998; DaConceicao

et al., 1998, 1999; Lonnqvist et al., 2000; Hansen et al., 2001a; Ivani, 2002). Controversy remains as to the potency of ropivacaine when compared with bupivacaine, and adult studies do not correlate with pediatric studies (Ivani, 2002). Although not confirmed, ropivacaine at 0.2% exhibits the same analgesic effect as 0.25% in children, perhaps because of the intrinsic vasoconstrictive activity that is evident at the lower concentrations used in children (Kopacz et al., 1989; Ivani, 2002). Ropivacaine has a lower risk for CNS and cardiac toxicity than bupivacaine. In fact, inadvertent intravenous ropivacaine in a 1-year-old child failed to produce neurotoxic or cardiotoxic signs or symptoms (Thong et al., 2000). In a pharmacokinetic study of ropivacaine in children ages 1 to 8 who were administered 1 mL/kg of 0.2% ropivacaine for caudal block, the free plasma concentrations were well below toxic levels (Lonnqvist et al., 2000). Clearance of the drug was 7.5 mL/kg per minute, and the terminal half-life was 3.2 hours. Hansen and associates (2001a) studied the pharmacokinetics of caudal ropivacaine in infants less than 1 year of age (see Table 16-1). In this study, infants less than 3 months of age were compared with infants 3 months to 1 year. Although the maximum free concentration of ropivacaine was significantly higher in the younger age group (99 mcg/L versus 38 mcg/L), the total and free plasma concentrations in all of the children less than 1 year were within the range of concentrations previously reported for adults and older children (Lonnqvist et al., 2000; Wulf et al., 2000).

Epidural ropivacaine in children aged 1 to 9 years was studied to determine pharmacokinetics and safety of 24- to 72-hour infusions (Berde et al., 2008). After a 2-mg/kg bolus, an infusion of 2 mg/mL at 0.4 mg/kg per hour was delivered and resulted in plasma concentrations that remained stable throughout the infusion and were well below toxic levels.

Levobupivacaine. Levobupivacaine is the S(–) enantiomer of bupivacaine and is less toxic to the CNS or heart than the racemic bupivacaine (Mazoit et al., 1993; Graf et al., 1997; Huang et al., 1998). The decreased risk for cardiotoxicity from levobupivacaine has been shown in healthy adult volunteers after intravenous administration of either levobupivacaine or racemic bupivacaine (Bardsley et al., 1998). Although similar intravenous studies have not been done in children, animal and human studies suggest less toxicity and equipotency of levobupivacaine compared with bupivacaine (Mather and Chang, 2001; McLeod and Burke, 2001; Gristwood, 2002). In pediatric studies, levobupivacaine has resulted in wide ranges of plasma concentrations when given in the caudal space (Chalkiadis et al., 2004, 2005). When levobupivacaine 0.25% was given in a single-shot caudal dose of 2 mg/mL in children less than 2 years of age, Chalkiadis and coworkers (2004) found that the time to peak plasma concentration ranged between 5 and 60 minutes and was reached later in children less than 3 months of age, and the plasma concentration ranged between 0.41 and 2.12 mcg/mL. In a similar study, but at a dosage of 2.5 mg/kg, the range was 0.62 to 2.4 mcg/mL, with the highest maximum concentration found in a 1-month-old infant (Cortinez et al., 2008). The authors suggested using caution when administering levobupivacaine at 2.5 mg/kg in the caudal space in this age group.

Toxicity Comparison among Commonly Used Local Anesthetics

Multiple studies have compared the risk for toxicity of various local anesthetics. Single high-dosage intravenous injection of

TABLE 16–1. Summary of Pharmacokinetics* of Local Anesthetics in Children

Block and Dosage	Age of Child	C_{max} (mg/L)	T_{max} (min)	Vd (L/kg)	Cl (mL/kg/min)	$t_{1/2}$ (hr)	Reference
Bupivacaine							
Caudal 2.5 mg/kg	1-6 mo	(0.55-1.93)	(10-60)	3.9 ± 2.0	7.1 ± 3.2	7.7 ± 2.4	Mazoit et al., 1988
Epidural infusion 0.2 mg/kg/hr	11 mo-15 yr	nm	nm	nm	6.49 (3.96-11.11)	3.36 ± 0.93	Desparmet et al., 1987
Caudal 2.5 mg/kg	0-5 mo	1.109 (0.6-2.195)	60 (30-240)	nm	nm	2.75 (1.7-4.4)	Hansen et al., 2001b
Caudal 2.5 mg/kg plus epinephrine 2.5 mcg/mL		1.102 (0.449-1.909)	60 (60-360)			6.05 (3.97-8.95)	
Ilioinguinal/iliohypogastric 2 mg/kg (0.5%)	2-16 yr	2.2 ± 1.0	24 ± 11.9	nm	nm	3.6 ± 1.8	Ala-Kokko et al., 2002
Ropivacaine							
Caudal 2 mg/kg	1-8 yr	0.47 ± 0.16	60 (12-249)	2.4 ± 0.7	7.4 ± 1.9	3.2 ± 0.8	Lonnqvist et al., 2000
Caudal 2 mg/kg	< 1 yr	0.73 ± 0.27	60 (15-90)	nm	nm	nm	Wulf et al., 2000
	1-5 yr	0.49 ± 0.21	52.5 (30-120)				
Caudal 2 mg/kg	0-3 mo	.748 (0.425-1.579)	nm	1.99 ± 1.7	4.8 ± 3.6	5.1	Hansen et al., 2001a
	3-12 mo	604 (0.41-1.278)		2.42 ± 2.03	6.5 ± 5.3		
Epidural 1.7 mg/kg	3-11 mo	0.61 (.55-.725)	60 (60-120)	2.37 (9%)	4.26 (9%)	nm	McCann et al., 2001
	1-4 yr	0.64 (.54-.75)	60 (30-90)	2.37 (9%)	6.15 (11%)	nm	
Epidural infusion 0.4 mg/kg/hr	0.3-7.3 yr	nm	nm	3.1 (2.1-4.2)	8.5 (5.8-11.1)	4.9 (3-6.7)	Hansen et al., 2000
Ilioinguinal/iliohypogastric 2 mg/kg (0.75%)	2-16 yr	1.5 ± 0.8	35 ± 15.4	nm	nm	6.5 ± 4.4	Ala-Kokko et al., 2002
Ilioinguinal/iliohypogastric 3 mg/kg (0.5%)	1-12 yr	1.5 ± 0.93	45 (15-64)	nm	nm	2.0 ± 0.7	Dalens et al., 2001

*Values are stated either with standard deviation (±), or with ranges or partition coefficients in parentheses.

Cl, Plasma clearance; C_{max}, peak plasma concentration; nm, not measured; T_{max}, time to peak plasma concentration; $t_{1/2}$, terminal half-life; Vd, volume of distribution.

TABLE 16-2. Local Anesthetics: Guidelines for Maximal Allowable Dosage

Local Anesthetic	Single Dose	Continuous Infusion Rate	Continuous Infusion Rate in Infants (< 6 mo)*
Bupivacaine	3 mg/kg	0.4-0.5 mg/kg/hr	0.2-0.25 mg/kg/hr
Levobupivacaine	3 mg/kg†	0.4-0.5 mg/kg/hr	0.2-0.25 mg/kg/hr
Ropivacaine	3 mg/kg†	0.4-0.5 mg/kg/hr	0.2-0.25 mg/kg/hr
Lidocaine	5 mg/kg	1.6 mg/kg/hr	0.8 mg/kg/hr
Lidocaine with epinephrine‡	7 mg/kg	NA	NA

Modified from Berde CB: Convulsions associated with pediatric regional anesthesia, *Anesth Analg* 75:164, 1992.
*For infants, rate should be reduced by an additional 30% after 48 hours.
†Maximal allowable may be up to 4 mg/kg (under investigation).
‡Epinephrine added to local anesthetic at 5 mcg/mL or 1:200,000.
NA, Not applicable.

the local anesthetics in the ewe model revealed that bupivacaine had the most pronounced changes in electrocardiographic and hemodynamic variables compared with ropivacaine, levobupivacaine, and lidocaine (Guinet et al., 2009). In addition, only the bupivacaine ewes experienced ventricular tachycardia. A recent review suggested that overall, ropivacaine has the greatest margin of safety of the long-acting local anesthetics that are currently available, partially because lipophilicity is a major determinant in local anesthetic toxicity (Zink and Graf, 2008).

Reducing Risks of Toxicity

Several safety measures can reduce the risks of toxicity from local anesthetics in children. One primary safety measure is to avoid overdosing by adhering to recommendations for maximal allowable dosages. For a bolus injection, the maximal recommended dosage of lidocaine is 5 mg/kg. Because epinephrine decreases uptake and absorption of local anesthetic, the dosage of lidocaine can be increased to 7 mg/kg when epinephrine (5 mcg/mL) is added to the local anesthetic. The maximal allowable bolus dosage for bupivacaine, ropivacaine, and levobupivacaine is 3 mg/kg, and the addition of epinephrine does not change the maximum (Agarwal et al., 1992; McCloskey et al., 1992). Recommendations for maximal dosing of continuous infusions (see Table 16-2) are the same for bupivacaine, levobupivacaine, and ropivacaine (Berde, 1992). For epidural infusions, the infusion rates should not exceed 0.4 to 0.5 mg/kg per hour for patients older than 6 months, and the recommendation for neonates is not to exceed 0.2 to 0.25 mg/kg per hour. Based on the clearance of bupivacaine and using the guidelines in Table 16-2, the plasma concentrations should remain below 2.5 mcg/mL and therefore below the toxic level of 4 mcg/mL (Tucker, 1986; Desparmet et al., 1987; Mazoit et al., 1988). These infusions assume a loading dosage of 2 to 2.5 mg/kg of bupivacaine and should be reduced by 25% in patients with risk factors for seizures (i.e., past history of febrile seizures, hypomagnesemia, and hyponatremia) (Agarwal et al., 1992; Berde, 1992).

Although there is extensive literature on maximal allowable dosing of local anesthetics, recommendations in children are mostly extrapolated from adults. Additionally, the recommendations for adults are not evidence based and are in turn extrapolated from animal experiences, blood concentration studies, local anesthetic toxicity case reports, and pharmacokinetics (Rosenberg et al., 2004). In the adult literature, it has

even been suggested that the idea of maximal blanket dosing be abandoned, as it is not scientifically valid or clinically relevant (Heavner, 2004). This criticism suggests that the maximum dosages that are quoted to be valid in all patients are not truly valid, and one blanket recommendation does not actually cover all types of patients or all types of blocks. Instead, block- and site-specific guidelines are needed so that dosing is tailored to the patient's situation. In addition, dosing must be based on children's per-kilogram weight; this is the only way to safeguard the risk of overdosing local anesthetics in different age groups.

The use of ultrasound, because the local anesthetic is deposited directly at the target location, has been shown to reduce overall amounts of local anesthetic needed for specific blocks. This will be discussed in more detail in the section on ultrasound.

In addition to dosing guidelines, the risk for toxicity is also affected by hypothermia, hypoxia, hypercarbia, acidosis, or hyperkalemia (Broadman, 1996). These factors enhance the toxicity of local anesthetics by different mechanisms. Another factor that leads to increased toxicity is the speed of injection of the local anesthetic agent. Rapid injections can cause toxicity by resulting in a rapid high peak that may not allow the sodium channels to adapt for the local anesthetic action.

When local anesthetics are combined, their toxicities are additive. Therefore, if the maximal allowable dosage of one local anesthetic has been reached, another local anesthetic agent should *not* be delivered (Giaufre et al., 1996). Although combining local anesthetics may be common at some centers, maximal allowable dosing should be calculated for each of the anesthetics used and decreased based on the relative percentage of each.

The choice of local anesthetic is a clinical decision. The risks for potential cardiotoxicity have been discussed and should help guide practitioners in choosing a local anesthetic that they feel has the greatest safety margin. After the local anesthetic is chosen, the concentration must be considered. In general, lower concentrations of local anesthetics such as 0.25% bupivacaine or levobupivacaine and 0.2% ropivacaine may be used in infants and small children, and higher concentrations such as 0.5% bupivacaine, levobupivacaine, or ropivacaine should be reserved for older children. Higher concentrations result in longer duration of action and increased motor block, but the total milligram dosage must be calculated carefully. Additionally, in young children there is a risk for direct local anesthetic toxicity on developing nerves (Selander, 1993; Lambert et al., 1994; Radwan et al., 2002). The age at which this is no longer a concern is unknown.

Test dosing. Before injecting local anesthetics, it is essential to determine that the agent will not be injected into the intravascular space. The absence of blood aspiration when administering a pediatric block is not a reliable indicator that the needle is not in a vessel. Infants, in particular, may be at greatest risk of intravascular injection (Freid et al., 1993; Ved et al., 1993; Flandin-Blety and Barrier, 1995). Although clinical practice has relied on a *test dose* to elicit a tachycardia when the test drug is inadvertently injected systemically, the test dose was often considered unreliable in the anesthetized patient and its usefulness continues to be questioned (Desparmet et al., 1990; Sethna and McGowan, 2005). In Desparmet's study of children anesthetized with halothane, only 16 of 21 children who received a test dose of 0.1% lidocaine with epinephrine 1:200,000 had an increase in heart rate that was greater than 10 beats per minute (bpm). Therefore, under halothane anesthesia, an increase of 20 bpm with prior administration of atropine improves the efficacy of the test dose. Sethna and associates (2000) determined that, with the patient under isoflurane anesthesia and after pretreatment of atropine, 0.75 mcg/kg epinephrine was more reliable than 0.5 mcg/kg. All patients in the 0.75-mcg/kg group had heart rate increases of 10 bpm or greater. Isoproterenol has also been used as a test drug, but although it is a more reliable indicator of an intravascular injection in patients anesthetized with halothane (Perillo et al., 1993; Kozek-Langenecker et al., 1996), its safety with neuraxial administration has not been determined, so it is not recommended for this use presently. The validity of test dosing has been studied and reviewed (Tanaka and Nishikawa, 1998, 1999; Tobias, 2001b). With the patient under sevoflurane anesthesia, Tanaka and Nishikawa (1998, 1999) were able to demonstrate that an increase in heart rate of 10 bpm, an increase in T-wave amplitude of 25%, or an increase in blood pressure of 15 mm Hg or more defines the criteria for a positive test dose. Prior administration of atropine did not affect these criteria. Varghese and coworkers (2009) had similar results when 0.1 mL/kg of intravenous 1% lidocaine with 5 mcg/mL epinephrine was injected in children under sevoflurane anesthesia to determine if T-wave amplitude would be visibly detectable on the monitor. An increase in T-wave amplitude in lead II was detected on the electrocardiographic (ECG) monitor in 91% of children and noted on the ECG strip in 94% of children. The amplitude change was considered more reliable for detecting intravascular injection than the increase in heart rate of 10 bpm, which occurred in 64% of children, or the increase of 15 mm Hg or greater in systolic blood pressure, which occurred in 76%. The increase in T-wave amplitude occurred within 30 seconds, as was found in other studies (Tanaka and Nishikawa, 1998; Kozek-Langenecker et al., 2000). Langenecker and associates (2000) delivered an epinephrine solution at 0.5 mcg/kg without being mixed in a local anesthetic and also concluded that the T-wave criterion was more reliable than hemodynamic criteria for a positive test dose.

A test dose can be a useful tool for identifying intravascular injection when the appropriate criteria are used. The test dose should not, however, be a replacement for slow incremental dosing of the total volume of the local anesthetic, with attention to vital sign and ECG monitoring throughout the drug administration. A recommended test dose under sevoflurane anesthesia is 0.1 mL/kg of the chosen local anesthetic with epinephrine 5 mcg/mL added, not to exceed 3 mL. A heart rate increase of 10 bpm, a systolic blood pressure increase of 15 mm Hg, a T-wave amplitude increase of 25% or greater from baseline, or bradycardia should alert the practitioner to possible intravascular injection (Freid et al., 1993; Fisher et al., 1997; Tanaka and Nishikawa, 1998, 1999; Tobias, 2001b).

Although it has not been extensively tested under total intravenous anesthesia (TIVA), there is evidence that the test dose criteria used for determining intravascular injection differ between TIVA and inhaled anesthesia (Polaner et al., 2010). Arterial blood pressure was the most consistent finding, with an increase in all patients of at least 30% within 2 minutes of injection. Heart rate increased by 10 bpm in only 73% of children, and t-wave amplitude was not reliable. Of note in this study, the injectate was 0.1 mL/kg bupivacaine 0.25%, with epinephrine 1:200,000.

Another advantage of epinephrine administration in regional anesthesia is that, in addition to its being a reliable marker for intravascular injection, its use decreases systemic absorption of the local anesthetic (Eyres et al., 1983, 1986). Children may be at increased risk for local anesthetic toxicity from increased systemic absorption because of their relatively higher cardiac output and regional blood flow. In a study comparing bupivacaine with epinephrine 5 mcg/mL to bupivacaine alone in children for fascia iliaca block, Doyle and coworkers (1997) demonstrated that the peak plasma concentration was lower in the bupivacaine-with-epinephrine group (0.35 mcg/mL versus 1.1 mcg/mL), and that the time to peak concentration was more gradual (20 minutes versus 40 minutes from injection). Similarly, the addition of epinephrine to caudal ropivacaine significantly lowers the maximal concentration of ropivacaine and delays the time to maximum concentration, thus improving the safety profile in children (Van Obbergh et al., 2003). In adults, this same delay in systemic absorption and a reduced peak plasma concentration have been shown when epinephrine was added to ropivacaine for paravertebral block (Karmaker et al., 2005). These findings do not suggest that the addition of epinephrine extends the duration of analgesia, but they do demonstrate the effects of epinephrine on the pharmacokinetics of local anesthetics, including those with intrinsic vasoconstrictive properties. Epinephrine (2.5 to 5 mcg/mL) should be added to local anesthetic doses, particularly when large volumes are used, to reduce the risks of local anesthetic toxicity (Rosenberg et al., 2004).

Management of Local Anesthetic Toxicity

Despite all efforts to safely deliver a local anesthetic to a child, it is still possible for local anesthetic toxicity to occur, either by undetected intravascular injection or from inadvertent overdose. When it is apparent that there is local anesthetic toxicity, the practitioner must act quickly to prevent the serious cardiac complications that may ensue. The first steps should focus on the basics, with attention to oxygenation, ventilation, and cardiovascular resuscitation. In particular, hypercarbia must be avoided when resuscitating a patient with local anesthetic toxicity, as an increased $Paco_2$ displaces local anesthetics from their plasma protein binding sites (Burney et al., 1978).

A significant change in the overall management of local anesthetic toxicity has been the introduction of the delivery of a lipid emulsion (Weinberg, 2006). In the clinical arena, lipid emulsion has been used to treat the neurotoxicity and cardiotoxicity that occur from bupivacaine, levobupivacaine, ropivacaine, and mepivacaine (Foxall et al., 2007; Litz et al., 2008; Warren et al., 2008; Marwick et al., 2009). These long-acting local anesthetics are highly soluble in lipid emulsion, and this high binding capacity explains the clinical efficacy of action, although several mechanisms of action have been proposed (Weinberg et al., 2006).

When comparing lipid emulsion (Intralipid) with epinephrine for bupivacaine-induced cardiotoxicity in a rat model, the lipid infusion resulted in better overall resuscitation hemodynamics than epinephrine (Weinberg et al., 2008). In addition, epinephrine resulted in higher lactate levels, hypoxemia, a mixed acidosis, and persistent ventricular ectopy. When compared with saline, epinephrine had similar hemodynamic and metabolic metrics during resuscitation.

Although several case reports in adults have shown success in resuscitation after local anesthetic–induced toxicity, little information related to children has been published (Ludot et al., 2008b). However, there has reportedly been successful resuscitation in at least one infant using lipid rescue for bupivacaine cardiotoxicity (personal communication at Seattle Pediatric Regional Conference, 2009).

Many questions remain regarding the use of Intralipid, and no clear consensus has been reached as to when Intralipid should be delivered (Weinberg, 2009). One school of thought is that the potential risks of administering the high dosages of Intralipid are yet uncertain, and therefore it should be used only after advanced cardiac life support has failed (Corman and Skledar, 2007). Potential risks include infection, intravenous thrombophlebitis, altered inflammatory responses, anaphylaxis, and fat emboli (Brull, 2008). Serum amylase increases and the risk for acute pancreatitis are concerns (Marwick et al., 2009). Certainly for the neonate, who is less likely to be able to handle a large Intralipid load, caution should be used and the risk-benefit ratio weighed prior to dosing. These risks certainly exist, but withholding Intralipid in the event of a local anesthetic–induced arrest would not be advised. The question remains whether it should be the first step in the resuscitation. Intralipid impairs return of cardiac function in the presence of profound hypoxia (Harvey et al., 2009). Likewise, Mazoit and associates (2009) found that a drop in pH, as might occur during resuscitative efforts, decreases the affinity of lipid emulsion for the local anesthetics ropivacaine and bupivacaine. Particularly after the use of epinephrine at dosages of 10 mcg/kg or higher, there is a decrease in successful resuscitation efforts in the presence of bupivacaine toxicity (Hiller et al., 2009). Although epinephrine results in a faster onset of spontaneous circulation than lipid rescue, the effect is not prolonged, and the overall inefficiency in resuscitation in the presence of this dosage of epinephrine probably results from high levels of lactate. These studies would support the early use of Intralipid for improved result.

To effectively use Intralipid, it should be immediately available with clear instructions attached for the practitioner. Dosing guidelines are presented in Box 16-1. As discussed, no specific guidelines have yet been established, and dosing relies only on a series of case reports and animal studies. Nevertheless, having some starting point is essential. A sufficient quantity of Intralipid must be immediately available, as it is possible for a patient to have recurrence of cardiotoxicity after lipid rescue that may require additional support (Marwick et al., 2009). It is important to distinguish that a 20% lipid emulsion has been

Box 16-1 Dosing Guidelines of Intralipid Infusion for Local Anesthetic Toxicity

INITIAL DOSE
1 to 1.5 mL/kg of 20% Intralipid over 1 minute

REPEAT DOSE
Every 3 to 5 minutes during resuscitation

1 to 1.5 mL/kg of 20% Intralipid over 1 minute, up to a total of 3 mL/kg

START INFUSION
On evidence of recovery 20% Intralipid at 0.25 to 0.5 mL/kg/min

effective for resuscitation, not propofol, which is 10% Intralipid and 1% propofol and would contribute further to cardiovascular depression in the arrest situation (Weinberg et al., 2004).

A website (http://lipidrescue.org) was developed to disseminate information about lipid rescue therapy and to allow practitioners to share their experiences.

Regional Anesthesia in the Anesthetized Child

A significant difference between adult and pediatric regional anesthesia is that children typically receive their regional anesthetic while they are under general anesthesia. This practice remains controversial outside of the pediatric arena (Bromage, 1996; Bromage and Benumof, 1998; Rosenquist and Birnback, 2003). Because of issues regarding patient cooperation, the practice of performing a regional anesthetic in children differs greatly from placing a block in an adult. Performing regional anesthetic blocks during general anesthesia in children, including thoracic epidural blocks, is an accepted practice as long as the individual has the proper training and expertise. Over 50 international pediatric anesthesiologists signed an editorial by Krane and coworkers (1998) to support the placement of blocks in anesthetized children. In fact, "It would be considered malpractice to perform such techniques in patients who were *not* fully anesthetized" (Dalens, 1999), and "Any performance of a block in an agitated and moving child is not only unethical, but could be dangerous when the needle approaches the delicate nervous structures" (De Negri et al., 2002). A large retrospective study of 4298 adult thoracic surgical patients who underwent epidural catheter placement while under general anesthesia revealed no neurologic complications including radicular symptoms or persistent paresthesias (Horlocker et al., 2003a).

In children who are under general anesthesia or who are heavily sedated, it may be difficult to recognize intravascular injection of a local anesthetic. Even in the awake child, recognizing the signs or symptoms of local anesthetic toxicity is challenging, and it would be optimistic to think that the child would be able to relay this information early in the injection phase. For this reason, the practice of test dosing with a local anesthetic with the addition of epinephrine has been readdressed, and this should be a common practice as it is more reliable than patient report for detecting or preventing intravascular injection (Tobias, 2001b; Bernards et al., 2008). It is also argued that an anesthetized child cannot warn the practitioner of a significant paresthesia and the potential risk for neurologic injury from intraneural placement of a needle or anesthetic. This is a hypothetical risk that has not been supported by reports of large series of pediatric regional anesthetics (Pietrapaoli et al., 1993; Goldman, 1995; Giaufre et al., 1996).

The American Society of Regional Anesthesia and Pain Medicine issued a practice advisory that was based on evidence and expert opinion as it pertains to performing procedures on anesthetized or heavily sedated patients (Bernards et al., 2008). These recommendations (see Box 16-2) differ somewhat from the recommendations set forth for adults.

An additional concern with regional anesthesia in an anesthetized child is that of "wrong-side block" for a unilateral extremity procedure. Universal protocols must be followed in the conscious child: the operative extremity must be appropriately marked by the surgical team with concurrence of a witness as well as the parent, and the consent must be checked for accuracy regarding the appropriate site. A time-out should occur before blocking the anesthetized child, to again check the consent and marked site. See related video online at www.expertconsult.com.

Direct Nerve Toxicity

The use of local anesthetics and neurotoxicity on the developing nerve is an area that continues to be addressed. Animal data have demonstrated that all local anesthetics are potentially neurotoxic, and this neurotoxicity parallels their anesthetic potency (Selander, 1993). The factors that contribute to the

---

Box 16-2 Recommendations* for Performing Regional Anesthesia in Anesthetized or Heavily Sedated Children

LIMITING LOCAL ANESTHETIC SYSTEM TOXICITY

The potential ability of general anesthesia or heavy sedation to obscure early signs of *systemic local anesthetic toxicity* is not a valid reason to forgo performing peripheral or epidural nerve blocks in anesthetized or heavily sedated patients. (Class I)

LIMITING NEURAL INJURY

There are no data to support the concept that peripheral nerve stimulation or ultrasound guidance, or injection pressure monitoring, reduces the risk for peripheral nerve injury in patients under general anesthesia or heavy sedation. (Class I)

The benefit of ensuring a cooperative and immobile infant or child may outweigh the risk of performing neuraxial regional anesthesia in pediatric patients undergoing general anesthesia or heavy sedation. The overall risk for neuraxial anesthesia should be weighed against its expected benefit. (Class II)

Regardless of wakefulness, infants and children may be unable to communicate symptoms of potential peripheral nerve injury. However, uncontrolled movement may increase the risk for injury. Therefore, the placement of peripheral nerve blocks in children undergoing general anesthesia or heavy sedation may be appropriate after duly considering the individual risk-to-benefit ratio. (Class II)

Modified from Bernards CM, Hadzic A, Suresh S, et al: Regional anesthesia in anesthetized or heavily sedated patients, *Reg Anesth Pain Med* 33:449, 2008.

*Level of evidence is reported in parentheses.

---

mechanism of the neurotoxicity include the concentration of the local anesthetic and the time of exposure of the nerve to the local anesthetic. This is important in children, particularly in neonates, who may be at greatest risk for direct neurotoxicity during nerve development and therefore should not receive the higher concentrations of local anesthetics. Studies on rabbit nerve fibers have demonstrated an increased sensitivity to the blocking effects of local anesthetics in young nerves (Benzon et al., 1988). Additional in vitro biological investigation has demonstrated that lidocaine, bupivacaine, mepivacaine, and ropivacaine are all capable of producing growth cone collapse and neurite degeneration (Radwan et al., 2002). However, the incidence of growth cone collapse with bupivacaine and ropivacaine is insignificant when compared with lidocaine and mepivacaine. This finding has not been consistent. When looking at cytotoxicity of local anesthetics on peripheral nerves by measuring viability and apoptotic activity, although all local anesthetics decreased cell viability in a concentration-dependent fashion, bupivacaine had the greatest effect (Castro-Perez et al., 2009). The order of the killing potency (based the concentration at which 50% of cells are killed, or the median lethal dose [LD_{50}]), from high to low, was bupivacaine, then ropivacaine, then chloroprocaine, then lidocaine, then mepivacaine, and finally, with much lower effect, procaine. Only bupivacaine and lidocaine killed all cells with increasing concentration and could cause apoptosis with either the increased concentration or time of exposure. The authors of the study concluded that cytotoxicity-induced nerve injury may have different mechanisms for the various local anesthetics, and that the targets may not be neurons, because they found that bupivacaine was the most toxic local anesthetic that they tested, but it has a history of having a low incidence of producing transient neurologic symptoms in the postoperative period.

Additional investigation in this area is needed to better understand the mechanisms behind neural injury and how it may affect nerves in children of different ages.

Risk of Infection

Another safety consideration concerns the risk for infection. An initial way to avoid infection is by preparing the skin prior to a regional block. Before placing any block, sterile preparation of the skin should be performed, but this is particularly important for central blocks, to reduce the risk for meningitis or epidural abscess. Chlorhexidine, despite its labeling, is the agent of choice for preparing the skin prior to regional anesthetic block (Hebl, 2006). It is recommended over the use of povidone iodine (Povidine), as it has been shown to decrease colonization when used in young children for epidural catheter placement (Kinirons et al., 2001; Wagner and Prielipp, 2003). In addition, povidone iodine may be harmful to the very sensitive skin of an infant. If used, the povidone iodine should be allowed to dry and not be carried centrally with the needle into the epidural or subdural spaces. After the block has been placed, the iodine should be washed from the skin to avoid iodine burns.

The actual risk for infection from regional techniques, however, is extremely low. For indwelling caudal catheters, the incidence of catheter tip colonization is 20%, as opposed to 4% for indwelling epidural catheters (McNeely et al., 1997b). No patients with bacterial colonization of the catheters exhibited systemic signs of infection. Strafford and associates (1995) studied 1620 children who received epidural catheters. There were no infections in the children who had the catheters placed for postoperative analgesia, and only one significant infection in an immunosuppressed child who received a long-term catheter for pain secondary to her malignancy (Strafford et al., 1995). Adult review has confirmed that infections are typically limited to long-term indwelling catheters in cancer patients (Ruppen et al., 2007). Giaufre and coworkers (1996), in a prospective study of over 24,000 regional techniques performed in children by members of the French-Language Society of Pediatric Anesthesiologists, reported no infections.

Compartment Syndrome

A concern often cited for failure to perform a regional anesthetic in pediatric patients for orthopedic procedures is the risk of an unrecognized compartment syndrome. Compartment syndrome puts the child at risk for muscle ischemia or loss of limb and must be recognized early so that decompressive fasciotomy may occur if necessary prior to these serious complications. The concern focuses on the possibility that the use of a local anesthetic in a regional block may mask the initial symptoms of the sensation of pressure in the limb that occurs with compartment syndrome (Dunwoody et al., 1997). Case reports in children have demonstrated that a successful epidural block with a low concentration of local anesthetic does not mask the symptoms of compartment syndrome. A literature review to assess the risk for compartment syndrome in children who have received epidurals revealed 12 cases (Johnson and Chalkiadis, 2009). In all cases, pain was the primary finding and was considered more severe than the clinical situation would explain. Five of the patients had compartment syndrome as a result of lithotomy position rather than operative site edema. The authors concluded that warning signs of compartment syndrome are the presence of increasing pain or pain that is remote to the site of surgery, an increase in analgesic requirements, paresthesia not due to analgesia, reduced perfusion, swelling, and pain on passive movement. They suggested that the presence of the epidural catheter did not result in delayed diagnosis but instead contributed to deficiencies in the system. Recommendations made included the following: educate staff as to the signs and symptoms of compartment syndrome, identify which patients are particularly at risk through discussion with the surgeon, use dilute local anesthetic solutions, site epidural catheters as close as possible to involved dermatomes, and assess distribution and density of block frequently. Serial examinations should be performed on children to assess the operated extremity in the presence of good analgesia. For the high-risk child, or if any question exists, measure compartmental pressures postoperatively, particularly in children who would clearly benefit from infusions of local anesthetic, such as those who have undergone microvascular surgery or amputation.

Consent Issues

Performance of a regional block must follow the same guidelines as performance of a surgical procedure with consideration of the risk-benefit ratio, a discussion of complications, and appropriate documentation to support its use. Not only should the more common complications be discussed, but the rare, serious complications should also be part of the preoperative consent process with regard to block placement in a

child (Domino, 2007). The manner by which this occurs varies with the country in which the procedure is performed, but some effort must be made to make the parents aware of the purpose, benefits, and risks of regional anesthesia for their child (Lonnqvist et al., 2009).

Reviews of Safety of Regional Anesthesia in Children

Despite the issues of the safety of regional anesthesia in children, studies have shown that the risks and complications of regional anesthesia in children are quite low and often preventable (Dalens and Hasnouai, 1989; Pietropaoli et al., 1993; Giaufre et al., 1996; Dalens and Mazoit, 1998). The largest of these studies was published by the French-Language Society of Pediatric Anesthesiologists (ADARPEF) (Giaufre et al., 1996). This prospective report included 24,409 regional blocks performed over 1 year in children. Central blocks accounted for greater than 60% of the blocks, whereas peripheral nerve blocks and local anesthetic techniques made up the remaining 38%. Only 25 complications occurred in the study, and all the complications occurred in children who received central blocks. Thus, the overall complication rate of regional anesthesia was 0.9 per 1000. The most common complications from regional blockade were inadvertent dural puncture ($n = 8$), inadvertent intravascular injection of local anesthetic ($n = 6$), technical problem ($n = 3$), and overdosing of local anesthesia leading to dysrhythmias ($n = 2$). In addition, two children had transient paresthesias, one child had apnea after central morphine, and one child had a skin lesion after a caudal anesthetic administration. There were no deaths secondary to any of the complications. The conclusion from this study of regional anesthesia in children was that complications were rare and minor, and that they occurred most often in the operating room where they were readily managed. In addition, when appropriate, a peripheral nerve block may be preferable to a central block.

The use of appropriately sized equipment for pediatric regional blocks cannot be overemphasized. The ease of performing a block in a small child is enhanced with the use of shorter, smaller-gauge needles that allow for exact placement. Eleven of the reviewed 23 complications in the large ADARPEF safety study could be attributed to the use of inappropriate equipment.

In a retrospective review of 24,005 regional anesthetics administered over a 10-year period, Flandin-Blety and Barrier (1995) reported 108 events without sequelae (0.45%). However, in this review, five events resulted in severe neurologic injury including tetraplegia in three children, paraplegia in one child, and one child with cerebral lesions. All five of the children were healthy and less than 3 months of age. Four of the five children had loss of resistance to air used in their technique to identify the epidural space. The true pathophysiologic causes for the neurologic injuries in these children are unknown, but the authors recommended that air not be used to identify the epidural space and a lower concentration of epinephrine (e.g., 2.5 mcg/mL) be used to avoid possible ischemic injury. In addition, the authors recommended that the indications for regional anesthesia be reconsidered in children less than 18 months of age because of their incomplete myelination of neuronal fibers.

Recent studies have also looked at new technology and whether these advances have improved the practice of regional anesthesia. Rubin and associates (2009) reviewed the literature on ultrasound-guided blocks and suggested that improved safety features included the need for a lower volume of local anesthetic, and better visibility. How these findings extrapolate to whether ultrasound improves overall safety of regional blocks in children is unclear and not adequately demonstrated except for ilioinguinal blocks.

INTRODUCTION TO ULTRASOUND

Before discussing specific blocks in pediatric anesthesia, the place of ultrasound in the practice of pediatric regional anesthesia should be appreciated. The use of ultrasound for regional anesthesia has experienced immense growth in recent years. The premise of image guidance for nerve localization could not have a better suitor than a developing pediatric anatomy that defies predictable landmarks and has a narrow margin of safety. Despite the demonstrated reduction in the volume of local anesthetic required, the faster onset and longer duration of sensory and motor blocks, and improved quality of sensory block, randomized, controlled studies examining the safety and efficacy of ultrasound-guided nerve blocks in children have been lacking (Marhofer et al.,1997, 1998, 2004; Willschke et al., 2005, 2006a). Therefore, this subject should be approached with the understanding of its evolving nature.

The development of ultrasound technology stems from the principles of piezoelectricity, the ability of crystals and certain other materials to generate an electric potential in response to applied mechanical stress. This effect was first described by brothers Pierre and Jacques Curie in 1880, shortly followed by the demonstration of the converse piezoelectric effect (strain to crystals when an electric field is applied) by Gabriel Lippmann in 1881. However, it took the military innovations of World War I, where ultrasound (sonar) was used to detect submarines, to fuel its use in the medical arena. The first Doppler-assisted nerve block was described in 1978 to locate the subclavian artery for placement of supraclavicular brachial plexus block, but it was not until 1994 that the two-dimensional imaging improved to allow for real-time visualization of the supraclavicular brachial plexus with observation of local anesthetic spread (la Grange et al., 1978; Kapral et al., 1994). Ultrasound guidance has since been used to visualize most remote peripheral and central nerves in both adults and children. This field continues to expand as portable machines with high-resolution capabilities are perfected and three-dimensional ultrasound delineates additional sonoanatomy (Clendenen et al., 2009).

Physics of Sonography

Medical ultrasound produces sound with frequencies in the range of 2 to 15 MHz, in contrast to the range of human hearing (20 to 20,000 Hz). The piezoelectric crystal in the ultrasound transducer propagates pulsed sound waves through the medium and at a regular interval switches to a receiver mode to detect echoes reflected off the tissue interface. Because the velocity of sound in human soft tissue is assumed to be constant at 1540 m/sec, the time lag for sound waves to return to the transducer infers the depth of the reflecting structure, which allows the ultrasound processor to construct an image. The speed of sound is a product of wavelength and frequency

$(v = f \times \lambda)$. Therefore, high-frequency sound waves have shorter wavelengths and generate higher image resolution, and as frequency is lowered, wavelength is increased with diminished image resolution.

Attenuation refers to loss in amplitude of the original signal as the depth of penetration increases. It results from acoustic energy loss to absorption, reflection, and scattering. The degree of attenuation is frequency dependent, with high-frequency waves experiencing a high degree of attenuation, resulting in poor tissue penetration, whereas low-frequency waves achieve deep tissue penetration. The absorption of energy by biological tissues can in theory result in warming of tissues and formation of cavitations. Although no adverse clinical effects have been observed from diagnostic ultrasound, it is prudent to restrict ultrasound use when possible.

Echogenicity is a function of the tissue's ability to reflect oncoming ultrasound beam. Strong reflectors, such as bone, diaphragm, and pericardium, block ultrasound wave transmission and appear as hyperechoic (or bright) images, whereas fluid- and blood-filled structures are ideal sound conduction media and return no reflection, resulting in anechoic (dark) spots. Intermediate reflectors such as solid organs produce hypoechoic (gray) images.

Doppler

When performing regional blocks, it is important to visualize and avoid vascular structures. Color Doppler ultrasonography uses the Doppler effect (a frequency shift that occurs when either a wave source or receiver moves) to assess blood flow and overlays the color velocity mapping on the two-dimensional gray image. The moving red blood cells act as a reflecting medium in the vessels and amplify the perceived signal frequency (red) when moving toward the transducer or diminish it when moving away (blue). The red and blue reflect the direction of the flow to the transducer, *not* whether the flow is arterial or venous. The image appears black when the wave hits red blood cells perpendicular to the flow. Power color Doppler is a recent alternative that enhances flow detection regardless of the angle of incidence, but it lacks directional information (Rubin et al., 1994).

Artifacts

The complex physics behind ultrasound image derivation frequently creates image distortions with no anatomic basis. Accurate interpretation not only avoids erroneous needle adjustment but also guides corrective action (Sites et al., 2007a, 2007b). Suspect structures can be confirmed by examining them in a second plane.

Air or contact artifact is most commonly encountered. It is caused by loss of acoustic coupling between transducer and skin, and it also results from trapped air bubbles under the sterile probe cover. Liberal use of conductive gel, probe cover adjustment, and firm pressure with the transducer corrects this phenomenon.

Acoustic enhancement artifact presents deep to the sonolucent structures (i.e. blood vessels) and results as the beam accelerated by high fluid conduction hits a tissue with a higher attenuation coefficient.

Acoustic shadow artifact results from high beam attenuation by a strongly reflecting surface (bone, kidney or gallbladder stones, and metallic implants) and appears as hypoechoic regions deep to the surface outline.

Reverberation artifact, or ghost images on the deep side of the needle, is caused by repetitive reflection of the ultrasound waves by the transducer–skin interface or another surface with different acoustical resistance. As the reverberated wave gets reflected by the same needle and returns to the transducer, it gives an erroneous impression of having traveled twice the distance of the original wave and is processed as a second needle twice the distance from the original.

Types of Ultrasound Transducers

Selection of transducer type, footprint size, and frequency are critical to successful nerve block performance (Fig. 16-2). Linear transducers produce rectangular images and offer superior sonographic views for superficial structures (<4 cm). This ability makes this type of transducer ideally suited for the majority of pediatric examinations. Hockey-stick probe configuration offers the additional advantage of smaller footprint (25 mm), ergonomic shape capable of navigating the pediatric landscape, and a broadband frequency (6 to 13 MHz) adequate to examine even deep pediatric blocks such as the psoas compartment block. Curvilinear probes create a wedge-shaped image capable of reaching deep structures, but they sacrifice lateral resolution as the beam disperses in the far field of the curved array. This type of transducer is useful for working with teenagers and obese children to perform deeper blocks or for epidural guidance. Phased-array transducers have the smallest footprint and electronically guide their beam to diverge distally. They produce deep panoramic views most suited for transthoracic echocardiography and hold little use for regional practice.

Ultrasound Handling and Image Adjustment

Four basic movements guide transducer handling and facilitate communication for training purposes. *Alignment* is a technique of sliding the transducer to follow the course of the target structure (nerve or needle). *Rotation* refers to clockwise or counterclockwise movement of the probe to capture the needle shaft in the narrow ultrasound beam or to switch from transverse to longitudinal structure sonodissection. Applying *pressure* to the transducer increases depth of the field and helps to differentiate vascular structures (arteries are pulsatile and veins are compressible). *Tilting* denotes angling of the transducer; it improves image quality by changing nerve anisotropy. As the transducer is tilted, scanning the distant field occurs faster than the proximal field. To avoid muscle fatigue and unintended

probe movements, it is helpful to stabilize the transducer by holding the hand against a fixed surface on the patient.

Gain adjustments change amplification of the returning wave and determine brightness of the echo. Both over- and under-gain reduce resolution and lead to loss of information. Modern ultrasound machines allow selective changes to gain in the near/far or entire field and may even be programmed to automatically adjust amplification.

Needle Handling and Tip Localization

Two simple nomenclatures describe needle advancement in relation to the ultrasound transducer. *Out-of-plane* or *cross-sectional* technique positions the needle transverse to the observed image. Although this approach offers the shortest skin-to-nerve distance, with a potential benefit of decreased patient discomfort, the needle shaft and tip are not clearly visualized and are deduced by transducer tilting or alignment, and by tissue movement. *In-plane* or *in-line* technique advocates longitudinal advancement of the needle. This allows complete shaft/tip imaging but requires training, may create reverberation artifact, and may be inappropriate for continuous catheter placement. Hydrolocation refers to injection of a small amount of liquid (0.5 mL) to find the needle tip on the ultrasound image. Needle visualization requires considerable training and is often a source of frustration for beginners. It is prudent to adjust the image by manipulating the transducer rather than by blindly advancing the needle.

Training and Safety

Inexperience is highly correlated with an increased complication rate, and in this age of heightened patient safety, awareness may preclude talented physicians from realizing the benefits of ultrasound-guided regional anesthesia. Recent publications have increasingly focused on optimizing the learning environment and on designing a learner-centered curriculum (Sites et al., 2007c; Smith et al., 2009). The most common novice behavior patterns that were associated with poor block outcomes are as follows: (1) advancement of the needle when the tip was not well visualized, (2) unintentional probe movements, (3) failure to recognize an intramuscular location of the needle tip before injection, (4) poor ergonomics, (5) failure to identify maldistribution of local anesthesia, (6) operator fatigue, (7) failure to correctly correlate ultrasound sidedness to patient's anatomy, and (8) inappropriate choice of needle insertion site and angle.

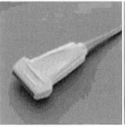 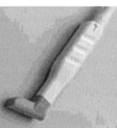 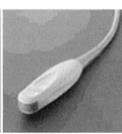 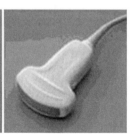

10–5 MHz	10–5 MHz	7–4 MHz	5–2 MHz
38-mm	25-mm	11-mm	60-mm
linear array	linear array	curved array	curved array

■ **FIGURE 16-2.** Types of ultrasound transducers.

Role of the Nerve Stimulator in the Age of Ultrasound

Regional anesthesia took a giant step forward when it abandoned paresthesia and field infiltration for nerve localization and developed a scientifically based, quantitative technique of nerve stimulation (NS). In its 30-year reign, NS has demonstrated a high degree of safety and success rates (Neal et al., 2002). Today, ultrasound guidance offers a qualitative anatomic endpoint, provides the ability to observe local anesthetic spread during injection, and can be used to identify abnormal anatomy. However, it is difficult to be a staunch proponent of solo methodology when both modalities offer complementary evidence of needle-to-nerve proximity and may reduce the time necessary for trainees to successfully reach the desired peripheral nerve block (Orebaugh et al., 2007). Pediatric regional anesthesia presents the additional challenges of working with anesthetized patients unable to report pain on injection, and smaller nerve size that is difficult to locate by NS alone, especially in patients less than 10 years of age (Gurnaney et al., 2007). In addition, NS may yield functional information on proximity to other nerves (phrenic stimulation in parascalene/supraclavicular nerve blocks) and alert to intrafascicular injection when evoked motor response is present with less than 0.2 mA, although this is not a uniform finding (Tsai et al., 2008). Thus, it is reasonable to advocate dual guidance in performing nerve blockade on nerves capable of NS (Gebhard et al., 2008).

The use of ultrasound and peripheral nerve stimulation will be discussed in more detail with regard to specific blocks.

CENTRAL NEURAXIAL BLOCKADE

Central blockade is performed in children for many of the same reasons that it is performed in adults, such as for bilateral lower extremity, abdominal, and thoracic procedures. The risks and benefits to performing central blocks are inherent to the type of block chosen. Central blocks performed in children include spinal blocks and epidural blocks, with the caudal technique being the most commonly used approach to the epidural space. Contraindications to central blockade include a child on anticoagulation therapy, a patient with a preexisting coagulopathy, and a patient or parent who refuses consent for the procedure. The guidelines for regional anesthesia and anticoagulation therapy in adults should be reviewed, as they may be useful for guiding the management of the child (Horlocker et al., 2003b).

Spinal Anesthesia

Spinal anesthesia was a very early form of regional anesthesia that was considered useful for children (Bainbridge, 1901; Tyrell-Gray, 1909). Since that time, spinal anesthetics have become an important anesthetic technique for reducing the incidence of postoperative apnea in premature and expremature infants (Harnik et al., 1986; Welborn et al., 1990; Krane et al., 1995; Somri et al., 1998). Infants who have continuing apnea at home, or a hematocrit of less than 30% are at particular risk for postoperative apnea (Cote et al., 1995; Welborn et al., 1991). Spinal anesthesia may also reduce the need for postoperative mechanical ventilation in infants who are less than 60 weeks of postconceptual age and after hernia repair (Huang and

Hirshberg, 2001). The ability of a spinal anesthetic to densely block the dermatomes involved in inguinal hernia repair has kept this regional technique a popular choice in pediatric anesthesia for inguinal surgery. Often, a spinal anesthetic combined with liberal clear liquids until 2 hours before the procedure, and a pacifier intraoperatively, are enough to keep an expremature infant comfortable while he or she undergoes inguinal hernia repair. However, any expremature infant up to 44 weeks of postconceptual age, and up to 60 weeks of postconceptual age if the infant has risk factors such as anemia or ongoing apnea, should be a candidate for overnight monitoring after the surgery, whether or not a pure regional technique was used.

Although spinal anesthesia may be used in any age group, there are relatively few true indications for a spinal anesthetic in older children, who may be at increased risk for post–dural puncture headaches (PDPHs) from the technique (Wee et al., 1996).

Anatomy

The anatomic differences between an infant and a young child or adult are clinically significant and must be taken into consideration when performing a spinal technique. Common teaching has always suggested that the dural sac in a newborn ends at S3, and the conus medullaris may be located at L3 (Fig. 16-3). Willschke and coworkers (2007), however, in a study of 145 neonates using ultrasound for epidural catheter placement, determined that the termination of the spinal cord in neonates actually ended at a median of L2. Likewise, Shin and associates (2009) found that the end of the dural sac was at a median level of the upper S2 in children less than 36 months of age. Even in children up to approximately 6 years of age, the dural sac ascended only slightly on sonographic examination, to remain near the level of S1 or S2 (Shin et al., 2009). This differs significantly from the final position in adults.

Technique

To administer a spinal anesthetic, one may position the infant on the side with the back flexed, but with the head extended to avoid airway compromise. Some practitioners prefer to have the awake neonate or infant in the sitting position to improve success of the block by increasing the chance of good cerebral spinal fluid (CSF) flow through the needle by increasing the

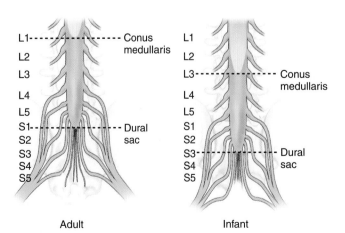

■ FIGURE 16-3. Levels of the conus medullaris and dural sac in infants, compared with the older child or adult.

hydrostatic pressure. In either position, it is important that an assistant keep a firm grasp of the awake infant during the placement of the spinal block. An assistant with a firm hold increases the likelihood of a successful block and decreases the chance of complications.

A sterile preparation and a clear plastic drape are used so that the anatomy may be seen (Fig. 16-4). For neonates and infants, a 1½-inch 22-gauge spinal needle is inserted at the L4-5 interspace. The stylet of the needle should be in place when it is passed through the skin. This avoids the remote risk for an epidermoid tumor (Shaywitz, 1972; Barnitzky et al., 1977). Using this size needle in this age group, a pop will be felt as the needle enters the ligamentum flavum, and another pop as the needle enters the dura. The stylet is removed to check for the flow of CSF. In a baby positioned in the lateral position, if no CSF is evident after what seemed to be appropriate needle placement, then the procedure may be repeated with the infant in the sitting position to improve CSF flow.

In children older than 2 years, a longer needle with a smaller gauge may be used. The smaller-gauge needle may decrease the incidence of PDPH, but it may also make it more difficult for the practitioner to feel the distinctive pop of the needle through the ligamentum flavum. The smaller size needle may inhibit the flow of CSF.

After confirmation of position into the subarachnoid space as evidenced by free flow of CSF through the needle, the local anesthetic solution is slowly injected. After the injection, the needle is removed and the child is placed in the supine position. It is extremely important that the child remain supine and that the legs not be raised for any reason, including placement of electrocautery pad. Lifting the legs will cause the local anesthetic to migrate and result in an undesirable high spinal blockade (Wright et al., 1990).

Dosing

The total volume of CSF in a neonate is 4 mL/kg, compared with 2 mL/kg in an adult, and the hydrostatic pressure is 30 to 40 mm H_2O, lower than that of an adult. In addition, almost half of the total CSF volume is in the spinal subarachnoid space, whereas only one fourth of the total volume in adults is found in the spinal region. These factors play an important part of dosing spinal blocks, as the local anesthetics are quickly diluted by the CSF in a neonate on injection. Infants require higher volumes based on weight, but the duration of action of spinal blocks are shorter than in adults (Rice et al., 1994).

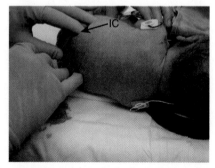

■ FIGURE 16-4. Performance of spinal anesthetic in the neonate. Note how the back is flexed, but the neck remains extended for airway patency. Drape was removed to show anatomy. *IC,* Iliac crest.

Although many different dosing regimens have been used, tetracaine either with or without epinephrine is a commonly employed local anesthetic for spinal anesthesia. Rice and associates (1994) studied 100 infants to determine the duration of spinal block, and the authors compared three groups: lidocaine 3 mg/kg with epinephrine, tetracaine 0.4 mg/kg plain, and tetracaine 0.4 mg/kg with epinephrine. The duration in the lidocaine with epinephrine group was 56 ± 2.5 minutes, the tetracaine plain group was 86 ± 4 minutes, and the tetracaine with epinephrine group was 128 ± 3 minutes.

When using 1% tetracaine for a spinal block in an infant, a dosage of 0.5 mg/kg mixed in an equivalent amount of 10% dextrose to make the solution hyperbaric should provide at least 90 minutes of surgical analgesia. Yaster and Maxwell (1989) suggested that regardless of the infant's weight, 1.5 to 2 mg of tetracaine is the minimal effective dosage. To achieve 5 mg/mL of tetracaine, mix 1 mL of 1% tetracaine with 1 mL of 10% dextrose in water (D10W). The delivered volume is then 0.3 to 0.4 mL for infants less than 10 kg in weight. If 0.01 mL/kg of epinephrine is added to 0.75 to 1 mg/kg of hyperbaric tetracaine, surgical analgesia can be extended up to 120 minutes. Similarly, the use of clonidine will extend a spinal block in a former preterm infant, but the risk for apnea may be increased (Rochette et al., 2005). When using bupivacaine for spinal block, 0.5 to 0.6 mg/kg of either isobaric or hyperbaric bupivacaine will provide an average of 80 minutes of surgical analgesia (Dalens, 2000). Dosing of bupivacaine should be reduced for infants and young children who are greater than 5 kg in weight, because of changes in CSF volume. For infants or toddlers 5 to 15 kg, the dosage of hyperbaric bupivacaine or tetracaine is 0.4 mg/kg or 0.08 mL/kg, and for children weighing more than 15 kg, the dosage of bupivacaine or tetracaine is 0.3 mg/kg or 0.06 mL/kg (Dalens, 1995).

Isobaric ropivacaine has been studied in children for spinal anesthesia at a dosage of 0.5 mg/kg up to 20 mg (Kokki et al., 2005). The mean highest sensory level of block was T6 and duration was 96 minutes with a range of 34 to 210 minutes. Additional study on intrathecal ropivacaine is warranted.

Complications

Complications during spinal anesthesia in children are uncommon. In the ADARPEF study, an intravascular injection during spinal anesthesia was the only reported complication in 506 cases (Giaufre et al., 1996). Although considered to be a rare occurrence in children, the incidence of PDPH is actually between 10% and 50% in children aged 10 to 18 years (Oliver, 2002; Wee, 1996). The onset of symptoms from a PDPH typically occurs within 48 hours, with the hallmark symptom being a frontal or occipital headache that is postural. The cause of PDPH is most likely a persistent leakage of spinal fluid that causes a net decrease in CSF volume and intracranial pressure. The supine position helps to alleviate the symptoms of PDPH by decreasing the effect of gravity on the CSF leak. The size of the dural perforation is the primary predictor of the development of PDPH. To reduce the risk for PDPH, smaller-gauge needles are used, and the needle is inserted with the bevel parallel to the dura's longitudinal fibers (Kokki and Hendolin, 1996). Electron microscopy has revealed that the collagen fibers of the dura are arranged in several layers, and that the thickness of the dura is more predictive of whether a leak will occur than the orientation of the needle's bevel (Turnbull and Shepherd, 2003). This explains the unpredictability of PDPH.

If a diagnosis of PDPH is made, simple measures such as bed rest and hydration can decrease the volume of CSF loss. In addition, analgesics to reduce the headache and intravenous caffeine may be administered. Caffeine is effective because of its ability to cause cerebrovascular vasoconstriction, resulting in decreased cerebral blood flow. In one study, when caffeine was used prophylactically in adults, visual analog pain scores and analgesic demand after PDPH were lower (Yucel et al., 1999). There is no current pediatric dosage recommendation for caffeine. The oral dosage for adult patients is 300 to 500 mg once or twice a day (Turnbull and Shepherd, 2003). The intravenous formulation of caffeine is administered with sodium benzoate. The adult intravenous dosage is 500 mg. This may be repeated within 2 to 4 hours if the headache is unchanged after the first dose (Janssen et al., 2003).

If conservative measures to treat PDPH are ineffective after 48 hours, an epidural blood patch should be considered. This requires that blood be drawn sterilely from a peripheral vein. The blood is then injected into the epidural space under aseptic technique. An epidural blood patch is most effective 48 to 72 hours after the dural puncture, and it may be ineffective if performed immediately after dural tap because high leakage of CSF may interfere with blood clotting (Oliver, 2002). If a child is awake during the placement of an epidural blood patch, the practitioner should stop the injection once the child feels either discomfort or pressure in the back. If a child is anesthetized during the performance of an epidural blood patch, no more than 0.3 mL/kg of blood should be injected into the epidural space (Ylonen and Kokki, 2002).

Total spinal block with respiratory arrest and bradycardia is another complication of spinal anesthesia (Desparmet, 1990). The preganglionic sympathetic blockade that is commonly seen in adults secondary to a high spinal is not typically seen in children, particularly in infants (Oberlander et al., 1995; Finkel et al., 2003; Somri et al., 2003). Dohi and coworkers (1979) were the first to describe the lack of hemodynamic changes after spinal block induced sympathetic blockade in children. They found that children less than 5 years of age had little or no hemodynamic response to a T3-level tetracaine spinal anesthetic, whereas children older than 8 years had cardiovascular responses that were more similar to adults. The mechanism for this lack of hemodynamic sympathectomy was postulated to be the immaturity of the sympathetic nervous system as well as differences in CSF volume and spinal cord surface area. In addition, it is also possible that the smaller blood volume that is present in the lower extremities of a young child compared with that of an adolescent or adult may account for less venous pooling and therefore less hemodynamic change (Dohi et al., 1979; Dohi and Seino, 1986). Despite the typical lack of cardiovascular compromise, neonates occasionally require ventilatory support or pharmacologic intervention because of a high spinal anesthesia with a resulting blockade of the cardiac accelerator fibers or a decrease in stimulation of the right atrial stretch receptors (Wright et al., 1990). Investigation has shown that even former premature infants in the absence of fluid loading tolerate high spinal anesthesia with minimal autonomic changes (Oberlander et al., 1995).

Caudal Anesthesia

Although regional anesthesia in children has a broader scope with the advent of ultrasound, a commonly employed regional block in pediatric practice remains the caudal epidural block. The reasons for the success of this regional technique include not only its extensive safety record for children but also the ease of performing the block and teaching of the technique. See related video online at www.expertconsult.com. Schuepfer and associates (2000) evaluated the technical skills of residents in anesthesiology to determine the learning curve for performing a caudal block in a child. They found that there was a high success rate after only a limited number of cases.

Caudal blocks have great utility in ambulatory surgical patients and for inpatients. They can be administered as a single injection or as a continuous infusion. A caudal block can be used for any surgery that is performed on the lower abdomen or lower extremities (i.e., procedures involving innervation from the sacral, lumbar, and lower thoracic dermatomes). Commonly performed pediatric surgery such as inguinal hernia repair and orchiopexy with their dermatomal distribution below T10 make the caudal block a useful adjunct to the anesthetic. Caudal blocks result in improved patient pain scores when compared with patients having general anesthesia alone (Londergan et al., 1994). Single-shot caudal anesthesia when combined with postoperative ketorolac administration allows children who have undergone intravesical ureteroneocystostomy to be discharged on the day of surgery (Miller et al., 2002). For outpatient urologic procedures, caudal block with light general anesthesia was superior to local nerve block or general anesthesia alone. Single-shot caudal anesthesia has also been used in expremature infants as the sole anesthetic, to decrease the incidence of postoperative apnea, and to avoid the use of general anesthesia and narcotics (Bouchut et al., 2001b).

The practice of placing a caudal block before the incision would seem likely to improve postoperative care by providing preemptive analgesia. The benefit of providing preemptive analgesia through regional block has not been confirmed in pediatric caudal studies. Holthusen and coworkers (1994) noted that there were no significant differences in cumulative postoperative analgesic requirements or cumulative pain scores between children having caudal blocks placed either before or after their circumcisions. In a separate study comparing two groups of children who received caudal blocks for clubfoot repair, Goodarzi (1996) noted that there were no significant differences in the time to first postoperative analgesic administration or in cumulative analgesic requirements for the first 48 hours between the group that received the block before the incision and the group that received the block after the incision. However, it should be realized that placing the caudal at the end of the procedure does not allow the benefit of lower inhaled anesthetic agent concentrations to be used intraoperatively.

Relative contraindications to performing caudal anesthetics in children include the presence of a pilonidal cyst or abnormal superficial landmarks at the sacral level. The presence of these may suggest that the dural sac and cord may not be in their normal anatomic positions. Hydrocephalus and intracranial tumors decrease intracranial compliance and should be considered, at the very least, relative contraindications to caudal or epidural anesthesia. Absolute contraindications include true meningomyelocele of the sacrum or meningitis. Progressive degenerative neuropathy is not an absolute contraindication, but it carries medicolegal implications.

Anatomy

The caudal space is the result of a defect caused by the nonfusion of the fifth sacral vertebral arch. This area of the nonfusion forms the sacral hiatus, the entry into the caudal epidural space. The landmarks around the sacral hiatus are the sacral cornua, the posterior superior iliac spines, and the coccyx (Fig. 16-5). To find the sacral hiatus, one palpates the sacral cornua and the indentation that is immediately caudal and in the midline. If the cornua are difficult to palpate, the general area of the sacral hiatus may be found by palpating the two posterior superior iliac spines, and assuming that a line between these would be the base of an equilateral triangle, the apex should be at the location of the sacral hiatus.

The caudal space itself lies underneath the sacrococcygeal ligament that runs through the sacral hiatus under the skin. At around 7 years of age, the child's caudal space begins to become more angulated and may be difficult to enter. Although it is possible to perform a caudal block in adolescents and adults, the formation of a presacral fat pad in puberty adds to the difficulty of placing the block. It should be remembered that the distance from the skin to the caudal space in neonates is minimal (Fig. 16-6), and because the dural sac may extend to S3 in neonates, the possibility of entering the dural sac in this age group is increased.

Technique

The choice of needle to be used depends on whether the caudal anesthetic is to be a single shot or whether additional dosing will be required. For a single-shot caudal, it is advantageous to use a short-beveled needle with a stylet. One may also use needles such as a blunt 22-gauge needle or an intravenous catheter that do not have stylets, but there is a remote risk of developing an epidermal inclusion cyst or tumor if the epidermis is carried through the shaft of the needle into the neuraxial space (Shaywitz, 1972). A Crawford needle is similar to an epidural Touhy needle, as it has a stylet and is blunt, but a Crawford needle's bevel is in alignment with the shaft of the needle so that a catheter will exit the needle in a straight line rather than at an angle, such as with a Touhy. The Crawford needle is ideal for either single-shot local anesthetic injection or for placement of a caudal epidural catheter.

With the child in the lateral position, flex the hips with the dependent leg less flexed than the top leg (Simm's position).

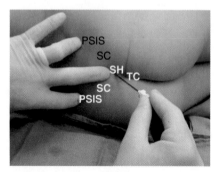

■ **FIGURE 16-5.** Caudal block. Note that an equilateral triangle is formed with the fingertips from the posterior superior iliac spine (*PSIS*) to PSIS to needle insertion at the sacral hiatus (*SH*). *SC*, Sacral cornua; *TC*, tip of coccyx.

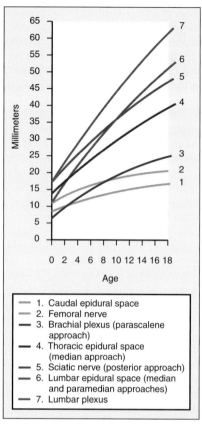

■ **FIGURE 16-6.** Depths to perineural, epidural, and subarachnoid spaces according to age. (*From Dalens B, editor:* Regional anesthesia in infants, children and adolescents, *Philadelphia, 1995, Williams & Wilkins, p 32.*)

Near the cephalad margin of the gluteal crease, feel for the sacral cornua and the sacral hiatus, a depression immediately inferior to these and in the midline. This is the sacral hiatus (see Fig. 16-5). After sterile preparation and draping, identify the sacral hiatus again with the nondominant gloved hand and place the needle into the skin in the midline at a 45-degree angle or less to the skin, aiming cephalad. Resistance might be felt as the sacrococcygeal ligament is penetrated with a pop once the needle has passed into the epidural space. If using a single-injection technique, local anesthetic may be delivered once the sacrococcygeal ligament has been pierced. Frequent aspiration for blood or CSF should occur, as small movements may result in misplacement of the tip of the needle. If using an intravenous catheter for entry into the caudal space, the angle of the needle must be dropped once the sacrococcygeal ligament has been pierced, to align the needle and intravenous catheter with the epidural space. The needle should then be advanced approximately 2 to 3 mm more, so that the catheter may be directly threaded into the epidural space. After a negative aspiration for blood and CSF, the local anesthetic should inject easily without resistance. A finger should palpate the skin cephalad to the injection to ensure that the agent is not being injected subcutaneously. Although air has been used to check for crepitus after injection, this practice is not recommended because of the risk for air embolism (Guinard and Borboen, 1993; Schwartz and Eisenkraft, 1993).

Technique Using Ultrasound

The superficial and mostly cartilaginous posterior vertebral segments of neonates and infants permit sonographic imaging of the neuraxial structures and have been applied to screen for the presence of spinal dysraphism (Kriss and Desai, 1998; Dick et al., 2002; Deeg et al., 2008). The ultrasound-guided caudal single-shot placement has been described in both children (Park et al., 2006; Roberts, 2006) and adults (Klocke et al., 2003; Chen et al., 2004). It decreases the failure rate by locating the sacral hiatus in the difficult-to-palpate patients (obese or older children), and by confirming the cannula placement in the caudal epidural space, thus limiting the incidence of intraosseous, intrathecal, and intravascular injections (Roberts et al., 2005).

A linear ultrasound transducer set at the highest operational frequency should be used to achieve maximal resolution of the superficial neuraxial anatomy. The child is positioned either prone or in a lateral position, with the operator next to or behind the patient, respectively, and with the ultrasound machine in the operator's direct line of view. The ultrasound transducer is placed in a longitudinal midline plane between the two sacral cornua, and the sacrococcygeal ligament is identified (Fig. 16-7, A). The sacral hiatus, visualized between the sacral and dorsal sacra, contains the dural sac and cauda equina. Progressive vertebral ossification limits midline neuraxial imaging in children older than 3 months, but a longitudinal paramedian angle may overcome this problem by scanning through a window lateral to the spinous processes (Marhofer et al., 2005). A needle is advanced in-plane via the sacrococcygeal ligament at approximately a 20-degree angle, and a saline test bolus of 0.1 to 0.3 mL/kg is administered to confirm correct needle position (Park et al., 2006). This injection should produce ventral displacement of the dura, and dilation of the caudal epidural space (see Fig. 16-7, B: Go to www.expertconsult.com to view this image online). In the absence of dural displacement, intrathecal or intravascular needle placement should be considered and the needle replaced. The needle may not be visible under real-time guidance if the insonating angle is misaligned, as may occur with paramedian scanning. If the sacral cornua are not palpable, scanning with the probe in a transverse plane starting at the coccyx and moving cephalad will identify these structures as two hyperechoic mounds connected by a hyperechoic sacrococcygeal ligament.

Dosing

For single-shot caudal anesthesia that will not involve repeat dosing, the goal is to provide the appropriate intraoperative level and a prolonged postoperative analgesia. Although formulas have been developed for determining levels for injection of a single-shot caudal, delivery of 1 mL/kg of local anesthetic with epinephrine (1:200,000) will provide thoracic level anesthesia with a duration of 4 to 6 hours depending on the local anesthetic chosen (Armitage, 1979) (Fig. 16-8). Although 1 mL/kg of local anesthetic would never be injected into the epidural space of an adult, the anatomy of the caudal epidural space in children is such that a high volume is needed to fill the loosely packed space and to spread to reach the appropriate dermatomes. The caudal space communicates freely with the perineural spaces of the spinal nerves, which allows a lower concentration of local anesthetic to be effective. Dosing guidelines are in Table 16-3. Although convention suggests that an increased volume of local anesthetic would be required for adequate block and duration of action, one study found that there was no advantage to increasing the volume of local anesthetic to greater than 0.7 mL/kg (Schrock et al., 2003). In children 1 to 6 years of age undergoing inguinal hernia repair, Schrock and associates (2003) compared three groups, all of whom received 0.175% bupivacaine administered at different volumes (0.7 mL/kg, 1 mL/kg, and 1.3 mL/kg). The durations of action as determined by the time of the first postoperative analgesic were similar for all three groups: 4.2, 3.6, and 4.8 hours, respectively. In addition, there were no differences among the groups with regard to first time to void, ambulate, or discharge. However, in another study, Verghese and coworkers (2002) noted that 1 mL/kg of bupivacaine 0.2% was more effective than a smaller volume (0.8 mL/kg) of 0.25% bupivacaine in blocking the peritoneal response of spermatic

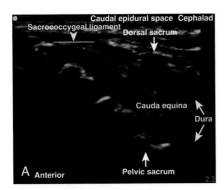

◀ FIGURE 16-7. A, Caudal sonoanatomy. **B,** Caudal sonoanatomy showing space after injection of local anesthetic. *(Go to www. expertconsult.com to view part B online.)*

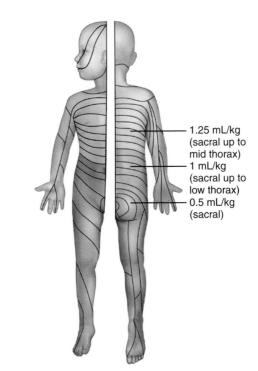

1.25 mL/kg (sacral up to mid thorax)
1 mL/kg (sacral up to low thorax)
0.5 mL/kg (sacral)

■ FIGURE 16-8. Dermatomal distribution of different volumes of local anesthetic for single-shot caudal block.

TABLE 16-3. Dosage Recommendations for Caudal and Epidural Blocks

	Concentration	Dose	Possible Additives
Single-dose caudal	0.175%-0.5%	0.75-1.25 mL/kg, not to exceed 3 mg/kg	Epinephrine 2.5-5 mcg/mL Clonidine 1-2 mcg/kg Morphine 30-70 mcg/kg
Continuous caudal or lumbar epidural catheters	0.1%-0.25%	0.4 mL/kg/hr or 0.2-0.4 mg/kg/hr	Fentanyl 2-5 mcg/mL Hydromorphone 5-10 mcg/mL
Continuous thoracic epidural	0.1%-0.25%	0.3 mL/kg/hr or 0.1-0.2 mg/kg/hr	Fentanyl 2-5 mcg/mL Hydromorphone 5-10 mcg/mL

Bupivacaine, levobupivacaine, or ropivacaine may be used. Greater concentrations and larger dosages should be reserved for levobupivacaine or ropivacaine. Dosages and concentrations should be reduced in infants. Children less than 2 years of age who receive morphine centrally require 24-hour monitoring after its delivery.

cord traction during orchiopexy. The quality of postoperative analgesia was similar in the two groups. When keeping the total dosage of local anesthetic consistent, a higher volume is much more effective than a higher concentration. Hong and associates (2009) demonstrated this effect by comparing a high-volume (1.5 mL/kg), low-concentration (0.15%) ropivacaine solution with a low-volume (1 mL/kg), high-concentration (0.225%) ropivacaine solution and found that the higher volume spread to T6 whereas the lower volume spread to T11. Although there were no differences in postoperative pain scores between the groups, the first time to oral pain medication was at 554 minutes for the high-volume group, compared with 363 minutes for the low-volume group, suggesting a longer analgesic duration when overall dosage is kept constant.

The recommended concentration of bupivacaine for a single-shot caudal is 0.125% to 0.25%, although Gunter and coworkers (1991) in a dose-range study concluded that 0.175% offered the best combination of analgesia and rapid recovery with the least number of side effects.

When performing a single-shot caudal in expremature infants for hernia repair, a combination of agents has been shown to be successful (Bouchut et al., 2001b). A mixture of 0.5 mL/kg of 1% lidocaine, along with 0.5 mL/kg of 0.5% bupivacaine, was used in 25 infants. This combination provided surgical analgesia for 60 minutes. However, one of the 25 infants developed a total spinal block and two children developed postoperative apnea.

Ropivacaine has been evaluated in children for caudal anesthesia and has been found to provide onset and analgesic duration similar to that of bupivacaine (Ivani et al., 1998). In some studies, when compared with bupivacaine, ropivacaine produced less of a motor block at 0.25% and 0.375% concentrations (DaConceicao and Coelho, 1998, 1999). When 0.2% ropivacaine, 0.25% levobupivacaine, and 0.25% bupivacaine were compared in children for caudal anesthesia, postoperative

analgesia was not significantly different among the groups, nor was the time for the first postoperative analgesic (Ivani et al., 2002b; Locatelli et al., 2005). The only difference was a slight reduction in the incidence of motor block in the ropivacaine group.

When using 1 mL/kg of 0.2% ropivacaine, free plasma concentrations were well below toxic levels (Lonnqvist et al., 2000). To determine the effective concentration of ropivacaine for single-shot caudal analgesia, Bosenberg and associates (2002b) compared 1 mL/kg of 0.1%, 0.2%, and 0.3% ropivacaine in 110 children aged 4 to 12 years. The median times to first analgesic were 3.3, 4.5, and 4.2 hours in the groups, respectively. Pain scores were significantly higher in the 0.1% group than in the 0.3% group. Motor block was 0%, 13%, and 28% in the 0.1%, 0.2%, and 0.3% groups, respectively. Bosenberg and coworkers concluded that 1 mL/kg of ropivacaine is effective for postoperative pain in children after inguinal surgery, and that the lower concentration of 0.1% is not effective, and the higher concentrations result in a higher rate of motor block.

In other dosing studies with ropivacaine, Koinig and associates (1999) compared 0.75 mL/kg of 0.5% ropivacaine, 0.25% ropivacaine, and 0.25% bupivacaine in children aged 1.5 to 7 years undergoing inguinal hernia repair. The remarkable finding in this study was the duration of analgesia afforded by 0.5% ropivacaine. The duration in the ropivacaine 0.5% group was 1440 minutes, whereas the 0.25% ropivacaine and 0.25% bupivacaine groups were 208 minutes and 220 minutes, respectively.

For neonates and infants up to 12 months, a single dose of 0.2% ropivacaine at 1 mL/kg resulted in plasma levels that were well below toxic dosages and followed a one-compartment open model (Rapp et al., 2004). The mean peak plasma concentration was 0.83 mg/L for total ropivacaine, and 0.042 mg/L for unbound ropivacaine. The time to first analgesic was 3.9 hours.

Levobupivacaine, the S(−) enantiomer of bupivacaine, has also been used clinically as an alternative to bupivacaine. Ivani and coworkers (2002b) compared 1 mL/kg of caudal 0.25% levobupivacaine with 0.2% ropivacaine and 0.25% racemic bupivacaine in children and noted no significant difference in intraoperative or postoperative analgesia among the three groups. In children less than 2 years of age, a dose of 2 mg/kg of 0.25% levobupivacaine had an efficacy similar to that of racemic bupivacaine, and levobupivacaine had a duration of action of 7.3 hours (Taylor et al., 2003). Ivani and associates (2003) noted the optimum concentration of levobupivacaine at 1 mL/kg for a single-shot caudal without any additive was 0.2%. This dosage provided 118 minutes of postoperative analgesia, compared with 60 minutes for 0.125% and 158 minutes for 0.25%. The advantage of using 0.2% instead of 0.25% was the decreased incidence of motor blockade. Dosing guidelines for levobupivacaine are similar to those for bupivacaine (see Table 16-3). The relative potencies of levobupivacaine and ropivacaine have been compared and found to be similar (Ingelmo et al., 2009). At one minimum alveolar concentration (MAC) of sevoflurane, the median effective dose (ED_{50}) for levobupivacaine was 0.069% and for ropivacaine it was 0.075% in boys aged 1 to 6 years receiving single-shot caudal anesthesia for unilateral groin surgery. The results of the study suggest that the ED_{95} for the local anesthetics would be 0.2% for levobupivacaine and 0.225% for ropivacaine.

Caudal Additives

One of the disadvantages of single-shot caudal anesthesia is the relatively short duration of postoperative analgesia in children, even when using long-acting local anesthetics. Many agents have been studied in an attempt to find an additive that would prolong the duration of analgesia for single-shot caudal anesthesia. Lonnqvist (2005a) addressed the use of adjuncts to caudal block in an editorial. In particular, the editorial pointed out that there are options such as clonidine and ketamine that enhance postoperative analgesia with acceptable safety profiles, and that anesthetists should adhere to existing literature and evidence-based medicine for the use of additives to the caudal space.

Epinephrine

The use of epinephrine for regional anesthetic techniques in children was discussed earlier. It is recommended that epinephrine be added to single-dose local anesthetics at a dosage of 5 mcg/mL or a concentration of 1:200,000. The hypothetical disadvantage of the use of epinephrine is vasoconstriction and possible cord ischemia from impaired flow to the artery of Adamkiewicz (Cook and Doyle, 1996). Therefore, an epinephrine dosage of 2.5 mcg/mL, or a concentration of 1:400,000 may be used as an additive for central blocks (Flandin-Blety and Barrier, 1995).

Epinephrine will serve as a marker for intravascular injection and decrease systemic absorption of local anesthetic. Additionally, epinephrine may prolong the duration of a regional block. Warner and coworkers (1987) compared children aged 3 months to 17 years receiving single-shot caudal block with 0.5 mL/kg bupivacaine 0.25%. One group received the bupivacaine plain, and for the other group, epinephrine 5 mcg/mL was added to the local anesthetic. Epinephrine prolonged the duration of the caudal block analgesia compared with the blocks that did not include epinephrine. The duration of analgesia decreased with increasing age, with the greatest effect on children less than 5 years of age. Children aged 5 years or less had a mean duration of analgesia 10 to 13 hours longer if epinephrine was in the solution. In children aged 6 to 10 years, epinephrine increased the duration of effect by 2 to 3 hours, whereas in children older than 11 years, epinephrine increased the block by 1 to 2 hours. However, in other studies, epinephrine was not shown to prolong a caudal block with bupivacaine (Fisher et al., 1993; Cook et al., 1995).

Ketamine

Preservative-free ketamine has been described for caudal use in children to prolong a bupivacaine block after hernia surgery. Naguib and associates (1991) compared three groups of children receiving either plain bupivacaine 0.25%, ketamine 0.5 mg/kg, or bupivacaine 0.25% plus ketamine 0.5 mg/kg. The group who received only 0.5 mg/kg ketamine had superior analgesia and longer duration of action than the group who had received plain 0.25% bupivacaine. The ketamine group also had similar analgesia and duration of action to the group who received the combination of ketamine and bupivacaine. No postoperative behavior changes were noted in the ketamine groups. These findings have been confirmed in subsequent

studies using 0.5 mg/kg ketamine as an additive to either 0.25% bupivacaine or 0.2% ropivacaine in the caudal space (De Negri et al., 2001a; Weber and Wulf, 2003). Cook and coworkers (1995) studied children aged 1 to 10 years who received caudal anesthesia using 1 mL/kg of 0.25% bupivacaine with the addition of either ketamine 0.5 mg/kg, clonidine 2 mcg/kg, or epinephrine 5 mcg/mL. The ketamine group had a mean duration of analgesia of 12.5 hours compared with 5.8 hours for the clonidine group and 3.2 hours in the epinephrine group. When used alone in the caudal space, ketamine at this dosage of 0.5 mg/kg had a shorter duration of action than bupivacaine 0.25% with 1:200,000 epinephrine, but ketamine 1 mg/kg provided surgical and postoperative analgesia that was equivalent to that of bupivacaine (Marhofer et al., 2000).

Another study using simply ketamine for caudal analgesia without local anesthetic compared a group who received ketamine 1 mg/kg with two other groups who received, in addition to ketamine, clonidine 1 or 2 mcg/kg (Hager et al., 2002). The ketamine group had a mean duration of postoperative analgesia of 13.3 hours. When clonidine 1 mcg/kg or 2 mcg/kg was added to the ketamine, the mean durations were 22.7 hours and 21.8 hours, respectively. This particular study prompted a letter to the editor by Eisenach and Yaksh (2003) that stressed concern over the performance and publications of studies that subjected healthy children to agents that have not had adequate preclinical toxicity studies. Eisenach and Yaksh further discussed the potential risks of neurotoxicity using S(+)-ketamine in the epidural space without significant benefits to the otherwise healthy child. The response to this letter from the authors of the study defended their position with a number of papers on ketamine in the epidural space (Marhofer and Semsroth, 2003). The issue remains controversial, as pointed out in a systematic review of nonopioid additives by Ansermino and associates (2003). This review summarized the findings of randomized control trials performed on children using nonopioid additives in the caudal space and concluded that although clonidine, ketamine, and midazolam increase the duration of analgesia, the potential for neurotoxicity remains a concern with ketamine and midazolam. They also concluded that the routine use of nonopioid adjuvants for elective outpatient surgery had not been shown to improve patient outcome.

What is clear from the studies and editorials is that only preservative-free ketamine should be used when administering it for regional blocks, particularly in the neuraxial space.

Clonidine

Clonidine, an α_2-adrenergic agonist, at 1 to 2 mcg/kg, has been used with success and may result in an additional 4 to 6 hours of analgesia when combined with bupivacaine (Jamali et al., 1994; Lee and Rubin, 1994; Constant et al., 1998; Tripi et al., 2005). Clonidine at 1 mcg/kg, when combined with bupivacaine for caudal block, provided a mean duration of 987 minutes compared with 377 minutes in a group of children who received bupivacaine with epinephrine, versus 460 minutes in children who received bupivacaine plain (Jamali et al., 1994). Ivani et al. (2000) demonstrated that 0.1% ropivacaine plus clonidine 2 mcg/mL provided superior analgesic quality to a caudal block compared with 0.2% ropivacaine without clonidine. The true mechanism of analgesic action of clonidine remains unknown, but there is evidence that it has both central and peripheral sites of action (Ivani et al., 2002a). Although clonidine may cause some sedation, particularly at the higher dosages, and although the sedation has not been considered clinically significant in controlled studies, caudal clonidine has been implicated in case reports as a cause of apnea in neonates (Breschan et al., 1999; Bouchut et al., 2001a).

De Negri and coworkers (2001a) compared ketamine with clonidine to determine which agent would more effectively prolong a ropivacaine caudal anesthetic. Children 1 to 5 years of age received 0.2% ropivacaine 2 mg/kg, ropivacaine plus clonidine 2 mcg/kg, or ropivacaine plus ketamine 0.5 mg/kg for caudal anesthesia. Postoperative analgesia was significantly longer in the ropivacaine with ketamine group (701 minutes) than in the ropivacaine with clonidine group (492 minutes) and the ropivacaine plain group (291 minutes). There were no clinically significant side effects in any of the groups. These findings were similar to the study by Cook and associates (1995) that compared clonidine 2 mcg/kg with ketamine 0.5 mg/kg as additives to 0.25% bupivacaine caudal anesthesia.

When clonidine is directly compared with opioids, its use offers comparable analgesia with fewer side effects. To illustrate this, Vetter and coworkers (2007) used single-shot caudal anesthesia for pediatric patients undergoing ureteral reimplantation. Each child received 1 mL/kg of 0.25% ropivacaine with epinephrine with a caudal additive. The three additive groups were 2 mcg/kg clonidine, 10 mcg/kg hydromorphone, or 50 mcg/kg morphine. Caudal morphine afforded the greatest duration of analgesia, although there was not a statistically significant difference overall. Clonidine appeared to be superior to either caudal morphine or hydromorphone because of its similar analgesic profile and lower incidence of postoperative nausea and vomiting.

Tramadol

Tramadol, an analgesic that acts centrally at opioid receptors, has been compared with bupivacaine alone and a tramadol-bupivacaine combination for caudal analgesia (Prosser et al., 1997; Batra et al., 1999; Gunduz et al., 2001). When 1 mg/kg of tramadol was added to bupivacaine, patients had lower pain scores and longer durations of analgesia than with bupivacaine alone (Batra et al., 1999). When 2 mg/kg of tramadol was added to bupivacaine, some children had sedative effects, but this was not considered to be clinically significant (Gunduz et al., 2001). Caudal tramadol 2 mg/kg provides reliable postoperative analgesia similar to caudal morphine 30 mcg/kg for children undergoing herniorrhaphy (Ozcengiz et al., 2001).

Neostigmine

The use of neostigmine in the epidural space in children is not yet common practice but shows promise. Its action may be attributed to either direct action on the spinal cord via inhibition of the breakdown of acetylcholine in the dorsal horn, or by peripheral antinociceptive effect (Shafer et al., 1998; Yang et al., 1998). A study in children compared three groups to determine the effectiveness of neostigmine (2 mcg/kg) as a caudal analgesic for hypospadias repair, either alone or in combination with bupivacaine (Abdulatif and El-Sanabary, 2002). The groups received 1 mL/kg of either 0.25% bupivacaine plain, bupivacaine with neostigmine 2 mcg/kg, or neostigmine

plain. The combination of bupivacaine and neostigmine provided superior analgesia to either of the other two groups, with a mean duration of 22.8 hours compared with 8.1 hours in the bupivacaine plain group and 5.2 hours in the neostigmine plain group. This prolonged duration when compared with plain local anesthetic has been demonstrated in other studies as well (Mahajan et al., 2004; Kumar et al., 2005). When compared in boys who received levobupivacaine caudal anesthetics for urologic surgery, the addition of neostigmine 2 mcg/kg compared with 4 mcg/kg provided similar duration of postoperative analgesia (15 hours and nearly 20 hours, respectively) and total analgesic consumption (Karaaslan et al., 2009). The higher dosage offered no advantage, and either dosage improved analgesia beyond levobupivacaine plain.

The combination of bupivacaine with neostigmine has been compared not only with plain bupivacaine, but also with other combinations of additives for single-shot caudal anesthetics (Kumar et al., 2005). Duration of analgesia with the bupivacaine-neostigmine group (19.6 hours) was similar to that of a group with bupivacaine and midazolam (16.8 hours), and longer than the bupivacaine plain group (7.6 hours) and bupivacaine-ketamine group (11.6 hours). The dosage of neostigmine used as an additive in this study was 2 mcg/kg. At dosages of 10 mcg/kg and higher, there may be an increased incidence of postoperative nausea and vomiting, which would make this an unattractive alternative as an adjunct to epidural anesthesia; however, no study has attempted to define whether antiemetics will decrease the incidence of nausea and vomiting in this population (Lonnqvist, 2005a; Almenrader and Passariello, 2006).

Note that neostigmine, which typically contains methylparabens and propylparabens as preservatives, should be used only in a preservative-free form when injected into the epidural space. Investigation as to its effect on neural structures is ongoing, and skepticism remains as to whether neostigmine is a viable option for pediatric caudal use (Lonnqvist, 2005a).

Opioids

Opioids have commonly been used in caudal blocks with or without local anesthetic agents. There are two distinct classes of opioids: hydrophilic and lipophilic. In general, hydrophilic opioids such as morphine are capable of rostral spread, whereas lipophilic opioids such as fentanyl remain more localized to the area of injection. This difference accounts for the greater incidence of sedation and respiratory depression that occurs with hydrophilic agents.

Opioids may be used to improve the quality and duration of a block, but there are advantages and disadvantages to spinal axis opioids (Lonnqvist et al., 2002). The major disadvantage of opioid additives is the risk for respiratory depression. In children less than 1 year of age, the risk for respiratory depression from caudal morphine is significantly higher than in children older than 1 year (Valley and Bailey, 1991). In this study of 138 children who had received 70 mcg/kg of caudal morphine, the incidence of clinically significant respiratory depression was 8%. Ten of the 11 children with respiratory depression were less than 1 year of age and weighed less than 9 kg. Seven of the 11 patients also received intravenous opioids. All episodes of respiratory depression occurred within 12 hours of the caudal morphine injection. Spinal axis opioids, because of the risk for delayed respiratory depression, are contraindicated in ambulatory surgical patients. Patients under 1 year of age and patients receiving supplemental intravenous opioids should be carefully monitored postoperatively.

Another disadvantage of neuraxial opioids is the increased incidence of postoperative pruritus, nausea, and vomiting. Although fentanyl 1 mcg/kg may prolong a caudal block, the incidence of pruritus and vomiting also increase (Constant et al., 1998). In one study, the investigation was actually halted because of the unacceptable incidence of postoperative vomiting in a group of children who had received caudal buprenorphine (Khan et al., 2002). Urinary retention is a side effect of caudal morphine and required urinary catheterization in 30% of children in one study using 70 mcg/kg morphine (Irving et al., 1993). Another reason to avoid neuraxial opioids is the availability of alternative additives. As previously discussed, additives such as clonidine and ketamine have been used as adjuncts for central blockade with success and result in fewer side effects compared with opioids.

Despite the pitfalls of using opioids as a component of central blockade, the practice continues because of the relative advantages these agents offer. Preservative-free morphine more than doubles the duration of a single-shot bupivacaine caudal (Krane et al., 1987). In a study of children aged 1 to 16 years, there was a slightly greater incidence of urinary retention, pruritus, and nausea in the group who received caudal morphine, but there was no evidence of delayed respiratory depression even at dosages of 100 mcg/kg in this age group. A caudal morphine dosage of 30 mcg/kg has been recommended for children to provide the advantage of increased analgesic duration with decreased incidence of side effects, particularly respiratory depression (Krane et al., 1989). In children who were undergoing open-heart procedures, a dosage of 70 mcg/kg morphine provided lower pain scores and decreased incidence of atelectatic changes on radiograph compared with a control group who had not received caudal morphine (Rosen and Rosen, 1989). Plasma levels of morphine given via the caudal route peak at 21 ± 4.8 ng/mL approximately 10 minutes after injection (Wolf et al., 1991). These levels are lower than those associated with systemic administration of morphine.

Lipophilic opioids do not offer the same risk for respiratory depression as hydrophilic agents. The disadvantage of the lipophilic agents is the shorter duration of postoperative analgesia than what is provided by morphine, and there may actually be no benefit to the addition of fentanyl to local anesthetic for a single-shot caudal. In most reports, caudal fentanyl 1 mcg/kg has not been shown to increase the duration of analgesia produced by 0.125% bupivacaine, 0.25% bupivacaine, 2% lidocaine, or 0.2% ropivacaine (Jones et al., 1990; Campbell et al., 1992; Joshi et al., 1999; Baris et al., 2003; Kawaraguchi et al., 2006). In contrast, Constant and associates (1998) demonstrated prolongation of analgesia in a study in which fentanyl 1 mcg/kg was added to a mixture of bupivacaine and lidocaine in children aged 6 to 108 months. The mean duration of analgesia in the group was 253 ± 105 minutes compared with 174 ± 29 minutes in the control group without fentanyl. Vomiting occurred in 4 of 15 children who had extradural fentanyl, and in none of the 14 children who had not received fentanyl.

Fentanyl and morphine were compared for efficacy and side effects in children aged 1 to 16 years (Lejus et al., 1994). The children all received a preincision epidural dosage of 0.5% bupivacaine, 0.75 mL/kg, and were then divided into two groups. The morphine group received a preoperative bolus of epidural morphine 75 mcg/kg and the same morphine bolus dose 24 hours later. The fentanyl group received 2 mcg/kg before incision, followed by a continuous infusion of 5 mcg/kg per day. The group who received the fentanyl infusion had comparable analgesia with the morphine group with less pruritus (20% versus 53%), and less nausea and vomiting (0% versus 33%).

Complications

Complications from caudal anesthesia include risks during the performance of the block, risks from injection of local anesthetic, and side effects from the agents used. During the performance of a caudal block, the needle could be accidentally placed into the intravascular space, the subarachnoid space, or the sacral marrow. The incidence of intravascular injection should be decreased with the use of a short-beveled needle, and a test dose should reveal whether the needle is intravascular or in the vascular marrow (Dalens and Hasnaoui, 1989). The detection of a subarachnoid injection may be difficult if CSF is not clearly seen on aspiration prior to local anesthetic injection. In the safety study of Giaufre and coworkers (1996), inadvertent dural puncture was the most frequent complication, but it was still uncommon. In the event the subarachnoid space has been entered, it is possible to reintroduce a needle for a caudal anesthetic; however, the agent should be injected very slowly to avoid the possible migration of local anesthetic solution into the subdural space through any previous puncture sites.

Children differ from adults in that hypotension secondary to centrally delivered local anesthetic is not generally a significant side effect from caudal or neuraxial regional anesthesia. Even without intravascular volume loading before the administration of a central blockade, hypotension is typically not observed in children less than 5 years of age (Dohi et al., 1979; Dohi and Seino, 1986). This may be because of the immature sympathetic nervous system, or because the lower extremities, in proportion to overall body size, do not provide a significant volume for venous pooling.

Studies have been performed in children to investigate the hemodynamic response to caudal analgesia. Doppler studies to investigate hemodynamic changes have demonstrated that cardiac output does not change during caudal anesthesia in infants (Payen et al., 1987). A study to investigate pulmonary Doppler flow revealed that the pulmonary flow velocity changes during caudal anesthesia, presumably secondary to an increase in pulmonary artery resistance (Ozasa et al., 2002). Because the change may have reflected local anesthetic–induced vasoconstriction, the authors concluded that caudal epidural anesthesia is not recommended in children with pulmonary hypertension.

Urinary retention, although a concern, is not considered a frequent side effect in single-shot caudal anesthetics. Fisher and associates (1993) reviewed the postoperative voiding interval in children who received either bupivacaine caudal anesthesia with and without epinephrine, or ilioinguinal hypogastric nerve blocks. They noted no significant difference in the time to micturition among these groups. Although the range of times to first micturition varied widely, from 25 to 630 minutes, no children required any intervention for urinary retention.

Complications from intravascular injection and accumulation of local anesthetics have previously been discussed.

Continuous Caudal Catheters

Intraoperatively, an indwelling catheter may be placed in the caudal epidural space. These catheters allow additional dosing of the local anesthetic agents at the end of the procedure or in the recovery area prior to catheter removal. A repeat or second dose of local anesthetic can be safely administered 90 to 120 minutes after the initial dose as long as the maximal allowable dosage is not exceeded in that time period. In addition, continuous caudal block may be used as an alternative to spinal anesthesia in the expremature infant who is at risk for postoperative apnea while undergoing inguinal hernia repair. This technique has been used with success with and without a concomitant general anesthetic (Henderson et al., 1993; Peutrell and Hughes, 1993; Tobias et al., 1996).

The presence of a caudal catheter allows continued postoperative pain management in children. Continuous infusions, although commonly used because of their ability to provide complete postoperative analgesia, have come under scrutiny because of a lack of prospective outcome studies that demonstrate benefit (Chalkiadis, 2003). Audits of postoperative infusions have demonstrated that 17% to 22% of patients require premature termination of the infusions. In 67% of these patients, the termination was because of an unacceptable rate of side effects or complication (Wilson and Lloyd-Thomas, 1993; Wood et al., 1994). This high rate leads one to question the benefit of neuraxial analgesia over intravenous analgesia (Chalkiadis, 2003). This side effect may be greater for lipophilic infused epidural opioids (e.g., fentanyl), because the catheter tip must be positioned at the interspace corresponding to the dermatomes of the surgical procedure. Another issue that argues against placing and maintaining a continuous epidural catheter includes the dissatisfaction of having a motor block in children. There may also be an increased incidence of postoperative urinary retention and pruritus in children who receive infusions of neuraxial opioids (Lloyd-Thomas and Howard, 1994). Although these side effects are not necessarily dangerous, they do result in increased workload for medical staff, additional medications, and child and parent distress. More serious issues with continuous caudal infusions include the rare risks of epidural hematomas, epidural infection and abscesses, and respiratory depression from central opioids. In addition, there is the cost of the epidural catheter kits, the operative time to insert the caudal and urinary catheters, and the postoperative costs for pharmacy, nursing, on-call staff, and a pain service. Therefore, it has been suggested that continuous infusions be reserved for those children who would truly receive a direct benefit.

Technique

The anatomy of and entry into the caudal space for placing a continuous catheter via the caudal route have already been described. In threading a caudal catheter, the space should first be dilated with a push of preservative-free normal saline. The catheter is then threaded through the needle until the tip of the catheter reaches the estimated desired level. The caudal approach to placing a lumbar or thoracic catheter in infants was described by Bosenberg and coworkers (1988). Because of the loosely packed fat in the epidural space, a catheter should be advanced easily. If resistance is felt, it is most likely because

the catheter has coiled or doubled back in the epidural space. In older children who may have more densely packed epidural fat, the use of a catheter with a stylet may increase the success rate (Gunter and Eng, 1992). In addition to using a catheter with a stylet, other means to improve success are dilating the space with preservative-free normal saline prior to catheter placement, flexing the hips to straighten the spine, and using fluoroscopy to ensure proper catheter tip position. If an angiocatheter has been used for insertion of the catheter, the catheter may be withdrawn, twisted, and advanced through the plastic introducer until the desired position as determined by radiography is obtained. Catheters should not be withdrawn through metal needles because of the risk of shearing the catheter into the epidural space.

Success in placing a thoracic catheter via the caudal route is variable. In a study of 86 infants who had caudal placement of a thoracic catheter that was confirmed by x-rays, the positions of 28 of these catheters were considered to be inadequate (Valairucha et al., 2002). Of the 28, 10 were determined to be in the high thoracic or cervical regions and were able to be pulled back, 17 were coiled in the lumbosacral area, and one was outside the epidural space in the presacral area. Thus, radiographic confirmation of catheter tip position for thoracic catheters that are threaded from the caudal route is essential, and 0.5 mL Omnipaque 180 (Amersham Health, Princeton, NJ) may be used for this indication. Rather than using radiographic evidence to help determine proper placement of the catheter tip, Tsui and associates (1998) described the use of low-current electrical stimulation during advancement of the catheter, resulting in muscle twitching at the corresponding dermatome. Although the immediate feedback on location of catheter tip helps to identify desired placement, it is unclear whether this method offers advantages over or higher success rate than conventional methods such as cutaneous landmarks and simple catheter measurement (Goobie et al., 2003).

Technique with ultrasound. The advancement of the epidural catheter from the sacral hiatus and tip positioning under the ultrasound guidance has been described (Chawathe et al., 2003; Roberts and Galvez, 2005). This technique avoids patient exposure to radiation and contrast injection and is independent of the neuromuscular blockade or local anesthetics use (Asato and Goto, 1996; Tsui et al., 1998; Valairucha et al., 2002). The catheter is introduced via a previously positioned caudal cannula and is advanced while being sonographically imaged. The catheter is followed cephalad with the ultrasound probe in the longitudinal paramedian plane by direct visualization, which is easiest with styletted catheters, or its level is inferred by the anterior dural displacement with saline injection. Scanning the neuraxial structures in the transverse plane allows direct catheter visualization and is less dependent on bony ossification (Fig. 16-9).

Dosing

Continuous caudal catheters that have their tip in the sacral or lower lumbar areas will be dosed differently from those that have been threaded to the low to mid thoracic levels. Suggestions for dosing are in Table 16-3. Continuous caudal catheters require large volumes of local anesthetic to fill the loose caudal epidural

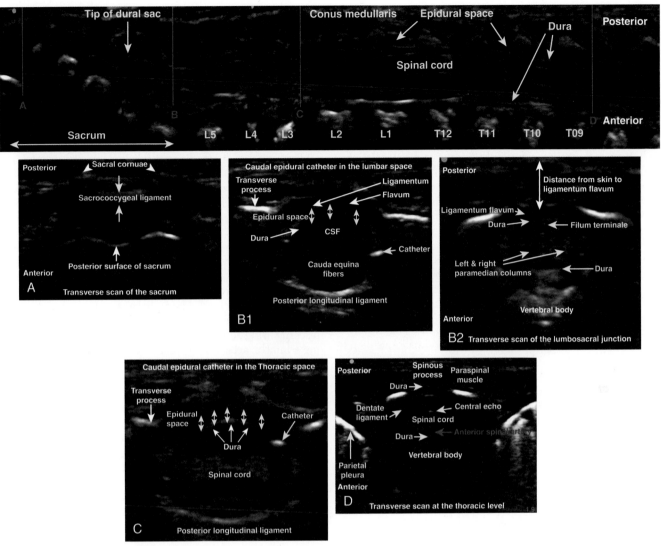

FIGURE 16-9. Panoramic view of epidural space. **A,** Cross-section at sacral cornuae. **B,** Cross-section at lumbosacral junction. **C,** Cross-section at lumbar spine. **D,** Cross-section at thoracic spine.

space and to spread the anesthetic cephalad to the desired dermatomal level. It is important to refer to the maximal allowable dosing recommendations so that these rates are not exceeded in an attempt to "drive up" the epidural block from the caudal space (see Table 16-2). Bupivacaine, ropivacaine, and levobupivacaine may be used for continuous caudal anesthesia, with or without additives. It is possible to improve the analgesia of a continuous caudal catheter by adding a hydrophilic opioid such as preservative-free morphine or hydromorphone to the infusion.

In addition to a continuous infusion, children can also benefit from patient-controlled epidural analgesia, which allows the patient to receive analgesia at the press of a button. Its popularity in children began in the late 1980s with intravenous opioids and has expanded to local anesthetic infusions for a variety of blocks. In a study of children who had undergone a total of 132 procedures and who used patient-controlled epidural analgesia postoperatively, more than 90% had satisfactory analgesia with no significant adverse effects (Birmingham et al., 2003). This study confirmed that children as young as 5 years have the cognitive ability to use of patient-controlled analgesia.

Complications

Complications of continuous caudal infusions are typically secondary to the agent that is being delivered. The risk for local anesthetic toxicity has been discussed, and there is ample evidence that the use of bupivacaine at dosages over 0.2 mg/kg per hour in infants and 0.4 mg/kg per hour in children older than 6 months may lead to neurotoxicity or cardiovascular collapse (Agarwal et al., 1992; Berde, 1992, 1993; McCloskey et al., 1992).

In addition to the risk for serious complications, minor complications such as urinary retention, muscle weakness, itching, or nausea and vomiting can occur. Lowering the concentrations of local anesthetics and avoiding opioids in the central infusion can reduce these risks. This regimen, however, puts the patient at greater risk of experiencing postoperative pain.

Continuous indwelling caudal catheters would seem to offer a risk for fecal contamination and infection. When caudal catheters have been compared with epidural catheters, caudal catheters were found to have a greater incidence of colonization of bacteria (20% versus 4%), with *Staphylococcus epidermidis* being responsible for the vast majority of colonizations (McNeely et al., 1997b). In addition, four of the nine caudal catheter tips that were colonized involved gram-negative bacteria. Caudal catheter tip colonization was not predicted by duration of catheterization, skin inflammation, or dressing contamination. None of the children developed signs of epidural infection, either in the hospital or during the 3-month follow-up. Another study demonstrated the absence of epidural abscess or clinically significant infection from indwelling catheters for postoperative pain (Strafford et al., 1995). An option for children who are to have prolonged analgesia provided by a continuous caudal or epidural catheter is to tunnel the catheter under the skin (Aram et al., 2001). This should allow a longer-term infusion of agents by decreasing the chance of catheter dislodgment and protecting against colonization and infection.

Epidural Anesthesia

Epidural anesthesia is commonly used for procedures that involve surgery of the mid to upper abdomen and thorax that are less amenable to a continuous caudal anesthetic. Children who have procedures that have higher morbidity rates such as Nissen fundoplication may benefit from perioperative epidural analgesia (McNeely et al., 1997a; Wilson et al., 2001). Postoperative complications and hospital stay may be reduced with the use of an epidural for this procedure compared with opioid analgesia alone (Miller et al., 2002). In addition, the use of epidural anesthesia is associated with a significantly reduced stress response to surgery in children, as determined by lower cortisol level and plasma epinephrine levels (Murat et al., 1988; Wolf et al., 1993).

Although lumbar epidurals are commonly employed, thoracic epidurals should be performed only by practitioners who are experienced in their use and should be reserved for children with pulmonary disease or who are to undergo a surgical procedure in the thoracic or upper abdominal area that is associated with significant postoperative pain. See related video online at www.expertconsult.com. As discussed, under continuous caudal anesthesia, a catheter may be threaded from the caudal space cephalad to the thoracic region to provide more site-specific analgesia without the risks associated with placing a needle in the thoracic spine. However, threaded catheters from the caudal space are frequently positioned poorly. In older children, a thoracic epidural inserted between T4 and T8 should attenuate the stress response associated with thoracic surgery and provide optimal postoperative analgesia (Hammer, 2001). Thoracic epidural catheters that are placed intraoperatively by the surgeon prior to wound closure for anterior spinal fusion and instrumentation for scoliosis have been shown to be safe and effective (Lowry et al., 2001).

Anatomy

The epidural space in children is divided into the sacral, lumbar, thoracic, and cervical levels. The caudal block enters at the sacral level. A lumbar epidural needle or catheter is typically placed at the L3-4 interspace, which in older children is found at the center of a line drawn between the two iliac crests. Although these landmarks are accurate in older children, the intercrestal line may actually cross the L5-S1 interspace in neonates, and the L4-5 interspace in infants up to a year of age because of the lag of the growth of the spinal cord (see Fig. 16-3). Because of the developmental changes that occur with the spinal cord and dural sac positions, placing an epidural catheter below the level of the intercrestal line (e.g., the caudal area) may decrease the risk of a wet tap in a neonate or young infant.

Epidural pressures differ depending on the age of the patient. Infants have narrow epidural spaces and are more likely to exhibit leak around an epidural catheter from a backflow of solution if injected too quickly (Vas et al., 2001). Even at slow injection rates, epidural pressures in infants are higher than in adults.

The anatomy of the thoracic spine is similar to that of the lumbar spine with some exceptions. The spinous processes in the thoracic area are longer and the interspinous spaces narrower. These differences necessitate that the epidural needle be placed at a sharper angle in a cephalad direction. The ligaments in the thoracic area are more lax and may be more difficult to discern during needle placement when compared with performing a lumbar needle insertion. Third, and most important, the spinal cord occupies most of the spinal canal in the thoracic area, leaving little margin for error once the needle reaches the epidural space.

The depth to the epidural space at the L2-3 level is approximately 10 mm at birth, and this depth increases linearly with age. The approximate expected distance from the skin to the epidural space in children aged 6 months to 10 years is approximately 1 mm/kg body weight (Bosenberg, 1995). See Figure 16-6 for approximate depths from the skin to the lumbar and thoracic epidural spaces at different ages.

Technique

With the child in the lateral position and knees and hips flexed, the line that joins the two iliac crests crosses the body of S1 in neonates, L5 in infants, L4-5 in young children, and L4 in older children and adolescents (Busoni and Messeri, 1989). After sterile preparation and draping, the needle should be placed in the midline between the spinous processes that are closest to the line that crosses the iliac crests. If performing a lumbar epidural puncture, the spinous processes require the needle to be directed slightly cephalad, but mostly perpendicular to the skin. The needle is advanced slowly, with one hand firmly against the child's back and holding the portion of the needle that is entering the child's skin. This is to avoid any inadvertent and rapid advancement of the needle. The needle will pass through skin, subcutaneous tissue, supraspinous ligament, interspinous ligament, and then ligamentum flavum before entering the epidural space (Fig. 16-10). Because of the risk for air embolus, a continuous-loss-of-resistance technique using saline rather than air to confirm the epidural space is the recommended approach (Sethna and Berde, 1993). The ability to feel entry into the ligamentum flavum and the loss of resistance as the epidural space is entered is subtler in infants than in adults. Once the catheter is threaded into the epidural space and there is negative aspiration for CSF or blood, the local anesthetic with epinephrine should be injected as an initial test dose before delivering the planned dose of local anesthetic. Compared with

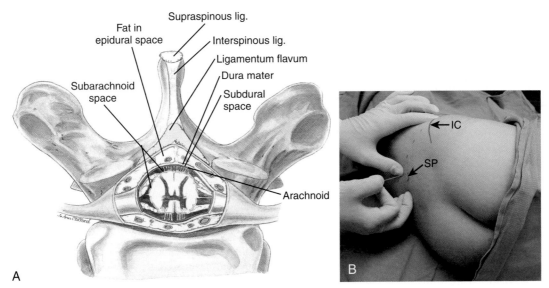

■ FIGURE 16-10. Epidural anesthesia. **A,** Anatomy of the epidural space. **B,** Performance of epidural block. *IC,* Iliac crest; *SP,* spinous process. (**A,** *Reproduced from Brown DL:* Atlas of regional anesthesia, *Philadelphia, 1992, Saunders, p 286.*)

adults, epidural pressures differ in children, particularly in infants (Vas et al., 2001). Based on the relationship between the volume and rate of injection of local anesthetics in infants and the epidural pressure, a slow rate of injection is used, perhaps 0.5 mL/min.

To place a thoracic epidural, the child is placed in the lateral decubitus position. After sterile preparation and draping, the point of needle insertion is chosen at the midpoint of the spinous processes. The needle should be at a 45- to 60-degree angle, aiming cephalad until resistance is felt as the spinous ligaments are encountered. A syringe to detect loss of resistance to saline is attached, and the needle is continuously advanced slowly with light pressure on the plunger of the syringe. A sudden loss of resistance indicates needle placement in the epidural space. One of the hallmarks of a successful thoracic epidural needle placement is the ease at which a catheter is threaded in this area. It should pass easily and without resistance.

Technique with Ultrasound

A preprocedural ultrasound scan of the vertebral column facilitates optimal site selection for the lumbar or thoracic epidural catheter insertion and allows measurement of the depth of the ligamentum flavum, thus estimating the depth at which loss of resistance will occur (Rapp et al., 2005; Willschke et al., 2007) (see Fig. 16-9). The longitudinal median view offers a slightly better correlation with actual depth than the transverse view by ultrasound (Kil et al., 2007). Real-time ultrasound-guided epidural placement has resulted in reduction in the catheter placement time and the frequency of bony contacts (Willschke et al., 2006c). This approach is challenging and requires two anesthesiologists experienced in the ultrasound-guided procedures and neonatal epidural techniques. To simplify the technique, perform a scout ultrasound scan to determine the depth of the epidural space, and then confirm catheter tip position by saline injection test once threading through the needle is completed.

Equipment

Appropriately sized equipment is readily available for epidural placement in children. Short Touhy needles and small-gauge catheters, with and without metal helixes, are available. The main disadvantage of a small-gauge catheter is that it increases resistance to continuous infusion of local anesthetic. Postoperatively, this can result in kinking and frequent alarms of the infusion pump.

Dosing

Epidural catheters are typically placed so that their use can be continued in the postoperative period. Because the tip of the epidural catheter should be in close proximity to the level of surgery, and because the lumbar and thoracic epidural spaces are more compact than the caudal space, the initial bolus of local anesthetic required for lumbar and thoracic epidurals is smaller (0.3 to 0.5 mL/kg) than the volumes required for a caudal injection. Approximately 90 minutes after the initial bolus, a continuous infusion may be initiated with care to stay within the maximal allowable dose (see Table 16-2). Recommendations for epidural dosing are in Table 16-3.

When using 0.25% bupivacaine at a rate of 0.08 mL/kg per hour in the lumbar epidural space in children aged 11 months to 15 years, Desparmet and coworkers (1987) demonstrated that the terminal half-life ranges from 164 to 270 minutes, and total body clearance is similar to that after single caudal injection. Larsson and associates (1994) studied bupivacaine infusions in 12 infants. In infants, bupivacaine infusions at rates of 0.5 to 0.83 mg/kg per hour for 12 hours resulted in marked increases in plasma bupivacaine concentrations. Larsson also noted possible toxic reactions in three of the 12 infants and suggested these infusion rates were excessive for this age group.

The pharmacokinetics of epidural ropivacaine were assessed after a single injection of 1.7 mg/kg via a lumbar epidural catheter (McCann et al., 2001). The median peak plasma concentrations of ropivacaine were 610 mcg/L in infants aged 3 to

11 months, and 640 mcg/L in children aged 12 to 48 months. In both groups of children, the median peak plasma concentration was reached in 60 minutes. The calculated clearance of ropivacaine was 4.26 mL/kg per minute in infants and 6.15 mL/kg per minute in older children. No ropivacaine toxicity was observed in either group. When ropivacaine 0.2% at 0.4 mg/kg per hour was delivered as a continuous lumbar or epidural infusion for 36 to 96 hours, Hansen and coworkers (2000) noted no clinically significant side effects in 18 pediatric patients aged 4 months to 7 years. In this study, the volume of distribution of epidural ropivacaine was 3.1 L/kg, total clearance was 8.5 mL/kg per minute, and the elimination half-life was 4.9 hours (see Table 16-1). In infants and neonates who received 48 to 72 hours of continuous ropivacaine epidural infusion, Bosenberg and associates (2005) found that plasma concentrations of unbound ropivacaine were not influenced by the duration of the infusion. Although the levels of unbound ropivacaine were higher in the neonates than in the infants, all were below the level of 0.35 mg/L, the threshold that is considered toxic in adults.

Epidural Additives

The advantage of adding clonidine to single-shot caudal blocks has been demonstrated, but there are also advantages to its use for continuous epidural analgesia. In a study of 60 children who received a low lumbar epidural catheter for hypospadias repair, a postoperative infusion of ropivacaine alone was compared with ropivacaine with varying dosages of clonidine. De Negri and coworkers (2001b) evaluated plain ropivacaine 0.1% at 0.2 mg/kg per hour, and ropivacaine 0.08% at 0.16 mg/kg per hour, plus either clonidine 0.04 mcg/kg per hour, 0.08 mcg/kg per hour, or 0.12 mcg/kg per hour. The children who received the ropivacaine with the higher clonidine dosages in the 0.08 to 0.12 mcg/kg per hour range had improved pain scores, longer time to first analgesic, and reduced total supplemental analgesics without increased sedation or other side effects.

The use of neuraxial opioids was discussed (see Caudal Analgesia, earlier). In a study designed to assess the efficacy of preoperative epidural morphine, 21 children were randomized to either a group that received 30 mcg/kg epidural morphine after induction of general anesthesia but prior to surgical incision, or to a group that did not receive an epidural injection (Kiffer et al., 2001). Both groups were given intraoperative infusions of sufentanil and postoperative patient-controlled analgesia with morphine. The group that had received preoperative epidural morphine, in comparison with the control group without epidural morphine, had lower pain scores and decreased total analgesic requirements postoperatively without increased side effects.

Epinephrine is a commonly used additive for single-shot epidural blocks because of its ability to decrease systemic absorption and perhaps prolong the block while adding an additional level of safety. For continuous infusions, these benefits must be weighed against the theoretical risks of vasoconstriction of spinal vessels. Kokki and coworkers (2002) compared a combination of ropivacaine and sufentanil with and without epinephrine 2 mcg/mL in a population of children. The children who had epinephrine in their postoperative epidural infusions had significantly lower infusion requirements and fewer side effects. In adults, the addition of epinephrine to a ropivacaine epidural infusion at 5 mcg/mL reduces the early systemic plasma concentrations of ropivacaine, and thereby may decrease the risk for toxicity from systemic absorption (Lee et al., 2002).

Complications

As discussed for caudal catheters, the risk for infection is very low. Although there have been case reports of epidural abscess, short-term epidural catheterization for postoperative courses do not appear to have the same risk for infection as those placed for chronic pain (Strafford et al., 1995). In 1620 children over a 6-year period who received epidural catheters, there were no infections or epidural abscesses in catheters that had been placed for postoperative pain management. There was only one epidural abscess found in this study, and that was in an immunosuppressed child with terminal malignancy who had *Candida* colonization of the epidural space that had been invaded by tumor and had an indwelling catheter for control of pain from her malignancy. When catheters have been removed and cultured, the incidence of catheter tip colonization in epidural catheters is 4%, lower than that found in caudal catheters (20%) (McNeely et al., 1997b).

A systematic review and pooled analysis of studies on the risk for infection of long-term epidural catheters estimated that one person in 35 may develop an epidural catheter infection (Ruppen et al., 2007). The populations reviewed were primarily adult cancer patients, and those who developed infections had catheters present for an average duration of 74 days. This population is certainly in a separate risk group from that of the typical pediatric surgical patient.

PERIPHERAL NERVE BLOCKS

The use of pediatric peripheral nerve blocks has seen the largest growth in practice and in the literature (Rochette et al., 2007). The goal of placing peripheral nerve blocks is to specifically target analgesia to the location of the surgery so that side effects are kept to a minimum (Ross et al., 2000). The safety of performing such blocks has been established, and it has been recommended by ADARPEF that peripheral blocks be used in place of central blocks when appropriate (Giaufre et al., 1996). In their safety study of regional anesthetics in children, there were no complications in the 9396 children who received peripheral nerve blocks or local anesthesia. Despite these findings, peripheral nerve blocks were often underused in children, probably related to inexperience and the perception that they may be difficult to perform or be hazardous. The use of ultrasound has changed the perception of safety and been responsible for a growth in literature on peripheral nerve blocks in children.

Success of placing peripheral nerve blocks is often a function of knowledge of the anatomy, and use of the appropriate equipment (Sethna and Berde, 1992). Insulated needles with a nerve stimulator have been used for peripheral nerve blockade in past years because the field of current is localized to the needle's tip. Unsheathed needles may be less expensive and result in successful blocks, but the current is distributed not only to the needle's tip but also along the shaft of the needle. Thus, the required stimulatory current is greater (up to 2 mA) (Bosenberg, 1995). For upper extremity nerve blocks, a 1- or 2-inch insulated needle will suffice. Lower extremity blocks may require the use of longer needles, particularly for sciatic blocks in adolescents. Another practical consideration in performing a peripheral nerve block with a nerve stimulator is that administration of neuromuscular blockers will abolish the ability to elicit muscle stimulation with a peripheral nerve stimulator. The peripheral nerve stimulator should be capable of delivering 0.1 to greater than 1.5 mA and be set to 2 Hz. The positive electrode of the nerve stimulator should be placed at least 10 cm from the nerve to be blocked and preferentially on the opposite limb. To locate a nerve or plexus, begin with the nerve stimulator set at 1 to 1.2 mA, and advance the needle until the desired motor response is achieved. The voltage may then be decreased. When the voltage is decreased to less than 0.5 mA, the motor response should be diminished but still present. One may need to make further fine adjustments in the needle's position in order to continue muscle stimulation of the appropriate muscle group at the lower voltage. However, an increase in voltage may be required to relocate the nerve if muscle stimulation is completely lost. Once the nerve stimulator's voltage is less than 0.5 mA and slight muscle stimulation results, the local anesthetic is injected. If the needle is in correct position, the muscle stimulation should cease immediately. If there is intense muscle stimulation with 0.2 mA, the possibility of intraneural needle placement must be considered. Consequently, the needle should be withdrawn and carefully readvanced. In anesthetized children, the placement of a needle into a nerve would not be detected, so this warning sign of intense muscle stimulation at lower voltage is significant. In animal studies, motor response to less than 0.2 mA occurred only when the needle tip was intraneural (Tsai et al., 2008). Unfortunately, motor response could also be absent with intraneural needle placement at currents up to 1.7 mA.

In addition to strong twitches at low voltage, one should look for other warning signs of intraneural injection, such as difficulty with injection and increased heart rate with injection. The routine use of a 5- or 10-mL syringe for local anesthetic injection may improve success by allowing the operator to have a consistent "feel" for the pressure on injection. Animal experiments suggest that pressures of greater than 20 psi suggest intraneural injection and neurologic sequelae.

As previously discussed, the use of ultrasound for peripheral nerve blockade in children is becoming increasingly common and has replaced the use of nerve stimulation at many high-volume centers. Ultrasonography allows the practitioner to visualize the anatomy and needle, presumably resulting in improved success of block with less risk for nerve injury, although this remains unproven. The technique of using the combination approach of nerve stimulation with ultrasound has been presented and may be valuable as part of the learning process in performing peripheral nerve blocks in children.

The ultrasonographic identification of peripheral nerves requires practice. Nerves come in many shapes depending on their anatomic location; however, with systematic examination, patterns emerge. Nerve roots and proximal segments have a hypoechoic core surrounded by a hyperechoic ring. Because nerve roots and trunks are clinically visualized only in the performance of the interscalene, parascalene, and supraclavicular blocks, it is generalized that nerves are dark above the clavicle. Peripheral nerves are hyperechoic with fascicular echotexture and exhibit anisotropy, which is a change in echogenicity depending on imaging angle (Crass et al., 1988; Grechenig et al., 2000). Directing the insonation angle perpendicular to the direction of the nerve fiber will optimize nerve appearance.

Although the practice has been replaced by ultrasound, surface nerve mapping was once recommended for use in children to improve the ability to locate a peripheral nerve or plexus (Bosenberg et al., 2002a). Nerve surface mapping is performed by setting the nerve stimulator at a frequency of 1 to 2 Hz and the current between 3 to 4 mA. The positive electrode should be at least 10 cm from the nerve to be mapped, and the negative electrode or alligator clamp that would normally be attached to the block needle is instead pressed against the skin at right angles across the suspected path of the nerve. Once a point of maximal motor response is found, a mark may be placed to indicate where the insulated needle may be inserted for regional blockade.

In children who are anesthetized, it is not possible to reliably test the success of a peripheral nerve block; however, one may increase the voltage of the nerve stimulator after local anesthetic injection to determine that there is loss of stimulation. Although subtle, it is also possible to determine the success of a motor block by comparing the flaccidity of the blocked limb to the muscle tone of the contralateral extremity. Vasodilation or increased skin temperature, when present in the blocked limb, may be a more reliable indicator of a successful block, but its absence does not mean that the block is unsuccessful. The absolute determinant of a successful block is the absence of response to the surgical incision. Most peripheral nerve blocks, regardless of the agent used, should provide total analgesia to the desired nerve or plexus within 20 minutes of the local anesthetic injection.

Dosing of peripheral nerve blocks will be discussed with regard to the individual block. Regardless of the local anesthetic delivered, the addition of epinephrine to the solution should provide additional safety when performing the block. Not only does the addition of epinephrine to the local anesthetic solution have the potential to serve as a marker for intravascular injection, it may also decrease overall absorption of the local anesthetic. In a study of 20 children who were to undergo unilateral surgery of the thigh, patients were administered a fascia iliaca block using 2 mg/kg bupivacaine either with or without epinephrine 5 mcg/mL (Doyle et al., 1997). The median maximal plasma bupivacaine concentration in the group without epinephrine was 1.1 mcg/mL, compared with 0.3 mcg/mL in the group of patients for whom epinephrine was added to the bupivacaine. Not only did the epinephrine group have a significantly lower peak plasma level, but the onset time to peak plasma concentration was more gradual for the group with epinephrine.

There is little information as to the use of adjuncts to local anesthetics in pediatric peripheral nerve blocks. In a database review of 435 patients at the Children's Hospital of Philadelphia, the use of clonidine 1 mcg/kg (up to 100 mcg) for peripheral nerve blockade resulted in a longer duration of sensory block of 17.2 hours versus 13.2 hours in the group who received either bupivacaine or ropivacaine with clonidine, and a prolonged motor block of 9.6 hours with clonidine versus 4.3 hours without (Cucchiaro and Ganesh, 2007). This increased duration occurred in children who had received either upper or lower extremity nerve blocks for a variety of surgeries, and it was also independent of which local anesthetic was used. These findings differ from adult studies, where the use of clonidine for peripheral nerve blocks has shown to be of benefit only for upper extremity blocks, particularly axillary block, and with intermediate-acting local anesthetics (McCartney et al., 2007a). The prolongation of sensory analgesia found by Cucchiaro and

Ganesh may have resulted from local effect from direct binding at α_2-adrenergic receptors. The use of clonidine in children was also in addition to low concentrations of local anesthetics versus higher concentrations that are typically used in adults. Additional investigation is necessary to determine the overall usefulness of clonidine for peripheral nerve blocks in children. Although the early work appears promising, no prolongation of analgesia was found when 1 mcg/kg clonidine was added to bupivacaine for ilioinguinal/iliohypogastric nerve blocks in children (Kaabachi et al., 2005).

The majority of peripheral nerve block techniques are similar to those of adults. The differences from adult practice are presented here, along with blocks that are more specifically for children. Although anatomy is stressed for most of the blocks using landmark techniques, many of the blocks also have a section describing the use of ultrasound for practitioners who are proficient in its use. Some blocks where ultrasound is clearly advantageous for success or safety of the block are presented with that as the sole technique.

Upper Extremity Nerve Blocks

Upper extremity blocks may be used for surgery of the shoulder, arm, and hand. Specifically, brachial plexus blocks below the clavicle including the axillary approach are suitable for surgery on the hand and those blocks above the clavicle are useful for surgery on the shoulder and upper arm. Depending on the approach to the plexus, it is also possible to provide total analgesia to the hand with blocks above the clavicle. See related video online at www.expertconsult.com.

Anatomy

The brachial plexus contains the anterior branches of spinal roots C5 through T1 (Fig. 16-11). In the neck, these branches run between the anterior and middle scalene muscles and are enclosed in a fascial sheath. They then form three trunks (superior, middle, inferior) that exit the interscalene groove and run behind the subclavian artery. As they exit the interscalene groove, these cords form an anterior and posterior division. The divisions then unite to form lateral, posterior, and medial cords, depending on their relation to the axillary artery. There is a natural separation between the supraclavicular and infraclavicular plexus at the coracoid process that ultimately affects spread of local anesthetic (Vester-Andersen et al., 1986).

Understanding of the medial neck anatomy and components at each level of the plexus is crucial to avoiding complications (Fig. 16-12). Because the brachial plexus may be blocked in a number of locations, it is important to know the anatomy at each level in the neck area for successful block (Fig. 16-13). Close anatomic relationship of the carotid artery and internal jugular vein should be observed to select the ideal location for local injection. The proximity of the phrenic nerve overlying the anterior scalene muscle with founding cervical nerve roots C3 to C5 and cervical sympathetic chain explains resulting diaphragmatic paresis and Horner's syndrome from the excessive spread of local anesthetic (Neal et al., 2009).

At the level of the axilla are the peripheral nerves that innervate the arm. The radial nerve supplies the dorsal aspect of the upper extremity below the shoulder including the thumb and dorsal aspects of the index, middle, and fourth fingers. The musculocutaneous nerve provides innervation to the biceps of the upper arm and cutaneous innervation to the lateral forearm. The median nerve innervates the majority of the forearm, as well as the ventral aspects of the second, third, and lateral portion of the fourth fingers, and the medial portion of the thumb. The ulnar nerve is more limited to the hand and innervates the lateral aspect of the fourth finger and all of the fifth (Fig. 16-14).

Interscalene Block

An interscalene block has been used for surgery of the shoulder and upper arm with success in children. It also anesthetizes the musculocutaneous nerve reliably, but there is less reliability of blocking the ulnar nerve than with the other nerve blocks because the ulnar nerve's origin is at the lower portion of the plexus. Interscalene blocks are infrequently used in children because of the perceived higher risk for complications and side effects, and they are not recommended for placement in the anesthetized child because of risk for spinal cord injury (Bernards et al., 2008). For this reason, the technique will not be described.

Complications

Complications of interscalene block are not insignificant and include pneumothorax, spinal cord injury, epidural injection,

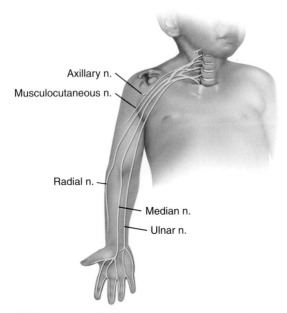

■ **FIGURE 16-11.** Brachial plexus anatomy.

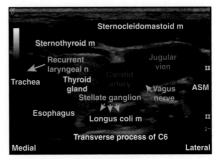

■ **FIGURE 16-12.** Medial neck anatomy.

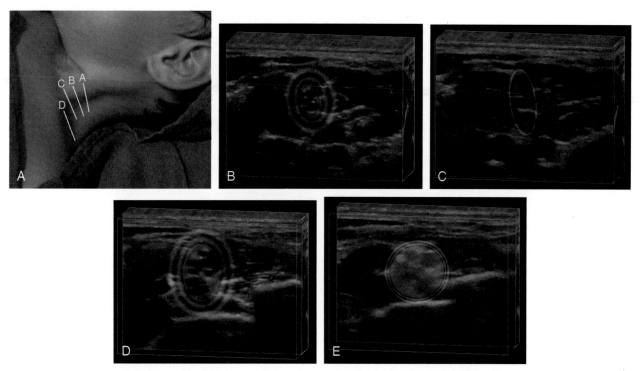

■ **FIGURE 16-13.** Brachial plexus in the neck. **A,** External landmarks. **B,** Plexus at level A *(encircled)*. **C,** Plexus at level B *(encircled)*. **D,** Plexus at level C *(encircled)*. **E,** Plexus at level D *(encircled)*.

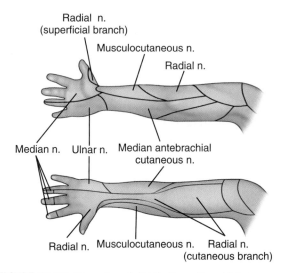

■ **FIGURE 16-14.** Dermatomal distribution of brachial plexus.

or intrathecal injection. Vertebral artery puncture may also occur, with a risk for local anesthetic delivery directly to the CNS resulting in CNS toxicity. In addition, there is a high risk for phrenic nerve block with paralysis of the hemidiaphragm. Phrenic nerve block is not well tolerated, especially in infants or patients with underlying respiratory compromise (Kempen et al., 2000). Unilateral vocal cord paralysis may also occur and result in airway compromise. Sympathetic blockade with Horner's syndrome is a common side effect of interscalene blocks.

Parascalene Block

The parascalene approach to the brachial plexus was developed by Dalens (1995) to provide effective analgesia to the shoulder and upper arm (Fig. 16-15, *A*) while minimizing the risks of vertebral artery puncture, dural puncture, and pneumothorax (i.e., the risks associated with an interscalene block). The parascalene block is similar to the interscalene approach, but by changing the insertion and direction of the needle, major structures in the neck are avoided. This block has been found to be easy to perform, with a 97% success rate in children on the first or second attempt (Dalens et al., 1987). See related video online at www.expertconsult.com.

Technique

With the child supine and a roll under the shoulders, the arm should be adducted next to the trunk and the head turned to the opposite side. The primary landmarks are Chassaignac's tubercle (transverse process of C6) and the midpoint of the clavicle. Draw a line between these two structures and insert a needle at the junction of the upper two thirds and lower one third of this line (see Fig. 16-15, *B* and *C*). This insertion spot should be at the level of the cricoid process near the external jugular vein. The approximate depth to the parascalene brachial plexus from the skin depends on the age of the child (see Fig. 16-6). Using low voltage, and once appropriate stimulation has been achieved, the local anesthetic solution is injected. Nerve stimulation for a parascalene block may result in muscle response in the biceps or triceps or with finger or hand movement. Shoulder muscle response suggests stimulation of the supraclavicular nerve, indicating that the needle is lateral to the plexus.

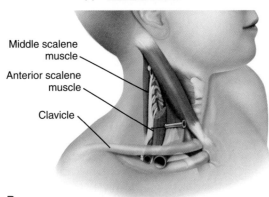

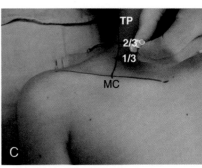

■ **FIGURE 16-15.** Parascalene block. **A,** Dermatomal distribution of parascalene block. **B,** Anatomy for parascalene block. **C,** Performance of parascalene block. *MC,* Midpoint of clavicle; *TP,* transverse process of C6.

Complications

Complications using the parascalene approach are rare but may include venous puncture, Horner's syndrome, and hemidiaphragmatic paralysis secondary to phrenic nerve paralysis.

Supraclavicular Block

The supraclavicular block has the advantage of providing analgesia to all portions of the arm and is useful for nearly all upper extremity procedures. Despite a pneumothorax-free application of the supraclavicular block in 200 pediatric patients by landmark technique, the close anatomic relationship of pleura to the brachial plexus justifiably deters many pediatric anesthesiologists (Pande et al., 2000). The ultrasound-guided approach was demonstrated to be safe in 40 pediatric patients, had a higher success rate, and was faster to perform than the infraclavicular block (De Jose Maria et al., 2008). The ability of ultrasound to

visualize the path and the tip of the needle, as well as the course of local anesthetic spread during injection, holds promise for using these blocks in a pediatric regional practice, and this has resulted in a pneumothorax-free application of supraclavicular block in pediatric patients. Because needle tip visualization is imperative to safe application of this procedure, only experienced ultrasound practitioners should attempt this block.

Technique with Ultrasound

A linear ultrasound transducer with the smallest available footprint, set at the highest operational frequency, should be used to achieve maximal resolution of the superficial supraclavicular structures (Fig. 16-16, *A*). The ultrasound machine should be positioned on the contralateral side in the direct line of view of the operator. The operator sits or stands by the patient's shoulder on the ipsilateral side with the ultrasound transducer held in the nondominant hand and positioned

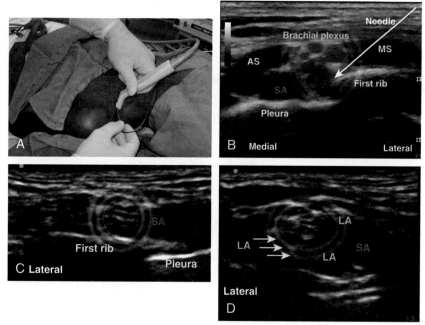

■ **FIGURE 16-16.** Ultrasound-guided supraclavicular block. **A,** Needle and transducer placement. **B,** Sonoanatomy. **C,** Before injection of local anesthetic. **D,** After injection of local anesthetic.

parallel to the clavicle in the supraclavicular groove. The subclavian artery is identified in the short axis as a round, pulsatile structure, and the cervical pleura and lung are imaged below. The brachial plexus is located posterosuperior to the artery between the insertion of the anterior and middle scalene muscle onto the first rib and has a cluster-of-grapes appearance (hypoechoic center with hyperechoic rim) (see Fig. 16-16, *B*). The block needle is inserted in-plane in a lateral to medial direction. Ideally, the needle tip is placed between the first rib and the most inferior aspect of the brachial plexus (see Fig. 16-16, *C*). Injection at this location prevents superficial image distortion; pushes the brachial plexus up and away from the pleura, thus creating a margin of safety if the needle tip needs to be repositioned; and ensures blockade of the inferior trunk (see Fig. 16-16, *D*). The needle should be repositioned around the middle and superior nerve structures to achieve complete envelopment of the plexus by local anesthetic. To avoid pleural puncture, the needle tip should be visualized throughout the block placement, and to rule out intravascular injection, separation of tissues with incremental local anesthetic injection should be observed.

Lateral Vertical Infraclavicular Block

A lateral vertical infraclavicular brachial plexus block was introduced for pediatric use because the block can be performed without arm abduction. In addition, the block is more reliable for anesthetizing the musculocutaneous nerve, and this block provides better analgesia of the upper arm than an axillary block (Fleischmann et al., 2003). Although other infraclavicular approaches were considered too hazardous because of the risk for pneumothorax, the more lateral and vertical approach developed by Kapral (1999) and associates provides a safe distance between puncture site and pleura. This technique has been used in adults and children and has been shown to provide a greater spectrum of block than the axillary approach (Kapral

et al., 1999; Fleischmann et al., 2003). The indications for a lateral infraclavicular block are the same as those for axillary block. See related video online at www.expertconsult.com.

Technique

With the child in the supine position, the upper arm should remain next to the trunk and the elbow flexed 90 degrees so that the forearm is on the abdomen. Palpate the coracoid process and using a nerve stimulator, insert a 1-inch 24-gauge insulated needle 0.5 cm distal to the coracoid process in a perpendicular or vertical direction while continuously aspirating for blood and/or air (Fig. 16-17). Once appropriate stimulation has been determined and continuous aspiration for blood or air has been negative, local anesthetic solution is injected. Obtaining wrist or finger movement predicts a successful block, whereas if only elbow twitches are seen, a failed block is likely to occur (Ponde and Diwan, 2009).

Complications

Complications with this approach are rare. There may still be a risk of inadvertent pleural or vascular puncture, but less so than with other approaches to the brachial plexus.

Infraclavicular Block

The infraclavicular block provides the same analgesia as can be expected from an axillary block, and it is suitable for distal upper extremity procedures. The ultrasound-guided infraclavicular block has been shown in children to offer shorter onset time, longer duration, and decreased discomfort during placement than nerve stimulation (Marhofer et al., 2004). In addition, the volume of local anesthetic needed to produce analgesia may be decreased with the ultrasound guidance, and the block can be successfully performed even in patients with altered response to

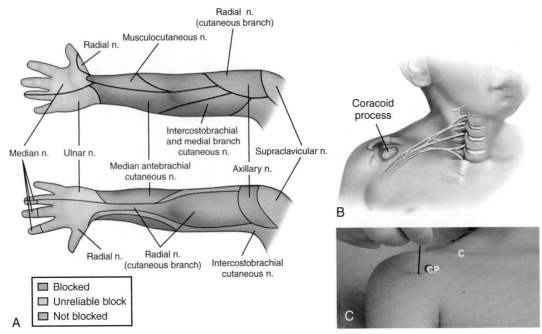

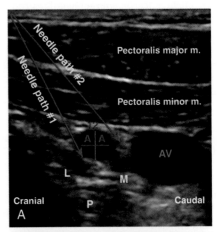

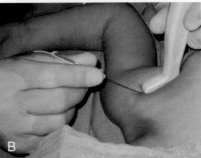

■ **FIGURE 16-17.** Lateral vertical infraclavicular brachial plexus (LVIBP) block. **A,** Dermatomal distribution of LVIBP block. **B,** Anatomy for LVIBP block. **C,** Performance of LVIBP block. *C,* Clavicle; *CP,* coracoid process.

nerve stimulation such as those with congenital abnormalities, trauma, or distal arm amputation (Sandhu et al., 2006; Ponde and Diwan, 2009). Because of the risk for pneumothorax, ultrasound-guided infraclavicular block is the preferred approach. See related video online at www.expertconsult.com.

Technique with Ultrasound

With the child in supine position and head rotated to the non-operative side, the operator stands or sits at the head of the bed and positions the ultrasound transducer below and perpendicular (sagittal plane) to the clavicle in the infraclavicular fossa, slightly medial to the coracoid process. A linear transducer with a small footprint should be used for this block, given the narrow anatomic relationship of the infraclavicular fossa. The frequency selection is size dependent: larger children with deeper anatomy benefit from medium frequency range (10 to 7 MHz), but superficial structures ae imaged best with a high frequency (13 to 10 MHz) in young children and toddlers. The ultrasound machine should be positioned in the direct line of view of the operator on the ipsilateral side of the patient. The child's arm can be kept at the side when block placement is attempted in an awake child with an injured extremity; however, if tolerated or in a sedated child, the arm is abducted to 90 degrees, and external rotation and flexion at the elbow raises the plexus closer to the skin and rotates the clavicle upward, thus creating additional space for probe positioning. Sonographic examination will reveal axillary vessels immediately deep to the pectoralis major and minor muscles, and the three hyperechoic cords surrounding the second part of the axillary artery at the 3-o'clock (medial cord), 6-o'clock (posterior cord), and 9-o'clock (lateral cord) positions (Fig. 16-18, *A*). The needle insertion site is determined by scanning the infraclavicular fossa in the mediolateral direction, and the ideal site is where the pleura is farthest separated from the plexus (see Fig. 16-18, *B*). The needle

■ **FIGURE 16-18.** Ultrasound scan of infraclavicular block. **A,** Sonoanatomy. **B,** Needle and transducer placement.

is advanced in-plane from the superior part of the transducer (cranial-caudal direction), and is positioned between the posterior cord of the brachial plexus and the axillary artery. Injection should produce circumferential spread around the axillary artery in young children; however, in older children, the median cord may be missed with a single injection and requires targeted injection to obtain a successful block. Maintaining continuous needle visualization may be challenging because of the acute angle of insertion, and it requires expertise in the ultrasound-guided techniques. Secondary confirmation of the needle tip can be gathered from tissue movement and hydro-locating with injection of 0.5 to 1 mL of normal saline.

Axillary Block

Axillary block is a common approach to the brachial plexus in children, as it is suitable for procedures on the hand such as syndactyly repair and finger reimplantation (Fig. 16-19, *A*). Advantages of performing an axillary block include the simplicity of the anatomy, ease of placement, and low risk for complications (Tobias, 2001a). Disadvantages include the need for a patient to be able to abduct the arm for access to the axilla, and the inability to block the musculocutaneous nerve 40% to 50% of the time because it branches higher in the axilla than the ulnar, median, and radial nerves. Because the musculocutaneous nerve innervates the lateral side of the forearm, it may need to be blocked separately for surgical procedures that involve that nerve's distribution. Many approaches for an axillary block have been described and used in children. In a study to compare a single injection versus multiple injection technique in

children, unlike in adults, there was no difference in block quality found between the two techniques (Carre et al., 2000). This study also confirmed that using either technique, separate block of the musculocutaneous nerve is still required if necessary for the surgical site.

In a study to assess the efficacy of the timing of an axillary block, 55 children received 2 mg/kg of 0.25% bupivacaine either prior to surgical incision, or immediately after surgery but before emergence (Altintas et al., 2000). In the presurgical group, 32% of the children required no additional analgesics within the first 24 hours, compared with 83% in the postsurgical group who required no additional analgesics. Although cumulative pain scores were higher in the presurgical group, nonetheless both groups had effective analgesia. See related video online at www.expertconsult.com.

Technique

A one-injection technique for axillary nerve block is accomplished by first palpating the axillary artery. The needle is then inserted immediately adjacent and superior to the artery high in the axilla, at a 30- to 45-degree angle aimed toward the midpoint of the clavicle (see Fig. 16-19, *B* and *C*). One may feel a pop as the plexus sheath is entered. Using a nerve stimulator, and after evidence of muscle stimulation in the hand is observed,

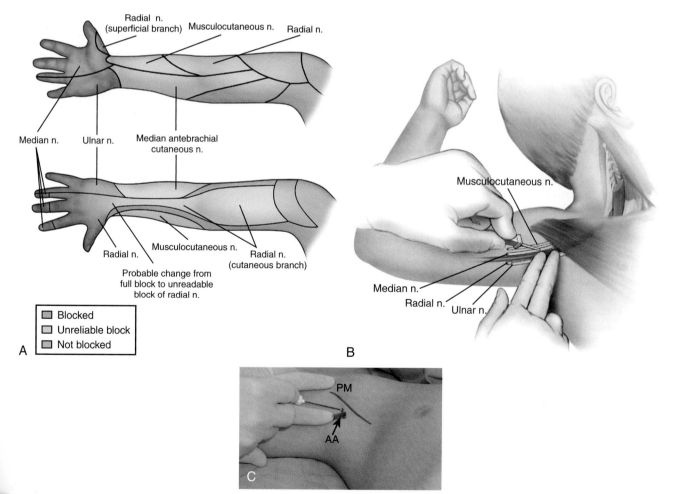

■ **FIGURE 16-19.** Axillary block. **A,** Dermatomal distribution of axillary block. **B,** Anatomy for axillary block. **C,** Performance of axillary block. *AA,* Axillary artery; *PM,* pectoralis muscle.

local anesthetic is injected. A longitudinal swelling immediately beneath the skin as the local anesthetic fills the sheath may appear, particularly in infants and young children. This swelling disappears quickly as the anesthetic spreads proximally into the sheath, and this swelling should not be confused with a subcutaneous injection, which would have a more circular distribution and not disappear quickly. After the local anesthetic has been delivered and the needle removed, the arm should be adducted, thus releasing the pressure of the head of the humerus from the fossa. This motion along with holding distal pressure at the site of injection will promote proximal spread of the local anesthetic into the sheath. With a single-injection technique, all of the local anesthetic is delivered in one location. With a multiple-injection technique, the nerves are individually anesthetized by locating at least two of them individually using the nerve stimulator or ultrasound. Either technique may miss the musculocutaneous nerve because it exits the sheath proximal to the other three distal nerves. For this reason, a separate block of the musculocutaneous nerve is generally required. The musculocutaneous nerve may be blocked by directly inserting the needle into the belly of the coracobrachialis muscle while looking for stimulation of the biceps. In addition, if a surgical tourniquet is to be used and the patient is not having a general anesthetic, the intercostobrachial nerve should be blocked. This is accomplished by placing a subcutaneous ring of local anesthetic high around the inner aspect of the arm.

Technique with ultrasound. In the adult literature, ultrasound guidance has been demonstrated to improve block success rate (Chan et al., 2007; Lo et al., 2008), diagnose abnormal anatomy (Manickam et al., 2008), and allow a decrease in the required volume of local anesthetic and the number of needle passes (Casati et al., 2007). Although not yet prospectively demonstrated in a pediatric model, and appreciating the degree of anatomic nerve variability in relation to the axillary artery, the sonographic ability to guide the needle direction should prove to be of benefit in children as well.

To use ultrasound for axillary block, the operator stands or sits by the child's ipsilateral shoulder and positions the ultrasound transducer transverse to the axilla at the crease formed by the pectoralis major and biceps muscles. A linear ultrasound transducer with the smallest available footprint, set at the highest operational frequency should be used to achieve maximal resolution of the superficial axillary plexus structures (Fig. 16-20, *A*). The ultrasound machine should be positioned in the direct line of view of the operator on the ipsilateral side of the patient. Sonographic examination will reveal a pulsatile axillary artery and a compressible axillary vein (or veins) surrounded by the coracobrachialis and biceps brachii (short head) muscle cranially and teres major and triceps brachii muscle caudally (see Fig. 16-20, *B*). The nerves of the axillary plexus exhibit fascicular appearance, appear in multiple shapes (round and oval most frequently), occupy varied locations around the axillary artery, and require dynamic distal tracing or neurostimulation to confirm the identity of each individual nerve (Retzl et al., 2001). The radial nerve is most frequently posterior or posteriocaudal (between 2 and 7 o'clock) to the axillary artery, deep to the ulnar nerve, and, when traced distally, it descends behind the triceps muscle into the spiral groove of the humerus accompanied by the radial collateral artery. The ulnar nerve is anterior or anteriocaudal (between 12 and 3 o'clock) to the axillary artery, and when traced distally, it remains superficial and slides

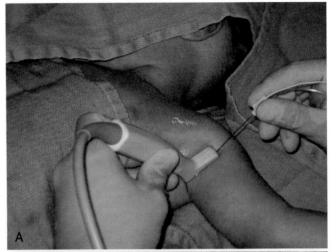

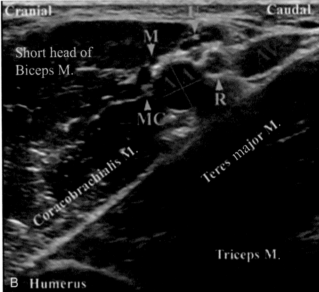

■ **FIGURE 16-20.** Ultrasound axillary block. **A,** Placement of needle and transducer. **B,** Sonoanatomy.

medially from the brachial artery on its way to the ulnar nerve sulcus. The median nerve is anterior or anterocranial (9 to 1 o'clock) to the axillary artery, and it remains close to the brachial artery as it is traced distally. The musculocutaneous nerve has a hyperechoic appearance, changes in shape from oval to triangular, is located posterocranial to the axillary artery adjacent to the median nerve in the proximal axilla, and separates cranially to lie in a fascial plane between the coracobrachialis and the short head of the biceps brachii muscles in the distal axilla. The needle is advanced in-plane from the superior part of the transducer and is repositioned to sequentially block the radial, ulnar, medial, and musculocutaneous nerves. Injection of local anesthetic around the radial nerve first prevents the distortion of the deep anatomy and may help to localize the ulnar nerve. Median and musculocutaneous nerves can often be surrounded by local anesthetic with minimal needle adjustment when performing the block proximally in the axilla.

Continuous axillary sheath catheter placement is feasible, but displacement is easy, especially in the frequently uncooperative pediatric patient, so it is not commonly performed.

Complications

There should be few complications when performing an axillary block. There is the rare risk for hematoma and nerve compression, and for this reason a transarterial approach may not be recommended in children. If inadvertent axillary artery puncture occurs, firm pressure should be held for at least 5 minutes to avoid formation of hematoma and subsequent vascular insufficiency (Merril et al., 1981). Other complications may include relative distortion of anatomy after the first injection of local anesthetic in the axillary region, or inadvertent overdose of local anesthetic when multiple injection techniques are used (Dalens, 1995). However, these complications were not reported in the pediatric study by Carre and coworkers (2000).

Dosing of Upper Extremity Blocks

Various local anesthetics either alone or in combination have been used for upper extremity blocks. For prolonged analgesia, bupivacaine, levobupivacaine, or ropivacaine should be used. Because the brachial plexus is not highly vascular, the uptake of local anesthetic is less than that of pleural or central blocks, but the maximal allowable dosages of local anesthetic must be determined and the block dosed accordingly. When concentrations were compared, bupivacaine 2 mg/kg versus 3 mg/kg delivered for axillary block in children resulted in plasma levels of 1.35 mcg/mL and 1.84 mcg/mL, respectively (Campbell et al., 1986). These values are well below the toxic range. To compare 0.2% ropivacaine with 0.25% bupivacaine, Thornton and associates (2003) administered 0.5 mL/kg to children for axillary block. There was no significant difference between the two groups in pain scores, time to first analgesic, or total analgesic in 24 hours. The median time to first dose of analgesic was 7.25 hours in the ropivacaine group and 9.3 hours in the bupivacaine group. In general, if using 0.25% to 0.5% bupivacaine or levobupivacaine, or 0.2% to 0.5% ropivacaine, the lower concentration should be used in children 5 years of age or younger at a volume of 0.5 mL/kg. Using this volume under ultrasound guidance will result in a faster onset (Marhofer et al., 2004). Epinephrine 5 mcg/mL should be added to the solution to assist in identifying intravascular injection and to decrease the absorption of the local anesthetic. Using these dosing guidelines, approximately 4 to 12 hours of analgesia should be achieved (Table 16-4).

Clonidine 1 mcg/kg may be added to extend the duration of block and was used successfully in a large series of children (Cucchiaro and Ganesh, 2007). The use of clonidine may allow lower concentrations of local anesthetic to be used with durations similar to those expected with higher concentrations, with less risk for local anesthetic toxicity.

Peripheral Nerve Blocks in the Forearm

Individual blockade of the peripheral nerves in the distal upper extremity offers selective analgesia for minor surgeries, avoids excessive motor blockade, and provides rescue for failed brachial plexus blocks. When performed using a landmark-only technique, these blocks are restricted to the superficial sites at the elbow or wrist. This may result in nerve ischemia from local anesthetic injection into a tightly bound space such as the ulnar nerve at the elbow or median nerve at the wrist, or vascular complications such as brachial artery puncture at the elbow

TABLE 16-4. Dosage Recommendations* for Peripheral Nerve Blocks

Regional Technique	Bolus Dose[†]	Continuous Infusion
Axillary	0.2-0.5 mL/kg	0.1-0.2 mL/kg/hr
Parascalene	0.2-0.4 mL/kg	0.1-0.2 mL/kg/hr
Femoral or LFC	0.3-1 mL/kg	0.15-0.3 mL/kg/hr
Fascia iliaca	0.5-1 mL/kg	0.15-0.3 mL/kg/hr
Lumbar plexus	0.5-1 mL/kg	0.15-0.3 mL/kg/hr
Sciatic	0.3-1 mL/kg	0.15-0.3 mL/kg/hr
ILIH	0.25 mL/kg	NA
Penile block	0.1 mL/kg	NA
Paravertebral	0.5 mL/kg	0.2-0.25 mL/kg/hr
TAP	0.3-0.5 mL/kg	0.25 mL/kg/hr

*Bupivacaine, levobupivacaine, or ropivacaine may be used. For bolus dosing, lower concentrations, such as 0.2% to 0.25%, should be used for infants and young children, whereas concentrations of 0.375% to 0.5% should be used in children older than 5 to 8 years. For continuous infusions, lower concentrations such as 0.1% to 0.2% of all agents are acceptable.
[†]Epinephrine 1:200,000 should be added to single-shot peripheral nerve blocks except for penile block.
ILIH, Ilioinguinal/iliohypogastric; *LFC*, lateral femoral cutaneous nerve; *NA*, not applicable; *TAP*, transversus abdominis plane.

and ulnar artery at the wrist, and thus these blocks have been reported to have a failure rate of 10% to 30% in adults (Delaunay and Chelly, 2001). Ultrasound imaging allows tracking of each nerve along its course in the arm and selection of the optimal block location (McCartney et al., 2007b). The aim is to visualize the target nerve at a site distant from the vascular structures and to accommodate local anesthetic without increased compartment pressures. Use of a linear ultrasound transducer with the smallest available footprint, set at the highest operational frequency, is advised for performance of these blocks.

(See www.expertconsult.com to view the complete text for the median, ulnar, and radial nerve blocks in the forearm, and to view Figs. 16-21 through 16-23.)

Lower Extremity Nerve Blocks

Although central axial blocks are commonly performed pediatric regional anesthetic techniques, lower extremity nerve blocks often provide analgesia to the lower limbs with a more direct effect (McNicol, 1986; Dalens, 1995; Ross et al., 2000; Tobias, 2003). Lower extremity blocks are performed by anesthetizing the lumbar or sacral plexus, or both. See related video online at www.expertconsult.com.

The lumbar plexus is located in the psoas compartment that lies in the paravertebral space (Fig. 16-24). The union of the anterior rami of lumbar nerves L1 to L4 constitutes the primary input of the lumbar plexus with a small portion of the 12th thoracic nerve. As the plexus emerges from the paravertebral space, it divides into three nerves, the femoral, the lateral femoral cutaneous, and the obturator. Although the iliac vessels run anterior to the iliac fascia, these three nerves remain posterior to the fascia. The femoral nerve is a mixed nerve with motor innervation to the quadriceps muscles and sensory innervation

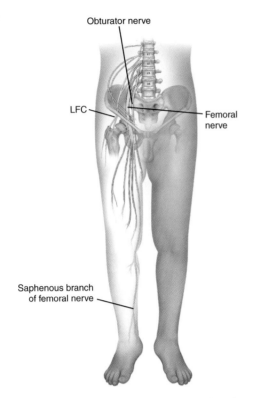

■ **FIGURE 16-24.** Anatomy and distribution of lumbar plexus.

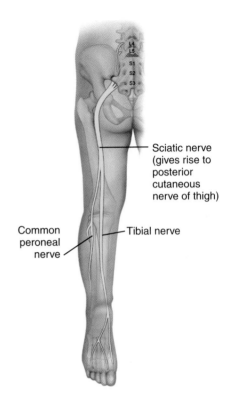

■ **FIGURE 16-25.** Anatomy and distribution of sacral plexus.

to the anterior and medial thigh. A branch of the femoral nerve, the saphenous nerve, provides innervation below the knee to the medial aspect of the lower leg and foot near the saphenous vein. The lateral femoral cutaneous nerve is a sensory nerve with innervation to the lateral thigh, and the obturator nerve is primarily motor to the leg adductors with some sensory to the lower medial thigh and knee.

The sacral plexus is derived from the anterior rami of L4, L5, and S1 to S3, and it gives rise to the sciatic nerve and the posterior cutaneous nerve of the thigh (Fig. 16-25). The sciatic nerve is a mixed nerve that provides motor and sensory innervation to the posterior aspect of the thigh and most of the lower leg. As the sciatic nerve travels down the posterior thigh, it branches into the common peroneal and posterior tibial nerves.

Specific blocks of the lower extremity will be described.

Lateral Femoral Cutaneous Nerve Block

Although an isolated block of the lateral femoral cutaneous nerve (LFC) is rarely needed, it may be blocked to provide analgesia for muscle biopsy of the vastus lateralis muscle during malignant hyperthermia testing (Wedel, 1989). An LFC block may also be used in combination with a femoral nerve block in high-risk children in place of a general anesthetic for complete analgesia for muscle biopsies of the thigh (Rosen and Broadman, 1986; Maccani et al., 1995). See related video online at www.expertconsult.com.

Anatomy

The lateral femoral cutaneous nerve arises from second and third lumbar nerves and travels deep to the iliacus fascia toward the anterior superior iliac spine until it emerges under the fascia lata in the upper thigh. It is a pure sensory nerve that

innervates the lateral thigh to the knee, including some terminal branches at the patellar plexus (Fig. 16-26, *A*).

Technique

No nerve stimulator is required to block the LFC, as it is purely a sensory nerve. In the infrainguinal approach, a blunt 22-gauge needle is inserted perpendicular to the skin, aiming in the direction of the nerve inferolaterally 0.5 to 1 cm below the inguinal ligament and medial to the anterior superior iliac spine (see Fig. 16-26, *B*). A pop will be felt as the needle pierces the fascia lata. Local anesthetic is then injected in a fanlike manner (McNicol, 1986).

Complications

There are no known serious complications from an isolated LFC except direct nerve trauma.

Femoral Nerve Block

A femoral nerve block may be used for any above-the-knee surgery of the lower extremity that requires analgesia of the majority of the thigh (Fig. 16-27, *A*). This includes analgesia for femur fracture (Ronchi et al., 1989). The block is simple to perform, either with or without a nerve stimulator, but a nerve stimulator should not be used in an awake child with a femur fracture because of the pain that may occur with muscle contraction from nerve stimulation. See related video online at www.expertconsult.com.

Anatomy

The femoral nerve, derived from lumbar nerves 1 to 3, enters the thigh in the femoral triangle below the inguinal ligament

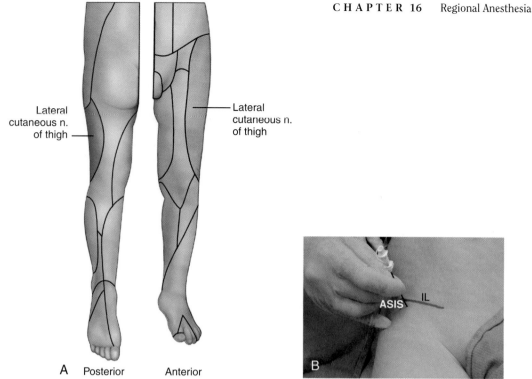

FIGURE 16-26. Lateral femoral cutaneous block. **A,** Dermatomal distribution of lateral femoral cutaneous block. **B,** Performance of lateral femoral cutaneous block. *ASIS,* Anterior superior iliac spine; *IL,* inguinal ligament.

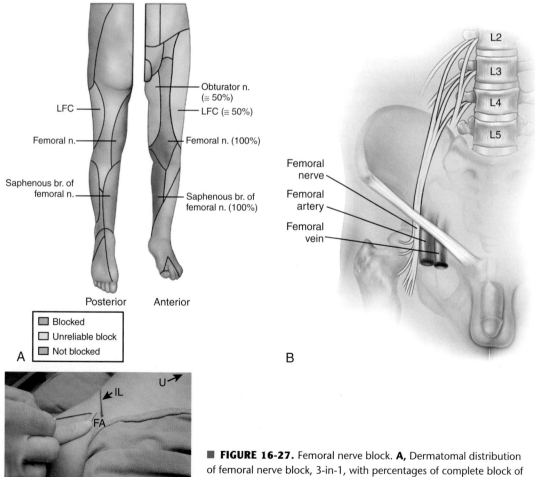

FIGURE 16-27. Femoral nerve block. **A,** Dermatomal distribution of femoral nerve block, 3-in-1, with percentages of complete block of individual nerves. **B,** Anatomy of femoral nerve block. **C,** Performance of femoral block. Needle insertion is 0.5 to 1 cm lateral to the artery. *FA,* Femoral artery; *IL,* inguinal ligament; *U,* umbilicus.

The approximate depth to the femoral nerve from the skin should be reviewed (see Fig. 16-6). The nerve is immediately lateral to the femoral artery and is covered by the fascia lata and fascia iliaca (see Fig. 16-27, *B*).

Technique

With the child supine and the feet rotated outward, the femoral artery is palpated immediately below the inguinal ligament. The needle is inserted at a slight cephalad angle to the skin at 0.5 to 1 cm below the inguinal ligament and 0.5 to 1 cm lateral to the artery (see Fig. 16-27, *C*). As the needle pierces the fascia lata, a distinct pop is felt. If a nerve stimulator is used, the desired muscle response should be contraction of the mid quadriceps with a "patellar kick" If there is muscle stimulation medial to the mid patella at the thigh adductors, the needle is slightly adjusted laterally. If there is lateral muscle stimulation, the needle is adjusted slightly medially. Because of the close proximity of the femoral vessels, continuous aspiration for blood should be performed to detect intravascular entry. Once the desired location of the needle is achieved, local anesthetic is then injected.

A 3-in-1 block is a modification of a femoral nerve block. This technique anesthetizes the lateral femoral cutaneous and obturator nerves, which lie more proximal in the sheath. The 3-in-1 technique is accomplished by performing a femoral nerve block and promoting proximal spread. The landmarks and needle insertion are exactly the same as for a simple femoral block, except that the volume of local anesthetic is increased and distal pressure is used to promote cephalad spread to the lumbar plexus with the femoral sheath as a conduit. When compared with a fascia iliaca compartment block (see later), a 3-in-1 approach can result in a higher failure rate (Dalens et al., 1989). Although it is effective in anesthetizing the femoral nerve 100% of the time, the LFC and obturator were successfully blocked in only 20% of the children. Dalens noted that the successful blocks of the LFC and obturator nerves in the 3-in-1 group were not the result of proximal spread of the local anesthetic but possibly of a fascia iliaca–like spread of the local anesthetic.

Technique with ultrasound. Ultrasound-guided femoral nerve block has been shown to improve the quality and lengthen the duration of the block while decreasing the required dose of the local anesthetic as compared with the nerve stimulation technique (Marhofer et al., 1997, 1998; Oberndorfer et al., 2007).

A linear ultrasound transducer set at the highest operational frequency should be used to achieve maximal resolution of the superficial inguinal anatomy. The patient is positioned supine with the leg slightly bent at the knee and externally rotated. The ultrasound machine should be positioned on the contralateral side in the direct line of view of the operator. The operator sits or stands by the patient's hip on the ipsalateral side, with the ultrasound transducer held in the nondominant hand and positioned transverse to the femoral artery, inferior to the inguinal ligament (Fig. 16-28, *A*). Femoral vessels are a readily recognized starting point for locating the nerve (see Fig. 16-28, *B*). The femoral nerve often has a triangular, hyperechoic appearance and is located lateral to the femoral artery, superficial to the iliopsoas muscle, and beneath the fascia iliaca. The block needle is inserted in-plane in a lateral-to-medial direction (see Fig. 16-28, *A*) and should be seen transversing the superficial fascia lata and immediately adherent fascia iliaca before the test dose is administered. Local anesthetic injection should produce circumferential spread around the nerve bundle below the fascia iliaca (see Fig. 16-28, *C*). Out-of-plane needle insertion is possible for the performance of this block once the inguinal sonoanatomy is appreciated, and for the placement of continuous catheters.

Complications

Complications from femoral or 3-in-1 blocks are uncommon, but they may include puncture of the femoral artery. In that event, pressure should be held for at least 5 minutes to avoid the formation of a large hematoma.

Fascia Iliaca Compartment Block

The fascia iliaca block provides analgesia of the femoral, lateral femoral cutaneous, and obturator nerves. A fascia iliaca block may be effective in more than 90% of children, compared with 20% effectiveness of the 3-in-1 technique (Dalens et al., 1989). Fascia iliaca blocks are useful for all above-the-knee lower

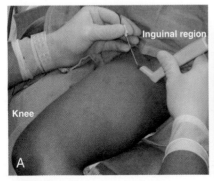
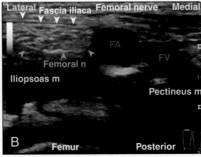
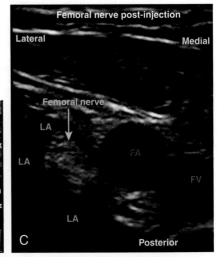

■ **FIGURE 16-28.** Ultrasound scan of femoral nerve block. **A,** Needle and transducer placement. **B,** Sonoanatomy before injection. **C,** Sonoanatomy after injection.

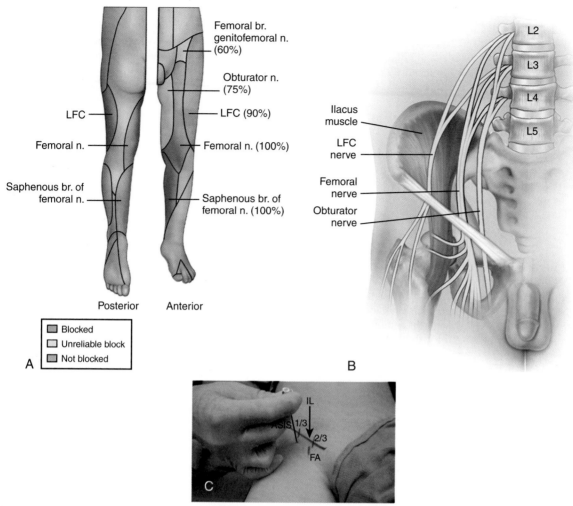

■ **FIGURE 16-29.** Fascia iliaca block. **A,** Dermatomal distribution of fascia iliaca block, with relative percentages of successful block of individual nerves by this approach. **B,** Anatomy of fascia iliaca block. **C,** Performance of fascia iliaca block. Needle insertion is 0.5 to 2 cm below inguinal ligament. *ASIS,* Anterior superior iliac spine; *FA,* femoral artery; *IL,* inguinal ligament.

extremity surgeries because of their ability to anesthetize this region in its entirety (Fig. 16-29, A). In addition, the fascia iliaca block reliably anesthetizes the femoral branch of the genitofemoral nerve, the sensory nerve supply to Scarpa's triangle. Because of its ability to block the upper leg, the fascia iliaca compartment block can be used in combination with intravenous sedation or nitrous oxide for children who are undergoing muscle biopsy of the thigh. See related video online at www.expertconsult.com.

Anatomy

The three distal nerves of the lumbar plexus, the femoral, lateral femoral cutaneous, and obturator nerves, all emerge from the psoas muscle and run along the inner surface of the fascia iliaca. A fascia iliaca compartment block delivers local anesthetic between the fascia iliaca and iliacus muscles where it spreads to bathe the three nerves (see Fig. 16-29, B).

Technique

With the child in the supine position, the inguinal ligament is located by drawing a line from the pubic tubercle to the anterior superior iliac spine. Divide the inguinal ligament into thirds.

At the junction of the lateral third and the medial two thirds of the inguinal ligament, drop a line inferiorly 0.5 to 2 cm and perpendicular to the ligament. This is the point of needle insertion (see Fig. 16-29, C). A blunt needle is inserted perpendicular to the skin. There is no need for a nerve stimulator, because the goal is to find the area behind the iliacus fascia for anesthetic injection, not to locate a specific nerve. Two pops are felt as the needle first pierces the fascia lata, then the fascia iliaca. If light pressure is held on the plunger of the syringe, a loss of resistance is felt as the fascia iliaca is pierced. With the needle in the correct position, local anesthetic solution is injected.

Complications

Complications during a fascia iliaca block might include isolated femoral block if the injection is too medial. Otherwise there are no known major complications from performing a fascia iliaca block.

Lumbar Plexus Block

Like the fascia iliaca compartment block, a lumbar plexus block provides analgesia to the three major nerves of the lumbar plexus. This block is useful for any surgery that may occur on the upper leg because it can completely anesthetize that region. This block also anesthetizes the distal branches of the lumbar plexus, including the iliohypogastric, ilioinguinal, and genitofemoral nerves that innervate the groin area applicable to many pediatric surgical procedures (Fig. 16-30, *A*). See related video online at www.expertconsult.com.

Anatomy

The lumbar plexus lies in the psoas compartment between the two masses of the psoas muscle that attach to the vertebrae, and it is surrounded by fascia derived from fascia iliaca (see Fig. 16-30, *B*). The approximate depth from the skin to the lumbar plexus at different ages is noted in Figure 16-6.

Technique

In a study of 50 children aged 6 months to 16 years undergoing hip and upper lower extremity procedures, Dalens and coworkers (1988) compared two techniques of lumbar plexus block. In group 1, a modification by Chayen of a psoas compartment block was used. A needle was inserted at the midpoint of a line connecting the spinous process of the fifth lumbar vertebra and the posterior superior iliac spine. There were difficulties with needle insertion in 7 of 25 children, and 23 of the 25 had epidural spread of local anesthesia. In the second group, a modification of Winnie's approach was used. In this technique, a needle was inserted at the intersection of the line drawn to connect the

iliac crests and a line drawn through the posterior superior iliac spine parallel to the spinous processes (see Fig. 16-30, *C*). There were no problems with needle insertion, and all 25 patients exhibited a unilateral lumbar plexus block distribution. Sacral distribution occurred in 23 of the 25 children, as these two plexuses are found in the same anatomic plane. Although both techniques provided effective analgesia to the lumbar plexus, the Chayen approach resulted in epidural spread rather than being isolated to the lumbar plexus. Because of the greater ease of performance of the modified Winnie technique, this technique will be further described for use in children.

Modified Winnie approach to the lumbar plexus. With the child in the lateral position, block side up, the knees and thighs are flexed. Two lines are drawn: (1) to connect the two iliac crests, and (2) from the ipsilateral posterosuperior iliac spine running cephalad and parallel to the spinous processes. The needle is inserted perpendicular to the skin at the intersection of the two lines (see Fig. 16-30, *C*) and then advanced through the quadratus lumborum. If contact is made with a transverse process, the needle is directed slightly more cephalad until a strong contraction of the mid (not lateral or medial) quadriceps with a patellar kick is apparent. If hamstring contractions are observed, the needle is directed slightly more laterally. If there is isolated hip movement, the psoas has been directly stimulated. If the quadriceps and hamstrings are contracting simultaneously, the needle should be directed more cephalad to stimulate the lumbar rather than sacral plexus.

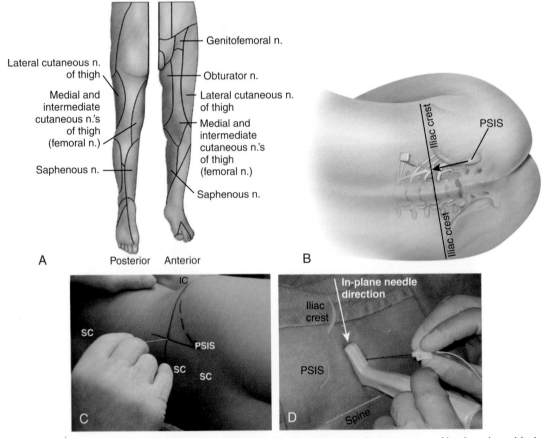

■ **FIGURE 16-30.** Lumbar plexus block. **A,** Dermatomal distribution of lumbar plexus block. **B,** Anatomy of lumbar plexus block. **C,** Performance of lumbar plexus block. Note that the needle is considerably lateral to the spinal column. **D,** Needle and transducer placement *IC,* Iliac crest; *PSIS,* posterior superior iliac spine; *SC,* spinal column.

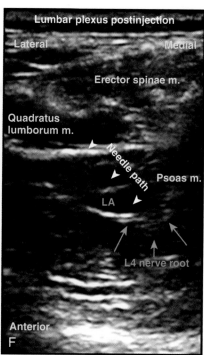

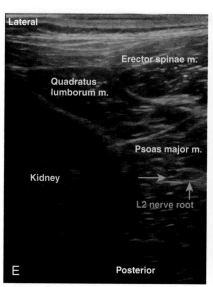

■ **FIGURE 16-30, cont'd. E,** Sonoanatomy prior to injection. **F,** Sonoanatomy after injection.

The needle is placed in the same location as in the landmark technique for ultrasonographic-guided lumbar plexus block (see Fig. 16-30, *D*). Sonoanatomy shows the relationship to the structures before (see Fig. 16-30, *E*) and after (see Fig. 16-30, *F*) local anesthetic injection.

Complications

Although complications are rare, they may be serious if the needle is advanced too deeply into the retroperitoneum. Retroperitoneal hematoma is a significant risk, and continuous aspiration for blood should be done while performing the block. The highest incidence of major bleeding after peripheral regional anesthetic techniques has been found to occur after a psoas compartment block (Horlocker et al., 2003a).

Saphenous Nerve Block

The saphenous nerve is the terminal branch of the femoral nerve and provides cutaneous innervation of the medial leg or foot. It enters the adductor canal lateral to the femoral artery, crosses it anteriorly, and lies medial to it at the farthest end of the canal. In the distal thigh, the saphenous nerve passes between the sartorius and gracilis muscles and pierces the deep fascia on the medial aspect of the knee. It descends down the medial side of the leg with the great saphenous vein.

Blocking the saphenous nerve provides analgesia to the medial portion of the foot immediately anterior to the medial malleolus and extending toward, but not reaching, the great toe. For procedures below the knee that include incisions on the medial anterior portion of the foot and leg, the saphenous nerve may be blocked to cover the small femoral component that has innervation below the knee.

Technique with Ultrasound

Multiple approaches to the saphenous nerve block have been described, but visualization of this nerve in a child can be challenging, so the transsartorial perifemoral artery approach is preferred (Benzon et al., 2005; Tsui and Ozelsel, 2009). A linear ultrasound transducer set at the highest operational frequency should be used. The patient is positioned supine with the leg slightly bent at the knee and externally rotated. The ultrasound machine should be positioned on the contralateral side in the direct line of view of the operator. The operator sits or stands by the patient's knee on the ipsilateral side with the ultrasound transducer held in the nondominant hand and positioned transverse to the longitudinal axis of the extremity at the mid thigh (Fig. 16-31, *A*). The femoral artery in the adductor canal is a reliable landmark for locating the nerve (see Fig. 16-31, *B*). The saphenous nerve appears hyperechoic and is located anterior to the artery below the sartorius muscle. The block needle is inserted in-plane in a lateral-to-medial direction toward the nerve, and circumferential envelopment by local anesthetic is the goal. If the nerve is not clearly visualized in the adductor canal, a perivascular injection will be adequate. As the practioner gains expertise in identifying and tracing the saphenous nerve, it may be advantageous to perform saphenous nerve blockade distally, as this will avoid motor blockade of the vastus medialis muscle because the nerve to the vastus medialis is located in the adductor canal.

Sciatic Nerve Block

A sciatic nerve block is indicated for surgical procedures that involve the lower extremity below the knee. When used in combination with blocks of the lumbar plexus, the lower extremity can be blocked in its entirety. See related video online at www.expertconsult.com.

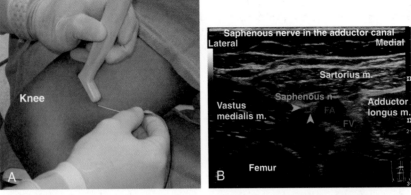

■ **FIGURE 16-31.** Ultrasound saphenous nerve block. **A,** Needle and transducer placement. **B,** Sonoanatomy.

Anatomy

The sciatic nerve is derived from the anterior rami of L4 to S3 and is the largest nerve in the body (see Fig. 16-25). It emerges through the greater sciatic foramen to run between the greater trochanter of the femur and the ischial tuberosity before taking its position in the thigh posterior to the quadriceps femoris. If the sciatic nerve is blocked in its proximal position, this will also anesthetize the posterior femoral cutaneous nerve (a branch of ventral rami of S1 to S3). This nerve innervates the posterior thigh above the knee and the hamstring muscles. The sciatic nerve primarily consists of two nerves, the tibial and common peroneal nerves, which travel in a common sheath in the posterior upper portion of the leg. These nerves typically divide near the popliteal fossa and innervate the leg below the knee.

Approaches to the Sciatic Nerve

Several approaches to the sciatic nerve have been described in children. The posterior, anterior, and lateral approaches have been compared with respect to ease of performance, efficacy of block, and rate of complications (Dalens et al., 1990). The overall success rate of all three approaches exceeded 90%. However, there were fewer difficulties reported with the posterior approach. The posterior approach resulted in an 88% success rate on first attempt, compared with 78% for the lateral approach and only 62% on the first attempt for the anterior approach. In addition, vascular punctures occurred only in children who underwent an anterior approach. Because of the higher success rate of the posterior approach and the completeness of analgesia of the sciatic nerve and posterior branches (Fig. 16-32, *A*), the posterior approach is described here.

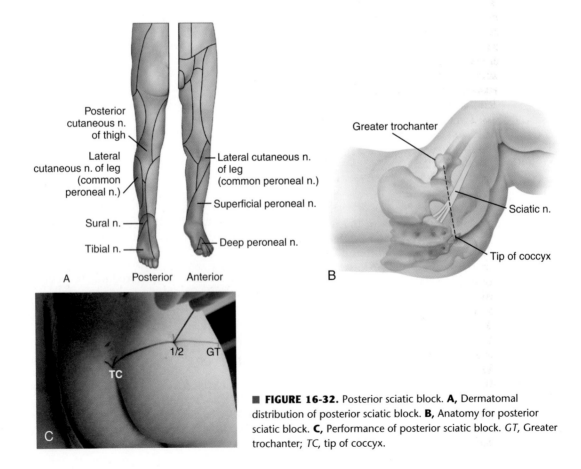

■ **FIGURE 16-32.** Posterior sciatic block. **A,** Dermatomal distribution of posterior sciatic block. **B,** Anatomy for posterior sciatic block. **C,** Performance of posterior sciatic block. *GT,* Greater trochanter; *TC,* tip of coccyx.

However, the reader is prompted to review the lateral approach, especially for use in children who are unable to be positioned for other approaches to the sciatic nerve (Dalens, 1995).

To block the sciatic nerve using the posterior approach, a modification of Labat's technique was developed by Dalens and associates (1990). The child is placed in the lateral position with the side to be blocked uppermost and the upper leg flexed at the hip and knee. Using a nerve stimulator and insulated needle, the point of needle insertion is at the midpoint of the line that extends from the tip of the coccyx to the greater trochanter of the femur. The needle should be perpendicular to the skin with slight angulation toward the lateral ischial tuberosity (see Fig. 16-32, B and C). The approximate depth to the sciatic nerve using the posterior approach depends on the age of the patient (see Fig. 16-6). Using a nerve stimulator, the motor response is a movement in the patient's foot. Plantar flexion indicates stimulation of the tibial nerve. Dorsiflexion or eversion at the ankle indicates stimulation of the peroneal nerve. Once the appropriate response is elicited, local anesthesia is injected.

Complications of the posterior approach to the sciatic nerve include vascular puncture of gluteal vessels. Constant aspiration for blood should be done during performance of the block to avoid this complication.

The Raj block was developed in 1975 and is similar to the posterior approach (Raj et al., 1975). This approach anesthetizes the sciatic nerve slightly more distal than in the classic posterior approach (Fig. 16-33, A). This block is performed in the supine child with the leg to be blocked lifted and flexed at the hip and knee. The needle is inserted at the midpoint between ischial tuberosity and greater trochanter in the sciatic groove (see Fig. 16-33, B and C). Once appropriate muscle stimulation with less than 0.5 mA is seen at the foot, local anesthetic is injected. The advantage to this block is the reliability of the landmarks and simplicity of the block itself. By flexing the hip, the Raj technique brings the sciatic nerve closer to the skin. This improves the likelihood of a successful block, especially in obese children and adolescents.

To use some of the principles of the posterior and Raj approaches, the ultrasound-guided subgluteal approach may be performed. A linear, high-frequency probe can be used in children, but as the depth of the imaged neural structure increases with age or obesity, use of the lower-frequency, curvilinear probe is required to achieve sufficient penetration. The child is positioned in a lateral decubitus position with the operative side uppermost and the knee flexed. The operator faces the patient with the ultrasound machine across in the direct line of view. A line connecting the greater trochanter and ischial tuberosity represents a starting point for the sonographic examination (Fig. 16-34, A). The sciatic nerve is visualized between the anterior surface of the gluteus maximus and the posterior surface of the quadratus femoris muscle. It is bounded medially by the ischial tuberosity and laterally by the greater trochanter. It has hyperechoic appearance and may be oval or triangular (see Fig. 16-34, B). Tracing the nerve cranially or caudally may allow for improved sonographic visualization. The posterior cutaneous nerve of the thigh is frequently observed medial to the sciatic nerve at this location (Karmakar et al., 2007). An in-plane approach is used to guide needle advancement, and circumferential spread of local anesthetic is sought. Medial envelopment of the sciatic nerve by local anesthetic ensures blockade of the

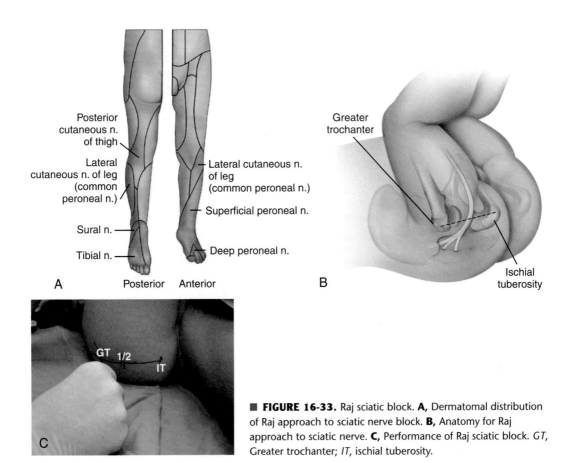

FIGURE 16-33. Raj sciatic block. **A,** Dermatomal distribution of Raj approach to sciatic nerve block. **B,** Anatomy for Raj approach to sciatic nerve. **C,** Performance of Raj sciatic block. *GT,* Greater trochanter; *IT,* ischial tuberosity.

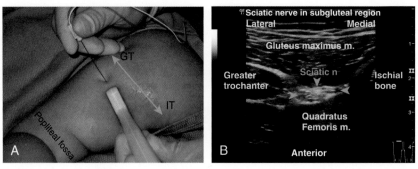

■ **FIGURE 16-34.** Ultrasound scan of subgluteal block. **A,** Needle and transducer placement. **B,** Sonanatomy. *GT,* Greater trochanter; *IT,* ischial tuberosity.

posterior cutaneous nerve of the thigh and may require needle repositioning when thigh incision or tourniquet use is planned. An out-of-plane approach is used for continuous catheter placement because it facilitates threading and fixation of the catheter (van Geffen and Gielen, 2006).

A popliteal fossa block may be used for procedures of the distal lower extremity and will anesthetize the sciatic nerve more distally in the leg and just proximal to the knee (Kempthorne and Brown, 1984) (Fig. 16-35, *A*). See related video online at www.expertconsult.com. Near the popliteal fossa, the sciatic nerve divides into the common peroneal nerve and the posterior tibial nerve (see Fig. 16-35, *B*). The common peroneal nerve runs anteriorly to wrap around the head of the fibula, and the posterior tibial nerve travels down the posterior lower

leg. In approximately 10% of the population, the branching of the sciatic nerve occurs more proximal to the popliteal fossa and high in the posterior thigh. Therefore, there may be a variable success rate in blocking the sciatic at this level, but both nerves are usually blocked by this approach because a common epineural sheath envelops the two nerves (Vloka et al., 1997). Advantages to the popliteal approach include the relatively superficial location of the sciatic nerve (i.e., near to the skin) and the decreased risk of intraneural injection, as the sciatic nerve is not fixed against any bony structures in this location. To easily access the popliteal fossa for a single-shot block, the patient may remain in the supine position and the leg to be blocked is lifted with the knee and thigh flexed. The child may also be turned to the lateral position and the leg to be blocked

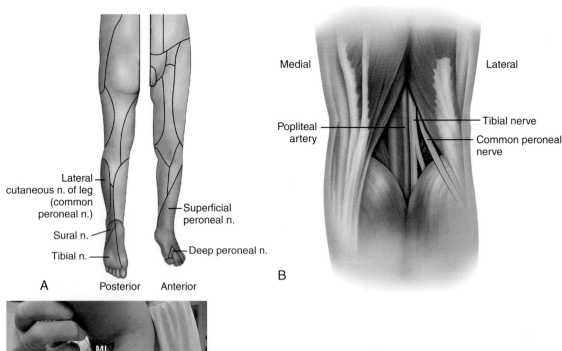

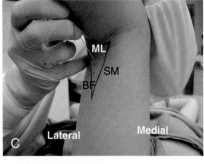

■ **FIGURE 16-35.** Popliteal block. **A,** Dermatomal distribution of popliteal fossa block. **B,** Anatomy of popliteal fossa block. **C,** Performance of popliteal block. *BF,* Biceps femoris; *ML,* midline; *SM,* semimembranous and semitendinosus tendons.

positioned uppermost. The superior triangle of the popliteal fossa has as its boundaries the semimembranosus and semitendinosus tendons medially, the biceps femoris tendon laterally, and the popliteal crease inferiorly. The needle is inserted 45 degrees to the skin, aiming cephalad and just lateral to the midline of the popliteal triangle (see Fig. 16-35, C). The distance from the popliteal fold to needle insertion is estimated based on weight. If the weight is less than 10 kg, the distance is 1 cm; if the weight is 10 to 20 kg, the distance is 2 cm (Konrad and Johr, 1998). Each 10 kg of body weight should move the needle cephalad in the triangle approximately 1 cm. Muscle stimulation of the foot in either the common peroneal or the posterior tibial distribution is a confirmation of an acceptable needle position, but stimulation of both branches suggests that the sciatic nerve has not yet separated into the two branches at this level. Local anesthetic is injected once appropriate stimulation is apparent at less than 0.5 mA.

Konrad and Johr (1998) sought to determine a system for standardization of popliteal fossa block. They performed the block in 50 children between the ages of 2 months and 18 years. They determined that the minimal distance to the sciatic nerve in the popliteal fossa was 13 mm, and the depth did not vary significantly in patients weighing less than 35 kg but did increase for children weighing more than 35 kg. All blocks in the study were successful, and there were no complications. Vascular puncture was avoided because of the lateral position of the needle in relation to the popliteal vessels.

Tobias and Mencio (1999) provided analgesia in 20 children for foot and ankle surgery by performing popliteal fossa blocks at the completion of the surgical procedure. When using 0.75 mL/kg of 0.2% ropivacaine, the duration of analgesia was between 8 and 12 hours.

The ultrasound-guided popliteal approach can also be performed with the linear ultrasound transducer set at the highest operational frequency. The child can be positioned supine with the leg elevated on a footrest or held by an assistant (Fig. 16-36, A) or lateral with the operative side uppermost and the knee flexed (see Fig. 16-36, B). The operator stands or sits by the child's ipsilateral limb with the ultrasound machine in the direct line of view. The sonographic examination begins by positioning the transducer over the popliteal fossa in an axial plane and locating the popliteal artery and vein. The tibial nerve is located superficial to the vein and has a round or fasciculated appearance. Dynamic cephalad tracing will identify the point of merger of the tibial and common peroneal components into the sciatic nerve (see Fig. 16-36, C and D). The level of the local anesthetic placement should be proximal to the division of the sciatic nerve to achieve complete blockade of the foot. The sciatic nerve exhibits a significant degree of anisotropy and is best visualized when the insonating ultrasound angle is directed caudally. An in-plane, lateral-to-medial approach is used to guide needle advancement for single-shot blocks, and the needle tip is guided posterior to the sciatic nerve to achieve the circumferential spread of local anesthetic (see Fig. 16-36, E and F). An out-of-plane approach is used for continuous catheter placement, because it facilitates threading and fixation of the catheter.

Ankle Block

An ankle block is a simple block that provides analgesia to the foot for procedures such as toe removal or simple reconstructive surgery. See related video online at www.expertconsult.com.

Anatomy

Five nerves that innervate the foot must be blocked for analgesia of the foot in its entirety (Fig. 16-37). The saphenous nerve is found near the saphenous vein on the medial side of

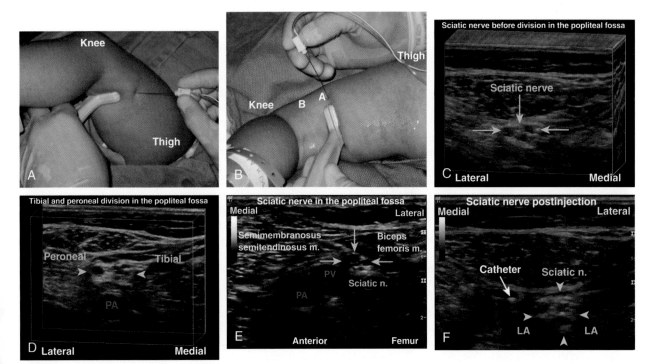

FIGURE 16-36. Ultrasound scan of popliteal block. **A,** Needle and transducer placement with leg up. **B,** Needle and transducer placement, lateral position. **C,** Sciatic before division. **D,** Sciatic after division. **E,** Before injection. **F,** After injection.

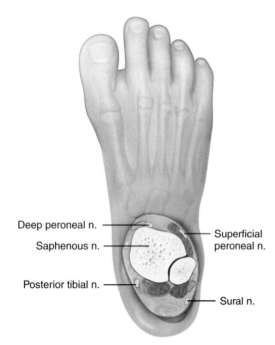

Deep peroneal n.

Saphenous n.

Posterior tibial n.

Superficial
peroneal n.

Sural n.

■ **FIGURE 16-37.** Anatomy for ankle block.

the dorsum of the foot and is somewhat superficial in its location. It innervates the skin surrounding the medial malleolus. Following the dorsum of the foot, and near the anterior tibial artery, runs the deep peroneal nerve, which is responsible for the innervation of the web space between the first and second toes. As the name implies, this nerve runs deep and is found near the tibia and between the extensor hallucis longus and anterior tibial artery. Immediately lateral to the deep peroneal nerve, but found superficially, is the superficial peroneal nerve. This nerve innervates the medial and lateral aspects of the dorsum of the foot. The plantar innervation of the foot is supplied by the tibial and sural nerves. The tibial nerve is found immediately posterior to the posterior tibial artery and medial malleolus, and the sural nerve is located posterior to the lateral malleolus.

Technique

To perform an ankle block, each of the five nerves is blocked using a 25-gauge needle. With the child supine, the saphenous nerve is blocked by injecting 1 to 5 mL of local anesthetic solution subcutaneously near the saphenous vein anterior to the medial malleolus. The deep peroneal nerve is blocked by inserting the needle lateral to the extensor hallucis longus tendon near the tibial artery and advancing it until it contacts the tibia. The needle should then be withdrawn slightly and 1 to 5 mL local anesthetic injected. The superficial peroneal nerve is blocked with a subcutaneous ring of local anesthetic across the lateral dorsum of the foot. The patient's foot then should be positioned so that the two posterior nerves can be blocked for complete analgesia of the foot. The tibial nerve is blocked midway between the medial malleolus and the calcaneus posterior to the tibial artery. The sural nerve is blocked midway between the lateral malleolus and the calcaneus. Each of the posterior nerves should receive 1 to 5 mL of local anesthetic solution.

Dosing

To ensure complete analgesia to the foot with a duration of action greater than 4 hours, bupivacaine, ropivacaine, or levobupivacaine 0.5% should be used. The volumes delivered at each nerve depend on the age and size of the patient. The larger volumes are reserved for adolescents, but the recommended maximal dosing should not be exceeded. Epinephrine should not be added to the solution because of the risk for peripheral vasoconstriction.

Complications

Risks during performance of an ankle block are rare. Because of the proximity of vessels, frequent aspiration for blood should be performed during injection. In addition, the use of epinephrine for an ankle block, particularly in an infant or young child, should be avoided to reduce the possibility of ischemia secondary to loss of perfusion to the distal foot.

Dosing of Lower Extremity Blocks

The volumes of local anesthesia depend on the nerves to be blocked. For femoral nerve blocks, 0.2 to 0.75 mL/kg is administered, whereas for plexus blocks, volumes of greater than 1 mL/kg are frequently needed (see Table 16-4). The duration of action of local anesthesia depends on the anesthetic concentration and age of the patient. When used in combination, local anesthetics are additive. It is important not to exceed maximal allowable dosing (see Table 16-2).

Continuous Peripheral Nerve Catheters

Indwelling catheters may be placed for peripheral nerve analgesia for those procedures that will result in significant and prolonged postoperative pain, or when vascular insufficiency is a risk. Commercially available continuous catheter kits allow catheter insertion after the plexus has been localized with a nerve stimulator or visualized by ultrasound. Kits that allow continuous catheter placement in children include a system using a short 18-gauge insulated Touhy needle through which a 20-gauge catheter may be threaded (B. Braun, Bethlehem, PA). Other systems use a catheter-over-needle approach, where a 20-gauge introducing catheter similar to an intravenous cannula fits over a 22-gauge insulated needle. Once the stimulation is achieved, the cannula is inserted into the sheath, the needle is removed, and a styletted 24-gauge catheter is threaded into the sheath for continuous infusion.

There is little information on the continuous infusions of local anesthetics in upper extremity catheters in children, but dosing of an indwelling catheter for brachial plexus anesthesia should adhere to maximal allowable dosing guidelines (see Table 16-2). Typical dosages should start at 0.1 to 0.2 mL/kg per hour of either bupivacaine or levobupivacaine (0.125% to 0.25%) or ropivacaine (0.1% to 0.2%) (see Table 16-4). Increases in the infusion rate may be made as needed as long as the maximal rate does not exceed 0.2 mg/kg per hour in infants less than 6 months, or 0.4 mg/kg per hour in children older than 6 months. It would be unusual, however, for peripheral nerve catheter infusions to reach maximal limits.

Continuous catheters have been used for the lower extremity in children, with early cases describing its use for femu fractures of patients in the intensive care unit (ICU) (Johnson, 1994; Tobias, 1994). Johnson used an epidural catheter in the femoral sheath and delivered 0.125% bupivacaine at 0.3 mg/kg per hour. In these patients, plasma bupivacaine concentrations were well below toxic levels. Using a Seldinger technique, and a 3-French, 8-cm, single-lumen central line catheter (Cook Critical Care, Bloomington, IN), Tobias administered continuous infusions at 0.15 mL/kg per hour of 0.2% bupivacaine to four children with femur fractures and closed head trauma. The catheters provided adequate analgesia in the ICU setting for 4 to 6 days and there were no complications. To provide more complete analgesia of the upper portion of the leg, catheters may also be placed in the lumbar plexus or fascia iliaca compartments. Sciard and coworkers (2001), using nerve stimulation, placed 20-gauge plexus catheters (Pajunk, Albany, NY) in the lumbar plexus of children and administered continuous infusions of 0.2% ropivacaine at 0.33 to 0.4 mg/kg per hour. Paut and associates (2001) inserted 20-gauge catheters (Contiplex, B. Braun, Melsungen, Germany) through 55-mm cannulae into the fascia iliaca compartment and administered continuous infusions of 0.1% bupivacaine at a rate of 0.5 mL/kg per year of age. After 48 hours, the mean delivered dosage of bupivacaine was 0.135 ± 0.03 mg/kg per hour, and the plasma bupivacaine levels at 24 and 48 hours were not significantly different at 0.71 mcg/mL and 0.84 mcg/mL, respectively. The authors concluded that the bupivacaine plasma concentrations at the rates used in their study for a continuous fascia iliaca block are within safety margins.

When compared with a continuous epidural catheter, a continuous popliteal catheter provides similar excellent postoperative analgesia without the side effects of urinary retention, nausea, and vomiting (Dadure et al., 2006). Children in this study received a popliteal catheter infusion of 0.2% ropivacaine at 0.1 mL/kg per hour for 48 hours and received a 100% parent satisfaction score. The subgluteal approach to the sciatic nerve has been used for continuous catheters by employing an ultrasound-guided approach to placement of a stimulating catheter (van Geffen and Gielen, 2006). These children received bupivacaine 0.25% at a rate of 0.1 mL/kg per hour and had excellent pain relief, with no children receiving morphine other than those who had undergone amputation. The children who had undergone limb amputation received intravenous morphine despite pain scores of less than 4 as part of their multimodal therapy.

The use of disposable pumps for continuous delivery via a peripheral catheter of local anesthetic solutions provides a great option for postoperative pain control after outpatient orthopedic surgery. Dadure and coworkers (2003) described the use of the disposable elastomeric pumps in 25 children aged 1 to 15 years receiving continuous infusion via catheters in the popliteal, femoral, or axillary sheaths. A continuous infusion of 0.2% ropivacaine was used at a rate of 0.1 mL/kg per hour. The median pain score for all children was zero up to 48 hours, and there were no adverse events. A larger study at Children's Hospital of Philadelphia reported on the use of 226 continuous peripheral nerve catheters in children aged 4 to 18 years (Ganesh et al., 2007). There was a 2.8% incidence of complications. Three patients had prolonged numbness that resolved spontaneously, one patient had cellulitis that was treated with antibiotics, one patient developed tinnitus that was reversed with clamping of the local anesthetic catheter, and one patient had difficulty removing the catheter at home. The conclusion of this report was that it is feasible to implement a program that provides continuous peripheral nerve catheters in children when appropriate expertise is available. Education of the patient and parents as well as frequent follow-up are important to recognize potential complications in a timely fashion.

Patient-controlled regional analgesia was investigated in 30 children who had undergone lower limb orthopedic surgery (Duflo et al., 2006). When comparing 0.2% ropivacaine delivered as a continuous infusion or by patient control, both groups had adequate analgesia, but the latter group achieved it with significantly less local anesthetic and, therefore, lower total plasma levels of ropivacaine.

TRUNCAL BLOCKS

Increased understanding of the abdominal wall anatomy has led to the introduction of new techniques capable of blocking sensory abdominal wall innervation (O'Donnell et al., 2006; Hebbard, 2008). Under sonographic guidance, the neurovascular plane housing various divisions of the thoracolumbar nerves can be safely blocked regardless of central neuroaxial abnormalities, bloodstream infections, or coagulopathy. These planes exist in continuity and can be precisely blocked at several anatomic locations depending on the area of analgesia required (Fig. 16-38).

Transversus Abdominis Plane Block

Transversus abdominis plane (TAP) block is the most recent addition in the field of abdominal wall blocks and holds the potential of blocking the sensory nerve supply of the entire anteriolateral abdominal wall with a single injection. Originally described in 2004 as a double-pop technique via the lumbar triangle of Petit (latissimus dorsi muscle [posterior], external oblique muscle [anterior], and iliac crest [inferior]), it has been demonstrated in the adult population to significantly decrease postoperative pain scores and opioid requirements after an open retropubic prostatectomy, cesarean delivery by Pfannenstein incision, and other major abdominal surgeries (O'Donnell et al., 2006; McDonnell et al., 2007a, 2007b, 2008). In a volunteer adult study, TAP block injection produced sensory deficit from the T7 to the L1 level and demonstrated radiographic evidence of contrast spread from the superior margin of the iliac crest to the costal margin and extending posteriorly to the quadratus lumborium (McDonnell et al., 2007b). However, the ability of TAP block to reliably produce sensory blockade above the T9 level was questioned in follow-up studies (Hebbard et al., 2007; Shibata et al., 2007). Ultrasound-guided TAP block dye injection

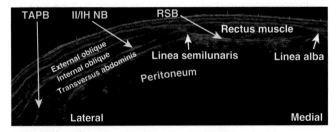

■ **FIGURE 16-38.** Sonoanatomy of truncal blocks.

into cadavers demonstrated involvement of only T10- to L1 nerve roots (Tran et al., 2009). An alternative subcostal TAP approach was suggested for the sensory blockade of the upper abdomen (Hebbard, 2008).

In pediatrics, this block has been successfully applied in small case studies with both landmark and ultrasound-guided techniques. TAP block via the triangle of Petit using 0.5 mL/kg of ropivacaine 0.375% was performed in 10 children aged 2 to 10 years undergoing elective unilateral inguinal hernia repair (Ludot et al., 2007). Anesthesia and postoperative analgesia were satisfactory in all children, and pharmacokinetic data determined peak plasma concentration to be 485 (±115) ng/mL at 50 (±15) minutes after block placement. This pharmokinetic behavior was similar to that described for ilioinguinal and iliohypogastric block, and it was thus concluded by the authors to be safe in children (Dalens et al., 2001). In a subsequent study by the same group, unilateral TAP block was performed by loss of resistance technique at the triangle of Petit in 25 children aged 2 to 13 years undergoing appendectomy with 0.5 mL/kg of 0.25% levobupivacaine (Ludot et al., 2008a). All of the blocks were considered successful, with good abdominal relaxation reported by the surgeons. Sensory block of the T7 to L1 region was described by the older children, and the duration of analgesia was 15 ± 2 hours, as defined by the time to the first opioid dose. Several ultrasound-guided TAP block case series have now been reported in children. The earliest was performed in eight children undergoing inguinal hernia repair (Fredrickson et al., 2008). A 50:50 mixture of 1% lidocaine and 1% ropivacaine with 1:200,000 epinephrine (0.3 mL/kg) was injected in-plane under ultrasound guidance between the internal oblique and transversus abdominis muscle 5 minutes before incision, and it was deemed successful in five out of the eight patients based on the hemodynamic response to incision. An alternative ultrasound approach to pediatric TAP block has been described advocating deposition of local anesthetic closer to the origin of the thoracolumbar roots, but no quantitative data were presented (Suresh and Chan, 2009). A recent report illustrated the use of ultrasound-guided TAP block in four neonates undergoing upper or mid-abdominal surgery (Fredrickson and Seal, 2009). Effective intraoperative analgesia was achieved with injection of 0.4 mL/kg of 0.25% ropivacaine, and three of the four patients were extubated without the use of narcotics. In another report, ultrasound-guided TAP block was performed on eight patients aged 2 days to 26 months undergoing a combination of lower abdominal (inguinal hernia repair), middle abdominal (colostomy closure, Ladd's procedure), and upper abdominal (Nissen, G-tube) surgeries (Bryskin, 2008). These patients were not considered neuroaxial anesthesia candidates for a variety of reasons and received ultrasound-guided TAP block at the origin of the transversus abdominis muscle with injection of 0.25 mL/kg of 0.25% bupivacaine with 1:200,000 epinephrine. Successful intraoperative analgesia was achieved in seven of the eight patients, with a duration of action of 9.6 hours (7 to 15.5 hours), as judged by the time to the first rescue dose, and a mean skin-to-TAP depth of 1.1 cm (0.8 to 1.6 cm). See related video online at www.expertconsult.com.

Anatomy

The abdominal wall is innervated by the thoracolumbar (T6 to L1) spinal segmental nerves. The anterior divisions of thoracolumbar nerve roots emerge anterior to the quadratus lumborum muscle, penetrate the neurofascial plane (i.e., the TAP)

between the transversus abdominis muscle and the internal oblique muscle, form complex anastomotic networks in the TAP, and emerge through the rectus muscle to supply the skin anteriorly. In the midaxillary line, these nerves send a lateral branch providing lateral abdominal wall innervation. The ilioinguinal and iliohypogastric nerves often enter the TAP in the anterior third of the iliac crest and may thus be missed by TAP block if local anesthetic is deposited too laterally. Deep circumflex iliac artery transverses TAP from below and forms anastomoses with the lower intercostal, subcostal and lumbar arteries anterior to the midaxillary line.

Technique

Although the original description of the TAP block was a loss-of-resistance/double-pop approach via the triangle of Petit, only the ultrasound-guided technique will be described in this text as it minimizes the risk of intraperitoneal needle placement and provides the endpoint for local anesthetic injection. No consensus has been reached regarding the ideal location in TAP for local anesthetic injection. A linear-array transducer set at the highest resolution frequency is used to perform this block. The operator stands on the side of the patient being blocked, with the screen directly across. The transducer is positioned transverse to the child's abdomen, midway between the anterior superior iliac spine (ASIS) and the subcostal border. It is then slowly moved laterally until the tendinous insertion of the transversus abdominis muscle is visualized just lateral of the midaxillary level. The internal oblique and external oblique muscles may also be approaching their aponeurotic insertion at this level. This position is chosen because the aponeurotic layer is easy to locate, allows greater longitudinal spread of local anesthetic (thus blocking upper abdominal segments), permits easier posterior diffusion (thus blocking the L1 nerve), and is always located posterior to the midaxillary line (thus guaranteeing blockade of the lateral branch) (Fig. 16-39, *A* and *B*). The block needle is inserted in the anterior-to-posterior direction, in-plane with the ultrasound transducer, until its tip is positioned between the internal oblique muscle and the tendinous insertion of the transversus muscle. After negative aspiration, local anesthetic should slowly be injected while visualizing separation of the two fascial layers (see Fig. 16-39, *C*). In small children and neonates, it may be necessary to slightly elevate the child's side off the bed to create space for the transducer to move laterally.

Catheter Insertion

The TAP block provides an ideal location for catheter placement in children who require prolonged infusion of local anesthetics and are not candidates for central neuraxial blockade. The child should be turned into a lateral decubitus position with the block side up. The leg should be flexed at the hip to allow greater subcostal-to-ASIS distance, and the transducer positioned longitudinally to the abdomen, just lateral to the midaxillary line (see Fig. 16-39, *D*). After visualization of the three layers, a Tuohy needle is introduced in-plane to the transducer in the caudal cranial direction, and a catheter is threaded 2 to 4 cm beyond the needle tip once negative aspiration and appropriate separation of fascial layers is visualized with ultrasound and with injection of a test dose (see Fig. 16-39, *E*). The approach for placement of the TAP catheter differs from the single-shot TAP injection in that the needle is introduced in the caudal-crania

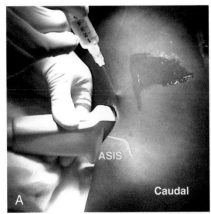
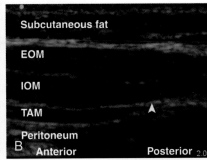
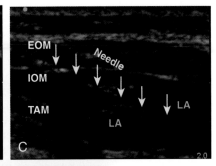
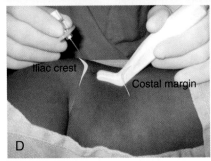
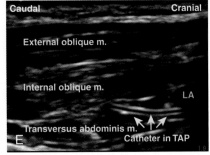

■ **FIGURE 16-39.** Ultrasound scan of transversus abdominis plane (TAP) block. **A,** Needle and transducer placement. **B,** Sonoanatomy. **C,** Ultrasonography of needle, local anesthetic. **D,** Ultrasound technique for TAP catheter placement. **E,** TAP catheter. *ASIS,* Anterior superior iliac spine.

direction as opposed to medial-lateral. This alteration ensures catheter placement in the TAP fascia before separation of the lateral nerve branches at the midaxillary line, extends anesthetic coverage toward superior abdominal dermatomes, and places the catheter outside the surgical field. Bilateral catheters can provide excellent pain relief in patients after major abdominal surgeries (personal experience).

Dosing

The optimal concentration and amount of local anesthetic necessary to produce complete abdominal wall blockade with TAP block in children is yet unknown. Successful outcomes after lower abdominal surgeries have been produced with the use of 0.5 mL/kg of 0.25% levobupivacaine or 0.375% ropivacaine by landmark technique, and 0.3 mL/kg of a 50:50 mixture of 1% lidocaine and 1% ropivacaine with 1:200,000 epinephrine by ultrasound-guided technique (Ludot et al., 2007, 2008a; Fredrickson et al., 2008). In the two case series describing upper abdominal surgeries, injection of 0.4 mL/kg of 0.25% ropivacaine and 0.25 mL/kg of 0.25% bupivacaine with 1:200,000 was deemed successful (Bryskin, 2008; Fredrickson and Seal, 2009). Since the injection of local anesthetic was performed into a different anatomic location in the TAP, it is difficult to draw quantitative conclusions regarding optimal dosage. In a pharmacokinetic adult study examining serum concentration of local anesthetic after a 400-mg injection of lidocaine via the triangle of Petit, a significant rise of serum concentration of local anesthetic was observed, with a maximal concentration of 3.7 to 5.5 µg/mL 15 to 60 minutes after the block, thus indicating that TAP block can potentially cause systemic toxicity with large dosage (Kato et al., 2009). Pediatric work indicates a safe

pharmacokinetic profile (Ludot et al., 2007). Although the data offer little conclusive evidence, it is clear that judicious use of local anesthetic is required and that the maximal dosage or concentration used in small children and neonates needs to be kept well below the toxic threshold. The use of epinephrine is advocated, as it may alert the operator to intravascular injection, whereas clonidine is unlikely to offer additional benefit judging by the ilioinguinal/iliohypogastric model (Dagher et al., 2006).

Complications

Because TAP block is essentially a lateral extension of the ilioinguinal/iliohypogastric nerve block, it is reasonable to assume that it will carry a similar complication profile. In the adult literature, a case of liver trauma has been reported during performance of TAP block in a 50-year-old woman with an enlarged liver (Farooq and Carey, 2008). In a neonatal patient with a frequently enlarged liver, this should be kept in mind, and hence performance of TAP block under ultrasound guidance is advocated. The presence of the deep circumflex iliac artery in the TAP suggests an increased risk of intravascular injection and hematoma formation, especially in patients with increased vascular congestion.

Ultrasound-Guided Rectus Sheath Block

Rectus sheath block provides analgesia to the anterior abdominal wall medial to the linea semilunaris, and it has been used for umbilical and epigastric hernia repairs, pyloromyotomy, and various laparoscopic procedures. With the advent of single-incision laparoscopic surgery via a large umbilical incision, this technique is likely to be increasingly used. An ultrasound-guided approach has been demonstrated to be efficacious in two studies for repair of umbilical hernia in children (Willschke et al., 2006b; de Jose Maria et al., 2007). See related video online at www.expertconsult.com.

Technique

A linear-array transducer set at the highest resolution frequency is used to perform this block. The operator stands on the side of the patient being blocked, with the screen directly across. The transducer is positioned transverse to the patient's abdomen just above the umbilicus (Fig. 16-40, *A*). Sonographic scan reveals the rectus muscle bordered laterally by tendinous insertions of the transversus abdominis, internal oblique, and external oblique muscles, and medially by the linea alba. It is enveloped by the rectus sheath, which is an aponeurotic extension of the three lateral muscles (see Fig. 16-38). Inferior epigastric vessels can frequently be visualized posterior to or in the rectus muscle belly and can be confirmed by color Doppler. The block needle is advanced in-line in the lateral-to-medial direction until the tip is visualized between the posterior border of the rectus muscle and the posterior rectus sheath (see Fig. 16-40, *B*). When anatomy allows, a needle path through the linea semilunaris is chosen, as this may avoid intramuscular vessel puncture and hematoma formation. After negative aspiration, a small volume of local anesthetic or saline is injected and should produce a lenslike separation between the rectus muscle and the posterior rectus sheath. Once an appropriate position of the needle tip is confirmed, injection of 0.1 to 0.2 mL/kg of local anesthetic per side should produce effective analgesia (Willschke et al., 2006b).

Ilioinguinal/Iliohypogastric Nerve Block

Ilioinguinal/iliohypogastric (ILIH) nerve block provides analgesia to the inguinal area and provides good perioperative pain relief for patients undergoing such procedures as inguinal hernia repair, orchiopexy, and hydrocelectomy (Hannallah

et al., 1987; Casey et al., 1990; Fisher et al., 1993). Early studies compared the use of an ilioinguinal/iliohypogastric block for children aged 1 to 7 years for inguinal hernia repair. The block was performed after induction of anesthesia but before surgical incision. When this was compared with general anesthesia without the block, the group of patients who received an ilioinguinal/iliohypogastric nerve block ambulated earlier and required less analgesia in the immediate postoperative period. The ilioinguinal/iliohypogastric block group also required less analgesia for the 48 hours after surgery (Langer et al., 1987). Hannallah and associates studied the efficacy of an ilioinguinal/iliohypogastric block for orchiopexy surgery (1987). They found no advantage to a caudal block over the ILIH block for orchiopexy surgery, as there were no significant differences between the groups in postoperative pain scores, postoperative vomiting, or time to meet discharge criteria. These results have been duplicated in other studies, with no differences found between the ILIH groups and caudal groups with respect to postoperative pain scores, analgesic requirements, or times to micturition (Fisher et al., 1993; Splinter et al., 1995). However, in a similarly designed study, Somri and coworkers (2002) noted that caudal anesthesia was significantly more effective than ILIH in decreasing plasma catecholamine levels after orchidopexy.

Casey and associates (1990) investigated the effectiveness of an ilioinguinal/iliohypogastric nerve block for inguinal hernia repair and compared this to simple installation of bupivacaine into the surgical wound. There was no difference between the ilioinguinal/iliohypogastric nerve block group and the wound installation group with regard to pain scores, analgesic requirements, recovery, or discharge times. In a study to assess the effectiveness of 0.5% bupivacaine in patients receiving an ilioinguinal/iliohypogastric nerve block, a wound infiltration, or a combination of wound infiltration and nerve block, Anatol and coworkers (1997) noted that all three patient groups had effective analgesia and that there were no differences in pain scores or analgesic requirements among the three groups. See related video online at www.expertconsult.com.

Anatomy

The ilioinguinal and iliohypogastric nerves originate from the lumbar plexus and pierce the transversus abdominis muscle. The iliohypogastric nerve then takes its course between the transversus and internal oblique muscles, and the ilioinguinal runs between internal oblique and external oblique. They pass superficial to the transversus abdominis near the anterior superior iliac spine, where they can be blocked before running their separate courses to innervate the inguinal region and upper scrotum (Fig. 16-41, *A*). The spermatic cord also receives innervation from the genital branch of the genitofemoral nerve that originates from lumbar plexus, usually at L1 or L2.

Technique

The ilioinguinal and iliohypogastric nerves may be blocked in their location near the anterior superior iliac spine. If performed before incision and after sterile preparation of the skin, a blunt 22- or 25-gauge needle is inserted 1 cm superior and 1 cm medial to the anterosuperior iliac spine (see Fig. 16-41, *B*). The needle is initially directed posterolaterally to contact the inner superficial lip of the ileum, then withdrawn while injecting local anesthetic during needle movement. Once the skin

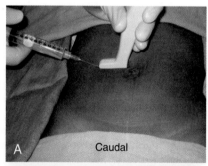

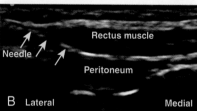

■ **FIGURE 16-40.** Ultrasound scan of rectus sheath block. **A,** Needle and transducer placement. **B,** Sonanatomy with needle.

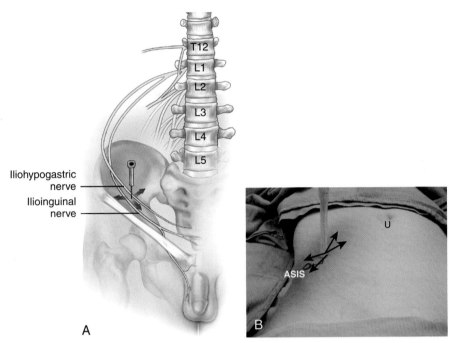

■ **FIGURE 16-41.** Ilioinguinal/iliohypogastric (ILIH) nerve block. **A,** Anatomy for ilioinguinal and iliohypogastric nerve block. **B,** Performance of ilioinguinal/iliohypogastric nerve block. A field block is performed in the direction of the *arrows* and inferiorly toward the inguinal ligament. *ASIS,* Anterior superior iliac spine; *U,* umbilicus.

reached, the needle is redirected toward the inguinal ligament (ensuring that the needle does not enter the ligament) and local anesthetic is injected after a pop is felt as the needle penetrates the oblique muscles. If the block is to be performed at the end of surgery, the surgeon may anesthetize the nerves under direct vision. The nerves lie at the lateral border of the incision. Lim and associates (2002) determined that there is no added advantage of a single-shot over a double-shot ilioinguinal/iliohypogastric nerve block.

Ultrasound-Guided Ilioinguinal/Iliohypogastric Nerve Block

Ultrasound-guided ILIH nerve block has been shown to increase accurate placement of local anesthetic around the ILIH nerves, decrease failure rate by 20% to 30%, and allow use of a smaller volume than the landmark-based ILIH nerve block technique (Willschke et al., 2005, 2006a; Weintraud et al., 2008).

In addition, continuous needle visualization under ultrasound should guard against complications that may occur with blind technique. Pharmacokinetic data indicated a faster absorption and higher local anesthetic concentration in serum when ultrasound-guided ILIH nerve block was performed, thus advocating reduction in the volume of local anesthetic when using this approach (Weintraud et al., 2009). See related video online at www.expertconsult.com.

Technique

A linear-array transducer set at the highest-resolution frequency is used to perform this block. The operator stands on the side of the patient being blocked, with the screen directly across. The transducer is positioned medial to the anterior superior iliac spine along the line connecting ASIS to the umbilicus (Fig. 16-42, *A*). The ilioinguinal and iliohypogastric nerves are found between the internal oblique and transversus abdominis muscle in close proximity to the ASIS and have an eliptical,

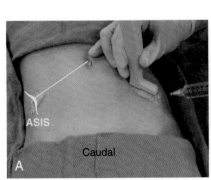

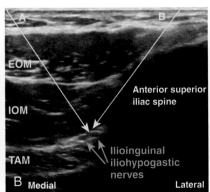

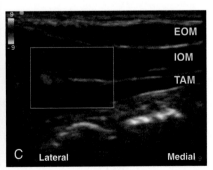

◀ **FIGURE 16-42.** Ultrasound scan of ILIH. **A,** Needle and transducer placement. **B,** Sonoanatomy. **C,** Sonoanatomy of vascular structures. *SIS,* Anterior superior iliac spine; *EOM,* external oblique muscle; *IOM,* internal oblique muscle; *TAM,* transversus abdominis muscle.

hypoechoic appearance (see Fig. 16-42, *B*). Doppler examination of the intended injection site should be performed first and may reveal vascular structures (branch of the deep circumflex iliac artery) that are not to be targeted (see Fig. 16-42, *C*). The block needle can be advanced in-plane either in the medial-to-lateral or lateral-to-medial direction, and it is positioned between the internal oblique and the transversus abdominis muscle. The medial-to-lateral approach is preferred as the needle tip is directed toward the ASIS, thus minimizing risk for intraperitoneal damage if the needle is inadvertently advanced outside of the ultrasound field. The lateral-to-medial needle direction can also be safely employed but requires continuous needle tip visualization. After negative aspiration, confirm needle location by hydro-dissection with 1 to 2 mL of normal saline and inject 0.2 mL/kg of local anesthetic while visualizing appropriate fascial spread.

Dosing

Bupivacaine 0.25% in a volume of 4 to 6 mL was used in a study by Hannallah and coworkers (1987) that included boys between the ages of 18 months and 12 years, and Casey and associates (1990) used 0.25 mL/kg of bupivacaine 0.25% for children 2 to 10 years for hernia repair. Both of these studies cited good postoperative pain relief for these children. Although the maximal duration of analgesia is unknown from these studies, in the study by Casey and coworkers (1990) effective analgesia was still present 180 minutes postoperatively. Levobupivacaine has been compared with placebo for patients 6 months to 12 years undergoing inguinal herniorrhaphy. In this study, Gunter and coworkers (1999) noted that 0.25 mL/kg of 0.5% levobupivacaine was effective for ILIH block and was associated with a longer time to rescue analgesic administration and lower pain scores when compared with children who had received no block. Dalens and coworkers (2001) evaluated the effectiveness and pharmacokinetic profile of 0.5% ropivacaine at 3 mg/kg for ILIH nerve block in children aged 1 to 12 years undergoing inguinal surgery. This dosage provided satisfactory pain relief, and peak ropivacaine plasma concentrations were 1.5 ± 0.93 mg/L. These levels were well below the toxic level.

Complications

Although complications from an ILIH nerve block are rare and generally minor, there have been case reports of colonic and small bowel perforation (Johr and Sossai, 1999; Amory et al., 2003). Inadvertent femoral nerve blockade and motor block of the quadriceps may occur if the local anesthetic solution spreads below the inguinal ligament during the block placement. This can yield a block similar to the fascia iliaca block (Roy-Shapiri et al., 1985). The use of ultrasound should avoid these complications.

Penile Nerve Block

A penile nerve block includes techniques such as subpubic nerve block, dorsal nerve block, and subcutaneous ring block and may be used for procedures on the distal penis including circumcision and uncomplicated hypospadias repair. Investigations have shown that newborns have a decreased stress response when undergoing circumcision with the benefit of a penile block. A ring block may be more effective than either a dorsal nerve block or local anesthetic cream (Maxwell et al., 1987; Stang et al., 1988; Lander et al., 1997; Butler-O'Hara et al., 1998; Hardwick-Smith et al., 1998). In addition, a subcutaneous ring block may result in a lower incidence of complications than a dorsal nerve block (Broadman et al., 1987). The subpubic nerve block blocks the nerves before they enter the base of the penis. This block is less likely to disrupt the vascular or penile structures. Holder and associates (1997) compared the subcutaneous ring block in boys undergoing circumcision with a group of boys who had a subpubic block. The group anesthetized with the subpubic block had significantly lower pain scores. In addition, three boys in the subcutaneous ring block group had tissue distortion from the block, which affected surgical conditions.

When using a penile block for boys undergoing hypospadias repair, Chhibber and coworkers (1997) showed that placing the block before incision and repeating the block at the end of surgery provided better postoperative pain control than placing the block only once (i.e., before or after the surgical procedure). See related video online at www.expertconsult.com.

Anatomy

The distal two thirds of the penis are supplied by the dorsal nerves, which are branches of the pudendal nerve (Fig. 16-43, *A*). The pudendal nerve arises from the sacral plexus. The dorsal nerves are located near the dorsal vessels and are surrounded by Buck's fascia.

Technique

Subcutaneous ring block. A simple approach for blocking the dorsal nerves to the penis is the subcutaneous ring block. A skin wheal of local anesthetic (without epinephrine) is injected circumferentially around the base of the penis but superficial to Buck's fascia.

Dorsal nerve penile block. A dorsal penile nerve block may be performed by injecting local anesthetic directly at the nerves as they run on each side of the penis at the level of the symphysis pubis (see Fig. 16-43, *B*). Using a 25-gauge needle, Buck's fascia is pierced and local anesthesia (without epinephrine) is injected at the clock positions of 10:30 and 1:30 at the base of the penis. Because of the close proximity of the dorsal vessels, frequent aspiration for blood during the local anesthetic injection is necessary. Ultrasound-guided dorsal penile nerve block has been demonstrated to be effective and may be used to visualize local anesthetic spread around the dorsal nerves (Sandeman and Dilley, 2007).

Subpubic block. To perform a subpubic block, the penis is gently pulled downward and the needle is inserted perpendicular to the skin 0.5 to 1 cm lateral to the midline and caudal to the symphysis pubis. As the needle is advanced, it is directed slightly medially and caudally until Scarpa's fascia is crossed. When "give" is felt and assuming a negative aspiration for blood, local anesthetic is delivered.

Dosing

The most important point to remember about dosing a penile block is to *never use epinephrine*. The penis is an end organ, and the use of epinephrine may lead to necrosis. For all techniques of providing penile nerve block, bupivacaine 0.25%, levobupivacaine 0.25%, or ropivacaine 0.2% may be used to provide

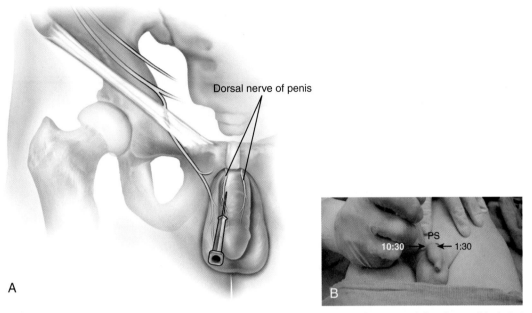

Dorsal nerve of penis

A

PS
10:30 → ← 1:30

B

FIGURE 16-43. Dorsal nerve penile block. **A,** Anatomy for dorsal nerve penile block. **B,** Performance of dorsal nerve block. Point of needle insertion is at clock referents 10:30 and 1:30 at the base of the penis. *PS,* Pubic symphysis.

analgesia with a duration of 4 to 6 hours. A subcutaneous ring block should be dosed so that there is subcutaneous evidence of local anesthetic injection around the base of the penis, but the dosage must not exceed the maximal allowable recommendations for single injection (see Table 16-2). For a dorsal nerve block or subpubic block, approximately 0.1 mL/kg of local anesthetic is injected at each site. Sfez and associates (1990) showed that for a penile block with 0.1 mL/kg at each injection site of either 0.25% bupivacaine or a 1:1 mixture of 0.25% bupivacaine with 1% lidocaine, serum local anesthetic concentrations were well below the toxic range.

Complications

Epinephrine should never be used when performing a penile block, as this may lead to significant vasoconstriction and ischemia (Berens and Pontus, 1990). An adult who received 0.75% ropivacaine for dorsal nerve block developed temporary ischemia of the glans, presumably from the intrinsic vasoconstrictive effects of the high concentration of ropivacaine, so this should be kept in mind when choosing local anesthetic and concentration (Burke et al., 2000). Hematoma formation may occur from puncture of the dorsal vessels during dorsal nerve block. This can result in necrosis of the tip of the penis (Sara and Lowry, 1984). When performed properly, a subcutaneous ring block should be void of complications with the exception of tissue edema at the base of the penis. Tissue edema may affect the surgical conditions if the block is performed before the surgical procedure.

Intercostal Nerve Block

Intercostal nerve block provides limited analgesia after thoracotomy, upper abdominal procedures, rib fractures, and indwelling chest tubes. An intercostal block may be useful for these indications in the perioperative arena or in an emergency room or ICU setting. See related video online at www.expertconsult.com.

Anatomy

The intercostal nerves arise paravertebrally from the first 11 thoracic spinal nerves and are located in a groove that is found underneath the corresponding rib and shared with the intercostal vessels. Gray and white rami communicantes branch off from the spinal nerves and adjoin the sympathetic ganglia before entering the intercostal space. The intercostal space contains the intercostal nerve, artery, and vein and is bordered by the intercostal muscles (Fig. 16-44, *A*).

Technique

To adequately anesthetize the intercostal nerves near their origin, the block is performed lateral to the paraspinous muscles toward the posterior axillary line. The child should be in the lateral decubitus position with the arm elevated so that the posterior axillary line is easily accessed (see Fig. 16-44, *B*). After sterile preparation, insert a 25-gauge needle (the length depends on the age of the child) through the skin, less than 1 cm below that the lower border of the rib and aiming cephalad to make contact with the rib itself. The needle is then withdrawn and advanced to "walk under" the inferior border of the rib until a slight loss of resistance is felt as the muscles are penetrated. The nerve is located immediately inferior to the vessels but in close proximity, and this requires frequent aspiration during injection of local anesthetic. To improve success of analgesia, the intercostal nerves two segments above and two segments below should be blocked in addition to the segment corresponding to the incision. Although a single injection of an increased volume of 10 mL per segment has been shown to spread to multiple intercostal spaces in adults, this is not a common practice in children (Moorthy et al., 1992).

Dosing

A dose of 0.1 to 0.15 mL/kg per interspace (maximum of 3 mL/ interspace) of local anesthetic agent is injected after negative

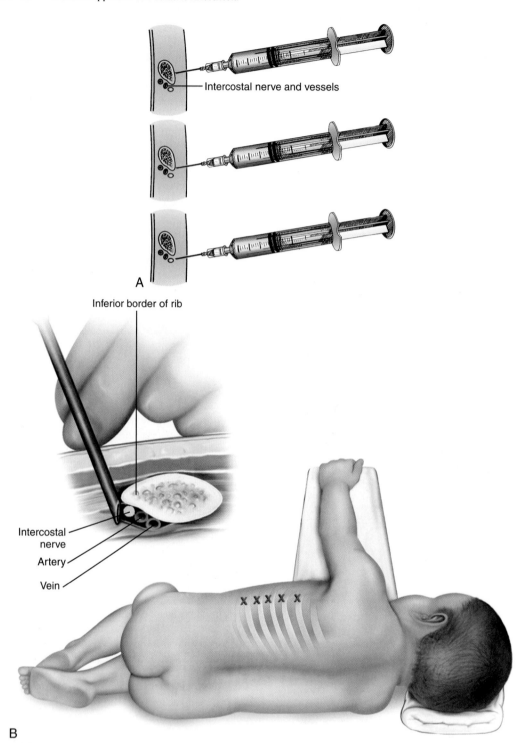

■ **FIGURE 16-44.** Intercostal block. **A,** Anatomy of intercostal nerves. **B,** Performance of intercostal block. The needle is directed to contact the inferior border of each rib to be blocked, then "walked off" posteriorly.

aspiration. Bupivacaine 0.25%, levobupivacaine 0.25%, or ropivacaine 0.2% should provide 8 to 12 hours of analgesia.

Complications

Complications of intercostal block include pneumothorax, vascular puncture, and epidural or spinal local anesthetic spread. Spread of local anesthetic to the epidural or spinal spaces may occur if the injection travels through a dural sleeve covering the spinal root and may be more common with the posterior approach than with more anterior approaches. In addition, there may be increased risk for local anesthetic toxicity from systemic uptake or inadvertent vascular puncture than with other peripheral nerve blocks because of the close proximity of the intercostal vessels to the nerve.

Paravertebral Nerve Block

Paravertebral nerve block provides analgesia at specific dermatomes, and it is generally used for children who undergo unilateral procedures. Its use has been established in children, and the main advantages include localized pain control and the ability to avoid large volumes of local anesthetic (Lonnqvist and Olsson, 1994; Lonnqvist et al., 1995; Richardson and Lonnqvist, 1998). Continuous paravertebral block has been shown to be effective for pain management for patients after thoracotomies, renal surgery, and cholecystectomy. Paravertebral blocks may be superior to epidural anesthesia in patients undergoing unilateral renal surgery, resulting in fewer morphine requirements in the postoperative period (Eng and Sabanathan, 1992; Lonnqvist, 1992; Lonnqvist and Olsson, 1994). Bolus injection of local anesthetic in the paravertebral space has been used successfully in children for inguinal surgery (Eck et al., 2002). Paravertebral blocks may be used in any patient where intercostal nerve blocks would be appropriate. Other advantages to performing paravertebral block include the spread of analgesia beyond one dermatome and the ease of catheter insertion for postoperative pain.

In the adult literature, preincisional paravertebral block resulted in a lower incidence of chronic pain after breast surgery, perhaps because of its preemptive analgesic effects (Lonnqvist, 2005b; Kairaluoma et al., 2006). There is evidence that the technique may even reduce the risk for recurrence or metastasis of breast cancer, and there is ongoing investigation (Exadaktylos et al., 2006; Sessler et al., 2008). See related video online at www.expertconsult.com.

Anatomy

The paravertebral space is a wedge-shaped area along the vertebral column that contains the intercostal nerve, its dorsal ramus, the rami communicantes, and the sympathetic chain. The anterior boundary of the paravertebral space is the parietal pleura, and posterior to it are the superior costotransverse ligament and posterior intercostal (Fig. 16-45, A). There are equations to determine the depth of the paravertebral space based on body weight (Lonnqvist and Hesser, 1992). The distance in millimeters from the spinous process to the paravertebral space is 0.12 times body weight (in kilograms) plus 10.2. The depth in millimeters from the skin to the paravertebral space is 0.48 times body weight (in kilograms) plus 18.7.

When local anesthetic is injected into the paravertebral space, it may spread several dermatomes because of the potential for free communication between adjacent spaces. The exception to this, however, may be at the T12 level, where the psoas major muscle inserts into the vertebral column. In human cadavers, the psoas muscle may be a limiting factor in spread of local anesthesia from the thoracic region to segments below T12 (Lonnqvist and Hildingsson, 1992). For this reason, in the study of children undergoing paravertebral blocks for inguinal surgery, Eck and coworkers (2002) administered two injections, one above T12 and the other below.

Technique

After sterile preparation and draping, with the child in the lateral position and the block side up, the spinous process of the level to be blocked is identified. The distance from the midline to the point of lateral puncture is approximately the same distance as the tip from one spinous process to another (see Fig. 16-45, B). If using a single-injection technique, a blunt spinal needle is used. If a catheter is to be threaded, a Touhy needle is necessary. Using a loss of resistance technique to saline, the needle is placed the proposed distance from the midline at the level of the spinous process. As the needle is inserted perpendicular to the skin, it will contact the corresponding transverse process. The needle is then "walked" over the cephalad margin of the transverse process. With gentle pressure on the syringe plunger, loss of resistance will occur once the needle crosses the costotransverse ligament and entry is gained into

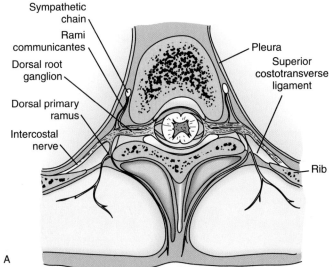
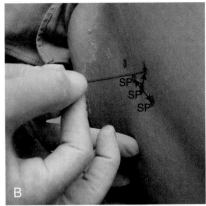

■ **FIGURE 16-45.** Paravertebral block. **A,** Anatomy of paravertebral space. **B,** Performance of paravertebral block. *SP,* Spinous process. Lateral distance to point of needle insertion from midline should be equal to distance between spinous processes *(arrows).* (**A,** *From Eason MJ, Wyatt R: Paravertebral thoracic block: a reappraisal,* Anaesthesia *34:638, 1979.)*

the paravertebral space. The loss of resistance is similar to, but less distinct than, that of going through the ligamentum flavum during epidural placement. Once the paravertebral space is identified, local anesthetic is injected into the space, and a catheter can be threaded if a continuous technique is desired. Threading a catheter through a Touhy needle into the paravertebral space may require some manipulation and cephalad angulation of the bevel of the needle. In a child, the catheter should not be threaded more than 2 to 3 cm. This avoids lateral placement of the catheter into an intercostal space and single-dermatome analgesia.

Technique with Ultrasound

The use of an ultrasound for the paravertebral nerve block placement has been described in several recent reports, with both an out-of-plane and in-plane needle advancement (Hara et al., 2007; Ben-Ari et al., 2009; Luyet et al., 2009; Shibata and Nishiwaki, 2009). Although the safety and reliability of these techniques is unknown, the in-plane technique offers the ability to visualize the block needle and may guide it away from the pleura and vascular structures.

A linear ultrasound transducer set at the highest operational frequency should be used to achieve maximal resolution. The child can be positioned either prone or in a lateral decubitus position with the operative side uppermost (Fig. 16-46, *A*). The operator stands or sits by the child's ipsilateral side for the prone position or faces the child for the lateral decubitus position. The ultrasound machine is positioned in the direct line of view. The sonographic examination begins by positioning the transducer in a transverse plane over the selected intercostal space and sliding it medially until the hyperechoic transverse process is visualized (see Fig. 16-46, *B*). The paravertebral space is located between the pleura below and the internal intercostal membrane above. The use of color Doppler, before needle placement, may help to avoid injuring the intercostal vessels. A Touhy needle is advanced in-plane from lateral to medial until the internal intercostal membrane is pierced. Local anesthetic injection should produce downward movement of the pleura as the paravertebral space is expanded (see Fig. 16-46, *C*). Care should be taken to ensure continuous sonographic visualization

of the needle tip, and aspiration is performed for blood or CSF before local anesthetic injection.

Dosing

For a unilateral paravertebral block, a bolus dosage of 0.5 mL/kg of local anesthetic provides reliable analgesia of four dermatomes (Lonnqvist and Hesser, 1993). Bupivacaine 0.25%, ropivacaine 0.2%, or levobupivacaine 0.25%, all with epinephrine (5 mcg/mL) may be used for single injection. If multiple levels are to be blocked, it is important not to exceed the maximal allowable dosing recommendations (see Table 16-2). For continuous infusions, bupivacaine 0.25%, ropivacaine 0.2%, or levobupivacaine 0.25% can be infused at a rate of 0.25 mL/kg per hour for most children, or lower concentrations at 0.2 mL/kg per hour for infants (Karmaker et al., 1996; Cheung et al., 1997).

Infants with a mean age of 5.3 weeks who received a bolus of bupivacaine 0.25% followed by infusion at 0.5 mg/kg per hour had bupivacaine serum levels that were suggestive of considerable bupivacaine accumulation. Some patients reached potentially toxic levels (Karmaker et al., 1996). In a similar study in younger infants (median age, 1.5 weeks), Cheung and associates (1997) used a lower concentration and a lower infusion rate and added epinephrine 1:400,000 in an attempt to decrease the uptake of local anesthetic. With an initial 1.25-mg/kg bolus of 0.25% bupivacaine, and an infusion of 0.125% at 0.25 mg/kg per hour, the mean serum concentration was 1.60 mcg/mL. Three patients had plasma bupivacaine measurements of greater than 3 mcg/mL between 30 and 48 hours. None of these patients had any sequelae.

Complications

In one series of 367 patients for paravertebral block, the failure rate was 10.7% for adults and 6.2% for children (Lonnqvist et al., 1995). Complications of the block included hypotension (4.6%), vascular puncture (3.8%), pleural puncture (1.1%), and pneumothorax (0.5%). Of these complications, all the patients who had hypotension were adults, none of the patients who had a vascular puncture demonstrated local anesthetic toxicity, and only one of the patients who had a pleural puncture had a pneumothorax. This study suggested that the failure rate was

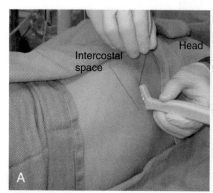

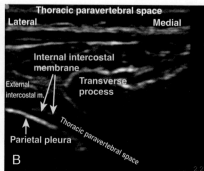

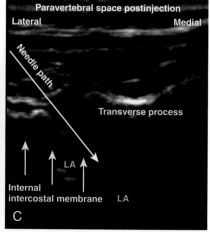

■ **FIGURE 16-46.** Ultrasound paravertebral block. **A,** Needle and transducer position. **B,** Sonanatomy. **C,** After injection.

comparable to that of epidural blocks, but with a much lower incidence of hypotension and little risk for dural puncture. Thus, the overall safety of paravertebral blocks has been established, although this technique should be limited to those who are experienced in its use.

BLOCKS OF THE FACE AND SCALP

Infraorbital Nerve Block

The infraorbital nerve consists of four branches, which innervate the upper lip and mucosa along the upper lip, the vermilion, the lateral inferior portion of the nose, and the lower lid of the eye. Blocking the infraorbital nerve provides effective analgesia for cleft lip repair (Bosenberg and Kimble, 1995; Prabhu et al., 1999). This block is also useful for nasal procedures such as endoscopic sinus surgery, nasal septal reconstruction, and rhinoplasty.

Anatomy

The infraorbital nerve is a purely sensory nerve derived from the second maxillary division of the trigeminal nerve. The infraorbital nerve is a terminal branch that exits the skull through the foramen rotundum to enter the pterygopalatine fossa. Here it emerges from the infraorbital foramen to divide into its four branches, the superior labial, internal nasal, external nasal, and inferior palpebral nerves.

Technique

The intraoral approach to block the infraorbital nerve is achieved by advancing a 27-gauge needle along the inner surface of the lip and cephalad to the infraorbital foramen parallel to the maxillary premolar. To perform this block, first palpate the infraorbital foramen and pull the upper lip superiorly to allow room for the needle and syringe (Fig. 16-47). Keep a finger on the

infraorbital foramen during needle advancement to provide accurate measurement to the desired space.

To block the infraorbital nerve transcutaneously, locate the infraorbital foramen and insert a 27-gauge needle toward, but not into, the foramen, in a lateral direction.

Dosing

A total volume of 0.5 to 1.5 mL of bupivacaine 0.25%, levobupivacaine 0.25%, or ropivacaine 0.2% with 1:200,000 epinephrine added is injected after negative aspiration for blood.

Complications

Hematoma, particularly using the transcutaneous approach, is not uncommon. To avoid this, pressure should be applied at the site of injection for 5 minutes. Other complications are rare as long as the foramen itself is not entered so that nerve compression does not occur.

Great Auricular Nerve Block

The mastoid and external ear are innervated by the great auricular nerve. Analgesia for otoplasty and tympanomastoidectomy is provided by blocking this nerve and leads to reduction in the perioperative use of opioids for these procedures (Cregg et al., 1996; Suresh and Wheeler, 2002).

Anatomy

The great auricular nerve is a sensory nerve branch of the superficial cervical plexus (C3). Its course at the level of the cricoid cartilage follows the posterior border of the belly of the clavicular head of the sternocleidomastoid muscle.

Technique

The great auricular nerve is blocked at the level of the cricoid cartilage at C6. The clavicular head of the sternocleidomastoid muscle is identified, and local anesthetic is injected superficially along the belly of the muscle approximately 5 to 6 cm below the ear (Fig. 16-48).

Complications

Complications from a great auricular nerve block may be significant and include intravascular injection because of the close proximity of the carotid artery and jugular veins. In addition, deep placement of the needle can result in phrenic nerve block, cervical plexus block, and Horner's syndrome.

Supraorbital and Supratrochlear Nerve Blocks

Anesthetizing the supraorbital and supratrochlear nerves can provide pain relief for procedures of the anterior scalp and forehead, including excision of skin lesions, neurosurgical procedures with incisions of the scalp or forehead, and laser therapy for hemangiomas (Suresh and Wheeler, 2002).

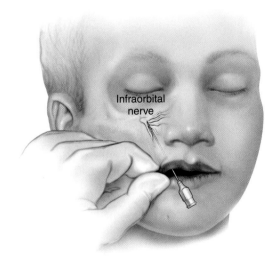

Infraorbital nerve

■ **FIGURE 16-47.** Infraorbital nerve block.

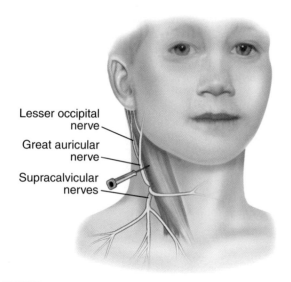

■ **FIGURE 16-48.** Anatomy for great auricular nerve block.

Anatomy

The supraorbital and supratrochlear nerves are terminal branches of the ophthalmic division of the trigeminal nerve (V₁). These nerves supply the forehead and the scalp anterior to the coronal suture. They are found immediately above the eyelid area, where the supraorbital nerve exits through the supraorbital foramen and the supratrochlear nerve exits the orbit between the trochlea and the supraorbital foramen (Fig. 16-49).

Technique

After identifying the supraorbital notch, a 27-gauge needle is inserted perpendicular to the skin at the notch until it contacts

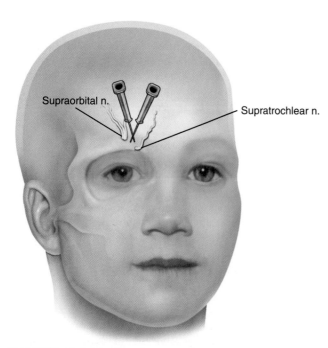

■ **FIGURE 16-49.** Anatomy for supraorbital and supratrochlear nerve blocks.

bone, then withdrawn slightly, and local anesthetic is injected after negative aspiration. The supratrochlear nerve is blocked by withdrawing the needle back to the skin and aiming slightly medially.

Complications

Periorbital edema and ecchymosis are common side effects when performing blocks around the eye. To avoid this side effect, pressure can be applied to the supraorbital area for 5 minutes after the block has been placed.

INTRAVENOUS REGIONAL ANESTHESIA

Intravenous regional anesthesia (IVRA), or Bier block, is a technique whereby an extremity is anesthetized by injecting local anesthetic intravenously and containing it within the extremity by using a tourniquet. This technique is useful only for intraoperative analgesia, as the effect of the local anesthetic dissipates with release of the tourniquet. Intravenous regional anesthesia has been used in children for forearm fracture reduction and is considered safe and effective for most procedures of distal extremities that require pain relief for a short period (Davidson et al., 2002). IVRA should not be used for procedures that have a potential of lasting greater than 90 minutes.

Technique

A separate intravenous line is placed in the limb that is to be blocked, and a double tourniquet is applied to this extremity. The limb should then be elevated and exsanguinated by wrapping the extremity with an elastic bandage, beginning with the digits and proceeding toward the tourniquets (Fig. 16-50: Go to www.expertconsult.com to view this image online). If the limb is fractured, exsanguination with the bandage should be deleted in an awake child to avoid excessive pain. The proximal tourniquet is then inflated to greater than 50 mm Hg above the baseline systolic blood pressure (Fitzgerald, 1976). If the operation is occurring on the lower extremity, inflation pressures should be closer to 100 mm Hg above systolic blood pressure. After proximal tourniquet inflation, local anesthetic is slowly injected into the venous cannula in the operative limb. Onset of block should occur within 5 minutes of injection. After testing for successful block, the procedure may begin. Once it is evident during the procedure that tourniquet pain is being experienced, the distal tourniquet is inflated. The proximal tourniquet may then be released. Tourniquet pain is typically not an immediate issue on inflation of the distal tourniquet because that area remains anesthetized. Most children require sedation in addition to the IVRA.

At the end of the procedure, the distal tourniquet may be released for 15 seconds, then reinflated. The tourniquet may be released and reinflated two additional times. This allows some of the local anesthetic into the systemic circulation at short intervals to avoid local anesthetic toxicity from a large amount of local anesthetic being released all at once. At least one cuff should remain inflated for at least 20 minutes after injection of the local anesthetic, regardless of the length of the procedure.

Dosing

Either lidocaine or prilocaine may be used for intravenous regional anesthesia. Bupivacaine is contraindicated because of its ability to produce cardiotoxicity if it reaches the systemic circulation. When using lidocaine 0.5% or prilocaine 0.5%, use 0.6 mL/kg for the upper extremity and 1 mL/kg for the lower extremity.

In a study of 249 children older than 3 years, either lidocaine 0.5% or prilocaine 0.5% was used for reduction of forearm fracture (Davidson et al., 2002). The dosage used in this study was 0.6 mL/kg (or 3 mg/kg of local anesthetic). The group who had received the lidocaine had better analgesia than the prilocaine group, with fewer cases of what was considered to be unacceptable pain during reduction of the fracture. There were no adverse events.

To improve block conditions, fentanyl 1 mcg/kg or pancuronium 0.01 mg/kg may be added to the local anesthetic solution. Although used in adults, these additives have not been proven to be beneficial in children.

Complications

Prilocaine can produce methemoglobinemia if injected systemically. Neurotoxicity and seizures may occur from lidocaine if the tourniquets fail or are released prematurely. For this reason, IVRA is not indicated for children with underlying seizure disorders. Children with sickle cell disease or vascular insufficiency should not receive IVRA because of the risk of prolonged tourniquet time.

TOPICAL ANESTHESIA

Topical anesthesia for a child may be applied as a cream, by local infiltration to anesthetize the skin, or by topical application of local anesthetic directly to mucous membranes.

Topical local anesthetic cream was developed in the 1990s and has found popularity in the pediatric population for anesthetizing the skin before minor procedures. Eutectic Mixture of Local Anesthetic (EMLA) cream, a mixture of prilocaine and lidocaine, was the first commercially available agent that anesthetized intact skin to a depth of 5 mm (Ehrenström et al., 1983). This mixture of prilocaine and lidocaine results in an oil-and-water emulsion that has a total local anesthetic concentration of 5%. It has been found to be effective for superficial procedures such as venipuncture, laser treatment of port wine stains, and neonatal circumcision (Mannuksela and Korpela, 1986; Ashinoff and Geronemus, 1990; Taddio et al., 1997). EMLA cream has been found to reduce the neonatal physiologic response to circumcision when compared with placebo, but it is not considered as effective as dorsal nerve block or penile ring block (Lander et al., 1997; Taddio et al., 1997; Howard et al., 1999).

EMLA cream is applied to intact skin at least 1 hour before the time of the procedure and covered with an occlusive dressing (Morgan-Hughes and Kirton, 2001). Heating the EMLA cream with an external heat pack after application has been shown to reduce the time to efficacy to 20 minutes, although a 60-minute waiting period is better (Liu et al., 2003). EMLA cream should not be applied to traumatized or inflamed skin or to mucosal membranes because of its potential for rapid absorption and systemic toxicity.

ELA-Max, which consists of 4% liposomal lidocaine, is commercially available for use as a topical anesthetic for minor procedures and is marketed as requiring only 30 minutes to be effective. In a study comparing ELA-Max with EMLA during venipuncture in 120 children, the local anesthetic creams were applied at either 30 or 60 minutes before the procedure (Eichenfield et al., 2002). Both were effective, and the study demonstrated that a 30-minute application of ELA-Max without an occlusive dressing was as effective as a 60-minute application of EMLA with an occlusive dressing.

Local infiltration prior to minor procedures is effective as a method to provide pain relief during needle puncture or superficial incision. Although any local anesthetic can be used for injection, there is no benefit to using higher concentrations for most indications. Lidocaine 0.5% will provide immediate analgesia to the site and be effective for 90 minutes. If a longer duration is desired for pain relief after the procedure, bupivacaine 0.25% can be used and will provide 2 to 3 hours of postprocedure analgesia. When using bupivacaine for local infiltration, one must be extremely careful to avoid injecting the local anesthetic into vascular structures. To decrease bleeding at the site during the procedure, epinephrine 2.5 to 5 mcg/mL is added to the local anesthetic solution. Plastic surgeons often increase the amount of epinephrine to 10 mcg/mL or 1:100,000 to keep the field clear of blood.

Maximal allowable dosage guidelines are the same for local infiltration as they are for other regional blocks. A total of 5 mg/kg of lidocaine, or 7 mg/kg lidocaine when epinephrine is added, can be used safely (Berde, 1993). When using bupivacaine with or without epinephrine, 3 mg/kg is the maximal allowable dosage. A simple rule of thumb when using bupivacaine 0.25% (2.5 mg/mL) is to not exceed 1 mL/kg of local anesthetic solution; therefore, the child never receives more than 2.5 mg/kg.

To use local infiltration in an awake child, measures should be taken to decrease the pain of the injection. The child should be secured to limit movement during the injection and the procedure. A small-gauge (e.g., 27-gauge) needle should be used, and the injection should be performed slowly to minimize the pain that occurs with dissection of the superficial layers of the skin during injection. To further minimize pain, sodium bicarbonate is added to the solution at 1 mL per 10 mL of lidocaine to increase the pH of the solution to physiologic values (Momson et al., 2000). This buffered solution will decrease the discomfort from the injection, because the lidocaine without buffer is more acidic (Christoph et al., 1988; Orlinsky et al., 1992).

Topical anesthesia may be applied by several methods to the *mucous membranes* of the nose and nasopharynx to decrease the discomfort associated with bronchoscopies, nasotracheal intubation, nasogastric tubes, or nasal airways. Lidocaine is available as a 5% ointment or a 2% jelly. For mucous membranes, the 2% jelly is easy to apply and can be used on a greater surface area because of its lower concentration. The jelly may be simply applied to the nares and the tube for passage into the nose, and pledgets with the lidocaine jelly applied to the tip can be gently placed posteriorly in the nasopharynx to anesthetize that region. Although there are methods of delivering lidocaine as a nebulizer or spray, it is difficult to control the amount delivered, and at concentrations of 4%, it is easy to overdose a small child with this method. Peak plasma concentrations that are greater than the toxic levels are reached within 1 minute after the application of the 4% lidocaine spray because of its fast absorption (Eyres et al., 1978). If this route is preferred by some practitioners, every attempt should be made to provide only the maximal allowable dosage and to be alert for the potential of local anesthetic toxicity that can occur because of the high uptake from this vascular area.

PRACTICAL CONSIDERATIONS TO PEDIATRIC REGIONAL ANESTHESIA

Despite the demonstrated benefits of regional anesthesia, there are many obstacles to its incorporation. Start-up regional programs face a multitude of challenges and require tools and education for success. The following are suggestions to incorporate regional anesthesia into your pediatric practice.

The dilemma of time: Regional anesthesia procedures in pediatrics are frequently performed in the operating room arena (whereas for adults, they usually occur in a presurgical block room), and are thus frequently met with resistance by surgeons who view them as an anesthesia delay. This misperception can be broken by starting the practice with the blocks that take the least time to perform, and by being efficient and demonstrating consistent results. Find simple approaches to each block, get proficient with these as you establish yourself and the regional program, and then branch out as the program grows. A satisfied parent and calm child will quickly convince the surgeons of the benefits of regional techniques.

Streamline the process: Any new undertaking has natural limiting steps, but by standardizing the process you will save time and energy. Patient and parent preoperative education can be simplified by distributing brochures describing the basic concepts of regional anesthesia, at their preoperative visit. A standardized form that adheres to documentation and billing criteria should help with the process (Gerancher et al., 2005). The steps required to gather equipment can be eliminated by devising block carts that contain all the necessary supplies. Postoperative block order sheets will improve patient care and minimize pain-related phone calls.

Money talks: Regional supplies and additional personnel consume departmental and hospital resources. To be appropriately reimbursed, review procedural coding and billing for the various blocks and postoperative pain management procedures.

Education: Regional anesthesia produces results only when a team approach is used. Involve and educate your surgeons, nurses, physical therapists, and pharmacists on the perioperative expectations for your patients. This includes benefits of techniques and adjunctive therapies, and how to recognize complications.

SUMMARY

Regional anesthesia for children continues to progress because of the development of improved local anesthetics and pediatric-sized equipment, the advent of ultrasound, improved patient safety, and efficacy. As the field grows, it may become the primary method of providing both intraoperative and postoperative analgesia if strategies continue to diminish the risks, and if studies are carried out to promote the benefits (Goldman, 1995; Dalens and Mazoit, 1998).

Experienced practitioners in pediatric regional techniques provide an important service to children. Additional research must be directed at outcome studies to determine the true risks and benefits of these techniques in large populations of children. With advanced training and appropriate use of agents and equipment, the practice of pediatric regional anesthesia as a means of providing superior analgesia will continue to be an essential part of the overall care of children in the perioperative period.

For questions and answers on topics in this chapter, go to "Chapter Questions" at www.expertconsult.com.

REFERENCES

Complete references used in this text can be found online at www.expertconsult.com.

Clinical Management of Specialized Surgical Problems

Neonatology for Anesthesiologists

George A. Gregory and Claire Brett

CONTENTS

Advances in obstetrics and neonatology have greatly improved neonatal survival, especially for preterm neonates (Fig. 17-1). Because the survival rate of premature infants is on the rise, so is the need for anesthesia and surgery for these patients. To safely care for newborns in the operating room, anesthesiologists must appreciate and understand the enormous physiologic variability that exists among infants born between 23 and 44 weeks of gestation, so they can better understand how immature organs respond to surgery and anesthetic agents. Fetal development is also relevant, because fetal surgery is a reality in many medical centers, and providing anesthesia for midgestation fetuses (20 to 23 weeks' gestation) via the mother poses a completely new set of challenges (Hirose et al., 2004). The purpose of this chapter is to present background information that will allow anesthesiologists to better understand the problems of neonates and to provide safe care for these patients based on an understanding of neonatal physiology. The preoperative evaluation of the neonate is arguably the most important part of anesthetic care.

Although some congenital anomalies are obvious at birth, others, such as gastrointestinal dysfunction, various central nervous system (CNS) malformations, or metabolic disorders, may not develop until later in life. In general, if one congenital anomaly is present, the anesthesiologist must be suspicious that there are others. Box 17-1 provides a list of disease entities and coexisting anomalies, and this list may be useful as part of a preoperative assessment (Jones and Pelton, 1976).

Neonatologists and the intensive care nurses are the best sources of information required for the anesthesiologist to understand a patient's clinical status. Because they have spent hours at the infant's bedside, the neonatal intensive care nursery (NICU) staff are able to provide critical insight about effective ventilatory strategies, positioning and its effect on oxygenation, responses to and requirements for intravenous fluids (e.g., blood pressure, heart rate, and urine output), tolerance to glucose administration, and temperature stability. Preparation for anesthesia and surgery requires detailed preoperative consultation with the NICU staff to establish the framework for temporarily transferring care to the operating room while avoiding dangerous and unnecessary alterations in care. In fact, developing an effective relationship with the NICU staff makes it easier to rapidly obtain intraoperative consultation with the primary medical team and communicate with the family. The anesthesiologist must understand the principles of neonatal anesthesia and surgery, the normal course of development, the pathophysiology of neonatal disease states, and the glossary of terms used to describe both neonates and their diseases

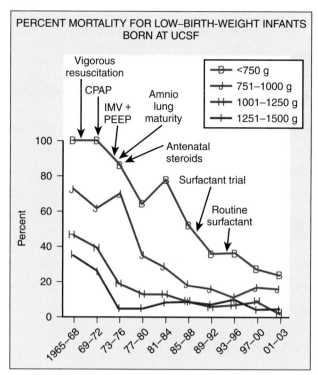

PERCENT MORTALITY FOR LOW–BIRTH-WEIGHT INFANTS BORN AT UCSF

■ FIGURE 17-1. Percent mortality for low–birth-weight infants born at University of California, San Francisco.

DEVELOPMENT OF THE FETUS AND THE INTRAUTERINE ENVIRONMENT

The intrauterine environment has dramatic effects on growth and on the ability of neonates to adapt to extra-uterine life. Although the impact of intrauterine events is most obvious during the first few hours and days of life, the effects of these events can last much longer. For example, phenytoin, thalidomide, alcohol, and maternal drug use has caused well-described syndromes, alterations in somatic growth, or drug-dependence and withdrawal (e.g., opioids or amphetamines). Exposure to drugs during pregnancy has been associated with anomalies of the heart, pulmonary circulation, brain, and other organs (e.g., cleft lip and palate) (Puhó et al., 2007).

During intrauterine life, fetuses expend little energy maintaining their body temperature. The placental circulation provides essential substrates and eliminates waste products. The fetus' primary activity is growth, which proceeds under conditions that at first glance appear hypoxic. However, fetal Pao_2 of no more than 20 to 30 mm Hg, plus a hemoglobin concentration of 18 to 20 g/dL, an oxygen dissociation curve that is shifted to the left (P50, 18 mm Hg), and a higher cardiac output (CO)/kg, provide sufficient oxygen content in blood to the fetal heart and brain. This can be demonstrated with the following formula:

$$([Hb \times 1.34 \text{ cc } O_2/g \text{ Hb}] \times Sao_2) + 0.03 \text{ cc } O_2 \times Pao_2$$

However, the fetus is at a great disadvantage—it has no store of oxygen beyond that in its blood, because the lungs are filled with fluid and not gas (Dudenhausen et al., 1997). After only a minute of umbilical cord occlusion, the fetus'

Box 17-1 Commonly Encountered Lesions in the Neonate

AIRWAY LESIONS
Choanal atresia
Pierre-Robin syndrome
Upper-airway obstruction
Cystic hygroma
Upper-airway cysts or webs
Laryngeal stenosis
Cleft lip and cleft palate

THORACIC LESIONS
Tracheoesophageal fistula
Diaphragmatic hernia
Eventration of the diaphragm
Pneumomediastinum, pneumothorax, pneumopericardium
Lobar emphysema
Congenital heart lesions
Mediastinal mass

ABDOMINAL LESIONS
Omphalocele
Gastroschisis
Intestinal atresia or stenosis
Pyloric stenosis
Malrotation and volvulus
Necrotizing enterocolitis
Imperforate anus
Extrophy of the bladder
Incarcerated hernia
Megacolon
Biliary atresia
Hirschsprung's disease

NEUROSURGICAL LESIONS
Myelomeningocele
Encephalocele
Craniostenosis
Intracranial mass
Skull fracture
Hydrocephalus
Subdural hemorrhage
Spinal tumor

Pao_2 is less than 5 mm Hg. At the same time, the $Paco_2$ steadily rises and the pH rapidly declines. The effects of intrauterine asphyxia can be sudden and profound, and they are often associated with severe hypoxia, hypotension, and acidosis (Fig. 17-2).

LABOR AND DELIVERY AND PERINATAL EVENTS

The neonate's respiratory rate increases briefly with the onset of asphyxia (see Fig. 17-2). Primary apnea quickly follows and lasts a variable amount of time. This is followed by slow gasping respirations and then by terminal apnea and death unless resuscitation is begun (Dawes, 1968). The heart rate and arterial blood pressure increase moderately, and bradycardia and

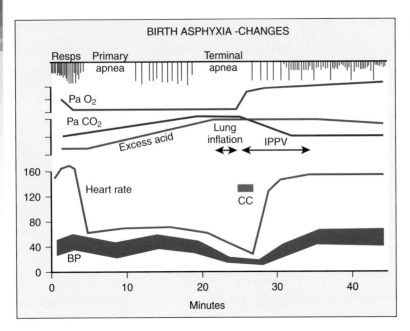

■ **FIGURE 17-2.** The effects of intrauterine asphyxia on vital signs and blood gases. *BP,* blood pressure; *CC,* cardiac compression; *IPPV,* intermittent positive pressure ventilation. *(From Sinha SK, Donn SM: Fetal-to-neonatal maladaptation, Semin Fetal Neonatal Med 11:166-2006.)*

hypotension follow. Because Cardiac Output (CO) is mostly dependent on heart rate in neonates, the severe, deep reduction in heart rate associated with asphyxia significantly reduces CO (Klopfenstein and Rudolph, 1978). To compensate for this reduction, blood flow is centralized to maintain blood flow and oxygen delivery to the brain, heart, and adrenal glands. The arterial blood pressure increases during gasping respirations and decreases markedly during terminal apnea. Heart rate, CO, and arterial blood pressure quickly improve with resuscitation. However, the metabolic component of acidosis may worsen as the pH_a is corrected, because fixed acids are washed out of the periphery by the improved peripheral perfusion. If the pH does not improve with ventilation alone, an infusion of tromethamine (Tham) or sodium bicarbonate may be necessary. The lungs should be ventilated if sodium bicarbonate is administered, because each milliequivalent of sodium bicarbonate (when fully reacted with hydrogen ion) produces 25 cc of CO_2 that must be removed via the lungs.

Labor and Delivery

Labor, fetal movements, and uterine contractions initiate removal of the 30 mL/kg of fluid that are normally present in the fetal lungs (Harding and Hooper, 1996). During labor, compression of the fetal chest by the uterus and vagina removes some of the lung fluid (Harding et al., 1990). After birth, breathing increases clearance of the lung fluid via the pulmonary capillaries and the lymphatics (see Pulmonary System, p. 518). The specific mechanism that initiates breathing at birth remains unclear, but several factors are known to play critical roles. First, placental factors that inhibit breathing in utero are removed by clamping the umbilical cord (Alvaro et al., 2004, 1997). Second, at birth the sudden release of the circumferential pressure around the chest allows the neonatal chest to recoil outward and draw gas into the lungs (Karlberg et al., 1962). Third, tactile stimulation and environmental thermal changes at birth stimulate breathing (Sinha and Donn, 2006). Lastly, the effects of hypoxia and hypercarbia on the chemosensors stimulate breathing (Taeusch et al., 2005).

Neonatal Asphyxia

Chronic intrauterine asphyxia affects placental blood flow, and placental infarction adversely affects fetal growth. In cases of chronic intrauterine asphyxia, labor may be poorly tolerated and neonatal resuscitation may be necessary. When neonatal resuscitation is required, primary or secondary consequences of asphyxia, including acidosis, seizures, transient cardiac dysfunction (e.g., cardiomyopathy or tricuspid insufficiency), pulmonary hypertension, renal insufficiency (e.g., acute tubular necrosis), gastrointestinal/hepatic insults (e.g., necrotizing enterocolitis [NEC]), or clotting abnormalities may occur.

Postnatal asphyxia is often the result of a continuum of intrauterine events, but it may also be caused by events that occur during labor and delivery. Immature respiratory control mechanisms can predispose neonates, especially premature neonates, to life-threatening responses to asphyxia. For example, the response to hypoxia during the first 3 to 4 weeks of life can be paradoxical, in that hypoxia produces a brief period of hyperpnea that is followed by bradypnea (Cross and Oppe, 1952; Brady and Ceruti, 1966). Hypothermia and hypercapnea blunt the initial hyperpnea (Ceruti, 1966; Rigatto et al., 1975). The ventilatory response to carbon dioxide increases with both postnatal and gestational age (see Chapter 3, Respiratory Physiology in Infants and Children) (Rigatto et al., 1975).

Although hypoxia may inflict long-term consequences on the fetus and newborn, hyperoxia can also cause significant morbidity, especially for preterm infants. For example, hyperoxia exposes preterm infants, especially those born before 32 weeks' gestation, to a significant risk for retinopathy of prematurity (ROP; see below) and, in some cases, blindness (see Chapter 27, Anesthesia for Ophthalmic Surgery) (Sylvester, 2008). The normal Pao_2 of a fetus is 20 to 30 mm Hg. After birth, a Pao_2 of 60 mm Hg is probably hyperoxic for infants born at 24 to 36 weeks' gestation. To avoid the effects of oxidative stress in the newborn, the oxygen saturation for premature infants is usually maintained between 88% and 93% (Pao_2 of 45 to 60 mm Hg) in the NICU, and similar Sao_2 levels are appropriate in the operating room. Continuous measurement of Sao_2 makes it easier to maintain the desired oxygen saturation. Of note is one preterm infant, who never had an elevated Pao_2 except in the operating room, but who developed ROP after surgery (Betts et al., 1977).

Metabolic Status: Early Postnatal Period

Thermal Environment

In a neutral thermal environment, neonates expend the least amount of energy to maintain their body temperature. The oxygen consumption ($\dot{V}o_2$) of normal neonates is 6 cc/kg per minute, twice that of resting adults. During the first week of life, $\dot{V}o_2$ increases to about 10 cc/kg per minute and may be twice that during heat-related stress. Because of their high oxygen consumption, greater CO, and smaller reserve of oxygen (i.e., smaller functional residual capacity [FRC]), neonates, especially preterm neonates, develop hypoxia more quickly than adults. In fact, hypoxia may develop in as few as 10 seconds in apneic neonates, whereas it takes several minutes for this to occur in adults (Peabody et al., 1978a, 1978b).

Sodium, Calcium, and Glucose

Box 17-2 contains common fluid and electrolyte requirements for neonatal infants. Because premature, large-for-gestational age (LGA), small-for-gestational-age (SGA), and asphyxiated neonates are often hyper- or hypoglycemic, intravenous glucose may be required to maintain normoglycemia (serum glucose concentration of 40 to 90 mg/dL; see Glucose Metabolism, p. 537) (Jain et al., 2008). Similarly, calcium homeostasis is often difficult to achieve in sick infants (Bass and Chan, 2006). Initial calcium administration is usually based on normal neonatal requirements and on need, as determined by serial ionized calcium measurements. Calcium should be infused into a well-functioning intravenous catheter to avoid extravasation of calcium into the tissues and severe tissue necrosis. During surgery the calcium infusion site is usually under the surgical drapes and hard to see. Therefore, calcium should be infused into a reliable intravenous catheter, preferably a central venous catheter.

For the first 2 to 3 hours of life, the neonate's electrolyte concentrations reflect those of the mother and of perinatal events (e.g., asphyxia, or placental or umbilical cord hemorrhage). Afterward, the electrolyte concentrations reflect a balance between normal metabolism, renal and hepatic function, and ongoing metabolic derangements (e.g., sepsis, inherited metabolic diseases, hemolysis, or inborn errors of metabolism). Until tissue perfusion is adequate, resuscitated neonates usually have ongoing metabolic acidosis.

In full-term and near-term infants, sodium is seldom added to intravenous fluids during the first 24 hours of life. Urine output is low, despite the fact that 30 mL/kg of fluid must be removed from the lungs during and after birth (Herin and Zetterström, 1994). On the second day of life, maintenance sodium (2 to 4 mEq/kg per day) is added to the intravenous fluids to replace renal and gastrointestinal tract sodium losses, to compensate for abnormal fluid metabolism, or to counter the effect of diuretics (e.g., furosemide). In the extremely low-birth weight (ELBW) infant, fluid that contains sodium is often administered to maintain adequate intravascular volume, especially when transcutaneous fluid losses are excessive. After the first few days of life, an adequate sodium intake is essential for infants of all gestational ages to permit normal growth.

GESTATIONAL AGE

The SGA Infant

In part, perinatal problems are related to gestational age and birth weight (Box 17-3). Infants who weigh less than the 10th

---

Box 17-2 Common Intravenous Fluid and Electrolyte Requirements in the Newborn

GLUCOSE
Most newborns require 2 to 4 mg/kg per minute.
SGA and LGA infants may require >15 mg/kg per minute on days 1 to 3 of life.
Glucose tolerance may fluctuate significantly in VLBW and ELBW infants.

SODIUM
Most newborns require no sodium for the first 24 hours of life.
On day 2 and beyond, most newborns receive 2 to 4 mEq/kg per day.
Sodium requirements may change dramatically in response to gastrointestinal, genitourinary, or transcutaneous losses, or drug or metabolic effects.
The ELBW infant may have huge transcutaneous fluid losses, requiring meticulous monitoring and replacement.

POTASSIUM
Requirements for potassium are minimal for the first 24 to 48 hours of life.
Subsequently, maintenance delivery is about 1 to 3 mEq/kg per day, always in the presence of a normal urine output.
Serum levels in the newborn, especially VLBW and ELBW infants, are higher than in older infants.
Replace gastrointestinal, genitourinary, or iatrogenic losses cautiously.

CALCIUM
Requirements for calcium range between 200 and 400 mg/kg per day (calcium gluconate).
Requirements for calcium vary with gestational age, history of asphyxia, and growth disturbances (SGA, LGA).
Serum levels can be obtained for total Ca^{2+} or ionized Ca^{2+}.

Box 17-3 Common Metabolic and Structural Problems in SGA and LGA Infants

SGA
Congenital anomalies
Chromosomal abnormalities
Chronic intrauterine infection
Heat loss
Asphyxia
Metabolic abnormalities (hypoglycemia, hypocalcemia)
Polycythemia and hyperbilirubinemia

LGA
Birth injury (brachial, phrenic nerve, fractured clavicle)
Asphyxia
Meconium aspiration
Metabolic abnormalities (hypoglycemia, hypocalcemia)
Polycythemia and hyperbilirubinemia

percentile of weight for gestational age at birth are usually considered to be small for their gestational age. SGA infants have different problems from those of preterm infants (fewer than 37 weeks' gestation) of the same weight (Lubchenco et al., 1963). Consequently, it is necessary to relate birth weight to gestational age. Although primary fetal (e.g., chromosomal disorders) and maternal (e.g., smoking or chronic disease) factors have been linked to intrauterine growth retardation, SGA is often the result of placental insufficiency. SGA newborns are often hypoglycemic because they have abnormally low glycogen stores. They commonly respond to placental insufficiency by increasing their red-blood-cell mass. Although an increase in red-blood-cell mass (polycythemia) increases the oxygen-carrying capacity of blood, polycythemia also has been associated with hyperviscosity, as well as renal failure, NEC, and CNS injury, especially if the hematocrit value exceeds 65% (Pallotto and Kilbride, 2006; Rosenberg, 2008). If the hematocrit value is higher than 65% in well-hydrated neonates, an exchange transfusion should be considered to reduce the hematocrit level to 55% or lower before surgery, although there is no evidence that doing so for patients who are not having surgery improves outcome (Dempsey and Barrington, 2006). However, the combination of polycythemia, hypotension, and dehydration that are common in sick SGA infants during anesthesia and surgery may increase their risk for hyperviscosity-related problems. Arterial blood pressure should be kept normal or slightly elevated throughout surgery. SGA infants may be relatively dehydrated at birth and usually do not lose the normal 200 to 300 g of weight that appropriate-for-gestational-age (AGA) neonates lose over the first 2 to 3 days of life. SGA neonates usually gain weight from birth. In spite of their low birth weights, the heart rates and blood pressures of SGA infants are similar to those of AGA infants of similar gestational ages. SGA neonates have similar incidences of hyaline membrane disease (HMD) to AGA babies of the same gestational age.

The LGA Infant

LGA infants are prone to birth injuries (e.g., fractures or intracranial bleeds) (Lawrence, 2007). Those born to diabetic mothers (a common reason for LGA) may have difficulty maintaining normal blood glucose concentrations and glucagon may be required to do so (Van Howe and Storms, 2008). On occasion, tracheal intubation may be difficult in LGA babies because of fat deposits in their mouth, tongue, and neck. Finding adequate insertion sites for intravenous fluid may be difficult because the veins are buried in tissue. It may be necessary to insert a central venous catheter or an external jugular vein catheter to ensure adequate intravenous access.

Very Low-Birth Weight and Extremely Low-Birth Weight Infants

Further subclassification of infants by both age and weight have been created and give further prognostic information regarding morbidity and mortality. In the 1960s, *low birth weight (LBW)* defined infants weighing less than 2500 g. As survival improved in these infants, the term *very low birth weight (VLBW)* was used to describe infants with birth weights of 1500 g or less. As survival of infants weighing less than 1000 g improved, the term *extremely low birth weight (ELBW)* was used to categorize these infants.

THE PREMATURE INFANT

Prematurity is defined as birth before 37 weeks of gestation. Premature infants account for 12.8% of all births in the United States (646,047 of 4,265,996), and the incidence has increased 21% since 1990 (Martin et al., 2008). The increase has been most dramatic between the gestational ages of 34 to 36 weeks (Davidoff et al., 2006). While the rates of VLBW (fewer than 1500 g) and ELBW (fewer than 1000 g) deliveries remained relatively unchanged from 2005 to 2006, the percentage of moderately low birth weight (1500 to 2499 g) deliveries increased slightly. In 2005, short gestation and low birth weight was the second leading cause of infant death (16.5%), ranked only below congenital malformations (19.5%) (Martin et al., 2008). However, in non-Hispanic black, and Puerto Rican infants, disorders related to short gestation and low birth weight were the leading causes of death. Today, the Centers for Disease Control (CDC) recognize prematurity, not birth defects, as the leading cause of infant mortality in the United States (Andrews et al., 2008).

Although premature infants share some common features, the physiologic variability between 24 and 36 weeks' gestation is enormous. An infant at 36 weeks' gestation is much more similar to a term infant than to infants born before 30 weeks gestation. For this discussion, premature infants are arbitrarily divided into subgroups based on gestational age.

Late Preterm (35 to 37 Weeks' Gestation)

In the absence of congenital anomalies or perinatal asphyxia, infants born between 35 and 37 weeks' gestation usually do well and have few of the common medical or surgical problems found in more premature infants. However, late preterm birth is associated with increased mortality (threefold higher than term infants), respiratory distress or apnea requiring support, and rehospitalization (Escobar et al., 2006; Tomashek et al., 2007). In addition, sepsis and intrapartum complications, centered on the placenta and cord, have contributed to increased mortality in late preterm infants (Tomashek et al., 2007). In addition, late-preterm infants may have some difficulty attaining full feeds, and the incidence of hyperbilirubinemia (not associated with Coombs' positivity or ABO/Rh incompatibility) occurs more commonly in late preterm infants than in term infants. Late-preterm infants born to diabetic mothers may have pulmonary immaturity and respiratory distress syndrome (RDS) (Deorari et al., 1991). Late-preterm infants born to nondiabetic mothers usually have similar lung function to that of term infants. Most surgical intervention in this group of patients is for treatment of congenital anomalies.

The rate of late preterm birth has increased 25% since 1990, and attention has been drawn to the increased mortality associated with late-preterm compared with term gestation (Escobar et al., 2006; Shapiro-Mendoza et al., 2006; Engle et al., 2007; Tomashek et al., 2007; Martin et al., 2008; McIntire and Leveno, 2008). The morbidity and mortality rates of late-preterm infants are particularly noticeable because of the large number of births at this developmental stage; in 2006, late-preterm births accounted for more than 71% of all preterm births (9.14%) (Martin et al., 2008). However, the long-term outcome of this group has not been well documented, in part related to the longstanding view of this group as "near term" rather than late preterm (Jain, 2007).

30 to 34 Weeks' Gestation

For the sake of this discussion, infants born between 30 and 34 weeks' gestation are considered to be similar, but the physiologic differences between a 30- and a 34-week gestation newborn can be significant. Infants at 30 weeks' gestation (≈1200 g) have more of the common problems of prematurity than infants at 34 weeks' gestation (≈2000 g).

Before the introduction of exogenous pulmonary surfactant into clinical practice, this group of infants often had RDS, also known as HMD (see Respiratory Distress Syndrome, p. 520). Complications of their respiratory care, including pneumothorax, pulmonary interstitial emphysema, chronic lung disease (CLD), and blood loss from repeated blood sampling, were common. Treatment of RDS with surfactant has dramatically reduced the incidence and severity of this disease and it complications. The sequelae of pulmonary immaturity and of the supportive care used to treat lung immaturity are fewer and less severe since the introduction of exogenous surface-active material (SAM). However, a new form of bronchopulmonary dysplasia (BPD), called *new BPD,* occurs in small preterm infants (Bancalari, 2001; Bancalari and del Moral, 2001). Approximately 20% to 25% of these infants have some form of CLD.

Although uncommon in infants after 34 weeks' gestation, newborns with a gestational age of 30 to 32 weeks often demonstrate temperature instability, especially if they are septic or asphyxiated. Feeding intolerance is also common, and it may take weeks before effective oral feeding and consistent weight gain occur. Before adequate enteral feeds are established, infants born at 30 to 34 weeks' gestation are often hypocalcemic or hypoglycemic. They are also prone to NEC, especially if they have a large patent ductus arteriosus (PDA) with significant left-to-right shunting of blood (Kitterman, 1980). Because enteral feeds must be advanced slowly, peripheral or central intravenous alimentation may be required for some time. Parenteral nutrition, for even 1 to 2 weeks, can cause hepatic and renal toxicity (Moreno Villares, 2008).

The incidence of a PDA is high (20% to 30%) in infants of this gestational age, but the hemodynamic consequences are often mild. Their PDA commonly closes spontaneously. If it does not close, chemical (with indomethacin) or surgical closure of the PDA may be necessary. The incidence of intracerebral hemorrhage (ICH) is higher in this age group and increases with decreasing gestational age, sepsis, asphyxia, or precipitous birth. Apnea is also more common at this developmental stage, especially in those infants who have sepsis, temperature instability, metabolic abnormalities (e.g., hypoglycemia or hypocalcemia), or anemia (Theobald et al., 2000).

27 to 29 Weeks' Gestation

The incidence and severity of pulmonary, cardiovascular, gastrointestinal, and neurologic complications are magnified in infants of this gestational age. A key feature is the variability of their disease processes. Some become "growing preemies" after 1 to 2 weeks, and others have multisystem dysfunction and poor growth and development for months.

The fragile skin and the absence of subcutaneous tissue in infants with fewer than 30 weeks' gestation result in temperature instability, enormous caloric expenditure to maintain body temperature, and significant transcutaneous fluid losses. Perioperative apnea is much more common in this group.

Fewer than 26 Weeks' Gestation

This group of patients is rapidly increasing because of increased survival rates, and they often have long-term pulmonary, neurologic, and gastrointestinal sequelae. The rate of progress in the NICU, in the incidence and severity of complications, and in the amount and urgency of surgical procedures is enormously variable at this gestation.

In this group of patients, the CNS is fragile, and ICH is common (Kadri et al., 2006). The severity of ICH is a common determinant of an infant's prognosis and long-term outcome, and it correlates with later neurologic injury (see The Central Nervous System, p. 528). Apnea and perioperative pulmonary insufficiency occur often and may persist for months. From the first few weeks to the first months of life, most infants of this developmental stage require mechanical ventilation, continuous positive airway pressure (CPAP), or an increased inspired oxygen concentration after surgery. Ventilatory support is often required, even if these interventions were not necessary preoperatively. Prolonged tracheal intubation is occasionally required and may lead to subglottic stenosis and lower airway obstruction.

REVIEW OF SYSTEMS AND DEVELOPMENTAL PHYSIOLOGY

Head and Neck

Anatomic differences of the head and neck between neonates and older patients make the management of the neonate's airway challenging (Dickison, 1987). The cricoid ring is the narrowest portion of the neonate's upper airway because the larynx has been thought to be cone shaped, rather than cylindrical as it is after 5 years of age (Coté et al., 1993). However, this concept has been challenged (Litman et al., 2003; Dalal et al., 2009; Motoyama, 2009). These newer studies indicate that the shape of the larynx is cylindrical, as it is in adults, but the cricoid ring remains the fixed and narrowest point of the upper airway system.

The narrowest portion of the cone is the cricoid ring. This is, in part, because the neonate's posterior larynx is more cephalad than the anterior larynx. When looking from above, the cricoid ring is really an ellipse and not a circle. By 5 years of age, the posterior larynx descends, the cricoid ring is circular, and the vocal cords are the narrowest portion of the airway (as they are in adults). These anatomic differences place the neonatal larynx in a more cephalad position than it is later in life. The epiglottis is relatively large, which makes it more difficult to lift with a laryngoscope blade. In fact it is easier to use a straight laryngoscope blade like a curved blade, place the tip in the vellecula, and pull up and out at a 45-degree angle to bring the glottic opening into view. The cephalad larynx and relatively large tongue also make it more difficult to maintain an airway or to intubate the trachea. However, the neonate's large occiput naturally places the head (when looking straight forward) in the "sniffing" position (i.e., an optimal position to ventilate the lungs and intubate the trachea). Extension or flexion of the head usually makes it more difficult to bag-and-mask ventilate the lungs and to intubate the trachea. A small jaw (micrognathia) or receding jaw (e.g., Pierre-Robin or Treacher-Collins syndromes) may make it difficult or impossible to directly visualize the vocal cords. A large tongue (as with hypothyroidism, Down syndrome, or Beckwith-Wiedemann syndrome) can also make tracheal intubation difficult or impossible. Techniques other than direct laryngoscopy may be needed to intubate the trachea of these infants (see Chapter 12, Airway Management).

Cleft lip, with and without a cleft palate, occurs in 1:600 to 1000 live births and is associated with other congenital defects in 13% to 50% of patients (see Chapter 25, Anesthesia for Plastic Surgery) (Arosarena, 2007). Tracheal intubation is occasionally more difficult in patients with a cleft palate because it may be difficult to fix the patient's tongue against the palate with the laryngoscope blade. If the tongue cannot be fixed against the palate, it may flop over the laryngoscope blade and block the view of the glottis. Choanal atresia occurs in 1:7000 to 1:8000 live births and is often diagnosed in the delivery room when a catheter cannot be passed through a nostril into the pharynx or when the neonate cannot breath and becomes cyanotic and bradycardic when the mouth is closed and the airway is totally obstructed (see Chapter 12, Airway Management) (Samadi et al., 2003). Thus, when using bag-and-mask ventilation on patients who have choanal atresia, the mouth must be kept open or an oral airway must be inserted. Some patients who have choanal atresia have the CHARGE association, which is defined through the anacronym as follows: C, Colobomatous malformation; H, Heart defect; A, Atresia choane; R, Retardation; G, Growth deficiency/Genital hypoplasia; and E, Ear anomalies (Sanlaville and Verloes, 2007).

Hemangiomas, lymphangiomas, and hygromas of the neck often obstruct the upper airway. Careful preoperative evaluation, including computerized tomography (CT) scan when appropriate, helps determine whether a lesion impinges on the airway. Patients with laryngeal or tracheal hemangiomas are of special concern, because tearing the hemangioma during tracheal intubation may result in airway hemorrhage and blood aspiration.

The Pulmonary System

Development

Lung development is divided into the following five stages:

1. The embryonic stage (weeks 4 to 6 of gestation), when early upper airways appear.
2. The glandular stage (weeks 7 to 16), when the lower conducting airways form.
3. The canalicular phase (weeks 17 to 28), when the acini develop.
4. The terminal sac period (weeks 28 to 36), when the first respiratory units for gas exchange (terminal air sacs and surrounding capillaries) make their appearance.
5. The alveolar phase, when alveoli develop.

The latter stage begins at about 36 weeks' gestation and continues until at least 18 months of age (Langston et al., 1984; Kotecha, 2000a, 2000b; Joshi and Kotecha, 2007). Knowledge of these phases of lung development allows estimation of when the various lung malformations occur in utero. For example, malformations of the conducting airways (e.g., cystic adenomatoid malformation) occur before 16 weeks' gestation. Upper airway abnormalities occur by 6 weeks' gestation, bronchial malformations between 6 and 16 weeks of gestation, and lung hypoplasia after 16 weeks' gestation. In general, extrauterine viability

is increased after 26 weeks' gestation, because the respiratory saccules have developed and the capillaries are in close approximation to the developing distal airways. Before this time, both the vascular network and surface area in the lungs may be inadequate for gas exchange. However, in the past decade many babies have survived after 24 to 25 weeks' gestation, usually with enormous effort and cost; these extremely premature infants often survive with severe CLD (Langston et al., 1984).

Most alveoli develop after birth, increasing from 20 million terminal air sacs at term to about 300 to 400 million alveoli at 18 months of age (Thurlbeck, 1982; Kotecha, 2000a, 2000b). Specific cell types are not recognizable in the lung until the canalicular stage of development (17 to 28 weeks' gestation). During the last 10% to 20% of gestation, type II pneumocytes are more commonly identified. Although present in the human fetus by 22 weeks' gestation, type II pneumocytes are more prominent after 34 to 36 weeks of gestation. The major distinguishing feature of type II cells is the presence of osmophilic lamellar bodies, which correlate closely with the presence of SAM in the lungs (Kotecha, 2000a, 2000b). The alveolar-capillary barrier is formed by type I pneumocytes (see Chapter 3, Respiratory Physiology in Infants and Children).

By 16 weeks' gestation, all subdivisions of the conducting airways have formed, including the main-stem bronchi and the conducting and terminal bronchioles. Preterm infants often require mechanical ventilation or CPAP and supplemental oxygen, which interfere with the normal, complex process of lung and airway development. The barotrauma, oxidative stress, and inflammatory injury associated with these life-saving interventions and the effects of superimposed infections predispose preterm infants to airway and lung injury and to abnormal airway resistance and reactivity (Van Marter, 2005).

The diaphragm arises in part from the third through fifth cervical somites, and myoblasts from these somites migrate into the septum transversum to form diaphragmatic muscle (Mitchell and Sharma, 2009). The central tendon of the diaphragm arises from the mesoderm of the septum transversum. Somites of the lateral chest wall form the lateral portions of the diaphragm. The nerve supply of the diaphragm is from the third through fifth cervical somites. Bilateral pericardioperitoneal canals, located lateral to the developing diaphragm, cause a Bochdalek hernia if the canals fail to close. Complete closure of the diaphragm normally occurs at 10 to 12 weeks' gestation, when the bowel is returning to the abdominal cavity from the amnion, where it resides in early gestation. If the diaphragm is incompletely formed, the returning bowel follows the path of least resistance and enters the chest. When this occurs lung growth ceases on the ipsilateral side. The mediastinum is then pushed into the opposite chest by the bowel and abdominal organs and contralateral lung growth is also reduced. Consequently, neonates who have a left-sided diaphragmatic hernia must survive with approximately two thirds of one lung or less (de Lorimier et al., 1967). In some cases, the amount of lung present is insufficient for survival (see Chapter 18, Anesthesia for General Surgery in the Neonate).

Failure of the lung buds to separate from the foregut causes a tracheal esophageal fistula (see Chapter 18, Anesthesia for General Surgery in the Neonate). The connection usually is found between the distal esophagus and the trachea, just above the carina. Failure of the distal and proximal ends of the esophagus to connect with each other results in esophageal atresia. Patients with esophageal atresia usually have copious secretions in the proximal esophageal pouch, and placing the patient flat without removing the secretions may cause aspiration of the secretions. Placing a suction catheter in the proximal esophageal pouch and connecting it to suction reduces this likelihood.

Early Postnatal Period: Changes in Oxygenation and Pulmonary Vascular Resistance

Although removal of fluid from the fetal lung begins during labor and delivery, the major transition to an air-filled lung occurs immediately after birth. The first active inspiration after birth produces a negative intrapleural pressure of 80 to 100 cm H_2O, which is required to overcome the high surface tension, low compliance, and high resistance of the liquid-filled lungs (Scarpelli and Mautone, 1984; Vyas et al., 2005). These pressures are not necessary when artificially ventilating neonatal lungs, however. In fact, delivering large tidal volumes and high airway pressures injure neonatal lungs (Bjorklund et al., 1997). In full-term neonates, the initial few spontaneous breaths are of 20 and 80 cc O_2 each. A small fraction of this volume is expired. The gas remaining in the lung forms the residual volume (RV) and the FRC, which are required for adequate gas exchange (Avery, 1974). If removal of lung fluid is delayed (e.g., with cesarean section) transient tachypnea of the newborn (TTN) develops (Guglani et al., 2008). Neonates with TTN breathe 60 to 150 times a minute and are often hypoxic and hypercarbic. Many of them require supplemental oxygen, and some require mechanical ventilation. Diuretics fail to induce a diuresis and improve lung function until a spontaneous diuresis occurs several days after birth (Lewis and Whitelaw, 2002).

Labor reduces pulmonary vascular resistance (PVR) by approximately 10%, but the most significant decrease occurs with the onset of breathing (Bland, 1983). Lung expansion increases alveolar and arterial Po_2, which dilates the pulmonary arterioles, decreases PVR and increases pulmonary blood flow (Dawes, 1974). These changes in PVR and blood flow are critical for conversion of the fetal circulation to the adult form of circulation (see Chapters 3, Respiratory Physiology, and 4, Cardiovascular Physiology). That is, transition to the gas-filled lung at birth, increased Fio_2 (air), and increased pH (decreased $Paco_2$) all interact to reduce PVR and increase pulmonary blood flow. Over the next 1 to 2 months, PVR decreases to adult levels. However, infants with cyanotic congenital heart disease (CHD) or large left-to-right shunts may have elevated PVR for months or longer (Rudolph, 2007).

The dramatic rise in pulmonary blood flow at birth increases the left atrial pressure and functionally closes the foramen ovale, preventing right-to-left shunting of deoxygenated blood through this structure. An increase in systemic vascular resistance that exceeds PVR dramatically reduces right-to-left blood flow through the ductus arteriosus. The rise in arterial oxygen tension at birth constricts and physiologically closes the ductus arteriosus in full-term but not in preterm neonates (Clyman et al., 1978). Nitric oxide (NO) and prostaglandins are important for anatomic closure of the ductus arteriosus, which usually occurs by 2 to 3 weeks of age (Born et al., 1956; Seidner et al., 2001; Clyman, 2006). If during this time hypoxia, acidosis, cold, or excessive airway pressures are present, the right atrial pressure increases and right-to-left shunting of blood can occur at both the atrial and the DA levels. When right-to-left shunting of blood occurs, hypoxemia ensues. The resulting pulmonary blood flow pattern mimics the pattern present in utero and is often referred to as persistent fetal circulation (PFC).

Establishing normal pulmonary blood flow and ventilation increases both arterial and mixed venous oxygen tensions. Although the transition to air breathing increases the oxygen content of blood, the Pao_2 of the neonate is usually 55 to 85 mm Hg for the first month of life, rather than the 95 to 100 mm Hg present after that. The lower Pao_2 is the result of a very compliant, cartilaginous neonatal chest wall that does not recoil outward at end-expiration, as it does in older children and adults (Koch and Wendel, 1968; Davis and Bureau, 1987). Failure to recoil outward produces a transpulmonary (intrapleural) pressure of 0 cm H_2O—not –5 cm H_2O pressure, as occurs in older patients. Because negative intrapleural pressures are important for maintenance of a normal FRC, neonates are predisposed to atelectasis and a lower Pao_2. In fact, application of sufficient negative pressure around the neonate's chest to produce a pleural pressure of –5 cm H_2O, increases the Pao_2 from about 65 mm Hg to nearly 100 mm Hg, indicating that the negative intrapleural pressure expands the lungs, increases FRC, reduces atelectasis, and improves the match of ventilation to perfusion (Thibeault et al., 1968). Application of negative intrapleural pressure, positive end expiratory pressure (PEEP), or CPAP also reduces the amount of atelectasis and improves oxygenation (Gregory et al., 1975).

In addition to its effects on transpulmonary pressure, the newborn's compliant rib cage has another unwanted effect on ventilation. That is, the cartilaginous, compliant chest wall tends to collapse inward (retract) during spontaneous inspiration, causing paradoxic chest-wall motion and limiting airflow (Knill et al., 1976). The circular configuration of the rib cage (rather than the ellipsoid rib cage of adults) and the horizontal angle of insertion of the diaphragm (rather than the oblique angle in adults) also distort the rib cage and make the diaphragm less efficient (Muller and Bryan, 1979).

Other factors also affect the infant's work and efficiency of breathing. For instance, the full-term infant's diaphragm is comprised of only 25% fatigue-resistant, slow-twitch, highly oxidative type I fibers, and the preterm infant has only 10% (the adult diaphragm has 55%). The lower percentage of type I fibers predisposes the diaphragm to fatigue (Keens et al., 1978). The intercostal muscles show a similar developmental pattern. Expression of various isoforms of the myosin heavy chains in muscle fibers of the diaphragm and the intercostal muscles of newborn and young infants may contribute to easier fatigability (Watchko and Sieck, 1993; Zhan et al., 1998). Less effective force-frequency, length-tension, and force-velocity relationships and a mismatch of energy supply and demand characterize diaphragmatic muscle and predisposes these newborns to fatigue, especially when there is widespread atelectasis (e.g., RDS) or poor chest wall compliance (e.g., anasarca) (Watchko et al., 1986; Watchko and Sieck,1993). Methylxanthines improve neonatal diaphragmatic function (Maycock et al., 1992).

Healthy neonates breathe 30 to 60 times per minute to maintain normal oxygenation and to remove the increased amount of CO_2 produced by an oxygen consumption of 6 to 10 cc/kg per minute. This respiratory rate also helps maintain the FRC by reducing the amount of time available for expiration and by trapping gas within the lung. At normal respiratory rates, the time constant of the lungs (compliance of lungs × airway resistance [C_L × R_{aw}]) is, on average, 0.25 seconds. A slow respiratory rate, apnea, or bradypnea can reduce the FRC, especially in preterm neonates (Fig. 17-3). A low level of PEEP

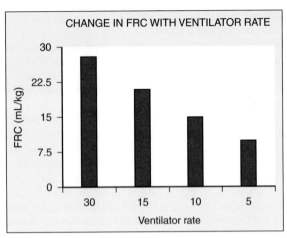

CHANGE IN FRC WITH VENTILATOR RATE

■ **FIGURE 17-3.** The change in FRC of a 1550 g infant that occurred with decreasing ventilator rates without PEEP. A PEEP of 5 cm H$_2$O maintained the FRC at about 25 mL/kg even at 5 breaths per minute (not shown).

TABLE 17-1. Changes in FRC Associated with Blood Transfusion in Five Term Infants*

Functional Residual Capacity (FRC) mL/kg	Blood Transfused mL/kg
15 ± 5	0
22 ± 4	5
27 ± 6	15

Gregory GA: Unpublished data.
*FRC was measured by helium dilution.

(5 to 7 cm H$_2$O) should always be added to maintain the FRC of infants and young children, especially when slow ventilatory rates are used.

Naturally occurring SAM or pulmonary surfactant is by far the most important mechanism for keeping alveoli of different sizes or diameters open. Initially, SAM appears in fetal lungs by 20 weeks' gestation, even though no functional alveoli exist (Clements, 1961). At about 35 to 36 weeks' gestation, the amount of SAM increases and is secreted onto the alveolar surface. The pulmonary surfactant monolayer creates a gas-liquid interface on the alveolar surface and drastically decreases surface tension during exhalation as the surface area decreases. During inspiration the monolayer is thinned, and the surface tension increases. SAM keeps the surface tension relatively constant regardless of the changes in the surface area and the radius of the alveoli. In neonates with RDS, there is loss of or inactivation of surfactant, and surface tension increases. The variability of surface tension normally occurring with changes in surface area is lost; alveoli develop higher pressures, collapse during exhalation, and remain collapsed (see Chapter 3, Respiratory Physiology in Infants and Children).

An additional mechanism that helps keep the alveoli open is the interdependence among alveoli, small airways, and lung parenchyma. Because the alveoli are attached to each other by connective tissues, the tendency of one alveolus to collapse during expiration pulls its neighbor open (Takishima and Mead, 1972). Millions of alveoli exerting this "pulling" effect help maintain FRC. Furthermore, blood-filled capillaries act as an exoskeleton for alveoli. If the pulmonary blood volume is inadequate, atelectasis develops. Increasing the blood volume increases FRC (Table 17-1) (Gregory, personal observation).

Thus, surfactant, intraalveolar forces, and pulmonary blood volume compensate for the lack of transpulmonary pressure at end expiration that is caused by the neonate's extremely compliant chest wall and are responsible for maintaining the infant's FRC, albeit smaller (30 cc/kg) than that of adults (50 cc/kg).

Surface Active Material

The demonstration by Avery and Mead (1959) that surfactant deficiency is the primary cause of RDS eventually led Phibbs et al. (1991) and Fujiwara et al. (1990) to use commercially available surfactant prophylactically after birth or in the rescue mode after the symptoms of RDS were apparent. Intubated infants of fewer than 28 weeks' gestation often receive 1 or 2 doses of surfactant 12 hours apart. During preoperative evaluation of a newborn with RDS, it should be determined when the last dose of SAM was given and if an additional dose is required before surgery because of progressive atelectasis or worsening blood gases and oxygen requirement.

Pulmonary gas exchange is only possible after a significant portion of the lung fluid present in utero is removed from the airways and alveoli. Increased pulmonary lymphatic flow and surface-active phospholipids and proteins facilitate this process (Humphreys et al., 1967; King, 1982). Surfactant reduces the surface tension of the gas-liquid interface of the alveoli, keeping the air spaces open at end expiration. This reduction of surface tension is critical for the maintenance of FRC and gas exchange.

Type I pneumocytes account for more than 90% of the alveolar surface cells; type II pneumocytes, the SAM-storing cells, populate most of the remaining surface. The total weight of SAM consists of about 10% protein, 90% lipids, and 0.1% carbohydrates. The lipids lower the surface tension, but the proteins allow absorption and dispersion of the lipids in the air-liquid interface. Proteins are also necessary for reuptake of SAM by type II cells. Congenital absence of these proteins leads to a chronic RDS-like state (Yurdakök, 2004). During inspiration SAM is spread over the alveolar surface. During expiration it is compacted to lower the alveolar surface tension. SAM also stabilizes small airways and is important for pulmonary defense mechanisms (Jarstarand, 1984).

Respiratory Distress Syndrome

Neonatal RDS occurs when the quantity of SAM is insufficient or when there is delayed synthesis or release of surfactant (e.g., in infants of diabetic mothers). Giving betamethasone to the fetus, by way of the mother, before 36 weeks' gestation accelerates the production and release of SAM from the type II alveolar epithelial cells and reduces the incidence of RDS (Liggins and Howie, 1972). Typical clinical features of RDS include: early onset of tachypnea; intercostal, sternal, and suprasternal retractions; grunting respirations; oxygen desaturation; respiratory and metabolic acidosis; and death if not treated. A chest radiograph shows a diffuse reticulogranular pattern and air bronchograms (Fig. 17-4). Unless SAM is given, the natural course of RDS includes worsening symptoms for 2 to 3 days, resulting in either improvement or death. In some cases, respiratory function may deteriorate, rather than improve, because of a superinfection

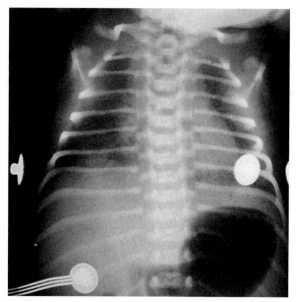

■ **FIGURE 17-4.** RDS. Note the ground-glass appearance and the presence of air bronchograms. *(From Brozanski BS, Bogen DL: Neonatology. In Zitelli BJ, Davis HW, editors:* Atlas of pediatric physical diagnosis, *ed 4, Philadelphia, 2002, Mosby.)*

or complications of ventilatory support. RDS-associated death is often the result of severe lung injury induced by mechanical ventilation, sepsis, renal or hepatic failure, or CNS injury. This severe clinical pattern occurs less commonly when pulmonary surfactant is provided early. About 5% of all babies with RDS are born at term.

Before the development of commercially available surfactant, lung injury (e.g., pneumothorax, pulmonary interstitial emphysema, or BPD), blood loss from repeated blood sampling, and sepsis and its secondary effects (e.g., renal and hepatic dysfunction) were relatively common. Since 1990, exogenous SAM administration has significantly reduced the need for mechanical ventilation and oxygen therapy in preterm infants because of its effects on lung mechanics, including distensibility of the lung and end-expiratory volume stability (Morley et al., 2008). However, volutrauma (high tidal volume), and barotrauma (high airway pressure) persist in causing lung injury despite recent decreases in the incidence and severity of classic RDS and a reduction in the complications of pulmonary immaturity and supportive care. Despite all of these changes, the incidence of BPD has remained stable at about 20% (higher in ELBW infants) over the last 20 years (Bancalari and del Moral, 2001). But the BPD now seen in surfactant-treated lungs is different from classic BPD and is called *new BPD*. New BPD most commonly develops in ELBW infants, is characterized by a more uniform pattern of injury, and seems to represent an arrest of lung growth. Persistence of BPD, in spite of surfactant, suggests that other factors beside SAM deficiency contribute to BPD (Bancalari, 2001). Inflammatory and oxidative injury caused by infection, oxygen therapy, and "gentle" ventilation during periods of rapid lung growth and development, especially in the ELBW infants, seem to cause long-term pulmonary dysfunction (Kramer et al., 2009). The increased number of survivors has enlarged the number of patients (with and without BPD) requiring surgical treatment for coexisting long-term sequelae of prematurity.

Recent efforts to minimize lung injury caused by mechanical ventilation of premature infants have included introducing nasal CPAP (nCPAP) in the delivery room to prevent or treat RDS (Morley et al., 2008). This tactic avoids endotracheal intubation in patients and has markedly reduced the use of SAM. On the other hand, some infants with RDS (especially those weighing less than 1000 g) often fail a trial of nCPAP and require endotracheal intubation. They are usually treated with surfactant when their trachea are intubated.

Oxidative Injury in the Newborn

Although the role of oxygen in ROP is well established, oxygen toxicity of other organs, especially those of more mature newborns, is being increasingly recognized. Despite its widespread use for more than a century and the recognition that oxygen can be toxic for at least 50 years, the precise molecular mechanism of oxygen toxicity remains unknown (Tin, 2002). The severity of BPD has been correlated with oxygen exposure and with the oxygen saturation level used. In addition, greater oxidative injury to the heart, brain, and kidneys has been reported when neonatal resuscitation is accomplished with supplemental oxygen (Munkeby et al., 2004; Martín et al., 2007).

ROP is a multifactorial disease, but two main factors are associated with its development—prematurity and oxygen (see Chapter 27, Anesthesia for Ophthalmic Surgery). As stated, the neonate is exposed in utero to an oxygen tension of 20 to 30 mm Hg. Birth raises the Pao_2 to 55 to 85 mm Hg that may represent hyperoxia, especially for preterm neonates. The retinal vessels grow radially outward from the center of the optic disc from about 16 to 40 weeks' gestation. Neonates born before term have incompletely developed retinal vessels (Roth, 1977). Two phases of ROP have been described. The initial phase, which occurs between 30 and 32 weeks' gestation, is associated with inhibition of growth and loss of retinal vessels. Growth of the retina under these circumstances leads to retinal hypoxia. The second phase of ROP is associated with effusive retinal neovascularization and occurs between 32 and 34 weeks' gestation. New vessels form in the avascular regions and send up fibrous bands to the vitreous gel and lens. These strands are responsible for retinal detachment in some premature infants (Chen and Smith, 2007). Vascular endothelial cell growth factor (VEGF) is required for new vessel growth in utero and afterwards. Administering oxygen after birth decreases VEGF during the first phase of ROP, which decreases vessel growth. In the second phase of ROP, retinal hypoxia increases VEGF expression, which causes exuberant vessel overgrowth. Insulin-like growth factor-1 (IGF-1) is required for VEGF to have its maximal effect. During gestation, serum concentrations of IGF-1 increase, and the severity of ROP is directly correlated with the level of IGF-1. In utero, IGF-1 is supplied by both the placenta and the amniotic fluid. This is withdrawn at birth, decreasing the effectiveness of VEGF, and vessel growth decreases. Excessive amounts of oxygen turn off VEGF. Thus, both VEGF and IGF-1, under appropriate circumstances, inhibit vessel growth and cause vessel regression. Because of the severe retinal hypoxia in phase I of ROP, VEGF and IGF-1 concentrations increase. Retinal vessels' growth causes the severe problems seen in the later stages of ROP. Avoidance of excessive oxygen concentrations in the operating room is therefore necessary (Betts et al., 1977).

Because there is evidence that supplemental oxygen causes a significant amount of injury, the use of supplemental oxygen should be limited to that required to maintain the oxygen saturation between 85% and 93%, both during resuscitation at birth and during the entire neonatal period (Rabi et al., 2007).

BPD in the Surgical Patient

Infants with moderate to severe BPD often require supplemental oxygen beyond 36 weeks' postconceptual age and often have evidence of lower-airway obstruction. Chest x-rays usually show hyperinflation or atelectasis and, on occasion, bronchopneumonia. Recurrent upper airway infections are common. If BPD is severe, hypercarbia and treatment with diuretics (e.g., furosemide) may complicate management of fluids, electrolytes, and nutrition. Maintaining normal pulmonary gas exchange in infants with BPD during anesthesia and surgery may be difficult. Consequently, many infants require increased respiratory support (including PIP, PEEP, and oxygen) to maintain baseline oxygenation and ventilation; however, use of these modalities also increases the risk of lung injury. Analyzing the infant's current and recent ventilatory history, including severity and treatment of airway reactivity, is necessary to guide intraoperative care. Imitating the care established in the NICU can minimize exposure to excessive pressures, tidal volumes, and oxygen concentrations. To minimize the risk of a pneumothorax, pneumomediastinum, or interstitial emphysema, high peak airway pressures should be avoided, and adequate expiratory times should be allowed, especially if a patient has obstructive lung disease. All of these factors can cause sudden deterioration of hemodynamic and respiratory function. Hyperreactivity of the small airways is a common feature of BPD, and bronchodilation should be maximized preoperatively. Stimulation of the airways by tracheal intubation and surgical manipulation can induce severe bronchospasm, even at surgical planes of anesthesia.

Perioperative nutritional deficits and increased fluid requirements during surgery affect pulmonary function and ventilatory management, especially during and after major surgery (e.g., laparotomy for NEC). Assessing an infant's acid-base status ($Paco_2$, pH, base deficit) and preoperative hepatic and renal function is essential for determining what kind and how much fluid to administer during surgery. Vigorous intravenous crystalloid and colloid administration during anesthesia and surgery, as well as postoperative hemodynamic instability, can dramatically affect pulmonary function, especially if the lungs were injured by BPD.

Preoperative Evaluation of the Pulmonary System

Evaluation of the pulmonary system begins with a review of the gestation, birth, and neonatal course. Was the infant hypoxic or asphyxiated in utero or at birth? Did the infant require artificial ventilation or other resuscitation at birth? If so, are there residual, active pulmonary symptoms, signs, or laboratory abnormalities? Does the infant presently require mechanical ventilation? If so, what are the current requirements for Fio_2, peak airway pressures, end-expiratory pressure, tidal volume, and ventilator rates? Have the ventilator settings increased or decreased over the previous 24 hours? What is the targeted oxygen saturation? What are the pH_a and $Paco_2$? If present, is hypercarbia chronic or acute, and is it intentional?

Physical Examination

Evaluating the chest movement and breathing pattern of patients from the foot of the bed often provides important information about ventilatory function. For example, do both sides of the chest move equally during inspiration? A difference in chest movement suggests a unilateral process, such as a pneumothorax, a pleural fluid collection, unilateral interstitial emphysema, or an endobroncheal intubation. Although auscultation of the chest may reveal decreased breath sounds on one side, it may not because breath sounds are readily transmitted from one side to the other in neonates. Consequently, the bilateral breath sounds of infants with a pneumothorax are often equal on each side. Percussing the chest or shining a high-intensity light through it may identify a pneumothorax when bilateral and equal breath sounds are present (Kuhns et al., 1975). Are intercostal, sternal, or suprasternal retractions present during spontaneous breathing? This is evidence of increased work of breathing and suggests collapse of lower airways (atelectasis), infiltration of air spaces (as with pneumonia, edema, meconium), pulmonary hypoplasia, or upper airway obstruction. Retractions are more prominent in preterm neonates because of the limited amount of fat and subcutaneous tissue surrounding their chests.

Does the nonintubated neonate grunt during expiration? Partial glottic closure during expiration (grunting) maintains a positive intrathoracic pressure, increases FRC, and improves oxygenation (Harrison et al., 1968). Grunting is common in patients who have reduced FRCs (as with HMD or pulmonary edema). Is expiration prolonged? Are the muscles of respiration actively used to expire? A prolonged expiratory phase of respiration suggests lower airway obstruction, for example, from secretions, masses (intrinsic or extrinsic to the airway), or bronchospasm. Additional details about treatment with bronchodilators (dose and frequency, response to various agents) and suctioning (frequency, quantity and quality of secretions, recent changes, results of cultures) are important for intraoperative planning for ventilatory care. An abnormal physical examination may suggest that further evaluation is required preoperatively (e.g., CT or magnetic resonance imaging [MRI] scan, fiber optic bronchoscopy, or pharmacologic intervention).

Stridor or a weak cry may be signs that the neonate has vocal cord injury (e.g., long-term intubation or congenital paralysis), subglottic stenosis, or subglottic granulomas (Hengerer et al., 1975). A smaller endotracheal tube may be required to prevent further laryngeal or tracheal injury, if tracheal intubation is planned in such patients. However, small endotracheal tubes are more easily occluded with secretions, and suctioning may be more difficult, especially during surgery. In addition, weaning patients from mechanical ventilation postoperatively may be difficult or impossible if the endotracheal tube is small for the infant's age. Mask or laryngeal mask airways (LMAs) or other airway devices may make the need for tracheal intubation unnecessary; however, LMAs increase dead space by adding large volumes above the glottis (Table 17-2). Most cases of neonatal stridor require the opinion of a pediatric pulmonologist, surgeon, or otolaryngologist to define the safest and most efficient means of providing adequate evaluation and treatment of the stridor (e.g., bronchoscopy, CT scan or MRI, or surgery). Clearly, planning for these evaluations must consider how to reduce the risk-to-benefit ratio of each diagnostic or therapeutic examination, especially if deep sedation or general anesthesia is

TABLE 17-2. The Dead Space of LMAs

Weight (Kg)	VT (mL)	VD (mL)	LMA (Size)	VD (Mask)	VD (Total)
1-5	1-35	2.5-11	1.0	6	8.3-17
6-10	42-70	18-21	1.5	7	25-28
11-20	77-140	23-42	2.0	10	33-52
21-30	147-210	44-63	2.5	13	57-76
30	221	65	3.0	22	87

LMAs and their connecting tubes were filled with water to determine the dead space. Tidal volume was assumed to be 7 mL/kg and the wasted ventilation (VD) to be 0.3. Based on these data, unless there is a leak around the mask, the PaCO$_2$ will be elevated, often above 60 mm Hg, in smaller patients.
VT, Tidal volume; *VD,* dead space volume; *LMA,* laryngeal mask airway.

required. The need for and timing of tracheostomy should be considered early and discussed with the parents before surgery, especially when general anesthesia is required.

Blood Gas Analysis

Analysis of pH$_a$, Paco$_2$, and base deficit provides valuable information about the neonate's pulmonary function. Hypercarbia is the usual, normal physiologic compensation for metabolic alkalosis (e.g., from chronic furosemide administration). The level of Paco$_2$ alone does not tell whether the child has respiratory compensation for a metabolic acidosis or a metabolic compensation for respiratory acidosis. Acute hypercarbia produces acidosis, and the pH$_a$ is appropriate for the level of Paco$_2$ (assuming there is no coexisting metabolic acidosis). Of course, mixed metabolic and respiratory abnormalities further complicate interpretation of the relationship between pH and Paco$_2$. If the Paco$_2$ is chronically elevated and the pH$_a$ is relatively normal, acutely reducing the Paco$_2$ to normal will precipitate an acute respiratory alkalosis, which may significantly reduce cerebral blood flow. Every 1 mm Hg change in Paco$_2$ between 20 and 80 mm Hg Paco$_2$ causes a 2% change in cerebral blood flow. Thus, if the Paco$_2$ is 60 mm Hg, and is acutely reduced to 40 mm Hg, cerebral blood flow will decrease by as much as 40%. If this occurs in conjunction with hypotension, cerebral perfusion may well be inadequate. Hypocarbia and severe alkalosis should be avoided when possible, because it can result in poor neurologic outcomes (Curry et al., 2008).

Mechanical Ventilation

Infants who require mechanical ventilation before surgery often require increased support of ventilation during and after surgery, and patients who are spontaneously breathing and treated with nasal CPAP before surgery, usually require tracheal intubation and mechanical ventilation for variable periods after surgery. The lungs of neonates, especially premature neonates, are sensitive to oxidative damage, volutrauma (high volume trauma) as a result of overdistention of the lungs, and shear stress injury (low volume trauma) caused by repetitive opening and collapse of alveoli and terminal airways. In particular, lungs are easily overdistended during hand ventilation. Interestingly, neonates treated with CPAP alone have less evidence of pulmonary inflammation and CLD (Jobe et al., 2002). Small tidal volumes, rapid respiratory rates, and permissive hypercapnea

seem to reduce the amount and severity of neonatal lung injury, suggesting that intraoperative ventilation strategies should use the lowest effective tidal volumes (inspiratory and end-expiratory pressures) and inspired oxygen concentrations possible (Thomas and Speer, 2008). The Sao$_2$ should be maintained between 85% and 93% in preterm neonates, which may require the use of room air. Mild hypercapnea (Paco$_2$ of 45 to 55 mm Hg) is acceptable if there is no evidence of increased intracranial pressure, pulmonary hypertension, or severe metabolic acidosis. Aggressive hyperventilation should be avoided, and no attempt should be made to reduce the Paco$_2$ to 40 mm Hg or less without a very good clinical reason for doing so. Although knowledge of the ventilator settings used in the NICU is important for setting the initial respiratory rate and airway pressures in the operating room, the less sophisticated ventilators used during surgery are rarely as effective as the NICU's ventilators. Furthermore, the impact of positioning for surgery (e.g., lateral or prone), the procedure itself, retractors, surgeon's hands, fluid administered, anesthesia, and other factors all affect the effectiveness of mechanical ventilation in the operating room.

Infants treated preoperatively with high-frequency ventilation (HFV) usually fare better if they undergo surgery and anesthesia in the NICU and have their HFV continued throughout the surgery. High-dose narcotics and muscle paralysis provide adequate anesthesia in the NICU and are used because infants' ventilators cannot deliver inhaled anesthetics. Performing surgery in the NICU also eliminates the risks of transporting sick neonates to and from the operating room and allows easy access to the expertise of the NICU nurses and neonatologists.

The Cardiovascular System

Transitional Circulation

The fetal circulation is characterized by increased PVR, decreased pulmonary blood flow, decreased systemic vascular resistance, and right-to-left blood flow through a PDA and foramen ovale (Rudolph, 2007). At birth, the onset of ventilation and the elimination of the placental circulation have dramatic effects on systemic and PVRs (see Chapters 4, Cardiovascular Physiology, and 21, Congenital Cardiac Anesthesia: Non-Bypass Procedures). Pulmonary vascular resistance (PVR) decreases and pulmonary blood flow increases. Simultaneously, systemic vascular resistance increases, and the left atrial pressure rises. This functionally closes the foramen ovale and stops right-to-left shunting at this level. However, bidirectional shunting through the ductus arteriosus often continues for the first 24 hours of extrauterine life in healthy infants. If the ductus arteriosus fails to close, blood is shunted left-to-right into the pulmonary circulation as the PVR declines after birth. Anatomic closure of the ductus arteriosus occurs after several days, and shunting of blood through this structure ceases. The neonate now has the circulation of an adult.

If arterial hypoxemia or acidosis occurs during the first few days of life, the neonate's circulation may revert to the fetal pattern (i.e., pulmonary arterial vasoconstriction, pulmonary hypertension, and reduced pulmonary blood flow). The resultant increase in right atrial pressure reestablishes right-to-left shunting of deoxygenated blood through the foramen ovale and ductus arteriosus, producing arterial hypoxemia (Rudolph and Yuan, 1966). This return to the fetal circulatory pattern, called PFC or persistent pulmonary hypertension of the newborn

(PPHN), further exacerbates the hypoxemia and acidosis. Although numerous treatments for PPHN (e.g., hyperventilation or vasoactive agents) have been used, a selective and highly effective vasodilator of the pulmonary circulation has not been identified. PPHN may be an isolated phenomenon, or it may be associated with a variety of clinical conditions, including meconium aspiration, sepsis, polycythemia, diaphragmatic hernia, hypoxemia, acidosis, and severe hypotension. An echocardiogram should be performed to exclude structural cyanotic heart disease (Peckham and Fox, 1978; Murphy et al., 1981). The primary treatment of PPHN is aggressive hemodynamic support, including maintaining intravascular volume, initiating inotropic support (especially if PPHN is associated with sepsis or asphyxia), correcting acidosis and electrolyte disturbances, and administering antibiotics when appropriate. Ventilatory strategies have moved away from hyperventilation (pH greater than 7.5) and hyperoxia to more gentle approaches, including maintenance of normal oxygenation, $Paco_2$, and pH with either conventional or high-frequency mechanical ventilators. Vasodilatory agents such as NO are often used, but the protocols vary from institution to institution. NO has significantly reduced the need for extracorporeal membrane oxygenation to treat PPHN (Field et al., 2007).

Nitric Oxide

Control of the pulmonary circulation, especially during the transition from fetal to postnatal life, is complex and depends on the interaction of a variety of mediators and factors, receptors, and neurologic, endocrine, and vascular control mechanisms, both in endothelial and smooth muscle cells (Kinsella and Abman, 1995). For example, increased oxygen tension and expansion of the lungs with the onset of breathing decreases PVR directly. The rise in blood flow imparts shear stress to the vessels, which distends them, flattening the endothelium and the smooth muscle cells, and promotes the release of various mediators (Haworth, 2006). The balance between the effects of vasodilators (e.g., NO and prostacyclin) vs. vasoconstrictors (e.g., endothelin-1 [ET-1], leukotrienes) significantly affects pulmonary blood flow. As noted by Haworth (2006), "The pioneering studies of Dr. Dawes and his colleagues in Oxford in the 1960s on fetal sheep showed that mechanical ventilation reduced PVR and that the response was enhanced when the inspired gas was enriched with oxygen" (Dawes, 1968). Fifty years later, no single factor has yet been identified as being primarily responsible for the initiation of pulmonary vasodilation at birth. Nor do we know whether the endothelial cell or the smooth muscle cell is the prime target (Haworth, 2006).

NO is produced by the pulmonary vascular endothelial cells and is important for pulmonary vasodilation. NO is used to treat PPHN and, in a less well-defined role, to stimulate angiogenesis and promote lung growth, primarily in the ELBW infant. Inhaled NO has a rapid onset of action, is potent, and is a selective pulmonary vasodilator. Unfortunately, up to 40% of infants with PPHN do not respond to NO, and with the use of this drug there has been no positive effect on the incidence of BPD or neurodevelopmental deficits, mortality, or long-term outcome (Steinhorn, 2008).

Soluble guanylate cyclase in vascular smooth muscle converts guanosine triphosphate (GTP) to cyclic guanosine monophosphate (cGMP). By stimulating guanylate cyclase, NO increases cGMP production, which decreases smooth muscle contractility and induces vasodilation.

Regulation of production and metabolism of NO occurs at multiple levels. First, NO production is subject to endothelial nitric-oxide synthetase activity (eNOS; lung eNOS is type III). eNOS has both reductase and oxygenase domains. When its substrate L-arginine is available, oxidation of NADPH and NO synthetase produce NO. On the other hand, when the concentration of substrates or cofactors (e.g., heat shock protein 90) is reduced, NOS is uncoupled and, instead of NO, reactive oxygen species such as peroxynitrite are produced. In fact, oxidative stress may contribute to the development of PPHN (Brennan et al., 2003). The balance between the vasodilating effects of oxygen and the injury caused by oxidative stress is a delicate one, and the injury may occur quickly. For example, ventilating the lungs of lambs with an Fio_2 of 1.0 for only 30 minutes blunted the subsequent response to NO (Lakshminrusimha et al., 2007). During high-dose NO administration, the deleterious effects of generating oxygen radicals must be balanced against its vasodilatory benefits.

Second, the activity of soluble guanylate cyclase and cyclic guanosine monophosphate (cGMP)-specific phosphodiesterase (PDE5) on smooth muscle cells contributes to NO's effectiveness in stimulating cGMP production. PDE5 hydrolyzes cGMP, which controls the duration and magnitude of cGMP's effect. Agents that inhibit PDE5, such as sildenafil, promote pulmonary vasodilation and have been used extensively to treat pulmonary hypertension in adults. There is less experience using these drugs in newborns with PPHN (Baquero et al., 2006; Martell et al., 2007). Development of a parenteral formula of these drugs may improve delivery of PDE5 antagonists for the treatment of PPHN (Mukherjee et al., 2009). Sildenafil has effectively diminished rebound pulmonary hypertension during weaning from NO (Atz and Wessel, 1999). Of note, both NO and sildenafil have been reported to stimulate lung growth. Ongoing trials of NO to minimize CLD may eventually define the role of this agent in the ELBW infant (Steinhorn and Porta, 2007). No agents are available that directly activate guanylate cyclase in patients.

The cyclic adenosine monophospate (cAMP) pathway is another mechanism by which pulmonary vasodilation can be induced. Prostacylin (PGI_2) stimulates adenylase cyclase and increases cAMP. However, intravenous infusion of this drug causes systemic hypotension, which often prevents the desired therapeutic effect from being achieved. Inhaled PGI_2 is a selective pulmonary vasodilator, but its efficacy in PPHN remains to be firmly established. Milrinone, on the other hand, inhibits cAMP metabolism by interfering with PDE3 and has been used clinically as adjunct therapy to NO (McNamara et al., 2006).

Antagonizing vasoconstriction is another strategy for treating PPHN. ET-1, a potent vasoconstrictor produced by the endothelium, and NO interact in a feedback loop. For example, NO decreases ET-1 production and ET-1 increases superoxide release, which impairs NO-induced vasodilation (Abman, 2007). In addition to directly antagonizing ET-1, other strategies to interrupt vasoconstriction offer promise. For example, a GTPase, RhoA, and its protein ρ-kinase are important for regulation of vascular tone, especially for maintaining the high PVR present in utero. Thus, inhibitors of both ET-1 and ρ-kinase may be useful for the treatment of PPHN. Finally, dysfunction of the signaling pathways of VEGF may be important in the pathogenesis of PPHN. For example, VEGF releases NO, and inhibition of VEGF receptors down-regulates eNOS. Reduced levels of VEGF have been reported in infants with PPHN (Lassu et al., 2001).

Myocardial Ultrastructure

The fetal and adult myocardia contract and relax using the same basic processes—increases in the cytosolic calcium concentration to cause force generation and decreases to cause relaxation (Crick et al., 1998). At all stages of maturation, the ventricle must develop force against a varying resistance or load (contraction and ejection) and then relax (filling). Membranes present in the adult myocardium that control both calcium flux and the contractile system are also present in the fetal heart; however, there are qualitative and quantitative age-related differences in these membranes. Progression toward adult myocardial function involves developmental changes in these structures associated with the mechanics of force generation (e.g., the sarcomere and myofibril), those involved with controlling calcium flux (e.g., the sarcoplasmic reticulum, receptors, channels, exchangers, transporters, and pumps), those related to myocardial compliance (e.g., extracellular matrix and cytoskeleton), and sympathetic innervation. In part, age-related differences in the response to calcium and various pharmacologic agents are the result of the developmental state of myocardial anatomy and function.

Force Generation

Sarcomere. The sarcomere is the functional unit of the myofilament. Sarcomeres consist of thick (myosin-containing) and thin (actin-containing) filaments and of regulatory proteins and a complex cytoskeletal matrix. All of these components undergo complex developmental changes during fetal and postnatal life.

The immature myocardium develops less force against a load than that of the adult (Anderson et al., 1984). For example, the premature and neonatal hearts are unable to maintain output against an arterial pressure that would be considered low in the adult. In part, this reflects a smaller myocardial mass and a thinner left-ventricular wall. In addition, the velocity and quantity of sarcomere shortening is less in isolated immature myocytes than it is in adult myocytes (Nassar et al., 1987).

Both the number and size of myocytes increase before and after birth. The shape of the myocyte changes from a smooth, spherical structure to a more irregular, rectangular one. With this change in shape, the surface area-to-volume ratio decreases. This process occurs more rapidly in the left ventricle than in the right. The neonatal period is characterized by significant development of the left ventricle and a shift from right-ventricular to left-ventricular predominance. There also is a marked increase in left-ventricular work that is the result of a higher stroke volume, systolic arterial pressure, and wall tension. Right-ventricular systolic pressure and work decrease. Relative to body weight, left-ventricular mass increases and right-ventricular mass decreases. The increase in the number (cell division) and size (hypertrophy) of the myocytes is more pronounced in the left ventricle than in the right. By the second month of life, increased cell size, rather than increased cell number, becomes the predominant developmental phenomenon. This has major implications for patients with CHD, especially those with lesions that obstruct outflow from either ventricle (Rudolph, 2000). Control of postnatal development is not completely understood, but α-agonist stimulation, cortisol, thyroid hormone, and a variety of growth factors seem to be important (Brown et al., 1985; Rudolph, 2000).

Myofibrils. The number of myofibrils per unit of intracellular volume increases, and their arrangement becomes more highly organized during myocyte maturation after birth. In the fetus, the myofibrils appear somewhat chaotic. In the adult they are in long, parallel rows that alternate with rows of mitochondria (and sarcoplasmic reticulum). In the immature myocardium, myofibrils are arranged in thin layers, and groups of nuclei and mitochondria reside in the center of the cell. In part, this difference in myofibril arrangement may be the anatomic basis for the differences in control of the intracellular calcium concentration and in sensitivity to calcium channel blockers in the neonate as compared with the adult (see Sarcoplasmic Reticulum, p. 526). That is, transsarcolemmal movement of calcium from the outside to the inside of the cell causes contraction of the immature myocardium, whereas intracellular release of calcium is responsible for contraction of the adult myocardium. The irregular arrangement of mitochondria in the immature myocardium is likely to prevent the organized contractile activity seen in the adult heart, where the mitochondria alternate regularly within sarcomeres.

Calcium Flux

Sarcolemma. The complex array of ion channels, pumps, exchangers, enzymes, and receptors of the plasma membrane (sarcolemma) of the sarcomere interact to maintain ionic homeostasis of the intracellular environment. Multiple age-related changes in the sarcolemma have been reported, and several of the most well-characterized and clinically important differences are included in the following list:

- Activity of the sodium-potassium adenosine triphosphatase (Na+, K+-ATPase) pump and expression of its subunits increases in number and activity with development. Digoxin binds to the α-subunit, and the reduced expression of this subunit is the reason digoxin has less inotropic effect in neonates.
- The sodium-calcium (Na+–Ca+) exchanger also undergoes developmental changes. The function of this exchanger is primarily to move calcium from the intracellular to the extracellular compartment after contraction. This site is also important for the movement of calcium into the myocyte. The sarcolemmal Na+–Ca+ exchanger apparently helps maintain intracellular calcium concentrations in some species of newborns (probably the human) but not adults. This exchanger may account in part for the sensitivity of the newborn myocardium to changes in extracellular calcium concentrations. For example, when blood is administered rapidly, serum calcium concentration can decrease and cause myocardial dysfunction (Sham et al., 1995). The higher density of the Na+–Ca+ exchanger in the immature heart may also be linked to differences in contraction and relaxation rates. Also, when digoxin inhibits the Na+, K+ ATPase pump, intracellular sodium increases, and it is the Na+–Ca+ exchanger that extrudes sodium. When sodium is transported extracellularly in exchange for calcium, the intracellular calcium concentration increases, which may in part be responsible for the effect of cardiac glycosides on contractility.
- Activity of the sodium-hydrogen (Na+–H+) exchanger is higher in the newborn myocardium and seems to be important for cell growth. In addition, this exchanger may be important for the well-described resistance of the newborn myocardium to acidosis.

- Developmental changes in structure and activity of the multiple types of potassium channels probably contribute to differences in the action potential (e.g., shortened action potential duration) measured in immature vs. mature myocytes.
- Density and distribution of the various types of calcium channels vary with maturation, but there is marked variability among species in the two general types of dihydropyridine-sensitive calcium channels (T [transient] type and L [long or slow] type).
- The T tubules are a network of invaginations of the sarcolemma into the center of the cell. These invaginations extend to the surface of the myocyte, thereby increasing its interaction with the extracellular environment (e.g., more rapid transmission of an action potential intracellularly). This system increases the ratio of cell surface-to-volume in the postnatal myocyte.

Sarcoplasmic reticulum. Various membranes surround the myofibrils and interact to control the intracellular calcium concentration. In the mature heart, the sarcoplasmic reticulum is the major intracellular organelle that controls cytosolic calcium concentrations during contraction; a small amount of extracellular calcium enters the myoctye and stimulates release of calcium form the sarcoplasmic reticulum (calcium-induced calcium release). The volume of sarcoplasmic reticulum, as well as its ability to pump calcium (i.e., uptake, longitudinal sarcoplasmic reticulum; storage and release, junctional sarcoplasmic reticulum), increases both before and after birth. The various subtypes of sarcoplasmic reticulum are less functionally differentiated in neonates.

Calcium flows through the calcium-release channel of the sarcoplasmic reticulum (i.e., ryanodine receptor) to initiate contraction. These channels form functional complexes with the L-type calcium channels of the sarcolemma and with various proteins (e.g., calsequestrin). Release channels interact with various immunosuppressive drugs (e.g., cyclosporine) and cause phosphorylation via the protein phospholamban during sympathetic stimulation. The concentration of phospholamban is reduced in the immature hearts of several species.

Caffeine, which releases calcium from the sarcoplasmic reticulum, has little effect on neonatal myocardial contractility. This suggests that extracellular, rather than intracellular, calcium controls contractility in the neonatal myocardium, probably through calcium entry via L-type channels of the sarcolemma. Also, extracellular calcium appears to more effectively activate myocardial contraction of the immature myocardium than of the adult myocardium. Compared with the adult heart, immature hearts are more sensitive to calcium-channel antagonists (Boucek et al., 1984). Furthermore, the newborn heart requires higher concentrations of extracellular calcium to achieve maximal contractility (Jarmakani et al., 1982). With maturation, the amount of sarcoplasmic reticulum and the number of specialized connections of sarcoplasmic reticulum with other membranes increases, as does the efficiency of pumping calcium. Finally, there is an increase in Ca+-ATPase activity, which has been linked to improved sarcoplasmic-reticulum function with maturation (Mahony and Jones, 1986; Mahony, 1988). Age-related increases in the amount and organization of the sarcoplasmic reticulum improve systolic and diastolic myocardial function with age (see Cardiovascular Function in the Newborn, p. 527).

Contractile proteins. Contractile proteins are arranged into regular strands that account for the typical appearance of the sarcomere. Sarcomeres are divided into units that are bordered by I bands, which are bisected by Z discs and A bands with a dark M in the center. I bands consist of thin actin filaments, troponin, and tropomyosin. Thick filaments are made up of myosin. The A band is composed of overlapping thin and thick filaments plus other proteins. Multiple age-related changes in the contractile proteins of the sarcomere have been reported, and several of the best-characterized and clinically important ones are briefly discussed in this section. Although actin is a prominent contractile protein, the significance of the expression of its various isoforms during development remains unclear.

- Myosin is the most abundant contractile protein and consists of two heavy and four light chains. Isoforms of each undergo developmental changes, and several have been associated with ventricular growth and development.
- Troponin consists of three distinct proteins: troponins T, I, and C. The roles and expression of the various isoforms are complex and vary with the stage of development. Myocardial expression of cardiac vs. slow skeletal muscle isoforms of troponin appear to be important in the immature myocardium, because it may be important for the relative resistance of the immature heart to acidosis (Solaro et al., 1988). Expression of slow skeletal muscle troponin I in the fetal heart is linked to the newborn's ability to tolerate higher levels of respiratory acidosis without myocardial depression. In contrast, the adult myocardium expresses cardiac troponin I. Response of the immature myocardium to sympathetic stimulation is correlated with expression of slow skeletal troponin I. Cardiac, but not slow skeletal muscle troponin, is phosphorylated by β-stimulation. Phosphorylation decreases sensitivity to calcium, which facilitates myocardial relaxation during diastole. The slow skeletal muscle isoform found in the immature heart is not phosphorylated by β-agonists, which may be one reason for the newborn's difference in diastolic function (Solaro et al., 1988). Finally, expression of specific isoforms of troponin T has been correlated with myofilament responsiveness to calcium. If newborn and adult myocardia respond differently to calcium and calcium-channel–mediated pharmacologic agents, this may affect the choice of cardiotropic agents in the presence of disease (Anderson et al., 1984).

Myocardial Compliance

Cytoskeleton. The cytoskeleton includes the contractile proteins, titan and extramyofibrillar filaments (i.e., microfilaments, intermediate fibers, and microtubules). This intricate matrix provides the structural framework that organizes the complex intracellular compartments. This multilevel organization provides the mechanism for the intra- and extracellular communication required for the movement of the individual sarcomeres for translation into effective contraction and relaxation. The cytoskeleton provides the system for mechanical signaling. From the general appearance of the immature sarcomere, it is evident that dramatic changes in organization must occur during early development. A and I bands are more irregular in the immature myocyte; th

M band is absent; and the Z band is variable in width. Several of the most well-characterized and clinically important age-related changes in the cytoskeleton (extracellular matrix) are briefly discussed here:

- Titin is a large protein that extends from the end of the Z band (the end of the sarcomere) to the M band at the center. Isoforms of this protein are developmentally regulated. Fetal hearts seem to express the more compliant isoform.
- Proteins in the Z disc interact with adjacent sarcomeres to communicate tension along the myofibril. Various developmental changes in this complex array of proteins have been linked to growth and remodeling of the heart in response to adaptation of the circulation at birth. For example, desmin, a protein important for linking Z bands of myofibrils, is distributed throughout the subsarcolemmal area. As the myocardium develops, organization of this protein improves the connection of myofibrils with mitochondria, thus facilitating the mechanics of contraction. The distribution of various proteins in the cytoskeleton and in the extracellular matrix probably explains the irregular A- and I-band patterns, as well as the indistinct or absent M band. Integrins, which are important for linking cell surfaces to extracellular matrix proteins, are distributed differently in the immature heart. The amount and types of collagen present in the myocardium also follow a developmental pattern that is associated with changes in the expression of various collagen isoforms. These isoforms improve the resting load and passive state of the myocardium. Many of the cytoskeletal and extracellular matrix changes occur rapidly after birth (Robinson et al., 1983).
- The extracellular complex of microfilaments, intermediate fibers, and microtubules and their components undergo postnatal development and mediate various activities, such as cell growth, migration, and adhesion. For example, the collagen network becomes progressively more organized with maturation, and the population of Type III (more elastic) collagen eventually exceeds that of Type I.

Sympathetic Innervation

The sympathetic nervous system modulates a wide range of critical events in the developing myocardium, including cell growth and differentiation and distribution of and sensitivity to calcium. With maturation of adrenergic innervation, the quantity of neurotransmitters and the number of receptors increase. At birth, adaptation to postnatal hemodynamics is mostly mediated by the α-adrenergic system. That is, an early high level of α-adrenoreceptors may be critical for left-ventricular growth in the early postnatal period. In fact, α-1-blockade interrupts the increase in protein synthesis in cultured myocytes exposed to α-stimulation (Robinson, 1996). For example, the increase in adrenergic fibers innervating the myocardium modulates widespread development and expression of the various contractile systems (e.g., expression of the contractile proteins, efficiency of the calcium channel, and expression of myosin ATPase isoforms). Finally, the activity of adenyl cyclase, an important enzyme involved in intracellular β-stimulation, increases in concert with the increase in catecholamine levels. The interaction of adrenergic innervation, catecholamine

concentrations, and functional changes in multiple proteins that regulate responses to various agonists is complex and difficult to accurately extrapolate to specific clinical scenarios.

Cardiovascular Function in the Newborn

In spite of the intense age-related changes in myocardial physiology and function, the qualitative characteristics of the fetal and neonatal heart are similar to those of the adult in that blood pressure is directly proportional to CO and systemic vascular resistance (Table 17-3). The primary determinants of CO are heart rate and stroke volume. Preload, afterload, and myocardial contractility interact to determine ventricular performance. At all times, oxygen delivery and oxygen demands are interdependent; oxygen delivery (CO) is regulated by oxygen consumption (metabolism).

The high collagen content and high ratio of Type I collagen to Type III collagen may be responsible for the relative noncompliance of the neonatal heart and its limited capacity to respond to volume loading (Klopfenstein and Rudolph,1978). This nondistensible heart has limited capacity to increase stroke volume and augment CO when faced with an increased preload. Thus, the Frank-Starling response appears to have a limited role, and heart rate is the primary means of increasing CO in the newborn. Over the first months of life, myocardial contractility gradually increases, which allows CO to be maintained over a wider range of preloads and afterloads. Similarly, the increase in contractile proteins and the shift in the expression of various isoforms; the development of sarcoplasmic reticulum and T tubules, adrenergic innervation, calcium recruitment and transport; and the overall response of the myocardium to stress or increased demands all contribute to complex changes in force development.

The newborn's CO per unit weight is the highest of any age group (approximately 200 mL/kg per minute). Teitel (1985) hypothesized that the greater increase in myocardial performance with adrenergic stimulation in older lambs is to the result of a "lesser resting β-adrenergic tone" in the older animals. That is, the baseline state of the newborn myocardium is at higher level of "β-adrenergic tone," and the high resting CO of the newborn limits its ability to further increase CO in response to increased demand or to adapt to wide variations in preload or afterload. Because the newborn's normal heart rate is high, increasing the heart rate has limited effect on CO, but decreasing the heart rate dramatically decreases output.

Volume loading of the immature ventricle increases CO, but the effect is less than that that seen at older ages (Klopfenstein and Rudolph,1978). Similarly, the tolerance of the immature myocardium to increases in afterload is less than it is at older ages. Thus, the impaired ventricular function of the fetus (i.e., preterm baby) and newborn are the result of fewer myofibrils;

TABLE 17-3. Comparison of Neonatal and Adult Myocardial Functions

	Neonate	Adult
Cardiac output	Rate dependent	Stroke volume and rate
Contractility	Reduced	Normal response
Starling response	Limited	Normal response
Catecholamine	Reduced	Normal response

decreased sympathetic innervation; decreased β-adrenoreceptor concentration; immaturity of the structure and function of the sarcoplasmic reticulum; maturation-specific mechanisms for calcium uptake, release, and storage; and a specific spectra of expression of various isoforms of contractile and noncontractile proteins, channels, exchangers, and enzymes.

Cardiovascular Evaluation

Preoperative evaluation of the newborn should focus on understanding "normal," because infants of the same gestational age can vary significantly in their baseline heart rates and blood pressures (Fig. 17-5). Acid-base status (electrolytes, pH, $Paco_2$), urine output, and rates of fluid administration must be interpreted in the context of "normal" blood pressure and heart rate and the interventions required to maintain normalcy. Trends in these data over the hour, 6 hours, and 12 to 48 hours prior to examination help clarify the infant's cardiac function. It is necessary to understand whether there were responses to fluid boluses and inotropic intervention, and if so, what those

responses were with respect to maintenance of cardiovascular stability. This critical insight is important when developing rational anesthetic plan. Finally, evaluation of the current level of sedation and the response to various agents also helps determine which drugs (e.g., morphine, fentanyl) and the amount of each drug that are required to achieve the desired effect. This knowledge will guide the anesthesiologist in determining which drugs may be most effective during surgery.

The Central Nervous System

During the third trimester, cortical gray and white matter volumes increase fourfold to fivefold. Growth and differentiation of dendrites and axons, proliferation of glia, synaptogenesis and myelination characterize this dramatic process. The proliferation in the cerebellum is even more rapid than the cerebral cortex and is characterized by intense migration of various populations of cells (Allin et al., 2001; Limperopoulos et al., 2005b; Limperopoulos and du Plessis, 2006).

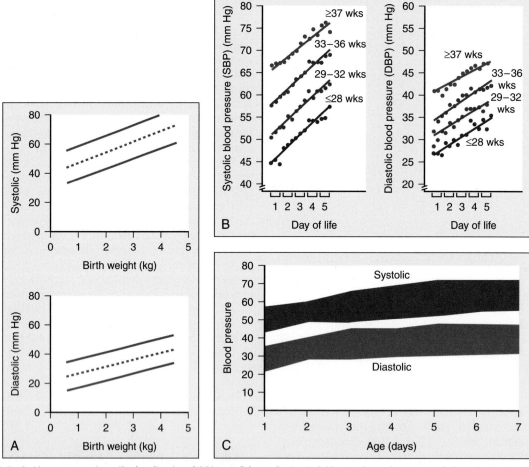

■ **FIGURE 17-5. A,** Linear regressions *(broken lines)* and 95% confidence limits *(solid lines)* of systolic *(top)* and diastolic *(bottom)* aortic blood pressures on birth weight in 61 healthy newborn infants during the first 12 hours after birth. For systolic pressure, y = 7.13x + 40.45; r = 0.79. For diastolic pressure, y = 4.81x + 22.18; r = 0.71. For both, n = 413 and P < 0.001. **B,** SBP and DBP are plotted for first 5 days of life with each day subdivided into 8-hour periods. Infants are categorized by gestational age into the following four groups: ≤28 weeks (n = 33); 29 to 32 weeks (n = 73); 33 to 36 weeks (n = 100); and ≥37 weeks (n = 110). **C,** Blood pressure ranges in premature infants during the first week of life, with a gestational age of 31.4 ± 2.6 weeks. (*A From Versmold HT, et al.: Aortic blood pressure during the first 12 hours of life in infants with birth weight 610 to 4220 grams,* Pediatrics *67:607, 1981; **B** From Zubrow AB, Hulman S, Kushner H, et al.: Determinants of blood pressure in infants admitted to neonatal intensive care units: a prospective multicenter study. Philadelphia Neonatal Blood Pressure Study Group,* J Perinatol *15:470, 1995; **C** From Hegyi T, Anwar M, Carbone MT, et al.: Blood pressure ranges in premature infants: II. The first week of life,* Pediatrics *97:336, 1996.)*

In parallel with the intense growth of the parenchyma, the vascular network of the late-gestation brain also develops rapidly. The long and short penetrators lengthen and arborize, leading to a decrease in end- and border-zone blood flow. Despite this rapid growth, cerebral blood flow in late fetal life (8 to 15 mL/g per minute) is remarkably low compared with that of the adult. Blood flow to the white matter is even lower, approximately 25% of the flow to the cerebral cortex (Khwaja and Volpe, 2008). The presence of a pressure-passive cerebral blood flow may further predispose the newborn, especially the premature newborn, to ischemic injury (Greisen, 2005).

In addition to the overall patterns of intense brain growth in late gestation, the development of specific cellular elements defines the unique susceptibility of the preterm brain to hypoxic and ischemic insults. Microglia are macrophages that are prominent in the normal human brain during development and are concentrated in the cortical white matter. This population of cells peaks during the third trimester, the period of highest vulnerability to the white matter injury that is common in the premature infant. Although microglia have a critical function in normal development, activation of these cells precipitates release of cytokine and glutamate, producing reactive oxygen and nitrogen species. Preoligodendrocytes (precursors to myelinating oligodendrocytes) are especially susceptible to injury from oxidative and excitotoxic stress. Neuropathologic studies have documented that an intense inflammatory response in the white matter accompanies periventricular leukomalacia (PVL), and specifically, microgliosis characterizes diffuse, noncystic PVL. Diffuse white matter injury on MRI correlates with neurodevelopmental delay in expremature infants (Woodward et al., 2006; Glass et al., 2008).

Another unique population of cells that is prominent during development is the so-called "subplate neuron" group. The subplate is three times thicker than the cortical plate between 22 and 36 weeks' gestation, but it is absent at term (McQuillen and Ferriero, 2005). These neurons express neurotransmitters and growth factors that seem to be critical in orchestrating the migration of cells from the germinal neuroepithelium to distant sites (e.g., the corpus callosum or thalamus). This layer receives synapses and organizes connections with distant structures, produces axons, and serves as a waiting zone for cells and axons as their final ultimate location in the cortex is defined (Leviton and Gressens, 2007). Injury to the subplate may disrupt the critical interaction and feedback between the cortex and thalamus, leading to long-term functional consequences. The connectivity among various distant structures during a time of critical brain development has been postulated to correlate with deficits identified in the expremature infant in the specific areas of behavior, cognition, and other complicated higher cortical functions (e.g., executive function) (Limperopoulos et al., 2005b; Boardman et al., 2006; Kapellou et al., 2006; Counsell et al., 2007).

Derangements of early brain development correlate with abnormalities in the two major structures of embryogenesis: the neural tube (future brain and spinal cord) and the prosencephalon (future forebrain) (Volpe, 2001). Primary development of the neural tube (3 to 4 weeks' gestation) and prosencephalon (2 to 3 months' gestation) are complete early in gestation. The term *primary neural tube* includes embryogenesis of both the brain and the spinal cord. The prosencephalon develops shortly after closure of the anterior neural tube and is related to both the telencephalon (future cerebral hemispheres) and the diencephalon (future thalamus and hypothalamus). Neural tube anomalies, such as anencephaly, craniorachischisis totalis, myeloschisis, and encephalocele, associated with these early events are dramatic and often fatal. Similarly, severe prosencephalic anomalies (holoprosencephalies) are often fatal, especially when they are associated with chromosomal abnormalities (e.g., trisomy 13-15 or trisomy/ring/deletion 18).

A less severe form of abnormal neural tube closure includes the lesions of spina bifida (incidence of 3 to 7 per 10,000 births). These neural tube anomalies are clinically important because affected infants often survive and have lifelong problems. The four primary types of spina bifida are categorized according to the severity of the defect. In the first type, spina bifida occulta, the divided vertebral arch, spinal cord, and meninges are covered with skin. Hair often protrudes from the skin overlying the defect, forming a sacral dimple. The presence of either hair or a dimple in this area should make anesthesiologists cautious of performing a caudal block without further information. In the second type, spina bifida cystica, neural tissue and its coverings protrude through the incompletely formed vertebral arch as a cystlike structure. In the third type, meningocele, the neural tube lies in its normal position but the meninges protrude through the defect; skin usually covers this lesion. In the fourth type, meningomyelocele, both the spinal cord and the meninges protrude, often without skin. These lesions can occur at any level of the spine. Hydrocephalus is a common accompaniment of myelomeningocele—60% in occipital, cervical, thoracic, or sacral lesions and about 90% in thoracolumbar, lumbar, and lumbosacral lesions (Lorber, 1961). In most infants, hydrocephalus is not evident before the meningomyelocele is closed, because cerebrospinal fluid leaks through the open lesion and decompresses the ventricles.

An Arnold-Chiari malformation is an abnormality of the hindbrain that occurs in most patients with meningomyelocele (Fig. 17-6). The medulla oblongata is flattened and elongated and, along with the fourth ventricle, protrudes into the spinal

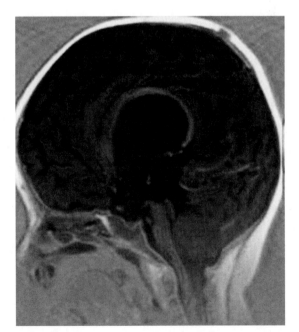

■ **FIGURE 17-6.** This MRI of Chiari's malformation shows the brain stem being pushed down through the foramen magnum. *(Courtesy Jim Barkovich, MD, University of California, San Francisco.)*

canal through the foramen magnum. The downward position of the medulla also elongates the lower pons and upper medulla and may compress brainstem nuclei and cranial nerves. If the cerebellar tonsils are displaced through the foramen magnum, aqueductal stenosis and hydrocephalus can occur. Whether it becomes necessary to decompress the posterior fossa depends on the severity of the anatomic abnormalities and the symptoms. For example, anomalies that are severe enough to cause apnea, vocal cord paralysis, or central and obstructive ventilatory disturbances require early correction (Kirk et al., 1999). Up to 20% of infants with myelomeningocele have sleep-disordered breathing, and some of these patients require a tracheostomy (Kirk et al., 2000). The anesthesiologist should be aware that a wide range of abnormalities associated with myelomeningocele exists beyond infancy, because this group of patients commonly requires ventriculoperitoneal shunt revision or urologic or orthopedic procedures.

Other disorders, such as agenesis of the corpus callosum and septum pellucidum, are less commonly fatal, but they are often associated with abnormal neuronal migration and significant clinical abnormalities. Agenesis of the corpus callosum is usually associated with a syndrome (e.g., Aicardi's or Andermann's syndrome) or a chromosomal abnormality (e.g., 8, 11, 13, 15, or 18). As many as 80% of patients without a corpus callosum have other brain anomalies, as well as non-CNS malformations (Parrish et al., 1979; Jeret et al., 1987). Partial agenesis of the brain probably occurs later in development and is associated with clinical syndromes that have migrational and structural disorders. Agenesis of the septum pellucidum is never an isolated lesion. It is often occurs in conjunction with optic nerve hypoplasia (septooptic dysplasia).

Once the structure of the neural tube and the prosencephalon are established (2 to 3 months of gestation), further development of the CNS is by proliferation and migration. Neurons proliferate from ventricular and subventricular regions at every level of the developing nervous system. From the second to the fourth month of gestation, some glia are formed, but most proliferating cells are neurons. From the fifth month of gestation into adulthood, glial multiplication is the primary process. Movement of cells from the ventricle to subventricular sites is important for our understanding of the pathophysiology of the preterm infant brain. For instance, the limited glial migration that occurs during early gestation is important for normal migration of other cells. Arterial and venous vessels develop at this same time. These developmental processes affect the prognosis of preterm infants, especially those born before 30 weeks' gestation (see Chapter 22, Anesthesia for Neurosurgery). The two diagnoses most commonly associated with CNS injury in preterm infants are periventricular hemorrhagic infarct (PVHI) and PVL.

Intraventricular/Periventricular Hemorrhage-Germinal Matrix/Intraventricular Hemorrhage

The pathophysiology of intraventricular hemorrhage (IVH) is related to the structure of the immature brain (Fig. 17-7) (Volpe, 2001). Proliferating ventricular and subventricular areas of the developing nervous system are very cellular and vascularized; neuroblasts (cerebral precursors for both gray and white matter) and glioblasts originate from these sites between 10 and 20 weeks' gestation. This region of the developing brain is gelatinous in midgestation, but the gelatinous nature of the area gradually decreases and is barely present in full-term infants.

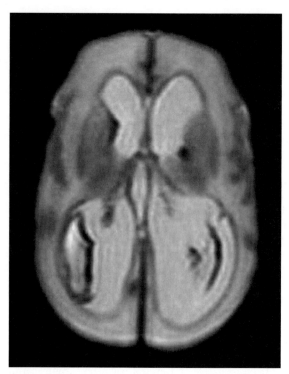

■ **FIGURE 17-7.** This MRI is of IVH that occurred in a 980-g infant. The ventricles are filled with blood, and there is blood in the interstitium of the brain. *(Courtesy Jim Barkovich, MD, University of California, San Francisco.)*

The dense, well-developed vascular network present in midgestation (which arises from the middle and anterior cerebral and anterior choroidal arteries) drains into a venous system that receives blood from the entire brain and terminates near the head of the caudate nucleus, where the veins join the Galen vein. The primary bleeding site in the premature brain is where veins and capillaries join, rather than where capillaries join to arteries or arterioles. Between 25 and 32 weeks' gestation, the germinal matrix is most prominent at the head of the caudate nucleus, and this is the usual site of germinal matrix hemorrhage.

IVH has been divided into categories that correlate with the severity and extent of the initial injury and with the clinical outcome (Papile et al., 1978). Grade 1 is a subependymal hemorrhage with minimal or no IVH. Grade II is an IVH without distention of the ventricles. Grade III is IVH with enlargement of the ventricles by intraventricular blood. Grade IV, the worst category of all, includes IVH, ventricular dilation, and extension of the bleeding into the parenchyma of the brain. Volpe (2001) revised the grading as follows:

Grade I: Germinal matrix hemorrhage is present, and ventricular enlargement is less than 10%.
Grade II: 10% to 50% of the ventricle is affected with IVH.
Grade III: More than 50% of the ventricle is involved, usually with enlargement of the lateral ventricles.

Echo density of the periventricular parenchyma falls into a separate classification.

The incidence and severity of IVH vary, but in general, they increase with decreasing gestational age and have an overall incidence of 7% to 23%. The incidence of grades III and IV IVH (10% to 12%) in VLBW infants has not changed during the last 10 to 15 years (Faranoff et al., 2003). In a group of ELBW infants, grade I IVH was present in 13%, grade II in 7%, grade III in 7%, and grade IV in 6% of neonates. The 13% incidence of grades III and IV IVH is similar to that reported by Fanaroff (Adams-Chapman et al., 2008). Mortality is high in infants with grade IV bleeds (at approximately 50%), but it is not increased in those with grades I and II bleeds (Vohr et al., 2000). While grades I and II IVH are not associated with severe neurologic sequelae, about 35% of survivors of grade III and 90% of grade IV IVH have poor neurodevelopmental outcomes (Whitelaw, 2001). Furthermore, posthemorrhagic hydrocephalus that is severe enough to require a ventriculoperitoneal shunt has the highest incidence of severe neurocognitive impairment in early childhood (78% in the group with grade III lesions and 92% in those with a grade IV IVH) (Adams-Chapman et al., 2008). Even though there is less significant neurodevelopmental delay in near-term infants with uncomplicated grade I or II IVH, they are reported to have lower developmental functioning, and their grey matter volumes are 16% smaller by MRI than predicted (Vasileiadias et al., 2004; Patra et al., 2006),

Periventricular Leukomalacia

This bilaterally symmetric, nonhemorrhagic lesion is the result of white matter necrosis that occurs dorsally and laterally to the external angles of the lateral ventricles (Fig. 17-8). In the past, this lesion was cystic and easily visualized on ultrasound. More recently, the most common form of PVL seen in ELBW infants on MRI consists of diffuse cerebral white matter injury without cyst formation. PVL is sometimes inappropriately thought to be a consequence of IVH, because both are commonly present on the same scan. However, PVL is a postischemic lesion, not a venous infarction (Takashima et al., 1986). While focal and tissue necrosis may cause cavitation and cyst formation, eventually the loss of oligodendrocytes and abnormal myelinization reduce the white-matter volume, causing ventriculomegaly. A consistent clinical correlate of PVL is spastic diplegia. More recently, a variety of neurodevelopmental and cognitive deficits have been associated with noncystic PVL in preterm infants.

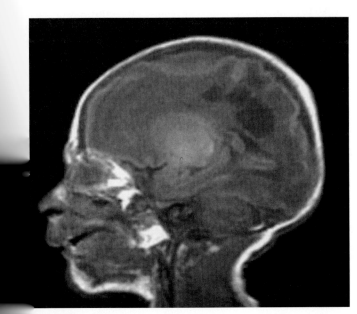

FIGURE 17-8. MRI of cystic PVL. *(Courtesy Jim Barkovich, MD, University of California, San Francisco.)*

Autoregulation of Cerebral Blood Flow

Critically ill newborns often require mechanical ventilation, airway suctioning, and intravenous fluid boluses, all of which can affect blood pressure, CO, heart rate, and cerebral blood flow. Hypoglycemia, hypercarbia, hypocarbia, hypoxia, hypo- or hypernatremia, and hypocalcemia can also dramatically affect the neonate's hemodynamic status. Fluctuations in blood pressure and CO often affect the newborn's CNS, since cerebral blood flow may change as a result of absent or attenuated cerebrovascular autoregulation. Cerebral blood flow autoregulation is present in both preterm and full-term newborns, but it is tenuous (Fig. 17-9). Also, the range of pressures over which blood flow is regulated is narrower for preterm infants. Cerebrovascular autoregulation is easily disrupted in neonates, and the normal blood pressure of preterm infants is close to the lower autoregulatory limit (Lou et al., 1979; Versmold et al., 1981; Tweed et al., 1983; Lou 1998). With decreasing gestational age, the lower limit approaches normal blood pressure. Similarly, the upper range of autoregulation may be approached during later gestational development (Papile et al., 1985). Furthermore, the normal range of autoregulation can be disturbed or disrupted by hypoxia, acidosis, seizures, and by the low diastolic blood pressures of patients with a PDA (Lou et al., 1979; Tweed et al., 1983; Lou, 1998). Rapid increases in arterial blood pressure can rupture the fragile vessels of the immature brain, while hypotension and low perfusion pressures may cause ischemia.

Hypoxic Ischemic Injury

If the amount of cerebral blood-flow is insufficient for cerebral oxidative metabolic needs, severe, long-term neurologic injury may occur. Asphyxia has three biochemical features: hypoxemia, hypercapnia, and metabolic acidosis. Some authors have suggested that the normal events occurring during labor and delivery, including uterine contractions, cause a degree of asphyxia in all fetuses. Although severe asphyxia can cause hypoxic-ischemic encephalopathy (HIE) and injure other organs, HIE often develops without injury to other organs. HIE is defined as abnormal levels of consciousness, the presence of seizures, and a history of severe asphyxia (e.g., umbilical cord pH < 7.0, Apgar score of 0 to 3 for longer than 5 minutes, neurologic

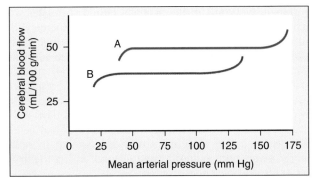

FIGURE 17-9. Autoregulation of cerebral circulation in neonates *(curve B)* and adults *(curve A)*. *(Redrawn from Harris MM: Pediatric neuroanesthesia. In Berry FA, editor: Anesthetic management of difficult and routine pediatric patients, ed 2, New York, 1990, Churchill Livingstone. Data from Hernandez MJ, Brennan RW, Vannucci RC, Bowman GS: Cerebral blood flow and oxygen consumption in the newborn dog, Am J Physiol 234:R209, 1878).*

dysfunction) (Leuthner and Das, 2004). Neurologic abnormalities caused by infections or metabolic causes should not be labeled HIE. HIE occurs in approximately 4 to 5 per 1000 live births. One study demonstrated a decrease in HIE between 1990 to 2000 (Wu et al., 2004a).

Hypoxic-ischemic injury is often multifactorial and can be traced to antepartum factors (e.g., infection, toxemia, or diabetes), intrapartum events (e.g., infection, abruption, or umbilical cord compression), and postpartum problems (e.g., CHD, diaphragmatic hernia, or sepsis). Regardless of its etiology, significant asphyxia results in depression at birth (e.g., apnea, bradycardia, or hypotonia) and a risk for HIE. Over the initial 24 hours of life, infants with HIE have depressed mental statuses and are difficult to arouse. They are often hypotonic and have temperature instability. In other cases, they may be "jittery." Multifocal or focal seizures are common during the first 4 to 12 hours of life. At times the seizures can be simply repetitive eye movements, blinking, tongue movements, or apnea. The Moro reflex, suck, grasp, and the deep tendon reflexes may be depressed or absent. By 24 hours of life, the Moro reflex is usually hyperactive, the cry is high-pitched and shrill, and generalized seizures or apnea are present. The subsequent course for these patients during the neonatal period is enormously variable and depends on the severity and etiology of the initial events.

Unfortunately, no specific clinical or biochemical markers of asphyxia accurately predict later neurologic function. Isolated low 1-minute Apgar scores (see Apgar Score), transient moderate acidosis, or other metabolic abnormalities, in the absence of encephalopathy, do not correlate well with long-term outcome. Neurodevelopmental outcome is best predicted by severity of the encephalopathy. Sarnat and Sarnat related encephalopathy to neurologic outcome. In stage 1 (first 24 hours), the infant is hyperalert with unimpaired Moro and sympathetic reflexes and an electroencephalograph (EEG) reading that is abnormal. Stage 2 includes obtundation, hypotonia, hyperreflexia, and seizures. In stage 3, infants are stuporous, flaccid, and have abnormal brain stem and autonomic reflexes (Sarnat and Sarnat, 1976). These investigators reported normal outcome in infants who were in stage 2 for less than 5 days, but when the symptoms persisted for more than 7 days, severe neurologic injury occurred. The presence of stage 3 at any time during the clinical course was predictive of injury or death. Although variations on this scheme have been described, the general trends indicate that a severe neurologic syndrome in the neonatal period correlates with high mortality or significant functional impairment. Miller and associates (2004) developed a simple, quantifiable neonatal encephalopathy score based on the criteria identified by Sarnat and Sarnat (1976). Miller et al.'s (2004) encephalopathy score includes feeding, alertness, tone, respiratory status, reflexes, and seizure activity. The score obtained on day 1 and the maximum score from the first 3 days of life were correlated with outcomes of patients (who had neonatal encephalopathy) at 30 months of age. Similar to earlier reports, severe encephalopathy and seizures during the first 3 days of life predicted poorer outcomes.

Metabolic abnormalities associated with multiorgan system dysfunction after severe asphyxia (e.g., hypoglycemia, hypocalcemia, and hyponatremia) can precipitate or exacerbate seizures. Consequently, fluid intake and output and electrolyte concentrations after an asphyxial event must be corrected. Renal or hepatic injury or a period of *nil per os* (NPO) may contribute

to metabolic instability and to the development of secondary electrolyte abnormalities, such as the syndrome of inappropriate antidiuretic hormone (SIADH). Neuroimaging (e.g., cranial ultrasound and CT or MRI scans) are used to detect underlying CNS anomalies (e.g., arterial or venous malformations and masses) and extent of injury (e.g., stroke, hemorrhage, or ischemia), and it may suggest a specific intervention (e.g., surgery, interventional procedure for arteriovenous malformation [AVM]), or further evaluation (e.g., clotting studies). Aggressively treating seizures pharmacologically and providing supportive care are essential.

After an initial period of stabilization after neonatal resuscitation, searching for multiorgan dysfunction is a priority, especially if the neonate has HIE. For example, myocardial ischemia may manifest as tricuspid insufficiency or hypotension (decreased contractility). Pulmonary hypertension may evolve (at times associated with meconium aspiration) and require invasive monitoring and ventilator support. Clearly, inadequate cardiorespiratory function may exacerbate HIE if the CO is reduced or hypoxemia persists. Concern for gastrointestinal ischemia often delays feeding of premature infants for 3 to 7 days because it is thought that this reduces the risk of NEC. However, recent data suggest that this may not be true (Schurr and Perkins, 2008). Severe hepatic insults can cause clotting abnormalities or disseminated intravascular coagulation (DIC) and predispose the newborn to hemorrhage. Finally, renal insufficiency has been associated with CNS injury (67% of patients studied) and death (33%) if oliguria persists longer than 24 hours (Perlman and Tack, 1988).

Apgar Score

The Apgar score was initially proposed as a means of rapidly assessing the status of newborns at 1 minute after birth and as a means of determining whether a neonate required respiratory support (Apgar, 1953) (Table 17-4). As Casey and others (2001) recently suggested, "Every baby born in a modern hospital in the world is looked at first through the eyes of Virginia Apgar." The Apgar score includes five variables with a range of scores from 0 to 2 (for a maximum of 10 points): heart rate, respiratory effort, muscle tone, reflex irritability, and color. Currently, the score is applied at 1 and 5 minutes, but in some cases the evaluation continues for as long as 20 minutes if continued resuscitative efforts are required.

The Apgar score has been demonstrated recently to be a predictor of mortality (Casey et al., 2001). In full-term infants,

TABLE 17-4. Apgar Score

Sign	0	1	2
Heart rate	Absent	Less than 100 beats per minute	More than 100 beats per minute
Respiratory effort	Absent	Slow, irregular	Good, crying
Muscle tone	Flaccid	Some flexion of extremities	Actie motion
Reflex irritability	No response	Grimace	Vigorous cry
Color	Pale	Cyanotic	Completely pink

these authors found a mortality rate of 244 per 1000 (24.4%) for infants with 5-minute Apgar scores of 1 to 3, compared with 0.2 per 1000 (0.02%) for infants with 5-minute Apgar scores of 7 to 10. Similarly, in preterm infants of 26 to 36 weeks' gestation, the mortality rate was 315 per 1000 (31.5%) for infants with 5-minute Apgar scores of 0 to 3 and 5 per 1000 (0.5%) for infants with 5-minute Apgar scores of 7 to 10. Thus, the incidence of neonatal death was highest when the 5-minute Apgar scores were 3 or lower, independent of gestational age. Neonatal death most commonly occurred during the first day of life, with the majority of infants dying before 3 days of age. These data indicate that the Apgar score is a valid predictor of neonatal mortality. In fact, the Apgar score better predicted outcome than umbilical-artery pH of 7.0 or less. Combining a 5-minute Apgar of 0 to 3 with an umbilical artery blood pH of 7.0 or less increased the risk of death in both preterm and full-term infants. An Apgar score of 0 for longer than 10 minutes suggests that resuscitative efforts should be suspended (Jain et al., 1991). Papile (2001) stated, "At present, there is no single measure of the fetal or neonatal condition that accurately predicts later neurodevelopmental disability...but, few will deny [the Apgar score's] application at 1 minute of age accomplishes Dr. Apgar's goal of focusing attention on the condition of the infant immediately after birth." Although outcomes vary with gestational age, with the etiology of neonatal depression, and with other factors, effective resuscitation of infants with low Apgar scores resulted in survival of about 40% to 60% of the patients and, approximately two thirds of survivors had normal neurologic function (Leuthner and Das, 2004). In 1964, the Collaborative Study on Cerebral Palsy reported a stronger relationship between the 5-minute Apgar score and neonatal mortality than the 1-minute score (Drage et al., 1964). Controversy about the Apgar score arises when people try to use the Apgar score to predict neurologic outcome. Dr. Apgar did not intend that the score be used to establish the diagnosis of asphyxia, to measure the severity of perinatal asphyxia, or to predict long-term neurologic outcome. In fact, 75% of children with cerebral palsy had normal Apgar scores at 5 minutes (Nelson and Ellenberg, 1981).

Pathophysiology of Hypoxic-Ischemic Injury

Asphyxia-related insults follow a pattern of early energy depletion and failure of the Na^+, K^+-ATPase pump, which disrupts normal transmembrane ion gradients. This loss of these gradients causes the release of excitatory neurotransmitters, such as glutamate, dopamine, serotonin, and aspartate. Although glutamate is important for normal brain development, excessive excitation of glutamate receptors (e.g., N-methyl-D-aspartate [NMDA], α-3-amino-hydroxy-5-methyl-4-isoxazole propionic acid [AMPA], and kainite) leads to excessive intracellular calcium concentrations and activation of a variety of phospholipases and proteases that cause the release of arachadonic acid and other mediators. Downstream production of xanthine and prostaglandins generates free radicals, in part via the NO synthase system. Although this is a condensed and simplified version of some of the pathways for cellular injury, the basic schema of hypoxic-ischemic injury is clearly one of disruption of membrane and intracellular function (Volpe, 2001). The clinical correlates of this intense cellular injury include seizures, abnormal mental status, eventual cell death, and long-term CNS deficits.

Neuroprotection

Gonzalez and Ferriero (2008) emphasized that treatment of neonatal brain injury should focus on both neuroprotection and after injury treatment. Optimal therapy may require intervening at multiple pathways to both prevent cell death and to induce cell growth and differentiation (Gonzalez and Ferriero, 2008). In general, therapies under evaluation attempt to decrease oxidative stress (e.g., inhibition of NO, melatonin, allopurinol, or deferoxamine), inflammation (e.g., minocycline), and excitotoxicity pathways (e.g., magnesium, MK-801, topiramate, or memantine). Other strategies include administering various growth factors, such as erythropoietin, a glycoprotein that has diverse CNS functions. These include vasogenic and immune responses that may provide neuroprotection during hypoxia and ischemia and modulate neurogenesis and neural differentiation. Primarily studies of VEGF in animals have shown that VEGF regulates both angiogenesis and neurogenesis. Cortical neurons are the primary site of VEGF-A activity early in development, but later its primary effect is on glial cells. VEGF seems to enhance the survival of neurons after hypoxia and after exposure to glutamate. Generating new neurons could play a major role in recovery after injury that results from perinatal stroke or hypoxia and ischemia.

Hypothermia is being used more often as a method of treating brain injury. It is hypothesized that hypothermia modifies apoptosis and necrosis of injured neurons by reducing their metabolic demands and by decreasing the release of excitotoxic mediators. Several studies have shown a significant reduction in CNS injury with cooling to 33° to 34° C for about 72 hours. Preliminary results suggested decreased mortality and improved neurodevelopmental outcome, although the differences in neurodevelopment after cooling are not large (Shankaran et al., 2005; 2008). Hypothermia plus another form of therapy may have greater therapeutic effect than either treatment alone (Alkan et al., 2001).

Seizures

Seizures occur commonly in neonates, especially after asphyxia (Silverstein and Jensen, 2007). Neonates with encephalopathy, stroke, intracranial hemorrhage, CHD, inborn errors of metabolism, and some syndromes are prone to develop seizures. Without an EEG, it may be difficult to tell if a neonate is having a seizure, because non–seizure-induced, repetitive movements are common. Cerebral palsy, low intelligence quotient (IQ), and epilepsy often accompany seizures and receptor expression, and neonatal seizures alter synaptic plasticity (Holden et al., 1982; Mellits et al., 1982; Swann and Hablitz, 2000; Stafstrom et al., 2006). Phenobarbital, diazepam, phenytoin, and valproate are commonly used drugs for the treatment of seizures, but these drugs can increase apoptotic neuronal death (Pereira de Vasconcelos et al., 1990; Schroeder et al., 1995). Furthermore, they fail to block neonatal seizures in as many as 50% of patients (Sankar and Painter, 2005). Hypoglycemia and hypocalcemia are other causes of seizures, and correcting these abnormalities usually terminates the seizures. The neonate's $Paco_2$ should be maintained within the normal preoperative range (not reduced), because alkalosis lowers the seizure threshold and may induce a seizure. Anesthesia obscures overt seizure activity, especially when paralytic drugs are used.

Perinatal Stroke

Perinatal stroke has been more commonly recognized during the past few years because of improved neuroimaging. The incidence is 1:2300 to 1:5000 infants born at term and 7:1000 in those born prematurely (Raju et al., 2007; Benders et al., 2008). Infants with CHD have significantly more ischemic perinatal strokes than other neonates (Sherlock et al., 2009). Approximately 40% of neonates with transposition of the great vessels (TGV) show evidence of preoperative stroke; an additional one third has evidence of a new stroke after cardiac surgery. Many of the patients who had a stroke before surgery underwent balloon septostomy to improve oxygen—the incidence of stroke is high after this procedure (McQuillen et al., 2006). Strokes are either detected in the first few days of life or after 28 days of age. Those detected early are found because patients have seizures or undergo an MRI. Despite the evidence of a stroke, many neonates have no signs of neurologic dysfunction. They may not show signs of focal lesions or encephalopathy (Miller, 2000). Perinatal strokes are classically located within the boundary of the area perfused by the middle cerebral artery, usually the left cerebral artery (Schulzke et al., 2005). The incidence of arterial perinatal stroke is similar in preterm neonates to that of term infants (de Veber et al., 1998). Cerebral venous thrombosis is another cause of perinatal strokes and is usually detected when the neonate develops seizures (Wu et al., 2003). Venous infarctions often become hemorrhagic.

Many infants with perinatal strokes show no evidence of injury in the neonatal period. The diagnosis is only made at 4 to 8 months of age when hemiplegia, seizures, or difficulty with locomotion or handedness are detected. Again, most of these injuries are the result of middle cerebral-artery occlusion.

The cause of a stroke in a given patient is almost never known. However, possible maternal factors include chorioamnionitis, prolonged rupture of the membranes, preeclampsia, and intrauterine growth retardation (Wu et al., 2004b). Twenty percent to 68% of infants with arterial ischemic stroke had prothrombotic states (Golomb et al., 2001). Polycythemia is also a cause of neonatal stroke, and suggested factors related to perinatal stroke include infection, inflammation, and hypoglycemia (Günther, et al., 2000; Benders et al., 2007).

Preoperative Neurologic Evaluation

Neurologically injured newborns often require surgery to treat CNS abnormalities (e.g., insertion of a ventriculoperitoneal shunt), to provide supportive care (e.g., insertion of a gastrostomy tube or central venous catheter for intravenous alimentation), or to treat associated anomalies and problems (e.g., repair of congenital diaphragmatic hernia [CDH], laparotomy to treat an intraabdominal crisis, repair of a meningomyelocele, or insertion of a vetriculoperitoneal shunt).

There are some important questions to answer as part of the preoperative evaluation of the nervous system of neonates. Does the neonate breathe spontaneously and is the heart rate relatively stable and normal (120 to 160 beats per minute)? Is the fontanel normal (i.e., skin even with the outer table of the skull), bulging (from increased intracranial pressure), or sunken (from dehydration or volume depletions)? Is the muscle tone normal for the infant's age? Differences in tone between the upper and lower extremities or between one side of the body or the other may suggest the presence of a neonatal stroke

(Ibrahim et al., 2008). Does the infant bring his hands and arms together in front of the chest (Moro reflex) when the arms are raised and suddenly released? Is the Moro reflex equal bilaterally? Does the infant grasp the examiner's finger when it is placed in a hand? When a finger is placed on the anterior sole of the foot, do the toes curl in a grasping motion? Is the Babinski reflex normal? Without experience it may be difficult to elicit deep tendon reflexes in neonates, especially preterm neonates. Do the eyes move normally when a flashlight is moved in different directions? The pupils should constrict to light, and there should be evidence of a gag reflex and a suck. A complete neurologic examination should be documented in the patient's chart to note neurologic abnormalities that predate surgery and anesthesia.

In addition to the above questions, infants with neurologic injury who are undergoing preoperative assessment are usually divided into three categories:

1. Stable infants with well-defined neurologic status who are scheduled for elective procedures,
2. Stable infants with evolving neurologic injuries, and
3. Acutely ill infants who require urgent surgery.

Preoperative evaluation of neurologically stable infants with no evidence of acute cardiorespiratory, hepatic, or renal problems and who require an elective surgical or diagnostic procedure should focus on determining what is normal for each patient. That is, what is the range of an infant's normal blood pressure, heart rate, respiratory rate, oxygen saturation (and F_{IO_2}), urine output, and nutritional status. These variables should be kept within this normal range if possible. The neurologic status should be documented, including evidence for gastroesophageal reflux and its treatment, as well as the incidence of seizures (if any) and their treatment. If available, electrolyte and calcium concentrations and liver function studies should be reviewed. If the neonate's course is stable and the procedure proposed is noninvasive, the most relevant laboratory value is a hematocrit.

Infants whose condition is stable except for ongoing neurologic problems (e.g., encephalopathy or seizures) require review of their vital signs, laboratory values, and medications, and they must have an appropriate physical examination. The hemodynamic responses to sedatives and analgesics and to painful procedures should be reviewed so the anesthesiologist can develop an anesthetic plan that will minimize wide variations in blood pressure. It should be determined whether the intravascular volume is adequate. Rapid administration of intravenous fluid during induction of anesthesia should be avoided because doing this may suddenly increase arterial and intracranial pressures, which can cause intracranial hemorrhage, especially in preterm neonates. The intracranial hypertension and increased intracranial volumes occur because cerebrovascular autoregulation is abnormal or absent. Both hypertension and hypotension can exacerbate neurologic injury. If available, near-infrared spectroscopy (NIRS) or EEG data should be reviewed. Do feeding, suctioning the trachea, medications (e.g., sedation), and fluid therapy alter cerebral oxygenation (Baserga et al., 2003)? If the patient is mechanically ventilated, understanding how oxygenation and ventilation are affected by various interventions may provide clues to the best ventilatory strategy to employ during surgery.

Finally, if the surgery is urgent or emergent, the overwhelming focus must be on the lesion that is making the surgery urgent, but the trends in cardiorespiratory and metabolic status must also be evaluated so that intraoperative management will have the least effect on the CNS injury and not make it worse.

Postanesthetic Apnea

Preterm and expremature infants undergoing elective surgery are prone to develop postoperative apnea (Steward, 1982; Gregory and Steward, 1983). Apnea is usually defined as cessation of breathing for 20 seconds or more. The likelihood of life-threatening postoperative apnea increases if the patient had apneic spells in the NICU (Liu et al., 1983). Twenty percent to 30% of preterm infants have apnea with cyanosis and bradycardia during the first month of extrauterine life. Steward (1982) reported the presence of apnea in 18% of preterm infants (with a gestational age of fewer than 38 weeks or a postnatal age of 3 to 28 weeks) during the first 12 hours after surgery.

A prospective study by Liu et al. (1983) found that a history of apnea and a postconceptual age of fewer than 44 weeks often resulted in apnea after surgery. Kurth and LeBard (1991) reported that postanesthetic apnea (defined as cessation of breathing for more than 15 seconds, not longer than 20 seconds) occurred commonly in expremature infants whose postconceptual ages varied from 32 to 55 weeks. The initial episode of apnea occurred as late as 12 hours after the termination of anesthesia. These authors recommended that infants who whose postconceptual age was younger than 60 weeks and who developed apnea after surgery be continuously monitored in the hospital until they were apnea free for at least 12 hours.

Welborn et al. (1986) found no evidence of apnea in a group of healthy premature infants who had a postconceptual age of 44 weeks or more at the time of surgery and who underwent general anesthesia for herniorrhaphy. Although many of these patients did not have apnea, 63.6% of the them had periodic breathing, a common finding in premature infants that is characterized by repetitive apneas of short duration (fewer than 5 to 10 seconds) without oxygen desaturation or cyanosis and is usually harmless. Malviya et al. (1993) noted that expremature infants younger than a postconceptual age of 44 weeks had significantly more apnea than older infants. Coté et al. (1995), using data from 255 patients garnered from previously published studies, found an incidence of apnea of 1% in infants of 55 to 56 weeks' postconceptual age. They also found an inverse relationship between postconceptional age and the incidence of apnea. Those who were 56 weeks' postconceptual age or younger had the greatest risk for apnea. Anemia (Hct < 30%) was also an important risk factor for apnea (Fig. 17-10).

Nearly all patients in these studies of postoperative apnea in prematurely born infants in the past were anesthetized with halothane or isoflurane, drugs that have higher blood-gas solubility coefficients than newer inhaled anesthetics such as sevoflurane and desflurane. These less soluble agents have been associated with a lower incidence of apnea in patients who do not have a history of preoperative apnea (William et al., 2001).

Other factors that predispose infants, especially premature infants, to apnea include hypoglycemia, hypoxia, hyperoxia, sepsis, anemia, hypocalcemia, and changes in the environmental temperature (Schulte, 1977). Postoperative apnea may also be the result of the interaction of general anesthesia with an immature CNS (including the respiratory center). For example, in low concentrations, halothane depressed the chemoreceptor

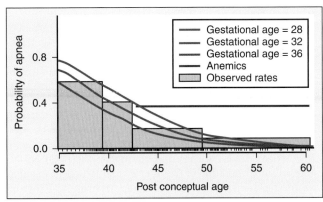

■ FIGURE 17-10. Predicted probability of apnea for all patients, by gestational age and weeks of postconceptual age. Patients with anemia are shown as the horizontal line. The bottom marks indicate the number of data points by postconceptual age. The shaded boxes represent the overall rates of apnea for infants within that range of gestational ages. The probability of apnea was the same regardless of postconceptual age or gestational age for infants with anemia. *(Redrawn from Coté CJ, et al.: Postoperative apnea in former preterm infants after inguinal herniorrhaphy: a combined analysis, Anesthesiology 82:807, 1995.)*

responses to hypoxia (Knill and Gelb, 1978). Inhaled anesthetics also depressed intercostal muscles function, thus reducing the FRC and increasing the risk of hypoxemia (Tusiewicz et al., 1977). These differences, coupled with an immature response to hypoxia and hypercarbia, predispose premature infants to erratic respiratory responses in the perioperative period (Rigatto et al., 1982).

Residual anesthesia in the postoperative period may also be an important factor in the development of apnea in preterm babies. This may be especially true when halothane, with its high lipid solubility, was the standard anesthetic in pediatric anesthesia. The cartilaginous upper airway of preterm infants may also predispose them to upper airway obstruction, and this obstruction may be made worse by the effects of residual anesthesia on pharyngeal muscles (Dransfield et al., 1983). Elective surgery should be delayed, if possible, until former preterm infants are beyond 44 weeks' postconceptual age (Gregory and Steward, 1983). Infants younger than 44 weeks' postconceptual age who require surgery must be individually evaluated. The type of surgery, the patient's gestational and postconceptual age, hematocrit, current cardiorespiratory function (i.e., oxygen or diuretic dependence, CLD, neurologic status) are all factors that must be taken into consideration when developing a perioperative plan for the expremature infant. These patients should be admitted to hospital for 24 to 36 hours for postoperative monitoring.

Thermoregulation

Newborns abruptly arrive into an environment that is approximately 20° C cooler than the one they just left. Living in this new, colder environment markedly increases the number of calories expended to regulate body temperature. Once born, neonates lose heat by evaporation, convection, conduction, and radiation. Extremely preterm infants can lose 15 times more heat by transdermal water loss than full-term babies (Hammarlund et al.,

1979). To compensate for increased heat losses, the sympathetic nervous system constricts skin blood vessels, which centralizes body heat (Asakura, 2004). Oxygen consumption and cell metabolism increase two- to threefold.

Many factors are responsible for heat loss, including cold environments (e.g., delivery rooms), a high ratio of surface area-to-body weight, reduced subcutaneous fat, and an underdeveloped ability to shiver in response to cold. Shivering is limited in part by the neonate's much smaller muscle mass (25% vs. 45% in the adult). The major compensatory mechanism for cold stress in neonates is nonshivering thermogenesis (NST). NST is the result of stimulation of triglyceride and fatty acid metabolism in energy-rich brown fat by norepinephrine and thyroid hormone (Stern et al., 1965). Brown fat, which is mostly deposited during the third trimester of pregnancy, is found between the scapulae and around major abdominal organs. Infants born before the third trimester have less ability to initiate NST and are prone to hypothermia. SGA neonates have NST but to a far lesser degree than AGA term infants.

Hypothermia (body temperature of less than 36° C) increases oxygen consumption, metabolic acidosis, and pulmonary and peripheral vascular resistance while reducing CO (Brady and Ceruti, 1966). Babies admitted to the NICU with a temperature of 35.5° C have a Pao_2 that is on average 18 mm Hg lower than neonates whose body temperatures are equal to 36.5° C. Warming cold infants to 36.5° C or higher increased Pao_2 (Stephenson et al., 1970). Neonates should reside in a neutral thermal environment (i.e., the environmental temperature at which their oxygen consumption is minimal). Normally, this occurs when the skin temperature is 36° C and the environment temperature is between 32° to 34° C (see Chapter 6, Thermoregulation: Physiology and Perioperative Disturbances, Fig. 6-2) (Adamson and Towell, 1965). Prematurity, hypoglycemia, and general anesthesia exaggerate the neonate's poor metabolic response to hypothermia (Swyer, 1975). Because preterm and asphyxiated or neurologically injured full-term neonates have limited ability to maintain normal body temperatures, their environmental temperature should be carefully controlled with overhead heaters, isolettes, and warm operating rooms.

Preoperative evaluation of temperature regulation should determine whether a neonate has difficulty maintaining body temperature. Preterm infants require servocontrolled devices to maintain normal body temperatures, whereas neurologically intact term infants usually require minimal assistance to maintain stable body temperatures (e.g., clothing and a blanket). AGA infants that have difficulty maintaining their body temperature should be evaluated for sepsis or neurologic injury. It is important to determine if the environmental temperature was increased or decreased to maintain a normal body temperature; having to do so is an indication of temperature instability and possible sepsis.

There are several methods of maintaining a neonate's body temperature, including covering the body with clear plastic, covering the head with a hat, placing a warming pad under the infant, increasing the environmental temperature, and wrapping the infant in warm blankets (see Chapter 6, Thermoregulation: Physiology and Perioperative Disturbances).

Maintenance of a normal body temperature is crucial, because hypothermia increases PVR, decreases pulmonary blood flow and causes right-to-left shunting of blood through the foramen ovale or PDA (see Transitional Circulation, p. 523, and Chapter 6, Thermoregulation: Physiology and Perioperative Disturbances, Fig. 6-8) (Brady and Ceruti, 1966; Stephenson et al., 1970).

Prolonged exposure to a hypothermic environment places demands on neonates that may exceed their ability compensate for these demands. If they cannot do so, hypoventilation, inadequate oxygen delivery, tissue acidosis, and cardiovascular collapse may occur (Adamsons et al., 1965).

The neonate's temperature can be maintained by wrapping the trunk and extremities with plastic wrap, using stockinet caps, and caring for the child in incubators and overhead heaters (Roberts, 1981; Vora et al., 1999). Other than a cap, it is difficult to use any of these devices in the operating room because their use makes it difficult or impossible to do the operation.

Overhead heaters allow access to the patient and are commonly used during the first few days of life and in the operating room before the surgical drapes are applied. Beside allowing access to the patient, these devices effectively maintain the baby's body temperature. Compared with incubators, overhead warmers increase insensible water loss by about 0.94 mL/kg per hour or 22.6 mL/kg per day (Flenady and Woodgate, 2003). More overhead warmer-treated patients had a serum sodium of greater than 150 mEq/L, compared with incubator-treated infants (Meyer et al., 2001). This increases the daily fluid requirements. The oxygen and energy consumption and the incidence of bradycardia are increased in overhead warmer-treated neonates (Long, 1980; Gorski et al., 1990; Hutchison, 1994). Nurses interact more often with infants who have been cared for in an overhead warmer than with those who were cared for in an incubator, which increases the opportunity for infections (Davenport, 1992). There are no reported differences in the rate of NEC, IVH, PVL, or death associated with overhead warmers and incubators.

Infants cared for in incubators have less insensible fluid loss, lower fluid intake, and lower body temperatures on the first 2 days of life. However, no difference in weight gain, maximum serum sodium, or serious complications (e.g., NEC, PVL, or ROP) was found in infants treated in the incubator vs. the overhead warmer (Meyer et al., 2001). More infants in the overhead-warmer group required phototherapy for hyperbilirubinemia. When evaluating neonates for surgery, anesthesiologists must be aware that patients cared for in overhead warmers may be hypovolemic more often than patients cared for in incubators and require correction of their intravascular volume preoperatively.

Liver

During the third to fourth week of gestation, epithelium of the posterior foregut forms an outpouching (liver bud) that invades the mesenchymal cells of the septum transversum of the diaphragm. Cells from both structures form hepatocellular tissue that is separated by sinusoids. The blood supply of the developing liver originates from the yolk sac. These vessels eventually become the hepatic and portal venous systems (Mitchell and Sharma, 2009). A connection between the hepatic bud and the duodenum forms the common bile duct, and an outgrowth from the common bile duct forms the gallbladder and the cystic duct. Endodermal cells occlude the extrahepatic bile ducts for the first 3 months of gestation. Failure to recannulate the ducts around this time results in extrahepatic biliary obstruction (i.e., biliary atresia), a common cause of liver failure during the first year of life. By the fourth week of gestation, hepatocytes produce and secrete some proteins, including α-fetoprotein and α_1-antitrypsin (Diehl-Jones and Askin, 2002). By the fifth week of gestation, hematopoietic stem cells are present in the liver, and these cells are the primary source of hematopoiesis throughout the first two thirds of gestation; the bone marrow assumes this role during the third trimester. To accomplish hematopoiesis, the liver mass increases fortyfold, and in early gestation, hematopoietic cells outnumber hepatocytes. Early in gestation hepatic cells differentiate into type II hepatocytes and intrahepatic bile ducts. Failure to develop intrahepatic ducts is another major cause of liver failure during infancy. Formation of the Golgi apparatus permits synthesis and secretion of albumin and other proteins. By the second month of gestation, bile is secreted. Glycogen synthesis occurs by the tenth week of gestation, and acini are present by the third gestational month. The umbilical vein, not the portal vein, supplies most of the blood flow to the left (90%) and the right (60%) lobes of the liver in utero (Bloom and Fawcett, 1975).

The liver serves a critical role in carbohydrate, protein, and lipid metabolism. It also synthesizes a wide array of compounds essential for coagulation; it stores iron (ferritin), and biotransforms a large number of endogenous (e.g., thyroxine and steroid hormones) and exogenous (e.g., drugs and toxins) substances. This discussion focuses on those aspects of liver function most relevant to the anesthetic care of the newborn: glucose metabolism, coagulation, and biotransformation of drugs. Because of its high incidence, hyperbilirubinemia is also discussed.

Glucose Metabolism

The fetal supply of glucose is abruptly interrupted at birth, requiring neonates to meet their glucose needs by glucose intake, by converting glycogen (which is stored in the liver and heart during the third trimester of pregnancy) to glucose, and by glycogenolysis. Glycogen breakdown is under the control of catecholamines and glucagon. The liver of infants born at term has a greater store of glycogen than the adult (Kalhan and Parimi, 2000). Glycogenolysis allows full-term infants to maintain normal serum glucose concentrations during a 10 to 12 hour fast. Since glycogen storage and the capacity for degradation mostly occur during the last trimester of pregnancy, preterm infants are predisposed to hypoglycemia. Gluconeogenesis is not active in fetal liver, but a variety of hepatic enzymes that are important in gluconeogenesis (e.g., glucose-6-phosphatase) undergo rapid development after birth (Kalhan and Parimi, 2000; Kalhan et al., 2001).

Preoperatively, most newborns receive an intravenous infusion containing 5% to 10% dextrose. In general, an infusion rate for dextrose of 4 to 7 mg/kg per minute (e.g., 10% dextrose at 4 mL/kg per hour equals 6.6 mg/kg per minute of dextrose) maintains normoglycemia in both full-term and preterm infants. Normal glucose levels are between 40 and 60 mg/dL. A blood sugar concentration of less than 40 mg/dL is defined as hypoglycemia. The symptoms of hypoglycemia are nonspecific and include jitteriness, cyanosis, apnea, lethargy, seizures, and hypotonia. The common causes of hypoglycemia include hypoxemia, sepsis, and high levels of circulating insulin. During a preoperative visit, the serum glucose concentration achieved with the current rate of intravenous glucose administration should provide the information needed to determine what glucose infusion rate is required during surgery. Occasionally administering this amount of glucose produces hyperglycemia, and the infused concentration of glucose must be reduced, usually to 2.5% dextrose.

Biotransformation

The liver is the primary site for metabolism of drugs and other xenobiotics, as well as for detoxification of nontherapeutic and environmental compounds. Because of this vital function, the liver is vulnerable to the toxic effects of these compounds. Because degradation pathways are immature, infants (especially newborns) may metabolize drugs and toxins less efficiently than older patients. Three main categories of hepatic-drug metabolizing systems include phase I (oxidation-reduction and hydrolysis), phase II (conjugation with glucuronic acid, glycine, acetate, or sulfate), and phase III (transport from liver) reactions. In general, the neonatal liver has less capacity to metabolize and excrete drugs because there are deficiencies of many of the enzymes involved in oxidation, reduction, hydrolysis, and conjugation.

Cytochrome P450 (CYP) enzymes are responsible for phase I processes. More than 50 CYP enzymes have been identified, and they are classified according to their nucleotide sequence (Wilkinson, 2005). Although the full clinical relevance of the relative expression of these enzymes in fetus and neonates is yet to be defined, their primary expression is in the liver, and their developmental expression has a major role in the pharmacokinetics and pharmacodynamics of drugs, including those used during anesthesia. The CYP3A family is responsible for metabolism of about 50% of all drugs (Hines and McCarver, 2002). Multiple patterns of developmental expression have been reported (Figs. 17-11 and 17-12). For example, although CYP3A7 is present in utero, its expression is negligible 1 week after birth. On the other hand, the concentration of CYP3A4 is low during fetal life but is about 50% of adult levels by 6 months of age. CYP2D6 has a multitude of polymorphisms and may be of particular relevance in the metabolism of psychotropic (and anesthetic) drugs (Blake et al., 2005). Clearly, as the ontogeny of metabolizing enzymes and transporters is understood, the dosing of drugs will be better adjusted for age-related differences, toxicity may be avoided, and clinical effectiveness will be improved.

Fewer data are available concerning the ontogeny of phases II and III. However, the uridine glucuronosyltransferases (UGTs) function at much lower levels in neonates than they do in adults. For example, glucuronidation of morphine reaches adult levels only at 2 to 6 months of age (de Wildt et al., 1999). Other conjugating enzymes with major roles in drug metabolism have been less well characterized (glutathione S-transferases, N-acetyltransferases, glucuronosyl transferases), but they are likely to play important roles in the unique drug handling commonly seen in the newborn.

Although the clinical implications of the genetic variability and developmental changes of hepatic metabolizing processes are not clearly identified, examples of age-related differences in drug responses are well documented. For example, the age-related pharmacokinetics of various muscle relaxants and narcotics were described more than 20 years ago (Cook, 1981; Fisher et al., 1982; Gauntlett et al., 1988). Caffeine and theophylline are metabolized by CYP1A2, which is expressed at low levels in the newborn and requires age-related considerations for therapeutic dosing (Hakkola et al., 1994). More recently, both postnatal age and postconceptual age were correlated with decreased and variable propofol clearance in preterm and full-term infants. Of note, multiple cytochrome P450 enzymes are required for metabolism of this drug. Consequently, altered expression of phases I and II hepatic metabolic enzymes may be responsible for these pharmacokinetic findings (Allegaert et al., 2007).

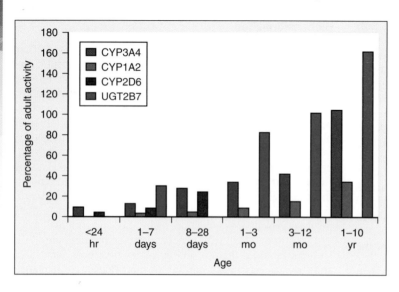

■ **FIGURE 17-11.** Changes in metabolic capacity. The activity of many cytochrome P-450 (CYP) isoforms and a single glucuronosyltransferase (UGT) isoform is markedly diminished during the first 2 months of life. In addition, the acquisition of adult activity over time is enzyme- and isoform-specific. *(From Kearns GL, et al.: Developmental pharmacology-drug disposition, action, and therapy in infants and children,* N Engl J Med *349:1157, 2003.)*

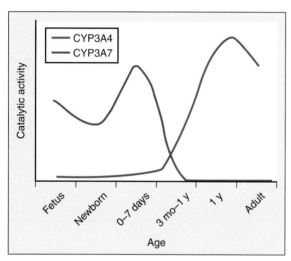

■ **FIGURE 17-12.** Ontogeny of cytochrome P450 (CYP) 3A4 and 3A7 activity expressed as activity measured using isoform-specific probes in human liver microsomes. *(From de Wildt SN, et al.: Cytochrome P450 3A: ontogeny and drug disposition,* Clin Pharmacokinet *37:485, 1999.)*

TABLE 17-5. Normal Values for Clotting Tests Appropriate for Gestational Age (AGA), Small for Gestational Age (SGA), and Premature Infants During the First Day of Life

Test	AGA	SGA	Premature
INR	1.3 ± 0.15	1.3 ± 0.2	1.3
Range	1.00-1.9	1.05-2.0	1.3
PT (Sec)	15.5 ± 1.4	16.2 ± 2.4	13
Range	13.4-19	13.3-23.6	10.6-16.2
aPTT (Sec)	42 ± 6.6	44 ± 8	53.5
Range	30-57	33-68	27.5-79.4
Fibrinogen g/l	2.83 ± 0.58	1.55	2.43
Range	1.25-3.0	0.2-2.2	1.5-3.73

Data from *Biol Neonate* 83-177-181, 2003; *Blood* 70:165-172, 1987; and *Blood* 72:1651-1657, 1988.

The preoperative evaluation of a newborn should include a review of current medications and determination of unexpected durations of action, toxicity, or side effects. In general, prolonged effects of these drugs can be expected in neonates because the enzymes of metabolism and elimination are immature.

Coagulation

The fetus produces coagulation factors because they inefficiently cross the placenta. Plasma levels of some coagulation proteins and factors and laboratory tests of clotting function (e.g., prothrombin time [PT] and activated partial thromboblastin time [APTT]) are markedly different in healthy full-term and preterm infants than in adults (Table 17-5).

Plasma concentrations of vitamin K–dependent proteins (e.g., factors II, VII, IX, and X), as well as factors XI and XII, prekallikrein, and kininogen, are about 50% lower than those of adults, but the concentrations of fibrinogen, factor V, and factor VIII are similar to those of adults (Andrew et al., 1987; 1988).

Disturbances in clotting caused by liver dysfunction correlate with decreased synthesis of both clotting and fibrinolytic factors and with abnormal platelet function. Hepatocytes synthesize factors 1 (fibrinogen), II (prothrombin), V, VII, IX, and X, and abnormal production of these factors is reflected in a prolonged PT. The PT mostly reflects availability of factor VII. Thrombin levels of newborns are about 50% those of adults. APTT primarily reflects the amount of thrombin generated (Green et al., 1976).

In spite of differences between newborn and adult liver function, clinically significant bleeding is uncommon in normal neonates who have adequate vitamin K levels. The association of vitamin K deficiency and hemorrhage in the newborn was initially described in 1894, is secondary to inadequate activity of vitamin K–dependent coagulation factors (i.e., II, VII, IX, and X), and is corrected by vitamin K replacement (Sutor et al., 1999). On the other hand, the newborn is predisposed to bleeding by infections and asphyxia, which may cause DIC. DIC is associated with prolonged PT and APTT that are caused by depletion of certain coagulation factors (e.g., fibrinogen and factors V and VIII), with increased fibrin degradation products and thrombocytopenia.

Preoperative evaluation should initially focus on whether or not there is a history of bleeding. If no clinical bleeding has been noted and the PT and PTT are normal for age, no further preoperative evaluation or treatment is indicated. Since many infants requiring surgery have significant physiologic derangements and nutritional deficiencies, laboratory studies, including a PT and APTT and a platelet count, should be obtained. If bleeding has occurred or if the laboratory studies are abnormal and there is clinical instability (e.g., sepsis or NEC), aggressive treatment is indicated. Preoperatively, interpretation of responses to fresh frozen plasma (FFP) (which contains adult levels of all coagulation proteins) or cryoprecipitate (which contains high levels of fibrinogen and factor VIII) will aid in planning to maintain intraoperative hemostasis. FFP is used sometimes for intraoperative volume repletion if hemostasis is also abnormal. However, rapid administration of FFP can cause hypotension because of the high concentrations of histamine present in some FFP and because of decreased ionized calcium concentrations caused by citrate. If large volumes of intravenous fluids are not needed, cryoprecipitate may be used to correct the fibrinogen and factor VIII deficiencies associated with DIC. Cryoprecipitate does not correct other clotting deficiencies.

Hyperbilirubinemia

Increased serum bilirubin concentrations are almost universal during the first postnatal week. (Kalhan and Parimi, 2000). In most cases, hyperbilirubinemia is transient and has been labeled *physiologic*. The primary source of bilirubin is hemoglobin, but other heme-containing proteins (e.g., cytochromes, catalases, and myoglobin) also contribute. Infants produce more bilirubin per kg of body mass than older patients because they have higher red cell masses and their red blood cells have shorter life spans. Bilirubin is the end product of hemoglobin breakdown and has also been reported to be an antioxidant and a free-radical scavenger (Sedlak and Snyder, 2004).

Because of its large nonpolar structure, bilirubin is lipophilic and requires biotransformation for excretion. Binding of bilirubin to albumin facilitates its delivery to the liver, and uptake of bilirubin into hepatocytes for conjugation requires glucuronic acid (i.e., organic anion transporter, [OATP2]) (Cui et al., 2001). Uridine diphosphate glucuronic acid provides the glucuronic acid. Most bilirubin is excreted in bile as bilirubin diglucuronides. Upon entry into the intestinal lumen, a variety of pathways exist for further disposal of bilrubin. As occurs in adults, bacteria metabolize bilirubin to urobilinogens for excretion in feces. Since the neonatal gastrointestinal tract lacks the same bacterial flora as adults, bilirubin may be reabsorbed and raise the serum bilirubin concentration. Beta-glucuronidase is also important for bilirubin metabolism, because it deconjugates bilirubin. Although this enzyme clears unconjugated bilirubin from the placenta, it increases bilirubin reabsorption from the gut after birth. Breast milk contains high level of β-glucuronidase and is partly responsible for "breast-milk jaundice" (Gourley and Arend, 1986).

Even if significant hemolysis occurs in utero, the normal placenta efficiently clears the bilirubin, and the newborn is seldom jaundiced. However, after birth the same bilirubin production would cause jaundice in most infants. With increasing bilirubin concentrations, the skin becomes progressively yellow (icteric) in a cephalocaudad pattern (Knudsen, 1990). The term *physiologic jaundice* refers to the common, transient, indirect

(unconjugated) hyperbilirubinemia in normal newborns. However, jaundice should be considered abnormal if it is present in the first 36 hours of life, persists beyond 10 days of life, is greater than 12 mg/dL, and the direct (conjugated) bilirubin is greater than 2 mg/dL or more than 30% of the total bilirubin concentration. Multiple disorders of increased bilirubin production (e.g., hemolysis secondary to maternal-fetal blood group incompatibility, other hemoglobinopathies, reabsorption of red blood cells from a hematoma, and polycythemia) or decreased excretion (e.g., as with genetic diseases, hypothyroidism, or infants of diabetic mothers) are recognized. Preterm infants more commonly develop elevated levels of bilirubin and are more vulnerable to bilirubin-induced CNS toxicity. CNS toxicity, or kernicterus, results from hyperbilirubinemia. Neuronal necrosis is the predominant feature and occurs mostly in the basal ganglia, brainstem, occulomotor nuclei, and cochlear nuclei.

During the preoperative visit, levels of total and direct bilirubin and their trends should be determined, as these levels and trends may reflect either normal postnatal development or sepsis and other anomalies. Hyperbilirubinemia, in association of other laboratory values, may provide an estimate of possible hepatic dysfunction and suggest the need for additional laboratory studies. Various tests evaluate direct injury to the liver; alanine aminotransferase (ALT), aspartate aminotransferase (AST), lactate dehydrogenase (LDH), and bilirubin concentrations may be increased as a result of asphyxia-ischemia-hypoxia ("shock liver"), sepsis, toxin-induced injury, or hepatitis. Direct bilirubin concentrations contribute to the hyperbilirubinemia that occurs with sepsis. Abnormalities in alkaline phosphatase, γ-glutamyltransferase (GGT), and 5-nucleotidase (5-NT) are more often to the result of impaired bile flow or cholestasis. Specific clearances of substances, such as indocyanine green and paraaminobenzoic acid (PABA), are measures of hepatic excretory function. While albumin is synthesized only in the liver, abnormal serum albumin levels may also result from protein lost in the gastrointestinal track or kidney or from chronic infection. Finally, abnormal ammonia concentrations should suggest the presence of specific urea-cycle defects. During preoperative assessment, the goal is to understand the functional status of the liver and to estimate the effect of current liver function on drug metabolism, blood loss, surgical trauma, and the need for coagulation factors.

Renal Function

Metabolic stability and electrolyte homeostasis are maintained in utero by the placenta; renal growth and development appear not to be linked or regulated by function during this time. Permanent kidneys appear during the fifth week of gestation, and nephrons appear during the eighth week, initially in the juxtamedullary region and cortex. A complex interaction of genes, such as Wilms' tumor gene 1 (WT1), and growth factors such as neurotrophic factor, (GDNF) orchestrate this process (Taeusch et al., 2005; Dziarmaga et al., 2006). By 20 weeks' gestation, one third of the final number of nephrons is present, and by 35 to 36 weeks' gestation, the adult number of nephrons is present (see Chapter 5, Regulation of Fluids and Electrolytes) (McDonald and Emery, 1959). During the second half of gestation, kidney growth is in direct proportion to gestational age. Infants born prematurely develop new nephrons until about 34 to 35 weeks' postconceptual age. Once the full complement of nephrons is present, further maturation of the kidneys occurs by increases in both glomerular and tubular size. Vascular growth and development parallel nephrogenesis. Anesthesiologists must understand renal development because of the kidneys' importance in maintaining acid-base homeostasis and fluid and electrolyte balance (see Chapter 5, Regulation of Fluids and Electrolytes).

Among healthy full-term infants, the number of nephrons varies up to fivefold (Merlet-Bénichou et al., 1999). Recent studies suggest that having fewer nephrons at birth correlates with hypertension later in life (Brenner et al., 1988; Keller et al., 2003). These authors suggest that hypertrophied, overworked nephrons slowly sclerose, leading to progressive renal dysfunction. The reduced number of nephrons is thought to result from both genetic and environmental factors (Lelièvre-Pégorier and Merlet-Bénichou, 2000). Recently, polymorphism of the RET gene was shown to reduce the number of nephrons (Zhang et al., 2008). A common variant of another gene, PAX2, is also associated with having smaller kidneys at birth (Quinlan et al., 2007). Both prematurity and fetal growth retardation have negative effects on postnatal renal growth (Huang et al., 2007; Rakow et al., 2008). Finally, oxidative injury during the neonatal period has been associated with decreased capillary density and fewer nephrons in adult rats (Yzydorczyk et al., 2008).

Urine is formed by 10 weeks' gestation, and urine production increases from about 2 to 5 mL/hour at 20 weeks' gestation to 10 to 12 mL/hr at 30 weeks', 12 to 16 mL/hr at 35 weeks', and to 35 to 50 mL/hr at 40 weeks' gestation (Rabinowitz et al., 1989). Because the fetal kidneys process large volumes of fluid, large quantities of hypotonic urine are produced. Fetal urine production is essential for the maintenance of normal amniotic fluid volumes, especially after 18 weeks' gestation. Oliguria causes oligohydramnios, which is associated with a specific facies, clubfeet, limb contractures, and in some cases, pulmonary hypoplasia. In essence, high fetal urine volumes are necessary for normal development of organs besides the urinary tract.

Fetal urine is initially hypotonic (100 to 250 mOsm/kg). Its tonicity decreases throughout gestation. For example, urinary sodium is 120 mEq/L at midgestation and decreases to 50 mEq/L by 32 to 35 weeks' gestation (Spitzer, 1996). Fetal and neonatal renal function is characterized by low renal blood flow, glomerular filtration rate (GFR), solid excretion, and concentrating power. Renal blood flow is low in utero because renal vascular resistance is high. After birth, renal blood flow increases markedly as a result of an increase in the arterial blood pressure and a decrease in renal vascular resistance. These changes allow more of the CO to be distributed to the kidneys (2% to 4% in utero, 10% at 1 week of age, 25% in the adult). Renal blood flow is about 20 mL/min per 1.73 m^2 at 30 weeks' gestation, 45 mL/min per 1.73 m^2 at 35 weeks' gestation, about 80 mL/kg per 1.73 m^2 at term, 250 mL/min per 1.73 m^2 at 8 days after birth, and 770 mL/min per 1.73 m^2 at 5 months of age (Heisler, 1993). Similarly, fetal GFR increases rapidly in utero as the number of nephrons increases. Because fetal kidney growth begins deep in the medulla, the juxtamedullary nephrons are more mature than other nephrons at birth and have greater tubular length than outer and inner cortical nephrons. Since the glomerulus is uniform, a "tubular-glomerular" imbalance exists. This imbalance explains, at least in part, why more of the solids presented to the proximal tubules of newborns are not reabsorbed.

The GFR of preterm infants is a function of both gestational and postnatal age. During the first 24 hours of extrauterine life, the GFR of infants born before 25 weeks' gestation may be as low as 2 mL/min per 1.73 m^2. Infants born between 25 and 28 weeks' gestation have a GFR of 10 to 13 mL/min per 1.73 m^2, and those born after 34 weeks' gestation have one of 20 to 25 mL/min per 1.73 m^2, which is similar to that of full-term infants (Svenningsen and Aronson, 1974). Although GFR increases at a slower rate in ELBW infants, all neonates without acquired renal insufficiency double their GFR by 2 weeks of age and triple it by 3 months of age. Thereafter, GFR increases more slowly. Adult values for GFR are reached by 12 to 24 months of age. Because there is rapid renal maturation after birth, a 3-week old infant with 27 weeks' gestation may have significantly more mature renal function than a healthy 6-hour-old full-term infant. Renal maturation apparently occurs in response to demand (separation from the placenta plus solute exposure). Renal filtration and concentrating ability increase when the kidneys are challenged.

The serum creatinine concentration is commonly used as a measure of glomerular function. At birth, it reflects maternal values and is higher than that of normal 1- to 2-week-old full-term neonates (0.4 mg/dL). For the first 4 weeks of life, the plasma creatinine concentration of preterm infants exceeds that of full-term infants (Bueva and Guignard, 1994). Interestingly, the serum creatinine concentration was the same at birth in infants born before 27 weeks' gestation as it was in those born at 31 to 32 weeks' gestation. Serum creatinine concentrations increased in all groups over the first 3 days of life and then gradually decreased to less than 0.5 mg/dL (Gallini et al., 2000). However, the maximum creatinine concentration reported was higher and occurred later (day 3.5 vs. day 1) in the most immature neonates. Creatinine clearance increased in all groups, but it increased more slowly in the infants who had fewer than 27 weeks' gestation. The variability in GFR and creatinine clearance, as a function of gestational and postnatal age, means that drugs primarily eliminated by the kidneys may be eliminated differently in different neonates.

Renal Tubular Function

Maintenance of normal extracellular fluid volume, water balance, sodium, and other electrolyte concentrations are interrelated and undergo significant postnatal changes. In addition to the marked changes in nephron number, glomerular function, and renal blood flow, developmental changes occur in the renal tubules throughout fetal and postnatal life. Coupled with tubular immaturity, metabolic demands of rapid growth and illnesses make managing fluids and providing nutritional support complicated in the newborn. The following factors should be considered:

1. Neonates, especially premature neonates, are less able to reabsorb and to excrete sodium (Fig. 17-13). Reabsorption of sodium by the proximal tubule increases with gestational age; 5% of the filtered sodium is excreted in the urine of infants with more than 30 weeks' gestation, but only 0.2% is excreted in full-term infants (Vanpeé et al., 1988). Hypoxia, respiratory distress, and hyperbilirubinemia may increase fractional sodium excretion.

2. Newborns have limited ability to concentrate their urine (245 to 450 mOsm/L in premature infants vs. 600 to 800 mOsm/L in full-term infants vs. 1200 to 1400 mOsm/L in adults).

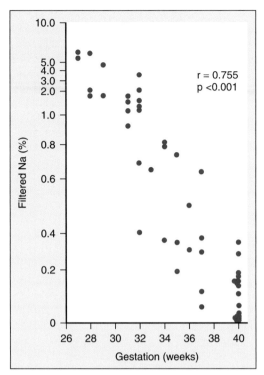

r = 0.755
p <0.001

■ FIGURE 17-13. Scattergram demonstrating the inversion correlation between fractional sodium excretion and gestational age. *(From Siegel SR, et al.: Renal function as a marker of human renal fetal maturation,* Acta Paediatr Scand *65:481, 1976.)*

3. Newborns of more than 35 weeks' gestation can dilute their urine to adult levels, about 50 mOsm/L. Infants born before 35 weeks' gestation can dilute it to about 70 mOsm/L. The maximum urinary osmolality attained after a dose of desmopressin (DDAVP) was about 520 mOsm/kg in infants with 30- to 35-weeks' gestation and 570 mOsm/kg in 4- to 6-week-old infants born at term. A 1- to 2-year-old child concentrates his urine to 1300 to 1400 mOsm/kg after a dose of DDAVP (Svenningsen and Aronson, 1974). The majority of infants still do not concentrate their urine that well at 6 to 12 months of life.

4. Newborns commonly have low serum bicarbonate concentrations (12 to 16 mEq/L in ELBW infants, 18 to 20 mEq/L in infants with 30 to 35 weeks' gestation, 20 to 22 mEq/L in term infants, and 25 to 28 mEq/L in adults) (Schwartz et al., 1979). The loss of bicarbonate increases urine pH.

5. The transport maximum (T_m) and the tubular reabsorption of glucose are both decreased (150 mg/dL in term neonates, 180 mg/dL in older children and adults). Glucosuria may occur in preterm infants at serum glucose concentrations below 100 mg/dL.

6. Calcium absorption occurs in the proximal tubules of the kidneys, primarily by passive diffusion. High renal sodium losses increase calcium loss. Sick neonates, especially premature neonates, require supplemental intravenous calcium to maintain normal ionized calcium concentrations.

7. Serum potassium concentrations that exceed 5.0 mmol/L are relatively common in newborns, particularly premature newborns that have a mild metabolic acidosis. Nonoliguric hyperkalemia, characterized by a rapid rise of serum potassium during the first 1 to 3 days of life, also occurs in ELBW infants, probably as the result of rapid shifts of potassium from intra- to extracellular compartments (Mildenberger et al., 2003). Treatment of this disorder includes insulin/glucose, calcium/bicarbonate, diuretics, and binding resins.

All renal tubular cells are polarized. The apical membrane faces the lumen of the tubule, and the basal membrane faces the capillaries. Sodium is actively reabsorbed along the entire tubular system. Most sodium-coupled transporters required to salvage amino acids, glucose, phosphate, and lactate are located on the apical membrane of the proximal tubules. The Na^+, K^+-ATPase pump, which is responsible for approximately 70% of renal oxygen consumption, is located on the basolateral membrane and is important for active transport of sodium. About 60% to 80% of sodium reabsorption occurs in the proximal tubules. Another 10% to 15% occurs in the distal (i.e., aldosterone responsive) and collecting tubules (antidiuretic hormone [ADH] determines water permeability). The amount of sodium in fluid presented to the distal tubules depends in part on the efficiency of the proximal tubules.

After birth, reabsorption of sodium in the proximal tubules increases five- to tenfold in response to increased Na^+, K^+-ATPase activity (Holtbäck and Aperia, 2003). Glucocorticoid hormones increase messenger ribonucleic acid (mRNA) for both subunits of this enzyme, and prenatal administration of betamethasone to mature the lungs may also mature renal function. Similarly, developmental changes in the Na^+–H^+ exchanger (NHE) may be responsible for differences in acid-base balance among newborns, older children, and adults. The kidneys both reabsorb bicarbonate and excrete fixed acids. Bicarbonate reabsorption occurs primarily in the proximal tubules, but it also occurs in the loop of Henle and the collecting ducts. Hydrogen is actively secreted, and the secreted hydrogen reacts with bicarbonate to produce carbonic acid and carbon dioxide. These substances enter the tubular cells through the action of carbonic anhydrase. Bicarbonate again forms and exits the cell via another transport mechanism. Several isoforms of NHE have been identified, and impaired function of this transporter has been described (Rodríguez-Soriano, 2000; Holtbäck and Aperia, 2003). Immature carbonic anhydrase activity and impaired NHE function explain in part the normal metabolic acidosis found in newborns.

Distribution of total body water changes throughout fetal life (Friis-Hansen, 1983; Brans, 1986). At 16 weeks' gestation, the total body water makes up 94% of the fetus' weight; at about 32 weeks' gestation it is 82%, and at term it is approximately 75%. The size of the extracellular compartment decreases from 65% at 16 weeks' gestation to about 60% at 24 to 25 weeks' gestation, to about 50% at term. At the same time the intracellular compartment increases from 34% in early gestation to 50% at term. Of note, most extracellular water is in the interstitial space (i.e., an extracellular compartment). This is exaggerated in preterm neonates, especially ELBW neonates, whose extracellular water compartments are very large.

During the first 3 to 7 days of extrauterine life, healthy term infants lose about 5% to 10% of their body weight, primarily through contraction of the extracellular water space (Fig. 17-14). Preterm infants follow a similar pattern, but they may lose more than 15% of their body weight; premature infants also take longer to establish steady growth than full-term infants do.

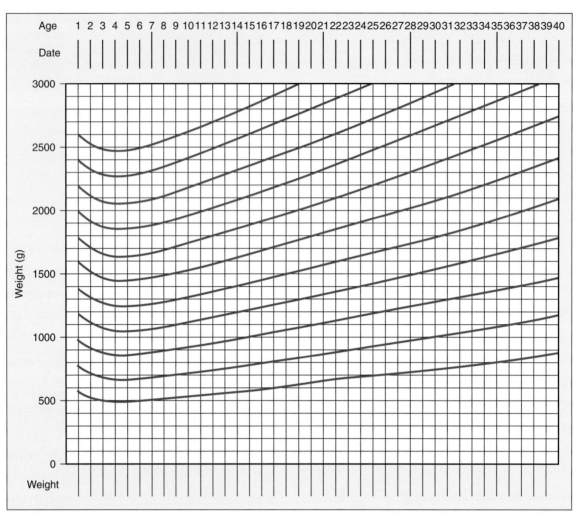

■ **FIGURE 17-14.** Extrauterine growth chart according to gestational age in weeks. *(Data from Schaffer SG, Quimiro CL, Anderson JR, Hall RT: Postnatal weight changes in low–birth-weight infants,* Pediatrics *79:702, 1987; Gleason CA, Taeusch HW, Ballard RA, editors: Avery's diseases of the newborn, ed 8, Philadelphia, 2005, Saunders, p. 1575.)*

Cardiorespiratory abnormalities and their treatment, infections and their side effects, and pharmacologic interventions so alter growth patterns that it is difficult to define normal growth patterns in preterm neonates.

Hormonal control of neonatal fluid and electrolyte homeostasis is complex, and some of its features are unique. The renin-angiotensin-aldosterone, atrial natriuretic peptide (ANP), vasopressin, and catecholamine (i.e., dopamine and noradrenalin) systems affect regulation of electrolytes and water balance. However, the overall effectiveness of each of these systems is less than it is later in development. For example:

1. Aldosterone, angiotensin, and plasma renin activity are elevated in both term and preterm infants and are inversely related to gestational age. Immature kidneys are less responsive to the sodium- and water-conserving effects of these hormones. The roles of these hormones in neonatal adaptation are not well established, but their concentrations are high for several weeks, especially in critically ill patients. Prostaglandins counterbalance the vasoconstrictive effects of these hormones. The high concentrations of these hormones cause vasoconstriction and may be responsible, at least in part, for the renal failure seen after a dose of indomethacin is given to close a PDA.

2. The plasma vasopressin (ADH) concentration is higher in newborns than it is later in life, especially after vaginal delivery, and it is thought to be responsible, at least in part, for low urine output during the first 24 hours of life. Vasopressin may also participate in the postnatal contraction of the extracellular volume immediately after birth. It may also be responsible for indomethacin-induced renal failure in premature infants. Hypoxia, atelectasis, IVH, and BPD increase urine ADH concentrations in both preterm and term infants, and this nonosmotic secretion of ADH partly accounts for the dilutional hyponatremia of newborns, especially premature newborns (Wiriyathian et al., 1986). Thus, the limited ability of fetuses and newborns to concentrate their urine is correlated with an immature concentrating ability of the medullary system, decreased response to ADH, and an immaturity of their aldosterone system.

3. ANP inhibits the production and action of both renin and aldosterone. High circulating concentrations of this peptide, plus prostaglandins and progesterone, are partly responsible for the negative sodium balance (Tulassay et al., 1986). Although few documented developmentally important actions of this compound have been reported, PEEP-induced oliguria can occur because less ANP is released.

TABLE 17-6. Maintenance Fluid Requirements During the First Month of Life

Birth Weight (g)	Insensible Water Loss (mL/kg/day)	Water Requirements (mL/kg/day) by Age		
		Day 1-2	Day 3-7	Day 8-30
<750	100-200	100-200+	150-200+	120-180
750-1000	60-70	80-150	100-150	120-180
1001-1500	30-65	60-100	80-150	120-180
>1500	15-30	60-80	100-150	120-180

Adapted from Veille JC: AGA infants in a thermoneutral environment during the first week of life, *Clin Perinatol* 15:863, 1988; Taeusch W, et al.: *Schaffer and Avery's diseases of the newborn,* ed 6, Philadelphia, 1991, Saunders; and Lorenz J, et al.: Phases of fluid and electrolyte homeostasis in extremely low birth weight infants, *Pediatrics* 96:484, 1995.

Based on the complex interactions of renal development, illness, prematurity, and therapy, fluid and electrolyte management in the newborn should take the following factors into account:

1. Postnatal diuresis contracts the extracellular space, and the amount of contraction is greater in preterm infants. During the first few days after birth, clinicians should allow the normal negative fluid and electrolyte balancing process of nonsurgical patients to take place while maintaining cardiorespiratory stability and providing sufficient fluid intake to keep up with transepidermal fluid losses (Table 17-6).

2. Transepidermal fluid loss is related to gestational age and can be as much as 60 to 100 mL/kg per day in ELBW infants. Over the first 5 days of life, fluid losses decrease dramatically from 45 to about 19 g/m^2 per hour in infants with 25 to 27 weeks of gestation (Fig. 17-15) (Sedin et al., 1983). During the first few postnatal days, naked preterm infants lose up to 15 times more water through evaporation than naked full-term infants (Hammarlund et al., 1983). Consequently, naked VLBW infants may lose as much as 10% of their body weight through evaporation during the first 24 hours of life. Premature neonates have increased respiration, which further increases water loss. Evaporation accounts for about 40% of total baseline water losses in children and adolescents. The insensible evaporative water loss is several magnitudes greater in premature neonates than it is in older patients, because preterm neonates have increased epidermal permeability for water and because they have a larger surface area-to-volume ratio. The larger relative surface area provides a larger surface from which preterm neonates can lose water. To maintain normal water and electrolyte balance, meticulous attention must be paid to intake and output of fluid, body weight, urine output, and electrolyte concentrations (especially in ELBW infants) during the first 3 to 5 days of life.

3. Providing a warm, humidified environment and inspired gases or using plastic shields reduces transepidermal fluid loss, especially in ELBW infants, but these methods are difficult or impossible to use during surgery.

4. Measurement of serum and urine electrolytes, serum glucose concentrations, hematocrit, body weight, and intake and output of fluids help guide fluid therapy. It has been suggested that PDA, NEC, and CLD are caused by overhydration or by hyper- or hyponatremia, but there is no conclusive evidence to support this contention.

5. An intravenous calcium infusion is usually required in preterm, asphyxiated, or LGA and SGA infants until they can take in adequate enteral nutrition.

The high anabolic rate associated with growth makes the neonate's limited ability to excrete solute a problem. Moreover, this increased solute load occurs at a time when the therapeutic index for fluid and electrolytes is narrow (especially in VLBW infants), when insensible water losses are enormous, when there is renal immaturity or insufficiency, and when multiorgan effects of prematurity and infection are common.

Hematology

Developmental hematopoiesis occurs in three stages and locations—the embryonic yolk sac, the fetal liver, and the bone marrow (Sacher and McPherson, 1986; Rappaport, 1997). Each stage is critical to survival.

Embryonic hematopoiesis begins at about 14 days' gestation when the mesodermal pluripotential stem cells of the ventral yolk sac form primitive megaloblastic nucleated red cells (mean corpuscular volume [MCV] 400), primitive macrophages, and megakaryocytes. At 5 weeks' gestation, pluripotential hematopoietic stem cells migrate from the aorta-gonad-mesonephros (AGM) region to populate the liver and spleen, the temporary sites of hematopoiesis. These uncommitted stem cells divide and produce progeny that either replenish the stem cell pool or mature to committed cell lines and then produce erythrocytes, macrophages, and myeloid and lymphoid cells. By 9 weeks, lymphopoiesis is present in the lymphoid plexuses and the thymus.

At 8 weeks' gestation, AGM stem cells begin to populate bone marrow, and the complex regulatory hematopoietic interactions that are sustained over a lifetime are initiated. As progenitor cells populate the maturing extracellular bone-marrow matrix, adhesion molecules such as integrins, selectins, and CD 14+ cells promote progenitor cell-stromal binding, creating protected microenvironments. The microenvironments allow the selective influence of growth factors (e.g., cytokines, colony stimulating factors, and interleukins) to promote cell growth and maturation. Generally, progenitor cells account for fewer than 1% of marrow cells, but at birth a much larger percentage of umbilical cord cells are progenitors. At term, hematopoietic capacity is comparable with that of adults.

Embryonic erythrocytes contain hemoglobin Gower-1 (unpaired globin chains, many forming tetramers), are nucleated, macrocytic (MCV 400), and not controlled by erythropoietin. Fetal erythrocytes are present and sensitive to erythropoietin

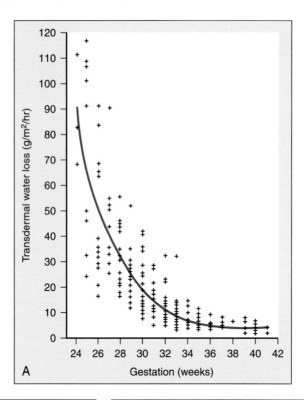

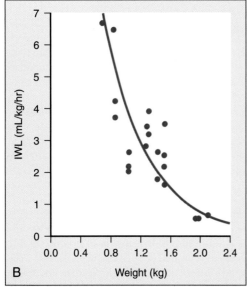

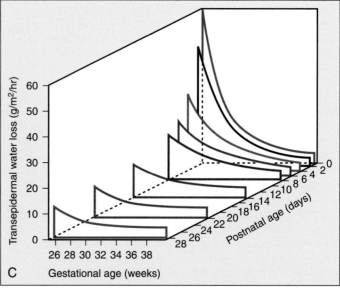

■ **FIGURE 17-15. A,** The effects of gestation on transepidermal water loss. Measurements were made from abdominal skin and carried out in the first few days of life. **B,** Insensible water loss *(IWL)* as a function of birth weight in premature infants nursed under radiant warmers. **C,** Transepidermal water evaporation from the skin of premature neonates with gestational ages of 25 to 40 weeks, followed longitudinally from birth over the first month of life. Dehydration is the most dangerous in the first week of life for the most immature babies of less than 28 weeks' gestation, before skin keratinization occurs. *(A, From Hammarlund K, et al.: Transepidermal water loss in newborn infants, III: relation to gestational age,* Acta Paediatr Scand *68:795, 1979. **B,** Adapted from Costarino AT, Baumgart S: Controversies in fluid and electrolyte therapy for the premature infant,* Clin Perinatol *15:863, 1988. **C,** From Sedin G, et al.: Measurements of transepidermal water loss in newborn infants,* Clin Perinatol *12:79, 1985.)*

by the sixth week of gestation. They contain mostly fetal hemoglobin ($\alpha 2\gamma 2$) with small amounts of hemoglobin A ($\alpha 2\beta 2$). At birth, erythrocytes are macrocytic (MCV 110) and contain primarily fetal hemoglobin (60% to 80%), which less effectively binds 2,3-diphosphoglycerate (2,3-DPG) and shifts the oxygen dissociation curve to the left, making it less difficult to take up oxygen but more difficult to release it to the tissues. Anti-A and anti-B isoagglutinins develop during the first 6 months of

life. Alloimmunization to red cell antigens is rare in neonates after transfusion. Myelopoiesis is active at 5 months' gestation, but granulocytopoiesis is half of that in adults and gradually increases to adult levels at term. Most of the increase in granulocytes occurs in the last trimester of pregnancy. The absolute number of granulocytes present at birth usually exceeds that of older children but decreases in the first few days after birth. Lymphocytes then become more numerous and remain more numerous for the first 4 years of life. Megakaryocytes are present in bone marrow, and platelets are present in blood by 11 weeks' gestation. At birth, the platelet counts of term and preterm infants are comparable to those of adults, but the newborn's ability to regulate thrombopoiesis and myelopoiesis is immature, causing inadequate cell production during severe stress.

Jopling et al. (2009) reported an increase in hemoglobin concentration from 14 g at 25 weeks' gestation, 16 g at 30 weeks, 17 g at 35 weeks, to 18 g at term in AGA neonates. A similar increase occurred in the hematocrit. The increases of hemoglobin and hematocrit were linear and not affected by gender. SGA infants have higher hemoglobin concentrations than full-term babies 3 hours after birth, and the concentration decreases about 10% over the first week of life. The higher hemoglobin concentration of SGA neonates is thought to be compensation for intrauterine hypoxia and elevated levels of erythropoietin (Snijders et al., 1993). Preterm infants have lower hemoglobin concentrations at birth than SGA or AGA infants, and the decrease in hemoglobin concentration is greater in premature infants after birth (Table 17-7) (Obladen et al., 2000).

The true hemoglobin of preterm infants may be difficult to determine, because many of these infants have intrauterine hypoxia before birth. This may stimulate hemoglobin production, as may steroid administration to the mother. The production of new erythrocytes decreased after birth as a result of lower concentrations of erythropoietin and fewer reticulocytes. Many preterm infants fail to respond to erythropoietin, because they have iron deficiency (Obladen et al., 2000). However, low iron concentrations may protect them from free-radical injury (Khawaja and Volpe, 2008).

The white blood count of neonates is variable at birth, especially in neonates who receive betamethasone or are infected in utero (Table 17-7) (Cohen et al., 1993). Some healthy infants have white blood cell (WBC) counts of 25,000 at birth. On the other hand, 21% of SGA neonates are neutropenic at birth but have normal cell counts by 7 days after birth (Ozyürek et al., 2006).

One third of SGA infants are thrombocytopenic on the first day of life, possibly because of consumption of platelets by placental infarcts. These infarcts may also be responsible for the polycythemia of SGA neonates. The platelet count of normal SGA infants is 102 to 292×10^9, and is usually greater than 250×10^9 after a few days (Table 17-7).

Preoperative Hematologic Evaluation

Several important questions must be answered during the preoperative evaluation. Is there evidence of bleeding? Are there petechiae or skin hemorrhages? Is there, or has there been, recent active bleeding into the bowels, lungs, or the brain? What is the platelet count, and has it decreased over the previous 24 hours? Were platelet transfusions required to maintain the desired platelet count, usually greater than $100,000/mm^3$? Are PT and PTT normal? If not, has the patient been treated with FFP? How many times? How much did FFP improve the PT, PTT, and international normalized ratio (INR)? For how long does it remain improved (normal)? When was FFP last administered? What is the WBC count? Is it increased or decreased from normal? Does an increase or decrease in the WBC count occur with sepsis? What are the patient's hemoglobin concentration and hematocrit value? Are they high? If so, is this because of overtransfusion or dehydration? Is the hematocrit value low? If so, is the low hematocrit value caused by bleeding or by excessive blood drawing? Is blood available for the patient in the blood bank? How many units have been cross-matched against the child? How old is the blood? Blood that has been in the blood bank for more than a few days has an elevated potassium concentration, often in excess of 10 mEq/L. If this blood is administered rapidly to replace blood loss in neonates, a potassium-induced cardiac arrest may occur, which may be difficult to treat (Brown et al., 1990). Because many infants have potassium concentrations of 5 mEq/L or more, rapid addition of potassium during blood transfusion may be disastrous or lethal.

TABLE 17-7. Normal Hematologic Values for Appropriate for Gestational Age (AGA), Small for Gestational Age (SGA), and Premature Infants

Test	AGA		SGA		Premature	
	Day 1	Day 7	Day 1	Day 7	Day 3	Day 12-14
Hb (g/dL)	17.0 ±0.4	16.2 ±0.4	18.2 ±0.4	15.4 ±0.3	15.5	14.4
(Range)	(17-23)	10,3-20.0	14-22.5	9.8-20.2		
Hct (%)	47.1 ± 1.0	44.6 ±1.0	53.3 ±0.8	44.4 ±1.0	47	44
(Range)	36.7-62.8	28.5 ±54.7	32.6-66.9	28.8-60.3		
RBC (109/uL	4.7 ±0.1	4.5 ±1.0	5.1 ±0.8	4.4 ±0.1	4.2	4.1
(Range)	(3.6-6.2)	(3.0-5.6)	(3.8-6.5)	(2.7-6.0)		
WBC (103)	15.0 ±7.0	10.6 ±3.3	13.3 ±0.9	9.6 ±0.4	9.5	12.3
(Range)	(7.1-25.4)	(6.6-15.4)	(4.6-16.5)	(3.8-15.5)		
Plts (109/L)	214.7 ±6.0	321.3 ±13.6	182 ±8.0	287.7 ±15.7	261	318
(Range)	(102-292)	(134-594)	(55.9-344)	(134-594)	(120-407)	

Data from *Pediatrics* 123:e333-e337, 2009; *Semin Perinatol* 33:3-11, 2009; *Clin Lab Haem* 28:97-104, 2006; and *Pediatrics* 106:707-711. 2000.

OUTCOMES

Survival

Precisely comparing data about preterm infants from various reports remains challenging because of factors such as differences in cohorts, single vs. multiple hospitals, differences in attitudes about survivability of ELBW infants, differing levels of available intensive care, and variable needs to transport mothers or infants. Infant mortality rates vary among and within countries and among ethnic and racial groups. Nevertheless, no doubt remains that gestational age imparts the most significant impact on both short- and long-term outcomes after preterm birth, although other factors must be considered. Tyson et al. (2008) noted that female gender, exposure to antenatal corticosteroid therapy, singleton birth, and increased birth weight (per 100-g increment) each showed improved outcomes similar to those associated with an increase in gestational age of approximately 1 week.

Comparing outcomes data across various decades continues to challenge experts. A "graduate" of the NICU in 1972 was exposed to a remarkably different set of standards than the infant who was a NICU patient in 2005 or later. The impact of prenatal steroids and postnatal surfactant on survival and morbidity is widely recognized and has been clearly documented since the 1990s (Hack et al., 1991, 1995; Stevenson et al., 1998; Horbar et al., 2002). In addition, definitions of diseases (e.g., CLD or BPD) and stratification of severity (e.g., IVH or NEC) evolve as outcomes are defined, but interpreting and comparing data among various decades is

challenging. Finally, the lag in understanding the impact of various therapies on long-term outcome requires years of analyzing serial evaluations of survivors that have been stratified according to birth weight and gestational age.

In spite of these challenges, certain patterns have emerged, and two of them deserve comment. First, no significant improvement in survival without neonatal and long-term morbidity has been measured between 1997 and 2002 (Fig. 17-16). Second, incurring three or more major morbidities (e.g., BPD, brain injury, ROP, and to a lesser degree, infection) predicts risk for death or survival with neurodevelopmental impairment (Bassler et al., 2009). Overall, 85% of inborn VLBW infants survive to be discharged from the NICU. Most deaths occur within the first week of life, and 87% of deaths happen within 28 days of extrauterine life (Fanaroff et al., 2007). Survival for an entire group of VLBW infants (501 to 1500 g) differed by only 1% when a cohort from 1995 to 1996 was compared with one from 1997 to 2002. In contrast, mortality decreased from 59% to 45% in a group of infants weighing between 501 and 750 g (1990 to 1991 vs. 1997 to 2002). As expected, mortality is strongly correlated with birth weight and gestational age, and less dramatic differences were noted when comparing the same time frames for other groups: 19% to 12% (751 to 1000 g), 7.7% to 6% (1001 to 1250 g), and 5% to 3% (1251 to 1500 g). Of greater significance, survival without major neonatal or long-term morbidity (e.g., BPD, IVH, or NEC) remained stable but differed as a function of gestational age (500 to 750 g, ≈20%; 751 to 1000 g, 50%; 1001 to 1250 g, 85%; 1251 to 1500 g, 90%) (Fanaroff et al., 2007; Eichenwald

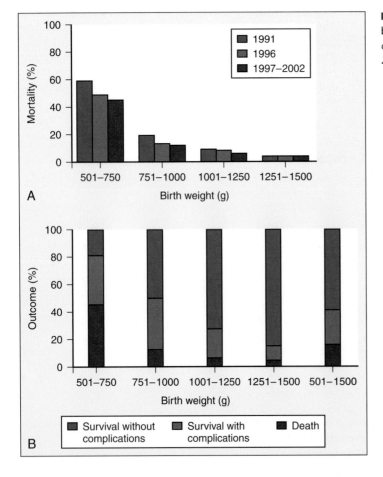

■ **FIGURE 17-16.** Short-term outcomes of VLBW according to birth-weight group. *(From Eichenwald E, Stark A: Management and outcomes of very low birth weight, N Engl J Med 358:1700, 2008.)*

and Stark, 2008). Data from other sources reveal similar findings and reinforce the concept that outcome of preterm infants must be meticulously analyzed within narrow ranges of gestational age (Costeloe et al., 2000; Wood et al., 2000; Fanaroff et al., 2003; Lucey et al., 2004; Markestad et al., 2005; Tommiska et al., 2007).

Although patterns of long-term outcome emerge with intense follow up of the expremature infant, accurately predicting outcome in the NICU during the first few days or weeks of life remains elusive. This is in part because the prolonged NICU course, especially for the ELBW infant, subjects the premature infant to repeated insults, including infection, PDA, and side effects of and complications from supportive therapy (e.g., oxygen toxicity, barotrauma, NEC, or drug effects). The cumulative impact of various morbidities has been reported, revealing that incurring just one of three common morbidities (i.e., BPD, brain injury, or ROP) doubled the incidence of death or neurosensory abnormality at 18 months. Identifying two of these morbidities tripled the incidence (Schmidt et al., 2003). Although less dramatic, the same investigators (as well as other groups), using the same cohort, reported that infection (e.g., sepsis, meningitis, or NEC) impacts death and neurodevelopmental outcome at the 18-month mark, although less dramatically (Glass et al., 2008; Bassler et al., 2009). The association of poor neurodevelopmental outcome with surgically treated NEC has been repeatedly noted (see The Expremature Infant: Neurologic Function, p. 552).

The perinatal factors that seem to dominate long-term pulmonary and neurologic outcomes seemed to be linked via the pathways of infection or inflammatory mediators and oxidative stress. Attempts to interrupt the injurious effects of inflammation and oxidative stress are challenging, because the injury is often an exaggeration of a normal process. For example, a variety of cellular damage is associated with production of reactive oxygen (ROS) and reactive nitrogen species (RNS) during hypoxic-ischemic events and reperfusion (e.g., peroxidation of membranes, structural proteins, and enzymes). However, these molecules have a critical role in regulating normal cellular function, immunity, circulation, and growth (Maltepe and Saugstad, 2008). Similarly, administering NO may have a role in preventing BPD in the ELBW infant, but results are controversial (Barrington and Finer, 2007; Arul and Konduri, 2009).

Chronic Lung Disease and Bronchopulmonary Dysplasia

Childhood CLD evolves from a variety of congenital and anatomic lesions (e.g., CDH, cystic adenomatoid malformation, and cardiac malformations) and acquired disorders (e.g., sepsis or meconium aspiration), but the overwhelming majority of infants and children acquire the disorder as a result of preterm birth and its supportive care, including oxygen and ventilatory support. BPD refers to CLD associated with prematurity. Although routine surfactant therapy has dramatically decreased the overall impact of BPD both in and after discharge from the NICU, residual lung disease persists as a critical factor that defines mortality and life-long morbidity associated with preterm birth. In fact, the incidence of BPD has remained steady over the last 20 years, recognized in approximately 20% of VLBW infants (Bancalari and del Moral, 2001). Additionally, BPD might be considered a systemic disease, because the retinitis and neurodevelopmental delay commonly coexist with this disorder.

The diagnostic criteria for CLD have been revised as the survival of preterm infants has improved. Northway et al. (1967) first described BPD as a CLD that developed in some preterm infants exposed to oxygen and positive pressure ventilation. In this original group of infants, none had fewer than 31 weeks' gestation, and only one weighed less than 1500 g.

Initially, the definition of BPD was based on the following clinical and radiographic criteria proposed by Bancalari et al. (1979):

1. Mechanical ventilation for more than 3 days in the first week of life.
2. Persistence of oxygen dependence after 28 days.
3. Radiographic abnormalities characterized by patchy density with areas of hyperlucency.

In 1988, CLD was redefined as oxygen dependence at 36 weeks' postconceptual age (rather than 28 days) (Shennan et al., 1988). More recently, pulmonary insufficiency after prematurity was defined as BPD rather than CLD, in order to distinguish it from other sources of neonatal respiratory disease. In addition, the definition of BPD has been revised as follows to include a system for grading its severity (Jobe and Bancalari, 2001):

1. Oxygen dependence for at least 28 postnatal days
2. Grading at 36 postmenstrual weeks for infants born with fewer than 32 weeks' gestation or at 56 days of life for infants born with more than 32 weeks' gestation.
   Mild-F_{IO_2}, 0.21
   Moderate-F_{IO_2}, 0.22-0.29
   Severe-F_{IO_2}, >0.30, CPAP, or mechanical ventilation

The definition of BPD continues to evolve as the mortality of infants of 28 weeks' gestation improves, and as the physiology and pathology of the new BPD is understood. The definition of BPD in the ELBW infant is likely to further change, as guidelines for oxygen administration and the target for oxygen saturation during resuscitation and in the NICU are standardized, ventilatory strategies are redefined, and effective or preventive pharmacologic interventions are identified for the premature and expremature infant.

CLD of infancy is simply defined as abnormal lung function, with an abnormal chest radiograph in the first 3 to 4 months after birth; abnormal function results from injury and repair with consequent maldevelopment of the lungs and respiratory dysfunction. This definition includes BPD. Initially, Northway et al. (1967) considered BPD to be caused by RDS, to evolve as a consequence of the repair process, and to lead to parenchymal fibrosis, chronic inflammation, airway epithelial metaplasia, injury to the large airways, and smooth muscle hypertrophy. Chest radiographs typically showed areas of overinflation as well as areas of volume loss consistent with fibrosis (Fig. 17-17, A,C).

Several factors, including increased survival rates and the possible unique susceptibility of the ELBW infant to lung injury, improved perinatal care to include the use of antenatal glucocorticoids and postnatal surfactant. Less aggressive ventilatory support and oxygen delivery also contribute to the current definition of BPD (Fig. 17-17, B,C) (Hussain et al., 1998). This "new" BPD is characterized by negligible epithelial lesions, injury to the large airways, fewer and larger alveoli, decreased and dysmorphic capillaries, and a variable amount of fibroproliferation. The characteristic fibroproliferative pattern of BPD is usually absent in the surfactant-treated lungs. Instead, the pathology is one of abnormal growth of both alveoli and vasculature (Hussain et al., 1998; Jobe and Bancalari, 2001).

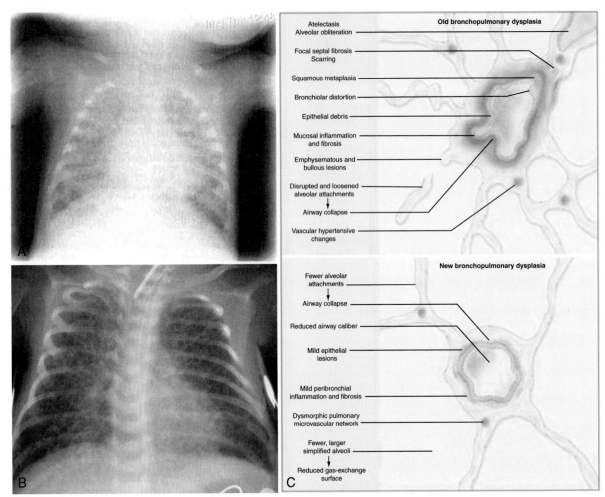

■ **FIGURE 17-17. A,** The pathologic description of classic chronic disease or "old BPD" is a fibroproliferative process with epithelial metaplasia, interstitial fibrosis, and air space obliteration from the fibrosis. This correlates with the radiologic findings of nonhomogeneity of the lung parenchyma with densities secondary to volume loss from fibrosis extending to the periphery coexisting with cystic emphysema (note cysts in both lung bases, right > left) and hyperinflation (note the flattened diaphragms). This is a pattern of repair of a response to injury. **B,** The abnormal pathology in the new BPD is abnormal growth of alveoli and vasculature, dilation of distal sites of gas exchange (alveolar ducts), but no prominent fibrosis. This correlates with a fine, hazy, uniform parenchymal pattern with modest hyperinflation but no cysts. This is a pattern of arrested development. **C,** Picture representation showing differences between old bronchopulmonary dysplasia and new bronchopulmonary dysplasia. (See text for specifics.)

Developmental delay and arrested growth, rather than severe epithelial injury with severe fibrosis and smooth muscle hyperplasia, characterize the lungs of the ELBW infant with new BPD (Fig. 17-17, *C*). As survival of ELBW infants has increased, the term *expremature* has evolved to refer to an infant who was born midgestation, with lungs in the canalicular stage of development (24 to 27 weeks' gestation), rather than in the saccular stage (31 to 34 weeks' gestation). Because of prenatal glucocorticoids and postnatal surfactant therapy, the expremature infant has less severe acute lung injury and requires less aggressive interventions.

Birth during the canalicular stage of lung development rather than the saccular stage seems to predispose ELBW infants to growth retardation of the lungs, perhaps secondary to interference with a variety of cell-signaling pathways that are essential for lung development. These signaling pathways can be affected by genetics, inflammation, infection, mechani-

cal ventilation, and oxygen toxicity. The role of genetics has not been clearly defined, but fibroblast growth factor-10, transforming growth factor-β (TGF-β), surfactant proteins, tumor necrosis factor a (TNF-a) converting enzyme, Hoxa-5 gene, epithelial sodium specific channel (ENaC), cytochrome P450 1A2, and glucocorticoid receptors have all been associated with the disease (Nogee et al., 1994; Ramet et al., 2000; Copland and Post, 2002; Hallman and Haataja, 2003; Kunzman et al., 2007; McDevitt et al., 2007; Kramer, 2008). Additional risks include sepsis or inflammation and the effects pharmacologic agents.

Some infants who have never had classic RDS develop BPD after minimal exposure to oxygen, ventilation, or infection. In these cases, despite seemingly minimal insult, the normal processes of alveolarization and microvascular development seem to be impaired. These infants are usually ELBW, develop oxygen dependency in the second or third (or later) week of life, may progress to requiring CPAP or mechanical ventilatory support, and subsequently develop BPD. Since 2000, approximately two thirds of infants with BPD were ELBW with fewer than 28 weeks' gestation (Baraldi and Filippone, 2007). A large number have long-term pulmonary insufficiency, are often hospitalized (especially during the first year of life), and have a higher incidence of developmental abnormalities than preterm infants without BPD (Short et al., 2003, 2007; Lamarche-Vadel et al., 2004; Vrijandt et al., 2007). Currently, no specific marker has been identified that predicts the development, course, or severity of BPD. Current evidence confirms that a variety of factors interact synergistically to disrupt normal lung growth and development. These factors include genetics, hypoxia, hyperoxia, mechanical ventilation, steroids, and inflammation (Baraldi and Filippone, 2007; Eichenweld and Stark, 2008).

Inflammation and BPD

Infection and inflammation play critical roles in the etiology of preterm delivery and subsequent BPD. Chorioamnionitis has been associated with preterm delivery, and several reports have suggested that an in utero inflammatory trigger initiates a cascade of injury that is sustained postnatally with the introduction of oxygen and positive pressure ventilation and by repeated bouts of infection (Yoon et al., 1999; Goldenberg et al., 2000; Schmidt et al., 2001; Speer, 2004, 2006; Kramer, 2008; Kramer et al., 2009).

TGF-1 has also been identified as a critical modulator in the development of BPD. TGF-1 regulates lung development, plays a role in inflammation and repair processes, and has been proposed as a key factor in inducing lung maturation associated with glucocorticoid administration (McDevitt et al., 2007).

Proinflammatory cytokines also appear critical in the initial postnatal response to lung injury in the preterm infant (Groneck et al., 1994; Tullus et al., 1996; Jonsson et al., 1997).

Mechanical Ventilation and BPD

The fluid-filled fetal lung must be inflated at birth to successfully transition to exchanging oxygen and carbon dioxide. Because of mechanical disadvantages (e.g., high chest wall compliance or inadequate surfactant), neurologic immaturity (e.g., immature control of breathing), and weakness of respiratory muscles, the preterm infant commonly requires ventilatory assistance (e.g., CPAP, mechanical ventilation, or supplemental oxygen) to achieve effective transition to breathing. In one report, 60% to 70% of newborns with fewer than 26 to 28 weeks gestation and all infants with fewer than 25 weeks' gestation were treated with positive pressure ventilation after intubation of the trachea (Morley et al., 2008). The premature lung has less collagen, so the chest wall is more compliant, and the airways are distensible; therefore, the response to stretch caused by the inflation pressure may be significant. Even after surfactant administration, mechanical ventilation initiates and sustains an inflammatory reaction (Ferreira et al., 2000). Lung neutrophils release cytokines and initiate an inflammatory cascade that is associated with a higher incidence of BPD. A recent report noted that ventilation at birth might initiate a systemic inflammatory response in addition to the local response in the lung (Hillman et al., 2007). Of note, PEEP does not seem to protect the preterm lung from this rapid injury (Hillman et al., 2008).

CPAP may be associated with less lung injury compared with positive pressure ventilation (Avery et al., 1987; Morley et al., 2008). However, many ELBW infants may not sustain adequate oxygenation or ventilation during CPAP and require mechanical ventilation.

Oxygen Therapy/Toxicity

The oxygen saturation of the fetus at term is approximately 50% to 60%, decreasing to as low as 30% intermittently during labor (East and Colditz, 2007). Immediately after birth, the full-term infant's oxygen saturation is approximately 60%, and 5 minutes after birth the lower limit of normal is approximately 70%. The healthy full-term infant may have oxygen saturation less than 90% for as long as 5 to 10 minutes after vaginal birth and longer after cesarean section (Kamlin et al., 2006; Rabi et al., 2006; Dawson et al., 2007). With these data in mind, oxygen treatment must be titrated to achieve what has been defined as normal in the first hour of life to avoid needless exposure to excess oxygen.

Pulse oximetry provides a constant, accurate reading of heart rate and oxygen saturation.

The Term Infant

Multiple studies and metaanalyses have provided evidence for revising recommendations for delivery of oxygen during resuscitation of the full-term infant, comparing short-term outcome as well as mortality after resuscitation with room air or 100% oxygen (Davis et al., 2004; Saugstad et al., 2005, 2008). Regardless of the specific physiologic mechanisms, infants who were resuscitated using room air recovered more quickly as assessed by Apgar score, time to first cry, heart rate at 90 seconds, and sustained pattern of respiration (Saugstad, 2005; Saugstad et al., 2008). Of importance, Davis and colleagues (2004) reported lower mortality at 1 and 4 weeks with no difference in the incidence of hypoxic-ischemic encephalopathy between the two groups.

Some published guidelines continue to recommend an FIO_2 of 1.0 during initial resuscitation (de Caen and Singhal, 2006). However, Canada and Australia have incorporated these data into their clinical practice by revising standards for resuscitation of the newborn, moving away from the tradition of administering an FIO_2 of 1.0 (de Caen and Singhal, 2006; Morley et al., 2008).

The Preterm Infant

Most experts will agree that oxygen plays a role in the most severe long-term consequences of preterm birth: BPD, ROP, and neurodevelopmental abnormalities. The question remains as to what oxygen saturation should be targeted during resuscitation and in the NICU (Tin and Gupta, 2007).

Hyperoxia produces lung injury at any stage of development, but it may be particularly damaging to the immature lung because of insufficiency of several systems that are important in protecting tissues from oxygen toxicity. This oxygen load may produce an excess of free radicals that induce inflammation and damage cellular lipids, proteins, and carbohydrates (Maltepe and

Saugstad, 2008). Antioxidant enzymes (e.g., superoxide dismutase [SOD], catalase, glutathione peroxidase, and glutathione reductase) develop on a time scale similar to surfactant, so that the level of these antioxidants normally rises rapidly just before birth (Frank and Sosenko, 1987). In addition to its effects on antioxidant systems, hyperoxia inhibits surfactant synthesis, normal protein synthesis, and DNA synthesis, as well as producing pulmonary vascular reactivity (Newman et al., 1983; Clement et al., 1985; Jornot et al., 1987).

Studies reported that targeting higher oxygen saturation was associated with higher incidence of CLD (STOP-ROP Multicenter Study Group, 2000; Askie et al., 2003).

The Expremature Infant: Pulmonary Function

Despite the vast amount of literature regarding pulmonary outcome after preterm birth, gestational age exerts the most critical influence on eventual pulmonary function. Nevertheless, the following generalizations can be made:

- BPD is common in ELBW infants, occurring in approximately 60% to 90% of infants at 23 weeks' gestation and approximately 50% to 70% of infants at 25 weeks' gestation. BPD is less common in infants with more than 30 weeks' gestation or who weigh more than 1500 g. Arrest of lung growth is the characteristic pattern of lung injury in the ELBW infant.
- Pulmonary dysfunction occurs in premature infants without BPD. This group often has spirometric finding that lie between those for healthy full-term infants and premature infants with BPD (Pelkonen et al., 1997).
- CLD commonly coexists with poor feeding and growth and prolonged neonatal hospitalization.
- Hospitalizations over the first year of life are common. Pulmonary function seems to improve over the first 6 to 8 years of life, but residual airflow abnormalities have been noted in expremature adolescents and adults.
- Routine surfactant therapy has not changed the incidence of BPD, especially in ELBW infants. New BPD is often milder in the neonatal period and later, but the ultimate pulmonary function in adult life remains unknown.
- Neurodevelopmental abnormalities are common in infants with BPD.

Prematurity with or without RDS and with or without BPD is associated with long-term pulmonary sequelae (Saigal and Doyle, 2008; Smith et al., 2008). In spite of recent dramatic changes to clinical care throughout the perinatal period, BPD persists as a major long-term health problem, especially for the ex-ELBW infant. As noted in the recent reports of the clinical trials of inspired NO in preterm infants, birth weight persists as the most predictive variable of outcome (e.g., death and BPD), although other factors (e.g., higher oxygen concentration, outborn status, or male gender) contributed to later pulmonary function (Arul and Konduri, 2009). In general, premature infants with BPD encounter the most severe long-term respiratory abnormalities compared to both gestationally matched expremature infants without BPD and control-group infants who were born at term. That is, expremature infants with BPD have more severe abnormalities of pulmonary function, especially those reflecting airflow, air-trapping, and hyperresponsiveness, than their counterparts without BPD, but even

this latter group has spirometric values below those of full-term infants. As noted by Doyle et al. (2006), "Tinier or more immature survivors have worse respiratory function than those who are more mature or larger at birth, whether they have BPD or not." Surprisingly, this general pattern has not changed since the introduction of surfactant (Halvorsen et al., 2004; Korhonen et al., 2004; Doyle et al., 2006).

In addition to spirometric pulmonary assessments, exercise tolerance and diffusion of gases during exercise have helped define the functional impact of residual respiratory abnormalities in the expremature infant (Jacob et al., 1997). Children aged 7 to 8 years old who had BPD after preterm birth had lower gas transfer compared with children who were born at term or were born prematurely but had no CLD (Mitchell et al., 1998). During exercise, only BPD survivors had wheezing or oxygen desaturation. In a study by Jacob et al. (1997), expremature infants with a history of severe BPD, expremature infants who had RDS but no BPD, and healthy term infants were studied at ages 9 to 12 years. The BPD group used a greater percentage of their ventilatory reserve (V_EMAX/40 FEV_1) during exercise, especially those children with the lowest forced expiratory volume at 1 second (FEV_1) (Jacob et al., 1997). Similar findings were noted in a group of 9- to 15-year-old ex-ELBW infants. In this study, in addition to having lower forced expiratory flow (FEF) rates and lower FEV_1, oxygen consumption was noted to be low in formerly ELBW infants. Of note, the values for the ELBW infants who had not had BPD were lower than infants of normal birth weight but better than those who had had BPD. Postexercise arterial oxygen saturation for both groups of ELBW infants was lower than in infants of normal birth weight (Kilbride et al., 2003).

Similarly, Smith et al. (2008) recently documented spirometric abnormalities (e.g., FEV_1, $FEF_{25\%-75\%}$, or peak expiratory flow rates [PEFR] values) in a group of 10-year old ex-ELBW infants as compared with a group of children born at term between 1992 and 1994. For example, 28.5% of the preterm group, compared with 11.8% of the controls, had an FEV_1 of less than 80% predicted; 41.5% of the preterm group had a $FEF_{25\%-75\%}$ of less than 67% predicted, but none in the control group did. The most striking results included the lower exercise capacity (44% of the control group) and lower predicted peak oxygen consumption. Other studies have suggested that children with a history of mild BPD do not have decreased exercise capacity compared with other survivors of neonatal mechanical respiratory support, but the BPD groups did have a greater incidence of oxygen desaturation during exercise (Bader et al., 1987; Parat et al., 1995; Santuz et al., 1995).

Postmortem assessment of morphometric lung development has documented the drastic restriction in the number of alveoli in survivors of BPD compared with that of normal infants. The total numbers of alveoli in a 22-month-old child (31.1 million) and in a 28-month-old child (40.4 million) were less than that in a healthy 1-week-old infant (67.2 million) (Margraf et al., 1991). Of course, infants who die from CLD may have more dramatic morphometric abnormalities than the less severely affected survivors.

These postmortem studies of infants with CLD also documented an abnormal architecture of elastic fibers, the framework on which new alveoli develop. Elastic fiber damage is primarily linked to oxygen damage and an increased activity of elastase (Bruce et al., 1985). With damage to the cellular matrix, further deposition of collagen and elastin is erratic. Although the effects of prematurity on the molecular mechanisms of lung growth are not clearly defined, the consequences of decreased alveolar surface area and airway hyperreactivity have significant clinical implications.

The First 6 Years

Chronic lung injury secondary to prematurity characteristically includes decreased vital capacity (VC), obstruction of small airways, chest hyperinflation, and reactive airways disease. Infants with BPD are more severely affected than those without BPD, and both have worse function than healthy infants born at term. Over the first 1 to 2 years of life, the expremature infant often has significant respiratory symptoms. Reactive airways disease is common and is exacerbated by a high incidence of infections (Greenough et al., 1990; Parat et al., 1995; Smyth et al., 1995; Tarpy and Celi, 1995; Walther et al., 1995; Tait et al., 2001). Oxygen therapy may be necessary for months to years in order to maintain oxygen saturation between 90% and 95%. Bronchodilators and diuretics are often mainstays of therapy. Significant hypoxemia often accompanies respiratory infections, and hospital admission and readjustment of medications are repeatedly needed. Finally, aspiration associated with gastroesophageal reflux can lead to acute or recurrent pulmonary deterioration (Greenough et al., 1990; Radford et al., 1996). These trends persist in the postsurfactant era, and similar data have been recently reported in ELBW infants (Baraldi and Filippone, 2007). Especially in the first 3 years of life, expreterm infants with a history of BPD are more likely to wheeze, cough, and require hospitalization for respiratory illness. (Hack and Fanaroff, 2000; Lamarche-Vadel et al., 2004; Greenough et al., 2005; Hennessy et al., 2008).

Some have noted that the conditions of patients with BPD may worsen over the first year, especially in the setting of acute viral infections, particularly respiratory syncytial virus (RSV). Preterm infants with BPD are at high risk for RSV infection because of the severity of their illness, their greater risk for respiratory failure, and the need for mechanical ventilation (Simon et al., 2007; Simoes, 2008). The impaired parenchymal and vascular development in the setting of new BPD may predispose this population to the inflammatory consequences of RSV that result in alveolar overinflation and pulmonary edema (Carpenter and Stenmark, 2004). Thus, expremature infants, even those without BPD, have been targeted to receive immunization with palivizumab (Lanctot et al., 2008).

After the First 6 Years—Adolescents and Adults

In 1990, Northway presented a follow-up study of 26 patients (ages 14 to 23 years) from his original cohort (Northway et al., 1967, 1990). Only one of the patients in the initial cohort had weighed less than 1500 g and was born at fewer than 30 weeks' gestation. On follow up, 76% of patients had pulmonary dysfunction (e.g., abnormalities on pulmonary function tests, reactive airways disease, or both). Airway obstruction was noted in 68% of patients, with 24% having fixed airway obstruction. Although all were leading normal lives and were usually asymptomatic, the former BPD patients had more incidences of wheezing and pneumonia, limitation of exercise, and long-term medication use.

Almost 20 years after the introduction of surfactant and with revised approaches to ventilation and oxygen therapy, studies have examined the pulmonary function of school-aged and older expremature infants. These infants can be divided into two groups: expremature infants who were treated with surfactant and expremature infants who were not. In one study, the pulmonary function of school-aged expremature infants with CLD who did not receive surfactant at birth was measured serially when the children were between 6 and 10 years of age and again between 11 and 18 years of age. At the final testing, pulmonary function tests revealed normal total lung capacity (TLC) and normal VC, but these values had improved over the course of the repeated pulmonary function studies. RV and RV/TLC decreased over time, suggesting gradual improvement in air trapping (Koumbourlis et al., 1996). The PEFR, FEV_1, and the ratio of FEV_1 to forced vital capacity (FVC) remained at or above the normal range in all patients. $FEF_{25\%-75\%}$, $FEF_{50\%}$, and $FEF_{75\%}$ were decreased in 50% of these patients. The lower values are suggestive of obstruction of relatively small airways. Regardless, most children in both groups responded to inhaled bronchodilator treatment.

Doyle (2006) has reported outcomes for patients at ages 8, 11, 14, and 19 years as part of a prospective longitudinal research study of VLBW survivors. Although the data in late adolescence reflect different neonatal practices than those currently followed, the report is notable in that it documents that airflow abnormalities at younger ages persisted into adulthood. Most subjects in the non-BPD group had normal lung function. In contrast, some variables reflecting airflow were lower in those with BPD compared with the non-BPD group. That is, 33% of the BPD group but only 8% of the non-BPD group had an FEV_1 greater than 75% predicted. Similarly, 42% and 16% of the BPD and non-BPD groups, respectively, had an FEV_1/FVC of less than 75%. However, when the non-BPD group was compared with a control group of normal birth weight, only 94% met their predicted FEV_1, compared with 99% of the control subjects. Similarly, FEV_1/FVC predicted values were met in 83% vs. 89% of the non-BPD group vs. controls. A significant finding in this study was that between 8 and 19 years of age, the BPD subjects had a greater decrease in the FEV_1/FVC ratio than the non-BPD group, and this difference was greater if the subjects were smokers. Similarly, Halvorsen et al. (2004) reported that in 17-year-old subjects, both FEV_1 and FEF were decreased in proportion to the severity of BPD. Those with moderate to severe BPD had greater decreases in FEV_1 and FEF than those with mild BPD, who in turn showed greater decreases than preterm infants without BPF. Those in the control group experienced the smallest about of decrease in rates.

Lung volume abnormalities tend to gradually normalize in groups of expremature infants with BPD, and the process of recovery continues well into adolescence. Chronic airflow obstruction is common but not present in all expremature infants who had BPD (Fig. 17-17). Of particular significance, expremature infants who had no BPD in the newborn period may actually suffer from obstructive airway disease that persists into adolescence and early adulthood.

The pulmonary function tests in school-aged expremature infants who received surfactant at birth reveal that FVC, FEV_1, and FRC are within normal limits (and similar to values obtained in a group who had not received surfactant) but lower than values in a control group of children born at term.

Airway resistance (Raw) was slightly elevated and maximum expiratory flow (MEF_{25}) was slightly decreased, suggestive of mild lower-airway obstruction. In addition, similar to studies in VLBW infants who were not treated with surfactant, exercise challenge elicited bronchial reactivity. Thus, these data reveal little effect of surfactant on VLBW infants (of 25 to 30 weeks' gestation) from the viewpoint of long-term pulmonary function at 6 to 7 years of age. Of note, surfactant has not dramatically altered respiratory function in ELBW infants (Pelkonen et al., 1998; Gappa et al., 1999).

The following observations can be made in summary:

- More than 90% of children diagnosed with BPD at 36 weeks' postconceptual age had documented airway obstruction in follow-up studies.
- The incidence of β-agonist responsive airway obstruction in expremature infants is striking—45% in those treated with surfactant and 67% in the placebo group, compared with 0% in those who were born at full term.
- The incidence of CLD did not differ after surfactant treatment.
- The duration of tracheal intubation and oxygen therapy, with or without surfactant therapy, correlated with pulmonary outcome (Pelkonen et al., 1998).

BPD and Neurologic Outcome

BPD is a well-recognized risk factor for adverse neurodevelopmental outcome in both the initial few years and at school age. For example, even with the changes in practices in the 1990s, rates of Mental Developmental Index (MDI) scores of less than 70 (severe disability) and overall developmental impairment at about 20 months of age in infants with BPD did not improve when a cohort from 1996 to 1999 was compared with one from 2000 to 2003 (Kobaly et al., 2008). In each group, 42% had an MDI of less than 70 and about 50% of each group had an overall developmental impairment. In another report, the incidences of enrollment in special education classes and scores lower than 70 on full-scale IQ tests (in the mental retardation range) were higher in a group of 8-year-old children who had been VLBW and had BPD (Short et al., 2003). In particular, speech and language problems and the need for occupational and physical therapy, as well as function on applied problems and motor skills, were all affected in the BPD group. Difficulty with mathematics seemed to be most pronounced.

In addition, Thompson et al. (2007), identified a uniform reduction in various cerebral volumes in premature infants with BPD. The common finding of arrested growth in both the brain and the lungs may eventually be linked via a specific molecular or physiologic pathway, extending understanding beyond the observational and shifting therapy toward prevention, rather than treatment, of complications.

The Expremature Infant: Neurologic Function

Injury to the brain in the perinatal period often can be linked to lifelong complications, including a higher risk for motor disorders, learning or developmental delays, seizures, and death. No specific therapy has been identified for long-term cognitive, sensory, and motor deficits. Minimizing or preventing neurologic complications from perinatal injury requires extensive knowledge of the precise cellular and molecular mechanisms of the developing brain's response to asphyxia, hypoxia, and inflammation. Such mechanisms have not been definitively mapped and cannot be definitely correlated with specific clinical scenarios, except in a very general way. Most agree that injury to the developing brain involves an initial insult from hypoxia or ischemia, followed by secondary damage from reperfusion that results in excitotoxicity and release of various cytokines; however, precisely connecting this principle to clinical care is often impossible (Perlman, 2006).

Schmidt et al. (2003) studied the rate of neurodevelopmental disability associated with a history of having between one and three of the following conditions: BPD, an abnormality visible on a head ultrasound, and severe ROP. The incidence of disability was 18%, 42%, 63%, and 88% with 0, 1, 2, or 3 of these complications, respectively.

Of significance, neonatal events associated with sepsis seem to be associated with a particularly high incidence of adverse neurodevelopment in preterm infants. The group with sepsis or NEC was noted to have delayed cognitive and motor development at 2 years (Shah et al., 2008).

Advances in neuroimaging techniques (e.g., diffusion-weighted MRI and spectroscopy) have dramatically advanced our knowledge about patterns of injury at various gestational and postnatal ages and allowed these to be correlated with the severity and nature of clinical events. Vulnerability to injury varies in different areas of the brain and for different cell populations at various maturational stages. For example, hypoxic-ischemic injury is most commonly associated with white-matter injury in premature infants but is associated with cortical or subcortical damage in term infants. In both groups, injury tends to evolve over days to weeks. The early, rapid necrotic death of cells is followed by the delayed neurodegeneration secondary to energy failure and membrane dysfunction, edema, massive neurotransmitter release, effects of oxygen free radicals and calcium release, and other complex cellular and molecular derangements. Thus, gestational and postnatal ages and severity of insult interact to define the neuropathology (e.g., region and extent of injury) of prenatal and neonatal brain injury and developmental outcome.

Brain Injury in the Preterm Infant

For simplicity, white-matter injury in the preterm infant can be divided into two main categories: PVHI and PVL. The effects of each are often difficult to separate, since they commonly coexist. In the past, cranial ultrasounds of the preterm infant identified focal necrotic lesions that evolved into cysts. These lesions seemed to correlate with the development of cerebral palsy (10% to 15% of VLBW infants). Although such severe lesions obviously define significant risk for abnormal development, most cases of abnormal neurologic outcome could not be correlated with the presence of cystic PVL or PVHI (Miller et al., 2003). Developmental deficits beyond what would be expected from focal white-matter injury are common in follow-up care of the ELBW infant. For example, the high incidence of cognitive deficits without prominent motor deficits among survivors of prematurity (approximately 50%) is more commonly attributed to neuronal abnormalities rather than white-matter abnormalities (Volpe, 2003).

Over the last decade, the nature of brain injury associated with prematurity has been identified as a more diffuse, noncystic white-matter injury and has been described in at least 50% of ELBW patients. Of major significance, studies using quantitative MRI have linked gray-matter injury to this diffuse white-matter injury (Volpe, 2003). That is, neuronal loss parallels the white-matter injury. Although the specific link between white- and gray-matter injury has not been clarified, the concept that prematurity disrupts the coordinated growth of the entire brain seems well accepted (Kepellou et al., 2006; Counsell et al., 2007).

Clinical Outcome

At least 50% of VLBW infants are diagnosed with white-matter injury based on MRI findings (Volpe, 2003; Dyet et al., 2006). Of significance, abnormalities persist and are seen in MRIs performed in late childhood and adolescence (Constable et al., 2008; Ment et al., 2009). Most studies of VLBW and ELBW infants note that although neurosensory deficits (e.g., hearing loss or blindness) have decreased, problems with cognitive and academic function and behavior (e.g., attention disorders, emotional control issues, or problems with social interaction) have increased. In addition, a higher incidence of anxiety and depressive disorders has been reported in expremature infants (Rickards et al., 2001; Saigal et al., 2003; Anderson and Doyle, 2004; Wilson-Costello et al., 2007; Constable et al., 2008; Kobaly et al., 2008; Ment and Vohr, 2008). In several reports, these problems have been noted to persist into adolescence and adulthood (Hack et al., 2004; Farooqi et al., 2006). Even with the pervasive incidence of intellectual, emotional, and academic disorders in expremature infants, lower rates of risky behaviors have been reported in young adults (Hack et al., 2004). Saigal et al. (2006) also reported that, in spite of lower levels of educational achievements, expremature infants display a high level of adapting and functioning as adults.

Cerebral Palsy

Cerebral palsy (CP) refers to a group of nonprogressive motor dysfunction syndromes related to CNS lesions encountered early in development, but they are usually without a clear-cut etiology. Cerebral palsy is diagnosed in approximately 1 infant per 1000 live births (Wu et al., 2006). The increase in motor tone observed with CP includes spasticity, rigidity, and dystonia; some patients have choreoathetosis. About half of the cases of CP are diagnosed in full-term infants.

A variety of lesions in neuroimaging studies accompany the clinical diagnosis. For example, Wu et al. (2006) noted a wide range of findings in a series of 273 patients (227 MRI; 46 CT), including focal infarction (22%), malformation (14%), periventricular white-matter abnormalities (12%), generalized brain atrophy (7%), hypoxic-ischemic brain injury (5%), and intracranial hemorrhage (5%). On closer examination, 45% of patients with spastic hemiparesis had evidence of focal arterial infarction. The brain malformations were diverse (e.g., schizencephaly, agenesis of the corpus callosum, polymicrogyria, septooptic dysplasia, and others). Of significance was the low incidence of

findings consistent with hypoxic-ischemic injury (5%) and the high incidence of a normal brain (31%).

SUMMARY

The medical and surgical history of the expremature infant is often characterized by a complicated medical and surgical history, often with superimposed persistent chronic disease. Preoperative assessment and integration of these chronic problems into the acute surgical and anesthetic setting require careful review of records and communication with multiple caregivers. As patients grow and develop, the relevance of their perinatal and neonatal course diminishes. Nonetheless, many of the events of early life can manifest as life-long disabilities, such as chronic pulmonary problems and developmental delay.

Reactive airways disease of the expremature has been reported to be less responsive to antiinflammatory agents and more prone to serious complications from RSV.

Developmental delay (and associated medical problems) is common in premature infants. Patients with neurologic disorders have a high incidence of autonomic neuropathy, which delays esophagogastric transit and gastric emptying. Neurologically impaired children are at high risk for symptomatic gastroesophageal reflux, especially when the patient is fed via nasogastric tube or gastrostomy. In addition, delayed gastric emptying has been documented in infants and children with neurologic disorders and symptoms of gastroesophageal reflux.

In addition to the medical issues of the expremature, parents of expremature infants are often over protective, have extensive experience with health care providers, and can provide encyclopedic data about their child's history (Wightman et al., 2007). Effectively interacting with parents of an expremature infant may require greater sensitivity and take more time than usual. Preoperative anxiety may be great in any child who requires repeated interaction with the operating room, but the challenge may be even greater in the setting of the patient with developmental delay and a variety of significant coexisting problems.

Various personality traits have also been associated with some older expremature patients, including anxiety and social isolation (Rickards et al., 2001; Allin et al., 2006; Wightman et al., 2007). Although evaluation of and attention to such traits in the preoperative setting are similar to others with a similar history, in the context of the expremature infant, focusing on the multitude of complex medical problems may allow the psychological concerns to be underappreciated.

For questions and answers on topics in this chapter, go to "Chapter Questions" at www.expertconsult.com.

REFERENCES

Complete references used in this text can be found online at www.expertconsult.com.

Anesthesia for General Surgery in the Neonate

Claire Brett and Peter J. Davis

CONTENTS

Surgical procedures during the neonatal period impose significant physiologic perturbations on the infant. With increasing regularity, diseases of adult life have been linked to events in early development (in utero, newborn, infancy, or childhood). For example, intrauterine growth retardation has been linked to an increased risk for a variety of adult disorders, including coronary heart disease, stroke, hypertension, type II diabetes, and even psychiatric illness (Barker and Osmond, 1986a; Barker, 1995, 2006; Ravelli et al., 1998; Singhal et al., 2003, 2004; Barker et al., 2005; Mittendorfer-Rutz et al., 2007). In addition, early postnatal and childhood nutrition and obesity have been associated with metabolic disorders such as dyslipidemia and glucose intolerance, growth abnormalities, and cardiovascular disease in adults (Huang et al., 2007; Mikkola et al., 2007; Rakow et al., 2008). These adult disorders with pediatric foundations were initially based on Barker and Osmond's epidemiologic study (1986b). However, subsequent research has expanded his original "thrifty-phenotype" hypothesis (i.e., survival of the undernourished fetus demands that nutrition be directed to vital organs such as the brain, resulting in insulin resistance in other tissues such as muscle and the pancreas) to include a "developmental plasticity" theory (Hales and Barker, 2001; Gluckman et al., 2005; McMillen and Robinson, 2005). These initial reports have spawned an entire focal point for research and a model termed the *developmental origins of health and disease* (Gluckman et al., 2005; Gillman et al., 2007; Silveira et al., 2007). Recently, the increased risk for cardiovascular and metabolic disease has been extended to include preterm infants, both those who are appropriate for gestational age (AGA) and those who are small for gestational age (SGA) (Hofman et al., 2004a, 2004b; Mikkola et al., 2007).

Perhaps the most obvious and irrefutable link between early events and adult diseases exists in the settings of major congenital anomalies and preterm birth. The full impact of the synergistic roles of the thrifty phenotype and developmental plasticity theories remains to be defined, but the critical long-term effects (from early postnatal development and beyond) of disease processes encountered after preterm birth and associated with congenital anomalies is already appreciated. This chapter addresses anesthetic pharmacology for the neonate, approaches to intraoperative monitoring of the neonate, and the more common neonatal general surgical procedures with respect to perioperative management, embryology, and long-term outcome.

ANESTHETIC PHARMACOLOGY IN THE NEONATE

Increasing evidence indicates that the physiologic response of neonates to painful stimuli is similar to that of adults (see Chapter 15, Pain Management). The response of the sympathetic nervous system to noxious stimulation includes tachycardia and hypertension, which in the setting of abnormal cerebral autoregulation predisposes the infant with a low birth weight (LBW) to intraventricular hemorrhage and possibly pulmonary hypertension. The goal during anesthesia is to avoid pain and its cardiovascular and neurologic consequences. The response of newborns to opioids and potent inhalation agents is variable, and meticulous titration is critical for neonates undergoing surgery, both to avoid cardiovascular collapse and to maintain acid-base balance and also to eliminate awareness and pain.

Pharmacokinetics and Pharmacodynamics

Pharmacokinetics and pharmacodynamics of drugs are affected by anatomic factors relating to body composition and distribution of water, as well as physiologic factors such as metabolism (i.e., hepatic biotransformation); protein binding; and pathologic factors (e.g., disease, anesthesia, and surgery) (see Chapter 7, Pharmacology of Pediatric Anesthesia). Maturational changes in distribution of total body water, tissue composition, and organ function contribute to the unique response of the newborn and young infant to various drugs. In early fetal development, water constitutes approximately 94% of body weight. As gestation continues, the total body water decreases so that at 32 weeks, 80% to 90% of body weight is water, and at term, total body water is approximately 70% to 75% of body weight. Adult proportions of fluid to body weight (55%) are reached between the ages of 9 months and 2 years. The distribution of water between the extracellular and intracellular compartments also changes during fetal growth. Extracellular water (interstitial fluid plus plasma volume) decreases from 60% of body weight at the fifth month of fetal life to approximately 45% at term. Intracellular water increases from 25% in the fifth month of fetal life to 33% at birth; therefore, the extracellular fluid compartment of the newborn is equal to or greater than the intracellular fluid space. In adults, the intracellular and extracellular fluid compartments are approximately 40% and 20% of body weight, respectively. Because the plasma component of the extracellular fluid compartment remains at approximately 5% of body weight throughout life, it is the interstitial water that is greater in infancy (40%) and declines to 10% to 15% in the adult (Friis-Hansen, 1971).

Age-dependent changes in body composition also occur. At term, fat constitutes 11% of body weight. Fat content doubles by 6 months of age and is approximately 30% at 1 year. Teenage girls remain with approximately 20% to 30% fat, whereas fat in teenage boys decreases to 10% to 15% fat. Moreover, the composition of fat tissue changes with age. Fat of the newborn may contain as much as 57% water and 35% lipids; adults have 26% water and 71% lipids (Friis-Hansen, 1971). Skeletal muscle comprises 25% of total body mass in a full-term newborn compared with 43% in an adult.

The binding of drugs to serum proteins depends on several factors, including the concentration of protein, the number of binding sites on these proteins, and the affinity of the binding sites. The concentration of total serum protein, albumin, and α_1-acid glycoprotein is lower in early infancy and reaches adult levels by approximately 1 year of age (Pacifica et al., 1986). Albumin primarily binds acidic drugs; α_1-acid glycoprotein binds basic drugs. The concentration of these two proteins and their binding affinities are deficient in the newborn (Piafsky and Woolner, 1982).

The primary organ for drug biotransformation is the liver, but the kidneys, intestines, lungs, and skin also have minor roles. Hepatic oxidation, reduction, and hydrolysis (nonsynthetic, phase I reactions) mature rapidly, achieving adult rates by 6 months (Niems et al., 1976). Drugs metabolized via this cytochrome P450-dependent monooxygenase system include phenobarbital and phenytoin. Conjugation reactions (synthetic, phase II reactions) convert drugs into more polar compounds to facilitate renal excretion. These systems also mature postnatally.

The renal excretion of drugs is a function of glomerular filtration rate (GFR), active secretion, and passive reabsorption. GFR and secretion increase in an age-dependent manner. Renal blood flow and GFR increase dramatically during the first postnatal week and more gradually during the next several months, and adult performance is achieved at approximately 6 to 12 months of age (Arant, 1978; Hook and Bailie, 1979). Tubular secretory and reabsorptive capacity also mature postnatally (Fetterman et al., 1965).

Cardiac output and its distribution to various organs contribute to drug elimination. The perinatal adaptation to extrauterine life demands rapid changes in the circulation. This process may be inhibited as a result of congenital heart disease or acid-base problems. Drug metabolism and elimination may be drastically affected when cardiovascular function is abnormal.

Inhaled Anesthetic Agents

Infants have a higher incidence of cardiovascular instability and cardiac arrest during induction of inhalational anesthesia than do older persons (Rackow et al., 1961; Friesen and Lichtor, 1982, 1983; Morray, 2000, 2002; Murat et al., 2004). This untoward effect of potent inhalational agents can be attributed to several factors, including faster equilibration, rapid myocardial uptake in infants, the increased anesthetic requirement, and sensitivity of the neonatal myocardium. Infants attain a higher concentration of inhaled anesthetic agents in the heart and brain than do adults at the same inspired concentration. Moreover, the neonatal myocardium has a smaller fraction of contractile mass, and the magnitude and velocity of fiber shortening are less than in the adult myocardium. These factors and the increased anesthetic requirement, which is inversely related to age, all produce a higher incidence of adverse cardiovascular effects in infants.

The rate of rise of the alveolar concentration of an inhaled anesthetic depends on several factors: the inspired concentration, alveolar ventilation, and uptake. The greater the alveolar ventilation, the faster is the rate of rise of the alveolar concentration. This effect of alveolar ventilation is affected by the size of the functional residual capacity (FRC). Infants and children have an FRC similar to that of the adult, 30 mL/kg per minute. In contrast, alveolar ventilation is much higher in the infant (100 to 150 mL/kg per minute) compared with the adult (60 mL/kg per minute). This difference parallels the greater oxygen consumption of the infant. Thus, in the normal term newborn who weighs 3.0 kg, the ratio of alveolar ventilation to FRC is approximately 5:1, compared with the adult, in whom the same ratio is 1.5:1. As a result of this difference, the time constant of the inhaled anesthetic equilibrium for infants is much shorter than for the adult. Consequently, changes in concentrations of inspired gas are reflected rapidly in alveolar levels. In fact, it has been demonstrated that alveolar levels of inhalational anesthetic agents reach equilibrium faster in infants that in adults (see Chapter 7, Pharmacology of Pediatric Anesthesia).

The rise of the alveolar concentration of an inhaled anesthetic is opposed by uptake of the agent into lung tissue and more importantly, blood. Three factors determine inhaled anesthetic uptake: cardiac output, the alveolar-to-mixed venous anesthetic partial pressure difference, and solubility. Each of these factors has unique aspects in the infant, compared with in the adult, and consequently affects the pharmacology of the uptake of inhaled agents.

The greater the cardiac output, the greater is the anesthetic uptake. The cardiac output of the newborn is 250 to 300 mL/kg per minute; by 8 weeks of age, the cardiac output has decreased to 150 mL/kg per minute. The cardiac output of young infants is approximately 3 to 6 times that of the normal adult (70 mL/kg per minute). By itself, this high cardiac output should significantly decrease the rate of rise of the alveolar concentration of the soluble anesthetic agents. However, the newborn distributes a greater proportion of this cardiac output to the vessel-rich group of organs and a smaller proportion to the muscle and fat group. The equilibrium between the inspired and alveolar concentrations of inhaled agent occurs more rapidly, because uptake decreases faster.

Because the cardiac output is predominantly distributed to the vessel-rich group and because the muscle group is small, the arterial-venous partial pressure difference narrows quickly in the young and thereby decreases uptake.

Both left-to-right and right-to-left shunting occurs in infants. A left-to-right shunt results in an increase in total cardiac output. However, the shunted blood does not lose anesthetic to tissue; instead it returns to the lung with the same anesthetic partial pressure. This recycled blood cannot accept more anesthetic agent unless the alveolar partial pressure has risen. Thus, a left-to-right shunt has no effect on anesthetic uptake. A right-to-left shunt slows the rate of rise of the alveolar concentration of an inhaled anesthetic. The anesthetic-deficient, shunted blood dilutes the concentration of the anesthetic in the blood, decreasing the partial pressure of anesthetic in the arterial circulation. This slows the rate of rise of the anesthetic by slowing tissue uptake and equilibration.

Blood-gas partition coefficients of isoflurane, halothane, and sevoflurane did not differ in preterm infants compared with full-term infants but were lower than in adults. Only serum cholesterol correlated with the blood-gas partition coefficients (Malviya and Lerman, 1990). The blood-gas partition coefficient is an important determinant of solubility and therefore the rate of rise of the alveolar concentration of an inhaled agent.

The effect of age on the solubility of the inhaled agents in tissue is also important in determining the rate of rise of the alveolar concentration of the agent—the rate of anesthetic induction. Data by Lerman et al. (1986) are consistent with earlier work documenting that anesthetic solubility in brain, heart, liver, and muscle increases with age. An increase in solubility may prolong uptake, delay equilibration of the tissue partial pressure of anesthetic, and prolong the time of induction. Lerman and others found that the rate of increase in tissue anesthetic partial pressure, and therefore alveolar anesthetic partial pressure, is approximately 30% more rapid in newborns than in adults.

Minimal alveolar concentration (MAC) is an estimate of anesthetic requirement and changes with age (Fig. 18-1) (Katoh and Ikeda, 1987, 1992; LeDez and Lerman, 1987). In the original study, Gregory et al. (1969) reported that infants in the first 6 months of life had the highest MAC. In a later study, newborns were noted to require approximately 25% less halothane at MAC compared with infants who are between 1 and 6 months of age (Lerman et al., 1983) (see Chapter 7, Pharmacology of Pediatric Anesthesia).

Intravenous Anesthetics and Analgesics

Several studies have shown an increased sensitivity to and more prolonged effects of barbiturates and morphine in the neonate and young infant (Kupferberg and Way, 1963; Way et al., 1965).

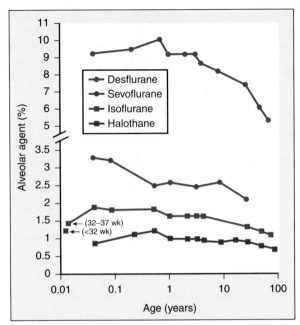

■ **FIGURE 18-1.** Effect of age on MAC of anesthetic gases. The MAC of anesthetic gases is dependent on age. MAC is higher at birth than in adults and increases until peaking at 3 to 6 months. The values at 1 year of age are closer to the adult values. *(From Greeley WJ: Pediatric anesthesia, In Miller RD, editor: Atlas of anesthesia, vol 7, Philadelphia, 1999, Churchill Livingstone.)*

These features have been attributed in part to the immaturity of the blood-brain barrier, allowing faster and greater penetration and therefore higher concentration of these drugs in the brain.

In 1981, Robinson and Gregory reported that after a 10 mL/kg bolus of lactated Ringer's solution, 30 to 50 mcg/kg of fentanyl was a safe anesthetic for premature infants undergoing ligation of a patent ductus arteriosus (PDA). Several years later, evidence was presented that infants who received fentanyl in combination with d-tubocurarine and nitrous oxide in oxygen had an improved perioperative course compared with those infants who did not receive analgesics (Anand et al., 1987).

Plasma levels of fentanyl are lower in infants vs. children vs. adults (newborns were not studied) after similar intravenous doses (Singleton et al., 1987). Gauntlett and others (1988) noted that clearance of fentanyl in newborns increased during the first few weeks of life. Elimination half-life and volume of distribution did not change. In a study of newborns who were administered continuous fentanyl infusions, Saarenmaa and others (2000) noted that plasma clearance correlated with maturity (gestational age) and weight, whereas Santeiro and others (1997) noted a correlation of clearance with postnatal age (Fig. 18-2). Koehntop et al. (1986) have shown a highly variable disposition and elimination of fentanyl in neonates. In addition, infants with increased intraabdominal pressure (e.g., omphalocele, gastroschisis, or septic ileus) appeared to have a further increase in the elimination half-life compared with infants undergoing repair of a PDA or myelomeningocele. Davis and others (1989) noted that the clearance of alfentanil in newborn premature infants was markedly reduced compared with older children (Fig. 18-3).

Koren and others (1985) have shown that the elimination half-life for morphine (13.9 hours) in human neonates is markedly prolonged compared with that in older children and adults (2 hours). They also showed reduced clearance and higher

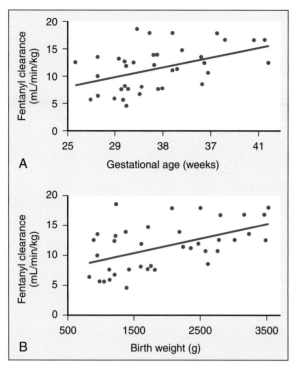

FIGURE 18-2. Plasma clearance of fentanyl correlates with **A,** gestational age (r = 0.46, P < 0.01), and **B,** birth weight (r = 0.48, P < 0.01). *(From Saarenmaa et al.: Gestational age and birth weight effects of plasma clearance of fentanyl in newborn infants,* J Pediatr *136:767, 2000.)*

serum concentration in neonates compared with those seen in older children after morphine infusion. Because of the large variability in clearance among neonates of different ages, the dose of opioids needs to be carefully titrated for each patient and each clinical setting.

Remifentanil is an ultrashort-acting opioid. Remifentanil is metabolized by plasma and tissue esterases, and its metabolism is independent of organ elimination. As a result, in neonates its pharmacokinetic profile is different from any other opioid. The remifentanil clearance rate in neonates is greater than in any other age group. Although its volume of distribution is large, its terminal elimination half-life does not change with age (Ross et al., 2001). Because remifentanil is metabolized in tissues and plasma, it does not accumulate, and consequently its context-sensitive half-time is flat (i.e., the time for 50% reduction at the effect site is independent of drug duration). Thus, remifentanil may be an ideal drug for anesthetic use in neonates.

Animal studies have shown a decreased median effective dose (ED$_{50}$) for thiopental in the early weeks of life. Also, arousal in newborn rats occurred at lower brain levels of thiopental than in adult rats (Mirkin, 1975). Although this may suggest that lower doses of thiopental are needed in young neonates, studies by Jonmarker and others (1987) suggest the contrary. Similarly, ketamine requirements are greater (mg per kg of body weight) in infants than in older children (Lockhart and Nelson, 1974). Ketamine has been shown to produce apnea in infants with increased intracranial pressure (Lockhart and Jenkins, 1972). Ketamine produces hypertension and tachycardia, which some anesthesiologists have taken advantage of in caring for infants and children with congenital heart disease, cardiovascular instability, or both.

Propofol is commonly administered to infants. Propofol clearance is dependent on hepatic blood flow (high extraction coefficient) with subsequent metabolism and glucuronidation. In population pharmacokinetic analysis, Allegaert et al. (2007) noted that postmenstrual age and postnatal age were predictive covariants for clearance and that developmental maturation occurs within the first two weeks of life (Fig. 18-4).

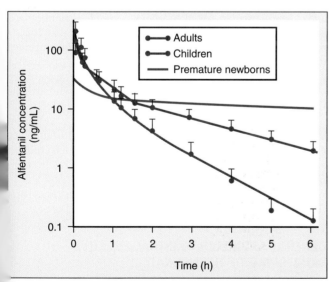

FIGURE 18-3. Age-related changes in alfentanil pharmacokinetics for premature infants, children, and adults. *(From Davis CM, Brando M: Pediatric pharmacology. In Greeley W, editor:* Atlas of anesthesiology, *vol 7, Philadelphia, 1999, Churchill Livingstone.)*

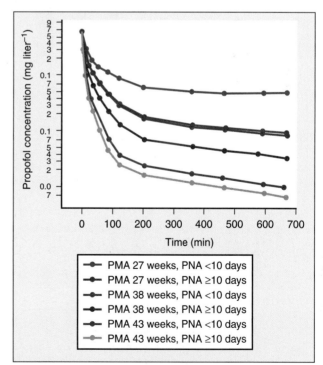

FIGURE 18-4. Simulated population propofol concentrations *(line)* in neonates aged 27, 38, and 43 weeks' gestation, with a postnatal age (PNA) of 10 days or less, after a bolus dose of 9 mg in 10 seconds. *(From Allegaert et al.: Interindividual variability in propofol pharmacokinetics in preterm and term neonates,* Br J Anaesth *99:864, 2007.)*

Midazolam is an extensively used drug in both full-term and preterm infants and is metabolized by the P450 3A subfamily. Midazolam clearance in preterm infants is less than in children and older infants, and it may reflect the pattern of CYP3A4 ontogeny (Fig. 18-5). DeWildt et al. (2001), in a study of 24 preterm infants, found no relationship between age (postconceptual, gestational, or postnatal) and midazolam clearance. Of note was that in infants exposed postnatally to indomethacin, plasma clearance was higher and the volume of distribution was larger than in those infants not exposed to indomethacin. Because CYP3A4 expression is actuated during the first week after birth regardless of gestational age at birth, the decrease in midazolam clearance probably represents a decrease in CYP3A activity.

Muscle Relaxants

Developmental pharmacologic changes influence the requirements for muscle relaxants in infants and older children. Synaptic transmission is slow at birth, the rate at which acetylcholine is released during repetitive stimulation is limited, and neuromuscular reserve is reduced (Fig. 18-6). In addition, the reported sensitivity of infants to the effects of neuromuscular blocking

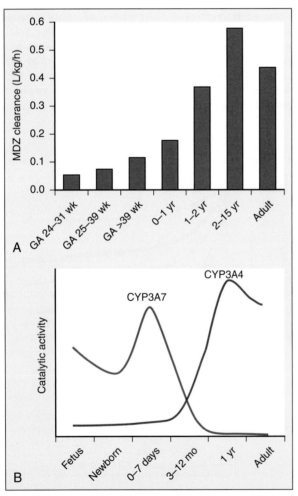

FIGURE 18-5. Developmental aspects of CYP3A activity. **A,** Clearance of the CYP3A4 probe midazolam. **B,** CYP3A7 and CYP3A4 expression. *GA,* Gestational age; *MDZ,* midazolam. *(From de Wildt SN et al.: Cytochrome P450 3A: ontogeny and drug disposition, Clin Pharmacokinet 37:485, 1999.)*

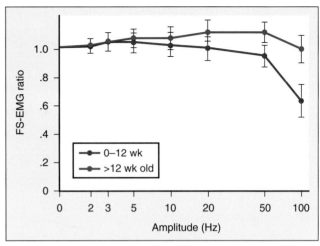

FIGURE 18-6. Tracings of the frequency sweep electromyogram (FS-EMG). *(From Crumrine RS, Yodlowski EH: Assessment of neuromuscular function in infants, Anesthesiology 54:29, 1981.)*

agents has differed depending on whether drug administration was indexed to body weight or to body surface area. Because most neuromuscular blocking agents are distributed in the extracellular space and the extracellular space is related to the body surface area, dosage requirements for neuromuscular blocking agents often correlate with surface area rather than with body weight. Neonates and infants have a higher sensitivity (lower ED_{50} and ED_{95}) for most nondepolarizing blocking agents.

Fisher et al. (1982) studied infants' sensitivity to nondepolarizing muscle relaxants using the pharmacodynamic and pharmacokinetic properties of d-tubocurarine. These investigators determined the steady-state plasma concentration associated with 50% neuromuscular blockade (CP_{ss50}) and noted that infants had a lower CP_{ss50} than older children. Because the volume of distribution of d-tubocurarine in infants is significantly larger than that in older children, the dose (mg per kg of body weight) required to achieve the same degree of neuromuscular blockade appeared the same for infants and older children. Although the pharmacokinetic data reveal similar clearance values for infants and older children, the infant's larger volume of distribution and consequently longer elimination half-life suggest that infants need less frequent and smaller supplemental doses for continued neuromuscular relaxation. Although these data are specific for d-tubocurarine, the general principles can be extrapolated to other hydrophilic compounds that are primarily distributed to the "central compartment" (i.e., small volume of distribution).

Studies of rocuronium in infants and children have shown that onset time in small infants is faster, and the occurrence of 100% block at lower doses compared with older children suggests a greater potency in infants. In addition, rocuronium has an age-dependent difference in duration of action and in recovery following 0.45 mg/kg and 0.6 mg/kg doses (Fig. 18-7) (Driessen et al., 2000; Rapp et al., 2004).

GENERAL APPROACH TO INTRAOPERATIVE MONITORING OF THE NEONATE

Safe and effective intraoperative management of the newborn depends on understanding basic principles of physiology and pharmacology, as well as understanding the technical aspects of monitoring and the anesthesia equipment.

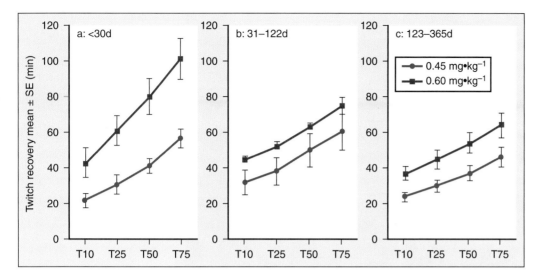

■ FIGURE 18-7. Recovery of twitch to 10%, 25%, 50%, and 75% of baseline value *(min)* in infants after single-dose relaxation with rocuronium bromide (n=61, mean ± SE). Note significant differences between 0 and 1 month and between 5 and 12 months. P = 0.05 (0.45 mg • kg⁻¹) and P = 0.05 (0.6 mg • kg⁻¹). *(From Rapp et al.: Neuromuscular recovery following rocuronium bromide single dose in infants, Pediatr Anesth 14:329, 2004.)*

Thermal Protection

As already described, the newborn infant loses thermal protection after birth, so measures must be taken to protect against heat loss during surgery (Box 18-1):

Attention must be paid to fine, seemingly insignificant details in the care of a sick neonate because the margin of safety is narrow. Although advanced electronic monitoring has contributed significantly to the safety of these babies, the anesthesiologists' clinical skills, judgment, and evaluation remain indispensable.

Monitoring in the Operating Room

General Observation

Color (e.g., cyanosis and pallor), chest mobility (e.g., bilateral expansion, respiratory pattern, and chest compliance), and palpation (e.g., warmth, pulses, and peripheral perfusion) are often difficult to assess because of the patient's position and draping on the operating room (OR) bed. The use of specific monitors depends on the planned surgical intervention and the underlying disease state.

Circulatory Monitoring

A precordial stethoscope is a simple and effective means to assess the quality of heart sounds, rate, and rhythm, as well as breath sounds. A change in the intensity of heart sounds

---

Box 18-1 Protection Against Heat Loss During Surgery

Transport the baby in a heated isolette
Warm the operating room to more than 27° C (80° F)
Use a warming mattress (water temperature of 40° C)
Heat and humidify gases to 36° C (at the trachea)
Use a radiant heat warmer with a servocontrol mechanism
Wrap noninvolved areas with plastic
Warm intravenous fluids and blood
Warm scrubbing and irrigation solutions
Monitor the temperature in the operating room

---

indicates a decrease in blood pressure and possibly cardiac output. Depending on the surgical procedure and the method of airway management (mask vs. laryngeal mask airway [LMA] vs. endotracheal tube), an esophageal stethoscope is an alternative monitor for noninvasive beat-to-beat cardiovascular monitoring. Although the sensitivity of the stethoscope has been discussed, the simplicity and accuracy of the precordial and esophageal devices to monitor heart tones and breath sounds during surgery involving pediatric patients cannot be denied (Hubmayr, 2004).

The primary role for continuous electrocardiography during anesthesia for the newborn is to detect arrhythmias, especially in the setting of electrolyte disturbance or as evidence of adverse effects of various drugs. Simple monitoring of heart rate is available via the pulse oximeter, now a routine monitor for all patients in the OR.

In most cases, the blood pressure can be accurately monitored with an automated device based on oscillometry (e.g., Dinamap) or ultrasonic flow (e.g., Arteriosonde) if the appropriate-sized cuff is available. Cuff inflation of the automatic devices should cycle no more frequently than every 3 to 4 minutes to avoid ischemia to the arm (Waugh and Johnson, 1984). Systolic blood pressure measurements correlate with the circulating blood volume and therefore are essential to monitor and guide fluid and blood replacement. Another alternative system is a Doppler ultrasonic transducer, which has a characteristic sound that decreases in intensity with a decrease in blood pressure.

An indwelling arterial cannula allows repeated blood sampling for cardiopulmonary and biochemical evaluation. A 22- or 24-gauge cannula can be inserted percutaneously or by cutdown into a variety of sites, including the radial, dorsalis pedis, or posterior tibial arteries. Before the insertion of the catheter, the adequacy of circulation to the hand should be assessed by applying a modified Allen's test (Brodsky, 1975). The axillary artery is rarely cannulated. In general, the umbilical artery can be cannulated in the first 4 to 7 days of life, but this is usually avoided after the first 2 days of life because of the risks of infection and vascular emboli. The umbilical catheter tip can be placed high (T10 to T12) or low, above the bifurcation of the aorta and below the level of the renal arteries (L4, L5). The placement of the catheter must be confirmed by a radiograph (Fig. 18-8).

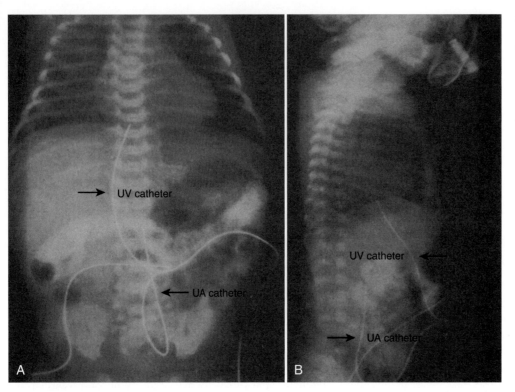

■ **FIGURE 18-8.** Umbilical artery-vein x-ray image. **A,** AP view. **B,** Lateral view. UA and UV catheters have different courses on plain films. The UV catheter goes directly up to the right atrium from the umbilicus, whereas the UA catheter goes down into the external iliac artery and up into the aorta.

The risk for retinopathy of prematurity necessitates meticulous monitoring of oxygen saturation in the neonate, especially the very low–birth-weight (VLBW) infant. Most neonatologists recommend adjusting the inspired oxygen to maintain oxygen saturation between 90% and 95%, depending on the underlying medical status, gestational age, hemoglobin, and postnatal age (i.e., quantity of HgF). Of importance, if blood is shunting right-to-left through a PDA, the oxygen saturation measured in the lower extremities or umbilical artery (postductal site) does not reflect the oxygen saturation in the retinal vessels (preductal site). To enable simultaneous monitoring of both preductal and postductal oxygen saturation, two pulse oximeters are placed—one on the right hand (preductal) and one on a lower extremity (postductal). During right-to-left shunting through the PDA, the preductal oxygen saturation is higher than the postductal value, and the difference depends on the amount of shunting. If blood is shunting right-to-left only via the foramen ovale or other intracardiac sites (e.g., ventriculoseptal defect), the preductal and postductal oxygen saturation are equal (see Chapters 3, 4, and 23, Respiratory Physiology in Infants and Children, Cardiovascular Physiology, and Anesthesia for General Abdominal, Thoracic, Urologic, and Bariatric Surgery).

An arterial cannula must be connected to a pressure transducer and slowly and continuously infused with a small volume of diluted heparin solution (0.1 to 1 units/mL) at the rate of 0.5 to 1 mL/hr. In the extremely low–birth-weight (ELBW) infant, the flush volume should be measured and included in calculating the total daily fluid intake. In addition, extreme caution is critical while flushing an arterial cannula, because retrograde embolization into the cerebral circulation is possible in the small infant, especially with a patent foramen ovale or PDA.

A central venous catheter may be indicated to administer blood, fluid, total parenteral nutrition (TPN) and medications, and to monitor central venous pressure (CVP). Using the Seldinger technique, a catheter can be inserted percutaneously into the subclavian, internal jugular, external jugular, or femoral veins. In emergencies or situations of difficult venous access, the umbilical catheter can be inserted and passed into the right atrium (Fig. 18-8). Its location must be verified by x-ray or by a CVP tracing. Umbilical vein catheters have been associated with portal vein thrombosis. All central venous catheters are associated with significant morbidity, including thrombosis, emboli, and infection. Central venous catheters in the LBW infant have additional risks, from malpositioning and from the disruption of venous flow (ratio of the size of vessel to the size of the catheter is low).

Ventilatory Monitoring

The combination of immature and fragile central nervous and cardiorespiratory systems coupled with unstable chest wall mechanics and variable responses to anesthetic agents are often indications for mechanical ventilatory support both during and after surgery for the newborn. For each patient and for each procedure, the anesthesiologist must evaluate the needs and the requirements for mechanical ventilation. For some infants, the ventilatory status might be so precarious that using a more advanced ventilator from the neonatal intensive care unit intraoperatively might offer additional options for responding to intraoperative events affecting ventilatory status. Of note, if an infant requires a specific mode of ventilatory support, such as high-frequency oscillation, the OR ventilatory strategy should be coordinated with the critical care team.

Manual ventilation has been proposed as a technique to allow the anesthesiologist to continuously sense changes in compliance of the chest and airways. However, Spears and others (1991) noted that manual ventilation can be extremely unreliable for sensing changes in airway compliance. In addition to monitoring heart sounds, the precordial or esophageal stethoscope is a simple system to monitor ventilation and quality of breath sounds. Peak airway and end-expiratory pressure should also be measured. End-tidal carbon dioxide devices (mass spectrometers or infrared analyzers) are now the "standard of care" to continuously monitor the adequacy of respiratory exchange. These devices provide a breath-to-breath level of carbon dioxide tension, and the waveform of this measurement can provide information about rebreathing, ventilator disconnection, suspected air embolism, and hypermetabolic states (see Chapter 10, Equipment).

The pulse oximeter provides a precise, continuous readout of the hemoglobin oxygen saturation. During the first 1 to 2 weeks of life and without transfusion of autologous blood, the oxygen dissociation curve of HgF is shifted to the left of the adult curve so that hemoglobin saturation of 95% to 97% corresponds to an arterial oxygen tension (Pa_{O_2}) of 52 to 77 mm Hg, assuming a Pa_{O_2} at 50% hemoglobin saturation (P_{50}) of 19 mm Hg. The hemoglobin saturation should be correlated with an arterial partial pressure of oxygen (Po_2) measurement to ensure valid interpretation of oxygen saturation data in the OR (see Chapter 3, Respiratory Physiology in Infants and Children).

Monitoring of the Neuromuscular Junction

Neuromuscular blockade can be monitored with a battery-operated nerve stimulator. The simple twitch and train-of-four are elicited by stimulating the ulnar nerve at the wrist or the posterior tibial nerve at the ankle. The neonate's neuromuscular response to nerve stimulation allows the anesthesiologist to titrate further doses of a muscle relaxant and avoid excessive neuromuscular blockade. However, neuromuscular monitoring is technically challenging for VLBW infants because of the small size of their muscles. Accurate data from the transcutaneous devices are often impossible to obtain. Inserting needles into a tiny infant's extremity should be justified because such trauma may cause bleeding or infection. Furthermore, even with needles in place, obtaining a reliable response using the standard battery-operated devices is unpredictable. Of significance, most of these infants require mechanical ventilation postoperatively, so that documenting full recovery to neuromuscular blockade is often unnecessary immediately after surgery.

Monitoring Urine Output

Devices that collect urine during surgery (specifically, Foley catheters or modifications) are helpful, because in the absence of glycosuria, urine output is a good indicator of hydration, circulating volume, and renal function. The desirable range of urine output in the neonate under anesthesia is 0.5 to 2.0 mL/kg per hour. Note that for a 1-kg infant, 0.5 to 2 mL of urine per hour is difficult to reliably collect in the setting of surgical drapes, lack of direct access to the patient, and easy kinking of drainage tubing secondary to pressure and positioning. Thus, in actual practice, accurately assessing urine output is difficult.

MINIMAL-ACCESS SURGERY IN THE NEONATE

The development and refinement of endoscopic tools, optical technology, and surgical skills have allowed even the most complex neonatal procedures, such as congenital diaphragmatic hernia (CDH), tracheoesophageal fistula (TEF), congenital cystic adenomatoid malformation, and lobar emphysema, to be routinely accomplished with minimal-access surgery (Georgeson, 2003; Al-Qahtani and Almaramhi, 2006; Ponsky and Rothenberg, 2008). The field of minimal-access surgery continues to evolve and expand into other arenas such as robotic techniques, "stealth surgery" (or "scarless surgery"), and natural orifice transluminal endoscopic surgery (NOTES) (Dutta and Albanese 2008; Dutta et al., 2008; Isaza et al., 2008).

Endoscopic surgical techniques improve surgical conditions and produce better outcomes for patients. Improved technology has created endoscopic tools and video equipment that produce a magnified image and consequently better visualization of the surgical field. In patients with TEF the thoracoscopic approach improves the surgeon's view, because the fistula is seen perpendicular to its connection to the membranous trachea; consequently the surgeon may more easily identify the exact site for ligation (Fig. 18-9) (Holcomb et al., 2005; Rothenberg, 2005b).

In addition to better visualization, minimally invasive surgery has also been associated with shorter postoperative recovery periods and decreased pain, inflammation, and scarring (Fujimoto et al., 1999). With less trauma to tissues, fluid therapy may be reduced as well. In some specific procedures, such as repair of a TEF, the avoidance of a posterior-lateral thoracotomy may prevent thoracic nerve damage, winged scapula, shoulder girdle weakness, fused ribs, chest wall asymmetry and muscular/soft tissue developmental abnormalities, and scoliosis (Jaureguizar et al., 1985; Rothenberg, 2005a;). In abdominal surgery, the use of minimally invasive techniques may decrease the incidence of adhesive injury after laparoscopy. This may be especially relevant in the newborn, in whom adhesive bowel obstruction after laparotomy ranges between 1% to 2% per year (Ponsky and Rothenberg, 2008).

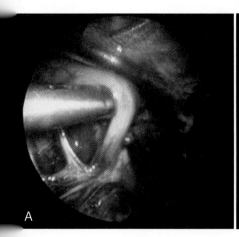
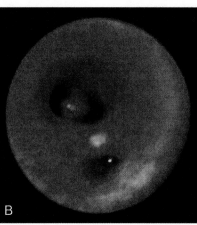

■ **FIGURE 18-9. A,** Thorascopic and **B,** bronchoscopic views of a TEF. In the bronchoscopic view the TEF is posterior *(bottom),* and the carina is more anterior *(top).* (**B** *From Barksdale EM, Jr: Surgery. In Zitelli BJ, Davis HW, editors: Atlas of pediatric physical diagnosis, ed 4, St. Louis, 2002, Mosby, p 562.)*

Minimal-access surgery in neonates also presents challenges and limitations. The small working space and small size of the newborn, coupled with the unique aspects of neonatal physiology, make thoracoscopic surgery and one-lung ventilation difficult. There is a learning curve to minimally invasive surgery. Procedure times, operative morbidity, and conversion rates to open procedures vary among centers and surgeons (Ponsky and Rothenberg, 2008).

Efficient and safe endoscopic surgery requires both surgical and biotechnical expertise, as well as highly skilled OR and anesthesia teams (Kalfa et al., 2007). Because of these technical challenges, the OR times in the early learning phase may be markedly prolonged compared with operating times for the open procedures (Rothenberg, 2005a; Tsao and Lee, 2005; Nguyen et al., 2006; Kalfa et al., 2007).

The newborn's small size, combined with the unique physiology of transitional and neonatal circulation, forces the pediatric anesthesiologist to analyze the risks of minimal access surgery. In particular, insufflation with carbon dioxide (CO_2) leads to increased pressure in either the thorax or the abdomen, as well as hypercarbia, and it may profoundly affect neonatal pulmonary physiology. In order to minimize complications, clear preoperative planning requires that both the surgeon and anesthesiologist ask the following questions as part of their assessment:

1. What contraindications exist to a laparoscopic approach? For example, weight less than 2 kg, long-gap esophageal atresia, severe lung disease, hemodynamic instability and pulmonary hypertension.
2. What intraoperative indications would occur to cause conversion to an open procedure? For example, a range of time limits and defining cardiorespiratory and blood-loss indications for converting to an open procedure should be at least tentatively established preoperatively.
3. What intraoperative access, monitoring, and anesthetic techniques are required? For example, some surgeons do not use routine bronchoscopic evaluation before TEF repair, whereas others would not proceed without it. In addition, the approach toward attempting one-lung ventilation should be addressed (i.e., bronchial blocker or mainstem intubation).
4. As with any surgery, informed consent, including risks and alternatives must be obtained. In this case, what should parents be told about the expertise of the surgeons, anesthesiologists, and OR team?

Minimal access surgery creates a unique set of operative conditions that may impose significant cardiorespiratory effects: positioning, insufflation, prolonged pneumoperitoneum or pneumothorax, and hypercarbia. The insufflation of any substance into the peritoneum or the thorax must be controlled to avoid excessive pressure in the cavity. The simple increase in pressure can dramatically affect hemodynamic and respiratory function. The development of low-flow devices and valved trocars has allowed surgeons to adopt specific approaches for the newborn or small infant (intrathoracic pressure greater than 10 mm Hg and intraabdominal pressure less than 15 mm Hg). CO_2 has become the most commonly used agent for insufflation because of its high solubility, low expense, and noncombustible nature. On the other hand, CO_2 is readily absorbed from both the peritoneum and the thoracic cavity. The cardiorespiratory effects of insufflation with CO_2 during laparoscopy and thoracoscopy have been well documented in adults but not in children, infants, and newborns. Although the hemodynamic and pulmonary effects of insufflation may be similar during laparoscopy and thoracoscopy, most of the data reported for thoracoscopy are derived during one-lung ventilation. However, one-lung ventilation in the newborn cannot be achieved with the same techniques used in the adult (e.g., double-lumen tubes or endobronchial blockers).

Laparoscopy Background

The cardiorespiratory effects of laparoscopy are often difficult to separate from those of anesthesia, surgery, and intraoperative positioning (e.g., Trendelenberg or reverse Trendelenberg). Although the enormous amount of data accumulated for adults, children, and older infants cannot be directly extrapolated to newborns, some of the trends noted in these studies are worth considering in the context of neonatal surgery and anesthesia.

In adults, intraoperative pulmonary catheter monitoring determined the hemodynamic effects of general anesthesia, the reverse Trendelenberg position, peritoneal insufflation, and their combined effects during laparoscopic cholecystectomy. After induction of anesthesia, mean arterial pressure and cardiac index decreased from baseline. Adding the reverse Trendelenberg position further decreased right atrial and pulmonary capillary wedge pressures, cardiac index, and mean arterial pressure. After peritoneal insufflation with CO_2 while in the reverse Trendelenberg position, mean arterial pressure increased as systemic and pulmonary vascular resistances increased. Right atrial and pulmonary capillary wedge pressures increased, and cardiac index decreased beyond the level associated with positioning.

These hemodynamic changes from insufflation, positioning, and hypercarbia are of minimal significance in a euvolemic, healthy adult, but the risks may become significant in patients with underlying cardiac disease (Grabowski and Talamini, 2009). Data documenting cardiorespiratory responses to laparoscopy in infants have been reported, but only about studies involving the use of noninvasive tools, and they differ from some of the results reported in healthy adults.

Using a transesophageal ultrasonic probe inserted after induction of general anesthesia in 12 healthy boys (23 ± 5 months of age), Gueugniaud et al. (1998) noted that pneumoperitoneum (10 mm Hg) decreased aortic blood flow and stroke volume and increased systemic vascular resistance. No effects on mean arterial pressure or end-tidal CO_2 were noted. Of importance, these patients remained supine (no reverse Trendelenberg positioning).

Manner et al. (1998) reported the pulmonary effects of pneumoperitoneum in 10 patients between the ages of 1 and 15 years who were undergoing a variety of laparoscopic procedures (intraperitoneal pressure, 12 mm Hg). In this study, the patients' pulmonary compliance decreased (17% with the reverse Trendelenberg position, 28% with the reverse Trendelenberg position plus insufflation); peak inspiratory pressure increased (25% with the reverse Trendelenberg position, 30% with the reverse Trendelenberg position plus insufflation) and end-tidal CO_2 tension (P_{ETCO_2}) concentration increased from 33 to 42 mm Hg at maximum insufflation pressure. In 17 infants (younger than 10 months) who were undergoing a variety of procedures that required at least 30 minutes of laparoscopy but experienced no change in position, Bannister et al. (2003) reported similar findings. Patients were divided into two groups: those weighing less than 5 kg (intraabdominal pressure less than 12 mm Hg), and those weighing more than 5 kg (intraabdominal pressure, less than 15 mm Hg). Again, peak inspiratory pressure increased (18%) and correlated with insufflation pressure, and dynamic compliance decreased (48%). Tidal volume decreased 33% and oxygen saturation fell 2% to 11% in 41% of the patients. Ventilation was adjusted to maintain PETCO$_2$ within 10% of baseline, and 20 adjustments were reported. Neither heart rate nor blood pressure changed with insufflation or ventilatory adjustments, and significant changes from baseline status were noted at insufflation pressures of 10 mm Hg and greater but not at pressures of 5 mm Hg. Similar minimal hemodynamic effects of low-pressure pneumoperitoneum have been documented in young children elsewhere (DeWaal and Kalkman, 2003).

Of note, inducing a pneumoperitoneum in the Tredelenburg position during gynecologic surgery in adults decreases the distance between the endotracheal tip and the carina as well as the tracheal length (Kim et al., 2007). Because the distance between the larynx and the carina is markedly less in the infant, this phenomenon may be of critical importance in the newborn undergoing laparoscopy.

Renal function is affected by pneumoperitoneum. However, data have primarily been acquired in the adult population. In adults, decreased urine production has been attributed to the decreased glomerular filtration rate and renal perfusion from the direct effects of pneumoperitoneum (e.g., compression of the renal artery, the inferior vena cava, or the parenchyma) or from secondary effects (e.g., decreased cardiac output and release of mediators) (Rosin et al., 2002). Renal blood flow and renal function decrease during pneumoperitoneum; the effects on blood flow are pressure dependent and exacerbated in the head-up position, but they return to normal after deflation (Demyttenaere et al., 2007).

The effect of pneumoperitoneum on intracranial pressure has been studied in adults. Although the newborn's cerebrovascular physiology and autoregulatory responses differ from those of the adult, newborns with limited autoregulatory responses may have more profound cerebral vascular responses from increased intraabdominal pressure. In adult animals, intraabdominal pressures of 15 and 25 mm Hg—but not 5 mm Hg—affected intracranial pressure, similar to findings by Rosenthal et al. (1998) (Rosin et al., 2002). Bloomfield et al. (1997) created models that linked intraabdominal, intrathoracic, and intracranial pressures. As with other studies, pleural, peak inspiratory, right atrial, and pulmonary arterial pressures increased as intraabdominal pressure increased above 10 mm Hg. The increases became especially significant at intraabdominal pressures of 25 mm Hg. At the same time cardiac index decreased, but systemic vascular resistance increased and blood pressure remained stable. Increased intracranial pressure accompanied the rise in intraabdominal pressure; however, these changes reversed when the abdomen was decompressed. Of significance, the increase in pleural and intracranial pressures with increased intraabdominal pressure was prevented in a group of swine with the chest opened (e.g., median sternotomy and pleuropericardotomy). However, in spite of the open chest, cardiac index decreased and systemic vascular resistance increased. The investigators suggested that the acuity of the increase in intrathoracic pressure secondary to an abrupt rise in intraabdominal pressure acutely increased central venous pressure,

preventing cerebral venous outflow. When they prevented the effect of intraabdominal pressure on the pleural pressure (open chest), venous and intracranial pressures did not change.

The absence of predictable autoregulation of cerebral perfusion in the newborn combined with the significant risk of injury secondary to oxygen and positive pressure ventilation may have unique implications for the anesthetic management of the newborn during either laparoscopy or thoracoscopy. Although indirect monitoring of cerebral blood flow is available (e.g., near-infrared spectroscopy, or *NIRS*), ideally a reliable, continuous method to accurately monitor cerebral perfusion pressure would be of critical benefit in this setting (Brady et al., 2007).

In summary, pneumoperitoneum in infants affects ventilation as well as cardiovascular, renal, and cerebrovascular function. With pneumoperitoneum, the upward displacement of the diaphragm affects intrathoracic pressure and lung volumes, ultimately affecting compliance, peak airway pressure, tidal volume, and effective minute ventilation. All of these changes result in a decrease in functional residual capacity, which can promote atelectasis and worsen the ventilation/perfusion mismatch abnormalities.

Laparoscopy and Thoracoscopy in the Newborn

The effects of insufflation during both laparoscopy and thoracoscopy are dramatic in the newborn. The impact of increased intrathoracic pressure and hypercarbia can profoundly influence the transitional circulation. Changes in patient oxygen saturation, hypotension, interruption of the procedure, and hypercarbia are common in the newborn (Kalfa et al., 2005, 2007; Krosnar and Baxter, 2005).

Insufflation in the newborn also decreases core body temperature. In 50% of newborns, the postoperative core temperature was less than 36° C. A long operative time (insufflation for more than 100 minutes) was associated with lower postoperative core body temperature (Kalfa et al., 2005).

Inaccurate end-tidal CO$_2$ values are common during laparoscopy, especially in the setting of cyanotic heart disease (Laffon et al., 1998; Wulkan and Vasudevan, 2001). At the same time, absorption of CO$_2$ from the peritoneum seems to be age-dependent (McHoney et al., 2003). The total amount of insufflated CO$_2$ and elimination of CO$_2$ correlated with age. Younger patients also demonstrated a short period of increased CO$_2$ elimination after desufflation, which may be related to increased venous return after the decrease in intraabdominal pressure.

Because one-lung ventilation is challenging to achieve and at times is not tolerated by a newborn, many pediatric surgeons suggest that insufflation of the chest with low flow of CO$_2$ (1 to 2 L/min, peak pressure of 4 to 6 mm Hg) in the 30- to 45-degree prone position induces adequate lung collapse (Rothenberg, 2002; 2005b; Holcomb et al., 2005).

Because many of the strategies to affect one-lung ventilation are not available for the newborn, adequate surgical exposure for thoracoscopy relies heavily on insufflation to collapse the lung. Lungs with abnormal distribution of ventilation impede uniform collapse with insufflation, so the newborn with abnormal lung function may not be eligible for thoracoscopic surgery. The effect of pneumoperitoneum on tracheal length implies that the risk for inadvertent endobronchial intubation may be increased in the newborn.

In spite of the myriad of critical physiologic challenges, endoscopic procedures have been conducted successfully in high-risk infants with conditions such as hypoplastic left heart syndrome, complex cyanotic heart disease, and patients with single ventricle physiology (Mariano et al., 2005; Rice-Townsend et al., 2007; Slater et al., 2007).

SPECIFIC NEONATAL SURGICAL LESIONS

Abdominal Wall Defects: Gastroschisis and Omphalocele

Gastroschisis and omphaloceles are the most common abdominal wall defects (ectopia cordis and cloacal and bladder extrophy are less common), but they are still rare, with an incidence of approximately 1:10,000 and 1:4000 to 7000 births (Paidas et al., 1994). Some have suggested that both ethnic and geographic origins affect the incidence, but overall the lesions seem sporadic (Mann et al., 2008).

Currently, fetal ultrasounds are routinely conducted to screen for high-risk conditions. For example, nuchal translucency and biochemical markers (free β-subunit of human chorionic gonadotropin and pregnancy-associated plasma protein A) are now measured to screen for aneuploidy or cardiac and other anomalies (Souter and Nyberg, 2001; Weiner et al., 2007). An abnormal value on screening prompts an evaluation that includes a detailed fetal ultrasound; in the case of abdominal wall defects, ultrasound confirms the presence of a lesion in approximately 95% of cases after as few as 10 to 14 weeks' gestation (Mann et al., 2008). The in utero diagnosis allows planned delivery at a medical center with resources for high-risk obstetric, surgical and anesthetic, and neonatal care.

Although omphalocele and gastroschisis appear to be similar in gross physical appearance, these lesions are distinct from each other. An omphalocele is a central defect of the umbilical ring; the abdominal contents herniate into the intact umbilical sac unless the sac ruptures in utero (Fig. 18-10). The umbilical cord is also inserted into the sac, which contains an internal peritoneal membrane and external amniotic membrane. The lesion has a fascial defect of more than 4 cm (fewer than 4 cm is often considered an umbilical hernia) and often as large as 10 to 12 cm. The sac often contains the stomach, loops of the small and large intestines, and in about 30% to 50% of cases, the liver. A gastroschisis, on the other hand, is an abdominal wall defect that usually occurs to the right of the umbilical cord, with evisceration of bowel through the defect (Fig. 18-11). This lesion is usually 2 to 5 cm in diameter, and in most cases there are only small and large bowel present. In rare cases the liver may exit through the abdominal wall defect as well. The bowel is exposed to the intrauterine environment with no sac, causing its loops to become matted, thickened, and often covered with an inflammatory coating or peel. Whether this exudative peel is secondary to a specific inflammatory pathway or just an effect of amniotic fluid is unclear. The umbilical cord is normal and separate from the defect. When the testes exit along with the bowel, cryptorchidism occurs with gastroschisis (Lawson and de La Hunt, 2001; Weber et al., 2002).

Embryology

Although experimental models have been described, the embryologic etiology of these lesions is not completely understood (Correia-Pinto et al., 2001). Omphalocele has been described as a failure of the cephalic, lateral, and caudal folds to fuse (closure of the exocelomic space) and as abnormal fusion and differentiation of myotomes to form abdominal wall musculature (7 to 12 weeks of gestation). That is, the abdominal cavity is primarily underdeveloped. During weeks 7 to 12 of development, the midgut elongates and herniates into the umbilical cord. By week 12, the abdominal cavity is large enough for the developing gut to exit the cord and reenter the abdomen. Some believe that the simple failure of this return to the abdomen is a developmental arrest that results in an omphalocele and a small abdominal cavity. The abdominal cavity is small only because the gut remains in the umbilical sac.

Gastroschisis is considered to be an earlier embryologic event, resulting from an abnormality of the development of the right omphalomesenteric artery or right umbilical vein, which in turn results in ischemia to the right paraumbilical area. More recently, abdominal wall defects have been ascribed to an

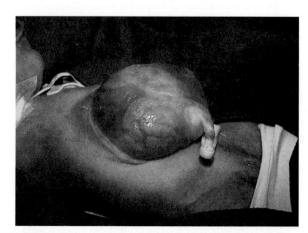

■ **FIGURE 18-10.** Newborn with large omphalocele, sac intact. Umbilical cord is seen emerging from mass. The major problem will be replacing the viscera in the small abdominal cavity.

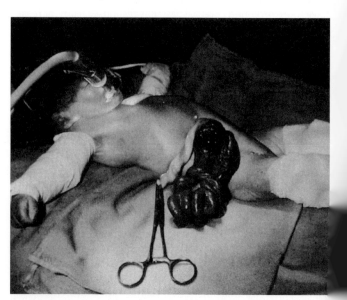

■ **FIGURE 18-11.** Gastroschisis, sometimes called ruptured omphalocele, with umbilical cord intact. Heat loss, rapid dehydration, and infection are added to problems of omphalocele.

abnormal relationship between cell proliferation and planned cell death (apoptosis) at the critical embryonic folding period (Robinson and Abuhamad, 2000). Inadequate mesoderm development may contribute to dysplastic abdominal wall growth. This underdeveloped site is commonly found just to the right of the umbilicus and ruptures with increased pressure of the growing intraabdominal organs. Similar defects in other areas may produce other lesions, such as extrophy of the bladder.

Gastroschisis is usually an isolated lesion, but recent reports raise the possibility of familial occurrence (Yang et al., 1992; Torfs et al., 1994). In utero exposure to acetaminophen, aspirin, and pseudoephedrine has been associated with an increased incidence of gastroschisis (Werler et al., 2002; Baerg et al., 2003). In the case of either an omphalocele or gastroschisis, rotation of the gut is incomplete in utero, resulting in various "malrotation" phenotypes. Intestinal atresias are common, especially in patients with gastroschisis.

Although neither gastroschisis nor omphalocele is considered to be familial, 50% to 75% of infants with an omphalocele have other anomalies, and 20% to 30% have chromosomal abnormalities (Robinson and Abuhamad, 2000; Weber et al., 2002; Mann et al., 2008). Only 15% to 20% of infants with gastroschisis have associated malformations, and only rarely is there a complex pattern of malformation (Stoll et al., 2008). For example, Beckwith-Wiedemann, Rieger's, and prune belly (Eagle-Barrett) syndromes are associated with omphaloceles, as are trisomies 13, 15, 18, and 21. If the omphalocele contains only bowel and if oligo- or polyhydramnios are present, the likelihood of an associated chromosomal abnormality increases. Others have noted that omphaloceles that contain liver and other viscera are more likely to have cardiac, renal, or limb anomalies, whereas the smaller omphaloceles are more likely to have gastrointestinal or central nervous system malformations (Mann et al., 2008). Syndromes of midline defects often include an omphalocele, and the lesion has been noted in the nonsyndromic multiple congenital anomalies (MCA) complex.

Single-gene mutations have been identified in omphaloceles with multiple anomalies, such as the filamin A, alpha (*FLNA*) gene in the otopalatodigital syndrome, which is characterized by abnormalities in the axial and appendicular skeleton plus extraskeletal anomalies such as omphalocele (Robertson, 2007). One syndrome, Pentalogy of Cantrell, includes an omphalocele, diaphragmatic hernia, sternal abnormalities, an ectopic and anomalous heart, and gene abnormalities at Xq25 to Xq26.1. Another syndrome (OEIS Complex) involving the lower abdomen includes omphalocele, bladder or cloacal extrophy, imperforate anus, colonic atresia, sacrovertebral anomalies, and meningomyelocele. No environmental or teratogenic associations have been proposed as etiologic causes. Allen et al. (2006) reported an association with assisted reproductive technology. Thus, identifying an abdominal wall defect in utero demands an intense evaluation for associated anomalies, which may be isolated, part of a recognizable malformation syndrome, or chromosomal. In addition, serial ultrasounds should be conducted to evaluate fetal growth and well being, as well as amniotic fluid volume. Of note, after 20 to 32 weeks' gestation, a higher incidence of fetal demise has been reported. The mode of delivery for infants with abdominal wall defects remains controversial, but recent studies have shown that in gastroschisis and nongiant omphaloceles (i.e., liver extracorporeal), outcome after vaginal delivery is no different than with caesarean section (Henrich et al., 2008). The controversy centers on delivery

with gastroschisis because of the unprotected viscera, but no advantages of cesarean section are consistently apparent when survival and incidence of complications are evaluated (Weber et al., 2002).

Preoperative Management

The preoperative management of abdominal wall defects is concerned primarily with fluid resuscitation, minimizing heat loss, treating sepsis, and avoiding direct trauma to the herniated organs. Rather than "rushing" to close the defect, careful assessment of associated defects, establishing smooth cardiorespiratory transition, and ensuring adequate intravascular volume comprise the critical aspects of preoperative management.

Normothermia should be maintained or achieved by preventing heat loss from the exposed viscera. A bowel bag may be used for this purpose (Towne et al., 1980). Emphasis should be placed on covering the lesion with gauze, nonadherent dressing, and a plastic cover rather than moist (saline-soaked) material, as moisture tends to exacerbate heat loss (Mann et al., 2008). It is critical to avoid distorting the sac or twisting at the base. Decompressing the stomach with an orogastric or nasogastric tube minimizes regurgitation, aspiration pneumonia, and further bowel distention. Broad-spectrum antibiotics are started and intravenous fluid therapy (e.g., lactated Ringer's solution) at as much as 3 to 4 times (150 to 300 mL/kg per day) the usual maintenance rate (80 to 100 mL/kg per day) is infused to provide adequate hydration and to compensate for a combination of peritonitis, edema, ischemia, protein loss, and significant third-space loss. Without such vigorous fluid resuscitation, hypovolemic shock, hemoconcentration, and metabolic acidosis may develop. A urine output of 1 to 2 mL/kg per hour suggests adequate hydration. Because of the large fluid requirements, acid-base status and electrolyte levels should be monitored carefully by serial arterial or venous blood-gas measurements. Rarely, severe metabolic acidosis develops in spite of aggressive fluid delivery (e.g., coexisting sepsis), and sodium bicarbonate (infusion or bolus) or sodium acetate infusion may be required to maintain the pH at greater than 7.20. In general, delivery of crystalloid and colloid provides adequate support.

Intraoperative Management

Surgical management aims to repair the abdominal wall defect and reduce the protruded viscera. If primary closure is not possible, a staged repair is planned, including the use of the silo chimney or the silastic silo prosthesis (Schuster, 1967). The "silo" consists of a silastic or Teflon mesh that is sutured to the fascia of the defect. The synthetic material used to cover the lesion and the specific mechanism for placing the organs into the abdomen (e.g., umbilical tapes or umbilical cord clamps) vary from center to center. After the silo is in place, the extraabdominal organs are gradually returned to the peritoneal cavity over 3 to 10 days (Fig. 18-12). Improved outcome using the delayed-repair approach after the nonoperative placement of a spring-loaded silo has been described by Schlatter et al. (2003). These authors state that this procedure is accomplished in the neonatal intensive care unit (NICU) or delivery room and requires no anesthesia. The prosthesis is then removed, the lesion is reduced under general anesthesia, and eventually the defect is closed. The authors also claim that the time to both first and full feeds was shorter in infants who underwent

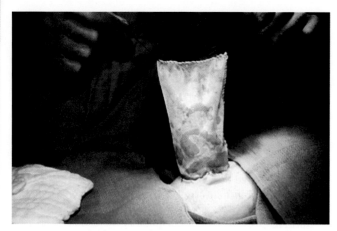

■ **FIGURE 18-12.** A silo is used to aid in the reduction of the abdominal contents when the abdominal cavity is too small. Over time, the intestinal contents are gradually reduced back into the abdominal cavity.

delayed closure. Similarly, Pastor et al. (2008) performed a prospective multicenter study of infants with gastroschisis. They noted that the routine use of a preformed silo was associated with similar outcomes as primary closure for infants; however, this method has not gained widespread acceptance.

Forcing the viscera into an underdeveloped abdominal cavity that cannot accommodate the herniated bowel and tight closure of the defect can restrict diaphragmatic excursion, possibly compress the lungs, and may produce abdominal compartment syndrome (ACS). ACS not only impairs respiratory function, but the high intraabdominal pressure can diminish blood flow to the kidneys and other viscera, impair venous return, and even increase intracranial pressure via effects on intrathoracic pressure (Rosenthal et al., 1998). Thus, during abdominal closure, the anesthesiologist must monitor airway pressures to identify decreased pulmonary compliance, as well as observe for evidence of decreased perfusion to the lower extremities (evidence of ACS). The surgeon and the anesthesiologist should cooperate to assess the feasibility of a primary closure. Yaster et al. (1988) noted that an increase in intragastric pressure of greater than 20 mm Hg and CVP of more than 4 mm Hg above baseline were often associated with reductions in venous return and cardiac index, requiring surgical decompression of the abdomen. The impact of ACS on hemodynamic function and its treatment with percutaneous drainage of the peritoneal cavity has been described in adults and older children, especially in the setting of trauma, and recently in a low–birth-weight infant with a sepsis and an intestinal perforation (Hunter and Damani, 2004; Hunter, 2008, Rasner et al., 2008).

An arterial catheter facilitates blood sampling and continuous monitoring of blood pressure. However, a CVP catheter might be equally valuable for evaluating changes in blood volume and the degree of visceral compression during abdominal closure, and to allow metabolic monitoring (e.g., serial intraoperative glucose levels in infants with Beckwith-Wiedemann syndrome) (Yaster et al., 1988). Intravenous fluids often consist of 5% to 10% dextrose in 0.2% saline to deliver the maintenance therapy and lactated Ringer's solution (8 to 15 mL/kg, or more, per hour) for third-space loss. Vigilant efforts at preventing heat loss should be sustained (see Chapter 6, Thermoregulation: Physiology and Perioperative Disturbances).

After decompression of the stomach, anesthesia may be induced with inhalation or intravenous agents. Because it distends the bowel, nitrous oxide is avoided. In most cases, neuromuscular blockade facilitates the abdominal decompression or closure. Ventilation with an air (or nitrogen) and oxygen mixture with low concentrations of an inhalation anesthetic plus intravenous opioids are titrated in response to the hemodynamic status. In neonates who have received transfusions of adult blood, the inspired oxygen concentration must be adjusted to maintain oxygen saturation between 85% and 95% and lower in the preterm infant (See Chapter 17, Neonatology for Anesthesiologists). In infants who have not received adult hemoglobin transfusions, the oxygen saturation should be maintained at 90% to 97%, and in preterm infants it should be kept at between 90% and 95%. In the infant who has had no transfusion, this assumes a P_{50} of 19 mm Hg, and an O_2 saturation between 90% and 97% results in a Pao_2 of 40 to 64 mm Hg. In the preterm infant, an O_2 saturation of 90% to 95% results in a Pao_2 of 40 to 52 mm Hg (See Chapter 3, Respiratory Physiology, Table 3-3). Vane et al. (1994) demonstrated that spinal anesthesia can be an effective anesthetic for the repair of gastroschisis in selected patients. Evaluating for associated intraabdominal anomalies (e.g., atresia) is worthwhile, but especially in the setting of gastroschisis the "matted" bowel is difficult to examine thoroughly for other malformations.

Postoperative Care

Postoperatively, after an uncomplicated primary closure of an abdominal wall defect, mechanical ventilation is usually required for 24 to 48 hours or longer; thereafter, respiratory compliance usually improves dramatically (Nakayama et al., 1991, 1992). Clearly, infants undergoing a gradual reduction after placement of a silo or similar device should be mechanically ventilated during this process. Infants with a small defect can sometimes be extubated at the conclusion of surgery. All patients must be carefully monitored for respiratory and infectious complications in an intensive care unit after closure of an abdominal wall defect. Inferior vena caval compression (evident by blueish lower limbs) or bowel ischemia (necrotizing enterocolitis) can occur as a result of increased abdominal pressure and may require surgical decompression.

The onset of peristalsis after repair of omphalocele or gastroschisis is usually delayed, and the resulting ileus may be prolonged so that total parenteral nutrition is generally required for days to weeks postoperatively (O'Neil and Grosfeld, 1974). Bowel hypomotility is most common in infants with gastroschisis. In anticipation of this, most infants with large lesions and especially gastroschisis should have appropriate intravenous access established in the OR to facilitate early postoperative nutritional support, which is essential for healing and recovery. Prolonged feeding intolerance should precipitate an evaluation for an associated intestinal atresia or other intestinal lesion.

Outcome

Survival of infants born with anterior abdominal wall defects has improved dramatically as a result of prenatal diagnosis; improved surgical, anesthetic, and perioperative intensive care; and nutritional support. The advent of accurate prenatal imaging has allowed termination of a pregnancy when a fetus with multiple anomalies, chromosomal lesions, or a huge defect is identified. When the defect exists in isolation from other anomalies or malformations, 95% to 97% survival is expected. Mortality and long-term outcome are related to associated anomalies (e.g., cardiac malfunction or intestinal atresia); complications of treatment (e.g., bowel perforation, necrotizing enterocolitis, sepsis, or short bowel syndrome); and the side effects of intravenous alimentation (e.g., liver failure or sepsis). In a single institutional report by Phillips et al. (2008), of the patients with gastroschisis and intestinal atresia about one third have significant intestinal dysmotility without short bowel syndrome or obstruction. Although specific data have been collected to stratify and predict outcomes of patients with abdominal wall defects, an obvious observation is that infants with a simple defect (i.e., no atresias, no extraintestinal anomalies, and defect smaller than 5 or 6 cm) and no postoperative complications (e.g., obstruction, necrotizing enterocolitis, or short gut syndrome) have a better prognosis than those with a complex lesion or difficult postoperative course (Molik et al., 2001; Henrich et al., 2008). Of course, outcomes in the setting of a giant omphalocele (i.e., a liver-containing lesion through an abdominal defect wider than 5 cm) are overshadowed by a significant incidence of long-term respiratory insufficiency that may be related to sequelae of abnormal chest wall development (Tsakayannis et al., 1996; Biard et al., 2004).

In a follow-up study of 23 infants born with gastroschisis between 1972 and 1984 and who survived more than 1 year (older than 16 years of age at the time of study), Davies and Stringer (1997) reported that 22 of these 23 infants were in good health and that their overall growth was normal. About one third of the patients with gastroschisis had undergone additional surgery for adhesions, bowel obstruction, or scar complications related to their defect. In a 30-year review of morbidity related to adhesions after an abdominal wall defect in the neonatal period, van Eijck et al. (2008) reported an incidence of small bowel obstruction of 25% in the gastroschisis group, but only 13% in the patients who had had an omphalocele. Of all the patients, 88% required a laparotomy, and 85% occurred in the first year of life. A history of sepsis or wound dehiscence was a factor for predicting the development of a small bowel obstruction. The authors suggest that pediatric surgeons should evaluate the relevance of adhesion-prevention techniques and materials at the time of the initial surgical treatment of abdominal wall defects (e.g., component separation technique or hyaluronate-based barrier) (van Eijck et al., 2008).

Of note, in 25% to 60% of patients with anterior wall defects, the absence of an umbilicus was a distressing physical sign, especially during adolescence (Tunell et al., 1995; Davies and Stringer, 1997). Studies involving shorter follow-up periods have noted patients with chronic abdominal pain and gastroesophageal reflux (Fasching et al., 1996). Recently, economic analysis of care of infants with gastroschisis emphasized that the cost of care is high and that on average 47 days of hospitalization were needed in order to establish full feeds (Sydorak et al., 2002).

Congenital Diaphragmatic Hernia

Congenital diaphragmatic hernia (CDH) is a defect in the diaphragm that develops early in gestation and is associated with extrusion of intraabdominal organs into the thoracic cavity (Fig. 18-13). The incidence of CDH ranges between 1:2500 and 1:3000 live births. CDH may be an isolated lesion, or it may

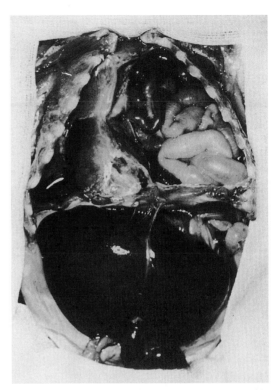

■ **FIGURE 18-13.** Diaphragmatic hernia at postmortem examination showing obliteration of left pleural cavity and severe compression of the heart and right lung. *(Courtesy of Dr. Arnold Colodny, Boston, Mass.)*

be associated with other anomalies. Although most cases are considered sporadic rather than part of a genetic syndrome, the nonisolated CDH has been linked to specific chromosomal anomalies including duplication of 1q24 to q31.2 and deletion of a portion of 6q, 8p23.1, and 15q26 (Holder et al., 2007; Clugston et al., 2008). In addition, CDH is a key feature of syndromes such as Beckwith-Wiedemann; coloboma, heart, atresia choanae, retardation, genital, and ear (CHARGE); Cornelia de Lange's; and Denys-Drash. Trisomies 13, 18, and 21 and 45 are the most common aneuploidies associated with CDH. Multiple examples of familial cases have been reported, but recurrence rates are low.

The most common defect is posterolateral (Bochdalek's hernia), occurring in 90% of cases, of which 75% are left sided. Morgagni (anteromedial) and paraesophageal hernias and eventrations make up the remainder (Fig. 18-14). This anomaly is much more than a hole in the diaphragm. CDH is also associated with the following conditions:

- Varying degrees of bilateral lung hypoplasia
- Pulmonary hypertension and arteriolar reactivity
- Congenital anomalies (e.g., cardiac, gastrointestinal, genitourinary, skeletal, neural, and trisomic)
- Significant morbidity and mortality

Since the 1980s, the survival of neonates with CDH has improved dramatically from 40% to 60% in the 1980s to 70% to 80% in the 1990s. The drastic improvement in the operative mortality rate of CDH has apparently resulted from the new strategy of delaying surgery, neonatal stabilization, and the adaptation of new a lung-protective, or "gentle ventilator," strategy with a small tidal volume, a higher and adequate positive end-expiratory pressure (PEEP) to keep the airways open, and

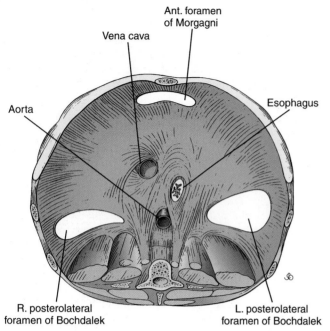

■ FIGURE 18-14. Diagram, with view from below, showing sites of congenital diaphragmatic hernia.

the acceptance of the resultant rise in P_{CO_2} (permissive hypercapnea) (Nakayama et al., 1991; Boloker et al., 2002; Harrison et al., 2003). The development of the lung-protective approach is based on the findings that the traditional ventilatory strategy of maintaining "normal" P_{CO_2} levels with large tidal volumes results in further damage to the lung tissues and exacerbates acute respiratory distress syndrome (ARDS) (Wada et al., 1997; Björklund et al., 1997) (see Timing of Surgery, p. 570).

CDH persists as a lesion with many unanswered questions; however, the impact of pulmonary hypoplasia and pulmonary hypertension on pathophysiology and clinical outcome is well recognized. For example, Dillon et al. (2004) correlated pulmonary artery pressure (measured via echocardiogram) with survival in a cohort of 47 full-term infants treated with delayed surgery and gentle ventilatory approaches such as high-frequency oscillatory ventilation (HFOV), permissive hypercarbia, nitric oxide (NO), or extracorporeal membrane oxygenation (ECMO). All 23 infants with estimated normal pulmonary artery pressure within the first 3 weeks of life (49% of study) survived. In contrast, none of the 8 patients with persistent systemic (or higher) pulmonary artery pressure survived. Of the remaining 16 patients with pulmonary artery pressure between these two extremes, 12 (75% of the 16) survived. Both in utero and postnatal optimum management strategies for these infants remains unclear (de Buys Roessingh and Dinh-Xuan, 2009).

Survival of inborn patients is lower (62.6%) than outborn patients (83.3%), suggesting that surviving transport to a tertiary care center occurs at a higher rate for those with less severe lesions. Since 2000, survival rates of patients who receive care at a NICU are at least 60% to 70% (Migliazza et al., 2007). Thus, institution-based reports that only include data about live-born infants cared for in an NICU may underestimate the total mortality of CDH and the incidence and severity of associated anomalies. Survival rates associated with an isolated congenital diaphragmatic hernia approaches 80% in those who do

not require ECMO (Sigalet et al., 1995; Reickert et al., 1998). Harrison first noted in the 1970s that mortality may be "hidden" when in utero deaths and early postnatal deaths are not included in calculating mortality associated with CDH (Harrison et al., 1978, 1994).

A population-based study of CDH in western Australia that included complete outcome data (i.e., miscarriages, stillbirths, and terminations of pregnancies) noted that of the 116 CDH cases studied, 61% of infants were born alive (Colvin et al., 2005). Of those born alive, 35% died before transport, and 52% survived beyond the age of 1 year. However, if the denominator includes all cases, only 32% survived past 1 year. Of these infants, only 16% of all prenatally-diagnosed and 33% of live-born, prenatally-diagnosed infants with CDH survived beyond the age of 1 year, whereas 92% of infants who had surgery and 80% of those who reached the referral center survived beyond 1 year of age. A major anomaly was identified in 47% of this cohort, and mortality reached 78% in this subgroup. In those pregnancies that were terminated, 71% had a major anomaly in addition to CDH. Similar to other reports, 53% of CDH cases were identified in utero; 49% of these were terminated. Of the 47% diagnosed postnatally, 74% were liveborn. Most deaths occurred in the first week of life. Eighty-eight percent of those with a preoperative pneumothorax died. Low birth weight and low Apgar scores at 1 and 5 minutes were also predictive of increased mortality. Thus, high mortality associated with this lesion persists, and prenatal termination dramatically confounds the accurate overall estimate of the outcome of CDH.

Similar findings have been reported from the United Kingdom's northern health region on all cases of CDH from 1991 to 2001, which included antenatal diagnoses and termination, associated anomalies, therapy, and outcome. Stege et al. (2003) claimed that in the era of gentle ventilation, various newer therapies (e.g., ECMO, HFOV, and NO) have had minimal impact on mortality when complete case ascertainment is included. The authors noted that the two factors that distort postnatal mortality include the rate of termination and the presence of other anomalies. Stege also reported that the mortality rate before ECMO was available was 68% total (57% of live births) and after ECMO was available, the mortality rate was 58% total (45% of live births). However, since discontinuing ECMO as a therapeutic option, mortality has remained at 58% overall (40% of live births). Similar patterns evolved for data about NO and HFOV. That is, changes in ventilator supportive care (i.e., gentle ventilation) of infants with CDH probably account for the decreased mortality and survival for CDH. The authors emphasize that only about 50% of CDH cases are identified on antenatal surveillance, leading to persistence of births of infants with this life-threatening lesion who are without the advantages of a tertiary level nursery care that has pediatric surgical and medical expertise.

Stillborn babies with CDH have a 95% incidence of other anomalies. A severe cardiac malformation combined with CDH implies a lethal outcome (Fauza and Wilson, 1994; Migliazza et al., 2007). Although various series' rank the incidence of associated malformations differently, Stege et al. (2003) reported that cardiovascular lesions were most common, followed by chromosomal, skeletal, facial dysmorphism (cleft palate, ear deformity), gastrointestinal, and syndromal. Rarely, CDH is a part of a complex set of anomalies called *Pentalogy of Cantrell*, which consists of omphalocele, sternal cleft, ectopia cordis, and an intracardiac defect (ventricular septal defect or diverticulum of the left ventricle) (Wesselhoeft and DeLuca, 1984). Although uncommon, CDH has been associated with several other syndromes including, Fryns' syndrome, Goldenhar's syndrome, Brachmann-deLange syndrome, and Beckwith-Weidemann syndrome (Thornburn et al., 1970; Fryns et al., 1979; Rollnick and Kaye, 1983; Jelsema et al., 1993).

Embryology

The diaphragm, lungs, and gastrointestinal tract develop synchronously. The lungs begin as a ventral bud of the foregut. Airway development and branching begin between the fourth and fifth weeks of gestation and progress until the terminal bronchioles are formed by the seventeenth week. The ventral (membranous) component of the diaphragm is formed between the third and fourth weeks of gestation. At about the eighth week of gestation, this portion envelops the esophagus, inferior vena cava, and aorta and fuses with the foregut mesentery to form the posterior and medial (membranous) portions of the diaphragm. The lateral margins of the diaphragm are considered to be derived from the muscular components of the body wall (recent investigations in rats have questioned the contribution of the body wall). The pleuroperitoneal canals close when all the membranous portions of the diaphragm fuse together, and by the ninth week of gestation, diaphragmatic closure is usually complete (Wells, 1954). If the closure (obliteration) of the pleuroperitoneal canals is delayed beyond the ninth to tenth weeks of development, or if the normal rotation and settling of the midgut occur before the tenth week or before the obliteration of the pleuroperitoneal canals, the midgut (abdominal viscera) herniates into the thoracic (pleural) cavity.

In the past, this defect has been attributed to an abnormal closure of the pleuroperitoneal canal, but investigations using the nitrofen-induced CDH model in the rat have used an innovative approach to reexamining the etiology of this lesion. CDH seems to be linked to a disordered formation of the pleuroperitoneal fold—a much earlier event (fourth week of gestation). An abnormal formation of the framework of mesenchyme, which inhibits muscular development of the diaphragm, has been linked to abnormalities in the retinoid signaling pathway. This suggests that vitamin A may play a role in the pathophysiology of CDH (Greer et al., 2003; Holder et al., 2007). CDH was found in 20% to 40% of offspring of rodents (dams) deficient in vitamin A, suggesting a critical role of the retinoid pathway. In addition, exposure to nitrofen (inhibitor of a key enzyme responsible for conversion of retinal to retinoic acid) was associated with development of CDH.

Preoperative Management

Pathophysiology

In the most common presentation, the herniated abdominal viscera (which includes the midgut but may also include the stomach, parts of the descending colon, the left kidney, and the left lobe of the liver) occupies the left thoracic cavity and interferes with the development of the lungs. In most cases, depending on the severity of the hernia, some degree of pulmonary hypoplasia exists, the severity of which depends on when the herniation and compression occurred during fetal development. The herniation of abdominal contents shifts the mediastinum to the right, compresses the contralateral lung and, in part, contributes to abnormal development of that lung. On the other hand, simple compression of the ipsilateral and contralateral lungs fails to explain the severe morphologic derangements in lung development, such as fewer alveoli with thickened walls, smaller alveolar and gas exchange surface area, decreased vasculature with medial hyperplasia, and extension of the muscle layer into intraacinar arterioles (Done et al., 2008).

The structural abnormalities of the pulmonary vasculature correlate with the pathophysiology, mortality, and morbidity of CDH. The low number of airways, the simple arterial branching pattern, the increase in smooth muscle mass at the level of the resistance vessels, and left ventricular abnormalities add to the severity of cardiorespiratory dysfunction produced by the hernia itself (Schwartz et al., 1994). Alveolar development does occur postnatally, but growth at the preacinar level is limited in that the number of airway generations remains constant after midgestation (Geggel and Reid, 1984). Postnatal vascular remodeling provides larger and less muscular arteries, so the pathology present at birth in the setting of CDH has been documented to reverse to some degree (Beals et al., 1992). Nonetheless, the degree of pulmonary hypoplasia and hypertension is predictive not only of mortality but of the development of long term sequelae in the survivor.

The anatomic abnormalities in the pulmonary vasculature of CDH imply that persistent pulmonary hypertension will commonly accompany this anomaly. The most consistent findings include a fewer number of pulmonary arteries per unit of lung volume and peripheral muscularization of small arteries leading to thickening of the medial and adventitial layers (Geggel et al., 1985). Although small arteries (equal to 200 mcm) predominantly determine pulmonary vascular resistance (PVR), other factors also influence the pulmonary circulation of the newborn.

The fall in PVR (approximately 80%, which normally occurs in the first 24 hours of life) and rise in pulmonary blood flow that is essential for the transition from placental circulation to the postnatal pattern is dependent on adequate function of the endothelial cell (see Chapters 3 and 4, Respiratory Physiology in Infants and Children and Cardiovascular Physiology). Imbalance in the production, release, and circulating levels of vasoconstrictors (leukotrienes C4 and D4, thromboxane A2, platelet activating factor) and vasodilators (NO, prostacylin) seems to be central to the right-to-left shunting observed with pulmonary hypertension associated with CDH (Furchgott and Zawadzki, 1980; Haworth, 2006). Endothelins are also involved in the persistence of high pulmonary vascular resistance. Persistently elevated levels of endothelin 1 (ET-1) have been described in infants with CDH (Rosenberg et al., 1993; Kobayashi and Puri, 1994). In utero, ET-1 contributes significantly to maintaining normal high PVR. Postnatally, various endothelially-derived vasoconstrictive peptides are produced in response to inflammation, ischemia, and other stimuli. Multiple receptors, both in the vascular smooth muscle and in the vascular endothelial cell, mediate response to these molecules. In part, the release of these vasoactive agents is also in response to ventilator-induced epithelial and endothelial damage from hyperinflation of the hypoplastic lungs. Active remodeling of the pulmonary vascular bed continues gradually over the first 2 to 4 weeks of life.

Diagnosis and Treatment

Diagnostic and therapeutic modalities have been developed for both the prenatal and postnatal periods.

Prenatal Diagnosis and Treatment

Prenatal diagnosis of CDH has increased from approximately 10% in 1985 to near 60% at present (Dillon et al., 2000). The most common findings include displacement of the heart and a fluid-filled bowel in the thorax. Both stomach and small bowel are often present (Garne et al., 2002). Ultrasound diagnosis of a large defect (e.g., dilated intrathoracic stomach, herniated left lobe of the liver, or polyhydramnios) suggests a severe lesion; however, prenatal ultrasounds can have a high incidence of false negatives (Lewis et al., 1997).

A variety of indices including lung-to-head circumference ratio (LHR), diameter of the proximal pulmonary artery indexed to the descending aorta, and others have been developed to estimate prognosis by evaluating the pulmonary circulation to estimate risk for severe pulmonary hypoplasia. Jani et al. (2009) noted that an LHR and intrathoracic position of the liver independently predicted poor outcome. In a study by Ruano et al. (2006), survival was estimated to be approximately 50% when the liver was herniated into the thorax. The LHR can also define extreme lung hypoplasia and predict 100% mortality (Albanese et al. 1998; Desfrere et al. 2000; Sbragia et al., 2000; Cacciari et al. 2001; Muratore et al. 2001; Boloker et al. 2002; Stege et al. 2003). However, differences in the specific method to generate the index may lead to confusion when interpreting results among various institutions. In addition to these indices, in utero magnetic resonance imaging (MRI) has been proposed as a method to define anatomy (e.g., position of the liver or volume of the lungs) and identify associated anomalies (Cannie et al., 2008).

Because the fundamental pathophysiology of CDH is pulmonary hypoplasia, various fetal surgical techniques to improve the growth of hypoplastic lungs in utero have been developed (Harrison et al., 1990, 1993, 1997). Starting with animal models in the 1980s, Harrison and colleagues gradually perfected some open fetal surgical procedures and introduced the ex utero intrapartum treatment (EXIT) procedure. The procedure was eventually abandoned in favor of a minimally invasive technique using fetoscopy to surgically occlude the trachea. Tracheal occlusion is aimed to manipulate the physiology of fetal lung development; that is, the fetal lung development is physiologically accelerated by the airway expansion that results from accumulation of lung fluid while the glottis is occluded. In a group of fetuses with moderate hypoplasia enrolled in a trial sponsored by the National Institutes of Health (NIH), the tracheal occlusion technique marginally improved the survival of the affected fetus. However, the procedure was associated with significant complications, including premature labor and delivery. At the same time, the survival of the infants with CDH with conventional postnatal managements improved (Harrison et al., 2003; de Buys Roessingh and Dinh-Xuan, 2009). Further studies of fetal endoscopic tracheal occlusion (FETO), in which the time of tracheal occlusion and release is adjusted, continue; however, the procedure remains investigational (Done et al., 2008).

Postnatal Diagnosis and Treatment

Clinical Presentation. Infants who are born with bilateral lung hypoplasia or severe unilateral hypoplasia exhibit symptoms immediately at birth. In the setting of a prenatal diagnosis, the delivery is deferred to a high-risk center with access to pediatric surgeons, NO, extracorporeal oxygenation, HFOV, and other advanced neonatal therapies.

The classic triad of CDH consists of cyanosis, dyspnea, and apparent dextrocardia. Physical examination reveals a scaphoid abdomen, bulging chest, decreased breath sounds, distant or right-displaced heart sounds, and bowel sounds in the chest. Radiographic examination of the chest shows a bowel gas pattern in the chest, mediastinal shift, and little lung tissue at the right costophrenic sulcus (Fig. 18-15).

Infants who weigh 1000 g, are born before 33 weeks' gestation, or who have an alveolar-to-arterial oxygen gradient (P[A-a]o_2) of more than 500 seldom survive (Raphaely and Downes, 1973). On the other hand, over the last two decades, antenatal diagnosis, neonatal stabilization and delayed surgery, and (most importantly) the avoidance of ventilator-induced lung injury have resulted in significant improvement in morbidity and mortality of infants with severe CDH.

Timing of Surgery. In the past, CDH was considered a neonatal emergency, and surgery to reduce the hernia was performed urgently. The infant's lungs were hyperventilated with 100% oxygen in an attempt to produce pulmonary vasodilation with hyperoxia and respiratory alkalosis. Although the combination of hyperoxia and respiratory alkalosis may produce transient pulmonary vasodilation, mechanical ventilation results in overdistension and damage to the alveolar and capillary membranes (volutrauma, previously called *barotrauma*), which induces an inflammatory reaction and the associated release of vasoactive mediators. Eventually, pulmonary vasoconstriction and hypertension occur, as the balance between vasodilation (oxygen plus alkalosis) and vasoconstriction (inflammatory mediators) shifts and secondary lung injury increases.

The goal of the initial management of CDH is to avoid a surgical intervention when the infant is hypoxic and acidotic and the cardiorespiratory status is labile. Optimizing hemodynamic and respiratory support rather than the specific timing of surgery contributes to improving outcome (Migliazza et al., 2007). Thus, medical management is directed to stabilizing the cardiorespiratory function by improving oxygenation to achieve a preductal saturation more than 90%, correcting any metabolic acidosis, reducing right-to-left shunting and increasing pulmonary perfusion using the least aggressive ventilation possible (Hazebroek et al., 1988). These goals underlie the rationale for some centers initiating HFOV immediately and introducing ECMO to allow pulmonary rest. Unfortunately, these maneuvers have not been predictably effective.

Surgery affects the respiratory system's compliance. Sakai et al. (1987) reported that the postoperative compliance of the respiratory system (CRS), as measured with a noninvasive, passive mechanic's technique, immediately decreased 10% to 77% from the preoperative value, suggesting that pulmonary dynamics often deteriorate after surgical repair of the hernia (Lesouef et al., 1984). These observations prompted a reevaluation of the practice of urgent surgery. Instead, surgery is delayed to allow transition to a stable postnatal cardiorespiratory status.

Nakayama and others (1991) evaluated pulmonary function and outcome of 22 infants with severe CDH treated either with traditional emergency repair or with preoperative stabilization for 2 to 11 days. Of 13 infants who underwent immediate repair of CDH, nine received ECMO support postoperatively, and six of the 13 infants (two after ECMO) survived (46% survival). Of nine infants whose surgery was delayed for preoperative stabilization, six immediately received ECMO support for 4 to 10 days;

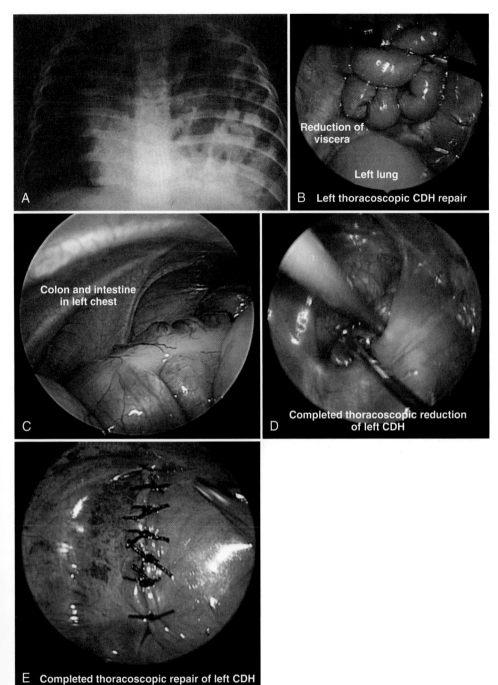

■ **FIGURE 18-15.** CDH. **A,** Chest x-ray showing small bowel. **B,** Laparoscopic view of herniated small bowel. **C,** Laparoscopic view of colon and intestine. **D,** Laparoscopic view of reduced abdominal contents. **E,** Laparoscopic view with completed repair.

one with extreme lung hypoplasia died before surgery after an intraventricular hemorrhage. The other eight infants survived after surgery (89% survival). Seven days after surgery, CRS of infants in the immediate repair group did not improve from the preoperative values. In contrast, CRS increased more than 60% from their baseline values in the infants who underwent preoperative stabilization. Although the duration of mechanical ventilation was similar in the survivors of the two groups, the preoperative stabilization group had higher postductal PaO₂, lower respiratory rates, lower peak and mean airway pressures, and lower fraction of inspired oxygen values (Fio₂). Based on the physiologic and clinical evidence, these researchers concluded that preoperative stabilization is beneficial before the repair of CDH. Surgery should be delayed as long as 5 to 15 days until

PVR has decreased and ventilation can be maintained with a low peak inspiratory pressure (less than 25 cm H₂O) and Fio₂ (about 0.50).

Preoperative care of an infant with severe CDH should start in the delivery room. Positive pressure ventilation by mask and bag has risks, because attempting to expand the noncompliant lungs may damage the hypoplastic lung by overdistention, as well as distend the stomach and intestines (which are in the left hemithorax), further decreasing chest compliance (Wada et al., 1997; Björklund et al., 1997). If spontaneous ventilatory efforts are inadequate, early intubation of the trachea and decompression of the stomach are important initial steps to prevent further distension of and pulmonary compression by the displaced abdominal viscera.

However, after intubation of the trachea, minimizing the trauma from positive pressure ventilation is an important ventilatory intervention. Björklund et al. (1997) found that six manual inflations with a tidal volume of 35 to 40 mL/kg in preterm lambs resulted in persistent respiratory failure and pneumothorax despite surfactant treatment. Wada and colleagues (1997) also found that ventilation of premature lambs at birth with a tidal volume of 20 mL/kg for only 30 minutes resulted in marked decreases in CRS, along with the development of poor gas exchange. In comparison, premature lambs ventilated with 5 or 10 mL/kg of tidal volumes maintained high CRS and normal gas exchange. Although most infants with CDH are born at term or near term, these data may be relevant in CHD where the pulmonary development is abnormal.

Animal studies suggest that ventilatory strategies that employ small tidal volumes maintain high CRS and better gas exchange (Björklund et al., 1997; Wada et al., 1997). Thus, current ventilatory strategies for an infant with CDH incorporate lower peak and end expiratory airway pressures and accept hypercapnea (Wung et al., 1985, 1995; Boloker et al., 2002). In general, HFOV serves as a rescue therapy; however, others advocate respiratory support with HFOV immediately at birth (Migliazza et al., 2007). Ventilation and F_{IO_2} are adjusted to maintain a preductal saturation of 90% to 95%. The Pa_{CO_2} is allowed to remain as high as 60 to 65 mm Hg (permissive hypercapnea). Crystalloid and blood products are administered to maintain intravascular volume and red–blood-cell mass. Adequate sedation is administered in efforts to minimize increase in PVR. Periods of right-to-left shunting are tolerated if the patient's underlying hemodynamic status is stable, and vasopressors (e.g., dopamine or milrinone) are infused to maintain hemodynamic stability. In the immediate postnatal period, some infants initially respond to stabilizing maneuvers (e.g., gentle ventilation or hemodynamic support), but in some cases this early stability represents a "honeymoon period" that is followed by a sudden, often unexplained return to a state of persistent pulmonary hypertension and clinical deterioration (e.g., acidosis, hypoxemia, severe hypercapnia, pulmonary hypertension, and right-to-left shunting through the foramen ovale, and patent ductus arteriosus). If a reversion to a state of persistent pulmonary hypertension occurs, then trials of NO and HFOV are initiated and ECMO is considered.

Nitric Oxide. NO is a free radical with a short half-life, produced endogenously but often administered as an inhaled agent to take advantage of its effects as a selective pulmonary vasodilator. Although a role for NO in the treatment of pulmonary hypertension with CDH is a logical extension from its effectiveness in infants with pulmonary hypertension associated with meconium aspiration, sepsis, or congenital heart disease, clear cut effectiveness in the setting of CDH has not been demonstrated (Kinsella et al., 1992; Roberts et al., 1992; Bloch et al., 2007).

NO diffuses across the alveolar capillary membranes and binds to and thereby stimulates enzymes with transition metal centers (e.g., heme), such as cyclic guanylate cyclase. This increases cyclic GMP, activates protein kinase, and causes vascular smooth muscle to relax (see Chapters 3, 4, and 17, Respiratory Physiology in Infants and Children, Cardiovascular Physiology, and Neonatology for Anesthesiologists). Phosphodiesterases quickly metabolize NO, thereby limiting its half-life. In addition to cyclic guanosine monophosphate (cGMP)-mediated action, NO also has non-cGMP actions. For example, NO interacts directly with proteins with active thiol groups, such as those in the heart. NO's modification of various myocardial proteins has been linked to regulation of contractility, but this action has not been well defined in the setting of CDH and neonatal pulmonary hypertension (Zimmet and Hare, 2006).

Toxic effects of NO are primarily attributed to its interaction with superoxide and the production of the highly reactive oxidant peroxynitrite. In addition, NO reacts with oxygenated hemoglobin to form methemoglobin. Although monitoring the concentration of methemoglobin is recommended if NO is administered for prolonged periods, significant methemoglobinemia is not commonly encountered during common clinical scenarios.

In a small series, Shah et al. (1994) noted that patients with CDH may be more resistant to the effects of inhaled NO, whereas Karamanoukian et al. (1994) noted that NO was effective in patients with hypoplastic lungs only after extracorporeal membrane oxygenation. In a study of patients treated with HFOV from birth, only 28% of those with severe pulmonary hypertension achieved reversal after NO. In general, most patients with intractable pulmonary hypertension plus lung hypoplasia do not have a predictable, dramatic response to NO. Nonetheless, because some patients do respond and the drug has limited toxicity in lower doses, NO is often used in infants with CDH who require therapy beyond gentle conventional ventilatory support (e.g., HFOV).

Even in the setting of respiratory failure without CDH, the long-term benefits of NO compared with other therapeutic interventions remain controversial. In a follow-up study of infants (with fewer and more than 34 weeks' gestation, treated and not treated with NO) who had been enrolled in the INNOVA trial (15 neonatal units in the United Kingdom, Republic of Ireland, Finland, and Belgium), respiratory morbidity was similar when the impact of NO was analyzed. For example, wheezing and rehospitalization were common in both term and preterm infants who received and did not receive NO (Hoo et al., 2009). Clearly, neonates with severe respiratory compromise are at high risk for long-term pulmonary dysfunction.

Extracorporeal Membrane Oxygenation. A notable series of 400 patients were reported in two manuscripts by Azarow et al. (1997) in Toronto and Wilson et al. (1997) in Boston. ECMO was used as rescue therapy in Boston, and HFOV was used in Toronto. Survival in the two cities was nearly identical (53% and 55%). A 2008 Cochrane review concluded that in spite of short-term efficacy, improved long-term survival without major sequelae was not apparent with ECMO (Mugford et al., 2008). Thus, many centers now reserve ECMO as a rescue therapy for infants who have persistent preductal hypoxemia in spite of inotropic and ventilatory support (including HFOV and NO) (Bohn, 2002, 2006).

A common set-up for ECMO is a venoarterial circuit where the patient's internal jugular vein and common carotid artery are cannulated. In this system, blood is drained by gravity from the right atrium, oxygenated through the membrane oxygenator, and returned to the patient through the arterial cannulae. During venovenous bypass, the patient's blood returns to the membrane oxygenator by gravity, is oxygenated in the membrane oxygenator, and is then returned to the venous system. Thus, in venovenous ECMO, adequate systemic oxygen delivery depends on an effective cardiac output, whereas in infants undergoing venoarterial ECMO the bypass system can compensate for both pulmonary and myocardial dysfunction. Significant risks are associated with ECMO, including bleeding at surgical or chest tube insertion sites, intracranial hemorrhage, sepsis, hypertension, and brain death. Clearly, the underlying disease (e.g., meconium aspiration without pulmonary hypoplasia vs. CDH with pulmonary hypoplasia) influences the success rates of ECMO (Dalton and Thompson, 1992). In general, because the mortality and the likelihood of intracranial hemorrhage are higher in low–birth-weight infants, ECMO is limited to infants weighing more than 2 kg and with more than 35 weeks' gestation, and to infants who have no evidence of prior intracranial hemorrhage.

The criteria for instituting ECMO vary, but guidelines generally include $P(A-a)o_2$ of greater than 600 mm Hg for more than 6 to 8 hours or an oxygen index ($Fio_2 \times$ mean airway pressure/Pao_2) of 51 for 5 hours. Nonetheless, no selection criteria appear to be accurate in predicting survival (Newman et al., 1990; Van Meurs, 1990; Steimle et al., 1994; Bohn, 2006; Mugford et al., 2008). In view of the improved survival with gentle ventilation (including HFOV), coupled with the significant morbidity associated with ECMO, ECMO intervention has been relegated a less central role in the setting of CDH.

Intraoperative and Postoperative Management: Open Repair

Although many centers now approach repair of CDH via minimal access techniques, open repair still remains common (Guner et al., 2008a). Severe pulmonary dysfunction limits the tolerance of thoracoscopy and one-lung ventilation, making minimal access surgery difficult or impossible (see Minimal-Access Surgery in the Neonate, p. 561).

In most cases, open surgical repair is approached through an abdominal incision, but a transthoracic or thoracoabdominal approach may be taken. Infants with large defects may not tolerate primary closure of the abdomen after the hernia is reduced. In such a case, a patch closure is attempted. In rare cases, a chimney prosthesis or silastic pouch is placed. In these infants, venous access in the lower extremities should be avoided because the inferior vena cava may be compressed after reduction of the hernia, limiting venous return. In all cases, an internal jugular cannula provides reliable access, allows CVP monitoring both intraoperatively and postoperatively, and may be essential to deliver TPN postoperatively.

With rare exceptions, infants with a moderate or large CDH require ventilatory support and sedation preoperatively, and many receive neuromuscular blockade. The goals of ventilation and oxygen delivery in the operating room are the same as the preoperative. Avoiding volutrauma includes a small tidal volume, appropriate PEEP (5 to 7 cm H_2O) to avoid atelectasis and shear stress trauma (low volume injury), adequate oxygenation without hyperoxia (oxygen saturation of hemoglobin, measured with pulse oximetry [SpO_2] 90% to 95%) and permissive hypercapnea as needed, while maintaining adequate pH (>7.25). In many cases, vigorously maintaining intravascular volume with crystalloid or colloid may be effective in minimizing right-to-left shunting. If a sudden deterioration occurs in ventilation or hemodynamic status, pulmonary hypertension must be quickly differentiated from a contralateral pneumothorax, because the treatment for a pneumothorax is needle thoracostomy and chest tube placement, and hyperventilation should be avoided to prevent air leak into a pneumothorax. NO treatment (10 to 20 ppm in inspired gas mixture) should be initiated if pulmonary hypertension with arterial desaturation is suspected, while ventilation with permissive hypercapnea and PEEP is maintained.

All newborns deserve meticulous attention to temperature stability in the operating room, but infants with a CDH have dramatic risks associated with hypothermia related to its effect on increasing PVR, which may increase right-to-left shunting through a PDA or the foramen ovale (see Chapter 6, Thermoregulation Physiology and Perioperative Disturbances). Hypothermia increases oxygen consumption, and in the setting of marginal cardiorespiratory function, may result in inadequate oxygen delivery and acidosis, which then further increases pulmonary vasoconstriction and worsens oxygen saturation.

The selection of specific anesthetic agents must be based on cardiorespiratory status, the location of the surgery (NICU or operating room), and the plans for intraoperative ventilatory support. Nitrous oxide is avoided in infants with CDH because many require high-inspired oxygen concentration and also because nitrous oxide can diffuse into the viscera and exaggerate lung compression. If an anesthesia machine is available, low concentrations of inhalation anesthetics (sevoflurane or isoflurane) may be advantageous in producing pulmonary vasodilation, but if effects on SVR are greater than PVR, right-to-left shunting may actually worsen. In most cases, high-dose opioids (usually fentanyl) are administered and the narcotic infusion continues into the postoperative period (Hickey et al., 1985; Hickey and Retzack, 1993).

Outcomes

The prolonged and complicated neonatal course of infants with CDH implies that these infants are at high risk for long-term pulmonary, gastrointestinal or nutritional, and neurocognitive disorders. Muratore et al. (2001) noted that therapy with ECMO and the need for a patch correlated with later significant pulmonary disease. However, non-ECMO survivors also required repeated treatment for respiratory problems secondary to ventilator-induced lung injury and the onset of reactive airways disease. For example, 52% of all CDH survivors required therapy with bronchodilators, and 41% received inhaled steroids. Approximately 25% of survivors had evidence of obstructive lung disease. Jaillard et al. (2003) noted significant long-term pulmonary complications, reporting a 22% incidence of chronic lung disease at two years of age, and the use of ECMO and need for patch repair predicted later respiratory illness. Others report higher incidence of chronic lung disease that seemed to improve over time. Nonetheless, exercise performance was described as abnormal in some survivors, and approximately 50% of adults in one study had abnormal pulmonary function (Vanamo et al., 1996). Finally, approximately 4% of survivors require tracheostomy (Muratore et al., 2001; Jaillard et al., 2003).

Growth failure, oral aversion, and gastroesophageal reflux occur in 45% to 90% of infants with CDH, and the incidence correlates with the size of the defect and need for patch repair (Committee on Fetus and Newborn, 2008). At least one third of these infants require nutritional supplements via gastrostomy or nasogastric tube. In these infants, reflux is often exacerbated by the presence of these devices.

Neurocognitive delay and behavioral disorders have been documented in the survivors of CDH, especially in those who had been supported with ECMO, with developmental delay noted in more than one third of some cohorts (Nobuhara et al., 1996).

In particular, motor and language problems are common and have been detected in 60% to 70% of patients with CDH at age 3 years (Friedman et al., 2008). In these and other series, the infants treated with ECMO may have a higher incidence of significant neurodevelopmental delays (Bernbaum et al., 1995). Sensorineural hearing loss has been described in as many as 50% of patients with CDH in later infancy, even after normal screening was documented in the NICU. Recurrent or prolonged hypoxemia, exposure to ototoxic drugs (e.g., lasix, aminoglycocides), and ECMO have been suggested as causative factors (Robertson et al., 2002; Fligor et al., 2005; Erikson et al., 2009).

In addition to neurologic, pulmonary, and gastrointestinal disorders, survivors of CDH often develop chest-wall deformities and scoliosis. The incidence is higher in those with large defects that required patching. Similarly, recurrence of a hernia is most common among those with large defects with a patch in place. Because survivors of CDH have undergone major invasive care in the NICU and multiple surgical interventions, long-term, structured, multidisciplinary follow-up care is essential to the future care of these patients.

Tracheoesophageal Fistula and Esophageal Atresia

The incidence of TEF and esophageal atresia (EA) ranges between 1:3000 and 1:4000 births (Sparey et al., 2000). Approximately 20% to 25% of these infants have additional congenital defects. The incidence of associated defects is particularly high (50% to 70%) in the group with isolated EA but least common in infants with the H-type fistula. The most common anomalies include congenital heart disease (approximately 35%, including ventricular septal defect, atrial septal defect, tetralogy of Fallot, atrioventricular canal, and coarctation of the aorta), genitourinary disorders (about 24%); gastrointestinal disorders (approximately 24%, including duodenal or ileal atresia, malrotation, and imperforate anus); skeletal anomalies (approximately 13%); and central nervous system disorders (about 10%) (Dave et al., 1999). The term *VACTERL (vertebral, anal, cardiac, tracheoesophageal, renal, limb) association* refers to these anomalies, because they commonly coexist in various combinations with TEF/EA. As many as 20% to 25% of infants with esophageal atresia have at least three of the lesions included in VACTERL (Rittler et al., 1996).

Recently, a significant incidence of non-VACTERL anomalies (single umbilical artery, 20%; genital defects, 23%; and respiratory tract anomalies, 13%) were retrospectively identified from two pediatric centers in the Netherlands (de Jong et al., 2008). In spite of the significant incidence of multiple anomalies, the risk of recurrence is less than 1% in nonsyndromal TEF/EA (Goyal et al., 2006; Ioannides and Copp, 2009). However, TEF and EA are known to be common in Trisomy 18 (about 25%), Trisomy 13, and to a lesser degree, Trisomy 21. As with CDH, the wide mining of databases and adaptation of techniques such as fluorescent in situ hybridization (FISH) and whole genome arrays have allowed identification of rare and small chromosomal abnormalities (e.g., partial trisomy 3p, partial deletion 5p, distal 13q deletion, interstitial deletions of 17q) in some cases of TEF/EA, but no specific regions have been consistently linked to these anomalies (Felix et al., 2007). Thus, at this point, the etiology seems to be multifactorial and sporadic in the nonsyndromic version. Familial and syndromic patterns

occur in fewer than 1% of the cases. Finally, exposure to various teratogens has not correlated consistently with TEF/EA.

A variety of other lung anomalies (e.g., lobar agenesis, pulmonary hypoplasia, horseshoe lung, and absence of a bronchus to the right upper lobe) have been reported in the context of TEF/EA, and some experts have proposed that the lesion should be termed "general foregut malformation" (Kovesi and Rubin, 2004). In addition, TEF/EA has been identified in the setting of DiGeorge's and Down syndromes as well as with CHARGE association.

Mortality associated with TEF/EA generally depends on the severity of the associated heart disease and birth weight. In 1994, Spitz linked survival rates to the following three categories:

Group 1: Birth weight more than 1500 g without a major cardiac anomaly (97% survival).

Group 2: Birth weight less than 1500 g or major cardiac anomaly (59% survival).

Group 3: Birth weight less than 1500 g and major cardiac anomaly (22% survival).

More recently, within the same three groups, survival rates improved to 98%, 82%, and 50%, respectively (Lopez et al., 2006). Clearly, the spectrum of presentation from an isolated TEF/EA to a multisystem or chromosomal disorder has major implications for mortality and morbidity, as well as for treatment options and surgical and anesthetic management.

Embryology

The embryogenesis of TEF/EA remains incompletely defined, but several theories have been proposed (Ioannides and Copp, 2009). It is known that the trachea and esophagus develop from the foregut in the first 4 to 5 weeks of gestation. One theory suggests that the respiratory system results from a rapid outgrowth from the foregut. That is, the tracheal primordium buds off the foregut and remains a separate structure during subsequent development. Another theory focuses on active growth of mesenchymal septum that divides the foregut into ventral (respiratory) and dorsal (gastrointestinal) structures. The septum has been considered to begin at the distal site (bronchopulmonary buds), but in fact such a structure has not been clearly identified in studies of tracheoesophageal development. Other theories seem to combine segments of each of these two theories, proposing that the trachea and esophagus separate as a result of foregut folds. Ioannides et al. (2002) suggested that the physical separation of the original foregut is a critical component of the organogenesis of the esophagus and trachea. On the other hand, differentiation of both respiratory and esophageal components usually does not occur in the setting of TEF/EA.

At the molecular level, aberrant signaling in the sonic hedgehog pathways and other regulatory genes has been linked to TEF/EA in several studies (Veraksa et al., 2000).

Hedgehog proteins are signaling glycoproteins involved in many processes of early development, including embryogenesis of the foregut as well as development of the craniofacial structures, heart, and great vessels. Of the multiple hedgehog proteins, only sonic hedgehog (Shh) is expressed in mammalian gut and lung. Mutants for Shh and for the Gli proteins (transcription factors) have been noted with tracheoesophageal malformations and various other well-described associated anomalies (e.g., VACTERL) (Kim et al., 2001).

In studies examining the expression of thyroid-transcription factor-1 (TTF-1) known to be specific to the respiratory tract, the distal esophagus in TEF/EA was proposed to be of tracheal origin. TTF-1 expression localizes to the lung bud but not to the esophagus early in gestation. TTF-1 is expressed in the fistula tract throughout gestation. Based on this work, the distal "esophagus" might be of embryonic lung origin. This finding, in part, could explain the pathophysiology and clinical findings of TEF/EA: poor esophageal motility, gastroesophageal reflux, esophageal stenosis, and pseudostratified columnar (respiratory epithelium) rather than squamous epithelium (esophageal epithelium) (Crisera et al., 1999a, 1999b). Other explanations for abnormal esophageal motor function in TEF/EA focus on the abnormal innervation of the esophagus. For example, dysplasia of both Meissner's plexus (submucosal nerves) and Auerbach's plexus (myenteric) occur along with an abnormal distribution of mitochondria, and high levels of vasoactive intestinal polypeptide and NO synthase (NOS) (Li et al., 2007).

Anatomy of TEF

The anatomic variations of TEF have been well described and, in most cases TEF and EA occur together (Types B, C, E) (Fig. 18-16). The most common lesion (more than 90% of cases) is type C, in which a fistula exists between the trachea and the lower esophageal segment at a point slightly above the carina, and the upper esophageal segment ends blindly in the mediastinum at the level of the second or third thoracic vertebra.

Prenatal Diagnosis and Clinical Presentation

TEF should be suspected in the presence of maternal polyhydramnios, which may result from esophageal obstruction that prevents the swallowing of amniotic fluid. Preterm labor may then develop as a result of the excessive intrauterine volume. However, in most cases polyhydramnios is a nonspecific sign and develops idiopathically; congenital anomalies account for only 10% to 20% of cases (Dashe et al., 2002). For example, polyhydramnios can develop secondary to impaired fetal swallowing because of abnormal central nervous system function, including weakness associated with neuromuscular dysfunction. Unfortunately, polyhydramnios and small or absent fetal stomach bubble are the most common ultrasound findings associated with TEF/EA. These have a low positive predictive value, and false positives are common (Houben and Curry, 2008). Similarly, when TEF accompanies EA, amniotic fluid can pass into the stomach from the trachea, usually enough to form a stomach bubble but not enough to prevent polyhydramnios. In addition, polyhydramnios is rarely identified before about 24 weeks' gestation (Pretorius et al., 1987). A dilated blind-ending upper pouch of the esophagus (upper pouch sign) has been described on ultrasound, but as with MRI studies, it has not been deemed an accurate prenatal method for diagnosing TEF/EA (Houben and Curry, 2008). Overall, the prenatal detection rate is 40% to 50%. The significant incidence of coexisting abnormalities and syndromes (e.g., Trisomy 18) implies that an in utero diagnosis should precipitate karyotyping and an intense search for other structural anomalies. As with other severe congenital anomalies, prenatal diagnosis of TEF/EA may improve outcome by allowing optimal prenatal counseling and postnatal treatment. Unlike with CDH, supportive interventions for TEF/EA are less urgent and the implications of birth outside a major medical center are less risky, so prenatal diagnosis, although ideal, is of somewhat less critical significance.

Postnatal diagnosis depends on the specific anatomy of the TEF/EA, except in the case of an H-fistula, when the newborn infant exhibits excessive salivation, drooling, cyanotic spells, swallowing problems, and coughing, which is relieved to some extent by suctioning. The diagnosis of EA can be confirmed in the delivery room by the inability to pass a catheter down the esophagus into the stomach. When a radiopaque catheter is used, a radiograph reveals the catheter in the blind upper pouch. If a TEF is present, a plain radiograph of the chest and abdomen reveals air or gas bubbles in the stomach and intestines that have entered through the fistula (Fig. 18-17).

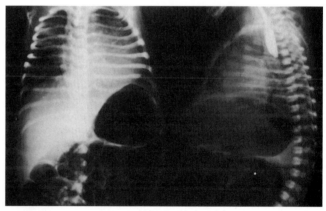

■ **FIGURE 18-17.** Gastric distention in type C lesion, may require prompt relief. Note blindly ending esophagus on lateral view. (*Courtesy of Dr. Arnold Colodny, Boston, Mass.*)

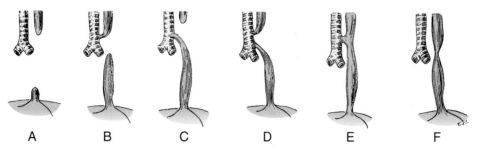

■ **FIGURE 18-16.** Types of congenital abnormalities of the esophagus. **A,** EA, no esophageal communication with the trachea. **B,** EA, upper segment communicating with the trachea. **C,** EA, lower segment communicating with the back of the trachea. More than 90% of all esophageal malformations fall into this group. **D,** EA, both segments communicating with the trachea. **E,** Esophagus has no disruption of its continuity but has a TEF. **F,** Esophageal stenosis. (*From Gross RE: The surgery of infancy and childhood, Philadelphia, 1953, WB Saunders.*)

Ultrasonography is important in the diagnosis of any associated cardiac, renal, or genitourinary abnormalities. Often, H-type fistulas escape diagnosis until an infant, child, or adult is evaluated for recurrent pneumonia.

Preoperative Management

The ligation of a TEF is urgent, but not emergent, except in the setting of respiratory insufficiency severe enough to require ventilatory support. In that setting, the presence of a TEF and poor lung compliance often prevent delivery of adequate tidal volumes (ventilation escapes into the esophagus and stomach via the fistula). In such cases, the dilation of the stomach may add to the respiratory compromise by elevating the diaphragm and worsening pulmonary compliance. Preoperatively, several interventions are undertaken promptly to protect the lungs from aspiration pneumonia, including:

- Avoiding feeding
- Upright positioning of the infant to minimize gastroesophageal reflux
- Intermittent suctioning of the upper pouch
- Administration of antibiotic therapy to treat sepsis or aspiration pneumonia

Intraoperative Management

Surgical Technique

Although thoracoscopic approaches have been adopted and are now the initial surgical approach at many centers, many infants with TEF/EA require the traditional open technique. Preoperative considerations are the same for either approach. Meticulous evaluation of pulmonary status helps determine whether one-lung ventilation will be tolerated and whether an intraoperative ventilator other than the device associated with the anesthesia machine should be available. Although considered routine by some surgeons, others may elect to reserve preoperative bronchoscopy only for infants with a confusing clinical picture. Along with careful consideration of the pulmonary status, assessment of the hemodynamic status and a search for associated anomalies dominate the preoperative evaluation.

Optimally, a total repair can be accomplished as a one-stage procedure, in which the fistula is ligated and the esophagus is primarily anastomosed. In infants with significant associated anomalies or sepsis, thoracotomy may be considered too risky, and instead a palliative procedure such as a gastrostomy may be performed. Because a gastrostomy would only be undertaken in the event that the infant is not able to tolerate a more definitive surgery, many of these infants receive preoperative mechanical ventilation. In many cases, a more definitive surgery can be performed within 24 to 72 hours, when the extent of other anomalies is defined, cardiovascular stability is established, and a clear surgical plan has been defined. The gastrostomy is kept patent to decompress the stomach and minimize regurgitation into the lungs, and in cases in which definitive surgery is delayed, it allows enteral feeds.

Unless the aortic arch is right-sided, the surgical approach for open repair is through a right thoracotomy using a posterolateral extrapleural approach. On occasion, the distal portion of the esophagus is either absent or too short to reach the proximal segment. Type C (EA with a TEF between the distal esophagus and the trachea) is most commonly associated with a gap short enough to allow a primary repair, and Type A (EA) is least commonly associated with such a gap. Usually, at some point preoperatively, the gap between the proximal and distal esophagus is measured. However, the methods to assess the gap range from simple radiographic contrast studies ("unstressed") to images with metal dilators inside the proximal and distal pouches (if a gastrostomy is present). In any case, the measurement only serves as an estimate for operative approach. In general, a gap smaller than two vertebral bodies is considered appropriate for a primary repair. If the gap is between two and six vertebral bodies, a delayed anastomosis might be considered, and if it is greater than six vertebral bodies, some would suggest that primary anastomosis is impossible. Others propose various methods to induce growth. In some series, EA with a long gap is defined in terms of centimeters between the ends. A gap of longer than 2.5 cm is sometimes considered the starting point for the category of long-gap EA (Foker et al., 2005). Thus, comparing approaches and results among series remains challenging because definitions and methods to measure the gap vary.

In cases in which a delayed surgery is planned, surgeons have traditionally ligated the fistula and inserted a gastrostomy, and some have also exteriorized the upper pouch through an esophagostomy. The baby can receive nutrition via the gastrostomy until surgery. In most cases, definitive repair is undertaken between 3 and 6 months of age, depending on the infant's status (e.g., growth and cardiorespiratory status) and the opinion of the surgeon. At that time, the two esophageal segments are either directly anastomosed or surgically bridged with an interposed bowel segment or gastric tube graft. In many centers, these traditional approaches have been replaced with those focused on inducing growth of the esophagus or simply waiting for spontaneous growth. The goal is to accomplish a primary anastomosis within the first few months of life, aiming to avoid the high incidence of reflux, dysmotility, and other associated complications using nonesophageal tissue to close the gap (see Outcomes, p. 578).

Techniques to lengthen the native esophagus in order to shorten the distance between the proximal and distal ends have remained controversial, but in some cases they have allowed primary anastomosis (Foker et al., 2009). Foker et al. (2005) described inducing esophageal lengthening by placing external or internal traction sutures to induce rapid growth, creating an anastomosis of the esophageal ends without disruption of the wall by myotomies, and placing the esophageal junction below the diaphragm. In most cases, normal growth of the esophagus has been induced, with traction allowing increases in width as well as length. Often at least two thoracotomies are required in this approach; the same small incision (3 cm) is used, thus sparing the seratus anterior muscle, minimizing the incidence of rib fusion, and decreasing both short- and long-term complications (Foker et al., 2009). Other techniques to induce growth of the esophagus have been proposed, and recently thoracoscopic elongation of the esophagus has been reported (van der Zee et al., 2007). In some cases, simply delaying the primary closures for several weeks or months allows adequate growth (i.e., no tension either internally or externally).

Airway Management

The awake intubation technique is considered by some to be the safest approach to secure the airway in infants with TEF. It allows appropriate positioning of the endotracheal tube without positive pressure ventilation, as well as minimizes the risk of gastric distention from inspired gases passing through the fistula. Often, titrating small doses of fentanyl (0.2 to 0.5 mcg/kg) or morphine (0.02 to 0.05 mg/kg) allows intubation of the trachea without excessive hemodynamic stimulation or depression. An alternative induction technique includes an inhalation anesthetic with or without muscle relaxation and with cautious, gentle positive pressure ventilation as needed.

Evaluating the upper airway via rigid or fiberoptic bronchoscopy remains integral to the presurgical planning of TEF/EA repair. Although some surgeons and anesthesiologists consider the procedure a fundamental part of the preoperative or intraoperative assessment (e.g., ensure that only one fistula is present, assess for tracheomalacia and other anomalies, and position the endotracheal tube), others reserve bronchoscopy for cases where the clinical status suggests that anatomy must be further defined. In fact, fistulas may be difficult to identify via bronchoscopy. In addition, if the bronchoscopy is conducted to ensure a precise positioning of an endotracheal tube, this goal may be difficult to sustain after the bronchoscopy (even with careful marking of the endotracheal tube, attention to flexion and extension of the neck, and other precautions) because of subsequent repositioning for surgery and normal movement of the endotracheal tube during positive pressure ventilation and repeated suctioning during surgery. Furthermore, the TEF is often located close to the carina, and attempts to position the endotracheal tube below the fistula may precipitate one-lung ventilation (intentional or unintentional).

A key decision for the surgeon and anesthesiologist involves whether one-lung ventilation would facilitate the surgical procedure, and if so, appropriately select those patients who are likely to tolerate the technique (see Minimal-Access Surgery in the Neonate, p. 561). If tolerated, collapse of the lung may improve surgical exposure, but in some cases an unacceptable fall in oxygen saturation (in spite of high Fio_2 and continuous positive airway pressure [CPAP] to the nonventilated lung) requires a return to two-lung ventilation. Thus, it may be illogical to commit significant time to bronchoscopy, and in some cases doing so may needlessly prolong the operative time. Finally, even with initial ideal positioning of the endotracheal tube, in some patients ventilation through the fistula still occurs, especially if high peak airway pressures are required.

After the endotracheal tube is in its "assigned" position (i.e., one- or two-lung ventilation), end-tidal carbon dioxide and oxygen saturation should be monitored, and the stomach and chest should be auscultated to ensure that the lung(s) are adequately ventilated. Ideally, the stomach is not distended with inspired gases (i.e., ventilation does not enter the stomach via the fistula, or the fistula itself has not been intubated). Salem et al. (1973) suggested distal positioning of the endotracheal tube, with the bevel facing anteriorly and the posterior wall of the endotracheal tube occluding the fistula, but this maneuver is challenging to achieve and maintain.

Although precordial stethoscopes have been relegated to secondary rank because monitoring oxygen saturation and end-tidal carbon dioxide have become standards of care, a precordial stethoscope can contribute importantly to intraoperative care during repair of TEF. The precordial stethoscope can be positioned in the left axilla (i.e., during a right thoracotomy) to allow breath-to-breath monitoring of adequate ventilation to the dependent lung. Ideally, in infants with unstable cardiorespiratory status or congenital heart disease, an arterial catheter (umbilical or radial) should be available. In the setting of right-to-left shunting via a patent ductus arteriosus, pre- and postductal oxygen saturation monitoring with two pulse oximeters may provide critical data about shunting and pulmonary hypertension (see Congenital Diaphragmatic Hernia, p. 567).

Few patients have a gastrostomy at the time of presentation for surgery for EA/TEF, but if one is present, the gastrostomy tube could be submerged in a container of water after the trachea is intubated to observe for gas bubbles, which would be evident during ventilation of the fistula. If bubbling occurs, the endotracheal tube should be repositioned. Alternatively, the gastrostomy tube can be connected to a capnograph. When the endotracheal tube is proximal to the fistula, carbon dioxide might be detected. When the endotracheal tube is distal to the fistula, no expiratory gases would be detected.

A gastrostomy may serve as a low-resistance vent through which some of the tidal volume escapes, especially if high peak airway pressures are needed to ventilate noncompliant lungs and the chest wall. Although inserting a Fogarty catheter (or other ballooned device) retrograde via the gastrostomy or via a bronchoscope into the TEF has been reported, this technique is often impractical in the setting of small infants (Filston et al., 1982; Karl, 1985). Precise positioning of a catheter so that the balloon is occluding only the fistula is difficult to achieve, and even if the positioning is perfect on initial attempt, maintaining this precise position of the catheter for any length of time is almost impossible. Furthermore, displacement of the balloon can be disastrous (e.g., occluding the trachea). Finally, a high-pressure balloon may impinge on small pulmonary vessels or airways, compromising pulmonary blood flow or ventilation.

Once satisfactory ventilation is assured, the chest is opened and the lungs are retracted. Lung retraction (or one-lung ventilation) may dramatically change oxygenation and ventilation, especially in infants with respiratory dysfunction from immature lungs, pneumonia, or congenital heart disease. Intermittent release of pressure by the surgeon to allow reinflation of the lungs often improves oxygenation and ventilation. Blood clots or secretions may block the endotracheal tube, and repeated endotracheal suctioning may be required. Because the trachea is a soft structure in the newborn, surgical manipulation may kink the airway and further obstruct the airway. Thus, interference with adequate oxygenation and ventilation can occur as a result of the patient's anatomy, operative positioning, and surgical manipulations. In many cases, the inspired concentration of oxygen and mechanical ventilation (sometimes manual ventilation) must be adjusted often, balancing the risks of oxygen toxicity and barotrauma with those of hypoxia. Of course, the surgeon and anesthesiologist must constantly communicate to minimize avoidable events.

Diaz et al. (2005) reported the incidence of intraoperative critical events (as well as overall survival) in open-surgical TEF/EA repair in patients with and without congenital heart disease (excluding patent ductus and or patent foramen ovale). In this report, all patients with ductus-dependent lesions were mechanically ventilated preoperatively, and the incidence of clinically important events was higher in this group, even when compared with infants who had less significant heart anomalies. Difficulty with intubation and oxygen saturation secondary to lung retraction, plugging of the endotracheal tube, and hypotension dominated the events. Perioperative mortality in the highest risk group was 23%, consistent with the survival rates (82% survival, even with a major cardiac lesion) as reported by Lopez et al. (2006), using a three-tiered risk assignment.

After the TEF is ligated and if primary esophageal anastomosis is planned, the anesthesiologist passes a catheter through the nose or mouth into the blind upper pouch to identify the upper esophageal structure. The surgeon passes a catheter into the lower part of the esophagus, and the anastomosis is made over the catheter. When the anastomosis is complete, the catheter is withdrawn just above the suture line, and the proximal end of the catheter is marked at the mouth. The distance from the mouth to the distal tip is noted to guide suctioning in the postoperative period.

Postoperative Management

Some full-term infants are extubated after simple ligation of a TEF, but this is rare. Tracheomalacia or a defective tracheal wall at the site of the fistula can cause collapse of the airway and preoperative aspiration may compromise pulmonary function. Treatment of postoperative pain, when combined with the host of other cardiorespiratory problems of the newborn, often requires a period of postoperative ventilation for at least 24 to 48 hours. Opioid infusions and regional anesthetic techniques have been successfully used for pain management. Most surgeons request that ventilation with a mask and bag be avoided for at least several days postoperatively, especially if the esophagus has been anastomosed. Infants who have had a "long-gap" atresia repaired often have tension at the anastomotic site that may be better protected with postoperative ventilatory support for 5 to 7 days. Deep sedation or neuromuscular blockade to eliminate spontaneous ventilation (i.e., eliminate negative intrapleural pressure transmitted to the anastomosis) are maintained as a function of the status of the infant, as well as bias of the surgeon or neonatologist. Babies whose lungs were contaminated preoperatively or intraoperatively, whose intraoperative course was complicated (e.g., trachea perforation), or whose underlying lung disease is associated with prematurity or other lesions are also mechanically ventilated postoperatively. In these cases, the approach to postoperative ventilatory support is often defined more by the pulmonary status than the surgical events. In part, the intraoperative anesthetic plan is tailored to meet the postoperative ventilatory requirements.

Outcomes

TEF/EA cannot be considered a simple anatomic problem that is easily cured by a surgical intervention. After surgery, structural and functional abnormalities commonly persist long term, even into adulthood. The design of the initial neonatal surgery must focus on the goal of achieving physiologically normal function, but this is difficult. To avoid the psychological overlay of "chronic disease," early repair is obviously ideal. In reality, multiple significant long-term problems should be anticipated in survivors of TEF/EA.

Early complications primarily consist of anastomotic leaks and strictures. Some anastomotic leaks spontaneously seal; others may require intensive medical or even surgical treatment. Strictures at the site of esophageal anastomosis or the fistula may develop in as many as 30% to 40% of infants, but early lesions often respond to two or three dilations. More significant strictures often develop in response to gastroesophageal reflux (GER) and are associated with a history of significant anastomotic leaks in the immediate postoperative period and after repair of long-gap lesions.

GER is probably the most common and significant long-term problem after TEF/EA. GER is recognized in at least 40% of patients (35% to 58%), and is more common after anastomosis under tension, after gastrostomy, and after delayed primary repair (Kovesi and Rubin, 2004; Spitz, 2006). GER seems to correlate with many of the long-term problems associated with TEF/EA: strictures; pulmonary disease (e.g., recurrent aspiration pneumonia, reactive airways disease, and parenchymal disease); feeding problems and oral aversion; and poor growth. Follow up and evaluation of GER are critical for all survivors of TEF/EA.

Esophageal dysmotility/disordered peristalsis and abnormal lower esophageal sphincter function is recognized in at least 75% of patients with EA and in all children who have undergone delayed repair with interposition procedures. In childhood, choking episodes are common. Many children eat slowly and often compensate by drinking water and other liquids during meals. Choking episodes may be associated with apnea and cyanotic spells. Esophageal obstruction may develop, and some patients require removal of impacted material. Although dysphagia may persist into adulthood in 10% to 30% of patients, symptoms seem to dissipate after the first decade of life (Kovesi and Rubin, 2004).

Symptoms of dysmotility correlate with reduced intrinsic innervation (e.g., myenteric plexus or Auerbach's plexus), disorganized muscle layers in the esophagus, tracheobronchial remnants, and a shortened intraabdominal segment of the esophagus (secondary to anastomosis). Feeding aversion develops more commonly in those with pure EA and in those who are exclusively fed via gastrostomy early in life. Feeding aversion, esophageal dysmotility, and GER may lead to growth failure. Furthermore, without aggressive medical or surgical therapy, esophagitis and eventually Barrett's esophagus, a precancerous lesion, may develop. Approaches toward performing antireflux surgery (e.g., Nissen fundoplication) vary from center to center, but surgery clearly plays a role in treating severe GER. Some surgeons recommend aggressive surgical intervention within the first 6 to 24 months of life to minimize the secondary complications of severe GER.

Tracheomalacia and other abnormalities of the trachea also define long-term outcome after TEF/EA. Although common, tracheomalacia appears to be clinically significant in only about 10% of patients (Spitz, 2007). Tracheomalacia tends to improve after the first 3 to 5 years of life, and is rare in isolated EA. Tracheomalacia is generally identified at or just above the site of the TEF, and therefore is most prominent in the lower one third of the trachea. The trachea seems to have an excessive membranous portion that is prone to instability. A brassy cough ("TEF cough") is common in infants and children but rarely persists into adulthood. When symptoms are severe, stridor may develop. Treatment for tracheomalacia is required only in patients with severe symptoms (e.g., apnea, recurrent pneumonia, or worsening stridor) and usually involves an aortopexy (i.e., suturing the aorta to the posterior surface of the sternum), which draws the anterior trachea forward as the posterior aspect of the aorta adheres to the trachea. Recently, a stenting procedure has been effective in treating tracheomalacia and may be less invasive than aortopexy (Kovesi and Rubin, 2004).

In addition to the major structural abnormalities, the epithelium at the site of the TEF (but at times in all the major airways) can be abnormal, lacking both cilia and goblet cells, and thereby decreasing mucociliary clearance (Goyal et al., 2006).

This lesion may be exacerbated by or be secondary to GER. Rarely, secretions may be retained to the point of inducing tracheal metaplasia. A blind pouch at the site of the former TEF can be a nidus for trapping secretions.

Recurrent upper and lower respiratory infections occur in 35% to 75% of infants and children, especially throughout the first 3 to 4 years of life, and they may be related to GER or impaired mucociliary clearance secondary to the abnormal tracheal epithelia (Dudley and Phelan, 1976; Spitz, 2007). Wheezing commonly accompanies these infections (Chetcuti and Phelan, 1993). Even with decreased symptoms over time, pulmonary function studies 6 to 37 years after repair show a high incidence of obstructive and restrictive forms of lung disease (Chetcuti et al., 1992; Robertson et al., 1995). Specifically, abnormal expiratory flow rates (e.g., low forced expiratory volume at 1 second [FEV$_1$] in 25%, low forced expiratory flow 25%-75% [FEF$_{25\%-75\%}$] in 14%), reduced lung volume (e.g., low vital capacity in 15%), and airway hyperreactivity have been documented in survivors.

Open posterolateral thoracostomy in infants has been associated with musculoskeletal malformations, including "winged" scapula and chest-wall asymmetry (see Minimal-Access Surgery in the Neonate, p. 561). Scoliosis has been attributed to both the thoracostomy and associated vertebral anomalies. Scoliosis would predictably reduce total lung capacity, so in survivors of TEF/EA, compromise may be exaggerated when a structural chest-wall deformity is added to other sources of pulmonary dysfunction.

As with other congenital anomalies, survivors of TEF/EA encounter lifelong disorders that require multidisciplinary, long-term supportive care and meticulous follow-up care to minimize complications induced by and secondary to their primary lesions.

Necrotizing Enterocolitis

Necrotizing enterocolitis (NEC) persists as a major source of perinatal and life-long morbidity and mortality, primarily affecting premature infants with a gestational age of fewer than 36 weeks (usually fewer than 32 weeks), and particularly virulent in ELBW infants. In its acute and severe phase, NEC is a gastrointestinal emergency. Although centered in the gastrointestinal tract, NEC is a systemic process primarily related to the sepsis that accompanies intestinal necrosis and increased mucosal permeability. Isolated intestinal perforation (IP) refers to a clinical scenario that some suggest is distinct from NEC (Pumberger et al., 2002). Of note, IP seems to occur earlier and with lower incidence of pneumatosis and pneumoperitoneum, and in the ELBW infant it may have a lower mortality (38.3%)

compared with that of NEC (55.2%) (Blakely et al., 2005). Others have reported that early exposure to indomethacin (but not prenatal steroids) plays a role in the etiology of IP (Attridge et al., 2006). The two entities are difficult to accurately differentiate preoperatively, so they are treated similarly—both medically and surgically. This discussion centers on "classic NEC."

In spite of intense basic, clinical, and epidemiologic research, the precise etiology of this life-threatening and common disease is unknown and considered to be multifactorial. The only clear-cut risk factor is prematurity. At least 90% of infants diagnosed with NEC are premature, and severity of symptoms, complications, and mortality are inversely related to gestational age (Hsueh et al., 2002). Of note, 11.5% of infants weighing 401 to 750 g, 9% of those between 751 and 1000 g, 6% of those between 1001 and 1250 g, and 4% of those between 1251 and 1500 g are affected (Guillet et al., 2006). As the survival rate of premature infants, especially ELBW infants, has improved, the incidence of NEC has increased in some populations. Although enormous progress in the delivery of neonatal care is apparent, estimates of incidence (10% to 20% in infants weighing less than 1500 g), requirement for surgery, and mortality associated with NEC have remained remarkably static. In part, the increased number of susceptible infants may explain the lack of improved overall survival in infants with NEC. Recent data note that 1 to 5 of every 1000 live births in the United States are diagnosed with NEC, and 1% to 7% of all patients admitted to the NICU and approximately 10% of VLBW infants are affected (Hsueh et al., 2002; Guillet et al. 2006; Holman et al., 2006; Lin and Stoll, 2006; Hunter et al., 2008; Lin et al., 2008b). Mortality ranges from 15% to 30% and is highest among the most immature and those treated surgically (30% to 50%). Between 20% and 40% of patients are treated surgically.

Bell et al. (1978) described three stages of NEC. Stage I refers to mild disease, with the infant having only nonspecific symptoms (e.g., vomiting, gastric residuals, apnea, bradycardia, and guaiac-positive stools). There is no definitive radiologic evidence for NEC, and the state of the bowel is completely unknown. Stage II includes infants with definitive NEC. They have clinical symptoms similar to the infants in Stage I, but radiographs show that they have pneumatosis intestinalis or portal venous air (Figs. 18-18 and 18-19). Stage II infants are suitable candidates for medical management. Stage III includes infants with advanced disease. These infants have evidence of intestinal necrosis or perforation along with clinical signs of hemodynamic, respiratory, and hematologic instability. Although these three stages are not distinct and represent a continuum of clinical disease, the three-stage concept helps define management strategies. Walsh and

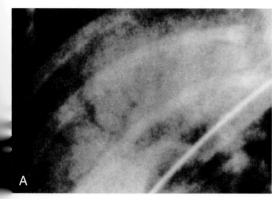
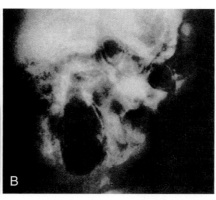

■ **FIGURE 18-18.** Air pattern in the portal venous system of the liver in an infant with NEC. *(From Rowe MI: Necrotizing enterocolitis. In Welch KJ et al., editors:* Pediatric surgery, ed 4, Chicago, 1986, Year Book.)

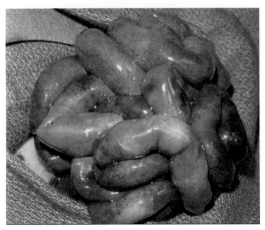

■ FIGURE 18-19. NEC at time of laparotomy. Patchy areas of small bowel involvement.

Kleigman (1986) expanded the classification, but the primary framework of suspected, definite, and advanced disease persists. Nonetheless, some have recommended abandoning Bell's criteria in favor of new guidelines, because NEC is not a uniform disease entity (i.e., does not have a specific etiology) and the pathophysiology remains incompletely defined (Table 18-1) (Gordon et al., 2007).

Pathophysiology

NEC is a paradoxical disease. Infants with milder disease usually recover with outcomes similar to those of other infants of the same gestational age, but severely affected infants who require surgery have high mortality, and those who survive usually develop significant gastrointestinal and neurodevelopmental morbidity. Although miniepidemics do occur, most cases of NEC are sporadic and cannot be correlated with any specific infectious agent. The disease only occurs postnatally (not in stillborns), and it is rare in full-term infants and infants who have never been fed (Hsueh et al., 2002). The full-term infant who does develop NEC tends to display symptoms and

signs in the first 1 to 3 days of life, sometimes before feeding has been initiated. There is usually a history of a hypoxic and ischemic events such as perinatal asphyxia, respiratory distress, or congenital heart disease. In contrast, the preterm infant tends to develop symptoms and signs after 2 to 3 weeks of life after feeding has been initiated, often without any preceding dramatic cardiorespiratory event.

Intestinal mucosal injury from ischemia caused by reduced mesenteric blood flow is commonly proposed as a physiologic mechanism for NEC. Mesenteric blood flow may be compromised by a decreased cardiac output in the presence of fetal asphyxia, a patent ductus arteriosus, apnea or bradycardia, heart failure, arrhythmia, severe cardiorespiratory instability, or hypoxemia. Immature regulation and autoregulation of the mesenteric circulation in response to a primary event (e.g., apnea, or patent ductus arteriosus) probably factors into the pathogenesis of NEC. Specific clinical events that seem to contribute to the pathogenesis of NEC include enteral feeding of small preterm infants, use of a hyperosmolar formula, bacterial infection, intestinal dysfunction (e.g., feeding intolerance or slow transit), infection, polycythemia, congenital heart disease, and a history of umbilical arterial catheterization or exchange transfusion.

The most common anatomic site for NEC is the ileocolic region. However, NEC is often discontinuous, with patchy distribution in both the small and large intestines in as many as 50% of cases (Fig. 18-19). Large bowel involvement is most common in the full-term infant. Perforations often are multiple and although commonly identified at the junction of a necrotic and normal bowel, perforations are also found within the affected areas.

The primary pathologic findings in NEC are coagulative or ischemic necrosis, as well as inflammation. The inflammatory response seems to be unique in that abscesses do not form, as seen in inflammatory bowel disease, infectious colitis, or acute arterial occlusion (Hsueh et al., 2002). The combination of ischemia and bacteremia seems to underline the pathophysiology of the disease. For example, NEC does not evolve after an episode of vascular injury in utero, when the bowel is sterile (Musemeche et al., 1986). Instead, an intestinal atresia or stenosis may develop. The formation of gas bubbles (pneumatosis intestinalis) reflects fermentation of an intraluminal substrate

TABLE 18-1. Modified Bell's Staging for NEC

Review of Bell's Stages	Clinical Findings	Radiographic Findings	Gastrointestinal Findings
Stage I	Apnea and bradycardia, temperature instability	Normal gas pattern or mild ileus	Gastric residuals, occult blood in stool, mild abdominal distention
Stage II A	Apnea and bradycardia, temperature instability	Ileus gas pattern with one or more dilated loops and focal pneumatosis	Grossly bloody stools, prominent abdominal distention, absent bowel sounds
Stage II B	Thrombocytopenia and mild metabolic acidosis	Widespread pneumatosis, ascites, portal-venous gas	Abdominal wall edema with palpable loops and tenderness
Stage III A	Mixed acidosis, oliguria, hypotension, coagulopathy	Prominent bowel loops, worsening ascites, no free air	Worsening wall edema, erythema and induration
Stage III B	Shock, deterioration in laboratory values and vital signs	Pneumoperitoneum	Perforated bowel

Adapted from Kleigman RM, Walsh MC: Neonatal necrotizing enterocolitis: pathogenesis, classification, and spectrum of disease, *Curr Probl Pediatr* 17(4):243–288, 1987; Gordon PV, Swanson JR, Attridge JT, Clark R: Emerging trends in acquired neonatal intestinal disease: is it time to abandon Bell's criteria? *J Perinatol* 27:661–671, 2007.

by bacteria; however, NEC is not associated with a specific organism or with particularly virulent bacteria. A wide range of organisms have been identified in the stool of infants with NEC, some who also have a bacteremia with the same organism: *Escherichia coli*; various strains of *Enterobacter*, *Klebsiella*, and *Pseudomonas*; coagulase-negative *Staphylococci*; and others. Viral agents have been associated with NEC but are not considered a major infectious etiology.

Classically, although the hypothesis for the etiology of NEC has focused on circulatory insufficiency or infection, the pathophysiology of NEC in the preterm infant also involves an exaggerated inflammatory response in the setting of abnormal bacterial colonization, an inadequate epithelial barrier (e.g., defects in mucus or immature tight junctions), an immature intestinal motility (e.g., disordered peristalsis), and an immature gastrointestinal immunity (Hunter et al., 2008). In fact, the immature gastrointestinal tract is characterized by inadequate secretion and production of mucin, which may predispose it to increased permeability to and adherence of bacteria. The immature immunity of the preterm intestine increases the susceptibility of an inadequate barrier to injury from uncontrolled inflammatory responses.

Activation of inflammatory and apoptotic pathways and antiapoptotic mechanisms relies on the interaction of systems in the invading organism with specific receptors in the host. So-called microbial-associated molecular patterns (MAMPs) interact with a specific pattern-recognition receptor (PRR) on host cells. A well-known PRR is the human toll-like receptor 4 (TLR4), a receptor for lipopolysaccharide (LPS), a substance in the cell walls of some bacteria. Of relevance to the preterm infant, hypoxia and exposure to infant formula may exaggerate expression of this receptor. Adult human intestine is characterized by minimal TLR4 expression, but expression in fetal intestine is high. The overexpression of the normal TLR4 receptor may predispose the immature intestine to enhanced proinflammatory injury; interaction with MAMPs of pathogenic bacteria leads to apoptosis and inhibition of healing from injury (Leaphart et al., 2007). Apoptosis of the intestinal epithelia has been noted in human infants with NEC (Ford et al., 1997). Thus the preterm infant may be predisposed to NEC via an inability to maintain adequate inflammatory responses while avoiding overactivation of proinflammatory responses (e.g., via TLR4 receptors), which lead to injury.

Although multiple inflammatory markers and various cytokines (IL-8, IL-10, liver and intestine fatty acid binding protein) have been associated with NEC, no single marker has been identified that allows early diagnosis and management of NEC (Young et al., 2009). Several "models" of NEC, emphasizing the role of inflammatory and vasoactive mediators, platelet-activating factor (PAF), and tumor necrosis factor-α (TNF α) have been developed (Fong et al., 1990; Sun and Hsueh, 1991; Sun et al., 1996; Wand et al., 1997; Tan et al., 2000). However, no experimental approach has been ideal, because models for this disease do not exactly mimic the clinical disease (Sodhi et al., 2008).

Nonetheless, by correlating clinical studies to experimental models, it appears that similar to sepsis, NEC is driven by the pathway of activation of cytokines, prostaglandins, and NO, which interact to initially induce intestinal injury via polymorphonuclear neutrophil (PMN) activation and PMN adhesion (Fig. 18-20). PAF and TNF α seem to play a central role in inducing intestinal injury.

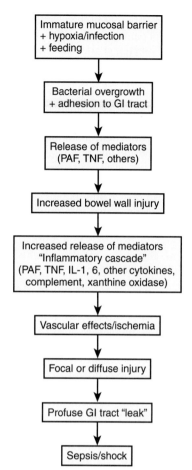

■ **FIGURE 18-20.** Schematic representation of the pathophysiology of NEC. *GI*, Gastrointestinal; *IL-1*, interleukin 1; *PAF*, platelet-activating factor; *TNF*, tumor necrosis factor.

One theory is that PAF induces cell injury after inducing production of various reactive oxygen species (ROS), but the precise mechanism is unclear. Of note, the xanthine dehydrogenase/xanthine oxidase system is abundant in the intestine and seems to generate superoxide during ischemia. Elevated levels of PAF have been measured in infants with NEC.(Rabinowitz et al., 2001). In addition, premature infants have low levels of the PAF-degrading enzyme acetylhydrolase (Caplan et al., 1990). Exactly how other mechanisms included in the pathogenesis of NEC (e.g., immature immunologic mechanisms, abnormal patterns of bacterial overgrowth, and deficient mesenteric blood flow regulation) interact with the intense inflammatory response is not completely understood. Finally, differences in the content of sialic acid and N-acetylglucosamine residues of the mucosa may affect anatomy and function of the microvilli, leading to certain types of bacterial colonization, bacterial adhesion, and eventually, permeation of the gastrointestinal tract (Claud and Walker, 2001).

Another pathway that plays a critical role in the pathophysiology of NEC centers on the interaction of NO, prostaglandins, and epidermal growth factor (EGF) in regulating epithelial function. Prostaglandins function in maintaining tight junctions. Normal low levels of NO regulated by endothelial nitric oxide synthase (NOS) activity enhance blood flow to the mucosa and maintain microvascular flow. However, high levels of NO in response to stimulation of inducible NOS may cause cytotoxicity as a result of damage to the epithelial barrier (disrupting epithelial tight junctions) and excessive apoptosis, as seen in early NEC (Ford et al., 1997; Chokshi et al., 2008). Thus, although NO seems to be critical in maintaining mucosal blood flow, high levels may have injurious effects, disrupting the tight junctions of the epithelium and inducing abnormal apoptosis. In addition, endothelin (a vasoconstrictor) is released in response to various pathologic conditions, such as NEC. EGF seems to induce migration and proliferation of epithelial cells in response to injury, but levels of this mediator are low in some preterm infants, specifically those with NEC. The cytoprotective effect of EGF, which is found in high levels in breast milk, may eventually be incorporated into nutritional strategies to prevent and treat NEC (Guner et al., 2008b; Nair et al., 2008).

Finally, various genetic factors (i.e., prematurity, respiratory distress syndrome, and periventricular leukomalacia) may interact either directly or indirectly in the development of NEC. For example, recent analyses of preterm twins uncovered a familial origin for NEC, as well as for intraventricular hemorrhage (IVH) and bronchopulmonary dysplasia (BPD) (Bhandari et al., 2006). That is, 52% of the variance for NEC could be explained by genetic and shared environmental factors. The *TLR4* gene and its products have been reported to be higher in an animal model of NEC, and the risk for NEC has been associated with a specific genotype of interleukin (CPS1 T1405N polymorphism, IL-18[607]) (Jilling et al., 2006). The incidence of the genotype was significantly higher in those with stage III compared with those who had stage I or II NEC (Moonen et al., 2007).

The observation that inflammation is the result of NEC, rather than the cause, has prompted a variety of interventions aimed at enhancing epithelial integrity, such as human milk feeds, various amino acid supplementations, and various probiotics, prebiotics, and postbiotics (Lin et al., 2008a). Although a specific role for any agents other than human milk remains unclear, any introduction of pharmacologic agents may have dramatic effects on other therapeutic agents used in the NICU and the operating room.

Preoperative Management

A typical infant with NEC is a preterm baby weighing less than 1500 g and often less than 1000 g. Some infants have had perinatal asphyxia or other respiratory complications in the early postnatal period. Prenatal complications associated with NEC may include events that are associated with asphyxia or prematurity, such as premature rupture of the membrane, placenta previa, maternal sepsis, toxemia, breech delivery, or cesarean section for fetal distress.

In "classic NEC," gastrointestinal signs appear between the first and tenth days of life in more than 90% of cases, and they include abdominal distention, retained gastric secretions and high gastric residuals after feeding (may be bile-tinged), vomiting, bloody or mucoid diarrhea, and occult blood in stools. Figure 18-21 shows the probability of a patient experiencing intramural gas, bloody stools, or portal venous gas when diagnosed with NEC vs. gestational age. In some cases, these signs are preceded by nonspecific abnormalities such as apnea, bradycardia, thermal instability, or lethargy, with a gradual development of gastrointestinal problems. In other infants, the course is fulminant with rapid onset of abdominal signs with acidosis, hemodynamic instability, and disseminated intravascular coagulation (i.e., septic shock), often with bowel perforation. In infants with acute onset of advanced NEC, surgical intervention is emergent. Many infants with obvious NEC have decreased platelet counts (50,000 to 75,000/mm³ or lower) and prolonged prothrombin and partial thromboplastin times. Some infants have leukocytosis with a high percentage of bands, but others develop profound leukopenia and neutropenia. Early in the disease process, abdominal radiographs may reveal dilated, fixed (adynamic ileus) loops of bowel, but in advanced NEC, pneumatosis (intramural air in the intestine), gas in the portal venous system, and pneumoperitoneum develop.

Without evidence of intestinal necrosis or perforation, the initial treatment for NEC is nonoperative. Decompressing the stomach with an orogastric tube, no feeding, administering fluid and electrolyte therapy (including parenteral nutrition),

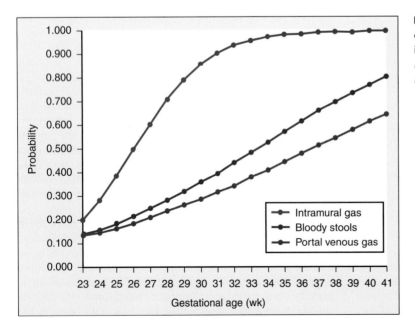

■ **FIGURE 18-21.** Probability curves for symptoms of bloody stools, intramural gas, or portal venous air in babies with NEC. *(From Sharma R et al.: Clinical manifestations of rotavirus infection in the neonatal intensive care unit,* Pediatr Infect Dis J *21:1099, 2002.)*

delivering broad-spectrum antibiotics after obtaining cultures of blood and urine, and correcting hematologic abnormalities are the main components of medical therapy. Supportive hemodynamic therapy, including inotropic agents and steroids, may be needed to treat septic shock. Bowel perforation is the only generally accepted indication for surgery, but relative indications may include peritonitis, air in the portal system, bowel wall edema, ascites, and a progressively deteriorating cardio-respiratory status (Box 18-2).

The role for primary peritoneal drainage in the surgical treatment of NEC and IP has been scrutinized. Peritoneal drainage was initially proposed as a method to treat the most unstable infants with NEC, usually ELBW infants (Ein et al., 1977). Some have reported that this intervention provides advantages in the ELBW infants but not in those weighing more than 1500 g (Azarow et al., 1997). Theoretically the ELBW infant may benefit from such a temporizing procedure that would allow resuscitation and stabilization. However, the effectiveness of peritoneal lavage in "buying time" for an infant to achieve hemodynamic, acid/base, and hematologic stability is actively debated.

In a prospective cohort of 16 NICUs (NICHD Neonatal Research Network), the overall in-hospital mortality associated with NEC in this group of ELBW infants was 49%. Poor prognosis was associated with lower gestational age and birth weight, preoperative vasopressors, and HFOV support. Mortality was 55% for patients with NEC and 38% for those with IP. However, in this study, initial treatment with a peritoneal drain vs. laparotomy was at the discretion of the surgeon (i.e., subject to bias), therefore mortality could not be accurately correlated with surgical management (Blakely et al., 2005). Subsequently, a multicentered randomized trial compared outcome of primary peritoneal drainage with laparotomy in another group of preterm infants. In this study, the infants were lighter than 1500 g and had fewer than 34 weeks' gestation (compared with a weight of less than 1000 g in the earlier study), who had free intraperitoneal air either on abdominal radiograph or by clinical examination (by both the surgeon and neonatologist),

or had stool, bile, or pus on paracentesis. Because of clinical deterioration, 5 of the 55 (9%) in the peritoneal drainage group underwent laparotomy. Because of stricture, obstruction, or feeding intolerance, another 16 (29%) underwent laparotomy. Mortality at 90 days was similar (peritoneal drainage, 34.5%; laparotomy, 35.5%), as was dependence on intravenous nutrition (peritoneal drainage, 47.2%; laparotomy, 40%). Length of hospitalization did not differ between the groups. Of note, the investigators did not uncover a difference in mortality when outcome was stratified according to gestational age subsets (younger than 24, 25 to 26, 27 to 30, and 30 to 34 weeks' gestation) (Moss et al., 2006).

In a multicenter randomized trial including 31 NICUs in 13 European countries, ELBW infants with pneumoperitoneum on radiograph either underwent laparotomy or placement of an intraperitoneal drain. Survival at 6 months was similar (51.4%, intraperitoneal drain; 63.6%, laparotomy). In contrast to Moss et al.'s (2006) study, 74% of infants underwent laparotomy between 0.4 and 21 days. These investigators suggest that peritoneal drainage is ineffective as a temporizing measure or as a definitive treatment. That is, if a drain is placed, a laparotomy should be performed soon afterward (Rees et al., 2008).

The preoperative assessment of infants with NEC focuses on evaluating and correcting the respiratory, circulatory, metabolic, and hematologic disorders. Trends in blood gases, glucose, electrolytes, hematocrit, and coagulation status (including platelet count) should be noted. Increased colloid and crystalloid therapy may be needed in hypovolemic infants with massive third-space fluid losses, bleeding, and disseminated intravascular coagulation. Electrolyte disturbances (including acidosis) are exaggerated in the setting of acute renal failure, which may evolve secondary to shock or abdominal compartment syndrome.

Respiratory support often must be increased as abdominal distention or metabolic and respiratory acidosis worsen. Thus, the anesthesiologist must decide whether a ventilator from the NICU would provide advantages, whether manual ventilation is necessary (possible need for more personnel), or whether the ventilator associated with the anesthesia machine is adequate. If the infant's status is so unstable that transport to the operating room seems too risky, a surgical procedure in the NICU should be considered.

Intraoperative Management

Intraoperative monitoring ideally includes arterial and central venous cannulae for continuous monitoring and blood gas and metabolic analysis. Fresh frozen plasma, platelets, and red blood cells may be administered early in surgery in response to clinical and laboratory evidence of coagulopathy. Inspired oxygen concentration should be adjusted to produce an arterial oxygen saturation of 85% to 90%. Nitrous oxide must be avoided, especially in the presence of free air in the gastrointestinal and portal venous systems.

Potent inhalation agents are often poorly tolerated and often are only introduced in low concentrations to supplement narcotics. High doses of fentanyl (e.g., 50 mcg/kg) or other narcotic can be slowly delivered, as tolerated hemodynamically, or delivered as an infusion to provide infants with analgesia and amnesia. Neuromuscular blocking agents facilitate surgical interventions. Inotropic agents are often needed to support the cardiovascular system when fluid therapy alone fails to maintain adequate perfusion. Glucose intolerance is common

---

Box 18-2. Indications for Surgery

ABSOLUTE INDICATIONS
Pneumoperitoneum
Intestinal gangrene (positive results of paracentesis)

RELATIVE INDICATIONS
Clinical deterioration
    Metabolic acidosis
    Ventilatory failure
    Oliguria, hypovolemia
    Thrombocytopenia
        Leukopenia, leukocytosis
Portal vein gas
Erythema of abdominal wall
Fixed abdominal mass
Persistently dilated loop

NONINDICATIONS
Severe gastrointestinal hemorrhage
Abdominal tenderness
Intestinal obstruction
Gasless abdomen with ascites

in septic infants. In all cases, fluid that does not contain glucose should be delivered to provide crystalloid resuscitation. Of note, the high glucose content of red blood cell products may eliminate any need for other glucose delivery. Ideally, glucose can be measured intraoperatively, especially in procedures longer than 45 to 60 minutes that require large quantities of blood, and in infants with major glucose instability preoperatively.

Because of the large fluid requirements, hypothermia is a common intraoperative complication. The operating room and infused fluids are warmed to assist in maintaining adequate body temperature. In the surgical treatment of NEC, necrotic bowel is resected, and usually, the marginally viable ends are exteriorized. The cardinal principles of surgery for NEC are to excise all necrotic bowel but preserve as much bowel length as possible by leaving "marginal" appearing bowel in place, decompressing the bowel, and removing pus, stool, and necrotic debris from the peritoneal cavity. Preserving the bowel may require multiple segmental resections and second-look operations to reassess bowel viability. Select patients may tolerate resection and primary reanastomosis. Bowel strictures may develop within days to months after the initial surgery, often necessitating further surgical intervention. Often enterostomies are closed within 4 weeks to 6 months after the initial surgery.

Postoperative Management

Postoperatively, mechanical ventilation and cardiovascular support are universally required in these infants. Central venous parenteral nutrition is essential after sepsis is controlled and metabolic stability is established.

Outcome

Mortality from NEC is high, ranging between 10% and 30% (or higher in surgically treated ELBW infants). Regardless of treatment (medical or surgical), approximately 30% of patients develop strictures. Recurrence of NEC is rare. Infants who initially respond to placement of an intraperitoneal drain may eventually require surgery, but some do not. Infants who develop an isolated intestinal perforation may be distinct from those with NEC and have a more benign course. The hospital course for preterm infants with NEC can be prolonged and characterized by repeated episodes of sepsis and long-term requirements for intravenous alimentation as enteral feedings are introduced slowly.

A devastating complication in survivors of NEC is short bowel syndrome, which develops in as many as 20% to 25% of surgically treated patients (Rees et al., 2008). In these cases, the bowel resection is so extensive that the infant is unable to establish enteral feedings, implying a need for long-term intravenous alimentation despite its high-risk morbidity (e.g., sepsis and hepatic failure). Although site and amount of resection seem to correlate with the development of short bowel syndrome, diffuse mucosal injury may persist in areas of bowel injured by NEC but not resected. Current interventions include intestinal lengthening procedures or even bowel transplantation. The use of tissue-engineered small intestine is under intense investigation (Guner et al., 2008b). Evidence suggests that breast milk decreases the incidence of NEC and its complications. The roles for treatment with probiotics, nonspecific (steroids, indomethacin, magnesium, copper) and specific antiinflammatory agents (PAF receptor blockers), growth factors (erythropoietin), or antibiotics remain speculative (Millar et al., 2003).

Beyond the gastrointestinal outcome, the risk for long-term neurodevelopmental problems was first reported in 50% of survivors almost three decades ago (Stevenson et al., 1980). Deficits in psychomotor and mental development have been confirmed in the VLBW survivors of NEC, especially those who have undergone surgery (Vohr et al., 2000; Stoll et al., 2004; Hintz et al., 2005; Rees et al., 2007; Schulzke et al., 2007). The risk for those treated surgically is approximately twice that of those treated medically. In fact, those treated medically have outcomes similar to those of the same gestational age without a history of NEC (see Chapter 17, Neonatology for Anesthesiologists).

Prevention strategies are now focused on feeding techniques and manipulating gut flora. However, definitive approaches for introducing probiotics, various amino acids, or agents such as epidermal growth factor have not been established. Clearly, identifying infants at risk to prevent progression to a disease that requires surgery may be critical in minimizing gastrointestinal and neurodevelopmental complications from NEC.

Imperforate Anus (Anal Atresia)

The incidence of anorectal malformations is 1:5000 live births. Miller et al. (2009) reported an association of anorectal atresia with caffeine intake, cigarette smoking, and environmental tobacco smoke. Imperforate anus can range from a mild stenosis to a complex syndrome with other associated congenital anomalies. The higher the anatomic relation of the terminal bowel to the puborectalis sling of the levator musculature, the greater is the incidence of associated anomalies. The incidence of additional genitourinary abnormalities is 48%, but it ranges from 14% in infants with perineal fistulas to 90% in infants with bladder fistulas. Twenty-four percent of infants have a tethered spinal cord (Levitt et al., 1997). Male infants with imperforate anus may require an operation soon after birth for relief of obstruction. In female infants, a rectovaginal fistula usually prevents total bowel obstruction so that surgical treatment is not an emergency.

Intraoperative Management

Anesthetic requirements vary depending on the severity of the abdominal distention and complexity of the surgery: a simple perineal anoplasty, a temporary colostomy, or an extensive abdominoperineal repair. Anorectal malformation can be classified by the presence or absence of a fistula and by the fistula's location (Pena and Hong, 2000) (Box 18-3). Perineal fistulas in both male and female infants represent the simplest defect, and treatment generally consists of an anoplasty performed in the neonatal period. Imperforate anus with no fistula is the least common, presentation, whereas rectourethral fistulas are the most common, with the exception of the perineal fistula. The standard surgical approach has generally involved the following three steps:

1. A diverting colostomy performed in the neonatal period,
2. The main repair done during infancy, and
3. A take-down colostomy performed later in infancy.

Surgical trends, however, have been aimed at performing the primary repair without a colostomy. The primary repair involves a posterior surgical approach. Laparoscopic techniques have been used to assist in the pull-through technique (Georgeson, 2000).

Box 18-3. Therapeutic Classification of Anorectal Malformations

MALES

Cutaneous fistula, no colostomy required
Anal stenosis
Anal membrane
Rectourethral fistula, colostomy required
    Bulbar
    Prostatic
Rectovesical fistula
Anorectal agenesis without fistula
Rectal atresia

FEMALES

Cutaneous (perineal), no colostomy required
Fistula
    Vestibular fistula, colostomy required
    Vaginal fistula
Anorectal agenesis without fistula
Rectal atresia
Persistent cloaca

Anesthetic considerations for neonates with intestinal obstruction from any etiology include airway management of a full stomach, assessment of fluid status, correction of electrolyte disturbances, treatment of sepsis, and cardiorespiratory evaluation. Marked abdominal distention secondary to intestinal obstruction can impede diaphragmatic excursion and impair ventilation. Gastric (or lower intestinal) contents often are incompletely emptied with nasogastric suction, so that the risk of aspiration is significant, especially during induction of general anesthesia.

Intubation of the trachea of infants with an apparently normal upper airway can be accomplished with an awake or rapid-sequence technique. If the anesthesiologist suspects that the upper airway will be difficult to visualize, the usual airway precautions should be observed. That is, neuromuscular blocking agents, deep sedation, and general anesthesia are avoided and an awake technique is attempted. Supplemental support systems for the difficult airway (e.g., neonatal bronchoscopes, light wand, and LMA) should be available (see Chapter 10, Equipment).

Anesthesia during the surgery can include potent inhalation anesthetics, narcotics, or both. In general, nitrous oxide is avoided because of the risk for increasing bowel distention. Intermediate-acting or long-acting nondepolarizing muscle relaxants often improve surgical conditions at lower inhaled anesthetic concentrations. If early postoperative extubation is planned, narcotics should be judiciously administered, but in many cases postoperative mechanical ventilation is required.

Imperforate anus is usually recognized early in the postnatal period, and massive distention may not develop in the group of infants without total bowel obstruction. Therefore the complications associated with intestinal obstruction are minimized, as are the complications from bowel ischemia, third-space fluid loss, electrolyte disturbances, and sepsis. Imperforate anus without a fistula can be associated with the development of total intestinal obstruction in utero, leading to severe abdominal distention, bowel perforation, sepsis, or a combination.

In addition, other congenital anomalies often have a dramatic effect on the management of these infants. For example, imperforate anus is associated with TEF, renal anomalies, and heart disease (VACTERL Association).

During surgery, the management of fluids, blood replacement, and electrolyte delivery are similar to the principles discussed for NEC and for intestinal obstruction. As with any intraabdominal surgery in the newborn, a major challenge is maintaining an adequate intravascular volume. The presence of radiopaque contrast agents, bowel manipulation, and peritonitis increases third-space fluid requirements. In such cases, 10 mL/kg per hour (or more) of isotonic saline solution or colloid is generally needed intraoperatively. Monitoring urine output, quality of heart tones, heart rate, and blood pressure is a basic requirement to assess continuing fluid needs. Invasive monitors such as an arterial catheter and a CVP catheter generally are reserved for those with marked cardiorespiratory instability.

Postoperative Management

The preoperative and intraoperative courses and the effects of associated congenital anomalies set the stage for the postoperative course. Many infants require postoperative ventilatory support, total parenteral alimentation, cardiovascular support, and treatment of sepsis. The function and recovery of the gastrointestinal system vary enormously among infants with imperforate anus and seem to be related to whether the lesion is isolated and whether the complications of total bowel obstruction have developed.

Outcome

Intestinal obstruction has historically been one of the major causes of death after neonatal surgery. With more skilled pediatric management and the development of parenteral alimentation, mortality is now limited primarily to infants whose condition is diagnosed late and who require extensive excision of the small and large bowels. Long-term complications from anorectal malformations, especially a high imperforate anus, can be lifelong and involve sequelae related to fecal soiling, constipation, and sexual inadequacy.

Intestinal Obstruction

Intestinal obstruction is a surgical emergency in the newborn, requiring swift intervention after diagnosis. Bowel obstruction has symptoms and signs similar to those seen at other ages, such as vomiting, abdominal distention, decreased bowel sounds, and radiologic evidence of gas-filled loops of bowel. However, in the newborn the list of etiologies includes a unique set of congenital anomalies.

Delay in the diagnosis and treatment of such lesions may lead to various complications that can increase morbidity and mortality. As described for the infant with imperforate anus, delay in diagnosis leads to disturbance of fluid and electrolyte balance and increased abdominal distention, with subsequent respiratory embarrassment and high risk for aspiration pneumonitis. Intestinal perforation, necrosis of the bowel, and septicemia are other secondary consequences if intestinal obstruction is not managed promptly.

Distended bowel forces the diaphragm into a high, fixed position, limiting excursion, causing severe ventilatory compromise, and increasing the risk of aspiration. Although prompt surgical repair is imperative, optimizing the patient's metabolic status is critical before surgery. Initiation of corrective fluid and electrolyte therapy should precede the induction of anesthesia. Nasogastric suction may decrease gastric distention and the risk for aspiration, but if the site of obstruction is below the duodenum, the abdominal distention is not drastically affected.

Although the underlying etiologies of intestinal obstruction are variable (annular pancreas, intestinal atresia or stenosis, duplication of intestine, meconium ileus, tumors, enterocolitis), the problems of anesthetic management for surgical correction of these lesions are similar.

Duodenal Obstruction

The incidence of duodenal obstruction in the neonate is 1:10,000 to 1:40,000 births and is often associated with other congenital anomalies such as Down syndrome, cystic fibrosis, renal anomalies, intestinal malrotation, and especially midline defects such as esophageal atresia and imperforate anus. An intraluminal diaphragm, a membranous web, or an annular pancreas can also be associated with obstruction of the duodenum. The degree of obstruction varies from severe or complete atresia to incomplete obstruction or stenosis (Mustafawi and Hassan, 2008). Air contrast films reveal a dilated stomach and a dilated proximal duodenum, resulting in the "double-bubble" appearance (Fig. 18-22).

Infants with complete obstruction exhibit copious vomiting of bile or bile-stained gastric contents and minimal abdominal distention. The infant may or may not pass meconium in the first day of life. Infants who have incomplete obstruction have intermittent bile-stained vomiting and usually pass meconium. A delay in the treatment of this condition can result in dehydration, weight loss, and hypochloremic alkalosis.

Jejunoileal Atresia

Jejunoileal atresia causes complete obstruction in 1:5000 live births. In contrast to duodenal atresias, jejunoileal atresias are associated with few other anomalies. Prematurity is associated with 50% of cases, polyhydramnios with 25%, and cystic fibrosis with 20%.

The etiology of jejunoileal atresia is uncertain but is thought to involve intrauterine vascular accidents. Four types of atresia have been identified (Fig. 18-23). Type I is not a true atresia but actually is a membranous obstruction of the lumen in an intestine of otherwise normal length and diameter. Type II, a true atresia, consists of two blind ends that are often connected by a fibrous strand with slightly shortened intestinal length. Type IIIA lesions have blind ends separated by a mesenteric defect. The type IIIB lesion is also called "apple peel" or "Christmas tree" deformity and consists of a long jejunal atresia with a very short remaining ileum. The superior mesenteric artery is missing, and the blood supply to the ileum is by retrograde flow via a branch of the ileocolic artery. Type IIIB lesions are rare but have a very high mortality rate. Type IV lesions involve multiple intestinal atresias.

Meconium Ileus

Meconium ileus is a luminal obstruction of the distal small bowel by abnormal meconium. Meconium ileus is found almost exclusively in patients with cystic fibrosis, but only 20% of patients with cystic fibrosis have meconium ileus. Because meconium ileus manifests in the neonatal period, respiratory symptoms of cystic fibrosis generally are not present. Both surgical and nonsurgical therapies are used to relieve the obstruction. The nonsurgical approach involves diatrizoate meglumine enemas, which can be both diagnostic and therapeutic. Diatrizoate meglumine, a water-soluble contrast agent, loosens and softens the meconium, thereby facilitating its evacuation. When medical management does not succeed, surgery is performed. After the peritoneal cavity is entered and the obstruction is located, diatrizoate meglumine or acetylcysteine is injected into the bowel lumen and allowed to mix with the meconium. When the meconium has loosened, it is massaged into the colon. If this is unsuccessful, an enterostomy is performed, and the sterile meconium is evacuated from the small bowel (Fig. 18-24).

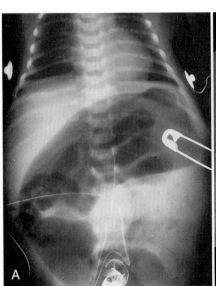

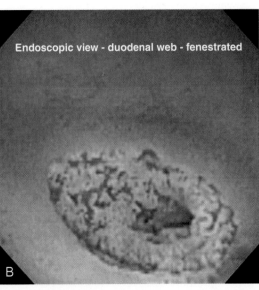

Endoscopic view - duodenal web - fenestrated

■ **FIGURE 18-22.** Duodenal obstruction. **A,** The classic plain-film sign of duodenal atresia. **B,** The endoscopic view of a duodenal web. *(From Barksdale EM, Jr: Surgery. In Zitelli BJ, Davis HW, editors: Atlas of pediatric physical diagnosis, ed 4, St. Louis, 2002, Mosby, p 572.)*

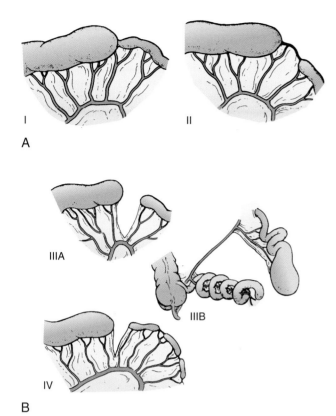

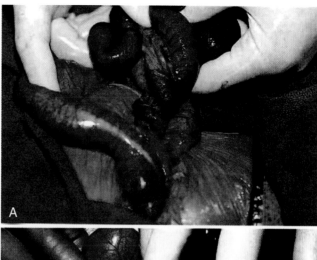

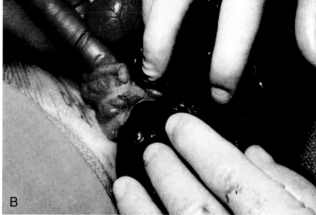

FIGURE 18-23. The various types of jejunal atresia. *(From Grosfeld JL: Jejunoileal atresia and stenosis. In Welch KJ et al., editors: Pediatric surgery, ed 4, Chicago, 1986, Year Book.)*

FIGURE 18-25. Malrotation with midgut volvulus without ischemia **(A)** and with infarction **(B).** *(From Barksdale EM, Jr: Surgery. In Zitelli BJ, Davis HW, editors: Atlas of pediatric physical diagnosis, ed 4, St. Louis, 2002, Mosby, p 572.)*

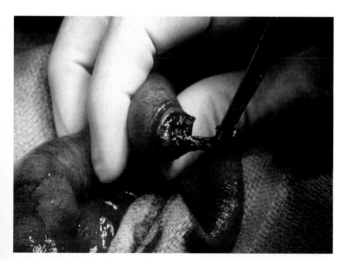

FIGURE 18-24. Thick tenacious meconium in a patient with meconium ileus.

Malrotations and Volvulus

Malrotations are rare and generally result from abnormalities in the rotation of the bowel, which usually occur during the tenth to twelfth weeks of gestation. Consequently, areas of ischemia and atresia develop, along with volvulus, resulting in strangulation of bowel, bloody stools, abdominal distention, peritonitis, and hypovolemic shock (Fig. 18-25). Nonrotation or malrotation is twice as common in boys as in girls and often produces symptoms of intestinal obstruction in the first 1 to 2 months after birth. In

other cases, symptoms do not appear until later, even adulthood. The diagnosis of malrotation cannot be excluded if diarrhea is present, if clinical symptoms are mild, or if x-rays are normal (Miller et al., 2003). In patients with intestinal malrotation without volvulus, surgery often involves Ladd's procedure, which can be performed either open or laparoscopically (Draus et al., 2007). Malrotations are often associated with duodenal stenosis or atresia or small intestinal atresia, as well as with cardiac, esophageal, urinary, and anal anomalies. Major anatomic defects of the abdominal wall (e.g., gastroschisis and omphalocele) and CDH universally have intestinal malrotation or nonrotation.

The operative procedure for a nonrotation complicated by volvulus consists of untwisting the intestine and then a short intraoperative period of observation to evaluate recovery of vascular perfusion to the involved intestine. Areas of frank necrosis are excised, and a primary anastomosis is performed. If the patient has peritonitis or poor perfusion of the remaining bowel, proximal and distal enteral stomas are formed. The surgical operation, Ladd's procedure, involves the following five steps: eviscerating the midgut, derotating the volvulus in a counterclockwise direction, lysis of Ladd's peritoneal band, appendectomy, and placing the caecum in the left lower quadrant.

Children with less than 30 to 40 cm of small bowel generally develop short-gut syndrome and ultimately require TPN. If marginal areas of intestinal viability are present at the operation, they may be left unresected in the hope that postoperative resuscitation improves the perfusion. Under these circumstances, a "second-look" operation usually is performed 24 to 48 hours later.

Sacrococcygeal Teratoma

Sacrococcygeal teratomas are the most common congenital neoplasm, occurring in 1:40,000 infants. Approximately 95% of infants are female.

Embryology and Diagnosis

The tumor is derived from pleuripotential cell lines and contains components consisting of all three germ layers. Perinatal mortality is high when the tumor is diagnosed antenatally. Postulated causes of death include high output cardiac failure, preterm delivery secondary to polyhydramnios, anemia from hemorrhage into the tumor, dystocia, and tumor rupture.

Sacrococcygeal teratomas receive their blood supply from the middle sacral artery and branches of the internal iliac artery. A steal syndrome can shunt blood from the placenta and lead to high output cardiac failure and hydrops. Approximately 2% to 10% of sacrococcygeal tumors are malignant before the infant reaches 2 months of age, and 50% are malignant by 1 year of age. Serum α-fetoprotein levels are elevated in 70% of children with malignant tumors.

Sacrococcygeal tumors generally arise from the tip of the coccyx and vary with the amount of internal and external extension. These tumors are classified into four types according to their locations (Box 18-4; Fig. 18-26).

Intraoperative Management

Surgical treatment involves complete resection of both the tumor and coccyx. Failure to remove the coccyx completely can result in local recurrence. In utero treatment options include open fetal surgery, endoscopic laser ablation, and radiofrequency ablation (Bullard and Harrison, 1995; Hecher and Hackeloer, 1996; Paek et al., 2001) (see Chapter 19, Anesthesia for Fetal Surgery).

Box 18-4   Sacrococcygeal Tumor Types

Type I: External with minimal pressure component
Type II: External with considerable intrapelvic extension
Type III: External with pelvic and intraabdominal extensions
Type IV: Presacral with no external presentation

Anesthetic management for removal of tumors in the neonatal period requires an understanding of neonatal physiology and an appreciation for the possibility of cardiovascular instability, massive blood transfusion requirements, hypothermia, and coagulation dysfunction. Death during resection is often related to hemorrhage, hypothermia, coagulopathy, and the inability to provide adequate cardiopulmonary support during the intraoperative manipulation of the tumor. For large tumors, adequate venous access, central venous access, and invasive arterial pressure monitoring are essential.

Outcome

Predictors of poor outcome have been associated with diagnosis before 20 weeks' gestation, delivery before 30 weeks' gestation, development of hydrops, low birth weight, and a 5-minute Apgar score of less than 7 (Chisholm et al., 1999). Long-term issues involve urologic complications, urinary incontinence, problems with defecation, and cosmetically unacceptable scars (Derikx et al., 2007; Tailor et al., 2009). Associated congenital anomalies are common in patients with congenital anorectal malformations (Stoll et al., 2007).

SUMMARY

For newborns to survive the transition from fetal to extrauterine life, critical multisystem developmental adaptation must occur. Congenital anomalies and acquired disease states requiring anesthetic and surgical intervention may deter this orderly physiologic transition. Those involved with anesthetic care of neonates must acquire and maintain an in-depth knowledge of developmental physiology as well as an understanding of the effects of immaturity on anesthetic and monitoring requirements. The pediatric anesthesiologist must assimilate this information and thoughtfully apply it to the practice of neonatal anesthesia.

For questions and answers on topics in this chapter, go to "Chapter Questions" at www.expertconsult.com.

REFERENCES

Complete references used in this text can be found online at www.expertconsult.com.

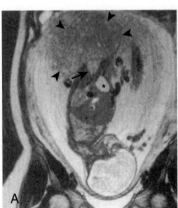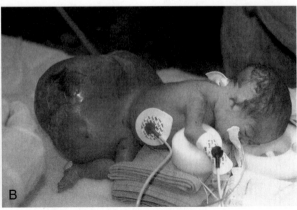

■ **FIGURE 18-26. A,** In utero diagnosis by MRI. **B,** Sacrococcygeal teratoma. *(From Avni FE, Guibaud L, Robert Y, et al.: MR imaging of fetal sacrococcygeal teratoma: diagnosis and assessment,* Am J Roentgenol *178(1):179–183, 2002.)*

Anesthesia for Fetal Surgery

CHAPTER 19

Kha Tran and David E. Cohen

Fetal interventions present a unique therapeutic opportunity. With advances in medical imaging technology, fetuses can be screened for anatomic congenital defects early in the course of a pregnancy. Although postnatal therapy is adequate for many fetuses, some congenital defects will not allow a successful transition to extrauterine life. Other birth defects may result in death in utero or serious disability after birth (Harrison, 1996). The logistics of fetal interventions can be quite challenging, but the ideas behind many of the treatments are conceptually quite simple. Some examples of interventions include bypass of fetal airway obstruction that would be fatal at birth, resection of a lung lesion causing hydrops fetalis, and repair of a myelomeningocele to minimize long-term disability (Table 19-1). Prenatal therapy opens new territory by making the fetus an active recipient of a given intervention. While the fetus is actively treated, the mother, by necessity, also receives medical care. Because of the high risk of these procedures, patient selection is an important consideration. The mothers must be at a sufficiently low anesthesia risk, and they must be highly motivated to comply with frequent follow-up and activity restrictions. Providing anesthesia for these patients requires a thorough understanding of maternal, fetal, and placental physiology. Familiarity with minimally invasive and open procedures and an understanding of the diseases amenable to fetal therapy are important. A list of key terms and acronyms is given in Box 19-1.

DISEASES

A common endpoint of many disease processes that are amenable to fetal therapy is hydrops fetalis leading to death in utero. This state is characterized by the accumulation of fluid in two or more of the following compartments: skin (e.g., scalp edema) or the pericardial, pleural, abdominal, or amniotic (i.e., in polyhydramnios) spaces. The placenta also becomes enlarged in this state. Just as in children and adults, these fluid collections are a manifestation of heart failure. Ultrasound examination readily reveals these fluid collections and the placentomegaly. Red cell alloimmunization is the most common cause of immune-mediated hydrops, whereas mechanical compression of cardiovascular structures is often the cause of nonimmune hydrops. Addressing the pathophysiology that gave rise to the hydrops is a goal of fetal therapy.

Nonimmune hydrops threatens the lives of both the fetus and mother (van Selm et al., 1991). The aptly named *maternal mirror syndrome* is a state of maternal edema that mirrors that of the fetus. The pathophysiology of this process is unclear, but it may involve a maternal inflammatory response to shedding of debris from a hydropic placenta (Redman and Sargent, 2000). In contrast to preeclampsia, the mother is hemodiluted rather than hemoconcentrated, and the fetus, by definition, must show signs of hydrops (Vidaeff et al., 2002). Pulmonary edema secondary to the mirror syndrome may be

TABLE 19-1. Fetal Interventions, Timing, and Therapy

Disease Process	Timing	Therapy	Rationale
Twin-twin transfusion	Early to mid gestation	Amnioreduction	Reduces polyhydramnios, less risk for preterm labor, may improve uterine blood flow
		Laser ablation of placental vessels	Ablation of vessels that are allowing unbalanced blood flow
		Bipolar umbilical cord cautery Radiofrequency ablation of the umbilical cord	In cases of imminent fetal demise
Twin reversed arterial perfusion	Early to mid gestation	Bipolar umbilical cord cautery Radiofrequency ablation of the umbilical cord	Prevents high output failure as pump twin supplies the acardiac cell mass
Cystic hygroma or airway teratoma	Late gestation	EXIT procedure	Secures airway or resects mass while umbilical cord is patent
Congenital high airway obstruction syndrome	Mid gestation	Tracheal decompression	Allows egress of lung fluid, prevents hydrops from cardiovascular compression by pulmonary hyperplasia
	Late gestation	EXIT procedure	Secures airway
Congenital cystic adenomatoid malformation or bronchopulmonary sequestration	Early, mid, or late gestation	Drain or thoracoamniotic shunt	Reduces size of cystic lesions or drains fluid collections causing fetal compromise
	Mid gestation	Pulmonary lobectomy	Resects large masses (not amenable to tap or shunt) causing fetal compromise
	Late gestation	EXIT for pulmonary lobectomy	Resects masses that will interfere with neonatal resuscitation
Congenital diaphragmatic hernia	Mid gestation	Tracheal occlusion	Prevents egress of lung fluid, stimulating lung growth
Aortic stenosis with evolving hypoplastic left heart	Mid gestation	Balloon dilation of aortic valve	Improves left ventricular outflow, which may allow better development of left ventricle
Hypoplastic left heart with intact or highly restrictive atrial septum	Mid gestation	Atrial septoplasty	Creates necessary communication between left and right atria
Myelomeningocele	Mid gestation	Closure of defect	Prevents exposure of neural elements to amniotic fluid
Bladder outlet obstruction	Mid gestation	Bladder decompression	Prevents renal injury, allows increased production of amniotic fluid
Sacrococcygeal teratoma	Mid gestation	Debulking or ablation of feeding vessels	Prevents high-output cardiac failure

life threatening, and treatment of maternal mirror syndrome involves either delivery of the fetus or treatment of the cause of the hydrops (Heyborne and Chism, 2000; Pirhonen and Hartgill, 2004; Livingston et al., 2007).

Complicated Multiple Gestations

Monozygotic twin gestations are at increased risk for complications. If a monozygotic cell mass splits within 3 days of fertilization, a dichorionic diamniotic twin gestation should result. If the mass splits later than 13 days after fertilization, conjoined twins will result. If the cell mass splits between days 3 and 13, the twins will be "conjoined" to varying degrees at the level of the placenta and placental vessels (Lewi et al., 2003). These conjoined placental vessels may result in a net flow of blood from one twin (donor) to the other twin (recipient). The donor will suffer from hypovolemia, oligohydramnios, and growth restriction, whereas the recipient will suffer from hypervolemia,

polyhydramnios, hydrops, and heart failure (Luks et al., 2005). Ultrasound and fetal echocardiographic changes may be used to describe the severity of disease (Quintero et al., 1999; Rychik et al., 2007). This process, twin-twin transfusion syndrome, places both twins at risk for preterm delivery, death, and neurologic disability.

Traditional treatment of twin-twin transfusion syndrome involves serial amnioreduction to relieve the polyhydramnios. This may decrease the risk of preterm labor and may allow better perfusion of the donor twin; however, this therapy does not target the physiologic problem, which arises from the connected placental vessels (Lewi et al., 2005). Newer therapies target the placental vessels, employing percutaneous placement of endoscopes into the amniotic fluid to allow visualization and ablation of the connected placental vessels (Fig. 19-1). Minimally invasive fetoscopic laser ablation of the vessels has been shown to be superior to amnioreduction in a randomized clinical trial (Senat et al., 2004). Another trial showed no difference between amnioreduction and laser ablation, but there

Box 19-1. Acronyms and Glossary

Amnioreduction: Percutaneous needle drainage of excess amniotic fluid

BPS: Bronchopulmonary sequestration, or lung tissues in the thoracic cavity that are not in communication with the pulmonary circulation or the pulmonary blood supply. These tissues are often supplied by a feeder vessel arising from the aorta.

CCAM: Congenital cystic adenomatoid malformation, a lung lesion formed by an overgrowth of terminal bronchioles

CDH: Congenital diaphragmatic hernia

CHAOS: Congenital high airway obstruction syndrome

EXIT: Ex utero intrapartum therapy

HLHS: Hypoplastic left heart syndrome

Hydrops fetalis: A manifestation of heart failure in the fetus, characterized by skin edema, pleural or pericardial effusions, ascites, or polyhydramnios

Maternal mirror syndrome: A potentially life-threatening state of maternal edema that may arise when the fetus suffers from hydrops fetalis

MMC: Myelomeningocele

Polyhydramnios: Excess amniotic fluid, which may be a sign of fetal pathology

SCT: Sacrococcygeal teratoma

TRAPS: Twin reversed arterial perfusion sequence

TTTS: Twin-twin transfusion syndrome

---

because it must supply cardiac output for itself and the acardiac cell mass (Tan and Sepulveda, 2003). In these cases, selective feticide of the acardiac cell mass will allow the normal pump twin to survive. This is accomplished by occlusion of blood flow to the umbilical cord of the acardiac mass either by bipolar cautery or radiofrequency ablation (Tsao et al., 2002). If the twins are monochorionic and monoamniotic, the umbilical cord of the acardiac cell mass must also be divided to prevent cord entanglement and death of the normal twin. These umbilical cord occlusions are accomplished with minimally invasive techniques, using ultrasound or fetoscopic guidance.

Neurologic

Fetal therapies for prenatally diagnosed hydrocephalus and myelomeningocele (MMC) have been described. Results for in utero treatment of hydrocephalus with ventriculoamniotic shunts have not been encouraging, and this therapy is no longer actively studied or offered (Manning et al., 1986; Bruner et al., 2006). However, in utero closure of MMC defects is more promising. This closure involves accessing the midgestation fetus via maternal laparotomy and hysterotomy (Fig. 19-2). The MMC is repaired, and uterine and abdominal incisions are closed. Pregnancy is continued with the goal of delivering as close to term as possible.

The rationale for in utero closure of MMC is based on animal models of fetuses with these lesions, where it appears that prolonged bathing of neurologic elements in the amniotic fluid worsens the neurologic outcome (Meuli et al., 1995; Meuli et al., 1996). In human studies, closure of fetal MMC decreases the need for postnatal ventriculoperitoneal shunting and the incidence of hindbrain herniation and Chiari malformation. Motor function may be somewhat improved, and cognitive behavioral testing does not appear to be adversely affected (Bruner et al., 1999; Tulipan et al., 1999; Johnson et al., 2003; Johnson et al., 2006). A randomized trial sponsored by the National Institutes of Health (NIH) is currently enrolling patients who are randomized either to standard postnatal closure of MMC or to in utero closure of MMC. Enrollment in the trial is, at this time, the only avenue for this surgery.

were differences in the studies that do not allow direct comparison (Crombleholme et al., 2007). More research is needed to fully define the role of minimally invasive laser therapy and amnioreduction in the treatment of twin-twin transfusion syndrome.

Twin reversed arterial perfusion sequence (TRAPS) is a similar clinical entity in which one of the twin cell masses may be acardiac, acephalic, or both. The normal or "pump" twin is at risk for death from high-output heart failure

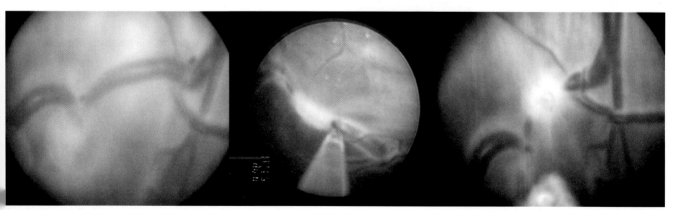

■ **FIGURE 19-1.** Three panels demonstrating the minimally invasive treatment of twin-twin transfusion. From *left to right*, fetoscopic image of the placenta, fiberoptic cable targeting a placental vessel, and a placental vessel after laser ablation. *(Photos courtesy Mark P. Johnson, MD, Children's Hospital of Philadelphia.)*

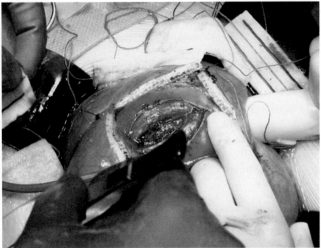

■ **FIGURE 19-2.** A fetus with myelomeningocele (MMC) exposed for in utero midgestation repair. The fetus is turned so that the MMC defect is exposed. Special uterine staples can be seen framing the hysterotomy. The red rubber catheter coming from the left side of the image is used to instill warmed crystalloid to maintain amniotic fluid volume. *(From Myers LB, Cohen D, Galinkin J, et al: Anaesthesia for fetal surgery,* Paediatr Anaesth *12:569, 2002, with permission from Wiley-Blackwell.)*

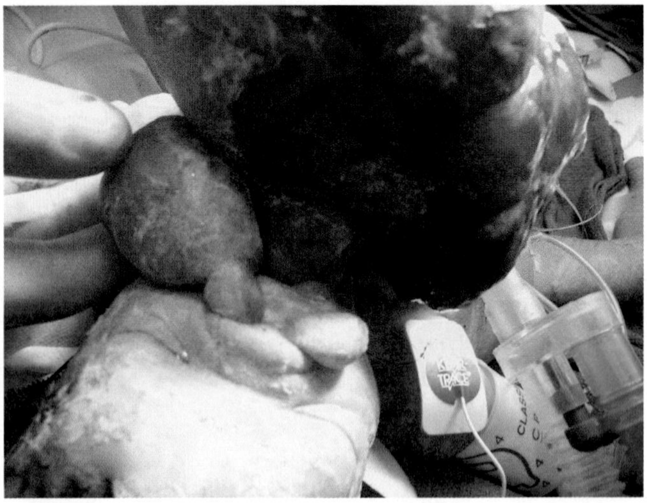

Airway

Airway obstruction is life threatening in the postnatal period, especially when airway patency cannot be established immediately on delivery by intubation. Extrinsic causes of airway obstruction include cystic hygroma and oral teratoma. Cystic hygroma is a type of lymphatic malformation that may develop in the neck, resulting in large, fluid-filled cystic masses (Fig. 19-3). Teratomas are germ cell tumors composed of tissues foreign to their normal location (Fig. 19-4). Polyhydramnios may result from an inability of the fetus to swallow amniotic fluid. Intrinsic causes of airway obstruction include laryngeal cysts, webs, and atresia. The spectrum of disease due to intrinsic compression has been called

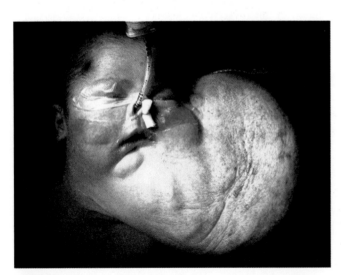

■ **FIGURE 19-3.** A newborn who underwent aspiration of a cystic hygroma and subsequent intubation during an EXIT procedure. *(Photo courtesy of Alan W. Flake, MD, Children's Hospital of Philadelphia.)*

■ **FIGURE 19-4.** A newborn with a massive oral teratoma. The infant was delivered via an EXIT procedure, during which she underwent an emergent tracheostomy. Tumor is protruding from the oral cavity and both nares. The anesthesia circuit is attached to a tracheostomy tube, which is obscured by the tumor. She was immediately taken to a second operating room for further debulking of the tumor. *(Photo courtesy Lynne G. Maxwell, MD, Children's Hospital of Philadelphia.)*

congenital high airway obstruction syndrome (CHAOS) (Hedrick et al., 1994; Lim et al., 2003).

Airway obstruction may be fatal in utero. This is not immediately intuitive, because the placenta serves as the organ of respiration, but complete airway obstruction will not allow egress of lung fluid into the amniotic space. This fluid will collect, and massive pulmonary hyperplasia may result. The fetal diaphragm may be flattened or even project into the abdominal space (Fig. 19-5). The intrathoracic pressure is presumably increased and will impede cardiovascular filling and function, resulting in nonimmune hydrops and fetal demise (Mong et al., 2008). If hydrops is not present, fetal airway obstruction is well served by the ex utero intrapartum therapy (EXIT) procedure. The EXIT procedure for a near-term fetus involves a maternal laparotomy and hysterotomy, exteriorization of the fetus, and securing of the fetal airway before clamping and division of the umbilical cord. After the cord is divided, the fetus is delivered and given to a neonatology team for further stabilization. If hydrops is present and the lungs are immature, midgestation tracheal decompression may be a treatment option (Kohl et al., 2006; Kohl et al., 2009).

Lung Lesions

Lung lesions that may be diagnosed in utero include congenital diaphragmatic hernia (CDH), congenital cystic adenomatoid malformation (CCAM), and bronchopulmonary sequestration (BPS). CDH has been a target for in utero therapy for decades. Results with both open and minimally invasive techniques have thus far been equivalent to those with optimal postnatal therapy. Thus, the risk-benefit analysis would support postnatal therapy. However, efforts at refining minimally invasive therapy continue and may prove to be of benefit in the future

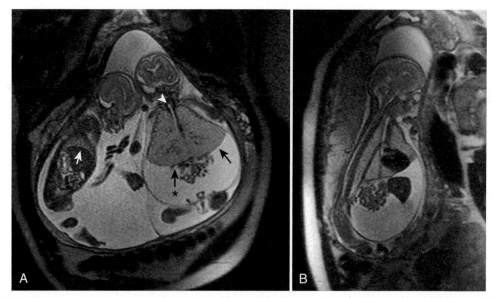

■ FIGURE 19-5. Magnetic resonance image of a maternal pelvis. The mother is pregnant with twins. **A,** Normal twin on the left with the *white arrow* pointing out the normal configuration of the fetal diaphragm. The *white arrowhead* marks the area of complete tracheal obstruction, the *black arrows* demonstrate the inverted diaphragms, and the *asterisk* demonstrates the massive ascites in this twin with congenital high airway obstruction syndrome (CHAOS). **B,** Sagittal view of the twin with CHAOS, clearly demonstrating massive ascites outlining both the bowel and the liver. *(From Mong A, Johnson AM, Kramer SS, et al: Congenital high airway obstruction syndrome: MR/US findings, effect on management, and outcome, Pediatr Radiol 38:1171, 2008, with permission from Springer.)*

(Harrison et al., 1997; Harrison et al., 2003; Deprest et al., 2005; Doné et al., 2008; Peralta et al., 2008).

The management of prenatally diagnosed CCAM is instructive because its natural history is variable (Fig. 19-6). CCAM results from an overgrowth of terminal bronchioles. These masses do not participate in gas exchange, may predispose to infection and malignancy, may cause mediastinal shift and cardiac compression, and may result in hypoplasia of the remaining lung tissue. Some CCAMs will grow and some will shrink—each at unpredictable, variable rates. Regular prenatal assessment is required. Lesion composition (microcystic or macrocystic) and size have varying physiologic effects. Taking pulmonary maturity into consideration, the treatment of CCAM may occur in early, mid, or late gestation. Therapies may be minimally invasive or require open fetal surgery. Compromise results mostly from mass effect or fluid collection, resulting in a tamponade physiology. Solitary lesions with a large single cyst may be treated minimally invasively with one-time or serial needle aspiration. Ultrasound-guided minimally invasive placement of a thoracoamniotic shunt may negate the need for serial procedures in large, cystic lesions.

In contrast to large lesions with a single cyst, microcystic lesions are not amenable to aspiration or shunting. If a mid-gestation fetus with immature lungs has significant physiologic compromise, an in utero fetal pulmonary lobectomy may be pursued. After the lobectomy is completed, the fetus is returned to the uterus for further growth and development (Adzick et al., 2003). If the fetus is late in gestation and the lesion is causing distress or may interfere with neonatal resuscitation, a delivery via the EXIT procedure can be undertaken, with fetal thoracotomy and pulmonary lobectomy before umbilical cord clamp (Hedrick et al., 2005). If the mass is asymptomatic, the child can be delivered normally, and a postnatal pulmonary lobectomy can be electively scheduled.

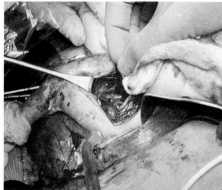

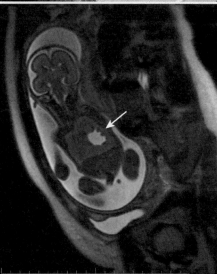

■ FIGURE 19-6. Fetal therapy for congenital cystic adenomatoid malformation (CCAM). **Upper:** The left chest of a fetus undergoing thoracotomy. **Lower:** MRI of a fetus with a large cystic CCAM (*white arrow*).

BPS is distinct from CCAM, because these lesions are composed of lung tissue that typically has no communication to the tracheobronchial tree or pulmonary circulation. Blood supply to a BPS typically comes from a feeder vessel originating from the aorta. Treatment of BPS is similar to that of CCAM and depends on multiple factors, such as size, location, and composition, which influence the physiology of the fetus.

Cardiac Disease

Most of the therapies for congenital cardiac malformations are minimally invasive and catheter based, with most of the reported literature describing fetal aortic valvuloplasty for treatment of severe aortic stenosis—a possible precursor to hypoplastic left heart syndrome (Tworetzky et al., 2004; Marshall et al., 2005; Wilkins-Haug et al., 2006). In utero atrial septoplasty (Fig. 19-7) has also been described for patients with hypoplastic left heart with an intact or highly restrictive atrial septum (Marshall et al., 2008). Pulmonary atresia with an intact ventricular septum may also be amenable to fetal cardiac intervention, as this is the "right-sided" equivalent of hypoplastic left heart syndrome (Tworetzky and

Marshall, 2004). Earlier surgical techniques involved a maternal laparotomy and exteriorization of the uterus. The necessary needles and catheters were then inserted through an otherwise intact uterus, and subsequently guided through the fetal chest wall and myocardium to the chambers or vessels of interest. Currently, an even less invasive approach to the fetal heart is performed. The approach is entirely percutaneous: through the maternal abdomen, uterus, and fetal chest wall. Great care and skill come into play as the trajectory of the needles, catheters, and wires is planned. Outcomes from fetal cardiac interventions have been encouraging but are not definitive yet.

Bladder Outlet Obstruction

Fetal urinary tract obstruction (Fig. 19-8) may result in a host of complications, such as pulmonary hypoplasia, renal dysplasia, bladder dysfunction, renal failure, skeletal abnormalities, and abdominal wall muscular abnormalities (Harrison et al., 1981; Harrison et al., 1982). Patient selection for therapy is challenging, because the disease process must be severe enough to warrant a prenatal surgical intervention, but not so far advanced that the renal damage is irreversible (Cendron et al., 1994). Fetal evaluation is quite involved and includes ultrasound examination of the urinary tract, measurement of amniotic fluid volumes, and analysis of fetal urine electrolytes and proteins (Crombleholme et al., 1990). Minimally invasive therapy may involve needle decompression of the

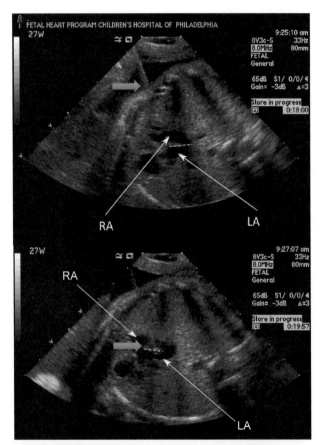

■ **FIGURE 19-7.** Ultrasound images of in utero fetal atrioseptoplasty. The *large arrows* demonstrate the tip of the introducer needle. **Upper:** The introducer needle is indenting the fetal chest wall. **Lower:** The needle is crossing the fetal atrial septum. The *dashed line* highlights the fetal atrial septum. The *thin arrows* demonstrate the right atrium (RA) and left atrium (LA), respectively. *(Images courtesy Jack Rychik, MD, The Children's Hospital of Philadelphia.)*

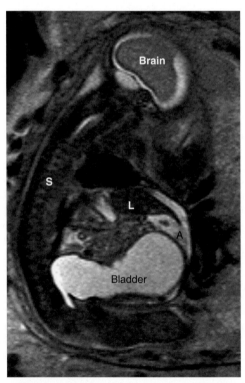

■ **FIGURE 19-8.** Magnetic resonance image of a fetus with lower urinary tract obstruction. The fetus is facing to the right of the image. Notice the massively distended bladder, proximal urethra, and fetal abdomen, and the distinct lack of amniotic fluid surrounding the fetus. *A,* Ascites in the fetal abdomen; *L,* liver; *S,* spine.

bladder, vesicoamniotic shunting, or ablation of posterior urethral valves. Open surgery for bladder marsupialization or ureterostomies has also been reported (Crombleholme et al., 1988). Decompression may reduce the severity of oligohydramnios and the resulting pulmonary hypoplasia, but it may not allow recovery of renal function. Placement of a vesicoamniotic shunt may be technically successful, but the shunt may become dislodged. Bladder function may still not be optimal, as the fetal bladder is not exposed to cyclic filling and emptying. Open fetal surgery has been performed, but the risks and benefits must be carefully considered (Crombleholme et al., 1988).

Sacrococcygeal Teratoma

Sacrococcygeal teratoma is a germ cell tumor arising from the coccyx (Fig. 19-9). Prenatal diagnosis is associated with much higher mortality than postnatal diagnosis (Flake, 1993). In utero, the teratoma places the fetus at risk of hydrops and death from high-output heart failure (Bond et al., 1990). Serial echocardiography is used to monitor the cardiac status of the fetus, and ultrasound is used to monitor tumor growth (Tran et al., 2008). The tumor may cause a vascular steal phenomenon, where much of the fetal cardiac output goes to supplying the tumor instead of the fetus. This is evidenced by increased flow in the descending aorta and increased diameter of the fetal inferior vena cava (Hedrick et al., 2004). The tumor may also rupture in utero, resulting in fetal anemia. Treatment may be minimally invasive in select cases of cystic tumors and involves aspiration of the cystic components. Therapy with radiofrequency ablation has not yielded consistent results (Paek et al., 2001; Ibrahim et al., 2003). In certain cases, midgestation debulking of the tumor may be attempted. An EXIT procedure for resection of a massive sacrococcygeal teratoma has also been performed. For large tumors, at the very least, a planned cesarean delivery is necessary, with provisions for immediate resection if necessary.

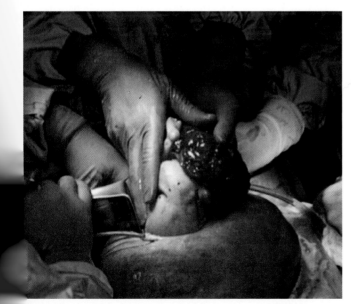

◀ **FIGURE 19-9.** Fetal sacrococcygeal teratoma for debulking.

PHYSIOLOGY

Maternal

The physiologic changes of pregnancy are well described and deserve mention, as these changes have an impact on anesthesia management. Although many organ systems are affected, the most relevant are the neurologic, respiratory, cardiovascular, gastrointestinal, and hematologic.

Sensitivity to anesthetic agents increases during pregnancy. Early in gestation, the minimum alveolar concentrations (MACs) for isoflurane and for halothane are approximately 30% lower in pregnant women than in nonpregnant women (Gin and Chan, 1994; Chan et al., 1996). CSF volume decreases, and the epidural venous plexus becomes distended (Kerr et al., 1964). Pregnancy enhances the spread of local anesthetics in the spinal fluid (Hirabayashi et al., 1995b); in the epidural space, the spread of small dosages of local anesthesia is increased, but the spread of large dosages is about the same in pregnant and nonpregnant women (Kalas et al., 1966; Grundy et al., 1978). Increased dermatomal spread of epidural anesthetics is likely to result from increased nerve sensitivity, hormonal changes, reduced protein levels, and pH changes in the CSF (Flanagan et al., 1987; Hirabayashi et al., 1995a; Hirabayashi et al., 1996; Popitz-Bergez et al., 1997).

Plasma cholinesterase activity decreases during pregnancy, but this decrease does not clinically affect the dosing of succinylcholine. Pregnancy also increases sensitivity to nondepolarizing muscle relaxants. Onset time is faster for vecuronium, and recovery time is longer for rocuronium (Baraka et al., 1992; Puhringer et al., 1997).

Airway management in a pregnant woman is potentially more difficult than in a nonpregnant woman. Capillary engorgement of the airway mucosal tissues has multiple implications. Resultant airway narrowing forces downsizing of endotracheal tubes, and nasal intubation is likely to cause epistaxis. The potential for difficult intubation is increased and airway complications are a significant factor in anesthesia-related morbidity and mortality (Cormack and Lehane, 1984; Samsoon and Young, 1987; Pilkington et al., 1995; Ezri et al., 2001; Ross, 2003; Munnur et al., 2005; Rudra et al., 2006; Goldszmidt, 2008). Respiratory and metabolic changes place the mother at increased risk of hypoxia. Oxygen consumption increases by as much as 60% (Spatling et al., 1992) and functional residual capacity (FRC) begins to decrease in the second trimester, reaching 80% of the nonpregnant volume at term (Alaily and Carrol, 1978). FRC decreases further in the supine position. Tidal volume and minute ventilation increase by 45% at term, and $Paco_2$ decreases to 30 mm Hg by the second trimester (Kelman and Templeton, 1975; Templeton and Kelman, 1976; Alaily and Carrol, 1978). The risk of pulmonary edema increases after open fetal surgery (DiFederico et al., 1998). This increased risk may be secondary to decreased plasma protein concentration, decreased colloid oncotic pressure, or medications used to terminate premature labor, or a combination of these (Mendenhall, 1970; Wu et al., 1983). In addition, surgical manipulation of the uterus and hysterotomy may release factors that increase pulmonary vascular permeability (DiFederico et al., 1998).

Pregnancy is a high cardiac output state. Heart rate and stroke volume increase as early as the first trimester, and at term cardiac output is increased approximately 50% from nonpregnant values (Laird-Meeter et al., 1979; Hunter and Robson,

1992). Cardiac output increases even more during labor and immediately postpartum (Robson et al., 1987). Systemic vascular resistance decreases by about 20% secondary to vasodilation and the addition of the placenta, which is a low-resistance vascular circuit (Clark et al., 1989). Supine hypotension may occur because of compression of the inferior vena cava by the gravid uterus. This compression results in a decrease of right atrial pressure in the supine position (Kerr, 1965). Compression of the aorta is most pronounced in the supine position and becomes negligible in the full lateral position (Eckstein and Marx, 1974). Human studies suggest a reduced response to arterial vasoconstriction by alpha agonists but an increased sensitivity to venous constriction (Nisell et al., 1985). Thus, any pressor response may be more likely to result from increased venous return and increased stroke volume. Plasma volume increases relatively more than red blood cell volume increases, and hemoglobin concentrations decrease in pregnancy.

The pregnant patient is at increased risk for pulmonary aspiration of gastric contents. Hormonal changes and displacement of the stomach with resultant reduction of tone in the lower esophageal high-pressure zone may allow reflux of gastric contents (Ulmsten and Sundstrom, 1978). Intragastric pressure is highest in the third trimester. Gastric emptying of solids and liquids is not slowed during pregnancy, but gastric emptying does slow down during labor (Davison et al., 1970; O'Sullivan et al., 1987; Macfie et al., 1991; Sandhar et al., 1992; Whitehead et al., 1993; Chiloiro et al., 2001; Wong et al., 2002). Although gastric acid production has not definitively been shown to be greater in pregnancy, acid aspiration is still a major concern.

The coagulation system is in a state of accelerated but compensated intravascular coagulation. This hypercoagulable state is suggested by an increase in the majority of coagulation factors, a decrease in prothrombin and partial thromboplastin times, and a decrease in antithrombin III. Increased fibrinolysis is suggested by an increase of fibrin degradation products. Particular attention must be paid to prophylaxis for venous thromboembolism, and a high index of suspicion for thromboembolic events must be maintained in a pregnant woman with shortness of breath.

Fetal

Fetal physiology is as complex as maternal physiology. Logistical considerations necessitate some extrapolation from animal studies. Neurologic pathways for cortical transmission of noxious stimuli in humans are still developing into the third trimester (Lee et al., 2005). Fetal sensitivity to volatile anesthetic agents is increased. With both isoflurane and halothane, the anesthesia requirement of fetal lambs is lower than that of a pregnant ewe (Gregory et al., 1983; Bachman et al., 1986). Perception and processing of pain are controversial, but noxious stimuli will elicit a physiologic response in the human fetus, as evidenced by increases in cortisol and β-endorphin, and decreases in the pulsatility index of the fetal middle cerebral artery (Fisk et al., 2001). These physiologic responses are attenuated by administration of fentanyl directly to the fetus. The pharmacokinetics and pharmacodynamics of fentanyl in the fetus remain to be studied.

The cardiopulmonary physiology of the fetus is not dependent on the lungs, because the placenta acts as the organ of respiration. A major role of the lungs in utero is the production of amniotic fluid. The lung epithelium actively secretes fluid, which fills the lungs. Excess fluid passes out the trachea and into the oropharynx. This fluid is then either swallowed or expelled into the amniotic space and becomes a component of amniotic fluid. Fluid in the lungs causes distention and allows lung development (Olver and Strang, 1974; Perks and Cassin, 1985; Harding and Hooper, 1996). Restriction of egress of this fluid from the lungs results in pulmonary hyperplasia, whereas continuous drainage results in pulmonary hypoplasia (Alcorn et al., 1977).

The fetal circulation is notable for being a parallel system prior to transitioning to a serial circulation at birth. The ductus venosus allows much of the blood from the umbilical vessels to bypass the liver and go directly to the inferior vena cava. The foramen ovale and ductus arteriosus allow mixing of blood between the left and right heart circulations. Oxygenated blood travels from the umbilical veins into the right atrium and preferentially across the foramen ovale to the left atrium. It then flows to the left ventricle to supply the most oxygen-rich blood to the brain and the preductal circulation. Deoxygenated blood returns from the superior vena cava and preferentially travels to the right ventricle via the right atrium. The majority of blood from the right ventricle travels out the pulmonary artery across the ductus arteriosus to supply the postductal circulation. Enough mixing occurs to supply the necessary oxygen to the lower extremities. Blood travels from the aorta to the iliac arteries to the umbilical arteries and then to the placenta, where oxygenation of this blood occurs.

When the pulmonary and systemic circulations are in a series, as in a normal adult heart, cardiac output can be quantitatively described by either the left or the right ventricular output. Because the fetus has a parallel circulatory system, fetal cardiac output is measured and reported as the sum of both the left and right ventricular output, or combined cardiac output (CCO). Echocardiographic studies have found that a normal human fetus has a CCO of 425 to 550 mL/kg per minute, with the right ventricle contributing 60% to 70% of the total output (De Smedt et al., 1987; Mielke and Benda, 2001; Rychik, 2004). The fetal myocardium has a greater proportion of noncontractile elements and is also stiffer with impaired relaxation compared with adult myocardium (Friedman, 1972; Rychik, 2004). Functioning close to the upper limit of the Starling curve, increases in preload provide only minimal, if any, incremental increases of stroke volume and cardiac output (Gilbert, 1980). Variation in heart rate provides a relatively greater contribution to variation in cardiac output. This lack of response to preload has been attributed to poor compliance of the myocardium, but it may also result from extrinsic compression of the fetal heart that is relieved with aeration of the lungs and clearance of lung fluid (Grant, 1999; Grant et al., 2001).

The blood volume of a fetus varies over gestation. At 16 to 22 weeks, blood volume of the fetoplacental unit has been estimated to be 120 to 162 mL/kg of fetal weight (Morris et al., 1974; Nicolaides et al., 1987). At 31 weeks, blood volume has been reported as 93 mL/kg of fetal weight (Nicolaides et al., 1987). It is important to note that about two thirds of the blood volume is contained on the placental side of the fetoplacental unit (Barcroft and Kennedy, 1939; Yao et al., 1969). A 16-week fetus weighs approximately 100 g, at 22 weeks 430 g, and at 31 weeks 1500 g.

Studying hemostasis is challenging because of the rapid evolution of the coagulation system in the fetal and neonatal period. The fetus produces coagulation factors independently of the mother, and these factors do not cross the placenta (Cade et al., 1969). The plasma concentrations of these proteins increase with increasing gestational age (Reverdiau-Moalic et al., 1996). A fetus at 19 to 23 weeks of gestation has a mean prothrombin time (PT) of 32.5 seconds with an International Normalized Ratio (INR) of 6.4 and a mean activated partial thromboplastin time (aPTT) of 168.8 seconds. At 30 to 38 weeks of gestation, mean PT is 22.6 seconds with an INR of 3.0 and an aPTT of 104.8 seconds (Reverdiau-Moalic et al., 1996).

While in utero, fetal temperature is closely linked to maternal variations in temperature. Fetal tissue is more metabolically active than adult tissue, and fetal heat production results in a fetal-to-maternal gradient of 0.5 °C. Excess heat flows from the fetus and is dissipated by the mother. After birth, an increase in heat production is required for homeostasis with the loss of the maternal "heat clamp," and with new evaporative and convective heat losses. The sympathetic nervous and endocrine systems generally activate and regulate this heat production. Shivering and nonshivering thermogenesis take a primary role in the generation of heat for the newborn (Power et al., 2004). A fetus removed from the uterus during open surgery has a similar need for increased heat production as a newborn, but it cannot increase its production adequately. Both fetal shivering and nonshivering thermogenesis responses are largely absent in utero if the umbilical cord is patent (Gunn et al., 1986). Maintenance of normothermia in a fetus exposed during open fetal surgery can be challenging, with a lack of shivering and nonshivering thermogenesis, immature skin barriers, and increased evaporative losses.

Uteroplacental Blood Flow

The fetus depends on intact uteroplacental blood flow and patent umbilical vessels for respiration and nutrition. Uterine blood flow, a surrogate for fetal oxygen delivery, correlates with fetal umbilical venous Po_2 (Skillman et al., 1985; Bilardo et al., 1990). Human uterine blood flow at term is extrapolated to be 700 mL/min (12% of cardiac output), compared with 200 mL/min in the nonpregnant uterus (Thaler et al., 1990).

Uterine blood flow is directly related to uterine perfusion pressure (the difference between uterine arterial pressure and uterine venous pressure) and inversely related to uterine vascular resistance (Box 19-2). Of note for fetal surgical procedures, maternal hypotension, aortocaval compression, and uterine contractions will decrease uterine blood flow. The effect of vasopressors, vasodilators, and anesthetic agents on uterine blood flow is variable because these agents affect uterine arterial pressure and uterine vascular resistance at the same time. Ephedrine has been suggested as the vasopressor of choice in obstetrics, as it may not cause as much uterine arterial vasoconstriction as phenylephrine. Several studies have shown no dramatic clinical differences in neonatal outcome and lend slightly more support to phenylephrine to support maternal blood pressure. When phenylephrine is compared with ephedrine to support blood pressure during cesarean section, newborn pH measurements are statistically but not clinically different (Thomas et al., 1996; Lee et al., 2002; Ngan Kee et al., 2008). Apgar scores are similar. In clinical practice, ephedrine would be a logical choice if the

---

Box 19-2   Uterine Blood Flow*

FACTORS THAT DECREASE UTERINE BLOOD FLOW
Hypotension
High uterine tone
Aortocaval compression

FACTORS WITH VARIABLE EFFECTS ON UTERINE BLOOD FLOW
Vasopressors
Vasodilators
Volatile anesthetic agents
Neuraxial anesthetics

*Uterine blood flow = (uterine arterial pressure − uterine venous pressure) ÷ uterine vascular resistance.

---

maternal heart rate were low, whereas phenylephrine could be used if the maternal heart rate were high. Local factors such as nitric oxide are released by the uterine vascular endothelium and modulate the effect of systemically administered vasoactive medications (Weiner et al., 1991).

Neuraxial and general anesthetics have variable effects on uterine blood flow. As long as maternal systemic pressure is maintained, epidural anesthesia does not seem to alter uterine blood flow in elective cesarean sections (Alahuhta et al., 1991). If a neuraxial technique causes significant hypotension, uterine blood flow will be decreased. In sheep models, pain and stress decrease uterine blood flow (Shnider et al., 1979). Relief of pain with an epidural may attenuate this reduction of flow. Barring resultant hypotensive decreases in blood flow, intravenous (IV) induction agents, thiopental, propofol, etomidate, and ketamine do not affect uterine blood flow dramatically. Volatile anesthetics decrease uterine tone and increase risk of bleeding (Cullen et al., 1970). Light and moderate levels of volatile anesthesia slightly depress blood pressure, but uterine vasodilation maintains blood flow. In a sheep model of fetal surgery, with deeper levels of volatile anesthesia, uterine vasodilation cannot compensate for the reductions in maternal blood pressure and cardiac output, and fetal acidosis occurs (Palahniuk and Shnider, 1974). It is important to note, however, that no medications were given to the pregnant ewes to support their blood pressure while undergoing general anesthesia with high dosages of volatile agent.

Although the studies are not entirely in agreement, maternal hypocapnia, with or without the mechanical effect of hyperventilation with positive pressure, is likely to decrease uterine blood flow, placental–umbilical blood flow, and fetal oxygenation in sheep, monkey, and human studies. In contrast, maternal hypercapnia is associated with an increase in fetal oxygenation and may be beneficial during labor and delivery (Motoyama et al., 1966, 1967; James, 1967; Rivard et al., 1967; Parer et al., 1970; Peng et al., 1972; Levinson et al., 1974).

Simple mechanical factors are important in the maintenance of uteroplacental perfusion and fetal oxygen delivery. Kinking or compression of the umbilical cord, either from loss of amniotic fluid volume or from surgical manipulation of the fetus, will cause a rapid deterioration in the condition of the fetus. Likewise, integrity of the uteroplacental interface must also be maintained. Separation of the placenta from the uterus results in catastrophic decreases in fetal perfusion.

Placental Anatomy and Transport

Maternal spiral arteries arise from the uterus and deposit oxygenated blood and nutrients into the intervillus space. The space is a cavernous expanse, into which the villous trees from the fetal circulation extend. The intervillus space contains maternal blood and is bounded on the maternal side by the basal plate, and on the fetal side by the chorionic plate. The villous trees and terminal villi contain the terminal umbilical arterioles and capillaries that arise from the umbilical arteries and transport the deoxygenated blood and waste products from the fetus for exchange in the intervillus space. These vessels return blood to the fetus via the umbilical veins (Fig. 19-10).

In maternal and fetal blood, the difference in partial pressures of oxygen drives oxygen across the placenta and into the fetal circulation. Fetal hemoglobin has a higher affinity for oxygen than maternal hemoglobin, and this affinity may also help with oxygen transport. Normal newborn umbilical arterial Po_2 is 17 mm Hg, and umbilical venous Po_2 is 29 mm Hg (Helwig et al., 1996). At term, fetal oxygen consumption is 6.8 ± 1.4 mL/kg per minute (Bonds et al., 1986). Fetal oxygen saturation has been shown to be 60% to 70% in term human fetuses (measured by scalp oximetry) and in fetal sheep (Johnson et al., 1991; Luks et al., 1998). Glucose is transported to the fetus by facilitated diffusion (Rice et al., 1979; Challier et al., 1985).

Passage of drugs across the placenta is influenced by size, lipid solubility, protein binding pKa, pH of fetal blood, and blood flow. Increased lipid solubility allows rapid transfer, but it may also result in trapping of the drug in the placenta. Drugs such as local anesthetics and opioids with higher acid dissociation constants may be trapped in ionized form in the fetal circulation if the fetal pH is lower than the drug's pKa. Protein binding has a variable effect, depending on the particular drug and protein combination.

Although the newer volatile anesthetics have not been studied as thoroughly as halothane and isoflurane, the low molecular weight and lipid insolubility of these medications should allow rapid transfer with relatively high fetal-to-maternal (F/M) ratios. A higher F/M ratio indicates that more of the agent in question is found in the fetal blood than in the maternal blood. Most human in vivo studies have been performed in patients undergoing elective termination of pregnancy or elective cesarean section. Isoflurane has an F/M ratio of 0.7 (Biehl et al., 1983b; Kangas et al., 1976; Dwyer et al., 1995), whereas the F/M ratio of desflurane is reported to be 0.5 (Schwarz et al., 2003). Cautious extension of the findings with halothane and isoflurane to desflurane and sevoflurane is reasonable (Fig. 19-11). After 3 minutes, nitrous oxide has an F/M ratio of 0.83 (Polvi et al., 1996).

Thiopental crosses rapidly into the fetal circulation, but F/M ratios range widely, between 0.4 and 1.1 (Levy and Owen, 1964; Finster et al., 1966). Propofol has been studied at term after bolus administration, with and without infusions. F/M ratios range between 0.5 and 0.85 (Dailland et al., 1989; Valtonen et al., 1989; Gin et al., 1990; Gregory et al., 1990). If used only for induction of general anesthesia for open fetal surgery, differences between propofol and thiopental are not likely to be clinically significant. Propofol infusions may be used for maternal sedation in early pregnancy for minimally invasive cases. In women between 12 and 18 weeks of gestation, the F/M ratio was 0.5 and was independent of time between 5 and 20 minutes of infusion (Jauniaux et al., 1998). Diazepam is a commonly used drug for maternal and fetal sedation; within minutes of injection, the F/M ratio approaches unity and ratios approach 2.0 after an hour (Erkkola et al., 1973; Mandelli et al., 1975). Although midazolam has a lower F/M ratio of 0.76, at term it is still frequently used as a sedative in noninvasive surgery (Wilson et al., 1987). No studies have shown any teratogenic relationship between oral clefts and benzodiazepines given in pregnancy (Koren et al., 1998). Morphine is hydrophilic, and

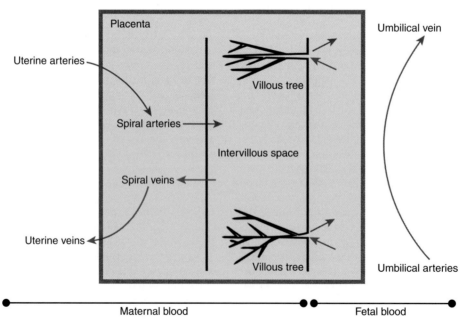

■ **FIGURE 19-10.** Diagram of placental circulation. The *arrows* demonstrate blood flow, and the *colors* signify relative levels of oxygenation. The villous trees contain umbilical arterioles and capillaries with fetal blood. These trees extend and branch into the intervillus space and form the interface for exchange of nutrients and waste between maternal and fetal blood.

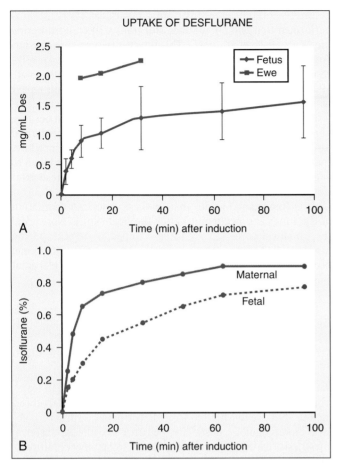

FIGURE 19-11. Comparison of fetal and maternal levels of volatile anesthetic agents in sheep models. **A,** Desflurane *(From Schwarz U, Galinkin JL, Biard JM, et al: The uptake of desflurane in fetal sheep preliminary results. Presented at the Annual Meeting of the Society for Pediatric Anesthesiology, Fort Myers, FL, Feb 20–23, 2003).* **B,** Isoflurane *(From Biehl DR, Tweed WA, Cote J, et al: Effect of halothane on cardiac output and regional flow in the fetal lamb in utero,* Anesth Analg *62:489, 1983).*

TABLE 19-2. Documented Fetal-to-Maternal Ratios of Medications Administered to the Mother

Drug	Fetal-to-Maternal Ratio
Halothane	0.7-0.9
Isoflurane	0.7
Nitrous oxide	0.83
Thiopental	0.4-1.1
Propofol	0.5-0.85
Diazepam	1-2
Midazolam	0.76
Morphine	0.61
Fentanyl	0.16-1.2
Remifentanil	0.29-0.88
Vecuronium	0.06-0.11
Glycopyrrolate	0.22
Ephedrine	0.7

cardia has been attributed to placental passage of neostigmine (Clark et al., 1996). Ephedrine crosses the placenta readily, with an F/M ratio of 0.7 (Hughes et al., 1985) (Table 19-2).

SURGICAL ISSUES

Minimally Invasive Interventions

Minimally invasive interventions are the most frequently performed fetal surgical procedures. The uterine cavity is accessed percutaneously with needles and small sheaths. Visualization of structures is provided by ultrasound guidance or fetoscopes inserted through the sheaths. Because minimally invasive techniques allow a wide range of therapeutic options via a wide range of operative techniques, a clear understanding of the surgical plan helps to shape the anesthesia plan. Placental vessels allowing unequal blood flow between monochorionic twins (twin-twin transfusion syndrome) may be ablated with lasers (Lewi et al., 2005; Habli et al., 2008). The umbilical cord of an acephalic acardiac twin mass (twin reversed arterial perfusion sequence) can be coagulated with radiofrequency to prevent harm to the normal twin (Tan and Sepulveda, 2003). With ultrasound guidance, fetal thoracoamniotic shunts can be placed to allow drainage of fluid from cystic lung lesions into the amniotic fluid (Adzick and Kitano, 1993). Tracheal occlusion can be performed to prevent egress of lung fluid, and this may attenuate the lung hypoplasia that results from congenital diaphragmatic hernia (Peralta et al., 2008). The efficacy of tracheal occlusion continues to be studied. Fetal cardiac catheterization and intervention may allow fetuses with evolving hypoplastic left heart syndrome to develop two ventricle circulations (Tworetzky and Marshall, 2003). Vesicoamniotic shunts have been placed in the bladders of fetuses with lower urinary tract obstruction to relieve hydroureter and hydronephrosis and perhaps allow improved bladder function (Crombleholme et al., 1990). Attempted treatment of fetal sacrococcygeal teratomas with radiofrequency ablation has been associated with

also quite commonly used for maternal and fetal analgesia and sedation. Intramuscular maternal administration of morphine (0.12 to 0.19 mg/kg) decreases fetal breathing movement; however, fetal tone and gross movement are not as affected by morphine, and the F/M ratio is 0.61 (Kopecky et al., 2000). In early gestation, fentanyl is detectable in fetal brain tissue between 10 and 30 minutes after maternal administration (Cooper et al., 1999). The F/M ratio of fentanyl varied from 0.16 to 1.2 in a small study of maternal IV administration (Shannon et al., 1998). Remifentanil, a short-acting potent opioid, is finding some use in both obstetric anesthesia and anesthesia for fetal surgery. With remifentanil infusions at term for cesarean section, umbilical vein to maternal artery ratio was 0.88, and umbilical artery to umbilical vein ratio was 0.29 (Kan et al., 1998). Succinylcholine in large (300 mg) or repeated doses crosses the placenta and affects the fetus. Nondepolarizing muscle relaxants and anticholinesterase agents are large, ionized molecules that do not easily cross the placenta. Vecuronium F/M ratios are 0.06 to 0.11 (Dailey et al., 1984; Iwama et al., 1999). Rocuronium has been used in mothers undergoing cesarean section with no adverse effects (Abouleish et al., 1994; Baraka et al., 1997). Atropine readily crosses the placenta, as opposed to glycopyrrolate, which has a mean F/M ratio of 0.22. A case of fetal brady-

too much morbidity at this time (Paek et al., 2001; Ibrahim et al., 2003). Techniques for endoscopic closure of fetal MMC also continue to be refined (Fichter et al., 2008).

Because of the wide range of therapeutic options, the requirements for surgical access to the fetus are also quite varied. The access may be as minimal as one small-gauge radiofrequency probe or may be as involved as multiple trocars for a robot-assisted MMC repair. Endoscopes range from 1.0 to 3.8 mm in external diameter (Klaritsch et al., 2009). The timing of these procedures is typically in early or middle gestation. However, given the varied pathophysiology of the disease processes to be treated and the varied nature of these interventions, it is possible that minimally invasive interventions may be done at any time in gestation. Tracheal balloons placed at around 26 weeks gestation to obstruct the egress of lung fluid are removed in late gestation before delivery (Deprest et al., 2005).

Open Midgestation Surgery

Open fetal surgery has been performed to relieve bladder outlet obstruction, repair congenital diaphragmatic hernia, resect lung lesions causing significant mass effect and hydrops, debulk sacrococcygeal teratomas, and close MMCs (Crombleholme et al., 1988; Harrison et al., 1997; Adzick et al., 2003; Hedrick et al., 2004; Fichter et al., 2008). Presently, open midgestation surgery is largely reserved for closure of MMC and resection of lung lesions causing hydrops. Open treatment for bladder outlet obstruction is also being performed at some institutions. Treatment of MMC in utero is currently restricted to patients enrolled in the NIH-sponsored Management of Myelomeningocele Study (MOMS trial).

After induction of anesthesia, a maternal laparotomy is performed. The location of this incision is transverse, but more cephalad than that performed for a low-segment transverse cesarean section, to allow easier access to the uterus and fetus. Once the uterus is exposed, the placental edges are mapped carefully with sterile ultrasound to plan for an appropriate hysterotomy. Implantation of the placenta on the anterior or posterior aspect of the uterus will influence the surgical approach, and an anterior placenta may necessitate exteriorization of the uterus for a posterior hysterotomy. Special uterine stapling devices are used to minimize blood loss (Bond et al., 1989). The fetus is exposed, but only the necessary anatomy is delivered via the hysterotomy. For example, in an MMC closure, the lesion is exposed while the rest of the fetus remains bathed in amniotic fluid in the uterus. If a fetal thoracotomy is planned, an arm is delivered, and the shoulder and chest are exposed while the rest of the fetus remains in the uterus (see Fig. 19-6). After surgery and skin closure, the fetus is placed back into the uterus, warmed crystalloid is infused to restore amniotic volume, and intrauterine antibiotics are given. The uterus is closed and a patch of omentum is sewn over a two-layer uterine closure to further prevent amniotic fluid leakage.

EXIT Procedure

The EXIT procedure is similar in approach to an open midgestation procedure, but with several key differences. Because the fetus will be delivered at the end of the case, these procedures are performed at or near term to optimize fetal lung maturity.

Before the umbilical cord is clamped, surgical intervention is performed that will allow successful transition to extrauterine life (Mychaliska et al., 1997). This intervention may involve laryngoscopy, rigid bronchoscopy, and intubation, or it may involve resection of airway tumors or tracheostomy (Liechty et al., 1997; Bouchard et al., 2002; Rahbar et al., 2005). Pulmonary pathology necessitating an EXIT procedure includes large lung lesions that would make neonatal resuscitation difficult because of mediastinal shift, air trapping, or compression of the normal lung (Hedrick et al., 2005). After completion of the procedure, the umbilical cord is clamped and cut. The newborn is taken to a team headed by a neonatologist for further neonatal resuscitation and management in an intensive care unit.

It is important to note that in these cases, no ventilation of the lungs can occur until after the fetal skin is closed and the umbilical cord is ready to be clamped. Ventilation of the lungs will initiate the cascade of events leading to a transitional neonatal circulation, and the benefits of operating on placental support are lost.

ANESTHETIC PLAN

Teamwork and Communication

Participation in fetal surgical cases is truly an exercise in teamwork and communication. The disciplines that may interact can include, but are not limited to, pediatric general surgery, pediatric otolaryngology, obstetrics, pediatric anesthesia, obstetric anesthesia, cardiology, radiology, neonatology, neonatal nursing, and operating room nursing. Weekly meetings are necessary to keep team members apprised of the new patients and new developments or progress of existing patients. Before any open surgical procedure, a multidisciplinary team meeting is held with the family in attendance to introduce the team members, discuss the details of the procedure, and address any concerns from any of the involved parties. Minimally invasive procedures also necessitate discussion to delineate special requirements, equipment, and issues.

Preoperative Preparation

The maternal preoperative preparation begins with the standard anesthetic history and physical, including a history of problems with anesthesia or difficult intubation. Specific questions for the mother would evaluate respiratory or circulatory compromise by the gravid uterus, as evidenced by symptoms of shortness of breath or lightheadedness. More-severe symptoms of aortocaval compression would call for meticulous left uterine displacement and would raise the level of suspicion in a mother with persistent hypotension after induction of anesthesia. Severity of gastroesophageal reflux may change the anesthesia plan in minimally invasive cases when maternal sedation is often considered. Examination of the airway and spine is particularly important. Maternal imaging and blood work will be guided by the history and physical examination. A blood type and screen is reasonable for most minimally invasive fetoscopic cases, but open cases should not proceed without cross-matched blood for the mother and type O, Rh-negative blood for the fetus immediately available. Maternal antibodies to blood antigens can cross the placenta, and the O negative blood for the fetus can be cross-matched with the maternal blood sample. A preoperative chest radiograph may be obtained if indicated.

More specific questions about the fetus are also necessary. Location of the placenta may alter surgical approach. The estimated fetal weight by ultrasound is used to determine dosage of drugs given directly to the fetus. The actual disease process and pathophysiology, and the extent of anatomic or physiologic derangement will give the providers an idea of the physiologic reserve of the fetus. Fetal studies to elucidate the lesion and extent of physiologic derangements include ultrasound, echocardiography, and fetal magnetic resonance imaging. Serial studies track the physiologic changes occurring in the fetuses. Lung lesions may grow or shrink, airway compression may worsen or resolve, combined cardiac outputs may change, hydrops fetalis may ensue, and polyhydramnios may develop at any time.

Aspiration prophylaxis in the obstetric population may include oral sodium citrate, histamine receptor blockers or proton pump inhibitors, and prokinetic agents such as metoclopramide.

Minimally Invasive Procedures

Because these cases are the most variable in terms of degree of invasiveness, need for maternal analgesia and anesthesia, and need for fetal analgesia or immobility, communication and understanding of needs of the case are vital. An anesthesia plan can range from local anesthetic infiltration to sedation to neuraxial technique to general anesthesia. Medications can be given directly to the mother by the anesthesia team and thus indirectly to the fetus by placental transfer (Van de Velde et al., 2005). Medications can also be given directly to the fetus by the surgical team. Route of direct administration can be variable, and intramuscular, IV, and intracardiac routes have been described (Fisk et al., 2001; Deprest et al., 2005; Mizrahi-Arnaud et al., 2007). Sheep models of intraamniotic opioid instillation have also been reported (Strumper et al., 2003). Maternal analgesia can often be accomplished with local anesthetic infiltration, whereas in other cases a neuraxial technique or general anesthesia may be necessary.

As instrumentation for treatment of twin-twin transfusion syndrome has shrunk and invasiveness has decreased, anesthesia techniques at some institutions have similarly changed. Initially, procedures were performed with general or neuraxial anesthesia techniques, but these procedures are now done with sedation. Routine use of magnesium sulfate tocolysis and severe IV fluid restriction are no longer needed. Pulmonary edema has been reported after fetoscopic surgery, but this was more likely the result of absorption of irrigation fluids through venous channels in the myometrium than a capillary leak phenomenon (Robinson et al., 2008). As surgical techniques vary, fluid restriction may be necessary, as well as close observation of irrigation fluids used during these cases.

At some institutions, the current practice for laser ablation of placental vessels includes maternal fasting, placement of one IV catheter, aspiration prophylaxis, and tocolysis with preoperative indomethacin. Light sedation and analgesia are administered to the mother to provide maternal comfort and decreased fetal movement to make the surgical procedure easier. Multiple regimens for sedation have been used successfully, including combinations of opioids and other sedatives such as benzodiazepines or propofol. In a randomized double-blind trial comparing diazepam and remifentanil for fetal immobilization in minimally invasive surgery, the remifentanil group (0.1 mcg/kg per minute) had significantly less fetal movement and surgeons reported better operating conditions (Van de Velde et al., 2005). The degree of maternal sedation needed often competes with the need to avoid paradoxical chest and abdominal breathing motions that make the surgical procedure impossible.

In contrast to the anesthesia for laser ablation of placental vessels, providing anesthesia for balloon dilation of fetal aortic stenosis involves maternal general endotracheal anesthesia and intramuscular administration of fentanyl, vecuronium, and atropine to the fetus (Tworetzky and Marshall, 2003). The potential risks of administration of general anesthesia in a pregnant woman are outweighed by the need for a completely immobile mother and fetus, along with the potential need for fetal analgesia as the catheters and needles are advanced through the fetal chest wall and heart. These different techniques for minimally invasive surgery illustrate the need for collaboration between the teams to prioritize needs and balance risks and benefits to arrive at an optimal anesthesia plan.

The location of the placenta plays an important role in determining the surgical approach. The approach selected needs to avoid trespass of the placenta with the instruments; careful mapping of the placenta with sterile intraoperative ultrasound guides safe instrument trajectories. If the placenta is implanted on the anterior surface of the uterus, trocars and curved instruments are inserted in the lateral aspect of the uterus if possible, or a laparotomy is made, the uterus exteriorized, and the instruments passed through the posterior aspect of the uterus. If instruments are to be introduced laterally, positioning the mother may involve "bumps" for left or right uterine displacement, or even placing the mother in full lateral decubitus position. It is conceivable that some approaches may preclude effective uterine displacement, and in these cases, the anesthesia and surgical teams must have a flexible plan if supine hypotension from aortocaval compression is clinically significant.

As with any minimally invasive procedure, the possibility of conversion to an open procedure exists. Conversion to an open procedure would probably involve a maternal laparotomy for exteriorization of the uterus, or for an exceedingly unlikely maternal hysterectomy for maternal hemorrhage. The fetus may also be manipulated more readily in cases of fetal cardiac catheterization. Strategies must be in place for failed procedures or fetal distress. These plans will depend on the gestational age of the fetuses, their projected viability, and preoperative discussion with the family. Plans may range from supportive or palliative therapy to emergent cesarean delivery.

Fetal monitoring is typically limited to measurement of the fetal heart rate by the obstetricians using ultrasound. Echocardiography may be used in cardiac interventions. Minimally invasive cases usually do not require the intense uterine relaxation required in open cases. Initial tocolytic regimens involved combinations of preoperative indomethacin with postoperative magnesium infusions and post-discharge oral nifedipine or subcutaneous terbutaline. Obstetricians are present for minimally invasive procedures, whereas both obstetricians and pediatric surgeons are present for open procedures. Post-discharge tocolytic requirement is rare.

Open Midgestation Procedures

Open midgestation surgery requires significant uterine relaxation. General endotracheal anesthesia with deep inhalational anesthesia (twice the minimum alveolar concentration) is most often used to achieve the necessary uterine relaxation for open surgery. Desflurane is the agent chosen at some institutions because its low solubility allows for timely emergence from deep levels of anesthesia, but isoflurane has also been used successfully. Nitroglycerin boluses can be used to further relax the uterus if sufficient relaxation cannot be achieved (Clark et al., 2004; George et al., 2007). Uterine relaxation allows easier fetal manipulation and decreases the likelihood of initiation of labor from uterine surgical manipulation. Uterine relaxation may allow increased uterine blood flow as long as maternal blood pressure is maintained, and it results in fetal exposure to some volatile anesthetic agents. The mother is at risk for hypotension both from the anesthetic agents and from aortocaval compression. With careful patient positioning and judicious use of vasopressors, a goal of systemic blood pressure within 10% of normal blood pressure should be achievable.

After fasting, placement of a peripheral IV catheter, and aspiration prophylaxis, a high lumbar epidural catheter is placed for postoperative analgesia. A test dose of local anesthetic is given, but a standard epidural dose is not given if volatile anesthesia is to be used. Oral tocolysis with indomethacin is also given. Standard monitors are placed, the mother is placed supine with left uterine displacement, and she is preoxygenated. After rapid-sequence induction of general anesthesia, she is intubated, and an orogastric tube and a Foley catheter are placed. Ventilation should maintain normocapnia. Hypocapnia should be avoided to prevent umbilical vasoconstriction and fetal hypoxia, but hypercapnia may be beneficial (Motoyama et al., 1966; Peng et al., 1972). Because of the risk for rapid bleeding and hemodynamic instability, a second large-bore peripheral IV line is placed, as well as an arterial catheter. Small changes in maternal blood pressure may have dramatic effects on the fetal oxygen saturation and heart rate and function. Swings in blood pressure are likely to be exacerbated by the restrictive administration of fluids and frequent use of vasopressors. Intravenous crystalloid administration is kept to a minimum because of the risk of maternal pulmonary edema after fetal surgery (DiFederico et al., 1998). Administration of 500 mL of crystalloid is typical. Restricting fluid administration may be more of an issue when nitroglycerin is used more liberally. Clinically, the maternal blood pressure improves with exteriorization of the uterus and with surgical manipulation. Phenylephrine and ephedrine should be prepared for use. Infusions of phenylephrine allow smoother blood pressure control and may allow more rigorous control of crystalloid administration. The anesthesia literature is still exploring the relative advantages and disadvantages of phenylephrine and ephedrine in the obstetric population, but no specific data exist to guide the choices in fetal surgery. Central venous pressure measurement has guided fluid therapy in the past but has not been used recently because it is very restrictive (500 cc), and hypotension is treated with either vasopressors or transfusion if bleeding is noted. Low central venous pressure would probably not trigger much change in fluid management.

When the uterus is exposed, some time is taken for mapping of the placenta to optimize the surgical approach. After hysterotomy and exposure of the fetus, an intramuscular injection of fentanyl (20 mcg/kg), atropine (20 mcg/kg), and vecuronium (0.2 mg/kg) is given by the surgical team. Amniotic fluid is lost through the hysterotomy, but it is replaced with a continuous pressurized infusion of warmed lactated Ringer's solution. If fetal IV access is deemed necessary, it is obtained at this time, and sterile IV tubing is handed over the surgical drapes to the anesthesia team. Monitoring of the fetus in these cases may include fetal heart rate by ultrasound, fetal echocardiography, and pulse oximetry (Fig. 19-12) (Luks et al., 1998; Keswani et al., 2005) in addition to direct fetal observation. The sterile pulse oximeter is placed by the surgical team, the hand is covered with sterile foil to prevent artifact from the operating room lights, and a sterile cable is passed to the anesthesia team over the surgical drapes. Values for fetal oxygen saturation range from 40% to 70% (Johnson et al., 1991; Helwig et al., 1996). Fetal echocardiography may be intermittent or continuous depending on the nature of the surgery. Cardiac filling, contractility, and rate, along with patency of the ductus arteriosus are helpful in intraoperative management of the fetus. Umbilical blood gas measurement may be used in select cases, although cord injury is a risk. Drugs may be given to the fetus intravenously or intramuscularly.

The anesthesia team must watch closely for fetal bradycardia, maternal or fetal bleeding, and maternal blood pressure changes. Careful observation and understanding of the events occurring in the surgical field are important. Maternal bleeding when the uterus is opened is often difficult to appreciate. A decrease in fetal oxygen saturation seems to be the most sensitive indicator of fetal distress (Luks et al., 1998). In the absence of a decrease in fetal oxygen saturation, the most common sign of fetal distress is bradycardia. Blood products should be readily available during this time. Prior to the resection of large chest lesions, a 10- to 20-mg/kg fluid bolus (usually packed red blood cells) to the fetus maintains fetal hemodynamic stability by preserving cardiac output when large shifts in mediastinal anatomy occur during the resection. With closure of the uterus, tocolysis is begun with a bolus of IV magnesium sulfate, the epidural block is initiated, and the volatile anesthetic is reduced. The maternal abdomen is closed, and the mother is extubated awake. Postoperative tocolysis continues with a magnesium infusion that is later transitioned to oral nifedipine.

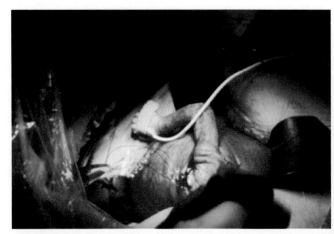

■ **FIGURE 19-12.** A pulse oximeter placed on the fetal hand during open surgery. This probe is covered by foil to prevent artifact from the surgical lights.

EXIT Procedure

Several key differences for the EXIT procedure result from the fact that the fetus is to be delivered at the conclusion of the case. Because magnesium tocolysis is no longer needed, pulmonary edema is less of a problem, so fluid management can be more generous. Another difference is the need for two operating rooms and a resuscitation area for the neonatal team. Although general endotracheal anesthesia is often used to provide high-dosage volatile anesthetics and is the technique of choice at some institutions, adequate uterine relaxation with nitroglycerin infusion is possible. Several reports have described neuraxial techniques for the EXIT procedure in conjunction with infusions of nitroglycerin (Clark et al., 2004; George et al., 2007).

After the patient has been adequately anesthetized, the surgical team passes sterile items off the field for the anesthesia team. These may include tubing for IV fluids, pulse oximeter cables, and oxygen tubing for a sterile Mapleson D circuit. Keeping fetal IV fluids and medication separate from maternal fluids and drugs is important to avoid confusion, especially in emergent or urgent parts of the procedure. Fetal well-being is monitored with pulse oximetry, heart rate, and possibly echocardiography. After maternal laparotomy, placental mapping, and hysterotomy, the fetus is externalized as little as possible to permit a surgical approach to the lesion while promoting placental circulation through the umbilical vessels. Once the airway is secured or the lesion resected, surfactant is aerosolized to the fetus and the lungs are ventilated. As mentioned previously, it is crucial that no ventilation take place until the umbilical cord is ready to be divided. Increases in oxygen saturation, the presence of end-tidal CO_2, and good chest movement are indicators of successful intubation. Fiberoptic bronchoscopy can also be used as confirmation. The baby is delivered for care by neonatologists.

Once the umbilical cord is cut and the placenta is delivered, uterine relaxation must be promptly reversed. Administration of oxytocin and rapidly decreasing the inspired concentration of volatile anesthetic is adequate in most cases, but methylergonovine and prostaglandin $F_2\alpha$ should be readily available. After uterine tone is established, the hysterotomy is closed. Epidural anesthesia is given after maternal hemodynamic stability is ensured, and the mother is extubated awake.

Additional considerations for the EXIT procedure include the presence of a neonatal resuscitation team and a second operating room team with separate anesthesia and surgical teams. The neonatal team receives the newborn if the EXIT is technically successful, and the operating room team is prepared to take the newborn and complete the surgery when the EXIT procedure is not successful. The neonatal team may receive the newborn in a variety of states, but always with a stable airway—either intubated or with a tracheostomy. If the fetus does not tolerate the procedure well, the umbilical cord must be cut, and the newborn taken immediately to the second operating room for further resuscitation and completion of the surgery if possible. The second anesthesia team must be immediately ready to receive a newborn in extremis. The airway may not be controlled, ventilation may not have been established, IV access may be lacking, and the newborn may be actively bleeding. The second operating room should also have a second set of nurses. The surgical team may easily be divided between two rooms, as the maternal operating room is staffed with obstetricians and pediatric surgeons. If the newborn is taken to the second room,

the obstetric team stays with the mother to control bleeding and close her uterus and abdomen, while the pediatric surgical team follows the newborn.

Because of the multiple teams that must be ready for multiple clinical pathways during an EXIT procedure, communication is important. The maternal room should have blood available for mother and fetus, but all parties should know how much blood is available for the fetus and where that blood is located. The blood for the fetus may be transfused while on placental support, after cord clamp while under care of the neonatal team, or after cord clamp while under care of the anesthesia team. All teams should have appropriate emergency resuscitation equipment and medications.

Intraoperative Fetal Resuscitation

Fetal distress may occur during any surgical procedure. Bradycardia or hypoxia may result from cord compression or kinking, placental separation, high uterine tone, maternal hypotension, hypoxia, or anemia. Fetal hypothermia, hypovolemia and anemia are also potential causes of fetal distress. Cardiac dysfunction may also result from prolonged exposure to high dosages of volatile anesthetic agents. As with any change in vital signs, the cause of the derangement must be sought as soon as possible.

The well-being and hemodynamic stability of the mother should be ensured. The umbilical cord must be patent, aortocaval compression should be avoided, and the integrity of the uteroplacental unit must also be confirmed. Placental abruption can be catastrophic if unnoticed. Signs of separation would include excessive, unexplained blood in the amniotic fluid; unexplained, new-onset maternal hypotension or anemia; fetal oxygen desaturation; or fetal bradycardia. Ultrasound can be used to confirm the diagnosis. Direct observation of the fetus can also assist with these diagnoses. The surgical team should be able to confirm adequate uterine relaxation, and fetal echocardiography will inform the team about cardiac filling and function, and patency of the ductus arteriosus.

Measures to resuscitate the fetus depend on how much access the surgical and anesthesia teams have to the fetus, and they range from simple measures, such as ensuring left uterine displacement or administration of maternal vasopressors, to more advanced measures, including administration of medications or blood directly to the fetus. In open cases, emergency medications such as atropine and epinephrine are given sterilely to the surgical team. Medications may be given via the intramuscular, IV, or even intracardiac route.

Pain and the Fetus

Controversy surrounds our understanding of the experience of pain by the fetus (Wise, 1997; Glover and Fisk, 1999; Lee et al., 2005; Lowery et al., 2007). Impeded by our inability to critically study human fetal physiology and neural development, a variety of contradictions drawn from available animal and human sources obfuscate our knowledge of this area. At what point, if ever, a fetus "feels" or experiences pain is unknown. The functional neurodevelopment of pain pathways in several experimental animal models is well described, although the exact correlation to human development and experience is unclear (Fitzgerald and Walker, 2009). Even less understood is the experience of pain. Some animal data imply that the fetus is unaware until birth; other data question the need for cortical function in the experience of pain (Mellor et al., 2005). Just as confusing is the relationship between pain and stress. A fetus in the second trimester can mount a stress response to a stimulus that is blocked by the administration of analgesics to the fetus; yet how this phenomenon relates to pain is unclear, especially because a similar stress response can be noted in an adult under deep anesthesia (Giannakoulopoulos et al., 1994; Teixeira et al., 1999; Fisk et al., 2001; Gruber et al., 2001; Baldini et al., 2008). The late effects of this stress response are worrisome, although these effects are as ambiguous and unsettled. Also ambiguous are the possible deleterious effects on the developing nervous system from the medications used to block this response and provide analgesia and anesthesia to the fetus (Jevtovic-Todorovic et al., 2003). In animal models, opioids have also been associated with adverse hemodynamic changes in fetuses (Sedgwick et al., 2005; Mizrahi-Arnaud et al., 2007). Finally, the significant risks to the mother when using her as a conduit to deliver medications to the fetus have to be considered (Golombeck et al., 2006). With the lack of clarity in this area, continued observation, research, and questioning are of paramount importance for the anesthesiologist caring for both mother and fetus.

Currently, transplacental administration of medications for fetal surgery is the norm. Procedures are performed either with maternal general anesthesia or with local anesthesia with maternal systemic anxiolysis and analgesia. Halothane and probably the other volatile anesthetics are transferred to the fetus through the placenta (Dwyer et al., 1995). Opioids and sedatives similarly pass through the placenta to the fetus (Bakke and Haram, 1982; Kan et al., 1998). Open procedures are often supplemented with IV or intramuscular analgesics, neuromuscular blockers, and anticholinergics. Until microsampling and microanalysis techniques are improved and long-term outcome studies are executed, the anesthesiologist will need to strive to provide the best possible conditions for the surgeon while subjecting the mother and fetus to as little risk or harm as possible.

SUMMARY

Fetal surgery is an exciting area for innovation and growth in medicine. The trends toward minimally invasive surgery are mirrored in the field of fetal surgery. Decreasing invasiveness is likely to mean decreased anesthesia and surgical risk, and this may allow an expansion of maternal eligibility criteria for fetal interventions. With decreasing invasiveness comes decreasing maternal risk of bleeding. A hysterotomy mandates a cesarean delivery for all subsequent pregnancies because of the risk of uterine rupture, but the use of needles and sheaths will allow for normal vaginal deliveries. Open fetal surgery is admittedly an undertaking that is intensive in its use of medical resources, and we can hope that decreasing invasiveness will allow more equitable distribution of limited resources. With improving therapy, neonatal care may be simplified, stays shortened, and outcomes improved.

More outcome studies are needed, as well as further studies to refine anesthesia techniques and methods. Some institutions are exploring the use of IV anesthesia to minimize fetal exposure to high-dosage volatile agents during portions of the case that do not require intense uterine relaxation (Boat, 2008). Research in this field is limited by practical, medicolegal, and ethical considerations, and the number of these cases is small in comparison with other fields. Protection of vulnerable populations such as pregnant mothers and fetuses is important, but these protections will limit flexibility in study design. Most anesthesia studies in this area are, however, still in the descriptive, hypothesis-generating stages, as compared with rigorous hypothesis testing. Many questions remain to be answered, and much progress remains to be made.

For questions and answers on topics in this chapter, go to "Chapter Questions" at www.expertconsult.com.

REFERENCES

Complete references used in this text can be found online at www.expertconsult.com.

Anesthesia for Congenital Heart Surgery

James A. DiNardo, Avinash C. Shukla, and Francis X. McGowan, Jr.

CONTENTS

his chapter describes the perioperative management of major forms of congenital heart disease (CHD) that require surgery with the use of cardiopulmonary bypass. Congenital cardiac lesions that are primarily addressed in the catheterization laboratory or without CPB are discussed in Chapter 21, Congenital Cardiac Anesthesia: Non-Bypass Procedures.

Congenital anomalies of the heart and cardiovascular system occur in 7 to 10 per 1000 live births. Congenital heart disease is the most common congenital disease, accounting for approximately 30% of all congenital diseases. CHD has become the principal cause of pediatric heart disease as the incidence of rheumatic heart disease has declined. Ten percent to 15% of children with CHD have associated congenital anomalies of the skeletal, genitourinary, or gastrointestinal system. The U.S. population of adults with CHD, surgically corrected or uncorrected, is estimated to exceed 1 million and is increasing steadily. As a result, it is not uncommon for adult patients with CHD to present for noncardiac surgery (see Chapter 21, Congenital Cardiac Anesthesia: Non-Bypass Procedures).

Transthoracic and transesophageal echocardiography has facilitated early, accurate diagnosis of congenital heart disease. Unlike in adults, who may have limited transthoracic echocardiographic windows, high-quality echocardiographic images in pediatric patients are easily obtained. Most neonates with CHD can have sufficient and thorough evaluation of their cardiac lesions by echocardiography and thus avoid catheterization studies for diagnosis and management. In some instances, catheterization and angiography are necessary to clearly delineate coronary or aortopulmonary collateral anatomy and other intracardiac defects, to assess pressure gradients, and to potentially intervene for palliative or reparative purposes. Fetal cardiac ultrasonography has permitted antenatal diagnosis of congenital heart defects, allowing subsequent perinatal management in specialized tertiary care centers. Imaging modalities such as cardiac magnetic resonance imaging (MRI) and three-dimensional echocardiography are being used with increasing frequency.

Advances in molecular biology have provided a new understanding of the genetic basis of CHD. Chromosomal abnormalities are associated with an estimated 10% of congenital cardiovascular lesions. Two thirds of these lesions occur in patients with trisomy 21; the other one third of lesions are found in patients with other chromosomal abnormalities, such as trisomy 13 and trisomy 18, and in patients with Turner's syndrome. Conotruncal lesions (tetralogy of Fallot, interrupted aortic arch, truncus arteriosus, ventricular septal defects) are commonly associated with a 22q11.2 chromosomal deletion. This defect is associated with DiGeorge syndrome, velocardiofacial syndrome, and conotruncal anomaly face syndromes. These syndromes can be associated with hypocalcemia, immunodeficiency, facial dysmorphia, palate anomalies, velopharyngeal dysfunction, renal anomalies, and developmental, speech, and feeding disorders. The remaining 90% or so of congenital cardiovascular lesions are currently without defined genetic association and are postulated to be the results of interactions of one or more genes with external or environmental factors (e.g., rubella, ethanol, lithium, maternal diabetes mellitus, folate deficiency).

Signs and symptoms of congenital heart disease in infants and children often include dyspnea, poor feeding, poor growth, delayed physical development, and the presence of a cardiac murmur. The diagnosis of CHD is apparent during the first week of life in about 50% of patients, and before 5 years of age in virtually all remaining patients. Echocardiography is the initial diagnostic step if CHD is suspected.

Congenital heart disease can be associated with specific complications. For example, infective endocarditis is a risk associated with most congenital cardiac anomalies. Sudden death occasionally occurs in patients who undergo surgical correction of CHD, presumably reflecting the effects of chronic abnormal hemodynamic loads, myocardial scarring and fibrosis, damage to the cardiac conduction system, or underlying (and presently occult) abnormal molecular and ion channel defects. Cardiac dysrhythmias are not usually a prominent presenting feature of CHD but can be more common as patients age and pathophysiologic sequelae of abnormal cardiac structure, function, and surgery accrue (see later and Chapter 21, Congenital Cardiac Anesthesia: Non-Bypass Procedures). Table 20-1 summarizes the pathophysiology and clinical picture associated with a wide variety of congenital heart defects. Table 20-2 summarizes the surgical repair options for each type of lesion.

PATHOPHYSIOLOGY OF CONGENITAL HEART DISEASE

Although some congenital heart defects involve purely obstructive or regurgitant valvular lesions, shunts (both physiologic and anatomic) are a hallmark of CHD. The concepts of shunting (both physiologic and anatomic), single-ventricle physiology, and intercirculatory mixing require discussion.

Shunting. Shunting is the process whereby venous return into one circulatory system is recirculated through the arterial outflow of the same circulatory system. Flow of blood from the systemic venous atrium or right atrium (RA) to the aorta produces recirculation of systemic venous blood. Flow of blood from the pulmonary venous atrium or left atrium (LA) to the pulmonary artery (PA) produces recirculation of pulmonary venous blood. Recirculation of blood produces a physiologic shunt. Recirculation of pulmonary venous blood produces a physiologic left-to-right (L-R), whereas recirculation of systemic venous blood produces a physiologic right-to-left (R-L) shunt.

Effective blood flow is the quantity of venous blood from one circulatory system reaching the arterial system of the other circulatory system. Effective pulmonary blood flow is the volume of systemic venous blood reaching the pulmonary circulation, whereas effective systemic blood flow is the volume of pulmonary venous blood reaching the systemic circulation. Effective pulmonary blood flow and effective systemic blood flows are the flows necessary to maintain life. Effective pulmonary blood flow and effective systemic blood flow are always equal, no matter how complex the lesions. Effective blood flow is usually the result of a normal pathway through the heart, but it may occur as the result of an anatomic R-L or L-R shunt, as in transposition physiology.

Total pulmonary blood flow ($\dot{Q}_P$) is the sum of effective pulmonary blood flow and recirculated pulmonary blood flow. Total systemic blood flow ($\dot{Q}_S$) is the sum of effective systemic blood flow and recirculated systemic blood flow. Total pulmonary blood flow and total systemic blood flow do not have to be equal. Therefore, it is best to think of recirculated flow (physiologic shunt flow) as the extra, noneffective flow superimposed on the nutritive effective blood flow. These concepts are illustrated in Figures 20-1 to 20-3.

Single-Ventricle Physiology. Single-ventricle physiology describes the situation in which there is complete mixing of pulmonary venous and systemic venous blood at the atrial or ventricular level, and the ventricle (or the ventricles) then distribute output to both the systemic and pulmonary beds. As a result of this physiology (1) ventricular output is the sum of pulmonary blood flow ($\dot{Q}_P$) and systemic blood flow ($\dot{Q}_S$), (2) distribution of systemic and pulmonary blood flow is dependent on the relative resistances to flow (both intracardiac and extracardiac) into the two parallel circuits, and (3) oxygen saturations are the same in the aorta and the pulmonary artery. This physiology can exist in patients with one well-developed ventricle and one hypoplastic ventricle, as well as in patients with two well-formed ventricles.

In the case of a single anatomic ventricle, there is always obstruction to either pulmonary or systemic blood flow as the result of complete or near-complete obstruction to inflow or outflow (or both) from the hypoplastic ventricle. In this circumstance, there must be a source of both systemic and pulmonary blood flow to assure postnatal survival. In some instances of a single anatomic ventricle, a direct connection between the aorta and the pulmonary artery via a patent ductus arteriosus (PDA) is the sole source of systemic blood flow (e.g., hypoplastic left heart syndrome [HLHS]) or of pulmonary blood flow (e.g., pulmonary atresia with intact ventricular septum). This is known as *ductal dependent circulation*. In other instances of a single anatomic ventricle, intracardiac pathways provide both systemic and pulmonary blood flow without a PDA. This is the case when tricuspid atresia occurs along with normally related great vessels, a nonrestrictive ventricular septal defect (VSD), and minimal or absent pulmonary stenosis.

In certain circumstances, single-ventricle physiology can exist in the presence of two well-formed anatomic ventricles: (1) tetralogy of Fallot (TOF) with pulmonary atresia (in which pulmonary blood flow is supplied via a PDA or multiple aortopulmonary collateral arteries), (2) truncus arteriosus, and (3) severe neonatal aortic stenosis and interrupted aortic arch (in which a substantial portion of systemic blood flow is supplied via a PDA).

Table 20-3 lists a number of single-ventricle physiology lesions. All patients with single-ventricle physiology who have severe hypoplasia of one ventricle will ultimately undergo the staged surgeries that comprise the single-ventricle pathway and result in Fontan physiology (described later). Patients with single-ventricle physiology and two well-formed ventricles are usually able to undergo a two-ventricle repair. In some cases, the two-ventricle repair will be complete. In others, significant residual lesions (VSD, aortopulmonary collaterals) will remain. In patients with single-ventricle physiology, the arterial oxygen saturation (Sao_2) is determined by the relative volumes and saturations of pulmonary venous and systemic venous blood flows that have mixed and reach the aorta (see Fig. 20-1).

TABLE 20-1. Pathophysiology and Clinical Picture of Congenital Heart Defects

Lesion Type	Pathophysiology	Clinical Signs and Symptoms
Shunt Lesion without Outflow Tract Obstruction		
• Atrial septal defects • Ventricular septal defects • Atrioventricular canal defects • Patent ductus arteriosus • Aortopulmonary window	• Intracardiac L-R shunt • Increased pulmonary blood flow	• CHF (systemic and pulmonary vascular congestion) • No cyanosis (unless high pulmonary blood flow leads to increased left atrial pressure, pulmonary edema, and intrapulmonary V/Q mismatch and shunt)
Shunt Lesions with Right Ventricular Outflow Tract Obstruction		
• Tetralogy of Fallot • Ebstein's anomaly • Pulmonary stenosis with atrial or ventricular septal defects • Eisenmenger's syndrome	• Intracardiac R-L shunt • Decreased pulmonary blood flow	• Cyanosis
Transposition Physiology (Intercirculatory mixing)		
• Dextro-transposition of the great arteries	• Intracardiac L-R and R-L shunts are equal	• Cyanosis
Single Ventricle Physiology		
One-Ventricle Lesions • Hypoplastic left heart syndrome • Tricuspid atresia • Double inlet left ventricle	• Mixing of systemic and pulmonary venous blood • Parallel distribution of pulmonary and systemic blood flow determined by relative circuit resistances	• CHF (systemic and pulmonary vascular congestion) • Cyanosis
Two-Ventricle Lesions • Truncus arteriosus • Tetralogy of Fallot with pulmonary atresia • Severe neonatal aortic stenosis		
Left Ventricular Obstructive Lesions		
Mitral Stenosis • Valvular • Cor triatriatum	• Left ventricular pressure overload from aortic lesions • Increased left atrial pressure from left ventricular systolic and diastolic dysfunction OR obstruction to left atrial emptying	• CHF (if high left atrial pressure leads to pulmonary vascular congestion) • No cyanosis (unless high left atrial pressure leads to pulmonary edema and intrapulmonary V/Q mismatch and shunt)
Aortic Stenosis • Valvular • Subvalvular (subaortic membrane) • Supravalvular (Williams-Beuren syndrome)		
Coarctation • Shone's syndrome (mitral stenosis, aortic stenosis, coarctation)		
Mixing of Systemic and Pulmonary Venous Blood with Series Circulation		
• Partial anomalous pulmonary venous return (PAPVR) • Total anomalous pulmonary venous return (TAPVR)	• Mixing of systemic and pulmonary venous blood • Increased pulmonary blood flow	*CHF* • Systemic and pulmonary vascular congestion; pulmonary vascular congestion is severe if pulmonary venous obstruction • No cyanosis *PAPVR* • Cyanosis *TAPVR* • Exacerbated if pulmonary venous obstruction leads to pulmonary edema and intrapulmonary V/Q mismatch and shunt

CHF, Congestive heart failure; *PAPVR,* partial anomalous pulmonary venous return; *TAPVR,* total anomalous pulmonary venous return.

Intercirculatory Mixing. Intercirculatory mixing is the unique situation that exists in transposition of the great arteries (TGA) (see Fig. 20-2). In TGA, there are two parallel circulations because of the existence of atrioventricular concordance (right atrium to right ventricle [RA-RV], and left atrium to left ventricle [LA-LV]) and ventriculoarterial discordance (right atrium to aorta [RV-Ao], and left ventricle to pulmonary artery [LV-PA]). This produces a parallel rather than a normal series circulation. In this arrangement, parallel recirculation of pulmonary venous blood in the pulmonary circuit

TABLE 20-2. Classification of Congenital Heart Lesions and Associated Repairs

Lesion Type	Repair
Shunt Lesions	
Left-to-Right	
• Atrial septal defects	Complete repair
• Ventricular septal defects	Complete repair
• Atrioventricular canal defects	Complete repair
• Patent ductus arteriosus	Complete repair
• Aortopulmonary window	Complete repair
Right-to-Left	
• Tetralogy of Fallot	Complete repair
• Ebstein's anomaly	Complete repair
• Pulmonary stenosis in conjunction with atrial or ventricular septal defects	Complete repair
• Eisenmenger's syndrome	No repair
Transposition Physiology	
• Dextro-transposition of the great arteries	Complete repair
Single-Ventricle Physiology	
One-Ventricle Lesions	
• Hypoplastic left heart syndrome	Staging to Fontan
• Tricuspid atresia	Staging to Fontan
• Double inlet left ventricle	Staging to Fontan
Two-Ventricle Lesions	
• Truncus arteriosus	Complete repair
• Tetralogy of Fallot with pulmonary atresia	Complete repair
• Severe neonatal aortic stenosis	Complete repair
Left Ventricular Obstructive Lesions	
Mitral Stenosis	
• Valvular	Complete repair
• Cor triatriatum	
Aortic Stenosis	
• Valvular	Complete repair
• Subvalvular (subaortic membrane)	
• Supravalvular (Williams-Beuren Syndrome)	
Coarctation	
• Shone's syndrome (mitral stenosis, aortic stenosis, coarctation)	Repair with likely residual lesions
Mixing of Systemic and Pulmonary Venous Blood with Series Circulation	
• Partial anomalous pulmonary venous return (PAPVR)	Complete repair
• Total anomalous pulmonary venous return (TAPVR)	

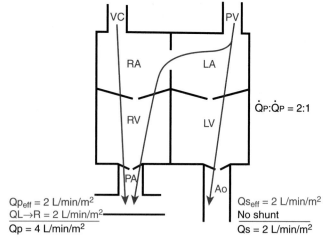

$$\dot{Q}_P : \dot{Q}_P = 2:1$$

Qp$_{eff}$ = 2 L/min/m^2
QL→R = 2 L/min/m^2
Qp = 4 L/min/m^2

Qs$_{eff}$ = 2 L/min/m^2
No shunt
Qs = 2 L/min/m^2

■ **FIGURE 20-1.** Blood flows in a nonrestrictive atrial septal defect (ASD). Effective pulmonary and effective systemic blood flows are equal (2.0 L/min/m^2). The $\dot{Q}_P : \dot{Q}_S$ (ratio of total pulmonary to total systemic blood flow) is 2:1. $\dot{Q}_P$ (4.0 L/min per meter-squared) is the sum of the effective pulmonary blood flow (2.0 L/min/m^2) and a L-R physiologic shunt (2.0 L/min/m^2). This L-R shunt is recirculation of pulmonary venous blood into the pulmonary artery that imposes a volume load on the left atrium, right atrium, and right ventricle.

Fontan Physiology. Fontan physiology (see also later) is a series (i.e., "normal") circulation in which one ventricle has sufficient diastolic, systolic, and atrioventricular valve function to support systemic circulation (Figs. 20-4 and 20-5). This ventricle must in turn be in unobstructed continuity with the aorta and pulmonary venous blood return; there must also be unobstructed delivery of systemic venous blood to the pulmonary circulation (total cavopulmonary continuity).

General Approach to Anesthetic Management

Preparation for Anesthesia

Preparation for anesthesia begins with a thorough assessment of the patient's medical and surgical conditions (as with any preoperative assessment). Also necessary is a complete understanding of the patient's "original" cardiac anatomy and physiology, any previous surgical or catheterization procedures and complications, the present status of the patient's anatomy and pathophysiology, current medications, and involvement of other organ systems (e.g., renal insufficiency). Also necessary is detailed knowledge of the anatomic and functional information contained in the most recent diagnostic studies (echocardiography or Doppler on most patients, and often catheterization and cardiac MRI data as well), as well as of the planned procedure and its acute physiologic consequences and potential complications.

Basic operating room preparation begins with the considerations common to all pediatric anesthesia, including the presence of appropriately sized airway; ventilator; monitoring; cardioversion, defibrillation, and external pacing (including external pads or paddles and internal paddles of appropriate sizes); temperature control (capability for warming and cooling); blood and fluid administration; and vascular

and systemic venous blood in the systemic circuit occurs. Therefore, the physiologic shunt or the percentage of venous blood from one system that recirculates in the arterial outflow of the same system is 100% for both circuits.

Thus, this lesion is incompatible with life unless there are one or more communications (atrial septal defect [ASD], patent foramen ovale [PFO], VSD, PDA) between the parallel circuits to allow intercirculatory mixing. In the presence of mixing, arterial saturation (Sao$_2$) is determined by the relative volumes and saturations of the recirculated systemic and effective systemic venous blood flows reaching the aorta (see Fig. 20-3).

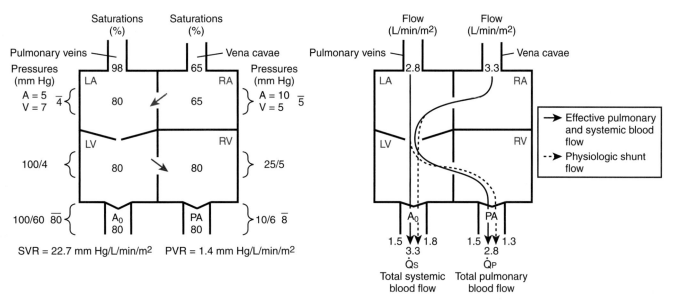

FIGURE 20-2. Saturations, pressures, and blood flows in tricuspid atresia with a mildly restrictive atrial septal defect (ASD), a small restrictive ventricular septal defect (VSD), and mild pulmonic stenosis (PS). Complete mixing or blending occurs at the atrial level. This complete mixing is the consequence of an obligatory physiologic and anatomic R-L shunting across the ASD. Effective pulmonary and effective systemic blood flows are equal (1.5 L/min/m²). Effective systemic blood flow occurs via a normal pathway through the heart. Effective pulmonary blood flow is the result of an anatomic R-L shunt at the atrial level, and an anatomic L-R shunt at the ventricular level. This illustrates the concept that when complete outflow obstruction exists and there is obligatory anatomic shunting, a downstream anatomic shunt must exist to deliver blood back to the obstructed circuit. Total pulmonary blood flow ($\dot{Q}P$) is 2.8 L/min/m² and is the sum of effective pulmonary blood flow (1.5 L/min/m²) and a physiologic and anatomic L-R shunt (1.3 L/min/m²) at the VSD. Total systemic blood flow ($\dot{Q}s$) is 3.3 L/min/m² and is the sum of effective systemic blood flow (1.5 L/min/m²) and a physiologic and anatomic R-L shunt (1.8 L/min/m²) at the ASD. Here, there is a small pressure gradient at the atrial level and a large pressure gradient at the ventricular level. In addition, there is a small additional gradient at the level of the pulmonic valve.

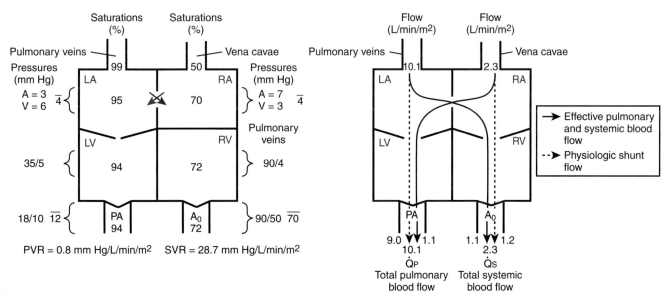

FIGURE 20-3. Saturations, pressures, and blood flows in transposition of the great arteries with a nonrestrictive atrial septal defect and a small left ventricular outflow tract gradient. Intercirculatory mixing occurs at the atrial level. Effective pulmonary and effective systemic blood flows are equal (1.1 L/min/m²) and are the result of a bidirectional anatomic shunt at the atrial level. The physiologic L-R shunt is 9.0 L/min/m²; this represents blood recirculated from the pulmonary veins to the pulmonary artery. The physiologic R-L shunt is 1.2 L/min/m²; this represents blood recirculated from the systemic veins to the aorta. Total pulmonary blood flow ($\dot{Q}P$ = 10.1 L/min/m²) is almost five times the total systemic blood flow ($\dot{Q}s$ = 2.3 L/min/m²). The bulk of pulmonary blood flow is recirculated pulmonary venous blood. Here, pulmonary vascular resistance is low (approximately 1/35 of systemic vascular resistance) and there is a small (17 mm Hg, peak to peak) gradient from the left ventricle to the pulmonary artery. These findings are compatible with the high pulmonary blood flow shown.

TABLE 20-3. Anatomic Subtypes of Single-Ventricle Physiology

	Aortic Blood Flow from:	Pulmonary Artery Blood Flow from:
HLHS	PDA	RV
Severe neonatal aortic stenosis	PDA	RV
IAA	LV (proximal) PDA (distal)	RV
PA with IVS	LV	PDA
Tetralogy of Fallot with pulmonary atresia	LV	PDA, MAPCAs
Tricuspid atresia, NRGA, with pulmonary atresia (type 1A)	LV	PDA, MAPCAs
Tricuspid atresia, NRGA, with restrictive VSD and pulmonary stenosis (type 1B)	LV	LV thru VSD to RV
Tricuspid atresia, NRGA, with non-restrictive VSD and no pulmonary stenosis (type 1C)	LV	LV thru VSD to RV
Truncus arteriosus	LV and RV	Aorta
DILV, NRGA	LV	LV thru BVF

BVF, Bulboventricular foramen; *DILV,* double-inlet left ventricle; *HLHS,* hypoplastic left heart syndrome; *IAA,* interrupted aortic arch; *LV,* left ventricle; *MAPCAs,* multiple aortopulmonary collateral arteries; *NRGA,* normally related great arteries; *PA with IVS,* pulmonary atresia with intact ventricular septum; *PDA,* patent ductus arteriosus; *RV,* right ventricle; *VSD,* ventricular septal defect.

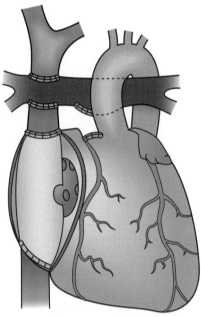

■ **FIGURE 20-4.** Total cavopulmonary connection (Fontan) using an intraatrial lateral tunnel or baffle. The tunnel is prosthetic graft material such as Gore-Tex. A fenestration has been placed in this prosthetic material allowing a physiologic R-L shunt to exist when baffle pressure exceeds common (pulmonary venous) atrial pressure. This pop-off allows systemic cardiac output to be maintained (at the expense of arterial saturation) when the resistance to pulmonary blood flow is high. *(Redrawn from Children's Hospital Boston, Boston, Mass.)*

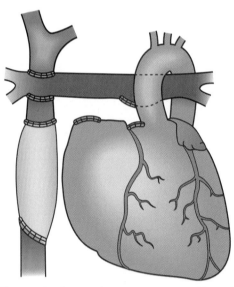

■ **FIGURE 20-5.** Total cavopulmonary connection (Fontan) using an extracardiac conduit or baffle. The conduit is prosthetic graft material such as Gore-Tex. In this example, no fenestration or pop-off is present to allow physiologic R-L shunting when baffle pressure exceeds common (pulmonary venous) atrial pressure. *(Redrawn from Children's Hospital Boston, Boston, Mass.)*

access equipment and supplies. In addition, an extra blood pressure cuff and pulse oximeter should be on hand in case the need arises for some specific lesions. Size-appropriate equipment and supplies (including vascular ultrasound devices and pressure monitoring transducers) to perform peripheral and femoral arterial and central venous cannulation and pressure monitoring are necessary. In addition to standard drugs, one should have predrawn and hence immediately available syringes con-

taining weight-appropriate concentrations of emergency drugs including epinephrine, calcium (gluconate or chloride salt), phenylephrine, and atropine. Other agents, such as sodium bicarbonate, glucose, potassium chloride, antiarrhythmics (e.g., adenosine, procainamide), β-blockers, heparin, and inotropes and other vasoactive drugs for infusion (e.g., dopamine, dobutamine, epinephrine, phenylephrine, milrinone, vasopressin, nitroglycerin, nitroprusside, esmolol) should be immediately available. Many find it helpful to complete a patient-specific emergency card for each patient that contains weight-based concentrations, dosages, and bolus volumes or infusion rates for the most frequently used agents before starting the case.

No one anesthetic induction technique is suitable for all patients with congenital heart disease. The patient's age, cardiopulmonary function, degree of cyanosis, and emotional state all play roles in the selection of an anesthetic technique. Intravenous administration of induction agents clearly affords the greatest flexibility in terms of drug selection and drug titration and allows prompt control of the airway. We believe that intravenous induction is the preferred technique in the majority of patients, including those with significantly impaired ventricular systolic function, significant obstruction to blood flow (e.g., severe aortic stenosis), and systemic or suprasystemic pulmonary artery pressures. In all patients, ensuring adequacy of the airway and gas exchange is a preeminent consideration.

Sevoflurane, halothane, isoflurane, and fentanyl plus midazolam do not change the ratio of pulmonary-to-systemic blood flow ($\dot{Q}_P:\dot{Q}_S$) in children with atrial and ventricular septal defects when cautiously administered with 100% oxygen (Laird et al., 2002). Sevoflurane (1 minimum alveolar concentration [MAC]) and fentanyl plus midazolam have no significant effect on myocardial function in patients with a single ventricle (Ikemba et al., 2004). Halothane (1 and 1.5 MAC) depresses cardiac index and contractility more than comparable levels of sevoflurane, isoflurane, and fentanyl plus midazolam anesthesia (Rivenes et al., 2001). In addition, halothane anesthesia may result in more severe hypotension and emergent drug use than sevoflurane anesthesia in children with CHD (Russell et al., 2001).

Mask Induction. Mask induction of anesthesia can be accomplished safely in the subset of children without severe cardiorespiratory compromise. However, reduced pulmonary blood flow in cyanotic patients will prolong the length of induction and the interval during which the airway is only partially controlled. In addition, in these patients, even short intervals of airway obstruction or hypoventilation may result in hypoxemia. Sevoflurane has probably become the inhalation induction agent of choice (halothane, even if desired, has become unobtainable in many places). Sevoflurane causes less myocardial depression, hypotension, and bradycardia than halothane. Isoflurane and particularly desflurane are unsuitable agents, as their pungency causes copious secretions, airway irritation, and laryngospasm.

Intravenous Induction. Many of these patients come to the operating room with functioning intravenous (IV) access. For those without it, effective premedication may facilitate IV placement and allow the attendant risks of mask induction in this population to be avoided. In some patients, oral midazolam (0.5 to 1.0 mg/kg) may suffice. Others have used oral combinations of meperidine (3 mg/kg) and pentobarbital (4 mg/kg) successfully in this group of patients (Nicolson et al., 1989). Ketamine (~3 to 6 mg/kg) and midazolam (1 mg/kg) given orally in combination can be quite effective in terms of producing deep sedation and conditions favorable for IV placement and subsequent intravenous induction (Auden et al., 2000).

High-dosage synthetic narcotics in combination with pancuronium (0.1 mg/kg) are commonly used for intravenous induction in neonates and infants. The vagolytic and sympathomimetic effects of pancuronium counteract the vagotonic effect of synthetic opioids. In patients with a low aortic diastolic blood pressure and a high baseline heart rate, vecuronium (0.1 mg/kg) or cisatracurium (0.2 mg/kg) may be used without

affecting heart rate. In older children with mild to moderately depressed systolic function, lower dosages of a synthetic opioid can be used in conjunction with etomidate (0.1 to 0.3 mg/kg) (Sarkar et al., 2005).

Ketamine (1 to 2 mg/kg) is a useful induction agent. For patients with both normal and elevated baseline pulmonary vascular resistance (PVR), ketamine causes minimal increases in pulmonary artery pressure as long as the airway and ventilation are supported (Morray et al., 1984). The tachycardia and increase in systemic vascular resistance (SVR) induced by ketamine may make it unfavorable for use in patients with systemic outflow tract obstructive lesions (Williams et al., 2007).

The myocardial depressive and vasodilatory effects of propofol and thiopental make them largely unsuitable as induction agents except in patients with simple shunt lesions in whom cardiovascular function is preserved (Williams et al., 1999b).

An alternative to IV induction in patients with difficult peripheral IV access is intramuscular induction with ketamine (3 to 5 mg/kg), succinylcholine (2 to 5 mg/kg), and glycopyrrolate (8 to 10 mcg/kg). Glycopyrrolate is used to reduce airway secretions associated with ketamine administration and to prevent the bradycardia that may accompany succinylcholine administration. The required dosage of succinylcholine per kilogram body weight is highest in infants. This technique provides prompt induction and immediate control of the airway with tracheal intubation. It is useful when it is anticipated that initial IV access will have to be obtained via the internal or external jugular vein or the femoral vein. One potential problem is that the short duration of action of succinylcholine limits the period of patient immobility. An alternative technique combines intramuscular ketamine (4 to 5 mg/kg), glycopyrrolate (8 to 10 mcg/kg), and rocuronium (1.0 mg/kg). This technique is limited by the longer time interval until attainment of adequate intubating conditions and the longer duration of action of rocuronium as compared with succinylcholine.

Maintenance of Anesthesia

Anesthesia is generally maintained using a synthetic opioid (fentanyl or sufentanil)–based technique. These opioids may be used in high dosages (25 to 100 mcg/kg fentanyl or 2.5 to 10 mcg/kg sufentanil) or in low to moderate dosages (5 to 25 mcg/kg fentanyl or 0.5 to 2.5 mcg/kg sufentanil). In either instance, opioids are typically used in combination with an inhalation agent (generally isoflurane 0.5% to 1.0% or sevoflurane 1.0% to 2.0%) or a benzodiazepine (generally midazolam 0.05 to 0.1 mg/kg), or both. Caution must be exercised because the combination of narcotics and benzodiazepines is synergistic in reducing systemic vascular resistance. The high-dosage opioid technique is particularly useful for neonates and infants. Patients in this age group presenting for surgery often have significant ventricular pressure or volume overload. In addition, many of these patients have tenuous subendocardial and systemic perfusion secondary to the volume overload in combination with runoff into the pulmonary circulation and associated low aortic diastolic blood pressure. Given the limited contractile reserve available in the immature myocardium, it is not surprising that the myocardial depressive and systemic vasodilatory effects of inhalation agents and the synergistic vasodilatory effects of benzodiazepines and opioids may be poorly tolerated in this patient group.

SPECIFIC LESIONS

Atrial Septal Defect

Atrial septal defect accounts for about one third of the congenital heart disease detected in adults, with the frequency in women two to three times that in men. See related video online at www.expertconsult.com. Strictly speaking, an ASD is a communication between the left and right atrium resulting from a defect in the intraatrial septum, which consists of a central membranous portion and a thicker inferior and superior fatty limbus. The central membranous portion is formed by tissue of the septum primum, ultimately forming the fossa ovalis. This membrane lies posterior to the superior aspect of the fatty limbus.

ASDs are classified by their location (Fig. 20-6). There are four morphologic types: ostium secundum defects, ostium primum defects, inferior and superior sinus venosus defects, and coronary sinus (CS) defects. Although they are classified as ASDs, sinus venosus and CS defects are not truly defects in the intraatrial septum. Secundum ASDs account for 80% of all ASDs. Whereas a PFO results from incomplete fusion of an intact fossa ovalis membrane with the superior aspect of the fatty limbus, an ostium secundum ASD is the result of actual deficiencies in the membrane (septum primum) of the fossa ovalis. Isolated ostium primum ASDs, also known as partial atrioventricular canal defects, are discussed later (see Atrioventricular Canal Defects). The isolated ostium primum defect extends from the inferior intraatrial septum fatty limbus, to the crest of the intact ventricular septum.

Both types of sinus venous defects are associated with partially anomalous pulmonary venous return. In the case of the superior defect, anomalous drainage of the right upper pulmonary vein into the junction of the superior vena cava (SVC) and the RA is the most common finding. In the case of the inferior defect, scimitar syndrome (anomalous drainage of the right upper and lower pulmonary veins to the junction of the inferior vena cava [IVC] and RA, aortopulmonary collaterals to the right lower lobe, and hypoplasia of the right lung) can be seen.

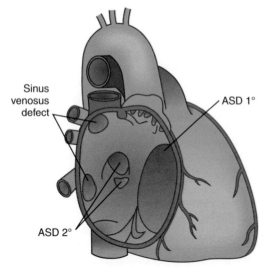

■ **FIGURE 20-6.** Location of atrial septal defects (ASDs). ASD 1°, primum ASD; ASD 2°, secundum ASD. Superior and inferior sinus venous defects are shown. (*Redrawn from Children's Hospital Boston, Boston, Mass.*)

Clinical Presentation

The physiologic consequences of ASDs are the same regardless of the anatomic location and reflect the shunting of blood from one atrium to the other; the direction and magnitude of the shunt are determined by the size of the defect and the relative compliance of the ventricles. A small defect (less than 0.5 cm in diameter) is associated with a small shunt and no hemodynamic sequelae. When the diameter of the ASD approaches 2 cm, it is likely that left atrial blood is being shunted to the right atrium (the right ventricle is more compliant than the left ventricle), resulting in increased pulmonary blood flow. A systolic ejection murmur audible in the second left intercostal space may be mistaken for an innocent flow murmur. The electrocardiogram (ECG) may reflect right axis deviation and incomplete right bundle branch block. Atrial fibrillation and supraventricular tachycardia may accompany an ASD that remains uncorrected into adulthood. The chest radiograph is likely to reveal prominent pulmonary arteries. Echocardiography is the mainstay of diagnostic imaging for these patients, with catheterization usually reserved for assessment of pulmonary artery pressures when indicated.

Because they initially produce no symptoms or striking findings on physical examination, ASDs may remain undetected for years. Symptoms resulting from large ASDs include dyspnea on exertion, supraventricular dysrhythmias, right heart failure, paradoxical embolism, and recurrent pulmonary infections. Prophylaxis against infective endocarditis is not recommended for patients with an ASD unless a concomitant valvular abnormality (mitral valve prolapse or mitral valve cleft) is present. Supraventricular dysrhythmias and pulmonary hypertension can increase in frequency, even for moderately sized defects, as patients enter the second and third decades of life.

Some small ostium secundum ASDs can be primarily closed, whereas larger defects are patched, usually with pericardium. An alternative is nonoperative device closure of secundum ASDs in the cardiac catheterization laboratory (see Chapter 21, Congenital Cardiac Anesthesia: Non-Bypass Procedures). Primum ASDs generally require patch closure and suture closure of the anterior leaflet mitral cleft. Sinus venous defects without partially anomalous pulmonary venous return can be closed primarily with a patch. An alternative procedure is performed when the pulmonary vein or veins anomalously enter the SVC. The SVC is transected above the origin of the anomalous vein or veins, and the SVC orifice is directed across the defect into the LA with a pericardial patch. The distal end of the SVC is then anastomosed in an end-to-end fashion to the roof of the RA appendage, recreating SVC-to-RA continuity.

Management of Anesthesia

The goals of anesthetic management for patients with ASD before cardiopulmonary bypass (CPB) follow from the aforementioned principles and are outlined in Box 20-1. The goals for these patients after CPB are outlined in Box 20-2.

Ventricular Septal Defect

Ventricular septal defect is the most common congenital cardiac abnormality in infants and children. See related video online at www.expertconsult.com. A large number of VSDs close

Box 20-1 Anesthesia Management Goals for ASD, VSD, AVC Defect, and PDA before Cardiopulmonary Bypass (CPB)

1. Maintain heart rate, contractility, and preload to maintain cardiac output.
   - A reduction in cardiac output compromises systemic perfusion, despite a relatively high pulmonary blood flow.
2. Avoid maneuvers that decrease the PVR-to-SVR ratio.
   - The increase in pulmonary blood flow that accompanies a reduced PVR-to-SVR ratio necessitates an increase in cardiac output to maintain systemic blood flow, thereby compromising systemic (e.g., coronary, cerebral, GI, renal) perfusion.
3. Maintain normoxia and normocarbia or mild hypercarbia.
   - Some patients overcirculate (excessive pulmonary blood flow) despite these measures, and it may be necessary to support systemic perfusion prior to CPB, with additional volume expansion or inotropes (or both).
   - The right pulmonary artery can be partially or completely occluded to mechanically control the magnitude of a left-to-right shunt and thus support systemic perfusion once adequate surgical exposure is attained.
4. Avoid large increases in the PVR-to-SVR ratio.
   - A substantial increase may result in production of a right-to-left shunt.
5. When a right-to-left shunt exists, ventilatory measures to decrease PVR should be entertained, and SVR must be maintained or increased.
   - These measures will reduce the magnitude of the right-to-left shunt.

ASD, Atrial septal defect; *AVC,* atrioventricular canal; *GI,* gastrointestinal; *PDA,* patent ductus arteriosus; *PVR,* pulmonary vascular resistance; *SVR,* systemic vascular resistance; *VSD,* ventricular septal defect.

Box 20-2 Management Goals for ASD, VSD, and AVC Defect after Cardiopulmonary Bypass (CPB)

1. Maintain heart rate (preferably sinus rhythm) at an age-appropriate rate.
   - Cardiac output is likely to be more heart rate dependent in the post-CPB period.
2. Reduce PVR through ventilatory interventions.
   - This is particularly important if PVOD is present.
3. Inotropic support of the right ventricle may be necessary, particularly if PVR is high. In patients with VSD or AVC, the left ventricle will no longer contribute to ejection of blood via the pulmonary artery, and the right ventricle will face a high afterload.
   - Dobutamine (5 to 10 mcg/kg per minute) or dopamine (5 to 10 mcg/kg per minute) provide inotropic support without increasing PVR.
   - Milrinone (0.5 to 1.0 mcg/kg per minute) after a loading dose of 50 mcg/kg has more-direct PVR-reducing effects in addition to inotropic, lusitrophic, and SVR reducing effects.
4. Infants with large VSDs or AVC defects, particularly in association with trisomy 21, are candidates for development of severe pulmonary hypertension and hypertensive crises after CPB.
   - Consider inhaled nitric oxide (iNO) when pulmonary hypertension and resultant RV dysfunction and low cardiac output persist.

From Bizzarro M, Gross I: Inhaled nitric oxide for the postoperative management of pulmonary hypertension in infants and children with congenital heart disease, *Cochrane Database Syst Rev* (4):CD005055, 2005. *ASD,* Atrial septal defect; *AVC,* atrioventricular canal; *PVOD,* pulmonary vascular occlusive disease; *PVR,* pulmonary vascular resistance; *SVR,* systemic vascular resistance; *VSD,* ventricular septal defect.

spontaneously by the time a child reaches 2 years of age. VSDs can be classified by their location in the septum (Fig. 20-7).

Subpulmonary or supracristal defects are located in the infundibular septum just below the aortic valve. Subpulmonary lesions may be associated with aortic insufficiency due to a lack of support for the right coronary cusp of the aortic valve and prolapse of this leaflet. Membranous or perimembranous defects comprise approximately 80% of all VSDs and are located in the subaortic region of the membranous septum, near or under the septal leaflet of the tricuspid valve, and they communicate with the LV just below the aortic valve. These defects are commonly partially closed by a collection of tricuspid valve and membranous septal tissue, giving an aneurysmal appearance to the septum. Conoventricular defects involve the same area as perimembranous defects, but they extend anteriorly and superiorly in the septum. Inlet- or canal-type defects involve the posterior septum near the atrioventricular (AV) valves. Muscular defects are located in the lower trabecular septum and may appear deceptively small on inspection from the right ventricular aspect of the septum because of heavy trabeculation. These defects may be apical, midmuscular, anterior, or posterior.

Clinical Presentation

The physiologic significance of a VSD depends on the size of the defect and the relative resistance in the systemic and pulmonary circulations. Restrictive VSDs have a substantial pressure gradient across them (i.e., left ventricular pressure signifi-

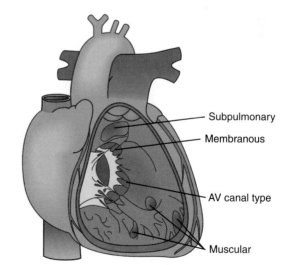

■ FIGURE 20-7. Locations of ventricular septal defects. *(Redrawn from Children's Hospital Boston, Boston, Mass.)*

cantly greater than the right) and, as the name suggests, are sufficiently small to limit the amount of flow (and pressure) entering the RV via the defect. In contrast, flow through unrestrictive VSDs is largely based on the relative resistance in the systemic and pulmonary circulations. If the defect is small, there is minimal functional disturbance, as pulmonary blood flow is only modestly increased. The newborn infant with a large VSD may have near-normal pulmonary blood flow as a result of the high PVR present at birth. However, by the second week of life and continuing into the second month, PVR begins to fall to near-normal levels and pulmonary blood flow increases dramatically. Continued decreases in PVR after birth may be delayed by the elevated left atrial pressure that accompanies increased pulmonary blood flow (PBF).

Patients with large VSDs present with one or more signs and symptoms of pulmonary overcirculation and congestive heart failure (CHF) that increase as PVR falls. These include tachypnea, other signs of increased work of breathing (including retractions and nasal flaring), poor feeding, poor growth, diaphoresis, delayed capillary refill, diminished pulses, and hepatomegaly. Patients can be managed medically with diuretics, at times in combination with digoxin; however, significant symptoms usually result in early surgery.

Large VSDs also predispose to the development of pulmonary vascular occlusive disease (PVOD) during the first few years of life as a result of exposure of the pulmonary vasculature to high flows and systemic blood pressures. The increases in PVR that accompany PVOD ultimately produce bidirectional and right-to-left shunts. Patients with advanced PVOD and markedly increased PVR (Eisenmenger's complex) are not generally candidates for VSD closure, because closure will result in an enormous increase in RV afterload and RV-afterload mismatch. For this reason, large VSDs ($\dot{Q}P:\dot{Q}S > 2:1$) are corrected early in childhood. Whether to close smaller, more restrictive VSDs (i.e., when the $\dot{Q}P:\dot{Q}S$ is < 1.5:1) remains controversial. Here, the major long-term risk is most likely subacute bacterial endocarditis, and much less likely the development of CHF or PVOD, which must be balanced against the risks of CPB and surgery.

The murmur of a moderate to large VSD is holosystolic and is loudest at the lower left sternal border. The ECG and chest radiograph remain essentially normal in the presence of a small VSD. When the VSD is large, there is evidence of left atrial and ventricular enlargement on the ECG. The chest radiograph in patients with larger VSDs typically demonstrates cardiomegaly and increased PBF; increased interstitial markings, enlarged central pulmonary arteries, and hyperinflation may also be seen, particularly as CHF worsens. If pulmonary hypertension develops, the QRS axis shifts to the right, and right atrial and ventricular enlargement are noted on the ECG. A significant finding on physical examination is a loud second single heart sound. Here again, echocardiography is the major diagnostic imaging modality. Cardiac catheterization is usually reserved to assess other potential lesions and the degree of pulmonary hypertension and its responsiveness to pulmonary vasodilators.

Treatment

VSDs are generally closed with a patch by a variety of approaches, depending on their location. To avoid postoperative compromise of a small ventricle, with its poor compliance and limited capacity for tension development, a ventriculotomy to approach and correct VSDs is usually avoided. Many defects are approachable through the right atrium and tricuspid valve, aorta, or pulmonary artery.

Management of Anesthesia

The before-CPB goals of anesthetic management for patients with VSD are outlined in Box 20-1. The goals for these patients after CPB are outlined in Box 20-2.

Atrioventricular Canal Defects

Embryologically, four endocardial cushions contribute to the development of the lower ostium primum portion of the atrial septum and the upper, posterior inlet portion of the intact ventricular septum (IVS), where the AV valves insert. See related video online at www.expertconsult.com. The endocardial cushions also contribute to the tissue that forms the septal leaflets of the mitral and tricuspid valves. Therefore, cushion defects, or atrioventricular canal (AVC) defects, can include abnormalities in all these structures. The terminology of these lesions can be confusing and is summarized as follows:

Partial AVC. This is an ostium primum ASD in association with a cleft mitral valve. There are two separate AV valve (mitral and tricuspid) annuli. No inlet VSD is present.

Transitional AVC. This is an ostium primum ASD, common AV valve orifice, common anterosuperior and posteroinferior bridging leaflets, with dense chordal attachments to the crest of the IVS creating functionally separate mitral and tricuspid valves. There is a very small or absent inlet VSD.

Complete AVC. This is an ostium primum ASD, common AV valve orifice, common anterosuperior and posteroinferior bridging leaflets, with varying chordal attachments to the crest of the IVS. There is a moderate to large inlet VSD.

Clinical Presentation

These defects can result in communication between all four heart chambers as well as in abnormalities of the mitral and tricuspid valves. Approximately 50% occur in patients with trisomy 21. Because the orifice between the four chambers is large, as with large VSDs, this results in (1) production of a large left-to-right shunt, (2) increased pulmonary blood flow, (3) transmission of systemic pressures to the right ventricle and pulmonary arteries, and (4) volume overloading of the right and left ventricles. The signs and symptoms are related mainly to pulmonary overcirculation and the development of CHF, and they are similar to those outlined previously for large VSD.

As with large VSDs, complete AVC defects predispose to the early development of PVOD. Advanced PVOD may increase the PVR:SVR ratio so that a bidirectional or right-to-left shunt develops. This is a particular concern for patients with trisomy 21, who appear to develop earlier and more significant irreversible PVOD than the patient without trisomy 21 who has a similar hemodynamic disturbance. In some complete AVC defects, the presence of severe mitral insufficiency results in regurgitation of left ventricular blood directly into the right atrium (LV to RA shunt). This increases the left-to-right shunt. In addition, mitral regurgitation increases the volume work of the LV. Use of echocardiography and catheterization are generally similar to that outlined for ASDs and VSDs.

Treatment

Repair of AV canal defects involves closure of the ostium primum ASD and inlet VSD, and septation of the common AV valve tissue into two separate, competent, nonstenotic tricuspid and mitral valves. This can usually be accomplished using a one-patch technique, wherein a single patch is used to close both the VSD and the ASD, and the reconstructed AV valves are resuspended by sutures to the patch. When the VSD is large and extends to other areas of the septum, two patches (atrial and ventricular) may be necessary. When the inlet VSD component is small, the AV valve tissue can be sutured down to the crest of the ventricular septum, essentially closing the VSD. A patch is then sutured to the crest of the ventricular septum and is used to close the ASD.

Management of Anesthesia

The before-CPB goals of anesthetic management for patients with AVC are outlined in Box 20-1. The goals for these patients after CPB are outlined in Box 20-2.

Tetralogy of Fallot

Tetralogy of Fallot is the most common cyanotic congenital heart defect. See related video online at www.expertconsult.com. It is characterized by a VSD, an overriding aorta, a right ventricular hypertrophy, and pulmonic stenosis (infundibular or subvalvular, valvular, supravalvular, or a combination thereof) (Fig. 20-8). The critical pathophysiologic malformation is underdevelopment of the right ventricular infundibulum and displacement of the infundibular septum, which together result in right ventricular outflow tract (RVOT) stenosis. Patients with TOF have displacement of the infundibular septum in an anterior, superior, and leftward direction. The posterior wall of the right ventricular outflow tract is formed by the infundibular septum, and its abnormal displacement results in narrowing of the right ventricular outflow tract. In addition, displacement of the infundibular septum creates a large malalignment VSD, with the aorta overriding the intraventricular septum. Abnormalities in the septal and parietal attachments of the outflow tract further exacerbate the infundibular stenosis.

Seventy-five percent of TOF patients have both infundibular and valvular stenosis. A small proportion of patients will have multiple muscular VSDs. The pulmonary valve is almost always bi-leaflet. At one end of the spectrum of TOF, the pulmonary valve may be mildly hypoplastic (reduced annulus size), with minimal fusion of the pulmonary valve leaflets. At the other end of the spectrum, the pulmonary annulus may be very small, with near fusion of the valve leaflets. In addition, there are varying degrees of main pulmonary artery and branch pulmonary artery hypoplasia. The most common associated lesion, present in 25% of patients, is a right aortic arch with mirror-image arch vessel branching (the innominate artery gives rise to the left carotid and left subclavian, and the right carotid and right subclavian arise separately).

In most patients with TOF, there is both a fixed and a dynamic component to RV outflow obstruction. The fixed component is produced by the infundibular, valvular, and supravalvular stenosis. The dynamic component (subvalvular pulmonic stenosis) is produced by variations in the caliber of the RV infundibulum. In patients with TOF, magnitude of the right-to-left shunt and resultant arterial saturation are a direct reflection of the effects of these fixed and variable obstructions on pulmonary blood flow. A small subset of TOF patients ("pink tet" patients) have minimal obstruction to pulmonary blood flow at the right ventricular outflow and pulmonary artery level and may have normal oxygen saturation. Some of these patients have a left-to-right shunt with increased pulmonary blood flow and symptoms of CHF. Another subset where the pulmonary valve is completely or largely absent ("tetralogy-absent valve") can have massive pulmonary artery enlargement and resultant prominent airway symptoms because of airway compression and tracheobronchomalacia.

Diagnosis

Echocardiography is used to establish the diagnosis and assess the presence of associated abnormalities, the level and severity of the obstruction to right ventricular outflow, the size of the main pulmonary artery and its branches, and the number and location of the VSDs. Right-to-left shunting through the VSD is visualized by color Doppler imaging, and the severity of the RVOT obstruction can be determined by spectral Doppler measurement. Cardiac catheterization and angiography is necessary only when echocardiography cannot rule out coronary artery abnormalities. Approximately 8% of patients have either the left main coronary artery or the left anterior descending artery as a branch of the right coronary artery. In these cases, a right ventriculotomy to enlarge the RVOT will endanger the left coronary artery. In such cases, an extracardiac conduit (RV to main PA) may be necessary to bypass the outflow tract obstruction and avoid injury to the coronary artery.

Clinical Presentation

Most patients with tetralogy of Fallot have cyanosis, frequently progressive, from shortly after birth or beginning during the first months to 1 year of life. The most common auscultatory finding is an ejection murmur heard along the left sternal border resulting from blood flow across the stenotic pulmonic valve.

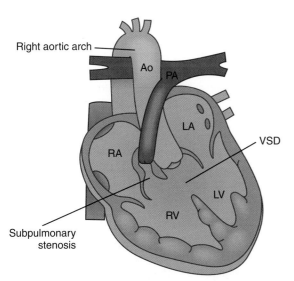

■ **FIGURE 20-8.** Anatomy of tetralogy of Fallot (TOF). The following features are notable: malalignment ventricular septal defect *(VSD)*, overriding aorta *(Ao)*, infundibular pulmonic stenosis, and small pulmonary arteries. There is a right aortic arch with mirror-image arch vessel branching, as occurs in 25% of patients with TOF. *(Redrawn from Children's Hospital Boston, Boston, Mass.)*

CHF rarely develops because of the RVOT obstruction limitation to PBF, and the large VSD permits equilibration of intraventricular pressures and cardiac workload. Chest radiographs show evidence of decreased lung vascularity, and the heart is "boot shaped" with an upturned right ventricular apex and a concave main pulmonary arterial segment. The ECG is characterized by changes of right axis deviation and right ventricular hypertrophy. Squatting is a common feature of in older children with tetralogy of Fallot. It is speculated that squatting increases the systemic vascular resistance by kinking the large arteries in the inguinal area. The resulting increase in systemic vascular resistance tends to decrease the magnitude of the right-to-left intracardiac shunt, which leads to increased pulmonary blood flow and subsequent improvement in arterial oxygenation.

Hypoxic or Hypercyanotic Episodes ("Tet Spells")

The occurrence of hypoxic episodes in TOF patients may be life threatening and should be anticipated in every patient, even those who are not normally cyanotic. Spells occur more frequently in cyanotic patients, with the peak frequency of spells between 2 and 3 months of age. The onset of spells usually prompts urgent surgical intervention, so it is not unusual for the anesthesiologist to care for an infant who is at great risk for spells during the preoperative period.

The etiology of spells is not completely understood, but infundibular spasm or constriction may play a role. Crying, defecation, feeding, fever, and awakening can all be precipitating events. Paroxysmal hyperpnea is the initial finding. There is an increase in rate and depth of respiration, leading to increasing cyanosis and potential syncope, convulsions, or death. During a spell, the infant appears pale and limp secondary to poor cardiac output. Hyperpnea has several deleterious effects in maintaining and worsening a hypoxic spell. Hyperpnea increases oxygen consumption through the increased work of breathing. Hypoxia induces a decrease in SVR, which further increases the right-to-left shunt. Hyperpnea also lowers intrathoracic pressure and leads to an increase in systemic venous return. In the face of worsening infundibular obstruction, this results in an increased RV preload and an increase in the right-to-left shunt. Thus, episodes seem to be associated with events that increase oxygen demand while simultaneous decreases in PO_2 and increases in pH and $Paco_2$ are occurring. Treatment of a Tet spell includes the following points:

- Administration of 100% oxygen.
- Compression of the femoral arteries or placing the patient in a knee-to-chest position, which transiently increases SVR and reduces the R-L shunt. Manual compression of the abdominal aorta is particularly effective for the anesthetized patient. After the chest is open, the surgeon can manually compress the ascending aorta to increase impedance to ejection through the LV.
- Administration of morphine sulfate (0.05 to 0.1 mg/kg), which sedates the patient and may have a depressant effect on respiratory drive and hyperpnea.
- Administration of 15 to 30 mL/kg of a crystalloid solution. Enhancing preload increases heart size, which may increase the diameter of the RVOT.
- Administration of sodium bicarbonate to treat the severe metabolic acidosis that occurs during a spell. Correction of the metabolic acidosis will normalize SVR and reduce

hyperpnea. Bicarbonate administration (1 to 2 mEq/kg) in the absence of a blood gas determination is warranted during a spell.
- Phenylephrine in relatively large dosages (5 to 10 mcg/kg IV as a bolus, or 2 to 5 mcg/kg per minute as an infusion) increases SVR and reduces R-L shunting. In the presence of severe RV outflow obstruction, phenylephrine-induced increases of PVR have little or no effect in increasing RV outflow resistance. It is important to point out that treatment with α-adrenergic agents to increase SVR does nothing to treat the underlying cause of the spell, although the decrease in unstressed venous volume induced by these agents may augment preload.
- β-Adrenergic agonists are absolutely contraindicated. Increasing contractility will further narrow the stenotic infundibulum.
- Administration of propranolol (0.1 mg/kg) or esmolol (0.5 mg/kg followed by an infusion of 50 to 300 mcg/kg per minute) may reduce infundibular spasm by depressing contractility. In addition, slowing of heart rate may allow improved diastolic filling (increased preload), increased heart size, and an increase in the diameter of the RVOT.
- Resuscitation by extracorporeal membrane oxygenation (ECMO) in refractory episodes, when immediate operative intervention is not possible.

Cerebral Complications

Cerebrovascular accidents are common in older children with severe tetralogy of Fallot. Cerebrovascular thrombosis or severe arterial hypoxemia may be the explanation for these adverse responses. Dehydration and polycythemia may contribute to thrombosis. Hemoglobin concentrations exceeding 20 g/dL are common in these patients. A cerebral abscess is suggested by the abrupt onset of headache, fever, and lethargy, followed by persistent emesis and the appearance of seizure activity. The most likely cause is arterial seeding into areas of prior cerebral infarction.

Infective Endocarditis

Infective endocarditis is a constant danger in patients with tetralogy of Fallot and is associated with a high mortality rate. Appropriate antibiotics should be administered whenever dental or surgical procedures are planned in these patients.

Treatment

Without surgery, mortality exceeds 50% by 3 years of age. Currently, most patients with TOF have an elective full correction between the ages of 2 and 10 months. In some centers, surgery is delayed as long as possible within this time interval, with the precise timing of repair dictated by the onset of cyanotic episodes. Definitive repair for TOF is being accomplished in neonates in some centers if favorable anatomy is present. Surgery is aimed at relieving the outflow obstruction by resection of hypertrophied, obstructing muscle bundles and augmentation and enlargement of the RVOT with a pericardial patch. In a somewhat older approach, unless the pulmonic annulus was near normal size, and the pulmonary valve only mildly stenotic, enlargement of the RVOT frequently included extension of the patch across the pulmonary valve annulus and into the main pulmonary artery (transannular patch). Because a transannular patch creates pulmonic insufficiency, which has been associated with a negative impact on long-term RV function and outcome, more recent data suggest it is best avoided when possible; as a result, the current approach for many is to enlarge the infundibular area with a patch (and resect interfering muscles bundles) and repair the pulmonary stenosis to the extent possible, thereby relieving most if not all of the outflow obstruction (and resultant RV hypertension) without creating significant pulmonary regurgitation. If stenosis of the pulmonary artery extends to the bifurcation of the pulmonary artery, a pericardial patch can be placed beyond the bifurcation of the pulmonary arteries (either de novo or as a continuation of the transannular patch). Finally, the VSD is closed. In neonates, this is usually done through the right ventriculotomy created for resection of RVOT obstruction, and with placement of the infundibular, pulmonary artery, or transannular patch. In infants and older children, the VSD can be closed via a trans–tricuspid valve approach, thereby avoiding the likely deleterious consequences of a right ventriculotomy. The overall goals of the surgery are to reduce RV pressure (ideally to below one half to three fourths of the systemic pressure), to avoid inducing RV volume overload (pulmonary regurgitation), and to successfully close the VSD (Apitz et al., 2009; Jonas, 2009; Khairy et al., 2009).

In the past, infants underwent palliative procedures that involved anastomosis of a systemic artery to a pulmonary artery in an effort to increase pulmonary blood flow and improve arterial oxygenation. These palliative procedures were the Waterston shunt (side-to-side anastomosis of the ascending aorta and the right pulmonary artery), the Potts shunt (side-to-side anastomosis of the descending aorta to the left pulmonary artery), the Blalock-Taussig shunt (end-to-side anastomosis of the subclavian artery to the pulmonary artery), and the modified Blalock-Taussig shunt (interposing a length of Gore-Tex tube graft between the subclavian or innominate artery and the branch pulmonary artery). Often, however, these procedures were associated with long-term complications such as pulmonary hypertension, left ventricular volume overload, distortion of the pulmonary arterial branches, reduced RV function, ventricular dysrhythmias, and sudden death.

Management of Anesthesia

The anesthetic management goals for patients with tetralogy of Fallot are summarized in Box 20-3. Preoperatively, it is important to avoid dehydration by maintaining oral feedings in infants and young children or by providing intravenous fluids before the patient's arrival in the operating room. Crying associated with intramuscular administration of drugs used for preoperative medication can lead to hypercyanotic spells in those prone to do so. β-Adrenergic antagonists (now used infrequently) should be continued until the induction of anesthesia in patients receiving these drugs, for prophylaxis against hypercyanotic attacks.

An IV induction may be desirable, particularly in patients with significant outflow obstruction. In patients without a pre-existing intravenous catheter, IV placement may be facilitated by administration of adequate premedication (see earlier).

Mask induction of anesthesia with either sevoflurane or halothane (if still available) is usually effective, as there is a parallel decrease in PVR and SVR. Interestingly, halothane may

---

Box 20-3 Goals of Anesthesia Management for Tetralogy of Fallot

1. Maintain heart rate, contractility, and preload to maintain cardiac output.
   - Euvolemia prevents exacerbation of dynamic RVOT obstruction from hypovolemia and reflex increases in HR and contractility.
2. Avoid increases in the PVR-to-SVR ratio.
   - Increases in PVR relative to SVR, and decreases in SVR relative to PVR, will increase R-L shunting, reduce pulmonary blood flow, and produce or worsen cyanosis.
3. Use ventilatory measures to reduce PVR.
   - Minimize mean airway pressure to avoid mechanical obstruction of pulmonary blood flow and effects to decrease preload.
4. Maintain or increase SVR.
   - This is particularly important when RV outflow obstruction is severe and changes in PVR have little or no effect on shunt.
5. Treat hypercyanosis promptly.
6. Avoid RV contractility depression with severe fixed RV outflow obstruction except in patients with dynamic infundibular obstruction (tet spell).
   - Reducing contractility during tet spells may reduce RV outflow obstruction via relaxation of the infundibulum.

HR, Heart rate; *PVR,* pulmonary vascular resistance; *RV,* right ventricle; *RVOT,* right ventricular outflow tract; *SVR,* systemic vascular resistance.

---

better attenuate the dynamic component of RVOT obstruction than sevoflurane, because of halothane's more potent negative inotropic effect. Regardless of induction technique, systemic hypotension should be avoided or treated promptly. Systemic hypotension is particularly likely to cause or increase right-to-left shunting when RV outflow obstruction is severe, because anesthesia-induced decreases in PVR have little effect on decreasing RV outflow resistance. Hypotension responds to intravascular volume expansion, and, if necessary, markedly reduced SVR and worsening hypoxemia can be treated with phenylephrine (0.5- to 1.0-mcg/kg intravenous boluses).

Ketamine is a useful induction agent in patients with TOF. Ketamine has been shown to cause no significant alteration in $\dot{Q}_P{:}\dot{Q}_S$ in these patients. Fentanyl or sufentanil provide very stable induction and maintenance hemodynamics and will blunt stimulation-induced increases in PVR. Maintenance of anesthesia with fentanyl or sufentanil, a muscle relaxant (perhaps avoiding pancuronium because of tachycardia, and because of its effects on RV preload and contractility), and modest amounts of benzodiazepine or inhalation agent is appropriate.

Regardless of the mode of induction, volume expansion with 10 to 15 mL/kg (or greater) of 5% albumin or normal saline should be initiated once intravenous access is obtained. This is particularly necessary in patients who have received nothing by mouth for a long interval before induction. This is the most effective first-line therapy in preventing and treating dynamic RVOT obstruction. In addition to the peri-induction period, pericardial incision and retraction and aortic and pulmonary artery manipulation are other frequent points of acute hypoxemia and tet spell–like behavior prior to CPB. In addition to aggressive volume expansion, phenylephrine may be needed to reverse precipitously declining systemic oxygen saturations; at times, rapid institution of CPB is the effective therapy.

After definite repair for TOF, several factors may contribute to impaired RV systolic and diastolic function. First, there is likely to be preexisting dysfunction as a result of hypertrophy, and perhaps cyanosis. Myocardial preservation of the RV in TOF is widely felt to be insufficient for several reasons, including difficulties protecting hypertrophic muscle, increased tendency to free radical injury, and increased washout of cardioplegia due to collaterals. There is likely to be a mechanical component of RV dysfunction because of the use of a right ventriculotomy and RVOT patch. Finally, there may be new or residual abnormal hemodynamic loads because of pulmonary regurgitation, created by enlargement of the RVOT with a transannular patch, which imposes a new volume load on the RV, or residual pressure load because of RVOT obstruction below (infundibular), at, or distal to (main or branch PA stenosis) the pulmonary valve.

A residual VSD is likely to be very poorly tolerated in the patient with TOF, with the most likely manifestation being low cardiac output syndrome associated with elevated central venous pressure, left atrial pressure (LAP), and pulmonary arterial pressure (PAP). RVOT obstruction should be nearly completely eliminated after repair. PVR is likely to be low and the pulmonary vasculature very compliant. As a result, there will be potential for a large left-to-right intracardiac shunt with a residual VSD. This will place a large volume load on the LV and RV. An acute volume load will not be well tolerated by the RV, which is likely to be concentrically hypertrophied and poorly compliant in response to the chronic pressure overload that existed preoperatively. The presence of pulmonary insufficiency will further exacerbate RV dysfunction by imposing an additional volume load. Any distal pulmonary artery stenoses, high mean airway pressures, and elevated PVR will all increase the regurgitant volume and subsequent RV volume load.

After complete repair of TOF with no residual lesions and minimal intrapulmonary shunt, the Sao_2 should be 100%, and most patients require only modest to moderate degrees of inotropic support with dopamine or dobutamine (3 to 10 mcg/kg per minute). The need for substantially higher levels of support should raise the suspicion of a residual anatomic defect. In infants and small children, particularly those left with pulmonary insufficiency as the result of a transannular patch and those expected to have RV dysfunction as a result of a ventriculotomy or extensive RV hypertrophy (this may be an especially prominent problem in repairs in infants < 3 to 4 months old), the surgeon may choose to leave a pop-off valve by leaving the PFO open or by creating a small (3 to 4 mm) atrial-level fenestration. This will allow physiologic intracardiac R-L shunting (there will be direct delivery of some desaturated venous blood to the LA), with the ability to augment systemic cardiac output at the expense of systemic oxygen saturation in the setting of RV dysfunction. In these patients, a Pao_2 of 40 to 50 mm Hg and a Sao_2 of 70% to 80% is acceptable until RV function improves over the course of days. A right bundle branch block is common. Rarely, heart block requiring temporary (or permanent) pacing can occur as a consequence of the VSD closure; a large VSD patch can also occasionally be associated with LV outflow tract obstruction.

Ebstein's Anomaly

Ebstein's anomaly is an abnormality of the tricuspid valve in which the septal and often the posterior valve leaflets are displaced downward into the right ventricle (Fig. 20-9). See related

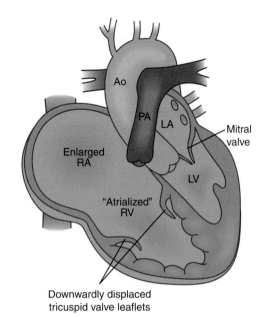

FIGURE 20-9. Anatomy of Ebstein's anomaly. There is apical displacement of the posterior and septal leaflets of the tricuspid valve. As a result, there is an atrialized right ventricle and an enlarged right atrium. The anterior tricuspid valve leaflet is not shown. An atrial septal defect or patent foramen ovale would be present. *(Redrawn from Children's Hospital Boston, Boston, Mass.)*

video online at www.expertconsult.com. In addition, the anterior tricuspid valve leaflet is abnormal. It is generally elongated and sail-like, with chordal attachments to the RV free wall. There may be RV outflow obstruction from the anterior leaflet. The result is a dilated right atrium with atrialization of the proximal RV and reduced effective RV cavity size and function. The tricuspid valve is usually regurgitant but may also be stenotic. Most patients with Ebstein's anomaly have an interatrial communication (ASD, PFO), through which there may be right-to-left shunting of blood, the magnitude of which depends on the severity of the tricuspid valve abnormality and degree of RV dysfunction.

Clinical Presentation

The severity of the hemodynamic derangements in patients with Ebstein's anomaly depends on the degree of displacement and the functional status of the tricuspid valve and RV. As a result, the clinical presentation varies from congestive heart failure in neonates to the absence of symptoms in adults in whom the anomaly is discovered incidentally. Neonates often manifest systemic venous congestion and cyanosis that worsens after ductus arteriosus closure reduces pulmonary blood flow. Older children with Ebstein's anomaly may be diagnosed as a result of an incidental murmur, whereas adolescents and adults are likely to present with supraventricular dysrhythmias that lead to CHF, worsening cyanosis, and occasionally syncope. Patients with Ebstein's anomaly and an interatrial communication are at risk for paradoxical embolization, brain abscess, CHF, and sudden death.

The severity of cyanosis depends on the magnitude of the right-to-left shunt. A systolic murmur caused by tricuspid regurgitation is usually present at the left lower sternal border. Hepatomegaly resulting from passive hepatic congestion due to increased right atrial pressures may be present. The ECG is characterized by tall and broad P waves (resembling right bundle branch block), and first-degree atrioventricular heart block is common. Paroxysmal supraventricular and ventricular tachydysrhythmias may occur; and as many as 20% of patients with Ebstein's anomaly have ventricular preexcitation by way of accessory electrical pathways between the atrium and ventricle (Wolff-Parkinson-White syndrome). In patients with severe disease (marked right-to-left shunting and minimal functional right ventricle), marked cardiomegaly is present that is largely the result of right atrial enlargement.

Echocardiography is used to assess right atrial dilation, distortion of the tricuspid valve leaflets, and the severity of the tricuspid regurgitation or stenosis. The presence and magnitude of interatrial shunting can be determined by color Doppler imaging studies. Enlargement of the right atrium may be so massive that the apical portions of the lungs are compressed, resulting in restrictive pulmonary disease.

Treatment

Treatment of neonatal Ebstein's anomaly is controversial and varies with the specific subtype of abnormality. Approaches range from tricuspid valve repair (for patients whose valve is amenable to repair and in whom the RV is likely to be able to support normal cardiac output), staging to a Fontan procedure (for those with significantly reduced RV size and function), and transplantation. In older patients, treatment is based on the prevention of associated complications, including antibiotic prophylaxis against infective endocarditis and administration of diuretics and digoxin for the management of CHF. Patients with supraventricular dysrhythmias are treated pharmacologically or with catheter ablation if an accessory pathway is present. Repair or replacement of the tricuspid valve in conjunction with closure of the interatrial communication is recommended for older patients who have severe symptoms despite medical therapy. Complications of surgery to correct Ebstein's anomaly include third-degree atrioventricular heart block, persistence of supraventricular dysrhythmias, residual tricuspid regurgitation after valve repair, and prosthetic valve dysfunction when the tricuspid valve is replaced (da Silva et al., 2007; Knott-Craig et al., 2007; Bove et al., 2009).

Management of Anesthesia

Delayed onset of pharmacologic effects can be expected after IV administration of an anesthetic, which may result in part from pooling and dilution in an enlarged right atrium. The major hazards during anesthesia in patients with Ebstein's anomaly include depression of RV function and reduced forward flow into the pulmonary artery, accentuation of arterial hypoxemia because of increases in the magnitude of the right-to-left intracardiac shunt, and the development of supraventricular tachydysrhythmias (Lerner et al., 2003). Increased right atrial pressures may indicate the presence of right ventricular failure. Both ventilatory and pharmacologic measures should focus on minimizing mechanical and metabolic effects of ventilation on RV afterload and on maintaining RV contractility. In the presence of a PFO, an increase in right atrial pressure above the pressure in the left atrium can lead to a right-to-left intracardiac shunt through the foramen ovale. Unexplained arterial hypoxemia or paradoxical air embolism during the

perioperative period may result from shunting of blood or air through a previously closed foramen ovale.

Tricuspid Atresia

Tricuspid atresia (TA) involves a lesion with single-ventricle physiology. See related video online at www.expertconsult.com. These patients are staged to a Fontan procedure. Patients with TA have complete obstruction to RV inflow and variable obstruction to RV outflow. A communication (ASD or PFO) results in an obligatory right-to-left shunt at the atrial level with complete mixing of systemic and pulmonary venous blood in the left atrium. When the ASD or PFO is restrictive, there is a large right atrial to left atrial pressure gradient, which results in poor decompression of the RA and systemic venous congestion. Pulmonary blood flow can be provided by a downstream shunt from intracardiac (VSD) and extracardiac (PDA, multiple aortopulmonary collateral arteries) sources. Anatomic classification is based on the presence or absence of transposition of the great arteries, the extent of pulmonary stenosis or atresia, and the size of the VSD. Approximately 70% of all patients with TA are type 1, and 50% percent of all TA patients are type 1B (Fig. 20-10, and see Fig. 20-2 and Table 20-3).

Treatment

Initial palliation depends on the anatomic variant. Infants with TA, adequate ASD, adequate VSD, and an "appropriate" amount of pulmonic stenosis can have a balanced circulation and require little or no intervention until later in infancy. Prostaglandin E_1 (PGE_1) is frequently necessary to augment PBF, and a balloon atrial septostomy may be necessary to allow adequate mixing and right atrial decompression. A Blalock-Taussig (BT) shunt may be required to provide a stable source of augmented pulmonary blood flow (e.g., TA with no VSD or with VSD but also with severe pulmonary stenosis or atresia). A staged approach to a Fontan procedure as described previously (see Figs. 20-4 and 20-5; Fig. 20-19) is the usual definitive treatment approach for TA.

Management of Anesthesia

Anesthetic management of patients with TA largely depends on their specific anatomy and where they are in their course of single-ventricle physiology. In general, IV induction techniques as outlined earlier are preferred for their reliability (e.g., uncertain uptake of inhaled agents in the presence of a "complete" right-to-left shunt) and hemodynamic stability; anesthetic maintenance typically uses "balanced" combinations of opioid, low-concentration inhaled agent, and muscle relaxation. The patient on PGE_1 presenting for balloon atrial septostomy or BT shunt creation is ductal dependent for PBF. As described previously, the major goals are to preserve overall cardiac contractility and output and to balance the relationship between PVR and SVR so that arterial oxygen saturations in the mid 70% to 80% range are maintained. Factors that raise PVR, decrease SVR, or reduce cardiac output can all contribute to increased hypoxemia by reducing ductal flow into the lungs. On the other hand, it may be possible to markedly compromise systemic perfusion by significantly reducing PVR (e.g., hyperoxic and hyperventilation or hypocarbia), thereby promoting increased left-to-right flow through the PDA. This occurrence may be signaled by increased arterial oxygen saturations, widened pulse pressure, and hypotension.

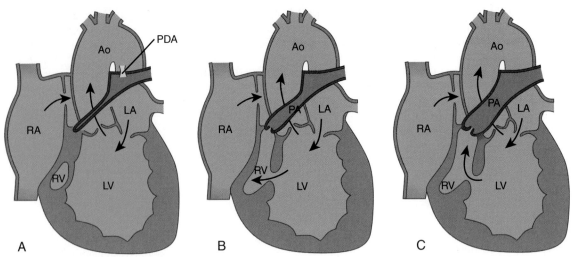

■ **FIGURE 20-10.** Anatomy and blood flow in tricuspid atresia type 1. Type 1A: pulmonary atresia with pulmonary blood flow via patent ductus arteriosus or major aortopulmonary collateral arteries (MAPCAs). Type 1B: small ventricular septal defect and pulmonary stenosis. Type 1C: large ventricular septal defect and no pulmonary stenosis.

Considerations after BT shunt creation have been discussed. In brief, one typically expects arterial oxygen saturations in the range of 75% to 85%. Substantially lower values may indicate shunt obstruction (arterial BP will be close to normal or high), low cardiac output or SVR, and, occasionally, high PVR. Pulmonary overcirculation (high arterial oxygen saturations, hypotension) may be managed by ventilatory maneuvers to increase PVR; at times, partial clipping of the shunt may be necessary. Controlled ventilation and inotropes are frequently required for several hours to days, as these infants adapt to the shunt-dependent circulation. The patient with TA, VSD, and no obstruction to PBF can be prone to pulmonary overcirculation and systemic hypoperfusion as PVR falls in the postnatal period. Initial management considerations are the same as those for other situations of potential excessive PBF—support systemic cardiac output and attempt to prevent increases in PBF by avoiding increased fraction of inspired oxygen (Fio$_2$) and hypocarbia; some patients will require palliation with a pulmonary artery band to mechanically control PBF before more definitive surgery.

Total Anomalous Pulmonary Venous Return

Anatomy

 Total anomalous pulmonary venous return (TAPVR) results in blood return from all of the pulmonary veins into the *systemic* venous system rather than directly into the left atrium. See related video online at www.expertconsult.com. The individual pulmonary veins usually drain into a common pulmonary venous confluence that has no direct connection to the LA; this confluence connects to the systemic venous circulation via one of four anatomic variants (Fig. 20-11):

1. Supracardiac TAPVR. Drainage of the pulmonary vein confluence is into a supracardiac venous structure. This occurs in nearly 50% of TAPVR cases, most often employing a "vertical

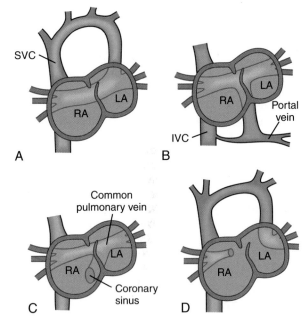

■ **FIGURE 20-11.** Types of total anomalous pulmonary venous return (TAPVR). **A,** Supracardiac (46%). Pulmonary venous blood returns to common pulmonary vein; the common pulmonary vein drains via a left vertical vein to the innominate vein, the superior vena cava *(SVC),* and finally to the right atrium. **B,** Infracardiac (22%). A common pulmonary vein passes through the diaphragm at the esophageal hiatus. The common vein then drains into the portal vein, hepatic vein, or ductus venosus. Obstruction of flow into the inferior vena cava *(IVC)* and right atrium may be caused by obligatory passage through the liver. **C,** Cardiac (24%). A common pulmonary vein directly enters the right atrium via the coronary sinus. **D,** Mixed (8%). The mixed type involves components of supracardiac, infracardiac, and cardiac drainage. Illustrated here is a combination of cardiac and supracardiac connections. *LA,* Left atrium; *RA,* right atrium. *(Redrawn from Children's Hospital Boston, Boston, Mass.)*

vein" that connects the pulmonary venous confluence with the innominate vein, which then drains into the SVC.

2. Infracardiac TAPVR. This next most frequent subtype, occurring in approximately 25% of patients, involves drainage of the pulmonary venous confluence into an infracardiac vessel, such as the IVC, portal vein, or hepatic vein, via an inferiorly directed vertical vein that goes through the diaphragm to connect to one of these infracardiac vessels.

3. Intracardiac TAPVR. Here, the pulmonary venous confluence drains directly into the RA via the coronary sinus.

4. Mixed TAPVR. In a small percentage (<10%) of patients, pulmonary venous drainage is some combination of types 1, 2, and 3.

Infracardiac TAPVR is most frequently associated with pulmonary venous obstruction, at least in part because of the long course of the vertical vein and its passage through the diaphragm. Some patients with supracardiac TAPVR exhibit compression of the vertical vein between the left main stem bronchus and left pulmonary artery.

Physiology

There is a complete mixing lesion where all of the systemic and pulmonary venous blood mixes in the right atrium. The return of all pulmonary venous blood to the right atrium results in a large L-R shunt. Thus, an anatomic R-L shunt (an ASD or a PFO) is necessary for left heart filing and postnatal survival. These patients usually have a nonrestrictive or only mildly restrictive atrial level defect; however, R-L flow across the atrial septum is usually hampered by poor LA and LV compliance, in part because the reduced blood flow to the left side of the heart in utero caused these chambers to be smaller and stiffer than normal.

Taken together, these factors have the following results. In the absence of pulmonary venous obstruction, newborn infants with TAPVR have a $\dot{Q}_P$:$\dot{Q}_S$ close to 1:1. The decrease of PVR that occurs shortly after birth, in combination with significantly decreased left-sided compliance, promotes delivery of the mixed systemic and pulmonary venous blood to the pulmonary circuit. Pulmonary artery pressures will then be near systemic because, although PVR is not markedly elevated, the $\dot{Q}_P$:$\dot{Q}_S$ is usually quite high (>2:1 to 3:1).

Compression of the vertical venous pathway produces obstructed TAPVR. This distinction and diagnosis are critical, because obstruction causes pulmonary venous hypertension, elevated PVR, and systemic or even suprasystemic RV and PA pressures. Some of these patients may develop PVOD in utero as well. In addition, pulmonary venous obstruction will produce pulmonary edema, further elevating PVR, much as it does with mitral stenosis. Obstructed TAPVR is a surgical emergency, one of the few remaining in the era of PGE_1 therapy

Clinical Presentation

Systemic cardiac output and organ perfusion can be severely compromised in these patients. Systemic or suprasystemic RV pressures can result in a leftward shift of the interventicular septum (known as ventricular interdependence) that pancakes the LV and further reduces the compliance and filling of the already small LV; a secondary effect of these alterations is to reduce R-L flow across the atrial septum (because the impedance to LA emptying has increased). There is also likely to be RV afterload mismatch, resulting in RV distention and tricuspid

regurgitation. Thus, systemic cardiac output largely depends on a physiologic R-L shunt across the ductus arteriosus, but one that is supplied by a failing RV. These patients have a small heart and congested lungs on chest radiograph, the latter appearing worse in the case of obstructed TAPVR. The diagnosis is usually confirmed by surface echocardiography.

Patients with TAPVR are hypoxemic because of complete mixing; their degree of hypoxemia is further exacerbated by low cardiac output (which reduces mixed venous oxyhemoglobin saturation [Sv_{O_2}] and hence the Sa_{O_2} that results from complete mixing), pulmonary edema (which causes intrapulmonary shunt and V/Q mismatch, leading to low pulmonary venous oxyhemoglobin saturation [Spv_{O_2}]), and reduced PBF arising from increased PVR. Efforts to increase pulmonary blood flow in these patients will only worsen the pulmonary edema (thus, e.g., inhaled nitric oxide [iNO], as well as other inhaled pulmonary vasodilators, are clearly contraindicated).

Patients with *obstructed* TAPVR present at birth with hypoxemia and poor systemic perfusion. In many, there is an ongoing metabolic acidosis and evidence of end-organ (hepatic and renal) dysfunction. In patients with severe pulmonary venous obstruction leading to suprasystemic RV and PA pressures and R-L shunting across the ductus arteriosus, ductal patency is necessary to maintain cardiac output (i.e., use of PGE_1 for temporary palliation may be indicated); frequently, inotropic support is required. In patients with less severe obstruction and subsystemic RV and PA pressures, ductal flow will be bidirectional or L-R. In these patients, ductal patency may exacerbate pulmonary edema.

Surgical Therapy

Definitive repair involves anastomosis of the pulmonary venous confluence to the posterior LA, ligation of the vertical vein, and closure of the ASD (Boger et al., 1999; Wang et al., 2004; Lacour-Gayet, 2006; Siles and Lapierre, 2008).

Anesthetic Management

General Considerations. The infant with TAPVR is frequently extremely ill and demonstrates both severe respiratory and circulatory compromise. This is especially true of TAPVR infants with pulmonary venous obstruction, in whom emergency surgery is the only viable therapeutic option. Efforts to increase pulmonary blood flow by ventilatory interventions will worsen pulmonary edema in these patients.

Overall, it is important to maintain heart rate, contractility, and preload so as to maintain systemic cardiac output. As noted previously, decreased cardiac output reduces systemic venous oxygen saturation, which, in a complete mixing lesion, will reduce arterial oxygen saturation. For patients with increased pulmonary blood flow, decreases in the PVR-to-SVR ratio should be avoided. The increase in pulmonary blood flow that accompanies a reduced PVR-to-SVR ratio necessitates an increase in cardiac output to maintain systemic blood flow, which will be difficult if not impossible in these patients for the reasons discussed previously. For patients with increased pulmonary blood flow and right ventricular volume overload, ventilatory interventions should be used to increase PVR, reduce pulmonary blood flow, and decrease the volume load on the right ventricle.

Induction and Maintenance. Neonates with pulmonary venous obstruction generally arrive in the operating room intubated, ventilated, and on inotropic support. Nonintubated patients are probably best managed by intravenous induction with etomidate or high-dosage potent opioid and muscle relaxation. The primary goals are to maintain systemic cardiac output and gain rapid control of ventilation without adversely affecting the tenuous relationships that affect the PVR-to-SVR ratio, systemic venous return, and cardiac output. Management of ventilation prior to CPB is therefore based on the aforementioned principles. These patients are best anesthetized with a high-dosage-narcotic technique that includes fentanyl or sufentanil and muscle relaxation. Patients with TAPVR, particularly those with venous obstruction, have a highly reactive pulmonary vasculature. High dosages of fentanyl and sufentanil may be useful for blunting increases in PVR associated with surgical stimulation.

Post-CPB Management

After surgical repair, the primary problems in these patients relate to left-sided filling and output compromise related to (1) small and noncompliant LA and LV, along with superimposed acute myocardial ischemia–reperfusion injury, and (2) reactive pulmonary vasculature, pulmonary hypertension, right ventricular hypertension, and RV dysfunction. The initial goals are to maintain heart rate (ideally, sinus rhythm) at an age-appropriate rate, using temporary pacing if necessary. Cardiac output is likely to be more heart-rate dependent in the post-CPB period.

Pulmonary hypertension (frequently at systemic or even suprasystemic levels of PA pressure) and limited systemic cardiac output are the major challenges after CPB. For patients' reactive pulmonary vasculature, blunting of stress-induced increases in PVR with narcotics is indicated. In addition, ventilatory interventions that reduce PVR and the use of selective pulmonary vasodilators such as iNO are frequently necessary; indeed, this group of patients with CHD are among those most likely to respond to iNO after CPB with a clinically significant decrease in PVR and improvement in cardiac function (Adatia and Wessel, 1994; Curran et al., 1995; Bizzarro and Gross, 2005; Roberts et al., 1993).

Despite maneuvers to decrease PVR, inotropic support of the RV may be necessary. Dobutamine (5 to 10 mcg/kg per minute) or dopamine (5 to 10 mcg/kg per minute) is useful in this instance because both agents provide potent inotropic support without increasing PVR. In the absence of systemic hypotension, milrinone (0.25 to 1.0 mcg/kg per minute after a 50-mcg/kg loading dosage, preferably administered on CPB) can be considered. Left-sided (e.g., LA) pressures are often high (~12 to 20 mm Hg) because of the combination of intrinsic, poor left-sided compliance, acute myocardial injury, and RV distention. It is easy to both underfill (resulting in low output) and overfill (acute distention and mitral regurgitation) the left heart. One, thus, needs to keep up with ongoing blood loss and replacement of clotting factors, but volume administration needs to be done with significant caution. The overall goal is to keep LA pressures within a reasonable target range while maintaining a reasonable (e.g., ~60 mm Hg systolic) blood pressure and evidence of adequate systemic perfusion (e.g., urine output, pH, cerebral oximetry, or SVC saturation).

Residual RV and PA hypertension can be caused by one or more of the following: (1) pulmonary venous obstruction, a technical (surgical) problem arising from the failure to construct a nonrestrictive anastomosis of the pulmonary venous confluence to the LA; (2) LA (and hence pulmonary venous) hypertension due to the small, noncompliant LA and LV and post-CPB LV dysfunction; and (3) labile increases in PVR due to reactive pulmonary vasoconstriction (capillary and precapillary). In the presence of postoperative pulmonary venous obstruction, efforts to increase pulmonary blood flow may worsen pulmonary edema. Surgical revision may be necessary (Lacour-Gayet, 2006).

The use of surgically placed PA and LA monitoring catheters, often in combination with echocardiography (surface "on-heart" or transesophageal echocardiography [TEE], depending on patient size and probe availability), can be helpful in sorting out these issues. For example, the presence of high PA pressure, elevated LAP, and a PA diastolic pressure of less than 5 mm Hg above the LAP suggests that LA hypertension is the primary cause of PA hypertension. In contrast, the presence of high PA pressure, low or normal LAP, and a PA diastolic pressure of greater than 15 to 20 mm Hg above the LAP suggests that reactive pulmonary vasoconstriction, PVOD, or anastomotic pulmonary venous obstruction exists. Similarly, the presence of reactive pulmonary vasoconstriction or PVOD is suggested by a pulmonary wedge pressure of less than 3 to 5 mm Hg above the LAP, whereas a wedge pressure of greater than 7 to 10 mm Hg above the LAP is consistent with pulmonary venous obstruction. Echocardiography can be helpful in assessing the status of the pulmonary venous connection to the LA, and in assessing ventricular function and filling.

Transposition of the Great Arteries

Anatomy

In patients with TGA, there is discordance of the ventriculoarterial connections and concordance of the atrioventricular connections. See related video online at www.expertconsult.com. In other words, a right-sided RA connects via a right-sided tricuspid valve and RV to a right-sided and anterior aorta. A left-sided LA connects via a left-sided mitral valve and LV to a left-sided and posterior pulmonary artery (Fig. 20-12). The coronary arteries in dextro- (D-)TGA arise from the aortic sinuses that face the pulmonary artery. In normally related vessels, these sinuses are located on the anterior portion of the aorta, whereas in D-TGA they are located posteriorly. In the majority of D-TGA patients (70%), the right sinus is the origin of the right coronary artery, whereas the left sinus is the origin of the left main coronary artery. In the remainder of cases, there is considerable variability in this coronary anatomy. The exact coronary anatomy must be delineated; variants can contribute significantly to operative difficulty and the success of surgical repair.

TGA can occur with an intact ventricular septum or with a VSD, with or without subpulmonic stenosis. In D-TGA, subpulmonic stenosis causes left ventricular outflow tract (LVOT) obstruction, which is present in about 25% of patients with VSD and is most often due to a subpulmonary fibromuscular ring or posterior displacement of the outlet portion of the ventricular septum (or both). In addition, the foramen ovale is almost always patent, whereas a true secundum ASD exists in only about 5% of patients; approximately 50% of patients with D-TGA present with a PDA. Although angiographically detectable VSDs may occur in 30% to 40% of patients, only about one

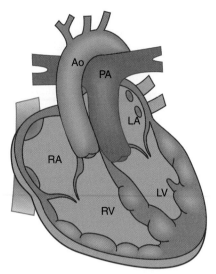

■ **FIGURE 20-12.** Anatomy of dextro-transposition of the great arteries (D-TGA). The aorta is in continuity with the right ventricle, and the pulmonary artery is in continuity with the left ventricle, producing a parallel rather than a series circulation. *Ao,* Aorta; *LV,* left ventricle; *RV,* right ventricle. *(Redrawn from Children's Hospital Boston, Boston, Mass.)*

third of these defects are hemodynamically significant. Thus, from a functional standpoint, 75% of patients will behave as if they have an intact ventricular septum (see later). Only 5% of patients with IVS have significant LVOT obstruction. Valvular pulmonary stenosis is rare in patients with TGA. Other less commonly seen lesions are tricuspid or mitral regurgitation (4% of each) and a coarctation of the aorta (5%). Bronchopulmonary collateral vessels arising from the aorta are visible angiographically in 30% of patients with D-TGA, more frequently and extensively to the right lung. These collaterals provide a site for intercirculatory mixing and have been implicated in the accelerated development of pulmonary vascular occlusive disease in TGA patients.

D-TGA produces two parallel circulations with recirculation of systemic and pulmonary venous blood. Short-term survival depends on the presence of one or more communications between the two parallel circuits to allow intercirculatory mixing; the potential sites in patients with D-TGA are both intracardiac (PFO, ASD, VSD) and extracardiac (PDA, bronchopulmonary collaterals). Several factors determine the amount of intercirculatory mixing and hence arterial oxygen saturation and delivery. One large, nonrestrictive communication provides better mixing than two or three restrictive communications. Reduced ventricular compliance and elevated systemic and pulmonary vascular resistance tend to reduce intercirculatory mixing by impeding flow across the anatomic communications. The location of the communications is also important. Poor mixing occurs even with large anterior muscular VSDs because of their unfavorable positions.

In TGA with VSD, some intercirculatory mixing can occur at the ventricular level, but there is predominantly anatomic R-to-L shunting (effective pulmonary blood flow) at the VSD (RV→LV→PA) and PDA (RV→Ao→PA) and anatomic L-to-R shunting (effective systemic blood flow) at the PFO or ASD

(LA→RA→RV→Ao). Clearly, the more severe the LVOT obstruction, the more dependent the effective pulmonary blood flow will be on the presence of a PDA.

Patients with pulmonary stenosis sufficient to limit PBF may be hypoxemic despite a relatively large intercirculatory communication. Patients with high pulmonary blood flow, particularly those with a large VSD, are at risk of developing both overcirculation and congestive symptoms and PVOD. In the presence of a good-sized intercirculatory communication and no obstruction to PBF, most of these patients will not initially be hypoxemic but will have a large volume load imposed on the LA and LV and develop signs and symptoms of pulmonary overcirculation and CHF. However, the progressive development of PVOD can eventually reduce pulmonary blood flow and produce hypoxemia.

In TGA with an intact ventricular septum, the anatomic mixing sites are typically restricted to a PDA and a PFO. The factors determining the degree of intercirculatory mixing in TGA/IVS are complex and potentially problematic clinically. Anatomic shunting at the atrial level is mainly determined by the size of the atrial communication and the cyclic pressure variations between the left and right atrial chambers. The volume and compliance of the atria, ventricles, and vascular beds in each circuit, as well as heart rate and respiration, all influence the result. Shunting is from the right atrium to the left atrium during diastole as a result of the reduced ventricular and vascular compliance of the systemic circuit. In systole, the shunt is predominantly from the left atrium to the right atrium, primarily because of the large volume of blood returning to the left atrium as a result of the high volume of recirculated pulmonary blood flow.

The direction of shunting across the PDA largely depends on the PVR and the size of the intraatrial communication. When the PVR is low and the intraatrial communication is nonrestrictive, shunting is predominantly from the aorta to the pulmonary artery via the PDA, and predominantly from the left to right atrium (and hence into the systemic right ventricle) across the atrial septum. When the PVR is elevated, shunting across the PDA is likely to be bidirectional, which would in turn encourage bidirectional shunting across the atrial septum.

When the PVR is high and pulmonary artery pressure exceeds aortic pressure, shunting at the PDA will be predominantly from the pulmonary artery to the aorta. This causes a phenomenon known as reverse differential cyanosis, where the preductal arterial oxygen saturation is lower than the postductal arterial oxygen saturation. This is usually the result of a restrictive atrial communication producing left atrial hypertension and is associated with poor mixing and hypoxemia. A balloon atrial septostomy can be lifesaving in this setting. Decompression of the left atrium promotes mixing at the atrial level and also reduces PVR and pulmonary artery pressure, thereby promoting mixing (bidirectional shunting) at the level of the PDA.

The majority of neonates with D-TGA and IVS are hypoxemic (arterial saturation ≤ 70%) immediately after birth, with some patients demonstrating severely reduced effective pulmonary and systemic blood flow. This can result in severe hypoxemia (Pao_2 < 20 mm Hg), hypercarbia, and increasing metabolic acidosis secondary to the poor tissue oxygen delivery. PGE_1 (0.01 to 0.05 mcg/kg per minute) is administered to dilate and maintain the patency of the ductus arteriosus and facilitate mixing at this level. This maneuver increases effective pulmonary and systemic blood flow and can improve Pao_2 and tissue oxygen delivery if PVR is less than SVR (see earlier) and there is a nonrestrictive or minimally restrictive atrial septal communication. PGE₁ infusion is associated with apnea, pyrexia, fluid retention, and platelet dysfunction, which are largely dosage dependent.

If PGE_1 does not improve tissue oxygen delivery, then an emergent balloon atrial septostomy can be performed in the catheterization laboratory (using angiography) or in the intensive care unit (ICU) (using echocardiographic guidance). These patients require tracheal intubation and mechanical ventilation if not already in place. This allows reduction of PVR via induction of a respiratory alkalosis and elimination of pulmonary V/Q mismatch; in addition, we have noted significant numbers of apnea episodes when trying to provide procedural sedation to neonates receiving PGE_1 infusions. In rare circumstances, the combination of PGE_1, a balloon atrial septostomy, and mechanical ventilation with sedation and muscle relaxation may be ineffective at improving oxygen saturation and systemic oxygen delivery. In this circumstance, ECMO (either veno-arterial or veno-veno) support to improve tissue oxygenation and to reverse end-organ insult and lactic acidosis prior to surgery may be necessary.

Surgical Therapy

Two general types of procedures have been performed to repair D-TGA, namely intraatrial baffle and arterial switch procedures.

Mustard and Senning Procedures. Both the Mustard and the Senning procedures are atrial switch procedures, which surgically create discordant atrioventricular connections in the presence of the preexisting discordant ventriculoarterial connections. As a result of atrial baffling, systemic venous blood is directed to the LV, which remains in continuity with the pulmonary artery, and pulmonary venous blood is baffled to the RV, which is in continuity with the aorta. This arrangement results in physiologic but not anatomic correction of D-TGA. After these procedures, the right ventricle remains the systemic ventricle and the tricuspid valve remains the systemic AV valve (Fig. 20-13).

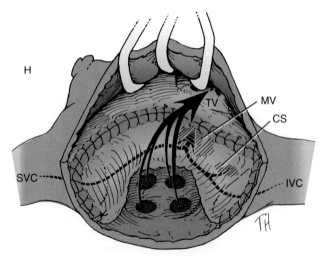

■ **FIGURE 20-13.** Interior of right atrium showing the baffle that rearranges and redirects atrial blood flow after the Mustard procedure. Pulmonary vein openings can be seen. *CS*, Coronary sinus; *IVC*, inferior vena cava; *MV*, mitral valve; *TV*, tricuspid valve. *(From Reed CC, Stafford TB, editors:* Cardiopulmonary bypass, *ed 2, Houston, 1985, Texas Medical Press, p 78.)*

The Mustard procedure redirects pulmonary and systemic venous return via an intraatrial baffle made from pericardium or artificial graft material that is created after excision of the interatrial septum. The Senning version uses autologous right atrial tissue instead of pericardium or synthetic material. As a result of either procedure, pulmonary venous blood is essentially guided over the top of the baffle and across the tricuspid valve, while systemic venous blood is directed beneath the baffle to cross the mitral valve.

Both systemic and pulmonary venous obstruction by baffle material may occur as the result of either procedure. Because of the extensive atrial suture lines and at times atrial distention, dysrhythmias occur frequently after these procedures: about 60% to 70% of patients have some form of dysrhythmia, 30% of which are serious (bradycardia, sick-sinus syndrome, atrial flutter). Long-term exposure of the right ventricle and tricuspid valve to systemic pressure can result in progressive and severe right ventricular dysfunction (Horer et al., 2008).

Anatomic Repair or the Arterial (Jatene) Switch Procedure. The arterial switch operation (ASO) surgically reverses the discordant ventriculoarterial connections so that after repair, the right ventricle is connected to the pulmonary artery and the left ventricle is connected to the aorta. This is now the most common procedure performed for D-TGA (DeBord et al., 2007; Gottlieb et al., 2008; Quinn et al., 2008). In brief, the pulmonary artery and the aorta are transected distal to their respective valves. The coronary arteries are excised from the ascending aorta with 3 to 4 mm of surrounding tissue and these sites repaired either with pericardium or synthetic material. The coronary arteries are reimplanted into the proximal pulmonary artery (neoaorta), the distal pulmonary artery is brought anterior (LeCompte maneuver) and reanastomosed to the proximal aorta (right ventricular outflow), and the distal aorta is reanastomosed to the proximal pulmonary artery (left ventricular outflow) (Fig. 20-14). As mentioned earlier, variants in coronary anatomy can complicate this scenario. Although most patients with D-TGA have coronary anatomy that is suitable for coronary reimplantation, some variants, such as a single right coronary artery, are at risk for postoperative myocardial ischemia and death because reimplantation can result in distortion of the coronary ostia or narrowing of the artery itself. Inverted, intramural, or parallel coronary arteries can also be a problem.

The ASO was originally described in patients with D-TGA and a large VSD or a large PDA, in whom the LV (the pulmonary ventricle prior to ASO) is exposed to systemic pressures, and the LV mass remains sufficient to support the systemic circulation. This situation requires that the ASO be performed within the first few months (usually within the first few weeks) of life to avoid the development of progressive CHF or PVOD. The VSD is usually closed via the tricuspid valve to avoid a right ventriculotomy and resultant RV dysfunction. A brief period (<15 minutes) of deep hypothermic circulatory arrest is often used to facilitate closure of the ASD.

In patients with D-TGA and IVS, the ASO can be performed primarily or as the second phase of a staged procedure. A primary ASO procedure is usual for these patients and is usually performed within the first week of life. This is because the LV mass (and thus its ability to support the systemic circulation after ASO) in these patients declines as the elevated PVR that is characteristic of the normal fetus and newborn declines in the days to weeks after birth. Adequate LV mass to support the

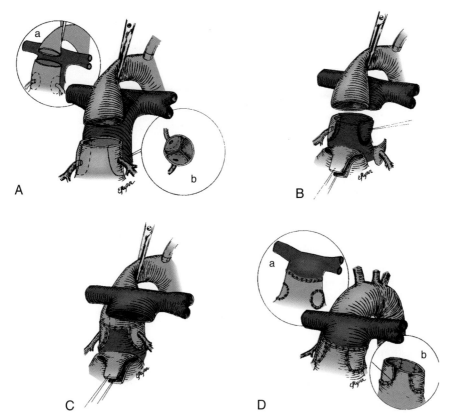

FIGURE 20-14. Arterial switch procedure. **A,** The aorta is transected, and left and right coronary arteries and their bases are excised. **B,** An equivalent segment of pulmonary arterial wall is excised, and coronary arteries are sutured to the pulmonary artery. **C,** The distal pulmonary artery is brought anterior to ascending aorta, and the proximal pulmonary artery is anastomosed to the distal aorta. **D,** Sites of coronary artery extraction are repaired with use of either (*a*) a patch of prosthetic material or (*b*) a segment of pericardium. Finally, the proximal aorta is sutured to distal pulmonary artery. *(Modified from Castaneda AR, Norwood WI, Jonas RA, et al: Transposition of the great arteries and intact ventricular septum: anatomical repair in the neonate,* Ann Thorac Surg *38:438, 1984, with permission from the Society of Thoracic Surgeons.)*

systemic circulation exists in these patients for only the first 2 to 3 months after birth, at most. Two-dimensional echocardiography is used to assess the LV-to-RV-pressure ratio and to quantify the adequacy of LV mass, size, and function.

A two-stage repair for D-TGA with IVS can be used for neonates and infants in whom significant regression of LV mass has occurred. These are generally infants on whom surgery was not performed during the first several weeks of life because of other factors (e.g., delayed diagnosis and referral, other anomalies, sepsis, or prematurity). To reestablish the ability of the LV to perform systemic workload, a pulmonary artery band is placed as a first stage; in addition, a BT shunt (one that enters the pulmonary artery distal to the band) is created to prevent hypoxemia. The goal of the band is to increase the LV (which is still the pulmonary ventricle) pressure to approximately one-half to two-thirds that in the systemic (right) ventricle to prevent further regression of LV mass and in fact promote a moderate degree of LV hypertrophy. These patients can initially be quite ill after the banding procedure, requiring mechanical ventilation and inotropic support as the adaptation occurs over several days; if the band is too tight, frank LV decompensation secondary to afterload mismatch can ensue.

After this first stage, the actual ASO can be performed as early as several days to 1 week after the pulmonary artery band procedure that was done to prepare the LV. The timing is often guided by noninvasive assessment of LV mass and function;

somewhat surprisingly, a marked increase of LV mass can be seen within a week or less of pulmonary artery banding in most patients. Nonetheless, some degree of impaired LV function after ASO should be anticipated in these patients (see later), and at times a period of ECMO support and "training of the LV" (where ECMO flows and support are slowly and progressively weaned over several days after ASO) are needed. In addition to the difficulties of obtaining appropriate band tightness and of its effects on LV function, the systemic-to-pulmonary artery shunt can distort the pulmonary artery, making the subsequent ASO more difficult.

Rastelli Procedure. The ASO is generally not performed on patients with significant anatomic and fixed LVOT obstruction (subpulmonic stenosis; patients with dynamic LVOT obstruction are likely to have no gradient across the LV outflow tract after the ASO). Correction of some types and severities of anatomic LVOT obstruction is possible and these patients are also potential candidates for ASO. For patients with D-TGA, VSD, and severe anatomic LVOT obstruction (subpulmonary stenosis), a Rastelli procedure is performed (Fig. 20-15).

Here, the VSD is closed via a right ventriculotomy using a more complicated patch, so that LV blood is directed through the aorta. The proximal pulmonary artery is ligated and a valved conduit is placed from the right ventriculotomy to the pulmonary artery, thereby bypassing the subpulmonic stenosis.

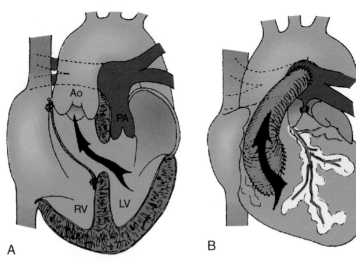

■ **FIGURE 20-15. A,** In the Rastelli procedure, closure of ventricular septal defect results in the left ventricle *(LV)* ejecting blood into the aorta *(Ao)*. **B,** An external right ventricle *(RV)*–to–pulmonary artery *(PA)* conduit is placed to provide pulmonary circulation. *(From Strafford M: Transposition of the great vessels. In Lake CL, editor:* Pediatric cardiac anesthesia, *Norwalk, Conn, 1988, Appleton & Lange, p 237.)*

Subaortic stenosis may result from placement of the complex VSD patch. Balloon dilations and eventual replacement of the valved RV-PA conduit are usually necessary because of calcification and patient growth.

Anesthetic Management

Several principles of anesthetic management pertain to all D-TGA infants, and some are specific for the individual subtypes. These will be discussed in turn.

For all patients, it is important to select drugs and other strategies that maintain cardiac output by their effects on heart rate, contractility, and preload. This is important because decreases in cardiac output decrease systemic venous saturation, with a resultant decrease in arterial saturation. Although this is true of all patients on PGE, it can be a critical consideration in patients with TGA and IVS, in whom optimizing preload and cardiac output may be the most reliable means to maintaining adequate intercirculatory mixing and avoid severe derangements in oxygen saturation (both systemic venous and arterial) and delivery.

When a patient has evidence of pulmonary overcirculation and congestive signs or symptoms, maneuvers (particularly ventilatory) that further decrease PVR should be avoided. It is also important to avoid significant increases in PVR relative to SVR, which will decrease pulmonary blood flow and reduce intercirculatory mixing. Similarly, reductions in SVR relative to PVR should also be avoided, because SVR promotes recirculation of systemic venous blood (and thus intercirculatory mixing) and decreases arterial saturation. Again, in general, promoting overall filling and ventricular output are the most reliable ways to maintain intercirculatory mixing, oxygenation, and oxygen delivery. Positive pressure ventilation needs to be sufficient to ensure adequate lung volume and gas exchange without promoting unwanted metabolic effects (e.g., hypocarbia and alkalosis in patients with already low PVR and evidence of pulmonary overcirculation) or substantial mechanical compromise of venous return, ventricular function, or mixing (e.g., increased PVR).

Induction and Maintenance. In prostaglandin-dependent neonates, the PGE$_1$ infusion (0.01 to 0.05 mcg/kg per minute) should be continued until shortly before CPB to ensure sufficient intercirculatory mixing. Anesthetic-related myocardial depression can occur on several counts and is more likely in these patients because of myocardial immaturity, the effects of positive pressure ventilation, and increased pulmonary blood flow with limited cardiac reserve. Therefore, this is another situation in which inhaled agent–based induction and maintenance techniques are not favored. Instead, anesthesia is usually induced and maintained using high-dosage fentanyl or sufentanil to provide hemodynamic stability and blunting of the stress response without adversely affecting intercirculatory mixing. In addition to muscle relaxation, judicious and divided doses of benzodiazepines (or low-concentration inhaled agent) can be added to promote amnesia.

In patients with reduced pulmonary blood flow or poor intercirculatory mixing, efforts to reduce PVR should be made to increase pulmonary blood flow and intercirculatory mixing (again with the caveat of not impeding PBF or cardiac output by excessive ventilatory maneuvers). Again, volume expansion and the addition of inotropic support (e.g., dopamine, 5 to 10 mcg/kg per minute) may be indicated to improve overall mixing and output and offset to some extent the alterations imposed by anesthetic agents and mechanical ventilation. In patients with PVOD, ventilatory measures to reduce PVR are useful if PVR is not fixed. Hypercarbia, acidosis, and hypoxemia further increase PVR and should be avoided because of limited myocardial reserve and deleterious effects on PVR (and therefore mixing as well). This is particularly true in neonates with TGA and IVS, where systemic oxygen delivery is tenuous, and in infants with TGA and VSD, in whom left ventricular volume overload is present. Indeed, it is not uncommon to see S-T segment changes on the ECG in these infants when systemic output and oxygenation are compromised, particularly in the face of LV volume overload. In addition, reactive increases in PVR are commonly seen in the immature pulmonary vasculature and may severely compromise pulmonary blood flow.

Post-CPB Management

After CPB and surgical repair, the most frequent problems include myocardial ischemia due to coronary insufficiency, decreased myocardial function, bleeding due to extensive and pressurized suture lines after neonatal CPB and hypothermia (i.e., clotting factor dilution, thrombocytopenia, and platelet dysfunction [see later]), and reactive pulmonary vasculature. Heart rate should be maintained at age-appropriate levels, using atrial pacing if necessary, as cardiac output is likely to be more heart-rate-dependent during the post-CPB period, particularly in these neonates and young infants. Although blood pressure should also be kept at age-appropriate norms (especially after hypothermic CPB or deep hypothermic circulatory arrest [DHCA] when cerebral autoregulation is likely to be impaired), at times reducing aortic or pulmonary artery pressure (or both) may be used to reduce suture line bleeding after the ASO. Systemic ventricular (RV after atrial baffle procedures and LV after arterial switch procedures) dysfunction may necessitate inotropic and vasodilator therapy to terminate CPB. Dobutamine (5 to 10 mcg/kg per minute) or dopamine (5 to 10 mcg/kg per minute) is most often used. Milrinone (0.25 to 1.0 mcg/kg per minute after a loading dose of 50 mcg/kg) may be used if SVR is high. Milrinone not only reduces LV afterload but may also contribute inotropic, lusitrophic, and PVR-reducing effects.

Obstruction of pulmonary or systemic venous return can occur after atrial baffle (Mustard or Senning) repairs. Systemic venous obstruction will produce evidence of systemic venous congestion and a measurable gradient between a catheter located in the SVC and one in the RA. Pulmonary venous obstruction may result in pulmonary venous and pulmonary arterial hypertension, pulmonary edema, and hypoxemia. Efforts to reduce SVR will reduce the RV afterload and help prevent tricuspid regurgitation. Therapy for atrial dysrhythmias also may be necessary. Echocardiography can help assess the presence of pulmonary or systemic venous obstruction, as well as atrial baffle leaks; any of these will require surgical revision if significant.

After the arterial switch procedure, there may be extensive bleeding from the aortic and pulmonary suture lines. Clotting factors (see later) and avoidance of hypertension are indicated. Myocardial ischemia after reimplantation of the coronary arteries is a potential and not infrequent problem after the ASO. In some circumstances, ischemia is caused by coronary air emboli and is transient. Maintenance of high perfusion pressures on CPB after aortic cross-clamp removal can promote distal migration and eventual dissipation of coronary air emboli. Echocardiography can help ensure adequate de-airing of the left atrium and ventricle prior to separating from CPB. It can also detect and distinguish between regional (i.e., potentially due to coronary insufficiency) and global (more likely due to ischemia–reperfusion injury) myocardial dysfunction and assess the presence of flow in the proximal portions of the reimplanted coronary arteries.

Evidence of myocardial ischemia after coronary reimplantation should be treated aggressively and should prompt immediate reevaluation of the anastomoses as well as the possibility of coronary kinking or external coronary compression by clot or hemostatic packing material. Such evidence is typically in the form of focal ECG abnormalities such as S-T/T wave changes, but it can also include various dysrhythmias and forms of AV block. Kinking of a reimplanted artery or obstruction of the implanted coronary ostia is likely to require immediate surgical intervention. If the quality of the repair is good and it was accomplished relatively swiftly (i.e., to limit myocardial ischemia–reperfusion damage), then it is unusual to require significant inotropic support or artificial pacing (for anything other than a relative sinus bradycardia) or experience much in the way of ECG abnormalities, dysrhythmias, or AV block. On the other hand, the need for AV pacing, the occurrence of dysrhythmias, or the need for unexpected degrees of vasoactive support (e.g., epinephrine) should lead to a search for a technical problem.

A sequence of LV dilation both initiating and exacerbating myocardial ischemia can occur in D-TGA patients after the ASO. Myocardial ischemia, afterload mismatch, or excessive volume infusion can result in LV distention and LA hypertension. This is particularly likely if there is mitral insufficiency from either (ischemic) papillary muscle dysfunction or dilation of the mitral valve annulus. LV distention may result in tension on and kinking of the coronary reanastomosis sites. LA hypertension produces elevations in pulmonary artery pressure and distention of the pulmonary artery. Because the LeCompte maneuver brings the distal pulmonary artery anterior to the ascending aorta, distention of the pulmonary artery may actually compress or place tension on the coronary ostia. The resulting myocardial ischemia produces further LV dilation, progressive elevations in LA and pulmonary artery pressures, and continuing compromise of coronary blood flow.

In some TGA patients, the LV may have limited ability to support the systemic circulation after the ASO. This may occur as the result of myocardial ischemia, inadequate LV mass, poor protection of the LV during aortic cross-clamping, or a combination thereof. Echocardiography can be useful in identifying both global and regional LV systolic dysfunction. It also detects mitral regurgitation, which may occur secondary to papillary muscle dysfunction or to dilation of the mitral valve annulus. Inotropic support of the LV and afterload reduction may be necessary to terminate CPB. Initial inotropic support is accomplished with dopamine (3 to 10 mcg/kg per minute). In rare instances when LV failure (that, again, has been proven not to be the result of a coronary problem) is severe, epinephrine (0.05 to 0.5 mcg/kg per minute) may have to be added. Milrinone (0.25 to 1.0 mcg/kg per minute after a 50-mcg/kg loading dose) can be a useful agent based on its inodilator properties (Hoffman et al., 2002, 2003). These patients are at particular risk for LV dysfunction in the immediate postoperative period secondary to afterload mismatch (insufficient contractility for the degree of systemic afterload). Although the vasodilation that accompanies milrinone administration in infants is substantially less than that seen in adult patients, it is nonetheless advisable to administer the loading dose of milrinone over 10 to 15 minutes or longer.

Truncus Arteriosus

Anatomy

A single great vessel arising from the base of the heart and giving rise to the pulmonary, coronary, and systemic arteries characterizes truncus arteriosus (Figs. 20-16 and 20-17). See related video online at www.expertconsult.com. There is a single semilunar valve, which is usually abnormal, and invariably a large (nonrestrictive) conoventricular septal VSD is present. The truncus straddles this large VSD (see Fig. 20-16). Truncus arteriosus is classified based on the origin of the pulmonary

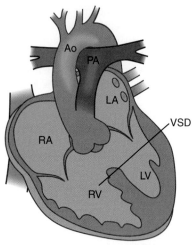

■ **FIGURE 20-16.** Anatomy of truncus arteriosus. Type 1 truncus arteriosus is illustrated here with a short pulmonary trunk arising from the truncus. There is a large conoventricular septal defect with truncal override. *(Redrawn from Children's Hospital Boston, Boston, Mass.)*

arteries. In type 1, a short pulmonary trunk originates from the truncus and gives rise to both pulmonary arteries. In type 2, both pulmonary arteries arise from a common orifice of the truncus, whereas in type 3, the right and left pulmonary arteries arise separately from the lateral aspect of the truncus. The VSD is usually of the infundibular or perimembranous infundibular type. The truncal valve is tricuspid in most patients, but multiple cusps (four to seven) are common, and the valve itself may be regurgitant or stenotic. Extracardiac anomalies are seen in approximately 30% of patients.

Physiology

Truncus arteriosus is a single-ventricle-physiology lesion amenable to a two-ventricle repair. The large (nonrestrictive) VSD allows equalization of pressures in the right and left ventricles. As a result, there is bidirectional shunting and complete mixing of systemic and pulmonary venous blood in a functionally common ventricular chamber. This blood is then ejected into the truncal root, which gives rise to the pulmonary, systemic, and coronary circulations. As with all simple shunts, $\dot{Q}p:\dot{Q}s$ is

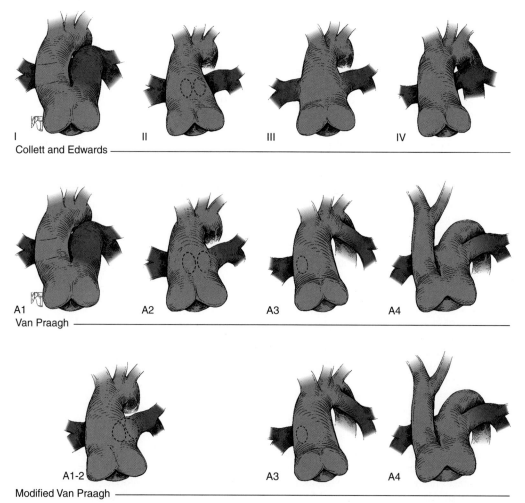

■ **FIGURE 20-17.** Truncus arteriosus. There are similarities between the Collett and Edwards and the Van Praagh classifications of truncus arteriosus. Type I is the same as A1. Types II and III are grouped as a single type A2, because they are not significantly distinct embryologically or therapeutically. Type A3 denotes a unilateral pulmonary artery with a collateral supply to the contralateral lung. Type A4 is truncus arteriosus associated with interrupted aortic arch (13% of all cases of truncus arteriosus). *(From Mavroudis C, Backer CL, editors:* Pediatric cardiac surgery, *Stamford, Conn, 1999, Appleton & Lange, p 340.)*

determined by the ratio of PVR to SVR. However, in truncus arteriosus, the pulmonary and systemic circulations are supplied in parallel from a single vessel, and for a given ventricular output, increases in flow to one circulatory system will produce reductions in flow to the other.

As with all single-ventricle lesions, a low $\dot{Q}_P{:}\dot{Q}_S$ reduces arterial saturation, whereas a high $\dot{Q}_P{:}\dot{Q}_S$ produces ventricular volume overload without a substantial increase in arterial saturation. Shortly after birth, the balance of PVR and SVR is such that pulmonary blood flow is high and the patient with truncus arteriosus has symptoms of CHF with mild cyanosis. After cardiac reserve has been exhausted, further decreases in PVR increase pulmonary blood flow at the expense of systemic and coronary perfusion. This produces a progressive metabolic acidosis. If truncal valve insufficiency is present, it imposes an additional volume load on the ventricles. Given the high pulmonary blood flow and the transmission of systemic arterial pressures to the pulmonary vasculature present in this lesion, development of PVOD is rapid. With development of PVOD comes a progressive decrease in pulmonary blood flow relative to systemic blood flow, and progressive hypoxemia.

Surgical Therapy

Because of the risk for early development of PVOD, surgical intervention in the first months of life is undertaken. Definitive repair of truncus arteriosus requires patch closure of the VSD, detachment of the pulmonary arteries from the truncus, and establishment of right-ventricular-to-pulmonary-artery continuity with a valved homograft. The RV-to-PA conduit requires placement of the proximal end of the conduit over a ventriculotomy in the RV free wall. The truncal valves must be assessed at the time of surgery. In some instances, valve repair or replacement is necessary to address valvular insufficiency or stenosis. Valvuloplasty is preferred over valve replacement. Valve replacement in a child necessitates subsequent replacements as the child grows. Management of the systemic anticoagulation necessary with a mechanical valve is also difficult in growing children. The RV-to-PA valved conduit eventually requires replacement as the child grows.

Anesthetic Management

These patients are managed according to the principles described later (see Hypoplastic Left Heart Syndrome and Single-Ventricle Physiology). This is a non–ductal-dependent lesion.

Post-CPB Management

Some degree of RV dysfunction is likely to exist because of the presence of a ventriculotomy and a large VSD patch. This is particularly problematic in patients with high PVR or early PVOD. Left ventricular volume overload may occur secondary to truncal valve insufficiency. The goals of management include maintenance of heart rate (preferably sinus rhythm) at an age-appropriate rate, as cardiac output is likely to be more heart rate dependent in the post-CPB period. PVR should be reduced when necessary through ventilatory interventions. Inotropic support of the left and right ventricles may be necessary for the reasons addressed previously.

Hypoplastic Left Heart Syndrome and Single-Ventricle Physiology

HLHS is characterized by hypoplasia of all left heart structures, and it is an example of single-ventricle physiology with ductal-dependent systemic blood flow. See related video online at www.expertconsult.com. In the most severe form, mitral and aortic atresia with hypoplasia of the left atrium, left ventricle, ascending aorta, and aortic arch (including coarctation) is present. Distal aortic blood flow occurs via the PDA. Proximal aortic blood flow and coronary blood flow occur by retrograde filling of a tiny ascending aorta via the PDA (Figs. 20-18 and 20-19). There is complete mixing of pulmonary venous and systemic venous blood in a single ventricle, which is connected in parallel to both the pulmonary and systemic circulations. Systemic blood flow is dependent on a PDA. Survival depends on a balance between systemic ($\dot{Q}_S$) and pulmonary ($\dot{Q}_P$) blood flow, because both circulations are supplied from the right ventricle in parallel. The major determinant of the distribution of $\dot{Q}_S$ and $\dot{Q}_P$ is their relative systemic and pulmonary vascular resistances (Barron et al., 2009).

The primary goal in the management of patients with HLHS, as for all patients with single-ventricle physiology, is optimization of systemic oxygen delivery and perfusion pressure. This is necessary if end-organ (myocardial, renal, hepatic, splanchnic) ischemia and injury are to be prevented. This goal is achieved by balancing the systemic and pulmonary circulations (Table 20-4). The term *balanced circulation* is used because both laboratory and clinical investigations have demonstrated that maximal systemic oxygen delivery (the product of systemic oxygen content and systemic blood flow) is achieved for a given single-ventricle

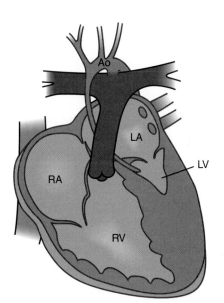

■ FIGURE 20-18. Anatomy of hypoplastic left heart syndrome (HLHS). There is severe mitral stenosis or mitral atresia, left ventricular hypoplasia, aortic valve atresia or severe stenosis, and hypoplasia of the ascending aorta (Asc. Ao) and transverse aortic arch. Pulmonary and systemic blood flows are both delivered via the right ventricle (*RV*). Aortic blood flow is provided via a large ductus arteriosus. There is antegrade flow from the patent ductus arteriosus to the descending aorta (Desc. Ao), and retrograde flow to the proximal aortic arch and cerebral circulation. The coronary arteries receive retrograde perfusion via the tiny ascending aorta. The left ventricle (*LV*) is diminutive. *(Redrawn from Children's Hospital Boston, Boston, Mass.)*

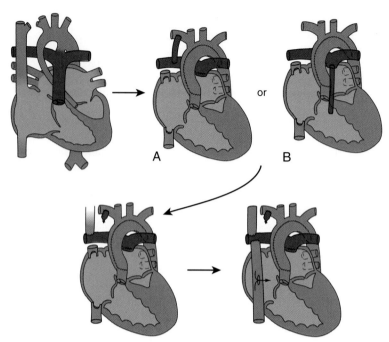

■ **FIGURE 20-19.** Sequence of repairs in the surgical staging of hypoplastic left heart syndrome (HLHS) to a fenestrated lateral-tunnel Fontan. *Upper left:* HLHS. *Upper right A:* Initial repair performed shortly after birth involving atrial septectomy, Damus-Kaye-Stansel (DKS) anastomosis of main pulmonary artery to ascending aorta, homograft augmentation of the aortic arch, and a right modified Blalock-Taussig shunt (BTS) to supply pulmonary blood flow. *Upper right B:* Alternate initial repair performed shortly after birth involving atrial septectomy, DKS anastomosis of main pulmonary artery to ascending aorta, homograft augmentation of the aortic arch, and a right ventricle–to–pulmonary artery conduit to supply pulmonary blood flow. *Lower left:* Superior cavopulmonary shunt or bidirectional Glenn (BDG), generally performed at 6 to 8 months of age. The right modified BTS has been taken down and ligated. *Lower right:* The completed total cavopulmonary connection or Fontan procedure generally performed at 2 to 3 years of age. A lateral-tunnel Fontan with a fenestration is shown. The *small arrows* indicate flow from the systemic venous baffle to the common pulmonary venous atrium, causing a small right-to-left physiologic shunt.

TABLE 20-4. Effects on Aortic and Mixed Venous Saturation of Pulmonary and Systemic Blood Flows in Patients with Single-Ventricle Physiology

Aortic Saturation (%)	Svo_2 (mm Hg)	$\dot{Q}P$:$\dot{Q}S$	Clinical Considerations
80	55	1:1	Balanced shunt
85	55	2:1	Mild reduction in systemic flow
90	55	4:1	Severe reduction in systemic flow
70	45	1:2	Mild reduction in pulmonary flow
70	70	1:4	Severe reduction in pulmonary flow
80	50	2:1	Decreased cardiac output, increased $\dot{Q}P$
80	30	>2:1	Decreased cardiac output, increased $\dot{Q}P$

$\dot{Q}P$, Pulmonary blood flow; $\dot{Q}S$, systemic blood flow.

output when $\dot{Q}P$:$\dot{Q}S$ is at or just below 1:1. Increases in $\dot{Q}P$:$\dot{Q}S$ in excess of 1:1 are associated with a progressive decrease in systemic oxygen delivery because the subsequent increase in systemic oxygen content is more than offset by the progressive decrease in systemic blood flow. There will be inadequate systemic oxygen delivery (systemic venous desaturation, a wide

difference in systemic arterial and superior vena caval oxygen saturation [Sa-vo_2], metabolic acidosis) and low perfusion pressure in the presence of a seemingly high arterial saturation of 85% to 90%. Decreases in $\dot{Q}P$:$\dot{Q}S$ below 1:1 are associated with a precipitous decrease in systemic oxygen delivery because the subsequent increase in systemic blood flow is more than offset by the dramatic decrease in systemic oxygen content. There will be inadequate systemic oxygen delivery (arterial and venous desaturation, metabolic acidosis) in the presence of a seemingly adequate arterial blood pressure. In either case, circulatory collapse will ultimately occur.

Treatment

Treatment can begin with interventions that temporarily stabilize the single-ventricle circulation in neonates, including PGE_1 infusion to maintain systemic perfusion via the ductus arteriosus. A balloon atrial septostomy may be performed if there is clinical and echocardiographic evidence of left atrial hypertension and significant restriction of circulatory mixing at the atrial level; however, a modest degree of restriction is felt by many to be desirable as it may help limit the tendency to pulmonary overcirculation (by maintaining a degree of left atrial hypertension) that can occur in these patients in the initial postnatal days while awaiting surgery. Usual management consists of spontaneous ventilation in room air and PGE_1 infusion prior to stage I palliative surgery. Inotropic agents may be required in some to support cardiac output and systemic perfusion. The use of different inspired gas mixtures to balance the single-ventricle circulation and in particular to improve systemic oxygen delivery remains fairly controversial (Tabbutt et al., 2001; Li et al., 2008; Barron et al., 2009).

Surgical correction of HLHS begins with a palliative procedure that eliminates the need for continued patency of the ductus arteriosus. This stage 1 procedure is performed during the first several days to a week of life using CPB in conjunction with 40 to 60 minutes of deep hypothermic circulatory arrest or low-flow selective cerebral perfusion during reconstruction of the aortic arch (see later) (Edwards et al., 2007; Pigula et al., 2007; Reemtsen et al., 2007; Silva et al., 2007). The procedures necessary are outlined in Figure 20-19. The first stage essentially consists of establishing unimpeded flow of venous return from both the systemic and pulmonary circulations into the right ventricle and then into the aorta and creating a stable conduit for pulmonary blood flow. In practice, this requires a freely patent atrial septum (an atrial septectomy is often necessary), a functioning tricuspid valve, construction of a proximal pulmonary artery–ascending aorta end-to-side anastomosis (the Damus-Kaye-Stansel procedure), so that the combined venous return is ejected by the right ventricle into the aorta, and reconstruction and enlargement of the aortic arch (using both the proximal pulmonary artery and homograft material. The distal PA is oversewn and the PDA ligated. Pulmonary blood flow is established via either a modified BT shunt (the proximal insertion of which is typically into the innominate artery) or an RV-PA conduit (the Sano modification). The completed stage 1 procedure leaves the infant with single-ventricle physiology.

Management of Anesthesia

Management of anesthesia is as described for patients with single-ventricle physiology (Box 20-4, and see earlier). An intravenous induction using a high-dosage synthetic narcotic technique in combination with a muscle relaxant is recommended. A benzodiazepine (usually midazolam) can be added as tolerated. Inhalation agents are generally poorly tolerated. Pancuronium is normally used. However, in patients with a low aortic diastolic blood pressure and a high baseline heart rate, consideration should be given to using one of the muscle relaxants that do not affect heart rate, such as vecuronium or rocuronium, so as to avoid iatrogenic subendocardial ischemia.

Post-CPB management is as summarized in Box 20-5. The major pathophysiologic perturbations after CPB include hypoxemia, hypotension, low systemic perfusion, difficulties with gas exchange, and significant bleeding (extensive suture lines and coagulopathy from hemodilution, hypothermia, coagulation factor and platelet consumption due to profuse bleeding [see Bleeding after Pediatric Cardiopulmonary Bypass]). End-organ injury, the result of CPB effects, preoperative or post-CPB hypoperfusion, and DHCA or selective perfusion strategies, is also relatively common, with myocardial, renal, and cerebral dysfunction and damage predominating (Mahle and Wernovsky, 2004; Wernovsky, 2007; Ohye et al., 2009; Aiyagari et al., 2010).

Myocardial dysfunction contributing to a low systemic cardiac output state is relatively common after stage I HLHS repairs. Given adequate filling pressures (common atrial pressure of ~8 to 15 mm Hg), dopamine (5 to 15 mcg/kg per minute) and at times α-agonist doses of epinephrine (0.03 to 0.05 mcg/kg per minute) may be necessary. The need for artificial pacing (for other than a relative sinus bradycardia), the presence of ST-T wave changes or dysrhythmias, or the need for substantially greater degrees

---

> ### Box 20-4 Goals of Anesthesia Management for Single-Ventricle (SV) Physiology before Cardiopulmonary Bypass
>
> 1. A continuous infusion of PGE_1 is used to maintain ductal patency in patients with ductal dependent blood flow (either systemic or pulmonary).
> 2. A target Pao_2 of 40 to 45 mm Hg and an Sao_2 of 70% to 80% are associated with adequate systemic O_2 delivery.
> 3. In SV patients with unrestricted pulmonary blood flow,
>   - -PVR manipulation is essential and $\dot{Q}p:\dot{Q}s$ is accomplished, most reliably with ventilatory interventions.
>   - -Hypercarbia in combination with a 21% Fio_2, and normocarbia in combination with a 17% Fio_2 (inspired N_2), is used to increase PVR and reduce $\dot{Q}p:\dot{Q}s$.
> 4. Hypercarbia ($Paco_2$ of 45 to 55 mm Hg) can be achieved with alveolar hypoventilation or with increased inspired CO_2 (3% $Fico_2$).
> 5. Avoid a high Fio_2 unless the Pao_2 is less than 35 to 40 mm Hg.
> 6. Because ventilatory interventions are incapable of reducing $\dot{Q}p:\dot{Q}s$ much below 2:1, increased cardiac output is often necessary to ensure adequate systemic oxygen delivery and coronary perfusion pressure.
>   - -Increased stroke volume with preload augmentation, limited
>   - -Increased heart rate (>140-150 bpm) can cause myocardial ischemia in patients with aortic diastolic blood pressures in the range of 20 to 30 mm Hg.
>   - -Inotropic support may be necessary
> 7. After sternotomy, the surgeon can limit pulmonary blood flow and reduce $\dot{Q}p:\dot{Q}s$ with a vessel loop around a PA (usually the right).
> 8. Infants with SV physiology who arrive in the operating room unintubated from the ICU have a balanced circulation, but after induction, intubation and mechanical lung expansion, these patients may have a precipitous decrease in PVR and immediate compromise of systemic circulation.
>
> *Fico₂*, Fraction of inspired CO_2; *Fio₂*, fraction of inspired oxygen; *ICU*, intensive care unit; *Pao₂*, arterial oxygen tension; *PGE₁*, prostaglandin E_1; *PVR*, pulmonary vascular resistance; *$\dot{Q}P:\dot{Q}S$*, ratio of pulmonary-to-systemic blood flow; *Sao₂*, arterial oxygen saturation of hemoglobin.

---

of vasoactive support should prompt consideration of potential technical problems with the repair (e.g., coronary insufficiency arising from the construction of the Stansel anastomosis).

In a somewhat oversimplified and artificial fashion, one can describe three general clinical situations in the post-CPB period after stage I repairs:

1. Too much PBF, or shunt too large. This is characterized by higher-than-expected arterial oxygen saturations (90% or higher), frequently in combination with low systolic and particularly diastolic blood pressure, systemic hypoperfusion, acidosis, and oliguria; ECG evidence of ischemia may also be present if of sufficient magnitude. This is perhaps the least common of the three because of the current use of smaller shunts placed more distally on the innominate artery. Although ventilatory maneuvers to increase PVR (e.g., hypoventilation, added inspired CO_2, or adding N_2 to create a hypoxic gas mixture [17% to 18% O_2]) or increased levels of inotropic support can be attempted, usually narrowing of the shunt is required.

Box 20-5 Anesthetic Management of Single-Ventricle Physiology after Cardiopulmonary Bypass (CPB)

1. After CPB, high PVR, reduced pulmonary blood flow, and hypoxemia (Pao₂ < 40 mm Hg) are common.
2. The modified Blalock-Taussig shunt or RV-PA conduit may be too large (resulting in pulmonary overcirculation and systemic hypoperfusion) or too small (inadequate pulmonary blood flow, excessive cyanosis) for prevailing physiologic conditions.
3. Ventricular dysfunction may exist. Low venous oxygen saturation may contribute to increased arterial desaturation, which can further exacerbate myocardial dysfunction.
4. Myocardial and tissue edema may be significant and preclude chest closure.
5. Bleeding may be significant.
6. Inhaled pulmonary vasodilators such as NO may be necessary to improve Sao₂ or reduce the transpulmonary gradient in these patients. This is particularly true in the subgroup of patients who have repair of partially obstructed pulmonary venous drainage at the time of their initial repair, and perhaps those with left atrial hypertension (e.g., restrictive atrial septum) prior to surgery.

NO, Nitric oxide; *PA,* pulmonary artery; *Pao₂,* arterial oxygen tension; *PVR,* pulmonary vascular resistance; *RV,* right ventricle; *Sao₂,* arterial oxygen saturation of hemoglobin.

2. Too little PBF or shunt too small. These patients display arterial oxygen saturations substantially lower than expected, often with normal or even elevated systemic blood pressures and perfusion (if myocardial performance is adequate). Causes include insufficient shunt diameter, narrowing at the proximal or distal insertion sites, more distal PA narrowing, increased intrinsic pulmonary vascular resistance, and lung disease (resulting from CPB or preoperative overcirculation or other processes). In the absence of technical difficulties or mechanical obstruction, maneuvers that decrease PVR, improve ventilation, or increase systemic arterial blood pressure and cardiac output can be attempted.

3. Low arterial oxygen saturation or low systemic blood pressure. This may be the most common symptom complex in most institutions, and it can be the most difficult to sort out. Some degree of myocardial injury occurs in all of these patients; significant myocardial dysfunction leads to low cardiac output, low shunt perfusion, and reduced venous oxygen saturation, which, taken together, result in low oxygenation. Alternatively, poor oxygenation (see #2) in at least some patients (perhaps including those who were not particularly cyanotic preoperatively and hence have less myocardial tolerance to reduced saturations postoperatively) results in compromised myocardial function, which then follows the low cardiac output scenario just described. Measuring SVC saturation can be helpful in making this determination, as a value that is more than about 25 saturation points lower than the arterial value (e.g., an SVC saturation of 25% when the arterial is 68% equals 43 saturation points) is indicative of some contribution of low oxygen delivery to the reduced arterial oxygen saturation. Echocardiography and measuring the saturation of pulmonary venous blood can at times be helpful in delineating myocardial versus pulmonary etiology. From a practical standpoint (once the possibility of

technical problems has been eliminated), treatment begins with ensuring appropriate ventilation parameters, oxygen-carrying capacity (hematocrit of 35% to 40%), and optimizing cardiac output (adequate filling, ionized calcium, and inotropic support) and arterial blood pressure (to ensure adequate PBF via the shunt).

The major differences between a BT and Sano-type shunt in the immediate postoperative period relate to these types of interactions between RV function, RV output, PBF, and oxygenation. In both situations, systemic and pulmonary blood flows and oxygenation are governed by RV function and output and the balance of SVR:PVR (with PVR affected by factors related to shunt- and lung-based resistances; the Sano, for example, is a wider [5 mm versus 3.5 mm] but substantially longer shunt). However, a major physiologic difference in the Sano is that there is no diastolic runoff from the aorta into the lungs. As a result, for a given degree of RV output, blood pressures (particularly diastolic) tend to be higher in the Sano than in the BT shunt patients, with resultant benefits to coronary perfusion and perhaps myocardial performance. Comparisons of the two types of shunts with regard to death, cardiac transplantation, cardiovascular interventions, and RV size and function have been reported in a large multicenter randomized study. Although transplantation-free survival at 12 months was better with an RV-to-PA shunt, after 12 months the difference between the two groups was not significant (Ohye et al., 2010). Questions about longer-term complications such as greater propensity to shunt and pulmonary artery narrowing and increased cyanosis, and perhaps RV dysfunction (perhaps at least in part due to the right ventriculotomy's being more prevalent after the Sano modification) are under study (Ohye et al., 2010).

Hybrid Procedure

The stage 1 hybrid procedure for HLHS is an alternative to the Norwood stage I procedure with either a modified BT shunt or an RV-to-PA conduit (Sano modification). The hybrid procedure obviates the need for CPB and the associated use of either DHCA or antegrade cerebral perfusion (ACP) in the neonate. This procedure must be done in a location (the hybrid operating room) that provides full cardiac catheterization infrastructure, including biplane cardioangiography, in a sterile operating room environment. The procedure (see Fig. 21-13 in Chapter 21, Congenital Cardiac Anesthesia: Non-Bypass Procedures) involves off-pump placement of a bare metallic stent in the ductus arteriosus, bilateral pulmonary artery banding, and dilation/stenting of the intraatrial septum. The balloon atrial septostomy is generally performed prior to discharge from the hospital unless there is obstruction of pulmonary venous blood delivery to the right ventricle and pulmonary venous hypertension detected earlier. The physiologic burden associated with CPB and DHCA or ACP avoided in the first stage is then incurred at the time of the comprehensive stage 2 (bidirectional Glenn [BDG] shunt, Stansel anastomosis, aortic arch reconstruction, and definitive atrial septectomy) performed at 3 to 6 months of age.

Superior Cavopulmonary Shunt or Bidirectional Glenn

Glenn's original description of a superior vena caval shunt was an end-to-side anastomosis of the cranial end of the transected superior vena cava to the distal end of the transected right pulmonary artery (RPA) performed through a right thoracotomy without the use of CPB. Both the proximal SVC and the RPA were oversewn. The current modified BDG procedure anastomoses the cranial end of the transected SVC in an end-to-side fashion to the RPA (which is left in continuity with the main and left PAs); the cardiac end of the SVC is oversewn. This creates SVC continuity with both the left and right pulmonary arteries and bidirectional pulmonary blood flow (i.e., the BDG directs systemic venous blood from the SVC directly into the pulmonary circulation). The BDG procedure is usually performed with the patient on CPB, and through a median sternotomy. If there were prior palliative procedures, the aortopulmonary shunt is ligated or the PA band taken down. The azygos vein is usually ligated so that the SVC does not decompress retrograde to the IVC, thereby reducing the quantity of blood delivered to the PAs (unless, e.g., the IVC is interrupted with azygous continuation, as occurs in frequently in patients with heterotaxy syndrome and some others). Normally, all upper extremity and cerebral venous return drains via the SVC. In some patients (particularly those with heterotaxy syndrome), there may be bilateral SVCs that are not in continuity via a connecting vein. In this case, a bilateral BDG must be done with one SVC anastomosed in an end-to-side fashion to the RPA and the other SVC anastomosed in an end-to-side fashion to the LPA.

The BDG is normally undertaken at about 3 to 8 months of age, at which point the PVR has decreased sufficiently such that systemic venous pressure (SVC pressure) is sufficient to drive pulmonary blood flow. Patients who have outgrown their PA band, their modified BT shunt, or their RV-to-PA conduit (as in the Sano-type stage I HLHS operation), or those who have a low Sao_2, as well as those who are not tolerating the additional volume load on their ventricle because of a loose PA band or large modified BT shunt, frequently undergo BDG at the earlier end of the spectrum.

There are physiologic differences between an aortopulmonary shunt and a BDG. Effective pulmonary blood flow in the aortopulmonary shunt and BDG circulations are essentially equal. However, for a given cardiac output, Sao_2, $Spvo_2$, and Svo_2, the volume load on the systemic ventricle is twice as large with an aortopulmonary shunt as it is with a BDG. This is because in the aortopulmonary shunt circulation there is recirculated pulmonary blood (physiologic L-R shunt), whereas in the BDG circulation there is no recirculated pulmonary blood flow. As a result, a child with a BDG will have the same Sao_2 as a child with an aortopulmonary shunt (typically in the range of 80% to 85%) but with a significant reduction in the volume load on the systemic ventricle.

Part of the confusion with these procedures arises from the large number of nomenclature and procedural modifications, many of which have been devised to simplify subsequent conversion to a Fontan. The *hemi-Fontan* is a procedure in which an atriopulmonary anastomosis is constructed between the dome of the right atrium at the RA/SVC junction and the inferior surface of the right pulmonary artery. A Gore-Tex baffle or plug is used to supplement the central pulmonary artery area and to isolate the cavopulmonary connection from the RA. Another modification involves creation of a double cavopulmonary anastomosis. The cranial end of the divided SVC is anastomosed to the superior surface of the RPA. The cardiac end of the divided SVC is anastomosed to the inferior surface of the RPA. The internal orifice of the SVC is closed with a Gore-Tex patch.

Anesthetic Management before BDG

The principles outlined previously regarding the management of single-ventricle physiology apply here, with some modifications. Most important, by the age of 3 to 8 months, when these infants present for BDG, they have generally grown and gained weight so that their $\dot{Q}P:\dot{Q}s$ is less likely to be (or to become) excessive—typically between 1.0:1 and 1.5:1. As a result, these patients are much less likely to develop an excess of pulmonary blood flow and hence compromised systemic O_2 delivery due to anesthetic induction and positive pressure ventilation (unless they are in the smaller subset being done early for excessive PBF and systemic ventricular volume overload). On the other hand, infants who have outgrown (or who have developed a narrowed shunt or RV-PA conduit) and thus have limited PBF and are more cyanotic as a result are at risk for significantly reduced PBF and arterial oxygen saturations if systemic ventricular cardiac output and SVR (the driving forces for flow through the narrowed or obstructed conduit) fall. As discussed previously, their baseline oxygen saturation is a reasonably good (albeit physiologically somewhat simplistic) indicator of which of the two general categories (pulmonary overcirculation versus limited PBF) they belong in.

In either case, an IV induction is generally preferred. Vascular access may be difficult, as many require prolonged ICU stays and other procedures (e.g., catheterizations, gastrostomy tubes) after the initial repair. In addition, some of these patients appear tolerant to opioids and benzodiazepines after their ICU stay. This should be considered if premedication is planned prior to IV placement. Once an IV line is in place, volume expansion (crystalloid or 5% albumin) is a reasonable consideration prior to induction. Induction techniques that favor prompt and reliable airway control as well as hemodynamic stability are preferable to ones associated with decreased myocardial contractility or SVR (e.g., propofol). Patients with significant ventricular dysfunction, ventricular volume overload, or critically narrowed sources of PBF may also benefit from the inclusion of inotropic support as part of the induction regimen.

Post-CPB Management of BDG Patients

The success of this circulation and the resultant arterial oxygen saturation depend not only on a technically satisfactory anastomosis but also on a number of hemodynamic and related parameters. The SVC return needs to flow unimpeded and at sufficient pressure to traverse the pulmonary vascular bed, where mechanical and intrinsic resistance must be low, followed by unimpeded egress via the pulmonary veins (here again without mechanical obstruction or increased pulmonary venous tone) to fill the common systemic ventricular atrium, traverse a nonstenotic, nonregurgitant atrioventricular valve, and fill a well-functioning systemic ventricle (for example, the mitral valve and LV in the case of tricuspid atresia, the tricuspid valve and RV in HLHS). It is therefore critical to maintain heart rate and sinus rhythm, contractility, and appropriate preload so as to maintain cardiac output. Decreases in cardiac output reduce IVC saturation; IVC and pulmonary venous blood mix in a common atrium, which will reduce arterial saturation.

A central line located in the internal jugular vein will measure SVC pressure (which also equals mean pulmonary artery pressure [mPAP] after a BDG). A surgically placed atrial catheter will measure common atrial pressure (a common atrium exists because of the large atrial septectomy). The difference between these two pressure measurements (SVC [or internal jugular] pressure and the common atrial pressure) is the transpulmonary gradient (TPG). A TPG of about 6 to 10 mm Hg is the norm in terms of driving adequate PBF and filling of the downstream systemic ventricle. Thus, with a common atrial pressure of 6 to 10 mm Hg (the expectation in the presence of preserved ventricular function, adequate arterial blood pressure, and other evidence of adequate systemic cardiac output), the proximal pressure in the SVC will be in the range of 12 to 18 mm Hg. Hypoventilation, lung disease, or increased PVR can widen the TPG; thus, to obtain a comparable degree of ventricular filling and cardiac output, the SVC pressure must increase (either by exogenous volume administration or by activation of adrenal and renal mechanisms that expand intravascular volume, which of course will be slower). Increased SVC pressure is also necessary to maintain preload and cardiac output in the case of systemic ventricular dysfunction. Here, the TPG is likely to be relatively normal (6 to 10 mm Hg), but the higher ventricular end-diastolic pressure (e.g., 12 to 16 mm Hg) results in an SVC pressure of 18 to 26 mm Hg to achieve comparable cardiac output.

In addition to adequate preload, inotropic support of the systemic ventricle may be necessary because of ventricular dysfunction induced by chronic volume overload, prior injury, and the acute effects of CPB and ischemia–reperfusion injury. Typically, dopamine (3 to 5 mcg/kg per minute, occasionally as high as 10 mcg/kg per minute) is used. Milrinone (0.25 to 0.5 mcg/kg per minute, at times up to 1.0 mcg/kg per minute) can benefit this circulation, although others reserve it for use in combination with dopamine or for patients who have hypertension or poor perfusion in the face of normal or elevated blood pressure.

In general, normocarbia should be the goal of post-CPB ventilatory management. Hypoventilation and atelectasis can compromise pulmonary blood flow and consequently systemic ventricular filling and cardiac output. High mean airway pressure will mechanically limit nonpulsatile pulmonary blood flow, thereby impairing it. After construction of the Glenn anastomosis, there is an acute increase in SVC pressure and presumably in intracranial pressure. The volume load reduction and elevated SVC pressure are believed to contribute to the (reflex) systemic hypertension and postoperative irritability that is commonly seen in these patients. The majority of pulmonary blood flow is supplied via venous blood from the brain, which is the largest single source of venous drainage from the upper body. Hyperventilation and hypocarbia, although beneficial in reducing PVR, also reduce cerebral blood flow (CBF) and cerebral venous drainage. Maintaining normocarbia after BDG has been demonstrated to provide maximal $\dot{Q}P:\dot{Q}S$ and Sao_2. These patients tend to have a large end-tidal-CO_2–$Paco_2$ gradient because of increased physiologic dead space. An increased portion of the lungs in these patients is ventilated but not perfused because of the low PA driving pressure (SVC pressure). Thus, mean airway pressure should be kept at the minimal level that is compatible with delivery of an adequate tidal volume and normal lung expansion. This can usually be accomplished with a relatively large tidal volume (10 to 12 mL/kg), slow respiratory rates (10 to 15 breaths/min), and short inspiratory times (inspiratory-to-expiratory ratio of 1:3 or 1:4) positive end-expiratory pressure (PEEP) can be used beneficially (i.e., for maintenance of functional residual capacity and gas exchange) but with caution.

BDG patients have an Sao_2 of about 76% to 85%, similar to that prior to their shunt. However, their $\dot{Q}P:\dot{Q}S$ ranges from 0.5:1 to 0.8:1, and as a result there is an acute reduction in volume load on the systemic ventricle. The most likely cause of a low Sao_2 after a BDG is low cardiac output with a low IVC saturation. Comparison of the SVC and common atrial pressures, perhaps in combination with surface echocardiography or TEE, may help delineate the cause (e.g., primary ventricular dysfunction, hypovolemia, AV valve dysfunction). If a low Sao_2 persists despite optimization of filling status and ventricular function, other causes of reduced pulmonary blood flow should be considered, such as a stenotic anastomosis or the presence of decompressing veno-venous collaterals (typically from the SVC to the IVC, or the SVC to the pulmonary veins or left atrium).

Reduced pulmonary venous oxygen saturation ($Ppvo_2$) may also be a source of low Sao_2. Ventilatory maneuvers to reduce V/Q mismatch and intrapulmonary shunt should be done. A high Fio_2 may be necessary in the presence of significant V/Q mismatch. Response to inhaled pulmonary vasodilators such as inhaled NO can be variable; the BDG (and Fontan) patients most likely to respond with improvements in arterial oxygen saturation and apparent cardiac output usually have significantly elevated proximal venous or TPG pressures (>18 to 20, and >10 mm Hg, respectively) (Gamillscheg, 1997; Agarwal, 2006).

Definitive Repair: The Fontan Procedure or Total Cavopulmonary Connection

Fontan Physiology

The Fontan procedure is generally performed at 2 to 3 years of age, and it is typically the final staged correction after one of the aforementioned palliative single-ventricle operations. See related video online at www.expertconsult.com. Fontan physiology is a series ("normal") circulation that is characterized by one ventricle with sufficient diastolic, systolic, and atrioventricular valve function to support the systemic circulation. This ventricle must be in unobstructed continuity with the aorta and receive unobstructed pulmonary venous return. In addition, there must be unobstructed flow of systemic venous blood to the pulmonary circulation (total cavopulmonary continuity).

The Fontan procedure was first performed in 1968 and was initially described for patients with tricuspid atresia. The original version included a Glenn shunt, which drained the SVC into the distal right pulmonary artery. The proximal end of the right pulmonary artery was joined to the right atrial appendage via an aortic valve homograft, and a pulmonary valve homograft valve was placed at the IVC–RA junction. The main pulmonary artery was ligated and the ASD was closed. In subsequent early iterations, creation of the Glenn shunt and placement of homograft valves at the RA–PA and IVC–RA junctions were eliminated, resulting in creation of a direct atriopulmonary connection. Since that time, many additional modifications have been described, but the goals of the procedure remain the same: to deliver all systemic venous blood directly to the pulmonary arteries in the absence of a reservoir or ventricular pump. This requires total cavopulmonary connection that is created either directly or via the systemic venous atrium. The most commonly performed procedures now are the lateral tunnel and extracardiac Fontan procedures (see Figs. 20-4, 20-5, and 20-19).

The lateral tunnel procedure incorporates a small amount of systemic venous atrium in the cavopulmonary pathway, whereas the extracardiac procedure does not incorporate any atrial tissue. These procedures are referred to as total cavopulmonary connections. Experience with direct atriopulmonary connections suggested that elevated systemic venous pressure leads to progressive and severe atrial dilation (volumes as large as 300 to 500 mL). The massive dilated atrium was believed to contribute to stasis (and hence thromboembolism) as well as being a source of atrial arrhythmias. In theory, the extracardiac procedure may offer additional protection from development of atrial arrhythmias because of a lack of suture lines in the atrium.

In the absence of any residual physiologic intracardiac or intrapulmonary R-L shunting, these patients should have an essentially normal Sao_2 (it may be depressed 3% to 5% as a result of drainage of coronary venous blood via the coronary sinus into the systemic ventricle). Although it is often stated that pulmonary blood flow is passive and driven by the components of the TPG (systemic venous pressure > mean pulmonary artery pressure > pulmonary venous atrial pressure), the systemic ventricle generates the energy necessary to provide flow through the pulmonary capillary bed because the systemic vascular bed and pulmonary vascular bed are in continuity, without an intervening atrium and ventricle to provide reservoir and pumping capacity. As a result, the single ventricle in a series Fontan circulation is faced with higher afterload than the systemic ventricle in a two-ventricle series circulation. Additional circulatory abnormalities that may contribute to impaired ventricular function, exercise capacity, and altered hemodynamic behaviors (e.g., in response to blood loss, stress, or exercise) include increased arteriolar tone and venous capacitance, limited preload augmentation ability, limited ability to increase heart rate, increased resistance across the total cavopulmonary connection, and decreased diastolic compliance of the systemic ventricle (Ghanayem et al., 2007; Sundareswaran et al., 2008; Krishnan et al., 2009; Goldstein et al., 2010).

Absolute contraindications to the Fontan procedure typically include early infancy, PVR greater than 4 Wood units/m², severe pulmonary artery hypoplasia, systemic ventricular ejection fraction (EF) less than 25% to 30%, and a ventricular end-diastolic pressure greater than 20 to 25 mm Hg. Many coexisting lesions previously believed to be at least relative contraindications (e.g., AV valve regurgitation or stenosis, significantly narrowed or distorted pulmonary arteries) are now corrected at the time of the Fontan (or prior palliative) procedure.

The acute reduction of systemic ventricular volume that occurs in the univentricular heart as a result of transitioning directly from stage I to Fontan physiology results in impaired ventricular compliance because wall thickness does not regress as quickly as ventricular volume. The result is impaired ventricular diastolic function and elevated end-diastolic pressure. This will impede pulmonary venous return, which is a liability in the Fontan procedure, because it subsequently reduces pulmonary blood flow. A low cardiac output state results because systemic ventricular output can only equal the quantity of blood that transverses the pulmonary vascular bed. One reason for interposing a BDG procedure in the staged single-ventricle pathway is that it results in reduced morbidity and mortality as compared with moving directly from single-ventricle to Fontan physiology. Performing the BDG shunt at 3 to 6 months of age allows early reduction in the volume overload to the systemic ventricle that accompanies univentricular physiology and thereby promotes remodeling of the ventricle at lower end-diastolic volume. As noted previously, the impaired ventricular

diastolic function that accompanies acute ventricular volume reduction is better tolerated in BDG or hemi-Fontan physiology than in Fontan physiology. When there is impairment of pulmonary venous return after the BDG or hemi-Fontan, blood from the IVC will continue to provide systemic ventricular filling and cardiac output at a lower pressure than that required to traverse the pulmonary bed; similar conceptual thinking underlies the creation of a fenestration in the Fontan pathway (see Fenestrated Fontan, later).

One risk of the staged procedures is the development of pulmonary arteriovenous malformations, which develop as a result of diversion of hepatic venous blood flow to another capillary bed (the systemic) before delivery to the pulmonary capillary bed. This of course is the blood flow pattern in BDG patients, approximately 10% of whom will develop significant pulmonary arteriovenous malformations and resultant increased arterial desaturation. These lesions usually resolve after the BDG is converted to a Fontan, and when hepatic-to-pulmonary blood flow "continuity" is restored.

Fenestrated Fontan

In patients with Fontan physiology, increased impedance to systemic venous blood flow return through the pulmonary capillary bed results in decreased delivery of blood to the pulmonary venous atrium, systemic ventricle, and aorta, producing a low cardiac output state with a normal or near normal Sao_2 ("pink but poor cardiac output"). This increased impedance is not uncommon in the initial days and weeks after Fontan surgery. Attempts to increase cardiac output by increasing systemic venous pressure may result in the development of refractory pleural effusions and ascites but does not necessarily improve ventricular filling and cardiac output. In many institutions, a 4-mm hole or fenestration is intentionally left in the cavopulmonary pathway or baffle. This allows systemic venous blood to "pop off" into the pulmonary venous atrium and ultimately into the systemic ventricle and aorta. This physiologic R-L shunt allows maintenance of systemic cardiac output at the expense of Sao_2 ("blue with cardiac output"—preferable) This fenestration can be easily closed in the cardiac catheterization laboratory with an occlusion device at a later date after demonstration of adequate hemodynamics, gas exchange, and cardiac output, with balloon occlusion of the fenestration (Bridges et al., 1998). Other practitioners do not believe in the need for routine fenestration of the Fontan pathway to reduce morbidity (e.g., low cardiac output, increased pleural effusions, increased volume requirements) in the postoperative period; some find the use of extracardiac conduits or inhaled NO to achieve similar benefits (Thompson et al., 1999; Harada et al., 2009).

Anesthetic Management, Pre-Fontan

The principles outlined in the section on managing BDG physiology after CPB generally apply here. These patients are typically 2 to 3 years of age with a superior cavopulmonary (BDG) shunt, generally with a stable cardiovascular system. Arterial Sao_2 is 76% to 85% unless there are significant decompressing venous collateral vessels from the SVC to either the IVC or the pulmonary venous system. These are usually addressed by coil occlusion in the cardiac catheterization laboratory prior to the Fontan.

Although these patients might tolerate an inhalation induction from a cardiovascular standpoint, it should be recognized that several factors might make a pure inhalation induction difficult: (1) venous congestion of the head and tongue resulting from a relatively high SVC pressure; (2) coughing, breathholding, or any other cause of high intrathoracic pressure impeding pulmonary blood, resulting not only in hypoxemia but altered uptake and distribution; and (3) significantly delayed rate of inhalation induction than expected in the typical child with $\dot{Q}_P:\dot{Q}_S$ of 0.5:1 to 0.7:1. Based on these factors, an IV induction is preferred by many. Premedication should be considered, because these patients and their families generally have had multiple hospital exposures and procedures. In addition, many of these patients are tolerant to opioids and benzodiazepines after neonatal and subsequent exposure. Midazolam, 0.75 to 1.0 mg/kg orally (maximum dosage, 20 to 30 mg by mouth [PO]), alone or with ketamine, 3 to 6 mg/kg PO, is usually effective for sedation and allowing IV placement.

The key physiologic principle in patients with BDG or Fontan physiology is maintaining filling and function of the systemic ventricle. *Optimal* physiology depends on adequate preload, unobstructed systemic venous return, low PVR, low mean intrathoracic pressure, normal lung parenchymal and alveolar ventilation, unobstructed pulmonary venous return, sinus rhythm (primarily resulting from the atrial contribution to ventricular filling, normal atrioventricular valve function and competency, normal ventricular function, and low ventricular afterload. Any significant departure from these requirements can result in severe compromise. Thus, considerations for anesthetic induction and pre-CPB management include (1) ensuring adequate preload, (2) avoiding significant myocardial depression, and (3) preventing mechanical or metabolic events that significantly increase PVR, including excessive stress response, airway obstruction, hypoventilation, hypoxemia, hypercarbia, acidosis, atelectasis, and excessive intrathoracic pressure. From a practical standpoint, volume expansion (isotonic crystalloid or colloid) followed by hemodynamically stable induction regimens such as etomidate (0.2 to 0.3 mg/kg) or opioid (e.g., fentanyl, 10 to 25 mcg/kg) supplemented with either etomidate or benzodiazepine and muscle relaxant are frequently used. Maintenance of anesthesia typically includes additional opioid, benzodiazepine, or low-concentration inhaled agent (or a combination of these), in combination with muscle relaxant. As with most other situations, an arterial catheter is placed after induction (usually in either radial artery, but at times guided by the location of prior arterial cutdown or systemic–pulmonary artery shunt procedures). Many centers also place an internal jugular multilumen catheter to measure proximal venous pressure and provide a reliable access site for drug infusions and other therapies; this catheter can provide useful information both before and after CPB (particularly in conjunction with a common atrial catheter) in terms of, for example, venous pressures, TPG, and potential anastomotic and cannulation issues. In addition, as discussed previously, measuring SVC saturation with an allowance for concurrent arterial oxygen saturation can provide a reasonable estimate of systemic oxygen delivery and cardiac output. Other centers, however, avoid SVC cannulation in most or all infants and in particular in Glenn and Fontan patients because of concerns about SVC thrombosis, as well as infection and other risks common to most forms of vascular access.

Post-CPB Management after the Fontan Procedure

Management goals immediately after a Fontan procedure also derive from the aforementioned principles (Table 20-5). It is

TABLE 20-5. Causes of Low Cardiac Output after Fontan Completion

	Systemic Venous Pressure	Common Atrial Pressure	Transpulmonary Gradient
Anatomic			
• Pulmonary artery stenosis or obstruction	↑	↓	↑
• Restrictive intraatrial septum	↑	↑	↓
• Systemic outflow tract obstruction	↑	↑	N to low
• Superior vena cava clot or obstruction*	↑	↓	↑
• Atrioventricular valve regurgitation or stenosis	↑	↑	N
• Systemic aortic valve stenosis or regurgitation	↑	↑	N
• Coarctation of the aorta	↑	↑	N
• Pulmonary venous obstruction	↑	↓	↑
Physiologic			
• Systemic ventricle dysfunction	↑	↑	N
• Pulmonary hypertension	↑	↓	↑

*Superior vena cava–to–pulmonary artery pressure gradient > 2 mm Hg. Note: After the cavopulmonary anastomosis, because inferior vena caval blood flow enters the systemic ventricle without first passing through the lungs, any anatomic obstruction through the lungs will result in low oxygen saturation but a preserved cardiac output.
N, Normal; ↑, increase; ↓, decrease.

important to maintain heart rate, contractility, and preload to maintain cardiac output. These patients frequently require substantial amounts of volume supplementation in the immediate postoperative period, even in the absence of significant bleeding. Low pulmonary blood flow produces low cardiac output because the systemic ventricle can pump only the volume of blood that is delivered to it across the pulmonary vascular bed. This differs from the situation after superior cavopulmonary shunts because there is a source of blood supply to the systemic ventricle that does not cross the pulmonary bed (i.e., IVC blood) in BDG patients.

It should also be emphasized that patients with Fontan physiology are expected to be fully saturated (with the aforementioned caveat regarding location and contribution of coronary sinus blood) and that low cardiac output will not result in a reduced Sao_2 unless there are significant sources of intrapulmonary, intracardiac (fenestration, baffle leak), or physiologic R-to-L shunting. In contrast, low cardiac output in a normal patient results in a low Sao_2 only if a significant quantity of intrapulmonary R-to-L shunt exists and low cardiac output produces a low Svo_2. When low cardiac output in a Fontan patient is caused by ventricular dysfunction, common (pulmonary venous) atrial hypertension may be sufficient to cause pulmonary edema and physiologic R-to-L intrapulmonary shunting. This situation is analogous to that in a normal patient with series circulation and no intracardiac lesions. The presence of a fenestration or baffle leak will exacerbate this Sao$_2$ decrease in the Fontan patient.

As discussed previously, a central catheter placed in the internal jugular vein will measure caval (baffle) pressure, which equals mPAP after a Fontan. A surgically placed atrial catheter will measure common atrial pressure. Allowing for individual variations, expected values can be summarized as follows:

- An mPAP of about 15 to 18 mm Hg is usually seen in the presence of reasonably good systemic ventricular function, absence of lung injury, appropriate ventilation, and so on.
- Reasonably good ventricular function will be associated with an EDP (and hence common atrial pressure) of about 5 to 10 mm Hg.
- The TPG (mPAP minus common atrial pressure) is usually less than 10 mm Hg with appropriate ventilation and no significant lung injury, mechanical or anastomotic obstructions, and so on.

Inotropic support of the systemic ventricle may be necessary as a result of ventricular dysfunction induced by chronic volume overload, prior surgical or ischemia–reperfusion injury, and the acute effects of CPB. Dopamine (3 to 5 mcg/kg per minute) is usually sufficient. Milrinone (0.5 to 1.0 mcg/kg per minute) may be useful for those patients who have high SVR and afterload/contractility mismatch. Occasionally, higher dosages of dopamine or the addition of other inotropes such as epinephrine (0.03 to 0.05 mcg/kg per minute) are needed to support systemic ventricular function.

There are several possible causes of reduced oxygen saturation after Fontan surgery. First, did the procedure include a fenestration? As noted earlier, the fenestration is meant to allow R-to-L shunting to preserve ventricular filling at the expense of some continued relative systemic oxygen desaturation. Thus, one expects at least a moderate decrease in Pao$_2$ compared with the completely separated two-ventricle circulation. For example, a newly fenestrated Fontan patient being ventilated with 100% oxygen, having relatively normal cardiac output and hemoglobin concentration, and with appropriate ventilation and minimal lung disease (after CPB) usually has a Pao$_2$ well below 100 mm Hg (50 to 70 mm Hg is not uncommon).

In Fontan patients with a patent fenestration, decreases in cardiac output will reduce Svo$_2$ and hence further reduce Pao$_2$ and Sao$_2$ (as a result of the R-to-L mixing via the fenestration); the magnitude of reduction depends on both the relative size of the shunt and the degree of venous desaturation. As noted previously, Svo$_2$ can be easily determined using a sample drawn from a central venous catheter. A difference of greater than 20% to 25% (e.g., 50% SVC saturation versus 88% arterial saturation) bewteen Sao$_2$ and Svo$_2$ is indicative of low cardiac output (assuming normal hemoglobin concentration). The relatively sudden occurrence of hypotension, increased SVC pressure, or increased Pao$_2$ (i.e., >150 to 200 mm Hg on 100% oxygen) should raise the possibility of acute fenestration closure.

As in the BGD circulation, low Ppvo$_2$ saturation is another cause of low Sao$_2$. Maneuvers to reduce V̇/Q̇ mismatch and intrapulmonary shunt should be undertaken. A high Fio$_2$ may be necessary in the presence of significant V̇/Q̇ mismatch. Ventilation and acid-base management should be optimized to keep PVR low. Mean airway pressure should be kept at the minimal level that is compatible with delivery of adequate minute ventilation and maintenance of normal lung expansion. This can usually be accomplished with a relatively large tidal volume (10 to 12 mL/kg), slow respiratory rates (10 to 15 breaths/min), and short inspiratory times (inspiratory-to-expiratory ratio of 1:3 or 1:4). Excessively high mean airway pressure will mechanically limit venous return, pulmonary blood flow, and potentially cardiac output (the severity of cardiac output effect will depend in part of fenestration presence/patency). Similarly, PEEP should be used with caution; however, it may be beneficial at levels sufficient to maintain functional residual capacity and support gas exchange without causing overdistention. As discussed previously, inhaled NO may benefit some patients with significantly increased SVC and TPG pressures (assuming the increased TPG is not the result of ventricular dysfunction) and low cardiac output, or desaturation resulting from V̇/Q̇ mismatch.

It is commonly stated that early tracheal extubation and spontaneous ventilation enhance pulmonary gas exchange and hemodynamics in Fontan patients (Morales et al., 2008; Hammer et al., 2000). On the other hand, positive pressure ventilation can improve the function of a dysfunctional systemic ventricle by reducing effective afterload (Laplace's law), as well as potentially reducing the work of breathing. In addition, low lung volumes, hypercarbia, and hypoxemia, along with potential resultant effects on ventricular filling and function, have the potential to negate any advantages produced by spontaneous ventilation.

CARDIOPULMONARY BYPASS IN INFANTS AND CHILDREN

The use of extracorporeal circulation to repair congenital cardiac defects began in the mid to late 1950s, following the conceptual development of CPB and the construction of heart-lung machines. The first report of use in children is attributed to Gibbon (1954), who repaired an atrial septal defect; this early CPB circuit required a dozen or more units of blood prime. At around the same time, Lillehei and coworkers used cross circulation to repair a variety of defects in relatively young infants and children, including ASDs, VSDs, AV canal defects, and TOF. Their reported overall survival was greater than 60%, which was remarkable considering the time frame and equipment available (Lillehei et al., 1986). Shortly thereafter, Kirklin et al. (1989) developed a bubble-type pump oxygenator that required approximately half the amount of fresh blood prime compared with the initial efforts of Gibbon and others. However, extreme blood foaming, which was lethal, was one major complication; nonetheless, survival was about 50% (Kirklin, 1989). These early reports prompted many subsequent investigations aimed at developing the scientific and technological knowledge needed to successfully undertake extracorporeal circulation in infants and children. In spite of these efforts, the morbidity and mortality of CPB remained high throughout the 1960s.

Continued attempts to understand the science and advance the technology to successfully perform CPB and complex congenital heart surgeries continued into the 1960s and 1970s, albeit with improvements that might best be characterized as necessary but incremental. In the early 1970s, Aldo Castaneda and others provided the next major conceptual advance when they described the use of deep hypothermic circulatory arrest in infants (Barratt-Boyes, 1973; Castaneda et al., 1974). These techniques relied primarily on surface cooling because difficulties and toxicities continued to be associated with infant CPB (which was typically limited to less than 20 to 30 minutes and used mainly to augment core cooling and rewarming). From the late 1970s to early 1990s, major advances in CPB science and technology were made so that the relative contribution of CPB per se to mortality in infants and children was progressively reduced to minimal levels, allowing the exploration and perfection of the complex surgeries required to approach lesions such as HLHS and TGA. Nonetheless, the morbidity associated with the use of CPB in infants and children is still widely held to be a major limitation to completely successful outcomes, and current research efforts include developing methods to operate on beating infant hearts without the use of CPB (Perrin et al., 2009).

Patient- and Lesion-Related Factors Affecting Infant and Pediatric CPB

The conduct and outcome of CPB in neonates, infants, and small children are particularly affected by patient-related variables as well as those linked to specific types of cardiac defects and pathophysiology. Neonates, in general, and particularly those who are premature or weigh less than 1.8 to 2.0 kg, comprise a high-risk group because of their immature organ function, as well as coexisting diseases such as sepsis, respiratory distress syndrome, or one or more other congenital anomalies (Pawade et al., 1993; Ungerleider and Shen, 2003; Oppido et al., 2004). There is increasing evidence that the central nervous system is more immature for a given postconceptual age in infants with CHD and that central nervous system injury may exist prior to surgery in many of these patients (Miller et al., 2004, 2007; Dent et al., 2006; McQuillen et al., 2006, 2007; Wheeler et al., 2008).

The immature myocardium may be similarly prone to CPB-related dysfunction for several reasons, including its relatively deficient (compared with adult) contractile protein mass and organization, the presence of fetal contractile protein isoforms, immature calcium cycling (which occurs primarily via the sarcolemmal membrane as opposed to the sarcoplasmic reticulum, which is less abundant and less well organized), and fewer mitochondria. Various features of congenital cardiac lesions can complicate CPB as well. For example, hypertrophic and cyanotic myocardium is more likely to be injured by ischemia–reperfusion and other consequences of CPB (del Nido, 1997; del Nido et al., 1988; Stamm et al., 2001; Friehs and del Nido 2003). Collateral vessels to the coronary circulation, perhaps most common in cyanotic patients, can wash out cardioplegia and thereby hinder effective myocardial preservation. Pulmonary dysfunction after CPB may be more prevalent in infants with other routes of high pulmonary blood flow (e.g., truncus arteriosus, hypoplastic left heart syndrome, transposition of the great arteries) and in cyanotic infants (Allen, 2003; Ungerleider and Shen, 2003). Aortopulmonary collaterals, which can be particularly significant in various lesions associated with cyanosis, may induce a steal phenomenon from the arterial compartment to the lungs, thereby promoting pulmonary dysfunction due to high flow on CPB while at the same time compromising arterial organ perfusion (low mean arterial pressures despite high flow rates while on CPB). Diffuse organ dysfunction is likely to be more common in patients who were severely cyanotic and hypoperfused at the time of delivery, or who required complex surgery in the early neonatal period.

For the neonate who suffered asphyxia or significant hypoperfusion and acidosis at the time of delivery or thereafter, most centers have found it beneficial to allow a period of stabilization of the circulation and recovery of organ function before undertaking CPB and cardiac surgery. Depending on the lesion (see later), interventions such as PGE_1, inotropic support, ventilatory strategies to balance systemic and pulmonary blood flow, and even extracorporeal circulatory support (ECMO or ventricular assist device [VAD]) are initiated preoperatively. Post-CPB organ dysfunction (e.g., renal, liver) can also be a source of morbidity for both neonates and infants, as well as for older (i.e., adult age) patients with various forms of CHD complicated by longstanding cyanosis, low cardiac output, and high systemic venous pressures.

Cannulation and Circuit Considerations

The cannulae used in infant and pediatric CPB are likely to be smaller than those used for adult cardiac operations. More significantly, their locations are likely to be different and more variable than in adults. It is therefore critical to understand potential cannulation locations for the different lesions and repairs and their potential effects on the conduct of the surgery and the locations and functions of venous and arterial pressure monitoring catheters.

Arterial cannulae for neonates and small infants must be of sufficient size to permit appropriate arterial inflow rates at reasonable line pressures, with minimal shear forces (which can damage the vessel intima, aortic valve, or blood elements), yet small enough to fit in small aortas without obstructing aortic flow. Small arterial cannulae (e.g., 8 Fr [Biomedicus]) with a thin-walled, reinforced design that prevents cannula kinking and allows a larger luminal diameter for a given external diameter have become popular. After insertion, it is important not to kink or compress the infant's pliable aorta by the location and orientation of the aortic cannula and its tubing, as well as to be aware that the cannula itself can significantly obstruct flow in the vessel. Location of the tip can direct blood flow toward or away from specific vessels; for example, locating and directing the tip more distally toward the transverse arch may reduce flow through the right carotid artery, or may favor lower body perfusion at the expense of cerebral perfusion and optimal brain cooling (Kern et al., 1992a).

Certain congenital cardiac lesions require unique aortic cannulation sites. For example, the aortic cannula is typically placed more distally in the aorta for repairs that involve extensive proximal aortic surgery such as the arterial switch procedure for transposition of the great vessels; this distal location may alter distribution of blood flow to the carotid vessels. Repair of interrupted aortic arch requires two arterial cannulae, one in each segment of the aorta (perfusing both the head and lower body). The aortic cannula is placed in the pulmonary artery at the beginning of CPB for stage I repair of HLHS because of the typically diminutive size of the ascending aorta in this lesion. The distal pulmonary arteries are occluded with tourniquets, and the aorta is perfused via the ductus arteriosus until the aortic reconstruction is completed, at which time the cannula is repositioned in the neoaorta; at times, the aortic cannula can be inserted into a surgically constructed shunt attached to the right carotid or innominate artery to allow perfusion of the head during parts of complicated aortic repairs.

In small infants (without recent sternotomy), the neck vessels are the preferred extrathoracic cannulation site for emergency access, or when there is concern about the proximity (and hence uncontrolled hemorrhage risk accompanying sternotomy) of major vascular or cardiac structures to the underside of the sternum. Unlike in adults, femoral arterial cannulation for CPB is not usually a viable option in infants and small children (weighing less than ~10 to 15 kg). This is because small vessel size precludes inserting an arterial cannula that is large enough to allow arterial inflow rates that are sufficient to completely meet metabolic needs. It is important to note, however, that in emergent situations (e.g., cardiopulmonary arrest in the cardiac catheterization laboratory, particularly when femoral vascular access is already in place), smaller perfusion cannulae located in the femoral vessels of small infants can allow a reduced but nevertheless life-saving amount of perfusion support. Femoral access is performed occasionally for older children, again either electively when there is concern that a cardiac chamber or vascular conduit lies immediately beneath the sternum, or emergently when one of these structures is entered inadvertently during the dissection.

The sizing and location of venous cannulae can also be fairly complex to take into account variations in venous anatomy and drainage as well as the operative approach. Venous cannulae are available in a variety of sizes and with design features for particular indications (Table 20-6). For example, thin-walled cannulae with multiple side holes enhance venous drainage; right-angled tips are frequently used in the SVC to improve alignment (and therefore drainage) and minimize impact on the surgical field; metal-tipped cannulae are used to prevent kinking; straight, short-tipped cannulae are used in the IVC to limit hepatic venous obstruction.

Overall, most repairs use separate SVC and IVC cannulae to achieve maximal collection of venous return and to minimize interference with the operative field. Common variations in venous anatomy that can complicate venous cannulation and must be taken into account include left or bilateral SVCs, azygous or hemiazygous continuation of the IVC, and direct drainage of the hepatic veins into the atrium. A single atrial cannula is frequently used when deep hypothermic circulatory arrest is

planned; in this instance, the venous cannula is removed after the patient is adequately cooled, to have a clear operative field.

Regardless of location, the cannula must be appropriately sited and must cause as little obstruction to venous drainage as possible. Poor venous drainage may be difficult to detect, and is more likely to occur in patients with complicated venous anatomy. The consequences of impaired venous drainage and increased venous pressures are likely to be magnified during CPB because arterial perfusion pressure is frequently reduced. Obstruction of the SVC may promote cerebral edema and otherwise increase the risk for brain injury by decreasing cerebral blood flow and hindering effective brain cooling. Many practitioners find monitoring of SVC pressure by a catheter placed in the internal jugular vein useful to detect possible SVC obstruction in this setting; the patient's head and face should also be inspected at regular intervals during CPB for the appearance congestion or swelling. It is likely that monitoring cerebral blood flow velocity using transcranial Doppler methodology might also be useful. IVC obstruction will increase lower body venous pressures and potentially decrease hepatic, renal, and mesenteric perfusion; isolated hepatic vein obstruction can also occur. Consequences can include hepatic dysfunction, renal dysfunction, ascites, and perhaps increased inflammatory consequences due to mesenteric congestion (Friesen and Thieme, 1987; Hickey and Andersen, 1987). Detection of IVC obstruction during CPB can be difficult, and it should be suspected whenever there is development of ascites, decreased urine output, or impaired venous return.

A sample schema for cannulae and other circuit components for the full size range of patients is shown in Table 20-7. Compared with adults, the surface area and volume of the CPB circuit relative to patient size and blood volume are much greater in neonates and infants. To minimize hemodilution, various circuit components and tubing diameters are kept as small as possible. Nonetheless, hemodilution that is equivalent to one to two blood volumes from the circuit prime and cardioplegia is fairly common in neonates and small infants. Pump flow rates can range from no flow for brief or extended periods (i.e., circulatory arrest) to more than 200 mL/min. Mean arterial pressures can vary from 10 to 20 mm Hg during low-flow CPB to more than 50 mm Hg at full flow rates. The temperatures used are typically lower for infant CPB and for complex repairs (15° to 18° C core temperatures for deep hypothermia, 22° to 28° C is frequently used for complex repairs, and 28° to 32° C is typical for ASDs and VSDs). Deep hypothermic circulatory arrest, although used much less frequently than even a few years ago (primarily because of increasing evidence of associated brain injury [see later]), is still employed occasionally. Different blood pH management strategies may be employed (i.e., alpha-stat versus pH-stat) depending on institutional practice, degree of cooling, and, in some cases, patient age and lesion type. Extensive use of cardiotomy suction and resultant blood trauma (including hemolysis) are common. In part because of the differences related to circuit area, bypass duration, blood trauma, temperature, and so on, the magnitude of neuroendocrine stress responses and systemic inflammatory responses to CPB, as well as their consequences, are generally believed to be more profound in neonates and infants than in adults.

Oxygenators

Membrane-type oxygenators are now used in virtually all instances. Oxygenators for infants and children must function

TABLE 20-6. Venous Cannula Sizes

Patient Weight (kg)	Cannula Size (for SVC/IVC) (French)
<3.5	12/12
3.5-6	12/14
6-8	12/16
8-12	14/16
12-16	14/18
16-23	16/18
23-28	16/20
28-36	18/20
36-48	18/22
48-60	20/22

IVC, Inferior vena cava; *SVC*, superior vena cava.

TABLE 20-7. Specifications for Oxygenators for Patients of Different Sizes

Oxygenator	Patient BSA (m²)	Oxygenator Prime (mL)	Total Circuit Prime Including Oxygenator (mL)	Arterial and Venous Tubing Diameter (inch)	Manufacturer Reference Flow (mL/min)
Terumo FX 05	<0.5	43	Neonate 240 Infant 255	³⁄₁₆ ¼	1500
Terumo FX 15-30	0.5-1.66	135	Toddler 555 Child 710	¼ or ³⁄₈ ³⁄₈	4000
Terumo FX 25	>1.67	250	Adult 1030	½	7000

BSA, Body surface area.

over a wide range of pump flow rates (maximal flow rates range between 800 and 4000 mL/min), temperatures, and hematocrits. These are of essentially two types: microporous (hollow-fiber or folded-membrane) and nonporous membrane oxygenators. The major advantage of microporous membranes is their ability to affect gas exchange with a relatively modest membrane surface area, typically in the range of 0.2 to 1.5 m², depending on the specific oxygenator and configuration. Major disadvantages of the microporous type include some blood-to-gas contact at the start of CPB (until protein accumulation blocks the sub-micron-sized pores) and protein leakage across the membrane, along with the potential for gas embolization if negative pressure develops on the blood side of the artificial membrane. Nonporous oxygenator membranes require a larger surface area to achieve gas exchange but do not accumulate or leak protein as readily, and are therefore more often the choice for longer-term applications such as ECMO.

Pumps

Most pediatric circuits use roller pumps, in which pump output (i.e., flow rate) is determined by the number of revolutions per minute (rpm) of the pump head, the degree of occlusion produced by the rollers, and the internal diameter of the tubing. A significant advantage is that pump flow is relatively independent of resistive and hydrostatic forces in the circuit. However, adequate flow is highly dependent on the proper setting of roller head occlusion (which also affects the degree of blood trauma and hemolysis), and on accurate knowledge of pump head revolution rate and tubing size. Failure to accurately account for any of these variables can lead to excessive or inadequate pump flow.

Tubing

The CPB pump is usually placed as close to the surgical field as possible to reduce tubing length, which is a major contributor to overall circuit volume. Choice of circuit tubing for infants (see Table 20-7) is based on having an internal diameter large enough to accommodate the required full flow rate (or greater) without inordinately increasing circuit line pressures, while simultaneously being as narrow and short as possible to minimize the contribution of priming volume. Some neonatal circuits use ¼-inch tubing on both the arterial and venous limbs, and most centers have further decreased the diameter of the arterial tubing to ³⁄₁₆ inch; some use ³⁄₁₆ inch for both arterial and venous limbs (although vacuum-assisted venous drainage may be required in this instance) (Ungerleider and Shen, 2003).

Priming volume is usually defined as the total volume of the oxygenator apparatus, tubing, and the minimal amount required for the venous reservoir. Typical priming volumes of commercial membrane oxygenators range from approximately 225 to 375 mL when used in the open configuration. Minimizing circuit priming volume is important to reduce hemodilution, blood product exposure, and the potential for fluid overload and edema. There are examples of membrane oxygenators with substantially smaller prime volumes (~70 mL; Dideco Lilliput hollow-fiber), but they are not yet available in an open system configuration. Various schemes for achieving low priming volume and thereby reducing or avoiding the need for blood products as a component of the priming solution have been described (Durandy, 2007, 2009; Miyaji et al., 2007, 2008).

Important Circuit Characteristics

Venous Drainage

As in adult circuits, venous blood usually flows from the patient to the venous reservoir of the CPB circuit by gravity. The level of blood in the venous reservoir serves as an important safety mechanism: it is a source of volume to increase arterial inflow, and to assess the adequacy of venous return. If venous return and the level in the venous reservoir decline, causes (e.g., unrecovered or lost blood in the surgical field, malpositioned venous cannulae, or excessive capillary leak) can be identified, and appropriate interventions (e.g., decreasing pump flow rate, adding volume, adjusting operating table height, or repositioning the cannulae) can be performed. Vacuum-assisted venous drainage is being used in larger (typically >30 kg) congenital heart surgery patients (Ojito et al., 2001; Ungerleider and Shen, 2003; Durandy, 2009). Potential advantages include reducing circuit volume by using lower venous reservoir volume and the ability to improve venous drainage (as opposed to gravity) through smaller (e.g., ³⁄₁₆ inch) venous tubing and venous cannulae (which decreases circuit volume and may improve visibility in the surgical field). An improvement in venous drainage could lead to reduced tissue and organ edema and congestion, improved organ function, and reduced inflammatory activation (e.g., via endotoxin release from congested, hypoperfused intestine). A major potential complication of vacuum-assisted venous drainage is venoarterial air embolism (Davila et al., 2001; Wang et al., 2008; Win et al., 2008).

Many venous reservoirs are rigid and open to the atmosphere. Some advantages include ease of removal of entrained venous air, free flow of venous drainage (i.e., no air lockage or buildup of pressure in the reservoir), integration of the cardiotomy reservoir (as opposed to having a separate reservoir for cardiotomy suction), and the ability to accurately measure reservoir volume via calibration lines on the side of the chamber. This last feature is a useful aid to assess the patient's intravascular volume and may therefore facilitate weaning from CPB. Major disadvantages of open (usually rigid) venous reservoirs include the presence of a blood-to-air interface, which may promote blood trauma and activation of the coagulation, fibrinolytic, and inflammatory cascades (see later), and the need for a larger priming volume. For these reasons, a soft, collapsible venous reservoir bag that expands and contracts in relation to overall blood volume, venous return, and arterial inflow rate is being used with increasing frequency in infant CPB. Advantages include the absence of direct blood-to-air contact and the fact that air is not entrained if the venous reservoir becomes empty, which collapses the bag. A major disadvantage can be the inability to accurately measure venous reservoir volume or recognize subtle but important changes in venous return. Other relative disadvantages compared with rigid reservoirs include the need for a removal mechanism if air is entrained, the need for a separate cardiotomy suction reservoir, and the fact that venous drainage will be significantly reduced if pressure builds up because of overfilling of the reservoir with blood or air.

Filters

Most but not all centers use an arterial filter (40 micron). Although filtering arterial inflow is believed by many to be required to reduce the amount of microemboli and other debris arising from cardiotomy suction, coagulation and fibrinolysis activation, and blood trauma, particularly as potential contributors to post-CPB neurologic and other end-organ injury, others omit arterial line filters, at least in part to reduce priming volume and hemodilution (Ungerleider and Shen, 2003).

Almost all pediatric CPB systems use 0.2-micron filters in the gas inflow lines to prevent bacterial or particulate contamination. Similarly, all crystalloid prime and cardioplegia solutions are passed through 0.2-micron filters prior to final addition to the CPB circuit. A 20- or 40-micron filter is usually used on the cardiotomy suction return line to remove macroaggregates and microaggregates and other debris from the blood returning from the surgical field. Specific removal of blood polymorphonuclear leukocytes using leukocyte-depleting filters placed in line on the CPB circuit (which typically reduce circulating leukocyte counts in the patient by ~75%) is advocated by some centers as a significant means of reducing reperfusion injury (Chiba et al., 1998; Allen, 2003).

CPB Prime Composition

Dilution of red cells, clotting factors, and other plasma constituents is usually greater in infant and pediatric CPB than in adult CPB, because the priming volume of even the smallest neonatal and infant CPB circuits is roughly equivalent to approximately 1.5 to 3 times the patient's blood volume. Physiologic crystalloid solutions (e.g., Normosol) are the major component of CPB priming solutions in infants and children; primes based on colloid are used infrequently. Packed red blood cells (or occasionally whole blood) are often required; fresh frozen plasma or other colloids such as albumin are also added by many centers.

Other agents that may be included in the pump prime include mannitol, steroids (see later), heparin, and buffers (e.g., sodium bicarbonate or tris[hydroxymethyl]-amino-methane [THAM]). Mannitol is used primarily for its osmotic properties and is intended to reduce organ and cellular edema as well as to promote diuresis and thereby contribute to renal protection. The osmotic diuresis may be particularly beneficial in those congenital cardiac operations in which a substantial amount of hemolysis from blood trauma due to cardiotomy suction and high pump flow rates occurs. Stabilization of cellular membranes and various antioxidant properties, including radical scavenging, have also been attributed to mannitol. The significance of any of these effects is not proven in pediatric CPB.

The use of albumin or other colloid to prime CPB circuits is also controversial (Myers, 1997; Tigchelaar et al., 1997; Boks et al., 2001). There is evidence that reduced plasma protein concentrations and diminished plasma oncotic pressure can reduce lymphatic flow and increase capillary leak in the lungs and other vascular beds (Byrick et al., 1977; Schupbach et al., 1978; Marelli et al., 1989; Riegger et al., 2002). Although fluid balance and weight gain were favorably influenced, a recent study that randomized pediatric CPB patients to crystalloid or colloid prime could not demonstrate significant differences in mortality or in length of mechanical ventilation, ICU, or hospital stay (Riegger et al., 2002). These results are similar to those obtained in adults, in whom albumin does prevent CPB-induced reductions in colloid oncotic pressure and lung water accumulation, but where it appears to have little effect on overall outcome or measures of pulmonary, myocardial, or renal function.

Hemodilution

As noted earlier, some centers have gone to substantial lengths to modify circuit design to reduce the degree of hemodilution associated with infant CPB and decrease the use of exogenous blood and others products. These modifications have included the use of the smallest possible tubing, cannulae, and oxygenators; altered orientation of the CPB circuit to decrease tubing length; vacuum-assisted venous drainage to improve return through the small cannulae and tubing; and omission of arterial filters. Resultant priming volumes in the 180- to 250-mL range have been reported. Ultrafiltration techniques (see later) are also used to offset the hemodiluting effects of CPB and thereby reduce the requirement for donor blood and blood products. With the possible exception of ultrafiltration, there is no evidence that edema, the inflammatory response to CPB, or overall outcome is improved by these measures and, at present, it remains difficult to avoid the use of exogenous blood or blood products in patients weighing less than approximately 10 to 20 kg.

Both packed red cells and whole blood have been used to ensure age-, lesion-, and temperature-appropriate hematocrit during CPB. Although packed red cells are readily available and increase and maintain the patient's hematocrit during CPB, questions about the actual oxygen carrying and delivery capacity of stored red blood cells have been raised (Spiess, 2002). Exogenous blood should also be filtered through a standard blood filter before adding it to either the pump circuit or cardioplegia. A major disadvantage of whole blood compared with packed red cells is the higher glucose load that accompanies whole blood: hyperglycemia may increase the risk for brain injury during cerebral ischemia. On the other hand, fresh whole blood more effectively maintains plasma factor concentrations, which can be significantly reduced by CPB in these patients (see later) and may have other outcome advantages as well (Mou et al., 2004; Gruenwald et al., 2008).

The optimal hematocrit for neonatal and infant CPB is uncertain. Perhaps the most important consideration is the combination of temperature and flow rate that is to be used (e.g., deep hypothermia, low-flow, or circulatory arrest). More profound degrees of hypothermia are used in pediatric patients to suppress metabolic demands and increase tolerance to periods of low flow (25° to 18° C) or absent flow (15° to 18° C). Although the oxygen-carrying capacity of hemoglobin increases at lower temperatures, its ability to off-load oxygen to the tissues is also reduced. Moreover, the increase in blood viscosity that accompanies hypothermia is a significant impediment to microcirculatory flow and can lead to sludging and regional ischemia. The nonpulsatile flow patterns typical of most CPB applications may also decrease microcirculatory flow, particularly in the setting of increased viscosity. It is also important to note that the oxygen-carrying capacity of the non–red cell fluid component of blood (i.e., plasma) increases at decreasing temperatures because of the increased solubility of gas in the liquid phase. This occurs as temperature declines, and, as a result, the net effect of hemodilution during hypothermia is to improve microvascular flow and oxygen delivery.

Despite these theoretical considerations, the optimal and maximal levels of hemodilution for a given degree of hypothermia are not established. The longstanding practice has been to target hematocrits in the 18% to 22% range during deep hypothermic CPB. The choice of this value was based on the aforementioned improvements in blood flow viscosity and overall oxygen-carrying capacity that accompany the combination of hemodilution and hypothermia. Normovolemic hemodilution with hematocrit levels down to 15% are believed to be well tolerated during normothermia in terms of cerebral and myocardial function, as long as blood pressure, oxygenation, and cardiac output are maintained (Spahn et al., 1993; Pua and Bissonnette, 1998). Animal studies and reports of children of the Jehovah's Witness faith undergoing hypothermic CPB suggest no detectable effect on overall outcome or cerebral or cardiovascular morbidity at hematocrits in the 10% to 18% range, as long as low temperature, perfusion pressure, and flow rate are maintained (Henling et al., 1985; Stein et al., 1991; Johnston et al., 1995; Pua and Bissonnette, 1998). Hematocrits of 10% or less in infants were associated with acidosis and other evidence of inadequate oxygen delivery.

More recent evidence has cast doubt on the safety of very low hematocrits during hypothermic CPB in infant patients. In experimental infant CPB models in animals, a higher hematocrit (in the 25% to 30% range) has been associated with enhanced preservation of brain high-energy phosphates, intracellular pH, tissue oxygenation, maintained capillary density and microvascular flow, reduced leukocyte activation, and reduced neurologic injury (Duebener et al., 2001, 2002; Jonas, 2002). A recent clinical study that randomized infants to either a low-hematocrit (mean hematocrit, 22% ± 3%) or high-hematocrit (28% ± 3%) strategy at the start of low-flow hypothermic CPB found lower postoperative cardiac index, higher serum lactate, and higher total body water in the low-hematocrit group. At 1 year, overall neurologic evaluations and Mental Development Index scores were similar in the two groups, but the low-hematocrit group had significantly lower Psychomotor Development Index scores (Jonas et al., 2003). A hematocrit level at the onset of low-flow cardiopulmonary bypass of around 25% was associated with higher Psychomotor Development Index scores and reduced lactate levels (Newburger et al., 2008; Wypij et al., 2008). In addition to any direct effects, it is likely that the somewhat higher hematocrit provides some degree of safety margin against other problems with perfusion, collaterals, and alterations in cerebral autoregulation and cerebral blood flow (Greeley et al., 1989; Greeley et al., 1991a, 1991b; Kern et al., 1993; Johnston et al., 1995; Newburger et al., 2008; Wypij et al., 2008). However, similar variations (e.g., in patient age, anatomy, collaterals, flow rate, pH strategy, cooling) make it impossible to proclaim a single optimal hematocrit for infants or children.

The optimal hematocrit for *weaning* from CPB is also controversial. The overall goal is adequate systemic oxygen delivery. Based on the preceding, hematocrits in the range of 30% or even somewhat higher (e.g., stage I repair of HLHS) are aimed for during rewarming and for termination of CPB. These levels (and perhaps even somewhat lower) are likely to be well tolerated by patients who have good myocardial function, minimal or no hemodynamic lesions, and a physiologic repair with normal oxygen saturation at the conclusion of the surgery. Consideration should be given to increasing hematocrit to improve oxygen-carrying capacity and oxygen delivery in patients with reduced myocardial function, or with palliative or staged operations that result in cyanosis. In these cases, hematocrits of 40% or even slightly higher may be beneficial, but here again definitive data are lacking.

Pump Flow Rates During Pediatric CPB

Optimal pump flow rates for pediatric CPB are, as for adults, based on furnishing appropriate systemic oxygenation, oxygen delivery, and organ perfusion as assessed by oxygen consumption and metabolic rate, mixed venous oxygen saturation, acid-base balance, and lactate production (Fox et al., 1982). These are typically indexed to body weight and are of course dependent on temperature. The higher metabolic rate of neonates and infants (approximately 1.5- to 2.5-fold greater than adults) mandates proportionately higher flow rates during normothermic CPB.

Heparinization

Heparin is usually given in a dosage of about 4 mg/kg (400 U/kg) prior to initiation of bypass, either directly into the right atrium or into a central venous catheter. Confirmation of heparin injection by blood aspiration, as well as the adequacy of heparin effect, should be performed before beginning CPB. The activated clotting time (ACT) remains the primary method of monitoring the efficacy of heparin anticoagulation (and reversal) in infants and children. Most centers mandate an ACT of greater than 400 seconds before initiating CPB, and maintaining ACTs between 400 and 600 seconds during CPB to prevent activation of blood coagulation pathways and clot formation. Inadequate concentrations of heparin are believed to be a major contributor to excessive activation of the coagulation and fibrinolytic systems (Chan et al., 1997). Other methods of monitoring heparin effect, anticoagulation, and clotting parameters such as blood heparin concentration and thromboelastography are adjunctive at present, and used mainly to assess residual heparin activity and diagnose and treat coagulopathies after termination of CPB (Miller et al., 2000; Guzzetta et al., 2008).

Neonates and young infants may be more sensitive to the effects of heparin administered for CPB, and the efficacy and duration of heparin-based anticoagulation is significantly more variable in neonates and young infants (Horkay et al., 1992; D'Errico et al., 1996a; Chan et al., 1997; Malviya, 1997). Potential mechanisms include the variable and generally lower levels of both procoagulant and anticoagulant factors present during the first few months of life and in some patients with CHD (Peters et al., 1985; Andrew et al., 1987; Odegard et al., 2002a, 2002b). The degree of hypothermia, amount of hemodilution, and relative immaturity of drug metabolism may also contribute to increased and a prolonged heparin effect in infants. Heparin resistance, on the other hand, is seen infrequently in infants, although examples resulting from recent heparin exposure or antithrombin III deficiency do occur. Heparin-induced thrombocytopenia and thrombosis appear to be less common in infants and children than in adult heart surgery patients, but the incidence may go up as the number of children who are repeatedly exposed in the operating room, catheterization laboratory, and other sites continues to increase (Severin et al., 2002; Newall et al., 2003; Mullen et al., 2008). There is at present only limited and anecdotal experience with the use of heparin alternatives such as the direct thrombin inhibitors for anticoagulation during pediatric CPB.

Heparin Reversal

Protamine sulfate is administered at the end of CPB to reverse the anticoagulant effects of heparin. Protamine dosing is usually based on body weight (3 to 4 mg/kg) or in a ratio to the heparin dosage (milligram-to-milligram) of 1:1 or 1.3:1; in vitro titration to neutralize heparin in a patient sample is also employed by some. In general, the target ACT after protamine administration should be within about 10% of the pre-CPB baseline. The first two dosing methods are likely to result in relative protamine excess, which is intentional because of greater heparin sensitivity and duration in infants and other factors that may potentiate heparinization, such as hemodilution, hypothermia, and delayed metabolic clearance. However, as for adults, there is evidence that empirical protamine dosing associated with excess protamine administration is possibly related to greater blood loss and transfusion requirements than with dosages that directly measure blood heparin using titration or other methods (Horkay et al., 1992; Martindale et al., 1996; Malviya, 1997; Guzzetta et al., 2008). Another argument against empirical dosing is that relatively small excesses of circulating protamine compared with heparin may have direct antiplatelet effects that can exacerbate bleeding after CPB (Griffin et al., 2001).

Typically, the drug is administered slowly over approximately 10 minutes. For unclear reasons, severe hypotensive, pulmonary vasoconstrictive, or anaphylactic/anaphylactoid reactions to protamine are uncommon in infants and children (Seifert et al., 2003). Of these, hypotension is most frequent, occurring in between about 1.5% to 3% of protamine administrations. It is dependent on dosage and rate of administration, most likely caused by histamine release, usually fairly mild and transient, and responsive to volume replacement or calcium administration. Severe pulmonary vasoconstriction appears to be much less common than in adults, may be caused by complement activation or pulmonary thromboxane release

(or both), and can be particularly problematic in patients with depressed contractile function (Lowenstein et al., 1983).

Conduct of Pediatric Cardiopulmonary Bypass

CPB is initiated once the arterial and venous cannulae are correctly positioned and connected to the circuit, the absence of air in the arterial line is confirmed, and adequate anticoagulation is demonstrated (usually by ACT). When it is important to keep the heart beating and possibly ejecting, the electrolyte concentration of CPB prime—specifically calcium and potassium—is usually normalized, along with solution temperature, so as to maintain myocardial function, prevent myocardial distention, and potentially allow an extended period of dissection and surgery, thereby potentially shortening the duration of aortic cross-clamping and myocardial ischemia that are required.

Large arterial collateral vessels (as may be seen in many forms of cyanotic heart disease, including TOF and pulmonary atresia), patent ductus arteriosus, and surgical aortopulmonary shunts can promote runoff from the systemic circulation at the start of CPB and thereby reduce cooling and perfusion pressure of critical organs despite seemingly adequate total pump flow. Thus, prompt surgical control and occlusion of large aortopulmonary collateral vessels, surgical shunts, and the PDA is accomplished immediately before or shortly after commencing CPB. Significant aortopulmonary collateral vessels that are not important sources of pulmonary blood flow or contributors to arterial oxygenation can be coil-occluded in the cardiac catheterization laboratory prior to surgery, which will also decrease the volume load on the systemic ventricle.

Monitoring During Pediatric CPB

Circuit Monitoring During Pediatric CPB

Arterial line pressure, pump flow rate, oxygenator gases, and temperature are important CPB variables that are usually monitored by the perfusionist. Arterial line pressure, measured via a pressure transducer placed in the arterial inflow limb, can be substantially higher than patient arterial pressure because of the driving pressure required to achieve adequate flow through the smaller diameter of infant arterial cannula and tubing; it will typically be in the range of 225 to 275 mm Hg at mean arterial pressures of 40 to 60 mm Hg. Excessively high arterial line pressures (>300 to 400 mm Hg) can be caused by tubing or cannula obstruction or cannula malposition and can result in circuit rupture. Many circuits include a sensor on the oxygenator reservoir to detect critically low volume levels and one on the arterial line to detect air.

Flow rate is critical. The flow produced by roller pumps is determined by roller head rpm, occlusion pressure, and the internal tubing diameter. It is important to know that pump flow rate on most CPB pumps is *calculated* by the perfusionist (or electronics on the pump) based on the aforementioned variables. Thus, because flow is not measured directly, incorrectly measuring or inputting rpm, tubing size, or occlusion, as well as possible shunts within the circuit, can lead to potentially harmful perfusion errors (either increased or decreased flow). Unexpectedly low or high mean arterial pressure for the calculated flow rate may be the first clue to these possibilities. In the case of low flow in particular, abnormal biochemical variables result if the condition is of sufficient magnitude and duration (see later).

The most common oxygenator gases are oxygen, air, and carbon dioxide. Continuous in-line monitors of pH, Po_2, and Pco_2 are used frequently. The gas "sweep speed" (flow rate) and oxygen concentration delivered to the oxygenator are controlled with a flow meter or blender and measured with appropriate electrodes. Variability in pump flow rates, temperatures, and blood gas management strategies leads to wide variations in the flow rates and composition of the gases administered during pediatric CPB. Use of pH-stat management (see later) can require altered gas sweep rates and the ability to widely vary and control CO_2 in the sweep gas.

Thermistors measure temperatures of the water bath and heat exchanger, along with arterial and venous blood temperatures. The temperature gradient between the patient and perfusate should not exceed $10°$ C; this may be especially important during rewarming to prevent formation of gaseous bubbles and emboli caused by decreased gas solubility as fluid temperature increases.

Patient Monitoring During Pediatric CPB

Monitoring of mean arterial pressure is required during CPB. This is most often accomplished via catheters in either the radial or femoral artery. Choice of arterial catheter location can occasionally be affected by issues that include the location of a previous surgery or shunt (e.g., BT) and the current lesion and planned operation. Femoral arterial pressure monitoring (with or without concomitant radial arterial monitoring) is preferred by some for aortic reconstructions and for increased reliability when very complex surgeries or deep hypothermia is planned, particularly in small infants. Left atrial (catheter placed intraoperatively) and central venous (SVC) or right atrial (intraoperatively placed) filling pressures are also measured routinely, depending on the surgery.

Nasopharyngeal, esophageal, and rectal temperatures are measured using appropriate thermistors. Nasopharyngeal or tympanic membrane temperatures are most often used and probably are the most accurate in terms of tracking brain temperature, although no extracranial site is truly reliable in this regard (Pua and Bissonnette, 1998). Rectal temperature is most often used to monitor core temperature. Esophageal temperature reflects aortic temperature and does not correlate well with core or brain temperatures.

Arterial and venous blood gases should be measured within 5 to 10 minutes after commencing bypass, and then at 15- to 30-minute intervals thereafter; more frequent measurements may be required if there is evidence of compromised perfusion. In addition to on-line measurements of pH, Po_2, and Pco_2, measurements include hematocrit, and serum electrolytes including sodium, potassium, and ionized calcium. Many centers favor allowing or even promoting (e.g., via the chelating effects of citrate in added blood products) reduced ionized calcium during CPB in an attempt to reduce the contribution of calcium to reperfusion injury. Ionized hypomagnesiumemia, another potential contributor to ischemia–reperfusion damage and dysrhythmias, has been found after pediatric CPB, although its clinical significance is uncertain (Munoz et al., 2000b; Mencia et al., 2002; Manrique et al., 2010). Increasing blood lactate concentrations before and after pediatric CPB has been suggested to correlate postoperative morbidity and mortality (Munoz et al., 2000a; Li et al., 2007; Wypij et al., 2008).

The oxygen saturation of venous blood (Svo_2) is an important index of tissue perfusion. It can be measured from venous blood samples at intervals as discussed earlier and also continuously via a calibrated in-line monitor on the venous catheter. Optimal and minimal acceptable values for Svo_2 during CPB, particularly as temperature and flow rate decrease, are not well defined. At normothermic or near normothermic temperatures, Svo_2 can be interpreted in a fashion similar to non-CPB situations, and hence low values (<~60% to 70%) should raise concern about inadequate tissue oxygen delivery (e.g., inadequate flow, low hemoglobin). As hypothermia progresses, dissolved oxygen contributes an increasing proportion of total oxygen delivery, and, more importantly, the increased affinity of hemoglobin for oxygen impairs transfer from hemoglobin to tissue (Dexter et al., 1997). As a result, the interpretation of Svo_2 during deep hypothermia becomes somewhat problematic. It may be prudent to assume that substantially higher levels of Svo_2 (~>90%) are required to infer the adequacy of perfusion during deep hypothermic CPB. The development of shunting around major vascular beds that may occur as a consequence of CPB, in addition to any preexisting collateral vessels, may also increase Svo_2 without indicating adequate perfusion of those tissues, meaning that organ hypoperfusion can exist despite what appear to be acceptable Svo_2 values.

Frequent monitoring of blood glucose and efforts to maintain it in the normoglycemic range are important during CPB in neonates, infants, and children. The major cause of hypoglycemia appears to be limited hepatic glycogen stores and gluconeogenic capability, especially in neonates, and perhaps also in cyanotic and malnourished (e.g., CHF) infants and young children. Failure to provide exogenous glucose can result in severe hypoglycemia and neurologic injury. The potential neurologic consequences of hypoglycemia may be exacerbated by hypocarbia, which seems to lower the threshold for hypoglycemic neuronal damage, and by patient lesions (e.g., aortopulmonary collaterals) and bypass strategies that independently reduce cerebral autoregulation and cerebral blood flow (Siesjo et al., 1983; Sieber et al., 1989; Glauser et al., 1990a).

Hyperglycemia can also be a frequent occurrence during pediatric CPB. Blood glucose may increase because of an increased supply from exogenous sources such as IV fluids and cardioplegia, as well as because of reduced glucose uptake, which is primarily the result of insulin resistance arising from the counter-regulatory effects of increases in stress hormones such as cortisol, growth hormone, and catecholamines (Anand et al., 1990; Furnary and Wu, 2006; Gandhi et al., 2007; Dickerson et al., 2008). Deep hypothermia can also suppress glucose-stimulated insulin secretion during hypothermic CPB and for at least a few hours thereafter. It has become well accepted that hyperglycemia can potentiate cerebral ischemia–reperfusion injury under a variety of circumstances in both infants and children (Lanier, 1991; Michaud et al., 1991; LeBlanc et al., 1994); a trend toward similar results occurs in pediatric CPB patients, although the data are largely retrospective and uncontrolled (Steward et al., 1988; Glauser et al., 1990a). Proposed mechanisms of hyperglycemic–ischemic brain injury include hyperosmolar cellular swelling from glucose loading, and promotion of lactic acidosis or increased intracellular acidosis caused by increased anaerobic glycolytic flux.

However, this issue remains controversial. There was only a weak correlation between blood glucose with creatine kinase-BB levels and no correlation with neurodevelopmental outcome in the Boston Circulatory Arrest study, and there was some evidence that post-CPB hyperglycemia was in fact protective, particularly against seizures, which were associated with worse neurodevelopmental outcomes (Burrows and McGowan, 1996; Rappaport et al., 1998). There are also substantial data in a variety of non-CPB animal models that preischemic hyperglycemia may protect the immature brain from hypoxia, asphyxia, or hypoxia–ischemia (Callahan et al., 1990; Hattori and Wasterlain, 1990; Vannucci, 1990; Vannucci and Mujsce, 1992). One important caveat is that these studies were conducted almost exclusively in immature rat models in which circulation and ventilation were unsupported, and some of the protective effect of hyperglycemia may have been the result of better maintenance of the circulation or ventilation in hyperglycemic animals (an effect that would be largely irrelevant during CPB). Further complicating this issue are reports that relatively modest degrees of hyperglycemia were associated with worse overall outcome in a variety of circumstances, including in adult cardiac surgery and in at least some adult and pediatric intensive care patients, and that tight glucose control could be beneficial (Van den Berghe, 2004, 2007; Dickerson et al., 2008; Lecomte et al., 2008; Oeyen, 2008; Patel, 2008; Rossano et al., 2008; Wiener et al., 2008; Levy and Rhodes, 2009). Particularly in the case of adult cardiac surgery patients, at least some of the benefit appeared to be obtained in diabetic (and perhaps prediabetic) patients and involve risks and complications not typically associated with infant congenital heart surgery (Furnary et al., 2004; Furnary and Wu, 2006; Lazar et al., 2009). However, additional and more recent analyses have called this conclusion into question, with a number of studies suggesting that moderate degrees of hyperglycemia are not associated with worse outcome and that tight control may in fact be detrimental (Gandhi et al., 2007; Rossano et al., 2008; Finfer et al., 2009; Inzucchi and Siegel, 2009; Levy and Rhodes, 2009).

Cardioplegia

The need to deliver cardioplegia is often a direct consequence of aortic cross-clamping, which is placed to enhance surgical exposure by excluding the heart from the circulation and providing a bloodless field. The heart must survive this interval of ischemia (the cross-clamp interval) without injury. Cardioplegia solutions arrest the heart in diastole, resulting in a profound reduction in metabolic demand. In addition, cardioplegia plays a restorative role, replenishing energy stores in ischemic hearts. Arrest in diastole can be induced by depolarized arrest (elevated potassium), polarized arrest (adenosine, potassium channel openers, procaine, lidocaine), or arrest by influencing calcium mechanisms (elevated magnesium, calcium antagonists).

Composition

There is considerable variability in the composition of cardioplegia solutions used in different institutions. Despite this wide variety of composition, there are certain properties all solutions must share:

- Potassium. Increasing extracellular potassium concentration to induce depolarized arrest is the primary method used to induce electromechanical arrest in most cardioplegia solutions. Cardioplegia solutions generally have a potassium concentration ranging from 15 to 30 mEq/L. This

concentration produces prompt electromechanical arrest. Concentrations of potassium higher than 40 mEq/L are detrimental because they increase calcium influx by increasing calcium conductance.

- Hypothermia. Hypothermia is an important component of cardioplegia solutions because it reduces myocardial oxygen consumption even in the arrested heart, reduces the degree of extracellular hyperkalemia needed to cause electromechanical arrest, and is additive with potassium-induced arrest in preventing ischemic damage.

- Calcium. Loss of calcium homeostasis is associated with cell dysfunction and death after ischemia. For this reason, one might assume that the addition of calcium to cardioplegia solutions is detrimental. In fact, a small amount of calcium is necessary to prevent the calcium paradox and to allow functional recovery after aortic cross-clamp removal. Calcium paradox is the massive cellular destruction that occurs when the myocardium is perfused with a calcium-containing solution after a period of calcium-free perfusion.

- Sodium. The optimal sodium concentration is unknown, but most cardioplegia solutions avoid extreme hyponatremia or hypernatremia relative to intracellular sodium concentration.

- Osmolarity. Because myocardial edema accompanies ischemia, cardioplegia solutions are formulated to minimize further accumulation of intracellular fluid. Cardioplegia solutions with osmolarities of greater than 400 mOsm/L exacerbate myocardial edema, probably by inducing increases in intracellular sodium. On the other hand, solutions with a low osmolarity will result in accumulation of intracellular water and further edema. The ideal osmolarity remains undetermined, but probably is approximately 370 mOsm/L. Mannitol and albumin are the additives commonly used to manipulate osmolarity in cardioplegia solutions.

- Buffering. Anaerobic metabolism accompanying ischemia results in cellular acidosis. Buffering allows anaerobic metabolism to continue and reduces ATP depletion in the ischemic myocardium. As myocardial temperature decreases, the appropriate uncorrected pH becomes more alkalotic. Therefore, the buffers chosen must be effective at the alkalotic pH found in the hypothermic myocardium. THAM, bicarbonate, phosphate, and histidine are all used as buffers in cardioplegia solutions.

Cardioplegia solutions are formulated as either a crystalloid or a blood medium. There are important differences between the two formulations. Crystalloid solutions are generally prepared by the hospital pharmacy in containers that are delivered to the perfusionist. Blood solutions are prepared by drawing off oxygenated blood from the CPB circuit into a separate reservoir and mixing it with a pre-prepared crystalloid base solution. The ratio of blood to crystalloid base varies from institution to institution (4:1 to 1:4). Potassium and other additives are then added to the blood in sufficient amounts to obtain the desired concentration. Both solutions can be temperature regulated.

Delivery

Cardioplegia is delivered under pressure to the heart via either a pressurized bag or a roller pump system. The advantages of roller pump system include easy incorporation of a continuous cooling system to maintain cardioplegia hypothermia, easy incorporation of the mixing apparatus necessary for blood cardioplegia systems, and second-to-second control of cardioplegia infusion pressure and flow rates. Optimal delivery of cardioplegia must be tailored to the operative procedure and operative technique. Cardioplegia delivery may be antegrade via the arterial system (aortic root or directly into the coronary ostia) or retrograde via the venous system (coronary sinus).

Hypothermia

Hypothermia continues to be the mainstay for protection of the brain and other organs during CPB, especially when reduced flow rates are required to facilitate the procedure. The major effect of hypothermia is a decrease in metabolic rate and consequently metabolic demand for oxygen and other substrates. During ischemia, hypothermia slows consumption of high-energy phosphate compounds and also maintains them intracellularly, thereby facilitating recovery of ATP and phosphocreatine during reperfusion. Hypothermia delays loss of ionic homeostasis during ischemia, particularly entry of sodium and calcium and resultant cellular edema, by energy-dependent, energy-independent, and membrane-stabilizing mechanisms (Kern et al., 1996). Reduced amounts of free radical generation, inflammatory cytokine production, white cell activation, and leukocyte adhesion molecule synthesis have all been associated with hypothermia or hypothermic CPB. Hypothermia suppresses release of excitatory amino acid neurotransmitters during ischemia and reperfusion, which is likely to be an important cerebral protective mechanism, especially in the neonatal and immature brain (Burrows and McGowan, 1996; Kern, 1996).

Hypothermic protection of the brain during periods of low or absent flow depends on homogenous cooling of all brain regions. There is evidence that this may not occur, based on the temperature or oxygen saturation of jugular bulb venous blood, which indicates the likelihood of ongoing cerebral metabolic activity despite low tympanic or nasopharyngeal temperatures (Kern et al., 1992a; Pua and Bissonnette, 1998). These data indicate that tympanic or nasopharyngeal temperatures may not identify subsets of patients with inadequately cooled brains. Risk factors for nonhomogeneous and delayed brain cooling in pediatric CPB patients may include the position of the aortic cannula, vascular anomalies, aortopulmonary and other collaterals, blood gas and pH management strategy (see later), and the duration of cooling. For example, using alpha-stat pH management, the duration of core cooling prior to a period of DHCA was the intraoperative variable most closely associated with postoperative cognitive outcome. Over cooling times between 11 and 18 minutes, increasing cooling time by 5 minutes increased development score by 26 points. It was speculated that shorter cooling times (<~15 minutes) permitted ongoing metabolism in nonhomogeneously cooled regions of the brain, making them more susceptible to injury during the period of DHCA (Bellinger et al., 1991). Also of interest, there was a trend for worse neurodevelopmental outcome (that did not reach not statistical significance) with cooling times longer than 20 minutes, perhaps due to the effects of prolonging exposure to the deleterious consequences of CPB, including microembolic events.

The reductions in metabolic rate produced by hypothermia allow CPB flow rates to be reduced, thereby reducing the amount of blood returning to the heart and improving surgical conditions. Most centers use values of approximately 50 mL/kg

per minute or 0.70 L/min per meter-squared for low-flow CPB. Studies in both adults and children have suggested the relative safety of low rates in this range, particularly in terms of the degree of cerebral protection afforded compared with deep hypothermic circulatory arrest (Fox et al., 1982; Miyamoto et al., 1986; Watanabe et al., 1989; Swain et al., 1991a; Pua and Bissonnette, 1998). Further reductions in pump flow to one fourth or less of normal may be used at deep levels of hypothermia (<18° C). However, there is no agreement on a "safe" degree of flow reduction for a given temperature in infants and children. Kern et al. (1993) have suggested that the critical pump flow rate in terms of the crucial juncture at which cerebral metabolism becomes flow dependent is between approximately 30 and 35 mL/kg per minute at moderate hypothermia (26° to 29° C), and 5 and 30 mL/kg per minute during deep hypothermia (18° to 22° C). The bulk of evidence suggests that cerebral autoregulation is markedly diminished or absent at temperatures below 20° C, and hence CBF becomes pressure passive at very low temperatures during CPB in infants (Pua and Bissonnette, 1998; Kern et al., 1993; Greeley, 1989). Burrows and Bissonnette (1993) showed that a significant percentage of neonates and infants who undergo low-flow CPB (<22% of normal pump flow) have no detectable CBF as measured by transcranial Doppler and require higher perfusion pressures to reestablish CBF.

Thus, it is possible that the result of low-flow CPB, at least in some infants, is the opposite of what is intended in terms of using low-flow techniques to avoid deep hypothermic circulatory arrest—that is, low-flow hypothermic CPB may result in, rather than prevent, cerebral ischemia. The development of critical closing and opening pressures may contribute to a no-reflow phenomenon and uneven brain cooling during low-flow CPB (Pua and Bissonnette, 1998). The notion of critical closing and opening pressures in the cerebral (and other vascular beds as well) also suggests that blood flow may be more dependent on arterial *pressure* than pump flow rate in these circumstances, and that a minimal mean arterial pressure is necessary to maintain adequate flow to the brain and other organs.

Antegrade Cerebral Perfusion

In an effort to prevent the potentially deleterious effects of DHCA on cerebral and somatic perfusion and oxygenation, some groups have directed efforts toward technical innovations to avoid the use of DHCA for aortic arch reconstruction in children with HLHS undergoing the Norwood procedure and in children with aortic hypoplasia or interruption undergoing biventricular repair. A number of techniques to provide continuous ACP or regional low-flow perfusion via the right innominate artery have been described and are used in conjunction with deep hypothermia (Pigula et al., 2000; Tchervenkov et al., 2000; Asou et al., 1996; Imoto et al., 1999). It is believed that these techniques provide both cerebral and somatic (subdiaphragmatic visceral) perfusion. Somatic perfusion is believed to be the result of the extensive network of arterial collaterals in the neonate that link the supradiaphragmatic and subdiaphragmatic viscera, such as the internal thoracic and intercostal arteries.

Access to the innominate artery can be obtained via placement of the arterial cannula into the open, distal end of a 3- or 3.5-mm Gore-Tex graft with the proximal end anastomosed to the distal right innominate or proximal right subclavian artery. In patients undergoing the Norwood procedure, this graft—when anastomosed distally to the right pulmonary artery—can constitute a modified BT shunt. In patients undergoing biventricular repair, the graft serves as the primary cannulation site. The graft is oversewn at its insertion site once separation from CPB has occurred.

When the ascending aorta is of reasonable size, the aorta cannula can be advanced up the innominate artery from the right side of the aortic arch during arch reconstruction. Alternatively, the cannula can be left in the ascending aorta with a cross-clamp applied just distal to the innominate artery for reconstruction of distal and descending aortic lesions.

The flow rates necessary to provide optimal cerebral and somatic perfusion during ACP have yet to be determined. An average flow rate of 63 mL/kg per minute was required to maintain cerebral blood flow velocity (as measured by transcranial Doppler) and cerebral oxygen saturation (as measured by near-infrared spectroscopy [NIRS]) within 10% of baseline during ACP in a group of 34 infants (Andropoulos et al., 2003).

Deep Hypothermic Circulatory Arrest

DHCA has been used since the 1970s for the repair of congenital heart defects, primarily in neonates and small infants, and occasionally in older children. Use of DHCA can decrease the length of time the patient is on CPB. This was an important advantage during the early congenital cardiac surgical experience, when limitations in CPB equipment and techniques put the neonate and small infant at increased risk. The impetus to minimize exposure to CPB has diminished as CPB methods for infants have improved. Continuous refinement of perfusion methods for neonates and infants and the increasing evidence of neurologic damage that may result have led to a reduction in the frequency of DHCA use in most centers. Nonetheless, DHCA can provide optimal surgical exposure in a small heart and chest by allowing removal of the perfusion cannulae, and its use (or similar alternatives such as DHCA alternated with periods of intermittent perfusion) remains unavoidable for some lesions. However, its use has become progressively restricted and reduced over time. Overall, DHCA has been found to result in greater short-term (1 year) and long-term (8 years) functional neurologic and neurodevelopmental deficits when compared with low-flow CPB. However, both strategies were associated with increased neurodevelopmental risk (Bellinger et al., 2003; Wypij et al., 2003).

When DHCA is required, both surface cooling and core cooling are used. Surface cooling is facilitated during the induction of anesthesia and surgical exposure and cannulation for CPB by lowering the room temperature (to <20° C), placing ice-filled bags around the head and neck, and positioning the patient on a cooling blanket set to about 10° C. Using these methods, the usual rectal temperature at the time of initiating CPB is about 33° C (temperature-related dysrhythmias or ventricular fibrillation are rare in neonates and small infants at core temperatures of greater than 28° to 30° C). For most cases of DHCA, an ascending aortic arterial cannula (the pulmonary artery is cannulated initially for HLHS) and a single right atrial venous cannula are inserted. As noted, extremely rapid cooling (core temperature decreasing to between 15° and 18° C in less than ~15 minutes) is usually avoided. Cooling is continued until both rectal and tympanic membrane temperatures are less than 18° C. Cardioplegia is administered and CPB then discontinued. Several pharmacologic adjuncts are usually given as part of DHCA. Many include an α-blocker such as phentolamine

or phenoxybenzamine in the pump prime to reduce vascular resistance, improve regional blood flow, and aid in homogeneous and effective cooling. High-dosage methylprednisolone (30 mg/kg) is given for reasons already discussed. Some administer sodium pentothal, 5 to 10 mg/kg, just prior to the start of DHCA to reduce cerebral electrical activity and metabolism; this is based in part on experience that up to 20% to 30% of neonatal brains will not be electrically silent despite tympanic and core temperatures of 18° C or less. As discussed, a higher hematocrit than used previously (~25% to 28% instead of 15% to 20%) is now favored by many, based on evidence that it does not impair the hypothermic cerebral circulation and may be associated with improved myocardial function, less total body water accumulation, and perhaps improved neurodevelopmental outcome (Duebener et al., 2001; Jonas, 2002; Newburger et al., 2008; Wypij et al., 2008). Finally, drainage of blood from the patient is promoted by several inflations of the lungs and manual compression of the abdomen. The venous cannula is then usually clamped and removed.

Prior to rewarming, initial steps are taken to remove air from the left ventricle, left atrium, and pulmonary veins. Cannulae are reinserted, and CPB is slowly resumed at 18° C. Because of concerns about cerebral injury *after* DHCA and the likely protective effects of hypothermia (and harmful effects of even mild hyperthermia *after* a cerebral injury), a period (~10 to 15 minutes) of 18° C perfusion on resumption of CPB after DHCA is initiated to limit both hyperthermic reperfusion (by keeping aortic perfusate temperatures lower) and post-CPB hyperthermia (Pua and Bissonnette, 1998; Shum-Tim et al., 1998; Scallan, 2003; Ungerleider and Shen, 2003). Similarly, efforts are made after CPB (cooling blankets and fans, acetaminophen) to keep core temperature at less than 36° C after DHCA or low-flow CPB. Frequently, before aortic cross-clamp removal, mannitol (0.25 to 0.5 g/kg) is given. Ionized calcium, which had been allowed to decrease to about 0.4 to 0.8 mmol/L during cooling and early rewarming, is normalized once the heart has had a period of reperfusion and the core temperature has increased to about 30 to 32° C. It is probably important to keep both flow rate and mean arterial pressure at age-appropriate normal values because of the loss of cerebral autoregulation and consequent pressure-flow dependence of CBF after DHCA. Once calcium is normalized and the patient rewarmed to about 34° C, pulsatile ejection is stimulated by restricting venous return into the pump, and ventilation is begun. Observation of the heart, intracardiac filling pressures, arterial blood pressure, and other available information (e.g., contractility and filling on TEE) are useful at this point to estimate the degree of inotropic support required when weaning from CPB. Typically, a low dosage of dopamine (~5 to 7.5 mg/kg per minute) is all that is required if the repair is technically satisfactory.

Management of Arterial Blood Gases During Pediatric CPB

Most centers adjust oxygen delivery to the CPB circuit so that arterial PO_2 values are in the range of approximately 400 to 600 mm Hg. This hyperoxic approach is based on evidence that brain injury is greater during normoxic CPB than with hyperoxic CPB (Nollert et al., 1999). Potential explanations for this effect include that the brain mainly uses dissolved oxygen during deep hypothermic CPB, that the amount of gas microemboli is decreased when nitrogen is omitted from the sweep gas, and that oxygen microemboli are resorbed much faster than those containing nitrogen (Dexter et al., 1997; Scallan, 2003). On the other hand, some centers favor significantly reducing P_{O_2} during CPB to reduce oxyradical production (Nollert et al., 1999; Allen, 2003). This mechanism may be especially important in cyanotic infants, in whom antioxidant reserves and scavenging enzyme systems may be downregulated (Cowan et al., 1992; Nollert et al., 1999; Allen, 2003). The issue remains unresolved, and it is likely that the relative benefits of the two oxygenation strategies depend in part on the organ system in question.

The optimal management strategy for pH and CO_2 during profound hypothermia, with or without DHCA, remains controversial. Both alpha-stat and pH-stat management strategies are used during pediatric CPB, and both have potential advantages and disadvantages. The biochemical basis of these two approaches bears some discussion. During hypothermia, the efficacy of the body's primary buffering systems (e.g., bicarbonate, phosphate) is markedly reduced, and amino acids become the most important intracellular buffers as temperature decreases. Of these amino acids, the α-imidazole ring of histidine is the most effective proton acceptor (i.e., buffer). Water is less ionized (into H^+ and OH^-) as temperature decreases, and thus the pH of water (the major fluid in the body) increases with falling temperature. The neutral point of water (i.e., the pH at which $[H^+] = [OH^-]$) also increases as temperature falls, and is about 7.4 at 37° C and about 7.7 to 7.8 at deep hypothermic temperatures. Alpha-stat management is based on preserving electrical neutrality at reduced temperatures and therefore the buffering capability of the α-imidazole ring of the amino acid histidine. Most enzyme, receptor, and metabolic systems function best at pH 7.4; several have been shown to function more efficiently at 20° C and at a pH of about 7.7 (Rahn et al., 1975; Somero and White, 1985). Blood from a normal patient cooled under alpha-stat methods will have a pH of about 7.4 and CO_2 at about 40 mm Hg when the sample is warmed to 37° C in the blood gas analyzer. Therefore, the alleged biochemical advantages of preserving electrochemical neutrality and intracellular buffering via alpha-stat management include better preservation of metabolism and of protein and enzyme function (by preserving intracellular pH [pH_i] and preventing abnormal charge accumulation on proteins), and a slowing of the diffusion of key charged intermediates such as ADP and AMP out of the cell. These facets promote faster recovery of oxidative metabolism and high-energy phosphates when oxygen and substrate supply are restored (Somero and White, 1985). Alpha-stat management is likely to be associated with better preservation of cerebral autoregulation at mild to moderate hypothermic temperatures, lower cerebral blood flow, and less brain swelling.

These features may have a net beneficial effect in adults, in whom microemboli and cerebral edema appear to be major components of the insult, as compared with the higher brain blood flow and greater microemboli load associated with pH stat (Murkin et al., 1987; Burrows and McGowan, 1996). On the other hand, the alpha-stat strategy causes a leftward shift in the oxyhemoglobin dissociation curve. In the setting of low flow, low perfusion pressures, and low temperatures, overall oxygen delivery under alpha-stat management may be marginal to meet metabolic needs, and cerebral blood flow may be inadequate to evenly and effectively cool the brain (Bove et al., 1987; Burrows and McGowan, 1996; Jonas, 1996).

In contrast, pH stat uses a mathematical correction for the effects of temperature on pH and then adds CO_2 to the circuit to correct the measured pH for the fall in temperature. The pH-stat strategy, therefore, attempts to normalize the patient's pH (i.e., make it ~7.4) and P_{CO_2} *at the hypothermic temperature*. In contrast to the alpha-stat example, a pH-stat sample analyzed at 37° C will be acidotic (pH ~7.1 to 7.2) and hypercarbic (P_{CO_2} at ~60 to 70 mm Hg). From a biochemical standpoint, the addition of CO_2 will theoretically lower pH_i and disrupt electrical neutrality. However, evidence suggests that the pH stat may only minimally reduce pH_i (Swain et al., 1991b; Aoki et al., 1994). On the other hand, the increase in cerebral blood flow associated with pH-stat management, along with the rightward shift in the oxyhemoglobin dissociation curve, may favor homogeneous and more rapid brain cooling and oxygen delivery as long as perfusion pressure and flow are maintained. Hypercapnia also decreases cerebral metabolic rate, energy use, glycolytic flux, and lactate production (Miller and Corddry, 1981; Tombaugh and Sapolsky, 1993; Vannucci et al., 1995; Burrows and McGowan, 1996). Hypercapnia and acidosis may decrease ischemia–reperfusion–related neurotoxic brain injury caused by excitatory amino acids by inhibiting N-methyl-D-aspartic acid receptor function, glutamate release, and neuronal calcium fluxes (Tombaugh and Sapolsky, 1993; Ou-Yang et al., 1994; Burrows and McGowan, 1996). Based on the work of the Aoki and Swain groups showing that cerebral pH_i becomes alkalotic during deep hypothermia even when pH-stat management is employed, it may be that the biochemical advantages of alpha stat are largely present during pH-stat management, and are supplemented by the effects of pH stat to increase CBF and oxygen availability as a result of its effect to rightward shift oxyhemoglobin dissociation (Swain et al., 1991b; Aoki et al., 1993).

The multiple potential beneficial effects of pH-stat management are likely to be particularly important in the neonate and infant exposed to low flow or no flow because hypoxic and ischemic injury probably pose the greatest risk to the infant (in contrast to the adult with significant atherosclerosis and vascular disease managed at mild or moderate hypothermia, in whom minimizing microemboli and preserving autoregulation—and therefore favoring alpha-stat management—are more pressing considerations). A small retrospective study using relatively brief cooling times (<15 minutes, average) suggested that pH stat might be preferable to alpha stat in terms of neurodevelopmental outcome when DHCA was used for Senning correction of arterial transposition (Jonas et al., 1993). In a larger, prospective, randomized, single-center study, no consistent improvement or impairment could be related to pH management strategy during deep hypothermic CPB (Bellinger et al., 2001). Based on this information, many centers choose pH-stat management for infant and pediatric CPB when deep hypothermia, low flow, and circulatory arrest are going to be employed (Aoki et al., 1993; Jonas et al., 1993; Kirshbom et al., 1995; Jonas, 1996, 2002; du Plessis et al., 2002; Forbess et al., 2002a, 2002b; Ungerleider and Shen, 2003). Patient factors can also influence this choice. The presence of cyanosis and aortopulmonary collaterals are considered by many to be indications for pH-stat management; CO_2 increases pulmonary vascular resistance, leading to improved systemic blood flow in these patients; cerebral perfusion is directly increased by CO_2 and also by the reduction in flow through the collaterals (Kirshbom et al., 1995; Kern, 1996; Scallan, 2003).

Bleeding after Pediatric Cardiopulmonary Bypass

Bleeding is one of the most significant problems after major cardiac surgical procedures in neonates, infants, and children.

Factors include difficulties surrounding heparinization and its antagonism by protamine (discussed previously), pathophysiology of the lesion, technical aspects of the operation, and multiple effects of CPB that perturb coagulation and promote blood loss. Most of the procoagulant and anticoagulant blood factors are present in reduced concentrations in neonates and infants; these concentrations approach adult values at varying rates over the first 6 to 12 months of life (Peters et al., 1985; Kern et al., 1992a; Odegard et al., 2002a, 2002b). When compared with age-matched controls, reduced levels of both procoagulant and anticoagulant factors have been found in many infants and children with congenital heart disease, particularly those with various forms of single-ventricle physiology (Odegard et al., 2002, 2003). The etiology is unclear at present, as is whether these abnormalities are linked to any functional disturbances (either increased or decreased) in ability to clot. Overall, however, the effects of hemodilution by CPB to lower clotting factor concentrations in infants, who appear to be functionally balanced albeit at a lower set point, will be increased.

Increased bleeding can occur in association with lesions that increase systemic venous pressures (e.g., Fontan physiology, Mustard or Senning atrial baffles, right ventricular dysfunction) resulting from hepatic dysfunction, development of large venous collateral vessels, and high venous pressures. Hepatic dysfunction can also occur in lesions with significant systemic hypoperfusion (large left-to-right shunt, left-sided obstructive lesion such as critical coarctation). Cardiac lesions that generate large shear forces such as aortic stenosis and VSDs can promote the degradation of active von Willebrand factor multimers to less active and inactive monomers, leading to an acquired form of von Willebrand's disease (Williams et al., 1999a; Yoshida et al., 2006; Vincentelli et al., 2003). PGE$_1$, used to maintain ductal patency preoperatively, can impair platelet function. Changes attributed to cyanosis that increase the risk for bleeding may include reduced platelet function, increased fibrinolysis, decreased total body amount of clotting factors (because of polycythemia and hence decreased plasma volume), and the development of collateral vessels. Compared with most adult cardiac surgery, many congenital cardiac operations require extensive suture lines and reconstructions using tissue or prosthetic graft materials, often on high-pressure vessels (e.g., stage I operation for HLHS, the arterial switch procedure). Reoperations also make up a substantial part of pediatric cardiac surgery.

The effects of CPB on blood activation, coagulation, and fibrinolysis are arguably greater in neonates and infants because of the greater degree of hemodilution, deeper degrees of hypothermia, higher shear forces caused by higher flow rates, more blood trauma and greater blood-to-air contact (higher flows, small tubing and cannulae, more cardiotomy suction), and a proportionately greater degree of blood contact with the foreign surface. CPB reduces platelet number and causes platelet dysfunction by several mechanisms, including hypothermia, contact activation from the CPB circuit, activation via coagulation mechanisms, and cleavage of platelet adhesive receptors by fibrinolytic proteases that are also activated by CPB. Platelet numbers in neonates and small infants are approximately halved at the end of bypass after protamine reversal, and platelet function is believed to be markedly impaired for the reasons outlined. Ongoing consumption of platelets and clotting factors resulting from bleeding at complex and pressurized anastomotic sites can add to thrombocytopenia. Neonates presenting for CPB are likely to have normal platelet counts but reduced (compared with age-matched subjects, who, as already noted, have lower clotting factor levels compared with adult values) concentrations of factors II, VII, VIII, IX, and X. A subset of neonates may also have significantly lower fibrinogen at the outset, which can then be critically low at the end of bypass and be a major contributor to postbypass bleeding (Kern et al., 1992b). Other significant abnormalities at the end of CPB after protamine administration include further reductions and functionally low concentrations of factors V, VII, and VIII. Low post-protamine platelet counts and fibrinogen concentrations correlate with bleeding in neonates and small infants (Miller et al., 1997).

The treatment approach to post-CPB bleeding in pediatric patients is based on the preceding coagulation considerations, coupled with the presence of complex surgical reconstructions and extensive vascular suture lines. Platelets are the initial therapy after adequate heparin reversal has been ensured. One to 2 units of platelets are typically administered to neonates and small infants to start, and up to 6 to 8 units in larger children. Each unit of platelets per 10 kg body weight usually increases the platelet count by approximately 50,000/mm^3. However, the actual platelet increase during and after pediatric CPB is frequently less, at least in part because of the consumption by ongoing bleeding and large exposed tissue and endothelial surfaces. When platelets are administered, they are in fluid that is essentially plasma, so that a fair amount of clotting factors is supplied simultaneously. Cryoprecipitate is usually the next blood component administered after platelets, and it is chosen in part because it is a good source of fibrinogen in a relatively small volume. This sequence of platelets followed by cryoprecipitate has been shown to restore hemostasis in a majority of pediatric patients after CPB (Miller et al., 1997). Fresh frozen plasma is usually reserved to replete measured factor deficiencies not amenable to cryoprecipitate, particularly because there is some evidence that it has little effect on, or may even be detrimental in, most post-CPB infants (Miller et al., 1997). Some pediatric cardiac centers prefer to use fresh whole blood as the primary therapy after protamine reversal. When used within 24 to 48 hours of collection, fresh whole blood contains active platelets and significant amounts of clotting factors, and it has been shown to reduce bleeding, transfusion requirements, and the use of other components in both neonates and adults (Mohr et al., 1988; Manno et al., 1991). A major limitation is the difficulty of obtaining reliable quantities within the 48-hour time frame, in part because of required blood banking procedures and testing for infectious agents.

Although truly accelerated fibrinolysis is probably uncommon during pediatric CPB (and largely resolves after protamine administration) (Miller et al., 1997, 2000), it is likely that the activation of the fibrinolytic system that accompanies surgical trauma, bleeding, and particularly CPB-induced activation of coagulation and inflammatory cascades has a significant role in consumption of clotting factors, generation of anticoagulant degradation products, and loss of adhesive receptors on platelets. For these reasons, antifibrinolytic agents such as ε-aminocaproic acid and tranexamic acid have become increasingly popular. Until recently, aprotinin was also used. Aprotinin is not available for clinical use now, because of reports of increased complications in *adult* cardiac surgery patients. These complications include stroke, renal failure, graft occlusion, and death. Interestingly, meta-analyses of adult aprotinin studies indicate a protective effect against neurologic injury, particularly stroke, which appeared to be due at least in part to reduced patient reinfusion of shed blood (Murkin, 2001; Smith et al., 2004).

At present, there is little controlled evidence that antifibrinolytic agents are beneficial in primary pediatric cardiac surgical operations in terms of, for example, blood loss, transfusion requirement, and platelet dysfunction, although many centers use them for complex first operations such as arterial switch and stage I hypoplastic left heart reconstructions. There is substantial evidence in favor of their use for reoperations, particularly of the complex variety (D'Errico et al., 1996b; Reid et al., 1997; Miller et al., 1998; D'Errico et al., 1999; Gruber et al., 2000; Carrel et al., 1998; McDonough and Gruenwald, 2003; D'Errico et al., 1996b). Theoretical concerns remain about potential deleterious prothrombotic consequences during low flow or deep hypothermic circulatory arrest and in tenuous anatomic or circulatory situations postoperatively (e.g., Fontan fenestration, coronary anastomoses, reconstructed HLHS ascending aortas, surgical shunts), although there are no direct reports of such, and one retrospective study was unable to identify any role for these agents in similar problems (Casta et al., 2000; Gruber et al., 2000). The role for activated factor VII in postcardiotomy bleeding continues to be controversial, and requires further study and definition (Pychynska-Pokorska et al., 2004; Agarwal et al., 2007; Guzzetta et al., 2009).

Because of concerns about inducing severe hypercoagulability and promoting the development of thombotic complications, the use of recombinant factor VIIa should be reserved for uncontrolled bleeding that persists despite administration of clotting factors; relative normalization of platelet count, prothrombin time (PT), partial thromboplastin time (PTT), and so on; and relative certainty that all surgical sites have been controlled (Pychynska-Pokorska et al., 2004; Agarwal et al., 2007; Guzzetta et al., 2009). It may be useful to note that efficacy may be preserved while reducing thrombotic risk by using "mini" or lower dosage protocols (in the range of 60 mcg/kg or even lower), although this too remains to be proven (Ekert et al., 2006).

Organ Injury During Pediatric CPB

The potentially damaging mechanisms of CPB include global (i.e., low-flow or DHCA) and regional (e.g., heart, lung, gastrointestinal tract) periods of ischemia and reperfusion, activation of multiple limbs of the systemic inflammatory response, and intramyocardial and systemic air and particulate microemboli. During hypothermic CPB at full flow rates, skeletal muscle functions as a large capacitance reservoir, and blood flow is to some extent shunted away from the vital organs. During low-flow hypothermic CPB, skeletal muscle vasculature constricts and flow to vital organs is preserved so that oxygen delivery is able to maintain oxygen consumption down to about 50% reduction in flow rate (Lazenby et al., 1981). The presence of large collateral vessels, arterial obstructive lesions, cannula position, and other shunts from the systemic circulation may further compromise vital organ blood flow, as previously discussed.

Pulmonary Effects

Lung injury is a variable but potentially significant problem after CPB in infants and children. Likely causes include hemodilution, inflammation, and ischemia–reperfusion (Seghaye et al., 1993; Brix-Christensen, 2001). Hemodilution promotes fluid extravasation by reducing oncotic pressure. Activated complement, leukocytes, cytokines, and leukotrienes induce alveolar and capillary membrane damage, augment capillary leak, increase

platelet and white blood cell plugging, and induce the release of additional mediators that further increase pulmonary vascular resistance and pulmonary parenchymal and vascular damage. Infants with current (e.g., infection, CHF, or pulmonary overcirculation) or prior (e.g., respiratory distress syndrome, bronchopulmonary dysplasia) pulmonary processes may be at greater risk. Measurable consequences of CPB-induced lung injury include loss of endothelium-dependent dilation and increased pulmonary vascular resistance, decreased compliance, decreased functional residual capacity, increased alveolar–arterial oxygen difference, leakage of fluid into the interstitial space, and reduced surfactant activity (McGowan et al., 1993; Gillinov et al., 1994; Dreyer et al., 1995; Morita et al., 1996; Schulze-Neick et al., 1999; Ozawa et al., 2000; Brix-Christensen, 2001; Chew et al., 2001). Facilitating lung cooling by allowing a period of pulmonary blood flow on CPB during core cooling (prior to occluding venous return) has been suggested as one means of reducing ischemic lung injury and its consequences (Chai et al., 1999).

Renal Effects

Glomerular filtration rate and renal diluting and concentrating abilities are immature in neonates and very young infants. Evidence of renal dysfunction after CPB in children can be common, in the range of 3% to 10% or more (Picca et al., 1995; Aiyagari et al., 2010). Preoperative renal dysfunction or injury and low cardiac output after CPB may be the best predictors of post-CPB renal dysfunction. Preoperative renal injury appears to be more likely in neonates, who may in fact have multiorgan dysfunction after delivery and initial stabilization (e.g., HLHS, arterial transposition), as well as in older patients with long-standing systemic ventricular dysfunction, chronically elevated systemic venous pressures, or cyanosis (e.g., failing Fontan circulations, TOF with severe right or biventricular dysfunction) (Price et al., 2008). Contributing factors are likely to include low flow and reduced mean arterial pressure, nonpulsatile perfusion, and hypothermia leading to the production and release of hormones such as endothelin, catecholamines, antidiuretic hormone, atrial natriuretic factor, and rennin/angiotensin (Anand and Hickey, 1987; Anand et al., 1990; Picca et al., 1995; Brix-Christensen, 2001). In addition to renal dysfunction, these factors may contribute to increased total body water, delayed fluid clearance after CPB, and related complications such as myocardial and pulmonary interstitial edema, delayed chest closure, and prolonged ventilatory support. At present, there is little information specifically devoted to infant and pediatric heart disease patients in terms of renal protection or preventive therapies. In larger patients, vacuum-assisted venous drainage has some obvious theoretical advantages. Several recent adult cardiac surgery studies (where much of the underlying pathophysiology may differ) suggest that relatively low dosages of fenoldopam or nesiritide can reduce renal-related morbidity in at-risk patients (Chen et al., 2007; Cogliati et al., 2007; Mentzer et al., 2007; Landoni et al., 2008; Roasio et al., 2008); one recent study suggests a benefit from N-acetylcysteine, perhaps related to its antioxidant properties (Aiyagari et al., 2010).

Brain Injury

Neurologic injury continues to be one of the most problematic aspects of surgery for CHD. Prevention of neurologic injury has become increasingly important as overall survival has increased and functional cardiopulmonary outcomes improve. Earlier retrospective series estimated the incidence of major neurologic injuries after pediatric heart surgery to be between 20% and 30% (Ferry, 1990; Pua and Bissonnette, 1998; Menache et al., 2002). Although there appears to have been a progressive decline in major complications such as seizures, persistent choreoathetosis, and severe developmental delay (for reasons that are largely unknown), more subtle but significant cognitive and neurodevelopmental delays in IQ, language and motor skills, attention, learning skills, visual and spatial skills, and working memory have recently been found in a number of different circumstances (Bellinger et al., 1999, 2003; Forbess et al., 2002a, 2002b; Wypij et al., 2003; Mahle et al., 2006; Mahle and Wernovsky, 2004; Tabbutt et al., 2008; Kussman et al., 2009). Cognitive development also appears to be lower in school-age survivors of HLHS and patients with Fontan physiology (Mahle et al., 2000; Wernovsky et al., 2000). Risks for lower achievement included surgery for HLHS, use of DHCA, and reoperation within 30 days.

Overall, it is clear that preoperative, intraoperative, and postoperative factors are all involved. The developing infant brain may be particularly susceptible to injury by hypoxia, ischemia–reperfusion, and the systemic inflammatory response, because of its relatively fragile vasculature, high metabolic activity, and the fact that is undergoing an intensive period of neuronal migration, axonal outgrowth, target finding and arborization, synaptogenesis, myelinization, astroglial development, and selective neuronal reduction (largely via apoptosis) (Burrows and McGowan, 1996). Most, if not all, of these processes are under the control of biochemical factors, neurotransmitters, and gene expression pathways that are likely to be affected by CPB and its consequences (e.g., cytokine and growth factor production, generation of oxyradical and nitroxyradical species, altered release and reuptake of excitotoxic amino acid neurotransmitters due to ischemia).

The developing brain of the newborn with CHD appears to be more immature (by MRI criteria) than that of the infant of comparable gestational age without CHD. In addition, increasing evidence suggests that various structural and developmental brain abnormalities are common in infants with congenital heart disease *prior* to any surgical interventions, or after balloon atrial septostomy alone. Interestingly, there is also some recent evidence that these preexisting brain abnormalities may not worsen after surgery, at least based on brain imaging criteria (Mahle and Wernovsky, 2004; Ikemba et al., 2004; Dent et al., 2005; Dent et al., 2006; McQuillen et al., 2006, 2007; Miller et al., 2007; Block et al., 2010). A substantial number of children with CHD have genetic syndromes associated with developmental delay of various sorts, including Down syndrome and the CATCH-22 syndrome (Gerdes et al., 1999). The latter is linked to microdeletions in the 22q11 region of chromosome 22; is associated with DiGeorge and velocardiofacial syndromes, developmental delays in language and speech, and mild hypotonia; and is present in 2% to 10% of children with CHD. It seems likely that other genetic abnormalities as yet undefined result in both neurologic problems and CHD. A sizable number of children with heart disease may have congenital brain malformations; more than 30% of infants with HLHS have evidence of brain dysgenesis or other anomalies before surgery (Glauser et al., 1990b; Miller and Vogel, 1999). Low cardiac output, high venous pressures, thromboemboli, and chronic cyanosis are all likely to contribute to both gross and subtle neurocognitive lesions prior to surgical interventions (Kern, 1996; Miller and Vogel, 1999; Scallan, 2003).

Intraoperative causes of brain injury include abnormalities of cerebral autoregulation and cerebral perfusion, ischemia–reperfusion mechanisms, and emboli. Many of these factors have been discussed. The "safe" period of DHCA remains controversial and in part depends on how it is defined, and under what conditions of flow, pH, temperature, cooling strategy, and patient population it is assessed. Clinical experience and some evidence suggests periods of DHCA as short as 20 minutes or as long as 45 minutes before major complications such as seizures or choreoathetosis begin to increase in frequency (Burrows and McGowan, 1996). In animal models, using ATP depletion or the cerebral metabolic rate for oxygen as the endpoint led to estimates of 20 to 30 minutes or 40 to 65 minutes, respectively (Greeley et al., 1991a, 1991b; Greeley and Ungerleider, 1991; Swain et al., 1991b). Overall, the consensus is that the risks for neurologic injury and developmental abnormalities increase and IQ decreases in direct proportion to the duration of DHCA (Wells et al., 1983; Jonas, 1996; du Plessis et al., 2002; Forbess et al., 2002a, 2002b; Bellinger et al., 2003; Wypij et al., 2003). As noted previously, these data in aggregate have led to reduced use or reduced duration of use of DHCA, realizing that in some anatomic circumstances, it cannot be avoided. The potential for neurologic dysfunction in association with low-flow hypothermic bypass has been discussed previously (Taylor et al., 1992; Burrows and Bissonnette, 1993; Pua and Bissonnette, 1998; Bellinger et al., 1999, 2003; Wypij et al., 2003); again, it is unclear how often and to what extent preexisting brain abnormalities and genetic factors contribute to impaired neurodevelopmental markers after CPB in infants and children.

These issues have spawned other technical modifications to reduce neurologic complications. Use of selective cerebral perfusion—for example, during stage I HLHS and other arch reconstructions—to avoid or reduce the use of DHCA appears to be an increasingly popular option. In many centers, the flow rates and perfusion pressures used during selective cerebral or arch perfusion are guided by continuous measurement of cerebral blood flow velocity or near-infrared spectroscopy (or both) (Langley et al., 1999; Pigula et al., 2001; Pigula, 2002, 2003; Williams and Ramamoorthy, 2007; Fraser and Andropoulos, 2008). These techniques have yet to be subjected to widespread and thorough appraisals, or to controlled comparisons with DHCA or other low-flow techniques, and there is evidence that selective perfusion of the cerebral circulation may in fact be harmful (Jonas, 2002; Goldberg et al., 2007; Ohye et al., 2009).

The postbypass period is also receiving increased attention as being vulnerable to neurologic injury. As discussed previously, both low-flow deep hypothermic CPB and DHCA techniques can lead to compromises in cerebral blood flow, autoregulation, and metabolism. Therefore, ensuring appropriate cardiac output, arterial blood pressure, cerebral perfusion pressure, and oxygen delivery (i.e., appropriate hematocrit for the level of oxygen saturation and cardiac output) in the postoperative period are likely to be important. In addition to standard volume replacement and inotropic therapies, more novel strategies to support cardiac output in this setting include delayed sternal closure and ready use of ECMO (Duncan et al., 1999; McElhinney et al., 2000; Ungerleider and Shen, 2003). Maintaining normothermic or even mildly hypothermic body temperatures in the first 24 to 48 hours postoperatively may also be beneficial (Shum-Tim et al., 1998).

The ability to assess various parameters of brain function and homeostasis and to use them to guide therapy are clearly critical but, unfortunately, still largely lacking. Although various forms of perioperative neurologic monitoring (e.g., electroencephalography, NIRS, cerebral Doppler blood flow velocity) are used and advocated with increasing frequency, no one technique or combination of techniques has emerged to fulfill this need (Hoffman et al., 2004; Ghanayem et al., 2006; Hoffman, 2006a, 2006b; Dickerson et al., 2008; Johnson et al., 2009). Most centers currently use some form of NIRS monitoring of cerebral (and often somatic as well) oxygen saturation. The NIRS value reflects tissue (arterioles, venules, capillaries) oxygen saturation and is algorithmically weighted to represent approximately 75% to 85% venous blood and 15% to 25% arterial blood. When the optodes are placed on the forehead, the NIRS value reflects frontal cortex oxygen content. The values measured most closely correlate with, in most patients, jugular bulb, jugular venous, or SVC oxygen saturation; thus, in some ways, it can function as a noninvasive monitor of mixed venous O_2 saturations. Some experimental data indicate that both the degree and duration of cerebral desaturation may predict neurologic injury (Kurth et al., 2002, 2009; Hirsch et al., 2009). However, human clinical data demonstrating a correlation between NIRS and neurologic injury or outcome are minimal, and data defining when intervention based on NIRS (i.e., level of desaturation) might be indicated, how to best intervene, and whether NIRS-driven interventions alter outcome remain to be seen (Kussman et al., 2007, 2009; Hirsch et al., 2009). There may also be a role for improved techniques to detect microemboli during CPB (Blauth et al., 1988; Miller et al., 2008; Win et al., 2008). It is clear the multiple and interacting genetic, maturational, procedural, and lesion-specific issues are likely to contribute to the overall neurodevelopmental outcome of CPB and surgery in infants with CHD. One theoretical advantage to hybrid-type procedures is that they avoid exposure to CPB and more complicated repairs in early infancy when neurodevelopmental vulnerability may be greatest (Gutgesell and Lim, 2007; Lim et al., 2006; Honjo, 2009).

The Stress Response to Cardiopulmonary Bypass

The stress response to CPB is characterized by the release of a large and diverse group of substances, including catecholamines, endothelin, various prostaglandins, cortisol, and growth hormone. The concentrations that have been measured in neonates and infants during or soon after CPB are some of the highest measured in humans, generally exceeding those measured in adult CPB patients by fivefold to 10-fold (Anand et al., 1990; Anand and Hickey, 1992). Stimuli include extensive and prolonged foreign surface contact, profound hypothermia, low flow, low perfusion pressure, and nonpulsatile perfusion. Clearance of many of these compounds by the liver, kidneys, or lungs may also be delayed. Possible deleterious consequences include vasoconstriction and reduced organ perfusion, direct tissue injury, pulmonary hypertension, endothelial damage, and increased pulmonary vasoreactivity. Decreased stress response hormones and possibly improved morbidity and mortality have been associated with high-dosage synthetic opioid administration to infants undergoing CPB and other stressful procedures (Anand et al., 1987; Anand and Hickey, 1992). On the other hand, the release of many of these compounds and the responses overall are likely to have adaptive benefits. It is unclear what level,

circumstances, or substances cause a net harmful response; to what extent acutely ill infants with CHD require some degree of stress response for hemodynamic stability, wound repair, and overall homeostasis; and to what degree the seemingly exaggerated response seen particularly in neonates and infants exposed to CPB is pathologic and should be attenuated. One follow-up study that attempted to clarify the role of high-dosage opioid regimens did not appear to confirm a major role for stress hormone suppression in outcome (Gruber et al., 2001).

The Systemic Inflammatory Response to CPB

Cardiopulmonary bypass causes a systemic inflammatory response via multiple mechanisms that include surgical trauma, blood contact with the CPB circuit, ischemia–reperfusion injury, and protamine administration (Butler et al., 1993; Plotz et al., 1993; Seghaye et al., 1993, 1994, 1996; Ashraf et al., 1997; Chew et al., 2001, 2002; Gessler et al., 2002). These triggers stimulate complex and interconnected cell- and humoral-based systems that include activation of the complement, coagulation, and fibrinolytic pathways; endotoxin release; cytokine production; endothelial activation and expression of leukocyte adhesion molecules; leukocyte and platelet activation; and production and release of oxyradicals, nitric oxide, prostanoids, eicosanoids, and proteolytic enzymes (e.g., myeloperoxidase and superoxide from activate neutrophils). The resultant tissue and organ injury, capillary leak, increased need for inotropic and ventilatory support, and perhaps effects on infection risk are widely believed to have a major impact on parameters affecting morbidity and duration of hospitalization (e.g., duration of ventilation, requirement for inotropic support) and overall outcome (Wheeler et al., 2008).

Complement activation occurs via the alternate (stimulated by foreign surface contact, endotoxin, and kallikrein), classical (protamine), and mannose-binding lectin pathways. Significant increases in activated complement fragments occur with initiation of bypass, and further still during rewarming, and these levels have correlated with post-CPB renal, cardiac, and pulmonary dysfunction (Butler et al., 1993; Seghaye et al., 1993, 1994; Li et al., 1994; Brix-Christensen, 2001; Busche et al., 2009). Various complement fragments cause white cell and platelet activation, white cell free radical production and degranulation, smooth muscle constriction, and capillary leak. Terminal complement fragments and the membrane attack complex can cause direct cell lysis.

Blood concentrations of bacterial endotoxin can increase because of its almost ubiquitous presence in sterile fluids and equipment, and also perhaps because of decreased intestinal perfusion, which can also augment reperfusion injury independent of endotoxin (Koike et al., 1994; Moore et al., 1994). Endotoxin can directly injure endothelial cells and cause capillary leak, as well as stimulate the production of proinflammatory cytokines such as tumor necrosis factor, interleukin (IL)-1, IL-6, and IL-8. Cytokine production can also be stimulated by foreign surface contact, complement fragments, and other cytokines. Mechanisms of cytokine-induced tissue injury are multiple. Cytokines such as IL-1 and TNF are directly toxic to endothelial and other cells, cause wasting and edema, cause myocardial contractile dysfunction, and stimulate a number of cytotoxic and cytoprotective signaling mechanisms such as inducible (high-output and potentially cytotoxic) NO production, various proapoptotic and antiapoptotic pathways and proteins, enhanced oxyradical injury, and induction of cellular antioxidant enzymes. Levels of TNF and IL-1 are inconsistently increased by CPB in neonates and infants. Cytokine-induced NO production can result in profound hypotension (it is the major mechanism of vascular depression in septic shock), myocardial depression, and inhibition of cellular respiration and metabolism. IL-6 has been demonstrated in some studies to be a good predictor of clinical outcome and may be related to the extent of tissue injury (Brix-Christensen, 2001). IL-8 is a potent neutrophil chemoattractant and also causes leukocytosis and activation of neutrophil proteases and free radical enzymes. Increased IL-8 has been found after pediatric CPB patients in proportion to ischemic and total bypass times (Journois et al., 1994; Seghaye et al., 1996; Ozawa et al., 2000; Brix-Christensen, 2001; Chew et al., 2001). Some children have increased levels of some cytokines preoperatively; the causes and significance of this finding are uncertain, but there is some evidence that neonates with a preoperative biochemical profile consistent with inflammation (e.g., increased plasma elastase and complement fragments) are more likely to manifest a capillary leak syndrome postoperatively (Seghaye et al., 1996; Wheeler et al., 2008; Allan, in press).

Neutrophil activation is believed to be a very important mechanism of cellular injury during and after CPB. It is produced by a wide variety of stimuli, including foreign surface contact, endotoxin, cytokines, complement, platelet-activating factor, and ischemia–reperfusion. Activated neutrophils express proadhesive molecules on their cell surface (which are complementary to ones induced on endothelial and other cell membranes), marginate into the tissue, have increased lipoxygenase and myeloperoxidase activities (the sources of superoxide and hypochlorous acid, respectively), and release neutrophil elastase. These products cause damage to lipids, proteins, and DNA. Elastase also causes endothelial damage, inactivates serine proteases in the coagulation pathway, and cleaves adhesive receptors from the platelet membrane (Wachtfogel et al., 1983, 1986, 1993; Burrows and McGowan, 1996). Both myeloperoxidase and elastase, as well as evidence of neutrophil-mediated oxidant injury, have been detected after pediatric CPB (Larson et al., 1996; Brix-Christensen, 2001; Allen, 2003).

It has recently become apparent that CPB also induces a corresponding increase in antiinflammatory cytokines such as IL-10 and IL-1 receptor antagonist (IL-1ra). C-reactive protein, an acute-phase protein that is a marker of inflammation and has antiinflammatory effects by decreasing neutrophil chemotaxis, also increases during and after pediatric CPB (Seghaye et al., 1993, 1996; Brix-Christensen, 2001; Chew et al., 2001, 2002; Tarnok and Schneider, 2001). Transient immunosuppression mediated by these events and others, such as loss of activated neutrophils and inhibition of cellular immune responses, have also been found after pediatric CPB (Tarnok and Schneider, 2001).

Overall, there is substantial variability in the release pattern and plasma concentrations of cytokines in infants and children undergoing cardiac surgery compared with adults (McBride and Booth, 1996; Seghaye et al., 1996; Ozawa et al., 2000; Chew et al., 2001; Allan, in press). Although increased elements of the systemic inflammatory response are generally associated with increased risk for postoperative organ dysfunction and morbidity and mortality, better-designed studies with direct assays and endpoints are necessary to truly define any cause-effect relationship between systemic inflammatory

response mediators and organ damage. It is also likely that the *balance* between proinflammatory and antiinflammatory stimuli and their diverse effects on a wide range of cellular types and functions must be taken into account (Chew et al., 2001; Appachi et al., 2007). Finally, the possibility that at least some of these substances are required to regulate the overall response and in fact potentially contribute to eventual repair and resolution should not be overlooked. For example, although the deleterious effects of substances such as TNFα and cyclooxygenase pathway derivatives have been demonstrated in numerous cellular and animal models, genetic or pharmacologic abrogation of these pathways can also lead to increased cell death and organ dysfunction under clinically relevant circumstances (e.g., ischemia–reperfusion). Similarly, other cytokines and chemokines, although mechanistically linked to the severity of acute tissue injury, are also required to contain and resolve the injury (genetic deletion results in reduced acute injury but worse overall outcome).

Steroids

Administration of relatively high dosages of steroids (either dexamethasone or methylprednisolone) prior to pediatric CPB may suppress the production of proinflammatory cytokines and improve organ function (Langley et al., 1999; Bronicki et al., 2000; Shum-Tim et al., 2001; El Azab et al., 2002). They are frequently administered by many pediatric congenital surgery programs, with notable differences in choice of drug, dosage, timing of administration (e.g., preoperatively, prior to CPB, during CPB), and patient selection (Checchia et al., 2005). Many believe that steroids are more likely to show a positive effect in neonates and infants because the magnitude and consequences of the systemic inflammatory response appear to be greater. Because the major mechanism of steroid action is to alter gene expression and cellular activation, maximal effect may require administration some time (up to 8 hours) before bypass and repeated dosing (Ungerleider and Shen, 2003). Improvements in body water accumulation, alveolar–arterial oxygen gradients, pulmonary artery pressure, and duration of mechanical ventilation and length of ICU stay have been observed (Bronicki et al., 2000; El Azab et al., 2002; Ungerleider and Shen, 2003). Results from more extensive investigations in adults confirm potential beneficial alterations in the balance of proinflammatory to antiinflammatory mediators (allowing for the caveats discussed earlier) (Chaney, 2002). However, there were no significant effects on fluid balance and possibly detrimental effects on pulmonary function, and glucose homeostasis (hyperglycemia) occurred as a result. Furthermore, as with the stress response, it remains unclear whether broad-spectrum and nonspecific suppression of the systemic inflammatory response by corticosteroids is beneficial. There is also some evidence that at least more prolonged periods of corticosteroid administration may be detrimental to the developing brain. Thus, caution is warranted until large, randomized, prospective, placebo-controlled studies with tightly regulated perioperative management are performed in pediatric patients.

Ultrafiltration

Conventional or modified ultrafiltration is being used with increasing frequency during pediatric cardiac surgery. Potential beneficial mechanisms include hemoconcentration, removal of various inflammatory mediators and vasoactive compounds in the ultrafiltrate, and decreased total body water and tissue edema. Significant clinical improvements in tissue edema, post-CPB weight gain, hematocrit, blood pressure, global left ventricular function, lung compliance, oxygenation, and duration of mechanical ventilation have been reported, along with decreased postoperative bleeding, decreased postoperative transfusion and blood product requirements, and decreased pulmonary vascular resistance. One or more of these benefits have been observed in many, but not all, studies (Elliott, 1993; Journois et al., 1994; Friesen et al., 1997; Bando et al., 1998; Chaturvedi et al., 1999; Gaynor, 2001, 2003; Maluf et al., 2001; Chew et al., 2002; Hiramatsu et al., 2002). Less certain are the mechanisms responsible for these effects, because significant reductions in blood concentrations of inflammatory cytokines, complement fragments, and prostanoids have not been universally identified (Chew et al., 2002; Gaynor, 2003; Huang et al., 2003). Although ultrafiltration techniques appear to be safe for infants and children, there is theoretical concern about removal of protective mediators and deleterious increases in viscosity and clotting factors (i.e., hypercoagulability). Additional studies are needed to define the mechanisms of ultrafiltration effect and identify the patients who are most likely to benefit.

HEART, LUNG, AND HEART-LUNG TRANSPLANTATION

Heart Transplantation

History

Christian Barnard conducted the first heart transplantation on December 3, 1967. The patient lived for 18 days before succumbing to a fatal bout of pneumonia (Barnard, 1967). The first pediatric cardiac heart transplantation was carried out within a week of this landmark achievement by a group led by Adrian Kantrowitz in a 3-week-old infant with Ebstein's anomaly and pulmonary atresia. The procedure used immersion of both the donor and recipient in iced water to achieve topical cooling. As the recipient's chest was opened, the heart fibrillated and thus open cardiac massage was undertaken until the patient's temperature was low enough to commence circulatory arrest (Kantrowitz et al., 1968). Over the next few years, about 100 more heart transplantations were conducted, with a mean survival of 1 month (Mendeloff, 2002). The poor outcomes probably resulted from inadequate technological advancements in key areas such as surgical techniques, CPB, immunosuppression, and the clinical diagnosis and management of rejection.

The preliminary understanding of the immunobiology of organ rejection and its role in transplantation failure, the development of the bioptome and a grading system for rejection, and the isolation of a fungal extract with immunosuppressive properties (later developed as cyclosporine) all helped spur renewed interest in transplantation (Caves et al., 1973, 1974). As adult transplantation programs began to be established, pediatric transplantation was mostly in adolescents and was conducted under the aegis of adult programs. Infant and pediatric cardiac transplantation did not become established as a separate entity until the mid 1980s, when transplantation was recommended as a primary therapy for lethal congenital

lesions, and a successful heart transplantation in an 8-month-old was performed by Cooley and colleagues (Bailey et al., 1986, 1989).

The number of pediatric patients undergoing heart transplantation steadily increased in the 1980s and early 1990s, with the rate peaking in the mid 1990s. Currently, procedures in infants and children account for up to 10% of all heart transplantations. Mortality figures have improved significantly, with an approximately 75% to 80% actuarial survival rate at 4 to 5 years (compared with less than 55% for the earlier era of pediatric heart transplantation). As indications have continued to expand (see later), continued growth in pediatric heart transplantation has been limited primarily by the availability of donor hearts. In response, particularly for neonates, most programs have opted whenever possible for staged palliation of congenital heart defects, to avoid the uncertainty (and potential death) that placement on the transplant waiting list entails. Increased use of ABO-incompatible donors is another, more recent attempt to increase the size of the useful donor pool (see later). The issue of transplantation versus palliation (for patients with congenital cardiac lesions) in early infancy is far from settled. Proponents of transplantation believe that infant transplantation may be associated with enhanced engraftment and induction of tolerance, reducing the amount of immunosuppression required. Neonates in particular may experience a window of immune tolerance, with a lower likelihood of rejection and the ability to use less aggressive immunosuppression (Mavroudis et al., 1988; Bailey et al., 1991). Heart transplantation is technically more difficult and may be associated with higher mortality in those who have undergone prior palliative cardiac surgery. Transplantation as a primary therapy also may reduce the risk for progressive organ deterioration, particularly of the pulmonary parenchyma and vasculature, that can result from some palliative procedures, or severe cardiac dysfunction arising after failed congenital procedures. On the other hand, the limited donor supply makes attempts at surgical correction the only option for many patients. Advocates of staged reconstruction argue that transplantation is a waste of resources when an alternative is available. In addition, transplantation carries the attendant complications of rejection, immunosuppression, drug toxicity, infection, malignancy, and the need for retransplantation.

HLHS is an example that outlines the nature of this conflict. The 5-year survival for this lesion after heart transplantation (including deaths while waiting for a donor) and the staged reconstruction procedures (stage I Norwood palliation, bidirectional Glenn cavopulmonary shunt, and modified Fontan procedure) are essentially the same. The transplanted heart is structurally normal but is associated with all of the complications of antirejection therapy and, when done in neonates, may require one or more retransplantations because of chronic rejection and graft failure. Staged reconstruction for HLHS mandates life with Fontan physiology, and thus a significant likelihood of severe dysrhythmias and late ventricular dysfunction, potentially resulting in a need for transplantation.

Patient Demographics

Children younger than 1 year continue to make up the majority of the transplantations performed (Fig. 20-20, A). There then appears to be a decreasing number of transplantations for the 5- to 7-year-old age group, followed by a second peak

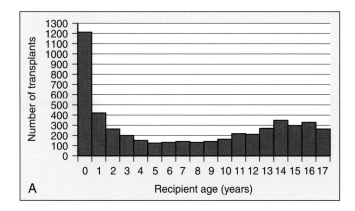

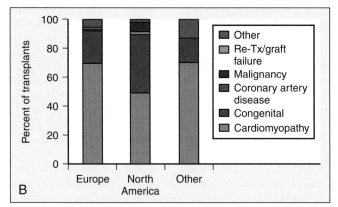

■ FIGURE 20-20. A, Age distribution of pediatric heart recipients for transplantations from January 1996 through June 2008. **B,** Diagnosis distribution by location for transplantations from January 2000 through June 2008. *(From Kirk R, Edwards LB, Aurora P, et al: Registry of the International Society for Heart and Lung Transplantation: twelfth official pediatric heart transplantation report—2009,* J Heart Lung Transplant *28:993, 2009.)*

in the teenage years. This distribution is closely linked to etiology, with CHD as the major indication for transplantation in the first year of life, and cardiomyopathy the primary indication in the older age groups. During the period from 1988 to 1995, 78% of pediatric transplantations in children less than 1 year of age were for CHD and 16% for myocarditis, whereas from 1996 to 2009, approximately 65% were in children with CHD and 30% for cardiomyopathies and myocarditis. In the other pediatric age groups, the ratios remained fairly constant. The majority of heart transplantations in older patients with CHD are performed as these patients' palliative or reconstructive surgeries become inadequate (e.g., ventricular failure, dysrhythmias). Valvular heart disease, coronary artery disease associated with hyperlipidemia, and myocardial tumors are less frequent (~2%) indications for heart transplantation in children. Drug-induced cardiomyopathy (especially anthracycline) is another infrequent indication, although there is some evidence that this may become a more frequent problem in pediatric patients as they age. Retransplantation accounted for 4% to 6% of all transplantations; this rate has not changed appreciably in the past several years (see Fig. 20-20, *B*). Overall, approximately 250 to 275 infant and pediatric heart transplantations are performed in the United States annually (Addonizio and Rose, 1987).

Surgical Indications for Heart Transplantation

The development of cyclosporine and other immunosuppressive agents has enabled heart transplantation to become a viable therapy for end-stage heart failure regardless of etiology. Indeed, according to the International Society for Heart and Lung Transplantation, survival at 4 years now exceeds 75%. It may thus be considered an alternative treatment to standard surgical procedures for certain congenital heart defects such as HLHS and pulmonary atresia with intact interventricular septum. The decision to perform transplantation is best made when patient survival is known to be unlikely or of short duration and other options have failed. As mentioned previously, the mortality rate of pediatric heart transplantation and concerns about long-term graft survival and immunosuppression must still be balanced against the natural history of the disease process and the results of alternative surgical repairs. For example, in the instance of dilated cardiomyopathy, particularly in children who are older than 2 years, heart transplantation may offer the only alternative to death. As noted earlier, the case for transplantation for HLHS is somewhat different. For infants with HLHS treated with heart transplantation, data indicate 1-year and overall survival rates of 84% and 63%, respectively (Bailey and Gundry, 1990), which are similar to current survival figures for staged reconstructive procedures initially described by Norwood and colleagues (Norwood et al., 1992). In the current era, both of these techniques are considered palliative. Of note, somewhat older (but likely still applicable) data from the Pediatric Heart Transplant Study Group suggest that if one were to list all neonates with HLHS for transplantation, less than 10% would receive a heart. It has been argued that using a scarce resource for conditions that can be palliated diverts donor organs from those for whom transplantation is the only option (Morrow et al., 1997; Fricker et al., 1999; Fricker, 1987).

Patient Selection

Congenital Heart Disease

Certain groups of infants have conditions that cannot be palliated—for example, the child with HLHS that consists of aortic atresia and a perforated mitral valve. These children have abnormal coronary artery anatomy and coronary myointimal hyperplasia that can predispose to systemic (right) ventricular dysfunction after staged reconstruction. Infants with this anatomic variant might therefore be better candidates for transplantation; HLHS infants with LV coronary fistulae may represent a similar group, although a hybrid procedure approach has also been recommended for this group (Weinberg et al., 1985; Pigott et al., 1988; Pigula et al., 2007; Chen and Parry, 2009). Needless to say, substantial controversy surrounds these sorts of considerations. Other lesions in neonates and infants that may be considered relatively strong indications in favor of heart transplantation include pulmonary atresia with intact ventricular septum (especially in the presence of right ventricular–dependent coronary perfusion via fistulous connections with the hypertensive RV), univentricular heart, and unbalanced forms of atrioventricular septal defect or double-outlet right ventricle. Although these conditions can usually be palliated with staged reconstructive techniques, transplantation is often favored for these infants because of the high perioperative mortality rates (the result of problematic cardiac anatomy or physiology) and because outcome studies have shown poor long-term results of the palliative procedures.

Patients with poor outcome after palliative or staged reconstructive attempts are another group with CHD who may require subsequent transplantation. Examples include (1) patients with univentricular heart physiology in whom ventricular dysfunction has developed, thus precluding a Fontan procedure (some of these patients will also develop pulmonary hypertension necessitating a heart-lung transplantation); (2) patients who had undergone a Fontan procedure and now present with end-stage ventricular dysfunction; (3) patients with significant myocardial damage in association with anomalous left coronary artery; and (4) patients with ventricular failure following an atrial baffle procedure (such as a Mustard or Senning procedure) for TGA.

Dilated Cardiomyopathy

Dilated cardiomyopathy is the most frequent type of cardiomyopathy encountered in children. Although most cases are believed to result from a viral or an inflammatory etiology, definitive proof is often lacking. Dilated cardiomyopathy can result from other metabolic and genetic defects as well. Potentially treatable causes of heart failure such as carnitine deficiency and other metabolic abnormalities should be excluded. Children diagnosed with dilated cardiomyopathy at ages greater than 2 years have a worse prognosis (Griffin et al., 1988; Chen et al., 1990); overall mortality exceeds 50% within 1 year of diagnosis. Factors other than age that are associated with poor outcome include severe cardiomegaly, decreased ejection fraction, and low cardiac output. These children usually present with systolic dysfunction (usually biventricular), CHF symptoms, or dysrhythmias. Occasionally, sudden death may be the first sign. Empirical treatment with, for example, diuretics, inotropes, vasodilators, pheresis, or immune modulators is usually initiated. Although these therapies may provide some symptomatic improvement, it is unclear whether even maximal medical management can alter the natural course of the disease process. A subset of patients with dilated cardiomyopathy presents with acute fulminant myocarditis, which further exacerbates their condition. Some patients (approximately one third) with dilated cardiomyopathy may substantially improve after a period of intensive medical or mechanical (e.g., ECMO or VAD) cardiac support.

Dilated cardiomyopathy can also occur after the use of doxorubicin in patients who have undergone chemotherapy regimens for a variety of pediatric leukemias and solid tumors. Doxorubicin is particularly toxic to cardiac muscle, at least in part because of free radical–mediated mitochondrial injury. In addition to the total dosage administered (especially in excess of 250 to 400 mg/m²), other risk factors appear to be female gender and an age less than 4 years when treated (Lipshultz et al., 1991a, 1991b, 1995, 2003). It appears that early myocyte loss results in an inability of the heart to successfully adapt to the demands of growth and increasing afterload. These patients frequently present for heart transplantation a decade or more after cancer treatment (Wallace, 2003). One major unresolved concern regarding transplantation for this group is the risk for cancer recurrence in the setting of intensive immunosuppression. It is believed that a candidate who has no evidence of the primary malignancy

1 year after treatment has an acceptable risk for the introduction of immunosuppression (Fricker et al., 1999).

Hypertrophic Cardiomyopathy

Hypertrophic cardiomyopathy is another major form of cardiomyopathy that occurs with some frequency in the pediatric population. One study found that hypertrophic cardiomyopathy made up 42% of all new presentations of cardiomyopathy during a 3-year period (Lipshultz et al., 2003). Left ventricular outflow obstruction and diastolic dysfunction as a result of increased ventricular mass secondary to left ventricular hypertrophy characterize this condition. Sudden death, most likely due to ventricular tachycardia, may also be the first manifesting feature. Increased risk may be associated with young age at presentation, a family history of hypertrophic cardiomyopathy, and a history of syncope (McKenna et al., 1981; Maron et al., 1987). There does not appear to be a good correlation between the severity of ventricular outflow obstruction and the risk for fatal arrhythmia (Wigle et al., 1985). Furthermore, although symptomatic improvement may occur with the use of β-adrenergic blockers or calcium channel antagonists, these therapies (as well as others that may be used to improve symptoms arising from outflow obstruction such as asynchronous biventricular pacing and ventricular myomectomy) do not appear to have a significant effect on mortality, thus making the identification of at-risk patients and the timing for transplantation extremely problematic. Use of implantable cardiac defibrillator technology in pediatric patients with some forms of increased risk for sudden death has increased and appears to be associated with a survival benefit (Stephenson et al., 2006; Berul et al., 2008).

Relative Contraindications to Pediatric Heart Transplantation

A number of variables must be assessed before referring any patient for heart transplantation. Increased PVR, active infection, irreversible organ damage, pulmonary emboli or infarction, other severe systemic disease, active malignancy, and significant psychosocial limitations are among the major factors to be considered.

Pulmonary Hypertension

Particular attention is given to the degree of pulmonary hypertension, as it is a key determinant of function of the donor right ventricle after transplantation and hence of overall outcome. The incidence of increased pulmonary vascular resistance in children who are admitted for heart transplantation is probably greater than that in adults because of the number of congenital pediatric lesions that can be associated with increased pulmonary blood flow or raised left atrial pressure. Increased left atrial pressure can also be a frequent contributor to elevated PVR in patients with cardiomyopathy. In adults, PVR of greater than 6 Wood units is usually considered to be a relative contraindication for heart transplantation. The upper limit of PVR that precludes successful heart transplantation in children has not been firmly established. It has been shown that right ventricular dysfunction or critical pulmonary hypertension after transplantation is unlikely in children whose preoperative PVR is less than 6 Wood units (Addonizio et al., 1987). This same group suggests that PVR index (PVRI) rather than PVR be used, as the former allows some correction for body size. Others suggest that the transpulmonary gradient is a more accurate predictor of early transplantation mortality than PVR, and that a TPG of greater than 15 mm Hg is associated with an increased risk, at least in adults (Murali et al., 1993). In the present era, most centers view increased PVR as only a relative contraindication, and successful heart transplantation has occurred in children with a PVRI between 7 and 15 Wood units. In such patients, one approach has been to attempt to distinguish a fixed, irreversible pulmonary vascular disease from pulmonary hypertension with a reactive component that resolves with insertion of a well-functioning heart. This distinction is frequently attempted on the basis of PVR response to vasodilators such as oxygen, nitroglycerin, PGE_1, or iNO in the catheterization laboratory, as well as assumptions based on the underlying pathophysiology.

Previously, children in whom the PVR was reduced to less than 8 Woods units after 1 to 2 weeks of prostaglandin therapy were also considered for transplantation (Baum et al., 1991; Benson et al., 1991). Evidence suggests that long-term (months rather than weeks) continuous intravenous prostacyclin (PGI_2) can significantly reduce PVR, thus reducing right ventricular afterload and allowing heart transplantation in a previously excluded group (Rosenzweig et al., 1999; Kao et al., 2001, Bush et al., 1987). Another approach to transplantation in the presence of pulmonary hypertension in infants and children is to use an oversized donor heart (1.5 to 2 times the size of the recipient heart). The oversized heart gives the recipient a greater right ventricular mass to respond to the elevated PVR. However, the usefulness of this approach has not been statistically confirmed.

Patients with truly fixed and overly severe pulmonary hypertension are not candidates for orthotopic heart transplantation. Options include either heterotopic transplantation (the recipient's heart remains in place to assist with right ventricular work) or heart-lung transplantation. Both alternatives are less desirable. The operative and long-term mortality rates of heterotopic transplantation are increased (5-year survival, 54%) compared with orthotopic transplantation (5-year survival, ~75%) (Kriett and Kaye, 1991). Survival after heterotopic transplantation is better compared with heart-lung transplantation.

Viral Infection

Cytomegalovirus (CMV) infection, in particular, is a significant cause of morbidity and mortality in transplantation patients, as well as being a likely major contributor to the manifestations and severity of chronic heart transplant rejection (see later) (Grattan et al., 1989). However, the limited donor pool has made it impossible from a practical standpoint to exclude the transplantation of hearts from CMV-positive donors into CMV-negative recipients. Use of anti-CMV therapies such as ganciclovir has become a standard component of most transplantation regimens. Whether hepatitis C viruses (HCVs) in the donor or recipient should be a contraindication remains undetermined. In an older survey of 72 thoracic transplantation centers, 64% did list HCV-positive patients for heart transplantation and 74% used HCV-positive organs (albeit in either HCV-positive recipients or UNOS 1 recipients) (Lake et al., 1997). Those in favor suggest that HCV acquisition is better than the alternative (i.e., death without transplantation). The argument against is that a significant proportion of infected posttransplantation patients begin to have progressive liver dysfunction within 5 to 10 years after transplantation. In addition, antiviral therapy appears to be less reliable; there also is an increased incidence

of hepatocellular carcinoma in this subgroup (Fishman et al., 1996). A full evaluation of liver function should be conducted on a potential HCV-positive recipient before listing, and the use of HCV-positive organs should follow the practice stated above (Fricker et al., 1999). There is a limited number of case studies of heart transplantation patients with preexisting or acquired human immunodeficiency virus (HIV) infection, making definitive recommendations problematic. Despite the fact that these individuals may be immunocompromised and more susceptible to opportunistic infections than other candidates, results in HIV-positive recipients seem to be encouraging (Calabrese et al., 2003; Morgan et al., 2003).

Psychosocial Disturbances

Psychosocial problems and noncompliance are significant issues in the pediatric population, particularly in adolescents. Severe psychiatric disorders that cannot be controlled are a contraindication to the procedure. However, postoperative noncompliance can be difficult to predict. Reliable caregivers and a stable family structure are extremely important to the success of transplantation in infants and children because of the requirements for and stresses of frequent hospital visits, procedures, numerous medications, and chronic illness.

Donor Selection

Donors are matched largely according to blood type and body size. Typically, donor weight approximates that of the recipient. As mentioned, if the PVR is increased, a donor up to 2.5 times the weight of the recipient may be sought. Human lymphocyte antibody (HLA) typing and donor lymphocyte cross-matching are usually done retrospectively.

Most infant and pediatric donors are trauma victims (motor vehicle accidents, child abuse); occasionally, they result from sudden infant death syndrome or intracranial hemorrhage. Hypotension requiring pressor support (catecholamines, vasopressin) is common in victims with severe brain injury or brain death; it should not be inferred that it indicates myocardial dysfunction. Significant myocardial damage can result directly from trauma or secondarily from hypotension, hemorrhage, or ischemia. Routine donor screening includes a chest radiograph, electrocardiogram, and echocardiogram; mild contractile dysfunction is usually not an absolute contraindication to donation. There is some evidence that increased blood concentrations of cardiomyocyte proteins such as the cardiac-specific isoform of troponin I in donor blood is predictive of graft failure. Many centers administer triiodothyronine (T_3) to the donor before harvest, based on evidence that it is associated with improved graft contractile function in the recipient; inclusion of insulin and vasopressin has also been advocated by some (Novitzky et al., 2006). Use of standardized donor management protocols and even donor management teams that, in addition to these measures, aggressively treat donor hypotension, diabetes insipidus or syndrome of inappropriate secretion of antidiuretic hormone (SIADH), neurogenic pulmonary edema, and coagulopathy have been recommended (Kutsogiannis et al., 2006; DuBose and Salim, 2008).

To expand the potential donor pool, some centers have extended the conventional limits for ischemic times. One study compared ischemic times of greater than 8 hours with less than 90 minutes in pediatric heart transplantations. They found no difference in early or late recipient outcome between the two groups (Scheule et al., 2002). Current practice recommendations suggest that limiting the ischemia time of the donor heart to less than 6 hours, and preferably to less than 4 hours, is likely to produce the least amount of myocardial preservation injury and acceptable graft function.

Infection, such as evidence of pneumonia, in the donor is relatively common. In general, rather than being a contraindication for the use of the organ, positive cultures in the donor are used to guide postoperative antibiotic management in the recipient.

Perioperative Management of the Pediatric Heart Transplant Recipient

Preoperative Considerations

In potential recipients, blood is typed to ensure ABO compatibility, and a panel reactive antibody test (PRA), which tests recipient reactivity to antigens in a panel of random, not donor, sera, is conducted. In children with a negative PRA test, matching is done solely on the basis of blood typing. In children who react to more than 10% of random sera, a negative prospective lymphocyte cross-match is ideal. However, this is not always possible, and strategies for the recipient with a highly reactive PRA include plasmapheresis of the recipient before and after transplantation, often in combination with intravenous pooled immunoglobulin (Leech et al., 2003); however, available data suggest that outcome is markedly reduced in highly reactive PRA recipients despite aggressive immunosuppression and plasmapheresis (Jacobs et al., 2004). In general, preoperative blood transfusions should be avoided whenever possible so as not to stimulate antibody production; transfused blood should be CMV negative for CMV-negative recipients, given the apparent increased risk for rejection and coronary vascular complications in transplant recipients who seroconvert.

Solid organ transplantation between donors and *adult* recipients with incompatible blood groups is contraindicated because of the high risk for hyperacute rejection, which occurs when preformed anti-A or anti-B antibodies (isohemagglutinins) in the recipient interact with A or B blood group antigens on vascular endothelial cells. The recognition that isohemagglutinin production is essentially absent in newborns and remains low until about 12 to 14 months of age has led to increasing and successful use of ABO-mismatched organs in this subgroup of pediatric patients (West et al., 2001a, 2001b; Foreman et al., 2004; Gambino et al., 2008; Patel et al., 2008; Roche et al., 2008). Key criteria for consideration for an ABO-mismatched organ include recipient age <15 months, low or absent isohemagglutinin levels, and satisfaction of all other transplantation criteria. In general, and preoperatively if necessary, patients should receive AB plasma products (i.e., cryoprecipitate or fresh frozen plasma) and AB platelets; red cells should be ABO-matched, and patients should never receive whole blood products. Use and matching of various donor, recipient, and blood product combinations in the ABO-mismatch situation are summarized in Table 20-8. Recipients typically receive a two- to three-blood-volume-plasma exchange transfusion while on CPB; this may need to be repeated one or more times in patients with measured preoperative isohemagglutinins until they reach undetectable levels prior to release of the cross-clamp and reperfusion of the new (donor) organ. The RBCs that are removed during these exchanges can be spun, washed, and reconstituted with AB or

TABLE 20-8. Blood Product Compatibility during ABO-Incompatible Heart Transplant

Donor's Blood Group	Recipient's Blood Group	Indicated Blood Group		
		Plasma	Packed RBCs	Platelets
AB	O	AB	O	AB
B	O	AB or B	O	AB or B
A	O	AB or A	O	AB or A
AB	B	AB	O or B	AB
A	B	AB	O or B	AB
AB	A	AB	O or A	AB
B	A	AB	O or A	AB

From West LJ, et al: ABO-Incompatible Heart Transplantation in Infants, *N Engl J Med* 344:793, 2001.

donor-type plasma. Similarly, isohemagglutinins are measured frequently in the postoperative period to guide the need for additional pheresis treatments. In terms of CPB prime, all plasma products administered intraoperatively should be blood group AB or *donor*-blood-group-type plasma. Packed RBCs administered intraoperatively should be blood group O or the recipient's blood group. Platelets should be group AB or donor blood type washed with saline. Again, whole blood use is avoided. Induction immunosuppression (see later) usually consists of mycophenolate mofetil, tacrolimus, methylprednisolone, and antithymocyte globulin.

Although the use of ABO-incompatible donors for infants and children is increasing, the use of hearts from donors after cardiac death continues to be relatively modest (Mazor and Baden, 2007; Harrison and Laussen, 2008; Pleacher et al., 2009). This is not only because of scientific issues related to donor heart injury and viability but also because of ongoing ethical and technical controversies. At the time of this writing, relatively few attempts have been undertaken in the pediatric community, although Ali and coworkers (2009) demonstrated recovery of cardiac function after application of extracorporeal perfusion in an adult.

Medical Management Considerations of the Potential Recipient

The anesthetic approach to the perioperative management of heart transplantation for patients with CHD should be based on a comprehensive understanding of the patient's cardiovascular pathophysiology. Outflow obstruction is characterized by increased pressure work, chamber hypertrophy, and a reduced ability to increase output. Optimal function is achieved by ensuring adequate preload and controlling the heart rate to allow adequate time for chamber filling and ejection. Left ventricular outflow obstruction requires the maintenance of SVR in the face of fixed cardiac output and coronary blood flow. Right ventricular obstruction may also benefit from reducing the afterload (PVR) where possible. In the instance of significant hypertrophy of either ventricle (or both ventricles), it is important to maintain coronary perfusion pressure (and hence aortic blood pressure) and oxygen-carrying capacity (i.e., hematocrit) to ensure adequate myocardial oxygen delivery to the hypertrophied muscle mass.

Valvular regurgitation may occur as a result of congenital lesions or severe dilated cardiomyopathy. Increased ventricular volume loading is the end result. Contractile function is best preserved by keeping the heart rate normal or somewhat increased so as to decrease ventricular filling time and volume and to optimize cardiac output. Other possible maneuvers include afterload reduction and inotropic support (inodilators such as milrinone or dobutamine), which tend to decrease chamber size and wall tension, increase forward flow, and reduce the regurgitant fraction.

Large left-to-right shunts impose both volume and pressure loads on the right ventricle and pulmonary circulation as well as a volume load on the left ventricle. Systemic hypoperfusion, ventricular dysfunction, acidosis, oliguria, and eventual circulatory collapse can be induced by maneuvers that increase the magnitude of the left-to-right shunt, $\dot{Q}_P/\dot{Q}_S$ (i.e., decrease PVR or increase SVR, or both). The increased pulmonary blood flow may also result in left atrial hypertension and pulmonary edema. Management involves the maintenance of PVR and preventing increased pulmonary flow with subsequent steal from the systemic circulation. Inotropic therapy may be required to maintain contractility and blood pressure.

Different principles apply to patients with cyanotic lesions associated with decreased pulmonary blood flow. Adequate oxygenation depends on the balance of PVR to SVR, as well as on overall cardiac output. Increasing PVR or decreasing SVR can severely compromise pulmonary blood flow. A subset of children admitted for heart transplantation are dependent on surgical systemic-to-pulmonary shunts for pulmonary blood flow. The flow through these shunts may be marginal at the time of transplantation, either because of growth or because of partial occlusion or narrowing of the shunt. Under these circumstances, systemic oxygen saturation is increased by increased cardiac output and SVR; significant increases in PVR should be avoided. The approach to shunts that are large with substantial pulmonary blood flow (best indicated clinically by high systemic oxygen saturation for the lesion [typically, ~85% to 90%] and wide pulse pressure) follows that described earlier for large left-to-right shunt lesions.

Cardiac function in end-stage dilated cardiomyopathy occurs at the extremes of the Laplace and Frank-Starling relation. This means that wall tension is maximal, subendocardial perfusion is easily compromised, and even minor changes in heart rate, contractility, preload, and afterload can lead to myocardial decompensation. The early addition of inotropic support may prevent bradycardia, augment contractility, augment myocardial blood flow, and minimize the negative inotropic effect of anesthetic agents. Positive-pressure ventilation can affect ventricular performance (Badke, 1982; Kaul, 1986). High intrathoracic pressure and large lung volumes can compress alveolar capillaries and thus increase PVR and right ventricular afterload. These effects can decrease right ventricular function. By the mechanism of ventricular interdependence, left ventricular filling and function can also be compromised by right ventricular dysfunction. Hypoventilation may also increase PVR by producing hypoxia, hypercarbia, and atelectasis. At appropriate lung volumes, positive pressure ventilation often improves function of the failing *systemic* ventricle by reducing afterload (ventricular transmural pressure is decreased by the increase in intrathoracic pressure, thereby reducing afterload as per Laplace's law) (Parmley, 1985).

The management of the child with HLHS awaiting transplantation merits specific discussion. To maintain systemic perfusion via the ductus arteriosus, an infusion of PGE$_1$ (0.05 to 0.10 mcg/kg per minute) is usually begun shortly after birth. Systemic perfusion may require further augmentation with inotropes and volume replacement. Any metabolic acidosis is monitored and also treated aggressively. A balloon atrial septostomy may be performed to ensure unimpeded left-to-right atrial flow.

The major goals of preoperative management of HLHS are to maintain systemic perfusion, promote optimal systemic oxygen delivery, and prevent excessive pulmonary blood flow; large increases in PVR are also to be avoided. Thus, a careful balance must be maintained between the ratio of pulmonary-to-systemic blood flow ($\dot{Q}_P:\dot{Q}_S$). Hyperventilation, alkalosis, and hyperoxia all decrease PVR and increase pulmonary blood flow ($\dot{Q}_P$), with a subsequent decrease in systemic blood flow ($\dot{Q}_S$). Therapeutic efforts are directed to maintaining normocarbia, normal pH, and the arterial oxygen saturation at approximately 75% to 80%. This range of SpO$_2$ is generally indicative of a balanced circulation (i.e., an acceptable $\dot{Q}_P:\dot{Q}_S$ ratio) and generally favors appropriate systemic oxygen delivery, adequate myocardial contractility, and blood pressure. If excessive pulmonary blood flow arises, nitrogen can be added to the inspired gas mixture (delivered via either endotracheal tube or head box) to provide a hypoxic gas mixture (<21%), with the caveat that this intervention may have a negative impact overall on systemic oxygen delivery. Intubation, paralysis, and induced hypercarbia (usually via CO$_2$ added to the breathing circuit in conjunction with normal minute ventilation) can also be used to decrease excessive pulmonary blood flow while improving systemic oxygen delivery and cerebral oxygenation (Tabbutt et al., 2001; Ramamoorthy et al., 2002).

Bridges to Heart Transplantation

A significant number of children die while awaiting heart transplantation. The number varies according to age, etiology, and degree of heart failure at the time of presentation but ranges from 23% to 70% (McGiffin et al., 1997a, 1997b, 1997c, 1997d; Morrow et al., 1997; Mital et al., 2003), although the advance of ABO-incompatible heart transplantation is having some effect to reduce the waiting list. Mechanical extracorporeal life support using either venoarterial ECMO or a paracorporeal VAD has been proven to minimize myocardial oxygen consumption and permit myocardial recovery (Kirshbom et al., 2002; Vashist and Singh, 2009). In children with end-stage heart failure awaiting transplantation, the major problem is the duration of mechanical support that is required and the increase in associated complications (e.g., infectious, thromboembolic, multiple organ dysfunction) that accrue. Nonetheless, these techniques have increasingly been successful in supporting the failing circulation as a bridge to transplantation (Kanter et al., 1987; Delius et al., 1990; del Nido et al., 1992; Tissot et al., 2009; Meliones et al., 1991). Additional indications for extracorporeal life support include postoperative ventricular or pulmonary failure that prevents weaning from CPB, severe pulmonary arterial hypertension despite maximal medical support (alkalinization, inotropic agents, inhaled NO), and refractory postoperative ventricular or pulmonary dysfunction.

The selection of technique depends on patient size and sites of dysfunction (see later). When using mechanical support in the postoperative setting, care must be taken to exclude anatomic causes of graft dysfunction that require operative intervention. The ability of mechanical support to facilitate recovery also requires that organ dysfunction be reversible. These factors mandate both appropriate patient selection and the institution of mechanical support before irreversible organ injury occurs. The importance of the latter consideration was demonstrated in early studies of ECMO treatment of respiratory failure in adults, where prolonged mechanical ventilatory support before ECMO use was associated with pathologic evidence of irreversible lung injury, minimal improvement during ECMO, and poor outcome (Gille and Bagniewski, 1976; Zapol et al., 1979).

Extracorporeal Membrane Oxygenation

ECMO reduces ventricular work by reducing wall tension, and it maintains systemic perfusion and oxygenation. It is the preferred means of mechanical support in very small infants with myocardial failure and in patients who require support of gas exchange. Arteriovenous cannulation is usually used, although venovenous bypass may be used in a patient requiring only ventilatory support. The most frequent cannulation sites are mediastinal, using single right atrial and ascending aortic cannulae, and in the neck, with cannulae in the internal jugular vein and carotid artery. Left atrial decompression is required in any patient whose left ventricular ejection fraction is inadequate or whose left atrium is not decompressed (i.e., via a PFO or ASD). This can be achieved via a separate left submammary approach to the apex of the heart or right anterior thoracotomy to the left atrium if the chest is closed. The femoral and iliac vessels in infants and young children (~10 to 15 kg) cannot usually accommodate cannulae of sufficient sizes to permit complete circulatory support. ECMO should be instituted early before significant nonthoracic end-organ damage has occurred, and complications such as pulmonary edema and infection should be treated aggressively.

The minimal circuit volume is usually 300 to 400 mL, and the complete system includes tubing, a reservoir, a membrane oxygenator, and a heat exchanger. Before cannulation, heparin (100 to 200 units/kg) is administered intravenously, with confirmation that systemic administration has occurred by measurement of the activated clotting time. The ACT is usually maintained between 180 to 200 seconds with a heparin infusion. Larger-than-usual dosages of heparin, as well as other drugs that are lipophilic (such as fentanyl or midazolam), may be required because of binding to the circuit and oxygenator (Rosen et al., 1990). Monitoring and treatment of anticoagulation during ECMO (and VAD therapies as well) continue to be difficult and imperfect. In addition to some form of ACT (which is a relatively imprecise and nonspecific measure of clot-forming capability at all times, especially in these lower ranges of test prolongation, as opposed to use in the >300- to 400-second range typical of CPB), many centers also measure heparin and antithrombin III concentrations, aiming for a heparin concentration of 0.4 to 0.6 IU/mL, and supplementing with fresh frozen plasma when ATIII activity is less than about 60%. ECMO perfusion flow rates range from 100 to as much as 150 mL/kg per minute or even somewhat greater for full circulatory support. An increased flow rate is required in the presence of a patent shunt, which also may need to be narrowed or occluded if systemic perfusion remains inadequate. Appropriate blood products are used to maintain the hematocrit between 35% and 45% and the platelet count greater than 100,00/mm³.

Fresh frozen plasma or cryoprecipitate may be needed to maintain adequate concentrations of clotting factors. If possible, the skin should be closed over the chest and cannulae, or a surgical membrane should be used instead. Echocardiography may be used frequently during ECMO to assess cardiac structure, global contractile function, and the need for left atrial venting or the evacuation of fluid and blood collections.

Once ECMO is established, levels of inotropic support are reduced. Ventilatory support and the Fio_2 are also decreased, although infrequent lung expansion (4 to 6 breaths/min) and low levels of PEEP are used to stabilize lung volumes, prevent alveolar collapse, and limit inactivation of alveolar surfactant. Greater amounts of PEEP may be indicated in the presence of significant pulmonary disease (Keszler et al., 1989). Mechanical ventilation of surfactant-deficient lungs may exacerbate lung injury (Jobe et al., 1985; Lewis and Jobe, 1993). Exogenous surfactant administration may have a role in improving pulmonary function and facilitating weaning from ECMO in patients with lung injury (Lewis and Jobe, 1993; McGowan et al., 1993).

ECMO has been used successfully as a bridge to cardiac transplantation, and as a mechanism to permit recovery in instances of severe postcardiotomy myocardial failure, including acute cardiac allograft failure (del Nido, 1996; Duncan et al., 1998). In one study (Delius et al., 1990), all threet patients placed on ECMO while awaiting transplantation died. Del Nido (1996) reported on 14 children who were considered candidates for heart transplantation and were placed on ECMO as a bridge to transplantation. In this series, eight children had postcardiotomy myocardial dysfunction, three had dilated cardiomyopathy, and three had acute viral myocarditis. Five of the 14 patients were placed on ECMO during cardiopulmonary resuscitation. Nine patients underwent a heart transplantation and seven patients had long-term survival. One patient with viral myocarditis recovered spontaneously. Four patients died of sepsis while on ECMO, and one late death occurred from posttransplant lymphoproliferative disorder (PTLD). Poor outcome associated with ECMO is usually the result of significant coexisting disease or injury. Complications from ECMO include hemorrhage, renal dysfunction, neurologic injury, infection, dysrhythmias, and difficulties maintaining adequate nutrition (Kanter et al., 1987; Weinhaus et al., 1989; Delius et al., 1990; Pennington and Swartz, 1993).

ECMO may also be used to support the failing heart after transplantation. Delius and coworkers (1990) reported on the early survival of two of three patients placed on ECMO postoperatively for acute rejection or graft dysfunction. In patients with CHD requiring postoperative ECMO support, overall survival was between 40% and 70% (Kanter et al., 1987; Rogers et al., 1989; Weinhaus et al., 1989). Outcome appears to be substantially better for children who are placed on ECMO postoperatively after an initial period without circulatory support than for those who require ECMO in the operating room to wean from CPB. Requiring ECMO to wean from CPB may reflect a more serious degree of irreversible cardiac injury. Major bleeding complications also appear to be less common in this setting if the patient has some period off CPB and before institution of ECMO. Sustained dysrhythmias are also likely to indicate severe myocardial injury and poor outcome. Left atrial decompression to reduce left ventricular end-diastolic pressure and increase subendocardial perfusion may improve myocardial and pulmonary function in these patients.

ECMO is not designed for long-term use, and after a period of greater than 6 weeks, the risk for bleeding, sepsis, and end-organ dysfunction becomes prohibitive. VADs have been demonstrated in the adult population to be capable of supporting patients for many months without end-organ damage (Farrar et al., 1988). The systems are not exclusive, and many children may be placed on ECMO in the emergent situation and converted to a VAD on an elective basis. Despite the successful use of small-size adult VADs in children (Helman et al., 2000; Reinhartz et al., 2001), until recently, the only choice for mechanical support in neonates was ECMO. However, the development of miniature pediatric-sized VADs has permitted the use of pulsatile mechanical support in neonates and children, and the numbers and types of these devices that are available for long-term ventricular support of infants and children are increasing (Hetzer et al., 1998; Stiller et al., 2003; Schweigmann et al., 2007; Bastardi et al., 2008; Gandhi et al., 2008; Rockett et al., 2008). In one outcome study following transplantation after VAD, Gandhi and colleagues (2008) noted eight of nine survivors without any acute negative neurologic outcome and only one episode of acute rejection in the survivors. However, other groups have, in fact, noted a significant level of neurologic morbidity in children with VADs (e.g., thromboembolic events, seizures), although the overall outcome has still been positive (Schweigmann et al., 2007; Bastardi et al., 2008; Rockett et al., 2008). Here again, monitoring and achieving appropriate anticoagulation remain major problems, as does occurrence of end-organ injury with long periods of support.

Another method that deserves mention as a bridge to transplantation is the use of partial ventriculectomy and mitral valve repair. This method has been used successfully to provide a biological rather than mechanical bridge in the period before transplantation in the child with dilated, end-stage cardiomyopathy (Hsu et al., 2002, 2003). Home or in-hospital inotropic therapy, using milrinone, dobutamine, or both in combination, may be effective in many patients with CHF awaiting transplantation (Berg et al., 2007; Skoyles et al., 1992). Children with ischemic cardiomyopathy (but not other conditions) may benefit from placement of an implantable defibrillator to reduce the risk for sudden death while awaiting a donor organ (Rhee et al., 2007).

Anesthetic Management

The anesthetic management of the pediatric heart transplant recipient requires a thorough understanding of the pathophysiology of the particular underlying condition. The first step is an analysis of the patient's anatomy and assessment of cardiopulmonary function. It is useful to next outline the events that will improve or destabilize contractile function, pulmonary blood flow, and systemic perfusion. An anesthetic plan can then be formulated based on these variables and the predicted responses to anesthetic agents, cardiovascular drugs, and ventilatory manipulations (Martin et al., 1989).

Premedication

Most children coming for heart transplantation, regardless of whether they have fasted, should probably be considered to have full stomachs because of their debilitated state and poor perfusion. Therefore, the administration of nonparticulate antacids or H2 antagonists and metoclopramide may be advisable. Sedative premedication is avoided or administered cautiously in patients

with severe ventricular dysfunction. In addition to limiting anxiety, judicious preoperative sedation can decrease PVR and myocardial oxygen demand and increase systemic saturations.

Monitoring

Standard noninvasive monitors, including a precordial stethoscope, pulse oximeter, three-lead ECG, and a noninvasive automated blood pressure monitor, are placed before induction. Arterial and central venous catheters and temperature monitors are generally placed after the induction of anesthesia and intubation of the patient's trachea. If the child has significant ventricular dysfunction, the arterial catheter may be placed using local anesthesia before induction. The avoidance of right internal jugular cannulation to preserve the vessel for subsequent endomyocardial biopsies is advocated by some. Routine pulmonary arterial catheterization before CPB has not been found to be beneficial. When such monitoring is warranted (e.g., for those with a potential for increased PVR), one practice is to insert the vascular sheath after induction. A thermodilution or oximetric catheter (4 Fr or greater) can then be passed into the pulmonary artery with surgical assistance before terminating CPB.

Induction and Maintenance of Anesthesia

Anesthetic agents should be selected according to their effects on heart rate, contractility, and vascular resistance (see Chapter 4, Cardiovascular Physiology, and Chapter 7, Pharmacology of Pediatric Anesthesia). Intravenous induction agents are almost always preferred. Among intravenous agents, ketamine, etomidate, and high-dosage synthetic opioids have all been used in pediatric patients undergoing heart transplantation. Ketamine or etomidate can be combined with succinylcholine or high-dosage rocuronium/vecuronium if a rapid sequence induction is required. Ketamine effectively preserves myocardial contractility and SVR in patients with relatively normal myocardial function and adrenergic tone. In patients with severe cardiomyopathy, the ability to increase stroke volume is absent, adrenergic receptors are downregulated as a result of increased circulating catecholamines, and sympathetic tone is already maximal. Ketamine may then reduce cardiac output as a result of its direct negative inotropic effects; if ketamine administration is accompanied by increased SVR, stroke volume, particularly by the myopathic heart, may be reduced further (Gutzke et al., 1989). Etomidate probably produces minimal effects on contractility and vascular resistances at standard induction dosages, although Pagel and coworkers (1998c) noted in experimental animals that etomidate-induced increases in aortic impedance could potentially reduce the contractility of the failing systemic ventricle. The opioids fentanyl and sufentanil are generally well tolerated in children. A delay in the time to peak effect of fentanyl, and perhaps increased sensitivity to the drug are apparent in patients with severely reduced ventricular function (Benowitz and Meister, 1976). These factors mandate slow administration and careful titration in children with congestive heart failure. Larger dosages of fentanyl (25 to 75 mcg/kg) and sufentanil (5 to 10 mcg/kg) can effectively blunt increases in PVR and provide extended hemodynamic stability (Tomicheck et al., 1983; Berberich and Fabian, 1987; Cirella et al., 1987; Hensley et al., 1987; Martin et al., 1989).

Pancuronium may be a useful muscle relaxant to offset the vagotonic and bradycardic effects of fentanyl and sufentanil. Vecuronium or rocuronium may be used when minimal effects on heart rate and blood pressure are preferred. Severe bradycardia and even asystole have been reported from the use of vecuronium and sufentanil in combination (Starr et al., 1986). Scopolamine may be useful for providing amnesia if a narcotic technique is used. Benzodiazepines can cause significant reductions in myocardial contractility and SVR when given in combination with potent opioids (Tomicheck et al., 1983; Reeves et al., 1984). Barbiturates decrease SVR and myocardial contractility. They should be avoided unless ventricular function is known to be preserved. Overall, one should expect delayed onset of sedation, induction, and muscle relaxation in patients with significant circulatory compromise, and often the appearance of increased effect (of sedatives, hypnotics, analgesics) as well.

Inhalation induction is used infrequently in this group of patients because of the hemodynamic side effects of myocardial depression and hypotension as well as the increased risk for aspiration (Borland, 1985; Demas et al., 1986). An inhalation induction with sevoflurane and careful airway management can be a satisfactory approach for the infant with CHD and preserved ventricular function. Nitrous oxide is usually avoided in older children with cardiomyopathy or increased PVR because of potentially significant reductions in myocardial contractility and uncertain effects on PVR (Lappas et al., 1975; Schulte-Sasse et al., 1982). However, in infants, Hickey and coworkers (1986) showed that N_2O does not produce the elevations in PAP and pulmonary artery resistance seen in adults. A right-to-left shunt will slow the rate of inhalation induction because less anesthetic is taken up from the lungs. The magnitude of slowing is less when using more soluble agents, because rapid uptake of soluble agents makes alveolar delivery the rate-limiting step. For insoluble agents such as nitrous oxide and sevoflurane, right-to-left shunts slow induction appreciably (see Chapter 7, Pharmacology). Of note, anesthetic removal rates and the ability to change anesthetic depth are similarly slowed, and thus inhaled anesthetic excess will be difficult to reverse in patients with significant right-to-left shunts. Left-to-right shunts do not affect the rate of inhaled induction in an appreciable manner (Tanner et al., 1985).

In summary, the potential for circulatory collapse during induction of anesthesia and conversion to positive pressure ventilation should be anticipated in the patient with severely compromised ventricular function or circulatory instability, regardless of the chosen anesthetic technique. In patients with relatively severe contractile dysfunction, it may be helpful to institute inotropic support before induction. A positive response to volume expansion, inotropic support, defibrillation, or other resuscitative measures is infrequent when acute cardiovascular collapse occurs in this setting in the severely compromised heart. The ability to proceed immediately to CPB should be available.

Operative Management

The surgical technique of pediatric heart transplantation is similar to that used in adults (Figs. 20-21 and 20-22). Increased technical difficulty and risk for hemorrhage before bypass should be expected in children who have had previous heart surgery. Hypothermic CPB is standard. A period of deep hypothermia, at times accompanied by a brief period of circulatory arrest, is

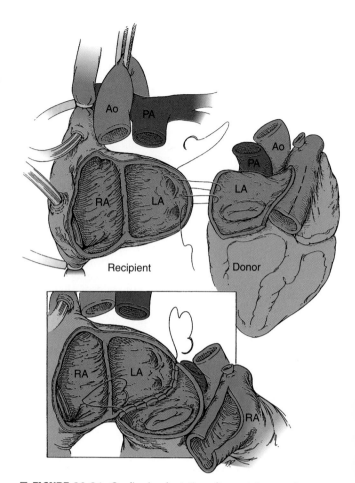

■ **FIGURE 20-21.** Cardiac implantation after recipient cardiectomy. The venous cannulae are shown entering the superior and inferior venae cavae with retained cuffs of the right and left atrial tissue. The pulmonary artery *(PA)* is transected and the aorta *(Ao)* is cross-clamped with the aortic cannula out of the field of view. *Inset:* The first atrial anastomosis along the inferior margin of the left atrium *(LA)*, showing the mitral valve of the donor heart. The aortic perfusion cannula is not shown. *RA,* Right atrium. *(From the Handbook of Cardiac Transplantation, 1995, with permission of the American College of Cardiology Foundation.)*

often required in young infants (e.g., those with HLHS) and those requiring extensive aortic or other vascular reconstruction (Mavroudis et al., 1988; Bailey et al., 1989).

For infants with unrepaired HLHS, the pulmonary artery is cannulated as the arterial inflow site for CPB (systemic blood flow occurs via the ductus arteriosus). Complicated repairs with extensive suture lines and anastomoses may be necessary in infants with HLHS (because of aortic hypoplasia), abnormalities of the pulmonary arteries (because of pulmonary atresia, truncus arteriosus, previous banding, or Fontan procedures), or abnormalities of the superior vena cava (after a Glenn anastomosis). Such reconstruction increases the overall risk of the procedure by prolonging the duration of bypass and circulatory arrest and also by increasing the severity of post-bypass bleeding.

Acute right ventricular dysfunction is one of the major problems in the transplanted heart immediately after CPB, with acute RV failure occurring in approximately 15% to 40% of pediatric

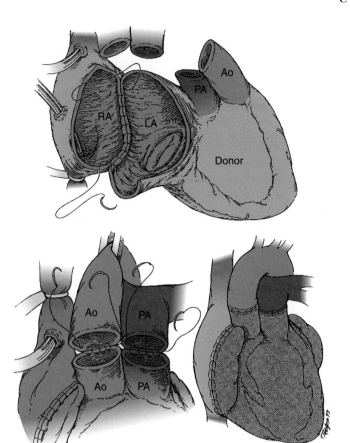

■ **FIGURE 20-22.** Anastomosis of the right atrial suture line. *Upper:* Right atrial anastomosis. *Lower:* After the anastomosis, the heart is swung over into position to complete the atrial free wall suture. The great artery anastomoses are made, after which the heart is de-aired and the cross-clamp is removed. The aortic perfusion cannula is not shown. *Ao,* Aorta; *LA,* left atrium; *PA,* pulmonary artery; *RA,* right atrium. *(From the* Handbook of Cardiac Transplantation, *1995, with permission of the American College of Cardiology Foundation.)*

heart transplant recipients (Hoskote et al., 2010). It appears to be more common in patients transplanted for restrictive or dilated cardiomyopathy and failed repairs of CHD, as well as elevated pretransplantation PVR. In infants, pretransplantation mechanical ventilation and high PVR index appear to predict acute graft RV dysfunction as well (Huang et al., 2004). The initial approach is to minimize PVR so as to reduce right ventricular afterload. Ventilatory manipulations are initially used to reduce PVR and optimize right ventricular (and consequently, left ventricular) performance. Before termination of CPB, the endotracheal tube is suctioned, and gentle inflations are performed to expand atelectatic lungs. Moderate hyperventilation with 100% oxygen is then used to maximize alveolar and arterial oxygen tension and achieve a $Paco_2$ in the range of 30 mm Hg. Although no specific mode of ventilation can be universally recommended, in general the use of larger tidal volumes (e.g., ≥10 mL/kg) and slower respiratory rates frequently appear to provide the best balance between minute ventilation and deleterious effects of PPV on right ventricular filling and function. The use of PEEP to improve gas exchange usually does not adversely affect PVR. In addition to hyperoxia and alkalinization (via both ventilation and supplemental sodium bicarbonate), inhaled NO can be a valuable therapy in the transplantation patient at risk for post-CPB pulmonary hypertension

(Hoskote et al., 2010). Other maneuvers to support the failing right ventricle include ensuring adequate coronary perfusion pressure, preload, and use of inotropes and inodilators (Costello and Pahl, 2002); occasionally, mechanical support (i.e., ECMO) and even retransplantation may be required. Usually, a modest level of inotropic support (e.g., 5 to 10 mcg/kg per minute of dopamine) is sufficient, unless there has been more extensive preservation or reperfusion injury, at which times epinephrine may be added. Acute RV dysfunction or failure can be another indication for increased levels of inotropic support, in conjunction with the aforementioned therapies to reduce RV afterload (Calvin et al., 1991). Most find limited need for agents such as norepinephrine or vasopressin in the absence of vasodilatory shock, which can occur, but infrequently, after CPB on neonates (Lechner et al., 2007; Wolf, 2008). Typically, right and left atrial filling pressures are similar; filling pressures in the range of 10 to 15 cm H_2O are necessary to support cardiac output. Higher values or significant discrepancies between right and left atrial pressures should arouse suspicion of pulmonary hypertension, right ventricular failure (increased right atrial pressure), or severe left ventricular dysfunction (increased left atrial pressure) (Banner and Yacoub, 1990).

A situation peculiar to infant and pediatric transplantation is the occasional use of hearts from donors of smaller body size than the recipient. Such undersizing of the donor may be associated with apparent graft insufficiency or failure, manifested by low cardiac output and systemic perfusion despite optimal or maximal filling pressures and inotropic support. Pulmonary hypertension and significant preservation injury exacerbate the hemodynamic instability. ECMO may be needed to permit a period of myocardial recovery in this setting of acute postoperative graft dysfunction.

In addition to developing ischemia–reperfusion injury, the donor heart is also denervated (Cannom et al., 1973). In the absence of sinus rhythm or if the chronotropic response to vasoactive drugs is insufficient, atrial or atrioventricular sequential pacing is often needed in the immediate postbypass period to facilitate adequate heart rate, cardiac output, and control of ventricular filling. It is unusual for pacing to be required for more than several days after transplantation. The continued need for pacing suggests that more significant myocardial injury has occurred.

Postoperative bleeding is another frequent problem with multiple potential causes. Extensive scarring and adhesions from previous palliative procedures are common. Pediatric patients may require some degree of aortic or pulmonary artery reconstruction at the time of transplantation, creating potentially extensive high-pressure suture lines that are not found in other heart transplantation settings. Chronic cyanosis may be associated with coagulation factor deficiencies, accelerated fibrinolysis, platelet function abnormalities, and an increased number and size of collateral vessels. Abnormalities in a variety of coagulation proteins have also been found in patients with single-ventricle physiology (Odegard et al., 2002a, 2002b, 2003, 2009). Many patients receive chronic anticoagulant therapy (e.g., aspirin, warfarin [Coumadin]), which cannot be discontinued in sufficient time to allow recovery of the coagulation profile before transplantation. Significant hemodynamic shear stress (e.g., aortic stenosis) can result in an acquired form of von Willebrand's disease by promoting degradation of active, high-molecular-weight von Willebrand multimers into inactive monomers. CPB induces bleeding in infants and small children. The causes for bypass-related bleeding are multifactorial and include hemodilution of coagulation factors, higher flow rates, higher shear stress (resulting in increased activation and consumption of platelets and coagulation and fibrinolytic proteins), greater blood trauma, use of colder temperatures, and an increased systemic inflammatory response.

In general, after protamine has been given to neutralize the heparin, platelets are given and can be followed by cryoprecipitate (Miller et al., 1997). Specific patients, such as those receiving warfarin preoperatively or with clinically significant preoperative coagulopathy due to hepatic dysfunction or malabsorption/protein-losing enteropathy, may also benefit from the administration of fresh frozen plasma. Use of antifibrinolytic agents such as tranexamic acid may also be beneficial, particularly in small infants and patients with a history of one or more prior thoracic procedures. The role for activated factor VII in postcardiotomy bleeding continues to be controversial and requires further study and definition (Pychynska-Pokorska et al., 2004; Agarwal et al., 2007; Guzzetta et al., 2009). At present, because of concerns about promoting hypercoaguability and thombotic complications, use of activated factor VII is probably best reserved for ongoing and uncontrolled bleeding that has been unresponsive to administration of the aforementioned clotting factors (and relative normalization of platelet count, PT, PTT, and so forth); there may be some ability to achieve effect while reducing thrombotic risk by using mini or lower dosage protocols (in the range of 60 mcg/kg, or even lower), although this too remains to be proven (Ekert et al., 2006).

Immunosuppression in Heart Transplantation

In brief, the rejection process begins when recipient CD4 T cells recognize foreign antigen in the donor heart. Recognition leads to activation of the larger T-cell pool, with subsequent IL-2 secretion, thereby triggering activation of monocytes/macrophages, B cells, and cytotoxic CD8 cells (Rose and Yacoub, 1990). Induction of immunotherapy is thus targeted toward the prevention of T-cell activation. This can occur by depleting the T-cell pool with monoclonal or polyclonal antibodies, or by using monoclonal antibodies to prevent IL-2 secretion. OKT3 is a murine monoclonal antibody used in clinical practice that binds to the CD3 molecule on the T-cell surface (Gay et al., 1988). This complex is closely linked to the antigenic recognition site of the T-cell receptor. Within minutes of beginning the administration of OKT3, the T-cell population decreases dramatically (Delmonico and Cosimi, 1988). T cells reappear within 3 to 5 days, but without the CD3 molecule. Although OKT3 was originally used in the context of acute rejection, its current use also includes induction of immunosuppression at the time of transplantation. When OKT3 is used in this fashion, the administration of cyclosporine or tacrolimus may be delayed by 5 to 7 days. This is particularly useful in the context of patients with borderline renal function, in whom calcineurin inhibitors and their nephrotoxic properties can further compromise renal function. Other side effects of OKT3 include chills, fever, diarrhea, dyspnea, and wheezing. Pulmonary edema and cardiac arrest have also been reported (Thistlethwaite et al., 1988).

ATG and ALG are polyclonal antibodies prepared from thymocytes and lymphoblasts, respectively. They are both IgG antibodies, and although the precise mechanism of action has yet to be elucidated, their administration causes profound lymphocytolysis. Side effects include chills, febrile reactions, erythema, and pruritus. Thrombocytopenia occurs in more than 50% of

patients, and serum sickness and Stevens-Johnson syndrome have also occurred secondary to ATG or ALG therapy.

Basiliximab and daclizumab are both monoclonal antibodies to the alpha chain of the IL-2 receptor. The receptor has three noncovalently bound chains. The alpha chain is specific for IL-2, and once activated by IL-2, the T cell begins its rejection amplification cascade (Kovarik et al., 1999). The binding of these monoclonal antibodies effectively and rapidly prevents activation of the cascade. Furthermore, the alpha chain is not present in inactivated T cells, and thus only activated T cells are targeted (Denton et al., 1999). There is some concern that these agents may be associated with an increased incidence of superimposed infections such as CMV and possibly the development of PTLD.

Maintenance of Immunosuppression

Three classes of drugs are available for maintenance of immunosuppression.

Corticosteroids. Corticosteroids are nonspecific antiinflammatory agents. Their effects are numerous and include inhibiting cytokine and cell-surface-molecule gene transcription in monocytes, inhibiting phospholipase A_2 enzyme activity and thus reducing the inflammatory cell activation, signaling, and inflammatory molecule production. Steroids also inhibit the nuclear transcription factor (NF)-κB, thus reducing IL-2 gene transcription and the production of several other proinflammatory cytokines and signaling and recognition molecules (Auphan et al., 1995). In general, most pediatric transplantation immunosuppressive regimens have moved toward trying to limit or even avoid routine steroid use due to the deleterious side effects on growth, glucose homeostasis, and so on.

Antiproliferative Agents. Antiproliferative agents prevent the expansion of activated T-cell and B-cell clones. The original agent used for this purpose, azathioprine, is being replaced by newer agents such as mycophenolate mofetil (MMF) and sirolimus (rapamycin). The toxic effects of azathioprine included bone marrow depression leading to marked leukopenia, possible liver damage, and the development of pancreatitis. MMF is a selective inhibitor of the de novo pathway of purine biosynthesis, thus inhibiting immune cell proliferation. It is administered as a morpholinoethylester prodrug of mycophenolic acid, which is metabolized to the active compound. Its mechanism of action is the result of reversible noncompetitive inhibition of inosine-monophosphate-dehydrogenase activity; it thereby targets proliferating lymphocytes. The lymphocytes are dependent on the availability of guanine nucleotides, which are no longer generated in the presence of the drug (Allison et al., 1993; Brazelton and Morris, 1996; Shaw et al., 1999). Side effects of MMF include nausea and vomiting, but it lacks significant bone marrow and renal toxicity. There is a concern, however, about the possible development of invasive CMV infection during the use of MMF. Rapamycin (sirolimus) is a newer antiproliferative agent that, despite binding to FK506-binding protein 12, confers its action by inhibiting cellular proliferation without inhibiting calcineurin (see later). Side effects appear to be dosage-dependent elevation of triglyceride levels and dosage-dependent bone marrow suppression.

Calcineurin Inhibitors. Calne's (1979) first published use of cyclosporine as an immunosuppressive agent was in 1979, and it continues to be one of the primary drugs used for the prevention of rejection in many transplantation programs. The mechanism of action of cyclosporine involves binding to cyclophilin in the T-cell cytosol. This cyclosporine–cyclophilin complex then binds to calcineurin and prevents calcineurin from promoting transcription of the IL-2 gene, thus preventing further IL-2 production (Schreiber and Crabtree, 1992; Schreier et al., 1993). The most significant side effect of cyclosporine therapy is nephrotoxicity; other significant side effects include liver dysfunction, hypertension, hyperlipidemia, and PTLD (Kahan et al., 1989).

Tacrolimus (FK506) is a macrolide that also acts as a calcineurin inhibitor. It forms a complex with an immunophilin, FK-binding protein, and this complex subsequently binds to calcineurin to prevent IL-2 gene transcription (Liu et al., 1991; Sigal and Dumont, 1992). Side effects include nephrotoxicity, glucose intolerance, and an increased incidence of PTLD.

Most pediatric heart transplantation programs use some form of triple immunosuppressive therapy, and calcineurin inhibitors, antimetabolites, and corticosteroids are the mainstays of antirejection therapies. Although cyclosporine is still used at times, tacrolimus use appears to be overtaking it. The nephrotoxicity of both drugs is significant. As noted earlier, use of azathioprine has decreased in favor of MMF or sirolimus. The use of sirolimus will increase further if suggestions of reduced transplantation vasculopathy associated with its use are confirmed (Mancini et al., 2003). The use of steroids remains at fairly constant levels, but increased acceptance of the newer agents is likely to lead to more rapid weaning and lower dosages of corticosteroids, thereby limiting the side effects of growth retardation, hypertension, and glucose intolerance; this is especially true in infant and pediatric transplantation. The roles of rapamycin and the IL-2 receptor antagonists continue to evolve, with the former being used with greater frequency to treat recurrent rejection, and the latter for induction and prevention of acute rejection (Sudan et al., 2007).

Data from the International Society for Heart and Lung Transplantation suggest that approximately 50% of children received induction immunotherapy between January 2001 and June 2009. The most common induction therapy included either ATG or ALG, followed by a specific IL-2 receptor antagonist. A small proportion of children also received OKT3. There are as yet no randomized multicenter studies to determine the benefits of induction therapy, but available evidence indicates that children given polyclonal ATG or other forms of induction therapy have lower mortality than those given no induction agent or OKT3 (Boucek et al., 1990, 2002; Sudan et al., 2007). In general, the use of induction therapy allows the initiation of calcineurin inhibitors to be delayed for a few days postoperatively, which may be most beneficial in patients with some degree of renal dysfunction.

Complications

Complications following heart transplantation can be divided into those associated with rejection and those arising from other causes (Behrendt et al., 1991; Steed et al., 1985). Acute rejection generally occurs in the first year after transplantation and is the most frequent cause of death during this time period. Late-onset acute rejection also occurs in a significant number of children beyond the first posttransplantation year. Acute rejection remains a major source of morbidity as well and correlates

with the ongoing need for immunosuppression (Chartrand et al., 2001; Azeka et al., 2002). Although specific risk factors for acute rejection have been sought, results have been conflicting (Kirklin et al., 1992; Webber, 2003). Overall, it appears that an older age at the time of transplantation increases the risk for acute rejection, and that an episode of acute rejection in the first year increases the risk for subsequent episodes (Webber, 2003).

Clinical detection of rejection remains difficult, as signs and symptoms are subtle and nonspecific; these include general malaise, fever, change in activity or appetite, tachycardia, and conduction or voltage changes on the surface ECG. More severe bouts may be accompanied by clinically symptomatic reductions in graft function. Other relatively noninvasive tests, such as various myocardial or inflammatory markers in blood, echocardiography, and cardiac MRI, continue to be investigated, but none of the tests has shown the necessary sensitivity and specificity. As a result, endomyocardial biopsy remains the gold standard for diagnosis of rejection (Boucek, 2000; Wagner et al., 2000; Atluri et al., 2008). It is performed at scheduled intervals as a surveillance tool, to guide immunosuppression regimens and dosing, and to diagnose acute rejection episodes.

Chronic rejection and associated posttransplantation coronary artery disease are the leading causes of death among late survivors of heart transplantation. According to data from the International Society for Heart and Lung Transplantation, approximately 20% of all pediatric transplantation patients have some degree of posttransplantation coronary artery disease at 5 years after transplantation. This accelerated vasculopathy can affect infants, children, and adults alike. The mortality after the diagnosis is substantial. The histologic appearance is that of concentric myointimal proliferation that ultimately results in luminal occlusion. In addition to repeated bouts of rejection, CMV infection is likely to be a contributing risk factor (Hussain et al., 2007; Mahle et al., 2009). Efforts have been made to more aggressively control other etiologic factors present in these patients that can contribute to the development of atherosclerosis, such as hypertension, hyperlipidemia, and glucose intolerance (Eich et al., 1991). At present, the effects of these efforts are uncertain. As the transplanted heart is denervated, chest pain caused by myocardial ischemia is a rare presenting complaint; progressive deterioration in graft function, heart failure, or sudden death are the primary evidences of rejection. For this reason, transplant recipients are routinely screened (usually on a yearly basis) for this development (Smart et al., 1991). Although coronary angiography was long thought to be the most sensitive means of detecting the development of graft vasculopathy, it underestimates the presence of early or mild disease. As a result, many centers have begun to use dobutamine stress echocardiography as the primary means of screening for coronary artery disease in transplant recipients (Pahl et al., 1999). Intracoronary ultrasound may also be useful (Dent et al., 2000; Schratz et al., 2002; Costello et al., 2003; Sudan et al., 2007).

Treatment of posttransplantation coronary artery disease is palliative coronary artery stenting (which is of limited benefit given the diffuse nature and involvement of distal vessels) or retransplantation. Rapamycin, which appears to slow the progression of transplantation vasculopathy, has shown some benefit, either as an additional immunosuppressive treatment or in the form of rapamycin-coated coronary stents (Morice et al., 2002; Mancini et al., 2003). Retransplantation for graft vasculopathy and resulting graft failure are usually felt to be associated with greater risk and diminished success, although there is some adult evidence that it can be accomplished with reasonable 1- and 5-year survival rates (Atluri et al., 2008; Kanter et al., 2004).

Infection after heart transplantation is usually caused by bacterial pathogens that do not cause disease in the immunocompetent host (Schowengerdt et al., 1997). Immunosuppression makes the severity of infections much worse, and even with early aggressive therapy, such infections are significant causes of morbidity and mortality in the transplantation patient (Dummer, 1990; Hoflin et al., 1987). In addition to bacterial pathogens, other opportunistic pathogens such as fungi and viruses (CMV, Epstein-Barr, and adenovirus) cause significant morbidity. Infection with Ebstein-Barr virus has been associated with the development of PTLD (Webber, 2003). This may be treated initially with reduction in immunosuppressive therapy and, failing this, with chemotherapeutic agents. Other complications in heart transplantation patients are mostly secondary to immunosuppressive regimens and include diabetes, growth retardation, hypertension, renal dysfunction, and malignancy (Groetzner et al., 2005; Kirk et al., 2009).

Outcome after Pediatric Heart Transplantation

Data from the International Society for Heart and Lung Transplantation show that the actuarial 10-year survival rate for all pediatric heart recipients exceeds 50% (Boucek et al., 2002; Kirk et al., 2009). The mortality rate is higher in infants in the first year of life, but this is followed by a slightly lower mortality rate of less than 2% per year in the 4- to 10-year period. If one excludes the first-year mortality rate, the conditional actuarial survival in infants exceeds 80%. Adolescents have a slightly higher average mortality—4% per year. In comparing the actuarial survival in the first 4 posttransplantation years by era, significant progress has occurred. There is some evidence that heart transplantation in adults with CHD may also be accomplished with reasonable short- and longer-term prognosis (Coskun et al., 2007a, 2007b).

From 1982 through 1987, the actuarial 4-year survival rate was just below 60%, whereas in the current era (2000 to 2008), the 4-year actuarial survival approaches 80%. The greatest risk factor for first-year mortality was the diagnosis of congenital heart disease. Recipient age was also found to be a risk factor. Patients younger than 6 years and older than 12 years were at increased risk. Other risk factors for poor first-year outcome may include ventilatory support or hospitalization before transplantation, high PVRI (>6 Wood units/m^2), hepatitis C positivity, PRA greater than 40%, low creatinine clearance (<40 mL/min), donor-to-recipient weight ratio less than 0.7, and the need for retransplantation; risk appears to increase as the number of these factors increases (Davies et al., 2008). The role for and success of cardiac retransplantation in pediatric patients remain controversial, with some data indicating worse outcomes, whereas others suggest that retransplantation can be accomplished in pediatric patients with 1- and 3-year survival rates that approximate those of primary transplantation (Mahle et al., 2005). Of note, recent data (based on adult heart transplantation results) suggest that low transplantation volume in a program (perhaps in the range of less than 2 to 10 transplantations per year) was an independent risk factor for worse short-term outcome (Weiss et al., 2008).

Acute primary graft failure is the major cause of death after infant cardiac transplantation, as well as a prominent cause in older patients (Huang et al., 2004). Anoxic brain death, prolonged cardiopulmonary resuscitation, and long cardiac ischemic time are prominent donor risk factors, with CHD (as opposed to cardiomyopathy), PVR index, and the need for preoperative mechanical support significant recipient risk factors. Recipient factors not associated with increased risk for death during the first year include the need for inotropic support, use of prostaglandin, use of ECMO, prior sternotomy, height, the need for dialysis, recent infection, and a history of malignancy. Although age did affect first-year mortality risk, weight as an independent factor posed no additional risk. Despite the increased risk for complications, use of ECMO appears to be associated with functional recovery and reasonable survival in pediatric heart transplant recipients suffering from acute graft failure and unresponsive to other therapies (Tissot et al., 2009).

Overall, the leading cause of death in transplant recipients under the age of 3 years is acute rejection. In addition to graft failure, other causes of early mortality include acute rejection and PTLD. In patients older than 3 years, coronary artery vasculopathy is a major source of morbidity and mortality, as are infections and neoplasms; hypertension and renal dysfunction can be prominent as well (Boucek et al., 2002; Gambino et al., 2007; Kirk et al., 2009). Adolescents represent a particularly problematic subgroup (for other types of transplantation as well) because of poor compliance. Among survivors, over 95% of patients report no limitation of activity at the 5-year follow-up. However, with formal exercise testing, as many as 50% may have mild to moderate limitations in exercise and aerobic capacity (Borow, 1985). In the absence of rejection, in general, myocardial and somatic growth are normal in most pediatric transplant recipients (de Broux et al., 2001; Sudan et al., 2007; Baum et al., 1991; Bernstein et al., 1992). A growing number of pediatric heart transplant recipients are entering their second and third decades after transplantation (Ross et al., 2006). There is also evidence of at least some degree of autonomic reinnervation of the cardiac allograft (Fallen et al., 1988; Stark et al., 1991).

Lung Transplantation

Demographics and Indications

At present, more than 2000 pediatric lung transplantations have been performed (Sweet, 2009). As with pediatric heart transplantation, available data suggest that the annual number of pediatric lung transplantations conducted since the late 1980s has plateaued since a peak in the late 1990s. Waiting times have increased overall; adolescents may wait as long as 1 or 2 years for cadaveric lungs (average waiting time, 20 months), whereas younger children (1 to 10 years old) wait an average of approximately 6 to 12 months. Organ donation number and viability continue to be major limitations (Burch and Aurora, 2004; Sudan et al., 2007; Sweet, 2009; Egan, 1989; Orens and Garrity, 2009), resulting in a consistent rate of approximately 50 pediatric lung transplantations per year in the United States. In 2005, the overall (adult) system of donor lung allocation was changed from one based primarily on waiting time to one based on survival models that attempt to estimate wait-list and posttransplantation survival. The effects (if any) of this change on wait times and outcome for adult and pediatric lung transplantation candidates are uncertain at the present time (Davis and Garrity, 2007; Iribarne et al., 2009; Hachem and Trulock, 2008a).

Early pediatric lung transplantation efforts emerged directly from adult experience (Egan, 1992), and the majority of the recipients were older children with cystic fibrosis (CF), primary pulmonary hypertension, secondary pulmonary hypertension (e.g., from CHD), and pulmonary fibrosis. With increasing experience and the development of pediatric lung transplantation centers, transplantations in infants and younger children have increased, and children younger than 2 to 3 years may now comprise 10% to 20% of lung transplant recipients. In infants and young children (without CF), the most common diagnoses include interstitial lung disease, primary pulmonary hypertension, severe pulmonary vein obstruction (which typically appears with severe pulmonary hypertension and varying degrees of airspace and ventilatory abnormalities), and alveolar proteinoses (Dandel et al., 2003). In contrast, CF accounts for greater than 50% of all lung transplantations in older children and adolescents, for whom 5-year survival rates range from about 50% to 65% (Waltz et al., 2006; Faro et al., 2007; Spahr et al., 2007; Aurora et al., 2009).

Contraindications

Absolute contraindications to pediatric lung transplantation include hepatitis B or C virus infection, HIV infection, active malignancy within the past 1 to 2 years, and irreversible neurologic or neuromuscular disorders. Significant liver, heart, or renal dysfunction (requiring dialysis) is also an absolute contraindication; lung-liver or heart-lung transplantation may be considered in the presence of the first two of these conditions. Some issues such as prior thoracotomies or pleurodeses, steroid dependence, or colonization with a variety of organisms (especially in patients with CF) are no longer absolute contraindications in most centers. Relative contraindications include significant musculoskeletal disease, invasive ventilation (which has been linked to increased risk in older patients, potentially less so in infants and young children), colonization with *Burkholderia cepacia,* various fungi or atypical mycobacteria, poor nutritional status (<70% or >130% of ideal body weight), and an inability to wean from or significantly reduce dependency on systemic corticosteroids (Hadjiliadis, 2007). As with heart transplantation, significant psychological and behavioral disturbances in the potential recipient, or social and familial circumstances that could hinder access to care or compliance with complex medical regimens, may also preclude transplantation.

Organ Preservation

Achieving successful lung preservation continues to be a difficult problem. Lung ischemic time is a major factor in the development of posttransplantation lung injury. The optimal duration of preservation is between 3 and 4 hours, although lungs with ischemic times as long as 9 hours have been implanted successfully (Kaiser et al., 1991). During organ harvest, the lungs and pericardium are exposed and a prostaglandin infusion is begun. Prostaglandin is believed to cause pulmonary dilation and thereby improves the distribution of preservation solution. The venae cavae are then transected, the left atrial appendage is incised, and then the aorta is cross-clamped. This harvesting sequence prevents any left atrial hypertension and thus reduces the risk for pulmonary edema. A cold crystalloid preservation solution (e.g., Euro-Collins') with a high potassium concentration is infused into the pulmonary artery while cardioplegia is administered into the aortic root. Ventilation is discontinued and the lungs are allowed to deflate. For single-

or sequential double-lung transplantation, the left atrium is divided so that a cuff of atrial tissue surrounds the right and left pulmonary veins. The pulmonary veins may be excised in a single atrial cuff for double-lung transplantation. If both the heart and lung (or lungs) are to be used (but in different recipients), adequate segments of the left atrium and pulmonary artery must be allocated to each (Griffith and Zenati, 1990). During transportation, the lungs are generally kept deflated, although there is some experimental evidence that intermittent inflation prolongs the allowable ischemic time (Toledo-Pereyra et al., 1977). In addition, some centers believe that donor cooling with CPB also extends the permissible ischemic time (Heritier et al., 1992).

Single-Lung Transplantation

Single-lung transplantation is performed infrequently in pediatric patients (Mal et al., 1989). One general reason is that the ability of the transplanted lung to grow remains uncertain. Most practitioners believe it is wise to implant as much normal lung tissue as possible to meet the demands of future somatic growth in children. Second, the most frequent indication for pediatric lung transplantation is CF, and there is great concern about the transplanted lung being contaminated by the chronically infected native lung.

When a single-lung transplantation is performed, the most important decision is the determination of laterality, usually determined by chest radiograph, chest computed tomography, or scans. The side that appears to have the less affected lung or that has a better ventilation/perfusion scan is kept; the opposite side is transplanted. If possible, implantation is done on the side opposite to any previous thoracotomy. Typically, a more emphysematous lung is removed (or its volume reduced) so as not to compress the allograft on the opposite side. A more fibrotic lung might remain, so as to favor ventilation and blood flow distribution to the transplanted lung. There is some evidence that outcomes from double-lung transplantation may be favored (compared with single) in patients with emphysematous-type processes (Hadjiliadis and Angel, 2006).

Omentum may be fashioned to provide a vascular cuff around the bronchial anastomosis to improve bronchial blood supply. In such cases, a midline laparotomy is performed first, to mobilize omentum with an attached pedicle. This is tunneled through the diaphragm and the incision is closed (Fig. 20-23). Single-lung ventilation is then instituted (see later). A thoracotomy is performed, and the pulmonary artery, pulmonary veins, and main stem bronchus are exposed. The pulmonary artery is then test-occluded while gas exchange, PAP, and hemodynamic status are observed. The lung is removed if the patient tolerates this procedure. Allograft implantation involves connecting the donor atrial flap containing the pulmonary vein orifices to an area of recipient left atrial tissue that is isolated within a clamp. The pulmonary artery anastomosis is completed. The technique of telescoping bronchial anastomosis is used frequently (Calhoon et al., 1991). To perform this, the smaller of the two bronchial ends is placed inside the other one to a depth of one cartilaginous ring, and then the connection is oversewn. This method provides sufficient blood flow for high-quality bronchial healing and precludes the need for an omental cuff. The lung is then gently inflated. Air in the vascular spaces is removed either via the pulmonary artery (with the left atrium partially occluded, the proximal end of

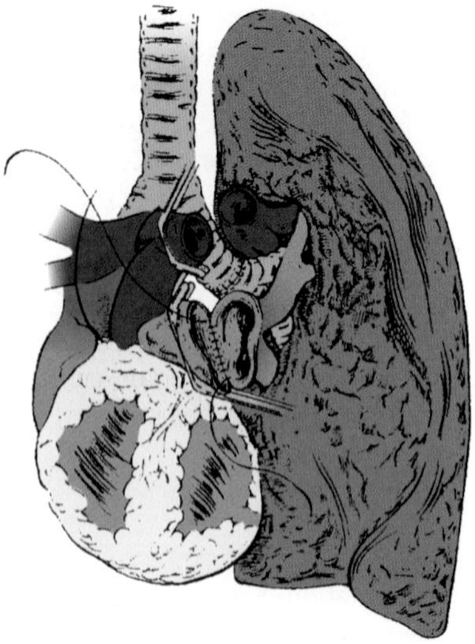

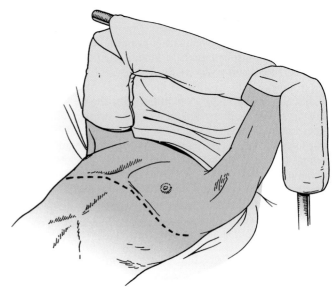

■ **FIGURE 20-23.** The bronchial anastomosis is completed first, followed by the vascular anastomoses. The vessel is reconstructed from posterior to anterior with the suture untied, allowing de-airing through the anastomosis later. *(From Kirby TJ, Birnbaum PL: Technique of single-lung transplantation. In Patterson GA, Couraud L, editors:* Current topics in general thoracic surgery, vol. 3: Lung transplantation, *Amsterdam, 1995, Elsevier Science.)*

■ **FIGURE 20-24.** Clam-shell position with the arms at a 90-degree angle.

the pulmonary artery is clamped, and its distal end vented) or via the left atrial cuff (with the pulmonary artery unclamped and the left atrial cuff vented). Pulmonary blood flow and ventilation are then established simultaneously.

Double-Lung Transplantation

Double-lung transplantation is the type of lung transplantation operation performed most frequently in pediatric patients. The technique most often used involves sequentially implanting each lung. This method has several advantages compared with en bloc implantation, which was done previously by some (Pasque et al., 1990; Kaiser et al., 1991). The lungs are harvested individually, each with a separate pulmonary artery, main stem bronchus, and two pulmonary veins encompassed within a cuff of the donor's left atrium. A bilateral anterior thoracosternotomy is performed extending across the midline by transverse sternotomy. This approach ("clamshell" incision) allows the anterior thoracic cage to be swiveled upward, providing full access to the bilateral hilar structures (Fig. 20-24). Each set of pulmonary arteries and main stem bronchi are anastomosed end to end, and each left atrial cuff is anastomosed to the recipient's left atrium. CPB is almost always used in pediatric patients, although it is possible to perform bilateral sequential lung transplantation without CPB. Omental flaps may be mobilized for each bronchial connection, although most current techniques use telescoping bronchial anastomoses. Both methods appear to result in improved healing of the airway connections, compared with tracheal anastomoses (as are used with the en bloc method). This is presumably because of enhanced blood flow. Volume reduction of the transplanted lungs may be required in infant and small child recipients from older or larger donors.

Living Donor Lung Transplantation

The shortage of donor organs has led to the development of living donor lobar lung transplantation, which requires that two separate donors each undergo lobectomies to provide right and left lower lobes. Outcomes of living donor lung transplantations have been comparable with cadaveric lung transplantations (Starnes et al., 1999; Toyooka et al., 2008). The technique of living related lung transplantations also overcomes some of the inherent difficulties of attempting to predict the clinical course of various types of lung disease and the appropriate timing for listing the patient for transplantation. Size limitations can be problematic: adult lobes are usually too large for children under 5 years, and, conversely, the amount of lung tissue may be insufficient for larger adolescents. The various anastomoses, particularly those of the pulmonary veins, can be technically difficult and prone to stenosis. The operation poses more than a minimal risk to the donors, and truly informed consent may be difficult to determine in such an emotionally difficult situation. The ethical issues are therefore complex, and this procedure is infrequently performed.

Non–Heart Beating Donors

Donation-after-cardiac-death (DCD) protocols have reemerged as a possible mechanism to increase the donor pool. This strategy remains in its infancy, and ethical issues are a significant limitation. As with the use of DCD hearts, there are technical issues relating to organ harvest and its effect on organ preservation and harvest regimens, ischemic time limitations, and resulting donor organ function. Some limited data show that this may be a useful technique that could modestly increase the donor pool with outcomes potentially similar to more conventional lung transplantation strategies (Erasmus et al., 2010; Oto, 2008; Snell et al., 2008a, 2008b).

Heart-Lung Transplantation

Because of early problems with the integrity of bronchial anastomoses, many patients with terminal lung disease received heart-lung transplants, with the possibility of their (normal) heart going to a heart transplant recipient in a "domino" procedure (Starnes, 1990). Since the development of techniques to promote healing of bronchial anastomoses, the frequency of heart-lung transplantation has decreased substantially. At present, in pediatric patients it is considered only for patients with pulmonary hypertension or other end-stage lung disease when there is also CHD that cannot be repaired, and for patients with end-stage lung disease and severe left or right ventricular dysfunction. Pulmonary hypertension with right heart dysfunction is no longer considered an indication, unless the right ventricular dysfunction is severe, as the right ventricular dysfunction often improves after successful lung transplantation.

Anesthetic Management of the Lung Transplant Recipient

These patients are often critically ill by the time they come for lung transplantation (Armitage et al., 1995). Reasons for this include the nature of the underlying disease, reticence on the parts of both physicians and patients (or families) to undergo such a procedure, and the long waiting time required for cadaveric organs. For example, the clinical course of CF is very unpredictable. Most centers initiate the transplantation process when a CF patient's forced expiratory volume at 1.0 second (FEV_1) falls below 30% to 40% of predicted value; however, most centers would not actually transplant patients at this point if the patient thinks that his or her quality of life is acceptable (Yankaskas and Mallory, 1998; Dellon et al., 2007). Thus, the CF patient is likely to be quite compromised (pulmonary function, nutrition, and so on) by the time of actual transplantation.

In children with pulmonary hypertension, survival has been inversely related to right atrial and pulmonary artery pressures, as well as to the product of right atrial pressure and PVR (Clabby et al., 1997). However, it is likely that prostacyclin therapy (and perhaps newer agents such as endothelin receptor antagonists or phosphodiesterase V inhibitors such as sildenafil) will improve survival and prevent, or at least delay, the need for lung transplantation in some children with pulmonary hypertension (Rosenzweig et al., 1999; Rubin et al., 2002; Landzberg, 2007; Bush et al., 1986, 1987). Similarly, patients with severe pulmonary venous obstructive disease, which can be a primary phenomenon or follow repair of totally anomalous venous return or other congenital cardiac lesions, may be palliated for prolonged periods with catheter balloon dilations and possibly chemotherapy (Peng et al., 2009). As seen in patients with CF, one consequence is that ventilatory or pulmonary hypertensive complications can be quite significant by the time they are referred for lung transplantation.

Patients with end-stage CF, idiopathic restrictive lung disease, pulmonary venous obstruction, or other lung parenchymal diseases (e.g., alveolar proteinosis) are often hypoxic or hypercarbic (or both) and may be dependent on supplemental oxygen. Their ventilatory effort is at least partially sustained by increased circulating catecholamine concentrations. Deep levels of sedation can reduce ventilatory drive and cause hypotension and are best avoided. If necessary, small increments of midazolam may be titrated until the desired effect is achieved. Although sedative medication may be useful as an adjunct to control pulmonary vascular responses during induction, this should be given only in the immediate preoperative period, with full monitoring in situ. If undertaken, small increments of midazolam are administered until the desired effect is achieved.

The preoperative assessment of the lung transplant recipient is focused on cardiopulmonary status as well as on dysfunction in other organ systems. The CF patient undergoing lung transplantation is usually already on maximal medical therapy. This may include oral or inhaled bronchodilators, supplemental oxygen, nebulized antibiotics, N-acetylcysteine or DNase, and chest physiotherapy. These are continued through the time of surgery. It is important to have recent information about right ventricular function and pulmonary artery pressures (both usually with echocardiography). Baseline liver and renal function, as well as coagulation status (potentially compromised by malabsorption in the CF patient), should also be determined.

Monitoring and Vascular Access

Noninvasive monitoring is instituted before induction. An arterial catheter may also be inserted under local anesthesia before induction. However, this is usually performed after induction in young children. Although cannulation of the central venous circulation may be difficult in the patient with severe obstruction or fibrosis because of the large negative intrathoracic pressures generated during spontaneous ventilation, it is usually possible before induction. Pulmonary artery catheterization before pneumonectomy is essential if assessment of the response to pulmonary arterial cross-clamping is required (i.e., single-lung transplantation or bilateral sequential transplantation without CPB). Either the catheter is floated into the appropriate artery using TEE guidance, or the surgeon places the tip by palpation. It is essential to withdraw the catheter tip into the main pulmonary artery before pneumonectomy in patients undergoing bilateral lung transplantation. If available, TEE may be used to visualize the effects of PA occlusion and mechanical ventilation on ventricular function (Triantafillou and Heerdt, 1991). TEE can also provide valuable information about ventricular function and volume status after transplantation.

Intraoperative and postoperative bleeding can be significant. This may be exacerbated by extensive adhesions, especially in patients with longstanding lung inflammation (e.g., CF) or those who have undergone prior thoracic surgery. Thus, it is important to have large-bore vascular access to facilitate rapid volume resuscitation. Often, the use of a rapid infusion device is quite helpful. Almost all pediatric lung transplantations are performed with the patient supine and the patient's arms raised over the head and flexed at the elbows (see Fig. 20-24). This position may occlude catheters placed in the antecubital fossae, and thus other sites are recommended. Epidural catheters can provide excellent postoperative analgesia and facilitate ventilatory effort and pulmonary toilet. Although the use of the lumbar or thoracic approach is adequate, the decision to place the catheter while the child is awake or after induction remains unresolved. In addition, the placement of an epidural catheter in a child who is to undergo lung transplantation using CPB is also contentious. An alternative approach is to place the epidural catheter on the first or second postoperative day, before extubation, when the coagulation status has normalized.

Induction and Maintenance of Anesthesia

A child who is to undergo lung transplantation has precarious physiology and minimal reserve and is usually frightened and thus has elevated levels of circulating endogenous catecholamines. Thus, it is important that the anesthetic induction have minimal effects on the pulmonary and cardiovascular systems. Myocardial depression and increased pulmonary vascular tone should be avoided, whereas bronchodilation and pulmonary vascular dilation are frequently desirable. Etomidate, ketamine, propofol, and thiopental have all been used successfully for IV induction (Triantafillou and Heerdt, 1991). However, should a rapid sequence induction be required, etomidate may provide the best overall combination of hemodynamic stability and rapid airway control. Ketamine is useful in those patients prone to airway reactivity. The effect of ketamine on PVR is controversial; it probably does not increase PVR if hypoxia and hypercarbia are avoided (Hickey et al., 1985). Ketamine does, however, have some direct negative inotropic effects, and it should be avoided in patients with severe pulmonary hypertension or significant right ventricular dysfunction.

Potent synthetic opioids such as fentanyl are frequently used for both induction and maintenance of anesthesia. In addition to providing relative hemodynamic stability, opioids are effective in attenuating sympathetic stimulation in those patients prone to pulmonary hypertensive crises. To avoid the chest wall rigidity (and limitation to ventilation) that may occur with these agents, it is usually preferable to perform an IV induction with etomidate, establish neuromuscular blockade, and then titrate the opioids to achieve the desired effect. Although the vagolytic effects of pancuronium may be useful in conjunction with synthetic opioid administration, vecuronium or rocuronium also may be used.

There is some evidence that nitrous oxide may increase PVR and impair hypoxic pulmonary vasoconstriction (Sykes et al., 1977; Schulte-Sasse et al., 1982), and thus it is probably best avoided. Inhaled anesthetics are usually used in moderate concentrations as anesthetic adjuncts and to provide amnesia; bronchodilation and perhaps some degree of pulmonary vasodilation secondary to abolishment of pulmonary vascular vasoconstriction may be other benefits. All volatile anesthetics are likely to impair hypoxic pulmonary vasoconstriction to some degree, which may be a particular problem if single-lung ventilation is used and also in patients with significant lung disease, V/Q mismatch, or intrapulmonary shunting (Benumof, 1985). In most situations, a standard single-lumen endotracheal tube of an appropriate size is used for lung transplantation with CPB. An appropriate double-lumen endotracheal tube is inserted after induction for single-lung transplantation or bilateral sequential transplantation without CPB. It is placed to provide differential lung isolation, and its position may be confirmed by flexible bronchoscopic examination (Benumof, 1985, 1991). At all times, the possibility of tube obstruction from inspirated secretions and blood clots must be kept in mind. If a double-lumen endotracheal tube is used, it is exchanged for a standard endotracheal tube at the completion of the procedure. Prior to lung replacement, the initial inspiratory oxygen concentration is usually set at 100%. This can then be adjusted according to pulse oximetry and blood gases. Ventilatory parameters are set according to the pathophysiology of the disease involved. The patient with restrictive lung disease is best ventilated with higher rates and lower-than-normal tidal volumes to minimize peak airway pressures, whereas the patient with obstructive lung disease may benefit from longer expiratory times to allow complete expiration and to prevent "stacking" of breaths. In some situations, it may be necessary to manually ventilate the patient to establish the optimal ventilatory pattern. The addition of PEEP may improve gas exchange, but excessive PEEP may compromise the patient's cardiovascular status. Volume resuscitation and inotropic support may be necessary to counter the negative hemodynamic effects of PEEP. In patients with CF, frequent suctioning of the endotracheal tube should be performed to keep it clear of copious and tenacious secretions, which in some patients can be voluminous.

Intraoperative Concerns

Patients undergoing lung transplantation have, by definition, severely compromised cardiorespiratory function. If the intention is to conduct either a single-lung or sequential bilateral lung transplantation without using CPB, there needs to be constant reassessment of the patient's underlying cardiorespiratory status, because single-lung ventilation frequently leads to unacceptable levels of CO_2 and cardiac instability (Triantafillou and Heerdt, 1991). If at any point the situation becomes untenable, the patient is placed on CPB to complete the procedure.

Two events must be critically evaluated. First, with the onset of single-lung ventilation, an immediate increase in airway resistance occurs in all patients. In patients with restrictive lung disease, these changes are more pronounced. High airway pressure will both inhibit venous return and reduce pulmonary blood flow. The initial respiratory management is an adjustment of the ventilatory setting and the possible addition of inotropic agents to augment support for right ventricular function. If gas exchange and hemodynamic status are not improved, then it is important to reinstitute two-lung ventilation while plans for CPB are instituted.

The second intervention that needs to be evaluated is when the pulmonary artery is occluded during single-lung ventilation. Occlusion of the pulmonary artery during one-lung ventilation leads to an improvement in gas exchange. This occurs because the shunt passing through the collapsed lung is removed and the V/Q matching in the perfused lung is improved by minimizing physiologic dead space. However, PAP is increased, with a concomitant increase in afterload. This increased afterload is best treated with pulmonary vasodilation using agents such as prostaglandin, milrinone, or NO. Maintaining coronary perfusion of the hypertensive right ventricle is essential to preserving its function. Thus, adequate preload and inotropic support (alone or in combination with β-adrenergic agonists) may also be necessary. If right ventricular failure cannot be managed with preload and inotropic support, then the pulmonary artery should be unclamped and CPB instituted.

In contrast, double sequential lung transplantation performed on CPB does not have these physiologic difficulties. The lungs are reperfused individually as soon as the anastomoses are complete. After the implantation of the first lung, there is often a "honeymoon" period of excellent gas exchange, but it may be short-lived. Gas exchange may worsen because of factors that include reperfusion injury and pulmonary edema, and reduced compliance. Pulmonary hypertension may also occur as a result of vascular injury triggered by ischemia–reperfusion, and hyperinflation in an open thoracic cavity. These two problems can usually be resolved with ventilatory adjustment and the use of moderate levels of PEEP. Inhaled NO (typically 20 to 40 ppm in oxygen) has become a mainstay of posttransplantation management in many centers (Date et al., 1996; Rea et al., 2005; Baez and Castillo, 2008; Yerebakan et al., 2009) to optimize PVR as well as V/Q matching. Inotropic support is frequently required.

Blood products, including platelets and clotting factors, may be required (occasionally in quite substantial amounts) to correct for ongoing bleeding at surgical sites, adhesions as a result of CPB, and preexisting coagulation abnormalities. The bronchial anastomoses are usually inspected toward the end of the procedure using flexible bronchoscopy, to verify integrity and patency of the airway anastomoses. Patients with "septic lungs" (e.g., CF patients) occasionally develop sepsis or a syndrome resembling septic shock, probably from bacteremia or release of inflammatory mediators during removal of their native lungs, in the early postbypass period. The outcome is frequently poor, despite intensive therapy with inotropes, antibiotics, and so on.

Early Postoperative Complications

Acute Graft Dysfunction

Acute dysfunction of the transplanted lung immediately after implantation or over the ensuing several hours continues to be a significant problem, occurring in up to 30% or 40% of recipients. The primary mechanism is believed to be related to ischemia–reperfusion injury, and in fact its appearance and severity are generally associated with a longer duration of ischemia. The contribution of other factors, such as duration of donor support and occult lung injury (e.g., trauma, infection, multiple transfusions), or recipient factors, such as chronic infection or colonization or use of CPB, is unclear. Acute graft dysfunction typically resembles an acute respiratory distress syndrome or noncardiogenic pulmonary edema, with key features that include markedly decreased lung compliance and impaired gas exchange (especially oxygenation), as well as frequently large amounts of pulmonary edema-like secretions.

The primary treatment is prevention, aiming to keep lung ischemic times to less than 5 to 6 hours whenever possible. The other major focus is on mechanical ventilation, with appropriate use of airway pressures and PEEP. In general, ventilatory parameters should be adjusted to maintain normocarbia or mild hypocarbia with adequate but not excessive lung expansion. Peak and mean airway pressures are kept at the minimum required to maintain gas exchange while protecting the bronchial anastomoses and limiting the possibility of volutrauma. Inspired oxygen concentration is kept as low as practical, so that Pao_2 is below 120 mm Hg, to limit oxygen toxicity and reperfusion injury. In the case of single-lung transplantation, the two differing cardiorespiratory requirements make hypoxia due to V/Q mismatch more likely (Triantafillou and Heerdt, 1991). It may, on occasion, be necessary to use differential lung ventilation to address the ventilatory requirements of the two lungs independently (Todd, 1990; Smiley et al., 1991). Fluid and blood product administration are limited as much as possible. As noted previously, inhaled NO may be beneficial in some circumstances to improve the V/Q matching and to reduce PVR (Rocca et al., 1997). ECMO has been used successfully in some cases of acute graft failure to allow recovery of lung function. As with some cases of acute cardiac allograft rejection, acute antibody-mediated rejection of lung allografts is being recognized with increasing frequency; treatment may include posttransplant plasmapheresis (Morrell et al., 2009). There is also emerging evidence that primary graft dysfunction is a significant risk factor for subsequent immune-mediated graft injury (Bharat et al., 2008).

Infection

Infection is a significant problem in the immediate postoperative period. There are multiple risk factors. In addition to extensive surgical sites and invasive catheters, the patient is often nutritionally compromised and has begun receiving high-potency immunosuppressive agents. The transplanted lung is denervated. The cough reflex is therefore lost below the level of the anastomosis. Airway ciliary function is also likely to be severely impaired in the posttransplantation period. It is essential that chest physiotherapy and tracheobronchial suction be performed routinely to prevent accumulation of blood and secretions, which can obstruct the endotracheal tube or airways and contribute to infection. Bronchoscopy may be necessary at times to clear the airway of the debris. An absence of lymphatic drainage from the donor lung (or lungs) contributes to the tendency to accumulate lung water and develop infection and acute graft dysfunction (Montefusco and Veith, 1986; Todd, 1990). Use of prophylactic antibiotics is routine and guided by the donor's and recipient's colonization status and by subsequent surveillance cultures in the recipient. Ganciclovir (for CMV) and antifungal agents are given when these pathogens exist in either donor or recipient. Infection with parainfluenza, adenovirus, and herpesvirus can be life threatening in pediatric lung transplant recipients (Razonable and Eid, 2009; Liu et al., 2010).

Other Acute Complications

Postoperative hemorrhage is one of the most frequent major complications, with the surgical anastomoses and adhesions in the chest being the most common sites. A high degree of suspicion must be maintained to quickly diagnose anastomotic obstruction or ischemia (bronchial anastomoses). Echocardiography and nuclear medicine perfusion scans can be effective in detecting obstruction of the pulmonary arterial or venous connections (the latter may be a particular problem in lobar transplantation, and in either setting can be heralded by copious amounts of pink, frothy secretions after reperfusion). Airway necrosis and dehiscence are frequently fatal. Increasing scarring and stenosis can also occur. Therefore, regular fiberoptic bronchoscopy is conducted after surgery to screen for these problems (Huddleston, 1996).

Rarely, recurrent laryngeal or phrenic nerve damage can become apparent in the postoperative period, most likely as a consequence of the surgical procedure. These are often transient, although permanent vocal cord or hemidiaphragmatic paralysis can occur; the latter may require plication of the diaphragm.

Later Complications

Although the principal cause of death during the first 30 days after transplantation is graft failure, infection in the setting of sustained immunosuppression is a leading cause of death in the first year, and it continues to be a significant cause of mortality after that (Boucek et al., 2002; Sudan et al., 2007; Kirk et al., 2009; Sweet, 2009). Symptoms of infection in the transplantation patient are often difficult to distinguish from those of rejection. Both can involve fever, dyspnea, decreased oxygenation, and pulmonary infiltrates. Definitive diagnosis for most entities requires bronchial lavage and culture; some patients may need a lung biopsy to rule out infection or rejection. Prevention of infection is a primary goal in the management of lung transplant recipients.

Cytomegalovirus is one of the most frequent causes of infection in the transplantation patient, especially in CMV-negative recipients who received organs from CMV-positive donors. CMV infection may be asymptomatic or symptomatic and may cause pneumonitis (where it is associated with fever, respiratory distress, decreased pulmonary function, hypoxemia, and patchy interstitial infiltrates), gastrointestinal disease (abdominal pain, fevers, and increased liver function enzymes), or viremia. It may also present a sepsis-like picture that can progress to multiple organ failure. CMV infection has been associated with acute cellular rejection and an increased frequency and severity of chronic rejection (Duncan et al., 1992; Razonable and Eid, 2009). Aggressive treatment with antiviral agents, with possible reduction in immunosuppressive therapy, is usually successful. Diagnosis is usually based on positive antibody staining in lung tissue specimens, although newer assays that detect antigenemia may allow earlier and less invasive diagnosis. The use of ganciclovir has decreased the incidence and severity of CMV-related disease in these patients. Prophylactic treatment is usually used in patients where either the donor or recipient is CMV positive.

Overall, patients are constantly at risk for bacterial lung infection. Patients with CF are more susceptible to bacterial infection with agents such as *Pseudomonas aeruginosa* or fungal organisms such as *Aspergillus*. These infectious agents should be actively sought (using bronchoalveolar lavage and transbronchial lung biopsy), especially in patients who do not respond to empirical therapy. Infection with Ebstein-Barr virus is of note because of its association with malignancy (see later).

Another significant and often insidious complication is the development of airway obstruction resulting from scarring and granuloma formation, usually at the bronchial anastomosis suture line. The lesion can progress over several months, and the patient typically presents with wheezing and shortness of breath. Flow-volume loops and large-airway flow rates are usually reduced. The diagnosis is confirmed by bronchoscopy and is treated with dilation or stenting (or both).

Delayed gastric emptying and gastroparesis frequently follows lung transplantation, perhaps as a result of surgical injury to the vagus nerve. In addition to the aspiration risk at the time of subsequent surgeries, gastroesophageal reflux has been linked to occult (or overt) aspiration, lung injury, graft failure, and bronchiolitis obliterans (Reid et al., 1990; Huddleston, 1996).

Acute Rejection

Acute rejection is the most frequent in the first year and particularly in the first several months after transplantation, declining substantially thereafter (Sweet et al., 1997; Waltz et al., 2006; Sweet, 2009). It is often initially asymptomatic. Symptoms include fever, dyspnea, and desaturation. Positive laboratory tests can include pleural effusions or perihilar infiltrates on chest radiography, and lower airway obstruction with decreased forced vital capacity and FEV_1 on spirometry. The diagnosis is made (and attempts are made to to differentiate it from infection) using bronchoalveolar lavage and transbronchial biopsy. The diagnosis of acute rejection requires the presence of lymphocytic bronchitis or bronchiolitis with associated perivascular mononuclear infiltrates. Acute rejection episodes are most

often treated with high-dosage steroids, to which patients usually respond rapidly with improvements in symptoms and pulmonary function tests. More persistent or severe episodes are typically treated with OKT3 or ATG. Although most lung transplantation patients experience at least one episode of rejection in the first year, additional episodes should prompt reevaluation of the immunosuppressive regimen. Acute rejection episodes are believed to be a major risk factor for the later development of bronchiolitis obliterans (Lawrence, 1990; Theodore et al., 1990).

Bronchiolitis Obliterans

The major manifestation of chronic rejection is obliterative bronchiolitis (bronchiolitis obliterans) (Wilkes et al., 2005; Huang et al., 2008). Bronchiolitis obliterans syndrome affects greater than 50% of all pediatric recipients more than 2 to 5 years after transplantation, and it is the most common cause of death after 1 year. All lung transplant recipients are followed with surveillance transbronchial biopsies, initially every 3 months and then at increasing intervals to evaluate for the presence of rejection. Pulmonary function tests are also performed to rule out, or to follow the progression of, bronchiolitis obliterans. Respiratory symptoms of bronchiolitis obliterans are not dissimilar to those of reactive airways disease involving the small airways; it sometimes responds mildly to bronchodilators. However, as time progresses, the airway obstruction becomes irreversible. Histologic examination confirms the diagnosis, with transbronchial biopsy results showing intraluminal occlusion and granulation of the respiratory and terminal bronchioles; high-resolution computerized tomography of the chest may have some diagnostic usefulness as well (Faro et al., 2007; Sudan et al., 2007). For many groups, progressive reductions in FEV_1 and maximum expiratory flow rates (FEF_{25-75}, FEF_{75}) are usually sufficient to make the diagnosis without histologic evidence. An association has been shown between bronchiolitis obliterans and increased episodes of acute rejection or infection (particularly CMV) and the onset of chronic rejection (Duncan et al., 1992; Sharples et al., 1996; Liu et al., 2010). The primary therapy is aimed at immunosuppressive prevention of acute rejection and prompt treatment of CMV. Although increased immunosuppressive therapy has been used to attempt to halt the progress of the disease, no solution except retransplantation has been shown to be beneficial.

Immunosuppression for Lung Transplantation

There is substantial variability among pediatric lung transplantation centers in terms of standard immunosuppressive regimens for preventing rejection. Currently, many if not most centers use induction therapy with an IL-2 receptor antagonist, usually in conjunction with one of the antilymphocyte preparations (see earlier) (Hachem et al., 2008a). Most maintenance immunosuppression regimens use MMF, steroids, and tacrolimus (Burch and Aurora, 2004; Waltz et al., 2006; Hachem et al., 2008; Sweet, 2009). Complications arising from the use of these agents were largely summarized earlier, and, as with heart transplantation, significant morbidity is associated with the use of these drugs. Hypertension, hyperlipidemia, diabetes, and renal dysfunction can all occur to varying degrees. Diabetes is a particular problem in CF patients who have undergone lung transplantation, most likely because of a contribution from pancreatic injury as a result of their underlying disease; as noted earlier, steroids (which cause insulin resistance) and tacrolimus (postulated to have a direct pancreatic effect) are additional risk factors. In addition, PTLD affects up to 15% of patients. Those treated with tacrolimus may have an even higher incidence of PTLD.

Outcome

The overall actuarial survival (adults and children) for single-lung transplantations is approximately 25% to 35% at 5 years, compared with 40% to 60% at 5 years with a double-lung transplantation. This difference reflects the better pulmonary reserve and larger pulmonary vascular bed in double-lung transplantations. Long-term survival in pediatric lung transplant recipients is approximately 50% and, unfortunately, does not appear to have improved significantly in the past decade (Fig. 20-25). When survival is compared by age group, children younger than 1 year of age have an actuarial survival at 7 years of greater than 40%, whereas those older than 1 year have an actuarial 7-year survival of less than 35%. Mortality in the first month after transplantation is usually secondary to graft failure, whereas mortality in the first year beyond the first month is predominantly the result of infection, both from more common organisms and from others such as *Aspergillus*. Interestingly, rejection, bronchiolitis obliterans, and infection may be less common in CF patients transplanted at an older age (Weiss et al., 2009).

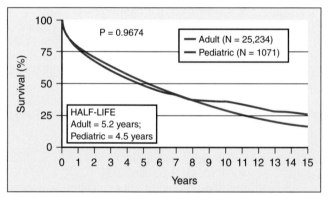

■ **FIGURE 20-25.** Kaplan-Meier survival by age group (pediatric versus adult) for lung transplantations performed between January 1990 and June 2007. *(From Aurora P, Edwards LB, Christie JD, et al: Registry of the International Society for Heart and Lung Transplantation: twelfth official pediatric heart transplantation report—2009,* J Heart Lung Transplant *28:1023, 2009.)*

Thereafter, bronchiolitis obliterans affects more than 50% of transplant recipients after the first year and becomes the main cause of death. On a slightly more optimistic note, of those patients who survive without significant bronchiolitis obliterans, more than 80% show no limitation of activity at 1, 3, and 5 years, and most report a markedly improved quality of life (Williams, 1992; Sweet, 2009). Clearly, much further work is needed in this arena to address donor organ insufficiency and preservation, acute and chronic graft failure, improved immunosuppression, and the prevention and treatment of bronchiolitis obliterans (Wilkes et al., 2005).

Limited data exist regarding the indications, contraindications, and success of lung retransplantation. It may be associated with increased risk, depending on donor selection, and it also raises ethical and resource utilization issues. Outcome appears to be worse in the case of emergent retransplantation because of acute graft failure or rejection, and in those less than 2 years removed from their initial transplantation (Shuhaiber et al., 2009); it may be somewhat better in those retransplanted for chronic rejection and obliterative bronchiolitis.

SUMMARY

In major pediatric cardiac centers, essentially every complex cardiac lesion is amenable to surgical intervention with the potential for substantial improvement in longevity and quality of life. At first glance, the complexity and anatomic variations of congenital cardiac lesions appear to present overwhelming challenges to the anesthesiologists caring for these patients in the perioperative period. Guided by the unifying, basic physiologic concepts outlined in this chapter, an individualized management plan can be developed and applied to each patient by an anesthesiologist in possession of solid pediatric anesthesia skills. As the surgical and medical management of CHD continues to rapidly evolve, it is incumbent on the pediatric anesthesia community—in conjunction with colleagues in cardiology, surgery, intensive care, perfusion, and nursing—to be intellectually agile and actively engaged in the process of refining and advancing the care of these patients.

For questions and answers on topics in this chapter, go to "Chapter Questions" at www.expertconsult.com.

REFERENCES

Complete references used in this text can be found online at www.expertconsult.com.

CHAPTER 21

Congenital Cardiac Anesthesia: Non-Bypass Procedures

Barry D. Kussman and Francis X. McGowan, Jr.

The population of children and adults who has undergone successful repair or palliation of congenital heart disease (CHD) continues to increase (Warnes and Deanfield, 2001; Warnes et al., 2001). Approximately 85% of infants born with CHD can expect to reach adulthood (Moller et al., 1994), and because children of parents with CHD have an increased incidence of CHD (Hoffman et al., 2004), the total incidence and prevalence of CHD are likely to increase generation by generation. Although CHD is synonymous with childhood, the number of adults with CHD currently equals, and is predicted to exceed, the number of children with CHD (Webb and

Williams, 2001); the total number in the United States alone may be approaching 500,000 individuals with significant versions of palliated CHD. The heterogeneous nature of the CHD population is made more so by the use of different treatment strategies for the same or similar lesions, in conjunction with advances in pediatric cardiac surgery, interventional catheterization, and electrophysiologic techniques. For example, in transposition of the great arteries (D-TGA), the majority of adults have had the *atrial* switch operation (the Mustard or Senning procedure), whereas most children have had the *arterial* switch operation (the Jatene). These two operations for the same underlying condition carry vastly different intermediate and long-term outcomes (Williams and Webb, 2000; Warnes, 2006).

Although it is common to differentiate between corrective and palliative surgery, *total correction or cure is not the rule* for the majority of children with CHD (Stark, 1989). *Cure or definitive repair,* in the strictest sense, means that normal cardiovascular structure and function are achieved and maintained; life expectancy is normal; further medical, surgical, and catheter-based treatments for the CHD are unnecessary; and noncardiovascular (e.g., renal, neurologic) consequences are nonexistent. With *cure,* there are no cardiac or vascular *residua* (abnormalities that were part of the original defect and are still present after repair), *sequelae* (disorders intentionally incurred at the time of reparative surgery and deemed unavoidable), or *complications* (unintentional aftermath) after surgery (Perloff, 1997). *Palliative repair* implies that future procedures are anticipated or necessary to maintain or restore the patient to a state of normal (or at least compensated) physiology and to improve life span. Lesions that lend themselves to cure are uncomplicated closure at an early age of an uncomplicated, nonpulmonary hypertensive patent ductus arteriosus (PDA), atrial septal defect (ASD), ventricular septal defect (VSD) (Talner et al., 1980), and in some instances catheter ablation of tachyarrhythmias (Walsh, 2007). Virtually all other forms of CHD require long-term surveillance. Many carry substantial risk for residual and potentially progressive structural, contractile, hemodynamic, electrophysiologic, and end-organ abnormalities.

CARDIAC FACTORS INFLUENCING OUTCOME AND ANESTHETIC RISK

The factors that determine the natural history and pathophysiologic consequences of congenital cardiovascular malformations also affect perioperative risk. Although the majority of anesthesiologists are not familiar with the natural history of each and every lesion, it is possible to develop a rational approach to the anesthetic management of this group of patients by focusing on the factors listed in Box 21-1. Identification of patients at increased risk, and development of an appropriate strategy to prevent adverse events is the cornerstone of anesthetic management.

Box 21-1 Factors Influencing Outcome and Anesthetic Risk

Defect and type of repair
Shunting
Ventricular dysfunction
Ventricular outflow obstruction
Hypoxemia and cyanosis
Rhythm and conduction abnormalities
Pulmonary hypertension and Eisenmenger's syndrome
Myocardial ischemia
Infective endocarditis
End-organ dysfunction and injury
Extracardiac anomalies
Heart transplant recipients

Defect and Type of Repair

In an *anatomic* repair, the morphologic left ventricle is connected to the aorta, the morphologic right ventricle is connected to the pulmonary artery, the circulation is in series, and cyanosis is corrected. An anatomic repair may be categorized as either a *simple* or a *complex* reconstruction. In a *simple anatomic repair,* the heart is structurally normal, and correction for the most part is "curative" without long-term sequelae. Repair of uncomplicated, nonpulmonary hypertensive PDA, ASD, or VSD would fall into this category. In a *complex anatomic repair,* anatomic correction is achieved, but because of the complex nature of the surgical repair there may be significant long-term sequelae. Complex repairs comprise extensive (right and/or left) ventricular outflow tract reconstruction, placement of conduits or baffles, and atrioventricular valve repair. Examples include TGA, tetralogy of Fallot (TOF) with or without pulmonary atresia, severe aortic stenosis (AS), severe pulmonary stenosis (PS), atrioventricular septal defects, mitral stenosis, truncus arteriosus, and interrupted aortic arch. Although patients may report few symptoms or limitations to activities of daily living, significant limitations (e.g., reduced exercise or aerobic capacity, heart rate and blood pressure response to exercise) may be evident on objective testing.

In a *physiologic repair,* the circulation is in series and the cyanosis relieved, but the heart is either univentricular (single ventricle) or biventricular with the morphologic *right* ventricle being the *systemic* ventricle and the morphologic left ventricle being the pulmonary ventricle. Single-ventricle repairs result in connection of the systemic venous return directly to the pulmonary artery, thereby excluding the pulmonary ventricle. By relieving hypoxemia, single-ventricle repairs are "functionally corrective." A physiologic biventricular repair is seen with the atrial switch operation (Mustard or Senning) for TGA, effectively resulting in a switch at the *atrial* level, with the right ventricle functioning as the systemic ventricle. One major clinical implication of a univentricular heart or systemic right ventricle is significant functional deterioration of the ventricle over time; progressive insufficiency of the systemic atrioventricular valve and dysrhythmias can be additional pathophysiologic features.

Anesthetic considerations: Patients with *simple anatomic repairs* who are asymptomatic have normal to near-normal hemodynamics and can generally be anesthetized in the same manner as patients with a structurally normal heart. *Patients with complex anatomic repairs,* because of the issues discussed later, are at increased perioperative risk. *Physiologic repairs* are always palliative and are associated with progressive ventricular dysfunction and other risk factors. Anesthetic management of patients with *single-ventricle physiologic repairs* is complex and can be associated with significant intraoperative problems if the pathophysiology is not well understood.

Shunting

A shunt is an abnormal communication between the systemic and pulmonary circulations, allowing blood to flow directly from one circulatory system to the other. A left-to-right shunt allows oxygenated pulmonary venous blood to return directly to the lungs rather than being pumped to the body, whereas a right-to-left shunt allows deoxygenated systemic venous blood to bypass the lungs and return to the body (Sommer et al., 2008). An increased workload is placed on the ventricles, with the degree (volume) of shunting determining the severity of symptoms. Factors influencing the direction and degree of shunting include the size of the shunt orifice, the pressure gradient between the chambers or arteries involved in the shunt, the relative compliance of the right and left ventricles, the ratio of pulmonary vascular resistance (PVR) to systemic vascular resistance (SVR), and the blood viscosity (hematocrit). Total pulmonary blood flow (Q_p) is the sum of effective pulmonary blood flow and recirculated pulmonary blood flow, whereas total systemic blood flow (Q_s) is the sum of effective systemic blood flow and recirculated systemic blood flow. Total Q_p and total Q_s do not have to be equal.

The lesions most likely to be encountered before repair that are associated with the potential for left-to-right shunting include large PDA, VSD, and atrioventricular canal defects; patients palliated with large, unobstructed modified Blalock-Taussig shunts (e.g., stage I repair of hypoplastic left heart syndrome) can behave similarly. Left-to-right shunting results in increased pulmonary blood flow, increased pulmonary vascular resistance, increased pulmonary artery pressures (PAP), increased left atrial volume or pressure, pulmonary edema, and volume overload of both the right and left ventricles leading to biventricular failure. Low aortic diastolic pressure accompanying large systemic-to-pulmonary artery shunts can lead to myocardial ischemia as well as organ hypoperfusion (e.g., bowel ischemia). Pulmonary overcirculation is associated with decreased lung compliance, increased airway resistance (Stayer et al., 2004), and airway compression (Berlinger et al., 1983). Alterations in pulmonary function lead to increased work of breathing (with increased energy expenditure), atelectasis, air trapping, and respiratory infections. The time course for developing pulmonary vascular occlusive disease (PVOD) with shunt reversal (right-to-left) and Eisenmenger's syndrome depends on the size and site of the shunt and age at repair; patients with underlying anatomic or genetic predisposition to the development of pulmonary hypertension—for example, trisomy 21 children—can develop earlier, more severe PVOD for a given shunt (Chi and Krovetz, 1975; Gorenflo et al., 2002).

Right-to-left shunting results in decreased oxygen content of the systemic arterial blood, with the decrease in proportion to the volume of deoxygenated systemic venous blood mixing with the oxygenated pulmonary venous blood. Even with normal cardiac output, the decrease in tissue oxygen delivery limits exercise tolerance (Sommer et al., 2008).

Anesthetic considerations: Avoidance of air bubbles in intravenous catheters to prevent systemic embolization and attention to pulmonary vascular tone and its influence on the PVR-to-SVR ratio are important considerations. Factors influencing PVR are discussed later in the pulmonary hypertension section. In patients with left-to-right shunts, the major perioperative concerns are threats to already limited *systemic* blood flow. Routine clinical monitoring tools are unlikely to indicate an evolving problem in this regard until severe hypotension and evidence of myocardial ischemia ensue; in patients with shunt physiology, it is important both to maintain myocardial pump function (i.e., avoid myocardial depression) and to try to limit decreases in PVR. Such decreases (e.g., those that can be produced by hyperventilation or hyperoxia) can lead to a steal phenomenon with increased pulmonary blood flow (PBF). The major *acute* consequence will be decreased Q_s with increased risk for significant systemic hypotension

and hypoperfusion; in the longer term, the increased Q_p that results can increase pulmonary congestion, lung water, and cardiac volume overload.

In patients who have or who are at risk for significant right-to-left shunting or who are dependent on a systemic-to-pulmonary artery shunt for pulmonary blood flow (e.g., after stage I repair of hypoplastic left heart syndrome [HLHS] or as the initial palliation for reduced blood flow lesions such a tricuspid atresia), primary management considerations are the maintenance of overall pump (cardiac) function and blood pressure and avoidance of factors that further increase PVR or decrease SVR (or both). It is important to note that the resultant arterial oxygen saturation in such patients will be affected by both the magnitude of the right-to-left shunting and the saturation of the shunted (essentially systemic venous return) blood.

Ventricular Dysfunction

Progressive ventricular dysfunction leading to congestive heart failure (CHF) is the most common cause of disability and death in patients with CHD (Warnes and Deanfield, 2001). The etiology is multifactorial and may result from the primary disease, many years of abnormal volume and pressure loading (which cause pathologic remodeling of numerous cardiomyocyte and nonmyocyte functions and processes), chronic hypoxemia, damage during surgical repair (inadequate myocardial preservation, scarring, poor repair, damage to coronary arteries), acquired disease (Graham, 1982), and arrhythmias (Shinbane et al., 1997; Deal, 2001). Ventricular *volume overload* occurs with intracardiac or extracardiac left-to-right shunts, valvular regurgitation, and single-ventricle lesions. The time course over which irreversible ventricular dysfunction develops is variable, but if surgical intervention to correct the volume overload is undertaken within the first year of life, residual dysfunction is uncommon (Cordell et al., 1976; Graham et al., 1976). Ventricular *pressure overload* results from residual or recurrent ventricular outflow obstruction or elevated PAP or PVR. The time to develop significant ventricular dysfunction is longer compared with a chronic volume load, so symptoms are uncommon unless the obstruction is severe and prolonged, or it is combined with a volume load (Graham, 1991). *Chronic hypoxemia and cyanosis* decrease ventricular oxygen supply and increase oxygen demand through increased work related to increases in pulmonary and systemic vascular resistance with associated polycythemia. Myocardial ischemia resulting from coronary artery anomalies or kinking or torsion after reimplantation may also cause ventricular dysfunction.

Anesthetic considerations: The chronic presence or potential to develop or exacerbate low systemic cardiac output is probably the single most important consideration in approaching the care of patients with CHD. Attempts to correlate clinical status and functional myocardial reserve can be unreliable. No single parameter or test is best to assist with this assessment. Rather, one is advised to carefully integrate historical, physical, and diagnostic test information pertaining to myocardial performance to arrive at an integrated assessment of the degree of ventricular dysfunction, as well as the potential for further decompensation that can occur as a result of anesthetic choices and procedural factors. Although there is no single recipe, key aspects of successful management include appropriate fluid administration, usually with maintenance of normal to modestly increased preload, and selection of suitable anesthetic induction and maintenance techniques most likely to maintain contractile function and hemodynamic stability. These techniques should also be chosen to minimize the possibility of airway obstruction and hypoventilation. Of note, positive pressure ventilation is likely to improve the function of a dysfunctional systemic ventricle according to Laplace's law, by the effect of increased intrathoracic pressure to decrease transmural myocardial pressure and hence decrease ventricular afterload. In instances of significant myocardial dysfunction, prophylactic inotrope administration before or soon after induction and also during the procedure may be beneficial.

Ventricular Outflow Obstruction

Ventricular outflow obstruction may be subvalvar, valvar, supravalvar, or a combination thereof, isolated or part of more complex malformations, residual or recurrent, and fixed or dynamic. Outflow obstruction results in pressure overload on the ventricle, ventricular hypertrophy, a "stiff" ventricle (diastolic dysfunction), and ultimately systolic ventricular dysfunction (Carabello, 2006). *Left ventricular outflow obstruction* may occur with aortic stenosis, coarctation of the aorta, interrupted aortic arch, and variants of HLHS and Shone's anomaly (Shone et al., 1963). *Right ventricular outflow obstruction* is seen with pulmonary stenosis, TOF, hypoplastic pulmonary arteries, right ventricle–to–pulmonary artery (RV-PA) conduits (performed in repair of pulmonary atresia, truncus arteriosus, TGA with pulmonary stenosis [Rastelli procedure], some double-outlet right ventricle defects), and pulmonary hypertension. Conduits calcify and narrow, and together with the increasing stroke volume that occurs with growth, significant obstruction can develop. The septal shift associated with severe right ventricular pressure overload can compromise left ventricular function via a reduction in left ventricular filling and systemic outflow obstruction.

Anesthetic considerations: Pressure-overloaded ventricles are at significant risk for myocardial ischemia during anesthesia, particularly in association with systemic hypotension and tachycardia. Subendocardial ischemia is a potential risk in patients with systemic or suprasystemic RV pressures as systolic coronary flow may be markedly diminished or absent. The overall goal of anesthetic induction and management is to optimize and maintain the major determinants of ventricular function in the face of a fixed outflow obstruction and often some degree of both diastolic and systolic dysfunction. Thus, dependency on sinus rhythm and preload to maintain cardiac output are increased. Adequate preoperative hydration in accordance with fasting guidelines or a bolus of intravenous fluid prior to induction is recommended. Volume infusion or replacement in the presence of a stiff left ventricle or mitral stenosis must be done judiciously, as it has the potential to cause an inordinate increase in left atrial pressure and consequent pulmonary edema. As severity of ventricular dysfunction increases, an intravenous induction with agents that maintain contractility and systemic blood pressure without significant alterations in heart rate is probably indicated. Although the majority of patients can tolerate at least modest concentrations of inhalational agent, a balanced technique employing a potent opioid

such as fentanyl in combination with low-concentration inhaled agent and muscle relaxant may offer greater hemodynamic stability. When feasible, relief of severe outflow tract obstruction, which can frequently be performed in the catheterization laboratory, should precede all but emergency surgery.

Hypoxemia and Cyanosis

Cyanosis is associated with decreased pulmonary blood flow or intracardiac mixing lesions, or both. Prior to repair, cyanotic lesions include tricuspid atresia, pulmonary atresia, tetralogy of Fallot, transposition of the great arteries, and truncus arteriosus; tricuspid atresia, pulmonary atresia, and TOF are all lesions that typically have reduced PBF. Increased PBF occurs in truncus arteriosus. In lesions with intracardiac mixing (e.g., TGA), cyanosis can occur with decreased or increased PBF depending on whether there is obstruction to the PBF. Cyanosis may also be found in the setting of very low cardiac output, increased arteriovenous oxygen difference, and respiratory disease. With the advent of early infant repair, chronic hypoxemia is now most frequently encountered in the young child undergoing staged repair, and in the adult with unrepaired or palliated CHD. Indeed, one stimulus for early, definitive repair is to eliminate hypoxemia and the compensatory polycythemia, with its rheologic, neurologic, hemostatic, renal, and metabolic consequences. Although the analyses are limited and imperfect for obvious reasons, the data that does exist suggests that chronic hypoxemia during infancy and early childhood is a significant risk factor for reduced cognitive performance. As blood viscosity increases, systemic (including coronary) and pulmonary vascular resistances increase markedly. Hemostatic abnormalities that can result from cyanosis and polycythemia include thrombocytopenia, platelet dysfunction, shortened platelet survival, disseminated intravascular coagulation, decreased production of coagulation factors, and primary fibrinolysis (Tempe and Virmani, 2002; Odegard et al., 2003, 2009). Sludging of red blood cells increases the risk for thromboembolism and stroke, particularly when the hemoglobin approaches or exceeds, 20 g/dL, and in conjunction with dehydration. Phlebotomy regimens are being used less frequently in the absence of symptoms, as they may be associated with an increased risk for cerebrovascular events (Ammash and Warnes, 1996). The duration and degree of hypoxemia and polycythemia are important historical factors in the evaluation of possible long-term residual cardiac muscle blood flow abnormalities.

Anesthetic considerations: It is important to maintain adequate preoperative hydration by encouraging liberal clear fluid intake in accordance with fasting guidelines or placement of an intravenous catheter and administration of maintenance fluids. Although the data are scant, preoperative hydration may be especially important as the hemoglobin concentration exceeds, 20 g/dL, and some consideration should be given to reducing red cell mass (pheresis, normovolemic phlebotomy) at higher hemoglobin values, perhaps particularly before more complicated procedures. There is an increased risk of bleeding in association with increased tissue vascularity, hemostatic abnormalities, and anticoagulants, and the risks of regional anesthesia in the presence of a hemostatic abnormality should be carefully considered. Of note, the effect of anemia on oxygen-carrying capacity is exaggerated as hemoglobin values "within the normal range" in cyanotic patients may represent a significant deficit. Other aspects of anesthetic management should be based on the underlying pathophysiology, as discussed later.

Rhythm and Conduction Abnormalities

Arrhythmias and conduction defects have a major impact on the prognosis and management of patients who have undergone palliation or repair of CHD (Warnes and Deanfield, 2001). Rhythm disturbances that may be well tolerated in a structurally normal heart may be life threatening in a structurally or functionally abnormal heart. The etiology is multifactorial and includes damage to the arterial supply or direct injury to the sinoatrial node, atrioventricular (AV) node, and conduction system, atrial or ventricular scarring, chamber dilation or hypertrophy with resultant pathologic remodeling, and myocardial ischemia.

Arrhythmias may occur in the postoperative period or many years after surgery, and they tend to vary with the type of underlying heart disease and surgical procedures that have been performed (Vetter, 1991). *Supraventricular tachycardias* (atrial flutter/intraatrial reentrant tachycardia, atrial fibrillation) and *sinoatrial node dysfunction* (bradycardia, tachy-brady syndrome, exit block, sinus arrest) are more common in lesions that required extensive intraatrial surgery or have residual elevations in right atrial pressure, such as the atrial switch (Mustard or Senning) procedure for TGA, the Fontan procedure, and TOF repair. Isolated *right bundle branch block* is frequent after ventriculotomy. The QRS duration may be an independent predictor of arrhythmia, right ventricular dysfunction, and sudden death risk in patients after TOF repair (Gatzoulis et al., 2000a). Whether aberrant conduction and ventricular dyssynchrony are independent causes of ventricular dysfunction and, consequently, whether using biventricular pacing to restore normal activation-contraction patterns can prevent or reverse ventricular function in patients with dyssynchrony is currently under investigation (Cecchin et al., 2009). *Ventricular arrhythmias* are more common in lesions with residual ventricular pressure or volume load, as in aortic stenosis, hypertrophic cardiomyopathy, and TOF repair. Tachyarrhythmias and ventricular dysfunction are a dangerous combination and a cause of late sudden death (Vetter, 1991).

Anesthetic considerations: Any new onset of palpitations or syncope should be investigated before elective surgery. Consultation with a pediatric electrophysiologist can be very helpful to understanding the risk factors and causes for various rhythm disturbances in the CHD population, the need for additional diagnostic procedures, and the preferred pharmacologic and electrical approaches to the rhythm disturbances likely to arise. Such discussions help ensure availability and appropriate use of antiarrhythmic agents and cardioversion/defibrillation devices. The availability of similar expertise consultation *during* procedures is also advisable. In patients with tachyarrhythmias, there is at least theoretical reason to avoid agents with vagolytic or sympathetic-stimulating properties (e.g., pancuronium). The electrophysiologic impact of most inhaled or intravenous agents is probably modest.

Existing pacemakers should be checked preoperatively and the appropriate precautions taken in patients with *complete AV block*. There is the need for preoperative evaluation and temporary resetting or shutting down of pacemakers and implantable cardioverter defibrillators (Practice advisory, 2005), as well as

backup pacing (transcutaneous pacing) in the event of pacemaker malfunction. For high-risk patients, an external pacing or defibrillator unit should be in the operating room and pads applied around the time of induction of anesthesia. The need for and use of electrocautery (monopolar versus bipolar) in pacemaker-dependent patients should be discussed with both the surgeon and electrophysiologist. Implanted pacemakers and cardioverter defibrillators typically need to be interrogated and reprogrammed after the surgical procedure. The electrophysiologist may also be helpful for patient optimization. For example, consideration should be given to temporary pacing in select unpaced patients with bradycardia, as well as to radiofrequency catheter ablation in patients with amenable tachyarrhythmias, especially before major procedures.

Pulmonary Hypertension

In the unrepaired child, unrestricted left-to-right shunting with increased pulmonary blood flow produces a volume load on the heart and structural changes in the pulmonary vascular bed (medial hypertrophy progressing to necrotizing arteritis [Heath and Edwards, 1958]), leading to decreased myocardial function and pulmonary hypertension (mean PAP greater than 25mm Hg). The time course for developing PVOD depends on the size and site of the shunt and age at surgery. Progression is more rapid when both the volume and the pressure load on the pulmonary circulation are increased, such as with a large VSD. For the majority of infants with an unrestrictive shunt, repair of the defect in the first year of life is usually associated with regression of the pulmonary vascular changes. Pulmonary hypertension develops more slowly with increased pulmonary blood flow in the absence of elevated pulmonary artery pressures, as with an ASD, where the absence of pulmonary hypertension into the third decade or beyond is not uncommon. Eisenmenger's syndrome is characterized by irreversible PVOD and cyanosis related to reversal of the left-to-right shunt (Wood, 1958).

Pulmonary hypertension and increased PVR can be reactive, fixed, or a combination of the two. The reactivity of the pulmonary vascular bed is determined during cardiac catheterization by the changes in PAP and PVR in response to vasodilators such as oxygen and nitric oxide (NO). Factors increasing PVR include hypoxemia, hypercarbia, acidemia, extremes of lung volume, hypothermia, and sympathetic stimulation associated with stress or light anesthesia. Acute dramatic increases in PAP or PVR result in increased RV afterload with decreased RV stroke volume; in addition, resultant RV dilation can cause a leftward shift of the interventricular septum, with further impairment of left ventricular (LV) function and filling, and decreased cardiac output. The ensuing hypotension can result in myocardial ischemia (particularly of the RV), bradycardia, and cardiac arrest. If an intracardiac communication (patent foramen ovale [PFO], ASD, VSD) is present, increases in PAP lead to right-to-left shunting and desaturation, albeit with better maintenance of LV filling and systemic cardiac output.

Anesthetic considerations: Severe pulmonary hypertension appears to impart major anesthetic risk, even for minor procedures (Ammash and Warnes, 1996; Raines et al., 1996; Daliento et al., 1998; Martin et al., 2002; Carmosino et al., 2007). This topic has been the subject of recent reviews (Subramaniam and Yared, 2007; Friesen and Williams, 2008). Suprasystemic pulmonary artery pressure is a significant predictor of major complications in children with pulmonary hypertension undergoing noncardiac surgery (Carmosino et al., 2007). It is not possible to recommend a specific anesthetic technique as all anesthetic techniques have been used successfully. Of note, many perioperative deaths occur in the postoperative period (Lyons et al., 1995; Martin et al., 2002). In older patients with Eisenmenger's syndrome, most deaths appear to occur either as a result of the surgical procedure and not of anesthesia, or in the postoperative period because of complications such as atelectasis, pneumonia, worsening hypoxemia, or other end-organ dysfunction (Martin et al., 2002). Preoperative knowledge of the degree of pulmonary hypertension, pulmonary vascular reactivity, right ventricular dysfunction, and the presence of an intracardiac communication is imperative. For example, patients with severe pulmonary arterial hypertension, significant RV dysfunction, and no "pop-off" communication (i.e., right-to-left shunt) are probably the most at risk.

Acute right ventricular dysfunction and resultant low systemic cardiac output are the major pathophysiologic consequences of acute exacerbations in pulmonary artery pressure. The overall goals of anesthesia, therefore, are to provide adequate analgesia and anesthesia while minimizing increases in PVR and depression of myocardial function (Friesen and Williams, 2008). Likely methods include providing adequate preoperative sedation, high inspired oxygen, hyperventilation (respiratory alkalosis) if possible, adequate depth of anesthesia, maintenance of a normal to increased preload, early use of an inotrope to support RV function and systemic blood pressure (i.e., RV perfusion), and use of induction and maintenance agents that do not significantly reduce contractility or systemic blood pressure. Endotracheal intubation as a potential mechanical trigger of pulmonary vasoreactivity should be recognized; this also applies to extubation on emergence from anesthesia. In addition to adequate anesthetic depth, lidocaine spray to the vocal cords and trachea may offer some degree of protection. Noninvasive ventilation may be an attractive alternative to support adequate gas exchange during anesthesia and surgery under some conditions. Although allowing better control of oxygenation and ventilation, positive pressure ventilation increases RV afterload and decreases RV filling so that excessive inspiratory pressures and volumes, and positive end-expiratory pressure (PEEP), should be avoided. It is critical that pulmonary vasodilator therapy not be interrupted perioperatively, particularly prostacyclin (Flolan) infusions, whose discontinuation can result in severe rebound pulmonary hypertension in as little as 10 to 15 minutes. With severe pulmonary hypertension and known responsiveness of the pulmonary vasculature to NO, it is advisable to have NO available for immediate or even prophylactic administration. The use of invasive monitoring (e.g., arterial blood pressure) is usually determined by the nature of the surgical procedure. Because of the significant morbidity and mortality of anesthesia and surgery for the patient with severe pulmonary hypertension, a risk-benefit analysis involving the cardiologist, surgeon, and anesthesiologist is essential before performing elective procedures.

Myocardial Ischemia

Coronary artery anomalies (e.g., intramural coronary, anomalous origin from the other sinus or pulmonary artery) or problems associated with coronary reimplantation in the arterial switch operation can result in myocardial ischemia. More commonly, in many patients with congenital defects and normal coronary arteries, ischemia is secondary to imbalances in myocardial oxygen supply and demand. There is some evidence, in lesions associated with abnormal load, including ones where the RV is the systemic ventricle, that coronary angiogenesis and capillary supply may not keep pace with increased muscle mass. This creates a relative supply-demand inequity. Subendocardial perfusion is largely determined by coronary perfusion pressure, which is the aortic diastolic pressure minus the ventricular end-diastolic pressure. In addition, the time interval available for perfusion (predominately diastole) is critical. As a result, the relationship between diastolic blood pressure, ventricular end-diastolic pressure, and heart rate determines whether subendocardial ischemia occurs. These three factors place patients with CHD at risk for ischemia in the following situations: (1) the *systolic pressure in the ventricles is abnormally elevated* (in some cases, the pulmonary ventricle may have suprasystemic pressures), thereby requiring elevated perfusion pressure; (2) the *aortic diastolic pressure* is compromised by diastolic runoff of aortic blood into the lower resistance pulmonary circuit in ductal-dependent and systemic-to-pulmonary artery shunts (coronary perfusion is further compromised if the coronary ostia are perfused with desaturated blood, as in patients with HLHS); (3) *elevated ventricular end-diastolic pressure,* which may be the result of impaired systolic function, impaired diastolic function (reduced ventricular compliance and relaxation, as seen with ventricular pressure overload), increased ventricular end-diastolic volume (volume overload), or a combination of these; and (4) *increases in heart rate,* which geometrically reduce the duration of diastole (the duration of systole stays relatively constant) so that the time available for coronary perfusion falls and consequently a higher diastolic pressure is necessary to maintain the same degree of subendocardial perfusion. In particular, the combination of a high heart rate and low diastolic blood pressure can produce significant ischemia.

Anesthetic considerations: Standard principles are followed to ensure that myocardial oxygen supply exceeds demand apply. In particular, maintaining aortic perfusion pressures, in combination with avoiding excessive tachycardia, frequently appears to be critical. With cyanotic lesions, a hemoglobin level above the normal acceptable range may be necessary.

Infective Endocarditis

The most recent guidelines of the American Heart Association concluded that only an extremely small number of cases of infective endocarditis could be prevented by antibiotic prophylaxis for dental procedures (Wilson et al., 2007). As a result, infective endocarditis prophylaxis for dental procedures is recommended only for patients with underlying cardiac conditions (Box 21-2) associated with the highest occurrence and risk for adverse outcome from infective endocarditis. Prophylaxis in this group is recommended for all dental procedures that involve manipulation of gingival tissue or the periapical region of teeth or perforation of the oral mucosa. The antibiotic is administered in a single dose before the procedure (Table 21-1). Administration of antibiotics solely to prevent endocarditis is not recommended for patients who undergo a genitourinary or gastrointestinal tract procedure.

Box 21-2 Cardiac Conditions Associated with the Highest Risk of Adverse Outcome from Endocarditis for Which Prophylaxis with Dental Procedures Is Recommended

Prosthetic cardiac valve or prosthetic material used for cardiac valve repair
Previous infective endocarditis
Congenital heart disease (CHD)*

- Unrepaired cyanotic CHD, including palliative shunts and conduits
- Completely repaired congenital heart defect repaired with prosthetic material or device, whether placed by surgery or by catheter intervention, during the first 6 months after the procedure[†]
- Repaired CHD with residual defects at the site or adjacent to the site of a prosthetic patch or prosthetic device (both of which inhibit endothelialization)

Cardiac transplant recipients with valve regurgitation resulting from a structurally abnormal valve

From Wilson W, Taubert KA, Gewitz M, et al: Prevention of infective endocarditis. Guidelines from the American Heart Association, *Circulation* 116:1736–1754, 2007.

*Except for the conditions listed above, antibiotic prophylaxis is no longer recommended for any form of CHD.

[†]Prophylaxis is recommended because endothelialization of prosthetic material occurs within 6 months after the procedure.

TABLE 21-1. Antibiotic Regimens for a Dental Procedure

Situation	Agent	Regimen: Single Dose 30 to 60 min Before Procedure	
		Adults	Children
Oral	Amoxicillin	2 g	50 mg/kg
Unable to take oral medication	Ampicillin OR cefazolin or ceftriaxone	2 g IM or IV 1 g IM or IV	50 mg/kg IM or IV 50 mg/kg IM or IV
Allergic to penicillins or ampicillin—oral	Cephalexin*[†] OR clindamycin OR azithromycin or clarithromycin	2 g 600 mg 500 mg	50 mg/kg 20 mg/kg 15 mg/kg
Allergic to penicillins or ampicillin and unable to take oral medication	Cefazolin or ceftriaxone[†] OR clindamycin	1 g IM or IV 600 mg IM or IV	50 mg/kg IM or IV 20 mg/kg IM or IV

From Wilson W, Taubert KA, Gewitz M, et al: Prevention of infective endocarditis. Guidelines from the American Heart Association, *Circulation* 116:1736–1754, 2007.

*Or other first- or second-generation oral cephalosporin in equivalent adult or pediatric dosage.

[†]Cephalosporins should not be used for an individual with a history of anaphylaxis, angioedema, or urticaria with penicillins or ampicillin.

IM, Intramuscular; *IV,* intravenous.

Rarely, patients scheduled for an invasive procedure have endocarditis, in which case the results of blood cultures should guide antibiotic therapy.

End-Organ Dysfunction and Injury

Unrestricted left-to-right shunting, in addition to increasing PAP and PVR, produces alterations in lung mechanics and airway compression. The primary effects on lung mechanics are a decrease in lung compliance and an increase in airway resistance (Bancalari et al., 1977; Stayer et al., 2004). Decreased compliance will necessitate higher than expected airway pressures, with care being taken not to insufflate the stomach during mask ventilation. Airway compression can result from dilated pulmonary arteries, left (or right) atrial dilation, massive cardiomegaly, or intraluminal bronchial obstruction (Berlinger et al., 1983). The pulmonary lymphatics are also compressed in these circumstances, perhaps explaining an increased incidence of pulmonary infectious symptoms in patients with large left-to-right shunts.

Neurologic injury and adverse neurodevelopmental outcome in CHD patients are multifactorial, with various contributions from genetic, lesion, and procedural elements (Newburger and Bellinger, 2006). Relatively pervasive issues include hyperactivity, diminished executive function, and various other neurocognitive abnormalities, especially in areas pertaining to speech and language and executive functions. Less commonly seen in the current era are seizures, stroke, and choreoathetosis. Structural brain abnormalities have been found with magnetic resonance imaging (MRI) in infants with CHD *before* any intervention, as well as after surgery or balloon atrial septostomy (Mahle et al., 2002; McQuillen et al., 2006; McQuillen et al., 2007; Miller et al., 2007; Andropoulos et al., 2010). Complex CHD may have anywhere from a mild to a profound impact on a child's psychosocial development (Horner et al., 2000). These issues necessitate additional sensitivity with the family, altering the amount of detail discussed in front of the child when obtaining informed consent, and precluding certain sedation or regional anesthetic techniques.

Chronic cyanosis, low systemic cardiac output, or high venous pressures (Damman et al., 2009) may over time contribute to the development of renal and hepatic insufficiency. This may not be evident on routine laboratory tests (e.g., serum creatinine or liver enzymes) but may predispose to perioperative dysfunction in response to relatively minor changes in organ perfusion and oxygen delivery, or to otherwise relatively mild toxic stresses (e.g., ketorolac). Cardiac catheterization (contrast nephropathy) increases the risk for perioperative renal dysfunction (Briguori et al., 2007).

Extracardiac Anomalies

Extracardiac anomalies occur in 25% of infants seen during the first year of life in patients with cardiac disease (Greenwood et al., 1975). The anomalies are often multiple and may result from chromosomal, genetic, teratogenic, or unknown causes.

Anesthetic considerations: A focused airway examination and thorough assessment of all organ systems is essential.

Heart Transplant Recipients

The worldwide annual transplant rate in children is around 400, with the major indications being cardiomyopathy and congenital heart disease (Kirk et al., 2008). Factors to consider in this population are cardiac physiology and functional status, cardiac allograft vasculopathy, rejection, the side effects of immunosuppressive agents, and the development of renal dysfunction, hypertension, and malignancy. Efferent denervation results in a resting tachycardia (withdrawal of vagal tone) and impaired chronotropic response to stress. Afferent denervation results in lack of angina during myocardial ischemia and alterations in cardiac baroreceptors and mechanoreceptors. Cardiac physiology is restrictive, with mildly elevated filling pressures and a low-normal ejection fraction (Cotts and Oren, 1997). There may be sinus node dysfunction and there is a shift from β_1 to β_2 receptors.

Anesthetic considerations (see Chapter 20, Anesthesia for Congenital Heart Surgery, for a more complete discussion): The response to hemodynamic instability is slower (dependence on circulating catecholamines) and less robust. The denervated heart is preload dependent, with a reduced chronotropic response to hypotension or sympathetic stimulation. Restrictive physiology, particularly with rejection, increases the risk for pulmonary edema when fluid administration is not judicious. Sensitivity is increased to direct-acting catecholamines, β-blockers, adenosine, and verapamil, and it is decreased to digoxin and indirect-acting sympathomimetic agents. Myocardial ischemia is an ever-present threat from coronary artery vasculopathy. A new onset of dysrhythmias or heart block is ominous, suggesting rejection or myocardial ischemia. Immunosuppression requires strict aseptic technique, and the hypertension and nephrotoxicity associated with some agents and possible need for stress-dose corticosteroids need to be addressed.

PREOPERATIVE ASSESSMENT

CHD adds significant risk for morbidity and mortality in patients requiring noncardiac surgery (Warner et al., 1998; Coran et al., 1999; Baum et al., 2000; Martin et al., 2002; Carmosino et al., 2007). The preoperative evaluation should be complete enough to provide a clear understanding of the pathophysiology of the cardiac defect, the implications of any corrective or palliative procedures, and the likely interactions with the planned surgical procedure. As a general rule, patients with CHD who are doing well clinically (i.e., have good functional status, few or no medications, and only routine medical examinations) tend to do well with anesthesia and surgery. Not surprisingly, the unrepaired or palliated patient presents a greater risk, as does the more complex and stressful surgical procedure. Broadly speaking, there are three categories of patients with CHD: those who have undergone a reparative (corrective) procedure, those who have undergone a palliative procedure, and those who have not undergone any procedure. The principles of anesthetic management are the same whether the patient is a child or an adult, and whether they have had a procedure or not.

History and Physical Examination

As the history may be incomplete or misleading with complex CHD (Colman, 2003), close collaboration with the patient's cardiologist is valuable. Additionally, the cardiologist can help identify patients at high risk, clarify pathophysiologic issues, establish if the current clinical status is the best possible, and provide the findings of recent cardiologic studies. The focus of the history should be on the type of lesion and factors listed in Box 21-1, prior surgical and catheterization procedures and complications thereof, anesthetic experience, medications, allergies, and current functional status. Specific symptoms that should be sought are feeding difficulties and sweating in infants, poor growth, cyanotic spells, decreased activity level such as inability to keep up with healthy peers, fatigue, dyspnea, palpitations, chest pain, and syncope. New or worsening symptoms require cardiology consultation. Recent respiratory tract infections can cause changes in pulmonary vascular resistance and airway reactivity, increasing anesthetic risk in the setting of decreased pulmonary compliance, pulmonary hypertension, systemic-to-pulmonary artery shunts, and cavopulmonary anastomosis.

The physical examination should include general appearance, level of activity, presence of distress, and vital signs. Arterial oxygen saturation (SpO_2) varies with clinical status, but is expected to be above 94% after definitive procedures and in the range of 75% to 85% after palliative interventions that create shunted or intracardiac mixing circulations. Evidence of tachycardia, cyanosis, tachypnea, labored breathing, congestive heart failure, and poor peripheral perfusion should be sought. Airway assessment is important, because extracardiac anomalies may be present in up to one quarter of patients with CHD (Friedman, 1997). Peripheral pulses and four extremity blood pressures should be assessed in the setting of known or suspected aortic arch obstruction, previous or present Blalock-Taussig shunts, or after multiple cardiac catheterizations.

Special Investigations

The extent of laboratory testing depends on the child's clinical status and the complexity of the planned procedure. General recommendations for blood testing include the following: (1) hematocrit or hemoglobin if the child is pale, cyanotic, or undergoing a procedure with the potential for significant blood loss; (2) serum electrolytes for patients with renal dysfunction or those receiving diuretics, angiotensin-converting enzyme inhibitors, or digoxin (although preoperative electrolyte disturbances in children and young adults presenting for cardiac surgery are uncommon [Hastings et al., 2008]); (3) platelet count and coagulation studies for cyanotic children or those on anticoagulants or antiplatelet agents; and (4) blood typing and cross-matching if significant blood loss is anticipated. A chest radiograph should be obtained with new cardiorespiratory symptoms or abnormal findings on clinical examination, or if dictated by the surgical procedure. Cardiologic studies should be coordinated with the child's cardiologist, because some tests will have been recently completed, and investigations such as cardiac catheterization, Holter monitoring, exercise stress tests, and cardiac MRI mandate the cardiologist's input. The electrocardiogram is reviewed for rhythm abnormalities, impaired conduction, chamber enlargement, and ischemia. Changes from prior studies need to be explained before proceeding. Preoperative consultation with the cardiologist is essential for patients with pacemakers, with evaluation of the pacemaker and a clear plan made for appropriate adjustment on the day of surgery (see earlier) (Practice advisory, 2005). In all but the simplest lesions, recent echocardiography is probably useful to document the current status of anatomy and ventricular function.

Procedure Scheduling

Institutional practices vary in the provision of anesthetic care for the highest-risk children with CHD. The aging of the CHD population has also resulted in adults with CHD undergoing noncardiac procedures at pediatric institutions (Warnes et al., 2001). In some institutions, anesthesia is provided by those who routinely practice pediatric cardiac anesthesia, and in others (including our own) pediatric anesthesiologists who do not practice cardiac anesthesia provide the care (Walker et al., 2009). The important point is that the case be assigned to an anesthesiologist who will understand the cardiac pathophysiology and know how to prevent and promptly deal with cardiac-related complications.

Ideally, patients with significant CHD should be scheduled for surgery early in the day. Clinical advantages include minimizing the effects of dehydration on hemodynamic function (particularly in infants and in cases of obstructive lesions, shunt-dependent circulations, cyanotic disease, single-ventricle physiology), possible reduction in the increased myocardial oxygen consumption associated with prolonged anxiety, provision of additional time to monitor patients in the postanesthesia care unit if discharge to home is being considered, greater availability of additional support if necessary, and avoidance of multiple care teams.

INTRAOPERATIVE MANAGEMENT

Premedication

The younger child will usually benefit from oral premedication before placement of an intravenous catheter. Premedication is especially beneficial for children with cyanotic CHD, particularly those with hypercyanotic spells, catecholamine-induced arrhythmias, and preexcitation syndromes. Although the potential effects of hypoventilation and hypoxemia on PVR need to be considered in the setting of pulmonary hypertension, sympathetic stimulation in a distressed patient may have a more deleterious effect.

Midazolam, 0.5 to 0.75 mg/kg orally, is usually sufficient, but for patients who have had multiple surgeries and catheterizations and thus are likely to be more anxious and perhaps more tolerant to sedative medications, it is often necessary to increase the dose to 1 mg/kg (Masue et al., 2003); sometimes oral ketamine, 3 to 10 mg/kg, is added as well (Auden et al., 2000; Funk, et al., 2000). Troublesome ketamine-stimulated secretions can usually be controlled with glycopyrrolate once intravenous access is established. If the patient has intravenous access in situ or after placement, a small bolus of midazolam, 0.05 mg/kg, repeated as necessary, will provide anxiolysis and facilitate separation from the parents. Intramuscular sedation with ketamine, 3 to 5 mg/kg, with or without midazolam, 0.05 to 0.1 mg/kg, may be necessary for the uncooperative or combative child who will not accept oral premedication and for whom an intravenous induction is most desirable. A combination of oral meperidine and pentobarbital for heavy premedication of CHD patients has been used with a substantial track record of safety and success (Nicolson et al., 1989), but insufficient effect and rage-like reactions (most likely attributable to pentobarbital) are known side effects. After any heavy premedication, the anesthesiologist should remain with the patient, and, particularly for patients with cyanotic CHD, oxygen saturation should be monitored and oxygen administered as needed (Stow et al., 1988; DeBock et al., 1990).

Anesthetic Technique

Standard principles of anesthetic management apply to patients with CHD who present for noncardiac surgery. The choice of anesthetic technique (local, regional, or general anesthesia), selection of pharmacologic agents, and requirement for invasive monitoring are determined by the physical (functional) status of the patient and the nature of the planned procedure. Cardiac medications, apart from diuretics, angiotensin-converting enzyme inhibitors, and angiotensin receptor antagonists (which are typically held), are generally administered on the morning of surgery. The patient's cardiologist should discuss with the surgeon the withholding of aspirin or other antiplatelet agents. Depending on the circumstances, the institution of an appropriate perioperative anticoagulation strategy may be necessary for patients on coumadin. In general, patients with prosthetic valves or a history of stroke and other thromboembolic events mandate the greatest degree of concern. Approaches to anticoagulation vary and depend to some extent on both the specific indication and the degree of concern regarding the relative risks. Management strategies vary from temporarily discontinuing coumadin (and usually following the prothrombin time and international normalized ratio [INR] and performing the surgery in the ensuing 24 to 48 hours), or discontinuing coumadin and instituting low-molecular-weight heparin prior to surgery, or discontinuing coumadin and administering periprocedural intravenous heparin.

For *general anesthesia,* an intravenous induction is recommended for patients with limited cardiac reserve, particularly those at risk for a marked decrease in cardiac output or circulatory instability with induction. Such high-risk cases include the more severe presentations of ventricular dysfunction, outflow tract obstruction, and pulmonary hypertension. Patients with cyanotic lesions resulting from right-to-left shunts have a slower inhalation induction because of the effects of reduced Q_p (Tanner et al., 1985). Dependency on a systemic-to-pulmonary artery shunt (and hence maintenance of adequate cardiac output and peripheral resistance) may also be better served by a hemodynamically stable intravenous induction, particularly if there is evidence (e.g., echocardiographic, history of decreasing arterial oxygen saturation or rising hemoglobin) of shunt narrowing or outgrowth over time.

Etomidate lacks significant hemodynamic effects in clinical dosages in children and adults (Gooding et al., 1979; Sarkar et al., 2005), and ketamine provides hemodynamic stability through sympathetically mediated increases in heart rate and systemic vascular resistance, albeit with direct myocardial depressant effects (Morray et al., 1984). There is no technique that guarantees preservation of myocardial function and hemodynamic stability during anesthetic induction at the extreme of ventricular dysfunction (e.g., severe end-stage dilated cardiomyopathy).

valvar obstruction, or pulmonary hypertension; reasons are multiple and include increased aortic impedance (both ketamine and etomidate) in the face of absent myocardial reserve to respond, deleterious effects of institution of positive pressure ventilation, and altered catecholamine tone. Clearly, only absolutely necessary or emergent procedures should be undertaken for such patients. Preoperative treatment with inotropes or inodilators (e.g., milrinone), or both, for patients with severe ventricular dysfunction or balloon dilation of severe valvar stenosis are examples of preoperative optimization techniques that should be considered. In addition to including inotropic support, the ability to rapidly convert to support with extracorporeal membrane oxygenation should be available (Duncan et al., 1998; Thiagarajan et al., 2007).

Although reports of the effect of ketamine on pulmonary vascular resistance are conflicting (Morray et al., 1984; Hickey et al., 1985; Berman et al., 1990; Maruyama et al., 1995), it can be used without risk of major increases in PVR in patients with CHD provided elevations in arterial CO_2 are prevented (Hickey et al., 1985). Opioid-benzodiazepine techniques are also suitable, particularly if postoperative mechanical ventilation is planned (Hickey and Hansen, 1984). Remifentanil provides profound analgesia with short recovery times, but it can be associated with bradycardia and hypotension in high dosages (Ross et al., 2001) and in association with sevoflurane (0.6 minimum alveolar concentration) (Foubert et al., 2002); bradycardia can be prevented with pretreatment with glycopyrrolate, 0.006 mg/kg (Reyntjens et al., 2005). Propofol use should probably be limited to children with adequate cardiovascular reserve who can tolerate mild to moderate decreases in systemic vascular resistance, contractility, and heart rate (Williams et al., 1999). Sevoflurane is associated with less myocardial depression and better hemodynamic stability than halothane, particularly in infants (Holzman et al., 1996; Wodey et al., 1997; Rivenes et al., 2001; Russell et al., 2001; Laird et al., 2002). Exposing neonates to large amounts of opioids and benzodiazepines can lead to tolerance that may persist (Mao and Mayer, 2001; Suresh and Anand, 2001), whereas inadequate analgesia for infants may lead to specific centrally mediated pain sensitization and thus increased sensitivity to pain and greater fear of painful procedures (Porter et al., 1999; Lowery et al., 2007). This has implications for premedication, opioid-benzodiazepine anesthesia, and postoperative pain control.

Regional anesthesia, alone or in combination with general anesthesia, has been used successfully in patients with CHD (Selsby and Sugden, 1989; Holzman et al., 1992; Martin et al., 2002; Sacrista et al., 2003; Katznelson et al., 2005; Walker et al., 2009), including those with shunt physiology and left-sided obstructive lesions. In infants and young children (<3 to 4 years of age), this success is likely to be at least in part due to minimal effects of regional blockade on α-adrenergic tone and SVR. As complex CHD can have a profound effect on emotional life and psychosocial development (Horner et al., 2000; Reid et al., 2006), substantial persuasion may be necessary in the older child or young adult when primarily regional or local anesthetic techniques are deemed to be indicated to reduce anesthetic risk.

Monitoring and Vascular Access

Standard monitoring according to the guidelines of the American Society of Anesthesiologists is recommended, with the need for invasive monitoring determined by the physical status of the patient and the complexity of the planned procedure. As discussed earlier, the site of previous Blalock-Taussig (BT) shunts, the presence of aortic arch obstruction, and a history of multiple cardiac catheterizations need to be considered when choosing a site for blood pressure cuff or arterial line placement. Classic BT shunts (subclavian artery–to–pulmonary artery anastomosis with ligation of distal subclavian artery) result in decreased or absent pulses on the side of the shunt. A modified BT shunt (synthetic graft between subclavian or innominate artery and pulmonary artery) may or may not result in stenosis of the subclavian artery with decreased pressure on the side of the shunt. The left subclavian artery is sometimes used as part of a flap in the repair of coarctation of the aorta. Lower limb blood pressures may be lower after narrowing or occlusion of the femoral arteries as a result of cardiac catheterization, or as a result of a technically inadequate repair (e.g., coarctation, arch reconstruction in patients with HLHS). Arterial access may be limited after radial artery cutdowns or femoral artery occlusion from multiple cardiac catheterizations.

Venous access may be limited as the result of multiple surgical procedures, cardiac catheterizations, and intensive care admissions. Multiple cardiac catheterizations can also lead to femoral vein occlusion. It is imperative to avoid the introduction of air into the venous system, leading to systemic air embolization in patients with intracardiac or intravascular communications and the potential for right-to-left shunting. For the more complex surgical procedures, central venous catheters allow monitoring of trends in central venous pressure and oxygen saturation (Dueck et al., 2005), as well as fluid and inotrope administration. Internal jugular or subclavian vein catheters can be quite useful but also carry a risk for thrombosis in the superior vena cava, as well as postoperative catheter-associated infection. The thrombotic complication can be disastrous in patients with a cavopulmonary anastomosis; consideration should be given to placing a femoral venous catheter if central access is necessary in such patients. Central venous catheters should be used for the shortest duration possible, access frequency limited, and special access ports and disinfection techniques employed to reduce the risk for catheter-associated infection. A low-dosage postoperative heparin infusion (10 IU/kg per hr) through the catheter can reduce the risk for thrombosis. Urinary catheters are placed as a guide to the adequacy of cardiac output and renal perfusion if major fluid shifts or blood losses are anticipated or if the procedure will be prolonged.

Transesophageal echocardiography (TEE) has been shown in adults to be useful for intraoperative assessment of ventricular preload and function (Schulmeyer et al., 2006), but the often complex anatomy in patients with CHD mandates additional expertise (Rivenes et al., 2001; Ikemba et al., 2004). TEE is likely to be used with increasing frequency in patients with and without CHD undergoing noncardiac procedures for monitoring of ventricular function and preload, particularly as the technology becomes more available and anesthesiologists become more practiced in its use (Mahmood et al., 2008). Intermittent transthoracic echocardiography is an alternative approach, provided that it is practical, there are adequate acoustic windows, and personnel with expertise are available.

Use of pulmonary artery catheterization (PAC) is controversial (Bernard et al., 2000), as added benefits have not convincingly been demonstrated with acquired heart disease. The risks are increased in the setting of pulmonary hypertension, and correct placement may be more difficult in some patients with

CHD (absence of pulsatile flow, need to traverse atrial baffles). PAC can be placed under fluoroscopic guidance in the cardiac catheterization laboratory before elective, major noncardiac surgery (e.g., spinal fusion) in patients with a Fontan circulation or severe ventricular dysfunction. In these circumstances, PAC can be useful as an indicator of systemic ventricular filling (pulmonary artery capillary wedge pressure) and oxygen delivery (pulmonary artery saturation). In the future, this role may be supplanted by TEE.

POSTOPERATIVE MANAGEMENT

The preoperative clinical status, nature of the surgical procedure, and intraoperative course determine whether postoperative admission will be to a general surgical ward, a cardiology ward, or an intensive care unit. Hemorrhage, hypoxia, hypoventilation, fever, uncontrolled pain, or myocardial ischemia may convert a well-tolerated surgical procedure into a crisis. Day surgery is possible for those patients whose cardiac status is well controlled, who have undergone a minor surgical procedure, and who have attained their baseline status prior to discharge. Higher-risk patients, particularly those undergoing major surgical procedures, are usually best managed in an intensive care setting. It is our practice to admit the child to the cardiology ward if changes in cardiac physiology pose a greater risk than complications from the surgical procedure. The healthier cardiac patient with a more complex surgical procedure is usually admitted to the appropriate surgical ward with cardiology consultation and follow-up. Standard fluid replacement guidelines are employed, and postoperative laboratory testing is guided by intraoperative blood loss, fluid shifts, and the child's preoperative status. Effective pain management is important and can be especially difficult if the patient is tolerant to sedatives and narcotics, or has recently been discharged after prolonged hospitalization and still on a withdrawal regimen. Involvement of colleagues with pediatric pain management expertise is recommended (see Chapter 15, Pain Management). Despite the best-possible anesthetic and procedure, it is in the postoperative period that complications are still likely to develop. In our experience, these are usually in patients with subtle or occult preexisting end-organ dysfunction, occurring as a consequence of chronic cyanosis, low cardiac output, or high venous pressures (or a combination of these). Certainly, the ability of various anesthetic agents, other drugs, and the surgical procedure to compromise organ blood flow or alter organ function plays a role as well.

OUTCOMES OF COMMON CONGENITAL HEART DEFECTS

Tetralogy of Fallot

Tetralogy of Fallot is the most common cyanotic lesion and accounts for approximately 10% of all CHD (Hoffman and Kaplan, 2002; Therrien and Webb, 2003). See related video online at www.expertconsult.com. The defect is characterized by anterocephalad deviation of the outlet septum, resulting in right ventricular outflow tract obstruction, a nonrestrictive VSD, aortic override, and right ventricular hypertrophy. The subpulmonary obstruction may be fixed or dynamic, it is invariably associated

with some degree of pulmonary valve stenosis, and there may be hypoplasia of the main and branch pulmonary arteries as well. Associated cardiac anomalies include a right-sided aortic arch (25%), a second VSD (3%), and coronary artery anomalies (anterior descending coronary artery arising from the right coronary artery and crossing the RV outflow tract [3%]). TOF is frequently associated with a 22q11 deletion, and DiGeorge and velocardiofacial syndromes.

Hypercyanotic episodes ("tet spells") are a hallmark of unrepaired TOF and can be life threatening, with increased cyanosis, syncope, and convulsions. Spells occur more frequently in cyanotic patients, with a peak frequency between 2 and 3 months of age. Infundibular spasm may play a role, and crying, defecation, feeding, fever, and awakening can be precipitating events. Spells are self-aggravating in that hypoxia induces a decrease in SVR, which further increases the right-to-left shunt. Paroxysmal hyperpnea increases oxygen consumption through increased work of breathing. Tet spells are managed as follows:

1. Nonanesthetized children are treated initially with 100% oxygen, knee–chest position, and morphine sulphate (0.05 to 0.1 mg/kg IM or IV) to relieve distress and air hunger. Ketamine is a suitable alternative (Tugrul et al., 2000).
2. Intravenous crystalloid (15 to 30 mL/kg) or colloid is used to increase preload and decrease the dynamic nature of the RV outflow tract spasm.
3. For continuing hypoxemia, an α-agonist (phenylephrine 0.5 to 2 mcg/kg) is used to increase SVR.
4. Judicious use of propranolol (0.1 mg/kg) or esmolol (0.5 mg/kg followed by an infusion of 50 to 300 mcg/kg per minute) slows the heart rate and relaxes the infundibulum. β-Adrenergic agonists are contraindicated.
5. Sodium bicarbonate (1 to 2 mEq/kg) can be administered to correct the metabolic acidosis, increasing the SVR and lowering the PVR.

If the spell persists, the child can be anesthetized, the trachea intubated, and mechanical ventilation instituted with 100% oxygen, low inspiratory pressures, and long expiratory times to promote venous return and antegrade flow across the RV outflow. An inhalation agent may be beneficial to reduce hyperdynamic right ventricular outflow obstruction. Manual compression of the abdominal aorta can be an effective means to temporarily increase SVR and decrease cyanosis in the anesthetized patient. In the operating room, there may be the need to proceed very rapidly to cardiopulmonary bypass (CPB) if the spell is severe and not resolving. Resuscitation with extracorporeal membrane oxygenation (ECMO) should be considered for refractory episodes when immediate operative intervention is not possible (Duncan et al., 1998; Thiagarajan et al., 2007).

Primary complete repair for the neonate or infant has largely replaced the traditional two-stage repair sequence of arteriopulmonary shunting in early infancy followed by later repair (Pigula et al., 1999). Thus, it is becoming fairly unusual to encounter an unrepaired or shunted infant with TOF. Right ventricular outflow obstruction is relieved by resection of hypertrophied muscle bundles and enlargement of the outflow tract with a pericardial patch. Although pulmonary valve-sparing techniques are increasingly being employed, a very small pulmonic annulus or a very stenotic pulmonary valve dictates placement of the patch across the annulus (transannular patch), resulting in pulmonary insufficiency. The VSD is closed with a Dacron patch. If a major coronary artery crosses the RV outflow tract (RVOT), or with long-segment pulmonary atresia, a right ventricle–to–pulmonary artery conduit rather than a pericardial patch is placed.

The majority of problems after TOF repair relate to chronic abnormal RV loading—that is, pressure loading from residual or recurrent RVOT obstruction and volume loading primarily from pulmonary regurgitation (issues shared by other lesions that require RVOT reconstruction or RV-PA conduit such as truncus arteriosus, pulmonary atresia, and the Rastelli procedure for TGA). In the long term, there is progressive RV dysfunction and the development of arrhythmias with increased risk for sudden death. Factors that have been associated with reduced long-term survival include older age (>4 years) at repair, initial palliative shunting procedures, significant RV hypertension, and volume loading of the RV (Gatzoulis et al., 2000a; Karamlou et al., 2006). Timely pulmonary valve replacement in children and young adults, before irreversible severe RV dilation and systolic ventricular dysfunction accrue, has become a major consideration (Therrien et al., 2000). Many patients after repair are asymptomatic with normal activity, although right ventricular dysfunction may progress and be evident only on exercise testing (decreased maximal aerobic capacity and endurance), stress echocardiography, or radionuclide techniques. Cardiac MRI is particularly useful to quantify RV systolic function, RV volume, the degree of pulmonary regurgitation, and sites of RVOT obstruction (Geva and Powell, 2008). The presence of tricuspid regurgitation is a likely surrogate for substantial RV dysfunction. Right bundle branch block is commonly seen after repair, whereas atrial tachyarrhythmias (atrial flutter or intraatrial reentrant tachycardia) arise in about one third of adults. Although the presence of premature ventricular contractions (PVCs) is common in asymptomatic patients (approximately 10% on routine electrocardiogram, 30% on exercise stress testing, and up to 50% during Holter monitoring), it is often of low grade and has not been a predictor of patients at risk for sudden death. Although a QRS duration of 180 msec or greater is a highly sensitive marker for sustained ventricular tachycardia and sudden death, its positive predictive value is low (Gatzoulis et al., 1995). LV dysfunction and dyssynchrony have been observed in patients with TOF and was associated with QRS duration, such that abnormal LV mechanics in combination with RV dysfunction may explain the relation between QRS duration and adverse cardiac outcomes (Tzemos et al., 2009).

However, the presence of monomorphic ventricular tachycardia in a symptomatic patient (syncope and palpitations) is significant and necessitates treatment. Electrophysiologic methods are to assess and ablate atrial or ventricular arrhythmias and for deciding on the need for an implantable cardioverter-defibrillator (Khairy et al., 2008b).

Anesthetic considerations: The degree of RV dysfunction needs to be defined and consideration given to preoperative interventional cardiac catheterization to reduce the impact of significant residual lesions (RVOT or PA obstruction, residual VSD, collaterals causing volume loading, arrhythmias). In the presence of pulmonary regurgitation or RV dysfunction, factors that increase PVR should be avoided, as should factors detrimental to RV myocardial supply-demand relationship (tachycardia, hypotension, anemia, and acidosis are detrimental). The role of pulmonary valve replacement in patients with severe pulmonary regurgitation, RV volume overload, and RV dysfunction (all best assessed by cardiac MRI) remains to be defined. Right ventricular filling should be maintained, understanding that excessive volume (or dysfunction) can lead to RV dilation and resultant LV dysfunction (ventricular interdependence). Prophylactic administration of an inotrope to improve RV contractile performance should be considered in patients with significant RV dysfunction. (See Pulmonary Hypertension, earlier.) A means for external defibrillation and pacing should be readily available. Late development of LV dysfunction is another consideration in patients with TOF as they age.

Transposition of the Great Arteries

Transposition of the great arteries (D-TGA) accounts for 3% to 10% of all CHD (Hoffman and Kaplan, 2002). See related video online at www.expertconsult.com. Ventriculoarterial discordance results in the aorta arising from the anatomic right ventricle and the pulmonary artery from the left ventricle. Associated defects include a VSD (40% to 45%), VSD with LV outflow tract obstruction (10%), or variability in coronary artery pattern (Mayer et al., 1990). A much less common form of TGA is congenitally (physiologically) "corrected" TGA (L-TGA), in which there is both ventriculoarterial and atrioventricular discordance (i.e., a series circulation in which the right atrium connects via the mitral valve to the LV and then the PA, and the left atrium connects via the tricuspid valve to the RV and then the aorta). Congenitally corrected transposition (without associated cardiac lesions) may go undetected for decades until the RV, which is the systemic ventricle, begins to fail. This group is at increased risk for the spontaneous development of complete heart block.

D-TGA produces two parallel circulations with recirculation of systemic and pulmonary venous blood. Adequate systemic oxygenation and survival are dependent on one or more communications between the two circuits to allow intercirculatory mixing; these communications can be intracardiac (ASD, VSD) or extracardiac (PDA, bronchopulmonary collaterals), or both. For initial palliation, the infant is maintained on a prostaglandin E_1 (PGE_1) infusion to support adequate intercirculatory mixing via the PDA. With adequate mixing and a good-sized PDA, excessive pulmonary blood flow can result, placing a volume load on the ventricle and inducing pulmonary congestion as a result of an increased Q_p:Q_s ratio, and causing decreased systemic perfusion. A general rule of thumb aims for arterial saturations in the 75% to 85% range in the nonintubated, spontaneously ventilating patient. With inadequate intracardiac mixing, frequently manifesting as excessive cyanosis and poor perfusion, a *balloon atrial septostomy* is performed in the catheterization laboratory or at the bedside to improve mixing and to reduce left atrial pressure. This can be an urgent or emergent procedure performed shortly after delivery. In patients with reduced pulmonary blood flow or poor intercirculatory mixing (most often those with an intact ventricular septum) despite PGE_1 and a widely patent atrial communication, volume loading often improves the situation, which at times requires further augmentation by inotropic support to increase overall myocardial function and venous blood saturation. In patients demonstrating significant overcirculation (e.g., tachypnea, pulmonary congestion on chest x-ray, systemic hypoperfusion, acidosis), reduced fraction of inspired oxygen (Fio_2) via blending of atmospheric air with nitrogen, or controlled ventilation with induced hypercarbia via added inspired CO_2, has been used to try to reduce excessive PBF. More frequently now, this situation is managed with circulatory support as needed (e.g., dopamine), controlled ventilation, and early surgical repair. Infants with evidence of multiple organ dysfunction after severe cyanosis and hypoperfusion are generally better managed with a period of stabilization and recovery, facilitated by the aforementioned measures to improve mixing and oxygen delivery, before undergoing corrective surgery.

D-TGA is currently repaired anatomically by the *arterial switch (Jatene) operation* (ASO) (Jatene et al., 1976). The pulmonary artery and aorta are transected distal to their respective valves. The coronary arteries are excised with a button of surrounding tissue and reimplanted into the proximal pulmonary artery (neoaorta). The great arteries are then switched, with the pulmonary artery brought anterior (Lecompte maneuver) and anastomosed to the proximal aorta (right ventricular outflow) and the aorta anastomosed to the proximal pulmonary artery (left ventricular outflow). Most patients with TGA have coronary anatomy that is suitable for coronary reimplantation. The variant of D-TGA with VSD and severe LVOT obstruction precludes the ASO. In this setting, the *Rastelli procedure* is performed, in which the VSD is repaired by a patch that directs blood from the left ventricle through the defect into the aorta (and also closes the VSD), and a valved conduit is placed from the right ventricle to the main pulmonary artery. With the Rastelli procedure, the LV functions as the systemic ventricle, but conduit degeneration and stenosis are inevitable (Warnes, 2006).

The *atrial* switch procedure (Mustard, Senning), which revolutionized the management of infants with TGA, is now rarely used. It is a physiologic repair in which a baffle in the atrium directs systemic venous blood to the mitral valve (and consequently to the LV and pulmonary artery) and pulmonary venous blood to the tricuspid valve (and consequently to the RV and aorta) (Fig. 21-1).

The *atrial switch* procedures provide excellent midterm results (15-year survival, 77% to 94%; 20-year survival, 80%)

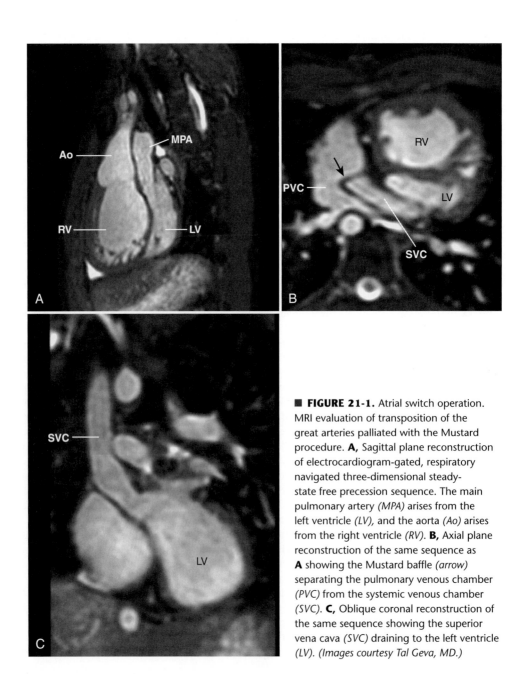

■ **FIGURE 21-1.** Atrial switch operation. MRI evaluation of transposition of the great arteries palliated with the Mustard procedure. **A,** Sagittal plane reconstruction of electrocardiogram-gated, respiratory navigated three-dimensional steady-state free precession sequence. The main pulmonary artery *(MPA)* arises from the left ventricle *(LV),* and the aorta *(Ao)* arises from the right ventricle *(RV).* **B,** Axial plane reconstruction of the same sequence as **A** showing the Mustard baffle *(arrow)* separating the pulmonary venous chamber *(PVC)* from the systemic venous chamber *(SVC).* **C,** Oblique coronal reconstruction of the same sequence showing the superior vena cava *(SVC)* draining to the left ventricle *(LV). (Images courtesy Tal Geva, MD.)*

(Merlo et al., 1991; Helbing et al., 1994; Wilson et al., 1998; Sarkar et al., 1999; Williams et al., 2003), with many patients able to lead fairly normal lives into their third and fourth decades. In the long term, there is progressive deterioration in RV function (Piran et al., 2002) and development of tricuspid regurgitation (which is the *systemic* atrioventricular valve in this circulation) with heart failure, arrhythmias, and risk for sudden death (Wilson et al., 1998). Even in asymptomatic patients, exercise testing demonstrates moderate to severe limitations in RV function and maximal aerobic capacity. Sinus rhythm is maintained in only 40% to 50% of patients (Deanfield et al., 1988), with the frequent occurrence of sick sinus syndrome. Atrial flutter parallels the development of ventricular dysfunction (Gatzoulis et al., 2000b) and is experienced in one third or more of patients, 20 years after surgery (Puley et al., 1999). Intraatrial baffle leaks can result in shunting and hypoxemia. Baffle obstruction of the systemic venous return can cause superior vena cava (SVC) syndrome, hepatic congestion, ascites, and peripheral edema, whereas pulmonary venous baffle obstruction can cause pulmonary edema and pulmonary hypertension. Subendocardial perfusion defects of the systemic (right) ventricle have been noted in a significant number of patients.

The ASO is associated with an early hospital mortality of less than 5% in experienced centers (Hutter et al., 2002; Warnes, 2006; Raisky et al., 2007). At 15 years, good LV function and sinus rhythm are maintained in 96.4% and 98.1% of patients, respectively (Losay et al., 2001). The ongoing risk for death is less than after the atrial switch operation, and it is related to coronary events and arrhythmias. In long-term follow-up, patients remain in good condition, and the majority are New York Heart Association functional class I (Hutter et al., 2002). The most frequent need for reintervention has been the development of supravalvar (anastomotic) pulmonary artery stenosis, less commonly supravalvar aortic stenosis. These are frequently amenable to balloon dilation, although reoperation may occasionally be necessary. Neoaortic insufficiency (i.e., the anatomic pulmonary valve now located in the aortic position) appears to be occurring with increasing frequency as more patients accrue and age. At present, it is usually of mild or lesser severity and thus far has infrequently required reintervention; however, the long-term implications of this problem are concerning. Another potential complication that is being found more frequently and requires ongoing attention is the development of coronary artery stenoses. Coronary obstruction is an infrequent clinical complication outside of the immediate perioperative period, where technical difficulties associated with coronary reimplantation can result in myocardial ischemia and problems related thereto. Overall, the incidence of coronary events has a bimodal pattern, with a high early incidence and low late incidence (Legendre et al., 2003). The arteries display varying degrees of proximal eccentric intimal proliferation (Pedra et al., 2004) and concentric intimal smooth muscle hyperplasia with preserved tunica media (Bartoloni et al., 2006), suggesting the potential for the development of early atherosclerosis in the reimplanted coronary arteries. Noninvasive tests are not sufficiently sensitive to detect delayed coronary artery stenosis, and coronary artery angiography or intracoronary ultrasound is required (or both); it is presently unclear whether such testing should be a mandatory component of surveillance in all patients who have undergone an ASO (Pedra et al., 2004). If needed, coronary revascularization can be achieved using coronary angioplasty in most cases (Raisky et al., 2007).

Anesthetic considerations: After an uncomplicated ASO, most patients can be managed in the same way as those with a structurally normal heart, but with an index of suspicion for coronary artery disease. Severe pulmonary artery stenosis can be managed with interventional cardiac catheterization prior to elective procedures. Anesthesia for patients after the *atrial switch* operation should be based on the knowledge that this can become an increasingly fragile circulation with limited physiologic reserve as patients age. The potential for decreased ventricular function is substantial, particularly of the systemic right ventricle, as well as for arrhythmias and end-organ dysfunction. Although some volatile anesthetic will be tolerated by most of these patients, many will benefit from the more hemodynamically stable induction and maintenance regimens that have been discussed earlier. As elsewhere, it may be prudent to start an inotrope infusion at the time of or shortly after induction in those with more severe degrees of ventricular dysfunction. A significant number of these patients have a pacemaker, and the appropriate guidelines need to be followed (see earlier) (Practice advisory, 2005). Baffle leaks can result in cyanosis and increase the risk for systemic embolization of air or debris; consideration should be given to device closure in the catheterization laboratory prior to elective procedures associated with a high risk for embolization.

Single-Ventricle Physiology

A single ventricle is defined as the presence of two atrioventricular valves with one ventricular chamber, or a large dominant ventricle with a diminutive opposing ventricle (Keane and Fyler, 2006c). See related video online at www.expertconsult.com. Single ventricle or *univentricular* hearts encompass a wide variety of lesions that include tricuspid atresia or severe tricuspid stenosis, double-inlet single ventricle (usually left), single ventricle with common atrioventricular valve (unbalanced complete AV canal, heterotaxy variants), HLHS, and some forms of double-outlet right ventricle and pulmonary atresia with intact ventricular septum. Initial management is aimed at optimization of systemic oxygen delivery and perfusion pressure. Subsequent management is aimed at reducing the volume load on the ventricle (superior cavopulmonary connection or Glenn procedure) and finally achieving a series circulation with fully saturated systemic arterial blood (Fontan procedure). This is usually achieved through a staged approach. Although, collectively, single-ventricle defects are relatively rare, they account for a disproportionate share of repeated procedures and resultant morbidity and mortality.

Unoperated *single-ventricle physiology* is characterized by complete mixing of systemic and pulmonary venous blood at the atrial or ventricular level (or both). If there is no obstruction to pulmonary or systemic outflow, the amount of flow to each circulation is determined by the relative resistances of the pulmonary and systemic vascular beds. With no obstruction to pulmonary blood flow and the normal postnatal regression in PVR, PBF gradually increases and results in congestive heart failure. Obstruction to PBF will result in progressive cyanosis in the absence of a patent ductus arteriosus. Systemic outflow obstruction will result in increased PBF, CHF, and systemic hypoperfusion. In patients with single-ventricle physiology, an arterial saturation of 75% to 80% is felt to be indicative of a relatively balanced circulation with a $Q_P:Q_S$ at or near 1:1 (assuming pulmonary venous saturation of 95% to 100% and mixed venous saturation of 50% to 55%) (Rudolph, 1974). However, even with a "balanced" $Q_P:Q_S$ of 1:1, the systemic ventricle is essentially pumping double the normal cardiac output. This gives some appreciation for the even greater degrees of systemic ventricular volume overload that is imposed by increased amounts of PBF.

The initial procedure in the neonatal period varies with the anatomy. In the presence of approximately the right amount of pulmonary obstruction to balance the circulations, no procedure will be required in the newborn period.

Norwood Operation

The Norwood procedure, also referred to as stage I single-ventricle palliation, is performed for patients with HLHS and its variants (Norwood et al., 1983) or when the pathway to the aorta from the systemic ventricle is obstructed. The pulmonary artery is transected just proximal to its bifurcation, and the pulmonary artery is anastomosed end to side, or side to side, to the ascending aorta, with reconstruction of the ascending and transverse aorta. In the neonatal period, PBF is supplied by a modified BT shunt or RV-to-PA conduit (Sano et al., 2003) (Fig. 21-2). When pulmonary venous blood must cross the atrial septum to reach the systemic ventricle, the atrial septum must be nonrestrictive. Creating a nonrestrictive atrial septum can be achieved in the cardiac catheterization laboratory with a Rashkind-Miller balloon atrial septostomy, or a surgical atrial septectomy can be performed at the time of initial palliation in procedures that require CPB.

Anesthetic Considerations for the Unoperated Neonate

A continuous infusion of PGE_1 is used to maintain ductal patency for lesions associated with ductal-dependent blood flow (either systemic or pulmonary). In right-sided obstructive lesions (e.g., pulmonary atresia), left-to-right flow through the duct is needed for pulmonary perfusion, whereas for left-sided obstructive lesions (e.g., HLHS, critical neonatal coarctation), an adequate amount of right-to-left flow through the duct is needed for systemic perfusion. In both settings, the underlying tendency is for excessive PBF, resulting in pulmonary overcirculation, pulmonary congestion, and systemic hypoperfusion.

Management principles are similar for patients whether they are dependent on the PDA or they have a surgically created shunt. A target arterial partial pressure of oxygen (Pao_2) of 40 to 45 mm Hg and an oxygen saturation of hemoglobin (Sao_2) of 70% to 80% are reasonable starting goals that are likely to approach achieving adequate systemic O_2 delivery and PBF. With unrestricted PBF, control and manipulation of PVR and subsequently of $Q_P:Q_S$ is accomplished most reliably through ventilatory interventions to increase PVR, usually hypercarbia in combination with 21% inspired oxygen to achieve a pH of 7.30 to 7.35; use of hypoxic (17% inspired O_2 achieved by addition of nitrogen to air) or hypercarbic ($Fico_2$, 2.7%) are alternatives (Tabbutt et al., 2001). In anesthetized patients, an appropriate degree of hypercarbia can usually be obtained with a tidal volume of 6 to 10 mL/kg, a PEEP of 3 to 5 cm H_2O, and a respiratory rate of 8 to 10 breaths/min. Higher Fio_2 is avoided unless the Pao_2 is less than 35 to 40 mm Hg and intrapulmonary $\dot{V}/\dot{Q}$

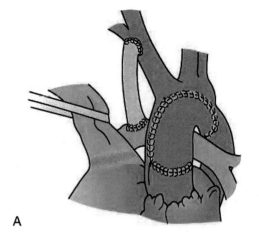

A

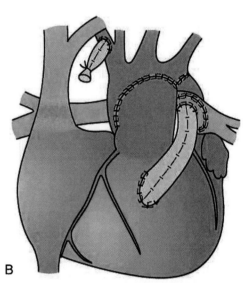

B

■ **FIGURE 21-2.** The Norwood operation for first-stage palliation of hypoplastic left heart syndrome. The pulmonary artery is transected just proximal to its bifurcation, and the pulmonary artery is anastomosed in an end-to-side or side-to-side fashion to the ascending aorta, with reconstruction of the ascending and transverse aorta. Pulmonary blood flow is supplied by a modified Blalock-Taussig shunt **(A)** or right-ventricle to pulmonary artery conduit **(B)**. *(Redrawn from Sano S, Ishino K, Kawada M, et al: Right ventricle–pulmonary artery shunt in first-stage palliation of hypoplastic left heart syndrome, J Thorac Cardiovasc Surg 126:504–510, 2003.)*

mismatch is suspected. Denitrogenation with 100% O_2 is recommended prior to laryngoscopy and tracheal intubation so as to prevent hypoxemia during this interval. Once the airway is secured, the Fio_2 can be reduced.

Because ventilatory interventions are usually incapable of reducing $Q_P:Q_S$ much below 2:1, additional measures to increase systemic cardiac output are often necessary to ensure adequate systemic oxygen delivery and coronary perfusion pressure; ensuring adequate preload and inotropic support with dopamine in the range of 3 to 10 µg/kg per minute is often sufficient to accomplish these goals. It should be noted that the ability to recruit stroke volume with preload augmentation is very limited in neonates, particularly in the presence of already volume-overloaded ventricles. Although cardiac output in these circumstances has increasing dependency on contractile state and heart rate, increasing heart rate much above normal (~140 to 160 beats/min) can potentially induce myocardial ischemia, particularly when aortic diastolic blood pressure is low (<20 to 30 mm Hg, caused by the large amount of runoff via the PDA).

An intravenous induction with ketamine, etomidate, or high-dosage narcotic (if postoperative ventilation is planned) and muscle relaxant is recommended. Inhalation agents should be used with caution, and a benzodiazepine (usually midazolam) can be added as tolerated. Use of invasive monitoring in shunt-dependent patients is usually determined by the nature of the surgical procedure.

Pulmonary Artery Band

Unrestricted PBF compromises systemic oxygen delivery, results in congestive heart failure, and ultimately leads to pulmonary artery hypertension and the development of pulmonary vascular occlusive disease. In this setting, a pulmonary artery band is placed to limit pulmonary blood flow, thereby controlling congestive heart failure and protecting the pulmonary vascular bed (Heath and Edwards, 1958).

Systemic-to-Pulmonary Artery Shunt

Infants with ductal-dependent pulmonary blood flow will require stabilization with PGE₁ followed by placement of a surgical aortopulmonary shunt (clearly, an intracardiac right-to-left shunt is also required). A *modified Blalock-Taussig shunt* is performed most commonly and involves placement of a Gore-Tex graft between the subclavian or innominate artery and the pulmonary artery on the side opposite to the aortic arch. The aim of this procedure is to establish a stable source of PBF as the PDA closes. In patients with HLHS, a right ventricle–to–pulmonary artery conduit is an alternative to a modified BT shunt (Sano et al., 2003). A superior cavopulmonary shunt cannot be performed in the neonatal period, because the high PVR necessitates a pumping ventricle or systemic blood pressure to drive blood through the lungs.

Anesthetic Considerations after Initial Palliation

After initial palliation, the same principles apply to balancing systemic and pulmonary blood flow as before (or immediately after) the initial operation. Surgically created shunts early in their course are typically large so as to allow for growth, and hence the major issues are controlling excessive PBF, ensuring adequate systemic perfusion, and managing congestive heart failure (see later). On the other hand, the child can outgrow the shunt or band (both involve fixed diameters) at around 3 to 6 months of age, so that the $Q_P:Q_S$ falls and eventually becomes less than 1:1 with a lower arterial oxygen saturation. Shunt calcification or stenosis also plays a role in limiting shunt flow, can occur at any time, and can result in increasing cyanosis. Clearly, severe or total shunt occlusion (thrombosis) can be catastrophic.

In patients with evidence of shunt flow that is beginning to be critically limited (decreased saturations, increasing hemoglobin, echocardiographic evidence), it is reasonable to assume that the effective resistance to PBF is relatively fixed (i.e., pulmonary overcirculation is unlikely to be possible), and primary attention is therefore directed toward maneuvers that maintain or in fact increase cardiac output and systemic blood pressure

in order to support adequate PBF. It is also reasonable to try to avoid increases in intrinsic and reactive components of PVR by using increased inspired oxygen concentrations and avoiding hypercarbia, acidosis, and other factors that increase PVR. An intravenous induction is generally preferred, as loss of the airway and hypotension can lead to profound hypoxia and cardiac arrest. Vascular access may be difficult, as many of these patients have had prolonged intensive care unit (ICU) stays. Many of these patients are tolerant to opioids and benzodiazepines, and this fact should be considered if premedication is planned prior to placement of an intravenous line. Intramuscular induction with ketamine can be a safe alternative.

Anesthetic Considerations after the Superior Cavopulmonary Connection

In the superior cavopulmonary connection or bidirectional Glenn operation, the SVC is transected and the cranial end is sewn in an end-to-side manner to the right pulmonary artery (which is in continuity with the left pulmonary artery); the distal (cardiac) end is oversewn (Fig. 21-3). Systemic venous return from the head and upper body thus passes directly from the SVC into the pulmonary circulation. The goal is to reduce the volume load on the ventricle and allow cardiac remodeling (compared with the prior shunted circulation) with maintenance of cardiac output at a lower ventricular filling volume. After the Glenn operation, the $Q_P:Q_S$ will be between approximately 0.5:1 and 0.8:1, as the inferior vena cava (IVC) blood does not pass through the lungs but mixes with pulmonary venous blood in a functionally common atrium. The arterial oxygen saturation will still be reduced (75% to 85%), with a typical SVC pressure of 10 to 12 mm Hg and an atrial pressure of 5 to 6 mm Hg. The transpulmonary gradient is thus 4 to 7 mm Hg. The physiology of PBF and anesthetic considerations are similar to the Fontan circulation and discussed later.

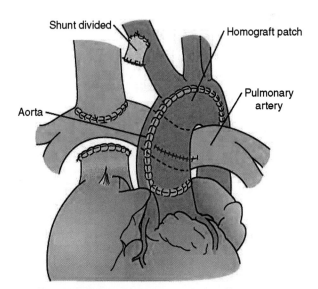

■ FIGURE 21-3. Bidirectional Glenn operation. The superior vena cava is transected and the cranial end is sewn in an end-to-side fashion to the right pulmonary artery (which is in continuity with the left pulmonary artery). The distal (cardiac end) is oversewn. *(Redrawn from Sano S, Ishino K, Kawada M, et al: Right ventricle–pulmonary artery shunt in first-stage palliation of hypoplastic left heart syndrome, J Thorac Cardiovasc Surg 126:504–510, 2003.)*

Anesthetic Considerations after the Total Cavopulmonary Connection or Fontan Operation

Patients with Fontan circulations are symbolic of how asymptomatic clinical status should not give the anesthesiologist a false sense of security about cardiovascular stability. The Fontan operation is usually performed within 1 to 2 years of a bidirectional Glenn (Jonas, 2004), and thus between 15 months and 2.5 years of age. The operative principle is diversion of the systemic venous return directly to the pulmonary arteries without the need for a subpulmonary ventricle, resulting in a series circulation with relief of cyanosis. Although many modifications of this procedure have been described, the total cavopulmonary connection (lateral tunnel Fontan) is currently the procedure of choice in most centers (Jonas, 2004) (Fig. 21-4). In the presence of a preexisting bidirectional Glenn anastomosis (the situation for most patients coming to Fontan surgery at present), an intraatrial baffle is placed to direct IVC flow from the IVC orifice along the side wall of the atrium up to the SVC orifice, with opening of the cardiac (distal) end of the SVC and anastomosis to the pulmonary artery.

The key physiologic principle in patients with Fontan physiology is maintaining filling and function of the systemic ventricle. In the absence of a pumping pulmonary ventricle, the initial consideration is to maintain an adequate pressure gradient between the systemic venous return circulation and the common atrium (i.e., the atrium that serves the systemic ventricle). The circulation can be viewed, in oversimplified fashion, as a waterfall, with the systemic venous pressure as the top, and the end-diastolic pressure in the systemic ventricle as the bottom. The ideal Fontan will have a mean systemic venous (pulmonary artery) pressure of approximately 10 to 15 mm Hg and a common atrial pressure of 7 to 10 mm Hg, resulting in a transpulmonary gradient of 3 to 8 mm Hg. Optimal physiology depends on adequate preload, unobstructed systemic venous return, low PVR, low mean intrathoracic pressure, normal lung parenchyma and alveolar ventilation, unobstructed pulmonary venous return, sinus rhythm (resulting primarily from the atrial contribution to ventricular filling [Penny et al., 1991]), atrioventricular valve competency, normal ventricular function, and low ventricular afterload. Any significant departure from these requirements can result in severe compromise. For example, ventricular dysfunction with an end-diastolic pressure of 15 mm Hg mandates a venous pressure of 20 to 25 mm Hg (i.e., the transpulmonary gradient is preserved but venous pressures must be proportionately higher) to achieve comparable pulmonary blood flow, ventricular filling, and cardiac output. Relatively *mild* acute lung disease (e.g., viral pneumonitis), if associated with increased PVR, can lead to an acute and severe decrease in systemic ventricular filling and cardiac output unless and until preload is restored sufficiently to restore ventricular filling (here, the transpulmonary gradient is increased)—that is, any downstream problem will necessitate a higher upstream pressure.

Because ventricular dysfunction and elevated PVR can contribute to early mortality after a Fontan operation, a fenestration (hole) is made in the intraatrial baffle at the time of the Fontan operation. This fenestration allows right-to-left shunting from the venous side of the baffle to the common atrial arterial side, and hence a portion of the cardiac output is able to avoid traversing the lungs; in the presence of an elevated PVR or elevated end-diastolic pressures (e.g., after cardiopulmonary bypass), flow through the fenestration maintains filling of the systemic ventricle and preserves cardiac output at lower systemic venous pressures, albeit at the expense of a physiologically acceptable reduction in systemic arterial saturation. The fenestration is a potential site for paradoxical embolism. In time, the fenestration either closes spontaneously or it can electively be closed with a device in the catheterization laboratory when adequate hemodynamics are achieved. Arterial oxygen saturations are usually in the range of 80% to 90% in the presence of a patent fenestration, depending on the magnitude of the shunt and the saturation of the shunted venous blood (and therefore systemic oxygen delivery and extraction). An SpO$_2$ of approximately 95% is expected with a closed fenestration, but saturations in the 90% to 95% range are common. This reduction from full saturation results in part from the fact that the coronary sinus is usually located on the common atrial side of the repair (causing mixing of highly desaturated coronary venous blood, about 20% of total cardiac output, with oxygenated blood in the systemic ventricle). Greater degrees of desaturation may reflect residual right-to-left shunt across a patent baffle fenestration, baffle suture line leaks, decompressing venous collaterals (typically between the SVC and the atrium or pulmonary veins), pulmonary arteriovenous malformations (can occur as a consequence of Glenn physiology), very low cardiac output, or intrinsic lung disease.

Complications after the Fontan operation are in part dependent on surgical technique and era, and partly on pathophysiologic sequelae of multiple factors such as multiple surgeries, long-standing systemic venous hypertension, cyanosis, and perhaps limited cardiac output as well. One can expect progressive

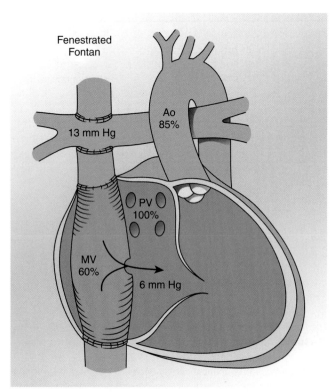

Fenestrated
Fontan

Ao
85%

13 mm Hg

PV
100%

MV
60%

6 mm Hg

■ **FIGURE 21-4.** Lateral tunnel Fontan with patent fenestration. *Ao,* Aortic saturation; *MV,* mixed venous saturation; *PV,* pulmonary vein saturation.

decline in the function of the systemic ventricle, an increasing risk for development of arrhythmias, and end-organ dysfunction as these patients age. Recent data suggest that diastolic dysfunction may be an early and persistent feature of Fontan myocardial physiology (Cheung et al., 2000; Olivier et al., 2003). Other specific issues include recurrent pleuropericardial effusions, peripheral edema, ascites, cirrhosis, and protein-losing enteropathy (3.7%) (Mertens et al., 1998; Khairy et al., 2007). Thrombosis in the venous pathway (6% to 33%) may occur early or late and result in both pulmonary and systemic embolic complications, particularly stroke. Sudden total obstruction appears as sudden death. It is unclear whether and to what extent specific hemostatic derangements such as increased factor VIII, dysregulation of other procoagulant and anticoagulant factor synthesis resulting from Fontan physiology, or the superimposition of this physiology on a "normal" background of thrombophilic polymorphisms (e.g., factor V Leiden, prothrombin mutations) might be responsible for the apparent increased thrombotic risk in these patients (Odegard et al., 2003, 2009).

Arrhythmias are associated with serious morbidity (especially the development of atrial thrombi) and can lead to profound hemodynamic deterioration. The combination of atrial incisions, multiple and extensive atrial suture lines, and increased right atrial pressure and size appear to be predisposing factors. The incidence of atrial tachyarrhythmias (atrial flutter or fibrillation, or both) is lower with the lateral tunnel Fontan (Stamm et al., 2001b) than in patients operated on in the 1970s and 1980s with direct atriopulmonary anastomosis (Fishberger et al., 1997). In the current era, freedom from new supraventricular tachyarrhythmia was 98% at 5 years and 95% at 10 years (Brown et al., 2010). A recent study found less atrial arrhythmia with extracardiac conduit than lateral tunnel Fontan (Robbers-Visser et al., 2009). Bradyarrhythmia (heart block and sick sinus syndrome), which may necessitate pacemaker implantation, also appears to be more frequent in the first 10 years than atrial tachyarrhythmias with the lateral tunnel version of the procedure (Stamm et al., 2001b). Freedom from late-onset bradyarrhythmia varies from 89% (Stamm et al., 2001b) to 96% (Brown et al., 2010) at 10 years.

The probability of survival after Fontan surgery has increased in more recent years (93.9% at 8 years in one study [Stamm et al., 2001b] and 95% at 15 years in another [Brown et al., 2010]), largely as a result of improved surgical techniques, patient selection, and perioperative management (Mitchell et al., 2006; Anderson et al., 2008; Khairy et al., 2008a; Robbers-Visser et al., 2009). Progressive deterioration of ventricular function (functional status) and gradual attrition occur, predominantly from thromboembolic, heart failure–related, and sudden (presumed arrhythmic) deaths (Khairy et al., 2008a).

Objective testing of functional status has indicated that patients with stable single-ventricle physiology are able to lead a fairly normal life with moderate exercise tolerance (Robbers-Visser et al., 2010). With exercise, maximal aerobic capacity was reduced, with only 28% of patients having peak oxygen consumption within the normal range (Paridon et al., 2008). Stroke volume reserve is the most important determinant of aerobic capacity, with exercise tolerance limited by peak blood flow in the pulmonary vascular bed. With exercise or other hemodynamic stress, a fall in cardiac index and oxygen saturation may occur because of an inability to increase stroke volume (Robbers-Visser et al., 2008). This inability probably results from multiple factors, including relatively fixed

myocardial contractile reserve and the fact that many Fontan patients are near-maximally venoconstricted, thereby limiting the amount of preload augmentation that can occur to support exercise-stimulated increases in cardiac output; a blunted heart rate response, for reasons discussed previously, may be an additional factor. In sum, the progressive and late decline in survival and functional status implies that these repairs are not curative and should be viewed as palliative at this time (Khairy et al., 2008a). A recent Pediatric Heart Network study found that sinus rhythm was present in 67% of patients; 13% used a pacemaker; semilunar and atrioventricular valve regurgitation was present in 49% and 74% of patients, respectively; 72% had abnormal diastolic function; and pulmonary reserve was below normal in 34% of cases (Anderson et al., 2008).

Anesthetic management: Management of Fontan physiology is summarized in Table 21-2. Hemodynamic goals are to maintain normal to increased preload, normal to slightly increased heart rate, normal to low pulmonary vascular resistance, and sinus rhythm (atrioventricular synchrony); to support ventricular function; and to avoid high ventricular afterload. In the hospitalized patient, maintenance intravenous fluids should be begun while the patient is fasting preoperatively. Particularly in outpatients, volume expansion may be necessary before induction to ensure adequate preload. A technique using sedation with local or regional anesthesia should be considered where feasible (recognizing that some patients will be on anticoagulants).

The use of mechanical ventilation deserves some consideration, as ventilation and acid-base management need to be optimized to keep PVR low. Although spontaneous ventilation enhances pulmonary blood flow (Penny and Redington, 1991), the accompanying hypoventilation likely to occur during anesthesia or procedures associated with abdominal or thoracic compression will increase PVR through atelectasis, hypoxic pulmonary vasoconstriction, and hypercarbia. In fact, increased PVR (and hence acutely reduced cardiac output) is more likely to occur during either relative hypoventilation (resulting primarily from increased Pco_2 and also from alveolar hypoxia and collapse) or excessive positive pressure ventilation (resulting from increased intrathoracic and pulmonary pressures that are transmitted to the vasculature, as well as from potential microvascular distention or compression [or both] caused by overinflation). For most surgical situations (all but the shortest of procedures), we believe that the sum of effects favors judicious use of positive pressure ventilation in order to provide an effective anesthetic while maintaining lung volumes and normal gas exchange. This can usually be accomplished with a relatively large tidal volume (~10 mL/kg), slower respiratory rates (10 to 15 breaths/min), and shorter inspiratory times (I:E of 1:3 or 1:4). Similar considerations apply to the use of PEEP: if it is targeted to maintain or improve functional residual capacity and lung compliance and thereby assist with gas exchange, it is likely to be helpful, whereas overdistention will favor deleterious effects. Additional fluid administration can be used to overcome the decrease in venous return associated with mechanical ventilation. Another benefit of positive pressure ventilation can be the decrease in afterload on the systemic ventricle (LaPlace's law) and consequent improvement in its function.

When choosing induction agents, etomidate or ketamine is likely to provide the greatest degree of hemodynamic stability, and either is preferred if functional status is diminished. Thiopental or propofol should be used with considerable caution. An inhalational induction in younger patients with

TABLE 21-2. Management of Fontan Physiology

Physiology	Causes	Clinical Presentation	Management
Low pulmonary blood flow and inadequate preload delivery to systemic (common) atrium TPG >> 10 mm Hg	Baffle obstruction Pulmonary artery obstruction Pulmonary vein obstruction Premature baffle fenestration closure	No fenestration Sao$_2$ 95%-100% Sa-vo$_2$ > 35%-40% Baffle pressure > 20 mm Hg Common atrial pres < 10 mm Hg Hypotension Tachycardia Poor distal perfusion	Volume replacement to keep baffle pressure stable Reduce PVR Correct acidosis Inotropic support Afterload reduction Consider catheterization Intervention to open or create baffle fenestration
Low pulmonary blood flow and inadequate preload delivery to systemic (common) atrium TPG >> 10 mm Hg	Fenestration patent or baffle leak present	Sao$_2$ 75%-80% Sa-vo$_2$ > 20 mm Hg Common atrial pressure < 10 mm Hg Hypotension Tachycardia Poor distal perfusion Metabolic acidosis	Volume replacement to keep baffle pressure stable Reduce PVR Correct acidosis Inotropic support Afterload reduction consider catheterization Intervention to open or create baffle fenestration
Systemic ventricular dysfunction TPG = 5-10 mm Hg	Systolic dysfunction Diastolic dysfunction AV valve regurgitation or stenosis Loss of AV synchrony Afterload-contractility mismatch	No fenestration or premature fenestration closure Sao$_2$ 85%-90% Sa-vo$_2$ > 35%-40% Baffle pressure > 20 mm Hg Common atrial pressure > 15 mm Hg Pulmonary edema Hypotension Tachycardia Poor distal perfusion Metabolic acidosis	Volume replacement to keep baffle pressure stable Correct acidosis PEEP may be necessary for pulmonary edema Inotropic support Afterload reduction Provide AV synchrony (antiarrhythmics or pacing) Mechanical support (postcardiotomy support or bridge to transplantation) Surgical intervention (takedown to BDG)
Systemic ventricular dysfunction TPG = 5-10 mm Hg	Systolic dysfunction Diastolic dysfunction AV valve regurgitation or stenosis Loss of AV synchrony Afterload-contractility mismatch	Fenestration patent or baffle leak present Sao$_2$ 70%-75% Sa-vo$_2$ > 35%-40% Baffle pressure > 20 mm Hg Common atrial pressure > 15 mm Hg Pulmonary edema Hypotension Tachycardia Poor distal perfusion Metabolic acidosis	Volume replacement to keep baffle pressure stable Correct acidosis PEEP may be necessary for pulmonary edema Inotropic support Afterload reduction Provide AV synchrony (antiarrhythmics/pacing) Mechanical support (postcardiotomy support or bridge to transplantation) Surgical intervention (takedown to BDG)

From DiNardo JA, Zvara DA: *Anesthesia for cardiac surgery*, ed 3, Malden, Mass, 2008, Blackwell.
AV, Atrioventricular; *BDG*, bidirectional Glenn shunt; *PEEP*, positive end-expiratory pressure; *PVR*, pulmonary vascular resistance; *TPG*, transpulmonary gradient.

well-preserved ventricular function and patent Fontan pathways is possible, keeping in mind that airway difficulty (e.g., prolonged obstruction or laryngospasm) is likely to be quite poorly tolerated, as are significant agent-induced negative inotropic effects. For maintenance of anesthesia, a balanced technique with moderate concentrations of inhaled anesthetic agents is usually tolerated. As previously stated, it is common to support patients with preexisting ventricular dysfunction with an inotropic agent (dopamine). Central venous catheters placed in the internal jugular or subclavian vein have a place in managing Fontan patients undergoing procedures associated with major blood loss or fluid shifts, providing information about proximal filling pressures and pulmonary artery pressure (the SVC is of course in direct continuity with the PA). In addition, oxygen delivery (and hence cardiac output) can be inferred from the oxygen saturation of SVC blood. A general guideline (not only in Fontan) is that the likelihood of reduced cardiac output increases (assuming reasonably normal hemoglobin concentration and tissue extraction) as the difference between arterial and SVC O$_2$ saturation exceeds ~25 (e.g., we would infer at least a component of low cardiac output in a fenestrated Fontan patient with an Sao$_2$ of 84% and an SVC saturation of 50%.) Because of the risk for thrombosis and caval obstruction of the Fontan pathway, a femoral venous catheter may be preferable when central venous access is needed only for infusions. Elevated venous pressures and coagulation defects may increase the risk of bleeding. For major surgery, especially in the setting of moderate to severely depressed ventricular function, referral to a specialized center with expertise in the care of patients with CHD is warranted.

Coarctation of the Aorta

The anatomy, pathophysiology, and anesthetic management for repair of aortic coarctation are discussed later (see Anesthesia for Closed Cardiac Procedures). The long-term consequences after coarctation repair are related to blood pressure and left ventricular mass. In long-term follow-up studies, persistent arterial hypertension in the absence of re-coarctation and type of repair is present in as many as one third of patients (de Divitiis et al., 2003; Rosenthal, 2005; Hager et al., 2007). Systolic blood pressure is positively associated with LV mass in this cohort, and elevated systolic blood pressure and LV mass are both important risk factors for late morbidity and mortality from heart failure, sudden death, and coronary and cerebrovascular disease (Toro-Salazar et al., 2002). Although it has been suggested that the risk of developing subsequent hypertension is reduced by repair in the first year of life (Seirafi et al., 1998), some series do not support this contention (de Divitiis et al., 2001). The etiology of this persistent hypertension is multifactorial and includes reduced pulsatility of the post-coarctation descending aorta (Pfammatter et al., 2004), reduced upper body vascular responses to reactive hyperemia and glyceryl trinitrate (possibly abnormal smooth muscle relaxation or structural abnormalities of the arterial wall [Murakami and Takeda, 2005]), aortic arch geometry (Ou et al., 2007, 2008), and abnormalities in baroreceptor reflexes and the renin-angiotensin-aldosterone system (Rosenthal, 2005). There is evidence to suggest that abnormalities in cardiovascular reflexes are already present in neonates with coarctation before repair (Polson et al., 2006).

These patients are at increased risk for premature coronary atherosclerosis, cerebral vascular disease, left ventricular hypertrophy with impaired diastolic function, congestive heart failure, aortic aneurysm and fistula formation, aortic dissections and rupture, and endarteritis at the repair site (Rosenthal, 2005; Hager et al., 2007). Bicuspid aortic valve and advanced age appear to be independent risk factors for aortic complications (Oliver et al., 2004).

Atrial Septal Defects

An atrial septal defect is a communication between the left and right atria, and it may be single or multiple, vary widely in size, be located anywhere in the atrial septum, and be isolated or associated with other congenital heart defects (50%). See related video online at www.expertconsult.com. There are four morphologic types: secundum ASD, primum ASD, sinus venosus ASD, and coronary sinus ASD. Patent foramen ovale is a normal interatrial communication during fetal life and is seen in almost all newborns. A probe-patent foramen ovale, present in up to 25% of adults, is not a true defect in the atrial septum but results from incomplete fusion of the septum primum and the superior limbic band of the fossa ovalis (septum secundum). Paradoxical embolism is a major anesthetic consideration in these patients.

ASDs allow shunts, and the amount of blood that passes through the defect is determined by the size of the defect, the pressure difference between the left and right atria, and the relative compliance of the right and left ventricles. Left-to-right shunting increases as the patient gets older (Campbell, 1970). Early in infancy, the right ventricle is less compliant, so that left-to-right shunting is minimal. With declines in pulmonary artery pressure and remodeling (increased compliance) of the right ventricle, shunting increases as the right atrial pressure becomes lower than left atrial pressure. The normally decreasing left ventricular compliance with age further increases left-to-right shunting. ASDs result in increased pulmonary blood flow and place a volume load on the right atrium, right ventricle, and left atrium.

Isolated ASDs are generally asymptomatic in infancy and childhood, but a few infants develop congestive heart failure as a result of pathophysiology that is incompletely understood. CHF is more common after 40 years of age. The incidence of atrial fibrillation (less commonly atrial flutter) also increases with advancing age (Murphy et al., 1990).

Spontaneous closure of secundum defects is related to defect diameter (<3 mm, 100%; 3 to 8 mm, 87%; 3 to 5 mm, 80%) (Radzik et al., 1993). Indications for closure are a pulmonary to systemic blood flow ratio greater than 2:1, with the second year

of life currently considered the optimal time for surgical closure. Normal ventricular function after repair is the rule, but ventricular dysfunction and atrial arrhythmias can occur with late repair. Pulmonary vascular occlusive disease will develop in approximately 5% to 10% of unrepaired ASDs, most commonly in the second decade or thereafter, and can result in shunt reversal and Eisenmenger's syndrome (Steele et al., 1987). Residua and sequelae are more commonly seen after repair of sinus venosus defects (loss of sinus node function, pulmonary venous obstruction, residual shunt) (Attenhofer Jost et al., 2005) and ostium primum defects (see Atrioventricular Septal Defects, p. 694).

Ventricular Septal Defects

A ventricular septal defect is an opening in the ventricular septum permitting communication between the left and right ventricles, and it is the most common congenital cardiac defect (2.5 per 1000 live births) after bicuspid aortic valve. VSDs are classified by their location in the septum, with multiple classifications existing. The physiologic effects are determined by the degree of shunting, which is influenced by the size of the defect and the relative pulmonary and systemic vascular resistances. Smaller (restrictive) defects limit shunting—there is a large pressure gradient across the defect. Large (nonrestrictive) defects have less pressure difference between the ventricles, so the magnitude and direction of shunting are more dependent on the relative pulmonary and systemic vascular resistances. The high PVR at birth limits left-to-right shunting, but the magnitude of the shunt increases over the first few months of life because of the normal postnatal decline in PVR; there is also a contribution from physiologic anemia of the infant (hematocrit has a disproportionately greater effect on PVR than SVR) (Lister et al., 1982). Excessive left-to-right shunting with increased pulmonary blood flow leads to pulmonary congestion, abnormal pulmonary mechanics (decreased compliance, increased airway resistance, airway compression), increased myocardial work, and pulmonary hypertension (Berlinger et al., 1983; Stayer et al., 2004). Congestive symptoms appear when the $Q_P:Q_S$ exceeds 1.4. Pulmonary hypertension is usually reversible initially but becomes increasingly fixed as PVOD develops; although the timing can be variable, irreversible pulmonary vascular disease is uncommon in infancy.

Most VSDs are small, and many will decrease in size or close spontaneously. Indications for surgical repair in infancy are poor growth, significant CHF, pulmonary artery pressure at or near systemic level, and multiple VSDs (Keane and Fyler, 2006d). Patients with advanced PVOD and pulmonary hypertension (Eisenmenger's complex) are generally not candidates for VSD closure. Device closure of muscular VSDs, particularly difficult-to-reach apical and anterior septal defects, is possible in the catheterization laboratory provided the device will not impinge on the atrioventricular or semilunar valves.

Anesthetic management: For unrepaired VSD, the focus should be on assessing the degree of systemic circulatory compromise and control of pulmonary vascular tone. Signs and symptoms of significant CHF in infants include (1) respiratory: tachypnea, grunting, flaring, retractions; pulmonary congestion on chest x-ray; (2) growth and nutrition: poor feeding, poor growth, failure to thrive; and (3) cardiovascular: tachycardia, diminished pulses, decreased peripheral perfusion, hepatic congestion (hepatomegaly). An inhalational induction should be reserved for patients with smaller defects, no worse than compensated CHF, well-preserved ventricular function, and no PVOD. The major concern is inducing significant decreases in PVR, resulting in decreased systemic flow and hypotension; less commonly, reactive elevations in PVR can result in right-to-left shunting with desaturation. Myocardial and pulmonary function are likely to be normal if complete repair is done within the first year or two of life (Kidd et al., 1993). Potential sequelae include residual defects, heart block, subaortic obstruction, and aortic regurgitation (Kidd et al., 1993; Chiu et al., 2007). Early and mid-term follow up of VSD closure by device found that complete atrioventricular block is a serious concern (Butera et al., 2007).

Atrioventricular Septal Defects

Atrioventricular septal defects (AVSDs), also referred to as canal defects or endocardial cushion defects, result from abnormal endocardial cushion development. See related video online at www.expertconsult.com. AVSDs may be *complete* (common AV valve with ostium primum ASD and moderate to large inlet VSD), *partial* (two distinct AV valves with ostium primum ASD and usually a cleft in the anterior leaflet of the mitral valve), or *transitional* (ostium primum ASD, restrictive VSD, common AV valve orifice with fused anterior and posterior bridging leaflets dividing the common AV valve into distinct mitral and tricuspid components). AVSDs are commonly associated with extracardiac defects and are present in approximately 60% of children with Down syndrome.

The physiology resembles that of atrial and ventricular septal defects, with the possible added feature of AV valve regurgitation. There is a left-to-right shunt with increased pulmonary blood flow and volume overloading of the right and left ventricles, with the magnitude of shunting largely determined by the size of the VSD component. Surgery for complete AV canal defects is usually undertaken in the first 2 to 3 months of life because of the risk for accelerated pulmonary vascular disease. Surgery is usually done later in infancy for partial and transitional AV canals because the pulmonary vasculature is protected and the normal AV valve tissue is thin and fragile (Jonas, 2004). The repair typically involves dividing the common AV valve and closing the ASD and VSD with either one or two patches, approximation and suspension of the valve apparatus, and suturing any cleft in the mitral valve.

Anesthetic management: For unrepaired canal defects, management is like that for left-to-right shunts. An inhalational induction should be reserved for patients with small defects, preserved ventricular function, no worse than compensated CHF, and no PVOD. Potential sequelae include residual septal defects, AV valve regurgitation or stenosis (especially mitral) (or both), AV block, subaortic obstruction, and occasionally pulmonary hypertension; the last is more likely in patients with Down syndrome.

Aortic Stenosis

Bicuspid aortic valve is the most common congenital cardiac defect. It occurs in 1% to 2% of the population and demonstrates a substantial male predominance (Hoffman and Kaplan, 2002). It may be an isolated lesion or associated with other left-sided obstructive defects (e.g., aortic coarctation), and it may be asymptomatic or become progressively obstructive or regur-

gitant. *Critical neonatal aortic stenosis* is frequently a ductal-dependant lesion, with an appearance similar to that of severe aortic coarctation. In its most severe forms, critical neonatal AS is poorly tolerated and produces left ventricular failure with poor systemic perfusion and pulmonary vascular congestion; factors that increase myocardial demand even modestly (e.g., mild fever, anemia) can markedly exacerbate the low cardiac output state and potentially precipitate cardiovascular collapse. In *supravalvar aortic stenosis* (SVAS), there is narrowing at the sinotubular junction, which may be associated with coronary artery stenoses, hypoplasia of the ascending aorta and arch, distal arterial tree, and pulmonary artery stenoses (Stamm et al., 2001a) (Fig. 21-5). *Subaortic stenosis* may comprise a discrete fibromuscular ridge or membrane, a long fibromuscular tunnel, or hypertrophy of the interventricular septum (hypertrophic cardiomyopathy). *Shone's anomaly* consists of aortic coarctation, subaortic stenosis, and mitral stenosis on the basis of both a parachute mitral valve and supravalvar mitral ring (Shone et al., 1963). Although the relief of coarctation is typically straightforward, patients with Shone's anomaly frequently have prolonged and recurrent left-sided obstruction arising from its other components, leading to reduced LV compliance and dysfunction despite one or more attempts at correction. The mitral stenosis (leading to pulmonary hypertension) and reduced ventricular function in particular can make these patients particularly difficult to manage in the perioperative period, because of associated fluid loads and shifts, anemia, fever, and stress response.

Balloon dilation of the aortic valve has replaced surgery as the initial procedure for significant *aortic valve stenosis,* effectively reducing the gradient and promoting growth of the valve annulus (Jonas, 2004). Aortic valvuloplasty or replacement becomes necessary when dilation of the stenosis is no longer effective or aortic regurgitation and consequent LV dilation become significant. *Subaortic stenosis* resulting from a discrete subaortic membrane is repaired by membrane resection. In addition to creating increased pressure within the LV, aortic valve damage and regurgitation caused by a jet arising from flow across the membrane is a common finding and an indication for surgery. Tunnel subaortic stenosis is managed by the modified Konno procedure in which LV septal tissue is excised and a patch placed to enlarge the LV outflow tract.

The pathophysiology and *anesthetic management* of left ventricular outflow obstruction were discussed earlier in this chapter.

Supravalvar aortic stenosis, specifically that associated with Williams (Williams-Beuren) syndrome, merits particular attention. Patients with SVAS are at significantly increased risk for cardiac arrest and death during anesthesia, cardiac catheterization, and surgery (Bird et al., 1996), and the anesthetic management has recently been reviewed (Burch et al., 2008). SVAS is associated with variable-sized deletions in the elastin gene and adjacent segments and can be accompanied by a diffuse and variable arteriopathy (Pober, 2010). Common manifestations of patients with Williams syndrome include SVAS, supravalvar pulmonic stenosis, more distal PA stenoses, and at times renal artery stenosis. The increased risk for sudden death appears to occur by at least two different but potentially interacting pathophysiologic features:

1. Significant ventricular hypertrophy as a consequence of severe outflow obstruction; the presence of severe, bilateral (i.e., supravalvar aortic and pulmonic) obstruction and hypertrophy poses the greatest risk.

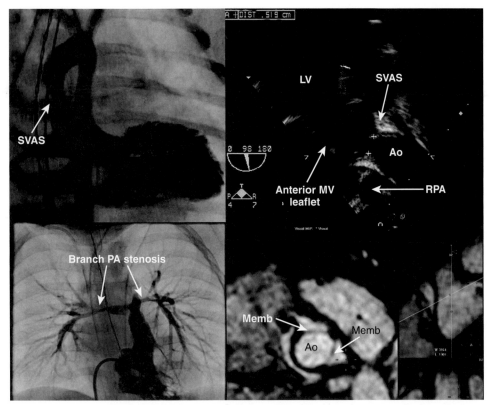

■ **FIGURE 21-5.** Supravalvular aortic stenosis (SVAS). *Top left:* Anteroposterior projection of a left ventricular angiogram demonstrating significant SVAS. *Top right:* Inverted transesophageal echocardiography of mid-esophageal aortic valve, long-axis view demonstrating SVAS. *Bottom left:* Anteroposterior projection of a right ventricular angiogram demonstrating significant proximal branch pulmonary artery stenoses. *Bottom right:* Cardiac MRI short-axis view of the ascending aorta demonstrating an obstructive membrane arising from the sinotubular junction and extending in front of both the right and left coronary ostia. *LV,* Left ventrical; *Ao,* aorta; *RPA,* right pulmonary artery; *MV,* mitral valve; *Memb;* membrane. *(From Burch TM, McGowan FX Jr, Kussman BD, et al: Congenital supravalvular aortic stenosis and sudden death associated with anesthesia: what's the mystery? Anesth Analg 107:1848-1854, 2008.)*

2. Various forms of coronary artery obstruction. It is noteworthy that the degree of coronary involvement may not be accurately imaged by echocardiography or predicted by the degree of supravalvar aortic obstruction.

Anesthetic management: Key features include avoidance of dehydration, hypotension, and other factors that compromise myocardial perfusion. Thus, minimizing the amount of time that the patient receives nothing by mouth, placing an intravenous catheter (aided by premedication as necessary), administering a fluid bolus, and administering intravenous induction with agents that maintain hemodynamic stability are important anesthetic management principles. Although uneventful inhalational inductions have been reported (Bragg et al., 2005; Medley et al., 2005; Astuto et al., 2007), we would advise against this, because significant hypotension can lead to cardiac arrest (especially when coronary artery obstruction is present) prior to establishing intravenous access; in many instances, resuscitation is unsuccessful (Bird et al., 1996). In the catheterization laboratory, both radiographic contrast injection (perhaps via its transient but significant ability to impair coronary oxygen delivery when injected into the aorta or left side of the heart) and cardiac rhythm disturbances (as might be induced by a wire or catheter) are possible events leading to decompensation. Although not based on evidence, it is our practice to have a norepinephrine infusion available for immediate administration should hypotension ensue or be predicted. The lesion itself is usually repaired by resection of the stenotic area and patch placement, although more extensive aortic (or supravalvar pulmonary) reconstruction may be necessary (Stamm et al., 2001a).

Truncus Arteriosus

Truncus arteriosus is a single arterial trunk from which the aorta and the pulmonary and coronary arteries arise, with a VSD present beneath the truncal valve. See related video online at www.expertconsult.com. Like tetralogy of Fallot, it is frequently associated with a 22q11 deletion, and with DiGeorge and velocardiofacial syndromes. It is the quintessential parallel circulation, with the $Q_P:Q_S$ ratio determined by the ratio of pulmonary to systemic vascular resistance (Hansen and Hickey, 1986; Wong et al., 1991). Surgical repair involves patch closure of the VSD and detachment of the pulmonary arteries from the truncus with establishment of right ventricle–to–pulmonary artery continuity with a conduit (valved homograft).

Anesthetic management: Control of pulmonary blood flow and support of ventricular function are central management tenets. Unrepaired truncus arteriosus poses a significant anesthetic challenge, because declines in PVR can be associated with increased left-to-right shunting, leading to systemic (in particular, diastolic) hypotension, coronary ischemia, and ventricular fibrillation. Increased PVR can result in right-to-left shunting with desaturation, systemic (and myocardial) hypoxia, myocardial depression, and cardiovascular collapse. Late sequelae after repair include obstruction of the right ventricle–to–pulmonary artery conduit, conduit regurgitation, truncal (aortic) valve regurgitation, residual VSD, and persistent pulmonary hypertension (for repairs done later in childhood). Anesthetic management for the repaired truncus is similar to that for right ventricular outflow obstruction (the most frequent sequela).

Ebstein's Anomaly

Ebstein's anomaly consists of displacement of the septal and posterior leaflets of the tricuspid valve toward the apex of the right ventricle. See related video online at www.expertconsult. com. The right ventricle between the true annulus and the level of attachment of the septal and posterior leaflets to the ventricular septum is thin and dysplastic ("atrialized") (Fig. 21-6). The anterior tricuspid leaflet at the annulus is larger than normal, whereas the other leaflets may be redundant, contracted, or thickened. The tricuspid valve is usually incompetent, occasionally stenotic. The right ventricular cavity beyond the atrialized portion ranges from small to large, whereas the right atrium is invariably enlarged. There is virtually always a PFO or an ASD, and an accessory AV conduction pathway (e.g., Wolff-Parkinson-White Syndrome) is present in 10% to 25% of cases (Watson, 1974; Smith et al., 1982).

The clinical spectrum of Ebstein's anomaly is extremely variable, ranging from the critically ill neonate with minimal to no anterograde flow out the right ventricle to the pulmonary artery, and with severe tricuspid regurgitation and heart failure, to the child with minimal or no symptoms (Brown et al., 2008). Atrial right-to-left shunting can produce cyanosis. Interventions for significant lesions include tricuspid valve

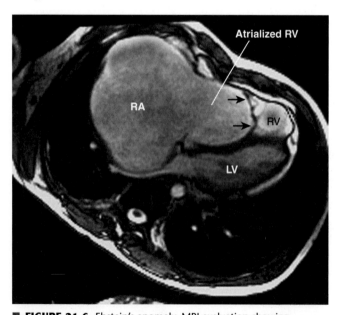

■ **FIGURE 21-6.** Ebstein's anomaly. MRI evaluation showing diastolic frame from electrocardiogram-gated steady-state free precession cine in the four-chamber plane. Note the markedly dilated right atrium (RA), the apically displaced tricuspid valve (arrows), and the hypoplastic functional right ventricle (RV) distal to the displaced tricuspid valve. LV, Left ventricle. (Image courtesy Tal Geva, MD.)

repair (cone procedure) (da Silva et al., 2007) or replacement, closure of interatrial communications, and ablation of accessory pathways.

ANESTHESIA FOR CLOSED CARDIAC PROCEDURES

Patent Ductus Arteriosus

The ductus arteriosus connects the origin of the left main pulmonary artery to the aorta and is a critical component of the fetal circulation. In utero, most of the blood from the RV bypasses the lungs via flow through the ductus to the descending aorta. In most newborns, the ductus closes within 72 hours of birth through contraction of a smooth muscle layer in response to an increase in postnatal systemic oxygen levels (Hermes-DeSantis and Clyman, 2006). The lumen is obliterated by 2 to 3 months of age, but if not fully obliterated, a connection remains between the systemic and pulmonary circulations. The PDA may be isolated (Fig. 21-7) or associated with almost any other congenital cardiac anomaly, in many instances of which it is lifesaving (ductal-dependent lesions). Isolated PDA is associated with increasing left-to-right shunting as the pulmonary vascular resistance falls.

A tiny or small PDA is asymptomatic and associated with normal life expectancy (Campbell, 1968); its closure may be controversial but is generally recommended because of the risk for endocarditis. With a hemodynamically significant ductus, excessive blood flow to the lungs, left atrium, left ventricle, and ascending aorta results in enlargement of these structures, and in large shunts, congestive heart failure. Elevation of left atrial pressure may cause enlargement of the foramen ovale with additional left-to-right shunting. In premature infants with respiratory distress, hypoxia promotes continued patency of the ductus, with the need for more aggressive ventilation. Runoff from the aorta into the pulmonary circulation during diastole reduces aortic diastolic pressure with decreased coronary, cerebral, and abdominal organ perfusion. Necrotizing enterocolitis and intracerebral and intraventricular hemorrhages are potential complications. Other cardiac anomalies determine the direction of shunting across a PDA. For example, with severe aortic coarctation or hypoplastic left heart syndrome, the shunting is predominantly right to left, and in fact necessary to support systemic perfusion until more definitive interventions are undertaken.

Closure of a PDA can be accomplished medically in the preterm infant with indomethacin, surgically, or in the catheterization laboratory. Surgical division is recommended in preterm infants with inadequate response to indomethacin and those with large communications (Ewert, 2005). Surgical management is typically via a small left posterolateral thoracotomy, but the video-assisted thoracoscopic (VAT) technique has become the surgical standard of care for infants and children with a small to moderate-sized ductus (Laborde et al., 1997; Jonas, 2004). Closure using interventional catheterization techniques has increased in frequency and is an attractive option because it can be done on an outpatient basis, it reduces surgical scarring, and it may be associated with less pain, faster recovery, and reduced risk for late thoracotomy complications (cosmetic defects, rib fusion, and scoliosis). It is best suited for a restrictive ductus with some length and an ampulla at the aortic end (Ewert, 2005; Keane and Fyler, 2006b).

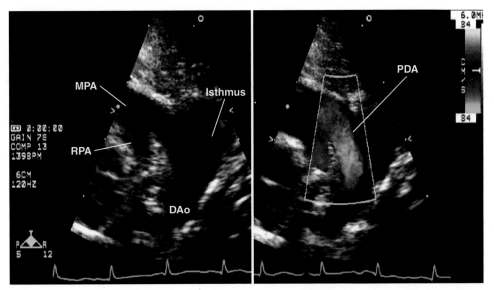

■ **FIGURE 21-7.** Patent ductus arteriosus *(PDA)*, oblique sagittal echocardiographic image. *Left panel:* Two-dimensional image showing the *PDA* connecting the aortic isthmus with the distal main pulmonary artery *(MPA)*. *Right panel:* Color Doppler flow map showing left-to-right flow through the *PDA*. *RPA,* Right pulmonary artery; *DAo,* descending aorta. *(Images courtesy Tal Geva, MD.)*

Anesthetic Management

Anesthetic management for PDA ligation depends on patient age and clinical status. Physiologic goals are similar to other patients with left-to-right shunts.

The majority of patients are sick, premature, ventilator-dependent neonates with respiratory distress syndrome and no better than borderline systemic blood pressure and perfusion. The major consideration is manipulations to balance the PVR and SVR. Maneuvers that decrease PVR, in particular, as well as those that reduce myocardial contractility and SVR, should be avoided. Dopamine is often already in use or may need to be added to maintain a blood pressure that is appropriate (one rule of thumb is mean arterial pressure approximately equal to the patient's gestational age). Although direct monitoring of arterial blood pressure can be helpful in the sicker patients, it can be technically challenging and is not part of our routine practice for neonates who arrive from the neonatal ICU without it. An anesthetic technique using high-dosage fentanyl (30 to 50 mcg/kg) and pancuronium is usually well tolerated (Robinson and Gregory, 1981). In the current era, although advisable to supplement this technique with low-dosage inhaled agent or benzodiazepine, the hemodynamics often do not allow for this. Transport of these neonates to the operating room can be hazardous, with the risks of accidental extubation, inadequate attention to ventilation, line disruption, and excessive cooling. Many centers perform PDA ligation in the neonatal ICU, either as routine practice or in cases where transport seems especially risky, but the unfamiliarity of the environment, available personnel, relative lack of surgical equipment should a complication arise, adequacy of lighting, and sterility need to be considered. Surgical dissection and the lung retraction necessary to expose the duct can result in hypoxemia, hypercarbia, and hypotension. If possible, blood pressure should be monitored in an upper and lower extremity; the right arm is preferable, because the surgeon may have to place a clamp on the aorta if control of the aortic end of the ductus is lost during dissection or ligation. A second pulse oximeter on a lower

extremity can provide reassuring information to the surgeon at the time the duct is clipped or ligated (the PDA can be larger than either the PA or the aorta). After ligation, there is an acute increase in blood pressure with an increase in LV afterload, so that increased inotropic support of the severely dysfunctional ventricle may be necessary. Other complications include accidental extubation, profound hemorrhage resulting from disruption or tearing of the ductus, inadvertent ligation of the left pulmonary artery or descending aorta, and recurrent laryngeal nerve (RLN) damage. One needs to be vigilant for plugging of the endotracheal tube, particularly during the surgery or after lung reexpansion, in very small infants with correspondingly small (≤ 3.0 mm) tubes.

Older infants and children with an isolated PDA undergoing surgical or catheterization procedures may be extubated at the end of the procedure, allowing a variety of anesthetic techniques. The incidence of RLN injury may be reduced by using direct intraoperative stimulation and evoked electromyogram monitoring (Odegard et al., 2000).

After repair of PDA, and in the absence of pulmonary hypertension, cardiovascular function should be normal so that anesthetic management is straightforward.

Coarctation of the Aorta

Coarctation of the aorta is a focal narrowing of the descending thoracic aorta consistent with a discrete posterior shelf or invagination just opposite the insertion of the ductus arteriosus (juxtaductal) and distal to the left subclavian artery (Fig. 21-8). In some instances, this shelf may be circumferential. The precise cause is unknown, but it is thought to be caused by extension of ductal tissue into the wall of the aorta or by abnormal fetal blood flow patterns associated with lesions that reduce antegrade flow into the ascending aorta. Not surprisingly, coarctation is associated with aortic valve stenosis or a bicuspid aortic valve (50%), ventricular septal defect (48%), hypoplasia of other left heart structures (mitral valve and left

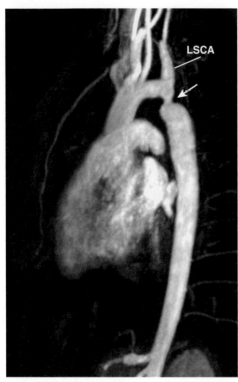

■ **FIGURE 21-8.** Coarctation of the aorta. Gadolinium-enhanced three-dimensional magnetic resonance angiogram showing coarctation of the aorta *(arrow)* distal to the left subclavian artery *(LSCA). (Image courtesy Tal Geva, MD.)*

ventricle), and aortic arch hypoplasia (Quaegebeur et al., 1994; Aboulhosn and Child, 2006).

The pathophysiology is varied and depends on the severity of the coarctation and the associated lesions. The ductus arteriosus plays a critical role as a source of systemic perfusion, so presentation is in infancy for all patients except those capable of tolerating ductal closure without overt hemodynamic compromise. In general, presentation beyond infancy is limited to patients with an isolated coarctation of mild to moderate severity. Critical neonatal coarctation with abrupt ductal closure results in profound circulatory collapse within the first days to a month of life, because perfusion to the lower body is dependent on patency of the ductus arteriosus and relatively high PVR. The presence of poor perfusion, acidosis, oliguria, and other signs and symptoms of acute systemic illness often results in these patients being seen emergently to rule out sepsis. Severe presentations typically involve some degree of acute myocardial dysfunction and can also include evidence of lung, liver, or renal injury. When a large VSD is also present, the aggravated degree of left-to-right shunting and heart failure (with elevated left atrial pressure and additional left-to-right shunting across the foramen ovale) results in presentation within days of birth. The initial treatment involves hemodynamic stabilization by reopening the ductus arteriosus with a PGE$_1$ infusion. Often, other resuscitative measures such as inotropic support, volume expansion, sodium bicarbonate, and, at times, intubation and controlled ventilation are needed. Of note, once the duct is open, it is possible for blood pressures in the upper and lower limbs to be similar despite severe aortic narrowing. Patients who presented with severe decompensation and evidence of

organ injury benefit from one or more days of restored systemic perfusion prior to surgical repair.

If the coarctation is not severe and closure of the ductus has occurred slowly, or if compensatory collaterals develop rapidly, presentation may be later in infancy, with tachypnea and failure to thrive. In such patients, the degree of coarctation commonly becomes more obstructive as the child grows. Blood pressure is elevated in the upper extremities, with an average gradient between upper and lower extremity sites of 30 to 40 mm Hg at rest (Keane and Fyler, 2006a). Collaterals may originate from the internal thoracic, intercostal, subclavian, or scapular arteries, and with extensive collateral development, patients may be asymptomatic with little difference in blood pressure between the arms and legs. Large collaterals can be a source of an auscultatable bruit over the rib cage or elsewhere, as well as rib notching on chest x-ray. Coarctation causes left ventricular hypertension and hypertrophy, as well as systemic hypertension. Symptoms (exercise intolerance, headache, chest pain, lower extremity claudication) are an absolute indication for surgical repair. For the asymptomatic patient, surgical indications include a blood pressure gradient between the upper and lower limbs of greater than 20 mm Hg, upper body blood pressure greater than two standard deviations above normal, or aortic diameter loss of 50% or greater.

The optimal treatment for neonates, infants, and children is currently felt to be complete excision of the area of coarctation and surrounding ductal tissue with end-to-end anastomosis (Dodge-Khatami et al., 2000). With a hypoplastic aortic isthmus, complete excision in conjunction with an extended end-to-end or end-to-side anastomosis is recommended (Backer, 2003). Although balloon angioplasty may be used for primary relief of coarctation (Golden and Hellenbrand, 2007), it is rather regarded as the standard of care for recurrent coarctation after previous surgical repair (Jonas, 2004). Paraplegia secondary to spinal cord ischemia is the most devastating complication associated with surgical repair. The incidence is quite low (0.14% to 0.4%), and several factors are associated with an increased risk of developing paraplegia: hyperthermia, prolonged aortic cross-clamp time, elevated cerebral spinal fluid pressures, low proximal and distal aortic blood pressures, and poorly developed collaterals to the descending aorta. In addition to recoarctation, long-term consequences of coarctation and its repair can include the development of essential hypertension (even in the absence of a residual coarctation gradient) and perhaps increased risk of premature or sudden death.

Anesthetic Management

The newborn with *critical* coarctation requires medical stabilization, as outlined earlier, prior to surgical repair. Anesthetic management includes continuation of PGE$_1$ infusion (0.01 to 0.05 mcg/kg per minute) to maintain ductal patency, inotropic support of left ventricular function, adequate preload, and preservation of increased PVR, as lower body perfusion is dependent on right-to-left flow across the ductus. Blood pressure above and below the coarctation should be monitored, with the arterial catheter preferentially in the right arm. The proximal aortic clamp may occlude or compromise the origin of the left subclavian artery, or the left subclavian artery may be sacrificed for the repair. A femoral arterial line and right arm cuff can be used if right radial artery cannulation is unsuccessful. Neonates and very young infants are not candidates for volatile-based anesthetics. A technique using high-dosage fentanyl in combination with a benzodiazepine or low inspired concentration of an inhalation agent is well tolerated by these patients. Ketamine may worsen hemodynamics in neonates with severe LV dysfunction by increasing SVR and should probably be avoided. In older children with only proximal systemic hypertension, intravenous or inhalational techniques are well tolerated. Regardless of the technique chosen, it should be appreciated that proximal blood pressure response to stimulation will be exaggerated.

The increase in proximal aortic pressure with application of the aortic cross-clamp in neonates and infants can usually be managed expectantly or with a volatile agent while continuing any inotropic support. In older children and adolescents, β-blockers and vasodilators may occasionally be necessary. However, a moderate increase in proximal aortic pressure during the cross-clamp period may be beneficial, as it is likely to encourage some degree of lower body perfusion via any existing collaterals. On the other hand, sodium nitroprusside results in further increases in cerebral spinal fluid pressure and further decreases in distal aortic blood pressure, reducing spinal cord blood perfusion pressure (Marini et al., 1998). In sum, we are unlikely to treat hypertension during the cross-clamp period unless it exceeds baseline arterial blood pressures by about 30% or more, or unless it approaches values that raise concern for cerebral toxicity. Spinal cord protection is accomplished with a short cross-clamp time (preferably <20 minutes) and mild induced hypothermia (34° C). Blood pressure is maintained at or a little higher than the preoperative level in the upper limbs. Removal of the cross-clamp will result in reactive hyperemia in distal tissues with vasodilation and transient hypotension, and release of acid metabolites will increase $Paco_2$. Anticipation by decreasing or discontinuing inhaled anesthetics or vasodilators in use, volume expansion, and appropriate ventilation are usually sufficient to limit these effects. Postoperatively, rebound hypertension may occur and persist for some time. Esmolol and sodium nitroprusside infusions are used in the early postoperative period. Older children without coexisting diseases can be additionally managed with lung isolation and may be candidates for early extubation.

Systemic-to-Pulmonary Artery Shunts

Systemic-to-pulmonary artery shunts (extracardiac shunts) are palliative procedures performed in neonates and infants with severely decreased pulmonary blood flow or ductal-dependent pulmonary blood flow when a corrective procedure is not possible (del Nido et al., 1988). With increased neonatal and infant repair of complex defects, fewer systemic-to-pulmonary artery shunts are being performed. The primary indications are single-ventricle, pulmonary atresia with intact ventricular septum, and some variants of TOF with pulmonary atresia.

The classic *Blalock-Taussig* shunt (end-to-side anastomosis of the transected subclavian artery to the branch pulmonary artery) has been abandoned because of resultant interruption of arm blood flow, and it has been replaced by the *modified Blalock-Taussig* (mBT) shunt in which a synthetic tube graft of polytetrafluoroethylene (PTFE; Gore-Tex) is interposed between the subclavian (or innominate) artery and the branch pulmonary artery (Gazzaniga et al., 1976a, 1976b; de Leval et al., 1981). With a median sternotomy approach, the shunt is placed more medially from the innominate artery. The shunt is usually performed on the side opposite the aortic arch, with a 3.5-mm shunt typically used in infants weighing 2 to 3.5 kg.

A *central* shunt, used when prior shunt procedures have failed, consists of a synthetic tube graft between the ascending aorta and the main or a branch pulmonary artery. The *Potts* shunt (side-to-side anastomosis of the descending aorta and left pulmonary artery) and *Waterston* shunt (side-to-side anastomosis of ascending aorta and right pulmonary artery) have largely been abandoned because of the high incidence of pulmonary artery distortion, the risk of too large a shunt, and the difficulty of closing the shunt at the time of subsequent repair.

Anesthetic Management

Anesthetic management for creation of a systemic-to-pulmonary artery shunt, as well as after shunt placement, necessitates control of the factors influencing the ratio of pulmonary to systemic flow across the shunt, usually in opposite directions from a physiologic standpoint. During *creation* of shunts to increase pulmonary blood flow (e.g., tricuspid atresia, and pulmonic atresia and its variants), pulmonary blood flow in most patients is clearly restricted, and concerns about increasing the degree of cyanosis are paramount. Thus, maneuvers to decrease PVR (high inspired oxygen concentration, induced respiratory alkalosis, avoidance of extremes of lung volume), to maintain or increase systemic cardiac output, and perhaps to increase SVR and blood pressure (volume administration, inotropic support) are most likely to be necessary to maintain oxygenation. In the presence of a widely patent PDA, there is the risk for pulmonary overcirculation prior to ligation of the ductus in some of these patients.

After shunt creation, pulmonary overcirculation is frequent. Such patients can be expected to demonstrate significant hemodynamic instability in the immediate postoperative period as they adapt to the shunt-dependent circulation. This situation is managed initially by lowering inspired O_2 to room air (or as low as tolerated based on SpO_2), allowing the $Paco_2$ to rise to at least moderate levels of hypercarbia, and adding PEEP to increase PVR. A major factor is that these shunts are intended to be large and therefore provide "excessive" amounts of PBF to accommodate patient growth (the duct may also be open for some period of time, and furthermore some surgeons do not ligate the duct initially so as to provide a margin of safety against acute shunt thrombosis). Shunts impose a volume load on the systemic ventricle, and together with any preexisting ventricular dysfunction, inotropic support may be necessary to ensure systemic and shunt perfusion after shunt creation. Thus, anticipation of significant hemodynamic instability and invasive monitoring of arterial pressure are required, and the need for significant inotropic support (dopamine, at times supplemented by epinephrine or norepinephrine) in the early postoperative period can be expected. Persistent and severe cyanosis after the shunt is opened should raise suspicions of inadequate shunt flow; arterial blood pressure in this instance may be either high or low, depending in large part on systemic cardiac output and the effect of hypoxia on myocardial function and SVR. Inadequate shunt flow may be caused by shunt occlusion (thrombus, stenosis, or compression), high PVR, low arterial blood pressure or SVR, low cardiac output (causing both decreased shunt flow and reduced venous saturations), or parenchymal lung disease.

The modified BT shunt can be performed via a thoracotomy or median sternotomy, and with or without CPB. Central shunts are usually performed through a median sternotomy. With a thoracotomy approach, unilateral lung retraction is necessary and the resulting atelectasis may compromise oxygenation and ventilation. The branch pulmonary artery will have to be partially occluded by a clamp to allow creation of the distal anastomosis, increasing physiologic dead space and further compromising oxygenation and CO_2 removal. The arterial-to-end-tidal CO_2 gradient will be further increased. Efforts to increase pulmonary blood flow by reducing PVR with ventilatory interventions and by increasing left-to-right shunting should be initiated before pulmonary artery occlusion. If persistent severe desaturation, bradycardia, or hypotension occurs with cross-clamping of the pulmonary artery, CPB will be required for shunt placement. A narcotic-based technique with muscle relaxant, supplemented with a volatile agent or benzodiazepine (or both) as tolerated, and a period of postoperative ventilation is the rule. Arterial catheter placement should preferably not be on the side of the subclavian artery to be shunted. Central venous access is recommended, but if it is not possible, a right atrial catheter can be placed by the surgeon for monitoring and inotrope administration. Heparin (50 to 100 IU/kg) may be requested by the surgeon to reduce the risk for shunt thrombosis. Complications include bleeding; desaturation during chest closure as a result of alterations in pulmonary mechanics or kinking, distortion, or compression of the shunt or pulmonary arteries; shunt thrombosis and profound hypoxemia; and pulmonary overcirculation with systemic hypotension if the shunt is too large or the PVR too low (see earlier). Postoperative ventilation is usually required to ensure adequate shunt function and attainment of a stable hemodynamic state.

Pulmonary Artery Banding

Pulmonary artery banding (PAB) is used to limit pulmonary blood flow in infants with a large left-to-right shunt not amenable to early corrective surgery, or as part of a staged palliation (Muller and Danimann, 1952). With the increase in early infant repair, PAB is performed less commonly, and it is currently most often indicated for very complex lesions (multiple VSDs, at times referred to as Swiss-cheese septum), in TGA for preparation of the left-ventricle prior to an arterial switch operation (Mee, 1986; Jonas et al., 1989), for double-inlet or double-outlet ventricles in the absence of pulmonary stenosis, or to temporize in neonates who are critically ill with significant noncardiac diseases. As congestive heart failure in the newborn period is atypical because of the high PVR, PAB is sometimes performed in the second or third month of life (del Nido et al., 1988). By reducing the extent of the left-to-right shunt, the band reduces the volume load on the ventricles, improves congestive symptoms, protects the pulmonary vascular bed against the development of pulmonary hypertension and PVOD, and improves respiratory mechanics. PAB may cause distortion of the main pulmonary artery or distortion of the branch pulmonary arteries by migration of the band distally. This distortion may complicate or even preclude subsequent attempts at definitive repair.

Anesthetic Management

The infant is usually in congestive heart failure with reduced systemic perfusion and excessive PBF. General endotracheal anesthesia with full cardiovascular monitoring and postoperative ventilation is usually required. Anesthetic management before band placement is conceptually the same as that for patients with large left-to-right shunts (i.e., focused on maintaining systemic perfusion and limiting further increases in PBF). It is usually opioid based, with inotropic support of the ventricle and systemic cardiac output as needed. The surgical approach may be via a left thoracotomy or sternotomy without CPB. The band is placed circumferentially around the main pulmonary artery. Techniques for determining the degree of band tightening vary by surgeon and are based on formula, the resultant level of arterial oxygen saturation (above 70% to 80%), the level of Pao_2 (>30 to 35 mm Hg), or the pulmonary artery pressure distal to the band (one third to one half of systemic pressure), the pressure proximal to the band (75% or greater of systemic, particularly when the indication is to "train" the LV prior to arterial switch), or some inexact combination thereof. An excessively tight band will severely reduce pulmonary blood flow, cause an intolerable degree of hypoxemia, and expose the ventricle to high afterload. Pulse oximetry has proved useful during pulmonary artery banding because arterial desaturation usually precedes hypotension and bradycardia when band tightness is excessive. Echocardiography can be valuable in assessing ventricular function and determining the pressure gradient across the band. Ventricular distention may require loosening of the band or initiation of inotropic support, or both. Postoperative ventilation is usually required to allow recovery of lung function.

Vascular Rings and Slings

A vascular ring is an aortic arch anomaly in which the trachea and esophagus are surrounded completely by vascular structures (Fig. 21-9, *A*). See related video online at www.expertconsult.com. Rings, which need not be composed entirely of patent vascular structures, are formed by abnormal persistence or regression of components of the aortic arch complex, and they can cause compression of the trachea, bronchi, and esophagus. In a vascular sling, the trachea and esophagus are not completely encircled but can be compressed. Although accounting for less than 1% of all congenital heart defects, vascular rings and slings represent an important source of airway and esophageal obstruction. Intracardiac defects are present in approximately 29% of patients with vascular rings (Humphrey et al., 2006).

The vast majority of patients with a vascular ring have either a double aortic arch with right arch dominance (see Fig. 21-9, *B*), a right aortic arch with mirror-image branching, or a right aortic arch with an aberrant left subclavian artery and left ligamentum arteriosum (Dodge-Khatami et al., 2002; Humphrey et al., 2006). With a double aortic arch with right arch dominance, the anteriorly located left aortic arch gives rise to the left carotid and left subclavian arteries. This left arch is generally atretic or severely hypoplastic beyond the origin of either the left carotid or left subclavian artery. A right aortic arch passes rightward and posterior to the trachea, and a left aortic arch passes leftward and anterior to the trachea. With mirror-image branching, the arch gives off, in order, the common trunk of the left common carotid and left subclavian, the right common carotid, and the right subclavian arteries.

Vascular rings and slings generally appear in childhood, with the most common symptoms being inspiratory stridor, dysphagia, wheezing, dyspnea, cough, and recurrent respiratory tract infections (Humphrey et al., 2006). Feeding problems are common. MRI is the diagnostic technique of choice in many

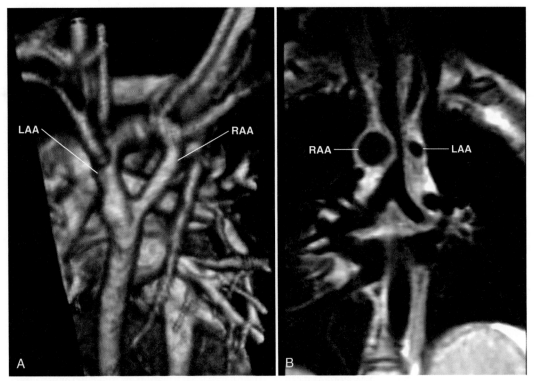

■ **FIGURE 21-9.** Vascular ring. **A,** Three-dimensional volume reconstruction of gadolinium-enhanced magnetic resonance angiogram showing a double aortic arch with nearly equal-sized left and right arches. **B,** Electrocardiogram-gated fast (turbo) spin-echo MRI in the coronal plane showing a double aortic arch with a large right aortic arch *(RAA)* and a small left aortic arch *(LAA)*. Note the severe compression of the trachea by the double aortic arch. *(Images courtesy Tal Geva, MD.)*

centers (van Son et al., 1994); other diagnostic tools include echocardiography (for evaluation of intracardiac defects), bronchoscopy, and barium swallow.

The goal of *repair* for vascular rings or slings is to divide the compressive ring, relieve the airway or esophageal compression, and maintain normal perfusion of the aortic arch. The surgical approach is typically via a left posterolateral thoracotomy, at times open, but more commonly using a video-assisted thoracoscopic technique (Burke and Chang, 1993). Simultaneous repair of vascular tracheobronchial compression syndromes and intracardiac defects carries a higher risk for morbidity and mortality (Sebening et al., 2000).

Anesthetic Management

Anesthetic management depends on the type of vascular ring, the type and severity of underlying CHD, and the planned surgical procedure. It is not clear how frequently, if ever, these lesions behave like anterior mediastinal masses (Kussman et al., 2004). The majority of these patients are best approached by careful induction, assurance of the ability to ventilate with positive pressure, and then muscle relaxation; the application of positive pressure and removal of respiratory effort usually result in improved airflow. With significant airway narrowing, the endotracheal tube tip should lie proximal to the stenotic segment to avoid edema and granulation tissue formation caused by tube impact on the narrowed area. Alternatively, cases of severe collapse may require stenting with an endotracheal tube or rigid bronchoscope to ensure adequate ventilation. For all of these reasons, previous characterization of tracheal narrowing with respect to mechanism (extrinsic compression, tracheomalacia,

complete tracheal rings), location, severity, and extent (length of segment) can critically inform intubation and other aspects of management in these patients. Airway radiography (plain film, MRI, computed tomography) and bronchoscopy (routine in some centers) (Chapotte et al., 1998) can also provide this information. In patients without a prior bronchoscopy, one can be performed after induction at the time of the ring or sling surgery. In older children, the surgical approach may benefit from single-lung ventilation techniques.

Successful tracheal extubation is possible in most patients with isolated vascular rings at the conclusion of the procedure. However, successful repair of the ring may not immediately relieve airway obstruction, so obstruction may recur immediately on extubation or as a remote problem after surgery. Persistent obstruction may result from residual compression, associated structural anomalies, and secondary airway wall instability (tracheomalacia, bronchomalacia) that can be exacerbated by posttraumatic edema and may persist for months after successful surgery. Bronchoscopy performed at the end of the surgical procedure may be helpful to assess residual airway compression and degree of dynamic airway collapse.

The potential for a variable course and relationship of the RLN to the ligamentum arteriosum and descending aorta makes the RLN susceptible to injury during either type of surgical approach to vascular ring. In the largest reported series, there was a 5.3% incidence of unilateral vocal cord paralysis (Geva et al., 2002). Intraoperative RLN monitoring may be useful (Odegard et al., 2000), in which case muscle relaxants should not be used or allowed to wear off prior to testing. When RLN injury occurs, there is a risk for stridor or hoarseness, and the potential for aspiration.

ANESTHESIA FOR CARDIAC CATHETERIZATION

The cardiac catheterization laboratory is one of the most challenging and unpredictable environments in which to provide anesthesia. Major advances in interventional catheterization techniques and imaging (echocardiography, cardiac MRI, cardiac computed tomography) in pediatric cardiology have led to fewer diagnostic or hemodynamic catheterizations and a concomitant increase in interventional or therapeutic procedures. Evolutions in the surgical management of CHD, together with the expanding role of interventional catheterization, has led to a larger and more complex population of children and adults with CHD undergoing one or repeated catheterizations, radiofrequency ablations, and imaging studies. Many congenital cardiovascular anomalies that previously required surgical management may now be corrected with transcatheter techniques, and some lesions that were previously inoperable can be effectively managed at cardiac catheterization (Lock, 2006). Surgical and interventional catheterization approaches complement one another so that the ability to treat patients with more complex CHD is enhanced (Mayer, 2000).

Anesthesia for cardiac catheterization mandates knowledge and understanding of the catheterization environment, indications for catheterization and procedures performed, the associated risks and complications thereof, and lesion- and procedure-specific principles of anesthetic management.

Catheterization Laboratory Environment

Cardiac catheterization laboratories are usually outside the operating suite, but provision of the same standards of care, patient monitoring, and equipment as in an operating room is mandatory (Stensrud, 2005) (see Chapter 10, Equipment). The development of hybrid procedures involving combined catheter and surgical approaches indicates that the modern catheterization laboratory is also an operating room (Bacha, 2008). Nonetheless, the laboratory is usually configured to accommodate the needs of the cardiologist, resulting in a confined space for the anesthesia machine, monitors, and other essential personnel and equipment. Access to the patient is limited by the radiology equipment, movable leaded-glass screens or partitions, and positioning of the patient's arms around the head (Fig. 21-10). These poor ergonomics are exacerbated by darkening of the room to facilitate viewing of images, repeated obstruction to observing the images by the anteroposterior and lateral cameras, and the relatively heavy lead apron and thyroid shield worn to limit radiation exposure. Extreme movement and positioning of the x-ray cameras to obtain greater magnification or different views are a danger to the patient and anesthesiologist, causing physical (positioning and compression) damage to the patient and anesthetic equipment or dislodgement of the anesthesia circuit, endotracheal tube, laryngeal mask airway, and intravenous catheters. The laboratory is kept cool to prevent overheating of the electronic equipment (and cardiologists), and the cold-flush solutions, wet drapes, exposure during positioning and groin preparation, large surface area–to–body mass ratio in neonates and infants, and general anesthesia additionally predispose to hypothermia.

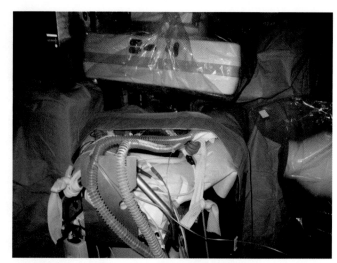

■ **FIGURE 21-10.** Catheterization laboratory environment showing limited access to the patient and obstruction to viewing the fluoroscopic images.

Indications for Cardiac Catheterization and Procedures Performed

Cardiac catheterization is indicated when precise physiologic measurements are required, when anatomic features are poorly visualized by imaging, when electrophysiologic studies are necessary, and when therapeutic catheterization is planned (Lock, 2006). Interventional procedures now account for greater than 50% of cardiac catheterization procedures at many centers (79% at Children's Hospital Boston) (Qureshi et al., 2000) and may be performed as the primary treatment of a defect, as an interim treatment prior to surgical repair, or for the treatment of a residual defect after surgery. Procedures performed in the catheterization laboratories are shown in Box 21-3. The anesthetic considerations for specific procedures are discussed toward the end of this section.

 Box 21-3 Types of Procedures Performed in the Cardiac Catheterization Laboratory

Diagnostic (hemodynamic) catheterization
Interventional catheterization
Endomyocardial biopsy
Valvotomy
Angioplasty with or without stent implantation
Device closure of cardiovascular communications
Creation of an atrial septal defect
Transcatheter implantation of pulmonary valves
Pericardiocentesis
Electrophysiologic
Diagnostic electrophysiologic studies
Catheter ablation of arrhythmias
Pacemaker implantation (including automatic implantable cardioverter defibrillators and testing)
Electrical cardioversion
Other imaging procedures
    Cardiac magnetic resonance imaging
    Echocardiography: transthoracic, transesophageal

Diagnostic or Hemodynamic Catheterization

Diagnostic or hemodynamic catheterization measures intracardiac (right and left atrial, ventricular end-diastolic) and intravascular (arterial, pulmonary artery, ventricular outflow gradient) pressures and oxygen saturation (arterial, mixed venous, pulmonary venous), from which the cardiac index (Fick principle with assumed or measured oxygen consumption), systemic and pulmonary blood flows and their ratio ($Q_P:Q_S$), and pulmonary vascular resistance can be calculated. The $Q_P:Q_S$ ratio is calculated according to the following formula: $Q_P:Q_S = (Sao_2 - S_{PA}o_2)/(S_{PV}o_2 - S_{PA}o_2)$; when an intracardiac shunt or intracardiac mixing is present, $S_{SVC}o_2$ is used rather than $S_{PA}o_2$. The methodology is concisely reviewed elsewhere (Lock, 2006; Bergersen et al., 2009). Arterial blood gas and activated clotting time are measured hourly, with analysis of the blood gas for hematocrit, acid-base status, electrolytes, and glucose. Hemodynamic measurements and calculations are usually performed with the patient breathing air (Fio_2, 0.21) to simulate baseline conditions. Normal hemodynamic data in children vary with age (Table 21-3). Angiography is performed when noninvasive imaging is inconclusive or fine vascular detail is needed. Most catheterizations are carried out percutaneously via the femoral vessels or umbilical vessels (newborns). The subclavian, internal jugular, and hepatic veins (transhepatic approach) may be used in patients with femoral vein occlusion, or as the preferred or necessary site for some procedures or anatomic situations (e.g., in setting of bidirectional cavopulmonary anastomosis).

Interventional Catheterization

Endomyocardial biopsy is used for evaluation of myocarditis or cardiomyopathy and remains the gold standard for detection of cellular rejection after heart transplantation. At least five biopsies of 1 mm or greater in diameter are obtained from the RV septum in all patients. The femoral vein is usually used in patients weighing 15 kg or less, and in bigger patients, the right internal jugular vein is the preferred access site (Lock, 2006).

Balloon valvotomy (valvuloplasty) is used in the management of valvar pulmonary stenosis, aortic stenosis, mitral stenosis, right ventricle–to–pulmonary artery conduits, and recurrent coarctation of the aorta. Indications for dilation are generally in the following ranges: valvar pulmonary stenosis, peak gradient greater than 50 mm Hg; aortic stenosis, peak gradient greater than 50 mm Hg; mitral stenosis, mean gradient greater than 10 mm Hg, taking into account morphology of valve apparatus and symptoms (poor growth, respiratory symptoms, hemoptysis, severe pulmonary hypertension); right ventricle–to–pulmonary artery conduits, when pressure in the right ventricle reaches three fourths of aortic pressure; aortic coarctation, peak gradient greater than 20 mm Hg. The principle involves placement of a guidewire across the valve, passage of a balloon catheter over the wire so that it straddles the valve, and then inflation of the balloon with resultant tearing of the fused leaflets (Kan et al., 1982). *Pulmonary valvotomy* is the treatment of choice for pulmonary valve stenosis, with excellent long-term results (Jarrar et al., 1999; Gudausky and Beekman, 2006). The procedure is performed in neonates with critical obstruction, or electively at 3 to 9 months of age when there is moderate obstruction, and it is generally associated with little hemodynamic instability. Although a sedation technique may be used, general anesthesia is recommended for the neonate with critical pulmonary stenosis or when radiofrequency catheterization is planned to perforate platelike pulmonary atresia (Justo et al., 1997), and in the older child with RV dysfunction and systemic or suprasystemic RV pressure. PGE_1 therapy appears to increase the incidence of apnea during procedural sedation of neonates, and hence elective intubation and general anesthesia is done for this subset of patients.

In contrast, *aortic valve dilation* provides short- to intermediate-term palliation (Pedra et al., 2004) of congenital aortic stenosis and is associated with greater risk than pulmonary valve dilation. It is undertaken in children and adolescents with a peak systolic gradient greater than 50 mm Hg without severe aortic regurgitation, and in infants with critical obstruction regardless of the gradient (Lock, 2006). An aim is to delay the need for surgical repair or valve replacement. Balloon inflation is associated with loss of cardiac output, arrhythmias, and the risk for coronary ischemia. Neonates with critical aortic stenosis are frequently hemodynamically unstable, have a ductal-dependent circulation, often have artificially low gradients because of decreased cardiac output, and are prone to ventricular fibrillation. General endotracheal anesthesia with inotropic support, PGE_1 infusion, and postoperative ventilation is frequently necessary. Sedation may be considered for older children with good ventricular function.

Mitral valvotomy, initially described for treatment of rheumatic mitral stenosis, is also now used for palliation of congenital valvar mitral stenosis (McElhinney et al., 2005). Indications include systemic or higher pulmonary artery pressures, failure to thrive, frequent respiratory infections, or mean mitral gradients greater than 15 mm Hg (Lock, 2006). In addition to resulting in arrhythmias and loss of cardiac output, balloon inflation can result in increased pulmonary venous pressure or acute mitral regurgitation, both of which can lead to significant pulmonary edema. Inotropic support is often necessary. For these reasons, general endotracheal anesthesia is recommended for most patients undergoing balloon mitral valve dilation, with consideration for postprocedure mechanical ventilation until resolution of the pulmonary edema. *Dilation of bioprosthetic valves* in right ventricle–to–pulmonary artery conduits is not usually successful, but it will allow postponement of conduit or valve replacement for 6 to 18 months.

TABLE 21-3. Normal Hemodynamic Data in Children

Right atrial pressure	3–5 mm Hg (mean)
Right ventricle pressure	20–30 or 3–5 mm Hg (systolic or end-diastolic)
Pulmonary artery pressure	12–15 mm Hg (mean)
Pulmonary capillary wedge pressure	8 mm Hg (mean)
Left atrial pressure	5–8 mm Hg (mean)
Left ventricular pressure	65–110 or 3–8 mm Hg (systolic or end-diastolic)
Aortic pressure	65–110 or 35–75 mm Hg (systolic or diastolic)
Pulmonary vascular resistance	<2 Wood units (indexed)
Systemic vascular resistance	15–20 Wood units (indexed)

Balloon angioplasty with or without stent implantation is most commonly employed for pulmonary artery stenoses, right ventricle–to–pulmonary artery conduits, and postoperative coarctation of the aorta, but it may also be used for pulmonary vein stenoses and dilation of atrial baffles. The procedure is similar to that of balloon valvotomy (balloon placement over a guide wire), with the goal being to create a controlled tear in the intima so that the vessel can heal in the newly created diameter (Moore and Lock, 2000). If the vessel (waist) is resistant to a conventional angioplasty balloon, a cutting balloon may be employed. *Stent implantation* in the dilated vessel is indicated with elastic recoil after dilation, for creation of an intimal flap, for occurrence of dissection or hematoma that may impair flow, or to control bleeding from a tear in the vessel wall. It is imperative that patients not move during balloon angioplasty and stent placement, as vessel rupture, stent malposition, or stent displacement (embolism) can occur. *Pulmonary artery balloon angioplasty* is the procedure of choice for hypoplastic noncentral pulmonary arteries after repair of tetralogy of Fallot, and in other arteriopathies (Noonan, Williams, Alagille, idiopathic). A successful relief of obstruction by pulmonary artery dilation frequently results in high-flow, high-pressure pulmonary edema, which may necessitate diuretic administration and in some cases a period of postoperative ventilation. Hemoptysis resulting from vessel tear can be brisk and life threatening, resulting in difficulty in securing the airway during a sedation technique and progressive difficulty ventilating and oxygenating once the airway is controlled; an acute respiratory distress syndrome (ARDS)–like process can occur after significant pulmonary hemorrhage (or at times after dilation-induced pulmonary edema, particularly in older patients). Balloon angioplasty has also been used postoperatively to dilate scar tissue at a sutured anastomosis (e.g., for relief of SVC syndrome), at the site of surgically created shunts, or because of vessel kinking or twisting.

Indications for general anesthesia in patients undergoing pulmonary artery dilation include moderate to severe right ventricular dysfunction, the presence of systemic to suprasystemic RV pressures, a previous history of significant pulmonary edema after reperfusion or bleeding from tears, or anticipation of a lengthy procedure. The presence of a "pop off" in the form of a VSD or an ASD confers some protection against acute RV dysfunction and systemic hypotension during PA dilation procedures. Elective creation of an ASD for this purpose via balloon atrial septostomy is done at times, particularly in the presence of systemic or suprasystemic RV pressures and RV dysfunction. Stent placement in bioprosthetic right ventricular conduits can interfere with pulmonary valve function or compress the coronary arteries.

Aortic balloon angioplasty is more useful for arch obstructions that recur or remain after repair of coarctation of the aorta, interrupted aortic arch, or hypoplastic left heart syndrome (Qureshi et al., 2007). Primary catheter therapy of native coarctation may be considered for the older child or adult, with less procedural success in neonates. *Pulmonary vein dilation* for pulmonary vein stenosis, although producing an acute improvement in the degree of obstruction and resultant pulmonary hypertension, almost invariably results in restenosis of the affected pulmonary vein within days or weeks after the procedure. These are some of the sickest children, and as pulmonary vein dilation can initially result in worsening of the pulmonary edema, general endotracheal anesthesia is recommended, and there is frequently the need for postprocedure ventilation.

Device closure of cardiovascular communications may be used for PDA, PFO, secundum ASD, VSD, Fontan fenestrations, periprosthetic valve leaks, and various other vessels (aortopulmonary collaterals, BT shunts, systemic arteriovenous fistulae, pulmonary arteriovenous fistulae, venous malformations). Devices approved by the U. S. Food and Drug Administration (FDA) include the Amplatzer (duct occluder, septal occluder, vascular plug), CardioSEAL, and various coils. Non-FDA approved at this time are the STARFlex (recent modification of CardioSEAL), BioSTAR (bioabsorbable), and HELEX (Fig. 21-11). Placement of devices for PDA, for PFO, for ASD, for Fontan fenestrations, and in vessels is usually associated with minimal hemodynamic instability and can often be done with a procedural sedation technique (Hickey et al., 1992). General endotracheal anesthesia is necessary when TEE will be used to guide device placement (e.g., device closure of a secundum ASD), and it is used because of the hemodynamic instability associated with closure of VSD (Laussen et al., 1995) and perivalvular leaks (Hourihan et al., 1992; Pate et al., 2006). Device closure of muscular VSDs is indicated for defects difficult to reach surgically, residual defects after surgery, and defects related to myocardial infarction or trauma (Lock et al., 1988; Knauth et al., 2004). Device closure for perimembranous defects has recently been reported (Hijazi et al., 2002; Holzer et al., 2006). Aside from preexisting ventricular dysfunction, device closure of VSDs is frequently associated with hemodynamic instability. The causes are multiple and include intracardiac manipulation of large, stiff catheters leading to arrhythmias, atrioventricular or aortic valve regurgitation from the stenting open of valves, blood loss (the result mainly of frequent catheter exchanges in and out of large sheaths), device malposition or displacement, and air embolus.

Creation of an atrial septal defect by balloon atrial septostomy was the first reported pediatric interventional procedure (Rashkind and Miller 1966), and is the procedure of choice to palliate the newborn with transposition of the great arteries. A catheter is passed across the atrial septum, and the balloon is inflated in the left atrium and then rapidly jerked two to three times across the septum to produce a tear in the septum primum of the fossa ovalis. An association with stroke has been reported (McQuillen et al., 2006). Balloon atrial septostomy is also used to facilitate adequate mixing in patients with HLHS and a restrictive atrial communication prior to stage I palliation. Beyond the neonatal period, the septum is too tough, so a blade is necessary. Creation of an ASD is also performed for severe pulmonary hypertension and for left atrial decompression during ECMO.

Transcatheter implantation of a pulmonary valve in a prosthetic RV outflow tract conduit is a relatively recent innovation (Bonhoeffer et al., 2002). The Melody Transcatheter Pulmonary Valve consists of an 18-mm bovine jugular vein valve mounted in a NuMed platinum iridium stent (Fig. 21-12). The valve is delivered via a 22-Fr balloon-in-balloon-sheathed delivery system, in a manner similar to that used for other RVOT stents. The hand-crimped valve is then delivered at a final diameter of approximately 18, 20, or 22 mm. The procedure is performed under general anesthesia with fluoroscopic imaging.

Pericardiocentesis may be diagnostic or performed to treat cardiac tamponade. It is frequently performed on an urgent or semiurgent basis in hemodynamically compromised postoperative patients, or as the result of misadventures in the catheterization laboratory (Zahn et al., 1992; Bergersen et al., 2009)

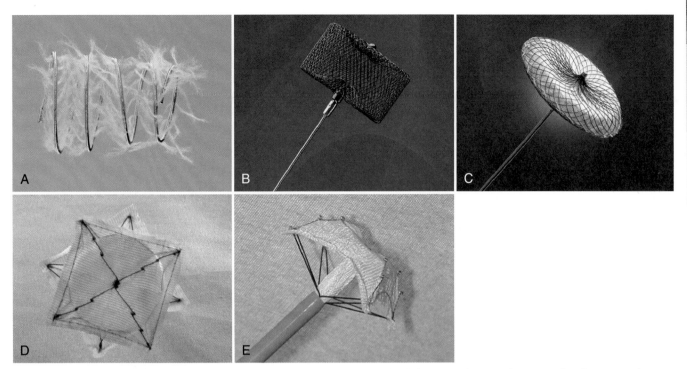

■ **FIGURE 21-11.** Devices for closing cardiovascular communications. **A,** MREye embolization coil. **B,** Amplatzer vascular plug. **C,** Amplatzer septal occluder. **D,** STARFlex septal occlusion system. **E,** STARFlex exiting sheath. (*A Courtesy Cook Medical; B and C Courtesy AGA Medical Corporation; D and E courtesy NMT Medical, Inc.*)

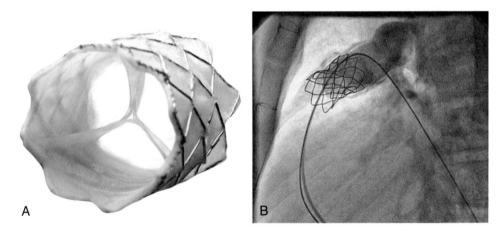

■ **FIGURE 21-12. A,** Melody® Transcatheter Pulmonary Valve. **B,** Melody valve placed in right ventricle-to-pulmonary artery conduit. (*Courtesy Medtronic, Inc.*)

A subxyphoid approach is used with echocardiographic and fluoroscopic guidance. Following standard management principles for this situation (volume loading as necessary, maintaining myocardial function and blood pressure) and titrating midazolam and ketamine with local anesthetic infiltration of the skin and subcutaneous tissues (while maintaining a natural airway with spontaneous ventilation) generally results in very satisfactory anesthesia and good hemodynamic stability (Morray et al., 1993; Jobeir et al., 2003)

Electrophysiologic Procedures

A *diagnostic electrophysiology study* (EPS) measures electrical activation of the heart in time and space (abnormal tissue has different conduction velocity and refractoriness) to determine the mechanism (automaticity versus reentry) and site of the arrhythmia generation or propagation. Standard electrode catheter recording sites for an EPS are high right atrium, across the tricuspid valve (bundle of His), the coronary sinus (left atrium and ventricle), and the right ventricular apex. Adenosine may be administered, often without warning to the anesthesiologist, to block the AV node in order to reveal a unidirectional retrograde accessory pathway or cryptic preexcitation during sinus rhythm, whereas an isoproterenol infusion may be used to induce tachycardia (Walsh et al., 2006a).

Catheter ablation of arrhythmias has dramatically altered the standards for clinical management of tachycardias in all age groups, resulting in a significant reduction in the use of pharmacologic antiarrhythmic drugs. Radiofrequency catheter ablation (RFCA) is the most widely used technique, with cryoablation (tissue freezing with a cryocatheter) selectively used for ablation in the vicinity of the AV node (Kirsh et al.,

2005). The majority of patients are otherwise healthy, present with well-tolerated supraventricular tachycardia (atrial flutter, AV nodal reentrant tachycardia, accessory pathways, atrial fibrillation), and have otherwise structurally normal hearts. Increasingly, patients who are to receive an EPS have had surgical repair of CHD, in which suture lines, damage to the conduction system, and pressure and volume overloading predispose to myocardial dysfunction and arrhythmias.

A sedation technique may be suitable for purely diagnostic procedures, but general anesthesia is used when EPS is combined with ablation. An exception to this is ablation of ectopic atrial tachycardia or ventricular tachycardia (automatic tachycardias) in older children and adults in whom the decrease in catecholamines associated with deep sedation or anesthesia may make mapping of the arrhythmia difficult or unachievable (Lai et al., 1999). Despite concerns by some and experimental evidence of various electrophysiologic alterations, propofol, isoflurane, sevoflurane, midazolam, alfentanil and fentanyl have little *clinically significant* effects on electrophysiologic studies (Lau et al., 1993; Sharpe et al., 1992, 1995, 1999; Lavoie et al., 1995; Erb et al., 2002b; Fujii et al., 2009) or the ability to map and ablate most arrhythmias. Interestingly, dexmedetomidine does significantly depress sinus and AV node function to an extent that might be relevant to EPS procedures (Hammer et al., 2008). Additional anesthetic considerations for ablation include prolonged procedures (3 to 9 hours); a need for absolute immobility during application of the ablative lesion, because permanent complete heart block can result if the focus is near or in the AV node or bundle of His; the occasional need for ventilation to be held at end-inspiration or during expiration to ensure adequate contact of the ablation catheter with the arrhythmic focus; and the potential for hemodynamic compromise caused by rhythm disturbances and possible need for electrical or pharmacologic cardioversion. As frequent episodes of tachycardia, even if hemodynamically stable, can produce cardiac remodeling and ventricular dysfunction, a preprocedure echocardiogram is typically done for this reason, as well as to look for structural abnormalities. Patients with structurally normal hearts usually tolerate the periods of rapid heart rate well.

In comparison with patients with structurally normal hearts, those with repaired CHD pose a much greater challenge. Patients following repair of Tetralogy of Fallot, the Mustard or Senning operation for TGA, and those with Fontan anatomy are among those with congenital heart disease that present frequently for ablation procedures. Preexisting ventricular dysfunction can limit the choice of anesthetic agents, the procedures are technically more difficult and thus much longer, and

invasive arterial monitoring and a urinary catheter are usually indicated. Inotropic support may be needed from very early in the procedure (sometimes with induction), and evidence of low cardiac output such as a developing metabolic acidosis should be sought with blood gas investigations. Low or falling SVC or mixed venous oxygen saturations can also indicate poor status or tolerance of the procedure. As induced arrhythmic episodes may be associated with significant hypotension, the duration may need to be short and terminated by pacing, drug, or cardioversion methods.

The incidence of postoperative nausea and vomiting with catheter ablation is high, even with little opioid use, and can be significantly reduced with a propofol-based anesthetic (Erb et al., 2002a). An antiemetic is routinely administered, but dexamethasone is avoided because of the theoretical concern of its antiinflammatory effects on the ablation lesion.

Pacemakers and Implantable Cardioverter Defibrillators

Although no pacemaker is specifically designed for use in children, pacemakers have become much smaller in size and weight. Pacemaker systems consist of a pulse generator and one, two, or three leads, with the functionality of the pacemaker described by a five-letter code (the NBG code) (Table 21-4) (Bernstein et al., 2002). The first letter (position I) refers to the chamber that is paced, the second letter (position II) refers to the chamber sensed, the third letter refers to the pacemaker response to sensing spontaneous cardiac depolarizations (or spurious interference signals), the fourth letter indicates the presence or absence of an adaptive-rate mechanism (rate modulation), and the fifth letter indicates whether multisite pacing is absent or present, and, if present, in which chambers. If adaptive-rate pacing and multisite pacing are absent, use of only the first three positions is sufficient.

Single-chamber atrial or ventricular pacemakers sense myocardial signals emanating from the corresponding cardiac chamber and deliver a pacing stimulus if no signal is sensed at the programmed lower rate (Kaszala et al., 2008). Dual-chamber pacemakers sense and pace both the atrium and the ventricle. Atrial-based pacing (e.g., AAI, DDD, AOO) is superior to simple ventricular-based pacing (such as VVI, VOO), as AV synchrony is preserved (see Table 21-4). Biventricular pacing activates both the right and left ventricles in a nearly simultaneous fashion to eliminate any delay or asynchrony between the two ventricles, and it is used in the setting of CHF and interventricular conduction delays.

The most common indications for permanent pacemaker implantation in children, adolescents, and patients with CHD are

TABLE 21-4. Revised NASPE/BPEG Generic Code for Antibradycardia, Adaptive-Rate, and Multisite Pacing

Position:	I	II	III	IV	V
Category:	Chamber(s) Paced	Chamber(s) Sensed	Responses to Sensing	Rate Modulation	Multisite Pacing
	O = None	O = None	O = None	O = None	O = None
	A = Atrium	A = Atrium	T = Triggered	R = Rate modulation	A = Atrium
	V = Ventricle	V = Ventricle	I = Inhibited	—	V = Ventricle
	D = Dual (A + V)	D = Dual (A + V)	D = Dual (T + I)	—	D = Dual (A + V)

From Bernstein AD, Daubert JC, Fletcher RD, et al: The revised NASPE/BPEG generic code for antibradycardia, adaptive-rate, and multisite pacing, *PACE* 25:260-264, 2002.
BPEG, British Pacing and Electrophysiology Group; *NASPE*, North American Society of Pacing and Electrophysiology.

symptomatic bradycardia, the bradycardia-tachycardia syndrome, and either congenital or postsurgical advanced second- or third-degree AV block (Epstein et al., 2008). Indications for implantable cardioverter defibrillators (ICD) include aborted sudden death, spontaneous sustained ventricular tachycardia, syncope with a positive ventricular stimulation study, and high-risk patients with hypertrophic cardiomyopathy or congenital long-QT syndrome. The transvenous route is preferred whenever possible, as a thoracotomy is avoided, pacing thresholds are lower, and there is a lower incidence of lead fractures. Disadvantages of transvenous leads are risk for venous occlusion and difficulties with length as the child grows. The primary indications for epicardial placement include small patient size, significant intracardiac shunting in which lead thrombus might impose an embolic risk, or lack of vascular access (Walsh et al., 2006b). Transvenous systems are placed with the patient under general anesthesia, either in the operating room or in the catheterization laboratory. The generator is usually placed in the left or right pectoral area with percutaneous puncture of the subclavian vein to introduce the leads. Miniaturization of ICD systems has led to implantation in smaller children and infants (Berul, 2008). It is standard practice to test the ICD by induction of ventricular fibrillation (defibrillation threshold testing). The patient is preoxygenated, and if the device fails the patient is defibrillated by previously placed external pads. While the device is recharging to administer a higher energy shock, the external defibrillator is charged, so that if the device fails a second time external defibrillation can be immediate (Berul et al., 2008). Clear communication between the anesthesia, cardiology, and nursing teams as to the planned sequence of events is essential.

Electrical cardioversion is usually performed in the catheterization laboratory. Anesthesia usually comprises rehydration with a fluid bolus, midazolam premedication if necessary, and titration of etomidate or propofol (the choice guided largely by underlying ventricular function) until loss of consciousness. The principles followed for anesthesia for noncardiac surgery apply.

Other Imaging Procedures

Cardiovascular Magnetic Resonance Imaging

Cardiovascular magnetic resonance (CMR) imaging is usually performed when echocardiography cannot provide the required diagnostic information, as an alternative to or to complement diagnostic cardiac catheterization, and to obtain diagnostic information for which CMR offers unique advantages (Geva and Powell, 2008). Specifically, CMR can provide high-resolution, three-dimensional images of cardiovascular anatomy and pathology, and can accurately quantify cardiac chamber volumes and mass, regional LV and RV myocardial function, and, with magnetic resonance angiography, determine ejection fraction, stroke volume, regurgitation volume and fraction, and systemic and pulmonary blood flows, as well as regional flow rates (Fogel, 2000; Geva, 2000). MRI-guided interventional cardiology for diagnostic and interventional applications is an emerging field (Lardo, 2000).

Anesthetic considerations for MRI in general are discussed in Chapter 33, Anesthesia and Sedation for Pediatric Procedures Outside the Operating Room; however, anesthesia for CMR has some unique requirements. Patients must remain immobile in the scanner bore for periods of 60 to 90 minutes at a minimum (Dorfman et al., 2007). As respiratory motion can degrade image quality, breath-holding sequences allow faster

data acquisition, shorter scan duration, and perhaps improved image quality. Factors that determine whether an examination can be done without sedation or anesthesia are the child's developmental age and maturity, level of anxiety, and experience with prior procedures; the parent's opinion of the child's ability to cooperate; and the anticipated length and complexity of the examination protocol. General anesthesia is used in neonates, infants, and children less than 6 to 8 years of age, as well as in developmentally delayed older children and adults. It has been shown to be relatively safe despite the complexity of many defects, the frequent breath-holding, and the MRI environment (Odegard et al., 2004). In a subsequent nonrandomized study, the group at highest risk for an adverse event was, not surprisingly the ICU patient undergoing general anesthesia (Dorfman et al., 2007).

Echocardiography

The anesthesiologist is frequently requested to provide sedation or anesthesia for transthoracic or transesophageal echocardiography. See related video online at www.expertconsult.com. A variety of techniques may be used for transthoracic echocardiography, including chloral hydrate (50 to 80 mg/kg), oral midazolam and ketamine, intramuscular ketamine, inhalational anesthesia, or a total intravenous technique, as determined by clinical status. Unlike in adult institutions, general anesthesia with endotracheal intubation is generally used for TEE. The anatomy is frequently more complex, resulting in longer studies, and many older children and adults with CHD strongly prefer general anesthesia to a sedation technique.

Risks and Complications of Cardiac Catheterization

All cardiac catheterizations involve definite risk, with the incidence of adverse events and complications influenced by definition, era, institution, patient, and procedural factors (Agnoletti et al., 2005; Bennett et al., 2005; Bergersen et al., 2008; Mehta et al., 2008). Although not all adverse events are preventable, the primary focus should be on anticipation rather than reaction. The complications frequently associated with cardiac catheterization are listed in Box 21-4. Many complications

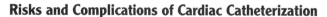

 Box 21-4 Complications Related to Cardiac Catheterization

Blood loss
Arrhythmias
Low cardiac output, hypotension
Vascular injury (tear, perforation, avulsion)
Valvular injury
Cardiac perforation and tamponade
Embolism (air, thrombus, device) and arterial or venous thrombosis
Pulmonary edema
Contrast toxicity
Hypothermia
Central nervous system and peripheral nerve injuries (particularly brachial plexus)
Apnea and airway obstruction (procedural sedation)
Cardiac arrest

are nonspecific, whereas others are exclusive to the procedure being performed. The majority of events are minor and either resolve spontaneously or with minimal intervention. Major life-threatening events can be sudden and include hemodynamic deterioration; cardiac arrest; bleeding; balloon or device damage to vessels, valves, and other cardiac structures; cardiac perforation and tamponade; and embolization of devices or thrombus with remote obstruction or damage. In a prospective series from Children's Hospital Boston, adverse events occurred in 19% of the cases performed, 9% being clinically significant, and 2.7% life threatening or catastrophic, with a mortality rate of 0.4% (Bergersen et al., 2008). Risk for any adverse event was associated with age less than 1 year, interventional procedures, procedure type, and the presence of hemodynamic vulnerability (suprasystemic pulmonary artery or right ventricular pressure, mean PAP greater than 30 mm Hg, systemic ventricle end-diastolic pressure greater than 20 mm Hg, cardiac index less than 2 L/min per m², systemic arterial saturation less than 75%, mixed venous saturation less than 50%, or case performed on ECMO). The low mortality rate attests in part to a dedicated anesthesia team working closely with the interventional cardiologists, nursing staff, and catheterization technicians to promptly manage critical events.

Blood loss with resultant hypovolemia and anemia is mostly the result of frequent sampling and ongoing leakage out the sheaths from around the catheters or with catheter exchanges. The amount of blood loss can be concealed by the drapes and darkened environment; although hematocrit is followed regularly as part of routine blood gas level tests, it will not (as is also the case in other operative blood loss settings) reflect the degree of blood loss given the relatively rapid rate at which blood can be lost, the correspondingly brief period for renal compensation, and limited fluid administration. Remote vascular injury, or less commonly injury at the cannulation site, can produce sudden and severe hemorrhage manifesting as blood in the airway or lung parenchyma, hemothorax, cardiac tamponade, or retroperitoneal hemorrhage (Pigula et al., 2000). A second intravenous catheter is placed if significant blood loss is anticipated or inotropic support is likely.

Arrhythmias secondary to catheter manipulation in the heart are extremely common and generally not clinically significant (West et al., 2006). Atrial or ventricular premature beats and sinus bradycardia are typically transient, terminating on their own or with repositioning of the catheter. Progression of ventricular extrasystoles to sustained ventricular tachycardia or fibrillation is more likely in critically ill infants, severe aortic stenosis, severe cardiomyopathy, or during extensive catheter manipulations in a ventricle. Radiolucent electrical defibrillator pads can be placed on every patient with the defibrillator turned on and the energy to be delivered set according to the patient's weight at the beginning of the procedure. Supraventricular tachycardia often terminates spontaneously or with catheter-induced atrial or ventricular extrasystoles, but may require adenosine or electrical cardioversion. Atrioventricular conduction disturbance is associated with direct trauma to the AV node or bundle of His, or balloon valvuloplasty, and is more frequent in patients with L-looped ventricles. The catheter is removed from the area and conduction allowed to recover; atropine may be administered for mild to moderate bradycardia in the presence of preserved cardiac output, and otherwise more aggressive therapy such as cardiopulmonary resuscitation (CPR) and epinephrine is indicated. Complete AV block may not be self-limited, and, as urgent placement of a transvenous pacing

catheter may be necessary, pacing catheters and a temporary pacemaker are standard equipment in each catheterization laboratory. Particularly in patients with poor functional status or depressed myocardial function, early and definitive interventions including CPR and associated therapies (e.g., inotrope infusion, epinephrine, cardioversion) are warranted.

Low cardiac output and/or *hypotension* may result from one or more of the following: (1) preexisting ventricular dysfunction; (2) hypovolemia related to prolonged preoperative fasting, diuretics, and blood loss; (3) anesthetic agents; (4) arrhythmias; (5) stenting open of valves by catheters and stiff guidewires causing temporary valvular regurgitation; (6) obstruction to flow across valves, conduits, or arteries by catheters, guidewires, and balloon inflation; (7) excessive left-to-right shunting resulting from hyperventilation or oxygen administration; (8) cardiac tamponade; (9) coronary emboli; (10) myocardial ischemia; and (11) hypothermia. Rehydration to achieve adequate preload, early administration of an inotropic agent, and attention to the interventions being performed are necessary. Low SVC saturations (see earlier) and metabolic acidosis on arterial blood gases are indications of low cardiac output, particularly in the presence of a normal blood pressure, and preservation of an appropriate intravascular volume, hematocrit, and inotropic support when indicated is important.

Vascular injury can occur at the cannulation site (small vessels, large sheaths, multiple catheter exchanges, previous vessel injury, improper technique) or centrally. Vessel injury, caused by perforation or balloon dilation, is more common with interventional procedures as the guidewires are larger, stiffer, and sharper, and they have relatively hard tips, and because of the intervention being performed. Successful balloon dilation of a stenotic area requires overstretching of the abnormal tissue causing an intimal tear with maintenance of vascular integrity by the adventitia (Moore and Lock, 2000). Damage to the *pulmonary arteries* is more common than to the systemic arteries, as the walls are thinner and there are more lesions that require therapeutic intervention. The initial indication thereof in unintubated patients is often cough and hemoptysis, which can be severe. A small perforation or tear in a pulmonary artery may appear as only a slight extravasation of contrast into the lung parenchyma, and this can often be managed expectantly. Major tears, particularly in the setting of high pulmonary artery pressures and abnormal vessel walls, can result in intrapulmonary hemorrhage, hemoptysis, hemothorax, or hemopericardium, and can lead to shock and cardiac arrest (Baker et al., 2000). Techniques available to the cardiologist to limit the hemorrhage include balloon inflation to occlude the leak and tamponade the bleeding, placement of a covered stent, and vessel occlusion with coils (distal pulmonary arteries); pleurocentesis and catheter drainage may be necessary. Anesthetic management comprises tracheal intubation and airway control (if a sedation technique was being used), administration of increased inspired oxygen concentrations and positive end-expiratory pressure, airway suctioning, avoidance of the patient coughing or bucking against the endotracheal tube, acute resuscitation often including blood, and a discussion with the cardiologist of the following: (1) heparin reversal, (2) need for urgent ECMO, and (3) need to go to the operating room. *Aortic tears* may result in catastrophic hemorrhage and the need for urgent surgical intervention, or they may be associated with extravasation of contrast and aneurysm formation without hemodynamic compromise. In the latter situation, the patient should be kept immobile and hypertension controlled with infusions of esmolol and sodium nitroprusside.

Valvular injury may occur with leaflet perforation or balloon dilation. Severe acute mitral and aortic regurgitation are not likely to be well tolerated in these patients, and urgent surgery may be indicated.

Cardiac perforation may be caused by or occur during catheter or wire manipulation; planned needle, radiofrequency, or blade transseptal puncture; balloon atrial septostomy; endomyocardial biopsy; mitral and aortic valvuloplasty; and during arrhythmia ablation procedures, especially when access to the left side of the heart is obtained via transseptal puncture. Although not all cardiac perforations lead to cardiac tamponade (Bergersen et al., 2008; Mehta et al., 2008), tamponade is an important cause of mortality (Bennett et al., 2005). Clues to the possibility of a new pericardial effusion are hypotension and an enlarged, less mobile cardiac silhouette on fluoroscopy. A transthoracic echocardiogram should be obtained immediately, and pericardiocentesis performed if necessary. With ongoing bleeding and hemodynamic lability, the cardiac surgeons should be notified early, as urgent surgical repair may become necessary. Anesthetic goals are volume administration, inotropic and vasopressor support, and consideration of the need for additional blood, platelets, and clotting factors, as coagulopathy can develop with reinfusion of pericardial blood and massive transfusion.

Embolism of air or thrombi is a constant threat and, if significant, can result in stroke, myocardial ischemia, cardiac arrest, and death. Predisposing factors are poor technique, large sheath size, indwelling sheaths, suction applied to the side port of the sheath (particularly with guidewire or catheter passing through the back-bleed valve), frequent catheter exchanges, contrast injection, marked negative intrathoracic pressure, balloon rupture, preexisting thrombi, and deployment of devices. The best treatment for air embolism is prevention. Precautions that reduce the risk of air embolism are meticulous technique, including frequent aspiration and flushing of catheters, inflation of catheter balloons with carbon dioxide, the use of a manometer to avoid burst pressures, and avoidance during sedation techniques of the marked negative intrathoracic pressures associated with airway obstruction. With air emboli, the cardiologist will usually ask that the inspired oxygen be increased. A large bolus of air may become trapped and seen as a radiolucent area in the least dependent parts of the heart (right atrial appendage, right ventricular outflow tract). Aspiration of visible air and support of the circulation with volume administration, cardiac massage, and vasoactive agents are likely to be necessary for hemodynamically significant air embolism.

Venous and arterial thrombi can preexist in vessels or cardiac chambers or develop spontaneously around catheters, sheaths, wires, or devices placed in the circulation. The risk for thrombus formation is reduced by systemic heparinization (50 to 100 IU/kg to maintain an activated clotting time of >200 sec) after placement of a sheath or catheter (Grady et al., 1995). Embolized or "displaced" stents, devices, or coils may be retrievable by the cardiologist, reducing the need for surgical intervention (Sheth et al., 2007; Mariano et al., 2008).

Pulmonary edema, apart from excess fluid administration in the susceptible patient, is commonly associated with balloon dilation of multiple peripheral pulmonary arteries. The increase in blood flow and pulmonary capillary hydrostatic pressure after successful angioplasty results in a change in Starling forces and unilateral pulmonary edema (Arnold et al., 1988). Risk factors

are an increase in vessel diameter greater than 70% at the site of the stenosis, a greater than 170% increase in distal pulmonary artery pressure, and mean distal PAP greater than 20 mm Hg immediately after dilation. Edema may be seen on fluoroscopy and accompanied by coughing and respiratory distress in the sedated or inadequately anesthetized patient, as well as hypoxemia, hemoptysis, or florid pulmonary edema that can flood the airway. Management includes securing the airway, controlled ventilation with positive end-expiratory pressure, increased inspired oxygen concentration, and diuretic therapy. Severe cases will require a period of mechanical ventilation until resolution of the edema. Dilation of stenotic pulmonary veins results in pulmonary edema because of increased pulmonary venous pressures, and it is managed similarly.

Contrast agents are water-soluble derivatives of triiodinated benzoic acid, with absorption of radiation attributable to the iodine component. Agents are classified on the basis of their osmolality and ionic strength, with four classes available for clinical use: high-osmolality ionic, low-osmolality ionic, low-osmolality nonionic, and isoosmolality nonionic (Esplugas et al., 2002). Adverse reactions may be idiosyncratic (anaphylactoid) or related to dose and physicochemical characteristics of the agent used (Thomsen and Morcos, 2000). Life-threatening hypersensitivity reactions have an incidence of 0.04% (nonionic agents) to 0.22% (ionic agents) (Katayama et al., 1990) and are more frequent in patients with an allergic history or a prior severe adverse reaction to contrast (Halpern et al., 1996). Cardiovascular effects are more prominent with the high-osmolality agents and include arteriolar vasodilation, ventricular dysfunction, intravascular volume expansion, pulmonary artery vasospasm, depression of atrioventricular nodal conduction, depression of sinoatrial automaticity, and decreased threshold for ventricular fibrillation or tachycardia (Esplugas et al., 2002). Nonionic low-osmolality agents (ioversol, iohexol, iopamidol) cause less patient discomfort (less warmth because of less arteriolar dilation), are probably safer overall, and are now used routinely for pediatric cardiac catheterization (Bergersen et al., 2009). Contrast-induced nephropathy may lead to increased morbidity and mortality in at-risk populations (preexisting renal dysfunction, dehydration, high-contrast dosing, concurrent nephrotoxic drugs) (Goldfarb et al., 2009). To date, preventive strategies have not been studied in children. Adult studies have found that intravenous volume expansion with a sodium bicarbonate–containing solution is superior than sodium chloride solution alone in reducing nephropathy associated with iopamidol (Merten et al., 2004; Masuda et al., 2007), and sodium bicarbonate plus *N*-acetylcysteine is superior to normal saline plus *N*-acetylcysteine with iodixanol (nonionic isoosmolar) (Briguori et al., 2007).

Hypothermia is a risk in all patients, especially small infants and debilitated patients. It can result in altered hemodynamics because of low cardiac output and vasoconstriction, pulmonary overcirculation in those at risk, prolonged recovery from general anesthesia or sedation, and increased oxygen consumption during rewarming. Fever during or after cardiac catheterization with no identifiable cause (malignant hyperthermia, bacteremia, overheating) is not uncommon and appears to be directly related to the number of angiocardiograms performed (Gilladoga et al., 1972) and perhaps also to a foreign body–type reaction to implanted coils or stents. The temperature elevation is usually to the range of 38.1° to 38.7° C and returns to normal by 24 hours after catheterization.

Central nervous system injury can result from embolization, low cardiac output states, extreme hypoxia, and reactions to contrast agents. Brachial plexus injury is the most common *peripheral nerve injury* and results from extreme extension or abduction of the arms above the head for long durations to improve visualization with extreme angles of the cameras. As much as possible, the arms should be internally rotated and minimally extended at the shoulder. Low cardiac output states and hypotension may increase the risk, which may be particularly exacerbated by underlying anatomic abnormalities (e.g., cervical rib). If such positioning is required by the cardiologist, it should be for the shortest time possible and noted on the anesthesia record. Although these injuries are usually transient, recovery can take months, and occasionally permanent paralysis results. Neurologic consultation should be obtained, and exercises under the supervision of a physical therapist should be used to reduce muscle atrophy during the disability. The brachial plexus may also be injured if the arm of a heavily sedated or paralyzed patient suddenly and violently falls off the side of the catheterization table.

The incidence of catheterization-related complications requiring emergency cardiac surgery is estimated to be 1.9%, so that presence of an in-house pediatric cardiothoracic surgeon is recommended policy (Schroeder et al., 2002). ECMO has been used successfully for resuscitation in the catheterization laboratory if the patient is unresponsive to conventional CPR (Allan et al., 2006). Occasionally, high-risk patients have been specifically placed on ECMO prior to the catheterization (Booth et al., 2002; Carmichael et al., 2002) or a primed circuit is placed in the laboratory if the planned intervention appears to have a high likelihood of cardiac arrest necessitating resuscitation with extracorporeal support. It is important to remember to use the acquired catheterization data to help guide resuscitation, and that the femoral (or other) sheaths can be used as a source of central venous access.

Anesthetic Technique

The shift from diagnostic catheterization to mostly interventional catheterization has required an increasing level of expertise in the provision of anesthesia care. Institutional practices vary from an anesthesiologist providing care for all procedures, to mixed models in which some patients are managed by anesthesiologists while others are managed by nurses trained in pediatric sedation in the cardiac catheterization laboratory, under supervision of the cardiologist (Andropoulos and Stayer, 2003; Guidelines, 2002; Practice guidelines, 1996, 2002). Whichever the model, it is very important that the anesthesiologist providing care or overseeing sedation have a high level of expertise in the management of children and adults with complex CHD, be immediately available to render assistance to the nonanesthesiologist, and be assigned regularly to the catheterization laboratory to better appreciate the procedures and potential complications.

The choice of technique or agents should be based on the child's functional status, the underlying heart disease, the type of procedure (with consideration of the risk for hemodynamic instability and complications), and the familiarity of the anesthesiologist with a specific technique. Although general endotracheal anesthesia with paralysis and controlled ventilation (GETA) is the rule in many institutions, the majority of hemodynamic and some interventional procedures can be performed with a spontaneously breathing patient, either with a laryngeal mask airway, a face mask with or without an oral airway, or a natural airway with intravenous anesthesia or sedation. Proximity to the radiation and the length of most procedures limit general anesthesia by face mask to short procedures (e.g., myocardial biopsy) in patients with preserved ventricular function. The major advantages of GETA are a secure airway, more precise control of oxygenation and ventilation (and thus the influence of Pao_2 and $Paco_2$ on pulmonary vascular resistance and shunting), reduced risk of patient movement, the propensity for prolonged procedures, the ability if necessary to suction edema fluid or blood from the trachea and large bronchi, and the degree of comfort for most anesthesiologists. A major disadvantage is the potential for wide fluctuations in hemodynamic parameters resulting from the effects of mechanical ventilation on right ventricular preload and afterload, the negative inotropic and vasodilatory effects of volatile agents, and decreased sympathetic tone. On the other hand, one can construct a convincing argument that a given patient is more likely to be closer to his or her baseline hemodynamic conditions under conditions of a well-conducted general anesthetic (which might include low-dosage inhaled agent and potent opioid, muscle relaxation, and controlled ventilation to normal blood gas values and lung volumes), than with procedural sedation requiring large amounts of opioids and benzodiazepines, with the possibility of the upper airway obstruction, hypoventilation, hypercarbia, and alveolar or arterial hypoxia that might result. GETA is generally indicated for procedures with a known risk for significant hemodynamic instability or complications (placement of VSD devices, balloon dilation of mitral stenosis, dilation of multiple peripheral pulmonary artery stenoses, dilation of severe pulmonary vein stenoses, transcatheter placement of a pulmonary valve), patients with limited cardiovascular reserve in whom the perturbations associated with catheterization place them at risk for severe cardiac compromise or arrest, patients who are unable to lie supine (severe CHF, limited diaphragm excursion secondary to hepatomegaly or ascites), planned intraprocedure transesophageal echocardiography, and the usual contraindications to sedation (difficult airway, obstructive sleep apnea, gastroesophageal reflux, previous adverse reaction to sedation). Some of the sickest patients undergoing diagnostic or minimally interventional procedures will best be served by generous reassurance and comfort maneuvers, appropriate use of local anesthetic infiltration, and low-dosage intravenous anesthesia or sedation with a natural airway.

The painful components of the catheterization procedure are vascular access, sheath changes at the access site, and balloon dilation of arteries and veins; pulmonary artery dilation can also induce coughing. Interspersed are periods of relatively little noxious stimulation. Although infiltration of the access site by the cardiologist with 1% lidocaine at the beginning of the procedure is routine, the child will experience pain when the analgesia has worn off and sheaths are exchanged. Reinfiltration may be necessary, particularly with sedation techniques, and good postprocedure analgesia can be obtained with reinfiltration prior to catheter removal at the conclusion of the procedure. It is important that pressure be applied to the access site during emergence from general anesthesia in order to reduce the risk of bleeding with coughing or straining.

Interventions associated with pain or noxious stimulation can be anticipated with good communication between the cardiologist and anesthesiologist.

Premedication

Premedication is similar to that used for patients with CHD undergoing noncardiac surgery.

Sedation Techniques

The transition from minimal (anxiolysis) to moderate (conscious) to deep (unconscious) sedation to general anesthesia is often difficult to control (Practice guidelines, 2002). Identifying potential patients at risk for sedation-related adverse events prior to the procedure is important. Conscious sedation in younger children is an oxymoron (Cote, 2001); the main considerations are airway maintenance, avoidance of significant respiratory depression, and a calm child. Maintenance of sedation during the procedure can be accomplished with a number of agents. Intermittent bolus doses of a benzodiazepine (usually midazolam) and opioid (fentanyl or morphine) are commonly used, particularly for diagnostic catheterization. Continuous intravenous infusions provide a more consistent and predictable level of sedation, and are especially useful for longer procedures and procedures for which interventions are planned. In patients with limited hemodynamic reserve, a combination of ketamine and midazolam can be very effective in maintaining a deep level of sedation with stable hemodynamic status and limited airway compromise or respiratory depression. A propofol infusion (50 to 100 mcg/kg per minute) provides a faster, better quality recovery, but it is more likely to be associated with hypotension and loss of the airway. A number of studies have examined the use of ketamine alone (Singh et al., 2000) or in combination with propofol (Kogan et al., 2003; Akin et al., 2005; Tosun et al., 2006; Gayatri et al., 2007), midazolam (Jobeir et al., 2003), or dexmedetomidine (Tosun et al., 2006). Combinations of ketamine and propofol tend to produce similar sedation with more stable hemodynamics than propofol alone (Akin et al., 2005). A dexmedetomidine-ketamine combination provided insufficient sedation when compared with a propofol-ketamine combination (Tosun et al., 2006). Remifentanil infusion has been used for sedation, but in many children supplementation with a hypnotic or amnestic agent is necessary (Donmez et al., 2001). Regardless of technique, hypoventilation, hypercarbia, and acidosis resulting from both peripheral (i.e., airway obstruction) and central respiratory effects can occur and, if of sufficient magnitude, mandate transition to some form of assisted or controlled ventilation. Supplemental oxygen is administered during establishment of sedation, and if possible is discontinued once access is achieved so that hemodynamic measurements can be done as close to baseline conditions as possible. Oxygen can be reinstituted if desired after the hemodynamic measurement phase.

General Anesthesia

An intravenous induction is recommended for patients with limited cardiac reserve, particularly those at risk for a marked decrease in cardiac output with induction. Such high-risk cases include patients with severe ventricular dysfunction, severe outflow tract obstruction, and severe pulmonary hypertension. Etomidate lacks clinically significant hemodynamic effects in children and adults (Gooding et al., 1979; Sarkar et al., 2005), whereas ketamine provides hemodynamic stability through sympathetically mediated increases in heart rate and systemic vascular resistance, albeit with direct myocardial depressant effects (Morray et al., 1984). Although reports of the effect of ketamine on pulmonary vascular resistance are conflicting (Morray et al., 1984; Hickey et al., 1985; Berman et al., 1990; Maruyama et al., 1995), it can be used provided elevations in arterial CO_2 are prevented. Opioid-benzodiazepine techniques are also suitable, particularly if postcatheterization mechanical ventilation is planned (Hickey and Hansen, 1984). Remifentanil provides profound analgesia with short recovery times, but it can be associated with bradycardia and hypotension in high dosages (Ross et al., 2001) and in association with sevoflurane at 0.6 minimum alveolar concentration (Foubert et al., 2002); the bradycardia can be prevented with pretreatment with glycopyrrolate, 0.006 mg/kg (Reyntjens et al., 2005). Propofol should probably be limited to children with adequate cardiovascular reserve who can tolerate mild decreases in contractility, heart rate, and systemic vascular resistance (Williams et al., 1999). Sevoflurane is associated with less myocardial depression and better hemodynamic stability than halothane, particularly in infants (Holzman et al., 1996; Wodey et al., 1997; Rivenes et al., 2001; Russell et al., 2001; Laird et al., 2002).

Monitoring and Vascular Access

Standard monitoring is used for all cases. Blood pressure cuffs should not be placed on the leg if the corresponding groin is to be used for cannulation; occasionally, noninvasive blood pressure measurements on the upper extremity become unreliable because of positioning. End-tidal CO_2 monitoring is possible in nonintubated patients with use of specifically designed nasal cannulas (or a butterfly cannula—the blunt end, after the needle is cut off, is inserted into a nostril or placed in front of the mouth, and the Luer-Loc end is attached to end-tidal CO_2 tubing) and correlates reasonably well with blood CO_2 values (Friesen and Alswang, 1996; Cote et al., 2007). In addition to respiratory rate and pattern, declines in end-tidal CO_2 could indicate decreases in pulmonary blood flow resulting from pulmonary artery obstruction or low cardiac output. Fluoroscopy allows assessment of endotracheal tube position, lung inflation, pneumothorax, hemothorax, extravasation of contrast, and pulmonary edema or hemorrhage. Arterial catheters are generally placed by the cardiologist in the femoral artery for their use. Because access to and measurements from these will be interrupted frequently during the procedure, consideration should be given to placement of a radial (or similar) arterial catheter in selected patients at risk for severe instability. Urinary catheters should be considered for prolonged procedures, particularly if significant volume administration, large dye loads, or administration of diuretics is anticipated.

A second peripheral intravenous cannula is recommended for most interventional procedures, particularly when administration of large fluid volumes or inotropic or vasoactive agents is anticipated. Groin access by the cardiologist could potentially influence the flow from venous catheters in the lower limbs. Although central administration of inotropic agents is recommended, it is possible to administer these agents peripherally for short durations, provided the peripheral venous site is reliable and accessible for repeated assessment. It can be useful to discuss with the cardiologist the possible need to use the side port of the venous sheath for drug or volume administration, particularly for rapid resuscitation. It is seldom necessary for the anesthesiologist to place a central venous catheter.

Postprocedure Care

Beside routine care after anesthesia, patients need to be monitored for events such as bleeding from the access sites, vascular occlusion with impaired limb perfusion, pulmonary edema after pulmonary artery dilations, and device displacement or embolization. As is apparent from the preceding discussions, some procedures should not be undertaken for some patients without the availability of a bed in the intensive care unit.

CURRENT AND FUTURE DIRECTIONS

Hybrid Transcatheter and Surgical Palliation

The hybrid strategy for neonates with hypoplastic left heart syndrome is a combined surgical and catheterization procedure (Gibbs et al., 1993). The procedure involves bilateral pulmonary artery banding, stenting of the ductus arteriosus, and atrial septectomy or septostomy when the atrial septum is restrictive (Fig. 21-13). The goals of the procedure are to provide unobstructed systemic cardiac output, unobstructed coronary blood flow, and control of pulmonary blood flow. Aortic arch reconstruction combined with bidirectional cavopulmonary connection is performed later in infancy—in one series, patients were a median age of 4.8 months (Akinturk et al., 2007). The proposed benefit of this approach rests on the assumption that avoiding major neonatal cardiac surgery (Norwood stage I operation)

and deferring aortic arch reconstruction will result in improved survival and superior neurologic and cardiac functional outcomes (Caldarone et al., 2007). Although this strategy is still evolving, indications include the need for an alternative to the Norwood operation, stabilization of patients before heart transplantation, and salvage of patients for hemodynamic instability not manageable with standard supportive measures. Other factors that may increase the favorability of neonatal hybrid approaches include ongoing evidence of cerebral injury related to cardiac surgery (Soul et al., 2009), particularly when associated with brain immaturity (Andropoulos et al., 2010), and the potential neurotoxicity of anesthetic agents on the developing brain (Patel and Sun, 2009).

The hybrid procedure may be performed in the catheterization laboratory (retrofitted or built as a hybrid suite), in the operating room (portable digital angiographic system), or with the PAB in the operating room and the ductal stenting in the catheterization laboratory (Galantowicz and Cheatham, 2005; Caldarone et al., 2007). In the largest series, management has evolved to the PAB's being performed prior to ductal stenting. Patient presentation can vary from the unintubated neonate breathing spontaneously on room air to the critically ill infant on mechanical ventilation, inotropic support, and with invasive monitoring catheters in situ. The anesthetic management of neonates undergoing the hybrid procedure has recently been reviewed (Naguib et al., 2010).

MRI-Guided Cardiac Catheterization

Cardiac catheterization guided by MRI has been shown to provide better anatomic visualization, reduced radiation exposure, and improved accuracy of some hemodynamic information (Razavi et al., 2003). The use of an interventional MR scanner and fluoroscopy system in a single suite still results in reduced radiation exposure. The technical and clinical considerations and current limitations have recently been reviewed (Ratnayaka et al., 2008), and increased use of these techniques can probably be eagerly anticipated in the not-too-distant future, especially as current investigations into development of MR-compatible catheters and other devices mature.

SUMMARY

Patients with congenital heart disease frequently require anesthesia for both diagnostic and therapeutic interventions. As survival rates for patients with congenital heart disease improve, these patients frequently have cardiovascular and neurologic sequelae from the reparative surgical process. Consequently, over time, myocardial structure and function undergo a remodeling process. As a result, anesthetic management and concerns change over time. Understanding the patient's underlying pathophysiology and the history of both repaired and unrepaired lesions allows the anesthesiologist to appropriately manage the perioperative needs of the patient.

For questions and answers on topics in this chapter, go to "Chapter Questions" at www.expertconsult.com.

REFERENCES

Complete references used in this text can be found online at www.expertconsult.com.

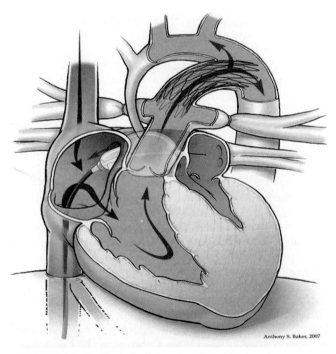

Anthony S. Baker, 2007

■ **FIGURE 21-13.** The hybrid stage I palliation. Note pulmonary artery bands on the left and right pulmonary arteries, stent in the patent ductus arteriosus, and balloon atrial septostomy. *(From Naguib AN, Winch P, Schwartz L, et al: Anesthetic management of the hybrid stage 1 procedure for hypoplastic left heart syndrome (HLHS),* Paediatr Anaesth *20(1):38–46, 2010.)*

Anesthesia for Neurosurgery

Monica S. Vavilala and Sulpicio G. Soriano

CONTENTS

T he perioperative management of pediatric neurosurgical patients presents many challenges to neurosurgeons and anesthesiologists. Many conditions are unique to small children, and an understanding of age-dependent variables and the interaction of anesthetic and surgical procedures is essential to minimize perioperative morbidity and mortality. This chapter will highlight the age-dependent physiologic and pathophysiologic changes relevant to the neurologic lesion, and their effects on the management of the pediatric neurosurgical patient.

DEVELOPMENTAL CONSIDERATIONS

Differences in cerebrovascular physiology and cranial bone maturation distinguish infants and children from adults. The central nervous system (CNS) undergoes a tremendous amount of structural and physiologic changes during the first 2 years of life, which influence the approach to the pediatric neurosurgical patient.

Intracranial Pressure

Normal intracranial pressure (ICP) is relatively low in premature infants and slightly higher in full-term infants (2 to 6 mm Hg) and children and adults (0 to 15 mm Hg). Intracranial compliance is defined as change in intracranial pressure relative to the intracranial volume (Fig. 22-1). At normal intracranial volumes (*point 1* in Fig. 22-1), ICP is low but compliance is high and remains so despite small increases in volume. As intracranial volume acutely rises, the ability to compensate is rapidly overwhelmed. This occurs even when the ICP is still within normal limits, but the compliance is low (*point 2* in Fig. 22-1). When ICP is already high, a threshold is reached, after which further volume expansion leads to rapid ICP elevation (*point 3* in Fig. 22-1). *Point 4* (see Fig. 22-1) reflects maximal intracranial volume and high ICP. Clinically, intracranial compliance can be assessed by a variety of devices that measure intracranial pressure (Wiegand and Richards, 2007).

The neonatal cranial vault is unique in that it is in a state of flux. Open fontanelles and cranial sutures lead to a compliant

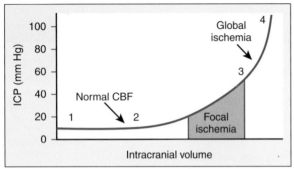

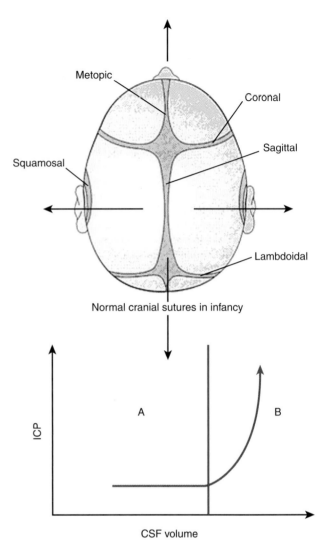

■ **FIGURE 22-1.** Intracranial compliance curve. At normal intracranial volumes *(point 1)*, intracranial pressure (ICP) is low but compliance is high and remains so despite small increases in volume. As intracranial volume acutely rises, the ability to compensate is rapidly overwhelmed. This only occurs when the ICP is still within normal limits but compliance is low *(point 2)*. When ICP is already high, a threshold is reached where further volume expansion leads to rapid ICP elevation *(point 3)*. *Point 4* reflects maximal intracranial volume and high ICP.

intracranial space (Fig. 22-2). The mass effect of a slow-growing tumor or insidious hemorrhage is often masked by a compensatory increase in intracranial volume accompanied by head growth. When ICP increases occur slowly, open fontanelles and cranial sutures separate and enlarge the intracranial space, and thus the mass effect of a slow-growing tumor or insidious intracranial bleeding is often shrouded by a compensatory increase in intracranial volume (widening of the fontanelles and cranial sutures). However, acute increases in cranial volume caused by massive hemorrhage or obstructed cerebrospinal fluid (CSF) flow cannot be attenuated by expansion of the cranial vault and frequently result in life-threatening intracranial hypertension in infants (Shapiro et al., 1980). Once the fontanelles and sutures have closed, children have a smaller cranial volume and lower intracranial compliance than adults. The posterior fontanelle is usually closed by 2 months of age. The anterior fontanelle closes after the posterior fontanelle. By 3 months of age, the anterior fontanelle is closed in 1% of infants. By 1 year it is closed in about 40%, and by 2 years it is closed in 96%. Contributory factors include a higher ratio of brain water content, less CSF volume, and a higher ratio of brain content to intracranial capacity (Arieff et al., 1992). Thus, children are at higher risk of herniation than adults.

Cerebrospinal Fluid Dynamics

Cerebrospinal fluid is produced by the choroid plexus and absorbed through arachnoid villi and the ependymal lining of the ventricles. The ventricular system consists of paired lateral ventricles, which connect to the third ventricle via the foramen of Monro; the third ventricle connects to the fourth ventricle through the aqueduct of Silvius. The fourth ventricle communicates via the paired foramina of Luschka and the foramen of Magendie to a system of cisterns. The rate of reabsorption of CSF increases as ICP increases. Intracranial hemorrhage, inflammation or infection, tumors, or congenital malformations can lead to decreased CSF absorption with possible elevations in ICP. In the adult, the normal volume of CSF is approximately 150 mL, of which 25% is in the ventricular system. CSF is formed at approximately 20 mL/hr.

Normal cranial sutures in infancy

■ **FIGURE 22-2.** Effect of cranial sutures and fontanelle in neonates and infants. Initially the compliant skull of the neonate minimizes insidious increases in intracranial volume. However, acute increases in intracranial volume (hemorrhage and obstructed ventriculoperitoneal shunt) lead to rapid rises in intracranial pressure.

Cerebral Blood Flow

The cerebral circulation is tightly regulated by a number of homeostatic mechanisms. The major influences of the cerebral circulation are metabolism, partial pressure of arterial carbon dioxide ($Paco_2$), partial pressure of oxygen in arterial blood (Pao_2) blood viscosity, and cerebral autoregulation. Coupling of flow and metabolism is the most significant regulator of the cerebral circulation and is preserved even during sleep (Madsen and Vorstrup, 1991; Lenzi et al., 2000) and during general anesthesia (Lam et al., 1995). Under normal conditions, cerebral blood flow (CBF) is tightly coupled to cerebral metabolism and cerebral metabolic rate of oxygen consumption ($CMRo_2$) at global as well as regional levels. However, during periods of CNS activation, CBF increases more than $CMRo_2$, resulting in a decrease in the cerebral oxygen extraction fraction (Fox and Raichle, 1986)

During development, CBF changes with age, mirroring changes in neural development. CBF increases during early childhood, peaking during early-to-mid childhood and plateauing at

7 to 8 years (Wintermark et al., 2004). The healthy brain receives about 15% of cardiac output, and normal adult CBF is approximately 50 mL/100 g per minute (Vavilala et al., 2002a). There are few data available from healthy children. Kennedy and Sokoloff (1957) found CBF to be much higher, in the order of 100 mL/100 g per minute, in conscious healthy children, and a study using arterial spin labeling found similar values in young children (Biagi et al., 2007), which then decreased and approached adult values during the teenage years. Even during low-dosage sevoflurane anesthesia, values for CBF in children are higher than those for adults, whose CBF ranges between 50 and 100 mL/100 g per minute (Settergren et al., 1980).

Transcranial Doppler (TCD) ultrasonography can be used to estimate CBF, assuming that changes in CBF are proportional to changes in cerebral blood flow velocity (CBFV), and that

mean flow velocities are used to represent mean CBF. Systolic and diastolic flow velocity parameters are often used to examine resistance of the cerebral vessels and also brain death. Studies using TCD show that in healthy newborns, CBFV is approximately 24 cm/sec, thereafter increasing with age until 6 to 9 years (97 cm/sec) (Bode and Wais, 1988) (Fig. 22-3). Beyond 10 years of age, CBFV decreases, approximating adult values of about 50 cm/sec (Aaslid et al., 1984; Vavilala et al., 2002a). Sex differences have also been observed and may result from differences in hematocrit, hormones, vessel size, or cerebral metabolism (Kennedy and Sokoloff, 1957; Tontisirin et al., 2007). The mean CBFV estimates for middle cerebral artery (V_{MCA}; anterior circulation) and basilar artery (V_{BAS}; posterior circulation) by age and sex are listed in Figure 22-3 and Table 22-1 (Bode and Wais, 1988; Wintermark et al., 2004; Vavilala et al., 2005).

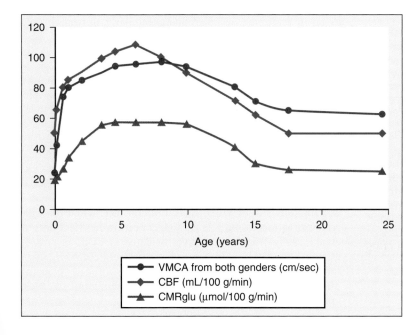

■ **FIGURE 22-3.** Age-related changes in mean flow velocity of middle cerebral artery *(VMCA)* in both sexes. cerebral blood flow *(CBF)* and cerebral metabolic rate of glucose *(CMRglu)* [14,22,27,39,40]. Adult values: VMCA, 50 cm/sec [15,16], CBF, 50 mL/100 g per minute [13], CMRglu, 19 to 33 μmol/100 g per minute [27].

TABLE 22-1. Age and Gender Differences in Mean Flow Velocity of Middle Cerebral (V_{MCA}, Anterior Circulation) and Basilar Arteries (V_{BAS}, Posterior Circulation)

Age	V_{MCA} (cm/sec)			V_{BAS} (cm/sec)		
---	Boys*	Girls*	Both†	Boys*	Girls*	Both†
0–10 days	—	—	24 ± 7	—	—	—
11–90 days	—	—	42 ± 10	—	—	—
3–11.9 mo	—	—	74 ± 14	—	—	—
1–2.9 yr	—	—	85 ± 10	—	—	51 ± 6
3–5.9 yr	92 ± 13‡	99 ± 11‡	94 ± 10	61 ± 9‡	70 ± 10‡	58 ± 6
6–9.9 yr	—	—	97 ± 9	—	—	58 ± 9
10–16.9 yr	75 ± 16‡	89 ± 16‡	81 ± 11	51 ± 12‡	59 ± 11‡	46 ± 8

Table adapted from Philip S, Chaiwat O, Udomphorn Y, et al: Variation in cerebral blood flow velocity with cerebral perfusion pressure >40 mm Hg in 42 children with severe traumatic brain injury, *Crit Care Med* 37:2973, 2009.
*From Vavilala MS, Muangman S, Waitayawinyu P, et al: Neurointensive care: impaired cerebral autoregulation in infants and young children early after inflicted traumatic brain injury—a preliminary report, *J Neurotrauma* 24:87, 2007; and from Tontisirin N, Muangman SL, Suz P, et al: Early childhood gender differences in anterior and posterior cerebral blood flow velocity and autoregulation, *Pediatrics* 119:610, 2007.
†Bode H, Wais U: Age dependence of flow velocities in basal cerebral arteries, *Arch Dis Child* 63:606, 1988.
‡*P* < .05.

Cerebral Metabolic Rate

Global cerebral metabolic rate (CMR) for oxygen and glucose is higher in children than in adults (oxygen, 5.8 versus 3.5 mL/100 g brain tissue per minute, and glucose, 6.8 versus 5.5 mL/100 g brain tissue per minute, respectively) (Kennedy and Sokoloff, 1957). Like $CMRo_2$, cerebral metabolic rate for glucose (CMRglu) is lower at birth (13 to 25 µmol/100 g per minute), increases during childhood, peaks by 3 to 4 years (49 to 65 µmol/100 g per minute), and remains high until 9 years of age. CMRglu decreases thereafter, approaching adult rates (19 to 33 µmol/100 g per minute) (Chugani et al., 1987); changes in $CMRo_2$ and CRMglu mirror age-related changes in CBF (see Fig. 22-3).

Adenosine and nitric oxide (NO) are two purported mediators of flow–metabolism coupling and CBF increase with neuronal activation. Although the effect of adenosine on human CBF is controversial (Stange et al., 1997; Sollevi et al., 1987), up-regulation of NO production has been reported to increase CBF (Endres et al., 2004). Antagonists of both adenosine and NO attenuate the rise in CBF associated with neuronal activation, although neither mediator antagonist, alone or in combination, completely abolishes the CBF increase in response to neuronal activation (Gotoh et al., 2001). Therefore, other mediators, such as H^+ ions, adenine nucleotides, potassium, prostaglandins, and vasoactive intestinal peptide, may also be involved in flow–metabolism coupling.

Hypothermia causes a reduction in $CMRo_2$, thereby decreasing CBF via flow–metabolism coupling. CBF decreases approximately 5% to 7% per degree Celsius, and reduction of the brain temperature to 15° C will reduce $CMRo_2$ to 10% of normothermic values (Vavilala et al., 2002). Hypothermia causes a reduction in both the basal metabolism required for maintenance of cellular integrity and the functional metabolism of the CNS.

Carbon Dioxide Vasoreactivity

Cerebral circulation is exquisitely sensitive to changes in $Paco_2$ (Harper and Glass, 1965; Padayachee et al., 1986). Like that of CBF and metabolism, the vasoreactivity of CO_2 may be higher in healthy children than in adults (13.8% and 10.3% change in mean CBFV per 1 mm Hg change in end-tidal CO_2) during propofol anesthesia (Leon and Bissonnette, 1991; Rowney et al., 2002; Karsli et al., 2003) The cerebrovascular response to changing CO_2 is attenuated at low blood pressure (Harper and Glass, 1965), increases in the presence of moderate hypoxia, decreases again during severe hypoxia (Quint et al., 1980), and may remain abnormally low after a hypoxic episode. Although there is an overall paucity of information regarding CO_2 reactivity in healthy children and in pediatric disease states, older studies suggest that reactivity to CO_2 is well developed even in healthy preterm infants (Pryds et al., 1990) and that CO_2 reactivity in newborns correlates with the lowest pH and may reflect the severity of perinatal asphyxia (Baenziger et al., 1999).

There are many potential control mechanisms involved in reactivity to carbon dioxide (CO_2R). Although neural regulation of CO_2R may be important (Meyer et al., 1971; Bates et al., 1977; Rovere et al., 1977), the most prominent proposed mechanism is the biochemical/metabolic control of cerebral vasoreactivity.

The brisk response of the cerebral vasculature to CO_2 *(the biochemical mechanism)* is caused by the rapid diffusion of arterial CO_2 across the blood-brain barrier (BBB) into the perivascular fluid and cerebral vascular smooth muscle. Changes in extracellular fluid pH by both CO_2 and bicarbonate ions lead to cerebral vasodilation and increased CBF (Kontos et al., 1977). Although CO_2 is a potent cerebral vasodilator, the role of arterial H^+ ions is more controversial. Although pH is not known to generally affect the cerebral vasculature, because arterial H^+ ions do not readily diffuse across the intact BBB (Harper and Bell, 1963), severe metabolic acidosis may cause vasodilation and increase CBF (Westerlind et al., 1994). Therefore, severe metabolic acidosis and alkalosis may affect cerebral vascular tone, as do respiratory acidosis and alkalosis.

During chronic hypercapnia maintained for 6 hours, an adaptive increase in the pH of the CSF occurs with a decrease in CBF (Warner et al., 1987). A decrease in pH is accompanied by an increase in CSF bicarbonate. Similarly, during chronic hypocapnia, CSF bicarbonate concentration decreases, CSF pH gradually decreases, and CBF increases (Muizelaar et al., 1988).

The mechanism of CO_2R also appears to be regulated by local mediators rather than by chemoreceptors in the periphery. NO is partially responsible for CO_2-mediated cerebral vasodilation. Schmetterer and coworkers (1997) demonstrated a significant reduction in mean V_{MCA} to hypercapnia in healthy humans after administration of an NO synthase (NOS) inhibitor. However, NOS inhibitors do not completely ablate CO_2R, and NO may be more important in regional than in global regulation of vasoreactivity. The cerebral cortex in primates was the only site in which NOS inhibitor attenuated the CBF response to increasing arterial CO_2 concentration (McPherson et al., 1995). Another putative mediator of CO_2R is prostaglandin (PG) E_2. In contrast, indomethacin (a cyclooxygenase inhibitor) was shown to inhibit prostanoid synthesis and completely abolished CO_2-induced cerebral vasodilation (Wagerle and Degiulio, 1994).

Hypoxic and Hyperoxic Control of CBF

Compared with $Paco_2$, the influence of Pao_2 on the cerebral circulation is of much less clinical significance. There are minimal changes in CBF with changes in Pao_2 to greater than 50 mm Hg. Below that threshold of 50 mm Hg, CBF increases to maintain adequate cerebral oxygen delivery. Unlike CO_2R, the equilibration of CBF is longer and takes approximately 6 minutes after the establishment of hypoxemia (Ellingsen et al., 1987).

Hypoxemia may induce cerebral vasodilation via anaerobic glycolysis and lactic acid production, causing decreased extracellular pH and subsequent vasodilation. However, pH changes during hypoxemia are only partially responsible for the increased CBF (Koehler and Traystman, 1982). Adenosine has been shown to be necessary for the vasodilatory response to hypoxemia (Morii et al., 1987; Brian et al., 1996; DiGeronimo et al., 1998). NO has also been implicated as a mediator, because NOS inhibitors attenuate the increase in CBF that occurs during hypoxemia (Hudetz et al., 1998). Opioids such as methionine enkephalin and leucine enkephalin have been observed to contribute to hypoxic pial artery dilation in the piglet. Vasopressin-induced CSF methionine enkephalin and leucine enkephalin release are attenuated in the presence of cyclic adenosine monophosphate (cAMP) and cyclic guanosine mono-phosphate (cGMP) antagonists. These data show that both cAMP and cGMP contribute to vasopressin-induced pial artery dilation and the release of the opioids methionine enkephalin and leucine enkephalin (Rossberg and Armstead, 1997).

Although hypoxemia produces cerebrovasodilation, the influence of increases in Pao_2 (hyperoxia) at normal atmospheric pressure is less well characterized and somewhat controversial (Armstead, 1998). Previous reports have documented both decrease in CBF (Kennedy et al., 1972) and no change in CBF (Busija et al., 1980) during hyperoxia. Animal studies demonstrate that hyperoxia elicits pial artery vasoconstriction during normocapnia, and that vasoconstrictor peptide endothelin-1 (ET-1) contributes to that vascular response (Armstead, 1999).

Effects of Viscosity on CBF

Viscosity of blood is primarily a function of hematocrit (Hct), and decrease in viscosity is usually secondary to hemodilution. During anemia, CBF increases as a result of improved rheology of the blood flow in the cerebral vessels and as a compensatory response to decreased oxygen delivery (Tomiyama et al., 1999). Although some data suggest that an Hct of less than 30% is associated with worse Glasgow Outcome Scale scores at discharge for adults with severe traumatic brain injury (TBI) (Carlson et al., 2006), neither the optimal duration for maintaining a specific hemoglobin (Hgb) level nor the relationship between target transfusion and neurologic outcome is fully known (Timmons, 2006). A recent study of critically ill children demonstrated that maintaining a Hgb of 7 g/dL rather than 9.5 g/dL can reduce requirements for blood transfusion, but none of these subjects had TBI (Lacroix et al., 2007).

Cerebral Autoregulation

Cerebral autoregulation is a homeostatic process: arterioles dilate and constrict to maintain CBF nearly constant over a range of blood pressures. In healthy adults, changes in mean arterial pressure (MAP) between 60 and 160 mm Hg result in little or no change in CBF (Fig. 22-4) (Lassen, 1959; Paulson et al., 1990). This adaptive mechanism maintains constant (adequate) CBF by vasodilation or decreasing cerebrovascular resistance. Beyond these limits of autoregulation, hypotension may result in cerebral ischemia, and hypertension may cause cerebral hyperemia.

Healthy infants appear to autoregulate CBF as well as older children during low-dosage sevoflurane anesthesia, but the long-held assumption that the lower limit of autoregulation (LLA) is lower in young than in older children may not be valid (same LLA range for younger and older children, 46 to 76 mm Hg) (Vavilala et al., 2003). There are no data on the LLA in healthy neonates. Because blood pressure increases with age, young children may be at increased risk of cerebral ischemia as a result of lower blood pressure reserve (mean arterial pressure to LLA); however, neonates are especially vulnerable to cerebral ischemia and intraventricular hemorrhage because of this narrow autoregulatory range (Pryds et al., 2005) (Fig. 22-5). Sick premature neonates have CBF pressure-passivity, resulting in a linear correlation between CBF and systemic blood pressure (Boylan et al., 2000). Therefore, tight blood pressure control

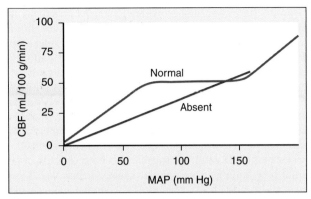

■ **FIGURE 22-4.** Normal and absent autoregulation curves. The "absent" curve indicates a pressure-passive condition in which cerebral blood flow (CBF) varies in proportion to cerebral perfusion pressure. The curve is drawn to indicate subnormal CBF values during normotension, as have been shown to occur immediately after head injury and subarachnoid hemorrhage. The potential for modest hypotension to cause ischemia is apparent. MAP, mean arterial pressure. *(From Miller RD, Eriksson LI, Fleisher LA, et al., editors: Miller's anesthesia, ed 7, Philadelphia, 2010, Churchill Livingstone.)*

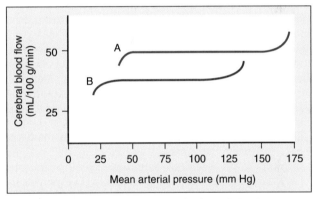

■ **FIGURE 22-5.** Autoregulation of cerebral circulation in neonates *(curve B)* and adults *(curve A)*. *(Redrawn from Harris MM: Pediatric neuroanesthesia. In Berry FA, editor: Anesthetic management of difficult and routine pediatric patients, ed 2, New York, 1990, Churchill Livingstone, p 341. After data of Hernández MJ, Brennan RW, Vannucci RC, et al: Cerebral blood flow and oxygen consumption in the newborn dog, Am J Physiol 234:R209, 1978.)*

is essential in the management of neonates to minimize both cerebral ischemia during hypotension and intraventricular hemorrhage with increased blood pressure. Techniques such as deliberate hypotension in very young children or infants may not be desirable. Age-related increased latency may also occur in cerebral autoregulatory response in young children (Vavilala et al., 2002a), but no data exist in neonates. Animal data suggest that although CBF pressure autoregulation and reactivity to CO_2 operate in the newborn rat, hypercapnia abolishes cerebral autoregulation (Pryds et al., 2005), that abolished autoregulation is associated with cerebral damage in asphyxiated infants, and that the combination of isoelectric electroencephalograms (EEGs) and cerebral hyperperfusion is an early indicator of very severe brain damage (Pryds et al., 1990).

Despite these clinical observations, the mechanisms of normal cerebral autoregulation in healthy children and adaptations in acute disease are not completely understood, and as occurs with changes in CBF, both anatomic and physiologic maturation might play a role in the development of a fully developed autoregulatory response. The mechanisms of cerebral autoregulation may involve a combination of myogenic, neurogenic, and metabolic processes. The metabolic mechanism stipulates that autoregulation is mediated by the release of a vasodilator substance that regulates the cerebrovascular resistance to maintain CBF constant. Although no specific substance fits all experimental observations, adenosine, a potent cerebral vasodilator, is formed from the breakdown of ATP when neuronal demand of oxygen exceeds supply (Winn et al., 1985). Adenosine can be found in increased concentration in cerebral tissue as systemic blood pressure falls toward the lower limit of autoregulation. In fact, brain adenosine concentration doubles within 5 seconds of decreasing blood pressure (Winn et al., 1980). Cortical activation via contralateral peripheral stimulation is also immediately followed by adenosine release and regional vasodilation (Ngai et al., 1998). It has been suggested that NO exerts an influence on basal and stimuli mediated cerebrovascular tone. The mechanism of NO-induced cerebral vasodilation probably involves cGMP and a decrease in intracellular calcium. It is unclear to what extent NO affects cerebral autoregulation in both healthy patients and in patients with TBI. Although earlier studies suggest that NO has no influence on cerebral autoregulation, Jones and coworkers (1999) described an increase in the lower limit of autoregulation with NOS inhibitors. Other transmitters or substances that have been proposed as mediators of autoregulation include protein kinase C (Jones et al., 1999), melatonin (Régrigny et al., 1999), prostacyclin, activated potassium channels, and intracellular second messengers (Faraci and Heistad, 1998).

Pressure-dependent myogenic tone in the systemic resistance vessels was first proposed by Bayliss in 1902 was not experimentally verified until approximately 50 years later. The myogenic theory states that the basal tone of the vascular smooth muscle is affected by change in perfusion or transmural pressure, and that muscle contracts with increased MAP and relaxes with decreased MAP. Studies suggest that there may be two myogenic mechanisms involved in cerebral autoregulation: a rapid reaction to pressure pulsations and a slower reaction to change in MAP. This adaptive process appears to be initiated within the first 400 msec (rapid and rate-dependent response) and is probably completed in a few minutes by the slower and rate-independent component of the autoregulatory process. The slower secondary component appears to be the dominant force in regulating CBF. Autoregulation might also be invoked by incremental increases in blood pressure. However, constant pressure elevation is probably not a sufficient stimulus to maintain sustained vascular contraction. Some investigators believe the myogenic mechanism sets the limits of autoregulation, whereas the metabolic mediators are responsible for cerebral autoregulation itself.

The Neurogenic Mechanism

Perivascular innervation of the cerebral resistance vessels and the specific neurotransmitter contained in the perivascular nerve fibers may also modulate vascular response to change in blood pressure. However, the specific mechanisms by which the CNS exerts control on the cerebral vasculature are poorly understood. Although acetylcholine is the most abundant perivascular neurotransmitter, the list of neurotransmitters involved in this neural response includes norepinephrine, neuropeptide Y, cholecystokinin, acetylcholine, vasoactive intestinal peptide, and calcitonin gene-related peptide (Yoon et al., 1997). Experimentally sympathetic stimulation can shift the autoregulatory curve to the right, thus protecting the brain against severe elevation of MAP.

EFFECTS OF DRUGS ON NEUROPHYSIOLOGY

The effects of the commonly used anesthetic agents on CBF, $CMRo_2$, and CSF dynamics are discussed here and summarized in Table 22-2. The data are scant on these effects in infants and children. The responses in children are assumed to be the same as those in adults.

Intravenous anesthetic drugs have varied effects on cerebral hemodynamics. Thiopental and propofol maintain autoregulation and coupling and potently reduce CBF, cerebral blood volume (CBV), and $CMRo_2$. Karsli and associates (2004) found that propofol maintained cerebrovascular reactivity to CO_2 at levels greater than 30 mm Hg end-tidal CO_2 in children. Furthermore, propofol, at high dosages, lowers CBFV and MAP values in children, which may be mediated by its cerebral vasoconstrictive properties (Karsli et al., 2002). Both thiopental and propofol have been touted as having neuroprotective properties, especially in preclinical studies, but their clinical efficacies in neurologically compromised pediatric patients have not been tested. Etomidate and ketamine are frequently used to induce anesthesia in hemodynamically compromised patients, as these drugs are less likely to cause hypotension than thiopental or propofol. However, CNS excitation and increased ICP have been associated with these drugs, respectively, and they may not be appropriate for many neurosurgical patients.

Intravenous Anesthetics

Propofol

Propofol is an intravenous (IV) induction agent with cerebrovascular properties similar to those of thiopental: both may depress systemic blood pressure but both potently decrease $CMRo_2$, CBF, and ICP (Van Hemelrijck et al., 1990). Cerebral autoregulation and cerebral responsiveness to changes in arterial CO_2 tension (Karsli et al., 2004) are well preserved during propofol anesthesia. Propofol is a good alternative to thiopental for induction of anesthesia for neurosurgery. In the presence of nitrous oxide and hypocapnia, propofol results in lower ICP, higher cerebral perfusion pressure (CPP), and less cerebral cortical edema than isoflurane or sevoflurane. In patients with or at risk for intracranial hypertension and decreased cerebral perfusion, maintenance of anesthesia with propofol is superior to inhaled halogenated anesthetics, at least until the dura has been opened.

Barbiturates

Barbiturates decrease CBF, CBV, and $CMRo_2$ in a dosage-dependent manner (Pierce et al., 1962; Michenfelder, 1974; Albrecht et al.,

TABLE 22-2. Anesthetic Agents and Their Effects on Cerebral Hemodynamics and Neurophysiologic Monitors

	MAP	CBF	CPP	ICP	CMRo$_2$	SSEP Amplitude Latency	CSF Production	CSF Absorption
Inhaled Agents								
Halothane	↓↓	↑↑↑	↑↑	↑↑	↓↓	↓↑	↑↓	↑↓
Isoflurane	↓↓	↑	↑↑	↑	↓↓↓	↓↑	↓↑	↑
Sevoflurane	↓↓	↑	↑	Ø–↑	↓↓↓	↓↑	↑	↓
Desflurane	↓↓	↑	↑	↑	↓	↓↑	↓↑	↑
N$_2$O	Ø–↓	↑–↑↑	↓	↑–↑↑	↓↑	↓Ø–↑	↓↑	↓↑
IV Agents								
Thiopental	↓↓	↓↓↓	↑↑↑	↓↓↓	↓↓↓	↓↑	↓↑	↑
Propofol	↓↓↓	↓↓↓	↑↑	↓↓	↓↓↓	↑↑	↓↑	↑
Etomidate	Ø–↓	↓↓↓	↑↑	↓↓↓	↓↓↓	↑↑	↓↑	↑
Ketamine	↑↑	↑↑↑	↓	↑↑↑	↑	↑Ø	↓↑	↓
Benzodiazepine	Ø–↓	↓↓	↑	Ø	↓↓	↓Ø–↑		↑
Opioids	Ø–↓	↓	↓↑	Ø–↓	↓	↓↑	↓↑	↑

CBF, Cerebral blood flow; *CMR,* cerebral metabolic rate; *CPP,* cerebral perfusion pressure; *CSF,* cerebrospinal fluid; *ICP,* intracranial pressure; *MAP,* mean arterial pressure; *SSEP,* somatosensory evoked potential; ↑, increased; ↓, decreased; Ø, none.

1977) and therefore reduce ICP. Neither CBF nor cerebral metabolism is significantly altered by subanesthetic dosages of barbiturates. When the EEG becomes isoelectric, CBF and CMRo$_2$ decrease to about 50% of normal, and additional doses of barbiturates have little further effect. Barbiturates may also be used to prevent increases in ICP that can occur with laryngoscopy and endotracheal intubation. Autoregulation and the cerebrovascular response to changes in Paco$_2$ remain intact during barbiturate anesthesia. The rate of CSF formation and the resistance to reabsorption of CSF are not altered by barbiturates (Mann et al., 1979). In dosages that suppress the EEG, barbiturates reduce cerebral damage in animal and human models of focal cerebral ischemia (Smith et al., 1974; Nehls et al., 1987). In animals, barbiturates also reduce the extent of cerebral edema after a cortical freeze injury. This decrease in edema is in contrast to the response observed with the volatile anesthetics (Smith and Marque 1976).

Opioids

Opioids have little effect on CBF, CBV, or ICP unless respiration is depressed and Paco$_2$ is increased (Miller et al., 1975; Misfeldt et al., 1976; Jobes, 1977; Moss et al., 1978).

Fentanyl

When combined with nitrous oxide, fentanyl decreases CBF by 47% and CMRo$_2$ by 18% (Michenfelder, 1974). Autoregulation and CO$_2$ responsiveness of the cerebral circulation are not altered. Fentanyl does not alter the rate of CSF formation, but it reduces the resistance to CSF reabsorption by 50% (Artru, 1984a, 1984c), the effect of which is to decrease CSF volume to a degree of unknown clinical significance. The neonatal cerebral circulation is also unaffected by fentanyl (Yaster et al., 1987). Sufentanil and alfentanil in high dosages (10 to 20 mcg/kg) reduce both CBF and CMRo$_2$ by 25% to 30% (Stephan et al., 1991), whereas at exceedingly high dosages (10 to 200 mcg/kg), sufentanil may transiently increase CBF while reducing CMRo$_2$

(Milde et al., 1990). However, at conventional dosages, sufentanil (Herrick et al., 1991; Weinstabl et al., 1991; Mayberg et al., 1993) does not appear to have adverse effects on the cerebral vasculature or on ICP in most patients. In a subset of patients with severe head injuries and very poor intracranial compliance, sufentanil may cause a small (e.g., <10 mm Hg) and transient increase in ICP that may be clinically significant in some settings (Sperry et al., 1992; Weinstabl et al., 1992; Albanese et al., 1993).

Remifentanil

Remifentanil is an ultra-short-acting to short-acting opioid that is rapidly metabolized by plasma and tissue esterases. The very short clinical duration of effect of remifentanil and its context-sensitive half-life, which is independent of the duration of infusion (Minto et al., 1997; Mertens et al., 2003), make it an appealing opioid for lengthy neurosurgical procedures after which rapid return of consciousness is desirable. As is the case with other opioids that have been studied, remifentanil does not increase CBF or ICP (Hoffman et al., 1993; Baker et al., 1997; Ostapkovich et al., 1998; Klimscha et al., 2003; Engelhard et al., 2004; Lagace et al., 2004). Return of consciousness is very rapid after remifentanil is discontinued, and the frequency of administration of naloxone to permit neurologic assessment is decreased (Guy et al., 1997). However, because remifentanil analgesia is very brief after its discontinuation, a long-acting opioid analgesic must be administered to prevent severe pain and rebound hypertension before or soon after remifentanil is discontinued (Gerlach et al., 2003; Cafiero et al., 2004).

Other Intravenous Anesthetics

Etomidate reduces ICP by decreasing CBF and CMRo$_2$ by 34% and 45%, respectively. It, too, preserves the CO$_2$ responsiveness of the cerebral circulation (Renou et al., 1978; Moss et al., 1979).

A side effect of etomidate administration is myoclonus, which has been reported after prolonged continuous infusion of etomidate (Laughlin and Newberg, 1985). *Lidocaine* in clinical dosages decreases CBF and reduces the increase in ICP associated with endotracheal intubation (Sakabe et al., 1974; Donegan and Bedford, 1980). The *benzodiazepines* (diazepam, lorazepam, and midazolam) decrease CBF and $CMRo_2$ by approximately 25% (Cotev and Shalit, 1975; Rockoff et al., 1980; Tateishi et al., 1981; Forster et al., 1982; Nugent et al., 1982; Nakahashi et al., 1991).

Dexmedetomidine

The neurophysiologic effects of dexmedetomidine (an α_2-agonist) have not been extensively studied in humans. In animals, it has been noted to decrease CBF but was not associated with a proportional decrease in the cerebral metabolic rate (Zornow et al., 1990). In human studies, CBFV decreases after dexmedetomidine administration (Zornow et al., 1993) and CBF—both global and regional—decreases by 30% at clinically relevant concentrations of dexmedetomidine (Prielipp et al., 2002).

The effect of dexmedetomidine on ICP in patients with space-occupying lesions is unclear. In patients undergoing transsphenoidal hypophysectomy, dexmedetomidine had no effect on lumbar CSF pressure (Talke et al., 1997). Its effect on the amplitude and latency of cortical somatosensory evoked potential is minimal.

Ketamine

In contrast to the other IV anesthetic agents, ketamine is a potent cerebrovasodilator. It increases CBF by 60% with little change in $CMRo_2$ (Dawson et al., 1971; Takeshita et al., 1972; Schwedler et al., 1982). The cerebrovascular response to administration of ketamine is thought to be the result of regional cerebral activation induced by the drug (Hougaard et al., 1974). Ketamine produces a marked increase in ICP, which can be reduced, but not prevented, by hyperventilation (Gardner et al., 1972; Takeshita et al., 1972; Wyte et al., 1972). The increase in CBF, and presumably in ICP, can be blocked by previous administration of thiopental (Dawson et al., 1971). Ketamine has been associated with sudden elevation of ICP and clinical deterioration when used in patients with hydrocephalus and other intracranial pathology (List et al., 1972; Lockhart and Jenkins, 1972; Wyte et al., 1972). Although ketamine is not currently used as a general anesthetic in patients with reduced intracranial compliance, a recent study in critically ill children reported a decrease in ICP following ketamine (Bar-Joseph et al., 2009), thereby challenging the notion that ketamine increases ICP.

Inhalational Anesthetics

Volatile anesthetic drugs are potent cerebrovasodilators and may produce uncoupling of $CMRo_2$ and CBF, and different volatile anesthetics may have varying uncoupling profiles (Hansen et al., 1989). Uncoupling may lead to increased CBV and can exacerbate intracranial hypertension. Children have increased sensitivity to the vasodilatory effects of volatile drugs. TCD measurements reveal that the following volatile agents increase CBFV in descending order: halothane, desflurane, isoflurane, and sevoflurane. Autoregulation is also blunted in the presence of volatile drugs in a dosage-dependent fashion. However, this perturbation is mitigated by hypocapnia. Nitrous oxide has vasodilatory effects alone and in combination with other anesthetics. Because isoflurane and sevoflurane significantly decrease $CMRo_2$ in children and maintain coupling, these two inhaled drugs are ideal anesthetics for the neurologically compromised patient. Sevoflurane does not significantly affect CBFV, and it preserves cerebral autoregulation in children anesthetized with up to a minimum alveolar concentration (MAC) of 1.5 (Fairgrieve et al., 2003; Wong et al., 2006).

Nitrous Oxide

Nitrous oxide is a weak cerebrovasodilator whose effects on CBF are offset by hyperventilation and barbiturate anesthesia (Algotsson et al., 1988). The variability of effects that nitrous oxide has on CBF and ICP in different reports results from differences in experimental species and background anesthesia. In many animals, nitrous oxide in subanesthetic dosages (60% to 70%) causes excitement and cerebral metabolic stimulation, with an accompanying increase in CBF (Theye and Michenfelder, 1968; Sakabe et al., 1978; Pelligrino et al., 1984; Drummond et al., 1987). Because nitrous oxide is not an adequate anesthetic in the absence of other inhalation or IV anesthetics, the modification of its cerebral effects by additional anesthetic drugs is particularly important. Nitrous oxide at 70% does not, for example, cause a change in CBF, but it does reduce $CMRo_2$ by 15% to 20% during barbiturate and narcotic anesthesia (Sakabe et al., 1978). However, when nitrous oxide is added to a volatile anesthetic such as isoflurane (Cucchiara et al., 1974; Manohar and Parks, 1984) or halothane (Sakabe et al., 1976), both CBF and $CMRo_2$ increase. When nitrous oxide is added to sevoflurane, cerebral hyperemia increases and autoregulation is impaired (Iacopino et al., 2003).

The cerebrovascular responses to changes in $Paco_2$ and MAP are preserved during nitrous oxide anesthesia. ICP may increase in response to nitrous oxide in patients with intracranial mass lesions and reduced intracranial compliance (Henriksen and Jörgensen, 1973; Moss and McDowall, 1979; Iacopino et al., 2003). The increase in ICP with nitrous oxide, however, is readily reversible by diazepam and barbiturate anesthesia and simultaneously initiated hyperventilation (Phirman and Shapiro, 1977).

The use of nitrous oxide for pediatric neuroanesthesia remains controversial. Some anesthesiologists prefer to avoid it because of its ability to increase $CMRo_2$ and reduce the cerebroprotective effects of barbiturates. Others are concerned because it readily diffuses into collections of intracranial air and may increase ICP in the presence of pneumocephalus (Artru, 1982; Skahen et al., 1986). Asymptomatic accumulation of intracranial air occurs commonly during craniotomies, especially those associated with posterior fossa surgery and drainage of CSF (Yates et al., 1994). Some anesthesiologists discontinue nitrous oxide before closure of the dura to reduce the incidence of tension pneumocephalus, and others administer nitrous oxide throughout the procedure without any obvious detrimental effects. Indeed, one randomized control trial comparing anesthetic techniques with and without nitrous oxide in patients undergoing sitting craniotomies showed no difference in the incidence or size of pneumocephalus between the three groups (Hernández-Palazón et al., 2003). It may be that nitrous oxide equilibrates with intracranial air before the dura is closed; if so,

ICP would not increase during craniodural closure because air pockets would already contain nitrous oxide. In addition, the discontinuance of nitrous oxide would decrease ICP, as nitrous oxide diffused back into the bloodstream (Skahen et al., 1986). Maintenance with nitrous oxide until the end of the surgery may be advantageous because it permits rapid awakening and may reduce the intracranial gas volume and the likelihood of delayed tension pneumocephalus. Nitrous oxide is generally not contraindicated during sitting craniotomies, even though the volume of a venous air embolus (VAE) expands in the presence of nitrous oxide. In fact, this phenomenon actually increases the sensitivity of monitoring for VAE by capnography, while at the same time nitrous oxide neither increases the risk of VAE (Losasso et al., 1992) nor increases the hemodynamic consequences of VAE, provided that nitrous oxide is discontinued when VAE is first detected (Losasso et al., 1992).

Isoflurane

Isoflurane is frequently used for neuroanesthesia. Its popularity is based on the fact that it affects CBF less than does halothane at equivalent MAC dosages (Todd and Drummond, 1984; Drummond and Todd, 1985; Algotsson et al., 1988), the fact that 1 MAC isoflurane preserves cerebral autoregulation (McPherson and Traystman, 1988) and CO_2 responsiveness (McPherson et al., 1989), and the belief that it may provide cerebral protection (Newberg and Michenfelder, 1983; Verhaegen et al., 1992). Cerebral autoregulation is less affected by isoflurane than by halothane (Todd and Drummond, 1984b). In addition, isoflurane does not change CSF production, and it reduces the resistance to reabsorption of CSF (Artru, 1984b). During hypocapnia, CBF is lower with 1.0 MAC isoflurane (with 75% nitrous oxide) than with nitrous oxide alone (Cucchiara et al., 1974; Drummond and Todd, 1985). In contrast, 1.0 MAC halothane (with 75% nitrous oxide) increases CBF. Despite their dissimilar effects on CBF, isoflurane and halothane increase ICP equally in an animal model of brain injury (Scheller et al., 1987). This is probably because isoflurane and halothane increase CBV to a similar degree (Artru 1984c; Archer et al., 1987). In patients with reduced intracranial compliance, isoflurane increases ICP. This increase can be attenuated by simultaneous initiation of hyperventilation (Adams et al., 1981).

Isoflurane may be safely used in patients with small supratentorial brain tumors (Madsen et al., 1987), but it may cause dangerous increases in ICP in patients with large intracranial mass lesions that are associated with a midline shift evident on a computed tomography (CT) scan (Grosslight et al., 1985). Like halothane, isoflurane should be avoided in patients with reduced intracranial compliance until the dura is open, if ICP is not being monitored. Isoflurane decreases $CMRo_2$ by 30%, and it causes an isoelectric EEG at concentrations above 2.0 MAC (Newberg and Michenfelder, 1983). It is unique among the volatile agents in that it preserves normal cerebral energy states and aerobic metabolism at very low blood pressure (40 mm Hg), in contrast to the findings observed with hypotension induced by halothane, trimethaphan, or sodium nitroprusside (Newberg et al., 1984). In studies of mice exposed to 5% oxygen, isoflurane increased survival time and thus may have provided some degree of cerebral protection. In studies of incomplete global ischemia in isoflurane-anesthetized dogs, cerebral energy stores were increased, presumably through depression of cortical electrical activity and cerebral metabolism (Newberg

and Michenfelder, 1983). Protective effects of isoflurane, however, were not observed in a primate model of regional cerebral ischemia (Nehls et al., 1987).

Sevoflurane

Sevoflurane is a fluorinated ether with a low blood-gas solubility. Studies in rabbits suggest that sevoflurane does not increase CBF at 0.5 to 1.0 MAC. Sevoflurane does cause increases in CBF and ICP and a decrease in cerebral oxygen consumption (Scheller et al., 1988) and CPP, similar to isoflurane (Petersen et al., 2003). Compared with isoflurane, sevoflurane allows more rapid emergence after lengthy neurosurgery, and thus more rapid neurologic assessment (Mönkhoff et al., 2001; Gauthier et al., 2002). Taken together, the available evidence suggests that sevoflurane is a more appropriate inhaled anesthetic than halothane during craniotomy, and that it is equivalent in its cerebrovascular effects to isoflurane, while allowing more rapid recovery after long anesthesia. As is the case with other halogenated agents, if ICP or intracranial compliance is compromised, sevoflurane should be withheld until the dura has been opened (Petersen et al., 2003).

Halothane

Halothane is a cerebral vasodilator that decreases cerebrovascular resistance and increases CBF in a dosage-dependent fashion (Wollman et al., 1964; Albrecht et al., 1977; Todd and Drummond, 1984; Brüssel et al., 1991). The increase in CBF is transient; CBF decreases to baseline levels after 150 minutes of halothane anesthesia (Albrecht et al., 1983). CBV, however, remains elevated by 11% to 12% over a 3-hour period of halothane administration (Artrub, 1983). Halothane reduces $CMRo_2$ by 17% to 33% (Albrecht et al., 1977). The cerebral vasculature remains responsive to changes in arterial $Paco_2$ (Alexander et al., 1964; Wollman et al., 1964; Drummond and Todd, 1985). Halothane in high concentrations (2.0 MAC) abolishes autoregulation of the cerebral circulation in response to changes in MAP in both adults (Miletich et al., 1976; Todd and Drummond, 1984) and infants (Messer et al., 1989). Halothane alters blood-brain barrier permeability, promoting the extravasation of plasma proteins into normal brain during periods of acute hypertension (Forster et al., 1978). Halothane reduces CSF formation by 30% in dogs and increases the resistance of reabsorption of CSF (Artru, 1983a, 1984b).

Because ICP is determined by CBV, CSF volume, and brain tissue volume, it is not surprising that ICP increases with halothane (Jennett et al., 1969; DiGiovanni et al., 1974). Peak increases are observed in 3 to 13 minutes, although the increase persists over 3 hours of halothane exposure (Artru, 1983b). The increase in ICP in patients with intracranial mass lesions can be attenuated, but not totally prevented, by establishing hyperventilation for 10 minutes before the introduction of halothane (Adams et al., 1981). If ICP is not being monitored, halothane should not be used in patients with reduced intracranial compliance until the dura is open and its effects on the brain can be seen.

Desflurane

Desflurane is an inhalation agent that is chemically similar to isoflurane. Its physicochemical properties are remarkable, with a blood-gas partition coefficient even lower than that of nitrous oxide, permitting rapid uptake and washout of the gas. The effects of desflurane on cerebral metabolism and hemodynamics are not as well studied as the effects of the other inhalation agents, but animal studies suggest that its effects are not unique in any way. Desflurane at clinical concentrations is a potent cerebral vasodilator, increasing ICP (Artru, 1994), increasing CBF by 50% at 1.5 MAC, and reducing autoregulation of CBF (Lutz and Milde, 1990). However, cerebrovascular responsiveness to hypocapnia is preserved during desflurane anesthesia in laboratory animals, protecting the animal from increases in ICP if hyperventilation occurs during the anesthesia (Lutz et al., 1991; Young, 1992). In patients with mass lesions, equivalent MAC dosages of desflurane and isoflurane are similar in terms of absolute CBF, the response to increasing dosages, and the preservation of CO_2 reactivity (Ornstein et al., 1993; Fraga et al., 2003). Desflurane effects seen on the EEG are also similar to those of isoflurane. At increasing concentrations, the electroencephalographic frequency decreases and the amplitude increases. Burst suppression appears at about 1.24 MAC (Rampil et al., 1991).

Muscle Relaxants

Succinylcholine

Succinylcholine is very infrequently used in pediatric anesthesia because of its association with life-threatening hyperkalemia and cardiac arrest in children with undiagnosed myopathies. This has led to a black-box warning by the U.S. Food and Drug Administration, reserving its use in children for emergency intubation when securing the airway is necessary. Most often, the use of even high-dosage nondepolarizing neuromuscular blockers is appropriate for emergently securing the airway in children, but in some cases a very rapid and immediate pharmacologic paralysis is required, and succinylcholine remains the drug of choice in these circumstances. Life-threatening hyperkalemia has also been associated with administration of succinylcholine after many types of CNS disorders, including closed-head injury, even without motor deficits (Mazze et al., 1969; Thomas, 1969; Smith and Grenvik, 1970), cerebral hypoxia caused by near-drowning (Tong, 1987), subarachnoid hemorrhage (Iwatsuki et al., 1980), encephalitis (Cowgill et al., 1974), cerebrovascular accidents (Cooperman et al., 1970), and paraplegia (Cooperman, 1970; Tobey, 1970). The onset of the period of vulnerability is not well defined. It may begin as early as 24 to 48 hours after injury and may last up to 1 to 2 years after injury (Cooperman, 1970). Because the period of risk for succinylcholine-induced hyperkalemia after cerebral injury is undefined, succinylcholine should be avoided in these patients, except in the period immediately after injury. Succinylcholine can increase CBF and ICP in patients with reduced intracranial compliance (Cottrell et al., 1983; Minton et al., 1986; Stirt et al., 1987a; Thiagarajah et al., 1988), probably because of cerebral stimulation from succinylcholine-induced increases in afferent-muscle spindle activity (Lanier et al., 1986.). The increases in CBF and ICP can be blunted by deep general anesthesia or by previous paralyzing or "defasciculating" dosages of nondepolarizing muscle relaxants (Minton et al., 1986; Stirt et al., 1987a). In contrast, most nondepolarizing relaxants have little effect on CBV and

ICP (Lanier et al., 1985; Minton et al., 1985; Stirt et al., 1987b; Rosa et al., 1991), unless associated with histamine release (D-tubocurarine, atracurium), which causes transient cerebrovasodilation and increased ICP (Tarkkanen et al., 1974). In dosages that do not release histamine, atracurium does not increase ICP, despite the accumulation of laudanosine, a major metabolic product of atracurium and a potential CNS arousal agent.

Nondepolarizing Muscle Relaxants

The presence of motor deficits or the administration of anticonvulsants may affect the dosage of nondepolarizing muscle relaxant necessary in neurosurgical patients. Hemiplegia from an upper motor neuron lesion (such as a stroke or a brain tumor) is associated with resistance to nondepolarizing relaxants on the paretic side (Graham, 1980; Moorthy and Hilgenberg, 1980; Shayevitz and Matteo, 1985). Excessive dosages of muscle relaxants may be given if the dosage is guided by a nerve stimulator monitoring a hemiplegic extremity. In contrast, an increased response to nondepolarizing muscle relaxants is observed in paretic-muscle lower motor neuron lesions (e.g., paraplegia and quadriplegia) (Brown et al., 1975). Acute administration of several anticonvulsants, including phenytoin, phenobarbital, trimethadione, and ethosuximide, enhances nondepolarizing neuromuscular blockade or delays its reversal (Gandhi et al., 1976; Spacek et al., 1999). Patients receiving chronic phenytoin or carbamazepine therapy are resistant to the effects of nondepolarizing relaxants, including pancuronium, (Roth and Ebrahim, 1987), metocurine (Ornstein et al., 1985), vecuronium (Ornstein et al., 1987; Alloul et al., 1996), and rocuronium (Spacek et al., 1999; Hernández-Palazón et al., 2001) but, interestingly, not mivacurium or atracurium (Ornstein et al., 1987; Spacek et al., 1996). The cause of phenytoin-induced resistance to nondepolarizing muscle relaxants and the reason for the lack of the same effect with mivacurium or atracurium are unclear. Finally, no data have yet been published describing the interactions of anticonvulsants (felbamate, gabapentin, levetiracetam, tiagabine, topiramate, sodium valproate, or valproic acid) with nondepolarizing neuromuscular blocking drugs (Fig. 22-6).

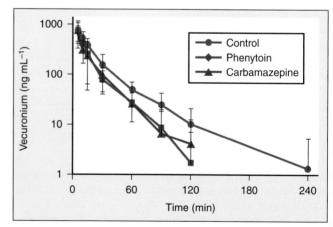

■ **FIGURE 22-6.** Effect of chronic anticonvulsant therapy on the half-life of the muscle relaxant vecuronium. Vecuronium plasma concentrations are plotted against time after a single bolus dose of vecuronium (0.15 mg/kg). Mean ± SD is plotted for all three groups.

Vasodilators

The direct-acting vasodilators, including sodium nitroprusside, ATP, adenosine, nitroglycerin, diazoxide, and hydralazine, are cerebrovasodilators and may increase CBF and ICP (Stoyka and Schutz, 1975; Turner et al., 1977; Marsh et al., 1979; Cottrell et al., 1980; McDowall, 1985). The calcium channel blockers also raise CBF and ICP (Griffin et al., 1983; Mazzoni et al., 1985). These drugs should therefore be avoided in patients with reduced intracranial compliance, unless the dura is open or ICP is monitored. Indirect-acting antihypertensives, including trimethaphan (a ganglionic blocker), propranolol and esmolol (β-adrenergic blockers), and labetalol (a combined α- and β-blocker), do not increase CBF or ICP (Magness et al., 1973; Turner et al., 1977; McDowall, 1985). These agents are useful for the control of blood pressure in patients with elevated ICP. Trimethaphan may interfere with the neurologic examination by causing mydriasis, cycloplegia, or anisocoria. Sodium nitroprusside lowers the range of cerebral autoregulation. Brain-surface oxygen tension is greater (Maekawa et al., 1977) and metabolic disturbances in brain biochemistry (e.g., lactate, pyruvate, and phosphocreatine levels) are less during nitroprusside-induced hypotension than with trimethaphan- or hemorrhage-induced hypotension (Michenfelder and Theye, 1977). In addition, cortical blood flow and electrical activity are better preserved at lower MAP with sodium nitroprusside (Ishikawa and McDowall, 1981). Nitroprusside, however, induces more pronounced blood-brain barrier dysfunction than does trimethaphan (Ishikawa et al., 1983). Because CBF, brain oxygen tension, neuronal function, and brain metabolism are better maintained with sodium nitroprusside than with trimethaphan at a MAP of 50 mm Hg, sodium nitroprusside is the preferred agent for deliberate hypotension.

Central Nervous System Toxicity of Anesthetic Agents

Preclinical studies have demonstrated that prolonged exposure of fetal and neonatal laboratory animals to anesthetic drugs leads to accelerated neurodegeneration (Ikonomidou et al., 1999; Jevtovic-Todorovic et al., 2003; Slikker et al., 2007). The data generated in these reports have provoked a heated debate on its relevance to the practice of pediatric anesthesia (Anand and Soriano, 2004; Olney et al., 2004). There is no doubt that this phenomenon is valid in the experimental paradigms used in these laboratory investigations. The same model has also implicated dexamethasone and magnesium sulfate in accelerating neuroapoptosis in the development of rat brain (Noguchi et al., 2008; Dribben et al., 2009). However, a number of factors make the extrapolation of these findings to humans in the daily practice of clinical pediatric anesthesiology questionable. For example, these animal and in vitro studies have significant limitations in terms of agent dosage and duration of exposure (both absolute and in comparison with human studies) (Loepke and Soriano, 2008). Furthermore, no defined clinical markers or syndromes are associated with neonatal exposure to general anesthetics. Unlike general anesthetic agents, exposure to alcohol or anticonvulsant drugs during gestational development has clearly characterized clinical syndromes. Although histologic evidence of accelerated neurodegeneration has been verified by several investigational groups, discrepancies in neurocognitive outcomes exist (Loepke et al., 2009). Prospective clinical investigations are underway to verify these observations. Finally, the majority of neonatal and infant surgery is urgent or emergent, and anesthetic care is essential to proceed safely. It has been clearly demonstrated that inadequate anesthesia leads to poor postoperative outcomes in infants (Anand and Hickey, 1987; Anand and Soriano, 2004), and it is crucial to attenuate the stress response associated with surgical stimulation.

Several retrospective reports have positively linked exposure to general anesthesia before the age of 4 with an increased chance of developing learning deficits. Wilder and colleagues (2009) examined the extensive medical and school records of 5358 children in Rochester, Minnesota, and determined that there was an association between learning deficits in school and having more than two surgeries before age 4. A cross-sectional study done by Kalkman and colleagues (2009) in Utrecht, The Netherlands, surveyed a small number of parents of children who had had surgery at a young age and determined that there was a trend toward greater prevalence of learning deficits in children who had had early surgery. However, these reports need to be reconciled with a recent report demonstrating no causal relationship between anesthesia exposure and subsequent learning behavior in twin cohorts (Bartels et al., 2009). Clinicians should be aware of the rapid developments in the area of anesthetic-induced neurodegeneration and keep in mind the degree of necessity of infant surgical procedures and the more significant effects of the hypoxic and cardiovascular mechanisms of brain injury and death during anesthesia and surgery in these patients.

PREOPERATIVE EVALUATION AND PREPARATION

A proper and thorough evaluation and preparation of the pediatric patient for anesthesia and surgery are essential components of minimizing perioperative morbidity and mortality. Because of the urgent nature of many pediatric neurosurgical procedures, a thorough preoperative evaluation may be difficult. The perioperative management of pediatric patients undergoing neurosurgical procedures should be based on the developmental stage of the patient and is discussed in Chapter 8, Psychological Aspects, and Chapter 9, Preoperative Preparation. Given the systemic effects of general anesthesia and the physiologic stress of surgery, an organ system–based approach is optimal for anticipating potential physiologic derangements and coexisting disease states that may increase the risk of perioperative complications (Ferrari, 1999). Many potential perioperative problems can be preemptively addressed with such an approach. Because some children are either preverbal or do not fully understand their medical condition, their parents or primary caregivers should be interviewed carefully to obtain information regarding coexisting medical problems. A thorough review of the patient's history can reveal conditions that may increase the risk of adverse reactions to anesthesia and perioperative morbidity and identify patients who need more extensive evaluation or whose medical condition needs to be optimized before surgery. There are also special perioperative concerns regarding children with neurologic abnormalities. However, certain aspects of this evaluation are of special relevance to neurosurgical patients. Specific concerns in these patients are listed in Table 22-3. Preoperative laboratory testing should be tailored to the proposed neurosurgical procedure.

TABLE 22-3. Common Perioperative Concerns for Infants and Children with Neurologic Lesions

Condition	Anesthetic Implications
Denervation injuries	Hyperkalemia after succinylcholine Resistance to nondepolarizing muscle relaxants Abnormal response to nerve stimulation
Chronic anticonvulsant therapy	Hepatic and hematologic abnormalities Increased metabolism of anesthetic agents
Arteriovenous malformation	Potential congestive heart failure
Neuromuscular disease	Malignant hyperthermia Respiratory failure Sudden cardiac death
Chiari malformation	Apnea Aspiration pneumonia Stridor
Hypothalamic and pituitary lesions	Diabetes insipidus or syndrome of inappropriate antidiuretic hormone Hypothyroidism or hyperthyroidism Adrenal insufficiency or adrenal excess

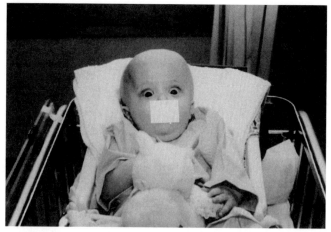

■ **FIGURE 22-7.** An infant with hydrocephalus. Note enlarged head and the downward gaze (the setting-sun sign). The latter suggests the presence of intracranial hypertension.

The chronicity and severity of the patient's neurologic condition vary greatly and should dictate the perioperative management. Special attention should be given to symptoms of allergy to latex products, because anaphylaxis has been reported in a number of children who have undergone multiple previous operations, especially patients with meningomyeloceles (Holzman, 1997). Severe dehydration and electrolyte abnormalities can be the result of protracted vomiting from intracranial hypertension. Patients with diabetes insipidus can develop hypovolemia as a result of polyuria. During the perioperative period, steroids are frequently initiated to palliate cerebral swelling in patients with intracranial tumors. Therapeutic levels of anticonvulsants should be verified preoperatively and maintained perioperatively. Patients on long-term anticonvulsants may develop toxicity, especially if seizures are difficult to control. This reaction frequently manifests with abnormalities in either hematologic or hepatic function, or both. Patients on chronic anticonvulsant therapy may also require increased amounts of sedatives, nondepolarizing muscle relaxants, and narcotics because of enhanced metabolism of these drugs (Soriano et al., 2000b; Soriano et al., 2001; Soriano and Martyn, 2004).

Physical Examination

The physical examination should include a brief neurologic evaluation that includes consciousness level, motor and sensory function, normal and pathologic reflexes, integrity of the cranial nerves, and signs and symptoms of intracranial hypertension (Fig. 22-7 and Table 22-4). It is essential to document these factors in the preoperative examination to be able to gauge postoperative neurologic function. Lesions of the brainstem can manifest with cranial nerve dysfunction such as respiratory distress, impaired gag reflex and swallowing, and pulmonary aspiration. Evidence of muscle atrophy and weakness should be noted, particularly if the patient is hemparetic, hemiplegic, or bedridden, because up-regulation of acetylcholine receptors may precipitate sudden hyperkalemia after succinylcholine administration and induce resistance to nondepolarizing muscle

TABLE 22-4. Signs of Intracranial Hypertension in Infants and Children

Infants	Children	Infants and Children
Irritability	Headache	Decreased consciousness
Full fontanelle	Diplopia	Cranial nerve (III and VI) palsies
Widely separated cranial sutures	Papilledema	Loss of upward gaze (setting-sun sign)
Cranial enlargement	Vomiting	Signs of herniation, Cushing's triad, pupillary changes

relaxants in the affected limbs. Body weight should be accurately measured to guide the administration of drugs, fluids, and blood products. Physical signs of dehydration should be noted, especially in patients who have been chronically ill or have received osmotic or diuretic agents.

Radiologic and Laboratory Evaluation

Most neurosurgical patients have a magnetic resonance imaging (MRI) or CT scan of the head as part of the preoperative assessment. These scans should be reviewed with the neurosurgeon to confirm the primary lesion and the presence of evolving neurologic conditions (hydrocephalus, compressed cisterns, midline shifts) (Fig. 22-8). Preoperative laboratory tests should be tailored to the proposed neurosurgical procedure. Given the risk of significant blood loss associated with surgery, the hematocrit, prothrombin time, and partial thromboplastin time should be obtained to uncover any insidious hematologic disorder. Patients with suprasellar pathology should have an endocrinology evaluation. Type- and cross-matched blood should be ordered before all craniotomies. Endocrinologists may be needed to help optimize the patient's condition before surgery and to assist in postoperative management. Liver function tests and a hematologic profile should be obtained if not recently reviewed for children taking long-term anticonvulsants.

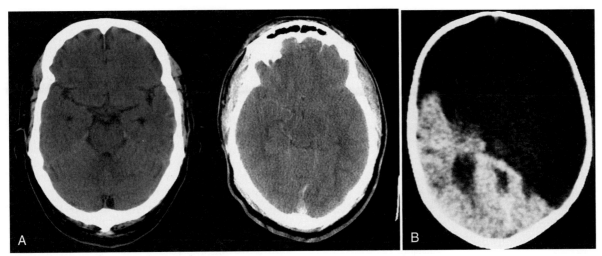

■ **FIGURE 22-8. A,** CT scan depicting normal *(left)* and compressed *(right)* basal cisterns. The basal, or perimesencephalic, cerebrospinal fluid space consists of the interpeduncular cistern (anterior), the ambient cisterns (lateral), and the quadrigeminal cisterns (posterior). In the patient *(right)* with diffuse cerebral swelling (caused by sagittal sinus thrombosis), the cisterns have been obliterated. **B,** Hydranencephaly. CT scan demonstrates replacement of the cerebral hemispheres by a large, water-dense cavity with residual islands of brain tissue in regions of the occipital poles and right inferior temporal lobe. *(**A,** Courtesy Ivan Petrovitch, MD; **B,** courtesy Division Neuroradiology, University of Health Center of Pittsburgh.)*

Premedication

Perioperative anxiety plays a significant role in the care of the pediatric neurosurgical patient. Anxiety issues are related to the cognitive development and age of the child (see Chapter 2, Behavioral Development). Preoperative sedatives given before the induction of anesthesia can ease the transition from the preoperative holding area to the operating room (Kain et al., 2004). Oral midazolam is particularly effective in relieving anxiety and producing amnesia. If an indwelling IV catheter is in place, midazolam can be slowly titrated to achieve sedation. Sedation is usually withheld from pediatric neurosurgical patients until they arrive in the preoperative area to avoid the problem of an oversedated, neurologically impaired patient with inadequate supervision; however, heavy premedication may be warranted to avoid agitation in patients with moyamoya disease or an intracranial aneurysm or arteriovenous malformation that has recently bled. Narcotics are best withheld preoperatively, as they may cause nausea or respiratory depression, especially in patients with increased ICP.

Sedatives are administered in the parents' presence to facilitate a smooth separation and induction. Midazolam (0.5 to 1.0 mg/kg) may be given orally; it usually requires 5 to 20 minutes to take effect. Alternatively, after application of EMLA (eutectic mixture of local anesthetics, 2.5% lidocaine, and 2.5% prilocaine) cream, an IV catheter can be inserted, into which incremental dosages of IV midazolam may then be carefully titrated.

GENERAL PRINCIPLES OF INTRAOPERATIVE MANAGEMENT

Induction of Anesthesia

The patient's preoperative status dictates the appropriate technique and drugs for induction of anesthesia. A modified Glasgow Coma Scale for infants and children is useful for assessing the mental status of the patient before the administration of anesthesia (Table 22-5). Somnolent patients with intracranial hypertension are at risk for aspiration pneumonitis and require a rapid-sequence induction of anesthesia.

In the presence of intracranial hypertension, the primary goal during induction is to minimize severe increases in ICP. The effects of anesthetic drugs on cerebral hemodynamics were discussed extensively earlier in this chapter and are summarized in Table 22-2. In general, most IV drugs decrease CBF, metabolism, and ICP. Thiopental (4 to 8 mg/kg) and propofol (2 to 5 mg/kg) have similar effects on cerebral hemodynamics and maintain tight coupling of CBF and cerebral metabolic rate. Patients at risk for aspiration pneumonitis (including certain patients with intracranial hypertension) should have rapid-sequence induction of anesthesia using cricoid pressure. An IV hypnotic drug, such as thiopental or propofol, is administered and followed immediately by a rapid-acting muscle relaxant. Rocuronium can be used when succinylcholine is contraindicated, such as for patients with spinal cord injuries or paretic extremities. In instances of preexisting neurologic injury (e.g., in a patient with a history of a stroke resulting in a weak extremity), succinylcholine can result in sudden, catastrophic hyperkalemia. Etomidate and ketamine are frequently used to induce anesthesia in hemodynamically compromised patients, because these drugs are less likely to cause hypotension than thiopental or propofol. However, CNS excitation and increased ICP have been associated with these drugs, respectively, and they may not be appropriate for many neurosurgical patients. Ketamine should be avoided because of its known ability to increase cerebral metabolism, CBF, and ICP.

General anesthesia can be induced with sevoflurane and nitrous oxide in patients who are neurologically stable. Although volatile anesthetic drugs are potent cerebrovasodilators and may produce uncoupling of cerebral metabolic requirement of oxygen, its use for induction of anesthesia is relatively brief. ICP can be lowered during induction by initiating controlled

TABLE 22-5. Glasgow Coma Scale and Modifications for Young Children

Glasgow Coma Scale	Pediatric Coma Scale	Infant Coma Scale	Score
Eyes: Best Response			
Open spontaneously	Open spontaneously	Open spontaneously	4
React to verbal command	React to speech	React to speech	3
React to pain	React to pain	React to pain	2
No response	No response	No response	1
Best Verbal Response			
Oriented and converses	Smiles, oriented, interacts	Coos, babbles, interacts	5
Disoriented and converses	Interacts inappropriately	Irritable	4
Inappropriate words	Moaning	Cries to pain	3
Incomprehensible sounds	Irritable, inconsolable	Moans to pain	2
No response	No response	No response	1
Best Motor Response			
Obeys verbal command	Spontaneous or obeys verbal command	Normal spontaneous movements	6
Localizes pain	Localizes pain	Withdraws to touch	5
Withdraws to pain	Withdraws to pain	Withdraws to pain	4
Abnormal flexion	Abnormal flexion	Abnormal flexion	3
Extension posturing	Extension posturing	Extension posturing	2
No response	No response	No response	1

hyperventilation and administering opioid and barbiturate supplements before laryngoscopy and intubation. A nondepolarizing muscle relaxant may then be administered after IV access has been established to facilitate intubation of the trachea. Pancuronium is an ideal muscle relaxant for neonates and infants because it produces tachycardia that counters the parasympathetic effect of laryngoscopy.

A common problem is an uncooperative toddler who has an intracranial tumor, has moderately decreased intracranial compliance, and is agitated and resistant to parental separation. Some clinicians advocate the use of rectal barbiturates with meticulous attention to airway maintenance to avoid obstruction and resultant hypercarbia and hypoxemia. However, others argue that a crying, agitated child has demonstrated a tolerance to increased ICP and that IV induction is safer. Fortunately (for the anesthesiologist), patients who have severe intracranial hypertension generally have a decreased level of consciousness, and it becomes easier to insert an IV catheter when it is most necessary.

Succinylcholine should be avoided in patients with denervating processes such stroke, or spinal cord injury, because it can result in life-threatening hyperkalemia.

Airway Management

Developmental changes in airway anatomy have a significant impact on management of the pediatric airway. Nasotracheal tubes may be best suited for situations when the patient will be prone, because orotracheal tubes can kink at the base of the tongue when the head is a flexed and result in airway obstruction. The timing of tracheal extubation may be challenging after neurosurgical procedures. Infants, particularly those with Chiari malformation (Cochrane et al., 1990) or older children after procedures in the posterior fossa (Cochrane et al., 1994), may exhibit intermittent apnea, vocal cord paralysis, or other irregularities before resuming a stable respiratory pattern. Significant airway edema and postoperative obstruction can complicate prone procedures or those involving significant blood losses and large volume replacement. Lingual or supraglottic swelling may require direct laryngoscopy to assess the airway. Head-up positioning and gentle forced diuresis usually improve airway edema within 24 hours.

Positioning

Patient positioning for surgery requires careful preoperative planning to allow adequate access to the patient for both the neurosurgeon and anesthesiologist. For the patient with altered physiologic states, various surgical positions can predispose to injury (Fig. 22-9 and Table 22-6). The prone position is commonly used for posterior fossa and spinal cord surgery. The sitting position may be more appropriate for obese patients, who may be difficult to ventilate in the prone position because of increased intrathoracic pressure. In addition to the physiologic sequelae of the sitting position, a spectrum of neurovascular compression and stretch injuries can occur. It is important to ensure free abdominal wall motion. Increased intraabdominal pressure can impair ventilation, cause venocaval compression, and increase epidural venous pressure and bleeding. Postoperative visual loss has been linked to surgery in the prone position. Therefore, the eyes must be free of any direct contact with the horseshoe or Mayfield head holder (Lee et al., 2006). Many neurosurgical procedures are performed with the head slightly elevated to facilitate venous and CSF drainage from the surgical site; however, superior sagittal sinus pressure decreases with increasing head elevation, and this increases the likelihood of VAE (Grady et al., 1986). Excessive rotation of the head can impede venous return via compression

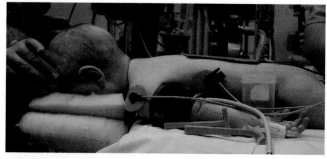

■ **FIGURE 22-9.** Positioning patients and padding them to prevent injuries is essential, especially for prolonged procedures with the patient in the prone position.

TABLE 22-6. Physiologic Effects of Patient Positioning

Position	Physiologic Effect
Head elevated	Enhanced cerebral venous drainage Decreased cerebral blood flow Increased venous pooling in lower extremities Postural hypotension
Head down	Increased cerebral venous and intracranial pressure Decreased functional residual capacity (lung function) Decreased lung compliance
Prone	Venous congestion of face, tongue, and neck Decreased lung compliance Increased abdominal pressure (can lead to venocaval compression)
Lateral decubitus	Decreased compliance of down-side lung

of the jugular veins and can lead to impaired cerebral perfusion, increased ICP, and venous bleeding. Flexion of the head can cause the tracheal tube to migrate into a main stem bronchus. Extreme head flexion can cause brainstem compression in patients with posterior fossa pathology, such as mass lesions or an Arnold-Chiari malformation and high cervical spinal cord ischemia. Likewise, extreme head extension may result in inadvertent tracheal extubation. Finally, all pressure points should be padded and peripheral pulses checked to prevent peripheral nerve and vascular compression and pressure injury.

Vascular Access

The routine use of central venous catheters in pediatric neurosurgical patients is controversial. The small bore and relatively long length of pediatric central catheters may produce too much resistance to high flow rates. Typically, two large peripheral venous cannulae are sufficient for most craniotomies. Should peripheral IV be difficult to secure, a cannulation of the femoral vein avoids the risk of pneumothorax associated with subclavian catheters, and it does not interfere with cerebral venous return as may be the case with jugular catheters. Because significant blood loss and hemodynamic instability can occur during craniotomies, an arterial catheter provides direct blood pressure monitoring and sampling for blood-gas analysis.

Maintenance of Anesthesia

Specific drugs used for the maintenance of anesthesia have not been shown to affect the outcome of neurosurgical procedures when properly administered (Todd et al., 1993). The most frequently used technique during neurosurgery consists of an opioid (i.e., fentanyl, sufentanil, or remifentanil) along with inhaled nitrous oxide (70%) and low-dosage (0.2% to 0.5%) isoflurane. Routine administration of a preoperative benzodiazepine such as midazolam (0.5 mg/kg orally, or 0.1 mg/kg intravenously) should provide some degree of amnesia of perioperative events as well as minimize anxiety.

Chronic administration of anticonvulsant drugs, such as phenytoin and carbamazepine, induces rapid metabolism and clearance of neuromuscular blockers and opioids because of the enhanced activity of the hepatic P450 enzymes (Soriano and Martyn, 2004). Patients receiving chronic anticonvulsant therapy require larger dosages of muscle relaxants and narcotics because of the induced enzymatic metabolism of these agents (see Fig. 22-6) (Soriano et al., 2001). Muscle relaxants should be withheld or permitted to wear off when assessment of motor function during neurosurgery is planned.

Fluid and Electrolyte Management

Meticulous fluid management is critical in the care of neurosurgical patients who are children. Diminutive size and immature renal function make fluid and electrolyte imbalances common. Water freely diffuses through the BBB and disruptions in tight junctions, and inequality of pressure gradients in osmolality, hydrostatic pressure, and colloid oncotic pressure facilitate the net movement of fluid across the BBB into the brain, resulting in increased ICP. Osmolar gradients are maintained only when the BBB is intact; when it is disrupted, large molecules that are typically excluded, such as albumin, enter the brain and can worsen edema.

There is no absolute formula for volume replacement in pediatric neuroanesthesia. Hemodynamic stability during intracranial surgery requires careful maintenance of intravascular volume, but preoperative fluid restriction or diuretic therapy may lead to blood pressure instability and even cardiovascular collapse if sudden blood loss occurs during surgery. Therefore, normovolemia should be maintained throughout the procedure. Estimation of the patient's blood volume is essential in determining the amount of allowable blood loss and when to transfuse blood. Blood volume depends on the age and size of the patient.

Normal saline is commonly used as the maintenance fluid during neurosurgery because it is mildly hyperosmolar (308 mOsm/kg) and should minimize cerebral edema. Isotonic crystalloid solutions are commonly used during anesthesia and for cerebral resuscitation. However, rapid infusion of large quantities of normal saline (>60 mL/kg) can be associated with hyperchloremic acidosis (Scheingraber et al., 1999). The calculated maintenance rate of fluid administration depends on the weight of the patient (Holliday and Segar, 1957). These rates are based on normal physiologic conditions. Increases in insensible losses, blood loss, or other conditions such as diabetes insipidus or the syndrome of inappropriate antidiuretic hormone excretion, as noted later, should be considered when determining the proper amount of fluid administration. Depending on the extent and length of the surgical procedure and the exposure of vascular beds, additional fluid administration (3 to 10 mL/kg per hour) may be necessary. Unlike adults, children can become hypovolemic from scalp injuries and isolated traumatic brain injury. Hypotonic crystalloids should be avoided, and the role of colloids is controversial. In 2007, the SAFE study reported that patients with TBI who received fluid resuscitation with albumin had higher mortality rates than those who received fluids with crystalloids (Myburgh et al., 2007). The use of hydroxyethyl starch is discouraged because of its role in exacerbating coagulopathy. Hypertonic saline (0.1 to 1.0 mL/kg) may be used to increase CPP, but, in this setting, well-conducted studies show that there is no advantage to hypertonic saline compared with conventional prehospital fluid protocols (Cooper et al., 2004), and the very large, randomized SAFE trial found that there was no difference in 28-day survival between albumin and saline resuscitation for intensive care patients. However, in a subgroup of patients with TBI, fluid resuscitation with albumin was noted to have higher mortality rates than resuscitation with crystalloid (Myburgh et al., 2007).

Because the potential for significant blood loss is likely in most craniotomies in infants and children, the maximum allowable blood loss should be determined in advance to know when blood should be transfused to the patient. However, there are no guidelines regarding an appropriate threshold for transfusing blood, as it is unclear what hematocrit is needed for optimal oxygen delivery for the pediatric brain and in different disease states. Thus, the decision to transfuse should be dictated by the type of surgery, underlying medical condition of the patient, and potential for additional blood loss both intraoperatively and postoperatively. Hematocrits of 17% to 25 % may warrant blood transfusion. Packed red blood cells (10 mL/kg) raise the hematocrit by 10%. Blood losses may be replaced with 3 mL of normal saline per 1 mL of loss blood, or a colloid solution such as 5% albumin equal to the volume of blood loss. It can be difficult to accurately estimate blood loss during intracranial procedures, as the anesthesiologist may have a compromised view of the surgical field, and blood loss may be hidden in the drapes or elsewhere.

Infants are at particular risk for perioperative hypoglycemia. Small premature neonates, with limited reserves of glycogen and limited gluconeogenesis, require continuous infusions of glucose at 5 to 6 mg/kg per minute to maintain serum levels. At the same time, the stress of critical illness and resulting insulin resistance can produce hyperglycemia that, in turn, is associated with neurologic injury (Jeremitsky et al., 2005; Van den Berghe et al., 2005) and poor outcomes in adults (Van den Berghe et al., 2001). However, it is unclear if tight glycemic control offers significant benefits to children (Branco and Tasker, 2007; Klein et al., 2007). Limited evidence now suggests that tight control may carry undue risk of hypoglycemia, and newer data are less supportive of very tight glycemic control (Van den Berghe et al., 2006). Retrospective studies from children suggest that both hyperglycemia (glucose level at 200 to 250 mg/100 mL) and hypoglycemia occur after TBI (Sharma et al., 2009), and that hyperglycemia is associated with poor outcome. Continuous intraoperative monitoring is not yet the standard of care. Hourly glucose checks are recommended.

Brain swelling can occur during neurosurgical procedures, with devastating consequences. Aggressive hyperventilation should be reserved for when herniation is impending and immediate life-saving maneuvers are required. However, a study in adults demonstrated that moderate hyperventilation may improve surgical conditions (Gelb et al., 2008). There is considerable evidence in patients with TBI that even mild hyperventilation leads to hypoperfusion (Coles et al., 2002). Although there are no data suggesting such a phenomenon in other neurosurgical patient populations, other methods of reducing intracranial pressure can be used. Elevation of the head above the heart and the use of hyperosmolar therapy (e.g., mannitol or hypertonic saline) are generally used initially.

Mannitol (0.25 to 0.5 g/kg) transiently alters cerebral hemodynamics and raises serum osmolality by 10 to 20 mOsm/kg (Soriano et al., 1996). However, repeated dosing can lead to extreme hyperosmolality, renal failure, and further brain edema. Hypertonic saline increases serum sodium, decreases ICP, and increases CPP titrated to a serum sodium rate change and brain edema (Khanna et al., 2000). Administration is typically 3 mL/kg

of 3% (hypertonic) saline targeted to a serum sodium rate change of 0.05 mEq/hr and serum sodium levels of 155 to 160 mEq/L. However, the endpoints depend on the initial serum sodium and the degree of brain edema (typically 155 to 160 mEq/L). Three percent normal saline is generally administered centrally to avoid phlebitis and tissue necrosis, but hypertonic saline concentrations of 2% may be administrated peripherally. Theoretical risks include central pontine myelinolysis and renal failure. Furosemide is a useful adjunct to mannitol for decreasing acute cerebral edema and has been shown in vitro to prevent rebound swelling caused by mannitol (McManus and Soriano, 1998; Thenuwara et al., 2002).

Nonosmotic secretion of antidiuretic hormone (ADH) makes hyponatremia common after neurosurgery. Elevated ADH levels can result from a variety of stimuli, ranging from pain and nausea to fluid shifts and intravascular hypovolemia. Acute hyponatremia can provoke seizures and can be treated with hypertonic saline, fluid restriction, and diuretics (Porzio et al., 2000). The syndrome of cerebral salt wasting is also common in children and can be seen after head trauma and all manner of neurosurgical procedures. The syndrome has been diagnosed with increasing frequency and reported in association with meningitis (Celik et al., 2005), calvarial remodeling (Levine et al., 2001; Byeon and Yoo, 2005), tumor resection (Jimenez et al., 2006), and even hydrocephalus (Table 22-7). Although it is easily confused with other entities (Singh et al., 2002), a recent retrospective review put its incidence at 11.3 per 1000 procedures (Jimenez et al., 2006). In these patients, the mean duration of symptoms was 6 days, with a range of 1 to 5. Cerebral salt wasting, the result of excessively high atrial or brain natriuretic peptide levels (Berger et al., 2002), is marked by hyponatremia, hypovolemia, and excessive urinary excretion of sodium. Although the classic treatment involves saline administration, more rapid resolution has been achieved with fludrocortisone (Papadimitriou et al., 2007).

Diabetes insipidus is a well-known complication of surgical procedures involving or adjacent to the pituitary and hypothalamus. It is most frequently seen in association with craniopharyngioma, where it can be a manifesting symptom in 40% of cases (Ghirardello et al., 2006). Diabetes insipidus is recognized by a rising serum sodium (>145 mg/dL) accompanied by copious (>4 mL/kg per hour) output of dilute urine. Severe

TABLE 22-7. Comparison of Syndrome of Inappropriate Antidiuretic Hormone (SIADH), Cerebral Salt Wasting (CSW), and Diabetes Insipidus

	SIADH	CSW	Diabetes Insipidus
CVP	High (>5)	Low(<5)	Low
UOP	Decreased	Increased	Increased
Urine sodium	High (>20 mmol/L)	High (>20 mmol/L)	< 20 mmol/L
Urine osmolarity	High	Low or normal	Low
Serum osmolarity	Low	Low or normal	High
ADH	High	Normal	—

ADH, Antidiuretic hormone; *CVP,* central venous pressure; *UOP,* urinary osmotic pressure.

dehydration and hypovolemia may develop. One effective protocol employs maximal antidiuresis with IV vasopressin and strict limitation of IV fluids (Wise-Faberowski et al., 2004). This strategy avoids the pitfalls of titrating drug to urine output and recognizes that renal blood flow remains normal in the normovolemic, but maximally antidiuresed, child. Because urine output can be minimal (0.5 mL/kg per minute), other clinical markers of volume status must be used.

MONITORING

Patients undergoing major craniotomies are at risk of sudden hemodynamic instability resulting from hemorrhage, venous air emboli, herniation syndromes, or manipulation of cranial nerves. The potential massive blood loss warrants placement of an arterial cannula for continuous invasive blood pressure monitoring as well as for sampling serial blood gases, electrolytes, glucose levels, and hematocrit. The usefulness of central venous catheterization remains controversial. Cannulation of the jugular or subclavian veins with multiorificed catheters in adults is often preferred, particularly when VAE is anticipated. However, these catheters are too large for infants and most small children. In infants, even when VAE occurred, a central venous catheter was frequently not successful for aspirating air, presumably because of the high resistance of the small-gauge catheters used in these patients (Cucchiara and Bowers, 1982). Therefore, the risks of a central venous catheter may outweigh its benefits.

Venous Air Embolus

Venous air embolus can occur during craniotomies in infants and children, primarily because the head of a small child is large in relation to the rest of the body, and it rests above the heart in either the prone or the supine position. Venous sinuses have dural attachments that impede their ability to collapse. Other conduits for VAE include bone, bridging veins, and spinal epidural veins. When air enters the central circulation, right ventricular output is impeded, leading to pulmonary edema and bronchoconstriction and cor pulmonale, cardiovascular collapse, and death in the most severe cases. Air may gain access to the systemic circulation through right-to-left intracardiac shunts. Potential cardiac shunts exist in many healthy infants and children and may become clinically significant if pulmonary hypertension develops acutely after a large air embolism. Paradoxical air emboli may cause cerebral or coronary artery obstruction, with subsequent cerebral infarction or ventricular fibrillation. Although the incidence of VAE is greatest in the sitting position, it has been reported in the lateral, supine, and prone positions. The incidence of VAE in children undergoing suboccipital craniotomy in the sitting position is not significantly different from that in adults, but children appear to have a higher incidence of hypotension and a lower likelihood of successful aspiration of central (intravascular) air (Cucchiara and Bowers, 1982).

Venous air emboli pose a risk during craniotomies in infants and children, primarily because the head of a small child is large in relation to rest of body and rests above the heart in both the prone and supine positions (Harris et al., 1987; Faberowski et al., 2000). Standard neurosurgical techniques may elevate

the patient's head even further by elevating the head of the table to improve cerebral venous drainage, which can increase the risk for air entrainment into the venous system through open venous channels in bone and sinuses (Grady et al., 1986). Patients with cardiac defects with potential for right-to-left shunting, such as patent foramen ovale or a patent ductus arteriosus, are at high risk for paradoxical air emboli leading to cerebral or myocardial infarction.

Prompt recognition of VAE is crucial to successful management (Fig. 22-10). Precordial Doppler ultrasonography has been demonstrated to be the earliest and most sensitive indicator of intracranial air. It enables diagnosis before the pathologic consequences occur. The Doppler probe is best positioned on the anterior chest, usually just over or to the right of the sternum at the fourth intercostal space (i.e., the nipple line). An alternative site between the scapulae on the posterior thorax can be used in infants in the prone position weighing approximately 6 kg or less (Soriano et al., 1994). Doppler positioning can be confirmed by listening for the characteristic change in sounds after rapid administration of a few milliliters of saline into a central or peripheral venous catheter. When VAE occurs, there is reflex pulmonary vasoconstriction and ventilation/perfusion mismatch caused by the air blocking passage of blood. This reflex results in increased dead-space ventilation and causes a sudden decrease in end-tidal CO_2 concentration. Monitoring the end-tidal CO_2 concentration is very useful in making the diagnosis and can be used to monitor the severity and duration of air emboli. An increase in end-tidal nitrogen concentration during continuous monitoring is a specific sign of air emboli, but it is usually of such small magnitude that it is difficult to detect with devices currently available in clinical practice. Increases in right atrial and pulmonary artery pressures correlate with the size of emboli, but these delayed findings alone should not be relied on for monitoring and diagnosis. Echocardiography (transthoracic or transesophageal) may be the most specific method for detecting small air emboli but is not easily used intraoperatively, especially in small infants and children. In addition to the

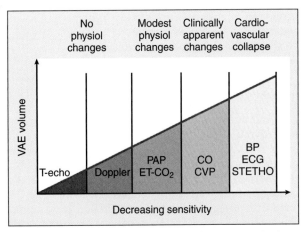

■ **FIGURE 22-10.** The relative sensitivities of various monitoring techniques to the occurrence of venous air embolism (*VAE*). *BP,* Blood pressure; *CO,* cardiac output; *CVP,* central venous pressure; *ECG,* electrocardiogram; *ET-CO₂,* end-tidal CO_2; *PAP,* pulmonary arterial pressure; physiol, physiologic; *T-echo,* transesophageal echo. (*From Miller RD, Eriksson LI, Fleisher LA, et al., editors: Miller's anesthesia, ed 7, Philadelphia, 2010, Churchill Livingstone.*)

characteristic changes in Doppler sounds, sudden decreases in end-tidal CO_2, dysrhythmias, and ischemic changes in the electrocardiogram can occur with VAE.

Aspiration of air from a central venous catheter is rarely successful unless massive amounts have been entrained. If small venous air emboli are detected by other devices (e.g., Doppler, end-tidal CO_2), the value of central venous catheter aspiration for air is quite limited. As soon as a change in Doppler sounds is noted during surgery (and not believed to be caused by administration of IV medications), the surgeon should be informed and nitrous oxide and inhalation agents discontinued. Attempts should immediately be made to identify and occlude the site of air entry, either by flooding the operative field with saline when appropriate (such as during a posterior fossa craniotomy) or by applying bone wax to bone edges. The head of the table can be lowered if necessary, which will have the effect of increasing cerebral venous pressure and stopping entrainment of air as well as augmenting the patient's peripheral venous return and increasing systemic blood pressure. Jugular veins can be compressed manually, although great care must be taken to avoid simultaneous compression of the carotid arteries. Attempts can be made to aspirate air through a central venous catheter if one is in place. The application of positive end-expiratory pressure increases central venous pressure but also decreases cardiac filling pressure, cardiac output, and blood pressure; extreme increases in positive end-expiratory pressure are usually unwarranted. One must be prepared to provide vasopressor support and fluid resuscitation.

Once the patient has been stabilized, the procedure is resumed and a revised anesthesia plan is instituted. The decision to administer nitrous oxide after successful treatment of VAE is controversial. If reinstitution of nitrous oxide is associated with another decrease in end-tidal CO_2 concentration or clinical deterioration, then residual air bubbles are probably present and nitrous oxide should be discontinued. If no changes occur, many clinicians reinstitute nitrous oxide unless repeated episodes of VAE occur. Hemodynamic support may be necessary to avoid hypotension, maintain adequate cerebral perfusion pressure, and minimize ischemic injury. Therefore, dopamine and epinephrine are effective in supporting systemic pressure and restoring cerebral blood flow, even in very low birth weight infants (Munro et al., 2004).

Neurophysiologic Monitoring

Recent advances in neurophysiologic monitoring have enhanced the ability to safely perform neurosurgical procedures in functional areas of the brain and spinal cord. However, the neurodepressant effects of many commonly used anesthetic agents limit the usefulness of these monitors. In general, electrocorticography (ECoG) and EEG can be used with low levels of volatile anesthetics. Somatosensory evoked potentials used during spinal and brainstem surgery can also be depressed by high levels of volatile agents and, to a lesser extent, nitrous oxide. An anesthetic technique using high-dosage opioids and minimal inhaled agents (<1 MAC) is the most appropriate type of monitoring. Alternatively, total IV anesthesia (TIVA) techniques can be used. Spinal cord and peripheral nerve surgery may require electromyography (EMG) and detection of muscle movement as an endpoint.

TABLE 22-8. Effect of Surgical Brainstem Manipulation

Brainstem Area	Signs	Changes in Monitor
CN V	Hypertension, bradycardia	Arterial pressure, ECG
CN VII	Facial muscle movement	EMG
CN X	Hypotension, bradycardia	Arterial pressure, ECG
Pons, medulla	Arrhythmias, hypotension or hypertension, tachycardia or bradycardia, irregular breathing pattern	ECG, arterial pressure, end-tidal CO_2 monitor

CN, Cranial nerve; *ECG*, electrocardiogram; *EMG*, electromyogram.

Therefore, muscle relaxation should be avoided or discontinued after tracheal intubation to facilitate monitoring. Table 22-2 lists common anesthetics and their effects on various neurophysiologic monitors. Motor evoked potential (MEP) can be used to monitor the integrity of the motor tracts of the spinal cord by stimulating the motor cortex and detecting the action potentials in the corresponding muscle groups (Table 22-8). Volatile anesthetic agents, including nitrous oxide, have a dosage-dependent depressant effect on the MEP. IV anesthetics (propofol, opioids, ketamine, and dexmedetomidine) preserve the MEP.

Monitors of Cerebral Oxygenation

The primary cause of cerebral ischemia in infants and children is cerebral hypoperfusion secondary to systemic arterial hypotension or sustained intracranial hypertension. The four major intraoperative modalities for monitoring cerebral ischemia are EEG, TCD, cerebral oximetry, and jugular bulb catheters.

Electroencephalography

The EEG is the most commonly used monitor for cerebral ischemia and has been intensively investigated during anesthesia. Electroencephalographic waveforms are the summation of excitatory and inhibitory postsynaptic potentials from the superficial layers of the cerebral cortex. Both regional and global ischemias result in profound depression of EEG activity, characterized by an attenuation of high-frequency activity and the appearance of slow waves in the corresponding area (Fig. 22-11). This feature makes the EEG the most reliable intraoperative monitor for focal cerebral ischemia. Direct analysis of the raw EEG by an electrophysiologist is the gold standard for monitoring cerebral ischemia. Conditions in which cerebral perfusion may be compromised can be monitored with scalp EEG electrodes or direct ECoG with subdural strip electrodes. Cerebrovascular disease is rare in infants and children, but two conditions in which EEG monitoring may be beneficial are temporary clipping of cerebral aneurysms and moyamoya disease. Cerebral aneurysm clipping can result in ischemia in the cerebral regions supplied by adjacent arteries. Direct ECoG in the region at risk can detect cerebral ischemic during test occlusion of the aneurysm and can serve as a guide for proper positioning of the aneurysm clip and institution of pharmacologic interventions to improve cerebral perfusion.

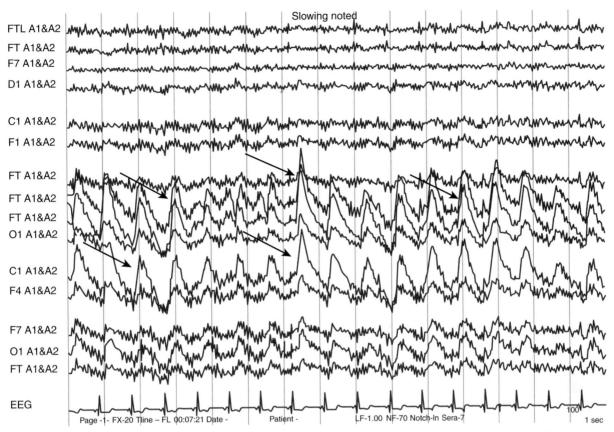

■ FIGURE 22-11. Slowing on the electroencephalogram (EEG). An intraoperative EEG of a child with impaired perfusion of the left hemisphere reveals characteristic waves with slow frequencies and high amplitudes *(arrows)* in the left-side leads.

Jugular Bulb Catheters

Jugular bulb catheters may also be inserted retrograde into the internal jugular using angiocatheters for intermittent sampling, or fiberoptic catheters for continuous readings, and are a useful tool for determining cerebral oxygenation via jugular venous oxygen saturation ($Sjvo_2$). Normal $Sjvo_2$ ranges from 50% to 75%; values at either extreme reflect global ischemia or hyperemia. $Sjvo_2$ monitoring can provide early diagnosis of global ischemia and is useful to guide decisions for optimizing hyperventilation therapy, perfusion pressure, fluid management, and oxygenation in head injury patients (Chan et al., 1992; Skippen et al., 1997). Matta and coworkers (1994) have demonstrated in adults that $Sjvo_2$ monitoring detects critical intraoperative cerebral desaturation that would otherwise have been untreated, and Moss and coworkers (1995) have used $Sjvo_2$ monitoring to determine the minimum blood pressure that should be maintained to avoid hypoperfusion during aneurysm surgery.

Transcranial Doppler

Transcranial Doppler ultrasonography measures cerebral blood flow velocity primarily from the first segment of the middle cerebral artery, and it uses fast Fourier and waveform analysis to provide relative values to flow and resistance. It has been used to detect decreases in CBFV during internal carotid occlusion and carotid endarterectomy, and to monitor for cerebral emboli during cardiopulmonary bypass and neurosurgery. Changes in cerebral hemodynamics caused by pharmacologic interventions can also be measured with the TCD. The major limitation of TCD is stabilization of the Doppler probe over the temporal bone and its inability to provide absolute values of CBF. Nevertheless, changes in systolic and diastolic velocities measured by TCD provide valuable indices and trends in cerebral perfusion and cerebral vascular resistance. Cycles of flow velocities measured in the brain correspond to the phases of the cardiac cycle (systole and diastole) and reflect changes in heart rate. For example, the number of pulses measured reflects the heart rate, and a decrease in diastolic CBFV may indicate altered cerebral vasoreactivity and excessive runoff or steal of CBF. Attention to cerebral venous drainage, pH, and arterial partial pressure of CO_2, mechanical ventilation, and hematocrit levels may be necessary in this circumstance. TCD ultrasonography estimates CBF assuming that changes in CBF changes are proportional to changes in CBFV, and mean flow velocities are used to represent mean CBF. Systolic and diastolic flow velocity parameters are often used to examine resistance of the cerebral vessels and also brain death.

Cerebral Oximetry

Near-infrared spectroscopy (NIRS) provides a noninvasive assessment of cerebral intravascular oxyhemoglobin and deoxyhemoglobin (oxyhemoglobin and deoxyhemoglobin) and mitochondrial cytochrome oxygenation by measuring the abilities of these two chromophores to absorb near-infrared light. Quantitative measurement of changes in cerebral chromophore oxygen (O_2) concentration is related to the overall optical attenuation of near-infrared light, and it has been used to assess O_2 delivery and extraction, cerebral blood volume, CBF (by an indicator dye technique), and the redox state of the brain. NIRS correlated with mean arterial pressure and is effective in identifying premature infants with impaired cerebrovascular autoregulation (Tsuji et al., 2000). The equipment used in these studies is primarily a research prototype and is not commercially produced. Therefore, this technique has yet to find a niche in routine intraoperative monitoring. Regional cerebral oximetry (rSo_2) (INVOS, Somanetics Corporation, Troy, MI) is a simpler NIRS modality that measures relative changes in oxygen extraction in the total blood volume of a small brain area. This technique uses two wavelengths to determine oxyhemoglobin and total cerebral hemoglobin concentrations. Because approximately 75% of the blood volume in the brain is venous, the cerebral oximeter measurement reflects venous oxyhemoglobin saturation and has been reported to correlate with jugular bulb saturation.

Nerve Root Monitoring

Neurosurgical procedures for tethered spinal cord syndrome and spasticity often use EMG monitoring to aid in identification and dissection of the nerve roots. The tethered spinal cord syndrome from spinal dysraphism is associated with conditions such as myelomeningocele, lipoma of the filum terminalis, spina bifida occulta, and adhesions from prior spinal surgery. Identification of functional nerve roots may be difficult and can result in an inadvertent injury during the surgical dissection. EMG monitoring can be helpful for identifying functional nerve roots. Placement of the EMG electrodes in the external anal and urethral (in females) sphincter allows continuous monitoring of the nerve roots supplying the pudendal nerves (S2 to S4). Movement and evoked action potentials of the anterior tibialis and sural muscles can also be detected both visually and by EMG, respectively. Muscle contractions can be readily observed by using clear sterile plastic drapes. Inserting a balloon manometer into the bladder and recording changes in pressure during stimulation can assess detrusor muscle function. Muscle relaxation must be discontinued before stimulation to accurately detect motor activity. The patient should be deeply anesthetized, because direct nerve root stimulation often elicits a significant sympathetic response and pain.

A specific modality for monitoring spinal cord reflexes is the Hoffman reflex (HR), which is a measure of motor neuron excitability and is significantly increased in children with spastic diplegia. This response can be evoked by directly stimulating the nerve root and recording the direct efferent muscle response and the HR (Fig. 22-12). The HR represents the reflex potential emanating from the motor neurons of the spinal cord (Logigian et al., 1994). An abnormal reflex would have an exaggerated HR amplitude. Inhalational agents, nitrous oxide, barbiturates, and benzodiazepines all depress the HR (Soriano et al., 1995). An opioid-based anesthetic with intermittent doses of ketamine or propofol does not appear to suppress the HR. Because the EMG is the observed endpoint of HR, muscle relaxation should be avoided.

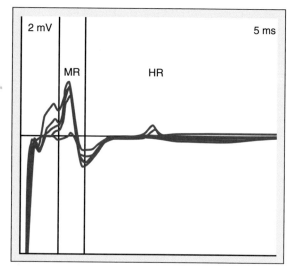

■ **FIGURE 22-12.** The Hoffman reflex *(HR)*. The initial biphasic wave represents the muscle response *(MR)* and is followed by the HR.

SPECIFIC PEDIATRIC NEUROSURGICAL CONDITIONS

Congenital anomalies of the CNS generally occur as midline defects. This dysraphism may occur anywhere along the neural axis involving the head (encephalocele) or spine (meningomyelocele). The defect may be relatively minor and affect only superficial bony and membranous structures, or it may include a large segment of malformed neural tissue.

Encephaloceles

Encephaloceles are neural tube defects that are protrusions of brain and CSF arising from the occiput to the frontal area (Fig. 22-13). They can even look like nasal polyps if they protrude through the cribriform plate. Large defects may present challenges to endotracheal intubation. Much blood loss can occur,

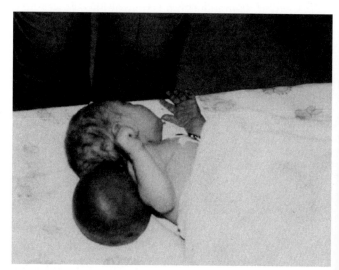

■ **FIGURE 22-13.** A newborn infant with an occipital encephalocele. Neurologic function was intact. The anesthesiologist's primary challenge is to control and intubate the airway in the lateral position to avoid traumatizing the lesion.

especially if venous sinuses are entered. Adequate IV access should be ensured, and blood products should be available.

Myelodysplasia

Defects in the spine are known as spina bifida. If a bulge containing CSF without spinal tissue exists, it is called a meningocele. When neural tissue is also present in the lesion, the defect is called a meningomyelocele. Open neural tissue is known as rachischisis. Hydrocephalus is usually present when paralysis occurs below the lesion and is usually associated with an Arnold-Chiari malformation (see later) (Figs. 22-14 and 22-15).

Most patients with a meningomyelocele present for primary closure within the first day or two of life to minimize the risk of infection. Many are now scheduled electively before birth for repair, because the defect is usually apparent on prenatal ultrasonography. Many neurosurgeons prefer to insert a ventriculoperitoneal shunt at the time of initial surgery. Alternatively, a shunt may be inserted a few days later or even occasionally deferred if there is no evidence of hydrocephalus at birth. A major anesthetic consideration is positioning the neonate for induction at surgery. In most cases, tracheal intubation can be performed with the infant in the supine position and the uninvolved portion of the patient's back supported with towels (or a "donut" ring), so that there is no direct pressure on the meningomyelocele. For very large defects, it is occasionally necessary to place the infant in the lateral position for induction and intubation. Succinylcholine is rarely necessary in these situations, yet it does not appear to cause problems with hyperkalemia because the defect develops early in gestation (Dierdorf et al., 1986).

Airway management, mask fit, and intubation may be difficult for infants with massive hydrocephalus or very large defects. Blood loss may be considerable during repair of a meningomyelocele when large amounts of skin are to be undermined to cover the defect.

Patients with myelodysplasia are at high risk of developing allergic reactions to latex (Holzman, 1997). This is probably a result of repeated exposures to latex products encountered during surgery, including nonneurosurgical procedures required to correct coexisting orthopedic and urologic problems, or repeated bladder catheterizations. Patients who develop latex allergy appear to have an increased incidence of allergic reactions to other substances, including some antibiotics and foods, so anaphylaxis should always be anticipated in these situations. Postoperatively, respiratory status should be carefully assessed. Pulse oximetry is valuable during recovery from anesthesia

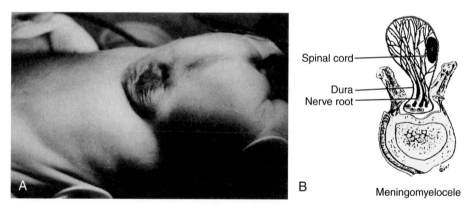

■ **FIGURE 22-14. A,** Newborn infant with a lumbosacral meningomyelocele. Note the partial epithelialization of the neural tissue, which is exposed to air centrally. Neurologic function was severely impaired distal to the defect. **B,** Schematic of meningomyelocele. *(**B,** From Carter S, Gold AP: Nervous system. In Rudolph AM, Barnett HL, Einhorn AH, editors: Pediatrics, ed 16, Norwalk, Conn, 1977, Appleton-Century-Crofts. Copyright 1977, McGraw-Hill.)*

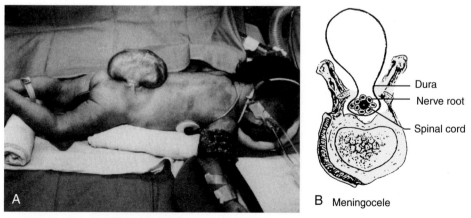

■ **FIGURE 22-15. A,** Newborn infant with a lumbar meningocele. No neural elements were in the sac, and neurologic function was normal distal to the lesion. **B,** Schematic of meningocele. *(**B,** From Carter S, Gold AP: Nervous system. In Rudolph AM, Barnett HL, Einhorn AH, editors: Pediatrics, ed 16, Norwalk, Conn, 1977, Appleton-Century-Crofts. Copyright 1977, McGraw-Hill.)*

because of difficulty with breathing after a tight closure, and because ventilatory responses to hypoxia are often diminished or absent in these patients when a Chiari malformation coexists (Waters et al., 1998).

Spinal dysraphism is the primary indication for laminectomies in pediatric patients. Patients with myelomeningocele suffer from multisystem diseases that result from a severe injury to the developing CNS early in gestation. The systems involved can include the musculoskeletal system, genitourinary system, and immune system in addition to the CNS. These patients suffer frequent exposures to latex products and are at high risk for developing a hypersensitivity to latex. All these patients should be treated with a latex alert, and a true anaphylaxis to latex must be considered when appropriate. Latex allergy can manifest itself by a severe anaphylactic reaction heralded by hypotension and wheezing with or without a rash and should be rapidly treated by removal of the source of latex and administration of IV fluid and vasopressors (Holzman, 1997). Insertion of an epidural catheter by the surgeon under direct vision can provide a conduit for the administration of local anesthetics and opioids for the management of postoperative pain.

Other spinal anomalies (lipomeningoceles, lipomyelomeningoceles, diastematomyelias, and dermoid tracts) may manifest themselves as tethered cords. Children who have had a meningomyelocele repaired after birth may also develop an ascending neurologic deficit from a tethered spinal cord as growth occurs.

The tethered spinal cord syndrome from spinal dysraphism is associated with conditions such as myelomeningocele, lipoma of the filum terminalis, spina bifida occulta, and adhesions from prior spinal surgery. Persistence of this anatomic anomaly can lead to cord or nerve root distortion and impaired perfusion of the spinal cord, resulting in progressive neurologic deficits and chronic pain. Early detection of a tethered cord is now more common with MRI. Visualization and identification of functional nerve roots may be difficult and may result in an inadvertent injury during the surgical dissection. This can lead to fecal and urinary incontinence and exacerbation of lower extremity neurologic dysfunction. EMG monitoring can be helpful for identifying functional nerve roots, as described earlier.

Severe spasticity associated with cerebral palsy can be surgically alleviated by a selective dorsal rhizotomy, which reduces spasticity by surgically dividing dorsal rootlets to diminish the afferent input to motor neurons in the spinal cord, thus decreasing the hyperactive active reflexes associated with spastic diplegia. Pathologic rootlets are identified by direct stimulation and noting the corresponding muscle action potential with EMG. Exaggerated action potentials can be elicited in innervated as well as other distal muscle groups. These abnormal rootlets are partially sectioned to decrease afferent nerve conduction. However, these rootlets may contain sensory and proprioceptive fibers. Spinal cord reflexes can be quantified by measuring the HR (as noted earlier). The postoperative care of these patients is completed by severe somatic incisional pain, dysesthesia, and hyperesthesia of the affected limb and muscle spasms. A variety of postoperative pain management techniques have been advocated in these patients. These include IV morphine, midazolam/diazepam infusions, and epidural opioids (Geiduschek et al., 1997).

Chiari Malformations

Chiari malformations are generally anatomic abnormalities of the posterior fossa leading to cephalad displacement of the cerebellar vermis through the foramen magnum. There are four types of Chiari malformations (Fig. 22-16 and Box 22-1). Type I occurs in healthy children without myelodysplasia. These patients, most of them adolescents, generally have much milder symptoms, sometimes presenting with only headache or neck pain. The Arnold-Chiari malformation (type II) almost always coexists in children with myelodysplasia. This defect consists of a bony abnormality in the posterior fossa and upper cervical spine with caudal displacement of the cerebellar vermis and lower brainstem below the plane of the foramen magnum. Medullary cervical cord compression can occur. Vocal cord paralysis with stridor and respiratory distress, apnea, abnormal swallowing and pulmonary aspiration, opisthotonos, and cranial nerve deficits may be associated with the Arnold-Chiari malformation and usually appear during infancy. Patients of any age may have abnormal responses to hypoxia and hypercarbia because of cranial nerve and brainstem dysfunction (Ward et al., 1986). Extreme head flexion may cause brainstem compression in otherwise asymptomatic patients. Type III Chiari malformations are associated with encephaloceles and have the

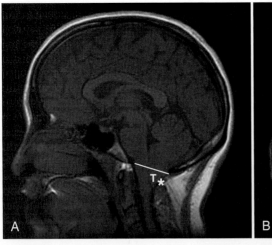
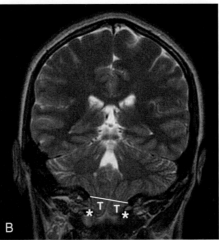

■ **FIGURE 22-16.** Sagittal and coronal MR images of Chiari type I malformation. Note descent of cerebellar tonsils (*T*) below the level of the foramen magnum (*white line*) to the level of the posterior arch (*).

Box 22-1 Chiari Malformations

CHIARI TYPE I

- Tonsillar herniation > 5 mm below the plane of the foramen magnum
- No associated brainstem herniation or supratentorial anomalies
- Low frequency of hydrocephalus

CHIARI TYPE II

- Caudal herniation of the vermis, brainstem, and fourth ventricle
- Associated with myelomeningocele and multiple brain anomalies
- High frequency of hydrocephalus and syringohydromyelia

CHIARI TYPE III

- Occipital encephalocele containing dysmorphic cerebellar and brainstem tissue

CHIARI TYPE IV

- Hypoplasia or aplasia of the cerebellum

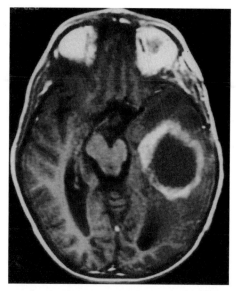

■ **FIGURE 22-17.** MR image of supratentorial tumor. High-grade gliomas are generally less well circumscribed, with irregular enhancement.

most severe symptoms and long-term disability. Type IV is associated with absent cerebellum, and large posterior fossa CSF spaces.

Tumors

Brain tumors are the most common solid tumors in children, which are exceeded only by the leukemias as the most common pediatric malignancy (Pollack, 1994). Supratentorial tumors account for about 25% to 40% of brain tumors in children. Supratentorial resection usually requires invasive monitoring and techniques to control elevated ICP (Fig. 22-17). The majority of brain tumors in children are infratentorial, in the posterior fossa. These include medulloblastomas, cerebellar astrocytomas, brainstem gliomas, and ependymomas of the fourth ventricle (Fig. 22-18). Because posterior fossa tumors usually obstruct CSF flow, increased ICP occurs early. Presenting signs and symptoms include early morning vomiting and irritability or lethargy. Cranial nerve palsies and ataxia are also common findings, with respiratory and cardiac irregularities usually

occurring late. Sedation or general anesthesia may be required for radiologic evaluation or radiation therapy.

Surgical resection of a posterior fossa tumor presents a number of anesthetic challenges. Children are usually positioned prone, although the lateral or sitting positions are used by some neurosurgeons. In any case, the head will be flexed, and the position and patency of the endotracheal tube must be meticulously ensured. A nasotracheal tube is preferred when the patient is prone, as it is easier to secure and less likely to be dislodged. Proper positioning of the endotracheal tube is initially done by confirmation of clear bilateral breath sounds with the head flexed as much as possible while the patient is still supine after intubation is performed. Care should be taken to ensure that all other nasal and oral tubes (e.g., gastric, esophageal) do not cause pressure on the nares or lips, which can lead to edema or erosion after lengthy procedures.

Arrhythmias and acute blood pressure changes may occur during surgical exploration, especially when the brainstem is manipulated, so careful observation of the electrocardiogram

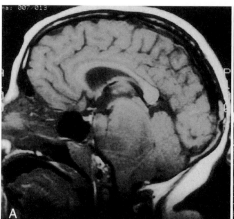
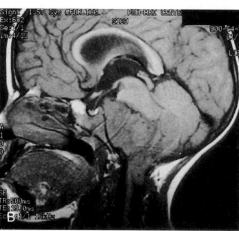

■ **FIGURE 22-18.** MR image of infratentorial tumors. **A,** Brainstem glioma. **B,** Ependymoma displacing the pons and medulla.

and arterial waveform tracing is important. Altered respiratory control is generally masked by muscle relaxants and mechanical ventilation. Intracranial compliance is presumed to decrease even when ICP is only marginally elevated, thus precautions to minimize increases in ICP should be taken. If ICP is markedly elevated or acutely worsens, a ventricular catheter may be inserted by the neurosurgeon prior to tumor resection to permit emergent drainage of CSF. Fixation pins used in small children can cause skull fractures, dural tears, and intracranial hematomas. Elevation of the bone flap can result in sinus tears, massive blood loss, or VAE. Surgical resection of tumors in the posterior fossa can also lead to brainstem and cranial nerve damage. Table 22-8 lists some of the signs of encroachment on these structures. VAE is a potentially serious complication that is not eliminated by the use of the prone or lateral position because head-up gradients of 10 to 20 degrees are frequently used to improve cerebral venous drainage. In infants and toddlers, large head size relative to body size accentuates this problem. Damage to the respiratory centers and cranial nerves can lead to apnea and airway obstruction after extubation of the patient's trachea.

Tumors in the midbrain include craniopharyngiomas, optic gliomas, pituitary adenomas, and hypothalamic tumors and account for approximately 15% of intracranial tumors (Fig. 22-19). Hypothalamic tumors (hamartomas, gliomas, and teratomas) frequently appear with precocious puberty in children who are large for their chronological age. Craniopharyngiomas are the most common perisellar tumors in children and adolescents and may be associated with hypothalamic and pituitary dysfunction. Symptoms often include growth failure, visual impairment, and endocrine abnormalities. Signs and symptoms of hypothyroidism should be sought and thyroid function tests measured. Steroid replacement (dexamethasone or hydrocortisone) is generally administered because the integrity of the hypothalamic-pituitary-adrenal axis may be uncertain. In addition, diabetes insipidus occurs preoperatively in some patients and is a common postoperative problem. A careful history usually reveals this condition preoperatively, especially if attention is focused on nocturnal drinking and enuresis. Evaluation of serum electrolytes and osmolality, urine-specific gravity, and urine output is helpful, because hypernatremia and

hyperosmolality, along with dilute urine, are typical findings. If diabetes insipidus does not exist preoperatively, it usually does not develop until the postoperative period. This occurs because the reserve of antidiuretic hormone in the posterior pituitary gland is enough to allow functioning for many hours even when the hypothalamic-pituitary stalk is damaged intraoperatively. Postoperative diabetes insipidus is marked by a sudden large increase in dilute urine output associated with a rising serum sodium concentration and osmolality. Treatment can initially be with dilute crystalloid solutions to replace the urine output, with careful attention to electrolyte measurements. However, urine output is usually so prodigious (up to 1 L/hr in an adult) that an infusion of aqueous vasopressin (1 to 10 mU/kg per hour) is best used, with fluid input then carefully restricted to match urine replacement and estimates of insensible losses. If diabetes insipidus persists, intranasal desmopressin can be used to replace IV pitressin, because desmopressin generally needs to be administered only twice daily. Return of antidiuretic hormone activity a few days postoperatively may cause a marked decrease in urinary output, water intoxication, seizures, and cerebral edema if desmopressin is not discontinued and fluid administration not adjusted appropriately.

Transsphenoidal surgery is generally performed only in adolescents and older children with pituitary adenomas. However, this procedure should be treated like other midbrain tumors in terms of monitoring and vascular access. Patients are usually intubated orally to give the surgeon optimal access to the nasopharynx, and preparations for an emergent craniotomy should be anticipated in case unexpected massive bleeding develops. Because nasal packs are inserted at the end of surgery, patients should be fully awake prior to tracheal extubation.

Approximately 25% of intracranial tumors in children involve the cerebral hemispheres. These are primarily astrocytomas, oligodendrogliomas, ependymomas, and glioblastomas. Neurologic symptoms are more likely to include a seizure disorder or focal deficits. Succinylcholine should be avoided if motor weakness is present, as it can cause sudden massive hyperkalemia. Nondepolarizing muscle relaxants and narcotics may be metabolized more rapidly than usual in patients receiving chronic anticonvulsants. Choroid plexus papillomas are rare but occur most often in children younger than 3 years. They usually arise from the choroid plexus of the lateral ventricle and produce early hydrocephalus as a result of increased production of CSF and obstruction of CSF flow. Hydrocephalus usually resolves with surgical resection. When lesions lie near the motor or sensory strip, a special type of somatosensory evoked potential monitoring called *phase reversal* may also be used to delineate these important eloquent locations (Hatipoğlu et al., 2009). If cortical stimulation is planned to help identify motor areas, muscle relaxants must be permitted to wear off. Nitrous oxide and narcotics are usually sufficient to prevent patient movement during these periods.

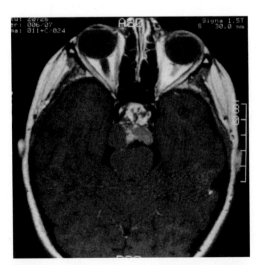

■ **FIGURE 22-19.** MR image of craniopharyngiomas, demonstrating both cystic and solid components.

Hydrocephalus

Hydrocephalus, the most common pediatric neurosurgical condition, involves a mismatch of CSF production and absorption, leading to increased intracranial CSF volume (Fig. 22-20). The majority of cases of hydrocephalus result from obstruction of CSF flow or inability to absorb CSF appropriately. Hemorrhage

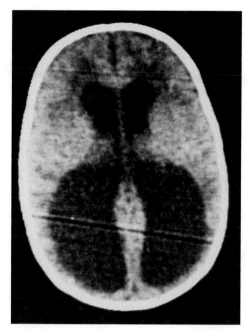

■ **FIGURE 22-20.** Infantile hydrocephalus. CT scan demonstrates a dilated ventricular system and thinning of the cortical mantle. *(Courtesy Division of Neuroradiology, University Health Center of Pittsburgh.)*

(neonatal intraventricular or subarachnoid), congenital problems (aqueductal stenosis), trauma, infection, or tumors (especially in the posterior fossa) can cause hydrocephalus. Hydrocephalus is classified as nonobstructive/communicating or obstructive/noncommunicating based on the ability of CSF to flow around the spinal cord in its usual manner. Unless the etiology of the hydrocephalus can be definitively treated, treatment entails surgical placement of a ventricular drain or ventriculoperitoneal shunt.

Intracranial hypertension or a decrease in intracranial compliance almost always accompanies untreated hydrocephalus in children. How much intracranial compliance exists and how acutely hydrocephalus develops are both instrumental in how severe the signs and symptoms of hydrocephalus will be. In the young infant, if hydrocephalus develops slowly, the skull will insidiously expand and the cerebral vault will expand. However, in older children, the cranial bones are fused or the cranium cannot expand fast enough, and signs of impending herniation rapidly become apparent. The patient may become progressively more lethargic and develop vomiting, cranial nerve dysfunction, bradycardia, and ultimately death.

The approach to patients with symptomatic hydrocephalus should be directed at controlling ICP and rapidly relieving the obstruction. These patients may be vomiting and at risk for pulmonary aspiration. A rapid-sequence induction of anesthesia with thiopental or propofol followed by a succinylcholine or rocuronium is indicated in these situations. Hyperventilation should be instituted as soon as the trachea is intubated.

Unless the etiology of the hydrocephalus can be definitively treated, treatment entails surgical placement of a ventricular shunt. Most shunts transport CSF from the lateral ventricles to the peritoneal cavity (ventriculoperitoneal shunts). Occasionally the distal end of the shunt must be placed in the right atrium or pleural cavity, usually because of problems with the ability of the peritoneal cavity to absorb CSF, as in peritonitis. VAE may occur during placement of the distal end of a ventriculoatrial shunt.

Endoscopic third ventriculoscopy by way of a percutaneous flexible neuroendoscope is an alternative to extracranial shunt placement (Goumnerova and Frim, 1997). During these procedures, a ventriculostomy may be made to bypass an obstruction (such as aqueductal stenosis) by forming a communicating hole from one area of CSF flow to another using a blunt probe inserted through the neuroendoscope (Fig. 22-21). Common locations for a ventriculostomy are through the septum pellucidum (so the lateral ventricles can communicate) or through the floor of the third ventricle into the adjacent CSF cisterns. Complications such as damage to the basilar artery or its branches or neural injuries can be life threatening, and the anesthesiologist should be prepared for an emergency craniotomy during these procedures. Bradycardia and other arrhythmias have also been reported in conjunction with irrigation fluids and manipulation of the floor of the third ventricle (El-Dawlatly et al., 2000).

There are a few special situations involving shunts that anesthesiologists should be familiar with. For example, children who develop a shunt infection usually have their entire shunt system removed and external ventricular drainage established. They return to the operating room for placement of a new system several days later after their infection has been treated with antibiotics. While an external drain is in place, care must be taken not to dislodge the ventricular tubing. In addition, to avoid sudden changes in ICP, the height of the drainage bag should not be changed in relationship to the patient's head. For example, suddenly lowering an open drainage bag can siphon CSF rapidly from the patient, resulting in collapse of the ventricles and rupture of cortical veins. When transporting patients with CSF drainage, or when moving them from a stretcher to an operating room table, it is best to close off the ventriculostomy tubing during these brief periods.

Slit ventricle syndrome develops in approximately 5% to 10% of patients with CSF shunts and is associated with overdrainage of CSF and small, slitlike lateral ventricular spaces. Patients with this condition do not have the usual amount of intracranial CSF to compensate for alterations in brain or intracranial blood volume. Administration of excess or hypotonic IV solutions should be avoided to minimize brain swelling, because postoperative cerebral herniation has been reported after uneventful surgical procedures in these children (Eldredge et al., 1997).

Postoperatively, the patient's mental status should be monitored because of the possibility of the reobstruction of the shunt, leading to life-threatening hydrocephalus.

Craniosynostosis

Craniosynostosis is a congenital anomaly in which one or more cranial sutures close prematurely. It occurs in approximately one of every 2000 births, with males affected more frequently than females. It can involve one suture, or it may be very complex and be associated with a variety of syndromes. If left uncorrected, the deformed cranium can result in increased ICP and compression of the brain, with potential neurologic consequences (Inagaki et al., 2007). Surgical correction is usually performed within the first months of life to achieve the best cosmetic results, because brain growth is very rapid during

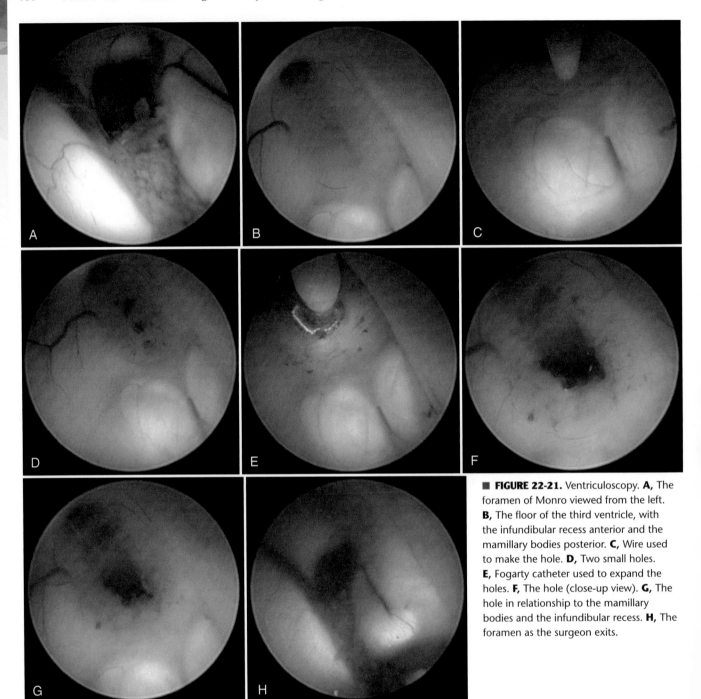

■ **FIGURE 22-21.** Ventriculoscopy. **A,** The foramen of Monro viewed from the left. **B,** The floor of the third ventricle, with the infundibular recess anterior and the mamillary bodies posterior. **C,** Wire used to make the hole. **D,** Two small holes. **E,** Fogarty catheter used to expand the holes. **F,** The hole (close-up view). **G,** The hole in relationship to the mamillary bodies and the infundibular recess. **H,** The foramen as the surgeon exits.

infancy, "pushing" the skull into a normal shape. Repair of craniosynostosis may involve removal of one small strip of bone from the skull, or it may entail a complete reconstruction of the calvarium (see Chapter 25, Anesthesia for Plastic Surgery).

Although these operations are extradural procedures, significant blood loss from the scalp and cranium make them challenging. It is essential that adequate venous access for rapid blood administration be secured, especially if multiple sutures are involved. Antifibrinolytic drugs (tranexamic acid) may have some usefulness in these procedures. The incidence of VAE is also significant during these procedures (Faberowski et al., 2000). Precordial Doppler ultrasonography and end-tidal

CO_2 monitoring are useful for early detection of VAE. Because neuroendoscopic techniques are designed to minimize surgical incision, dissection, and blood loss, less aggressive fluid replacement and invasive hemodynamic monitoring is becoming the norm. The application of endoscopic techniques for craniosynostosis repair has resulted in significantly less morbidity. Endoscopic strip craniectomies are associated with decreased blood loss, decreased surgical time, and improved postoperative recovery time for neonates and infants (Jimenez and Barone, 1998; Jimenez et al., 2002). Tobias and colleagues (2001) reported a significant decrease in the incidence of VAE during this procedure.

Epilepsy

Epilepsy remains one of the most common neurologic disorders in children. Although new pharmacologic interventions have shown promise in the medical management of childhood epilepsy, a large number of children continue to have intractable seizures, and physicians resort to surgical interventions in such situations. Chronic administration of anticonvulsant drugs, such as phenytoin and carbamazepine, induces rapid metabolism and clearance of neuromuscular blockers and opioids by up-regulating hepatic P450 enzymes (Soriano and Martyn, 2004). General anesthetics can compromise the sensitivity of intraoperative neurophysiologic monitors that are used to guide the actual resection of the epileptogenic focus (Eldredge et al., 1995). If cortical stimulation is used to mimic the seizure pattern or identify areas on the motor strip, neuromuscular blockade should be antagonized.

Advances in neurophysiologic monitoring have enhanced the ability to safely perform more definitive neurosurgical resections in functional areas of the brain. A variety of techniques are used during the entire perioperative period to aid in localization of seizure foci. A major part of preoperative planning should include a thorough discussion of the modality and type of neurophysiologic monitoring to be used during the surgical procedure. In general, ECoG and an EEG can be used when the patient is on low levels of volatile anesthetics. Cortical stimulation of the motor cortex necessitates observation of motor movement of the specific area of the homunculus. Therefore, muscle relaxation should be avoided, or permitted to dissipate, during the monitoring period. ECoG is typically recorded continuously on a polygraph via a grid and strip electrodes placed on the surface of the brain after dural opening. Because some epileptogenic foci are in close proximity to cortical areas controlling speech, memory, and motor or sensory function, monitoring of patient and electrophysiologic responses is frequently used to minimize iatrogenic injury to these areas (Adelson et al., 1995; Ojemann et al., 2003). Cortical stimulation of the motor strip in a child under general anesthesia will require either EMG or direct visualization of muscle movement. Neuromuscular blockade should not be used in this situation. Cortical stimulation is possible using a dual channel stimulator. Epileptogenic activity may be evident by either clearly documented electrographic seizures or EEG spike activity, which consists of either interictal spikes of 50 to 80 msec or sharp waves of 80 to 200 msec. During anesthesia, the use of low concentrations of volatile anesthetics or nitrous oxide and opioids alone should avoid attenuating ECoG and EEG recordings.

In patients with generalized seizures, precise localization of the seizure focus is essential to minimize postoperative functional deficits. This involves serial craniotomies. The first is insertion of an intracranial grid and strip electrodes. EEG grids or strips are placed on the exposed cortical surface to accurately create a map that will localize the seizure focus. The patient is then observed in an electrophysiology unit to map the location of the seizure foci and provide a road map for the neurosurgeon for the resection. In some cases, the patient is monitored over several days. Once a seizure map is generated, the patient returns to the operating room for definitive resection. Depending on the location of seizure foci, age, and development of the patient, the resection is performed under general anesthesia or by an awake craniotomy technique. It is important to avoid administration of nitrous oxide until the dura is opened, because intracranial air can persist up to 3 weeks after a craniotomy, and nitrous oxide in these situations can cause rapid expansion of air cavities and result in tension pneumocephalus (Reasoner et al., 1994).

Neural function is best assessed in an awake and cooperative patient (Penfield, 1954). Positioning of the patient is critical for the success of this technique, as the patient must remain still for an extended period of time. The patient should be in a semilateral position to allow patient comfort as well as surgical and airway access to the patient. Motor and sensory cortices are localized by inducing motor movements or sensory changes with cortical stimulation. Language function is tested by eliciting speech arrest with cortical stimulation. Verbal memory is tested by stimulating the hippocampus or lateral temporal cortex. A variety of techniques have been advocated to facilitate intraoperative assessment of motor-sensory function and speech. These range from no sedation with local anesthesia, to asleep-awake-asleep techniques involving general anesthesia induced before and after functional testing (Sarang and Dinsmore, 2003; Brunson and Mayhew, 2005). The asleep-awake-asleep technique entails induction of general anesthesia. The airway is secured either by tracheal intubation or by placement of a laryngeal mask airway. General anesthesia is maintained during the craniotomy. The anesthetic is discontinued to permit functional neurophysiologic testing. Once the testing is completed, general anesthesia is reinstituted and the airway is secured. The advantage of this technique is that the patient is completely anesthetized during the most painful segments of the surgery. However, a major drawback is the depressant effects of residual anesthetics and the inability to predict the patient's response to emerging from anesthesia under the surgical drapes. Therefore, monitored conscious sedation is the most frequently used technique in pediatric patients. Deep levels of sedation with a variety of IV anesthetic and sedative drugs (propofol and dexmedetomidine) combined with an opioid (fentanyl or remifentanil) have been shown to be efficient in several clinical reports (Ard et al., 2003; Keifer et al., 2005; Everett et al., 2006). An important factor in the choice of anesthetic drugs is its effect on the intraoperative ECoG. Therapeutic levels of propofol can potentially depress the ECoG. Propofol, when discontinued 20 minutes before monitoring, did not interfere with the ECoG, in awake cooperative children older than 10 years (Soriano et al., 2000a). However, it is imperative that candidates for an awake craniotomy be mature and psychologically prepared to participate in this procedure. Therefore, patients who are developmentally delayed or have a history of severe anxiety or psychiatric disorders should not be considered appropriate for an awake craniotomy.

Postoperative seizures are an uncommon but devastating complication. Prophylaxis in the perioperative period and aggressive treatment of new convulsions are well-recognized mainstays of care. Phenytoin is the agent used most commonly for prophylaxis, but maintaining therapeutic serum levels can be a challenge (Wolf et al., 2006). Levetiracetam (Keppra) is becoming increasingly common and in many instances supplants phenytoin as the choice for prophylaxis. Both drugs can be administered intravenously, but unlike phenytoin, administration of levetiracetam does not require following serum drug levels to monitor for toxicity. Alternative agents frequently used in pediatrics include phenobarbital, carbamazepine, and valproic acid. Status epilepticus can be treated effectively with lorezepam (0.1 mg/kg IV bolus over 2 minutes) or diazepam

(0.5 mg/kg rectally). Lorezepam may be repeated after 10 minutes and accompanied by fosphenytoin (20 mg/kg IV or IM) if initial doses are ineffective. Phenobarbital (20 mg/kg) is also an effective first-line antiepileptic drug.

Vascular Malformations

Vascular anomalies are rare in infants and children. Most are congenital lesions that appear early in life. Large arteriovenous malformations (AVMs) in neonates may be associated with high-output congestive heart failure and require vasoactive support. Initial treatment of large AVMs often consists of several treatments involving intravascular embolization in the interventional radiology suite (Burrows and Robertson, 1998). Operative management is commonly associated with massive blood loss. Ligation of an AVM can lead to sudden hypertension with hyperemic cerebral edema (Morgan et al., 1999) and should be treated with vasodilators such as labetalol or nitroprusside.

Moyamoya syndrome is a rare chronic vasoocclusive disorder of the internal carotid arteries that appears as transient ischemic attacks or recurrent strokes (or both) in childhood. The etiology is unknown, but the syndrome can be associated with prior intracranial radiation, neurofibromatosis, Down syndrome, and a variety of hematologic disorders including sickle cell disease. Medical management consists of antiplatelet medications (e.g., aspirin or calcium channel blockers) and surgical management aims to improve blood flow to the ischemic area. The operation involves suturing a scalp artery onto the pial surface of the brain (pial synangiosis). The anesthetic management of these patients is directed at optimizing cerebral perfusion (Soriano et al., 1993); this includes ensuring generous preoperative hydration and maintaining the blood pressure close to the patient's preoperative levels. Maintenance of normocapnia is essential as well, because both hypercapnia and hypocapnia can lead to steal from the ischemic region and further aggravate cerebral ischemia (Kuwabara et al., 1997). A nitrous oxide and narcotic-based anesthetic provides a stable level of anesthesia for these patients and is compatible with intraoperative EEG monitoring. Once the patient emerges from anesthesia, the same maneuvers that optimize cerebral perfusion should be extended into the postoperative period.

Neurotrauma

Neurotrauma primarily includes TBI and spinal cord injury (SCI). TBI is the leading cause of death and disability in children over 1 year of age. Approximately half of children with cervical spine injury have concomitant TBI, and the presence of TBI increases the risk of spine injury. After TBI, mortality is lower for children than for adults (10.4% versus 2.5%), but certain factors predict worse outcomes (Box 22-2). Because secondary injuries can progressively worsen outcome, basic life support algorithms, such as Pediatric Advanced Life Support (PALS) and Advanced Trauma Life Support (ATLS), and the principles of ATLS, including primary and secondary surveys, should be immediately applied. The spine cannot be "cleared" by radiographic examination alone; a child with normal cervical spine radiographs should be maintained with cervical spine immobilization until a thorough examination can be performed.

Box 22-2 Predictors of Poor Outcome after Traumatic Brain Injury in Children

- Age < 4 years
- Cardiopulmonary resuscitation needed
- Multiple trauma
- Hypoxia (Pao_2 < 60 mm Hg)
- Hyperventilation ($Paco_2$ < 35 mm Hg)
- Hyperglycemia (glucose > 250 mg/dL)
- Hyperthermia (temperature > 38° C)
- Hypotension (systolic blood pressure < 5th percentile for age)
- Intracranial hypertension (intracranial pressure > 20 mm Hg)
- Poor rehabilitation

In children, cervical spine fractures can occur without neurologic deficit, and neurologic deficit can occur without fracture. Neurologic deficit without fracture has been termed SCIWORA (SCI without radiologic abnormalities). Most children undergo an MRI evaluation. Blunt abdominal trauma and long-bone fractures may occur with TBI/SCI and can be major sources of blood loss. Craniotomies for the evacuation of either epidural or subdural hematomas are at high risk for massive blood loss and VAE. Infants with inflicted trauma often present with a myriad of chronic and acute subdural hematomas (Duhaime et al., 1998). Most inflicted injuries involving death involve TBI. Children with inflicted TBI (iTBI) commonly present with altered consciousness, coma, seizures, vomiting, or irritability, and either injuries out of proportion to history or developmental milestones or incomplete histories. Types of injuries include subdural hematoma, subarachnoid hemorrhage, skull fractures, and diffuse axonal injury with or without cerebral edema. Outcome is poor after iTBI.

Cerebral Hemodynamics after TBI

Cerebral Metabolic Rate, Blood Flow, Autoregulation, and CO₂ Reactivity

During the first 6 to 12 hours after TBI, the brain may suffer poor perfusion and cerebral ischemia. This may be followed by hyperemia and ICP. Finally, vasospasm occurs in up to 19% of patients with TBI, and poor perfusion may occur (White et al., 2001). Compared with children without TBI, children with TBI have a lower V_{MCA}, and cerebral hypoperfusion (CBF < 25 mL/100 g per minute) is associated with cerebral ischemia and poor outcome (Adelson et al., 1997; Skippen et al., 1997). However, after TBI, CBF and $CMRo_2$ may not be matched, resulting in either cerebral ischemia or hyperemia. As noted before, there are age-related changes in V_{MCA}, CBF, and CMRglu (see Fig. 22-3) (Kennedy and Sokoloff, 1957; Ogawa et al., 1987; Bode and Wais, 1988; Vink et al., 1988). One study of 30 children showed CO_2 vasoreactivity changes of less than 2% to be associated with poor outcome (Adelson et al., 1997). Cerebral autoregulation is impaired more often after severe (42%) than after mild (17%) pediatric TBI (Stoyka and Schutz, 1975; Bouma et al., 1998; Vavilala et al., 2004, 2007), and autoregulation may be more impaired in children with iTBI (Vavilala et al., 2007). Hemispheric differences in cerebral autoregulation are common (40%) after focal TBI (Vavilala et al., 2008). If cerebral autoregulation is impaired, lower blood pressure may passively

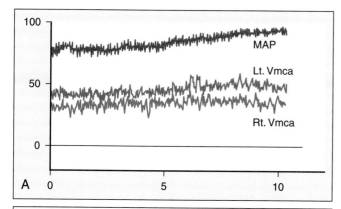

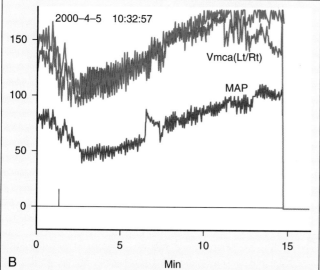

■ **FIGURE 22-22. A,** Intact cerebral autoregulation. There is relatively little change in cerebral blood flow velocity (CBFV) with increase in mean arterial pressure (*MAP*). **B,** Impaired cerebral autoregulation. There is a linear increase in CBFV with increase in MAP.

result in diminished CPP and CBF (Fig. 22-22). Autoregulation is not a static condition and may deteriorate in patients with initially intact autoregulatory capacity. Empirically increasing MAP to prevent cerebral ischemia in the presence of unilaterally impaired cerebral autoregulation in the presence of hyperemia could result in cerebral hemorrhage (Bruce et al., 1981; Aldrich et al., 1992; Mandera et al., 2002). Impaired cerebral autoregulation has been associated with poor outcome after pediatric TBI (Vavilala et al., 2006, 2007).

Cerebral Perfusion Pressure

In 2003, pediatric guidelines issued by a number of organizations recommended that a CPP of less than 40 mm Hg be avoided after severe TBI to prevent cerebral hypoperfusion leading to cerebral ischemia (Adelson et al., 2003). However, although it is not well understood, there is probably an age-dependent CPP threshold, with older children with TBI requiring higher CPP (Chambers et al., 2005, 2006). Furthermore, there may be variability (low and high) in CBFV, despite a CPP of greater than 40 mm Hg (Philip et al., 2009). These data suggest that empirical CPP management may not have predictable effects on

CBF. However, today, either systolic blood pressure or CPP is used clinically to estimate cerebral perfusion. The presence of Cushing's reflex and autonomic dysfunction might be the only indicators of increased ICP. Although hypotension is defined by a systolic blood pressure below the fifth percentile, in the absence of ICP monitoring and suspected increased ICP, supranormal systolic blood pressure may be needed to maintain CPP. At a minimum, MAP should not be allowed to decrease below values normal for age by using vasopressors. IV phenylephrine infusion is often used to maintain CPP above 50 mm Hg.

Intracranial Pressure and Intracranial Pressure Monitoring

The management of increased ICP in children is similar to that in adults (Fig. 22-23). The indications for ICP monitoring and the treatment threshold for increased ICP are given in the 2003 pediatric guidelines (Adelson et al., 2003). The use of ICP monitoring for infants and children with severe TBI and a Glasgow Coma Scale of 8 or less varies, but it is supported by several clinical studies (Adelson et al., 2003). Symptoms of increased ICP (>20 mm Hg) are nonspecific in children, and intermittent apnea may be its first sign in infancy (Sharples et al., 1995). ICP measurements from ventricular catheters and fiberoptic intraparenchymal transducers have a good correlation (Gambardella et al., 1993). Ventricular catheters also provide a conduit for withdrawing CSF.

Intracranial hypertension can be initially managed through elevation of the head, neuromuscular blockade, and hyperosmolar therapy. Mannitol can be given at a dosage of 0.25 to 1.0 g/kg intravenously. All diuretics interfere with the use of urine output as a guide to intravascular volume status. Hypertonic saline (3% NaCl) decreases ICP and increases CPP (Khanna et al., 2000). High-dosage barbiturate therapy can be titrated to produce a burst suppression pattern on the EEG, which results in a reduction in CMR. Refractory ICP can be treated with thiopental infusions, but volume loading and inotropic support may be needed to counter myocardial depression and hypotension (Adelson et al., 2003). If these maneuvers fail to control elevated ICP, decompressive craniectomy should be considered. Careful monitoring of blood gasses, minute ventilation, and end-tidal CO_2 tensions are recommended. Current guidelines recommend maintaining normocapnia (Pa_{CO_2}, 35 to 40 mm Hg) except in the presence of impending herniation.

Anesthetic Management

The anesthetic approach to the traumatized child is based on the principles outlined in the 2003 pediatric guidelines for managing children with severe TBI (Table 22-9; see Fig. 22-23) and on ATLS guidelines and as previously described. Children with a Glasgow Coma Scale score of less than 9 require tracheal intubation for airway protection, and management of increased ICP. The most common approach to tracheal intubation is direct laryngoscopy and oral intubation with cricoid pressure after induction of anesthesia, ventilation with 100% oxygen, and neck in-line stabilization, without traction. Nasotracheal intubations are contraindicated in patients with basilar skull fractures. If increases in ICP occur despite hyperosmolar therapy during surgery, changing from less than 1 MAC volatile anesthesia to TIVA may be considered. Invasive arterial blood pressure monitoring should be used to guide blood pressure management and for hourly sampling of blood gases,

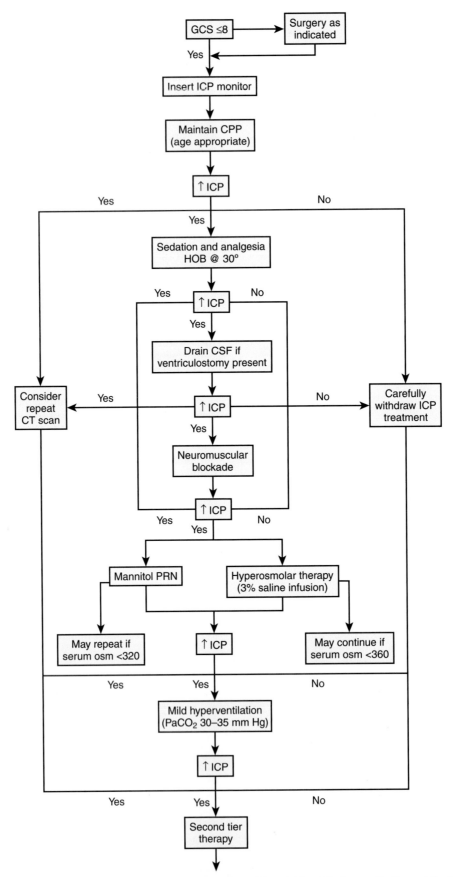

■ **FIGURE 22-23.** Algorithm for intracranial pressure management. *(Adapted from Adelson PD, Bratton SL, Carney NA, et al: Guidelines for the acute medical management of severe traumatic brain injury in infants, children, and adolescents: critical pathway for the treatment of established intracranial hypertension in pediatric traumatic brain injury, Pediatr Crit Care Med 4[3 Suppl]:S65, 2003.)*

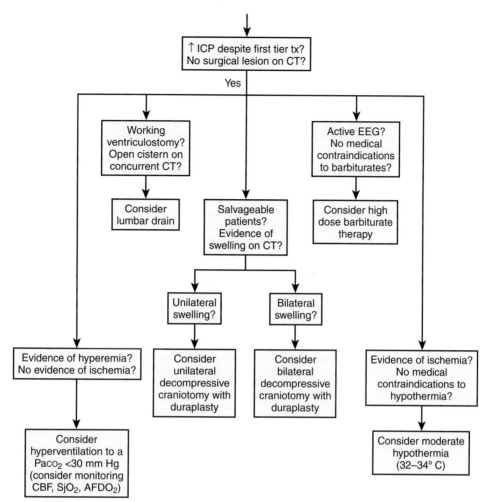

■ **FIGURE 22-23—cont'd.**

TABLE 22-9. Selected 2003 Pediatric Guidelines for the Management of Severe Brain Injury

Physiologic Parameter	Recommendations
Blood glucose	Avoid dextrose-containing solutions Keep blood glucose level at < 200 to 250 mg/dL
Temperature	Avoid hyperthermia: cool patients to 36° to 37° C Hypothermia (32° to 34° C) may be considered for refractory ICP
Cerebral blood flow (CBF) and $Paco_2$	Avoid mild or prophylactic hyperventilation ($Paco_2$ < 35 mm Hg) Mild hyperventilation if acute brainstem herniation exists Mild hyperventilation may be considered for refractory ICP
Systolic blood pressure (SBP)	Hypovolemia should be corrected ASAP SBP should be maintained at the 5th percentile, at least, for age May be beneficial to maintain SBP in normal range (≥50th percentile)
Cerebral perfusion pressure (CPP)	Keep CPP >40 mm Hg CPP 40 to 65 mm Hg may represent an age-related continuum for best treatment
Intracranial pressure (ICP)	Monitor if Glasgow Coma Scale score < 9 Treat ICP ≥20 mm Hg Ventriculostomy or intraparenchymal catheter
Hypertonic solutions	3% saline, 0.1 to 1.0 mL/kg/hr Mannitol, 0.25 to 1.0 g/kg

Adapted from Adelson PD, Bratton SL, Carney NA, et al; American Association for Surgery of Trauma; Child Neurology Society; International Society for Pediatric Neurosurgery; International Trauma Anesthesia and Critical Care Society; Society of Critical Care Medicine; World Federation of Pediatric Intensive and Critical Care Societies: Guidelines for the acute medical management of severe traumatic brain injury in infants, children, and adolescents. Chapter 8: Cerebral perfusion pressure, *Pediatr Crit Care Med* 4(3 Suppl):S31, 2003.

glucose, and coagulation. Central access should be attempted by experienced personnel; intraosseous access is a second-line option if immediate vascular access is required (see Chapter 30, Anesthesia for the Pediatric Trauma Patient). Muscle relaxants should be used in unstable patients, and opioids should be used sparingly in patients with TBI if tracheal extubation is planned for the end of the case. For SCI, when neuromonitoring (including motor evoked potentials) is used, TIVA should be used to maintain anesthesia. Normothermia is currently maintained unless refractory ICP is present.

Indications for Surgery

The major goal of surgery for patients with TBI is to optimize the recovery of viable brain. Most operations deal with the removal of mass lesions to prevent herniation, intracranial hypertension, or alterations in CBF. In general, unless small and deemed likely venous, epidural hematomas should be evacuated in comatose patients. Subdural hematomas that are associated with herniation thicker than 10 mm, or that produce a midline shift of greater than 5 mm, should be removed. Indications on intraparenchymal mass lesions include progressive neurologic deterioration referable to the lesion, signs of mass effect on CT, or refractory intracranial hypertension. Penetrating injury can often be managed with local débridement and watertight closure if not extensive, and if there is minimal intracranial mass effect (see Intracranial Pressure, earlier). Patients with severe brain swelling as manifest by cisternal compression or midline shift on CT, or intracranial hypertension by monitor, are potential candidates for decompressive craniectomy (Taylor et al., 2001). The relatively increased frequency of diffuse swelling in the pediatric population makes children more frequently candidates for such treatment. Generous decompressive craniectomy with duraplasty should be considered when intracranial hypertension reaches or approaches medical refractoriness in salvageable patients when the ICP elevation and its effects are believed to be the major threat to recovery. Unilateral craniectomy is appropriate for lateralized swelling; bifrontal decompression is selected for diffuse disease. In general, surgical removal of mass lesions in comatose patients should be performed as early as safely feasible. As this often involves incompletely resuscitated patients, close collaboration between surgery and anesthesia is critical. Bidirectional communication should be maintained regarding issues such as the stage of the procedure, anticipated and ongoing blood loss, systemic stability, and unanticipated events, so that the procedure can be altered or even terminated if necessary.

Induced Hypothermia

Head cooling and mild hypothermia have been demonstrated to be protective in asphyxiated neonates (Wyatt et al., 2007).

However, induced hypothermia in adult with TBI has mixed results (Clifton et al., 2001). Recently, Adelson and colleagues (2005) demonstrated in a phase II trial that induced hypothermia can be a safe therapeutic option for children with TBI. A National Institutes of Health–sponsored phase III trial is underway. An international multicenter trial of induced hypothermia in pediatric patients reported that hypothermia did not improve the neurologic outcome and may increase mortality (Hutchison et al., 2008). Interestingly, the International Hypothermia in Aneurysm Surgery Trial failed to demonstrate any advantage of hypothermia over normothermia intraoperatively during surgical clipping of intracranial aneurysms (Todd et al., 2005).

Neuroendoscopy

Technological advances in minimally invasive endoscopic surgery have entered the neurosurgical arena. The anesthetic considerations for these evolving techniques are the same as those for other neurosurgical procedures discussed in this chapter. (See the discussion of neuroendoscopic techniques under Craniosynostosis, earlier.) Endoscopic third ventriculostomy is another approach for the treatment of obstructive hydrocephalus in infants and children (Rekate, 2004). A flexible fiberoptic scope inserted through a trocar provides a working channel that allows the neurosurgeon to insert a ventricular catheter or make fenestrations. Despite the relative safety of this procedure, bradycardia and other arrhythmias have been reported in conjunction with lack of egress of irrigation fluids and manipulation of the floor of the third ventricle (El-Dawlatly et al., 2000, 2001).

SUMMARY

The role of the pediatric neuroanesthetist is to provide comprehensive care to children with neurologic pathologies. The cerebral physiology is influenced by the developmental stage of the child. The understanding of the effects of anesthetic agents on the physiology of cerebral vasculature in the pediatric population has significantly increased in the past decade, allowing more rationale decision making in anesthesia management. Although no single anesthetic technique can be recommended, sound knowledge of the principles of cerebral physiology and anesthetic neuropharmacology will facilitate the care of pediatric neurosurgical patients.

For questions and answers on topics in this chapter, go to "Chapter Questions" at www.expertconsult.com.

REFERENCES

Complete references used in this text can be found online at www.expertconsult.com.

Anesthesia for General Abdominal, Thoracic, Urologic, and Bariatric Surgery

CHAPTER

23

Gregory Hammer, Steven Hall, and Peter J. Davis

CONTENTS

In this chapter, the anesthetic considerations of the most common general abdominal, thoracic, urologic, and bariatric procedures are summarized. Practical suggestions and discussions of anesthetic techniques and anesthetic concerns for common surgical problems are offered.

For the most part, anesthetic considerations for pediatric general surgery are similar to those for adults. Inhalation anesthesia supplemented with muscle relaxants can provide adequate operating conditions. Nitrous oxide should be avoided in the presence of a bowel obstruction and when one-lung anesthesia may render the patient hypoxemic. When aspiration of gastric contents is a major concern, either rapid-sequence induction or awake intubation should be performed. Because children about to undergo urgent emergency surgery frequently have fluid and electrolyte imbalances as well as underlying hemodynamic instability, a thorough preoperative assessment of the patient is essential. Anesthetic agents are selected to render the patient unconscious, but, in addition, regional anesthesia is used to provide the child with perioperative pain relief. The details of the regional techniques of caudal, lumbar epidural anesthesia, ilioinguinal/iliohypogastric nerve block, penile nerve block, and intercostal nerve block are discussed in Chapter 16, Regional

Anesthesia. The planned operative approach influences anesthetic management. As the frontiers of minimally invasive surgery expand, these new techniques can markedly influence the patient's cardiorespiratory stability and, consequently, the choice of anesthetic agents.

VIDEO ENDOSCOPY

With the development of smaller instruments, the technological progress in video imaging, and the increasing experience among pediatric surgeons, video endoscopic surgery is being performed for a growing number of pediatric surgical indications. Benefits of video laparoscopy and thoracoscopy include small incisions and scars, reduced surgical intervention and postoperative pain, earlier return of bowel function, and more rapid recovery (Box 23-1) (Reddick and Olsen, 1989; Soper et al., 1992; Rogers et al., 1992; Rodgers, 1993; Soper et al., 1994; Steiner et al., 1994; Sawyers, 1996; Hunter, 1997; Danelli et al., 2002). Fiberoptic endoscopes that can be passed through a needle are now manufactured, and digital video signals can be electronically modified to yield sharp, detailed, color images

Box 23-1 Advantages of Video Endoscopic Surgery in Infants and Children

Improved visualization
Decreased surgical stress
Decreased postoperative pain
Decreased ileus, and earlier return to enteral feeding
Shorter hospitalization
Quicker return to normal activity (parents and patient)
Fewer long-term complications
Cosmetically superior

Box 23-2 Common Pediatric Abdominal Surgical Conditions

Intestinal obstruction
Atresia
Stenosis
Duplication
Volvulus
Meconium ileus
Tumor
Pyloric stenosis
Appendicitis
Meckel's diverticulum
Regional enteritis
Acute necrotizing enterocolitis
Inguinal or umbilical hernia
Biliary atresia
Liver cysts or tumors
Neuroblastoma
Wilms tumor
Hirschsprung's disease
Portal hypertension
Splenomegaly
Ruptured viscus
Exstrophy of the bladder
Tumors of the bladder
Adrenogenital syndrome
Ovarian cysts or tumors

with a minimum light intensity. Digital cameras are designed to maintain an image in an upright orientation regardless of how the telescope is rotated. They are also equipped with an optical or a digital zoom to magnify the image or give the illusion of moving the telescope closer to the object of interest. The smallest of telescopes use fiberoptics and are less than 2 mm in diameter. Two-millimeter disposable ports, mounted on a Veress needle, are used for introduction of these small instruments. Larger instruments and ports are used in larger patients and for more complex cases.

Another major advance in video endoscopic surgery is the development of the endoscopic suite in which all necessary wiring is in equipment booms, ceilings, and walls. The manipulation of digital images is controlled by voice or touch-screen command, either from the operative field or at a conveniently located station nearby. High-quality digital images are displayed on flat-panel monitors that can be positioned within a comfortable viewing range. Remote-controlled cameras can direct any view in the room to any of the monitors or to a remote site. Digital radiographs can be routed from the radiology department to the operating room, and consultants in remote locations can be viewed on monitors in the operating room so that the surgeon can see with whom they are speaking.

An additional feature of newer endoscopy suites is voice-controlled bed positioning. Robotic tools can be vocally directed to position telescopes in the surgical field for optimal viewing; these surgical telemanipulators facilitate microsurgery in confined spaces even in small infants. Other endoscopic robots are being developed for a wide range of surgical applications.

GENERAL ABDOMINAL SURGERY

Abdominal and thoracic pathologic conditions requiring surgical intervention can be caused by metabolic or endocrine disturbances, tumors, inflammatory processes, or embryologic disorders. Box 23-2 lists abdominal conditions commonly encountered in pediatric general surgery.

Laparoscopy

Laparoscopic surgery involves the intraperitoneal or extraperitoneal insufflation of carbon dioxide (CO_2) through a Veress needle. A variable-flow insufflator terminates flow at a preset intraabdominal pressure of up to 15 mm Hg. Once the abdomen is filled with CO_2, the Veress needle is replaced by a cannula

through which a video laparoscope is inserted. Additional ports are placed according to the surgical procedure undertaken.

The laparoscopic procedures that can be performed in infants and children are virtually unlimited. A list of operations currently being performed is shown in Box 23-3. As surgeons gain more experience with laparoscopic surgery, the time required to complete these operations decreases (Fig. 23-1). The safety and efficacy of commonly performed laparoscopic procedures compared with alternative approaches (e.g., endoscopic, open surgical techniques) have been compared (Mattei, 2007; Chertin et al., 2007; Perger et al., 2009).

Laparoscopic gastrostomy involves placement of an umbilical port and a left subcostal cannula (the future site of the gastrostomy). The stomach is pulled to the abdominal wall and the gastrostomy is performed using the Seldinger technique (Fig. 23-2). Operative time is approximately 30 minutes (Tomicic et al., 2002). The risks may be lower than in percutaneous endoscopic gastrostomy in small children, because the procedure is done under direct vision. There is less trauma than with open surgery, and feedings are initiated within 24 hours. Laparoscopic fundoplication for the treatment of gastroesophageal reflux disease is associated with a complication and recurrence rate comparable with or less than that for open surgery (Esposito et al., 2000).

The laparoscopic treatment of appendicitis in children has been controversial, particularly in complicated cases (e.g., gangrene, perforation). Experience indicates, however, that laparoscopic appendectomy is not associated with an increased risk compared with open surgery, even in the presence of perforation (Meguerditchian et al., 2002). The incidence of wound infections and intraabdominal abscesses may be less in laparoscopic than in open appendectomy (Paya et al., 2000). Surgical times are comparable, and postoperative pain and length of

Box 23-3 Laparoscopic Procedures in Infants and Children

ABDOMINAL EXPLORATION
- Infection
- Mass
- Trauma
- Abdominal pain
- Adrenalectomy
- Appendectomy

ABDOMINAL SURGERY
- Diaphragmatic hernia repair
- Fundoplication
- Gastrostomy
- Herniorrhaphy
- Intestinal atresia repair
- Intussusception repair
- Jejunostomy
- Kasai procedure
- Ladd's procedure
- Liver resection
- Nephrectomy
- Oophorectomy
- Orchidopexy
- Orchiectomy
- Ovarian cystectomy
- Pancreatectomy
- Posterior urethral valve repair
- Pull-through
- Hirschsprung's disease procedure
- Imperforate anus
- Splenectomy
- Tenckhoff catheter placement
- Ventriculoperitoneal shunt placement
- Vesicoureteral reimplantation

BARIATRIC PROCEDURES
- Biopsy
- Abscess
- Mass

LIVER AND KIDNEY
- Cholecystectomy
- Colectomy
- Drainage
- Abscess
- Cyst
- Biliary tract

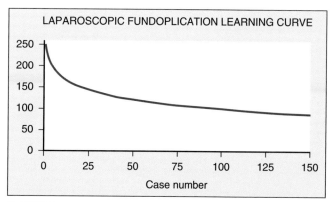

■ **FIGURE 23-1.** The learning curve for laparoscopic fundoplication. *(Adapted from Georgeson KE, Inge TH, Albanese CT: Laparoscopically assisted anorectal pull-through for high imperforate anus: a new technique,* J Pediatr Surg *35:927, 2000.)*

Laparoscopic tumor ablation or curative resection may have a role in selected cases. Open surgery may be required when complete resection of the intact specimen with delineation of surgical margins is part of the protocol design in patients enrolled in multicenter studies. Although advocates of laparoscopic surgery maintain that it can reduce hospital costs, promote earlier patient discharge, produce less postoperative pain, improve cosmetic results, and allow patients a more rapid return to full activity, evidence for this is questionable so far (Rangel et al., 2003).

Anesthetic Considerations

Although regional anesthesia may be used alone in older children, general anesthesia is nearly always used for laparoscopic procedures. The use of the laryngeal mask airway (LMA) has been described in adults undergoing laparoscopy. The reliability of the standard LMA to provide adequate gas exchange during positive pressure ventilation is controversial (Maltby et al., 2000; Lu et al., 2002). More favorable ventilation and a reduction in inadvertent gastric insufflation have been reported with the LMA-ProSeal (Laryngeal Mask Company Limited, Henley on Thames, UK) (Maltby et al., 2002). The pediatric ProSeal LMA has been shown to be effective for short laparoscopic procedures (Sinha et al., 2007). In infants and children, however, endotracheal tube (ETT) placement remains the standard.

After tracheal intubation, the stomach is suctioned with an orogastric tube to decrease the risk for visceral injury during trocar insertion. The surgeon may prefer to place the patient near the foot of the table, especially for procedures in infants. The table position may need to be changed repeatedly during the operation, and both the Trendelenburg and the reverse Trendelenburg positions are often used. Accordingly, care must be taken to secure the patient to the table (e.g., using rolls of gauze and tape) while ensuring that the extremities are well padded and are not subject to inadvertent movement and untoward pressure during the operation. Inadvertent endobronchial intubation may occur as a result of cephalad displacement of the diaphragm associated with the Trendelenburg position or abdominal insufflation with gas. As a part of routine monitoring, a precordial stethoscope should be placed over the left sternal border at the nipple line of the chest to detect this complication readily.

hospital stay are diminished (Canty et al., 2000; Lintula et al., 2001). Comparable results have been reported for laparoscopic cholecystectomy (Esposito et al., 2001) and laparoscopic splenectomy in pediatric patients (Danielson et al., 2000; Park et al., 2000). Infants undergoing laparoscopic pyloromyotomy have shorter times to enteral feeding and hospital discharge (Hall et al., 2009). Diagnostic laparoscopy and laparoscope-guided cholangiography are being used in the evaluation of neonatal conjugated hyperbilirubinemia, avoiding the need for laparotomy and operative cholangiography (Hay et al., 2000).

The role of laparoscopy in the treatment of solid neoplasms is evolving. Indications include biopsy of suspected malignancies, staging or determination of resectability, second-look procedures to help determine response to chemotherapy, and diagnosis of recurrent or metastatic disease (Sailhamer et al., 2003).

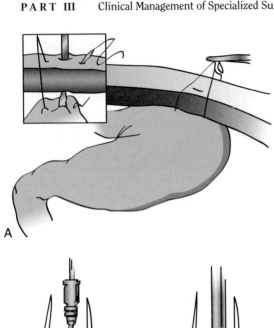

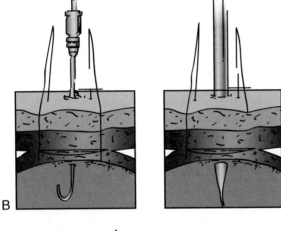

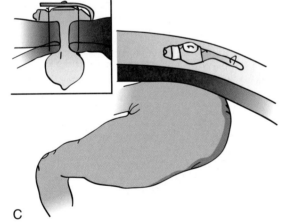

■ **FIGURE 23-2.** Laparoscopic gastrostomy. The stomach is entered and pulled up to the anterior abdominal wall **(A)** and is sutured in place **(B)**. The gastrostomy tube is then placed **(C)**. See related video online at www.expertconsult.com.

A variety of general anesthetic techniques have been used for laparoscopic surgery. Regional anesthesia is not commonly used as an adjunct to general anesthesia in pediatric patients unless the laparoscopy is converted to an open procedure. The use of nitrous oxide is controversial. Concerns have been raised that nitrous oxide may cause bowel distention, compromising visibility and exposure during surgery (Eger and Saidman, 1965; Cunningham and Brull, 1993). In addition, nitrous oxide may exacerbate the already increased incidence of nausea and

vomiting after laparoscopy (Lonie and Harper, 1986; Divatia et al., 1996; Tramer et al., 1996), although the findings of several studies have failed to confirm these effects of nitrous oxide (Taylor et al., 1992; Jensen et al., 1993). However, nitrous oxide can also support combustion. Because of its antiemetic effect, propofol has been recommended for maintenance of anesthesia during laparoscopy (Martin et al., 1993; Song et al., 1998). The combination of propofol and remifentanil has been advocated because the patient emerges rapidly and without an increase in postoperative nausea and vomiting compared with the use of inhalation anesthesia (Grundmann et al., 2001). Because of the increased incidence of postoperative nausea and vomiting associated with laparoscopy, prophylactic treatment with antiemetics and histamine blockers (droperidol, metoclopramide) have been commonly used. Orogastric suctioning at the end of the operation may also help reduce the risk for postoperative nausea and vomiting.

For most surgical procedures, postoperative pain is reduced with laparoscopy compared with open surgery, and postoperative analgesia can usually be achieved with intravenous (IV) and oral agents. Although diminished compared with open surgery, pain after laparoscopic surgery is associated with the incision, visceral manipulation, irritation and traction of nerves, vascular traction and injury, the presence of residual gas in the abdomen, and inflammatory mediators (Alexander, 1997). Pain is frequently localized to the back or shoulder. Laparoscopic repair has been associated with more postoperative pain than open hernia repair (Koivusalo et al., 2009).

A variety of approaches to prevent and treat pain after laparoscopy have been described. Bupivacaine infiltration at incision sites before skin incision has been shown to decrease postoperative pain (Kato et al., 2000; Moiniche et al., 2000). Bupivacaine infiltration has been found to be superior to IV fentanyl or tenoxicam in reducing postoperative pain (Salman et al., 2000). Low-dosage intrathecal morphine and bupivacaine also decrease postoperative pain (Motamed et al., 2000). Intraperitoneal local anesthetic instillation and mesosalpinx block may diminish postoperative pain after laparoscopy and may be beneficial in reducing postoperative shoulder pain (Kiliç et al., 1996). Intraperitoneal instillation of both bupivacaine and meperidine has been shown to be more efficacious than the combination of intraperitoneal bupivacaine and intramuscular meperidine (Colbert et al., 2000).

Caution must be used to avoid toxic plasma concentrations of local anesthetics due to systemic absorption in infants and children, however. Perioperative acetaminophen, nonsteroidal antiinflammatory agents, and other nonopioid analgesics should be used in combination with opioids as needed for postoperative analgesia. Clonidine has been shown to reduce the requirement for postoperative opioids, and it has the advantage of decreasing the tachycardia associated with pneumoperitoneum (Yu et al., 2003).

Physiologic changes during laparoscopic surgery are related to positioning (Trendelenburg, reverse Trendelenburg), increased abdominal pressure resulting from gas insufflation, and increased arterial CO_2 tension associated with insufflation. The magnitude of physiologic changes associated with laparoscopic surgery is influenced by the patient's age, underlying myocardial function, and anesthetic agents. The reverse Trendelenburg position may cause hypotension, especially in the anesthetized patient with intravascular hypovolemia. The Trendelenburg position causes cephalad displacement of the diaphragm, restricting lung excursion and posing a risk for endobronchial intubation. In addition, central venous pressure and heart rate increase, and systemic arterial pressures and cardiac output decrease (Hirvonen et al., 1995). The pulmonary effects depend on the patient's age, weight, pulmonary function, extent of Trendelenburg position, anesthetic agents, and ventilation technique (Sprung et al., 2002). Atelectasis and a decrease in functional residual capacity and pulmonary compliance may be observed. Ventilation/perfusion mismatch may result in decreased arterial oxygen tension. Neuromuscular blockade, endotracheal intubation, and positive pressure ventilation may help to reduce the pulmonary effects of the Trendelenburg position. As long as intraabdominal pressure is kept below 15 mm Hg, oxygen saturation can generally be maintained during position changes and pneumoperitoneum despite adverse changes in respiratory mechanics (Sprung et al., 2003). Significant hypercarbia may occur despite adjustments in mechanical ventilation, especially in infants.

Both pneumoperitoneum and the Trendelenburg position reduce femoral venous flow, increasing the risk for thrombotic complications (Rosen et al., 2000). Cardiovascular instability associated with laparoscopy has also been attributed to hypercarbia-induced arrhythmias, venous gas embolus, compression of the vena cava, pneumothorax, and pneumomediastinum (Lalwani and Aliason, 2009). Insufflation to an intraabdominal pressure of 12 mm Hg can cause septal hypokinesis and left ventricular wall motion abnormalities (Hoymork et al., 2003; Huettemann et al., 2003). The increase in intraabdominal pressure associated with gas insufflation results in increased intrathoracic pressure and increased pulmonary and systemic vascular resistances and decreased cardiac output (Hirvonen et al., 1995, 2000). Arterial blood pressure may be decreased, maintained, or even elevated by an increase in systemic vascular resistance. Reduction in splanchnic, hepatic, and renal blood flow and increases in the plasma concentrations of catecholamines, cortisol, prolactin, growth hormone, and glucose levels have been reported with CO_2 pneumoperitoneum (Hashikura et al., 1994; Mikami et al., 1998; Ishizuka et al., 2000).

Hypothermia is avoided by warming the insufflating gas or by maintaining insufflating flows of less than 2 L/min.

A new technique, known as gasless laparoscopy, eliminates the risks of pneumoperitoneum by using mechanical retraction (Canestrelli et al., 1999). Reduced visualization is associated with this technique, but its application to pediatrics remains uncertain (Lukban et al., 2000).

Inguinal Herniorrhaphy and Umbilical Herniorrhaphy

During the seventh month of gestation, the testicle descends from the abdomen through the inguinal wall into the scrotum. The processus vaginalis, a peritoneal covering, encloses the testicles during their descent. In term infants, the processus vaginalis is usually closed at birth, but it remains patent in 15% to 37% of people. In premature infants, the incidence of closure is much higher, depending on the gestational age at the time of birth. The continued patency of the processus vaginalis is the principal factor in the development of congenital hernias and hydroceles.

Inguinal hernia repair is the most frequent general surgical procedure performed by pediatric surgeons. Males are more frequently affected than females, and the incidence of inguinal

hernia is highest in the first year of life. Right-sided hernias (60%) occur more frequently than left-sided (30%) and bilateral (10%) hernias. Other risk factors associated with inguinal hernias are prematurity, chronic respiratory illness, and excessive intraperitoneal fluid (ventriculoperitoneal shunts, ascites, peritoneal dialysis).

The surgical technique for this procedure is well described (Rowe and Lloyd, 1986). Laparoscopic techniques have also been described (Lobe and Schropp, 1992; Lee and Liang, 2002; Schier et al., 2002), as well as needleoscopic techniques (Prasad et al., 2003). The overall complication rate after an elective hernia repair is about 2%, and it increases to 14% after operations for incarcerated hernia. A major surgical issue in patients with a unilateral inguinal hernia is whether the contralateral side should be explored, thereby subjecting the patient to possible unnecessary damage to the contralateral vas deferens and spermatic cord. In a number of studies, a patent contralateral processus vaginalis occurs about 60% of the time. However, this patency appears to be age related, with the highest rate occurring in infants (63%), and with the incidence decreasing until 2 years of age, when it appears to plateau at 41% (Rowe and Lloyd, 1986). Despite the high incidence of patent processus vaginalis, the incidence of contralateral hernias is about 15%. The development of a contralateral hernia is also age dependent. If the initial hernia developed in the first year of life, there is a fourfold greater chance that a contralateral hernia will develop compared with children whose initial hernia manifested after 1 year of age. In girls with unilateral inguinal hernias, the incidence of positive explorations for contralateral hernias is 60%. Consequently, girls almost always undergo contralateral exploration. Laparoscopy without a separate incision has been advocated to examine the contralateral side for a patent process vaginalis when the ipsilateral hernia sac is of sufficient width to allow passage of a laparoscope (Yerkes et al., 1998) (Fig. 23-3).

Herniorrhaphies are commonly performed as an elective procedure; however, in children with incarceration and signs of bowel obstruction, a rapid-sequence induction with application of cricoid pressure is needed.

The following discussion pertains to elective, uncomplicated hernias. Anesthesia can be induced by mask inhalation of volatile agents or by IV or rectal technique. Endotracheal

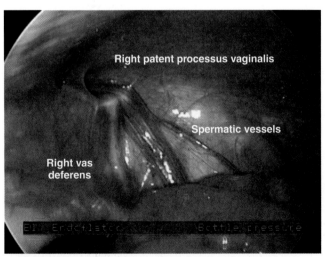

■ **FIGURE 23-3.** Laparoscopic hernia repair with patent process vaginalis.

intubation is usually unnecessary for herniorrhaphy, except in infants younger than 1 year, in whom it may be difficult to maintain an adequate airway with bag and mask ventilation without distending the stomach. However, the use of the LMA in these patients may make tracheal intubation unnecessary. The patient must be well anesthetized when the spermatic cord is being manipulated. Inadequate depth of anesthesia at this stage can result in laryngospasm or bradycardia. Caudal epidural anesthesia or ilioinguinal/iliohypogastric nerve block can be quite effective, both in providing postoperative pain relief and in diminishing the intraoperative anesthetic requirements (Markham et al., 1986). Premature infants have a particularly high incidence of inguinal hernias. In these infants, for whom an inhalation anesthetic may have increased risks, spinal anesthesia (Harnik et al., 1986) and caudal epidural (Spear et al., 1988) anesthesia have been used successfully to avoid general anesthesia and endotracheal intubation (Williams et al., 2006).

Orchiopexy

Cryptorchidism affects approximately 0.8% of 1-year-old boys. The undescended testicle may lie within the abdomen, the inguinal canal, or the external ring just proximal to the scrotum. Although the undescended testicle is usually associated with a hernia, the most significant medical risk for the patient is the chance of developing a malignancy, which is 10-fold greater than in a normally descended one.

The objectives of repair for undescended testicles are to alter the course of the spermatic artery from the renal pedicle to the internal ring to the external ring, and to create in its place a direct line from the renal pedicle to the scrotum. However, the surgical approach to patients with undescended testes is not uniform (Hinman, 1987; Heiss and Shandling, 1992). The general approach to patients with a nonpalpable testis is inguinal exploration. If neither the testis nor proof of its absence is found, the lower posterolateral surface of the peritoneal cavity is explored. When the testis is found, it is either removed or surgically placed in the scrotum. This can be accomplished by a staged orchiopexy, autotransplantation of the testis, or Fowler-Stephens procedure. The Fowler-Stephens approach takes advantage of the vascular arcades between the deferential and spermatic arteries in the cord. Because of this collateral blood flow, high ligation of the testicular vessels can preserve the testicular blood supply and provide the surgeon with mobility in bringing the testicle down into the scrotum. The Fowler-Stephens approach has undergone modification and is now generally done in two stages. The first stage involves clipping the spermatic vessel, whereas the second stage, performed months later, involves the formal orchiopexy. With the advent of laparoscopic surgery, both stages of the Fowler-Stephens approach can be done with the aid of a laparoscope (Atlas and Stone, 1992; Bogaert et al., 1993).

The anesthetic considerations are similar to those for inguinal hernia repair. Because of the traction and manipulation of the spermatic cord and testicle, the incidence of intraoperative bradycardia and laryngospasm is somewhat increased. Consequently, a deeper level of anesthesia is required. However, the need for a deeper plane of anesthesia and the risk for bradycardia and laryngospasm can be lessened by the use of intraoperative nerve blocks or regional anesthesia. If an intraabdominal exploration or the use of laparoscopy is anticipated, the trachea is generally intubated. Because the incidence of postoperative nausea and pain is significant, caudal nerve blocks and prophylactic antiemetics, such as ondansetron (0.1 mg/kg) are recommended.

Surgery for Pyloric Stenosis

Pyloric stenosis is one of the most common gastrointestinal abnormalities appearing in the first 6 months of life. This disorder has a polygenic mode of inheritance and occurs four times more commonly in males and more frequently in white infants. The frequency of this disorder ranges from 1.4 to 8.8 per 1000 live births (Zeidan et al., 1988; Dubé et al., 1990; Saunders and Williams, 1990; Bissonnette and Sullivan, 1991; Murtagh et al., 1992). Some controversy exists regarding the associated risk for pyloric stenosis with the maternal postnatal exposure to macrolides (Louik et al., 2002; Sorensen et al., 2003). Pyloric stenosis has been associated with cleft palate and esophageal reflux.

The cardinal features of pyloric stenosis are projectile vomiting, visible peristalsis, and a hypochloremic, hypokalemic, metabolic alkalosis. Although hypokalemia is a frequent finding, Schwartz and colleagues (2003) reported in a retrospective chart review that 36% of patients with pyloric stenosis were noted to have hyperkalemia. Nonbilious vomiting is the classic presenting symptom and generally occurs between 2 and 8 weeks of age. Jaundice occurs in less than 5% of patients and is thought to be associated with caloric deprivation and hepatic glucuronyl transferase deficiency. The jaundice resolves after successful treatment. Diagnosis is made by palpation of an olive-sized mass in the upper abdomen and is frequently confirmed by radiographic studies. Although false-positive studies are rare, false-negative findings can occur in up to 19% of the ultrasound examinations and in 10% of the contrast studies. Preoperative ultrasound measurements of the pylorus correlate well with intraoperative surgical measurements (Muramori et al., 2007).

The pathologic condition involves gross thickening of the circular muscles of the pylorus, resulting in a gradual obstruction of the gastric outlets. Vanderwinden and coworkers (1992) noted a deficiency of nitric oxide synthetase in the muscle layers of infants with pyloric stenosis. The pathophysiology of pyloric stenosis frequently leads to hypovolemia and a hypochloremic metabolic alkalosis.

Winters (1973) outlined the pathophysiology that leads to hypochloremic, hypokalemic, metabolic alkalosis. In pyloric stenosis, persistent vomiting results in a loss of gastric juices rich in hydrogen and chloride ions and, to a lesser extent, sodium and potassium ions. Because the obstruction is at the level of the pylorus, the vomitus does not contain the usual alkaline secretions of the small intestine; the patient develops a metabolic alkalosis. As an increased bicarbonate load is presented to the kidneys, the resorptive capacity of the proximal tubule is overwhelmed, and an increased amount of $NaHCO_3$ and water is delivered to the distal tubule. Because $NaHCO_3$ cannot be reabsorbed in the distal tubule, aldosterone secretion occurs. Increased aldosterone increases sodium reabsorption and kaliuresis. Potassium loss is further exacerbated by potassium being exchanged in the tubule for hydrogen in an effort to maintain normal plasma pH.

With persistent vomiting and intravascular volume depletion, the renal response shifts to maintain the patient's intravascular volume, and sodium conservation occurs. Increased secretion of aldosterone promotes sodium conservation and potassium excretion. In the distal tubule, sodium is also conserved in exchange for hydrogen ions. This may result in a paradoxical aciduria and worsening metabolic alkalosis.

Surgical pyloromyotomy, a relatively simple procedure in the hands of skilled pediatric surgeons, is curative (Fig. 23-4). The operative mortality rates of 10% has declined to less than 0.5%. The surgery can be performed either as an open procedure or laparoscopically. In a comparative study, Campbell and colleagues (2002) noted that laparoscopic pyloromyotomy has become the dominant approach. See related video online at www. expertconsult.com. Hall and coworkers (2009) have shown that laparoscopically performed procedures have shorter times for patients to achieve full enteral feeds and faster hospital discharge times than patients having open pyloromyotomy. However, laparoscopic pyloromyotomy is associated with an increased rate of complications, higher hospital charges, and a reduction in the general surgical resident's operating experience (Campbell et al., 2002). Pyloromyotomy for pyloric stenosis is not a medical emergency that requires immediate surgical intervention. The major anesthetic considerations are recognizing and treating dehydration and acid-base abnormalities before beginning anesthesia. In addition, the patient is at risk for aspirating gastric contents.

The initial therapeutic approach is aimed at repletion of intravascular volume and correction of electrolyte and acid-base abnormalities (e.g., 5% dextrose in 0.45% NaCl with 40 mmol/L of potassium infused at 3 L/m^2 per 24 hours). Most children respond to therapy within 12 to 48 hours, after which surgical correction can proceed in a nonemergent manner. The use of cimetidine has also been shown to rapidly normalize the metabolic alkalosis in patients with hypertrophic pyloric stenosis (Banieghbal, 2009).

Once the child is satisfactorily hydrated and after the appropriate monitors (precordial stethoscope, electrocardiogram, pulse oximeter, and blood pressure cuff) are placed, the infant is ready for induction of anesthesia. The obstructed pylorus and associated vomiting increase the possibility of aspirating gastric contents during induction of anesthesia. A thorough evacuation of stomach contents through a nasogastric or orogastric tube, with proper preoxygenation and monitoring, greatly reduces the chance of regurgitation during induction, although it does not completely eliminate the possibility of aspiration (Cook-Sather et al., 1997). Infants with pyloric stenosis are thus considered by some anesthesiologists to have a status equivalent to that of infants with a full stomach; therefore, a rapid-sequence induction is preferred to secure the airway and minimize the risks of aspiration (Dierdorf and Krishna, 1981; Battersby et al., 1984). On the other hand, mask inhalation induction preceded by careful emptying of the stomach has been used safely in several pediatric centers (MacDonald et al., 1987). In a prospective nonrandomized observational study of 76 infants with pyloric stenosis, Cook-Sather and colleagues (1998) compared three techniques: awake intubation, rapid-sequence intubation, and modified rapid-sequence intubation (ventilation through cricoid pressure). In this study, awake intubation was not superior to anesthetized, paralyzed intubations. Awake intubation prevented neither bradycardia nor oxygen desaturations.

After induction and intubation of the trachea, a nasogastric or an orogastric tube is reinserted and left in place during the operative procedure. This allows the surgeon to test the integrity of the pyloric mucosa after pyloromyotomy. A small volume of air is injected down the nasogastric tube, and the surgeon manipulates the air bubble into the duodenum and occludes the bowel lumen both proximal and distal to the incision. Mucosal perforation is indicated if there is air leakage. After the operation, which usually requires less than 30 minutes, the effects of any nondepolarizing muscle relaxant are reversed. The infant can then be safely extubated when fully awake and with intact protective airway reflexes. Some believe that opioid analgesia is seldom necessary (Battersby et al., 1984) and may predispose patients to a prolonged emergence from anesthesia (MacDonald et al., 1987). It is not unusual to encounter lethargy or drowsiness in these infants in the immediate postoperative period. Respiratory depression has been noted to occur postoperatively and is possibly related to cerebrospinal fluid pH and hyperventilation (Andropoulos et al., 1994). Rare occurrences of hypoglycemia, apnea, convulsions, and cardiac arrest in the early postoperative period have also been cited. These events have been ascribed to the cessation of IV glucose infusions and the depletion of liver glycogen (Shumake, 1975). Infants usually begin oral feedings 8 hours after the procedure. The choice of maintenance anesthetic agent for infants with pyloric stenosis has been studied (Wolf et al., 1996; Chipps et al., 1999; Davis et al., 2001; Galinkin et al., 2001).

Wolf and coworkers (1996) found that clinical postoperative apnea occurred in 3 of 11 infants anesthetized with isoflurane, and in none of the nine infants anesthetized with desflurane. In a multicenter study comparing halothane and remifentanil, where both drugs were administered to similar clinical endpoints, remifentanil was not associated with postoperative respiratory depression. In this study, all infants received both preoperative and postoperative pneumograms, and remifentanil (as opposed to halothane) was not associated with new pneumogram abnormalities in the postoperative period (Davis et al., 2001; Galinkin et al., 2001).

Wilms Tumor Procedures

Wilms tumor is the most common childhood abdominal malignancy, occurring with an incidence, consistent throughout the world, of 5.0 to 7.8 per 1 million children less than 15 years of age. Wilms tumor accounts for about 6% of all malignancies in childhood. The incidence is equal in the two genders. The peak age at diagnosis is between 1 and 3 years. Wilms tumor occurs bilaterally in 5% of patients. Patients with Wilms tumor frequently have associated anomalies (aniridia, 1%; hemihypertrophy, 2%; genitourinary abnormalities, 5%; ectopic and solitary kidneys [horseshoe kidneys, ureteral duplications, hypospadias]). Other associated conditions include Beckwith-Wiedemann syndrome and neurofibromatosis. The signs and symptoms associated with Wilms tumor are variable. The most frequent finding is an increasing abdominal girth with a palpable abdominal mass (85%). Hypertension occurs in 60% of patients, and hematuria is present in 10% to 25%. Acquired von Willebrand's syndrome with Wilms tumor occurs infrequently (Baxter et al., 2009).

Wilms tumor is generally located in the upper or lower renal pole. It may involve the renal vein (10% of cases) and extend up the vena cava to the right atrium (5% of cases) (Fig. 23-5). Prognosis for patients with the disease is related to its staging (Table 23-1). Patients with favorable staging have an 80% to 90%

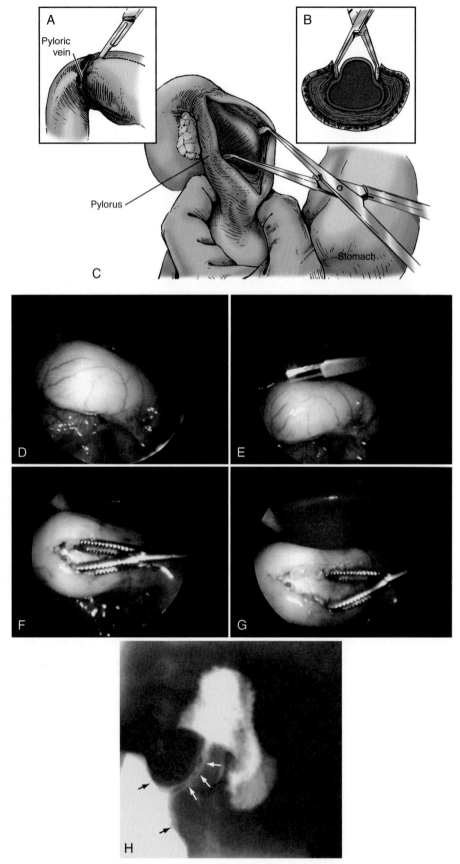

■ **FIGURE 23-4.** Pyloric stenosis. Operative technique of pyloromyotomy: **A,** Incision made on anterosuperior surface through avascular area. **B,** Cross-section of hypertrophied pylorus after operation has been completed. **C,** Circular muscle is separated, allowing submucosa to bulge. Laparoscopic view of pyloromyotomy: **D,** Hypertrophied pyloris. **E,** Incision. **F** and **G,** Spreading the incision to the mucosae. **H,** Upper GI study demonstrates the antral "teat:" shouldering *(black arrows),* and the elongated, narrowed, double-tracked pyloric channel *(white arrows). (**A** to **C,** From Benson CO: Infantile hypertrophic pyloric stenosis. In Welch KJ, et al., editors:* Pediatric surgery, *ed 4, Chicago, 1986, Year Book Medical;* **H** *from Blickman JG, Parker R, Barnes PD:* Pediatric radiology, *St Louis, 2009, Mosby.)*

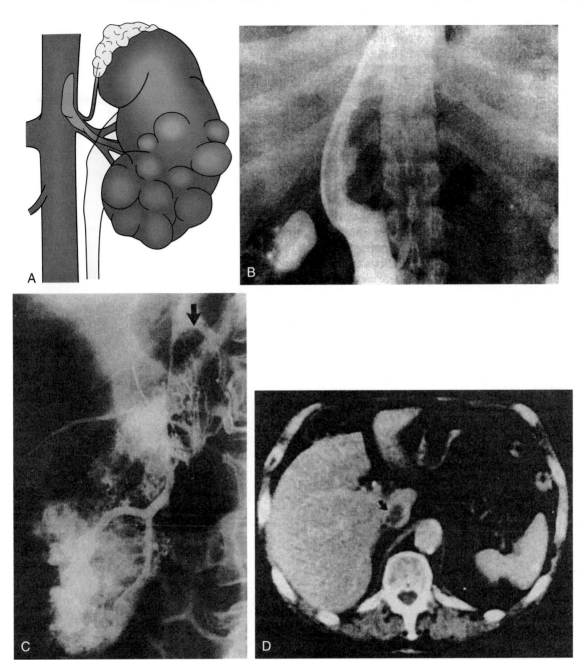

■ **FIGURE 23-5.** Wilms tumor. **A,** Tumor extension into renal vein and inferior vena cava (IVC). **B,** Inferior vena cavagram showing IVC displacement and possible invastion of tumor. **C,** Renal arteriogram feeding vessels into tumor thrombus in IVC. **D,** CT scan of intraluminal thrombus in the IVC. (**A,** From Ehrlich PF: Wilms tumor: progress and considerations for the surgeon, Surg Oncol 16:157, 2007. **B, C,** and **D** from Marks WM, Korobkin M, Callen PW, et al: CT diagnosis of tumor thrombosis of the renal vein and inferior vena cava, Am J Roentgenol 131:843, 1978.)

TABLE 23-1. Wilms Tumor Staging

Stage	Description
I	Tumor limited to the kidneys and excised
II	Tumor extending beyond the kidneys, but completely excised
III	Residual nonhematogenous tumor confined to the abdomen
IV	Hematogenous metastases Lymph node involvement
V	Bilateral renal involvement at diagnosis

chance of cure, whereas patients with metastasis have a 50% chance of long-term survival. Risk factors for local recurrence of Wilms tumor include an advanced local stage (involvement of the paraaortic lymph nodes), unfavorable histology, and spillage of tumor at the time of resection (Shamberger et al., 1999). Overexpression of HER2, an oncoprotein, has been shown to be a good predictor of overall survival and longer recurrence-free survival (Ragab et al., 2010). Therapy for Wilms tumor includes surgery, chemotherapy, and radiotherapy. Depending on the size of the tumor and the staging, chemotherapy may be started either before or after surgery. Chemotherapy generally involves vincristine, actinomycin, and anthracycline (doxorubicin).

Preoperative evaluation of the patient is related to the presence of metastases and the patient's cardiopulmonary function. If the patient has had prior chemotherapy with Adriamycin, cardiac function should be assessed by echocardiography (see Chapter 4, Cardiovascular Physiology, and Chapter 36, Systemic Disorders). Serum electrolyte levels should be assessed if there is a history of vomiting. Renal dysfunction is unusual even in patients with bilateral Wilms tumor. Although the surgical approach is generally an open incision, laparoscopic nephrectomy has been reported for the unilateral removal of tumor (Barber et al., 2009; Duarte et al., 2009). Anesthetic considerations revolve around the issue of abdominal distention with delayed gastric emptying and potentially large intraoperative blood losses. Abdominal distention may place the patient at risk for aspiration of gastric contents, so full-stomach precautions should be taken at the induction of anesthesia. Intraoperative blood loss can be a significant factor because of the tumor's location and possible involvement of the renal vein and vena cava (Cristofani et al., 2007). Two large-bore IV catheters are recommended. Because of the possibility that the vena cava may be cross-clamped (either to be explored for extension of tumor or to control hemorrhage), the large-bore catheters should be inserted above the diaphragm.

Pulmonary function may be compromised because of metastasis, tumor embolization, abdominal distention, or surgical traction. Monitoring of the patient should include pulse oximetry and capnography, as well as the standard monitors of electrocardiography, blood pressure, and esophageal stethoscope. Arterial catheters are generally reserved for patients with large tumors, patients with previous intraabdominal surgery (increased number of adhesions), and patients with significant cardiorespiratory depression.

After induction, anesthesia is maintained with potent inhalation anesthetic agents. Nitrous oxide is avoided because of bowel distention, and opioids are administered to reduce the anesthetic requirements. An alternative approach that provides excellent operative conditions and postoperative pain control is the use of combined general anesthesia with either a continuous epidural infusion or paravertebral catheters.

Neuroblastoma Procedures

Neuroblastoma, the most common extracranial solid tumor of childhood, involves the postganglionic sympathetic nervous system. Fifty percent of tumors arise in the adrenals, 30% occur below the diaphragm, and 20% occur in cervical or thoracic sites. Neuroblastoma accounts for 8% to 10% of pediatric cancer malignancies. The median age at presentation is 22 months, with 37% of patients presenting at less than 1 year of age, and 51% of new patients being less than 4 years of age. Clinical presentation may be related to the primary tumor, to its metastasis, or to the associated paraneoplastic syndromes (Table 23-2). Metastases from neuroblastoma occur in lymph nodes, liver, cortical bone, bone marrow, orbits, and skin. The paraneoplastic syndromes can exhibit hypertension secondary to catecholamine release, or kidney displacement with renal artery stretching and renin-angiotensin stimulus. The gastrointestinal symptoms (diarrhea, flushing, abdominal distention) are attributed to vasoactive intestinal peptides (VIPs), whereas the etiology of opsoclonus and ataxia is unclear.

TABLE 23-2. Presenting Signs and Symptoms of Neuroblastoma

Primary tumor	Abdominal mass or pain
	Respiratory distress or dysphagia
	Vocal cord paralysis
	Bowel or bladder dysfunction
	Horner's syndrome
	Heterochromia of iris on affected side
	Incidental finding on chest radiograph
Metastatic disease	Hepatomegaly
	Lymphadenopathy
	Bone pain
	Periorbital ecchymoses
	Subcutaneous nodules
	Marrow replacement with anemia, fever, or bruising from low blood counts
	Systemic illness
	Failure to thrive
	Fever of unknown origin
Paraneoplastic syndromes	Vasoactive intestinal peptide syndrome (chronic watery diarrhea and abdominal distention)
	Opsoclonus-myoclonus or cerebellar ataxia syndrome
	Excessive catecholamine syndrome (hypertension, headaches, flushing, sweating, tachycardia, palpitations)

Tumor prognosis has been related to age at presentation, extent of disease (staging), degree of tumor differentiation, amount of catecholamine metabolites, serum ferritin level, lactate dehydrogenase level, neuron-specific enolase level, serum lymphocyte count, ganglioside presence, N-myc amplification, deletion of chromosome 1p, additional copies of chromosome 17q, and TRKA expression (Smith et al., 1989; Hiyama et al., 1991; Berthold et al., 1992; Eckschlager, 1992; Murakami et al., 1992; Qualman et al., 1992; Shuster et al., 1992; Haase et al., 1999). However, patient age and tumor stage are the two most important independent variables (Fig. 23-6). The Evans staging system uses tumor location, lymph node involvement, and presence of metastases, whereas the Pediatric Oncology Group system emphasizes tumor resectability and identification of residual disease to predict survival and treatment.

Treatment involves surgical resection and chemotherapy. Although neuroblastoma is radiosensitive, 45% of patients present with metastasis, so the use of radiation is sometimes limited in primary therapy. In a series of adrenal neuroblastomas less than 6 cm not associated with adjacent vessel or organ involvement, DeLagausie and colleagues (2003) reported successful tumor removal with laparoscopic techniques. The anesthetic considerations depend on the planned surgical procedure, the location and size of the tumor, and the metabolic effects of the tumor. Electrolyte imbalance may result from vomiting and diarrhea caused by excessive production of VIP. Despite the production of catecholamines, significant hypertension has been reported in 9% to 30% of patients (Weinblatt et al., 1983; Haberkern et al., 1992).

Intraoperatively, blood loss and third-space fluid losses can accompany the resection of tumor. Haberkern and coworkers (1992) noted in a retrospective review that 45% of patients had hypotension after the tumor excision, whereas fewer than 3% of the patients had cardiovascular signs of increased

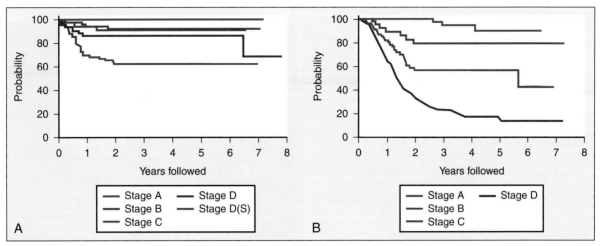

■ **FIGURE 23-6.** Prognoses for patients with neuroblastoma as related to age and staging. **A,** Children less than 1 year of age. **B,** Children older than 1 year. Staging is according to the Pediatric Oncology Group (POG) system. *Stage A:* Complete gross resection of primary tumor, with or without microscopic residua. Intracavitary lymph nodes that are not adhered to and removed with primary (nodes adhered to or within tumor resection may be positive for tumor without upstaging patient to stage C) are histologically free of tumor. If primary is in abdomen or pelvis, liver is histologically free of tumor. *Stage B:* Grossly unresected primary tumor. Nodes and liver are the same as for stage A. *Stage C:* Complete or incomplete resection of primary. Intracavitary nodes not adhered to primary histologically are positive for tumor. Liver as in stage A. *Stage D:* Any dissemination of disease beyond intracavitary nodes: extracavitary nodes, liver, skin, bone marrow, bone. *Stage D(S):* Would be Evans stage I or II except for metastatic tumor in the liver, bone marrow, or skin. *Evans stage I:* Tumor confined to the organ of structure of origin. *Evans stage II:* Tumor extending in continuity beyond the organ or structure of origin but not crossing the midline. Regional lymph nodes on the ipsilateral side may be involved. *(Data courtesy Dr. Jonathan J. Shuster and the Pediatric Oncology Group. From Brodeur GM: Neuroblastoma and other peripheral neuroectodermal tumors. In Fernbach DJ, Viett TJ, editors:* Clinical pediatric oncology, *St Louis, 1991, Mosby.)*

catecholamine release during tumor resection. Although in patients with mediastinal neuroblastoma, airway complications are rare because of the tumor's location in the posterior mediastinum, airway compromise can occur, and evidence of airway compression by the tumor should be evaluated before starting the anesthetic induction. IV or inhalational inductions may be performed. Both volatile agents and opioids have been safely used along with combined regional and general anesthetic techniques (Haberkern et al., 1992).

Anti-Gastroesophageal Reflux Procedures

Gastroesophageal reflux (GER) involves a dysfunction of the esophageal sphincter mechanism that allows gastric contents to return into the esophagus. Thus, GER may place an anesthetized patient at risk for aspiration. The clinical spectrum of GER can range from patients who are completely asymptomatic to patients with severe esophagitis, esophageal bleeding, esophageal stricture, malnutrition, and respiratory compromise. In the pediatric population, GER can be physiologic, secondary to immature maturation of the lower esophageal sphincter mechanism; however, this aspect of GER generally resolves by 15 months of age. GER is also seen in children who are neurologically compromised, as well as in patients who have survived diaphragmatic hernias, tracheoesophageal fistula, and esophageal atresia repairs (Barry and Auldist, 1974). GER has also been noted in about 10% of patients who have undergone successful treatment of pyloric stenosis.

In normal children, reflux of gastric contents is prevented by the gastroesophageal junction. This junction is composed of a lower esophageal sphincter (LES). The LES is a high-pressure zone in the distal esophagus that lies in both the mediastinum and the abdomen and becomes functionally mature by 6 weeks of postnatal age. Factors that affect the valve mechanism of the LES include the cardioesophageal angle of His, the esophageal hiatus (a sling of muscle that is part of the diaphragm), and the phrenoesophageal ligament. The degree of reflux, the duration of acid exposure in the esophagus, the ability of the esophagus to clear its contents, and the extent of mucosal damage are the primary factors that determine the degree of esophagitis and consequently its clinical and pathologic significance.

In pediatric patients, the complications of GER include respiratory compromise (bronchospasm, chronic aspiration with pneumonitis, reactive airways disease, and apnea) and esophagitis (esophageal metaplasia, Barrett's esophagus, stricture, dysphagia). Diagnostic evaluation includes an upper gastrointestinal series, a nuclear scan, an upper endoscopy, and an esophageal pH probe.

Treatment of GER may involve both medical and surgical therapies. Medical therapy consists of both conservative and pharmacologic interventions (thickened feedings, avoidance of overfeeding, postcibal position therapy). The use of medication is aimed at blocking acid secretions using histamine (H_2)-blocker agents (e.g., ranitidine) and improving gastroesophageal motility and gastric emptying (e.g., metoclopramide, bethanechol). Cisapride, a dopamine antagonist, is also used as a motility drug. Its mode of action is postulated to increase the release of acetylcholine from the myenteric plexus and to increase receptor sensitivity to acetylcholine.

Surgical procedures are aimed at establishing an intraabdominal segment of esophagus and creating a physiologic angle of His (Fig. 23-7). The two common procedures are the 360-degree fundoplication of Nissen and the partial wrap of Thal-Nissen. To avoid the gas bloat syndrome (aerophagia, gastric distention, inability to belch or vomit) associated with Nissen fundoplications, the Thal-Nissen partial wrap is frequently used.

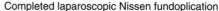
Completed laparoscopic Nissen fundoplication

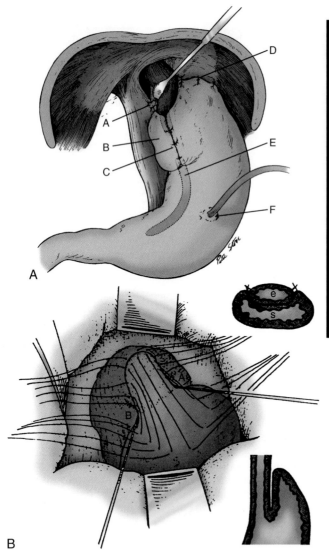

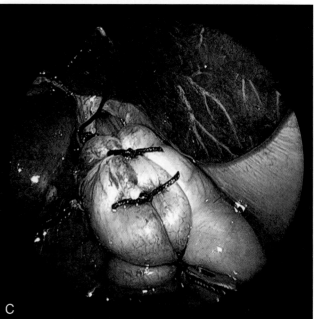

■ **FIGURE 23-7. A**, Salient features of Nissen fundoplication in infants. Crural sutures to reduce hiatus *(A)*. Generous loose, adequate tissue in the wrap *(B)*. Sutures placed through seromuscular depth of both gastric and esophageal walls *(C)*. Sutures to fix the fundus to the diaphragm *(D)*. Appropriately sized mercury-filled dilator to ensure adequate lumen *(E)*. Gastrostomy in all infants and whenever there is any question of gastric outlet problems *(F)*. **B**, The Thal fundoplication. A partial wrap of the fundus is performed anteriorly around the lower esophageal segment. **C**, Laparoscopic view of completed Nissen fundoplication *(A, From Randolph JG: Experience with the Nissen fundoplication for correction of gastroesophageal reflux in infants, Ann Surg 198:579, 1983; illustrated by Peter Stone. B, from Ashcraft KW: Thal fundoplication. In Ashcraft KW, Holder TM, editors: Pediatric esophageal surgery, Orlando, 1986, Grune & Stratton.)*

The surgical procedure can be performed as either an open or a laparoscopic procedure (Randolph, 1983; Georgeson, 1993; Rothenberg, 1998; Bourne et al., 2003; Esposito et al., 2003; Steyaert et al., 2003). See related video online at www.expertconsult.com. The failure rates of the surgical approaches appear to be similar (Lopez et al., 2008), and laparoscopic fundoplications can be performed in children who have had previous open procedures (Barsness et al., 2009). In children undergoing laparoscopic antireflux procedures, the physiologic perturbations of pneumoperitoneum, increased intraabdominal pressure, and the associated absorption of carbon dioxide need to be considered.

Surgical success rates approach 95% in pediatric patients with normal neurologic development, but in children who are neurologically impaired, morbidity and mortality remain high. It is important to determine if the underlying symptoms of these patients result from GER as opposed to nasopharyngeal incoordination or esophageal or antral dysmotility; (Martinez et al., 1992; Smith et al., 1992). The presence of GER places the patient at risk for aspiration during induction of anesthesia. Preoperative preparation with H_2-blockers and motility drugs should be continued. A rapid-sequence induction should be used if a difficult airway is not anticipated. At least one large-bore IV

catheter should be placed, although fluid and blood losses are minimal. However, pneumothorax, lacerated spleen, puncture, or compression of the vena cava or aorta, and lacerated hepatic veins can occur.

Other anesthesia concerns in patients with GER are the degree of neurologic and respiratory compromise of the patient. Because these children frequently have seizure disorders, preoperative concern should be directed at proper anticonvulsant therapy. Oral anticonvulsants generally cannot be administered for 48 to 72 hours in the postoperative period. Consequently, patients requiring carbamazepine and valproic acid need alternative medicines so that breakthrough seizures do not occur. In addition, a significant number of patients with neurocompromise may also have ventricular-peritoneal shunts. However, the Nissen fundoplication does not appear to increase the risk for shunt infection to more than the risk of placing a shunt (Bui et al., 2007).

For children with severe respiratory compromise or neuromuscular disease, postoperative ventilatory support may be necessary. In children without significant preoperative pulmonary compromise, extubation may be delayed after surgery and supplemental oxygen given as needed. After surgery, the use of antireflux medication decreased. Within 1 year of surgery, 75% were reported on antireflux medication (Lee et al., 2008).

Surgery for Biliary Atresia

Biliary atresia, characterized by a lack of gross patency of the extrahepatic bile duct, occurs in 1:15,000 live births (Shim et al., 1974). In 10% to 15% of patients, other abnormalities associated with embryologic development are seen, including absent inferior vena cava, intestinal malrotation, polysplenia, and preduodenal portal vein (Lilly and Chandra, 1974). Although biliary atresia is often considered a congenital lesion, it has dynamic properties as well. In microscopic studies of the biliary anatomy obtained from patients at 2 and 4 months of age, the histologic results suggest that biliary structures gradually disappear and are replaced by fibrous tissue. In addition, the success rate for the palliative surgical procedure has been reported as 50% in infants operated on before 4 months of age and 80% in those undergoing surgery before 2 months of age (Ohi et al., 1985). In a study by Serinet and colleagues (2009), among 695 patients who underwent the Kasai procedure, the 2-, 5-, 10-, and 15-year survival rates were 57.1, 32.9, 32.4, and 28.5%, respectively. Increased age at the time of Kasai procedure has been associated with decreased survival rates (Serinet et al., 2009).

Kasai and coworkers (1989), in a review of 245 patients undergoing corrective procedures over a 35-year period, noted that 10-year survival was 74% in infants operated on before 60 days of life. However, Tan and colleagues (1994) have questioned whether earlier corrective surgery is associated with ductal patency. In a series of 205 patients, they noted that survival may be more closely related to the severity of intrahepatic biliary cholangiopathy.

In a 27-year review of 81 patients with biliary atresia, Wildhaber and coworkers (2003) noted that direct bilirubin of less than 2.0, the absence of bridging liver fibrosis, and the number of cholangitis episodes were predictive factors in the success of the Kasai portoenterostomy. Popovic and colleagues (2003) noted that cholinesterase levels can be a useful index of liver function (protein synthesis) early after the Kasai procedure and is independent of albumin synthesis.

Clinically, biliary atresia presents in infants from 1 to 6 weeks of age. About 50% are anicteric until the second or third week of life. The diagnosis of biliary atresia is confirmed either by liver biopsy or by exploratory laparotomy. Surgical palliation for biliary atresia involves hepatic portoenterostomy (Kasai procedure) (Fig. 23-8).

Complications of the surgical repair and from the underlying disease state include cholangitis, portal hypertension, and fat-soluble vitamin deficiency (Kasai et al., 1975). For the anesthesiologist, these complications take on greater significance in patients who return to the operating room for further surgical revision of biliary drainage, treatment of intraabdominal sepsis, or relief of an intestinal obstruction. Because these complications occur frequently and because end-stage liver disease can follow the Kasai procedure, the role of liver transplantation as a primary treatment of biliary atresia has been raised. Kasai and coworkers (1989) suggested that liver transplantation as a primary form of treatment may be indicated for patients older than 3 months with an enlarged, hard liver. Laurent and colleagues (1990) noted that although Kasai's

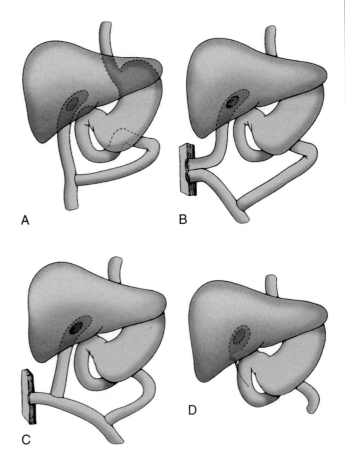

■ FIGURE 23-8. The Kasai procedure and its various modifications. **A,** Original Kasai. **B,** Kasai H-double-barreled vent. **C,** Bishop-Koop vent. **D,** Gallbladder Kasai. *(From Filston HC, Izant RJ Jr: The surgical neonate, evaluation, and care, Norwalk, Conn, 1985, Appleton-Century-Crofts.)*

operation does improve the prognosis of biliary atresia, it is not a definitive cure, and 80% of these patients become candidates for liver transplantation.

Anesthetic management for a Kasai procedure (Kasai, 1974) in patients with biliary atresia follows the basic principles of pediatric anesthesia. In infants in whom venous access is already present, induction is achieved with a hypnotic agent, such as propofol (2 to 3 mg/kg), and a muscle relaxant (cisatracurium, 0.2 mg/kg). In infants without an IV catheter in place, inhalation induction is performed with oxygen, nitrous oxide, and sevoflurane. Once the child is adequately anesthetized, an IV catheter is inserted and a muscle relaxant is administered to facilitate endotracheal intubation and to decrease the concentration of potent inhalation anesthetic. After induction, anesthesia is maintained with an oxygen-air-isoflurane mixture along with IV opioids. Because of bowel distention, nitrous oxide is avoided.

Gelman and coworkers (1984) have shown that hepatic blood flow and oxygen supply are better maintained during isoflurane than during halothane anesthesia. Consequently, isoflurane in an oxygen and air mixture is most commonly administered to patients undergoing surgery for biliary atresia.

Anesthesia monitoring for the patient undergoing a Kasai procedure is similar to that used for other pediatric surgical procedures. Arterial cannulation and central venous pressure monitors are rarely used and are generally reserved for patients with coexisting problems, such as sepsis, pneumonia, cholangitis, and severe cirrhosis. In general, hemodynamic stability is well maintained and the need for intraoperative vasoactive agents is rare. Sometimes the surgical approach involves dividing the triangular and coronary ligaments and displacing the whole liver anteriorly. Although this technique may facilitate exposure, it may compress the inferior vena cava and thereby result in hypotension by decreasing venous return. Ventilation is controlled and end-tidal gases are monitored for carbon dioxide, oxygen, and volatile anesthetic agents. Adequacy of oxygenation is monitored by the pulse oximeter.

The operative procedures generally last 3 to 4 hours, and major blood loss does not occur. Perioperative fluid therapy involves replacement of maintenance and deficit fluids as well as provision for the calculated third-space losses. Third-space losses may vary from 6 to 10 mL/kg per hour. Generally, lactated Ringer's solution is used to restore third-space losses.

Prevention of hypothermia is a major concern for the anesthesiologist. The large surface-to-volume ratio of infants, their relative lack of insulation tissue, coupled with the cold operating room, exposure of body cavities to low environmental temperatures, infusions of cold fluid, and ventilation with dry gases, all increase the potential for hypothermia during surgery. Consequently, great effort must be applied both before and during surgery to protect against heat loss. Methods of preventing heat loss are discussed in Chapter 6, Thermoregulation: Physiology and Perioperative Disturbances.

The pharmacology of anesthetic agents in infants and children with hepatic disease has not been fully evaluated. Although the liver is the major site of drug biotransformation, the effects of hepatic dysfunction on drug elimination and disposition are inconsistent. The degree of liver dysfunction and the drug's ability to bind to plasma proteins are important variables in determining drug kinetics in patients with liver disease.

In general, liver function is fairly well preserved in the first few months of life in children with biliary atresia. As the children get older and ductal fibrosis begins, liver dysfunction ensues. Consequently, in children who return for repeat surgical procedures, the pharmacology of IV anesthetic agents and adjuncts may be altered.

In infants with biliary atresia undergoing the Kasai procedure, if major fluid shifts have not occurred, blood loss has been minimal, and the patient has remained warm, all efforts are made to reverse the muscle relaxation and extubate the trachea at the end of the procedure. In children with other organ system failures (specifically sepsis, cholangitis, or pneumonia), those who are cold at the end of the procedure (<35° C), or those who have undergone transfusion of more than one blood volume, extubation is delayed until warmth and hemodynamic stability are restored. In these children, postoperative recovery and monitoring are carried out in an intensive care setting. The long-term (5-, 10-, and 20-year) survival rates for 80 children after a Kasai procedure, without transplantation, were 63%, 54%, and 44%, respectively. By age 20, almost half had cirrhosis and its sequelae (Shinkai et al., 2009).

Liver Tumor Procedures

Liver tumors in children are uncommon, but 72% of pediatric primary hepatic tumors and 1.1% of all childhood tumors

TABLE 23-3. Malignant Hepatic Tumors

Tumor Type	Tumor	Cases Reported
Hepatomas	Hepatoblastoma	129
	Hepatocellular carcinoma	98
Other	Mixed mesenchymal tumor	9
	Rhabdomyosarcoma	6
	Angiosarcoma	4
	Undifferentiated sarcoma	3
	Teratocarcinoma	1
	Cholangiosarcoma	1
	Malignant histiocytoma	1

From Exelby PR, Filler RM, Grosfeld JL: Liver tumors in children in the particular reference to hepatoblastoma and hepatocellular carcinoma: American Academy of Pediatrics Surgical Section Survey—1974, *J Pediatr Surg* 10:329, 1975.

are malignant. Of these malignant tumors, hepatoblastoma and hepatocarcinoma are the predominant tissue types (Table 23-3). Hepatoblastoma commonly affects white boys less than 2 years of age. An abdominal mass that has increased in size is usually the presenting symptom. Anemia, jaundice, and ascites are infrequent findings. Liver function test results are frequently normal. From 2% to 3% of patients may have an associated hemihypertrophy (Geiser et al., 1970). Hepatoblastoma has also been associated with isosexual precocity as a result of the liver's ectopic gonadotropic production and the Beckwith-Wiedemann syndrome (Sotelo-Avita et al., 1976), polyposis coli, Wilms tumor, and fetal alcohol syndrome. An increased incidence of hepatoblastoma has been associated with low birth weight (Ikeda et al 1997; Feusner et al., 1998) (Box 23-4). Between 1973 and 1997, the rate of hepatoblastoma increased. This is in contrast to the decreased incidence observed for hepatocarcinoma (Darbari et al., 2003).

Hepatoblastomas are derived from primitive epithelial parenchyma and are classified by the predominant epithelial component. Among the variants are fetal, embryonal, macrotrabecular, and anaplastic. Survival is related to the histology and complete-

Box 23-4 Clinical Antecedents of Hepatoblastoma and Hepatocellular Carcinoma in Childhood

Extreme prematurity (especially weight < 1500 g)
Hepatitis B virus
Beckwith-Wiedemann syndrome
Familial adenomatosis polyposis
Glycogen storage diseases (mainly type I)
Hereditary tyrosinemia
Cholestatic conditions
- Biliary atresia
- Progressive familial intrahepatic cholestasis type 2 (ABCB11 disease)
Alagille syndrome

From Finegold MJ, Egler RA, Goss JA, et al: Liver tumors: pediatric population, *Liver Transpl* 14:1545, 2008.

TABLE 23-4. Children's Oncology Group Staging for Hepatoblastoma

Stage	Comments
Stage I	Complete resection Favorable histology Purely fetal histology with a low mitotic index
Stage II	Gross total resection with microscopic residuals or with preoperative or intra-operative rupture
State III	Unresectable tumors as determined by the attending surgeon partially resected tumors with macroscopic residual, or any tumor with lymph node involvement
Stage IV	Measurable metastatic disease to lungs or other organs

From Finegold MJ, Egler RA, Goss JA, et al: Liver tumors: pediatric population, *Liver Transpl* 14:1545, 2008.

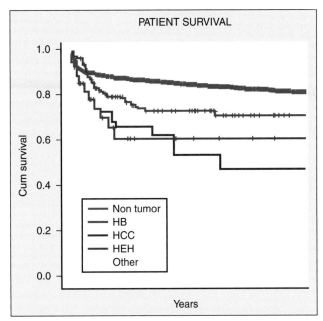

■ **FIGURE 23-9.** One-year patient survival: United Network for Organ Sharing (UNOS) standard transplant and research file 1989–2007. A total of 8047 patients (age, <18 years) who underwent orthotopic liver transplant between 1989 and 2007 were analyzed from the UNOS database. Of these patients, 237 underwent transplantation for hepatoblastoma, 58 for hepatocellular carcinoma, 35 for hemangioendothelioma, and 36 for other tumors. *HB,* Hepatoblastoma; *HCC,* hepatocellular carcinoma; *HEH,* hemangioendothelioma. *(From Finegold MJ, Egler RA, Goss JA, et al: Liver tumors: pediatric population,* Liver Transpl *14:1545, 2008 [fig. 6].)*

ness of the surgical resection (Table 23-4). Fetal histology has a greater than 90% survival rate, compared with a 50% survival rate for embryonal histology. A few survivors have anaplastic histology. Patients with resectable stages I and II hepatoblastomas have better survival (95%) than patients with unresectable stage III (69%) or metastatic disease (37%). For patients with resectable disease, a 5-year survival rate is 83%, as opposed to 41% for those who had residual tumor after surgery (Finegold et al., 2008) (see Box 23-4). Complete surgical resection offers the only chance for cure in patients with hepatocellular carcinoma, because the tumor is chemoresistant. In patients requiring a liver transplant, the 1-, 5-, and 10-year survival rates are 86%, 67%, and 58%, respectively (Fig. 23-9).

Liver transplantation has been used as both a primary surgical therapy and a rescue for incomplete resection or recurrence of disease. Patients who were rescued had a 30% disease-free survival compared with 82% in the primary treatment group (Otte et al., 2004).

Hepatocellular carcinoma appears to have two age peaks: one at less than 4 years of age and the other between 12 and 15 years of age (Leventhal, 1987). As in adults with hepatocellular carcinoma, the prognosis of survival in children with the disease is 5% to 10%. Typically, patients with hepatocellular carcinoma have the systemic symptoms of weight loss, jaundice, fever, and lethargy. As opposed to adults with this tumor, only about 5% of children have associated cirrhosis (Jones, 1960). Other associated diseases include von Gierke's disease, type I glycogenesis, cystinosis, extrahepatic biliary atresia, α_1-antitrypsin deficiency, hypoplasia of intrahepatic bile ducts, Wilson's disease, giant cell hepatitis, and Solo's syndrome (Zangeneh et al., 1969; Palmer and Wolfe, 1976; Weinberg et al., 1976; Dehner, 1978) (see Box 23-4). Complete surgical resection offers the only chance for a cure for patients with hepatocellular carcinoma, because the tumor is chemoresistant. In patients requiring a liver transplant, the 1-, 5-, and 10-year patient survival rates are 86%, 67%, and 58%, respectively (see Fig. 23-9).

Anesthetic management for pediatric patients undergoing hepatic lobe resection or tumor resection involves the same principles as for patients with biliary atresia. Efforts at maintaining adequate alveolar ventilation, temperature homeostasis, cardiovas-

cular stability, and fluid management have been described. Some patients receive adjunct chemotherapy before surgery. The chemotherapeutic protocol must be reviewed. Frequently, Adriamycin, an anthracycline, is a major component of hepatic cancer chemotherapy and has been associated with a dosage-dependent irreversible cardiomyopathy. All patients receiving anthracycline chemotherapy should be studied by history, physical examination, electrocardiography, chest radiography, and echocardiography to further evaluate signs and symptoms of cardiac toxicity and cardiac reserve (see Chapters 4 and 36, Cardiovascular Physiology and Systemic Disorders).

Because the potential for massive blood loss exists in patients undergoing hepatic resection, adequate venous access and invasive monitoring are essential to patient management. Two or three large-bore peripheral IV catheters are inserted, and a central venous pressure catheter is placed to monitor cardiac filling pressures. Either the radial or the femoral artery is cannulated, not only to monitor blood pressure but also to determine blood gas levels, chemistry, and coagulation profile. Because of the potential for large fluid shifts, a Foley catheter is placed to measure urine output and assist in assessing the adequacy of fluid resuscitation.

Massive blood volume replacement is a frequent component of the anesthetic resuscitation in children undergoing hepatic resection. Massive blood volume replacement may create physiologic derangements that have anesthetic and surgical consequences. These physiologic alterations include disorders of coagulation, acid-base imbalance, electrolyte imbalance, hypothermia, and decreased tissue oxygen delivery.

Many children undergoing tumor resection require postoperative ventilatory support. The anesthetic plan should permit early tracheal extubation in the operating room. However, in the event that intraoperative findings reveal unresectable tumor, postoperative care should include observation in the pediatric intensive care unit and attention to changes in intravascular volume and blood pressure. Continued bleeding may require transfusion of blood or fresh frozen plasma, or even return to the operating room for surgical control.

Hirschsprung's Disease Procedures

The basic pathology underlying congenital megacolon, or Hirschsprung's disease, is aganglionosis, or total absence of ganglion cells, in the intrinsic nerve supply of the bowel. The aganglionic area extends proximally from the anal sphincter and involves varying lengths of colon. The normal nerve supply, consisting of Auerbach's plexuses and Meissner's plexuses, which together form the myenteric nerve complex of the bowel, usually becomes an increasingly diffuse network in the descending and terminal portions of the bowel. Absence of the ganglion cells, which occurs in approximately 1 in 10,000 infants, causes a condition resembling spasm in the area without ganglion cells, and the normal bowel proximal to the spastic portion undergoes tremendous distention, with retention of feces and intestinal obstruction or, in less serious cases, prolonged bouts of constipation. Although the cause of Hirschsprung's disease is unknown, defects in nonadrenergic, noncholinergic innervations may prevent relaxation of the aganglionic segment. Bealer and colleagues (1994) demonstrated that nitric oxide synthetase is deficient in the aganglionic colon of patients with Hirschsprung's disease, and that this deficiency may prevent smooth muscle relaxation of the aganglionic segment. On a molecular level, mutations in the RET protooncogene have been found (Sancandi et al., 2000).

In 10% to 20% of patients with Hirschsprung's disease, it is clinically present at birth. Symptomatic infants have delayed passage of meconium, irritability, failure to thrive, and abdominal distention. Older children may present with constipation, fecal soiling, and diarrhea. The major complication from Hirschsprung's disease is acute enterocolitis, a potentially life-threatening event. Diagnosis of Hirschsprung's disease is made by radiographic examination and confirmed by suction biopsy specimens from the rectum. Surgery is usually a two-stage procedure, with the initial procedure being a colostomy. The definitive surgical procedure is generally performed when the child is older (>1 year). The surgical approaches are varied and over time have undergone modifications (Fig. 23-10). Attention has focused on the use of a one-stage transanal endorectal pull-through approach (Elhalaby et al., 2004). Each surgical technique has its own associated intraoperative and perioperative complications, but enterocolitis, wound dehiscence, anastomotic leakage, intestinal obstruction, and fecal soiling are common to all. All of these surgical procedures aim either to excise or to bypass the aganglionic portion of the bowel and to free and advance the remaining normal portion of bowel toward the rectum. These procedures are often long (6 to 8 hours) and involve surgical explorations through the perineum and abdomen.

Laparoscopic surgery has also been used in the treatment of Hirschsprung's disease (Jona et al., 1998; Wulkan and Georgeson, 1998; Georgeson et al., 1999). The minimally invasive assisted pull-through technique is generally used for patients when

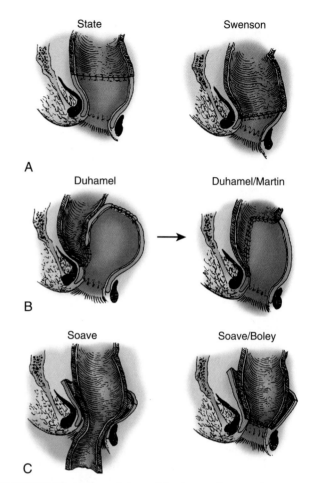

■ **FIGURE 23-10.** Lateral views of the three major operative procedures for Hirschsprung's disease. Evolution of each occurs from *left* to *right*. *Unshaded* native rectum is aganglionic. *Shaded,* pulled-through bowel contains ganglion cells. **A,** State's procedure was a prototypical anterior resection of dilated rectosigmoid. Lengthy aganglionic segment remained. In Swenson's procedure, an oblique anastomosis resulted in ganglion cells within 1 cm of the verge posteriorly. **B,** In the original Duhamel's operation, the oversewn native rectum enlarged as a blind loop, which resulted in a fecaloma that caused partial obstruction. In Martin's modification, the blind loop is obviated by complete division of the septum and anastomosis of the anterior walls of the native rectum and pulled-through colon. Bowel that contains ganglion cells reaches within 1 cm of the anal verge posteriorly. **C,** In the original Soave's procedure, full-thickness colon that contained ganglion cells was advanced through the demucosalized native rectal sleeve. Excess colon extended from the anus for several weeks before transection and delayed anastomosis. In the Boley modification, a primary anastomosis is done 1 cm above the verge. Ganglion cells are present circumferentially at that level. *(From Philappart AI: Hirschsprung's disease. In Ashcraft KW, Holder TM:* Pediatric surgery, *ed 2, Philadelphia, 1993, Saunders.)*

the aganglionic segment is confined to the rectum sigmoid or proximal left colon (Georgeson, 2002). Anesthetic concerns for patients with Hirschsprung's disease are similar to those for any child having surgery. Maintaining body temperature and providing appropriate fluid therapy (for replacement of large third-space losses) are the major challenges for the anesthesiologist.

Anesthesia induction can be either by inhalation or IV means. Because of the surgical bowel manipulation and the relatively obstructive nature of the underlying disease, nitrous oxide is discontinued after induction, and anesthesia is maintained with a mixture of air, oxygen, and potent inhalation agent. Long-term follow-up of patients with Hirschsprung's disease suggests that 25% of patients will require reoperation, and that 19% to 25% of patients will develop enterocolitis (Fortuna et al., 1996).

Surgery for Appendicitis

Acute appendicitis is a common condition in children. Although the mortality from acute appendicitis is rare (case-fatality ratio, 0.3%) (Addiss et al., 1990), morbidity (peritonitis, abscess formation, wound infection) is related to the state of the appendix at the time of the operation. The highest incidence of appendicitis is found in patients aged 10 to 19 years. The incidence of perforation of the appendix in children appears to be about 30% to 45%, but in preschool children and infants it can be as high as 80%. The incidence of appendicitis appears to be affected by race and gender. The incidence of appendicitis is 1.4 to 1.6 times greater in whites than nonwhites, whereas the perforation rate for nonwhites is 22% compared with 18% for whites (Addiss et al., 1990).

The signs and symptoms of appendicitis are variable. The incidence of negative appendectomy (surgery performed without positive appendicitis) is significant. In males, the negative appendectomy rate is about 9%, whereas in females it is about 22%. In females, diagnostic accuracy decreases during child-bearing years, whereas in males, diagnostic accuracy does not appear to be affected by age. Classically, the patient presents with periumbilical pain that eventually localizes to the right lower quadrant. Anorexia, nausea, and vomiting are frequent, as is a low-grade fever. Continued progression of the inflammatory course results in increased tenderness in the right lower quadrant as well as pain referred to the right lower quadrant on palpation of other areas of the abdomen. With advanced disease, gangrene and perforation of the appendix occur, with ensuing peritonitis and possible abscess formation. Both ultrasound and computed tomographic (CT) imaging have been used to evaluate appendicitis in children. The advantages of ultrasound include cost, lack of exposure to radiation, and its ability to assess ovarian pathology, but CT affords a higher diagnostic accuracy and better delineation of extent of disease where the appendix is perforated.

The pathophysiology of appendicitis is thought to be related to an obstruction of the lumen of the appendix, with subsequent bacterial overgrowth and distention of the appendix (Fig. 23-11). In untreated cases, distention and overgrowth lead to gangrene and rupture. Although there is some urgency in making the diagnosis and surgically removing the appendix, the operation is never so urgent that a proper review of the patient's medical history and physical assessment cannot be performed.

Preoperative anesthetic management of the child with diagnosed appendicitis includes concerns regarding fluid and electrolyte disorders. Because these children may have been vomiting and may be febrile, signs and symptoms of dehydration should be assessed and any fluid or electrolyte deficits corrected.

Once the child has been adequately volume-resuscitated and a normal airway is anticipated, an IV rapid-sequence induction with cricoid pressure is performed. Anesthetic technique (inhalation agents versus opioid-based techniques) may depend on the surgical technique used to remove the appendix. Although frequently the appendix is removed by laparotomy, the role of laparoscopy (especially in female patients) in both diagnosis and management is increasing (Gilchrist et al., 1992; Kuster

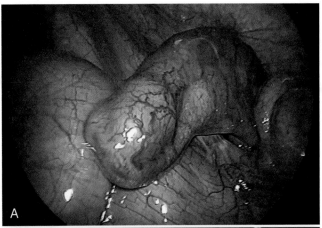
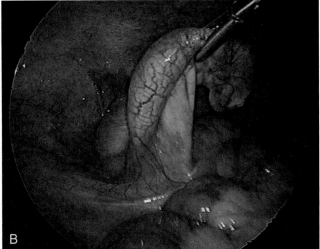

■ **FIGURE 23-11.** Laparoscopic acute appendicitis.

and Gilroy, 1992; Olsen et al., 1993). See related video online at www.expertconsult.com. In a study by McAnena and coworkers (1992), the median postoperative hospitalization stay was one half and the rate of wound infection one third in patients undergoing laparoscopic appendectomy compared with patients undergoing open appendectomy. In a study involving 30 pediatric hospitals, Newman and colleagues (2003) noted significant variability in practice and resource utilization among the institutions. In addition, the length of stay did not differ between those patients who underwent an open or a laparoscopic appendectomy.

Regardless of surgical technique, monitoring of the patient includes electrocardiogram, pulse oximeter, temperature probe, blood pressure cuff, precordial stethoscope, and end-tidal gas measurements. Depending on the patient's body temperature, active cooling techniques (cooling blanket, rectal acetaminophen suppositories, cool IV fluids, and cool intraabdominal irrigations) may be needed to help lower the patient's temperature. The addition of inhalational anesthetics may also augment cooling by promoting cutaneous vasodilation with subsequent increased heat loss.

Intussusception Repair

Intussusception is the invagination or telescoping of one portion of the intestine into another (Fig. 23-12). It tends to occur more frequently in males than females. Over 50%

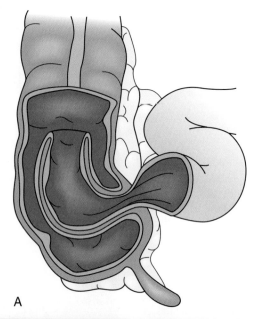

A

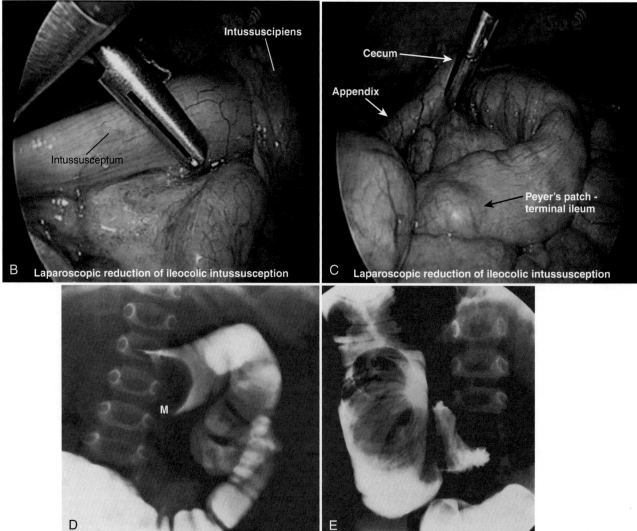

■ **FIGURE 23-12. A,** Intussusception. **B,** Laparoscopic view of intussusception, **C,** Laparoscopic view of reduced intussusception with hypertrophid Peyer's patch at the lead point. **D,** Diagnostic enema encounters the intussusceptum in the mid-transverse colon (M). **E,** The coiled-spring appearance of an ileocolic intussusception: the contrast material has interdigitated between the intussusceptum and the intussuscipiens (**A,** From deLorimier AA, Harrison MR: Pediatric surgery. In Dunphy JE, Way LW: Current surgical diagnosis and treatment, Los Altos, Calif, 1979, Lange Medical. **D** and **E,** From Blickman JG, Parker R, Barnes PD: Pediatric radiology, St Louis, 2009, Mosby, p 73.)

of cases occur in children less than 1 year of age, and less than 10% of cases occur in children older than 5 years. Ninety percent of cases have idiopathic causes—frequently seen in children less than 1 year of age. Older children are more likely to have Meckel's diverticulum, intestinal polyps, lymphoma, adhesions, trauma, hemolytic uremic syndrome, or ectopic pancreatic nodule as an etiology. Intussusception has also been reported postoperatively and after blunt abdominal trauma (Komadina and Smrkolj, 1998; Linke et al., 1998). In addition, an association between rotavirus vaccine and intussusception has been reported (Zanardi et al., 2001).

The clinical presentation of acute intussusception involves sudden paroxysms of abdominal pain, bloody stools, and an abdominal mass, although in one series of patients, 18% of the children had painless intussusception (Hutchison et al., 1980). In a review of 14 published reports, Losek (1993) noted that bloody stools were present in 42% of patients. Occult blood was noted in 43% and abdominal masses were present in 62% of patients. Intussusception can also manifest with neurologic findings (lethargy, apnea, seizures, hypotonia, opisthotonus) similar to a picture of septic encephalopathy (Conway, 1993). Other symptoms and signs may include diarrhea, vomiting, fever, and dehydration. In other children, intussusception can be a chronic entity that may mimic gastroenteritis (Shekhawat et al., 1992), whereas in neonates, intussusception may mimic necrotizing enterocolitis (Price et al., 1993).

About 90% of intussusceptions are ileocolic, and the remainder are ileoileal and colocolic. Treatment for intussusception involves the administration of appropriate fluids to combat dehydration, and radiologic or surgical attempts to reduce the invaginated bowel. Hydrostatic enemas with barium or air have been reported to be successful in 80% of patients. However, enemas are contraindicated in patients with evidence of peritonitis, shock, and intestinal perforation. Surgical laparotomy with manual reduction or resection (or both) as well as laparoscopic approaches have been described for surgical management in patients with unsuccessful radiologic reduction and in patients with signs of intestinal perforation, peritonitis, and shock (Hay et al., 1999).

Anesthetic considerations include restoring electrolyte and fluid deficits. Shock should be treated before commencing anesthesia. The intravascular deficits may be further exacerbated by the presence of barium in the gastrointestinal tract. The child with an intussusception should also be considered at risk for aspiration, and because of the intestinal obstruction, nitrous oxide should be avoided. Anesthesia should be induced with IV agents. If hemodynamic instability is a concern, ketamine or etomidate should be used as the hypnotic agent for induction.

GENERAL THORACIC SURGERY

Thoracic surgery in children is performed for a wide variety of congenital, neoplastic, infectious, and traumatic lesions (Box 23-5). The patient may be a few hours old with a congenital cystic adenomatoid malformation (CCAM) and life-threatening respiratory distress or an adolescent with an asymptomatic mediastinal tumor. Regardless of age or disease, four principles are common to all patients undergoing general anesthesia for thoracic surgery, as follows:

- Preoperative evaluation and preparation can minimize intraoperative problems and improve the safety of the anesthetic.

Box 23-5 Childhood Lesions Requiring Thoracic Surgery

Empyema
Chest wall deformities
Chest wall masses
Lung abscess
Bronchiectasis
Lobar emphysema
Tumor (primary or metastatic)
Pulmonary sequestration
Congenital adenomatoid malformation
Congenital cysts of the lung
Bronchogenic cysts
Esophageal lesions
Mediastinal masses
Scoliosis

- The anesthesiologist must be aware of potential intraoperative problems.
- Modern monitoring techniques have increased safety with regard to anesthetic management.
- Surgical approaches and techniques are constantly changing as efforts are made by surgeons to use minimally invasive procedures.

A thorough preoperative evaluation is essential in caring for the pediatric patient scheduled for thoracic surgery. Appropriate imaging and laboratory studies should be performed preoperatively according to the lesion involved. Guidelines for fasting, choice of premedication, and preparation of the operating room are used as for other infants and children scheduled for major surgery. After induction of anesthesia, placement of an IV catheter, and tracheal intubation, arterial catheterization should be performed for most patients undergoing thoracotomy as well as for those with severe lung disease having thoracoscopic surgery. This facilitates monitoring of arterial blood pressure during manipulation of the lungs and mediastinum, as well as monitoring of arterial blood gas tensions during single lung ventilation (SLV). For thoracoscopic procedures of relatively short duration in patients without severe lung disease, the insertion of an arterial catheter is not required (Rao et al., 1981). Placement of a central venous catheter is generally not indicated if peripheral IV access is adequate for projected fluid and blood administration.

Inhaled anesthetic agents are commonly administered in 100% O_2 during maintenance of anesthesia. Isoflurane may be preferred because there is less attenuation of hypoxic pulmonary vasoconstriction (HPV) than with other inhaled agents, although this has not been studied in children (Benumof et al., 1987). Nitrous oxide is avoided. Use of IV opioids may facilitate a decrease in the concentration of inhaled anesthetics used and thereby limit impairment of hypoxic pulmonary vasoconstriction. Alternatively, total IV anesthesia may be used with a variety of agents. The combination of general anesthesia with regional anesthesia and postoperative analgesia is particularly desirable for thoracotomy, but it may also be beneficial for thoracoscopic procedures, especially when thoracostomy tube drainage, a source of significant postoperative pain, is used after surgery. A variety of regional anesthetic techniques have been described for intraoperative anesthesia and postoperative analgesia, including intercostal and paravertebral blocks, intra-pleural infusions, and epidural anesthesia (see Chapter 16, Regional Anesthesia).

In awake patients, except for young infants, ventilation is normally distributed preferentially to dependent regions of the lung, so that there is a gradient of increasing ventilation from the most nondependent to the most dependent lung segments. Because of gravitational effects, perfusion normally follows a similar distribution, with increased blood flow to dependent lung segments; therefore, ventilation and perfusion are normally well matched. However, controlled ventilation under general anesthesia with decreased functional residual capacity and absent diaphragmatic contractions results in a reverse distribution of ventilation (see Chapter 3, Respiratory Physiology in Infants and Children). During thoracic surgery, these and other factors act to increase ventilation/perfusion (V/Q) mismatch. Compression of the dependent lung in the lateral decubitus position may cause atelectasis. Surgical retraction, SLV, or both result in collapse of the operative lung. Hypoxic pulmonary vasoconstriction (HPV), which acts to divert blood flow away from underventilated lung regions, thereby minimizing V/Q mismatch, may be diminished by the use of inhaled anesthetic agents and other vasodilating drugs. These factors apply similarly to infants, children, and adults. The overall effect of the lateral decubitus position on V/Q mismatch, however, differs in infants compared with older children and adults.

In adults with unilateral lung disease, oxygenation is optimal when the patient is placed in the lateral decubitus position with the healthy lung dependent (down) and the diseased lung nondependent (up) (Bachland et al., 1975; Remolina et al., 1981). Presumably, this is related to an increase in blood flow to the dependent, healthy lung and a decrease in blood flow to the nondependent, diseased lung as a result of the hydrostatic pressure (i.e., gravitational) gradient between the two lungs. This phenomenon promotes V/Q matching in the adult patient undergoing thoracic surgery in the lateral decubitus position.

In infants with unilateral lung disease, however, oxygenation is better with the healthy lung up (Heaf et al., 1983). Several factors account for this discrepancy between adults and infants. Infants have a soft, easily compressible rib cage that cannot fully support the underlying lung. Functional residual capacity, especially in the lower lung, is closer to or at residual volume, making airway closure likely to occur in the dependent lung even during tidal breathing (Mansell et al., 1972).

Finally, the infant's increased oxygen requirement, coupled with a small functional residual capacity, predisposes to hypoxemia. Infants normally consume 6 to 8 mL of O_2/kg per minute, compared with a normal O_2 consumption in adults of 2 to 3 mL/kg per minute (Dawes, 1973). For these reasons, infants are at increased risk for significant oxygen desaturation during surgery in the lateral decubitus position.

Thoracoscopy

During the past decade, the use of video-assisted thoracoscopic surgery has dramatically increased in both adults and children (see Video Endoscopy, p. 745). As with laparoscopy, reported advantages of thoracoscopy include smaller chest incisions, reduced postoperative pain, and more rapid postoperative recovery compared with thoracotomy (Weatherford et al., 1995; Angelillo Mackinlay et al., 1996; Mouroux et al., 1997).

Box 23-6 Thoracoscopic Procedures in Infants and Children

Anterior spinal fusion
Aortopexy
Biopsy
- Abscess
- Interstitial lung disease
- Mass
Cyst excision
Decortication or debridement of empyema
Diaphragmatic plication
Diaphragmatic hernia repair
Drainage
- Abscess
- Cyst
Esophageal atresia repair
Exploration
- Infection
- Mass
- Trauma
Foregut duplication resection
Hiatal hernia repair
Lobectomy
Mediastinal mass excision
Patent ductus arteriosus ligation
Segmentectomy
Sequestration resection
Sympathectomy
Tracheoesophageal fistula ligation
Thymectomy
Thoracic duct ligation

Thoracoscopic surgery is being used extensively for pleural débridement in patients with empyema, lung biopsy, and wedge resections for interstitial lung disease, mediastinal masses, and metastatic lesions. More extensive pulmonary resections, including segmentectomy and lobectomy, have been performed for lung abscess, bullous disease, sequestrations, lobar emphysema, CCAM, and neoplasms. Thoracoscopic procedures used in infants and children are listed in Box 23-6.

Thoracoscopy can be performed while both lungs are being ventilated using CO_2 insufflation and a retractor to displace lung tissue in the operative field. However, SLV is extremely desirable during thoracoscopy, because lung deflation improves visualization of thoracic contents and may reduce lung injury caused by the retractors (Benumof, 1995).

Surgery for Chest Wall Deformities

Pectus excavatum (funnel chest) (Fig. 23-13) and the less common pectus carinatum (pigeon breast) deformities are congenital abnormalities of the sternum, ribs, and costal cartilages. These deformities are usually minimal at birth but progress with age. A higher incidence of both deformities occurs in children with Marfan syndrome or congenital heart disease, and in families in which other children have the defect (Shamberger and Welch, 1987; Robicsek and Lobato, 2000). These children often appear asymptomatic but occasionally have cardiac or pulmonary abnormalities related to the deformity (Malek et al., 2003). Patients with pectus excavatum generally present with normal

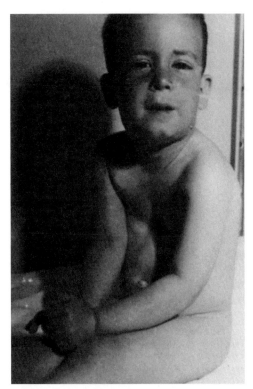

■ **FIGURE 23-13.** Pectus excavatum deformity becomes most obvious when the child is in the sitting position.

or modestly reduced forced vital capacity and total lung capacity and, in severe cases, V/Q mismatch. The heart is displaced to the left and compressed, lending to arrhythmias, right-axis deviation on electrocardiogram, a functional murmur, and reduced stroke volume—most noticeable in the standing position and during exercise, explaining the mild exercise intolerance experienced by some patients. The cardiac and pulmonary abnormalities are in most instances benign and may worsen as the child ages but may be improved by surgical repair. There also is an increased incidence of mitral valve prolapse in patients with pectus deformities (Shamberger et al., 1987).

Preoperative assessment focuses on exercise tolerance and other signs of cardiopulmonary compromise, such as lung infections. Laboratory evaluation includes a chest radiograph; pulmonary function tests, arterial blood gases, and electrocardiogram are added only if there is clinical evidence of significant underlying disease. Echocardiography is now commonly performed to detect the presence of mitral valve prolapse, and, if the child has it, prophylaxis for subacute bacterial endocarditis is administered. Patients are often emotionally distressed by the appearance of a chest deformity and may benefit from preoperative counseling and, if needed, premedication.

Classic operative repair involves extrapleural excision of the sternocostal cartilages and mobilization of the sternum and ribs. The most common complications of operative repair are pneumothorax, flail chest, and postoperative atelectasis; blood loss is usually minimal to moderate. Intraoperative monitoring includes temperature, blood pressure, pulse, heart and breath sounds, airway pressure, and oxygen saturation or tension. Capnography is also useful, but arterial catheterization is needed only if there is a specific indication. General anesthesia

with controlled ventilation is the method of choice, with no agents specifically indicated or contraindicated because of the operation itself. Oxygen by face mask is administered in the recovery room, but it is usually not needed after the child fully awakens. Although patient-controlled analgesia is commonly used for postoperative analgesia, both intercostal nerve blocks and thoracic epidural analgesia have become increasingly popular for children undergoing pectus repair (Robicsek, 2000).

A thoracic epidural catheter provides more reliable analgesia to the operative area than a lumbar epidural that has been threaded a great distance. However, thoracic epidural catheters are not as easy to insert as lumbar catheters, and many practitioners are not comfortable with their routine use. Although a technique using electrocardiographic guidance and insertion from the caudal space has been described, it is not widely used (Tsui et al., 2002). An additional issue with the thoracic catheters is the safety of their insertion under general anesthesia (Horlocker, 2003). Although some children allow insertion before induction (McBride et al., 1996), many younger children are not likely to remain cooperative for the procedure, mandating insertion after induction (Hammer, 2002; Birmingham et al., 2003). Moreover, several centers have actively and successfully used thoracic epidural techniques in anesthetized children for thoracic and cardiac procedures without complications related to insertion after induction (Cassady, 2000; Birmingham, 2003). Solutions of both bupivacaine with fentanyl and fentanyl alone have been used successfully, including in the patient-controlled mode for appropriately mature children (Caudle et al., 1993; Birmingham et al., 2003) (see Chapter 16, Regional Anesthesia).

Another approach is to use a minimally invasive technique in which the costal cartilages are preserved and the sternum is elevated with a bar. Under direct vision and through a thoracoscope, a transmediastinal tunnel is created and a prebent bar is passed behind the sternum with the convex side down. The bar is then rotated 180 degrees to elevate the sternum (Fig. 23-14) (Nuss et al., 1998; Nuss, 2002). Borowitz and coworkers (2003) have shown that static pulmonary function and ventilatory response to exercise was normal both before and after surgery, thereby suggesting that placement of the bar does not result in an increased chest wall restriction. In addition, Lawson and colleagues (2003) noted that the surgical repair of the pectus excavatum after the Nuss procedure had a positive impact on the patient's physical and emotional well-being. Complications of this minimally invasive approach include atelectasis, subcutaneous emphysema, pericardial and pleural effusions, myocardial perforation, diaphragmatic perforation, and dislocation of the stabilizing bar (Willekes et al., 1999; Hebra et al., 2000; Molik et al., 2001; Moss, 2001; Hosie et al., 2002; Uemura et al., 2003). Postoperative pain after the Nuss procedure is significant. Thoracic epidural analgesia for 2 to 3 days, followed by oral opioid and nonsteroidal antiinflammatory drug therapy, is appropriate.

Thoracotomy, Lobectomy, and Pneumonectomy

Thoracotomy in the infant or child may be indicated for congenital abnormalities (cysts), tumors (mediastinal teratomas), trauma (gunshot wounds), or infective lesions (bronchiectasis). Subsegmental resection is used for biopsy and removal of

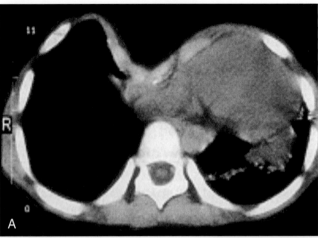

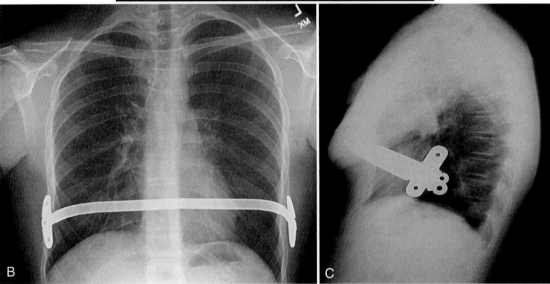

■ **FIGURE 23-14.** CT scan of a patient undergoing Nuss procedure **(A)**. AP **(B)** and lateral **(C)** radiographs of a patient with a Nuss bar in place.

metastatic tumors, whereas lobectomy is most commonly used for removal of congenital anomalies and extensive tumor metastasis. Pneumonectomy in children is done for various tumors, congenital abnormalities, and inflammatory lesions such as bronchiectasis. Perioperative management differs dramatically depending on the indication for surgery.

Surgical Lesion

If a space-occupying lesion is present, the patient is examined for signs of decreased cardiac output, diminished lung volume and reserve, and airway compression (Keon, 1981). History focuses not only on general exercise tolerance but also on signs of intermittent airway obstruction (stridor, cyanosis, or wheezing). Physical examination includes checking for a shift in the trachea, asymmetric chest movement, wheezing, and any signs of respiratory distress. Laboratory assessment should include a chest radiograph, but additional studies such as tomography, angiography, or computed tomography often provide more exact data about vascular or airway compression and compromise. It is crucial to determine the extent of airway compression and physiologic compromise, because impairment may worsen with induction of anesthesia as sympathetic and muscular tones are reduced.

If the intrathoracic lesion is a primary or metastatic tumor, the history concentrates on previous treatment (Baldeyrou et al., 1984). Previous treatment for the tumor, especially chemotherapy and radiation, is important to know about. Special attention is given to anthracycline (cardiac toxicity), bleomycin (pulmonary toxicity), and steroid (adrenal suppression) therapy. If there is any question about functional disability caused by this treatment, consultation with the child's oncologist is useful. Anemia, thrombocytopenia, and malnutrition are common in these patients and should be improved before surgery (Beattie, 1984). A special consideration is the immunocompromised patient with an unknown pulmonary infiltrate. This is usually assumed to be an opportunistic infection, but because it may represent metastasis, a biopsy is occasionally requested. These patients are often in poor general condition and may require postoperative ventilatory support, especially if they had only marginal compensation before surgery (Imoke et al., 1983; Prober et al., 1984).

Assessment

General assessment of the child starts with vital signs and overall appearance. Because children tolerate the loss of large amounts of usable lung tissue without obvious distress, the appearance of dyspnea or diminished exercise tolerance is an ominous sign. The history in older children focuses on complaints of dyspnea, cyanosis, wheezing, coughing, and weight loss. Infants often show less specific signs, such as poor feeding, irritability, choking, or change in sleep habits. If the child has had previous surgery, the perioperative course should be examined. The chest is inspected for asymmetric expansion and use of accessory muscles and then is auscultated for wheezes, rales, rhonchi, and absent breath sounds in both the supine and sitting positions. Physical assessment of the cardiovascular system concentrates on the presence of a gallop, murmurs, arrhythmias, and adequate peripheral pulses.

Preparation

Preparation for surgery starts with a discussion of the proposed anesthetic with the parents and, if appropriate, with the child. The anesthetic plan, including monitoring, possible complications, and potential for postoperative ventilation, is discussed. It is best to delay surgery until any infection or bronchospasm has been brought under optimal medical control with antibiotics, chest physiotherapy, and bronchodilators, as needed (Sutton et al., 1983). It may be difficult or impossible to eradicate infections or bronchospasm completely in destructive lesions such as bronchiectasis. If this is the case, it is acceptable to proceed after reasonable medical therapy has optimized the patient's status so that no further improvement is anticipated.

Monitoring

At a minimum, thoracotomy requires monitoring of inspired oxygen, blood pressure, heart and breath sounds, airway pressure, and temperature, as well as an electrocardiogram. Oxygen saturation by pulse oximeter or, less commonly, by transcutaneous oxygen tension (Po_2) monitor (Harnick et al., 1983) is vital for detection of sudden changes in oxygenation from lung compression or kinking of the airway. Capnography is particularly useful for detecting sudden changes in effective ventilation. Arterial cannulation for pressure and arterial blood samples is useful and is needed if extensive blood loss or resection of lung tissue is expected or if the child is already critically ill. Percutaneous arterial cannulas (24 gauge in neonates, 22 gauge in children up to 8 to 10 years of age, and 20 gauge in preadolescents and older) can be inserted in children and should be used whenever indicated. Central venous monitoring is used less commonly but can be helpful for guiding extensive volume replacement. Urinary drainage is a consideration for particularly long procedures.

Positioning

Positioning of the patient has often been used to minimize spillage of lung contents because double-lumen tubes are impractical in smaller patients (Conlan et al., 1986). Suction through the ETT may not be adequate to control the large quantities of pus freed during surgical manipulation. The prone and lateral positions are the most commonly used. Positioning can cause significant ventilatory changes in children. Functional residual capacity (FRC) decreases during general anesthesia (Motoyama et al., 1982), and it falls dramatically once the pleura is opened (Larsson et al., 1987).

The practical problems of dislodgment of the ETT with movement and adequate padding in these positions are especially important in children. Open-celled foam with adhesive backing (Reston; 3M, St. Paul, MN) can be applied to the thorax, pelvic rim, and other pressure points to minimize the effects of positioning. Also, the tube position must be rechecked each time the patient is moved.

Anesthesia

General endotracheal anesthesia presents various challenges to the anesthesiologist. A quiet, smooth inhalation induction is often used in infants and smaller children, whereas an IV induction is used in the older child. If there is concern about spillage of lung contents, rapid securing of the airway with IV induction is preferred to minimize coughing. The choice of appropriate anesthetic agents depends on both the patient's status and the surgical lesion. Nitrous oxide can accumulate in cysts with air-fluid levels and should be avoided in these patients or in patients requiring a high fraction of inspired oxygen (Fio_2). Volatile agents are especially useful in patients with bronchospastic disorders. The rate of rise of inhalational anesthetics may be slowed in the presence of intrapulmonary shunting. Precipitous hypotension is another potential problem with volatile agents in patients with low cardiac reserve. Muscle relaxants are routinely used along with controlled ventilation employing humidified gases. Although mechanical ventilators are usually acceptable, manual ventilation provides useful information to the anesthesiologist about changes in compliance or airway resistance, especially in infants or in procedures where there is recurrent obstruction of the airway.

Single-Lung Ventilation Techniques

Single-Lung Ventilation Using a Single-Lumen Endotracheal Tube. The simplest means of providing SLV is to intentionally intubate the ipsilateral main stem bronchus with a conventional single-lumen ETT (Baraka, 1987; Kubota et al., 1987; Rowe et al., 1994). See related video online at www.expertconsult.com. When the left bronchus is to be intubated, the bevel of the ETT is rotated 180 degrees and the patient's head is turned to the right (Bloch, 1986; Kubota et al., 1987). The ETT is advanced into the bronchus until breath sounds on the operative side disappear. A fiberoptic bronchoscope (FOB) may be passed through or alongside the ETT to confirm or guide placement (Watson et al., 1982). When a cuffed ETT is used, the distance from the tip of the tube to the distal cuff must be shorter than the length of the bronchus so that the ETT does not occlude the upper lobe bronchus (Lammers et al., 1997) (Fig. 23-15). This technique is simple and requires no special equipment other than a FOB. This may be the preferred technique of SLV in emergency situations such as airway hemorrhage or contralateral tension pneumothorax.

Problems can occur when using a single-lumen ETT for SLV. If a smaller, uncuffed ETT is used, it may be difficult to provide an adequate seal of the intended bronchus. This may prevent the operative lung from adequately collapsing, or it may fail to protect the healthy, ventilated lung from contamination by purulent material from the contralateral lung. The operative lung cannot be suctioned using this technique. Hypoxemia may occur because of obstruction of the upper lobe bronchus, especially when the short right main stem bronchus is intubated.

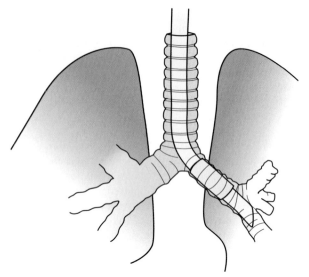

■ **FIGURE 23-15.** Obstruction of the left upper lobe bronchus with a cuffed endotracheal tube used for left-sided, single-lung ventilation.

TABLE 23-5. Diameters of Pediatric Endotracheal Tubes

Inner Diameter (mm)	Outer Diameter* (mm)
3.0	4.3
3.5	4.9
4.0	5.5
4.5	6.2
5.0	6.8
5.5	7.5
6.0	8.2
6.5	8.9
7.0	9.6

From Sheridan Tracheal Tubes, Kendall Healthcare, Mansfield, Mass.
*Cuffed tubes add approximately 0.5 mm to the outer diameter.

Single-Lung Ventilation Using a Balloon-Tipped Bronchial Blocker. A Fogarty embolectomy catheter or an end-hole, balloon-wedge catheter may be used for bronchial blockade to provide SLV (Fig. 23-16) (Ginsberg, 1981; Lin and Hackel, 1994; Hammer et al., 1996; Turner et al., 1997). Placement of a Fogarty catheter is facilitated by bending the tip of its stylet toward the bronchus on the operative side. A FOB is used to reposition the catheter and confirm appropriate placement. When an end-hole catheter is placed outside the ETT, the bronchus on the operative side is initially intubated with an ETT. A guidewire is then advanced into that bronchus through the ETT. The ETT is removed and the blocker is advanced over the guidewire into the bronchus. An ETT is then reinserted into the trachea alongside the blocker catheter. The catheter balloon is positioned in the proximal main stem bronchus under fiberoptic visual guidance. With an inflated blocker balloon, the airway is completely sealed, providing more-predictable lung collapse and better operating conditions than with an ETT in the contralateral bronchus.

A potential problem with this technique is dislodgment of the blocker balloon into the trachea. The inflated balloon then blocks ventilation to both lungs or prevents collapse of the operated lung, or both. The balloons of most catheters currently used for bronchial blockade have low-volume, high-pressure properties, and overdistention can damage or even rupture the airway (Borchardt et al., 1998). One study, however, reported that bronchial blocker cuffs produced lower cuff-to-tracheal pressures than double-lumen tubes (Guyton

et al., 1997). When closed-tip bronchial blockers are used, the operative lung cannot be suctioned, and continuous positive airway pressure (CPAP) cannot be provided to the operative lung if needed.

When a bronchial blocker is placed outside the ETT, care must be taken to avoid injury caused by compression and resultant ischemia of the tracheal mucosa. The sum of the catheter diameter and the outer diameter of the ETT should not exceed the tracheal diameter. Diameters for pediatric ETTs are shown in Table 23-5.

Adapters have been used that facilitate ventilation during placement of a bronchial blocker through an indwelling ETT (Arndt et al., 1999; Takahashi et al., 2000). For use in children, a 5-F endobronchial blocker designed with a multiport adapter and FOB has been described (Cook Critical Care, Bloomington, IN) (Hammer, 2001; Hammer et al., 2002). The balloon is elliptical, so it conforms to the bronchial lumen when inflated. The blocker catheter has a maximal outer diameter of 2.5 mm (including the deflated balloon), a central lumen with a diameter of 0.7 mm, and a distal balloon with a capacity of 3 mL. The balloon has a length of 1.0 cm, corresponding to the length of the right main stem bronchus in children approximately 2 years of age (Scammon, 1923). The blocker is placed coaxially through a dedicated port in the adapter, which also has a port for passage of an FOB and ports for connection to the anesthesia breathing circuit and ETT (Fig. 23-17). The FOB port has a plastic sealing cap, whereas the blocker port has a Tuohy-Borst connector, which locks the catheter in place and maintains an airtight seal. Because oxygen can be administered during passage of the blocker and FOB, the risk for hypoxemia during blocker placement is diminished, and repositioning of

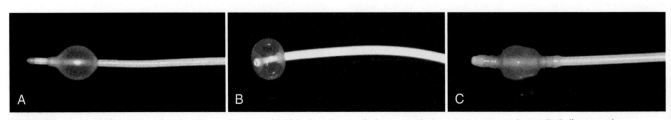

■ **FIGURE 23-16.** Balloon-tipped catheters used as bronchial blockers for single-lung ventilation. **A,** Fogarty catheter. **B,** Balloon wedge catheter. **C,** Cook endobronchial blocker. *(From Hammer GB: Pediatric thoracic anesthesia, Anesthesiol Clin North Am 20:153–180, 2002.)*

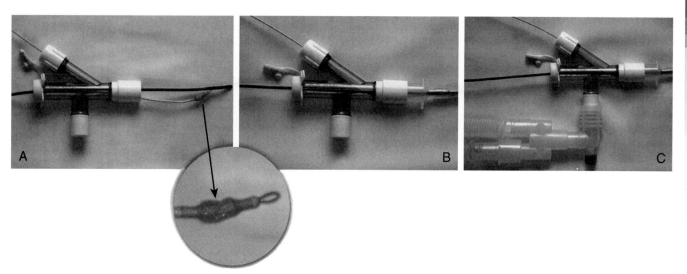

■ **FIGURE 23-17.** The Cook 5-F endobronchial catheter is shown inserted in the multiport adapter (Cook Critical Care, Bloomington, IN). The adapter has four ports for connection to (clockwise from bottom) the breathing circuit, fiberoptic bronchoscope (FOB), endobronchial catheter, and endotracheal tube **(A)**. After the FOB and endobronchial catheter have been inserted through the multiport adaptor, the FOB is placed through the monofilament loop at the distal end of the catheter *(arrow)*. The multiport adaptor is then attached to the indwelling endotracheal tube **(B)** and the breathing circuit **(C)**. The FOB is directed into the main stem bronchus on the operative side. The catheter is then advanced until the monofilament loop slides off the end of the FOB into the bronchus. *(From Hammer GB: Selective bronchial blockade in small infants,* Anesth Analg *93(6):1624–1625, 2001.)*

the blocker may be performed with fiberoptic guidance during surgery (Bird et al., 2007).

When placement of a bronchial blocker inside the ETT is guided by an FOB, both the blocker catheter and the FOB must pass through the indwelling ETT. The inner diameter of the ETT through which the catheter and FOB are to be placed must be larger than the sum of the outer diameters of the catheter and the FOB. The 5-F blocker catheter and an FOB with a 2.2-mm diameter, for example, may be inserted through an ETT as small as 5.0 mm in inner diameter. For children with an indwelling ETT smaller than 5.0 mm in inner diameter, a blocker catheter can be positioned under fluoroscopy (Fig. 23-18).

Single-Lung Ventilation Using a Univent Tube. The Univent tube (Fuji Systems Corporation, Tokyo, Japan) is a single-lumen ETT with a second lumen containing a small blocker catheter that can be advanced into a bronchus (Fig. 23-19) (Kamaya and Krishna, 1985; Kawande, 1987; Gayes, 1993). A balloon located at the distal end of this small tube serves as a blocker. Univent tubes require a FOB for successful placement. Univent tubes are now available in sizes as small as 3.5- and 4.5-mm inner diameter for use in children older than 6 years (Table 23-6) (Hammer et al., 1998). Because the blocker tube is firmly attached to the main ETT, displacement of the Univent blocker balloon is less likely than when other blocker techniques are used. The blocker of the 4.5-mm Univent tube has a small lumen, which allows egress of gas and can be used to insufflate oxygen or to suction the operated lung.

A disadvantage of the Univent tube is the large amount of cross-sectional area occupied by the blocker channel, especially in the smaller-sized tubes. Smaller Univent tubes have a disproportionately high resistance to gas flow (Slinger and Lesiuk, 1998). The Univent tube's blocker balloon has low-volume, high-pressure characteristics, so mucosal injury can occur during normal inflation (Benumof et al., 1992; Kelley et al., 1992).

Single-Lung Ventilation Using a Double-Lumen Tube. All double-lumen tubes (DLTs) are essentially two tracheal tubes of unequal length, molded longitudinally together. The shorter tube ends in the trachea, and the longer tube, in the bronchus. Marraro (1994) described a bilumen tube for infants (Pawar and Marraro, 2005). DLTs for older children and adults have cuffs located on the tracheal and bronchial lumens. The tracheal cuff, when inflated, allows positive pressure ventilation. The inflated bronchial cuff allows ventilation to be diverted to either or both lungs and protects each lung from contamination from the contralateral side.

Conventional plastic DLTs, once available only in adult sizes (35-F, 37-F, 39-F, and 41-F), are now available in smaller sizes (Table 23-7). The smallest cuffed DLT is 26-F (Rusch, Duluth, GA) and may be used in children as young as 8 years. DLTs are also available in sizes 28-F and 32-F (Mallinckrodt Medical, St. Louis, MO), suitable for children 10 years of age and older.

DLTs are inserted in children using the same technique used in adults (Brodsky and Mark, 1983). The tip of the tube is inserted just past the vocal cords and the stylet is withdrawn. The DLT is rotated 90 degrees to the appropriate side and then advanced into the bronchus. In the adult population, the depth of insertion is directly related to the height of the patient (Brodsky et al., 1996). No equivalent measurements are yet available in children. If fiberoptic bronchoscopy is to be used to confirm tube placement, an FOB with a small diameter and sufficient length must be available (Slinger, 1989).

A DLT offers the advantage of ease of insertion and the ability to suction and oxygenate the operative lung with CPAP. Left DLTs are preferred to right DLTs because of the shorter length of the right main bronchus (Benumof et al., 1987). Right DLTs are more difficult to accurately position because of the greater risk for right upper lobe obstruction. DLTs are safe and easy to use. There are very few reports of airway damage from DLTs in adults, and none in children. Their high-volume, low-pressure cuffs should not damage the

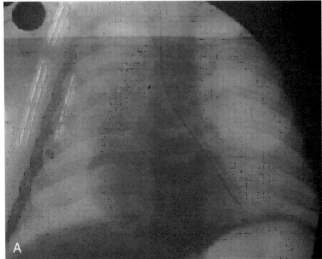

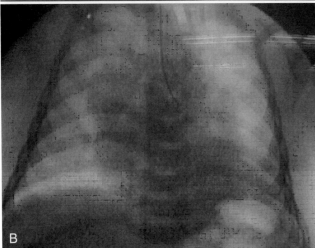

■ FIGURE 23-18. Positioning a bronchial blocker under fluoroscopy. **A,** The catheter has been advanced into a segmental bronchus on the left. **B,** The catheter has been pulled back so that the balloon is in the left main stem bronchus.

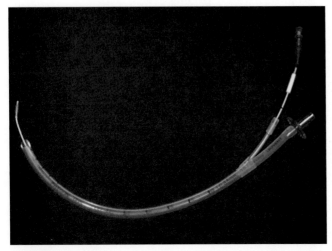

■ FIGURE 23-19. The Univent tube is a single-lumen endotracheal tube with a second lumen containing a small blocker catheter.

TABLE 23-6. Univent Tube Diameters

Inner Diameter (mm)	Outer Diameter* (mm)
3.5	7.5/8.0
4.5	8.5/9.0
6.0	10.0/11.0
6.5	10.5/11.5
7.0	11.0/12.0
7.5	11.5/12.5
8.0	12.0/13.0
8.5	12.5/13.5
9.0	13.0/14.0

*Sagittal/transverse.

TABLE 23-7. Tube Selection for Single-Lung Ventilation in Children

Age of Child (yr)	ETT (mm, inner diameter*)	BB (F)	Univent†	DLT (F)
0.5 to 1	3.5 to 4.0	2‡	—	—
1 to 2	4.0 to 4.5	3‡	—	—
2 to 4	4.5 to 5.0	5§	—	—
4 to 6	5.0 to 5.5	5§	—	—
6 to 8	5.5 to 6	5§	3.5	—
8 to 10	6.0 cuffed	5§	3.5	—
10 to 12	6.5 cuffed	5§	4.5	26‖ to 28¶
12 to 14	6.5 to 7.0 cuffed	5§	4.5	32¶
14 to 16	7.0 cuffed	5§	6.0	35¶
16 to 18	7.0 to 8.0 cuffed	9§	7.0	35¶

BB, Bronchial blocker; *DLT,* double-lumen tube; *ETT,* endotracheal tube; *F,* French.
*Sheridan Tracheal Tubes, Kendall Healthcare, Mansfield, MA.
†Fuji Systems Corporation, Tokyo, Japan.
‡Edwards Lifesciences LLC, Irvine, CA.
§Cook Critical Care, Inc., Bloomington, IN.
‖Rusch, Duluth, GA.
¶Mallinckrodt Medical, Inc., St. Louis, MO.

airway if they are not overinflated with air or distended with nitrous oxide while in place. Guidelines for selecting appropriate tubes (or catheters) for SLV in children are shown in Table 23–7. There is significant variability in overall size and airway dimensions among children, particularly among teenagers, and these recommendations are based on average values for airway dimensions. Larger DLTs may be safely used in adult-size teenagers.

Postoperative Care

Tracheal extubation at the completion of surgery is often possible after simple subsegmental resection or lobectomy. However, the patient's underlying cardiopulmonary reserve, the course of the surgery, and the expected postoperative course may preclude extubation. Although postoperative pain can cause significant splinting, intercostal or epidural blocks, coupled with judicious parenteral opioids, can minimize the discomfort (see Chapters 15 and 16, Pain Management and Regional Anesthesia). Whether in the operating room or in the intensive care area, before extubation the patient must be awake, breathing well, able to cough and maintain an airway, and able to maintain acceptable oxygenation with no more than 40% inspired oxygen. A chest radiograph should be obtained as soon as possible after surgery to detect any significant pneumothorax or atelectasis. Atelectasis is common and usually responds to humidity, encouragement to cough, CPAP, and if necessary, endotracheal suction.

The expected postoperative course depends on both the surgical procedure and the underlying diseases. After simple lobectomy, most children develop normally and have normal exercise tolerance (McBride et al., 1980). Children who have undergone pneumonectomy may have more problems (Buhain and Brody, 1973). With time, overinflation of the remaining lung occurs, with a demonstrable decrease in vital capacity. These children may have significant exercise intolerance for a prolonged period after surgery.

Surgery for Congenital Lobar Emphysema, Pulmonary Sequestration, and Cystic Lesions

Congenital Lobar Emphysema

Congenital lobar emphysema is a rare cause of sudden respiratory distress in infants (Leape and Longino, 1964; Raynor et al., 1967). Hyperinflation and progressive air trapping cause expansion of the affected lobe, along with compression of other lung tissue, mediastinal shifting, and impaired venous return. The most commonly affected is the left upper lobe, followed by the right middle and upper lobes. Occasionally, more than one lobe is affected. The cause of the obstruction is unknown in most cases, although many show evidence of deficient and disordered bronchial cartilage. In some cases, there are identifiable causes of bronchial compression, such as aberrant blood vessels, bronchial cysts, and bronchial stenosis. Finally, some patients have widespread lung disease with poor elastic recoil throughout (Ryckman and Rosenkrantz, 1985). See related video online at www.expertconsult.com.

Congenital lobar emphysema usually appears clinically between the newborn period and the first 6 months of life (Murray, 1967) with tachycardia and retractions. The child may have rapid, progressive accumulation of gas in the affected lobe. Physical examination reveals asymmetric expansion of the thorax, wheezing, displacement of the cardiac impulse, hyperresonance to percussion, and diminished breath and heart sounds. Chest radiographs (Fig. 23-20) show overdistention of the affected lobe, mediastinal shift, and atelectasis in other lobes. The chest radiograph can help differentiate lobar emphysema from pneumothorax or congenital cysts by the presence of faint bronchovascular markings and herniation of the affected lobe across the midline.

Infants who show rapid deterioration constitute a surgical emergency to relieve the expanding lobe with its ventilatory and cardiac impairment. Many patients do not have a clear clinical picture, however, but rather have a vague history of intermittent cyanosis or respiratory distress, failure to thrive, or unusual respiratory distress with feeding or a cold. Lobar emphysema is also seen in preterm infants with respiratory distress who are undergoing mechanical ventilation, and it most frequently develops in the right upper lobe.

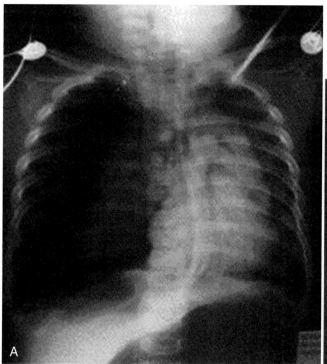

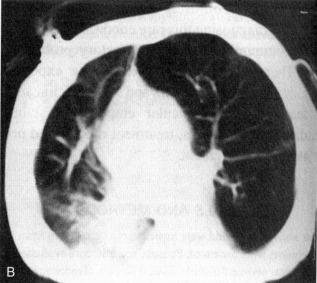

■ **FIGURE 23-20.** Right-sided congenital lobar emphysema. **A,** The right lung appears hyperinflated and lucent and may be mistaken for a pneumothorax. **B,** CT scan reveals markedly hyperexpanded right lung, mediastinal shift to the left, and compression of the left lung.

Preoperative evaluation depends on the degree of patient distress (Payne et al., 1984). If there is rapid deterioration, evaluation is limited. Chest tube placement, needle aspiration of the trapped air, and vigorous mechanical ventilation have been tried as palliative procedures but are associated with a much higher mortality than thoracotomy and lobectomy. If the patient is stable and there is any question about the diagnosis, procedures such as radioisotope perfusion scans, angiography, or CT imaging can be used before proceeding with definitive surgery. During preanesthesia evaluation, cardiopulmonary stability of the patient is the prime concern. The degree of distress, its progression, and the need for supplemental oxygen are key components of the examination. Cardiac evaluation is important because these patients have a higher incidence of congenital heart disease, especially ventricular septal defect.

Monitoring includes pulse oximetry to detect rapid changes in oxygenation, especially with induction. In deteriorating patients, there may be little time to establish intraarterial monitoring before incision. Doppler-assisted or automated blood pressure cuffs increase the accuracy of measurements and are especially useful in infants. After intubation, capnography is helpful.

Induction of anesthesia in infants with congenital lobar emphysema is a critical phase in the management of anesthesia. The crying, struggling infant can increase the amount of trapped gas, whereas positive-pressure ventilation or positive airway pressure by the anesthesiologist can also increase the emphysema. A smooth inhalation induction with sevoflurane and oxygen is often used, with positive pressure ventilation minimized until the chest is open (Coté, 1978). Controlled or assisted ventilation is added if unacceptable hypoventilation develops, whereas intubation is performed with or without muscle relaxants, depending on the patient's tolerance of positive pressure ventilation. High-frequency ventilation has been used successfully in infants with lobar emphysema (Goto et al., 1987) and should be considered if the practitioner is familiar with the technique. The low airway pressures are especially suitable for these patients. Nitrous oxide is avoided because it can expand the emphysematous areas (Payne et al., 1984). If the lobe expands suddenly, the surgeon should be ready to open the chest immediately and relieve the pressure. Raghavendran and coworkers (2001) described a technique involving a caudal epidural catheter threaded to the thoracic level in spontaneously breathing patients who were anesthetized with potent inhaled anesthetic agents.

An alternative induction approach, especially for unstable infants, is sedation with IV ketamine (1 to 2 mg/kg) and local anesthetic infiltration of the incision site (Coté, 1978). After the intrathoracic pressure has been relieved, general anesthesia can proceed with any technique appropriate to the patient's underlying status. Older children who are stable often undergo bronchoscopy before thoracotomy to rule out a foreign body or other correctable lesions. After induction with oxygen and a volatile agent, thorough topical anesthesia with 2% to 4% lidocaine (not more than 4 to 6 mg/kg) smoothes the course. As with the younger patient, rapid surgical decompression may be needed as the case proceeds.

In most patients, the trachea can be extubated at the end of the lobectomy. Humidity, coughing, and early increases in activity or ambulation minimize atelectasis in the immediate postoperative period. These children do well clinically after surgery but have reduced forced vital capacity and delayed forced expiration, not only in the immediate postoperative period but throughout childhood (Eigen et al., 1976; McBride et al., 1980).

Pulmonary Sequestrations

Pulmonary sequestrations (Fig. 23-21) result from disordered embryogenesis producing a nonfunctional mass of lung tissue supplied by anomalous systemic arteries. Signs include cough, pneumonia, and failure to thrive and they often appear during the neonatal period, usually before the age of 2 years. Diagnostic studies include CT scans of the chest and abdomen and arteriography. Magnetic resonance imaging may provide high-resolution images, including definition of vascular supply. This may obviate the need for angiography. Surgical resection is performed after the diagnosis. Pulmonary sequestrations do not generally become hyperinflated during positive pressure ventilation. Nitrous oxide administration may result in expansion of these masses, however, and should be avoided.

Congenital Cystic Lesions

Congenital cystic lesions in the thorax fall into three categories: bronchogenic, dermoid, and cystic adenomatoid malformations (Fig. 23-22) (Stocker et al., 1977; Nishibayashi et al., 1981; Kravitz, 1994). Bronchogenic cysts result from abnormal budding or branching of the tracheobronchial tree. They may cause respiratory distress, recurrent pneumonia, or atelectasis due to lung compression. Dermoid cysts are clinically similar to bronchogenic cysts but differ histologically, as they are lined with keratinized, squamous epithelium rather than respiratory (ciliated columnar) epithelium. They usually appear later in childhood or adulthood. CCAMs are structurally similar to bronchioles but lack associated alveoli, bronchial glands, and cartilage (Ryckman and Rosenkrantz, 1985). Because these lesions communicate with the airways, they may become overdistended as a result of gas trapping, leading to respiratory distress in the first few days of life. When they are multiple and air filled, CCAMs may resemble congenital diaphragmatic hernia radiographically. Treatment is surgical resection of the affected lobe. As with the diaphragmatic hernia, prognosis depends on the amount of remaining lung tissue, which may be hypoplastic because of compression in utero (Adelman and Benson, 1976; Schwartz and Ramachandran, 1997).

Surgery for Diseases of the Mediastinum

Surgical problems of the mediastinum fall into three major categories: masses, infections, and pneumomediastinum. The mediastinum is functionally divided into anterior, middle, and posterior segments. This classification is useful diagnostically in evaluating defects, because of the propensity of lesions to develop primarily in only one of the divisions (Table 23-8 and Box 23-7).

Masses in the anterior portion of the mediastinum tend to be lymphomas, lymphangiomas (cystic hygroma), and teratomas. See related video online at www.expertconsult.com. Thymomas and thymic cysts can appear here but are rare in childhood. Lymphomas are primarily of the Hodgkin's type, and biopsies of them are done only for diagnostic purposes. The survival of the child with mediastinal lymphoma depends on the systemic spread of the tumor and not on the amount of

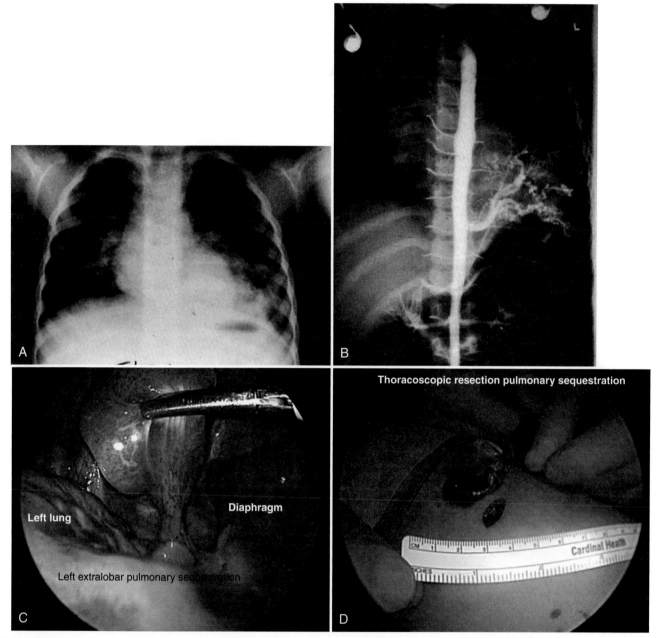

■ FIGURE 23-21. Extralobar pulmonary sequestration. **A,** Chest radiograph of pulmonary sequestration. **B,** Aortogram of pulmonary sequestration of arterial blood supply coming from aorta. **C,** Thoroscopic resection of sequestration. **D,** Resected sequestration. *(From Zitelli BJ, Davis HW, editors: Atlas of pediatric physical diagnosis, ed 4, St Louis, 2002, Mosby, p 539.)*

lymphoma present in the mediastinum. Lymphangiomas are often extensions of cystic hygromas from the cervical region into the mediastinum. If not all of the lymphangioma is removed at the initial resection, further extension may occur. Anterior mediastinal masses can appear in various ways. Although they may be asymptomatic and detected incidentally on a chest radiograph, they may also present as compression of pulmonary or vascular structures. Superior vena cava syndrome, cardiac tamponade, and both tracheal and lung compression can be prominent characteristics (Levin et al., 1985; Northrip et al., 1986).

Bronchogenic cysts, granulomas, and lymphomas predominate in the middle division. Bronchogenic cysts make up 7.5%

of all mediastinal masses (Fig. 23-23). They may be asymptomatic or exhibit symptoms of airway obstruction or recurrent pulmonary infection (Birmingham et al., 1993; Landsman et al., 1994). Bronchogenic cysts are usually next to the trachea or main stem bronchi at the level of the carina, but they can also be intrapulmonary. They can produce sudden, life-threatening airway obstruction at any age. Lesser degrees of obstruction appear initially as wheezing, stridor, or unilateral obstructive emphysema (Azizkhan et al., 1985; Azarow et al., 1993).

In the posterior division, enteric cysts and tumors of neurogenic origin (neuroblastoma, ganglioneuroma, neurofibroma) predominate. See related video online at www.expertconsult. com. Enteric cysts and duplications are lined with secretory

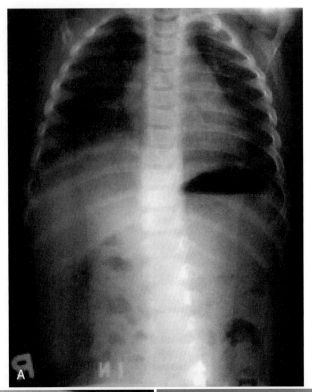

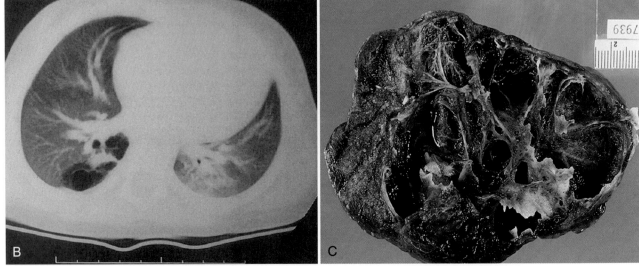

■ **FIGURE 23-22.** Microcystic adenomatoid malformation seen on plain film **(A)**, CT scan **(B)**, and surgical specimen **(C)**. *(From Zitelli BJ, Davis HW, editors:* Atlas of pediatric physical diagnosis, *ed 4, St Louis, 2002, Mosby, p 565.)*

epithelium and can enlarge rapidly and cause dysphagia, ulceration, or bleeding. In rare cases, they can ulcerate directly into the tracheobronchial tree. Neurogenic tumors are usually asymptomatic and detected on a routine chest radiograph, although they can be responsible for tracheobronchial compression, recurrent pneumonias, and, rarely, stigmata of pheochromocytoma.

Mediastinal infections and inflammation are less common today than in the past (Campbell and Lilly, 1983). Modern antibiotic therapy dramatically reduced the incidence of suppurative mediastinitis caused by *Staphylococcus* and other organisms, whereas the incidence of tuberculosis and other similar infections in the general population has diminished. Although mediastinitis can result from extension of cervical node infections

or hematogenous spread, the more likely cause is perforation of the trachea or esophagus. Foreign bodies can be responsible for perforation of the larynx, trachea, or esophagus; instrumentation of the trachea (endotracheal intubation or suction) or esophagus (esophageal dilation) can also be responsible.

Pneumomediastinum is an accumulation of air, usually in the superior anterior division. This occurs in trauma patients and as a result of mechanical ventilation, especially in newborns who undergo long-term ventilation and children with severe asthma. Pneumomediastinum is usually asymptomatic, but it may be responsible for tamponade and hypotension. These patients need urgent decompression by thoracostomy. Pneumomediastinum can be accompanied by pneumopericardium, which may need

TABLE 23-8. Mediastinal Masses

Location	Presentation
Anterior Division	
Lymphomas	Superior vena cava syndrome
Lymphangiomas (cystic hygroma)	Cardiac tamponade
Teratomas	Tracheal and lung compression
Thymomas and thymic cysts	Thymomas and thymic cysts
Middle Division	
Bronchogenic cysts	Airway obstruction
Granulomas	Stridor
Lymphomas	Obstructive emphysema
Posterior Division	
Enteric cysts, duplications	Airway obstruction
Neuroblastoma	Recurrent pneumonias
Ganglioneuroma, neurofibroma	Dysphagia

Box 23-7 Mediastinal Masses

ANTERIOR
Thymus: normal, rebound hypertrophy, thymoma
Teratoma (three layers), dermoid (two layers)
Lymphoma
Thyroid tumor
Bronchogenic cyst

MIDDLE
Inflammatory lymph nodes or lymphoma
Foregut abnormalities (esophageal duplication, bronchogenic cysts)
Prominent pulmonary vessels, aortic dilation, or aneurysm
Pericardial abnormalities

POSTERIOR
Neurally based tumors: ganglioneuroma, ganglioneuroblastoma, neuroblastoma
Congenital pulmonary or pleural lesions: sequestration, bronchogenic or neurenteric cyst

SUPERIOR
Cystic hygroma
Bronchogenic cyst
Neurally based tumors
Rare vascular lesions

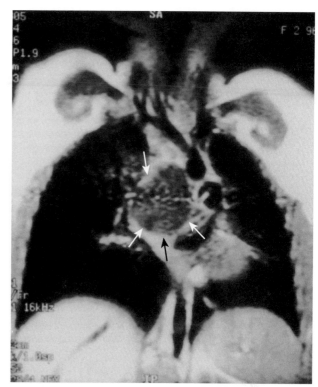

■ **FIGURE 23-23.** Magnetic resonance imaging of the chest; coronal section through the trachea and bronchogenic cyst *(black arrows)* located in the subcrinal area. The cyst is shown compressing the right main stem bronchus *(white arrows)*. *(From Landsman IS, et al: Fluoroscopy as an aid to anesthetic management for bronchogenic cyst resection, Anesth Analg 79:803, 1994.)*

to be drained urgently as well. The intrathoracic pressure generated by pneumomediastinum can impede venous drainage of the head and result in increased intracranial pressure (Fig. 23-24).

Anesthetic management of children with mediastinal diseases demands careful preoperative evaluation (Mackie and Watson, 1984). The location and nature of the disease are crucial to both preparation and management (see Fig. 23-24). The airway is considered first (Todres et al., 1976; Keon, 1981). If there is evidence of obstruction, the site and degree must be assessed. History and physical examination should focus not only on signs such as cyanosis and stridor but also on maneuvers or circumstances that change the signs. The practitioner should determine if sleep, excitement, position, movement of the head and neck, or coughing changes the degree of obstruction. Although chest radiographs and barium studies provide some information, CT scans are best at delineating the obstruction of vascular and airway structures (Anghelescu et al., 2007). These scans have the added advantage of demonstrating extension of infection or tumor into structures such as the pericardium.

Signs of lower airway disease can be caused by mediastinal tumors (Sibert et al., 1987). Compression of the lower airways and lung tissue can be responsible for wheezing, atelectasis, obstructive emphysema, and recurrent pneumonias. This is important because wheezing caused by compression of lower airways and lung tissue usually does not respond to bronchodilators, nor will atelectasis caused by compression respond to chest physical therapy. Repeat chest radiographs or pulmonary function tests can help delineate the degree of functional impairment. In older, more cooperative children, maximal inspiratory and expiratory flow-volume loops obtained with the patient upright and supine can quantitate the functional degree of impairment and help distinguish fixed from variable obstructions (Fig. 23-25).

Cardiovascular involvement may be related to direct compression of the heart or of the great vessels. Echocardiography or CT scanning can delineate impingement. The important determination is assessment of functional impairment. If the child has arrhythmias, pulsus paradoxus, hypotension, or superior vena cava syndrome, the risk of general anesthesia increases dramatically.

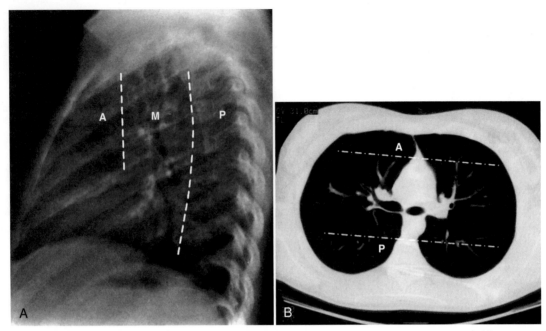

■ **FIGURE 23-24.** Mediastinal compartmentalization on lateral radiograph **(A)** and CT scan **(B).** *A,* Anterior; *M,* Middle; *P,* Posterior. *(From Blickman JG, Parker R, Barnes PD: Pediatric radiology, St Louis, 2009, Mosby.)*

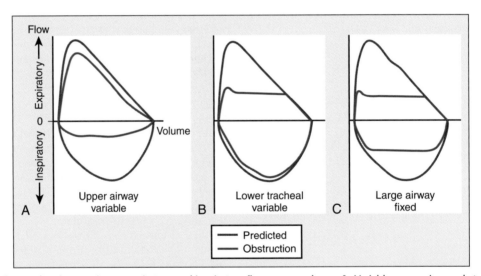

■ **FIGURE 23-25.** Curves showing maximum expiratory and inspiratory flow versus volume. **A,** Variable upper airway obstruction caused by papillomatosis of the larynx. **B,** Variable central (intrathoracic) airway obstruction caused by tracheomalacia. **C,** Fixed-type obstruction caused by tracheal stenosis. *(From Motoyama EK: Physiologic alterations in tracheostomy. In Myers EN, Stool SE, Johnson JT, editors:* Tracheostomy, *New York, 1985, Churchill Livingstone.)*

Induction of anesthesia may remove compensatory efforts by the patient (Neuman et al., 1984). The child's position, pattern of ventilation, or sympathetic tone while awake may have been responsible for barely maintaining adequate cardiopulmonary function (Bray and Fernandes, 1982; Prakash et al., 1988) (Fig. 23-26). In these situations, the anesthesiologist and surgeon must determine alternative approaches to the lesion (Mackie and Watson, 1984). If the child has a better airway, easier ventilation, or less hypotension in one position, efforts are made to keep him or her in this position. Although respiratory compromise is a significant complication in patients with an anterior medial mass undergoing general anesthesia, this complication is more likely in patients with a tracheal cross-sectional area less than 50% of normal (as predicted by CT) and a peak expiratory flow rate less than 50% of predicted (Shamberger, 1999). Biopsy of accessible lesions under local anesthesia should be considered if there is significant cardiopulmonary compromise. In extreme cases, radiation therapy quickly shrinks the tumor mass, allowing a biopsy to be done later with less risk to the patient (Piro et al., 1976). If general anesthesia is used, the surgeon should be present at induction and prepared for interventions such as passage of a rigid bronchoscope or immediate release of a pneumomediastinum via subxiphoid thoracostomy. Of utmost importance is that the patient, family, pediatrician,

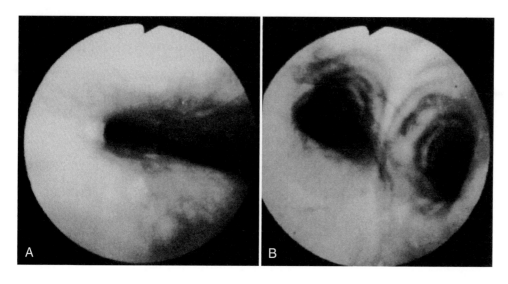

■ **FIGURE 23-26.** The effects of anesthesia on tracheal compression in a patient with a mediastinal mass. *(From Prakash UBS, Abel MD, Hubmayr RD: Mediastinal mass and tracheal obstruction during general anesthesia, Mayo Clin Proc 63:1004, 1988.)*

and surgeon all understand the risk for cardiovascular and respiratory compromise that exists in performing tissue biopsies under general anesthesia (Fig. 23-27).

Mask induction with a volatile agent and 100% oxygen is appropriate if there is concern about airway obstruction. The negative intrathoracic pressure of spontaneous breathing and any beneficial effect this has on maintenance of airway patency are preserved (Sibert et al., 1987). In some cases, airway obstruction worsens with positive pressure ventilation; it may be necessary to maintain spontaneous or assisted ventilation. Two important monitors during induction are breath sounds from the precordial stethoscope and continuous oxygen saturation monitoring from a pulse oximeter. Nitrous oxide is avoided in all cases of pneumomediastinum or obstructive emphysema and in patients who have significant V/Q abnormalities

from lung compression (Mackie and Watson, 1984). The role of nitrous oxide in patients with asymptomatic bronchogenic cysts is unclear. Because these cysts are air filled, they may expand on exposure to nitrous oxide and cause airway compromise. In rare cases of severe airway impingement, intubation in the awake, sedated patient may be necessary to secure the airway safely for general anesthesia. If cardiac compression is of primary concern, narcotic-based anesthesia with or without ketamine for induction is a useful technique.

Thoracotomy or thoracostomy is usually the operative procedure performed in these patients. Major complications include massive blood loss, further obstruction or perforation of the airway, and lung compression (Barash et al., 1976; Neuman et al., 1984). There continue to be sporadic reports of death during the induction and maintenance of anesthesia in children

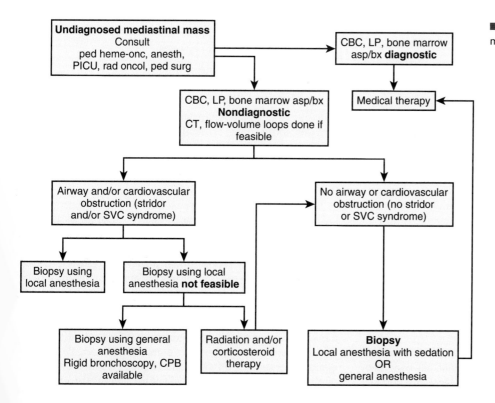

■ **FIGURE 23-27.** Algorithm for mediastinal mass.

with mediastinal masses, emphasizing the need for meticulous preoperative evaluation and intraoperative care. After reviewing 44 pediatric patients with mediastinal masses, Ferrari and Bedford (1990) noted that significant anesthesia-related problems occurred in the patients who were symptomatic before surgery. They noted that general anesthesia could be administered with the following caveats: spontaneous ventilation must be performed, induction of anesthesia should be in the sitting position, IV access should be in the lower upper extremity, and a rigid bronchoscope and experienced bronchoscopist must be available. The anesthesiologist not only must be prepared for each complication but also must notify the surgeon immediately if there is loss of airway, difficulty in ventilation, or sudden hypotension.

UROLOGIC SURGERY

A wide range of surgical lesions require the expertise of a pediatric urologist (Box 23-8 and Table 23-9). Although the anesthetic requirements for the different surgical lesions vary, the preoperative anesthetic assessment focuses on several important considerations. First, does the child have a known syndrome that has multiple anesthetic considerations? Second, does the child have other congenital anomalies, such as cardiac abnormalities, that require evaluation? Last, does the child have signs or symptoms of any underlying renal insufficiency? In general, renal failure is divided into acute and chronic components. Acute renal failure is the sudden loss of the kidneys' ability to excrete water, electrolytes, and waste products in sufficient quantities to maintain the body's homeostasis. The causes of acute renal failure are numerous and can be divided into four broad categories: prerenal, renal parenchymal, renal tubule, and obstructive. Regardless of its cause, management of acute renal failure is aimed at ensuring that the patient has an adequate circulating blood volume, and at avoiding fluid overload.

Congestive heart failure occurs when more than insensible fluid losses and urinary output are replaced. Although either a normal or reduced urinary output can occur with acute renal failure, with the onset of anuria or oliguria, hyperkalemia and hypocalcemia can occur. Hyperkalemia is the major life-threatening complication of acute renal failure and therefore must be treated immediately. Because of the kidneys' inability to excrete cellular waste products, acidosis also develops in acute renal failure. Although for most patients, acute renal failure is reversible, some patients go on to develop chronic failure (see Chapter 5, Regulation of Fluids and Electrolytes).

Chronic renal failure or end-stage renal disease results in a 95% loss of creatinine clearance. A 50% loss of nephrons generally results in no biochemical abnormalities and a glomerular filtration rate of about 80%. The biochemical manifestations of end-stage renal disease result in the inability of the kidneys to regulate water and electrolytes and to excrete acid waste products. Because the kidney is also an exocrine organ, progressive renal failure is accompanied by abnormalities in the excretion of vitamin D, parathyroid hormone, and erythropoietin. End-stage renal disease, through its biochemical and hormonal mediators, affects all organ systems (see Chapter 28, Anesthesia for Organ Transplantation).

In addition to being aware of the pathophysiologic problems that accompany patients with renal and urologic abnormalities, the anesthesiologist must be cognizant of potential emotional

Box 23-8 Genitourinary Conditions Requiring Surgery During Infancy and Childhood

CONGENITAL ANOMALIES
- Ureteral valves
- Double renal pelvis and ureters
- Ectopic ureter
- Megaureter
- Ureterocele
- Neurogenic bladder
- Exstrophy of bladder
- Undescended testes
- Hypospadias, epispadias
- Phimosis
- Vaginal anomalies

CYSTS AND TUMORS
- Wilms tumor
- Cystic kidney
- Neuroblastoma
- Ganglioneuroma
- Adrenogenital tumors
- Pheochromocytoma
- Retroperitoneal teratoma
- Ovarian tumor

TRAUMA
- Ruptured kidney
- Ruptured bladder
- Urethral injuries

RENAL FAILURE (OPERATIVE PROCEDURES)
- Renal biopsy
- Nephrectomy
- Shunt and fistula creation
- Parathyroidectomy
- Renal transplantation

INFECTIONS
- Cystitis
- Urethritis
- Paraphimosis

OTHER
- Renal and bladder calculi and stones

difficulties that children have when faced with genitourinary surgery. Not infrequently, some of these patients have deep-seated emotional problems, and the anesthesiologist should be sensitive to their needs. Issues involving the psychological preparation of the patient are explored in Chapter 8, Psychological Aspects of Pediatric Anesthesia.

In the child with normal renal function, anesthesia for urologic surgery is similar to anesthesia for most other types of surgery. In patients with renal insufficiency, nephrotoxic drugs should be avoided or their dosage reduced. The differences in distribution and excretion of drugs that are renally excreted should be remembered. This primarily applies to neuromuscular blockers, because there is little evidence that the volatile agents are materially different in patients with renal insufficiency. There is a well-known risk of prolongation of action with morphine and, especially, meperidine, but the synthetic opioids are used more commonly in this population. Among the muscle relaxants, a delayed onset of and slight resistance to vecuronium have been reported in renal failure patients (Hunter et al.,

TABLE 23-9. Signs and Symptoms of Patients with Renal Insufficiency

Other System Involved	Signs and Symptoms
Cardiovascular	Hypertension Increased cardiac output or high output failure Atherosclerosis or hyperlipidemia Pericarditis Variable increase in 2, 3-diphosphoglycerate levels
Pulmonary	Hypoxemia Pulmonary edema Pleuritis
Hematologic	Anemia secondary to erythropoietin deficiency Anemia secondary to blood loss, decreased iron absorption, and folic acid deficiency Platelet dysfunction Decreased antithrombin III levels Increased factor VIII and fibrinogen
Neurologic	Irritability, confusion, anxiety, memory loss, encephalopathy, and psychosis Seizures, coma Peripheral neuropathy
Gastrointestinal	Anorexia, nausea, vomiting, gastroparesis
Metabolic/endocrine	Renal osteodystrophy secondary to hyperparathyroidism, hyperkalemia, hypocalcemia, metabolic acidosis, hypernatremia, and hyponatremia
Infectious	Hepatitis B or non-A, non-B hepatitis Cytomegalovirus and human immunodeficiency virus

1984), as well as delayed onset of rocuronium (Driessen et al., 2002). However, these differences are modest, even in children with complete renal failure.

Urologic procedures frequently require patients to be positioned in the lateral, prone, or lithotomy position. Each of these positions can be associated with compression-type injuries, as well as with compromise of ventilation and venous return. Consequently, anesthetic management requires not only diligence to patient monitoring but also attention to appropriate patient positioning, padding, and rechecking of positioning.

Cystoscopy

Cystoscopy is commonly performed in children under general anesthesia to evaluate abnormalities of the urethra, bladder, and ureters. This is a relatively brief procedure; however, positioning the patient away from the anesthesia machine, extending the anesthetic tubing and monitor cables, maintaining a possibly difficult airway at the far end of the operating table, and exposing the patient to a cold room and irrigating solutions may complicate the delivery of anesthesia. Mask inhalation anesthesia is usually satisfactory, and endotracheal intubation or laryngeal mask airway is not necessary beyond infancy, as long as a satisfactory airway can be maintained. It is important, however, to maintain a relatively deep plane of anesthesia before insertion of the cystoscope, because the urethral stimulation may precipitate laryngospasm (Breuer-Lockhart reflex) (Stehling

and Furman, 1980). Regional anesthesia is infrequently used as the primary anesthetic for cystoscopy, but it can be used for postoperative analgesia. However, most children experience little discomfort on awakening.

Circumcision

Circumcision is the most frequently performed surgical procedure in the world (Klauber and Sant, 1985). Most circumcisions are performed during the newborn period, and many are done without any anesthesia. However, there is increasing attention paid to providing analgesia for the procedure, including the use of the simple penile nerve block by obstetricians, family practitioners, and pediatricians (Maxwell et al., 1987; Howard et al., 1998). Simple techniques can significantly decrease cardiovascular and behavioral responses to pain in these neonates (Holliday et al., 1999). With increased education, especially at the resident level, there should be an increase in these techniques being used by primary care practitioners.

Beyond the newborn period, circumcision is usually performed under general anesthesia. Mask inhalation anesthesia with sevoflurane or isoflurane in nitrous oxide and oxygen is commonly used. A penile nerve block can be performed either immediately after anesthetic induction or at the end of the operation. It may be advantageous to place the block before the circumcision because the anesthetic requirement is decreased and emergence is more rapid. Caudal epidural anesthesia is also efficacious, although penile nerve block is preferred by some because less local anesthetic is given and less time is taken to perform the block. Others have suggested that the time, expense, and risk of caudal block are not justified for circumcision, because parenteral opioid administration is equally effective (Martin, 1982).

A comparison of different modalities for analgesia, with a focus on caudal analgesia, found that although the need for rescue analgesia is reduced in the early postoperative period when caudal block is compared with parenteral analgesia, there the data in the literature are not sufficient to accurately compare both the short- and long-term effectiveness of caudal block versus other modalities such as parental analgesia, penile block, or topical anesthetic gel or cream (Allan et al., 2003). This analysis points out a problem in analyzing almost all the work on analgesia for urologic procedures—there are insufficient studies available that compare all available modalities in a consistent, uniform manner, thereby allowing direct comparison of risks and benefits.

Ureteral Reimplantation and Bladder Neck Surgery

Reimplantation of one or both ureters is performed for treatment of vesicoureteral reflux, whether it occurs congenitally or results from repeated urinary tract infections. Vesicoureteral reflux occurs in up to 2% of children, and its severity is based on a voiding cystourethrogram. The need for surgical reimplantation is based on the patient's age, gender, grade of reflux, degree of renal scarring, and anatomic abnormalities. In addition to reimplantation, some patients may be amenable to deflux procedures (Fig. 23-28). Deflux procedures involve cystoscopy and injection of compounds (Teflon, and, more recently, polydimethylsiloxane and dextranomer polymer) into the terminal

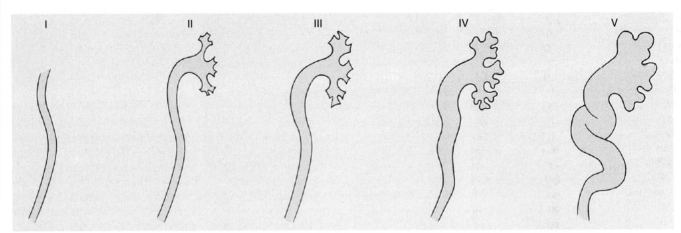

■ **FIGURE 23-28.** *Grade I:* Reflux into the ureter only. *Grade II:* Complete reflux into the ureter, pelvis, and calices without any dilation of the structures. *Grade III:* Complete reflux with mild dilation or tortuosity of the ureter, and mild dilation of the renal pelvis but only slight blunting of the caliceal fornices. *Grade IV:* Complete reflux with moderate dilation of the ureter, renal pelvis, and calices; complete obliteration of the sharp angle of the fornices with maintenance of the papillary impressions of the calices. *Grade V:* Gross dilation and tortuosity of the ureter with gross dilation of the renal pelvis and calices; obliteration of the papillary impressions of the calices. Grades I through III have a high rate of spontaneous resolution and often require surgical correction. *(From Zitelli BJ, Davis HW, editors:* Atlas of pediatric physical diagnosis, *ed 4, St Louis, 2002, Mosby, p 464.)*

submucosal area of the ureter as it enters the bladder (Schlussel, 2004). This injection causes a mechanical obstruction just inferior to the ureteral opening and thereby prevents urine from the bladder from refluxing back into the ureter. The duration of the procedure may vary from 2 to 5 hours, so general anesthesia and endotracheal intubation are indicated. A caudal or lumbar epidural catheter can be used to provide supplemental regional anesthesia intraoperatively, minimizing the general anesthetic requirement as well as providing for postoperative analgesia and prevention of bladder spasm. The surgical procedure usually precludes the ability to measure urine output accurately. In those patients for whom the surgery is anticipated to take a long time, a central venous pressure catheter can be placed. For shorter surgical procedures, losses can be estimated by observation of the surgical field and vital signs. Serial hematocrit values should be measured whenever blood loss appears excessive. As with other urologic procedures, regional anesthesia

via the caudal or epidural approach can be very useful for both intraoperative and postoperative pain relief.

Procedures for Prune-Belly Syndrome

The prune-belly syndrome (Eagle-Barrett syndrome) occurs in 1 in 40,000 births, mostly in boys, and results from distal urinary tract obstruction that leads to multiple secondary organ dysfunction (Jones, 1988). Figure 23-29 outlines the proposed sequence of events in the urethral obstruction malformation complex that leads to the classic manifestations—namely, abdominal muscular deficiency, renal dysplasia, excess abdominal skin, and cryptorchidism. Other variable features include colonic malrotation, persistent urachus, and lower limb abnormalities. Figure 23-30 shows the typical physical appearance of a child with prune-belly syndrome.

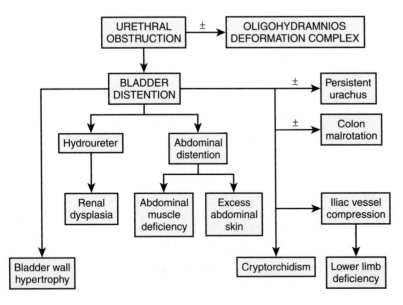

■ **FIGURE 23-29.** Developmental pathogenesis of early urethral obstruction sequence. *(From Jones KL, editor:* Smith's recognizable patterns of human malformation, *Philadelphia, 1988, Saunders.)*

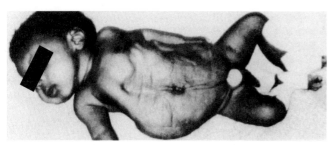

■ **FIGURE 23-30.** Infant with prune-belly syndrome. Note lax abdominal skin. *(From Jones KL, editor:* Smith's recognizable patterns of human malformation, *Philadelphia, 1988, Saunders.)*

A classification system has been devised according to the severity of disease in prune-belly syndrome (Woodhouse et al., 1982). Children in group I have severe renal disease, pulmonary hypoplasia, or both, which is incompatible with survival. Children in group II are seen as neonatal emergencies with severe uropathy and urinary tract infection and require multiple corrective surgical procedures. Patients in group III have minimal problems in the newborn period but are prone to infections in later childhood. The prognosis for children in groups II and III is good, with as many as half of the children in group II developing normally and exhibiting good renal function.

These patients have a depressed cough mechanism resulting from deficient abdominal musculature, so preoperative sedation is best avoided. Because aspiration is a risk, administration of an H_2-antagonist (such as ranitidine) and sodium citrate may be indicated to raise gastric pH, and rapid-sequence induction may be recommended. Controlled ventilation is necessary intraoperatively to prevent hypoventilation. Anesthesia can be maintained with inhalation agents or IV techniques, although muscle relaxation is usually unnecessary. Tracheal extubation should be performed only when the patient is awake and meets appropriate criteria. A review of 120 anesthetic cases suggested that intraoperative morbidity was rare, despite allowing spontaneous breathing in half of the cases (Henderson et al., 1987).

Postoperatively, respiratory infections occurred in approximately 7% of cases; one patient died from postoperative aspiration pneumonitis (Henderson et al., 1987). These patients require close observation and aggressive pulmonary toilet. Caudal, epidural, or spinal anesthesia in awake or mildly sedated patients may be useful for procedures such as cystoscopy or herniorrhaphy. After abdominal procedures, caudal or lumbar epidural administration of local anesthetic may be indicated to minimize postoperative pain. Postoperative mechanical ventilation may be required for patients who undergo extensive abdominal procedures or when significant pulmonary disease is present.

A wide variety of urologic abnormalities are found in prune-belly syndrome, including renal dysplasia, dilated and tortuous ureters, enlarged and dysfunctional bladder, urethral obstruction, and prostatic hypoplasia (Barratt and Manzoni, 1987). Despite severe urologic abnormalities, renal function may be well preserved. The surgical approach has become more conservative with the appreciation of the relatively good outcome in these patients. The standard surgical approach includes acceptance of the dilated upper urinary tract without extensive ureteral remodeling procedures, and maintenance of adequate bladder drainage with urethral surgery (Barratt and Manzoni, 1987).

Repair of Exstrophy of the Bladder

Exstrophy of the bladder is a rare anomaly, occurring in 1 in 30,000 births, most commonly in boys. This anomaly can be subdivided into classic exstrophy, cloacal exstrophy, and epispadias. Classic exstrophy is most common, with an absence of the anterior wall of the bladder and overlying abdominal wall, epispadias, and separation of the symphysis pubis (Fig. 23-31). Many urologists prefer to perform a staged repair, with the initial stage scheduled during the newborn period. This allows approximation of the symphysis pubis without the need for iliac osteotomies. Multiple procedures are usually necessary in the first years of life to achieve complete repair. To formulate an appropriate anesthetic plan, including an accurate prediction of blood loss, the anesthesiologist must discuss the surgical plan preoperatively with the urologist.

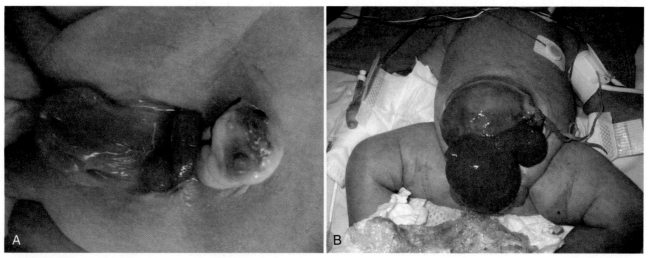

■ **FIGURE 23-31. A,** Bladder exstrophy. The bladder extrudes from the abdominal wall and the mucosa is exposed. **B,** Cloacal exstrophy, which occurs along with an omphalocele, as well as anomalies of the colon and rectum.

During the newborn period, blood loss, evaporative losses, and third-space fluid losses can be excessive during bladder exstrophy repair. It is recommended that two IV catheters or a central venous catheter be placed before surgery. An arterial catheter may be useful for monitoring blood pressure and allowing the sampling of blood for measurement of glucose levels, hematocrit, and blood gas analysis. In addition, significant heat loss is common during these procedures, demanding close attention to temperature levels and active warming, usually through a forced-air heating system. A combined general anesthetic-and-epidural technique is increasingly popular for these cases, with the epidural catheter providing excellent analgesia into the postoperative period (Wee et al., 1999). Bupivacaine or ropivacaine is commonly used, but an opioid is not often added in the neonatal period because of the risk for respiratory depression, unless prolonged mechanical ventilation is anticipated. Postoperatively, careful attention must be focused on maintaining fluid and electrolyte homeostasis, as well as on preventing anemia, hypotension, and hypoxia, as in any other case.

Hypospadias Repair

Hypospadias occurs in approximately 8 per 1000 male births (Belman, 1985). Associated anomalies that cause difficulties for the anesthesiologist are rare. Hypospadias is repaired either as a single-stage or a multistage procedure, depending on the complexity of the anatomic abnormality (Fig. 23-32). The surgical procedure usually requires several hours, so most anesthesiologists prefer endotracheal intubation rather than mask anesthesia for patient safety and for convenience. The laryngeal mask airway may also be useful in these procedures. Blood loss is usually not significant, and transfusion is rarely required. Induction of anesthesia can be achieved by any of the techniques commonly used in children. Intraoperatively, anesthesia can be maintained using either an inhalation or a balanced technique. General anesthesia combined with a conduction block provides excellent intraoperative conditions and postoperative pain relief.

Caudal epidural block may be the optimal choice because it provides complete intraoperative and postoperative analgesia. Penile block is less effective than caudal epidural anesthesia for postoperative analgesia after hypospadias repair, especially in cases of proximally located hypospadias (Blaise and Roy, 1986). When only a distal penile hypospadias is present, penile nerve block may be as effective as caudal epidural anesthesia. In children less than 1 year of age, a single caudal epidural injection of bupivacaine (0.25% with 5 mcg/mL epinephrine; 1.2 mL/kg) is administered after the induction of general anesthesia (Hannallah, 1987). Some practitioners prefer 0.2% or 0.125% bupivacaine to give greater volume with less risk for motor blockade. The caudal block is repeated at the end of the surgery if more than 1 hour has elapsed since the first caudal epidural injection. For children older than 1 year, it can be worthwhile to place a catheter for continuous caudal block using a commercially available epidural catheter kit. With the availability of smaller epidural catheters, a continuous infusion of local anesthetic may also be practical for younger patients (see Chapter 16, Regional Anesthesia).

BARIATRIC SURGERY

Obesity in Children and Adolescents

Obesity is the most common health problem facing U.S. children today. Data suggest that the prevalence of obesity continues to increase rapidly. Results from the National Health and Nutrition Examination Survey III reveal that approximately 14% of children in the United States are obese, as defined by body mass index (BMI) greater than the 95th percentile (Centers for Disease Control, 1997). The prevalence is increasing approximately 47% to 73% faster among black and Hispanic children than among non-Hispanic white children. As of 1998, the prevalence of obesity in children had increased to 21.5% among African Americans, 21.8% among Hispanics, and 12.3% among non-Hispanic whites (Strauss and Pollack, 2001).

Childhood obesity has been defined variously by absolute weight, weight-for-height percentiles, percentiles of ideal body weight, triceps skinfolds, and BMI (weight in kilograms divided by height in meters squared). The most recent recommendations from the Centers for Disease Control and Prevention suggest that BMI is the most appropriate and easily available method to screen for childhood obesity. Age and gender cutoffs for BMI have been published (Kuczmarski et al., 2000); patients with a BMI of greater than 30 are considered obese, and those with a BMI of greater than 40 are considered morbidly obese.

Although many of the adverse effects of childhood obesity may not become apparent for decades, even young children may suffer from severe morbidity. Psychological problems include low self-esteem, self-consciousness, helplessness, and depression. Hypertension, hypercholesterolemia, and hyperinsulinism all occur in young, obese children, leading to coronary artery disease and diabetes in adulthood. Obese children may develop gallstones, hepatitis, obstructive sleep apnea, and increased intracranial pressure resulting from pseudotumor cerebri (Strauss, 2002). Obese children are more likely to be admitted to the hospital than their normal-weight peers. In addition, obese children have higher hospital charges and longer lengths of stay (Nafiu et al., 2008). The adverse effects of obesity in childhood are shown in Box 23-9. These complications may result in the need for surgery (e.g., gallstones, slipped epiphysis, bariatric surgery) and complicate anesthetic management during surgery (airway obstruction or reactivity, hyperglycemia, systemic or intracranial hypertension) (Nafiu et al., 2007).

Physiologic Considerations

Obesity is associated with many physiologic disturbances of concern to anesthesiologists. Work of breathing is increased, and fatty chest and abdominal walls decrease chest compliance. FRC is significantly reduced, leading to lower airways closure and atelectasis, causing hypoxemia due to intrapulmonary shunting. Exacerbations of hypoxemia caused by sleep apnea may lead to pulmonary hypertension, cor pulmonale, and heart failure. A small number of morbidly obese patients have somnolence, cardiac enlargement, polycythemia, hypoxemia, and hypercapnia (Pickwickian syndrome). Morbidly obese patients with preoperative pulmonary dysfunction have higher morbidity after bariatric surgery but may subsequently have significant improvement in sleep apnea, gas exchange abnormalities, pulmonary hypertension, and cardiac function (Sugerman et al., 1992).

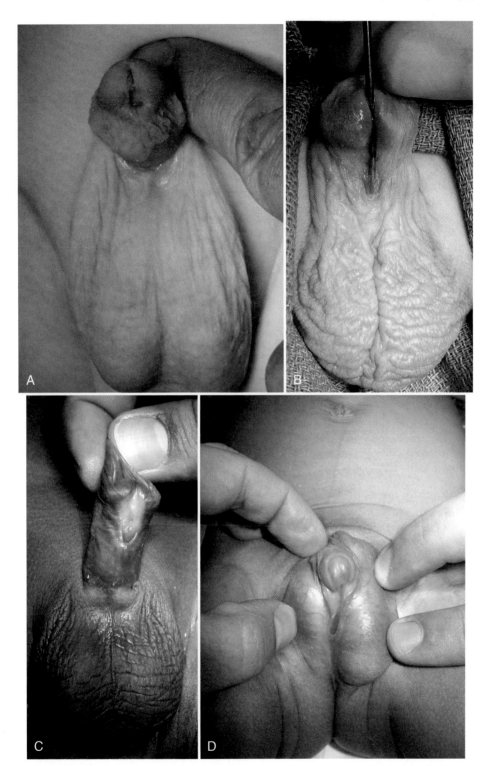

■ **FIGURE 23-32.** Different locations of hypospadias. **A,** Glans. **B,** Proximal. **C,** Midshaft. **D,** Scrotum.

Cardiac reserve is decreased in obese patients. Even normotensive morbidly obese patients have increased preload and afterload, increased pulmonary artery pressures, and elevated right and left ventricular stroke work compared with nonobese patients. The degree of cardiac abnormality correlates with the degree of obesity. Left ventricular dysfunction is often present in young, asymptomatic obese patients. Right ventricular failure is common in older patients (Brodsky and Vierra, 2000).

Weight loss, whether through diet or bariatric surgery, can reverse cardiac dysfunction and hypertension (Jones, 1996). Hypertension is common among morbidly obese adolescents and adults.

The gastric contents of unpremedicated, nondiabetic, fasting obese patients (BMI ≥ 30) without GER are not increased in volume or acidity compared with nonobese surgical patients (Harter et al., 1998). However, morbidly obese patients (BMI ≥

> **Box 23-9 Adverse Effects of Obesity in Childhood**
>
> Hypertension
> Dyslipidemia
> Orthopedic problems
> - Slipped capital femoral epiphysis
> - Blount's disease (tibia vara)
> Endocrine problems
> - Diabetes
> - Insulin resistance
> - Polycystic ovary syndrome, irregular menses
> Gastroenterologic problems
> - Gallstones
> - Steatohepatitis
> Respiratory problems
> - Asthma
> - Sleep apnea
> Neurologic problems
> - Pseudotumor cerebri

40) do have large gastric volumes and low pH (Vaughan et al., 1975). Morbid obesity is also associated with a high incidence of GER, with 70% of patients complaining of heartburn (Hagen et al., 1987).

Other gastrointestinal abnormalities in morbidly obese patients include steatohepatitis, cirrhosis, and gallstones (Clain and Lefkowitch, 1987). Approximately 30% of patients who do not have gallstones at the time of bariatric surgery develop gallstones within 3 to 6 months after surgery, prompting many surgeons to perform a cholecystectomy at the time of the bariatric procedure.

Endocrine and genetic abnormalities are associated with obesity and short stature. Hirsutism, increased muscle mass, and acanthosis nigricans are associated with polycystic ovary syndrome. Obesity associated with mental retardation may signify a congenital syndrome such as Prader-Willi, Laurence-Moon-Biedl, or Cohen's syndromes. Female patients with short stature and obesity may be diagnosed with Turner's syndrome. Recurrent headaches, especially if associated with vomiting, may be caused by pseudotumor cerebri; papilledema may be seen on fundoscopic examination.

Bariatric Surgical Procedures

Gastric bypass and other types of bariatric surgery have been considered appropriate for select adults with a BMI of 40, or of 35 in the presence of comorbid conditions (Consensus Development Conference Panel, 1991; National Institutes of Health, 1998). Few data and no guidelines exist for bariatric surgery in adolescents. In 1975, Soper and colleagues reported on 18 morbidly obese adolescents and young adults (age, >20 years) who underwent either gastric bypass or gastroplasty. The median weight loss was approximately 25% of body weight by 3 years after surgery. A similar report in 1980 described an average weight loss of 40 kg at 3 years and 26 kg at 5 years after surgery (Anderson et al., 1980). Major early postoperative complications occurred in more than a third of the patients, including one death from an anastomotic leak. Since these early reports, the gastric bypass procedure has undergone significant modifications. Surgical stapling devices

allow compartmentalization of the stomach without complete transection (Kellum et al., 1998). "Long limb" gastric bypass has also been used in patients with a BMI of greater than 50, with improved weight loss compared with conventional bypass procedures (Brolin et al., 1992).

Strauss and coworkers (2001) reported their results in 10 adolescents, aged 15 to 17 years, who underwent gastric bypass surgery. All patients were highly motivated and had demonstrated serious attempts at weight loss by diet and behavior modification programs. All adolescents were behaviorally and genetically normal and were more than 100% and 100 pounds above their ideal body weight. Obesity-related morbidities included sleep apnea, hypertension, vertebral fracture, and severe school avoidance. No perioperative complications were reported. Satisfactory weight loss was achieved in 9 of 10 patients, with a mean weight loss of greater than 50 kg. Late complications included protein-calorie and micronutrient malnutrition in one patient, an abdominal wall hernia requiring surgical repair in one patient, cholecystectomy in two patients, and small bowel obstruction requiring surgery in one patient.

Abu-Abeid and colleagues (2003) reported their experience with 11 adolescents, aged 11 to 17 years, who underwent laparoscopic adjustable gastric banding (LAGB). Unlike gastric bypass operations, LAGB involves no anastomoses and no bypass of functional bowel, and the operation is reversible. The authors cited no perioperative or late complications; the mean decrease in BMI was from 46.6 to 32.1 kg/m². One patient with heart failure and pulmonary hypertension had significant functional improvement during the 23-month follow-up period.

Anesthetic Management

Preoperative Considerations

In preparation for surgery, a thorough history and physical examination should be performed. Review of systems is focused on medical complications of obesity shown in Box 23-9. Medications taken for weight loss and other conditions are noted. Blood pressure and oxygen saturation should be recorded. Airway examination may reveal large tonsils and a small pharyngeal airway. Cardiac and lung auscultation may reveal signs of heart failure, pulmonary hypertension, wheezing, and low lung volumes. An electrocardiogram may show findings of cor pulmonale. An echocardiogram should be considered if cardiac dysfunction is suspected. In association with frequent urination, nocturia, and fatigue, blood glucose values may confirm the diagnosis of diabetes.

Administration of premedication should be followed by monitoring of oxygen saturation, as ventilatory depression and airway obstruction may occur. An H₂-receptor antagonist and metoclopramide may be given 60 to 90 minutes before anesthetic induction to decrease gastric volume and acidity. A nonparticulate oral antacid may be given immediately before induction.

Intraoperative Management

Many obese patients become hypoxemic in the supine position because of upper airway obstruction and diminished FRC. Elevating the head of the operating room table may diminish these changes.

Noninvasive blood pressure measurements may be inaccurate, prompting the need for intraarterial monitoring. Measurement of arterial blood gases at baseline and during general anesthesia is recommended, especially for lengthy surgeries. Because venous access may be limited, placement of a central venous catheter, although technically challenging, may be required. Meticulous attention to positioning and padding of the head, neck, and extremities is essential to prevent injury during surgery. Patients must be well secured to the operating table in anticipation of the use of the Trendelenburg and reverse Trendelenburg positions, as well as lateral rotation of the operating table.

Because the risk for aspiration is high in morbidly obese patients, tracheal intubation should be performed when general anesthesia is administered even for brief procedures. Rapid-sequence induction or awake fiberoptic-guided intubation should be performed to minimize the risk for pulmonary aspiration of gastric contents. Although most patients can be intubated with appropriate body positioning and direct laryngoscopy, two anesthesiologists and a "difficult airway" cart should be present during induction and intubation. Preoxygenation should be performed until the oxygen saturation has been 100% for several minutes. Patients should be ventilated with 100% oxygen, with 10 to 15 mL/kg tidal volumes based on ideal weight. Moderate levels of positive end-expiratory pressure (PEEP) should be added to minimize airway closure, atelectasis, and oxygen desaturations. High levels of PEEP may depress cardiac output. Hypoxemia may occur as a result of placement of abdominal packs or retractors, gas insufflation during laparoscopic procedures, and use of the lithotomy or Trendelenburg position. In extreme cases, the panniculus may need to be mechanically displaced to improve compliance and reduce physiologic shunt during surgery (Wyner et al., 1981).

Drug and fluid administration should be based on ideal body weight. Dosages of select drugs may need to be increased compared with those administered to lean patients, however, because of increases in blood volume and cardiac output in the obese patient (Brodsky and Vierra, 2000). Thiopental and midazolam have increased volumes of distribution in obese patients. Dosing regimens based on ideal body weight for propofol have been recommended (Servin et al., 1993). A nerve stimulator should be used to guide the dosing of muscle relaxants and to monitor complete reversal of their effect. Excessive fat overlying the nerves may render surface electrodes ineffective, and needle electrodes may occasionally be required.

Although technically more difficult in obese patients, regional anesthetic techniques should be considered with or without general anesthesia. Local anesthetics may eliminate the need for muscle relaxants and their reversal. Even when general anesthesia is used in combination with regional anesthesia, decreased concentrations and dosages of inhalation and IV agents allow more rapid awakening and spontaneous airway control. Postoperative analgesia with epidural infusions facilitates improved pulmonary function.

Regional blocks can be difficult because important anatomic landmarks are often obscured. Long spinal or epidural needles are needed. The depth of insertion is difficult to predict; BMI alone is not an accurate predictor for depth of the epidural space (Watts, 1993). Accordingly, the incidence of inadvertent dural puncture is increased in obese patients. Morbidly obese patients, however, have a decreased incidence of postdural puncture headache. Because the spread of local anesthetics is directly related to BMI, local anesthetic dosages should be reduced by 20% to 25% for both epidural and subarachnoid blocks in obese patients (Pitkanen, 1987; Taivainen et al., 1990). Insulated needles and a nerve stimulator may be helpful in identifying the appropriate nerves for peripheral nerve blocks.

Postoperative Care

Postoperative mechanical ventilation is infrequently needed except in the presence of significant cardiac disease, massive intraoperative fluid resuscitation, sepsis, or airway trauma during intubation. Tracheal extubation in hemodynamically stable, morbidly obese patients should be performed with the upper body elevated 30 to 45 degrees. The patient should be maintained in this position for transport to maximize FRC and oxygenation (Vaughan et al., 1976). Supplemental oxygen should be administered via nasal cannula or mask for at least 3 days after abdominal or thoracic procedures (Taylor et al., 1985). Nasal CPAP or bilevel positive airway pressure (BiPAP) via nasal mask is used for patients with sleep apnea; these modalities may normalize breathing during sleep and prevent nocturnal oxyhemoglobin desaturation (Series et al., 1992; Rennotte et al., 1995). Nasogastric tubes used during surgery must be removed before the application of nasal CPAP or BiPAP. A potential complication of these therapies is gastric distention and disruption of bowel anastomoses, although this risk appears to be small.

Thromboembolism is a major cause of postoperative morbidity in obese surgical patients. Pulmonary emboli occur in as many as 5% of obese patients after laparotomy (Brodsky and Vierra, 2000). The risk for thromboembolism can be reduced with heparin, pneumatic compression devices, or both (Fasting et al., 1985). If an epidural catheter is to be used, it should be placed before initiation of heparin therapy and removed at least 12 hours after the last dose of heparin (Horlocker et al., 2003).

Deep breathing, coughing, and early ambulation must be encouraged, and effective postoperative analgesia is essential. Patient-controlled analgesia with an IV opioid or epidural opioid with or without local anesthetic may be used. Analgesic drugs should be dosed according to ideal body weight. Vigilant monitoring for signs of excessive sedation and respiratory depression is required.

SUMMARY

The pediatric patient presenting for abdominal, genitourinary, or thoracic surgery spans the pathophysiologic spectrum. Both acute and elective clinical presentations, coupled with age-related nuances of the disease, dictate the perioperative anesthetic care of the patient. Advances in intraoperative techniques and postoperative pain management have enabled the surgical frontiers in those specialties to advance.

For questions and answers on topics in this chapter, go to "Chapter Questions" at www.expertconsult.com.

REFERENCES

Complete references used in this text can be found online at www.expertconsult.com.

Anesthesia for Pediatric Otorhinolaryngologic Surgery

Ira S. Landsman, Jay A. Werkhaven, and Etsuro K. Motoyama

CONTENTS

T he care of children requiring anesthesia for otorhinolaryngologic, or ear, nose, and throat (ENT), surgery is described in this chapter. Most pediatric otorhinolaryngologic surgical procedures are of short to intermediate duration, and most of the children who are the patients are in reasonably good health. However, the anesthesiologist often encounters children with potentially life-threatening upper airway obstruction (e.g., acute epiglottitis) or with severe pulmonary insufficiency requiring diagnostic or therapeutic ENT procedures. New surgical techniques, such as laryngeal laser surgery, have challenged pediatric anesthesiologists to develop innovative approaches for the protection and maintenance of the patent upper airway.

The art and science of anesthesia must be well integrated in caring for the child undergoing ENT anesthesia. Many procedures, including adenoidectomy, rigid bronchoscopy, and laser removal of papillomas, require short intervals of deep planes of anesthesia and limited movement of the patient. To effectively manage operating room services, the patient must awake in a timely manner without airway irritability. One of the major changes in pediatric anesthesia over the past decade has been the abandonment of halothane in favor of sevoflurane. Although sevoflurane appears to be a safer anesthetic agent than halothane, sevoflurane-induced postoperative delirium continues to challenge the pediatric anesthesiologist (Vlajkovic and Sindjelic, 2007; Kuratani and Oi, 2008).

Propofol has many properties that make it a useful anesthetic agent for ENT surgery. It causes less airway irritability than thiopental. Propofol may be protective against and therapeutic for laryngospasm (Brown et al., 1991; Scanlon et al., 1993; Allsop et al., 1995; Afshan et al., 2002). Propofol also has useful antiemetic properties and a low incidence of emergence delirium (Uezono et al., 2000; Moore et al., 2003; Voepel-Lewis et al., 2003), making this anesthetic a good choice for ENT anesthesia.

ANESTHESIA FOR OTOLOGIC PROCEDURES

Otitis media is the most frequently diagnosed childhood malady, with the highest incidence occurring among children between the ages of 6 and 18 months. Its frequency decreases after the first year of life. By age 7 years, otitis media is a less frequent pediatric diagnosis. Otitis media is inflammation of the middle ear, without reference to pathogenesis or cause. The other areas of the temporal bone that are contiguous with the middle ear, including the mastoid, petrous apex, and perilabyrinthine air cells, also may be involved. In those who have had a single episode of acute otitis media, residual middle ear fluid remains in up to 40% of patients at 1 month, 20% at 2 months, and 10% at 3 months (Pelton et al., 1977; Teele et al., 1980; Gluckman, 1990).

Many children with persistent middle ear effusion continue to be clinically symptomatic with recurrent acute otitis media, pain, fever, vertigo, disturbed sleep, or significant hearing loss. These symptoms are the most common indications for middle ear effusion drainage by myringotomy and tympanostomy tubes. Myringotomy and insertion of tympanostomy tubes may also be helpful in patients with recurrent acute otitis or atelectasis of the tympanic membrane. Tympanostomy tubes may prevent permanent structural damage and cholesteatoma. Myringotomy with aspiration of the middle ear effusion, but without tube placement, may be appropriate in children with severe otalgia or when culture of the middle ear fluid is required in the evaluation of a child with fever of unknown origin. If the patient requires multiple myringotomy procedures, placement of a tympanostomy tube may be considered.

Many patients with congenital anomalies are candidates for myringotomy tubes. Patients with cleft palate, craniofacial malformations, Down syndrome, Turner's syndrome, and human immunodeficiency virus (HIV) infection have a higher incidence of otitis media and therefore have a greater need for myringotomy and insertion of tympanostomy tubes than the general population (Bluestone and Klein, 2003). These children have other airway and medical issues that complicate the usual approach to the healthy child requiring myringotomy tubes. Critically ill patients with a history of prolonged nasotracheal intubation have a high incidence of persistent middle ear effusions requiring middle ear ventilation.

Adenoidectomy for chronic otitis media with effusion may benefit some children. The effectiveness of adenoidectomy for chronic otitis media with effusion is not directly related to adenoid size. For children who have recurrent or chronic otitis media with effusion and who had one or more myringotomy and tympanostomy tube insertion procedure in the past, adenoidectomy may be a reasonable option (Paradise et al., 2003). Upper airway obstruction, recurrent acute or chronic adenoiditis, and sinusitis are additional indications for adenoidectomy in children who have chronic otitis media with effusion.

Myringotomy and Insertion of Tympanostomy Tubes

Candidates for myringotomy and tube insertion present with subacute or chronic upper respiratory tract infection with or without fever. In these children, surgical intervention appears to improve the symptoms of upper respiratory infection postoperatively (Tait and Knight, 1987). However, the finding by these investigators is applicable only to myringotomy for children with middle ear effusion; it should not be generalized or applied to children with upper respiratory infection (especially in its acute phase with fever) who are scheduled for other surgical procedures (Hinkle, 1989).

In expert hands, the performance of uncomplicated bilateral myringotomies and tube insertions requires only 5 to 10 minutes of operating time; the procedure, however, may take considerably more time when performed by inexperienced trainees or in patients with narrow ear canals. Myringotomy is almost exclusively performed on an outpatient basis.

Preoperative sedation should be administered based on the child's anxiety level. Mask induction of anesthesia with nitrous oxide, oxygen, and sevoflurane provides effective and smooth induction and maintenance anesthesia with prompt emergence. Preoperative or intraoperative analgesia is advocated for early postoperative pain relief. Because these children are usually anesthetized without intravascular access, preoperative administration of oral acetaminophen or nonsteroidal antiinflammatory drugs (NSAIDs) (Watcha et al., 1992) and intraoperative intranasal fentanyl or butorphanol (Bennie et al., 1998; Galinkin et al., 2000; Finkel et al., 2001) or intramuscular ketorolac (Pappas et al., 2003) has been studied and recommended. It appears that intraoperative ketorolac (0.5 mg/kg, up to 30 mg) administered by the intramuscular route provides better analgesia than oral or rectal acetaminophen. Ketorolac is associated with less vomiting and minimal sedation compared with intranasal butorphanol and perhaps with fentanyl. However, ketorolac, along with other NSAIDs, should be used with caution because ketorolac affects platelet function, and increased postoperative bleeding during tonsillectomy or adenoidectomy has been reported (Dahl and Kehlet, 1994; Nikanne et al., 1997).

Because children undergoing myringotomy commonly have adenoidal hypertrophy, they may exhibit signs of nasal and upper airway obstruction (Bluestone and Klein, 2001). These children often require continuous positive airway pressure (CPAP) during inhalational induction and insertion of an oropharyngeal airway after reaching a surgical plane of anesthesia to maintain a patent airway (see Chapter 3, Respiratory Physiology, and Chapter 13, Induction, Maintenance, and Recovery). Although myringotomy and tube insertion may last less than 10 minutes, it should be performed with standard monitoring (i.e., using a precordial stethoscope, pulse oximeter, electrocardiogram, thermometer, and automated blood pressure cuff). Myringotomy is one of a few exceptions in modern pediatric anesthesia practice in the United States for which intravenous infusion is not routinely administered.

Postoperative hypoxemia occurs frequently in infants and children during transport and in the recovery room, even after minor surgical procedures such as myringotomy (Motoyama and Glazener, 1986). After myringotomy, patients are prone to upper airway obstruction, and these children should be transferred to the recovery room in the lateral position while receiving supplemental oxygen (see Chapter 13, Induction, Maintenance, and Recovery).

Mastoidectomy and Tympanoplasty

The clinical importance of the mastoid process is related to its contiguous structures, which include the posterior and middle cranial fossa, sigmoid and lateral sinuses, facial nerve, semicircular canals, and petrous tip of the temporal bone. The distal part of the middle ear and mastoid are connected by the aditus ad antrum, making the mastoid susceptible to infection by infectious processes from the middle ear. With improved medical and surgical management of otitis media, mastoidectomy for mastoiditis has declined considerably over the past several decades. However, mastoidectomies may also be performed in association with cholesteatoma removal and tympanoplasty. Tympanoplasty is performed in patients with chronic perforation or atelectasis of the tympanic membrane (Bluestone and Klein, 2003). Deep retraction pockets may lead to squamous epithelium proliferation in the middle ear and mastoid cavities, causing a cholesteatoma that may grow by the enzymatic activity of the skin tissues and accumulation of squamous debris.

Tympanoplasty is an operation to reconstruct the tympanic membrane with or without grafting. Its primary indications are repair of tympanic perforation; stabilization or improvement of hearing; removal or prevention of congenital, iatrogenic, or primary or secondary acquired cholesteatoma; and removal of atelectatic or diseased areas of the tympanic membrane (Haynes and Harley, 2002). Grafting materials include fat, fascia, perichondrium, periosteum, cartilage, vein, and paper patch.

Mastoidectomy involves the surgical exposure and removal of mastoid air cells. There are several types of mastoidectomy (Bluestone and Klein, 2003). In a complete simple cortical mastoidectomy, the mastoid air-cell system is removed, but the canal wall is left intact. The operation is performed for acute or chronic mastoid osteitis, and it is frequently part of the surgical procedure advocated by some surgeons for cholesteatoma.

Posterior tympanotomy or facial recess tympanotomy involves removal of mastoid air cells, followed by formation of an opening between the mastoid and middle ear created in the posterior wall of the middle ear lateral to the facial nerve and medial to the chorda tympani. This procedure allows better visualization of the facial recess without removing the canal wall, and it is primarily advocated for ears in which a cholesteatoma has formed.

With a modified radical mastoidectomy, a portion of the posterior ear canal wall is removed, and a permanent mastoidectomy cavity is created, but the tympanic membrane and some or all of the ossicles are left intact. The procedure is usually performed when a cholesteatoma cannot be removed without removing the canal wall; some function may be preserved.

Radical mastoidectomy involves removal of all mastoid air cells, the posterior ear canal wall, the tympanic membrane, and the ossicles except part or all the stapes. No attempt is made to preserve function. Removal of the posterior ear canal wall allows communication among the exenterated mastoid cellular area, middle ear, and external auditory canal, forming a common single cavity. The procedure is indicated when there is extensive cholesteatoma in the middle ear and mastoid that cannot be removed by a less radical procedure. The operation may be indicated for a suppurative complication of otitis media.

Tympanomastoidectomy with tympanoplasty is the term used when a tympanoplasty is performed in conjunction with a mastoidectomy. Mastoidectomies that leave the posterior ear canal wall intact are closed cavity, canal wall up, or intact canal wall procedures, whereas those in which the posterior canal is partially removed are open cavity or canal wall down procedures.

Anesthetic Management

All children should be monitored with standard monitoring that includes a pulse oximeter, a capnograph for end-tidal carbon dioxide (CO_2) monitor, precordial stethoscope, electrocardiogram, thermometer, and automated blood pressure cuff. Often, electromyography is used to avoid injury to the facial nerve. In these circumstances, neuromuscular blockade is avoided. Standard no oral intake (NPO) guidelines should be followed in nonemergent situations.

For mastoidectomy and tympanoplasty, the patient is positioned supine, with the head laterally rotated away from the affected side. It is important to carefully rotate the neck of a patient under general anesthesia because of the risk for atlanto-axial rotational subluxation (Brisson et al., 2000).

Induction of anesthesia can entail inhalational or intravenous induction. The anesthesiologist should consider endotracheal intubation without muscle relaxation or with a short-acting muscle relaxant so the facial nerve can be monitored during surgery. The use of nitrous oxide may be contraindicated during and after placement of the tympanic graft, because nitrous oxide accumulates in a closed gas space and increases the ambient pressure; some surgeons believe this tends to lift the graft away from its new site (Koivunen et al., 1996; Doyle and Banks, 2003).

The most common postoperative complication requiring unscheduled admission to the hospital for children who have undergone tympanomastoidectomy is postoperative nausea and vomiting (PONV) (Megerian et al., 2000). PONV has been attributed to surgical stimulation of the vestibular labyrinth, anesthetic techniques, or a combination of the two (Jellish et al., 1995; Dornhoffer and Manning, 2000). Propofol has antiemetic properties (Ved et al., 1996; Erb et al., 2002b). It appears that propofol used for induction and maintenance of anesthesia is superior to isoflurane or sevoflurane in reducing PONV after middle ear surgery (Jellish et al., 1995, 1999; Moore et al., 2003). The use of intravenous dexamethasone during surgery appears to decrease PONV in patients after undergoing tympanomastoid surgery (Liu et al., 2001).

Cochlear Implantation

Cochlear implantation has become a feasible choice for profoundly hearing-impaired children (Figs. 24-1 and 24-2). Profoundly deaf children's auditory nerve fibers remain intact, but the sensory neuroepithelium in the cochlea is absent. This damage occurs because of a genetic defect, infection, cochlear ossification, or aging (Fischetti, 2003). Cochlear implants bypass the damage by receiving and converting sound into signals sent along electrodes to cells adjacent to the auditory nerve. Hearing aids are ineffective because sound cannot be converted into an electrical impulse. Cochlear implants have eight to 22 electrodes that are placed through a cochleostomy. Sounds received from an external microphone are converted to an electrical signal that is received and transmitted by the cochlear nerve (Balkany et al., 2001; Miyamoto and Kirk, 2003). Because the cochlea is full size at birth, there is no anatomic difficulty with electrode insertion in very young children.

Surgery requires 2 to 3 hours, and it is performed through an extended postauricular incision along with a mastoidectomy. Anesthetic considerations are the same as those for mastoidectomy, including the avoidance of muscle relaxants so the facial nerve can be monitored. The anesthesiologist should establish the patient's level of hearing dysfunction so that a method of communication can be established. It is helpful to have a parent or sign language specialist accompany the child to the operating room. If the child reads lips, masks should be kept down from the anesthesiologist's mouth until after induction of anesthesia.

Otoplasty

Otoplasty is a cosmetic procedure to reconstruct or restructure the auricle. Anesthetic considerations are similar to those in other head and neck cosmetic procedures, with one minor

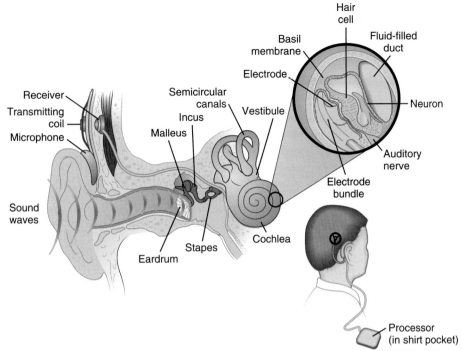

■ FIGURE 24-1. The outer ear collects the pressure waves of a sound, which the eardrum converts into mechanical vibrations in tiny bones in the middle ear. The oscillating stapes sets off pressure waves in the fluid in the cochlea, which stimulates nerve cells on the auditory nerve that leads to the brain. The cochlea transmits pressure waves through its duct fluid, displacing the basilar membrane, which bends hair cells to varying degrees. The cells release neurotransmitters that cause attached neurons to fire, telling the brain where along the duct the bending has occurred, which corresponds to the frequency of the original sound, and communicating the amplitude of the bending, which indicates the loudness. The cochlear implant uses a microphone worn behind the ear to pick up sound and send it to a processor, where integrated circuits and algorithms amplify, digitize, and filter the sound into a coded signal sent to the transmitter coil. The coil sends the signal by radio waves through the skin to an implanted receiver. The receiver converts the waves into electrical impulses that travel along electrodes that end at cells at certain points along the cochlea. A magnet in the transmitter holds it against the implanted receiver. *(From Fischetti M: Cochlear implants: to hear again,* Sci Am *288:82, 2003.)*

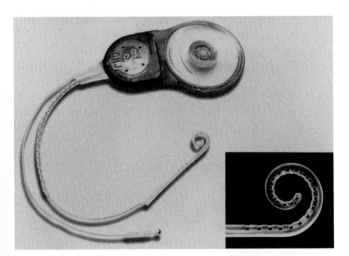

■ FIGURE 24-2. In the Nucleus 24 Counter implant, the active intracochlear electrode array is precurved to wrap around the modiolus. A stylus is used to straighten the electrode during insertion. *(From Miyamoto RT, Kirk KI: Cochlear implants in children. In Bluestone CD, Stool SE, Alper CM, et al., editors:* Pediatric otolaryngology, *ed 4, Philadelphia, 2003, Saunders, p 809.)*

modification. Otoplasty is frequently bilateral, requiring both sides to be simultaneously prepared and draped. To ensure symmetry, simultaneous visualization requires frequent head motion, and the endotracheal tube must be well secured. PONV is frequent.

ANESTHESIA FOR RHINOLOGIC PROCEDURES

Reduction of Nasal Fracture

A nasal fracture may cause considerable bleeding, and the blood may be swallowed into the stomach. These patients therefore are assumed to have a full stomach, regardless of the time of last food intake. Reduction of a nasal fracture may take only a few moments, but in the acute situation, an oral endotracheal tube is mandatory to protect the airway from pulmonary aspiration. More commonly, surgery is delayed for several days after an isolated nasal fracture to allow swelling to subside. In these cases, a flexible laryngeal mask airway (LMA) can be substituted for an endotracheal tube. The LMA cannot prevent aspiration of stomach contents into the lungs, but it can prevent blood from the nose from passing through the vocal cords (John et al., 1991; Williams and Bailey, 1993). The LMA may be removed either when the patient is deeply anesthetized or when awake.

Nasal Polypectomy

Nasal polypectomy is performed under general anesthesia, often using a preformed Ring, Adair, Ellwyn (RAE) endotracheal tube, which was originally developed by Ring and associates (1975) (see Chapter 10, Equipment). Packing of the pharynx is indicated in most intranasal procedures. One end of the oropharyngeal gauze packing should be tagged with a hemostat and left hanging externally at one corner of the mouth. A note should be prominently placed in the room for all to see, or a labeled tape should be placed across the exit door, reminding all operating room personnel that a throat pack is in place and needs to be removed. Historically, as much as 10 mcg/kg of epinephrine, usually in a 1:200,000 solution (5 mcg/mL), can be used in children for hemostasis under halothane anesthesia without apparent myocardial irritability (Karl et al., 1983; Ueda et al., 1983). More recently, however, our anesthesia practice has decided to use isoflurane, sevoflurane, desflurane, propofol, or remifentanil as maintenance anesthetic, without changing the epinephrine dosage (see Chapter 13, Induction, Maintenance, and Recovery).

Special consideration should be given to the management of children with cystic fibrosis, in whom nasal polyps often occur (Hulka, 2000) (see Chapter 36, Systemic Disorders). The polyps are multiple and recur after removal. These children often have severe obstructive lung disease with recurrent pulmonary infection and thick, tenacious secretions. They are frequently hypoxemic in room air. During general anesthesia, the cystic fibrosis patient may require frequent endotracheal lavage with saline and deep suctioning. Secretions can hamper oxygenation and ventilation; a rise in the peak inspiratory pressure intraoperatively may indicate that the endotracheal tube requires suctioning. An inhaled bronchodilator should be immediately available to treat bronchospasm. Inhaled anesthetics and nitrous oxide or opioids and a relaxant may be used for patients with mild to moderate airway obstruction. Nitrous oxide should be avoided in those with severe lower airway obstruction with air trapping, because of possible hyperinflation of trapped air spaces. These patients with lower airway obstruction should be ventilated with an oxygen-air mixture, and appropriate positive end-expiratory pressure (5 to 7 cm H_2O) should be added throughout the procedure to minimize airway closure and atelectasis (see Chapter 3, Respiratory Physiology in Infants and Children). Because of the association of nasal/ethmoidal polyposis with asthma and aspirin sensitivity (Samter's triad), NSAIDs should be used with caution.

In addition to pulmonary pathology, upper airway obstruction frequently occurs in these patients. During induction, the mouth must be kept open because nasal air passages may be completely blocked by the polyp. Nasal packing, usually placed at the completion of the surgical procedure, may lead to further problems in ventilation and oxygenation in the postoperative period. This situation is partially relieved if the surgeon first introduces a nasopharyngeal airway and then packs around it. If preoperative pulmonary function is poor, the physician should consider transferring the patient to the intensive care unit (ICU), with the endotracheal tube in place, for immediate postoperative respiratory care.

Sinus Surgery

Sinus surgery is indicated for children who have failed maximal medical therapy. Children with allergy or gastroesophageal reflux disease should receive maximal medical therapy and should rarely require surgery (Goldsmith and Rosenfeld, 2003). Children with immune deficiency, immotile cilia syndrome (i.e., Kartagener's syndrome), or cystic fibrosis (Gysin et al., 2000) are at high risk for chronic sinusitis. Unfortunately, because of their underlying disease, these children have a significant surgical failure rate (Herbert and Bent, 1998).

In children with recurrent sinusitis without chronic disease, adenoidectomy should be the initial procedure if the quantity of adenoid tissue visualized on endoscopy is considered sufficient to serve as a reservoir of bacterial pathogens. Adenoidectomy or adenotonsillectomy is usually the first-line surgical intervention for preschoolers, and it is often appropriate in older children. The expected rate of improvement is 70% to 80% (Goldsmith and Rosenfeld, 2003).

Endoscopic sinus surgery (ESS) should be performed only when children have failed previous therapies. In contrast to older traditional techniques of sinus surgery, ESS focuses on enlarging the natural ostia of the maxillary and ethmoid sinuses, while preserving most or all of the sinus mucosa (Goldsmith and Rosenfeld, 2003). In addition to children with chronic sinusitis who fail medical management, Lusk (2003) lists the accepted indications for ESS as complete nasal obstruction in patients with cystic fibrosis, antrochoanal polyps, intracranial complications, mucoceles and mucopyoceles, orbital abscess, traumatic injury in the optic canal, dacryocystorhinitis resulting from sinusitis, fungal sinusitis, certain neoplasms, and meningoencephalocele. In properly selected children, the results are good, with an expected improvement of 80% (Lusk, 2003). Preoperative computed tomography (CT) is essential in defining the specific diseased sinuses and in looking for anatomic abnormalities that need to be addressed, including septal deviation, concha bullosa cells, obstructing Haller air cells, and abnormal middle turbinates (Goldsmith and Rosenfeld, 2003).

ESS is performed under general anesthesia using an oral preformed (RAE) or standard endotracheal tube. Many of these children have chronic disease or upper airway obstruction. The anesthetic approach is similar to that described for nasal polypectomy and adenotonsillectomy. The surgeon may elect to use topical oxymetazoline (0.25% to 0.50%) for initial vasoconstriction and then infiltrate the tissue with lidocaine (0.5%) and epinephrine (1:100,000 solution) for hemostasis. The surgeon and the anesthesiologist should be aware that the duration of vasoconstriction usually does not last longer than 1.5 hours, and when surgical procedures are not completed within this period, mild bleeding may make visualization of the surgical site difficult and present a potential problem postoperatively. Some surgeons routinely pack the nose with gauze after the procedure for hemostasis, and the patient becomes an obligate mouth breather. Other surgeons may elect to use Surgicel or FloSeal to obtain hemostasis, and each of these materials has the potential for migration into the lower airway.

Choanal Atresia

Choanal atresia is a congenital malformation in which no connection exists between the nasal cavity and the aerodigestive tract (Prasad et al., 2002); it has an incidence of 1 in 7000 births. The atresia is bony (30%) or mixed membranous and bony (70%). The existence of purely membranous atresia has come into question (Brown et al., 1996). Choanal atresia is unilateral in 50% to 60% of patients. Syndromes associated with choanal atresia include Apert's syndrome, DiGeorge syndrome, trisomy 18, Treacher Collins syndrome, camptomelic dysplasia, and CHARGE association (i.e., coloboma, heart defects, atresia choanae, retardation of growth and development, genitourinary problems, and ear anomalies) (Tewfick et al., 1997).

The symptoms caused by choanal atresia depend on whether the obstruction is unilateral or bilateral. Because neonates are obligatory nasal breathers, those with bilateral disease present with acute respiratory distress. Respiratory distress can be attenuated if the mouth is kept open with an oral airway strapped in place or by a large rubber nipple with a large hole cut in it and kept in place with an umbilical tape around the neck (McGovern, 1961; Hengerer and Wein, 2003). For the neonate with bilateral choanal atresia, surgical nasal correction or tracheostomy must be performed within the first few days of life. Other infants may have only unilateral atresia, with minimal symptoms that can go undiagnosed for months or even years. The most common complaint is intractable unilateral anterior nasal discharge.

A number of surgical procedures have been described for the correction of choanal atresia, including endoscopic, transnasal, transseptal, and transpalatal procedures (Holland and McGuirt, 2001). Timing of surgery for bilateral choanal atresia varies and depends on the infant's ability to adapt to oral breathing and acquire adequate nutrition. Hengerer and Wein (2003) state that some surgeons advocate "a rule of tens" to guide the timing of surgical intervention. The child must reach 10 weeks of age, weigh 10 pounds, and have a hemoglobin level of 10 g/dL. Other surgeons have demonstrated routine success in newborns 48 to 72 hours old and weighing as little as 1900 g (Werkhaven J, 2003, personal communication).

The anesthetic approach depends on the child's condition. In general, intravenous induction with a muscle relaxant of intermediate duration, endotracheal intubation with an oral RAE tube, and maintenance with an inhaled agent and opioid or propofol and remifentanil infusion suffice. Rarely, algorithms for difficult neonatal intubation must be used for securing the airway in infants with bilateral choanal atresia. After the atresia is surgically corrected, the surgeon is often faced with the problem of restenosis (Pirsig, 1986); however, recent innovations have created optimism that the restenosis rate can be reduced. Newer endoscopic techniques with powered instrumentation have enhanced the safety and efficacy for choanal atresia repair (Prasad et al., 2002). Mitomycin-C, an aminoglycoside and alkylating agent used as an intravenous antineoplastic agent, can be used topically after choanal atresia repair. Topical application inhibits fibroblast growth and migration and granulation tissue formation responsible for restenosis (Holland and McGuirt, 2001). Topical mitomycin has not caused systemic effects and has not contributed to anesthetic complications. Patients with unilateral obstruction usually do well in the postoperative period and require no special monitoring. However, infants undergoing bilateral repair can exhibit partial or intermittent upper airway obstruction that persists for some time. The infant should be observed closely in the ICU with appropriate monitoring until breathing dynamics have normalized.

ANESTHESIA FOR PHARYNGEAL AND LARYNGEAL PROCEDURES

Tonsillectomy and Adenoidectomy

Tonsillectomy and adenoidectomy (perhaps with the exception of myringotomies) are the most common pediatric surgical procedures performed in the United States. Although tonsillectomy and adenoidectomy are frequently performed procedures, the benefits in relation to cost and risk are still hotly debated (Paradise, 2003). Just about every indication has its advocates and detractors (Bluestone, 2001; Paradise, 2003).

Nocturnal upper airway obstruction, with or without obstructive sleep apnea (OSA), is a common indication for adenotonsillectomy. A mild, partial obstruction in otherwise healthy children is exacerbated by conditions such as achondroplasia, Down syndrome, mucopolysaccharidosis, and obesity. Adenotonsillectomy is considered curative when adenotonsillar hypertrophy is the primary cause of childhood sleep-related breathing disorders (Schechter, 2002). Indications for tonsillectomy include recurrent pharyngotonsillitis, chronic tonsillitis, hemorrhagic tonsillitis, peritonsillar abscess, streptococcal carriage, dysphagia, abnormal dentofacial growth, halitosis, and suspicion of malignant disease (i.e., tonsil asymmetry) (Darrow and Siemans, 2002). Additional indications for adenoidectomy include recurrent or chronic rhinosinusitis or adenoiditis, and recurrent otitis media (Darrow and Siemans, 2002). Adenotonsillar hypertrophy with resultant upper airway obstruction is the most frequent cause of OSA in children (Fig. 24-3).

Obstructive Sleep Apnea Syndrome

Obstructive sleep apnea syndrome (OSAS) is a disorder of breathing during sleep characterized by prolonged partial upper airway obstruction (obstructive hypopnea) or intermittent complete obstruction (OSA) with or without snoring and associated with moderate to severe oxygen desaturation that disrupts normal sleep-time breathing and normal sleep patterns (American Thoracic Society, 1996). The most common cause of OSAS among children is upper airway narrowing with adenotonsillar hypertrophy. OSAS also occurs in infants and children with upper airway narrowing resulting from craniofacial anomalies, and in those with neuromuscular diseases, including cerebral palsy and muscular dystrophy (Marcus, 2001; Schwengel et al., 2009) (Box 24-1). See related video online at www.expertconsult.com.

In recent years, the epidemic increase in the prevalence of obesity during childhood seems to be contributing to substantial changes in the cross-sectional demographic and anthropometric characteristics of the children being referred for evaluation of OSAS. Although less than 15% of all symptomatic habitually snoring children were obese (i.e., >95th percentile for age and gender) in the early 1990s, more than 50% fulfilled the criteria for obesity among all referrals to a Kentucky sleep center by the mid 2000s (Gozal et al., 2006; Schwengel et al., 2009).

Adenotonsillar hypertrophy is the most common cause of OSAS in children. Many published papers, primarily case reports

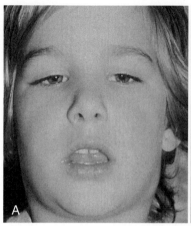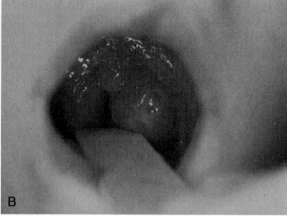

■ **FIGURE 24-3.** Adenoidal and tonsillar hypertrophy. **A,** Dull expression of a child with marked adenotonsillar hypertrophy and nasal obstruction (i.e., adenoid facies). He must keep his mouth open to breathe and shows signs of fatigue as a result of obstructive sleep apnea caused by upper airway obstruction. **B,** On examination of the pharynx, his enlarged tonsils are seen meeting in the midline. *(From Yellon RB, McBride TP, Davis HW: Otolaryngology. In Zitelli BJ, Davis HW, editors:* Atlas of pediatric physical diagnosis, *ed 4, St Louis, 2002, Mosby, p 836.)*

Box 24-1 Some Congenital and Medical Conditions Associated with Obstructive Sleep Apnea Syndrome

Achondroplasia
Apert syndrome
Beckwith-Wiedemann syndrome
Cerebral palsy
Choanal stenosis
Cleft palate patients after repair
Crouzon syndrome
Cystic hygroma
Down syndrome
Hallerman-Streiff syndrome
Hypothyroidism
Klippel-Feil syndrome
Mucopolysaccharidosis
Obesity
Osteopetrosis
Papillomatosis (oropharyngeal)
Pierre Robin syndrome
Pfeiffer syndrome
Pharyngeal flap surgery
Prader-Willi syndrome
Sickle cell disease
Treacher Collins syndrome

From Sterni LM, Tunkel DE: Obstructive sleep apnea in children: an update, *Pediatr Clin North Am* 50:427, 2003.

---

and case series, support the idea that tonsillectomy with or without adenoidectomy is often the cure for OSAS (Schechter et al., 2002; Garetz, 2008).

The peak prevalence of OSAS in children occurs between 2 and 8 years, which is the age when the tonsils and adenoids are large in relation to the child's upper airways. The site of collapse is most commonly at the level of the adenoids or velopharynx (Isono et al., 1998; Isono, 2006). Although OSAS is associated with adenotonsillar hypertrophy, there must be other neuromuscular factors involved. These patients usually do not obstruct while awake, implying that sleep induces another dimension to OSAS. Some otherwise normal children with OSAS but with smaller tonsils and adenoids are cured by adenotonsillectomy, whereas others with larger tonsils and adenoids are not (Marcus, 2001). The patency of pharyngeal airway is maintained by tonic and phasic contractions of the upper airway dilator muscles, such as the genioglossus, geniohyoid, and velopalatine muscles (Isono, 2006). Compared with other inspiratory muscles (i.e., diaphragm and intercostal muscles), these upper airway muscles are preferentially depressed with sleep, sedatives, and general anesthetics (Ochiai et al., 1989, 1992) (see Chapter 3, Respiratory Physiology in Infants and Children). It is hypothesized that children with OSAS may have abnormal centrally mediated activation of their airway muscles, leading to a more collapsible upper airway (Marcus et al., 1994).

Fatty deposits of the upper airway structures, and subcutaneous fat deposits in the anterior neck region are the direct causes of airway obstruction in obese children (mostly adolescents), as well as in obese adults, with OSAS. In addition, increased adipose deposits in the chest wall and abdomen can reduce chest wall compliance as well as cephalad displacement of the diaphragm, causing inefficient ventilation by mass loading and decreased functional residual capacity of the lung (Dayyat et al., 2007; Schwengel et al., 2009). Obese patients have symptoms that differ from those in children with OSAS caused by adenotonsillar hypertrophy. Obese patients tend to have a significantly greater incidence of daytime sleepiness, insulin resistance, and systemic as well as pulmonary hypertension than children with adenotonsillar hypertrophy (Tauman et al., 2004). Furthermore, Tauman and coworkers recently observed a high failure rate for obese children with OSAS undergoing adentotonsillectomy.

Dayyat and colleagues (2007) differentiated between children with OSAS into two types. The type 1 child with OSAS is not obese but has disordered breathing secondary to marked lymphadenoid hypertrophy. The type 2 patient is obese with minimal lymphadenoid hyperplasia. Table 24-1 compares the common symptoms experienced by the two types of patients (Dayyat et al., 2007).

One of the most interesting areas of childhood OSAS research has been on the effects that OSAS has on systemic inflammation. Children with OSAS are at risk for developing inflammatory responses that may lead to endothelial dysfunction and

TABLE 24-1. Clinical Presentation of Pediatric Obstructive Sleep Apnea Types I and II

Symptoms and Findings Seen with Similar Frequencies in Types I and II

- Snoring
- Difficulty breathing during sleep, with snorting episodes
- Restless sleep and frequent awakenings
- Excessive sweating
- Night terrors
- Enuresis
- Breathing pauses reported by parents
- Mouth breathing and limited nasal airflow
- Chronic rhinorrhea
- Frequent visits to primary care physician for respiratory-related symptoms
- Retrognathia
- Pulmonary hypertension and cor pulmonale

Symptoms and Findings that Differ Between Types	Type I	Type II
Excessive daytime sleepiness	+	++++
Weight gain	−	++
Hyperactive behavior	++++	− or +
Truncal obesity	− or +	+++
Enlarged neck circumference	− or +	+++
Enlarged tonsils or adenoids	++++	++
Depression and low self-esteem	+	+++
Shyness and social withdrawal	+	+++
Left ventricular hypertrophy	++	++++
Systemic hypertension	+	++++
Recurrent ear infections	+++	− or +
Insulin resistance	−	++++
Dyslipidemia	+	++++
Elevated C-reactive protein	++	++++
Elevated liver enzymes	−	++

From Dayyat E, Kheirandish-Gozal L, Gozal D: Childhood obstructive sleep apnea: one or two distinct disease entities? *Sleep Med Clin* 2:433, 2007.
−, Absent; + infrequent to ++++ very frequent.

TABLE 24-2. Polysomnographic Characteristics of Obstructive Sleep Apnea in Children and Adults

Characteristic	Adults	Children
Apnea duration	10 sec	2 breaths
Hypopnea desaturation	≥4%	≥3%
Hypopnea duration	10 sec	2 breaths
Hypopnea nasal pressure drop	>30%	≥50%
Cortical arousals	Common	Uncommon
Normal apnea-hypopnea index	<5	<1

From Karlson KH Jr: What's new in pediatric obstructive sleep apnea? *Clin Pulm Med* 15:226, 2008.

Many of these children experience a growth spurt after surgery. Children with OSAS may have neurocognitive deficits such as poor learning, behavioral problems, and lower grades in school than non-OSAS children. Adenotonsillectomy improves functioning in these children (Marcus, 2001). Recent studies demonstrate that despite negative polysomnographic findings, the benefits of adenotonsillectomy are still observed in children with symptomatic airway obstruction, including improvements in behavior and quality of life (Leong and Davis 2007).

The diagnosis of OSAS is based on a thorough history and physical examination along with appropriate sleep studies, including polysomnography (Table 24-2 and Boxes 24-2 and 24-3). Snoring, increased respiratory efforts, periodic obstructive apnea, and oxygen desaturation while sleeping are the universal features of OSAS, which must be differentiated from the benign condition referred to as primary snoring.

Box 24-2 Key Questions to Ask Parents

- Does your child have difficulty breathing during sleep?
- Have you observed symptoms of apnea?
- Have you observed sweating while your child sleeps?
- Does your child have restless sleep?
- Does your child breathe through his or her mouth when awake?
- Are you worried about your child's breathing at night?
- Do you have any family history of obstructive sleep apnea, sudden infant death syndrome, or apparent life-threatening events?
- Does your child have behavioral problems?

Box 24-3 Facial and Airway Features Suggestive of Obstructive Sleep Apnea

- Small triangular chin
- Retro position of the mandible
- Steep mandibular plane
- High palate
- Long, oval face
- Long soft palate
- Large tonsils in association with the aforementioned facial features

atherogenesis (Gozal et al., 2008). School-aged children with OSAS have a higher serum C-reactive protein level than controls, and the elevation correlates with the severity of OSAS, and levels decrease after adenotonsillectomy (Gozal et al., 2007). Serum proteomic patterns in children with OSAS differ significantly from those in children who have primary snoring but do not have OSAS (Shah et al., 2006). In the Shah group's study, proteomic profiling of serum samples in children with OSAS revealed differential expression of circulating proteins. Proteomics may play a future role in diagnosing OSAS in the snoring child.

Symptoms of OSAS include nocturnal snoring, breathing pauses, gasping, use of accessory muscles of respiration, enuresis, and excessive sweating (Messner, 2003). In addition, children with OSAS have a host of sequelae, which are usually reversible after adenotonsillectomy but can lead to perioperative complications during and after surgery. Children with OSAS may present with failure to thrive, although the cause of this growth failure is unclear (Sterni and Tunkel, 2003).

Polysomnography

Pediatric polysomnography includes measurement of end-tidal CO$_2$, electroencephalogram, chin EMG, chest wall movement, airflow through the nose and mouth, leg movement, and oxygen saturation via pulse oximetry (Box 24-4). After all events are reviewed and scored, several indices can be calculated. These include the apnea index and the apnea-hypopnea index, which are calculated for the entire sleep period, for both rapid eye movement sleep and non–rapid eye movement sleep. The term *index* refers to the number of events divided by the number of hours of sleep (Table 24-3). This calculation allows the comparison of polysomnograms of varying time lengths. The apnea index is determined using only apneas, whereas the apnea-hypopnea index includes both apneas and hypopneas (Wagner and Torrez, 2007).

It is helpful to divide the scores into severity-based categories (Table 24-4). OSAS severity can be used to determine the appropriate surgical center where the surgery should be performed and whether the child requires overnight observation (Box 24-5).

Although definitive diagnosis of OSAS is made by a positive polysomnogram, many children are not tested because the polysomnography laboratories specializing in children are few, and the tests are expensive and require an overnight stay (Sterni and Tunkel, 2003). Most children are diagnosed by recommendations set forth by the section of Pediatric Pulmonology Subcommittee

---

Box 24-4 Components of Polysomnography*

- Respiratory effort—assessed by abdominal and chest wall movements
- Airflow at nose, mouth, or both
- Arterial oxygen saturation
- End-tidal CO$_2$ or transcutaneous CO$_2$ (recommended specifically for pediatric polysomnography to detect hypoventilation)
- Electrocardiography
- Electromyography (tibial) to monitor arousals
- Electroencephalography, electrooculography, and electromyography for sleep staging

From American Thoracic Society: Standards and indications for cardiopulmonary sleep studies in children, *Am J Respir Crit Care Med* 153:866, 1996.
* As recommended by the American Thoracic Society.

TABLE 24-4. Proposed Classification and Severity Criteria of Pediatric Sleep-Disordered Breathing

	OAHI (per hour TST)	Nadir SpO$_2$ (%)	P$_{ETCO_2}$ > 50 mm Hg (% TST)	RAI (per hour TST)
Normal	≤1	>94	<10	<1
Habitual snoring	≤1	>94	<10	<2
Upper airway resistance syndrome	≤2	>92	10-15	≥2
Obstructive alveolar hypoventilation	≤2	>92	>20	≥2
Obstructive sleep apnea				
Mild	2-5	88-92	10-15	2-5
Moderate	5-10	80-88	15-20	5-8
Severe	>10	<80	>20	>8

OAHI, Obstructive apnea-hypopnea index; *P$_{ETCO_2}$*, end-tidal carbon dioxide tension; *RAI*, respiratory arousal index; *SpO$_2$*, oxyhemoglobin saturation by pulse oximetry; *TST*, total sleep time.

TABLE 24-3. Respiratory Events that Can Be Seen During Polysomnography

Event	Definition
Central apnea	Pause in airflow with absent respiratory effort, scored when >20 sec or 2 missed breaths and a >3% drop in oxygen saturation
Obstructive apnea	>90% reduction of airflow despite continuing respiratory effort, scored when event lasts at least 2 missed breaths in children
Obstructive hypopnea	>50% reduction of airflow with associated respiratory effort, scored when at least 2 missed breaths and >3% drop in oxygen saturation or arousal
Mixed apneas	≥90% reduction in airflow, lasting at least 2 missed breaths, and containing absent respiratory effort initially (a central apneic pause), followed by resumption of respiratory effort without a resumption of airflow (an obstructive apnea)
Obstructive hypoventilation	End-tidal CO$_2$ > 50 mm Hg for >25% of the total sleep time, with paradoxical respirations, snoring, and no baseline lung disease

---

Box 24-5 Clinical Features that Predict Respiratory Compromise after Adenotonsillectomy and, in Some Cases, Persistent Obstructive Sleep Apnea

- Severe obstructive sleep apnea on polysomnography
- History of prematurity, especially with respiratory disease
- Age less than years
- Morbid obesity
- Nasal problems (deviated septum, enlarged turbinates)
- Mallampati score of 3 or 4
- Neuromuscular disorders or disordered pharyngeal tone
- Genetic or chromosomal disorders
- Craniofacial disorders
- Enlarged lingual tonsils
- Upper respiratory infection within 4 weeks of surgery
- Cor pulmonale
- Systemic hypertension
- Marked obstruction on inhalational induction
- Disordered breathing in the postanesthesia care unit
- Difficulty breathing during sleep
- Growth impairment resulting from chronic obstructed breathing

Data from McGowan et al., 1992; Gerber et al., 1996; Blum et al., 2004; Fricke et al., 2006; Guilleminault et al., 2007.

on Obstructive Sleep Apnea, sans Polysomnography. This committee's recommendations for otherwise healthy children older than 1 year are as follows (Schechter, 2002):

- All children should be screened for snoring. As part of routine health care maintenance for all children, pediatricians should ask whether the patient snores. An affirmative answer should be followed by a more detailed evaluation.
- Complex, high-risk patients should be referred to a specialist.
- Patients with cardiorespiratory failure cannot await elective evaluation. It is expected that these patients will be in an intensive care setting and will be treated by a specialist; these patients are not covered in this practice guideline.
- A thorough diagnostic evaluation should be performed. History and physical examination have been shown to be poor in discriminating between primary snoring and OSAS. Polysomnography is the only method that quantifies ventilatory and sleep abnormalities, and it is recommended as the diagnostic test of choice. Other diagnostic techniques, such as videotaping, nocturnal pulse oximetry, and daytime nap studies, may be useful in discriminating between primary snoring and OSAS. However, they do not assess the severity of OSAS, which is useful for determining treatment and follow-up.
- Adenotonsillectomy is the first line of treatment for most children. CPAP is an option for those who are not candidates for surgery or do not respond to surgery.

Severe, untreated OSAS may lead to pulmonary hypertension and cor pulmonale caused by nocturnal hypoxia and hypercarbia, resulting in compensatory changes in the pulmonary vasculature. Pulmonary vascular resistance increases, causing increased right ventricular strain. Severe cases may progress to pulmonary hypertension, arrhythmias, and cor pulmonale, which are reversible by performing early adenotonsillectomy (Miman et al., 2000). Children with OSAS also tend to have higher diastolic blood pressures. The cardiovascular changes appear to be the result of an increase in sympathetic tone that results from obstructive respiratory events (Marcus et al., 1998). Fortunately, few children develop clinically significant heart failure. It is prudent to pursue an aggressive cardiac evaluation if the child has a loud second heart sound, exercise intolerance, or diastolic hypertension. Because children are diagnosed earlier today, significant heart disease is rarely an issue (Marcus, 2001).

Preoperative Preparation

A careful review of the history, laboratory data, and physical examination results are essential for the optimal outcome of adenotonsillectomy. Careful evaluation of coagulation status is important before performing this procedure. If there is a history of easy bruising, frequent epistaxis, or positive family history, the prothrombin time, partial thromboplastin time, and platelet count should be obtained to rule out coagulopathies. In many pediatric institutions, a coagulation profile is obtained routinely for patients scheduled for adenotonsillectomy. However, in a prospective study of hemostatic assessment of patients before tonsillectomy, routine measurements of a coagulation profile were not useful predictors of postoperative bleeding (Close et al., 1994).

Although relatively mild, von Willebrand's disease (i.e., reduced factor VIII, decreased platelet adhesiveness because of

deficient von Willebrand factor) is the most common coagulopathy seen among patients scheduled for adenotonsillectomy. Children with von Willebrand's disease or mild hemophilia A are treated preoperatively with desmopressin (1-desamino-8-D-arginine vasopressin [DDAVP]) (Prinsley et al., 1993). DDAVP is a synthetic analogue of vasopressin, which, in addition to its antidiuretic effect, stimulates endothelial cells and releases stored factor VIII and von Willebrand factor (Mannucci, 1988). The intravenous dosage of DDAVP is 0.3 mcg/kg, given over 20 minutes before anesthetic induction.

Patients who receive DDAVP are at increased risk for hyponatremia because of the retention of free water that occurs with DDAVP. Anesthesia care providers need to remember that intravenous fluids for these patients should be isotonic (preferably normal saline) and should be administered at one-half to two-thirds maintenance dosage. Patients who require intravenous fluids postoperatively should have their sodium monitored to assess for the development of hyponatremia.

The examiner should elicit a history of drug ingestion, especially acetylsalicylic acid. If the patient was given such drugs recently, surgery should be postponed, because these drugs cause platelet dysfunction for as long as 10 days and may cause excessive bleeding intraoperatively and postoperatively (Davies and Steward, 1977; Paradise, 2003).

During the preoperative visit, the patency of oral and nasal air passages is carefully examined. The patient's mouth should be inspected for the degree of tonsillar hypertrophy or inflammation. The examiner should also have the child breathe with the mouth closed to evaluate the degree of nasal airway obstruction and estimate adenoidal hypertrophy. It is important to inspect the teeth routinely, because tonsillectomy is often performed on children who are losing their primary dentition. Any teeth missing preoperatively should be noted carefully. A tooth that is loose should be pointed out to the parent and child, with the explanation that it may be necessary to remove it while the child is anesthetized (it must then be saved). It is also possible for the surgeon to dislodge or chip teeth in the application of a mouth gag or during other intraoperative manipulations.

Anesthetic Management

All children should be monitored with a pulse oximeter, endtidal CO_2, precordial stethoscope, electrocardiogram, thermometer, and automated blood pressure cuff. Oxygen saturation is determined in room air before the induction of anesthesia to establish the baseline value. If neuromuscular blockade is required, a nerve stimulator should be used to track the depth of paralysis. Standard NPO guidelines should be followed in nonemergent situations.

Children who are anxious preoperatively may receive sedation with oral midazolam. In older children scheduled for intravenous induction, EMLA cream (i.e., eutectic mixture of local anesthetics, 2.5% lidocaine and 2.5% prilocaine) is applied to the dorsum of both hands and sealed with plastic adhesives at least 1 hour before intravenous catheter insertion (see Chapter 9, Preoperative Preparation, and Chapter 13, Induction, Maintenance, and Recovery).

Adenoidectomy is a relatively short procedure (15 to 45 minutes), and many centers perform anesthesia without neuromuscular blockade and with less opioid than suggested in the following descriptions. Anesthesia is induced most commonly with oxygen, nitrous oxide, and sevoflurane. As with those undergoing myringotomies, children with adenotonsillar hypertrophy often have partial or complete nasal airway obstruction. The mouth must be kept open during the induction of anesthesia until the gag reflex is abolished and the oral airway is inserted. If necessary, moderate CPAP (10 to 15 cm H_2O), with jaw thrust during induction (before the patient is deep enough for oral airway insertion) helps to prevent the pharyngeal airway collapse that results from the relaxation of upper airway muscle tone (Reber et al., 2001; Bruppacher et al., 2003).

After the intravenous route is established, atropine or glycopyrrolate may be given for its anticholinergic effects. The patient's trachea is intubated with a preformed oral (RAE) tube under deep inhalational anesthesia supplemented with a topical lidocaine spray to the vocal cords under a direct vision, an intravenous bolus of propofol, or an intermediate-acting, nondepolarizing muscle relaxant (e.g., cisatracurium, vecuronium). In older children, anesthesia may be induced intravenously with propofol (2 to 3 mg/kg) mixed with lidocaine (1 to 2 mg/mL of propofol) to reduce pain at the injection site, with or without anticholinergic agent or a muscle relaxant. Inhalation anesthetic or propofol infusion is continued thereafter with spontaneous or controlled ventilation. A cuffed endotracheal tube is recommended to reduce the chance of aspiration of blood and secretions and to reduce gas leaks around the tube. A cuffed endotracheal tube, 0.5 to 1.0 mm (inner diameter) smaller than the age-appropriate size, should be chosen to accommodate the passage of the cuff through the subglottis (Khine et al., 1997; James, 2001; Fine and Borland, 2004). The endotracheal tube is immobilized with adhesive tape over the middle of the lower lip (Fig. 24-4). The breath sounds on both sides of the chest should be auscultated carefully to avoid endobronchial intubation. The endotracheal tube is then held in place by the groove-bladed tongue depressor that is a part of the Ring adaptation of the Brown-Davis mouth gag (Fig. 24-5).

Anesthesia is maintained with supplemental opioids to reduce the requirement of the anesthesia maintenance agent and to provide postoperative analgesia. The physician may start with a loading dose of 1 to 2 mcg/kg of fentanyl, 50 to 100 mcg/kg of morphine, or 10 to 20 mcg/kg of hydromorphone given intravenously, with additional doses administered as needed. Children with moderate and severe OSAS should receive lower

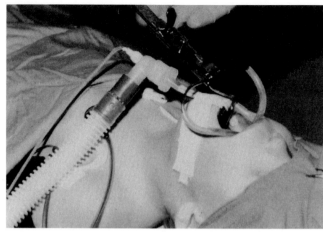

FIGURE 24-5. Patient in position for tonsillectomy. A Brown-Davis mouth gag holds the mouth open. An oral Ring, Adaire, Ellwyn (RAE) endotracheal tube is fixed to the middle of the lower lip and is held in the groove of the tongue blade.

dosages of opioids to minimize the risk for prolonged apnea during emergence and postoperative upper airway obstruction. Brown and coworkers (2004) have shown that young age and low preoperative oxygen saturation were associated with lower postoperative morphine requirement. It appears that children with a minimal oxygen saturation of 85% or less during preoperative sleep required half the postoperative analgesic dosage required by children whose saturations were 85% or greater (Brown et al., 2006).

The use of NSAIDs during or after tonsillectomy is controversial. A meta-analysis suggested that there is an increased risk for bleeding and increased return to the operating room when NSAIDs such as ketorolac are used (Marret, 2003). Criticism of this meta-analysis focuses on the small number of patients evaluated, the varying types and dosages of NSAID, and the varying surgical techniques used for the tonsillectomy. A Cochrane database review evaluated the role of NSAIDs in posttonsillectomy bleeding and found no significant correlation between NSAID use and increased risk for posttonsillectomy bleeding (Cardwell et al., 2005). Practice among pediatric anesthesiologists varies. Some centers do not use NSAIDs during adenoidectomy or tonsillectomy, whereas others use them routinely (Allford, 2009).

There is evidence that high dosages of dexamethasone (up to 1 mg/kg, 25 mg maximum) reduce postoperative swelling and pain and decrease the incidence of PONV without apparent adverse effects attributable to dexamethasone (Pappas et al., 1998). Children receiving dexamethasone are more likely to advance to a soft-solid diet on the first postoperative day (Steward et al., 2003).

Bleeding during tonsil and adenoid surgery is seldom excessive, but massive hemorrhage has occurred with tearing of the carotid vessels (Smith, 1972, 1980). Homeostasis is usually obtained using electrocautery. There have been several reports of fires due to electrocautery-induced ignition of the endotracheal tube or packing during tonsillectomy. Fires are caused by combustible material in an oxygen-rich environment (Mattucci and Militana, 2003); management of airway fires is discussed later.

Children with OSAS tend to emerge from anesthesia more slowly than children without OSAS. This may be explained by their deficit in sleep arousal mechanisms. They seem to have elevated sleep arousal mechanisms in response to hypercarbia

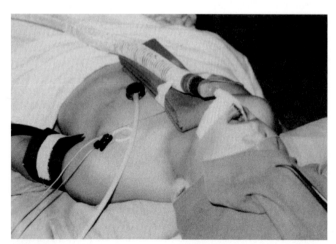

FIGURE 24-4. For tonsillectomy or adenoidectomy, an oral Ring, Adaire, Ellwyn (RAE) endotracheal tube is fixed over the middle of the lower lip.

and increased upper airway obstruction (Marcus et al., 1998, 1999). Other subtle disturbances of sleep architecture may also be present (Bandla et al., 1999).

Techniques of Tonsillectomy and Adenoidectomy

A myriad of surgical techniques are used to perform tonsillectomy and adenoidectomy, and they use a mouth gag to give oropharyngeal exposure. The surgeon should use caution when placing and removing the mouth gag to avoid displacement of the endotracheal tube.

The adenoidectomy is performed either with a mechanical or a thermal technique (Hesham, 2009). Mechanical removal of the adenoids may be performed using curettes, adenotomes, or a micro-debrider. These mechanical techniques require nasopharyngeal packing to prevent bleeding, and the surgeon must remember to remove the packing at the end of the procedure. Thermal removal of adenoid tissue may employ electrosurgical cautery, radiofrequency ablation, or lasers, and it usually results in little bleeding.

Tonsillectomy can also be performed via mechanical or thermal techniques. Intracapsular removal of tonsil tissue is a newer approach that preserves the integrity of the tonsil capsule, and will be discussed later.

Mechanical removal of the tonsil has many technical variations. In general, an incision is made in the anterior pillar mucosa to expose the tonsil capsule, and using sharp or blunt dissection, the tonsil and capsule are removed together. Alternatively, a guillotine, or snare, is occasionally used to remove the tonsil without making an incision. This results in exposure of the underlying pharyngeal musculature with the perforating vascular supply to the tonsil, and hemostasis must be established. At the turn of the previous century, snare tonsillectomy with ether anesthesia was the standard, and hemostasis was achieved after prolonged observation of the surgical field to ensure passive wound clotting. This was less than ideal, and the mortality rate was unacceptably high. Today, active hemorrhage control is performed after removal of the tonsils. Some surgeons use dissolvable suture to ligate the bleeding points, but this is becoming less common. More often, electrosurgical cautery is used for hemostasis. This technique completes an electrical arc between the patient and the surgical instrument and has the potential to ignite flammable gases and combustible materials (such as the sponges in the nasopharynx used for tamponade of the adenoid bleeding). Case reports of airway fires have been reported with the use of electrosurgical cautery in tonsillectomy (Mattucci and Militana, 2003). It is suggested that the inspired oxygen levels be maintained as they are for the use of lasers in the airway (see Laser Surgery of the Larynx, later).

Thermal removal of the tonsil uses the electrosurgical unit or a radiofrequency unit for tonsil dissection. The most common radiofrequency unit in use is Coblation (ArthroCare, Austin, TX). Thermal removal of the tonsils and adenoids generally results in less blood loss, but it may be accompanied by slightly more postoperative pain than other techniques. A cuffed endotracheal tube, using moist throat packing and inspired oxygen levels of less than 40%, will minimize the risk for an airway fire (Johnson et al., 2002).

Intracapsular tonsillectomy is a newer technique that uses either the micro-debrider or the radiofrequency ablator to remove the tonsil tissue while preserving the tonsil capsule (Koltai et al., 2002). In effect, this may be considered a selective removal of the tonsillar mass, which is believed to be the most common cause of OSAS. Preservation of the capsule protects the underlying pharyngeal musculature, resulting in less postoperative pain and hemorrhage. Because the vascular supply is interrupted at a more terminal point, the muscular bed can contract around the vessels, providing better hemostasis. Initially, this technique was recommended only for those patients with OSAS. Recurrent infection is considered a contraindication, because this technique leaves behind residual tonsil tissue that may become reinfected. This technique is especially appropriate in those OSAS children 3 years of age and younger because of the lower postoperative pain scores and thus less opioid need (Solares et al., 2005; Colen et al., 2008). In general, the only risk of an intracapsular tonsillectomy is the rare (<1 in 1500) need to return for a complete tonsillectomy because of tissue regrowth leading to recurrent infectious tonsillitis.

At the conclusion of surgery, the surgeon usually suctions the pharynx and larynx under direct vision to prevent bleeding caused by agitation of raw mucosal surfaces by a suction catheter. Suctioning of the stomach contents may also remove swallowed secretions, blood, or residual preoperative sedative medications. Removal of these preoperative medications may decrease excess sedation in the postoperative period. Some surgeons elect to infiltrate 0.25% bupivacaine or other local anesthetic medications into the tonsillar fossa to aid in postoperative pain relief (Naja et al., 2005), whereas others feel that this analgesic technique may lead to premature discharge of patients who will then experience rebound pain when the local anesthetic wears off. This practice has occasionally been associated with airway obstruction after extubation.

After tonsillectomy, the anesthesia provider should always use a tonsil suction tip and should never blindly suction the nasopharynx or oropharynx after adenoidectomy or tonsillectomy. Suctioning should be directed toward the midline to avoid the lateral tonsil fossa. A soft nasopharyngeal airway may be inserted to facilitate airway patency for extubation. If adenoid hemostasis is adequate prior to insertion of the nasopharyngeal airway, usually no additional bleeding is encountered. Toward the completion of surgery, before a child regains active reflexes, the anesthesiologist should auscultate both sides of the chest to rule out the presence of aspirated blood or secretions and, under direct laryngoscopic visualization, examine the mouth and pharynx for blood and other debris that could cause airway irritation after extubation.

Laryngospasm may occur when the patient is extubated after tonsillectomy. Methods for avoiding this problem include extubating the trachea while the child is deeply anesthetized (not recommended for children with OSAS) or almost completely awake (see Chapter 13, Induction, Maintenance, and Recovery). Although intravenous lidocaine has not consistently proved helpful in preventing laryngospasm, application of local anesthetic before intubation or manipulation of the airway can reduce the incidence of laryngospasm during intubation and after extubation (Leicht et al., 1985; McCulloch et al., 1992; Landsman, 1997). It appears that lidocaine deposited locally in the laryngeal area suppresses laryngeal mucosa neuroreceptor transmission. However, lidocaine's duration of action at laryngeal receptor sites is only 30 minutes, and its administration before intubation may not protect against laryngospasm at the time of extubation (Warner, 1996).

Before extubation, the lungs should be well expanded with an oxygen-air mixture at sustained high positive pressure (35 to 40 cm H_2O) several times (the vital capacity maneuver), to reopen intrathoracic airways and reverse atelectasis, which frequently develops during anesthesia and surgery; the patient should then be extubated under positive pressure (Benoit et al., 2002; Tusman et al., 2003) to prevent postoperative oxygen desaturation. Positive airway pressure at the moment of extubation causes a coughing motion, which helps to expel secretions around the vocal cords. Positive extending pressure on the upper airway walls also attenuates the excitation of the superior laryngeal nerve and may diminish the risk for laryngospasm (Suzuki and Sasaki, 1977; Sasaki, 1979) (see Chapter 3, Respiratory Physiology in Infants and Children, and Chapter 13, Induction, Maintenance, and Recovery).

Postoperative Management

Children with hypertrophic tonsils and adenoids tend to have increased airway obstruction in the immediate postoperative period. The presence of blood and secretions in the pharynx and larynx may provoke upper airway reflexes, leading to laryngospasm. These patients tend to become hypoxemic more often and perhaps more severely during the first several hours after surgery than patients undergoing procedures not involving the upper airways (Motoyama and Glazener, 1986). However, they seem to maintain their preoperative levels of oxygen saturation in room air thereafter, as determined with pulse oximetry (Motoyama and Borland, unpublished observations). Fortunately, serious complications after adenotonsillectomy are infrequent. Postoperative hemorrhage, however, does occur and can become a life-threatening catastrophe (discussed later). Postoperative emesis is relatively common because of pharyngeal mucosal irritation from surgery, which may stimulate the glossopharyngeal nerves, or from bloody secretions that are swallowed. It is therefore prudent for the anesthesiologist to administer antiemetics (e.g., ondansetron or metoclopramide) prophylactically, in addition to dexamethasone before the end of surgery (Pappas et al., 1998). Pain after tonsillectomy is mild to moderate and may be controlled by opioids given intraoperatively as part of anesthetic management or by supplementation (morphine, 50 mcg/kg; fentanyl, 0.5 to 1.0 mcg/kg; hydromorphone, 10 mcg/kg) in the postanesthetic care unit. Postoperative pain after adenoidectomy is relatively mild. Acetaminophen is a good adjunct to pain control in these patients.

It has been reported that children with OSAS have reduced opioid requirements after adenotonsillectomy. In addition, children with OSAS spontaneously breathing during halothane anesthesia are more likely to become apneic than non-OSAS children when treated with the same dosage of fentanyl (Waters et al., 2002). However, others have found no morbidity from opioid or benzodiazepine treatment in OSAS pediatric patients undergoing adenotonsillectomy (Helfaer et al., 1996; Sanders et al., 2006; Leong and Davis, 2007).

Preoperative sedation with benzodiazepines and postoperative treatment with opioids should be tailored to meet the needs of the patient. It would be prudent to titrate opioids, anticipating that the more severe the OSAS, the higher is the risk of opioid and benzodiazepine sensitivity. For patients with moderate or severe OSAS, many anesthesiologists prefer not to administer opioids until the patient has fully emerged from the anesthetic, has regained spontaneous ventilation, has been extubated, and is able to maintain an open airway with spontaneous ventilation. The patient's opioid therapy may then be titrated carefully to achieve analgesia without respiratory compromise (Leong and Davis, 2007). During the immediate postoperative period, monitoring these patients in a postanesthetic care unit staffed with pediatric recovery room nurses allows a safe postoperative recovery with pain control.

Children with OSAS have a higher incidence of postoperative respiratory complications, including prolonged oxygen requirements, airway obstruction requiring nasal airway, and major respiratory compromise requiring airway instrumentation, than children without OSAS (Biavati et al., 1997; Wilson and Robertson 2002). Because OSAS is a disorder of anatomic and dynamic factors of upper airway function, it is not surprising that a procedure that is curative in many of these children would cause significant postoperative respiratory complications. Because these children are presumed to have impaired neuromuscular control of upper airway patency, residual anesthetic effects combined with blood, edema, and residual lymphoid tissue obstructing the postsurgical airway can lead to postoperative respiratory events (Wilson et al., 2002). McColley and colleagues (1992) reported a 58% incidence of severe respiratory compromise in children younger than 3 years that was associated with severe oxygen desaturation (SpO_2, $\leq 70\%$) or hypoventilation from upper airway obstruction. Among children with OSAS undergoing adenotonsillectomy (mean age, 5 years), intraoperative and postoperative complications are particularly high among those who were born prematurely (85% versus 25% to 34% in full-term infants).

Nixon and coworkers (2005) demonstrated that, not infrequently, children with OSAS continue to have polysomnogram-documented airway obstruction the night after adenotonsillectomy. Obstructive apneas and hypopneas were four times as frequent and associated with greater oxygen desaturation in the severe OSAS group as opposed to the mild OSAS group.

The subpopulation of children with OSAS who must be monitored in the hospital is still unknown. Children who are most likely to experience postoperative respiratory complications and have a higher postoperative respiratory disturbance index on their postoperative polysomnogram include children 3 years of age and younger, children with severe OSAS diagnosed by preoperative polysomnography, and those with associated medical conditions such as hypotonia, morbid obesity, failure to thrive, or severe structural airway abnormalities (Statham et al., 2006; Karlson 2008). These children are not candidates for outpatient surgery facilities and should receive medical care in centers with pediatric inpatient facilities and pediatric intensive care support. High-risk patients should be monitored overnight with continuous pulse oximetry, because standard apnea monitoring is unable to detect obstructive apnea and hypopnea. Patients can be discharged when significant oxygen desaturation during sleep has resolved.

A rare complication of adenotonsillectomy in children with severe OSAS is pulmonary edema resulting from relief of upper airway obstruction (Mehta et al., 2006). The exact cause is unknown. Galvis and colleagues (1980) hypothesized that during obstructed breathing, extreme negative pressures occur in the intrapleural and intrathoracic compartments. Intubation results in sudden equalization of pressure. The pulmonary venous pressure is suddenly much higher than intrathoracic pressure, resulting in pulmonary hyperemia and edema.

Furuhashi-Yanaha and colleagues (2000) hypothesized that the abrupt switch from nasal to oral breathing during emergence from anesthesia might create acute obstruction, which creates an increase in negative intrapleural pressure, leading to pulmonary edema. Regardless of the cause, these children require oxygen and possible reintubation to provide CPAP or positive end-expiratory pressure. This condition usually resolves in 24 to 48 hours (Carcillo, 2003), and the use of diuretics is controversial.

Bleeding after Tonsillectomy

Occasionally, bleeding continues or recurs after tonsillectomy, and the child must be anesthetized to suture or pack the bleeding area. Posttonsillectomy bleeding is classified as primary or secondary bleeding. Primary bleeding occurs within the first 24 hours after surgery and is usually more brisk and profuse than secondary bleeding. Most fatal hemorrhages occur within the first 24 hours after surgery (Randall and Hoffer, 1998). Most posttonsillectomy bleeding, however, occurs within the first 6 hours after surgery (Crysdale and Russel, 1986; Carithers et al., 1987; Guida and Mattucci, 1990).

Secondary bleeding usually occurs 24 hours to 5 to 10 days after surgery, when the eschar covering the tonsillar bed sloughs (Verghese and Hannallah, 2001). Allen and coworkers (1973) reported a 0.1% incidence of posttonsillectomy bleeding necessitating repeat exploration in the operating room. Crysdale and Russel (1986) reported a 2.15% incidence of bleeding during the overnight stay in the hospital for 9400 children undergoing tonsillectomy with or without adenoidectomy. Of these, 3% (0.06% of all patients) required reexploration under general anesthesia.

The child with tonsillar bleeding may be brought back to the anesthesia service several hours or even days or weeks after the surgery. Because primary bleeding tends to be more rigorous, bleeding may obstruct the view of the larynx, and emergent tracheostomy may be needed. The otolaryngologist should be present before anesthetic induction. Whether the bleeding is primary or secondary, several issues must be addressed before induction of anesthesia; the child usually is hypovolemic, anemic, agitated, or in shock, with a stomach full of blood clots and often without an intravenous catheter. This is one of the most dangerous and challenging situations in pediatric anesthesia practice, and the failure to initiate prompt action has been one of the main causes of death associated with tonsillectomy (Alexander et al., 1965).

Under these circumstances, intravenous access must be reestablished, unless it is still in place, to rehydrate or transfuse without delay. It is frequently difficult to find a suitable vein for insertion of a large-enough catheter (at least 22 gauge for infants, 20 gauge for children) for rapid hydration and transfusion in an agitated and hypovolemic child with extreme cutaneous vasoconstriction. An intraosseous infusion or surgical cutdown may be indicated in some patients.

It may be difficult to estimate the extent of blood loss and dehydration. The patient may be tachycardic and have an elevated blood pressure caused by the release of endogenous catecholamines from hemorrhage, hypovolemia, or fear and excitement. If the child is sitting up and talking without feeling dizzy, hypovolemia is only mild to moderate; there is enough time to evaluate volume status and to determine hemoglobin, hematocrit, and urine specific gravity and obtain additional information on overall physical status. The child who is lying down and has pale conjunctivae, hypotension, and diminished consciousness may be on the verge of hypovolemic shock, and volume resuscitation must begin without delay. In most cases, tonsillar bleeding is not massive, and the child should be rehydrated and transfused as needed before the induction of anesthesia. Hematocrit values should be rechecked after rehydration to have a more accurate estimate of blood loss.

The anesthesiologist must be aware that the child and parents are extremely frightened. If the condition permits, the patient may be sedated with intravenous midazolam to relieve anxiety. Before the induction of anesthesia, precautions for a patient with a full stomach should be taken. These include at least one, but preferably two, well-functioning suction apparatuses with large-bore suction tubes, extra laryngoscope handles and blades, and several cuffed endotracheal tubes with lubricated stylets in place. An experienced assistant should always be available to help the anesthesiologist and to apply cricoid pressure during the rapid-sequence induction (see Chapter 13, Induction, Maintenance, and Recovery).

After preoxygenation, atropine (0.02 mg/kg), and a defasciculating dosage of nondepolarizing muscle relaxant in older children, the child is intubated, most commonly with a rapid-sequence technique using propofol (2 mg/kg), sodium thiopental (3 to 6 mg/kg), etomidate (0.3 to 0.4 mg/kg), or ketamine (2 mg/kg), with dosages guided by the patient's hemodynamic status, and succinylcholine (2 mg/kg) with cricoid pressure. Alternatively, rocuronium (1.2 mg/kg) may be used. When using thiopental and rocuronium for induction, significant precipitation occurs if they are given together without flushing the intravenous tubing between the two drugs. If the child is still anemic or dehydrated before induction, ketamine (2 mg/kg) may be used instead of propofol or thiopental, because the latter two drugs may cause profound myocardial depression and hypotension. A cuffed endotracheal tube is used in these cases to prevent blood from entering the trachea around the uncuffed tube.

Management of anesthesia during maintenance and emergence in these patients focuses on hypovolemia and a full stomach. A large-bore gastric tube is introduced through the mouth to decompress the stomach, although it is not possible to evacuate all blood clots and solid food. Both sides of the chest are carefully auscultated, and the endotracheal tube is suctioned to rule out aspiration of blood or gastric contents. When there is doubt, fiberoptic bronchoscopy may be performed before extubation, and a portable chest radiograph is taken in the operating room or in the postanesthetic care unit. The endotracheal tube is left in place until the child is fully awake and normal gag and cough reflexes have returned.

The death of a child as a consequence of hemorrhage after tonsil and adenoid surgery is particularly tragic because the operation in most cases is elective and the child is in relatively good health. Mortality rates reported in the literature range from 1 in 1000 to 1 in 27,000 (10 to 0.37 per 10,000) in old reports (Bluestone et al., 1975; Avery and Harris, 1976). The anesthesia-related mortality unadjusted for age is reported to be 1 in 14,000 (Avery and Harris, 1976). A more recent survey in Europe shows the posttonsillectomy mortality rates of 0.62 to 0.63 per 10,000 (Windfuhr et al., 2009). Windfuhr and colleagues (2008a, 2008b) also reported life-threatening posttonsillectomy hemorrhage in 79 patients between 1980 and 2006. There were 36 children involved in the study. Out of

29 deaths, 18 were children. Nearly 90% of the life-threatening crises were related to secondary hemorrhage (>24 hours), and all deaths were directly or indirectly attributable to posttonsillectomy hemorrhage.

Peritonsillar Abscess

Peritonsillar cellulitis and abscesses occur more frequently in older children and adults than in young children. Most infections appear to originate in the tonsils and spread to the peritonsillar space between the tonsillar capsule and the superior constrictor muscle. The infection may spread upward into the palate, but it usually does not invade the posterior tonsillar pillar or the posterior pharyngeal wall (Teele, 1983). The patient presents with complaints of severe sore throat, difficulty in swallowing, and high fever. Progressive difficulty in opening the mouth may develop because of spasm of the pterygoid muscles. It is therefore imperative to determine the extent of limitation of mouth opening preoperatively. The affected tonsillar area is markedly inflamed and swollen, and the uvula is displaced to the opposite side (Cook, 1982). In older children and adolescents, it is possible to perform incision and drainage of a peritonsillar abscess with intravenous sedation using an opioid and topical or local anesthesia, with the patient in a head-down position and the head turned to the side of the abscess. If this is not possible, general endotracheal anesthesia is necessary.

The child should be well sedated. Anesthesia is induced with oxygen, nitrous oxide, and sevoflurane by mask or with intravenous sodium thiopental or propofol. Anesthesia is deepened in oxygen without nitrous oxide, while spontaneous breathing is maintained and assisted with a head-down tilt and with the head turned toward the affected side. Under deep inhalational anesthesia, the larynx is exposed carefully with the laryngoscope blade for intubation with a cuffed endotracheal tube. It is advantageous to let the patient breathe spontaneously to maintain the upper airway muscle tone and airway patency. Muscle relaxants should not be given until the anesthesiologist is certain that the airway can be maintained by mask and bag. Two large-bore suction catheters and tonsil suction tips should be on hand in case the abscess ruptures during the process of laryngoscopy and intubation.

Use of the Laryngeal Mask Airway During Adenotonsillectomy

Since the early 1990s, several reports (but no scientific studies) have described the use of the armored LMA rather than an endotracheal tube for airway support during tonsil or adenoid surgery. The armored LMA can be held within the Boyle-Davis gag and remain patent (Alexander, 1990) (Fig. 24-6). A reported benefit of using the LMA is avoiding tracheal intubation and its associated complications (trauma, cardiovascular stimulation, endobronchial intubation, coughing, laryngospasm, and subglottic edema) (Hatcher and Stack, 1999). The disadvantages of the armored LMA include the risk for aspiration of stomach contents and the risk of inadequate positioning (Hatcher and Stack, 1999).

Hern and coworkers (1999) reported the surgeon's perspective on the use of LMA for tonsillectomy. In their study, 44 children were anesthetized using an LMA, and 47 patients were anesthetized using an endotracheal tube before tonsillectomy. There was an 11.4% failure rate for the LMA, requiring

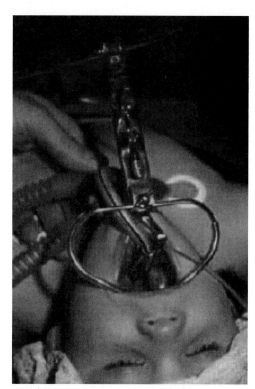

■ **FIGURE 24-6.** Armored laryngeal mask airway used for adenotonsillectomy in a child. *(From Kretz FJ, Reimann B, Stelzner J, et al: The laryngeal mask in pediatric adenotonsillectomy: a meta-analysis of medical studies [in German]. Anaesthesist 49:706, 2000. With permission of Springer Science and Business Media.)*

change to an endotracheal tube before the end of the procedure. The LMA was reported to hamper the surgeon's visualization of the field and might have led to removal of less tonsillar tissue in the LMA group. It is difficult to suggest that the LMA is a superior choice for airway management during tonsillectomy. Additional objective data must be accumulated before recommending this technique.

Laser Surgery of the Larynx

The laser (light amplification by stimulated emission of radiation) has been used increasingly in otolaryngology since the introduction of the CO_2 laser for laryngeal surgery (Strong et al., 1973). The laser is a beam of coherent electromagnetic radiation that can be focused to a very small spot with precision, resulting in controlled coagulation, incision, or vaporization of the target tissue without affecting the neighboring tissues (Geffin et al., 1986; Keon, 1988). Clinical uses of the laser for upper and lower airways and its anesthetic implications have been reviewed elsewhere (Beamis et al., 1991; Rampil, 1992; Pashayan, 1994).

The principal components of a laser system include a lasing medium (gaseous or solid) that holds the molecules whose electrons create the laser light, resonating mirrors to boost lasing efficiency, and an energy source that pumps the lasing molecules into producing laser light (Rampil, 1992) (Fig. 24-7). Some lasers use a gaseous lasing media, such as CO_2, argon, or helium-neon, whereas others use solid rods of laser-passive material that contain small quantities of ionic impurities, such

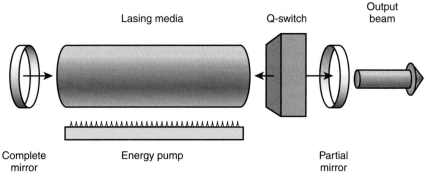

■ **FIGURE 24-7.** The central component is the lasing medium itself. This may be, for example, a solid crystal of yttrium-aluminum-garnet (YAG) with a small concentration of neodymium (Nd), or a tube containing carbon dioxide. The energy pump provides the means of obtaining a population inversion of orbital electrons. It may consist of a xenon flash lamp or an electric spark generator. A pair of axial mirrors allows separated passes of collimated photons through the media, enabling maximal amplification by stimulated emission. The mirror on the right is not 100% reflective, allowing the beam to escape eventually. The optional Q-switch increases efficiency of pulsed lasers by allowing a small delay to increase the pumping. *(Adapted from Rampil IJ: Anesthetic considerations for laser surgery,* Anesth Analg *74:424, 1992.)*

as chromium (for ruby laser) and neodymium (Nd). A synthetic gem crystal, yttrium-aluminum-garnet (YAG), is commonly used as a passive host matrix (Rampil, 1992). Fiberoptic bundles are used for beam delivery of lasers of visible and near-infrared wavelengths. For the CO_2 laser with invisible far-infrared wavelength, the most common delivery system is an articulated arm containing front-surface mirrors at each junction, which is used together with a low-powered visible helium-neon gas laser beam through the same optical path as a beam guide (Rampil, 1992; Pashayan, 1994). Recently, a flexible, hollow waveguide for delivery of the CO_2 has become available. Physical characteristics of commonly used lasers are described in Table 24-5.

The most commonly used laser for laryngeal surgery is the CO_2 laser. This has a long, far-infrared wavelength and is completely absorbed by the bending frequency of the water molecules; it is absorbed completely in the first few layers of cells and produces very little scatter of energy. The powerful, focused CO_2 laser beam therefore produces explosive vaporization of the target tissue surface with minimal damage to the underlying tissues (Beamis et al., 1991; Rampil, 1992). The thermal effect (i.e., coagulation lateral to the zone of vaporization) can be varied between 80 and 400 mcm and is diminished with increasing water content or vascularity of the tissue or by the use of less power. Thermal coagulation also decreases with shorter pulse duration. The CO_2 laser beam is delivered to the target tissue by means of an articulated arm and a micromanipulator attached

to the microscope or a bronchoscope coupler for tracheobronchial applications (Werkhaven, 1995). The micromanipulator allows surgical precision on the order of 250 mcm.

The potassium (kalium) titanyl phosphate (KTP) laser and argon laser operate in the green and blue-green wavelength range of the spectrum. The KTP and argon laser beams are transmitted through clear substances and are well absorbed by pigments in the tissues, especially melanin and hemoglobin. They therefore have widespread application for certain lesions, such as hemangiomas and granulation tissue (Werkhaven, 1995). The energy scatter is intermediate between the CO_2 and Nd:YAG laser beams. Because the depth of thermal damage produced by a laser beam beyond the immediate vaporization site partially depends on scatter, it produces vaporization (but less than that of the CO_2 laser) in addition to coagulation and cutting (Beamis et al., 1991). The depth of tissue penetration is 0.5 to 2 mm (Pashayan, 1994). KTP and argon laser beams, as well as the Nd:YAG beam, can be transmitted by means of fiberoptic bundles through the rigid or flexible bronchoscope to vaporize or coagulate lesions in the tracheobronchial lumen (Geffin et al., 1986; Ward, 1992).

The Nd:YAG laser has a near-infrared wavelength, is transmitted through clear fluids, and is readily absorbed by proteins. It is absorbed much less by water, and the beam is transmitted and scattered through much larger volumes of tissue. The energy of the Nd:YAG laser beam is therefore widely disseminated and produces less vaporization and more thermal coagulation. The depth of tissue penetration may range from 2 to 6 mm (Pashayan, 1994). The Nd:YAG laser is transmitted by means of flexible optic fibers that can be directed through the side suction port of ventilating bronchoscope. The ablation of granulation tissue, mixed capillary-cavernous hemangioma, or obstructive vascular tumor in the tracheobronchial wall may be accomplished successfully with the Nd:YAG laser (Werkhaven, 1995).

Risks Associated with Laser Surgery

Because of the potential danger with the use of laser beams in the operating room, the users and other operating room personnel should follow the safety guidelines established by the American National Standard for the Safe Use of Laser in Health

TABLE 24-5. Lasers Commonly Used for Airway Surgery

Laser Medium	Color	Wavelength (nm)	Tissue Penetration (mm)
CO_2	Far infrared	10,600	<0.25
Nd:YAG	Near infrared	1064	2 to 6
KTP	Green	532	0.5 to 2
Argon	Blue/green	488/515	0.5 to 2

Data from Rampil IJ: Anesth Analg 74:424, 1992; and Pashayan AG: Anesthesia for laser surgery, Annual Refresher Courses, No. 221, 1994, ASA.
KTP, Potassium (kalium) titanyl phosphate; *Nd:YAG,* neodymium–yttrium-aluminum-garnet.

Care Facilities and published by the American National Standard Institute (the ANSI Z136 Standard) (ANSI, New York). Doors to operating rooms where laser surgery is in progress should be clearly marked to prevent unprotected personnel from accidentally straying into the path of laser beams. Warning signs should specify the class and type of the laser being used as well as appropriate protective measures specific for the wavelength (Rampil, 1992; Pashayan, 1994).

All laser beams for medical use are transmitted through air and are well reflected by smooth metal surfaces. Patients and health care personnel involved in laser surgery are at risk for laser injury, particularly of the eyes. The nature and extent of eye injury depend on the wavelength of the laser beam and its energy. Because the laser beam of far-infrared wavelength is absorbed by the surface it first encounters, errant CO_2 laser beams can cause serious corneal ulcerations and scar formation (Liebowitz and Peacock, 1980). Visible and near-infrared lasers (e.g., KTP, argon, Nd:YAG) penetrate through the transparent cornea and anterior chamber of the eye, are absorbed by the retina, and cause serious damage. The anesthetized patient's eyes should be taped closed and covered with saline-soaked eye pads or metal shields, or both (Keon, 1988). Operating room personnel must wear safety goggles that are specific for the laser wavelength in use. Safety goggles should provide wraparound protection from reflected beams (Rampil, 1992). For CO_2 lasers, any plastic or regular eyeglasses (not contact lenses or thin plastic splash protection shields) will suffice as protection (provided that lateral aspects of the eye are also covered), because far-infrared beams are completely absorbed. Visible and near-infrared lasers require specific filters for particular laser wavelengths.

Incandescent debris resulting from the explosive vaporization of the tissue in contact with the laser beam produces a plume of smoke with fine particulates (0.1 to 0.8 mcm), which may contain infectious or mutagenic viral particles (Nezhat et al., 1987; Kokosa and Eugene, 1989). Fragments of DNA have been found in the smoke plume, but only one study has found viral transmission from the laser plume (Garden et al., 2002). The same risk exists for the smoke plume from electrocautery. Ordinary surgical masks do not effectively filter particles smaller than 3.0 mcm; special high-efficiency masks are therefore needed to filter laser plume particles (Rampil, 1992).

A laser beam can ignite inflammable materials used for general anesthesia, such as endotracheal tubes, anesthesia circuits, oil-based lubricants, ointments, sponges, and drapes (Snow et al., 1976; Cozine et al., 1981; Hermens et al., 1983). All materials used for endotracheal tubes, with the exception of special metallic tubes, are quite vulnerable to laser impact (Geffin et al., 1986; Sosis, 1989a, 1989b). Polyvinyl chloride (PVC) tubes appear to be more easily punctured and ignited by CO_2 laser than red-rubber tubes, and to produce more toxic combustion fumes (Ossof et al., 1983), although black smoke from burning rubber is probably just as damaging to the airway mucosa. Wolf and Simpson (1987) found that once PVC is ignited, it is less flammable than silicone or red rubber, with a flammability index (i.e., the fraction of inspired oxygen [Fio_2] at which the material ignites) of 0.26, compared with silicone (0.19) and red rubber (0.18); this means that silicone and rubber tubes continue to burn in room air, whereas PVC tubes do not. Red-rubber tubes, however, are more resistant to puncture than PVC tubes (41 versus 0.8 seconds with PVC, at the same power density) and intramural fires are less likely to occur (Ossof, 1989). For these reasons, metal tubes are preferred overall.

During laser surgery, when a nonmetallic endotracheal tube is used, the Fio_2 should be reduced to 30% or less, as long as the patient is adequately oxygenated, to reduce combustibility of endotracheal tubes (Hermens et al., 1983). Oxygen may be diluted by nitrogen or helium to reduce the flammability of endotracheal tubes (Pashayan and Gravenstein, 1985; Simpson et al., 1990). Oxygen concentrations up to 60% may be used if helium is the diluent gas. Nitrous oxide supports combustion above 450° C and should therefore be avoided (Wolf and Simpson, 1987; Keon, 1988). It is imperative that the patient be immobilized during laser surgery. The choice of anesthetics depends largely on the technique of ventilation during the laser surgery.

Airway Fire

An airway fire is potentially the worst complication to occur with the use of the laser. Although uncommon, the risk should be appreciated by the anesthesiologist and surgeon, and appropriate responses should be planned before the procedure. Airway fires also have been reported with the use of electrocautery for tonsillectomy and tracheotomy.

Although fires can occur in the operating room environment if the laser accidentally contacts flammable material, airway fires may occur only if flammable materials are present in the airway. Materials such as endotracheal tubes or cottonoid pledgets in the airway are the most common sources of combustion. In the absence of flammable materials, an airway fire cannot be sustained. Although the use of the laser on tissue may generate combustible breakdown products such as methane, the amounts are too small to produce enough heat to self-generate other combustible products. As noted, the concentration of oxygen should be kept as low as possible in the presence of combustible materials.

In the unfortunate event of an airway fire, a mnemonic of the 4 Es—extract, eliminate, extinguish, and evaluate (Box 24-6)—may help guide management. In the event of an airway fire, immediately extract all combustible materials from the airway such as pledgets or endotracheal tubes, even if they are still burning. Second, eliminate the source of oxygen being delivered to the endotracheal tube. The continued delivery of oxygen to a combustible source produces a blowtorch effect that can further ignite material in the vicinity. Third, extinguish any other fires in the vicinity. If a combustible material such as a pledget is still in the airway and cannot be removed, saline flush should be used to extinguish the fire. Fourth, evaluate any damage that may have been caused by the fire or the combustion byproducts. The operative field needs to be examined along with the lower tracheobronchial tree. Standards and guidelines for the management of surgical fires, including airway fires, have been published (A Clinician's Guide to Surgical Fires, 2003).

Box 24-6   Airway Fire—the Four Es

- Extract
- Eliminate
- Extinguish
- Evaluate

Ventilatory Management During Laser Surgery

Numerous anesthetic approaches have been reported for airway management during laryngeal laser surgery. General transtracheal anesthesia, through a preexisting tracheostomy, is the easiest and probably the safest method. It is performed by replacing the preexisting tracheostomy cannula with a metal tracheostomy tube. Manually operated intermittent jet ventilation (Rontal et al., 1980; Scamman and McCabe, 1986; Ravussin et al., 1987) or high-frequency jet ventilation (Smith et al., 1975) by means of a needle or a catheter through the cricothyroid membrane has been used. These techniques, however, have a potential risk for barotrauma to the upper airways and overdistention of lungs (e.g., pneumothorax, pneumomediastinum), particularly when the laryngeal airway is obstructed. Subcutaneous emphysema and pneumomediastinum also may occur because of needle misplacement or a direct leak at the tracheal puncture site (Borland and Reilly, 1987). Without tracheostomy or transtracheal puncture, the maintenance of airways and pulmonary ventilation during laser surgery can be accomplished by means of manual jet ventilation (i.e., Saunder's jet) without an endotracheal tube. A combination of intravenous propofol, topical lidocaine, and small dosages of opioids (i.e., fentanyl or remifentanil infusion) has been used successfully with the patient breathing spontaneously (Borland LM, unpublished data).

Nonflammable Endotracheal Tubes

Red-rubber tubes wrapped with reflective aluminum or copper adhesive-backed tape, originally described by Snow and colleagues (1974), have been used effectively (Norton et al., 1976), but the use of these homemade, laser-resistive tubes has decreased considerably over the past decade with the advent of commercially available nonflammable endotracheal tubes. Before wrapping a red-rubber tube with a metal tape, the tube should be wiped with alcohol to remove greasy or oily residues that interfere with adhesion. It should also be wiped with tincture of benzoin or an equivalent before spiral wrapping with a metal tape (Rampil, 1992). There should be no windows of exposed tube; care should be taken to prevent wrinkles, which may cause abrasion of the laryngotracheal mucosa.

Certain metallic tapes do not sufficiently prevent the CO_2, Nd:YAG, or KTP laser beams from penetrating the endotracheal tube and igniting a blowtorch fire. The CO_2 laser can ignite the adhesive backing of all these tapes and perforate the aluminum tapes within 0.1 second (Sosis, 1989a). Other aluminum tapes (3M No. 425 and 433; 3M Corp., St. Paul, MN) and a copper foil tape (Venture Tape Corp., Rockland, MA; 3M Corp.) are effective in shielding at least 60 seconds of direct exposure (Sosis and Dillon, 1990). A metallic foil wrap for endotracheal tubes, specifically manufactured for the laser, is also available (Laser Guard, Merocel Corp., Mystic, CT) and is approved by the U.S. Food and Drug Administration. This metal-based surgical sponge provides protection against CO_2, argon, and KTP lasers but not against Nd:YAG lasers, according to the study by the Emergency Care Research Institute (ECRI, 1990). It also provides a smoother surface than metal tapes on the endotracheal tube for better airway mucosal protection, but it is bulky, adding about 2 mm to the diameter of the endotracheal tube.

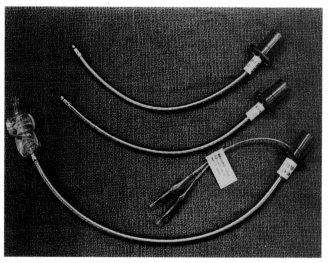

■ **FIGURE 24-8.** Flexible stainless steel (Laser Flex) tubes. *Top to bottom:* A 3.5-mm-ID, uncuffed tube; a 4.0-mm-ID, uncuffed tube; and a 5.0-mm, double-cuffed tube. ID, inner diameter. *(Courtesy Mallinckrodt Medical, Inc., St Louis, MO.)*

A number of laser-resistant endotracheal tubes with metal exteriors have become available for clinical use. The Laser Flex tube (Mallinckrodt, St. Louis, MO; Bivona, Gary, IN) is a stainless steel spiral with a PVC tip, with or without two distal saline-inflatable cuffs (Fig. 24-8). This tube is resistant to CO_2 and the Nd:YAG laser. The Fome Cuff tube (Bivona) is an aluminum spiral tube with an outer coating of silicone that is approved by the manufacturer for the CO_2 laser only. This tube has a self-inflating foam sponge–filled cuff. The foam in the cuff prevents deflation of the cuff after puncture, but damage to the filling tube may cause difficulty in deflating the cuff (Rampil, 1992). The Laser Shield II (Medtronic/Xomed, Jacksonville, FL) is silicon-based endotracheal tube wrapped with metal foil and then wrapped in polytetrafluoroethylene tape to smooth the tube. These tubes are available only in two sizes, and the smaller size (5.0) has an outside diameter with a cuff roughly equivalent to a size 5.5 endotracheal tube.

Anesthesia with Nonflammable Endotracheal Tubes

For laser resections of laryngeal papillomas in a child, anesthesia may be induced by mask with nitrous oxide and sevoflurane with the standard monitors, including a precordial stethoscope, pulse oximeter, capnography, electrocardiography, blood pressure cuff, and nerve stimulator. After intravenous access is secured and an intermediate-acting muscle relaxant is given, the child is intubated with a laser-resistant endotracheal tube. Nitrous oxide is then replaced with air or a helium-oxygen mixture (i.e., heliox). Anesthesia is maintained with a volatile anesthetic or propofol infusion with nitrogen and oxygen, and inspired oxygen concentration is kept at 30% or less as long as oxygen saturation can be maintained at or above 98%. The patient's eyes are taped closed and then covered with saline-soaked gauze pads; the portion of the endotracheal tube not metal coated is also covered with saline-soaked towels to avoid the fire hazard of the laser beam while a Jako-type suspension laryngoscope is being positioned. The child is paralyzed, and ventilation is controlled manually or mechanically with a ventilator. Supplemental opioids may be added intravenously to

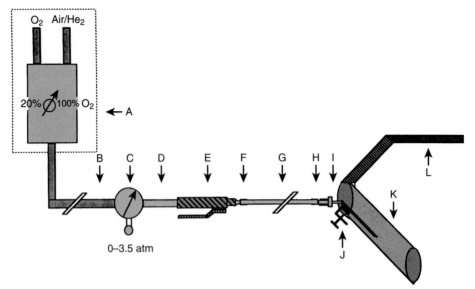

FIGURE 24-9. The Venturi ventilation apparatus with injector needle-on-clamp. *A,* High-pressure gas source with optional oxygen–nitrous oxide or helium blender. *B,* High-pressure tubing. *C,* Reducing valve and pressure gauge. *D,* Short piece of high-pressure tubing. *E,* Manual, all-or-none trigger valve. *F,* Tapered metal connector of the pop-off type. *G,* Low-pressure plastic tubing. *H,* Optional Luer-Loc fitting on tapered metal connector of the pop-off type. *I,* An adapted, curved stainless steel needle, 12 to 18 gauge. *J,* Screw clamp to fit on the edge of the operating laryngoscope. *K,* The operating laryngoscope. *L,* Laryngoscope handle that fits the suspension apparatus. It should be possible for fittings *F* and *H* to pop off when high pressure is inadvertently transmitted through the low-pressure tubing (i.e., when *C* or *E,* or both, are failing) or when an obstruction occurs distally. *(Adapted from Van Der Spek AF, Spargo PM, Norton ML: The physics of lasers and implications for their use during airway surgery,* Br J Anaesth *60:709, 1988.)*

reduce the need for the inhaled anesthetic. Dexamethasone (0.4 mg to 1 mg/kg) may be used prophylactically to minimize postoperative mucosal swelling.

Anesthesia with Manual Jet Ventilation

A more commonly accepted and practiced method for ventilation during laryngeal laser surgery is the use of a Venturi apparatus (i.e., Saunders' jet injector), originally described by Saunders (1967) and Spoerel and coworkers (Donlon and Benumof (1996) and applied in pediatric patients by Miyasaka and colleagues (1980) as well as others (Johans and Reichert, 1984; Scamman and McCabe, 1986; Borland and Reilly, 1987). The apparatus consists of an injector and tubing, a toggle switch, a reducing valve or regulator, and tubing with a connector to a high-pressure wall oxygen supply (50 psi) (Figs. 24-9 and 24-10). After a precordial stethoscope, a pulse oximeter sensor, electrocardiogram leads, and a blood pressure cuff are positioned on the child, and anesthesia is induced, usually by mask with nitrous oxide, sevoflurane, and oxygen. An intravenous catheter is inserted, an axillary or rectal temperature probe is placed, and a nerve stimulator is positioned. Cisatracurium (or other intermediate-acting muscle relaxant), fentanyl (2 to 3 mcg/kg), and lidocaine (1 mg/kg) are injected intravenously. Midazolam may be given to ensure amnesia during the laser surgery. Alternatively, anesthesia may be switched to intravenous propofol with or without a small dosage of fentanyl. Nitrous oxide is discontinued, and the patient is ventilated with 100% oxygen for several minutes before the mask is removed. The surgeon positions the child's head and inserts a Jako suspension laryngoscope to secure a patent laryngeal airway.

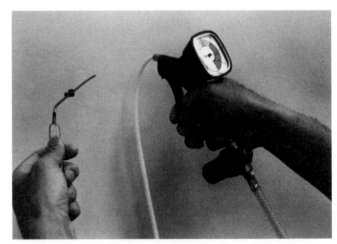

FIGURE 24-10. A Saunders-type, hand-held jet ventilation apparatus. *(Courtesy Manujet III, VBM Medizintechnik, Sulz am Neckar, Germany.)*

In children, supraglottic jet ventilation is used. Subglottic jet ventilation is rarely used in children, because it requires extremely delicate skills to access adequate egress of air between pulses, and if this is not accomplished, pneumothorax or pneumomediastinum results (Hunsaker, 1994).

For supraglottic ventilation, a 10-French metal injector is inserted into the side channel of the suspension laryngoscope and secured with the distal end 1 to 2 cm above the glottic opening; the metal injector is readjusted as needed to obtain the optimal distance and direction. Oxygen concentration of the jet injector is adjusted with an oxygen blender to reduce the inspired oxygen concentration with room air entrainment to 30% or less, provided that oxygen saturation on the pulse oximeter is 98% or higher. The anesthesiologist begins jet ventilation by intermittently squeezing the toggle switch. Short bursts of inspiration with air entrainment (1 to 2 seconds) with a driving pressure of 15 psi or less (the pressure may vary with different setups), followed by enough expiration time (2 to 4 seconds) to complete exhalation, provides adequate pulmonary ventilation. Close observation of the child's chest motion during each breath is crucial to prevent air trapping, hyperinflation, and volutrauma to the lungs (Borland and Reilly, 1987). Inspired oxygen concentration is decreased as low as possible by adjusting the oxygen-blender to maintain SpO_2 between 98% and 100% throughout the procedure. If passive exhalation is unusually prolonged, measures to improve airway patency must be taken immediately. This can usually be accomplished by readjusting or redirecting the injector. Occasionally, when papillomatous growth about the glottis is extensive, the child may require intubation with a small tube and manual ventilation while the surgeon improves the glottic aperture by debulking papillomas on and around the vocal cords.

After the laryngeal surgery is completed, ventilation is maintained with 2:1 or 1:1 ratio of oxygen and air by mask and bag, or the airway is secured by intubation with a small cuffed or uncuffed orotracheal tube. Neuromuscular blockade is reversed in the usual manner. The endotracheal tube is removed after neuromuscular blockade is completely reversed and the child is breathing satisfactorily.

The manual jet ventilation technique offers several advantages in laryngeal laser surgery, including adequate ventilation, excellent surgical access to the larynx (especially to the anterior and posterior commissures where an endotracheal tube obliterates the exposure), and the absence of ignitable material in the surgical field (Norton et al., 1976; Goforth et al., 1983). Potential risks of this technique include pneumothorax, pneumomediastinum, distention of the stomach and regurgitation, aspiration of resected material, and dehydration of mucosal surface (Lines, 1973; Norton et al., 1976; Rontal et al., 1980; Ruder et al., 1981; Keon, 1988).

Anesthesia with Spontaneous Breathing

Anesthesia for airway laser surgery can be managed by experts with a combination of carefully administered intravenous anesthesia and topical lidocaine. Anesthesia may be induced with inhalation of sevoflurane with a nitrous oxide–oxygen mixture while the patient is allowed to breathe spontaneously. After an intravenous catheter is inserted and the patient positioned with a suspension laryngoscope, topical lidocaine is sprayed under the direct vision. Inhaled anesthetics are turned off and an infusion of propofol is started. During laser surgery, high-dosage propofol (300 to 400 mcg/kg per minute) is supplemented with intermittent doses of morphine (up to 0.1 mg/kg) or an infusion of fentanyl (2 to 3 mcg/kg per hour) to prevent tachypnea. The concentration of oxygen insufflations should be limited to less than 30% for safety, while the patient's breathing is continuously monitored with a precordial stethoscope, and oxygen saturation is monitored with a pulse oximeter. A manual jet ventilator (Sanders) should be readily available for supraglottic jet ventilation as needed if the patient's breathing is too depressed or he or she becomes apneic. Alternatively, total intravenous anesthesia

may be administered with a combination of remifentanil and propofol infusions. This combination appears to make spontaneous breathing more difficult to maintain.

Laser Bronchoscopy

The laser may be used coupled with a ventilating bronchoscope. If the CO_2 laser is used with the rigid ventilating laser bronchoscope, higher oxygen concentrations can be employed, because there is no flammable material in the airway. The fibers used for KTP and Nd:YAG laser delivery may support combustion, and when used through a bronchoscope, the inspired oxygen concentration should be less than 40%. The newer CO_2 laser waveguide has not been tested for combustibility, so prudence suggests limiting the inspired oxygen concentration to less than 40%.

Tracheostomy

Tracheostomy is indicated in numerous situations before development of respiratory distress (Stool and Eavey, 1990). The three primary indications for the creation of an artificial airway are airway obstruction, chronic assisted ventilation, and pulmonary toilet (Wetmore et al., 1999; Carron et al., 2000). Table 24-6 lists the conditions for which tracheotomy has been advocated in pediatric patients (Wetmore, 2003).

The ideal tracheotomy tube conforms to the trachea and neck without causing undue pressure or injury to the skin or tracheal mucosa. Plastic tracheotomy tubes are commonly used because they cause minimal tissue reaction. Tracheotomy tubes should be manufactured in metric sizes that correspond to endotracheal tube sizes. However, metal tracheotomy tubes are still measured in French sizes (Wetmore, 2003). Table 24-7 compares the sizes of the endotracheal tubes and commonly used tracheotomy tubes in infants and children (Wetmore, 2003).

Anesthetic Approach for Tracheostomy

The need for tracheotomy may occur emergently, urgently, or electively. It is essential for the surgeon and anesthesiologist to establish a plan before surgery. Some situations, including laryngeal trauma, massive facial injuries, upper airway obstruction, and oropharyngeal distortion, require emergency tracheostomy for airway management. This procedure is usually performed outside the operating room and, fortunately, rarely in the pediatric population.

Urgent tracheotomy may be required in neonates for congenital airway defects and for older children because of upper airway trauma, corrosive ingestion, infections, and tumors (see Table 24-6). Although these children may initially maintain oxygenation and ventilation, they are at risk for acute respiratory failure. They may have airway anomalies that contribute to difficult or impossible tracheal intubation. The location of the obstruction dictates the surgical and anesthetic approach. The anesthesiologist must establish whether the child can maintain a patent airway under anesthesia and whether they can be intubated by standard laryngoscopy or fiberoptic bronchoscopy. Sedation with ketamine may also be an option. Otherwise, anesthesia is induced with an inhaled anesthetic agent after preoxygenation in the position in which the child is most comfortable, often

TABLE 24-6. Conditions for Which Tracheotomy Has Been Advocated

	Allergic	Metabolic	Prophylactic	Degenerative or Idiopathic	Sleep Disorders
Upper airway obstruction	Angioneurotic edema Anaphylaxis	—	Head and neck surgery Neurosurgery Cardiac surgery Prolonged endotracheal tube placement	Vocal cord paralysis	Pharyngeal musculature collapse Tonsilloadenoid hypertrophy
Pulmonary toilet, assisted ventilation	Asthma	Cystic fibrosis Coma due to diabetes, Reye's syndrome, uremia, etc. Respiratory distress syndrome	—	Central nervous system or neuromuscular failure, as in Guillain-Barré syndrome, polymyositis, myasthenia gravis, botulism, cardiac arrest, respiratory arrest	—
	Congenital	Traumatic	Toxic	Infectious	Neoplastic
Upper airway obstruction	Choanal atresia Macroglossia Cleft palate Pierre Robin syndrome Laryngomalacia Laryngeal stenosis Vocal cord paralysis Laryngeal webs, cysts Subglottic stenosis Vascular ring Tracheal hypoplasia	Facial injury Oral injury Foreign body Burns (steam, smoke, thermal) Laryngeal edema Recurrent laryngeal nerve injury Laryngeal fracture	Corrosives	Epiglottitis Laryngotracheitis (croup) Gingivostomatitis Diphtheria Retropharyngeal abscess Ludwig's angina Neck cellulitis Tetanus Rabies Plague	Laryngeal tumors Tracheal tumors Tumors of pharynx and tongue: papilloma, hemangioma, lymphangioma, sarcoma
Pulmonary toilet, assisted ventilation	Congenital heart disease Congenital heart failure Esophageal atresia due to tracheoesophageal fistula Hypoplastic lung due to diaphragmatic hernia Adjunct to craniofacial surgery	Head trauma Crushed chest Shock lung Intrapulmonary hemorrhage Pneumothorax After lung bypass	Coma due to toxins (e.g., phenobarbital) Hydrocarbon lung Aspiration syndromes (e.g., from meconium)	Meningitis Encephalitis Brain abscess Pneumonia Bronchiolitis Poliomyelitis Pulmonary aspiration necessitating laryngeal closure	Brain tumors Spinal cord tumors

From Werkhaven J: Laser surgery. In Bluestone CD, Stool SE, Alper CM, et al, editors: *Pediatric otolaryngology*, ed 4, Philadelphia, 2003, Saunders, p 1573.

the sitting position. If no intravenous catheter is in place, one is inserted, and atropine (0.01 to 0.02 mg/kg) or glycopyrrolate (0.01 mg/kg) may be injected intravenously as indicated after induction of anesthesia. Unless a normal, unobstructed airway can be maintained, muscle relaxants should not be used because total upper airway obstruction may result. After the child is anesthetized but spontaneously breathing, topical lidocaine (up to 5 mg/kg) may be sprayed on the larynx to ablate laryngeal reflexes before laryngoscopy. If intubation is impossible, an LMA may be used to maintain an airway until the tracheotomy is performed. Tracheostomy is best performed in infants with an endotracheal tube or a rigid bronchoscope in place to ensure adequate pulmonary gas exchange. The endotracheal tube also helps the surgeon to identify the trachea. Many surgeons prefer to use a rigid bronchoscope held in place rather than an endotracheal tube. The rigid bronchoscope allows a firmer anatomic reference for the trachea, but it cannot be taped in place and must be held by hand. Elective tracheotomy is usually performed in children already intubated for chronic ventilation or pulmonary toilet or performed in combination with tumor removal or repair of tracheal abnormalities.

For tracheotomy, the patient is positioned with the shoulders elevated by placing a roll under the neck so that the neck is hyperextended. Some surgeons request that the anesthesiologist hold the chin with the left hand to keep the neck stretched so that soft tissue over the trachea is stabilized (Fig. 24-11) (Stool and Eavey, 1990). The surgeon palpates the neck to identify the thyroid and cricoid cartilages, sometimes with difficulty. The trachea is palpated down to the sternal notch, guided by the presence of an endotracheal tube. A skin incision is made about one fingerbreadth above the sternal notch, either horizontally or vertically. When the fascial layer is incised under the subcutaneous fat and the trachea is identified, a pair of stay sutures, one on each side of the tracheal incision, is placed for traction during the cannulation of the tracheotomy tube. The stay sutures also serve to prevent asphyxiation in the event that the tracheotomy tube becomes displaced in the immediate postoperative period before the tract has formed (Myers et al., 1985). Before the tracheotomy cannula is inserted in the tracheal incision, the endotracheal tube or bronchoscope is slowly pulled back to accommodate the insertion. The endotracheal tube or bronchoscope should not be removed completely until successful

TABLE 24-7. Size Comparisons of Endotracheal and Plastic Tracheostomy Tubes

Cannula	Approx French	Inner Diameter (mm)	Outer Diameter (mm)	Overall Length	Cannula	Approx French	Inner Diameter (mm)	Outer Diameter (mm)	Overall Length
Endotracheal Tube*					4.5	—	4.5	6.7	48 mm
2.5	—	2.5	3.6	12 cm	5.0	—	5.0	8.0	51 mm
3.0	—	3.0	4.3	14 cm	5.5	—	5.5	8.5	54 mm
3.5	—	3.5	4.9	16 cm	6.0	—	6.0	9.3	57 mm
4.0	—	4.0	5.6	18 cm	**Portex**				
4.5	—	4.5	6.2	20 cm	3.0	—	3.0	5.0	36 mm
5.0	—	5.0	6.9	22 cm	3.5	—	3.5	5.8	40 mm
5.5	—	5.5	7.5	25 cm	4.0	—	4.0	6.5	44 mm
6.0	—	6.0	8.2	26 cm	4.5	—	4.5	7.1	48 mm
Bivona†					5.0	—	5.0	7.7	50 mm
2.5	12	2.5	4.0	30 mm	5.5	—	5.5	8.3	52 mm
2.5	12	2.5	4.0	38 mm	**Shiley§**				
3.0	14	3.0	4.7	32 mm	00 Neonatal	—	3.1	4.5	30 mm
3.0	14	3.0	4.7	39 mm	00 Pediatric	—	3.1	4.5	39 mm
3.5	16	3.5	5.3	34 mm	0 Neonatal	—	3.4	5.0	32 mm
3.5	16	3.5	5.3	40 mm	0 Pediatric	—	3.4	5.0	40 mm
4.0	18	4.0	6.0	36 mm	1 Neonatal	—	3.7	5.5	34 mm
4.0	18	4.0	6.0	41 mm	1 Pediatric	—	3.7	5.5	41 mm
4.5	20	4.5	6.7	42 mm	2 Pediatric	—	4.1	6.0	42 mm
5.0	22	5.0	7.3	44 mm	3 Pediatric	—	4.8	7.0	44 mm
5.5	24	5.5	8.0	46 mm	4 Pediatric	—	5.5	8.0	46 mm
Franklin‡									
3.5	—	3.5	5.0	44 mm					
4.0	—	4.0	6.0	44 mm					

From Werkhaven J: Laser surgery. In Bluestone CD, Stool SE, Alper CM, et al., editors: *Pediatric otolaryngology,* ed 4, Philadelphia, 2003, Saunders, p 1573.
*The endotracheal tubes are marked with the inner diameter, usually with the outer diameter, and with the length.
†The Bivona tube is manufactured by the Bivona Corporation of Gray, IN. Both the inner and outer diameters are marked on the tubes.
‡The Franklin tube is of the Great Ormond Street design, manufactured in England and distributed by Inmed Corporation, Norcross, GA. The tubes are stamped with just the inner diameter.
§The Shiley tube is manufactured by Shiley Laboratories, Irvine, CA. The tubes are stamped with the size and inner and outer diameters.

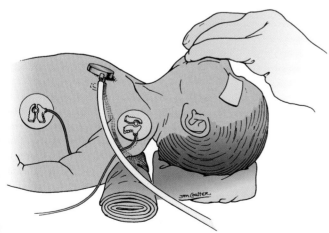

■ **FIGURE 24-11.** A child positioned for tracheostomy with the shoulders elevated, the neck hyperextended, and the chin pulled up by hand.

ventilation is demonstrated after placement of the tracheotomy tube. The anesthesia delivery tube is then disconnected from the endotracheal tube under the drapes and reconnected to the proximal universal adapter end of the tracheotomy tube over the operative field.

An esophageal stethoscope or a nasogastric tube has occasionally been misidentified as an endotracheal tube in the trachea by the surgeon, and inadvertent esophageal incision has been made (Schwartz and Downes, 1977); esophageal stethoscopes therefore should be avoided during tracheotomy. The child is monitored with a precordial stethoscope, pulse oximeter, capnography, electrocardiography, automated blood pressure cuff, and rectal or skin thermometer.

Major intraoperative and postoperative complications of tracheotomy include hemorrhage, subcutaneous emphysema, pneumothorax, and pneumomediastinum. The neck and shoulders of the child should be palpated for the typical crepitus to rule out subcutaneous emphysema. Then both sides of the chest are auscultated. In most hospitals, the patient is transferred to the ICU for observation and a chest radiograph to ensure proper tracheotomy tube positioning and the absence of pneumothorax.

Laryngeal Stenosis

Laryngeal stenosis may occur in the supraglottis, glottis, or subglottis. Clinically, subglottic stenosis is most common. Supraglottic stenosis is rare in children. It usually is a consequence of thermal or chemical injury or iatrogenic injury after previous reconstructive airway surgery.

Subglottic Stenosis

Neonatal subglottic stenosis can be categorized as congenital or acquired. The incidence of congenital subglottic stenosis is 5%; the remaining cases are acquired. Subglottic stenosis in the full-term infant is defined as a subglottic airway diameter of less than 4 mm at the level of the cricoid cartilage, and less than 3 mm in the premature infant (Walner et al., 2001). This narrowing can be compared with the reference point of a neonatal endotracheal tube. The outer diameter of a 2.5 endotracheal tube is 3.6 mm, and the outer diameter of a 3.0 endotracheal tube is 4.2 mm (Rutter et al., 2003). The diagnosis of subglottic stenosis is made by rigid endoscopy while the patient is anesthetized. The extent of the subglottic stenosis is determined by placement of an endotracheal tube that allows an airway leak between 10 and 25 cm H_2O (Table 24-8). This leak allows accurate measure of the airway size. The airway stenosis is then graded as follows: grade I, less than 50% obstruction; grade II, 51% to 70% obstruction; grade III, 71% to 91% obstruction; and grade IV, no detectable lumen (Gerber and Holinger, 2003).

In the absence of trauma, an abnormality of the cartilage or subglottic tissues is usually considered congenital. The cause of congenital subglottic stenosis is thought to be a failure of the laryngeal lumen to recanalize after completion of normal epithelial fusion at the end of the third month of gestation (Walander, 1955). Congenital subglottic stenosis lies on a continuum of embryologic failure that includes laryngeal atresia, stenosis, and webs. In its mildest form, congenital subglottic stenosis merely represents a normal-appearing cricoid with a smaller-than-average diameter, usually with an elliptical shape. Infants and children with mild subglottic stenosis may present with a history of recurrent upper respiratory infections, often diagnosed as croup, in which minimal glottic swelling precipitates airway obstruction. The location of the stenosis is usually 2 to 3 mm below the true vocal cords (Rutter et al., 2003).

Severe congenital subglottic stenosis can be a life-threatening airway emergency manifesting immediately after the infant is delivered. See related video online at www.expertconsult.com. If endotracheal intubation is successful, the patient may require intervention before extubation. In more severe cases, tracheotomy can be life saving at the time of delivery. Infants with congenital subglottic stenosis may have surprisingly few symptoms and may not present for treatment for weeks or months after birth (Rutter et al., 2003). After the initial management of congenital subglottic stenosis, the larynx will grow with the patient and may not require further surgical intervention.

Laryngomalacia is a congenital condition of excessive flaccidity of the laryngeal structures, especially the epiglottis and arytenoids, most likely caused by the lack of neural control of laryngeal muscles. See related video online at www.expertconsult.com. Laryngomalacia accounts for more than 70% of persistent stridor in neonates and young infants (Fig. 24-12); the remaining 10% of neonatal stridor is caused by vocal cord paralysis (Yellon et al., 2002) (Fig. 24-13).

In the mid-1960s, long-term intubation was introduced as the preferred artificial airway in neonates (McDonald and Stocks, 1965). As neonatal survival rates increased with the advent of neonatology and improved neonatal intensive care, subglottic stenosis occurred as a frequent morbidity caused by long-term tracheal intubation. Acquired subglottic stenosis results from intubation trauma and accompanying inflammatory responses. Factors suspected of contributing to this problem include prematurity, the size and amount of movement of the endotracheal tube, duration of intubation, laryngeal or tracheal injury during intubation, and presence of infection during the course of

TABLE 24-8. Obstruction of Laryngotracheal Stenosis Estimated by Endotracheal Tube Size

Age of Patient	ID 2.0	ID 2.5	ID 3.0	ID 3.5	ID 4.0	ID 4.5	ID 5.0	ID 5.5
Premature	40*	—	—	—	—	—	—	—
	58	30	—	—	—	—	—	—
0-3 mo	68	48	26	—	—	—	—	—
3-9 mo	75	59	41	22	—	—	—	—
9 mo to 2 yr	80	67	53	38	20	—	—	—
2 yr	84	74	62	50	35	19	—	—
4 yr	86	78	68	57	45	32	17	—
6 yr	89	81	73	64	54	43	30	16

Adapted from Gerber ME, Holinger LD: Congenital laryngeal anomalies. In Bluestone CD, Stool SE, editors: *Pediatric otolaryngology*, New York, 2003, Saunders, p 1460.
*Endotracheal tube size is used for characterizing firm, mature subglottic stenosis. The size is determined by placement of an endotracheal tube that leaks 10 to 25 cm H_2O.
The numbers in the columns indicate the percentage of obstruction.
ID, Internal diameter of the endotracheal tube.

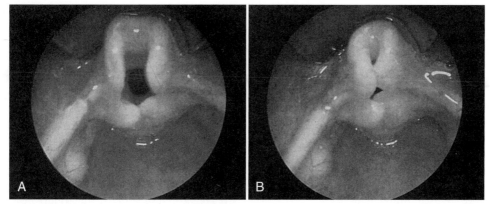

■ **FIGURE 24-12.** Laryngomalacia. **A,** The larynx during expiration. The omega-shaped epiglottis and the arytenoid cartilages appear normal. **B,** The larynx during inspiration. The force of the inspiratory airflow leads to collapse of the laryngeal inlet. Infolding of the epiglottic surface and the arytenoids causes severe upper airway obstruction. *(From Yellon RF, McBride TP, et al: Otolaryngology. In Zitelli BJ, Davis HW, editors:* Atlas of pediatric physical diagnosis, *ed 4, St Louis, 2002, Mosby, p 863.)*

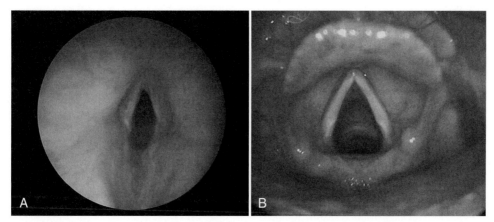

■ **FIGURE 24-13. A,** Congenital bilateral vocal cord paralysis. The marked narrowing of the aperture between the vocal cords stems from the loss of ability to abduct on inspiration. **B,** Normal neonatal vocal cords with a wide opening during inspiration. *(From Yellon RF, McBride TP, Davis HW: Otolaryngology. In Zitelli BJ, Davis HW, editors:* Atlas of pediatric physical diagnosis, *ed 4, St Louis, 2002, Mosby, p 863.)*

tracheal intubation. The incidence of acquired subglottic stenosis has been decreased over the past decade by minimizing the issues known to exacerbate subglottic injury (Walner et al., 2001). Patients presenting to the otolaryngologist for diagnosis or treatment of subglottic stenosis are former preterm infants who were intubated in the neonatal ICU for extended periods and have a tracheotomy in place with an established diagnosis, or are examined on an outpatient basis for symptoms suggesting subglottic stenosis (Cotton, 2000).

Surgical Management of Acquired Subglottic Stenosis in the Neonate

Neonatal subglottic stenosis unresponsive to nonoperative therapy may require tracheotomy or an anterior cricoid split procedure. Tracheotomy is performed if, in addition to severe subglottic injury, there is substantial glottic or tracheal involvement. After tracheotomy and without the endotracheal tube to act as a stent, the stenosis becomes more severe. Over the next 2 years, the airway may heal, allowing for decannulation, but more often, surgical reconstruction of the trachea will be necessary (Rutter et al., 2003).

The anterior cricothyroidotomy, or cricoid split, is an effective treatment for some cases of acquired neonatal subglottic stenosis in the absence of substantial glottic or tracheal or pulmonary pathology (Rutter et al., 2003). The neonate must meet the following criteria (Cotton, 2000):

- Failure of extubation on at least two occasions
- Body weight greater than 1500 g
- Absence of assisted ventilation for 10 days
- Supplemental oxygen requirement of less than 30%
- Absence of heart failure for at least 1 month
- No evidence of an upper or lower respiratory infection
- No antihypertensive medication required

The procedure is performed under general anesthesia with muscle relaxation. The shoulders are elevated, and the neck is extended as in the tracheotomy position (see Fig. 24-11). A horizontal incision is made in the skin over the cricoid cartilage. The cricoid cartilage, upper trachea, and lower edge of the thyroid cartilage are exposed. An incision is made through the cricoid ring and underlying mucosa through the first two tracheal rings and the lower one third of the thyroid cartilage. Stay sutures are placed on both severed edges of the cricoid cartilage, as in a tracheotomy (Healy, 1995b). The endotracheal tube that was used for anesthesia and airway management is then removed. It is replaced, while the larynx is still split, with a nasotracheal tube that is one size (0.5 mm) larger than that predicted for the patient's age and body size. The surgeon helps guide the nasotracheal tube into position through the open incision, and the wound is closed loosely, with a drain. The nasotracheal tube is left in place for 7 days to stent the subglottic aperture. The patient is kept well sedated with or without mechanical ventilation in the pediatric ICU. A modification of the anterior cricoid split is to place a cartilage graft over the split in an effort to allow the airway to seal more rapidly, leading to earlier extubation. Thyroid alar cartilage and occasionally auricular cartilage are used (Rutter et al., 2003).

Laryngotracheal Reconstruction in Children

Chronically ventilated infants who have undergone tracheotomy because of prolonged intubation and subglottic stenosis will most likely require laryngeal reconstructive surgery. Children with greater than 70% obstruction of their laryngeal lumen usually require this surgery to allow decannulation (Rutter et al., 2003).

Laryngotracheal reconstruction has become the standard of care for symptomatic subglottic stenosis in the pediatric age group. There are five stages: characterization of the stenosis, expansion of the tracheal lumen, stabilization of the framework, healing of the airway, and decannulation (Rothschild et al., 1995). The procedure has evolved to include a variety of techniques for expanding the laryngotracheal complex to provide a stable airway of sufficient size. These include, but are not limited to, anterior cartilage graft with the tracheotomy left in place without stent, long-term (several months) stenting with or without cartilage grafts, and short-term (4 to 6 weeks) stenting with anterior or posterior cartilage grafts (Cotton, 2000).

Anterior cartilage graft with a tracheotomy left in place without a stent is indicated primarily for isolated anterior subglottic stenosis with no or relatively mild posterior subglottic components. A variation of this procedure is to remove the tracheotomy at the time of surgery and perform a single-stage laryngotracheoplasty. Posterior division of the cricoid plate and the introduction of a cartilage graft between the cut ends are indicated particularly for children with persistent posterior glottic pathology or primarily posterior subglottic pathology (Cotton, 2000).

Single-stage laryngotracheal reconstruction (LTR) uses cartilage grafts to obtain stability of the reconstructed airway. Single-stage LTR may include an anterior cartilage graft, a posterior cartilage graft, or both, and reconstruction often includes a cartilage graft at the former stoma site. The grafts are supported temporarily by a full-length endotracheal tube fixed in position through the nasal route (Cotton, 2000). The optimal time for extubation has not been established definitively. In general, children remain intubated for 7 to 10 days for anterior cartilage grafts alone, and 12 to 14 days if a posterior and anterior graft is required (Cotton, 2000).

The patient may be anesthetized by the intravenous route or with inhalation anesthesia through a tracheotomy cannula. Standard monitoring includes pulse oximetry, precordial stethoscope, capnography, anesthetic gas monitoring, electrocardiography, blood pressure apparatus, peripheral nerve stimulator, and axillary or rectal temperature monitor. The patient is placed in the tracheotomy position with the shoulders elevated and the neck hyperextended. A tracheotomy tube is replaced with a sterile cuffed armored (anode) endotracheal tube through the tracheostomy stoma and is covered under an adhesive drape to minimize contamination of the surgical field.

Through a horizontal skin incision over the cricoid cartilage, laryngeal structures are exposed. A vertical incision is made through the lower thyroid cartilage, the cricoid cartilage, and the upper tracheal rings (Fig. 24-14, A). The rib cartilage graft, which had been taken from the anterior chest wall with the external perichondrium intact, is used for the anterior or posterior grafts (see Fig. 24-14, B). Auricular cartilage and septal cartilage have also been used as graft materials. Toward the conclusion of surgery, the armored tube is removed from the tracheotomy stoma and replaced with a cuffed nasotracheal tube, one size larger than is appropriate for the patient's age and size, to stent the larynx. This intraoperative transition needs to be carefully coordinated between the anesthesiologist and the surgeon.

One requirement of single-stage LTR is meticulous postoperative management of the patient's condition in the ICU. The nasotracheal airway must be maintained securely during the time of extended stenting without accidental extubation. The postoperative management of patients with single-stage LTR is not standardized (Cotton, 2000). Some centers use sedation to prevent agitation and accidental self-extubation and to avoid pharmacologic paralysis (Rothschild et al., 1995). However, many children do not tolerate nasotracheal intubation and require prolonged sedation and neuromuscular blockade to ensure maintenance of an airway

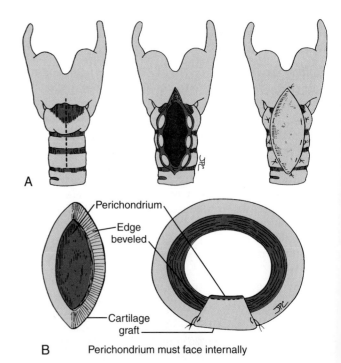

■ FIGURE 24-14. Schematic of laryngotracheoplasty for subglottic stenosis. **A,** Laryngotracheal incision with upper and lower extension, depending on the extent of stenosis, and a cartilage graft. **B,** Cartilage graft is shown with the perichondrium internalized. A graft is sutured in position. *(From Licameli GR, Healy GB: Surgery of the larynx and trachea. In Bluestone CD, Stool SE, editors: Atlas of pediatric otolaryngology, Philadelphia, 1995, Saunders, pp 597–632.)*

with minimal trauma during healing (Brandom, 1997; Yellon et al., 1997). If neuromuscular blockade is used, daily recovery of neuromuscular function and the avoidance of prolonged use of corticosteroids will be associated with less muscle weakness after extubation (Yellon et al., 1997). Prolonged sedation with benzodiazepines or opioids can lead to withdrawal syndrome, and close observation after weaning from these agents is paramount. The role of dexmedetomidine in pediatric patients for prolonged sedation in the ICU setting continues to be investigated (Chrysostomou et al., 2006, 2009; Bejian et al., 2009).

Acute Supraglottitis or Epiglottitis

Acute infectious epiglottitis or supraglottitis is a relatively uncommon but truly life-threatening disease of childhood. See related video online at www.expertconsult.com. Acute epiglottitis is an acute bacterial infection principally involving supraglottic structures, including the lingular surface of the epiglottis, the aryepiglottic folds, and the arytenoids, with little or no involvement of subglottic structures, including the laryngeal surface of the epiglottis. It is therefore more appropriate to call it *supraglottitis*. Until the late 1980s, before the vaccination became available, *Haemophilus influenzae* type b (Hib) was the causative organism in more than 75% of cases. Group A β-hemolytic streptococci account for most of the rare cases of epiglottitis (Gorelick and Baker, 1994). With the advent of effective Hib conjugate vaccines in 1988, the incidence of Hib disease declined dramatically in the United States (Adams et al., 1993; Hoekelman, 1994). The age-specific incidence of Hib disease among children younger than 5 years old decreased by 71%, and that of Hib meningitis by 82%, between 1985 and 1991 (Adams et al., 1993). Similarly, the incidence of acute supraglottitis, one of the most dreaded childhood emergencies, has declined by 84% (Gorelick and Baker, 1994).

Until the late 1980s, before the era of Hib conjugate vaccination, preschool children between the ages of 2 and 6 years had the highest incidence of supraglottitis, although it occurred in infants, older children, and occasionally adults (Schloss et al., 1979; Blackstock et al., 1987; Crysdale and Sendi, 1988). The highest number of cases is reported in the spring and fall, but sporadic cases are reported in other seasons as well. The condition usually begins with complaints of severe sore throat associated with dysphagia and a thick, muffled voice without a preceding history of runny nose. Rarely is there a croupy or barking cough, except in atypical cases in infants (Blackstock et al., 1987). The symptoms rapidly progress, and typical pathognomonic signs of dysphagia, dysphonia, dyspnea, and drooling (the 4 Ds) appear (Diaz, 1985).

In most children presenting with stridor in the emergency room, the most common symptoms found in those with acute supraglottitis are drooling, agitation, and absence of spontaneous cough (Mauro et al., 1988). The child looks toxic and usually has a high fever and tachycardia. The disease progresses very rapidly and may be fatal, with severe airway obstruction within 6 to 12 hours, unless immediate steps are taken to restore the patient's upper airway patency. Classically, the child is sitting up, is dyspneic with the mouth open and drooling, and resists attempts to get him or her to lie down. There is forward chin thrust, slight cervical flexion, and forward flexion at the waist, together with tripod placement of the arms to support this posture. The inspiratory phase is slow, with stridor and retraction, whereas the expiratory phase is unobstructed. The inspiratory sound has been compared with that of a quacking duck.

As soon as acute supraglottitis is diagnosed in the emergency room, a pediatric anesthesiologist, an intensive care physician, and an otolaryngologist should be called. The child should never be left unattended by one of these physicians, because the disease can progress so rapidly that complete upper airway obstruction may ensue within minutes. The patient is kept in a sitting or tripod position with an oxygen mask in place and with pulse oximetry monitoring. The child is transferred to the operating room without delay and is accompanied by an anesthesiologist or an intensivist and a otolaryngologist.

A laryngoscope with several blades, endotracheal tubes with stylets, a bronchoscope, and a self-inflating bag with face mask and oxygen must accompany the patient for emergency intubation (Oh and Motoyama, 1977). Throat examination should not be attempted in the emergency room, because the risk for complete airway obstruction is great. If the child's condition permits or when the diagnosis is questionable, the patient may be transferred to the pediatric ICU, where a radiograph of the lateral neck is taken with a portable x-ray machine (Butt et al., 1988). In the ICU, all the help and expertise needed for an emergency should be readily available. In most patients, a swollen epiglottis obstructing the air space (shadow) is seen on the lateral neck radiograph (Fig. 24-15, *A*). Negative radiographs, however, do not necessarily rule out supraglottitis.

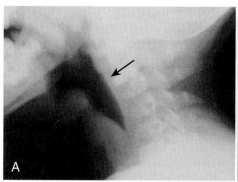
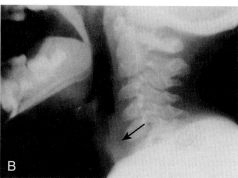

■ FIGURE 24-15. Radiographs of the lateral area of the neck. **A,** Supraglottitis. The upper airway is obstructed by marked swelling of the epiglottis and other supraglottic structures. Notice the loss of normal curvature of the cervical spine. **B,** Laryngotracheitis. *Arrows* point to airway constriction below the vocal cords. (*Courtesy Dr. K. S. Oh, Department of Radiology, Children's Hospital of Pittsburgh.*)

Compared with acute supraglottitis, the onset of laryngo-tracheobronchitis (subglottic croup) is insidious. The child starts with the symptoms of upper respiratory infection, with rhinorrhea, cough, sore throat, and low-grade fever for several days before developing the symptoms of upper airway obstruction characterized by inspiratory stridor and barky or seal-like coughs (i.e., croup). The symptoms may last for a few days to more than a week, with varying degrees of severity that is worse at night in the supine position. In severe cases, endotracheal intubation under general anesthesia is required.

A lateral neck radiograph typically shows a narrowing of the airway shadow below the vocal cords (see Fig. 24-15, *B*). An anteroposterior radiograph of the neck may show a long area of airway narrowing resembling the steeple of a church ("steeple sign") (Fig. 24-16).

Anesthetic Management of Acute Supraglottitis

In the operating room, anesthesia is induced with sevoflurane and oxygen while the child is in a sitting position and monitored with a precordial stethoscope, pulse oximeter, and electrocardiogram. The child in respiratory distress usually breathes continually, uninterrupted by breath-holding. A moderate continuous positive pressure (10 to 15 cm H_2O) must be maintained to minimize the inspiratory collapse of laryngeal airways by the Venturi effect, and ventilation must be assisted with moderate continuous positive airway pressure while avoiding inflating the stomach with excessive pressure. An intravenous access is established as soon as the child is sufficiently obtunded, and atropine (0.02 mg/kg) is given to block vagally mediated slowing of the heart; bradycardia in an atropinized child is a sign of severe hypoxia.

The induction may take much longer, even with a higher concentration of an anesthetic, to reach the state where relaxation and centrally fixed pupils indicate that the child is ready for intubation. A moderate CPAP should be applied to expand inflamed pharyngeal soft tissues and prevent the collapse of the airway, especially during the inspiratory phase of assisted ventilation. The use of muscle relaxants is contraindicated, even when the maintenance of the airway with mask and bag seems reasonable, because their use often results in the relaxation of pharyngeal muscles and complete obstruction of the laryngeal airway; frantic attempts to ventilate the child with high pressure cause gastric distention, regurgitation, and further asphyxia.

Endotracheal intubation is performed orally with a styletted tube one or two sizes smaller than usual. Visualization of the classic cherry-red epiglottis under direct laryngoscopy confirms the diagnosis (Fig. 24-17). However, the picture may be

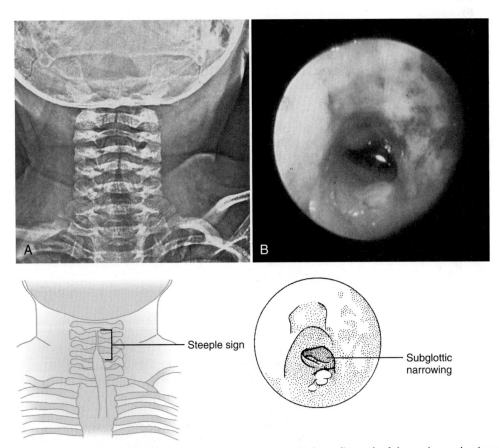

■ **FIGURE 24-16.** Subglottic croup (i.e., laryngotracheobronchitis). **A,** Anteroposterior radiograph of the neck reveals a long area of the airway *(shadow)* narrowing and extending well below the normally narrowed area at the level of the vocal cords. This finding often is called the steeple sign. **B,** In this child, direct visualization using a bronchoscope revealed subglottic narrowing that was so severe that it would require endotracheal intubation or tracheostomy to establish an adequate airway. *(From Yellon RF, McBride TP, Davis HW: Otolaryngology. In Zitelli BJ, Davis HW, editors: Atlas of pediatric physical diagnosis, ed 4, St Louis, 2002, Mosby, p 860; and courtesy Sylvan Stool, MD, Children's Hospital of Pittsburgh.)*

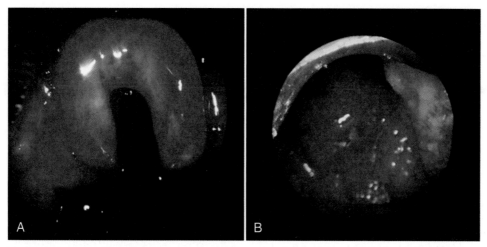

■ **FIGURE 24-17.** A bright red and swollen epiglottis in a patient with acute supraglottitis. It may retain its omega shape **(A)** or resemble a cherry **(B)**. *(From Yellon RF, McBride TP, Davis HW: Otolaryngology. In Zitelli BJ, Davis HW, editors:* Atlas of pediatric physical diagnosis, *ed 4, St Louis, 2002, Mosby, p 858.)*

atypical or only part of the epiglottis may be inflamed or swollen. Inflammatory swelling of other supraglottic structures, including the uvula, arytenoids, aryepiglottic folds, and false vocal cords, also causes severe obstruction. To visualize the vocal cords for intubation, the epiglottis is lifted by the curved tip of a straight laryngoscope blade (e.g., Phillips 1). In children with severe obstruction and mucosal swelling, identification of supraglottic structures and glottic opening with a laryngoscope blade may be extremely difficult. Under these circumstances, forcible manual chest compression by the assistant may open up the expiratory passages momentarily (or produce a few bubbles of expired air). By aiming the tip of the endotracheal tube at that spot and advancing the tube with a gentle twisting motion, the physician may be successful in inserting the tube in the glottis (Smith, 1980). In case intubation proves to be impossible, a surgeon who can perform an emergency tracheotomy in the operating room with the surgical instruments and various tracheotomy tubes should be immediately available.

After the endotracheal tube is in place, breath sounds are checked on both sides of the chest, and the tube is fixed with adhesive tape. The breath sounds are monitored carefully with the precordial stethoscope while continuous positive pressure (10 to 15 cm H$_2$O) is maintained, because pulmonary edema may occur after the relief of severe upper airway obstruction (Travis et al., 1977; Galvis et al., 1980), with an incidence of about 7% (Davis et al., 1981). Throat and blood cultures are taken during this period of stabilization but not before the intubation and restoration of adequate pulmonary gas exchange.

After the child's condition is stabilized and adequate alveolar ventilation is reestablished, some anesthesiologists replace the orotracheal tube with a nasotracheal tube that has a leak, at or below 30 cm H$_2$O, for postoperative management in the ICU with minimal sedation of the patient (Oh and Motoyama, 1977). This is not a necessary step, and the physician should be confident that the switch could be made without losing the airway. Because acute epiglottitis has become an uncommon phenomenon, many anesthesiologists are happy with the oral intubation and leave the tube in place. The child can be deeply sedated for 24 hours to avoid premature extubation.

Since the mid 1970s, the management of epiglottitis with tracheotomy has been replaced by the less invasive long-term nasotracheal or orotracheal intubation as the standard treatment of choice. This has significantly reduced the duration of hospital stay for children with acute supraglottitis (Oh and Motoyama, 1977; Schloss et al., 1983). Accidental or self-extubation is a potentially disastrous complication. Careful taping of the tube and proper restraint of elbows and hands can prevent untimely extubation. Because most children are bacteremic, antimicrobial therapy, consisting of ampicillin with sulbactam, cefotaxime, or ceftriaxone, is started after blood and throat cultures are obtained. Any fluid deficits should be corrected parenterally. After emergence from anesthesia, the child often falls back to sleep for some time because of sleep deprivation and exhaustion. After this period, most patients require minimal or no sedation (Oh and Motoyama, 1977), although deep sedation has been used in some centers. Usually, it is possible to extubate these patients in 24 to 48 hours. A return of normal body temperature and increased leaks around the nasotracheal tube are major signs of recovery. The epiglottis may be examined under direct vision, with intravenous propofol to determine the time for extubation. Alternatively, a flexible fiberoptic bronchoscope may be used transnasally with intravenous sedation.

ANESTHESIA FOR ENDOSCOPY

Anesthesia for rigid and flexible bronchoscopy in infants and children requires meaningful cooperation and communication between the endoscopist and anesthesiologist (Donlon and Benumof, 1996). The surgeon and the anesthesiologist are both working in the same anatomic field. The anesthesiologist is concerned about maintaining a patent airway, oxygenation, adequate ventilation, preventing aspiration, minimizing laryngeal motion, and preventing cardiac dysrhythmias, and the surgeon needs a clear view of a motionless field for a reasonable time. Sometimes, these goals conflict. Donlon and Benumof (1996) described the anesthetic goals during bronchoscopy:

- Control of the airway
- Decreased airway reflexes
- Topical anesthesia
- Amnesia

- Unobstructed view of immobile surgical field
- No time restriction on surgeon inherent in the anesthetic technique
- Prevention of aspiration
- Smooth emergence
- Safe extubation
- Minimization of secretions
- Prevention of adrenergic reflexes

To achieve these goals, anesthetic management must be individualized based on the patient's age, concurrent illnesses, goals of endoscopy, skill of the anesthesiologist, and the proven track record of the anesthetic technique.

Rigid bronchoscopy has broad applications in the diagnostic and therapeutic arenas. Common indications for pediatric patients include investigation of stridor, upper and central (tracheobronchial) airway obstruction, gastroesophageal reflux disease, and removal of airway foreign bodies (Hoeve and Rombout, 1992; Cohen et al., 2001). Flexible bronchoscopy is frequently used for examination of the nasal cavity, nasopharynx, larynx, trachea, and bronchi in motion. Technological advances, such as smaller instruments and improved forceps, will continue to expand the diagnostic and therapeutic role of the flexible bronchoscopy (Cohen et al., 2001). Flexible and rigid bronchoscopies are used complementarily, and these procedures are often performed during the same examination. Box 24-7 lists the common indications for fiberoptic and rigid bronchoscopy. In many scenarios, either instrument can be used for the same indication.

The Storz-Hopkins rigid bronchoscope, with a ventilating sidearm, provides excellent visibility for pediatric bronchoscopy (Szekely and Farkas, 1978; Johnson et al., 1986). This bronchoscope consists of several components: Storz bronchoscope (sizes 3.0 to 6.0); Hopkins glass rod telescope (2.8 and 4.0 mm outer diameter); antifog sheath for the telescope; adapter for anesthesia circuit connecting to the sidearm, which shares the same narrow channel for aspiration and instrumentation; glass obturator cap; and the light source attached to the telescope and prism (Fig. 24-18). Pediatric Storz rigid bronchoscopes are available in three lengths and various diameters (Fig. 24-19). A variety of forceps is available for biopsy and foreign body removal.

It is important to use the smallest optical telescope through the rigid bronchoscope to not completely occlude or unduly increase airflow resistance. For example, use of the standard optical telescope (4-mm outer diameter), as recommended in the literature (Szekely and Farkas, 1978), almost completely occludes the lumen of small bronchoscopes (sizes 3.5 and smaller). The total airway resistance increases sixfold to sevenfold (Widlund, et al., 1982) unless a smaller telescope (2.8-mm outer diameter) is used (Table 24-9). When airway resistance is too high, neither spontaneous nor controlled ventilation is sufficient for adequate gas exchange during rigid bronchoscopy. High airway resistance would be expected to cause hyperinflation of the lungs, and hypercapnia or respiratory acidosis (Rah et al., 1979). Spontaneous breathing during rigid bronchoscopy, especially in neonates and infants, should be limited primarily to evaluations of the larynx and documentation of tracheobronchomalacia in the patient with stridor. The high resistance caused by the telescope in the bronchoscope, together with central respiratory depression caused by general anesthesia, makes spontaneous breathing nearly impossible in these young children (Motoyama, 1992).

With the advances in fiberoptic technology, diagnostic bronchoscopy can be performed with a flexible fiberoptic bronchoscope

Box 24-7 Indications for Flexible or Rigid Bronchoscopy

INDICATIONS FOR FIBEROPTIC LARYNGOSCOPY
- Evaluation of stridor
- Hoarseness or weak cry
- Difficult preextubation of epiglottitis

INDICATIONS FOR RIGID MICROLARYNGOSCOPY AND BRONCHOSCOPY
- Stridor
- Tracheotomy surveillance
- Foreign body evaluation or management
- Interval evaluation after laryngotracheal reconstruction
- Chronic cough
- Severe hemoptysis
- Management of severe laryngotracheal infections
- Airway trauma
- Assessment of toxic inhalation or aspiration
- Evaluation of laryngeal pathology
- Management of mass lesions of the airway, including recurrent respiratory papillomatosis

INDICATIONS FOR FIBEROPTIC BRONCHOSCOPY
- Diagnosis
- Stridor
- Tracheotomy surveillance
- Persistent wheezing
- Persistent atelectasis
- Persistent pneumonia or diffuse infiltrates
- Chronic cough
- Infiltrates in the immunocompromised host bronchoalveolar lavage
- Mild hemoptysis
- Lung lesion of unknown cause
- Selective bronchography
- Assessment of toxic inhalation or aspiration
- Monitoring after lung transplantation
- Therapeutic
- Confirmation of endotracheal tube position
- Acute lobar atelectasis
- Cystic fibrosis management
- Removal of mucus plugs

From Hartnick CJ, Cotton RT: Stridor and airway obstruction. In Bluestone CD, Stool SE, Alper CM, et al., editors: *Pediatric otolaryngology*, ed 4, Philadelphia, 2003, Saunders, p 1437.

during spontaneous breathing with topical anesthesia and minimal sedation even in the sick premature infant. Bronchoscopy also may be performed under general anesthesia through an endotracheal tube or LMA by means of a right-angle adapter with a diaphragm (Maekawa et al., 1981; Wood and Postma, 1988). The use of the flexible fiberoptic bronchoscope for difficult intubation is described in Chapter 13, Induction, Maintenance, and Recovery, and Chapter 12, Airway Management.

Laryngoscopy and Bronchoscopy for Stridor

Stridor in pediatric patients may be congenital or acquired (Fig. 24-20). Most cases are of extrathoracic origin, but some originate in the large intrathoracic airways (i.e., trachea or

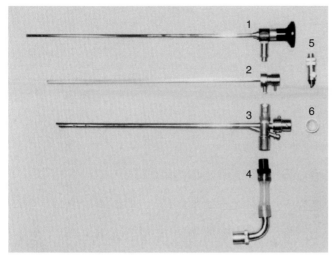

■ **FIGURE 24-18.** Storz-Hopkins pediatric bronchoscopy assembly. *1,* Hopkins glass rod telescope. *2,* Antifog sheath for the telescope shown in 1. *3,* Storz ventilation bronchoscope, which accommodates the telescope and antifog sheath. *4,* Adapter for the anesthesia circuit. *5,* Prism. *6,* Glass obturator cap.

TABLE 24-9. Flow Resistance of Storz Bronchoscope in Relation to Estimated Airway Resistance in Infants and Children

Age	Airway Resistance (Raw) (cm H_2O/L per sec)	Bronchoscope Size (mm)	Bronchoscope Resistance		Ratio Rsa-2/Raw
			Rsa-1*	Rsa-2†	
1 wk	29	3.0	17	31	4.1
6 mo	19	3.5	12	134	7.0
3 yr	10	4.0	14	37	5.7
5 yr	8	5.0	10	17	3.1
10 yr	5	6.0	16	19	4.3

Based on data from Widlund B, Walczak S, Motoyama EK: Flow-pressure characteristics of pediatric Storz-Hopkins bronchoscopes, *Anesthesiology* 57:A417, 1982.
*Flow resistance through breathing sidearm (Rsa) at 0.4 L/sec without telescope.
†Rsa at 0.4 L/sec with telescope (4.0-mm outer diameter) engaged in bronchoscope.

major bronchi) (Maze and Bloch, 1979) (Box 24-8). See related video online at www.expertconsult.com. Stridor may be caused by fixed obstruction (i.e., airway cross-section does not change with transmural pressure) or varying degrees of obstruction (i.e., airway caliber responds to changes in transmural pressure). These children must be examined while they are actively breathing to document underlying pathophysiology.

The anesthesia approach should be individualized, with good communication between the endoscopist and anesthesiologist. All children should be monitored with a pulse oximeter, end-tidal CO_2 monitor, precordial stethoscope, electrocardiogram,

and automated blood pressure and thermometer. Oxygen saturation is determined in room air before the induction of anesthesia to establish the baseline value. Standard NPO guidelines should be followed.

In the newborn infant, flexible and rigid forms of bronchoscopy are used to determine the cause of stridor. Flexible bronchoscopic examination of the infant's larynx by the nasal approach is possible when the child is awake. The infant should be swaddled for restraint. Information about cord mobility and laryngeal dynamics can be made without much stress to the infant. Atropine or glycopyrrolate can be used as an anti-sialagogue

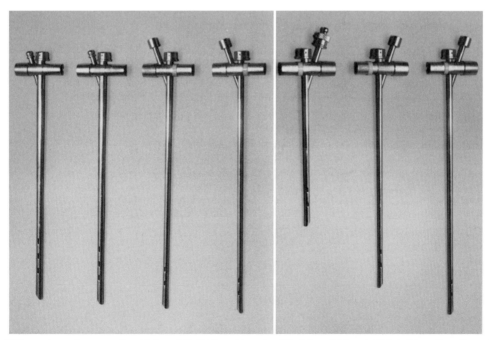

■ **FIGURE 24-19.** Different bronchoscope sizes (3.5 to 6.0) *(left)* and lengths (20, 26, and 30 cm) *(right). (From Casselbrant ML, Alper CM: Methods of examination. In Bluestone CD, Stool SE, editors: Pediatric otolaryngology, ed 4, New York, 2003, Saunders, p 1379.)*

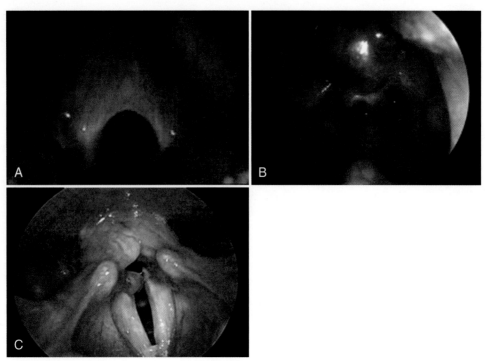

■ **FIGURE 24-20.** Causes of stridor are numerous. More common causes include laryngeal web **(A)**, supraglottic or glottic cyst **(B)**, and postextubation granulomas **(C)**.

Box 24-8 Causes of Stridor in the Pediatric Patient

Congenital stridor
Craniofacial dysmorphology (with micrognathia and
  glossoptosis)
Pierre Robin syndrome
Treacher Collins syndrome (mandibulofacial dysostosis)
Hallerman-Streiff (oculomandibular) syndrome
Moebius' sequence
De Lange's syndrome
Freeman-Sheldon syndrome (whistling face)
Macroglossia
Beckwith's syndrome
Congenital hypothyroidism
Glycogen storage diseases
Down syndrome
Diffuse muscular hypertrophy of the tongue
Localized lingual tumors
Laryngomalacia
Congenital subglottic stenosis
Congenital laryngeal webs
Laryngotracheoesophageal cleft
Congenital vocal cord paralysis
Vascular rings and slings
Congenital tracheal anomalies

Congenital tumors and cysts
Congenital subglottic hemangioma
Laryngeal lymphangioma and cystic hygroma
Cysts and laryngoceles
Miscellaneous congenital tumors
Birth trauma: edema
Metabolic stridor: laryngismus stridulus
Immunologic stridor: hereditary angioneurotic edema
Neurogenic stridor: reflex laryngospasm
Acquired stridor
Infectious stridor
Supraglottitis
Subglottic group
Acute spasmodic laryngitis
Diphtheria
Retropharyngeal abscess
Immunologic stridor—juvenile rheumatoid arthritis
Foreign bodies
Postintubation stridor
Laryngeal trauma: mechanical, thermal, chemical
Neoplasia
Laryngeal papillomatosis
Miscellaneous tumors and nodes

Modified from Maze A, Bloch E: Stridor in pediatric patients, *Anesthesiology* 50:132, 1979.

---

and to prevent vagally mediated bradycardia. The nasal mucosa can be anesthetized with topical lidocaine to prevent discomfort during the transnasal approach, but the vocal cords should not be sprayed, because topical anesthesia affects their motion. Midazolam, dexmedetomidine, or low-dosage propofol may be helpful to reduce the infant's excessive movement while still maintaining breathing dynamics. Because the upper airway muscles, including the vocal cords (i.e., cricoarytenoid muscles), are extremely sensitive to the depressant effect of sedatives and anesthetics (Ochiai et al., 1989, 1992), anesthesia should be maintained at a minimal level; otherwise, the vocal cord motions will cease.

Alternatively, anesthesia is induced with an inhaled agent (i.e., sevoflurane or halothane) without assisted ventilation, and intravenous access is established. After atropine or glycopyrrolate is infused and a nasal topical decongestant (e.g., oxymetazoline) and lidocaine are sprayed, the anesthetic is discontinued while flexible nasopharyngoscopy is performed. As the infant starts to wake up and the motion of the vocal cords begins to return, the diagnosis of vocal cord paralysis can be made. This approach is superior, especially for the diagnosis of laryngomalacia. The infant breathes actively and may move but is still unconscious during the flexible laryngoscopy. The patient is then reanesthetized with an inhaled anesthetic or with propofol for rigid tracheobronchoscopy.

Only by rigid bronchoscopy under the controlled conditions of general anesthesia can a magnified clear view of the larynx and lower airways be achieved (Hartnick and Cotton, 2003). The use of the rigid bronchoscope allows lower airway inspection while maintaining complete and secure control over oxygenation and ventilation. After airway dynamics are inspected by fiberoptic or rigid bronchoscopy, the child may be paralyzed with an intermediate muscle relaxant. Anesthesia can be maintained with an inhaled anesthetic agent or total intravenous anesthesia. Communication must continue with the bronchoscopist to maintain adequate oxygenation and ventilation. When the lower airways are explored, the endoscopist may need to be reminded to intermittently to return to above the carina for the anesthesiologist to ventilate and oxygenate both lungs. In older infants and children, spontaneous breathing may be maintained during the entire procedure.

This technique for laryngoscopy and bronchoscopy with spontaneous breathing is useful for the evaluation of stridor, laryngomalacia, and tracheobronchomalacia. It is also a technique some anesthesiologists advocate for foreign body removal from the airway. Maintenance of spontaneous breathing can be achieved with an inhalational or an intravenous anesthetic technique. For example, after inhalational induction, the concentration of sevoflurane in oxygen is maintained at a minimum alveolar concentration (MAC) of 2 or 3 for about 5 minutes to establish a sufficient tissue level of anesthesia to allow endotracheal instrumentation (Smith, 1980). An alternative is to discontinue the inhaled anesthetic, slowly provide a bolus (2 to 3 mg/kg) of propofol, and begin a propofol infusion between 200 and 400 mcg/kg per minute while maintaining spontaneous breathing. Supplementation with fentanyl or morphine can further ablate laryngeal responses. Before endoscopy, the glottis and trachea are topically anesthetized with 2% to 4% lidocaine (up to 5 mg/kg) under direct vision.

The otolaryngologist then proceeds, using a ventilating bronchoscope and a telescope in situ. Initially, the endoscopist inspects the appearance and motion (widening) of vocal cords with inspiration and the motion of the soft tissues surrounding the inlet to the larynx. The tip of the bronchoscope is held above the inlet to the larynx without touching the pharyngeal or laryngeal soft tissues. After the bronchoscope is introduced past the vocal cords, the anesthesia circuit is connected to the side arm of the bronchoscope, allowing continued assisted ventilation or controlled ventilation. At the end of bronchoscopy, the bronchoscope is removed, and the anesthetic agents are discontinued. If the patient has been spontaneously breathing throughout the anesthesia, the patient can be maintained with oxygen by means of a mask and CPAP. If the patient is apneic or

neuromuscular blockade was required, the child may be intubated and ventilated until clinically ready for extubation.

Bronchoscopy for Foreign Body Aspiration

Foreign body aspiration occurs most frequently in children between 1 and 3 years of age. See related video online at www.expertconsult.com. Commonly aspirated objects include peanuts, seeds, and other food particles and less frequently plastic and metal particles (Baraka, 1974; Blazer et al., 1980). Foreign bodies are embedded more commonly in the right main bronchus than in the left, and less frequently in the larynx and trachea (Blazer et al., 1980; Cohen et al., 2001). Symptoms and signs associated with bronchial aspiration include coughing, wheezing, dyspnea, and decreased air entry in the affected side, whereas dyspnea, stridor, coughing, and cyanosis are more common with laryngeal or tracheal foreign bodies (Blazer et al., 1980).

In addition to the usual preoperative assessment, physical examination should focus on the location, degree of airway obstruction, and gas exchange. A review of the latest chest radiographs is helpful in determining the location of the foreign body and for evidence of secondary pathologic changes such as atelectasis, air trapping, or pneumonia (Fig. 24-21). If significant hyperinflation of one lung or lobe exists, nitrous oxide should be withheld because of the potential danger of further increase in gas volume and possible rupture of the affected lung. Although it is desirable to keep the child NPO (waiting 6 or more hours for solids and 2 hours for clear liquids), the patient's condition determines the timing of the bronchoscopic examination. If foreign body aspiration causes life-threatening respiratory distress, its removal takes precedence over NPO guidelines.

A major controversy in the anesthetic management of patients undergoing bronchoscopy for foreign body removal

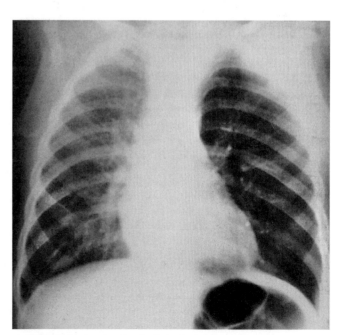

■ FIGURE 24-21. Foreign body in the left bronchus with hyperinflation of the ipsilateral portion of the lung. *(Courtesy Dr. K. S. Oh, Department of Radiology, Children's Hospital of Pittsburgh.)*

is whether to control ventilation or to maintain spontaneous ventilation (Verghese and Hannallah, 2001; Chen et al., 2009). There are few data to justify one technique over the other. Woods (1990) prefers spontaneous ventilation, and Kosloske (1982) advocates neuromuscular blockade and controlled ventilation. The risk of controlled ventilation is to force the foreign body deeper into the small airways, and the risk for the spontaneously breathing patient is unexpected movement or cough (Donlon and Benumof, 1996). In a report of four patients in whom the bronchoscopist had the foreign body slip from the forceps back into the airway, neither controlled ventilation with muscle paralysis nor spontaneous breathing under a deep plane of anesthesia played a role in the mishaps. It was thought that the experience of the endoscopist and the availability of proper equipment were more important factors than the method of ventilation (Pawar, 2000).

Muscle relaxation is particularly useful for bronchoscopy involving the removal of a foreign body distal to the carina, especially because the duration of these procedures can extend to more than an hour. If the spontaneous ventilation technique is employed, meticulous topical anesthesia of the vocal cords with lidocaine can decrease the risks for coughing and laryngospasm. Propofol-based total intravenous anesthesia would be a better choice than inhalational anesthesia because propofol provides a steady level of anesthesia regardless of ventilation and perfusion mismatches (Verghese and Hannallah, 2001).

The anesthetic approach to the child who has aspirated a foreign body must be individualized. All children should be monitored with a pulse oximeter, end-tidal CO_2 precordial stethoscope, electrocardiogram, thermometer, and automated blood pressure. Oxygen saturation is determined in room air before the induction of anesthesia to establish the baseline value. If neuromuscular blockade is required, a nerve stimulator should be used to track the depth of paralysis.

Foreign bodies in the larynx are more likely to cause total airway obstruction than foreign bodies below the glottis. Foreign bodies located in the bronchi may dislodge from cough or change in position and cause total obstruction (Woods, 1990). In case of acute respiratory distress and hypoxemia with a laryngeal foreign body, anesthesia is induced with the patient in a sitting position with an inhaled anesthetic and oxygen while the patient is monitored with a precordial stethoscope, pulse oximeter, and electrocardiogram. Spontaneous breathing is preferable; positive pressure ventilation may cause the foreign body to be displaced and further obstruct the airway (Darrow and Holinger, 2003). After inhalational induction, intravenous access is established (if not already available), and a vagolytic dose of atropine (0.02 to 0.03 mg/kg) is administered. After intravascular access is established, inhalational anesthesia may be switched to total intravenous anesthesia with propofol with or without opioids (e.g., fentanyl, remifentanil). For children in stable condition with a foreign body presumed to be in the bronchus, an intravenous catheter is inserted before the induction, and the child is monitored in the usual manner. If a full stomach is suspected, the physician must weigh the risk for aspiration against loss of a patent airway before rapid-sequence induction with succinylcholine and cricoid pressure is considered.

As soon as the child is anesthetized, the endoscopist must ensure that no foreign body is present above the vocal cords. If the laryngeal outlet is clear, the larynx is sprayed with 2% to 4% lidocaine, and a bronchoscope is inserted through the laryngeal inlet. Fortunately, it is rare for an anesthesiologist to encounter a foreign body in the larynx and upper trachea that causes dyspnea and life-threatening hypoxia.

Immediately after the bronchoscope passes the glottis, the anesthesia circuit is connected to the breathing sidearm of the bronchoscope, and manual ventilation, or spontaneous breathing with manual assist, is resumed. It is important to remember that, with extremely high flow resistance through the side arm of the bronchoscope, spontaneous breathing is all but ineffective and the respiratory rate (especially the expiratory phase) must be kept very slow to allow sufficient time for passive exhalation. Inspiratory gas flow is adjusted to accommodate for the leak around the bronchoscope.

During the procedure, the anesthesiologist's attention should be focused on the breath sounds detected by the precordial stethoscope, the symmetry of respiratory excursion, and oxygen saturation measured by a pulse oximeter. Close communication and cooperation between the bronchoscopist and the anesthesiologist are essential throughout bronchoscopy. It is important to remember that the lumen of the bronchoscope is narrowed by the telescope and other instruments, especially when a suction catheter is inserted through the side port, the same narrow channel through which the patient must be ventilated (Cotton and Reilly, 1990). The rate of rise in end-tidal P_{CO_2} in apneic infants and young children is extremely high—approximately 9 mm Hg/min (Motoyama et al., 2001). The period of apnea or severe hypoventilation therefore should be closely observed and communicated to the endoscopist. The physician must make sure that after each period of hypoventilation or apnea the telescope, forceps, and endobronchial suction catheter through the bronchoscope's side arm are removed. The distal end of the bronchoscope should be pulled above the carina, and the proximal open end of the bronchoscope is occluded with the endoscopist's thumb or a glass obturator cap (see Fig. 24-18), so that the child can be hyperventilated before instrumentation is resumed. During the crucial moment of foreign body retrieval, ventilation must sometimes be held until the oxygen saturation begins to fall.

When the foreign body or its fragment is successfully grasped with the forceps, the forceps and the bronchoscope are carefully pulled out of the trachea and the larynx together as a single unit. It is imperative that the upper airway and glottis be totally relaxed, allowing the foreign body to pass through without being dislodged prematurely. The patient is mask ventilated until the bronchoscope is reintroduced into the trachea. This maneuver can be repeated when the foreign body is fragmented. If a large, obstructive foreign body is removed from the bronchus but is dislodged into the trachea or larynx during the process of retrieval, it can cause serious obstruction of the entire respiratory system unless it is removed immediately. If prompt removal is not possible, the foreign body should be pushed back into one of the main bronchi so that ventilation can be resumed with at least one lung.

Intraoperative complications include laryngospasm, bronchospasm, hypoxia, arrhythmias, and pneumothorax. They are preventable by maintaining adequate anesthesia, oxygenation, ventilation, and muscle relaxation. Premature ventricular contraction, although rare (and most commonly associated with halothane anesthesia in the past), can usually be treated with oxygenation, hyperventilation, and intravenous lidocaine (1 mg/kg), and by reducing the anesthetic concentration. Pneumothorax, although infrequent, must be considered if acute deterioration of ventilation and gas exchange occurs. A portable chest radiograph is diagnostic, and a chest tube is inserted to reexpand the lung.

After the completion of bronchoscopy for foreign body retrieval, the child is usually intubated with an endotracheal tube. Tracheal intubation allows tracheobronchial suction, lung expansion, and oxygenation and ventilation until adequate reversal of muscle relaxation and return to spontaneous breathing. Dexamethasone (0.4 to 1.0 mg/kg, up to a total of 20 mg/kg) is given prophylactically to prevent laryngeal edema (Tunnessen and Feinstein, 1980; Postma et al., 1987). Postoperative croup is treated with inhalation of racemic epinephrine (0.5 mL of 2.25% solution diluted in 3 mL of saline solution) (Adair et al., 1971).

Endoscopy for Foreign Body Ingestion

According to the National Safety Council, suffocation from foreign body ingestion and aspiration is the third leading cause of accidental death in children younger than 1 year and the fourth leading cause in children between 1 and 6 years old. Ingestions are often asymptomatic, unrecognized, and self-resolving. Because retained esophageal foreign bodies are so much more common than aspirations, procedures for their removal outnumber those for aspirated foreign bodies (Manning and Stool, 2003). The most commonly ingested foreign body is a coin, followed by food or bones. Other foreign bodies include buttons, batteries, pins, safety pins, thumbtacks, and small toys (McGahren, 1999). Once in the stomach or bowel, coins usually pass through the remainder of the gastrointestinal tract. Many coins, however, become lodged in the esophagus. The most frequent symptoms of upper esophageal foreign body include dysphagia, drooling, gagging, retching, and vomiting. The child may also experience coughing, choking, and significant airway compromise. Serious complications, such as esophageal erosion, caused by retained esophageal coins are rare and occur only after a coin has been lodged for more than 24 hours. Soprano and coworkers (1999) recommend that children with a single coin in any part of the esophagus who have no history of esophageal disease, or respiratory compromise on presentation to the emergency department, be observed for 12 to 24 hours. These authors found that within 24 hours there is a 28% chance of spontaneous passage of the coin into the stomach, regardless of esophageal location.

A chest radiograph should be obtained in all cases of suspected foreign body ingestion. Ingested foreign bodies are predisposed to lodge in three areas of anatomic constriction in the esophagus: the proximal esophagus at the level of the cricopharyngeal muscle and thoracic inlet (the foreign body is seen at the level of the clavicles on chest radiograph), the middle esophagus at the level of the carina and the aortic arch, and the distal esophagus just proximal to the esophageal gastric junction (the foreign body is seen two to four vertebral bodies above the stomach bubble on chest radiography). The most common site for foreign bodies to lodge is at the upper esophagus at the level of the thoracic inlet. If the foreign body is a coin, it will be oriented in a transverse position because the opening of the esophagus is widest in a transverse position (McGahren, 1999).

Removal of a foreign body from the esophagus is not usually a complicated procedure. As long as the child is not

dyspneic, the physician should wait 4 to 6 hours after the last meal, depending on the child's age, until the stomach is empty. The child should be well sedated, and anesthesia is induced with inhaled or intravenous anesthetics. During esophagoscopy, the mucosa over the cricoid cartilage may be traumatized by compression between the endotracheal tube anteriorly and the rigid esophagoscope posteriorly. A prospective review involving more than 50,000 general pediatric anesthetic cases revealed that the incidence of postintubation croup after esophagoscopy was 20 times higher than that of the general pediatric surgical population during the same time period (Moro, Borland, and Motoyama, unpublished observations). A reduced-size endotracheal tube may be helpful to minimize subglottic swelling (Smith, 1980). Dexamethasone (0.4 to 1 mg/kg, up to 20 mg) may also reduce the incidence of postoperative stridor.

The only potential major hazard with foreign body ingestion is when the foreign body, usually a coin, is held in the hypopharynx, and on gagging and coughing, it dislodges and slips into the larynx, completely occluding the airway. When a radiograph of the neck demonstrates a foreign body high in the esophagus (Fig. 24-22), the child is sedated heavily with an opioid and a sedative to avoid excitement, gagging, and coughing. After intravenous access is established and atropine is given, the trachea is intubated under deep sevoflurane anesthesia or propofol, with or without muscle relaxation. The use of neuromuscular blockade is determined by the ability to ventilate the child with positive pressure. Cricoid pressure is avoided under these circumstances because it may irritate the upper airway or dislodge the foreign body.

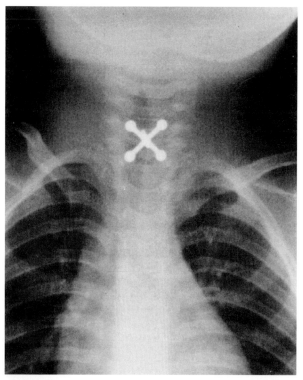

■ **FIGURE 24-22.** A jack is lodged high in the esophagus of a 4-year-old boy. (*Courtesy Dr. J. Medina, Department of Radiology, Children's Hospital of Pittsburgh.*)

SUMMARY

Surgical procedures involving the ear, nose, and throat are the most frequently performed procedures requiring general anesthesia in infants and children. Most procedures are of short duration and involve relatively healthy patients. However, there is a subset of patients with congenital abnormalities and OSAS who present with difficult airways and significant upper airway obstruction. Improved monitoring technology, newer anesthetic agents (e.g., sevoflurane, propofol), and shorter-acting muscle relaxants have made care of these patients safer and more efficient.

Over the past two decades, a drastic decline of acute supraglottitis, the most dreaded of childhood emergencies for pediatric anesthesiologists, has been witnessed with the development of the Hib vaccine. Technological advances in laser surgery and laryngoplasty have continued to challenge pediatric anesthesiologists to develop approaches to meet the needs of advancing otolaryngologic technology.

For questions and answers on topics in this chapter, go to "Chapter Questions" at www.expertconsult.com.

REFERENCES

Complete references used in this text can be found online at www.expertconsult.com.

Anesthesia for Plastic Surgery

Franklyn P. Cladis, Lorelei Grunwaldt, and Joseph Losee

CONTENTS

Plastic and reconstructive surgery for the pediatric patient can involve any part of the body, and some of the children have pathologies related to coexisting diseases and syndromes. They may require surgery on the face, skull, thorax, and extremities, sometimes involving other surgical specialties such as pediatric neurosurgery and otolaryngology. This chapter focuses on reconstruction as it relates to the craniofacial skeleton, extremities, and skin defects involving nevi and vascular malformations.

For the pediatric plastic surgeon, a significant portion of reconstructive surgery involves pathologies of the craniofacial skeleton and soft tissue, and these may be of significant concern for the pediatric anesthesiologist. In this chapter, the pathologies that result in surgery are set in the framework established by Whitaker and associates in 1979. The anesthesiologist who cares for these children will find it easier to organize the varied syndromes and sequences when they are structured in this manner.

CRANIOFACIAL SURGERY

Craniofacial anomalies are characterized by congenital or acquired deformities of the cranial or facial skeleton. Although rare, they comprise a diverse group of defects, and the goal of surgical intervention is to restore both form and function. The classification of craniofacial anomalies is difficult because of their variability, rarity, and degree of severity, and often because of our lack of understanding of their etiology and pathogenesis. The Committee on Nomenclature and Classification of Craniofacial Anomalies of the American Cleft Palate Association has proposed the following categories: synostosis, clefts, hypoplasia, hyperplasia, and unclassified (Whitaker and Bartlett, 1990).

Craniosynostosis

Craniosynostosis is defined as premature closure of one or more of the cranial sutures. It is a relatively common defect, occurring in one in 2000 to 2500 live births (Posnick, 2000). It can result in abnormalities in the size and shape of the calvarium, cranial base, and orbits, and can cause dental occlusion, and thus it constitutes a diverse group of deformities. Craniosynostosis is not only a cosmetic issue, for it can also affect brain growth, intracranial pressure (ICP), and vision, resulting in developmental delay and vision impairment (Slater et al., 2008).

Premature fusion of a cranial suture results in an abnormal head shape. Growth of the skull perpendicular to the suture is impaired. Compensatory growth parallel to the suture creates the characteristic abnormal skull shape. The shape of the skull defines craniosynostosis. Figure 25-1 shows the different types of abnormal skull shapes and the corresponding synostotic sutures.

Craniosynostosis can occur by itself (simple) or as a major component of a syndrome (complex, or syndromic). Over 100 craniosynostosis syndromes have been described, but six are more common than the others (Slater et al., 2008). These are Apert, Pfeiffer, Saethre-Chotzen, Carpenter's, Crouzon, and Muenke's syndromes. Of these, Apert and Crouzon syndromes are the most common. Table 25-1 lists the various syndromes and their associated anomalies and anesthetic concerns. The timing of surgery usually occurs before 1 year of age. The importance of early intervention is related to improved ability of the infant to reossify, the malleable nature of the calvaria during infancy, and the rapid brain growth that occurs during the first year of life (Panchal and Uttchin, 2003). The motivation for and goal of surgical intervention are to reduce ICP, prevent brain injury, and enhance appearance. Repair of syndromic craniosynostosis may be more complicated and appears to be associated with increased blood loss. The etiology of the increased bleeding is unclear, but it might be related to the length of surgery (Fearon and Weinthal, 2002).

Apert Syndrome

Apert syndrome, also referred to as acrocephalosyndactyly, occurs at a frequency of 1 in 160,000 live births (Cohen et al., 1992). Acrocephalosyndactyly, a defect involving the cranium

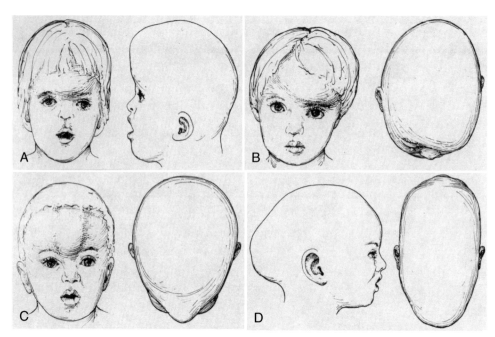

■ FIGURE 25-1. Skull shapes and their associated synostotic sutures. Note the abnormal growth parallel to the fused suture. **A,** Turribrachycephaly. Bilateral coronal sutures are fused. **B,** Plagiocephaly. Unilateral coronal suture is fused. **C,** Trigonocephaly. The metopic suture is fused. **D,** Scaphocephaly. The sagittal suture is fused. *(From Whitaker LA, Bartlett SP: Craniofacial anomalies. In Jurkiewicz J, Krizek T, Mathes S, et al, editors:* Plastic surgery: principles and practice, *St Louis, 1990, Mosby, p 99.)*

TABLE 25-1. Anesthetic Considerations for Craniofacial Syndromes

Syndrome	Suture(s)	Clinical Features	Anesthesia Issues
Apert syndrome	Coronal	HEENT: Turribrachycephaly, midface hypoplasia, orbital hypertelorism, cleft palate in 30%, occasional choanal atresia and tracheal stenosis, airway obstruction. Cardiac: Congenital heart disease occurs in 10%; may include VSD, pulmonary stenosis. Genitourinary: Hydronephrosis in 3%, cryptorchidism in 4.5%. Musculoskeletal: Syndactyly of the hands and feet, fusion of digits 2 to 4, fusion of the cervical vertebrae can occur. Neurologic: Mental retardation common, may have elevated ICP. Dermatologic: Acne vulgaris common.	Preoperative labs: HCT, blood type and screen. Airway management: Mask ventilation may be very difficult because of midface hypoplasia, choanal, atresia, and tracheal stenosis. Intubation may be difficult because of facial anomalies and decreased neck mobility. Cardiac: Emphasis on balancing pulmonary and systemic blood flow, de-air IV lines, endocarditis prophylaxis. Musculoskeletal: Cervical fusion may decrease neck extension; syndactyly may make vascular access difficult. Neurologic: Caution with premedication if ICP elevated.
Pfeiffer syndrome	Coronal and occasionally sagittal	HEENT: Tower skull, midface hypoplasia, orbital hypertelorism, proptosis; choanal atresia is uncommon. Pulmonary: Obstructive sleep apnea Cardiac: May have cardiac defects. Musculoskeletal: Usually mild syndactyly involving broad thumbs and great toes, rarely ankylosis of the elbow occurs, fusion of cervical vertebrae reported. Neurologic: Generally normal but mild developmental delay can occur, may have increased ICP.	Preoperative labs: HCT, blood type and screen. Airway management: No reported cases of difficult intubation, airway obstruction may occur intraoperatively or postoperatively. Cardiac: Emphasis on balancing pulmonary and systemic blood flow, de-air IV lines, endocarditis prophylaxis. Musculoskeletal: Cervical fusion may decrease neck extension, syndactyly may make vascular access difficult. Neurologic: Caution with premedication if ICP elevated, eyes require protection if ocular proptosis present.
Saethre-Chotzen syndrome	Coronal and others	HEENT: Brachycephaly, maxillary hypoplasia, orbital hypertelorism, beaked nose, occasional cleft palate. Genitourinary: Renal anomalies and cryptorchidism. Musculoskeletal: Short stature, mild syndactyly, cervical fusion possible. Neurologic: Mild developmental delay, rare increased ICP.	Preoperative labs: HCT, blood type and screen Airway management: No reported cases of difficulty with ventilation or intubation. Musculoskeletal: cervical fusion may decrease neck extension, syndactyly may make vascular access difficult. Neurologic: Caution with premedication if elevated ICP.

TABLE 25-1. Anesthetic Considerations for Craniofacial Syndromes—cont'd

Syndrome	Suture(s)	Clinical Features	Anesthesia Issues
Carpenter's syndrome	Coronal and others	HEENT: Tower skull, down thrust eyes, orbital hypertelorism, low set ears, small mandible. Cardiac: cardiac defects common (VSD, ASD). Genitourinary: hypogonadism. Musculoskeletal: Syndactyly of hands and feet. Neurologic: Developmental delay common but variable, may have increased ICP. Other: Obesity.	Preoperative labs: HCT, blood type and screen. Airway management: The small mandible may make intubation difficult. Obesity may make ventilation difficult. Musculoskeletal: Syndactyly may make IV access difficult. Neurologic: Caution with premedication if elevated ICP.
Crouzon syndrome	Coronal, lambdoid, others	HEENT: Frontal bossing, tower skull, midface hypoplasia, beaked nose, hypertelorism, ocular proptosis, airway obstruction can occur. Neurologic: Occasional mild developmental delay, may have increased ICP.	Preoperative labs: HCT, blood type and screen. Airway management: May be a difficult intubation (uncommon), airway obstruction with sedation or anesthesia, caution with premedication. Neurologic: Caution with premedication if elevated ICP, eyes require protection if ocular proptosis present.
Muenke's syndrome	Coronal	HEENT: Wide-set eyes, hearing loss. Neurologic: Developmental delay uncommon.	Preoperative labs: HCT, blood type and screen. Neurologic: Caution with premedication if elevated ICP.

ASD, Atrial septal defect; *HCT,* hematocrit; *HEENT,* head ears eyes nose throat; *ICP,* intracranial pressure; *IV,* intravenous; *VSD,* ventricular septal defect.

and the extremities, occurs in Apert, Pfeiffer, Carpenter's, and Saethre-Chotzen syndromes. The characteristic features of Apert syndrome include turribrachycephaly (high steep flat forehead and occiput), mid-face hypoplasia, and orbital hypertelorism (Fig. 25-2). Cleft palate occurs in approximately 30% of these patients. Choanal atresia and occasionally tracheal stenosis have been reported and can cause airway obstruction. Congenital cardiac disease is one of the more common associated visceral anomalies, occurring in approximately 10% of patients. Genitourinary anomalies (hydronephrosis, cryptorchidism) also occur in 10% of patients with Apert syndrome (Cohen and Kreiborg, 1993). Severe synostosis can result in increased ICP and, if uncorrected, developmental delay. Syndactyly of the hands and feet with the fusion of digits two to four can occur and can make intravenous (IV) access difficult. Kreiborg and

coworkers (1992) have reported cervical spine fusion, and they have suggested that cervical spine films prior to anesthesia may help predict difficult intubation. Although infants and children with Apert syndrome are often difficult to intubate, many have been intubated uneventfully. In some cases, suboptimal laryngoscopic views secondary to abnormal anatomy may require flexible fiberoptic intubation. The laryngeal mask airway (LMA) may be a reasonable adjunct in those patients who are difficult to ventilate or intubate. However, to date there are no reported instances of their use in infants and children with Apert syndrome. The clinical features and anesthetic implications of Apert syndrome and the other acrocephalosyndactylies are outlined in Table 25-1. Unlike Apert syndrome, the other acrocephalosyndactylies are not typically associated with difficult airways. However, midface hypoplasia is common in these infants and may cause significant upper airway obstruction intraoperatively and postoperatively (Perkins, 1997).

Pfeiffer Syndrome

Pfeiffer syndrome is another example of an acrocephalosyndactyly. The incidence of Pfeiffer syndrome is approximately 1 in 100,000 live births. This syndrome is characterized by bicoronal synostosis, proptosis, midface hypoplasia, and broad thumbs and great toes (Moore et al., 1995). Patients with Pfeiffer syndrome can also present with hydrocephalus, which may contribute to increased intracranial pressure. There are three types of Pfeiffer syndrome, and typically the clinical features, degree of airway obstruction, and mortality rates increase with types 2 and 3 (Moore et al., 1995).

Saethre-Chotzen and Carpenter's Syndromes

The clinical features of Saethre-Chotzen include brachycephaly, facial asymmetry, low hairline, proptosis, beaked nose, large halluces (great toes), and pectus excavatum. Some patients may have renal anomalies, cryptorchism, developmental delay, and epilepsy. It can be difficult to differentiate it from the other acrocephalosyndactylies because there can be significant clinical

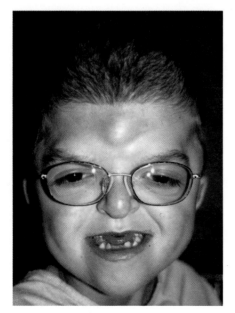

■ **FIGURE 25-2.** Apert syndrome.

variability (Nascimento et al., 2004). Carpenter's syndrome is the most rare of the syndromic craniosynostosis, with only 45 reported cases since the mid 1990s. As with all of the syndromic craniosynostosis, patients with Carpenter's syndrome have synostosis, midface hypoplasia, and musculoskeletal deformities. They may also have hypogonadism, developmental delay, and obesity (Idestrand et al., 2009).

Crouzon Syndrome

Crouzon syndrome, also known as craniofacial dysostosis, is one of the syndromic craniosynostoses. These infants present with craniosynostosis, proptosis, and midface hypoplasia but without visceral or extremity involvement (Fig. 25-3). As in other patients with midface hypoplasia, significant airway obstruction can occur and may require early tracheostomy (Sirotnak et al., 1995). Table 25-1 outlines the main clinical features and anesthetic issues as they relate to patients with Crouzon syndrome. During infancy, patients with Crouzon syndrome may come to the operating room for tracheostomy or cranial vault remodeling.

Surgical Management

Cranial Vault

Surgical correction for craniosynostosis can be performed with an open or an endoscopic procedure. The calvarial vault reconstruction typically involves both plastic surgery (by craniofacial surgeons) and neurosurgery. The surgical approach for an open cranial vault reconstruction is through a bicoronal incision (Fig. 25-4, *A*). A blocking stitch or clips may be applied to the skin flaps to minimize blood loss. The clips may be more effective in preventing bleeding, but some surgeons have expressed concern about the risk for ischemia of the underlying hair

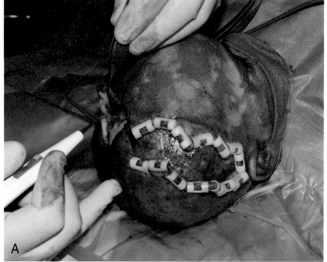

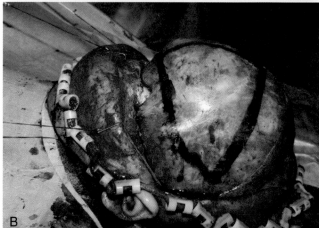

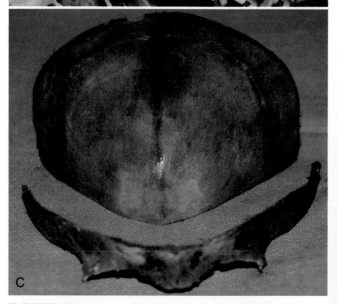

■ **FIGURE 25-4.** Bicoronal skin incision. **A,** A bicoronal incision is made for access to the calvarium. Note the skin clips on the scalp flap to minimize bleeding. **B,** The skin flap is mobilized off the forehead to expose the orbits. **C,** The calvarium and the supraorbital rim are seen in approximation.

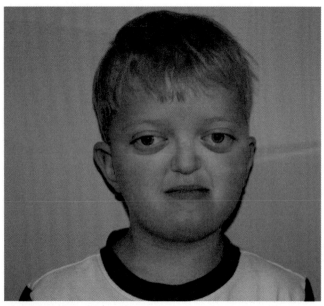

■ **FIGURE 25-3.** Crouzon syndrome.

follicles (Ray Harschberger, personal communication, 2009). The scalp flap is dissected off the forehead and mobilized down to expose the superior orbital rim (see Fig. 25-4, *B*). The calvarium is typically removed by the neurosurgeons in one or several pieces. A bandeau osteotomy is then performed along the lateral temporal bones and the nasion to mobilize the superior orbital rim (see Fig. 25-4, *C*). Once the osteotomies are complete, the surgical field is protected with moist gauze. The calvarium and the orbital bandeau are sectioned and the pieces are reshaped and replaced in a manner that replicates a normal head shape. The bone is secured with a craniofacial plating system, the scalp flaps are replaced, and the coronal incision is closed.

Strip Craniectomy with Helmet

The endoscopic approach is less invasive and has been reported to cause less blood loss (Jimenez et al., 2002). This procedure is more commonly used for sagittal synostosis, although it has been described for the repair of other single suture and even multiple-suture synostosis. The surgical approach is through smaller incisions. As with open approaches, significant blood loss can occur if the sagittal sinus is entered. Jiminez reported a small percentage of patients who required transfusions, and most were discharged on the first postoperative day. Unlike those who had an open calvarial reconstruction, these patients do require helmet therapy after this repair.

Midface Advancement

Midface advancements are performed to correct midface hypoplasia. The different types of advancements include the Le Fort I maxillary advancement, the Le Fort III maxillary and upper face advancement (Fig. 25-5), and the monobloc advancement, which includes the maxilla, upper face, orbits, and forehead. The

Le Fort I osteotomy is typically performed for patients with midface hypoplasia secondary to cleft lip and palate. The Le Fort III and monobloc osteotomies are typically performed for patients with midface hypoplasia secondary to syndromic craniosynostosis (Apert, Pfeiffer, Crouzon syndromes). The surgical approach for the Le Fort III and monobloc osteotomies are through bicoronal, intraoral, and often eyelid incisions. Significant blood loss can occur during the surgical dissection and osteotomies. Once the midface is mobilized, the advancement can be performed immediately with rigid fixation or gradually with internal or external distraction osteogenesis. Distraction osteogenesis became a common in craniofacial surgery in 1997, and the advantages include less morbidity, more long-term stability, and improved aesthetic outcome (Fearon, 2001; Shetye et al., 2007). The external distraction device has a frame that is anchored to the skull, with a distraction bar positioned perpendicular to the face. The distraction bar is anchored to the newly mobilized midface with wires (Fig. 25-6). Once in place, the midface may be distracted at a rate of 1 to 2 mm a day.

Anesthesia Management

The anesthetic management of infants with craniosynostosis begins with a complete preoperative evaluation. The history should define the cranial sutures involved, the planned surgical procedure, and previous craniofacial reconstruction, and it should identify any associated syndrome. Infants and children with syndromes may have difficult airways, other organ involvement, and more complicated surgical repair with more bleeding. Associated anomalies that can present a challenge to the anesthesiologist include facial and airway features that make mask ventilation and intubation difficult. Airway pathology can also cause obstruction, and some of these children have obstructive sleep apnea (OSA) (Mixter et al., 1990; Pijpers et al., 2004).

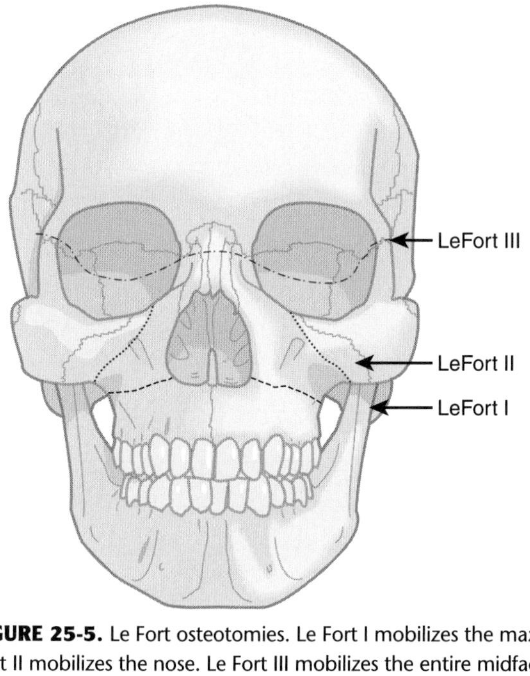

■ FIGURE 25-5. Le Fort osteotomies. Le Fort I mobilizes the maxillae. Le Fort II mobilizes the nose. Le Fort III mobilizes the entire midface.

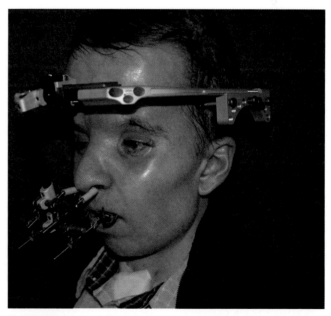

■ FIGURE 25-6. Midface distraction. An adolescent boy with Apert syndrome, in a midface distractor.

Children with OSA may present with daytime somnolence, enuresis, behavioral changes, and snoring. As many as 40% to 50% of infants and children with syndromic craniosynostosis have clinical features of OSA. This compares with the 0.2% to 0.7% incidence of OSA in the general pediatric population (Lo and Chen, 1999; Pijpers et al., 2004). The most common treatment for OSA is adenotonsillectomy. If this fails to reduce the symptoms, the sequence of recommended steps in this population includes nasal continuous positive airway pressure (CPAP), Le Fort III osteotomy with midface advancement, and as a last resort, tracheostomy. Several studies have demonstrated a reduction in the symptoms of OSA after midface advancement. In one study by Nelson and colleagues (2008), all of the patients reported a decrease in snoring, and five of the six patients with a tracheostomy could be decannulated.

A history of fatigue (or sweating with feedings), cyanosis, and syncope are suggestive of an underlying cardiac anomaly. Cardiac pathology is associated with some of the syndromes (e.g., Apert, Pfeiffer, Carpenter's). Congenital heart disease is most common in Apert syndrome, and the most common cardiac defect is ventricular septal defect (Hidestrand et al., 2009). Infants and children with clinical signs or symptoms suggestive of heart disease or a heart murmur should be preoperatively evaluated by a pediatric cardiologist.

Some infants and children with craniosynostosis may have increased ICP. The incidence of increased ICP in nonsyndromic craniosynostosis varies from 8% to 47%, depending on the number of sutures involved (Arnaud et al., 1995; Renier et al., 2000; Mathijssen et al., 2006). The incidence appears to be higher in syndromic craniosynostosis, with approximately 50% having funduscopic evidence of papilledema (Bannink et al., 2008). This may manifest as headaches, vomiting, and somnolence. However, infants and children with chronically elevated ICP may be asymptomatic. Elevations in ICP manifest as papilledema on ophthalmologic examination, so all patients with craniosynostosis should have a funduscopic examination by an ophthalmologist.

A thorough airway examination may be difficult to perform on an infant. Features that predict difficulty with mask ventilation include midface hypoplasia and enlarged tongues. In addition, a small mandibular space, decreased jaw opening and translocation, and decreased neck flexion and extension predict difficult intubation. The rest of the examination should focus on identifying heart murmurs and, in infants with syndactyly, identifying potential IV and arterial access sites. For reconstructions that involve significant blood loss (cranial vault reconstruction, midface advancement), a preoperative hematocrit level should be obtained, and blood typing and crossmatching should be performed. Former premature infants and infants less than 2 month old should have perioperative glucose monitoring. Premedication can be performed for most children over the age of 1 year but is rarely necessary in those less than 9 months old. Children with evidence of airway obstruction or acute elevations in ICP should not receive a premedicant agent. Endocarditis prophylaxis is not necessary in those patients with congenital heart disease.

Airway

Airway management in these patients can be very challenging during attempts at ventilation, intubation, or both. Fortunately, difficult airways are not common. However, the incidence is higher in those patients with syndromes and in those patients who have had previous reconstruction. Successful techniques described for infants and children include using the Bullard laryngoscope, laryngeal mask airway, flexible fiberoptic scope, and retrograde intubation (Cooper and Murray-Wilson, 1987; Blanco et al., 2001; Brown et al., 1993, 2004) (see Chapter 10, Equipment, and Chapter 12, Airway Management). A combination of techniques may be required to secure the airway. For example, the LMA has been used to facilitate the passage of the fiberoptic scope and endotracheal tube (Inada et al., 1995) (Fig. 25-7). Although those authors report this technique in a patient with Treacher Collins syndrome, it could be used for any craniofacial patient with a difficult airway. An endotracheal tube and LMA size chart helps in choosing the appropriate equipment (Table 25-2, and see also Table 10-3 in Chapter 10, Equipment). Cuffed endotracheal tubes may be more challenging, because the cuff on the endotracheal tube may not fit through the smaller LMAs. However, the air-Q (Trudell Medical Marketing, London, Ontario, Canada) has its short stalk and detachable adapter that make it easy to pass a cuffed endotracheal tube with the pilot balloon. If an uncuffed endotracheal tube is used, it can be secured while removing the LMA by telescoping a smaller

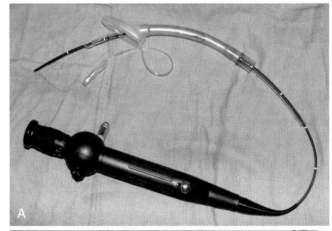

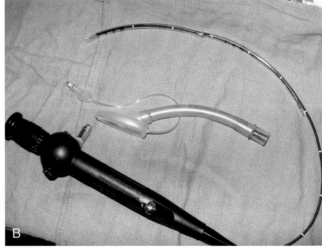

■ **FIGURE 25-7. A,** Once the laryngeal mask airway (LMA) is positioned in the mouth, the fiberoptic scope is placed through it, and the endotracheal tube is fed over the fiberoptic scope into the trachea. **B,** Another uncuffed endotracheal (one-half size smaller) is used as a pusher to facilitate LMA removal without extubation.

TABLE 25-2. Equipment Sizes for Airway Management

Laryngeal Mask Airway (size)	Endotracheal Tube (mm)
1.0	3.0 uncuffed
1.5	4.0 uncuffed
2	4.5-5.0 uncuffed
2.5	5.5 uncuffed
3	6.0 uncuffed
4	6.0 cuffed

endotracheal tube through the top of the larger tube (see Fig. 25-7, *B*). When passing an endotracheal tube through an LMA that is a size 3 or smaller, an uncuffed endotracheal tube is easier to use, but it runs the risk for creating a large air leak.

The airway for patients having craniosynostosis surgery can be secured with a standard oral endotracheal tube. For these patients, a nasal intubation may be easier to perform when using the flexible fiberoptic scope. A standard endotracheal tube may be preferred to a nasal RAE (Ring, Adaire, Ellwyn) tube because of the surgical approach, which involves a bicoronal incision.

Patients having Le Fort osteotomies require a nasal or an oral intubation depending on the type of Le Fort. Those having a Le Fort I osteotomy (for clefts) will need a nasal endotracheal tube so the maxillae and the mandible can be aligned properly. Nasal endotracheal tubes have been damaged during Le Fort osteotomies, resulting in difficulty with ventilation (Bidgoli et al., 1999), so care must be taken by the surgeons when mobilizing the maxillae. Patients having a Le Fort III osteotomy for midface distraction can be intubated orally with an oral RAE tube.

Some infants with craniofacial anomalies require tracheostomy because of significant upper airway obstruction (Perkins, 1997; Sculerati et al., 1998). Adequate preparation entails having all the necessary equipment available and having personnel who are trained and experienced in the use these airway instruments. It may also mean having a pediatric otorhinolaryngologist immediately available.

Intracranial Pressure

Patients with craniosynostosis may develop intracranial hypertension. Typically this is diagnosed by the presence of papilledema during an ophthalmologic examination. Clinically, increased ICP may range from being asymptomatic to complaints of visual changes, headaches, somnolence, and vomiting. Children with chronically elevated ICP may be relatively asymptomatic and active. Chronically elevated ICP can have anatomic and physiologic consequences that may affect the surgical and anesthetic management. Computed tomography scans and magnetic resonance imaging (MRI) will show a beaten-copper-pot appearance of the skull in patients with chronically elevated ICP. The close proximity of the brain to the skull may make removal of the calvarium difficult. Mannitol (0.25 to 0.75 g/kg) and mild hyperventilation may facilitate this process.

Hemodynamic instability can occur in patients with chronically elevated ICP after the calvarium is removed. The probable physiologic cause is the sudden reduction in blood pressure required to maintain cerebral perfusion pressure once the calvarium is removed and the ICP equilibrates with atmospheric pressure. Patients may require transient hemodynamic support with vasoactive medication (e.g., epinephrine or phenylephrine).

Blood Conservation and Transfusion Medicine

Craniofacial procedures are often long, exposing infants to the risks of hypovolemia, hypothermia, blood loss, and venous air emboli. The craniofacial procedures typically performed during the first year of life include cranial vault remodeling (including fronto-orbital, posterior, and total vault advancement) and strip craniectomy. One of the most pressing concerns related to anesthesia care in craniofacial surgery is the management of intraoperative bleeding. The cranial procedures can involve significant blood loss because of the duration of the procedure, the many exposed skin and bone surfaces, and the rare complication of entering large vessels such as the sagittal sinus. Blood loss during these procedures has remained an issue since Whitaker and colleagues' description of perioperative blood loss in 1979. Blood loss is often as high as half to one blood volume, and nearly 90% to 100% of the infants undergoing these procedures may require a blood transfusion (Faberowski et al., 1999; Tuncbilek et al., 2005; Stricker et al., 2010). Even the strip craniectomy, which is typically performed to correct nonsyndromic isolated sagittal synostosis and results in less blood loss, can produce significant hemorrhage. In a recent study by White and others (2009), predictors of blood loss during craniofacial surgery included surgery time greater than 5 hours, age less than 18 months, the presence of multiple-suture craniosynostosis, and syndromic craniosynostosis. Infants undergoing strip craniectomy usually experience less blood loss, but this population may be at increased risk because they come to the operating room at the nadir of their physiologic anemia (i.e., at 2 to 3 months of age). Preparation for these procedures requires a baseline hematocrit, and blood typing and cross-match. Some centers also obtain coagulation studies. Adequate IV access needs to be obtained for resuscitation. In an infant, at least two large-bore (22- to 20-gauge) peripheral IV catheters should be placed to provide adequate access. Arterial pressure monitoring is recommended for beat-to-beat analysis of blood pressure and intravascular volume status, as well as for blood gas monitoring. A central venous catheter may be placed for central venous pressure monitoring, or in patients with difficult IV access.

Recently, some centers have reported significant success with minimizing blood loss and exposure to allogeneic blood products during craniofacial surgery. Surgical techniques that minimize blood loss include infiltrating subcutaneous epinephrine, needle tip cautery, scalp clips for the scalp flap, and bone wax for the osteotomy edges. Several medical and pharmacologic blood conservation techniques have been described in the older pediatric patient, but less information is available for the infant having cranial vault reconstruction.

Preoperative blood donation has been described in children as small as 8 kg (Mayer et al., 1996), but this technique has significant limitations in the infant. Their young age, small size, and lower hematocrit may make blood collection more challenging and less feasible. Acute normovolemic hemodilution has been described in older children and adolescents and may be effective. Hemodilution is relatively contraindicated in the infant less than 6 months old. The normal physiologic advantage with hemodilution (increased preload, increased stroke volume, and decreased systemic vascular resistance, increased tissue oxygenation) may be lost in the infant because of fetal hemoglobin, which more avidly binds oxygen, and a naturally less compliant myocardium.

Because most infants presenting for cranial vault reconstruction have a normal physiologic anemia, erythropoietin was proposed as a therapy to address this concern. Preoperatively, recombinant erythropoietin decreases the transfusion requirements in infants having craniosynostosis repair. Fearon and Weinthal (2002) reported the dosage of erythropoietin as 600 units/kg given subcutaneously once per week along with oral iron supplementation. Erythropoietin was started 3 to 4 weeks before surgery, and the incidence of blood transfusions in infants having craniosynostosis repair decreased from 93% to 57%.

In March of 2007, the U.S. Food and Drug Administration placed a black-box warning on synthetic erythropoietin because of the concern of increased death, deep venous thrombosis, and cancer spread in adult patients receiving synthetic Epogen (Singh et al., 2006; see also www.fda.gov/for consumers). These concerns have occurred only in the adult population, but some centers have stopped using synthetic erythropoietin for craniofacial surgery. A multicenter retrospective review of 396 pediatric craniofacial patients receiving erythropoietin did not reveal an increase in perioperative complications, specifically death or deep venous thrombosis (Naran et al., 2010).

Antifibrinolytic therapy has been described in pediatric surgery, but the data for craniofacial surgery are limited. Aprotinin, a serine protease inhibitor, decreases perioperative blood loss and transfusion requirements during craniofacial procedures. In a prospective, randomized, and blinded placebo-controlled study evaluating the effect of aprotinin in infants and children having cranial vault remodeling and frontal orbital advancements, D'Errico and colleagues (2003) noted a reduction in the amount of packed red blood cells being transfused intraoperatively and postoperatively in those receiving aprotinin. However, aprotinin did not reduce the number of patients requiring transfusion. Although no adverse events were reported, the option of aprotinin has been curtailed with its removal from the market. Tranexamic acid and aminocaproic acid are two antifibrinolytics that remain available for potential pediatric use. The data to guide the use of tranexamic acid and aminocaproic acid in this population are limited, but a small study by Durán de la Fuente and colleagues (2003) demonstrated a reduction in estimated blood loss and transfusion requirements. The tranexamic acid was not infused continuously but instead was administered every 8 hours at a dosage of 15 mg/kg. Table 25-3 shows standard dosage regimens for tranexamic acid and aminocaproic acid.

In the past, the use of a cell saver was reported as being impractical for small pediatric patients because of the size of the collection reservoir (De Ville, 1997). Recently, the cell-saver reservoirs are available in sizes as small as 25 mL. This technology may reduce the rate of autologous blood transfusion in infants having craniofacial surgery. In fact, the most significant

benefit may occur when cell-saver technology is combined with erythropoietin pretreatment. In a prospective analysis evaluating the use of cell saver with a 55-mL pediatric bowl for patients pretreated with erythropoietin, only 30% of those infants having cranial vault remodeling required allogeneic blood (Fearon, 2005). Krajewski and coworkers (2008) in a prospective randomized trial describe a 5% transfusion rate in infants having elective craniosynostosis surgery when both cell saver (25-mL collection reservoir) and erythropoietin were used, compared with a 100% transfusion rate for those not receiving cell-saver techniques or erythropoietin.

Temperature and Positioning

Craniofacial procedures can be very long—sometimes several hours. Complications resulting from long surgical procedures include skin breakdown, neuropathic injury, and hypothermia. Attention must be paid to the initial setup to ensure adequate positioning and padding to minimize these intraoperative injuries. Infants having cranial vault remodeling may be positioned prone, and attention to protecting the face and eyes is important. Patients with midface hypoplasia and proptosis may present a challenge when placed prone, because adequately protecting the face and eyes may be more difficult. The infant is placed on a full-access forced-hot-air blanket to minimize hypothermia, and the surgical site (head) is then isolated from the body using plastic drapes (Fig. 25-8). This not only minimizes convective and radiant heat losses but also prevents conductive heat loss to a bed wet from irrigation and blood. Blood products should be warmed through a fluid warmer before administration (except for platelets). Intravenous fluid warmers may be used, particularly if large volumes of cold allogeneic blood are being administered.

Venous Air Embolism

Venous air embolism (VAE) is a potential complication of craniofacial and neurosurgical procedures (see Chapter 22, Anesthesia for Neurosurgery). VAE can present with hemodynamic instability

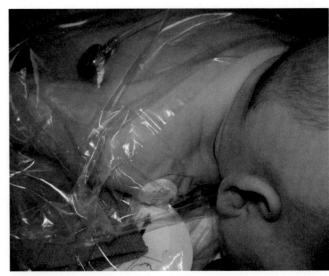

■ **FIGURE 25-8.** The head is isolated from the torso with plastic drapes. The drapes are placed in opposite directions and sealed to minimize moisture and thus hypothermia from blood and irrigation fluids.

TABLE 25-3. Dosage Guidelines for Antifibrinolytic Therapy

Drug	Dosage
Aminocaproic acid (Amicar)	Load 100 mg/kg Infuse 10 mg/kg per hr
Tranexamic acid	Load 10-100 mg/kg Infuse 1-10 mg/kg per hr

and can result in death. VAE occurs commonly in pediatric patients having cranial procedures. A prospective study using precordial Doppler in infants and children having craniosynostosis repair detected VAE in 82% of the patients; 31% percent developed hypotension secondary to VAE, but none developed cardiovascular collapse (Faberowski et al., 2000). This is higher than the previously reported incidence of 66% (Harris et al., 1987). Infants may be at increased risk for VAE, because significant hemorrhage during cranial vault remodeling can result in low central venous pressures. In addition, the relatively large size of the infant head may raise the surgical site above the level of the heart, thereby increasing the pressure gradient for air entrainment. Some advocate the placement of central venous catheters to monitor the trend of central venous pressures and minimize the risk for air embolism. However, no data suggest that central venous pressure monitoring decreases the risk for VAE.

Management of VAE begins with preventing hypovolemic states by providing adequate volume resuscitation and using a precordial Doppler for early detection of VAE. The precordial Doppler should be placed over the left or right parasternal border between the third and sixth intercostal spaces (Schubert et al., 2006). Lowering the head of the bed, left lateral positioning, flooding the surgical field with saline, applying bone wax, discontinuing nitrous oxide, and providing inotropic support are all measures that have been used to acutely manage VAE. Pediatric advanced life support with chest compressions and epinephrine is required for patients who develop symptomatic low blood pressure, bradycardia (heart rate < 60 bpm), or pulseless electrical activity.

Postoperative Care

The postoperative treatment of infants having craniofacial surgery depends on coexisting morbidities and the procedure performed. Most infants and children presenting for cranial vault reconstruction or midface advancement can be extubated in the operating room at the completion of surgery. Factors that may preclude extubation include intraoperative complications resulting in hemodynamic instability, known difficult airway, significant tongue swelling, and intranasal cerebrospinal fluid drainage after Le Fort III osteotomy. Infants in whom distractors were placed may have a more difficult airway after extubation (Fig. 25-9). Mask ventilation can be very difficult with mandibular distractors and impossible with midface distractors. Airway equipment, including oral and nasal airways and appropriately sized LMAs, should be available after extubation. Equipment and personnel to remove part of the distractor device are also important in the operating room (Wong et al., 2004).

Infants having cranial vault remodeling and frontal orbital advancements can experience significant blood loss intraoperatively. If these patients are adequately resuscitated and are hemodynamically stable, they can often be extubated in the operating room. Infants with difficult airways or significant airway obstruction, or those who have experienced intraoperative complications, may benefit from delayed extubation in the intensive care unit (or in the operating room) after their condition has stabilized. Ongoing blood loss is common after major craniofacial surgery, and infants may require repeat transfusions in the immediate postoperative setting. Other complications include cerebral edema (Levine et al., 2001), visual changes (Lo et al., 2002), cerebrospinal fluid leak (Fearon, 2003), infection (Fialkov et al., 2001), metabolic acidosis, and transfusion reactions.

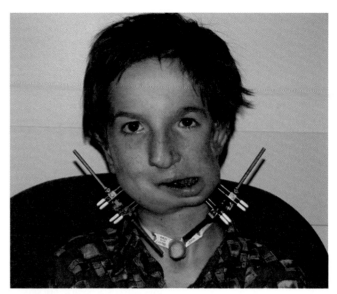

■ FIGURE 25-9. Mandibular distractors.

Hyponatremia has been reported after major intracranial procedures in pediatric patients. This was originally attributed to syndrome of inappropriate diuretic hormone (SIADH). However, this diagnosis has come into question. Although it is not entirely clear, cerebral salt wasting syndrome (CSW) may be the more likely cause. Both SIADH and CSW manifest with hyponatremia. CSW is differentiated from SIADH by hypovolemia, high urine output, and low or normal antidiuretic hormone levels (Levine et al., 2001) (Table 25-4). The proper diagnosis is important because the two are managed differently. SIADH is treated with free water restriction, whereas CSW is managed with isotonic fluid replacement (normal saline) to cover maintenance requirements and urine losses. Frequent sodium evaluations are important to guide therapy.

Hypoplasia

Hypoplasia of the craniofacial skeleton is a category of craniofacial anomalies characterized by hypoplasia or atrophy of a portion of the craniofacial soft tissue and skeleton. Pierre Robin sequence, hemifacial microsomia (including Goldenhar syndrome), and Romberg's disease are examples of these anomalies.

TABLE 25-4. Comparison of Syndrome of Inappropriate Antidiuretic Hormone (SIADH) and Cerebral Salt Wasting (CSW)

Monitoring	SIADH	CSW
Central venous pressure	High (>5)	Low (<5)
Urine output	Decreased	Increased
Urine sodium level	High (>20 mmol/L)	High (>20 mmol/L)
Urine osmolality	High	Low or normal
Serum osmolality	Low	Low or normal
Antidiuretic hormone	High	Normal

Pierre Robin Sequence

Pierre Robin syndrome (PRS) is characterized by retrognathia, glossoptosis (tongue falling to the back of the throat), and airway obstruction. It is referred to as a sequence rather than a syndrome because the small mandible and subsequent airway obstruction is secondary to a fixed fetal position in utero that inhibits mandibular growth. PRS occurs with an incidence of 1 in 20,000 to 50,000. The sequence is often associated with a syndrome such as Stickler syndrome, the syndrome most commonly associated with PRS, which is characterized by micrognathia, poor vision, and a collagen disorder with hyperflexible joints. Other syndromes and facial anomalies seen with PRS include velocardiofacial syndrome, fetal alcohol syndrome, and bilateral hemifacial microsomia.

Neonates and infants with PRS will have some degree of airway obstruction. They often also present with significant reflux and feeding difficulties. Mild airway obstruction may require only lateral or prone positioning to relieve the airway obstruction; however, as many as one quarter of infants with PRS have more severe obstruction, necessitating surgical intervention (Bijnen et al., 2009). The optimal surgical intervention is not clear, and there is significant regional variation. Preoperative evaluation by a pediatric plastic surgeon and pediatric otolaryngologist is essential to completely evaluate the airway and identify coexisting airway pathology. The management options include tongue-lip adhesion, mandibular distraction, and tracheostomy. A tongue-lip adhesion involves suturing the inferior portion of the tongue to the lower lip to prevent the tongue from falling to the back of the pharynx and causing obstruction (Fig. 25-10). Once the mucosal flaps from the tongue and the lower lip are approximated, a temporary retention suture with a button is placed through the floor of the mouth and around the mandible to secure the repair. The infant is intubated postoperatively for several days to ensure the success of the adhesion. The goal of the tongue-lip adhesion is to relieve the airway obstruction and improve feeding until the mandible has had a chance to grow. Some evidence suggests that this repair is effective at decreasing airway obstruction and improving feeding (Kirschner et al., 2003). Bijnen and coworkers

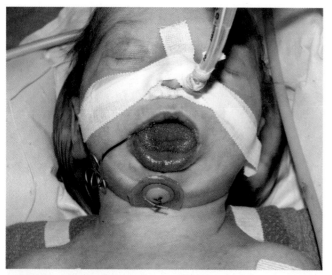

■ FIGURE 25-10. An infant after a tongue-lip adhesion. Note the temporary retention suture placed through the floor of the mouth and fixed in place with a button.

(2009) found that 73% of their patients had improved airway patency, based on sleep studies, and improved feeding. The tongue-lip adhesion is left intact until the patient is approximately 1 year old. At that time, the mandible has had time to grow and the adhesion can be taken down.

An alternative therapeutic approach involves mandibular distraction. In infants with severe obstruction, mandibular distraction can be performed to rapidly distract the jaw. It can be performed in infants less than 6 months old. Genecov and colleagues (2009) recently described their 10-year experience with mandibular distraction for PRS. Of the 67 patients that had preoperative polysomnography, 65 experienced an improvement. Also, several of the patients who required tracheostomy for PRS could be decannulated after their mandibles were distracted.

Tracheostomy is a final option for those patients who fail conservative treatment, tongue-lip adhesion, or distraction. Some have advocated for early tracheostomy for PRS, but there is evidence that it involves increased morbidity and mortality. Also, once infants receive a tracheostomy, it takes on average 3 years for decannulation to occur (Tomaski et al., 1995).

Anesthesia Management

Airway management in the infant with Pierre Robin sequence can be very challenging because of difficulty with mask ventilation and intubation. The laryngeal mask has been successfully used to ventilate and to assist in the intubation of these patients (Markakis et al., 1992). The LMA has even been placed in the awake patient with PRS after regional nerve blockade (Stricker et al., 2008). Nasal intubation with the flexible fiberoptic scope has also been described (Blanco et al., 2001). Other airway devices used for patients with PRS and difficult intubation include the Storz video laryngoscope (KARL STORZ Endoscopy-America, Inc.) and the Airtraq optical laryngoscope (PRODOL MEDITEC S.A.). In addition, when infants have significant difficulty with ventilation or intubation, aside from oral pharyngeal and nasal airways, a suture (0-silk) can be placed at the base of the tongue to displace the tongue anteriorly to assist with ventilation or intubation.

Infants presenting for tongue-lip adhesion or mandibular distraction will require nasal intubation. After inhalation induction with spontaneous ventilation, a flexible fiberoptic nasal intubation can be performed. After the tongue-lip adhesion is completed, infants typically recover in the intensive care unit, where they remain intubated, relaxed, and sedated for several days. Extubation can be performed in the operating room when both the anesthesiologist and pediatric otorhinolaryngologist can be present. When extubation fails, patients may require direct laryngoscopy, bronchoscopy, and tracheostomy. After mandibular distraction, the airway may become even more challenging because once the distractors are in place they may prevent effective mask ventilation.

Hemifacial Microsomia

Hemifacial microsomia is characterized by unilateral or asymmetric development of the facial bones and muscles and frequently involves the ear. This manifests as hypoplasia of the malar-maxillary-mandibular region and usually involves the temporomandibular joint. The vertebral pathology can involve the cervical vertebrae and can significantly reduce the cervical range of motion. Other associated anomalies of hemifacial microsomia include cardiac (ventricular septal defect, tetralogy of Fallot, coarctation), renal, and neurologic defects (hydrocephalus). Patients with hemifacial microsomia can have significant upper airway obstruction and OSA. Most patients with hemifacial microsomia are nonsyndromic, but a small percentage have Goldenhar syndrome, which is characterized by hemifacial microsomia, eye colobomas, and vertebral or scapular anomalies. These patients may be very difficult to intubate.

Anesthesia Management

As with PRS, the most significant anesthetic challenge with hemifacial microsomia is airway management (see Pierre Robin Sequence, Anesthesia Management, earlier). Mask ventilation may be difficult because of facial asymmetry. Intubation may be more challenging because of micrognathia and asymmetric mandibular hypoplasia, and also potentially because of decreased cervical range of motion. This difficulty may decrease with age, but it may increase after surgical reconstruction. Successful ventilation and intubation of the infant have been reported with an LMA and fiberoptic laryngoscopy (Johnson, 1994).

Parry-Romberg Syndrome

Parry-Romberg syndrome is a rare disorder characterized by progressive hemifacial atrophy. Many believe this is a form of linear scleroderma. The process often starts in infancy or later childhood as a pigmented line *(coup de sabre)* on the forehead, and then progressive atrophy (which ultimately burns itself out) affects the subcutaneous tissues and skeleton of the hemiface. Reconstruction, which occurs after the atrophy is complete, is often complicated and may require multiple surgeries. Microvascular flaps and fat injections are surgical options (Hunt and Hobar, 2003).

Clefting

Historically, repair of the cleft lip and palate was performed with no anesthesia (Jones, 1971). It consisted of reapproximating pared tissue edges. These simple and quick procedures were performed on older children or adults who could tolerate the pain and inconvenience of the procedure. At most, patients were allowed to gargle with ice water to produce local numbing. In 1847, Snow described using ether for a cleft lip repair. Later in 1850, chloroform was reported for the repair of a bilateral lip and palate in a 7-year-old (Jones, 1971). The airway was unprotected, and blood could drain into the posterior pharynx. In 1921, Magill provided the first endotracheal insufflation technique on an infant and later applied this technique for the repair of a cleft palate in 1924 (Jones, 1971).

Today, general anesthesia is routinely and safely used for infants, children, and young adults having cleft lip or palate repairs. Typically, surgical repair of the cleft lip is performed at 3 to 6 months and the repair of the cleft palate at 9 to 18 months. Pharyngoplasty, performed for velopalatal insufficiency, is usually performed later, at 5 to 15 years of age. The safe age for cleft lip repair was established to be 6 to 12 weeks in 1964 by an audit of American plastic surgeons (Lewin, 1964) and later supported in 1966 by a large retrospective review (Wilhelmsen and Musgrave, 1966) that showed an increased rate of complications in children with a weight of less than 10 lb, hemoglobin level

less than 10 g/dL, and white cell counts higher than 10,000. More recent studies have highlighted the safety of anesthesia for full-term and preterm neonates (Rudolph, 1974; Van Boven et al., 1993). The authors of these studies stress the importance of having a team of surgeons, anesthesiologists, and nursing staff that are experienced and comfortable with the intraoperative and postoperative care of the neonate. The preoperative preparation of the infant for cleft lip and palate surgery begins with a sound understanding of their anatomy, physiology, and associated anomalies.

Lip and Palate

Surgical Management

Palatoplasty. Many techniques describe the repair of a cleft palate, but all include a hard palate procedure and a soft palate (velar) procedure. Palatoplasties are performed with the intention of obtaining velopharyngeal (VP) competence and normal speech and are typically performed before the first year of age. Hard palate repairs include raising oral mucoperiosteal flaps and mobilizing them to the midline of the cleft defect. These oral flaps are raised on the greater palatine neurovascular bundles. Nasal lining flaps, often harvested from the vomer (the posterior bony portion of the nasal septum), are used to repair the nasal lining of the hard palate. After the nasal lining repair, the oral mucoperiosteal flaps are closed in a straight line.

Velar repairs include straight line and z-plasty techniques. Modern velar repairs include dissecting free the abnormally positioned levator palatini muscle and reconstructing the muscular sling in the velum, thus performing an intravelar veloplasty. The soft palate tissue is mobilized to the midline by use of lateral relaxing incisions, which are left open at the conclusion of the procedure. These raw areas are expected to heal by granulation during the first few postoperative days, with serosanguineous drainage during the early postoperative period. At the conclusion of the procedure, a tongue stitch is often placed, as well as a nasopharyngeal airway for prophylaxis, should postoperative tongue swelling result from pressure placed by the mouth retractor.

Pharyngoplasty. Pharyngoplasties are performed to treat an incompetent velopharyngeal sphincter that allows inappropriate nasal air escape during speech, or hypernasality, defined as VP insufficiency. Pharyngoplasties, often performed as secondary speech procedures after a palatoplasty that failed to result in VP competence, alter the anatomy of the posterior pharynx and the VP port. The VP port is the muscular sphincter connecting the posterior nasal cavity and pharynx, and it is made up anteriorly by the posterior free edge of the soft palate (velum), posteriorly by the posterior pharyngeal wall, and laterally by the tonsillar pillars or lateral pharyngeal walls. Pharyngoplasties include the posterior pharyngeal flap and the sphincter pharyngoplasty.

The *posterior pharyngeal flap* (PPF) is a superiorly based flap of tissue raised off the posterior pharyngeal wall. It includes pharyngeal mucosa and a portion of the superior constrictor muscle. The PPF is superiorly based at the level of C2 or the adenoid pad, and it is inset into the posterior free edge of the velum. The PPF is sewn to the middle of the velum creating VP ports on either side of the PPF. These VP ports function as nasal airways.

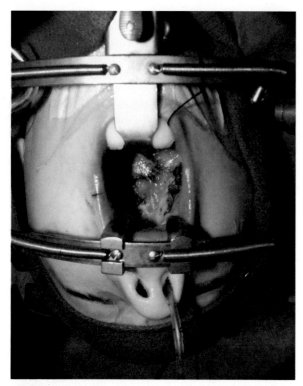

FIGURE 25-11. Cleft palate repair complete. The mouth retractor is in place. Cotton rolls are placed on either side of the oral RAE tube to prevent compression from the metal tongue blade of the mouth retractor.

The *sphincter pharyngoplasty* significantly narrows the VP port by elevating the anterior tonsillar pillar bilaterally with the underlying palatopharyngeus muscle. The bilaterally elevated anterior tonsillar pillars are rotated 90 degrees medially and sewn to a horizontal incision made in the posterior pharyngeal wall. Because the tonsillar pillars are a continuation of the posterior free edge of the velum, this technique creates a much smaller muscular sphincter, thereby greatly narrowing the natural VP port.

Because pharyngoplasties alter the anatomy of the VP port and posterior pharynx, they carry the lifetime risk for overcorrection, hyponasality, and, more importantly OSA.

Anesthesia Management

Most patients with a cleft lip or palate can be induced with a standard inhalational induction. If an IV catheter is in place, an IV induction can also be performed. Induction for patients with orofacial clefting can be achieved with an inhalation agent such as sevoflurane. Airway management for most of these children is straightforward, but difficulty with mask ventilation and intubation can occur in infants with craniofacial anomalies or retrognathia. Airway obstruction can usually be managed with the insertion of an oropharyngeal airway and CPAP.

For the patient with an isolated cleft lip and palate, difficulty with laryngoscopy is common. Some studies have described the incidence of difficult laryngoscopy (laryngoscopic view of Cormack and Lehane laryngoscope view grades 3 and 4) to be as high as 4% to 7% (Xue et al., 2006). Factors predicting a more difficult laryngoscopic view include bilateral clefts and retrognathia. Despite this high percentage of poor laryngoscopic view,

only 1% of the patients were difficult to intubate, and only one patient had a failed intubation (Gunawardana, 1996).

Cleft patients with associated craniofacial anomalies or retrognathia may be difficult to ventilate or intubate. In these patients, preparations for alternative airway management need to be made. If general anesthesia is induced, the patient should remain spontaneously ventilating until the trachea is secured with an endotracheal tube. Successful intubation through a laryngeal mask with the aid of a fiberoptic scope has been described for pediatric patients with difficult airways (Inada et al., 1995). Other intubating devices include the Shikani Optical Stylet (Shukry et al., 2005; Clarus Medical). Surgical repair of the cleft palate using an LMA has even been described (Beveridge, 1989). However, disruption of a previous cleft palate repair during the placement of an LMA has also been described, suggesting that care should be taken when placing an LMA in a patient with a history of cleft palate repair (Somerville et al., 2004).

The oral RAE preformed tracheal tube is routinely used for the intubation because the preformed bend in the tube facilitates the use of the mouth retractor. Care should be paid to securing the tube and protecting it from unintentional extubation. Surgical preparation of the field can result in removal of the tape from the tube if it is not secured well (Fig. 25-12). Because of the fixed length of the preformed oral RAE tube, there is a risk of main stem intubation in a smaller infant. Cotton rolls can be placed in the Dingman-Dott retractor to minimize this risk. There is also an increased risk of extubation if an unexpectedly small endotracheal tube is required. An armor-reinforced endotracheal tube (see Fig. 10-11 in Chapter 10, Equipment) can be used to secure the airway in this situation. These reinforced endotracheal tubes do not kink with flexion, making them ideal for infants or children who require a smaller than expected endotracheal tube. Breath sounds should be reevaluated after the mouth gag is in place because of possible compression of the tube, and because advancement may cause single-lung ventilation.

There is no standard technique for the maintenance of anesthesia. Both inhalation and total IV anesthetics have been described for patients having cleft lip and palate surgery. A balanced anesthetic of an inhalation agent (with or without nitrous

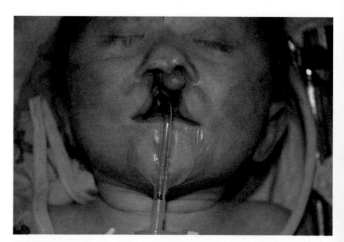

FIGURE 25-12. Securing an oral RAE endotracheal tube for cleft lip or palate surgery. Note the normal midline position of the oral RAE tube. The tube is initially secured with a double-sided adhesive sticker or adhesive tape. A Tegaderm dressing is placed over the tube and the double-sided adhesive stickers (or tape) to protect against the liquid preparation.

oxide), an opioid, and a muscle relaxant (optional) is effective and safe. For patients having palate surgery, keeping the mean arterial pressure at 50 to 60 mm Hg may prevent excessive bleeding from the surgical site. This can be achieved by deepening the anesthetic with inhalation agents, opioids (remifentanil), or α_2-agonists (clonidine or dexmedetomidine). Some studies (Rolla et al., 2003; Steinmetz et al., 2007) have attempted to determine whether the IV or the inhalation technique is better. However, there does not appear to be a clear benefit of either one.

The surgeon infiltrates the palate with epinephrine to prevent excessive bleeding and to facilitate mucosal dissection. It has been demonstrated that inhaled anesthetics sensitize the myocardium and decrease the arrhythmia threshold of epinephrine. Katz and others (1962), almost 50 years ago, described ventricular dysrhythmias when epinephrine was infiltrated during halothane anesthesia. The safe dosage of epinephrine is different for adults and for children. Dosages as low as 1 mcg/kg were found to be arrhythmogenic in adults under halothane anesthesia (Katz et al., 1962). In contrast, a 1983 study found that 10 mcg/kg was safe in children under halothane anesthesia (Karl, 1983). The children in this study ranged from 3 months to 17 years old and were ventilated to maintain an end-tidal CO_2 of 40 mm Hg. The other inhaled anesthetics appear to be as safe or safer than halothane. In adults, the arrhythmogenic dosage of epinephrine was greater than 5 mcg/kg and did not differ between isoflurane, sevoflurane, or desflurane (Moore et al., 1993; Navarro et al., 1994). In children, 10 mcg/kg appears to be a safe maximal dosage of epinephrine for infiltration (see Box 7-3 in Chapter 7, Pharmacology of Pediatric Anesthesia).

Positioning and padding are critical during long periods of anesthesia. In particular, attention should be paid to protecting the infant's chest wall and extremities from the breathing circuit and the tight monitoring leads. The patient is often rotated 90 to 180 degrees, and a straight adapter can facilitate the positioning of the circuit.

Precautions with the airway management should be taken before extubation, especially for patients with difficult airways. Airway obstruction has been described after palatoplasties (Anthony and Sloan, 2002). Patients undergoing a palatoplasty who have a history of a difficult airway or have an associated congenital anomaly should have a nasopharyngeal airway placed by the surgeon before emergence. This may help maintain a patent airway and decrease the work of breathing after extubation (Fig. 25-13). Throat packs can result in airway obstruction if unintentionally left in place, and confirmation of their removal must take place before extubation.

Tongue edema is a particular concern for the anesthesiologist taking care of an extubated patient after cleft palate surgery. Profound tongue, palate, and pharyngeal edema can occur from venous engorgement after use of the Dingman-Dott mouth retractor. It is prudent for surgeons to release the retractor repeatedly throughout the procedure to minimize this risk (Anthony and Sloan, 2002; Oste et al., 2004). Patients experiencing respiratory distress need to be reintubated and mechanically ventilated (Fig. 25-14). It may take several for days for the edema to resolve (Anthony and Sloan, 2002).

Postoperative pain management for cleft lip and palate repair should provide analgesia without respiratory depression, nausea, or vomiting. The best solution seems to be a combination of different medications, usually acetaminophen with the occasional addition of an opioid. Acetaminophen, when

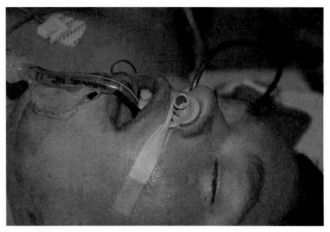

■ **FIGURE 25-13.** Nasopharyngeal airway for airway patency for emergence from cleft palate repair.

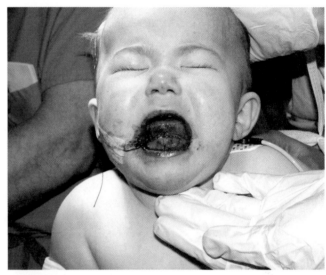

■ **FIGURE 25-14.** Tongue edema secondary to the Dingman-Dott retractor. Note the tongue stitch placed to help displace the tongue anteriorly and relieve the airway obstruction.

administered rectally, is given at an initial dosage of 20 to 40 mg/kg, followed by 20 mg/kg every 6 hours. The oral dosage is 10 to 15 mg/kg every 4 to 6 hours (Birmingham et al., 1997, 2001). Acetaminophen may have an opioid-sparing effect, and some infants after cleft lip repair require none, or very small amounts, in the postoperative period (Stephens et al., 1997).

Nonsteroidal antiinflammatory agents have been described for analgesia after cleft palate surgery (Sylaidis and O'Neill, 1998). Although some evidence suggests there may be no increased risk for bleeding, many surgeons and anesthesiologists choose not to use them routinely. Dosages of opioids, if administered, should be appropriate for weight, to minimize the risk for respiratory compromise in infants. A safe starting dosage of morphine for infants is 0.02 mg/kg every 3 to 4 hours, as needed. Infants undergoing cleft surgery and being given postoperative parenteral narcotics should be appropriately monitored (e.g., for apnea and bradycardia, electrocardiography, oxygen saturation).

The bilateral infraorbital nerve block works very well as an adjunct or as the sole analgesic technique for cleft lip repair

(Eipe et al., 2006). The block, which can be performed by anesthesiologists or surgeons, provides better analgesia than periincisional infiltration or opioids alone (Pradeep et al., 1999; Rajamani et al., 2007). The infraorbital nerve block has been described for all age groups including neonates (Bosenberg and Kible, 1995).

The maxillary division of the trigeminal nerve exits from the infraorbital foramen. The nerve provides the sensory supply to the upper lip, the choana, the maxillary sinus, and part of the nasal septum. This block can be used to provide analgesia for cleft lip surgery, nasal septal repair, and endoscopic sinus surgery. There are two approaches to the maxillary division of the trigeminal nerve: extraoral (percutaneous) and intraoral. For the extraoral approach, the needle is directed toward the infraorbital foramen externally through the skin. The location of the foramen varies with the age. In children and adults, the foramen is located approximately 5 to 10 mm below the infraorbital rim in a vertical line from the pupil of the eye (Fig. 25-15). The thumb or a finger of the hand not holding the syringe can be placed on the inferior orbital rim as a guide and to protect the eye during the injection. The needle is placed just inferior to finger. Once it makes contact with the bone, it is withdrawn slightly and the local anesthetic is injected.

The intraoral route is accessed through the subsulcal area in the buccal mucosa. The point of insertion is the upper incisor or the second bicuspid on the side to be blocked. A needle is passed through the subsulcal route toward the location of the

infraorbital foramen. As with the transcutaneous approach, it is suggested that the thumb or a finger of the hand not holding the syringe be placed on the infant's inferior orbital rim and used as a guide and to protect the orbit and eye. Infants scheduled for cleft lip repairs require 0.5 to 1 mL of local anesthetic solution on each side; for older children and adolescents, 1.5 mL to 2 mL can be used. Bupivacaine (0.125%, 0.25%, or 0.5%, with or without epinephrine [5 mcg/mL]) or ropivacaine (0.2% or 0.5%) can be used for the block.

The duration of postoperative analgesia depends on the local anesthetic and its concentration. For children and adults, 0.125% bupivacaine provided analgesia for approximately 4 to 8 hours (Pradeep et al., 1999). Bupivacaine (0.5%) provides analgesia for 6 to 24 hours (Nicodemus et al., 1991; Eipe et al., 2006). In neonates, the block may be shorter (2 to 3 hours) (Bosenberg and Kible, 1995).

Anesthesia in Developing Countries. Medical missions are performed in developing countries for a variety of procedures including cardiac, orthopedic, and genitourinary. Cleft lip and palate missions are some of the most common and are carried out by multiple organizations around the world. The barriers to providing safe effective surgical and anesthesia care in developing countries include lack of hospital resources (electricity, lighting), medical resources (anesthesia machines, ventilators, oxygen, surgical equipment, medications), personnel resources (lack of training, temperament), standards of care, language skills, and cultural and social differences (Ward and James, 1990; Hodges and Hodges, 2000; Fisher et al., 2001). Despite these barriers, many health care providers volunteer their time and skills to help children with cleft deformities.

There is no standard of care for anesthetizing patients in a developing country, so care must be tailored to the limited available resources. Difficulties include limitations in preoperative evaluations, number of anesthetizing agents, ventilators, monitoring, and postanesthesia care units. The preoperative screening process should identify children with obvious cardiovascular and respiratory pathologies. Because of the high volume and limited ability to preoperatively prepare these patients, many are not selected for surgery.

Pathologies that occur in developing countries and complicate anesthesia care include malnutrition, anemia, and parasitic infections, to name a few. Unfortunately, many of these pathologies are not identified, and it is not clear what impact this has on outcomes. Also, families may withhold information for fear of having the surgery cancelled, which may result in increased morbidity and even mortality (Fisher et al., 2001).

The induction of, maintenance of, and emergence from anesthesia need to be tailored to the available resources. Patients who present for isolated lip repair, and who are old enough, can have the procedure under local anesthesia (Hodges and Hodges, 2000). Patients who require general anesthesia are induced with either an inhalational or an IV technique. Halothane is a commonly used inhalational agent because of its cost. The airway is secured with an endotracheal tube in most circumstances; however, endotracheal tubes may have to be reused. Muscle relaxants in some practices (Fisher et al., 2001) are rarely used because of the lack of mechanical ventilation. In this population, spontaneous ventilation may be safer for the patient, and the anesthetist's hands are free. Some groups preferred muscle relaxants because it facilitated rapid recovery in a setting that had no recovery area (Ward and James, 1990).

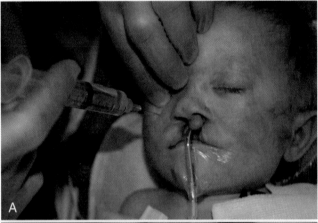

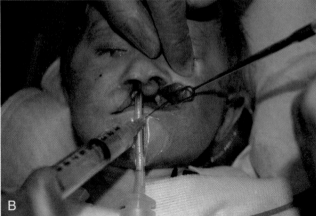

■ **FIGURE 25-15.** Infraorbital nerve block. **A,** The extraoral route. **B,** The intraoral route.

Outcome data for patients having cleft repairs in developing countries are limited. In a recent survey, (Fisher et al., 2001) identified complications associated with surgical patients from Operation Smile. Most of the surgeries were for cleft lip and palate repair, but other common plastic and orthopedic procedures were included. The data, collected from voluntary submission of perioperative data sheets, were collected on 6037 of the 9422 patients. Complications in the operating room, which included laryngospasm, bronchospasm, and unintentional extubation, occurred in 5% of these patients. In the recovery area, complications such as upper airway obstruction, postextubation croup, bronchospasm, and delayed discharge (pain, agitation) occurred in 3.3%. Cardiovascular complications including ventricular ectopy and supraventricular tachycardia occurred in 1.5%. The complications from arrhythmias are most likely underreported because not all patients had electrocardiographic monitoring. Significant negative events that occurred in 1.8% of the patients included return to the operating room for bleeding, intraoperative reintubation, cancellation of surgery after induction, blood transfusion, cardiac arrest, and death. The age of the patient predicted respiratory complications. A significantly larger percentage of children less than 1 year old experienced intraoperative respiratory complications. Death was an uncommon event; during the 18-month collection period, there were four deaths among all of the Operation Smile patients. This death rate of 0.4 per 1000 (Fisher et al., 2001) is higher than some other reports of pediatric perioperative deaths (<1 per 10,000) (Tiret et al., 1988; Morray et al., 2000), but it is difficult to compare the different patient populations. Despite this information, countless lives have benefited from medical missions to developing countries, and most of these procedures are accomplished safely. However, it must be recognized that performing surgery and anesthesia in these environments poses unique cultural, patient care, and system-based challenges for the entire surgical team.

Facial Clefting

Craniofacial clefts involve a defect of the underlying cranial or facial skeleton (or both), as well as the soft tissue envelope, and they can involve the entire face. Tessier classified these defects by the location of the facial clefts. In his classification, the orbit is the center of the defect, and the clefts radiate out like the spokes of a wheel (Whitaker and Bartless, 1990) (Fig. 25-16).

Treacher Collins Syndrome

Treacher Collins syndrome (TCS), also know as mandibulofacial dysostosis, is an example of a bilateral 6, 7, and 8 craniofacial cleft (Fig. 25-17). It was first described in 1846 by Thompson and was further elaborated on by Treacher Collins. Inheritance is as an autosomal dominant pattern with variable penetration. The syndrome is characterized by poorly developed supraorbital ridges, aplastic/hypoplastic zygomas, ear deformities, hearing loss, cleft palate (in one third), and mandibular and midface hypoplasia. From birth, the adequacy of the airway is of primary concern. The degree of airway obstruction is related to the degree of maxillary and mandibular hypoplasia, choanal atresia, and glossoptosis. Tracheostomy may be required during infancy for those at highest risk for OSA and sudden infant death syndrome. The morbidity associated with tracheostomy is significant and some have advocated distraction osteogenesis or tongue-lip adhesion for these patients (Genecov et al., 2009; Thompson et al., 2009). Approximately 50% of patients with

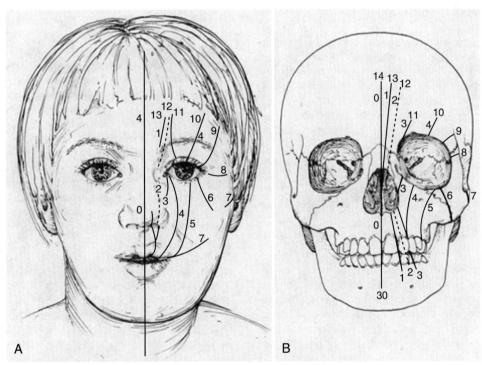

A   B

■ **FIGURE 25-16.** Topographic map of craniofacial clefting. Treacher Collins syndrome is a facial cleft located at 6, 7, and 8. *(From Whitaker LA, Bartlett SP: Craniofacial anomalies. In Jurkiewicz J, Krizek T, Mathes S, et al, editors: Plastic surgery: principles and practice, St Louis, 1990, Mosby, p 99.)*

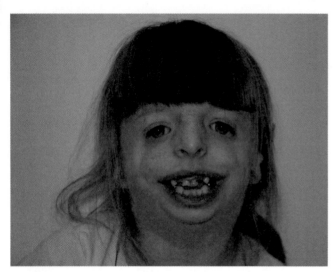

■ **FIGURE 25-17.** Treacher Collins syndrome.

TCS have hearing loss, which occurs secondary to anomalies of the inner ear. They also suffer from external ear anomalies (microtia) (Marres, 2002). Congenital heart disease has been described in patients with TCS but it is uncommon (Gollin, 1976). Developmental delay is also uncommon in this population. These patients are followed by a multidisciplinary craniofacial team and can come to the operating room for a variety of procedures. Aside from cleft lip and palate repair, the timing of major reconstruction typically occurs during childhood or adolescence when the cranioorbital zygomatic bony development is nearly complete.

Surgical Management. The focus of care of the patient with TCS during the first 1 to 2 years of life is on the airway and feeding. These patients may have significant airway obstruction and may require positioning, tongue-lip adhesion, mandibular distraction, or tracheostomy. Patients with an associated cleft palate ideally have it repaired before 1 year of age. After 2 years of age, the surgical care of these patients focuses on restoration of hearing, and on reconstruction of the upper face. Ear surgery can involve the external ear (microtia repair) for cosmesis and the middle ear for hearing. Several surgical procedures have been described to reconstruct the upper face. Autologous and vascularized bone flaps are used to reconstruct the zygoma and orbits, and local flaps have been described to repair the eyelid defects. Unfortunately, good cosmetic results are very difficult to achieve and do not last long. Repeat surgery is common. Once dental development is complete, orthodontic and orthognathic surgery is scheduled. These procedures usually involve a sagittal split osteotomy, with or without a Le Fort I (Thompson et al., 2009).

Anesthesia Management. Anesthetic concerns specific to this syndrome primarily involve the airway. Infants and children with Treacher Collins syndrome may be very difficult or impossible to mask ventilate or intubate, and this airway difficulty may increase with age (Nargozian, 2004). Several techniques have been successfully used to manage the airway safely in these patients. Direct laryngoscopy regardless of the blade used may be difficult. However, the Bullard laryngoscope has been used to successfully intubate a child with TCS (Brown et al., 1993). The LMA has also been used successfully to assist in the

intubation of these children (Ebata et al., 1991; Inada et al., 1995). In one series, the LMA was placed in neonates with PRS and TCS awake, and it was then used to guide intubation (Asai et al., 2008). The LMA has even been used successfully to ventilate a newborn with TCS for an extended period of time (Bucx et al., 2003). Other techniques used to intubate infants and children with TCS include the GlideScope (Verathon) (Bishop et al., 2009), a video-assisted laryngoscope (Sugawara et al., 2009), and the Airtraq optical stylet (PRODOL MEDITEL S.A.) (Hirabayashi et al., 2009). Given the potential for difficult mask ventilation and intubation, this population may be best managed with a sedated fiberoptic intubation. Successful sedation in a 6-year-old with TCS using dexmedetomidine and ketamine has been described (Iravani and Wald, 2008).

Another concern for the anesthesiologist is protecting the patient's eyes. Because of the maxillary and zygomatic hypoplasia, prone positioning may increase the risk for orbital compression and perioperative blindness. Infants and children with TCS can have congenital cardiac defects and require prophylaxis for subacute endocarditis when indicated. Those most affected by upper airway obstruction and OSA may have reduced opioid intraoperative and postoperative requirements (Brown et al., 2004).

Hypertrophy and Vascular Anomalies

Vascular anomalies—disorders of the arteries, veins, capillaries, and lymphatics—were classified by Glowacki and Mulliken (1982). They are divided into two groups: vascular tumors and vascular malformations. The most common vascular tumor is the hemangioma. Vascular malformations are further divided into arterial, venous, capillary, and lymphatic malformations.

Hemangiomas

Hemangiomas, the most common vascular tumor, are characterized by endothelial proliferation and angiogenesis and then postnatal regression. Examples include "strawberry" and capillary hemangiomas. Hemangiomas develop after birth and can be common, with 4% to 12% of infants having one by the first year of life. There is a higher incidence in female children. By 9 years of age, most have involuted. A rule of thumb is that 50% involute by 5 years of age, 70% by 7 years of age, and 90% by 9 years of age (Bruckner and Frieden, 2003). Most hemangiomas appear on the head and neck (60%) or the trunk (24%) (Finn et al., 1983). Airway hemangiomas, although rare, can be seen in infants. The typical clinical findings are cough and stridor. Many airway hemangiomas (60%) have associated cutaneous lesions on the preauricular region, chin, lower lip, and neck (Orlow et al., 1997).

Observation is the most common treatment for hemangiomas, as most resolve on their own, but 10% to 20% require some treatment. Medical therapy includes steroid injections or systemic steroids. Laser therapy with flashlamp pulsed dye lasers can be used for superficial hemangiomas. The neodymium yttrium-aluminum-garnet (Nd:YAG) laser can be used for deep hemangiomas. Lesions that involve the airway, affect vision, or cause a consumptive coagulopathy may need to be embolized. Embolization may also be indicated for hemangiomas that need to be surgically removed, because it may facilitate surgical excision.

Some hemangiomas have associated anomalies. For example, facial hemangiomas can be associated with central nervous system vessel anomalies, coarctation of the aorta, right-sided aortic arch, and eye abnormalities. Some hemangioma-associated syndromes are of importance to the anesthesiologist. PHACES syndrome occurs with facial hemangiomas and is composed of *p*osterior fossa abnormalities (Dandy-Walker), *h*emangiomas, *a*rterial anomalies (coarctation), *c*ongenital heart disease (patent ductus arteriosus, ventricular septal defect), *e*ye abnormalities (cataracts), and *s*ternal defects (Poetke et al., 2002).

Vascular Malformations

Vascular malformations occur because of an error in the embryonic vascular structure. Unlike vascular tumors, these malformations are present at birth and grow with the child. The malformation can be arterial, venous, capillary, or lymphatic. Arterial vascular malformations are referred to as high-flow lesions, whereas capillary, venous, and lymphatic malformations are low-flow lesions. MRI is one of the best ways to define the internal structure of these malformations.

Arterial. Arterial malformations are often asymptomatic. However, when they do become symptomatic they may have systemic sequelae. These malformations may cause limb hypertrophy or if extensive may result in a consumptive coagulopathy or congestive heart failure. Treatment is more effective with staged excision and embolization (Upton et al., 1985).

Capillary. Capillary malformations occur in 0.3% to 0.5 % of infants. They often appear on the face and neck. Port-wine stains and nevus flammeus are examples. Facial port-wine stains typically occur in the trigeminal nerve distributions V1 (ophthalmic) and V2 (maxillary). Glaucoma and retinal arterial venous malformations are associated findings, and these patients need to be evaluated by an ophthalmologist. Head and brain MRI may also be required to identify underlying leptomeningeal malformations and choroidal angioma. Associated syndromes of capillary malformations include Sturge-Weber and Klippel-Trénaunay. Sturge-Weber syndrome consists of port-wine stain in the V1 trigeminal nerve distribution, glaucoma, overgrowth of the facial skeleton, leptomeningeal malformations, choroidal angiomas, and seizures (Fig. 25-18). Klippel-Trénaunay syndrome consists of capillary, venous, and lymphatic malformations. These lesions may involve the trunk and the extremities (Fig. 25-19). Treatment for capillary vascular malformations consists of multiple treatments with flashlamp pulsed dye lasers (Garzon et al., 2007).

Venous. Venous malformations are low-flow lesions that typically appear on the extremities and are often asymptomatic. However, they may occur in the gastrointestinal tract and can cause bleeding. Because most venous malformations are asymptomatic, treatment is conservative and consists of compressive garments. Treatment for symptomatic lesions includes embolization, sclerotherapy, and surgical excision (Hein et al., 2002).

Lymphatic. Lymphatic malformations are low-flow lesions that can involve the skin and underlying muscle. They typically appear on the head, neck, axillae, and chest. Lesions in the neck can be massive and can cause airway compromise, especially if they become infected and enlarged (Greinwald et al., 2008). These lesions do not regress spontaneously. They can be associated with

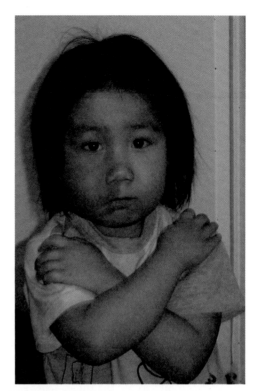

■ **FIGURE 25-18.** Sturge-Weber syndrome.

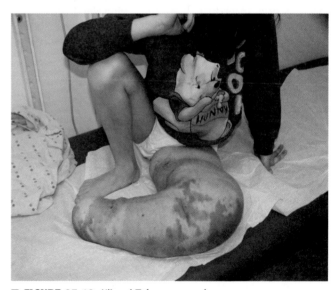

■ **FIGURE 25-19.** Klippel-Trénaunay syndrome.

syndromes including Klippel-Trénaunay, Turner's, Noonan's, and trisomies 13, 18, and 21. Intralesional sclerotherapy, laser treatment (CO_2, Nd:YAG), and surgical excision have been described for their treatment (Padwa et al., 1995).

Anesthesia Management

Anesthesia for patients with vascular tumors or malformations can range from routine and uncomplicated to difficult and life threatening. For many patients with a small vascular malformation in an anatomic location of minimal clinical consequence, anesthesia for radiologic evaluation, radiologic intervention, or surgery can be safe and uneventful. However, anesthesia for vascular malformations can be more complicated because of anatomic location (airway), size and systemic involvement (congestive heart failure, thrombocytopenia, blood loss), and sequelae from therapeutic interventions (ethanol sclerotherapy).

Patients with hemangiomas or capillary malformations such as the port-wine stain may present for repeat laser treatments. For those patients with few or no comorbidities, these treatments can be performed in the outpatient setting. Typically, an inhalational anesthetic via a mask with or without IV access is all that is required. Lesions on the face or back may require an LMA or an endotracheal tube to secure the airway (Isago et al., 2006). Nitrous oxide, although safe for induction, may pose a fire hazard when laser treatments are near the face. Postoperative analgesia can be achieved with acetaminophen.

Vascular malformations involving the airway can lead to respiratory obstruction and OSA (Arneja and Gosain, 2008). In the anesthetized patient, there may be problems with ventilation and intubation (Nargozian, 2004; McLoughlin and McBrien, 2009). Some of the vascular malformations may not initially be obstructing lesions, but after sclerotherapy treatment or dependent positioning may swell dramatically leading to an obstructed airway (Sun et al., 2009). These patients may require alternative techniques to secure the endotracheal tube, such as a fiberoptic scope, the GlideScope, esophageal intubating devices, or intubating through an LMA. A hallmark of the management of the difficult pediatric airway is to secure the airway under general anesthesia while preserving spontaneous ventilation. When preservation of spontaneous ventilation under general anesthesia is not feasible, an awake or sedated intubation or tracheostomy is required. Patients with a consumptive process (Kasabach-Merritt syndrome) may be predisposed to intraoperative bleeding secondary to thrombocytopenia, and they may not be candidates for a regional anesthetic technique. However, regional anesthesia (intrathecal block) has been described in patients with Kasabach-Merritt syndrome when their platelet count is stable (Holak and Pagel, 2010).

Congenital Melanocytic Nevi

Congenital melanocytic nevi are pigmented, plaquelike skin lesions that are typically present at birth and persist and become more pigmented with age. They are classified by their size, which ranges from small to giant. Small nevi are 1.5 cm or less in diameter. Medium-sized nevi measure 1.5 to 19.9 cm in diameter, and large nevi have a diameter of greater than 20 cm. The giant nevi are significantly larger, with a diameter of greater than 50 cm. Small and medium nevi are more common and occur in approximately 1 in 1000 live births. Large nevi are less common and occur in 1 in 20,000 live births. Giant nevi are far less common and occur in only 1 in 50,000 births (Zaal et al., 2005). Besides the cosmetic concerns about congenital melanocytic nevi, there is the risk for malignant transformation, and this is an important consideration for removing these lesions. (Zaal et al., 2005) demonstrated in a large Dutch study that patients with congenital melanocytic nevi have a higher risk for developing malignant melanoma (15 cases in 19,253 person-years versus 1.2 expected cases), and the risk appears to be even higher in those with giant congenital melanocytic nevi. Some have reported melanoma rates as high as 10% in large

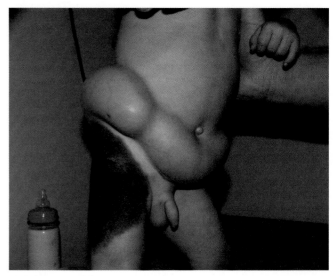

■ **FIGURE 25-20.** Tissue expanders placed circumferentially around the waist.

nevi, with the majority of the malignant transformations in the largest lesions occurring by puberty (Tromberg et al., 2005).

Prophylactic removal of large nevi is typically performed early in life. The complexity of the surgical management of congenital nevi depends on the size and the location of the lesion. Large nevi may require a staged excision or the use of tissue expanders (Fig. 25-20). Placement of tissue expanders may occur at as early as 6 months of age. The expanders can be placed in the scalp, forehead, trunk, back, and lower extremities. Expansion is performed gradually over weeks to months and may allow complete closure after the nevi is surgically removed. Other treatment modalities include dermabrasion, lasers (CO_2), and curettage. All of these techniques typically require general anesthesia. Patients with large congenital nevi may also require anesthesia for MRI evaluation for neurocutaneous melanosis. Patients with large nevi in axial locations (head, neck, back) are at increased risk for having melanocyte proliferation in the leptomeninges (pia and arachnoid mater). These melanocytes may malignantly transform and require radiologic surveillance (Lovett et al., 2009).

Anesthesia Management

Many surgical excisions for small and medium nevi in children and adolescents can be performed under local anesthesia in an office setting. Younger patients, or patients who are uncooperative, may require a general anesthetic to facilitate excision. For healthy patients, excisions can typically be performed in an office setting or an ambulatory surgical center. An inhalational anesthetic will achieve appropriate surgical conditions. Depending on the size of the lesion and its location, an IV and an LMA or endotracheal tube may be required. Larger lesions are more likely to require a general anesthetic because of the degree of tissue resection and undermining, the duration of the procedure, and the location of the lesion. Regional anesthesia can be combined with general anesthesia to ensure a pain-free postoperative course. The regional technique can be a neuraxial (single-shot caudal) or peripheral block, depending on the location and size of the surgical excision.

Trauma

Facial Fractures

Trauma to the facial skeleton may result in one or more fractures and may require surgical fixation. Typical facial fractures include zygoma fractures, Le Fort II, Le Fort III, mandible, orbital, nasal, and panfacial fractures. Depending on the mechanism of injury, there may be associated injuries, the most concerning of which is traumatic brain injury. In one study, 25% of patients diagnosed with facial fractures had associated injuries, including limb, brain, chest, spine, and abdominal injuries. Up to 10% of these patients had a brain injury (Thoren et al., 2010). Although only 2.7% of the patients had spinal injuries, almost all of these involved the cervical spine. Another study demonstrated that up to 69% of patients with mandible fractures had an associated traumatic brain injury. Although most of these patients had mild traumatic brain injury, up to 40% of them had a moderate to severe injury (intraparenchymal hemorrhage, epidural or subdural hemorrhage). Of concern, 20% of the patients with mild brain injuries had minimal signs or symptoms (Glasgow Coma Scale [GCS] 15, or no loss of consciousness), but they had an injury documented by computed tomography scan (Czerwinski et al., 2008). The hazard is that these brain injuries may be missed.

Anesthesia Management

Anesthesia management for the pediatric facial fracture patients begins with a complete trauma assessment to identify airway pathology and then to identify associated injuries. Patients at risk for a brain injury with an underlying intracranial lesion (mandible, facial fracture with GCS < 15 or loss of consciousness) should have a neurosurgical evaluation prior to anesthesia for their facial fractures.

Facial fractures involving the midface commonly result in airway compromise because of the displacement of the midface posteriorly into the oropharynx. Blood and secretions may also contribute to airway obstruction. One third of adult patients in one study with midface fractures required intubation (Ng et al., 1998). Patients with Le Fort III fractures developed more severe airway obstruction than patients with Le Fort I or II fractures. In fact, up to 40% of Le Fort III fractures required tracheostomy in one study of adults, compared with 9% of Le Fort I and II fractures (Bagheri et al., 2005).

The airway management of pediatric patients with facial fractures can be challenging. Those with mild injuries like an isolated zygoma or orbital floor fracture typically do not present a significant challenge. However, those patients with complicated midface fractures (Le Fort III) or panfacial fractures can present a dilemma. Children not properly fasted require either a rapid-sequence induction or a sedated fiberoptic intubation. All patients with suspected or known cervical injuries require cervical immobilization.

Facial fractures that result in malocclusion (mandible or Le Fort I) require maxillomandibular fixation (MMF). Intubation options that allow MMF include nasal or retromolar intubation. If there is concern for a full stomach and aspiration, the airway can be initially secured with an oral endotracheal tube after a rapid-sequence induction. The oral endotracheal tube can then be changed to a nasal endotracheal tube using direct laryngoscopy or fiberoptic guidance. The nasal endotracheal tube can also be placed initially in the awake patient with sedation and topical local anesthetic.

This technique, however, is not an ideal option for the injured pediatric patient. The retromolar approach has been described for patients requiring MMF. This technique requires placing the endotracheal in the retromolar space, and it is meant for short-term intubation. The endotracheal tube can be sutured or wired in place by the surgeon. A smaller tube is recommended, and the anesthesiologist needs to be aware of the peak airway pressures once the tube is manipulated into this space (Lee et al., 2009).

The airway options for the patient with midface fractures or panfacial fractures include the placement of an oral endotracheal tube, submandibular airway, or tracheostomy. If MMF is not required, an oral intubation can be performed. In the patient who requires either MMF or long-term intubation, a submandibular airway or tracheostomy is recommended. A nasotracheal intubation is relatively contraindicated in patients with significant midface fractures (Le Fort II and III) because of concern for neurologic injury in those with a skull base (cribriform plate) fracture.

Traditionally, a short-term tracheostomy was recommended for patients with panfacial fractures because of the prolonged intubation in a patient with a potentially difficult airway or MMF. However, tracheostomy has an associated morbidity, and some have advocated a submental or submandibular approach to the airway (Amin et al., 2002; Anwer et al., 2007). The technique is performed after the patient is anesthetized and orally intubated. An armor-reinforced tube is recommended to prevent kinking. A small submandibular incision is made by the surgeon and bluntly dissected until it communicates with the floor of the mouth. The endotracheal tube cuff and then the end of the endotracheal tube (without the adaptor for the circuit) can be passed through this opening with the assistance of curved forceps or hemostats. The tube is sutured in place (Fig. 25-21). The submandibular airway can be removed at the end of surgery or can be left in place for several days (Amin et al., 2002; Anwer, 2009). This technique has been described for young adolescents (12 years old) (Eipe et al., 2005) and children as young as 6 years (Amin et al., 2002). Patients that are placed in MMF should have wire cutters at the bedside to release the fixation in case of an airway emergency. Even in skilled hands, this may

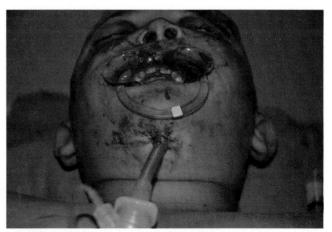

■ **FIGURE 25-21.** Submandibular intubation.

not be quick. In one study, surgeons were able to remove the fixation in 30 seconds, but nonsurgical hospital staff took more than 2 minutes (Goss et al., 1979).

EXTREMITY SURGERY

Hand Surgery

Congenital hand anomalies are numerous and varied. A classification of hand anomalies and descriptions of specific defects follow. Approximately 1 in 600 infants is born with some form of congenital hand anomaly. The terminology of hand anomalies (Table 25-5) reflects the type, classification, and degree of the defect (Netscher and Baumholtz, 2007). Surgical correction is needed for many of them. The American Society of Surgery of the Hand has created a classification of these anomalies (Box 25-1).

Most anomalies can be surgically managed after the first year of life, but there are a few indications for neonatal hand surgery. Neonates with a superficial extra digit (attached by skin) can have it removed easily with local anesthesia and ligation without general anesthesia or sedation. Constriction bands that compromise circulation or lymphatic drainage often require urgent surgical correction in the neonatal period.

Anomalies that require surgical correction after the neonatal period but before 1 year of age are the syndactylies that occur between fingers of unequal length (Fig. 25-22). Hands exhibit a growth spurt by 2 years of age. Digits of unequal length that are fused together may need to be separated before significant hand growth occurs, because the anomalous growth of one of

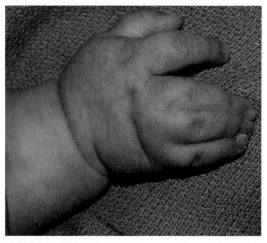

■ **FIGURE 25-22.** Hand syndactyly.

the digits may alter the growth of the other digit if they remain tethered together. Also, surgeries that affect critical hand function, such as opposition, need to be performed early so the development of grasping skills is not delayed. Thus, pollicization, movement of the index finger into the thumb position for a baby without a thumb, may be done on the early side, so that the child can grasp things with the thumb and perform the critical function known as opposition.

Brachial Plexus Palsy

Obstetric brachial plexus palsy is defined as an injury or a disruption to one or more of the trunks (C5 to T1) of the brachial plexus. The injury occurs at an incidence of 0.4 to 4 per 100 vaginal births and decreases significantly for cesarean sections but does not decrease to zero. Usually the injury occurs during passage through the birth canal. Perinatal risk factors for a brachial injury are thought to include large size for gestational age, shoulder dystocia, breech presentation, prolonged labor, and history of previous brachial plexus injuries (Waters, 2005). Patients present with varying degrees of motor and sensory loss of the upper extremity, depending on the type of injury.

The injuries are categorized into four groups, and the groupings predict outcome and guide recommendations for surgical intervention. Group one, involving an injury to the C5 to C6 trunks only, is the most common injury and accounts for approximately 50% of brachial plexus injuries. This upper trunk lesion is commonly called an Erb's palsy. This group has the best prognosis. Group two involves an injury or disruption to the C5 to C7 trunks. Nearly 30% of patients with brachial plexopathy have this injury, and its prognosis is worse than for group one. Group three involves the entire brachial plexus (C5 to T1), with complete loss of function of the entire upper extremity. This injury pattern is seen in 20% of patients. Group four is the most severe, with injury to the entire brachial plexus, including the sympathetic chain. This injury most likely involves an avulsion at or near the spinal cord. These patients have complete loss of motor function of the upper extremity and Horner's syndrome (ptosis, miosis, and anhydrosis). They may also have other motor injuries involving the phrenic, long thoracic, dorsoscapular, and suprascapular nerves (Hale, 2010).

TABLE 25-5. Terminology for Hand Anomalies

Term	Definition
Brachy-	Short
Clino-	Bent
Campto-	Flexed
Phoco-	Shortened or "seal-like"
-Melia-	Extremity
Syn-	Side-to-side fusion
Sym-	Longitudinal fusion

From Netscher DT, Baumholtz MA: Treatment of congenital upper extremity problems, *Plast Reconstr Surg* 119:101e–129e, 2007.

Box 25-1 Types of Congenital Hand Anomalies

Failure of formation of parts (amelia, phocomelia)
Failure of differentiation (syndactyly, clinodactyly)
Duplication (polydactyly)
Overgrowth (macrodactyly)
Undergrowth (hypoplastic thumb)
Constriction band syndrome
Generalized skeletal deformity (dwarfism)

From Netscher DT, Baumholtz MA: Treatment of congenital upper extremity problems, *Plast Reconstr Surg* 119:101e–129e, 2007.

Most brachial plexus injuries are transient and resolve with time alone. Physical therapy often helps to keep the shoulder joint supple while the nerves are recovering. Surgical repair is recommended for patients with group four injuries who are less than 3 months old. The timing and role of brachial plexus surgery become more controversial in those patients in groups one to three who do not demonstrate clinical recovery by 6 to 9 months of age. Surgical repair often involves exploration and resection of the neuroma and placement of a nerve graft. Nerve grafts can be harvested from several locations but the sural nerve is most often used (Waters, 2005; Hale et al., 2010). Neurolysis may be performed if the nerve appears completely normal but is encased by scar (Clarke, 2007).

Anesthesia Management

The anesthesia management of the pediatric patient presenting for upper extremity surgery begins with a thorough preoperative evaluation. Infants and children with hand anomalies may have underlying systemic disorders. Some of the syndromic craniofacial anomalies (Apert and Pfeiffer syndromes) may have associated upper extremity anomalies that need hand surgery. The anesthesia issues concerning these syndromes are outlined in Table 25-1. Patients with epidermolysis bullosa present for hand surgery because of the pseudosyndactyly from dermal loss. Anesthesia for these patients is described in Chapter 36, Systemic Disorders.

Other syndromes involving the hand may also involve the heart. Holt-Oram syndrome, otherwise known as hand-heart syndrome, exhibits varying degrees of congenital cardiac disease and arrhythmias (Shono et al., 1998). The degree of hand pathology does not predict the degree of cardiac involvement. A history consistent with cardiac pathology (poor feeding, sweating with feeding, cyanosis, syncope) or a heart murmur on examination warrants a cardiac evaluation before surgery. Patients with radial anomalies (aplasia) may have an associated VATER (vertebral defects, imperforate anus, tracheoesophageal fistula, radial and renal dysplasia) association. These patients require a preoperative evaluation to identify cardiac, renal, and vertebral anomalies. Radial anomalies also occur with the TAR (thrombocytopenia–absent radius) syndrome. The Poland sequence, also associated with upper extremity anomalies, starts with an initial chest wall deformity and then subsequent ipsilateral upper extremity anomalies. These patients may have significant thoracic insufficiency (Sethuraman et al., 1998).

Patients with brachial plexus injury should be evaluated for the degree of injury. Many patients presenting for surgery have a group four injury, which involves injury to the entire brachial plexus and the sympathetic chain. Horner's syndrome should be noted preoperatively. A small number may have injury to the phrenic nerve as well. This may affect respiratory reserve, and the anesthesia team should be aware of this preoperatively. Often the surgeon will have obtained a preoperative ultrasound of the diaphragm to diagnose this before the operation.

When patients having hand surgery are otherwise healthy, general anesthesia can be used, with or without peripheral nerve blockade. Older patients can have hand procedures with a regional technique as the primary anesthetic (see Chapter 16, Regional Anesthesia). Anesthesia can be achieved with an inhalation or IV induction. Airway management depends on the size of the patient, coexisting disease, and duration of surgery. Infants having procedures with surgical field avoidance most likely require endotracheal intubation. Otherwise, larger healthy children can have their airway managed with an LMA. Patients with congenital heart disease do not require subacute endocarditis prophylaxis for hand surgery.

Patients presenting for surgical repair of the brachial plexus require a general anesthetic. The airway is managed with an endotracheal tube, as the surgery is long and the surgical field is close to the airway. It is important to secure the endotracheal tube well, because the head and shoulder may be moved during the operation. Use of a transparent drape for the uppermost sterile drape can help the anesthesiologist monitor the endotracheal tube position (Clarke, 2007). Neuromuscular blockade may be used for intubation, but a short- or intermediate-acting agent should be used and should not be repeated if the surgeons are using neuromuscular monitoring. Remifentanil with an inhalation or IV anesthetic will help produce a profound level of anesthesia and akinesis in those patients where neuromuscular blockade is avoided. The surgical repair of the brachial plexus may be lengthy and may require exposure of large areas of the infant. Sometimes both lower extremities are exposed and prepared so as to harvest the sural nerve. Proper padding is essential to minimize risk for pressure injuries, and multiple warming devices (forced hot air devices and warming lamps) may be required to maintain normothermia.

SUMMARY

The anesthetic management of the pediatric patient receiving plastic surgery can be varied and complex. Many of these patients have minimal coexisting disease and can be treated in an outpatient or third-world setting. However, some have multisystem involvement and life-threatening pathologies requiring intensive intraoperative and postoperative care. Also, these patients are cared for by multiple pediatric subspecialties including neurosurgery and otorhinolaryngology. Having an appreciation of the range of clinical disease states and surgical interventions required for the pediatric plastic surgery patient is essential for the pediatric anesthesiologist.

For questions and answers on topics in this chapter, go to "Chapter Questions" at www.expertconsult.com.

REFERENCES

Complete references used in this text can be found online at www.expertconsult.com.

Anesthesia for Orthopedic Surgery

Aaron L. Zuckerberg and Myron Yaster

CONTENTS

The topic of anesthesia for pediatric orthopedic surgery encompasses the entire age and medical spectrum of pediatrics and includes the newborn and adolescent, the otherwise normal, the chronically ill, the patient with multiple complex congenital anomalies, the patient with emergent trauma, the elective inpatient, and the outpatient. Orthopedic surgeons operate on virtually every area of the body from the cervical spine to the pelvis to the toes. In many instances, the perioperative anesthesia plan for pediatric orthopedic patients depends more on their ages, on the site and emergent nature of surgery, and on the need for perioperative analgesia and sedation, than it does on the underlying disease or the specifics of the surgical procedure. In other cases, the underlying medical condition, associated anomalies, pathophysiology, and surgical procedure dictate the anesthesia plan. Positioning the patient on the operating room table may be difficult because of deformities or contractures, and often patients require special operating tables or frames to achieve the best posture for surgery. The anesthesiologist must be aware of unusual associated syndromes that have clear orthopedic implications, and syndromes with underlying clinical significance unrelated to the orthopedic condition. Conditions that are commonly encountered in pediatric orthopedic surgery and their anesthesia implications are listed in Table 26-1, but the list is by no means comprehensive (Campbell, 2009). The Online Mendelian Inheritance in Man website (www.ncbi.nlm.nih.gov/omim) is a good source for this information.

Orthopedic surgery is among the most common types of surgery performed in the United States. Technological advances permit more sophisticated orthopedic diagnoses, and they have vastly expanded the range of treatment options and operations available to the orthopedic surgeon. Moreover, technological, physiologic, and pharmacologic advances in anesthesiology have allowed the orthopedic surgeon to contemplate longer, more extensive, and more innovative operations on younger and sicker patients than were ever before possible. Regardless of the underlying condition, almost all orthopedic surgical procedures have recurring anesthesia concerns, including positioning, airway management, blood loss and fluid replacement, conservation of body temperature, and postoperative pain and sedation management.

A common feature of children with orthopedic diseases, particularly patients with congenital anomalies, generalized constitutional diseases of bone and cartilage, or connective tissue disorders, is the significant disability that affects their everyday lives. Some of these children must undergo multiple hospitalizations, anesthesias, and surgical procedures. A single bad anesthesia experience can have an impact on care for years, and an individualized approach is necessary. Sometimes, these children are overwhelmingly fearful and may be completely terrorized by the hospital experience. Simply approaching these children in hospital clothing may elicit screams of terror. Others are seasoned veterans and have

TABLE 26-1. Anesthetic Implications of Commonly Encountered Orthopedic Disorders

Disease	Surgical Interventions	Anesthetic Implications
Congenital Malformations		
Amniotic band constriction	Soft tissue release	May have facial clefts
Clubfoot	Tendon lengthening, release	Dictated by associated malformations
Klippel-Feil syndrome	Release, scoliosis	Hemifused or fused vertebra; limited cervical spine mobility; possible difficult intubation; heart defects
Radial dysgenesis	Tendon lengthening, pollicization release	Episodic thrombocytopenia; congenital heart disease
Sprengel's deformity	—	Associated only with Klippel-Feil syndrome
Trisomy 21 (Down syndrome)	Cervical spine fusion	Large tongue; usually easy intubation; in-line stabilization during intubation; congenital heart disease; opioid sensitivity
Acquired Conditions		
Charcot-Marie-Tooth disease	Tendon transfer	Possible sensitivity with nondepolarizing muscle relaxants; succinylcholine may result in hyperkalemia
Legg-Calvé-Perthes disease	Osteotomies, pinning	None known
Osteomyelitis	Culture, aspiration	Systemic bacterial infection
Septic arthritis	Culture, irrigation	Systemic bacterial infection
Slipped femoral capital epiphysis	Pinning	Obesity
Tumors, benign	Excision, curettage	Possible significant blood loss; pathologic fracture
Tumors, malignant	Radical excision, amputation	Blood loss; metastasis: CNS, lung; chemotherapy; cardiotoxicity
Syndromes, Inherited Conditions		
Apert syndrome and Crouzon disease	Syndactyly repair; craniosynostosis; hypertelorism	Airway usually normal, but occasional mandibular hypoplasia; cardiac defect
Ellis-van Creveld syndrome	Polydactyly	Cardiac defects; bronchial collapse
Holt-Oram syndrome	Tendon lengthening, pollicization release	Cardiac defects (ASD, VSD)
Jeune syndrome (asphyxiating thoracic dystrophy)	Chest reconstruction, scoliosis	Respiratory failure, prolonged mechanical ventilation; renal failure
Marfan syndrome	Scoliosis	Cardiac (AI, MR), aortic aneurysm
Moebius sequence	Syndactyly	Micrognathia; cleft palate; cranial nerve palsy
Osteogenesis imperfecta	Pathologic fractures, scoliosis	Fractures on positioning or intubation; hypermetabolic fever, platelet dysfunction; blood pressure cuff may cause fractures
VATER (vertebral, anal, tracheal esophageal fistula, renal, cardiac)	Tendon lengthening, pollicization release	Cardiac defects; tracheoesophageal fistula
Short-Stature Syndrome		
Achondroplasia	Spinal fusion, cervical decompression, Ilizarov	Poor cervical mobility, difficult arterial catheterization
Morquio-Ullrich disease	Cervical spine fusion	Poor cervical mobility, difficult airway
Mucopolysaccharidoses (Hurler's, Hunter's, Morquio's syndromes)	Kyphoscoliosis, bony abnormalities	Very difficult intubations; unstable necks; respiratory failure perioperatively
Systemic Disease		
Juvenile rheumatoid arthritis	Varies	TMJ ankylosis; cervical spine immobility or instability; carditis; occasional pulmonary involvement; difficult airway
Neurofibromatosis	Scoliosis	CNS tumors; occasional pheochromocytoma
Sickle cell anemia	Osteomyelitis, Legg-Calvé-Perthes disease, pathologic fracture	Anemia; vasoocclusive crisis; acute chest syndrome; stroke; hypothermia; hypoxia; hypovolemia; immunocompromised host; avoid tourniquet when possible

(Continued)

TABLE 26-1. Anesthetic Implications of Commonly Encountered Orthopedic Disorders—cont'd

Disease	Surgical Interventions	Anesthetic Implications
CNS Diseases		
Arthrogryposis multiplex	Tendon releases (multiple congenital contractures), scoliosis	Difficult intubation (TMJ ankylosis, cervical spine immobility); GE reflux; postoperative upper airway obstruction; congenital heart disease
Cerebral palsy	Tendon releases	GE reflux; postoperative upper airway obstruction
Myelomeningocele	Lower extremity tendon releases, scoliosis, kyphosis	Hydrocephalus
Werdnig-Hoffmann disease	Scoliosis	Respiratory insufficiency; bulbar involvement (poor secretion handling); succinylcholine-induced hyperkalemia
Myopathies		
Duchenne's muscular dystrophy	Tendon releases, scoliosis	Respiratory insufficiency; cardiomyopathy; succinylcholine-induced hyperkalemia; anesthesia induced rhabdomyolysis
Myotonia dystrophica	Tendon releases	Succinylcholine-induced myotonic spasm; cardiac conduction system involvement; avoid direct muscle stimulation

AI, Aortic incompetence; *ASD,* atrial septal defect; *CNS,* central nervous system; *GE,* gastroesophageal; *MR,* mitral regurgitation; *TMJ,* temporomandibular joint; *VSD,* ventricular septal defect.

very specific desires about who should treat them and how they are to be anesthetized. For example, some may prefer an intravenous (IV) induction to a mask induction, or have specific sites in which they want their IV placed. Thus, the anesthesiologist must have knowledge of the particular surgeon, the procedure, the positioning of the patient, and the expected duration of the procedure.

SCOLIOSIS

Scoliosis, derived from the Greek root meaning "crooked," is a lateral and rotational deformity of the thoracolumbar spine. With progression of the lateral spinal curvature, the spinous processes rotate toward the concave side of the curve. The ribs on the convex side are pushed posteriorly by the rotating spine, forming the characteristic gibbous deformity. The ribs on the concave side become prominent anteriorly and are crowded together. Occasionally, scoliosis is associated with kyphosis ("humpback") or lordosis ("bent backward") (Fig. 26-1).

The progression of scoliosis and the severity of its systemic manifestations correlate with the angle of curvature measured by the Cobb method (Table 26-2)—that is, the angle between the upper surface of the top vertebra and the lower surface of the bottom vertebra. The end vertebrae are those that are maximally tilted. Perpendicular lines are extended from these end vertebrae to the center of the curve. The angle formed by the intersecting perpendiculars determines the angle of curvature (Fig. 26-2). The curve is defined as facing to the right or to the left, depending on the convexity of the curve. A lateral curve of greater than 10 degrees is abnormal. Respiratory impairment rarely occurs with a curvature of less than 60 degrees.

Epidemiology and Etiology

The overall prevalence of spinal deformities in the North American population is between 1% and 2% (Weinstein et al., 2003). Curves can be described on the basis of their anatomic configurations, age of onset, and associated pathology. In the past, polio and tuberculosis infection were the most common causes. Today, most cases of scoliosis are classified as idiopathic because the basic pathophysiology is unknown. Pedigree analysis suggests that scoliosis is a sex-linked trait with variable expression and incomplete penetrance (Xiong and Sevastik, 1998; Lowe et al., 2000). The most common types of scoliosis are listed in Box 26-1.

Congenital scoliosis is a curvature of the spine that is the result of a rib or vertebral anomaly. *Idiopathic scoliosis* is the most common of the spinal deformities and has three periods of onset, all coincident with periods of rapid growth spurts: infantile (<3 years old), juvenile (3 to 10 years old), and adolescent (>10 years old). Progression of the deformity depends on the age of onset. *Infantile idiopathic scoliosis* is associated with an increased incidence of mental retardation, inguinal hernias, congenital dislocation of the hip, and congenital heart disease. *Juvenile idiopathic scoliosis* can usually be managed conservatively (Lowe et al., 2000). *Adolescent idiopathic scoliosis* is the most common form of scoliosis and occurs most commonly in girls (Weinstein et al., 2003). The curve may resolve, remain stable, or progress in severity. The most significant prognosticators of curve progression in girls are age at onset, premenarchal status, and bone age (Table 26-3) (Lowe et al., 2000; Ahn et al., 2002). Postulated mechanisms for the progression of adolescent idiopathic scoliosis include abnormal vertebral ossification, leptin-induced increased sympathetic nervous system activity, and increases in platelet-derived calmodulin (Lowe et al., 2004; Burwell et al., 2008; Burwell et al., 2009; Gu et al., 2009). *Exotic*

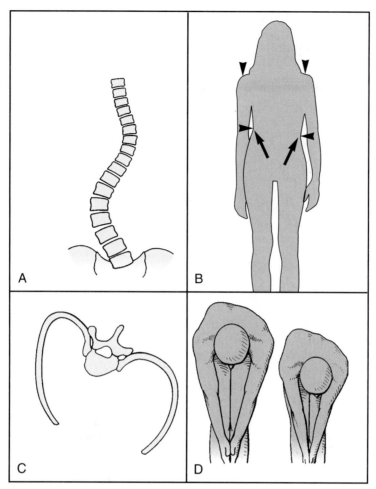

■ **FIGURE 26-1.** Structural changes in idiopathic scoliosis. **A,** As curvature increases, alterations in body configuration develop in the primary and compensatory curve regions. **B,** Asymmetry of shoulder height, waistline, and elbow-to-flank distance are common findings. **C,** Vertebral rotation and associated posterior displacement of the ribs on the convex side of the curve are responsible for the characteristic deformity of the chest wall in scoliosis patients. **D,** In the school screening examination for scoliosis, the patient bends forward at the waist. Rib asymmetry of even a small degree is obvious. *(From Scoles PV: Spinal deformity in childhood and adolescence. In Behrman RE, Vaughn VC III, editors: Nelson textbook of pediatrics, ed 5, Philadelphia, 1989, Saunders, pp 925–933.)*

scoliosis is a term introduced by Campbell and Smith (2007) to describe the spinal deformity found in rare pediatric conditions that pose special challenges beyond simply correcting the spinal curve. These very complicated patients with early-onset spinal deformity often tax the multisubspecialty resources of even the

most sophisticated pediatric centers. Examples include patients with Jeune and Marfan syndromes.

Natural History

The natural history of scoliosis varies according to the cause and the pattern of vertebral involvement. Uncorrected, scoliosis results in curve progression, cosmetic deformity, back pain, and physiologic compromise (Weinstein et al., 2003). In most cases of idiopathic scoliosis, the spinal curvature remains small, and conservative nonoperative management is appropriate (Richards et al., 1976). In 0.2% to 0.5% of cases, the curve increases, necessitating surgical intervention (Ahn et al., 2002). In patients with idiopathic scoliosis, only those with thoracic apices and curves of greater than 100 degrees are at increased risk for death from cor pulmonale and right ventricular failure (Asher and Burton, 2006). The grim prognosis of early death and respiratory failure is untrue in most patients with idiopathic scoliosis (Weinstein et al., 1981). The timing of surgery for this condition is controversial. The worse the curve and the more compromised the cardiorespiratory function, the greater

TABLE 26-2. Correlation of Angle of Curve and Symptoms in Patients with Scoliosis

Angle of Curvature	Significance
<10	Normal
>25	Echocardiographic evidence of increased pulmonary artery pressures
>40	Surgical intervention
>65	Restrictive lung disease
>100	Symptomatic lung disease, dyspnea on exertion
>120	Alveolar hypoventilation

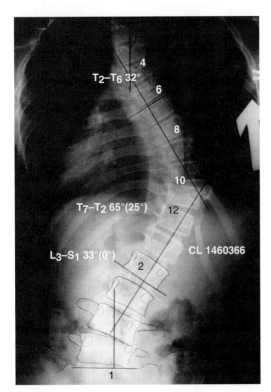

■ FIGURE 26-2. Standing posteroanterior radiograph from a 13-year-old girl with a severe right thoracic section. Notice the Cobb measurement technique. The Cobb angle is derived by drawing lines parallel to the superior surface of the proximal-end vertebra and the inferior surface of the distal-end vertebra. Perpendiculars to these lines are erected, and the angle of intersection of these lines is measured. The numbers in parentheses indicate the degree of correction of the deformity on side-bending radiographs. *(From Thompson GH: The spine. In Behrman RE, editor: Nelson textbook of pediatrics, ed 16, Philadelphia, 2004, Saunders, pp 2280–2284.)*

Box 26-1 Classification of Scoliosis

CONGENITAL SCOLIOSIS
- Vertebral anomalies
- Rib anomalies
- Spinal dysraphism
- Idiopathic scoliosis
- Infantile (<3 years of age)
- Juvenile (3 to 10 years of age)
- Adolescent (>10 years of age)

SCOLIOSIS ASSOCIATED WITH NEUROMUSCULAR DISEASE
- Cerebral palsy
- Poliomyelitis
- Myopathies
- Muscular dystrophies
- Syringomyelia
- Friedreich's ataxia

TRAUMATIC SCOLIOSIS
- Fractures
- Irradiation
- Burns
- Surgery

SYNDROMES ASSOCIATED WITH SCOLIOSIS
- Neurofibromatosis (von Recklinghausen's disease)
- Marfan syndrome
- Osteogenesis imperfecta
- Mucopolysaccharidosis
- Rheumatoid arthritis

NEOPLASTIC DISEASE

TABLE 26-3. Incidence of Scoliotic Curve Progression at Time of Diagnosis of 10-Degree Curve

Age	Menarchal Status	Bone Maturity
<11 yr (88%)	Premenarche (53%)	Immature (68%)
>15 yr (29%)	Postmenarchal (11%)	Mature (18%)

---

the risk for perioperative morbidity and mortality. The pulmonary hypertension of progressive uncorrected idiopathic scoliosis often results in life-compromising respiratory failure in the fourth or fifth decade (Taylor and Gropper, 2006).

Respiratory Sequelae

Even asymptomatic scoliotic patients have demonstrable abnormalities in pulmonary function. As the degree of curvature progresses, vertebral rotation leads to thoracic cage asymmetry and deformation; lung volumes and pulmonary compliance are often but not always inversely related to the degree of this curve (Newton et al., 2005). When the scoliotic curve is greater than 65 degrees, pulmonary function tests demonstrate the characteristic pattern of restrictive lung disease. The first manifestation of this restrictive lung disease is a reduction in vital capacity; in many cases, the vital capacity (normal, 60 mL/kg) is *severely* reduced, often to less than 60% of predicted. Of the subdivisions of vital capacity, inspiratory capacity is affected to a greater extent than expiratory reserve volume. Functional residual capacity and residual volume are not as severely affected. These alterations in lung volumes are referable to the scoliotic changes in chest wall compliance and the resting position of

the thoracic cage, rather than to parenchymal changes. The thoracic deformity of early-onset scoliosis damages pulmonary vascular development and inhibits physiologic alveolar growth, also producing decreases in pulmonary volumes (Charles et al., 1976; Fernandes and Weinstein, 2007).

The pulmonary impairment that results from the scoliosis of neuromuscular disease is exacerbated by coexisting abnormalities in central respiratory drive, coordination of swallowing, and innervation of the upper airway and respiratory musculature. Pulmonary dysfunction in these patients is exacerbated by an increased frequency of respiratory infections, a predilection to aspiration, and an impaired ability to clear pulmonary secretions. Patients who have abnormal results on their pulmonary function test, particularly a forced vital capacity (FVC) of less than 30%, or those who have hypercapnia preoperatively will probably require postoperative (or chronic) ventilation (Almenrader and Patel, 2006). Maximum inspiratory and expiratory mouth pressures (Pi_{max}, Pe_{max}) that the patient can generate against airway occlusion are the important indices for his or her ability to reexpand the lungs (sighs, $Pi_{max} \leq 40$ cm H_2O)

and to expel secretions (coughs, $Pe_{max} > 40$ cm H_2O). Unless the patient can generate more than these threshold pressures preoperatively, postoperative admission to the intensive care unit for ventilatory support should be anticipated.

Cardiovascular Sequelae

Mitral valve prolapse is found in 25% of patients with scoliosis but in less than 10% of age-matched controls. Echocardiographic evidence for increased pulmonary artery pressures has been demonstrated in individuals with only modest degrees of scoliosis in the absence of abnormal pulmonary function. Patients with angles of curvature greater than 70 degrees develop pulmonary hypertension on exercise; those with curves greater than 110 degrees have mean pulmonary artery hypertension at rest. Kafer (1980) proposed that this increase in pulmonary vascular resistance is not just the result of lung compression from thoracic cage abnormalities but is also the result of an increased incidence of hypoxic pulmonary vasoconstriction (Schur et al., 1984). In addition, development of the pulmonary vascular bed may be impaired, resulting in a fundamental reduction in the number of functional vascular units per lung (Kafer, 1980; Schur et al., 1984). Chronic hypoxia induces pulmonary vascular remodeling, which contributes significantly to the pulmonary hypertension in these patients (Morrell et al., 2009).

Any child with a myopathy or borderline respiratory status should have an electrocardiogram and an echocardiogram performed to assess the presence of cor pulmonale, ventricular wall motion, ejection fraction, and ventricular wall thickness. Many myopathies, particularly Duchenne's muscular dystrophy, involve cardiac muscle and skeletal muscle (Manzur and Muntoni, 2009; Strehle, 2009). Duchenne's muscular dystrophy is the most common muscular dystrophy in children who present for surgery. An X-linked recessive disorder, this progressive, debilitating disease affects skeletal, cardiac, and smooth muscle. Typically, afflicted boys become wheelchair dependent by the age of 10 years, and in the past, death from respiratory or cardiac failure occurred in this population before the age of 20. With the introduction of contemporary cardiopulmonary interventions, including noninvasive home ventilation, these men are living to previously unprecedented ages (Birnkrant et al., 2007; Birnkrant, 2009). Scoliosis is common, and surgery is often performed to improve the quality of life (see Chapter 3, Respiratory Physiology in Infants and Children).

Numerous anesthesia challenges are presented by patients with Duchenne's muscular dystrophy. Clinically significant cardiomyopathies and rhythm disturbances manifest by 10 years of age (see Chapter 36, Systemic Disorders). Many of these children are obese because of muscle weakness, fatty degeneration of muscle fibers, and lack of exercise. Succinylcholine can cause a fatal hyperkalemia in these patients, who may present for surgery before the diagnosis has been definitively made; therefore, the routine use of this muscle relaxant is no longer recommended in all children (Birnkrant et al., 2007; Birnkrant, 2009; Gurnaney et al., 2009).

Preoperative Evaluation

The most important aspects of the preoperative evaluation include determination of the location and degree of spinal curvature, the cause of the scoliosis, the patient's history of exercise tolerance, respiratory symptoms, and the presence of coexisting diseases. A directed physical examination of the cardiorespiratory system should evaluate the presence of tachypnea, crackles, wheezing, and signs of right heart failure, such as hepatomegaly, jugular venous distention, and peripheral edema. Any preoperative neurologic deficits should be recorded. Based on the severity of the curve and the degree of respiratory impairment, the preoperative laboratory studies listed in Box 26-2 should be requested.

Right heart involvement is reflected in the findings of right ventricular hypertrophy and right axis deviation on the electrocardiogram. Estimates of the degree of pulmonary hypertension may be made by evaluating the right systolic time interval and the velocity of tricuspid regurgitation on the echocardiogram. Pulmonary function tests are useful in establishing the risk for pulmonary complications in the immediate postoperative period. An FVC of less than 30 mL/kg (or <50% of predicted), or a forced expiratory volume at 1 second (FEV_1) that is less than 50% of predicted, usually indicates postoperative respiratory insufficiency and the need for prolonged postoperative mechanical ventilation. With the airway occluded, peak inspiratory and expiratory forces of at least –30 cm H_2O and +40 cm H_2O, respectively, are necessary for effective sighs and postoperative coughing and expulsion of secretions.

Children with myelodysplastic syndromes are likely to develop an allergy to latex products (Kelly et al., 1994; Maxwell, 2004; Dewachter et al., 2009). All children with any of these syndromes should be considered allergic to latex, and nonlatex products (e.g., tourniquets, sterile and nonsterile gloves) should be substituted for the latex equivalents. Corticosteroids and antihistamines are not administered prophylactically.

Surgical Techniques

The treatment of spinal curvature is dictated by the type of scoliosis and by the surgeon's expertise and preferences. Very few cases of congenital scoliosis can be managed conservatively. The mainstay of therapy is posterior spinal fusion without instrumentation, followed by prolonged immobilization.

Box 26-2 Preoperative Tests for Scoliosis Surgery

Chest radiography
Electrocardiography
Echocardiography
Pulmonary function tests
- Arterial blood gas
- Spirometry
- Forced vital capacity (FVC)
- Forced expiratory volume at 1 second (FEV1, FEV1/FVC)
- Peak expiratory flow rate (PEFR)
- Peak inspiratory pressure (Pi_{max})
- Peak expiratory pressure (Pe_{max})
Coagulation studies
- Platelet count
- Prothrombin time, partial thromboplastin time
- Electrolyte panel
- Liver function tests

Instrumentation in these patients has been associated with a prohibitively high rate of paraplegia, which is presumed to be the result of coexisting cord and vertebral anomalies. Although conservative therapy is the most frequently used treatment for idiopathic scoliosis, when rapid curve progression is anticipated, surgical intervention is used for severe truncal deformities and for pain unrelieved by medical therapy (Weinstein et al., 2003).

Posterior Spinal Fusion

The goal of scoliosis surgery is to achieve a spinal fusion and stabilization of the curve. After incision through the supraspinal ligament, the paraspinous musculature is reflected. The vertebral laminae are decorticated, the facet joints are destroyed, and the spinous processes are removed so that raw cancellous bone is exposed. Bone graft obtained from the iliac crest, ribs on the convex side, or the bone bank is cut into matchstick-size strips and packed over the decorticated surfaces, mainly on the concave side. The fusion extends from one vertebra above the curve to the second vertebra below. Instrumentation is usually inserted to hold the spine in the best possible position while fusion is accomplished. Without a properly performed fusion, the instrumentation ultimately fatigues.

Several instrumentation techniques are available for treatment of the scoliotic spine. The *Harrington rod,* the original instrumentation system, consists of a stainless steel rod that is connected to the inferior facets and pedicles of the spine by multiple ratchet hooks placed at the terminal aspects of the curve. Distraction is adjusted using the ratchet principle (Harrington and Dickson, 1976; Harrington, 1988). The incidence of neurologic complications after this technique is 0.23%. The disadvantages of the Harrington rod include two-dimensional correction, curvature distraction by the end hooks, and the need for prolonged postoperative immobilization. Because of these problems, this technique is rarely used.

Segmental spinal instrumentation was introduced to provide three-dimensional correction and to achieve differential distraction at multiple levels. The *Luque instrumentation system* consists of sublaminar wires on each side of the spinous process and a long, L-shaped rod that can be contoured three dimensionally. The curve is corrected as the wires are tightened (Luque, 1986; Luque and Rapp, 1988). The internal fixation achieved is more rigid than that obtained with the Harrington system, and it can be extended to the pelvis. The most common deficit after Luque rod instrumentation is a dysesthesia, which is usually observed late (2 to 6 days) in the postoperative period. The proposed mechanism for these findings is expansion of an epidural hematoma in the area of the sublaminar wires (Johnston et al., 1986).

The *Cotrel-Dubousset segmental spinal instrumentation system* uses multiple laminar and pedicular hooks attached to a double-rod frame (Richards and Johnston, 1987). This system enables three-dimensional correction of complex curves and obviates the need for postoperative immobilization. It is more time consuming than the Harrington system, increases intraoperative blood loss, and has a lower incidence (0.6%) of neurologic complications than Luque rods. Double-curve patterns are more complex and require multiple hooks at multiple fixation sites, necessitating more extensive decortication and contributing to additional blood loss.

Pedicle screws are the most recent advance in posterior spinal fusion (Kim and Noonan, 2009). Initially used for lumbar curves, they are now used for total curve correction. The limitation of posterior spinal fusion with or without instrumentation is that the anterior growth plates, which play a major role in the development of the deformity, are not affected. Late torsional deformities can result.

Anterior Spinal Surgery

The anterior approach to spinal deformities has been advocated for several specific deformities, including severe kyphosis and lordotic paralytic curves in patients with cerebral palsy. Surgery consists of discectomies with or without instrumentation, performed alone or in combination with a posterior spinal fusion. Video-assisted thoracoscopic surgery can be used for this procedure if instrumentation is not being used (Sucato, 2003). The surgical approach used to expose the anterior portion of the spine depends on the exact spinal deformity. Thoracic curves are usually approached through a left thoracotomy, and the procedure is facilitated by insertion of a double-lumen endotracheal tube and one-lung ventilation. Alternatively, single-lung ventilation in young children is performed by advancing a tracheal tube into the main stem bronchus opposite the side of surgery, or by positioning a bronchial blocker into the main stem bronchus on the operative side.

Many techniques for placing a variety of bronchial blockers outside the tracheal tube have been described for use in children (see Chapter 23, Anesthesia for General Abdominal, Thoracic, Urologic, and Bariatric Surgery) (Hammer, 2001, 2004; Hammer et al., 2002). The combined curve of the thoracolumbar spine is exposed transdiaphragmatically by means of a high subcostal incision that necessitates taking the diaphragm down from its bony insertion. Lumbar curves can be approached extraperitoneally or transabdominally. In general, complications of the anterior approach include great vessel disruption, hemothorax, pneumothorax, paralytic interruption of spinal cord perfusion, and excessive angulation or compression of the spinal cord by rapid distraction of the curvature. Spinal cord injury can result from mechanical damage by a screw or disruption of segmental spinal arteries. At the beginning of the 21st century, performance of anterior scoliosis surgery diminished because of the corrective power of pedicle screw constructs and better surgical methods designed to improve flexibility, such as posterior release, posterior osteotomy, and vertebral resection (Kim and Noonan, 2009).

As an alternative to open thoracotomy, a video-assisted thoracoscopic surgery (VATS) approach is being used to perform anterior thoracic spine release in patients who require both anterior and posterior procedures to correct their scoliosis. The appropriate use of pedicle screws has resulted in a 50% to 66% curve correction, with good maintenance of the curve correction for a minimum of 3 years (Lehman et al., 1976).

Anesthesia Management of Scoliosis Surgery

Overview

Dramatic hemodynamic instability and substantial blood and heat loss are the hallmarks of scoliosis surgery. In addition to the monitors routinely used in conducting pediatric general anesthesia, large-bore IV access and intraarterial, central venous, and bladder catheterization are recommended. These invasive catheters allow monitoring of beat-to-beat changes in blood pressure, adequacy of oxygenation, ventilation, organ perfusion, and intravascular volume. Additionally, central venous catheterization provides a direct route for administering cardiotonic medications. Body temperature will decrease during the course of a spinal procedure, and continuous monitoring and meticulous thermoprotective strategies are required to prevent intraoperative hypothermia.

Monitoring and Intraoperative Complications

Scoliosis surgery is very high-risk surgery. Common intraoperative problems are listed in Table 26-4. Complications are related to the surgery (blood loss and its therapy), the prone position, and cardiovascular collapse from myriad causes. Practiced crisis management is essential if patient survival is to be ensured.

Hypotension and cardiovascular collapse are common during this surgery, making it among the highest-risk procedures performed in pediatric surgery and anesthesia. *Physicians should always presume that hypotension is caused by hypovolemia until proven otherwise.* Other causes are far less common and include latex (or rarely, drug) anaphylaxis, anesthetic overdose,

pneumothorax or hemothorax (particularly in a single-staged anterior posterior procedure), and impaired venous return resulting from the prone position, surgical manipulation, and venous air embolism. Air embolism can occur because the epidural veins are exposed during surgery and are above the level of the heart. The outcome from a massive air embolus is almost uniformly fatal.

Because cardiopulmonary resuscitation is virtually impossible to perform with the patient in the prone position, a plan to turn the patient supine must be well established and rehearsed. As in any emergency, it is the anesthesiologist's responsibility to declare the emergency and to call for help. Because the surgeon needs time to pack and cover the open wound with sterile towels and adhesive plastic, it is always better to begin the process early rather than waiting until the last possible moment.

Neurologic Monitoring

Postoperative paralysis or sensory loss is the most feared, devastating, and often unpredictable complication of scoliosis surgery (Owen, 1999). Neurologic injury may result from direct injury to the spinal cord or nerves during instrumentation, from excessive traction during distraction, or from compromised perfusion of the spinal cord. Because the ramifications

TABLE 26-4. Potential Intraoperative Complications During Scoliosis Surgery

Problem	Monitoring Solution

Endotracheal tube malposition	Securely tape tube before turning
	   Benzoin
	   Waterproof tape
	   Bite block (rolled 4×4 gauze pads)
	After turning prone
	   Hand ventilate and listen to both lung fields
	   DO NOT ALLOW STRETCHER TO LEAVE THE OPERATING ROOM until you are satisfied that the
	     endotracheal tube has not migrated
	Hourly arterial blood gas determinations
	Esophageal stethoscope

Alteration in pulmonary compliance in the prone position	Proper position on bed frame: ensure chest can expand unimpeded Hourly arterial blood gas determinations
Alteration in cardiac function in the prone position	Proper position on bed frame to ensure that venous return is not compromised Indwelling arterial catheter Central venous catheter Bladder catheter
Hypotension	*Blood loss until proven otherwise* Ensure that typed and cross-matched blood is available when surgery starts. Two large-bore peripheral IV catheters and blood warmer Central venous catheter Hourly measurement of hemoglobin/hematocrit Consider Amicar
Coagulopathy	Platelet count Prothrombin time, activated partial thromboplastin time, fibrin split products Thromboelastogram
Electrolyte abnormalities (usually from blood transfusions)	Frequent measurements of sodium, potassium, and ionized calcium Avoid using "old" packed red blood cells NEVER use hypotonic solutions (including for maintenance fluid requirements)
Excessive heat loss	Measure core temperature Heat conservation Active warming (forced air)
Neurologic injuries	Proper positioning, with particular attention to eyes and elbows (brachial plexus) Intraoperative assessment of cord function (e.g., sensory and motor evoked potentials)

associated with motor deficit are significantly greater than those associated with sensory deficit, surgically induced paraplegia has always been the major concern of scoliosis surgery.

Spinal Cord Blood Flow

The organization of the spinal cord blood supply is segmental in a cross-sectional and rostral-caudal fashion (Fig. 26-3). The intrinsic spinal cord vasculature consists of the *anterior median* and the *paired posterior spinal arteries*. The vasculature supplying these vessels arises from the segmental arteries of the aorta and branches of the subclavian—the vertebral arteries—and the internal iliac arteries. The solitary anterior median spinal artery runs along the entire length of the cord in the anterior sulcus, giving off penetrating branches that supply the ventral two thirds of the spinal cord. Blood flow in the anterior spinal artery is not continuous throughout its span; instead, the anterior spinal artery functions as an anastomotic channel between the terminal branches of successive radicular arteries. Blood that leaves the terminal aspects of

these radicular arteries courses upward and downward in the anterior spinal artery. At points between adjacent radicular arteries, blood flows in either direction. The paired posterior spinal arteries, which supply the dorsal third of the cord, also have discontinuous segments and appear more like a plexus of pial vessels than paired arteries.

The three perimedullary vessels give rise to the intramedullary arterial system: the central arteries that supply the gray matter and the deep portions of the white matter and the radial arteries that supply most of the white matter. Nonfunctional anastomotic links exist between the central arterial supply and the radial arterial supply at a given spinal segment. This border zone and the radial circulation appear to be at highest risk for ischemic insult.

The regional circulation of the spinal cord is divided into four segments. The cervical and lumbosacral regions each receive double the blood flow received by the thoracic region (see Fig. 26-3). Although each vertebral level has paired segmental arteries, only six to eight important medullary arteries are formed. These medullary arteries join the spinal arteries.

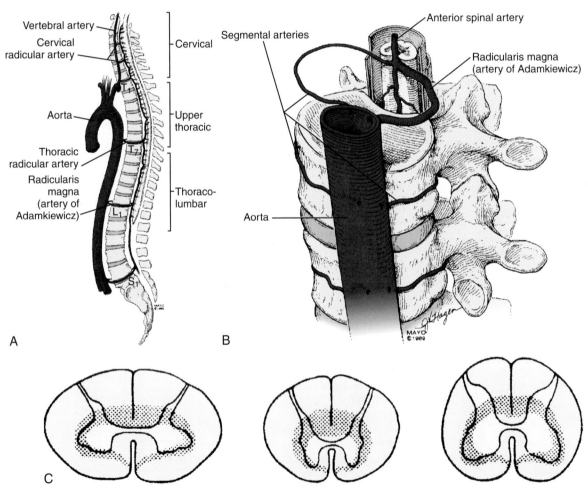

■ **FIGURE 26-3.** The anatomy of blood flow to the spinal cord is distinctive in the vertical and horizontal distributions. **A,** Segmental blood flow along the cord axis. **B,** The thoracic cord depends on flow from a number of thoracic radicular arteries, principally the artery of Adamkiewicz. **C,** The cross-sectional distribution of blood flow is distinctive. The outer zone of the cord (white matter) is supplied by the radial arteries; the inner zone (gray and white matter) is supplied by the central arteries. Tissue in the *shaded region* is supplied by both sources. (*A and B,* From *Cucchiara RF, Michenfelder JD, editors:* Clinical neuroanesthesia, *New York, 1990, Churchill Livingstone;* **C** *from Vinken PJ, Bruyn GW, editors:* The handbook of clinical neurology, *vol 12, New York, 1972, North Holland.*)

The segmental arteries at all other levels are functionally non-suppliers of blood to the spinal cord itself. The vertebral arteries form the rostral origins of the anterior and posterior spinal arteries and represent the principal supply to the cervical cord. Branches of the thyrocervical and costovertebral arteries supply the lower cervical and upper thoracic cord. A radicular artery arising from T7 provides perfusion for the middle thoracic cord. The most consistent and important of the anterior medullary arteries is the artery of Adamkiewicz—the arteria radicularis magna—which usually joins the anterior spinal artery between T8 and L3. This artery is the predominant source of blood supply to the lower two thirds of the spinal cord. The implications of this design dictate the clinical manifestations of impaired cord perfusion. Watershed areas, which are subject to ischemia during low-flow states, exist between the anterior and posterior circulations and between the four different spinal segments. The segments of T4 to T7 appear to be highly susceptible to injury during periods of hypoperfusion. The dependence of the lower two thirds of the cord on the artery of Adamkiewicz puts this region at particular risk during surgical manipulation of the thoracolumbar aorta and spinal column, and this is referred to as the *lumbar artery enlargement syndrome.* Although the clinical picture of this syndrome is not constant, it is marked by the development of flaccid paraplegia or quadriplegia (depending on the level of the lesion) and dissociated sensory impairment in which heat and pain sensations are affected but deep sensation is spared.

The same principles that regulate the cerebral blood flow apply to spinal cord blood flow. Thus, cord blood flow depends on the perfusion pressure (i.e., mean arterial pressure [MAP] minus cerebrospinal fluid pressure), integrity of the circulation, microcirculatory autoregulation, and intrinsic regulation. If the perfusion pressure falls below 50 mm Hg, spinal cord blood flow is reduced. Spinal cord blood flow autoregulates within the range of a MAP of 60 to 150 mm Hg. Spinal cord blood flow is also regulated on an intrinsic basis in response to arterial oxygen and carbon dioxide tensions, pH, and cord temperature in a fashion identical to that of the cerebral circulation. Hypercapnia increases flow, whereas a Pao_2 below 60 mm Hg results in a vasodilation that overrides the effects of hypocarbia and autoregulation (see Chapter 22, Anesthesia for Neurosurgery).

Minimizing Postoperative Neurologic Complications

The estimated risk for postoperative neurologic injury in patients undergoing spinal instrumentation is 0.72% to 1.6% (Cervellati et al., 1996). In a study of 7885 patients who underwent instrumentation or fusion without instrumentation, 87 patients developed acute neurologic changes, and 36% of these patients recovered without sequelae. Individuals with nonidiopathic scoliosis are at higher risk for neurologic injury. Children with congenital scoliosis suffer neurologic complications disproportionately (Cervellati et al., 1996).

To minimize the risk for these devastating neurologic injuries, a variety of methods of intraoperative neurologic monitoring have been used. The goal of this monitoring is to identify and herald the onset of neurologic impairment and to provide the surgeon and anesthesiologist with the opportunity to implement appropriate interventions that may minimize permanent damage. These approaches include wake-up tests and neurophysiologic monitoring.

Wake-Up Test

Vauzelle and colleagues (1973) first described the use of the wake-up test to assess the integrity of the spinal cord. In this technique, patients are awakened intraoperatively to assess spinal cord motor function. The wake-up test requires an anesthetic that allows rapid recovery of consciousness and motor function. Ideally, the test is rehearsed preoperatively. During rehearsal, patients are informed that they will be momentarily awakened at the time of rod insertion to test the function of the spinal cord. Patients must be reassured that they will neither remember the event nor experience pain while they are "awake." Preoperative preparation increases the speed and success of the test. The effectiveness of neurophysiologic monitoring during spinal deformity surgery is now so well established that the wake-up test is rarely used except to confirm monitoring changes (Schwartz et al., 2007).

When a wake-up test is performed, the operating room must be quiet, the surgeon must stop operating, and an observer is positioned (usually under the drapes) to look for foot movement. After discontinuation of the anesthetic, the patient is first asked to move the hands ("squeeze my fingers") to evaluate the level of consciousness and is then asked to move the feet ("wiggle your toes"). If the patient is unable to move the feet but can move the hands, spinal cord compromise is presumed, and the spinal rod instrumentation is removed immediately. Spinal cord perfusion is maximized by raising the MAP, increasing the hemoglobin concentration, and normalizing arterial carbon dioxide and oxygen tensions. In one series of 166 patients in whom the wake-up test was used, three patients had demonstrable neurologic deficits when awakened (Hall et al., 1978). These deficits disappeared immediately on release of the distracting force (i.e., rods) (Hall et al., 1978).

Hazards associated with the wake-up test include dislodgment of spinal instrumentation rods and vascular catheters, accidental extubation, air embolization produced by deep inspirations, the patient falling off the operating room table, and recall with subsequent psychological trauma. This test has many other limitations: it tests only the anterior spinal cord (motor function) and not the dorsal column (sensory); it requires patient cooperation and has limited use in patients with baseline cognitive dysfunction; it provides a snapshot of a single moment of spinal cord function and can realistically be performed only once or twice during a procedure; a spinal injury may be missed because it occurred after the wake-up test was performed; depending on the anesthesiologist's skill and the anesthesia technique employed, it may take 5 to 45 minutes after a wake-up test is requested by the surgeon before wake-up status can be achieved.

Neurometric Monitoring

Sensory-Evoked Potentials. Electrophysiologic (neurometric) monitoring provides real-time, continuous assessment of spinal cord function and does not require patient movement, arousal, or cooperation (see Chapter 11, Monitoring) (Gonzalez et al., 2009). The most common technique uses somatosensory evoked potentials (SSEPs), in which the cortical and subcortical responses to peripheral nerve stimulation are monitored (Banoub et al., 2003). Typically, a peripheral mixed nerve (i.e., posterior tibial nerve, peroneal nerve, or median nerve) is stimulated at fixed intervals during a procedure. SSEPs are recorded repeatedly during surgery, and their amplitude (height) and latency (time of occurrence) are compared with baseline values (Gonzalez et al., 2009; Menditta and Emerson, 2009). Based on changes in these characteristics, it is possible to determine the functional status of the spinal cord sensory tracts. SSEP monitoring requires specialized technology and expertise. To resolve the very low amplitude evoked potentials from background, random, or spontaneous cortical activity, computer signal averaging of repetitive sensory responses is required. The processed evoked-potential waveform is plotted as voltage against time and is characterized by the poststimulus latency and amplitude. The poststimulus latency reflects the time required for impulse transmission from the site of sensory stimulation. A reduction in amplitude of greater than 50% or an increase in latency of less than 10% relative to baseline values is generally considered significant (Banoub et al., 2003; Gonzalez et al., 2009; Menditta and Emerson, 2009).

SSEPs monitor only the dorsal columns of the spinal cord and provide no direct evidence of loss of motor function or anterior spinal cord injury. Motor deficits may occur in the absence of alterations in SSEPs, and numerous case reports have recorded the postoperative finding of paralysis despite unchanged intraoperative SSEPs (i.e., false-negative results). In the setting of spinal cord ischemia, the time to loss of SSEPs was almost three times longer than the time to motor evoked potential (MEP) loss (Banoub et al., 2003; Shine et al., 2008). The most comprehensive information regarding the false-negative rate of SSEPs comes from a survey of spine surgeons by the Scoliosis Research Society and the European Spinal Deformity Society, in which definite neurologic deficits, despite stable SSEPs, occurred during surgery in 0.063% of patients (Nuwer et al., 1995). Children with neuromuscular scoliosis frequently have unreliable SSEP data. Despite these limitations, SSEP monitoring reduces postoperative paraplegia by more than 50% (Nuwer et al., 1995). When SSEP monitoring is equivocal, many recommend an intraoperative wake-up test to assess motor function (Grundy, 1983).

Many pharmacologic and physiologic variables affect the latency and amplitude of SSEPs and have been estimated to account for up to 44% of intraoperative SSEP changes. The most important of these are the anesthesia agents, blood pressure, and body temperature (Table 26-5) (Grundy, 1983; Banoub et al., 2003; Gonzalez et al., 2009). All of the potent inhaled anesthesia agents produce dosage-dependent increases in latency and decreases in amplitude. These effects are less for sevoflurane and desflurane, permitting dosages of 1.5 minimum alveolar concentration (MAC) with minimal SSEP changes. Nitrous oxide compounds the effects of volatile anesthetics on cortical SSEPs (Banoub et al., 2003). Alone, nitrous oxide has no effect on SSEP latency but does decrease its amplitude by 50% (Schwartz et al., 2007). Substantial recovery of latency and amplitude is achievable with discontinuance of nitrous oxide and the inhaled vapors (da Costa et al., 2001). In general, the IV agents affect SSEP less than inhaled agents do; at high dosages, they produce slight to moderate decreases in amplitude and increases in latency. Midazolam has no effect on latency (Laureau et al., 1999; Banoub et al., 2003). Ketamine (Langeron et al., 1997) and etomidate (Thakor et al., 1991) augment SSEP amplitude. Propofol has no effect on amplitude or latency and is highly recommended as a component of total IV anesthesia for scoliosis surgery (Laureau et al., 1999; Boisseau et al., 2002). Opioids given in either analgesic or anesthetic dosages

TABLE 26-5. Effects of Anesthesia Agents on Somatosensory Evoked Potentials

Agent	Amplitude	Latency
Desflurane	↓	↑
Isoflurane	↓	↑
Sevoflurane	↓	↑
Nitrous oxide	↓	↔
Barbiturates	↓	↑
Etomidate	↑	↔
Ketamine	↑	↔
Midazolam	↓	↔
Opioids	↔	↔
Propofol	↔	↔
Dexmedetomidine	↔	↔

↓, Decreases; ↑, increases; ↔, remains the same.

produce minimal SSEP effects (Banoub et al., 2003). In a very small study, dexmedetomidine had no effect on SSEP or MEP (Tobias et al., 2008).

The amplitude and latency of the waveform are also affected by age, preexisting neurologic deficits, body temperature, $Paco_2$, hypoxia, and blood pressure (Fig. 26-4) (Banoub et al., 2003). The reliability of spinal cord monitoring may be dramatically affected by the variability of the evoked responses. Muscle relaxants have no direct deleterious effects on the SSEP but may produce a more reliable recording by providing "quieter" conditions.

An anesthesia milieu that is compatible with adequate neurometric monitoring and that allows rapid awakening can be created using a variety of approaches. Combining desflurane or sevoflurane with a remifentanil infusion produces ideal SSEPs and still allows for rapid wake-up if a wake-up test is required. Alternatively, the physician can substitute a continuous propofol infusion for the potent inhaled anesthetics in combination with an opioid (Kalkman et al., 1991a; Kalkman et al., 1991b). Because etomidate augments SSEP amplitude, it is particularly useful in patients with abnormal preoperative SSEPs. These individuals are at greatest risk for the development of postoperative neurologic catastrophes (Sloan et al., 1988; Samra and Sorkin, 1991).

Baseline SSEP recordings are made after turning the patient to the prone position. After the patient is prone, the anesthesia depth, end-tidal carbon dioxide (CO_2) levels (35 to 45 mm Hg), temperature, and blood pressure (MAP >60 mm Hg) should be maintained to minimize their effects on the SSEPs during surgery. Throughout the surgical procedure, a physiologic and pharmacologic steady state must be maintained so that SSEPs can be used effectively as monitors of spinal cord function. Deepening the anesthesia depth during critical operative moments when the risk for neurologic compromise is highest must be avoided to minimize the potential for pharmacologically induced false-positive changes. The intraoperative changes of increased latency, decreased amplitude, or complete loss of waveform must be attributed to spinal cord injury rather than to an anesthetic-induced effect.

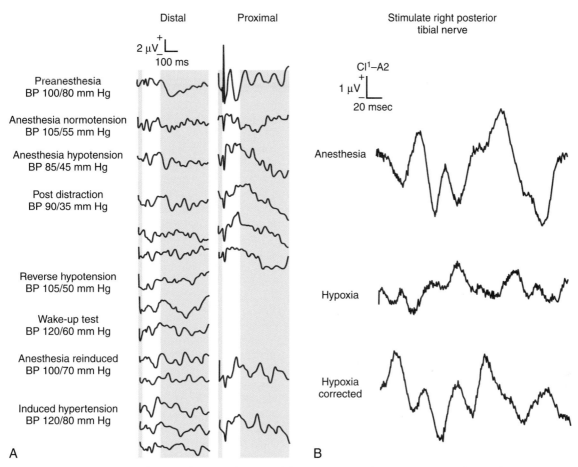

FIGURE 26-4. Somatosensory evoked potentials (SEPs) change with hypotension and hypoxia. **A,** During the combination of distraction and hypotension, distal SEPs were unchanged. Resumption of normotension restored the SEP to baseline. **B,** SEP responses are exquisitely sensitive to hypoxia (Po$_2$ ≤ 41 mm Hg). Resumption of normoxia restored the SEP to baseline.

When the baseline is being established, knowledge of the various effects of anesthesia drugs on SSEPs can be advantageously used to produce optimal signal acquisition. In the setting of less-than-optimal baseline SSEP acquisition, a strategic change in the anesthesia regimen may result in improvement of the quality of the SSEP signal. For example, discontinuing nitrous oxide or desflurane, or both, and substituting an etomidate or propofol infusion can significantly improve SSEP acquisition.

Using the criterion of a decrease in amplitude of greater than 40% amplitude as a significant change, excellent specificity and sensitivity are achievable. In patients with idiopathic scoliosis (i.e., neurologically intact), SSEPs are reliable and can be obtained in more than 98% of patients (Padberg et al., 1998). However, in patients with preexisting diseases such as neuromuscular scoliosis, the reliability of the SSEP is less than 75% but can be improved with the addition of MEP monitoring (Sarwark and Sarwahi, 2007). Precise communication and coordination of efforts among the surgeon, anesthesiologist, and neurometric specialist are imperative when a change in SSEP is observed. Normalization of the SSEPs may occur spontaneously with relaxation of the distraction instrumentation or by improving spinal cord perfusion (e.g., increasing blood pressure and Paco$_2$ levels).

Motor Evoked Potentials. SSEPs are not the modality of choice for monitoring motor tract function or for detecting the presence of a surgically induced motor deficit. The motor pathways can be activated by transcranial stimulation of the motor cortex or by spinal cord stimulation. Transcranial MEPs (TcMEPs) are exquisitely sensitive to compromised spinal cord function and should be used in combination with SSEPs to improve the accuracy of spinal cord monitoring. In a series of 1121 adolescents with idiopathic scoliosis, nine children awoke with a postoperative neurologic deficit, seven had motor or sensorimotor deficit, and two had pure sensory impairment. All seven patients with motor impairments had significant TcMEP changes; only three of the seven had significant SSEP changes. When changes were detected by both modalities, SSEPs lagged behind TcMEPs by approximately 5 minutes (Schwartz et al., 2007). As a result, some centers have abandoned using SSEPs entirely. Finally, the false-positive rate attributed to MEP monitoring during spinal surgery is less than 10% (Langeloo et al., 2003).

Anesthesia agents have profound effects on MEP recordings. Volatile anesthetics, benzodiazepines, etomidate, barbiturates, and even high-dosage propofol affect MEP fidelity (Sloan and Heyer, 2002; Sloan et al., 2008). A maintenance anesthesia that is based on a continuous infusion of propofol and remifentanil is titrated to maintain a MAP of at least 65 mm Hg, and that avoids nitrous oxide and muscle relaxants, provides adequate conditions for uncompromised TcMEP monitoring. Alternatively, high-dosage remifentanil in combination with low-dosage sevoflurane (0.4 to 0.7 MAC), or continuous infusions of propofol, fentanyl, and dexmedetomidine, are also regimens compatible with reliable monitoring (Joseph et al., 1976; Langeloo et al., 2003, 2007; Anschel et al., 2008).

Blood Loss

Exposure of a vast area of decorticated, raw, cancellous bone during spinal surgery results in extensive blood loss that can exceed 25 mL/kg, even in uncomplicated surgery. Children with neuromuscular scoliosis often require more extensive procedures, including pelvic stabilization, than children with idiopathic scoliosis and can easily have blood loss that exceeds a blood volume (Kannan et al., 2002; Meert et al., 2002). However, even if the extent of surgery is controlled, patients with neuromuscular diseases have an almost seven times higher risk for losing greater than 50% of their estimated total blood volume during scoliosis surgery than do normal controls (Edler et al., 2003).

An estimation of circulating blood volume should be made before the induction of anesthesia. The estimated blood volume (EBV) is calculated by multiplying the patient's weight by the approximate blood volume based on age (Table 26-6). From the EBV, the initial hematocrit, and the minimum acceptable hematocrit, the maximum allowable blood loss can be estimated before packed red blood cell transfusion is indicated.

The decision to transfuse red blood cells should be based on the balance between oxygen supply and demand, which depends on the oxygen content of the blood, cardiac output, regional distribution, and metabolic needs. The trigger to transfuse is then based on the patient's risk of developing inadequate oxygenation. Because blood loss may be difficult or impossible to assess accurately, blood loss is estimated by measuring the hemoglobin concentration hourly and by assuming that changes in central venous pressure reflect ongoing blood loss. As blood loss progresses and exceeds a blood volume, it becomes increasingly important to know the medical causes of bleeding (e.g., dilutional thrombocytopenia or loss of clotting factors V and VIII) so as to account for the inability of the surgeon to achieve hemostasis. Platelet counts and coagulation profiles (i.e., prothrombin time, partial thromboplastin time, fibrinogen, and fibrin split products) should be obtained at regular intervals when extensive blood loss occurs.

Multiple strategies have been described to reduce intraoperative blood loss and the need for blood transfusions of homologous blood in the perioperative period (see Chapter 14, Blood Conservation). Techniques that may decrease intraoperative blood loss include induced hypotension, alteration of the operative position, changes in surgical technique, and administration of antifibrinolytic agents such as ε-aminocaproic acid (Amicar) or tranexamic acid (Cyklokapron). Techniques aimed at decreasing the use of homologous blood products include intraoperative blood salvage, preoperative autologous blood donation, and perioperative normovolemic hemodilution and apheresis (Joseph et al., 1976). Each of these techniques has demonstrated efficacy in some clinical situations.

Preoperative autologous donation with and without erythropoietin treatment has been used extensively in children (Helfaer et al., 1998; Vitale et al., 1998). As this has become more widespread for pediatric scoliosis, 70% of children and adolescents have been able to donate sufficient units for their procedures, a figure similar to that for adults (Murray et al., 1997). Using preoperative autologous donation as the sole blood conservation method limited the number of adolescents undergoing scoliosis surgery who required allogeneic transfusions to 11% to 23%. The addition of autologous donation to deliberate hypotension further reduced allogeneic exposure to 10% (Murray et al., 1997).

Alternatively, perioperative hemodilution and apheresis, isovolemic hemodilution, or acute normovolemic hemodilution can substitute for or augment autologous blood donation (Bryson et al., 1998; Copley et al., 1999). Before incision, the patient's blood is withdrawn through a large-bore peripheral IV cannula or through a central venous catheter and replaced with an isotonic balanced salt solution or colloid in a ratio of 3:1. When using this technique, cardiac index and oxygen extraction increase, and systemic vascular resistance, oxygen delivery, and mixed venous saturation decrease. Lactic acidosis develops when oxygen delivery falls to critical. Moderate acute normovolemic hemodilution, with a minimum hematocrit of 17%, did not result in changes in either oxygen delivery or oxygen consumption in healthy children. The removed blood is stored in anticoagulated bags and is administered as needed to maintain the hematocrit at a predetermined level, usually greater than 20%. Complications of this technique include postoperative pulmonary edema, anasarca, and prolonged postoperative mechanical ventilation.

Perioperative salvage of blood (i.e., use of a cell-saver system) allows blood lost in the operative field to be returned to the patient during the perioperative period (Huet et al., 1999). The efficiency of this technique, its benefits in limiting blood transfusion, and the survivability of red blood cells are unclear (Vitale et al., 2002). When using salvaged blood, it is imperative that the blood be processed and washed adequately to avoid life-threatening bleeding and pulmonary complications caused by transfusion of cellular and tissue debris. Salvaged blood can also cause profound hypotension (e.g., citrate, air embolism) and hemolytic and bleeding complications from centrifugation, cellular debris, or anticoagulant overdose.

Pharmacologic manipulation of the hemostatic mechanism is effective in limiting perioperative blood loss. A series of prospective, randomized, double-blind studies demonstrated that the antifibrinolytic agent ε-aminocaproic acid significantly reduces perioperative blood loss and transfusion requirements in patients with either idiopathic or neuromuscular scoliosis who are undergoing spinal fusion (Florentino-Pineda et al., 1976; Thompson et al., 1976a, 1976b). Similarly, tranexamic acid, 100 mg/kg over 15 minutes, followed by an

TABLE 26-6. Approximate Blood Volume Based on Age

Age	Total Blood Volume (mL/kg)
Premature infant	90-105
Term newborn	80-85
1 to 12 months	70-80
Older child	70-80
Adult	55-65

infusion of 10 mg/kg per hour, significantly reduces blood loss during posterior spinal surgery in children and adolescents with idiopathic and secondary (congenital and neuromuscular) scoliosis but may not affect the actual amount of blood transfused (Sethna et al., 2005). The main safety issues related to antifibrinolytic drugs are hypersensitivity reactions, effects on the kidneys, potential for thrombotic events, and effect on mortality.

Deliberate Hypotension

The most common blood-preservation technique is deliberate hypotension (see Chapter 14, Blood Conservation) (Yaster et al., 1986; Tobias, 2002). Numerous techniques to reduce blood pressure have been used, typically with drugs that are direct venous and arterial vasodilators such as nitroprusside and nitroglycerin. Ganglionic blocking drugs (e.g., trimethaphan), α_2-adrenergic agonists (e.g., clonidine), β- and α_1-antagonists (e.g., propranolol, esmolol, prazosin, hydralazine), dopamine agonists (e.g., fenoldopam), inhaled anesthetics (e.g., halothane, isoflurane, sevoflurane, desflurane), major conduction blockade (i.e., epidural), and calcium-channel blockers (e.g., nicardipine) are used alone or in combination with the direct-acting venous and arterial vasodilators to lower blood pressure (Yaster et al., 1986; Tobias, 2002; Hammer et al., 2008).

Deliberate hypotension can be used in any patient who is otherwise healthy. It is contraindicated in the presence of evidence of end-organ injury or ischemia. Blood pressure is usually lowered to an MAP of 60 mm Hg. In the past, the most commonly used technique was a continuous infusion of nitroprusside (1 to 8 mcg/kg per minute) combined with β-blockade, using propranolol (1 to 2 mg), labetalol, or an esmolol infusion. β-Blockade is necessary when hypotension is induced with nitroprusside, because nitroprusside produces a reflex tachycardia and increases cardiac index. These effects combine to limit the ability of nitroprusside to lower blood pressure (Yaster et al., 1986). Nitroglycerin, which is often used for deliberate hypotension in adults, fails to reduce MAPs to below 60 mm Hg in children when administered in dosages as high as 40 mcg/kg per minute (Yaster et al., 1986). Potent inhalation agents such as sevoflurane can also be used to induce hypotension in children and adolescents, but they interfere with intraoperative monitoring and delay the ability to rapidly perform a wake-up test. When combined with low-dosage sevoflurane or desflurane, remifentanil is extremely effective. Regardless of the technique used to induce deliberate hypotension, the appropriate use of adjuvants in the anesthesia technique can aid in achieving the desired effect of hypotension (Tobias, 2002). Children can be premedicated with oral clonidine (4 to 8 mcg/kg) 2 hours before surgery to reduce anxiety and to facilitate the induction and maintenance of hypotension during surgery (Hackmann et al., 2003).

Although deliberate hypotension clearly reduces blood loss, provides a relatively bloodless surgical field, and facilitates surgical dissection, its use in scoliosis surgery is controversial. Animal studies have suggested an additive effect of hypotension and surgical pressure on the spinal cord in producing neurologic injury (Brodkey et al., 1972). In dogs, Griffiths and colleagues (1979) showed that cord compression can alter dorsal column conduction at perfusion pressures that did not affect blood flow. Use of deliberate hypotension mandates normocarbia and adequate oxygen-carrying capacity.

Invasive monitoring is essential when deliberate hypotension is used. An arterial catheter for beat-to-beat monitoring of blood pressure and for frequent hematocrit determinations and sampling of arterial blood gas are essential. Because patients must remain normovolemic at all times, a central venous pressure catheter is a useful monitor. Nitroprusside has been shown to decrease arterial oxygen tension in children and to increase the alveolar to pulmonary artery (Pao_2-to-Pao_2) pressure difference (Yaster et al., 1986). We can assume that the lowered oxygen-carrying capacity of low-hematocrit blood, when coupled with hypoxemia and hypocapnia from overzealous ventilation, can only exacerbate the cord ischemia caused by surgical traction or hypotension. Other end organs that must be protected from hypotension include the heart and kidneys. The heart is easily monitored by following the ST segment of the V_5 lead of the electrocardiogram. The kidneys are monitored by bladder catheterization and hourly measurement of urine output. Renal perfusion pressure can be assumed to be inadequate if urine output falls to less than 1 mL/kg per hour.

Positioning

Anesthetized patients are extremely vulnerable during positioning for scoliosis surgery because of their inability to feel the extreme discomfort of certain positions that alter the normal mechanics of the body. Vulnerable parts that must be especially protected to avoid injury by pressure or stretching include the peripheral (ulnar) nerves, the male genitalia, the nipples, and the anterior superior iliac spine (to protect the lateral femoral cutaneous nerve of the thigh). Of the peripheral nerves, the brachial plexus is most vulnerable to stretch in the prone position (Martin and Warner, 1997). Stretching of the lower trunks of the brachial plexus is most likely to occur when the head is turned to the contralateral side, the ipsilateral shoulder is abducted, and the ipsilateral elbow is bent. Although efforts to prevent neuropathies are frequently debated, there is little hard evidence to support specific management recommendations.

The patient's eyes are vulnerable to corneal abrasion, optic vein engorgement, and retinal ischemia. Postoperative visual loss is a devastating and poorly understood injury. Over the past decade, speculation has grown that the frequency of perioperative blindness has been increasing among patients undergoing major spine surgery. Roth and colleagues found a much higher incidence of blindness (1 in 600) among patients undergoing complex spinal surgery (Roth et al., 1996, 1997; Roth and Barach, 2001). However, a report from the Mayo Clinic did not support this finding (Nuttall et al., 2001). In an effort to help analyze the risk factors involved, the American Society of Anesthesiologists has established an anonymous postoperative visual loss registry (www.asaclosedclaims.org).

Ischemic optic neuropathy, which affects the anterior or posterior portions of the optic nerve, is the most common cause of postoperative visual loss. Visual loss may also be caused by retinal arterial occlusion and cortical blindness. Awaking with visual impairment is one of the most frightening and catastrophic postanesthesia complications that a patient may sustain. It is also an enormous medicolegal liability problem. Commonly cited risk factors in patients who undergo scoliosis surgery in the prone position include hypotension, anemia, and external compression of the eye. Unfortunately, blindness has occurred even when these risk factors were not present (Lee and Lam, 2001; Roth and Barach, 2001).

Decreased perfusion pressure in the retina or optic nerve may be caused by decreased MAP or increased pressure in the venous drainage of the retina or optic nerve. Prolonged decreases in blood pressure, especially in patients with disturbed autoregulation, may be deleterious. Increased venous pressure (i.e., with internal jugular vein compression or ligation, prolonged head-down position, or large quantities of fluid infusion) also decreases perfusion. With prone positioning, increases in intraocular pressure might be potentiated by these factors. The combination of decreased blood pressure and increased venous pressure seems to pose the greatest risk.

The prone position increases intraabdominal pressure, which impairs ventilation by decreasing chest compliance and by limiting chest expansion. It also engorges epidural veins, which increases intraoperative bleeding and potentially increases the risk for postoperative epidural hematoma formation. Increased intraabdominal pressure leads to compression of the inferior vena cava, which impedes venous return to the heart, thereby decreasing cardiac output and engorging epidural veins. In an effort to facilitate venous return and avoid increased intraabdominal pressure, specially designed frames have been developed that allow the abdomen to hang free and facilitate respiratory movement (Relton and Hall, 1967).

Turning the anesthetized patient from the supine to the prone position requires careful orchestration by the entire surgical and anesthesia team. Cervical spine injury, dislodgment of intravascular and urinary catheters, accidental extubation or dislodgment of the endotracheal tube, inability to ventilate once prone, and dramatic changes in cardiac output can easily occur. During the turn, monitoring, except with an esophageal stethoscope, is difficult. Once the patient is turned, immediate restoration of pulse oximetry monitoring and auscultation of both lung fields is imperative. Adequate pressure-point padding (e.g., elbows, breasts, scrotum, feet) must be ensured to avoid peripheral nerve compression (i.e., ulnar nerve) and soft tissue damage.

The surgical plan and preference determine the patient's position and the device used to stabilize the patient's head. A pin-type or horseshoe-shaped holder may be employed and requires careful application and padding to avoid catastrophic oculofacial injuries. Alternatively, the head may be rested on a securely arranged stack of pillows to avoid exaggerated neck flexion or rotation, or ear trauma.

Anesthesia Techniques

Given the potential complications of neurologic injury and profound hemorrhage associated with spinal surgery, the anesthesia technique used should have minimal effects on neurophysiologic monitoring, allow for a wake-up test, and provide hemodynamic stability to minimize complications. The combination of remifentanil with either desflurane or propofol allows SSEP and MEP monitoring and a rapid wake-up response if necessary.

Patients with preexisting neurologic deficits such as cerebral palsy, paralytic scoliosis, and congenital scoliosis have variable SSEP waveforms of weak amplitude. The use of a ketamine or an etomidate infusion in these patients can augment

the amplitude of the evoked responses and increase the reliability of SSEP monitoring (Banoub et al., 2003; Lotto et al., 2004).

Postoperative Management

Although pulmonary failure and the need for postoperative ventilation are the primary problems of scoliosis surgery, other common postoperative concerns include ongoing blood loss, disseminated intravascular coagulation, hypovolemia, and development of syndrome of inappropriate secretion of antidiuretic hormone, paralytic ileus, and pain. The most important initial decision at the conclusion of surgery is whether to extubate the trachea. This decision is based in large part on the patient's preoperative pulmonary function and on the intraoperative course. Scoliosis surgery produces an immediate and transient decrease in pulmonary function of up to 60% of baseline values. The nadir of pulmonary function occurs on the third postoperative day, and it remains at approximately half of baseline values through the first postoperative week. These changes can resolve within 6 months of the procedure (Yuan et al., 1976). Patients with preoperative FVC levels of less than 50% of predicted and patients with nonidiopathic scoliosis should be extubated in the pediatric intensive care unit after cognitive faculties and respiratory muscle strength have returned to baseline. After spinal fusion, 18 children with severe restrictive lung disease (FVC < 45%) required a mean of 9 days of postoperative ventilation (Wazeka et al., 1976). Other common pulmonary complications in the postoperative period include atelectasis, pneumothorax, and pleural effusions.

Syndrome of inappropriate secretion of antidiuretic hormone is common and manifests as hyponatremia, hypoosmolality, decreased urine output, and increased urine osmolality. The increased plasma volume reduces the hemoglobin concentration and can be identified by following the red blood cell's mean corpuscular volume. As the level of antidiuretic hormone increases, plasma water increases, resulting in free water entry into red blood cells. The mean corpuscular volume increases, and the hemoglobin and mean corpuscular hemoglobin content decrease. The mean corpuscular volume should not change in the face of postoperative blood loss (Mason et al., 1989).

Because the surgery is so extensive, pain is an expected complication in all scoliosis patients. Furthermore, if remifentanil was used intraoperatively without loading the patient with a longer-acting opioid, an exaggerated pain response is to be expected on awaking. Remifentanil produces opioid-induced hyperalgesia, a paradoxical process by which opioid administration, even for short periods of time, increases the sensitivity to pain and worsens pain when the opioid is discontinued (Crawford et al., 2006). Postoperative pain can be treated with IV opioid therapy (i.e., patient-controlled analgesia [PCA]), regional anesthesia techniques, or both (Tobias, 2004). To use PCA, patients are started on a basal infusion of morphine (0.02 mg/kg per hour) or hydromorphone (0.004 mg/kg per hour) combined with a low-dosage naloxone infusion (0.25 mcg/kg per hour) (Maxwell and Yaster, 2003). The patient or nurse can trigger the PCA machine's bolus button, which provides an additional dose of morphine (0.02 mg/kg) or hydromorphone (0.004 mg/kg) (Monitto et al., 1998). Many centers are using neuraxial techniques for postoperative analgesia (Tobias, 2004).

Typically, a single epidural catheter is inserted by the surgeon at the T8 or T9 level before wound closure. Alternatively, two catheters are placed at the top and bottom of the wound by the surgeon. These catheters are intermittently or continuously infused with opioids (i.e., morphine, hydromorphone, or fentanyl), local anesthetics (i.e., 0.625% to 1.25% bupivacaine solutions), or both.

Nonsteroidal antiinflammatory drugs (NSAIDs) such as ketorolac have a morphine-sparing effect and result in fewer opioid-induced side effects such as somnolence, constipation, and pruritus (Reuben et al., 1997, 1998). The use of ketorolac does not increase bleeding, the need for transfusions, or reoperation (Reuben et al., 1997; Vitale et al., 2003). Nevertheless, for reasons that are discussed later, the use of ketorolac in scoliosis patients should be avoided, because NSAIDs significantly inhibited spinal fusion in human and laboratory studies (Glassman et al., 1998; Martin et al., 1999). NSAIDs such as ketorolac are thought to have deleterious effects on bone healing and fracture repair, although the actual clinical effects appear to be controversial at this point. In some studies, chronic NSAID use for more than 3 months was associated with lower fusion and success rates (Deguchi et al., 1998; Harder and An, 2003).

NSAIDs are thought to principally affect the bone morphogenetic proteins (BMPs) (Harder and An, 2003), which are a class of osteoinductive proteins that play an important role in bone growth and are essential for the growth and development of skeletal tissue and for bone regeneration during fracture repair (Kanakaris and Giannoudis, 2008; Dean et al., 2009). Martin and colleagues (1999), using a rabbit model of spinal fusion, investigated the effects of ketorolac on graft healing. Compared with a saline control group, less than half of the rabbits receiving ketorolac had a stable bone graft. However, the coadministration of a recombinant BMP with ketorolac to a third group of rabbits resulted in a 100% successful fusion rate. The investigators concluded that the effects of the NSAID could be completely reversed by the administration of a BMP (Martin et al., 1999). Clinical trials using recombinant BMPs to improve graft healing are in only the preliminary stage (Khan et al., 2002; Sandhu and Khan, 2003). Initial efforts to evaluate the effects of cyclooxygenase-2 (COX-2)–specific inhibitors of bone healing have produced similar results (Gilron et al., 2003). The healing of stabilized tibial fractures in COX-2–deficient mice was significantly delayed, as was intramembranous calvarial bone formation. These bone-healing deficiencies were reversed by the administration of prostaglandin E_2 and BMP-2 (Zhang et al., 2002; Clark et al., 2009). In some studies, COX-2 inhibition seemed to have less severe effects on bone healing than nonspecific COX-1 and COX-2 NSAIDs (Gerstenfeld et al., 2003).

Clinically, because of limited data, the effects of NSAIDs on bone healing remain controversial (Vuolteenaho et al., 2008). In a retrospective analysis of more than 300 patients undergoing spinal fusion who received a COX-2 inhibitor (ketorolac) or no NSAIDs for the first 5 postoperative days, patients who received ketorolac had a threefold increase in nonunion rate compared with COX-2 recipients or controls (Maxy and Glassman, 2001; Gajraj, 2003). On the other hand, in a retrospective study of 405 patients undergoing spinal fusion, no difference was noted in fusion rates between those who received ketorolac for the first 48 hours postoperatively and those who did not (Pradhan et al., 1976).

JOINT DISORDERS

Arthrogryposis Multiplex Congenita

Arthrogryposis multiplex congenita (AMC) consists of a heterogeneous group of disorders characterized by nonprogressive congenital joint contractures. Fetal akinesia results in the birth of a baby with multiple curved, rigid joints. The incidence is 1 in 3000 live births. Because of their extensive contractures, tense skin, and minimal muscle mass and subcutaneous tissue, these children have been described as looking like thin wooden dolls. Arthrogryposis is a clinical finding that is characteristic of a vast number of disorders (Bamshad et al., 2009). In the past, an in utero, self-limited anterior horn cell disease was proposed (Bonilla-Felix, 2004). AMC is now recognized as resulting from fetal neurogenic, myogenic, or connective tissue abnormalities, as well as maternal disorders such as maternal myasthenia gravis. The child's neurologic examination is fundamental to determining the etiology of AMC. The AMC of children with normal neurologic examinations results from amyoplasia, a distal arthrogryposis, a generalized connective tissue disorder, or fetal crowding. Children with amyoplasia frequently have midfacial hemangiomata, and 10% have gastroschisis or intestinal atresia. The distal arthrogryposes are a group of 10 autosomal dominant disorders with mutations in the genes that encode proteins of the contractile apparatus of fast-twitch myofibers (Sung et al., 1993). Children with these disorders have characteristic congenital contractures of two or more different body areas. The AMC of children with abnormal neurologic examinations is the result of developmental central nervous system abnormalities, spinal muscular atrophies, peripheral neuropathies, and myopathies (Takano et al., 2001). Mutations in the genes that encode for the neuromuscular junction's acetylcholine receptor proteins appear as AMC (Burke et al., 2003). AMC has also been associated with spinal cord dysplasia, lung hypoplasia, renal tubular dysfunction, and micrognathia (Narkis et al., 2007a, 2007b).

Most children with AMC have quadrimelic limb involvement. Joint involvement is symmetric, increases distally, and results in severe contractures and joint rigidity. The most common orthopedic deformities include talipes equinovarus, dislocated hip, dislocated patella, and scoliosis. Intelligence is usually normal. Surgical management is directed at correcting all lower extremity deformities that delay ambulation, and surgery is ideally performed before the patient is 2 years old. Upper extremity surgery is designed to improve hand function.

The anesthesia management of children with AMC is complicated by associated congenital abnormalities, an abnormal upper airway, and positioning difficulties (Martin and Tobias, 2006). Arthrogryposis is associated with congenital heart disease, pulmonary hypertension, cor pulmonale, and urogenital anomalies. The distal arthrogryposis disorders can be associated with Freeman-Sheldon syndrome, as well as the presence of trismus, cleft palate, or pulmonary hypertension (Laishley and Roy, 1986; Stevenson et al., 2006; Toydemir et al., 2006; Toydemir and Bamshad, 2009). Decreased pulmonary reserve that results from pulmonary hypoplasia and scoliotic restrictive lung disease may potentiate hypoxemia and may necessitate postoperative ventilatory support.

Patients with arthrogryposis have micrognathia, a high arched palate, and a short and rigid neck, making tracheal intubation difficult and at times impossible (Szmuk et al., 2001).

Direct laryngoscopy and intubation become more difficult as the patient ages, because craniofacial involvement often progresses with growth. Alternative strategies to direct laryngoscopy and tracheal intubation, such as the use of the laryngeal mask airway with or without the use of a tube exchanger, or fiberoptics, have been employed successfully in this disorder (Szmuk et al., 2001). The extensive contractures, tense skin, and minimal muscle mass and subcutaneous tissue pose challenges for intraoperative positioning and IV access.

Children with arthrogryposis may have altered responses to neuromuscular relaxants and are akin to other patients with anterior horn cell diseases. Although hyperkalemic responses to succinylcholine have not been reported, prudence mandates avoiding the routine use of depolarizing muscle relaxants.

Children with Freeman-Sheldon syndrome, in particular, are prone to hyperthermia and muscular rigidity responses to inhaled anesthetics and a neuroleptic malignant syndromic response to metoclopramide (Madi-Jebara et al., 2007). Although the response to nondepolarizing relaxants has been reported to be extremely variable, the use of short-acting nondepolarizing agents in association with careful monitoring of neuromuscular function has been successful in these patients.

The association of intraoperative hyperthermic crises with AMC has been sporadically reported. Hopkins and colleagues, in reporting three cases of hyperpyrexia, reviewed the literature of nine additional cases (Hopkins et al., 1991). In nine cases, hyperthermia, tachycardia, and hypercarbia were observed intraoperatively. Six episodes were assumed to be malignant hyperthermia, and dantrolene therapy was immediately instituted. Two cases responded rapidly to aggressive cooling. One patient received a nontriggering anesthetic. The halothane contracture test was not performed in any of these reported cases. In two large series of children with AMC who were anesthetized with triggering agents, no confirmed cases of malignant hyperthermia were reported (Baines et al., 1986). In light of the absence of laboratory confirmation, the occurrence of a hyperthermic crisis without exposure to triggering agents, and a large number of affected patients without hyperthermic response, Hopkins and colleagues (1991) concluded that these hypermetabolic responses are distinct from malignant hyperthermia. Patients with AMC are not considered to be at an increased risk for malignant hyperthermia (Laishley and Roy, 1986; Benca and Hogan, 2009).

Juvenile Idiopathic Arthritis (Formerly Juvenile Rheumatoid Arthritis)

Juvenile idiopathic arthritis (JIA) is the most common autoimmune disease of childhood, affecting 20 to 150 per 100,000 children (Helmick et al., 2008). It is defined as the presence of joint pain, stiffness, and swelling that persists for longer than 6 weeks, first occurring when the patient is younger than 16 years. The estimated incidence is 14 cases per 100,000 children per year. The International League of Associations for Rheumatology reclassified this disease as juvenile idiopathic arthritis to distinguish it from adult-onset rheumatoid arthritis (Weiss and Ilowite, 2005; Hayward and Wallace, 2009).

JIA is divided into three subsets based on the symptoms at onset. *Oligoarticular arthritis*, representing approximately 50% of all JIA cases, is common in girls, with the peak age of onset at 2 years. During the first 6 months of the disease, fewer than five joints are affected—typically the knees and less commonly the ankles and wrists. Approximately 75% of these patients have a positive antinuclear antibody (ANA) titer. Uveitis occurs in 15% to 45% of children with oligoarticular JIA. Oligoarticular arthritis is rarely destructive. *Polyarticular JIA*, representing 20% to 40% of JIA cases, is also more common in girls, with a peak age of onset of 3 years. In this variant, five or more joints are affected—commonly the small joints of the hand. Only 40% of these patients have a positive ANA titer, and 10% have positive test results for rheumatoid factor. Polyarticular JIA has associated subcutaneous nodules and erosions. The arthritis is destructive in 15% of patients. Moderate systemic manifestations of anemia and growth retardation are seen. *Systemic JIA*, also known as *Still disease*, manifests with fever, macular rash, leukocytosis, lymphadenopathy, and hepatomegaly. Symmetric polyarthritis is seen in these children. Boys and girls are affected equally, and they can present for treatment at any age. The cervical spine, jaw, hands, hips, and shoulders can be involved. Only 10% of these children have positive ANA results. The arthritis can be destructive in 25% of cases. Patients with systemic JIA can have pericarditis (30%), pleuritis, uveitis, splenomegaly, and abdominal pain. Although spontaneous disease remission can occur in patients with JIA, the therapeutic goals are to control pain, preserve joint range of motion, minimize systemic complications, and optimize growth and development.

Patients with juvenile ankylosing spondylitis and arthritis associated with inflammatory bowel disease are included in the enthesitis-related arthritis (ERA) subtype. ERA has a prevalence of 12 to 33 per 100,000 and is most common in boys older than 8 years. It has a strong genetic predisposition, as evidenced by a positive family history and the high frequency of the presence of HLA-B27 in affected patients. The hallmarks of the disease are pain, stiffness, and eventual loss of mobility of the back. ERA should be suspected in any child with chronic arthritis of the axial and peripheral skeleton, enthesitis (inflammation at points where tendons insert to bone), and rheumatoid factor and ANA seronegativity.

Therapy

Physical and occupational therapies are important adjuncts to medication in the management of JIA, because they help to maintain and improve range of motion, muscle strength, and skills for activities of daily living. Splints may be used to prevent contractures and to help in the work of improving range of motion. Arthroplasty may be needed for patients with severe deformities. Medications used to achieve these goals include NSAIDs, glucocorticoids, and disease-modifying antirheumatic drugs (methotrexate, sulfasalazine, leflunomide, cyclophosphamide, gold). Finally, biological agents, including tumor necrosis factor inhibitors (etanercept, infliximab, adalimumab, the interleukin-1 inhibitor anakinra, and the B-cell depleter rituximab), have all been added to the treatment armamentarium with great success (Hashkes and Laxer, 2005, 2006; Weiss and Ilowite, 2005).

Common surgical procedures include various joint arthroplasties and synovectomies, correction of uveitis, scoliosis surgery, limb-length discrepancy surgery, and limb and mandibular osteotomies.

Anesthesia considerations in the child with JIA are principally focused on airway management. JIA involvement of the mandibular head and the temporomandibular joint (TMJ), which limits mouth opening, occurs in over 60% of children (Pedersen et al., 2001; Sidiropoulou-Chatzigianni et al., 2008). As a result of TMJ disease, the mandible's growth is stunted, producing micrognathia in as many as 30% of children with JIA (Arabshahi and Cron, 2006). Magnetic resonance imaging (MRI) and ultrasound are useful imaging modalities to detect TMJ disease. Cervical spine disease is commonly seen in the systemic and the polyarticular forms of JIA, sometimes resulting in spinal fusion, which reduces cervical mobility (Fig. 26-5). Cervical stiffness is reported in 46% to 60% of patients. Radiographic changes are usually seen in the late stages of the disease and only in children with severe involvement. As a component of atlantoaxial rotatory subluxation or as a solitary manifestation, torticollis can develop, further increasing the degree of difficulty in airway management in these patients (Subach et al., 1998). Cricoarytenoiditis, an unusual manifestation of systemic JIA, can result in airway obstruction and severe distortion of the glottic anatomy (Jacobs and Hui, 1977; Vetter, 1994). Children with JIA should undergo a complete preoperative evaluation of the TMJ and cervical spine to assess for evidence of limited range of motion. The assessment should include dynamic radiographs.

Marfan Syndrome

Marfan syndrome (MFS) is an autosomal dominant connective tissue disorder caused by mutations of the gene *FBN1* on chromosome 15q21, which is responsible for the production of fibrillin-1, a complex glycoprotein that is a major constituent of various connective tissue types (Dietz et al., 2005; Judge and

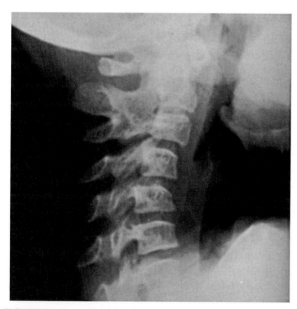

■ FIGURE 26-5. Radiograph of the cervical spine of a patient with active juvenile rheumatoid arthritis, showing fusion of the neural arch between joints C2 and C3, narrowing and erosion of the remaining neural arch joints, obliteration of the apophyseal space, and loss of the normal lordosis. *(From Miller ML, Cassidy JT: Juvenile rheumatoid arthritis. In Kliegman RM, Behrman RE, Jenson HB, et al, editors: Nelson textbook of pediatrics, ed 18, Philadelphia, 2007, Saunders, p 1004.)*

Dietz, 2005). Mouse models of MFS have revealed that fibrillin-1 mutations perturb the signaling of local transforming growth factor-β (TGFβ), in addition to impairing tissue integrity. This discovery has led to the identification of a new disorder (Loeys-Dietz syndrome), which has significantly worse cardiovascular consequences than MFS, and which has led to new avenues of therapeutic intervention (Dietz et al., 2005; Judge and Dietz, 2005; Ramirez and Dietz, 2007). Cardiovascular (mitral valve prolapse), ocular, craniofacial, and musculoskeletal systems are frequently affected in these patients. The cardiovascular complications of MFS and Loeys-Dietz syndrome, specifically aortic root disease (dilation, aneurysm), aneurysms and dissections throughout the arterial tree, and generalized arterial tortuosity, are the major causes of morbidity and premature death of these patients (Dietz et al., 2005; Judge and Dietz, 2005; Ramirez and Dietz, 2007). The clinical features of the musculoskeletal abnormalities of MFS include scoliosis, joint hypermobility, and craniofacial abnormalities. The prevalence of MFS is 2 to 3 cases per 10,000 individuals; about 25% of patients have no family history.

Aortic size appears to correlate with central pulse pressure, and historically, children with MFS were maintained on β-blockade to slow aortic root growth. Recent literature is in conflict as to the efficacy of this approach. Ladouceur and colleagues (2007) found that children treated with β-blockade had decreased aortic root growth; however, Selamet Tierney and colleagues (2007) found that the rate of aortic root dilation was no different between treated and untreated children. A promising new approach to slow the progression of aortic root dilation uses the angiotensin II–receptor blocker losartan, an antihypertensive medication known to inhibit TGFβ signaling (Brooke et al., 2008). The long-term survival of patients with MFS and ascending aortas greater than 50 mm is increased with long-term medical therapy in combination with prophylactic cardiac surgery.

In addition to the cardiovascular anomalies, patients with MFS have a high incidence of pectus deformities and spontaneous pneumothoraces. The inward depression of the sternum that results from excessive growth of costochondral cartilages, in combination with severe scoliosis, produces a precarious physiologic state in which respiratory compromise can result from lung compression, or cardiovascular collapse can occur from impeded venous return, distortion of the great vessels, or diminished coronary perfusion. Operative alteration of the complex three-dimensional geometry of a patient with MFS can result in sudden cardiovascular collapse.

MFS affects the spine in several ways. The prevalence of scoliosis in MFS is greater than 50%; only 10% to 20% of these patients require any treatment. The scoliosis of MFS progresses at a faster rate than in the general population. Sagittal plane spinal deformities are also common in MFS; 40% of patients with MFS have a kyphosis greater than 50 degrees (Demetracopoulos and Sponseller, 2007). These patients are at risk for atlantoaxial translocation with neck flexion and extension (Hobbs et al., 1997). Patients undergoing seemingly routine, uneventful direct laryngoscopy and endotracheal intubation can develop atlantoaxial rotatory subluxation, manifested as unresolved torticollis and neck pain in the postoperative period. These events are thought to result from abnormal bone morphology, the abnormal shape of the atlantoaxial facet, or the laxity of ligaments (Herzka et al., 2000). In a series of 100 patients with MFS, greater than 50% had evidence of increased atlantoaxial translation. The preadolescent population had a greater range of motion than did the adolescent or adult groups (Hobbs et al., 1997). Atlantoaxial subluxation has been reported as a cause of sudden death in patients with MFS (MacKenzie and Rankin, 2003). MFS is also associated with dural ectasia, a widening of the dural sac and nerve roots in the caudal portion of the spine. The MRIs of children with MFS suggest dural ectasia in 40% of cases. Dural ectasia can manifest as headache, proximal leg pain, leg weakness and numbness, and abdominal, genital, and rectal pain. Bony erosion can lead to myelomeningocele formation (MacKenzie and Rankin, 2003). As demonstrated in Figure 26-6, the presence of a dural ectatic segment (dilation of the dural sac) could have dramatic implications for neuraxial regional anesthetics, and MRI of the lumbosacral spine should be obtained preoperatively when this technique is contemplated in patients with MFS.

Anesthetic management of patients with MFS starts with a preoperative cardiovascular and cervical spine evaluation. Patients who are destined to undergo prone procedures should have the effects of sternal compression evaluated preoperatively by echocardiography. The anesthesiologist should consult with the patient's cardiologist to determine whether the dosages of β-blockade are appropriate. To minimize the risk for aortic dissection or rupture, the anesthesia technique should aim to decrease myocardial contractility and avoid sudden increases in blood pressure. In the setting of mitral valve prolapse, hypovolemia and tachycardia should be avoided. Nasotracheal fiberoptic intubation may be useful in patients with underlying disease and in those with atlantoaxial instability. The differential diagnosis of sudden intraoperative cardiovascular collapse in these patients with MFS should be expanded to include both a tension pneumothorax and a thoracic distortion that results in cardiac failure.

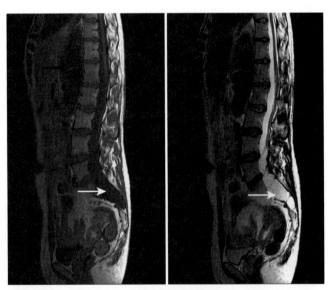

FIGURE 26-6. T1- and T2-weighted sagittal MR images of the lumbar spine of a 29-year-old man with Marfan syndrome reveal enlargement of the thecal sac *(yellow arrow)* with mild scalloping of the lumbar vertebral bodies and marked focal thinning of the sacrum *(white arrow)*. An enlarged flow void anterior to the spine *(red arrow)* is related to dilation of the descending aorta. *(From Sánchez I, Concepción L, Cortés JJ, et al: Dural ectasia in Marfan syndrome, Neurology 71:1378, 2008.)*

SYNDROMES OF DISPROPORTIONATE SHORT STATURE: DWARFISM

Children with dwarfism are unified solely by their phenotype of disproportionate short stature and associated limb deformities. More than 35,000 dwarfs are estimated to live in the United States, and the individual osteochondrodysplasias and mucopolysaccharidoses that produce this phenotype number well over 350 (Berkowitz et al., 1990). Achondroplasia is the most common form of dwarfism, with an incidence of 1 in 30,000 live births. It affects more than 250,000 individuals worldwide (Shirley and Ain, 2009). More than 95% of patients have the same point mutation in the *FGFR3* gene, on chromosome 4p16. *FGFR3* codes for fibroblast growth factor receptors, which normally function as an inhibitor to linear bone growth; achondroplastic mutations exaggerate this normal physiologic function (Horton et al., 2007). The mucopolysaccharidosis (MPS) syndromes (i.e., Hurler's syndrome [MPS I-H], Hunter's syndrome [MPS II], Morquio's syndrome [MPS IV], and Scheie's syndrome [MPS V]) are few in number but pose significant anesthesia challenges. Limb-lengthening techniques, cervical decompression, joint replacement, limb realignment, and bone marrow transplantation for patients with mucopolysaccharidoses are but a few of the procedures that are increasingly being performed on these patients. The number of diseases that constitute the dwarfing syndrome is enormous, and the limited anecdotal anesthesia experience for many of these precludes an encyclopedic review of all of the syndromes. Nevertheless, the common pathologic conditions to a large number of the dwarfing syndromes listed in Box 26-3 should be evaluated in the preoperative preparation of an affected patient.

Airway Abnormalities

The anesthesia management of dwarfs is frequently complicated by anatomic abnormalities of the upper airway and by difficulty in visualization of the larynx during direct laryngoscopy. Inability to intubate is the major cause of morbidity and mortality when anesthetizing dwarfs (Berkowitz et al., 1990). Upper airway obstruction is frequently a result of thickened pharyngeal and laryngeal structures, narrowed nasal passages, micrognathia, copious secretions, pharyngeal hypoplasia, and tracheal narrowing. It is seen most frequently in patients with mucopolysaccharidoses, diastrophic dysplasia, camptomelic dysplasia, severe diastrophic dysplasia, and Russell-Silver syndrome. Some patients demonstrate upper airway obstruction even in the awake state. Airway patency can be severely affected by positional changes alone. Some patients with achondroplasia, Morquio's syndrome, and metatropic dysplasia maintain a patent airway with the neck extended but completely obstruct when the neck is flexed. Sedation and general anesthesia often result in complete upper airway obstruction. Direct laryngoscopy and tracheal intubation are extremely difficult to perform in many dwarfs. Children with mucopolysaccharidoses have been described as presenting the worst airway problem in pediatric anesthesia; 54% of patients with MPS I are difficult intubations, and 23% are intubation "failures" (Martins et al., 2009). Endotracheal intubation is often hampered by inadequate laryngeal exposure from a shortened neck and protruding tongue, infiltration of the glottic and epiglottic structures with abnormal mucopolysaccharide, enlarged tonsils and adenoids,

Box 26-3 Systemic Manifestations of the Dwarfing Syndromes

Upper airway abnormalities: mucopolysaccharidosis (MPS), achondroplasia
- Macroglossia
- Micrognathia (mesomelic dysplasia, diastrophic dysplasia, Russell-Silver dwarf)
- Small oral opening
- Temporomandibular joint immobility
- Tonsillar and adenoidal hypertrophy
- Narrow nasopharynx
- Laryngomalacia

Difficult laryngoscopy: MPS ("most difficult intubations bar none")
- Abnormal, unrecognizable glottic structures
- Short neck, cervical scoliosis (Morquio's syndrome, metatropic dysplasia, diastrophic dysplasia, spondyloepiphyseal dysplasia)
- Copious secretions

Upper airway obstruction: MPS
- Abnormal neck position
- Abnormal upper airway
- Laryngomalacia
- Copious secretions

Pulmonary dysfunction: MPS, achondroplasia, asphyxiating thoracic dystrophy (Jeune's syndrome)
- Restrictive lung disease
- Thoracic dystrophy
- Scoliosis
- Pulmonary hypertension
- Obstructive sleep apnea

Cardiovascular dysfunction: osteogenesis imperfecta (OI), MPS, asphyxiating thoracic dystrophy, achondroplasia
- Congenital heart disease
- Acquired valvular disease
- Cor pulmonale
- Restrictive lung disease
- Obstructive sleep apnea

Neurologic complications: achondroplasia, OI
- Atlantooccipital instability, odontoid hypoplasia
- Cervicomedullary compression
- Intracranial hypertension
- Deafness

Hematologic dysfunction: OI
- Platelet aggregation disorder

Other: OI
- Propensity for bony fractures
- Hypermetabolism

---

and subglottic, tracheal, and bronchial narrowing. In contrast, the patient with achondroplasia, who may also have narrowed nasal passages and pharyngeal hypoplasia because of cranial base angulation and midface hypoplasia, rarely develops peri-induction airway obstruction and can be easily managed with a face mask (Monedero et al., 1997).

Anesthesia Management

Preoperative sedative drugs should be avoided in patients prone to upper airway obstruction. Before induction, IV access is obtained, and an antisialagogue is administered. If the potential for severe upper airway obstruction and difficult intubation is anticipated, the equipment and personnel required to establish an emergency airway should be present before the induction of anesthesia (see Chapter 13, Induction, Maintenance, and Recovery, and Chapter 12, Airway Management). Spontaneous ventilation is mandatory. Often, the only way to identify the glottis is by observation of the air bubbles during spontaneous ventilation. An inhalational induction with high concentrations of oxygen and sevoflurane or a continuous IV infusion of propofol or ketamine are equally effective approaches in this situation. After an adequate anesthesia plane is achieved, endotracheal intubation can be accomplished by direct laryngoscopy or by fiberoptic-guided bronchoscopy. Alternatives include insertion of the lightwand and fiberoptic intubation by means of a laryngeal mask airway. Neuromuscular relaxants are avoided until the airway is secured. Rarely, a tracheostomy performed while the patient is awake may be the safest approach. The examiner must avoid neck manipulation, particularly neck flexion during laryngoscopy, in patients with atlantoaxial instability or foramen magnum stenosis.

Pulmonary Dysfunction

The pulmonary dysfunction common to children with a dwarfing syndrome is multifactorial in origin. Restrictive lung disease is a consequence of thoracic cage dystrophy (e.g., Jeune's syndrome) or scoliosis, and it results in reduced lung volumes, ventilation/perfusion mismatching, progressive hypoxemia, and hypercarbia. Obstructive or central sleep apnea causes pulmonary hypertension, behavioral disorders, substantial morbidity, and sudden death (Sisk et al., 1999). Structural abnormalities, particularly in patients with MPS, may cause intrathoracic obstruction. Children with MPS frequently suffer from chronic sinus infections that result from mucosal alterations and an increased viscosity of their secretions, a combination that produces a milieu of chronic airway inflammation (Martins et al., 2009). The preoperative assessment of these patients must include an evaluation of pulmonary function and a sleep study. The finding of central apnea necessitates a neuroradiologic evaluation of the cervical spine and foramen magnum. The presence and severity of pulmonary hypertension can be determined by an electrocardiography and echocardiography.

Anesthesia Management

The degree of pulmonary dysfunction discovered during preoperative evaluation has profound implications on intraoperative and postoperative management. Severe obstructive sleep apnea may preclude an inhalational induction of anesthesia or the use of premedication. Significant restrictive lung diseases with attendant ventilation/perfusion mismatch, proclivity to atelectasis, and development of an increased $Pao_2–Pao_2$ gradient may necessitate placement of an indwelling arterial catheter to ensure adequate gas exchange throughout the perioperative period. The severity of restrictive lung disease dictates the necessity for continued intubation and ventilation postoperatively.

Cardiac Dysfunction

Children with dwarfing syndromes have a variety of causes for cardiac dysfunction. A high incidence of coexisting structural heart disease, such as atrial septal defects, occurs in a number of the dysplasias. Acquired valvular heart disease is a common complicating feature of children with MPS and is occasionally found in osteogenesis imperfecta. Ischemic heart disease may result from infiltrative mucopolysaccharides or from the consequences of cor pulmonale and longstanding pulmonary hypertension. Cardiomyopathy is a severe problem for children with MPS (Mohan et al., 2002; Rigante and Segni, 2002). Physical examination, chest radiography, electrocardiography, and especially echocardiography are useful in diagnosing the extent of cardiovascular involvement. The most reliable indicators of pulmonary hypertension are the presence of tricuspid regurgitation and prolongation of the right systolic time interval. The electrocardiogram should be reviewed for evidence of myocardial ischemia, particularly in patients with Hurler's syndrome or Hunter's syndrome.

Anesthesia Management

The anesthesia management of a patient with dwarfism, impaired myocardial dysfunction, and pulmonary hypertension must be meticulously planned and executed. Invasive monitoring of arterial, central venous, and, in severe cases, pulmonary artery pressures is frequently necessary. The use of intraoperative transesophageal echocardiography may be warranted in patients with severe valvular dysfunction or those who have evidence of ischemic heart disease. Modest hypoxemia and hypovolemia can exacerbate preexisting pulmonary hypertension and borderline right ventricular function, and must be avoided. The need to maintain an adequate anesthesia depth, crucial in avoiding intraoperative pulmonary hypertensive crises, must be balanced by the limitations imposed by compromised ventricular function. Attention must also be directed to the effects of changes in heart rate, blood pressure, filling pressures, and systemic vascular resistance on myocardial function. In light of these challenges, an opioid-based anesthetic in combination with adrenergic-modulating agents may provide the most stable intraoperative milieu for this subset of patients. The use of opioids in patients at risk for postoperative airway obstruction may result in postoperative intubation and mechanical ventilation.

Neurologic Dysfunction

Cervicomedullary compression and hydrocephalus are the main neurologic concerns in patients with dwarfism. The causes of cervical cord compression include atlantooccipital instability, odontoid process hypoplasia, foramen magnum stenosis, abnormal meningeal glycosaminoglycan deposition, and, infrequently, cervical scoliosis (Kachur and Del, 2000). Foramen magnum stenosis is a frequent complication of achondroplasia. Physical findings or a history consistent with upper motor neuron weakness (e.g., progressive weakness, hyperreflexia, abnormal plantar response), sleep apnea, cyanosis, or respiratory distress is suggestive of cervicomedullary compression. Flexion and extension neck films should be obtained to determine the degree of cervical spine instability in affected patients. Achondroplasia and MPS are associated with increased intracranial pressure; hydrocephalus arises from the impaired absorption of cerebrospinal fluid by the arachnoid granulations (Sheridan and Johnston, 1994).

Anesthesia Management

Improper positioning of the head, neck, and shoulders during the induction of anesthesia, laryngoscopy, and surgery may lead to catastrophic intraoperative cord ischemia. Patients with Morquio's syndrome, diastrophic dysplasia, or achondroplasia are at greatest risk. The maintenance of neck stabilization during intubation or fiberoptic intubation may be advisable. Cervical stabilizing devices such as a halo cast or a Milwaukee brace may be applied before anesthesia to avoid cervical subluxation and dislocation. Unfortunately, these devices may make direct laryngoscopy impossible. Succinylcholine should be avoided when there is evidence of pyramidal tract signs, muscle wasting, or paresis. Autonomic hyperreflexia may be a problem in patients with cervical cord compression or myelopathy.

The coexistence of intracranial hypertension and a difficult airway is particularly challenging to the anesthesiologist. The conventional approaches of inhalational or intravascular induction may have salutary effects on one element of management but catastrophic consequences on another. These conflicting requirements must be balanced on a case-by-case basis. One approach is to use an IV infusion of propofol to place a laryngeal mask airway, through which a fiberoptic bronchoscope is passed. Once identification of the glottic structures is ensured, an intubating dose of propofol is administered to blunt the intracranial pressure response to endotracheal intubation.

OSTEOGENESIS IMPERFECTA

Osteogenesis imperfecta (OI) is another of the dwarfing syndromes that involves unique problems. It is a heritable disorder of collagen production with varying degrees of severity. Its cardinal manifestation is bone fragility, and it frequently appears in childhood with multiple fractures after little or no trauma. Ninety percent of individuals with OI have mutations of the pro-α1 or pro-α2 chains of type I collagen (*COL1A1* or *COL1A2*) genes. A number of those without collagen mutations have mutations involving the enzyme complex responsible for posttranslational hydroxylation of the position 3 proline residue of COL1A1. Two of the genes encoding proteins involved in that enzyme complex, *LEPRE1* and cartilage-associated protein, when mutated, have been shown to cause autosomal-recessive osteogenesis imperfecta, which has a moderate to severe clinical phenotype, often indistinguishable from OI types II or III (Basel and Steiner, 2009; Shapiro and Sponsellor, 2009). The pathogenetic molecular mechanism of these deletions dictates the severity of the clinical features. Chain exclusion, in which the abnormal chain is not incorporated into the collagen triple helix, produces a milder phenotype. Chain inclusion, in which the abnormal chain is incorporated into the collagen triple helix, results in a defective helix and a more severe phenotype (Basel and Steiner, 2009). The effects of OI manifest as abnormalities of bone, teeth, sclera, and ligaments. The four clinical subtypes are listed in Table 26-7 (Cohen, 2002).

The hallmarks of this disease are bony fragility and multiple fractures after even innocuous trauma. Scoliosis and kyphosis are common, producing significant restrictive lung disease and pulmonary hypertension, especially in OI type III. A majority of patients with OI develop valvular regurgitant lesions. Medical management includes the use of bisphosphonates, which are anti-bone-resorptive drugs (Phillipi et al., 2008; Castillo and

TABLE 26-7. Types of Osteogenesis Imperfecta

Type	Features
I	Mildest form Mild bone fragility; bimodal fracture curve (first peak: between 1 year and puberty; second, smaller peak: postmenopausally in women and after 70 years in men); normal stature; blue sclerae; deafness in some cases, most commonly occurring in second decade; dominant inheritance
II	Most severe form: perinatal lethal form Half do not survive day 1, and 90% are dead by 1 week; extreme short stature; short, bowed long bones, particularly lower limbs; ribs have beaded appearance from recurrent fractures; respiratory insufficiency; absence of calvarial mineralization; dominant mutation
III	Progressively deforming type Many fractures; thin ribs with discrete fractures; curvature of spine that may be severe enough to reduce pulmonary reserve; severe short stature; deafness; dentinogenesis imperfecta; dominant mutation; rare recessives unlinked to type I collagen genes
IV	Mild-to-moderate bone fragility; short stature; deafness in some cases; dentinogenesis imperfecta; dominant inheritance

Adapted from Cohen MM Jr: Some chondrodysplasias with short limbs: molecular perspectives, *Am J Med Genet* 112:304, 2002.

Samson-Fang, 2009). Some data suggest their efficacy in reducing fracture frequency, increasing bone density, promoting remodeling of previously crush-fractured vertebrae, reducing chronic pain, and improving mobility in children and infants with osteogenesis imperfecta (Cheung and Glorieux, 2008; Phillipi et al., 2008; Castillo and Samson-Fang, 2009).

Anesthesia Management

The mainstay of OI management is orthopedic surgery and rehabilitative physiotherapy (Cheung and Glorieux, 2008; Basel and Steiner, 2009). The hallmark of anesthesia management is to handle these patients very gently. Indeed, fractures may occur from simple procedures such as applying a tourniquet or measuring blood pressure or while positioning the patient on the operating room table. Airway management may cause fractures, and the physician must pay particular attention to the teeth, mandible, and cervical spine. Occasionally, visualization of the airway is difficult, and the use of a laryngeal mask airway, as in other patients with difficult airways, may be very helpful (Kostopanagiotou et al., 2000; Asai and Shingu, 2001). Patients with OI have a hypermetabolic state and become hyperthermic during anesthesia (Benca and Hogan, 2009). This condition is not malignant hyperthermia, even though a few case reports of true malignant hyperthermia have been reported in these patients (Rampton et al., 1984; Porsborg et al., 1996). Many have recommended the use of a total IV anesthesia technique (Karabiyik et al., 2002). The routine pediatric anesthesia practice of preventing intraoperative hypothermia, such as using warming blankets and heated, humidified gasses, should be tempered, and antimuscarinics such as atropine and glycopyrrolate should be used judiciously. Some patients with OI bruise easily as a result of a presumed platelet abnormality. Bleeding

and hemorrhage are rare, but approximately 30% of these patients have abnormal bleeding times, capillary fragility, and reduced levels of factor VIII.

OSTEOPETROSIS

Osteopetrosis (i.e., marble bone disease) is an inherited disease with diminished bone resorption resulting from osteoclastic abnormalities, whose clinical hallmark is hard and brittle bones that fracture very easily (Balemans et al., 2005; Del et al., 2008). The metabolic disorders in this group are genetically heterogeneous. Autosomal-dominant osteopetrosis is the result of either abnormal osteoclast resorption or abnormal low-density lipoprotein receptor–related proteins (Balemans et al., 2005; Del et al., 2008). Clinically, osteopetrosis appears in three forms: infantile autosomal recessive ("malignant"), intermediate autosomal recessive, and autosomal dominant. Children with the severe form of osteopetrosis have insufficient bone marrow to support normal hematopoiesis; thrombocytopenia, anemia, and infectious complications are life threatening in the first decade of life. Patients with all forms of osteopetrosis are at risk for pathologic fractures (Tolar et al., 2004). Stem-cell transplantation is the only curative treatment for malignant osteopetrosis (Driessen et al., 2003). Patients with osteopetrosis frequently require anesthetics for bone marrow examinations and for treatment of their pathologic fractures.

Airway and cervical spine issues dominate the perioperative concerns of those caring for a child with osteopetrosis. Burt and coworkers (1999), in a series of 65 anesthesias for children with osteopetrosis, reported that the rate of airway management difficulties was much higher for this group of children than for the other children anesthetized at their institution. Mandibular abnormalities and TMJ immobility contributed to the difficulty of orotracheal intubation, and abnormalities of the nasal turbinates made nasotracheal intubation difficult. Cervicomedullary stenosis limited optimal head positioning, and concurrent thrombocytopenia exacerbated airway instrumentation and limited the options of a regional anesthetic. Afflicted children are also at risk for spontaneous cervical fractures. Children with the malignant infantile osteopetrosis variant have obstructive sleep apnea and nocturnal hypoxemia (Kasow et al., 2008). No particular anesthesia technique was deemed superior, but there was an emphasis on meticulous preoperative airway preparation with the ready availability of the resources for emergency airway management. Placement of intraosseous needles for emergency vascular access is difficult and nearly impossible in patients with this disease.

CEREBRAL PALSY

Cerebral palsy (CP) is a static encephalopathy defined as a nonprogressive disorder of posture and movement that manifests as poor muscle control, weakness, and increased muscle tone (Rosenbaum, 2007). Epilepsy and abnormalities of speech, vision, and intellect that result from a defect or lesion of the developing brain are often associated. It is the most common childhood motor disability, occurring in 2 of 1000 live births (Paneth et al., 2006). The CP phenotype results from multiple etiologies. In premature infants, periventricular leukomalacia is commonly associated with the development of CP. In term

TABLE 26-8. The Four Classification Systems of Cerebral Palsy

Physiology	Topography	Etiology	Functional Capacity
Spastic	Monoplegia	Prenatal	Class 1–No limitation of activity
Athetoid	Paraplegia	(e.g., infection, metabolic, anoxic, toxic, genetic)	
Rigid	Hemiplegia		Class II–Slight to moderate limitation
Ataxic	Triplegia		
Tremor	Quadriplegia	Perinatal	
Atonic	Diplegia	(e.g., anoxic)	Class III–Moderate to great limitation
Mixed	Double hemiplegia	Postnatal	
Unclassified		(e.g., toxins, trauma, infection)	Class IV–No useful physical activity

infants, early antenatal insults are attributed to be the cause of CNS injury and can manifest as events at the time of delivery. The most common etiologic factors are prematurity and birth weight greater or less than ideal weight for gestational age (Pharoah et al., 1996; Paneth et al., 2006; Rosenbaum, 2007).

CP can be classified by a description of the motor handicap in terms of physiology (major motor abnormality), topography (extremity involved), etiology, and functional capacity (Table 26-8). Although the CNS lesion is static, the degree of impairment can change with time. CP is commonly associated with a spectrum of developmental disabilities, including mental retardation, epilepsy, and visual, hearing, speech, cognitive, and behavioral abnormalities. The motor handicap may be the least of the child's problems. The necessity to treat each patient's problems uniquely and to avoid generalization cannot be overemphasized. Some children with CP may be of normal intelligence but limited in their ability to communicate. Others with marked developmental delay may be difficult to separate from their parents because of natural fear and an inability to reason in a way expected of children with normal intelligence (see Chapter 9, Preoperative Preparation).

Patients with CP often require multiple surgical procedures. Orthopedic operations to improve function of the extremities are common, and some patients require surgical correction of progressive spinal deformities. Common procedures include surgical soft tissue procedures that reduce muscle spasm around the hip girdle, including an adductor tenotomy or psoas transfer and release.

Several drugs are commonly used in treating spasticity, athetosis, dystonia, and seizures in patients with CP, and many of these drugs have significant anesthesia implications. Drugs used to treat spasticity include dantrolene, benzodiazepines, and baclofen. Incapacitating athetosis is treated with levodopa; dystonia, with carbamazepine and trihexyphenidyl. Seizures are commonly treated with phenobarbital, phenytoin, clonazepam, carbamazepine, and sodium valproate. The muscle spasticity of CP is thought to be caused by inadequate release of the inhibitor γ-aminobenzoic acid (GABA) in the dorsal horn of the spinal cord, resulting in a relative excess of excitatory glutamate on the alpha motor neurons, which produces simultaneous contraction of agonist and antagonist muscle groups. The symptoms of spastic diplegia can be treated surgically with rhizotomy, a procedure in which the roots of the spinal nerves are divided (Albright, 1992). Spasticity can also be treated medically by administering a continuous intrathecal infusion of baclofen or

by local intramuscular injection of botulinum toxin (Albright, 1996a). Baclofen is a GABA agonist that binds to the GABA(B) receptor located in the dorsal horn of the spinal cord, where the primary sensory fibers end, producing presynaptic inhibition of monosynaptic and polysynaptic reflexes. Continuous intrathecal baclofen infusions are used to manage intractable and generalized spasticity while minimizing side effects (Albright, 1996b; Verrotti et al., 2006). Most patients will have improved range of motion, decreased painful muscle spasms, and improvements in independent function.

Intramuscular botulinum toxin A (BTX-A) is also used to relieve dynamic deformities that result from muscle spasticity. After injection, BTX-A is taken up in presynaptic terminals, inhibiting acetylcholine release and functionally denervating muscle fibers within 2 to 3 cm of the injection site. Focal controlled muscle weakness is produced, which reduces spasticity for up to 6 months (Bjornson et al., 2007). Tight heel cords may be treated conservatively with serial casting, with botulinum injection, or surgically with an Achilles tenotomy. The child's particular spasticity and resulting joint contractures require vigilant positioning and padding in the operating room to avoid neurovascular compromise and skin ulcerations.

Preoperative concerns for children with CP focus on their pulmonary, gastrointestinal, and neurologic problems. This population is prone to aspiration pneumonia from gastroesophageal reflux and nasopharyngeal aspiration, as demonstrated by the finding that 75% of children with gastroesophageal reflux and delayed gastric emptying are neurologically impaired (Gisel et al., 2003; Ceriati et al., 2006). Many have chronic lung disease with a reactive component, and they suffer from frequent respiratory infections. Obstructive sleep apnea, seen in 20% to 50% of this patient population, has many causes, including bulbar dysfunction, neurogenic laryngomalacia, and decreased pharyngeal tone (Schwengel et al., 2009). Children with developmental disabilities are more than three times more likely to develop sedation-related hypoxia (Kannikeswaran et al., 2009).

Airway management can be complicated by restricted TMJ range of motion and by poor and malpositioned dentition. Patients with CP commonly have gastroesophageal reflux disease, dysfunctional swallowing, and severe food refusal, all contributing to suboptimal nutritional status that portends increased perioperative complications. Children with severe CP have a significant narrowing of their palates, placing them at increased risk for airway obstruction. Children with CP have a higher incidence of latex allergy than the general population. Thirty percent of children with CP require antiepileptic medications (Singhi et al., 2003).

Perioperative seizure management in the patient with CP is the same as for any patient with a seizure disorder. Most anesthesia agents are anticonvulsants, and they can be used safely in patients with underlying seizure disorders. A few anesthesia agents, such as enflurane, etomidate, ketamine, methohexital, EMLA (i.e., eutectic mixture of local anesthetics, 2.5% lidocaine and 2.5% prilocaine), and normeperidine (an active metabolite of meperidine) are proconvulsants and should be avoided if alternatives are available. Most of these proconvulsant anesthesia agents actually raise the seizure threshold in normal patients and are proconvulsant only in patients with underlying seizure disorders. Patients should take their chronic anticonvulsants on the day of surgery. Virtually all anticonvulsants have a long half-life of elimination (24 to 36 hours), and if blood anticonvulsant levels are within the therapeutic range, a 24-hour period can elapse without the patient having to take the anticonvulsant and without increasing the risk for a seizure.

In most orthopedic surgical procedures performed in patients with CP, almost any anesthesia technique and combination of drugs can be used. Potent inhaled anesthetics, muscle relaxants (including succinylcholine), hypnotics, sedatives, opioids, and local anesthetics have been used safely. Children with CP appear to have a lower MAC than unaffected children (Frei et al., 1997). Succinylcholine does not cause hyperkalemia, and it can be safely administered to patients with CP. They have a slightly increased sensitivity to succinylcholine compared with normal children (Dierdorf et al., 1985; Theroux et al., 1994). Resistance to nondepolarizing muscle relaxants and rapid recovery from neuromuscular blockade have been reported in this patient population, which may be explained by the increase in extrajunctional acetylcholine receptors (Theroux et al., 2002). Propofol requirements are significantly lower in noncommunicative CP children than in their unaffected peers (Saricaoglu et al., 2005).

Postoperative pain management is important in the care of patients with CP. The surgical procedures, particularly those for relieving spasticity, are extremely painful. The child severely affected with CP may be unable to communicate his or her pain, and health care providers are often unable to accurately assess the severity of postoperative pain. Parents and other routine caregivers are invaluable in assessing the pain of these patients. The Non-Communicating Children's Pain Checklist–Postoperative Version has been validated for children with intellectual disabilities (Breau et al., 2002, 2003). Postoperative pain is treated with continuous epidural (caudal or lumbar) infusions. Lidocaine (1.5 to 2.0 mg/kg per hour) plus fentanyl (0.5 mcg/kg per hour), chloroprocaine (3 mg/kg per hour) plus fentanyl (0.5 mcg/kg per hour), and bupivacaine (0.625 to 1 mg/mL, 0.2 to 0.4 mg/kg per hour) with or without fentanyl (0.5 mcg/kg per hour) or hydromorphone

(2 to 4 mcg/kg per hour) have all been used. Muscle spasms are virtually universal and are treated prophylactically with IV diazepam. The addition of clonidine to the postoperative epidural infusion at a dosage of 0.08 to 0.12 mcg/kg per hour is also effective at relieving muscle spasm. The management of posterior rhizotomy requires special attention. Often used in severe spasticity, this surgical procedure requires stimulation of the dorsal roots intraoperatively and observation of muscle response (see Chapter 22, Anesthesia for Neurosurgery) (Farmer and Sabbagh, 2007).

ILIZAROV METHOD

Professor G. A. Ilizarov introduced the concept of distraction osteogenesis in the 1950s (Herbert et al., 1995). Working as a general practitioner in Siberia, he found himself treating many patients with chronic osteomyelitis associated with bone loss and many veterans of World War II who had developed fracture nonunions. Using materials from the metal factories at which many of his patients were employed, he fashioned external fixators and transosseous wires to induce the formation of new bone between freshly cut osseous surfaces that are gradually pulled apart. Using this technique, he was able to salvage limbs that otherwise would have been amputated. For many years, he worked in isolation, with his techniques remaining unknown in most of the world (Fig. 26-7).

Over the past 20 years, this method has undergone significant refinements, and it is now employed in the treatment of congenital limb and other skeletal deformities, acquired short limbs, and angular deformities, and in the reconstruction of large bony defects that result from trauma, tumor excision, infection, and fracture nonunions (Herbert et al., 1995). Distraction osteogenesis has also been used to treat the numerous syndromes associated with micrognathia and retrognathia,

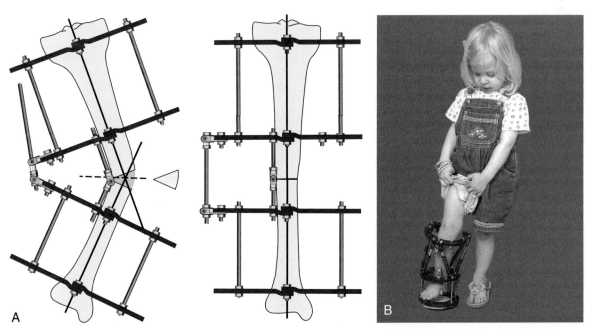

■ **FIGURE 26-7. A,** Wedge osteotomy *(right)* after application of an Ilizarov apparatus to correct a rotational deformity. With the external fixator in place *(left)*, the rotational deformity has been corrected, and the bone is ready for lengthening by slow adjustment of the diaphyseal rings. **B,** Children with external fixators are encouraged to resume as much normal function as possible.

such as the Pierre Robin syndrome, Treacher Collins syndrome, Nager's syndrome, velocardiofacial syndrome, and Pfeiffer's syndrome, all of which can result in airway obstruction (McCarthy et al., 2001; Sidman et al., 2001).

The success of the Ilizarov technique of distraction osteogenesis depends on adherence to the principles of tension-stress phenomena. These include a low-energy osteotomy to preserve periosteal blood supply; a slow, incremental distraction rate to preserve soft tissue blood supply; and maintenance of full function of the extremity. Bone healing is promoted by the biological stress of walking on or flexing a broken limb, causing a trampoline-like effect of pulling and contracting that stimulates bone growth and healing. Using a corticotomy that preserves blood flow to the periosteum and the medullary canal, a gap between healthy, vascular-sufficient bone is created. Wires are inserted into the bone above and below the osteotomy and are attached under tension to an external fixator at 90-degree angles to the plane of the deformity. After an initial latency period, the osteotomy is gradually distracted at a rate of 1 mm/day in four incremental steps. The external fixator serves as the distracting device and provides optimal mechanical stability so that weight bearing and range of motion on the operative limb are possible on the second hospital day. The early functional use of the affected limb stimulates callus formation and osteoblastic activity (Birch and Samchukov, 2004).

Anesthesia Considerations

Because the Ilizarov procedure is applied to children with a wide spectrum of diseases, including those with complex congenital musculoskeletal anomalies, the anesthesia implications of their coexisting diseases often take precedence over those of the operative procedure. These operative procedures are often long and complex but are associated with few hemodynamic perturbations and only modest blood loss. The perioperative complications of the Ilizarov procedure that are affected by anesthesia management include nerve injury and the need for intact motor function and optimal analgesia in the postoperative period. Nerve injury can occur during pin placement and during the distraction process. To recognize inadvertent surgical trauma to nerves in the operative field, neuromuscular relaxation is avoided so that muscle contractions can be recognized. Postoperative surgical pain can be intense in the first 48 hours, and these patients are encouraged to begin physical therapy on the first postoperative day, with an emphasis on passive range of motion and weight bearing (Paley, 1990).

Children undergoing an Ilizarov procedure are often anesthetized with a general anesthetic supplemented with an epidural or peripheral nerve catheter. In most cases, endotracheal intubation is accomplished with short-acting neuromuscular blockade or with deep inhalational or IV anesthesia. Children with concurrent airway or cervical spine anomalies are intubated with a fiberoptic bronchoscope or with a laryngeal mask airway–guided approach during spontaneous breathing. After the induction of general anesthesia, an epidural or peripheral nerve catheter is placed. If an epidural is used, a continuous epidural infusion of 0.8 to 1 mg/mL of bupivacaine with 1 mcg/mL of fentanyl can be started in the operating room at an infusion rate of 1 mL/kg per hour. Anesthesia is maintained with small amounts of opioids and a low concentration of inhaled anesthesia agents. The epidural infusion of bupivacaine and fentanyl is continued for the first 24 to 36 hours postoperatively

and augmented with acetaminophen (see Chapter 16, Regional Anesthesia). In patients who do not have a neuraxial or peripheral nerve catheter in place, IV PCA can be used.

TOURNIQUETS

Pneumatic tourniquets are commonly used to provide a dry operative field and limit intraoperative blood loss during extremity surgery (Kam et al., 2001). Modern pneumatic tourniquets consist of three basic components: a cuff that is similar to a blood pressure cuff and is wrapped around a patient's limb and then inflated, a compressed gas source, and a mechanism with a pressure gauge that is designed to maintain pressure in the cuff at a set value. After elevation and application of an Esmarch's bandage to exsanguinate the limb, the tourniquet is applied over smooth padding and inflated. Older methods inflate the tourniquet to a pressure based on the patient's systolic pressure. Recent practice is to determine the limb occlusion pressure and add a margin of 75 mm Hg for lower extremity surgery and 50 mm Hg for upper extremity procedures. Limb occlusion pressure, first suggested by Cushing, is the minimum pressure necessary to occlude arterial blood flow, as determined automatically or via palpation or pulse oximeter. To prevent accidental injury, the cuff should have a width that is greater than one half of the limb's diameter and an accurate pressure gauge, and the cuff should be inflated to the lowest possible inflation pressure recommended. The duration of inflation should also be carefully monitored (Tuncali et al., 2006; Reilly et al., 2009).

The length of time that the tourniquet can remain safely inflated is controversial. The most common recommendation, 2 hours, is based on the finding that cellular ischemic changes such as mitochondrial swelling, myelin degeneration, glycogen storage depletion, and Z-line lysis are reversible if the tourniquet is inflated for no more than 1 to 2 hours (Patterson and Klenerman, 1979). The deleterious effects of tourniquet inflation include pain while the tourniquet is inflated ("tourniquet pain"), metabolic and hemodynamic changes that occur during tourniquet inflation and deflation, and damage to blood vessels and muscle if the tourniquet is inflated for excessive periods. The use of pneumatic tourniquets has been associated with perioperative neuropathy (Welch et al., 2009).

In awake patients undergoing extremity surgery under regional anesthesia blockade, tourniquet pain is described as a dull, ill-defined ache that occurs approximately 45 to 60 minutes after a tourniquet is inflated. Over time, this pain becomes unbearable, but it subsides immediately after tourniquet deflation. This pain occurs despite adequate regional anesthesia for the surgical procedure itself. The cause of tourniquet pain remains uncertain, and early intervention is imperative. IV opioids have limited efficacy, and induction of general anesthesia or deflation of the cuff is the only effective solution to this problem. Prophylaxis may be possible. The addition of opioids to local anesthesia solutions at the time of neural blockade appears to decrease the incidence of tourniquet pain in patients undergoing a regional anesthesia.

The hemodynamic consequences of tourniquet application include increases in blood and central venous pressures. Kaufman and Walts (1982) reported an overall 30% increase in blood pressure during tourniquet inflation. The blood pressure response is more exaggerated in patients under general anesthesia than in those undergoing regional blockade (Valli et al., 1987). Tourniquet-induced hypertension can be prevented by the preoperative administration of 0.25 mg/kg of ketamine (Satsumae et al., 2001). Limb exsanguination and tourniquet inflation can redistribute 15% of the total blood volume to the general circulation rapidly. Central venous pressure increases of up to 14 mm Hg have been reported in adults with the application of bilateral tourniquets. The clinical significance of central venous pressure reduction that accompanies tourniquet deflation primarily depends on the presence of preexisting cardiac dysfunction.

The metabolic changes that accompany tourniquet use include an increase in core temperature during tourniquet inflation and the development of transient metabolic acidemia and hypercarbia after tourniquet release. The increased output of CO_2 and lactic acid from the ischemic limb causes a transient decrease in arterial pH, with a maximum decrease within 4 minutes, returning to baseline values within 10 to 30 minutes. The sudden release of CO_2 into the circulation when lower limb tourniquets are released can markedly increase intracranial pressure in patients with head trauma. Normocapnia maintained by hyperventilation after tourniquet deflation can prevent increased cerebral blood flow velocity and intracranial pressure.

Tourniquet-induced hyperthermia, usually 1° to 2° C, occurs within 90 minutes of tourniquet inflation and appears to be the result of decreased cutaneous heat loss from skin distal to the tourniquet. The effect is more profound if bilateral tourniquets are used (Estebe et al., 1996). The combination of metabolic acidosis and hypercarbia that occurs after tourniquet release is the result of reperfusion and the washing out and reentry into the central circulation of lactic acid, potassium, and other toxic substances that accumulated in tissues during tourniquet-induced limb ischemia. Accompanying hemodynamic effects include hypertension and hypotension, tachycardia, bradycardia, and, rarely, ventricular dysrhythmias. These effects are self-limited and usually resolve over a few minutes. Other than increasing minute ventilation in patients who are being mechanically ventilated, most pediatric patients rarely or never require specific therapy for tourniquet deflation.

CLUBFOOT

Clubfoot (talipes equinovarus) is a relatively common congenital deformity that occurs in 1 of 1000 live births (Alvarez et al., 2008; Dobbs and Gurnett, 2009). Most clubfoot deformities are bilateral and can occur in otherwise normal children who have no syndrome, cytogenetic abnormality, or extrinsic cause for the deformity (Drvaric et al., 1989; Cummings et al., 2002). Clubfoot is also commonly seen in patients with neuropathies and myopathies such as myelodysplasia, CP, arthrogryposis, spinal muscular atrophy, and muscular dystrophy (Drvaric et al., 1989; Cummings et al., 2002). Clubfoot has degrees of severity, and the treatment is individualized in each patient. In some patients, manipulation and casting can restore the bony architecture. In others, surgery is required. When to perform surgery is controversial. Some surgeons prefer to operate on neonates; others operate when the affected child is 3 months, 6 months, or older than 1 year.

The patient is positioned prone (for Cincinnati and two-incision techniques) or supine (for Turco incision), and the procedure is performed with a tourniquet. The surgery involves soft tissue release, including posterior, medial, plantar, and lateral releases; tendon transfer and lengthening; and pin fixation (Drvaric et al., 1989; Cummings et al., 2002). At the completion of surgery, the foot and the calf to the middle thigh are well padded and casted. Postoperatively, patients experience intense pain. Virtually any general anesthesia technique can and has been used for this surgery. Because postoperative pain is such an important aspect of the care of these patients, a combined regional (epidural or sciatic nerve block) and general anesthesia technique is commonly used. The epidural catheter is used intraoperatively and postoperatively.

The percutaneous Ponseti approach to the clubfoot involves weekly stretching of the deformity, followed by application of a long leg cast. By 4 to 5 weeks, all components of the deformity are corrected, with the exception of the equinus. The equinus is addressed with a percutaneous Achilles tenotomy, followed by a final long leg cast (Herzenberg et al., 2002; Janicki et al., 2009).

DEVELOPMENTAL DYSPLASIA OF THE HIP

Developmental dysplasia of the hip (i.e., congenital hip dislocation) is a spectrum of abnormalities of the developing hip joint that ranges from shallowness of the acetabulum to capsular laxity and instability to frank dislocation (Eastwood, 2003; Scherl, 2004). Developmental dysplasia of the hip is relatively common, occurring in 1.5 to 20 of 1000 live births (Swaroop and Mubarak, 2009). Previously known as congenital hip dislocation, it is now understood to be a condition that is not purely congenital but one that develops over time. It is common in children born by breech delivery. Screening in the newborn period consists of looking for asymmetries in skin folds, range of abduction, and height of the knees, as well as using provocative testing. The latter, known as the Ortolani test, elicits a click or clunk as the femoral head is moved in and out of the acetabulum. In the absence of other developmental disabilities, developmental dysplasia of the hip does not cause significant functional disability even if the diagnosis is missed or delayed; however, if untreated, it can lead to degenerative hip arthritis. Ultrasound and MRI are useful for detecting hip dysplasia within the first weeks of life and valuable in following the course of treatment (Harding et al., 1997; Dwek, 2009).

Treatment is designed to relocate and stabilize the femoral head in the acetabulum. Bracing with the Pavlik harness (which prevents extension and adduction of the hip joint while allowing movement in the safe zone) and body casting are used for the first 6 months to 1 year of life. Virtually any general anesthesia technique, including caudal epidural blockade, can and has been used for casting and surgery (Castillo-Zamora et al., 2005).

SLIPPED CAPITAL FEMORAL EPIPHYSIS

Slipped capital femoral epiphysis (SCFE) is a displacement of the femoral head in relation to the femoral neck through the growth plate during a period of rapid growth in adolescence (Aronsson et al., 2006). SCFE is common in obese teenagers and manifests with pain localized to the groin, the knee, or the distal thigh (Kocher et al., 2004). On physical examination, these children limp, and diagnosis is made by obtaining anteroposterior and frog-leg lateral radiographs of the pelvis. In 20% of patients, SCFE is bilateral on presentation, although only one side may be symptomatic.

Surgical management consists of placing one or two screws across the growth plate of the affected hip to prevent further slippage (Kocher et al., 2004; Aronsson et al., 2006). The pinning is done in situ, meaning that no attempt is made to reduce the epiphysis back to its original position; such maneuvers damage the blood supply to the femoral head and lead to avascular necrosis (Boero et al., 2003). Virtually any general anesthesia technique can and has been used for this surgery. Many of these patients have full stomachs when they present emergently; therefore, patients are at risk for pulmonary aspiration of gastric contents, necessitating a rapid-sequence induction of general anesthesia.

FRACTURES

Children with fractures are among the patients most commonly seen by orthopedic surgeons. Most fractures are simple and treated without an anesthesiologist present. However, major blunt trauma often involves fractures of the long bones in children. These patients should be carefully examined for evidence of trauma that involves other organ systems, particularly the cervical spine. In very young infants, fractures are rare; when they are present, child abuse must be considered in the differential diagnosis.

The method by which to anesthetize a patient with a fracture depends on the urgency of the procedure, the risk for vomiting and aspiration, the child's maturity, and the wishes of the parents and surgeon. Regional or general anesthesia is possible. Regional anesthesia may make it impossible to evaluate motor function even if dilute concentrations of local anesthetics are used. With general anesthesia, full-stomach precautions should be taken to minimize the risks of vomiting and pulmonary aspiration of gastric contents; thus, rapid-sequence induction and airway protection with an endotracheal tube are in order. A complete discussion on how to perform blocks of the upper and lower extremity, and how to manage peripheral nerve catheters, can be found in Chapter 16, Regional Anesthesia.

FAT EMBOLISM SYNDROME

Fat embolism develops in nearly all patients with bone fractures, or during orthopedic procedures, but is usually asymptomatic (Akhtar, 2009). Fat embolism syndrome (FES) is a collection of respiratory, hematologic, neurologic, and cutaneous symptoms and signs that are associated with trauma and other disparate surgical and medical conditions such as sickle cell acute chest syndrome and acute pancreatitis (Georgopoulos and Bouros, 2003). The incidence of the clinical syndrome is low (<1% in retrospective reviews), and embolization of marrow fat appears to be an almost inevitable consequence of closed long-bone fractures (Mellor and Soni, 2001; Parisi et al., 2002). Multiple fractures increase the incidence of FES to 30%. FES is characterized by the triad of hypoxemia, neurologic abnormalities, and a petechial rash (Box 26-4). The challenge to the pediatric anesthesiologist is to recognize the intraoperative manifestations of FES in a multiple-trauma patient or in a patient with an isolated long-bone fracture.

> ### Box 26-4 Diagnostic Criteria in Fat Embolism Syndrome
>
> **MAJOR CRITERIA**
> Pulmonary insufficiency
> - Pao_2 < 60 mm Hg
>
> Neurologic dysfunction
> - Confusion
> - Disorientation
> - Lethargy
> - Focal deficits
> - Seizures
> - Coma
>
> Petechiae
>
> **MINOR CRITERIA**
> Fever
> Thrombocytopenia
> Anemia
> Tachycardia
> Elevated erythrocyte sedimentation rate
> Retinal changes

Pathophysiology

The pathophysiologic mechanisms that produce the FES remain controversial. In the most accepted mechanical hypothesis, bone injury disrupts the medullary canal, the adipose tissue, and the bone's vasculature; a hematoma forms at the site of this injury. When the intramedullary pressure exceeds venous pressure, fat globules are forced into the circulation (Arai et al., 2007). Chylomicrons are destabilized by the effects of fat intravasation and form very large, circulating fat globules. Fat can be detected in pulmonary arterial samples in up to 70% of patients with long-bone or pelvic fractures, especially if the pulmonary artery catheter is wedged (Byrick et al., 1989). The embolic particles can then obstruct right ventricular outflow or, in the setting of a patent foramen ovale, the systemic circulation. The biochemical hypothesis attributes the manifestations of the FES to the toxic effects of free fatty acids on the pulmonary microcirculation. In the pulmonary vascular bed, these fat particles are hydrolyzed to free fatty acids, which produce pulmonary vasculitis and hemorrhagic pneumonitis—a combination physiologically indistinguishable from acute respiratory distress syndrome. Surfactant activity is compromised, functional residual capacity is decreased, and endothelial integrity is violated, producing a large Pao_2–Pao_2 gradient and increased pulmonary vascular resistance. Fat particles and free fatty acids can enter the systemic circulation through pulmonary arteriovenous shunts to generate the central, renal, and cutaneous manifestations of this syndrome. As compared with air, the volume of fat associated with cardiopulmonary failure is 20-fold less (Husebye et al., 2006).

FES can be demonstrated in 90% of patients with long-bone fractures, but symptomatic FES occurs in only 10% to 22% of patients with long-bone or pelvic fractures. Classically, it develops 24 to 72 hours after an injury and is characterized by acute respiratory insufficiency with diffuse pulmonary infiltrates, global neurologic dysfunction, and petechiae. The pulmonary compromise is usually followed by the neurologic changes. If a petechial rash develops, it occurs 48 to 72 hours after the onset of FES. This complete presentation is seen in less than 10% of cases. Respiratory insufficiency may be the only manifestation of this syndrome, and it may occur in only one third of patients. This unexplained hypoxia is how FES manifests during general anesthesia (van Besouw and Hinds, 1989). Few patients with FES have a fulminant course, in which severe pulmonary hypertension and progressive right heart failure develop within hours of the injury. Vasopressor infusions and cardiopulmonary bypass support may be necessary to treat these sequelae.

The diagnosis of FES is a clinical one, and it may be difficult to establish (Georgopoulos and Bouros, 2003). Supportive laboratory tests include an inexplicable drop in Pao_2, hematocrit, platelet counts, and fibrinogen levels. The characteristic radiograph of bilateral fluffy pulmonary infiltrates may not be apparent for 24 to 48 hours after the onset of FES. Fat is seen in the urine in 50% of patients within 3 days. The usefulness of serum and urinary measurements of fat and lipase activity is limited by their poor sensitivity and specificity and by a lack of availability. Identification of fat droplet cells in bronchoalveolar lavage is the only rapid and specific method of identifying the development of this syndrome (Mimoz et al., 1995). The retinal changes of bilateral cotton-wool spots and intraretinal hemorrhages are seen in 60% of patients with FES.

In the operating room, the time of highest risk for the development of FES occurs when transferring a patient with a fracture from the stretcher to the operating room table. Fulminant FES can manifest within 30 minutes of this transfer, and it is recognized by inexplicable progressive oxygen desaturation and increasing peak inspiratory pressures. A high index of suspicion is necessary to make the diagnosis. Other manifestations of FES during anesthesia include sudden hypotension, tachycardia, bradycardia, dysrhythmia, decreased lung compliance, pulmonary edema, and severe unexplained surgical bleeding or oozing from multiple sites that results from disseminated intravascular coagulation.

End-tidal CO_2 monitoring does not seem to be as sensitive to fat emboli as it is in other embolic states. Although end-tidal CO_2 does change with a massive fat embolism, monitoring it has not been as effective as echocardiography in detecting smaller emboli. Transesophageal echocardiography can detect fat emboli during surgical manipulation of the operative bone, and it can demonstrate the regional wall motion abnormalities and right ventricular dilation that are harbingers of the FES physiologic perturbations (Capan and Miller, 2001).

After FES develops, treatment is nonspecific and supportive. It consists of early resuscitation and stabilization, administration of 100% oxygen, application of positive end-expiratory pressure, and the use of inverse-ratio ventilation. Bronchoscopy and bronchoalveolar lavage are useful in establishing a diagnosis and in removing the intraluminal debris and hemorrhagic exudate that accompany a fulminant presentation. An adequate intravascular volume must be maintained, and inotropic infusions and red blood cell transfusions are often required. Historically, advocated therapies have included IV alcohol, heparin, low-molecular-weight dextrans, and steroids. Limited data support the efficacy of any of these therapies once FES has begun. Early administration of methylprednisolone may decrease the incidence of FES (Lindeque et al., 1987). A 10% mortality rate has been reported for all patients; among children, the mortality rate is 33%.

SUMMARY

The orthopedic patient presents multiple challenges to the anesthesiologist. In many instances, the perioperative anesthesia plan for pediatric orthopedic patients depends more on the child's age and on the site and emergent nature of surgery than on the underlying disease or the specifics of the surgical procedure. In other cases, the underlying medical condition, associated anomalies, pathophysiology, and surgical procedure dictate the anesthesia plan. The anesthesia plan must address these issues and the recurring themes of positioning, airway management, blood loss and fluid replacement, conservation of body temperature, and postoperative pain management. In the future, the continued technological, physiologic, and pharmacologic advances in our specialty will allow longer, more extensive, and more innovative operations on younger and sicker patients than was possible in the past.

For questions and answers on topics in this chapter, go to "Chapter Questions" at www.expertconsult.com.

REFERENCES

Complete references used in this text can be found online at www.expertconsult.com.

CHAPTER 27

Anesthesia for Ophthalmic Surgery

Lori T. Justice, Robert D. Valley, Ann G. Bailey, and Michael W. Hauser

CONTENTS

Anesthesia for ophthalmologic procedures in children requires an understanding of several physiologic and pharmacologic concepts that are unique to this population. The majority of ophthalmic procedures are brief and noninvasive, but the spectrum extends to more invasive procedures in patients with significant comorbid disease. Caring for otherwise healthy children undergoing nasolacrimal duct probing or strabismus surgery may be relatively straightforward, but the pediatric anesthesiologist is also required to care for vulnerable infants born prematurely or with congenital disorders and associated pathology of the eye. In 2005 there were 2.2 million procedures performed on patients younger than 15 years of age; 12,000 of these were operations on the eye (Defrances and Hall, 2007). Most of these procedures are performed in the ambulatory setting. In an analysis of ophthalmic procedures performed in surgery centers, the reasons for cancellation of surgery within 24 hours were explored. The pediatric group (0 to 9 years of age) had the highest rate of cancellation when compared with those in other age groups. The majority of cancellations, however, were because of unpreventable causes such as patient illness (Henderson et al., 2005). The information contained in this chapter will give anesthesiologists the information needed to plan for and safely perform anesthesia for ophthalmic procedures.

Anesthesiologists with a particular interest in ophthalmologic anesthesia can find valuable resources through the Ophthalmic Anesthesia Society (http://www.eyeanesthesia.org) and the British Ophthalmic Anaesthesia Society (http://www. boas.org). A glossary of terms is given in Box 27-1.

ANATOMY AND PHYSIOLOGY

Knowledge of the anatomy and physiology of the eye is paramount to understanding the array of ophthalmic procedures performed, the influence that anesthesia may have on normal and abnormal ocular physiology, and the systemic effects that surgical manipulation of the eye may have on the patient (McGoldrick, 1992a).

Anatomy Overview

The eye is an extension of the central nervous system (the diencephalon) that rests in the orbit, is cushioned by fat, and is suspended by ligaments and fascial structure.

The orbit is formed by a complex arrangement of seven cranial bones: frontal, zygomatic, sphenoid, maxilla, palatine, lacrimal, and ethmoid (Fig. 27-1). The optic foramen transmits the

Box 27-1 Glossary of Ophthalmologic Terms

Blepharospasm: Tonic spasm of the orbicularis oculi muscle, producing more or less complete closure of the eyelids

Buphthalmos: Enlargement and distention of the fibrous coats of the eye

Cyclocryotherapy: Freezing of the ciliary body, performed for the treatment of glaucoma

Epiphora: Abnormal overflow of tears, also known as illacrimation

Episcleritis: Inflammation of tissues overlying the sclera, also inflammation of the outermost layers of the sclera

Gonioscopy: Examination of the angle of the anterior chamber of the eye

Goniotomy: Operation for glaucoma characterized by an open angle and normal depth of the anterior chamber; consists of the opening of Schlemm's canal under direct vision secured by a contact glass

Tonometry: Measurement of tension or pressure commonly assessed by the applanation

Tonometer: Instrument that measures intraocular pressure by determination of the force necessary to flatten a corneal surface of constant size

Trabeculectomy: Creation of a fistula between the anterior chamber of the eye and the subconjunctival space by surgical removal of a portion of the trabecular meshwork

From *Dorland's illustrated medical dictionary*, Philadelphia, 2000, Saunders.

The globe is composed of three contiguous layers: the sclera, uveal tract, and retina. The sclera is the dense outer covering that provides the fibrous structure necessary for maintaining the shape of the globe. The anterior portion of the sclera (the cornea) is transparent and avascular, permitting transmission of light to the retina. The highly vascular uveal tract is composed of the iris, ciliary body, and choroid, enveloping the posterior aspect of the globe. The iris divides the anterior segment of the eye into the anterior and posterior chambers. The ciliary body is the site of aqueous humor production and contains the ciliary muscles that are responsible for accommodation of the lens. The choroid is the highly vascular layer of the globe that provides blood supply to the retina. The retina is a delicate membrane composed of 10 distinct layers that are involved in the conversion of light to neural impulses. The axons of the retinal ganglion nerves converge at the optic disc and pierce the sclera to form the optic nerve.

The aqueous humor occupies the anterior and posterior chambers of the eye and is responsible for providing nutrients to the avascular lens and the endothelial aspect of the cornea (Fig. 27-2). The volume of aqueous humor (0.3 mL in the adult) is primarily responsible for intraocular pressure (IOP) regulation. The vitreous humor, created embryologically between 1 and 4 months' gestation, is a hydrophilic gel that accounts for 80% of the volume of the globe. The vitrous humor is 99% water, although in the presence of hyaluronic acid (a mucopolysaccharide), its viscosity is twice that of water. The volume of the vitreous humor is more constant than that of the aqueous humor, although it may be slightly influenced by hydration status and osmotically active medications.

The optic nerve (cranial nerve II) is the nerve of vision and may be thought of as a diverticulum of the forebrain. The oculomotor nerve (cranial nerve III) provides motor innervation to four of the six extraocular muscles and the levator palpebrae superioris, as well as parasympathetic innervation to the pupillary sphincter (miosis) and ciliary muscles (accommodation). The two other extraocular muscles are innervated by the trochlear and abducens nerves. The ophthalmic division of the

optic nerve, the ophthalmic artery and vein, and the sympathetic contributions from the carotid plexus. The superior orbital fissure transmits branches from four other cranial nerves (oculomotor, trigeminal, trochlear, and abducens) and the superior and inferior ophthalmic veins. The infraorbital fissure (representing the weakest aspect of the orbit) transmits the infraorbital and zygomatic nerves. The infraorbital foramen (located below the orbital rim) transmits the infraorbital nerve, artery, and vein.

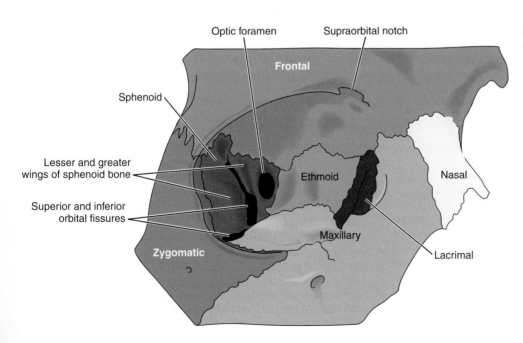

Optic foramen   Supraorbital notch

Frontal

Sphenoid

Lesser and greater wings of sphenoid bone

Ethmoid

Nasal

Superior and inferior orbital fissures

Maxillary

Zygomatic

Lacrimal

■ **FIGURE 27-1.** Skeletal anatomy of the orbit.

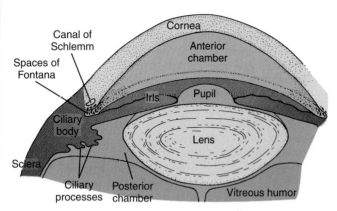

■ FIGURE 27-2. Anatomy of the anterior eye. *(From McGoldrick KE: Anesthesia for ophthalmic surgery. In Motoyama ES, Davis PJ, editors: Smith's anesthesia for infants and children, ed 6, Philadelphia, 1996, Mosby.)*

trigeminal nerve (cranial nerve V) transmits all of the nonvisual sensory innervation from the eye and orbit and provides sympathetic innervation to the pupillary dilators (mydriasis). The temporal and zygomatic branches of the facial nerve (cranial nerve VII) innervate the orbicularis oculi (Ellis and Feldman, 1997).

Blood is supplied to the eye and orbit through branches of the internal and external carotid arteries. The first branch of the intracranial carotid artery, the ophthalmic artery, divides into the central retinal artery, as well as the long and short posterior ciliary arteries, to nourish the retina. The long and short posterior ciliary arteries converge to supply the choriocapillaris, the capillary layer within the choroid that supplies 60% to 80% of the oxygen to the retina. The anterior portion of the optic nerve is perfused by the posterior ciliary arteries. It is this network of arteries that is subject to significant individual variation, predisposing some patients to anterior ischemic optic neuropathy after periods of hypotension. The posterior optic nerve is perfused by pial vessels branching from the ophthalmic artery. Superior and inferior ophthalmic veins drain the orbit, and the central retinal vein provides ocular drainage. All venous drainage is subsequently transmitted to the cavernous sinus (Williams, 2002).

Physiology Overview

The physiology of the eye is quite complex, but an understanding of the physiologic and pharmacologic control of IOP is of primary importance to the anesthesiologist. The ability to avoid deviations in IOP is key to providing satisfactory anesthesia for all intraocular procedures and in caring for the patient with glaucoma and traumatic injury to the globe.

Normal IOP varies between 10 and 20 mm Hg and may differ by as much as 5 mm Hg between the two eyes. Normal pressures are somewhat lower in the newborn (average, 9.5 mm Hg) but approximate adult pressures by 5 years of age (Pensiero et al., 1992). A pressure above 25 mm Hg at any age is considered abnormal (Johnson and Forrest, 1994). Transient changes in IOP are well tolerated in the intact eye, although chronic elevations may be detrimental to normal retinal perfusion and vision.

Three primary determinants of IOP are external pressure, venous congestion, and changes in intraocular volume. The volume and exertional pressure of the aqueous humor are carefully regulated in the normal eye to maintain normal IOP. As mentioned previously, the volume of the vitreous humor is usually constant.

The aqueous humor is formed primarily by the ciliary bodies, where secretion is facilitated by the carbonic anhydrase and cytochrome oxidase systems. The feedback control of aqueous humor formation is poorly understood, although production of aqueous humor is known to be augmented by sympathetic stimulation and suppressed by parasympathetic control. Variations in the osmotic pressure of the aqueous humor and plasma influence aqueous humor formation, as illustrated by the following equation:

$$IOP = k[(OPaq - OPpl) + Pc]$$

where *k* is the coefficient of outflow, *OPaq* and *OPpl* are the osmotic pressures of the aqueous humor and plasma, respectively, and *Pc* is the capillary perfusion pressure. The benefit of hypertonic solutions in lowering IOP is realized through an understanding of this equation.

Most of the aqueous humor produced in the posterior chamber flows through the pupil into the anterior chamber, exiting the eye through Schlemm's canal (a thin vein that extends circumferentially around the eye) and into the orbital venous system.

Fluctuations in aqueous humor outflow also dramatically alter IOP. The prime factor determining outflow of aqueous humor is the diameter of Fontana's spaces, as illustrated by the following equation based on the Hagen-Poiseuille Law:

$$A = \frac{r^4(Piop - Pv)}{8\eta l}$$

where *A* is the volume of aqueous humor outflow per unit of time, *r* is the radius of Fontana's spaces, *Piop* is IOP, *Pv* is venous pressure, *η* is viscosity, and *l* is length of Fontana's spaces.

With mydriasis, Fontana's spaces narrow, resistance to outflow is increased, and IOP rises. Mydriasis is a threat in both closed-angle and open-angle glaucoma.* Hence, a miotic agent such as pilocarpine hydrochloride is often efficacious when applied conjunctivally before surgery in patients with glaucoma.

Stimulation of α_1-sympathetic receptors leads to mydriasis, a decrease in aqueous outflow, and an increase in IOP. Most of the agents used to produce mydriasis also modestly increase IOP. β-stimulation has no effect on pupillary diameter, but paradoxically, both β-agonists and β-antagonists may decrease IOP. Cholinergic stimulation or parasympathetic stimulation produces miosis and a decrease in IOP such that glaucoma patients are commonly treated with miotic agents.

The arterial circulation of the eye is autoregulated. Only marked deviations in systemic arterial pressures affect IOP. Elevated venous pressures, on the other hand, can dramatically increase IOP, primarily by augmenting the choroidal blood volume and tension of the orbit. Coughing, vomiting, and Valsalva maneuvers may increase IOP to 40 mm Hg or more. Respiratory acidosis increases IOP, whereas metabolic acidosis has the opposite effect. Conversely, respiratory alkalosis decreases IOP, whereas metabolic alkalosis increases IOP (Calobrisi and

---

*Open-angle glaucoma, also known as chronic simple glaucoma, is a condition of elevated IOP in an eye with an anatomically open anterior chamber angle. The trabecular meshwork is thought to be sclerosed, resulting in inefficient aqueous filtration and drainage. Closed-angle glaucoma is a mechanical closing of the pathway for aqueous egress for the eye. The iris may move into direct contact with the posterior surface of the cornea, impeding the aqueous outflow path, or the crystalline lens may swell, resulting in papillary blocking. In the latter case, the lens blocks the route for aqueous humor to travel from the posterior to the anterior chamber.

Lebowitz, 1990). Hypoxia is capable of increasing IOP by dilating intraocular vessels, whereas hyperoxia appears to decrease IOP (Johnson and Forrest, 1994).

Three ophthalmic reflexes that should be recognized by the anesthesiologist caring for the ophthalmic patient include the oculocardiac reflex (OCR), the oculorespiratory reflex (ORR), and the oculoemetic reflex (OER). All three reflexes are elicited by pressure or torsion on the extraocular muscles transmitting afferent impulses through the ophthalmic division of the trigeminal nerve.

The OCR, through its vagal efferent pathway, may manifest as sinus bradycardia, ectopy, and sinus arrest. Death secondary to the OCR in otherwise healthy children has been described (Lang and Van der Wal, 1994; Smith, 1994). A more thorough description of this reflex, prophylaxis, and therapy are provided later in the discussion on intraoperative complications.

The ORR has also been recognized for nearly 100 years but is less often appreciated with the use of controlled ventilation. Through a postulated connection between the trigeminal nerve, the pneumotaxic center of the pons, and the medullary respiratory centers, pressure on the extraocular muscles may result in tachypnea or respiratory arrest (Johnson and Forrest, 1994). This reflex is not inhibited by the use of atropine or glycopyrrolate. A review of the ORR and its potential for causing hypercapnia and hypoxia (potentially aggravating the OCR) has heightened awareness of the reflex and led some investigators to recommend controlled ventilation during strabismus surgery (Blanc et al., 1988).

The OER is admittedly more theoretic than the other two reflexes but would explain the high incidence of nausea and emesis after strabismus surgery. An association between the OCR and the OER has been demonstrated such that patients who exhibit the OCR intraoperatively are 2.6 times more likely to experience postoperative vomiting than those without OCR manifestations (Allen et al., 1998). Anticholinergic therapy does not decrease the incidence of postoperative nausea and vomiting (PONV). Appropriate prophylaxis and treatment of PONV have been studied extensively and are thoroughly reviewed later in this chapter.

GENERAL CONSIDERATIONS IN CARING FOR THE OPHTHALMOLOGIC PATIENT

The anesthesiologist caring for the ophthalmologic patient should be familiar with the disorders and syndromes commonly associated with ocular pathology, the effects of ophthalmic medications used preoperatively and intraoperatively, and the ocular effects of the anesthetic agents to be used during the perioperative period.

Associated Congenital and Metabolic Conditions

Ophthalmologic disorders may be inherited as isolated defects in autosomal recessive, autosomal dominant, and X-linked recessive fashion. An additional large number of metabolic defects, congenital syndromes, and chromosomal abnormalities are also associated with ocular pathology. The anesthesiologist caring for the ophthalmologic patient must be aware of these associations. An overview of the commonly encountered syndromes and disorders along with their ocular manifestations and potential anesthetic implications is provided in Table 27-1 (McGoldrick, 1992d; Butera et al., 2000; Baum and O'Flaherty, 2006).

TABLE 27-1. Congenital Syndromes and Chromosomal Abnormalities with Associated Ocular Manifestations

Disorder or Syndrome	Ocular Manifestations	Anesthetic Implications
Acute intermittent porphyria	Cataracts, retinal degeneration, optic atrophy	Various medications, including barbiturates and etomidate, may trigger attacks.
Apert's syndrome	Glaucoma, cataracts, strabismus, hypertelorism, proptosis	Possibly difficult intubation, possible choanal stenosis, cervical spine fusion, CHD (10% incidence)
Cri du chat syndrome	Strabismus	Micrognathia and possibly difficult intubation, hypotonia, prone to hypothermia, CHD (33% incidence)
Crouzon's disease	Glaucoma, cataracts, strabismus, hypertelorism, proptosis	Possibly difficult intubation, possible elevated intracranial pressure
Cystinosis	Corneal clouding, retinal degeneration	Chronic renal failure, possible diabetes mellitus, esophageal varices, recurrent epistaxis, hyperthermia
Down syndrome	Cataracts, strabismus	Trisomy 21, airway obstruction, atlantoaxial instability, CHD (50% incidence), may be more sensitive to atropine
Ehlers-Danlos syndrome	Retinal detachment, blue sclera, ectopia lentis, keratoconus	Laryngeal trauma possible with intubation, careful positioning, avoid arterial and central venous lines
Goldenhar's syndrome	Glaucoma, cataracts, strabismus, lacrimal drainage defects	Hemifacial microsomia and possible cervical spine abnormalities, possible difficult mask and intubation, rare CHD, and hydrocephalus
Hallerman-Streiff syndrome	Congenital cataracts, coloboma, microphthalmia, glaucoma	Major craniofacial abnormalities with likely difficult intubation, upper airway obstruction, chronic lung disease
Homocystinuria	Ectopia lentis, pupillary block glaucoma, retinal detachment, central retinal artery occlusion, strabismus optic atrophy,	Marfanoid habitus with kyphoscoliosis and sternal deformity, prone to thromboembolic complications and hypoglycemia
Hunter's syndrome	Retinal degeneration, optic atrophy	Often difficult intubation, copious secretions, macroglossia, stiff temporomandibular joint, limited neck mobility, possible ischemic or valvular heart disease

Continued

TABLE 27-1. Congenital Syndromes and Chromosomal Abnormalities with Associated Ocular Manifestations—cont'd

Disorder or Syndrome	Ocular Manifestations	Anesthetic Implications
Hurler's syndrome	Corneal clouding, retinal degeneration, optic atrophy	Often difficult intubation and difficult mask, possible cervical spine instability, possible ischemic or valvular heart disease
Jeune syndrome	Retinal degeneration	Limited thoracic excursion, pulmonary hypoplasia, possible renal and hepatic insufficiency
Lowe's syndrome	Cataracts, glaucoma (hydrophthalmia)	Renal failure, renal tubular acidosis
Marfan syndrome	Ectopia lentis, glaucoma, retinal detachment, cataracts, strabismus	Aortic or pulmonary artery dilation, aortic and mitral valve disease, pectus excavatum, risk for pneumothorax
Moebius sequence	Strabismus, ptosis, congenital nerve VI and VII palsy	Possibly difficult intubation, micrognathia, copious secretions, possible cervical spine anomalies
Myotonia congenita	Cataracts, blepharospasm	Prone to myotonic contractions, sustained contraction with succinylcholine
Myotonic dystrophy	Cataracts, ptosis, strabismus	Prone to myotonic contractions, succinylcholine-associated contractions and hyperkalemia, cardiac conduction abnormalities, sensitive to central nervous system depressants
Rubella syndrome	Cataracts, microphthalmos, glaucoma, optic atrophy	Neonatal pneumonia, anemia, and thrombocytopenia; CHD, hypopituitarism, diabetes mellitus
Sickle cell disease	Retinal detachment, vitreous hemorrhage, retinitis proliferans	Tendency for sickling occurs with high hemoglobin S concentrations, hypoxemia, cold, stasis, dehydration, and infection
Smith-Lemli-Opitz syndrome	Congenital cataracts	Possibly difficult intubation, micrognathia, pulmonary hypoplasia, CHD, gastroesophageal reflux, seizure disorders
Stickler syndrome	Vitreous degeneration, retinal detachments, cataracts, strabismus	Possibly difficult intubation, micrognathia, mitral valve prolapse, marfanoid habitus, scoliosis, kyphosis
Sturge-Weber syndrome	Choroidal hemangioma, glaucoma, ectopia lentis	Angiomas of the airway, CHD and high output failure, seizure disorders, hyperkalemic response to succinylcholine in those with hemiplegia
Treacher Collins syndrome	Lid defects, microphthalmia	Often difficult intubation, mandibular hypoplasia, CHD
Turner's syndrome	Ptosis, strabismus, cataracts, corneal scars, blue sclera	Possibly difficult intubation and intravenous access, CHD
von Hippel–Lindau syndrome	Retinal hemangioma	Possible increased intracranial pressure, possible pheochromocytoma, cerebellar tumors may also produce episodic hypertension
von Recklinghausen's disease	Ptosis, proptosis, optic glioma and meningioma, optic atrophy, glaucoma, Lisch nodules	Possibly difficult mask ventilation and intubation, possible airway tumors, restrictive lung disease, renovascular hypertension, possible pheochromocytoma, sensitive to neuromuscular blockers
Zellweger syndrome	Glaucoma, cataracts, optic atrophy, optic nerve hypoplasia	Micrognathia, possible CHD, renal and adrenal insufficiency

CHD, Congenital heart disease.

Ophthalmologic Medications and Their Systemic Effects

There are a variety of medications used by pediatric ophthalmologists in the outpatient and perioperative settings that may have important anesthetic ramifications. As with all medications, the ophthalmic agents have both desirable and undesirable effects that may be more pronounced and ominous in the pediatric patient by virtue of greater systemic absorption or higher dosing relative to body weight and pharmacologic compartment. The anesthesiologist must be familiar with every medication used in the perioperative period and pay particular attention to the total dose administered and potential for deleterious effects. An overview of the ophthalmic medications is provided (Table 27-2).

Topical ophthalmologic agents have greater use than systemic agents in the pediatric and adult populations, primarily because most of the side effects that would be consequential to systemic administration are diminished. Nevertheless, the excess from ocular application invariably enters the lacrimal system, reaching the nasopharyngeal mucosa where systemic absorption is greatly enhanced compared with that at the conjunctival sac. Whereas a single drop from a commercial eye dropper may have a volume ranging between 50 and 75 μL, maximal ocular bioavailability is reached by instillation of only 20 μL (McGoldrick, 1992b). It has been recommended that digital pressure over the lacrimal duct for 5 minutes after instillation may reduce systemic absorption by 67% (Zimmerman et al., 1984). Keeping the eye gently closed for 5 minutes may afford similar benefit, yet both techniques are understandably difficult in the conscious and fretful child.

Cycloplegic and Mydriatic Agents

Those agents used most commonly in the perioperative setting include cycloplegic and mydriatic agents. The agents are necessary for performing certain procedures, cycloplegic refraction,

TABLE 27-2. Commonly Used Ophthalmic Medications

Type	Medication	Concentration	Pertinent Systemic and Ocular Effects
Cycloplegic			
	Cyclopentolate	0.5%, 1%, 2%	Muscarinic antagonist; side effects include gastrointestinal disturbance, atropine-like toxicity, and inhibition of plasma cholinesterase (in vitro).
	Tropicamide	0.5%, 1%	Muscarinic antagonist; side effects are minimal.
	Atropine	1%	Muscarinic antagonist with the most potent ocular effects and a duration of action of longer than 1 week; side effects are numerous.
	Homatropine	2%, 5%	Muscarinic antagonist with a shorter onset and duration of action than atropine; side effects are numerous.
	Scopolamine	0.25%	Muscarinic antagonist that is not commonly used for diagnostic cycloplegia and mydriasis and for the treatment of iridocyclitis; side effects include an increase in intraocular pressure such that IV or IM scopolamine as a premedication should not be used in the patient with glaucoma.
Mydriatic			
	Phenylephrine	2.5%, 10%	α-Agonist used for maximal mydriasis and vasoconstriction without cycloplegia; potential side effects include hypertension, tachycardia or reflex bradycardia, pulmonary edema, cardiac arrhythmia, cardiac arrest, and subarachnoid hemorrhage.
	Hydroxyamphetamine	1%	Sympathomimetic used in combination with tropicamide primarily for differentiating preganglionic and postganglionic lesions producing Horner's syndrome.
Miotic			
	Acetylcholine	1%	Cholinergic agonist used intraocularly to produce complete miosis after cataract surgery, keratoplasty, other anterior segment surgery; side effects include bradycardia, hypotension, and bronchospasm.
Glaucoma Agent			
	Pilocarpine	1% to 8%	Cholinomimetic or parasympathomimetic agent used to produce miosis and a decrease in intraocular pressure for chronic and acute angle-closure glaucoma; side effects include gastrointestinal disturbance, diaphoresis, and brow pain.
	Echothiophate iodide	0.125%	Long-acting anticholinesterase agent used to produce miosis for open-angle glaucoma; side effects include bradycardia, hypotension, nausea, vomiting, diarrhea, weakness, and inhibition of plasma cholinesterase for up to 6 weeks after discontinuation.
	Timolol, levobunolol	0.25%, 0.5%	Nonselective β-antagonists that reduce intraocular pressure by decreasing aqueous humor production and possibly outflow; side effects include bronchospasm, bradycardia, hypotension, and apnea in neonates.
	Betaxolol	0.5%	Selective β_1-antagonist; side effects are possible but less commonly observed in contrast to the nonselective β-antagonists.
	Apraclonidine	0.5%, 1%	Selective α_2 agonist incapable of crossing the blood-brain barrier and used to reduce aqueous secretion; side effects are minimal.
	Brimonidine	0.15%, 0.2%	Selective β_2-agonist capable of crossing the blood-brain barrier; side effects include apnea, bradycardia, hypotension, hypothermia, and somnolence with an incidence as high as 83%.
	Latanoprost, bimatoprost, travoprost	Varies	Prostaglandin F2 analogues that increase aqueous humor outflow and decrease intraocular pressure in open-angle glaucoma; side effects are minimal and usually limited to ocular side effects.
	Acetazolamide	Varies	Systemic competitive inhibitor of carbonic anhydrase that reduces formation of aqueous humor; side effects include acidosis, hypokalemia, hyponatremia, and allergic reactions.
	Dorzolamide, brinzolamide	Varies	Topical carbonic anhydrase inhibitors that reduce the production of aqueous humor; side effects are uncommon.
	Mannitol	25%	Inert sugar that increases plasma osmotic pressure and decreases the volume of aqueous humor; side effects include transient hypervolemia followed by hypovolemia and potential for hypotension.

Continued

TABLE 27-2. Commonly Used Ophthalmic Medications—cont'd

Type	Medication	Concentration	Pertinent Systemic and Ocular Effects
Miscellaneous			
	Proparacaine, tetracaine	0.5%	Ester local anesthetics commonly used intraoperatively and during examination; side effects are minimal and usually limited to burning and possible epithelial damage.
	Cocaine	4%, 10%	Ester local anesthetic with vasoconstrictive properties; side effects include tachycardia, hypertension, dysrhythmias, hyperthermia, and seizures.
	Naphazoline	0.01%, 0.1%	α-Agonist used primarily for intraoperative vasoconstriction.
	Fluorescein	NA	Intravascular dye used to evaluate the integrity of retinal vasculature; side effects include hypertension, nausea, and vomiting.
	Sulfur hexafluoride	NA	Intraocular gas known to persist for up to 4 weeks after injection.
	Perfluoropropane, carbon octofluorine	NA	Intraocular gases known to persist for up to 6 weeks after injection.
	Botulinum toxin	NA	Neurotoxin produced by *Clostridium botulinum*, which inhibits release of acetylcholine used for treatment of strabismus and blepharospasm.

and funduscopy. The cycloplegic agents act via parasympatholytic action to block the muscarinic receptors of the ciliary body, paralyze the ciliary muscles, and inhibit accommodation. Outside of the perioperative period, the cycloplegic agents are also used to decrease the discomfort of ciliary body spasm common to a variety of inflammatory conditions.

Cyclopentolate, a commonly used cycloplegic agent, has a peak effect within 20 to 45 minutes and residual effects that persist for as long as 36 hours (Cooper et al., 2000). Mild gastrointestinal discomfort and feeding intolerance are the most commonly encountered side effects, although more severe atropine-like toxicity with symptoms ranging from vomiting, ileus, hyperthermia, delirium, and grand mal seizures (Kennerdell and Wucher, 1972; Bauer et al., 1973) has also been reported.

Tropicamide is a belladonna alkaloid that is also used as a topical cycloplegic agent. Maximal cycloplegic effect takes place within 20 to 40 minutes, and residual effects may persist for 6 hours. Because tropicamide is less reliable than cyclopentolate, it is most often used in combination with cyclopentolate or phenylephrine.

Atropine and homatropine are extremely potent anti-accommodative agents that are rarely used for pediatric patients in the perioperative setting. These agents are more commonly used for intraocular inflammation and amblyopia therapy; they may also be used for prolonged mydriasis after cataract extraction to prevent the formation of synechiae. Common side effects include thirst, tachycardia, and hyperthermia, although more severe symptoms may result after overzealous administration (McGoldrick, 1992b).

Mydriasis is usually produced as a secondary effect of the cycloplegic agents (by paralyzing the constrictors of the iris), yet additional mydriatic agents are often used to maximize peripheral and anterior retinal visualization. The mydriatic agents are sympathomimetic agents that mimic the effects of endogenous epinephrine and norepinephrine.

Ophthalmic phenylephrine (available in 2.5% and 10% concentrations) is commonly used for mydriasis and vasoconstriction during various procedures. Maximal effects are usually observed within 15 minutes, and residual effects may persist for 4 hours after administration. The generally accepted dosing limit for pediatric patients is one drop of the 2.5% solution in each eye per hour (Borromeo-McGrail et al., 1973). One drop (50 μL) of the 2.5% solution contains approximately 1.25 mg of phenylephrine. The potential for severe hypertension, pulmonary edema, cardiac arrhythmia, cardiac arrest, and subarachnoid hemorrhage with topical phenylephrine is well appreciated by surgeons and anesthesiologists alike. With careful application of the 2.5% solution, systemic effects are typically mild, well tolerated, and generally observed within 1 to 20 minutes after application (Fraunfelder et al., 2002). Although one study demonstrated no significant difference in the mydriatic effects of cyclopentolate vs. phenylephrine (both administered in combination with tropicamide), many ophthalmologists still rely on the medication either primarily or when additional dilation is needed after the administration of other preparations (Rosales et al., 1981).

Glaucoma Pharmacologic Therapy

Unlike the management of adult glaucoma, the primary treatment for pediatric glaucoma is surgical. Medical therapy may occasionally be instituted perioperatively in an effort to minimize IOP. There are an expansive number of medications and combination products available, but none is formally approved for pediatric use. Convenient classifications for the glaucoma medications include the direct- and indirect-acting parasympathomimetics, sympathomimetics, β-antagonists, selective α$_2$-agonists, carbonic anhydrase inhibitors, prostaglandin analogues, and hypertonic solutions.

Pilocarpine is a parasympathomimetic agent that produces miosis and a fall in IOP that is thought to result from an increase in aqueous humor outflow. It is rarely used for temporary treatment before surgery in children but should be discontinued on the evening before surgery for adequate assessment of pressure (Khaw et al., 2000). At recommended dosages, side effects are thought to be rare but may include gastrointestinal disturbances and diaphoresis. More severe cardiovascular effects (e.g., hypotension, bradycardia, and atrioventricular block) are occasionally observed in the geriatric patient (Everitt and Avorn, 1990).

The long-acting anticholinesterase drugs (echothiophate iodide and demecarium bromide) are uncommonly used in the pediatric patient. They are occasionally used in the adult refractory to other glaucoma therapy. These agents are of particular interest to the anesthesiologist because of their ability to profoundly inhibit the metabolism of succinylcholine, mivacurium, and the ester anesthetics for up to 6 weeks after discontinuation of therapy.

Topical epinephrine and its prodrug, dipivefrin, are sympathomimetic agents historically used in the treatment of glaucoma. Topical epinephrine is occasionally used by ophthalmologists in the intraoperative setting and is known to potentiate dysrhythmias in the myocardium sensitized by the volatile agents. Of all the potent inhalation agents, halothane clearly has the greatest dysrhythmogenic potential, although one study has demonstrated that the pediatric heart may be more resistant to the interactions between halothane and exogenous epinephrine (Karl et al., 1983; Ueda et al., 1983). At equipotent concentrations, isoflurane has three times less dysrhythmogenic potential than halothane (Marshall and Longnecker, 2001). Desflurane and sevoflurane are thought to be similar to isoflurane in this regard (Moore et al., 1993; Navarro et al., 1994).

The β-blocking agents timolol, levobunolol, and betaxolol act by decreasing the production of aqueous humor and are occasionally used postoperatively in children. The agents should not be used in the neonatal and infant populations in light of several reports of apnea with the use of timolol (Olson et al., 1979; Bailey, 1984). In older children and adults, the use of betaxolol, which is selective for the β_1-receptors, is associated with fewer complications involving the pulmonary system, although dyspnea and bronchospasm have been reported (Everitt and Avorn, 1990). Lethargy, bradycardia, and heart block are possible with all of the topical β-blocking agents (Gross and Pineyro, 1997).

Apraclonidine and brimonidine are topical α_2-agonists that decrease sympathetic tone and subsequently reduce aqueous humor production. Brimonidine, unlike apraclonidine, is capable of crossing the blood-brain barrier and should be used with great caution in young children. Bradycardia, hypotension, hypothermia, hypotonia, and apnea have all been reported with the use of brimonidine (Enyedi and Freedman, 2001).

Newer topical agents, including the prostaglandin analogues (latanoprost, bimatoprost, and travoprost) and the topical carbonic anhydrase inhibitors (dorzolamide and brinzolamide), are generally very safe in the pediatric population but are believed to be less effective than they are in adults (Beck, 2001). The topical carbonic anhydrase inhibitors, like systemic acetazolamide, are sulfonamide derivatives that should be avoided in the patient with sulfa sensitivity.

Miscellaneous Ophthalmologic Agents

Topical anesthetics, including cocaine, tetracaine, and proparacaine, are occasionally used by ophthalmologists in the perioperative setting. Cocaine is rarely used, but it is unique among the local anesthetics because of its vasoconstrictive properties. The potential for serious cardiovascular and central nervous system effects should be recognized by both the surgeon and anesthesiologist. The accepted maximum dose is 3 mg/kg, 1.5 mg/kg in the presence of volatile anesthetics. One drop of the 4% formulation contains approximately 1.5 mg of cocaine (McGoldrick, 1992b). The drug should not be used in patients with cardiovascular disease or in the presence of additional adrenergic-modifying medications such as monoamine oxidase inhibitors or tricyclic antidepressants.

Intraocular gases, including sulfur hexafluoride, perfluoropropane, and carbon octofluorine, are poorly diffusible inert gases that may be injected during certain vitreoretinal procedures. When nitrous oxide is present during injection, the nitrous oxide equilibrates with these new gas spaces to increase the volume and pressure of the intraocular injection, potentially compromising retinal perfusion. Animal studies, case reports, and mathematic models have demonstrated the necessity of discontinuing nitrous oxide no less than 15 minutes before intraocular gas injection and avoiding subsequent use of nitrous oxide for at least 4 weeks after the use of sulfur hexafluoride and 6 weeks after the use of perfluoropropane or carbon octofluorine (Wolf et al., 1983; McGoldrick, 1992b; Seaberg et al., 2002).

Effects of Various Anesthetic Agents on Intraocular Pressure

It is important to understand the ocular effects of the various anesthetic agents. An anesthetic plan should be chosen that provides optimal surgical conditions for intraocular procedures and minimizes risk of morbidity in those patients with preexisting intraocular hypertension and traumatic injury to the globe.

The central nervous system depressants (benzodiazepines, barbiturates, and opioids) commonly used by the anesthesiologist decrease IOP in both normal and glaucomatous eyes. The agents commonly used for preoperative anxiolysis in the pediatric population are associated with minor decreases in IOP that should not affect diagnostic measurements and likewise should not be relied on to attenuate the increase in IOP attributable to the use of succinylcholine and laryngoscopy. Effects specific to the use of oral or rectal midazolam in the pediatric population have not been delineated, although two studies of the use of intravenous (IV) midazolam in adults demonstrate minimal effects on IOP (Virkkila et al., 1992; Carter et al., 1999).

With the possible exception of ketamine, all of the IV induction agents are associated with a significant decrease in IOP. Thiopental and propofol reduced IOP by 40% and 53%, respectively, in one study, although both agents are unable to completely attenuate increases that are secondary to succinylcholine and laryngoscopy (Mirakhur and Shepherd, 1985; Mirakhur et al., 1987). Etomidate diminished IOP more profoundly than thiopental in one adult study (Calla et al., 1987). Etomidate-related myoclonus could be hazardous to the patient with traumatic injury and bothersome to the ophthalmologist. Early studies of the effects of ketamine uniformly demonstrated an increase in IOP, but subsequent studies in adults and children have demonstrated either insignificant changes or minor decreases in IOP (Peuler et al., 1975; Ausinsch et al., 1976). There is no clear consensus regarding the effects of ketamine on IOP, although its association with blepharospasm and nystagmus makes other induction agents more useful for ophthalmologic surgery.

All of the volatile anesthetics are associated with a dose-dependent decrease in IOP. Various postulated mechanisms include a reduction in aqueous humor production with a concomitant increase in outflow, relaxation of the supporting musculature, and depression of the central nervous system control center for IOP (McGoldrick, 1992c). As was previously demonstrated with halothane, reliable measurements of IOP may be made for approximately 10 minutes after mask induction with sevoflurane (Watcha et al., 1990; Yoshitake et al., 1993).

The deleterious effects of succinylcholine on IOP and the various methods of attenuating these effects have been evaluated by numerous investigators for several decades. The augmentation of IOP is thought to be mediated not only by tonic contractions of the extraocular muscles but also by dilation of the choroidal vasculature and relaxation of the orbital smooth muscle (Calobrisi and Lebowitz, 1990). In a study of patients undergoing elective enucleation, it was noted that the change in IOP after succinylcholine administration was the same in the normal eye as in the eye where the extraocular muscles were detached; therefore, it does not appear that extraocular muscle contraction significantly contributes to the increase in IOP after succinylcholine administration (Kelly et al., 1993). In adult patients with normal IOP, succinylcholine at doses between 1.5 and 2 mg/kg increased pressures by no more than 9 mm Hg, with peak effects demonstrated within 3 minutes after administration (Pandey et al., 1972). In patients who were not intubated, IOP was restored to baseline within 6 minutes, although other studies have demonstrated mild elevations that may persist for 30 minutes after succinylcholine administration. Whereas these effects of succinylcholine are significant in comparison with the effects of the nondepolarizing agents, they are clearly insignificant in comparison with the increase in IOP that is possible with laryngoscopy, coughing, and retching.

Numerous methods of blunting the rise in IOP secondary to succinylcholine and laryngoscopy have been evaluated, although none has demonstrated consistent or reliable efficacy. The results of early studies of pretreating patients with small doses of the nondepolarizing agents were promising but later refuted (Miller et al., 1968; Meyers et al., 1978). In two adult studies, the use of alfentanil was demonstrated to significantly attenuate the response to succinylcholine and intubation (Polarz et al., 1992; Eti et al., 2000). Another study comparing the effects of fentanyl and alfentanil demonstrated that although both agents were effective in attenuating the response to succinylcholine, fentanyl did not significantly attenuate the increase in IOP secondary to laryngoscopy (Sweeney et al., 1989). Early studies concerning the benefit of lidocaine before succinylcholine were discouraging, but lidocaine had favorable effects on IOP during laryngoscopy and intubation in subsequent investigations (Smith et al., 1979; Mahajan et al., 1987; Warner et al., 1989). The opioids and lidocaine may also facilitate gentle extubations after intraocular procedures and in patients with elevated IOP.

More contemporary methods of controlling IOP with the use of succinylcholine and laryngoscopy have been promising. Premedication with sublingual nifedipine and oral clonidine has demonstrated efficacy in the elderly population (Ghignone et al., 1988; Indu et al., 1989; Polarz et al., 1993). Intramuscular (IM) dexmedetomidine also effectively reduced IOP during regional anesthetic procedures in adults (Virkkila et al., 1994). None of these methods has been evaluated in the pediatric population.

More information regarding airway management and the effects on IOP are discussed in Chapter 30, Anesthesia for the Pediatric Trauma Patient. In addition, Vachon and others (2003) review the use of succinylcholine and the open globe.

GENERAL ANESTHETIC CONSIDERATIONS

Premedication

The value of premedication is well appreciated by all physicians providing anesthetic care to children. Premedication is useful to ease separation from parents and to provide for a smooth induction. Children between the ages of 1 and 6 years commonly benefit from premedication. Older children, especially those subject to repeated procedures, may also benefit from premedication or having a parent present during induction of anesthesia (Kain et al., 2006). Parental presence has also been shown to enhance the effects of oral midazolam on induction and emergence behavior (Arai et al., 2007). Oral midazolam (0.25 to 0.5 mg/kg) is commonly used and is generally effective within 10 to 20 minutes after administration (Coté et al., 2002). Nasal midazolam (0.2 mg/kg) may be useful in the patient refusing oral administration, but the acidity of the formulation is associated with a 71% incidence of burning and crying on administration (Karl et al., 1993). Oral clonidine (2 to 4 mcg/kg) also provides adequate anxiolysis within 30 minutes and has been demonstrated to decrease the incidence of PONV after strabismus surgery in two investigations (Mikawa et al., 1995; Handa and Fujii, 2001). In one study, oral clonidine was more effective than oral midazolam in multiple aspects of premedication, including acceptance by patients, more effective sedation, and better recovery from anesthesia (Almenrader et al., 2007). Neither midazolam nor clonidine consistently decreases the incidence of emergence delirium (Fazi et al., 2001; Valley et al., 2003). At recommended doses, neither of the agents should prolong the time required for discharge from the postoperative recovery unit.

General Anesthesia

General anesthesia for ophthalmologic procedures in children is similar to that provided for other brief surgical procedures. Many ophthalmologic procedures may be performed on an outpatient basis when the age of the patient does not mandate postoperative monitoring. Mask induction with nitrous oxide and sevoflurane is common for young patients who do not require rapid-sequence induction. Clear communication with the ophthalmologist can delineate which procedure may be performed with mask anesthesia or requires the use of a laryngeal mask airway or endotracheal tube. Consideration should be given to the proposed duration of the procedure and the possibility that access to the airway may be difficult.

Anesthesia can be maintained with any of the volatile agents, but the incidence of emergence delirium may be higher with the newer, less-soluble agents (Welborn et al., 1996; Lapin et al., 1999). Nitrous oxide is avoided if inert gas is to be injected into the eye. Nitrous oxide has been associated with an increased incidence of PONV in some adult studies, although similar effects cannot be demonstrated in the pediatric population (Hartung, 1996; Tramer et al., 1996, 1997). One study demonstrated no correlation between the use of nitrous oxide and the incidence of PONV in pediatric patients with strabismus (Kuhn et al., 1999). Maintenance with propofol may also be used, but three studies have demonstrated a higher incidence of dysrhythmias attributable to the OCR with propofol anesthesia (Watcha et al., 1991; Larsson et al., 1992; Tramer et al., 1998). Neuromuscular blockade is often indicated for intraocular procedures to ensure that the field remains motionless and that coughing or bucking does not result in damage to the eye and untoward increases in IOP.

A smooth emergence from anesthesia is desired after ophthalmologic procedures. This may be facilitated by deep extubation in the lateral position. Any of the inhaled agents may be safely used for deep extubation, although slightly more airway complications may occur with the use of desflurane (Valley et al., 2003). Small doses of IV lidocaine (0.5 to 1 mg/kg) may be administered before extubation if the depth of anesthesia is unclear.

Local and Regional Anesthesia

The primary methods of administering local anesthetics for ocular procedures include topical application, infiltration, and regional blockade. Conjunctival injection is often used to provide anesthesia for the treatment of retinopathy of prematurity (ROP). Topical application or infiltration may be useful in the cooperative older child to perform otherwise uncomfortable examinations and simple procedures such as foreign body removal and laceration repair. Regional techniques, including retrobulbar, peribulbar, and sub-Tenon's blocks, are useful in adults as the primary anesthetic for a variety of ophthalmologic procedures, but they are less likely to be used as the sole anesthetic in children younger than 18 years of age (Johnson and Forrest, 1994). The benefits of regional techniques as adjuncts to general anesthesia in children are controversial.

The retrobulbar or intraconal block was first described in 1884. The block involves injection of local anesthetic into the posterior cone of the extraocular muscles and is effective in producing anesthesia and akinesia by blocking the ciliary ganglion and the oculomotor and abducens nerves. Hyaluronidase is a commonly used adjuvant that decreases the time for onset. The retrobulbar technique is not often used in the pediatric population. Complications of the retrobulbar block include stimulation of the OCR, retrobulbar hemorrhage, penetration of the optic nerve, intravascular injection, and brainstem anesthesia (McGoldrick, 1992e). One study evaluating the efficacy of retrobulbar blocks in combination with general anesthesia for pediatric strabismus surgery demonstrated no significant benefit, although the sample size was relatively small (Ates et al., 1998). An additional study of 45 patients showed a significant decrease in incidence and severity of OCR with retrobulbar block, and a decrease in PONV with retrobulbar block or topical local anesthesia (Gupta et al., 2007).

The peribulbar or periconal block has been used increasingly since it was first described in 1986. Because the cone of the extraocular muscles is not entered, the potential for intraocular and intradural injection is minimized, and the risk of retrobulbar hemorrhage and direct nerve injury is virtually eliminated (McGoldrick, 1992e). Disadvantages of the peribulbar block include a slightly higher failure rate (10% incidence) and an increased forward pressure on the globe secondary to the larger volumes of local anesthetic required (Zahl, 1992). Two pediatric studies that compared peribulbar blocks with IV meperidine for vitreoretinal and strabismus surgery demonstrated superior analgesia and significantly less PONV for up to 24 hours after surgery (Deb et al., 2001; Subramaniam et al., 2003). Parental satisfaction was also greater for those patients receiving adjunctive regional blocks.

The sub-Tenon's block was first reported in adults in 1992 as a blunt-needle alternative to the sharp needle peribulbar or retrobulbar blocks (Stevens, 1992). Tenon's capsule is a fascial sheath that envelops the eyeball and separates it from the orbital fat. The inner surface is separated from the outer surface of the sclera by a potential space called the episcleral or sub-Tenon's space (Fig. 27-3). Typically, a blunt, curved cannula is inserted in the inferonasal quadrant under the Tenon's capsule and 3 to 5 mL of local anesthesia are deposited in adults. In pediatric patients the volume is considerably less. The advantages include relatively painless insertion of the block and the ability to use a blunt needle with less opportunity to inject into unwanted areas of the eye. This block is associated with a higher incidence of chemosis and subconjunctival hemorrhage (Guise, 2003).

The sub-Tenon's block in conjunction with general anesthesia has been reported to decrease PONV, improve postoperative pain control, and reduce intraoperative analgesia requirements in patients having strabismus surgery (Steib et al., 2005). Ghai et al. (2009) in a prospective, randomized, blinded study of pediatric cataract patients compared sub-Tenon's block (0.06 to 0.08 mL/kg 2% lidocaine with 0.5% bupivacaine [50:50 mixture]) to IV fentanyl (1 mcg/kg) and found significantly less pain and lower incidence of oculocardiac reflex. There was no statistically significant reduction in PONV, but parent satisfaction scores were higher with the sub-Tenon's block. Additionally, it has been proposed as a technique in conjunction with sedation to perform laser surgery for ROP in neonates at the bedside (Parulekar et al., 2008).

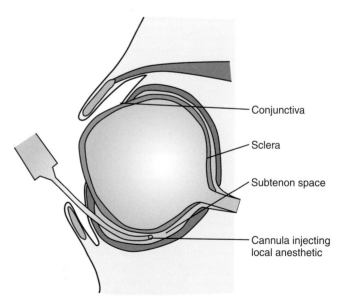

Conjunctiva

Sclera

Subtenon space

Cannula injecting local anesthetic

■ **FIGURE 27-3.** Anatomy of the sub-Tenon's space *(From Ghai B et al.: Subtenon block compared to intravenous fentanyl for perioperative analgesia in pediatric cataract surgery,* Anesth Analg *108:1132, 2009.)*

Although pediatric ophthalmologic patients are not often candidates for a pure regional anesthetic, its use in combination with general anesthesia will likely increase as benefits are measured. Although it is unlikely that most pediatric anesthesiologists will perform such procedures, a general understanding of the techniques and potential complications is important when caring for these children.

INTRAOPERATIVE AND POSTOPERATIVE COMPLICATIONS

Oculocardiac Reflex

The OCR was first described by two independent observers in 1908. The OCR is reported to occur at an incidence as high as 70% to 79% during pediatric ophthalmologic surgery (particularly strabismus surgery) without the use of prophylaxis (Ruta et al., 1996; Allen et al., 1998). The reflex is most often elicited by traction on the extraocular muscles but is also elicited by pressure on the eye and after intraorbital or retrobulbar injections. The reflex has been observed in the child who is congenitally anophthalmic and in the patient with an empty orbit after enucleation (Kerr and Vance, 1983; Ward and Bass, 2001). The anesthesiologist should be aware of the OCR and its potential consequences.

The OCR is mediated by the afferent ophthalmic division of the trigeminal nerve and the efferent vagal nerve (Fig. 27-4). The most common manifestation of the reflex is sinus bradycardia, but more ominous manifestations, including atrioventricular block, ventricular bigeminy, ventricular tachycardia, and asystole, have been described. Most studies define significant

OCR-related bradycardia as a 10% to 20% decrease in the resting heart rate that is sustained for 5 seconds or longer. With sustained traction on one of the extraocular muscles, a counterregulatory adrenergic phase and restoration of heart rate occurs, which may be followed by a further increase in heart rate once traction is released (Braun et al., 1993). Most often, the initial bradycardia is associated with a variable degree of hypotension, although bradycardic hypertensive responses are also possible (Hahnenkamp et al., 2000).

When the reflex occurs intraoperatively, release of the stimulus is usually effective in ablating dysrhythmias within 10 to 20 seconds. If bradycardia persists or is worrisome, the patient may be given atropine (10 to 20 mcg/kg, IV) or glycopyrrolate (10 mcg/kg, IV). The initial effects of atropine should be evident within 20 seconds, and the maximal response is observed after 80 seconds (Braun et al., 1993). In the event that IV access is not available or is unreliable, one study has determined that intraglossal administration is superior to the IM route and in fact may be superior to IV administration (Arnold et al., 2002). It is generally safe to proceed with surgery once normal sinus rhythm at a rate within 10% of baseline is restored.

The value of prophylaxis has been debated for many years. There clearly is no method of completely eliminating the occurrence of the OCR. The consensus is that most pediatric patients (but not adults) undergoing strabismus surgery should be treated with IV atropine at a dose of 20 mcg/kg before manipulation (Steward, 1983). IV glycopyrrolate at a dose of 10 mcg/kg also has demonstrated efficacy with slightly less pronounced tachycardia. One randomized study of 120 children demonstrated a reduction in the incidence of OCR to 5% with glycopyrrolate and 2% with atropine given immediately after induction (Chisakuta and Mirakhur, 1995). Preoperative treatment by

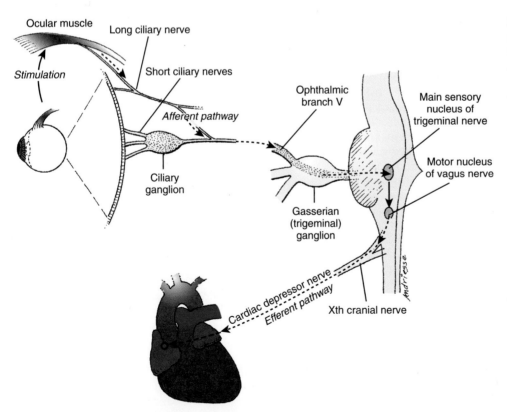

■ **FIGURE 27-4.** Anatomy and physiology of the oculocardiac reflex. *(From Vassallo SA, Ferrari LR: Anesthesia for ophthalmology. In Coté CJ et al., editors: A practice of anesthesia for infants and children, ed 2, Philadelphia, 1993, Saunders.)*

oral or IM routes is generally not warranted and is probably less effective (Mirakhur et al., 1982; Mirakhur, 1991). Opponents to prophylaxis with atropine maintain that possible dysrhythmias secondary to atropine itself (e.g., ventricular tachycardia, ventricular fibrillation, and left bundle branch block) may be more ominous and difficult to treat than the dysrhythmias associated with the OCR (Massumi et al., 1972; McGoldrick, 1992f). These effects are much more common in the adult patient. In otherwise healthy children, the tachycardic effects of atropine or glycopyrrolate should be safe and well tolerated.

Retrobulbar blocks are effective in preventing the OCR (Taylor et al., 1963; Braun et al., 1993; Deb et al., 2001); regional blocks are not commonly used during pediatric procedures and have triggered the reflex during placement. Topical lidocaine, applied directly to the medial rectus at 1 mg/kg, decreased the incidence of the OCR to 19% (vs. 79% in the control population); this technique has not been investigated since the initial study of 36 pediatric patients (Ruta et al., 1996).

The reflex may occur during regional and general anesthesia, and the depth of anesthesia has been thought to be irrelevant. However, there is one study using bispectral index (BIS) to estimate the depth of anesthesia that suggests a BIS of 40 to 50 seems to adequately prevent the OCR, compared with a BIS greater than 60 (Yi and Jee, 2008). Hypercarbia and hypoxemia, which may be more likely in the spontaneously breathing patient, are associated with a greater incidence of the bradycardic response. At least six studies have demonstrated that the choice of maintenance agents may influence the incidence or severity of the OCR. In one study of 39 pediatric patients who were mechanically ventilated through laryngeal mask airways, propofol anesthesia was associated with the greatest decrease in heart rate during a standardized traction of an extraocular muscle. Ketamine was associated with the least decrease in heart rate, whereas halothane and sevoflurane were associated with intermediate effects (Hahnenkamp et al., 2000). In another study of spontaneously breathing normocarbic patients who were not pretreated with atropine, sevoflurane was associated with a 38% incidence of OCR, whereas halothane was associated with an incidence of 79% (Allison et al., 2000). There is no discernable difference between the OCR provoked with desflurane vs. sevoflurane (Oh et al., 2007). Remifentanil appears to have an effect on the incidence of OCR. During strabismus surgery on children between 1 and 9 years of age without anticholinergic prophylaxis, those with maintenance of anesthesia using remifentanil had twice the incidence of OCR compared with those in the group receiving sevoflurane (Chung et al., 2008).

Postoperative Pain

Many of the common ophthalmologic procedures have minimal postoperative analgesic requirements. Examinations under anesthesia, nasolacrimal duct probing, and cataract extraction are associated with negligible postoperative discomfort. The various procedures performed for glaucoma and strabismus are associated with moderate postoperative pain. The requirements for analgesia should be reviewed with the surgeon, the patient, and the family during the formulation and general discussion of the anesthetic plan.

For patients requiring minimal analgesia, rectal acetaminophen (30 to 40 mg/kg) may be administered after induction and followed with subsequent doses (20 mg/kg) at 6-hour intervals

(Birmingham et al., 2001). Up to 120 minutes may be required to achieve peak serum levels. IV ketorolac (0.5 mg/kg) yields consistent analgesia for those procedures resulting in moderate postoperative pain (Dsida et al., 2002). Two studies of ketorolac administered for strabismus surgery have demonstrated analgesia equivalent to that provided by fentanyl (1 mcg/kg) or morphine (0.1 mg/kg) with a substantial reduction in PONV (Munro et al., 1994; Mendel et al., 1995). Another more recent study investigated the effect of topical tetracaine on postoperative pain control and emergence delirium. Although they were unable to make conclusions about emergence agitation, they did demonstrate that tetracaine drops improved pain control in the early postoperative period (Anninger et al., 2007).

Opioid analgesics should not be withheld from patients requiring more intensive analgesia. More painful procedures include cryotherapy (for various disorders), ablation, and enucleation for patients with retinoblastoma. Nausea, vomiting, and respiratory depression can complicate postoperative recovery, but the opioid agents provide greater facility for titration, may minimize coughing and bucking at extubation, and attenuate the incidence of emergence delirium.

Postoperative Nausea and Vomiting

Nausea and vomiting after ophthalmologic procedures are so common that they often serve as a model for the evaluation of various prophylactic techniques. Because nausea is subjective and difficult to measure in children, most studies look only at postoperative vomiting (POV). Several large scale studies report POV in children to occur at an incidence ranging from 13% to 42% after general anesthesia for all procedures (Rose and Watcha, 1999). The incidence of POV in untreated children after strabismus surgery ranges from 40% to 88% (Lerman, 1995). Older children and those receiving opioid analgesics are at greater risk. Whereas prophylaxis vs. symptomatic treatment is debated for low-risk procedures in children, it is generally accepted that prophylaxis should be provided for children undergoing strabismus surgery and all intraocular procedures regardless of demographics and the anesthetic technique employed. Retching and vomiting may be particularly detrimental after surgical or traumatic trespass of the globe. A summary of prophylactic measures is provided in Box 27-2.

One simple measure that does not involve the administration of any drug prophylaxis is the use of IV fluid therapy. In a

---

Box 27-2 Prophylaxis for Postoperative Nausea and Vomiting

DEMONSTRATED BENEFIT
Avoiding opioid analgesics
Avoiding nitrous oxide (controversial)
Dexamethasone 0.15-1 mg/kg, IV
Ondansetron 50-200 mcg/kg, IV
Other 5-HT$_3$–receptor antagonists (if available)
Adequate IV hydration
Withholding oral intake postoperatively

NO DEMONSTRATED BENEFIT
Anticholinergic therapy

comparison of pediatric patients undergoing strabismus surgery, the amount of fluid resuscitation was shown to make a difference in the incidence of PONV. POV was reported in 54% of the control group, who received 10 mL/kg per hour of lactated Ringer's solution, vs. only 22% of the "superhydration group," who received 30 mL/kg per hour of lactated Ringer's solution (Goodarzi et al., 2005).

The efficacy of droperidol, a butyrophenone, has been demonstrated in numerous studies over the past 20 years. Low doses (20 mcg/kg) given after induction are as effective as higher doses (75 mcg/kg) and are less likely to prolong recovery time (Brown, et al., 1991). Lower doses (15 mcg/kg) in combination with ondansetron (100 mcg/kg, IV) are more effective than either drug given individually (Shende et al., 2001). The Food and Drug Administration (FDA) issued a black box warning in 2001 regarding the potential for fatal dysrhythmias associated with prolonged QTc intervals in rare instances when patients were given droperidol (Gan et al., 2002). No significant complications have been reported in children with the use of low-dose droperidol. However, considering a recent study showing doses of 25 mcg/kg of droperidol and 150 mcg/kg of ondansetron administered at induction of anesthesia to be equally effective in reducing the incidence and severity of POV, the pediatric anesthesiologist may find it easier to use alternative drugs than to comply with the rigorous monitoring recommendations made by the FDA (Bharti and Shende, 2003).

Ondansetron is a serotonin 5-HT$_3$–receptor antagonist commonly used for prophylaxis and rescue therapy at doses ranging from 50 to 200 mcg/kg, IV. The half-life in children is slightly shorter than it is in adults (2.5 vs. 3.8 hours), and side effects are unusual in all populations (Culy et al., 2001). Administration either before or after surgical manipulation is acceptable with equivalent benefit (Madan et al., 2000). It has been demonstrated that doses of 75 mcg/kg are as effective as higher doses in the immediate postoperative period (Sadhasivam et al., 2000). Two studies have demonstrated that higher doses (150 to 200 mcg/kg) are required for significant benefit carried through the initial 24-hour postoperative period (Rose et al., 1994; Bowhay et al., 2001).

Other 5-HT$_3$–receptor antagonists have been developed since 1991, primarily in an effort to provide a longer duration of action. Granisetron (20 to 40 mcg/kg, IV or orally [PO]) and dolasetron (12.5 mg or 350 mcg/kg, IV) have demonstrated efficacy in the pediatric strabismus population (Munro et al., 1999; Wagner et al., 2003). Tropisetron (200 mcg/kg up to 2 mg) has also been used in pediatric patients. As costs fall on these newer agents, their use may become more common.

Studies of dexamethasone as an antiemetic have been favorable, primarily in light of the agent's low risk, low cost, long duration of action (up to 48 hours), and potential for augmenting postoperative analgesia (Splinter and Rhine, 1998). Many studies demonstrate its efficacy both alone and in conjunction with other antiemetics. In a dose response study, 250 mcg/kg, IV was found to be as effective as higher doses (Madan et al., 2005). The greatest reduction in POV after surgery for strabismus was reported in a study using low-dose dexamethasone (150 mcg/kg, maximum 8 mg) in combination with ondansetron (50 mcg/kg) after induction (Splinter, 2001). These results were upheld in a more recent study using 0.15 mg/kg of ondansetron and 0.2 mg/kg dexamethasone, resulting in only a 10% incidence of POV (Bhardwaj et al., 2004). One study comparing high-dose dexamethasone at 1 mg/kg (maximum of

25 mg) to ondansetron at 100 mcg/kg (maximum 4 mg) demonstrated a similar incidence of PONV during the initial 6 hours but significantly less during the subsequent 18 postoperative hours in those treated with dexamethasone (Subramaniam et al., 2001). The severity of POV and the number of patients requiring rescue medication were also significantly less in the dexamethasone group. Facial flushing is possible after dexamethasone, but there is no evidence in the literature for more detrimental side effects (e.g., hyperglycemia, delayed wound healing, or adrenal suppression) after single dose therapy (Subramaniam et al., 2001; Madan 2005).

Metoclopramide is a dopaminergic antagonist that provides central antiemetic action as well as increased gastric emptying and increased tone at the lower esophageal sphincter. There is inconsistent support in the literature for the use of metoclopramide for POV prophylaxis. Two randomized studies have demonstrated moderate benefit with metoclopramide at a dose of 250 mcg/kg given after induction, although two more recent studies failed to demonstrate any significant benefit (Broadman et al., 1990; Lin et al., 1992; Shende and Haldar, 1998; Kathirvel et al., 1999). A recent consensus panel failed to find evidence to recommend metoclopramide as a routine antiemetic (Gan, 2007).

Four early studies comparing propofol with halothane demonstrated a significant attenuation of POV after strabismus surgery when propofol was used (Watcha et al., 1991; Larsson et al., 1992; Reimer et al., 1993; Weir et al., 1993). The benefit was demonstrated primarily during the immediate postoperative period. A more recent study comparing propofol with isoflurane failed to demonstrate any significant benefit with propofol (Hamunen et al., 1997).

Other modalities of prophylaxis for POV will continue to emerge in response to an appropriate focus on cost effectiveness and patient and parental satisfaction. It is left to each clinician to determine what risk is tolerable and which patient population may derive the greatest benefit from therapy.

SPECIFIC PATHOLOGY AND SURGICAL AND ANESTHETIC MANAGEMENT

Examination under Anesthesia

Although some centers perform simple examinations and minor procedures for young children under procedural sedation, many ophthalmologists prefer general anesthesia to perform more thorough and accurate examinations. Common evaluations include tonometry, funduscopy, and the assessment of visual evoked potentials. Most examinations take no more than 5 to 10 minutes, but a sufficient depth of anesthesia must be provided. Premedication and anxiolysis are most beneficial to children who require a series of examinations over time.

For healthy children, mask induction and maintenance of spontaneous ventilation provide adequate conditions for the ophthalmologist and affording accurate control of anesthetic depth and a smooth emergence from anesthesia. Accurate measurements of IOP can be made for the initial 10 minutes after induction and maintenance with both sevoflurane and halothane (Watcha et al., 1990; Yoshitake et al., 1993). More lengthy examinations, including photographic retinal mapping and assessment of visual evoked potentials, may be performed with either propofol sedation or spontaneous ventilation with inhaled anesthetic agents and a laryngeal mask airway.

Retinopathy of Prematurity

ROP is a multifactorial disease initiated by delayed retinal vascular growth after premature birth (phase 1) followed by abnormal retinal vessel growth (phase 2). The infant with ROP may require anesthetic care for procedures both related and unrelated to ocular pathology. ROP is of particular interest to the pediatric anesthesiologist, because the routine management of the infant at risk may alter the development or progression of the disease itself.

Conditions associated with ROP include low birth weight, prematurity, oxygen exposure, mechanical ventilation, blood transfusions, intraventricular hemorrhage, sepsis, and vitamin E deficiency. ROP occurs in approximately 70% of infants who weigh less than 1000 g at birth. Fortunately, 80% to 90% of these infants have spontaneous regression of their retinal changes (Simons and Flynn, 1999; Moore, 2000). The greatest risk of oxidative damage to the developing retina appears to be in the first few weeks of life (Gaynon, 2006). It is clear that supplemental oxygen and relative hyperoxia are not the only factors responsible for development of the disease. Nevertheless, the immature retina is indisputably more susceptible to damage from the higher ex utero concentrations of oxygen and subsequent elevated levels of vascular endothelial growth factor (VEGF).

The immature retina responds to elevated oxygen tension (or another insult) by arrest of normal vasculogenesis and later by neovascularization and fibrous-tissue formation in the retina and vitreous humor. Retinal tears and detachment may occur secondary to contraction of the vitreous humor. Vasculogenesis takes place between 16 and 44 weeks' postconception. In the normal developing retina, there is no clear border dividing the vascular and avascular tissue. This border becomes more prominent in those patients with ROP and forms the basis for staging the disease. The International Classification of Retinopathy of Prematurity (ICROP) was established in 1984 to uniformly describe the anatomic zone involved and the severity or stage of disease (Committee for the Classification of Retinopathy of Prematurity, 1984). This was revisited in 2005 with some modifications, including a description of a more virulent form of retinopathy in the tiniest babies (International Committee for the Classification of Retinopathy of Prematurity, 2005). Definitions for the various stages are provided in Box 27-3 and can be seen Figure 27-5. Threshold ROP, defined by specific ICROP criteria, is the stage of progression that is amenable to treatment.

Investigations have demonstrated the benefit of extremely limited oxygen supplementation in premature infants without ROP and the potential benefit of more liberal oxygen therapy in older infants with established prethreshold disease (Sinha and Tin, 2003). At one institution, rigorous guidelines restricting the use of oxygen greatly diminished the occurrence of advanced ROP and abolished the need for laser therapy over a 5-year period (Chow et al., 2003). The STOP-ROP multicenter controlled trial revealed that patients with established prethreshold disease are not harmed by oxygen supplementation and that a subset of these patients may benefit from higher arterial saturations (STOP-ROP Multicenter Study Group, 2000).

> ### Box 27-3 International Classification of Retinopathy of Prematurity Stages
>
> **Stage 1:** Fine demarcation line is visible between vascular and avascular regions.
> **Stage 2:** Broad ridge divides the vascular and avascular regions.
> **Stage 3:** Neovascularization is noted at the ridge, on the posterior surface and anteriorly toward the vitreous cavity.
> **Stage 4:** Subtotal retinal detachment has occurred.
> **Stage 5:** Total retinal detachment in an open or closed funnel configuration has occurred.
>
> From Committee for the Classification of Retinopathy of Prematurity: An international classification of retinopathy of prematurity, *Pediatrics*, 74:127, 1984.

It is prudent to the anesthesiologist to limit oxygen supplementation in those infants without a diagnosis of ROP during the period of retinal vascularization. Older infants (older than 44 weeks' postconceptional age) and those with established prethreshold disease are probably less vulnerable to higher oxygen tensions commonly provided during transports and general anesthesia. Anesthesia provided for nonophthalmologic procedures was once believed to increase the risk of ROP, but controlling for other risk factors has revealed that such a population is at no greater risk (Flynn, 1984).

Infants with threshold ROP are treated by cryotherapy or laser photocoagulation, depending on specific clinical findings. Cryotherapy involves placement of a probe chilled with nitrous oxide on the outer surface of the globe. Cryonecrosis of the underlying retinal tissues results in a decrease in the incidence of retinal detachment. Laser procedures (diode and argon lasers) are the preferred modality of therapy and are easier for the infant and the therapist than the cryotherapy technique. In many hospitals, these procedures are performed at the bedside in the neonatal intensive care unit. Both procedures may be performed with atropine, analgesics including opioids and ketamine, and local anesthesia that includes the sub-Tenon's block (Lyon et al., 2008). Infants who are not intubated for the procedure may experience respiratory or hemodynamic instability, leading some neonatologists to electively intubate these infants for the procedure (Sullivan TJ et al., 1995). Cardiorespiratory disturbances may occur in 5% to 9% of all cases (Brown et al., 1990; Haigh et al., 1997). Some ophthalmologists prefer the benefits of general anesthesia in an operating-room setting. In a recent survey of pediatric ophthalmologists, 50% preferred general anesthesia with a controlled airway, whereas the rest used IV or oral sedation with local anesthesia (Chen et al., 2007). Variation in practice is because of the ophthalmologists' beliefs and experiences, and also because of resource allocation, such as the availabilty of pediatric anesthesia. Once ROP progresses to stage 4 or 5, scleral buckle or vitectomy are performed to attempt to prevent blindness. These surgeries are almost always performed with general endotracheal anesthesia.

Strabismus

Strabismus has a prevalence of 3% to 5% in the pediatric population (Vivian, 2000). The disorder is most often idiopathic but may be associated with poor vision, cataracts, trauma, neuromuscular

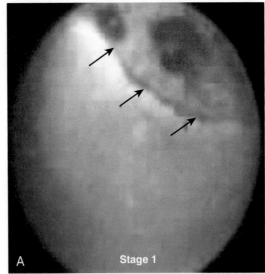

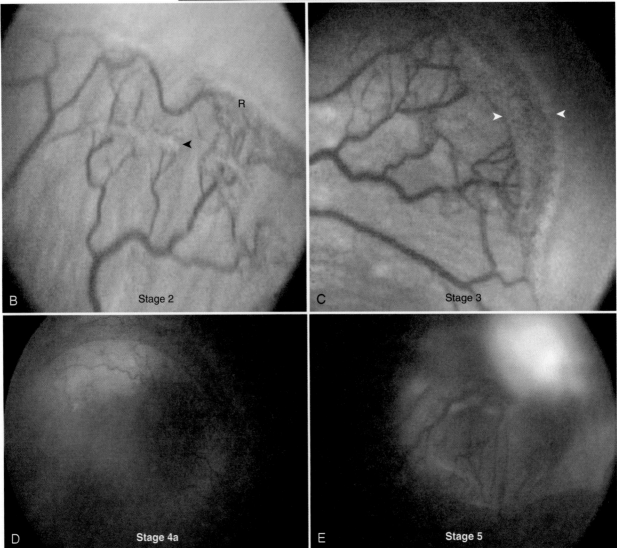

■ **FIGURE 27-5.** Retinopathy of prematurity. **A,** *Stage 1:* Demarcation line—a line that is seen at the edge of vessels *(black arrows),* dividing the vascular from the avascular retina. Retinal blood vessels fail to reach the retinal periphery and they multiply abnormally where they end. **B,** *Stage 2:* Ridge *(R)* of scar tissue and new vessels in place of the demarcation line. The white line now has width and height and occupies some volume. Small tufts of new vessels ("popcorn vessels") may appear posterior to the ridge *(white arrowhead).* **C,** *Stage 3:* Increased size of the vascular ridge *(between white arrowheads),* with growth of fibrovascular tissue on the ridge and extending out into the vitreous. Fibrous scar tissue is beginning to form in this stage, with attachments between the vitreous gel and the ridge. **D,** *Stage 4a:* Partial retinal detachment; detachment does not include the macula, and the vision may be good. In Stage 4B (not shown) the macula is detached, and visual potential is markedly decreased. **E,** *Stage 5:* Complete retinal detachment. *(Courtesy of Dr. Richard Hertle, The Children's Hospital of Pittsburgh.)*

disorders, or one of several congenital syndromes (see Table 27-1). Surgical correction involves isolation of one or more of the extraocular muscles with subsequent recession (transection and reinsertion) or resection (shortening) of the muscle. Contemporary techniques involving botulinum toxin injection and postoperative adjustable sutures are not commonly used in the pediatric population. Amblyopia develops in approximately 50% of all patients with congenital esotropia and should be treated with occlusion therapy before surgical correction for strabismus (Guthrie and Wright, 2001).

General anesthesia may be provided by a flexible laryngeal mask airway, although endotracheal intubation with controlled ventilation may lessen the risk of hypercarbia and hypoxemia, which are known to increase the incidence and severity of the OCR (Blanc et al., 1988). Many ophthalmologists request the use of paralytic agents for performance of the forced duction test to more clearly differentiate paretic and restrictive disorders before surgical correction. This possibility should be discussed with the surgeon before formulating the anesthetic plan. Prolonged contractions of the extraocular muscles associated with the use of succinylcholine interfere with interpretation of the forced duction test for at least 15 minutes after administration (France et al., 1980). Its use is relatively contraindicated.

Masseter muscle rigidity after succinylcholine administration is four times more common in children anesthetized for strabismus surgery than in the general pediatric surgical population (Carroll, 1987). Because of the association of masseter muscle rigidity with malignant hyperthermia and an increased incidence of malignant hyperthermia in patients undergoing strabismus surgery, these patients are thought to be at a greater risk for the development of malignant hyperthermia (Strazis and Fox, 1993) (see Chapter 37, Malignant Hyperthermia).

Prophylaxis for both the OCR and PONV are critical for the patient undergoing strabismus repair. Postoperative pain is generally mild and of conjunctival origin. Acetaminophen, IV ketorolac, or both are usually effective. Topical analgesics (ketorolac, diclofenac, and benoxinate [oxybuprocaine]) have been evaluated in the strabismus population, and clear advantages over systemic agents and uniform efficacy have not been demonstrated (Morton et al., 1997; Bridge et al., 2000).

Lacrimal Apparatus Dysfunction

Congenital nasolacrimal duct obstruction is present in 60% to 70% of all infants at birth; spontaneous resolution is observed in 96% of these children by 1 year of age (Freitag and Woog, 2000). Congenital obstructions are most often isolated findings, but they may be associated with a variety of syndromes and craniofacial defects (Table 27-1). Acquired nasolacrimal duct obstruction is uncommonly encountered in the pediatric population but may be secondary to trauma, granulomatous disease, and systemic neoplasms (leukemia and lymphoma). The anatomy of the nasolacrimal duct system is illustrated in Figure 27-6.

The initial surgical management of congenital obstruction usually requires only simple probing to establish patency. A small Bowman probe is inserted through one or both of the puncti, through the lacrimal sac, and subsequently into the nasolacrimal duct to pierce the valve of Hasner beneath the inferior turbinate (Freitag and Woog, 2000). The procedure is often atraumatic, requires no more than 5 to 10 minutes, and has been performed successfully in the office setting in children younger than 6 months of age. Usually the procedure is performed with general mask anesthesia. As with similar noninvasive procedures, IV access is not absolutely required for patients who are

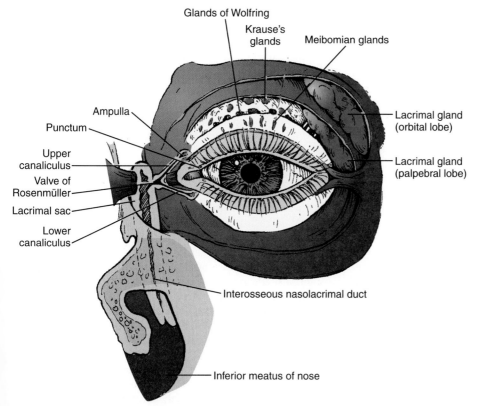

Glands of Wolfring
Krause's glands
Meibomian glands
Ampulla
Punctum
Upper canaliculus
Valve of Rosenmüller
Lacrimal sac
Lower canaliculus
Lacrimal gland (orbital lobe)
Lacrimal gland (palpebral lobe)
Interosseous nasolacrimal duct
Inferior meatus of nose

■ **FIGURE 27-6.** Anatomy of the lacrimal duct apparatus. *(From Nowinski TS: Anatomy and physiology of the lacrimal system. In Bosniak S, editor: Principles and practice of ophthalmic plastic and reconstructive surgery, vol 2, Philadelphia, 1996, Saunders.)*

easily ventilated with a mask. Patients with significant comorbidities may be more safely cared for with IV access (Eippert et al., 1998). Although transient bacteremia has been demonstrated after nasolacrimal duct probing, the benefit of antibiotics to prevent endocarditis is questionable (Wilson et al., 2007).

The lacrimal system may be irrigated with saline or fluorescein after the procedure to demonstrate patency. Preventing excessive pooling, possible laryngospasm, and aspiration may require only head-down positioning and careful suctioning through the ipsilateral naris or oropharynx. Some anesthesiologists believe that patients are better managed with intubation to provide optimal protection of the airway (Johnson and Forrest, 1994). Analgesic requirements after nasolacrimal probing and irrigation are negligible.

Secondary surgical management of nasolacrimal obstruction may include infracture of the inferior turbinate, placement of silicone tubing that remains in place for 3 to 12 months, and dacryocystorhinostomy (Freitag and Woog, 2000). Dacryocystorhinostomy is a procedure used to bypass the nasolacrimal duct by creating an anastomosis between the lacrimal sac and the nasal mucosa beneath the middle turbinate. A small incision is made just medial to the medial canthus and overlying the lacrimal sac. These more complex procedures may require up to 2 hours to perform and may be complicated by appreciable blood loss. They require general anesthesia with endotracheal intubation. Topical vasoconstrictors may be used to minimize bleeding at the highly vascular nasal mucosa, and pharyngeal packing is usually beneficial. Acetaminophen, ketorolac, or small doses of opioids should provide adequate postoperative analgesia.

Cataracts

The prevalence of pediatric cataracts is between 1.2 and 6:10,000 live births. Bilateral cataracts are most commonly associated with systemic disease (see Table 27-1), whereas unilateral cataracts are more often idiopathic (Russell-Eggitt, 2000; Fallaha and Lambert, 2001). Surgery for bilateral congenital cataracts must be performed within the first several weeks of life to allow for normal retinal development. Unilateral congenital disease requires surgical attention within the first 4 months of life to prohibit the development of irreversible amblyopia.

Lens extraction is performed after maximal mydriasis with one or more of the topical agents. Ultrasonic phacoemulsification (commonly used in adults) is not often used in the pediatric population because of the pliable nature of the immature lens. Vitrectomy instrumentation is the preferred method of extraction in young children; the entire procedure is typically performed with only one intraocular instrument. Capsular opacification occurs often in children, and a capsulectomy is usually performed at the time of primary surgery. Intraocular lens implants are commonly provided to children older than 6 months with unilateral disease and children older than 1 year with bilateral disease (Fallaha and Lambert, 2001).

Anesthesia for lens extraction should provide complete akinesia and meticulous control of IOP. Because most of these patients are infants, controlled ventilation with muscle relaxants provides optimal operating conditions. The anesthesiologist should be aware of associated systemic disease and the potential systemic effects of the topical preparations used by the ophthalmologist. Rarely (1:200,000), maximal pupillary dilation requires an infusion of epinephrine delivered and then continuously aspirated from the anterior chamber. Attention to the electrocardiogram tracing permits detection of systemic absorption, which fortunately is uncommon (McGoldrick, 1992b). Analgesic requirements are usually minimal and under normal circumstances may be met with acetaminophen.

Postoperative apnea has been reported in the otherwise healthy full-term infant after cataract surgery (Tetzlaff et al., 1988). Speculation has associated ocular pathology or procedures with postoperative apnea in the otherwise healthy infant, but this association has yet to be clearly described.

Surgical postoperative complications include the formation of secondary membranes, glaucoma, and endophthalmitis (Fallaha and Lambert, 2001). Endophthalmitis may be avoided by treating nasolacrimal duct obstruction before cataract surgery and postponing cataract surgery in children with evidence of upper respiratory tract infection.

Glaucoma

Pediatric glaucomas are a diverse group of disorders with a prevalence of 1:10,000 live births (Khaw et al., 2000). Pediatric glaucoma is most often a congenital abnormality inherited in an autosomal recessive pattern that is slightly more prevalent in males (McGoldrick, 1992f). Only 10% of pediatric glaucoma diagnoses are associated with systemic disease, congenital disorders, or other ocular abnormalities. The diagnosis may be suspected in the patient who has buphthalmia, epiphora, photophobia, or corneal clouding (Khaw et al., 2000). The definitive diagnosis is made only by tonometry, corneal examination, funduscopy, and gonioscopy (examination of the iridocorneal angle).

Open-angle glaucoma is diagnosed when a normal trabecular meshwork is visible via gonioscopy. Closed-angle glaucoma is diagnosed when the iridocorneal angle is obstructed by the iris. Infantile glaucoma develops before the age of 3 years and is a primary disorder in approximately 50% of all cases. Juvenile glaucoma refers to disease that develops after the age of 3 years and is most often secondary to or associated with other ocular or systemic disorders.

Surgical management varies between patients and is dependent on the measurements and observations made under general anesthesia. Corrective procedures include goniotomy, trabeculotomy, trabeculectomy, and cyclocryotherapy (Beck, 2001). Goniotomy is a relatively brief procedure, whereas the other surgical techniques may require longer periods of general anesthesia. Patients often require repeated evaluations, because surgical correction is typically incremental and performed in carefully monitored stages.

The anesthetic management is quite similar for all procedures. A careful review of the past medical history, comorbid conditions, and concurrent pharmacologic therapy is crucial (see Tables 27-1 and 27-2). Premedication with atropine or glycopyrrolate is acceptable, but the use of scopolamine is generally contraindicated in the patient with glaucoma. Mask inductions are acceptable and followed by gentle laryngoscopy and placement of an oral Ring-Adair-Elwyn (RAE) endotracheal tube. Stable IOP and complete akinesia must be maintained throughout the surgical procedure. Neostigmine with glycopyrrolate or atropine may be safely administered for reversal of neuromuscular blockade; both agents have only minimal ocular effects at the routinely recommended doses. Unlike many other ocular procedures, surgery for glaucoma (particularly cyclocryotherapy) may be associated with moderate to severe postoperative pain. Opioids, in conjunction with prophylaxis for PONV, should be incorporated into the anesthetic plan.

Retinoblastoma

Retinoblastoma is the most common intraocular malignancy in the pediatric population with a prevalence of 1:20,000 live births. Fifty percent of all cases are secondary to mutations of the retinoblastoma gene, although only 25% of patients with the heritable form of the disease have a positive family history (Moore, 2000). The diagnosis is generally made by 3 years of age. Children with a positive family history have a 5% risk for developing retinoblastoma; these patients require regular examinations until the age of 5 years.

Therapy for retinoblastoma varies according to the severity of disease and has evolved dramatically since the 1970s. Treatment modalities may include combinations of enucleation, external beam radiation, localized radiotherapy, laser ablation, thermotherapy, cryotherapy, and chemotherapy (Uusitalo and Wheeler, 1999). Enucleation of the affected eye (or the more involved eye in bilateral disease) followed by external beam radiation was the cornerstone of treatment in the 1990s, leading to survival of over 90%. However, the risk of second cancers in the field of radiation began to appear with the risk increasing by 10% per decade of life. Through chemoreduction and focal ablation methods, many children with retinoblastoma are spared enucleation and serial external beam radiotherapy (Shields and Shields, 1999). Candidates for external beam radiotherapy include patients with bilateral disease that requires enucleation of the more involved eye and patients with diffuse vitreous and subretinal seeding.

Anesthetic requirements for enucleation are similar to those for other moderately complex ophthalmic procedures. The incidence of OCR-mediated dysrhythmias is high, and appropriate prophylaxis with atropine or glycopyrrolate is warranted. Contemporary surgical techniques effectively minimize blood loss such that the need for transfusion is uncommon. Postoperative pain is often significant.

External beam radiotherapy may require as many as 24 radiation sessions and anesthetics over the course of 4 to 6 weeks. Each session is of a few minutes' duration, but the session requires the patient to remain motionless. Various anesthetic methods have been used, including rectal or IM methohexital, IV or IM ketamine, and brief inhalation anesthetics by insufflation methods, laryngeal mask airway, and endotracheal intubation (McGoldrick, 1992f). When a central venous catheter has been placed for adjuvant chemotherapy, a single bolus of propofol is probably the most effective method of providing the required 2 to 3 minutes of anesthesia with minimal recovery requirements.

Vitreoretinal Disorders

Retinal tears and detachment in the pediatric population are most often secondary to ROP but may also result from trauma and vitreous degeneration common to certain syndromes (see Table 27-1). Small tears may be amenable to laser therapy or cryopexy, but more significant tears and detachment often require complex surgical management and up to 3 hours of general anesthesia. Surgical options include scleral buckling (in combination with cryopexy), closed vitrectomy, and open-sky vitrectomy (Hunter et al., 2000).

The scleral buckle procedure involves the attachment of a tiny sponge or silicone band that constricts the sclera and holds the retina in position (Fig. 27-7). The scleral buckle remains permanently attached to the eye and may restrict normal growth of the child's eye if tension is not released with subsequent surgery. Vitrectomy may be considered in the presence of a failed scleral buckle, for high retinal detachment, and for media opacification. The closed vitrectomy is slightly more difficult in the pediatric population and involves lensectomy for segmentation and removal of the vitreous by microvitreoretinal blades and vitrectomy instruments. The open-sky technique involves complete removal of the cornea, lensectomy, and en bloc removal of the fibrous mass filling the funnel of the detached retina (Hunter et al., 2000).

Anesthetic considerations for such procedures include prophylaxis for the OCR (the extraocular muscles are often bridled to permit optimal positioning), complete neuromuscular blockade, and the potential need to lower IOP with agents such as mannitol and acetazolamide. Silicone oil or one of the long-acting inert gases may be injected into the vitreous chamber at the conclusion of the procedure in an effort to improve surgical success (see Table 27-2). Should reoperation be necessary within a month of injection of an inert gas, nitrous oxide may be contraindicated because of its potential to expand the gaseous space.

Traumatic Injury and Ruptured Globe

The optimal management for the patient with ocular injury has been widely debated for many years, although many contemporary pundits consider the controversy mundane. Ophthalmic

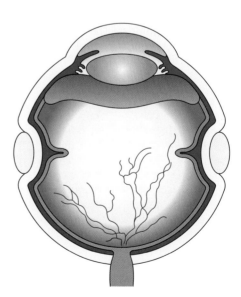

■ **FIGURE 27-7.** Scleral buckle. *(From Sears J, Capone A: Retinopathy of prematurity. In Yanoff M, Duker JS, editors:* Ophthalmology, *Philadelphia, 1999, Mosby.)*

injuries are most often superficial, but a disproportionate number of serious penetrating injuries occur in children (Johnson and Forrest, 1994). It is often difficult to differentiate the emergent case (penetrating injury) from the nonemergent (nonpenetrating injury) case in children without examination under general anesthesia.

The pressure in the ruptured globe becomes atmospheric, and any external pressure or increase in internal pressure may lead to prolapse of the intraocular contents and a diminished possibility for recovery of vision. The possibility of salvaging the eye after penetrating injury requires surgical intervention within several hours of the injury. Traditional periods of fasting are not acceptable.

The importance of maintaining a quiet environment in the preoperative period cannot be overemphasized. Crying and thrashing can have devastating effects on IOP. Forceful eyelid closure may increase IOP by as much as 70 mm Hg (McGoldrick, 1993). Venous cannulation can be facilitated by pentobarbital, oral or rectal midazolam, and transdermal anesthetics. Access subsequently permits the administration of additional anxiolytics, analgesics, and prophylaxis for aspiration. Once sedation is adequate, the injured eye should be patched to provide comfort and minimize ocular movement.

When IV access is available, the anesthesiologists must consider the risks and benefits of succinylcholine (Vachon et al., 2003). Current consensus remains in favor of succinylcholine for rapid provision of optimal intubating conditions and reliable attenuation of coughing and bucking immediately after the endotracheal tube is secured. It is widely accepted that succinylcholine increases IOP despite various methods of blunting the response, but it is also clear that the succinylcholine-induced rise in IOP is inconsequential in relation to the possible rise with laryngoscopy and intubation (Cunningham and Barry, 1986). Support for the use of succinylcholine is derived from feline models of both anterior and posterior segment trauma and retrospective chart reviews and testimonials from the Wills Eye Hospital and the Massachusetts Eye and Ear Infirmary (Libonati et al., 1985; Donlon, 1986; Moreno et al., 1991).

Some anesthesiologists use nondepolarizing neuromuscular blockers for modified rapid sequence inductions in patients with penetrating ocular injuries. The nondepolarizing agents provide either no effect on or a slight decrease in IOP. Three described methods for accelerating the onset of the older nondepolarizing agents are divided doses of pancuronium, high-dose vecuronium, and synergism with d-tubocurarine and pancuronium (Mehta et al., 1985; Abbott and Samuel, 1987; Abdulla, 1993). Most anesthesiologists concede that none of these techniques provides the speed and reliability of succinylcholine. Rocuronium (1.2 mg/kg) has been demonstrated to have no effect on IOP and may provide intubating conditions comparable to succinylcholine within 60 seconds (Mazurek et al., 1998; Mitra et al., 2001; Perry et al., 2003). For patients with comorbid conditions that mandate avoidance of succinylcholine, rocuronium is probably the most effective alternative.

Although isolated ocular injuries are more common in children, the anesthesiologist should be aware of other injuries that may compromise the patient's condition. Liberal doses of either propofol or thiopental, adjuvant agents, and neuromuscular monitoring are paramount before attempted laryngoscopy and placement of the endotracheal tube. A gastric tube should be placed to evacuate the contents of the stomach only after the airway is protected and paralysis is complete. Complex surgical repairs may not be performed during the initial presentation, and surgical time may vary from 1 hour to several hours. Complete paralysis and attention to IOP are mandatory throughout the procedure. Deep extubation is an option for patients not considered at risk for aspiration.

SUMMARY

The pediatric population provides the anesthesiologist with a wide variety of ophthalmologic pathology. The anesthetic challenges are considerable. An understanding of the pertinent physiologic and pharmacologic principles, as well as an appreciation of the continued advancement in surgical therapy, affords optimal patient management and favorable outcomes.

For questions and answers on topics in this chapter, go to "Chapter Questions" at www.expertconsult.com.

REFERENCES

Complete references used in this text can be found online at www.expertconsult.com.

Anesthesia for Organ Transplantation

Victor L. Scott II, Kerri M. Wahl, Kyle Soltys, Kumar G. Belani,
David S. Beebe, and Peter J. Davis

CHAPTER

28

CONTENTS

S ince the inception of the United Network of Organ Sharing (UNOS) in 1987, nearly half a million solid organ transplants have been performed in the United States. Of these, 375,000 have been from deceased donors, or donation after cardiac death (DCD), and 103,000 have been from living donors (UNOS 4-2010) (Tables 28-1 and 28-2). The total number of pediatric transplants has reached nearly 37,000, and the total number of living donors is 9200 for all pediatric patients. In 2009, the yearly totals for pediatric organ transplants increased significantly for the first time in 6 years, to a total of 2019, from a low of 1964 transplants in both of the years 2005 and 2008. Unfortunately, the yearly total of pediatric living donors decreased from a decade high of 560 in 2001, to 387 in 2009. The incidence of end-stage organ disease increases with age, and children still account for only a small fraction (7.60%) of the total number of transplant recipients.

In 1973, the U.S. Congress recognized organ donation as a legal voluntary gift by adopting the Uniform Anatomical Gift Act. In addition, the Omnibus Budget Reconciliation Act (implemented in October 1987) stipulates that hospitals will not receive reimbursement from Medicare or Medicaid unless written protocols for the identification of potential organ donors are established. Physicians are now routinely expected to approach families of brain-dead patients and request organ donation. UNOS established uniform policies and standards, with a guarantee of equitable access of member institutions to

TABLE 28-1. Donor Transplant Data: Pediatric versus Adult, 1985 to April 2010

	To Date*	2009	2008	2007	2006	2005
All Donors						
All Ages	478,347	28,464	27,965	28,369	28,940	28,116
Pediatric	36,530 (7.6%)	2019	1964	1959	1984	1964
Adult	441,808	26,445	26,000	26,410	26,956	26,152
Unknown	9	0	1	0	0	0
Deceased Donor						
All Ages	374,926	21,854	21,747	22,056	22,208	21,213
Pediatric	27,336	1632	1600	1589	1603	1476
Adult	347,581	20,222	20,146	20,467	20,605	19,737
Unknown	9	0	1	0	0	0
Living Donor						
All Ages	103,421	6610	6218	6313	6732	6903
Pediatric	9194	387	364	370	381	488
Adult	94,227	6223	5854	5943	6351	6415

From the United Network for Organ Sharing (UNOS) and Organ Procurement and Transplantation Network (OPTN) data, 2010. Available at http://optn.transplant.hrsa.gov/data.
*Includes patients who received transplants since 1988.
Total of all solid organ transplants 1985 to 2010.

TABLE 28-2. Solid Organ Transplantations: Pediatric Data, 2005 to 2010

		To Date*	2009	2008	2007	2006	2005
All Ages	All organs	475,978	26,095	27,965	28,369	28,940	28,116
Pediatric	All organs	36,367	2019	1964	1959	1984	1963
	Kidney	15,867	792	773	796	893	892
	Liver	11,958	525	613	605	577	569
	Pancreas	396	54	67	61	39	27
	Kidney and pancreas	43	5	2	4	3	7
	Heart	5905	333	365	327	314	313
	Lung	931	56	45	52	55	54
	Heart and lung	176	3	6	3	7	5
	Intestine	1091	89	93	111	96	96

From the United Network for Organ Sharing (UNOS) and Organ Procurement and Transplantation Network (OPTN) data, 2010. Available at http://optn.transplant.hrsa.gov/data.
*Includes transplants from 1985.

all available donor organs. UNOS revised and reviewed a number of their inclusion criteria for both donors and recipients in November 2009.

With the new changes, Organ Procurement Organization (OPO) members must submit data to the Organ Procurement and Transplantation Network (OPTN) under the directorship of the U.S. Department of Health and Human Services through the use of standardized forms and electronic databases. There are 11 OPTNs in the United States and Puerto Rico (Fig. 28-1). In addition to providing data on all deceased donors, living donors, potential transplant recipients, and actual transplant recipients, all OPOs must also submit of the total number of reported deaths by donor hospital.

As of January 2010, there are 486 transplant centers or hospitals in the United States that operate one or more organ transplant programs. These centers house 1136 types of solid organ transplantation programs, managed by the 11 OPTNs (UNOS-OPTN, April 2010), as reported by the Health Resources and Services Administration of Health and Human Services. Data extracted from the UNOS database suggest that there are currently over 100,000 candidates awaiting transplantation. Table 28-3 demonstrates the numbers of pediatric and adult candidates awaiting organ transplantation by organ type. Pediatric patients outnumber these adults only in the category of intestinal transplantation.

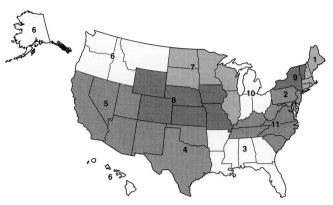

■ **FIGURE 28-1.** A map of the 11 organ procurement and transplantation networks in the United States in 2010. *(From the United Network for Organ Sharing (UNOS) and Organ Procurement and Transplantation Network (OPTN) data, 2010. Available at http://optn. transplant.hrsa.gov/data.)*

TABLE 28-3. Organ Transplant Waiting List

Waiting List Candidates 4/25/2010		Pediatric	Adult
All	115,818	1953	113,865
Kidney	90,068	799	89,269
Pancreas	1470	60	1410
Kidney and pancreas	2253	1	2252
Liver	16,652	539	16,113
Intestine	247	175	72
Heart	3177	264	2913
Lung	1873	103	1770
Heart and lung	78	12	66

From the United Network for Organ Sharing (UNOS) and Organ Procurement and Transplantation Network (OPTN) data, 2010. Available at http://optn. transplant.hrsa.gov/data.

The number of pediatric candidates awaiting organ transplantation pales in comparison with the total number of available organs. In fact, for the past 5 years, the total number of patients awaiting transplantation (~100,000) is one fifth of the total number of patients transplanted since 1985 (~500,000). Although organ transplantation procedures are relatively infrequent compared with the over 50 million surgical procedures performed per year in the United States, perioperative care for these patients has become highly specialized. Maintenance of physiologic homeostasis during the removal of a failed native organ and the subsequent allograft reperfusion period are challenging for both anesthesiologists and surgeons. This chapter focuses on the current body of knowledge for each type of major solid organ transplantation, with a specific focus on special considerations for the management of children. In addition, cellular transplantation, stem-cell transplantation, immunosuppression, complications, graft-versus-host disease, and posttransplant lymphoproliferative disease will be addressed. Information on artificial assist devices being used in the treatment of end-organ failure or as a bridge to

transplantation, and information on xenotransplantation. See related video online at www.expertconsult.com.

DETERMINATION OF BRAIN DEATH IN CHILDREN

The medical and legal aspects of determining brain death have evolved over the past 3 decades. The need for special criteria for determination of brain death in infants and children was clear as early as 1967 when the first successful heart transplantation took place. The organ came from a brain-dead, beating-heart donor, and the first U.S. committee met to form a consensus opinion.

The pediatric central nervous system (CNS) may be more resilient to certain forms of injury, a fact that should be considered when interpreting diagnostic evidence and confirming brain death in infants and children. Brain death is defined as the absence of cortical and cerebral function without preservation of brainstem function. When measured in this setting, cerebral blood flow (CBF) is absent. Publication of brain death criteria specifically addressing findings in infants and children has clarified most of the ambiguities created by age-related neurologic differences. The Task Force for the Uniform Determination of Brain Death in Children was assembled in 1987 *(Report of Special Task Force, Pediatrics, 1988).* Box 28-1 summarizes the currently accepted guidelines for determination of brain death in neonates, infants, and children.

Box 28-1 Guidelines for Brain Death in Children

1. Diagnosis of irreversible coma
   a. Exclude all potentially reversible causes of coma: drug intoxication (barbiturates, sedatives, hypnotics, and alcohol).
2. Physical examination
   a. Coma
   b. Apnea (determined by standardized testing)
   c. Absence of brainstem function (no cough, gag, sucking reflexes; no oculocephalic or cold caloric–induced eye movement)
   d. Normothermia
   e. Normotension
   f. Flaccid tone, absence of spontaneous movement
   g. Atropine resistance (failure to increase the heart rate by more than 5 beats/min after atropine sulfate is given intravenously at a dosage of 40 mcg/kg)*
3. Consistent physical examination during period of observation, as follows:
   a. For ages 7 days to 2 months: two examinations and isoelectric electroencephalograms (EEGs) 48 hours apart
   b. For ages 2 months to 1 year: two examinations and isoelectric EEGs 24 hours apart, or one examination and isoelectric EEG, plus radionuclide angiogram showing absence of cerebral blood flow
   c. For ages greater than 1 year: two examinations 12 to 24 hours apart, EEGs, and isotope angiography.

*From Hosenpud JD, Novick RJ, Breen TJ, et al: The Registry of the International Society for Heart and Lung Transplantation: eleventh official report–1994, *J Heart Lung Transplant* 13:561–570, 1994.

If hypoxic encephalopathy is present, observation for 24 hours is recommended. This time may be reduced if an electroencephalogram shows electrocortical silence, or if a radionuclide study is negative for CBF. In patients with electrocortical silence, metabolic coma must be excluded. Detailed reviews of these guidelines and their applications have been published (Ashwal and Schneider, 1991; Ashwal, 1993; Koszer and Moshe, 2010). Prospective donors must fully meet the age-appropriate criteria and be declared legally brain dead before attempting to obtain consent for organ donation from their family. A physician must record the official time of death in the chart before transferring the donor to the operating room for the organ procurement procedure. Although the donor is officially dead, the care of an anesthesiologist is needed during these procedures to continue efforts to maintain cardiac output, at least until the viscera have been flushed with the cold preservative solution. At this point, ventilation can be discontinued and the responsibility of the anesthesiologist is concluded.

One area that remains particularly controversial is the appropriateness of organ donation from anencephalic newborns. This developmental anomaly results in absence of the cerebral cortex and upper brainstem, so these infants possess no potential for normal neurologic development. Despite the uniformly fatal outcome in these cases, such infants never meet the usual criteria for brain death (Baird and Sadovnick, 1984).

DONOR STRATEGIES

Successful donor-directed strategies for the 21st century focus on increasing the size of the donor pool through expansion of acceptable donor criteria, adoption of comprehensive donation management guidelines, and innovative surgical techniques that allow organ sharing. Here, the term *pediatric organ donors* refers to critically ill children, from the newborn to the 17-year-old, with cessation of neurologic function. Unique challenges may limit the number of deceased pediatric donor organs available for transplantation, including size and weight constraints, as well as the lack of expertise required for declaration of brain death and management of the pediatric donor at some institutions. Thus, organ availability for transplantation (kidney, liver, lung, small bowel, and pancreas) is becoming increasingly dependent on living donors, on split-liver transplantation, and on asystolic, non-heart-beating (DCD) donors.

Organ donation in the pediatric population has decreased by almost 25% in the past 15 years, from 1201 in 1995, to 919 in 2009, with a low in 2008 of 879, the lowest number of pediatric donors since the inception of UNOS data collection (Table 28-4). Additionally, living donation has also decreased significantly in the past 5 years, a result of the ethics controversy and the complications that are now apparent with respect to living donation. The distribution of pediatric donor ages has remained consistent, with close to 60% being between the ages of 11 and 17 (Table 28-5). Although the number of adult donors is significantly greater than the number of pediatric donors, the percentage of recovered organs in the pediatric age range is generally greater than the percent of adult transplanted organs. For deceased kidney donors, 94.7% of the pediatric kidneys recovered were transplanted compared with 91.6% of the kidneys recovered from donors aged 18 to 49 years. There was a similar trend for pancreas donors (81.4% versus 72.2%), liver donors (96.0% versus 91.4%), and intestine donors (94.7% versus 85.7%). For heart and lung donors, the percentage of recovered organs transplanted was high, and it was similar for both

TABLE 28-4. Donors of Organs Recovered in the United States between January 1, 2001 and January 31, 2010

	To Date	2009	2008	2007	2006	2005	2004	2003	2002	2001
All Donor Types										
All ages	235,826	14,630	14,208	14,400	14,751	14,495	14,154	13,285	12,820	12,696
Pediatric	22,423	919	879	927	967	899	979	887	934	990
Adult	213,386	13,710	13,329	13,472	13,782	13,596	13,175	12,398	11,886	11,706
Pediatric Donor %*	9.6%	6.3%	6.2%	6.4%	6.6%	6.2%	6.9%	6.6%	7.3%	7.7%
Unknown	17	1	0	1	2	0	0	0	0	0
Deceased Donor										
All ages	131,675	8021	7990	8085	8019	7593	7150	6457	6190	6080
Pediatric	22,370	916	879	926	966	899	979	886	932	989
Adult	109,303	7105	7111	7159	7053	6694	6171	5571	5258	5091
Unknown	2	0	0	0	0	0	0	0	0	0
Living Donor										
All ages	104,151	6609	6218	6315	6732	6902	7004	6828	6630	6616
Pediatric	53	3	0	1	1	0	0	1	2	1
Adult	104,083	6605	6218	6313	6729	6902	7004	6827	6628	6615
Unknown	15	1	0	1	2	0	0	0	0	0

From the United Network for Organ Sharing (UNOS) and Organ Procurement and Transplantation Network (OPTN) data, 2010. Available at http://optn.transplant.hrsa.gov/data.
*Percent of all donors.

TABLE 28-5. Donor Organs Recovered in the United States as of January 31, 2010

Age (yr)	All Organs	Kidney	Liver	Pancreas	Kidney and Pancreas	Heart	Lung	Heart and Lung	Intestine
All ages	107,022	84,573	15,981	1450	2177	3169	1851	77	246
<1	115	1	56	5	0	42	1	0	20
1-5	494	152	176	38	0	90	14	2	106
6-10	362	134	128	7	0	53	20	2	31
11-17	832	499	170	9	1	79	68	8	17
18-34	10,381	8765	781	190	410	343	217	21	24
35-49	27,973	23,357	2638	778	1248	632	349	26	22
50-64	48,660	36,363	9842	407	511	1435	895	16	20
65+	18,222	15,315	2193	16	7	495	287	2	6

From the United Network for Organ Sharing (UNOS) and Organ Procurement and Transplantation Network (OPTN) data, 2010. Available at http://optn.transplant.hrsa.gov/data.

pediatric donors and adult donors aged 18 to 49 years (98.9% versus 99.0% for heart and 98.1% versus 96.4% for lung) (OPTN/SRTR, 2010).

Over the past decade, the number of pediatric DCD donors increased from six (less than 1%) in 1997, to 77 (8%) in 2006. Although the percentages of DCD donors currently are similar in the adult and pediatric populations, there is probably an unmet potential of DCD donors in the pediatric population.

Recovery of organs from deceased donors requires continuing care of the patient's preexisting condition, with a shift in primary emphasis from minimizing neurologic injury and preserving life to protection of specific organs. Principles of pediatric donor care are comparable with those of adults, but meticulous adjustments are necessary because of the special physiologic needs of children. The leading causes of death in children are asphyxia and trauma, so a history of cardiac resuscitation, hypotension, and hypoxemia is frequent in this donor population (Fischer-Froehlich et al., 2002).

Pediatric donation management goals and dosing guidelines are available for reference from NATCO (Nakagawa, 2008b), the UNOS Critical Pathway for the Pediatric Organ Donor (www.unos.org), and the Canadian Council for Donation and Transplantation (www.ccdt.ca) (Shemie et al., 2006). In 2001, a Consensus Conference made specific recommendations for management of cardiac donors (Zaroff et al., 2002). See also Kutsogiannis (2006), Braunfeld (2004), Wood et al. (2004), and Ullah et al. (2006).

Ultimately, the management of the pediatric organ donation is dictated by regional standards of care and the physicians caring for the child. The primary responsibilities of the pediatric intensive care specialist and anesthesiologist are to anticipate the normal physiologic sequelae of brain death (Table 28-6), and to direct therapy toward normalizing gross alterations in physiologic and biochemical parameters.

Organs from deceased donors may be injured or damaged from many things: the preexisting comorbid factors; hemodynamic instability (autonomic surge, hypotension, cardiac ischemia, metabolic acidosis, and use of vasopressors); endocrine, metabolic and electrolyte imbalances; hypoxemia (acute respiratory distress syndrome [ARDS]); coagulopathy; thrombocytopenia; renal failure; endotoxin release; and immune activation inherent in the brain death process (Jawan et al., 2002; Zaroff et al., 2002). The presence of brain death–related complications has been reported to have no effect on the number of organs donated if an aggressive donation management protocol is instituted (DuBose and Salim, 2008).

Organ Retrieval

Organ procurement is usually completed in 4 hours or less, depending on the operating team's experience, the number of organs intended for retrieval, and the presence of variations in the vascular anatomy. In the face of worsening hypoxemia, coagulopathy, or refractory hypotension, the organ recovery surgery should be expedited to prevent warm ischemic injury to transplantable organs. The specific organs to be retrieved determine the type of fluid management, the ideal central venous pressure (CVP), the fraction of inspired oxygen (Fio$_2$), and the choice of inotropic or vasopressor support and maximum allowable dosages. Management decisions depend on the organs being considered; for example, hemodynamic goals preferred by abdominal transplant surgeons occasionally differ from those of cardiothoracic transplant surgeons. Pediatric donation management goals are summarized in (Table 28-7) (Nakagawa, 2008b).

Preoperative donor evaluation includes the determination of hemodynamic stability and vasopressor support, electrolytes and therapy for diabetes insipidus, pulmonary status, renal function and urine output, coagulopathy, and the degree of hypothermia. Routine anesthesia monitoring is supplemented with the placement of an intraarterial catheter in an upper extremity to facilitate sampling and monitoring of the arterial blood pressure. Measuring CVP is especially important if the heart and lungs are being considered for donation. Arterial blood gases, hematocrit, electrolytes, blood glucose, and osmolality are usually assessed every hour, or more frequently as needed.

Strict asepsis is observed, prophylactic antibiotics are administered, and the donor is positioned and prepared surgically. If the corneas are to be harvested, the eyelids are taped shut and covered with cold saline compresses or ice packs for corneal protection. After 300 U/kg of heparin is administered and cardioplegia is achieved, the liver, intestines, pancreas, and kidneys are flushed with cold preservation solution, and sequential removal of organs can proceed. The spleen and omental lymph nodes are removed for tissue typing, and the aorta, inferior vena cava, and common carotid and iliac vessels are taken for vascular grafts. Anesthesia support of the organ donor is necessary

TABLE 28-6. Normal Physiologic Sequelae of Brain Death

Sequela	Cause	Management
Hypotension	Neurogenic shock, hypovolemia, hypothermia, electrolyte disorders, endocrine abnormalities, myocardial dysfunction	Mean arterial pressure > 60 mm Hg CVP 4 to 12 mm Hg PCWP 8 to 12 mm Hg SVR 800 to 1200 dyne/sec per cm^5 Cardiac index > 2.4 L/min per m^2 Inotropic support in order of preference (in mcg/kg per min): 　Dopamine <10 　Dobutamine <10 　Epinephrine <0.1 　Norepinephrine and renal-dose dopamine
Endocrine abnormalities	Disruption of the hypothalamic pituitary axis, resulting in adrenal insufficiency, hypothyroidism, or diabetes insipidus	Volume replacement; correct electrolytes; inotropic support Steroids: methylprednisolone (15 mg/kg) T$_3$: 4-mcg bolus and 3 mcg/hr infusion Arginine vasopressin: 1-U bolus, then continuous infusion at 0.5 to 4 U/hr, titrated to a systemic vascular resistance of 800 to 1200 dyne/sec per cm^5 Insulin: 1 U/hr minimum. Titrate to maintain blood sugar 120 to 180 mg/dL
Hypothermia	Loss of hypothalamic, neural, or endocrine regulation; resuscitation with cold fluids or blood products	Early aggressive warming to maintain temperature at >36° C At <30° C, may be unresponsive to ACLS, drug therapy, defibrillation, or pacing
Anemia	Hemorrhage, hemodilution	Transfuse, hemoglobin 7-10 g/dL
Coagulopathies	DIC, fibrinolysis, dilutional, hypothermia	Factor replacement, transfusion rewarming, early organ retrieval

From Rosengard B, Feng S, Alfrey E, et al: Report of the Crystal City meeting to maximize the use of organs recovered from the cadaver donor, *Am J Transplant* 2:701, 2002.
ACLS, Advanced cardiac life support; *CVP,* cerebrovascular pressure; *DIC,* disseminated intravascular coagulation; *PCWP,* pulmonary capillary wedge pressure; *SVR,* systemic vascular resistance.

TABLE 28-7. Pediatric Donation Management Goals

Hemodynamic Support			Blood Pressure*		
• Normalization of blood pressure Systolic blood pressure appropriate for age Note: Lower systolic blood pressures may be acceptable if biomarkers such as lactate are normal • CVP < 12 *(if measured)* • Dopamine < 10 mcg/kg per min • Normal serum lactate			**Age**	**Systolic**	**Diastolic**
			Neonate/Infants (6 mo)	60-90	35-60
			Toddler (2 yr)	80-95	50-65
			School age (7 yr)	85-100	50-65
			Adolescent (15 yr)	90-115	60-70
				110-130	65-80

Oxygenation and Ventilation	Fluids and Electrolytes	
• Maintain Pao$_2$ > 100 mm Hg • Fio$_2$ 0.40 • Normalize Paco$_2$ 35-45 mm Hg • Arterial pH 7.30-7.45 • Tidal volumes 8-10 cc/kg • PEEP 5 cm H$_2$O	• Serum Na$^+$ • Serum K$^+$ • Serum glucose • Ionized Ca^{+2} (if measured)	130-150 meq/L 3-5.0 meq/L 60-150 mg/dL 0.9-1.2 mmol/L

Thermal Regulation

• Core body temperature 36° to 38° C

From Nakagawa TA: Updated pediatric donor management and dosing guidelines. NATCO, Organization for Transplant Professionals, 2008. Available at www.natco1.org/prof_development/index.htm#guidelines; accessed September 2008.
*For children, normal systolic blood pressure = 80 + 2 × age in years.

until the proximal aorta is surgically occluded and in situ flushing of organs has begun. Subsequently, the ventilator should be disconnected and monitoring discontinued, as electrocardiographic (ECG) activity may persist for up to 70 minutes after cardiac arrest (Oaknine, 1975; Logigian and Ropper, 1985).

To avoid reflex muscular contractions and facilitate surgical exposure, a long-acting muscle relaxant is administered intravenously. Complex movements of the limbs and trunk can be confused with reflex movements of cerebral origin and may create tremendous anxiety for the operating room personnel because, although the declaration of brain death requires the loss of cerebral and brainstem reflexes, spinal reflexes may remain intact.

In addition to spinal reflexes, a reflex pressor response to nociceptive stimuli is sometimes observed. This vasopressor response may lead to excessive operative blood loss and damage to the renal grafts. Management requires a reduction in preload or afterload, or both, while minimizing any possible adverse drug toxicity, especially to the liver and kidneys. Thus, antihypertensive agents such as nitroglycerin or nitroprusside may be required if the volatile anesthetic, preferably isoflurane, is not successful in ablating this response.

Because brain death results in the loss of central mechanisms that control the endocrine and autonomic nervous systems, cardiac death usually occurs within 48 to 72 hours despite maximal physiologic support. Up to 25% of potential brain-dead organ donors are lost each year in North America because of cardiovascular collapse (Jenkins et al., 1999). Hypotension and hemodynamic instability secondary to neurogenic shock, dysrhythmias, and hypovolemia, all resulting from the absence of brainstem function, should be anticipated and treated in all donors.

Intravascular Fluid Management

Brainstem injury produces a sequence of hemodynamic events, beginning with an increase in parasympathetic tone and evolving to a massive autonomic surge with hypertension (systolic blood pressure > 200 mm Hg) and tachycardia (>140 beats/min) (Audibert et al., 2006). The pathophysiology of neurocardiogenic injury involves an initial neural phase (catecholamine surge and mixed venous oxygen saturation [MVo$_2$] supply-demand imbalance) within hours, followed by a humoral phase and release of inflammatory cytokines. Depletion of thyroid hormones and cortisol, and decreased coronary perfusion pressure may also impair myocardial function. Coronary vasoconstriction, subendocardial ischemia, focal myocardial necrosis, and endothelial injury are factors that contribute to accelerated cardiac allograft vasculopathy in the recipient (Segel et al., 2002; Szabo et al., 2002; Mehra et al., 2004). Systolic and diastolic dysfunction has been reported in 10% to 28% of pediatric donors and 71% of adult donors. It is reversible in the majority of cases (Banki and Zaroff, 2003). Despite normal or increased perfusion pressure, the resulting vasoconstriction may cause tissue ischemia that disrupts the production of ATP, generates oxygen free radicals, increases cytosolic calcium concentration, and activates various enzymatic cascades such as endonucleases and nitric oxide syntheses (Kunzendorf et al., 2002). A subsequent hypotensive phase caused by loss of autonomic regulation of the peripheral vasculature and unopposed vasodilation may further reduce oxygen supply to the tissues. Hypovolemia is seen with diuresis and fluid restriction during brain resuscitation, inadequate volume replacement after trauma, and diuresis resulting from diabetes insipidus or hyperglycemia.

Brain death is a dynamic inflammatory process. The activation of inflammatory mediators leads to a nonspecific immune response, which may be associated with accelerated acute graft rejection and poor long-term outcomes (Kunzendorf et al., 2002). In addition, a significant factor in organ injury after storage and cold ischemia is caused by reperfusion, initiated by leukocyte adhesion to endothelial cells and the production of oxygen-derived free radicals and peroxides.

Fluid replacement therapy with colloid or crystalloid solutions and cytomegalovirus (CMV)-negative blood products directed at restoring and maintaining the intravascular volume is the first step in resuscitation of the hemodynamically unstable donor. Use of lactated Ringer's solution, normal saline, Plasmalyte, or 5% albumin, is recommended, starting with a 20-mL/kg intravenous (IV) bolus and followed by hemodynamic

reassessment of the donor and two additional boluses as needed. The lowest acceptable systolic blood pressure can be calculated by multiplying the patient's age in years by 2, and adding 70. Hypotonic and dextrose-containing crystalloid solutions should never be used for fluid resuscitation. Hetastarch (Hespan) or other artificial plasma expanders should be avoided for fluid resuscitation because of their inherent risk for coagulopathy and renal impairment. Volume loading with crystalloid- or colloid-containing solutions usually depends on institutional preference and the sensitivity of the liver and lungs to low osmotic pressure–mediated tissue edema. When only the kidneys are to be procured, the donor can be maximally volume loaded. For lung or heart-lung retrieval, fluid restriction (CVP ≤ 6 mm Hg) is preferred. Infusion of colloids is recommended, with limited use of crystalloid and early initiation of inotropic support to maintain a mean arterial pressure of 60 mm Hg or greater.

If the initial two-dimensional echocardiographic evaluation reveals that the left ventricular ejection fraction is less than 45%, management with invasive monitoring, fluids, inotropes, vasopressors, hormonal, replacement therapy (with hydrocortisone, levothyroxine, or triiodothyronine), and treatment of diabetes insipidus (with desmopressin [DDAVP] or vasopressin infusion) is strongly recommended (Table 28-8).

Hourly maintenance fluids are calculated according to the 4-2-1 rule; that is, for the first 10 kg, use 4 mL/kg; for the second 10 kg, use 2 mL/kg; when the weight is greater than 20 kg, use the weight in kilograms plus 40. Guidelines for transfusion therapy are listed in Table 28-9. Packed red blood cells (RBCs) are transfused to maintain the hemoglobin at 10 g/dL for unstable donors, with the lowest acceptable being 70 g/L. Platelets, International Normalized Ratio (INR), and partial thromboplastin time (PTT) have no predefined targets, with transfusion indicated in cases of clinically evident bleeding or coagulopathy. The recommended hemodynamic endpoints are mean arterial pressure (MAP), 60 mm Hg or greater; CVP and pulmonary capillary wedge pressure (PCWP), 12 mm Hg or less; systemic vascular resistance (SVR), 800 to 1200; cardiac index, 2.5 or

TABLE 28-8. Maintaining Mean Arterial Pressure in the Pediatric Organ Donor

Hemodynamically Stable	Hemodynamically Unstable

• Hydrocortisone
• Levothyroxine OR triiodothyronine
• For patients with diabetes insipidus, administration of the following should be considered:
 1. Desmopressin acetate
  a. Continuous infusion (preferred)
  b. Intermittent doses OR
 2. Vasopressin administered by continuous infusion
	• Volume loading with crystalloid or colloid
	• Inotropic support
	 • Dopamine
	 • Dobutamine
	 • Epinephrine
	 • Phenylephrine
	 • Norepinephrine
	 • Hydrocortisone
	• Bolus dose of levothyroxine followed by continuous infusion OR triiodothyronine infusion
	• For patients with diabetes insipidus, vasopressin administered by continuous infusion

From Nakagawa TA: Updated pediatric donor management and dosing guidelines. NATCO, Organization for Transplant Professionals, 2008. Available at www.natco1.org/prof_development/index.htm#guidelines; accessed September 2008.

TABLE 28-9. Transfusion Therapy for the Organ Donor

Component	Quantity (mL/kg)	Administration
Packed red blood cells	10-15	Administer over 2-3 hours. May be administered faster if hypotension or bleeding requires more aggressive correction of anemia.
Fresh frozen plasma	10-15	Administer over 1-2 hours. May be administered faster if correction of coagulopathy is associated with volume depletion or hypotension.
Cryoprecipitate	5-10 or 1 unit for every 10 kg of body weight	Administer for hypofibrinogenemia.
Platelets	<15 kg: 10-20 >15 kg: single unit of platelets	Administer slowly over 2-3 hours.

From Nakagawa TA: Updated pediatric donor management and dosing guidelines. NATCO, Organization for Transplant Professionals, 2008. Available at www.natco1.org/prof_development/index.htm#guidelines; accessed September 2008.

TABLE 28-10. Causes of Hypotension in the Potential Organ Donor

Hypovolemia	Cardiac Dysfunction	Vasodilation
Initial injury	Preexisting disease	Spinal shock
Inadequate resuscitation	Initial injury	Catecholamine depletion
Third spacing	Myocardial contusion	Loss of vasomotor
Decreased intravascular oncotic pressure after crystalloid resuscitation	Pericardial tamponade	control and autoregulation
	Myocardial ischemia/infarct	"Relative" adrenal insufficiency of
	Brain death process	trauma or critical
Dehydration from treatment of intracranial pressure	Catecholamine damage	illness
	Ischemia-reperfusion injury	Endocrinopathy of brain death
Fluid restriction	Metabolic depression	Acquired sepsis
Urea	Acidosis	
Diuretics	Hypothermia	
Mannitol	Hypophosphatemia	
Hyperglycemia-induced osmotic dieresis	Hypocalcemia	
	Hypoxia	
Diabetes insipidus	Endocrinopathy of brain death	
Hypothermic "cold" diuresis	Volume overload congestive heart failure	
Venodilation	Arrhythmias	
Loss of vasomotor tone and pooling in venous capacitance bed	Catecholamines	
	Ischemia	
	Hypokalemia	
Rewarming of hypothermia	Hypomagnesemia	

From Jalili M: Organ donor management: intensivist's role. Pediatric Summit Powerpoint presentation, Los Angeles, March 2008. Available at www.onelegacy.org.

greater; left ventricular stroke work index, 15 or greater; and dopamine dosage, 12 mcg/kg per minute or less (UNOS Critical Pathway for the Pediatric Organ Donor).

Cardiovascular Management

Hypotension in the potential organ donor most commonly results from hypovolemia (absolute or effective with a reduction in venous return), cardiac dysfunction, or arterial vasodilation from neurogenic shock (Table 28-10). The goals of hemodynamic support are to correct hypovolemia, to adjust vasoconstrictors and vasodilators to maintain a normal afterload, and to optimize cardiac output and maintain perfusion pressure gradients without relying on high dosages of β-agonists or other inotropes. Proposed adverse biochemical, histopathologic, and functional effects of catecholamine infusions on the myocardium include high-energy substrate depletion, intramyocardial noradrenaline depletion, and myocardial β-adrenoceptor down-regulation (Sakagoshi et al., 1992; Pinelli et al., 1995; Zaroff et al., 2002). With persistent hypotension despite volume replacement, vasopressor therapy should be initiated.

Dopamine up to 10 mcg/kg per minute is the drug of choice because the glomerular filtration rate (GFR) is increased as well as cardiac output while dilating the renal, mesenteric, and coronary vasculature. Inotropic agents should be titrated to maintain a normal blood pressure for the patient's age (normal systolic blood pressure mm Hg = 80 + 2 × age in years). Blood pressure alone does not indicate adequate tissue perfusion. Therefore, serum biomarkers such as base deficit and lactate should be followed as inotropic support is titrated (Table 28-11).

Echocardiography should be performed early, followed by insertion of a pulmonary artery catheter, especially if the ejection fraction is less than 40% or the donor requires high-dosage inotropes. According to Zaroff (2004), ejection fraction is the most significant predictor of nonuse of potential donor hearts, with an odds ratio of 1.48 per 5% decrease in ejection fraction.

When dopamine is used for inotropic support in infants, dosages significantly higher than those needed in the adult may be

TABLE 28-11. Inotropic Infusions

Drug	Dosage
Milrinone (Primacor)	0.25-0.75 mcg/kg per min IV Loading dose: 50 mcg/kg
Dopamine	2-20 mcg/kg per min IV
Dobutamine (Dobutrex)	2-20 mcg/kg per min IV
Epinephrine	0.1-1 mcg/kg per min IV
Norepinephrine (Levophed)	0.05-2 mcg/kg per min IV
Phenylephrine (Neosynephrine)	0.1-0.5 mcg/kg per min IV Bolus: 5-20 mcg/kg
Vasopressin (Pitressin)	0.3-2 mU/kg per min IV Note: Dosage is different for treatment of patients with diabetes insipidus

From Nakagawa TA: Updated pediatric donor management and dosing guidelines. NATCO, Organization for Transplant Professionals, 2008. Available at www.natco1.org/prof_development/index.htm#guidelines; accessed September 2008.

required, presumably because of catecholamine receptor immaturity or deficiency (Kelly et al., 1984). At these higher dosages (15 mcg/kg per minute), no adverse effects on GFR or urine output are apparent (Outwater and Rockoff, 1984). Dopamine at α-agonist dosages has not been shown to influence outcomes in liver, kidney, or heart in pediatric donors (Finfer et al., 1996). There is evidence that dopamine may reduce allograft rejection, not only through support of blood pressure but possibly also through more complex immunomodulatory effects that inhibit expression of adhesion molecules, which are required for leukocyte migration into the graft to produce acute rejection (Carlos et al., 1997; Schnuelle et al., 1999).

An infusion of an α-adrenoceptor vasoconstrictor, epinephrine or phenylephrine, may be useful to increase peripheral vascular tone, but they have the inherent risk of causing marked peripheral vasoconstriction and/or an increase in pulmonary artery pressure (PAP) or oxygen consumption. Jhanji and colleagues (2009) have shown norepinephrine to be protective of global oxygen consumption, without affecting the splanchnic circulation or producing significant deleterious renal effects. An infusion of vasopressin starting at 0.3 mU/kg per minute and titrated to the desired blood pressure, with a maximal infusion rate of 2 mU/kg per minute, may be efficacious in the setting of hypotension and low SVR, especially in combination with an inotropic infusion such as epinephrine. Vasopressin is not recommended as first-line therapy, as there are limited data available in children. Recent studies, however, suggest it is most efficacious when coupled with corticosteroids (Büchele et al., 2009). Dobutamine (IV, at 2 to 20 mcg/kg per minute) should be used when cardiac output is decreased because of reduced myocardial contractility and pulmonary hypertension. ECG abnormalities are common during the brain-death process, manifested as marked ST-T wave abnormalities, ischemic changes, inverted T waves, widened QRS complexes, and prolonged QT interval. In addition, atrial and ventricular arrhythmias and varying degrees of conduction abnormalities may occur. These arrhythmias usually result from autonomic instability (catecholamine storm and loss of the vagal motor nucleus) compounded by oxygenation, acid-base, temperature, and electrolyte (e.g., low magnesium and potassium) disturbances or increased intracranial pressure (ICP) (Cushing's reflex) (Powner and Allison, 2006). The difficulty lies in differentiating these transient findings from those of catecholamine-induced myocardial injury or irreversible ischemia, which can produce global myocardial dysfunction. Bradycardia is not a problem unless it contributes to hypotension. It may be treated with any inotropic agent or temporary transthoracic or venous pacing.

Eventually, the heart stops. Despite all therapeutic efforts, the arrhythmias encountered are usually resistant to therapy (Table 28-12). Bradyarrhythmias leading to asystole rather than ventricular fibrillation (as seen in adults) are the terminal cardiac rhythms in pediatric patients. The propensity for this particular dysrhythmia may be related to the immature autonomic nervous system and small muscle mass in the pediatric donor (Walsh and Krongrad, 1983). In the event of a sudden cardiac arrest during the procurement procedure, cardiopulmonary resuscitation should be started to facilitate organ perfusion, and liver, pancreas, intestines, and kidney procurement should proceed rapidly with cross-clamping of the aorta at the diaphragm and infusion of cold preservation solution into the distal aorta and portal vein.

Pulmonary Management

All potential organ donors require mechanical ventilation, usually for a period of several days. Progressive pulmonary dysfunction may result from pulmonary contusions resulting from trauma, aspiration pneumonitis, fat emboli, and pulmonary edema (cardiogenic and neurogenic). Any of these may result in hypoxia, placing all perfuseable organs at risk for ischemia. In addition, infectious complications, oxygen toxicity, barotrauma or volutrauma, pulmonary embolism, and atelectasis may contribute to an increase in the alveolar-arterial oxygen gradient. High-dosage methylprednisolone administration has been shown to significantly improve oxygenation and increase donor lung recovery (Follette et al., 1998). The beneficial effects of steroids probably result from attenuation of the effects of proinflammatory cytokines released as a consequence of brain death (Glasser et al., 2001). Interleukin (IL)-8 expression and neutrophil infiltration of the donor lungs may result in impairment of graft oxygenation, development of severe early graft dysfunction, and early recipient mortality (Fisher et al., 2001). As the total lung water increases

TABLE 28-12. Antiarrhythmic Agents and Correction of Metabolic Acidosis

Drug	Dosage	Route	Comments
Adenosine (Adenocard IV)	100 mcg/kg	Rapid IV push	Repeat dose: 200 mcg/kg Max. single dose: 12 mg
Amiodarone (Cordarone)	5 mg/kg infused over 5-60 min	IV	Repeat dose: 5 mg/kg Infusion: 5-15 mcg/kg per min Monitor for hypotension
Atropine	0.02 mg/kg	IV	Min. dose: 0.1 mg Max. dose: 0.5-1.0 mg
Lidocaine	1-2 mg/kg	IV	Infusion: 20-50 mcg/kg per min
Magnesium sulfate	30 mg/kg infused over 10 min	IV	Max. dose: 2.5 g Repeat dose: 10 mg/kg
Sodium bicarbonate	1 mEq/kg	IV	May increase plasma osmolarity. Hypernatremia can occur or be aggravated with repeated dosing.
Tromethamine (THAM)	Base deficit × wt (kg) = mL of 0.3M solution of THAM	IV	Does not increase osmolarity or CO_2 production. Hypoglycemia can occur. Contraindicated in renal failure; may increase coagulation time.

From Nakagawa TA: Updated pediatric donor management and dosing guidelines. NATCO, Organization for Transplant Professionals, 2008. Available at www.natco1.org/prof_development/index.htm#guidelines; accessed September 2008.

from a combination of pulmonary capillary leakage and disruption of the Starling forces in the lungs, pulmonary compliance decreases, with resultant impedance of alveolar gas exchange. Neurogenic pulmonary edema is best managed with positive end-expiratory pressure (PEEP), diuresis, and small volume fluid resuscitation. Lung-protective strategies include maintenance of an arterial saturation of 95% or a Pao_2 greater than 100 mm Hg, with the lowest possible Fio_2 setting preferably being no higher than 40%, and with Pao_2/Fio_2 greater than 300. Limiting high distention pressures in the lung during volume-controlled modes of ventilation using tidal volumes of 6 to 8 mL/kg, low peak inspiratory pressure (28 to 30 cm H_2O), and avoiding PEEP in excess of 5 cm H_2O is desirable. $Paco_2$ should be normalized to 35 to 45 mm Hg, and serum pH to 7.35 to 7.45. The maintenance of a mild to moderate alkalemia has been reported by some to reduce the likelihood of ventricular fibrillation (programmed ventilator sigh) (Becker et al., 1981). Pulmonary hygiene, bronchodilators, and lung-expansion techniques every hour or two may help in preventing atelectasis and improve the quality of donor lungs. Recruitment maneuvers for oxygenation impairment include periodic increases in PEEP (up to 15 cm H_2O) and sustained inflations (peak inspiratory pressure at 30 cm H_2O for 30 to 60 seconds).

Endocrine Management

Diabetes insipidus (DI) occurs in the vast majority of brain-dead donors. It is a direct result of hypothalamic-pituitary dysfunction, with a resultant deficiency of antidiuretic hormone from the posterior lobe of the pituitary. Typically, DI is clinically manifested by a massive urine output that bears no relationship to the intravascular fluid volume, with decreasing urine osmolarity (≤ 200 mOsm), rising serum osmolarity (≥ 300 mOsm), and normal sodium excretion. This massive hypotonic diuresis (urine output, >4 mL/kg per hour) then leads to hypovolemia and rising serum sodium (≥ 145 mmol/L), as well as loss of potassium, calcium, magnesium, and phosphate.

Once the diagnosis is confirmed, therapeutic intervention should consist of pharmacologic management to decrease urine output to 3 mL/kg per hour or less. Replacement of urine output with 0.2% one-fourth or 0.45% normal saline should be used in conjunction with desmopressin (intermittent IV DDAVP, 0.25 to 1 mcg every 6 hours) or vasopressin (0.5 to 0.7 mU/kg per minute IV to a maximum dosage of 2.4 U/hour) infusion to maintain serum sodium levels between 130 and 150 mEq/L. DDAVP is an analogue of arginine vasopressin, which is highly selective for the vasopressin V_2 receptor subtype found in the renal collecting duct, and without the vasopressor activity in humans that is mediated by V_1 receptors on vascular smooth muscle. DDAVP has a long half-life of 75 to 120 minutes, so an IV infusion may be discontinued 2 to 3 hours before organ recovery. Several mechanisms regulate the release of arginine vasopressin (AVP). Hypovolemia resulting from hemorrhage or any other cause results in a decrease in atrial pressure. Specialized stretch receptors in the atrial walls and large veins (cardiopulmonary baroreceptors) entering the atria decrease their firing rate when there is a fall in atrial pressure. Afferent nerve fibers from these receptors synapse in the nucleus tractus solitarii of the medulla, which sends fibers to the hypothalamus, a region of the brain that controls AVP release by the pituitary gland. Atrial receptor firing normally inhibits the release of AVP by the posterior pituitary. With hypovolemia or decreased AVP, the decreased firing of atrial stretch receptors leads to an increase

in AVP release. Hypothalamic osmoreceptors sense extracellular osmolarity and stimulate AVP release when osmolarity rises, as occurs with dehydration. Finally, angiotensin II receptors located in a region of the hypothalamus regulate AVP. Therapy should always be guided by serum electrolyte and osmolality measurements made every 2 to 4 hours. Several investigators have demonstrated prolonged hemodynamic stability in donors, with the addition of an infusion of AVP to existing pressor support. Donors without clinically apparent DI may demonstrate a baroreflex-mediated defect of vasopressin secretion and pressor hypersensitivity to exogenous hormones. In these patients, low-dosage vasopressin significantly increases blood pressure (Chen et al., 1999). Absence of AVP may be a predominant contributing factor to the eventual cardiac arrest in all brain-dead patients.

Vasopressin is a potent vasoconstrictor. Its hemodynamic effects are dosage dependent and include generalized systemic vasoconstriction; increased blood pressure; decreased cardiac output; diminished coronary, splanchnic, and renal blood flows; bradycardia; and arrhythmias. These effects may cause irreversible ischemia to donor organs. Therefore, it is desirable to avoid and discontinue its use at least 1 hour before surgery.

Endocrine and Metabolic Functions

Despite disruption of the hypothalamic-pituitary-adrenal axis, hormone production from the anterior lobe of the pituitary gland persists in most brain-dead patients. The prevalence of anterior pituitary dysfunction is estimated at 30% (Schneider et al., 2005), with evidence of at least one abnormal hormonal function in 53% (Dimopoulou et al., 2004). More recently, Nicolas-Robin and colleagues (2010) noted in 31 brain-dead donors older than 18 years that the incidence of adrenal insufficiency was 87% and that the administration of 50 mg of hydrocortisone enhanced cardiovascular stability and decreased the requirement for norepinephrine. The incidences of hormonal reduction are estimated as follows: adrenal, 15%; thyroid, 5% to 15%; growth hormone, 18%; gonadal, 25% to 80%; and vasopressin, 3% to 37%. Endocrine failure is associated with basilar skull fracture, hypothalamic edema, prolonged unresponsiveness, hyponatremia, and hypotension (Powner and Allison, 2006).

Rapid depletion of vasopressin, cortisol, insulin, thyroxine (T_4) and free triiodothyronine (T_3) occurs in experimental animal models of brain death (Novitzky et al., 1984, 2006), but endocrine dysfunction in humans is usually manifested solely as DI (Wijdicks, 2001). Novitzky and others (1987) claim that true hypothyroidism exists, as evidenced by a decrease in free T_3. They have shown that hormonal replacement therapy (T_3, cortisol, and insulin with glucose) improves cardiac output and reduces the need for pressor support. Brain death is also associated with global mitochondrial dysfunction with a change to anaerobic metabolism and lactic acidosis. It leads to depletion of myocardial high-energy phosphates and cellular dysfunction. Thus, many organ procurement groups administer thyroid hormones to hemodynamically "rescue" unstable donors who show evidence of anaerobic metabolism or profound hypotension refractory to volume resuscitation and therapy with multiple vasopressors. In a landmark paper published in 1995, Wheeldon and colleagues (1995) showed that by using invasive hemodynamic monitoring and a standard donation management protocol (steroids, insulin, vasopressin, and T_3), the Papworth Hospital Group in Cambridge, United Kingdom, was able to functionally resuscitate 92% of initially unacceptable donors into acceptable donors. Hormonal replacement therapy (methylprednisolone, T_4) has been shown to decrease the need for inotropic support and improve metabolic stability in critically ill children with cessation of neurologic function and hemodynamic instability (Powner, 2001; Salim et al., 2001; Zuppa et al., 2004). Rosendale and colleagues (2003) compared non–hormone replacement with a three–hormone replacement protocol (methylprednisolone bolus and infusions of vasopressin and T_3 or T_4) in brain-dead donors, with 30-day mortality and early graft dysfunction used as measures of outcome. Multivariate results demonstrated a 46% reduced odds of death within 30 days and a 48% reduced odds of early graft dysfunction in the three–hormone replacement donor group.

An infusion of nitroglycerine or nitroprusside is occasionally recommended to prevent myocardial ischemia and the potential untoward renal effects of diminished renal perfusion with the use of vasopressin. Vasopressin supplementation (2 to 10 mcg/kg per minute continuous infusion) in a porcine model of brain-dead potential organ donors resulted in physiologic levels of the hormone, with normal plasma osmolarity and serum sodium levels and decreased urine output, potassium needs, and fluid requirements, without effects on peripheral vascular resistance and without microscopic evidence of organ ischemia (Blaine et al., 1984).

North American Transplant Coordinators Organization (Nakagawa, 2008a) currently recommends that hormonal replacement therapy (T_4 or T_3, steroids, insulin) be considered early in the course of pediatric donation management to improve donor heart function. Levothyroxine (Synthroid) is administered as a bolus dosage of 1 to 5 mcg/kg followed by an IV infusion of 0.8 to 1.4 mcg/kg per hour, with infants and smaller children requiring a larger bolus and infusion dosage. IV T_4 has the disadvantage of a slower and unpredictable onset of action. Alternatively, T_3 may be replaced as an infusion 0.05 to 0.2 mcg/kg per hour IV. Although T3 may rescue the donor heart, it may have detrimental effects, including tachycardia, arrhythmia, metabolic acidosis, and profound hypotension. Methylprednisolone (Solu-Medrol), 20 to 30 mg/kg IV bolus, is administered and may be repeated in 8 to 12 hours. An IV insulin infusion (0.05 to 0.1 units/kg per hour) is titrated to control blood glucose levels to 60 to 150 mg/dL, with monitoring for hypoglycemia (Table 28-13).

Electrolyte disturbances are routine, most being iatrogenic, resulting from treatment of the original injury or in response to physiologic perturbations during the brain-death process. Hypernatremia is inevitable as a result of DI, and a variety of strategies are used to treat elevated ICP. The liver is exquisitely sensitive to hypernatremia (>155 mEq/L) with increased levels correlating with primary graft loss after transplantation (Figueras et al., 1996). Serum potassium, magnesium, calcium, and phosphate levels are often depleted and require prompt replacement therapy. Hyperglycemia may be caused by glucose intolerance (steroids) or administration of large amounts of a dextrose-containing solution for fluid resuscitation.

Hypothermia

Although hyperthermia is common in the early phase of the sympathetic storm, the donor rapidly becomes hypothermic as a result of vasodilation and the loss of thermal regulation by the CNS. The patient becomes poikilothermic, with the body temperature determined by the environmental temperature. Although a mild degree of hypothermia may be beneficial to organ protection and preservation, the undesirable consequences of hypothermia, which are clinically significant, include diuresis and hypovolemia, hyperglycemia, coagulopathy, arrhythmias, myocardial depression, pulmonary hypertension, and eventually cardiac arrest (Reuler, 1978). Hypothermia further complicates the process of certification of brain death by causing the pupils to appear fixed and dilated. Active rewarming measures to maintain a core body temperature 36° to 38° C should be initiated early.

Organ Preservation

The field of organ preservation includes in situ core cooling, organ preservation fluids, and machine perfusion techniques. Traditionally, optimal organ preservation has been achieved by the combination of maximizing donor hemodynamics, using improved surgical procurement techniques with minimal dissection of vascular structures, cannulating the abdominal aorta

TABLE 28-13. Pharmacologic Agents for Hormonal Resuscitation

Drug	Dosage	Route	Comments
Desmopressin (DDAVP)	0.5 mcg per hr	IV	Half-life, 75-120 min Titrate to decrease urine output to 3-4 mL/kg per hr May be beneficial in patients with an ongoing coagulopathy
Vasopressin (Pitressin)	0.5-1 mU/kg per hr	IV	Half-life, 10-35 min Titrate to decrease urine output to 3-4 mL/kg per hr Hypertension can occur
Levothyroxine (Synthroid)	0.8-1.4 mcg/kg per hr	IV	Bolus dose of 1-5 mcg/kg can be administered. Infants and smaller children require a larger bolus and infusion dosage.
Triiodothyronine (T_3)	0.05-0.2 mcg/kg per hr	IV	—
Methylprednisolone (Solu-Medrol)	20-30 mg/kg	IV	Dose may be repeated in 8-12 hours Fluid retention Glucose intolerance
Insulin	0.05-0.1 U/kg per hr	IV	Titrate to control blood glucose levels to 60-150 mg/dL Monitor for hypoglycemia

From Nakagawa TA: Updated pediatric donor management and dosing guidelines. NATCO, Organization for Transplant Professionals, 2008. Available at www.natco1.org/prof_development/index.htm#guidelines; accessed September 2008.

for rapid in situ core cooling, removing abdominal organs en bloc with separation of graft components on the back table, employing cold storage techniques with a hyperkalemic hyperosmolar solution at a temperature of 4° C, and treating the donor or recipient (or both) pharmacologically. Most centers use static cold storage to preserve organs, and this is useful for younger donors with good-quality organs (Southard and Belzer, 1995; Marshall, 1997). With the introduction of extended donor criteria, the limitations of cold storage have probably been reached. Kidneys can be preserved for up to 72 hours but seldom do well in the recipient after 36 to 48 hours with cold ischemia. The heart and lungs should be transplanted within 4 to 6 hours, and the pancreas preferably within 6 to 12 hours.

The preservation solution introduced by the University of Wisconsin (UW solution) in 1987 allowed extension of the safe preservation time of the donor livers from 8 to 24 hours (Jamieson et al., 1988) and kidneys for up to 72 hours. Iced storage and core cooling result in a slowing of cellular metabolism and energy consumption; glucose or hydrogen ion buffers prevent cellular acidosis; donor heparinization (30,000 U, or 300 U/kg) prevents microvascular thrombosis and promotes a more even organ flushing and reperfusion. Effective impermeants are saccharides and nonsaccharide anions. Molecular weight determines the effectiveness of saccharides to prevent cell swelling, with larger saccharides being more effective (Sumimoto et al., 1990; Hart et al., 2002). The UW solution, histidine-tryptophan-ketoglutarate (HTK), and Celsior are the primary solutions used currently for organ preservation (Table 28-14).

HTK, originally introduced for cardioplegia in 1980, has gained popularity in clinical transplantation for cold perfusion and organ storage since the U.S. Food and Drug Administration (FDA) approved its use for kidney and liver preservation (Lam et al., 1989). Early experiences with HTK have demonstrated that it compares favorably with the UW solution in kidney and liver organ preservation. Growing clinical experience with living donor liver transplantation has shown comparable clinical performances of UW solution and HTK (Lange et al., 1997; Testa et al., 2003). UW solution and HTK also show clinical equivalence for deceased donor liver transplants, although UW solution remains the gold standard for longer preservation times (Guarrera and Karim, 2008).

The non–heart-beating (DCD) kidney perfusion protocols of Hoffman and D'Alessandro (Wisconsin), Koostra (Maastricht, The Netherlands), and Gage and Light (Washington, DC) have increased the donor pool of organs. The expansion of organ perfusion from kidneys to other solid organs became a reality in 2004, when Guarrera, Arrington, and Kinkhabwala became the world's first team to successfully transplant a machine-perfused liver into a human.

In the early 1970s, hypothermic machine perfusion (HMP) was used by many centers in the United States and Europe to preserve kidneys, allowing transportation to distant transplantation centers. Although modern HMP systems are smaller, lighter, and more sophisticated than the original machine used by Belzer and coworkers, the principles of HMP have not changed. Machine perfusion generates a controlled continuous or pulsatile recirculating flow of preservation solution at 0° to 4° C. This continuous flow allows complete perfusion of the organ, promoting a thorough washout of blood and subsequent tissue equilibration with the preservation solution. Beneficial effects of machine perfusion are a low incidence of delayed graft function, the possibility of real-time organ viability assessment, the ability to provide metabolic support during perfusion, and the potential to add pharmacologic

agents to the perfusate. A meta-analysis reported by Wight and coworkers noted that HMP produced a 20% reduction in delayed graft function compared with cold storage (Guarrera and Karim, 2008). Most experience with HMP involves the kidneys (Henry, 1997), and clinical application of HMP in human liver transplantation has been limited to the recent pioneering work of Guarrera and colleagues (2004).

LIVING RELATED ORGAN DONOR

Over the past several years, a consistently widening gap has become evident between the demand for and supply of transplantable organs. At the end of 2009, there were 1907 pediatric

TABLE 28-14. Organ Preservation Solutions

	University of Wisconsin Solution	Histidine-Tryptophan-Ketoglutarate Solution	Celsior
Year of introduction	1987	1975	1994
Source	Belzer (USA)	Bretschneider (Germany)	Pasteur-Merieus (France)
Components			
Na⁺ (mmol/L)	25-30	15	100
K⁺ (mmol/L)	125-130	10	15
Mg²⁺ (mmol/L)	5	13	4
Ca²⁺ (mmol/L)	—	0.025	0.015
Mannitol (g/L)	—	30	60
Lactobionic acid (mmol/L)	100	—	80
HES (g/L)	50	—	—
Raffinose (mmol/L)	30	—	—
Hisidine (mmol/L)	—	180	30
H₂PO₄/HPO₄ (mmol/L)	25	—	—
OH (mmol/L)	—	—	100
Glutathione (mmol/L)	3	—	3
Allopurinol (mmol/L)	—	1	—
Adenosine (mmol/L)	5	—	—
Acetone dicarboxylic acid (mmol/L)	—	1	—
Tryptophan (mmol/L)	—	2	—
Amnioglutamnic acid (mmol/L)	—	—	20
Properties			
mOsm/L	320	310	320
pH	7.4	7.2	7.3

From Guarrera JV, Karim NA: Liver preservation: is there anything new yet? *Curr Opin Organ Transplant* 13:148, 2008.

transplant candidates on the waiting lists for various organs, out of a total of 113,702 candidates of all ages awaiting all organs. Of the pediatric candidates, approximately 50% were from 11 to 17 years old. This reflects a decline in the past 10 years and a decrease in the size of the liver and lung waiting lists, with the majority of children wait-listed for liver and kidney organs. The number of pediatric deceased donors over the past decade has steadily decreased (OPTN/UNOS, January 1988 to June 2010). Compared with adult deceased donors, pediatric deceased donors are more likely to donate a specific organ, as evident in data reported up to 2010: kidneys (92%), livers (87%), lungs (16%), heart (50%), pancreas (40%), and intestine (9%) (OPTN/UNOS, December 2009). With this serious shortage of donor organs of appropriate size and suitability for infants and small children, the waiting times for some organs has increased dramatically. For example, with only 20% of lungs from deceased donors meeting stringent donor criteria, the waiting period varies from 42% of pediatric patients waiting less than 1 year, to 15% listed for 5 or more years. This chronic shortage has prompted the development of programs for living related organ donation. The original concept was developed for renal transplantation in the early 1950s, and, currently in the United States, 25.2% of pediatric transplants are from living donors (OPTN/UNOS, 2009) (Table 28-15). Justification was relatively easy, as healthy relatives could "safely" donate one of their two kidneys without jeopardizing renal function in their remaining solitary kidney, and the results from living related pediatric renal transplantation have, until recently, been superior to deceased donor transplantation, at all ages. Later, techniques were developed to use one or more left-lateral segments of a parent's liver, which would be suitable for a small child with chronic liver disease (Broelsch et al., 1991; Lang et al., 2004). Lessons learned from split or reduced-size deceased adult livers for implantation into children were used in the development of living related liver transplantation programs, which can accommodate large children and small adults using the right lobe of the liver. From 1987 to 2009 in the United States, 1264 of the total 3967 pediatric liver transplants were from living donors (see Table 28-15). With similar methods, living donor transplantation has been successfully developed for pancreas, lung (unilateral and bilateral lower lobes), and small bowel transplantation.

Living-related organ donation has, for the most part, been performed from parent to child. The use of children for living kidney donation remains highly controversial, and in general, most transplant programs do not use a donor younger than 18 years except in very limited circumstances, such as identical twins or an emancipated minor for his or her own child (Abecassis et al., 2000). Living-related donor procedures have several advantages, including the fact that they can be electively scheduled when the recipient is in optimal condition. However, with the exception of living related renal transplantation (which has excellent outcomes, with 1-year graft survival in children older than 1 year ranging from 94% to 96%), the long-term functional outcome of living-donor lung, pancreas, and small intestine transplants remains to be established because of the relatively small number of transplants performed. Currently, the risk for mortality and graft loss is *less* for children younger than 2 years if they receive a liver allograft from a living donor compared with a deceased donor (Reding et al., 2003). In addition, many troubling ethical issues arise, such as the risk to the donor and recipient, the validity of informed consent, and concerns about donor privacy and confidentiality. Uncomplicated unilateral nephrectomy has an exceedingly low mortality (less than 0.1%), but the same is *not* true for right lobe liver donors (0.2% to 1%, or 4 to 10 of 2000 cases), left segment/lobe liver donors (0.06% to 0.2%, or 2 to 6 of 3300), and right lobectomy of the lung, less than 5% mortality (Hayashi and Trotter, 2002; Trotter et al., 2002). Additionally, Hashikura and colleagues (2009) reported an 8.4% complication rate in 299 donors undergoing living related liver donation. Postoperative donor

---

TABLE 28-15. Pediatric Organ Transplant Data for Individual Organs, from 1985 to April 20, 2010

Donor Type	All Organs			Kidney			Liver		
	All Tx	1° Tx	Repeat Tx	All Tx	1° Tx	Repeat Tx	All Tx	1° Tx	Repeat Tx
ADT	36,368	31,769	4599	15,867	13,768	2099	11,958	9977	1981
DCD	27,218	23,350	3868	8099	6623	1476	10,694	8806	1888
LD	9150 (25.2 %)	8419	731	7768	7145	623	1264	1171	93

Donor Type	Pancreas			Kidney-Pancreas			Heart		
	All Tx	1° Tx	Repeat Tx	All Tx	1° Tx	Repeat Tx	All Tx	1° Tx	Repeat Tx
ADT	396	380	16	43	43	0	5905	5573	332
DCD	396	380	16	42	42	0	5902	5570	332
LD	0	0	0	1	1	0	3	3	0

Donor Type	Lung			Heart-Lung			Intestine		
	All Tx	1°Tx	Repeat Tx	All Tx	1° Tx	Repeat Tx	All Tx	1° Tx	Repeat Tx
ADT	932	862	70	176	169	7	1091	997	94
DCD	836	778	58	176	169	7	1073	982	91
LD	96	84	12	0	0	0	18	15	3

From the United Network for Organ Sharing (UNOS) and Organ Procurement and Transplantation Network (OPTN) data, 2010 (http://optn.transplant.hrsa.gov/data).
ADT, All donor types; *DCD,* deceased donor; *LD,* living donor; *Tx,* transplant; *1° Tx,* primary transplant.

complications included biliary complications (3.0%), reoperation (1.3%), severe aftereffects in two cases (0.06%), and death (apparently related to donor surgery) in one donor (0.03%). The incidences of postoperative complications in left- and right-lobe donors were 8.7% and 9.4%, respectively.

In addition, there have been increasing interest and use of DCD, with the hope of expanding this pool from 200 to 1000 donors per year in the United States. Although pediatric donors constitute approximately 20% of the total DCD donor pool, very few of the kidneys recovered are allocated to pediatric recipients (OPTN/UNOS, 2009). This practice may reflect concerns about long-term graft function, given the limited outcomes data available.

IMMUNOSUPPRESSION

Since the early 1980s, organ transplantation has emerged from an experimental therapy to a highly successful treatment for end-organ failure of multiple causes. The single most important factor in this progression has been the development of effective immunosuppressive regimens. The following discussion focuses on the immunosuppressive agents used, complications, and the emergence of newer agents.

History

The idea of organ transplantation is a century old, and only with the development of immunosuppressive agents has the viability of this field reached its zenith today. Before 1981, patient survival was poor because of inadequate immunosuppressive regimens. Corticosteroids and azathioprine were the mainstays of therapy, with graft survival in the range of only 30% to 50%. The introduction of the calcineurin inhibitors cyclosporine (in 1981) and then tacrolimus revolutionized the field of solid organ transplantation, with 1-year graft and patient survival rates as high as 90%, and greater for some organ systems. The main goal of any effective immunosuppression regimen is the prevention of organ rejection with minimal side effects and complications. Various immunosuppressive agents are used for induction (primary) therapy, maintenance therapy, and treatment of rejection after organ transplantation, but, regardless of the organ system, the applied principles are almost identical. The major agents used by most transplant centers worldwide are the calcineurin inhibitors cyclosporine and tacrolimus. Although steroids were always part of the induction therapy, they are now commonly eliminated.

Immunosuppression Medications

Corticosteroids

Corticosteroids were the initial mainstay of therapy for organ transplantation, but their use is on the decline. They are particularly effective in both the prevention and treatment of acute rejection episodes. Their predominant mechanisms of action include the inhibition of IL-1 and IL-2 production, suppression of helper and suppressor T cells, suppression of cytotoxic T cells, and reduction in the migration and activity of neutrophils (Cohen, 2002). The long-term use of corticosteroids has been questioned because of their adverse side effects, particularly in the pediatric population. The trend during the past decade and a half is to use fewer steroids for maintenance therapy (Margarit et al., 1989; Ascher, 1995). Many centers do not now use steroids as part of their long-term regimens. The first report of steroid withdrawal after transplantation was published in 1989 (Margarit et al., 1989). Everson and associates (1999) published a literature review, which demonstrated that greater than 50% to 85% of patients can be withdrawn from steroids without changes in acute rejection episodes, patient survival, or graft survival rates (Stegall et al., 1997). This percentile difference depends on the antirejection agent used for maintenance therapy (e.g., tacrolimus versus cyclosporine or serolimus). Steroid withdrawal is preferable, as it is associated with significantly less hypertension, hypercholesterolemia, and diabetes mellitus, and, moreover, it is less likely to result in cushingoid features and delayed development and obesity in the pediatric patient. Despite controversy over their use in maintenance therapy, corticosteroids remain the first-line agents for the treatment of acute rejection. The response rates vary depending on the organ system and whether the patient is maintained on cyclosporine or tacrolimus (U.S. Multicenter FK506 Liver Study Group, 1994).

Azathioprine

Azathioprine, the imidazole derivative of 6-mercaptopurine, was introduced in the late 1950s and early 1960s. Its mechanism of action is the inhibition of differentiation and proliferation of T and B lymphocytes by blocking DNA and RNA synthesis. The effect is a reduction in the numbers of circulating white cells, both lymphocytes and granulocytes. One notable advantage of this agent is its steroid-sparing effect, allowing lower dosages of steroids to be used with equal efficacy and fewer side effects. The use of this agent is limited, however, by side effects, particularly hematologic and gastrointestinal (GI). Its use may result in as many as 50% of patients exhibiting bone marrow suppression and a profound leukopenia or thrombocytopenia (Cattral et al., 2000). Gastrointestinal side effects include pancreatitis, nausea, vomiting, and hepatotoxicity. Patients are at increased risk for opportunistic infections. An increased risk for malignancy, especially lymphoma, however, remains controversial. The primary pathway of metabolism is inactivation by xanthine oxidase, an enzyme blocked by allopurinol. The recommended dosage of azathioprine is 1 to 2 mg/kg per day. Plasma levels are not monitored for this agent.

Mycophenolate Mofetil

Mycophenolate mofetil (MMF) (CellCept) is a morpholinoethyl ester of mycophenolate. It is well absorbed orally and hydrolyzed to its active form, mycophenolic acid, which acts by competitively inhibiting inosine monophosphate dehydrogenase and hence blocks de novo synthesis of purines, primarily guanine. Lymphocytes, unlike other rapidly replicating cells, depend entirely on this pathway for purine synthesis. Hence, the primary mechanism of action of MMF is the selective inhibition of lymphocyte proliferation. This drug is one of the newer agents introduced in the past 10 years and has been shown to be more efficacious than azathioprine in combination therapy (Fisher et al., 1998). There is also some experimental evidence to suggest that MMF may reduce the risk for chronic allograft rejection, which has been attributed to its antiproliferative activity against B lymphocytes and arterial smooth-muscle cells (Azuma et al., 1995; Schmid et al., 1995). The most common side effects are GI, including nausea, abdominal pain, anorexia, gastritis, and diarrhea. Diarrhea affects as many as 30% of patients but usually responds to a decrease in dosage. MMF also causes leukopenia and thus should be avoided in combination with azathioprine. The usual dosage is 1 to 3 g/day orally in two divided doses. Like azathioprine, blood levels are not monitored with this agent. The antivirals acyclovir and ganciclovir increase MMF levels, and antacid decrease the absorption of MMF (Cohen, 2002).

Calcineurin Inhibitors

Calcineurin inhibitors are the primary immunosuppressives agents that have been developed to date; they include tacrolimus and cyclosporine and are effective by their interaction with calcineurin. The most important cytokine in the immunology of transplantation rejection appears to be IL-2. It is produced through a sequence of events, which commence when a recipient antigen-processing cell comes into contact with the donor cells' major histocompatibility (MHC) antigens. The donor MHC fragment is processed and placed on the antigen-processing cell surface. When an appropriate recipient T cell is encountered, the T-cell receptor and the donor MHC bind. This initiates a cascade of intracellular enzymatic reactions via phosphorylation, and calcium stores are released, which then combine with calmodulin. This calcium-calmodulin complex then activates calcineurin. Calcineurin appears to be directly involved in the pathway that induces the production of the IL-2 molecule. Cyclosporine and tacrolimus act primarily by binding calcineurin via the cyclosporine-cyclophilin complex or the tacrolimus-FK binding protein complex, respectively. Binding of calcineurin by either of these complexes inhibits its enzymatic action, preventing the dephosphorylation of nuclear factor of activated T cells. This nuclear factor of activated T cells must be dephosphorylated to enter the nucleus, where it is required for IL-2 gene transcription.

Cyclosporine

Cyclosporine is a neutral lipophilic cyclic endecapeptide extracted from the fungus *Tolypocladium inflatum* in the early 1970s. Cyclosporine is poorly absorbed from the GI tract, and there is considerable variation in its bioavailability, as biliary output is essential for its absorption. Neoral (Novartis Pharmaceutical Corp., East Hanover, NJ), the microemulsion formula of cyclosporine, is much less dependent on bile production and flow than Sandimmune (Novartis Pharmaceuticals Corp.), the standard preparation. Neoral gives a more consistent level of cyclosporine and is associated with less evidence of rejection (Graziadei et al., 1997; Pinson et al., 1998), so it has replaced Sandimmune in most major transplant centers worldwide.

Cyclosporine is metabolized by the cytochrome P450 3A system (Cantarovich et al., 1998). Agents that induce these enzymes increase the metabolism of cyclosporine, resulting in lower blood levels, whereas agents that inhibit P450 activity result in higher circulating cyclosporine levels. In addition, cyclosporine can interfere with the metabolism of other medications. Digoxin, lovastatin, and prednisolone can have significantly decreased clearance with resultant toxicity.

The side effects associated with cyclosporine are numerous. Nephrotoxicity is one of the most significant, and it may involve acute or chronic renal pathologic alterations. The acute nephrotoxicity, which often resolves on reducing or discontinuing the medication, probably results from afferent arteriolar vasoconstriction with resulting decreased GFR. The chronic nephrotoxicity, which does not appear to be reversible, is associated with arteriolar hyalinosis, tubular vacuolization, interstitial nephritis, and cortical atrophy. Neurotoxicity is another common side effect, seen in as many as 50% of patients. This can range from headaches and tremors to seizures and coma. Because of variations in absorption and metabolism, cyclosporine levels tend to fluctuate. Dosages should be determined on the basis of the formulation used (i.e., Neoral versus Sandimmune) and serum or blood levels. Techniques to measure cyclosporine levels include radioimmunoassay and high-pressure liquid chromatography. The levels can be measured in whole blood, serum, or plasma. Most centers use whole blood trough levels by the radioimmunoassay technique. A level of 100 to 200 ng/mL is generally desirable in the first 3 to 6 months after transplantation, depending on the organ transplanted. The level can usually be maintained at lower levels thereafter, depending on the organ transplanted.

Tacrolimus

The calcineurin inhibitor tacrolimus, initially researched and brought to the market under the name FK-506, is a novel immunosuppressant that was isolated from *Streptomyces tsukubaensis* in 1985 (Kino et al., 1987; Starzl et al., 1989). Tacrolimus (FK506, Prograf) shares many similarities with cyclosporine, including its basic mechanism of action and metabolism by cytochrome P450 3A, in addition to its side-effect profiles. However, significant differences between these drugs have been elucidated in the past decade. Tacrolimus is 10 to 100 times more potent than cyclosporine, it possesses hepatotrophic properties, and it does not rely on bile for its absorption. Renal impairment, neurotoxicity, and hypertension occur with similar frequencies in both cyclosporine- and tacrolimus-based regimens. Tacrolimus is associated with more hyperglycemia. Reportedly, as many as 20% of tacrolimus recipients become insulin-dependent diabetics because of the agent's direct effect on pancreatic beta cells and peripheral insulin receptors. Tacrolimus appears to have a higher incidence of posttransplant lymphoproliferative disease. Considering that accelerated atherosclerosis is an important issue after solid organ transplantation, it is important to note that tacrolimus produces less hyperlipidemia and thus a less adverse cardiovascular risk profile than cyclosporine. Statistically significant improvements have been seen in total cholesterol, low-density lipoprotein cholesterol, and triglyceride levels when patients were switched from cyclosporine to tacrolimus (Manzarbeitia et al., 2001). Tacrolimus levels are usually measured in whole blood specimens by enzyme immunoassay techniques. Drug levels of 5 to 15 ng/mL are desirable in the first few months after transplantation, depending on the organ system transplanted.

Efficacy of Cyclosporine and Tacrolimus

After its introduction, cyclosporine became the drug of choice for the prevention of allograft rejection. Tacrolimus, initially reserved for use as rescue therapy in refractory rejection, has now become a first-line immunosuppressive agent in many centers worldwide. Large multicenter U.S. and European randomized clinical trials have been performed to compare tacrolimus and cyclosporine (Sandimmune) for primary and maintenance immunosuppression (European FK506 Multicenter Liver Study Group, 1994; U.S. Multicenter FK506 Liver Study Group, 1994, Wiesner, 1998). In the European trial, patient and graft survival rates were similar; however, significantly lower rates of acute rejection were seen in the tacrolimus group in some organ systems. More episodes of acute and steroid-resistant rejection were seen in the cyclosporine group. The tacrolimus group had a lower cumulative steroid exposure and fewer requirements for monoclonal antibody therapy (European FK506 Multicenter Liver Study Group). Patients on tacrolimus, however, had significantly more medication-related adverse effects. At the 5-year follow-up, tacrolimus showed less rejection but no overall improvement in patient or graft survival for all solid organ transplants. Many of these large trials used Sandimmune as the cyclosporine preparation, hence confounding some of the data to date. Neoral has been shown to be superior to Sandimmune (Freeman et al., 1995; Mirza et al., 1997). Tacrolimus appears to be superior to cyclosporine for the treatment of periodic rejection. These episodes of acute rejection, even steroid-resistant events, may resolve when patients are switched from cyclosporine- to tacrolimus-based therapy (Jonas et al., 1996; Millis et al., 1996a, 1996b, 1998; Doria et al., 2003; Mazariegos, 2010). Additionally, chronic rejection was responsive in more than half of patients converted from cyclosporine to tacrolimus for some solid organ transplants (Klintmalm et al., 1993). Hence, the choice of calcineurin inhibitor tends to be a matter of institutional preference. Many institutions are now using tacrolimus-based therapy, citing less rejection, less steroid use, reduced metabolic derangements (including reduced rates of hyperlipidemia), diminished neurologic complications, and less OKT3 needed for immunosuppression. However, many centers still advocate the use of cyclosporine (usually Neoral) based on equivalent patient or graft survival rates and a lower incidence of diabetes mellitus and posttransplant lymphoproliferative disease.

Rapamycin

Rapamycin (Sirolimus) is a macrolide antibiotic isolated from the fungus *Streptomyces hygroscopicus*. It effectively inhibits both B- and T-cell activity (Poon et al., 1996; Poston et al., 1999). Rapamycin is structurally similar to tacrolimus. It uses the same intracellular binding protein as tacrolimus but blocks B- and T-cell activation at a later stage than the calcineurin inhibitors. Rapamycin and cyclosporine appear to act synergistically to inhibit lymphocyte proliferation (Kimball et al., 1991). The oral bioavailability of rapamycin is variable. Like the calcineurin inhibitors, it is metabolized by the cytochrome P450 3A system. The efficacy of rapamycin in solid organ transplantation was initially shown in the renal transplant population (Groth et al., 1999; Kahan et al., 1999; McAlister et al., 2000). Small studies in liver transplant patients have shown rapamycin to be an effective agent when combined with a calcineurin inhibitor (Watson et al., 1999; Trotter et al., 2001). Most of these patients could be maintained on steroid-free regimens. Acute rejection episodes were significantly decreased compared with historical controls (30% versus 70%) (Kahan for the Rapamune U.S. Study Group 2000). A primary role of rapamycin is to facilitate a dosage reduction of calcineurin inhibitor in those patients with evidence of

tacrolimus or cyclosporine toxicity (Brattstrom et al., 1998; Groth et al., 1999). The most frequent dosage-related adverse effects include hyperlipidemia, leukopenia, thrombocytopenia, oral ulcerations, and joint pains. Both cholesterol and triglyceride levels can significantly increase and should be monitored while on therapy. Calcineurin inhibitor levels, especially those of cyclosporine, have been shown to significantly increase while on rapamycin therapy and should be closely monitored.

Antilymphocyte and Antithymocyte Globulins

Antilymphocyte globulin (ALG) and antithymocyte globulin (ATG) are produced by extracting immunoglobulins from animals (usually horse or rabbit) that have been immunized with human lymphocytes or thymocytes, respectively. The IV administration of these polyclonal antibodies causes rapid and profound depletion of peripheral lymphocytes. A major limitation of all polyclonal antilymphocyte preparations is batch-to-batch heterogeneity, which results in unpredictable side effects and more importantly, variable efficacy. ALG and ATG are not typically used as first-line agents for immunosuppression. They appear to delay the onset of the first episodes of organ rejection, but the overall rates of rejection are similar to those seen with calcineurin inhibitors (Neuhaus et al., 2000). The focus of this form of therapy is as the primary immunosuppression in patients unable to tolerate calcineurin inhibitors (i.e., because of significant pretransplant renal insufficiency) and in the treatment of steroid-resistant (and possibly OKT3-resistant) rejection. Commonly observed side effects include allergic reactions, serum sickness, fever, and thrombocytopenia, as with OKT3 and other systemically infused immunoglobulins. Cytokine release syndrome (cardiovascular collapse with a hemodynamic profile similar to septic shock, noncardiogenic pulmonary edema, seizures, hyperpyrexia and renal insufficiency) may be seen with the administration of these agents, which is similar to that sometimes seen with OKT3 or any other immunoglobulin. The incidence of lymphoproliferative disease is also increased among patients who have received ALG and ATG.

OKT3

OKT3 (Orthoclone OKT3, muromonab-CD3) is a monoclonal antibody directed against the CD3 complex of the cell membrane of lymphocytes (Fung et al., 1987); it is an antibody specifically directed at the T3 antigen of human T cells—the cells that directly attack the transplanted organ—and it is unlike the polyclonal antibody preparations. IV infusion results in tremendous lymphocyte depletion. Induction with OKT3 has not shown any significant benefit over the calcineurin inhibitors (McDiarmid et al., 1991). Because of its toxicity and the availability of less toxic agents, OKT3 is generally reserved for patients with severe steroid-resistant rejection (Portela et al., 1995; Wall and Adams, 1995). OKT3, ALG, and ATG provide 60% to 90% graft salvage rates for acute rejection in various organ system transplants. The side-effect profile of OKT3 is similar to that of ALG and ATG, including the cytokine release syndrome, infectious complications, and malignancy potential. This protein, like ALG and ATG, should be administered to a patient who is monitered. Lymphocyte and platelet counts must be closely monitored. CMV infection should be anticipated in all patients treated with OKT3 if they have not received CMV prophylaxis.

Interleukin-2 Receptor Antagonists

As discussed earlier, IL-2 is the most noteworthy cytokine known to be involved in the rejection of transplanted solid organs. Although calcineurin inhibitors decrease the amount of IL-2 produced, competitive inhibition by IL-2 receptor antagonists prevents the protein itself from binding to the active lymphocytes. Unlike ALG, ATG, and OKT3, which target the entire lymphocyte population, IL-2 receptor antagonists specifically target the actively dividing cells by binding to the IL-2 receptor's CD25 moiety, which is expressed only in active cells (Langrehr et al., 1998). The two available IL-2 receptor antagonists are basiliximab and daclizumab. Early studies indicated that these agents need to be combined with calcineurin inhibitors to be effective (Vincenti et al., 1998). These agents should probably be used for induction of immunosuppression (Eckhoff et al., 2000) in those patients at high risk for calcineurin inhibitor–related toxicity. Additionally, they appear to be well tolerated without significant adverse effects. Dosages and timing of administration of these agents vary, depending on the organ system to be transplanted. Moreover, it appears that IL-2 receptor antagonists are needed immediately at the time of the transplantation (immediately before or after reperfusion of the transplanted organ), with a second dose at approximately 4 days in the immediate immunosuppressive induction period.

Belatacept

Belatacept is a fusion protein composed of the Fe fragment of a human IgG1 immunoglobulin linked to the extracellular domain of CTLA-4, which is a molecule crucial for T-cell costimulation, selectively blocking the process of T-cell activation. It is intended to provide extended graft survival while limiting the toxicity generated by standard immune suppressing regimens, such as calcineurin inhibitors.

In a phase II multicenter study comparing the safety and efficacy of belatacept and cyclosporine A in 218 patients who had undergone renal transplantation with deceased- or living-donor kidneys, Vincenti and colleagues (2005) noted that at 6 months after transplantation, there were no significant differences in the incidence of clinically suspected, biopsy-proved acute rejection between the two treatment groups. In addition, investigators noted that renal function and chronic allograft nephropathy were significantly better in patients receiving belatacept, and the cardiovascular and metabolic endpoints of hypertension, hyperlipidemia, and posttransplantation diabetes were also better in patients receiving belatacept.

Alemtuzumab (Campath-1H)

The use of alemtuzumab (Campath-1H) in organ transplantation goes back to 1986, when Hale and colleagues (1986) in Europe reported on the preliminary results of a pilot study in renal, liver, and pancreas transplant recipients. Alemtuzumab is a humanized immunoglobulin IgG1 monoclonal antibody directed against CD52, a cell-surface glycoprotein expressed on circulating T and B cells and to a lesser extent on natural killer cells, monocytes, and macrophages. It has been suggested that after binding to its target, alemtuzumab causes cell death through complement-mediated cell lysis and antibody-mediated cellular cytotoxicity (Hale et al., 1986; Nuckel et al., 2005; Weaver and Kirk, 2007). Alemtuzumab was approved by the FDA for the treatment of lymphoid malignancies in 1999. It has been used off-label in bone marrow transplantation to prevent graft-versus-host disease and to treat various autoimmune diseases such as rheumatoid arthritis, scleroderma, and multiple sclerosis. Because of its rapid and profound lymphocyte-depleting effects, alemtuzumab was initially used off-label as induction therapy in renal transplantation to allow safe avoidance or minimization of steroid or calcineurin-inhibitor therapy. Retrospective analysis of the OPTN/UNOS database revealed that alemtuzumab induction was associated with a lower rate of acute rejection during the first 6 months after transplantation compared with no induction. Other studies have shown that antibody preconditioning with alemtuzumab without maintenance immunosuppression failed to achieve tolerance in clinical transplantation. Campath-1H also has an associated cytokine-release syndrome, which reportedly has been prevented completely by coadministration of solumedrol (2 mg/kg), Benadryl (2 mg/kg), and other antiinflammatory agents. Most patients who are pretreated still become febrile with the induction dose of the medication. The treatment for this hyperpyrexia is discontinuation of the agent. The usual pediatric induction dose is 0.3 to 0.4 mg/kg infused over 8 hours. Opportunistic infections and malignancies are of grave concern with a potent lymphocyte-depleting agent such as this, but an excessive frequency has not been reported.

LIVER TRANSPLANTATION

The first successful pediatric liver transplantation was performed in 1967 (Starzl et al., 1968). Before 1980, with the use of the immunosuppressive agents azathioprine and prednisone, the 5-year survival rate in the pediatric patient after liver transplantation was 20% (Gordon and Bismuth, 1991; Gordon et al., 1991). After the introduction of cyclosporine in 1980, long-term survival after liver transplantation became a reality. For the first time, 5-year patient survival began to exceed that of the life expectancy related to the specific disease process. Graft survival has progressively improved since 1992, with, for example, a 1-year graft survival of 81% in the 6- to 10-year-old recipient, compared with 68% a decade ago (UNOS, 2009). Patient survival for this age group is estimated to be 90.5% at 1 year, 85.9% at 3 years, and 83.8% at 5 years. Patient survival in the first year after transplantation is similar for all age groups except children younger than 1 year, who have the highest annual death rate. For these infant recipients transplanted between 2003 and 2004, there was a marked decline in 1-year death rate, a trend also seen for children ages 1 to 5 years and those ages 11 to 17 years. Improvements in patient and graft survival rates have been attributed to new immunosuppressive regimens consisting of tacrolimus Campath, mycophenolate, and rapamycin, with diminished use of cyclosporine, azathioprine, and corticosteroids and improved access to the donor pool using reduced grafts, living donors, and a new UNOS pediatric end-stage liver disease (PELD) scoring system for estimating medical urgency.

The majority of pediatric liver transplantations are performed in children less than 5 years of age. In children, 28% of grafts have been transplanted in patients less than 1 year of age, 37% in patients 1 to 5 years of age, and 35% in children 6 to 17 years of age. From 1988 to 2010, a total of 11,958 pediatric liver transplantations have been performed in the United States, of which 1264 (approximately 10%) have been living related (UNOS, 2009) (see Table 28-15).

General Indications and Contraindications

The recognition of orthotopic liver transplantation (OLT) as a viable alternative for pediatric patients with liver failure has increased the number of potential recipients. The indications for OLT can be classified in general as follows:

- End-stage liver disease (ESLD) expected to progress to death
- Secondary disease confined to the liver
- Prevention of the complications of major metabolic disorders
- Nonprogressive liver disease in which mortality is greater than the risk of OLT
- Fulminant hepatic failure

Disease-specific indications for OLT are shown in Box 28-2.

With improvements in surgical and medical expertise, the absolute and relative contraindications to pediatric OLT continue to evolve. There are very few absolute contraindications to OLT: the presence of any active, untreated bacterial, fungal, or viral infection at the time of transplantation; cancer outside the liver or those liver tumors not meeting cure criteria; actively replicating hepatitis B virus infection; acquired immune deficiency syndrome; or surgery that is technically not feasible. The relative contraindications are more variable and tend to be transplantation center–specific. Examples include a child with ESLD and advanced cardiopulmonary disease, epilepsy, or multisystem organ failure states; or human immunodeficiency virus (HIV)-positive serology.

Box 28-2 Disease-Specific Indications for Orthotopic Liver Transplantation

BILIARY ATRESIA
- Biliary hypoplasia
- Alagille's syndrome
- Extrahepatic

METABOLIC DISEASES
- Tyrosinemia
- Glycogen storage disease types I and II
- α_1-Antitrypsin deficiency
- Wilson's disease
- Primary oxalosis/oxaluria
- Hemochromatosis/hemosiderosis
- Hyperlipidemia II, homozygous
- Cystic fibrosis
- Maple syrup urine disease
- Urea cycle defects

CHOLESTATIC AND NONCHOLESTATIC CIRRHOSIS
MALIGNANT NEOPLASMS AND BENIGN TUMORS
ACUTE HEPATIC NECROSIS
MISCELLANEOUS
- Budd-Chiari syndrome
- Liver disease induced by total parenteral nutrition or hyperalimentation
- Neonatal hepatitis
- Congenital hepatic fibrosis
- Familial cholestasis
- Trauma
- Graft-versus-host disease secondary to transplantation (other than liver)

Pathophysiology of End-Stage Liver Disease

ESLD is an irreversible process that results in diffuse fibrosis and cirrhosis with loss of functional hepatocytes. The clinical manifestations are independent of the etiology but are primarily related to the degree of liver dysfunction. This dysfunction is secondary to structural changes that the liver undergoes after it sustains any type of significant damage. Irrespective of the cause of the hepatic injury, cell necrosis is followed by an attempt at regeneration. If the damage is of a chronic nature, this regeneration leads ultimately to fibrosis, further necrosis, and micronodular or macronodular cirrhosis (or both). Interestingly, the liver is the only solid organ in the body that can fully regenerate after sustaining up to 80% destruction of its functional capacity.

The two main mechanisms through which structural changes lead to hepatic failure are cellular dysfunction and portal hypertension. In cellular dysfunction, liver cell mass decreases as hepatocytes become necrotic. As the liver attempts to regenerate, fibrosis develops, with the eventual disruption of the portal triads. The result is formation of intrahepatic shunts, sinusoidal thickening, and an overall increase in the resistance to blood flow. This constellation of abnormalities results in the development of portal hypertension and varices. Similarly, biliary drainage becomes abnormal, leading to the intracellular accumulation of by-products that are normally secreted (proteins, bile). Together, these changes lead to abnormal hepatocyte energy metabolism, defects in protein and lipid synthesis, and alterations in substrate clearance.

Portal hypertension develops as a result of the increased resistance to blood flow through the disrupted sinusoids. In addition to this increase in resistance, there is an increase in splanchnic arterial blood flow caused by the development of arteriovenous shunts and vasodilation as liver failure progresses. Worsening portal hypertension is manifested by ascites, splenomegaly, and portosystemic shunts (varices, hemorrhoids, telangiectasia). These portosystemic shunts lead to decreased clearance of previously metabolized substrates by the liver. Cellular function is further compromised as oxygen is shunted away, leading to a potentially dysoxic hepatocellular environment. Regardless of the cause of the underlying liver failure, the pathophysiologic derangements are manifested similarly in the cardiovascular, pulmonary, renal, neurologic, and hematologic systems.

Child-Pugh Classification

The Child-Pugh classification is a universal scoring system of the degree of liver failure in patients with cirrhosis. Traditionally, the Child-Pugh class (A, B, or C) has been used as a predictive index for operative mortality rate in adult patients undergoing portosystemic shunting procedures. The estimated 1- and 5-year survival rates are 95% and 75% for patients with Child-Pugh class B, and 85% and 50% for patients with Child-Pugh class C. After the onset of the first major medical complication (ascites, variceal bleeding, jaundice, or encephalopathy), survival rates for these patients are significantly reduced. Variables measured by this system include ascites, encephalopathy, serum albumin, bilirubin, and prothrombin time (PT). Points are then assigned to different degrees of each variable, and the total points are used to assign a grade in the Child-Pugh scoring system (Table 28-16). Although a liver

TABLE 28-16. Child-Pugh Scoring System* for Cirrhosis

Score (points)	Bilirubin (mg/dL)	Albumin (g/dL)	Prothrombin Time (sec > control)	Hepatic Encephalopathy	Ascites (grade)
1	<2	>3.5	<4	None	None
2	2 to 3	2.8 to 3.5	4 to 6	1 to 2	Mild
3	>3	<2.8	>6	3 to 4	Severe

*Child class A = 5 to 6 points, class B = 7 to 9 points, class C = 10 to 15 points.

biopsy is often helpful in assessing histologic activity and the amount of fibrosis in patients with chronic hepatitis, it is not essential for the determination of the Child-Pugh class. Until February 2002, the Child-Pugh score was used by transplantation centers to group patients into one of four medical urgency categories. Blood type, patient size, medical urgency and waiting time determined liver allocation.

Pediatric End-Stage Liver Disease Scale

The PELD numerical scale is currently used by UNOS for liver allocation for children less than 12 years old. (PELD replaced the previous status 2B and 3 for pediatric patients, but status 1 is not affected by PELD.) PELD is based on bilirubin, INR, albumin, growth failure, and age when the patient is listed for transplantation, and it is used to calculate a numerical value that is an accurate predictor of 3-month mortality, independent of the complications of portal hypertension and the etiology of the liver disease. The MELD (model for end-stage liver disease) scale is a similar numerical scale ranging from 6 (less ill) to 40

(gravely ill) that is used for patients 12 years old and older. The score indicates how urgently the patient needs a transplant in the next 3 months. The number is calculated from three routine laboratory test results: bilirubin, INR, and creatinine. The measures used are as follows:

- Bilirubin, which measures how effectively the liver excretes bile
- INR (prothrombin time), which measures the liver's ability to make blood clotting factors
- Albumin, which measures the liver's ability to maintain nutrition
- Growth failure
- Whether the child is less than 1 year old

Systemic Manifestations of End-Stage Liver Disease

ESLD is associated with unique systemic physiologic alterations (Box 28-3) (Robertson, 1998).

Box 28-3 Cardiovascular, Pulmonary, and Renal Complications of Advanced Cirrhosis

CARDIOVASCULAR
- "Hyperdynamic" circulation
  - Increased cardiac index and stroke volume
  - Decreased systemic vascular resistance
  - Low to normal mean arterial pressure (widened pulse pressure)
  - Increased heart rate
- Central hypovolemia
  - Increased circulating blood volume
  - Decreased effective plasma volume
  - Increased sympathetic tone
- Hyporesponsiveness of the vasculature to pressor therapy
- Flow-dependent oxygen consumption
- Hepatic and splanchnic vasculature
  - Portal hypertension
  - Portosystemic collateral circulation
  - Decreased hepatic blood flow
- Alcoholic cardiomyopathy (reduced left-ventricular ejection fraction)
- Cirrhotic cardiomyopathy (impaired cardiac contractility, defective excitation contraction coupling, impaired systolic and diastolic function, prolonged QTc interval, autonomic dysfunction, impaired β-adrenergic function and postreceptor defect, decreased responsiveness to catecholamines, conductance abnormalities)
- Arrhythmias

PULMONARY
- Arterial hypoxemia (Pao_2 < 70 mm Hg)
  - Hepatopulmonary syndrome
  - Portopulmonary hypertension
  - Impaired hypoxic pulmonary vasoconstriction
  - Increased pulmonary blood flow
  - V/Q Mismatch
- Parenchymal abnormalities
  - Restrictive ventilatory pattern resulting from ascites limiting diaphragmatic excursion, pleural effusions, or chest wall deformity caused by osteoporosis
  - Obstructive airway disease, emphysema, bronchitis/bronchiectasis
  - Interstitial lung disease (infection, pneumonitis, pulmonary edema)

RENAL
- Renin-angiotensin-aldosterone activation: impaired sodium handling, water excretion, potassium metabolism, and concentrating ability
- Impaired renal acidification
- Prerenal insufficiency (ascites or diuretics)
- Acute renal failure (acute liver failure, biliary obstruction, sepsis)
- Hepatorenal syndrome
- Glomerulopathies

Cardiovascular System

Progressive liver failure is characterized by a hyperdynamic circulation with a left ventricular (LV) ejection fraction of greater than 65%, fixed low total peripheral resistance, and a compensatory rise in cardiac output, impaired circulatory reserve, and diminished response to catecholamine infusions. High-risk patients have cardiomyopathy and dysrhythmias, congestive heart failure from fluid and electrolyte imbalances, and moderate to severe pulmonary hypertension.

Systemic vascular resistance is low because of peripheral vasodilation and shunting (cutaneous, splanchnic, intrapulmonary, portopulmonary, lumbrical, and pleural). This profound vasodilation may result from abnormal levels of vasodilator substances, possibly originating in the splanchnic circulation, which would otherwise be cleared by the liver, or from the lack of a substance produced by the liver. The most likely mediators include nitric oxide, tumor necrosis factor-α, and endothelium-derived relaxing factor. Activation of the renin-angiotensin-aldosterone system causes an increase in extracellular fluid volume through salt and water retention, and release of AVP results in a decrease in free-water excretion. Similarly, the sympathetic nervous system is activated in an attempt to cause peripheral vasoconstriction to maintain an adequate MAP. Mixed venous oxygen saturation (Svo_2) measured in the pulmonary artery outflow tract is markedly elevated (usually ≥85%). The increase in Svo_2 presumably results from poor oxygen extraction capacity and correlates somewhat with cardiac index (Jugan et al., 1992; Steib et al., 1993). Yet there is no evidence of tissue dysoxia or increased serum lactate with the patient at rest.

Respiratory System

Cirrhotic patients are predisposed to arterial hypoxemia from intrapulmonary shunting because of capillary vasodilation, restrictive lung disease caused by ascites or pleural effusions, impaired hypoxic pulmonary vasoconstriction, increased pulmonary blood flow, and a rightward shift in the oxygen-dissociation curve resulting from decreased levels of 2, 3-diphosphoglycerate. Respiratory compromise may also result from the hepatopulmonary syndrome (HPS), portopulmonary hypertension, defects in alveolar oxygen diffusion, or pulmonary manifestations of systemic disease (e.g., cystic fibrosis, autoimmune disease, α_1-antitrypsin deficiency). These defects are seemingly compensated for by an increase in Svo_2 and resting cardiac output (Schott et al., 1999; Teramoto et al., 2000). Arterial hypoxemia usually responds to supplemental oxygen and positive pressure ventilation suggestive of a V/Q mismatch. Depressed airway reflexes, delayed gastric emptying, hiatus hernia, and massive ascites increase the risk for aspiration. Pulmonary edema, atelectasis, and pneumonia are also common findings in patients with ESLD.

The frequency of HPS (chronic liver disease, increased alveolar-arterial gradient while breathing room air, and intrapulmonary vasodilation) is reported to be between 4% and 29% (Naeije, 2003; Mazzeo et al., 2004). Patients with liver disease may develop progressive and refractory hypoxemia when abnormal intrapulmonary vascular dilation causes anatomic shunting and diffusion-perfusion abnormalities (Hoeper et al., 2004). The prognosis for patients with HPS is poor, and a mortality rate of 41% within 2 to 5 years has been reported (Krowka et al.,

1993). In contrast, up to 20% of cirrhotic patients are at risk of developing portopulmonary hypertension (portal hypertension and increased pulmonary vascular resistance). Severe pulmonary hypertension may cause acute right ventricular failure and sudden cardiac death (Scott et al., 1999). Preoperative therapy with epoprostenol and nitric oxide may improve outcome in this group if right ventricular function is preserved and treatment results in a decrease in pulmonary pressures and vascular remodeling.

Renal System

Renal dysfunction is common in patients with ESLD, and the kidneys are very susceptible to injury and prone to failure. Fluid and electrolyte imbalances are secondary to diuretic therapy, hypoalbuminemia, and portal hypertension causing generalized ascites, progressive edema, hypovolemia, dilutional hyponatremia, and hypokalemic metabolic alkalosis resulting from renin-aldosterone activation. Three main mechanisms, singularly or in combination, contribute to renal insufficiency: prerenal causes, acute tubular necrosis, and hepatorenal syndrome. Renal insufficiency not only complicates the management of liver failure but, more importantly, may increase patient mortality. Thus, it is important to evaluate and treat reversible causes of renal insufficiency (Box 28-4). Renal function is often difficult to assess in these patients because reduced muscle mass and hepatic synthesis of creatine reduces the serum creatinine level. Creatinine clearance will overestimate the GFR.

Prerenal azotemia is most commonly associated with aggressive use of diuretic therapy in the treatment of ascites. With a decreased effective arterial volume, patients are more susceptible to the volume depletion effects of diuretics and

---

Box 28-4 Strategy for Optimizing Renal Function and Preventing Hepatorenal Syndrome

INITIAL MANAGEMENT

- Homeostatic environment (electrolytes, acid-base status, hematocrit)
- Cardiovascular stability (euvolemia, mean arterial pressure > 60 mm Hg)
- Identify intrinsic renal parenchymal disease
- Treat bacterial infections and complications related to liver disease (i.e., ascites, dilutional hyponatremia, and variceal bleeding)
- Avoidance of nephrotoxic agents (e.g., nonsteroidal antiinflammatory drugs or aminoglycosides)

OPTIMIZE RENAL PERFUSION

- Intravascular volume expansion
- Drug therapy (splanchnic vasoconstriction or renal vasodilators): vasopressin analogues, α-adrenergic agonists, endothelin antagonists, antioxidants

STRATEGIES

- Transjugular intrahepatic portosystemic shunt
- Albumin and antibiotic therapy for spontaneous bacterial peritonitis

Adapted from Gines P, Guevara M, Arroyo V, Rodes J: Hepatorenal syndrome, *Lancet* 362:1819, 2003.

large volume paracentesis without adequate intravascular volume replacement. As with other types of prerenal azotemia, the urine sodium level is low (<10 mEq/L), with a fractional excretion of sodium (FENa) of less than 1%. This type of renal failure is amenable to careful volume replacement.

The kidneys in patients with liver failure are also at increased risk for developing acute tubular necrosis (ATN) as a result of decreased renal perfusion. This decreased perfusion is a consequence of a relative decrease in central blood volume caused by splanchnic pooling, which activates secretion of vasopressin, in combination with other compensatory mechanisms attempting to restore MAP, such as increased sympathetic tone and renin-angiotensin activity. Renal perfusion is further compromised because prostaglandin synthesis is reduced in advanced liver disease. Prostaglandins are potent renal arteriolar vasodilators (Govindarajan et al., 1987; Claria and Arroyo, 2003). Hence, tubular function is much closer to an ischemic threshold in patients with liver failure. This low ischemic threshold renders the kidneys more susceptible to nephrotoxic drugs such as IV contrast dye or aminoglycosides. Additionally, in the patient with tense ascites, renal cortical perfusion may also be diminished as a result of elevated intraabdominal pressure. Urine sodium in this setting is usually greater than 20 mEq/L, with a FENa of greater than 1% (Epstein, 1985). Treatment should be directed at minimizing additional renal injury, optimizing renal perfusion, and maintaining urine output, with some form of dialysis possibly introduced until the ATN resolves. This usually occurs within 10 to 14 days. It is not uncommon, however, for the hepatorenal syndrome to become superimposed once the patient develops ATN.

The most consequential form of renal dysfunction is the hepatorenal syndrome, and it has a very poor prognosis. It is characterized by a rapid deterioration in renal function associated with profound sodium retention and low urinary sodium excretion. It is usually precipitated by a major physiologic event, such as GI hemorrhage, sepsis, or surgery. It is differentiated from prerenal azotemia by the lack of responsiveness to volume expansion. The pathogenesis is severe renal vasoconstriction with absence of renal cortical blood flow. Interestingly, this vasoconstriction is reversible if the kidney is transplanted into a host with normal hepatic function (Koppel et al., 1969). This form of renal failure requires dialysis to sustain life, but it may be reversible with liver transplantation (Iwatsuki et al., 1973).

Hematologic Complications

Anemia, thrombocytopenia, and coagulopathy are the expected findings in the patient with liver failure. Anemia is usually a result of bone marrow suppression, vitamin deficiency, hemorrhage, and diminished erythropoietin production caused by renal insufficiency. Thrombocytopenia (platelet count < 100,000/mm³) is seen in 70% of patients with liver disease (Kang et al., 1985) and is primarily a result of diminished thrombopoietin production and portal hypertension with platelet sequestration in the spleen (Kaushansky, 1995; Martin et al., 1997). However, bone marrow suppression, abnormalities in platelet metabolism or autoimmune causes may also be contributing factors (Peck-Radosavljevic, 2000). Impaired platelet aggregation and clot retraction caused by qualitative platelet defects are also seen in patients with liver disease and renal failure.

The tissue factor pathway of coagulation is classically assessed by measuring PTT and PT. The liver is the main site

TABLE 28-17. Clotting Factors: Activity and Half-Life

Factor	Biological Half-Life	Vitamin K Dependent	Plasma Concentration
Fibrinogen	90 hr	No	300-400 mg/dL
Prothrombin	60 hr	Yes	10-15 mg/dL
Factor V	12-36 hr	No	0.5-1.0 mg/dL
Factor VII	4-6 hr	Yes	0.1 mg/dL
Factor VIII:C	12 hr	No	1-2 mg/dL
Factor IX	20 hr	Yes	4 mcg/mL
Factor X	24 hr	Yes	0.75 mg/dL
Factor XI	40 hr	No	1.2 mg/dL
Factor XII	48-52 hr	No	0.4 mg/dL
Prekallikrein	48-52 hr	No	0.29 mg/dL
High-molecular-weight kininogen	6.5 day	No	0.70 mg/dL
Factor XIII	3-5 day	No	2.5 mg/dL
Protein C	8-12 hr	Yes	4-5 mcg/mL
Protein S	—	Yes	25 mg/L

From the United Network for Organ Sharing (UNOS) and Organ Procurement and Transplantation Network (OPTN) data, 2010. Available at http://optn.transplant.hrsa.gov/data.

of synthesis of all coagulation factors except von Willebrand's factor, which is produced primarily in the vascular endothelium. Failure of bile salt secretion results in poor absorption of vitamin K, which is a cofactor necessary for the post-transcriptional γ-carboxylation and activation of factors II, VII, IX, and X (Table 28-17). In cirrhotic patients, the levels of fibrinogen and factor VIII are usually supranormal, and the production of all other clotting factors is diminished. Additionally, approximately 80% of patients with liver failure produce an abnormal fibrinogen molecule (dysfibrinogenemia) (Martinez et al., 1978; Cunningham et al., 2002). Control of coagulation therefore depends on the balance of hepatic synthesis of clotting factors and the clearance of activated clotting factors, plasminogen activators, and fibrinolytic proteins.

Neurologic Complications

Hepatic encephalopathy is a frequent metabolic complication of acute or chronic liver disease. The neuropsychiatric abnormalities are often reversible, with the clinical presentation ranging from subtle personality changes to frank coma. Neuromuscular symptoms include tremor, hyperreflexia, and decerebrate posturing. The three theories regarding the pathogenesis of hepatic encephalopathy are (1) ammonia toxicity with accumulation of toxins in the brain, (2) an alteration in plasma amino acid composition with accumulation of false neurotransmitters, and (3) an increase in neuroinhibitory substances, such as manganese, monoamines, and endogenous opiates. Various studies have supported aspects of each hypothesis, yet none has been conclusively established. In patients who have died in hepatic coma, neuropathologic findings occur in the astrocytes rather than in the neurons. Positron emission tomography studies show decreased glucose use in the cerebral cortex, which may explain some neuropsychiatric abnormalities (Butterworth, 1996).

Forty percent of ammonia is generated in the intestine from ingested nitrogenous substances, and it is subsequently metabolized in the liver into urea, which is excreted through the kidneys and into the colon. With liver failure and portosystemic shunting, ammonia, which is a known neurotoxin, accumulates and readily diffuses into the brain, where it exerts its neurotoxicity. Arguments against ammonia being the sole factor in the pathogenesis have been based on (1) the lack of a strong correlation between blood ammonia levels and the degree of hepatic encephalopathy, (2) the presence of this condition in the absence of elevated ammonia levels, and (3) the neuroexcitatory effects of low ammonia concentration. Other metabolic by-products, such as mercaptans and short-chain fatty acids, have also been implicated.

With progressive liver failure, the ratio of branched-chain amino acids to aromatic amino acids decreases. These aromatic amino acids cross the blood-brain barrier and may competitively inhibit normal neurotransmitters and favor the generation of false neurotransmitters (e.g., octopamine) that have an inhibitory effect on cerebral function.

Gamma-aminobutyric acid (GABA), a major inhibitory neurotransmitter in the CNS, regulates the chloride channel. It has been suggested that elevated ammonia levels enhance GABA-ergic neurotransmission and synergistically augment the action of benzodiazepine receptor agonists (Basile and Jones, 1997). This theory is supported by the fact that hepatic encephalopathy can at times be improved by the benzodiazepine receptor-antagonist flumazenil.

Among the multiple precipitating factors of hepatic encephalopathy are azotemia, drugs (sedatives, tranquilizers, analgesics), GI bleeding, excess dietary protein, metabolic alkalosis, infection, and constipation (Abou-Assi et al., 2001). Treatment consists of reducing dietary protein, avoiding sedatives, administering antibiotics such as neomycin or Bactrim, administering lactulose (which converts ammonia to nonabsorbable ammonium and modifies the colonic flora), correction of hypokalemia, discontinuation of diuretics, treating infection, and volume expansion.

Endocrine dysfunction is common in ESLD. Oversecretion of growth hormone and glucagon leads to peripheral and hepatic insulin resistance and impaired glucose metabolism, with lipids as a preferred energy substrate. Hypoglycemia is an ominous sign indicative of depletion of glycogen stores in the liver and survival is limited to days without IV glucose supplementation and transplantation. It is often seen with infections or sepsis.

Pathophysiology of a Few Uncommon Genetic Disorders

Although liver transplantation is performed for a myriad of metabolic disorders, a few conditions merit special mention because of their unique pathophysiology. Two important features are common among them. First, patients have no intrinsic hepatic dysfunction and thus have not developed the portosystemic collaterals that afford the visceral protection from mesenteric venous hypertension during portal vein clamping. These patients also do not have the compensatory increase in hepatic arterial flow seen in patients with parenchymal liver disease and portal hypertension. In addition, these patients are generally

not coagulopathic and it is often necessary to begin anticoagulant therapy after reperfusion so as to prevent thrombotic complications. The second feature is that patients with metabolic disorders cannot become catabolic. Dextrose-containing solutions and careful avoidance of stress are necessary for successful outcomes. Given the known risk for metabolic stroke and coma, allograft selection for these patients is imperative, and any possibility of primary nonfunction should be avoided with careful attention paid to cold and warm ischemic times.

Urea-Cycle Disorders

Urea-cycle disorders are one of the common inborn errors of metabolism that are clinically cured by liver transplantation (Morioka et al., 2005). As the urea cycle is the final pathway for the elimination of nitrogen. Enzymatic defects or errors in the pathway lead to the accumulation of nitrogen as ammonia, alanine, glutamate, and other intermediate metabolites. The urea cycle contains five enzyme systems, and the clinical manifestations depend on the enzyme that is deficient (Fig. 28-2). These enzyme deficiency syndromes are carbamoyl phosphate synthetase I deficiency, ornithine transcarbamylase deficiency (OTCD), argininosuccinate synthetase deficiency (citrullinemia), argininosuccinate lyase deficiency, and *N*-acetylglutamate synthetase deficiency. OTCD is the most common urea-cycle disorder, with a prevalence of 1 in 40,000 live births, and it is inherited as an X-linked, partially dominant chromosomal defect. Ornithine transcarbamylase is a mitochondrial enzyme that catalyzes the conversion of ornithine (the product of carbamoyl phosphate synthetase–catalyzed ammonia and bicarbonate) and carbamylphosphate to citrulline. OTCD thus results in the accumulation of ammonia, carbamylphosphate, and glutamate, with diminished production of citrulline, arginine, and urea. Because of the X-linked, partially dominant inheritance of OTCD, the phenotypical expression of OTCD is varied. In the severe form, which affects homozygous males, hypothermia, lethargy, and vomiting follow a 24- to 72-hour asymptomatic period. Symptoms are progressive and severe and are related to accumulation of glutamine and ammonia and secondary cerebral edema. In heterozygous females, the expression is more varied and can range from neonatal expression to clinically imperceptible disease. Accumulation of ammonia is exacerbated by protein breakdown at times of stress (surgery, sepsis, dehydration, anesthesia) or fasting, and also with the ingestion of high-protein foods or parenteral nutrition. Anesthesia management in these children focuses on avoidance of catabolic states through infusion of physiologic fluids containing at least 10% dextrose. Avoidance of emotional stress is imperative, with liberal use of perioperative benzodiazepines and analgesics. Hypothermia should be prevented with the use of warm room temperatures, irrigation, and warming blankets. Some centers also use continuous intraoperative IV infusions of sodium benzoate (300 to 500 mg/kg per day) for nitrogen binding. OTCD may also be independently associated with a hypercoagulable state, with documented thrombotic complications in four children (Venkateswaran, 2009).

Maple Syrup Urine Disease

Maple syrup urine disease (MSUD) is an inborn error of amino acid metabolism caused by the autosomal recessive–mediated deficiency in branched-chain α-ketoacid dehydrogenase (BCKD)

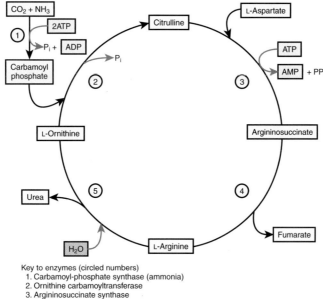

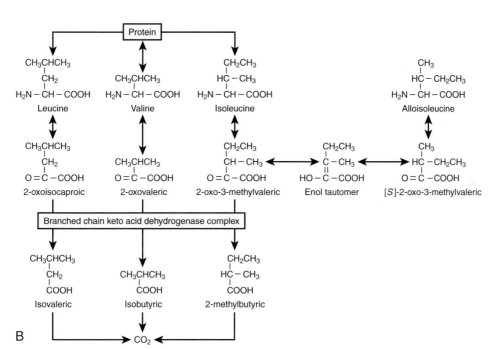

FIGURE 28-2. A, Urea cycle, showing the reactions by which excess nitrogen in the form of ammonia is converted to soluble urea, using l-ornithine as a recyclable carrier. **B,** Pathway of branched-chain amino acid (BCAA) catabolism. Note that the branched-chain organic acids are derived from the BCAAs by deamination, and the site of the defect in maple syrup urine disease (MSUD) is the dehydrogenase complex. The asymmetry of the β-carbon of isoleucine and the reversibility of the keto-enol interconversion give rise to alloisoleucine, which is virtually pathognomonic for MSUD. *(From Khanna A, Hart M, Nyhan WL, et al: Liver transplantation in maple syrup urine disease,* Liver Transplant *12:876, 2006.)*

activity. BCKD is the second enzyme in the pathway used in the degradation of the branched-chain amino acids leucine, isoleucine, and valine (Morton et al., 2002) (see Fig. 28-2). The pathophysiology of MSUD is primarily explained by the accumulation of leucine in the plasma and in the organs. Similar to the urea-cycle disorders, severe metabolic decompensation is associated with catabolism of tissue proteins at times of starvation and stress. The disease usually manifests within

48 hours of birth with ketonuria, irritability, and dystonia that progresses to seizures and coma by the fourth day of life (Felber et al., 1993). Diagnosis is confirmed by testing for the presence of branched-chain 2-ketoacids in the urine and by quantification of branched-chain amino acids in the plasma. Children are treated with dietary restriction of branched-chain amino acids and avoidance of catabolic states. Despite strict dietary control, severe metabolic crises can still develop suddenly

during intercurrent illnesses and can be associated with life-threatening cerebral edema. In addition to facing the dangers of acute metabolic decompensation, patients with MSUD often suffer from neurocognitive disorders, probably from imbalances of branched-chain amino acids in the brain. Because of their protein-restricted diet, MSUD patients can also develop essential-amino-acid deficiencies, resulting in immunodeficiency, growth failure, and global developmental delays. Patients undergoing liver transplantation for MSUD are carefully selected, and successful outcomes depend on a multidisciplinary approach to their management in the perioperative period (Strauss, 2006). A careful neurologic examination should be documented before sedation to serve as a baseline, and a careful history of past metabolic crises and neurologic deficits should be obtained. Baseline levels of branched-chain amino acids should be recorded, and, if they are excessive, transplantation should be deferred and medical treatment initiated. Like patients with urea-cycle disorders, patients with MSUD cannot be fasted without catabolic consequence. In addition, specialized total parenteral nutrition (TPN) should be used that include concentrated dextrose infusions. MSUD patients should never receive hypotonic infusions, and plasma osmolarity should be carefully monitored and kept in the normal range. Perioperative sedation and analgesia should be optimized to avoid catabolism, and physiologic stress should be kept to a minimum (Kahraman, 1996; Fuentes-Garcia, 2009). Leucine levels are generally followed after reperfusion of the liver and daily after the transplantation. Patients are immediately fed an unrestricted diet or are given enteral feedings with standard protein compositions.

Domino Liver Transplantation

Domino liver transplantation is a procedure in which an index patient (e.g., one with MSUD) with a genetic defect receives a hepatic allograft, and that index patient's liver is then carefully resected and removed, maintaining anatomic integrity, and it is then flushed and used as an allograft for a second patient (Khanna, 2006; Wilczek, 2008). The hepatectomy of the index donor must preserve adequate vascular and biliary cuffs for use in implantation into the second recipient. Because of the anatomy of the hepatic veins, this often requires the hepatectomy to be performed in the standard manner, which involves removal of the retrohepatic vena cava together with the hepatectomy specimen. As the index patients do not have portal hypertension or parenchymal liver disease, portal and caval clamping is not well tolerated and venovenous bypass (VVB) is often required in older patients to avoid significant mesenteric venous hypertension, associated visceral edema, and hemodynamic instability.

The index liver can then be transplanted into a patient with ESLD, who must not be a carrier of the genetic defect that results in MSUD. The liver removed from the patient with MSUD can function as a normal liver because the genetic defect, α-ketoacid dehydrogenase deficiency, is not present in any of the recipient's cells or organ systems. Hence, cellular metabolism and degradation of the branched-chain amino acids leucine, isoleucine, and valine occurs without consequence. Thus, in this case, the index liver is not disposed of but used in another recipient without that particular genetic defect, who can now live normally. Domino transplantation is initiated only when there is a donor organ offered for the MSUD index patient.

Alagille's Syndrome

Alagille's syndrome (AS) is an autosomal disorder characterized by bile duct paucity, cholestasis, and progression to cirrhosis, requiring transplantation in 30% of patients. The syndrome is also associated with characteristic facial features, ocular manifestations, vertebral anomalies, and pancreatic insufficiency. Renal disease is another important feature of this syndrome with structural and functional disorders in up to 50% of patients including renal artery stenosis, dysplastic or ectopic kidneys, and tubulointerstitial nephropathy. Idiopathic intracranial hemorrhage occurs in up to 15% of patients and is often fatal. Patients with AS should be screened with magnetic resonance angiography (MRA) of the head prior to transplantation to identify any cerebral vascular malformations. Cardiac anomalies are also a component of AS, with the most common manifestation being central or peripheral pulmonary arterial stenoses. Up to 24% of patients also have associated intracardiac anomalies. Tetralogy of Fallot, aortic coarctation, septal defects, patent ductus arteriosus, pulmonary atresia and pulmonary stenosis have also been reported with AS (Perlmutter and Shepherd, 2002). In patients with right ventricular outflow obstruction, the severity of the outflow gradient is a major factor in the perioperative morbidity and mortality.

Wilson's Disease

Wilson's disease (hepatolenticular degeneration) is an autosomal recessive disorder characterized by progressive or acute liver decompensation in the first 2 decades of life, although its appearance later with neuropsychiatric symptoms is also common. Wilson's disease represents a mutation in the *ATP7B* gene, which causes a progressive accumulation of copper in the liver as a result of impaired copper excretion into the bile. As time passes, the capacity of the liver to accumulate copper is exceeded, and copper is released into the circulation. In addition to liver decompensation, copper accumulation also affects the CNS, with a myriad of neuropsychiatric symptoms. Severe Coombs-negative (non-immune-mediated) intravascular hemolysis is frequent and is the presenting symptom in up to 15% of patients. Arrhythmias, autonomic dysfunction, and LV hypertrophy are seen in up to 25% of patients (Hlubocká et al., 2002).

α₁-Antitrypsin Deficiency

α_1-Antitrypsin deficiency (A1AT) is a relatively common autosomal recessive disorder. It is a serine protease inhibitor that inhibits destructive neutrophil proteases, and it limits the destructive effects of neutrophil effectors during times of inflammation. In the homozygous form, there is a 90% reduction in circulating concentrations of A1AT. α_1-Antitrypsin has a reported incidence of liver involvement in 10% to 20% of patients, primarily those who are PIZZ homozygotic (Psacharopoulos et al., 1983). The incidence of this phenotype is 1 in 7000 in the United States and 1 in 2000 in Scandinavia (Schwarzenberg and Sharp, 1990). Males are affected more frequently than females. Some 10% to 20% of PIZZ individuals develop neonatal cholestasis, and jaundice is often the first sign of this disease. The liver disease associated with A1AT deficiency can become clinically apparent at any time from infancy to late adulthood. Of note for anesthesiologists, patients with homozygous A1AT deficiency develop progressive emphysematous lung disease; however, these changes are generally not severe until well into adulthood.

Fulminant Hepatic Failure

Fulminant hepatic failure (FHF) is the most severe, life-threatening complication of liver failure. See related video online at www.expertconsult.com. Differentiating acute fulminant liver failure from an acute exacerbation of chronic liver disease has important therapeutic and prognostic implications, as not all patients with acute liver failure are the same. Fulminant hepatic failure is usually defined as rapidly progressive liver failure, with the onset of encephalopathy within 8 weeks of the onset of jaundice in patients without a previous history of liver disease. However, no uniform definition of FHF in children has been established yet. One definition that is widely accepted is the sudden onset of liver failure with altered mental status and coagulopathy in an otherwise healthy child (Nazer and Nazer, 2004). FHF was the primary diagnosis in 15% of pediatric patients transplanted from 1995 to 2000. Viral hepatitis and drug-induced hepatotoxity are the two most common causes, but in most cases, the etiology is unidentified. For the majority of patients with fulminant failure, survival ultimately depends on medical stabilization and urgent liver transplantation, as mortality rates may reach 80%.

The etiology of FHF is quite varied. In approximately 50% of patients, FHF is caused by acute viral hepatitis (A, B, C, D, E, or non A–E). Hepatitis C virus infection is not a significant cause of FHF in children. Many other viruses are also recognized, including Epstein-Barr virus, CMV, paramyxovirus, varicella-zoster virus, herpesvirus types 1, 2, and 6, parvovirus, and adenovirus. Less common causes include hepatotoxic drugs (acetaminophen, salicylates, chlorinated hydrocarbons, halothane, isoniazid, IV tetracycline, sodium valproate, and methanol), *Amanita* mushroom poisoning, ischemia, vascular obstruction (Budd-Chiari syndrome), massive steatosis (Reye's syndrome), and metabolic causes (Wilson's disease in older children; inborn errors of metabolism and hemochromatosis in neonates).

Jaundice is the most common presenting symptom, with mental changes occurring over the next two weeks in most patients. The condition then progresses to coma in as many as 80% of patients, with the development of ascites, cerebral edema, decortical and decerebrate posturing, severe coagulopathy, GI bleeding, respiratory failure, pulmonary edema, and hemodynamic instability.

Cerebral edema appears to be the major cause of morbidity in patients with FHF and contributes to the high mortality. Early signs and symptoms include increased muscle tone, arterial hypertension, seizures, agitation, and sluggish papillary response to light. Infants may present with poor feeding, irritability, and altered sleep patterns. The mechanism of cerebral edema is unknown, although vasogenic and cytotoxic etiologies have been proposed. Whatever the cause, cerebral edema ultimately leads to intracranial hypertension, impairment of cerebral perfusion, irreversible neurologic brain injury, uncal herniation, and death (Hanid et al., 1979). Encephalopathy may be classified according to the scheme in Table 28-18. This is useful to judge the effects of treatment and assess the progression of the disease process.

TABLE 28-18. Staging (Grading) of Hepatic Encephalopathy

Stage	Mental Status	Tremor (Asterixis)	Electroencephalography
I	Euphoria, altered sleep, slurred speech	Slight	Δ and α irregularities
II	Drowsiness, incontinence	Marked	Slow α and Δ
III	Arousable from sleep, confused	Diminished	τ wave prevalent
IV	Responsive to painful stimuli	Absent	Slow Δ to flat
V	Unresponsive to pain	Absent	Flat

Medical treatment is generally supportive until either recovery with hepatocyte regeneration, liver transplantation (deceased, split, or living related donor), hepatocyte transplantation, or death. See related video online at www.expertconsult.com. Experimental approaches have been attempted using liver-assist devices. Supportive measures are directed at minimizing morbidity and mortality from serious complications. This includes a critical care unit, monitoring, endotracheal intubation for airway protection, infusions of 10% to 20% dextrose to prevent hypoglycemia, replacement of calcium phosphorous and magnesium, antibiotic treatment of infections, maintenance of adequate urine output, avoidance of nephrotoxic drugs with surveillance for renal insufficiency, and H_2-blockers for stress ulcer prophylaxis. Correction of coagulopathy is with vitamin K and plasmapheresis. In general, platelets and fresh frozen plasma are reserved for patients with active bleeding. Normalization of the patient's PT is often used as a prognostic indicator for recovery of synthetic function. Avoiding volume overload and management of intracranial hypertension are crucial in the management of FHF. Protein intake is restricted. Lactulose enemas and oral neomycin are administered to decrease enteric bacteria that produce ammonia If a causative agent is identified, specific treatment should be initiated early (e.g., *N*-acetylcysteine for acetaminophen overdose).

Initial management of cerebral edema should begin with a computed tomography (CT) scan of the brain to assess cerebral blood flow with xenon (Aggarwal et al., 1994). If there is evidence of cerebral edema and compromise of cerebral blood flow without CO_2 responsiveness, continuous monitoring of intracranial pressure is vital, especially in stage 3 or 4 encephalopathy. Therapeutic measures to reduce ICP include head-up positioning, ventilatory support with moderate hyperventilation, and mannitol for a documented ICP greater than 30 mm Hg and for progressive edema. It may be efficacious to place a jugular bulb catheter so that adequate assessment of cerebral metabolism is possible (Lassen and Lane, 1961). The important parameters that aid in management are the measured arteriovenous oxygen content difference ($AVDo_2$), glucose, and lactate differences across the brain (Aggarwal et al., 1993, 1994). Mild hypothermia (to 34° C) and barbiturate coma remain controversial topics with respect to the management of hepatic coma. Barbiturate coma should be reserved until all therapeutic interventions have failed to reduce ICP. However, hypothermia should be initiated early in stage III coma. Continuous EEG monitoring is essential, as the goal is to achieve EEG silence with IV barbiturates.

Serial abdominal CT scans may be useful in assessing the hepatic size and morphology. A transjugular liver biopsy may be necessary but may not provide a definitive diagnosis. Histologic findings are usually of two types: extensive necrosis of the peripheral hepatocytes with little or no regeneration (drugs and viral hepatitis), and microvesicular steatosis and centrilobular necrosis (Reye's syndrome and metabolic disorders). Serum levels of liver enzymes do not correlate with the severity of the disease. Typically, conjugated hyperbilirubinemia is present, with hyponatremia, hyperkalemia, respiratory alkalosis, and metabolic acidosis.

Prognostic criteria include the patient's age, cause of liver disease, onset and degree of encephalopathy relative to the appearance of jaundice, serum bilirubin level, PT and INR, serum creatinine, factor V level, and arterial pH. A sensitive predictor of outcome is the INR value. With an INR of 4 or more, the mortality rate reaches 86%; with an INR of less than 4, it may be as low as 27% (Nazer and Nazer, 2004).

Preoperative Evaluation

Risk assessment of the patient scheduled for OLT is still in its evolutionary stage. The primary focus for the anesthesiologist is to evaluate the *whole* patient for systemic manifestations of ESLD as well as predictable disease-specific extrahepatic manifestations (such as pulmonary involvement with cystic fibrosis).

Cardiovascular Evaluation

Cardiac evaluations of pediatric candidates for OLT should be tailored to the underlying cause of cirrhosis. Inherited metabolic liver disorders rank second behind biliary atresia as an indication for OLT in children, so possible myocardial involvement should be considered in patients with oxalosis, glycogen storage disease types III and IV, Gaucher's disease, Niemann-Pick disease, Wilson's disease, neonatal iron storage disease, and amyloidosis. The physical examination and diagnostic work-up should focus on cardiac auscultation, the presence or absence of cyanosis (arterial oxygen saturation SpO_2 and Pao_2), or clubbing and transthoracic echocardiography. Detection of a cardiac anomaly may then require cardiac catheterization.

Cardiac function in adults with cirrhosis has been extensively investigated, but there is little information available on children. A study of 22 children with cirrhosis compared with a control group of healthy age- and gender-matched children (mean age, 4.1 ± 3.5 years) reported that pediatric OLT candidates have normal LV systolic function unless their heart was primarily involved in the underlying disease. In advanced liver failure, LV systolic function may be impaired. These children also had increased systolic LV posterior wall thickness, which may reflect LV hypertrophy and impaired diastolic function. LV ejection fraction is usually normal or increased at rest in adults with cirrhosis unaccompanied by ascites (Grose et al., 1995; Laffi et al., 1997). The presence of ascites adversely affects cardiac function in adults (Valeriano et al., 2000). In contrast, most

pediatric patients with ascites have normal LV systolic function. Cyanosis is not a reliable sign of hypoxemia in children because of changes caused by crying, anemia, and jaundice. Clubbing in patients with chronic liver disease is a common finding, with a prevalence ranging from 23% to 32% (Ozcay et al., 2002). Given the physiologic stresses inherent in liver transplantation surgery, cardiac problems may emerge perioperatively that contribute to significant morbidity and mortality in patients with cirrhosis and mild or latent cardiomyopathy (Myers and Lee, 2000).

Pulmonary Evaluation

Patients with FHF have varying degrees of pulmonary impairment, including normal Pao_2 and reduced diffusion capacity of the lung for CO (D_Lco), significant arterial hypoxemia, HPS, portopulmonary hypertension, and preexisting lung disease. It is not known whether the high-risk pediatric patient scheduled for liver transplantation surgery can be identified by obtaining values for forced expiratory volume at 1 second (FEV_1), D_Lco, and Pao_2. Investigative studies include chest radiography, pulmonary function studies, a high-resolution CT lung scan, contrast echocardiography, a technetium-99m radionuclide scan, arterial blood gas measurements, and a multiple inert gas elimination technique (MIGET) study when indicated.

Cirrhosis affects the pulmonary circulation, lung parenchyma, and pleural spaces. Reduced alveolar-capillary diffusion (D_Lco) may be seen in the absence of significant hypoxemia, especially in patients with hepatitis C virus (HCV) cirrhosis. This anatomic derangement of the alveolar-capillary membrane worsens with disease progression, with the measured D_Lco becoming abnormal at less than 80% of predicted value. A reduced diffusion capacity may persist up to 15 months after transplantation (Ewert et al., 1999). Of interest, the Hepatitis C Association supports a no-smoking policy for teens and adults, as smoking has been determined to be an independent risk factor associated with elevated ALT levels among anti-HCV-seropositive patients (Wang et al., 2002; Hezode et al., 2003).

Mild Arterial Hypoxemia. Mild arterial hypoxemia is common in patients with cirrhosis and primarily caused by a decrease in functional residual capacity (FRC) and total lung capacity (ascites, pleural effusions), impaired diffusion capacity, and pulmonary arteriovenous shunting (Liu and Lee, 1999). In advanced liver diseases, ventilation-perfusion ($\dot{V}/\dot{Q}$) defect is an important cause of hypoxemia. The arterial blood gas analysis with the patient standing and breathing 100% Fio_2 is of particular importance, because severely hypoxemic patients with at least a moderate response to breathing 100% oxygen on standing ($Pao_2 > 150$ mm Hg) are thought to have an adequate pulmonary reserve and may be safely oxygenated intraoperatively (Krowka et al., 1997; Mohamed et al., 2002). Unresponsive patients should be suspected of having a fixed shunt, and transplantation should be delayed pending further evaluation.

Hepatopulmonary Syndrome. Hepatopulmonary syndrome was once considered a contraindication to transplantation, but now it is considered an indication for early liver transplantation, as there is no successful long-term medical treatment. Patients typically present with progressive exertional dyspnea and hypoxemia. HPS is characterized by the triad of chronic liver disease, hypoxemia, and intrapulmonary shunting in the absence of primary cardiac or pulmonary disease. The incidence in the pediatric patient population is unknown. The pathologic defects causing arterial hypoxemia include intrapulmonary vascular dilation resulting from dilated precapillaries, direct arteriovenous communications, portopulmonary communication, and pleural arteriovenous malformations. This results in decreased oxygen diffusion into the dilated vessels, along with decreased intrapulmonary transit time and decreased hypoxic pulmonary vasoconstriction. This is not a true anatomic shunt, as the patient with the more common type I lesion demonstrates a significant Pao_2 response to 100% oxygen. Appropriate preoperative evaluation should include a chest radiograph, an arterial blood gas measurement with the patient breathing room air and then 100% Fio_2, and one of several imaging techniques: perfusion lung scanning, contrast-enhanced (microbubble) transthoracic echocardiography, lung scintiscan, and, rarely, pulmonary angiography (which identifies type I O_2 reactive versus type II O_2 nonreactive lesions). With liver transplantation, HPS is reversible (Liang et al., 2001), but regression of vascular abnormalities in patients with true anatomic shunts and those with marked precapillary dilation and evidence of poor response to supplemental oxygenation is not predictable (Lange and Stoller, 1995). Treatment of HPS type II presents a dilemma, although liver transplantation with concomitant lung transplantation is a possible choice (Yuan et al., 2003).

Portopulmonary Hypertension. Pulmonary arterial hypertension as a consequence of liver dysfunction is termed portopulmonary hypertension (PPH). This is a pulmonary vasoproliferative and vasoconstrictive process leading to pulmonary hypertension (increased peripheral vascular resistance and normal PCWP or LV end-diastolic pressure) and right heart failure frequently not reversible by liver transplantation. This disorder is uncommon (20% of patients with cirrhosis of the liver), and its existence in the pediatric population is not well described. How rapidly PPH can develop varies, as reports indicate anywhere from 3 weeks to 5 years. Remarkably, a review of published PPH cases through 1999 documented that 65% of diagnoses were first recognized during the liver transplantation procedure (Krowka et al., 2004). The clinical presentation is subtle and includes exertional dyspnea, fatigue, ankle edema, chest pain, and syncope. Arterial hypoxemia is reported in 80% of patients with moderate to severe disease, with an increased alveolar-arterial oxygen gradient, reduced diffusion capacity, and accentuated respiratory alkalosis (Kuo et al., 1997; Cotton et al., 2002). Transthoracic contrast-enhanced echocardiography is the screening procedure of choice, with right heart catheterization the gold standard for making the diagnosis and assessing right ventricular function. The best prognosis is in patients with mild symptoms, preserved right heart function, and pulmonary arteries responsive to vasodilator therapy. Treatment options include inhaled nitric oxide, sildenafil (Viagra), calcium channel blockers, anticoagulation, digoxin, diuretics, supplemental oxygen, and IV prostacyclin. The significance of this disease entity is its high perioperative morbidity and mortality in patients undergoing OLT. The available data indicate a perioperative mortality of greater than 70% with a mean pulmonary artery pressure of 45 mm Hg or higher, and up to 100% if the mean pressure is greater than 50 mm Hg at the time of transplan-

tation. The national liver transplantation database reports an overall mortality perioperatively of 36%. The key to survival is preserved right ventricular function. Even after OLT, however, the pulmonary vascular abnormalities may progress unless long-term pulmonary vasodilator therapy is instituted.

Pulmonary involvement in the pediatric patient with α_1-antitrypsin deficiency or cystic fibrosis is not uncommon. A1AT deficiency is also associated with cirrhosis and primary liver cancer and may be associated with coexisting obstructive lung disease. Therefore, appropriate assessment should be obtained in this particular group of patients with liver failure.

Renal Evaluation

Renal dysfunction in conjunction with worsening hepatic function is common. Acute renal failure requiring hemodialysis is a strong predictor of mortality in these patients. Bartosh and colleagues (1997) reported abnormal renal function in one third of children after liver transplantation, with acute renal failure requiring dialysis (in 6.2%) being a predictor of a high mortality rate (85%). The etiology of renal insufficiency in the patient with ESLD is usually multifactorial. Possible causes include hepatorenal syndrome, disturbances of salt and water clearance, acute tubular necrosis, renal pathology associated with the underlying liver diseases, and diminished intravascular volume causing prerenal azotemia. Exposure to nephrotoxic drugs such as IV contrast dyes, aminoglycosides, or nonsteroidal antiinflammatory agents may also contribute to ATN.

Urine sodium handling is an important variable during evaluations. Both prerenal azotemia and hepatorenal syndrome are characterized by normal urinary sediment, very low urine sodium concentrations (<10 mEq/L), azotemia, and oliguria; it is therefore important to exclude hypovolemia. Specifically, hepatorenal syndrome does not respond to a fluid challenge with diuresis, whereas the expected response in the patient with prerenal azotemia is diuresis and a subsequent decrease in the serum creatinine and urea nitrogen levels. ATN tends to be salt wasting at its initial presentation, with urine sodium concentrations characteristically greater than 20 mEq/L. An important diagnostic test is the FENa, which also aids in the distinction between these two disease processes (FENa $\le$ 1% for HRS and prerenal azotemia, and greater than 1% for ATN). Obtaining an accurate GFR using creatinine clearance rate values in patients with cirrhosis and ascites may give spurious results, as GFR measurements may range from high values to those diagnostic of end-stage renal disease despite the presence of a normal serum creatinine level (Papadakis and Arieff, 1987).

Renal ultrasonography is a simple (noninvasive), useful adjunct in the evaluation of azotemia. Kidney size and structural abnormalities should be ascertained for evidence of obstructive uropathy. If a renal biopsy demonstrates irreversible renal disease, a combined liver and kidney transplantation should be considered.

Prerenal azotemia caused by hypovolemia usually resolves with judicious volume replacement. ATN is usually self-limited, with resolution in 4 to 6 weeks with appropriate support. However, the hepatorenal syndrome is usually not reversible without liver transplantation (Gonwa et al., 1989).

Surgical Technique

The technique used for liver transplantation in children has evolved over the past two decades and varies greatly between different centers, but the physiologic changes that occur during the procedure can be divided into four distinct stages. Here, we review the operative considerations during each stage, and a little later, the anesthesia management during each stage will be discussed. In general, open communication between the surgical and anesthesia teams is essential to avoid difficulty in the progression between the different stages. See related video online at www.expertconsult.com.

Stage I: Preanhepatic Stage

Stage I begins at the time of incision and, from an operative standpoint, is dominated by the careful dissection of the liver from surrounding structures. In reoperative cases, this stage can be of considerable length and can involve a significant amount of blood loss because of the presence of portal hypertension and collateralized mesenteric venous circulation. Meticulous dissection of the hilum is imperative in this stage, as preservation of the vascular inflow to the new liver is crucial to successful transplantation. The adequacy of the flow in the native hepatic artery and portal vein is assessed at this point, and if flow is believed to be inadequate, several techniques can be used either to augment flow in the native vessels or to bypass them altogether. Sufficient portal flow is a requisite to successful reperfusion of the liver. In cases of inadequate portal flow, the vein is dissected to the level of the confluence of the superior mesenteric vein and the splenic vein. Major collaterals shunting blood away from the portal vein are ligated, including the left gastric vein. If flow remains poor, a careful search for collaterals from the splenic vein to the renal vein is undertaken and these are ligated if present. In some cases, the portal vein is relatively atretic in the hilum, but the flow and caliber of the vein dramatically improve at the level of the confluence. In such cases, extension grafts of donor iliac vein can be anastomosed at the level of the confluence. If flows are still inadequate for inflow, the superior mesenteric vein (SMV) should be carefully dissected below the level of the middle colic vein. This thin-walled vein is often surrounded by multiple collateral vessels, requiring meticulous dissection to avoid significant blood loss. An appropriately oriented vein graft is then anastamosed in an end-to-side manner with the SMV, and this can be tunneled through the transverse mesocolon to the hepatic hilum. The hepatic arterial inflow is then assessed for adequacy. If the native hepatic artery is diminutive, an aortic graft is often used to deliver arterial flow from the infrarenal aorta to the hepatic artery of the donor liver. It can be expected that hemodynamic changes will be encountered during the several minutes of aortic occlusion needed to fashion an end-to-side anastomosis between an appropriate arterial conduit and the native infrarenal aorta.

The second portion of stage I entails the dissection of the inferior vena cava (IVC), culminating in the hepatectomy. This can be performed in two ways. The standard complete hepatectomy (Starzl et al., 1984; Starzl and Iwatsuki, 1987) (Fig. 28-3) is performed with complete excision of the retrohepatic vena cava along with the liver. The alternative approach is the one primarily used for the pediatric patient: the "piggyback" hepatectomy (Tzakis et al., 1989). With the standard technique, during stage I, the infrahepatic cava is circumferentially dissected with careful control of adrenal vasculature, and the suprarenal cava is prepared for clamping. Similarly, the suprahepatic cava is isolated. The standard procedure requires careful preparation for complete caval occlusion. IV infusions should be limited to the tributaries of the superior vena cava (SVC), as those infused below the diaphragm encounter upstream obstruction once the IVC is clamped. Most children tolerate complete caval occlusion well; however, the surgical team should always perform a brief test clamp before structures are divided to allow proper fluid resuscitation to begin. If hemodynamic stability is not achieved with clamping, the use of VVB to augment preload during caval clamping should be considered (see later). Although the standard hepatectomy generally affords some usefulness in tumor cases and can be done relatively quickly, excision of the native cava requires a separate, lower caval anastomosis to be performed prior to reperfusion, possibly extending the warm ischemic time and adding an additional site of potential complication.

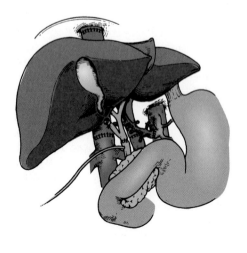

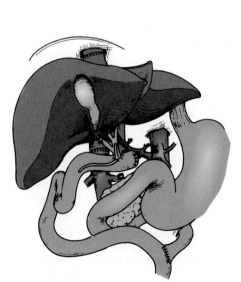

■ **FIGURE 28-3.** Biliary tract reconstruction with choledochojejunostomy, using a Roux-en-Y limb. *(From Starzl TE, Iwatsuki S, VanThiel DH, et al: Evolution of liver transplantation,* Hepatology *2:614, 1982.)*

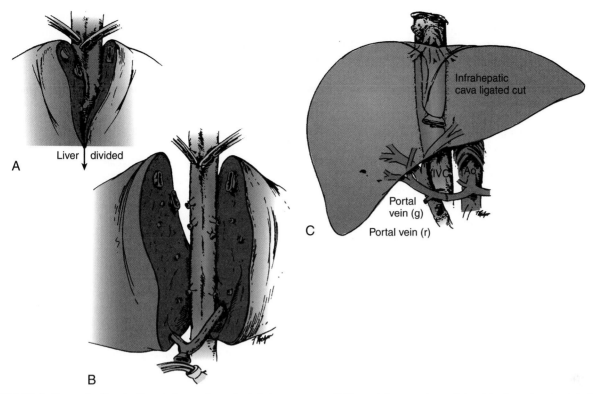

A   Liver | divided

B

C   Infrahepatic cava ligated cut

Portal vein (g)

Portal vein (r)

■ **FIGURE 28-4.** The native liver is dissected away from the inferior vena cava (IVC), and the vascular pedicle of the hepatic veins is isolated. The native liver, after being devascularized, may then be transected to allow intraparenchymal exposure of the hepatic veins (**A** and **B**). The final appearance of the recipient liver, with the native IVC intact and the confluence of the recipient's hepatic veins at the suprahepatic cava, being anastomosed to the donor's intact IVC (**C**). *(From Tzakis A, Todo S, Starzl TE: Orthotopic liver transplantation with preservation of the inferior vena cava,* Ann Surg *210:649, 1989.)*

The piggyback hepatectomy (Tzakis et al., 1989) (Fig. 28-4) involves careful dissection of the liver from the retrohepatic vena cava with preservation of the native vena cava. Briefly, the hepatic veins connecting the posterior liver and the cava are isolated and divided, allowing the liver to be lifted off the vena cava. The main hepatic veins are also circumferentially dissected and readied for clamping. Although the piggyback procedure can take some additional time, avoidance of caval division and the need for one less anastomosis makes it an attractive option in children. Hemodynamic instability is usually insignificant because of the retroperitoneal collateralization of vessels with the azygous system. However significant blood loss can occur with accidental injury to the vena cava, the short hepatic veins, or the main hepatic veins. Although complete caval occlusion is not needed, partial obstruction of the cava generally occurs and can result in some instability (Moreno-Gonzalez et al., 2003).

Stage I is completed with the removal of the native liver. This requires occlusion and division of the portal vein in the hilum (usually at the level of the bifurcation) and subsequent clamping of the hepatic veins in the piggyback technique or the division of the suprahepatic and infrahepatic venae cavae in standard cases. Immediately on ligation of the hepatic artery and removal of the liver, the anhepatic stage begins. In general, there is no value in correcting coagulation defects in this stage, as most of this correction will immediately be subject to extensive fibrinolysis associated with allograft reperfusion. In addition, as inflow structures are occluded at this point, formation of intravascular thrombi is a realistic concern.

Stage II: Anhepatic Stage

Stage II is a crucial time in pediatric transplantation, and errors made during this relatively brief period can significantly alter the patient's course. From a surgical standpoint, the anhepatic stage begins with creation of an upper caval cuff to sew by invagination to the donor suprahepatic cava. This is accomplished by careful occlusion of the cava just above the level of the confluence of the hepatic veins. In the standard operation, the entire suprahepatic cava is clamped and the anastomosis is between the donor and the entire recipient suprahepatic vena cava. In the piggyback method, a clamp is placed just above the level of the hepatic veins, only partially occluding the vena cava. A common cuff of the three ostia of the hepatic veins is then created and prepared for anastomosis with the upper cava of the donor liver. Once the upper caval anastomosis is completed, in standard cases, a separate anastomosis is performed between the infrahepatic cava of the donor liver and the suprarenal vena cava of the recipient. Once the vena cava has been addressed, a vascular anastomosis is fashioned between the portal vein and the mesenteric inflow vessel of the recipient (either the native portal vein or a mesenteric vein graft).

Stage II is completed with the resumption of flow to the hepatic allograft by either the hepatic artery (HA) or the portal vein (PV), or by both vessels. Most often it is with the portal vein only. Anesthesia management in the second stage represents a careful preparation for the instability associated with reperfusion. Concerns about hyperkalemia, acidosis, and hemodynamic lability should all be addressed during the terminal portion of the second stage. Close communication between the surgical and anesthesia teams accomplishes a smooth transition through graft reperfusion. Stage II is also the proper time to administer immunosuppressive dosages of corticosteroids.

Stage III: Reperfusion Stage

Surgical considerations early after hepatic reperfusion focus on the rapid achievement of necessary surgical hemostasis. The initial attempt at hemostasis should be judicious, as relatively severe coagulopathy is the rule before the allograft function recovers from the stress of ischemia and reperfusion. Careful rotation of the liver should allow a rapid assessment of the caval and portal anastomoses, and, once immediate hemostasis is achieved and the patient is stabilized, attention can be turned to the hepatic arterial anastomosis. Because the vessels used in pediatric liver transplantation are small, this anastomosis is often time consuming and can involve the use of either the native hepatic artery or an aortic graft as inflow. Maintenance of an adequate perfusion pressure and avoidance of procoagulants is imperative to the success of this anastomosis. Some centers also employ low dosages of IV anticoagulants during this stage. Once hepatic arterial inflow is established, it is evaluated with intraoperative Doppler ultrasound.

The second portion of stage III (sometimes referred to as stage IV) involves the establishment of biliary continuity. In adults and larger children, this can be performed with a standard duct-to-duct anastomosis. In smaller children and in patients with diseased native bile ducts, creation of a biliary-enteric anastomosis is required. Although several possibilities exist, this is generally achieved with a Roux-en-Y limb of jejunum, and either the hepatic or the common bile duct of the donor. With the newly implanted denervated liver, optimal hepatic arterial flow is essential as the biliary system now becomes 100% of its blood supply from the HA. Careful surgical technique is imperative in this stage to avoid biliary and enteric leaks, which can lead to significant morbidity and mortality in both the early and late postoperative stages.

The final consideration in stage III involves abdominal closure. Because of the greater donor-to-recipient size ratios in pediatric liver transplantation, accidental creation of an intraabdominal compartment syndrome is possible and must be avoided. In addition to the reperfusion-associated inflammation of the allograft, visceral edema from mesenteric venous clamping and tissue edema often makes closure difficult. Even slight increases in abdominal pressure and associated hemodynamic instability can cause allograft vascular thrombosis in the early postoperative period. Careful attention should be paid to changes in ventilatory compliance, peak airway pressure, and hemodynamics with abdominal closure, and any significant changes should be rapidly communicated to the surgical team. Abdominal closure is often achieved with temporary prosthetic mesh, with gradual closure over several days after careful diuresis and diminished edema. Indeed, temporary closure of skin alone, leaving a large ventral hernia, is often needed. Formal closure of fascia, often requiring component separation and use of prosthetic mesh, is often deferred for several months, even up to 1 year after the transplantation.

Venovenous Bypass

The routine use of VVB during the anhepatic phase of OLT, with or without preservation of the cava, remains controversial. In early experiments of OLT in a noncirrhotic dog model, it was discovered that clamping of the portal vein or IVC resulted in death of the animal within 30 minutes (Shaw et al., 1985). Although it was later found that most patients can tolerate caval and portal vein clamping remarkably well, Shaw and colleagues (1984) reported a 10% intraoperative mortality due to hemodynamic instability in adults during the anhepatic phase. Therefore, a bypass system was developed consisting of heparin-bonded tubing and a centripetal-vortex pump, allowing cannulation of the femoral and portal veins and diversion of mesenteric and IVC blood to the SVC through the subclavian or axillary veins (Griffith et al., 1985) (Fig. 28-5). There are no published randomized clinical trials of specific outcomes to evaluate its potential benefits.

It is difficult to use VVB in patients weighing less than 40 or 45 pounds (~20 kg) (Shaw et al., 1984, 1985). The prerequisite VVB blood flow is usually 20% to 40% of the cardiac output, or greater than 1 L/min (Griffith et al., 1985). As patients are not heparinized, the extremely low-flow states (<500 to 700 mL/min) that result in children weighing less than 20 kg would predispose to almost certain formation of emboli. Despite these findings, VVB still has some specific value in pediatric liver transplantation—notably in larger children with FHF or in older pediatric recipients who are being used as donors for living-donor domino transplantations.

Anesthesia Management

Anesthesia management can be categorized into four distinct stages corresponding to the four surgical stages previously described. Thus, an understanding of the pathophysiologic changes that occur in each stage of the surgery allows the anesthesiologist to anticipate and appropriately diagnose, manage,

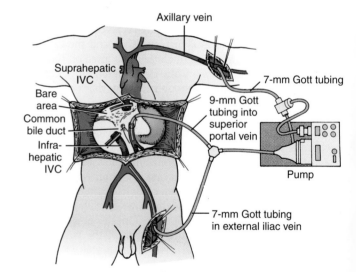

■ **FIGURE 28-5.** This technique was developed to augment cardiac output and diminish vascular congestion during the anhepatic stage of the surgery. Note the placement of the cannulas, joined by a connector, into the portal vein and the femoral veins. Blood drained from the splanchnic and systemic venous systems is then returned to the right heart through the axillary vein with the aid of a pump. *(From Kang Y, Gelman S: Liver transplantation. In Gelman S, editor: Anesthesia and organ transplantation, Philadelphia, 1987, Saunders, pp 139–185.)*

and treat the cardiovascular, hematologic, metabolic, and other derangements encountered throughout the surgery (Borland et al., 1985; Carlier et al., 1987; Kang and Gelman, 1987; Lindop and Farman, 1987; Carton et al., 1994a, 1994b). Liver transplantation in the pediatric patient is very similar to that in adults from a technical point of view, but there are distinct differences in transfusion requirements and strategies for minimizing blood loss, perioperative coagulation, hemodynamic consequences of caval clamping and reperfusion of the liver, monitoring, vascular access, incidence of thrombosis of the hepatic artery, retransplantation rate, and postoperative pain relief.

Induction and Maintenance of Anesthesia

Liver transplantation has essentially become a semiurgent or elective procedure. The recipient is premedicated with oral, IV, or intranasal midazolam. In the operating room, standard monitors are placed and the patient is preoxygenated. Patients without serious cardiac disease or multisystem organ failure can tolerate routine induction of anesthesia followed by endotracheal intubation. Rapid-sequence IV induction includes atropine (0.01 to 0.02 mg/kg); a sedative hypnotic agent using thiopental (3 to 5 mg/kg), propofol (2 to 5 mg/kg), etomidate (0.2 to 0.3 mg/kg), or ketamine (1 to 2 mg/kg); and rocuronium (1.0 mg/kg) or succinylcholine (1 to 2 mg/kg). The airway is secured with an oral endotracheal tube (preferably cuffed) with tincture of benzoin and adhesive tape. Placement of an uncuffed tracheal tube of insufficient diameter may result in inadequate alveolar ventilation (especially as chest compliance is reduced during surgery by upper abdominal retraction), tissue edema of the lung parenchyma, surgeons accidentally leaning on the chest wall, and placement of a large liver graft. Additionally, the postoperative risk for silent aspiration must be considered.

Succinylcholine has traditionally been used for intubation in pediatric patients at risk for aspiration. Today, this practice is controversial because of its black-box warning. Because it is difficult to identify which patients are at risk, it is recommended that the use of succinylcholine in children should be reserved for emergency intubation or for when immediate securing of an airway is necessary, as succinylcholine has a faster onset (30 to 60 seconds) than other muscle relaxants. Liver disease, especially if chronic and severe, may be associated with decreased plasma levels of pseudocholinesterases, which will result in prolongation of the duration of action of succinylcholine or drugs requiring ester hydrolysis for degradation (Khoury et al., 1987). However, this effect is of little clinical significance when one considers the duration of perioperative ventilation and the dilutional effect of blood replacement during massive intraoperative bleeding.

Preoperative hyperkalemia may be seen in patients with episodes of acute rejection, sepsis, or poor renal function, or in those taking oral cyclosporine who have chronic rejection or hepatic artery thrombosis. Administration of succinylcholine may increase the serum potassium concentration by 0.5 to 0.7 mmol/L, predisposing the patient with already high serum potassium levels to cardiac arrhythmias and hemodynamic instability. ECG abnormalities and arrhythmias typically do not appear until the serum potassium level is greater than 6.5 mEq/L. Common ECG signs include widened QRS, peaked T-waves, prolonged PR interval, loss of P waves, and atrial systole. ST-segment elevation may mimic acute myocardial infarction. First-degree block may ultimately lead to complete heart block. Late signs include prolonged QRS complex that can lead to sine wave ventricular arrhythmia, ventricular fibrillation, or asystole. Treatment for succinylcholine-induced hyperkalemia focuses on direct cardiac antagonism, intracellular shift, and removal of potassium from the body. Arrhythmia and hypotension are treated with either calcium gluconate or calcium chloride. Intracellular shifting of potassium can be accomplished by administering sodium bicarbonate, glucose, and insulin and hyperventilation ($Paco_2$, 25 to 30 mm Hg). Kayexalate, furosemide, peritoneal dialysis, or hemodialysis can decrease the total body potassium level.

Alternatively, using a relatively large dosage of a nondepolarizing muscle relaxant (e.g., rocuronium) permits securing the airway rapidly without placing the patient at risk for hyperkalemia. Cisatracurium is the ideal drug for patients with end-stage liver or kidney disease, as it undergoes spontaneous breakdown at physiologic temperature and pH (Hoffmann elimination), as well as ester hydrolysis. However, the dosage required for a rapid onset of action may result in hypotension. In patients with hepatorenal syndrome, nondepolarizing muscle relaxants should be administered cautiously and titrated to effect. Muscle relaxants requiring significant renal excretion include pancuronium (40%), doxacurium (30%), and pipecuronium (38%). Vecuronium and pancuronium also have 3-hydroxy metabolites, which accumulate in renal failure. The 3-hydroxy metabolite of vecuronium is 50% as potent as the parent compound, and that of pancuronium has two-thirds the potency of the parent compound. Muscle relaxants that are metabolized in the liver include pancuronium, vecuronium, rocuronium, and pipecuronium. Vecuronium and rocuronium also have significant biliary excretion. Pancuronium has an increased volume of distribution, prolonged elimination half-life, and decreased plasma clearance in patients with cirrhosis. Therefore, these patients may need more pancuronium initially to achieve muscle relaxation, and they have a prolonged recovery of blockade between doses (Duvaldestin et al., 1978). In patients with biliary obstruction, the initial dosage of pancuronium required is unchanged, but the duration of action of each dose is similarly prolonged (Duvaldestin et al., 1978). This may be advantageous because the operative procedure is lengthy and ventilation is usually required for at least 24 hours postoperatively.

Following induction, the patient is positioned on the operating table supine with the arms abducted and elbows flexed. It is essential to keep the patient covered, warm, and dry. Strategies include the use of a warming blanket, heated humidified gases, or IV fluid warmers; wrapping the extremities; mylar foil wrapping; and use of a thick cotton mattress pad below with a U-shaped surround Bair Hugger forced-air warming device. Care should be taken to avoid stretch injury of the brachial plexus or pressure necrosis of the occiput, ears, heels, sacrum, or elbows. After the induction of anesthesia, additional monitoring is established, using end-tidal CO_2, rectal and esophageal temperature probes, an esophageal stethoscope, an indwelling urinary catheter, a peripheral nerve stimulator, and systemic arterial and CVP cannulas. Access to arterial pressure monitoring above the diaphragm is ideal because cross-clamping of the abdominal aorta may be necessary during the hepatic arterial anastomosis. A femoral arterial catheter can also be used during surgery if there is concern about the accuracy of the radial arterial blood pressure (Kamath et al., 2001). One or two additional large IV cannulas (preferably 20- or 18-gauge) are then inserted in the upper extremities, either percutaneously or by surgical cutdown. The use of VVB in larger children may preclude use of the left arm for venous access. If vascular access in the arms is difficult to obtain, the lower extremities may be used, with the understanding that during the anhepatic stage, venous return to the heart depends on collateral flow or VVB. A central venous catheter is placed in the external or internal jugular vein. In smaller children, the surgeon will often insert a Hickman catheter (large-bore, double-lumen central venous line). The use of a sheath-type catheter in larger children allows the rapid infusion of large volumes of blood components and, in rare circumstances, the insertion of a flow-directed, balloon-tipped pulmonary artery catheter. Technical difficulties in placing a pulmonary artery catheter and subsequent displacement or migration by surgical maneuvers generally preclude its routine use in pediatric patients.

The patient is ventilated with a tidal volume and respiratory rate adjusted to maintain a normal end-tidal CO_2 and arterial CO_2 level of 35 to 40 mm Hg. Tidal volume and minute ventilation can be improved by using a pressure-limited mode. Air oxygen is used with an inspiratory oxygen concentration sufficient to maintain adequate oxygenation. A PEEP of 5 cm H_2O is routinely added because progressive atelectasis is common. Nitrous oxide is avoided because of its sympathomimetic effects, its propensity to cause bowel distention (which may make surgical exposure and closure of the abdomen difficult), and its limiting effect on increasing the inspiratory concentration of oxygen.

During anesthesia, all factors inducing arterial hypotension should be avoided. General anesthesia and surgery decrease hepatic blood flow and jeopardize oxygen supply to the liver. Intraoperative reductions in the arterial blood pressure and cardiac output decrease portal blood flow. Contributing factors include anesthesia drugs (inhalational anesthetics, vasodilators, β-blockers, α-1-agonists, histamine receptor-2 (H_2) blockers, and vasopressin), hypovolemia, ventilatory mode, hypoxemia, hypercarbia, and acidosis. Surgical manipulation in the right upper quadrant can reduce hepatic blood flow up to 60% from sympathetic activation or direct compression of the vena cava and splanchnic vessels. Compensatory vasodilation of the hepatic artery in response to decreased portal inflow is diminished by volatile anesthetic agents in a dosage-related manner (and absent in a denervated liver), and consequently blood flow becomes pressure dependent. Isoflurane has the least detrimental effect on hepatic blood flow. A simultaneous decrease in the liver's metabolic demand tends to balance the oxygen supply-uptake ratio. A study of hepatic circulation in pigs during surgical stress and anesthesia suggested that fentanyl and light isoflurane provided adequate hepatic oxygen supply, whereas anesthesia with concentrations of isoflurane that decreased blood pressure more than 30%, or with halothane in any concentrations studied, resulted in inadequate hepatic oxygen supply (Gelman et al., 1987). Matsumoto and colleagues (1987) examined the effects of various anesthetic agents on hepatic oxygen supply and hepatic oxygen consumption in the presence of hypoxia. Their results showed that during exposure to mild hypoxia, a dosage of isoflurane less than the minimum alveolar concentration (sub-MAC) maintained the relation of hepatic oxygen supply to hepatic oxygen consumption better than thiopental, halothane, or enflurane.

When administering drugs to patients with chronic liver disease, all dosages should be decreased and carefully titrated until the desired effect is achieved. Current practice is to administer

isoflurane alone or in combination with small dosages of fentanyl. The anesthesia management protocol used at the Children's Hospital of Pittsburgh, and the anesthesia management problems encountered during the four stages of the surgery, can be found online at www.expertconsult.com.

Physiologic Alterations during Liver Transplantation

Cardiovascular Changes

During stage I, hypotension results from major fluid shifts, bleeding, and ionized hypocalcemia (Jawan et al., 2003). Transient decreases in MAP are not unusual in this stage and result from surgical manipulation of the liver and compression of the IVC, which transiently preclude venous return to the heart. Drainage of ascites may result in hypotension if the patient is not adequately hydrated prior to incision of the peritoneum. Factors contributing to blood loss include adhesions from prior operations, coagulopathy (factor deficiency, low platelet count, abnormal fibrinogen, or disseminated intravascular coagulation), portal hypertension and collateral venous circulation, and lack of surgical hemostasis (especially a laceration to the IVC). Placement of the suprahepatic caval clamp may be associated with arrhythmia and hypoxemia because of acute right ventricular outflow tract obstruction, as the pericardium and a portion of the RV may be included in the clamp. Hypotension that is unresponsive to IV pressors should raise suspicions of absolute or relative hypovolemia (limited preload caused by vascular clotting or torsion of the liver on its vascular pedicle), acidosis, sepsis, or vasoparesis.

During stage II, classic OLT requires a trial of portal vein and IVC clamping. The hemodynamic response is characterized by a decrease in cardiac output, CVP, and PAP and compensatory increase in heart rate and SVR (Eyraud et al., 2002). Hemodynamic instability may result from decreased venous return (modified by VVB or piggyback technique) and insufficient physiologic compensation by the patient for this acute change. Therapeutic strategies include colloid or crystalloid boluses, and vasopressor support with dopamine or norepinephrine (phenylephrine or epinephrine). The goal is to maintain the lowest filling pressures compatible with an acceptable MAP in anticipation of an increase in PAP with removal of the caval and portal vein clamps. Pulmonary hypertension may result because of an increase in venous return from the gut and lower extremities and reactive changes in PVR with the release of vasoactive hormones that are recirculated systemically. The donor liver is flushed with crystalloid or colloid, or by backwashing (backflushing) the liver. The procedure for backwashing involves insertion of a red rubber cannula into the recipient/donor IVC, and then removal of the clamp from the portal vein allows washing of the liver with autologous blood retrograde from the portal vein through the donor liver, exiting through the cannula into a stainless steel graduated cylinder. If the patient become immediately and dramatically hypotensive, the surgeon must be notified immediately. Hypotension associated with this maneuver can be ameliorated with the prophylactic administration of phenylephrine or epinephrine boluses, gentle fluid administration, or transfusion of packed RBCs if the hematocrit is low. The elimination of air bubbles, hyperkalemic preservation solution, hormones, or other "evil humors" has been credited for decreasing the incidence, in adult patients, of subsequent reperfusion syndrome that may occur with reperfusion of the liver (Fukuzawa et al., 1994). The goal for warm ischemia time is usually less than 60 minutes, so managing hypotension and preparing for reperfusion occurs over a relatively short period. Reactivation of HCV has been shown to be less if the warm ischemia time can be kept under 35 minutes, which shortens the target time for completing this portion of the operation even further (Clavien et al., 2004).

During stage III, profound hemodynamic instability may occur immediately after graft reperfusion. This instability includes severe hypotension, bradycardia, supraventricular and ventricular arrhythmias, variable cardiac output, and occasionally cardiac arrest (0% to 0.5%). These changes are caused by recirculation of the residual cold, acidotic, hyperkalemic preservation solution from the donor liver directly into the recipient's heart. The incidence of this postreperfusion syndrome (defined as a decrease in MAP and heart rate > 30% from baseline for at least 1 minute within 5 minutes of reperfusion) in adults may be as high as 30%, and epinephrine boluses are usually required to prevent cardiovascular collapse (Aggarwal et al., 1987). Immediately after reperfusion, LV function may be impaired, and PCWP, CVP, and PAP usually increase with a major decrease in SVR, and transesophageal echocardiogram (TEE) monitoring shows a stable or even decreased LV end-diastolic volume. These contradictory findings may be result from a period of deteriorated LV compliance, or cardioplegia, on reperfusion (Suriani et al., 1996; De Wolf, 1999). The etiology of PRS remains unclear, but it may be caused by the release of vasoactive mediators from the ischemic liver or decompressed portal circulation, changes in the rate of venous return (volume overload), and perhaps an increase in serum potassium. Possible mediators that are highly suspect include nitric oxide and tumor necrosis factor-α, with demonstrably increased levels after graft reperfusion (Nishimura et al., 1993), and xanthine oxidase, a generator of cytotoxic oxygen radicals, which may produce myocardial dysfunction and cellular damage. Vasoactive drugs for pressor support (norepinephrine, epinephrine, dopamine) may be required, and a balance is reached between a lowered MAP and often a very low SVR permitting increased flow to perfusable organs at a lower perfusion pressure. High filling pressures should be avoided, as they may cause congestion of the donor liver, bleeding from surgical sites, and biventricular dysfunction with pulmonary edema. Therapies for reducing filling pressures include limiting IV infusions, furosemide-induced diuresis, vasodilation (IV nitroglycerine or morphine), nitric oxide, or prostaglandin E_1.

Blood Loss, Coagulation, and Hemostasis

During liver transplantation surgery, the effects of fibrinolysis, thrombocytopenia, decreased coagulation factors, and fibrinogen deficiency on clinical bleeding are not always predictable, and transfusion requirements are variable. Portal hypertension with fragile venous collaterals, adhesions from prior operations, and lack of surgical hemostasis contribute to blood loss. Independent predictors of increased transfusion requirements include the severity of liver disease or Child-Pugh classification (especially for those hospitalized for inpatient support), preoperative PT, history of abdominal operations, preoperative hematocrit, and factor V levels. In addition, portal vein hypoplasia, the use of a reduced-size liver graft, and increased operative time make surgery technically challenging (Ozier et al., 1995;

Maurer and Spence, 2004). Usually, the greatest operative blood loss occurs during vascular dissection and the hepatectomy phase (stage II). During this stage, there is a progressive degradation of the coagulation cascade, and a dilutional coagulopathy with a progressive thrombocytopenia. The blood loss can range from 0.5 to 25 times the patient's blood volume (Borland et al., 1985).

Alterations of coagulation in the pediatric patient during OLT have been studied (Kang et al., 1989). Classic hourly monitoring of the PT, activated PTT (aPTT), and platelet counts demonstrates a progressive prolongation of the PT and PTT, as well as a significant decrease of all clotting factors. On graft reperfusion, there may be profound prolongation of the PTT, usually to greater than 100 seconds. Besides the standard coagulation tests (PT, aPTT, fibrinogen, platelets, and D-dimer), the thromboelastogram (TEG) and Sonoclot (coagulation and platelet function analyzer) are used in the evaluation of coagulation. The TEG is performed using whole blood; it assesses clot formation until an endpoint of clot lysis or retraction is determined. TEG findings have correlated with clinical bleeding and can assist in treating intraoperative hemorrhage by identifying the cause of the bleeding diathesis (factor deficiency, fibrinolysis, heparin effect, thrombocytopenia, or platelet dysfunction) (Zuckerman et al., 1981; Kang, 1986) (Fig. 28-6). Abnormalities of the reaction time (r), the alpha angle (a), or the maximum amplitude (MA) may indicate decreased clotting factors, diminished factor VIII and fibrinogen, or diminished platelet function or number, respectively (Kang et al., 1989). In contrast, a short reaction time is indicative of a hypercoagulable state. This has occasionally been observed in patients who have developed thrombosis after graft reperfusion (Kang, 1995a, 1995b; Gologorsky et al., 2001; Planinsic et al., 2004).

Increased fibrinolytic activity is observed in patients with ESLD as a result of increased tissue plasminogen activator activity and reduced synthesis of fibrinolysis inhibitors. Tissue plasminogen activator further increases during the anhepatic stages and peaks immediately after graft reperfusion. Various antifibrinolytic agents have been used to counter this accelerated fibrinolysis (evident immediately on graft reperfusion in up to 80% of patients), but their precise role remains undefined. These include aprotinin, ε-aminocaproic acid (EACA), and tranexamic acid. Aprotinin, a serine protease inhibitor that prevents the lysis of fibrinogen by inhibiting plasmin, kallikrein, and leukocyte elastase, is no longer available. EACA (Kang et al., 1987) and tranexamic acid prevent fibrinolysis by inhibiting plasminogen and plasmin, thus preventing the eventual degradation of fibrin. In addition, a significant heparin effect may be seen immediately on graft reperfusion for up to 30 minutes. This effect is caused by the release of endogenous heparinoids from the liver, as well as residual heparin from the preservation solution. Calcium is an important coenzyme in the coagulation cascade. During the dissection and anhepatic phases of liver transplantation, hypocalcemia may develop, especially when large amounts of fresh frozen plasma have been given. In many transplantation centers, continuous calcium infusions and magnesium supplements are routine therapy.

The approach to blood product replacement in children differs from that in adults because of two important concerns: thrombosis of the hepatic artery and postoperative hypercoagulability. Thrombosis of the hepatic artery is the most common serious complication after liver transplantation in children, so less fresh frozen plasma and platelets are routinely administered.

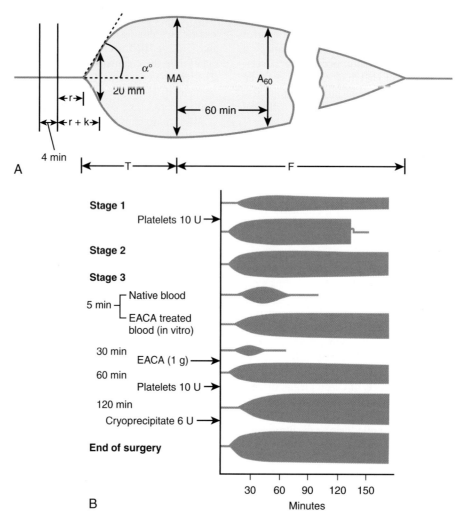

■ **FIGURE 28-6.** Thromboelastogram (TEG). **A,** The normal parameters measured and analyzed for interpretation of the TEG. **B,** The coagulation alterations noted during OLT. Note the elements of low platelets (and the improvement in the maximum amplitude after administration of platelets), and the development of fibrinolysis, which is treated by ε-aminocaproic acid (EACA) and detected early on the TEG (at the time of graft reperfusion). Also, the diminished alpha angle in stage 3 is treated with administration of cryoprecipitate, with noted improvement of coagulation. *(From Kang Y, Gelman S: Liver transplantation. In Gelman S, editor:* Anesthesia and organ transplantation, *Philadelphia, 1987, Saunders, pp 139–185.)*

After reperfusion, the hematocrit should ideally be maintained at 20% to 30% to minimize the increase in blood viscosity and to limit the risk for thrombotic complications (Tisone et al., 1988). Children may be at greater risk for hepatic artery thrombosis than adults because their arteries are smaller, and because of their postoperative hypercoagulable state (Heffron et al., 2003). The incidence of hepatic artery thrombosis has been reported in 15% of the mixed-age; pediatric series (Otte et al., 1990); however, it appears to be directly related to the size of the hepatic artery (smaller arteries and livers from neonates or infants having a higher incidence of this complication) (Mazzaferro et al., 1989; Jurim et al., 1995; Mas et al., 2003; Martin et al., 2004) and to technical complications during the vascular reconstruction. When a split liver is used, thrombosis is relatively rare (5% to 8%) and is similar to the adult rate (Gridelli et al., 2003). Thus, in some institutions, aggressive correction of coagulation is pursued only when there is diffuse bleeding after graft reperfusion or if monitoring reveals fibrinolysis that was not reversed by the new liver. Many transplantation centers use normalization of the PT and platelet count as indicators of recovery of donor

liver graft function. Persistent hypothermia, coagulopathy with bleeding, increased serum lactate, hypocapnia, hyperkalemia, acidosis, absence of bile production, hyperglycemia, renal insufficiency, and hemodynamic instability may suggest suboptimal graft function.

After liver transplantation in children, levels of protein C and antithrombin III decrease to below 50% of normal and stay there for 10 days. These prolonged decreases are not seen in adults. Immediately after surgery, a 10-fold increase in plasminogen activator inhibitor occurs, with a further increase 6 to 9 days later. Therefore, in the immediate postoperative period, between days 4 and 10, children are at increased risk for thrombosis (Harper et al., 1988). To minimize this, anticoagulation therapy has been administered (IV heparin, dextran 40, aspirin, and antithrombin III) (Abengochea et al., 1995). There are also differences in coagulation between the infant and adult. In the normal neonate, there is a deficiency of vitamin K–dependent clotting factors (II, VII, IX, X) for several weeks. Protein C is significantly reduced for at least 6 months (Andrew et al., 1987), and protein S concentrations do not increase to within the normal adult range until 3 months of age (Donaldson et al., 1991). Protein C inhibits the function of factors VIII and V and enhances fibrinolysis, which is enhanced by protein S.

When the child's body weight is greater than 20 kg, use of the rapid infusion system facilitates the rapid replacement of blood products. In this instance, however, blood product replacement is similar to that for an adult. A unit each of RBCs and fresh frozen plasma, and 250 mL of either normal saline solution or neutral pH balanced salt solution (Plasmalyte) is mixed in the cardiotomy reservoir of the rapid infusion system. This mixture mimics whole blood with a hematocrit of 28% to 30%. Blood replacement may occur at a rate of up to 1500 mL/min if needed.

Hypothermia and hypocalcemia are known to contribute to coagulopathy (Kang, 1995a), and they affect platelet function and increase the incidence of fibrinolysis. Thus, temperatures below 35° C are best avoided. Finally, cell salvage may be beneficial in the patient undergoing OLT. Blood recovery of up to 30% is expected, but the need for rapid volume replacement limits its use. In addition, the use of the cell saver is contraindicated in patients with viral or bacterial infections, tumors, or FHF without an identifiable cause of the liver failure. Massive blood transfusion has an associated morbidity of more frequent bouts of sepsis, a prolonged stay in the intensive care unit (ICU), a higher rate of severe CMV infection, and higher rates of graft failure and patient mortality (Maurer and Spence, 2004).

Metabolic Function

Hepatic failure can result in impairment of numerous complex metabolic functions that may significantly impact anesthesia care. The liver plays a critical role in maintaining a normal blood glucose level; hypoglycemia frequently results from failure of gluconeogenesis, insufficient insulin degradation, and a depletion of glycogen stores. Most patients with chronic liver disease are undernourished, and fat stores are diminished with impairment of lipid transport and the integrity of cellular membranes.

Altered Glucose Metabolism

Hypoglycemia is rarely seen except in patients who present with acute FHF or have exhausted their liver glycogen stores. Patients may also be at risk during catecholamine infusions or if they require insulin for the management of hyperkalemia. During the anhepatic phase, several sources of glucose are available to the patient, such as packed RBCs (which contain a significant amount of free glucose: 84 mg/dL by day 35 of storage) (Miller, 2000), 5% dextrose in water (D_5W, used as a carrier for drug infusions), and IV methylprednisolone (used for induction of immunosuppression during the portal anastomosis). Hyperglycemia after graft reperfusion is common because of glucose release from ischemic hepatocytes, steroid-induced insulin resistance, and decreased glucose metabolism in hypothermic patients (DeWolf et al., 1987). Thus, hourly monitoring of blood glucose levels is essential (Fig. 28-7).

Acute Ionized Hypocalcemia and Hypomagnesemia

Ionized hypocalcemia results from the rapid transfusion of large volumes of blood products containing citrate, especially during periods of hypothermia and acidosis. Citrate chelates calcium and magnesium and other divalent cations. Hypotension is the usual consequence and becomes significant at an ionized calcium level

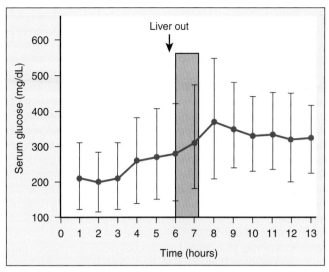

FIGURE 28-7. Glucose levels during liver transplantation, as plotted against time. Mean and standard deviation (SD) values are shown. *Shaded area* represents the anhepatic phase. *(From Borland LM, Roule M, Cook DR: Anesthesia for pediatric orthotopic liver transplantation, Anesth Analg 64:117, 1985.)*

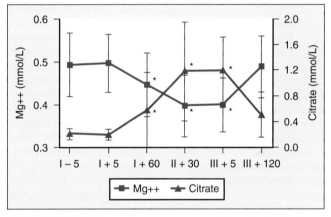

FIGURE 28-8. Changes in magnesium and citrate levels during liver transplantation.

of 0.56 mmol/L, at which point the patient may develop cardiovascular collapse (Marquez et al., 1986; Martin et al., 1990).

The consequence of acute ionized hypomagnesemia (Scott et al., 1996) is not yet apparent, but it may result in a higher incidence of atrial arrhythmias and decreased myocardial contractility (Fig. 28-8).

Replacement of calcium is effective with either calcium chloride or gluconate in equivalent calcium dosages. Administration of calcium chloride in the central catheter may result in transient arrhythmia, but deposition into tissues from an extravasated peripheral catheter will result in severe tissue necrosis. The recipient routinely receives sodium bicarbonate and calcium chloride about 1 minute before reperfusion to counteract anticipated hyperkalemia and hypotension.

Hypokalemia

Hypokalemia is the norm in chronic liver failure. It results from the use of diuretics, altered aldosterone metabolism, and metabolic alkalosis. If ventricular arrhythmias are noted during stages I and II, magnesium replacement is recommended. Potassium replacement is avoided because there is an expected transient twofold to threefold increase in potassium concentration immediately on graft reperfusion. Hypokalemia is common after graft reperfusion, usually as a result of diuresis, receptor stimulation with epinephrine, and uptake of potassium by the new liver (Xia et al., 2006). Cautious replacement during the biliary reconstruction phase is appropriate if the patient has no preexisting renal insufficiency and has evidence of adequate urine output.

Hyperkalemia should be treated aggressively at any point during the surgery. This electrolyte disturbance usually results from massive transfusion of RBCs, which have an estimated potassium content of 76 mEq/L by day 35 of cold storage, or from renal failure (Miller, 2000). The judicious use of diuretics as well as an infusion of glucose and insulin may be of benefit in reducing the potassium load (De Wolf et al., 1993). This is most crucial before revascularization of the donor liver. Postreperfusion hyperkalemia (7 to 12 mEq/L) is transitory, with redistribution occurring in 1 to 2 minutes, which seldom needs pharmacologic intervention other than prophylactic sodium bicarbonate and calcium intravenously (Nakasuji and Bookallil, 2000). Washed RBCs prevent the further development of this problem. When hyperkalemia is life threatening, the use of venovenous hemofiltration or removal of part of the patient's blood volume and washing by the cell saver may be beneficial.

Metabolic acidosis is progressive during OLT and peaks during graft reperfusion. It results from transfusion of blood products and becomes accentuated during the anhepatic stage when liver metabolism of citrate, lactate, and other acids is absent. Whether tissue hypoperfusion is a contributing factor remains unclear; however, this should be balanced by the fact that overall body oxygen consumption is reduced during the anhepatic stage. The threshold for bicarbonate administration is a base deficit (<5 mEq/L). Associated morbidity includes hypernatremia, hypercarbia, and hyperosmolality. Acidosis usually resolves after reperfusion of the graft. Sodium bicarbonate should be administered as indicated and any ongoing problem identified (poor perfusion with lactic acidosis, or delayed primary function or nonfunction of the graft). Metabolic alkalosis is common postoperatively as a result of diuretic therapy and metabolism of citrate or lactate. This may delay weaning of the patient from mechanical ventilation, but it is another useful marker of resumption of hepatocellular function.

Hyponatremia and Hyperosmolarity

Dilutional hyponatremia is common and worrisome at serum sodium levels less than 125 mEq/L. Central pontine myelinolysis (CPM) is a frequently symmetric, noninflammatory demyelinating disorder in the brainstem pons. In at least 10% of patients, demyelination also occurs in extrapontine areas. Clinical manifestations are postoperative confusion or weakness, or a "locked-in" syndrome, after transplantation (Estol et al., 1989; Wszolek et al., 1989). The most frequent findings are delirium, pseudobulbar palsy, and spastic quadriplegia, which may result in permanent neurologic deficits. CPM occurs inconsistently as a complication of severe and prolonged hyponatremia, particularly when the sodium is corrected too rapidly. A study by Singh and coworkers (1994) demonstrated that CPM was present in 29% of postmortem examinations of

adults after liver transplantation. Risk factors included serum sodium less than 120 mEq/L for more than 48 hours, aggressive IV fluid therapy with hypertonic saline solutions, and hypernatremia during treatment.

Empirical data show that CPM is likely to occur when the total perioperative increase in sodium concentration is above 15 to 20 mEq/L (Estol et al., 1989; Yu et al., 2004). In these patients, the choice of crystalloid solution should be Plasmalyte or 0.45% NaCl. Hyperosmolality has also been considered a contributor to the development of CPM. In the presence of either of these metabolic derangements, the judicious use of tris(hydroxymethyl)aminomethane (THAM) is recommended because its osmolality is 308 mOsm/L, whereas that of sodium bicarbonate is 2000 mOsm/L. In addition, the sodium content of bicarbonate buffer is 8.4% compared with 0.9% NaCl in IV solutions.

Temperature Regulation

Surgical procedures that place these patients at risk for unintentional hypothermia involve exposure of large skin, serosal, and mucosal surfaces during lengthy procedures under general anesthesia in a cold operating room, especially with no humidification of gases and with infusion of cold IV fluids. The most significant contributors to hypothermia in the pediatric patient undergoing OLT are radiant and evaporative heat losses. In addition, the use of VVB may result in a temperature loss of 0.5° to 1.0° C when a heat exchanger is not used. Preservation of the donor liver depends on rendering the organ metabolically inert by reducing the core temperature to 4° C with cold preservation techniques. To further extend this cooling period while performing the vascular anastomosis in the recipient, the liver may be wrapped in cold compresses or ice, which will further reduce the core temperature of the patient. With reperfusion, a hypothermia-induced cardiac arrhythmia and arrest may result if the perfusate of the liver is allowed to further cool the sinus node. Modest hypothermia (to 35° C) is well tolerated with minimal effects on coagulation, but platelet dysfunction, fibrinolysis, and bleeding begin to increase in a linear fashion as the core temperature decreases. Mild hypothermia may be beneficial, as a reduction in metabolic oxygen requirements may limit warm ischemia and cerebral and myocardial injury. In pediatric patients, the detrimental physiologic effects of mild hypothermia (32° to 35° C) and the increased risk for infection clearly outweigh these minimal benefits.

Attention should be directed to aggressively maintaining a normal body temperature. This may be achieved by using forced-air warming (Bair Hugger) or raising the ambient temperature of the operating theater. In addition, protective barriers should be strategically placed to prevent the operating room table from becoming wet, because this will result in conductive cooling of the patient. Heating of the humidified gases is also an important maneuver. In some cases, intraperitoneal lavage with warmed irrigation after the completion of the arterial anastomosis can be undertaken to assist in warming. Concerns about hypothermia should be communicated with the surgical team, as hypothermia-induced coagulopathy can result in unnecessary nonsurgical hemorrhage, and time spent in warming maneuvers could result in reduced blood loss and improved hemostasis. In the patient receiving Compath, however, hyperthermia is the norm. In this instance, care should be taken to avoid temperatures of 38° C or higher, as this may serve to augment ischemic reperfusion injury of the graft.

Pulmonary Function

Hypoxemia is common in pediatric patients with ESLD because ascites and pleural effusions cause a decrease in FRC and total lung capacity, impaired diffusion capacity, and pulmonary arteriovenous shunting. After the induction of anesthesia, difficulties in ventilation and oxygenation may occur, and diaphragmatic paralysis can result in an acute restrictive lung effect. The increased alveolar-arterial oxygen gradient usually improves after the abdominal cavity is opened. If relative hypoxemia persists, other causes of venous admixture should be sought.

Factors that may worsen oxygenation during the surgical procedure include clot or air emboli, progression of ARDS, transfusion-related acute lung injury, HPS, and pulmonary edema from excessive fluid administration. Finally, extubation of the patient at the end of the procedure is not recommended, no matter how short the duration of the surgery, because 50% to 55% (McAlister et al., 1993) of patients develop right diaphragmatic paralysis postoperatively and 25% will have pleural effusions, which compromise pulmonary function. The fast-track approach to anesthesia care may reduce the requirement for postoperative mechanical ventilation, but it does not reduce the length of stay in the ICU after liver transplantation (Findlay et al., 2002).

Renal Function

Renal insufficiency, a common finding in patients undergoing OLT, contributes significantly to postoperative morbidity, and it is an independent predictor of postoperative mortality (Gonwa, 2005). The patient who comes to the operating room with hepatorenal syndrome or ATN should not be expected to show improvement of renal function until after the graft functions (McCauley et al., 1990). Information collected by the National Institute of Diabetes and Digestive and Kidney Diseases Liver Transplantation Database support the conclusion that renal insufficiency in patients with FHF and in those requiring preoperative dialysis or liver-kidney transplantation for cirrhosis predicts lower posttransplantation patient and graft survival rates (Brown et al., 1996).

A progressive decline in urine output is expected, with little or none during the anhepatic portion of the surgery without preservation of the IVC or use of VVB. This physiologic alteration has been thought to be secondary to congestion of the kidneys from increased renal venous pressures with total cross-clamping of the infrahepatic IVC (Gunning et al., 1991). Whether the incidence of postoperative renal insufficiency is as frequent when the piggy-back technique is used remains unclear. Thus, the judicious use of the diuretics (mannitol and furosemide) is recommended in the patient who develops oliguria (Polson et al., 1987). It should be noted that furosemide may be ineffective in the patient with a low albumin level (average albumin in the patient with liver failure for OLT is 2.5 to 1.8 mg/dL). Although a renal dosage of dopamine not exceeding 1.5 mcg/kg per min is often recommended, there is no clear benefit from its use as a renal protective agent (Polson et al., 1987; Gray et al., 1991; Swygert et al., 1991; Kellum and Decker, 2001). The incidence of renal complications postoperatively in all patients undergoing OLT remains the same with or without the use of VVB or diuretic therapy (Schwarz et al., 2001; Cabezuelo et al., 2003). Acute renal insufficiency is estimated to occur after liver transplantation in up to 67% of recipients (Rimola et al., 1987). Contributing factors include preexisting renal insufficiency, intraoperative complications (suboptimal renal perfusion associated with hypotension, massive transfusion, increased caval pressures), early graft dysfunction, sepsis, and administration of cyclosporine or tacrolimus and other nephrotoxic drugs in the immediate posttransplantation period.

Graft Reduction and Split-Liver Transplantation

With the plateau in organ availability in the past 5 years and the increased number of indications for OLT, creative techniques have been developed to increase organ availability to pediatric patients. Three techniques, living related (see Living Related Organ Donor, p. 900), split livers, and graft reduction, now account for up to 30% of all pediatric OLTs in some centers. See related video online at www.expertconsult.com.

Reduced-size liver transplantation (graft reduction) was first performed by Bismuth and Houssin (1984; Broelsch et al., 1988). This procedure involves the dissection of the graft at the back table with preparation of either the right lobe, the left lobe, or the left-lateral segment graft, depending on the size of the recipient. With a recipient-to-donor size ratio of 1:2, a right lobe graft is chosen. Similarly, if the recipient-to-donor size ratio is 1:4 or 1:8 (Thistlethwaite et al., 1991), a left lobe graft or a left-lateral segment graft is chosen, respectively. Because this technique, as with split livers, requires the preparation of the graft at the back table, it lends itself to an increased cold ischemic time of the liver. Vascular anastomoses for this procedure are usually of the end-to-end type, with the occasional need for a piggy-back technique or the direct anastomosis of the hepatic veins to the vena cava.

In split-liver transplantation, the liver is divided into left and right lobes and transplanted into two recipients (Emond et al., 1990; Otte et al., 1990; Renz et al., 2004) (Fig. 28-9). As a result, the right lobe contains the portal vein, hepatic artery, IVC, and common bile duct, and the left lobe includes the left lobar branches of the vessels and the left hepatic duct. Transplantation of the left lobe may necessitate the use of interposition vascular grafts, whereas the right lobe is transplanted in a fashion similar to that used for the whole organ. Most frequently, biliary reconstruction is by the Roux-en-Y technique because of the size discrepancy of the donor and recipient bile ducts.

Living related liver transplantation from parent to child, described in 1989 by Broelsch and coworkers (1991), has the potential advantages of increasing the availability of organs, reducing the waiting times and deaths on the recipient waiting list, allowing medical optimization of the recipient while minimizing the risk for clinical deterioration, and limiting immunosuppressive therapy by decreasing the immunogenicity of the transplanted organ. In addition, societies whose criteria for death differ from those previously described (Tanaka et al., 1993) are now able to offer organ transplantation in a socially acceptable manner. Until 1998, the majority of all living donor grafts in the United States went to children under 1 year of age. Living donation is not without risk. Mortality among healthy donors is low, but complications in the donor are relatively common. These findings then raise the issues of safety and ethics. Potential risks to the donor include transfusion complications,

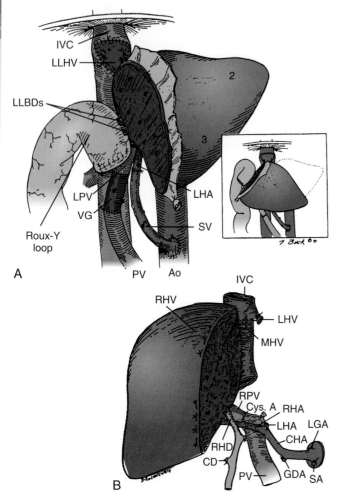

■ **FIGURE 28-9. A** and **B,** Split-liver transplantation. Demonstrated here is the use of either a right (**B**) or left (**A**) hepatic lobe. Note that the right lobe retains the native donor IVC, whereas the left lobe is connected to the recipient IVC by the use of the left hepatic vein. (**A,** *From Broelsch CE, Whitington PF, Emond JC, et al.: Liver transplantation in children from living related donors,* Ann Surg *214:428, 1991;* **B,** *From Broelsch CE, Emond JC, Thistlewaite JR, et al: Liver transplantation, including the concept of reduced-size liver transplants in children,* Ann Surg *208:410, 1988.)*

biliary complications, negative psychosocial aspects (out-of-pocket expenses, loss of income, stress on the donor and donor family, change in body image, inability to work for at least 4 to 8 weeks after donation, and poor recipient outcome), and death. Up to 20% of donors experience complications related to major abdominal surgery, including pneumonia, atelectasis, wound infection, small-bowel obstruction, incisional hernia, pressure ulcers, phlebitis, neuropraxia or peroneal nerve palsy, and reoperation. Until 1994, all living-donor liver transplantations were performed with a left-lateral segmentectomy of one or more lobes, or with a left lobectomy (20% of liver) from parent to child, or adult to small adult. Adult-to-adult transplantation of the right hepatic lobe (60% of liver) was first reported in Japan in 1994. An estimated 5% of patients on the transplant waiting list would be able to identify a suitable donor, resulting in approximately 750 living-donor liver cases in the United States each year. Adult-sized pediatric patients undergoing adult-to-adult living-donor liver transplantation may require a

right hepatic lobe to provide sufficient liver mass for the recipient. The donor is left with approximately half or less of their hepatic mass after hepatectomy, but because of the large functional reserve of the liver and its regenerative capacity, clinical evidence of hepatic insufficiency is rare. Prolonged PT, elevated serum aminotransferase levels, and increased bilirubin levels normalize after 1 week. The donor's native liver can regenerate to its original size within several weeks. The greatest concern for donor safety is the risk for donor death, which has been estimated to be between 0.28% and 2% to 3%, with ten reported cases caused by technical errors, sepsis, and pulmonary embolism (Hayashi and Trotter, 2002; Trotter et al., 2002). The actual mortality rates are probably higher than those reported.

All three of these techniques have associated complications, with split-liver grafts having the highest rates of associated complications and mortality. Because the integrity of the transected surface of the liver cannot be fully assessed until after reperfusion of the graft, these procedures have a greater associated blood loss than whole organ transplantation (Moreno et al., 1991). In addition, bile duct leaks and seroma formations are not uncommon in the transected liver. Although this specific complication was initially associated with split-liver transplantations, alterations of the surgical techniques have resulted in bile leak complications similar to those seen with reduced-size liver transplantation.

The incidence of hepatic artery and portal vein thrombosis is clearly reduced with the use of these three techniques. Survival of grafts and of patients at 1 year is better after living related liver transplantation (81%) (Epstein, 1985) than after split-liver transplantation (67%) (Broelsch et al., 1991). However, overall 5-year survival rates with all these procedures are similar.

Outcomes

In the 2006 report from Studies of Pediatric Liver Transplantation, Ng and colleagues (2008) reported on a cohort of 5-year survivors for whom the 1- and 5-year Kaplan Meier estimates of survival rates were 89.8% and 84.8%, respectively. Among the 5-year survivors, first allograft survival rates at 1, 3, and 5 years were 93%, 90%, and 88%, respectively. There was no difference in graft survival by donor type (Figs. 28-10 and 28-11). However, Diamond and colleagues (2007) reported that graft survival in 2192 children undergoing liver transplantation was decreased, and the relative risk for graft loss was increased in all of the technical variants compared with whole-organ recipients (Table 28-19, and Figs. 28-12 and 28-13). Survival also appears to be influenced by the underlying disease (Fig. 28-14).

Early studies in children undergoing OLT for a variety of conditions reported that infants less than 1 year of age had lower graft and patient survival rates than older children. However, recent trends suggest that survival rates for younger patients now approach those for older children. In children undergoing OLT for metabolic reasons, 1-, 5-, and 10-year survival rates for children older than 1 year were better than for children less than 1 year of age (Sze et al., 2009).

In a single-center study of 638 children receiving 745 grafts, Bourdeaux and coworkers (2009) noted in their 21-year experience that single liver transplantations had 5- and 10-year patient survival rates of 86% and 85%, respectively, versus 66% and 61% for recipients who needed to be retransplanted. Not

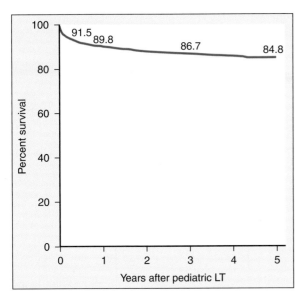

■ **FIGURE 28-10.** Kaplan-Meier probability of patient survival after pediatric liver transplantation. *(From Ng VL, Fecteau A, Shepherd R, et al: Outcomes of 5-year survivors of pediatric liver transplantation: report on 461 children from a North American multicenter registry,* Pediatrics *122:e1128, 2008.)*

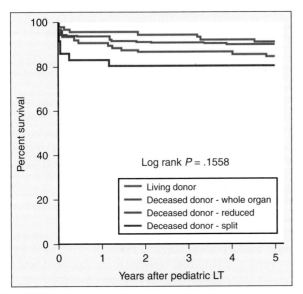

■ **FIGURE 28-11.** Kaplan-Meier probability of first allograft survival by graft type among 5-year survivors of pediatric liver transplantation. *(From Ng VL, Fecteau A, Shepherd R, et al: Outcomes of 5-year survivors of pediatric liver transplantation: report on 461 children from a North American multicenter registry,* Pediatrics *122:e1128, 2008.)*

TABLE 28-19. Multiple Variable Predictors of Graft Loss

Factor	A	B	Relative Risk*	95% Confidence Interval
Graft type	Whole	Split	1.74[†]	1.17-2.58
		Reduced	1.77	1.30-2.41
		Live donor	1.19	0.77-1.84

Adapted from Diamond ER, Fecteau A, Millis JM, et al: Impact of graft type on outcome in pediatric liver transplantation, *Ann Surg* 246:301, 2007.
*Relative risk >1 implies patients in group B have higher risk of outcome compared with group A. Relative risks and the corresponding confidence intervals are adjusted for other factors in the model.
[†]P < .05.

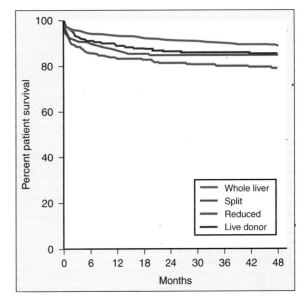

■ **FIGURE 28-12.** Kaplan-Meier probability of patient survival after pediatric liver transplantation. *(From Diamond ER, Fecteau A, Millis JM, et al: Impact of graft type on outcome in pediatric liver transplantation,* Ann Surg *246:305, 2007.)*

With improved outcomes, the population of survivors has grown, and the number of survivors is more than 10-fold greater than the number of children and adolescents who undergo liver transplantation each year (Ryckman et al., 2008). Thus, the study of outcomes should focus on the side effects of immunosuppression and on quality of life issues, in addition to patient and graft survival and surgical technical issues.

Hepatic artery thrombosis (HAT) and portal vein thrombosis (PVT) are the most common vascular complications after liver transplantation, reported to occur after 4% to 15% of liver transplantations, and more frequently after pediatric liver transplantations. Factors associated with HAT include dissection of the hepatic arterial wall, technical imperfections, celiac stenosis, aberrant donor or recipient arterial anatomy, complex back-table arterial reconstruction, and organ rejection (Duffy et al., 2009). In pediatrics, type of organ graft, whole versus split, and deceased versus living donor, as well as age less than 1 year, also affect the incidence of HAT. Overall, HAT decreases both patient and graft survival.

surprisingly, these authors also noted that the era in which the child received the transplant also affected survival. Patients recently transplanted had better survival rates and less need to be retransplanted than patients who received their transplant in an earlier era (Fig. 28-15). The rate of retransplantation was less (3%) for patients who received a living-donor graft than for children who received a whole (15%), reduced-size (20%), or split (12%) liver at first transplantation (Bourdeaux et al., 2009).

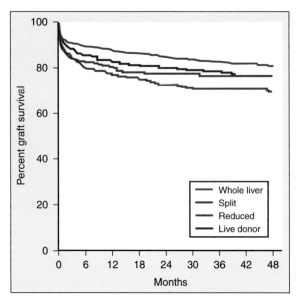

FIGURE 28-13. Kaplan-Meier probability of graft survival pediatric liver transplantation. *(From Diamond ER, Fecteau A, Millis JM, et al: Impact of graft type on outcome in pediatric liver transplantation, Ann Surg 246:305, 2007.)*

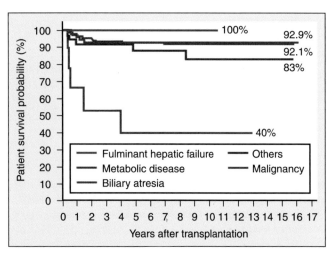

FIGURE 28-14. Kaplan-Meier survival curves of 376 pediatric primary liver allograft recipients who survived more than 3 months after transplantation. Survival in patients undergoing transplantation for malignancy was significantly lower than in the children undergoing transplantation for other diseases (P < .0001). *(From Wallot MA, Mathot M, Janssen M, et al: Long-term survival and late graft loss in pediatric liver transplant recipients: a 15-year single-center experience, Liver Transpl 8:615, 2002.)*

PVT occurs about 2% of the time but is usually more detrimental to patient and graft survival. As with HAT, pediatric patients are at greater risk than adult patients. Risk factors for PVT include small portal vein size, portal vein redundancy, pretransplantation PVT, and prior splenectomy (Duffy et al., 2009). Type of graft may also influence the incidence (Diamond et al., 2007). Life-long immunosuppression with reduction in therapy remains the practice. Thus, immunosuppression balances the preservation of graft function with its side effects. Posttransplant lymphoproliferative disease occurs in 3% to

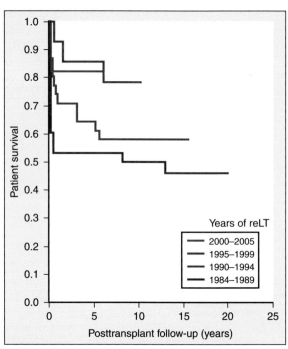

FIGURE 28-15. Patient survival after retransplantation according to transplant era, in a series of 638 pediatric liver recipients transplanted between March 1, 1984, and December 31, 2005. The rate of retransplantation decreased from 18% to 6% between 1984 and 2005 (P = .1218). *(From Bourdeaux C, Brunati A, Janssen M, et al: Liver retransplantation in children: a 21-year single-center experience, Transplant Int 22:416, 2009.)*

28% of children after liver transplantation. Nephrotoxicity is a well-known complication of the immunosuppressive agents. Chronic renal disease increases with increased survival. Renal insufficiency was reported as 33% and 77% in 3- and 10-year survivors, respectively (Starzl and Kaupp, 1960).

Growth is also adversely affected by both disease and immunosuppressive therapy. In children, approximately 73% were below average in height and 29% below the 10th percentile (Ng et al., 2008). Quality-of-life issues for children frequently focus on school performance. Ng reported that almost 18% of 5-year survivors had either repeated a grade or been held back more than one school year. Learning disabilities were reported in 21% of 5-year survivors.

MULTIVISCERAL AND INTESTINAL TRANSPLANTATIONS

Liver, multivisceral, and small bowel transplantations have now become widely accepted therapies for organ failure of the abdominal viscera. Small bowel transplantation has gained recognition as an acceptable therapy for intestinal dysfunction of various etiologies. As of 2010, 1091 intestinal transplantations have been performed in patients of all ages.

The technical feasibility of intestinal transplantation was first described in 1905 by Alexis Carrel (1905). After early successes with kidney transplantation in identical twins during the early 1960s, Lillehei and colleagues (1967) described experimental transplantation of the stomach, intestine, and pancreas.

Simultaneously, Starzl and colleagues described transplantation of multiple abdominal viscera in dogs and, many years later, in humans (Starzl et al., 1989). Until the late 1980s, there were no long-term (>6 months) survivors of small bowel transplantation (SBT). With the introduction of cyclosporine and tacrolimus, and with an improved understanding of graft rejection in pigs, successful long-term survival became possible (Grant et al., 1990). This procedure has a high rate of morbidity and mortality. The major cause of graft failure is acute or chronic rejection (SBT, 79%; small bowel in combination with liver transplantation [SB/LT], 71%; multivisceral transplantation, 56%). Infection, CMV enteritis, lymphoproliferative disease, and multisystem organ failure are major causes of death. The rate of graft-versus-host disease after intestinal transplantation is 0% to 16% (Abu-Elmagd et al., 1998; Reyes et al., 1998; Sudan et al., 2000; Pirenne et al., 2007). Patient and graft survival rates are lower for intestinal transplantation than for solid organ transplantation, with approximately half of the patients receiving intestinal transplants surviving 5 years.

Multivisceral transplantation may include SBT in isolation, in combination with liver transplantation, or in combination with multiple abdominal organs (Starzl et al., 1991a, 1991b). An isolated SBT is typically recommended for patients on home parenteral nutrition (HPN) who have exhausted their venous access. Combined SB/LT is recommended for patients with irreversible cirrhosis when HPN has failed, or those who have intestinal failure associated with a hypercoagulable state that can be corrected by a simultaneous liver transplantation. Multivisceral transplantations are for patients with locally aggressive tumors that necessitate evisceration of the abdominal organs (duodenal fistulae, locally aggressive tumors, multiorgan failure with a nonreconstructible GI tract) or for the patient with benign conditions involving the liver, pancreas, or stomach (Tzakis et al., 1989).

The Health Care Financing Administration's clinical indications for intestinal transplantation (implemented in 2001) includes impending liver failure because of failure of HPN, thrombosis of major central venous channels, frequent line infection and sepsis, and frequent episodes of severe dehydration. Significant bone disease, metabolic disorders, failure to thrive, and significant limitations on social and personal activities are not considered indications. As most patients function well on HPN, the risks of intestinal transplantation are warranted only with failure of HPN therapy. The goal of intestinal transplantation is to eliminate the need for TPN and to reverse or prevent TPN-associated liver disease. The first year of wait-listing candidates for intestinal transplantation with UNOS was 1993.

General Indications

In the pediatric population, chronic intestinal failure results from massive bowel resection (short bowel syndrome) or functional impairment of the bowel caused by disturbances in motility or extensive parenchymal disorders (Okada et al., 1994). Necrotizing enterocolitis, intestinal atresia (Todo et al., 1994a, 1994b), midgut volvulus, gastroschisis, microvillous inclusion disease, Hirschsprung's disease, and intestine pseudoobstruction are the primary causes of isolated small intestinal failure. This is in marked contrast to the adult population, in which intestinal failure is caused primarily by Crohn's disease and thrombotic episodes involving the major splanchnic vessels.

If the length of the small bowel is less than 60 or 70 cm, parenteral nutrition is required (normal length of a small bowel in the infant being 200 to 250 cm). For the patient to survive, HPN is essential. HPN has significant metabolic sequelae, the foremost being liver failure and bone disease (Bowyer et al., 1985; Colomb et al., 1994; Sondheimer et al., 1998; Chan et al., 1999; Wasa et al., 1999; Cavicchi et al., 2000). The hepatic dysfunction in the patient on long-term TPN most commonly includes hepatic steatosis, as well as cholestasis, phospholipidosis, or cirrhosis, which is observed in 15% to 40% of patients after 3 years. Up to 100% of patients have biliary sludge or gallstones after 6 weeks. In the pediatric population, this is a reversible form of liver dysfunction (Grosfeld et al., 1986) if the bilirubin level is less than 30 mg/dL and the patient is returned to total enteral feeding. Patients are followed through the North American Home Parenteral and Enteral Nutrition Patient Registry supported by the Oley Foundation (formerly the OASIS registry, started in 1984) (Howard et al., 1991). This registry reports survival for patients on long-term HPN to be 87% to 96% at 1 year, and 70% to 90 % at 3 years. The majority of deaths are related to progression of the underlying disease.

Since 2000, over 1900 intestinal transplantations have been performed in only five centers in the United States. Over half of these intestinal transplantations have been performed in children, and more than half of the children were less than 6 years of age. Outcomes for children with isolated SBT are similar to those children undergoing SB/LT.

In patients with isolated SBTs, graft survival rates at 3 months and at 1, 3, 5, and 10 years were 83%, 68%, 57%, 36%, and 25% respectively, and patient survival rates at these same intervals were 94%, 81%, 71%, 56%, and 46%, respectively. In patients with SB/LT, patient survival rates at 3 months and at 1, 3, 5, and 10 years were 88%, 73%, 61%, 55%, and 38%, respectively.

Preoperative Assessment

The patient should be evaluated specifically for progressive liver disease and evidence of portal hypertension. Extrahepatic manifestation of the primary disease causing the patient's intestinal failure should be identified. Complications of TPN should be elucidated (infection, catheter occlusion, hepatic disease). Comorbid conditions such as infection, renal disease, electrolyte abnormalities, and gastroparesis predisposing to regurgitation and aspiration should be considered. Appropriate evaluation of patency of the large vessels of the neck (subclavian and internal jugular veins) is essential, because repeated central vein cannulation or long-term indwelling catheter use for the administration of HPN may lead to loss of vascular access resulting from venous thrombosis (Grosfeld et al., 1986). Doppler ultrasonography is sometimes useful to find central venous access, but the gold standard is a venogram.

Knowledge of the patient's prior surgeries as well as the abdominal vascular anatomy is important, particularly in a patient scheduled for a multivisceral transplantation, because these are the most technically complex surgical procedures. A discussion with the surgical team regarding the planned approach is essential, particularly because multiple blood vessels may be partially or fully crossed-clamped during the operation.

Because of the high rate of postoperative infectious complications, broad-spectrum antibiotics, antifungal drugs, and ganciclovir prophylaxis are routinely administered.

Surgical Technique: Recipient Surgery

The final decision to proceed with either a multivisceral or an intestinal transplantation is made after a laparotomy and a meticulous inspection of the native vessels and abdominal organs. Thus, continuous communication between the donor and recipient teams is essential. In addition, procurement of the donor iliac artery and vein (Starzl et al., 1991a, 1991b), as well as the thoracic aorta, is essential for vascular reconstruction of the graft. The graft is usually preserved with cold UW solution. The length of time the organ is kept in the preservation solution should be minimized because intestinal mucosal damage occurs in UW solution as a result of increased lipid peroxidation (Takeyoshi et al., 2001).

The operation begins with a midline incision, which is extended to either a unilateral or bilateral transverse subcostal incision. The choice of incision depends on the planned operation, with a bilateral incision used preferentially in the multivisceral transplantation. The procedure continues as described by Todo and coworkers (1992) (Fig. 28-16). In the patient receiving an isolated intestinal transplantation, the superior mesenteric artery is anastomosed exclusively to the infrarenal aorta. Venous blood from the isolated small bowel graft is drained into the mesenteric venous system at one of three sites: the donor SMV to the distal end of the recipient SMV, SMV to the hilar portion of the main portal vein, or donor SMV to the confluence of the SMV and splenic vein (Todo et al., 1994a, 1994b).

In the recipient of liver-intestine or multivisceral graft, the use of VVB is usually impossible because of vascular thromboses of the major vessels seen with the long-term use of HPN.

The liver is usually placed in a piggy-back fashion, and occasionally a temporary portacaval shunt is used to decompress the abdominal viscera. Vascular anastomoses are performed as illustrated in Figure 28-16.

The arterial and venous anastomoses are performed before reperfusion of the graft. Arterial anastomoses in this instance are usually with a Carrel patch (Fig. 28-17), containing both the celiac and superior mesenteric arteries for the combined intestinal and multivisceral graft to the infrarenal abdominal aorta. In some instances, an aortic conduit may be used to facilitate the anastomoses of the superior mesenteric artery and celiac axis to the abdominal aorta. If a portacaval shunt is performed, it is subsequently converted to a portaportal anastomosis to facilitate perfusion of the liver with the splanchnic hepatotropic factors.

After completion of the vascular anastomoses, the GI continuity is reestablished by anastomosing the appropriate donor intestine to recipient bowel. In the multivisceral recipient, proximal intestinal reconstruction is accomplished by anastomosing the distal esophagus to the anterior wall of the donor stomach. A pyloroplasty is routinely preformed, followed by a gastrostomy, the first of three essential enterotomies, which helps to prevent delayed gastric emptying and decompress the intestine. A jejunostomy is performed for enteral feeding. The final enterotomy is achieved by exteriorization of the distal end of the donor intestine in a chimney fashion. The recipient ileum or colon is then anastomosed to the side of the graft distal to the stoma. Finally, a cholecystectomy follows, as well as biliary reconstruction by a choledochojejunostomy or Roux-en-Y procedure.

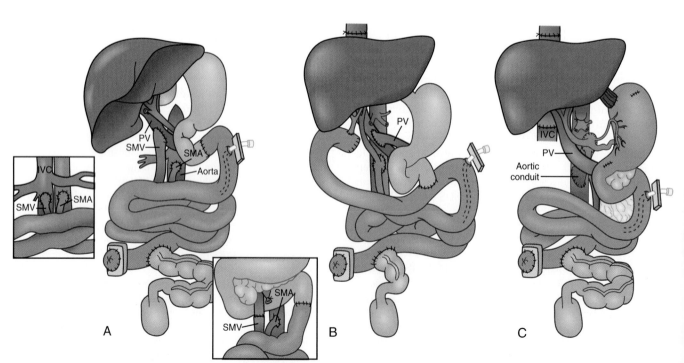

■ **FIGURE 28-16.** Intestinal and multivisceral transplantations. **A,** Isolated intestinal transplantation. **B,** Combined liver-intestine transplantation. **C,** Full multivisceral transplantation with resection of the native retrohepatic vena cava. IVC, inferior vena cava; PV, portal vein; SMA, superior mesenteric artery; SMV, superior mesenteric vein; VC, vena cava. *(From Todo S, Tzaki AG, Abu-Elmagd K, et al: Intestinal transplantation in composite visceral graft or alone, Ann Surg 216:223, 1992.)*

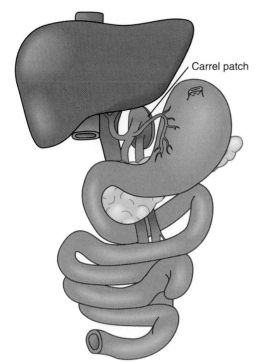

■ **FIGURE 28-17.** Multivisceral allograft using the Carrel patch. In this case, a Carrel patch with superior mesenteric artery and celiac axis origins has been used to cap a free graft of the donor thoracic aorta that has been used as a conduit. This is one of the several options for the surgeon. *(From Todo S, Tzakis A, Abu-Elmagd K, et al: Current status of intestinal transplantation,* Adv Surg *27:295, 1994.)*

Anesthesia Management

Small Bowel Transplantation

In the patient scheduled for isolated SBT, the anesthesia management is similar to that for other major abdominal surgeries. The patient usually has a central venous catheter, although it is sometimes placed in an unconventional site if the subclavian and internal jugular veins are thrombosed (right atrial, transhepatic, or direct inferior vena caval catheters). These procedures are lengthy and lend themselves to significant third-space losses and major fluid shifts. Two large-bore IV catheters above the diaphragm and a radial arterial catheter are recommended. CVP should also be monitored as a guide for fluid replacement. If central vein cannulation is impossible, it is best to proceed without its use; femoral vein cannulation can be used for volume replacement. All blood products should be CMV negative and irradiated, to minimize the risk for graft-versus-host disease.

The choice of anesthesia agent depends on the patient's underlying disease and hemodynamic status. Nitrous oxide should be avoided because it may cause additional bowel distention. The choice of fluids remains controversial in patients undergoing bowel surgery. Not infrequently, significant bowel swelling and distention are noted after reperfusion of the graft. Frequently, diuresis is recommended as a means to treat this problem, although it is often ineffective. Moreover, the etiology of the intestinal edema is most likely related to the preservation of the organ. The use of colloids, preferentially albumin, is recommended when the patient had a low albumin level preoperatively,

Reperfusion of the isolated small bowel graft usually has minimal hemodynamic effects. The reperfusion syndrome seen

with liver transplantation is absent because of the relatively low potassium load and the low volume of effluent extruded from the graft. Hemodynamic stability is the norm, and coagulopathy or metabolic derangements are unusual.

Multivisceral Transplantation

Anesthesia considerations for the patient scheduled for multivisceral transplantation are identical to those for the patient undergoing OLT. There are, however, unique and specific considerations with respect to planned vascular anastomoses (Starzl et al., 1993; Todo et al., 1995) (see Fig. 28-16). The liver is usually placed in piggy-back fashion in this instance. A partial cross-clamping of the abdominal aorta should be anticipated for the placement of the arterial anastomosis using a Carrel patch (see Fig. 28-17). The surgical procedure is divided into three stages, similar to those with solitary liver transplantation. Completion of the abdominal viscera exenteration during the preanhepatic stage is the period of greatest blood loss (De Wolf, 1991). Hemodynamic alterations during this period are related to complications of massive transfusion and manipulation of the abdominal viscera. Ionized hypocalcemia, lactic acidosis, and progressive hypothermia should be anticipated. In addition, a progressive coagulopathy, as seen in patients undergoing OLT, is expected. Thus, monitoring of coagulation is essential. The anhepatic stage of the surgery is usually performed without the use of VVB. The liver is placed in piggy-back fashion, and vascular anastomosis of the intestine follows. A significant difference with respect to reperfusion of the multivisceral graft from that of the liver is that the arterial anastomoses must be performed before graft reperfusion. The graft is flushed with 50 mL/kg of cold saline or lactated Ringer's solution before reperfusion, to reduce the potassium load from the preservation solution.

Reperfusion of the multivisceral graft is similar to that of the hepatic graft. Hypotension and bradycardia are the usual observations secondary to the release of a large volume of hypothermic, hyperkalemic, acidotic preservation solution into the right heart. These changes are usually short lived, with normalization of the hemodynamics within minutes after reperfusion. The incidence of the postreperfusion syndrome in this group of patients is not well defined.

KIDNEY TRANSPLANTATION

Michon and colleagues in Paris performed the earliest kidney transplantation in a child on Christmas Eve in 1952. A 16-year-old boy had just undergone nephrectomy for a right ruptured kidney after a fall, when the surgeons made the unfortunate discovery that he had no left kidney. An ABO-compatible kidney from his mother was placed in the iliac region. Initially, the kidney excreted urine and had good renal function; however, abrupt anuria occurred on posttransplant day 21 (indicating rejection), and the patient died. Two years later, Murray and colleagues performed the first successful kidney transplantation between two identical twins. Goodwin, Mims, and Kaufman at the University of Oregon performed the first successful pediatric transplantation in 1959 between identical twins, one of whom had glomerulonephritis. Eighteen years after transplantation, the kidney was still functioning with normal morphology by biopsy (Papalois and Najarian, 2001).

Routine kidney transplantation in pediatric patients, however, awaited the development of effective immunosuppressive agents. Potent corticosteroids, calcineurin inhibitors such as cyclosporine or tacrolimus, monoclonal antibodies, antimetabolites such as azathioprine, and the purine synthetase inhibitor mycophenolate mofetil (MMF) have all been used successfully in pediatric patients to prevent rejection (Papalois and Najarian, 2001). Superior survival and improved long-term growth and development can be obtained with kidney transplantation compared with chronic hemodialysis or peritoneal dialysis. Newer immunosuppressive regimens relying less on high-dosage corticosteroids have further improved the growth and development of children receiving a renal transplant. Tan and others (2008) reported that, in 42 pediatric patients undergoing living related kidney transplantation after monoclonal antibody (alemtuzumab) pretreatment and tacrolimus monotherapy, the use of corticosteroids could be eliminated and the actuarial 1-, 2-, 3-, and 4-year patient end-graft survival rates were 97.7% and 97.6%, 93.5% and 85.4%, 93.5% and 85.4%, and 93.5% and 85.4%, respectively. In addition, pediatric patients who receive a kidney transplant are much more likely to have a normal lifestyle than those requiring hemodialysis (So et al., 1987; Beebe et al., 1991; Turenne et al., 1997; Benfield et al., 1999; Elshihabi et al., 2000; Healy et al., 2000; McDonald et al., 2000; Qvist et al., 2000, 2002; Papalois and Najarian, 2001; Smith et al., 2002, Gillen et al., 2008).

Finally, kidney transplantation using infants or small children as donors has a lower success rate because of the small size of the donor vasculature. Therefore, infants and small children usually receive a transplant from someone who is an adult or a larger child, often much larger than the recipient. In recipients who are infants or small children, the kidney may be many times larger than they would normally have (Miller et al., 1983; Beebe et al., 1991; Healy et al., 2000; Chavers et al., 2007). Nephron mass can be an important nonimmunologic factor in long-term graft survival. Giuliani and coworkers (2009) have shown that the donor-to-recipient body surface area affects 5-year graft survival.

Infants less than 2 years of age are an important subset of pediatric patients because they are at higher risk for graft loss. Unlike older children or adults, rejection in infants is not the primary cause of failure of the transplanted kidney. One of the main reasons for graft loss in the younger recipient is vascular thrombosis (Beebe et al., 1991; Singh et al., 1997; Healy et al., 2000; Neipp et al., 2002; Chavers et al., 2007).

Infants also have a higher incidence of delayed function of the renal allograft. This is important because infants and children with delayed graft function have an increased incidence of graft loss in the years after transplantation. Kidneys with delayed function are likely to have sustained permanent injury and are susceptible to failure after rejection or other insult. Providing adequate perfusion of a very large kidney relative to the recipient size to prevent vascular thrombosis and delayed graft function is one of the main challenges for the pediatric anesthesiologist caring for an infant or a small child undergoing renal transplantation (Tejani et al., 1999).

Epidemiology

End-stage renal disease (ESRD) is less common in the pediatric age group than in adults. Its overall incidence in children aged 0 to 19 is approximately 14 per million, and this has been relatively stable since 1981. The incidence is lower at 0 to 4 years of age (approximately 10 per million) than older children (15 to 19 years old) (approximately 28 per million). In contrast, the incidence of ESRD in adults 20 to 24 years of age is approximately 120 per million (Chavers et al., 2007).

Pediatric recipients of renal transplants differ from their adult counterparts in several ways. Obstructive nephropathy or hypoplastic kidneys are common causes for transplantation in the pediatric age group. Glomerulonephritis is less common, and, in contrast to adults, diabetes as a cause of renal failure in this age group is rare (North American Pediatric Renal Transplant Cooperative Study, 2007) (Table 28-20). Consequently, many of the diseases that cause renal failure in children do not recur, and successful transplantation could, in theory, be a permanent solution. Also, although most adults have received dialysis before transplantation, approximately 30% of children who receive a transplant have never had dialysis before. Of the children who are on dialysis, approximately half are receiving peritoneal dialysis, and the other half, hemodialysis (Elshihabi et al., 2000; McDonald et al., 2000; NAPRTCS, 2007).

Approximately 300 pediatric patients undergo living related kidney transplantation each year in the United States, and an equal number receive a deceased donor transplant. There has been a recent increase in the number of teenagers and older children who now receive a deceased-donor transplant, probably because a higher priority has been given to children requiring a kidney over the past decade (Magee et al., 2008). Infants and small children (<15 kg) constitute between 10% and 15% of both deceased-donor and living related transplantations in the pediatric age group (Elshihabi et al., 2000; McDonald et al., 2000). Pediatric living-donor kidney transplantations have been shown to have increased half-lives and graft survival in patients 2 to 5 years of age when compared with transplants from deceased donors (Shapiro, 2006; Hardy et al., 2009) (Figs. 28-18 and 28-19). Factors affecting graft survival in both living and deceased donors that are associated with worse outcomes include African American race of the recipient, no antibody induction, more than five transfusions, and retransplantation and pretransplantation dialysis (Shapiro et al., 2006). Of note, laparoscopically obtained donor nephrectomies may have a higher rate of delayed graft function and 6-month rejection rates (Troppman et al., 2005).

Pathophysiology of Renal Failure

The effects of chronic renal failure on infants and children result from the kidney's role as a filter of metabolic waste products and fluid regulation and its active role in hormone production. As the glomerulofiltration rate becomes reduced, the kidney's ability to clear acids, urea, and potassium diminishes, and overall poor nutrition is the result. Therefore, infants and children with renal failure have growth retardation and often developmental delay. Chronic metabolic acidosis, hyperkalemia, and hyperphosphatemia develop. The elevated phosphorus binds to the serum calcium and magnesium, resulting in hypocalcemia and magnesemia. Fractures in active children can occur as calcium is leached from the bones. Chronic uremia can result in CNS depression and congestive heart failure and can impair platelet function. Seizures and permanent neurologic damage may be a consequence of electrolyte imbalances and fluxes

TABLE 28-20. Primary Diagnoses in Pediatric Kidney Transplant Recipients

Recipient and Transplant Characteristics	Patients (N)	Patients (%)
Total	9506	100.0
Aplastic/hypoplastic/dysplastic kidney	1521	16.0
Obstructive uropathy	1486	15.6
Focal segmental glomerulosclerosis	1110	11.7
Reflux nephropathy	500	5.3
Chronic glomerulonephritis	324	3.4
Polycystic disease	281	3.0
Medullary cystic disease	263	2.8
Hemolytic uremic syndrome	254	2.7
Prune belly syndrome	249	2.6
Congenital nephrotic syndrome	246	2.6
Familial nephritis	211	2.2
Cystinosis	195	2.1
Pyelo/interstitial nephritis	173	1.8
Membranoproliferative glomerulonephritis type I	170	1.8
Idiopathic crescentic glomerulonephritis	168	1.8
Systemic lupus erythematosus nephritis	145	1.5
Renal infarct	130	1.4
Berger's (IgA) nephritis	123	1.3
Henoch-Schönlein nephritis	110	1.2
Membranoproliferative glomerulonephritis type II	81	0.9
Wegener's granulomatosis	52	0.5
Wilms tumor	51	0.5
Drash syndrome	50	0.5
Oxalosis	49	0.5
Membranous nephropathy	42	0.4
Other systemic immunologic diseases	32	0.3
Sickle cell nephropathy	15	0.2
Diabetic glomerulonephritis	11	0.1
Other	897	9.4
Unknown	567	6.0

Adapted from North American Pediatric Renal Transplant Cooperative Study, annual report, p 25, 2007. Available at https://web.emmes.com/study/ped/annlrept/annlrept/annlrept2007.pdf; accessed June 2009.

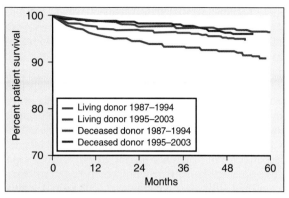

■ **FIGURE 28-18.** Survival of pediatric patient recipients after kidney transplantation. *(From Shapiro R: Living donor Kidney transplantation in pediatric recipients,* Pediatr Transpl *10:845, 2006, with data from the North American Pediatric Renal Transplant Cooperative Study [NAPRTCS].)*

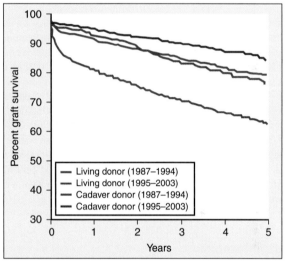

■ **FIGURE 28-19.** Graft survival after living- and deceased-donor pediatric kidney transplantation. *(From Shapiro R: Living donor Kidney transplantation in pediatric recipients,* Pediatr Transpl *10:845, 2006, with data from the North American Pediatric Renal Transplant Cooperative Study [NAPRTCS].)*

These changes occur in infants and small children to various degrees despite adequate dialysis and the administration of exogenous erythropoietin and vitamin supplementation. The net effect is a child who is small and frail, hypertensive, and chronically acidotic (Beebe et al., 1991; Belani and Palahniuk, 1991).

Indications for Transplantation

Any medical condition listed in Table 28-20 is an indications for potential transplantation. Educational guidelines were published in 1998 by the Pediatric Committee of the American Society of Transplantation on the indications for pediatric transplantation. They suggested that the following pediatric patients with renal disease receive a kidney transplant: patients with ESRD unresponsive to medical management, patients with growth failure

from renal insufficiency and dialysis therapy. Volume overload can result as the kidney's ability to clear sodium and free water diminishes (Belani and Palahniuk, 1991).

Hormone function of the kidneys is affected by renal failure as well. Erythropoietin production may be severely reduced and cause anemia. Renin production becomes elevated as the kidney senses diminished perfusion, resulting in hypertension. Similarly, parathyroid hormone levels become elevated as the parathyroid gland responds to a reduced serum calcium level.

in spite of optimal nutritional management, patients with developmental delay, children with progressive renal osteodystrophy in spite of optimal medical management, and patients who fail to thrive (Chavers et al., 2007).

The optimal age for transplantation in an infant or small child is controversial. Infants less than 2 years of age are technically more difficult to transplant and have a higher incidence of arterial thrombosis and delayed graft function. Many surgeons prefer to wait until the infant is at least 2 years of age or weighs more than 15 to 20 kg (Glessing et al., 2007). On the other hand, infants who receive kidney transplants have better growth and development than those managed on dialysis. Also, the increased risk for graft loss compared with older children and adults was mainly seen in infants who received a deceased-donor rather than a living related kidney transplant (Chavers et al., 2007). Centers that perform kidney transplantation in infants on a regular basis report graft and patient survival rates that are similar to those seen in older children or adults. Therefore, transplantation in an infant, particularly with a living related organ, is optimal as soon it is technically feasible at a center experienced with the procedure (Humar et al., 2001; Becker et al., 2006; Chavers et al., 2007).

Also controversial is whether kidneys from deceased pediatric donors should be given preferentially to pediatric recipients. Initially, kidneys from donors less than 5 years of age were not used because they had a high incidence of vascular thromboses secondary to technical difficulties. Some studies have shown that kidneys from younger donors can be successfully transplanted into pediatric patients, and they may have the advantage of being able to grow along with the recipient (Becker et al., 2006; Pape et al., 2006). Kidneys from donors weighing less than 10 kg are usually transplanted en bloc to avoid small vessel anastomosis and to increase nephron mass. The en bloc technique comprises end-to-side anastomosis of the infrarenal donor vena cava and aorta to the recipient vessels.

Surgical Technique

The surgical technique has been described in detail elsewhere (Miller et al., 1983). In larger children (>20 kg), the kidney is placed in the pelvis as in an adult renal transplant. A lower flank incision is used with a retroperitoneal approach. Systemic heparinization is usually not required because heparin can be applied directly by the surgeon through the arteriotomy and venotomy, and the anastomoses are performed quickly. The renal artery is anastomosed to the common iliac or hypogastric artery. The renal vein is usually attached to the common iliac or external iliac vein. The ureter is then anastomosed to the bladder (Fig. 28-20, A). In this approach, only one lower extremity is without circulation before reperfusion. Occasionally, hypotension results from revascularization of the kidney in the older child or teenager. In general, the hemodynamic changes are minimal.

In contrast, when transplanting an adult kidney into an infant or small child (<20 kg), the kidney is sewn directly onto the aorta and vena cava (see Fig. 28-20, B). A retroperitoneal approach to the aorta and vena cava is advocated by some surgeons, to potentially avoid bowel complications such as adhesions and bowel atony. It also maintains the possibility of peritoneal dialysis. However, the graft may be compressed by this approach, particularly if an adult kidney is used (Becker et al., 2006). Therefore, in many centers the peritoneum is opened to expose the aorta and vena cava (Chavers et al., 2007). Currently,

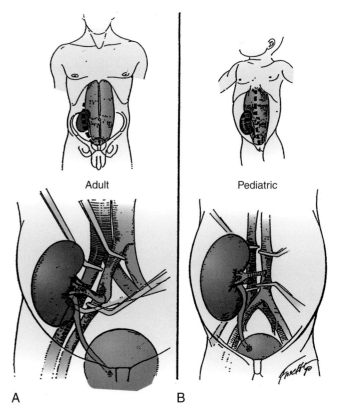

Adult   Pediatric

A   B

■ **FIGURE 28-20.** Surgical placement of renal allograft in adults and older children (**A**) versus infants (**B**). The vascular anastomosis of an adult-size organ in the pediatric patient is to the aorta and vena cava. *(From Belani KG, Polahniuk RJ: Kidney Transplantation,* Internat Anesth Clin *29:17–40, 1991.)*

there are no differences in initial graft function, graft survival, or surgical complications between the approaches (Becker et al., 2006). In both approaches, the aorta and inferior vena cava are cross-clamped. Because the major vessels are clamped, low-dosage heparinization (50 to 100 mg/kg) is often used. The lower extremity is deprived of both arterial perfusion and venous drainage during the anastomoses. Because the kidney is much larger relative to the recipient than in the older child or adult, the hemodynamic changes in an infant on reperfusion can be profound (Beebe et al., 1991; Chavers et al., 2007).

Infants and small children usually require other concurrent operations in addition to the kidney transplantation. For example, if the cause of renal failure is vesicoureteral reflux with recurrent urinary tract infections, bilateral nephrectomies are often performed simultaneously to prevent graft sepsis. Concurrent splenectomy, although no longer routine, is occasionally performed if the spleen is enlarged, to allow room for the kidney. A large-bore Hickman dialysis catheter is also placed in infants before beginning the transplantation if not already present for IV access and CVP monitoring (Beebe et al., 1991).

Anesthesia Concerns

All systems are affected by ESRD. Attention must be paid to the extent of renal failure and its effects on organ function, and to the child's growth and development. Smaller tracheal tube sizes and intravascular catheters may be needed if the child has not been growing adequately. The cause of renal failure, if a systemic disorder such as oxalosis exists, also affects the function of other organs. Agenesis or dysplasia of the kidneys may be associated with other congenital disorders such as ventricular septal defects. The presence of cardiac failure or congestive heart disease should be determined. Although most children with renal failure have a hyperdynamic circulation from chronic anemia, some do develop cardiac insufficiency from concurrent congenital heart disease, uremia, or chronic volume overload. The parents should be asked about frequent episodes of dyspnea or asthma attacks. In addition to usual reactive airways disease in children, asthma attacks in children with renal insufficiency may suggest volume overload. The presence of wheezing, rales, dyspnea, an enlarged liver, and hypertension on physical examination suggests fluid overload that may require dialysis before surgery. A history of frequent fractures suggests the child may have brittle bones from hypocalcemia and be at risk for dental injury during anesthesia. Finally, the parents or patient should be asked if the child has symptoms of acid reflux or delayed gastric emptying, because those conditions are quite common with renal insufficiency (Beebe et al., 1991; Belani and Palahniuk, 1991).

When examining the airway, the anesthesiologist must pay particular attention to the teeth, which may be fragile from chronic hypocalcemia. Vascular access is also often difficult in these patients because of frequent hospitalizations and repeated blood drawing and catheterizations. The extremities should be examined to plan where to obtain vascular access for an arterial catheter, if indicated (Beebe et al., 1991; Belani and Palahniuk, 1991).

Preoperative Dialysis

Before surgery, the anesthesiologist and surgeon should ascertain if the patient needs dialysis. The day of the last dialysis and type of dialysis, hemodialysis or peritoneal, should be determined. Some patients who have not previously been dialyzed are chronically hyperkalemic. Potassium can be transfused from the donor kidney as it is reperfused, particularly if it has been filled with a high-potassium preservative, such as the UW solution. It is therefore best to reduce the potassium to normal levels either via dialysis or ion exchange resins (Kayexalate) before transplantation in the chronically hyperkalemic patient (Beebe et al., 1991; Belani and Palahniuk, 1991).

If the patient is hyperkalemic (potassium > 6.0 mmol/L), acidotic, or volume overloaded, the surgery should be delayed and dialysis performed. Although peritoneal dialysis may be adequate for the daily treatment of patients and is commonly used in children, it may be inadequate to prepare children for surgery. Therefore, children are sometimes converted from peritoneal to hemodialysis several weeks before transplantation to ensure adequate dialysis. The large-bore (2 mm inner diameter) Hickman catheters are usually used for hemodialysis in infants and young children; they also provide excellent vascular access for the renal transplant procedure (Beebe et al., 1991).

Anesthesia Management

Many anesthesia techniques have been used successfully in the anesthesia management of renal transplantation in children. However, when planning the anesthesia, several items unique to renal transplantation must be kept in mind (Beebe et al., 1991; Belani and Palahniuk, 1991):

- The patient suffers from chronic renal failure and may present with many of its effects, including anemia, hyperkalemia, and hypervolemia.
- The transplanted kidney may not function effectively initially. Therefore, muscle relaxants, such as pancuronium, and other drugs dependent primarily on the kidney for excretion should not be used.
- Immunosuppressive drugs need to be administered. Allergic reactions and hypotension may occur with some of the agents.
- The kidney has been ischemic before transplantation, which may increase its vulnerability to further injury.
- Adequacy of the intravascular volume status before and after reperfusion of the allograft must be ensured.
- The anesthesiologist must be prepared to deal with hyperkalemia, hyperglycemia, hypocalcemia, and other electrolyte disorders that may arise over the course of the operation and perioperative period.

Induction and Maintenance of Anesthesia

In general, most children without an IV catheter in place receive preoperative sedation with either oral or rectal midazolam (0.5 mg/kg). Ketamine (3 mg/kg) and atropine (20 mcg/kg) may be added to rectal midazolam if a greater level of sedation is desired (Beebe et al., 1992). If an IV catheter is in place, IV midazolam (0.1 to 0.2 mg/kg) may be administered for sedation.

An inhaled induction of anesthesia with sevoflurane with or without nitrous oxide may be used in stable patients with normal gastric function who have been NPO for an adequate length of time.

Often an IV induction of anesthesia is used in children undergoing renal transplantation, particularly if there is a concern that the patient may be unstable and require vasopressors or other drugs. Also, transplant surgeons often order oral immunosuppressive agents preoperatively. Sometimes the children take the drugs only with milk or juice. If the medications are necessary and the surgery cannot be delayed, an IV induction and aspiration precautions are required (Beebe et al., 1991; Belani and Palahniuk, 1991).

Intravenous propofol or thiopental may be used in healthy children. Ketamine (1 to 3 mg/kg) has proved useful as an induction agent in infants and children suspected to be hypovolemic from recent dialysis. Ketamine maintains the autonomic tone and blood pressure while the volume status is corrected. Maintenance of the blood pressure and a strong pulse with ketamine is also useful when attempting to place an arterial catheter (Beebe et al., 1991; Belani and Palahniuk, 1991).

Tracheal intubation and skeletal muscle relaxation are always provided by an agent not dependent on the kidneys for excretion, such as cisatracurium. Intermediate-acting steroidal muscle relaxants such as vecuronium or rocuronium may also be used, but their action may be prolonged because of partial renal excretion. Succinylcholine is usually not administered except in emergencies, because it can raise the serum potassium concentration by 0.5 to 0.7 mmol/L. This could be dangerous in patients who are already hyperkalemic. Also, drugs dependent on renal excretion, such as pancuronium, should not be used because prolonged neuromuscular blockade can result if the kidney does not function properly in the perioperative period (Beebe et al., 1991; Belani and Palahniuk, 1991).

After the induction of general anesthesia and tracheal intubation, anesthesia is maintained with isoflurane or desflurane. Even if sevoflurane has been used for inhaled induction of general anesthesia, it is usually not used for maintenance because of concerns about nephrotoxicity with sevoflurane from fluoride ion or compound A production. Although nephrotoxicity in normal kidneys from sevoflurane in humans has never been demonstrated, its effects on transplanted kidneys are unknown (Artru, 1998).

Nitrous oxide was used frequently in the past and may still be used in older children. An air-oxygen mixture is usually used in infants to prevent the bowel distention that may occur with nitrous oxide in an abdomen that will be quite full with an adult kidney. Opioids such as fentanyl are also administered in moderate dosages to reduce the amount of inhaled agent required and to provide postoperative pain relief (Beebe et al., 1991; Belani and Palahniuk, 1991).

Monitoring

In addition to standard monitors (ECG, pulse oximetry, noninvasive blood pressure, end-tidal gas analysis, temperature), all children undergoing renal transplantation need monitoring of their CVP. This helps ensure that an adequate volume is administered before perfusion of the allograft, and it provides a means to administer immunosuppressive agents that can be given only centrally (e.g., thymoglobulin, OKT3). As noted earlier, in infants, the CVP is often monitored through a large-bore Hickman catheter. This also serves as an excellent, high-flowing catheter to allow transfusion directly into the central circulation as well as a means to provide dialysis should the kidney initially fail (Beebe et al., 1991; Belani and Palahniuk, 1991).

Arterial catheters are also useful in infants and small children who require cross-clamping of the aorta. Reperfusion of the kidney in this situation can result in profound hypotension. The beat-to-beat data provided by an arterial catheter allow more rapid correction of hypotension and greater stability. Arterial blood gases obtainable from an arterial catheter are also often helpful. However, because the lower extremity is not perfused during anastomosis, the arterial catheter must be placed in an upper extremity (Beebe et al., 1991; Belani and Palahniuk, 1991).

In older children who receive a kidney that is the appropriate size for their body weight, patient care during reperfusion is relatively straightforward. The hemoglobin level and electrolytes are checked after induction of general anesthesia. Older children usually do not require blood unless the hemoglobin level is less than 8 mg/dL. Similarly, children with renal failure often have a chronic metabolic acidosis; sodium bicarbonate is rarely required unless the pH is less than 7.25 despite mild hyperventilation. To ensure adequate hydration before reperfusion, normal saline or albumin is administered, provided the hematocrit is adequate until the CVP is 12 to 14 mm Hg. The systolic blood pressure is also allowed to rise to approximately 100 to 120 mm Hg before reperfusion to prevent hypotension when the clamps are released. Sodium mannitol (0.5 g/kg) and furosemide (1 mg/kg) are also administered to stimulate a diuresis. Sodium mannitol administration prior to release of the cross clamps has also been shown to reduce the requirement of posttransplantation dialysis, perhaps by releasing vasodilatory

prostaglandins in the kidney or by acting as a free-radical scavenger (Schnuelle and Johannes van der Woude, 2006). If the systolic blood pressure falls below 90 mm Hg, administration of a vasopressor such as ephedrine may be necessary. Rarely, dopamine or other vasopressors may be administered by infusion for persistent hypotension (Belani and Palahniuk, 1991). In the past, dopamine was commonly administered at low dosages in renal transplantations in children in an attempt to increase renal perfusion and blood flow. However, no long-term benefit was found in terms of graft, and its use at low dosages for renal perfusion is no longer recommended in kidney transplantation (Schnuelle and Johannes van der Woude, 2006).

Managing the perfusion of an adult kidney in an infant is more challenging. Unlike in older children or adults, both the aorta and the inferior vena cava are cross-clamped. Also unlike in adults, low-dosage systemic heparinization (50 U/kg) is required before clamping the vessels. Because blood pools in the unperfused lower extremities while the kidney is being sutured into place, release of the cross clamps causes ischemic by-products in both the kidney and lower extremities to enter the central circulation. The adult kidney itself can initially absorb up to 300 mL of blood. Vasodilation from ischemia can cause a large fraction of the infant's cardiac output to shunt through the new kidney. Occasionally, potassium from the preservative solution in the new kidney is transfused rapidly into the central circulation of the infant, resulting in cardiac arrhythmias, hypotension, and sometimes arrest. Surgeons try to prevent this by perfusing the kidney with normal saline to wash out the hyperkalemic preservative solution (UW solution), but they are not always successful. Also, in all cases, the kidney has been kept cold to preserve the organ while ischemic. Revascularization can result in significant hypothermia. Hypothermia may subsequently depress cardiac function and interfere with cardiac contractility that is needed to increase the cardiac output to perfuse the new kidney. Hypothermia also interferes with platelet and coagulation function, thereby predisposing the infant or child to increased perioperative bleeding (Beebe et al., 1991; Belani and Palahniuk, 1991).

In the past, infants receiving this operation had a high incidence of profound hypotension with perfusion of the allograft. This was often followed by vascular thrombosis or ATN. Subsequent experience in infants receiving an adult kidney has been much more successful (Beebe et al., 1991; Healy et al., 2000; Humar et al., 2001; Becker et al., 2006; Chavers et al., 2007).

The main difference in reperfusion of the kidney received by an infant compared with an older child or adult is that the CVP must be raised to a much higher level, at least 18 mm Hg, before reperfusion (Beebe et al., 1991; Chavers et al., 2007). Although there is no evidence that colloid solutions such as 5% albumin are superior to crystalloid solutions in renal transplantation, it is difficult to achieve volume expansion to CVP as high as 18 mm Hg with crystalloid solution alone because of its extravasation into the extracellular fluid (Schnuelle and Johannes van der Woude, 2006). Therefore, packed RBCs and colloids (5% albumin or fresh frozen plasma, or both, if clotting parameters are diminished) are usually required before reperfusion (Beebe et al., 1991). The use of synthetic colloid solutions such as Hetastarch has not been studied in this patient population (Schnuelle and Johannes van der Woude, 2006). The systemic blood pressure must also be at least 20% higher than the preoperative value, for the infant to tolerate cross-clamp release. Often this is achieved with transfusion to elevate the

CVP and lowering the anesthetic concentration to 0.5 MAC. However, some infants require an infusion of dopamine (3 to 5 mcg/kg per min) or other vasopressor to increase the blood pressure. As in older children and adults, sodium mannitol (0.5 to 1.0 g/kg) is administered before cross-clamp release, as well as Lasix (1 mg/kg) (Beebe et al., 1991).

The amount of volume required to raise the CVP to 18 mm Hg is often impressive. Many times, greater than 100% of the infant's calculated blood volume is administered before reperfusion of the kidney. Additional volume is often required after reperfusion to replace ongoing blood loss or to support the blood pressure if still inadequate (Beebe et al., 1991).

All blood products administered through the Hickman catheter during kidney transplantation in children require warming, because transfusion of cold blood into the central circulation can result in myocardial depression as well as worsen hypothermia (Beebe et al., 1991).

Forced-air surface warming with a device such as the Bair Hugger is also helpful to prevent hypothermia in kidney transplantation in children. However, the lower extremities should not be warmed until unclamping of renal vessels has been accomplished. Warming of the lower extremities using forced-air surface warming during aortic cross-clamping in animals resulted in hypotension, pulmonary hypertension, and myocardial depression. This was thought to result from greater production of ischemic by-products in lower extremities warmed during aortic cross-clamping (Beebe et al., 1993).

Immediately before cross-clamp release, atropine (20 mcg/kg) and calcium chloride (10 mg/kg) are administered. Atropine is administered because infants can occasionally develop vagally mediated profound bradycardia with the sudden loss of SVR. Calcium is important because potassium may be immediately transfused into the central circulation from the kidney if it has not been flushed of the high-potassium preservative solution (UW solution) before reperfusion. Often, sodium bicarbonate is administered as well (1 mmol/kg) to neutralize the acid that develops in the ischemic lower extremities and new kidney. The dopamine infusion may need to be increased, and other inotropes (e.g., epinephrine 1 mcg/kg as single aliquots) may be necessary immediately after reperfusion, but generally the pressure stabilizes at the initial, preoperative value (Beebe et al., 1991) (Fig. 28-21).

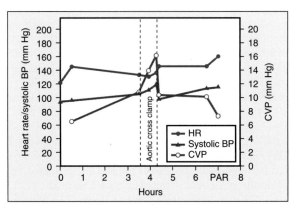

■ FIGURE 28-21. Systolic blood pressure (BP), heart rate (HR), and central venous pressure (CVP) during renal transplantation in infants. *(From Beebe DS, Belani KG, Mergens P, et al: Anesthetic management of infants receiving an adult kidney transplant,* Anesth Analg *73:725, 1991.)*

In both infants and older children, the urine output is replaced milliliter per milliliter with one-half normal saline solution as soon as it can be measured. This solution is chosen because this is the concentration of sodium excreted by a kidney with some degree of ATN or one that received large dosages of diuretics. Replacement of all the urine output with IV fluid ensures a brisk diuresis, and it is continued for up to 2 days after surgery. Dextrose is not added to the replacement solution because, if large volumes are administered because of a brisk urine output, hyperglycemia often results (Beebe et al., 1991; Belani and Palahniuk, 1991).

Postoperative Management

After closure of the wounds, virtually all older children can have skeletal muscle relaxants reversed and can be extubated as soon as they are awake and strong. Infants can usually be extubated in the operating room or recovery room as well, despite the presence of a large adult kidney, which causes obvious abdominal distention. Pain relief is usually achieved by means of patient-controlled analgesia with morphine, fentanyl, or hydromorphone. Recently, some anesthesiologists have reported successfully using epidural analgesia for postoperative analgesia, as well as part of a combined technique of epidural and general anesthesia intraoperatively. This is controversial because many children receive heparin intraoperatively or in the postoperative period, and this subjects children to a risk for epidural hematomas (Bhosale and Shah et al., 2008).

Most older children are cared for in the transplantation unit or ward. Rarely is ICU admission required, although most infants and small children require care in the pediatric ICU overnight. Urine is replaced milliliter per milliliter with half-normal saline for 2 days postoperatively. In infants, fluid management is similar to that in older children, but the amount of urine output from the adult kidney can be profound (i.e., 80 mL/kg per hr). Electrolytes therefore must be closely monitored. Eventually, over several days, the kidney adjusts to the smaller size of the recipient and produces the proper amount of urine (Beebe et al., 1991). Then, these children are allowed to begin oral intake, and diuresis is no longer forced. Discharge to home varies with the patient's ability to tolerate oral feedings, but it is usually within 1 week of surgery (Beebe et al., 1991; Belani and Palahniuk, 1991).

Postoperative Complications

Chest radiographic evidence of pulmonary edema caused by the large amounts of fluid administered to infants is present in at least 25% of patients in the recovery room. Despite this, less than 10% of infants require mechanical ventilation in the ICU postoperatively because diuresis from the new kidney occurs rapidly (Beebe et al., 1991).

Delayed graft function, defined as a need for dialysis within 1 week after surgery, can be a serious complication in pediatric patients. The incidence varies from 3% to 10% in recipients of living related kidneys in the pediatric age group, and it may be three times more common in recipients of deceased-donor kidneys (Tejani et al., 1999; Troppmann et al., 2005). Patients with delayed graft function have both an increased early incidence of graft loss and more rapid long-term graft failure in both deceased-donor and living related recipients

(Tejani et al., 1999). Of concern is a study by Troppmann that suggests that pediatric recipients of grafts harvested laparoscopically may be at increased risk for delayed graft function compared with those who received a kidney harvested by the open technique. Whether this is a true complication of the procedure or a complication of surgeons learning this new technique remains to be determined (Troppmann et al., 2005).

Graft thrombosis remains the primary cause of graft loss in the first year of transplantation in the pediatric age group. The rate of thrombosis is approximately 2%, and is more common in those who received a deceased-donor rather than living related donor organ and in recipients who were receiving peritoneal dialysis. Recently, the thrombosis rate appears to have declined, perhaps because of newer immunosuppressive agents and the improved technical skill of the surgeons (Smith et al., 2006). Kidney transplantation has now been successfully performed with outcomes comparable with those in normal children with renal failure in a series of patients with thrombotic risk factors (Kranz, 2006).

Finally, rejection is still the primary cause of graft loss over the long term. In recent years, the incidence of both acute and chronic rejection resulting in graft loss has declined as a result of more potent immunosuppressive agents. However, this decline in rejection has been accompanied by an increase in the number of posttransplantation infections (Dharnidharka et al., 2004).

Outcomes

Numerous studies have shown that the overall success rate for renal transplantation in children and teenagers is similar to that in adults (Elshihabi et al., 2000; McDonald et al., 2000; Smith et al., 2002; Magee et al., 2008). The 5-year patient survival rates in patients receiving living related kidney transplants for different pediatric age groups ranged from 94.7% to 96.3%. The patient survival rates were slightly lower for recipients of deceased-donor transplants (see Figs. 28-18 and 28-19). The 5-year graft survival rates over the same time period ranged from 74% to 89% in recipients of living related transplants, and 63% to 75% in those receiving a deceased donor organ (Magee, 2008). Rejection is the main cause of graft loss (Elshihabi et al., 2000). Until recently, most reports showed that the 1-year patient survival rate after transplantation was lower if the recipient was less than 2 years of age compared with older children after living related transplantation (89%). Graft survival was also less (85%). Both the mortality and graft loss were greater in deceased-donor transplantations as well (Elshihabi et al., 2000; McDonald et al., 2000). Vascular thrombosis was much more likely to be a cause of graft loss in infants than in older recipients. However, recent reports from selected centers demonstrate results in infants and small children with success rates similar to those in older children or adults (Becker et al., 2006; Chavers et al., 2007). Although infants and small children constitute a high-risk group, kidney transplantation can still lead to a good outcome. Although corticosteroids have been an essential cornerstone of immunosuppression after organ transplantation, the side effects of steroids are significant, and in children their effects on growth can be devastating. Steroid-free immunosuppression in children after kidney transplantation has been reported (Sarwal et al., 2003), and Sutherland and colleagues (2009) have reported that in a 5-year follow-up period, 87% remain steroid-free with patient and allograft survival rates of 96.4% and 94.1%, respectively.

ISLET CELL, PANCREAS, AND KIDNEY-PANCREAS TRANSPLANTATIONS

Diabetes mellitus (DM) has reached epidemic levels in the United States, probably related to the increased incidence of obesity, estimated at 67% in both the pediatric and adult populations. In 2009, an estimated 23.6 million people were living with type 2 DM, and an estimated 5 million undiagnosed or untreated patients in the United States (CDC Diabetes Public Health Resource, 2009). Although only 3% of type 2 DM develops in persons younger than 20 years (Fagot-Campagna et al., 2000), individuals who develop type 2 DM in childhood and adolescence are affected in early adulthood by the microvascular complications of DM (Krakoff et al., 2003; Le et al., 2008).

Based on 2005 to 2007 data from the Centers for Disease Control and Prevention and the National Institute of Diabetes and Digestive and Kidney Diseases, 15,000 youths in the United States were newly diagnosed with type 1 DM annually, and about 3700 were newly diagnosed with type 2 DM annually.

DM is one of the top five causes of morbidity and mortality in the industrialized world. The first clinical pancreas transplantation was performed in 1966 with a simultaneous kidney transplantation in a uremic, diabetic patient at the University of Minnesota, by Kelly, Lillehei, and colleagues (Lillehei et al., 1970; Sutherland et al., 1979). Since that initial event, simultaneous kidney-pancreas (SKP), pancreas after kidney (PAK), pancreas transplantation alone (PTA), and islet cell transplantations have increased dramatically. In 2008, a total of 126 U.S. centers (and nearly the same number worldwide) reported that they had performed at least one pancreas transplantation. Only three centers (2%) reported more than 50 pancreas transplantations, but 81 centers (64%) reported fewer than 10 (Gruessner and Sutherland, 2008).

Pediatric patients, however, account for a very small percentage (less than 3%) of all the pancreas transplantation procedures, which is the smallest percentile group of any solid organ transplantation (see Table 28-15). As of April 1, 2009, UNOS reported a total of 396 pancreas (PTA + PAK) and 43 SKP transplantations performed since 1988 in the pediatric patient population (UNOS, 2010); interestingly, one of these was listed as a living related transplantation. The total numbers of pediatric candidates on the UNOS waiting list, as of April 2010, are 62 for PTA and one for SKP. These numbers are markedly less than the numbers of adults on the UNOS waiting list, which currently are 1407 for SKP and 2497 for PTA.

In the United States between 1988 and 2010, 90.2% of these transplantation patients underwent SKP. The 1-year graft survival for SKP is approximately 86% to 91%; for PTA, it is 83.8%; and for PAK, it is 78.4%. The 1-year patient survival data are 95.9%, 99.2%, and 96.6% for SKP, PTA, and PAK, respectively. Long-term insulin independence is achieved in 70% to 80% of pancreas transplant recipients (Kahl et al., 2001; Bland, 2003; UNOS, 2010).

Islet Cell Transplantation

Islet cell transplantation was first performed in 1974. This procedure, like bone marrow transplantation, is dependent on the total mass or number of transplanted islet cells. Most notably, islet allotransplantation was not consistently successful until the early 1990s (Gruessner and Sutherland, 2003) in terms of the ability of patients to achieve sustained insulin independence. The number of procedures performed worldwide to date has been reported to be more than 412, with patient and graft survival rates at 75% and 65%, respectively (CITR Research Group, 2009). Islet cell transplantation as the dominant form of islet beta-cell replacement may occur in the near future; however, the needs for SKP, PTA, and PAK will remain, because of the need for exocrine pancreatic function. In addition, patients may not be able to achieve insulin independence without the critical mass of beta cells provided by a solitary pancreas transplantation. Although only a small percentage of patients are insulin independent after islet cell transplantation, graft survival is achieved in the majority of islet transplant recipients, with greater than 70% of them retaining C-peptide levels, normalized hemoglobin A1c, nearly absent severe hypoglycemia, and significantly reduced insulin requirements (compared with pretransplantation dosage) at 5 years under the Edmonton Protocol (Ryan et al., 2001, 2005a; Vantyghem et al., 2009). Insulin independence is improved after performing islet allotransplantation after kidney transplantation (IAK), 45% at 1 year, and simultaneous islet and kidney transplantation (SIK), 74% at 1 year with normalized glycosylated (glycated) hemoglobin (Ichii and Ricordi, 2009).

Islet Cell Transplantation Procedure and Anesthesia Considerations

Recent progress in the understanding of enzymatic digestion process of the pancreas, along with novel immunosuppression strategies have led to successful clinical trials of islet transplantation in humans (Ricordi et al., 2005). Automated islet cell isolation using a computerized centrifugation system and continuous enzymatic digestion of the pancreas for islet purification in discontinuous gradients has increased the yield of islet cells (Ricordi et al., 1988, 1992a, 1992b; Linetsky et al., 1997; Fiorina et al., 2008; Faradji et al., 2007; Kahl et al., 2001). Currently, the recommendations are for 10,000 cells/kg to be infused into the donor. Islet cell infusion into the liver is the most common and successful technique for this procedure (Ricordi, 1996).

Implantation of the islets is performed via a seemingly minimally invasive radiologic procedure. The portal vein is cannulated by a transhepatic percutaneous approach with angiographic guidance. General anesthesia is usually required for children. Alternatively, for SIK transplantation, an open procedure may be performed after completion of the kidney transplantation via a midline incision. In this case, the portal system is usually accessed by catheterization of a mesenteric vein. The purified islet suspension is slowly infused with continuous monitoring of the intraportal hydrostatic pressure (Oberholzer et al., 1999). Because it is necessary to cannulate the portal vein percutaneously and there is the potential for massive blood loss, central venous access and a large-bore IV catheter are usually recommended. Additionally, arterial cannulation may be necessary to monitor electrolytes and

glucose every 30 to 60 minutes after the infusion of the beta cells. Infusions of insulin and glucose may be equally necessary to maintain the serum glucose between 80 and 120 mg/dL, which is best for cell viability. The morbidity and mortality associated with intraportal islet infusion are minimal (Hering and Ricordi, 1999; Ricordi et al., 1997; Hogan et al., 2008). However, as with all allogeneic cellular infusions, foreign antigen recognition by the recipient means the possibility of a reperfusion-type syndrome, which may require bolus doses of epinephrine or phenylephrine and an infusion of a vasoactive agent (e.g., dopamine). These hemodynamic changes have been noted in 14.6% of patients undergoing autologous islet cell transplantation (Manciu et al., 1999).

Through December 2010, more than 450 islet allografts have been performed worldwide, including 306 since 1990 (Oberholzer et al., 1999; Thierry and Ricordi, 2000). Cumulative 1-year patient and graft survival rates of 96% and 35%, respectively, were obtained in 200 C-peptide negative, type-1 diabetic patients transplanted from 1990 through 1997. The persistence of graft function can be assessed by measurable levels of basal serum C-peptide, at a threshold of 0.5 ng/mL. The observation that 32% of recipients lose graft function within 1 month of transplantation (and 46% within 3 months) indicates that primary nonfunction might be a major cause of islet graft loss (Meyer et al., 1998; International Islet Transplant Registry Newsletter, 1999, 2000).

Although the evidence of measurable C-peptide in the serum indicates survival of the islet graft, it does not necessarily imply that patients can survive long term without supplemental insulin. However, islet graft function in the absence of insulin-independence is still associated with markedly improved metabolic control, glucose counterregulation, and hypoglycemia awareness (Meyer et al., 1998).

In 2000, the Edmonton Protocol introduced several modifications to the transplantation procedure, such as the use of a steroid-free immunosuppression regimen and transplantation of a mean islet mass of 11,000 islet equivalents per kilogram. These modifications improved 1-year outcomes. Although the results of a 5-year follow-up in 65 patients demonstrated improvement in glycemic stability in a significant portion, only 7.5% of the patients have reached insulin independence. In addition to the scarcity of organs available for transplantation, islet transplantation still faces major challenges, especially those related to cell loss during the process of islet isolation and the losses related to the graft site, apoptosis, allorejection, autoimmunity, and immunosuppression. The function of transplanted islets has often been defined on the basis of C-peptide values, (Ryan et al., 2005a, 2005b) the presence of which in before-transplantation C-peptide–negative patients seems to be the best function marker for engrafted islets. C-peptide is also correlated with the reduction of exogenous insulin requirement, confirming that it may be representative of engrafted cell mass and function (Shapiro and Ricordi, 2004; Shapiro et al., 2006).

Pancreas and Kidney-Pancreas Transplantations

Pathophysiology of Pancreatic Failure

Type 1 DM (insulin-dependent diabetes mellitus [IDDM]) is usually the result of the synergistic effects of genetic, environmental, infectious, and immunologic factors leading to pancreatic beta cell destruction and the resultant absolute absence of insulin production or secretion (Powers, 2001). Its U.S. incidence appears to be about 30,000 new-onset cases per year, and it has been the predominant cause of DM in the pediatric population for the past decade.

Type 2 DM (noninsulin-dependent diabetes mellitus [NIDDM]) is most often associated with obesity and is seen in the elderly population, albeit not exclusively. It has, however, been noted to be occurring with increasing frequency in the pediatric population and is linked to the increased incidence of childhood obesity. Furthermore genetic differences exist between IDDM and NIDDM, as evidenced by twin studies (Barnett et al., 1981). In this classic publication by Barnett and coworkers, the concordance rate (both twins affected) of IDDM was 50%, as contrasted with a concordance rate of greater than 90% for twins having NIDDM, demonstrating that genetic factors play a much larger role in this variant of the disease.

The primary objective of pancreas or islet beta-cell transplantation is to restore endogenous insulin secretion to a diabetic individual, by the provision of the missing normal beta cell function. Achieving euglycemia, as well as the release of glucagon in response to hypoglycemia, allows patients to be insulin free and to eat a regular diet, and it ultimately prevents the multisystem organ complications of diabetes. Occasionally, exocrine pancreatic function is also desired to restore both types of pancreatic hormonal function, possibly lost as a result of total pancreatectomy or in patients with cystic fibrosis (Kiberd et al., 2000; Kahl et al., 2001; Paty et al., 2001; Powers, 2001; Coosemans and Pirenne, 2003; Hakim, 2003). Carbohydrate, fat, and protein metabolism is expected to normalize after pancreas transplantation and may eventually stabilize and even prevent the development of microvascular disease (Coosemans and Pirenne, 2004).

For diabetic patients with imminent or established ESRD who have had or plan to have a renal transplantation, the American Diabetes Association now recommends pancreas transplantation as an acceptable therapeutic alternative to exogenous insulin therapy (American Diabetic Association, 2000). Additionally, diabetic patients should be considered for pancreas transplantation (PTA) in the absence of indications for kidney transplantation in the setting of frequent, acute, and severe metabolic complications, incapacitating clinical and emotional problems with exogenous insulin therapy, and consistent failure of insulin-based management to prevent complications. In the majority of cases, pancreas transplantation is performed in patients with type 1 DM and ESRD. Patients eligible for PTA or PAK procedures must have stable and adequate kidney function at the time of transplantation, as both the operative procedure and the immunosuppressive agent may produce a further decline in the patients' renal function.

Absolute contraindications to transplantation include active malignancy or infection, recently treated malignancy not meeting the minimum disease-free observation period as suggested by the Clinical Practice Guidelines of the American Society of Transplantation (Diabetes Control and Complications Trial Research Group, 1993), psychiatric disease so severe or unstable that the stress of a large surgery would probably result in marked decompensation, and inability or unwillingness to take immunosuppressant medications regularly so that graft failure would be certain.

Preoperative Evaluation

As with kidney transplantation, patients with pancreatic failure for any of the group of procedures for islet-beta cell replacement will require a thorough evaluation given the constellation of hyperglycemic complications seen in the diabetic patient; these include ischemic heart disease, cardiomyopathy, renal failure, autonomic neuropathy and gastroparesis, hypertension, and cerebrovascular, ophthalmologic, and macrovascular diseases. In addition, a meticulous review of the current list of medications and allergies must be undertaken. The patient selected to receive a deceased donor organ requires urgent attention, evaluation, and preparation for the procedure, as the procured organ has a limited life in the preservation solution, usually not to exceed 24 hours. Hence, the anesthesia evaluation, if not previously completed as part of the pretransplantation evaluation, requires a de novo thorough evaluation in a timely manner.

The degree of renal dysfunction, if any, is of particular importance, as it will dictate the particular type of procedure that the patient should receive (i.e., SKP versus PTA). SKP transplantations account for 79% of pancreas transplantations, whereas PAK transplantations account for 14%. Most often, this decision has been made as part of the preoperative evaluation so as to have the patient placed on the waiting list. Moreover, a determination of the patient's acid-base status, daily serum glucose, electrolyte concentrations, and time of last hemodialysis is of great importance. Anemia associated with ESRD, resulting from diminished production of erythropoietin and chronic bone marrow suppression, is often associated with an increased morbidity and diminished graft success (Koehntop et al., 2000).

The principal cause of perioperative mortality in adult pancreas recipients is coronary artery disease (Bland, 2003). Thus, mandatory screening tests for the preoperative cardiovascular evaluation include coronary angiography in addition to the usual noninvasive studies, which often include a dobutamine stress echocardiogram (Rabbat et al., 2003). Moreover, depending on the findings, pretransplantation coronary revascularization reduces the risk for subsequent cardiac events (Rabbat et al., 2003).

The pediatric patient facing pancreas transplantation, however, is usually devoid of cardiovascular or significant renal complications, as the disease process is usually of a shorter duration than in the adult population. Nonetheless, all end-organ damage must be fully assessed and excluded.

A history of gastroparesis needs to be addressed appropriately in the pediatric patient, as it may warrant an IV rapid-sequence induction as opposed to an inhalation induction. Aspiration prophylaxis with H_2 antagonists, metoclopramide, and possibly a nonparticulate antacid should be considered. Additionally, autonomic neuropathy, which results in gastroparesis, may predispose these patients to episodes of hypotension during the transplantation or any anesthesia.

Airway evaluation is of special importance, because diabetics have an increased incidence of difficult intubations (Hogan et al., 1988). This finding has been correlated with the stiffness of the interphalangeal joints, which results in difficulty in opposing the fingers (Hogan et al., 1988). This too correlates with longevity of the disease and may prove irrelevant in the pediatric population.

Surgical Procedure

Several surgical techniques for pancreas transplantation have been described, and the approach depends on whether the procedure is an SKP or a PTA. After appropriate blood and tissue typing for human lymphocyte antigen (HLA) markers and ABO compatibility, the organ is prepared on the back table. Vascular grafts, if needed, are anastomosed at this time, and the organ is maintained in cold preservation solution (to minimize warm ischemic preservation injury).

After induction of general anesthesia and the placement of monitors and arterial and central venous catheters, a surgical midline incision is made to facilitate implantation of the pancreas graft and the kidney if necessary. The right colon is mobilized by incising the peritoneal reflection, allowing positioning of the right colon cephalad. The right iliac vessels are then dissected, and in patients undergoing bladder drainage (BD), the right iliac vein is completely mobilized by ligating and dividing all posterior branches. Mobilizing the sigmoid colon and reflecting it medially exposes the left iliac system. Ligating and dividing the posterior branches as on the right side then allow mobilization of the iliac vein. The graft is then implanted with the head of the pancreas and the duodenum directed toward the pelvis. In BD grafts, the site for the vascular anastomosis is usually the common iliac vein and the common iliac artery. The graft, with a duodenal "button," is then anastomosed to the bladder (Fig. 28-22).

Compared with BD pancreatic allografts, the vascular anastomoses of enteric drainage grafts are achieved using the more proximal iliac vasculature. Usually, the venous anastomosis is performed in the area of the distal IVC, and the arterial anastomosis is to the proximal right common iliac artery. The organ is then anastomosed to a proximal portion of the jejunum (Fig. 28-23).

A crucial element at the time of graft reperfusion is the sequence of slow releases of the vascular clamps. Over the course of several minutes, the clamps are removed in the following sequence: proximal venous clamp, distal arterial clamp, proximal arterial clamp, and distal venous clamp. After each clamp is removed, careful hemostasis of bleeding vessels on the surface of the pancreas and at each vascular anastomosis, if necessary, is accomplished before any further clamps are removed.

The surgical approach to pancreas engraftment depends on whether exocrine secretions will be managed by enteric or by

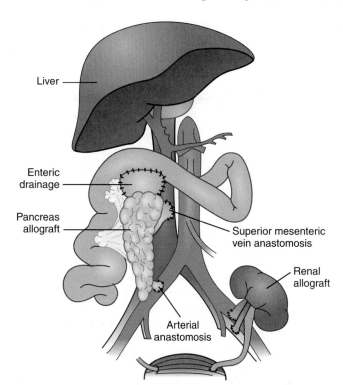

■ **FIGURE 28-23.** Pancreas and kidney transplants (PAK or SKP) with the donor pancreas vascularized to facilitate enteric exocrine drainage to a proximal portion of the jejunum (enteric drainage technique). The donor kidney is implanted in the left iliac fossa anastomosed to the femoral vessels, and a ureteroneocystostomy is performed (see text). *(From Larson-Wadd K, Belani KG: Anesthesiol Clin North America 22:663, 2004.)*

bladder drainage. Between 1987 and 1995, more than 90% of pancreas transplantations were performed using BD, initially described by Sollinger and colleagues, (1998) and later modified by Corry and associates to include the duodenal button, which acts as a reinforcement of the anastomosis of the graft to the bladder. This approach allows serial measurements of urinary amylase, one method of monitoring graft rejection (Bloom et al., 1997; Cattral et al., 2000; Bland, 2003; Coosemans and Pirenne, 2003). Additionally, pancreatic biopsies are less risky, as the organ is placed lower in the pelvis.

Chronic loss of pancreatic secretions into the bladder can result in associated complications of metabolic acidosis, a finding in the majority of patients with BD, and perhaps dehydration. Electrolyte abnormalities, which are the results of the loss of sodium bicarbonate–rich pancreatic secretions, are not infrequent. Moreover, local bladder irritation, hematuria, urethritis, bladder leak, neurogenic bladder, chemical cystitis and uretheritis, allograft pancreatitis, duodenitis, bladder calculi, urethral erosions, prostatitis, urethral strictures, and infections are all possible complications (Bloom et al., 1997; Cattral et al., 2000; Kahl et al., 2001). In fact, the frequency of urologic complications is high, 50% to 77%, with this approach, but this rarely results in either patient mortality or graft loss.

The kidney, if implanted as in the SKP procedure, is positioned in the left iliac fossa and an ureteroneocystostomy performed. Vascular anastomoses are to the dissected left iliac vessels in the child weighing more than 20 kg (see Fig. 28-23).

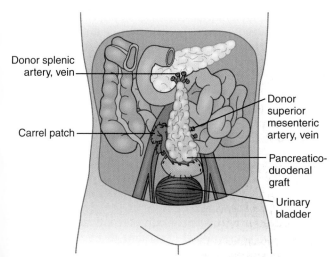

■ **FIGURE 28-22.** Solitary pancreas transplant (PTA), with the urinary bladder being used for exocrine drainage (bladder drainage technique). Note the native pancreas is in situ (see text).

However, in the infant weighing less than 20 kg, the graft is implanted with anastomoses of the vasculature to the aorta and vena cava.

More recently, the enteric drainage technique has become the surgical technique of choice (Bloom et al., 1997; Cattral et al., 2000; Bland, 2003; Coosemans and Pirenne, 2003), although initially it was associated with a high morbidity rate because of peritoneal leakage and the need for frequent reoperations. In this procedure, the pancreatic duct is inserted into the small bowel using a button of duodenum, or with a Roux-en-Y limb (see Fig. 28-17). Although Roux-en-Y was once used predominantly for enteric drainage at most centers, its role has diminished, primarily as a result of the reduced need for monitoring of graft rejection as immunosuppressive regimens have improved and the frequency of rejection episodes has decreased. Over 55% to 77% of pancreas transplantations are with enteric drainage, as reported to UNOS for the period from 1999 to 2002.

Enteric drainage avoids the complications associated with BD (Bloom et al., 1997; Cattral et al., 2000; Coosemans and Pirenne, 2003). Vascular management of the pancreatic graft has also evolved. Venous graft effluent can be drained into either the systemic or the portal circulation. Portal venous drainage was used in approximately 25% of pancreas transplantations from 1996 to 2002 (Bland, 2003). Both portal and systemic drainage is associated with excellent glycemic control; however, fasting serum insulin levels are significantly lower in portal drainage, without effect on graft survival rates at 1 year for SKP or PAK (Cattral et al., 2000; Bland, 2003); and PTA has a slightly higher graft survival rate with portal drainage (Bland, 2003). A postulated advantage of portal venous drainage is the avoidance of hyperinsulinemia, which has been associated with advanced atherosclerosis and vasculopathy. Pancreas grafts have been associated with the highest surgical complication rate of all routinely transplanted solid organs. Causes for technical failure of the deceased-donor primary pancreas transplantations include vascular thrombosis, pancreatitis, anastomotic leak, bleeding, rejection, and infections (Laftavi et al., 1998; Troppman et al., 1998; Humar et al., 2000a, 2000b; Sutherland et al., 2001; Michalaka et al., 2003).

Vascular thrombosis is the most commonly sited cause of graft failure, and it was assumed to be associated with technical complications of the operation. However, after a thorough pathologic evaluation of sequential cases of massive thrombosis, it is now evident that unrecognized hyperacute rejection is far more common than had been appreciated in this setting. Thus, organ rejection may in fact be the most common cause of graft loss. Significant risk factors for graft loss include older donor age, retransplantation, and relaparotomy for infection, leakage, or bleeding (Troppman et al., 1998; Humar et al., 2000a, 2000b). The quality of a deceased-donor graft can directly affect graft performance. As experience with pancreas transplantation has increased, the incidence of relaparotomy has decreased (Humar et al., 2000a, 2000b). Risk factors for recipient death include older recipients, retransplantation, and relaparotomy for thrombosis, infection, leakage, or bleeding (Troppman et al., 1998).

Anesthesia Management

After appropriate positioning and placement of the standard monitors, anesthesia is induced either with an IV technique or an inhalation technique with agents appropriate for the patient's baseline metabolic condition, followed by orotracheal intubation. In children, a central venous catheter and preferably a radial arterial catheter are inserted (as both iliac arteries may potentially be used for vascular anastomoses). After the induction, the volatile anesthesia agent should be isoflurane or desflurane for patients with renal dysfunction, as they appear to be virtually devoid of nephrotoxicity and physiologically do not diminish renal arteriolar blood flow. Nitrous oxide is avoided because it increases the size of gas-containing spaces such as the bowel. A balanced anesthesia technique may also be used to maintain general anesthesia.

Morphine-6-glucuronide and normeperidine, the metabolites of morphine and meperidine, respectively, may lead to toxicities, with seizures in the case of normeperidine in the setting of renal failure, and hence should be avoided. Hydromorphone may be used in preference to these agents, as it is less dependent on renal excretion. However, intraoperatively and immediately postoperatively, fentanyl is the narcotic of choice, because it has minimal associated hemodynamic alterations. The choice of muscle relaxant depends on the degree of renal impairment.

In patients with significant cardiovascular disease, direct arterial pressure monitoring and right heart monitoring with a pulmonary artery catheter should be considered, as well as continuous TEE monitoring as needed. This, however, is rarely necessary in the pediatric patient. Serum glucose levels must be carefully monitored at least hourly during general anesthesia, particularly after graft reperfusion, with maintenance of the serum glucose between 100 to 200 mg/dL (Koehntop et al., 2000), as hyperglycemia triggers early islet cell dysfunction (Clark et al., 1982; Imamura et al., 1988). Maintaining serum glucose levels in an acceptable range is accomplished by continuous infusion of regular insulin at a rate of 1 to 5 U/hr, with concurrent dextrose infusion when serum glucose levels are 150 mg/dL. The addition of dextrose ensures uninterrupted intracellular fuel to avoid perioperative ketosis. Pancreatic beta cells may function as early as 5 minutes after reperfusion with the release of insulin (Troppmann et al., 1996, 1999; Jung et al., 2009; Koh et al., 2008). Delayed graft function may be treated postoperatively with an insulin infusion titrated to keep blood glucose levels 150 mg/dL (Sealey, 1988; Kin, 2010; Anazawa; 2009). Somatostatin may also be administered to decrease exocrine pancreatic secretion (Bloom et al., 1997).

Prior to allograft reperfusion with release of the vascular clamps, the hemodynamics are optimized to ensure adequate perfusion and prevent hypotension. IV fluids, either crystalloid or colloid, are administered to achieve a CVP in the range of 12 to 14 mm Hg and a systolic blood pressure of at least 140 mm Hg (Koehntop et al., 2000). Alternatively, in patients with a pulmonary artery catheter, careful titration of volume versus filling pressures and cardiac output can be used to optimize intravascular fluid status before vascular unclamping. Additionally, the end-tidal concentration of the inhaled agents may need to be reduced, because reperfusion of both grafts may result in short-lived hypotension as a result of vasodilation, cytokine release, transient myocardial dysfunction, and metabolic acidosis. This may require the administration of fluids, the use of a vasopressor (preferably dopamine), IV bicarbonate or thamasol, and blood products when appropriate.

It is imperative to maintain adequate and even supranormal perfusion pressure and blood flow to the new allograft (see Kidney Transplantation, earlier). This may help to prevent graft vessel thrombosis, the most common cause of technical pancreatic graft failure (Bland, 2003). However, as noted previously, this complication is probably related to organ rejection.

Most patients should be extubated in the operating room at the end of surgery, if the usual criteria are met for this. Serum glucose, hemoglobin, electrolytes, and troponin levels should be checked, along with a baseline arterial blood gas for the determination of any residual acidosis immediately on arrival in the ICU or the recovery room. Patients with a bladder anastomosis often require supplemental sodium bicarbonate to treat the metabolic acidosis caused by the loss of pancreatic secretions into the bladder (Sudan et al., 2000; Kahl et al., 2001; Coosemans and Pirenne, 2003; Troppmann et al., 2004). Postoperatively, patients receive 5% dextrose in normal saline as maintenance fluid. Nasogastric and urine output losses are replaced in equivalent amounts with normal saline. Pancreas transplant recipients have a higher incidence of acute rejection and immunologic graft loss than any other solid organ recipients. They are at risk of developing infection for numerous reasons, including immunosuppression, contamination from the duodenal segment of the graft, and serum glucose irregularity because of DM (Troppmann et al., 2004). Infection prophylaxis with broad-spectrum antibiotics targeting *Staphylococcus,* gram-negative bacteria, anaerobes, and CMV is routine in many centers (Bloom et al., 1997; Humar et al., 2000a, 2000b; Coosemans and Pirenne, 2003). Prophylaxis against vascular thrombosis consists of either low-dosage IV heparin (300 to 500 U/hr) or subcutaneous administration of heparin followed by aspirin (Humar et al., 2000a, 2000b; Coosemans and Pirenne, 2003).

HEMATOPOIETIC STEM-CELL TRANSPLANTATION

The first hematopoietic stem-cell transplantation (HSCT) was an allograft procedure performed in 1968 in a 2-year-old boy who received HLA-matched bone marrow from his sister to treat Wiskott-Aldrich syndrome (Bach et al., 1968). *Stem-cell transplantation* is a generic term that includes several different techniques. When an allogeneic transplantation is performed, hematopoietic stem cells are taken from the bone marrow, peripheral blood, or umbilical cord of a healthy donor matched for HLA type (either a family member or an unrelated volunteer). During cord blood harvesting, cord blood is collected from an umbilical vein under sterile conditions, without physical risk to the mother or infant donor, from the delivered placenta (ex utero) or during the third stage of labor (in utero). An experienced collector can harvest an average of 110 mL of blood. This contains approximately 1×10^9 nucleated cells from a single placenta (Kurtzberg, 2009). When an autologous transplantation is performed, the child's own stem cells are taken from either the bone marrow or peripheral blood, and preserved for later transplantation. In both instances, the child is prepared prior to transplantation, by a process known as conditioning, with either chemotherapy or chemoradiotherapy. The term *syngeneic* transplantation refers to transplantation of stem cells obtained from an identical twin (Stein et al., 1990; Beebe et al., 1995). Figure 28-24, from the Center for International Blood and Marrow Transplant Research registry, provides information about the source of stem cells used for HSCT in children. As seen in the figure, there is an increase in the use of cord blood and peripheral blood as a source for stem cells in the pediatric age group. Bone marrow as a source of stem cells is usually used for autologous transplantation, whereas mobilized peripheral blood stem cells are used in the majority of cases in

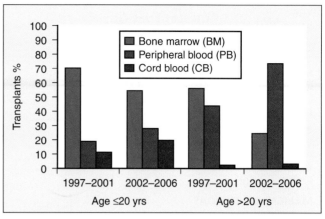

FIGURE 28-24. Allogeneic stem-cell sources used in different eras. *(From the Center for International Blood and Marrow Transplant Research (CIBMTR): Newsletter. 13(2), Dec 2007 [see www.cibmtr.org]. Also see www.marrow.org/PHYSICIAN/Outcomes_Data/index.html.)*

allogenic settings (Machaczka et al., 2009). Banked cord blood is usually used for unrelated donor transplantation (Kurtzberg, 2009). Cord blood has several advantages: prompt availability of stem cells, decrease of graft-versus-host disease (GVHD), and better long-term immune recovery resulting in equivalent long-term survivals even when compared with HLA-matched bone marrow–obtained stem cells (Gluckman, 2009). Bone marrow harvesting from both adult and pediatric donors is usually done under general anesthesia. The harvesting of mobilized peripheral blood stem cells on the other hand requires a deep venous catheter for performing a plasmapheresis procedure (Demeocq, 1994; Kanold et al., 1999). This is usually done under sedation and requires processing of one to three blood volumes (Kanold et al., 1999), and the procedure can take up to 8.5 hours (Demeocq, 1994). During autologous harvest of bone marrow, Perez de Sa and colleagues (1991) were able to avoid the use of RBC transfusion by performing hemodilution with 6% dextran during the removal of 24 ± 6 mL/kg of bone marrow. However, in some instances, autologous or allogenic blood may be required (Machaczka et al., 2009).

HSCTs are now performed for various illnesses, ranging from hematologic and oncologic disorders to metabolic and genetic defects (Kurtzberg, 2009). Most commonly, HSCT is performed in patients with leukemia, lymphoma, neuroblastoma, and multiple myeloma (Box 28-5). HSCT was performed to treat children with epidermolysis bullosa dystrophica (Tolar et al., 2009). An 18-month-old boy with recessive dystrophic epidermolysis bullosa was one of the first patients transplanted for this disease. He received umbilical cord blood and bone marrow in 2007 from a perfectly matched sibling, at the University of Minnesota. Epidermolysis bullosa dystrophica is a progressive disease of the skin that is ultimately fatal. The children are a challenge for the anesthesiologist. No adhesive tape can be used on the skin, and the skin has to be carefully protected with lubricants and steroid cream. Scarification can result in significant difficulties in mouth opening and can also result in lesions in the mouth and pharynx, making airway care a challenge (Karabiyik et al., 2009) (see Chapter 36, Systemic Disorders).

Although the death rate from graft failure, infection, and GVHD is still high (approximately 40%), the success rate of

Box 28-5 Illnesses that Qualify for Hematopoietic Stem-Cell Transplantation

MALIGNANT HEMATOLOGIC DISORDERS
- Acute myelogenous leukemia
- Chronic myelogenous leukemia
- Acute lymphoblastic leukemia
- Hodgkin's lymphoma
- Non-Hodgkin's lymphoma
- Plasma cell disorders
- Histiocytic disorders
- Other malignancies

MALIGNANT TUMORS
- Neuroblastoma
- Medulloblastoma
- Ewing's sarcoma

NONMALIGNANT HEMATOLOGIC DISORDERS
- Immunodeficiency syndromes
- Acquired bone marrow failure syndromes

GENETIC DISORDERS
- Congenital immunodeficiency disorders
- Inherited erythrocyte abnormalities
  - Hemoglobinopathies
- Inherited platelet disorders
- Inborn errors of metabolism
  - Mucopolysaccharidoses
  - Leukodystrophies
- Epidermolysis bullosa dystrophica
- Congenital bone marrow failure syndromes

From the United Network for Organ Sharing (UNOS) and Organ Procurement and Transplantation Network (OPTN) data, 2010. Available at http://optn.transplant.hrsa.gov/data.

TABLE 28-21. Noninfectious Pulmonary Complications after Hematopoietic Stem-Cell Transplantation

Complication	Interval after Transplantation
Diffuse alveolar hemorrhage	1 day to 3 mo
Idiopathic pneumonia syndrome	1 day to 15 mo
Pulmonary cytolytic thrombi	15 day to 11 mo
Peri-engraftment respiratory distress syndrome	3rd to 4th wk
Bronchiolitis obliterans organizing pneumonia	1 mo to 13 mo
Bronchiolitis obliterans	3.5 mo to 15 mo
Delayed pulmonary toxicity syndrome	4 mo to 5 mo

From Afessa B, Litzow MR, Tefferi A: Bronchiolitis obliterans and other late onset non-infectious pulmonary complications in hematopoietic stem cell transplantation, *Bone Marrow Transplant* 28:425, 2001.

HSCT has improved over time with advances in immunosuppression, chemotherapy, antibiotics, and supportive care (Beebe et al., 1995). Between 1989 and 2006, the number of children receiving bone marrow transplantation for various disorders has reached a steady number—between 4000 to 4500 per year (CIBMTR, 2007).

The cord blood of newborn donors has become popular as a marrow source for both pediatric patients and adults (Tse et al., 2008). There is minimal risk for viral exposure with cord blood, and the donor is not at risk. The primary benefit to cord blood transplantation, however, is for reasons related to the immaturity of the newborn stem cell, and the incidence of GVHD is markedly lower than with standard bone marrow or peripheral stem cell transplantations (Cohena and Nagler, 2003; Kurtzberg, 2009).

Before receiving HSCT, children require bone marrow ablation with chemotherapy and occasionally total body irradiation (TBI). The intensity of this protocol varies and is dependent on several factors (Riordan et al., 2007). After successful preparation, the processed donor marrow or stem cells from peripheral or cord blood are administered intravascularly into the HSCT recipient, where they circulate and settle into the patient's bone marrow beds. Occasionally, engraftment fails to occur. Even if engraftment is successful, complications are frequent and include infection, GVHD, toxicity from chemotherapy or radiation therapy, and venoocclusive disease of the liver (Gentet et al., 1988; Stein et al., 1990; McDowall, 1993; Beebe et al., 1995; Schure and Holzman, 2000; Wah et al., 2003; Thiruvenkatarajan and Rebecca, 2007). Furthermore, several noninfective pulmonary complications (Table 28-21) can occur soon after HSCT and even up to 15 months after transplantation (Afessa et al., 2001).

Infection is one of the main causes of morbidity and mortality in bone marrow transplant recipients. Ablation of the bone marrow renders a child neutropenic for as long as several weeks before full engraftment occurs. T- and B-cell function may also be depressed for several months after HSCT, causing recipients to be susceptible to viral and fungal infections (Stein et al., 1990; Beebe, 1995).

GVHD occurs when the T lymphocytes derived from the donor's bone marrow react against the host. Acute GVHD has an incidence of 40% to 60% and occurs within 100 days after transplantation and may manifest with skin rash, watery or bloody diarrhea, or hepatic involvement with hyperbilirubinemia. Fever is common. Chronic GVHD has an incidence of 20% to 40% and occurs after day 100 following allogenic HSCT. It occurs most commonly in patients who have previously had acute GVHD. Chronic GVHD may manifest with scleroderma, oral mucositis, interstitial pneumonitis, polymyositis with contractures, and thrombocytopenia (Stein et al., 1990; Schure and Holzman, 2000; Wah et al., 2003; Thiruvenkatarajan and Rebecca, 2007).

The TBI used in preparation for HSCT may cause pneumonitis, restrictive cardiomyopathy, pulmonary fibrosis, and oral mucositis. Chemotherapeutic agents such as doxorubicin can result in cardiomyopathy and other toxicities (see Chapter 36, Systemic Disorders). In addition, venoocclusive disease of the liver may develop after intensive chemotherapy and radiation therapy. This complication, which is most often fatal, occurs approximately 2 weeks after transplantation, when the small hepatic venules become fibrotic and develop pericentral hepatocyte necrosis and congestion (Gentet et al., 1988).

Before receiving HSCT, pediatric patients often require anesthesia for indwelling central venous catheterization, bone marrow biopsies, baseline diagnostic testing (eye examinations, magnetic resonance imaging, CT, pulmonary washing for macrophage function evaluation) and TBI. After HSCT, children often require anesthesia for (1) biopsies to evaluate the status of the transplanted graft and to determine if GVHD has developed, and (2) treatment of the surgical complications that may follow the HSCT procedure and for complications related to GVHD.

Most children tolerate anesthesia for these procedures without difficulty. However, complications can occur, particularly in recipients less than 2 years of age and those with metabolic and storage diseases, so anesthesia providers must keep in mind the unique medical problems associated with children undergoing HSCT (Stein et al., 1990; Beebe et al., 1995; Thiruvenkatarajan and Rebecca, 2007).

Preoperative Assessment

Before anesthesia is administered, HSCT recipients must be examined for potential difficulties from the patient's underlying disease and for the complications arising from HSCT. For example, tracheal intubation and airway care are often difficult in patients with Hurler's syndrome (Belani et al., 1993). Before anesthesia, especially when mucositis is present, the airways in all children before and after HSCT must be examined for feasibility of the approach, and for the presence of mucositis. Mucositis usually develops when these patients become neutropenic prior to the marrow's becoming functional. This leads to oral infections and mucositis, which can lead to difficulty in visualizing the laryngeal inlet. Mucositis is also associated with an increased incidence of postextubation laryngeal edema in the postoperative period. Cardiopulmonary evaluation must be undertaken in all children before HSCT. Cardiac disease is common in many children with mucopolysaccharidosis (Belani et al., 1993), and anthracycline therapy used in children needing HSCT can exert detrimental cardiopulmonary effects (Uderzo et al., 2007). Thus, all children need an ECG evaluation, an echocardiogram, and pulmonary function tests (PFTs) when indicated. Uderzo and associates (2007) suggest that after 5 years, the cumulative incidence of respiratory function abnormalities is 35%, and impairment of the cardiac shortening fraction occurs in 26% of children. Similarly, thrombocytopenia and other coagulopathies resulting from liver dysfunction may require attention prior to anesthesia care. Because of GVHD, there may be significant pulmonary involvement, which needs to be defined before anesthesia for potential intraoperative complications and for planning a postoperative ventilation strategy. Chemotherapy-related cardiac dysfunction needs to be documented but is usually not a big concern in pediatric HSCT patients. Both radiation and chemotherapy are associated with a higher likelihood of nausea and vomiting, and the need for airway protection may favor endotracheal intubation (Stein et al., 1990; Beebe et al., 1995; Schure and Holzman, 2000; Wah et al., 2003; Thiruvenkatarajan and Rebecca, 2007).

Anesthesia Management

A variety of anesthesia techniques can be safely used to anesthetize a child for HSCT. No drug, agent, or technique is absolutely contraindicated (Stein et al., 1990; Beebe et al., 1995; Thiruvenkatarajan and Rebecca, 2007). Several anesthesia providers have raised concern about the use of nitrous oxide in HSCT recipients because it suppresses methionine synthetase, which is required for nucleotide synthesis (Thiruvenkatarajan and Rebecca, 2007). However, a randomized study of cellular function and marrow engraftment of stem-cell recipients exposed to short-term use of nitrous oxide anesthesia failed to show any deleterious effects (Lederhaas et al., 1995). One of the major concerns of anesthesia care for HSCT recipients is the anatomic morbidity from their underlying problems (mucopolysaccharidosis, epidermolysis bullosa dystrophica) and the acquired mucositis that they develop after HSCT. The incidence of mucositis is quite high, and it occurs when the patient becomes severely neutropenic. Techniques should thus be chosen to minimize mucosal damage in the oropharynx. For example, IV propofol and, more recently, dexmedetomidine with or without ketamine are suitable choices to provide sedation for simple procedures. Propofol has proved useful for anesthesia for TBI using spontaneous ventilation without airway instrumentation. It not only has a rapid recovery profile but is also an antiemetic and therefore promotes adequate nutritional intake when compared with thiopental or ketamine (Beebe et al., 1995). In some instances, the laryngeal mask airway may be used to provide a more secure airway during TBI or other procedures when children have a preexisting condition such as Hurler's syndrome and a difficult upper airway. Significant lubrication and caution must be used when using the laryngeal mask airway in these children, because trauma can occur with it (Marjot, 1991).

Patients who have already developed mucositis and require anesthesia present a challenge to the pediatric anesthesia provider. Most of these children require tracheal intubation to prevent aspiration of infected mucus. The preoperative airway examination may be difficult because of significant discomfort. For the same reason, awake intubation is less likely to be an available option. Movement and struggling during the procedure may initiate bleeding and edema and obscure the laryngeal inlet. Unless the mouth is anatomically fixed and unable to be opened, a rapid-sequence induction often provides the best option for atraumatic access to the trachea, and this approach also minimizes the time in which aspiration of infected secretions can occur.

In other cases, especially when stridor or other signs of airway obstruction are evident, an approach that is often practiced in children with supraglottitis is favored. This often requires that the child be transported to the operating room for ideal intubating conditions, the presence of a trained pediatric otolaryngologist, and all the necessary tools to handle a difficult airway. After an effective dosage of an anticholinergic and carefully titrated sedation, the child is allowed to breathe sevoflurane in oxygen in the position that best promotes spontaneous breathing. Controlled breathing is attempted at the appropriate time, and when this is possible, a decision is made about whether the use of neuromuscular blockers is appropriate.

Care must be taken with extubation as well. Most patients with mucositis can be extubated when fully awake. Often these patients develop croup in the postoperative period, which may require treatment with dexamethasone (0.5 to 1.0 mg/kg) and one or more courses of racemic epinephrine treatment. However, patients with mucositis and severe edema of the laryngeal inlet may require prolonged intubation until the edema has resolved (Beebe et al., 1995; Thiruvenkatarajan and Rebecca, 2007).

Outcome

Outcome after HSCT depends on numerous factors and is related to disease type, response to chemotherapy, phenotype,

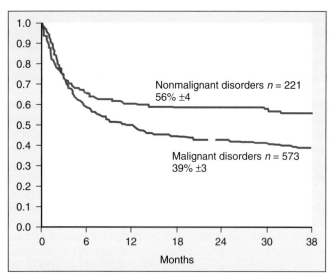

■ **FIGURE 28-25.** Three-year survival curves after stem-cell transplantation for malignant and nonmalignant disorders. *(From Gluckman E: History of cord blood transplantation, Bone Marrow Transplant 44:621, 2009.)*

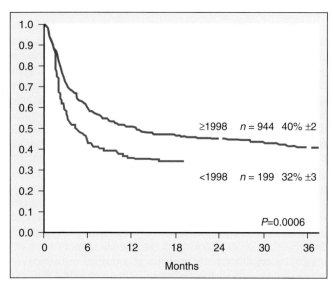

■ **FIGURE 28-26.** Survival curves comparing patients transplanted before and after 1998. *(From Gluckman E: History of cord blood transplantation, Bone Marrow Transplant 44:621, 2009.)*

molecular genetics, and conditioning protocols (Buchholz and Ganser, 2009). The Center for International Blood and Marrow Transplant Research (CIBMTR) publishes a newsletter that provides survival and outcomes information for transplantations facilitated by the National Marrow Program. The 3-year overall results for survival after transplantation in children with non-malignant disorders are better than for those with malignant disorders (Fig. 28-25) (Gluckman, 2009), and the results significantly improved after 1998 (Fig. 28-26).

HEPATOCYTE TRANSPLANTATION

Since the development of techniques for the isolation of individual cells from the liver, transplantation of isolated hepatocytes has been considered a potential therapy for the treatment of liver disorders. Over the past decade, several investigators have shown that hepatocyte suspensions can successfully engraft into the liver or splenic parenchyma or into the peritoneal cavity and other extrahepatic sites. These hepatocytes have been shown to function after transplantation, have partially corrected liver-based errors of metabolism, and have reproducibly prolonged survival of animals with liver failure. Although hepatocyte transplantation (HT) is in its infancy, abundant preclinical studies and small series of patients suggest great value in acute liver failure and in the treatment of liver-based metabolic diseases, such as urea cycle disorders. From a technical standpoint, HT is begun with cannulation of the portomesenteric circulation. This can be performed using open exploration and isolation of mesenteric venous tributaries or by percutaneous access to the intrahepatic portal vein. Slow infusion of the hepatocyte suspension occurs over several hours. Infusion-related complications include transient reductions of portal venous flow and hemodynamic instability. In addition, portosystemic embolization of hepatocytes into the pulmonary circulation can result in transient increases in pulmonary pressures and hypoxia (Fox, 1998; Horslen and Fox, 2004; Strom, 1997, 1999).

To date, human HT has been attempted in patients with acute and chronic liver failure, and in some patients with liver-based metabolic disease. Clinical experience suggests that in contrast to animal studies, transplanted hepatocytes have a markedly diminished regenerative ability in humans (Strom, 1997, 1999; Fox, 1998; Horslen, 2003). Despite this, HT remains an alternative experimental therapy that has been used to bridge patients to orthotopic liver transplantation with potential reductions of the preoperative morbidity and mortality associated with severe liver failure and poorly controlled metabolic deficiencies.

POSTTRANSPLANTATION SIDE EFFECTS

Posttransplantation Lymphoproliferative Disease

Posttransplantation lymphoproliferative disease (PTLD) is one of the most life-threatening complications of immunosuppressive therapy in this era of organ transplantation, even with the use of newer immunosuppressive agents and regimens for induction and maintenance. It is seen after both solid organ and bone marrow transplantation. Patients receiving bone marrow, liver, or kidney transplants have an estimated incidence of PTLD of 1% to 3%; heart and heart-lung recipients, 5% to 13%; and intestinal transplantations, 30%. Recently, the incidence of PTLD has been reduced to 8% in intestine and 3% in liver transplantations (Bond et al., 2008). Mortality is reported to be as high as 50% (Faye and Vilmer, 2005). Epstein-Barr virus (EBV) is confirmed in greater than 50% of pediatric and 85% of adult patients. The interval to presentation of this disease ranges from months to years after transplantation.

The most common sites of involvement are the lymph nodes and GI tract, with homograft involvement dependent on the organ transplanted. The heart is usually spared from involvement with heart transplantation. However, with heart-lung transplantation, the lungs are the most frequently involved sites (Sklarin, 1991). Similarly, the liver is a frequent site of involvement in recipients of bone marrow transplantation.

Because lymphoproliferative disease requires active viral infection of the B cell, it seems that pediatric patients have a higher likelihood for the development of lymphoproliferative disease, the rationale being that pediatric patients have not been exposed to the virus and thus have no antibodies for the prevention of infection. The risk for PTLD is five times greater in patients who are EBV seronegative at the time of transplantation (Kirk et al., 2007). Cyclosporin A (CyA)-induced suppression of the suppressor T lymphocyte is responsible for continued uncontrolled polyclonal proliferation of the transformed B lymphocyte, infected with the episomal EBV DNA. Tumors generated in response to the virus are varied. Non-Hodgkin's lymphomas are the usual lymphomas.

Treatment of PTLD is by several modalities, with reduction of the immunosuppressive agent being the most efficacious. This allows the improvement of immunosurveillance; however, the reestablishment of the host defense may exacerbate organ rejection. Approximately two thirds of patients will be responsive to this maneuver in EBV-related PTLD. Alternatively, cytokines and immune globulin have been used to enhance the immune response. Fischer-Froehlich and coworkers (2002) reported the use of anti–B-cell antibodies in controlling B-cell lymphomas. Interferon-γ in conjugation with gamma globulin has also proved to be efficacious. Surgical resection of tumors has also improved survival in selected cases, with survival reported at 74%, relative to the 31% overall survival after the presentation of PTLD (Stieber et al., 1991). Acyclovir inhibits EBV replication. Prophylaxis with this agent may prove to be beneficial because the drug does not prevent proliferation of EBV-infected cells already transformed.

Immunosuppression under tacrolimus apparently does not appear to confer protection from the development of PTLD. The time to development of the disease with its use appears to be similar to CyA.

For the anesthesiologist, perioperative concerns of children with PTLD involve the airway. Tonsillar hypertrophy is a frequent presentation of this disease in the pediatric patient and often requires bilateral tonsillectomy for diagnosis of the disease as well as management of upper airway obstruction. Occasionally, these patients have been treated with chemotherapeutic agents, which may result in additional organ dysfunction.

Infectious Diseases

The risk for infection in the transplant patient is directly influenced by two factors: the patient's environmental exposure and the patient's immunosuppressive regimen. The spectrum of viral causative agents included CMV, the most deleterious (Ho, 1991; Patel et al., 1996). Antirejection therapy is the most important contributor to the development of infection, with CyA at the top of the list of implicated agents. A clear example is the incidence of CMV infection, which has increased from 15% in the pre-CyA era to greater than 50% (Rubin and Tolkoff-Rubin, 1991).

Patients who experience increases in immunosuppression for acute and chronic rejection are at increased risk for all types of infection (Fishman, 2007). Opportunistic viral infections can affect both patient and graft survival. Ganciclovir and valgoncycloroxin are used in the treatment of CMV and in EBV infections. The spectrum of presentation of CMV infection is bimodal and has two sources. The virus may be reactivated from a latent phase, or there may be active infection. Although prior infection confers acquired immunity, this may also be the source of latent infection in the immunosuppressed patient. The donor

organ has been shown to act as a source of latent infection. The effects of CMV infection may be quite devastating, and damage to the grafted organ is frequently encountered. Obliterative bronchiolitis, chronic coronary atherosclerosis, and vanishing bile duct syndrome are often attributed to CMV infection of the lungs, heart, and liver, respectively. The greatest risk for both CMV and EBV infections occurs in seronegative patients who receive allografts from seropositive donors. Completion of vaccination series with virus vaccines is important in children. Live-virus series (e.g., mumps, measles, and rubella [MMR], and varicella) should ideally be completed before transplantation.

Other viral infections with significant consequence to the host are hepatitis viruses B and C and HIV infection. There is a significant reinfection rate of the hepatic graft in patients known to be ε-antigen positive before transplantation. This has raised the question of whether this group of patients should have transplants. Hepatitis B is devastating to all graft recipients, and a higher than normal rate of overwhelming hepatic failure is the rule. Hepatitis C is also a significant problem, with approximately 10% of solid organ recipients acquiring the virus. Data suggest that up to 50% of organ recipients from donors who are antibody positive progress to develop active infection.

Fungal infections remain a major concern in organ transplantation (Castaldo et al., 1991a, 1991b). Divided into two categories, these infections may be invasive and opportunistic, or represent geographically restricted systemic mycoses. Amphotericin, the mainstay of therapy for systemic infections, has now been joined by fluconazole. Fluconazole is far less toxic than amphotericin and represents a significant advance in antifungal therapy.

Bacterial infections have a devastating consequence, cover a wide spectrum, and include atypical agents such as *Nocardia asteroides* and *Mycobacterium*. Prophylactic therapy for several infections has gained wide acceptance. For example, low-dosage trimethoprim-sulfamethoxazole has been quite efficacious in the prevention of *Pneumocystis carinii* infection in all organ transplantations, as well as in the prevention of urosepsis in the renal transplantation patient.

Chimerism and Tolerance

In the past three decades, a particular subgroup of patients who no longer required immunosuppression, along with the apparent development clinical immunotolerance, gave genesis to the idea of chimerism. It became evident that solid organ transplant recipients could be, and were, transformed into chimeras, to varying degrees irrespective of the organ transplanted. A chimera was thus defined as the acquisition by the recipient of the donor leukocytes, lymphocytes, and dendritic cells, which spread via vascular conduits to the host's lymphoid tissue and organ systems from the transplanted organ.

In the early stages after transplantation, donor antigen–presenting cells, mainly immature dendritic cells, migrate out of the allograft toward secondary lymphoid organs, where they mature and encounter recipient alloreactive naive T cells and resting or central memory T cells, a direct pathway for normal tissue allorecognition. Furthermore, the engrafted organ acquires the recipient's immune system and a population of the recipient's leukocytes. This was clearly demonstrated in liver transplantation, when the entire macrophage system, including the Kupffer cells of the graft (one component of the liver's

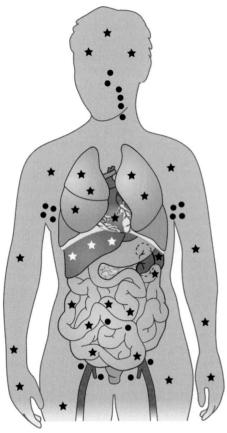

dendritic cells), is replaced by that of the host (Starzl et al., 1992). This became the first actual biochemical realization of a chimera (Fig. 28-27).

Transplantation tolerance indeed refers to a state of sustained specific nonresponsiveness of the recipient's immune system to donor alloantigens, allowing long-term allograft survival in the absence of potentially harmful chronic immunosuppressive therapy. More specifically, it is the unambiguous evidence of normal graft function without features of graft rejection and the need for any immunosuppressive agents. Since the pioneering work of Billingham, Brent, and Medawar (1953) more than half a century ago, many experimental animal models, as well as some clinical data in specific settings, support the concept that transplantation tolerance could be an achievable target for selected patients.

The early thoughts and dismissal of leukocyte chimerism–associated mechanisms were diversionary, in view of the early recognition that implanted organ allografts promptly become mixtures of donor and recipient cells (i.e., organ chimerism). The evidence was first presented in 1968 by karyotyping studies of livers that had been transplanted to female recipients from male deceased donors (Kashiwagi et al., 1969). Whereas the rest of the allograft remained male, the bone marrow–derived

passenger leukocytes including Kupffer cells were largely replaced with recipient female cells within 100 days of transplantation. These alterations were incorrectly assumed to be a unique feature of the transplanted liver until it was demonstrated that most of the lymphoid tissues of the engrafted rat (Murase et al., 1991) and human intestine (Iwaki et al., 1991) were replaced by recipient cells of the same lineages. An epiphany occurred when comparable findings were confirmed in successfully transplanted human kidney, pancreatic (Randhawa et al., 1993; Starzl et al., 1993), and thoracic organ allografts (Randhawa et al., 1993), and thus it became unambiguously clear that all engrafted organs were chimeric structures.

Chimerism and tolerance can be viewed as central or peripheral. The concept of *central tolerance* and mixed chimerism involves the recognition of the critical important role the thymus plays in the maintenance of tolerance to self-antigens, and many experimental data support its role in the induction of sustained robust tolerance to alloantigens. During the physiologic maturation process in the thymus, central tolerance is achieved by intrathymic deletion of T cells with high avidity for thymic expressed self-antigens (negative selection), so that potentially deleterious antigen-reactive T cells will not reach the periphery. In the transplantation setting, this process can be exploited by the delivery of donor alloantigens to the thymus prior to solid organ transplantation. This can be achieved either experimentally by direct intrathymic injections of donor- derived allopeptides or by the induction of a state of hematopoietic mixed chimerism in the recipient's repertoire (the presence of cells from both recipient and donor origin) allowing donor antigen–presenting cells to migrate to the recipient's thymus and induce negative selection of donor-reactive T cells. For mixed chimerism to occur in the recipient, the infused bone marrow cells from the donor and recipient must engraft, implying the need for preconditioning treatments that allow the creation of "space" for engraftment, combined with deletion of preexisting cross-reactive peripheral T cells that could reject the donor bone marrow.

T cells are crucial in the initiation and coordination of the rejection response and to promote *peripheral tolerance.* The alloreactive effector T-cell pool must be minimized, and regulatory mechanisms enhanced. Various strategies have been explored to achieve peripheral tolerance to alloantigens in experimental transplantation models:

● Deletion of peripheral effector T cells (lymphocyte-depleting protocols)
● Inhibition of T-cell activation by blocking or modifying costimulatory signals (costimulatory blockade, manipulation of dendritic cells)
● Interference with the effector function or homing of activated T cells (anticytokines, antichemokines)
● Active regulation of effector T cells by antigen-specific CD4 and CD25 cells

Most of these approaches have been extensively studied in experimental models and are now being progressively transposed to the clinical arena.

Calne and colleagues (1998) first divulged interesting clinical data using lymphocyte depletion with alemtuzumab (Campath), which provided long-term rejection-free allograft survival with minimal maintenance therapy (low-dosage cyclosporine) in most patients. Because these recipients did not exhibit true operational tolerance, Calne and colleagues coined the term *prope tolerance* (near tolerance) to describe this immunologic state. The targeted immunomodulation has led to the development of several immunomodulating agents, which are targeted at a number of the cell-surface markers of T and B lymphocytes. These agents offer real prospects for the realization of the holy grail of successful long-term transplantation. The model of HLA matching in kidney and bone marrow transplantation has helped to establish the role of these cell-surface markers for all solid organ transplantation, which is important if success is to be achieved with respect to chimerism, tolerance, and the reduction if not elimination of GVHD.

Selective immune tolerance of alloantigens and transplanted tissues will improve significantly in the future. The strategies to induce tolerance to foreign tissues may include clonal T- and B-cell deletion, induction of bone marrow chimerism, manipulation of regulatory cytokines, and blockade of T-lymphocyte-specific–mediated costimulation. Additionally, newer pharmacologic agents have certainly enhanced our understanding and the advancement of this field. Induction of selective immune tolerance could make it possible to minimize, or dispense with, immunosuppressive regimens that now cause end-organ toxicity, life-threatening infections, and neoplasm development. With the exponential growth in the area of stem-cell and xenotransplantation, the dream to have a transgenic pig for every human who needs a specific organ or multivisceral transplantation may become reality in the not too distant future.

SUMMARY

In the past 25 years, solid organ transplantation has gained acceptability as a viable form of medical therapy for many forms of end-stage organ disease in the pediatric patient, as well as early therapy for congenital anomalies and varied inherited genetic diseases otherwise without a cure. Advances in immunosuppression protocols have enhanced the survival of children from otherwise deadly diseases. The challenge for the future is the development of more specific immunomodulation, and better understanding of chimerism.

Improved patient survival will probably come not from advances in surgical technique but from advances in immunology, and from advances in hepatocyte and stem-cell transplantation. Consensus protocols with randomized arms of immunosuppressive therapies need to be considered to further advance the specialty. The effects of anesthesia agents during organ harvest need to be further explored. Finally, in addition to the medical and surgical challenges, organ transplantation imposes ethical and quality-of-life issues that must constantly be assessed and reassessed.

For questions and answers on topics in this chapter, go to "Chapter Questions" at www.expertconsult.com.

REFERENCES

Complete references used in this text can be found online at www.expertconsult.com.

Anesthesia for Conjoined Twins

Jennifer Thomas

CONTENTS

A nesthesia for conjoined twins may range from a very straightforward pediatric anesthetic procedure to one of the most daunting and challenging procedures faced by any pediatric anesthesiologist.

This rare but fascinating congenital problem is of considerable importance to anesthesiologists. In recent medical literature, there are ever-increasing reports of anesthesia for conjoined twins, both general and regional. From the twins' initial admission, anesthesiologists should be involved in the care and decision-making procedures planned for these infants. At any stage of their time in the hospital, anesthesiologists may be called on to provide resuscitation for the infants or to anesthetize them for investigations or procedures. These may be related to their conjoined state or for some other pathology in one or the other twin, such as pyloric stenosis, or adenoidectomy for upper airway obstruction (Thomas, 2004). Management of conjoined twins is a multidisciplinary exercise involving many specialties, and the anesthesiologist is an integral part of this team. Likewise, it is essential that the anesthesiologists establish a team approach within their own discipline, so that each specialist knows precisely the roles of all individuals at the various stages of the procedures. The separation of a set of conjoined twins is the best example of teamwork that any hospital staff will experience.

Four major centers in the world have described their experiences and outcomes in their management of conjoined twins (Spitz and Kiely, 2003; O'Neill, 1998; Rode et al., 2006; Millar et al., 2009; Rabeeah, 2006) (Table 29-1). Many of the cases and examples used and described in this chapter are from the Red Cross War Memorial Children's Hospital in Cape Town, South Africa, where over a period of 44 years (1964 to 2009) 49 sets of symmetric and asymmetric conjoined twins have been managed.

INCIDENCE

Because of the significant number of conjoined twins who are aborted or who are stillborn, the exact incidence is not known, but the reported incidence worldwide is estimated at 1:50,000 to 1:100,000 live births, with a higher incidence of 1:14,000 to 1:25,000 experienced in Africa and Asia (Hoyle, 1990). Of those that are born, many may have congenital abnormalities that are incompatible with life. The presence of associated congenital anomalies in live twins is common. Congenital diaphragmatic hernia, pulmonary hypoplasia, congenital heart disease, anomalous hepatic arterial and venous drainage, biliary tree anomalies, bowel atresia, Meckel's diverticulum, complex urogenital anatomy, and spinal dysraphism have all been reported.

TABLE 29-1. Summary of Symmetric Conjoined Twins Managed in Four Centers

			Operated			
			Emergency Surgery		Elective Surgery	
	Number of Sets	Not Operated Sets	Number of Sets	Number of Individual Survivors (%)	Number of Sets	Number of Individual Survivors (%)
Spitz and Kiely, 2000	22	6	7	4/14 (29)	9	15/18 (83)
O'Neill, 1998	18	5	5	1/10 (10)	8	13/16 (81)
Rode et al., 2006	33	16	3	2/6 (33)	14	20/28 (72)
Millar et al., 2009	34	17	3	2/6 (33)	15	22/30 (73)
Rabeeah, 2006	29	18	0	—	11	20/22 (90)

HISTORICAL PERSPECTIVES

Conjoined twins are one of nature's greatest enigmas. Cave drawings, pottery, figurines, and folklore indicate that conjoined twins have occurred since prehistoric times. Embryonic duplication also occurs in plant and other animal forms of life (Fig. 29-1) (Thomas and Lopez, 2004). The famous and most celebrated pair of conjoined twins, Chang and Eng Bunker, who were joined at their xiphisterna, was born in Siam (now Thailand) in 1811. Because of their fame and the rarity of this pathology, the term *Siamese twins* has become synonymous with conjoined twins. Over time, the bridge of skin and tissue between them stretched, and they were able to stand side by side. The twins were taken to America, where they were on

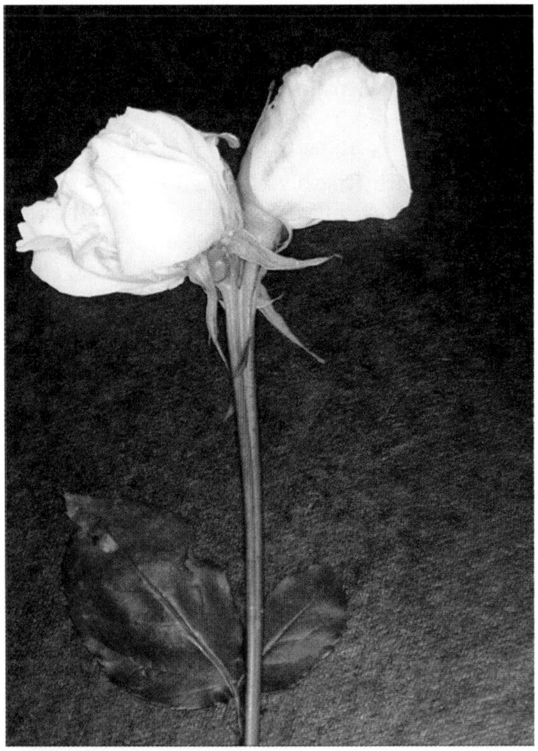

■ FIGURE 29-1. Conjoined twinning occurs in plants and animals, as well as in human life. This photograph is of twin roses of the Double Delight variety.

display by Phineas T. Barnum in his circus. Surgery for separation was deemed too risky unless one of the twins was to die. The Bunker twins lived very interesting lives—they married sisters and fathered 22 children between them. They died within hours of each other at the age of 63 (Spitz, 2003). Interestingly, the twins who have become most famous have all remained conjoined, whereas there is very little literature on the lives of those who have been separated. Votteler and Lipsky (2005) have reported on the long-term results of ten separations, as have Hoyle and Thomas (1989) with their experiences studying ischiopagus twins over 23 years. The first set of omphalopagus twins separated at the Red Cross Children's Hospital now each has children of their own (Cywes and Louw, 1967; Cywes et al., 1982).

The first successful separation of conjoined twins was performed by Konig in 1689, when he separated omphalopagus twins by slowly tightening an encircling band around the connection until it necrosed the connecting bridge. The first successful separation of thoracopagus twins with a conjoined heart was reported in 1979 when, after the interatrial bridge was interrupted, there was a single survivor (Synhorst et al., 1979).

During the 1960s and 1970s, emphasis in the perioperative management of conjoined twins was on preoperative discussions and planning, dress rehearsals, and on the then-new techniques of invasive intraoperative monitoring for blood loss and hemodynamic status (Diaz and Furman, 1987). From the 1980s onward, most improvements have occurred in obstetric and fetal ultrasound; fetal and neonatal surgery; magnetic resonance imaging (MRI); contrast computed tomography (CT); numerous radiographic technological options to help delineate anatomic variations in different twins; in the anesthetic advances of oximetry, capnography, agent analysis; and in techniques for monitoring brain oxygenation and blood flow.

For the induction of omphalopagus twins, Allen et al. (1959) described the use of cyclopropane and oxygen, supplemented by ether via the open-drop method. He describes the attempts at intubation by holding one infant above the other to facilitate easier intubation as a "near fatal mistake." In this position, the upper twin became pale and apneic, whereas the condition of the lower infant rapidly deteriorated and it became plethoric. Once they were returned to their normal position, they were successfully intubated. He comments that "there are few vital signs available for monitoring infants of this size. The most important signs are respirations, color, and muscle tone." Both infants survived the surgical separation.

The anesthesia provided to separate the first set of twins in 1967 in Cape Town, South Africa, was described as "uneventful" (Cywes and Louw, 1967). Preoperative investigations in these omphalopagus twins indicated that there was no cross-circulation between the infants and this was confirmed at the induction of anesthesia, when the pancuronium given to one infant had no effect on the other.

In Furman's report (Furman et al., 1971), intubation on a set of xiphopagus twins was performed when both infants were awake, and vascular cannulation was done when they were under local anesthetic. Jarem (Jarem et al., 1977), in his classic paper, describes the double breathing circuit fashioned from readily available parts of anesthetic equipment.

Roy (1980) described his experience with craniopagus twins. His group used two anesthetic teams, but only one anesthetic machine with a non–rebreathing Jackson-Rees breathing system from the gas outlet leading to two T pieces. Monitoring included: electrocardiograph (ECG), Doppler arm-cuff pressures, esophageal stethoscopes, and rectal telethermometers. Each infant received preoperative atropine, and they were induced simultaneously with halothane, nitrous oxide, and oxygen. He continued to describe the 15-month preparation time before their separation. This was successfully achieved, but he describes the anesthetic challenges as severe hemorrhage and maintenance of a clear airway with obstruction from secretions, kinking, or accidental extubation. Harrison and his team (1985) commented on the need for modification of the breathing circuit to accommodate the process of ventilating neonatal conjoined twins simultaneously and stated that adequate intravascular fluid replacement was essential to prevent hypotension at separation. They also commented on the intraoperative challenges of these infants.

Diaz and Furman, (1987), in their well-known paper on the perioperative management of conjoined twins, highlighted many factors that are now integral to the care of these patients. Advances in anesthetic equipment, monitoring, and drugs (inhalational or intravenous) give us options for anesthesia that earlier anesthetic specialists did not have. Similarly, outcomes for surgical procedures in these patients have improved. The developments in pediatric intensive care have had a positive impact on both the preoperative and postoperative care and outcomes of these children.

EMBRYOLOGY

Two theories have been proposed as to the etiology of conjoined twins: fusion and fission. Although the differences between these theories have yet to be resolved, fission is the generally accepted and older theory, where the fertilized egg fails to split completely (Kaufman, 2004). The theory of fusion, proposed by Spencer (2000a, 2000b, 2003), suggests that the fertilized egg splits completely, but a secondary union of two separate embryonic discs at the dorsal neural tube or ventral yolk sac takes place at 3 to 4 weeks' gestation. This theory was also held by Aristotle (Millar et al., 2009).

Monozygotic twins are the result of one ovum being fertilized by one sperm and then dividing into two embryos. In conjoined twins, this division, at the 13th to 17th day of the blastocyst stage, is incomplete.

Conjoined twins are identical, with what has always been thought to be an identical chromosomal pattern. With new

molecular genetics, this has been shown to not necessarily be the case, and the twins may neither be completely identical nor have the same chromosome pattern (Hall, 2003). It has been hypothesized that monozygotic twinning occurs at four possible phases: up to 3 days' postconception, after 4 to 6 days, after 7 to 12 days, and finally after 13 to 17 days. It is during this latter period that conjoined twins, fetus-in-fetu, or a teratoma may arise (Hall and Lopez-Rangel, 1996). Parasitic twins are thought to result from the embryonic death of one twin, with the remaining parts of the body vascularized by the surviving autocyte. Fetus-in-fetu are asymmetric monozygotic diamniotic intraparasitic twins (Hall and Lopez-Rangel, 1996). Conjoined triplets and quadruplets have been documented, although all have been aborted (O'Neill, 1998; Rode et al., 2006). These cases are exceptionally rare, with an even more obscure pathogenesis.

Conjoined twins are always the same gender. There is a 3:1 female-to-male incidence in live births, but more males are stillborn (Hoyle, 1990; Rejjal et al., 1992). They are monozygotic, monoamniotic, and monochorionic. Despite this, the infants usually vary in size, appearance, personality, internal anatomy, and degree of organ-sharing and duplication. Many of the challenges for all disciplines relate to the vast diversity in the anatomic variations that may possibly occur. Organs may be conjoined, duplicated, or absent. Investigations are crucial to clarifying these differences in order to make decisions about surgery, interventions, and survival. Even then, surprises occur at the time of surgery, and innovative techniques may be necessary.

Survival depends on the site and complexity of conjunction, the degree of organ sharing, and the presence of other congenital anomalies, with the extent of cardiac fusion and lung development being major determining factors (Andrews et al., 2006).

CLASSIFICATION, NOMENCLATURE, AND TERMINOLOGY

Conjoined twins are typically classified by the anatomic site of conjunction (which may be complex) followed by the suffix -pagus—the Greek word meaning *that which is joined* (Box 29-1). There is an international collaboration attempting

Box 29-1 Nomenclature and Classification of Conjoined Twins

VENTRAL UNION (87%)	DORSAL UNION (13%)
Rostral (48%)	Craniopagus (5%)
Cephalopagus (11%)	Rachipagus (2%)
Thoracopagus (19%)	Pygopagus (6%)
Omphalopagus (18%)	
Caudal (11%)	
Ischiopagus	
Lateral (28%)	
Parapagus	
Dipagus	
Dicephalus	

VENTRAL CONJUNCTIONS

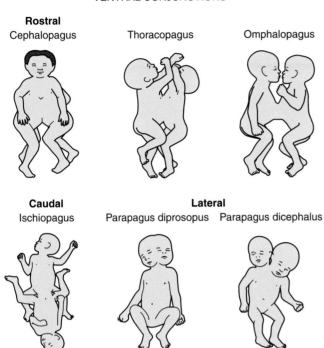

Rostral

Cephalopagus   Thoracopagus   Omphalopagus

Caudal   **Lateral**

Ischiopagus   Parapagus diprosopus   Parapagus dicephalus

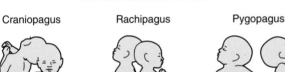

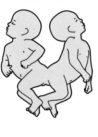

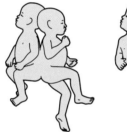

DORSAL CONJUNCTIONS

Craniopagus   Rachipagus   Pygopagus

■ **FIGURE 29-2.** Illustrations depicting the anatomic relationships of the different types of symmetric conjoined twins. (*Modified from Spencer R: Conjoined twins: developmental malformation and clinical implications, Baltimore, 2003, John Hopkins University Press.*)

to create a more uniform classification of conjoined twins (Spencer, 1996). This considers a ventral (front, caudal, or lateral) or dorsal (back-to-back, sacrum-to-sacrum, or head-to-head) fusion, with further classification described in the following paragraphs (Fig. 29-2).

Twins are described as being *symmetric* or *asymmetric,* although these terms are often misleading, because even when the twins are fully formed they are seldom truly symmetric. According to the most prominent site of conjunction, the following sites of conjunction are the most common: the chest (thoracopagus twins), the abdomen (omphalopagus twins), sacrum (pygopagus twins), pelvis (ischiopagus twins), and back (rachipagus twins) (Table 29-2).

Symmetric twins are two anatomically identifiable infants with a physical appearance suggestive of two possible survivors. With asymmetric, or parasitic, twins, one twin is a potential survivor and usually appears normal, but the other is incomplete and attached as a parasite. This may be externally visible,

or it may be internal. Where there is an attachment of an anatomically identifiable part, but not of a total individual, the term *heteropagus* is used. It is in this group, that regional anesthesia is particularly useful. Within a classified group, especially with complex conjunctions, the external physical appearance and spatial arrangement of the infants may be very different (Figs. 29-3 and 29-4).

Conjoined twins are further classified by the number of limbs present and the internal organs that are involved in the conjunction. The following list shows this classification system:

> Two arms: dibrachius
> Three arms: tribrachius
> Four arms: tertrabrachius
> Two legs: bipus
> Three legs: tripus
> Four legs: tetrapus

The degree of cardiac fusion, or degree of cardiopagus, can be considered as follows (Andrews et al., 2006):
A: Separate hearts and pericardium
B: Separate hearts and a common/shared pericardium
C: Fused atria and separate ventricles
D: Fused atria and ventricles
Outcomes for separation in groups C and D are poor.

Twins Joined at the Head

There are three types of twins joined at the head (Spencer, 2003).

Parapagus twins have two faces lateral to each other on the same side of one head, with a single neck and body.

Cephalopagus twinning is a rare form of conjoined twins in which the infants are united from the tops of the heads down to the umbilicus, with two separate lower abdomens and pelvises (also referred to as *cephalothoracopagus*). The two fused faces are on opposite sides of the head, so named after the two-faced god Janus, this type of conjunction is sometimes referred to as *Janiceps.* The brains and spinal cords are abnormal, and the number and type of limbs vary. This type of conjoined twins is not separable, and early diagnosis allows for termination of the pregnancy.

Craniopagus twins are united only at the cranial vault, with two completely separate faces and bodies. O'Connell (1976) described a practical approach to classifying craniopagus twins—partial and total. In the partial form, union is limited and separation is feasible with a good chance of survival; however, in the total form, significant intracranial abnormalities may be present and make attempted separation hazardous. Blood loss may be considerable, making death(s) on the operating table highly likely. Bucholz et al. (1987) reported higher perioperative mortality in the temporoparietal and occipital junctions, with parietal junctions having an intermediate mortality, and frontal craniopagus having the lowest mortality. Winston (1987) described a classification based on the deepest structures shared:

> Type A: Share only scalp and subcutaneous structures
> Type B: Share dura mater
> Type C: Share dura mater and arachnoid and pia mater
> Type D: Share brain structures as well as structures from types A, B, and C

In predicting the outcome, the extent of fusion of venous structures is almost as important as the degree of brain conjunction. For twins who come to surgery, this also has considerable impact on intraoperative blood loss.

TABLE 29-2. Types of Symmetric Conjoined Twins

Type	Area(s) Conjoined	Consequences
Thoracopagus Thoracoomphalopagus	Upper to lower chest Heart and pericardium always involved Chest and abdomen	High mortality Usually face-to-face Complex anatomy of heart, diaphragm, GI tract
Thoraco-omphaloischiopagus	Chest, abdomen, and pelvis	Face-to-face Four arms; two, three, or four legs; variable genitalia
Xiphopagus	Xiphoid cartilage, upper abdomen	Possible liver fusion Simple conjunction
Omphalopagus	Lower chest, upper abdomen	Heart not involved Liver, proximal GI tract, diaphragm, other organs variable
Ischiopagus	Fused lower bodies, spinal and urogenital system involvement	Four arms; two, three, or four legs
Pygopagus (pyopagus/ileopagus)	Back-to-back at pelvis Sacrum and coccyx fused	Spine often involved, distal GI tract often fused
Parapagus	Fused side-by-side with a shared pelvis **Dithoracic:** fused abdomen pelvis, not thorax **Diprosopic:** one trunk, one head, two faces with varying fusion **Dicephalic:** one trunk, two heads, two, three, or four arms	Organ sharing variable Limbs variable
Craniopagus	Fused skulls, separate bodies Fused back (occipital), front (frontal), side (temporoparietal) or top (parietal) of head, not face or base of skull	Extent of brain fusion variable Venous connections important
Rachipagus	Dorsal fusion, back to back Face away from each other	Extremely rare Spine involvement variable; fusion terminates above sacrum Occiput possibly involved

GI, Gastrointestinal.

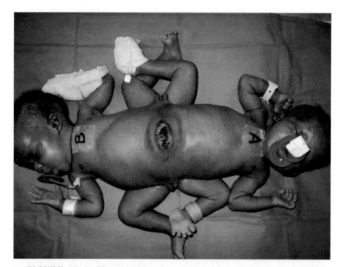

■ **FIGURE 29-3.** These ischiopagus twin girls were born via vaginal delivery to a very surprised mother and her midwife.

ETHICS

In broad terms, ethics are a set of standards of professional conduct (Atkinson, 2004). Whenever planned separation of conjoined twins takes place, and when there is a possibility or probability that one twin may not survive the procedure, moral, ethical, and legal arguments are raised. Many of these issues have been addressed in the literature (Pearn, 2001; Unknown

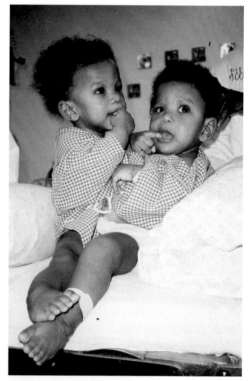

■ **FIGURE 29-4.** This set of twin boys has a complex conjunction at the thoracic, abdominal and pelvic levels, and despite also being ischiopagus, show no physical resemblance to the twins in Figure 29-3.

author, 2000; Spitz and Kiely, 2000; Spitz, 2000; Bratton and Chetwynd, 2004). The Hastings report identified three cardinal issues (London and Knowles, 2001):

- If one twin would not (be able to) survive, surgical separation is justified to provide life for the other twin.
- Survival is determined by the premorbid condition and not by surgery.
- Parents have the right to refuse separation.

In his review of this subject, Atkinson (2004) commented that the birth of a handicapped child is an immense burden to any parents. If they are to avoid greater challenges, the clinicians require sensitivity and patience as they steer the family along a pathway to survival. The question most often asked is whether it is justified to sacrifice one life to save another, or should both infants be allowed to die? Answers are seldom simple, and each case should be assessed on its own merits. Decisions depend on the type and complexity of the conjunction, the overall health of both infants, the laws of the country, and the religion and beliefs of the parents. If the sacrifice of one twin is necessary for the other twin to survive, it is important to recognize that both would die without separation. If they were separated, at least one would live (O'Neill et al., 1988).

Especially in centers where these operations are done more often, medical staff is more confident of their ability to provide insightful management decisions pertaining to these care of conjoined twins. They are supported by investigations that provide valuable information, allowing rational decisions to be made about the immediate and long-term futures of these infants. These investigations, performed to clarify anatomic structures include radiologic imaging, ultrasonography, CT, MRI, radioisotope studies, echocardiography, cardiac catheterization, and neuroradiologic imaging. As a consequence, in the perioperative period the pediatric surgeons and anesthesiologists in these centers have reported much higher rates of success in operating on these infants. Developments in intensive care also have a positive impact on these improved outcomes.

Ian Aird (1954, 1959) wrote that if there was a possibility of at least one twin surviving, surgery should be performed. The operation does not decide which twin will survive; this is determined by their relative conditions (O'Neill et al., 1988).

Great Ormond Street Ethical Guidelines for Conjoined Twin Separation has been adopted by a number of units. Where separation is feasible with a reasonable chance of success, it should be carried out. When surgery is not possible, custodial care should be offered, and nature should be allowed to take its course. When one twin is dead or has a lethal abnormality and cannot survive independently from its normal twin, and if there is no surgery both twins would die, separation to save the healthy twin should be attempted (Rode et al., 2006; Millar et al., 2009).

PERINATAL CONSIDERATIONS

Improved techniques of antenatal diagnosis and fetal imaging have allowed the diagnosis of conjoined twins to be made during pregnancy, so that counseling of the parents may allow them the option to have the pregnancy terminated. Conjoined twins can be identified as early as 11 weeks' gestation, and in this series of cases studied by Sebire et al. (2000), all the parents opted for termination. Complex craniopagus and cardiopagus anatomy in particular may tilt the decision in this direction. Conjoined hearts are easier to study via ultrasound in utero, because the amniotic fluid acts as a buffer, whereas after birth the lungs inflate with air and prevent optimal visibility (Kingston et al., 2001).

Obstructed labor with difficult vaginal delivery may necessitate an emergency cesarean section, but this can be avoided by antenatal diagnosis and elective cesarean section at 36 to 38 weeks' gestation (Millar et al., 2009). In many developing countries, the birth of conjoined twins may come as a surprise to the mother and the attending midwife or medical practitioner (Thomas, 2004; Thomas and Lopez, 2004).

Perinatal management of conjoined twins involves a close collaboration between anesthesiologists, obstetricians, and pediatricians so that birth trauma for both the mother and the infants can be minimized. Unborn conjoined twins may be referred to pediatric surgeons for advice in order to plan the delivery and the immediate perinatal management.

Careful prenatal investigations may identify cases in which emergency separation at birth is life saving (MacKenzie et al., 2002). Advances in prenatal ultrasound, as well as the use of color-flow Doppler and prenatal MRI, have improved the antenatal diagnosis of conjoined twins. In particular, prenatal and postnatal echocardiography has been shown to accurately delineate the extent of cardiac fusion, the intracardiac anatomy, and the ventricular function (Andrews et al., 2006). Planning of the antenatal course and the perinatal management of twins can be facilitated by identifying those twins at particular risk, such as twins with twin reversed–arterial perfusion sequence. In this situation, vascular communications between the two fetuses allows deoxygenated blood from one fetus (the pump twin) to perfuse the other fetus (the perfused twin), resulting in reversed flow in the umbilical vessels and the development of multiple anomalies, including acardia, in the perfused twin (Norwitz et al., 2000). Antenatal surgical intervention, removing the acardiac twin in utero, may allow for the survival of the remaining (pump) twin. If they are conjoined, however, this is not possible, and immediate surgical intervention at birth is necessary. In order to make rational and sound decisions as to the anesthetic management, anesthesia for fetoscopic fetal surgery requires knowledge of the pathophysiology of the fetus, the fetoplacental unit, and the condition of the mother (Galankin et al., 2000).

Plans may be necessary, in those units providing that option, for an ex utero intrapartum treatment (EXIT) procedure (Bouchard et al., 2002). In this operation, access to the fetus is achieved when the fetus is brought into the surgical field while it is still attached to the mother's placenta. The planned procedure, whether for access to the fetal airway in the case of an airway tumor, or to allow separation of a conjoined twin from its non–survivable twin, is then carried out. Once it has been completed, the infant is then delivered from the mother and separated from its placenta. This procedure has also been used for airway control of both twins when the antenatal airway and cardiopulmonary status of the twins was not known (Ossowski and Suskind, 2005).

At delivery, it is optimal to have two sets of all neonatal resuscitation equipment available and a pediatrician (or anesthesiologist) present for each infant. A conventional open incubator usually provides a large enough surface area to accommodate both infants. If one twin is doing poorly, it should be attended to first. Especially with thoracopagus twins, over-vigorous ventilation of one may compromise the other because of the chest contents moving across into the chest cavity of the other. If intubation is necessary, this should be performed on one infant at a time, with the other twin being supported, if necessary, with bag face-mask oxygen and ventilation. A T piece and small mask is easier to use than an Ambu bag. While laryngoscopy is being performed on one twin, care must be taken to protect the infant who is not being intubated from trauma to the face and eyes by the laryngoscope. The aim of immediate postnatal management should be the resuscitation and stabilization of both infants, thorough physical examination and special investigations that will allow for definition of the relevant anatomy, and subsequent medical and surgical management.

Cardiopulmonary resuscitation (CPR) in conjoined twins has significant limitations. Not only can it be physically challenging, but it may also be unreliable because the anatomy is distorted and access to the heart, especially in thoracopagus twins, is limited. Damage to other organs, particularly the upper gastrointestinal tract and liver, may occur (Millar et al., 2009). The basics of neonatal and pediatric resuscitation should be followed.

MEDICAL AND SURGICAL MANAGEMENT

Spitz and Kiely (2002) describe the management of conjoined twins in the prenatal and postnatal stages. When complex thoracopagus or craniopagus twins are diagnosed, termination of pregnancy is recommended. The postnatal management involves the following options:

- Nonoperative care: palliative care until the twins die or raise the twins in their conjoined status (i.e., no attempt is made to separate them).
- Emergency operative care: surgery that may include separation is performed.
- Operative or surgical management aimed at elective separation: elective separation may be performed as a staged procedure, or separation may occur with a single operation.

Some overlap occurs when the twins arrive for emergency surgery before the results of all the investigations have enabled decisions around survival to be made (e.g., when intestinal obstruction develops). Emergency surgery is then performed, but later findings may indicate that other anomalies that are incompatible with life are present. In all studies, emergency surgery for separation is associated with a poor prognosis.

Indications for emergency separation include the following (O'Neill, 1998, Millar et al., 2009; Rode et al., 2006; Cywes et al., 1997):

- Where there is damage to a connecting bridge (e.g., omphalopagus). This may occur at the time of delivery.
- When the condition of one twin threatens the survival of the other (e.g., complex congenital heart disease, cardiomyopathy, sepsis).
- Deterioration of both twins because of hemodynamic and respiratory compromise. This occurs typically in thoracopagus twins.
- When the condition of one twin is incompatible with life (e.g., anencephalic, acardiac, stillborn, or complex congenital anomalies) but the other twin has a good chance of survival.

Elective separation for simple conjunctions can be performed in the neonatal period with minimal problems. No benefit is gained from waiting for the infants to grow or for further investigations to be done. The maternal hormonal influences are still present; thus, the skin is more pliable to cover the wound defect. In general, separation is planned for some time between 4 and 11 months of age when the infants are bigger and their investigations are more meaningful and when they have had adequate tissue expansion to allow closure of the skin defect (O'Neill et al., 1988).

INVESTIGATIONS

Accurate preoperative imaging is essential to surgical planning and prognosis, and the area(s) of fusion determine the imaging modality used. MRI and CT provide very good anatomic and bone detail and show organ positions, shared structures, and limited vascular anatomy (Kingston et al., 2001). Radiography with contrast material provides excellent gastrointestinal and urogenital evaluation. When there is liver conjunction, its anatomy, the vascular supply, and assessment of the biliary tree are required. Angiography helps clarify the vascular supply of organs and determine blood supply between the twins. Careful use of contrast material is important, because there may be overenthusiastic administration of this in an attempt to achieve better views. Evaluation of vascular shunts and cross circulation is vital for anesthesiologists—loss of blood from these during surgery can be catastrophic.

Cardiac catheterization is required to identify intracardiac connections and to clarify cardiac chambers. Echocardiographic technology is constantly improving, so the need for catheterization (and therefore anesthesia) is becoming less common. When cardiac surgery is required, however, this is the preferred investigation (Fig. 29-5).

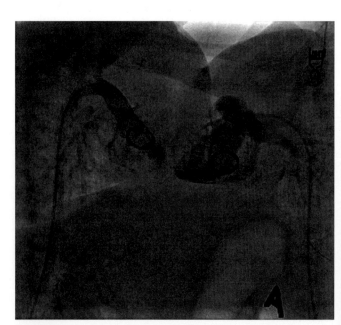

■ **FIGURE 29-5.** A cardiac catheterization image of complex cardiopagus thoracopagus twins with a catheter and contrast material in each heart. These twins could not be separated.

Results of these tests clarify anatomic variations in each infant. Understanding the complexity of organ conjunctions enables investigators to identify those structures that are present or missing. The results of complex investigations are best evaluated by a multidisciplinary team, because many factors are raised that anesthesiologists do not consider but that are important for both anesthetic management and good overall care of the infants. Each test has its own role for all of these requirements. Box 29-2 details investigations for craniopagus twins. The order in which procedures occur is also determined by the results of the investigations.

Sedation Techniques for Investigations

The anatomic evaluations of conjoined twins require multiple tests that commonly require the administrations of sedative medications or anesthetic agents. These techniques or options may vary from a simple feed to a full general anesthetic. Regardless of the choice, a full and comprehensive presedation evaluation should be carried out. The choice of technique depends on the following factors:

- Age and size of the twins
- Site and complexity of the twins' conjunction
- Airway anatomy of the twins
- Venue for the investigation
- Accessibility to the twins
- Level of pain caused by procedure
- Length of time taken for the investigation
- Availability and achievability of an intravenous catheter line

Options for simple sedation used include a feeding before CT or MRI, sucrose on a pacifier, swaddling and physical support, chloral hydrate, trimeprazine (with or without droperidol), and midazolam (Thomas, 2004; Thomas and Lopez, 2004). Two pediatric anesthesiologists should be present from the beginning of these investigations, rather than them having to be called in an emergency situation.

Commonly used agents include propofol, ketamine, fentanyl, dexmedetomidine, and inhalational agents. For MRI evaluations, the safest option may be a general anesthetic to ensure airway control for the procedure (Sury et al., 1994). The use of laryngeal mask airways may not always provide the ideal

airway management, and rescue maneuvers in this environment are fraught with potential complications (Shank et al., 2005; Szmuk et al., 2005).

Whether simple or advanced techniques are used, monitoring should include pulse oximetry, ECG, blood pressure, and where possible, capnography. For CT scanning in particular, a capnography limb attached to the nasal cannula providing oxygen has been a very useful monitor for these twins. Again, there should be at least two anesthesiologists present—one for each infant.

PLANNING BEFORE SURGERY

Preparation of Parents

Congenital abnormalities in singleton children are challenging enough for parents; parenting a set of conjoined twins can be daunting, with the burden of decision making being overwhelming (Atkinson, 2004). This is especially problematic when one infant is not expected to survive or when both may die. Even for infants with a simple conjunction, every effort should be made to make this experience as atraumatic as possible. This may include the involvement of child-life specialists, play therapists, physiotherapists, occupational therapists, and social workers. Where physical challenges and deformities will be present after surgery, involvement of these caregivers before surgery is essential. These principles of care are often overlooked, and it may be necessary during planning meetings to remind the multidisciplinary team of their importance.

Preparation of the Environment and Equipment

An important emphasis for anesthesiologists is the adequate preparation of the area where the procedure will occur. This may involve sites distant from the anesthesia suite or operating rooms (and will thus present all the problems of this type of pediatric anesthesia), or surgery may take place in the operating room environment.

This stage of the planning should also include involvement of the hospital management, the public relations department, and plans to avoid extensive media involvement. Privacy of patients and parents should be protected.

When procedures on these twins are to be performed outside the operating rooms, these venues or areas should be visited and scrutinized for suitability for sedation, general anesthesia, and appropriate monitoring. If general anesthesia is planned, the supply of two sources of oxygen, medical air, nitrous oxide, suctioning, and scavenging must be available. It may be necessary to have the maintenance department make up equipment to facilitate this, such as splitters from the wall gas supply. Innovative techniques have been devised to provide ventilation of both twins with one ventilator using a Carlen's Y-adaptor for ECG-gated MRI angiography (Szmuk et al., 2006). The use of bispectral index (BIS) for detecting cross circulation in thoracopagus twins is also described (Szmuk et al., 2006).

Total intravenous anesthesia (TIVA) may be the preferred option in these circumstances. Space for anesthesia and other personnel is often a limiting factor, because it may be necessary to bring two anesthesia machines into a small area (e.g., the cardiac catheterization laboratory). Meticulous attention to detail

---

Box 29-2 Investigations for Craniopagus Twins

Routine blood tests and urinalysis
Neuroimaging and neurointerventional radiologic procedures
3-Dimensional CT imaging
MRI scan and angiography
Cerebral echography; color Doppler echo via the fontanels
Cerebral angiography
Preoperative neuroendovascular techniques to occlude shared vascular anastomotic channels allow for safer surgery for separation as a one-staged operation.
CT angiography reconstruction
Neurophysiology: electroencephalograms, visual evoked potentials, and somatic sensory evoked potentials

is essential. Previous experience in these scenarios is extremely valuable. When space is an issue, instead of two full anesthesia teams, a team leader (coordinator) and two pediatric anesthesiologists or hands-on anesthesia care providers (fellows, residents, or certified registered nurse anesthetists [CRNAs]) (one each per infant) are usually sufficient. Investigations for MRI and CT scan are particularly challenging, but with planning and insight as to the possible problems, many potential catastrophes can be avoided.

Temperature control should be as for any pediatric anesthesia procedure, and all facilities to prevent heat loss and provide warmth should be available. To maintain their heat, the infants should be appropriately covered for transportation. The anesthetic should be started in a warm operating room (28° C), and the operating room should be cooled as soon the infants are draped. Intraoperative use of plastic drapes prevents the infants from getting wet and cold. Fluids may be warmed, and warm-air convection devices are very beneficial.

Multidisciplinary Team Preparation

Although the surgeons take the primary responsibility for the twins, it is often the anesthesiology team that assumes the role of the perioperative operating room organizers. Anesthesiologists are the caregivers who are present from the very beginning of the anesthesia, through each stage of surgical intervention (especially when more than one or two surgical disciplines are involved), until the end when handover to the intensive care unit staff occurs. Communication with the nursing personnel is imperative. The following list details all the disciplines that should be present at preparatory meetings:

Anesthesiology: Head of department team leader, specialists, technologists (especially when technical assistance is anticipated), trainees, and anesthesia nurses
Surgeons: General, plastic and reconstructive, cardiothoracic, orthopedic, neurosurgical, urologic, and ophthalmologic
Nursing: Operating-room manager or operating nurse leader
Intensive Care: Head of department or representative, nursing staff, pediatricians, cardiologists, and pulmonologists
Other Disciplines: Physiotherapist, occupational therapist, child life specialist
Hospital Management
Public Relations

In multidisciplinary meetings, the following should be discussed: the results of all investigations of all disciplines; an assessment of how they overlap in the different specialties; the order in which these surgical specialties will operate; any planned changes in the positions of the infants; locations where intravenous lines may or may not be placed; any anticipated problems or concerns; and whether or not intensive care will be necessary after the procedure. An example to illustrate the importance of such a discussion is a pair of ischiopagus twins who require defunctioning colostomies for intestinal obstruction. The pediatric general surgeon needs to perform the colostomies, the urologist needs to do an examination of the urogenital system under anesthesia, the orthopedic surgeons and neurosurgeons may require input for assessment of the sacrum and pelvis, and finally, the otolaryngologic surgeon has to assess one of the twins for upper airway obstruction and possible adenoidectomy. The use of diagrams of the anatomy,

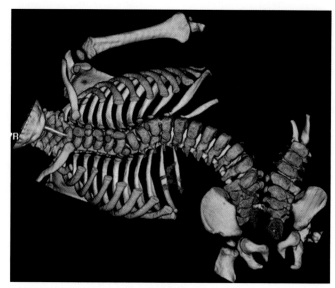

■ **FIGURE 29-6.** This is a CT reconstructed image of a surviving ischiopagus twin's spine after emergency separation when the other twin did not survive. This twin has required a number of surgical procedures to correct the abnormal anatomy of both the spine and pelvis.

three-dimensional or CT-reconstructed models, and rehearsals in the operating room allow the process to proceed as smoothly as possible (Fig. 29-6).

ANESTHETIC CARE OF CONJOINED TWINS

General Principles

Anesthesia services for conjoined twins are required for various situations (Box 29-3). Anesthetizing conjoined twins is demanding and complex. The anesthesiologists must treat each

Box 29-3 Anesthesia Services for Conjoined Twins

Obstetric anesthesia for the mother
Mother and infants for the EXIT procedure
Resuscitation of the newborn infants
Airway management
Acquisition of vascular access
Intensive care management, neonatal or pediatric
Examinations under anesthesia
To facilitate investigations, cardiac catheterization, MRI, CT scans
Emergency surgery: intestinal obstruction, palliative heart surgery on one twin (Tirotta et al., 2005).

SURGERY FOR NON–SEPARATION PROCEDURES
Related to their conjoined state
Not related to their conjoined state

SURGERY FOR SEPARATION
Reconstruction and rehabilitation procedures
Chronic pain syndromes

child as a separate individual. The general principles of pediatric anesthesia, including factors predicting a difficult anesthesia, apply in all of these cases. Any deterioration in the condition of the twins should be anticipated, so intubation and emergency resuscitation measures can be taken in a controlled manner. Two anesthetic teams are always involved in the management of the two patients, with duplication of all equipment necessary for their care.

If an urgent resuscitation is required in the ward, two anesthesia providers must attend, with one provider for each infant. No induction agent, especially a muscle relaxant, should be administered to one infant until the airway of the second twin can be maintained and supplemental oxygen and ventilation can be provided.

Reviews of operative procedures before separation provide ideal dress rehearsals for the management of these patients.

Anesthetic Challenges in the More Common Types of Conjoined Twins

Thoracopagus Conjunctions

Thoracopagus conjunctions are the most common form of conjunction. They are associated with a significant risk of complications, either when they are an isolated abnormality or when they are part of a complex cephalad or caudal conjunction. Sudden unexpected deterioration in respiratory and cardiovascular function in the preoperative period may occur, resulting in the untimely demise of both infants. Early intubation and ventilation with cardiac support may be necessary. Sudden death in this group is not uncommon.

Airway management is difficult because of the extreme lordosis and hyperextension of the infants, with variability of the proximity of their faces (Fig. 29-7). The higher the conjunction, the more difficult airway access becomes. This improves as they grow. Emergency intubation in either or both twins should be avoided. Their deterioration and the need for intervention should be anticipated, and the procedures should be carried out in a quiet and controlled way. Intubation should be done on

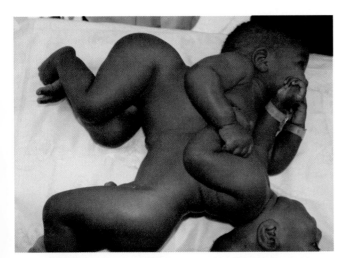

■ **FIGURE 29-7.** This lateral photograph of a thoracopagus twin demonstrates the typical hyperextension of the head and neck and the exaggerated lordosis of this group of conjoined twins.

one infant at a time, taking care not to damage the other twin in the process. It is not advisable to paralyze either infant until there is airway support and control in both infants. Except in moribund patients, awake intubation may be very difficult. It is usually easier to intubate the infants when they are on their sides, turned with the face upward. Positioning one infant above the other causes adverse hemodynamic and respiratory consequences in both infants and is not recommended.

The use of laryngeal mask airways is not as successful in this group as in those twins whose heads face away from each other or in twins whose heads are at opposite ends of the body. Once the infants have been anesthetized, fiberoptic intubation has been used with success, but most intubations can be performed without it. It may be useful to insert a nasopharyngeal tube (a short endotracheal tube [ETT]) into one nostril to provide oxygen and an inhalational agent while attempting to intubate the trachea, either orally or nasally. Direct laryngoscopy and distal airway evaluation may be of value in the work-up before separation, but it is often difficult to insert a rigid bronchoscope without causing damage to the infants (Strocker et al., 2005). A fiberoptic technique is easier. There is little emphasis placed on investigating the respiratory systems of these infants. Lung abnormalities have been identified and include tracheomalacia and the presence of aberrant bronchi (Strocker et al., 2005).

Cardiac complications, especially cardiac failure in the neonatal period, are common. Anatomic possibilities include twins with a single normal heart, twins with two conventional hearts, or twins with compound hearts. The anatomy of major vessels may be extremely variable. With compound hearts, the extent of sharing may vary from minimal to almost complete (Gerlis et al., 1993). Coronary artery sharing usually coexists, even with minor venous sharing, and fusion may occur at the level of the sinus venosus, at the atrial level, or at the atrial and ventricular levels. Cruciate connections from the right atrium of one infant to the right atrium of the other, or from the left ventricle of one to the left ventricle of the other, may be present (Gerlis et al., 1993). Many of the components may only be determined at surgery (or postmortem). For technical reasons, it is often difficult to differentiate whether the ventricles are contiguous or fused.

Electrocardiograms (ECGs) in these infants are interesting, but are not conclusive. The presence of two complexes does not rule out significant abnormalities, and a single complex does not necessarily mean significant sharing of heart structures. Reciprocal complexes, or those appearing as a mirror image, usually indicate shared hearts. (Fig. 29-8)

Cardiovascular and respiratory instability may occur with any maneuver that alters the intrathoracic pressures and moves the hearts and lungs of each infant back and forth between them. Coughing, crying, and breath-holding are all contributing factors. Positive pressure ventilation should be timed in both infants to avoid this complication. This can be achieved with manual ventilation, synchronized intermittent positive pressure ventilation, or with the use of circuits made up to ventilate both infants with a single ventilator. With the latter method, good chest movement (and capnography) is a vital clinical indicator of adequate ventilation.

Central vascular access, whether subclavian, internal jugular, or femoral, is difficult because of variable anatomic differences, which make the usual anatomic landmarks unreliable. Ultrasound has been helpful in identifying these vessels. Blood loss, as with most conjoined twins, may be significant (two to three times the estimated blood volumes).

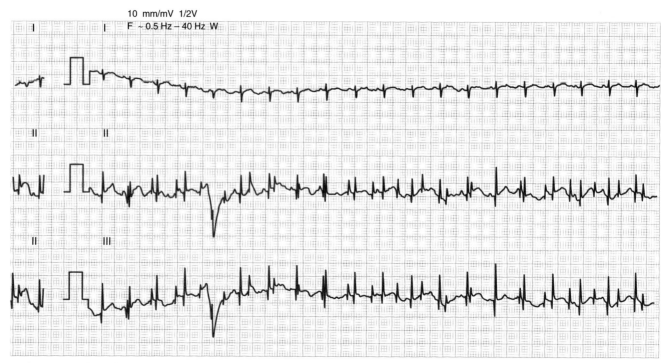

■ FIGURE 29-8. This is the ECG of thoracopagus twins who share a pericardium but have separate hearts. The complex of one twin is superimposed on that of the other.

After separation, postoperative ventilation is generally the rule rather than the exception. The repair of deficits in the anterior chest wall needs to be planned, because most require some sort of structural support to facilitate normal ventilatory mechanics and to avoid the development of a flail segment (Hoshina et al., 1987).

Omphalopagus Conjunctions

Omphalopagus twins range from a very simple conjunction containing fibrous tissue or a sliver of liver, to an extremely complex conjunction. If the livers are extensively fused, blood loss may be considerable. Complex hepatobiliary fusion and proximal gastrointestinal sharing of organs may complicate surgery. Airway access may be difficult but not as hazardous as it is in thoracopagus twins. In more complex conjunctions, ventilatory challenges are the same as those for thoracopagus twins (i.e., coughing and straining in one twin affects the other's ability to breathe properly).

Ischiopagus and Pygopagus Conjunctions

Airway management is not usually a problem except in those cases where a compound or complex conjunction is present. In general, the twins' faces, heads, and necks are easily accessible for intubation. As with thoracopagus twins, if their abdomens are joined, abdominal contents can move between the infants with Valsalva maneuvers and may compromise the ventilation and diaphragmatic excursion of the other infant. In ischiopagus twins before separation, bowel surgery for intestinal obstruction may be necessary.

Especially in twins where posterior osteotomies are required for pelvic ring closure, blood loss may be extensive. This may also occur suddenly and unexpectedly with dural incision and when vascular structures are unpredictable (Fieggen et al., 2004).

Tethering of the cord, spinal dysraphism, cord fusion, and syringomyelia, in association with anorectal and urogenital abnormalities, are often encountered in ischiopagus, pygopagus, and dipagus twins (Peter et al., 1996). This may preclude the use of spinal or epidural anesthesia in these twins unless ultrasound views clearly identify the anatomy.

If nerve stimulation is required by the surgeon to identify the nerve routes, muscle relaxation should not be used. Preoperative documentation of the neurologic status is essential.

Preoperative bowel preparation may cause fluid losses that need to be factored into preoperative and intraoperative fluid-administration requirements.

Neurosurgeons are experts in the management of craniopagus twins, but their expertise is also required for both ischiopagus and pygopagus conjoined twins who may have a variety of spinal abnormalities (Peter and Fieggen, 2004). These may present challenges both at the time of separation as well as for long-term management. In the presence of hemivertebrae, asymmetric or small chest cavities, or spinal anomalies, progressive scoliosis may develop and will require diligent follow-up care and possible intervention (Fig. 29-9) (Fieggen et al., 2004; Rode et al., 2006).

Duplication of an anatomic area (e.g., ischiopagus dipagus, a single trunk but four legs) is amenable to surgical correction with a good outcome (Fig. 29-10). Anesthetic problems in this group are similar to those that would be experienced with tumors of that region, namely vagal stimulation with manipulation of the mass and blood loss.

Craniopagus Conjunctions

Because of the proximity of the infants' heads and faces, airway management of these twins is often a challenge. Stabilization of the ETT requires particular attention, and fluid or blood from

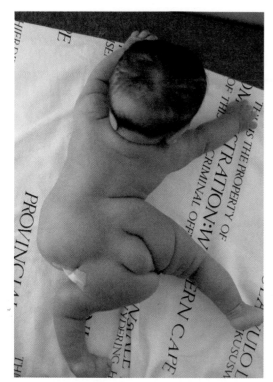

■ FIGURE 29-9. This is the surviving infant of ischiopagus twins with spinal deformities who requires follow-up surgery. His CT is shown in Figure 29-6.

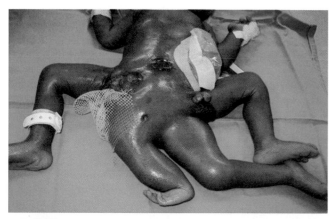

■ FIGURE 29-10. Ischiopagus dipagus twins are seen here. One with lower extremity duplication, where the abnormal segment comprises the middle two limbs. A pelvic osteotomy is usually performed to facilitate rotation of the legs into a normal position. If a heteropagus parasite occurs at this site, an osteotomy is not usually necessary.

the surgical field can result in dislodgement or displacement during surgery with potentially catastrophic consequences. Especially if significant flexion is anticipated, a reinforced ETT may be the best option. Many of the principles of pediatric neurosurgery apply, including the potential for venous air embolism, and these are affected by the complexity of the conjunction (Girshin et al., 2006). Walker and Browd (2004) provide a comprehensive approach to the embryology, classification, surgical anatomy, and separation of craniopagus twins.

If the venous sinuses of the twins are in communication in the fusion, blood loss may be enormous, and it is often this factor that limits the possibility of surgery for separation. The abnormal development of the arteriovenous system is one of the greatest challenges faced during the separation procedure. To reduce blood loss and allow each child to develop adequate independent vascular drainage and to prevent perioperative cerebral edema, staged separation may be indicated (Walker and Browd, 2004; Girshin et al., 2006). These staged operations have been attempted to encourage the development of a collateral circulation before final separation and to improve outcome.

The preoperative neurologic status needs meticulous documentation, because the degree of neurologic deficit after surgery depends on the extent of brain, vascular, and meningeal conjunction and the complexity of the procedure.

Central vascular access may be limited to the femoral route.

Preoperative Evaluation

Each type of conjoined twins has challenges specific to their type of conjunction. A comprehensive knowledge and understanding of the pathophysiology of conjoined twins is essential to good anesthetic management. Procedural planning sessions and rehearsals are invaluable to identifying potential or actual stumbling blocks.

The preoperative visit should be as that for any pediatric patient, but there should be particular emphasis on a number of the factors previously described. For urgent operations or separation, rapid preoperative evaluation and assessment before transportation to the operating room is necessary. Prior experience with conjoined-twin management provides considerable advantages at this time.

A thorough goal-directed review that includes the history of perinatal events and growth since birth, exposure to infectious diseases (e.g., human immunodeficiency virus), and whether or not and what prophylaxis was taken (mother-to-child transmission medication), as well as previous intubation experience for respiratory or cardiovascular pathology, is required. An understanding of the complexities of each investigation and the implications of these for surgery (and therefore anesthesia) is vital. It is especially important to understand the degree of cross circulation between the twins and at what anatomic level this may be present (e.g., heart, liver, brain, or bowel) (Table 29-3).

Especially in thoracopagus twins, signs of cardiovascular decompensation should be sought. These include tachypnea, tachycardia, decreasing saturations, loss of appetite, and failure to thrive.

Regardless of the degree of cross-circulation, drugs should be administered as they would be for two separate individuals. The weight of a heteropagus infant, however, should include the weight of the parasitic part until it is removed and can be regarded in the same light as a pediatric patient who has a tumor that requires resection. For most symmetric twins, the two infants are more or less the same size, so it is appropriate to take their combined weight and halve it to arrive at the weight of each infant.

Careful consideration should be given to where catheter lines should be placed, which cannulae should be used, and how many will be necessary for the particular procedure. Doppler ultrasound has been useful in identifying the site of central vessels, but because of space limitations in some sets of twins, it is not always easy to insert the catheter lines under direct vision. In these infants, it is easier to identify the vessels, place the ultrasound

TABLE 29-3. Summary of Multidisciplinary Investigations Commonly Required for Conjoined Twins

System	Investigation
Cardiorespiratory Cross circulation	Radiography: total body X-ray Electrocardiogram Echocardiography/Doppler ultrasound in all conjoined twins MRI/CT with contrast Angiogram Radioisotope scan Tc-99-DMSA, radiolabeled albumin, or red blood cells45
Alimentary tract	Contrast meal and enema Ultrasound Radioisotope scans53 (liver); technetium Tc-99m-(Sn), colloid and excretion Tc-99m mebrofenin Radioisotope scintigraphy
Genitourinary	Ultrasound Isotope renography Micturating cystourethrography Genitogram
Skeletal system	Radiography MRI (spinal cord) Ultrasound
Vascular	Doppler ultrasound Angiography

Modified from Di Rocco C, Caldarelli M, Tamburrini G, et al: Craniopagus: the Thessaloniki-Rome experience, *Childs Nerv Syst* 20:576–586, 2004; Mann M, Coutts JP, Kaschula ROC, et al: The use of radionucleotides in the investigation of conjoined twins, *J Nucl Med* 24:479–484, 1984; Rode H et al: Four decades of conjoined twins at Red Cross Children's Hospital: lessons learned, *S Afr Med J* 96(9):931, 2006; Rutka JT, Souweidane M, ter Brugge K, et al: Separation of craniopagus twins in the era of modern neuroimaging, interventional neuroradiology, and frameless stereotaxy, *Childs Nerv Syst* 20:587–592, 2004.

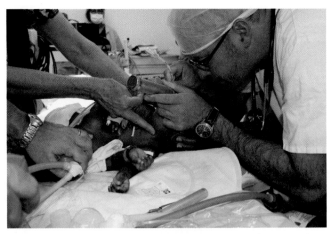

■ **FIGURE 29-11.** Intubation of thoracopagus twins demonstrating the use of an assistant's finger to bring the vocal cords into view. This photograph also shows the airway of the other twin being managed while the intubation is taking place.

probe aside, and then attempt cannulation, or to have an assistant hold the probe while cannulation is attempted.

Physical Examination

Importance must be given to assessing the following:

The Airway

Managing the airway is crucial to good anesthetic management, and certain types of patients have predictably more difficult airways than others. In general, airway management of ventrally conjoined twins is more difficult. Problems with the airway in conjoined twins include:

- Access to the mouth and larynx is difficult.
- Visualization of the vocal cords may be impossible. Close faces leave little room to move to insert instruments in the airway.
- Placement of the ETT through the cords is challenging, because it tends to get caught on the subglottis. Rotation of the tube through 180 degrees as it passes through the cords facilitates this maneuver. Fiberoptic intubation, either directly or via a laryngeal mask, may be a valuable adjunct. Other techniques that may help include all the usual pediatric anesthetists' tricks to bring the larynx into view: the use of one's little finger, having an assistant provide rotational pressure on the larynx; and the use of a stitch into the infant's

tongue to pull the hypomandibular structures forward and allow visualization of the epiglottis and cords (Fig. 29-11). The successful use of the Magill's forceps is often compromised by lack of space both inside and outside the mouth, but oral intubation is usually easier than the nasal route. Once placed correctly, secure strapping of the ETT is critical.

Thoracopagus Twins. Thoracopagus twins have difficult airways until proven otherwise. There is invariably some degree of opisthotonus and hyperextension of the head and neck, making visualization of the vocal cords very difficult. Plans for fiberoptic-assisted intubation may be necessary. In order to facilitate long-term ventilation, tracheostomy has been described in one set of twins, but this should not be regarded as the routine recommendation of airway management (Mair and Mair, 2006). Depending on the relative positions of the heads and faces, craniopagus airway access may also be problematic.

Mechanisms of Ventilation

It is important to ascertain whether or not the diaphragm is involved in the junction, or whether its function will be affected by surgery. In those twins where conjunction involves the chest wall and its contents, serious consideration needs to be given to breathing and ventilation. Lung compliance is affected, areas of atelectasis develop because of the limited space between the two infants and the abnormal anatomy of thoracic structures, the hearts are usually abnormal, and cardiac failure is common in thoracopagus twins. As one twin develops cardiorespiratory compromise with tachycardia, tachypnea, and coughing, the other is also affected. This has significant short- and long-term consequences and should be a major consideration when planning for separation. New synthetic substances that enable reconstruction of an unstable sternum and anterior chest wall are now available. Muscle flaps and skin grafts may be needed (Rabeeah, 2006). In the postoperative period, these grafts avoid the development of a flail chest, which causes significant respiratory compromise and affects long-term survival and quality of life. In cases where one twin has not survived, autologous tissue has been used to cover the deficit caused at separation (Rode et al., 2006; Spitz and Kiely, 2002; Fisherman et al., 2002).

Cardiovascular System

Assessment of the heart and major vascular anatomy is crucial, because this impacts anesthesia and vice versa. Craniopagus twins may, as with thoracopagus twins, have cardiac failure. Because many of these infants will have spent considerable time in the hospital, venous access may be a challenge, and ultrasound guidance for central venous access may be necessary. Intravenous catheters within the surgical field should be avoided.

Disability

In craniopagus twins or any of the types where the spinal cord may be involved in surgery, a full neurologic examination is required. This is especially the case if any neuroaxial intervention or procedure is planned as part of the anesthetic. Bowel and bladder function must be documented. It may not always be possible to place a urinary catheter, and urine output may not always come from the kidneys of that infant. This problem occurs when one or both ureters cross over from one infant to the other's bladder.

Gastroesophageal Reflux

Gastroesophageal reflux is most common in thoracopagus twins, although it may occur in any type of conjoined twins. Nursing the infants with their heads up is helpful, and the use of antireflux medication should be considered.

While they are waiting for separation, good nutrition is crucial to the infants' growth. The body composition differs between the two twins, as does their resting energy expenditure and caloric intake. This difference stabilizes after separation, with both twins having similar requirements (Powis et al., 1999; Spitz and Kiely, 2002).

Skin Cover: Tissue Expanders

Tissue expanders are inserted to facilitate skin closure when surgery will leave a significant area uncovered. There are numerous reports in the literature of the use of tissue expanders in many sets of all types of conjoined twins. The advantage of their use includes the provision of autologous tissue to cover the defect, thus avoiding the need for the use of foreign material. The disadvantages are the effects of pressure exerted by the expanders in all directions on contiguous tissue where pressure is not desirable. Areas of skin covering the expanders may become necrotic or infected, and the expanders may need to be removed. The inward pressure may affect cardiorespiratory function and result in twins with preexisting lung disease requiring ventilation before separation (Losee et al., 2009). Immediately after insertion, intraabdominal tissue expanders may initially cause an ileus, and they may cause anorexia as the volume in the expanders increase. For craniopagus twins' skin expansion, especially in younger infants, the pressure effects may impact the growth of underlying bone, resulting in a deformed skull. Depending on the age of the infants, the site chosen for placement of the expanders, the number of expanders inserted, the length of time they will be in place vary, as does the volume of fluid injected (100 to 1,000 mL) to expand the tissue sufficiently. The smaller the infant, the more critical is the volume injected. The shape of the expanders are determined by the age of the infants and the sites chosen for their placement. Depending on the decision of the surgeon, the expanders may remain in situ for anything from 6 weeks to several months.

Wound closure in craniopagus twins is critical, because skin, dura, and bone cover are necessary to prevent perioperative wound breakdown, cerebrospinal leaks, and meningitis. Skull defects may be left to granulate closed, or bone from other sites such as ribs may be used. Fascia lata may be used for dural cover, and prosthetic material (e.g., a titanium plate) may be considered. Malformation in the skull configuration may not allow or accommodate tissue expanders. The risks associated with the prolonged time necessary for tissue expansion may preclude their use (Walker and Browd, 2004).

The site(s) for tissue expanders need to be chosen carefully, and everything possible should be done to avoid complications that may necessitate their removal because this leaves areas of fibrosis and scarring, thus limiting availability of suitable skin for cover later. Skin sepsis and wound breakdown are the most common reasons for the removal of expanders, and this delays surgery for separation.

An important consideration for all medical staff caring for children with tissue expanders is that of pain at the injection port when injecting fluid into the expanders. The port(s) may be on only one or on both of the infants, and before injection of the expanders local anesthetic should be used on the skin covering the port. In one set of twins, this problem was ignored, and at the time of each injection the twin with the port developed significant anxiety, whereas the other remained unconcerned. This also impacted on the management of postoperative pain and anxiety of the same twin.

Alternatives to the use of tissue expanders include the use of pedicle flaps, periosteal flaps, and skin grafts. Methods for reconstruction of the deficit caused by separation continue to be explored.

The size of the deficit can be measured preoperatively by physical assessment of the size of the potential defect (measuring with a tape measure and three-dimensional CT reconstruction), as well as by the use of acrylic models (Campbell, 2004). This information may then be used to facilitate reconstruction.

Anesthetic implications of the use of tissue expanders include preoperative assessment of the pressure effects of the expanders on the different organ systems. This includes the effects on the skin and the cardiovascular system. The need to remove the expanders may present significant logistic implications for the operating room staff. All of the challenges of anesthetizing these infants, albeit for a relatively small operation, present themselves—two teams, two sets of equipment, and the need for vascular access are just a few to mention.

ANESTHESIA FOR NON–SEPARATION PROCEDURES

A variety of preseparation or palliative procedures and investigations can be expected. These may include surgery to remove an inappropriately sited limb, place tissue expanders, perform laparotomy for intestinal obstruction, divert stomas, repair an inguinal hernia in one twin, perform gastroschisis, complete urologic procedures such as vesicostomy, do an adenoidectomy for adenoidal hypertrophy and obstructive sleep apnea in one twin, and to repair necrotizing enterocolitis (Hoyle, 1990; O'Neill, 1998; Jaffray et al., 1999; Seefelder et al., 2003; Lonnee et al., 2007). The possible investigations are listed in Table 29-3. Anesthesia preparation and preoperative evaluation for these

Box 29-4 Preoperative Questions About Conjoined Twins

What procedure(s) is/are the surgeons planning?
Will the surgery affect both infants?
Will the anesthetic impact each infant equally?
Will the procedure necessitate the insertion of invasive monitoring?
In what position will the infants be placed?
Will it be necessary for the infants to be moved or have their positions changed during the operation?
Will they require admission to the intensive care unit?

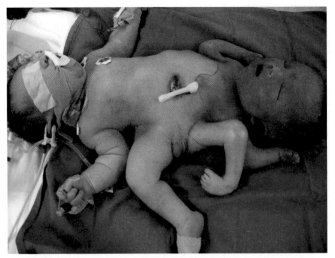

■ **FIGURE 29-12.** A set of ischiopagus twins where one twin deteriorated rapidly before surgery, necessitating emergency separation. To minimize the metabolic consequences, the dying twin should also have been intubated and ventilated.

procedures should be based on the same principles of management as for separation, but the planning for separation involves a more comprehensive approach to the intraoperative and postoperative care.

To prevent confusion and to allow all medical staff to understand the procedure, simple but accurate diagrams of the anatomy should be provided at preoperative discussions.

The questions that need to be answered preoperatively are listed in Box 29-4. Routine pediatric anesthetic preoperative blood tests are required, and blood should be cross-matched according to the procedure planned.

The size, age, and state of health of the infants; the site and complexity of their conjunction; the anatomy of organs involved; the organs or structures that are missing; the presence of other congenital anomalies; and the degree and location of cross circulation are all vital factors in planning for anesthesia and surgery. Regardless of the procedure or operation, neonatal conjoined twins are a considerable challenge. The younger and smaller the patients are, the more complex the conjunction, and the presence of associated congenital anomalies may complicate all aspects of the anesthetic management. Thoracopagus and craniopagus twins have a higher perioperative morbidity and mortality. The greater the extent of the junction, the more organs are affected by fusion or by being absent.

A dead or dying twin, if not quickly separated from its twin, aggravates the acidosis and causes deterioration and death of both infants (Fig. 29-12). That error was made in one set of twins. By the time they were prepared for surgery nearly 24 hours after birth, one of the twins was regarded as moribund and was not resuscitated or ventilated in the intensive care unit, and this nearly resulted in the death of his brother. As the ill twin deteriorates and dies, there is extensive vasodilation and acidosis, so the intravascular volume of the surviving infant transfuses into the dead twin, causing the healthier twin to succumb. The biochemical challenges are similar to those of a reperfusion syndrome.

Airway difficulties are more common in those infants where the conjunction is high on the chest, where the heads face each other and are close together, where the head and facial anatomy is abnormal, when hyperextension of the head and neck with exaggerated lordosis is present, and where the parasite of a heteropagus twin is around the head, neck, or upper chest (Fig. 29-13). Vascular access is anticipated to be difficult in this group.

Vascular access, especially central venous access, is challenging, because deviation from normal anatomic relationships of arteries and veins is common. When available, ultrasound guidance is recommended.

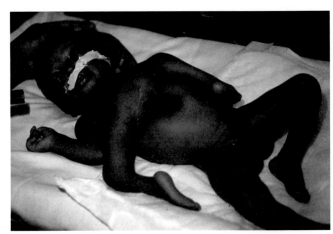

■ **FIGURE 29-13.** A heteropagus conjunction of the upper chest may have an impact on airway management. This one did not cause any problems.

The greater the extent of the fusion, and the more complex the organ involvement, the greater is the propensity for significant blood loss (more than one estimated blood volume) at the time of separation. Blood loss may be obvious (e.g., with thoracopagus or craniopagus), but it may also be covert, as occurs in ischiopagus twins, where posterior osteotomies result in a slow, constant ooze under the dressing and out of sight of the anesthetist. Appropriate preoperative cross-matching of blood and products for intraoperative use is essential.

The need for cardiopulmonary bypass brings with it technical difficulties in inserting cannulae, space in the operating room, and all the consequences and complications of open heart surgery (Suan et al., 1998). Preoperative planning is critical for successful outcomes.

During the week before surgery, in order to ascertain whether the infants will fit onto the operating table, their length and width must be measured. This is especially important in larger, older sets of twins, who will have grown since their previous procedure. In consultation with each of the surgical specialties (especially if the positions need to be changed) and nursing staff, positioning of the infants for surgery must be defined and accommodated. All catheter lines, monitoring, and diathermy should be placed accordingly.

Support materials, such as sponge supports for upright twins or a special chair, may take time to prepare (Fig. 29-14) (Mair and Mair, 2006). When extra limbs or abnormally sited limbs are present, careful protection of these limbs during surgery should be ensured.

Anesthesiologists should prepare for numerous changes in position. When conjunctions are very complex and a number of surgical specialties are involved, the changes in position require forethought and planning. Color coding is of particular value at this time. Meticulous care of the ETTs is essential. Arterial and venous lines need to be moved in an orderly fashion so as to avoid the otherwise inevitable tangle that takes a long time to unravel. Certain equipment, such as diathermy, may need a new site after each change in position.

A rehearsal in the operating room may be very useful to all concerned. Infants should be handled gently and safely; as they grow, they are heavier and more active. If they are fed immediately before their arrival for this exercise, the infants are usually very cooperative.

A preoperative discussion with all role players is necessary, but especially among those anesthetists involved in the procedure; they should display a diagram of the anatomy and the planned surgery and discuss the extent of circulatory mixing, the positions required, and the order of the procedures. This discussion allows rational ordering of blood and blood products based on

calculations of anticipated blood and fluid losses. It is also useful to have a written agenda to follow during the procedures.

Anesthesia providers should be sure to have a double supply of all necessary equipment: anesthesia machines, monitoring, infusion devices, blood warmers, and temperature control modalities. Point-of-care blood analyzing facilities must be checked and ready for use.

As space is often a problem, a drug cart may be shared between the two anesthesiology teams, but drugs should be drawn up independently for each infant. The routine drugs available should include analgesics, anesthetic agents, muscle relaxants, inotropes, and other specific requirements of any of the surgical specialties. Emergency drugs include epinephrine, phenylephrine, norepinephrine, sodium bicarbonate, calcium, and steroids. Aggressive cardiac resuscitation may be necessary in all but the simplest conjunctions.

The operating room should be arranged to suit the type of twins; thoracopagus and craniopagus twins tend have the anesthetic machines at the same end of the table, whereas ischiopagus twins' surgery necessitates that the machines be at opposite ends of the operating room table (Fig. 29-15).

Color coding of each infant's equipment with all the lines, monitors, equipment, and drugs is very useful (Fig. 29-16). Color coding for each team is also valuable, especially when there are two surviving infants to be operated on in two operating rooms or on two separate operating tables.

At the separation of ischiopagus or pygopagus twins, posterior osteotomies may be performed to facilitate pelvic ring closure (Verrier et al., 2000). The approach to the iliac spines is from the back of each infant, and appropriate positioning may be a problem. Positions are rehearsed when the infants are awake, and innovative plans may be necessary to achieve the correct positioning of the infants for surgery (Fig. 29-17). Postoperatively, the legs of the infants are anteromedially rotated and strapped in position for 6 weeks; this will impact their diaphragmatic excursions with the potential for atelectasis and pneumonia (Fig. 29-18). Physiotherapy is crucial to their recovery.

Drug pharmacokinetics and pharmacodynamics may be inconsistent. The use of contrast, radioisotopes, and drugs have all been used to determine the extent of cross circulation, but

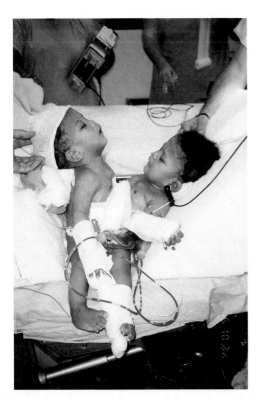

■ **FIGURE 29-14.** Thoracoomphaloischiopagus twins, with tissue expanders in the upper abdomen and lower chest. Because of the unusual positioning during surgery, careful attention to blood pressure, oxygen delivery, and cerebral perfusion is necessary.

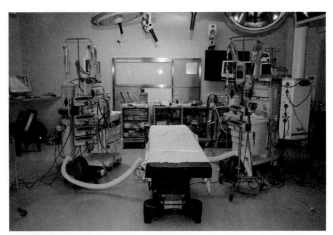

■ **FIGURE 29-15.** The arrangement of the operating room for thoracopagus twins' separation is shown here. A single operating table but duplicate anesthetic machines, monitoring and warm air devices, syringes drivers, and drug carts were used.

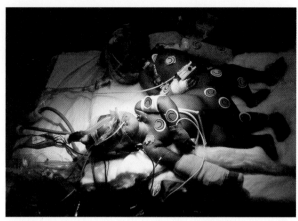

■ **FIGURE 29-16.** Color coding of each child, equipment, lines, and monitoring provides easy identification and prevents drug and fluid administration errors.

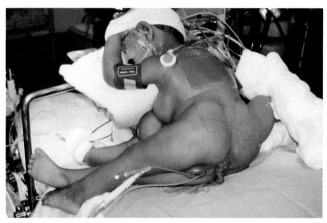

■ **FIGURE 29-17.** For many of the surgical procedures on conjoined twins, innovative positioning for the operation may be necessary. Because of their complex conjunction, this was the most ideal position possible to expose the back of each infant for its posterior osteotomies.

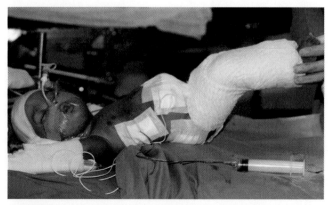

■ **FIGURE 29-18.** After pelvic ring closure in ischiopagus twins, the legs need to be kept in the same position for up to 6 weeks after surgery. This requires firm bandaging of the legs and pelvis, as shown in this photograph.

it is safest to assume some degree of it until proven otherwise. In practical terms, thoracopagus and craniopagus twins have a considerable degree of cross circulation, and few have none at all. The option of local and regional anesthesia use should always be considered, and it should be used whenever possible. Where there is the potential for considerable blood loss, or where there are other contraindications, these techniques should be used with caution.

Control of traffic in the operating room is essential. Noise and congestion are distracting and not in the patients' best interests. Strict guidelines, drawn up by operating room staff and hospital management, must be in place well before embarking on any surgical procedure. Advances in communication technology allow for operations to be viewed via constant in-operating room camera feed, to a distant venue where interested parties can observe proceedings. This also provides a valuable teaching experience for students of all disciplines who cannot be directly involved in the anesthesia and surgery.

Everyone should take time to check everything as a team just before the twins are brought into the operating room.

ANESTHESIA FOR SEPARATION

Nonemergency surgical separation is usually planned for between 4 and 11 months, when the infants are larger and the investigations have given information that is clearer and more meaningful. After this age, psychological issues with separation become more problematic (O'Neill et al., 1988). This operation is the culmination of a multidisciplinary preparation that hopefully will end in the successful separation of a pair of conjoined twins.

Premedication

Sedative or anxiolytic premedication is generally not required, but when the infants are older this may be a consideration. Each set of twins should be assessed individually. In older sets of twins, sedation options include midazolam, trimeprazine, chloral hydrate—each of these has been used successfully in some twins over 6 months of age (Thomas and Lopez, 2004). Atropine has been used for neonatal twins, but this is only necessary when vagal stimulation is likely to occur (e.g., with laryngoscopy or bronchoscopy) or when the use of ketamine is planned.

If an intravenous induction is planned, the use of a topical local anesthetic cream before venipuncture should be encouraged and placed before the twins are transported to the operating room.

Transport

Transportation of the infants to operating room may well be a simple process, and they may be brought to the operating room door by the parents and accompanied by a nurse. In ill twins who have been in intensive care and who are intubated with all invasive catheter lines in place, transportation to the operating room involves the use of a transport monitor and a ventilator for each twin, and the accompaniment of two anesthesiologists. Maintaining normothermia in transit is essential, and meticulous attention to the airways and intravascular lines reduces the possible risk of disconnection or dislodgement at this time. Each anesthesiologist must clearly understand his or her role during this process. Box 29-5 gives a preparatory checklist for the anesthesiologists before caring for conjoined twins.

Box 29-5 Preoperative Conjoined Twin Checklist

- Preparation of operating room (duplicates of all equipment): anesthetic machines; infusion pumps; temperature of operating room set between 26° and 28° C; warm air devices and blankets; grounding pads (one between two at the beginning of surgery is acceptable and changed to one each after separation); a second operating room table to be brought into the operating room (or preparation of another operating room if one of the twins is to be moved); invasive monitoring equipment ready for use; egg-box sponge; silicone pads or rings or an equivalent for pressure protection during the procedure (Fig. 29-19); labels to distinguish drugs and equipment for each twin
- Vascular access devices (central and peripheral)
- Ultrasound machine for intravenous access
- All drugs, routine and emergency, drawn up in duplication for each infant
- Intravenous fluid and blood administration sets for each twin
- Blood cross-matched and immediately available
- Techniques to minimize blood loss, such as the use of cell savers or a protocol for major blood loss, should be considered when massive or sudden blood loss is anticipated (Paterson, 2009)
- Confirmed availability of intensive care beds

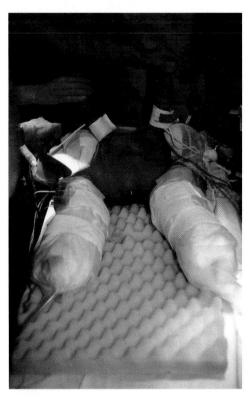

■ **FIGURE 29-19.** The use of soft bandages and plastic protect the legs during surgery and prevent heat loss.

Induction

Techniques for induction of anesthesia are determined by the airway, the availability of intravenous access at induction, the state of health of each infant, the drugs available, and the preferences of the attending anesthesiologists. In those twins with potentially difficult airways, spontaneous respiration with inhalational induction with sevoflurane or the intravenous use of ketamine is helpful (Fig. 29-20) (Thomas, 2004; Thomas and Lopez, 2004; Diaz and Furman, 1987). In this same group, a lidocaine "gargle" before induction to partially anesthetize the airway is a useful technique (2% lidocaine sprayed into the infant's mouth before starting the anesthetic). In infants with cyanotic congenital heart disease or in those with complex anatomy, intravenous ketamine is a safe option (Thomas and Lopez, 2004; Diaz and Furman, 1987).

Muscle relaxation must not be used until airway access is assured. Rapid sequence induction is often not possible in ventrally conjoined twins. Ideally, intravenous access should be established in the ward before transfer to the operating room, but because many of the infants have been in the hospital for some time, this may not always be possible. When this is the case, inhalational induction may be followed by the use of topical local anesthetic spray (2% lidocaine) to the vocal cords to facilitate intubation. The type of ETT and the route used (oral or nasal) are determined by the type of conjunction (nasal is not suitable for craniopagus twins surgery, and this route is often very difficult in thoracopagus twins), whether or not postoperative ventilation is planned, whether the surgical position requires the use of a reinforced tube, and how accessible the infants' faces and ETTs are during surgery. To facilitate postoperative ventilation, oral tubes may be changed to nasal tubes at the end of the procedure. Good securement of the ETT is crucial, and inadvertent extubation during surgery may be disastrous.

In cases when the airway is not a problem and the infants are hemodynamically stable, any agent commonly used for pediatric anesthesia is suitable. Intravenous inductions using propofol, etomidate, thiopentone, and ketamine have all been used successfully.

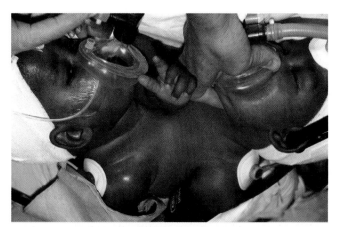

■ **FIGURE 29-20.** This inhalational induction in thoracopagus twins with a high conjunction demonstrates the close proximity of the airways of many of these infants.

Intraoperative Management

Intraoperative care of these twins should aim to provide ideal surgical conditions in a safe and appropriate way for the type of conjoined twins undergoing the procedure. Analgesia, amnesia, and muscle relaxation should be provided, with control of the airway, ventilation, hemodynamic stability, and temperature regulation as for any pediatric anesthetic. Challenges with cardiovascular depression, difficult ventilation in thoracopagus twins, and unpredictable drug absorption and responses with uncertain degrees of cross circulation all necessitate regular adjustments in anesthetic agents and muscle relaxation. Especially if extubation is planned after anesthesia, short-acting drugs by constant infusion to each infant may well be the preferred option. This may also be the case with operations that have significant blood loss and a constantly changing hemodynamic status. For most operations, long-acting drugs such as pancuronium may be used.

During anesthesia, vasodilation in one infant may result in blood being diverted to this infant, causing a significant drop in the blood pressure of the other twin. Vigilant attention to each twin compared with the other is essential. This function is often best performed by the coordinator, as the other anesthesiologists are each busy with their own infant.

Cardiac support may be required early in any twins, but thoracopagus twin are at particular risk for this intervention. Early use of inotropes may be required.

All techniques, such as color coding of patients and their infusions, cannot be overstated. When positions are changed, the process should be carried out slowly to avoid dropping or damaging the infants or inadvertently pulling out catheters or ETTs.

The use of local anesthesia should always be considered. Epidural, caudal, and combined epidural-spinal anesthesia have all been used successfully for surgery and postoperative pain relief (Greenberg et al., 2001). There are definite advantages and disadvantages to the use of neuroaxial blocks and regional anesthesia, and each set of twins needs to be assessed individually as to the feasibility of this option. Where regional anesthesia is not possible, the use of infiltration of local anesthetic, together with a vasoconstrictor, should be considered and also helps reduce blood loss.

Blood loss is always mentioned in both the surgical and anesthetic literature with good reason. Vascular structures may not always be predictable, and blood loss may be sudden. Fluid and blood loss may be anything from half to more than five times each infant's estimated blood volume. Blood loss may be massive in craniopagus or cardiopagus twins, in those whose livers are extensively fused, and in those where a significant bony fusion is to be separated. This should be anticipated and monitored, with blood products immediately available. The blood bank and the laboratories should be informed of the surgery, and all point-of-care monitors checked and functioning. Fluid administration is determined by many aspects, but in general, a balanced electrolyte solution with the possible addition of 1% dextrose for neonatal surgery is most suitable. Colloids and blood products should be used early rather than later in the procedure and administered as required.

Circulatory collapse at separation was described in early reports, and adrenal suppression was cited as the cause. This led to the recommendation for use of perioperative steroids (Hoyle and Thomas, 1989; Synhorst et al., 1979; Aird, 1959), but this is no longer relevant, and steroids are only advised for specific surgical specialties such as neurosurgery. Other causes of circulatory collapse at separation are considered to be unappreciated blood loss resulting in an inadequate intravascular volume a vagal response (especially with bony separations of ischiopagus, pygopagus, or dipagus twins) and undiagnosed cardiac abnormalities. Where intravascular blood volume replacement is sufficient and vagal responses is preempted, this has not been a problem.

Monitoring

Routine noninvasive neonatal or pediatric monitoring is used until invasive lines are inserted. Urinary output from each infant is monitored, recognizing that in some twins with urogenital abnormalities the kidney function may not be accurately reflected by this test. For each infant, temperature monitoring is essential.

For control of the airway and breathing, routine pediatric ventilatory monitoring is required, with special attention being given to those infants in whom synchronized ventilation prevents hemodynamic consequences. Cardiovascular invasive monitoring is required in all but the simplest of conjunctions. This takes time to place, because the anatomic relations in most twins are unpredictable.

Monitoring of neurologic function is crucial in all cases. Recent developments in the use of BIS, near infrared spectroscopy (NIRS), and transcranial Doppler (TCD), makes these attractive options in monitoring cerebral blood flow and oxygenation during separation.

Arterial blood gases, electrolytes, and clotting parameters should be regularly checked. If it is available, a thromboelastogram (TEG) should be used.

Temperature monitoring should aim at normothermia, and all techniques available should be used to ensure proper temperature control. The use of plastic drapes, padded bandages around the limbs, and waterproof plastic bandages makes a significant difference to temperature control during the surgery. After each surgical group has operated and the positions have changed, these measures also need to be moved.

Reconstruction after Separation

For all disciplines of surgery, this phase is of the utmost importance for immediate and long-term outcomes. This surgery takes a long time, and blood loss may be covert and prolonged. It is vital to stabilize all aspects of both infants physiologically and to optimize their conditions before transfer to the intensive care unit. Primary closure that is too tight may compromise cardiac, pulmonary, gut, or renal function. Maintaining normothermia during this phase may be difficult.

Postoperative Care

Problems in the immediate postoperative period relate to the consequences of massive blood transfusion, tight closure, prolonged surgery, and alterations in preoperative anatomy. Cardiovascular and respiratory complications remain the most common causes of death. Monitoring for bleeding, hypoxia, hypercarbia, acidosis, hypothermia, hypotension, and electrolyte imbalance is mandatory. Ongoing volume losses, cardiac instability, and respiratory impairment are common at this time. When weaning the infants from mechanical ventilation, attention must be paid to sternal insufficiency, diaphragmatic dysfunction, and to the mechanics of breathing. Gastroesophageal reflux may be an additional complication. Sepsis is both a short- and long-term problem and may impact morbidity and mortality.

Good pain relief is obligatory and may include the use of intravenous acetaminophen (paracetamol), which can be given orally or rectally, as well as the more traditional options of morphine or clonidine. If chronic pain syndromes are anticipated, the early use of gabapentin should be considered. Further anesthetics may be required for vascular access, secondary wound closure, and wound dehiscence (Rode et al., 2006).

Especially in older sets of twins, nursing care in the same bed as soon as is practical and safe attends to the problems of separation anxiety.

Prognosis

Immediate and long-term survival of conjoined twins is extremely variable. Outcomes are better in twins who do not share vital organs, but many of these children still have considerable rehabilitation requirements. Despite tissue expansion, the use of prosthetic materials, skin grafts, complex plastic surgical flaps, and innovative methods to provide skin cover to close those areas exposed by the separation remains an ongoing challenge.

Hidden long-term morbidity and mortality occur with unresolved aspiration after thoracopagus separation; bronchopneumonia, arrhythmias, and embolic cerebrovascular pathology occurred in one survivor when the entire cardiac complex had been assigned to one infant (Rode et al., 2006; Millar et al., 2009).

For many years after their separation, some patients must undergo further surgery to reconstruct shared pelvises and urogenital systems, to improve wound closure with skin grafts, and to revise their anatomic abnormalities in an ongoing effort to improve the quality of their lives. Some survivors will be disabled and require lifelong follow-up care. For many others, life goes on with minimal sequelae (Figs. 29-21 and 29-22).

CONCLUSION

Many lessons have been learned over generations, and these include the need to consult widely—locally and internationally. The Internet makes this extraordinarily easy. It is important to search using both the American and English spellings of *anesthesia* and *anaesthesia,* because different references appear as the result of a search, and there is very little overlap. Descriptions of anesthetic challenges are being reported from all over the world in different socioeconomic and political circumstances, and each article teaches something of value (Bloch and Karis, 1980; Norsidah et al., 1996; Huanc et al., 2004; Leelanukrom et al., 2004). Whether surgery for separation is an option or not, an experienced multidisciplinary team approach to the management of these infants results in the overall improved handling of the patients and their parents. Success requires an

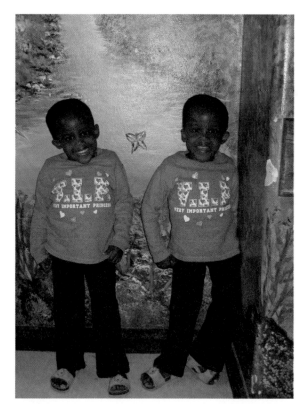

■ **FIGURE 29-21.** The ischiopagus twin girls from Figure 29-3, 5 years later.

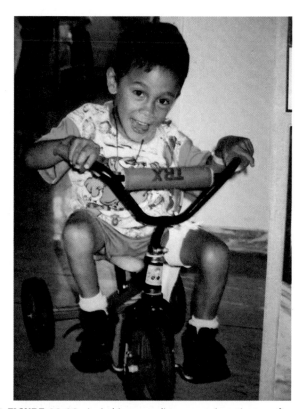

■ **FIGURE 29-22.** An ischiopagus dipagus survivor, 4 years after surgery to remove the duplicate segment, riding his tricycle in the ward.

experienced team functioning in a tertiary referral center with the full range of medical, surgical, and anesthetic specialties (Spitz and Kiely, 2003).

As technologies improve, anesthesia and intensive care will continue to positively impact the surgical outcomes of this fascinating and challenging group of patients. Some of these infants and children will grow up to become adults, so a greater understanding of the long-term outcome of this extraordinary pathology is essential. Although the physical needs of these children are usually addressed, the emotional consequences of their pathology should always be kept in mind and addressed.

Many of the basic principles of anesthetic care have not changed much in 60 years, but advances in anesthetic equipment, monitoring, investigative technology, pharmacology, and surgical materials make the desirable outcome of surgery, as well as the long-term prognosis for a good quality of life for conjoined twins, an attainable reality.

ACKNOWLEDGMENTS

Numerous colleagues, both past and present, have contributed to our knowledge of this extraordinary group of patients. The importance of a multidisciplinary team with good communication cannot be overemphasized. This includes sharing of patient data and photographs, and I thank all those surgeons and anesthesiologists who have allowed me to use their information. These include Professors Syd Cywes, Heinz Rode, Alastair Millar, Jonathan Peter, and Graham Fieggen, who are inspirational in their knowledge, technical skills, and teaching; Drs. Rob Dunn, John Lawrenson, and Jonathan Karpelowsky for clinical material; and Dr. Mike Porter for his assistance with the manuscript. To all those anesthesiologists who have assisted me over the years, and to those who have reported their experiences in the literature, I thank you. Most of all, I am deeply indebted to those parents and their children who have contributed so much and have enabled us to learn much of what we now know about this fascinating and challenging subject.

REFERENCES

Complete references used in this text can be found online at www.expertconsult.com.

Anesthesia for the Pediatric Trauma Patient

**Paul Reynolds, Joseph A. Scattoloni, Peter Ehrlich,
Franklyn P. Cladis, and Peter J. Davis**

CONTENTS

Trauma is the forceful disruption of bodily homeostasis that affects physical, psychological, and family functioning, and it remains the number one pediatric public health problem worldwide (Jurkovich et al., 2004). Each year injuries kill more children in the United States than the combined number of pediatric deaths from cancer, congenital anomalies, heart and chronic respiratory diseases, influenza, pneumonia, septicemia, and cerebrovascular disease (Centers for Disease Control and Prevention [CDC], 2002). Over 6 million children are evaluated and treated annually in emergency departments for their injuries, and of these, 500,000 children require hospitalization. Approximately 92,000 children annually become permanently physically disabled as a result of their injuries (Baker et al., 1992; Department of Rehabilitation Medicine, 1995; Tuggle, 1998; CDC, 2002; National Center for Injury Control and Prevention, 2005). Many children who survive their injuries are burdened with lifelong physical limitations or disabilities. For every 400 pediatric injuries, 250 require treatment in the emergency room, 16 are admitted to the hospital, and 1 dies as a result of the injuries (National Center for Injury Control and Prevention, 2005). Trauma care for children includes prevention, treatment and resuscitation, and rehabilitation.

Risk of death from injury can occur during any of three critical times. The first occurs at the time of injury, the second is within the first few hours after trauma, and the third is some time later as a result of complications from the injuries sustained at the time of the traumatic event. Development of effective regional trauma systems and educational programs, such as the Advanced Trauma Life Support for Doctors course, has contributed significantly to the reduction in mortality during the second and third of these critical periods (Tuggle, 1998; Rogers et al., 1999). Unfortunately, however, over 70% of mortality from trauma occurs at the time of injury.

EPIDEMIOLOGY

In 2006, approximately 6 million children received treatment in emergency departments for nonfatal injuries, and of these over 500,000 children needed hospitalization (Child Trends Data Bank, 2005). Injuries can be classified as either intentional or unintentional; most children's injuries are unintentional. Falls (32.4%) are the leading cause of nonfatal, unintentional injuries among hospitalized children 1 to 14 years of age, followed by injuries sustained as a result of being an occupant in a motor vehicle crash (12.3%) (National Center for Injury Control and Prevention, 2006). The rate of injury and the morbidity and mortality rates remain relatively stable until age 14, when they begin to increase substantially. Males are injured more commonly than females. Motor vehicle accidents are responsible for 75% of pediatric traumatic deaths (DiScala, 2002). Intracranial injuries are the cause of most pediatric traumatic deaths. Unintentional injuries are more prevalent among children who are male, poor, and black or Native American (Safe Kids USA, 2005). In 2004, there were 654,647 (715/100,000 population) nonfatal intentional injuries and 4738 (5.8/100,000 population) fatal intentional injuries in children 19 years and younger. Abuse (physical and sexual), followed by self harm were the major causes of intentional injuries (National Center for Injury Control and Prevention, 2005).

Injuries can be classified as either blunt or penetrating. Blunt injures far outnumber penetrating injuries (12:1), and whereas most are unintentional, up to 7% of injuries are a result of physical assault or abuse (DiScala, 2002). See related video online at www.expertconsult.com.

PEDIATRIC TRAUMA SYSTEMS

Historical Development

In North America, improvements to trauma care began in the 1960s and 1970s (Trunkey, 1983; Haller, 1995; Mullins, 1999; Morrison et al., 2002). Pediatric trauma systems did not develop in isolation but in concert with adult care. Trauma care was advanced in both the Korean and Vietnam wars, with the military experiences of treating injured soldiers. A report by Howard (1966) highlighted the enormity of the injury problem and stressed its significance as a neglected public health problem. Furthermore, a series of "preventable death studies" was published that provided fodder for community and political support of coordinated care for injured patients. Funding for emergency medical services first became available in 1966 with the National Highway Safety Act, and further support followed with the Emergency Medical Services System Act in 1973 (Mullins, 1999). In 1968, Cook County hospital in Chicago (for adult care) and Kings County hospital in Brooklyn (for pediatrics) were recognized as the first specialized centers for civilian trauma care in the United States. In 1969, the University of Maryland and the Maryland State police developed a coordinated transport system for injured patients to preferentially take them to a hospital with specific interest in caring for injured patients (Cowley et al., 1973; Cowley and Scanlan, 1979). Illinois is credited as the first state to develop a comprehensive state-wide trauma system that included categorization of trauma hospitals and the establishment of a communication system and a trauma registry (Boyd et al., 1973). In 1984, the Department of Health and Human Services, in conjunction with the National Highway Traffic Safety Administration, began the Emergency Medical

Services for Children Program in the United States. This funding has been a critical resource for developing programs and research to improve emergency service systems for children.

The American College of Surgeons Committee on Trauma (ACSCOT) has also strived to improve trauma care in North America. This has been accomplished through the publication of standards for trauma systems, the creation of educational courses for health care professionals, and the establishment of and verification programs to ensure published standards are met. In 1976, the first version of the Optimal Resources for Care of Seriously Injured was released (Committee on Trauma: American College of Surgeons, 1999). The most recent version of this publication (2006) is currently in use and has been retitled "Resources for the Optimal Care of Injured Patient." It remains a dynamic and important document. This publication established criteria for defining levels of trauma centers (I through III) and trauma systems (I and II), and it defined resource requirements for prehospital care through discharge, as well as specific pediatric needs. Level I centers offer the widest range of services for the most severely injured patient, whereas level III centers allow for stabilization and triage. With respect to trauma system development, eight criteria were defined and have become accepted benchmarks for trauma care (Boxes 30-1 and 30-2). Recently, designation of a level IV trauma center has occurred in some states where the resources do not exist for a level III trauma center. Level IV trauma centers are able to

---

Box 30-1 American College of Surgeons Trauma Center Levels and Descriptions

LEVEL I

The center provides comprehensive trauma care, serves as a regional resource, and provides leadership in education, research, and system planning.

A level I center is required to have immediate availability of trauma surgeons, anesthesiologists, physician specialists, nurses, and resuscitation equipment.

American College of Surgeons' volume performance criteria further stipulate that level I centers treat 1200 admissions a year or 240 major trauma patients per year or an average of 35 major trauma patients per surgeon.

LEVEL II

The center provides comprehensive trauma care either as a supplement to a level I trauma center in a large urban area or as the lead hospital in a less populated area.

Level II centers must meet essentially the same criteria as those for level I, but volume performance standards are not required and may depend on the geographic area served.

Centers are not expected to provide leadership in teaching and research.

LEVEL III

The center provides prompt assessment, resuscitation, emergency surgery, and stabilization with transfer to a level I or II center as indicated.

Level III facilities typically serve communities that do not have immediate access to a level I or II trauma center.

From MacKenzie EJ, Hoyt DB, Sacra JC, et al: National Inventory of Hospital Trauma Centers, *JAMA* 289(12):1515–1522, 2003.

Box 30-2 American College of Surgeons Criteria for Trauma System Development

1. State authority to designate, certify, identify, or categorize trauma centers
2. Existence of a formal process to designate or otherwise identify trauma centers
3. Use of the ACS standards to designate and identify trauma centers
4. Inclusion of onsite verification during the designation and identification process and use of out-of-area surveyors
5. Authority to limit the number of trauma centers based on the need for trauma services
6. Existence of a process for monitoring trauma-center performance
7. State-wide coverage of a trauma system

From Adler P: *Directorate for epidemiology*, Washington, DC, 1994, U.S. Consumer Product Safety Commission.

provide initial evaluation, stabilization, preliminary diagnoses, and transportation to a center with a higher level of care. These centers may also provide surgery and critical care services (as defined in the scope of services of trauma care). A trained trauma nurse and physicians are available on the patients' arrival to the emergency department.

In 1986, the ACSCOT established its consultation and verification program to ensure that these standards were being met. At present in North America, there are 94 verified level I centers for adult care and 46 level I centers for pediatrics.

Another valuable contribution by the ACSCOT is the Advanced Trauma Life Support course (ATLS). First released in 1979, the course is now taught all over the world (American College of Surgeons Committee on Trauma, 1997). The first pediatric chapter was introduced in 1983. Although initially designed for surgeons, a wide variety of health care professionals involved in trauma care participate today. The ATLS course provides a common language, framework, and approach to injured patients that facilitate communication between health care professionals in order to optimize and prioritize care. Regular recertification is mandated to keep physicians current with new advances in trauma management. Similar to other ACSCOT programs, the ATLS course is constantly evolving. The current version is the seventh edition.

Trauma System Components

A trauma system is not simply an isolated hospital that cares for injured patients but a broad coalition of participants that includes an integrated approach to trauma. This includes prevention, prehospital care, and hospital care through rehabilitation (Ehrlich et al., 2001, 2002).

A primary step in developing an effective trauma system is a needs assessment of the community that it serves. For example, rural trauma systems differ from those in urban settings—each have different mortality rates, injury patterns, geographic areas, available resources, and expertise (Rogers et al., 1999; Ehrlich et al., 2004). Community responsibility and involvement (particularly with injury prevention) are essential for political support and funding. Studies support the concept that community-based injury-prevention programs play a substantial role in reducing morbidity and mortality (Hulka et al., 1997; Nathens et al., 2000).

A second important consideration in developing a regional trauma system is to understand that all facilities have a role in treating injured patients. A tiered approach (e.g., Levels I through IV) with specific hospitals designated to care for the varied complexity of injured patients is essential. Level I hospitals are tertiary or quaternary centers, with levels II and III centers having fewer capabilities and resources. Level IV hospitals are distinct because of their remote nature (rural trauma). A list of recommended requirements for each level of care can be found in the ACSCOT publication *Resources for the Optimal Care of the Injured patient: 2006* (Committee on Trauma: American College of Surgeons, 1999). A basic tenet and overarching requirement for this tiered system is a central communication (central command) structure and a well-developed triage system so that the most severely injured patients go first to the appropriately designated hospital. In addition, a trauma registry system is essential for outcomes analysis and quality-assurance programs.

A third point is that a trauma system is not an isolated surgical program but a multidisciplinary team of physicians, nurses, technicians, and allied health professions. A large trauma program uses a significant percentage of hospital resources for everything from the blood bank to social work. Regular meetings of all stakeholders are needed to solve problems and respond to changing injury patterns and community needs.

Anesthesiologists play a variety of roles in trauma response. These roles span from assisting as primary responders in airway management and vascular access to coordinating operating-room resources to ensure that patients are treated in a timely and effective fashion. A pediatric anesthesiologist is an invaluable resource when treating injured children. A 1993 report from the Institute of Medicine identified specific pediatric emergency medical service deficiencies in rural states (Institute of Medicine, 1993), including the pediatric airway management, vascular access, and special resuscitation needs of injured children. Airway control is a primary tenet of trauma care, and proper endotracheal intubation (ETI) is recognized as a definitive method to achieve airway control. ETI, however, in injured children is required less often than in adults; hence, maintaining skills can be difficult for health care providers (Baker et al., 2009). Several studies have looked at airway management in pediatric trauma and examined significant aspects, including how success and complication rates of ETI vary by location (e.g., field, transferring hospital, or trauma center) and personnel, whether bag-mask ventilation is effective with respect to oxygenation and ventilation before ETI, and whether multiple attempts at intubation adversely affect patient care or outcomes (Cooper et al., 1992; Gausche et al., 2000; Glaeser, 2000; Ehrlich et al., 2004). These studies have demonstrated that field intubation success rates are poor. Successful pediatric intubations relate to the skill of the person performing the intubation, and anesthesiologists' airway management skills are considered superior to those of all other health care professionals. Failed attempts at ETI appear to produce a spiral effect that results in multiple failed attempts and delayed transfer to definitive care. Complications resulting from ETI seem far more common when the intubation is attempted in the field and the risk of complication is exacerbated with each attempt. Increased complication rates do impact patient recovery, as shown by longer durations of hospitalization (Cooper et al., 1992; Gausche et al., 2000; Glaeser, 2000).

TRAUMA SCORING SYSTEMS

Trauma scoring systems form an integral component of the trauma care structure. Many scoring systems have been described in the literature, and understanding the differences between each can be confusing. To further complicate matters, most trauma scoring systems for pediatric care are derived from adult data. Some of the most commonly used scoring systems are discussed in this chapter.

Trauma scoring systems serve two specific functions. The first is to help determine where is best for an injured patient to be treated. These scores help "triage" the injured child, and therefore help determine the necessity of requiring a trauma center to care for the injury. The best-known and most widely used is the Glasgow Coma Scale (GCS). The second type of scoring system quantifies the severity of illness (SOI), or the risk of mortality. These are typically determined retrospectively and serve as markers for quality assurance, benchmarking, and research, particularly for health services and outcome studies. Triage scores can also form a component of an SOI tool. For example, the GCS is used both as a triage tool and in outcome models. These models rely on a variety of variables, including the diagnosis (using the International Classification of Diseases [ICD-9-CM]), the demographic of the injured patient, and anatomic, physiologic, and laboratory variables. Triage scoring systems are designed to help make quick decisions; they tend to have few data points to assess and are therefore simple to use. Alternatively, the SOI scoring systems have many variables, are more cumbersome, and are often computer generated.

Triage Scores: Where is the Injured Child Best Treated?

An ideal triage scoring system would have few data points, be easy to apply, have limited subjective assessments, and have a high sensitivity and specificity. Unfortunately, no triage score accomplishes all of these tasks, but each system does have strengths and limitations. For example, studies have shown that assessments made in the field by paramedics are less accurate and reliable for pediatric trauma patients when compared with adults (Engum, 2000). Alternatively, comparisons between adult and pediatric trauma triage scores have not shown that a pediatric specific trauma score provides a significant advantage over the original adult measure.

Glasgow Coma Scale

In 1974, Teasdale and Jennett first introduced the GCS. A lower score reflects a lower level of consciousness and therefore a potentially more serious head injury. Scores can range from 3 to a maximum of 15 (normal). The GCS measures three specific components of consciousness (eye movement, verbal, and motor responses) with higher scores (up to 5) given to the best response. A patient with a GCS of 13 to 14 is considered to have a mild head injury; 9 to 12 indicates a moderate injury; and a score of 8 or lower indicates a severe insult. Adaptations of the GCS for the pediatric population have occurred, and a Pediatric GCS is now widely used (Table 30-1).

GCS scores determined in the field are less predictive of outcome than those generated at a hospital (Meredith et al., 1995). When each individual component of the GCS is evaluated, the motor component is the strongest predictor of outcome.

Revised Trauma Score

The revised trauma score (RTS) is a physiologic-based triage score (Table 30-2). The RTS was derived from two earlier versions of a triage scores, the Triage Index and the Trauma Score (Champion et al., 1980, 1981, 1989). The RTS has three variables—respiratory rate, systolic blood pressure, and GCS. The RTS is the sum of each variable multiplied by a weighted coefficient.

TABLE 30-1. Glasgow Coma Scale Adult and Pediatric Variables

Best Response	Adult GCS	Pediatric GCS	Score
Eye	No eye opening	No eye opening	1
	Eye opening to pain	Eye opening to pain	2
	Opening to verbal command	Eye opening to speech	3
	Open spontaneously	Open spontaneously	4
Verbal	No verbal response	No vocal response	1
	Incomprehensible	Inconsolable, agitated	2
	Inappropriate	Inconsistently consolable,	3
	Confused conversation	moaning	4
	Orientated	Cries but is consolable, inappropriate interactions	5
		Smiles, orientated to sounds, follows objects, interacts	
Motor	No motor response	No motor response	1
	Extension to pain	Extension to pain	2
	Flexion to pain	Flexion to pain	3
	Withdrawal from pain	Withdrawal from pain	4
	Localizing pain	Localizing pain	5
	Obeys commands	Obeys commands	6

From Brown RL et al.: Cervical spine injuries in children: a review of 103 patients treated consecutively at a level 1 pediatric trauma center, *J Pediatr* Surg 36:1107, 2001.

TABLE 30-2. Revised Trauma Score*

Clinical Measurement	Parameter	Score
Respiratory rate	10–24	4
	25–35	3
	>35	2
	<10	1
	0	0
Systolic blood pressure	>90	4
	70–89	3
	50–69	2
	<50	1
	0	0
Glasgow Coma Scale	14–15	4
	11–13	3
	8–10	2
	5–7	1
	3–4	0

From Centers for Disease Control and Prevention: *Traumatic brain injury in the United States: a report to Congress,* Atlanta, 1999, Department of Health and Human Services National Center for Injury Control and Prevention.
* The Revised Trauma score is the sum of the weighted variables (see formula in text). The higher the score, the better the prognosis.

$$RTS = 0.9368(GCS) + 0.7326(SBP) + 0.22908(RR \text{ value})$$

where *GCS* is the Glasgow Coma Scale; *SBP* is systolic blood pressure; and *RR* is respiratory rate. These variables were determined to correlate statistically with survival and mortality. A higher RTS is associated with a better chance of survival. An injured patient with a RTS score of 11 or lower is recommended to be treated at a designated trauma center. Eichelberger established and developed pediatric coefficients for the RTS that was then validated in the pediatric population (Engum et al., 2000). The RTS is also recommended as one of the triage tools in the American College of Surgeons trauma guidelines, *Resources for the Optimal Care of the Injured Patient* (Committee on Trauma: American College of Surgeons, 1999).

Alert, Verbal, Painful, or Unresponsive Scale

This is a simple scale that categorizes a patient's condition as alert, verbal, painful, or unresponsive (APVU). No numeric scores are given, but an injured child with a P or U should be taken to the designated trauma center. Subjective interpretation is inherent in this score, so it is best used as a component of the triage process, especially for children in whom the age and development of the child can impact the response. There is a significant risk of undertriaging patients when using this score.

Pediatric Trauma Score

The Pediatric Trauma Score (PTS) was first introduced by Tepas in 1987 (Tepas et al., 1987; Nayduch et al., 1991). Its design was thought to be more reflective of pediatric injuries (Table 30-3). Six variables comprise both physiologic and injury attributes. After a number for each variable is totaled, a score of 8 or lower is considered to be a marker for children requiring care at a designated trauma center. A limitation of the PTS

TABLE 30-3. Pediatric Trauma Score

Clinical	Parameter	Score*
Weight (kg)	>20	2
	10-19	1
	<10	−1
Airway	Normal	2
	Maintainable	1
	Unmaintainable	−1
Systolic blood pressure	>90	2
	50-89	1
	<50	−1
Central nervous system	Awake	2
	Obtunded or loss of consciousness	1
	Coma or decerebrate	−1
Open wound	None	2
	Minor	1
	Major or penetrating	−1
Skeletal	None	2
	Closed fracture	1
	Open or multiple fractures	−1

Data from Tepas JJ III, Mollitt DL, Talbert JL, et al: The pediatric trauma score as a predictor of injury severity in the injured child, *J Pediatr Surg* 22:14–18, 1987; Tobias JD, Ross AK: Intraosseous infusions: a review for the anesthesiologist with a focus on pediatric use, *Anesth Analg* 110:391–401, 2010.
*A total score of 8 or less suggests care at a designated trauma center.

is that some variables are subjectively scored, particularly the central nervous system (CNS) assessment. Therefore, there is a risk of interrater and intrarater variability. The PTS has been compared with the RTS with surprisingly few apparent differences or inherent advantages (Tepas et al., 1987, 1988; Nayduch et al., 1991).

Age-Specific PTS

The most recent proposed triage score is the Age Specific PTS (Table 30-4). First described by Potoka et al. in 2001, the main addition is the use of age-specific physiologic variables.

TABLE 30-4. Age-Specific Pediatric Trauma Score*

GCS	SBP	Pulse	RR	Score
14-15	Normal	Normal	Normal	3
10-13	Mild to moderate hypotension (SBP < −2SD)	Tachycardia (pulse > mean + SD)	Tachypnea (RR > mean + SD)	2
4-9	Severe hypotension (SBP < −3SD)	Bradycardia (pulse > mean − SD)	Hypoventilation (RR < mean −SD)	1
3	0	0	0 or intubated	0

From Potoka DA, et al.: Development of a novel age-specific pediatric trauma score, *J Pediatr Surg* 36:106, 2001.
* Age-specific variables are stratified by degree of severity, and coded values (0-3) are assigned to each variable. The integer scores are then added (maximum score is 12).

To date, long-term data are lacking and only a single study suggests that it is better than traditional adult scores; therefore, the clinical utility as a triage score still remains to be proven. This score is, however, a pediatric-specific tool that addresses areas where other adult scores become less accurate (e.g., extremes of age).

Abbreviated Injury Scale

$$\text{AIS Score} = \sum (\text{AIS body region 1 to 9})$$

The Abbreviated Injury Scale (AIS) emerged from the automotive industry in 1969 (JAMA, 1971; Association for the Advancement of Automotive Medicine, 1990). It was initially designed as an epidemiologic tool to describe motor-vehicle crashes but has been adapted to all types of trauma (JAMA, 1971; Association for the Advancement of Automotive Medicine, 1990). Revised and updated several times over the years, the first version published was the AIS-90 (for the year 1990) in 1998 (Association for the Advancement of Automotive Medicine, 1990). This score evaluates nine body regions. A scale from 1 to 6 is used to define injuries (1, minor; 2, moderate; 3, serious; 4, severe; 5, critical; and 6, maximal.) The underlying premise is an association of injury with threat to life. A body region with a score of 6 is considered an unsurvivable injury. The scores are determined retrospectively and based primarily on ICD-9-CM codes. A significant amount of expertise is required to assign these ratings, and interrater and intrarater variability is common. To help limit this phenomenon, software has been developed to convert the ICD-9-CM codes directly to an AIS score. Unfortunately, ICD-9-CM coding itself is inherently variable (MacKenzie et al., 1985, 1989).

Injury Severity Score

$$\text{ISS} = (\text{AIS body region 1})^2 + $$
$$(\text{AIS body region 2})^2 + (\text{AIS body region 3})^2$$

The Injury Severity Score (ISS) is one of the most widely used scoring systems in the trauma literature. It correlates well with several important trauma outcomes such as mortality and duration of hospitalization. Developed in 1974, the ISS is a method of characterizing the trauma patient with multiple injuries (Baker et al., 1974; Baker and O'Neill, 1976). The ISS is based on the AIS, which describes the severity of injury to different body regions (see the previous section). For example:

$$\text{ISS} = (A)^2 + (B)^2 + (C)^2$$

The above formula shows AIS scores of the three most injured of the following body regions: A, the head, neck, and face; B, the thorax and abdomen, and C, the extremities (including the external pelvis). The ISS takes scores from 0 to 75 (i.e., AIS scores of 5 for each category). However, if any of the three scores is a 6, the score is automatically set at 75, because a score of 6 indicates that an injury is unsurvivable.

Two modifications have been reported to the ISS score—the modified ISS (MISS) incorporating the GCS, and the New ISS, focusing on injuries over body regions. However, evaluations of both the MISS and new ISS have not shown advantages over the standard ISS; therefore, in many centers and registries the AIS-90 still remains the standard severity of injury scoring system.

Survival Probability: Trauma Score and Injury Severity Score

The Trauma Score and Injury Severity Score (TRISS) is not a score but rather a method of predicting mortality. It was first proposed in 1987 and combines the physiologic variables of the RTS with the anatomic severity-of-injury scores generated by the ISS (Boyd et al., 1987). The final result is that a probability of survival (Ps) is generated.

$$\text{Ps} = 1 / (1 + e - b)$$

Where e is the base of the natural log 2.72183, and b is derived from the following formula:

$$b = b0 + b1(\text{RTS}) + b2(\text{ISS}) + b3(\text{age factor})$$

The age factor is 0 for those younger than 55 years of age, and 1 for those who are 55 years of age. The variables $b0$, $b1$, $b2$, and $b3$ are blunt and penetrating trauma coefficients for adult and pediatric populations (Eichelberger et al., 1993).

TRISS is the most widely used predictor of survival in the trauma literature. As with other statistical processes, limitations exist. These are specifically noted in patients older than 55 years of age (extremes of age), and with trauma patients whose ISS is greater than 25. In fact, some authors suggest that because of the TRISS deficiencies, this method of calculating survival probabilities should be abandoned completely, particularly in urban centers (Cayten et al., 1991; Demetriades et al., 1998).

Application of the TRISS Results (W and Z Scores)

A common application of the TRISS and Ps is to compare practice-based outcomes with population-based outcomes. Typically, this comparison uses a group of national norms that were identified in the Major Trauma Outcomes Study (MTOS) (Champion et al., 1990b). The MTOS data set is derived from 160,000 hospitalized patients at 139 centers between 1982 and 1989. Children represented 11% of this population. From 80,544 adult patients in this data set, regression coefficients for predicting mortality were derived based on the revised trauma score and ISS (TRISS methodology). A single data set can be compared with the MTOS. A "Z score" is generated, whereby

$$Z = (A - E) / S$$

where A equals the actual outcomes, E equals expected outcomes ($E = \Sigma Pi$), and S is a scale factor that accounts for statistical variation ($S = \sqrt{\Sigma Pi [1 - Pi]}$). Pi is the TRISS survival probability for each patient. Z norms should be between 1.96 and −1.96. If the Z statistic is greater than 1.96, survival is better than the MTOS norms, whereas if it is less than −1.96, survival is less than MTOS norms.

A probability slope (PRE) is calculated using the RTS vs. the ISS. A Ps_{50} slope can be calculated that represents a 0.50 probability of survival (based on MTOS data). Survivors whose data fall above this line and those with fatal injuries whose data fall below this line represent statistically unexpected outcomes.

W Scores

W is used when the Z score is found to be significant. W measures the statistical differences between the actual (A) and expected (E) survivors in a patient group. Sample size plays an important role in delineating the clinical significance of the difference between the actual and expected numbers of survivors (Taylor et al., 1986). Consider the following formula:

$$W = \frac{(A - E)}{(N / 100)}$$

A and *E* carry the same values as they did for the Z score. *N* represents the number of children analyzed, and *W* represents the number of survivors[+/-] that would be expected per 100 children.

Both the W and Z scores are limited by the same factors that limit TRISS data.

A Severity Characterization of Trauma Score

A Severity Characterization of Trauma (ASCOT) score is an attempt to revise and fix the limitations found using TRISS methodology (i.e., severely injured patients and extremes of age) (Champion et al., 1990b). ASCOT uses individual components of the RTS (not totaled) and incorporates a modification of AIS entitled *The Anatomic Profile*. Furthermore, it excludes those patients with either very severe or nonserious injuries (a maximum AIS score of less than 2 and an RTS score of greater than 0; an AIS score of 6 and an RTS score equal to 0). The Anatomic Profile categorizes the AIS scores that are greater than 2 into three groups: head, brain, and spinal cord injuries; thorax or neck injuries; and all other serious injuries. A comparison of ASCOT vs. TRISS with a pediatric population did not provide more reliable or accurate scoring over the TRISS.

Pediatric Age-Adjusted TRISS

This is a recent tool used to describe mortality that applies the pediatric-specific, age-adjusted PTS. Although it may be a more promising predictor of mortality, its data are limited and it has not been validated by other investigators (Schall et al., 2002).

The multitude of scoring systems reflect the reality that no single approach addresses all aspects of pediatric trauma accurately or provides the necessary tools to effectively answer all research questions. Many scoring systems suffer from inherent inaccuracies of coding (e.g., related to discharge diagnoses, ICD-9-CD diagnoses, and data on death certificates). Although physiologic variables generally seem to outperform anatomic variables in these systems, codification requires experience and training. Finally, certain elements of the laboratory data have been shown to be a strong predictor of mortality, yet these variables are not included in the prediction models.

PRIMARY AND SECONDARY SURVEYS

Although children have unique characteristics that distinguish them from adults, the principles of initial management of the injured child and adult are identical.

The first priority is to save a life through identifying and treating all life-threatening illnesses and injuries. To understand and acquire the necessary clinical skills for the management of injured adults and children, it is best to become certified by completing the ATLS course designed by the American Colleges of Surgeons (Schall et al., 2002). The ATLS course is a well-recognized certification for trauma care and is now used worldwide to teach physicians and other health care providers. The ATLS course gives a common approach and language to the care of injured patients, thus allowing a framework for physicians and allied health personnel to communicate.

The initial management of the injured child can be divided into two phases. The first is the primary survey that incorporates the "ABCs" and where all life-threatening injuries are identified and treated. The second phase is the secondary survey, where other injuries that contribute significantly to illness and deaths are identified and treatment is instituted. The ABCs are defined in the following list, and the priorities of the primary survey are further detailed in Box 30-3.

A: Airway — Ensure a patent airway.
B: Breathing — Assess and provide adequate respiration.
C: Circulation — Assess and assist the circulation with intravenous (IV) fluids and cardiopulmonary resuscitation (CPR) as needed.

During the resuscitation of the injured child, many processes are conducted concurrently (Fig. 30-1). It is important to continually assess, intervene, and reassess within the priorities of the primary survey. The final components of the primary survey are the placement of a Foley catheter and gastric tube unless contraindicated. The contraindications to placing a Foley catheter include pelvic fracture and blood at the tip of the meatus.

The secondary survey is comprised of a complete physical examination, patient history, laboratory tests, and radiologic imaging. This phase may be delayed or completed in the operating room in patients who require urgent interventions. Historical information about the patient and the event should be collected during the secondary survey. The acronym SAMPLE (standing for *Symptoms, Allergies, Medications, Past illnesses, Last meal, Events,* and *Environment*) may be helpful in guiding the trauma team. Definitive care occurs in the intensive care unit or operating room and often involves care by pediatric surgical subspecialists (e.g., neurosurgeons or orthopedic surgeons). Patients may also require transfer to comprehensive trauma centers during this phase (Krantz, 1996).

Airway

The first step in trauma resuscitation is to assess the airway and then secure it when necessary to assure respirations. Indications for ETI include inability to oxygenate and ventilate and the need to protect the airway against aspiration.

Box 30-3 ABCs of Resuscitation

A = Airway with cervical spinal control
B = Breathing and ventilation, pulse oximetry and oxygen
C = Circulation with hemorrhage control
D = Disability and neurologic control
E = Exposure/environmental control

Data from Tepas JJ 3rd, Mollitt DL, Talbert JL, et al: The pediatric trauma score as a predictor of injury severity in the injured child, *J Pediatr Surg* 22:14–18, 1987; Tobias JD, Ross AK: Intraosseous infusions: a review for the anesthesiologist with a focus on pediatric use, *Anesth Analg* 110:391–401, 2010.

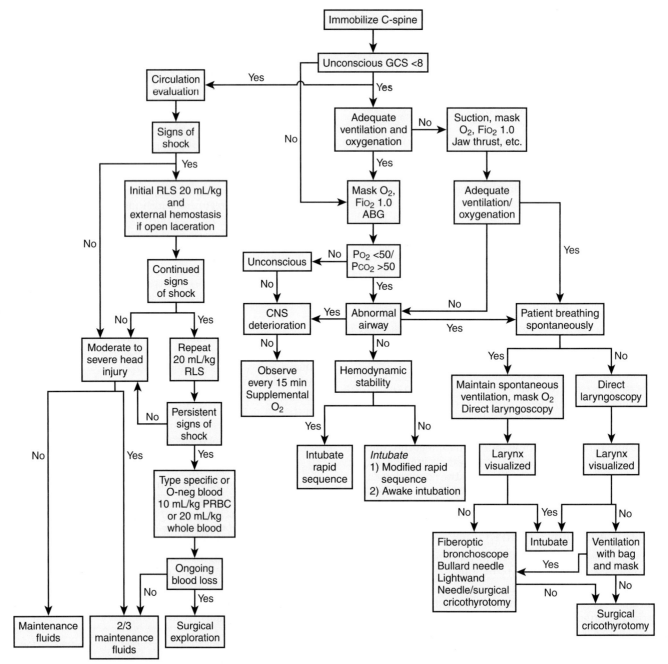

■ FIGURE 30-1. Guidelines for airway and cardiovascular assessment in the traumatized pediatric patient.

Appropriate management of the airway may be challenging or difficult without proper preparation and familiarity with the unique characteristics of the pediatric airway. In a young child or infant, the tongue is relatively large and the larynx and glottic opening are more anterior. A child's airway has a smaller diameter and a shorter length. Airway edema occurring in an already small airway results in significant changes in the internal diameter of the airway and in increased resistance to airflow. The short length of the trachea makes right mainstem intubations more likely and increases the likelihood of extubation from small positional changes of the ET tube. Because the pediatric mid-face is small compared with the tongue, airway obstruction is common. Blood, vomit, teeth, and foreign bodies are common causes of airway obstruction. In addition, children are often placed in cervical collars that may be too large for

them. This can make it hard see a child's face and can present a challenge to identifying an airway obstruction. The first step to making the obstructed airway patent (while keeping the cervical collar on) is a jaw thrust with suction. Oral or nasal airways may be required if a jaw thrust is unsuccessful. If the airway is still not patent after these maneuvers, there should be consideration of a possible airway foreign body.

The initial management of the pediatric airway involves bag-valve-mask ventilation with a jaw-thrust maneuver. Intubation is indicated in patients with respiratory or cardiac compromise or an altered level of consciousness. All pediatric trauma patients should be considered to have a full stomach and possible cervical spine injury. See related video online at www.expertconsult.com. Because of this, the airway should be secured after a rapid-sequence induction (RSI) (that may include cricoid pressure) with manual inline stabilization and an oral ETI. Nasotracheal intubation may be suboptimal and difficult because of the small size and acute angle of the nasopharynx and the more anterior and cephalad position of the glottic opening.

The RSI for pediatric trauma patients can be accomplished with an induction agent that is immediately followed by a muscle relaxant. Standard induction agents for trauma patients include etomidate (0.2 to 0.3 mg/kg) and ketamine (2 to 4 mg/kg) or the combination of fentanyl (2 to 3 mcg/kg), midazolam (0.05 to 0.1 mg/kg) with lidocaine (1 mg/kg). Sodium thiopental (STP) and propofol should be reserved for patients who are not hemodynamically unstable. STP is an ideal induction agent for patients with head trauma, provided they are not hypovolemic. Ketamine is relatively contraindicated in patients with increased intracranial pressure (ICP). Although etomidate provides hemodynamic stability in trauma patients who are hypovolemic, it may decrease survival in patients with sepsis secondary to adrenal suppression (Annane et al., 2002). Muscle relaxation can be achieved with rocuronium (0.8 to 1.2 mg/kg) or succinylcholine (1 to 1.5 mg/kg). Succinylcholine is contraindicated in crush injuries, long-bone fractures, and patients susceptible to malignant hyperthermia. In patients who are hemodynamically stable, the combination of propofol (4 mg/kg) and remifentanil (3 mcg/kg) can be used for rapid-sequence intubation and has an onset and offset similar to propofol and succinylcholine (1 mg/kg) (Crawford et al., 2005).

ETIs have been deemphasized in the prehospital setting, because they are often unsuccessful. Gausche and others (2000) reported a success rate of only 57%. All intubated trauma patients that come to the emergency department should have the placement of their endotracheal tubes (ETTs) confirmed with either end-tidal carbon dioxide (CO_2) or direct laryngoscopy.

If initial intubation attempts are unsuccessful after an RSI, the patient should be ventilated with bag-mask ventilation. If a patient cannot be ventilated or if it is very difficult, a laryngeal mask airway (LMA) can be placed to facilitate ventilation and subsequent intubation. However, it must be recognized that the LMA does not protect the airway from aspiration and must be replaced by an ETT as soon as skilled personnel become available. The stomach should be decompressed with a nasogastric or orogastic tube after intubation, and a chest x-ray should be obtained to verify the ETT position (Fig. 30-2).

Depending on the nature of the underlying injury, securing the airway in a patient who has sustained multiple injuries or even isolated facial injuries can be extremely complicated, as illustrated in Figure 30-3. The management of such cases calls upon the resourcefulness and skills of the anesthesiologist and requires careful consideration of damage to surrounding structures such as major blood vessels and the airway structures themselves. The ability to maintain a patent airway via face mask, and the potential for an expanding hematoma that may subsequently compromise an airway that may be patent at the current time, must be anticipated. Additional considerations include the risks of increased ICP with concomitant head trauma, exacerbating an existing cervical spine injury, and aspiration during airway manipulation. The presence of rhinorrhea, otorrhea, or ecchymoses around the eyes should raise suspicion about a possible basilar skull fracture, and any instrumentation of the nasal passages, including passage of a nasal ETT or an N/G tube, should be avoided. Similarly, crepitus at the neck may herald the presence of a tracheal disruption, and intubation under direct vision using a fiberoptic scope should be considered to avoid false passage of the ETT. See related video online at www.expertconsult.com.

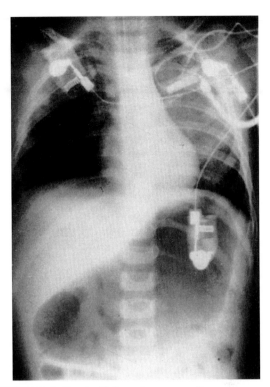

FIGURE 30-2. Gastric dilation often occurs after crying or positive-pressure ventilation by gas and mask.

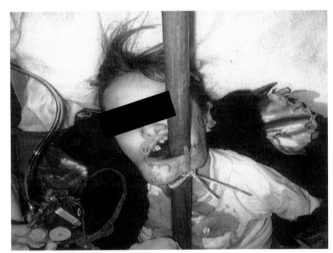

FIGURE 30-3. An 11-year-old girl fell 10 to 15 feet while sliding down the school banisters onto a plant supported by a thick wooden pole. She eventually was intubated orally with direct laryngoscopy. *(From Melillo EP, et al: Difficult airway management of a child impaled through the neck, Paediatr Anaesth 11:615, 2001.)*

In cases in which airway difficulty is anticipated, it may be prudent to transport the child to the operating room with an anesthesiologist and otolaryngologist once the child has been stabilized hemodynamically and additional injuries have been ruled out. The airway may then be secured with preparations to perform an emergent tracheostomy in case of failed laryngoscopy. An inhalational induction may be tolerated by the patient who has been volume resuscitated. This permits direct laryngoscopy or flexible fiberoptic intubation while the patient is breathing spontaneously. In patients who have suffered loss of consciousness or head injury, there should be a high index of suspicion for cervical

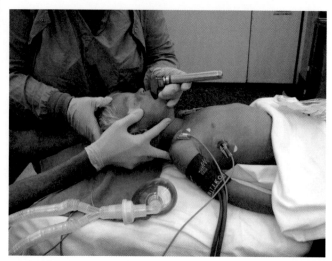

■ **FIGURE 30-4.** Manual axial inline stabilization during direct laryngoscopy.

spine injury, even with the absence of radiologic evidence. When performing laryngoscopy, inline axial stabilization must be performed (Fig. 30-4). Inline axial stabilization is performed by an assistant during laryngoscopy. The assistant should place both arms on either side of the patient's head while gripping the patient's shoulders. The assistant's function is to maintain the patient in a neutral position during laryngoscopy, avoiding flexion, extension, or rotation of the cervical spine. The use of muscle relaxants is best avoided until the airway is secured. If intravenous agents are required to induce anesthesia, it is preferable to use short-acting agents such as propofol and remifentanil that effectively blunt ICP responses to direct laryngoscopy yet permit return of spontaneous respiration in case of failed intubation.

Breathing

Assuring adequate ventilation is the next task after securing the airway. Breathing is best assessed by auscultation and observation of chest motion. During the primary assessment the patient should be assessed for the presence or absence of breathing, respiratory rate, and work of breathing. The chest should also be observed for symmetry of chest motion and breath sounds. The chest wall should also be observed for evidence of direct chest trauma resulting in abrasions, penetration, or chest-wall instability. The back needs to be assessed as well for posterior chest wall trauma. Although there are no concrete recommendations to guide intubation, pediatric patients with increased work of breathing or life-threatening injuries (head injuries) may require ETI. Immediately after ETT placement, the position should be confirmed with end-tidal CO_2. Patients in cardiac arrest or very small patients may require direct laryngoscopy. A portable chest x-ray and arterial blood gas should be obtained before leaving the trauma bay to determine the position of the ETT and its adequate delivery of oxygenation and ventilation. Continuous end-tidal CO_2 monitoring and pulse oximetry are useful adjuncts. Many injuries that impair respiration include simple, tension, and open pneumothorax; massive hemothorax; flail chest; and pulmonary contusion. A sudden change in the respiratory status after successful intubation should prompt an immediate evaluation for a reversible cause. An enlarged pneumothorax or development of a tension pneumothorax can occur after converting from spontaneous ventilation to positive pressure ventilation. Other causes for a decline in respiratory status include a displaced ETT (e.g., extubation or right mainstem intubation), obstruction in the ETT (e.g., blood or secretions), and equipment failure.

Circulation and Access

Children who sustain multiple injuries often arrive in hypovolemic or hemorrhagic shock that must be promptly recognized and treated. Unlike adults, children maintain an almost normal blood pressure until 25% to 35% of their circulating blood volume is lost (Fig. 30-5). This is likely because of their high sympathetic tone that causes peripheral vasoconstriction in an effort to maintain blood pressure in the face of a diminished blood volume. Therefore, tachycardia is an earlier sign of impending shock than hypotension. Additionally, signs of poor peripheral perfusion such as delayed capillary refill (more than 2 seconds), weak or thready pulses, mottling or cyanosis of the skin, and impaired consciousness are earlier indicators of shock than low blood pressure. The presence of hypotension as a result of hypovolemia should be considered an ominous sign that usually heralds impending cardiovascular collapse. Table 30-5 describes the stages of pediatric shock and clinical signs seen at these stages.

It is imperative to rapidly assess the pediatric trauma patient for signs of shock upon arrival in the trauma center and at regular intervals thereafter. The initial fluid bolus administered in the trauma setting is warmed isotonic crystalloid (lactated Ringer's solution or normal saline) in a bolus of 20 mL/kg, IV (see Fig. 30-1). The pulse, capillary refill, and blood pressure are

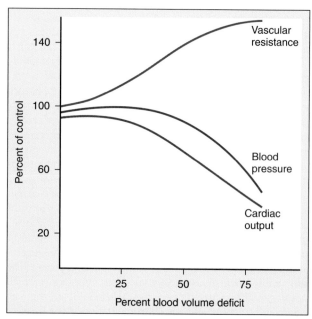

■ **FIGURE 30-5.** Increase in systemic vascular resistance in response to hypovolemia preserves blood pressure until 25% of blood volume is lost. Hypotension is a late sign of hypovolemia. (*From Rasmussen GE, Grandes CM: Blood, fluids, and electrolytes in the pediatric trauma patient,* Int Anesthesiol Clin *32:79, 1994.*)

TABLE 30-5. Stages of Pediatric Blood Volume Loss (Shock) and Associated Clinical Signs

Blood Volume Loss	Clinical Signs
<20%	CV: Tachycardia; weak, thready pulses Skin: Cool to touch, capillary refill 2-3 sec Renal: Slight decrease in urine output, increase in specific gravity CNS: Irritable, may be combative
25%	CV: Tachycardia; weak, thready distal pulses Skin: Cold extremities, cyanosis, and mottling Renal: Decrease in urine output CNS: Confusion, lethargy
40%	CV: Frank hypotension; tachycardia may progress to bradycardia Skin: Pale, cold Renal: No urine output CNS: Comatose

From Rasmussen GE, Grandes CM: Blood, fluids, and electrolytes in the pediatric trauma patient, *Int Anesthesiol Clin* 32:79-101, 1994.
CV, Cardiovascular; *CNS,* central nervous system.

reassessed. A second bolus of 20 mL/kg is administered if there is no significant response or only a transient improvement in these parameters. A third crystalloid bolus may be given if necessary to maintain appropriate vital signs and circulation. Blood (10 mL/kg) should be administered next if additional fluid resuscitation is required. The need for blood transfusion initially is uncommon and usually signals surgical bleeding that may require an operation.

If shock persists and fails to respond to fluid therapy, other causes should be sought. Such causes may include long bone or pelvic fractures. Pericardial effusion and tamponade are less common occurrences in blunt trauma compared with penetrating injuries. The classic clinical signs of cardiac tamponade are shock, muffled heart sounds, pulses paradoxus, electrical alternans, and distended neck veins. Treatment requires immediate pericardiocentesis.

Pneumothorax is a common complication of blunt chest injury in children, with nearly one fourth of pneumothoraces under tension (Nakayama et al., 1992). Unilateral or bilateral tension pneumothoraces may produce hypotension and hypoxemia. The classic signs of tension pneumothorax are ipsilateral tympany, shift of the trachea to the contralateral side, and distended neck veins.

Significant occult blood loss may be overlooked on the initial examination of the small child and infant. Because the absolute blood volume of a child is small, the significance of external blood loss may be underestimated. In addition, blood accumulation in the infant's large, expandable head and open fontanels can produce shock. Careful assessment of the abdomen is also central in the evaluation of the injured patient in shock.

Adequate large-bore IV access must be established as early as possible in the course of the resuscitation. Although peripheral routes offer the most rapidly accessible sites, such access may be difficult or impossible to obtain in the child with depleted intravascular volume or shock and resultant peripheral vasoconstriction. In such cases, a central venous catheter may be placed in the femoral or neck vessels if personnel with the necessary skills are available. Delays in establishing vascular access may be lifethreatening; therefore, if the above routes fail,

intraosseous (IO) access should be rapidly initiated to expedite the administration of volume expanders and necessary pharmacologic agents. Once the child has been resuscitated, additional vascular access should be obtained.

IO access is placed in the medial surface of the proximal tibia 1 to 3 cm below the tibial tuberosity or the distal femoral metaphysis. IO has been used as a lifesaving measure to establish short-term vascular access in critically ill or injured children (Fig. 30-6).

The use of IO infusions in the algorithm of trauma and cardiopulmonary resuscitation has evolved over the years and now takes a more prominent role for providing vascular access to children. The subject of IO has been reviewed by Tobias and Ross (2010).

Access needles for IOs include manual devices such as butterfly needles, spinal needles, bone marrow biopsy needle such as Susfast (Cook Critical Care; Bloomington, Indiana) and the basic Jamshidi needle (Baxter Healthcare Corporation; Deerfield, Illinois). More recently, automated devices have been marketed (Fig. 30-7). The EZ-IO (Vidacare; San Antonio, Texas) functions like a battery-powered drill, with a beveled drill and a preset depth. It is designed to be used in the tibia. The Bone Injection Gun (BIG; Waismed; Kansas City, Missouri) is a spring-locked device also designed to be used in the tibia. It comes in a range of sizes for use in infants, small children, and adults. A device specifically designed for entry into the bone marrow of the sternum is the FAST1 (First Access for Shock and Trauma, PYN6 Medical Corporation; Vancouver, British Columbia). It is approved for patients ages 12 and older. Table 30-6 summarizes these devices. Details regarding instructions on the use of these devices can be viewed on the manufacturers' websites.

A review of the use of IO access in pediatric trauma patients up to 10 years of age reported successful placement of access in 28 out of 32 attempts in the prehospital setting and in the trauma care center (Guy et al., 1993). In this study, IO access was placed successfully by paramedics, nurses, and physicians with only one incident of minor extravasation of fluid and no long-term complications in the survivors. The commonest complication of IO access is subperiosteal infiltration that in most cases resolves spontaneously without further problems. The most feared complication—osteomyelitis—occurs in 0.6% cases (Rosetti et al., 1985). Other rare complications include fractures and emboli. Although few complications have been

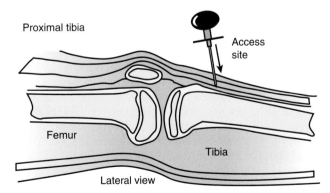

■ **FIGURE 30-6.** Appropriate placement of the IO infusion needle on the medial surface, distal to tibial tuberosity. *(From Ellemunter H: Intraosseous lines in preterm and full-term neonates,* Arch Dis Child Fetal Neonatal Ed *80:74F, 1999.)*

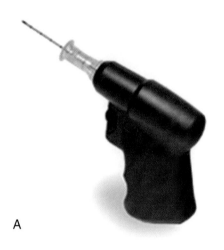
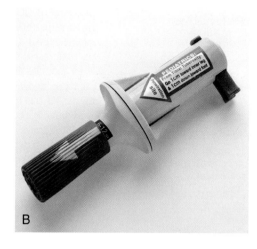

■ **FIGURE 30-7.** Automated devices.
A, EZ-IO. **B**, Bone Injection Gun.
(**A**, *Courtesy Vidacare, San Antonio, TX;*
B, *Courtesy Waismed, Kansas City, Mo.*)

TABLE 30-6. Comparison of Intraosseous Devices

Device	Summary of Features	Recommended Ages for Use	Sizes Available
Butterfly needles	Simple needle design	All ages	Variety of lengths and gauges
Spinal needles	Straight needle with stylet	All ages	Variety of lengths and gauges
Bone marrow biopsy needles	Hand-held hollow needle with stylet and handle	All ages	16- and 18-gauge needles; varying lengths
EZ-IO	Lithium-powered drill leaving metal catheter in place	All ages down to 3 kg	15-gauge needles; length 25 mm (>40 kg) and 15 mm (<40 kg)
Bone injection gun (BIG)	Spring-loaded device using "position and press" action	All ages	15-gauge needles (≤12 years), 18-gauge needles (>12 years); varying lengths
FAST1	Sternal needle device that inserts plastic catheter	No pediatric device at present	

From Tobias JD; Ross AK: Intraosseous infusions: a review for the anesthesiologist with a focus on pediatric use, *Anesth Analg* 110:391–401, 2010.

reported with this technique, it must be recognized that the high mortality in patients who require IO access prevents the assessment of long-term complications.

Disability (Neurologic Assessment)

A brief rapid neurologic evaluation is performed as part of the primary survey. It should include assessment of the patient's level of consciousness and pupillary function. The AVPU method or the more detailed GCS should be performed. If AVPU is selected, the GCS calculation is performed during the secondary survey with a detailed neurologic examination. Periodic reassessment of the level of consciousness is necessary to detect neurologic deterioration caused by progression of traumatic brain injury (TBI), hypoxemia, or hypovolemia. Changes in mental status require prompt reevaluation of the ABCs. If they are adequately managed, then deterioration in mental status should be considered to be a result of TBI, prompting further brain imaging and consultation with a neurosurgeon.

Exposure

Exposure involves removing the trauma patient's garments, usually with shears, to allow detailed physical examination and detect injuries. Rolling the patient, while maintaining

cervical spine precautions, is necessary to identify injuries to the dorsal surface of the body that would otherwise be occult. Padding should be placed on the backboard at this time to prevent decubitus ulcer formation. This assessment should be rapid, and the patient should be covered in warmed blankets or with a warming device to prevent hypothermia. In addition, IV fluids should be warmed, and the room temperature should be raised. This is especially important in small children, who are more prone to hypothermia because of their larger surface area-to-volume ratio.

Secondary Survey

Diagnostic Evaluation

The diagnostic evaluation of the injured child involves clinical examination supplemented by radiologic examinations and laboratory testing. Imaging plays a major role in the evaluation of the injured child (Vane, 2002). Improvements in imaging techniques have allowed progress in the nonoperative management of abdominal and thoracic trauma, supplanting exploratory laparotomy and diagnostic peritoneal lavage in many hemodynamically stable patients.

Initial plain-film screening examinations in children with mechanisms that may cause significant injuries are generally limited to a chest x-ray, pelvis x-ray, and lateral cervical spine films obtained in the emergency department trauma bay. Further plain films are directed by physical findings (e.g., extremity deformity or spine tenderness). Spine films are obtained when spine tenderness, deformity, neurologic deficits, or inadequate examination with significant mechanisms prevent clinical spine clearance.

Computed tomography (CT) is widely used in the evaluation of pediatric trauma. CT scans of the head are routinely obtained in children with a history of loss of consciousness, altered mental status, and focal neurologic deficits. CT scans of the neck are obtained to supplement cervical plain-film studies or when a cervical-spine injury may exist on clinical grounds. Whenever cervical-spine injuries may exist based on clinical grounds or the mechanism of injury, cervical-spine precautions should be maintained. Cervical-spine clearance in the patient with brain injury may not be possible until the patient's mental status has improved.

The most common cause of a distended abdomen in a child is swallowed air (see Fig. 30-2). Distention can be massive and can appear as if the child has an acute abdomen condition. Placement of a nasogastric tube is imperative. Often that alone improves both abdominal and respiratory status. Abdominal distention or tenderness despite nasogastric-tube decompression suggests a possible solid-organ or hollow-viscus injury. Hemodynamic instability with abdominal tenderness or distension mandates immediate surgical consultation and or operation. Ultrasound is increasingly being used in the emergent assessment of injured patients. Focused Assessment by Sonography in Trauma (FAST) is used to detect intraabdominal blood; however, the clinical significance in children of this finding and the management are unclear. FAST has largely replaced the diagnostic peritoneal lavage that has no role in the diagnosis of pediatric abdominal injury. CT scanning of the abdomen is still the most effective method to diagnosis solid-organ injuries and intraabdominal blood. FAST may not add much to the care, because most stable patients with or without blood loss are managed conservatively (Thourani et al., 1998; Miller et al., 2003; Soundappan et al., 2005). Unstable patients may require surgical intervention.

Pelvic fractures are assessed clinically by pressing on both anterior superior iliac spines at the same time to see if the wings spread apart and with the pelvic radiograph. Pelvic fractures can be a significant source of bleeding, although most bleeding can be controlled with fixation and interventional radiology. The presence of a pelvic fracture with blood at the tip of the meatus or a high-riding mobile prostate is a contraindication to placing a Foley catheter. An urethrogram should be performed before placement of a catheter. In rare situations a suprapubic catheter is needed. The pediatric bladder is more susceptible to injury, because it rides higher and there is a shallow pelvis. A pelvic fracture increases the risk of a bladder injury.

Because most injured children are generally healthy and take few or no medications, laboratory screening examinations are limited and focused. Children with minor injuries (e.g., upper extremity fractures) may require limited or no laboratory testing. In more significantly injured patients, laboratory testing may generally be safely limited to specific clinical indications rather than a generalized routine trauma panel (Chu et al., 1996). A complete blood count, blood gas, blood type and screen, and urinalysis are suggested for initial testing in significantly injured patients. Routine testing of liver functions, pancreatic enzymes and coagulation parameters is of limited value and should only be obtained when clinically indicated.

ANESTHETIC PERIOPERATIVE MANAGEMENT

Children with multiple injuries often arrive with an unusual combination of anesthetic problems that present a challenge to the anesthesiologist. It must be emphasized that the likelihood of a successful outcome is greatly enhanced by the initial stabilization efforts that must include early initiation of critical-care management in the emergency department based on appropriate and rapid physical examination and diagnostic studies rather than an urgent rush to the operating room for emergency surgical interventions (Meyer, 1999). Respiratory stabilization and suitable hemodynamic support, including volume resuscitation can prevent further decompensation as well as the development of secondary injuries. This in turn requires a well-coordinated effort by all members of the health care team including the anesthesiologist, the emergency department physician, surgeons of the relevant specialties, respiratory therapists, and critical-care nurses. Only in rare instances is there little time for initial stabilization and a child must undergo emergency surgery to ensure a favorable outcome. In such cases there must be clear communication between the anesthesiologist and surgeon regarding the time available for resuscitation, securing vascular access, and placement of invasive monitoring catheters, keeping in mind the need for immediate surgical intervention.

Ideally, the role of anesthesiologists in the care of the child who has sustained significant trauma should begin with securing the airway in the emergency department when necessary. However, failing this, it is imperative that they become familiar with the immediate resuscitative efforts, the extent and nature of the injuries, and details regarding the use of analgesics, sedatives, and neuromuscular blocking agents so that the intensive care may be continued throughout the perioperative period. This section addresses the anesthetic management of the child who comes for emergency surgery after multiple traumatic injuries.

Fasting Duration

It is common practice to consider all trauma patients at risk for aspiration regardless of the time of last oral intake. The rationale for this approach is that major injury, the presence of pain and anxiety, and the administration of opioid analgesics delay gastric emptying. Additionally, bag-and-mask ventilation at the scene of the accident or in the emergency department that leads to gastric distention and the use of oral contrast solutions for diagnostic imaging studies may further increase the risk for aspiration. Indeed, previous investigators have demonstrated that patients who come for emergency surgery are at five times the risk for aspiration compared with those who undergo elective surgery (Olsson et al., 1986). Other investigators reported a 17% incidence of vomiting and 3% incidence of aspiration in 60 children younger than 19 years of age who required emergency ETI after they sustained a severe traumatic injury (Nakayama et al., 1992). Interestingly, residual gastric volume has been previously found to have a greater correlation with the interval from oral intake to injury than with actual fasting interval (Bricker et al., 1989).

These data raise two questions regarding the management of anesthetic induction for the trauma patient: whether it is possible to predict the safe interval between oral intake, injury, and induction of anesthesia, whether imposing a fasting duration once the trauma has already occurred offers any benefit in terms of reduction in aspiration risk. Goodwin and Robinson (2000) surveyed 167 practicing anesthesiologists in the United Kingdom regarding their practice in three different scenarios after a forearm fracture in a child. Approximately one third of the respondents did not believe there was any benefit in delaying the procedure and would perform a RSI and ETI regardless of the fasting duration, whereas almost two thirds of the respondents would delay the procedure if it was not emergent and then use a LMA or face mask as they would for elective cases. Such variability in clinical practice related to the management of the trauma patient is likely because of the difficulty in predicting a safe interval between oral intake, injury, and induction of anesthesia with regard to aspiration risk. A conservative and practical approach would be to proceed with surgery when an operating room becomes available and do a RSI and intubation if airway difficulty is not anticipated.

Induction of Anesthesia

Anesthetic induction techniques should be individualized according to the nature of the injuries, whether the airway has been secured before arrival in the operating suite, anticipated airway difficulty, hemodynamic status of the patient, and the presence of ongoing hemorrhage. The child with head trauma merits special consideration because of the risk of increased ICP during induction of anesthesia. Selection of an induction technique in these patients must be made with the goal of avoiding secondary brain injury. IV-induction agents such as thiopental, propofol, or etomidate may be preferred because of their beneficial effects on ICP and cerebral oxygen consumption (CMR_{O_2}). On the other hand, a child with an anticipated difficult airway may be better managed with an inhaled route of induction so that spontaneous respiration is assured. Induction of anesthesia in a patient with dehydration or hypovolemia may lead to cardiovascular collapse. It is therefore imperative to have adequate IV access and rehydrate these patients before induction of anesthesia. A brief description of commonly used induction agents and pitfalls with the use of each in a child with trauma follows. Additional details about anesthetic agents are described in Chapters 7 and 22, Pharmacology of Pediatric Anesthesia and Anesthesia for Neurosurgery.

Thiopental

The barbiturates have a long history of use as neuroprotectants. Thiopental has been extensively used as an induction agent in patients with head-injuries, because it is a cerebral vasoconstrictor and decreases cerebral blood flow (CBF), CMR_{O_2}, and ICP in a dose-dependent manner. Another beneficial CNS effect is reduction in epileptiform activity. Furthermore, thiopental reliably attenuates the increase in ICP caused by noxious interventions, such as direct laryngoscopy and ETT placement. However, thiopental should be used with caution in a child with multiple traumatic injuries, because it is a direct myocardial depressant and may produce a decrease in cardiac output and systemic blood pressure, with a resultant decrease

in cerebral perfusion pressure (CPP). These effects are more pronounced in patients who have been inadequately volume resuscitated, and the use of alternative induction agents such as etomidate should be strongly considered in patients with a questionable volume status or with uncontrolled, ongoing hemorrhage.

Propofol

Induction of anesthesia with propofol in healthy children is commonly associated with a significant (10% to 20%) decrease in mean arterial pressure (MAP) because of its direct relaxant effects on vascular smooth muscle that cause a reduction in systemic vascular resistance and preload (Aun et al., 1993). It should, therefore, be used with caution, if at all, in patients with depleted intravascular volume. Its beneficial effects of cerebral vasoconstriction, reduced CBF, and CMR_{O_2} in patients with head trauma are offset to an extent by a reduction in CPP because of a decrease in systemic blood pressure. It has been further hypothesized that the decrease in CPP may lead to reflex cerebral vasodilation to maintain CBF, thereby also negating its beneficial effects in reducing ICP (Spitzfaden et al., 1999).

The literature evaluating the use of propofol in adult neurosurgery patients has yielded conflicting results. Previous studies have demonstrated that whereas propofol effectively lowered ICP in patients with elevated ICP after TBI and during cerebral aneurysm surgery, there was a significant reduction in overall CPP because of a greater decrease in MAP than ICP (Herregods et al., 1988; Ravussin et al., 1988; Pinaud et al., 1990). Other investigators reported no reduction in ICP with propofol sedation in adults with head trauma (Stewart et al., 1994).

Etomidate

Etomidate provides both hemodynamic stability as well as cerebral protection, making it the ideal anesthetic induction agent for emergency surgery in a child with multiple traumatic injuries. Although it does cause a direct myocardial depressant effect, it does so to a significantly lesser extent than equipotent doses of other induction agents, including thiopental, propofol, and ketamine (Stowe et al., 1992). Etomidate, however, maintains sympathetic outflow and produces no significant changes in blood pressure, making it the agent of choice in the hemodynamically unstable patient. Similar to thiopental and propofol, it is a cerebral vasoconstrictor and causes a reduction in ICP, CBF, and CMR_{O_2}. However, because MAP is maintained with etomidate, CPP is also maintained. Perhaps the only concern with its use has been adrenal suppression; however, this is believed to have questionable clinical significance with brief use (Crozier et al., 1987). A recent retrospective review reported successful fracture reduction in 52 of 53 patients who received etomidate alone or in combination with midazolam or opioids (Dickinson et al., 2001). This study found a low incidence of minor side effects, including nausea and vomiting, mild hypotension, and prolonged sedation in one patient each.

Ketamine

Ketamine is a dissociative anesthetic that is commonly selected for induction in children who are hypovolemic, because its sympathomimetic actions result in increases in blood pressure and heart rate. However, like the other induction agents described above, ketamine has direct myocardial depressant effects as well as direct vasodilatory effects. In fact, significant hypotension has been reported after ketamine administration in critically ill patients, likely as a result of its direct myocardial depressant effects predominating in the presence of depleted catecholamine stores (Waxman et al., 1980).

Ketamine, however, is a potent cerebral vasodilator and causes a marked increase in CBF. Although $CMRo_2$ usually remains unchanged after ketamine administration, ICP may increase, especially in patients with intracranial pathologic conditions. However, data regarding the effects of ketamine on ICP remain inconclusive, with some studies demonstrating modest decreases in ICP after ketamine administration, particularly when they are administered concomitantly with other sedatives (Mayberg et al., 1995; Albanese et al., 1997). A recent controlled, randomized, double-blind trial found no differences in mean daily values of ICP, CPP, and the number of episodes of ICP elevations in patients with severe TBI who were sedated with ketamine and midazolam compared with those who were sedated with sufentanil and midazolam (Bourgoin et al., 2003). Yet, its cerebral vasodilatory effects preclude the use of ketamine as an induction agent in patients with head trauma.

Maintenance of Anesthesia

Selection of agents for maintenance of anesthesia should be based on the nature and duration of the proposed procedure; the extent of injuries; the child's ventilatory, hemodynamic, and neurologic status; and whether postoperative mechanical ventilation is anticipated. In hemodynamically stable patients, a standard general anesthetic may be used, including volatile agents, opioids for postoperative pain relief, and muscle relaxants as needed to provide good operating conditions. On the other hand, a technique using an opioid, a hypnotic, muscle relaxant, and oxygen may be more suitable in a child with unacceptably low blood pressure and who may not tolerate the negative inotropic effects of potent volatile anesthetics. In such cases, fentanyl or sufentanil are the preferred opioids, because they do not significantly alter hemodynamic parameters especially blood pressure. In children whose injuries are not completely determined, nitrous oxide is best avoided because it may diffuse into closed air spaces such as the pleural cavity.

In a child with severe head trauma, efforts must be directed at preventing secondary brain injury and protecting the injured brain from further ischemic injury by selecting anesthetic techniques that maintain blood pressure while reducing ICP. All volatile anesthetics cause cerebral vasodilation, which has been correlated with increasing minimum alveolar concentration (MAC) in children (Vavilala and Lam, 2002). Isoflurane affects CBF and cerebral autoregulation to a lesser extent than halothane. Sevoflurane offers greater advantages in that CBF velocities do not increase significantly with less than 1 MAC, and cerebral pressure autoregulation is maintained up to 1.5 MAC sevoflurane (Gupta et al., 1997; Monkhoff et al., 2001). For these reasons, sevoflurane may be the preferred volatile anesthetic for the child with TBI, and it would be prudent to limit its use to 1 MAC.

Opioids (fentanyl, sufentanil, or remifentanil) are often administered as intermittent bolus doses or infusions to supplement volatile anesthetics, for postoperative analgesia, and

as additional measures to lower ICP. However, increased ICP has been reported in an 11-year-old child with closed head injury after bolus doses of fentanyl that responded to hyperventilation and barbiturates (Tobias, 1994). In addition, recent studies in adults have reported a transient but significant increase in ICP accompanied by a decrease in MAP and CPP after bolus doses of morphine, fentanyl, sufentanil, and alfentanil (Albanese et al., 1999; de Nadal et al., 2000). The exact mechanism of these changes remains unknown; however, impaired cerebrovascular autoregulation and direct cerebral vasodilatory effects of opioids have been implicated. Such effects may have significant implications in the management of the child with traumatic head injuries; however, until additional data become available, the judicious use of opioid infusions with careful monitoring of hemodynamic parameters is recommended.

Monitoring

In addition to routine monitors, placement of invasive monitors, including arterial and central venous catheters and a urinary catheter must be placed in the child with extensive injuries and in children with head trauma. Placement of monitoring catheters should be efficient, and in some cases when the surgery must be performed expeditiously, invasive catheters may need to be placed when the procedure is already underway. An arterial catheter is invaluable for continuous blood-pressure monitoring and frequent monitoring of arterial blood gases, acid base status, electrolytes, and serial hematocrits. Central venous pressure monitoring is useful when large fluid shifts are expected and in cases of rapid ongoing blood loss. Urine output is an important measure of fluid status. Additional monitors, such as ICP monitors in cases of head trauma and somatosensory evoked-potential monitors as a measure of spinal-cord function in a child with spinal injury, must be individualized. In some cases of chest trauma, transesophageal echocardiography may be useful in diagnosing injury and guiding surgical repair.

Temperature Maintenance

Temperature maintenance is an important part of trauma resuscitation but one that is often overlooked because of other priorities, such as resuscitation. In the traumatized child, several factors contribute to ongoing heat loss, including exposure to a cold environment at the scene of the accident, large open wounds, rapid infusion of fluids and blood, and exposure of body cavities during operative procedures. Hypothermia has significant deleterious effects that may hinder resuscitative efforts. Such effects include myocardial dysfunction, cardiac irritability, and dysrhythmias. Other effects of hypothermia include acid-base disturbances, a leftward shift of the oxyhemoglobin dissociation curve, and coagulopathies that can exacerbate ongoing hemorrhage. Continuous temperature monitoring in all pediatric trauma patients is therefore essential. Every effort should be made to maintain temperature, including the use of warm IV fluids, keeping the child covered once initial evaluation is completed, maintaining a warm environment, use of radiant warmers for infants, and forced-air warming devices.

Fluid Resuscitation

Shock is defined as a metabolic demand that exceeds either oxygen supply or oxygen delivery (Rasmussen and Grandes, 1994). When a child who has sustained multiple injuries arrives for surgical intervention, the fluid status must be assessed quickly (before induction of anesthesia) based on a physical examination as well as a history of fluid resuscitation received before arrival in the operating suite. The anesthesiologist must be prepared to continue the resuscitation in case of ongoing blood loss or third spacing of fluid. The goals of fluid resuscitation should be to maintain normovolemia as well as the osmolar and oncotic pressures in the intravascular space. Isotonic crystalloid solutions such as lactated Ringer's solution or normal saline are most commonly used in the initial stages of resuscitation. Hypertonic saline solutions have also been used in this setting, based on the premise that they increase serum osmolality and thereby maintain intravascular volume for longer periods and with smaller volumes administered than isotonic solutions (Rasmussen and Grandes, 1994). However, the data that support these arguments are inconclusive and further work in this area is needed. The decision to administer glucose-containing solutions must be based on serial blood-glucose values (Sharma et al., 2009). This is of greatest importance in the presence of head trauma, because elevated blood-glucose levels have been found to correlate significantly with indicators of the severity of brain injury and poor neurologic outcomes in children with severe brain injuries (Michaud et al., 1991).

Colloid solutions such as 5% albumin and hydroxyethyl starch have also been used for fluid resuscitation. Hydroxyethyl starch may exacerbate existing coagulopathy by interfering with platelet function, decreasing fibrinogen activity, and interfering with factor VIII. It is therefore unsuitable for the pediatric trauma patient. The purported benefits of colloid solutions include their ability to increase colloid oncotic pressure and prolonged maintenance of intravascular volume and smaller volumes required compared with crystalloid solutions (Rasmussen and Grandes, 1994). For these reasons, colloids may also be beneficial in children with head trauma because the smaller volume of fluids administered may reduce the likelihood of cerebral edema. One of the major concerns with the use of colloids has been the cost. In most patients who require massive fluid resuscitation, the cost of using colloids to supplement crystalloids may be justified. The Saline vs. Albumin Fluid Evaluation (SAFE) study, a randomized, controlled trial conducted in 16 intensive care units in Australia and New Zealand, concluded that albumin and saline should be considered clinically equivalent treatments for volume resuscitation in intensive care patients (Finfer et al., 2004). Further discussion of crystalloid and colloid use in pediatrics has been reviewed by Bailey et al. (2010).

Blood Product Transfusion

The primary purposes for transfusion of blood products in a pediatric trauma patient are to maintain oxygen delivery and to ensure hemostasis (see Chapter 36, Systemic Disorders). Packed red blood cells are required when oxygen-carrying capacity is inadequate to meet tissue demands and metabolic rate. Losses of up to 40% of blood volume can usually be replaced with isotonic crystalloid solutions or colloids without physiologic signs of inadequate oxygen delivery (Solheim and Wesenberg, 2001). When estimated blood volume losses exceed 40%, the decision to transfuse blood should be based on an overall assessment of the patient, including the hemodynamic status, the extent of ongoing blood loss and the underlying comorbidity. Some children may require blood transfusion with blood-volume losses of less than 40% if the blood loss has been rapid or if they have significant underlying medical conditions such as congenital cyanotic heart disease or blood dyscrasias. Although there can be no fixed numeric transfusion trigger in all trauma patients, Box 30-4 presents formulas that may be used as general guidelines to calculate allowable blood losses (Rasmussen and Grandes, 1994). Blood banks in most centers supply blood components rather than whole blood. The primary advantage of component therapy is more efficient and cost-effective use of resources by eliminating the transfusion of unnecessary components and making components from a single blood donation available to several patients. It also permits improved preservation of individual components (Table 30-7).

Packed Red Blood Cells

The reason to transfuse packed red blood cells (PRBCs) is to increase oxygen carrying capacity. PRBCs are supplied in units of approximately 250 mL with hematocrit values ranging from 60% to 80%. The units are preserved either in citrate, phosphate, and dextrose (CPD) with a shelf life of 21 days or in citrate, phosphate, dextrose, and adenine CPD-A with a shelf life of 35 days. The citrate in the preservative chelates calcium, therefore, calcium chloride must be readily available when transfusing PRBCs especially at a rapid rate. The usual starting dose of PRBCs is 10 to 20 mL/kg, depending on rapidity of blood loss.

Fresh Frozen Plasma

Fresh frozen plasma (FFP) must be separated from whole blood within 6 to 8 hours of collection. It generally takes approximately 45 minutes to thaw, because it is stored at –18° C, and it must be used within 24 hours once it has been thawed. FFP provides factors II, V, VIII, IX, X, XI, and antithrombin III. In general, FFP should be transfused when clotting studies become abnormal with a prolonged prothrombin time (PT) or activated partial thromboplastin time (APTT). Nonsurgical bleeding in

---

Box 30-4 Formulas to Use as a General Guideline to Calculate Allowable Blood Loss

Calculation 1: ABL = EBV × (HCT initial – HCT target) HCT initial*
Calculation 2: ERCM = EBV × HCT starting
  ERCM target = EBV × HCT target
  ARCL = ERCM – ERCM target
  ABL = ARCL × 3

From Rasmussen GE, Grandes CM: Blood, fluids, and electrolytes in the pediatric trauma patient, *Int Anesthesiol Clin* 32:79, 1994.
* The ABL, in milliliters, must be multiplied by 3 if replacement is by crystalloid and replaced, 1:1 if blood is to be used.
ABL, Allowable blood loss; *EBV,* estimated blood volume; *HCT,* hematocrit; *ERCM,* estimated red cell mass; *ARCL,* allowable red cell loss.

TABLE 30-7. Differences in the Compositions of Major Blood Products

	Normal Whole Blood (in vivo)	Citrated Whole Blood (2 Weeks Old) CPD	Citrated Packed Red Blood Cells*	Frozen Packed Red Blood Cells	FFP
pH	7.4	6.6-6.9	6.6-6.9	6.6-7.2	6.6-6.9
P_{CO_2}	35-45	180-210	180-210	0-10	180-210
Base deficit (mmol/L)	0	9-15	9-15	?	9-15
Potassium (mmol/L)	3.5-5.0	18-26	18-26 mmol/L	1-2 mmol/L	4-8
Citrate	None	++++	++	None	++++
Factors V and VIII	Normal	20%-50%	20%-50%	None	85%-100%
Fibrinogen	Normal	Normal	Normal	None	Normal
Platelets	240,000-400,000	None	None	None	None
2, 3-DPG	Normal	3% of normal	3% of normal	Nearly normal	—
Hematocrit	35-45	35-45	60-70	50-95	—
Temperature	37° C	4°-6° C	4°-6° C	4°-6° C	Cold

From Coté CJ et al.: A practice of anesthesia for infants and children, ed 2, New York, 1993, Grune and Stratton; modified from Miller RD: *Refresher courses in anesthesiology* 1:101, 1973.
* Citrated whole blood and citrated packed red blood cells have the same chemical composition, but citrated red blood cells have considerably less plasma volume.
CPD, Citrate-phosphate-dextrose; *FFP,* fresh frozen plasma.

children who receive more than one blood volume of PRBCs often require FFP because of factors V and VIII deficiency. The recommended initial dose of FFP is 10 to 15 mL/kg (see Chapter 36, Systemic Disorders, Table 36-25).

Platelets

Platelets are prepared by centrifugation and recentrifugation of fresh whole blood. Dilutional thrombocytopenia is the most likely cause of nonsurgical or microvascular bleeding after massive blood transfusion, and usually platelets are required before FFP for this condition. To raise the platelet count by approximately 20,000, 0.1 units/kg of platelets are needed. Because platelet counts of 50,000 are adequate to achieve surgical hemostasis, doses in excess of 0.2 units/kg are rarely required (see Chapter 36, Systemic Disorders, Table 36-25).

Cryoprecipitate

Cryoprecipitate that is produced by refreezing the insoluble portion of plasma is rich in factor VIII and fibrinogen. The residual component from 1 unit of FFP yields 100 units of cryoprecipitate. The primary indications for cryoprecipitate in the trauma patient are bleeding abnormalities after massive transfusion, disseminated intravascular coagulation (DIC), and decreased fibrinogen levels. The recommended initial dose of cryoprecipitate is 0.1 units/kg (see Chapter 36, Systemic Disorders, Table 36-25).

Massive Blood Replacement

Massive blood replacement is defined as the administration of one blood volume or more within 24 hours. It causes a number of physiologic derangements that can be detrimental in the child with multiple injuries, including coagulation defects, electrolyte and acid-base abnormalities, and hypo-

thermia (see Chapter 36, Systemic Disorders). Dilutional thrombocytopenia and clotting factor deficiencies have been primarily implicated in the etiology of nonsurgical bleeding after massive blood transfusion. However, mathematical models have demonstrated that a third of the patient's own blood remains after a single blood volume exchange, thereby retaining sufficient platelets and clotting factors to permit hemostasis (Marsaglia and Thomas, 1971). Therefore, other factors, such as incompatibility of transfused blood and DIC, have also been implicated in the etiology of nonsurgical bleeding in the trauma patient.

The ratio of fresh frozen plasma to PRBCs may be an important determinant of outcome in trauma patients who receive massive transfusions. Sperry and others (2008) demonstrated in adults that during massive transfusions, an FFP/PRBC ratio of greater than or equal to 1:1.5 decreased the number of transfusions and one-day mortality more than did an FFP/PRBC ratio of less than 1:1.5. This means that those patients who received close-to-equal volumes of FFP and PRBCs had decreased 24-hour mortality rates over those who received significantly more PRBCs than FFP, although patients receiving larger quantities of FFP had a higher incidence of ARDS. The likely explanation for the reduction in mortality is the early correction of coagulopathy and reduction in hemorrhage.

Monitoring the coagulation status is vital in patients who require massive transfusions. Hypothermia, acidosis, and hemodilution with hypofibrinogenemia further exacerbate any coagulopathy. Massive transfusions decrease fibrinogen, decrease platelets, and dilute coagulation factors. Intraoperative evaluation of the bleeding patient can be assessed by classic tests (PT, PTT, and platelet count). However, the coagulation system, including clot formation and clot dissolution, can also be assessed by thromboelastography. Thromboelastography is a global measure of hemostasis and is further described in Chapter 36, Systemic Disorders.

Factor VIIA

Recombinant Factor VIIA (rFVIIA) is currently approved by the FDA for treatment and prevention of bleeding disorders in patients with hemophilia A or B who have developed inhibitors to factor VIII or factor IX, respectively (Novo Nordisk, 2005). However, rFVIIa is increasingly being used as an off-label drug for patients, both children and adults, when conventional therapies have failed to control bleeding after trauma. A retrospective case series published in *Pediatrics* in 2009 concluded that administration of rFVIIa to bleeding surgical trauma patients is associated with a significant decrease in blood-product administration, with low associated mortality and adverse events (Alten et al., 2009).

SPECIFIC INJURIES

Head Injuries

TBI is the leading cause of morbidity and mortality resulting from trauma in children (Langlois et al., 2006). A TBI is caused by a blow or jolt to the head or a penetrating head injury that disrupts the normal function of the brain. Severe TBI often includes an extended period of unconsciousness or amnesia after the injury and is associated with the poorest outcomes (Adelson et al., 2006). Among children ages 0 to 19 years, TBI results in an estimated 7441 deaths, 62,000 hospitalizations, and 564,000 emergency-department visits annually (CDC, 1999). The leading causes of TBI in children are falls (39%) and motor-vehicle crashes (11%) (Fig. 30-8) (National Center for Injury Control and Prevention, 2005).

Most preventable deaths and deficits after pediatric head injury are secondary to subsequent complications, including diffuse brain swelling and resultant elevated ICP, which are independent predictors of mortality (Jurkovich et al., 2004). Poor CPP, often related to elevated ICP and trauma related systemic hypotension, are also known to worsen outcome. See related video online at www.expertconsult.com.

Problems that result from TBI, such as diminished cognition and memory loss, are often not visible (Langlois et al., 2006). TBI can cause a wide range of functional changes that affect thinking, sensation, language, and emotion (CDC, 2003). TBI can also cause epilepsy and increase the risk for conditions that become more prevalent with age, such as Alzheimer's or Parkinson's disease (CDC, 2003). The impact of a TBI not only affects the child but the whole family. The two age groups at highest risk for TBI are children between the ages of 0 and 4 years and those between 15 and 19 years old. Males are 1.5 times more likely to sustain a TBI, and African Americans have the highest death rate from TBI. The outcomes and the treatment of children with a severe TBI remain a great challenge. The CDC estimates that at least 5.3 million Americans, approximately 2% of the U.S. population, currently have a long-term or lifelong requirement for assistance with daily living activities as a result of a TBI (Langlois et al., 2006). Each year, 56,000 children are discharged home with a permanent disability from a TBI, whereas another 5000 require intensive inpatient rehabilitation facilities. The economic burden of head injury to patients is substantial—estimated to be $56.3 billion, with the highest rate of injuries reported among the lower socioeconomic classes. TBI is the most common reason a child requires intensive care or develops a significant life-long disability.

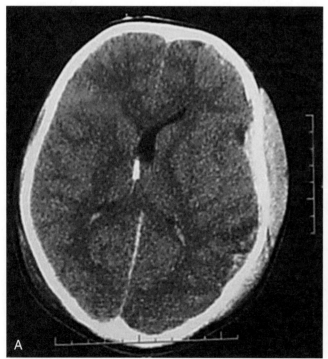

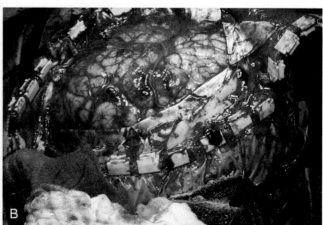

■ **FIGURE 30-8. A,** CT scan of the head a 15-year-old girl who fell off a motor vehicle while "car surfing." Note the skull fracture, epidural hematoma, and the midline shift of the brain before surgery. **B,** Same patient during craniotomy after drainage of her epidural hematoma; she was noted to have cerebral contusions in the area of her injury.

There are important differences between a TBI in a child compared with a TBI in an adult (Luerssen, 2006). Because of the smaller body mass of children, the energy received from an injury (e.g.,. fall) results in a greater force applied per unit body area and to a body with less fat and less connective tissue that might absorb or diminish the energy. The brain of a child is also anatomically different from that of an adult; the subarachnoid space is smaller and offers less protection because there is less buoyancy. Thus, head momentum is more likely to impart parenchymal structural damage. Additionally, the brain is proportionately larger to the rest of the body and therefore a bigger target for injury. Children are particularly susceptible to the effects of secondary brain injury that may be produced by hypovolemia with reduced cerebral profusion, hypoxia, seizures, or hyperthermia. Alternatively, the young child with open fontanels and mobile cranial suture lines is more tolerant of an expanding intracranial mass lesion. Overall, children with a TBI have better outcomes than adults with a TBI.

Monitoring of ICP and CBF are essential in the head injured patient. ICP can be measured with intraventricular catheters, subarachnoid bolts, and epidural sensors. CBF can be assessed by Doppler, and brain metabolic demands can be evaluated with the use of internal jugular bulb catheters and near-infrared measurements of mixed venous oxygen saturation $S\bar{v}o_2$ (see Chapter 22, Anesthesia for Neurosurgery). In general, efforts are made to insure adequate venous drainage (30-degree, head-up position), adequate oxygenation, avoidance of hypotension, and maintenance of slight hypocarbia (partial pressure of CO_2 [$Paco_2$] of 35 to 38).

At present, there is insufficient evidence-based medicine to provide standards of care in children with head injuries. However, a number of interventions have become mainstay as guidelines for treatment of the pediatric patient with head injuries. Most of these guidelines emanate from data in adults (Krantz, 1996; Gupta et al., 1997). An algorithm for the treatment of intracranial hypertension in children is shown in Figure 30-9.

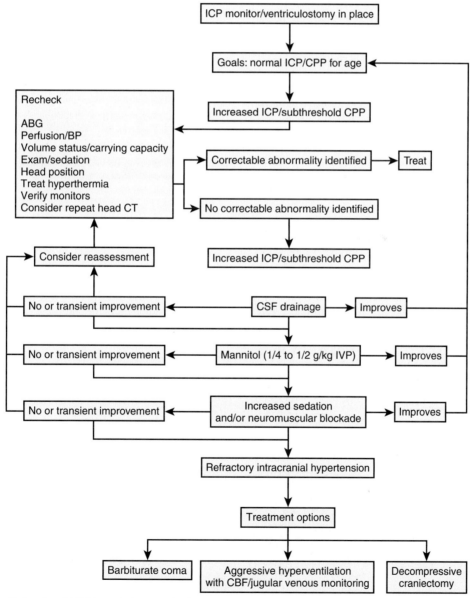

■ **FIGURE 30-9.** The University of Michigan C. S. Mott Children's Hospital algorithm for the treatment of intracranial hypertension in children. *(Courtesy C. S. Mott Children's Hospital, Ann Arbor, Mich.)*

Primary and secondary brain injuries are the major variables affecting outcomes. Primary injury describes the immediate disruption of neuronal, axonal, and supportive structures and vascular tissue and is essentially untreatable except by prevention (Luerssen, 2006). If the primary injury is not fatal, it triggers a cascade of intracellular and extracellular biochemical changes that can augment and accelerate the injury. This is known as secondary injury. Secondary injury produces new damage to the tissue at the primary injury site as well as in other areas of the brain (Luerssen, 2006). For example, hypermetabolic responses related to neuronal tissue injury occur that may outstrip local or regional substrate supply. Ischemia is the final pathway that produces brain-tissue damage and poor clinical outcomes; it is caused by hypoxia, hypotension, seizures, hyperglycemia, and hyperthermia. Despite a lack of systematic evidence, there has been a trend toward improved outcomes by aggressively treating ischemia. The key features of such therapy are support of MAP, reduction of ICP to ensure CPP, and surgery for compressive lesions (such as epidural hematoma) (Alberico et al., 1987; Downard et al., 2000). Figure 30-10 depicts changes in MAP, CPP, and ICP with age. In addition to basic interventions of normal-to-slight hypocapnea, adequate perfusion pressure and oxygenation, the use of hyperosmolar therapy and hypothermia to treat increased ICP has been examined. Table 30-8 lists some of the commonly used interventions (excluding hyperosmolar therapy, discussed in the next section) and the strength of supporting data.

Hyperosmolar Therapy

In areas where the blood brain barrier (BBB) is disrupted, the flow of proteins and electrolytes across the membrane is facilitated. Hydrostatic pressure becomes the dominant driving force for fluid movement from the intravascular space to brain tissue (Klatzo, 1967; Harukuni et al., 2002). This leads to brain swelling with an increase in ICP, a decrease in CPP, cerebral hypoxia, and secondary brain injury.

The beneficial effects of osmotherapy on ICP are thought to result from brain shrinkage after the shift of water out of brain parenchyma. This has been confirmed in animal studies

TABLE 30-8. Evidence-Based Medicine for Pediatric Trauma

Condition	Standards	Guidelines	Evidence
BP and O_2	None	Rapid correction of hypotension SBP > than 70 mm Hg + (2 × age in years)	Class II Class III
ICP monitoring	None	None (vs. adult) Options: ICP monitoring appropriate Children with GCS < 9 Children with GCS > 8 (selected)	Class III
CPP	None	Maintain CPP > 40 mm Hg	Class III
Sedation/paralytics	None	None	Class II
CSF fluid drains	None	None	Class III
Hyper-ventilation	None	None Options: avoid prophylactic mild hyperventilation (P_{CO_2} < 35 mm Hg); Consider therapeutic mild hyperventilation (P_{CO_2} = 30-35 mm Hg) for refractory ICP; Consider aggressive therapeutic hyperventilation (P_{CO_2} < 30 mm Hg) for refractory ICP Suggest monitoring for ischemia	Class II

Class I data are based on randomized controlled trials, and class II trials are prospective nonrandomized and retrospective studies based on "clearly reliable data." These are typically observational, cohort, and case-control trials. Class III data, the weakest source of data, are retrospective studies based on clinical series, registry surveys, and expert opinion.

where osmotherapy after brain injury led to shrinkage of normal, but not injured, brain tissue (Wisner et al., 1990; Shackford et al., 1992).

Mannitol and hypertonic saline (3% normal saline) are the two most commonly administered osmotic agents. Mannitol is used in 70% of pediatric intensive care units (two class III studies); however, it has not been subjected to controlled clinical trials vs. placebo or other osmolar agents in children (Wakai et al., 2007). Mannitol lowers cerebral blood volume and ICP by reducing blood viscosity while maintaining CBF. It osmotically dehydrates the brain parenchyma to decrease intracranial volume and pressure, and therapy can be titrated to a serum osmolality of 320 mOsm/L. Although it has been the predominant osmotherapeutic drug for the past four decades, mannitol has several limitations. Hyperosmolality is a common problem, and a serum osmolarity greater than 320 mOsmol/L is associated with adverse renal and CNS effects (Dorman et al., 1990; Roberts et al., 2003). The osmotic diuresis that accompanies mannitol administration may lead to hypotension, especially in hypovolemic patients. Although controversial, accumulation of mannitol in cerebral tissue may lead to a rebound phenomenon and increased ICP. A 2007 Cochrane Database review evaluated mannitol for acute TBI in adults. Only four studies met the eligibility criteria. The review concluded that compared with

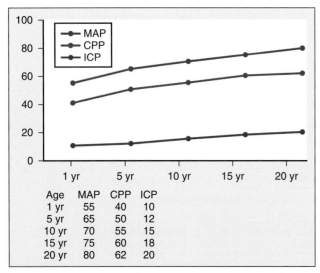

■ **FIGURE 30-10.** Age-related increases in MAP, CPP, and ICP.

Age	MAP	CPP	ICP
1 yr	55	40	10
5 yr	65	50	12
10 yr	70	55	15
15 yr	75	60	18
20 yr	80	62	20

pentobarbital, mannitol may have a beneficial effect on mortality in patients with raised ICP, but mannitol may have a detrimental effect on mortality when compared with hypertonic saline (Wakai et al., 2007).

Hypertonic saline (3% normal saline) has a similar mechanism of action as mannitol with the added theoretic benefits of restoration of normal cellular resting membrane potential and cell volume, stimulation of atrial naturietic peptide release, inhibition of inflammation, and enhancement of cardiac output (Moss and Gould, 1988; McManus and Soriano, 1998; Dickinson et al., 2001). It has also been suggested that it may help patients who are refractory to mannitol infusions. The serum osmolarity may be allowed to rise as high as 360 mOsm/L. Proposed beneficial effects of hypertonic saline in TBI may result because the permeability of the BBB to sodium is low (Betz, 1983). Hypertonic saline produces an osmotic gradient between the intravascular and intracellular/interstitial compartments, leading to shrinkage of brain tissue (where BBB is intact) and therefore a reduction in ICP; the reflection coefficient (selectivity of the BBB to a particular substance) of NaCl is more than that of mannitol, making it potentially a more effective osmotic drug (Fenstermacher and Johnson, 1966). Hypertonic saline also augments volume resuscitation and increases circulating blood volume, MAP, and CPP, and it restores the neuronal membrane potential, maintains the BBB integrity, and modulates of the inflammatory response by reducing adhesion of leukocytes to endothelium (Schmoker et al., 1992; Hartl et al., 2002). The detrimental effects of hypertonic saline include central pontine myelinolysis, coagulopathies, excessive intravascular volume, and electrolyte abnormalities. Electrolyte abnormalities are common. Careful monitoring is required, because hyperkalemia and natriuresis may develop after intravascular administration. Hypertonic saline also tends to reduce the plasma strong-ion difference, and a nonanion-gap metabolic acidosis may result (Bruegger et al., 2005). A number of studies suggest that hypertonic saline may be more effective than mannitol in reducing ICP and have a longer duration of action (Berger et al., 1994; Mirski et al., 2000). Whether this leads to improved outcomes is not known. Clinical studies in children using 3% normal saline are limited (Berger et al., 2004; Vialet et al., 2003).

Cervical Spine Injuries

Cervical spine injuries remain one of the most devastating consequences of trauma. The incidence of cervical spine injury in pediatric trauma patients is low (1% to 2%), but the morbidity and mortality of these injuries are substantial. Kokoska et al. (2001), in a 5-year review from the National Pediatric Trauma Registry, reported a 1.6% incidence (408 out of 24,740, 17% mortality) of blunt cervical spine injuries. Injury patterns were different by age with children less than 10 years of age having a higher incidence of C1-C4 injuries vs. C5-C7 injuries (85% vs. 57%; p < .01) (Kokoska et al., 2001). Brown et al. (2001) reviewed the experience of 103 pediatric cervical spine injury patients over 9 years and found an 18% mortality rate. Subluxation of cervical vertebrae and odontoid fractures are more common in children (Fig. 30-11). See related video online at www.expertconsult.com. Distinguishing between a true subluxation and a pseudosubluxation in a young child can be challenging (Table 30-9). In 40% of children younger than 7 years of age, pseudosubluxation-anterior displacement of C2 on C3 less than 3 mm is a normal variant. Pseudosubluxation becomes more prominent when a child is supine (i.e., on a backboard). Another normal variant is an increased distance between the dens and the anterior arch of C1 found in 20% of children (Bohn et al., 1990). The combination of a child's proportionately large head, elastic interspinous ligaments, and horizontal position of the vertebrae is thought to explain both the pattern of injury and the normal variations (Bohn et al., 1990).

Current issues that relate to pediatric cervical spine issues include identifying who needs to be imaged, how that imaging should be performed, and what combination of imaging and clinical examination constitutes a "cleared" cervical spine.

One method to reduce excess and unnecessary imaging is to use Clinical Decision Rules (CDRs). CDRs are developed to reduce the uncertainty of medical decision-making by standardizing the collection and interpretation of clinical data (Laupacis et al., 1997; Stiell and Wells, 1999; McGinn et al., 2000).

The National Emergency X-Radiography Utilization Low Risk Criteria (NLC) and the Canadian C-spine Rule (CCR) are two clinical decision rules developed to assist with cervical spine imaging after a trauma. Their goals are twofold: to identify patients at risk for a cervical spine injury and to reduce unnecessary imaging. The NLC criteria were developed and then validated in a mixed population of adults and children; however, only 9% of the patients were considered pediatric.

Studies have shown that although CCR and NLC criteria may reduce the need for cervical spine imaging in children 10 years old and younger, the criteria are not sensitive or specific enough to be used as currently designed (Viccellio et al., 2001; Stiell et al., 2003; Ehrlich et al., 2009). Neither clinical decision rule is performed at a high enough level to be used with confidence.

A second issue pertaining to cervical spine clearance revolves around determining which imaging modality to use to assess the cervical spine. Physical examination in alert patients has been proven to be reliable; however, controversy remains as to which imaging studies to perform on pediatric CSI patients when the patient has altered mental status or is intubated (Marion et al., 2008). Most data for the diagnosis of cervical spine injures have been derived from the adult literature. Griffen et al. described a retrospective study of 3,018 blunt trauma patients of whom 1199 (40%) were at risk for CSI (Griffen et al., 2003). Plain radiographs (3 views) and a CT cervical spine were performed. Of 116 patients with spinal injuries, there were 41 patients whose injuries were missed by plain films, but diagnosed by CT scan. More significantly, all of the 41 patients with missed injuries required treatment. A prospective study from Schenarts et al. (2001) compared the use of cervical-spine CT for the upper cervical spine (C_1-C_3) to plain films for adult trauma patients with altered mental status. Plain films identified only 54% of the injuries to the upper cervical spine in their series, compared with 96% diagnosed with CT scan. In contrast to the previous study, a different study found that three injuries seen on plain films were missed on CT, including one atlantooccipital dislocation in a patient with quadriplegia and two subluxations (Schmoker et al., 1992).

Rana et al. (2009) recently examined their experience with cervical-spine imaging using either CT or conventional films in cervical-spine clearance with intubated children. Plain

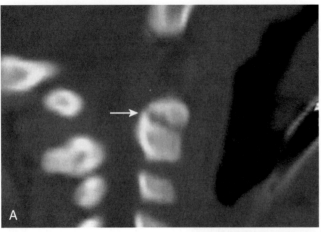
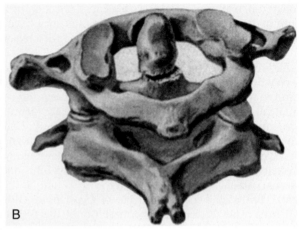
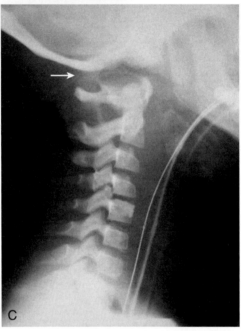

■ **FIGURE 30-11. A,** MRI of a 22-month-old boy who fell off of a grocery cart onto his head. *Arrow* points to a nondisplaced fracture of the odontoid process in C2. **B,** Posterior view of C2 odontoid (dens) fracture. **C,** Lateral cervical spine radiograph of a 9-year-old involved in an automobile accident. *Arrow* points to an occipitoatloid (C1) dislocation. The patient died. (*B, From Netter F, editor:* The Ciba collection of medical illustrations, vol 1: nervous system, *Summit, NJ, 1953.*)

TABLE 30-9. Upper Normal Limits of Cervical Spine Measurements in Adults and Children

	Adults	**Children**
Predental space	2.5 mm	4 to 5 mm
C2-3 override (flexion)	3 mm	4 to 5 mm
Prevertebral space	7 mm	½ to ⅔ AP distance (extension) vertebral body

From Eichelberger MR: *Pediatric trauma prevention, acute care, rehabilitation,* St. Louis, 1993, Mosby.

radiographs missed injuries and had a significantly lower sensitivity compared with CT scan (61% vs. 100%). In addition, all patients who remained intubated for 24 hours received flexion and extension views, but no new injuries were detected.

This result is supported in adult trauma literature; Insko et al. (2002) reviewed the use of flexion-extension films and demonstrated that 30% of the patients were unable to flex and extend adequately, leading to further imaging with CT or MRI. They concluded that these films are of limited diagnostic utility in the acute setting for evaluation of the cervical spine at a Level I pediatric trauma center (Insko et al., 2002; Rana et al., 2009).

Radiation exposure from CT scans is an important concern and driving force for the rational use of imaging in children. Adelgais et al. (2004) examined this issue in a prospective study reviewing the differences of radiation exposure between conventional radiographs and CT. In this study, the patients receiving CT had 1.25 times the effective radiation dose compared with plain films. However, the comparison groups were markedly different; the patients undergoing CT scan were significantly more ill than the patients who only received plain films. The CT group had higher numbers of abnormal head CT (41% vs. 20%), intubation (20% vs. 2%), and transfer to intensive care or operating rooms (46% vs. 23%), compared with the group only receiving plain films. Keenan et al. (2001) examined this issue from another perspective by reviewing the number of excess radiographs required to clear the cervical spine of injury compared with the use of CT scan. Patients who underwent CT of the neck on initial evaluation had significantly fewer repeated radiographs than patients without cervical-spine CT (mean, 2.1 ± 2.6 vs. 3.6 ± 2.7 repeated radiographs, p = 0.04). The amount of radiation exposure was also determined, and the authors concluded that the children with initial CT did receive a higher effective dose (p < 0.001); however, patients with a GCS of less than 8 received equivalent doses compared with those not undergoing early cervical-spine CT (p=0.15) (Keenan et al., 2001). Although radiation exposure is increased in patients undergoing CT imaging, the actual increased risk of cancer above the natural background rate is low at 0.25% (Bier, 1990).

Child Abuse

The CDC defines child maltreatment as any act of commission (abuse) or omission (neglect) by a parent or other caregiver that results in harm, potential for harm, or threat of harm to a child. Unfortunately, such harm perpetrated on children permeates society. Even worse, child abuse remains to a great extent concealed or inadequately appreciated. Many experts believe that the number of annual referrals filed probably represent less than one third of actual cases; in fact, some sources describe as much as a tenfold difference between victim or parental self-reports and official estimates of incidence (Coté et al., 2009; Gilbert et al., 2009). Whether participating in the resuscitation and stabilization of a victim of acute pediatric trauma or assisting in the serial procedures required of more chronic medical conditions, anesthesiologists should step back and view their pediatric patients in a larger context that includes the possibility of child maltreatment.

Epidemiology

The U.S. Department of Health and Human Services collects and publishes data on child abuse in an annual report (U.S. Department of Health and Human Services, 2006). Of the estimated 3.2 million referrals made to Children's Protective Services (CPS) in 2007, 61.7% progressed to investigation or assessment. Approximately 25% of these investigations indicated or substantiated child maltreatment, leading to an estimated 794,000 children being counted as victims of abuse or neglect. The most recognized forms of maltreatment are generally categorized as physical abuse, sexual abuse, psychological or emotional abuse, and neglect. During 2007, 59% of the victims suffered from neglect, whereas 11% were physically abused, 8% were sexually abused, and 4% were psychologically maltreated. Maltreatment is inversely related to age, as victimization is most prevalent among children under 1 year of age.

Perhaps even more disturbing is the high recidivism rate for perpetrators, because maltreatment often develops into a repetitive pattern of offense. In one study, 75% of victims younger than 24 months of age demonstrated evidence or history of previous trauma or injury (Kellogg, 2007). Children who

are prior victims are 96% more likely to experience a repetition of abuse compared with those who are not previous victims. These trends are also inversely related to age, as adolescents from 16 to 21 years old are 51% less likely to experience recurrence compared with infants (U.S. Department of Health and Human Services, 2006).

Clearly, the most tragic outcome associated with maltreatment is a child's death. Such cases often go unrecognized and unreported because of poor coordination and communication between various agencies, as well as a lack of standardized terminology and investigation techniques. Nevertheless, in 2007, 1760 children's deaths were attributed to maltreatment. Again, the most fragile and defenseless children endure the greatest risk. Children younger than 1 year old accounted for 42% of fatalities, and 76% of the deaths attributed to maltreatment were associated with children under 4 years old (U.S. Department of Health and Human Services, 2006).

Many of these children have already been seen by various branches of the health care system, but the practice of pediatric anesthesiology provides a further level of screening for some of the most at-risk children. Children with disabilities, chronic illnesses, or special needs are at an increased risk for maltreatment and make up 8% of all child abuse victims (U.S. Department of Health and Human Services, 2006). It has been observed that compared with children who are not disabled, children with disabilities are 3.76 times more likely to be neglected, 3.79 times more likely to be physically abused, and 3.14 times more likely to be sexually abused (Hibbard and Desch, 2007).

Although child abuse affects children of all ages, genders, cultures, and socioeconomic strata, certain children are statistically predisposed to increased risk. Some of the indicative characteristics include the child's age (infants and preschoolers) and whether the child was born premature, is developmentally delayed, possesses special health needs, or succumbs to behavioral problems. Also, given that greater than 80% of documented abuse cases are perpetrated by parents or caregivers, these victims' home or care environments demonstrate other clear risk factors (Box 30-5) (Hornor, 2005; Kellogg, 2007). Obviously, bias should be avoided, because these risk factors in isolation do not indicate child abuse. Such characteristics should instead aid and guide further investigation as well as prevention strategies and treatment plans.

Box 30-5 Risk Factors for Child Abuse

PARENTAL OR CAREGIVER CHARACTERISTICS
Poverty
Unemployment
Lack of or minimal education
Social isolation
Single parenting or unrelated caregivers

CAREGIVER HISTORY
Substance abuse
Domestic violence
Mental illness
Their own neglect or abuse as children

For the anesthesia provider, a patient's preoperative or preprocedure evaluation is often streamlined and focused on the impending operative physiology and risks; however, certain information should raise a level of concern for possible abuse:

- There is a lack of or inadequate explanation for the injury or condition.
- The details of the explanation change.
- There are differing accounts from witnesses.
- The explanation does not fit the pattern, age, or severity of the injury.
- The explanation does not fit the child's developmental capacity.
- There are delays in seeking medical attention for the injury or condition.
- The concern expressed by caregivers is inappropriate for the condition or injury sustained.

It must be noted that children may be naturally prone to injury as they test the limits of their autonomy. Most childhood injuries are not the result of maltreatment; hence, common sense should apply when considering each child's ability to sustain observed bruising or trauma (Fig. 30-12). The same injury in a mobile 4-year-old child may be diagnostic of physical abuse in an infant. Likewise, outside of infancy, superficial injuries or bruising should be consistent with the hazards of daily living activities. Bruising to skin over bony prominences (e.g., shins, knees, forehead, chin, and forearms) is more consistent with normal activities, whereas injuries to protected, padded areas (e.g., neck, abdomen, buttocks, genitalia, cheeks, and ears) should always be suspect.

Anesthesiologists are perfectly positioned to routinely complete a full-body survey in the course of each patient's positioning in the operating room and for anesthesia. The key is to recognize a pattern or constellation of physical findings that may point to possible abuse or neglect. Some compelling or indicative findings are noted in Table 30-10. Complete documentation of injuries, including diagrams and photographs, is paramount to facilitate peer review as well as CPS and law enforcement intervention and court proceedings.

If abuse is suspected, other tests may be appropriate to assess for additional injuries or to elucidate other medical etiologies for injuries. These diagnostic studies may be more easily determined in consultation with child-abuse specialists. Regardless, the younger the child or the more severe the injury, the greater the need exists to evaluate for other injuries. And if one child is a suspected victim, other siblings or children in contact with the caregivers should also be assessed.

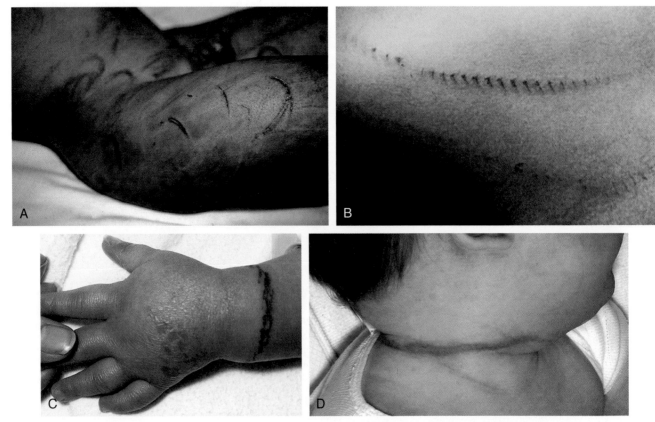

■ **FIGURE 30-12. A,** Severe bruising with underlying muscle damage. This toddler was covered from head to toe with severe looped-cord contusions and lacerations. He had secondary myoglobinuria, necessitating intensive care management to prevent renal failure. **B,** This boy was struck with a chain, leaving a clear imprint of the links. **C,** A deep, circumferential rope burn on the wrist with considerable edema and early skin breakdown of the hand is seen in this infant, who was tied to the siderails of her crib. **D,** This circumferential cord burn was the result of an attempted strangulation.

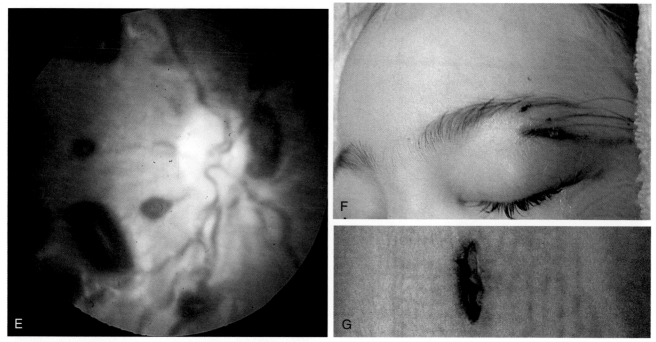

■ **FIGURE 30-12—cont'd. E,** Multiple retinal hemorrhages are seen on funduscopic examination of this infant who was a victim of the shaken-baby syndrome. Subdural hematoma and multiple metaphyseal "shake" fractures are typical associated findings. **F,** A superficial laceration is seen over the left eyelid. **G,** A deeper stab wound over the right flank penetrated into the subcutaneous tissue. *(From Zitelli BJ, Davis HW, editors: Atlas of pediatric physical diagnosis, ed 4, St. Louis, 2002, Elsevier.)*

TABLE 30-10. Physical Examination Findings Associated with Maltreatment

General	Notes
Extensive dental caries	Examples of general neglect
Severe diaper dermatitis	
Derelict wound care	
General uncleanliness	
Failure to thrive (may manifest in nutritional neglect)	
Anxiety and reluctance when the child is asked about abuse	
Skin	In groups or patterns, especially around soft, protected, padded areas
Bruises	
Bites	
Lacerations	
Burns • Immersion: genital, "stocking," or "glove" pattern from dipping the afflicted body part • Contact: from cigarettes, irons, curling irons, etc. (especially branding pattern) • Chemical: ingestion (may indicate neglect or abuse)	
Head	
Bruising or injury to ears, nose, or mouth	
Fontanel: fullness or asymmetry (may indicate step-off fracture or intracranial pathology)	
Eyes not tracking: may indicate head injury	
Retinal hemorrhage (by funduscopic exam)	
Thorax/Abdomen	
Any significant bruising or trauma, especially in infant or nonambulatory child	

Continued

TABLE 30-10. Physical Examination Findings Associated with Maltreatment—cont'd

General	Notes
Skeletal	
Specific fractures carry higher specificity for abuse (especially in infants)	
• Posterior ribs fractures	
• Sternum fractures	
• Scapular fractures	
• Spiral long-bone fractures (from torsion or twisting of extremities)	
• Metaphyseal fractures (from whole traction forces on limbs; may be seen with shaking)	
Genitalia/Anus	
Should be examined in any child when abuse is suspected	

Management Issues

Laws mandating the report of suspected abuse and neglect exist in all 50 states. Proof is not required before reporting, and good-faith reporting has immunity in some form or another (Kellogg, 2007).

Almost all states have what are nominally called *child-protection teams*. Such teams are composed of specialists who are well versed and trained in the medical, social, and legal aspects involved with these cases. The members of these teams are composed of social workers and physicians or medical providers with specific experience in the field. In fact, the American Academy of Pediatrics has recently implemented and accredited a new board subspecialty in Child-Abuse Pediatrics. Such child-protection teams should be available to concerned clinicians and typically work in conjunction with emergency departments, primary care practitioners, law enforcement agencies, and county CPS. These teams may offer onsite assistance and provide consultation on specific case questions.

In most tertiary care or academic centers, assistance may be readily available. However, in other health care facilities, there may not be any familiarity with these processes, so providers should solicit assistance from hospital social workers, administrators, or regional tertiary care centers. In the absence of any other source or after normal business hours, law enforcement and CPS are available to provide information and assure child safety. The U.S. Department of Justice also furnishes applicable information (http://www.ojp.usdoj.gov/ovc/help/ca.htm) and advertises a child-abuse hotline (1-800-4-A-Child) for referral information.

In order to recognize child maltreatment, anesthesia providers must understand and acknowledge that abuse and neglect occur on a regular basis, that such victimization occurs in any segment of society, and that maltreatment must be considered as part of the differential diagnosis when assessing any instance of childhood trauma.

Facial Trauma

Although severe facial trauma in children is a relatively uncommon event, it does occur, and it can make ETI challenging if not impossible (Fig. 30-13) (Zerfowski and Bremerich, 1998). Blood, secretions, hematomas, damaged tissues, or dentition may all obstruct the airway during respiration, ventilation, direct laryngoscopy, and fiberoptic intubation. Facial injuries can be categorized (in order of decreasing incidence)

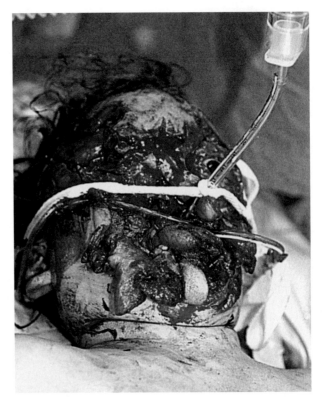

■ FIGURE 30-13. Photograph of a 3-year-old child who was backed over by a riding lawnmower and sustained massive facial trauma and amputation of the left foot.

as soft-tissue injuries, dental injuries, and facial fractures. As depicted in Figure 30-14, the incidence of these injuries varies with the age of the child. See related video online at www.expertconsult.com. In all instances, injuries are more common in males than females. Facial trauma in children under 5 years of age is less severe because of the protective environment supported by parental supervision (Kaban, 1993). However, Shaikh and Worrall (2002) found that 42% of the pediatric population sampled with facial injuries were younger than 5 years of age, where soft-tissue injuries were more common. The vast majority of these injuries were caused by falls, where insecurity of motion and lack of coordination prevented victims from shielding their faces or turning their heads. In such cases, the injury is then focused on a relatively small area of the face, from the nose to the mentum, which is referred to as *the falling zone* (Zerfowski and Bremerich, 1998). The rates

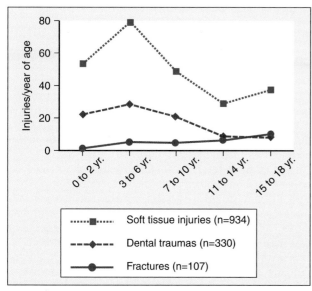

■ **FIGURE 30-14.** Type of injuries per year of age, demonstrated separately for soft-tissue injuries, dental trauma, and fractures. *(From Ferfowski M, Bremerich A: Facial trauma in children and adolescents,* Clin Oral Invest *2:120, 1998.)*

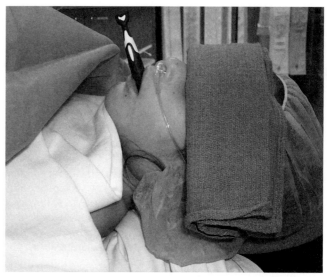

■ **FIGURE 30-15.** The left tonsillar bed of a 6-year-old girl was impaled after she fell with a toothbrush in her mouth. She was intubated orally with direct laryngoscopy.

of soft-tissue injuries increase in adolescence. This trend may be explained by more aggressive, risky behavior that may be related to alcohol consumption or sports activities. Compared with soft-tissue injuries, the incidence of dental injuries is diminished throughout childhood. It should nevertheless be noted that accidental aspiration of teeth before or during resuscitation can complicate care and necessitate removal via bronchoscopy. Facial fractures were the least common form of pediatric facial trauma. Facial fractures accounted for only 8% of patients in the study by Zerfowski and Bremerich (1998). Nasal fractures are the most common facial fractures in children. Anderson (1995) noted that nasal fractures accounted for over 50% of all facial fractures, followed by mandibular fractures and lastly maxillary fractures.

Another form of pediatric facial injury that can pose a challenge to anesthesiologists is laceration or impalement of oropharyngeal structures or tissues. It is not uncommon for children to fall with foreign objects in their mouths (e.g., pencils or toothbrushes), sometimes sustaining abrasions or lacerations to the soft palate or oropharynx. Most of such injuries are mild and spontaneously heal without intervention (Hellmann et al., 1993). However, some injuries raise concerns of vascular involvement and require angiographic studies before surgical extraction of the foreign body (Fig. 30-15). Carotid artery thrombosis and stroke have been reported after blunt pharyngeal trauma (Moriarty et al., 1997).

Extrusion of eye contents through a full-thickness–penetrating ocular laceration may result in permanent loss of vision (Fig. 30-16). Intraoperative anesthetic management of open globe injuries is discussed further in Chapter 27, Anesthesia for Ophthalmic Surgery.

Dog Bites

Dog-bite victims represent another common instance of facial injury in children. In a study by McHeik et al. (2000), the

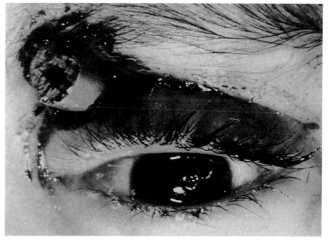

■ **FIGURE 30-16.** Open-eye injury in children is often caused by a projectile object.

majority of children suffering dog bites (68%) were younger than 5 years of age. It was believed that the increased rate of dog bites in this age group was as a result of young children's lack of caution and comprehension regarding animals, coupled with the fact that their heads and necks are on the same level as that of a dog. A study by Bernardo et al. (2002) revealed that younger children (younger than 6 years old) commonly sustained dog bites from their family dogs in their own homes and confirmed that these injuries typically involve facial structures. The goals of immediate surgical repair are to diminish scarring and decrease the rate of wound infection.

As with other trauma, facial injuries in children should be evaluated in the field or the emergency room during the primary survey. If there is any evidence of airway obstruction or respiratory insufficiency, the airway should be secured immediately with LMA, ETT via direct laryngoscopy, LMA, or surgery. As mentioned previously, special attention to cervical spine stability during direct laryngoscopy should be accomplished with inline stabilization of the neck. Once the airway is secured, a secondary survey can be performed to ascertain the extent of the facial injury and the need for surgical intervention.

Soft-Tissue Neck Trauma

Soft tissue injuries to the neck can occur in children. As mentioned earlier in the chapter, blunt trauma is much more common than penetrating trauma in the pediatric patient. Although rare, penetrating trauma can occur in this area also. Atta and Walker (1998) divided the neck into three anatomic zones. Zone I is the area between the thoracic outlet and the cricoid cartilage and contains the proximal common carotid, vertebral, and subclavian arteries, the trachea, the esophagus, the thoracic duct, and the thymus (Fig. 30-17). Zone II is between the cricoid cartilage and the angle of the mandible. Contents include the internal and external carotid arteries, jugular veins, pharynx, larynx, esophagus, recurrent laryngeal nerve, spinal cord, trachea, thyroid, and parathyroids. Zone III is between the angle of the mandible and the base of the skull. Its vascular structures include extracranial carotid and vertebral arteries and the uppermost segments of the jugular veins. Zone I injuries have the worst prognosis with regard to morbidity and mortality. Zone II injuries are the most prevalent but have the best prognosis because of their accessibility (Levy and Gruber, 2008).

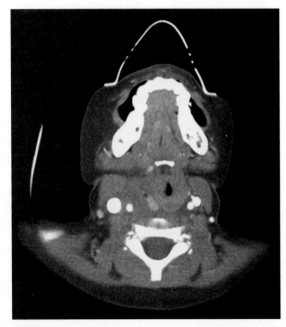

■ **FIGURE 30-17.** Neck CT angiography of a 4-year-old girl who was accidentally shot in the neck (zone I) with a BB gun. She suffered an aneurysm of her right common carotid artery, with a midline shift of her trachea (because of a hematoma) in both zones I and II. She underwent successful repair of this injury without sequelae.

Chest Trauma

Pulmonary contusions are the most common thoracic injury in children (Vane, 2002; Miller et al., 2003; Soundappan et al., 2005). Because most of the bony support or rib cage in a child is cartilaginous, significant forces may be transmitted to the lung and mediastinum without external signs. Pulmonary contusions may signal a simple isolated lung injury that includes pneumothorax, hemothorax, and rib fractures. Life-threatening injuries that impair ventilation include open or tension pneumothorax, flail chest, or injuries to the trachea or bronchi. A thoracotomy is rarely required, although chest tubes have been placed in up to 50% of reported case series. Injuries to the heart, diaphragm, great vessels, bronchi, and esophagus are rare. A chest tube stabilizes most life-threatening pulmonary lesions (e.g., tension pneumothorax). An important consideration when managing pulmonary trauma in children is that when a child suffers a significant pulmonary injury the mortality rate increases tenfold (Chu et al., 1996; Thourani et al., 1998; Soundappan et al., 2005). Tension pneumothorax is an urgent yet manageable complication of chest injury that produces diminished breath sounds, tracheal deviation, hypotension, and increased ventilation pressure. It occurs because of accumulation of needed air in the pleural space under pressure. An area in the injured lung acts as a one-way valve, leaking air into the pleural space. The leaked air becomes trapped in the pleural space, and each successive breath introduces more air under progressively increasing pressure. This impairs ventilation and venous return to the heart. It should be treated immediately with decompression by bore-IV catheter insertion in the midclavicular second intercostal space and followed by chest tube placement.

Open pneumothorax occurs when injury has produced a chest-wall defect. This equalizes the pressure between the pleural space and the environment, causing collapse of the lung and movement of air through the chest-wall defect rather than the trachea. It is managed by covering the defect with an occlusive dressing taped on three sides. This allows ventilation and prevents the air accumulation consistent with a tension pneumothorax.

Another consequence of a cartilaginous rib cage is that rib fractures and flail chest are less common in children than adults; however, significant intrathoracic injury, such as pulmonary contusion, may occur in the absence of a rib fracture. Flail chest occurs when four or more ribs are each fractured in two places by blunt trauma. The floating fracture segments produce paradoxical movement of the chest wall so that spontaneous ventilation is impaired. Any underlying pulmonary contusion further impairs gas exchange or ventilation. Although penetrating chest wounds in children are rare, as in an adult they can be immediately life threatening (Fig. 30-18). Hemothorax can occur when intercostal vessels or lung parenchyma are injured. It is important to have a high index of suspicion because blood in the pleural space can be asymptomatic; however, a hemothorax can cause significant hemodynamic compromise, because each hemithorax can hold 40% of a pediatric patient's blood volume (Grisoni and Volsko, 2001).

Although the chest cavity is compliant, the child is still at risk for tension pneumothorax, mediastinal shifts, and cardiac tamponade leading to respiratory and circulatory collapse. Because of the mobility of the mediastinum, aortic tears in children are

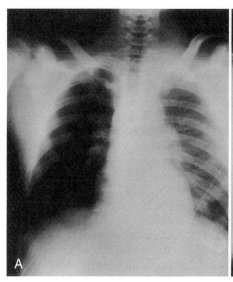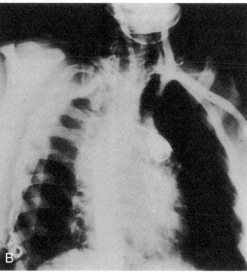

■ **FIGURE 30-18. A,** This child came to the hospital with a widened mediastinum after blunt chest trauma. **B,** An immediate arteriogram revealed a disrupted aortic arch.

rare. A widened mediastinum, fracture of the first rib, and presence of an apical pleural cap on the left side all raise concerns about an aortic disruption.

Abdominal Trauma

A rapid deceleration or shearing injury (e.g., motor vehicle crash) is the mechanism most commonly associated with abdominal injuries. Solid organs (e.g., the liver, spleen, and kidneys) are the most commonly injured, followed by the hollow visceral organs (Baker et al., 1992; Soundappan et al., 2005; Adelson et al., 2006; Langlois et al., 2006). Among these visceral injuries, the third and fourth parts of the duodenum, terminal ileum, and sigmoid colon are most at risk to injury because of their relative fixation. Death from abdominal injuries is usually secondary to hemorrhage. Injuries to the great vessels, genitourinary tract, pancreas, and pelvis are rare and account for proportionately fewer deaths. The body of the pancreas as it crosses the vertebrae column is the most susceptible portion of the pancreas injured by blunt force or compression (e.g., from a bicycle's handle bar or seat belt) (Fig. 30-19).

The abdomen of a child is vulnerable to injury for several reasons. The liver and spleen are less protected by the lower thoracic cage, and the bladder rides higher in the immature shallow pelvis. Gastric dilation in children is commonly encountered after trauma as a result of crying or swallowing air. It is important to recognize, because it can simulate peritonitis, limit diaphragmatic excursion (thereby hindering breathing), increase the risk of aspiration, and inhibit the vagally mediated tachycardia response to hypovolemia.

The management of solid-organ injuries in children has evolved over several years from an operative to a nonoperative approach (CDC, 1999). Success rates for nonoperative management of liver, spleen, and kidney trauma now exceed 90%. The relatively new use of interventional radiology techniques has further decreased the need for emergency surgery in children with solid abdominal injuries (CDC, 2003; Jankowitz and Adelson, 2006; Wakai et al., 2007). Furthermore, evidence-based guidelines now exist for critical care, radiographic procedures, follow-up care, and return to activity (CDC, 1999). The extent of the injury is scored on a scale from 1 to 5, based on radiographic findings, with a higher number representing increasing severity. However, the decision to operate is solely determined by the clinical situation. The only indication for operative intervention is hemodynamic instability—not the radiographic stage.

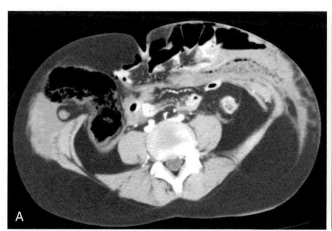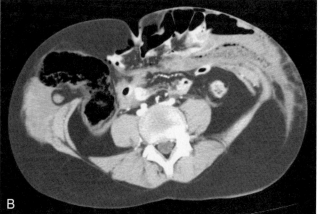

■ **FIGURE 30-19. A,** CT of a child with a disrupted rectus muscle and lateral-wall hematoma after a lap-belt injury. **B,** The same child with a perforation in the anterior abdominal wall.

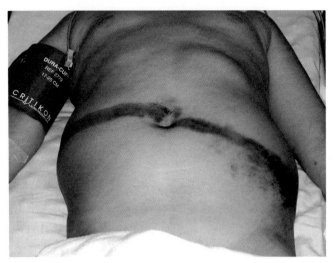

■ **FIGURE 30-20.** The same child after repair. Note the abdominal bruising pattern from the lap-belt injury.

A common mechanism of injury in children is motor-vehicle crashes. The lap-belt complex is a pattern of injury commonly encountered after a motor-vehicle crash (Fig. 30-20). The lap-belt complex describes a pattern of injury to intestinal viscera and its mesentery, with concomitant fracture, dislocation, or subluxation of the thoracic, lumbar, sacral spine, or the iliac wing. It was first described by Garrett and Braunstein (1962) to denote distinctive pattern of injury resulting from the use of lap-style safety belts (Luerssen, 2006). The lap-belt complex is characterized by soft-tissue injury, intraabdominal injury, and orthopedic injuries. The soft-tissue injury may be a slight bruise, ecchymosis, or a degloving injury with fascial dehiscence. The abdominal injury may be a solid organ, hollow viscus hematoma or perforation, mesenteric bleeding, or a bladder or aortic injury. Orthopedic injuries may include fractures, dislocation, or subluxation of the lumbar, sacral, thoracic spine or the iliac wing.

The orthopedic and abdominal injuries may be subtle and hard to detect at first. Paraspinal tenderness is suggestive of a spinal injury and mandates further radiographic investigations. Hollow-viscus injuries may appear clinically or radiographically (despite contrast) for a few days. Repeated physical examination is needed. In some situations, a healing hematoma may result in scarring and bowel obstruction 4 to 6 weeks after the injury.

Lawnmower Related Injuries

Lawnmowers cause more than 9400 injuries annually in the United States in children younger than 18 years of age, with almost one quarter of these injuries occurring in children younger than 5 years of age (U.S. Consumer Product Commission, 1990–1999). The age distribution is bimodal, with peaks at 2 and 15 years, probably representing injuries to bystanders vs. operators. Over 7% of children who incur mower-related injuries require hospitalization, a higher rate than injuries incurred from any other consumer product (U.S. Consumer Product Commission, 1990–1999). Riding mowers, commonly used for lawn and field maintenance in this country, are more powerful and complex to operate than walk-behind mowers. They carry a much higher risk of injury

and possible death than walk-behind mowers (more than three times higher) (Adler, 1994). In 1993, a U.S. Consumer Product Safety Commission report identified four mechanisms of injury caused by riding mowers: loss of mower stability, blade contact, layout and function of the mower controls, and running over or backing over young children (Adler, 1993). Back-over injuries occur approximately twice as often as run-over injuries, with about 85% of these injuries occurring in children between 15 months and 10 years of age. Typically, this occurs when the child is playing in the area, following the mower, or falls off the back of the mower (Deppa, 1994). The type of injuries children incur from lawnmowers range from lacerations (41%) to amputations and avulsions (7%) (U.S. Consumer Product Commission, 1990–1999). Aside from initial stabilization and treatment, children with these injuries may require repeated anesthetics for wound débridement, reductions of bony fractures, skin grafts, or reconstructive surgery. A child with a lower extremity injury may benefit from combined epidural and general anesthesia, with continued epidural analgesia in the postoperative period. Because of infection, consideration for antibiotic prophylaxis and tetanus must be considered. In addition, emotional trauma both to the patient and family is considerable. The following list shows some of the recommendations of the American Academy of Pediatrics Committee on Injury and Poison Prevention (Smith, 2001):

- Manufacturers of riding lawnmowers should only sell tractors that will not mow in reverse without a manual override.
- Children younger than 6 years of age should be kept indoors when lawnmowers are being operated.
- Children must not be allowed to ride as passengers on mowers.
- Children should not operate lawnmowers until they have displayed the necessary levels of judgment, strength, skill, and maturity. Most children will not be ready to operate a walk-behind mower until 12 years of age, and a riding mower until at least 16 years of age.

Skeletal Injuries

Musculoskeletal injuries are rarely life threatening, except when they are associated with ongoing severe hemorrhage. Still, they are a leading cause of morbidity and long-term disability, and if not managed appropriately and in a timely manner, long-term sequelae may result, including limb deformities, permanent neurologic and joint dysfunction, and loss of limb viability. See related video online at www.expertconsult.com. Additional considerations in children include premature growth arrest and potential for growth-plate injuries. In the child with multiple injuries, it is important to identify the priorities of treatment. Control of bleeding as a result of skeletal injuries should occur as part of the primary survey. Once life-threatening injuries such as head and chest injuries are addressed and initially stabilized, the extent of skeletal injuries should be carefully assessed based on symptoms, physical examination, and radiography. Appropriate initial measures include functional bracing or splinting to alleviate pain and immobilization of bone fragments to prevent further injury of adjacent neurovascular structures, allow safe transport of the patient, and minimize impairment of limb function. In patients with adequate alignment of fracture segments, this may be the only necessary treatment. Other interventions that may be needed in case of displaced fractures include external traction, external fixation, and internal fixation.

Urgent or emergent surgical interventions are usually indicated in the case of complex or displaced fractures associated with vascular damage and potential for limb ischemia, neurologic dysfunction, open fractures, joint dislocations that cannot be reduced, and compartment syndromes (Musgrave and Mendelson, 2002). Vascular injuries in conjunction with limb fractures are, fortunately, rare in children. Although the majority of vascular injuries are associated with supracondylar distal humerus fractures, they may also occur in conjunction with fractures of the distal femur, proximal tibia, displaced pelvic fractures, and knee dislocations. Children with suspected vascular injuries may require an angiogram to delineate the extent of the injury and to determine the need for revascularization. In the case of open fractures, wound irrigation and débridement with extensive removal of contaminated and necrotic tissue are required. Children with open fractures often require repeated débridement under general anesthesia every 48 to 72 hours until all of the devitalized tissue has been removed. Pain out of proportion to the extent of the injury should raise concern about compartment syndrome. In these cases, emergent fasciotomies of all involved compartments is indicated because significant muscle necrosis can occur if intracompartment pressures exceed 30 mm Hg for longer than 8 hours (Musgrave and Mendelson, 2002).

Fractures of the femur in children most commonly involve the femoral shaft or the distal femoral physis. Femoral-shaft fractures can result in significant blood loss from the fracture segments, and such blood loss may not be readily recognized because the blood accumulates in the large thigh compartments. Serial hematocrits should be obtained in children with femur fractures, and they should be adequately volume resuscitated before the induction of anesthesia to avoid cardiovascular collapse on induction. A high index of suspicion for compartment syndrome should be maintained, particularly in the patient with concomitant head trauma who may be difficult to evaluate. Children with distal femur fractures are at risk of arterial injury and compartment syndrome; attention should be focused on the neurovascular status of the limb (Musgrave and Mendelson, 2002).

The issue of early vs. delayed stabilization of femur fractures in children with closed head injuries remains contentious. Interpretation of the existing literature is confounded by variability in study design, small sample size of patients studied, differences in severity of head injury in the early vs. late treatment groups, and variable definitions of early vs. late treatment. Previous studies in adults have found that early fixation significantly reduced the incidence of severe pulmonary complications, including respiratory distress syndrome, pneumonia, and pulmonary emboli (Bone et al., 1989; Behrman et al., 1990). Pediatric studies found that early stabilization did not lessen the risk of pulmonary complications in the child with multiple injuries. A retrospective study by Hedequist and others (1999) identified 25 children with femur fractures and CNS injury (GCS score of 8). Seven of these children underwent early stabilization, of whom 4 (57%) experienced a respiratory complication compared with 8 complications out of 18 (44%) who underwent delayed fixation. In another retrospective study in children, Mendelson and others (2001) reported twice the number of respiratory complications in the late treatment group (4 out of 13 vs. 2 out of 12, p = ns). This difference may be clinically significant, but the groups were dissimilar in that children in the late-treatment group had a higher incidence of increased ICP. Other purported benefits of

early fixation include early patient mobilization, shorter hospital and intensive care unit stays, improved predictability of fracture outcome, and decreased costs.

Proponents of late stabilization argue that minor hemodynamic changes, including shifts in blood pressure and volume status, may potentiate secondary brain injury and lead to adverse neurologic outcomes. Previous investigators have reported a greater incidence of intraoperative hypotension and hypoxemia and lower mean GCS scores in patients undergoing early fracture stabilization (Jaicks et al., 1997; Townsend et al., 1998). Other studies have found no relation between timing of fracture fixation and head trauma outcome (McKee et al., 1997; Kalb et al., 1998; Mendelson et al., 2001). The Committee on Trauma of the American College of Surgeons has recommended that femoral fractures be treated early provided hemodynamic stability has been achieved (Burgess and Cates, 1993). The appropriate timing of fixation for a femur fracture in a child with a head injury remains open to further investigation. Until more definitive data become available, it may be prudent to delay operative fixation of femur fractures until stabilization of hemodynamic and neurologic status are achieved. Also, adequate volume resuscitation and careful monitoring of end-organ perfusion and pressure, including blood pressure and ICP monitoring, should be strongly considered to guide intraoperative interventions that reduce the risk of secondary brain injury.

Another potential complication of long-bone fractures is compartment syndrome. Acute compartment syndrome can be both a limb- and life-threatening surgical emergency. Compartment syndrome is defined as a condition where the circulation of blood through tissue is compromised within a closed space by increased pressure within that space (Matsen, 1975). Fractures that are most commonly associated with compartment syndrome are of the tibia and forearm (Namias, 2007). The classic signs and symptoms of compartment syndrome are the seven "Ps": pain, pallor, parasthesias, paralysis, pulselessness, pressure, and poikilothermia. Patients exhibit pain out of proportion to the clinical situation. Treatment should include elevation of the extremity, removal of restrictive dressings, and maintenance of normotension. Definitive surgical management of compartment in the extremity is fasciotomy (Fig. 30-21).

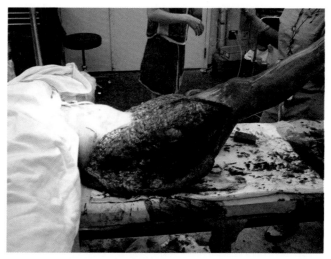

■ **FIGURE 30-21.** A 12-year old girl who was crossing the freeway as a shortcut to school and was hit by a semi truck. Note extensive bilateral thigh swelling that resulted in bilateral compartment syndromes.

SUMMARY

Pediatric trauma accounts for 25% of all traumas in the United States. Advanced trauma life support should be thought of as a continuum, beginning with the traumatic event; continuing through resuscitation and stabilization in the emergency room, diagnostic areas, and the operating room; and ending with the discharge of a stable patient into the recovery room or intensive care unit. Careful evaluation with good teamwork and meticulous attention to detail can contribute to a positive outcome.

For questions and answers on topics in this chapter, go to "Chapter Questions" at www.expertconsult.com.

REFERENCES

Complete references used in this text can be found online at www.expertconsult.com.

Anesthesia for Burn Injuries

Thomas Romanelli

31

CONTENTS

EPIDEMIOLOGY

The most recent edition of the American Burn Association's National Burn Repository includes a comprehensive analysis of data from acute burn admissions within the United States that were collected between 1998 and 2007. Pediatric burn patients account for almost one third of the total projected volume. Burn-related trauma is the second leading cause of accidental death in children between 1 and 4 years of age and remains the third leading cause of accidental death in individuals younger than age 18 years, exceeded only by motor vehicle accidents and drowning. Approximately 70% of pediatric burns up to the age of 4 years old are the result of scald injuries, whereas flame burns are the most common pattern among children 5 years of age and older (American Burn Association, 2007). In general, younger children are at higher risk for sustaining burn injuries, and abuse or neglect may account for as much as 15% to 20% of these cases (Tucker, 1986; Sheridan et al., 1997a).

The mortality previously associated with severe burn trauma has been significantly reduced since the 1980s. Current survival expectations associated with management of burn wounds may be attributed to improved access to emergency medical care and targeted resuscitation, advanced ventilation modalities and a more comprehensive understanding of the pathophysiology of inhalation injury, rigorous infection control practices, enhanced nutritional support, early burn wound excision and grafting, and the attenuation of the hypermetabolic response (Herndon and Spies, 2001). The development of evidence-based practice guidelines and multidisciplinary care models available at regional burn care centers have aided these efforts. Long-term outcomes have subsequently improved, and pediatric burn survivors are able to report a satisfying quality of life as measured by several psychometric tools (Sheridan et al., 2000; Baker et al., 2007, 2008).

BURN-WOUND ASSESSMENT

Injury depth, size, and location are the three components that contribute to the overall severity of burn wounds and are the direct results of exposure to thermal, chemical, electrical, ultraviolet, and radiologic sources. Regardless of the medium, the protective functions of the skin are impaired or destroyed. Burn wounds are dynamic, in that dermal changes evolve over time with damage extending to adjacent or deeper tissues (Palmieri and Greenhalgh, 2002).

The traditional classification of burn depth (first through fourth degrees) has been supplanted by the use of more

TABLE 31-1. Burn Injury Characteristics

First degree	Superficial	Epidermal layer only Mild pain No scarring Barrier functions preserved (Sunburn)
Second degree	Superficial/partial thickness Deep/partial thickness	Epidermal layer with varying degree of dermal extension Wet appearance Hyperemic Edematous Blistering Painful Heals in 7 to 10 days Scar formation is uncommon (Scald) Dry May appear red or pale Moderate-severe blistering Less pain (nerve damage) May advance to full-thickness injury Heals in 2 to 8 weeks Probable scar formation without surgical therapy (Flame/chemical exposure)
Third degree	Full thickness	Epidermal and complete dermal layer involvement Dry Waxy white or leathery appearance Painless (nerve destruction) Evolving wound site Excision and grafting required (Prolonged flame contact)
Fourth degree	Full thickness	Epidermal/dermal loss Fascia violation down to tendon or bone Muscle necrosis (Electrical injury)

Modified from de Campo T, Aldrete JA: The anesthetic management of the severely burned patient, *Int Care Med* 7:55, 1981.

comprehensive terminology to include the superficial, partial-thickness, and full-thickness categories, although there remains considerable overlap between these designations (Table 31-1). First-degree (superficial) burns are restricted to the epidermis and generally heal quickly without scarring, pigmentation changes, or contractures. Sunburn is the most common example and is associated with erythema, mild pain, and possible minor blistering (Fig. 31-1, *A*). Second-degree (partial-thickness) burns involve the epidermis and variable portions of underlying dermal structures and are further categorized as superficial or deep partial-thickness injuries, with different implications for the progression of tissue damage and the level of anticipated care. A superficial partial-thickness burn poses minimal risk of scar formation, because the dermal structures (e.g., nail beds, hair follicles, sebaceous glands, and nerves) are largely unaffected, allowing for injuries to heal within 2 weeks (Fig. 31-1, *B*). In contrast, deep partial-thickness injuries disrupt portions of the dermal matrix, and epithelial regeneration is commonly associated with scar formation. Pain may not be severe, despite extensive injury, which probably reflects variable degrees of nerve dysfunction or loss. Many of these wounds require excision and grafting in order to heal properly (Fig. 31-1, *C*). Full-thickness burns (formerly third-degree burns) are characterized by deep-tissue destruction where the necrotic debris adheres tightly to the dermal-matrix remnant as a thick, waxy layer of eschar (Fig. 31-1, *D*). In the absence of normal regenerative capabilities, wound healing can only occur by prolonged peripheral granulation and contraction, with a significantly increased incidence of infection and debilitating scar formation. Surgical intervention is required to reestablish normal barrier functions and prevent infectious sequelae (Sheridan, 2002). Even with early excision and grafting, hypertophic scarring persists years after the original injury. Fourth-degree burns are full-thickness burns with extensions beyond the fascia and include the destruction of gross muscle mass or the disruption of major joint-capsule integrity (Fig. 31-1, *E*). Injuries of this type are often a precursor to surgical amputation.

Reassessments of burn-wound size and depth are necessary, because injuries have the potential to evolve from their initial presentation (dermal dysfunction worsens and affects a broader and deeper area than originally observed). Therapeutic fluid administration, nutritional requirements, and prognostic determinations are dependent on the physician's ability to perform consistent serial evaluations and can be influenced to varying degrees by a clinician's experience and subjectivity. Several methods have been developed to minimize potential inaccuracies and include laser Doppler, thermography, vital dye fluorescence, and video angiography (Mandal, 2006; McGill et al., 2007; Monstrey et al., 2008). These techniques are used to identify viable tissue by documenting the presence of adequate vascular flow to the site of injury.

Estimates of dermal involvement are recorded as a percentage of total body surface area (TBSA), and several clinometric instruments are available (Wachtel et al., 2000; Jose et al.,

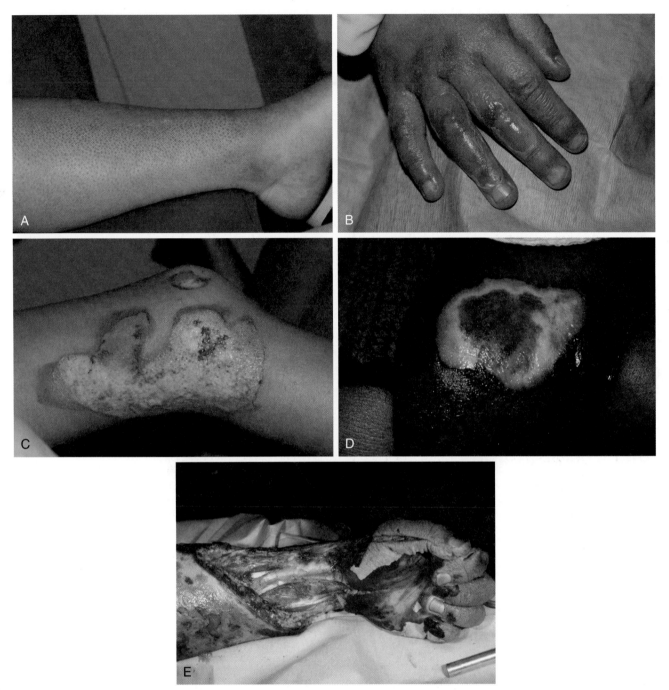

■ **FIGURE 31-1.** Depth of thermal injury. **A,** Patient with sunburn of the lower extremity (superficial or first-degree burn with associated blister on anterior tibial surface). **B,** Partial-thickness injury of the hand (superficial second-degree burn). **C,** Partial-thickness injury extending beyond subcutaneous layers (deep second-degree burn). **D,** Full-thickness (third-degree) burn. **E,** Full-thickness injury with extensive tissue loss (fourth-degree burn).

2004). Each method seeks to balance ease of use with consistent assessments among different care providers. The Lund-Browder diagram remains a commonly used tool, because it addresses the differences observed with patient size and body proportions in relation to growth (Fig. 31-2) (Lund and Browder, 1994). It has been adapted for the evaluation of pediatric patients. The "rule of nines" is well-suited for a rapid field-estimate of burn injuries to facilitate prehospital management and identify criteria for transfer to a regional burn center. This technique has also been modified to appropriately account for the alterations in body proportions observed with infants, small children, and the morbidly obese (Livingston and Lee, 2000; Smith et al., 2005).

Pediatric burn patients have also been evaluated using the palmar method, in which the size of the patient's palm represents the equivalent of 1% TBSA (Sheridan et al., 1995b; Rossiter et al., 1996). Complex burn wounds often have highly irregular distributions across multiple body segments, introducing additional inaccuracies to surface-area assessments. Newer techniques have been pioneered to improve the precision and reproducibility of clinician assessments. They include a flexible single-use nomogram that can be applied directly to the patient's wound sites and an advanced graphics software platform that creates a three-dimensional virtual display (Neuwalder et al., 2002; Dirnberger et al., 2003; Malic et al., 2007).

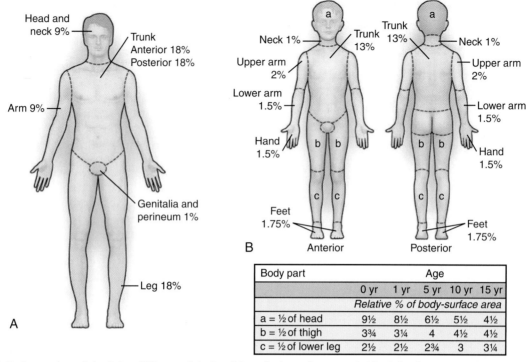

■ **FIGURE 31-2.** Comparison of the Rules of Nines and the Lund-Browder burn diagrams. **A,** The Rule of Nines is applicable to most adult burn patients. **B,** The Lund-Browder charts improve the accuracy of burn estimates for infants and young children, because body-surface area values correlate well with the patient's age. *(Modified from Orgill DP: Excision and skin grafting of thermal burns,* N Engl J Med *360:893, 2009.)*

TABLE 31-2. Burn Wound Severity

Minor	Superficial burns <15% TBSA
Moderate	Superficial burns = 15%-25% TBSA Superficial burns = 10%-20% TBSA in children Full-thickness burns <10% TBSA and burns not involving eyes, ears, face, hands, feet, or perineum
Major	Partial-thickness burns >25% TBSA Full-thickness burns >10% TBSA Concomitant inhalation injury Electrical burns Any complicated burn injury, i.e., patients with co-morbid conditions, patients with burns to the eyes, ears, face, hands, feet, or perineum Burns involving the face, eyes, ears, hands, feet, or perineum that may result in functional or cosmetic impairment

Modified from the American Burn Association: Guidelines for service standards and severity classifications in the treatment of burn injury, *Am Coll Surg Bull* 69:24, 1984.
TBSA, Total body surface area (%).

Burns are further classified by their overall severity (minor, moderate, or major) as defined by the American Burn Association and the American College of Surgeons Committee on Trauma (Table 31-2). These parameters may serve as useful indicators of the anticipated degree of physiologic derangement, but their prognostic value has not been validated.

PATHOPHYSIOLOGY

An evidence-based, multidisciplinary approach directed by a pediatric specialist is the most effective way to minimize mortality and improve long-term, functional outcomes among pediatric burn-trauma victims (Thombs et al., 2006; Gore et al., 2007). The spectrum of burn-related physiologic abnormalities includes, but is not limited to, loss of thermal insulation and antimicrobial barriers, distortions of airway anatomy and pulmonary derangements, fluctuating intravascular volumes and the need for individualized fluid replacement, hypermetabolism accompanied by grossly elevated caloric needs, septicemia, altered responses to common anesthetic agents, and a prolonged inflammatory response to systemic trauma. Most patients benefit from the capabilities of a regional burn unit to deal with these complex pathophysiologic changes, and the American Burn Association has forwarded selection criteria to facilitate referrals (Box 31-1).

Dermal Barrier Disruption

The epidermis is an effective barrier to heat loss, evaporation, and infection; the dermis and its supporting neurovascular structures provide elasticity, flexibility, and the mechanism for epithelial regeneration. Burn trauma induces localized tissue coagulation and microvascular reactions in the underlying dermis that can lead to injury extension (Aggarwal et al., 1994a, 1994b). Protective functions are immediately lost with dermal disruption and result in significantly increased risk of infection and hypothermia. The risk of hypothermia is particularly high in infants and young children because of their disproportionate surface area/body mass ratio; burn patients benefit from aggressive control of ambient temperature and humidity to restrict heat loss and limit the caloric expense of shivering.

The severity of skin damage is a function of temperature and its duration of contact. Burn wounds have three zones

Box 31-1 Burn-Center Transfer Criteria

Partial- and full-thickness burns on more than 10% TBSA in patients under 10 or over 50 years of age

Partial- and full-thickness burns on more than 20% TBSA in other age groups

Partial- and full-thickness burns affecting the face, hands, feet, genitalia, perineum, and major joints

Partial- burns on more than 5% TBSA in any age group

Electrical burns, including lightning injury

Chemical burns

Inhalation injury

Burn injuries in patients with comorbid conditions that could complicate management, prolong recovery, or affect mortality

Any patient with burns and concurrent trauma (e.g., fractures) in which the burn injury poses the greatest risk of morbidity or mortality; in such cases, if trauma poses the greater immediate risk, the patient may be treated initially in a trauma center until stable before being transferred to a burn center; physician judgment is necessary is such situations and should be in concert with the regional medical control plan and triage protocols

Hospitals without qualified personnel or equipment for the care of children with burns should transfer children with burns to a burn center with these capabilities

Burn injury in patients who require special social, emotional or long-term rehabilitative support, including cases involving suspected child abuse and substance abuse

Modified from the American Burn Association: Hospital and Prehospital Resources for Optimal Care of Patients with Burn Injury: Guidelines for development and operation of burn centers, *Burn Care Rehab* 11:980, 1990; American College of Surgeons: *Resources for optimal care of the injured patient*, 1993, American College of Surgeons, p 64.

of heterogeneous tissue damage, radiating from the epicenter of maximal tissue destruction (Jackson, 1953). The zone of edema and stasis is of particular importance, because it represents affected tissues that are potentially salvageable with supportive care. Successful management helps reduce the final TBSA measurement (Fig. 31-3) (Hettiaratchy and Dziewulski, 2004). During the first 24 to 48 hours, systemic hypotension, acidosis, and developing sepsis contribute to injury extension. These conditions are likely to exacerbate tissue edema, impaired microcirculation, and perfusion deficits. Serial examination is the most prudent method to address the variability of burn-wound progression. Early detection of nonviable areas with subsequent surgical excision and grafting has been consistently demonstrated to decrease morbidity and mortality in this patient population (Ong et al., 2006).

Respiratory Abnormalities

It is often difficult to definitively distinguish respiratory insufficiency caused by the toxic products of combustion from the pulmonary derangements that are commonly observed with systemic responses to severe burn trauma. *Inhalational injury* is a term that encompasses both the direct thermal and subsequent inflammatory damage to the upper and lower airways. Several studies have demonstrated that inhalation injury associated with burns increases mortality, although no specific indicators are reliably predictive of the overall degree of pulmonary dysfunction (Shirani et al., 1987; Hollingsed et al., 1993; Ryan et al., 1998; Edelman et al., 2006; Endorf and Gamelli, 2007).

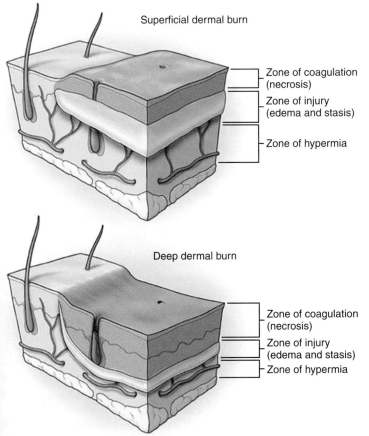

Superficial dermal burn

Zone of coagulation (necrosis)

Zone of injury (edema and stasis)

Zone of hypermia

Deep dermal burn

Zone of coagulation (necrosis)

Zone of injury (edema and stasis)

Zone of hypermia

■ **FIGURE 31-3.** Zones of thermal injury. Burn injuries create three distinct zones of tissue reaction. The zone of necrosis is caused by tissue-protein denaturation. The zone of injury is associated with edema and reduced blood flow. The extent of this zone is variable, and appropriate burn management may limit its progression to necrosis. *(Modified from Orgill DP: Excision and skin grafting of thermal burns,* N Engl J Med *360:893, 2009.)*

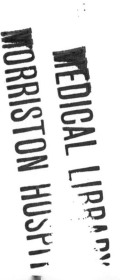

Upper-Airway Effects

Direct-heat injury caused by superheated gas inhalation and toxic smoke exposure may manifest as rapidly progressive edema of the tongue, epiglottis, and aryepiglottic folds (Pruitt et al., 1970). Macroglossia, micrognathia, and tonsillar hypertrophy are common findings in previously healthy children, and the normal presence of these features may further restrict airway patency (Benjamin and Herndon, 2002). Reduced cross-sectional area and increased flow resistance are poorly tolerated by infants and young children because of their elevated baseline minute ventilation, oxygen consumption, and limited endurance of the major respiratory muscle groups (Keens et al., 1978). Large-volume intravenous fluid administration is likely to accelerate oropharyngeal edema and convert a marginal airway into a severely compromised one, with subsequent anatomic distortions that make successful direct laryngoscopy challenging or impossible. Avoiding the "lost airway scenario" in the pediatric burn patient is a critical step during initial management, and the clinician should be guided by serial examinations to avoid airway catastrophe. Early, definitive control of the airway using context-appropriate methods is preferable for patients with evidence of progressive respiratory distress. This principle also applies to other clinical circumstances where the oropharyngeal architecture has been altered (e.g., ingestion of caustic agents such as lye).

Lower-Airway Effects (Smoke-Inhalation Injury)

Lower-airway injury is a clinical diagnosis supported by the presenting history and serial examination. Chest radiographs and bedside pulmonary function tests usually remain normal until infectious complications arise, and then their results often show an underestimation of the severity of lung damage (Lee and O'Connell, 1988; Wittram and Kenny, 1994). Fiberoptic bronchoscopy and bronchoalveolar lavage can be used to document the presence of carbonaceous debris and mucosal sloughing, although the absence of these findings should not preclude the diagnosis (Hunt et al., 1975). Technetium scanning is an assessment of pulmonary vascular endothelium damage represented as abnormal lung/liver uptake ratios of the isotope. In the future, this method may be accepted as a more objective diagnostic tool to detect lung injury in those patients with pulmonary signs and symptoms (but negative chest radiographs or pulmonary function test [PFT] findings), although it will require additional study (Shiau et al., 2003).

Toxicologic analysis of the victims with smoke-inhalation injury has demonstrated exposure to many poisonous aerosols, including carbon monoxide (CO), hydrogen cyanide, various aldehydes, hydrogen chloride, and other aromatic hydrocarbons (e.g., benzene). Even a brief exposure has significant adverse effects on the ciliated respiratory epithelial cells; toxic gases induce separation of cells from basement membranes, leukocyte migration, and exudate formation with severe impairment of the mucociliary-clearance mechanism (Fein et al., 1980). Severe ciliary dysfunction permits the accumulation of cellular debris, secretions, and bacteria. Endobronchial sloughing and edema contribute to small airway narrowing. Diminished flow capacity promotes widespread atelectasis that is magnified by surfactant loss (Herndon et al., 1985). Leukocytes aggregate in the affected lung tissue and release potent inflammatory mediators and other chemotaxins that increase endothelial

TABLE 31-3. Pulmonary Dysfunction Evolving from Burn Injury

Early resuscitation phase (0-48 hours)	Upper-airway compromise Persistent bronchospasm Conducting-airway obstruction Impaired ciliary clearance Decreased lung and chest-wall compliance
Late resuscitation phase (48+ hours)	Surfactant loss Increased dead space Increased closing volume Decreased functional residual capacity Tracheobronchitis ARDS/pulmonary edema/pneumonia

ARDS, Acute respiratory distress syndrome.

permeability (Wright and Murphy, 2005). Dyspnea, tachypnea, diffuse rhonchi, and bronchospasm are common clinical signs observed with evolving pulmonary insufficiency and impaired gas exchange in the presence of persistent aerosolized irritants (Table 31-3).

The cascade of endobronchial cell destruction and protracted inflammatory changes predispose the patient to barotrauma (lung injury secondary to elevated ventilatory pressures and air trapping in the smaller airways), significant ventilation-perfusion distortions, and the potential for bacterial infection that leads to bronchopneumonia after several days (Pruitt et al., 1975; Rue et al., 1993). Lower-airway injuries also substantially increase systemic fluid requirements. Paradoxically, efforts to minimize pulmonary edema with fluid restriction increase mortality in these patients because inadequate intravascular volume invariably results in systemic hypoperfusion and multiorgan dysfunction (Ansermino and Hemsley, 2004).

During this period, clinical efforts must focus on the maintenance of effective gas exchange to provide time for the resolution of pulmonary tissue injury. Vigorous pulmonary toilet is needed to clear accumulated endobronchial debris, purulent exudates, mucous plugs, and residual particulates (Demling, 2008). A number of studies have reported that the administration of aerosolized heparin and mucolytics may reduce cast formation and attenuate respiratory failure (Desai et al., 1998; Holt et al., 2008). Ventilation modalities should be selected to minimize barotrauma and reperfusion injury, because elevated peak inspiratory pressures and hyperoxygenation worsen pulmonary insufficiency (Shapiro et al., 1980; Slutsky, 1993). Low-volume, pressure-limited ventilation with permissive hypercapnia (allowing for the deliberate elevation of measured arterial carbon dioxide tension [$Paco_2$] while maintaining pH greater than 7.25 and an arterial oxygen saturation of hemoglobin [SpO_2] of greater than 90%) is one method that may preserve tissue oxygenation in the presence of severe pulmonary dysfunction and is associated with a reduction in short-term mortality (Hickling et al., 1994; Sheridan et al., 1995a). Other methods (e.g., high-frequency percussive ventilation) have also been used, but outcomes data remain unclear (Rodeberg et al., 1994; Micak et al., 1997; Sheridan et al., 1997b; Cortiella et al., 1999; Silver et al., 2004).

Infection is the most common complication after the accumulation of denuded endobronchial tissue, small-airway obstruction, persistent edema, and extended intubation intervals (Rue et al., 1995). The incidence has been reported as high as 30% in pediatric burn patients, with infection occurring after the loss of antimicrobial barriers and the onset of generalized immunosuppression that follows severe burn trauma (Fitzpatrick et al., 1994). Fever, mucopurulent secretions, and lobar consolidation documented by chest radiographs support the diagnosis of pneumonia (or tracheobronchitis if no x-ray changes are noted). Bronchoalveolar lavage and brushings may help support the diagnosis (Ramzy et al., 2003; Wood et al., 2003; Goldberg et al., 2008; Malhotra et al., 2008). Culture-guided and Gram-stain–guided antibiotic therapies should be reevaluated often and adjusted to optimize bacteriocidal effects and limit the development of antibiotic resistance.

Tracheostomy for pediatric patients has been advocated as a useful adjunct for airway and ventilatory management, but its application is not without risk (Sellers et al., 1997; Coin et al., 1998; Palmieri et al., 2002). The typical challenges encountered during pediatric direct laryngoscopy are made considerably more difficult in the presence of facial burns and progressive edema. Tracheostomy provides a stable, definitive airway and should be considered when the treatment plan requires multiple transports to and from the operating room or frequent repositioning of the patient for wound care. Improved secretion clearance, dead-space reduction, decreased airway resistance, and facilitation of the weaning process are also perceived benefits of a tracheostomy. However, surgical airways in small children may be associated with a greater incidence of structural abnormalities (e.g., subglottic stenosis and tracheoesophageal fistula), and subsequent life-long restricted tolerance of exercise. The routine use of this technique is not recommended (Calhoun et al., 1988; Desai et al., 1993; Barret et al., 2000).

Carbon-Monoxide Exposure

CO is a by-product of incomplete organic combustion and a persistent toxin of heme-containing species because of its strong binding affinity. Although CO reversibly binds hemoglobin, it does so at approximately 200 times the strength of oxygen, producing a functional anemia. Only a brief exposure is necessary to produce clinical symptoms (Fig. 31-4). A person exposed to

1% CO vapor attains measured carboxyhemoglobin (COHb) levels of 30% within 2 minutes. Severe CO poisoning may occur even without evidence of overt burn trauma, and delayed diagnosis contributes to significant morbidity and mortality after exposure (Cone et al., 2008; Stefanidou et al., 2008). The half-life of CO in a patient breathing room air approaches 200 minutes, but by applying 100% oxygen therapy this time can be reduced to approximately 40 minutes (Weaver et al., 2000). The clinician should always maintain a high index of suspicion for occult CO intoxication.

CO binding of hemoglobin and cytochrome P450 produces a leftward shift of the oxygen-hemoglobin dissociation curve and subsequently interferes with erythrocyte transport and oxygen use within the mitochondria (Fig. 31-5). CO-induced alterations of oxygen delivery and cellular usage have the greatest impact on those organ systems with the highest baseline oxygen requirements (i.e., the brain and heart). Ambient levels of 100 ppm are sufficient to produce acute neurologic symptoms (e.g., agitation, dizziness, lethargy, and seizures) in addition to chest pain, dyspnea, and noncardiogenic pulmonary edema. In animal models, CO has been observed to have direct myocardial depressant properties that are independent from the effects of global hypoxemia (Suner and Jay, 2008). The classically-described cherry-red appearance of patients with CO toxicity is rare and should actually be considered a late sign associated with high mortality ("when you're cherry red, you're dead"). Most patients have pallor that reflects the functional anemia previously described.

Standard peripheral oximetry overestimates oxygen saturation in the patient with acute CO intoxication and masks profound hypoxemia (Kao and Nañangas, 2004). Arterial sampling of Pa_{O_2} is also misleading, because this technique quantifies plasma levels of dissolved oxygen rather than actual hemoglobin saturation. COHb may be assayed with blood samples

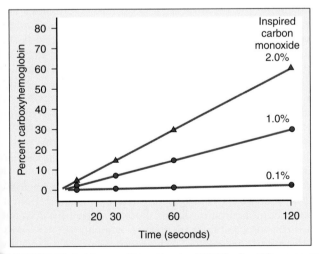

FIGURE 31-4. Measured blood levels of COHb after CO exposure. COHb accumulates rapidly after minimal exposure to CO. This effect becomes more pronounced with higher inspired concentrations of CO. *(Modified from Stewart RD, et al.: Rapid estimation of carboxyhemoglobin level in fire fighters,* JAMA *235:390-392, 1976.)*

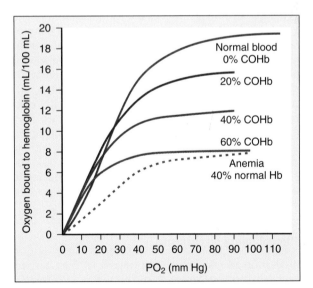

■ **FIGURE 31-5.** Leftward shift of hemoglobin dissociation curve. Accumulating levels of COHb interfere with normal oxygen transport and create a functional anemia with subsequent reduction of tissue oxygen delivery. *(Modified from Fein A, et al.: Pathophysiology and management of complications resulting from fire and the inhaled products of combustion: review of the literature,* Crit Care Med *8:94, 1980.)*

or measured directly with a noninvasive cooximeter (Masimo Rad-57, Masimo Corporation; Irvine, Calif) that measures and compares multiple light wavelengths to identify COHb and methemoglobin levels (Suner and McMurdy, 2009).

Long-term sequelae may manifest as chronic headaches, memory disturbances, learning disabilities, and neuromotor dysfunction in as many as 10% of those patients who experience severe exposure (Ginsberg, 1985). Some studies suggest that CO induces brain-lipid peroxidation and leukocyte-mediated inflammation, which culminate in white matter demyelination or focal necrosis (Wang et al., 2009). Neuropsychiatric effects may appear days to weeks after the initial exposure, and although most patients eventually achieve complete clinical recovery, radiographic evidence of CO-induced changes persist for far longer.

Currently, it is difficult to determine the precise risk of long-term neurologic effects, although some clinicians have advocated the use of hyperbaric oxygen therapy (HBOT) to limit neuropsychiatric changes. There is conflicting evidence pertaining to the efficacy of HBOT, in part because the neurocognitive symptoms may be attributable to several factors other than CO exposure (Chou et al., 2000; Gilmer et al., 2002). The benefits of this treatment remain controversial, and HBOT is often impractical for those patients with severe comorbid injuries.

Cyanide Toxicity

Cyanide inactivates cytochrome oxidase and prevents mitochondrial oxidative phosphorylation, even in the presence of adequate oxygen; therefore, normal cellular aerobic metabolism is altered to an anaerobic state (Geller et al., 2006). Toxicity manifests as supranormal venous oxygen levels with a concurrent metabolic lactic acidosis that does not resolve with oxygen therapy. The patient displays many similar neurologic and cardiovascular symptoms as observed with CO poisoning, and in fact may require treatment for the toxic effects from both vapors. Treatment involves the administration of agents that scavenge intracellular cyanide and promote its conversion to nontoxic metabolites. Sodium thiosulfate donates a sulfur group to cyanide and increases its conversion rate to thiocyanate, which then undergoes renal elimination (Gracia and Shepard, 2004). Nitrites (e.g., amyl nitrite and sodium nitrite) induce methemoglobin, which then interacts with cyanide to release it from cytochrome-oxidase binding sites. Nitrites should be used with caution in children because concurrent methemoglobin and carboxyhemoglobinemias significantly reduce oxygen-carrying capacity (Fidkowski et al., 2009). Hydroxocobalamin combines with cyanide to form nontoxic cyanocobalamin (vitamin B_{12}), and this compound is excreted by the kidneys (Borron et al., 2007).

Additional Injury Mechanisms

Acute dermal necrosis from burn trauma is characterized by protein denaturation, loss of elasticity, and tense contractures of the dermal remnant. The rigid layer of eschar that accompanies circumferential full-thickness burns of the abdomen and thorax may severely restrict diaphragmatic movement and chest-wall expansion, quickly progressing to respiratory failure within the first hours after trauma (Quinby, 1972). Markedly elevated intraabdominal and intrathoracic pressures impair venous return, with subsequent reduction of cardiac output

(Demling, 1986). Compressive effects of circumferential burns involving the upper or lower extremities lead to neurovascular compromise and render the limbs nonviable. Abdominothoracic and extremity escharotomies are performed to relieve compartment syndromes and restore effective chest wall compliance and limb perfusion.

Cardiovascular Abnormalities

Pediatric burn patients experience profound changes in intravascular fluid dynamics and impairments of systemic organ perfusion. Hypotension is the result of volume deficits and low peripheral vascular resistance that lead to diminished measures of cardiac output, central venous pressure, and pulmonary artery occlusion pressure. Additionally, pediatric patients often experience varying degrees of the systemic inflammatory response syndrome (SIRS), a complex milieu of cytokines, chemokines, and proinflammatory mediators that alter capillary permeability, depress myocardial contractility, and impair the normal function of many other organ systems (Table 31-4).

The release of tumor necrosis factor-α (TNFα) from cardiac myocytes has been demonstrated to contribute to progressive cardiac contractile dysfunction in several models of trauma, thermal injury, and sepsis (Horton et al., 2004; Niederbichler et al., 2006). TNFα is a well-recognized inflammatory mediator that normally modulates the antimicrobial and metabolic response to tissue injury. In the context of burn trauma, this mediator recruits additional neurohumoral agents that exacerbate organ injury and initiate cellular apoptosis. Interleukins (IL-1β, IL-6, and others) also possess negative inotropic effects and may act synergistically with TNFα to perpetuate postburn myocardial cardiac depression (Maass et al., 2002a, 2002b). Nuclear factor κβ (NFκβ) is a transcription agent involved in the regulation of many of the cytokines and chemokines that contribute to the progression of SIRS. Burn trauma appears to activate myocardial NFκß, which promotes the secretion of TNFα (Maass et al., 2002a). Prolonged hypotension that is resolved with volume replacement may result in reperfusion injury and the formation of oxidized free radicals and lipid peroxidation by-products. These agents exacerbate the tissue damage incurred during the low-flow state (Parihar et al., 2008). Free radical generation is accompanied by impaired antioxidant mechanisms and the up-regulation of inducible nitric oxide synthetase (iNOS). This cascade promotes peripheral vasodilation, enhanced NFκβ release, and production of additional reactive tissue injury mediators such as peroxynitrite (Horton, 2003). Leukotrienes, platelet activation factor, thromboxane A$_2$ and complement are other factors that potentially modulate burn-induced inflammatory responses. Cellular oxidative stress is an important component of burn-mediated injury with a complex and extensive impact on organ function. Further studies are needed to fully describe the interactions of many neurohumoral mediators detected during the systemic burn response, and their appropriate manipulation may result in therapeutic benefits.

Burn shock is the clinical summation of intravascular fluid deficits and cellular ischemia that is initially characterized by decreased cardiac output, impaired contractility, and hypoperfusion of organ systems. Thermal injury also creates significant alterations in endothelial permeability, resulting in pronounced

TABLE 31-4. Systemic Effects of Thermal Injury

System	Early	Late
Cardiovascular	↓ CO caused by decreased circulating blood volume, myocardial depression (TNFα)	↑ CO caused by sepsis or hypermetabolism Hypertension
Pulmonary	Upper- and lower-airway obstruction ↓ FRC ↓ Pulmonary compliance ↓ Chest-wall compliance	Bronchopneumonia Tracheal stenosis Restricted chest-wall expansion
Renal	↓ GFR caused by: • ↓ Circulating blood volume • Myoglobinuria • Hemoglobinuria Tubular dysfunction	↑ GFR caused by ↑ CO Tubular dysfunction
Hepatic	↓Synthetic function caused by • ↓ Circulating blood volume • Hypoxia • Hepatotoxins	Hepatitis ↑ Synthetic function caused by • Hypermetabolism • Enzyme induction • ↑ CO Dysfunction caused by sepsis or drug interaction
Hematopoietic	↓ Red cell mass, anemia Thrombocytopenia ↑ Fibrin split products Coagulopathies	Thrombocytosis Coagulopathies Transfusion reactions Transfusion-related infection
Neurologic	Encephalopathy Seizures ↑ ICP	Encephalopathy Seizures ICU disorientation
Skin	↑ Thermal, fluid, electrolyte loss	Contractures and scarring
Metabolic	↓ Ionized calcium	↑ Oxygen consumption ↑ CO_2 production ↓ Ionized calcium
Pharmacokinetics	Altered volume of distribution Altered protein binding Altered pharmacokinetics Altered pharmacodynamics	↑ Opioid/sedative tolerance Enzyme induction Altered receptor function Drug interactions

Modified from Szyfelbein SK, et al.: Burn injuries. In Coté CJ, et al., editors: *A practice of anesthesia for infants and children*, ed 2, Philadelphia, 1993, Saunders.
TNFα, Tumor necrosis factor-α; *GFR*, glomerular filtration rate; *ICU*, intensive care unit.

fluid translocation and generalized edema formation (Warden, 2002). Transcellular electrolyte shifts and the loss of circulating plasma proteins further impair tissue perfusion. Pediatric burn patients possess limited compensatory responses to systemic hypotension and vasoactive infusions (e.g., dopamine or norepinephrine) may be needed to supplement intravenous fluid administration to achieve adequate blood pressure and cardiac output. Resuscitation guidelines have evolved to become goal-oriented rather than formula-driven; current recommendations advocate periodic reassessment and adjustment of individual fluid requirements to restore organ perfusion and tissue oxygenation.

Survivors of the acute injury phase often develop a hyperdynamic circulation that is characterized by marked elevation of cardiac output and lowered peripheral vascular resistance. Hypertension has been observed with increased incidence in patients who have sustained more than 20% TBSA thermal injuries (Falkner et al., 1978). Elevations of plasma renin, aldosterone, and catecholamines have been noted. Untreated hypertension may manifest as seizures, encephalopathy, and ultimately, end-organ dysfunction in up to 7% of pediatric patients with severe burns (Popp et al., 1980). Although desirable, antihypertensive therapy may have adverse side effects

in this setting and should be guided by clinically relevant measures of systemic perfusion.

Renal Abnormalities

Acute renal dysfunction occurs in the context of hypoperfusion, intravascular depletion, myoglobin-induced tubular damage, and mechanical obstruction secondary to cast formation by the products of hemolysis (Aikawa et al., 1990). Hyperglycemia is a function of the stress response and may add to intravascular volume depletion by promoting an osmotic diuresis. Efforts to maintain urine output within a recommended range of 1 to 1.5 mL/kg per hour should be confirmed with serial urimeter measurements that demonstrate ongoing evidence of adequate fluid resuscitation. Tubular dysfunction in the form of altered responses to plasma renin and aldosterone may also contribute to renal derangements (Mariano et al., 2008).

Significant interpatient differences concerning the pharmacodynamics and pharmacokinetics of commonly used antibiotics have been reported (Weinbrem, 1999; Kiser et al., 2006; Conil et al., 2007). Alterations of creatinine clearance and glomerular filtration rates impact drug-dosing schedules and effective plasma concentrations, necessitating customized dosing regimens guided by serum plasma levels (Boucher et al., 1992). Antibiotics with nephrotoxic properties are likely to exacerbate renal dysfunction.

Perturbations of extracellular water and macromolecules affect electrolyte composition, and rapid changes of serum sodium, potassium, and calcium concentrations are associated with increased morbidity; serial monitoring and correction of these alterations is an essential component of acute burn management. Elevated levels of stress hormones (e.g., aldosterone, angiotensin, catecholamines, and plasma renin) also contribute to renal dysfunction observed in the early postburn period. Patients with thermal injuries release elevated levels of atrial natriuretic peptide (ANP), which may mitigate the adverse effects of low-flow states by improving renal blood flow and urine output (Onuoha et al., 2000). Animal studies have shown intrarenal redistribution of blood flow with the preservation of inner cortical perfusion. Reductions in urinary chloride and sodium concentration reflect the increased perfusion of the juxtaglomerular nephrons that possess significant salt-retention capacity (Carter and Well, 1975).

Hepatic Abnormalities

Burn-related hepatic dysfunction is a significant contributor to morbidity and mortality. Hepatic blood flow is compromised in the early burn phase secondary to blood loss, large-volume fluid shifts, and compensatory vasoconstriction. The extent of hepatocellular derangement is also influenced by the onset of sepsis, toxic drug interactions, and the potential infectious risks of multiple blood product transfusions. Liver dysfunction is likely modulated by cytokines IL-1β and TNFα, both of which are potent inflammatory mediators (Jeschke et al., 1999). Elevations of serum transaminases, reduced synthesis of constitutive proteins (e.g., albumin, transferrin, and retinol-binding protein), and focal hypertrophy are all clinical markers of evolving hepatic dysfunction (Jeschke et al., 2007a).

Restoration of hepatic blood flow precedes an extended phase of hypermetabolism and initiates a catabolic cascade with adverse systemic effects. Acute phase protein production occurs at the expense of albumin synthesis, and subsequent reductions of the protein binding capacity result in unpredictable drug plasma levels. The acute-phase process may continue for months, prolonging systemic organ dysfunction and delaying efforts to restore lean body mass (Jeschke et al., 2004). The duration and severity of hepatic dysfunction are variable and ultimately dependent on the ability to reconvert the patient's hepatic function to an anabolic state; this process requires successful wound closure, infection control, and adequate nutritional support.

Metabolic and Gastrointestinal Abnormalities

The severity of burn trauma correlates directly with the anticipated degree of inflammatory and hypermetabolic responses, and these physiologic derangements are associated with increased mortality for those patients who have experienced more than 60% TBSA burn (Jeschke et al., 2007b). Endogenous catecholamines and other stress hormones (e.g., glucagon and glucocorticoids) act synergistically to produce metabolic

changes that include a hyperdynamic circulation, sharply elevated basal energy expenditure, and the catabolism of skeletal muscle proteins. Additional clinical findings include refractory tachycardia, increased cardiac output and oxygen consumption, hyperpyrexia, and increased carbon dioxide production (Tredget and Yu, 1992).

The prolonged catabolic phase of thermal injury is also marked by accelerated gluconeogenesis, glucose intolerance, lipolysis, glycogen mobilization, and insulin resistance. Increased amino-acid oxidation causes urea formation and nitrogen loss. These processes manifest as delayed wound healing, muscle wasting, and long-term rehabilitative failure if they are not adequately treated. Recent experimental efforts have examined the pharmacologic attenuation of burn-related metabolic disturbances with the administration of exogenous β-adrenergic blockade, human growth hormone, insulin, synthetic testosterone analogues, and nutrient-specific enteral formulae to restore systemic anabolic balance (Herndon and Tompkins, 2004; Pereira and Herndon, 2005; Mayes et al., 2008; Jeschke et al., 2008).

Gastroduodenal ulceration is a common complication of extensive burns that can be prevented with the early administration of proton-pump inhibitors, H_2-receptor antagonists, and neutralizing agents such as sulcrafate. Acid prophylaxis is an important adjunctive therapy, because thermal injury is strongly associated with disruptions of the mucosal intestinal barrier. Severe burns induce enlargement of the mucosal gap junctions and are followed by bacterial translocation and systemic absorption of endotoxins; these two factors contribute to an increased risk of sepsis (Ziegler et al., 1988). Enteral feeding is superior to intravenous caloric administration as a means of preserving gastrointestinal motility and mucosal barrier integrity and reducing the incidence of enterogenic infection (Chen et al., 2007).

Hematologic Abnormalities

The immediate postburn period features a significant contraction of red blood cell mass secondary to destruction by heat-induced denaturation, lysis by circulating free radicals, and sequestration in the extravascular space. Hemoglobinuria (particularly after electrical injury) and the accumulation of cellular debris promote cast formation and impair renal function. Normal erythrocyte deformability may also be affected with a subsequent decrease in functional half-life and an increased risk of thrombosis (Schachar et al., 1974). During the acute phase, normal or supranormal hemoglobin measurements may represent hemoconcentration—an indirect indicator of inadequate resuscitation. After restoration of intravascular volume, anemia can persist despite elevated levels of erythropoietin; persistent bone marrow suppression is likely mediated by circulating inflammatory factors (Jelkmann et al., 1990). Repetitive excisional procedures, gastroduodenal ulceration, and phlebotomy are other important factors to consider during assessment of ongoing blood loss. Because of the limited circulating blood volumes of infants and small children, these may become disproportionately significant sources of anemia.

Platelet abnormalities initially manifest as thrombocytopenia secondary to platelet aggregation, microemboli consumption, and dilution secondary to large-volume fluid administration. A biphasic pattern is seen when thrombocytosis occurs 10 to

14 days postburn and continues for several months (Heideman, 1979). Qualitative platelet function may be altered after thermal injury, and clinical evidence of coagulopathy should be treated with platelet transfusions. Persistent thrombocytopenia in the immediate postburn period is associated with sepsis and is considered to be a poor prognostic indicator.

Elevations of factors V, VII, VIII, fibrinogen, and fibrinogen split products normally occur with burn trauma and indicate thrombotic and fibrinolytic pathway activity. Despite increased factor levels that may continue for months, there does not seem to be a higher incidence of hypercoagulable states (Simon et al., 1977). The response to extensive burn trauma may include disseminated intravascular coagulation (DIC); the clinical diagnosis is supported by thrombocytopenia, decreased fibrinogen, prothrombin time (PT)/partial thromboblastin time (PTT) prolongation, and elevated levels of fibrin split products. Underlying etiologies (e.g., sepsis, hypoxemia, and burn shock) need to be identified and aggressively treated using blood product transfusions as supportive therapy.

Neurologic Injury

Varying degrees of neurologic dysfunction may occur through multiple mechanisms, and the evaluation of these deficits remains particularly challenging in infants and young children. Direct nerve trauma from crush or electrical injuries and compartment syndromes often appear as peripheral neuropathies and profound sensorimotor loss. Neurologic dysfunction may also arise from the acute or delayed toxic effects of hypoxia, metabolic derangements, and potential drug interactions. Burn encephalopathy is a complex syndrome characterized by a variable course of delirium, hallucinations, seizure activity, coma, and behavioral changes that afflict as many as 1 in 7 pediatric burn patients (Antoon et al., 1972). One third of all pediatric burn patients are predisposed to acute stress disorders, and the incidence increases with burn severity (Stoddard et al., 2006). Additional neuropsychiatric disturbances may arise from the complex interactions of stress, anxiety, anticipated procedural pain, and generalized sleep deprivation that often occurs in the intensive care environment but remains underappreciated.

Children with severe burn injuries often become obtunded in the first hours after trauma as a result of rapid fluid shifts, side effects of analgesia, and stress-related exhaustion. CO intoxication must always be suspected and promptly treated; diagnostic delays may manifest as persistent neurologic deficits in the survivors (Meert et al., 1998). Occult brain trauma should be investigated with computerized axial tomography when the elicited patient history supports a mechanism of injury.

Increased intracranial pressure from cerebral edema may occur within 72 hours postinjury (Gueugniaud et al., 1997). Patients requiring massive volume resuscitation may be subject to electrolyte shifts that potentiate the risk of cerebral edema and subsequent seizure activity. Aggressive correction of iatrogenic hyponatremia results in central pontine demyelination (Cohen et al., 1991). Serial monitoring of electrolyte concentrations and correcting imbalances help avert undesirable consequences.

In addition to direct nerve trauma, metabolic derangements, and tissue hypoxia, peripheral neuropathies may evolve secondary to constrictive dressings complicated by progressive edema (Dagum et al., 1993). Careful attention to patient positioning and periodic documentation of peripheral pulses by Doppler ultrasound helps detect vascular compromise.

The pediatric burn patient is exposed to varying degrees of polypharmacy during efforts to achieve clinically adequate sedation and analgesia, often through the use of supranormal doses of benzodiazepines, narcotics, and other drugs for extended periods. Burn-related derangements of hepatic and renal function alter the normal pharmacodynamics and kinetics of these agents and contribute to unpredictable plasma concentrations. The clinician should be aware that these agents may be associated with transient or sustained neurocognitive impairments observed in some pediatric burn patients. Several animal studies have identified the potential for premature apoptotic neurodegeneration with the use of drugs that interact with N-methyl-D-aspartate (NMDA) and γ-aminobutyric acid (GABA) receptors (Jevtovic-Todorovic et al., 2003; Young et al., 2005). Many of the anesthetic agents expected to be used throughout the conduct of pediatric burn procedures (e.g., midazolam and ketamine) act at one or both receptor sites and are implicated as potential sources for neuroapoptosis; there are data suggesting that some combinations of these agents may possess greater neurotoxic potency. No information is currently available to reliably identify the least harmful pharmacologic choice (Mellon et al., 2007) (see Chapter 7, Pharmacology).

Immunosuppression

The child with major burn trauma suffers from epithelial barrier loss and a dynamic proinflammatory cascade that creates a grossly immunocompromised state. Absence of the normal dermal functions is further complicated by the infectious potential of invasive monitoring devices and passive exposure to drug-resistant organisms (Weber et al., 1997). Bacterial translocation secondary to gastrointestinal-permeability changes increases the incidence of sepsis. Common inflammatory mediators have been demonstrated to impair neutrophil chemotaxis and cytotoxic activity (Church et al., 2006). Strict observance of sterile technique, early burn wound excision, restoration of dermal barriers, and targeted antibiotic administration are all important components to limit infectious complications.

PHARMACOLOGIC ALTERATIONS

Pediatric burn patients experience a spectrum of metabolic and organ-system derangements, with implications for the pharmacodynamics and kinetics of commonly-used anesthetic drugs. Significant interpatient variability observed with drug uptake and elimination necessitates the titration of all prescribed medications toward a desirable clinical endpoint, and each individual should be frequently reassessed for developing side effects. The more extensive the burn injury, the more pronounced this phenomenon (Martyn, 1986).

Intravascular depletion, transcompartmental fluid shifts, and blood-flow deficits in organs are factors that alter the distribution volume and clearance mechanisms of the drugs used throughout the acute burn admission. Major organ perfusion is preserved at the expense of blood flow to the gastrointestinal tract and extremity muscle groups and thereby renders oral and intramuscular administration routes of uptake unreliable. Organ blood flow improves with the onset of the hypermetabolic phase, but it is not clear if there is a concurrent increase in the rate of drug metabolism (Wilmore et al., 1980; Aulick et al., 1981). Hepatic protein synthesis shifts from albumin to α_1-acid glycoprotein during the hypermetabolic phase. Albumin binds acidic drugs (e.g., benzodiazepines), and a reduction of circulating protein levels increases the pharmacologically active fraction. Conversely, α_1-acid glycoprotein provides competitive binding sites for basic drugs (e.g., muscle relaxants) and reduces muscle bioavailability (Martyn et al., 1984).

Neuromuscular Relaxants

Succinylcholine is normally an appropriate drug selection to facilitate rapid sequence inductions and establish a definitive airway; however, in the context of the acutely burned patient, the risk of a severe hyperkalemic response must be carefully considered (Tolmie et al., 1967; Gronert and Theye, 1975). Excessive succinylcholine-induced potassium efflux may be observed as early as 12 hours postinjury and can persist for up to 2 years (Gronert, 1999). It has been posited that extensive proliferation of acetylcholine receptors and multiple isoforms occur throughout the muscle membrane, even at sites distant from the original injury (Martyn et al., 2006). As large masses of extrajunctional tissues are depolarized, serum potassium levels rapidly increase to induce lethal cardiac arrhythmias. Some controversy remains concerning the onset and duration of receptor proliferation with the subsequent risk of hyperkalemic responses, but the availability of rapid-acting nondepolarizing alternatives (e.g., rocuronium) obviate the need for succinylcholine in acute burn management.

Resistance to a variety of nondepolarizing muscle relaxants (NDMRs) has been previously reported (Martyn et al., 1983a, 1983b; Mills and Martyn, 1989). Although there are notable distinctions concerning the pharmacokinetics and protein-binding capacities between patient cohorts with and without burns, these factors probably do not contribute significantly to observed clinical differences. Increases in receptor density are believed to be the predominant mechanism attributable to developing NDMR tolerance, and this effect correlates with burn severity (Martyn et al., 1982). Studies of vecuronium and rocuronium in adults with thermal injuries demonstrated the clinical effects of this resistance phenomenon; longer onset times and shorter recovery profiles were observed and attributed to decreased drug saturation of an enlarged receptor population (Fig. 31-6) (Mills and Martyn, 1989; Han et al., 2004). Burn patients generally require larger doses of NDMRs to produce clinically relevant responses for airway manipulation and surgical procedures (Table 31-5). The serum half-lives of the short- and intermediate-acting relaxants do not appear to be prolonged, and appropriate reversal of neuromuscular blockade is successful using the normal dosing ranges of neostigmine and glycopyrrolate (Martyn et al., 2006).

Analgesics

Effective pain management for pediatric burn patients is highly desirable but difficult to achieve consistently because of the varying intensities of pain associated with recurrent

débridement, dressing changes, and physical therapy occurring throughout treatment. Previously, insufficient analgesic administration was often because of unsupported but lingering reservations concerning the risk of addiction to potent narcotics (Perry and Heidrich, 1982). Additional confounders included patient- or family-held misconceptions concerning dependence and associated social stigma, clinicians' fear of potential litigation, and individual variations of nociception attributable to cultural differences. Frequent assessment with age-appropriate rating systems, education, and candid discussions about reasonable expectations for pain relief have largely eliminated opiate underuse.

In addition to their analgesic properties, opiates attenuate metabolic demands and help reduce the anxiety that is encountered during extended stays in an intensive care unit. Rapid-dose escalation is a consequence of thermal-injury–induced changes observed in protein binding, distribution volume, altered clearance, and hypermetabolism. Consequently, individual titration of opioid analgesic agents to appropriate clinical endpoints is a consistent and effective analgesic technique (as opposed to arbitrarily recommended dosing regimens) to making patients comfortable.

Morphine sulfate is widely used, and although its metabolism to active glucuronidated metabolites suggests a prolonged duration of action, this has not been substantiated (Furman et al., 1990; Perreault et al., 2001). Fentanyl is another common choice, and kinetics studies in adults have demonstrated increased distribution volumes and clearance; these changes have partially explained observed increases in opiate requirements (Han et al., 2007; Kaneda and Han, 2009). Agonist-antagonist drugs (e.g., nalbuphine) theoretically offer the advantage of analgesia without significant respiratory depression; when administered to adult patients for limited debridement procedures, results have compared favorably with morphine (Lee et al., 1989). Methadone has been used for patients who were unresponsive to other analgesics, but its duration of action may be variable in the context of burn-related drug kinetics (Concilus et al., 1989). Methadone also possesses weak NMDA antagonism and as such may be an appropriate drug selection to minimize opioid tolerance and pathologic hyperalgesia (the paradoxical sensitization to painful stimuli) (Callahan et al., 2004). With its ultrashort half-life (7 to 10 minutes), remifentanil has no practical utility in the burn unit.

Tolerance develops in pediatric burn patients, but this fact should not preclude opioid administration. Addiction and the subsequent abuse of narcotics are rare when opiates are prescribed to achieve clinically appropriate endpoints (Porter and Jick, 1980; Goodman and McGrath, 1991). The supranormal dosing ranges commonly needed to provide effective analgesia in burn patients are the consequence of thermal-injury–induced quantitative and qualitative changes of receptor populations. After skin wound closure, opioid requirements rapidly decline. Undesirable withdrawal symptoms can be avoided by prescribing a gradual taper that parallels the decreasing frequency of procedures conducted during the acute injury phase (see Chapter 15, Pain Management).

Although opioid addiction has not been observed with regularity among the pediatric burn population, some animal studies cite potential adverse effects from exposure to high-dose narcotic regimens. Hyperalgesia has been observed in burn patients who have been the recipients of opiate-dose escalation, and this

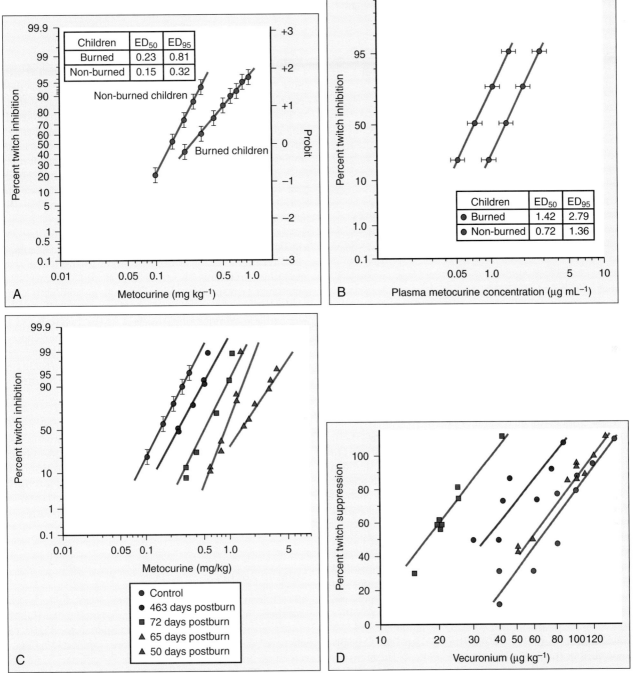

■ FIGURE 31-6. These four figures illustrate the neuromuscular effects of nondepolarizing agents in burn patients. Figures **A** and **B** show the increased dose requirement for metocurine on a mg/kg and plasma-concentration basis, respectively. Figure **C** demonstrates the effect of age of burn on neuromuscular blockade. Even after 1 year, patients with burns are still resistant to neuromuscular blocking agents. Figure **D** shows the effects of burn area on neuromuscular blockade resistance. Group 1 *(purple square)* is comprised of patients in a control group with burn injuries that occurred 3 years before the study. Group 2 *(red circle)* is made up of patients with less than 40% burn area. Group 3 *(blue triangle)* includes patients with 40% to 60% burn area, group 4 *(brown circle)* has patients with more than 60% burn area. *(From Martyn JAJ, et al.: Unprecendented resistance to neuromuscular locking effects of metocurine with persistence after complete recovery in a burned patient,* Anesth Analg *61:61, 1982; Martyn JAJ, et al.: Metocurine requirements and plasma concentrations in burned paediatric patients,* Br J Anaesth *55:263, 1983; and Mills AK, Martyn JA: Neuromuscular blockade with vecuronium in paediatric patients with burn injury,* Br J Clin Pharmacol *28:155, 1989.)*

condition is thought to be secondary to neuroplastic changes in nociception pathways (Chu et al., 2008). Modulations of spinal receptors may produce hyperalgesic conditions secondary to inhibitory neuron apoptosis (Angst and Clark, 2006). Tolerance and opioid-induced hyperalgesia are clinically similar (both show evidence of decreased analgesic efficacy) but the molecular mechanisms are distinct. Other studies have examined opioids and their contribution to postburn immunosuppression, possibly through cytokine modulation (Alexander et al., 2005; Schwacha et al., 2006).

TABLE 31-5. Emergency-Department Values of Vecuronium in Burn Patients and Control Patients

(% TBSA Burn)	Study Group	
	ED$_{50}$ (mcg/kg)	ED$_{95}$ (mcg/kg)
Controls	17.6 (15.4-19.9)[†]	35.3 (30.6-42.3)
<40	34.0* (29.3-38.7)[‡]	68.2* (59.8-79.9)
40-60	55.4* (48.1-62.1)	111.1* (99.8-126.2)
>60	64.5* (57.4-71.9)	129.4* (113.0-154.0)

From Mills AK, Martyn JA: Neuromuscular blockade with vecuronium in paediatric patients with burn injury, *Br J Clin Pharm* 28:155, 1989.
*Significantly different from controls, p < 0.01.
[†]Numbers in parentheses represent lower and upper 95% confidence limits.
[‡]ED$_{50}$ and ED$_{95}$ for vecuronium are significantly increased in burned children compared with controls; the shift in the dose-response curve is related to the magnitude of burn.
TBSA, Total body surface area; *ED$_{50}$* and *ED$_{95}$*, effective doses for 50% and 95% twitch suppression.

Anxiolytics

Adequate sedation improves acceptance of prolonged mechanical ventilation, decreases narcotic requirements, and reduces anxiety associated with dressing changes or other bedside procedures. Benzodiazepine infusions are administered concurrently with opioids, and patient requirements are elevated in the presence of developing tolerance and altered pharmacokinetics. Daily background infusions up to 0.1 mg/kg per hour are typical for severely burned patients and may be titrated to desired clinical effect throughout the weaning period (Sheridan et al., 2001). Clinicians should be aware of potential side effects; in one pediatric study, neurocognitive and behavioral changes attributed to midazolam fully resolved with drug cessation (Sheridan et al., 1994).

Dexmedetomidine is an α_2-agonist with analgesic, anxiolytic, and sedative properties that has been used successfully as a supplement for mechanically ventilated children with opiate and benzodiazepine resistance (Walker et al., 2006). It is insufficient for primary analgesia but offers minimal respiratory depression and reasonable hemodynamic stability. In contrast to other sedative agents, treatment with dexmedetomidine mimics a physiologic sleep state that may attenuate sleep-related disorders observed in the intensive-care environment. Hypotension and bradycardia are potential side-effects of dexmedetomidine, presumably mediated through unopposed vagal stimulation (Carroll et al., 2008).

Patients treated with protracted opioid and benzodiazepine infusions are required to metabolize several half-lives worth of drug. In this setting, it is often difficult to balance the need for clinically effective sedation with the desire for the prompt return of protective airway reflexes. Short-term infusions of propofol have been used in the hours preceding extubation, so that opiate and benzodiazepine administration may be adequately weaned (Sheridan et al., 2003). Extended infusions of propofol are not suitable for pediatric burn patients, because there is an ill-defined risk of refractory acidosis and myocardial depression specific to the lipid-based emulsion (Parke et al., 1992; Vasile et al., 2003). Additionally, bacterial contamination of a centrally-infused sedative would be poorly tolerated in the setting of postburn immunosuppression (see Chapter 7, Pharmacology).

Ketamine

Some animal models that studied thermal injury have demonstrated an increase in NMDA receptors, which suggests that ketamine (a noncompetitive antagonist) may be a more effective analgesic than opioids for burn patients. Ketamine may also prove useful in reducing the incidence of opioid-induced hyperalgesia. Its analgesic potency is enhanced by several metabolites, the most active of which is norketamine (which possesses one third of the potency of ketamine). Used in combination with benzodiazepines, its half-life increases 20% to 30% (Reich and Silvay, 1980).

Ketamine produces a dose-dependent shift of the carbon dioxide response curve but unlike other hypnotic agents, does not alter the slope; hypercarbic respiratory drive remains intact at clinically relevant doses (Bourke et al., 1987). Preservation of spontaneous respiratory drive is complemented with a degree of hemodynamic stability secondary to centrally mediated sympathetic stimulation. However, in the hypovolemic burn patient who has exhausted the compensatory endogenous catecholamines, ketamine acts as a direct myocardial depressant (Owens et al., 2006). Dosing should be adjusted to avoid hemodynamic collapse in these patients or a vasoactive infusion (e.g., norepinephrine) can be used to provide a background level of sympathomimetic support.

Because concurrent benzodiazepine administration is so prevalent in burn patients, the unpleasant psychomimetic residua attributed to ketamine have not been clinically significant. Ketamine has been used as an adjunct for other drugs, and multiple delivery routes make it particularly suitable for those burn patients with behavioral difficulties or developmental delay (Allison and Smith, 1998; Heinrich et al., 2004; Tosun et al., 2008).

Volatile Agents

All of the common volatile agents have been successfully used for anesthetic maintenance in pediatric burn patients. Halothane is inexpensive and possesses some residual anesthetic effect, whereas sevoflurane promotes more rapid awakening and return of protective airway reflexes. Sevoflurane is an appropriate choice for inhalation induction, but its rapid taper may be associated with an increased incidence of emergence delirium (Kain et al., 2005). Patients with acute injuries and decompensated burn shock generally do not tolerate the vasodilation associated with potent volatile agents; concurrent vasoactive support may be needed. Pediatric burn patients with residual pulmonary injury and elevated metabolism demonstrate variable degrees of dead-space ventilation and elevated cardiac output that may alter the speed of inhalation inductions.

CONSIDERATIONS FOR INITIAL MANAGEMENT

After admission of the pediatric burn patient, there are three immediate goals that should be addressed simultaneously: the clinician should conduct a prompt airway assessment and judge the perceived risk of impending compromise; the burn process should be arrested to prevent further tissue destruction; and burn shock and its treatment with volume resuscitation should be evaluated. A brief review of conditions at the scene and pertinent transport events is also prudent.

Airway

Supraglottic edema has the potential to evolve rapidly and severely reduce airway patency. Aspiration of scalding liquids or caustic agents may have a presentation similar to that of epiglottitis (Sheridan, 1996). A focused history should identify factors supporting possible inhalational injury; prolonged extrication from a confined space is consistent with increased risk (Box 31-2). Preexisting pulmonary disease and prior intubation attempts in the field by paramedic personnel should also be reviewed.

Fiberoptic bronchoscopy has been used to support the diagnosis of inhalation injury but should not supersede clinical judgment (Hunt et al., 1975). Arterial blood gas values and chest radiographs are often normal with initial presentation and may therefore provide false reassurance of patient stability. The absence of overt thermal injury does not preclude significant CO poisoning and 100% fraction of inspired oxygen (Fio_2) should be empirically applied. Although it is not always possible to avoid the "lost airway scenario," the clinician should be aware that the American Society of Anesthesiologists' (ASA) difficult-airway algorithm has practical limitations when applied to pediatric burn patients. Fiberoptic intubation performed when the patient is awake is rarely feasible for injured children who are not profoundly sedated, and the presence of oropharyngeal debris or edema reduces the likelihood of success. See related video online at www.expertconsult.com. Small ketamine boluses titrated to maintain spontaneous ventilation provide a reasonable margin of safety over the protocolized administration of rapid-sequence hypnotics and muscle relaxants. Ketamine is thought to leave protective airway reflexes intact; however, this may not be the case depending on the level of sedation (Drummand, 1996; Peña and Krauss, 1999).

A semielective surgical airway created early may be considered for facial burns, because ensuing edema alters anatomy and renders endotracheal tube stabilization difficult at best (Fig. 31-7) (Palmieri et al., 2002). Perceived advantages of early tracheostomy in the setting of prolonged mechanical ventilation remain controversial (Saffle et al., 2002). Laryngeal mask airways have been used as a bridging technique to definitive airway control, but direct injuries to the oral cavity and unpredictable

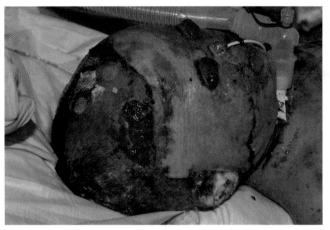

■ **FIGURE 31-7.** Full-thickness facial burn. The patient required autografts to produce biological wound closure. A tracheostomy provides improved safety during multiple surgical procedures and patient transports.

swelling may prevent an adequate seal and preclude delivery of sufficient tidal volumes. Progressive edema distorts facial and neck circumference, leading to inadvertent malposition or extubation; the endotracheal tube must be thoroughly stabilized (often using nonconventional methods such as dental anchoring with sutures or wire). Potentially catastrophic dislodgement may be minimized with frequent reassessments and secondary confirmation by chest radiographs.

Volume Resuscitation

Adequate intravenous access is problematic with extensive tissue destruction, and patients often require central venous catheters (femoral or subclavian) for extended periods. Intraosseous routes offer a safe and reliable alternative in the presence of severe injury and are suitable for large-volume infusions (Horton and Beamer, 2008) (see Chapter 30, Anesthesia for the Pediatric Trauma Patient). Bladder catheterization is performed to accurately quantitate urine output and continuously evaluate the efficacy of ongoing resuscitation.

Treatment of burn shock initially depends on weight-based calculations for crystalloid administration. There are several formulas in use, but none is ideal or suitable for every patient and should only provide guidelines; actual fluid volumes need to be based on the patient's clinical response (Warden, 2002). The Parkland formula recommends 4mL/kg per percentage of burn over 24 hours, with half of the calculated volume delivered during the first 8 hours of treatment, followed by the projected balance over the remaining 16 hours. The Brooke formula uses a combination of crystalloid and colloid delivered over the same time period (Table 31-6). However, a recent adult study demonstrated that volume requirements based on accepted values of minimal hourly urine output were higher than those predicted by the either formula (Blumetti et al., 2008). The formulas are inadequate when calculating resuscitation requirements for children who weigh less than 10kg. A suggested guideline for these patients is to administer the sum of normal hourly maintenance fluids and the volumes derived from the Parkland or Brooke formula over a 24-hour period (Graves et al., 1988).

Capillary permeability increases in patients with burns more than 20% TBSA, and the degree of change correlates with burn

---

Box 31-2 Indicators of Lower-Airway Injury*

Victim extricated from enclosed environment
Burns noted on face, lips, nares, or intraoral cavaties
Carbonaceous debris in mouth, nose, or sputum
Stridor or hoarseness
Dyspnea, retractions, or nasal flaring
Hypoxia
CO confirmed by cooximeter

*Symptom onset and severity are highly variable.

TABLE 31-6. Parkland and Brooke Formulas for Fluid Management in Burn Patients

	Crystalloid (mL/kg)	Colloid	(mL/kg)
Parkland	4.0	0	X% Burn
Brooke	1.5	0.45	X% Burn

Half of the calculated volume is administered in first 8 hours. The remainder is administered over the next 16 hours.

severity. Some centers advocate the use of colloids as the primary fluid choice during early resuscitation, because colloids offer improved intravascular retention and may decrease the total volume requirements while minimizing tissue edema (Sheridan, 2002). There has been no definitive demonstration of improved outcomes when isotonic crystalloid- and colloid-resuscitation regimens have been compared (Bowser-Wallace and Caldwell, 1986). Hypertonic saline has been proposed as an alternative choice for resuscitation fluids, but the outcomes data are unclear and there is a potential risk of iatrogenic hypernatremia (Huang et al., 1995; Junger et al., 1997). Normal vascular integrity is usually restored within 24 to 36 hours if resuscitation efforts are adequate.

Hypoglycemia may occur during the resuscitation of infants and children weighing less than 20 kg. Lactated Ringer's solution with 5% dextrose delivered at a maintenance rate helps preserve appropriate serum-glucose levels, but frequent monitoring is recommended during the first 24 hours after injury. Myoglobin and hemoglobin released from damaged tissues may impair renal function, and pigmented urine should be cleared with adequate intravenous fluids. Severely compromised individuals may require sodium bicarbonate or mannitol to avoid mechanical obstruction from cast formation.

Achieving clinometric targets consistent with normal organ perfusion (goal-oriented resuscitation) has prove superior to the fulfillment of rote volume algorithms, and this principle has been an important advance of modern burn care (Box 31-3). Urine output (1 to 1.5 mL/kg per hour) has been cited as an indicator of systemic normoperfusion, and the maintenance of target outputs often requires intravenous volumes that exceed the initial formulaic predictions (Yowler and Fratianne, 2000; Hoskins et al., 2006). Closed-loop and decision-assist algorithms have been introduced to manage infusion rates directed by desired levels of urinary flow and have the potential to reduce total volume requirements and minimize edema (Salinas et al., 2008). Despite these advances, there

is growing controversy concerning the suitability of accepted invasive monitors and clinical endpoints as valid indicators of adequate cellular perfusion (Ahrns, 2004). Further research is needed to refine monitoring strategies and identify physiologic markers that accurately reflect oxygen derangements and perfusion deficits.

Nutritional Supplementation

Early enteral feeding via a nasoduodenal tube provides caloric support and helps maintain the integrity of the intestinal mucosal barrier that restricts bacterial translocation (McDonald et al., 1991). These devices offer the opportunity for continuous feeding throughout surgical procedures without the risk of aspiration. Patients with extensive burns or inadequate volume replacement may not tolerate these feedings because of splanchnic hypoperfusion (Jenkins et al., 1994). Poor caloric replacement results in delayed wound healing, an increased risk of sepsis, and resistance to ventilator weaning from catabolic loss of lean body mass. Modulation of hormonal, adrenergic, and inflammatory mediators continues to be the focus of therapeutic research (Ipaktchi and Arbabi, 2006).

Surgical Excision

The goal of current surgical techniques is to remove necrotic debris and achieve biological wound closure. The early reestablishment of a physical barrier, which provides protection from bacteria, mechanical trauma, and insensible water loss, improves long-term outcomes even for those patients who have experienced significant thermal injury. Variable mesh sizes may expand harvested autograft coverage, but staged procedures are to be expected in patients with more than 50% TBSA as suitable donor sites are rapidly depleted. Split-thickness cadaveric allograft provides physiologic protection similar to native skin (Sheridan and Tompkins, 1999). A number of dermal analogs have been manufactured and used clinically. Integra (Integra Life Sciences; Plainboro, New Jersey) is a bovine-derived acellular dressing that promotes fibroblast migration and growth. Alloderm (LifeCell Corporation; The Woodlands, Texas) is an acellular collagen matrix procured from screened cadaveric donors. These dermal substitutes restore protective barriers and provide a structural framework for the rapid revascularization and fibroblast repopulation of the recipient sites (Sheridan, 2002). As wound healing progresses, temporary biological dressings are resurfaced with autograft. Physiologic closure is most advantageous when performed within the first 24 hours of injury to circumvent wound colonization and reduce the systemic inflammatory response.

Excisional procedures have been refined so that blood loss is minimized through the use of extremity tourniquets, subcutaneous deposition of diluted epinephrine, and controlled operative times. These operations are still associated with hemorrhage in the range of 3% to 5% of estimated blood volume for each 1% TBSA excised (Budny et al., 1993; Housinger et al., 1993). Intraoperative fluid selection and replacement should be guided by oxygen delivery needs and serial lab analysis.

Circumferential burns are notable for the inelastic eschar that can quickly induce neurovascular compromise, possibly leading to limb loss. Patients with thoracic-wall involvement

---

Box 31-3 Clinical Endpoints for Volume Resuscitation

Intact sensorium
Normothermia
Age-appropriate hemodynamics
Sustained urine output (= 1 mL/kg/hr; negative glucose or protein)
Minimal systemic acidosis, base deficit less than 2

Adapted from Sheridan RL: Burns, *Crit Care Med* 30:S500, 2002.

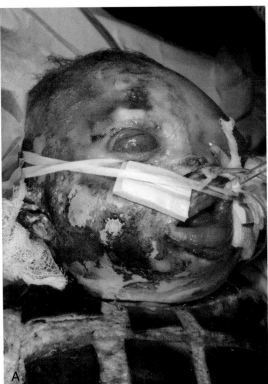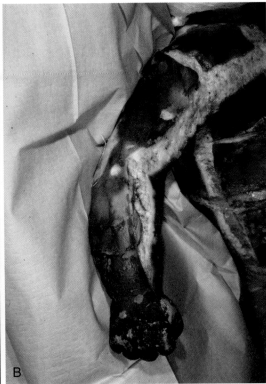

■ FIGURE 31-8. Escharotomies. The patient experienced more than 60% full-thickness burns and required escharotomies of the chest **(A)** and upper extremities **(B)** to relieve compartment syndrome and reduce neurovascular compromise.

develop a restrictive form of respiratory insufficiency. Extensive burns involving the trunk may be complicated by abdominal compartment syndrome, which has symptoms of diminished venous return, cardiac output, and urinary flow (Jensen et al., 2006). Escharotomies decompress these insults to restore perfusion (Fig. 31-8).

Concurrent Trauma

All pediatric patients should be evaluated as multitrauma victims because of the increased morbidity associated with missed injuries. Falling debris from destabilized structures and explosions associated with transmitted overpressure may complicate burn management with varying degrees of neurologic trauma, fractures, and internal hemorrhage. In older children and adolescents, there is also the possibility of alcohol or drug ingestion that adds further layers of complexity to treatment. A focused history and complete secondary survey help guide pertinent labwork, x-ray studies, and other diagnostics for treatment of concurrent injuries.

PERIOPERATIVE CONSIDERATIONS

After initial resuscitation efforts, the pediatric burn patient is likely to need repetitive excision and grafting procedures to achieve appropriate wound closure. Volume replacement continues throughout the conduct of serial operations and the usual physiologic insults associated with surgical trauma add to those resulting from thermal and traumatic injuries.

Preoperative Assessment

The clinician should assess the resuscitation efficacy by examining current trends of hemodynamics, urinary output, and use of vasoactive support. Airway evaluation includes the confirmation of endotracheal tube position and ventilator settings. Electrolyte balance, serial hematocrit, and arterial blood gas results should also be reviewed.

The proposed procedure is discussed with the burn surgeon to address anticipated blood and fluid requirements. Ideally, both the surgeon and anesthesiologist should agree on parameters for abbreviating the surgical plan if the patient's condition deteriorates unexpectedly. The parents also need to be briefed about potential surgical and anesthetic risks to establish informed consent.

Induction and Airway Management

The transfer of a patient to the operating room presents opportunities for inadvertent extubation, intravenous catheter displacement, hypothermia, and respiratory insufficiency after separation from the ventilator in the intensive care unit. Additional personnel need to be recruited for safely transporting multiple infusion sets, as well as providing assisted ventilation and uninterrupted hemodynamic monitoring. The patient must be kept warm, and it is advisable to continue adequate sedation during the transfer process.

Standard monitor application is often problematic with extensive burn injury and concurrent trauma. Noninvasive blood-pressure cuffs may not provide reliable data, necessitating the placement of an arterial catheter. Oximetric signal degradation often occurs with poor peripheral perfusion; oximeters have been creatively applied to many locations (e.g., tongue, cheek wall, nose, and ear lobe) for improved signal capture. Redundant monitors in this setting are recommended, because surgical manipulation and patient repositioning further deteriorate signal transduction. Electrocardiogram pads may not adhere to burned tissue, and adequate lead contact may be accomplished with needle probes.

Performing the induction with the patient in the intensive-care bed is reasonable, because discomfort caused by transferral to the operating room table and positioning is common. Selection of the induction drug is based predominantly on hemodynamic status, and volume-repleted patients are likely to tolerate most intravenous induction agents. The suitability of ketamine for hemodynamically compromised individuals relates to its moderate sympathomimetic effect and preservation of cardiac output. Caution is warranted for select patients who already function at the limit of their sympathetic response; exogenous catecholamine support with epinephrine or norepinephrine may be required to avoid sudden cardiovascular decompensation.

Mechanical trauma and edema may sufficiently alter facial features to impair mask fit and assisted ventilation. Tight eschar restricts mandibular mobility and mouth opening despite effective muscle relaxation. Mask-seal maintenance may require the participation of a second anesthesia provider. In general, difficult airways should be anticipated for the first 24 to 48 hours, with alternative techniques and necessary equipment immediately available. The surgeon should be physically present to perform an emergent tracheostomy in the event of an unrecoverable airway. In rare circumstances, the use of extracorporeal membrane oxygenation has been used as the initial technique to maintain oxygenation in a patient who had surgery for delayed closure with gross neck deformity that was judged sufficient to preclude tracheostomy rescue (Sheridan et al., 2008). Primary tracheostomy might be considered in the presence of gross deformities of the face, neck or head, but there are risks of long-term sequelae (Palmieri et al., 2002).

Fiberoptic-assisted endotracheal intubation is the preferred method for securing a potentially difficult pediatric airway. Appropriate sedation and maintenance of spontaneous respirations may be accomplished by the judicious use of low-dose ketamine or dexmedetomidine infusion. Manual distraction of the tongue, jaw thrust, and antisialogue therapy improve conditions. The success of additional methods such as retrograde wire, light wand, and GlideScope video laryngoscopy (Verathon; Bothell, Washington) have been reported (Hsu et al., 2007, 2008). Some practitioners have advocated the use of laryngeal mask airways to avoid the potential trauma of repetitive intubations, but this method is impractical if an adequate seal cannot be maintained secondary to anatomic distortion (McCall et al., 1999). Laryngeal mask airways may also be used as an assist-device to facilitate fiberoptic intubation as previously described (see Chapter 12, Airway Management). All airway devices possess positive qualities and disadvantages, and the specific use of any technique should be guided by the anticipated needs of the patient and the clinician's experience.

Endotracheal tube stabilization is often difficult and must be tested repeatedly as the patient is repositioned throughout the procedure. Various tapes, staples, and wiring of the endotracheal tube to the teeth have all been successfully employed to maintain a secure airway. If postoperative mechanical ventilation is anticipated, a nasotracheal tube offers stability, improved patient comfort, and the capacity to better deliver oral care.

Ventilator settings should mimic those delivered in the intensive care unit, with the stipulation that surgical manipulation and repositioning require repeated adjustment of ventilatory parameters. Noncompliant lung tissue and restricted thoracic-wall expansion dictate the delivery of elevated pressures and the application of positive end-expiratory pressure (PEEP) to provide adequate gas exchange. Cuffed endotracheal tubes, sometimes avoided in small children, ensure an effective subglottic seal for the transmission of adequate inspiratory pressures. As edema resolves, cuff inflation can be adjusted to maintain an appropriate air leak while preserving delivered tidal volumes. Periodic assessment of arterial blood gases is recommended, because the end-tidal carbon dioxide (E_{TCO_2}) may not accurately reflect arterial carbon dioxide secondary to increased dead-space ventilation and shunt.

Maintenance of Anesthesia

Many techniques (e.g., nitrous oxide and oxygen [N_2O/O_2], total intravenous anesthesia [TIVA], volatile agents, and various combinations) have been used, and selection is often based on the patient's physiologic status and surgical procedure. Preoperative infusions should be continued in the operating theater, including caloric replacement delivered via nasoduodenal tube feeds. Opiate and benzodiazepine infusions can be supplemented with additional doses titrated to the level of clinical effect, and the provider should be aware of the generalized increase of these drug requirements. Antibiotic dosing schedules are often accelerated as a result of alterations of distribution volume and fluid loss. Resistance to NMDRs has been discussed previously; individual dosing regimens are adjusted according to monitored twitches.

The maintenance of normothermia is vital in the prevention of caloric wastage and coagulation defects during débridement. Increasing the ambient temperature and humidity is the most effective conservation method, although providers find prolonged exposure to these conditions to be personally uncomfortable. Wrapping exposed body segments in impermeable sleeves and other thermal barriers also reduces heat and evaporative losses, as does the incorporation of heated humidifier systems into the breathing circuit. All fluids and blood products should be delivered through heat-exchange devices. Forced–warm-air blankets have marginal utility because of the limited coverage of exposed body surfaces.

Hemostasis

Tangential excisions are invariably associated with hemorrhage, although the amount of blood loss during the procedure is difficult to quantitate, because blood is distributed among the drapes, table, and floor. Excisions of the face, neck, and head involve greater losses attributable to the increased vascularity of these areas. One study offered guidelines suggesting that 3% to 5% of estimated blood volume (EBV) will be lost for every 1% TBSA excised; increasing the precision of anticipated blood-volume loss may improve the efficiency of product ordering (Housinger et al., 1993). Where significant volume depletion is expected, transfusion therapy should begin preoperatively to maintain adequate oxygen delivery. Despite the known inaccuracies involved with blood-loss estimates, some practical intraoperative recommendations have been forwarded; the surgical time should be limited to no more than 2 hours, with the planned excision restricted to 15% TBSA. The procedure should be aborted if blood loss exceeds 50% EBV (Engrav et al., 1983).

Transfusion volumes that exceed the calculated EBV often cause dilutional thrombocytopenia and coagulation factor loss. The avoidance of unnecessary blood-product administration is desirable for the pediatric burn patient and relates to issues of cost, infectious potential, and risks of transfusion complications. There is no substantiated "transfusion trigger" for the pediatric burn patient, but the maintenance of a hematocrit value of 27% to 30%, guided by periodic intraoperative measurement and hemodynamic trends, is likely to be prudent in the context of hypermetabolism and elevated oxygen consumption.

Multiple blood conservation techniques have been described and include the injection of a saline solution mixed with diluted epinephrine, epinephrine-soaked compressive wraps, topical sealants, extremity tourniquets, and preoperative acute normovolemic hemodilution (Gomez et al., 2001; Losee et al., 2005). The tumescent technique uses a solution (consisting of isotonic crystalloid with 1:100,000 epinephrine) that is subdermally injected to facilitate eschar débridement and donor-site harvest by creating a smooth, tense skin surface (Robertson et al., 2001). Blood loss from freshly debrided areas can be further reduced by the liberal application of fibrin sealants or thrombin sprays that promote hemostasis and graft adherence (Nervi et al., 2001; Foster, 2007). Few adverse affects have been noted.

Postoperative Pain Management

Significant pain is to be expected, and opiate and benzodiazepine infusions should be continued in the immediate postoperative period, with additional bolus doses of narcotics titrated to clinical response. Developing tolerance and elevated baseline drug requirements often confound pain assessments but need not delay monitored dose escalation (Abdi and Zhou, 2002). Pain tends to be most intense from freshly harvested donor sites. The tumescent solution may be supplemented with bupivicaine (2 to 2.5 mg/kg) or lidocaine (5 to 7 mg/kg) for locoregional analgesia (Jellish et al., 1999; Bussolin et al., 2003). Serum measurements of local anesthetic absorption have demonstrated that this technique is safe and effective. Intravenous lidocaine infusion has also been used to improve analgesia and may possibly modulate nociceptive pathways in burn patients (Cassuto and Tarnow, 2003). However, the experience with local anesthetic infusion is limited to case reports and has yet to be validated in well-designed clinical trials (Wasiak and Cleland, 2007).

CONSIDERATIONS FOR OTHER BURN INJURIES

Electrical Injury

Low voltage events (those less than or equal to 500 volts) typically occur in the residential setting and are associated with full-thickness burns at the point of contact (most commonly the hands and oral cavity of young children). The voltage is

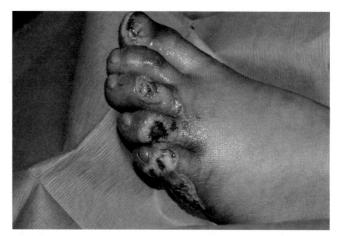

■ FIGURE 31-9. Electrical burn. The patient experienced a contact burn with an exposed electrical wire across the dorsa of the toes.

insufficient to traverse large body segments, so that deep tissue damage is generally limited to the area demarcated by the contact burn (Fig. 31-9). These injuries can still present significant trauma and airway management challenges, such as when an unfortunate young child suffers bilateral oral commissure burns from biting into an electrical cord. New-onset cardiac conduction abnormalities have also been documented (Garcia et al., 1995). Low-voltage burns are treated using the same principles as previously described for the care of thermal injuries.

High-voltage events (of 1000 volts or more) are generally encountered in commercial or industrial environments and involve catastrophic neurovascular and skeletal muscle damage that follows the conductive path from its source to the ground. Several distinct forms of trauma occur with these events: plasma arcing and its associated flash create localized heat in excess of 2000° F that often ignites clothing; high-energy electrical transfer produces acute cardiac and neurologic injury; and loss of coordination and profound muscle spasm is associated with falls, potential fractures, or organ rupture. Energy that passes through the axis of the trunk and limbs affects muscle, nerves, and vasculature. Unlike the entrance and exit wounds that demarcate the path of current flow, these devastating internal injuries are not immediately apparent. Victims of high-voltage electrical exposure should therefore be evaluated as polytrauma patients because there can be such a variety of resulting systemic manifestations (Edlich et al., 2005).

Initial treatment is focused on airway support and the identification of cardiac conduction abnormalities. The risk of delayed and unpredictable cardiac arrhythmias increases when the presenting history supports transthoracic current propagation, tetany, loss of consciousness, and abnormal electrocardiography results from admission (Bailey et al., 2007). Early fasciotomy is often necessary to preserve the extremities, as myonecrosis causes severe edema with subsequent compartment syndrome. Myoglobin and hemoglobin are released in large quantities, and their precipitation as glomerular casts impairs renal function. Urine output should be maintained with fluids, sodium bicarbonate-induced alkalinization, and osmotic diuretics. Global and focal neurologic dysfunction resulting from electrical exposure and its associated trauma is variable and may continue to affect the patient throughout the rehabilitation course (Cherington, 2005).

Chemical Exposure

Caustic liquids continue to damage adjacent tissues until the offending agent is neutralized, and clinician safety may be compromised if these active residuals are not properly handled (Fig. 31-10). Before definitive treatment begins, decontamination requires the removal of the patient's clothing and copious irrigation of affected surfaces with warm water until the efficacy of rinsing is confirmed with litmus paper applied to the wound (Sheridan, 2002). Consultation with a poison-control center is warranted if there is a potential risk of systemic toxicity from chemical absorption. Many caustic agents are potent respiratory irritants, and concurrent inhalation injury should be considered and treated appropriately.

REHABILITATION AND RECONSTRUCTIVE PROCEDURES

The medical and technical advances of modern burn care have reduced mortality and improved expectations concerning long-term functional outcomes and cosmesis. Physical therapy is a key element in preventing debilitating contractures, which may begin to form in young patients within days after their injury. Passive range of motion, antideformity positioning, and the application of therapeutic splints are all necessary but uncomfortable techniques; an adequate level of sedation and analgesia is needed to facilitate patient and family participation.

Many pediatric burn patients return to the operating room over the course of several years to reduce hypertrophic scarring and reestablish function, particularly with injuries that encompass the major joints, hands, and face. Children may have contractures and scar distortions in anatomic locations that provide limited intravenous access options. Inhalation induction is commonly used to permit multiple intravenous

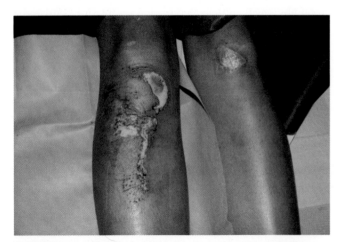

■ **FIGURE 31-10.** Chemical burn. The irregular, pitted appearance of this injury as a result of caustic lye exposure is characteristic of chemical burns. Early decontamination and treatment allow for limited injury progression.

attempts without discomfort, but intramuscular ketamine (and rectal methohexital for some small children) are also effective. Hypertrophic scarring of the face, neck, or head may present challenges to airway management and should be reviewed with the burn surgeon to plan appropriate alternatives in the event of sudden airway compromise.

Anxiety and fear are often problematic, because many children retain unpleasant memories of their admission and previous procedures. Parental participation during induction, the liberal use of comfort objects, and nontraditional methods of reducing patient anxiety (e.g., music and video games) have all been used to ease the transition from the holding area to the operating room. The choice of anesthetic is based on the patient's current physiologic status and residual cardiopulmonary dysfunction as well as procedural requirements. No single method is suitable for all circumstances, and the anesthesiologist needs to be sensitive to the patient's emotional and physical maturation, as well as to the patient's perception of the perioperative experience over time. Consideration of persistent psychosocial issues and the potential for increased analgesic requirements should be continued during emergence and recovery in the postanesthesia care unit.

SUMMARY

The applied principles of modern pediatric burn management have achieved an overall decline in morbidity and mortality accompanied by improvements in long-term functional outcomes and the assisted reintegration of the patient into their familial and social environments. However, treatment of the pediatric burn patient continues to test the skill set of the anesthesia provider and the multidisciplinary team. Initial management remains focused on targeted resuscitation, caloric replacement, and the delivery of effective anxiolysis and analgesia both in the intensive care unit and during a multitude of surgical excisions. There are continuing research efforts evaluating the pharmacologic mediation of the catabolic state and protracted inflammatory response. Although the acute burn phase requires an intense commitment to identify and address evolving physiologic derangements, the anesthesiologist is also challenged by the sequelae of the original injury as this unique patient population revisits the operating room over the course of several years.

ACKNOWLEDGMENTS

The author would like to thank Drs. John McCall and Carl Fischer for their previous contributions to this chapter. I would also like to express my gratitude to Sue Brogna of the Shriners Burn Hospital, Boston, for her patience and tireless assistance during the illustration-selection process for this edition.

For questions and answers on topics in this chapter, go to "Chapter Questions" at www.expertconsult.com.

REFERENCES

Complete references used in this text can be found online at www.expertconsult.com.

Anesthesia for Pediatric Dentistry

Andrew Herlich, Brian P. Martin, Lisa Vecchione, and Franklyn P. Cladis

CONTENTS

I n light of the advances in health care, dental disease is still among the most prevalent of diseases, according to the Centers for Disease Control and Prevention (CDC). Although dental caries (tooth decay) is largely preventable, it remains the most common chronic disease of children aged 6 to 11 years, and of adolescents aged 12 to 19 years. Tooth decay is more common than many other common chronic diseases of childhood including asthma. It is four times more common than asthma among adolescents aged 14 to 17 years (CDC Division of Oral Health). Maternal nutritional and behavioral influences are very strong factors that propagate transmission of caries from the mother to her infant (American Academy of Pediatrics, 2003). The impact of caries is pervasive; poor nutrition may cause them or be the result of them. However, fluoridation of community water supplies, use of children's vitamins containing fluoride, and increased awareness of dental hygiene have produced a significant reduction in dental caries in the general population.

Despite advances in preventive dentistry, some conditions still require more than local anesthesia to facilitate dental treatment. General anesthesia may be required to treat children with severe systemic disease or disabling congenital anomalies, as well as infants and toddlers with milk-bottle caries who require partial or complete oral rehabilitation. General anesthesia may also be required for children and adolescents with severe developmental delay who require a safe and effective environment to render the necessary dental treatment. In addition, the fearful or combative child may require procedural sedation when behavior modification techniques have not succeeded. Proper care for these populations necessitates a care team approach, consisting of properly trained anesthesia and dental providers. A glossary of commonly used dental terms is shown in Table 32-1.

HUMAN DENTITION

Dental Development

Initial calcification of the primary tooth buds may be seen in the fourth month of prenatal life. In general, by the end of the sixth prenatal month, all of the primary teeth have begun to develop. The newborn infant is edentulous, with the rare exception of a mandibular central incisor. This natal or neonatal tooth tends to be quite mobile, and in the past it was thought to require immediate extraction. Recent data suggest that by the end of the neonatal period, this mobile tooth becomes quite stable and capable of normal masticatory function. This is indeed fortunate for the infant, because these neonatal teeth are frequently the only primary teeth that develop in that position (King and Lee, 1989; Cunha et al., 2001).

The sequence of eruption of human teeth may critically affect infant feeding, behavioral, and masticatory skills. Major changes in the appearance of the dentition in the oral cavity probably alter important aspects of neurobehavioral development (Wright, 2000). As an example of eruption sequence alterations, premature infants and neonates requiring prolonged orotracheal intubation have significant defects in both oral and dental structures that may persist past age 5 years, even after removal of the orotracheal tube (Fadavi et al., 1992).

The order of appearance of the teeth in the oral cavity tends to follow generalized patterns (Table 32-2). Usually the teeth erupt in pairs. A mandibular right central incisor erupts at approximately the same time as the mandibular left central incisor, at approximately 6 to 7 months of age. The mandibular teeth usually precede their maxillary counterparts; the maxillary incisors erupt approximately 1 month later than the mandibular incisors. The eruption sequence continues and is usually complete

TABLE 32-1. Glossary of Common Dental Terms

Proper Name	Common Name or Definition
Abutment	Tooth or teeth on either side of an edentulous area supporting a bridge
Amalgam	Silver-coated restoration
Bicuspid	Premolar tooth (older term)
Bitewing	Dental radiograph that views several adjacent maxillary and mandibular teeth simultaneously; especially useful in evaluating dental caries
Bruxism	Involuntary tooth grinding
Burr	Drill bit used to prepare a tooth for caries restoration
Caries	Dental cavity or cavities
Composite	Tooth-colored restoration
Crown	Portion of the tooth seen in the mouth above the gum line; also, term used for the dental restoration of the same anatomic region; popularly known as a cap
Cuspid	Canine tooth (older term)
Diastemata	Separations between the teeth; commonly seen between the maxillary central incisors
Dry socket	Nonhealing extraction site
Endodontic therapy	Root canal therapy
Exfoliation	Spontaneous loss of a tooth
Exodontia	Dental extraction
Eye tooth	Canine tooth (familiar term)
Gingivitis	Inflammation of superficial aspects of the peridontium
Handpiece	Dental drill
Ludwig's angina	Dental infection of the floor of the mouth involving the submandibular, submaxillary, and submental spaces bilaterally
Milk tooth	Primary or baby tooth
Occlusion	Patient's "bite"
Oral prophylaxis	Dental cleaning
Overbite	Degree of vertical overlap of the maxillary teeth over the mandibular teeth
Overjet	Degree of horizontal projection of the maxillary teeth beyond the mandibular teeth
Periapical	Area surrounding the apex of the root; a periapical dental radiograph also includes the clinical crown of the tooth
Periodontium	Soft and hard tissues surrounding and supporting teeth
Pulpotomy	Therapeutic removal of the coronal portion of the dental pulp
Pyorrhea	Common name for periodontal inflammation, or gum disease; except for gingivitis, periodontal disease is rare in children
Rubber dam	Square latex or vinyl sheet used to isolate the teeth from the oral cavity during dental treatments

TABLE 32–2. Eruption Sequence of the Human Dentition

	Approximate Age Eruption Begins	Approximate Age Eruption Is Completed
Primary Dentition		
Maxillary		
Central incisor	7½ mo	1½ yr
Lateral incisor	9 mo	2 yr
Cuspid	18 mo	3¼ yr
First molar	14 mo	2½ yr
Second molar	24 mo	3 yr
Mandibular		
Central incisor	6 mo	1½ yr
Lateral incisor	7 mo	1½ yr
Cuspid	16 mo	3¼ yr
First molar	12 mo	2¼ yr
Second molar	20 mo	3 yr
Permanent Dentition		
Maxillary		
Central incisor	7–8 yr	10 yr
Lateral incisor	8–9 yr	11 yr
Cuspid	11–12 yr	13–15 yr
First bicuspid	10–11 yr	12–13 yr
Second bicuspid	10–12 yr	12–14 yr
First molar	6–7 yr	9–10 yr
Second molar	12–13 yr	14–16 yr
Mandibular		
Central incisor	6–7 yr	9 yr
Lateral incisor	7–8 yr	10 yr
Cuspid	9–10 yr	12–14 yr
First bicuspid	10–12 yr	12–13 yr
Second bicuspid	11–12 yr	13–14 yr
First molar	6–7 yr	9–10 yr
Second molar	11–13 yr	14–15 yr

From Schour I, Massler M: The development of the human dentition, *JADA* 28:1153, 1941. Reprinted by permission of ADA Publishing.

by age 2 to 2½ years. The last tooth to erupt is the deciduous second molar, called the 2-year molar because of its appearance at age 2 years.

When completed, the primary dentition totals 20 teeth (Wright, 2000). As the toddler's growth continues, the mandible and maxilla enlarge, causing separations, also known as diastemata, between the primary teeth (Zwemer, 1993). The diastemata increase as the primary teeth are beginning to exfoliate and the permanent or succedaneous teeth begin to erupt. The separations also permit sufficient room for the proper alignment of the permanent dentition.

The maintenance of the health and hygiene of the primary teeth is essential to avoid premature tooth loss. When primary teeth are prematurely lost as a result of decay or trauma, the space needed for the permanent tooth eruption is also lost because the natural tendency of the tooth is to tip mesially (toward the midline) in the oral cavity. Subsequently, dental malocclusions tend to occur. Finally, the primary teeth may also function as the permanent teeth if the permanent analogous tooth fails to develop (Wright, 2000).

The transition period between exfoliation of the primary teeth and eruption of the permanent teeth is called the mixed-dentition phase. This phase continues until the last primary tooth is normally exfoliated or extracted. Unlike the primary teeth, the permanent teeth normally erupt so that there is tooth-to-tooth contact.

Development of the secondary, or permanent, dentition begins at birth with calcification of the buds of the permanent first molars. The permanent dentition begins its eruption pattern with the permanent first molar, usually at approximately 6 years of age. Like their primary counterparts, the mandibular teeth usually precede the maxillary teeth, with the permanent mandibular incisors beginning to appear at approximately age 6 to 7 years. Unlike the primary dentition, where there is usually a variability of several months in the timing of eruption, the permanent teeth may vary as much as 1 to 2 years in eruption sequence. After eruption of the permanent first molars, eruption of the remaining permanent teeth then occurs in this sequence: mandibular central incisors, maxillary central incisors, mandibular lateral incisors, maxillary lateral incisors, mandibular cuspids, maxillary and mandibular first premolars, maxillary and mandibular second premolars, maxillary cuspids, and mandibular and maxillary second molars (see Table 32-2). At the completion of the eruption sequence, the permanent dentition consists of 32 teeth (Wright, 2000).

The third molars, commonly known as wisdom teeth, have the least predictable eruption sequence of any of the human dentition. They may erupt as early as age 15 to 16 years, as late as age 25 years, or not at all. Quite commonly, the third molars fail to erupt because of dental germinal pattern alterations or impactions in the soft or hard tissues. Impactions usually occur because of insufficient bony growth of the maxilla or mandible in proportion to the individual's full dental complement.

In addition to the frequently absent third molars, two other permanent tooth forms are sometimes congenitally absent. The mandibular premolars and the maxillary lateral incisors may be congenitally absent, either singly or in symmetric pairs (Neville et al., 2002). Occasionally, a tooth that is thought to be congenitally absent is actually impacted in the soft tissues or alveolar bone.

Just as there are congenitally absent teeth, there are supernumerary or accessory teeth. The most common supernumerary tooth is the mesiodens, a conically shaped tooth consistently located in the midline between the maxillary central incisors. Other supernumerary teeth are the third premolars and fourth maxillary molars (Neville et al., 2002).

Identification of mobile primary versus transitional, or mixed, dentition can be of importance to anesthesia personnel. It is often recommended that mobile primary teeth be removed prior to airway instrumentation, as they may be at risk for dislodgment and airway obstruction. Likewise, it is important to note that newly erupted permanent teeth are often slightly mobile, with incomplete root formation. For this reason, extra care should be taken during laryngoscopy, oral airway placement, or other jaw manipulation, as immature permanent teeth may be predisposed to luxation or avulsion trauma if too great a force is placed on them.

Dental Identification

There are two principal universal dental identification systems. In both systems, the primary teeth are designated by letters, and the permanent teeth are designated by numbers. These systems differ in the way that the dental arches (mandible and maxilla) are divided. The first system uses a sequential means for identification, with the primary maxillary right second molar designated as tooth A and followed sequentially around the contralateral side of the maxilla to the left second molar, which is tooth J. The primary mandibular left second molar is tooth K, and the sequence is completed on reaching the mandibular right second molar, tooth T. Similarly, the numbering system for the permanent dentition starts with the maxillary right third molar as tooth 1 and continues to the maxillary left third molar, tooth 16. The sequence continues with the mandibular left third molar, tooth 17, and is completed with the mandibular right third molar, tooth 32 (Herlich, 1990). Both pediatric and general dentists commonly use this system of tooth identification.

The second designation system divides the dental arch into quadrants. All primary central incisors are tooth A and follow distally or posteriorly, so that all primary second molars are tooth E. To make the designation more specific, the quadrant is also named. For example, the primary maxillary right lateral incisor is designated maxillary right B. Similarly, the permanent dentition is divided into quadrants. All central incisors are tooth 1 and continue posteriorly, so that all third molars are tooth 8. This system is most commonly used by orthodontists (Fig. 32-1).

Dental Anatomy and Physiology

The tooth is composed of a crown, which is usually visible for clinical examination, and a root, which is not seen during routine clinical examination. They are separated by the cementoenamel junction or cervical region of the tooth (Fig. 32-2). The cementoenamel junctions are seen more commonly in adult dentition if gingival ("gum") recession occurs. The crown is responsible for the slicing, ripping, and grinding of foodstuffs (incisors, canines, and molars, respectively). The root structure imparts stability to the tooth in its surrounding tissues. The anterior teeth, the incisors and the canines, are single rooted with a conical shape. The posterior teeth, the premolars and molars, are multirooted and impart most of their stability by both the number of roots and the subtly divergent directions in which the roots may grow.

Surrounding the root structure of the tooth is the periodontium, which is composed of three structures as follows:

● The most external portion is a combination of the gingival and alveolar mucosa, which constitute the soft tissue covering for the remainder of the periodontal structures.
● The periodontal ligament attaches the external surface of the root to the alveolar bone, acting as a shock absorber and anchor during masticatory function.

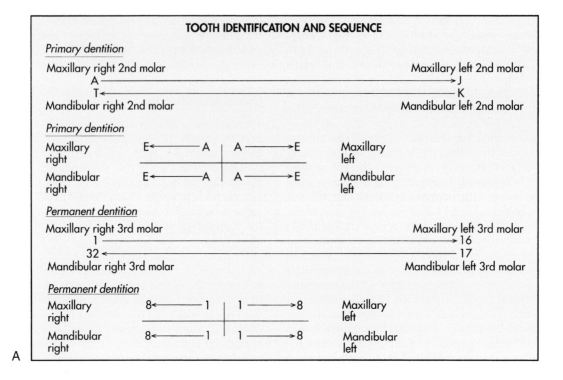

TOOTH IDENTIFICATION AND SEQUENCE

Primary dentition

Maxillary right 2nd molar   Maxillary left 2nd molar
A ————————————————————————————→ J
T ←———————————————————————————— K
Mandibular right 2nd molar   Mandibular left 2nd molar

Primary dentition

Maxillary   E ←——— A | A ———→ E   Maxillary
right   left

Mandibular   E ←——— A | A ———→ E   Mandibular
right   left

Permanent dentition

Maxillary right 3rd molar   Maxillary left 3rd molar
1 ————————————————————————————→ 16
32 ←——————————————————————————— 17
Mandibular right 3rd molar   Mandibular left 3rd molar

Permanent dentition

Maxillary   8 ←——— 1 | 1 ———→ 8   Maxillary
right   left

Mandibular   8 ←——— 1 | 1 ———→ 8   Mandibular
right   left

A

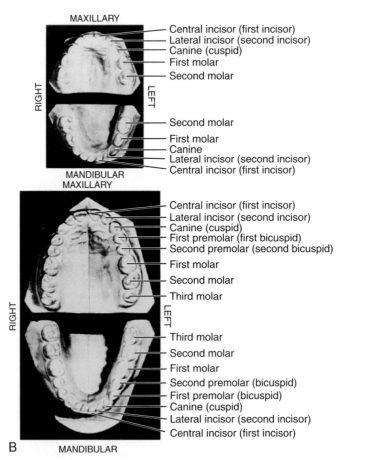

MAXILLARY
— Central incisor (first incisor)
— Lateral incisor (second incisor)
— Canine (cuspid)
— First molar
— Second molar

RIGHT   LEFT

— Second molar
— First molar
— Canine
— Lateral incisor (second incisor)
— Central incisor (first incisor)
MANDIBULAR

MAXILLARY
— Central incisor (first incisor)
— Lateral incisor (second incisor)
— Canine (cuspid)
— First premolar (first bicuspid)
— Second premolar (second bicuspid)
— First molar
— Second molar
— Third molar

RIGHT   LEFT

— Third molar
— Second molar
— First molar
— Second premolar (bicuspid)
— First premolar (bicuspid)
— Canine (cuspid)
— Lateral incisor (second incisor)
— Central incisor (first incisor)
B   MANDIBULAR

■ **FIGURE 32-1. A,** Tooth identification and sequence. **B,** Cast models of the primary dentition *(upper)* and permanent dentition *(lower).* (*A, From Herlich A: Dental complications of anesthesia,* Prog Anesthesiol 11:250, 1990. *B, From Ash MM Jr, editor:* Wheeler's dental anatomy, physiology, and occlusion, *ed 7, Philadelphia, 1993, Saunders, p 2.)*

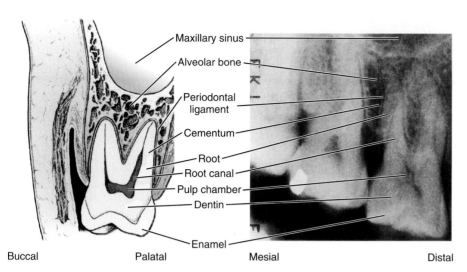

Maxillary sinus
Alveolar bone
Periodontal ligament
Cementum
Root
Root canal
Pulp chamber
Dentin
Enamel

Buccal   Palatal   Mesial   Distal

FIGURE 32-2. Schematic *(left)* and radiographic *(right)* views of a right maxillary molar. *(Modified with permission from Ash MM Jr, editor:* Wheeler's dental anatomy, physiology, and occlusion, *ed 7, Philadelphia, 1993, Saunders, p 6.)*

- The bony component is called the alveolar bone or tooth socket. Beneath the alveolar bone rests the supporting basal or skeletal bone. Basal bone, the part seen in edentulous patients, forms the skeletal support for full or partial dentures. When the tooth structure is lost, alveolar bone is also lost and is not naturally regenerated.

The individual teeth are composed of enamel, dentin, dental pulp, and cementum (Wright, 2000) (see Fig. 32-2). The enamel covers the external surface of the dental crown. It is the hardest substance in the human body and, unlike bone, has no living cells. When intact, enamel functions as a thermal insulator and an impervious barrier to chemicals and microorganisms.

On the internal surface of the enamel lies the dentin. It is composed of microtubules and has living cells in the dentinal structure. When tooth decay is advanced, noxious stimuli are readily transmitted via the dentinal tubules to the underlying dental pulp. The neurovascular supply of the individual teeth is contained in the dental pulp. Pain is easily elicited by many different stimuli—thermal, tactile, or liquid. The pain is transmitted from the dental pulp through the root apices to the alveolar bone and subsequently to the body's pain receptors.

The final portion of the tooth structure is the dental cementum, which covers the external surface of the roots. Because it is not nearly as hard and impervious to the surroundings as is enamel, noxious stimuli are perceived when the cementum is exposed. The cementum is similar to the dentin of the tooth. Patients who enjoy good dental health usually do not have exposed cementum. However, with gingival and alveolar recession, root structure and its investing cementum may be exposed to the external environment.

Some morphologic differences exist between deciduous and succedaneous teeth. The most obvious difference exists in the size of the teeth in general. The deciduous teeth are significantly smaller than their permanent counterparts. With respect to the molars, the buccal-lingual dimensions are proportionately narrower. In contrast, the mesial-distal dimensions are proportionately larger.

Another difference between the sets of dentition rests in the color of the enamel. The primary teeth are milky white, or opalescent; hence, the name *milk teeth*. The permanent teeth, on the other hand, are significantly less "milky" because pigment absorption has occurred during their development or has been acquired during the intraoral lifetime of the tooth (Wright, 2000). Two examples are tetracycline staining (developmental) and caffeine staining (acquired).

The pulp chambers of the primary teeth are larger than the permanent teeth because of the relative thinness of the deciduous enamel and dentin (Wright, 2000). Less than meticulous dental restorations or large carious lesions may predispose the primary teeth to pulpal or endodontic therapy earlier than their permanent counterparts.

The root structures of the primary molars are more saber shaped and extend laterally beyond the crown width. This unique root structure allows adequate room for the permanent tooth bud to develop and mature until the exfoliative process is completed for the primary tooth (Wright, 2000).

DENTAL PATHOPHYSIOLOGY

Despite declines in the overall caries rate of the general population, dental caries remains a common chronic disease of childhood. The high incidence is related to several risk factors, including consumption of fermentable carbohydrates (sugar-containing beverages), lack of adequate oral hygiene practices and fluoride exposure, and socioeconomic status. *Early childhood caries* specifically refers to severe caries involving multiple teeth in the preschool age group.

In the presence of fermentable carbohydrate, the metabolic by-products of microorganisms (particularly *Streptococcus mutans*) result in the acidic demineralization of enamel of the teeth. If the body's capacity for remineralization of the affected tooth is is overwhelmed, a microscopic cavity will form in the surface of the enamel. Topical fluoride exposure in toothpaste is an important resource for remineralization of these initial lesions. If remineralization capacity is inadequate, the carious lesion will progress through the enamel into the dentin, or the inner layer of tooth structure. Further progression will involve the neurovascular bundle or pulp in the tooth. Bacterial contamination of the pulp will result in pulpal inflammation (toothache) or outright necrosis. An acute or chronic dental abscess may then develop. Localized signs of dental abscess include gingival edema, and pain during mastication or palpation. Treatment of dental abscess is accomplished with either endodontic therapy (root canal) or extraction of the tooth.

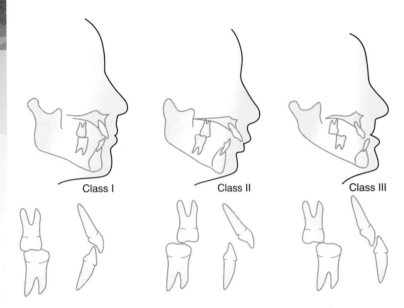

■ **FIGURE 32-3.** Angle classification system for malocclusion.

Class I   Class II   Class III

Treatment of dental caries is surgical. Using a burr, the carious portion of the tooth structure is removed. The tooth is then restored to form and function using an appropriate dental restorative material, such as amalgam (traditional silver filling material), composite resin (mixture of plastic and silicate particles), or stainless steel (for crowns).

Orthodontic Pathology

Teeth erupt into the alveolar processes of the maxilla and mandible and are held into bone by the periodontal membrane and gingival fibers. Together, the teeth and the jaws provide structure to the lower third of the face. In a normal bite, the maxilla and maxillary teeth are larger, which allows the maxillary arch to overlap the mandibular arch. *Occlusion* describes how maxillary and mandibular teeth fit together during chewing or at rest.

Malocclusion is the improper alignment of the teeth and jaws or bad bite. A skeletal malocclusion describes a malalignment between the jaws. A dental malocclusion describes the interarch relationship between the upper and lower teeth. A malocclusion may be caused by both hereditary and environmental factors. Crowding, spacing, supernumerary teeth, hypodontia, and asymmetric jaw growth are determined mostly by inheritance. Environmental factors such as thumb sucking, dental caries, premature loss of primary teeth, and trauma also can contribute to malocclusion (Mossey, 1999). An untreated malocclusion can lead to tooth decay, periodontal disease, abnormal wear of teeth, difficulty in chewing and speaking, and poor self-image.

Edward H. Angle, who is regarded as the father of orthodontics, developed a classification system for malocclusion based on the sagittal (anteroposterior) relationship of the teeth and jaws (Angle, 1899). Angle believed the upper first molars were critical to occlusion, and that the upper and lower molars should meet so that the mesiobuccal cusp of the upper molar contacts in the buccal groove of the lower molar. If this molar relationship existed and the teeth were arranged on a smoothly curving line of occlusion, then

normal occlusion would result (Fig. 32-3). Angle's classification system is as follows:

Class I: Malocclusion, in which jaws are aligned well, but teeth are crowded, rotated, or missing.

Class II: Overbite, in which the maxilla may be too large and protrude, or the lower jaw may be too small and retruded. The maxillary molar is anterior to the mandibular molar.

Class III: Underbite, in which the upper jaw is too small or the lower jaw is too large and protrudes. The maxillary molar is posterior to the mandibular molar.

Discrepancies in the vertical or transverse dimension can also contribute to a malocclusion. An openbite or deepbite describe how teeth fit together in the vertical dimension.

Whether orthodontic treatment should occur in one or two phases of treatment is a source of controversy. Phase I, or early orthodontic treatment, may correct a problem when the patient still has primary teeth or has a combination of primary and permanent teeth. Some practitioners believe it may keep more serious problems from developing, and it may make treatment at a later age shorter or less complicated. Typically, early treatment involves the use of materials and techniques to guide or modify growth as adult teeth are erupting (Kluemper et al., 2000)

Appliances used in early treatment may be removable or fixed (cemented). They may be made of metal, ceramic, or acrylic. Examples of appliances used to address transverse discrepancies include palatal expanders, quad helixes, and transpalatal arches (Fig. 32-4). Headgear therapy may be used to treat anteroposterior discrepancies (class II or class III malocclusions) and are composed of a removable and fixed component. A lower lingual holding arch is a banded appliance used to maintain space for the eruption of permanent teeth in the mandibular arch (Fig. 32-5). Functional appliances change the position of the lower jaw to produce movement of teeth and modification of growth. Examples of functional appliances include the Twin block, Herbst appliance (Fig. 32-6), and Bionator.

Phase II or active treatment involves placement of fixed appliances (braces) or Invisalign in the permanent dentition

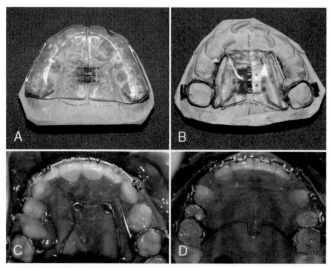

■ FIGURE 32-4. Appliances used to address transverse discrepancies include bonded palatal expander (**A**), banded palatal expander (**B**), quad helix (**C**), and transpalatal arch (**D**).

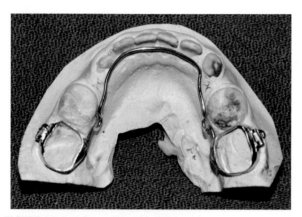

■ FIGURE 32-5. A lower lingual holding arch.

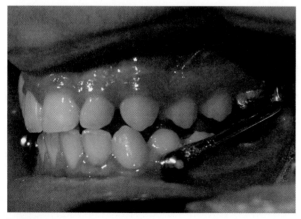

■ FIGURE 32-6. Herbst appliance, used to change the position of the lower jaw.

(Boyd, 2008). Treatment times vary with several factors, including the severity of the problem being corrected, patient response to treatment, and patient compliance. Temporary anchorage devices (Fig. 32-7) are implants used to provide absolute anchorage and help move teeth (Cope, 2005). Patients use retainers to keep teeth in their new positions after treatment.

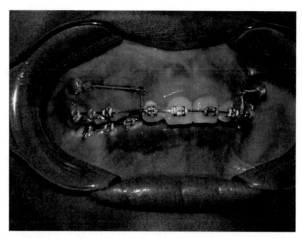

■ FIGURE 32-7. Temporary orthodontic anchorage devices.

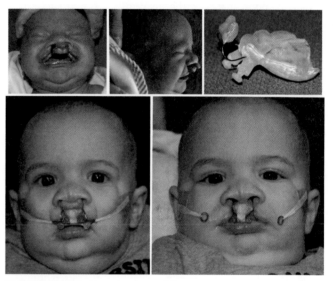

■ FIGURE 32-8. Nasoalveolar molding.

Combined surgical orthodontic treatment is used to treat patients with severe malocclusions or craniofacial anomalies. Presurgical orthodontic treatment is used to prepare patients for surgery by removing dental compensations and upright teeth over basal bone (Proffit and Miguel, 1995). In a traditional orthognathic procedure, a surgical splint may be fabricated and wired to the patient's teeth. This splint may help the surgeon determine the final position of the jaws.

Nasoalveolar molding (NAM) is a presurgical orthopedic technique used to reduce the severity of the cleft deformity in infant patients with complete unilateral or bilateral cleft lip and palate (Grayson et al., 1999). The appliance is composed of a removable acrylic plate fabricated from an intraoral impression, and a nasal stent (Fig. 32-8). The amount of acrylic is sequentially reduced to decrease the separation between the greater and lesser alveolar segments. Once the gap between the alveolar segments is 5 mm or less, the nasal stent is added to mold the nasal cartilage. Lip or nasal repair occurs at 4 to 6 months of age. Patients with NAM can present for cleft lip surgery or ear, nose, and throat procedures such as myringotomy and tubes. The NAM appliance can be left in place during inhalation induction and mask ventilation, or it can be removed before the beginning of induction. The device should be removed before airway instrumentation for a laryngeal mask airway (LMA) or endotracheal tube.

Facial Cellulitis

Bacterial abscess can spread from the apex of the root of the primary or permanent tooth into the surrounding alveolar bone and periosteum into deep tissue planes of the face or neck, resulting in an odontogenic facial cellulitis. Fever, dysphagia, leukocytosis, trismus, and dehydration are common physical findings. The lateral pharyngeal, retropharyngeal, masticator, buccal, submandibular, and submental spaces may be involved. Appropriate antibiotic therapy and prompt surgical drainage and extraction of the infected tooth are critical components of care.

Careful preoperative airway evaluation is critical in patients with facial cellulitis. Involvement of the masticator space or other anatomic spaces of the neck may threaten the airway. Ludwig's angina, with bilateral involvement of the submandibular space and with associated superior displacement of the tongue base can cause airway compromise.

PATIENT SPECTRUM

The population base of the pediatric dentist or pedodontist is generally composed of healthy children who are able to comprehend and follow simple directions by the pedodontists and their staff. However, pediatric dentists are trained (2 years or longer) to treat the following patient groups:

- Physically handicapped adolescents and adults
- Neonates, young infants, and toddlers too young to cooperate with routine dental care
- Fearful, unmanageable, or psychologically challenged children
- The entire spectrum of medically compromised children
- Children with dental problems in a hospital critical care unit
- Children with orofacial trauma
- Children requiring interceptive or minor orthodontic care

The physically handicapped patient most likely to appear for pedodontal treatment has athetoid cerebral palsy, postencephalitis syndrome, profound mental retardation, or autistic behavior (Dougherty et al., 2001; Shenkin et al., 2001; Waldman and Perlman, 2001). For example, patients with cerebral palsy may be wheelchair bound and have significant difficulty in controlling athetoid motion. The use of nitrous oxide, which depresses involuntary movement, may ensure a higher success rate in dental treatments for patients with cerebral palsy (Kaufman et al., 1991). The pedodontist is specially trained to deal with these problems in the kindest and most expedient methods available regardless of the clinical setting (Rosenstein, 1978; Pope and Curzon, 1991).

The pedodontist may be called on to fabricate a presurgical appliance for cleft lip and cleft palate in newborn infants. These presurgical appliances facilitate surgical closure of the palate. They also improve sucking and feeding in the cleft lip and palate patient. Toddlers who have circumoral burns from child abuse or domestic accidents may need an acrylic prosthesis to protect their circumoral tissues from shrinkage.

Emotionally impaired children or those who are too fearful to undergo routine treatment by a general dentist are frequently referred to the pediatric dentist who is both familiar with and comfortable in the treatment of such patients.

The pediatric dentist is routinely called on to treat the medically compromised child or adolescent when the general practitioner is reluctant to get involved in treatment. For example, the pediatric dentist primarily treats the child with congenital heart disease, the insulin-dependent diabetic, the patient with craniofacial anomalies, or the child with oncologic diseases in conjunction with the pediatrician or primary care physician. Both fear and lack of training may cause the general dentist to feel quite uncomfortable in treating the compromised child or adolescent. In addition, the general dental practitioner frequently lacks the physical resources, such as specialized equipment, to care for these patients. The pediatric dentist is usually quite comfortable in recommending and prescribing antibiotic prophylaxis for subacute bacterial endocarditis (SBE), for example, and keeps current with appropriate timing in dosage, effectiveness, and relative risks (Wahl, 1994; Hayes and Fasules, 2001; American Academy of Pediatric Dentistry, 2002e).

A few unfortunate children develop such severe illnesses or injuries that they require prolonged admissions in critical care units. These children also need dental care, which takes place at the bedside. For example, the child who has sustained significant head injuries may develop neuropathic chewing, which damages dental tissues (wearing down of teeth via grinding action) or soft tissues (tongue or cheek maceration). The pedodontist can fabricate an intraoral acrylic appliance to prevent further damage to oral tissues.

Finally, the pediatric dentist may be called to the emergency department of a hospital to treat orofacial trauma. This situation is more common in pediatric hospitals, where pediatric dental house officers are on 24-hour call with attending supervision. In general, in hospitals without specific pediatric dental services, the oral and maxillofacial surgeon handles pediatric dental trauma.

DENTIST'S NEEDS AND TECHNIQUES

The pediatric dental patient requiring anesthesiology services usually needs many dental procedures during a single anesthetic administration. The quality of dental restorations is probably improved under general anesthesia (Tate et al., 2002; Al-Eheideb and Herman, 2003). In addition, the parents of children who have had general anesthesia for pediatric dental care have greater satisfaction than parents of children who did not have general anesthesia (Acs et al., 2001). After induction of general anesthesia and protection of the airway, the anesthesiologist, the anesthesia machine, and the anesthesia equipment cart are positioned at either the patient's head or side.

The dentist's first step is to obtain necessary intraoral radiographs of the teeth (periapical, bitewing, and occlusal radiographs). The dentist then performs a clinical examination. After placement of a pharyngeal pack (which should be noted on the anesthesia record), dental impressions may be taken if future orthodontic treatment is anticipated. Also, the dentist usually places a rubber dam around the dental arch to be treated. Despite its name, the rubber dam is not usually latex. Nevertheless, if the patient is latex sensitive, care must be taken to ensure that nonlatex products are being used. The rubber dam is held in place by a metal clamp that grasps the dental crown. A substantial length of dental floss or umbilical tape is tied around the clamp before its placement, to prevent inadvertent loss in the aerodigestive tract. Except for extractions and oral prophylaxis, the remainder of the treatment is performed with the rubber dam in place. Caries removal and tooth restoration take place with silver amalgam, tooth-colored composite, or preformed crowns. The rubber dam affords the dentist a dry environment in which the dental materials can cure optimally and achieve their greatest compressive and tensile strength. The rubber dam is also a barrier to protect the patient from iatrogenic dental trauma, including the accidental loss of dental materials or broken instruments and their possible entrance into the aerodigestive tract. The application of topical fluorides takes place after all of the restorative dentistry is completed with the rubber dam still in place (Mathewson and Primosch, 1995).

When severe malocclusion, facial skeleton dysmorphism, or tooth loss prevents rubber dam placement, the dentist still needs to maintain a dry intraoral environment. Injection of glycopyrrolate (0.005 to 0.01 mg/kg) or atropine (0.01 to 0.02 mg/kg) immediately after the placement of the intravenous cannula affords satisfactory intraoral conditions. The pedodontist places cotton rolls along the buccal and lingual or facial and palatal margins of the adjacent soft tissues to assist in the achievement of a dry oral cavity.

Pediatric dentistry may also encompass the need for oral and maxillofacial surgery. Oral and maxillofacial surgeons frequently perform these procedures after extensive training. Many oral and maxillofacial surgeons have dual dental and medical training, as well as fellowship training in head and neck surgery or plastic and reconstructive surgery. Because children may have craniofacial anomalies, including orofacial clefts, orthognathic problems, tumors, and blunt or penetrating trauma, such surgical management requires the ability to combine cosmesis, restoration of normal occlusion, and the promotion of normal growth and development of the entire facial skeleton (Kaban, 1993; Vig and Fields, 2000; Ord et al., 2002; Oza et al., 2002; Zeltser et al., 2003).

Clinical Settings for Pediatric Dentists

Most pediatric dental treatment occurs in the dental office without the need for psychological or pharmacologic intervention to address the child's fear and anxiety. The hallmark of dental pain management is a kind practitioner and staff and the responsible use of adequate local or topical anesthesia, or both. For some patients, simple behavior modification techniques improve the level of cooperation in the dental chair. These techniques include the tell-show-do method and voice control for the fearful, hostile, or disruptive child. The tell-show-do technique involves explaining before the procedure, demonstrating the procedure outside of the child's mouth, and then actually performing the procedure on the patient. This technique removes the fear of the unknown from the procedure (Lenchner and Wright, 1975). Voice control involves modulation of both the volume and tone of the dentist's voice to achieve positive behavioral results (Wilson, 1994; American Academy of Pediatric Dentistry, 2008). When behavior modification is deemed necessary for a preschool child, it should be scheduled during the morning, because the child's longest

attention span and optimal level of cooperation are early in the day. Additional techniques include positive reinforcement, distraction, and parental presence (American Academy of Pediatric Dentistry, 2008). Additional behavior modification techniques have been used by the dentist to physically restrain frightened children. This *protective stabilization* is the restriction of the patients' freedom of movement, with or without their permission, to decrease the risk of injury and to allow the safe completion of the treatment. Included in these techniques are passive physical restraint with a rigid board (papoose board), and active physical restraint by dental personnel. These techniques are controversial because of their potential psychological trauma and legal implications (Nathan, 1989; Wilson, 1994; Wright, 1994). Continuous monitoring of the patient is essential during protective stabilization.

Most analgesia for pediatric dental procedures is achieved by local anesthetic block. Most blocks are local infiltration in the maxillary region, or mandibular nerve blocks in the mandible. Adverse reactions to local anesthetics seldom occur when they are administered alone. Most commonly, they are related to a relative overdose or lapse in technique. However, even a low dosage, inappropriately injected, can cause palpitations, diaphoresis, or even dizziness (Kaufman et al., 2000). Rarely does vasomotor collapse occur. True allergic reactions, including allergy to metabisulfite or other preservatives of local anesthetics (e.g., paraaminobenzoic acid), are probably the smallest proportion of untoward reactions (Campbell et al., 2001).

Behavior modification may include such novel approaches as hypnosis or music therapy. Highly motivated, intelligent, attentive, or anxious children may have a good emotional and analgesic response to hypnosis when other forms of behavior modification, including pharmacologic forms, are precluded (Kleinhauz and Eli, 1993). Children as young as 3 to 4 years may be successfully hypnotized in the dental office (Lampshire, 1975). Music did not diminish pain, anxiety, or disruptive behavior in a recent study (Aitken et al., 2002), despite anecdotal beliefs of pediatric dentists and parents. Nevertheless, in this study, the patients enjoyed listening to the music and chose to listen to music in subsequent visits.

Electroanesthesia (transcutaneous electronic nerve stimulation [TENS]) has been used successfully for children in the dental office setting. TENS is reported to be effective based on several interrelated theories. These pain control theories include gate control, endorphin release, and serotonin release. For dental procedures, disposable electrode pads are placed bilaterally in the treated dental arch after drying the buccal mucosa. Using a dentally specific TENS device, a pulse rate of 110 Hz, and a pulse width of 225 microseconds in the normal mode, amplitude is slowly increased until the desired response is obtained. Twitching of the lower lip is the amplitude end point in the mandibular arch, and twitching of the orbicularis oculi is the amplitude end point in the maxillary arch. Children are instructed to raise a hand if the amplitude is too uncomfortable, and it is then diminished (te Duits et al., 1993). This technique works best in the area of restorative dentistry in the teeth that have relatively shallow lesions with respect to the dentoenamel junction (Quarnstrom, 1992; te Duits et al., 1993).

The spectrum of use of sedation is illustrated by the fact that medication, including nitrous oxide, is being used less than in previous years and studies. A study by Houpt (2002) suggests that, although more sedation is being used, it is being used by fewer practitioners on more patients in the United States.

A retrospective review of pediatric sedation management suggests that at one U.S. dental school pediatric dental clinic, nonpharmacologic behavioral management is favored more frequently because of its greater success (Eid, 2002). One British study estimated that more than 300,000 general anesthesias are still being administered for dentistry each year in Great Britain, mostly for children. The authors suggest that fewer general anesthetics are available for dentistry now than in the 1970s (Blayney et al., 1999). It is implied that most general anesthesias in Great Britain, however, as opposed to in the United States, are provided in a hospital setting.

Most pediatric dentists and those treating handicapped patients are experienced in the use of nitrous oxide and oral premedication when necessary in the dental office. The reported advantages of nitrous oxide delivered via a Goldman nasal mask include analgesia and sedation (Nathan et al., 1988). The incidence of diffusion hypoxia is minimal after the use of nitrous oxide and oxygen alone, as opposed to nitrous oxide supplementation to parenteral or oral sedatives (Quarnstrom et al., 1991; Dunn-Russell et al., 1993). Hypoxemia may occur when 30% to 50% nitrous oxide is added to chloral hydrate sedation (Litman et al., 1998b). In a recent study, nasal midazolam and nitrous oxide resulted in satisfactory sedation in 96% of the pediatric patients without any clinically relevant oxygen desaturation (Wood, 2010). However, in children with enlarged tonsils, oral midazolam (0.5 mg/kg) and 50% nitrous oxide resulted in significant upper airway obstruction and implied hypoxia (Litman et al., 1998a).

Patients classified by the American Society of Anesthesiologists (ASA) as having physical status I or II are appropriate candidates for treatment with pharmacologic adjuncts in the dental office setting. If a child's physical status is III or beyond, the hospital setting is probably a wiser choice. It must be emphasized that the pediatric dentist should use local anesthesia to optimize analgesia and anesthesia for the patient. Local anesthesia may add to the potential complications of polypharmacy if attention is not paid to dosages that are age and weight appropriate. This is especially true in the pediatric age group. The pediatric dentist rarely uses intramuscular or intravenous sedation while serving as both the operator and the practitioner administering the sedation.

The reports of severe adverse outcomes include hypoxic brain damage and occasional deaths, with the use of nitrous oxide, local anesthesia, and other premedicants. Anesthesiologists should have an active role in the training of pediatric dentists in techniques of anxiolysis and moderate sedation. Adverse outcomes will likely be diminished under these circumstances (Herlich, 2010; Costa et al, 2010). Invariably, these adverse outcomes result from relative or absolute overdosage of one or a combination of nitrous oxide, local anesthetic, and parenteral medication (Goodson and Moore, 1983; Doyle and Goepferd, 1989; Coté et al., 2000a). Because of the widely publicized adverse outcomes of dental office sedation and general anesthesia, the trend in this type of care has been to move away from the dental office unless guidelines for deep sedation and anesthesia by the American Academy of Pediatric Dentistry are followed. These guidelines were promulgated in 1985 and restated in 2006 to promote and ensure that the public is aware and the pediatric patient is protected. The guidelines describe that the anesthesia care provider must be a separate individual with appropriate licensing, credentialing, and training to perform deep sedation and general anesthesia.

In the United Kingdom, a group of investigators performed several retrospective analyses during the 1970s and 1980s.

Retrospective data obtained from a national data bank indicated that dental office deaths were infrequent, and the number decreased substantially in the second survey. The decreases in deaths probably result from two factors. First, fewer general anesthesias were being administered in the dental office. Second, the practice of the single individual being both dental practitioner and anesthetist is becoming less frequent because of warnings and suggestions from the General Dental Council of Great Britain. The anesthetist and dental practitioner are more commonly two individuals, each of whose attention is directed toward a single task. Also, the British survey indicated that the person providing anesthesia is more commonly a physician (Coplans and Curson, 1982, 1993). In the United States, closed claims morbidity and mortality involving oral surgeons show that during the period of 1988 to 1999, there were 22 deaths in the office and 136 anesthesia-related claims in total. It was calculated that the death rate was 1 in every 747,732 (0.013 in 10,000) administrations of anesthesia in the dental office (Deegan, 2001). D'Eramo and colleagues (2008) in a survey of oral maxillofacial surgeons in Massachusetts found the adult death rate to be 1 in 1,733,055 from office-based anesthesia. Data from the Pediatric Sedation Research Consortium indicated no mortality in over 49,000 propofol sedations, of which 307 were for dental procedures (Cravero et al., 2009).

In the United States, opposing forces create difficulties for the pediatric dental patient. Economic issues tend to restrict hospital-based procedures, including payment for the dental service only, without payment for the anesthesia service; payment for the anesthesia service only, without payment for the dental service; and frequently no payment or only partial payment for the hospital service. Frequently, the patient's family is faced with a significant out-of-pocket expense, which many cannot afford. On the other hand, the litigious nature of our society has prevented the rational expansion of anesthesia services in the office environment beyond sedation. Mandated equipment and monitors and the cost of liability insurance may be prohibitive for the office practitioner.

Another issue with significant economic ramifications is the cost of multiple treatments in the dental office with procedural sedation as opposed to a single session in the operating room of the hospital under general anesthesia. In studying healthy patients aged 24 to 60 months, Lee and colleagues (2001) found that a patient who required more than three treatment visits with procedural sedation had more cost-effective treatment when all of the treatments were provided in a single visit under general anesthesia.

A reasonable compromise may be a well-equipped hospital or surgicenter dental clinic with standard monitoring devices and resuscitation equipment. Pediatric patients with ASA status I or II may be suitable candidates. With the use of proper equipment and appropriately trained personnel, a large diversity of patients may be safely and satisfactorily treated on an outpatient basis. If the clinic is rationally designed, including recovery areas equipped with oxygen, suction apparatus, and essential monitoring devices, the anesthesiologist can safely administer the anesthetic outside of the traditional operating room setting. It allows more efficient use of time and space as well as reduced cost. From the perspective of the parent and child, outpatient treatment permits a more rapid return to familiar surroundings and activities of daily living (Zuckerberg, 1994). Only the patients with disease or physical conditions that preclude off-site clinical practice need to be treated in the operating room in today's environment. Some examples of the patients who may need the traditional operating room setting include those with difficult airways, those with coagulopathies, and those with complex anomalies or cardiovascular disease for whom more than standard monitoring is necessary.

SEDATION AND ANESTHESIA FOR DENTAL PROCEDURES

The key to success in anesthetic management is a good patient history and physical examination. The parent or caregiver of the child should be able to relate relevant data such as previous anesthetic successes and failures. These anesthetic experiences should also be related for any family members. Birth history, growth, and development, including psychological issues and the child's emotional status, may be helpful in conducting a safe and pleasant dental experience. If the child has significant fears or behavioral problems that warrant premedication, the historical background permits the anesthesiologist to select an appropriate premedication agent.

The physical examination of the child must include the airway. Despite plans for nasotracheal intubation, the oral cavity must also be examined, because nasotracheal intubation may not be successful. Loose teeth, enlarged tonsils and adenoids, or herpes labialis all affect the anesthesiologist's management of the airway. Issues of nasal obstruction or sinus disease also have a great impact on the decision-making process for airway management. Cardiac murmurs should be investigated as to their relative seriousness. Most cardiac murmurs are in fact innocent flow murmurs; however, reasonable percentages are pathologic conditions and warrant prophylaxis for endocarditis. Other factors, such as coagulation status, neurologic history, and recent viral syndromes, may also affect the anesthesiologist's decision-making process.

Procedural Sedation

In 1985, The American Academy of Pediatric Dentistry established goals for sedation of the pediatric dental patient. These goals were updated in 2006 and are as follows:

1. To guard the patient's safety and welfare
2. To minimize physical discomfort and pain
3. To control anxiety, minimize psychological trauma, and maximize the potential for amnesia
4. To control behavior and/or movement so as to allow the safe completion of the procedure
5. To return the patient to a state in which safe discharge from medical supervision, as determined by recognized criteria, is possible

With these goals in mind, procedural sedation of the pediatric dental patient may be considered. The foundations of pharmacologic sedation for the pediatric dental patient are monitoring standards to which all practitioners should adhere (Wilson, 2000). Minimum or moderate procedural sedation intended in the sensitive patient may become deep sedation or general anesthesia if vigilance is not applied. These standards have been promulgated by several organizations, including the ASA (2002), The American Academy of Pediatric Dentistry and American Academy of Pediatrics (McGuire, 2007), and the American Academy of Pediatric Dentistry (2002d) (Consensus

Conference, National Institutes of Health, 1985; Rosenberg and Campbell, 1991; Council on Scientific Affairs, AMA, 1993). The American Academy of Pediatric Dentistry guidelines suggest that children who are status ASA III or IV should have treatment that necessitates sedation performed in a hospital environment.

The use of precordial/pulse oximetry for nitrous patients is not supported for nitrous oxide alone in the 2009 American Academy of Pediatric Dentistry Guidelines (American Academy of Pediatrics and American Academy of Pediatric Dentistry, 2006). Additionally, a full E-cylinder of oxygen and a self-inflating bag and mask capable of delivering 15 L/min of oxygen must be available in the care facility. An important monitor is a trained individual whose sole duty is to pay attention to the electronic and mechanical monitors in place and who is prepared to act on untoward events. As mentioned, the treating dentist should not be the person administering the anesthetic.

Before any sedation is administered, including nitrous oxide with oxygen, appropriate fasting guidelines must be given to the parents or guardians of the patient. Data suggest that prolonged fasts meant to reduce the likelihood of vomiting and aspiration are somewhat deleterious to patient outcome. Guidelines for fasting from solid foods, milk, and milk products remain at a minimum of 8 hours. However, clear liquids, including pulpless juices, plain gelatin, and ice popsicles, are encouraged and acceptable until 2 hours before the anticipated arrival in the care facility. The pediatric patient is more cooperative and the parents are more satisfied as a result of these suggested guidelines (Schreiner, 1994). All of these guidelines are predicated on normal gastrointestinal function. If the patient has abnormal gastrointestinal function, more conservative fasting orders must be considered.

Oral, intranasal or transoral, parenteral, and rectal routes for administration of sedative medications are used during procedural sedation. Pediatric dentists have traditionally and preferentially used the oral route to administer premedication (Primosch and Bender, 2001). The old practice of having the parents administer a prescribed oral medication at home has been fraught with danger to the toddler and young child. Airway obstruction and emesis with aspiration were real complications of that practice. For reasons of safety, the practice has changed. Children are now brought to the treatment facility or dental office 1 hour ahead of the scheduled procedure time, and the oral premedication is administered under the guidance of the pediatric dentist. Two of the most popular agents have been hydroxyzine (1 to 2 mg/kg) and chloral hydrate (50 to 75 mg/kg; maximal dosage, 2 g). These agents have had a good success rate and a reasonable margin of safety. In addition, nitrous oxide may be given in conjunction with the usual administration of local anesthetic blocks (Moore et al., 1984; Shapira et al., 1992). More potent oral agents, such as ketamine, diazepam, and midazolam, are also given in the treatment facility or dental office. The practitioner must allow a reasonable time for onset of action before dental treatment (Sullivan et al., 2001). Oral midazolam has gained widespread popularity because of its reasonable margin of safety in addition to its rapid onset for either premedication before general anesthesia or as the main agent for procedural sedation (Kupietzky and Houpt, 1993; Levine et al., 1993). These agents may be given alone or with another agent (Dallman et al., 2001; Bui et al., 2002; Nathan and Vargas, 2002).

Mild oxygen desaturation has been noted and is easily treated with supplemental oxygen and repositioning of the patient's airway. In some cases, when nitrous oxide was added to the oral premedication, the degree of hypoxemia increased (Litman et al., 1998a). The use of traditional monitors such as clinical observation, blood pressure, and pulse was clearly insufficient to assess the degree of hypoxemia. Pulse oximetry, capnography, and precordial stethoscopes have become necessary to adequately assess and prevent poor outcomes despite limitations in the pediatric dental environment (Anderson and Vann, 1988; Poiset et al., 1990; Wilson, 1990; Dunn-Russell et al., 1993). The use of supplemental oxygen also helps to reduce hypoxemia. Novel means of improving oxygenation include the delivery of supplemental oxygen via the saliva injector and the use of external nasal dilators (Milnes, 2002; Moses and Lieberman, 2003).

Intranasal or transoral administration of water-soluble agents such as ketamine, midazolam, or sufentanil produces effective sedation and premedication for procedural sedation. However, sufentanil produces a significantly high incidence of respiratory depression, even in relatively small dosages (1.0 mcg/kg) and is not recommended (Abrams et al., 1993). Midazolam (0.5 mg/kg orally, or 0.2 to 0.3 mg/kg intranasally) is ideal for creating a milieu in which the child is easily separated from the parent. It also transforms a disruptive child into a quiescent child in the dental chair with minimal desaturation (Abrams et al., 1993; Levine et al., 1993). However, once the handpiece (dental drill) was activated, the noise distracted the child sufficiently that the pediatric dentist could not efficiently treat the child (Theroux et al., 1994). Despite the popularity of oral sedation, one group of investigators found that there was no relationship between oral sedation and behavior of the children in the dental office on subsequent visits (McComb et al., 2002).

The rectal route of administration for procedural sedation and premedication has enjoyed popularity with only a small number of practitioners. Midazolam (1.0 mg/kg or even higher dosages) has been used for procedural sedation and for premedication. Onset of action usually occurs within 15 to 30 minutes (Roelofse and Van der Bijl, 1991). The main drawback to rectal administration of these agents is the risk of expulsion of the sedative and the unreliable uptake from the distal colonic mucosa.

Many drugs have been used as parenteral agents for procedural sedation in pediatric dentistry. Opioids, benzodiazepines, antihistamines, ultra-short-acting barbiturates, and dissociatives have been used successfully. All have had some negative features as well. Short-acting agents with acceptable margins of safety in dental sedation include methohexital, meperidine, ketamine, diazepam, and midazolam. Respiratory depression and concomitant hypoxia have been the recurrent theme in parenteral sedation by pediatric dentists (Allen, 1992; Coté et al., 2000a, 2000b). As previously mentioned, clinical observation was insufficient and the airway was subsequently lost. Because of the fine line between moderate procedural sedation, deep sedation, and general anesthesia, the dentist and assistant who administer procedural sedation must be experienced in recognizing and handling cardiorespiratory depression. Electrocardiography, pulse oximetry, blood pressure, capnography, and precordial stethoscope are essential monitors (American Academy of Pediatrics and American Academy of Pediatric Dentistry, 2006).

Other drawbacks to intravenous sedation in pediatric dentistry have been the potential for inflicted pain to achieve intravenous access and the lack of familiarity with drug combinations on the part of the practitioner. The child's fear of pain from a needle puncture has been successfully addressed by inhalation of nitrous oxide in oxygen or the transmucosal administration of midazolam. Use of EMLA (eutectic mixture of local anesthetics, 2.5% lidocaine, and 2.5% prilocaine) cream or topical (ELA-Max) lidocaine cream before venipuncture has been successful in reducing or eliminating needle puncture pain (Nilsson et al., 1994; Koh et al., 2004). Also, EMLA- and lidocaine-impregnated patches have been used intraorally with varying success before local anesthetic blocks and local procedures before the insertion of rubber dam clamps (Stecker et al., 2002). The main disadvantage of the use of the transdermal local anesthetics in EMLA cream is that it requires application at least 45 minutes to 1 hour before a painful procedure. ELA-Max is faster and requires approximately 30 minutes to take effect (Koh et al., 2004).

General Anesthesia

The American Academy of Pediatric Dentistry (2002d) has issued guidelines for the indications for general anesthesia for children having dental procedures (Box 32-1). Nunn et al. (1995) also described the indications for general anesthesia in 265 pediatric patients. These indications include extensive treatment needs, behavior management issues, medically compromised children, extreme anxiety, and physical disabilities. The most common indication, accounting for 30.6% of the anesthesias, was intellectual impairment and autism. Dental phobia accounted for 21.4% of the patients.

Behavioral issues are a very common indication for sedation or general anesthesia in children. The behavioral issues may stem from fear and anxiety or an abnormality in development such as autism, autism spectrum disorders, cerebral palsy with mental retardation, and Down syndrome.

Fear of dental procedures affects all ages. For some it may be so strong that dental visits are avoided altogether. In children, anxiety prior to a surgical or dental procedure centers on the fear of pain, loss of control, and separation from the parent or guardian. Preoperative anxiety and its risk factors are discussed in Chapter 8, Psychological Aspects of Pediatric Anesthesia, and Chapter 9, Preoperative Preparation. Children most at risk

Box 32-1 American Academy of Pediatric Dentistry Guidelines for the Elective Use of Sedation and General Anesthesia

- Patients who are unable to cooperate due to a lack of psychological or emotional maturity and/or mental, physical, or medical disability
- Patients who are extremely fearful, anxious, or non-communicative or in instances where it may protect the developing psyche.
- Patients who require significant surgical intervention or in instances where local anesthetic may be ineffective like an acute infection, anatomic variation, or allergy or patients needing immediate comprehensive care.

From the American Academy of Pediatric Dentistry: Guidelines for the elective use of conscious sedation, deep sedation and general anesthesia in pediatric dental patients, *Pediatr Dent* 24:74, 2002.

for heightened anxiety are between 1 and 5 years old and have divorced parents, previous negative medical experiences, and heightened emotionality (Kain et al, 2007).

Autism is an abnormality in neurodevelopment that results in abnormal social interactions and recurrent repetitive behavior. The diagnostic criteria include age of onset of less than 3 years old, severe abnormality of social reciprocity, severe abnormality of communication development, and restrictive, repetitive patterns of behavior and imagination (Klein and Nowak, 1998). The incidence of autism is increasing and is now estimated to be 1 to 2 per 1000 (Newschaffer et al., 2007). Autism spectrum disorders are a heterogeneous group of disorders that include autism, Asperger's syndrome, Rett syndrome, and Pervasive Developmental Disorder-Not Otherwise Specified (PDD-NOS). Children with autism and autism spectrum disorders can be uncooperative and often require behavioral interventions, sedation, or general anesthesia to complete a dental examination or procedure.

The child with significant medical disorders may require the assistance of an anesthesiologist during dental care. Some of these medical disorders may include the child with a known difficult airway, congenital cardiac disease, or multiple coexisting disorders. Children with cyanotic congenital heart disease may require SBE prophylaxis (Box 32-2). The appropriate antibiotic selection is summarized in Table 32-3. Patients with one of the cardiac conditions in Box 32-2 having dental procedures that manipulate the gingival tissue or periapical region of the teeth or perforate the oral mucosa require SBE prophylaxis. Procedures that do not require prophylaxis include routine anesthetic injections through noninfected tissue, taking dental radiographs, placement of removable prosthodontic or orthodontic appliances, adjustment of orthodontic appliances, placement of orthodontic brackets, shedding of deciduous teeth, and bleeding from trauma to the lips (Wilson et al., 2007).

Premedication

Patients presenting for general anesthesia often require a premedication to reduce anxiety and enhance cooperation.

Box 32-2 Indications for the Use of Subacute Bacterial Endocarditis Prophylaxis

- Presence of a prosthetic cardiac valve or prosthetic material for cardiac valve repair
- Previous infective endocarditis
- Congenital heart disease (CHD), including the following:
  - Unrepaired cyanotic CHD, including palliative shunts and conduits
  - Completely repaired congenital heart defect with prosthetic material or device, whether placed by surgery or by catheter intervention, during the first 6 months after the procedure
  - Repaired CHD with residual defects at the site or adjacent to the site of a prosthetic patch or prosthetic device (which inhibit endothelialization)
- Cardiac transplantation recipients who develop cardiac valvulopathy

Adapted from the AHA SBE guidelines, 2007.

TABLE 32-3. Antibiotic for Subacute Bacterial Endocarditis (SBE) Prophylaxis

Indication	Agent	Single Dose 30 to 60 min before Procedure	
		Adults	Children
No contraindications	Amoxicillin (oral)	2 g	50 mg/kg
Unable to take oral medication	Ampicillin (IM or IV)	2 g	50 mg/kg
	OR cefazolin or ceftriaxone (IM or IV)	1 g	50 mg/kg
Allergic to penicillins or ampicillin	Cephalexin (oral)	2 g	50 mg/kg
	OR clindamycin (oral)	600 mg	20 mg/kg
	OR azithromycin or clarithromycin (oral)	500 mg	15 mg/kg
Allergic to penicillins or ampicillin and unable to take oral medication	Cefazolin or ceftriaxone (IM or IV)	1 g	50 mg/kg
	OR clindamycin (IM or IV)	600 mg	20 mg/kg

Adapted from the AHA SBE guidelines 2007, Table 4.
IM, Intramuscular; *IV,* intravenous.

Benzodiazepines are a very effective anxiolytic. Adults or adolescents can be given diazepam. In one study, patients with autism were sedated more effectively with midazolam (0.5 mg/kg) than with diazepam (0.3 mg/kg) (Pisalchaiyong et al., 2005). In younger children, midazolam can be administered orally in a commercially flavored liquid or the concentrated intravenous solution can be given intranasally. The recommended dosage for midazolam is 0.5 mg/kg and 0.2 mg/kg for oral and nasal administration, respectively (Davis et al, 1995; Kain et al, 2000). Buccal midazolam (0.2 mg/kg) was described for dental procedures but found not to be effective (Hosey et al., 2009). Ketamine can also be administered alone or in combination with midazolam. This combination is effective and provides both anxiolysis and analgesia. The dosage of oral ketamine is 3 to 10 mg/kg. When combined with oral midazolam, the dosage is typically 3 to 6 mg/kg. This combination has been described to be very effective in patients with developmental delay. In this case report, the authors suggest using a flavored soda such as Dr. Pepper to mask the bitter flavor of the medication (Shah et al., 2009).

Clonidine has also been described as a premedicant for anxiolysis for children prior to surgical procedures. There are some significant advantages. It has no bitter taste, it may provide some analgesia, and it may decrease the incidence of emergence agitation, and it may decrease postoperative nausea and vomiting. A significant disadvantage is its slow onset time (30 to 45 minutes) (Almenrader et al., 2007; Dahmani et al., 2010). α_2-Agonists have been used in patients with autism, autism spectrum disorders, and attention deficit hyperactivity disorder (ADHD) and have been shown to have some benefit (Ming et al., 2008; Scahill, 2009). Clonidine may be an effective premedication for these patients when they present for dental procedures. The dosage of oral clonidine for sedation is 4 mcg/kg.

Induction and Maintenance

There is no standard anesthetic for children having dental procedures. Patients that require a general anesthetic require medications that will allow them to remain motionless during repeated painful stimuli without feeling pain or having recall. This can be achieved with intravenous or inhalational anesthetics. The principles that guide the selection of anesthetics depend on the underlying medical disorders and the procedure being performed. In the United States, the traditional induction technique for general anesthesia in the pediatric age group has been inhalational anesthesia. The anesthesia mask is coated with a pleasant scent such as a fruit-scented lip balm. Sevoflurane, nitrous oxide, and oxygen is administered using high flows and concentrations while the anesthesiologist tells a story or employs another distraction technique. Intravenous induction techniques may include the use of a transdermal local anesthetic (ELA-Max), followed by the insertion of an intravenous cannula and subsequent administration of an appropriate intravenous agent, most commonly propofol or thiopental (Zuckerberg, 1994). Propofol can be mixed with lidocaine (1 mL of 1% lidocaine added to 9 mL of 1% propofol) to minimize local irritation and pain (see Chapter 13, Induction, Maintenance, and Recovery). Other, less commonly used techniques for the induction of general anesthesia include rectal administration of methohexital, thiopental, ketamine, or midazolam (Martone et al., 1991; Roelofse and Van der Bijl, 1991; Zuckerberg, 1994). The nasal or oral transmucosal administration of water-soluble agents such as ketamine or midazolam has also been used (Levine et al., 1993).

When all other attempts have been futile for a child with intellectual or emotional handicaps, an intramuscular injection of ketamine and glycopyrrolate with or without midazolam is used. These techniques should be attempted only with appropriate monitoring and when oxygen, self-inflating resuscitation bag, and suction are available.

Once general anesthesia is induced, intravenous access and the airway are secured. All monitors may be placed before or after induction of anesthesia, depending on the cooperation of the patient. When possible, the first monitors that are placed, regardless of the timing of their placement, should be pulse oximetry and a precordial stethoscope. Careful positioning, padding, and application of thermal conservation devices must be accomplished before beginning dental treatment (see Chapter 13, Induction, Maintenance, and Recovery).

Maintenance of anesthesia for the pediatric patient having dental surgery can be accomplished with either an inhalation technique or an intravenous technique. Sevoflurane is used very commonly as an inhaled anesthetic for outpatient anesthesia. Its use has been described in children having dental procedures. Desflurane is also commonly used for outpatient procedures because of its relatively low blood gas solubility. There does not appear to be a significant advantage of either of these agents over the other for ambulatory anesthesia in terms of clinically significant discharge times. A potential concern for desflurane is its effect on airway reactivity. Patients recovering from desflurane may experience more coughing than those receiving sevoflurane (White et al., 2009). This occurs because, unlike sevoflurane, desflurane increases airway resistance in children having anesthesia. Patients with bronchial hyperreactivity (asthma, upper respiratory tract infections, and bronchopulmonary dysplasia) may be particularly prone to the bronchospastic effects of desflurane and should probably avoid this agent (von Ungern-Sternberg et al., 2008). If an intravenous agent is chosen for maintenance, an ideal agent may be propofol. It has the advantage of a short duration

of action along with its antiemetic benefits (Coté, 1994). Remifentanil is also an appropriate choice.

Studies have not demonstrated benefit of one anesthetic technique over another for dental procedures. Konig et al, (2009), in a double-blind study, compared a sevoflurane-based anesthetic with a propofol-based anesthetic and found no difference in emergence delirium or postoperative pain. However, there was significantly less postoperative nausea and vomiting in the propofol group. Children with autism may have increased propofol requirements when compared with other children with intellectual impairments. In a retrospective study, Asahi and others (2009) found that an increased amount of propofol was required to achieve adequate sedation in children with autism.

Postoperative pain management for children having dental surgery is best accomplished with a multimodal technique. Intraoperatively, the dentist can place dental nerve blocks prior to dental extractions. Nonsteroidal antiinflammatory agents such as ketorolac are very effective for dental pain. The pharmacology of ketorolac has been established in infants and children. A dosage of 0.5 mg/kg provides adequate analgesic plasma levels, and it is cleared at a faster rate in infants, even in those less than 6 months old, than in adults (Lynn et al., 2007; Zuppa et al., 2009). Analgesia may also be supplemented with morphine (0.05 to 0.10 mg/kg), or fentanyl (1 to 4 mcg/kg).

Airway Management

Management of the airway during general anesthesia for dentistry begins with mask ventilation. If the patient has a NAM device in place, it can be removed before initiating mask ventilation. If the device does not interfere with mask ventilation, it can be left in place until the airway is instrumented. Intubation for dental procedures is typically performed nasally to keep the mouth clear for the dentist or oral surgeon. During the preoperative examination, a history of epistaxis should be elicited, and the nares should be inspected for evidence or recent nosebleeds. A child who is old enough may be able to breath through the nares individually to determine which one is more patent. Despite these preoperative tests, epistaxis may still be a significant issue.

Preparation of the nasal cavity is essential to minimize the risk of bleeding and to optimize the laryngoscopic or fiberoptic view. Once the child has been anesthetized, a mucosal vasoconstrictor such as oxymetazoline (Afrin) is applied to the nasal mucosa in both nares. The dosage for the child between 2 to 5 years of age is 2 to 3 drops of a 0.025% solution in each nostril (Mcgee et al., 2009). Oxymetazoline can be administered as drops or it can be applied via nasal cottonoids. There is controversy regarding the use of topical vasoconstrictors. Some pediatric anesthesiologists choose not to use topical vasoconstrictors (phenylephrine or oxymetazoline) because of concern about cardiac complications (e.g., pulmonary edema and cardiac arrest) (Thrush, 1995; Groudine et al., 2000). Systemic absorption of the vasoconstrictor can result in profound systemic vasoconstriction and hypertension. Pulmonary edema occurs secondary to β-blockade treatment of the hypertension.

Before introduction of the nasal endotracheal tube, each naris should be assessed to determine which is the most patent. A lubricated nasal pharyngeal airway can be passed into each naris to accomplish this. The most effective way to determine the best anatomic route for nasal intubation is to fiberoptically inspect each nares. Previously unidentified anatomic abnormalities are most likely to be found with this technique (Smith and Reid, 1999).

Other techniques to minimize bleeding during nasotracheal intubation in children include reducing the size of the endotracheal tube (ETT) by a half to a full size, warming it in warmed saline, and telescoping its end into a rubber catheter (Elwood et al., 2002; Watt et al., 2007). The incidence of bleeding appears to be reduced when the ETT is warmed in saline. The reduction in bleeding is even more pronounced when its tip is covered with a rubber catheter prior to introduction into the naris. In Watt's study, 56% of children who had a room temperature ETT placed had clinically significant bleeding. This was reduced to 39% if the ETT was exposed to warm saline, and it was reduced even further (to 5%) when the tube was telescoped with a rubber catheter. A final technique is to use an obturator, which can be an esophageal stethoscope (Seo et al., 2007), a suction catheter (Herlich et al., 1996), or a fiberoptic scope. Beside bleeding, complications of nasotracheal intubation include bacteremia, dislodgment of adenoidal tissue, and laceration of aerodigestive mucosa with subsequent false passage. Turbinate ulceration may also occur. Fiberoptic guidance of nasotracheal intubation may reduce some of the attendant comorbidities that the anesthesiologist may face (Herlich, 1991). Once the tip of the ETT is positioned in the posterior pharynx, it can be guided into the larynx with direct laryngoscopy or with a flexible fiberoptic scope.

Nasotracheal tubes need to be secured in a way that avoids alar pressure (Fig. 32-9). Prolonged alar pressure can result in tissue ischemia and loss. In addition, the eyes must be protected and the forehead padded.

Fiberoptic intubation may become the rule rather than the exception in patients with facial trauma (Kaban, 1993), mandibulofacial dysostosis (Treacher Collins syndrome), and other congenital craniofacial anomalies (Pierre Robin sequence, Goldenhar's syndrome). These patients frequently have palatal clefts and severe dental problems that require dental therapy and possibly orthognathic surgery (Gendelman and Herlich, 1993).

Patients with a history of recurrent epistaxis, recent nasal trauma, or recent head trauma should potentially not have a nasal intubation performed. In these patients, a straight ETT or an oral RAE tube can be used. A preformed orotracheal tube, such as the oral RAE tube, may be disadvantageous because it is designed to be a midline tube. Moving the preformed tube to either side of the mouth may cause an eccentric positioning in the trachea. An endobronchial intubation may create difficulties in ventilation. If orotracheal intubation is needed, a conventional ETT easily moves to either side of the mouth and oropharynx with the compensatory eccentric tracheal position of the tube. Another concern with moving an oral ETT from side to side is the increased risk of unintentional extubation. An oral tube also decreases the ability of the dental operator to place a rubber dam and complete the dental treatment efficiently. Suboptimal position and placement of dental instruments may also occur when an orotracheal tube is in place. A pharyngeal pack reduces the likelihood that blood and debris are introduced into the aerodigestive tract. Noting the times of insertion and pack removal from the pharynx on the anesthesia record reduces the risk of airway embarrassment postoperatively.

The armored version of the LMA, or flexible LMA, may be indicated for some pediatric dental patients who need dental care under general anesthesia. The advantages of the LMA are its ease of placement and tolerance in the spontaneously ventilating patient. Like an orotracheal tube, it has disadvantages, including its presence in the oral cavity, the interference with rubber dam placement, and its larger size in comparison with a standard orotracheal tube. With a skilled pediatric dentist performing restorative dentistry or surgical procedures, minimal hemorrhage may be seen on the LMA at the end of the procedure (Alexander, 1990; Webster et al., 1993).

Despite meticulous technique on the part of the pediatric dentist who is placing a rubber dam, dental materials may lodge in the oropharynx and subsequently enter the laryngotracheobronchial tree. Hence, a gentle but thorough cleaning and suctioning of the oropharynx before extubation are mandatory.

POSTOPERATIVE PROBLEMS

Most postoperative problems related to pediatric dentistry are common to many other surgical procedures. Postoperative pain, prolonged emergence difficulties with voiding and ambulation, and nausea and vomiting are all seen in pediatric dental patients. However, even after brief general anesthetics for dental procedures, significant hypoxemia may be encountered that is not relieved by administering supplemental oxygen alone. A British study demonstrated that experienced postanesthesia nursing after dental procedures was the most effective means of preventing and treating hypoxemia (Lanigan, 1992).

Postoperative pain may be obviated by the early intraoperative administration of analgesics such as morphine (0.05 to 0.1 mg/kg) or fentanyl (1 to 2 mcg/kg). In addition, an acetaminophen suppository (30 to 40 mg/kg), given shortly before the end of the procedure, confers additional analgesia with minimal side effects. Oral acetaminophen (10 to 15 mg/kg) may be even more effective if given preoperatively (Yaster et al., 1994).

Postoperative nausea and vomiting have numerous causes in the pediatric dental population. A common cause is swallowed blood. Once intraoral bleeding has ceased, the nausea and vomiting from this cause usually abate. Opioid use and abdominal distention caused by bag-mask ventilation with upper airway obstruction or with excessive pressure may also produce postoperative nausea and vomiting. Nitrous oxide is a controversial

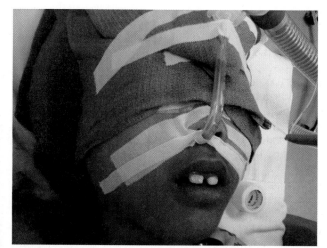

■ **FIGURE 32-9.** One method of taping a nasotracheal tube. Note there is no alar pressure.

cause of postoperative nausea and vomiting. A cause of emesis or nausea unique to dentistry is the inadvertent ingestion of intraoperatively administered topical fluorides to reduce dental caries (Mathewson and Primosch, 1995).

With prolonged postoperative nausea and vomiting, increased hydration and antiemetics may be administered with their attendant caveats, including bladder distention, extrapyramidal effects, and prolonged sedation (Herlich et al., 1996). Ondansetron (100 to 150 mcg/kg) is effective at lessening the severity of postoperative nausea and vomiting when administered prophylactically. Dexamethasone (0.1 to 0.2 mg/kg, up to a maximum of 10 mg) is another highly effective medication for the prevention and treatment of postoperative nausea and vomiting, especially in conjunction with ondansetron (see Chapter 13, Induction, Maintenance, and Recovery). Moderate dose metoclopramide (0.5 mg/kg) has been described prophylactically in children having tonsillectomies, but it is less effective than ondansetron (0.1 mg/kg) (Bolton et al., 2007). If the emesis is severe enough to warrant admission to the hospital for control and rehydration, the pediatric dentist requires the services of a primary care physician (presumably a pediatrician) to assume the overall management of the pediatric dental patient. Fluid and electrolyte management, as well as general patient welfare issues, may be beyond the scope and comfort level of the pediatric dentist. Patients with refractory vomiting requiring admission should have their serum sodium measured to look for hyponatremia.

Some postoperative problems appear more frequently among patients who have had dental rehabilitation, surgical removal of impacted teeth, or other surgical lesions. Postoperative hyperpyrexia seems to occur with greater frequency in patients in whom intraoral dental procedures have been performed. One group investigated preschool-age children to ascertain the etiology of such febrile states. In a randomized fashion, some children were given oral antibiotics 1 hour before their procedure. All children received general anesthesia with nasotracheal intubation and subsequent packing of the oropharynx to reduce the incidence of aspiration of gastric contents and blood. Ventilation was controlled to reduce the likelihood of atelectasis as a cause of postoperative temperature elevation. Intravenous fluid therapy was administered to both groups to reduce the contribution of dehydration as a cause of postoperative temperature elevation. The two groups were found to have equal rates of significant postoperative temperature elevation. The authors suggested that other perioperative etiologies should be investigated, including anesthetic effects on temperature regulation during dental procedures (Holan et al., 1993). There may be certain dentally induced pyrogens, or an antibiotic with a broader spectrum may be needed to cover the organism causing the hyperpyrexic bacteremia.

Nasotracheal intubation, as previously described, is the preferred method of airway protection. However, transient postoperative epistaxis is not uncommon in patients with boggy turbinates, traumatic intubation or extubation, or relatively stenotic nares (Herlich et al., 1996). Usually, direct pressure adequately treats the problem. Rarely, vasoconstrictors and intranasal packing are needed to treat the epistaxis.

Other sequelae of traumatic intubations or extubations, such as croup or generalized laryngeal edema, may need to be treated with intravenous dexamethasone (0.4 mg/kg) immediately after a traumatic or oversized intubation, and possible vasoconstrictors such as racemic epinephrine may be used after extubation.

Postobstruction or negative pressure pulmonary edema may be seen in children with large muscle mass or obesity. The patients are usually adolescents, but this can occur in children as young as 5 years (Van Kooy and Gargiulo, 2000; Ciavarro and Kelly, 2002).

Postoperative oral bleeding should be treated with direct intraoral pressure if a site can be located. Generalized oozing of blood may be treated with gauze dental packs that have large extraoral tails for retrieval. The oral packs act as compression dressings, which should be left in place for 2 hours and not be replaced unless there is significant ongoing hemorrhage. Premature removal or replacement dislodges clots that have not sufficiently matured and retracted into the dental socket. Persistent, minor oral hemorrhage after extraction may also be created. Dislodgment of recently cemented crowns or appliances, inadvertent movement of dental packs, or avulsion of loose teeth not previously extracted may require the presence of the dentist in the postanesthesia care unit to treat the problem.

Dental Complications of Anesthesia

The dental complications of anesthetic care are varied, usually minor, but a frequent source of malpractice claims. Most minor injuries are settled without going through malpractice litigation. The incidence of periperative dental injury is based on retrospective data and varies from 0.02% to 0.05% (Lockhart et al., 1986; Warner et al., 1999; Newland et al., 2007). In one study of a large tertiary medical center, the frequency of perianesthetic dental trauma requiring repair, stabilization, or removal of the tooth was approximately 1 in 4500 cases (Warner et al., 1999). Nevertheless, the anesthesiologist must be aware of the potential pitfalls and take appropriate safeguards. If a dental complication of anesthesia does occur, a dental consultation should be obtained as soon as possible. Also, the chief of the anesthesia department, the hospital's risk manager, and the patient's family should be notified. Patients old enough to understand what has transpired should also be informed.

The neonate is not immune from the dental complications of anesthesia. Laryngoscopy of the neonatal oral cavity may result in excoriation or laceration of the gum pads. Unilateral right- or left-sided hypoplastic enamel defects may be seen in the primary maxillary incisors as a result of laryngoscopy during the neonatal period (Angelos et al., 1989). Oropharyngeal airways, as well as suction devices, may also cause lacerations or excoriation of the intraoral soft tissues. Prophylactic use of water-soluble lubricants or saline solution applied to any of these devices before their placement reduces the likelihood of intraoral trauma.

Many children and their parents are aware of loose primary teeth during the preoperative visit. However, a careful examination, including a mobility check of each primary tooth before induction of general anesthesia, is appropriate (Maxwell et al., 1994).

If an excessively loose primary tooth is noted during the exfoliative phase, the parents should be informed, and it may be safely removed by the anesthesiologist once general anesthesia has been induced. In this increasingly litigious society, a separate, written consent may be necessary for removal of the loose primary tooth by the anesthesiologist. A gauze barrier is placed lingually to prevent inadvertent introduction of the tooth into more distal locations in the respiratory or gastrointestinal tract. Subsequently, a second gauze is wrapped around the loose tooth to be extracted. With a twisting and snapping action, the tooth is easily removed. The tooth is usually missing most or all of its root structure. The reason for the root structure loss is the natural resorptive processes that occur from the underlying permanent tooth that is beginning to erupt. If some of the root structure remains in the extraction site, no attempt should be made to retrieve it. The retrieval process may cause damage to the erupting permanent tooth bud. Also, the remaining root fragment naturally and harmlessly sequesters into the oral cavity (Herlich et al., 1996).

Conditions that may predispose the pediatric patient to dental avulsions under general anesthetic conditions include the scissors-like action of the anesthesiologist's fingers in the mouth opening before laryngoscopy. If this maneuver is accomplished using the incisors, the likelihood of inadvertent avulsion is increased. The mouth-opening maneuvers should be accomplished by using the molars whenever possible to take advantage of their inherent dental stability as well as to effect the largest opening possible. The use of oropharyngeal airways in the pediatric or adult patient as a bite block should be avoided for similar reasons. The anterior teeth are single rooted. If the patient closes the mouth with excessive force, the force transmitted by the tooth is essentially perpendicular to the airway and leads to increased risk of avulsion or fracture. The ideal technique uses gauze bite blocks with a long retrieval tag placed along the molar teeth. The forces are now directed toward softer material and the multirooted molar teeth, which are more likely to sustain and evenly disperse the vertical, shear forces (Herlich, 1990; Herlich et al., 1996).

The inadvertent avulsion of loose primary teeth may nevertheless be unavoidable during airway manipulations. If a primary tooth is avulsed, it is imperative that it be retrieved. The tooth is usually found elsewhere in the mouth or outside of the oral cavity. It may also be found on the patient's gown or bed sheets or on the floor. If it cannot be located in these likely places, anteroposterior and lateral thoracoabdominal radiographs are necessary to locate the tooth. If the tooth is found in the digestive tract, it should pass without incident within several days. If the tooth is found in the tracheobronchial tree, however, it must be retrieved by whatever means necessary, including thoracotomy. The sequelae of leaving a foreign body in the tracheobronchial tree are extremely dangerous (Herlich, 1990; Herlich et al., 1996).

If a primary tooth was lost and then retrieved, it should not be reimplanted. Such attempts are usually futile because of its advanced root resorption before exfoliation. Reimplantation of a primary tooth may also cause significant damage to the underlying permanent tooth bud. However, if the avulsed tooth is a permanent tooth and morphologically intact, attempts should be made to reimplant it as soon as possible. The success of dental reimplantation depends on early reimplantation. Because the periodontal ligament has remnants attached to the tooth that are crucial to the success of reimplantation, the avulsed tooth should not be scrubbed with any material. Ideal preparation consists of gentle rinsing of the tooth in cool physiologic saline solution to remove crude debris and gross clots. Then the tooth should be placed in a cool saline-soaked gauze pad until a dentist can reimplant it, either in the operating room or as early as possible during the postoperative period.

Reimplantation also includes splinting of the tooth to one or two adjacent teeth on each side of the reimplanted tooth to confer stability. Despite early reimplantation, failures exist and may necessitate root canal therapy or extraction at an unspecified later date. The time course of reimplantation failure is unpredictable (Herlich, 1990), but if reimplantation occurs within 30 minutes, success may be as high as 90% (Kainuma et al., 1996).

Pediatric dentistry has made many advances to conserve tooth structure and space if deciduous teeth are lost prematurely. Various polymer and metal crown structures may be bonded or cemented in place. Normal intraoral forces or untoward unnatural forces may cause these prosthetic devices to be loosened or avulsed during airway manipulations. For the most part, they may be easily recemented or bonded postoperatively. Most hospital dental consultants are able to rebond or recement these prostheses in place without difficulty.

Interceptive orthodontic appliances, such as mandibular lingual arch wires or maxillary segmental orthodontic wires, or both, are bonded by brackets to the teeth. These appliances may become loosened or avulsed during airway maneuvers. Like other prosthetic devices, they may also be recemented or bonded postoperatively with little harm to the patient or dentition (Herlich, 1990).

In general, a thorough preoperative history and examination and prudent warnings to the parent reduce dissatisfaction when inadvertent dental complications do occur. Congenital craniofacial anomalies, such as palatal clefts, mandibulofacial dysostosis (Treacher Collins syndrome), Pierre Robin sequence, and hemifacial microsomia, may indeed increase the likelihood of dental complications because of intubation difficulties. Congenital dental anomalies, such as amelogenesis imperfecta or dentinogenesis imperfecta, may subject the patient to dental fracture with even the most trivial airway manipulations.

Acquired dental problems, such as milk-bottle caries syndrome, occur on the lingual surfaces of teeth in children who are regularly put to bed with a bottle of milk, formula, or glucose water. These carious lesions tend to require extensive pediatric dental rehabilitation in very young patients for whom prolonged dental visits are not feasible. As mentioned, those lesions may also be subject to the dental complications of anesthesia.

Pharmacologic agents such as oncologic chemotherapy, chronic inhaled or systemic steroids, diphenylhydantoin, and nifedipine may also cause intraoral or dental damage. A child with a blood dyscrasia or one who has had head and neck radiotherapy may also be subject to dental complications of anesthesia. Blood dyscrasias predispose the child to increased intraoral hemorrhage even during daily oral hygiene activities such as tooth brushing.

Head and neck radiation result in significant xerostomia (dry mouth) because of the destruction of the salivary glands. Because normal salivary flow has been eliminated, these children are at a very high risk for cervical (gumline) caries and possible dental complications during anesthesia. Regardless of the severity or nature of the injury, any head, neck, and oral trauma may predispose a patient to dental complications of anesthesia. With proper planning and care, the patient will have fewer and less severe dental complications (Herlich et al., 1996).

SUMMARY

A diverse and potentially challenging pediatric population requires dental care. For the most part, the dental needs of children are largely unappreciated by physicians, short of their personal experience in the dental chair. This chapter addresses dental issues from the viewpoint of anatomy, physiology, and dental growth and development. The dentist's needs and technical refinements are elaborated to prepare the anesthesiologist to deal with the spectrum of dental procedures. Particular attention is paid to the behavioral and physiologic needs of the pediatric dental population. Nonpharmacologic, pharmacologic, and practical technical strategies are suggested for both the dental operatory and the operating room settings. The pitfalls and complications of each anesthetic technique are given to reduce the learning curve and the anesthesiologist's anxiety when problems do arise, as well as to provide a background for future clinical research. Gentleness and understanding of the pediatric dental patient are required to meet the challenges facing the anesthesiologist and to ultimately improve patient care.

For questions and answers on topics in this chapter, go to "Chapter Questions" at www.expertconsult.com.

REFERENCES

Complete references used in this text can be found online at www.expertconsult.com.

Anesthesia and Sedation for Pediatric Procedures Outside the Operating Room

Keira P. Mason and Robert S. Holzman

Advances in imaging and endoscopic technology requests from medical colleagues for support during prolonged or high-risk procedures and concern about liability exposure have led to increasing demands for anesthesiologists' professional services outside the operating room. In the 14 years since the first publication of this chapter, anesthesia services outside the operating room have increased more than sixfold at Children's Hospital Boston to over 7000 anesthetic procedures annually. As the demand for sedation services has increased nationally, so also have nonanesthesiologists expressed an interest in providing these services and are often using anesthesia billing codes. Indeed, pediatric radiologists, oncologists, dentists, gastroenterologists, pulmonologists, pediatricians, hospitalists, and intensivists are all able to supervise and deliver sedation. Monitoring techniques, sedative choices, and sedation guidelines vary between specialty organizations. Although the American Academy of Pediatrics (AAP) recently updated its guidelines, the recommendations of the American College of Gastroenterology and the American College of Emergency Physicians differ from those of the AAP (AAP et al., 2008).

Anesthesia departments may be reluctant or unable to commit limited financial resources to providing state-of-the-art anesthesia equipment and monitors to extramural locations with limited caseloads. Historically, anesthesia equipment and monitors designed for the outfield environment—small, portable, or safe for use with magnetic resonance imaging (MRI)—are at least double the costs of their operating-room counterparts. In addition, insurance reimbursement may be dif-

ficult, because insurers do not always understand the need for an anesthesiologist. Nonsurgical colleagues and support personnel may have little experience with anesthesia care, delivery, and needs, particularly in urgent situations. Even anesthesiologists are challenged, as few are familiar with the specific requirements associated with interventional, endoscopic, or radiologic procedures. Conflicts may inevitably arise between physicians, administrative personnel, and insurers, particularly because each group has different priorities and expectations. This chapter explores the requirements for anesthetic administration outside the operating room, the available anesthetic techniques, and some specialty-specific considerations. It concludes with current and important safety issues.

REQUIREMENTS FOR EXTRAMURAL LOCATIONS

Organization and Administration

A collaborative relationship between extramural and anesthesiology departments is critical to providing safe patient care. At a minimum, safe patient care requires appropriate anesthesia equipment and monitors, adequate space, and experienced ancillary providers who are knowledgeable in anesthesia and facile in providing assistance if needed. Each off-site area has its own needs, goals, and guidelines. It is ideal to designate a team of anesthesiologists committed to providing extramural anesthesia care and troubleshooting the logistical challenges in the various locations. Each member should rotate regularly through the different extramural sites in order to maintain familiarity with the procedures, to foster a relationship with the physicians and ancillary personnel, to understand the anesthesia demands unique to each site, and sharing information about ongoing advances. Technological advances are particularly expanding in the field of radiology, and complicated imaging studies challenge the anesthesiologist to have an understanding of the unique conditions that each study requires. Understanding these requirements will guide the anesthesiologist in developing a management plan (Lee et al, 2008).

In the past, extramural locations were not designed with the anesthesiologist in mind. The need for anesthesia had not been anticipated when off-site locations were planned. It is only within the past decade that the demand for anesthesia services in these sites has burgeoned. Thus, most off-site locations have not been configured to support the capabilities for anesthesia. Ideally, anesthesiologists should be involved in the early stages of site design to ensure that minimum standards for anesthesia delivery are met and to troubleshoot engineering issues and advocate for adequate space for anesthetic induction and emergence (Committee on Drugs, 1992; American Academy of Pediatrics Section on Anesthesiology, 1999). Physical plant considerations for MRI-site planning have been previously described (Koskinen, 1985). When anesthesia services are requested, these sites may not meet minimum standards and may require reengineering to meet minimum requirements of the American Society of Anesthesiologists (ASA) (House et al., 1994). The anesthesia machine should be equipped with back-up supplies of E cylinders filled with oxygen and nitrous oxide. If pipeline oxygen is not available, then oxygen should be supplied from H cylinders (6600 L) rather than the smaller E tanks (659 L).

Scavenging systems should be carefully evaluated in the extramural location. Unlike the operating room, passive scavenging systems may not always be possible. A safe means of active scavenging may be provided by the vacuum at the wall or wall suction canisters. A scavenging system should be dedicated solely to waste gases. Many MRI scanners do not have wall suction because MRI-compatible wall suction is not widely available. If the suction is located outside the MRI suite, then a mouse-sized hole may be created in the suite's wall to allow suction tubing to be passed inside (Koskinen, 1985).

Electrical circuitry and lighting in extramural locations may not be up to operating room standards, even if the outlets are grounded and up to hospital grade. Although some extramural locations carry minimal risk of electrical shock or electrocution, these sites do not have line-isolation monitors (LIMs) and therefore do not warn of excess leakage of current. Supplemental lighting for recordkeeping, label verification, establishment of intravenous (IV) access, and visualization of the patient is critical. Even under the best circumstances, for example, lighting is dim in the MRI scanner, and monitoring by simple clinical observation can be limited. Anesthesia personnel may not always remain in the imaging suite, particularly during ionizing radiation imaging, computerized tomography (CT) scanning, and radiation therapy. Monitoring capabilities via remote television or hardwiring through reinforced walls can allow video display of the patient and the physiologic monitors within.

A storage area large enough to stock anesthesia equipment and supplies must be easily and quickly accessible. This area should be routinely checked, restocked, and kept locked when anesthesia services are not required. The need for redundancy of nondisposable supplies is a matter of philosophy. Are two laryngoscopes enough, or should there be a third? Is one electrocardiograph (ECG) monitor enough, or should there be a battery-operated monitor for back-up and transport? Drugs should be checked according to the usual operating-room routine, and expired medications should be replaced. Gas-cylinder supplies must be reliable, especially in areas without piped oxygen. A code cart should be conveniently located in an area known to all physicians and ancillary personnel. This cart should be routinely checked and restocked. With larger volumes of patients necessitating significantly sized critical care areas, strong consideration should be given to having a difficult-airway cart available at extramural locations.

Finally, extramural anesthetizing locations are often distant from the operating room. Patients may need to remain anesthetized during transport to or from the extramural location. For these circumstances, assured elevator access with key-controlled emergency overrides is a must. All anesthesiologists who deliver extramural services should be familiar with their surroundings. Checklists are invaluable to guarantee consistent patient care, anesthesia monitoring, equipment, documentation, and back-up assistance.

Personnel, Support, and Logistics

Support and medical personnel in nonsurgical areas may not be familiar with the requirements of an anesthesiologist, thus providing an important educational and training opportunity. Proper training facilitates teamwork and minimizes chaos in critical situations. A standard anesthesia cart at each anesthetizing location should be fully stocked with essential medications, necessary additional equipment, a spare self-inflating bag, endotracheal tubes, laryngeal mask airways (LMAs), suction catheters, IV supplies, laryngoscope handles and blades, and a variety of oral and nasopharyngeal airways.

Leadership is crucial; a director of anesthesia services at an extramural location can orchestrate, facilitate, and coordinate anesthesia services. This director can also serve as a consultant for the other medical and nursing staff. By being available to answer questions, do on-site consultations, examine patients, and provide back-up support or emergency-airway expertise, the anesthesiologist can also support a nurse-administered sedation program. Nurses who provide sedation under the supervision of the ordering extramural physician (e.g., gastrointestinal, radiologic, or dental) should have Pediatric Advanced Life Support (PALS) and Basic Life Support (BLS) certifications. The Joint Commission on Accreditation of Healthcare Organizations (JCAHO) (2009) requires that individuals who administer sedation are able to rescue patients from whatever level of sedation or anesthesia is achieved, whether intentional or unintentional. All children scheduled for nursing sedation during a scan should receive a prescreening telephone call from a radiology nurse the day before the scheduled scan. Often, these telephone calls are made after business hours to ensure that a parent is home. The nurse reviews the medical history, relays fasting instructions, and reminds the parent to administer the child's routine medications with a sip of clear fluid. The supervising physician must give final approval for sedation after reviewing the child's medical history and current medical status and before ordering the medications. To minimize the chance of drug-delivery error or miscalculation, it is helpful to have preprinted order sheets or a computerized order-entry template.

It is crucial to know whom to call for assistance if a problem arises. A speed-dial system should be available from all extramural anesthetizing location sites in order to immediately request emergency back-up help.

PERIPROCEDURAL PATIENT CARE: STANDARDS OF PRACTICE AND QUALITY ASSURANCE

The practice standards adopted by the American Society of Anesthesiologists (ASA) in 1986 for basic intraoperative monitoring apply to extramural locations as well. Practice standards and guidelines promulgated by the AAP are exceeded by established practice standards in anesthesiology (Committee on Drugs, 1992; Anesthesiology and Pediatrics, 1999). Significant variances may exist when practitioners who are not anesthesiologists administer sedation (Keeter et al., 1990). Practice Standards for Non-Anesthetizing Locations were adopted by the ASA in 1994 (ASA House of Delegates, 1994).

As recommended by the JCAHO, sedation-related policies and procedures should be part of a quality-assurance initiative that should accompany all sedation programs. Ideally, adverse events such as failed or prolonged sedations, paradoxical reactions, hypoxia, emesis, unscheduled admissions, or cardiac and respiratory events should be identified and entered into a computerized database. In addition, the extramural nurse should call all patients and families within 24 hours in order to follow-up care on patient outcome and identify any delayed adverse events.

Scheduling and Preparation of Patients

Appropriate planning for an anesthetic begins with a familiarity with the procedure. The requesting service orders the procedure and then leaves the logistics of scheduling to the extramural service. Radiologists recognize that involvement with anesthesia lengthens their total time commitment to a patient and potentially limits the number of procedures accomplished in a day (Winter, 1978; Cremin, 1990). A well-coordinated system to screen patients on the day of the procedure is important. Experienced personnel, ideally a certified pediatric nurse practitioner (CPNP), should be designated to take initial vital signs, review recent medical history, begin IV lines if necessary, and familiarize the family with the upcoming procedure, including anesthesia.

Screening patients for extramural procedures may be challenging and time consuming. Many children are chronically ill, nutritionally impaired, and have complicated medical conditions. These issues must be carefully addressed through attention to the patient's history, physical examination, old medical records, outside consultations, and close communication with other medical colleagues. Several consultants may need to confer in order to fully understand the patient's current state of health. Not every procedure is elective. Urgent procedures may be required despite an upper respiratory tract infection (URI), ongoing pneumonia, deteriorating physical status, untreated gastroesophageal reflux, sepsis, or hemodynamic instability. In these situations, consultation between the anesthesiologist, the requesting physician, and the radiologist should confirm urgency. Anesthesia plans should be adjusted to accommodate the requirements of the procedure (e.g., holding breath for a CT scan of the chest) and the patient's medical condition.

It is not always possible for an anesthesiologist to provide sedation and anesthesia for all children when there is a large volume of cases. A structured nursing sedation program can provide safe and effective sedation. In many hospitals, the extramural department (gastroenterology, radiology, cardiology) outsources responsibility for sedation to another department, which could include pediatrics, hospital medicine, anesthesiology, intensive care, or emergency medicine. After screening the patient, an appropriate referral for either general anesthesia or procedural sedation is the usual result. Because MRI is a unique environment, it is more efficient to have the MRI nurses screen patients before and on the day of the procedure. To ensure consistent decision making, the anesthesiology and radiology departments should develop a set of guidelines and easily identifiable "red flags" to help in this triaging process (Table 33-1). If any questions arise, additional medical history needs to be clarified, or additional studies need to be performed, the nurse and anesthesiologist confer before making the final decision regarding general anesthesia or procedural sedation. In addition, chronically ill children often have electrolyte disturbances, coagulation and hematologic abnormalities, and hemodynamic instability. A consent for the administration of general anesthesia or procedural sedation must be obtained in parity with policies established for anesthesia in the operating room.

Because gastroesophageal regurgitation is common in infants, a detailed clinical history should be taken with regard to the incidence and timing of the regurgitation. If the reflux is predictable (i.e., only associated with mealtimes or soon thereafter) infants are usually approved for procedural sedation. Fasting guidelines are adjusted to minimize the risk of reflux. For example, if the infant has refluxes within 2 hours of eating solid food but never after 3 hours, the fasting guidelines for this infant may be extended to 6 hours for solids.

TABLE 33-1. Red Flags for Sedation

Red Flag	Indications
Apnea	Documented by sleep study, strong clinical history, or on an apnea monitor
Unstable cardiac disease	Cyanotic, depressed myocardial function, or significant stenotic or regurgitation lesions
Respiratory compromise	Recent (<8 weeks) pneumonia, bronchitis, asthma, or respiratory infection
Craniofacial defect	Potential for difficult airway
History of a difficult airway	
Active gastroesophageal reflux or vomiting	In poor control, with or without medical or surgical treatment
Hypotonia and lack of head control	Patient may not be able to maintain own airway without assistance
Allergies to barbiturates	Usually the mainstay of a sedation protocol; also allergies to other sedatives to be administered
Prior failed sedation	Unable to be sedated or unsuccessful imaging study because of excessive movement
Tremors	Unlikely to be ablated with sedation

Selection of Agents and Techniques

The selection of an anesthetic technique in an extramural location depends on the patient's underlying medical condition, age, drug tolerance, and anticipated procedure. The airway management may be influenced by the procedure itself, anticipated postprocedure course (e.g., intensive care unit [ICU] or postprocedure intubation) and past anesthetic course (e.g., difficult intubation). The assistance of an anesthesiologist is often sought when sedation administered by the radiologist has failed in the past; it is important to be aware that parents and radiologists may have the expectation that anesthesia will provide ideal conditions and guarantee successful completion of the procedure (Hubbard et al., 1992).

Premedication has many purposes: the relief of anxiety, easy separation from parents, sedation, analgesia, amnesia, reduction of salivary and gastric secretions, elevation of gastric pH, and decreased cardiac vagal activity. Medications should be adjusted to the psychological and physiologic condition of the patient and family. Parent-present inductions may be offered when the presence of a parent has a calming effect on the child. In the event of potentially detrimental parent anxiety, premedication may be preferable to a parent-present induction (Kain et al., 2001).

Barbiturates may be useful as the sole method of providing sedation. Pentobarbital, for example, has the advantage of providing sedation, causes minimal respiratory and circulatory depression, and is rarely associated with adverse events (Karian et al., 2002). Barbiturates have no analgesic properties. They can produce paradoxical reactions, especially in children. No antagonist to barbiturates is available, thus dosing should be carefully titrated. IV pentobarbital by titration has been used successfully by radiologists while monitoring oral and nasal air flow, oxygen saturation with a pulse oximeter (SpO_2), end-tidal carbon dioxide, and cardiac rate and rhythm, with transient decreases in SpO_2 in up to 7.5% of patients; interventions have included stimulation and head repositioning (Strain et al., 1988; Rooks et al., 2003).

Other studies have described the use of pentobarbital both in the oral and IV forms (Chung et al., 2000; Mason et al., 2001a). For infants younger than 1 year of age, oral pentobarbital is more successful and carries a lower rate of adverse events compared with chloral hydrate (Rooks et al., 2003). The long half-life of pentobarbital (approximately 24 hours) requires careful and conservative recovery and discharge guidelines. The dosage of oral pentobarbital is 2 to 6 mg/kg and up to 9 mg/kg in patients who are receiving barbiturate therapy.

Sodium thiopental in a mean induction dose of 6 mg/kg and a mean total dose of 8.5 ± 3 mg/kg has been used successfully as the sole anesthetic for CT and MRI in 200 children from 1 month to 12 years of age (Spear et al., 1993). Methohexital has a shorter recovery time than thiopental and is more effective than oral chloral hydrate (Manuli and Davies, 1993). Methohexital-induced seizures in patients with temporal lobe epilepsy have been reported. Thiopental or pentobarbital are alternatives for these patients (Rockoff and Goudsouzian, 1981). For patients taking barbiturate-containing anticonvulsant medications, a higher dose limit is generally more successful. Methohexital has also been used intramuscularly (IM) for radiotherapy in doses of 8 to 10 mg/kg. The onset time via this route is often twofold to threefold longer than rectally administered methohexital (Jeffries, 1988).

Although propofol does not have a labeled indication for children younger than 3 years of age, propofol has been used extensively in this age group as a means of providing sedation or anesthesia. Propofol sedation by bolus or continuous infusion for MRI scans of the brain can provide successful imaging conditions but with the risk of need for airway intervention and respiratory compromise (Vangerven et al., 1992; Cravero et al., 2009). Fatal metabolic acidosis and myocardial failure associated with lipemic serum have been reported in five children who were admitted to the ICU for respiratory support for upper respiratory tract infections while being sedated with continuous infusion propofol (Parke et al., 1992). Bloomfield and others (1993) have suggested a continuous infusion beginning at a rate of 99 mL/hr until the patients fall asleep (usually over 1 to 3 minutes) and then a decreasing rate during treatment, a strategy that works very well. Patients were typically awake, alert, and taking clear liquids 20 minutes later (Bloomfield et al., 1993).

Opiates reduce anesthetic, preprocedure, and postprocedure analgesic requirements. They are reversible with naloxone. Whereas narcotics may be unnecessary for diagnostic procedures that are not painful, they may be very useful for therapeutic interventions, especially for patients with postprocedural pain. They are also useful after anthracycline chemotherapy, with documented impaired myocardial function (Burrows et al., 1985). Because narcotics depress the ventilatory response to carbon dioxide (CO_2), this respiratory depression may be of particular concern for children with increased intracranial pressure. Narcotics may also worsen preexisting nausea and vomiting.

Benzodiazepines have the advantage of anxiolysis with minimal vomiting and cardiorespiratory depression. Diazepam is painful during IV injection and may lead to thrombophlebitis; midazolam is water soluble and therefore may be more suitable intravenously or intramuscularly. The elimination half-life of midazolam averages 2.5 hours, compared with 20 to 70 hours for diazepam (Greenblatt et al., 1981; Reves et al., 1985). Young patients or patients with significant liver disease may have prolonged duration and exaggerated effect of the benzodiazepines.

Preparation of the stomach and aspiration prophylaxis are of particular concern for urgently scheduled cases (outside of fasting guidelines) or when the medical history suggests aspiration risk. If using H_2-receptor antagonists, bronchospasm may occur in patients with asthma because of the relative increased availability of H_1-receptors. H_2-blockers may also inhibit metabolism of other concurrently administered medications. Metoclopramide accelerates gastric emptying and increases tone in the lower esophageal sphincter, but it is associated with a significant incidence of extrapyramidal side effects in children (Sledge et al., 1992). Ondansetron works synergistically with other agents through its vagal blocking actions in the gastrointestinal tract, as well as through its inhibition of the chemoreceptor trigger zone via serotonin receptor antagonism, particularly for patients undergoing radiation therapy with pulses of chemotherapy (Burnette and Perkins, 1992; Figg et al., 1993).

Ketamine has enjoyed great popularity during the past 30 years for sedation, analgesia, or anesthesia outside the operating room because of its support of the cardiovascular and respiratory systems. Ketamine-induced nightmares, hallucinations, delusions, and agitation are rare in children (Sussman, 1974; Hostetler and Davis, 2002). Karian and others (2002) have reported on a ketamine-sedation program for use in interventional radiology. In this program, IV or IM ketamine was administered in the interventional radiology suite by credentialed nurses and radiologists to patients undergoing select procedures. This protocol has allowed painful procedures to be tolerated by patients who previously would have required general anesthesia (Karian et al., 2002).

Dexmedetomidine, although not approved by the Food and Drug Administration (FDA) for pediatric use, obtained approval in October 2008 for adult procedural sedation in areas outside of the ICU. Particularly for pediatric sedation for radiologic imaging studies, dexmedetomidine alone in high dosages can achieve immobility for MRI and CT examinations (Mason et al., 2006, 2008a, 2008b). Its use for procedural sedation has still to be explored further, because its clinical application has been examined only in small studies and often in combination with ketamine (Barton et al., 2008).

Some patients require general anesthesia because of previous sedation failures, the need for a secure airway, or procedural logistics. Newer, less-soluble anesthetic agents such as sevoflurane and desflurane have pharmacokinetic profiles that compare favorably with propofol in adults; there seems little reason to think that this would not be the case with children, although pediatric anesthesiologists often avoid using desflurane because of its pungency and associated airway irritability (Van Hemelrijck et al., 1991). Since its introduction to clinical practice in the mid-1990s, sevoflurane has become the volatile anesthetic of choice in children. Its lack of airway irritability as a side effect and its ability to provide children with stable hemodynamic function, together with its rapid onset and offset make sevoflurane a useful agent for children (Furst et al., 1996).

Regional anesthesia, rarely administered outside the pediatric operating room, nevertheless remains a valid choice in some circumstances. Intercostal nerve blocks may be useful for lung or rib biopsies, chest tubes, biliary or subphrenic drainage procedures, and insertion of biliary stents. Nerve block of the brachial plexus by the axillary, interscalene, or supraclavicular route has been reported for the brachial approach to catheterization and neuraxial block of the lower extremities for femoral catheterizations and percutaneous approaches to the kidneys (Eggers et al., 1967; Ross, 1970; Lind and Mushlin, 1987). Spinal anesthesia in conjunction with regional hyperthermia and limb exsanguination has been successfully used for repeated painful radiotherapy on lower extremities (Spencer and Barnes, 1980).

Indwelling central catheters are implanted in the majority of radiotherapy patients and can be used for induction and maintenance of anesthesia, blood draws, IV fluid administration, and chemotherapy. Dressing changes are often accomplished in conjunction with the sedation or anesthesia. Antiseptic preparation of all injection sites with povidone-iodine and alcohol is critical. At the end of the session the catheter should be carefully flushed with heparinized saline. An alternative to central catheters is the use of a heparin-lock peripheral IV port, changed weekly, with careful parental instruction. Smoothness of emergence is particularly important after angiographic procedures because of the risk of a dislodged clot or bleeding at the puncture site. Some patients have been heparinized without protamine reversal. Unlike adults, sand bags and weights are not routinely applied to angiographic cannulation sites of children.

Occasionally, the loss of self-control with sedation results in dysphoria, and some patients fare better when they are completely awake. Minimal medication may be preferable in patients with complicated and unstable medical conditions who may not tolerate the anesthesia or sedation. Some procedures (e.g., unilateral carotid barbiturate injection or the Wada test) may require conversation, interaction, and responsiveness of the patient. In these situations, no sedation may be the best alternative.

POSTANESTHESIA CARE

Recovery criteria and the postanesthesia care unit (PACU) environment in an extramural location must be no different than the postanesthesia care delivered to children after an operative procedure. Each site must have sources of supplemental oxygen, the ability to deliver positive pressure ventilation, the availability of suction and monitoring equipment, and a nursing staff trained in postanesthesia care. Discharge criteria should be established by an anesthesiologist in conjunction with the extramural service and its nursing staff.

Postprocedure analgesic requirements are extremely variable. Whereas a groin puncture may be only mildly annoying for adults, the inability to move about and the ache of blood dissecting subcutaneously causes considerable discomfort in children. All children who have undergone angiography require a minimum PACU stay of 4 hours to ensure that the puncture site does not bleed or develop a hematoma. Ideally, a patient should be free of pain and resting supine and motionless in order to minimize the risk of a groin-puncture bleed or hematoma. An experienced member of the nursing staff should be able to recognize and manage unexpected agitation, delirium, or an unanticipated or undesired change in mental status and know to call for extra help.

The anesthesiologist may be asked to participate in the perioperative care of patients who have had embolization procedures. These patients often experience pain or swelling after the procedure, with the severity of discomfort depending on the extent of embolization, the agent used for embolization, postembolic swelling, and the amount of tissue necrosis. A variety of analgesic techniques are available, and the use of steroids perioperatively, although they do not directly decrease pain, may be of benefit in reducing edema and postembolic neuritis. Postembolic swelling influences perioperative airway management for procedures in the head and neck. Pediatric patients may need to remain intubated after such procedures, particularly when visible edema in the floor of the mouth, tongue, hypopharynx, oropharynx, or anterior neck could compromise the airway.

Nausea or vomiting may increase venous blood pressure because of the Valsalva maneuver, which can aggravate bleeding and swelling in puncture sites or after head and neck procedures. Hypothermia is a risk at some extramural locations because the MRI, CT, and interventional radiology equipment require a cool environment. Heating lamps and forced air heaters may be used when it is safe and appropriate to do so. Finally, with the use of iodine-containing radiocontrast media, as well as sclerosing and embolizing agents, consideration must be given to adequate volume resuscitation, the risk of a contrast reaction, and bladder catheterization for detection of oliguria, polyuria, or hematuria.

RESUSCITATION

Each extramural anesthetizing location is unique with regard to conducting resuscitation. Redundancy of monitoring devices and equipment is important; a provider should not be limited to a single item that could malfunction at the time of resuscitation. Patients with multiple allergies, shellfish allergies, or atopic disease are at increased risk of exhibiting anaphylaxis to iodine-containing contrast. These patients may benefit from pretreatment with steroids and antihistamines. Areas with restricted access (MRI in particular) should have designated adjacent locations to perform full resuscitation. These areas should be equipped with wall oxygen, suction, and full monitoring and resuscitation capability. A self-inflating silicone bag (no ferromagnetic working parts) or nonferrous Jackson-Rees circuit should always be kept inside the MRI suite.

The physicians, nurses, anesthesiologists, technologists, and support personnel must know the location of a readily accessible code cart. In addition, a hard board to be placed under the patient during resuscitation should be available. Mock codes should be performed regularly to ensure adequate flow, teamwork, and delineation of responsibilities in the event of an emergency. The MRI scanner poses a special problem. Codes should never be conducted in the scanner because as support personnel rush inside to assist, ferrous materials that are not removed will become projectile and create an even more hazardous situation. Quenching a magnet should not be an alternative, because it requires a minimum of 3 minutes to eliminate the magnetic field. In addition, inadequate exhaust during a quench has been known to produce hypoxic conditions in the scanner and has resulted in patient death. A "black quench" could melt the MRI coils and require replacement of the scanner, a costly and time-consuming undertaking. Defibrillators are not compatible with MRI and may not function properly when they are exposed to the magnetic field (Snowdon, 1989). In an emergency, a patient should be removed from the scanner to an area outside of the magnetic field. This designated area is a safe place for resuscitation and should have not only a wall oxygen source for a self-inflating bag but also access to appropriate monitors.

SPECIFIC EXTRAMURAL SITES

Radiology

Computerized Tomography Scan

CT differentiates between high-density (e.g., calcium, iron, bone, and contrast-enhanced vascular and cerebrospinal fluid [CSF] spaces) and low-density (e.g., oxygen, nitrogen, carbon in air, fat, CSF, muscle, white matter, gray matter, and water-containing lesions) structures. Because the scan time is quick, CT may be preferable for patients who are medically unstable and in need of rapid diagnosis—for example, with the child being evaluated for abuse, an intracranial hemorrhage, or abdominal or thoracic mass. Other indications for emergency CT scans may include encephalopathy and a change in neurologic status. In these situations, the issues of a full stomach and increased intracranial pressure usually necessitate a rapid-sequence induction with tracheal intubation. A CT scan of the head is often the preferred study in emergency situations where head trauma is involved (Blankenberg et al., 2000).

The actual scanning sequences are short and can range from 10 to 40 seconds. These short scan times enable many children to complete a CT scan without any sedation, especially with parental presence and distraction techniques. When an anesthesiologist is involved, it is often for airway or failed-sedation issues or for a medically complicated patient. An important aspect of some CT scans is to visualize the sinuses, ears, inner auditory canal, and temporomandibular bones and to evaluate for choanal atresia or craniofacial abnormalities. These scans may require direct coronal imaging with extreme head extension (off the end of the table at an angle between 40 and 70 degrees) or absolute immobility for three-dimensional reconstruction, so it is critical for the treatment team to have a thorough understanding of the specifics of the study. Three-dimensional airway and cardiac studies have evolved and have unique anesthetic requirements. The airway studies require breath holding on inspiration and expiration in order to allow visualization of areas with airway collapse (Lee et al., 2008). The cardiac studies are often done in collaboration with cardiologists and radiologists who are able to make structural and functional assessments of the heart. These scans can also be challenging, because adenosine is often requested in order to briefly pause heart function so that image quality is maximized (Woodard et al., 2006).

Any patient who is at risk for cervical instability should be properly screened before neck extension. Children with Down syndrome are at risk for atlantoaxial instability. The incidence of instability varies from 12% to 32% (Blankenberg et al., 2000). Many children with Down syndrome require cervical spine radiographs before entering grade school or participating in Special Olympics. Usually, the parents are well aware of the radiologic findings. The cervical spine films, however, do not indicate whether or not a child is at risk for dislocation (Davidson, 1988). Rather, those children who exhibit neurologic signs or symptoms such as abnormal gait, increased clumsiness, fatigue with ambulation, or a new preference for sitting games are at risk. In infants, developmental milestones (e.g., crawling, sitting up, and reaching for objects) should be verified. Physical signs of Down syndrome may include clonus, hyperreflexia, quadriparesis, neurogenic bladder, hemiparesis, ataxia, and sensory loss. The asymptomatic Down syndrome child with radiologic evidence of instability may be approved for procedural sedation; however, unnecessary neck movement should be avoided. Any child who displays neurologic signs or symptoms should not be sedated until a neurosurgical or orthopedic consultation is obtained.

Radiologists employ Gastrografin when evaluating abdominal masses. Gastrografin diluted to a concentration of 1.5% is usually considered a clear liquid. The volume that is administered orally is significant; newborns younger than 1 month of age receive 60 to 90 mL, infants between 1 month and 1 year of age may receive up to 240 mL, and children between the ages of 1 and 5 years receive between 240 and 360 mL. Because sedation or anesthesia should usually be accomplished within a window of 1 to 2 hours after ingestion of the contrast, most "elective" fasting guidelines would be violated; however, the scan must be completed while the Gastrografin is still in the gastrointestinal tract. There are no published data to guide optimal induction or sedation techniques as they relate to aspiration risk in these circumstances. Full strength (3%) Gastrografin is hyperosmolar and hypertonic. All Gastrografin should be diluted to an isosmolar and isotonic 1.5% concentration of neutral pH. There is one case report of 1.5% Gastrografin aspiration in a child with no adverse sequelae; therefore, the risk of using a 1.5% concentration of Gastrografin seems low (Friedman et al., 1986; Wells et al., 1991).

Embolization Procedures

Interventional techniques include nonvascular and vascular interventions (Towbin and Ball, 1988). In vascular interventions, embolization and sclerotherapy have become important techniques for treating vascular malformations, aneurysms, fistulas, and hemorrhage; for accomplishing renal ablation; and for presurgical embolization of hypervascular masses. Percutaneous transluminal angioplasty and fibrinolytic therapy are increasing in pediatric institutions; great success is being reported, even in the smallest infants, and the important contribution that adequate sedation and analgesia can make to ultimate outcome has been recognized (Diament et al., 1985).

Vascular malformations are congenital aberrant connections between blood vessels and may be composed of lymphatic, arterial, and venous connections. These lesions, although present at birth, are often discrete and not clearly visible. As the child grows, the vascular malformation may expand rapidly, growing with the child. This rapid proliferative phase may occur in response to hormonal changes (e.g., pregnancy or puberty), trauma, or other stimuli (Jackson et al., 1993). Vascular malformations may be high-flow or low-flow lesions, depending on which vessels are involved. High-flow lesions include arteriovenous fistulas, some large hemangiomas, and arteriovenous malformations. Particularly with large lesions, high-output cardiac failure and congestive heart failure with the potential for pulmonary edema should be anticipated and sought out in the medical history and physical examination. Low-flow lesions consist of venous, intramuscular venous, and lymphatic malformations. Surgical resection of symptomatic vascular malformations may be hazardous as well as unsuccessful—any vascular element not resected may enlarge and cause further problems.

Because vascular malformations enlarge over time, even asymptomatic lesions may require intervention. Patients with symptoms may suffer from pain, tissue ulceration, disfigurement, airway or cardiovascular compromise, impairment of limb function, coagulopathy, claudication, hemorrhage, and progressive nerve degeneration or palsy. Because large vascular lesions require multiple embolizations, parents and patients are often comforted by seeing familiar anesthesiologists, another benefit of having a core group of anesthesiologists in the radiology suite. Vascular embolization is also used as a bridge to surgical resection. Successful embolization and sclerotherapy decrease the size of the malformation and reduce blood flow to the lesion, thereby decreasing surgical risks.

When embolizing vascular malformations, radiologists often aim to cut off not only the feeding vessels but also the central confluence (nidus) where much of the arterial shunting occurs. Embolic agents include stainless-steel minicoils, absorbable gelatin pledgets and powder, detachable silicone balloons, polyvinyl alcohol foam, cyanoacrylate glue, and ethanol. The choice of agent depends on the clinical situation and the size of the blood vessel. When permanent occlusion is the goal, polyvinyl alcohol foam and ethanol are often employed. Both occlude at the level of the arterioles and capillaries. Medium to small-sized arteries may be occluded with coils, the equivalent of surgical ligation. Particularly in trauma situations, when only tempo-

rary occlusion (days) is the goal, absorbable gelatin pledgets or powder are used (Coldwell et al., 1994).

Large hemangiomas may be associated with the coagulopathy of Kasabach-Merritt syndrome. In this condition, the hemangioma traps and destroys platelets and other coagulation factors, resulting in thrombocytopenia and an increased risk of bleeding. As the hemangioma involutes, the coagulation status improves (Mulliken and Young, 1988). A condition described as systemic intravascular coagulation (SIC) can occur after the embolization of extensive vascular malformations. This condition is marked by an elevated prothrombin time (PT) with a decrease in coagulation factors and platelets.

Absolute (99.9%) ethanol is injected in vascular malformations to promote sclerosis. Ethanol may produce a coagulum of blood and cause endothelial necrosis (Becker et al., 1984). Sclerotherapy or embolization with absolute ethanol increases the risk of developing a postprocedure coagulopathy marked by positive D-dimers, elevated PT, and decreased platelets (Mason et al., 2001b). Ethanol causes thrombosis, because it injures the vascular endothelium. Ethanol also denatures blood proteins. Extensive ethanol injections can cause hematuria, and urinary catheters should be inserted to monitor urine output, diuresis, and hematuria. Especially with children scheduled for outpatient surgery, liberal fluid replacement ensures that the hematuria clears before discharge. Ethanol can cause neuropathy and tissue necrosis if it is not injected selectively. Using selective catheterization and direct percutaneous puncture, care is taken not to expose normal blood vessels to the ethanol. In addition to the risk of hematuria, ethanol also can produce significant serum alcohol levels. Mason and others (2000) note that up to 1 mL/kg of ethanol can be administered and that serum ethanol levels have been greater than the intoxication level of .008 mg/dL (Fig. 33-1). Patients with high serum-ethanol levels may be either sedated or extremely agitated, depending on their particular response to intoxication.

Embolization or balloon occlusion of arterial venous malformations, vascular tumors, intracranial aneurysms, and fistulae carries considerable risk of catastrophic results. Risks include a sudden intracranial hemorrhage, acute cerebral ischemia, or catheter or balloon migration. If sedated, the patient may require urgent airway management. Long cases require a urinary catheter, especially if contrast material is used.

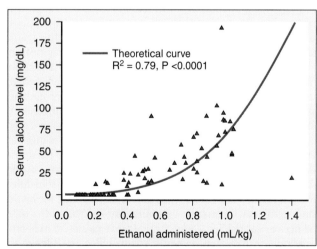

■ **FIGURE 33-1.** Relationship between ethanol administered (mL/kg) and serum ethanol level (mg/dL).

Cerebral angiography requires motionlessness as well as exquisite control of ventilation. Anesthetic technique, in choice of agent as well as in control of arterial CO_2 tension, may affect cerebral blood flow and hence the quality of the scan. Cerebral angiography may be performed in children for the diagnosis or follow-up study of Moyamoya disease, and these children should have anesthetic techniques that minimize the risk of transient ischemic attacks (TIAs) and stroke during the procedure (Soriano et al., 1993). Other considerations include controlled hypercarbia to promote vasodilation and facilitate access and visualization of the vasculature for the radiologist. In the event of vasospasm or difficult access of small, torturous vessels, locally administered (through the catheter) nitroglycerin in small doses (25 to 50 mcg) may facilitate visualization and access. Occlusion of the venous portion of the arteriovenous malformation (AVM) without complete occlusion of the arterial inflow vessels could result in acute swelling and bleeding. Vascularity reduction through occlusion of major feeder vessels is the goal of embolizing large AVMs before planned surgical excision. This may be accomplished as a staged procedure over several days, involving repeated anesthetics or sedation sessions.

Angiographic imaging may be enhanced through the use of glucagon. Glucagon is efficacious for digital subtraction angiography, visceral angiography, and selective arterial injection in the viscera. When needed, glucagon is administered intravenously in divided doses of 0.25 mg to a maximum of 1 mg. Risks include glucagon-induced hyperglycemia, vomiting (particularly when given rapidly), gastric hypotonia, and provocation signs of pheochromocytoma (McLoughlin et al., 1981; Chernish et al., 1990; Jehenson, 1991). Children who receive glucagon should routinely receive prophylactic antiemetics.

The ability to intermittently assess neurologic function and mental status is invaluable during embolization procedures, but it may not be practical in children because of fear, pain, and movement. General anesthesia permits easier control of blood pressure and ventilation and eliminates the concern about patient movement. For children, general anesthesia is often preferred when performing high-risk procedures that require immobility and periods of breath-holding. Preprocedural assessment should include any history of seizures, bleeding, treatment with anticonvulsants or anticoagulants, neurologic symptoms, and evaluation of intracranial-pressure status. It is important to determine whether the patient has had any TIAs or has evidence of cerebrovascular occlusion. Vasodilator agents (calcium channel blockers) or nitrate derivatives may need to be administered after embolization. Because many patients are anticoagulated during the procedure, a preoperative coagulation profile should be obtained. A variety of anticoagulants may have to be on hand as well to prophylaxis for thrombosis (Bidabe et al., 1990).

Morbidity associated with embolization is not negligible. Arteriovenous malformations (AVMs) involving the head and neck often require cannulation of the external carotid artery branches and the thyrocervical trunk. All patients scheduled for embolization should be typed and cross-matched for blood. Those patients who undergo embolizations of AVMs of the head and neck are at risk for stroke, cranial nerve palsies, skin necrosis, blindness, infection, and pulmonary embolism (Riles et al., 1993). It is important to assess and document full return of neurologic status after the patient is extubated.

Ultrasound-Directed Procedures

Needle biopsies and drainage procedures are directed with ultrasound guidance for diagnostic examination (e.g., of the kidneys, liver, lungs, muscle, unknown mass, or unknown fluid). Percutaneous drainage of abscesses, cysts, pancreatic pseudocysts, and other fluid-containing structures can often be accomplished with ultrasound guidance. Ultrasound is useful for placement of difficult central venous-line (CVL) catheters and peripherally inserted central catheters (PICCs). The requirement for general anesthesia vs. sedation for ultrasound-guided procedures depends in part on the duration of the procedure, the location involved, the risks associated with the procedure, and any procedural requirements. The need for controlled ventilation with breath holding may require an endotracheal tube and general anesthesia. Associated secondary effects of the end-organ disease must be kept in mind in the overall anesthetic care plan.

Magnetic Resonance Imaging

Atoms with an odd number of protons or neutrons are capable of acting as magnets. When they are aligned in a static magnetic field, they can be subjected to radiofrequent energy that alters their original orientation. With removal of the radiofrequency pulse, the nuclei rotate back to their original alignment (relaxation), and the energy released can be detected and transformed into an image. Hydrogen is the atom most often used for imaging, because it is present in most tissues as water and long-chain triglycerides.

MRI is employed for the evaluation of neoplasms, trauma, skeletal abnormalities, and vascular anatomy (Barnes, 1992). MRIs of the brain are often performed to evaluate developmental delay, behavioral disorders, seizures, failure to thrive, apnea and cyanosis, hypotonia, and mitochondrial or metabolic disorders. Magnetic resonance angiography and venography (MRA and MRV) are especially helpful in evaluating vascular flow and can sometimes replace invasive catheterization studies for follow-up or initial evaluations of vascular malformations, interventional treatment, or radiotherapy (Edelman and Warach, 1993). Functional MRI (fMRI) is an evolving technology that measures the hemodynamic or even metabolic response related to neural activity in the brain or spinal cord. fMRI is often able to localize sites of brain activation and is now dominating brain-mapping techniques because of its low invasiveness and lack of radiation exposure. Some fMRI studies require cognitive facility and are typically interactive with a conscious and responsive patient. fMRI studies on children who are unable to respond appropriately either because of age or cognitive compromise are challenging—how that will evolve in pediatric anesthesiology practice is not yet clear.

Historically, the anesthetic management of children in the MRI suite has been highly dependent and somewhat limited by MRI-compatible monitors and anesthesia gas machines. (Karlik et al., 1988; Menon et al., 1992; Tobin et al., 1992). The American College of Radiology (ACR) established guidelines to minimize the risk of MRI-related mishaps but did not address the needs of the anesthesiologist (Kanal et al., 2007). These guidelines were written in response to fatalities that had occurred when loose, nonferrous oxygen cylinders became projectiles when brought inadvertently into the MRI suite with a patient in the bore of the magnet (Chaljub et al., 2001). In 2008 the ASA assembled a task force composed of anesthesiologists and a radiologist with MRI expertise. This Task Force on Anesthetic Care for Magnetic Resonance Imaging created a document entitled the *Practice Advisory on Anesthetic Care for Magnetic Resonance Imaging* (ASA Task Force on Anesthetic Care for MRI, 2009). This document establishes important recommendations for safe practice as well as consistency of anesthesia care in the MRI environment. Most important, the Practice Advisory includes all sedation, including monitored anesthesia care, general anesthesia, critical care, and ventilatory support. Conditions of high-risk imaging were defined as imaging in patients with medical or health-related risks or as equipment-related, procedure-related, or surgery-related risks. MRI-guided interventions, cardiac imaging, and airway imaging were all identified as high-risk procedures. The Task Force was designed to promote patient and health care provider safety, prevent MRI mishaps, recognize limitations in physiologic monitoring, optimize patient management, and identify potential equipment and health risks (ASA Task Force on Anesthetic Care for MRI, 2009).

Anesthetic management also depends on the availability of support personnel, equipment and monitors; the personal style and comfort level of the anesthesiologist; and the patient's particular medical history. Requiring a general anesthetic solely to ensure motionless conditions for a radiologic imaging study is often a frightening concept for parents. Parents often equate pain and surgical interventions with the need for anesthesia and are reluctant to expose their child to a general anesthetic for the sake of an MRI study. Children under the age of 5 years most commonly require moderate or deep sedation or an anesthetic to ensure motionless conditions. Ketamine, narcotics, or benzodiazepines are generally unsuccessful. Pentobarbital, propofol, and dexmedetomidine offer successful alternatives to inhalation anesthesia (Mason et al., 2001a, 2004, 2008a, 2008b; Guenther et al., 2003, Yamamoto, 2008). One technique for general anesthesia is to perform an inhalation induction followed by placement of an LMA. During the scan, the patient maintains spontaneous ventilation. Lidocaine gel (2%) on the LMA cuff is a useful adjunct, because it decreases the incidence of sore throat and retching (Chan and Tham, 1995; Keller et al., 1997). A retrospective study of 200 patients demonstrated the usefulness of this approach (Brimacombe et al., 1995). In children with upper respiratory infections, there was a lower incidence of mild bronchospasm, laryngospasm, breath-holding, and major oxygen desaturation (less than 90%) in the group with LMAs compared with the group that received endotracheal anesthesia (Tait et al., 1998). Temperature monitoring can be accomplished by liquid crystal display (skin temperature). There is still no means of monitoring core temperature, because any temperature probe would risk heat generation and thermal burns to the patient.

Anesthesiologists must be aware of many personal items taken for granted—clipboards, pens, watches, scissors, clamps, credit cards, eyeglasses, and paper clips that should not be in the MRI field (Karlik et al., 1988; Menon et al., 1992; Tobin et al., 1992). Conventional ECG monitoring is not possible, because as the lead wires traverse the magnetic fields, image degradation occurs and, most importantly, the ECG leads heat and cause burns on the patient. Fiberoptic ECG monitoring is necessary to minimize the risk of patient burn. Even with fiberoptic cables, it is important to recognize that the connections between the ECG pads and the telemetry box are still hardwired, and careful attention must be paid to prevent frays,

overlap, exposed wires, and knots in the cables (Shellock, 1989). In order to prevent injury to the patient, care must be used to avoid creating a conductive loop between the patient and a conductor (e.g., ECG monitoring and gating leads, plethysmographic gating wire, and fingertip attachments). During the scan, no exposed wires or conductors can touch the patient's skin, and no imaging coil can be left unconnected to the magnet. Pulse oximeters are also not conventional to the operating room environment; rather they are fiberoptic. Failure to remove the conventional pulse oximeter probes and adhesives has resulted in second- and third-degree burns (Shellock, 1989; Brow et al., 1993).

Current advances in physiologic monitoring and anesthesia machines for the MRI environment have optimized the ability of the anesthesia care provider to provide safe care in the MRI suite. The Dräger Fabius MRI (Dräger Medical AG; Lübeck, Germany) was designed for MRI and approved by the FDA in 2008 for use within both a 1.5-Tesla (T) and 3-T magnetic field up to a field strength of 400 gauss. The Dräger Fabius MRI, equipped with two vaporizers, is an electronically controlled ventilator and the first one able to deliver multiple modes of ventilation in the MRI suite. Advances in physiologic monitoring now offer the ability to monitor ECG and pulse oximetry in a 1.5-T and 3-T MRI scanner via wireless, fiberoptic communication (Invivo Precess, Inviv; Orlando, Florida).

Average noise levels of 95 dB have been measured in a 1.5-T MRI scanner; this level of noise is comparable with the noise level of very heavy traffic (92 dB) or light road work (90 to 110 dB). Exposure to this level of noise has not been considered hazardous if it is limited to less than 2 hours per day (Gangarosa et al., 1987). There are case reports, however, of both temporary and permanent hearing loss after an MRI scan (Brummett et al., 1988; Kanal et al., 1990). Three-Tesla magnets offer the advantage of less image degradation and improved neuroskeletal and musculoskeletal imaging. As the field strength increases, so does the noise (Hattori et al., 2007). In fact, the peak sound-pressure level of a 3-T magnet exceeds 99 dB, the level approved by the International Electrotechnical Commission. Noise reduction did not differ between earplugs and headphones, although the combination of both was more effective at reducing sound (Hattori et al., 2007). Earplugs or MRI-compatible headphones should be offered to all pediatric patients and are required for all patients imaged in the 3-T MRI scanner. fMRI provides additional challenges in the 3-T environment; the noise of the 3 T can interfere with the acoustic stimulation generated for purposes of obtaining the fMRI (Ravicz et al., 2000; Menendez-Colino et al., 2007). Video goggles compatible with the 1.5-T and 3-T environments (Resonance Technology; Los Angeles, California) may be worn by the patient during MR imaging to provide a three-dimensional virtual reality system complete with audio integration. The introduction of this integrated audio-video headset has revolutionized the ability to offer distraction to patients, many of whom are able to tolerate imaging without adjuvant sedation or anesthesia.

Although studies in mice and dogs suggest that exposure to magnetic fields may increase body temperature, it is unlikely that static magnetic fields up to 1.5 T have any effect on core body temperature in adult humans (Sperber et al., 1984; Shellock et al., 1986; Shuman et al., 1988). However, this may be of greater concern in infants and small children, especially in cases like cardiac MRI studies that require a long scan time. The specific absorption rate (SAR) is measured in watts per kilogram and is used to follow the effects of radiofrequency heating. The FDA allows an SAR of 0.4 W/kg averaged over the whole body (Department of Health and Human Services, FDA, 1982). Ex vivo exposure of large metal prostheses to fields over six times that experienced in MRI have not revealed any appreciable heating (Davis et al., 1981). To date, there has been no conclusive evidence that radiofrequency is a significant clinical issue in magnets up to 3 T.

The biological effect of MRI should be considered when offering parent-present induction; however, there are no reports implicating MRI-caused chromosomal aberrations. Studies in amphibians demonstrate that exposure to a 4-T magnetic field does not cause any defects in embryologic development (Prasad et al., 1990). Most hospital's MRI machines are 1.5 T. Despite these studies, pregnant patients or family members are not usually allowed into the MRI scanner. MRI scans during pregnancy are discouraged by the ACR during the first and second trimesters unless fetal imaging is required or the MRI is necessary for emergent medical care (Woodard et al., 2006).

Additional safety issues for MRI include implanted objects (i.e., cardiac pacemakers), ferromagnetic attraction that causes objects to become projectile, noise, biological effects of the magnetic field, thermal effects, equipment issues, and claustrophobia. Some stainless steel may contain ferritic, austenitic, and martensitic components (Dujovny et al., 1985; Persson et al., 1985). Martensitic alloys contain fractions of a crystal phase known as martensite, which has a body-centered cubic structure, is prone to stress corrosion failure, and is ferromagnetic. Austenite is formed in the hardening process of low carbon and alloyed steels and has ferromagnetic properties. Iron, nickel, and cobalt are also ferromagnetic. For this reason, the components of any implanted device should be carefully researched before entering the magnet. Stainless steel or surgical stainless objects interacting with an external magnetic field may produce translational (attractive) and rotational (torque) forces. Intracranial aneurysm clips, cochlear and stapedial implants, shrapnel, intraorbital metallic bodies, and prosthetic limbs may move and potentially dislodge. Special precaution should be taken with cochlear implants in the 3-T environment, because unremovable magnets may suffer demagnetization in the scanner. These patients should only undergo imaging in the 3-T scanner after special precautions are taken (Majdani et al., 2008). Some eye makeup and tattoos may contain metallic dyes and therefore cause ocular, periorbital, and skin irritation (Scherzinger and Hendee, 1985; Prasad et al., 1990). Some tissue expanders employed in reconstructive surgery have a magnetic port to help identify the location for intermittent injections of saline (Liang et al., 1989). Bivona tracheostomy tubes usually contain ferrous material (although it is not specified in the package insert) and should be replaced with Shiley tracheostomy tubes before patients enter the MRI environment.

Cardiac pacemakers present a special hazard in and around the MRI scanner, especially in patients who are dependent on pacemakers. Most pacemakers have a reed relay switch that can be activated when they are exposed to a magnet of sufficient strength (Pavlicek et al., 1983). This activation could convert the pacemaker to the asynchronous mode. There are at least two known cases of patients with pacemakers who died from cardiac arrest while in an MRI scanner. The autopsy of one patient determined that the death was the result of an interruption of the pacemaker in the magnetic environment (Center for Disease and Radiological Health, 1989).

In addition to the risk of pacemaker malfunction, there is also the chance that torque on the pacer or pacing leads may create a disconnect or microshock (Erlebacher et al., 1986). Recent studies demonstrate that with careful preparation, select patients with permanent pacemakers and implantable cardioverter defibrillators may safely undergo imaging in the 1.5-T environment without any inhibition or activation of their device (Nazarian et al., 2006). The ACR formed a Blue Ribbon Panel on MRI Safety in 2001 to review existing MRI safety practices and issue new guidelines. The *ACR Guidance Documents for Safe MR Practices* was published in 2002 and updated in 2004 and again in 2007 (Kanal et al., 2007). Safety concerns related to pediatric MRI were specifically addressed in the 2007 document, with specific emphasis on patient screening, sedation, and monitoring issues. Implanted cardiac pacemakers or implantable cardioverter defibrillators were considered a relative contraindication to MRI and only scanned in locations staffed with radiologists and cardiologists of appropriate expertise. The recommendation was for radiology and cardiology personnel, along with a fully stocked crash cart, to be readily available, as well as a programmer to adjust the device if necessary. After the MRI, a cardiologist should confirm function of the device and recheck it within 1 to 6 weeks. In general, heart valves are not ferromagnetic and are not a contraindication to MRI. It is critical that everyone entering the vicinity of the MRI scanner fills out a screening form that specifically lists every possible implantable device, alerting the MRI staff to any potential hazards.

The magnetic field may affect the electrocardiogram. The changes in the T wave are not the results of biological effects of the magnetic field but rather to superimposed induced voltages. This effect of the magnetic field on the T wave is not related to cardiac depolarization, because no changes to the P, Q, R, or S waves have ever been observed in patients exposed to fields up to 2 T. There are no reports of MRI affecting heart rate, ECG recordings, cardiac contractility, or blood pressure (Beischer, 1969; Tenforde et al., 1983; McRobbie and Foster, 1985; Gulch and Lutz, 1986). One study, however, found that humans exposed to a 2-T magnet for 10 minutes developed a 17% increase in the cardiac cycle length (CCL). The CCL represented the duration of the RR interval. The CCL reverted to preexposure length within 10 minutes of removing the patient from the magnetic field (Jehenson et al., 1988). The implications of this finding are unclear. This change in CCL in patients with normal hearts may be of no consequence. The implications of this finding for patients with fragile dysrhythmias or sick sinus syndrome, however, have yet to be determined.

In the presence of an external magnetic field, a ferromagnetic object can develop its own magnetic field and become a projectile object. The attractive forces that are created between the intrinsic and extrinsic magnetic fields can propel the ferromagnetic object toward the MRI scanner. Special note should be made of the magnet's strength. Over the past few years, 1.5-T magnets have been supplanted by 3-T magnets. The field strength and magnetic force generated by a 3-T MRI scanner are unforgiving to the careless or inadvertent introduction of a ferrous object into the environment. Placing a magnet outside the MRI scanner can be a helpful but crude and sometimes inaccurate way to test any objects. If the object is not attracted to the magnet, this is not an absolute indication that there is no ferrous material present. A positive attraction, however, provides critical information to the anesthesiologist. Some unusual objects that have found their way into the MRI suite only to become projectile objects include a metal fan, a pulse oximeter, shrapnel, a wheelchair, a cigarette lighter, a stethoscope, a pager, a hearing aid, a vacuum cleaner, a calculator, a hair pin, an oxygen tank, a prosthetic limb, a pencil, an insulin infusion pump, keys, watches, and steel-tipped or heeled shoes (Kanal, 1992). Small objects can usually be easily removed from the magnet, but large objects may have so much attractive force to the MRI scanner that it is impossible to remove them by manual force. In these circumstances, quenching the magnet may be the only way to release the object once it is attached to the scanner. Quenching the magnet eliminates the magnetic field over a matter of minutes. This process is not without substantial risk; as helium gas is vented, condensation and considerable noise fill the suite. All personnel are required to vacate the suite during a quench, because there is a risk of hypoxic conditions if the helium should inadvertently enter the room.

In 2008, the JCAHO recognized the potential and existent hazards of the MRI environment when they published the *Sentinel Event Alert* (The Joint Commission, 2009). This alert identified 5 MRI-related cases of injury and 4 MRI-related deaths—one from a projectile and three cardiac events. The alert was designed to prevent accidents and injuries in the MRI suite, specifically identifying eight types of possible injuries (Box 33-1).

Special attention has recently been devoted to the topic of the IV gadolinium contrast that is used to enhance MR images. Gadolinium (in the form of gadopentetate dimeglumine) was approved by the FDA in 1998 as a contrast agent for MRI. With an elimination half-life of between 1.3 and 1.6 hours, gadolinium is excreted via the kidneys after forming a complex with chelating agents (Baker et al., 2004). Adults and children have similar elimination half-lives of gadolinium, with 95% excreted within 72 hours (Weinmann et al., 1984; Van Wagoner et al., 1990). Because gadolinium does not contain iodine, it does not produce an osmotic load and is generally considered safer and less allergenic than iodine (Brasch, 1993; Murphy et al., 1996; Dorta et al., 1997). Important warnings from the FDA suggest that patients with advanced kidney failure are at risk of developing nephrogenic systemic fibrosis or nephrogenic fibrosing dermopathy after gadolinium-based MR contrast agents. The FDA first notified health care professionals and the public about this risk in June 2006. There are currently five gadolinium-based contrast agents approved for use in the United States: Magnevist (gadopentetate dimeglumine), Ominiscan (gadodiamide); OptiMARK (gadoversetamide); MultiHance (gadobenate dimeglumine); and Prohance (gadoteridol). To date there are no reports of nephrogenic systemic fibrosis in those with normal kidney function or those with mild-to-moderate kidney insufficiency. The FDA suggests that gadolinium only be used when absolutely necessary in those with advanced kidney failure and that these patients undergo dialysis after vascular studies that require a large amount of gadolinium contrast.

Some patients experience claustrophobia and have difficulty cooperating during the study. Anxiety reactions are estimated to occur in 4% to 30% of patients (Granet and Gelber, 1990; Melendez and McCrank, 1993). As already discussed, new advances in technology now offer patients with anxiety or claustrophobia distraction with MRI-safe video goggles (Resonance Technology; Los Angeles, California). Patients with extreme skeletal abnormalities such as advanced scoliosis or flexion contractures, although motivated, may be unable to lie motionless

Box 33-1 The Joint Commission Sentinel Event Alert

PREVENTING ACCIDENTS AND INJURIES IN THE MRI SUITE

"Missile effect" or "projectile" injury in which ferromagnetic objects (those having magnetic properties) such as ink pens, wheelchairs, and oxygen canisters are pulled into the MRI scanner at rapid velocity.

Injury related to dislodged ferromagnetic implants such as aneurysm clips, pins in joints, and drug infusion devices.

Burns from objects that may heat during the MRI process, such as wires (including lead wires for both implants and external devices) and surgical staples, or from the patient's body touching the inside walls (the bore) of the MRI scanner during the scan.

Injury or complication related to equipment or device malfunction or failure caused by the magnetic field. For example, battery-powered devices (laryngoscopes, microinfusion pumps, monitors, etc.) can suddenly fail to operate; some programmable infusion pumps may perform erratically; and pacemakers and implantable defibrillators may not behave as programmed.

Injury or complication because of failure to attend to patient support systems during the MRI. This is especially true for patient sedation or anesthesia in MRI arenas. For example, oxygen canisters or infusion pumps run out and staff must either leave the MRI area to retrieve a replacement or move the patient to an area where a replacement can be found.

Acoustic injury from the loud knocking noise that the MRI scanner makes.

Adverse events related to the administration of MRI contrast agents.

Adverse events related to cryogen handling, storage, or inadvertent release in superconducting MR imaging system sites.

From The Joint Commission: *Preventing accidents and injuries in the MRI suite*, 2008. Available at http://www.jointcommission.org/SentinelEvents/SentinelEventAlert/sea_38.htm.

or supine on the solid, uncushioned MRI table for the extended duration of a spinal MRI. These patients may require general anesthesia for positioning and comfort or may need adjunctive pain medication.

Nuclear Medicine

Nuclear medicine is one of the oldest functional imaging disciplines. Scans obtained through nuclear medicine are useful for identification of epileptic foci in refractory epilepsy, evaluation of cerebrovascular disease (e.g., Moyamoya disease), and the evaluation of cognitive and behavioral disorders (O'Tuama and Treves, 1993). Anesthesiologists become involved when the child's medical history suggests that procedural sedation would not be appropriate. In order to complete these scans, the child must remain motionless for at least 1 hour.

The two most common nuclear medicine studies that require the administration of an anesthetic are single-photon emission computed tomography (SPECT) scans and positron emission tomography (PET) scans. SPECT scans use single-photon gamma-emitting radioisotopes and rotating gamma cameras to produce three-dimensional brain images. SPECT scans involve the use of radiolabeled technetium-99 (half-life, 6 hours), which has a high rate of first-pass extraction as well as intracellular trapping in proportion to regional cerebral blood flow (Chiron et al., 1989). SPECT scans are ideal when seeking seizure foci, and they often precede surgical resection of an identified focus. The technetium radionuclide is ideal because it remains intracellular and can be visualized on scan hours after a seizure has occurred. Ideally, the child should be scanned within 1 to 6 hours of the seizure. The radionuclides are physiologically harmless and not allergenic. Caregivers should, however, wear gloves to minimize contact with radiation-containing secretions.

PET scans use positron emission tomography and radionuclide tracers of metabolic activity, such as oxygen or glucose metabolism (Chugani, 1993; Griffeth et al., 1993). Unlike SPECT scans, PET scans should be performed during the seizure itself. Because of the short half-life of the glucose tracer (110 minutes), the scan is best completed during the seizure or within 1 hour thereafter.

Radiation Oncology

Pediatric radiation oncologists use ionizing photons to destroy lymphomas, acute leukemias, Wilms tumor, retinoblastomas, and tumors of the central nervous system. Multiple sessions are typical, requiring reliable motionlessness in order to precisely aim the beam at malignant cells while sparing healthy cells. A planning session in a simulator is often scheduled before the initiation of radiation therapy so that fields to be irradiated can be plotted and marked.

Radiation therapy is usually brief, nonpainful, and may be approached with a variety of plans for rendering the patient temporarily motionless. The key issue is the anesthesiologist's limited access to the patient. Remote video monitoring, as well as ECG and pulse oximeter use, are crucial. Two, or in some locations three, video cameras are used to look at the monitors, the chest, and the face of the patient. A central venous catheter in young children undergoing a long course of radiation therapy helps immensely. It is important to remember that infants undergoing radiation therapy after a prolonged fast are at risk for hypoglycemia; delayed awakening, or tremulousness, any of which should prompt a glucose determination.

Fractionated radiation therapy is the strategy of dividing the total radiation therapy course into discrete daily sessions, allowing normal tissue repair between sessions while the tumor burden is lessened or destroyed. Hyperfractionated, or multiple-session daily radiation therapy, is a modality reported primarily in adults for head and neck cancers. The rationale for twice-daily fractionation in children is that fractionation to growing bone in rats reduces the growth deficit by 25% to 30%; the hope is that other normal tissues may be similarly spared during growth (Eifel, 1988; Eifel et al., 1990). Whereas one successful approach has been to give infants an initial formula feeding 6 hours before their first treatment and keep them fasting until recovery from their second anesthetic (6 hours after the first), with the current liberalization of fasting guidelines it is preferable to give children clear liquids during their recovery from the first anesthetic and keep them fasting thereafter for 4 hours before the second anesthetic (Menache et al., 1990).

Stereotactic radiosurgery (with a Gamma Knife) is a major advance in the treatment of select intracranial arteriovenous malformations and tumors in children (Loeffler et al., 1990). Stereotactic radiosurgery differs from external-beam radiotherapy in several important ways. A focused, single, large fraction of radiation is used instead of smaller, daily fractions. Stereotactic radiosurgery uses gamma rays of relatively weak intensity that are produced by 201 cobalt-60 sources that intersect at a single point where all 201 beams converge to destroy tumors, vascular malformations, or abnormal tissue sites within the brain. Normal brain tissue surrounding the abnormality is therefore relatively protected from radiation effects. In pediatrics as well as in adults, most radiosurgery originally concentrated on treatment of small, histologically benign lesions such as vascular malformations, acoustic neuromas, and pituitary adenomas. This has more recently been expanded to include malignant tumors such as solitary metastases, ependymomas, glioblastomas, and several other tissue types. For optimal results, the tumor's volume should be small (14 cm^3) (Coffey et al., 1992).

Stereotactic radiosurgery requires coordination between departments of radiology, radiation therapy, neurosurgery, and anesthesiology. The stereotactic procedure begins either during the CT or MRI scan. The child is placed in a stereotactic head frame that is screwed into the cranium. Most adults are able to tolerate this entire procedure with local anesthesia or sedation. The neurosurgeon infiltrates the skin with a local anesthetic before applying the head frame. Adults and older children who tolerate this procedure with sedation alone may vomit as a result of anxiety, headache, or the location of the tumor itself. Because the head frame is heavy and cumbersome, it is difficult for the vomiting patient to turn his or her head in order to protect his or her airway. Pediatric patients (including most adolescents) typically require a general anesthetic. General anesthesia with tracheal intubation is induced before placement of the head frame. The key for removal of the head frame is taped to the frame itself. A nasogastric tube is placed for the day's anesthetic.

Calculations for dose and the three-dimensional coordinates for the beam may take several hours to compute after the initial radiologic study and head-frame placement. Some patients do well with sedation and spontaneous breathing; however, younger patients are usually mechanically ventilated. An initial CT scan is followed by computer calculations. Once the calculations are complete, the patient is transferred to the radiosurgery suite. After the irradiation, the patient is allowed to emerge from the anesthetic (Loeffler et al., 1990). The most common perioperative problem is nausea and vomiting, probably because of radiation sensitivity of the chemoreceptor trigger zone.

Stereotactic radiation therapy is a more precise localization of the fractionated radiation dose over the same duration of time as conventional radiation therapy, with the adjunctive use of a head frame. Considerations for the head frame include ease of application, reliability, ability to deliver supplemental oxygen and support the airway with a face mask if needed, and rapid removal of the facial restraint should it become necessary.

Total body irradiation (TBI) is generally performed twice a day over a 6-week period. It is usually in preparation for a bone-marrow transplant. For those patients who require anesthesia, the commitment is large—not only for the twice daily anesthetic but also for the coincident fasting status required. As these patients progress with their TBI treatment and become more immunocompromised, there is an increased risk of acquiring an illness during the course of treatment. Vomiting, respiratory illness, poor nutrition, or hypovolemia are all possible. Cancelling a TBI treatment because of an associated illness is discouraged, because it disrupts the course of treatment and could compromise the patient's overall prognosis. Although anesthesiologists are wary of the risks of aspiration, both sedation and general endotracheal anesthesia have been found to decrease the incidence of vomiting with TBI (Westbrook et al., 1987; Whitwam et al., 1978).

Clinic and Office Procedures

Endoscopic Procedures

Gastrointestinal endoscopy has become a routine part of patient care, and as such it constitutes the bulk of procedures performed by a pediatric gastroenterologist (Fox, 1998). Depending on the patient and the type of procedure contemplated (therapeutic vs. diagnostic), children may require no sedation, minimal to moderately deep sedation, or general anesthesia. Minimal sedation may impair cognitive function and coordination while ventilatory and cardiovascular functions are relatively unaffected. However, pediatric patients often are uncooperative and do not tolerate endoscopic procedures with minimal or moderate sedation, necessitating deeper sedation or general anesthesia to successfully accomplish the procedure (American Society of Anesthesiologists Task Force on Sedation and Analgesia by Non-Anesthesiologists, 2002). Over the past 15 years, the volume of endoscopic procedures has increased by twofold to fourfold in the adult community, and has most likely increased at a similar rate in children (Cohen et al., 2006).

The inability to independently maintain ventilatory function and to respond purposefully increases the risk involved with deep sedation. Although some recommend that deep sedation be limited to anesthesiologist delivery only, gastroenterologists have demonstrated that they too are able to safely administer sedation (Saint-Maurice and Hamza, 1992; Wolfe and Rao, 1992; Hassall, 1993, 1994; Dillon et al., 1998; Bouchut et al., 2001; Koh et al., 2001; Paspatis et al., 2006). Propofol, considered by the ASA to be within the scope of anesthesia practice only, is considered by the American Society for Gastrointestinal Endoscopy (ASGE) to be an acceptable sedative for gastroenterologist administration (ASGE, 2002; Walker et al., 2003; Rex et al., 2005; Perera et al., 2006; Rex, 2006; Abu-Shahwan and Mack, 2007). Propofol is an important sedative for gastroenterologists, and it is estimated that one quarter of all adult endoscopies are performed with propofol sedation (Cohen et al., 2006). Children with more complex medical problems, anticipated airway difficulties, morbid obesity, or behavioral problems can undergo their procedures in the operating room. Regardless of the site of the procedure, all patients scheduled for endoscopy should be evaluated in advance to confirm that they are appropriate candidates. In addition, the anesthetic technique depends on the procedure, the patient, and the skill of the endoscopist, as well as the limitations and capabilities of the endoscopy suite. There is a wide range of sedation agents for children as well as adults, and there is no optimal sedation regimen for either age group (Lightdale et al., 2007).

Procedural sedation is readily achieved with an IV anesthetic combining a sedative (e.g., midazolam), opioid (e.g., fentanyl, alfentanil, remifentanil, or dexmedetomidine), and a hypnotic (e.g., propofol). Spontaneous ventilation without the patient's airway being intubated has been shown to be a safe and effective technique (Bouchut et al., 2001; Koh et al., 2001; Koroglu et al., 2006). The majority of complications are respiratory and usually occur during an esophagogastroduodenoscopy (EGD). These complications include apnea, laryngospasm, bronchospasm, and airway obstruction. Bradycardia has been observed with dexmedetomidine use in children. Most problems resolve after withdrawal of the endoscope and positive pressure ventilation with a tightly-fitting mask; however, some patients may require endotracheal intubation to secure an airway and safely complete the procedure.

Esophagogastroduodenoscopy

Access to the airway is obviously limited once a transoral endoscope is in place. It is important to maintain spontaneous ventilation during deep sedation, because any airway intervention needed typically requires the removal of the endoscope. The two most stimulating portions of the EGD are transoral and transpyloric passage of the endoscope. A smooth endoscope insertion can be aided by topical spray of local anesthesia to the oropharynx to help eliminate coughing and gagging.

A majority of the respiratory complications noted previously occur during EGD when compared with colonoscopy, especially in infants and younger children. It has been suggested that this results from a combination of factors, including the large size of the endoscope and partial airway obstruction resulting in hypoxemia. Abdominal distention as a result of air introduced into the stomach may impair diaphragmatic excursion, leading to hypoventilation. This has led several groups to select 6 months of age, as a result of the higher respiratory complication rate in this age group, as the time before which general anesthesia with endotracheal intubation is required for the procedure (Wolfe and Rao, 1992; Koh et al., 2001).

Colonoscopy

Access to the airway is unimpeded during a colonoscopy. Deep sedation can be achieved more readily, and if respiratory problems occur, airway interventions are straightforward to manage. Patients undergoing colonoscopy also experience increased stimulation during certain parts of the procedure, such as when traversing the colon to the cecum. Also, at times, abdominal pressure is applied to help guide the colonoscope. The depth of the anesthetic should be adjusted accordingly.

Endoscopic Retrograde Cannulation of the Pancreas

Although many institutions report success of procedural sedation in pediatric patients undergoing endoscopic retrograde cannulation of the pancreas, general anesthesia with endotracheal intubation may make the procedure easier to perform, especially if the procedure is of long duration, the patient has significant comorbid diseases, or the procedure is performed with the patient in the prone position (Teng et al., 2000; Prasil et al., 2001).

Psychiatric Interviews

IV sodium amobarbital has a long history as an adjunct to psychotherapy, having found its peak use during World War II and immediately thereafter in helping soldiers deal with the stresses and trauma of combat (Zonana, 1979). Although this technique has enjoyed a resurgence for diagnostic and therapeutic interventions in adults, pediatric reports are rare. Weller et al. (1985) described the successful use of sodium Amytal in psychiatric interviews in prepubescent children. The induction of a tranquil state and sedation (e.g., slurred speech, a sense of fatigue, difficulty counting backwards, and basal vital signs) is similar to the anxiolysis achieved during monitored anesthesia care. A bispectral index (BIS) monitor may prove to be a useful adjunct as well (Palmer et al., 2001). The psychiatric interview process under these conditions is fascinating to participate in, if only as an observer. Memory retrieval, for instance the uncovering of relationships between current psychopathology and earlier traumatic life events, or symptom removal via therapeutic suggestions, are examples of interventions facilitated by the pharmacologically induced relaxed state made possible by the anesthesiologist during the interview.

SAFETY ISSUES FOR PATIENTS AND THEIR ANESTHESIOLOGISTS

As anesthesiologists find themselves participating in the care of patients who require increasingly sophisticated imaging technology, it is appropriate to examine the risks for patients and staff exposed to the types of high energies and contrast agents used.

Use of Intravascular Contrast Media

In a comprehensive review, Goldberg (1984) noted that approximately 5% of radiologic examinations with radiocontrast media (RCM) are complicated by adverse reactions, with one third of these being severe and requiring immediate treatment. Reactions occur most commonly in patients between 20 and 50 years of age and are relatively rare in children. The male/female ratio is about 2.5:1, not dissimilar to the gender distribution of other allergies such as latex, aspirin, and neuromuscular blocking agents. With a history of atopy or allergy, the risk of a reaction is increased from 1.5- to 10-fold. Reactions vary from mild, subjective sensations of restlessness, nausea, and vomiting to a rapidly evolving, angioedema-like picture accompanied by respiratory distress, bronchospasm, arrhythmias, and cardiac arrest. Because of the high osmolar concentrations of these agents (often higher than 1000 mOsm, and sometimes more than 2000 mOsm), caution should be exercised with patients who have a limited cardiovascular reserve (such as patients in congestive heart failure or those with cardiomyopathy). In addition, volume-depleted young children who have been kept fasting for prolonged intervals or who have had bowel preparations should be prehydrated before RCM administration. Those patients who are dependent on a full intravascular volume status (e.g., patients with sickle cell disease or restricted pulmonary circuit volume with cyanotic congenital heart disease and patients with arteriovenous shunts) should be monitored carefully for an initial rise in filling pressures and intravascular volume and subsequent diuresis after an osmolar load. Patients with impaired excretory mechanisms, such as those in renal failure, must be monitored closely after high osmolar loads. Low-osmolar RCM administrations are relatively safe with regard to life-threatening reactions, but moderate non–life-threatening

reactions requiring some treatment occur 0.2% to 0.4% of the time, and a severe life-threatening reaction can occur in 0.04% of patients (Thomsen and Bush, 1998).

RCM contains iodine, because iodine's high density and low toxicity make it an ideal agent for visualization and differentiation. The iodine is filtered through the glomeruli and is not reabsorbed by the glomeruli or the tubules. Because the contrast agent is hypertonic relative to plasma, an initial hypertensive response is usually followed by a hyperosmotic diuresis with the potential for hypotension. Equilibration with the extracellular fluid compartment occurs within 10 minutes, heralded by the onset of diuresis. Special attention should be paid when administering RCM with iodine to any child with a history of congestive heart failure. Patients with hepatic or renal dysfunction should be observed closely for signs of impaired excretion of the RCM. In sickle cell disease, the increase in blood osmolarity may precipitate shrinkage, clumping, and ultimately sickling of erythrocytes and vascular occlusion. Sickled cells are known to align with external magnetic fields to which they are exposed; it is unknown how this theoretic concern compares, for example, with the normal forces of deformation imposed on red cells of patients with sickle cell disease in their normal course through the vascular tree (Kanal et al., 1990).

Gadolinium diethylenetriaminepentaacetic acid (DTPA) is a low osmolar ionic contrast medium used for MRI, with a slower clearance in neonates and young infants than adults, yielding longer windows for imaging (Elster, 1990). Free gadolinium has a biological half-life of several weeks, with uptake and excretion taking place in the kidneys and liver. Unfortunately, free gadolinium is quite toxic and is therefore chelated to another structure that restricts the ion and decreases its toxicity. The most common adverse reactions are nausea, vomiting, hives, and headache. Local injection site symptoms include irritation, focal burning, or a cool sensation. Transient elevations in serum bilirubin (3% to 4% of patients) have been reported, and a transient elevation in iron for Magnevist and Omniscan (15% to 30% of patients) occurs, which tends to reverse spontaneously within 24 to 48 hours (Van Wagoner and Worah, 1993). Anaphylactoid reactions occur on the order of 1:100,000 to 1:500,000 and are more rare (< 1:100,000 doses) in children.

The older literature states that patients who have had anaphylactic reactions to shellfish are at increased risk of anaphylactoid reaction to RCM. The irony of the statement is that it may be correct, but not for obvious reasons. The original rationale was that shellfish contain high quantities of iodine, and therefore it was assumed that there would be a risk of cross-reactivity. However, neither shellfish allergy nor RCM reactions are caused by iodine. Atopy is a risk factor; therefore, the association between atopy, anaphylactic reactions to shellfish, and a possible predisposition to a RCM reaction may indeed be valid.

The treatment of severe allergic reactions, whether anaphylactoid or anaphylactic, is no different than for any other allergic reaction. Epinephrine, aminophylline, atropine, diphenhydramine, and steroids have all been employed in order to control varying degrees of adverse reactions. A patient who requires RCM administration and who has had a previous reaction to RCM has an increased (35% to 60%) risk for a reaction on reexposure. Pretreatment of these high-risk patients with prednisone and diphenhydramine 1 hour before RCM administration reduces the risk of reactions to 9%; the addition of ephedrine 1 hour before RCM administration further reduces the rate to 3.1% (Kelly et al., 1978; Greenberger, 1984).

In 2007, the ACR updated their practice guidelines for the use of intravascular contrast media that they published in the *Manual on Contrast Media* (ACR, 2008). Iodinated low-osmolality contrast media have a lower incidence of adverse effects as compared with ionic high-osmolality contrast media. The management of acute reactions in children is clearly outlined by the ACR (Box 33-2).

Allergic reactions rarely occur with oral agents. The incidence of severe anaphylactoid reactions to gastrointestinally administered agents is approximately 1:2,500,000, and the causes remain unknown. There are no pretreatment protocols established for these types of reactions and no well-defined risk factors. Gastrointestinal complications include nausea, vomiting, and diarrhea. One of the factors that may protect against having an allergic reaction is the poor absorption of oral iodinated contrast agents. Indeed, disruption of the GI mucosa is recognized as causing an increase in absorption of oral contrast, and the urinary excretion of contrast in a gastrointestinal study is a well-recognized sign. However, these signs are rarely associated with bronchospasm, flushing, periorbital edema, pruritis, rash, rhinitis or urticaria.

Ionizing Radiation

Radiation exposure is directly proportional to the duration of the procedure and inversely proportional to the square of the distance from the source. Henderson et al. (1991) monitored the radiation exposure of 16 pediatric anesthesia fellows during a - month period. Fellows assigned to the cardiac catheterization laboratory had a fluoroscopy exposure time of 14 to 85 minutes per case, typically for two to three cases per day. For these anesthesiologists, badge readings ranged from 20 to 180 mrem/month. All noncardiac anesthesia fellows had undetectable (<10 mrem/month) levels. All fellows wore lead aprons, 50% wore a thyroid shield, and one stepped at least 10 feet away from the source during every exposure; this latter fellow had a reading of 30 mrem, despite having spent 26 hours in the catheterization laboratory. The annual maximum permissible dose (MPD) for nonradiation workers (including anesthesiologists) is 100 mrem or 1 mSievert (mSv, Systeme Internationale Units). For comparison, the MPD for radiation workers is 50 mSv annually and 10 mSv times age cumulatively. MPD during pregnancy for radiation workers (per gestation) is 5 mSv. Limits of exposure and comparative sources of exposure are listed in Table 33-2.

High-Intensity Magnetic Fields

MRI exposes the patient (and the health care workers surrounding the patient) to a static magnetic field, a rapidly switched spatial-gradient magnetic field, and radiofrequency magnetic fields. The static magnetic field, which causes alignment

---

Box 33-2 Management of Acute Reactions in Children

URTICARIA

No treatment needed in most cases

Give H_1-receptor blocker: diphenhydramine PO, IM, or IV 1 to 2 mg/kg, up to 50 mg.

If severe or widely disseminated: give α-agonist, epinephrine SC (1:1000) 0.01 mL/kg.

FACIAL EDEMA

Give O_2 6 to 10 L/min (via mask, face tent, or blow-by stream). Monitor electrocardiogram, O_2 saturation (pulse oximeter), and blood pressure.

Give α-agonist: epinephrine SC or IM (1:1000) 0.01 mL/kg, up to 0.3 mL/dose. Repeat in 15 to 30 minutes as needed.

Give H_1-receptor blocker: diphenhydramine IM or IV 1 to 2 mg/kg, up to 50 mg.

If not responsive to therapy, seek appropriate assistance (e.g., cardiopulmonary arrest response team).

LARYNGEAL EDEMA OR BRONCHOSPASM

Give O_2 6 to 10 L/min (via mask, face tent, or blow-by stream). Monitor electrocardiogram, O_2 saturation (pulse oximeter), and blood pressure.

Give β-agonist inhalers: bronchiolar dilators, such as metaproterenol, terbutaline, or albuterol, 2 to 3 puffs. Repeat as necessary.

Give epinephrine SC or IM (1:1000) 0.01 mL/kg, maximum 0.3 mL/dose or IV epinephrine (1:10,000) 0.1 mL/kg, maximum 3 mL/dose. Repeat in 3 to 5 minutes as needed.

Call for assistance (e.g., cardiopulmonary arrest response team) for severe bronchospasm or if O_2 saturation <88% persists.

PULMONARY EDEMA

Give O_2 6 to 10 L/min (via mask, face tent, or blow-by stream). Monitor electrocardiogram, O_2 saturation (pulse oximeter), and blood pressure.

Give diuretic: furosemide IV 1 to 2 mg/kg.

Call for assistance (e.g., cardiopulmonary arrest response team).

HYPOTENSION WITH TACHYCARDIA

Give O_2 6 to 10 L/min (via mask). Monitor electrocardiogram, O_2 saturation (pulse oximeter), and blood pressure.

Legs elevated 60 degrees or more (preferred) or Trendelenburg position.

Keep patient warm.

Give IV or IO normal saline or lactated Ringer's solution 20 mL/kg over 5 to 10 minutes. Bolus infusion over 10 to 20 minutes in patients with myocardial dysfunction.

Seek appropriate assistance (e.g., cardiopulmonary arrest response team).

HYPOTENSION WITH BRADYCARDIA (VAGAL REACTION)

Give O_2 6 to 10 L/min (via mask). Monitor electrocardiogram, O_2 saturation (pulse oximeter), and blood pressure.

Legs elevated 60 degrees or more (preferred) or Trendelenburg position.

Keep patient warm.

Give IV or IO normal saline or lactated Ringer's solution 20 mL/kg over 5 to 10 minutes. Give infusion over 10 to 20 minutes in patients with myocardial dysfunction.

Give atropine IV 0.02 mg/kg if patient does not respond quickly to steps 2, 3, and 4. Minimum initial dose of 0.1 mg. Maximum initial dose of 0.5 mg (infant/child), 1 mg (adolescent). Atropine dose may be doubled for second administration.

Seek appropriate assistance (e.g., cardiopulmonary arrest response team).

From American College of Radiology 2008 "Manual on Contrast Media." Version 6. Reston, Va, p 75-76.

IM, Intramuscular; *IO*, intraosseous; *IV*, intravenous; *SC*, subcutaneous; *PO*, orally.

TABLE 33-2. Limits and Sources of Radiation Exposure

Limits for Exposures	Exposure	Range
Occupational dose limit (U.S. NRC)	5000 mrem/year	
Occupational exposure limits for minors	500 mrem/year	
Occupational exposure limits for fetus	500 mrem	
Source of exposure		
Average dose to U.S. public from all sources	630 mrem/year	
Average dose to U.S. public from natural sources	330 mrem/year	
Average dose to U.S. public from medial sources	53 mrem/year	
Chest x-ray	8 mrem	5-20 mrem
Extremities x-rays	1 mrem	
Dental x-ray	10 mrem	
Head/neck x-ray	20 mrem	
Cervical spine x-ray	22 mrem	
Lumbar spinal x-rays	130 mrem	
Pelvis x-ray	44 mrem	
Hip x-ray	83 mrem	
Upper GI series	245 mrem	
Lower GI series	405 mrem	
CT (head and body)	1100 mrem	
Expected 50% death without medical attention	400,000 mrad	300,000-500,000 mrem
Doubling dose for genetic effects	100,000 mrad	
Doubling dose for cancer	500,000 mrad	(8% per mSv, natural level at 20%)
Dose for increase cancer risk 1:1,000	1250 mrem	(8% per mSv)
Consideration of therapeutic abortion threshold (dose in utero)	10,000 mrem	

1 mrem = 10 mSv; 1 rad is the amount of radiation to deposit 0.01 joules of energy per kilogram.
NRC, Nuclear Regulatory Commission; *U.S.,* United States.

of unpaired tissue protons, may cause movement of ferromagnetic devices such as vascular clips, ventricular shunt connectors, casings for pacemakers, and control devices for pacemakers. Metallic devices in other areas, particularly when invested with fibrous tissue, are less problematic (Shellock and Crues, 1988; Shellock, 1989). As mentioned previously, tissue expanders may have magnetic ports to facilitate identification of the injection site. Despite their low mass, such ports have a potential for torque and movement in the presence of a strong magnetic field; therefore, the specific type of tissue expander should be identified before patient evaluation in an MRI (Liang

et al., 1989). Assessment of risk in patients with implants or other possibly ferromagnetic devices or objects consists of a careful history including penetrating wounds, physical examination to look for scars, and possibly a plain radiograph of the region in question (Pohost et al., 1992). Other concerns have been increased blood pressure, cardiac arrhythmias, and impaired mental function. Although described or theorized on an experimental basis, little clinical documentation is available.

The magnetic field generates an electrical current two to three orders of magnitude less than a defibrillator (10 mA/M^2, compared with, 000 to 10,000 mA/M^2). This current strength may nevertheless reprogram a programmable pacemaker and interfere with its function (Erlebacher et al., 1986). Exposure to a strong external magnetic or electromagnetic field can lead to conversion of a demand pulse generator from synchronous to asynchronous mode, damage to the reed switch (that activates the fixed-rate pulse generator), reprogramming of pacemaker parameters, induction of currents in the electrode wires, or displacement of the generator itself. Indeed, it is the sensitivity of some reed switches that has determined the safety boundary of MRI devices as being 5 Gauss (5×10^{-4} T). Patients with implantable defibrillators or cardioverters, implantable infusion pumps (e.g., for insulin), cochlear implants, and neurostimulators are all at risk for having the implant device reprogrammed on exposure to the magnetic field. Defibrillator failure has been reported in the MRI environment (Snowdon, 1989).

Radiofrequency pulses cause heat production in metallic implants and coiled wires such as ECG cables or pulse oximeter cables if they are looped and laying on the patient's skin. Patients with compromised thermoregulatory abilities, such as those with cardiac problems, fever, or taking certain drugs, may be at particular risk. Included in this group are infants, whose SAR is greater than that of adults because of the greater ratio of body surface area to body mass, and whose thermoregulatory abilities may be interfered with during a general anesthetic (Kussman et al., 2004). SAR refers to the energy absorption (e.g., increasing body temperature) with an increase in the total amount of radiofrequent energy absorbed (Fitzsimmons, 1992).

Increased reports of vertigo, nausea, and a metallic taste have been found in a study on human exposure to the 4-T magnetic field of a whole-body scanner (Schenck et al., 1992). Fertilized frog embryos exposed to a 4-T magnetic field did not demonstrate any adverse effects on early development (Prasad et al., 1990). An increase in CCL of 17% was found in healthy volunteers in a 2-T environment after 10 minutes of exposure, causing speculation about the effect of the 2-T environment on the sinus node (Jehenson et al., 1988). This may be of particular concern in patients with a preexisting arrhythmia history. Of more significant concern in pediatric patients is the potential for hypothermia, because of the air flow directed through the scanner cavity and the inability to control room temperature or use radiant warmers. The use of warm IV fluid bags, thermal packs, and blankets can decrease heat loss. Excellent reviews of monitoring considerations and equipment choices in the MRI environment, as well as patient safety principles are available, and the ACR (with a representative from the ASA) has published a recent white paper on MRI safety (Kanal et al., 1990, 2007; International Non-Ionizing Radiation Committee of the International Radiation Protection Association, 1991; Fitzsimmons, 1992; Menon et al., 1992; Patteson and Chesney, 1992; Pohost et al., 1992).

MRI and spectroscopy do not employ ionizing radiation. However, secondary harmful effects, such as magnetic objects becoming projectiles within the magnetic field as they approach the bore of the magnet and potentially causing injury, are a consideration (Chu and Sangster, 1986; Chaljub et al., 2001). Patients (and anesthesiologists) with metallic implants such as vascular clamps, hemostatic clips, dental devices, heart valve prostheses, intravascular coils, filters and stents, ocular implants, orthopedic implants, otologic implants, shrapnel, penile implants, and vascular access ports must be individually evaluated for their risk in the MRI environment (Cahalan et al., 1987; Shellock and Curtis, 1991).

As with individual precautions, equipment precautions should be taken for all ferromagnetic objects such as IV stands, oxygen, and nitrous oxide cylinders, and monitoring equipment. The anesthesia machine, if used in the scanning room, should be outfitted with aluminum gas cylinders and kept in the corner of the room. Anesthesia machines especially designed to be MRI-compatible are now readily available.

DIFFICULT-AIRWAY MANAGEMENT IN THE RADIOLOGY SUITE

If a child with a known difficult airway requires endotracheal intubation in order for the scheduled procedure to be completed, it is wise to perform the anesthetic induction in the operating room, an area where access to difficult-airway equipment is readily available. Regardless of an anesthesiologist's comfort level and familiarity with extramural environments, the same depth of back-up coverage is simply not available.

The unrecognized difficult airway is problematic in a remote location; therefore, it is important to have LMAs stocked in all extramural anesthesia carts. If a child cannot be intubated or ventilated with a mask, LMAs can provide a successful alternative. Case reports describe the successful use of LMAs in children with difficult craniofacial anomalies, such as Goldenhar's syndrome and even Pierre Robin sequence (Fan et al., 1995; Hansen et al., 1995; Haxby and Liban, 1995). Similarly, a light wand may facilitate endotracheal intubation in the child with a difficult airway (Holzman et al., 1988). Recently introduced rigid laryngoscopes with video in infant through pediatric sizes (e.g., Glidescope), should be strongly considered for availability in offsite locations.

It is important to recognize that an airway that was not difficult on induction may become difficult on emergence after sclerotherapy with alcohol and subsequent tissue edema, particularly at the base of the tongue, neck, or the mediastinum (Furst et al., 1996; Ohlms et al., 1996; Fishman, 1999). These patients often require several days of airway support and ongoing evaluation in the ICU until airway swelling is no longer a concern.

BLOOD-LOSS MANAGEMENT OUTSIDE OF THE OPERATING ROOM

Transfusion requirements are rare in extramural locations, yet preprocedural anemia, accidental perforation of vascular structures, or medical transfusion requirements such as sickle cell disease or prematurity may require transfusion therapy. Equipment familiar to the anesthesiologist and identical to that available in the operating room is a welcome sight in a life-threatening emergency. Calling for additional help, establishing additional vascular access, and coordinating with the blood bank is crucial. Having a runner available may be critical when there is no equivalent to a circulating nurse. In an emergency, it may become necessary to involve a surgeon and transport the patient to the operating room, in which case it would be optimal for another anesthesia team to set up the operating room while the patient is being prepared for transport.

SUMMARY

The demand for anesthesia and sedation services in sites distant to the operating room is continuing to increase. Providing patient services in locations remote to the operating room can be challenging and poses risks that may not exist in the operating-room setting. Although the incidence of adverse outcomes for anesthesia and sedation in these remote areas has never been prospectively studied, we can look at office-based and ambulatory surgery centers to extrapolate the risk. Comparative outcomes analysis in Florida reveals that the incidence of adverse events is higher in the office-based setting when compared with outpatient surgical centers (Vila et al., 2003). Although these outcomes cannot be directly compared, it raises the question of added risk in the off-site anesthetizing location. Sedation, monitored anesthesia care, and general anesthesia are all choices that carry risks. Historically, an avoidance of a general anesthesia has been thought to minimize the risk of adverse outcome. Closed-claims analysis has shown, however, that monitored anesthesia care poses an equal risk to general anesthesia with respect to severity of injury, death, and permanent brain damage. Furthermore, 24% of all monitored anesthesia care claims involve oversedation and respiratory depression (Bhananker et al., 2006). In summary, anesthesia care providers must recognize that as the demand for off-site services increases, so also should their ability to understand the environment and do careful risk analysis when selecting patients and formulating a plan of care.

REFERENCES

Complete references used in this text can be found online at www.expertconsult.com.

CHAPTER 34

Anesthesia for Same-Day Surgical Procedures

David M. Polaner

Outpatient procedures continue to account for the majority of anesthetics given to children in the United States. It is estimated that more than 60% of anesthetics in children are performed on outpatients, and this number is considerably higher in some practice settings. Although the practice of outpatient anesthesia and surgery for children is not new—reports in the medical literature have documented the practice for over 100 years—advances in drugs and techniques are transforming the care given to day-surgery patients. Procedures that previously required overnight stays can often be performed on a same-day basis. It is possible to reduce the incidence of troubling side effects of anesthetics that may have prevented the discharge of patients in the past, and better postoperative analgesic regimens may allow for earlier discharge. Changes in facility designs have improved our ability to provide outpatient care in an efficient and cost-effective manner, while simultaneously enhancing and simplifying the perioperative experience for patients and their families. Nevertheless, along with these advances have come new challenges. The envelope of

what patient and procedure is appropriate for same-day surgery has continued to stretch, whereas resources may be shrinking. The pressure to increase performance and throughput places greater stresses on the perioperative system, and great care must be taken to avoid cutting corners for the illusionary benefits of efficiency and cost-containment alone.

Historical reports of outpatient surgery date back to the early twentieth century, when Nicholl reported nearly 9000 operations on ambulatory children at Glasgow's Royal Hospital for Sick Children (Nicholl, 1909). Other early reports from the United States soon followed, but it was not until the 1970s that studies looking at same-day surgery from a systems perspective were published. In addition to examining the patient population, complication rates and surgical procedures, these reports began to look at issues such as cost and delivery of care, as well as the optimization of the nursing and support staff, organization, and physical plant for outpatient surgery. Attention to these details continues to play a central role in the increased use and success of outpatient surgery. In the current economic climate of health care in the United States, there is and will continue to be a major emphasis on cost savings. In addition to the economic advantages of savings on hospital resources, a primary driving force in the popularity of outpatient surgery is satisfaction of the patient's parents. There are obvious advantages for many parents and children to avoid overnight hospitalization and to have the child back in a familiar home environment on the same day. The decisions that are made in planning the outpatient system will have a major impact on how parents perceive ease of use and quality of care of the entire system, and, as a result, its success. Factors that are not medical at all (e.g., ease of parking, efficiency of check-in procedures, waiting time, parental presence during induction of anesthesia, and early admission to the postanesthetic recovery unit [PACU]) may make impressions on the parent that are equal to the obvious medical issues, such as complication rates, management of postoperative analgesia, postoperative nausea and vomiting (PONV), and rapid return to the preoperative mental state.

PROCEDURES AND PATIENTS AMENABLE TO OUTPATIENT SURGERY AND ANESTHESIA

Many operative procedures are well suited to be performed on pediatric outpatients and all share several common characteristics. They all are peripheral procedures that do not involve major violation of a body cavity. They all have limited duration, generally lasting less than 2 hours, and have minimal or moderate amounts of postoperative pain that can easily be managed after discharge from the PACU with oral analgesics, or by either a single-injection regional block placed at the time of surgery or continuous regional analgesia at home. They do not result in major physiologic perturbations or blood loss, nor do they disturb the ability to take oral fluids and nutrition in the immediate postoperative period. They do not require postoperative monitoring beyond the capability of the parents and home. Commonly performed outpatient procedures are listed and categorized in Table 34-1.

CONTRAINDICATIONS FOR OUTPATIENT ANESTHESIA

There are few firm contraindications to outpatient surgery for amenable procedures, but there are some patients who have medical issues that make it advisable to consider an overnight ("23-hour") admission rather than discharge on the day of surgery. In the majority of these cases, monitoring is required because of anesthetic-related risks or because of exceptional risks related to the operative procedure or postoperative care in susceptible individuals.

Expremature Infants and Apnea

The risk of postanesthetic apnea in former premature infants has been well described since the early 1980s, when Liu et al. (1983) published the first prospective study of premature infants anesthetized between 41 and 46 weeks' postconceptional age (postconceptual age equals the gestational age at birth plus an infant's current age in weeks). The authors compared a group of premature infants with a control group of term infants of similar

TABLE 34-1. Operations Commonly Performed as Outpatient Surgical Procedures by Specialty

Specialty	Procedures
Otolaryngology	Myringotomy and ventilating tubes, adenoidectomy (see text), tonsillectomy (see text), frenulectomy, branchial cleft cysts, endoscopic sinus surgery, examination under anesthesia including some bronchoscopy
Ophthalmology	Examination under anesthesia, strabismus repair, nasolacrimal duct probe, intraocular lens implantation, trabeculectomy
General pediatric surgery and urology	Herniorrhaphy and hydrocelectomy, orchiopexy, uncomplicated hypospadias, cystoscopy and cystoscopic surgery, circumcision, esophogoscopy, lumps and bumps
Gastroenterology	Endoscopy
Plastic surgery	Cleft lip and some cleft palate repair, placement of tissue expanders, scar revision, minor reconstructive procedures (otoplasty, septorhinoplasty, etc.)
Orthopedics	Hardware removal, casting, percutaneous tenotomy, arthrograms Percutaneous pinnings and simple OFIF
Radiology	Imaging studies, radiation therapy
Dentistry	Extractions, restorations, examinations Nerve treatments, crowns, sealants, and fillings

ages. The incidence of apnea, defined as pauses in breathing lasting greater than 15 seconds, was 20%. Subsequent studies have approximated this incidence, although some have placed the at-risk period as far out as 60 weeks' postconceptual age (Welborn et al., 1986; Kurth et al., 1987; Warner et al., 1992). It is now established that infants born before 36 weeks' conceptional age are at some risk of apnea after general anesthesia. It appears that this risk is because of immaturity in the brainstem's control of breathing after exposure to general anesthetics, and there may be similar risks after exposure to sedative-hypnotic agents and neuroleptic agents such as ketamine. Numerous studies have tried to define the period of susceptibility in the at-risk population. Several investigators have stratified the risk according to postconceptual age and gestational age at birth, and a meta-analysis of eight studies has reported that the postconceptual age required to reduce the risk to less than 1% with 95% confidence was 54 weeks in infants born at 35 weeks' gestational age and 56 weeks in those born before 32 weeks' gestation (Malviya et al., 1993; Coté et al., 1995). In this meta-analysis, anemia was also associated with increased apnea risk, particularly in infants older than 42 weeks' postconceptual age. The patients in the numerous studies that were included in this meta-analysis may not have all been comparable in terms of underlying state of health, so these data (as in all meta-analyses) must be approached with some caution. Several investigators have suggested that the use of regional anesthesia may eliminate the risk, and a few even advocate discharge of these patients on the day of surgery if no other agents have been administered (Veverka et al., 1991; Webster et al., 1991; Sartorelli et al., 1992; Krane et al., 1995). However, uncontrolled case reports of apnea after spinal anesthesia have been published (Watcha et al., 1989; Tobias et al., 1998). Because these are case reports and there were no control pneumograms, it is unknown if the apnea was related to the anesthetic or not, but these reports have still prompted most clinicians and consultants to continue to recommend admission and monitoring of these patients for 24 hours after any anesthetic. Krane et al. (1995), in a prospective randomized controlled study, compared former premature infants receiving general or spinal anesthesia with preoperative and postoperative impedance respirometry, oxygen saturation, and electrocardiography (ECG). In this small sample of 18 patients, no central apnea differences were detected, but the group receiving spinal anesthesia had fewer desaturations and bradycardic events than those receiving general anesthesia. Caffeine, which has a long history of effective use in apnea of prematurity, has also been suggested to increase central respiratory drive after anesthesia in these patients, although it is still not commonly used (Welborn et al., 1988, 1989).

Obstructive Sleep Apnea

One of the most common indications for tonsillectomy is upper-airway obstruction during sleep. In many centers, obstructive sleep apnea (OSA) accounts for 50% or more of all children who come for tonsillectomy and adenoidectomy (Messner, 2003). These children may have abnormal ventilatory responses to both hypoxia and hypercarbia as a result of the chronic exposure to hypoxic and hypercarbic conditions during sleep (Strauss et al., 1999; Kerbl et al., 2001). These responses can take up to several weeks to revert to normal after resolution of the obstruction. There are concerns, therefore, about the ability to maintain adequate ventilation and oxygenation in the period immediately after the exposure to general anesthetics and to opioids given for postoperative analgesia. A study of 15 otherwise healthy children, ages 1 to 18, with mild OSA used preoperative and postoperative pneumograms to assess respiratory status on the night after adenotonsillectomy. Nine of these children received a halothane-based anesthetic, and six received a fentanyl-based technique. The number of obstructive events decreased, and the nadir of oxygen saturation improved from 78% to 92%. The authors concluded that in cases of mild OSA without other underlying disorders, intensive postoperative monitoring is not necessary (Helfaer et al., 1996). In another group of 134 children selected for outpatient tonsillectomy, 83% of whom carried the diagnosis and indication for surgery for OSA, 11 (8.2%) were admitted for inpatient observation after experiencing respiratory problems in the postanesthetic care unit (Lalakea et al., 1999). These patients as a group were significantly younger than those discharged home (an average age of 4 vs. 6.3 years). Preoperative evaluation and assessment of OSA was not described. Most otolaryngologists consider significant (as opposed to mild or moderate) OSA to be a relative contraindication to outpatient management of adenotonsillectomy, especially in children younger than 3 years of age, although in one small study the postoperative complications in these younger children were not related to obstructive events (Slovik et al., 2003). Those investigators suggested that the severity of OSA, rather than a patient's age, may be a more predictive factor, but this is in conflict with other reports that recommend that an age younger than 3 years should be considered an independent discriminator (Shott et al., 1987; Biavati et al., 1997). One large retrospective analysis of 2315 patients younger than 6 years of age undergoing adenotonsillectomy for

OSA found a higher rate of respiratory complications in those younger than 3 years (9.8% vs. 4.9%) (Statham et al., 2006). The only criterion that appears to be unequivocally accurate in the diagnosis and stratification of severity in OSA is polysomnography; neither the history nor pulse oximetry alone is specific or sensitive enough (American Thoracic Society 1996; Schechter, 2002; Subcommittee on Obstructive Sleep Apnea, American Academy of Pediatrics, 2002). In the absence of objective data, it is worthwhile to elicit a history of significant snoring or sleep-disordered breathing during the preoperative interview with the parent. Even though such historical data may not be accurate in all cases, it serves to alert the anesthesiologist to the potential for problems (Sinha et al., 2008).

Recent data on opioids in the patient with chronic hypoxemia are particularly relevant to the child with OSA, whether the child is to undergo tonsillectomy or another surgical procedure. In an animal model, rats exposed to chronic hypoxic conditions had greater respiratory sensitivity to opioids, exhibiting diminished respiratory drive (Moss et al., 2006). Confirming these animal data, children who experienced significant hypoxia during sleep had lower opioid requirements to achieve analgesia after tonsillectomy (Brown et al., 2006). In this prospective study of 22 children with OSA undergoing tonsillectomy, the opioid dose required to achieve equal analgesic scores on a behavioral pain scale was directly correlated with the nadir of their oxygen saturation on the preoperative polysomnogram. Those with the lowest saturations required the least opioid, demonstrating that chronic recurrent hypoxemia during sleep was associated with increased analgesic sensitivity to morphine. The key implication is that not only are ventilatory responses to hypoxia and hypercarbia with opioids blunted, but actual analgesic requirements are less, and lowering opioid and other sedative medication doses still results in adequate analgesia while potentially reducing the risk of untoward effects.

PREOPERATIVE EVALUATION AND PLANNING

The evaluation of outpatients for surgical procedures presents a significant organizational challenge to the anesthesiologist. Because one of the primary goals of outpatient surgery is both efficiency and rapid throughput, there is a great disincentive to require preoperative visits before the day of surgery itself. At the same time, an efficient system demands an absolute minimum of cancellations on the day of surgery. Such pressures put both the anesthesiologist and the system as a whole at significant risk of proceeding with cases in which the patient may not be optimally prepared for surgery and anesthesia. There is also the stress of "production pressure"—the urgency to move patients rapidly through the preoperative queue and into the operating room on schedule. This, too, is in competition with the need to provide the best and most complete evaluation and care of the patient. In order to avoid these situations, a system of preoperative screening must be instituted that provides the most accurate, up to date, and complete information so the anesthesiologist may make well-informed decisions about patient management. Fortunately, both technological and nontechnological aids exist to streamline this process.

The implications of cancellation, particularly on the day of surgery, go far beyond the efficiency of the operating room. A survey by Tait et al. (1997) found that nearly half of parents whose children's operations were cancelled on the day of scheduled surgery missed a day of work, and about half of these went unpaid as a result. Many drove long distances to get to the hospital, and nearly 25% were frustrated or angry as a result of the cancellation. A small number of dissatisfied or angry parents can have an adverse impact on the success of an outpatient surgery program well out of proportion to their numbers, and great attention must be paid to minimizing these events by using systems that work effectively.

In many cases, a preoperative visit to the anesthesiologist is neither practical nor necessary. Because the majority of children who come for same-day surgery are relatively healthy, screening tools that employ methods such as telephone interviews and self-reporting can often be employed. Coordination with the surgeon's office may reduce both redundancy in paperwork and repeated questioning of the patient's family. The efficiency in combining surgical, anesthetic, and nursing evaluations can be greatly enhanced if a computerized record is used. With these systems, which are finally beginning to reach maturity after years of development, data from one evaluation can automatically populate another linked database; however, at times implementation of these systems still remains limited, and lack of universal interoperability and poor interface and database design remain major impediments to their acceptance. Nevertheless, at the start of the second decade of the 2000s, progress is being made and it can be expected that increased use of electronic medical records will greatly streamline the evaluation process. Even in the majority of institutions, where paper records still remain the standard, systems using secure e-mail, facsimile, or even common forms can be designed to eliminate redundancy. The elimination of needless paperwork or data entry can be a great aid in increasing patient throughput, as well as reducing the frustration of staff and parents alike.

The initial step in preoperative planning and evaluation begins when the surgeon books the case. This is the first opportunity for the system to alert the anesthesiologist of any unusual conditions or underlying illnesses that the patient may have. A short list of check-boxes on the booking form suffices and need not have any great detail. This information can be reviewed by an anesthesiologist (or, in an electronic system, automatically trigger an alert to a consulting anesthesiologist) to detect any cases that might benefit from especially extensive consultation or planning before the day of surgery.

The surgeon's office, because it is the initial contact point of the patient's family with the perioperative system, also provides an excellent opportunity to present the parents with introductory information about the anesthetic. A pamphlet describing generalities such as the role of the pediatric anesthesiologist in caring for the child, fasting instructions, contact numbers, and other information specific to the hospital or outpatient surgical center can be a useful reference for the family. Having a written reference for fasting guidelines is especially helpful, because lack of adherence to these instructions is a common cause of case delay or cancellation. The language should be clear and uncomplicated, and a place for the actual times that the child in question should cease eating and drinking should be provided to eliminate confusion and misinterpretation. It is advisable to set the fasting time based not on the scheduled time of operation but rather on the time of arrival at the preoperative unit. This permits the case to go forward early if the operating room runs ahead of schedule. Parents should be given a number to call both for questions about the anesthetic that they feel cannot wait until the preoperative assessment, and for consultation with an anesthesiologist should an intercurrent illness develop between the time of the visit to the surgeon and the day of surgery.

A preoperative visit to the surgeon alone, however, will not optimize the preoperative evaluation process for the anesthesiologist or for the same-day surgery process as a whole. A case-control study of pediatric outpatient cancellations found that 10% of all day surgery patients at a children's hospital were cancelled on the day of surgery, and half of those were for preventable reasons. Cancelled patients who had inadequate preoperative preparation were more likely to have been seen only in the surgeon's office and not in the hospital's preoperative program (Macarthur et al., 1995). It is clear that further screening is optimal to address general medical and anesthetic concerns.

Background

A short telephone interview with the patient's parent before scheduled surgery, whether conducted by the anesthesiologist, a physician's assistant, or a nurse practitioner, can be not only a source of clinical information about the patient and about the parent's concerns, but can also forestall unanticipated problems that can cause delays, cancellations, or complications on the day of surgery. Knowing in advance, for example, that a child with asthma had a mild upper respiratory infection (URI) the week before surgery, can allow the anesthesiologist to prescribe a short preoperative course of steroids with ample time for the drug to take effect. The child who has sickle cell disease with an active URI, on the other hand, might have surgery postponed, thus saving the parents a trip to the hospital and allowing the schedule to be rearranged before the day begins. A well-organized system for conducting these calls should be established, so patients are not missed and communications with the anesthesiologist scheduled to care for a particular patient can be easily accomplished. It is important to organize the system so that calls are most effective. A study of over 5000 patients conducted at National Children's Hospital in 1992 found that calls made during the evening were far more likely to successfully reach the parents—not an unexpected finding (Patel and Hannallah, 1992). In Great Britain and in some hospitals in the United States, preoperative clinics rather than telephone screening are used, but this may necessitate an additional visit by the family. The inconvenience may outweigh the advantages of a face-to-face visit for some families, and success may be predicated on ease of use of the system. Preoperative screening and evaluation can also improve throughput on the day of surgery, particularly if there is a long list of short cases, such as myringotomy and ventilation-tube placement. The duration of those cases is so short that the time it takes to do a preoperative evaluation may be longer than the operative time. Saving even 10 or 15 minutes per hour might allow the team to perform an additional operative procedure each hour.

Other methods of communication, including secure websites and e-mail, have been used for similar purposes. The ability for a family to access a secure server and enter preoperative interview information will likely become increasingly attractive in coming years. Although the personal interaction with a knowledgeable professional can never be replaced, certain "boilerplate" data can be entered with great efficiency in this manner, permitting rapid and efficient review by the anesthesiologist. Intranet-based kiosks at the hospital, where patients' families can use either keyboard or touch-screen technology to enter information that is now entered on paper questionnaires at the time of admission, will become increasingly important modalities as hospitals move from paper-based records to digital ones.

It is particularly important that reports of previous operative procedures or consultations by specialists be made available to the anesthesiologist during the preoperative assessment. A computerized repository of this information is the best solution, because it allows immediate access from any location. However, many institutions have not yet migrated to completely digital medical records, and legacy data from the paper chart must be entered into the electronic chart as scanned documents. Unless all electronic documents are properly tagged or archived in a appropriate folders, they may be difficult to locate. Knowledgeable database professionals, in consultation with the anesthesiology department, must carefully determine a scheme for labeling and retrieving archived documents in advance. If an electronic medical record is not in place, a day-surgery coordinator should have the responsibility of ensuring that necessary outside and internal records are readily available the day before surgery in order to avoid delays. Such information must be immediately accessible to the anesthesiologist on the day of surgery as well.

In some locations, it is common for a child's pediatrician to be responsible for "clearing" the child for surgery. This can be a considerable help, because the pediatrician often has the best knowledge of the child's underlying illnesses and conditions. The pediatrician, however, often has little understanding of the issues that are of greatest concern to the anesthesiologist and may actually miss or ignore problems that can impact anesthetic management, to the detriment of the preoperative evaluation process. The anesthetic implications and preoperative optimization of airway anatomy and function, gastroesophageal reflux, upper respiratory illness, and asthma, as well as of syndromes and chronic conditions such as Trisomy 21 and the former premature infant, all may be underappreciated by pediatricians who do not work in the operating room or administer anesthetics and have usually had little or no training in perioperative medicine (Fisher, 1991). Several recent reviews (written by pediatric anesthesiologists) in the pediatric literature have discussed the preoperative screening process and what the pediatrician needs to know about preparing the child for anesthesia (Fisher, 1991; Fisher et al., 1994; Maxwell et al., 1994; Section on Anesthesiology, 1996). If a hospital or surgery center relies on pediatricians as a major link in the preoperative assessment chain, pediatricians must be familiar with this literature and should have ongoing communication with their anesthesiology colleagues. Collaborative efforts, such as continuing medical education conferences and residency training about these topics, can reap significant rewards.

Policies on preoperative testing have been completely reassessed in recent years, and abandonment of the routine use of tests has become the norm. This is driven by both the growing number of studies that demonstrated little or no value in such testing, as well as by economic concerns that mandate the elimination of unnecessary expenditures.

Urinalysis

A 1990 study of nearly 500 children scheduled for elective surgery found abnormalities in 15% of children; however, more than 80% of those were historically known, clinically insignificant, or false positives. The authors concluded that preoperative urinalysis should not be routinely performed on healthy children for preoperative assessment (O'Conner and Drasner, 1990).

Hematocrit and Complete Blood Count

Unless a surgery is expected to result in significant blood loss (highly unlikely for outpatient surgery), the complete blood count (CBC) screening has little or no value (Roy et al., 1990, 1991; Hackmann et al., 1991). Several studies have demonstrated that the presence of mild to moderate anemia has little to no effect on the conduction of anesthesia or outcome in children undergoing same-day surgical procedures. The presence of anemia in former premature infants of fewer than 54 weeks' postconceptual age has been found to correlate with an increased risk of postanesthetic apnea, and screening for anemia in this population may detect those at increased risk (Welborn et al., 1991). It is not known, however, if the anemia is the cause of increased apnea or only an associated finding. There are no data to determine whether correction of anemia in these patients reduces the risk of apnea. All former premature infants who are at risk should be admitted for postoperative monitoring in any case, thus screening may not alter clinical practice. Children with sickle cell disease (not trait) need to have their hemoglobin level measured, because both management and outcomes of these patients are dependent on an adequate level of hemoglobin A or F (see the following section).

Sickle Cell Testing

In many states, newborns in at-risk populations are screened for sickle cell disease, thus the sickle cell status of all infants and children in those locations is known. In locations where such newborn screening is not universal, it is prudent to obtain sickle cell testing in any infant or child under the age of 3 years of at-risk ethnicity whose status is unknown. Children older than this are likely to have had symptoms if they are affected. In children who do have sickle cell disease, a preoperative hemoglobin level is mandated to determine the need for preoperative transfusion. A large multicenter trial found that simple transfusion, if the hemoglobin was less than 10g/dL, is as effective as exchange transfusion in these patients (Vichinsky et al., 1995) (see Chapter 36, Systemic Disorders). One study has reported that minor surgical procedures like those usually performed on outpatients could be safely performed in patients with sickle cell disease without preoperative transfusion; complication rates were significantly higher in children undergoing abdominal, thoracic, or airway procedures (Griffin and Buchanan, 1993). However, sickle cell trait, which usually does not cause any symptoms or illness, has rarely been associated with the complications of surgery and anesthesia, and hemoglobin determination in these patients is unnecessary (Konotey-Ahulu, 1969; McGarry and Duncan, 1973; Atlas, 1974; Gibson and Love, 1974).

Heart Murmurs and Cardiology Consultation

At least 25% of healthy children have an audible heart murmur at some time during childhood, and the question of when to refer a child to a pediatric cardiologist for the evaluation of a new murmur is often raised during the preoperative evaluation. The vast majority of these are functional ("innocent") murmurs, not associated with any structural heart disease. Innocent murmurs are soft (less than grade 3), blowing, and loudest along the left sternal border. They tend to decrease or disappear during inspiration. Most congenital heart lesions appear before the first several months of life, so an asymptomatic murmur in an older child is less likely—but not entirely impossible—to be significant. Exceptions include atrial septal defects, small ventricular septal defects, coarctation of the aorta, some valvular lesions that have no hemodynamic symptoms during normal activity, and in rare instances, other lesions. The ability of a pediatric cardiologist to distinguish between a functional murmur and one caused by a structural heart lesion by examination alone was evaluated and found to be high, so more extensive (and expensive) evaluation, such as echocardiography, is rarely necessary (Newburger et al., 1983). If the child is older than 6 months of age, without any symptoms referable to the cardiac system, most skilled clinicians should be able to evaluate these murmurs and rule out hemodynamically significant congenital heart disease. Cardiomyopathy can also bring on a new murmur, so a previously undetected murmur accompanied by symptoms suggestive of impaired myocardial performance or irritability, such as dysrhythmias, especially if it follows a viral illness, should be evaluated by a cardiologist.

Children with some congenital heart lesions require antibiotic prophylaxis for the prevention of endocarditis when undergoing operations during which they will be at risk. In 2007 there was a major revision in the recommendations for antibiotic prophylaxis of congenital heart disease that significantly reduced the number of conditions that require treatment (Box 34-1). The current American Heart Association recommendations are available online at *http://circ.ahajournals.org/cgi/reprint/CIRCULATIONAHA.106.183095*. It should be noted that for optimal treatment, the intravenous (IV) antibiotic should be administered 30 minutes before the procedure's start, which can pose a considerable problem in day surgery when an IV port is not present before induction. Antibiotic prophylaxis is no longer recommended for routine procedures of the gastrointestinal (GI) or genitourinary (GU) tract, but it is still advisable for dental and oral procedures during which there is manipulation of the gingivae and periapical region of the teeth or perforation of the oral mucosa, procedures of the respiratory tract, and procedures on infected skin or musculoskeletal tissues. For these procedures, oral antibiotics can be given 1 hour before the procedure, thereby eliminating the problem of timing. When IV antibiotics are desired, our current practice is to begin their administration as soon as IV access is obtained.

UNDERLYING ILLNESSES AND COMPLICATING FACTORS

There are numerous underlying conditions that exist commonly in relatively healthy children that do not preclude outpatient surgery but have implications regarding the preoperative preparation and anesthetic management.

Upper Respiratory Tract Infections

Probably the most common problem to confront the anesthesiologist caring for children in outpatient surgery is the child with a URI. Viral respiratory tract illness is virtually ubiquitous in children, particularly during the winter months when close indoor contact in schools and daycare facilities with other children with colds is impossible to avoid. The average preschool child contracts between 6 and 8 URIs per year. Both upper and lower respiratory tract viral infections can increase airway inflammation, irritability, and respiratory tract secretions by mechanisms as diverse as increased production and decreased degradation of tachykinins and other neuropeptides, viral induced damage to M2 muscarinic receptors in the airways leading to vagal-mediated hyperreactivity, and increased volume and viscidity of airway secretions causing subsegmental atelectasis (Empey et al., 1976; Dusser et al., 1989; Williams et al., 1992). Increased airway reactivity and hyperresponsiveness occur in the lower airways even in patients with respiratory viral illness clinically limited to the upper airway and even in those with no history of asthma (de Kluijver et al., 2002). After the apparent resolution of the URI, increased airway hyperresponsiveness and irritability may persist for as long as 8 weeks (Empey et al., 1976; Empey, 1983). In children with underlying respiratory disease, such as asthma, bronchopulmonary dysplasia, or other chronic lung diseases, these responses may be further exaggerated. Other risk factors that may be associated with more serious or common complications are age younger than 1 year and sickle cell disease (Cohen and Cameron, 1991). In what is perhaps one of the most comprehensive investigations of URI and anesthesia, 1078 infants and children were prospectively studied (Tait et al., 2001). Independent risk factors for respiratory complications were endotracheal intubation, history of prematurity, reactive airways disease, parental smoking, airway surgery and nasal congestion, and the presence of copious secretions. Of interest is that a history of prematurity was a risk factor even in children who were several years old and no longer had ongoing problems referable to their premature birth.

Box 34-1 AHA Recommendations for Antibiotic Prophylaxis for Endocarditis: Cardiac Conditions Associated with a High Risk of Adverse Outcome

Prosthetic cardiac valve
Previous history of infectious endocarditis
Unrepaired cyanotic congenital heart disease, including palliative shunts or conduits
Completely repaired congenital heart disease with prosthetic material or devices, whether placed surgically or by catheter intervention, during the first 6 months after the procedure
Repaired congenital heart disease with residual defects or shunts at the site or adjacent to the site of a prosthetic patch or prosthetic device (that inhibit endothelialization)
Cardiac transplant recipients who develop cardiac valvulopathy

Adapted from Wilson et al.: Prevention of infective endocarditis: guidelines from the American Heart Association, *Circulation* 115:1736–1754, 2007.

Numerous studies have documented that children who either have URIs or who have recently recovered from one have more minor airway complications during or after anesthesia compared with healthy children. Mild oxygen desaturation and coughing, as well as more potentially serious complications such as bronchospasm, laryngospasm, and respiratory failure are particularly likely to occur if the airway is stimulated. Tait and Knight (1987) prospectively studied a large cohort of children undergoing myringotomy and ventilating-tube placement for chronic or recurrent otitis media under general mask anesthesia with halothane. The group that had URIs had no difference in the incidence of respiratory problems, no increase in the severity of respiratory illness, and no increase in the duration of URI symptoms. When compared with matched unanesthetized controls, URI symptoms actually decreased in the group receiving halothane anesthesia. These beneficial results may have been influenced by the effects of myringotomy on the course of the infection, but there is also some laboratory evidence that halothane has viricidal properties in tissue-culture preparations. It is not known if the newer volatile anesthetics have similar effects.

Coté et al., in their investigation of the utility of capnometry and pulse oximetry in detecting adverse events during anesthesia and in a subsequent paper further analyzing these data, found that children with URIs commonly had mild oxygen desaturation both during surgery and in recovery (Coté et al., 1991; Rolf and Coté, 1992). Others have noted that postoperative oxygen requirements in these children are commonly transiently increased (Levy et al., 1992). It is possible that the cause is related to subsegmental atelectasis from increased quantity and viscidity of secretions, and that with deep breathing and coughing after emergence, reexpansion of these segments occurs. In the prospective study previously cited, patients with current or recent URIs had a greater incidence of respiratory complications, including breath-holding and desaturation less than 90%, although none of the complications was associated with long-term sequelae. Both the authors and an accompanying editorial concluded that most children with URIs who were not overtly ill and had no other complicating medical issues could, with judicious attention to anesthetic technique, be safely anesthetized with increased risk for only mild transient sequelae (Coté, 2001; Tait et al., 2001).

Although most children with clinically mild URIs can undergo anesthesia safely, the potential for more serious complications in children with URIs should not be overlooked. A prospective study of over 15,000 children found that children who developed laryngospasm were twice as likely to have a URI (Schreiner et al., 1996). The investigators found that the incidence of laryngospasm was most clearly related to the parent's subjective assessment of a URI, and that younger age and surgeries involving the airway were additive risk factors. A prospective case-controlled study of 1283 children with URI who underwent general anesthesia found a two- to sevenfold increase in respiratory complications during the perioperative course when compared with their counterparts without URIs (Cohen and Cameron, 1991). The incidence was 11-fold higher if the patient was intubated. A very small minority of children with URIs who do not appear to be ill during the preoperative examination may develop acute respiratory failure after the induction of anesthesia or some time during the anesthetic course. Severe hypoxia, bronchospasm, ventilatory insufficiency, and reduced compliance may occur and may even require postoperative ventilation and critical-care management. Some of these children have an unrecognized underlying lower tract disease, such as pneumonia, and others may experience shunt and ventilation-perfusion mismatching from atelectasis and pulmonary collapse as a result of inspissation of secretions and mucus plugging (Campbell, 1990; Williams et al., 1992). In rare instances, cardiomyopathy may follow viral illness. There are several reports of cardiac dysrhythmias or collapse occurring after induction of general anesthesia that were attributed to postviral myocarditis. The onset of abnormal rhythms on the ECG tracing or sudden deterioration of blood pressure or perfusion should alert the anesthesiologist to this possibility (Brampton and Jago, 1990; Terasaki et al., 1990).

It should be kept in mind that all of the ill patients who are included in these studies had mild to moderate URIs—children who were more severely ill had their surgery cancelled by the clinicians responsible for their care and were never enrolled in the study. Thus, clinical judgment remains crucial in deciding whether or not to cancel a case. Firm criteria for when to proceed and when to cancel are hard to discern, but the most current data suggest that there are several guidelines that can be applied:

- Laboratory tests are usually not useful; clinical impression is more reliable, such as noting the presence of toxicity, fever, purulent nasal discharge, productive cough, or wheezing. If physical examination suggests pneumonia, a chest radiograph may be confirmatory.
- There should be a lower threshold for postponing surgery in patients at increased risk, such as former premature infants, children with underlying pulmonary disease (e.g., asthma or bronchopulmonary dysplasia), infants younger than 1 year of age, and children with sickle cell disease.
- Patients who are to undergo surgery involving the airway should be considered at increased risk.
- If endotracheal intubation can be avoided, it is likely to decrease the risk of complications. Data suggest that the risk of airway complications in children with URIs is least with a conventional face mask, intermediate with a laryngeal mask airway (LMA), and greatest with an endotracheal tube (Tait et al., 1998, 2001). A logistic regression based on retrospective data did not identify any specific clinical factors that were associated with a higher incidence of adverse respiratory events during anesthesia in children with URIs, it but did find an association with endotracheal intubation and to a lesser degree with the use of an LMA, as compared with mask anesthesia (Rachel Homer et al., 2007).
- If a child is deemed too ill for anesthesia and surgery to proceed, it is best to wait 3 to 4 weeks from the resolution of the URI to reschedule the operation to allow for resolution of airway hyperresponsiveness. The aforementioned logistic regression found an increased incidence of adverse airway events if the peak symptoms of the URI had occurred within 4 weeks of the anesthetic (Rachel Homer et al., 2007).
- One should anticipate that the child with a URI might have a modest prolongation in PACU stay because of transient oxygen requirements or other mild respiratory symptoms that can delay discharge.

Asthma

The prevalence and severity of asthma, especially in children, remains a significant health problem in the United States. As of 1998, 6.4% of the U.S. population carried the diagnosis; two thirds of those were children. A more recent assessment of prevalence rates from 1980 to 2007 found that the prevalence plateaued in 1997, but that 9.1% (or 6.7 million) of American children carried the diagnosis (Akinbami et al., 2009). Nearly one-half million patients are hospitalized yearly with exacerbations of asthma, and almost half of those are children. The prevalence has increased by about 60% in the past 20 years before leveling off in the past 10 years. The death rate, although small, more than doubled from 1975 to 1995, but it appears to have stabilized in the past decade. Children with asthma can be safely and effectively anesthetized for same-day surgery, but careful preoperative preparation and evaluation, as well as intraoperative management, are crucial to avoid exacerbations and complications. Although it was previously common to think of asthma in terms of bronchospasm, current definitions of the disease emphasize the role or airway inflammation in pathogenesis, progression, and management. Recent consensus conferences of the National Institutes of Health (NIH) National Heart, Lung, and Blood Institute have defined asthma as a chronic inflammatory disorder of the airways that comprises many cells beyond those structural elements of the airways themselves, including mast cells, eosinophils, and T lymphocytes. The inflammatory processes that are involved in both the pathogenesis of the disorder, as well as in the progression of disease, are now addressed much more effectively in therapy for all patients with asthma and not only those with severe disease. The mainstay of therapy in the past was the chronic use of bronchodilator therapy, with antiinflammatory drugs reserved for the more severe cases; current thinking is that the first line of treatment should target inflammation with drugs such as inhaled steroids and newer drugs targeting inflammatory mediators (see Chapter 36, Systemic Disorders).

Anesthetizing the child with asthma for outpatient surgery involves the same general principles as for inpatient procedures (Pradal et al., 1995). It is critical for the asthmatic patient to closely adhere to their medication regimen before surgery. Inhaled steroids and agents like leukotriene inhibitors and cromolyn all require regular use for efficacy. The patient must use these medicines regularly and faithfully in the days (and weeks) before undergoing anesthesia. For those who have required systemic steroids in the past, a short course of steroids, beginning 24 hours before induction of anesthesia, may be advisable, particularly if intubation of the trachea will be required. Preoperative treatment with a short acting β-agonist such as albuterol may be helpful as well, even if the patient is not symptomatic, because events may occur during surgery that are likely to provoke airway irritability, especially intubation (Maslow et al., 2000). Much like the child with a URI, avoidance of intubation and airway stimulation, if possible, reduces the potential for exacerbation of airway irritability.

Volatile anesthetics, which have bronchodilatory properties, have obvious advantages in the child with asthma. Propofol, which has been shown to relax tracheal smooth muscle in vitro and to decrease airway resistance in subjects with and without asthma during induction of anesthesia, is an excellent choice when an IV induction is used (Pizov et al., 1995; Eames et al., 1996). This effect on airway smooth muscle has been shown to be even greater than that of ketamine and was also demonstrated during maintenance when an infusion was continued during the anesthetic (Pedersen et al., 1993). A propofol-based anesthetic, combined with either regional anesthesia or a non–histamine-releasing opioid, is a good alternative to volatile anesthesia when a total IV technique is indicated or desired. Some

caution must be taken with the sulfite-containing preparation of propofol, as one study in adults has demonstrated a significant increase in airway resistance with this formulation compared with the non–sulfite-containing drug, although adverse clinical events have not been often reported despite widespread use (Rieschke et al., 2003).

Emergence from anesthesia is perhaps the most vulnerable period that is faced during the case. Although the stimulation of intubation at induction is unquestionably a time of increased risk, the ability to treat bronchospasm by deepening the anesthetic in response to airway hyperreactivity is not present at emergence. There is, therefore, a significant advantage to deep extubation when a volatile technique is used, because the patient can awaken without the endotracheal tube (a highly potent stimulus to the airway) in place. Judicious timing of extubation during emergence from total IV anesthesia can accomplish the same goal.

The risk from anesthesia in a child with an active exacerbation of asthma is certainly increased, and careful attention must be given to postponing procedures in these patients until baseline control of the disease is regained. The child with severe asthma who is never fully "clear" can still be a suitable candidate for outpatient surgery if the clinical management is optimized; there is aggressive preoperative treatment, such as a short course of systemic steroids, increased bronchodilator therapy, and strict avoidance of airway irritants like tobacco smoke is instituted; and contingency plans for admission are made in the event of an exacerbation.

Diabetes

Type I diabetes in children is relatively common, occurring in approximately 1 in 500 school-aged children, but data on the optimal intraoperative management of children with this disease are scant. Although there are no prospective investigations published in the English language literature on the subject, there are two recent reviews and consensus guidelines on the perioperative management of insulin-dependent diabetes in children that offer excellent and well-reasoned guidance on their care (Rhodes et al., 2005; Betts et al., 2007). Although many of the problems in anesthetizing adults relate to the late complications of this condition (e.g., damage to many end-organ systems and autonomic dysfunction), these problems are less prevalent in children, and the most common issue is that of glucose control. Children with diabetes can be safely anesthetized as outpatients if great care is taken to maintain good glucose homeostasis. The child should observe the usual fasting guidelines for elective surgery and should be scheduled for surgery early in the day. If the child is receiving a split-dose insulin regimen with short- and intermediate-acting insulins, the child may receive half of the usual intermediate- or long-acting insulin dose on the morning of surgery and omit any short-acting insulin (McAnulty et al., 2000; McAnulty and Hall, 2003). For children receiving a basal insulin regimen, there should be no short-acting insulin administered at all on the morning of surgery, but they should be given the usual dose of insulin glargine, an insulin for basal control with no true peak and a very long duration of action of about 24 hours (Chase et al., 2008; Hirsch, 2005). In all cases, the blood glucose level should be checked upon awakening and again 2 to 3 hours later. Intravenous infusions containing 5% glucose have often been recommended for intraoperative fluid management, but it has generally been found easier to use a non–glucose-containing IV fluid into which a glucose-containing IV is "piggybacked." In this manner, the patient's fluid requirements and glucose requirements can be independently regulated. Because the most potentially catastrophic complication of diabetes during surgery is unrecognized hypoglycemia, and symptoms of hypoglycemia may be undetectable during anesthesia, blood glucose levels should be checked every 30 to 60 minutes during the procedure. Hypoglycemia should be treated promptly by reducing or stopping any insulin administration and increasing the IV glucose rate, and hyperglycemia (blood glucose levels over 250 mg/dL) should be treated with a continuous insulin infusion titrated to effect, usually beginning at a rate of 0.05 units/kg per hour. The very short duration of action of IV regular insulin (about 5 minutes) makes glucose control much easier with this method (Barnett et al., 1980). The same management scheme is continued in the PACU until the patient is awake and taking oral fluids without difficulty. At that time, a dose of subcutaneous regular insulin can be administered and an oral diet begun. The patient should check blood glucose levels often during the postoperative day, because the stress of surgery often alters insulin requirements. The dose should be adjusted accordingly. The usual insulin regimen can often be restarted on the day after surgery.

Malignant Hyperthermia

The advent of improved and short-acting IV anesthetics has made the management of patients with malignant hyperthermia (MH) considerably simpler. Current recommendations for the care of patients with MH no longer includes prophylactic therapy with dantrolene, and the use of nontriggering techniques coupled with proper preparation of the anesthesia machine can assure that these patients are not exposed to triggering agents. A 10-year review of 303 patients with the diagnosis of MH who underwent trigger-free anesthesia found that none developed fever in the perioperative period that was attributable to an MH crisis, and none required treatment with dantrolene (Yentis et al., 1992). The authors concluded that patients with MH are suitable candidates for outpatient anesthesia (see Chapter 37, Malignant Hyperthermia).

Sickle Cell Anemia

Children with sickle cell disease have increased risks in the perioperative period; however, they can usually undergo anesthesia and surgery as outpatients. Preoperative testing and management of transfusion was discussed above. The major risk factors for inducing a crisis in the perioperative period are dehydration, hypoxia, diminished perfusion, and acidosis. If close attention is paid to avoiding these risk factors, most patients with sickle cell disease can be managed as outpatients for suitable operations. In particular, good hydration and analgesia are important for stable recovery. Caregivers must be more strict than usual in ensuring that the child can take oral fluids without difficulty before discharge to home. The use of surgical tourniquets for orthopedic surgery in patients with sickle cell disease is controversial, but they should probably be avoided in outpatient surgery where postoperative acid-base status, perfusion, and the development of late-onset complications cannot be closely

monitored (Adu-Gyamfi et al., 1993). Tonsillectomy and adenoidectomy in patients with sickle cell disease and OSA appear to entail increased risks and probably should not be performed on an outpatient basis (Sidman and Fry, 1988; Derkay et al., 1991; Halvorson et al., 1997) (see Chapter 36, Systemic Disorders).

PREOPERATIVE PREPARATION OF THE CHILD AND FAMILY

Family-Centered Care

There has been increasing emphasis in pediatric medicine on the care of the child within the context of the family. This is in part behind the current vogue for including the parents of the patient in the experience of induction of anesthesia and early admission to the PACU. When one considers outpatient surgery, however, this concept is extended even further, because the family is more intimately involved in the postoperative care of the child than ever before. The parent or primary caregiver becomes the surrogate nurse once the child is discharged home and therefore must be involved to a greater degree in the postoperative experience even before discharge from the day-surgery unit. It has become the norm in most pediatric institutions and general hospitals that have sizable pediatric surgical programs for parental involvement to include preoperative tours of the operating room and PACU, parental presence during induction of anesthesia, and admission of the parents to the PACU very soon after the child's arrival and emergence from anesthesia. In most cases, experience with these programs have found them to ease, not complicate, the care of the child, and disruptive parents are the rare exception (Schofield and White, 1989).

Preoperative Teaching and Parental Presence

Outpatient surgery is an intense experience for both parents and children. Many things happen within a short time span, and the emphasis on efficiency and throughput can limit the time that staff can spend in preparing each parent and child for all that will happen. Preoperative teaching programs have become common methods of education to help families understand what to expect on the day of surgery. These programs include preoperative tours of the outpatient surgery center, preoperative telephone calls, written brochures, and videotapes (Karl et al., 1990; Kleinfeldt, 1990; O'Byrne et al., 1997; Cassady et al., 1999; Bellew et al., 2002; Koinig, 2002). Whereas the explicit goals of these programs are education and the efficient transmission of information, an implicit goal is reduction of anxiety and undesirable behavioral consequences of the stress of the perioperative experience (Margolis et al., 1998). The first objective can be met by many, if not all of these programs, but the more far-reaching ones may be more difficult to attain. A study of 143 2- to 6-year-old children who were randomized to receive either an interactive teaching book or no intervention found more, not less, preoperative anxiety in the children who had received the book, but less aggression during induction and fewer behavioral changes 2 weeks after surgery (Margolis et al., 1998). A well-controlled and designed study found that preoperative teaching programs of various modalities had an effect of anxiolysis only in the holding area on the day of surgery; that effect did not extend effectively to the induction period itself (Kain et al., 1998b). Although parental satisfaction was clearly increased by parental presence during induction, and highly anxious children benefited from presence of a parent during induction, children's anxiety and behavior were more effectively modulated by the use of premedication (Kain et al., 1996; Kain et al. 1998a). Although these data might suggest that the expense and effort of elaborate teaching programs, when examined in a critical and rigorous manner, may not be as cost-effective as more modest programs combined with premedication, one must recognize that limited benefits have value as well. For the parent and child who are waiting for an hour in the preoperative area, a reduction in stress for that period alone is meaningful. Furthermore, the norm in many communities is that such programs are welcomed and expected by many parents; they can also serve as opportunities to educate and improve compliance with preoperative procedures and thereby reduce the incidence of case cancellation.

Part of the art of pediatric anesthesia, of course, is the ability to rapidly establish effective and reassuring communication with the parent and child. The rapport and trust that the anesthesiologist creates during the preoperative interview is also an important and effective method of reassurance and anxiolysis that can enhance the transition to the operating room. In the outpatient setting, where time is more constrained, the value of a quick game, magic trick, kind word, or even brief induction of hypnotic suggestion should not be underestimated. Bringing a security item, such as a blanket or favorite toy into the operating room, can provide additional comfort to the child. Having this item immediately available at the time of emergence may also be helpful (see Chapter 8, Psychological Aspects of Pediatric Anesthesia).

Premedication

As was noted above, the use of sedative premedication has been shown to be the most effective means of reducing preoperative anxiety, postoperative recall, and maladaptive behavior in children undergoing outpatient surgery. Oral midazolam has become the most commonly used premedicant in the United States since 2000 (Kain et al., 2004). Significant reduction in postoperative recall and establishment of anterograde amnesia has been demonstrated with 0.5 mg/kg of midazolam administered orally as little as 10 minutes before induction (Kain et al., 2000). Oral doses as low as 0.25 mg/kg have been demonstrated to be as effective as larger doses with only a slightly slower time of onset (Coté et al., 2002). Of particular concern in the outpatient setting, however, is the problem of delayed emergence. Several studies using 0.5 mg/kg of oral midazolam have found that the drug delayed recovery, but the actual time of discharge from the hospital was not prolonged (Bevan et al., 1997; Viitanen et al., 1999a, 1999b). In institutions where the PACU is divided into phase I (initial recovery from the operating room until the child has reached an awake state with stable vital signs and is ready to take oral fluids) and phase II (less intensive observation and readying for discharge to home) areas, this translates to a longer stay in phase I recovery only. Such delays have the potential to affect throughput and cause bottlenecks for patients arriving from the operating room, but they do not effect total hospital time. The use of lower doses may reduce this problem, but data are not yet available. Young children who return to the operating room for repeated procedures (e.g.,

those with recurrent laryngeal papillomas) may especially benefit from premedication, even with relatively low doses. In this population the benefits largely outweigh any disadvantage of delayed emergence.

The benefits of oral administration, fairly rapid onset, and reliability of effect give midazolam considerable advantage over other agents. It does have several disadvantages, however, that must be considered. Midazolam has an extremely bitter, unpleasant taste. Although both the commercially available oral product and products compounded by the hospital mask the flavor to some degree, acceptance by some children remains poor. Alternative nonparenteral routes of administration have been studied, including nasal (0.2 to 0.3 mg/kg), transmucosal (0.2 mg/kg), and rectal (0.3 mg/kg), but each of these also has disadvantages, so that the oral administration remains the most commonly used and best-tolerated method for the majority of children (Saint-Maurice et al., 1986; Karl et al., 1993; Pandit et al., 2001).

Other agents and routes of administration, although less commonly used, have a place in the armamentarium. Other medications have been used in conjunction with midazolam, notably ketamine (Funk et al., 2000). Its advantage over a single-drug regimen appears to be in the child who is exceptionally uncooperative and requires a deeper level of sedation resulting from a dissociative state. Oral and transmucosal fentanyl has been used with success as well. Both the oral administration of the IV preparation and the commercially available oral transmucosal fentanyl "lollipop" have been shown to be effective; however, postoperative nausea may be increased compared with other agents, limiting its usefulness in the outpatient setting (Howell et al., 2002; Tamura et al., 2003). Similar results have been seen with nasally administered sufentanil, which also may cause nasal burning and chest wall rigidity. This agent appears to be less useful than others for these reasons and has largely fallen out of favor with most pediatric anesthesiologists. Intramuscular administration of premedication is uncommonly used in children for obvious reasons—children have an intense dislike and fear of needles. In some cases, however, when a child is exceedingly uncooperative and unmanageable, there may be no better alternative, and it is safer and more humane to administer a quick intramuscular injection with a small needle than to force the anesthesia mask on the face of an awake struggling child for what will surely appear to be a very long 60 seconds. Ketamine, often in combination with midazolam and glycopyrrolate, is the most commonly used agent. The usual doses range from 3 to 5 mg/kg; the lower doses are administered in combination with 0.1 mg/kg of midazolam. A high concentration (100 mg/mL) of ketamine should be used to minimize the injected volume. The anterior thigh is the most common site of administration (see Chapter 9, Preoperative Preparation).

ANESTHETIC TECHNIQUES

The operative procedure and underlying condition of the patient remain the primary decisive factors when choosing an anesthetic plan, but the disposition of the patient (i.e., discharge on the day of surgery) is an important consideration as well. An outpatient anesthetic has, in addition to all of the other usual goals, the additional priorities of rapid return to baseline function with minimal untoward effects and effective postoperative analgesia that can be sustained after leaving the hospital. It is only by achieving all of these objectives that patients can be effectively discharged home in a timely fashion.

Induction

Although clinical indications may on occasion dictate the safest induction technique, in many instances the older child may be given a choice, usually between inhalation and IV induction. Although the great majority of children seem to prefer an inhalation induction, there are a few who find the mask intolerable and prefer to have an IV line with local anesthetic, sometimes while breathing nitrous oxide. In cooperative school-aged children this can often be accomplished without difficulty, and it may be offered to appropriate children as an option. IV cannulation is often best accomplished in the operating room itself, where in the event of difficulty the plan can be easily and seamlessly changed.

The vast majority of children in the United States have an inhalation induction of anesthesia for outpatient procedures. The advantages are obvious—relatively rapid induction without any painful stimulus. Most children are needle-phobic, and are quite relieved when informed that they need not have anything painful done to them while they are conscious. The technique of inhalation induction is described in detail in Chapter 13, Induction, Maintenance, and Recovery. If the child uses a pacifier, it may be kept in the mouth until consciousness is lost, and the face mask may be placed over it. Scented lip gloss, such as bubble gum or fruit flavors, may be added to the facemask to disguise the odor of the volatile agent. The room should be otherwise quiet and free from conversation or other disruptions; the anesthesiologist should maintain continuous verbal contact with the child, telling a story in a soft, soothing modulated voice until the child falls asleep. Distracting modalities, such as movies or cartoons projected on the operating room's video monitors or on hand-held video devices can be used to good effect as well.

Sevoflurane has replaced halothane, which is no longer available in the United States, as the agent of choice for inhalation induction. Induction is rapid, and because sevoflurane is nonpungent, it causes very little airway irritation and coughing. It is possible to quickly increase the inspired concentration or even begin with the vaporizer set at 8% and still avoid coughing. Sevoflurane does have a mildly unpleasant odor, but it is still relatively easy to breathe. Sevoflurane, however, causes some interference with ventilatory drive and respiratory muscle function, reducing the effectiveness of spontaneous ventilation (Brown et al., 1998). In many cases, even if a total IV anesthetic is planned, an inhalation induction with sevoflurane is performed until IV access can be established.

Intravenous induction is a less commonly used technique. Propofol (3.5 to 5 mg/kg) has many attributes that make it an ideal IV induction agent for outpatient anesthesia. Not only does it have a very rapid onset of action, but its termination of action is similarly fast, with a characteristic rapid return to baseline function. The drug also has antiemetic properties, a highly desirable asset in outpatient anesthesia. Its only drawback is pain on injection. Although this may be moderated with lidocaine (1 to 2 mg/kg), injected before or mixed with the propofol, it can be quite painful, especially if it is injected into a small vein.

Rectal induction with a barbiturate such as methohexital, thiopental, or thiamylal has largely fallen out of favor, despite its advantage of being able to be performed in the parent's presence in an induction area outside of the operating room. Rectal induction and barbiturates in general have a significant disadvantage in outpatient anesthesia—a very prolonged elimination half-life—and for this reason they are not recommended.

Airway Management

There are numerous options for management of the airway in outpatient anesthesia. In many cases, an anesthesia mask alone is used—for example, during myringotomy and tube placement. This minimizes the risk of airway irritation but requires at least one of the anesthesiologist's hands be occupied. It is contraindicated in the event of a full stomach and may be problematic in patients who easily obstruct their airways, such as those with adenotonsillar hypertrophy.

The endotracheal tube remains the gold standard for the secured airway. Most pediatric anesthesiologists intubate their patients "deep," or without the use of neuromuscular relaxants. This eliminates the need for reversal or for concerns of residual neuromuscular blockade, but mandates skillful judgment of anesthetic depth to avoid cord injury or laryngospasm. Just as in any anesthetic, one must choose the tube's size carefully so as to avoid producing injury or irritation to the vocal cords and trachea. This is especially critical in a patient who is going to be discharged home the same day. Supraglottic airway devices, although useful, have not supplanted the need to intubate a patient for many outpatient surgery cases that may still benefit from the placement of an endotracheal tube. Intracavitary operations, including laparoscopic operations, are generally best performed with an endotracheal tube, although brief laparoscopic examinations, such as laparoscopic examination of the contralateral side during herniorrhaphy, can be effectively performed with a supraglottic airway device. Surgery in or near the airway (including tonsillectomy, adenoidectomy, and upper GI endoscopy) can be performed with a LMA, but this remains somewhat controversial.

Supraglottic airway devices may cause less laryngeal irritation than endotracheal tubes and can be placed without visualization of the airway (Brimacombe, 1995). The LMA, developed by Dr. Brain, is the first of these devices and is available in multiple pediatric sizes. Several competitors, including the COBRA Perilaryngeal Airway and the COPA Oropharyngeal Airway, are now marketed (Figs. 34-1 and 34-2). All of these devices offer a less stimulating means of maintaining the airway while freeing the hands of the anesthesiologist for other tasks. As was mentioned above, a number of studies have demonstrated that the ability to maintain a stable airway without stimulating the larynx and trachea can decrease the incidence of adverse respiratory events in children with active or recent URIs (Tait et al., 1998). The same might be true for patients with asthma, where the airway is also hyperirritable, although there are no data in children at this time. Airway pressure and resistance in anesthetized adults without lung disease have been shown to be lower with the LMA compared with an endotracheal tube, and it has been shown to induce less bronchoconstriction (Berry et al., 1999). Although the LMA may diminish lower respiratory tract stimulation, it does not appear to decrease the incidence of postoperative sore throat (Splinter et al., 1994). The findings by Tait et al. that endotracheal tubes are more stimulating than LMAs, which are in turn more stimulating than a face mask, may serve to guide the decision of how to manage the airway if all other factors are equal.

Infants appear to have a greater incidence of problems with supraglottic airway devices than older children. There is a high incidence of infolding of the epiglottis and malposition in children under 10 kg and a significantly higher incidence of airway complications such as laryngospasm, breath-holding, obstruction, and coughing when compared with a conventional mask with oral airway (Harnett et al., 2000; Bagshaw, 2002; Polaner et al., 2006).

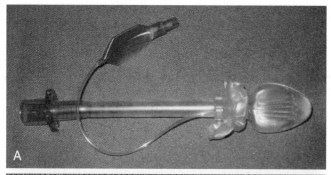

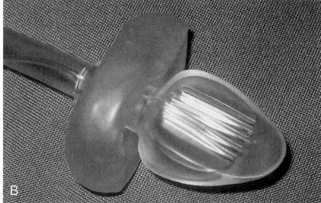

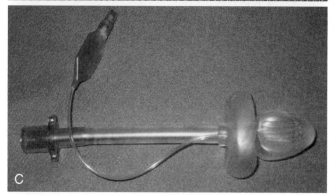

■ **FIGURE 34-1.** COBRA Perilaryngeal Airway. **A,** The device with the cuff deflated and ready for insertion. **B,** A view of the laryngeal surface of the device. **C,** The inflated cuff, which fills and conforms to the pharynx when in place.

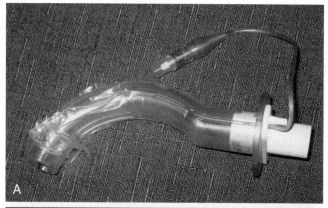

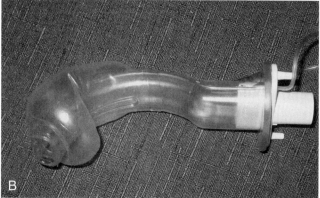

■ **FIGURE 34-2.** Cuffed COPA Oropharyngeal Airway. The device is sized and inserted like a conventional oropharyngeal airway with the cuff deflated **(A)** and the cuff inflated **(B).** The end of the device has a standard 15-mm connector to attach to the breathing circuit.

Anesthetic Maintenance

The ideal maintenance regimen for outpatient anesthesia would have three defining characteristics: ease of titration, rapid offset, and minimal residual side effects. Although it can be argued that several techniques or contemporary agents fit this definition, none is entirely free of all side effects, or are ideal agents in every situation.

Inhalation anesthesia is still the most commonly used maintenance technique and has numerous advantages to commend it. No organ or enzymatic metabolism is necessary for its elimination—it is simply breathed away. Volatile agents are easily titrated to effect, and anesthetic depth can be adjusted with relative rapidity. They are relatively economical, especially when low fresh gas flows are used, and they have beneficial effects on reactive airways, a common problem in children. There are several disadvantages, however, that may temper the claim for

volatile agents as the ideal agents for outpatient anesthesia in all circumstances. Total IV anesthesia, as will be discussed, has numerous benefits for outpatients in many instances as well.

Halothane is no longer available in the United States and has been replaced by sevoflurane as the primary volatile anesthetic for inhalation induction. It has been argued that sevoflurane's lower blood-gas solubility and blood:gas partition coefficient give it significant advantage over older, more soluble agents such as isoflurane for emergence, where a more rapid return to consciousness is desired in the outpatient setting. Whereas return to wakefulness may indeed be quicker with sevoflurane (and is even more rapid with desflurane), for short cases the speed to awakening with isoflurane can approach that of the less soluble agents if the isoflurane is turned off sooner. Perhaps more importantly, time to awakening has no relationship to time to discharge from the hospital (Lerman et al., 1996; Sury et al., 1996; Welborn et al., 1996). The latter is the metric that reflects both day-surgery unit efficiency and cost savings, and anesthesia with sevoflurane has not been shown to produce shorter discharge times, which is generally related not to speed of emergence but more to other factors, including premedication, complications of recovery such as postoperative nausea and vomiting, emergence agitation, and analgesic needs (Bacher et al., 1997).

Sevoflurane has one additional characteristic that limits its effectiveness as a maintenance agent in outpatient anesthesia—the problem of emergence agitation. Several investigators have studied this problem, which can be exceedingly disruptive and disturbing for PACU caregivers and parents. With the increased use of sevoflurane, it became apparent that there was an increase in emergence agitation or delirium in the PACU, and the majority of studies, including a recent meta-analysis (see Chapter 13, Induction, Maintenance, and Recovery, Figure 13-4), support this clinical impression (Mayer et al., 2006; Rieger et al., 1996; Beskow and Westrin, 1999; Cravero et al., 2000; Kuratani and Oi, 2008; Bortone et al., 2006). However, there are a few studies that have not found an increased incidence compared with isoflurane (Meyer et al., 2007; Voepel et al., 2003). The child with emergence agitation appears wild and incoherent; he is inconsolable and does not appear to recognize familiar people. This phenomenon has clearly been distinguished from inadequate analgesia. Cravero et al. (2000) compared emergence characteristics of sevoflurane to halothane anesthesia in children undergoing magnetic resonance imaging. This prospective randomized study design effectively eliminated pain or dysphoria of neural blockade as potential confounding variables, leaving only the choice of volatile agent as a factor (Cravero et al., 2000). Using either low- or high-threshold criteria to define agitation and delirium, the investigators found much higher rates (33% vs. 0% with high-threshold criteria and 88% vs. 12% applying low-threshold criteria) with sevoflurane as compared with halothane. Any time advantage gained by more rapid emergence was eliminated by the difficulty in caring for the agitated child in the PACU, and hospital discharge times were not different. Another study of sevoflurane in 100 children undergoing myringotomy and tube placement found that even with very short times under anesthesia, the incidence of emergence agitation was unacceptably high (Lapin et al., 1999). Although discharge times in this study were faster in the sevoflurane group, 67% demonstrated emergence agitation, leading them to conclude that sevoflurane was unsuitable for use as a sole agent for this procedure. They found that the addition of midazolam reduced this problem while lengthening recovery but not discharge times. Other investigators have found that midazolam does not prevent emergence agitation, and have found better responses to opioids, dexmedetomidine, low-dose ketamine, and propofol and ketorolac (Guler et al., 2005; Hung et al., 2005; Aouad et al., 2007; Breschan et al., 2007; Tsai et al., 2008; Davis et al., 1999). It is possible that the cause is related to the different effects of these agents on brain function that has been noted on electroencephalogram; speed of emergence does not seem to be a cause (Constant et al., 1999; Cohen et al., 2003; Oh et al., 2005).

Desflurane is another new volatile agent with rapid onset and offset characteristics caused by an exceptionally low blood: gas partition coefficient and solubility. It, too, appears to have a higher incidence of emergence agitation than older agents, although less than has been reported with sevoflurane (Mayer et al., 2006; Davis et al., 1994; Welborn et al., 1996; Valley et al., 2003). Emergence is significantly faster than with sevoflurane, however. This is because of its low solubility in tissues such as muscle and brain as compared with sevoflurane. Because sevoflurane is similar to halothane in its solubility in vessel-rich tissue groups, after discontinuance of the agent, significant blood concentrations are maintained as the agent returns from these depot storage sites to the bloodstream along its concentration gradient. This does not occur to a significant degree with desflurane because of its low tissue solubility, thereby speeding emergence time. Desflurane has also been found to decrease the ability to maintain spontaneous ventilation at concentrations greater than 1 MAC (Behforouz et al., 1998). Although desflurane is a potent airway irritant and is contraindicated for inhalation induction because of a very high incidence of severe laryngospasm, it does not appear to cause problems with deep extubation, although the incidence of coughing and other symptoms of airway irritability appear to be somewhat higher with desflurane (Zwass et al., 1992; Sneyd et al., 1998; Valley et al., 2003).

Nitrous oxide continues to be used as an adjunctive agent for outpatient anesthesia in combination with both volatile and IV agents. It is useful as a sedative when placing IV cannulae in situations where a pure IV technique is used, and it can ease the introduction of the pungent volatile agents when performing inhalation induction. Its utility as an agent for maintenance, however, is limited by its capacity to increase the incidence of postoperative nausea and vomiting. For this reason, its use in the outpatient setting should be constrained (Divatia et al., 1996).

The development of propofol heralded a new era in the maintenance of anesthesia in outpatients. It is not hyperbole to suggest that it thrust total IV anesthesia (TIVA) into the mainstream of anesthetic techniques, allowing rapid titration of anesthetic depth and prompt emergence without the use of volatile agents. Propofol is a potent antiemetic and can reduce the incidence of nausea and vomiting when used in combination with both other anesthetic agents and other antiemetics (Sneyd et al., 1998; Barst et al., 1999). Despite its rapid emergence characteristics when used for anesthetics of short or moderate duration, the incidence of delirium and agitation is very low when compared with sevoflurane or desflurane (Nakayama et al., 2007). Propofol's major limitation is its lack of analgesic properties, and it must be used with an opioid or regional technique to provide adequate depth of anesthesia for most stimulating procedures. It is an excellent (and perhaps the ideal) agent for use in imaging, radiation treatment, or interventional radiologic procedures where there is a minimum or absence of stimulation (Aldridge and Gordon, 1992; Martin et al., 1992; Vangerven et al., 1992; Frankville et al., 1993). It is particularly attractive for anesthesia for radiation therapy, where children require daily repeated general anesthetics for up to 6 consecutive weeks. In this situation, children are able to be ready for discharge to home within 20 minutes of the end of the treatment session, and in contrast to other agents such as barbiturates, children receiving propofol have no evidence of either drug accumulation or development of tolerance and dose escalation (Glauber and Audenaert, 1987; Mills and Lord, 1992; Fassoulaki et al., 1994).

Remifentanil is a unique IV opioid with rapid onset and elimination. In contrast to other opioids, its degradation is independent of organ metabolism, instead relying on hydrolysis by plasma esterases. The drug permits the anesthesiologist to provide intense intraoperative levels of opioid analgesia with no residual respiratory depression after emergence (Roulleau et al., 2003). Other postoperative side effects usually associated with opioids, such as nausea and vomiting, excessive sedation, and respiratory depression are absent or extremely rare (Pinsker and Carroll, 1999; Eltzschig et al., 2002). Intraoperative conditions are notable for hemodynamic stability, although both bradycardia and hypotension can occur at higher infusion rates. The most significant caveat to the use of remifentanil is that its rapid degradation provides no postoperative analgesia whatsoever (Davis et al., 2000). It is essential, therefore, to use another agent or technique for this purpose, such as a long-acting opioid, a regional block, or a nonsteroidal such as ketorolac, and to administer it with adequate time for action before the patient's emergence and the dissipation of remifentanil's effect.

Perhaps the most effective manner in which to use remifentanil is to combine it with propofol. The combination of the two agents provides a balanced anesthetic that is easily titratable and results in significant reductions in the dose of both (Grundmann et al., 1998; Keidan et al., 2001). The two drugs can be mixed in the same syringe and administered via syringe pump. Because remifentanil degrades in propofol over time, aliquots small enough to be infused within 1 hour should be used (Stewart et al., 2000). For procedures of mild to moderate stimulation, 10 mcg of remifentanil per 1 mL (10 mg) of propofol is used, with infusion rates beginning at 100 mcg/kg per minute of propofol (0.1 mcg/kg per minute of remifentanil). This concentration permits the maintenance of spontaneous ventilation in most patients (Peacock et al., 1998; Reyle-Hahn et al., 2000). In particular, spontaneous ventilation is well maintained in children younger than 3 years old, even at higher infusion rates and even though remifentanil requirements to block the somatic response to skin incision are close to twofold higher in children than in adults (0.15 vs. 0.08 mcg/kg) (Barker et al., 2007; Munoz et al., 2007). For more stimulating procedures, the remifentanil concentration is doubled to 20 mcg/mL of propofol, and the infusion begins at the same rate of 100 mcg/kg per minute of propofol (0.2 mcg/kg per minute of remifentanil). Many patients breathe spontaneously with this concentration as well, although slow respiratory rates are common, and clinicians must be vigilant to avoid hypoventilation. This technique provides a stable intraoperative course, combined with an exceptionally smooth emergence and rapid return to baseline function, especially for patients undergoing procedures such as bone marrow aspirations, lumbar punctures, interventional radiology, upper and lower GI endoscopies, and incision and drainage of abscesses (Glaisyer and Sury, 2005).

Regional anesthesia (usually in combination with a general anesthetic) can be used to great advantage in outpatients. Although the prime advantage and reason for its use is the provision of postoperative analgesia (as is later discussed in more detail), the modest reduction in the depth of general anesthesia can speed recovery and reduce the incidence of opioid-related untoward effects. Motor blockade is, in most cases, not a contraindication to discharge to home and can be reduced or eliminated by the use of low concentration local anesthetics. Most children have their motor block resolved before discharge from the PACU, although this may not be the case for longer-acting peripheral nerve blocks (Burns et al., 1990). For those who are discharged with residual blockade, clear and explicit instructions to the parents as to how to guard the limb and good follow-up inquiry via telephone are critical. Other reported advantages of regional blockade include decreased intraoperative blood loss and improved operating conditions during hypospadias repair (Gunter et al., 1990). For operations shorter than 1 hour in duration, preoperative blockade did not affect the duration of postoperative analgesia compared with blockade administered at the end of the case (Rice et al., 1990).

Nearly all regional anesthetics in children in the United States are administered after the induction of general anesthesia, although Marhofer and others (2004) reports the extensive use of regional anesthesia with sedation in Austria. See Chapter 16, Regional Anesthesia, for details on performing the various regional blocks. In most cases, regional blockade for ambulatory surgery is performed with local anesthetics only, omitting opioids and adjunctive agents, although there is growing experience with caudal clonidine (2 mcg/kg or less) in outpatient anesthesia in children over 6 months of age. The risks of respiratory depression that can occur with those additives must always be considered, an important safety factor in the patient who will not be monitored after discharge from the PACU.

Neuromuscular Blockade

In most outpatient procedures in infants and children, neuromuscular blockade is not necessary. The majority of surgical procedures that are done in this setting can be performed without it, and intubation can most commonly be achieved with inhalation anesthesia, sometimes combined with a single dose of propofol in older children. Alternatively, a single dose of remifentanil can be administered in combination with propofol for intubation and has been shown to facilitate rapid sequence induction without muscle relaxants (Batra et al., 2004). When muscle relaxants are employed, it is best to avoid any of the longer-acting nondepolarizers and rely on intermediate acting drugs such as atracurium or cisatracurium, rocuronium or vecuronium. These agents are discussed in detail in Chapter 7, Pharmacology of Pediatric Anesthesia. When a muscle relaxant is used, adequacy of reversal must be assured. A recent investigation in adults found that incomplete reversal and mild degrees of residual neuromuscular blockade were common (Debaene et al., 2003). At least with some agents, children are less prone to inadequate spontaneous reversal. In children receiving mivacurium (no longer available in the United States), residual weakness was not observed, whereas the finding was present in the adults (Bevan et al., 1996). Stringent criteria for adequacy of spontaneous reversal must be sought, and reversal agents administered if necessary (Baurain et al., 1998; Ali, 2003).

Fluids

As fasting times become shorter, the consequences of preoperative fasting are less problematic, but there remain occasional patients who come to surgery with varying degrees of dehydration (Coté, 1990; Cook-Sather et al., 2003). Additionally, the patient who is to be discharged home may not be interested in drinking large amounts of fluids in the hours immediately after surgery. It is useful, therefore, to provide adequate hydration not only to correct the fluid deficit but also to provide a cushion for the postoperative period. This is particularly the case for operations that may disrupt the ability to drink easily, such as tonsillectomy. Isotonic fluids should be administered, and the IV catheter may be kept in place until just before discharge. It is rarely necessary to provide glucose supplementation in the IV fluids in children outside the neonatal period (Sandstrom et al., 1993). The deficit plus current maintenance requirements should be repleted within 2 to 3 hours. In some cases, children are discharged home before that, but those are generally the ones at least risk for inadequate intake.

Emergence

The management of emergence from anesthesia in the outpatient is largely a question about the intubated child, and whether the endotracheal tube should be removed when the patient is deep or awake. Certainly the contraindications to deep extubation (e.g., full stomach, difficult airway, and blood in the pharynx) are no different in outpatients or inpatients. Those who argue for awake extubation are primarily concerned about the loss of airway and of the development of laryngospasm. These concerns are magnified if the PACU staff is not adept and experienced at dealing with the patient who has been extubated deep. The advantages of deep extubation are numerous. The patient awakens from anesthesia in the PACU without the noxious stimulus of an endotracheal tube in place and may have a smoother emergence. The child with reactive airways disease does not have the airway stimulation that may precipitate a potentially severe episode of bronchospasm. Operating-room efficiency is enhanced, because the patient is able to leave within a minute of the end of the surgery, and room turnover can proceed at a more rapid pace. Several practices, in addition to the contraindications mentioned above, are crucial to increase the safety of this practice. The tube should not be withdrawn unless the patient is breathing spontaneously and has been demonstrated to have no alteration in breathing pattern with stimulation of the trachea (usually accomplished by gently moving the endotracheal tube). This may require at least a 2-MAC value of inhaled anesthetic; however, the concomitant administration of an opioid or propofol or topicalization of the vocal cords significantly reduces this value. The patient should be placed on the side after extubation and once airway patency is confirmed to prevent oropharyngeal secretions from collecting in the hypopharynx and either stimulating the larynx or causing aspiration and to promote the forward prolapse of the tongue, which improves airway patency and helps prevent the tongue from falling back to the palate and obstructing the airway. Supplemental oxygen and close attention to airway patency are necessary during transport to the PACU.

POSTOPERATIVE ANALGESIA

If there is any issue that has the potential to completely sabotage the success of an outpatient surgery it is inadequate postoperative analgesia. No child can be discharged to home if the parents cannot adequately manage their pain using simple interventions. Inadequate analgesia has been identified in several studies as one of the most common causes for unanticipated admission to the hospital after surgery (Grenier et al., 1998). In another study, postoperative pain was identified by parents as the major problem they encountered after discharge to home (Kokinsky et al., 1999). Only 28% of the patients in that study had received regional blocks, however.

Regional and Local Anesthesia

Regional and local anesthesia has become one of the key modalities for postoperative analgesia for amenable procedures. Among the commonly performed operations in pediatric outpatient surgery that are associated with significant postoperative pain, only adenotonsillectomy and tympanostomy tube placement are not suitable for local or regional anesthesia. A prospective randomized study of glossopharyngeal nerve block, previously reported as an effective technique in adults, was stopped before its completion because of a 50% incidence of upper airway obstruction in the treatment group. The authors

terminated the study and concluded that glossopharyngeal block is dangerous in children after tonsillectomy because of the common occurrence of inadvertent blockade of the vagus and recurrent laryngeal nerves (Bean-Lijewski, 1997).

Strict attention to the limits of local anesthetic dose must be observed with any regional block, and aspiration should precede any injection. When large volumes of local anesthetic are injected for any regional block, both a test dose and incremental injection technique should be employed to minimize the risk of intravascular injection. A maximum of 2.5 mg/kg of bupivacaine can be administered to children over 6 months of age; younger infants should have the dose reduced by 30% (1.8 mg/kg) because of decreased levels of plasma binding proteins (Lerman et al., 1989; Luz et al., 1998). In addition, there appears to be an increased toxicity risk during general anesthesia with volatile agents (Badgwell et al., 1990). In these younger infants an additional margin of safety may be gained by the use of ropivacaine or levobupivacaine (no longer available in the United States), which appear to have less toxic potential (Bardsley et al., 1998; Kohane et al., 1998; Gunter et al., 1999; Morrison et al., 2000).

Although usually performed by the surgeon rather than the anesthesiologist, the value of wound infiltration with local anesthetic should not be underestimated. There are numerous limited procedures for which a regional nerve block would be more intervention than necessary, such as simple hardware removals in orthopedics or excisional biopsies of small lesions, where infiltration of the wound can be used to great advantage. Local anesthetic blood levels with this technique have been found to be low when dose limits are adhered to (Mobley et al., 1991). When a peripheral nerve or regional block can be performed, however, those techniques may offer superior analgesia. A study of caudal analgesia compared with wound infiltration for analgesia after inguinal herniorrhaphy found better analgesia and quicker emergence times, fewer pain-related behaviors, and earlier hospital discharge times with the caudal block. Less supplementation with systemic analgesics was required (Conroy et al., 1993).

Caudal anesthesia is probably the most commonly performed block in pediatric anesthesia practice. It is usually easy to administer, has an acceptably low incidence of complications, and is highly effective for surgical procedures below the level of the umbilicus (Dalens and Hasnaoui, 1989). The duration of effective analgesia is considerably longer than one would expect based on the usual length of action of the local anesthetic alone. A study that compared 0.25% bupivacaine with and without epinephrine found that the addition of epinephrine markedly prolonged the analgesia, and that prolonged duration of analgesia was correlated with both younger age and lower surgical site (penoscrotal vs. inguinal) (Warner et al., 1987). Duration of analgesia ranged from as short as 5 hours (inguinal surgery in patients older than 11 years of age) to as long as 23 hours (penoscrotal operation in patients 1 to 5 years of age) as judged by the time to first requirement for supplemental analgesia. In a study of caudal blockade for analgesia after club foot repair, analgesia lasted at least 8 hours (Foulk et al., 1995). The addition of clonidine to the local anesthetic has been found by some, but not all, investigators to prolong the duration of caudal analgesia (Constant et al., 1998; Ansermino et al., 2003; Tripi et al., 2005; Wheeler et al., 2005). Controversy remains, however, regarding the safety of this drug for outpatient use, particularly in smaller infants and at higher doses because of the risk of oversedation (Hansen and Henneberg, 2004). It appears prudent to limit the dose to less than 2 mcg/kg if caudal clonidine is used in a patient who will be discharged home and to avoid it altogether in infants younger than 6 months of age.

Side effects of caudal blockade in children are unusual. Multiple studies have confirmed that urinary retention does not occur after caudal block using local anesthetic without central neuraxis opioids (Warner et al., 1987; Fisher et al., 1993). No differences in side effects were seen between caudal blockade and ilioinguinal-iliohypogastric nerve block; PACU stays were longer by less than 5 minutes and hospital stays by less than 10 minutes with the caudal block (Splinter et al., 1995). Motor function is not significantly impaired at the time of discharge and does not preclude or delay discharge (Burns et al., 1990).

Although one study found that placing the block at the end of the case resulted in better analgesia, other well-controlled studies have shown that there is no decrement in the duration of analgesia with blocks administered at the beginning or end of surgery for procedures lasting less than 1 hour (Rice et al., 1990; Holthusen et al., 1994). A study of 0.5 mL/kg vs. 1 mL/kg of 0.125% bupivacaine with epinephrine for penile and scrotal surgery found no difference in the duration of analgesia up to 8 hours postoperatively (Malviya et al., 1992).

Peripheral nerve blocks can be used with considerable efficacy for outpatient surgery in children and can be administered either by the anesthesiologist or by the surgeon on the operative field. Ilioinguinal-iliohypogastric nerve block combined with wound infiltration showed similar efficacy to a caudal block for analgesia after inguinal herniorrhaphy in two randomized studies (Schindler et al., 1991; Splinter et al., 1995). Paraumbilical block was shown to provide excellent analgesia for umbilical herniorrhaphy, although the duration of analgesia was less than 8 hours in three of 11 subjects (Courreges et al., 1997). The transverse abdominis plane block, which can be reliably placed under ultrasound guidance, has been shown to be effective for prolonged analgesia after abdominal operations, including herniorrhaphy (Suresh and Chan, 2009). Fascia iliaca block is an effective and easy to place block for surgery of the leg above the level of the knee (Dalens et al., 1989). Ophthalmic surgery is often associated with considerable postoperative pain. Placement of a peribulbar block or a subconjunctival injection has been shown to provide long-lasting analgesia with a minimum of side effects in pediatric patients (Ates et al., 1998; Coppens et al., 2002; Subramaniam et al., 2003). Penile nerve blocks are often used in older patients undergoing distal hypospadias repairs or for circumcision. The dorsal nerve block has been shown to result in better postoperative analgesia than a penile ring block (Holder et al., 1997). Greater auricular nerve block has been shown to be efficacious after tympanomastiod surgery (Suresh et al., 2002). Many peripheral blocks of the extremities are very useful for analgesia after ambulatory surgery because of their long duration of action (Marhofer et al., 2004). If children have residual motor blockade at the time of discharge, follow-up care is necessary until the block has completely resolved.

An emerging practice in regional anesthesia is the use of continuous ambulatory peripheral nerve blocks and field blocks for postoperative analgesia (Ganesh et al., 2007). This has been facilitated by two technological innovations: the increased use of ultrasound to accurately place peripheral nerve or plexus cannulae, and the development of elastomeric infusion devices that permit delivery of local anesthetic at a controlled rate without

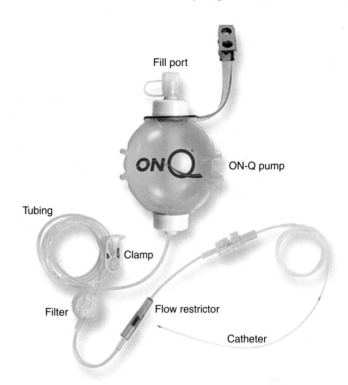

■ **FIGURE 34-3.** Elastomeric infusion device.

the use of high-cost pumps. These devices contain a reservoir of local anesthetic large enough to last several days. The reservoir is surrounded by a balloon-like bulb that when filled with air compresses the reservoir and infuses the drug. A flow limiter in the tubing controls the infusion rate (Fig. 34-3). Children can be sent home, and with daily telephone follow-up conversations, can receive either a long-acting nerve block or the infusion of the local anesthetic into their wound for several days. The parent can easily remove the catheter when the infusion is complete.

The development of parenterally administered nonsteroidal antiinflammatory drugs, principally ketorolac, has allowed the anesthesiologist to administer long-acting nonopioid analgesics so that they have taken effect by the time the patient awakens. There is a sizable literature on the use of ketorolac in pediatric patients over the age of 1 year, but no randomized studies to date of COX-2 type drugs in pediatrics. Many of these studies have specifically examined the role of ketorolac in outpatient surgery. Ketorolac has been shown to have several advantages over opioid analgesics for postoperative analgesia in pediatric outpatients. There is a significant reduction in nausea and vomiting in patients receiving ketorolac as compared with morphine, fentanyl, or other opioids (Mendel et al., 1995; Purday et al., 1996). The duration of a single dose of ketorolac is longer (6 hours) than most of the commonly used opioid analgesics (Dsida et al., 2002). Lack of respiratory depression, of course, is one ketorolac's major advantages over opioids. Ketorolac's major problem for use in outpatient analgesia is that it causes reversible dysfunction of platelet adhesion, and bleeding problems have been noted to be more common in children undergoing adenotonsillectomy (Gallagher et al., 1995; Judkins et al., 1996; Splinter et al., 1996; Splinter and Roberts, 1996). Bleeding problems have not been reported in other types of surgery, but caution should be used when administering ketorolac after other oral surgical procedures. Ketorolac appears to offer significant benefits to the pediatric outpatient after select operations.

Opioids remain the gold standard for postoperative analgesia for moderate to severe pain, and they are still commonly prescribed for pediatric outpatients, both parenterally during anesthesia and by oral, transmucosal, and other routes for postoperative analgesia. Their principal disadvantages are the side effects of nausea and respiratory depression; at the doses prescribed for outpatients, ileus is rarely a problem. Even a single dose of morphine administered for postoperative analgesia after inguinal hernia surgery has been reported to increase the incidence of PONV (Weinstein et al., 1994). Adjunctive nonopioid analgesics such as acetaminophen have an opioid-sparing effect and can reduce the amount of opioid necessary to achieve analgesia, thereby reducing the risk of side effects.

Intranasal fentanyl (2 mcg/kg, administered intraoperatively) has been used primarily for analgesia after myringotomy and tube surgery. Because these procedures are commonly performed without obtaining IV access, this provides an easy route for the administration of a potent analgesic. In a study comparing intranasal fentanyl to placebo, postoperative conditions were superior with fentanyl (Henderson et al., 1988). Children who received intranasal fentanyl were not only more comfortable and less agitated, but they did not have an increase in PONV, a problem that has been noted with intranasal sufentanil (Henderson et al., 1988; Galinkin et al., 2000).

Numerous oral opioid analgesics are used for postoperative analgesia in children. The surgeon and not the anesthesiologist often prescribes these drugs, but the anesthesiologist's expertise in the use of analgesics should be sought or offered when protocols are devised. Commonly used agents include oxycodone, hydrocodone, and tramadol (Table 34-2). All of these agents can be given in combination with acetaminophen and nonsteroidal antiinflammatory drugs for added efficacy. These agents are generally administered for 1 to 3 days; operations that result in more severe pain are less commonly performed on outpatients and require analgesic inpatient management. Codeine is still commonly prescribed for pain, but its use should be discouraged. Codeine is actually a prodrug—methylmorphine—that must be demethylated to its active form. Bioavailability varies widely depending on genetic variants of demethylation ability. Because of these pharmacogenetic differences, some patients achieve no analgesia at all as a result of an inability to demethylate the drug, whereas some suffer from increased side effects or even achieve potentially toxic drug levels because of more extensive demethylation (Quiding et al., 1992; Fagerlund and Braaten, 2001; El-Tahtawy et al., 2006) (see Chapter 15, Pain Management).

PACU, RECOVERY, AND DISCHARGE ISSUES

Nausea and Vomiting

PONV is perhaps the most common complication after anesthesia, although the reported incidence varies widely from approximately 8% to 50% (Heyland et al., 1997; Villeret et al., 2002). The

TABLE 34-2. Outpatient Analgesic Agents

Oxycodone	0.1-0.2 mg/kg	PO q3-4 hours
Hydrocodone	0.5 mg/kg	PO q3-4 hours
Tramadol	1-2 mg/kg	PO q4-6 hours

TABLE 34-3. Common Causes of Postoperative Nausea and Vomiting in Outpatients

Surgical Factors	Anesthetic Factors	Patient Factors
Adenotonsillectomy	Use of volatile agents	Prior history of PONV
Middle ear surgery	Use of nitrous oxide	History of motion sickness
Testicular surgery	Use of opioids	Age over 2 years
Laparoscopic surgery	Insufflation of the stomach (difficult mask ventilation)	Girls > boys
Insufflation of the bowel (endoscopy)	Reversal of neuromuscular blockade (cholinergics)	
	Unrelieved pain	

PONV, Postoperative nausea and vomiting.

variance is most likely because of study methodology and definitions. It is usually not an intractable problem, but it certainly is the cause of considerable distress, and if not well controlled may be a cause of unanticipated admission (Patel et al., 1997; Rose and Watcha, 1999). Numerous factors have been identified as increasing the risk of postoperative vomiting, some related to the surgical procedure, some to the anesthetic agents and some to the patient (Eberhart et al., 2004; Gan et al., 2007; Kranke et al., 2007). The most common of these are listed in Table 34-3. Eberhart et al. (2004) noted the following risk factors for pediatric PONV: surgery lasting longer than 30 minutes, age older than 3 years, family or patient history of PONV, and strabismus surgery. The incidence of postoperative vomiting was 9%, 10%, 30%, 55%, and 70% if zero, one, two, three, or four risk factors were present. Because discharge to home is so dependent on the child returning to a baseline condition that allows the intake of fluids and nutrients, it is essential that nausea and vomiting be kept to a minimum for outpatient surgeries.

Anesthetic technique has been correlated with the incidence of PONV, with propofol-based techniques having the lowest incidence (Sneyd et al., 1998; Barst et al., 1999; Gurkan et al., 1999). The use of volatile agents, opioids, nitrous oxide, and cholinergic drugs for the reversal of neuromuscular blockade all increase the risk, although one study found that desflurane had less PONV than reported with other volatile anesthetics (Mendel et al., 1995; Divatia et al., 1996; Kuhn et al., 1999). Remifentanil, in contrast with other opioids, does not appear to increase PONV (Pinsker and Carroll, 1999).

There have been studies of both treatment and prophylaxis of PONV in children undergoing outpatient surgery and anesthesia. One of the drugs commonly studied, droperidol, is no longer in common use because of a rare association with prolonged QT interval, so it will not be discussed here. The most commonly used drugs for treatment and prophylaxis are currently the HT_3-antagonists (ondansetron and granisetron), dexamethasone, and metaclopramide. All have been shown to be effective for both prophylaxis and treatment.

Dose-response studies of ondansetron suggest that for maximal efficacy, prophylactic doses of 0.1 to 0.15 mg/kg up to 4 mg should be administered (Rose et al., 1996; Patel et al., 1997; Sadhasivam et al., 2000). Lower doses were either not as effective, or were no more effective than placebo. Timing the dose before or after manipulation of the extraocular muscles in strabismus surgery (one of the most emetogenic operations) did not appear to make a difference, although the best effect has been reported when the drug is given at the end of the procedure (Madan et al., 2000). Another HT_3-antagonist, granisetron, was effective when 0.2 mg/kg was administered orally before induction of anesthesia (Munro et al., 1999). When a single dose was not adequate, controversy exists as to whether a second dose is efficacious (Rose and Martin, 1996; Kovac et al., 1999). Dexamethasone is effective at preventing PONV, and has the additional advantage of costing substantially less than the 5–HT_3-antagonists (Splinter and Roberts, 1996; Subramaniam et al., 2001). Dosing recommendations vary widely, but two-dose ranging studies found no additional benefits to using more than 0.25 mg/kg for decreasing postoperative nausea and vomiting; higher doses may be justified after tonsillectomy for the additional benefit of improving the ability to take oral fluids (Madan et al., 2005; Kim et al., 2007; Karaman et al., 2009). Despite a recent controversial study that found an increased incidence of bleeding after a single dose of dexamethasone, a Cochrane Database meta-analysis found benefit with no adverse effects of this therapy (Steward et al., 2003; Czarnetzki et al., 2008).

Metaclopramide is thought to act by increasing gastric emptying. Although it appears to be effective, several investigators have found it to be less so than ondansetron; in a recent meta-analysis, metaclopramide was found to be less effective than either the 5-HT blocking agents or dexamethasone (Broadman et al., 1990; Furst and Rodarte, 1994; Bolton et al., 2006). It has a higher incidence of side effects, primarily sleepiness and occasional extrapyramidal effects, than either of the other agents; therefore, it should be viewed as a second-line therapy. Cisapride, which also is a prokinetic agent, was found to be ineffective at treating PONV (Cook-Sather et al., 2002).

Several investigators recommend the use of multiple agents in combination for those at greatest risk of PONV. It appears that combining multiple drugs with different mechanisms of action yield the best results (Rose and Watcha, 1999; Gan et al., 2007). A factorial analysis comparing the use ondansetron, metaclopramide, and dexamethasone alone and in combination found that although each of the drugs decreased the odds of vomiting, and the addition of dexamethasone to ondansetron further decreased the odds of postoperative emesis, the combination of metaclopramide and ondansetron actually had a negative effect, and the authors therefore recommend against that particular combination (Gunter et al., 2006). Similarly, the use of a low-risk anesthetic, especially propofol, which appears to have antiemetic properties of its own, in combination with prophylaxis, may result in the lowest incidence of all (Barst et al., 1999). Low infusion rates of propofol as an anesthetic adjunct have been shown to have similar effects (Erdem et al., 2008).

An additional factor that has been found to promote PONV is the insistence on oral intake in the PACU before discharge. Although it appears sensible to want to demonstrate that a child is able to take and retain oral intake before discharge to home, investigators found that insistence on oral intake before discharge increased the incidence of PONV and lengthened hospital stay (Schreiner et al., 1992; Schreiner and Nicolson, 1995). This common practice probably deserves a critical reexamination.

Inadequate Analgesia

One of the most common reasons for unanticipated admission, acceptable levels of analgesia are a necessity before discharge. No child can leave the hospital unless one is sure that the caregivers at home will be able to manage postoperative pain. More potent oral analgesics are often adequate to enable discharge, but in the event that it is not the case, admission and parenteral agents may be necessary. When the level of pain seems out of proportion to either the procedure performed or the experience of the clinicians, causes other than the obvious ones should be sought, although it must also be remembered that pain is a subjective experience and pain thresholds can vary widely.

Excessive Somnolence

This is rarely a cause for admission, but may be a cause for a prolonged PACU stay. Common reasons include excessive narcosis, sedative, or opioid drug errors (unintentional or patient sensitivity), unusual sensitivity to inhaled anesthetics, and drug interactions.

COMPLICATIONS AND UNANTICIPATED ADMISSION

Even when all care issues have been optimized, there inevitably are patients who develop complications that prevent discharge to home and require hospitalization. Inadequate analgesia, inability to take adequate oral fluids, PONV, excessive somnolence, respiratory deterioration in children with URI or occult lower tract disease, or surgical complications all occur at some point. What is most important is that there is a system in place to streamline these admissions. In some institutions, this is overnight admission to a short-stay unit, which may be on the ward, in the PACU, or in the emergency room. In others, it means a bed on the regular ward. In all cases, it is essential that adequate follow-up care be maintained by both the surgical and anesthetic teams so that the issues that mandated admission are properly and adequately addressed.

FACILITY DESIGN AND PATIENT THROUGHPUT

Because such a large percentage of children undergoing surgery are cared for as outpatients, it is common that their surgery takes place not in a separate outpatient facility but in the main operating room. Even though these facilities are not usually designed with outpatients in mind, there are still numerous changes in organization and structure that can reap benefits both in parent and patient satisfaction and in efficiency and throughput.

Many hospitals care for a very large volume of outpatients in their main operating suites and have modified older designs or planned new facilities to enhance the simultaneous throughput of inpatients, same-day admissions, and outpatients. In addition to the obvious efficiencies this produces, it also permits surgeons to operate on a mix of patients without changing operating rooms. Inpatients, outpatients, and same-day admissions can share a common preoperative area with different "regions" where intake and preparation for surgery are done; all patients are then brought postoperatively to a common phase I PACU. Whereas inpatients and same-day admissions are discharged from phase I directly to the floor, outpatient-surgery patients are routed to a phase II recovery area immediately adjacent to the PACU, where they are able to complete their recovery in preparation for discharge to home. This enables "fast tracking" and more rapid discharge of these patients. The same concept is used for anesthesia in procedure and imaging centers, where ideally a satellite preoperative area and PACU should be established so that those patients may have their preoperative preparation done directly on site and tailored for their specific case flow and then may be discharged directly to home without having to relocate to the main PACU. Focusing on these system issues can enable more patients to be cared for in a smoother, more professional manner.

To complement the large volume of outpatients who are cared for in the main hospital, many large children's hospitals have opened satellite outpatient-surgery centers in suburban areas. These facilities are staffed by anesthesiologists and nurses who meet the same standards of care as the main facility. Although satellite outpatient-surgery centers offer advantages in efficiency and costs, transfer protocols and arrangements must be established to cover the rare emergency or complication that may develop. In addition, an anesthesiologist must remain in the outpatient center until the last child is discharged home from the PACU and leaves the facility.

SUMMARY

The number of children in the United States undergoing outpatient anesthesia has surpassed the number of inpatient cases. Many of the considerations for the care of these patients are identical to that of inpatients, but there are unique issues that must be addressed to enable children to go home on the day of surgery and anesthesia. Careful case selection, both on the basis of the child's underlying condition and for the planned surgical procedure, is critical in ensuring the success of an outpatient program. Whether these procedures are performed in the day surgery unit of a hospital or in a freestanding surgical center, the same level of same-day perioperative services for children should be available. One must have a well-designed systematic approach to organization, throughout, and clinical care to achieve both efficiency and safety.

REFERENCES

Complete references used in this text can be found online at www.expertconsult.com.

Anesthesia for Office-Based Pediatric Anesthesia

Richard Berkowitz and David Barinholtz

CHAPTER

35

CONTENTS

"A pediatrician's dream of the ideal world would be to have individuals knowledgeable about the special needs of infants and children assembled wherever children are to be treated" (Avery, 1975). Little did Dr. Avery know back in 1975, as she wrote these words in the journal *Anesthesiology* as a guest editor introducing a symposium on pediatric anesthesia, to what extent and in what places children were to be anesthetized and by whom. The prophetic nature of her question, "Where will pediatric surgery be done in the future?" and her statement, "Surely the anesthetist should contribute to the definition of what can be done in what setting," is astounding when considering how rapidly the surgical and anesthetic care of children has progressed from the hospital to the ambulatory surgery center to the office-based setting since Dr. Avery's remarks (1975).

The concept of office-based anesthesia and surgery is not a novel one, because dentists, oral surgeons, and plastic surgeons have been using office-based procedures for decades. In fact, dentists and oral surgeons have been at the forefront of office anesthesia and surgery dating back to one of the first office-based anesthetics, involving Colton and Wells in 1844, for an extraction of a wisdom tooth (Jacobsohn, 1995; Yagiela, 1999).

Surgical practice has now come full circle, because before the early 1900s many surgical procedures were performed in offices. Subsequently, because surgical procedures became more complex, the hospital became the major site for surgery (Yagiela, 1999). Despite this shift, the development of ambulatory anesthesia continued throughout the twentieth century with the development of the first free-standing surgical center in 1916, by Waters, and ultimately with the first ambulatory surgery center established by Reed and Ford in the late 1960s (White, 1997).

Over the past several years, the concept of office-based anesthesia and surgery has become well publicized. In addition to the increasing number of clinical reports, professional society publications, review articles and texts looking at the efficacy or regarding the subject of office-based anesthesia, there are unfortunately numerous reports of significant morbidity and mortality, as well as near misses both in the medical and dental literature and in the lay press (LaMendola, 1998; Laurito, 1998; Schulte and Bergal, 1998; de Jong, 1999; Neergaard, 1999; Rao et al., 1999; Tang et al., 1999; Arens, 2000; Morrell, 2000; Stoelting, 2000; Vogt, 2000; Hilton, 2001; Joshi, 2003; Gooden, 2006; Kaushal et al., 2006; Hussain, 2006; Hausman and Frost, 2007; Shapiro, 2007; ASA, 2008a, 2008b, 2008c; Coldiron et al., 2008; Heard et al., 2009; Sherry, 2009). The initial reports of mortality in the office-based setting have been highlighted by the unexpected death of the mother of music celebrity Kanye West and consequent legislation in California (Carter, 2007; McGreevy, 2009).

Resident training in office-based anesthesia has also recently been advocated by some within the field of anesthesia. This information, along with the fact that there is an ongoing closed-claim analysis of office-based anesthesia and surgery within the American Society of Anesthesiologists (ASA) (lending itself to the knowledge that this entity does exist and that improvements to existing procedures have been started), must be compelling evidence for the anesthesiologist to realize that office-based surgery and anesthesia are here to stay (Domino, 2001; Hausman et al., 2006; Hausman, 2008; Posner, personal communication, January 2009).

Interest in office-based anesthesia is also manifesting in the increasing number of societies—specifically, the Society for Ambulatory Anesthesia (SAMBA), and the Anesthesia Patient Safety Foundation (APSF)—that promulgate educational and

TABLE 35-1. Specialty-Specific Guidelines for Sedation and Analgesia and Office-Based Anesthesia and Surgery*

Organization	Document	Adopted	Revised
American Society of Anesthesiologists (ASA)	Guidelines for Ambulatory Anesthesia and Surgery	1973	2008
	Statement on Nonoperating Room Anesthetizing Locations	1994	2008
	Practice Guidelines for Sedation and Analgesia by Non-Anesthesiologists (DVD)	1995	2009
	Guidelines for Office-Based Anesthesia	1999	2009
	Continuum of Depth of Sedation	1999	2009
	Qualifications of Anesthesia Providers in an Office-Based Setting	1999	2009
American College of Surgeons (ACS)	Guidelines for Optimal Ambulatory Surgical Care and Office-Based Surgery[†]	1994	2005
American Academy of Pediatrics (AAP)	Guidelines for Monitoring and Management of Pediatric Patients During and After Sedation for Diagnostic and Therapeutic Procedures[‡]	1985	2006
	Guidelines for the Pediatric Perioperative Environment	1999	NA
American Academy of Pediatric Dentistry (AAPD)	Guideline on the Use of Anesthesia-Trained Personnel in the Provision of Gen Anesthesia/Deep Sedation to the Peds Dental Patient	2001	2009
American Dental Association (ADA)	ADA Policy Statement: The Use of Sedation and General Anesthesia by Dentists	2007	NA
	Guidelines for the Use of Sedation and General Anesthesia by Dentists	2007	NA
American Society of Dentist Anesthesiologists (ASDA)	Ascribe to ADA guidelines	2007	
American Society of Plastic Surgery (ASPS)	Patient Safety in Office-Based Surgery Facilities. I. Procedures in the Office-Based Setting	2001	NA
	Patient Safety in Office-Based Surgery Facilities. II. Patient Selection[§] Practice Advisory on Liposuction[¶]	2003	NA
American Association of Nurse Anesthetists (AANA)	Standards for Office-Based Anesthesia Practice	1987	2009

From American College of Surgeons: Guidelines for optimal ambulatory surgical care and office-based surgery, ed 3, Chicago, 2005, American College of Surgeons; American Dental Association: ADA policy statement: the use of sedation and general anesthesia by dentists, 2007. Available at http://www.ada.org/prof/resources/positions/statements/statements_anesthesia.pdf; accessed October 26, 2009; American Dental Association: Guidelines for the use of sedation and general anesthesia by dentists, 2007. Available at http://www.ada.org/prof/resources/positions/statements/anesthesia_guidelines.pdf; accessed October 26, 2009; American Society of Anesthesiologists: Practice guidelines for sedation and analgesia by nonanesthesiologists, 2009. Available at http://www.asahq.org/publicationsAndServices/sedation1017.pdf; American Society of Anesthesiologists Office of Governmental and Legal Affairs: Office-based surgery and anesthesia, statutes, regulations, and guidelines, rev. ed., Washington, D.C., 2009, American Society of Anesthesiologists; American Society of Plastic Surgery (ASPS) Committee on Patient Safety: Practice advisory on liposuction: executive summary, Arlington Heights, Ill, 2003, ASPS; American Association of Nurse Anesthetists : Standards for office-based anesthesia practice, 2009. Available at http://www.aana.com/WorkArea/showcontent.aspx?id=23028; accessed October 26, 2009.

*Not a complete list, as other professional societies may also have related guidelines.
[†]These guidelines specify surgery by facility class (A, B, C) depending on the invasiveness of the surgery and type of anesthesia used.
[‡]Joint statement with the American Academy of Pediatric Dentistry.
[§]Practice advisory only.
[¶]In this practice advisory, the ASPS recommends that in the event that sedation or analgesia is used, the surgeon follow the ASA Guidelines for Sedation and Analgesia by Non-Anesthesiologists.

safety-related literature in this relatively new arena for anesthesiologists. Also, the ASA, as well as other groups including, but not limited to, The American College of Surgeons and various surgical subspecialty societies, the American Dental Association, the American Academy of Pediatric Dentistry, and the American Association of Nurse Anesthetists, have published guidelines specifically addressing office-based anesthesia or surgery or both (Table 35-1). Furthermore, the ASA Committee on Ambulatory Surgical Care and SAMBA have published a "how-to" manual for setting up a safe office environment (ASA, 2008d).

In an effort to establish consistency in the safe administration of sedation and anesthesia to children, some societies have established joint guidelines or updated guidelines outlining the use of anesthesia personnel to its membership (American Academy of Pediatrics, 2006; American Academy of Pediatric Dentistry, 2009). All of these societies have developed their guidelines or policies in response to the overwhelming interest

and growing participation by their memberships in this area, as well as an overall common concern for patient safety.

Also significant, and perhaps legitimizing the presence of office-based anesthesia and surgery in present-day medicine, is the ever-increasing number of states developing legislation that specifically address this area. Consequent to this dynamic period of law making and law revision is that the ASA Office of Legal Affairs continues to compile information pertinent to the states that have developed and those that are developing legislation regulating office-based anesthesia and surgery.

Simply stated, office-based anesthesia is the practice of anesthesia in the free-standing physician's office and is defined as the provision of anesthesia service in an operating area or a procedure room that is not licensed as an ambulatory surgery center. The most important distinctions are that it occurs within the four walls of a physician's office where surgery is offered as a secondary service, and only physicians who are members of the practice perform procedures in this space. It is the most "liberated" form of anesthesia practice and is at the most extreme end of the spectrum of "out-of-the-operating-room" or "off-site" anesthesia. In a sense, it is anesthesia for the most remote location (except, perhaps, for those individuals delivering anesthesia care in isolated areas of Third World countries).

Traditionally, office-based anesthesia has been the realm of various specialists, including but not limited to dentists, oral surgeons, plastic surgeons, podiatrists, certified registered nurse anesthetists (CRNAs), and in some instances, gastroenterologists. Until recently, few anesthesiologists dared to venture out of their conventional roles as hospital-based or ambulatory surgery–based physicians.

To what extent is the office-based surgical volume increasing that it requires or necessitates the continued evolution of this new "subspecialty" of ambulatory anesthesia?

Estimates of the actual number of surgical cases completed, pediatric or otherwise, in an office setting, are difficult to ascertain. It is estimated that there were 10 million office-based surgical procedures performed in 2005, consistent with one marketing study from several years ago, that estimated that by 2006 the total number of outpatient procedures performed would be approximately 40 million, with 11 million of these being office-based procedures (Fig. 35-1) (SMG Marketing-Verispan, L.L.C., 2002; Twersky, 2008). In 2009, these numbers are holding steady; however, the dynamic nature of the reimbursement environment and the development of minimally invasive surgical technologies may make the number of office-based procedures skyrocket over the next several years.

According to a 2009 report from the National Center for Health Statistics, in 2006 there were approximately 35 million ambulatory surgery visits in the United States, with most of these being in hospital-based facilities vs. free-standing facilities (Cullen et al., 2009). Just over 7% of these reported ambulatory surgery visits were by children younger than 15 years of age. Although the total number of ambulatory surgery visits for this age group went up in 2006, the percentage decreased from the 8.5% reported for 1996 (Hall and Lawrence, 1998). As is suggested, without mandatory reporting of all ambulatory surgery procedures requiring anesthesia to a central agency, office-based anesthesia data will remain obscure (Perrott, 2008).

Although many different types of surgical procedures, including otolaryngologic, urologic, cosmetic, ophthalmologic, and radiologic (including single-photon emission computed tomography [SPECT]) scanning are performed on children in the office-based setting, the majority of procedures requiring anesthesia or sedation in the office setting for children are dental procedures (Cartwright et al., 1996; Goldblum et al., 1996; Grevelink et al., 1997; Yagiela, 1999; Siegel et al., 2000; Smith and Smith, 2000; Garin et al., 2001; Friedman et al., 2002; Ross and Eck, 2002; Barinholtz, 2009; Gravningsbraten et al., 2009).

The most common reason for children to require dental procedures is related to early childhood caries (ECC), with an incidence in primary teeth of 41% in children between ages 2 and 11 years (Beltrán-Aguilar et al., 2005). Furthermore, a majority of ECC in the United States occurs in children from low-income households. (Vargas et al., 1998; Nunn et al., 2009). Yagiela (1999) reports that a survey by the American Academy of Pediatric Dentistry estimated in 1995 that the number of children who received anesthesia for dental procedures was close to 200,000. Presently, the actual number of dental procedures performed with patients under general anesthesia is

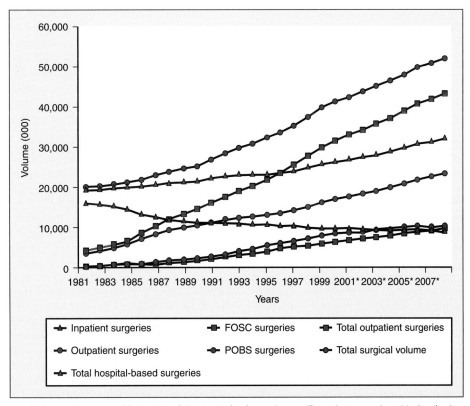

■ **FIGURE 35-1.** This graph represents past and future trends in surgical volumes in specific patient-care sites. Notice the increasing surgical volumes in the free-standing outpatient surgery center (FOSC) and physician office-based surgery (POBS) center. *(Courtesy SMG Marketing-Verispan, LLC., 2002, Chicago, Ill.)*

difficult to determine because of underreporting, and because estimates are generated from Medicaid-provided information of hospital-based care (Casamassimo et al., 2009). The actual number of children requiring anesthesia for these procedures may be significantly greater than this, with the discrepancy being because of a paucity of access to the appropriate care secondary to a lack of primary-care access and as important, a lack of insurance coverage. Significantly, this access to care can be positively impacted by state legislation. White and others (2008) report that non–Medicaid and Medicaid dental visits increased by approximately 60% and 30% (p < .05), respectively after the State of North Carolina introduced general-anesthesia legislation for preschool-aged children.

In a 2006 survey of Illinois dentists licensed to give some form of sedation or anesthesia, close to 116,000 cases were performed with some form of sedation and general anesthesia (Flick et al., 2007). Most of these sedation and anesthesia cases (90%) were performed by oral and maxillofacial surgeons (63% of survey respondents); however, general dentist and pediatric dentist respondents (29%) accounted for most of the remaining sedation and anesthesia. The number of pediatric patients cared for, however, was not specified.

WHY OFFICE-BASED SURGERY AND ANESTHESIA?

As one can see from the information presented in Figure 35-1, there is a compelling need to be able to provide quality surgical and anesthesia services in the office-based setting. The actual reasons as to why this boom has occurred and continues to evolve and why anesthesiologists are more aggressively entering this arena are severalfold.

Ostensibly, the most persuasive argument for a paradigm shift to the office-based setting is financial. Potential and realized limitations and reductions in reimbursement because of health care reform and economic constraints are causing physicians to become more creative in facilitating cost-effective approaches to surgery. Costs can be reduced by reducing or eliminating facility fees that ordinarily accompany the cost-sharing charges at hospital-based and ambulatory surgery-based centers. Much of office-based surgery, especially cosmetic surgery, is performed on a cash-payment, fee-for-service basis, and therefore cost containment by limiting facility-fee overhead becomes crucial to patient affordability. This affordability is critical in the case of pediatric dental procedures, where in many instances, neither dental nor medical insurance covers out-of-office dental procedures and anesthesia costs (Ross and Eck, 2002).

Although the lack of a facility fee is ideal and helps provide the surgeon with a cheaper alternative for the patient, the reality of the situation is that surgeons often include a facility fee in their global fee to the patient to offset the overhead required to run an office-based practice (e.g., personnel and supplies). In some instances, insurance companies may reimburse physicians a facility fee, but the cost to the third-party payers may still be less than if the procedure is performed in a hospital- or surgery center-based setting. Consequently, the procedure becomes financially advantageous for the surgeon, the anesthesiologist, the insurance company, and the patient.

One surgical study from the United States as early as 1994 compares the cost of performing an inguinal herniorrhaphy in the hospital with that of the cost in an office setting. This study finds the latter a more cost-effective alternative with a reduction

in cost of a laparoscopic approach or an open approach of approximately 70% and 60%, respectively when compared with the hospital outpatient setting (Schultz, 1994). In one pediatric study, Lalwani and others (2007) show a per-patient savings of close to $5000 when patients with special health care needs who require anesthesia or sedation undergo dental rehabilitation procedures in an office-based setting when compared with those receiving care in a hospital operating room.

Operating in the office affords the surgeon not only financial but also logistic advantages. Office-based surgical practice virtually eliminates the lost time caused by turnover delays, bumping cases secondary to emergencies, overscheduled cases, and travel times between facilities. In the office-based setting, whatever turnover delays do occur can be quickly remedied by the surgeon, because he or she has total control over the personnel and the facility.

The ability of the surgeon to schedule on-site clinic visits between surgical cases allows for the efficient use of time. This eliminates the usual routine of having to rush back to the office between procedures or having office hours at the conclusion of a long and busy day at the hospital or surgery center.

Another advantage of office-based procedures is the more private, less stressful, and more familiar environment. For the anesthesiologist, office-based anesthesia may allow for an enhanced income, a better work environment (working with a limited number of surgeons or, in some instances, the same surgeon), and in most practices, the lack of a nighttime call schedule. Furthermore, this type of practice provides the anesthesiologist with the opportunity to have complete control over all aspects of practice for which he or she is ultimately responsible. Whether these potential advantages of establishing or taking part in an office-based practice prevail over the relative disadvantages of working in an extremely remote environment, routinely providing anesthesia care for cases of decreased complexity (compared with those cases in a hospital setting, but this may be changing), providing anesthesia services under itinerant conditions, and perpetually competing with other anesthesiologists and anesthesia providers for business, become individual decisions.

SAFETY AND OUTCOME

With the government, medical community, third-party payers, and the consumers (patients) pushing for more expeditious and cost-effective (and hence potentially more profitable) ways in which to provide surgical and anesthesia services, the anesthesia services provided are moving further away from the hospital safety net. Dr. Ervin Moss (1998), the impetus behind tighter regulation of office-based anesthesia and surgery in the state of New Jersey and perhaps beyond, stated, "Some say the major difference between the office-based and hospital-based anesthesiologist is that the former must be more courageous or foolhardy."

Whether or not Dr. Moss's characterization of the office-based anesthesiologist holds true, the fact remains that anesthesia care must be provided safely, if not more vigilantly, than hospital-based or surgery center-based anesthesia. Although some have questioned whether the convenience of office-based surgery and anesthesia is worth the risk, consensus opinion, as this specialty area continues to develop, is that it must be done correctly and consistently (Arens, 2000; Bridenbaugh, 2005).

Although anesthesia-related mortality risk continues to be difficult to assess, perhaps because of methodologic issues, it has nevertheless decreased over the past several decades (Lagasse,

2009). Anesthesia-related mortality risk in the United States has recently been quoted to range from 0.1: 10,000 to approximately 0.8:10,000 procedures performed (Biboulet et al., 2001; Lagasse, 2002, 2009; Newland et al., 2002; Li et al., 2009). These numbers appear slightly lower than the rate published outside the United States, at 1.12:10,000 cases (Braz et al., 2006).

In children, the incidence of cardiac arrest from anesthesia is reported to range from 1.4:10,000 to 4.6:10,000 with the incidence of anesthesia-related mortality being reported by some as between 1.2:10,000 and 7.7:10,000 cases in ASA Physical Status (PS) I-II and ASA PS III-IV, respectively (Morray et al., 2000). This disparity seen between patients of lower and higher ASA PS is consistent with morbidity statistics presented by Murat and others (2004) in a report of over 24,000 anesthesia cases over 2½ years and by Kakavouli and others (2009) in a study comparing adverse events for patients receiving anesthesia in the operating room (2.5%) with those outside the operating room (3.5%). Respiratory events were the leading cause in both studies, 1.7% and 1.9%, respectively (Zuercher and Ummenhofer, 2008; Bharti et al., 2009).

Interestingly, the number of pediatric arrests related to medications decreased almost 20% from 1994 to 1997 (37%) and from 1998 to 2004 (18%) as reported in an update on the pediatric perioperative cardiac arrest (POCA) registry (Bhananker et al., 2007). The authors suggest that this may be because of the decreased use of halothane in pediatric anesthesia. This is important in that the relatively newer, faster onset and offset (desirable characteristics in the office-based setting) volatile agents, sevoflurane and to a lesser extent desflurane, may confer a larger therapeutic index in the office-based setting. Furthermore, these authors report that airway causes for pediatric arrest still occur with a high incidence (27%), reemphasizing the importance of having superior airway management skills in pediatric anesthesia regardless of location.

Despite this information, an accurate assessment of the safety profile of office-based anesthesia and surgery relative to the pediatric population is difficult secondary to the paucity of site-specific information. Until across-the-board mandatory reporting for morbidity and mortality related to office procedures exists, in order to make an assessment of the relative safety of office-based anesthesia and surgery, it is imperative to continue to analyze data reviewing the safety of pediatric ambulatory and in-patient surgery, pediatric dental office surgery, and pediatric sedation and analgesia, as well as the adult literature that reviews this topic.

Many of the cases brought to the attention of the medical, dental, and lay community involve children undergoing dental procedures (Morell, 2000; Hussain, 2006; Sherry, 2009). This information is not only tied intimately to the present topic but also is the point of origin for much of the controversy over the safety and efficacy of office-based anesthesia for children.

In two reports from the United States, Coté and others (2000a, 2000b) retrospectively analyzed information obtained from the Food and Drug Administration, the United States Pharmacopoeia, and a survey of pediatric specialists to report on contributing factors to critical incidents and medications used in sedation as they relate to adverse sedation events in children undergoing diagnostic and therapeutic procedures.

In the first report, Coté and others (2000a) reported on 95 incidents. Over half of these incidents resulted in death (n = 51) or permanent neurologic injury (n = 9). The remaining patients either had prolonged hospitalization without injury (n = 21) or sustained no harm as a result of the adverse event (n = 14). Of note

was that those children who were cared for in non–hospital-based facilities (older and healthier) had a much higher rate of death and permanent neurologic injury (93%) than did those cared for in hospital-based facilities (37%). The authors also reported that inadequate resuscitation was a major factor in the non–hospital-based facilities (57%) compared with the hospital-based setting (2.5%) and that patients cared for in the nonhospital setting were more likely to sustain a cardiac arrest as the second or third event compared with those in the hospital setting (p < .001).

In the second report, Coté and others (2000b) used the same 95 incidents to determine whether there was a relationship between medications and adverse events. Although the authors noted no relationship between the class of drug used, the route of administration, and the incidence of death and permanent neurologic injury, they did note that adverse outcomes were associated with the administration of drug overdoses and administration of three or more sedating medications. Furthermore, 11 of 12 patients (all younger than 6 years of age) sustained adverse outcomes either at home or in a car. Two of the 12 patients, who had received sedative medication at home before their procedure, sustained an adverse event at home before the scheduled procedure.

Of note was that over one third of the reported events occurred during sedation for dental procedures (n = 32). Twenty-nine of these resulted in death or permanent neurologic injury. Most of the involved practitioners were either oral surgeons or dentists, three were pedodontists, and one was a nurse anesthetist under the supervision of a dentist. None of the practitioners was an anesthesiologist (Coté et al., 2000b).

The dental practices were the only sites in these reports to have used nitrous oxide. In addition to the greater tendency toward the use of nitrous oxide, there was a greater tendency for these practitioners to use multiple drugs (more than three) compared with other practitioners: 39% and 13%, respectively. The authors conclude that many of these adverse events may have been prevented by consistency between monitoring guidelines (as now exists with sedation guidelines promulgated by the American Academy of Pediatrics and the American Academy of Pediatric Dentistry) and by practice and training requirements among health care professionals of differing specialties who administer sedation and anesthesia.

Although these conclusions may seem intuitive to those who regularly care for children, they are reinforced by recent reports suggesting that severe adverse outcomes in pediatric sedation or analgesia outside the operating room may be improved by consistency in guidelines, training, and adverse-event reporting across institutions and specialties that are implemented through well-designed sedation services (Cravero et al., 2006, 2009; Bhatt et al., 2009). In the latter study, Cravero and others (2009) show that whereas the incidence of pulmonary events (e.g., stridor, laryngospasm, excessive secretions, and central and obstructive sleep apnea) is high, they report a low incidence for cardiopulmonary resuscitation (0.4:10,000) and no mortalities in approximately 50,000 sedation procedures performed by various nonanesthesiologist pediatric specialists. Lightdale and others (2006) advocate the use of microstream capnography to enhance the safety of pediatric patients undergoing procedures under sedation or analgesia via early detection of hypoxemia caused by alveolar hypoventilation.

Although there are anecdotal reports and studies of adverse outcomes, complications, and side effects related to sedation and anesthesia in the dental literature, others have reported on a safety record that is as good as, if not better than, that of the anesthesia community (Denman et al., 1968; Yee et al., 1985; Blayney et al., 1999; Girdler and Smith, 1999; Laskin, 1999; Saxen et al., 1999; Whitmire, 1999; Johnson et al., 2001; Manoharan et al., 2001; Yagiela, 2001; Perrott et al., 2003). The incidence of mortality rates in dental anesthesia is reported to be anywhere from 1:250,000 in the United Kingdom to 1:300,000 to less than 1:1 million in the United States (Cartwright, 1999; Brandom and Herlich, 1999; D'Eramo, 1999; Laskin, 1999).

As if there is not enough controversy within the anesthesia community, within the dental community there is also debate over who can best serve the patient requiring anesthesia for a dental procedure. Yagiela (2001) points out that members of the American Society of Dental Anesthesiologists, those who provide "approximately 25,000 pediatric general anesthetics per year," subscribe closely to the American Academy of Pediatrics and American Society of Anesthesiologists guidelines for sedation and anesthesia. He also states that "since the organization's inception 2 decades ago, there have been no known incidents of mortality or significant morbidity in children managed in the dental office by a dentist anesthesiologist" and intimates that safety may be improved in dental offices with a greater adherence to these guidelines by the dental community as a whole (Yagiela, 2001).

In contrast to the paucity of information about the safety and outcomes related to office-based anesthesia, the efficacy of anesthesia in pediatric ambulatory surgery in general is well known. As reported by Willetts and others (1997), outpatient surgery may date back to James H. Nicoll, a Glasgow surgeon who in the early 1900s successfully performed several thousand ambulatory procedures on young children at the West Graham Street Dispensary for Children. Contemporary literature continues to confirm over the past 50 years that for a growing variety of surgical procedures, the ambulatory setting for surgery and anesthesia is safe, cost effective, and therefore preferable to inpatient surgery (Postuma et al., 1987; Patel and Hannallah, 1988; Hannallah, 1991; Ghosh and Sallam, 1994; Blacoe et al., 2008; Shah et al., 2008; Mattila et al., 2009).

In one prospective study examining the efficacy of pediatric day surgery at the Children's Hospital of Eastern Ontario, the overall complication rate was very low. The investigators, over 5 years, prospectively studied children undergoing various outpatient procedures, including myringotomy, tonsillectomy and adenoidectomy, dental procedures, and inguinal hernia repairs. Most of the children were between 2 and 7 years old, and the total number of cases approached 25,000. The reported complication rate was 1.6% per year. The most common complication was postoperative bleeding, primarily secondary to tonsillectomy and adenoidectomy. None of the complications resulted in permanent disability (Letts et al., 2001). In a retrospective study from Children's National Medical Center focusing on pediatric otolaryngology procedures, Shah and others (2008) report that in close to 5000 cases (55% of total surgical cases) over 7 years, the rate of unanticipated outcomes was 0.2%. Similar to the previous study, the majority of adverse outcomes were related to posttonsillectomy and adenoidectomy bleeding.

Most of the information relative to the outcomes for office-based anesthesia and surgery is related to adult patients. In a retrospective report specifically looking at outcomes for plastic surgical procedures, Hoefflin and others (2001) reported no significant morbidity and no mortality over 18 years in more than 23,000 procedures in which general anesthesia was used. The anesthesia was provided by a board-certified anesthesi-

ologist, and the single facility was accredited by the American Association for Accreditation of Ambulatory Surgical Facilities (AAAASF) (Hoefflin et al., 2001). In this report, most of the patients underwent cosmetic surgery, with some patients having multiple procedures. The only incidents reported as significant by the authors were the rare occurrence of electrocardiograph and oxygen-monitor failure. None of these events resulted in any patient complications, although three patients were hospitalized for custodial care. Minor anesthetic complications included nausea and vomiting (fewer than 5%), postextubation sore throat (fewer than 5%), shivering, one case of dental damage, one case of delayed (10 days) deep vein thrombosis, and one case of carpal tunnel syndrome after intravenous catheter infiltration.

In a retrospective study comparing outcomes in physician offices and ambulatory surgery centers in Florida, Vila and others (2003) found that despite new regulations imposed by the Florida Board of Medicine in the year 2000, between 2000 and 2002 there was a significantly increased risk of adverse incidents and deaths in offices (65.8:100,000 and 5.3:100,000, respectively) compared with ambulatory surgery centers (9.2:100,000 and 0.8:100,000, respectively). Furthermore, the authors estimated that a significant number of injuries and at least six deaths per year could have been prevented had all surgical cases been performed in an ambulatory surgery center.

In another report and as a follow-up study to previous reports, Coldiron and others (2008) reviewed critical surgical incidents that occurred in physicians' offices in the state of Florida from 2000 to 2007 subsequent to mandatory reporting that began in February 2000 (Coldiron 2001, 2002). This mandatory reporting initially resulted from several newspaper accounts of poor patient outcomes and questions of whether office anesthesia and surgery were safe. Those incidents requiring reporting are listed in Box 35-1.

In the data obtained from Florida's Agency for Health Care Administration, there were 31 deaths and 143 procedure-related complications and hospital transfers. Most of the bad outcomes occurred during "nonmedically-indicated" cosmetic surgery such as liposuction or liposuction with abdominoplasty. Plastic surgeons were responsible for 48% of all deaths and 52% of hospital transfers. Interestingly, most of the deaths (78%) occurred in ASA PS I patients. These authors note that the reported deaths and complications were unrelated to whether the physician was board certified or whether the physician had similar surgical

---

Box 35-1 Incidents in Surgical Offices Requiring Reporting by the State of Florida

- Death
- Brain damage
- Wrong patient surgery
- Wrong site surgery
- Wrong procedure
- Surgery to remove an unplanned foreign object from a surgical procedure
- Transfer of a patient to a hospital
- Spinal damage
- Surgical repair of injuries or damage resulting from a planned surgical procedure

From Coldiron B: Office surgical incidents: 19 months of Florida data, *Dermatol Surg* 28:710, 2002.

privileges in a hospital (the latter being a mandatory requirement in some states). However, only 40% of facilities reporting adverse events were accredited by an independent agency. Despite the latter data, there are those who suggest that rigid state regulations and licensing laws along with accreditation of office-based surgical and anesthesia practices will help ensure patient safety (Kaushal et al., 2006).

Bitar and others (2003) retrospectively reviewed close to 5000 office-based plastic surgery procedures that were performed under monitored anesthesia care with sedation. The procedures in this study were performed by board-certified plastic surgeons, and anesthesia was provided by a CRNA. Nearly all patients were reported to be ASA PS I or II (99.9%), and the majority of patients were adult females (92%). The most common complications reported in this study were dyspnea (0.05%, n = 2), protracted nausea and vomiting (0.2%, n = 6), and unplanned hospital admission (0.05%, n = 2). One patient required intubation without prolonged sequelae. The author reported no cardiac arrests, deaths, or any incidence of deep vein thrombosis or pulmonary embolus. The author concluded that office anesthesia and surgery were safe when using appropriate protocols and patient selection.

One Pittsburgh-based office dental anesthesiologist practice, delivering approximately 30,000 anesthetics from between 2004 and 2009, reports no mortality or major morbidity, including central nervous system injury. Furthermore, this practice reports no instances of aspiration, pulmonary embolism, local anesthetic toxicity, or malignant hyperthermia. There was one unplanned hospital admission, not related to anesthesia, involving massive bleeding from a mandibular arteriovenous malformation from which the patient made a full recovery after transfer to an acute care hospital (Finder, personal communication, January 2010).

In another office-based dental anesthesia practice in Seattle, 4321 pediatric (younger than 12 years old) dental procedures have been completed since the year 2000 (Isackson, personal communication, 2010). Dr. Isackson reports no serious adverse events. There were no unplanned hospital admissions, although one patient was referred to a primary care physician for cardiac evaluation. Minor respiratory events and immediate and delayed postoperative nausea and vomiting (PONV) each occurred in 0.07% of cases, with one patient in the group who experienced nausea and vomiting requiring office assessment by a primary care physician.

Koch and others (2003) reported on several office-based anesthesia practices from various regions of the United States that were performed between 1981 and 2002. In this report, the authors noted no intraoperative deaths in over 64,000 anesthesia cases. Furthermore, in a subset of pediatric patients that comprised this report, one Chicago-based office anesthesia practice reported no intraoperative deaths, significant perioperative morbidity, or emergent hospital transfers in over 600 pediatric anesthesia cases. This number is now approximately 1200 cases and includes only one pediatric emergent hospital transfer (a possible malignant hyperthermia case). All complications continue to be minor, with a reported incidence of immediate and delayed PONV of less than 0.07% and 1%, respectively. Children in this subset ranged in age from 18 months to 17 years. Most of the children were younger than 6 years old and were classified as ASA PS I or II patients (Barinholtz, personal communication, 2009). These safety results are consistent with those reported by others caring for special-needs dental patients in the office-based setting (Caputo, 2009).

TABLE 35-2. Patient Characteristics in Analysis of Claims Made in Office-Based Anesthesia Incidents

	Ambulatory (n = 753)	Office Based (n = 14)
Age (mean yr)	41	45
Female (%)	58	64
ASA PS class I/II (%)	82	89
Elective surgery (%)	97	100
Anesthesia type		
General (%)	66	71
MAC (%)	10	14
Surgical procedure		
Dental (%)	3	21
Plastic surgery (%)	32*	64*
Other (%)	64[†]	14[†]

From Domino KB: Office-based anesthesia: lessons learned from the Closed Claims Project, *ASA Newsletter,* 2001, American Society of Anesthesiologists.
*p < 0.05, Ambulatory vs. office based.
[†]p < 0.01, Ambulatory vs. office based.
MAC, Monitored anesthesia care.

In a review of the ASA's Closed Claims Project database, Domino (2001) compared claims (all age populations) made against anesthesiologists in the office setting (n = 14) with those made in other ambulatory surgery settings (n = 753). Claims for dental damage and for nonoperative pain management were excluded from this analysis. Although patient demographics were similar in both groups (Table 35-2), most of the claims in the office-based setting were related to plastic surgery or dental procedures, whereas in the ambulatory setting, most claims were related to procedures other than plastic or dental. The severity of injury appeared greater in the office-based setting compared with other ambulatory sites. In this initial report, most of the claims made in other ambulatory sites (62%) were for "temporary or nondisabling injury," whereas most of the claims from the office-based setting were for death (64%). The author pointed out, however, that without a denominator, a true risk assessment for each site cannot be ascertained. Subsequent data from the ASA Closed Claims Analysis, with more claims in both the ambulatory (total, n = 877) and office-based settings (total, n = 29), continue to show a preponderance of death and brain damage in the office-based setting, although at a reduced (40%) incidence (Posner, personal communication, 2009). Likewise, Jimenez and others (2007), in a closed claims analysis of 532 pediatric cases from 1973 to 2000 (not exclusively ambulatory or office-based, but from 1990 to 2000 the highest percentage of the claims involved dental, otolaryngologic, and maxillofacial surgeries), found that death and brain damage were also the dominant injuries in malpractice claims, although the proportion of these claims decreased in the 10 years before 2001.

In both office-based settings and ambulatory settings, Domino (2001) noted that respiratory events were most common. A summary of airway-related complications and drug-related complications in office-based claims is shown in Table 35-3. Although the timing for injury was similar for both

TABLE 35-3. Damaging Events in Office-Based Anesthesia Claims

Type of Event	Ambulatory Anesthesia (n = 666)		Office Based (n = 12)	
	Number	%	Number	%
Respiratory	150	22	6	50
Cardiovascular	67	10	1	8
Equipment	74	11	1	8
Drug related	58	9	3	25
Block-needle trauma	41	6	1	8

From Domino KB: Office-based anesthesia: lessons learned from the Closed Claims Project, *ASA Newsletter,* 2001, American Society of Anesthesiologists.

sites, there tended to be fewer claims for events occurring after discharge in the other ambulatory claims (7%) than for the office-based claims (21%).

The Closed Claims Project analysis also discloses that a greater number of office-based claims continue to be potentially preventable with better monitoring (Posner, personal communication, 2009). In the earlier report, a greater percentage of office-based claims involved substandard care compared with other ambulatory settings (not statistically significant), and payment was made in a higher percentage of claims (92% vs. 59%) and for a higher median payment ($200,000 vs. $85,000) for office-based claims than for other ambulatory settings (Domino, 2001).

LEGISLATION AND REGULATIONS

There are many entities presently imparting their influences on the practice of office-based anesthesia and surgery. These include, but are not limited to, state regulatory bodies; federal regulatory agencies such as the Centers for Medicare and Medicaid Services (CMS) and the Office of the Inspector General (OIG); national medical professional societies; national medical and safety organizations such as the Federation of State Medical Boards (FSMB, 2002), the National Committee for Quality Assurance (NCQA), and the National Patient Safety Foundation (NPSF); accrediting organizations such as the American Association for Accreditation of Ambulatory Surgery Facilities (AAAASF), the Accreditation Association for Ambulatory Health Care (AAAHC), and The Joint Commission; and the insurance industry. Also, in 2003, the AMA published the *Core Principles for Office-Based Surgery* that are currently endorsed by government agencies, the accrediting bodies, and specialty societies.

The main problem with regulation and legislation concerning office-based surgery and anesthesia is the wide regulatory variability that exists among states. Some states are highly regulated, whereas other states have no regulations (Fig. 35-2). In the states that do have regulations, these regulations are often ambiguous. State regulations regarding facility structure, personnel, equipment, and credentialing of individual practitioners differ widely. A more complete compendium of state regulations is available through the ASA Office of Governmental and Legal Affairs (ASA, 2009). In addition to state agencies and legislation,

professional societies can regulate practice by establishing practice guidelines, practice standards, and advisories. The disadvantage of professional societies is that they run the risk of being self-interest groups. Consistent regulatory control could also be achieved by recognizing established accrediting bodies as oversight organizations. The organizations most commonly involved in the accreditation of ambulatory surgery centers are AAAASF, AAAHC, and The Joint Commission.

Historically, AAAASF, known until the early 1990s as the American Association for Accreditation of Ambulatory Plastic Surgery Facilities (AAAAPSF), was created to accredit only outpatient plastic surgery facilities. However, as other medical specialties moved procedures to free-standing outpatient settings, this organization became active in accrediting these facilities as well (AAAASF, 2003).

In contrast to AAAHC and The Joint Commission, AAAASF accredits facilities over a much narrower spectrum of medical specialties. The surgical specialties include colon and rectal surgery, obstetrics and gynecology, ophthalmology, orthopedic surgery, otolaryngology, plastic surgery, general surgery, and urology. AAAASF is particularly restrictive in its practitioner credentialing. This organization requires all surgeons to be certified by the American Board of Medical Specialties (ABMS) and requires all of its surgeons practicing at an ambulatory or office-based facility to have hospital privileges for the same procedures being performed in the office facility (AAAASF, 2003). AAAASF will only accredit a practice where the surgeons practice in their area of board certification. Furthermore, the AAAASF will not accredit an organization if propofol is not administered by an anesthesiologist or a properly supervised CRNA or anesthesia assistant.

The Joint Commission and AAAHC, in addition to the facilities mentioned for AAAASF, approve facilities where oral and maxillofacial, dental, dermatologic, podiatric, cosmetic, vascular, and pain procedures are performed. Although these two organizations are not as restrictive on the practitioner-privilege issue as the AAAASF, their credentialing policies are complete.

In addition to defining requirements for surgical personnel, all three organizations offer accreditation processes that outline expectations for the facilities as they relate to meeting standards for the facility physical plant (e.g., by ensuring that state, local, Occupational Safety and Health Administration [OSHA], and National Fire Protection Association regulations are followed), anesthesia administration, monitoring, equipment and personnel, ancillary staff, patient transfer policies, patient safety and emergency resuscitation issues, quality improvement, and patient satisfaction issues. A summary of some of the similarities and differences between the three most visible accrediting organizations is given in Table 35-4.

Whether accreditation affects outcomes in office-based surgery and anesthesia is uncertain. In a survey study, the AAAASF sent a questionnaire to its accredited facilities that addressed patient safety in plastic surgery office facilities. Two hundred forty-one of 418 facilities responded to the questionnaire. Over 5 years 400,000 surgical procedures were studied, and the authors reported the risk of significant complications to be 1:213 and the risk of death to be 1:57,000 cases. They concluded that overall risk in an accredited office is comparable with that of other ambulatory surgery sites (free-standing or hospital based) (Morello et al., 1997). In a retrospective review of an accredited office-based plastic surgery facility, Byrd and others

2009 OFFICE–BASED SURGERY AND ANESTHESIA REQUIREMENTS

This table was current as of the time of the publication, however state health statutes, regulations, health department, and medical licensure regulations are different for each state and should be reviewed and updated accordingly. A summary of state regulations is provided by the ASA Washington Office that can be found at www.asahq.org/Washington/rulesregs.htm. This site is maintained by the ASA and contains a state by state summary of Office-Based Anesthesia legislative activity.

	AL	AZ[4]	CA	CO	CT	FL	IL	IN	KS	LA	MA	MS	NJ	NC	NY	OK	OH	OR	PA	RI	SC	TN	TX[47]	VA
Accreditation of Facility	X[1]		X		X	X		X[11]		X[15]	X[18]			X[27]	X[30]		X[32]	X[35]	X	X[36]	X[39]	X[43]	*[48]	
Physician Supervision of CRNAs	X[2]	X*	X*	X		X	X	X[12]		X	X		X	X	X*	X	X		X	X	X	X	X	X*
CME for Surgeons Supervising CRNAs						X[7]	X[10]					X[21]	X[24]				X[33]				X[40]			
Hospital Privileges to Perform Procedures				X[6]		X[8]	X	X[13]		X[16]	X[19]		X[25]	X[28]			X[34]			X[37]	X[41]	X[44]		
Reporting Requirements	X[3]		X[5]			X[9]			X[14]	X[17]	X[20]	X[22]	X[26]	X[29]	X[31]					X[38]	X[42]	X[45]	X[49]	X[51]
Transfer Agreement	X	X	X	X	X			X	X	X	X	X[23]	X	X		X		X	X		X	X[46]	X[50]	X

*Physician supervision or direction requirements derived from other sources of state law, not from OBA requirements.

[1]AL: Encouraged for Levels 4 (deep sedation) and 5 (general).

[2]AL: Direction of the general and regional anesthesia should be provided by a physician who is immediately and physically present.

[3]AL: Report within 3 business days surgical related deaths and events resulting in emergency transfer to hospital, anesthetic surgical events requiring CPR, unscheduled hospitalization related to surgery, and surgical site deep wound infection.

[4]AZ: A physician who uses general anesthesia when performing office-based surgery using sedation must obtain a health care institution license as required by the Department of Health Services.

[5]CA: Report within 15 days after occurrence death or transfer to hospital for period exceeding 24 hours.

[6]CO: Surgeon should have staff privileges or document satisfactory completion of training such as Board certification or certify comparable background, training and experience.

[7]FL: Level I: Surgeon's CME should include proper dosages; management of toxicity or hypersensitivity to regional anesthetic drugs.

[8]FL: Level II, IIA: Surgeon must have staff privileges or be able to document satisfactory completion of training such as Board certification or comparable background, training and experience. Level III: Physician must have staff privileges.

[9]FL: Send incident report by certified mail within 15 calendar days after occurrence of the adverse incident.

[10]IL: An operating physician must either maintain clinical privileges to administer anesthesia in a hospital or ASC or have CMEs in anesthesia to administer anesthesia or enter into a practice agreement with a CRNA to provide anesthesia. Training and experience may be met by completing CME hours: 8 hours for conscious sedation, 34 hours for deep sedation, regional anesthesia and/or general anesthesia. No training and experience requirements when an anesthesiologist administers or supervises the administration of anesthesia. (upheld by Illinois Appellate Court)

[11]IN: Effective January 1, 2010

[12]IN: CRNAs must administer anesthesia under the direction of and in the immediate presence of a physician.

[13]IN: Privileges at either an accredited hospital or ASC. Alternatively, the governing body of the office is responsible for a peer review process for privileging practitioners based on nationally recognized credentialing standards.

[14]KS: Report withing 15 calendar days of discovery of event: transfer to ER; unscheduled hospital admission withing 72 hours of discharge: death within 72 hours of surgery; unplanned extension of surgery (more than 4 hours); foreign object remaining in patient; wrong surgical procedure, site, or patient.

[15]LA: Accreditation not required, but offices accredited by JCAHO, AAAASF, or AAAHC and those that are part of but physically separated from a licensed hospital are exempt from the regulations.

[16]LA: Physician performing surgery must have current staff privileges or board certification in specialty encompassing office procedure and possess current hospital admitting privileges.

[17]LA: Report within 15 days after occurrence resulting in transfer to ER, office readmission with 72 hours of discharge, unscheduled hospital admission within 72 hours of discharge, death within 30 days of surgery.

[18]MA: Level II, III: Pre-accrediting suvey prior to surgical procedures; definitive accreditation survey 6 months after procedures begin.

[19]MA: Level II, III: Surgeon must have staff privileges at hospital or accredited outpatient facility or document satisfactory completion of training such as Board certification/Board eligibility or comparable background, formal training, or experience as determined by MA BRM.

[20]MA: Reporting requirements are not specific; guidelines recommend following all BRM adverse incident rules.

[21]MS: Level I: Surgeon's CME should include proper dosages and management of toxicity or hypersensitivity to regional anesthetic drugs.

[22]MS: Report within 15 days after occurrence any surgical event in the immediate peri-operative period that is life-threatening, or requires special treatment or hospitalization that is related to anesthesia or surgery.

[23]MS: Level II, III: required of surgeon who does not have privileges at hospital within reasonable proximity.

[24]NJ: A physician who administers or supervises the administration of general anesthesia must complete at least 60 Category I hours of CME in anesthesia; regional and conscious sedation-8 hours. (upheld by NJ Supreme Court)

[25]NJ: Physician who performs surgery should have hospital privileges or seek Board-approved privileges.

[26]NJ: Report within 7 days death, transfer to hospital exceeding 24 hours., untoward event occurring within 48 hrs. of surgery.

[27]NC: Level II or III should show substantial compliance with guidelines or obtain accreditation.

[28]NC: MD should be credentialed by hospital, ASC or comply with Board criteria to perform surgical or special procedures that require administration of anesthesia.

[29]NC: Should report complications.

[30]NY: Effective July 14, 2009.

[31]NY: Effective January 14, 2008, licensees (physicians, physician assistants, and special assistants) must report adverse events to the Department of Health's Patient Safetley Center within one business day of the occurrence.

[32]OH: Required if using moderate sedation/analgesia or anesthesia services (deep sedation/analgesia, regional or general anesthesia)

[33]OH: Moderate sedation/analgesia: Hold privileges to provide moderate sedation/analgesia from hospital or ASF or complete at least 5 hours of Category I CME; Deep sedation/analgesia, regional or general anesthesia; Hold privileges to provide anesthesia services from hospital or ASF; Completed a residency training program in anesthesia; or complted at least 20 hours of category I CME. Qualifications apply whether a CRNA or anesthesiologist administers anesthesia.

[34]OH: Holding current privileges at hospital or ASF, among other qulifications, demonstrages sufficient certification, training, experience.

[35]OR: Accreditation by a Board-recognized national or state orgainization. Facilities where office surgeries are already being performed, accreditation by August 1, 2009; new offices must be accredited within 1 year of the start date of the procedures being performed.

[36]RI: Office shall apply within 9 months of initial licensure; attain within 24 months.

[37]RI: Surgical procedures shall only be performed by physicians or podiatrists who have current surgical privileges for the same or similar class of procedures at a nearby hospital.

[38]RI: Within 72 hrs. of receipt of information, notify of death within 30 days, transfer to ER, hospital admission within 72 hrs. of discharge, extension of surgical procedure beyond 4 hrs., unplanned readmission to office operatory within 72 hrs., subjecting patient to procedure not offered or intended by pysician, incidents reported to malpractice insurer.

[39]SC: Level II, III

[40]SC: Level I: Surgeon is encouraged to pursue CME in proper dosages, management of toxicity or hypersensitivity to local anestthetic and other drugs.

[41]SC: Surgeon must have staff privileges or document satisfactory completion of training such as Board certified or Board eligibilty, or comparable background, formal training, experience.

[42]SC: Report within 3 business days anesthetic or surgical mishaps requiring resuscitation, emergency transfer, or death.

[43]TN: Level III by AAAHS, AAAASF, or JCAHO.

[44]TN: Level III; Physician performing office procedure must have staff privileges to perform same procedure at hospital within reasonable proximity.

[45]TN: Applies to Level II surgeries; report within 15 calendar days following physician's discovery of event.

[46]TN: Level II: required if physician performing procedure does not have staff privileges at hospital withing reasonable proximity.

[47]TX: Physicians shall follow ASA standards and guidelines.

[48]TX Offices accredited by AAAHC, JCAHO, and AAAASF and those that are part of a licensed hospital or ASC are exempt from the guidelines.

[49]TX: Notify BME within 15 days if procedure resulted in unanticipated and unplanned transport to hospital for period exceeding 24 hrs., death intraoperatively or within 72 hrs. of procedure.

[50]TX: If physician does not have hospital privileges must have written transfer agreement.

[51]VA: Report within 30 days incidents resulting in death within 72 hr. post-operative period or transport to hospital exceeding 24 hrs.

■ **FIGURE 35-2.** 2009 Office-based surgery and anesthesia requirements. *(From ASA Office-based anesthesia: considerations for anesthesiologists in setting up and maintaining a safe office anesthesia environment. American Society of Anesthesiologists, 2008d.)*

TABLE 35-4. Similarities and Differences Between Various Accreditation Organizations

Accreditation Body	AAAASF	AAAHC	TJC
Medicare deemed status	Yes	Yes	Yes
Requires board certification of surgeon	Yes	No	No
Requires physician supervision of anesthesia*	Yes	Yes	Yes
Additional educational requirements for nonanesthesiologists supervising	Yes	No	No
Accreditation cycle	3 Years	6 Months, 1 year, or 3 years	3 Years
Approximate base cost†	$4265	$3000-$5000	$6950
Corporate website	www.aaaasf.org/	www.aaahc.org/	www.jointcommission.org

From Accreditation Association for Ambulatory Health Care (AAAHC): *Summary of state activities on office-based surgery, August 2003 update,* accessed, September 29, 2003.

*This requirement may not apply in the event a state's governor has opted out of the physician supervision of nonanesthesiologist anesthesia providers requirement.
†Cost for an accreditation survey may be influenced by the number of offices to be accredited, the number of surgeons and surgical specialties, and whether a facility is asking for Medicare "deemed" status.
AAAASF, American Association for Accreditation of Ambulatory Surgical Facilities; *AAAHC,* American Association for Ambulatory Health Care; *TJC,* The Joint Commission.

(2003) reported no deaths in over 5000 cases. However, these authors noted that several patients required hospital admission for various medical problems.

Another dynamic that is and will continue to influence the push toward accreditation is the recognition by payers of the significant cost savings that can be realized in the office-based setting. Although the payers want to leverage these savings, they have to be reassured and be able to reassure their subscribers that they will only sanction care in a safe environment. Because the industry standards have been established by the accrediting bodies, it wouldn't be surprising if this fueled the push toward uniform requirement for accreditation more quickly than the state legislatures or the federal government.

CLINICAL ASPECTS

Particular attention must be paid to patient and case selection, preoperative preparation, special problems related to anesthetic administration, and postoperative care. Absence of a plan specifically related to these issues by the anesthesiologist caring for a child in the office can lead to a practice that is fraught with safety dilemmas and logistic and scheduling problems that negatively impact the success of an office-based anesthesia practice. Time constraints are the rule rather than the exception in office-based practice.

Patient and Procedure Selection

The decision process that occurs when determining which patients are appropriate to care for in the office-based setting does not differ greatly from that of caring for patients in the "free-standing" ambulatory surgery center. The factors that most commonly determine whether a child is an appropriate candidate for office-based anesthesia and surgery are patient age, associated medical illnesses and ASA physical status, type of surgery, potential for blood loss, potential for significant postoperative complications, and duration of surgery.

Because most office-based procedures for pediatric patients involve dental procedures, a majority of the children undergoing these procedures are older than 1 year of age. However, as the realm of office surgery for children expands (including tonsillectomies), and because there are no prospective studies as yet in the office-based anesthesia literature looking at outcomes and patient age for children undergoing office-based surgery, it seems that the present guidelines for other ambulatory surgery venues should be used (Gravningsbraten et al., 2009). When taking this latter point into consideration, the minimum age requirement (other parameters such as type of procedure not withstanding) for children undergoing office-based procedures can be determined by whether a child requires prolonged postoperative monitoring based on postconceptual age or the administration of opiate analgesics and other respiratory depressant agents (Welborn and Greenspun, 1994; Galinkin and Kurth, 1998). Although postanesthesia care unit (PACU) complications resulting from respiratory complications may be more common in neonates and infants, any other minimum age requirements are often arbitrary and may reflect the comfort level of the surgeon, office staff, and anesthesia personnel caring for the child (Westman, 1999; Ross and Eck, 2002; Murat et al., 2004). Adherence to policies and guidelines set forth for minimum age requirements for outpatient anesthesia in ambulatory surgery centers and hospital-based ambulatory surgery departments is critical.

Most children cared for in the office-based setting are ASA PS I and II patients. In some situations, it may be acceptable to provide anesthesia care for those children with stable comorbidities who are ASA PS III patients despite the fact that these patients in general may be more susceptible to adverse outcomes from anesthesia (Morray, 2002; Murat et al., 2004; Jimenez et al., 2007). Not surprisingly, getting consensus from pediatric anesthesiologists as to which comorbidities are appropriate for hospital-based or free-standing ambulatory surgery is difficult, but some of the pediatric comorbidities considered high risk for the office-based surgical suite are listed in Box 35-2 (Abu-Shahwan, 2007).

In an early prospective study looking at prolonged recovery stay and unplanned hospital admission after ambulatory surgery in pediatric patients, the authors reported annual rates of approximately 4% and 2%, respectively. PONV and respiratory complications were the most common factors leading to prolonged recovery stay, whereas respiratory complications (32%) and surgical reasons (30%) were the factors most commonly responsible for unplanned hospital admission. These authors also found that higher ASA physical status had a direct relationship to unplanned hospital admission and adverse respiratory events (D'Errico et al., 1998).

Subsequently, Dornhoffer and Manning (2000), in a retrospective chart review, evaluated unplanned hospital admission

---

> ### Box 35-2 Pediatric Comorbidities Considered High Risk for the Office-Based Surgical Suite
>
> - Obstructive sleep apnea
> - Labile asthma and other significant pulmonary disease
> - Complex congenital heart disease
> - Labile diabetes mellitus
> - Significant neurologic and neuromuscular disorders
> - Sickle cell disease
> - Upper respiratory tract infection
> - Increased body mass index

---

after four types of otologic procedures (not including myringotomy tube placement) in adult and pediatric outpatients. The unplanned hospital admission rates for children and adults were 5.7% and 2.3%, respectively. The most common reason for unplanned hospital admission was PONV. These findings are relatively consistent over time, and in a more recent study, Blacoe and others (2008) in Scotland found an overall unplanned admission rate of 1.8% in over 13,000 day-surgery cases. The combined percentage of admissions for two surgical complications (postoperative bleeding, 13.9%, and more extensive surgery than planned, 11.8%) exceeded that for the most common anesthesia-related cause for admission, PONV (23.5%).

Dornhoffer and Manning (2000) also noted that tympanomastoidectomy with ossicular reconstruction, procedures lasting longer than 2 hours, and asthma were risk factors predicting the need for postoperative admission. In contrast to this study, Mingus and others (1997) reported that surgical cases lasting as little as 1 hour may be associated with a higher rate of unplanned hospital admission.

In a study by Fortier and others (1998) involving over 15,000 patients, unplanned hospital admission after ambulatory surgery was related to longer duration of anesthesia and surgery, higher ASA PS (classes II and III), postoperative bleeding, excessive pain, and nausea and vomiting. Of note, and similar to the more recent study of Blacoe and others (2008), is that surgical reasons are identified to be more commonly responsible for hospital admission than are anesthesia-related issues (38% and 25%, respectively). The fact that the office-based setting is best suited for those children who are healthy without significant comorbidity and are undergoing minimally invasive procedures may inherently result in few postoperative complications.

Preoperative Preparation

Preanesthetic Interview

As is the case with ambulatory surgery in general, rarely is the preanesthetic interview for office-based surgery for pediatric patients conducted in person. For the anesthesiologist who works in a limited number of offices, preanesthetic interviews may be possible during the patient's presurgical office visit if the anesthesiologist should be attending that particular office on the same day. This is the exception rather than the rule when anesthesiologists provide itinerant care for a multitude of offices. Although some authors have advocated presurgical

evaluation in certain instances on the same day of surgery (Overdyk et al., 1999; Mangia et al., 2009), citing economic and logistic advantages for practitioners and patients, most preanesthetic interviews will be initiated by telephone before the day of surgery.

The preanesthetic interview for office-based procedures does not differ much from that described for other ambulatory settings (Ferrari, 2004; Polaner, 2006). However, there are caveats relative to the preanesthetic interview for an office-based procedure.

First, the anesthesiologist should make some initial contact with a child's parents or guardian before the day of surgery. Unlike the ambulatory surgery center or hospital-based ambulatory surgery department, the parents often cannot associate their child's scheduled procedure with the community-acquired reputation of a particular private or academic institution. An anesthesiologist's reputation in the office-based environment is based on the advocacy of the child's private physician, surgeon, or dentist and unfortunately is only as good as the anesthesiologist's last case (or self-advocacy literature). The initial telephone interview must be used as a way to instill confidence in his or her abilities and to alleviate parental anxiety by relating one's level of experience or training background or by discussing a cogent and acceptable anesthetic plan. These few "public relations" minutes are invaluable.

Second, the interview process must elicit enough of a history to determine whether a child is a candidate for the scheduled office-based procedure or whether the procedure needs to be delayed. The dreaded same-day cancellation leaves an undesirable block of open time for the anesthesiologist and the surgeon. Finally, in many instances, the preanesthetic telephone interview is used not only as the mechanism by which parents receive final preoperative instructions (e.g., NPO guidelines, medication instructions) but also to make final financial arrangements.

Preoperative Laboratory Testing

Because most children receiving office-based anesthesia services are healthy and are undergoing minimally invasive procedures, the necessity for preoperative laboratory testing is rare. As is advocated by other authors, any laboratory testing should be determined on an individual patient basis by clinical need after the preanesthetic interview (Meneghini et al., 1998; Friedberg, 2003; Maxwell, 2004; Polaner, 2006). Despite agreement on the lack of clinical utility and increased cost of routine preoperative laboratory screening among anesthesia professionals, an anesthesiologist providing office-based anesthesia services must be aware of any state and local government mandates for such testing. Additionally, each practitioner must establish a policy for determining the cost-to-benefit yield (especially in the office setting where cost savings are a key advantage) on more controversial laboratory testing such as pregnancy testing, especially in adolescents and teenagers (Wheeler and Coté, 1999; Hennrikus et al., 2001; Kahn et al., 2008; Bodin et al., 2010).

Preoperative Sedation

Despite the ostensibly less intimidating environment of the office, the anxiety that pediatric patients (and their parents) undergoing office-based procedures experience is probably no less than that in other surgical environments. The need for preoperative sedation or some other useful mechanism by which the anesthesiologist can reduce preoperative anxiety is critical for a couple of reasons. First, parents are becoming more educated about the perioperative process via the Internet and the lay press, and second, the space-limited environment of many office practices and the close proximity to office waiting rooms and other patients may make preoperative sedation of children most at risk for preoperative anxiety even more important (Baldauf, 2009).

The group of children most likely to undergo a mask induction of anesthesia is also the age group of children most likely to experience preoperative anxiety (Kain et al., 1996, 2002; McCann et al., 2001; Watson and Visram, 2003). Most children receiving preoperative sedation receive midazolam (McCann et al., 2001; Rosenbaum et al., 2009). Although various routes of administration are advocated, including intranasal and rectal, oral administration of midazolam is the most common (Levine et al., 1993; Davis et al., 1995; Griffith et al., 1998; McGraw and Kendrick, 1998; Marhofer et al., 1999). Ease of administration as determined by acceptance by the child, in most instances, dictates the route of administration. Most often in practice, a dose of 0.5 to 1 mg/kg (maximum dose, 20 mg) orally is effective.

Although some have found that certain routes of administration of midazolam have no impact on discharge times (Davis et al., 1995; Kain et al., 2000), others find that there are significant delays in recovery or discharge times with the use of orally administered midazolam in combination with various anesthetic techniques (Viitanen et al., 1999).

Despite a report on the decreased efficacy in the levels of preoperative sedation using oral melatonin compared with oral midazolam, Kain and others (2009) did show a significant (p < 0.05) dose-related lower incidence of emergence agitation (another office undesirable) in those patients receiving melatonin. Furthermore, the use of combination preoperative sedation, such as intramuscular ketamine and midazolam, in uncooperative children may be inappropriate for the office-based setting because of prolonged discharge times (Verghese et al., 2003).

For children tolerating preoperative intravenous catheter placement (with or without application of local anesthetic cream), the use of midazolam may not be necessary. Small repeated doses (0.25 to 0.5 mg/kg) of intravenous propofol under constant monitoring provide excellent preoperative anxiolysis without respiratory depression and in most instances will provide excellent amnesia to the immediate preoperative period. This technique is especially advantageous in short surgical procedures. However, propofol is associated with pain on injection, and lidocaine may have to be added to the bolus syringe or infusion.

The benefit of parental presence in reducing preoperative anxiety remains questionable (to the child and parent), especially compared with other nonpharmacologic and pharmacologic approaches to preoperative anxiety reduction (McCann et al., 2001; Kain et al., 2003; Chundamala et al., 2009; Yip et al. 2009). Whatever a practitioner's personal preference, the office-based environment may provide an excellent opportunity for parental presence during induction of anesthesia, especially in cases where sterility concerns are minimal, such as for dental restoration or radiologic procedures.

When choosing parental presence as the sole method of anxiety reduction, it is important to consider the information available that may enhance the success of this approach. Some authors report that specific patient behavior profiles, specific parent-child anxiety level combinations (e.g., calm parent and anxious child), and the presence of a child's mother as opposed to the father may have the most impact on reducing the anxiety level of the child (Messeri et al., 2004; Kain et al., 2006a; Chorney and Kain, 2009).

If the administration of a preoperative sedative is indicated, the anesthesiologist must take into consideration whether the benefit of sedation (to the patient, parents, waiting patients, and office staff) outweighs the chance that the sedative will delay discharge after anesthesia. This is particularly true in instances where a physician must be present until the patient is discharged to home.

Intraoperative Care

The intraoperative care of the pediatric patient in the office-based setting relative to induction and maintenance of anesthesia does not differ much from that in other ambulatory settings. Despite the minimal standards set forth by most states relative to office-based anesthesia, from the anesthesiologist's perspective, monitoring and equipment standards and guidelines must not be different for the office than for other surgical and anesthesia sites. The anesthesiologist should adhere to the *Standards for Basic Anesthetic Monitoring* and *Guidelines for Office-Based Anesthesia* (ASA, 2005, 2009b) (see Chapters 10 and 11, Equipment and Monitoring). With this in mind, anesthetic technique is limited only by the equipment, supplies, and resources of the physical plant that are available.

Most office-based surgical procedures using anesthesia require intravenous access and hydration. The child's fluid deficit is based on the fasting period and is replaced with lactated Ringer's solution.

Despite liberalizing the fasting period (clear liquids 2 to 3 hours before anesthesia), administration of intravenous fluids both during and after the surgical procedure is important. There is evidence in both adult and pediatric populations that aggressive intraoperative fluid management may in fact decrease the incidence of PONV (Holte et al., 2007; Goodarzi et al., 2009).

Anesthetic Technique

The concepts of "rapid onset, rapid recovery, and minimal side effects," used often to describe the important characteristics of an appropriate anesthetic technique in an ambulatory setting, is equally important for the office setting. Although all types of anesthesia, including regional anesthesia, can be used in the office setting, general anesthesia and varying levels of sedation are most often used in children (Hausman, 2008).

Even though anesthesiologists debate the clinical (safety and outcome) and cost efficacy of relatively newer anesthetic agents (e.g., sevoflurane, desflurane, remifentanil, and propofol) compared with some of the older agents (e.g., halothane and isoflurane), these newer agents offer a distinct advantage as it relates to their predictability and perhaps their safety (Tang et al., 1999; Moore et al., 2002; Fishkin and Litman, 2003; Bhananker et al., 2007). All levels of the continuum of anesthesia (minimal sedation to general anesthesia) are used in the office setting. The type of anesthesia is determined by the age and cooperation level of the child, the type of procedure, the ease with which local anesthetic can be administered, its efficacy in a particular surgical procedure, the specific routine of the anesthesiologist, and as stated previously, the available equipment.

General anesthesia can be accomplished by using a pure volatile technique, a total intravenous technique, or a combination of the two (volatile induction with intravenous maintenance) techniques. The first and latter obviously depend on the availability of an anesthesia machine and on whether a specific office can comply with OSHA requirements relative to appropriate gas scavenging. Some surgical offices, depending on surgical volume and cost efficacy, may provide the anesthesiologist with a standard anesthesia machine; in other instances, the anesthesiologist may transport a single-vaporizer-equipped portable anesthesia machine to each office (Barinholtz, personal communication, 2009).

All of the newer volatile agents are efficacious in pediatric ambulatory surgery (Moore et al., 2002; Polaner 2006). However, if the anesthesiologist is transporting a machine with single-vaporizer capability, then sevoflurane may be the agent of choice because of its efficacy in both induction and maintenance of anesthesia, as well as its rapid onset and offset characteristics. Although some advocate the use of desflurane for maintenance of anesthesia for ambulatory surgery because of its predictability relative to emergence, it is impractical as a complete office-based anesthetic agent in children because of its lack of efficacy for inhalation induction (Zwass et al., 1992; Olssen, 1995; Smiley, 1996; Fishkin and Litman, 2003). Similarly, the intravenous agents propofol and remifentanil have been shown to be useful in the ambulatory setting (Hannallah et al., 1994; Davis et al., 1997, 2000; Pinsker and Caroll, 1999; Cohen et al., 2001).

Although remifentanil can be used successfully in an ambulatory setting when the airway is secured with an endotracheal tube, evidence suggests this narcotic should be used cautiously when the airway is not secured. Litman (1999) evaluated the use of remifentanil for moderate sedation in 17 patients (20 procedures) aged 2 to 12 years who were undergoing short, painful procedures. All patients received intravenous midazolam, 50 mcg/kg, in combination with remifentanil 1 mcg/kg followed by an initial infusion of remifentanil of 0.1 mcg/kg per minute. The remifentanil infusion was then titrated every 5 minutes to provide adequate sedation and analgesia. The average appropriate dose of remifentanil used was 0.4 mcg/kg per minute. Although the author reported successful use of this technique in 17 of 20 procedures, 1 child became unresponsive and required assisted ventilation, and hypoxemia was avoided in 10 of 13 children by continuous stimulation during the procedure.

In adults, the combination of a propofol infusion, titrated to bispectral analysis (BIS) number, and intermittent ketamine boluses has been reported (Friedberg and Sigl, 2000; Friedberg, 2003). In children undergoing dental restoration procedures, Barinholtz (2009) noted that combining propofol (100 to 200 mcg/kg per minute, titrated by BIS) with ketamine (0.5- to 1.0-mg/kg boluses) completely avoided the need for opiate analgesics. In contrast to these latter two reports, successful implementation of sevoflurane for maintenance of anesthesia for dental restorations has been reported by multiple authors (Abu-Shahwan and Chowdary, 2007; König et al., 2009).

Although it appears that any agent can be safely implemented in the office-based setting, it is imperative that the office-based anesthesiologist develop an anesthetic routine that allows for an expeditious induction with appropriate maintenance levels of anesthesia while at the same time affording a rapid emergence. It is also essential that this anesthetic routine minimize the incidence of postoperative side effects such as nausea and vomiting.

Another critical aspect of intraoperative anesthesia care in the office-based setting is airway management. Although multiple factors determine the type of airway, any type of airway from a mask to laryngeal mask airway to an endotracheal tube may be appropriate. For some procedures, especially when using only sedation, airway intervention is usually minimal; on the other hand, deciding on the appropriate airway intervention may be difficult in other cases. This is particularly true when providing anesthesia for dental or other intraoral procedures.

Many dental cases are performed with oral sedation and nitrous oxide; however, longer dental restoration procedures may necessitate the use of an endotracheal tube (Saxen et al., 1999; Ross and Eck, 2002; Barinholtz, personal communication, October 2009). This is most prevalent in offices where the anesthesiologist may have limited access to the patient's airway because of positioning or cramped quarters. Subsequently, ventilation is controlled by hand or mechanical means or the patient is allowed to breathe spontaneously. The anesthesiologist must be judicious in the use of muscle relaxants to facilitate intubation. Prolonged effects of these agents may lead to delayed emergence and consequently delayed discharge and turnover for subsequent cases.

Another concern for the anesthesiologist practicing in an office-based setting is emergence agitation. The incidence of emergence agitation is reported to be approximately 12% to 18%, but Faulk and others (2010) report an incidence of approximately 30% in 400 patients undergoing dental procedures under general anesthesia with sevoflurane. The etiology of emergence agitation appears to be multifactorial and is associated with inadequate postoperative analgesia, high preoperative anxiety levels, rapid emergence, and the newer volatile agents, and it is reported to occur with both intravenous and volatile anesthetic techniques (Kain et al., 2006b; Vlajkovic and Sindjelic, 2007; Kuratani and Oi, 2008; König et al., 2009).

There may be some benefits, although inconsistent, to preoperative sedation with various agents such as midazolam, clonidine, and melatonin in reducing the incidence of emergence agitation (Cox et al., 2006; Almenrader et al., 2007; Kain et al., 2009). The incidence of emergence agitation is also shown to be reduced by the intraoperative use of regional anesthesia, opiates, 5-HT$_3$ receptor antagonists and dexmedetomidine, as well as the administration of ketamine or propofol at emergence from sevoflurane anesthesia (Cohen et al., 2002; Ibacache et al., 2004; Weldon et al., 2004; Lankinen et al., 2006; Abu-Shahwan and Chowdary, 2007; Abu-Shahwan, 2008; Kim et al., 2009).

Depth of Anesthesia Monitoring

The central theme of office-based anesthesia is to accomplish excellent, safe, time-efficient, and cost-effective anesthesia. Hence, the anesthesiologist can look favorably on any technology that can possibly aid in achieving these goals simultaneously.

The BIS monitor (Aspect Medical; Newton, Massachusetts) was originally described as able to determine the level of sedation, predict the loss of consciousness, and thereby diminish intraoperative awareness when used with various anesthetic agents (Glass et al., 1997). Although in some early reports BIS was shown to minimize awareness, decrease anesthetic use, or hasten recovery in adult patients, a more recent report of a prospective study of 2000 adult patients by Avidan and others (2008) describes no advantage to using accepted target values for BIS (40 to 60) over target values of end-tidal anesthetic concentrations in preventing anesthesia awareness or in reducing the administration of volatile agent (Glass et al., 1997; Song et al., 1997). Consequently, these authors did not recommend routine use of BIS monitoring during anesthesia.

The use of the BIS monitor is also controversial in pediatric anesthesia. A standard BIS number or range of numbers that precludes anesthesia awareness and simultaneously minimizes the amount of anesthesia delivered is difficult to establish, because subgroups of pediatric patients may have different baseline BIS numbers as is reported by Valkenburg and others (2009). In this report, intellectually challenged patients are found to have significantly lower BIS numbers while awake and while under anesthesia compared with patients in a controls group. This inconsistency is relevant, because care for intellectually challenged and special-needs children is commonplace in one of the higher volume areas using pediatric office-based anesthesia, the dental office. (Lalwani et al., 2007).

In a report on an electronic mail survey of members of the British and French pediatric anesthesia societies, over 60% of respondents feel that intraoperative awareness is an important issue in pediatric patients, whereas 10% of respondents report using BIS routinely (Engelhardt et al., 2007). Thus, the vast majority of respondents still continue to use clinical monitoring and end-tidal agent concentrations to assess depth of anesthesia.

There are also pediatric-anesthesia studies reporting advantages to BIS monitoring in patients receiving various types of anesthesia for a range of diagnostic and surgical procedures (Denman et al., 2000; Bannister et al., 2001; McCann et al., 2002; Religa et al., 2002; Messieha et al., 2005; Powers et al., 2005).

Denman and others (2000) found that in children ages 0 to 12 years who were anesthetized with sevoflurane, the BIS value correlated to the depth of anesthesia. Furthermore, this study also found that for a particular level of anesthesia (BIS = 50), children younger than 2 years had a significantly higher end-tidal concentration of sevoflurane than did children ages 2 to 12 years (1.55% vs. 1.25%, respectively). Bannister and others (2001) studied the effect of BIS on anesthetic use and recovery in 240 children. They noted that in patients aged 0 to 6 months the BIS had no effect on anesthetic emergence. However, in older children, BIS was associated with less anesthetic administration and an earlier emergence time.

Religa and others (2002) evaluated the association between BIS and level of consciousness in pediatric patients (aged to 6 years) undergoing dental procedures using a sedation protocol. These authors find that there is a significant association between behavioral responses and levels of sedation. However, the authors note that BIS offered no advantage over routine clinical monitoring and behavioral assessment in this setting.

Messieha and others (2005) report earlier times to extubation (5 ± 2 minutes sooner, p = .04) and PACU discharge (47 ± 17 vs. 63 ± 17 minutes, p = .02) in BIS-monitored patients receiving standardized doses of preoperative sedation with oral midazolam and sevoflurane for induction, with maintenance of anesthesia for dental procedures. Whereas these few "saved" minutes may seem germane to the office-based setting, the cost effectiveness and clinical utility of level-of-consciousness monitoring across pediatric subpopulations still need to be elucidated.

Postanesthesia Care

As in any ambulatory setting, the patient undergoing office-based surgery must meet established criteria before discharge to home, with the goal being to discharge the patient as quickly and as safely as possible (Patel et al., 2001). Actual discharge criteria include an adequate level of consciousness, good pain control, good hydration, minimal to no nausea, and a defined period of time since the last emesis (Ross and Eck, 2002; Fishkin and Litman, 2003). Furthermore, the appropriate personnel (at the minimum that which is outlined by the *ASA Guidelines for Office-Based Anesthesia*, 2009b) must remain with the child until discharge-ready status is reached.

The causes for delayed discharge can be related to either anesthesia or surgery, but in the ambulatory setting two of the most common non–life-threatening causes are inadequate pain control and PONV. Unlike the typical ambulatory setting, where there exists the capability to care for patients with a prolonged recovery period, the office-based setting has little margin for error relative to these two problems.

Postoperative Pain Control

The undertreatment of pain in pediatric patients in traditional surgical and hospital settings continues to be an issue (Stamer et al., 2005; Segerdahl et al., 2008; Fortier et al., 2009). In fact, one study that compared oral ibuprofen (10 mg/kg) with oral acetaminophen with codeine (1 mg/kg per dose of the codeine component) for the emergency room treatment of acute arm fractures found that ibuprofen was more preferable to (because of its side-effect profile) and at least as effective (analgesia) as acetaminophen with codeine; however, the high incidence of treatment failure in both groups, 20.3% and 31.0%, respectively, although not statistically significant between the groups, is clinically relevant to the previous point of potential undertreatment of pain in pediatric patients (Drendal et al., 2009).

With this latter point in mind, the goals for postoperative pain control in the office setting are not dissimilar from the overall goals for office-based anesthesia and surgery. In situations where the use of local anesthesia is not possible or feasible, the anesthesiologist must attempt to use analgesic agents that are efficacious, have minimal side effects, and do not delay patient discharge.

Although various opiate analgesics are routinely used in pediatrics and can be administered via conventional (e.g., intravenously, intramuscularly while asleep, or orally) and less conventional (e.g., intranasally) routes in traditional ambulatory surgery settings, their use in the office setting is often minimized or eliminated to help avoid postoperative sedation and PONV that are specific to drugs, dose, and perhaps patients (Weinstein et al., 1994; Anderson et al., 2000; Galinkin et al., 2000; Finkel et al., 2001; Duedahl et al., 2007; Howard et al., 2008a, 2008b; Voronov et al., 2008). Furthermore, because a preponderance of complications leading to unplanned hospital admission after ambulatory surgery in infants is related to the respiratory system, opiate use, which can cause respiratory depression in this age group, could potentially increase these numbers (Westman, 1999).

Because most office-based procedures in children are minimally invasive (at least for now), standard use of nonopioid analgesics such as the nonsteroidal antiinflammatory drugs (NSAIDs) and acetaminophen, when not contraindicated, is advocated. Ketorolac is found to be useful with an excellent safety profile for postoperative analgesia in a variety of pediatric surgical procedures, and it can be administered intravenously in a dose of 0.5 to 0.8 mg/kg (maximum dose, 30 mg) (Lynn et al., 2007).

Relative to pediatric dental procedures, Needleman and others (2008) report that 95% of 90 children undergoing dental rehabilitation under a standardized general anesthesia regimen without local anesthetic infiltration experience postoperative pain. Increased postoperative pain was reported to be more likely in children who had dental extractions, those at least 4 years of age, and those who had experienced a greater number of procedures. It seems intuitive, then, that local anesthetic infiltration should be an excellent analgesic supplement for children undergoing dental rehabilitation. However, Townsend and others (2009) report that in children, 3 to 5½ years old, undergoing oral rehabilitation while under general anesthesia and receiving local anesthetic infiltration in addition to intravenous ketorolac did no better relative to postprocedural pain than those children receiving intravenous ketorolac alone. In fact, these authors report a greater (but not statistically significant) incidence of lip and cheek biting in those children receiving local anesthetic infiltration.

In some pediatric dental rehabilitation cases done under general anesthesia, patients receive 0.5 mg/kg of intravenous ketorolac with supplemental fentanyl (1 to 2 mcg/kg only when extractions are performed) after induction of anesthesia. More than 95% of patients qualify to bypass phase I recovery and rarely require supplemental analgesics before discharge. Those receiving intraoperative fentanyl receive prophylactic ondansetron, 0.15 mg/kg.

This experience with ketorolac is similar to those of Purday and others (1996) who found ketorolac, 0.75 mg/kg, 1.0 mg/kg, and 1.5 mg/kg to be as efficacious with statistically less PONV as 0.1 mg/kg of morphine sulfate in treating postoperative pain in patients aged 2 to 12 years undergoing dental restoration procedures. Similarly, Maunuksela and others (1992) noted ketorolac to be as efficacious as morphine after pediatric eye surgery. In contrast, Kim and others (2003) report that topical ketorolac is ineffective in treating the pain associated with strabismus surgery. Ibuprofen can also be used to treat postoperative pain, but reports on its effectiveness for some surgical procedures are mixed. Kokki and others (1994) showed that preoperative administration of rectal ibuprofen, 40 mg/kg, divided into four equal doses, was effective in the treatment of postoperative pain in children aged 1 to 4 years in that it reduced the need for supplemental morphine postoperatively. In contrast, Bennie and others (1997), in a double-blind, placebo-controlled study of children older than 6 months who were undergoing bilateral myringotomy and tube placement, found no benefit to the preoperative oral administration of ibuprofen (10 mg/kg) or acetaminophen (15 mg/kg) in the treatment of postoperative pain compared with a placebo group. Joshi and others (2003) reported success with preoperatively administered oral rofecoxib, a cyclooxygenase-2 NSAID, given in a dose of 1 mg/kg, in treating postoperative pain and reducing PONV in children (3 to 11 years old) undergoing tonsillectomy.

Acetaminophen administration is also effective for postoperative analgesia, especially in procedures resulting in mild or moderate pain (Tobias, 2000). Although high-dose acetaminophen (40 mg/kg) administered rectally has been shown to be effective and has opiate-sparing effects, the restrictive quarters of some offices may make this route of administration somewhat prohibitive (Korpela et al., 1999). Similarly, preoperative high-dose acetaminophen (40 mg/kg), administered orally in a one-time dose is shown to be effective in the treatment of postoperative pain after myringotomy and tube placement in children ages 17 months to 6 years, without reaching toxic plasma levels (Bolton et al., 2002). This is contrary to the aforementioned studies, where oral acetaminophen in standard doses (15 mg/kg) was shown to be ineffective (Bennie et al., 1997).

Although NSAIDs alone, or in combination with acetaminophen are opiate-sparing in certain types of surgical procedures, opiate analgesics are not totally precluded from office-based surgery and may in fact at times be necessary (Purday et al. 1996; Hiller et al., 2006; Riad and Moussa, 2007). When either NSAIDs or acetaminophen is inadequate in the treatment of postoperative pain, then traditional combination drugs such as acetaminophen with codeine (0.5 to 1.0 mg/kg of the codeine component) may be appropriate.

Whether interesting alternatives or adjuncts to traditional analgesia regimen, such as innovative nerve blocks and acupuncture, for specific surgical procedures can be time efficient and efficacious in the office setting warrants further study (Voronov et al., 2008; Lin et al., 2009).

Postoperative Nausea and Vomiting

The etiology of PONV is multifactorial, with perhaps a genetic component in some individuals, and remains a major cause of prolonged discharge time and unanticipated hospital admission after ambulatory surgery in children (Awad et al., 2004; Blacoe et al., 2008; Rueffert et al., 2009). Adequate treatment of this side effect may play a significant role in improving patient satisfaction with the perioperative experience (Eberhart et al., 2002). Furthermore, the incidence of postdischarge nausea and vomiting (PDNV) is also significant after ambulatory surgery and has risk factors that do not totally mirror those of PONV. In fact, PDNV occurs in a significant number of individuals who do not experience immediate postoperative vomiting before discharge (Wu et al., 2002; Kolodzie and Apfel, 2009). The optimal treatments of both PONV and PDNV, whether prophylactic or rescue, are essential because of the negative influence these entities can have on an office-based practice (Tang et al., 1999; Kolodzie and Apfel, 2009).

Prophylactic and rescue treatment of PONV and PDNV may not be completely effective, but Engelman and others (2008) show significant risk reduction in postoperative vomiting in a meta-analysis of 11 reports of the use of single- and multiple-drug pharmacologic prophylaxis regimens in children. With this in mind and in addition to the information previously provided on the low incidences of PONV and PDNV anecdotally reported in children and adults by those practitioners intimately involved in the practice of office-based anesthesia, several studies examining the incidence and treatment of PONV and PDNV in this setting are available.

Tang and others (2001) compared the use of propofol-N_2O anesthesia with the use of desflurane-N_2O anesthesia plus antiemetic prophylaxis on the incidence of PONV in patients undergoing brief, superficial surgical procedures in an office setting. Patients in the propofol group received no PONV prophylaxis, whereas those in the desflurane group received ondansetron (4 mg), droperidol (0.625 mg), and metoclopramide (10 mg) intravenously at the end of surgery. Neither group received opiate analgesics or muscle relaxants, and all patients received local anesthetic at the surgical site and ketorolac for postoperative pain management. The overall incidence of nausea and vomiting was very low in both groups (less than 10%) and did not differ statistically. Patient satisfaction in both groups was excellent.

In another office-based study, Tang and others (2003) compared the addition of 5-HT$_3$ receptor antagonists to a control regimen in patients receiving desflurane-N$_2$O maintenance anesthesia after propofol induction. All patients received droperidol (0.625 mg) and dexamethasone (4 mg) as baseline antiemetic prophylaxis. Subsequently, patients were randomly assigned to receive placebo, dolasetron (12.5 mg), or ondansetron (4 mg) intravenously before emergence from anesthesia. The results of this study show that the incidence of nausea and vomiting was the same in all groups.

It is obviously advantageous to the office-based practitioner to be able to predict which children are more likely to experience PONV and PDNV. A scoring system, included in management guidelines published by the Society for Ambulatory Anesthesia, predicting the risk of postoperative vomiting in children was presented several years ago and prospectively validated in another report (Eberhardt et al., 2004; Gan et al., 2007; Kranke et al., 2007). In this scoring system, the presence of one or more specific risk factors (surgery lasting longer than 30 minutes, strabismus surgery, age older than 3 years, and an immediate family with history of postoperative vomiting or PONV) increases the likelihood of postoperative vomiting.

Although the best regimen for the prophylaxis and rescue treatment of PONV/PDNV in children is not known, the approach to management is multimodal (Kovac, 2007). Treatment includes reducing baseline risk factors (e.g., regional vs. general anesthesia and avoiding opiates, nitrous oxide, volatile agents, and neostigmine) when possible (Gan et al., 2007). Other authors show that appropriate hydration and superhydration decrease the incidence of postoperative vomiting in certain surgeries (Scuderi et al., 2000; Goodarzi et al., 2009). On the other hand, interventions such as routine use of an intraoperative nasogastric tube and its inherent difficulties and routine postoperative fasting may not be effective (Kerger et al., 2009; Radke et al., 2009).

Pharmacologically, a multidrug approach to PONV prophylaxis in children is advocated, and medications from several drug classes are effective in prophylaxis and rescue treatment (Gan et al., 2007; Kovac, 2007). Dexamethasone is shown to be an excellent choice for various procedures in the pediatric and adult populations either by itself or in combination with 5-HT$_3$ receptor antagonists (Splinter, 2001; Subramaniam, 2001; Negri and Ivani, 2002; Sukhani et al., 2002; Liechti et al., 2007). Although the optimal dose for dexamethasone is unknown and reported to be from 0.1 mg/kg when used with ondansetron to 1.5 mg/kg when used alone, Kim and others (2007) report that a dose of 0.0625 mg/kg is as effective as 1 mg/kg (maximum dose, 24 mg) in the treatment of PONV in children undergoing tonsillectomy and adenoidectomy (Splinter and Rhine, 1998; Henzi et al., 2000). Although in a quantitative systematic review, Henzi and

others (2000) found the use of dexamethasone to be safe in otherwise healthy patients, a report by Czarnetzki and others (2008) shows that despite a dose-dependent decrease in PONV, there is an increased risk of bleeding in children receiving dexamethasone who undergo tonsillectomy and adenoidectomy.

Rescue treatment should focus on using agents from different classes of medications from those used for prophylaxis in a particular patient, and there is evidence that ondansetron in oral disintegrating tablets may be effective in preventing PONV and PDNV, specifically in those children who do not require rescue therapy before discharge (Wagner et al., 2007; Davis et al., 2008).

Whether prophylactic treatment of PONV and PDNV, either through a single-drug or multiple-drug approach, in low-risk patients undergoing office-based surgery and anesthesia is clinically and economically efficacious, as opposed to only treating patients who are at moderate and high risk, needs to be determined.

ESTABLISHING AN OFFICE-BASED PRACTICE

The individual or hospital-based surgery-center group must decide whether committing resources to this type of practice is a worthwhile endeavor. The initial investment for this type of practice in the United States can be prohibitive, because the cost may run as high as $100,000 to $200,000 (Barinholtz, personal communication, 2009). These costs include, but are not limited to, costs for equipment, supplies and drugs, professional accreditation as discussed earlier, legal services for incorporation of the group, malpractice coverage, professional staff (i.e., physician, nurses, biomedical technicians, and secretarial and billing staff), policy and procedure development, and marketing. Of course, an office to house all of these things is also a necessary expense.

It is also important to consider the type of office-based practice that should be initiated. The group or individual can be committed to one surgeon's office, depending on case volume, or to several surgeons, traveling to various office locations. From a logistic perspective, the former is easier because it allows for centralization of resources, the most important of which are equipment and medications. However, from a business perspective, if an individual or group is going to commit significant resources to establishing an office-based anesthesia practice, it makes sense to diversify among many different clients and across multiple specialties.

A group practice considering an office-based venture must decide whether it can designate a specific number of full-time equivalent staff to this site and still be able to provide sufficient clinical coverage to fulfill its contractual obligation to its home facility. If not, the group must then decide whether the cost of hiring new staff (e.g., physicians, recovery nurses, and technical staff) will be offset by the potential revenue generated by the new practice. As customer service is essential in office-based anesthesiology, the single biggest mistake large practices make when delving into an office-based practice is failure to give the client the personal attention required. For the solo practitioner who may be caught up in the excitement of a new practice, overcommitment to too many surgeons may result in scheduling nightmares and a failure to meet obligations.

The individual or group must also meet the challenge of being able to market against other physicians or physician groups, as well as alternative and perhaps less expensive anesthesia providers in this competitive arena. Can the group provide a unique service, such as pediatric anesthesia coverage, that will make it more attractive to a particular surgeon or dentist?

Finally, and probably as important as any of the other issues related to establishing an office-based practice, the potential political fallout related to a new practice cannot be overemphasized. An anesthesia group with obligations to specific hospital or surgery center facilities must be ready to justify to administrators its practice of providing office-based anesthesia services to surgeons who typically operate in these administrators' facilities. This diversion of income-generating surgical procedures may be construed as a violation of a group's service agreement and consequently prompt administrators to solicit the services of a new group.

For a busy hospital or surgery center, however, there are now many procedures where the profit margin for the hospital or surgery center is narrow, and the ability to divert these cases from the overcrowded operating rooms to physicians' offices may be looked upon favorably by administrators. Furthermore, this could be an opportunity for a joint venture between the hospital (that owns the equipment) and physician group (that doesn't want to outlay capital dollars).

Equipment and Supplies

Essentially all of the standard anesthesia equipment that is required in hospital ambulatory facilities (operating room and off-site) and surgery centers is required for office-based practice. All monitoring standards must be met in the office-surgical suite. Monitoring equipment must have battery back-up capability, because some offices may not have emergency generator capabilities in the event of power failure. Working in one facility where the equipment is capitalized by the surgeon or capitalized by the anesthesiologist and stored in the surgeon's office is much easier to deal with than the more common alternative of the anesthesiologist bringing the anesthesia workroom from place to place. Box 35-3 outlines general categories of supplies, standard and emergency, that must be transported to surgical sites by the office-based anesthesiologist. The array of portable equipment that exists these days is more than adequate to meet standards.

> **Box 35-3 General Categories of Required Supplies Transported by the Office-Based Anesthesiologist**
>
> Anesthesia supply box
> Defibrillator (with appropriate-sized paddles)
> Recovery supply box
> Anesthesia drug box
> Pediatric supply box
> Recovery drug box
> Airway box
> Emergency airway equipment (e.g., LMAs, fiberoptic bronchoscope, and cricothyrotomy kits)
> Portable suction equipment
> Monitoring equipment with disposables
> Malignant hyperthermia tray
> Portable anesthesia machine with vaporizer
> Positive pressure ventilation system
> Oxygen "E" cylinders
> Miscellaneous (e.g., batteries, records, other helpful items)
>
> Courtesy D. Barinholtz, Mobile Anesthesiologists, LLC, 2003.

For those practitioners who provide total intravenous anesthesia, an anesthesia machine is not necessary, but the presence of equipment capable of delivering positive-pressure ventilation with oxygen is mandatory. For those anesthesiologists providing care to pediatric patients, a vaporizer-equipped anesthesia machine is invaluable. Most anesthesia machines are moveable, but there are a few machines that are truly portable and available for care of pediatric and adult patients in the office setting. One such machine is the OBA-1 (OBAMED, Cardinal Medical Specialties; Louisville, Kentucky), which weighs approximately 35 pounds, is vaporizer equipped, and is compatible with magnetic resonance imaging (MRI) devices (Fig. 35-3). The OBA-1 allows only spontaneous or manually controlled ventilation, because it is not equipped with an internal ventilator. The Magellan-2200, Model 1/M (Oceanic Medical Products; Atchison, Kansas) and the Narkomed-Mobile (Draeger Medical; Telford, Pennsylvania) are also marketed for office anesthesia, and both contain an internal ventilator. The latter machine, despite its ability to be rolled, is a much heavier

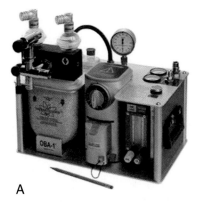
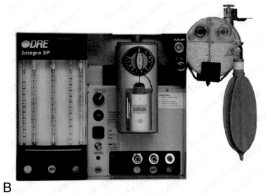

■ FIGURE 35-3. Two types of portable anesthesia machines. **A,** The OBA-1 portable, MRI-compatible anesthesia machine. **B,** The DRE Integra portable anesthesia machine. *(Courtesy Charles A. Smith, Vice-President of Operations, Research and Development, Cardinal Medical Specialties, Louisville, Ky.)*

unit and may not be practical for the anesthesiologist who is changing office venues on a daily basis.

Regardless of the type of machine one chooses to use, caution must be used during transport; maintaining the machine's vaporizer in an upright position is essential to avoid spillage and the administration of an inappropriately high concentration of volatile agent. Often, draining the vaporizer before transport minimizes this risk. Furthermore, familiarity with state and federal safety guidelines relative to the transportation of medical gases is critical.

Whenever a volatile agent or succinylcholine is to be used, one must be prepared to treat malignant hyperthermia. A stock supply of dantrolene must be available, and it is the responsibility of the anesthesiologist or a representative of the practice to proactively educate the surgeon and the surgeon's office personnel on appropriate protocol in the event of a malignant hyperthermia episode (see Chapter 37, Malignant Hyperthermia).

Finally, the office-based anesthesiologist must become aware of and be in compliance with the rules and regulations (federal and state-specific) relative to the delivery, transport, clerical requirements (e.g., related to dispensing and wastage), and storage of opiates and other controlled substances that are used in the office setting.

Staffing

In the United States, the providers of office-based anesthesia services presently fall into one of three major categories (exclusive of the operator-anesthetist scenario): physician anesthesiologists, dentist anesthesiologists (two years of anesthesia training after completion of dental school), and CRNAs. The conditions under which each of these three groups can practice are determined by state regulations regarding the administration of anesthesia in dental and surgical offices. Consequently, the composition of office-based anesthesia groups may vary by geographic location and can be comprised of and owned by all physicians, all dentist anesthesiologists, CRNA groups with and without collaborating physician medical directors, or various combinations of these individuals.

Beyond the anesthesia providers, however, are the ancillary personnel who are necessary to make a busy office-based practice successful. The individuals who are often required include nursing staff, biomedical and technical staff, credentialing personnel, and billing and clerical staff. The number of anesthesia sites a practice covers simultaneously and the volume of cases usually determine the staffing for a particular organization.

In some practices, an anesthesiologist or a CRNA may travel alone to a site. In this instance, the anesthesia provider is responsible for preoperative, intraoperative, and postanesthesia care of the child and requires the assistance of the surgical nursing staff. When multiple cases are performed at a single site, then a surgical office nurse is responsible for monitoring a patient during recovery.

In anesthesiologist-only practices, the preferred scenario is to have a staff nurse, employed by the group, available to assist with induction of anesthesia and to be responsible for monitoring the postanesthesia care of the child. Nurses with critical care or PACU experience, who are certified in advanced cardiac life support and pediatric advance life support (ACLS-PALS), are best suited for this type of position. Anesthesia practices are

sometimes able to procure reimbursement for the professional services rendered by these nurses for the care of patients in the PACU.

Having such personnel relieves the surgical ancillary staff from any anesthesia-related patient care responsibility and facilitates timely turnover when multiple cases are being performed in a single office. Experienced nurses may also be used to initiate telephone screening to provide patients with their preoperative anesthesia and surgical instructions, coordinate anesthesia scheduling, assist in purchasing supplies and equipment, and educate surgical staff on the specifics of the anesthesia process.

Reimbursement

Mentioned earlier is the potential for cost savings by moving surgical cases from hospital outpatient or ambulatory surgical facilities to the office. Unfortunately, in some arenas, anesthesia-requiring office procedures are the rule because of the lack of insurance coverage for these procedures. This is especially true in pediatric dentistry. With few exceptions in the United States, dental and medical insurance policies traditionally fail to cover the cost of anesthesia or hospitalization for children requiring dental procedures (Saxen et al., 1999; Yagiela, 1999; White et al., 2008). This has forced dentists to minimize costs for these children and their families by performing procedures in the office with or without the aid of an anesthesia provider.

However, the American Dental Association reports that there are at least 31 states that have passed laws since 1995 (Medically Necessary Care or Special Needs Legislation) requiring that medical insurance plans pay for hospital and connected medical expenses (e.g., general anesthesia services) when the dental treatment occurs in the hospital, ambulatory surgery center, or dental office (Box 35-4) (O'Connor, personal communication, January 2010).

Some of the elements of these state laws are similar and often determine which children are eligible to receive coverage based on minimum and maximum age and medical or behavioral conditions. Many of these laws, despite mandating coverage, also outline that any provisions of the existing policy, such as meeting prior authorization requirements by showing medical necessity or payable deductibles, still hold true.

Some states also determine the acceptable facilities where the procedure can be performed by mandating insurance coverage only for procedures performed in the hospital or surgery center. Some laws also exempt dental-only insurance plans from their provisions. The number of states requiring coverage for the anesthesia portion of dental care may continue to increase, resulting in increased access to care for those children having the greatest need, regardless of qualified surgical site.

Reimbursement and collections for anesthesia and surgery in offices are somewhat complex and often work differently for the surgical provider and the anesthesia provider (Koch et al., 2003). Fee-for-service reimbursement can be lucrative for the anesthesiologist in a high-volume cosmetic surgeon's office. However, because patients undergoing cosmetic surgery are often charged a set global fee for a specific procedure, some surgeons may look toward a lower-cost anesthesia provider, so the surgeon may recover a greater amount of the preset fee. This may intensify competition among anesthesia providers for these types of procedures.

Box 35-4 States (Some) Adopting Associated Medical Cost Laws Requiring Medical Plans to Pay for Hospitalization/General Anesthesia When Dental Treatment Must Be Performed in the Hospital or Medical Expenses Incurred When Treatment Is in the Dental Office

Arkansas (2005)	Louisiana (1997)	North Carolina (1999)
California (1998)	Maine (2001)	North Dakota (1999)
Colorado (1998)	Maryland (1998)	Oklahoma (1998)
Connecticut (1999)	Michigan (2001)	South Dakota (1999)
Florida (1998)	Minnesota (1995)	Tennessee (1997)
Georgia (1999)	Mississippi (1999)	Texas (1997)
Illinois (2002)	Missouri (1998)	Virginia (2000)
Indiana (1999)	Nebraska (2000)	Washington (2001)
Iowa (2000)	New Hampshire (1998, 2003)	West Virginia (2009)
Kansas (1999)	New Jersey (1999)	Wisconsin (1997)
Kentucky (2002)		

Courtesy the American Dental Association, Department of State Government Affairs, January 20, 2010.

Reimbursement from third-party payers is at negotiated rates that usually vary by geographic location and payer. Despite the fact that some payers reimburse anesthesia practices for professional fees and supplies or equipment, there are those that invoke the CMS policy that a facility be licensed by the state in order to bill for the latter. Consequently, this may mean a greater cost burden to the patient (Barinholtz, personal communication, 2003). Koch and others (2003) point out that office-based anesthesia practices may become even more ubiquitous and successful by duplicating cost-recovery strategies of surgeons—namely, better collection of facility fees and site-of-service differentials that provide for greater reimbursement for procedures performed in offices.

The reimbursement landscape for office-based surgery and anesthesia is improving significantly over the past several years. Payers are recognizing the significant cost savings that can be realized in the office compared with hospitals and surgery centers. Anthem in Virginia recently launched a program that pays facility fees in offices for over 2000 outpatient procedures. Blue Cross of Illinois is going to launch a similar program in 2010. The caveat to collecting these facility fees is that the facility must be accredited by the AAAHC, AAAASF, or The Joint Commission.

SUMMARY

Anesthesiologists are heavily involved in the practice of office-based anesthesia and surgery. Consequently, anesthesiologists must be proactive in ensuring that patient safety is the principal concern for all professionals providing anesthesia services in the office setting. Although there is some progress in this arena, it seems unlikely that the various professional societies, whose memberships are actively involved in office anesthesia and surgery, will agree on a specific set of anesthesia-delivery guidelines. Consistency between states in the regulation of this practice, perhaps in the form of accreditation of both office-based facilities and anesthesia practices, is imperative and may be the only viable alternative in helping to ensure that "the standard of care is the standard of care." This standard should be applicable regardless of surgical setting or patient age. Only further study will assist in determining whether the safety and cost profiles for office-based anesthesia are comparable with those of other ambulatory settings and ultimately whether office-based anesthesia will continue to be a worthwhile venture.

REFERENCES

Complete references used in this text can be found online at www.expertconsult.com.

Associated Problems in Pediatric Anesthesia

Systemic Disorders

Lynne G. Maxwell, Salvatore R. Goodwin, Thomas J. Mancuso,
Victor C. Baum, Aaron L. Zuckerberg, Philip G. Morgan,
Etsuro K. Motoyama, Peter J. Davis, and Kevin J. Sullivan

CONTENTS

A mong patients who present special problems for anesthesiologists are children whose underlying conditions complicate anesthetic management and may be associated with an increased risk of morbidity. The number of rare diseases that may be encountered in infants and children is great, although only a few are mentioned here. Chosen for discussion are the diseases most commonly seen, those carrying an increased risk related to anesthetic management, and a few of unusual interest. Modifications to the understanding of mechanisms of coagulation are included, along with consideration of coagulopathic states, and there is a comprehensive review of the anesthetic implications of pediatric syndromes associated with genetic, metabolic, and dysmorphic features (Baum and O'Flaherty, 2006). A partial list of syndromes with possible anesthetic implications is included in Appendix D, which can be accessed online at www.expertconsult.com

ENDOCRINE DISORDERS

Diabetes Mellitus

The endocrine condition most commonly dealt with in the perioperative period is the management of glucose homeostasis in children with diabetes mellitus. The prevalence of type 1 (insulin-dependent) diabetes in the United States has remained stable for the past 15 years at 1 in 400 to 600 school-aged children, whereas the incidence of type 2 diabetes is increasing, especially among American Indian, Black, and Hispanic children and adolescents (CDC, 2007c). Diabetes mellitus is the result of an absolute or functional deficiency of insulin production by the pancreas. In type 1 diabetes, this deficiency is caused by an autoimmune pathophysiologic process. Insulin deficiency results in abnormalities of glucose transport and storage and of lipid and protein synthesis. Over time, these metabolic derangements result in the vascular pathology that leads to end-stage complications of renal, cardiac, and eye disease—diseases that typically do not occur before adulthood. The anesthetic implications of type 1 diabetes in children differ from those in adults with the same disease, for whom the primary concern is the type and severity of end-organ disease.

Children with type 1 diabetes may be treated with various types of insulin on a daily basis to maintain tight glucose control with the aid of frequent blood-glucose monitoring. Since 1982, most newly approved insulin preparations have been produced using recombinant DNA technology with laboratory-cultivated bacteria or yeast. This process allows the bacteria or yeast cells to produce complete human insulin. Recombinant human insulin has mostly replaced animal-derived insulin (e.g., pork and beef insulin) in diabetes management (Plotnick and Henderson, 1998). Insulin products called *insulin analogues* are produced so that the structure differs slightly from human insulin (by one or two amino acids) to change onset and peak of action. An example of an analogue is human lispro, an ultra–short-acting insulin that is given only 15 minutes before a meal. Its peak and duration of action parallel the glucose rise that results from carbohydrate ingestion.

Another new insulin is glargine, which almost mimics an insulin pump, providing a continuous, 24-hour, low background

TABLE 36-1. Kinetics of Commonly Used Insulins

Insulin	Route	Onset (hr)	Peak (hr)	Effective Duration (hr)
Human				
Lispro (Humalog)	SC	0.25	0.5–1.5	3–4
Regular	IV/SC	0.5–1.0	2–3	3–6
NPH	SC	2–4	4–10	10–18
Glargine (Lantus)	SC	1	2–3	24
Animal				
Regular	IV/SC	0.5–1	2–5	4–6

IV, Intravenous; *SC*, subcutaneous; *NPH*, neutral protamine Hagedorn.

level of insulin. The kinetics of some of the insulin preparations most commonly used in children are listed in Table 36-1. Some children's diabetes may be managed with an external insulin pump, which provides a low, background, subcutaneous infusion of insulin and the ability to give small boluses before meals. Most children with diabetes administer insulin at least three times each day and check their blood sugar at least four times each day. Type 2 diabetes in children and adolescents may be controlled with diet and exercise, but these children also may be taking metformin. Metformin was recently shown to decrease gluconeogenesis by directly modulating copper-binding protein (CBP) in the liver much as insulin itself does, rather than by overcoming the liver's decreased sensitivity to insulin (He et al., 2009).

Because of the effects of surgical stress on glucose homeostasis, children with type 1 diabetes are at risk for significant perioperative difficulties, even when their preoperative glucose control is good. Brittle or noncompliant patients with diabetes have additional problems, including an increased risk of perioperative hypoglycemia or hyperglycemia, osmotic diuresis with resultant hypovolemia, and altered mental status. The physician must document the child's current insulin regimen, degree of compliance, preoperative glucose control, and risk of hypoglycemia from preoperative fast. Much of this information can be obtained from the patient's endocrinologist or by examination of the child's blood-glucose monitoring log. A recent growth history can indicate how well controlled the child's diabetes may be. Coordination and cooperation among the patient, parents, pediatrician, endocrinologist, and anesthesiologist are essential if the goal of optimal perioperative glucose homeostasis is to be achieved. The anesthesiologist must particularly heed the recommendations of the child's primary physician.

Insulin is an anabolic hormone that promotes glycogen and triglyceride storage and protein synthesis. Present in small amounts even in the fasting state, it decreases glycogenolysis, gluconeogenesis, and lipolysis, with resultant ketogenesis and protein breakdown. Its complete absence at the time of surgery puts the patient in a state of starvation, in which caloric intake is greatly restricted and substrate demands (e.g., for healing) are at their highest. The risk of a catabolic state is increased by the release of stress hormones, including catecholamines, cortisol, and glucagon. Perioperative insulin administration is essential to control glucose and to promote an anabolic state, which is most conducive to speedy healing and metabolic homeostasis. Preoperative anesthesia evaluation for elective procedures, informed by contemporaneous endocrine assessment of adequacy of glucose control, should be completed 7 to 10 days before the scheduled date of surgery to allow adjustment of treatment regimen or delay of procedure if control is not optimal. Rhodes and colleagues (2005) published a comprehensive review of concerns and perioperative management of pediatric patients with diabetes; it features an extremely useful clinical practice guideline that incorporates both preoperative assessment and choice of preoperative insulin regimen.

Preoperative Evaluation

The preoperative evaluation should include measurements of the hematocrit, electrolyte levels, and glucose levels. A hemoglobin (Hb) A1c level (i.e., glycosylated Hb assay), although a useful index of long-term glucose control, is unlikely to affect the anesthetic plan and is not a necessary preoperative test (Nathan et al., 1984). If glycohemoglobin results are available, it is important to remember that different laboratories have different ranges for Hb A1c in normal subjects. Even in the same laboratory, the normal range may change from time to time. It is therefore important to know the laboratory's normal range to interpret results in patients with diabetes. The normal range of Hb A1c is 4.5% to 6.1%, but the normal range also varies with age (Rhodes et al., 2005; Custer and Rau, 2009).

Several systemic abnormalities may be present in the child with diabetes. Nineteen percent of children with diabetes have a vital capacity two standard deviations below the predicted mean value, suggesting the presence of restrictive lung disease (Buckingham et al., 1986). No apparent association exists between decreased vital capacity and duration of diabetes or presence of other diabetic complications. Abnormal lung elasticity and thickening of the alveolar basal laminae have been reported in children with diabetes (Schuyler et al., 1976; Vracko et al., 1980). Routine preoperative pulmonary function tests are not indicated in the asymptomatic child who has diabetes.

Decreased atlantooccipital joint mobility, resulting in difficult intubation, may be present in a subset of adolescents with a syndrome of diabetes mellitus, short stature, and tightness of small joints of the fingers, wrists, ankles, and elbows (Salzarulo and Taylor, 1986). Abnormal cross-linking of collagen by nonenzymatic glycosylation is the postulated cause of this syndrome (Chang et al., 1980).

Perioperative Management

Various regimens for managing insulin therapy perioperatively have been proposed, three of which are discussed in the following sections and in Table 36-2: a classic regimen, the subcutaneous infusion insulin pump, and intravenous (IV) insulin infusion. Essential to optimal management, regardless of regimen, is the scheduling of elective surgery for the child with diabetes as early as possible in the day (first case) to minimize time that the patient must fast. The fasting interval should be the same as that recommended for patients who do not have diabetes: no solid food or milk for 8 hours, and clear liquids are permissible until 2 hours before the scheduled time of surgery (Schreiner et al., 1990). Children with diabetes should be encouraged to continue taking clear liquids until 2 hours before surgery. If this is not possible, an

TABLE 36-2. Protocols for Perioperative Insulin Therapy

Regimen	Morning of Surgery Procedure
Classic regimen	Start IV infusion of 5% dextrose in 0.45% saline or Ringer's lactate solution at 1500 mL/m²/day. Administer half of usual morning insulin dose as regular insulin. Check blood glucose before induction, during and after anesthesia
Continuous insulin infusion	Start IV infusion of 5% dextrose in 0.45% saline or Ringer's lactate solution at 1500 mL/m²/day. Add 1-2 units of insulin per 100 mL of 5% dextrose. Starting insulin dose = 0.02 units/kg/hr. Check blood glucose before induction, and during and after anesthesia
Insulin- and glucose-free regimen (for operative procedures of short duration)	Withhold morning insulin dose. If indicated for procedure, give glucose-free solution (e.g., Ringer's lactate) at maintenance rate. Check blood glucose before induction, and during and after anesthesia.

IV fluid infusion should be started (described later). As recommended in adult patients with type 2 diabetes, metformin should be stopped 48 hours before surgery, based on reports of lactic acidosis in patients who remain on the drug and are in a fasting state perioperatively. Other orally administered medications (e.g., thiazolidinediones or sulfonylureas) may be continued through the day before surgery.

Although some investigators have recommended the withholding of preoperative sedation from patients with diabetes to better monitor for signs of hypoglycemia, premedication is recommended in children. The use of agents such as benzodiazepines, opioids, or barbiturates does not alter glucose metabolism, and the failure to use such agents may elevate the blood sugar level as a result of anxiety, which causes a stress response with catecholamine release.

Based on the blood-glucose level determined on arrival to the preoperative facility and before implementation of the regimens discussed in the following sections, glucose or insulin should be administered according to the scheme outlined in Table 36-3.

TABLE 36-3. Preoperative Glucose and Insulin Management for Diabetic Patients

Blood Glucose Level	Management
<80 mg/dL	2 mL/kg D10W followed by glucose infusion
80-250 mg/dL	D5/0.45 NS or D10/0.45 NS solution at maintenance if insulin is to be administered; 0.9 NS if short case; no insulin
>250 mg/dL	Administer rapid-acting (lispro) or short-acting (regular) insulin SC to reduce blood sugar; use correction factor from patient's endocrine provider or 0.2 unit/kg SC
>350 mg/dL	Consider canceling or postponing surgery, especially if ketonuria

NS, Normal saline; *SC,* subcutaneously.

Classic Regimen

On the morning of surgery, one half of the usual dose of long-acting insulin (e.g., Neutral Protamine Hagedorn [NPH]) is administered subcutaneously after establishing an IV infusion of 5% glucose-containing solution at a rate of 100 mg/kg per hour of glucose (Table 36-2). Plasma-glucose concentrations should be maintained between 100 and 180 mg/dL. This target range is chosen because mild to moderate hyperglycemia (without ketosis) usually does not present a serious problem to the child, whereas hypoglycemia has devastating consequences. Hyperglycemia greater than 250 mg/dL should be avoided because of associated mental status changes, diuresis, and subsequent dehydration, which can occur because of the hyperosmolar state. Hyperglycemia has been associated with poorer outcomes in patients at risk for central nervous system (CNS) ischemia, including those undergoing cardiopulmonary bypass (Lanier et al., 1987; Lanier, 1991). Hyperglycemia has also been shown to impair wound healing and has adverse effects on neutrophil function in vitro. (Marhoffer et al., 1992; Delamaire et al., 1997). When the classic regimen is employed, supplemental subcutaneous doses of short-acting insulin can be given on a sliding scale postoperatively to maintain the desired plasma glucose level. This regimen should be restricted to patients who are scheduled for short surgical procedures, after which they are expected to resume eating promptly.

Subcutaneous Infusion Insulin Pump

Increasing numbers of pediatric patients with type I diabetes are being managed with an external insulin pump that is capable of subcutaneous administration of both continuous and bolus doses of insulin. Such pumps afford excellent control, with changes in administration coordinated with eating, exercise, and stress. At this time, the proliferation of pumps from multiple manufacturers precludes the easy acquisition of knowledge and familiarity with their use in the perioperative setting. Some clinicians and institutions allow continued use of insulin pumps for short, uncomplicated procedures (e.g., less than 2 hours), whereas most recommend transition to a continuous insulin infusion, as described in the next section (Glister and Vigersky, 2003; Rhodes et al., 2005).

Intravenous Insulin Infusion

If a long procedure or a prolonged period of postoperative fasting is anticipated, the continuous IV infusion of glucose and insulin may provide the best control. On the morning of surgery, a glucose infusion is begun at a maintenance rate of 100 mg/kg per hour, with an insulin infusion of 0.02 to 0.05 unit/kg per hour "piggy-backed" into the glucose infusion. The glucose infusion can be D5 or D10 in half-normal saline with 10 to 20 mEq/L of potassium chloride. These infusions should be started 2 hours before surgery to minimize the duration of fasting and decrease the risk of the development of a catabolic state. Insulin is absorbed by IV bags and tubing. When the insulin solution is prepared, the first portion of the solution should be run through the tubing and discarded to saturate the sites in the tubing that bind insulin (Kaufman et al., 1996). Blood glucose levels should be checked hourly for the first few hours, and adjustments of 0.01 unit/kg per hour in the insulin rate should be made to keep the blood sugar in the acceptable range of 100 to 180 mg/dL. This continuous-infusion regimen has been shown to yield better control of glucose concentrations than the regimen in which intermittent subcutaneous insulin is administered (Kaufman et al., 1996). The administration of intermittent large IV-insulin doses has no role, as it can result in large swings in glucose concentration (high and low) and a greater chance of lipolysis and ketogenesis. Patients with insulin pumps should have them turned off in the perioperative period, and pumps should be replaced by the continuous-infusion regimen, as most anesthesiologists are not familiar with the details of operation of such pumps. Fifty-percent dextrose solution should be available for administration in case of the development of hypoglycemia; 0.1 g/kg of dextrose raises the blood-glucose level by approximately 30 mg/dL.

The glucose and insulin should be infused through a dedicated IV cannula to enable it to be well regulated apart from the non–glucose-containing crystalloid solutions that are administered to replace blood or fluid losses—especially important if the maintenance glucose solution contains potassium. Many institutions avoid potassium-containing solutions to prevent their inadvertent rapid administration in the setting of rapid administration of fluid for blood or fluid replacement. Most investigators believe that lactated Ringer's solution should not be used for blood and fluid replacement, because lactate is a glycogenic precursor and may result in higher blood-glucose levels.

Alternative Procedure (Insulin- and Glucose-free Regimen)

For extremely brief procedures, after which prompt resumption of oral intake is expected, an alternative protocol involves the administration of no insulin or glucose before or during surgery. When oral intake is established postoperatively, 40% to 60% of the usual daily insulin dose is given (Stevens and Roizen, 1987). Myringotomy with tube placement is an example of a procedure for which this regimen would be appropriate. The surgical procedure should be performed as the first case on the morning schedule to avoid prolonged fasting and excessive delay in insulin administration.

The most serious perioperative complication that can occur in the diabetic child is hypoglycemia. Common signs of low blood-glucose levels include tachycardia, tearing, diaphoresis, and hypertension. In the anesthetized patient, these signs may be misinterpreted as the result of inadequate anesthesia. Because the clinical signs of hypoglycemia are masked by sedation or anesthesia, frequent (every hour) measurement of the serum-glucose level is critical for the prevention of hypoglycemia, independent of the glucose-insulin regimen chosen. Glucose test strips, with or without the use of a reflectance photometer, provide quick, convenient, and reliable bedside blood-sugar measurements to guide therapy. Blood-glucose determinations performed with reflectance photometers provide results that are generally within 10% of clinical laboratory glucose determinations done on the same specimen (Chen et al., 2003). Visual evaluation of blood-glucose strips is less accurate (Arslanian et al., 1994). Postoperative insulin administration is determined by the time of resumption of oral or enteral feeding and by the postoperative blood-glucose concentration. The endocrinologist and surgeon should be active partners in the choice of an appropriate insulin regimen, because they are responsible for monitoring glucose homeostasis after the patient leaves the recovery room. For day-surgery patients, contingency planning for insulin management and mechanisms for follow-up care and consultation should be clearly defined for members of the care team and family.

Anesthetic Management

Regional or general anesthesia is appropriate for the child with diabetes mellitus. If tolerated with minimal sedation, regional anesthesia might be argued to offer the advantage of allowing for observation of the level of consciousness as a monitor of hypoglycemia. Practically speaking, most children require general anesthesia, even when regional techniques are employed. The ease and availability of point-of-care glucose determination from venous or finger-stick specimens obviate the need for monitoring of cerebral function.

Perioperative Management of Diabetic Ketoacidosis

Occasionally, patients with diabetes require surgery for trauma or infection while they are in a state of ketoacidosis. Diabetic ketoacidosis includes hyperglycemia (plasma-glucose concentration greater than 300 mg/dL) with glucosuria, ketonemia (ketones strongly positive at greater than 1:2 dilution of serum), ketonuria, and acidemia (pH lower than 7.30, serum bicarbonate lower than 15 mEq/L, or both). It is common for intraabdominal catastrophes with infection (e.g., appendicitis) to precipitate ketoacidosis. Foster and McGarry (1983) have succinctly summarized the pathophysiology of diabetic ketoacidosis. The initiating event is usually cessation of insulin therapy or onset of stress that renders the usual dose of insulin inadequate. Glucagon, catecholamines, cortisol, and growth hormone levels increase. A catabolic state is produced as substrates are mobilized, resulting in hepatic production of glucose and ketone bodies, which causes hyperglycemia and ketoacidosis. Subclinical brain swelling nearly always occurs during diabetic ketoacidosis therapy, although most patients remain asymptomatic (Krane et al., 1985). Fatalities from cerebral edema do occur, and some studies suggest that high rates of fluid administration early in treatment (more than 50 mL/kg in the first 4 hours) greatly increase the risk of herniation (Mahoney et al., 1999). Studies using 4 L/m² for the first 24 hours followed by 1 to 1.5 times maintenance resulted in clearance of ketoacidosis equal to that in patients who were given more fluid, but a low but persistent incidence (0.35% to 0.5%) of symptomatic cerebral edema remained (Felner and White, 2001). The best methods to prevent the development of this devastating complication are administration of isotonic fluid only and frequent monitoring of serum osmolality (by direct measurement or calculation) to ensure that elevated osmolality is reduced gradually. Insulin therapy should be tailored to decrease the blood glucose concentration at a rate not greater than 100 mg/dL per hour. To prevent a more rapid decrease in blood glucose concentration, 5% dextrose and if necessary, 10% dextrose, should be added to the rehydration solution to slow the rate of fall, rather than decreasing the rate of insulin infusion (Arslanian et al., 1994). Fortunately, the anesthesiologist is rarely called on to administer anesthesia during this severe metabolic derangement. If an anesthetic is required during diabetic ketoacidosis, preoperative attention should be directed toward the correction of hypovolemia and hypokalemia, along with beginning an insulin infusion. Invasive hemodynamic monitoring may be indicated preoperatively to optimize the patient's fluid and electrolyte balance and to monitor the patient's hemodynamic status accurately. Surgery should not be delayed inordinately because it may be impossible to correct the metabolic derangements before the underlying source of infection or organ dysfunction is corrected. For patients with signs of cerebral edema, monitoring of intracranial pressure may be necessary.

Diabetes Insipidus

Diabetes insipidus (DI) is a clinical syndrome of hypotonic polyuria in the face of elevated plasma osmolality that results from inadequate production of, or inadequate response to, antidiuretic hormone (ADH). Central DI results from inadequate production or release of ADH from the posterior pituitary gland. ADH is synonymous with arginine vasopressin. Nephrogenic DI (also referred to as *vasopressin-resistant DI*) is characterized by partial or complete renal tubular unresponsiveness to endogenous ADH or exogenously administered arginine vasopressin. Congenital nephrogenic DI is caused by mutations in either the vasopressin receptor or aquaporin-2 gene. Inheritance is X-linked in the former and autosomal recessive or dominant in the latter (Sasaki, 2004). A combination of hydrochlorothiazide and a nonsteroidal antiinflammatory drug (NSAID) has been effective for the treatment of nephrogenic DI. Both cyclooxygenase-1 (COX-1; i.e., tolmetin and indomethacin) and cyclooxygenase-2 (COX-2; i.e., rofecoxib) drugs have been effective (Jakobsson and Berg, 1994; Pattaragarn and Alon, 2003). Toxic drug effects may also lead to acquired nephrogenic DI. Anesthetic implications of nephrogenic DI have been reviewed by Cramolini (1993) and Malhotra and Roizen (1987).

The causes of DI are outlined in Box 36-1. This discussion focuses on central DI and its clinical manifestations, which are

---

Box 36-1 Causes of Diabetes Insipidus

VASOPRESSIN DEFICIENCY (NEUROGENIC DI)
Acquired
    Idiopathic
    Traumatic (accidental, surgical)
    Neoplastic (craniopharyngioma, metastasis, lymphoma)
    Granulomatous (sarcoid, histiocytosis)
    Infectious (meningitis, encephalitis)
    Vascular (Sheehan syndrome, aneurysm)
Familial (autosomal dominant)

EXCESSIVE WATER INTAKE (PRIMARY POLYDIPSIA)
Acquired
    Idiopathic (resetting of the osmostat)
    Psychogenic

VASOPRESSIN INSENSITIVITY (NEPHROGENIC DI)
Acquired
    Infectious (pyelonephritis)
    Postobstructive (urethral, ureteral)
    Vascular (sickle cell disease or trait)
    Infiltrative (amyloid)
    Cystic (polycystic disease)
    Metabolic (hypokalemia, hypercalcemia)
    Granulomatous (sarcoid)
    Toxic (lithium, demeclocycline)
    Solute overload (glucosuria, postobstructive)
Familial (X-linked recessive)

DI, Diabetes insipidus.

polyuria and polydipsia. The urine is hypotonic relative to the plasma. The urine osmolality is usually less than 200 mOsm/L, and urine specific gravity is less than 1.005 (Custer and Rau, 2009). When the patient has had inadequate access to water, severe dehydration and hypernatremia ensue, because a large volume of dilute urine is continually produced.

Patients with preexisting DI may need incidental surgery. They are usually taking maintenance doses of vasopressin, which for relatively short, uncomplicated, elective procedures, should be continued through the perioperative period (Wise-Faberowski et al., 2004). Desmopressin (1-desamino-8-D-arginine vasopressin, or DDAVP), a longer-acting (8 to 20 hours) vasopressin analogue, has a decreased vasopressor effect relative to its antidiuretic effect (Hays, 1990). DDAVP is usually given intranasally (2.5 to 10 mcg once or twice daily) or orally (25 to 200 mcg once or twice daily) to prevent diuresis (Lee et al., 1976). DDAVP also may be given subcutaneously or intravenously (1 to 2 mcg twice daily). An algorithm for the management of DI, whether preexisting or developing intraoperatively or postoperatively, is presented in Figure 36-1.

The most common situation encountered by the anesthesiologist, however, is the new onset of DI intraoperatively or postoperatively in patients who are having surgery for pituitary or hypothalamic tumors, most commonly craniopharyngiomas; 70% to 90% of these patients develop DI (Lehrnbecher et al., 1998; Ghirardello et al., 2006;). Perioperative DI may present in one of four ways:

1. Transient polyuria probably is related to the onset and resolution of transient cerebral edema rather than to injury to the pituitary stalk. It usually resolves in 24 to 36 hours.
2. A triphasic pattern with an interval of normal urine output reflects the release of stored vasopressin from the posterior lobe or median eminence of the pituitary, followed by resumption of polyuria when the stored supply of vasopressin is exhausted.
3. Mild polyuria reflects partial DI, which is exaggerated by local edema and corticosteroid administration.
4. Permanent DI is caused by destruction or removal of all cells capable of producing and storing vasopressin.

If any degree of DI is going to occur, the onset is most commonly within 18 hours after the operation. Recommendations for therapy are reviewed by Wise-Faberowski and colleagues (2004).

The goal of perioperative management of DI is to maintain normal fluid and electrolyte balance, urine output, and hemodynamic stability. Urine output may be prodigious (10 to 20 mL/kg per hour). Care must be taken to differentiate polyuria caused by DI (urine specific gravity of less than 1.005) from diuresis caused by mannitol administration, hyperglycemia (urine specific gravity that is usually greater than 1.015), or simple excessive administration of crystalloid (urine specific gravity of greater than 1.005). Patients with partial ADH deficiency usually do not require supplemental aqueous vasopressin perioperatively, because large quantities of ADH are produced in response to surgical stress (Malhotra and Roizen, 1987). However, serum osmolality should be measured often, and aqueous vasopressin should be given if the plasma osmolality exceeds 300 mOsm/L (Wise-Faberowski et al., 2004).

If central DI is present preoperatively and the planned surgery is prolonged, an infusion of aqueous vasopressin is begun preoperatively and continued intraoperatively. The recommendations for adults include a bolus of 100 milliunits of aqueous vasopressin followed by a continuous infusion of 100 to 200 mU/hr. This should be accompanied by the intraoperative administration of isotonic saline at two thirds of the maintenance rate, with additional fluid given for blood loss replacement and for maintaining hemodynamic stability (Malhotra and Roizen, 1987). Hypotonic fluids should be avoided, as hyponatremia may result. For the pediatric population, an infusion is begun at 0.5 mU/kg per hour and increased in 0.5 mU/kg per hour increments until a urine osmolality twice that of plasma and a urine output of less than 2 mL/kg per hour are achieved. It is rarely necessary to use more than 10 mU/kg per hour (Weigle, 1987). Side effects from vasopressin administration are minimal at doses used for antidiuresis; at larger doses, generalized vasoconstriction can occur and has resulted in tissue ischemia and myocardial infarction.

DDAVP, rather than aqueous vasopressin, may also be used for treatment of perioperative DI because of its potent antidiuretic effect with minimal pressor activity or other side effects. In the perioperative period, it may be given intravenously until intranasal administration can be started or resumed. The suggested IV dose is 0.5 to 4 mcg, with a single dose having a duration of action of 8 to 12 hours (Muglia and Majzoub, 2008). It is important to note that this dose of DDAVP is one fortieth to one fourth of that used to prevent bleeding in patients with von Willebrand's disease (vWD). The ease of intermittent dosing with DDAVP with low incidence of side effects must be balanced against the ability to titrate the continuous vasopressin infusion cited earlier. The long half-life of DDAVP (6 to 24 hours) in combination with intraoperative fluid administration may incur an increased chance of hyponatremia. In either case, careful monitoring of fluid balance is essential.

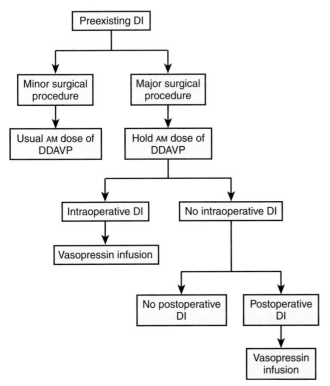

■ **FIGURE 36-1.** Perioperative management of patients with preexisting DI.

The anesthesiologist may occasionally encounter children who are receiving nightly nasal DDAVP for the treatment of enuresis. A review of its use reveals a negligible incidence of water intoxication (and no permanent effect on enuresis when treatment is stopped) (van Kerrebroeck, 2002). Given the known duration of action, DDAVP administered the night before outpatient surgery should not affect the urine output on the day of surgery.

Syndrome of Inappropriate Antidiuretic Hormone Secretion

Just as central DI is caused by ADH deficiency, syndrome of inappropriate ADH secretion (SIADH) is caused by an excess production of ADH that is inappropriate with respect to the state of the intravascular volume. The most common causes of SIADH are listed in Box 36-2. The hallmark of SIADH is hyponatremia in the face of high urine osmolality and sodium levels. A comparison of the urine and serum electrolyte status seen in DI and SIADH is presented in Table 36-4. The treatment for mild cases of SIADH is fluid restriction (50% to 60% of maintenance fluid requirement) or insensible loss (400 mL/m² per day), plus one half to three fourths of the urine output. If hyponatremia is severe enough to cause coma or seizures, treatment with hypertonic saline (3%) solution may be indicated, but caution should be employed because the administration of hypertonic saline may cause circulatory overload because the intravascular volume is already increased. A too-rapid rise of osmolarity (more than 20 mOsm/kg or more than 10 mmol/L of sodium in 24 hours) carries a risk of central pontine myelinolysis, a condition that can result in death (Laureno and Karp, 1997). This syndrome is thought to be caused by the sudden shrinkage of brain cells in response to rapidly increasing extracellular osmolality.

TABLE 36-4. Comparison of Diabetes Insipidus and SIADH

Laboratory Test	Diabetes Insipidus	SIADH
Urine specific gravity	≤1.005	≥1.005
Urine osmolality	50-200 mOsm/L	>200 mOsm/L
Serum osmolality	>280 mOsm/L	<280 mOsm/L
Serum sodium	High (usually >148 mEq/L)	Low (usually <132 mEq/L)
Urine sodium	<20 mmol/L	>20 mmol/L

Adrenal Insufficiency

Adrenal Insufficiency as a Result of Primary Abnormalities of the Hypothalamic-Pituitary-Adrenal Axis

Adrenal insufficiency is an uncommon disease in children, but when it occurs it is associated with significant implications for the anesthesiologist. The causes of adrenal insufficiency are listed in Box 36-3. Adrenal insufficiency may include glucocorticoid deficiency with or without mineralocorticoid deficiency (Box 36-4). Isolated hypoaldosteronism is rare. In the perioperative period, children with congenital adrenal insufficiency require glucocorticoid and mineralocorticoid replacement.

Chronic deficits in adrenal function result in the classic findings of Addison disease, including hyperpigmentation, weakness, and hyponatremia. The hyperpigmentation results from high levels of adrenocorticotropic hormone (ACTH) and unopposed melanophore-stimulating hormone caused by cortisol insufficiency. The additional presence of aldosterone insufficiency may produce hyponatremia, hyperkalemia, hypotension, and a small cardiac silhouette that results from hypovolemia (Keon and Templeton, 1993).

Box 36-2 Causes of Syndrome of Inappropriate Antidiuretic Hormone Secretion

CENTRAL NERVOUS SYSTEM
Infection
  Meningitis
  Encephalitis
  Abscess
  Guillain-Barré syndrome
Neoplastic
  Tumor
Trauma
  Subarachnoid hemorrhage

INFECTIOUS
Pneumonia
Tuberculosis
Shigellosis
Infant botulism

POSITIVE-PRESSURE VENTILATION

DRUGS
Vincristine
Vinblastine

Box 36-3 Causes of Adrenal Insufficiency

PRIMARY ADRENOCORTICAL INSUFFICIENCY
Congenital

ENZYME DEFICIENCY
Adrenal aplasia
Adrenocortical unresponsiveness to ACTH
Adrenoleukodystrophy or adrenomyeloneuropathy

TRAUMA OR SEPTIC
Adrenal hemorrhage of newborn
Adrenal hemorrhage of acute infection
Chronic hypoadrenocorticism (Addison disease)

SECONDARY TO DEFICIENT ACTH SECRETION
Hypopituitarism
Cessation of glucocorticoid therapy
Resection of unilateral cortisol-producing tumor
Infants born to steroid-treated mothers
Respiratory distress syndrome
Anencephaly
Inanition, anorexia nervosa

RELATED TO END-ORGAN UNRESPONSIVENESS
Pseudohyopoaldosteronism
  Cortisol resistance

Box 36-4 Signs and Symptoms of Adrenal Insufficiency

GLUCOCORTICOID DEFICIENCY
Fasting hypoglycemia
Increasing insulin sensitivity
Decreased gastric acidity
Gastrointestinal symptoms (nausea, vomiting)
Fatigue

MINERALOCORTICOID DEFICIENCY
Muscle weakness
Weight loss
Fatigue
Nausea, vomiting, anorexia
Salt craving
Hypotension
Electrolyte disturbance
Hypokalemia
Hyponatremia
Acidosis

ADRENAL ANDROGEN DEFICIENCY
Decreased pubic and axillary hair
Decreased libido

INCREASED β-LIPOPROTEIN LEVELS
Hyperpigmentation

Perioperative Steroid Management

The preoperative recognition of adrenal insufficiency and appropriate preoperative therapy minimize the likelihood of significant perioperative complications. Ninety percent of patients with congenital adrenal hyperplasia with adrenal insufficiency have 21-hydroxylase deficiency (Migeon and Donohoue, 1994). Virilization of the external genitalia occurs in female patients, and they often require surgical revision of their external genitalia. An abnormal genital pigmentation occurs in male patients, but this finding may be subtle. Infants with undiagnosed congenital adrenal hyperplasia may undergo exploratory laparotomy for acute abdomen because of nausea and vomiting. It is important to be attuned to the signs and symptoms in the history, physical examination, and laboratory evaluation that point to this diagnosis to prevent or treat shock, which may occur because of failure to administer steroid replacement.

Mineralocorticoid deficiency can be managed by administering saline solution and avoiding potassium in IV fluids. Mineralocorticoid secretion rates in children are similar to those in adults, and the replacement dose is independent of age and weight. Desoxycorticosterone acetate may be administered intramuscularly in a dose of 1 mg/day. The intramuscular injection may be replaced by a single daily oral dose of 9-fluorocortisol (Florinef, 0.05 to 0.1 mg) when it is clear that an oral medication can be tolerated and absorbed. When cortisol is administered perioperatively, it has sufficient mineralocorticoid activity to obviate the need for any other replacement; 20 mg of hydrocortisone has mineralocorticoid activity equivalent to 0.1 mg 9a-fluorocortisol (Miller et al., 2008).

Glucocorticoid deficiency is treated with cortisol (hydrocortisone) replacement. The importance of cortisol replacement for patients with known adrenal insufficiency should not

be underestimated, although vastly excessive doses are unwarranted. In the normal individual, the adrenal gland secretes 12 ± 2 mg of cortisol per square meter of body surface area every 24 hours (Kenny and Preeyasombat, 1966). The normal replacement dose prescribed for unstressed children is 25 mg/m^2 per day; the dose is double the normal production because of factors of bioavailability and half-life (Migeon and Donohoue, 1994). In response to stress (e.g., fever, acute illness, surgery, and anesthesia), the normal adrenal gland secretes 3 to 15 times this amount. Consequently, in the past, the recommendations for "stress" steroid coverage in the perioperative period ranged from 36 to 180 mg/m^2 per day.

More important than just the dose of steroid to be given, consideration should be devoted to the type of glucocorticoid administered, its half-life, the route of administration, and the timing of doses. The equivalencies for steroid preparations in terms of their relative glucocorticoid and mineralocorticoid effects are presented in Table 36-5. The most commonly cited recommendation for perioperative steroid coverage is hydrocortisone hemisuccinate (Solu-Cortef), given intravenously as 2 mg/kg immediately preoperatively and every 6 hours on the day of surgery, with reductions in the postoperative period depending on the degree of stress. Some practitioners feel that the half-life of hydrocortisone is so short that a 6-hour dosing interval may lead to periods of inadequate "coverage." These practitioners recommend a preinduction dose of 25 mg/m^2 of hydrocortisone given intravenously, followed by a continuous infusion of 50 mg/m^2 administered during the estimated period of anesthesia. Postoperatively, 50 mg/m^2 by continuous infusion is administered over the remainder of the first 24 hours. The total dose for the first 24 hours is 125 mg/m^2, or 10 times normal physiologic production (Migeon and Donohoue, 1994). The first bolus dose must be administered before induction of anesthesia rather than waiting for an IV cannula to be placed after inhalational induction because of the stress associated with anesthetic induction itself. In the postoperative period, the steroid dose is tapered to a level commensurate with the residual stress. It is replaced with the child's usual oral preparation when the child clearly can tolerate and absorb oral medication.

Hypothalamic-Pituitary-Adrenal Axis Suppression Caused by Exogenous Steroid Therapy

In addition to the diseases discussed previously, suppression of the hypothalamic-pituitary-adrenal (HPA) axis can also occur after exogenous steroid usage, such as that administered for the treatment of inflammatory conditions (e.g., Crohn disease and asthma) or autoimmune disease (e.g., lupus and juvenile rheumatoid arthritis). Nearly 60 years ago, it was reported that two patients developed irreversible shock perioperatively after glucocorticoid administration was stopped preoperatively (Fraser et al., 1952; Lewis et al., 1953). Both patients were found to have adrenal atrophy and hemorrhage at autopsy. These two cases led to suggestions for "stress" steroid coverage in the perioperative period. HPA suppression places steroid-dependent children at increased risk for complications in the perioperative period, because they may be unable to respond to stress with an appropriate increase in the adrenal secretion of glucocorticoid. Dosages of cortisol or its equivalent that exceed 15 mg/m^2 per day for more than 2 to 4 weeks invariably produce HPA suppression. A study in children with relatively short-term exposure to

TABLE 36-5. Potency of Commonly Used Steroid Preparations

Generic Name	Trade Name	Glucocorticoid Effect (= 100 mg Cortisol)	Sodium Retention Effect (= 0.1 mg Fludrocortisone [Florinef])	Duration of Action
Hydrocortisone	Hydrocortisone Solu-Cortef	100	20	S
Cortisone	Cortone	125	20	S
Prednisolone	Delta-Cortef	20	50	I
Prednisone	Deltasone Meticorten	25	50	I
Methylprednisolone	Medrol Solu-Medrol	15	No effect	I
Triamcinolone	Aristacort Kenacort	10	No effect	I
Dexamethasone	Decadron Hexadrol	1.5	No effect	L
Betamethasone	Celestone	3	No effect or salt loss	L
Aldosterone	NCA	300	0.1-0.04	—
9-Fluorocortisol	Florinef	6.5	0.1	I
Desoxycorticosterone acetate	NCA	0	1 (IM)	I

Adapted from Migeon C, Donohoue PA: Adrenal disorders. In Kappy MS et al., editors: *The diagnosis and treatment of endocrine disorders in childhood and adolescence*, Springfield, Ill, 1994, Charles C. Thomas.
S, Short (8-12 hr biological half-life); *I,* intermediate (12-36 hr biological half-life); *L,* long (36-72 hr biological half-life); *IM,* intramuscularly; *NCA,* not commercially available.

prednisolone or dexamethasone (5 and 3 weeks, respectively) for treatment of acute lymphoblastic leukemia showed that recovery of normal adrenal function (in response to ACTH stimulation) had a very wide range, occurring between 2 weeks and 8 months (Petersen et al., 2003).

Although high dosages, prolonged therapy, and short duration between discontinuance of therapy and the surgical procedure increase the likelihood of HPA suppression, no practical test is available that unequivocally identifies patients who will need intraoperative steroids. Metyrapone depresses the production of cortisol by the adrenal glands and can be used to test the capacity of the pituitary gland to respond to decreased plasma cortisol concentrations by increasing ACTH secretion (Haynes, 1990). However, this test takes 3 days, is expensive, and has the risk of inducing adrenal insufficiency. Similarly, an ACTH-stimulation test can be performed at great expense to test adrenal responsiveness. However, even if cost and time were not issues, a study has shown a poor correlation between tests that indicate normal HPA function and dose or duration of glucocorticoid therapy or basal cortisol levels (Schlaghecke et al., 1992). Clinically significant events rarely occur during the perioperative period in unsupplemented patients who were receiving steroid medications for diseases other than adrenal insufficiency. Nevertheless, the potential for symptomatic adrenal insufficiency, although rare, coupled with the low risk of steroid-induced complications for short-term administration, suggests that steroids should be given in uncertain cases. If steroid therapy has been discontinued within the previous year, Donohoue (2005) makes the following recommendations:

- If the dose of the glucocorticoid administered was less than replacement levels, independent of the duration of

administration, there will be no major HPA suppression and therefore no need for supplementation.
- If the dose of glucocorticoid administered was greater than replacement levels, HPA suppression will occur. If treatment lasted fewer than 2 weeks, suppression is transient, with prompt recovery (fewer than 2 weeks). If treatment lasted longer than 2 weeks, HPA suppression may persist for 1 week to 6 months, with 50% of patients recovering function within 6 weeks. This is the case even if the glucocorticoid was administered on an every-other-day basis.

HPA suppression also can result from modes of steroid administration other than oral, including topical, nasal spray, and inhalers. Although adrenal suppression is rarely symptomatic with these modes of administration, some drugs, especially fluticasone propionate, in high doses have been associated with growth failure and adrenal suppression (Duplantier et al., 1998). With surgical stress, patients with adrenal suppression may become symptomatic, as has been reported for other kinds of stress. The patients reported by Drake et al. (2002) all had been taking fluticasone and had hypoglycemia at times of stress from intercurrent illness. Numerous cases of acute adrenal crisis have been reported in children receiving inhaled corticosteroids (ICS) for prolonged periods (Randell et al., 2003). Anesthesiologists should have a high index of suspicion of adrenal suppression if an asthmatic child on inhaled steroids develops hypotension or hypoglycemia in the perioperative period.

For children who have been on prolonged courses of high-dose steroids (e.g., for asthma or treatment of acute lymphocytic leukemia), the glucocorticoid regimen should follow that described earlier for patients with adrenal insufficiency. The dose given should be commensurate with the normal physiologic corticosteroid production in response to stress (as described) and does not need to be a multiple of the pharmacologic dose being administered for the underlying medical illness.

The dose administered should also be proportional to the perceived degree of surgical stress. For brief procedures, such as upper endoscopy, a single preoperative dose of steroids is suggested (50 mg/m^2 of hydrocortisone); for more complicated cases, such as appendectomy or major intraabdominal operations, 100 mg/m^2 is administered as a continuous infusion or divided into 4 doses per day. This dose is usually continued for 1 to 3 days after more complex surgical procedures (Krasner, 1999). The dose is tapered postoperatively and replaced with the patient's usual oral steroid preparation and dose when the child is able to tolerate oral medications. The dose that these patients commonly take for the underlying disease often exceeds even maximum "stress" doses described for congenitally adrenal insufficient patients, and treatment required for the underlying disease may limit further tapering of the steroid dose. A small study of adults comparing "stress steroids" with saline showed no adverse effects in patients who continued their usual steroid dose for their underlying disease (Glowniak and Loriaux, 1997).

Thyroid Disorders

Hypothyroidism

Hypothyroidism occurs because of abnormally low production of thyroid hormone. It may be caused by primary thyroid dysfunction or result from pituitary failure with decreased production of thyroid-stimulating hormone (TSH). Normal values for routinely performed thyroid function tests are presented in Table 36-6, and the interpretation of these test results with regard to diagnosis is presented in Table 36-7.

Primary thyroid dysfunction may be congenital or acquired. Congenital hypothyroidism usually appears in infancy. Classic features in the infant include large fontanels, wide sutures, large tongue, umbilical hernia, and decreased deep tendon reflexes. In the older child, manifestations include slow heart rate, narrow pulse pressure, growth failure, hypothermia, and cold intolerance. Severe hypothyroidism is rare but may be associated with coma, cardiovascular collapse, hyponatremia, hypothermia, and respiratory failure. Keon and Templeton (1993) reviewed the anesthetic management of patients with hypothyroidism and stressed the importance of correcting hypothyroidism gradually over a 2-week period. Sudden death has been reported in children with myxedematous heart disease 2 to 3 weeks into therapy (LaFranchi, 1979). It is suggested that these children receive one fourth of the maintenance dose of thyroid hormone (6 to 8 mcg/kg per day for an infant), with gradual incremental increases over 2 to 4 weeks until a maintenance dose is reached (Custer and Rau, 2009). Patients who are adequately treated will have normal thyroid hormone and TSH levels. Patients who do not respond to oral thyroid replacement may be given IV triiodothyronine (T3; loading dose of 0.7 mcg/kg), followed by an infusion titrated to T3 and TSH levels. Severe cardiac dysfunction in such a patient improved with T3 therapy (Mason et al., 2001). Patients with incompletely restored thyroid hormone levels may require hemodynamic monitoring and support to maintain hemodynamic stability. Patients with severe hypothyroidism may have

TABLE 36-6. Thyroid Function Tests

Test	Age	Normal
T$_4$ RIA (mcg/dL)	1-3 days	11-21.5
	1-4 weeks	8.2-16.6
	1-12 months	7.2-15.6
	1-5 years	7.3-15
	6-10 years	6.4-13.3
	11-15 years	5.6-11.7
	16-20 years	4.2-11.8
T$_3$ RU		25%-35%*
T index		1.25-4.20†
Free T$_4$ (ng/dL)	1-10 days	0.6-2
	>10 days	0.7-1.7
T$_3$ RIA (ng/dL)	1-3 days	100-380
	1-4 weeks	99-310
	1-12 months	102-264
	1-5 years	105-269
	6-10 years	94-241
	11-15 years	83-213
	16-20 years	80-210
TSH RIA (mIU/mL)	1-3 days	<2.5-13.3
	1-4 weeks	0.6-10
	1 month-15 years	0.6-6.3
	16-20 years	0.2-7.6
TBG (mg/dL)	1-3 days	—
	1-4 weeks	0.5-4.5
	1-12 months	1.6-3.6
	1-5 years	1.3-2.8
	6-20 years	1.4-2.6
Reverse T$_3$‡ (mg/dL)	Newborns	90-250
	Adults	10-50

Modified from Johnson KB, editor: *The Harriet Lane Handbook*, St. Louis, 1993, Mosby.
*Measures thyroid hormone binding, not T$_3$.
†T$_4$ RIA × T$_3$ RU.
‡Reverse T$_3$.
RIA, Radioimmunoassay; *RU,* resin uptake; *T$_3$,* triiodothyronine; *T$_4$,* thyroxine; *TBG,* thyroid-binding globulin; *TSH,* thyroid-stimulating hormone.

TABLE 36-7. Interpretation of Thyroid Function Tests

	T$_4$ RIA	T$_3$ RU	T Index	Free T$_4$	TSH
Primary hypothyroidism	L	L	L	L	H
Secondary hypothyroidism	L	L	L	L	L, N, or H
TBG deficiency	L	H	N	N	N
Hyperthyroidism	H	H	H	H	L

Modified from Siberry GK, Iannone R, editors: *The Harriet Lane handbook,* St. Louis, 2000, Mosby.
L, Low; *H,* high; *N,* normal; *RIA,* radioimmunoassay; *RU,* resin uptake; *T$_3$,* triiodothyronine; *T$_4$,* thyroxine; *TBG,* thyroid-binding globulin; *TSH,* thyroid-stimulating hormone.

associated adrenal insufficiency, and if so, they should receive stress steroid coverage as outlined earlier.

The anesthetic care of the symptomatic patient with hypothyroidism can be problematic and requires caution when any depressant medications are given. Prolonged effects may result

TABLE 36-8. Anesthetic Implications of Hypothyroidism

System	Anesthetic Considerations
Pharmacologic	Possible lower MAC value; prolonged recovery from opioid anesthesia
Cardiovascular	Decreased cardiac output, heart rate, and stroke volume; increased PVR and decreased intravascular volume; myocardial depression resulting from impaired cellular metabolism or myxedematous infiltration; baroreceptor dysfunction
Respiratory	Abnormal response to hypercapnia and hypoxia
Thermal regulation	Hypothermia resulting from reduced basal metabolic rate; reduced ability to increase core temperature
Endocrine	Increased incidence of adrenal insufficiency; consideration for stress steroid coverage
Metabolic	SIADH; hypoglycemia with prolonged fasting
Gastrointestinal	Delayed gastric emptying; consideration for full stomach precaution

MAC, Minimum alveolar concentration; *PVR*, peripheral vascular resistance; *SIADH*, syndrome of inappropriate antidiuretic hormone.

from decreased drug metabolism. Important considerations in the management of hypothyroidism as described by Keon and Templeton (1993) are outlined in Table 36-8. Invasive monitoring may be indicated when significant blood loss or fluid shifts occur. Care should be taken intraoperatively to minimize heat loss. Postoperative care should include monitoring of oxygen saturation, blood pressure, heart rate, and respiratory rate; postoperative ventilation may be necessary in the patient with delayed emergence from anesthesia.

Hyperthyroidism

Hyperthyroidism is a syndrome produced by excess levels of circulating thyroid hormone. The most common causes are congenital hyperthyroidism and Graves disease (i.e., toxic goiter). Less commonly, acute suppurative thyroiditis, hyperfunctioning thyroid carcinoma, thyrotoxicosis factitia (i.e., exogenous administration of thyroid hormone), and toxic uninodular goiter (i.e., Plummer disease) may produce this syndrome. McCune-Albright syndrome (i.e., precocious puberty with polyostotic fibrous dysplasia) is also commonly associated with hyperthyroidism (Jones, 1988).

Congenital Hyperthyroidism

Congenital hyperthyroidism is a transient phenomenon seen in newborns that results from the transplacental transfer of thyroid-stimulating antibody from mothers who commonly have a history of Graves disease. Most of these infants have a goiter and typically appear anxious and restless or irritable. Signs of hypermetabolism, including tachycardia, tachypnea, and elevated temperature, may be present. In the severely affected infant, symptoms may progress to weight loss, severe hypertension, and high-output cardiac failure with hepatomegaly (Smith et al., 2001). Appropriate medical therapy (methimazole) should be instituted early. Because maternal immunoglobulins have a short half-life in infants, the hyperthyroid state resolves in a few weeks to a few months, and it sometimes may be followed by a period of hypothyroidism (Higuchi et al., 2001).

Graves Disease

Diffuse toxic goiter (Graves disease) is the most common cause of hyperthyroidism in children. Its peak incidence occurs during adolescence, and it is five times more common in girls than in boys. The clinical course is generally gradual, with symptoms developing over 6 to 12 months. Early signs include motor hyperactivity, emotional disturbances, and nervousness. Affected children are progressively more irritable and restless and may have increased sweating, increased appetite, palpitations, and tremors of their fingers. Most children have obvious exophthalmos and an enlarged palpable thyroid. The cardiopulmonary symptoms of hyperthyroidism include systolic hypertension, tachycardia, palpitations, dyspnea, and cardiac enlargement, which may progress to frank cardiac decompensation. On rare occasions, atrial fibrillation or mitral regurgitation may also be present.

Thyroid Storm

An acute onset of hyperthermia, severe tachycardia, and restlessness comprises the syndrome of acute uncompensated thyrotoxicosis, or "thyroid storm." Without appropriate and timely therapy, the patient's condition may deteriorate to delirium, coma, and death. Therapy includes treatment of hyperthermia by cooling, maintenance of intravascular volume with balanced salt solutions, and β-adrenergic blockers such as propranolol titrated to ameliorate the cardiovascular response. Specific thyroid suppression therapy with propylthiouracil should be instituted. The clinical presentation of thyroid storm may occur intraoperatively, and this hypermetabolic state may be mistaken for malignant hyperthermia (Peters et al., 1981). The use of dantrolene mitigated the clinical signs in a patient who turned out to have thyroid storm (Bennett and Wainwright, 1989). It is well known that perioperative surgical stress can trigger the development of thyroid storm in a patient with previously unrecognized thyrotoxicosis (Stevens, 1983). For this reason, patients with signs and symptoms that may indicate the presence of hyperthyroidism should be carefully evaluated. Patients should be rendered euthyroid before any elective surgery, even if it is minor.

Laboratory Evaluation

Serum levels of thyroxine (T4) and T3 are usually elevated in hyperthyroidism. TSH secretion is suppressed and may be unmeasurable. T3 toxicosis (elevated T3 level with normal amounts of T4) is more common in adult patients and rarely seen in children. For borderline cases, thyrotropin-releasing hormone (TRH) stimulation tests may be needed. Many patients with Graves disease of recent onset may have elevated levels of thyroid-stimulating immunoglobulin. Radionuclide scans can also be helpful in making a diagnosis. If a large goiter is present, neck radiographs, computed tomography (CT) scans, or magnetic resonance imaging (MRI) may be used to evaluate the degree of tracheal compression and deviation.

Treatment

The management of hyperthyroidism is aimed at controlling the cardiovascular effects. β-adrenergic receptor blockade, usually with propranolol (1 to 2 mg/kg per day), is titrated to effect. Antithyroid medications include propylthiouracil and methimazole, both of which inhibit the incorporation of inorganic iodide into organic compounds. Propylthiouracil inhibits the conversion of T4 to T3. Although early studies suggested that these agents might inhibit the formation of thyroid antibodies, later studies that included careful histopathologic analysis have shown this to be false (Paschke et al., 1995). The Food and Drug Administration (FDA) has recently recommended that propylthiouracil not be administered to pediatric patients because of reports of liver failure associated with its use. Methimazole is the antithyroid medication recommended for use in infants, children, and adolescents (FDA, 2009). Saturated solutions of potassium iodide may be administered orally (1 drop every 8 hours) to suppress thyroid hormone secretion. The clinical response to therapy is evident in 1 to 3 weeks, and the patient may require up to 3 months for adequate control to be achieved. Patients must have appropriate, regular surveillance to ensure that the T3 and T4 levels are in the normal range and that TSH concentrations are normal. Clinically, the patient demonstrates a euthyroid state by return of the heart rate, blood pressure, and reflexes to normal.

Radioactive iodine is often used to treat hyperthyroidism in adults. However, such therapy is avoided in children because of side effects such as thyroid cancer, genetic damage to germ cells, and a higher incidence of hypothyroidism than occurs with pharmacologic therapy.

Anesthetic Management

Preoperatively, patients should be pharmacologically euthyroid. Any residual cardiovascular signs and symptoms should be well controlled through the use of a β-adrenergic receptor blocker. Esmolol is an excellent choice for intraoperative use. A large goiter may produce tracheal deviation or compression, and the possibility of airway compromise should be evaluated preoperatively with radiographic studies. Any commonly used sedative may be given for premedication. Atropine and other anticholinergics should be avoided or used with extreme caution, because they decrease sweating and may interfere with thermoregulation. Medications, including antithyroid drugs and β-adrenergic blockers, should be administered through the morning of surgery.

Intraoperative Management of Patients for Thyroidectomy

In children with large goiters who have a compromised airway, anesthesia should be managed with caution, as in any other child with upper airway obstruction. A sedated fiberoptic intubation may be chosen, or an inhalational induction performed, with maintenance of spontaneous ventilation until the airway is secured. If a large goiter has caused prolonged tracheal compression, a segment of tracheomalacia may exist, and an armored endotracheal tube (ETT) may be indicated.

For patients without issues of tracheal compression, anesthesia may be induced with thiopental or propofol. However, if the patient's laboratory evaluation indicates a continued hyperthyroid state, ketamine should be avoided because of its effect on catecholamine release. Mask inductions may be prolonged in these patients because of increased cardiac output, resulting in a slower rise in the alveolar concentration of the anesthetic if the ventilation is kept constant. Minute ventilation may be reduced if significant airway obstruction resulting from goiter or tracheomalacia is present. Care should be taken to lubricate, pad, and appropriately protect the eyes, especially if they are protuberant because of Graves disease.

With respect to choice of drugs, muscle relaxants with few cardiovascular side effects, such as cisatracurium, vecuronium, or rocuronium, provide a potential benefit by minimizing the occurrence of tachycardia. Similarly, for the maintenance of general anesthesia, anesthetics that have sympathomimetic effects should be avoided. If the child is in a hypermetabolic state, drug biotransformation may be accelerated; therefore, agents such as halothane, which has toxic metabolic products, are potentially more hazardous. Another reason to avoid halothane is its sensitization of the myocardium to catecholamines. If the patient is in a hypermetabolic state, controlled ventilation should be employed during the surgical procedure to minimize the development of hypercapnia, which can contribute to further sympathetic stimulation.

Anesthetic management at the conclusion of surgery may include deep extubation, with direct or fiberoptic laryngoscopy performed to evaluate the presence or absence of vocal cord paralysis, which may result from surgical trauma to the recurrent laryngeal nerve (traction or transection). Care should be taken after extubation to observe for signs of airway obstruction as a result of residual tracheomalacia. The decision to evaluate the airway prospectively at the time of extubation should be made jointly by the anesthesiologist and surgeon and should be based on the likelihood of residual tracheal obstruction caused by tracheomalacia or of vocal cord paralysis because the surgeon thinks that surgical trauma is likely.

Postoperative Care

Children who have undergone thyroidectomy require close observation in the postoperative period (Fewins et al., 2003). They may develop postextubation croup or upper airway obstruction as a result of paralysis of the vocal cords, tetany (hypocalcemia), residual tracheomalacia, or tracheal compression resulting from a hematoma. Patients with postextubation croup may respond to supportive measures, including humidified supplemental oxygen, nebulized racemic epinephrine, and possibly, continuous positive airway pressure (CPAP) or bilevel positive airway pressure (BiPAP). Occasionally, these patients require brief reintubation before they can be successfully extubated. Unilateral vocal cord paralysis may go unnoticed or be associated with only mild stridor. Bilateral vocal cord paralysis, on the other hand, may manifest as severe stridor and upper airway obstruction. The child with bilateral vocal cord paralysis requires reintubation for airway support. A muscle relaxant such as rocuronium should be used to facilitate reintubation to avoid damage to the abducted cords. If the paralysis is prolonged, the child may subsequently require tracheostomy. Compression of the trachea by a hematoma may occur immediately after the operation or over the course of several hours. The child requires reintubation and surgical evacuation of the hematoma to relieve tracheal compression. Opening the wound in the recovery room may be necessary and lifesaving. After the extrinsic obstruction has been relieved and the incision closed again (if necessary), the child may be safely extubated.

Inadvertent resection of the parathyroid glands during thyroidectomy may result in acute hypoparathyroidism after surgery. Clinical signs of hypocalcemia may become manifest within the first postoperative day or take as long as 72 hours to develop. A low serum-ionized calcium level and a low concentration of parathyroid hormone are diagnostic. Clinical hypocalcemia, including tetany, is treated with IV calcium therapy. Surgical manipulation of the trachea and neck tissues can also lead to subcutaneous emphysema and the more serious possibility of pneumomediastinum or pneumothorax. Postoperative evaluation should include radiologic examination of the chest if respiratory distress occurs.

Pheochromocytoma

Pheochromocytoma is a catecholamine-secreting tumor of chromaffin cells that most commonly arises in the adrenal medulla (DiGeorge, 1987). It may be found anywhere along the abdominal sympathetic chain, but it is most commonly near the aorta at the inferior mesenteric artery or the aortic bifurcation. Other sites include the neck, the mediastinum, and the walls of the bladder or ureters. Pheochromocytoma is a rare neoplasm in the pediatric population. Fewer than 5% of reported cases occur in children. The tumors may occur bilaterally or at multiple sites. This condition can be inherited as an autosomal-dominant trait (most often in association with von Hippel–Lindau syndrome) or as part of a multiple endocrine neoplasia (MEN) type II or III (Table 36-9).

The abnormally high plasma levels of epinephrine and norepinephrine produce a clinical syndrome with signs and symptoms related directly to the level of each hormone present in the patient. Hypertension is common and often leads to hypertensive encephalopathy and seizures. In particular, paroxysmal hypertension is most suggestive of pheochromocytoma. The patient may also complain of headaches and palpitations, pallor, sweating, and vomiting. In severe cases, patients develop chest pain that radiates to the arms, pulmonary edema, and cardiac decompensation. The catecholamine-induced hypermetabolism also can cause patients to have a voracious appetite but still lose weight and become cachectic. Polyuria, polydipsia, and abdominal pain may occur and be confused with diabetes mellitus.

Diagnosis

It is extremely important to establish the diagnosis of pheochromocytoma before induction of anesthesia and start of surgery. The significant cardiovascular effects of excess catecholamines can pose difficulties for the anesthesiologist and endanger the patient during the perioperative period if an appropriate diagnosis is not made preoperatively. These tumors can produce paroxysms of hypertension and other symptoms. Between paroxysms, the patient may be totally asymptomatic, making diagnosis extremely difficult. The demonstration of increased levels of catecholamines is the most specific diagnostic test. Although pheochromocytomas can produce norepinephrine and epinephrine, the predominant catecholamine produced in children is norepinephrine, which leads to chronic hypertension. Urine catecholamine concentrations are directly proportional to circulating levels, and determination of 24-hour urinary excretion of the primary catecholamines and their metabolites (i.e., 3-methoxy 4-hydroxy vanillyl-mandelic acid [VMA] and metanephrine) used to be the primary means of establishing the diagnosis. The plasma free metanephrine determination has better sensitivity (100%) and specificity (94%). Because normal values differ with age, it is important to use age-specific norms when interpreting results (Weise et al., 2002).

The differential diagnosis includes renal vascular disease, hyperthyroidism, Cushing syndrome, coarctation of the aorta, adrenal cortical tumors, and essential hypertension. Cerebral disorders, diabetes mellitus, and DI may produce similar symptoms. Neoplasms of neural origin (e.g., neuroblastoma or ganglioneuroma) may also secrete catecholamines.

Before any contemplated anesthesia and surgery, the patient must undergo a complete evaluation to localize the tumor, including CT and MRI scans. Magnetic resonance angiography (MRA) and venography (MRV) may be used to identify vascular supply. A radionuclide (I-131 metaiodobenzylguanidine [MIBG]) scan may also help to localize the tumor. Differential venous catheterization may be needed to obtain blood from various sites for catecholamine levels if multiple tumors are suspected. Sedation or anesthesia may be required to perform these studies in infants and children. Before sedation for these diagnostic studies, hemodynamic abnormalities must be normalized. Drugs that induce catecholamine secretion or histamine release should be avoided. General anesthesia for the diagnostic procedures must be conducted with the same extreme caution one would exercise for resection of the tumor itself.

Preoperative Preparation and Evaluation

Preoperative evaluation should include the measurement of serum electrolytes, determination of renal function, and fasting blood glucose. Excessive serum epinephrine levels may be associated with hyperglycemia and hypokalemia. An electrocardiogram and echocardiogram are important to evaluate cardiac rhythm, size, and function. Some patients with pheochromocytoma have a catecholamine-induced cardiomyopathy with decreased left ventricular contractility. The patient should be evaluated for associated endocrinopathies that may be present as part of MEN type II or III.

Symptomatic treatment includes the administration of phenoxybenzamine over a period of several days to weeks before surgery. Phenoxybenzamine is a long-acting, orally administered α-adrenergic blocking agent that attenuates the effects of catecholamines on the peripheral circulation by blocking excessive vasoconstriction (Hoffman and Lefkowitz, 1990). The starting dose of phenoxybenzamine is 0.2 mg/kg once daily (maximum adult dose, 10 mg) (Taketomo et al., 2008). Then both dose and frequency are gradually increased (up to 3 times a day)

TABLE 36-9. Multiple Endocrine Neoplasia Syndromes

MEN Syndrome	Affected Organs	Disorder
Werner syndrome (type I, familial)	Parathyroid gland; pancreas; pituitary gland	Hypercalcemia; hypoglycemia; peptic ulcer
Sipple syndrome (type II, autosomal dominant)	Thyroid and parathyroid glands; adrenal medulla	Medullary carcinoma; hypercalcemia; pheochromocytoma
Type III	Nervous system; thyroid gland; adrenal medulla	Multiple neuromas; medullary carcinoma; pheochromocytoma

MEN, Multiple endocrine neoplasia.

until a clinical effect is obtained; that is, the patient's hematocrit decreases (because of vasodilation and increased blood volume), and the patient develops orthostatic changes in vital signs. Long-standing vasoconstriction produced by chronically high catecholamine levels causes decreased intravascular volume. Although the use of phenoxybenzamine restores vascular capacity to normal, increased oral fluid intake should accompany administration of phenoxybenzamine to avoid severe orthostatic changes. In some children, β-adrenergic blocking drugs such as propranolol may be needed to control heart rate and blood pressure. However, β-blocking agents should never be used without concurrent α-blockade therapy because of the deleterious effects of unopposed α-agonism, which may result in cardiac failure as a result of increased afterload. Labetalol may have a role in the management of pheochromocytoma, because it has α- and β-adrenergic blocking properties (Blom et al., 1987). It can be useful in minimizing the cardiovascular effects of excess catecholamines during the perioperative period, but it is not as potent an a blocker as is phenoxybenzamine for preoperative treatment.

In addition to pharmacologic preparation, children with pheochromocytoma benefit from preoperative sedation to reduce the release of catecholamines caused by anxiety. Oral or IV midazolam alone or in combination with an opioid provides a good level of sedation.

Anesthetic Induction

Induction of anesthesia is accomplished with IV anesthetics. Ketamine is specifically contraindicated, because it induces catecholamine release. Halothane should be avoided, because it may sensitize the myocardium to catecholamines and produce dysrhythmias. Mask induction with sevoflurane is well tolerated if hemodynamic parameters are well controlled, and IV cannula placement can be deferred until after induction. Intubation may proceed in the usual fashion, facilitated by a hemodynamically neutral nondepolarizing muscle relaxant such as vecuronium. Pancuronium, which causes muscarinic blockade and tachycardia, should be avoided. Despite the fact that atracurium causes histamine release and vasodilation, it has been used safely in adult patients with pheochromocytoma (Prys-Roberts, 2000). Before intubation, IV lidocaine (1 mg/kg), fentanyl (2 to 5 mcg/kg), or both are effective in minimizing the hemodynamic response to intubation.

Intraoperative Management

After induction of anesthesia, an intraarterial catheter is placed to monitor the blood pressure continuously. Before induction, a reliable automated blood pressure device can provide frequent, accurate blood pressure measurements. A central venous catheter provides direct and reliable access for the assessment of intravascular volume and for infusions of fluids and emergency medications.

Anesthesia may be maintained with isoflurane or sevoflurane, air, and oxygen. Both anesthetic agents have been used without exacerbation of hypertension, despite the fact that they do not blunt the production of norepinephrine in response to surgical stimulation (Suzukawa et al., 1983). Desflurane should be avoided because of its tendency to cause tachycardia and hypertension. The addition of moderately large doses of fentanyl (10 mcg/kg) or remifentanil (0.3 to 1 mcg/kg per minute) minimizes the stress response and provides stable hemodynamics. If remifentanil is chosen, it is important to give a longer-acting opioid before the end of surgery to avoid hypertension as a result of pain on awakening. Adjunctive use of epidural anesthesia (i.e., local anesthetic with or without a small dose of fentanyl) is an excellent method of reducing the stress response and catecholamine release caused by usual surgical stimulation. However, none of these anesthetic strategies blocks catecholamine release that results from direct surgical manipulation of tumor tissue.

Historically, controlling blood pressure during the induction and maintenance of anesthesia has been accomplished by an infusion of sodium nitroprusside or phentolamine. However, resection is increasingly being performed using a laparoscopic technique, and either nicardipine or magnesium sulfate infusions are used to maintain vasodilation and normotension during this type of surgery (Pretorius et al., 1998; Minami et al., 2002). In addition to propranolol use preoperatively, esmolol has been effective as a continuous infusion titrated to the level of surgical stimulation (Nicholas et al., 1988). Infusions of only short-acting vasodilators are recommended for control of hypertension before tumor resection, because with removal of the tumor, vasodilation caused by a persistent blockade and loss of excess catecholamines may lead to precipitous hypotension. Phenoxybenzamine has a long half-life; therefore, some physicians recommend discontinuing it 24 hours before surgery to decrease the likelihood that persistent vasodilation caused by a blockade will cause severe hypotension after the tumor is removed because of withdrawal of the catecholamines of tumor origin (Prys-Roberts, 2000). Hypotension is best treated with discontinuation of vasodilator infusions, titration of anesthetic agents, and administration of crystalloid or colloid and blood products, if it is indicated by the magnitude of blood loss. If these measures are ineffective, vasopressors may be necessary, but the patient may be relatively resistant to α-agonists as a result of persistent α-blockade. If this occurs, judicious use of small doses of more potent, direct-acting vasoconstrictors (e.g., norepinephrine or epinephrine) may be necessary. Recently, vasopressin infusion has been effective in this situation (Deutsch and Tobias, 2006).

During surgery, arterial blood gases, serum glucose, urine output, and body temperature should be closely monitored. Hyperglycemia may occur in response to high catecholamine levels. Hypoglycemia may occur when the tumor is removed and catecholamine levels decrease. Because of the potential for dysrhythmias, the electrocardiogram should also be vigilantly observed. At the end of surgery, the muscle paralysis is reversed. Extubation can be accomplished when the patient meets all normal extubation criteria.

Postoperative Care

Postoperatively, the patient should be observed in an intensive care unit, with continuous monitoring of the arterial blood pressure and electrocardiogram. Hypertension usually resolves within 24 to 48 hours after surgery. If symptoms persist beyond this period, further investigation for residual pheochromocytoma is warranted. Good postoperative analgesia is provided with epidural infusion (if an open procedure was performed) or IV patient- (parent- or nurse-) controlled analgesia.

RESPIRATORY DISORDERS

Upper Respiratory Tract Infection

Viral upper respiratory tract infections (URIs) are mild processes that do not preclude school attendance and other routine activities. However, URIs hold much greater significance for anesthesiologists. For many anesthesiologists, it is standard practice to avoid general anesthesia for elective surgery in children with URIs because of the respiratory complications during and after anesthesia reported in multiple small case series (McGill et al., 1979; Cohen and Cameron, 1991; Konarzewski et al., 1992; Williams et al., 1992). Unfortunately, the vexing problem of runny noses in children is accentuated by the difficulty in differentiating URIs from other causes, such as allergic rhinitis, which does not increase the risk of complications.

Pathophysiology of Upper Tract Respiratory Infection

Many investigators suggest that complications, including bronchospasm, intraoperative hypoxemia with an increased alveolar-arterial oxygen gradient, and postoperative hypoxemia, occur more often in children who undergo anesthesia while they have URIs (McGill et al., 1979; Olsson, 1987; DeSoto et al., 1988). The proclivity for these complications may be related to peripheral airway abnormalities, which have been demonstrated experimentally in adult humans and animals infected with viral respiratory pathogens (Johanson et al., 1969; Fridy et al., 1974; Dueck et al., 1991). These abnormalities include decreased diffusing capacity and increased closing volume—factors that can predispose patients to intrapulmonary shunting and hypoxemia, especially when they are combined with the effect of general anesthesia on lung volumes (decreased functional residual capacity) (see Chapter 3, Respiratory Physiology in Infants and Children) (Murat et al., 1985). These studies were done in adults who had infections involving their entire respiratory tracts rather than isolated URIs, and their results may support separation of treatment of patients with truly isolated URIs from those with any symptoms of more global airway or pulmonary parenchymal involvement (lower respiratory tract infection). Although the mechanisms by which viral respiratory infections lead to alterations in airway function are unclear, these experimental studies support the clinical impression that increased risk of perioperative hypoxemia occurs in patients with recent viral respiratory infection.

Empey et al. (1976) demonstrated in adult patients that acute viral respiratory tract infection (influenza) produced marked bronchial reactivity to experimental bronchoconstrictor challenge that may persist for 6 weeks. Mechanisms by which viral infections lead to increased airway reactivity include the release of immunologic and inflammatory mediators such as leukotrienes, bradykinin, and histamine, which cause bronchoconstriction. Vagal-mediated mechanisms may be involved, because viral infections have been associated with changes in muscarinic receptors on airway smooth muscle (Fryer et al., 1990). Tissue concentrations of important enzymes such as neutral endopeptidase, which break down the neuropeptides that cause bronchoconstriction, are also decreased in viral infections (Jacoby et al., 1988; Dusser et al., 1989). However, these patients and animals cannot be said to have only URIs, because the airways below the larynx are also clearly affected. Patients whose infections are truly uncomplicated URIs or those with noninfectious causes of runny nose should be differentiated from those who have evidence of lower respiratory involvement.

Perioperative Risk

Many case reports in the literature document that in the perioperative period children with URIs have respiratory complications, including bronchospasm, stridor caused by subglottic edema, hypoxia, and atelectasis (McGill et al., 1979; Konarzewski et al., 1992; Williams et al., 1992). Three prospective studies have shown that patients with an active or recent URI had a 2- to 10-fold higher risk of bronchospasm or laryngospasm (Olsson and Hallen, 1984; Olsson, 1987; Cohen and Cameron, 1991). The incidence was higher among younger children, especially those younger than 2 years and those whose tracheas were intubated (Cohen and Cameron, 1991). Retrospective studies of much larger numbers of patients show a higher risk of respiratory complications may actually exist in asymptomatic children with history of URI within the 2 to 4 weeks preceding surgery than in those with acute URI (Tait and Knight, 1987b; Tait et al., 2001). Other studies found that the factors that increase the risk of adverse events were history of prematurity or reactive airways disease (RAD), parental smoking, copious secretions, nasal congestion intubation, and airway surgery (Tait et al., 2000, 2001). Despite this increased risk of adverse events, complications usually were easily treated and were not associated with any significant prolonged morbidity (Rolf and Cote, 1992; Tait et al., 2000, 2001). However, some patients in one study developed atelectasis severe enough to require bronchoscopy and prolonged postoperative mechanical ventilation. Although most of these studies evaluated children undergoing relatively minor elective surgery, another study reported that children with URI symptoms at the time of cardiac surgery also had increased risks for respiratory and other complications, including nonrespiratory infection (Malviya et al., 2003). Despite these findings, patients' hospital stays were not prolonged, and the incidence of long-term sequelae was not increased.

One study found that children with URIs who undergo mask halothane-nitrous oxide-oxygen anesthesia for myringotomy surgery had reduced severity and duration of URI symptoms in the postoperative period (Tait and Knight, 1987a). However, this reduction in symptoms may have resulted from the drainage and removal of infectious foci by the surgical procedure rather than from the beneficial effects of general anesthetics. Other investigators have reported no significant respiratory complications when children with URI were anesthetized (Hinkle, 1989; Jacoby and Hirshman, 1991). It is extraordinarily difficult to integrate the contradictory conclusions of these various series of patients to develop a logical algorithm for dealing with the child with a URI.

Anesthetic Decision Making

It is apparent that no consensus has been reached in the literature or in the general anesthesia community with regard to the wisdom and safety of anesthetizing children with active or recent URIs. The bulk of the literature, clinical and experimental, suggests that recent viral infection increases the perioperative risk for respiratory complications, albeit mild and treatable, when the surgical and anesthetic plans require intubation. In children with underlying RAD, the risk for pulmonary complications immediately after acute URI is much greater than in the normal patient population, making intraoperative broncho-spasm much more likely. The threshold for postponing surgery in the asthmatic child with a recent URI who requires intuba-tion is much lower. These risks must be weighed against the physiologic, psychological, and financial implications of delay-ing surgery.

The most conservative approach to the child with a URI or recent URI is to postpone elective procedures for 1 to 2 weeks for uncomplicated rhinorrhea, congestion, and nonproduc-tive cough and for 4 to 6 weeks for patients with lower-airway involvement (e.g., wheezing or productive cough). However, this may be an overly cautious and somewhat unrealistic rec-ommendation. Children without other health conditions have an average of 3 to 8 colds per year, and children whose mothers smoke, who live in crowded conditions, and who attend day-care centers have a 61% incidence of URIs over a 2-week period (Fig. 36-2) (Fleming et al., 1987). It may be nearly impossible to find a time when the child does not have a URI or is not recov-ering from one. The needs of the family must be considered. Often, parents have traveled significant distances, taken time off from work, and made alternative childcare arrangements for their other children. Because the available data do not clearly indicate a single best approach to these patients, each anesthe-siologist should develop a consistent approach appropriate to the individual practice.

The following is a summary of an approach to the child with symptoms of URI. First, many children undergo operations directed at ameliorating their chronic upper respiratory tract symptoms. In cases such as myringotomy with tube placement, tonsillectomy, adenoidectomy, and cleft palate repair, the pro-cedures are not automatically canceled or postponed unless the child's signs and symptoms are clearly "different from base-line" or clearly involve more than the upper respiratory tract. Children who undergo the procedures just listed have a high incidence of upper respiratory tract symptoms and may always have manifestations consistent with URI. Most parents can advise whether their child is more congested than usual.

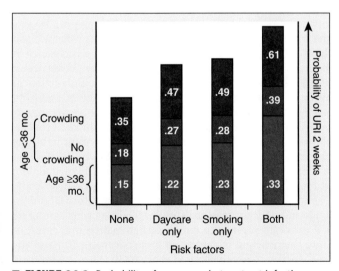

■ FIGURE 36-2. Probability of upper respiratory tract infection according to age, crowding, maternal smoking, and daycare status. *(From Fleming DW, et al.: Childhood upper respiratory tract infections: to what degree is incidence affected by daycare attendance? Pediatrics 79:55, 1987.)*

Box 36-5 Signs and Symptoms of Upper Respiratory Infection

1. Mild sore or scratchy throat
2. Mild malaise
3. Sneezing
4. Rhinorrhea
5. Nasal congestion or stuffiness
6. Nonproductive cough
7. Fever higher than 101° F (38° C)
8. Laryngitis

To make a diagnosis of URI, two of any of the above signs or symptoms are required. If 1 and 2, 3 and 4, or 5 and 6 are combined, one additional sign or symptom is required.

Modified from Tait AR, Knight PR: The effects of general anesthesia on upper respiratory tract infections in children, *Anesthesiology* 67:930, 1987a.

Elective surgeries other than those cited previously are postponed if any of the following are present: "croupy" cough; rectal temperature higher than 38.3° C associated with any URI sign or symptom; malaise or decreased appetite; and any evi-dence or recent history of lower respiratory tract involvement such as rales, wheezes, productive cough, or abnormal chest radiograph (Box 36-5). Laboratory and radiographic tests are usually not helpful in the decision-making process, although some investigators recommend obtaining a chest radiograph and a white blood cell count to evaluate the child with a URI. The white blood cell count is neither sensitive nor specific in identifying a URI, and chest radiography associated with a nor-mal auscultative examination is unlikely to identify abnormali-ties (Brill et al., 1973). The presence of rales or wheezes should lead to postponement of elective surgery, regardless of find-ings on the chest radiograph. A suggested algorithm for mak-ing decisions about proceeding with surgery is presented in Figure 36-3.

Anesthetic Management

Several major principles of anesthetic management can be sug-gested for dealing with children with acute or recent URIs (Tait and Malviya, 2005). These are especially important in anesthe-tizing children when surgery is urgent and cannot be delayed. In elective situations, it is best to avoid intubation if possible (if the surgical procedure allows), instead using regional anes-thesia or general anesthesia by mask or laryngeal mask airway (LMA). A randomized, prospective study demonstrated a much lower incidence of bronchospasm in children with URI managed with LMA rather than ETT (0% vs. 12.2%) (Tait et al., 1998). The incidence of all respiratory complications was reduced by 50% for the LMA group (19% vs. 35%). LMA may be an excel-lent alternative for airway management for patients with URI if the planned surgical procedure and fasting status are compat-ible with its use. If intubation is indicated, it should be accom-plished when the patient is at a deep plane of anesthesia using an ETT at least 1 size (0.5 cm) smaller than age would determine. Any IV induction agent is acceptable, with the most important guiding principle being that enough should be given to achieve a deep level of anesthesia. An alternative is mask induction of inhalation anesthesia with sevoflurane, with or without nitrous oxide, and oxygen. If the procedure is expected to be prolonged,

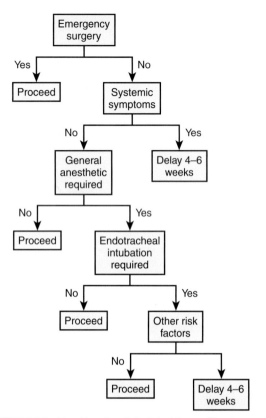

■ FIGURE 36-3. Algorithm for clinical decision making for a patient with upper respiratory tract infection. *(From Martin LD: Anesthetic implications of an upper respiratory tract infection in children,* Pediatr Clin North Am *41:121, 1994.)*

heated humidification should be used, because use of dry gas may lead to inspissation of secretions.

Adjunctive agents, such as IV lidocaine (1 mg/kg), an opioid, or both, decrease airway reflexes (Hirshman, 1983). The preoperative use of anticholinergic agents (i.e., atropine and glycopyrrolate) theoretically may block muscarinic receptors, thereby interrupting the airway reflex arc (Jacoby and Hirshman, 1991). Their properties as antisialogogues may be helpful; however, these agents have not been shown to be beneficial in prospective studies (Tait et al., 2007). The use of glucocorticoids experimentally has decreased viral-associated, tachykinin-induced airway edema formation, although glucocorticoids are not routinely prescribed in this clinical situation—in contrast to their use in the patient with RAD (Piedimonte et al., 1990). Dexamethasone, however, has been used in an effort to prevent postextubation croup, but these studies have been performed in critically ill children who had undergone prolonged intubation and mechanical ventilation in the intensive care unit, rather than in children with respiratory infections who are undergoing surgery. In this high-risk population, dexamethasone may be effective (Markovitz and Randolph 2002; Lukkassen et al., 2006). If intubation is necessary, tracheal suction of URI-associated secretions after intubation and before extubation may decrease the chance of atelectasis and mucus plugging, although this hypothesis has not been studied.

Management of children with URI requires a logical approach. When this issue arises in the preoperative period, the patient, parents, surgeon, and anesthesiologist must participate in an informed fashion in the decision-making process; however, "in the final analysis, the name of the game is clinical judgment and a degree of good fortune" (Berry, 1990).

Reactive Airways Disease (Asthma)

RAD, or asthma, the most common chronic disease of childhood in industrialized countries, has received wide public attention in recent years because of increases in morbidity and mortality. Asthma is the major cause of restricted activity, absence from school, and hospital admission in children, and it is responsible for significant health care costs in the United States (Newacheck and Halfon, 2000). The prevalence of asthma among children is greater than among adults, and it has increased by an average of 4.3% each year between 1980 and 1996 (Akinbami and Schoendorf, 2002). Beginning in 1997, the survey questions used to determine the prevalence of asthma were changed, which resulted in a slightly lower prevalence than in previous years, but the increasing trend has remained constant (MMWR, 2000).

Etiologic Factors and Pathophysiology

Asthma is a chronic inflammatory disorder of medium and small airways in which many cell types play a role, including mast cells and eosinophils. These cells release mediators of inflammation that, in susceptible individuals, cause symptoms associated with variable airway obstruction and airway hyperreactivity that is partially or completely reversible spontaneously or with appropriate treatment. Understanding the important role of inflammation in the immunopathogenesis of asthma in recent years has changed the focus to a newer therapeutic approach using antiinflammatory agents. Among the immune regulatory pathways involved in the pathogenesis of asthma, 2 cytokines—interleukin-4 and interferon-γ—appear to be important in controlling immunoglobin E (IgE) production, which is critical in the allergic inflammatory process. In individuals with asthma, mast cells and eosinophils are attracted to airways and release cytokines and lipid mediators that cause inflammation (Goldstein et al., 1994). The interplay of allergens and irritants, mast cells, eosinophils and their mediators, and the end effects on pulmonary vessels and airways is depicted in Figure 36-4. These mediators include histamines, leukotrienes, prostaglandins, kinins, and cytokines. Airway obstruction in asthma results from a combination of several factors, including airway smooth muscle spasm, airway mucosal edema, hypersecretion, and mucus plugging of small bronchi and bronchioles (Djukanovic et al., 1990). These changes result in airway obstruction, increased work of breathing, uneven distribution of ventilation, and in severe disease, air trapping, hyperinflation, and ventilation-perfusion imbalance, which leads to hypoxemia, diaphragmatic fatigue, hypercapnia, and respiratory failure. In longstanding RAD, mast cells infiltrate airway smooth muscle and in combination with chronic inflammation may result in airway remodeling, potentiating bronchoconstriction and airway hyperreactivity (Brightling et al., 2002).

A strong association exists between asthma and allergy. Up to 90% of children with recurrent wheezing respond positively to bronchoconstrictor challenge, especially when associated with atopy (Clough et al., 1991). An increased prevalence of asthma is reported among first-degree relatives of asthmatic

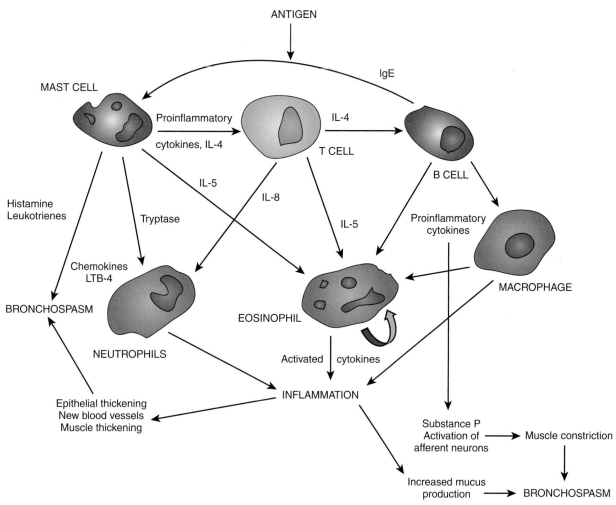

■ **FIGURE 36-4.** Pathophysiology of asthma.

subjects; over two thirds of children with asthma appear to have a familial predisposition (Clifford et al., 1989). Various environmental factors precipitate airway hyperreactivity and trigger asthma. Recent evidence has shown that obesity is associated with a proinflammatory state and is an independent risk factor for the development of asthma (Visser et al., 2001; Guerra et al., 2004).

The onset of asthmatic symptoms is often associated with viral infection of the lower respiratory tract, particularly respiratory syncytial virus (RSV) infection in infants and children (Rooney and Williams, 1971). Severe viral bronchiolitis in infancy is significantly associated with the subsequent development of airway hyperreactivity and asthma, although familial factors cannot be ruled out (Gurwitz et al., 1981; Gern et al., 2005; Lemanske et al., 2005). The development of IgE antibody to RSV may have an important role in inducing an allergic response to the virus (Welliver et al., 1989; Rakes et al., 1999). Children who experience respiratory failure and mechanical ventilation during infancy and early childhood, such as those with bronchopulmonary dysplasia (BPD), neonatal repair of congenital diaphragmatic hernia, or severe viral bronchiolitis, develop and sustain airway hyperreactivity even without a family history of asthma (Mallory et al., 1989; Nakayama et al., 1991). Prematurity alone may be associated with a higher incidence of asthma in preadolescent children (von Mutius et al.,

1993). The primary site of airway obstruction and hyperreactivity in children with a history of neonatal respiratory failure appears to be in relatively small airways—in contrast to relatively large central airway obstruction and hyperreactivity in those with typical allergic (i.e., IgE antibody-mediated) asthma (Mallory et al., 1991). In these patients, airway spasm is characterized by a rapid drop in oxygen saturation of Hb (SpO_2) without audible wheezing by auscultation.

In children with RAD, parental smoking (passive smoking) increases the severity of symptoms and exacerbates airway hyperreactivity (Soussan et al., 2003). Intrauterine exposure to maternal smoking also increases the incidence of airway hyperresponsiveness in infants (Singh et al., 2003). Infants with gastroesophageal reflux and chronic esophagitis often develop airway hyperresponsiveness with or without chronic aspiration and resultant tracheobronchial inflammation (Sheikh et al., 1999). Contributing factors responsible for the development of airway hyperreactivity and asthma are listed in Figure 36-5.

Precipitating Factors for Reactive Airways Disease

Viral lower respiratory infections, particularly those caused by RSV and influenza, sensitize airways and provoke airway hyperreactivity even in individuals who are nonasthmatic and nonallergic for as long as 6 weeks (Empey et al., 1976). Exposure

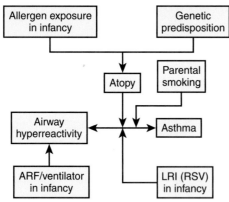

■ **FIGURE 36-5.** Contributing factors to the development of RAD. *ARF,* Acute renal failure; *LRI,* lower respiratory tract infection; *RSV,* respiratory syncytial virus.

to dry, cold air can precipitate tracheobronchial constriction in subjects with asthma, presumably in response to reduced tracheal temperature caused by evaporative heat loss (Gilbert et al., 1988). The same mechanism appears to be responsible for exercise-induced bronchospasm and precipitation of asthma with excitement, anxiety, and hyperventilation (McFadden and Gilbert, 1994).

The time before and during the induction of anesthesia is uniquely suited to trigger bronchospasm in susceptible individuals because of the patient's emotional stress, fear, and excitement. Hyperventilation results, with mouth breathing of dry anesthetic gas mixtures, airway irritation by volatile anesthetics, and mechanical stimulation of the pharyngeal and laryngeal mucosa by laryngoscopy and endotracheal intubation (Box 36-6).

Pharmacologic Agents for Asthma

The pharmacologic management of asthma consists of bronchodilators and antiinflammatory drugs and includes six different classes of drugs: corticosteroids, leukotriene inhibitors, β-adrenergic agonists, theophylline, cromolyn (or nedocromil), and anticholinergics. Recently published guidelines for treatment of asthma in children include a useful algorithm (Fig. 36-6) (Bacharier et al., 2008). Initial treatment for asthma most commonly consists of inhaled corticosteroids (ICSs) and leukotriene-receptor antagonists, with ICSs usually being the first-line drugs. Montelukast has been used widely in children. Other first-line alternatives are cromolyn

Box 36-6 Precipitating Factors for Bronchospasm

Lower respiratory infection (adenovirus, RSV)
Irritants (cigarette smoke, inhaled anesthetics)
Allergens (inhaled)
Emotional stress; fear and excitement
Exercise, hyperventilation
Cold or dry gas (anesthetic gases without humidification)
Manipulation/mechanical stimulation of pharynx and larynx
Gastroesophageal reflux

ALGORITHM FOR PHARMACOLOGIC
TREATMENT OF REACTIVE AIRWAYS DISEASE

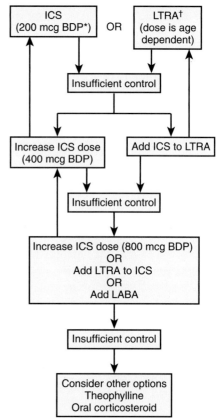

■ **FIGURE 36-6.** Algorithm for treatment of RAD. Once control is achieved, therapy may be stepped down to previous level. *ICS,* Inhaled corticosteroid; *BDP,* beclomethasone equivalent; *LTRA,* leukotriene receptor antagonist, for dose, see Table 36-10. *(Modified from Bacharier LB, et al: Diagnosis and treatment of asthma in childhood: a PRACTALL consensus report,* Allergy 63:5, 2008.)

(or nedocromil). Because of safety concerns, long-acting β₂-agonists such as salmeterol are now reserved for patients with poor control despite use of an ICS and leukotriene-receptor antagonists (Martinez, 2005). Theophylline has reentered the treatment algorithm if patients have exacerbations despite ICS and β-adrenergic agonists. Oral corticosteroids in brief high-dose pulses are reserved for patients with moderate to severe asthma that is unresponsive to combinations of the other drugs (Stempel, 2003). Drugs commonly used in children are listed in Table 36-10.

Corticosteroids

ICSs have become popular for the treatment of asthma because of their potent antiinflammatory effect on the airways with limited systemic effects (as compared with oral steroids) and are a first-line regimen recommended in treatment guidelines. Regular use of an ICS allows effective control of symptoms and improvement in lung function, reduces airway inflammation, and results in a gradual reduction in airway hyperreactivity (Konig, 1988; Juniper et al., 1991). Although corticosteroids inhibit the in vitro proliferation of airway smooth muscle

TABLE 36-10. Drugs Used for Asthma

Drug	Formulation	Dosage
Antiinflammatory Drugs		
Inhaled Corticosteroids		
Beclomethasone dipropionate (QVAR)	MDI, 40, 80 mcg/puff	2-4 puffs bid (5-11 yr)
Budesonide (Pulmicort)	DPI, 90, 180 mcg/inhalation	1-2 inhalations bid (6-17 yr)
Flunisolide (AeroBid)	MDI, 250 mcg/puff	2 puffs bid (6-15 yr)
Fluticasone proprionate (Flovent)	MDI, 44, 110, or 220 mcg/puff	1-2 puffs bid (max, 440 mcg/d) (4-11yr)
Fluticasone proprionate (Flovent Diskus)	DPI, 50 mcg/inhalation	1-2 inhalations bid (4-11 yr)
Triamcinolone acetonide (Azmacort)	MDI, 75 mcg/inhalation	2-4 inhalations bid (6-12 yr)
Oral Corticosteroids		
Prednisone/prednisolone	Oral tablets (1, 2.5, 5, 10, 20 mg)	Acute: 1 mg/kg q d/bid × 5-14 d
Prednisone/prednisolone (Prelone, Pediapred)	Oral liquid (1 mg/mL)	Chronic: 0.25-2 mg/kg qod Preoperative: 1 mg/kg/d × 3 d Max, 60 mg/d
Leukotriene Receptor Antagonist		
Montelukast (Singulair)	Oral granules, 4 mg; chewable tablets, 4.5 mg	12 mos-5 yrs: 4 mg qd; 6-14 yrs: 4.5 mg qd
Cromolyn Sodium (Intal)		
Cromolyn (generic)	Solution for nebulization (10 mg/mL)	1-2 inhalations tid-qid
Inhaled β-2 Agonists (Bronchodilators)		
Short-acting (SABA)		
Albuterol (Proventil, Ventolin)	MDI, 90 mcg/inhalation	2 puffs q 4-6 hr prn
Albuterol (generic)	Nebulized solution (0.63, 1.25, or 2.5 mg/3 mL; 2.5 mg/0.5 mL)	0.63 or 1.25 mg tid-qid prn
Levalbuterol (Xopenex)	Nebulized solution (0.31, 0.63, or 1.25 mg/3 mL)	0.31-0.63 mg tid prn (6-11 yrs)
Long-acting (LABA)*		
Salmeterol (Serevent)	DPI, 50 mcg/blister	50 mcg bid (≥4 yrs)
Theophylline (generic)	Oral solution, 80 mg/15 mL	<1 yr: max, 0.2 × (age in weeks) + 5 = dose in mg/kg/d
	Tablet (immediate release), 100 mg	>1 yr: 10 mg/kg/d; max, 16 mg/kg/d
	Capsule (sustained release), 125, 200, 300 mg	
Anticholinergics		
Ipratropium bromide (Atrovent)	MDI, 17 mcg/puff	3-14 yr: 1-2 puffs qid (for acute exacerbation); >14 yr: 2 puffs qid
Ipratropium bromide (generic)	Nebulized solution (500 mcg/2.5 mL)	125-250 mcg q 6-8 hr mixed with albuterol (5-12 yr) 250-500 mcg q 6-8 hr (>12 yr)†

*Recommended only for use in combination with inhaled corticosteroid for children >4-5 years of age. Data from Bacharier LB et al.: Diagnosis and treatment of asthma in childhood: a PRACTALL consensus report, *Allergy* 63:5, 2008; modified from *Treatment guidelines from the medical letter* 6:86, 2008.
†Zorc JJ et al.: Ipratroprium bromide added to asthma treatment in the pediatric emergency department, *Pediatrics* 103:748, 1999.
DPI, Dry powder inhaler; *MDI*, metered-dose inhaler; *prn*, as needed

cells from subjects without asthma, they do not do so in airway smooth muscle cells from patients who have asthma (Roth et al., 2004). Recommended doses of ICS generally have minimal effects on the HPA axis; however, high doses, especially of fluticasone, have resulted in reduction of cortisol levels and symptomatic adrenal insufficiency in children (Barnes and Pedersen, 1993; Todd et al., 2002; Sim et al., 2003). Oral or parenteral corticosteroids are most effective for acute exacerbations of asthma unresponsive to maximal bronchodilator therapy (Chapman et al., 1991; Schuh et al., 2000).

Leukotriene-Receptor Antagonists

Leukotriene-receptor antagonists are a class of drugs developed for the prevention and treatment of bronchial asthma. They are an alternative first-line treatment or may be added if ICSs do not provide adequate control. The formation of leukotrienes through the 5-lipoxygenase pathway depends on lipoxygenation of arachidonic acid, a major constituent of cell membrane phospholipids, detached by phospholipase A_2 activity. Leukotrienes are potent bronchial smooth muscle constrictors; on a molecular basis, leukotrienes C4 and D4 (LTC4 and LTD4) are approximately 1000 times more potent than histamine (Undem and Lichtenstein, 2001). Bronchial smooth muscle constriction by leukotrienes is considered a major cause of asthmatic symptoms. Leukotriene-receptor antagonists (e.g., zafirlukast, montelukast) are selective high-affinity LT1-receptor antagonists (Jones et al., 1995). Their use is associated with increased exhaled nitric oxide (NO) (Straub et al., 2005). Montelukast has been reported to be effective as maintenance therapy in children with moderate to severe asthma, with or without concomitant steroid therapy, with minimal side effects (Knorr et al., 2001; Phipatanakul et al., 2003).

β_2-Adrenergic Agonists

β_2-adrenergic agonists initiate their action on the receptor sites of airway smooth muscle cells and increase adenylate cyclase activity, which produces cyclic adenosine monophosphate (cAMP) from adenosine triphosphate (ATP) and results in smooth muscle relaxation and bronchodilation.

For maintenance therapy in more severe RAD and for the prevention of exercise-induced bronchoconstriction, long-acting β_2-agonists (LABAs) are recommended (Bacharier et al., 2008). Studies suggest a small risk of increased asthma-related deaths in patients older than 12 years of age who take LABAs, especially if they are used regularly without an ICS; thus, the FDA requested that a "black box warning" be added to the labels of salmeterol and salmeterol/fluticasone in 2003 (Nelson et al., 2006). An FDA meeting was later convened to consider safety concerns regarding LABAs in adults and children. Although few children younger than 12 years of age have been studied, the risk of asthma exacerbations and hospitalizations was higher in children 4 to 11 years of age who received a combination drug with LABA and ICS when compared with patients who received ICS alone (Bisgaard and Szefler, 2006; Kramer, 2009). Until further studies are undertaken, it has been recommended that LABA not be given as monotherapy but only in combination with ICS (Drazen and O'Byrne, 2009). This concern does not apply to the use of short-acting β_2-agonists (SABAs), which are the drugs of choice for the treatment of intermittent episodes, acute exacerbations, and prevention of exercise-induced asthma in patients with RAD. The recommended doses of commonly used β_2-agonists are listed in Table 36-10.

Methylxanthines

Methylxanthines (e.g., theophylline) produce bronchodilation by inhibiting adenosine-induced bronchoconstriction in asthmatic patients—not as was formerly thought, by competitively inhibiting phosphodiesterase, which metabolizes cAMP (Holgate, 1984). Although theophylline was the mainstay of pediatric asthma therapy in the 1970s and 1980s, it is no longer used for therapy in acute exacerbations of RAD (Rooklin, 1989). Theophylline still has a role in decreasing the severity of persistent bronchospasm, especially that which occurs at night. Theophylline has a narrow therapeutic index, with greatest efficacy at serum levels of 5 to 15 mcg/mL. Levels greater than 20 mcg/mL are associated with symptoms of toxicity, such as nausea, gastroesophageal reflux, irritability, learning difficulties in children, and headache (Creer and Gustafson, 1989; Ellis, 1985). Vomiting, tachyarrhythmias, and seizures can occur at higher levels. The great variability of drug metabolism and the necessity for monitoring of blood levels are two reasons the use of theophylline has declined (Drugs for Asthma, 2002).

Anticholinergics

Ipratropium bromide is an atropine derivative and is available as a metered-dose inhaler and as a nebulizable solution. Ipratropium has a slower onset of action than β_2-agonists, but the duration of action is longer (up to 8 hours). Side effects are uncommon.

Cromolyn Sodium and Nedocromil Sodium

Cromolyn sodium does not have a bronchodilator effect; therefore it is exclusively a prophylactic agent and has no bearing on anesthetic practice. It attenuates bronchoconstriction caused by allergen, exercise, and bronchial challenge (Stempel, 2003). Nedocromil sodium has similar chemical and biological properties to cromolyn, which became available in the early 1990s (van Bever and Stevens, 1992). Cromolyn and nedocromil are thought to act on pulmonary mast cells and stabilize cell membranes. They reduce IgE antibody-induced release of inflammatory mediators, including histamine and leukotrienes, from activated mast cells (Douglas, 1985). Maintenance therapy with cromolyn or nedocromil is recommended in children with moderate to severe asthma.

Preanesthetic Consideration

The goal of the preoperative assessment of children with asthma is to ensure that each patient receives optimal treatment before reaching the operating room. The patient's history, physical examination, and laboratory tests are all helpful to determine whether the patient's condition is adequately managed. Children with RAD rarely require preoperative pulmonary function testing, but they are commonly monitored by pulmonology or allergy and immunology services with frequent assessment of pulmonary function testing (i.e., spirometry with flow-volume curves). Some families use the peak expiratory flow rate for home assessment. If this is so, the family should be queried to ensure that the peak expiratory flow rate is maximized.

Careful history taking is the single most important element of the preoperative evaluation of children with asthma. The profile of a typical acute episode, precipitating factors, and time of the most recent episode of asthma should be obtained. Previous and current drug therapy, dosages, effectiveness, and side effects, if any, should also be documented. Specific points of importance in the history include the following:

1. Determine whether the child has had episodes of bronchospasm and bronchodilator treatment in the previous 4 to 6 weeks. Ideally, elective surgery should be postponed for at least 4 to 6 weeks after an episode of symptomatic asthma, because airway hyperreactivity may be worsened after acute exacerbations, and pulmonary gas exchange may still be impaired because of bronchoconstriction, mucosal edema, and mucus plugs.
2. Determine whether the patient has a recent history of a URI or if the symptoms of URI still exist. URI in children with RAD is often associated with the exacerbation of bronchospasm and requires a more conservative approach

than in children who do not have asthma. Optimally, the child with a history of RAD should be free of URI symptoms for 4 to 6 weeks before an elective procedure, unless the URI symptoms recur so often that an asymptomatic period is difficult to attain. If the child has had a lower respiratory infection, such as influenza, within the previous 6 weeks, the postponement of scheduled surgery should be seriously considered, because airway hyperreactivity would be exaggerated as long as 6 weeks, even in nonasthmatic patients.

3. Ascertain the child's steroid requirements over the previous year and the possible need for perioperative stress-dose steroid coverage (see preceding discussion). Children who often have bronchospasm that is poorly controlled with maximal therapy and require repeated courses of oral steroids may benefit from a short preoperative course of prednisone (1 mg/kg per day to a maximum of 60 mg once daily for 3 days, including the day of surgery), especially if endotracheal intubation is planned.

Physical examination should be focused on careful auscultation of the chest for clinical evidence of bronchoconstriction (i.e., expiratory wheezing), use of the accessory muscles of respiration, and a prolonged expiratory phase. During severe episodes of bronchospasm, air movement may become so limited that wheezing may be barely audible. Patients with a history of BPD and asthma are most likely to have lower-airway obstruction and small airway hyperreactivity; wheezing and rhonchi may not be present (see Chapter 17, Neonatology for Anesthesiologists). The preanesthetic level of oxygen saturation should be obtained with a pulse oximeter while the child is breathing room air to determine the baseline oxygen saturation and assess for any preexisting hypoxemia. This information is exceptionally valuable for the postoperative assessment of lung function and gas exchange.

Anesthetic Management

The anesthesiologist must get to know the child with asthma and his or her parents and gain their confidence to minimize the child's anxiety before anesthesia induction. The child should be well sedated to avoid struggle and hyperventilation, which can provoke exercise-induced asthma. Midazolam, which may be administered transmucosally (i.e., orally, nasally, or rectally) in infants and young children and orally or intravenously (if IV access is present) in older children, works well for sedation. A β_2-adrenergic agonist may be given prophylactically using a metered-dose inhaler or nebulizer before induction (Table 36-10). Otherwise, the drug can be given after the induction of anesthesia through the ETT using the metered-dose inhaler and an aerosol chamber inserted in between the ETT adapter and the anesthesia circuit.

The anesthetic approach is similar to that for children with URIs. After applying standard monitors (a minimum of a pulse oximeter and precordial stethoscope if the child is uncooperative), the inhalation induction should be smooth and progress swiftly with sevoflurane and nitrous oxide (see Chapter 11, Monitoring). For infants and young children, heated humidification should be used if available; the dry gas mixture from the anesthesia machine is a perfect environment for provocation of bronchospasm secondary to irritation and reduced tracheal

temperature from evaporative heat loss of the tracheal mucosa in a child with asthma (McFadden and Gilbert, 1994).

For IV induction, propofol may be a better agent of choice than thiopental because it suppresses airway reflexes as compared with barbiturates, although thiopental, despite risk of histamine release, is not necessarily contraindicated in patients with asthma (Brown et al., 1992; Gal, 1994). Propofol may also produce bronchodilation in patients with other types of airway disease (Conti et al., 1993). Regardless of the drug chosen, it is important to give sufficiently large IV doses to blunt the reflex response, and sevoflurane should be added before the peak effect of the IV agent is lost.

Whenever possible, endotracheal intubation should be avoided in patients with asthma, because the ETT stimulates large airway irritant receptors and can trigger bronchospasm (Hirshman, 1983). When no contraindications exist, an LMA is a good choice for patients with RAD, as its use avoids the laryngeal and tracheal stimulation of intubation (Groudine et al., 1995). It may also be prudent to avoid anesthetic agents that might release histamine (e.g., atracurium and morphine), although clinical evidence that such drugs actually cause intraoperative bronchospasm is limited.

An anesthetic technique using a volatile anesthetic may be preferable to a balanced technique (i.e., nitrous oxide, opioid, and muscle relaxant) for patients who have asthma because of the salutary bronchodilating properties of volatile agents. Regional anesthesia can be combined with inhalation anesthesia with sevoflurane or isoflurane. Desflurane may cause more airway irritation in patients with RAD and lead to bronchospasm and associated coughing, especially during emergence (von Ungern-Sternberg et al., 2008).

Intraoperative Wheezing

The differential diagnosis of intraoperative wheezing includes "light anesthesia," kinked ETT, mainstem bronchial intubation, increased airway secretions, foreign body in the airway, pulmonary edema, embolus, and aspiration. In the child with RAD, wheezing can result from exacerbation of airway hyperreactivity and requires immediate attention. The treatment of intraoperative bronchospasm is detailed in Box 36-7. Treatment should begin after chest auscultation to confirm that there are bilateral breath sounds and therefore no mainstem intubation. The first step includes increasing the inhaled concentration of oxygen and deepening the level of anesthesia with volatile anesthetics, or administering IV propofol or

Box 36-7 Treatment of Intraoperative Bronchospasm

Confirm diagnosis (exclude mainstem bronchus intubation, mucus plug, pneumothorax, anaphylaxis, and congestive heart failure).
Deepen anesthesia with volatile agent.
Administer inhaled β-agonists and ipratropium.
Consider propofol or ketamine to further deepen anesthesia.
Consider IV lidocaine, atropine, or both.
Administer an IV corticosteroid.
Modify ventilation to avoid stacking breaths, gas trapping, and barotrauma.

ketamine (0.5 to 2 mg/kg), a known bronchodilator (Corssen et al., 1972; Hirshman et al., 1979). Lidocaine (1 mg/kg) may also be given intravenously to reduce airway reactivity at the earliest sign of bronchospasm. Administration of muscle relaxant and suctioning of the ETT may be performed if the patient is intubated. The second step consists of the administration of β_2-agonists given by a metered-dose inhaler and adapter through the ETT, followed by the squeezing of the anesthesia bag manually to provide a vital-capacity maneuver to distribute the bronchodilator mist to the tracheobronchial tree. Because only 5% to 10% of the administered dose may reach the end of the ETT and contact the airway, 4 to 8 puffs of the β_2-agonist should be administered through the ETT. This maneuver may be repeated two or three times. Parasympatholytic agents (atropine, 0.02 to 0.03 mg/kg) or antihistamines (diphenhydramine, 0.5 mg/kg) are indicated when wheezing is associated with increased vagal tone or histamine release, respectively. The development of hypotension, urticaria, or flushing should lead to the consideration of anaphylaxis. Corticosteroids (e.g., 2 mg/kg of IV hydrocortisone) should be given, and circulation should be supported with appropriate vasoactive agents.

Techniques of Extubation

At the conclusion of surgery and anesthesia, the patient with asthma can be extubated "deep" or "awake" to avoid laryngospasm. Upper airway obstruction caused by soft-tissue collapse in the pharynx is the major disadvantage of deep extubation. Deep extubation can be accomplished safely provided the maintenance of upper airway patency was satisfactory during the induction of anesthesia before intubation and that no excessive secretions or blood are in the airway. If maintaining airway patency was difficult during induction, the patient's airway may become obstructed during emergence. If this is the case, airway patency may be facilitated by prophylactic placement of an oropharyngeal or nasopharyngeal airway, well lubricated with lidocaine or lubricant jelly, when the patient is still deeply anesthetized. Successful deep extubation is facilitated by the attainment of spontaneous breathing before attempted extubation.

For a successful "awake" extubation, prophylactic treatment with the inhalation of a β_2-agonist must be given even if a dose was previously given during or after the induction of anesthesia. Tracheal suction of any secretions before emergence may decrease coughing caused by migration of mucus plugs. Lidocaine (1 mg/kg) given intravenously on emergence is helpful in minimizing tracheal stimulation as the patient awakens. The use of IV atropine (0.02 mg/kg), given for its vagolytic and bronchodilator effects, may be an additional safety precaution before extubation.

Bronchopulmonary Dysplasia

BPD is a chronic disease of lung parenchyma and small airways with chronic respiratory insufficiency that occurs in prematurely born infants (see Chapter 17, Neonatology for Anesthesiologists). As originally described by Northway's group (1967), BPD develops after a period of acute and subacute ventilator-induced lung injury and oxygen toxicity, in prematurely born infants with severe respiratory distress syndrome (Hazinski, 1990). Although Northway's original series

involved infants born at a mean gestational age of 34 weeks, all of whom had received excessive concentrations of oxygen during mechanical ventilation with a primitive ventilator by modern standards, over time, BPD has been seen in infants who had prolonged barotrauma (or volutrauma) in the absence of "excessive" oxygen. Early series were characterized by a high incidence of mortality with persistent respiratory symptoms and oxygen requirement beyond 4 weeks of age. Chest radiographs were abnormal and characterized by hyperinflation of the lungs with focal areas of increased density. Northway et al. called this condition BPD to "emphasize the involvement of all the tissues of the lungs in the pathologic process" (Northway et al., 1967; Northway, 2001).

The number of infants with BPD has not decreased over the past two decades despite improved neonatal intensive care, probably because of the survival of more infants who are premature. However, the clinical picture has changed with the advent of antenatal steroids, the use of surfactant therapy, and advances in ventilatory strategies for reducing volutrauma and ventilator-induced lung injury, including noninvasive techniques such as nasal continuous positive airway pressure (Geary et al., 2008, Greenough et al., 2008). Currently, most infants who develop BPD are born at 24 to 28 weeks' gestation and are rarely born later than 32 weeks' gestation, whereas the mean gestational age of Northway's original series was 34 weeks (Hazinski, 1990). Because of changes in neonatal intensive care and affected patient population, many aspects of BPD have changed, including the definition, theories of pathogenesis, pathology, and clinical picture (Jobe and Ikegami, 2000; Jobe and Bancalari, 2001).

Infants with BPD today are likely to have a minimal respiratory distress syndrome that does not progress after surfactant administration. The reason for prolonged ventilation in these premature infants is more commonly apnea or poor respiratory effort, which may be related to immaturity of central respiratory control mechanisms. These infants rarely require the high airway pressures and high oxygen concentration that led to the "old BPD." This newer clinical picture had been referred to as chronic lung disease or "new BPD," but it is now simply called BPD. The current definition of BPD is oxygen dependence for at least 28 postnatal days. Evaluation for the presence of BPD and grading of severity is assessed at 36 weeks' postconceptual age in infants born at fewer than 32 weeks' gestation and at 56 days after birth in infants born at or after 32 weeks' gestation (Jobe and Bancalari, 2001). BPD is graded as mild, moderate, or severe, based on oxygen requirement and the need for ventilatory support (Table 36-11). Prevalence ranges from 67% in the smallest weight group to 1% in the largest, with an overall prevalence of 20% of infants born at less than 1500 g (Lemons et al., 2001; Bancalari et al., 2003).

Pathogenesis

In the past, the development of BPD was associated with a condition that caused respiratory failure in the neonatal period (e.g., prematurity with respiratory distress syndrome, meconium aspiration syndrome, or congenital diaphragmatic hernia). Mechanical ventilation with high concentrations of oxygen (i.e., an acute insult to immature lungs) was employed, usually lasting longer than 1 week. Oxygen free radicals, which are not well handled by an immature antioxidant host-defense system in the neonatal lungs, can cause direct cellular injury (Ackerman, 1994). Although much lower concentrations of oxygen are now used

TABLE 36-11. Assessment of the Severity of Bronchopulmonary Dysplasia*

Grade	Fio₂ and Ventilatory Support	
	GA at Birth <32 wks Assessed at 36 Weeks' PCA	GA at Birth ≥32 wks Assessed at 56 Days Postnatally
Mild	0.21	0.21
Moderate	0.22-0.30	0.22-0.30
Severe	>0.30 and/or continuous positive airway pressure or mechanical ventilation	>0.30 and/or continuous positive airway pressure or mechanical ventilation

Modified from Baraldi E, Filippone M: Chronic lung disease after premature birth, *N Engl J Med* 357:1946, 2007.
*Applies to patients who have been treated with >21% oxygen for at least 28 days.
GA, Gestational age; *PCA*, postconceptual age.

than in the past, even room air (21% oxygen) is relatively hyperoxic for a premature infant whose in utero Po₂ is less than 30 mm Hg (Hazinski, 1990). Excessive hydration and patent ductus arteriosus with increased pulmonary fluid have been recognized as additional important factors contributing to the development of BPD (Gerhardt and Bancalari, 1980; van Marter et al., 1992). The current theory of the mechanism of injury in BPD also emphasizes the role of infection and inflammation (Gonzalez et al., 1996; Sadeghi et al., 1998). Recurrent bacterial or viral infections in these infants may cause persistent alveolitis, which worsens alveolar and airway damage (Rojas et al., 1995; Hannaford et al., 1999). Multiple markers of inflammation (e.g., lipid mediators, proteases, oxygen free radicals, and cytokines) are elevated (Bose et al., 2008; Ryan et al., 2008). Nutritional deficiencies may also play a role (Sosenko et al., 2000; Geary et al., 2008).

Immature, inflamed lungs with decreased compliance are most susceptible to high-volume (i.e., volutrauma) and low-volume (i.e., shear stress trauma) trauma with marked distortion and distention of terminal bronchioles at high positive pressures (Hazinski, 1990). In earlier pathologic examination of lungs of infants dying with BPD, peribronchiolar fibrosis and smooth muscle thickening were seen. They were also found in animal models exposed to prolonged positive pressure ventilation and hyperdistention (Coalson, 1999). The pathology now seen in extremely premature infants reflects the immature state of their pulmonary parenchyma, with enlarged and simplified alveolar structure and reduced numbers of capillaries that are dysmorphic in appearance. Therefore, the new BPD is now regarded primarily as a disorder of lung development with superimposition of mechanical factors. Fibroproliferation may still occur but is more variable. Changes in larger blood vessels are less prominent with less indication of pulmonary hypertension than seen in old BPD. Airway smooth muscle hyperplasia may still occur, but it is also more variable (Coalson, 2006). After this damage has occurred to immature lungs, infants may require prolonged mechanical ventilation and high oxygen concentration for weeks or months, despite having not required high oxygen concentrations in the first few weeks of life. Although less common than with old BPD, progressive respiratory failure with associated pulmonary hypertension, with or without cor pulmonale, may follow.

Even after the perinatal period, RAD persists in infants with BPD. Mallory et al. (1991) studied lung function longitudinally in infants with moderate to severe BPD during the first 4 years of life with the forced deflation technique and found that airway hyperresponsiveness or hyperreactivity continued to be present in all children studied. They postulated that airway hyperreactivity is an important etiologic factor for the pathogenesis of lower airway obstruction in BPD. Attributing the cause of RAD to BPD is confounded by the recent evidence that antenatal steroid therapy to hasten lung maturation is a risk factor for the development of RAD between the ages of 3 and 6, as well as by the fact that the rates of RAD-like symptoms occur more often in prematurely born children than in those born at term (Doyle, 2006; Pole et al., 2009). Most long-term studies of lung function are reports of infants who had the old form of BPD. Little information is available regarding long-term outcomes of infants with new BPD.

Preanesthetic Considerations

Most infants with moderate to severe BPD remain dependent on oxygen, with or without CPAP, or dependent on a ventilator beyond 4 weeks of age. They have persistent lower airway obstruction and airway hyperreactivity (Mallory et al., 1991). Tachypnea and dyspnea may be intermittently or chronically present. Growth failure because of chronic hypoxia despite oxygen therapy may occur, as well as cor pulmonale associated with pulmonary hypertension (Hazinski, 1990). Wheezing may or may not be present on auscultation, because the site of airway hyperreactivity is primarily in the periphery of the lungs as a result of increased thickness of the airway wall (Tiddens et al., 2008). In addition to lower airway obstruction primarily involving small airways, infants who have been intubated for prolonged periods sometimes develop large airway disease such as subglottic stenosis (that may or may not be recognized), tracheomalacia, and bronchomalacia (Miller et al., 1987; McCubbin et al., 1989). A later study also found a greater degree of upper airway obstruction in children with history of BPD, as compared with age-matched children with asthma (Sadeghi et al., 1998).

Infants with mild forms of BPD improve with age and may become asymptomatic, but airway hyperreactivity may persist. Parents of such an infant may not be aware of the history of BPD even when their child received prolonged mechanical ventilation as a neonate. It is appropriate, therefore, to assume that a child has or had BPD and has RAD if he or she was born prematurely and was mechanically ventilated for more than 1 week during the neonatal period. Inguinal hernia is often present in infants with BPD, probably owing to prematurity and continually increased abdominal pressure that results from airway obstruction and increased inspiratory effort. Prematurely born infants may require postoperative admission for monitoring, because they have an increased risk of postoperative apnea as discussed in Chapters 3, Respiratory Physiology in Infants and Children; 17, Neonatology for Anesthesiologists; and 18, Anesthesia for General Surgery in the Neonate.

As with asthmatic patients, careful history taking is of utmost importance before anesthetizing an infant with BPD or a history of BPD. These patients may have failure to thrive (a sign of chronic hypoxia). With lower respiratory tract infection, worsening of symptoms or even respiratory failure may occur. The patient may be taking SABAs or other treatments for asthma. Other medications may include diuretics. A family history of allergy and asthma is significant, because premature birth may be linked to smooth muscle hyperresponsiveness and asthma (Bertland et al., 1985). Relatively common surgical conditions in infants and children with BPD or a history of BPD include inguinal hernia, direct laryngoscopy and bronchoscopy for subglottic stenosis, and surgical procedures of the larynx for the complications of prolonged intubation or tracheostomy (e.g., excision of granuloma or laryngotracheoplasty).

Anesthetic Management

Anesthetic management of infants and children with BPD or a history of BPD is similar to that for those with asthma. Before anesthetizing a child in this population, it is imperative to obtain a baseline oxygen saturation measurement with a pulse oximeter (SpO_2), although a normal oxygen saturation level does not necessarily guarantee the absence of lung dysfunction. Many infants and young children with a history of BPD maintain remarkably good SpO_2 values, presumably because of hypoxic pulmonary vasoconstriction (HPV). The infant with BPD with near-normal SpO_2 in room air may develop marked desaturation after induction with sevoflurane, presumably because of a loss of HPV under general anesthesia, although HPV in healthy human volunteers may be insignificant (Benumof, 1994). In these patients, oxygen saturation may be maintained better with IV induction and maintenance techniques using opioids and propofol; however, no evidence supports this management protocol. Preoperative prophylactic treatment with a β_2-adrenergic agonist by a metered-dose inhaler or handheld nebulizer may be beneficial for patients with potential airway hyperreactivity to prevent perioperative bronchoconstriction. In intubating a child with a history of mechanical ventilation, it is prudent to start with an ETT one size (0.5 mm inner diameter) smaller than the appropriate size for the age in anticipation of subglottic narrowing, which may be the result of prolonged intubation. If rapid sequence intubation is required because of fasting violation or intestinal obstruction, desaturation may be rapid when apnea occurs, and gentle ventilation by mask with maintenance of cricoid pressure may be necessary to maintain saturation if intubation is not rapidly accomplished.

Cystic Fibrosis

Cystic fibrosis (CF), an autosomal-recessive disorder, is the most common life-limiting inherited disorder among whites (Rosenstein and Cutting, 1998). In the United States, the gene frequency (heterozygotes) in whites is approximately 1 in 28; it is uncommon among Hispanics (1 in 46) and African Americans (1 in 65) and lowest among Asians and Native Americans (1 in 90) (Hamosh et al., 1998). The disease incidence among whites is approximately 1 in 2500 live births. Owing to early diagnosis and aggressive treatment over the past 40 years, in 2007 the median survival of a CF patient had increased to 37 years (Cystic Fibrosis Foundation, 2007).

In 1985, Tsui et al. localized the gene responsible for the manifestation of CF to 250 kilobases on the long arm of chromosome 7. The deletion of three base pairs, removing a phenylalanine residue at position 508 (d508) from a 1480-amino acid protein called *CF transmembrane conductance regulator (CFTR),* a cAMP-dependent chloride ion channel, accounts for approximately 70% of CF chromosome abnormalities (Moskowitz et

al., 2008). Of the other 1000 documented mutations, 20 account for most of the remaining 30% of cases, with the prevalence of mutations varying among ethnic groups (Tsui and Zielenski, 2007). Although the type of CFTR mutation does correlate with pancreatic function, poor correlation exists between the type of mutation and the severity of lung disease. Evidence suggests that other genetic polymorphisms influence the severity of lung disease (Drumm et al., 2005).

Pathogenesis

CF is characterized by exocrine gland dysfunction that results in chronic pulmonary disease, pancreatic dysfunction, and abnormalities in electrolyte reabsorption in the sweat duct, with increases in sweat sodium and chloride concentrations and electrolyte imbalance. The fact that CF patients have sweat chloride levels in excess of 60 mEq/L (normal is less than 40 mEq/L), as measured by pilocarpine iontophoresis, is the basis of the sweat chloride test, which is still the gold standard for making the diagnosis of CF. Increasingly, the diagnosis of CF is being made earlier because of newborn screening techniques that are designed to detect elevated serum levels of immunoreactive trypsinogen and the most common CFTR mutations (Comeau et al., 2007). Such screening accounted for 21.6% of the diagnoses of CF in the United States in 2006 (Cystic Fibrosis Foundation, 2007). Even if these screenings are found to be positive, two sweat chloride test results of greater than 60 mEq/L are necessary to make the diagnosis of CF. Significant clinical manifestations of CF, other than pulmonary disease, include those listed in Table 36-12.

Pulmonary disease is the most common cause of morbidity and death. Enhanced absorption of sodium across the airway

TABLE 36-12. Organ System Involvement in Cystic Fibrosis

Organ System	Incidence (%)
ENT	
Pansinusitis	90-100
Nasal polyps	20
Gastrointestinal	
Pancreatic	
Enzyme deficiency	85-90
Diabetes secondary to pancreatic failure	15
Intestinal	
Meconium ileus (newborn)	7-20
Distal intestinal obstruction syndrome (includes intussusception)	10-30
Rectal prolapse	20
Gastroesophageal reflux disease	50
Liver	
Hepatic failure	5-20
Coagulopathy caused by vitamin K deficiency	100 if untreated
Pulmonary	
Pneumothorax caused by bleb rupture	5-8

epithelium and failure to secrete chloride and fluid toward the airway lumen is thought to lead to dehydration and thickening of airway mucus and abnormal mucociliary clearance with subsequent bronchial inflammation and infection. Patients are initially colonized with *Haemophilus influenzae* and then by *Staphylococcus aureus*, and eventually by the mucoid variant of *Pseudomonas aeruginosa*. Colonization with *Aspergillus* and atypical mycobacteria may occur. The chronic infection in the periphery of the tracheobronchial tree results in bronchiolitis, which may lead to airway hyperresponsiveness, bronchiectasis, lobar or segmental atelectasis, and pneumothorax. Advanced disease is associated with destruction of airway architecture, fibrosis of lung parenchyma, and development of abscesses. Hemoptysis and eventually, cor pulmonale and respiratory failure ensue (Eckles and Anderson, 2003).

Small airway obstruction, hyperinflation, and ventilation-perfusion imbalance are the most common and important pulmonary changes in children with moderate-to-severe CF. The early signs of lung dysfunction include a reduction in maximum expiratory flow rates at low lung volumes (e.g., FEF_{25-75}, FEF_{50}, and FEF_{75}) and an increase in the ratio of residual volume to total lung capacity (RV/TLC) (see Chapter 3, Respiratory Physiology in Infants and Children). Airway hyperreactivity is often present, probably in response to airway inflammation. Some patients have a good response to bronchodilators, but others have inconsistent or even paradoxical responses, sometimes worsening airway function because of the relaxation of airway smooth muscles and resultant increases in airway collapsibility (Brand, 2000).

Treatment

Patients with CF take multiple medications. In 2007, a committee organized by the Cystic Fibrosis Foundation published guidelines for long-term medication used for optimal pulmonary symptom control in CF patients older than 6 years (Flume et al., 2007). Patients with a prominent bronchospastic component are on long acting β_2-agonist therapy (Hordvik et al., 2002). They often take inhaled or oral antibiotics for prophylaxis or treatment of pulmonary infection. Patients infected with *P. aeruginosa* often take aerosolized tobramycin, which when administered on a bimonthly basis has been shown to preserve pulmonary function and reduce hospitalization (Ramsey et al., 1999). Patients with infectious exacerbations are treated with IV antibiotics in a hospital or at home. Chest physiotherapy several times per day is a mainstay of CF treatment. Inhaled mucolytics (N-acetylcysteine) have long been used to decrease the viscosity of pulmonary secretions, but little is found in the literature documenting their efficacy (Duijvestijn and Brand, 1999). Inhaled hypertonic saline, which is thought to improve fluidity of pulmonary secretions, has been shown to decrease the frequency of pulmonary exacerbations (Flume et al., 2007). Dornase alfa (i.e., human recombinant DNase), which dissolves deoxyribonucleic acid (DNA) released from neutrophils, has improved pulmonary function and reduced the frequency of infection (Jones et al., 2003; Flume et al., 2007). High-dose ibuprofen therapy has been found to slow the decline of forced expiratory volume during the first second of measurement (FEV_1) in children and adolescents if started when the FEV_1 is greater than 60% of that predicted (Lands and Stanojevic, 2007). This effect is related to reduction in inflammation (Nichols et al., 2008). Doses between 20 and 30 mg/kg every 6 hours are administered to achieve plasma concentrations of 50 to 100 mcg/mL

(Arranz et al., 2003). Ibuprofen treatment has been associated with a significant increase in gastrointestinal (GI) bleeding compared with patients who are not taking ibuprofen, although the absolute number of patients affected is small (Konstan et al., 2007). Patients with pancreatic impairment require pancreatic enzyme replacement.

Preanesthetic Considerations

Common surgical indications in infants and children with CF are listed in Table 36-13. Although some patients with CF require surgery in the neonatal period for meconium ileus, no special anesthetic considerations are necessary. Management of children with CF is a challenge to the anesthesiologist. These patients are often frail and malnourished. Decreased plasma albumin levels may affect anesthetic potency. Intravascular volume may be diminished because of chronic diarrhea, poor oral intake, and diuretic therapy. Electrolyte imbalance may result from excessive chloride and sodium losses. Pulmonary function ranges from near normal without airway obstruction to severe obstruction, air trapping, hypoxemia, and hypercapnia. Copious thick secretions and resultant ventilation-perfusion imbalance may prolong mask induction with volatile anesthetics. Secretions may irritate the larynx and precipitate laryngospasm. Nasal polyps may block the nasal airway completely during mask induction. Pathophysiologic considerations in patients with CF that may affect anesthetic management are listed in Table 36-14.

The preoperative evaluation should include the assessment of pulmonary function by history, physical examination, and pulmonary-function testing. Pulmonary-function testing should include assessments of maximum expiratory flow-volume curves, lung volume measurements, and response to bronchodilators. An increase in TLC and the RV/TLC ratio with decreased vital capacity indicates the presence of hyperinflation and air trapping. Lower airway obstruction with small airway involvement is demonstrated when FEF_{25-75}, FEF_{50}, and especially FEF_{75} are markedly decreased from predicted values. A recent preoperative chest radiograph is needed in patients with moderate to severe pulmonary disease. Preoperative oxygen saturation should be obtained by means of pulse oximetry in room air for postoperative comparison. Recent tracheal

TABLE 36-13. Surgical Indications for Patients with Cystic Fibrosis

Conditions	Typical Age Range
Meconium ileus or equivalent	1 d-3 yr
Nasal polyp/sinusitis	10-18 yr
Other procedures	10-18 yr
Bronchoscopy	
Feeding gastrostomy; central venous access (port or PICC)	
Lobectomy or thoracoplasty/thoracoscopy	
Organ transplantation (double lungs; heart-lungs)	

PICC, Peripherally inserted central catheter.

TABLE 36-14. Pathophysiology of Cystic Fibrosis: Effect on Anesthetic Management

Pathophysiology	Possible Outcome
Pulmonary Dysfunction	
Airway obstruction V/Q imbalance	Prolonged mask induction
Copious secretions Airway hyperreactivity	Laryngospasm, bronchospasm
Nasal polyp	Upper airway obstruction
Gastrointestinal and Hepatobiliary Disorders	
Decreased serum albumin levels	Increased drug potency
Coagulopathies	Increased bleeding
Diabetes or glucose intolerance	Hyperglycemia, acidosis
Abnormal sweat gland function	Electrolyte imbalance
Cor pulmonale	Hemodynamic instability; dysrhythmia

culture results should be reviewed as a guide to choice of perioperative antibiotic therapy. In patients with significant lower airway obstruction and air trapping, preoperative arterial blood gas measurement is recommended to assess the degree of hypoxemia more accurately and to evaluate the presence of hypercapnia and acid-base status. In those with long-standing hypoxemia, pulmonary hypertension and cor pulmonale should be suspected. These patients should have preoperative electrocardiography and echocardiography to evaluate myocardial function and reserve. Blood sugar, liver-function tests, and coagulation studies may be indicated. Eight percent of CF patients between the ages of 11 and 17 develop CF-related diabetes mellitus as a result of fibrosis and fatty infiltration of the pancreas (Cystic Fibrosis Foundation, 2007). Some, but not all, may require insulin, because some insulin continues to be produced. Malabsorption and liver disease may be associated with abnormal coagulation. Additional vitamin K supplementation may be necessary to correct coagulopathy. The patient's pulmonary physician should be consulted to ensure that the patient's condition is optimized as much as is possible before surgery. Ibuprofen should be stopped 2 days before surgery to allow its inhibitory effects on platelet aggregation to dissipate.

The child with CF and his or her family are exceedingly knowledgeable regarding the pathogenesis and treatment of the disease. A lack of knowledge of CF in general, and of the patient's past history and present conditions in particular, at the time of the preoperative visit could quickly undermine the confidence of the family in the anesthesiologist. More importantly, the patient with CF is often petrified by the thought of death under anesthesia, in part because of a long-held belief in the pulmonary medicine community that general anesthesia leads to prolonged deterioration of pulmonary function (Price, 1986). It is therefore prudent for the anesthesiologist to gain the patient's and the parents' confidence and administer preoperative sedation such as oral midazolam (Della Rocca, 2002). Opioid premedication should be avoided in severe cases because of possible respiratory depression and hypoxemia.

Anesthetic Management

Because of copious secretions in affected patients, it is preferable to schedule surgery later in the day to allow enough time for ambulation and chest physiotherapy in the morning to facilitate expectoration of secretions retained overnight. The baseline oxygen saturation in room air is measured with a pulse oximeter before administering oxygen and anesthetics.

In patients with significant pulmonary involvement, IV access should be established before the induction of anesthesia because of prolonged mask induction and possible nasal obstruction from nasal polyps. An anticholinergic may be given during induction. Concern about excessive drying of secretions is unfounded, because atropine decreases secretions without changes in viscosity and has not been a significant problem in clinical practice (Lamberty and Rubin, 1985). IV propofol may be preferred to thiopental because it is less irritating to the upper airways and actually causes bronchodilation. Ketamine, despite its bronchodilating properties, is relatively contraindicated because it tends to increase secretions and may cause laryngospasm. Fifty percent of children with CF have gastroesophageal reflux disease and may require rapid-sequence intubation, although chronic treatment with H_2-blockers and or a proton-pump inhibitor along with an adequate fasting interval mitigates the risk of aspiration. Inhalation induction is usually satisfactory in young children with mild lung disease. Anesthetic gases should be heated and humidified to prevent irritation of the upper airways and laryngospasm and to avoid drying and inspissation of secretions. When trapped gas volume is suspected or proven by pulmonary function test, nitrous oxide should be avoided to prevent expansion of the emphysematous area and the potential danger of bleb rupture.

Endotracheal intubation with muscle relaxation is mandatory in patients with severe respiratory involvement, although the anesthesiologist should be exceedingly careful not to overdistend already air-trapped lungs. When a nondepolarizing muscle relaxant is chosen, the effect of aminoglycoside antibiotics to prolong the duration of action of such drugs must be kept in mind, and monitoring of train-of-four should be used to guide relaxant administration. It is also mandatory to carefully monitor end-tidal carbon dioxide to prevent hyperventilation and to maintain preoperative arterial partial pressure of carbon dioxide (Pco_2) levels, which may be elevated. Sudden hypocapnia in a chronically hypercapnic patient can disrupt the patient's ventilatory control mechanisms, increasing the chance that the patient might require postoperative ventilation. After intubation, tracheobronchial suction should be performed and repeated at intervals throughout surgery and before extubation to improve pulmonary gas exchange. Although the use of an LMA might be an option for short cases, disadvantages include the inability to suction secretions, obstruction of the LMA by thick secretions, risk of laryngospasm, and risk of aspiration in patients with gastroesophageal reflux disease. For bronchoscopy for the purpose of removal of secretions for culture and bronchial lavage, the LMA has been safely used in patients with CF (Nussbaum and Zagnoev, 2001). Intraoperatively, glucose should be monitored in patients with glucose intolerance. Care should be taken to conserve heat in these patients with reduced body fat.

Regional anesthesia should be considered whenever applicable. Although regional anesthetic techniques without general anesthesia might be useful in some situations, these techniques should be carefully considered in children with severe pulmonary disease. Depression of abdominal and intercostal muscle function by thoracic levels of spinal or epidural anesthesia may not be tolerated. Pediatricians and pulmonologists often request regional anesthesia instead of general anesthesia because of fear that severely affected patients with CF will not tolerate general anesthesia or may become dependent on a ventilator after endotracheal intubation. However, most of these sick patients with CF, dyspneic or orthopneic with hypercapnia and oxygen dependence, may not tolerate even a short surgical intervention, such as insertion of a central venous catheter or MediPort, with local anesthesia and sedation. Instead, general endotracheal anesthesia with an inhaled agent, supplemented by caudal, lumbar, or thoracic epidural anesthesia for abdominal or thoracic procedures, is much better tolerated, safer, and provides good operative conditions, rapid emergence, and a pain-free postoperative state (Dalens et al., 1986). If epidural anesthesia is to be used, coagulopathy should be ruled out, and the appropriate concentration of local anesthetic drugs should be chosen to minimize motor block. Continuous caudal or epidural anesthesia with local anesthetic with or without carefully chosen doses of an opioid provides prolonged postoperative pain relief and facilitates coughing and deep breathing after upper abdominal or thoracic procedures. If regional anesthesia is not appropriate, judicious use of inhalation agents and short-acting opioids and wound infiltration with local anesthetic by the surgeon should facilitate early extubation, which is desirable in most cases. After surgeries without a high risk of postoperative bleeding, the use of NSAIDs may be effective in reducing the amount of opioid needed for analgesia.

Cystic Fibrosis and Hemoptysis

Hemoptysis may occur in older children with more severe lung disease. These children may come to the hospital for angiography and bronchial artery embolization. Preanesthetic considerations as described above should be evaluated, and the patient's pulmonary status should be optimized to the greatest extent. Pulmonary hemorrhage has been reported after induction of general anesthesia, intubation, and institution of positive-pressure ventilation (McDougall and Sherrington, 1999). It is possible that airway and parenchymal distention associated with positive pressure ventilation results in the breach of relatively thinwalled vessels. These authors have recommended that sedation and local anesthesia may be safer in this situation (McDougall and Sherrington, 1999; Barben et al., 2002)

Cystic Fibrosis and Lung Transplantation

For patients with end-stage pulmonary disease, lung transplantation may be the final surgical option. Fifty percent of patients with CF and FEV$_1$ of less than 30%, partial pressure of oxygen (Pao$_2$) less than 55 mm Hg, or partial pressure of carbon dioxide (Paco$_2$) greater than 50 mm Hg will survive for 2 years and may be candidates for lung transplantation (i.e., double-lung or heart-lung procedure) (Belkin et al., 2006). Approximately 175 patients with CF per year undergo bilateral lung transplantation in the United States, of whom the minority are children (Cystic Fibrosis Foundation, 2007). The 3-year survival rate is 60%, which is similar to that seen in patients who do not have CF (Sweet et al., 1997). Some (27%) lungtransplant patients develop bronchiolitis obliterans, which is

responsible for 40% of deaths that occur more than 1 year after transplantation (Boucek et al., 2004). Among the survivors of lung transplantation, no recurrence of CF in the transplanted lungs has been reported, as measured by the transepithelial potential differences (Alton et al., 1991). The management of end-stage CF patients for lung transplantation is described in Chapter 3, Respiratory Physiology, and Chapter 28, Anesthesia for Organ Transplantation.

CARDIOVASCULAR DISORDERS

Cardiovascular disorders are commonly encountered in the pediatric population. The baseline incidence of congenital heart disease in the population is approximately 0.8 in 100 births, on which is superimposed an incidence of acquired heart disease. However, more and more congenital cardiac defects have been appreciated to have either a genetic or an environmental basis, either alone or in combination, such that incidence and risks in offspring may be higher in selected populations (Jenkins et al., 2007). Both congenital and acquired diseases have the ability to affect myocardial function, valve function, and conduction tissue, all of which can also be affected by anesthetics. In addition, anesthetic effects on vascular tone can have a positive or negative impact on myocardial function and shunting of blood through intracardiac defects.

Patients with cardiac disease should be identified preoperatively. Although children with congenital heart disease who undergo noncardiac surgery should generally do well with appropriate anesthetic and perioperative care, preliminary information suggests that in the aggregate, congenital cardiac disease of even a moderate degree can increase mortality and adverse events during and after noncardiac surgery (Baum et al., 2000). Even hemodynamically insignificant lesions may necessitate perioperative endocarditis prophylaxis (Table 36-15). However, not all surgical procedures or all children with cardiac disease require endocarditis prophylaxis. Recommendations for endocarditis prophylaxis were significantly changed in 2007, with a general decrement in the use of prophylaxis, because previous recommendations were recognized to be lacking in validity or efficacy or were overly complicated (Wilson et al., 2007). Current recommendations are outlined in Boxes 36-8 and 36-9.

Anesthetic Management

Although the specifics of the anesthetic management of individual cardiac problems are discussed in Chapters 20, Anesthesia for Congenital Heart Surgery, and 21, Anesthesia for Children with Congenital Heart Disease Undergoing Non-Cardiac Surgery, the following comments are generally applicable.

Preoperative Period

Prolonged preoperative fasting should be avoided in children who have cyanotic heart disease with significant erythrocytosis to avoid dehydration and further increase of elevated hematocrit and blood viscosity. Small infants with significant heart failure and failure to thrive can have inadequate glycogen reserves and are at risk for hypoglycemia if they fast for many hours. Otherwise conventional age-appropriate preoperative sedation is

TABLE 36-15. Endocarditis Prophylaxis Regimens for Dental Procedures

Reason	Agent	Regimen
Standard general prophylaxis	Amoxicillin	50 mg/kg orally (adults: 2 g)
Unable to take orally	Ampicillin	50 mg/kg IM or IV* (adults: 2 g)
	OR	
	Cefazolin or ceftriaxone	50 mg/kg IM or IV* (adults: 1 g)
Allergic to penicillin	Clindamycin	20 mg/kg orally (adults: 600 mg)
	OR	
	Cephalexin	50 mg/kg orally (adults: 2 g)
	OR	
	Azithromycin or clarithromycin	15 mg/kg orally (adults: 500 mg)
Allergic to penicillin and unable to take orally	Clindamycin	20 mg/kg IV* (adults: 600 mg)
	OR	
	Cefazolin or ceftriaxone	50 mg/kg IM or IV* (adults: 1 g)

Modified from Wilson W et al: Prevention of infective endocarditis: guidelines from the American Heart Association, *Circulation* 116:1736, 2007.
*It is appreciated that many children do not have IV access prior to surgery. IV antibiotics should be given as soon as possible and before surgical incision. Children's dose should not exceed adult dose.
IM, Intramuscularly; *IV,* intravenously.

in no way contraindicated in children with cyanotic or acyanotic heart disease unless the child is in profound heart failure.

Intraoperative Period

Although much discussion is appropriately devoted to the specifics of cardiac pathophysiology, most children with congenital heart disease who develop problems during anesthesia do so for primarily noncardiac reasons, particularly airway compromise (Strafford and Henderson, 1991). Infants who are cyanotic, in particular, begin with decreased oxygen saturation and can rapidly desaturate with transient interruption in ventilation, whether as a result of apnea or airway obstruction. Children with severe congestive failure or cyanosis have a decreased margin of safety and tolerate failures of respiratory or hemodynamic management poorly.

Much time is spent discussing the effects of left-to-right and right-to-left shunts on the onset time of IV and volatile anesthetics. Although differences exist, with currently available anesthetic gases of relatively low solubility, these differences are almost always so small as to be clinically irrelevant. In the absence of a complication such as loss of the airway or the development of a hypercyanotic "tet" spell in children with tetralogy of Fallot or variants, oxygen saturation in children with cyanotic disease almost invariably increases with induction of anesthesia (Laishley et al., 1986; Greeley et al., 1986). Several reasons are possible, one of the most likely being a decrease in oxygen

Box 36-8 Changes in Most Recent Endocarditis Prophylaxis Recommendations

- The number of cardiac conditions that require prophylaxis has been reduced. Moderate- and high-risk groups are not differentiated.
- Dental prophylaxis is reserved solely for conditions in Box 36-9 and solely for manipulation of gingival tissues or the periapical region of teeth, or for perforation of oral mucosa.
- Prophylaxis is reasonable for patients with conditions in Box 36-9 for invasive procedures of the respiratory tract that involve incision or biopsy, such as tonsillectomy and adenoidectomy. For patients who have an established infection of the respiratory tract, treatment with an agent active against *Viridens streptococci* is recommended, unless the infection is known or suspected to be caused by staphylococcus, in which case the regimen should include an appropriate agent such as an antistaphylococcal penicillin, cephalosporin, or vancomycin.
- Prophylaxis for procedures on infected skin or musculoskeletal tissue is indicated only for patients with conditions in Box 36-9. As tissue is already infected, it is reasonable to use an antibiotic such as an antistaphylococcal penicillin or a cephalosporin that is active against those organisms (staphylococcus and β-hemolytic streptococci) that cause these infections and may lead to endocarditis. Vancomycin or clindamycin can be substituted in case of allergy or antibiotic resistance.
- Antibiotic prophylaxis is not recommended for GI or genitourinary procedures, including vaginal delivery and hysterectomy. For patients in a high-risk group with established infections of the GI or genitourinary tracts who require surgery or cystoscopy, an appropriate antibiotic effective against enterococci, such as penicillin, ampicillin, piperacillin, or vancomycin, can be used, without empirical evidence of clinical efficacy in preventing endocarditis (Box 36-9).
- Prophylaxis is not required for endotracheal intubation.
- Prophylaxis is no longer required for patients with mitral valve prolapse.
- Timing is simplified to 30 to 60 minutes before incision for all regimens.

Data from Wilson W, et al: Prevention of infective endocarditis: guidelines from the American Heart Association, *Circulation* 116:1736, 2007.

Box 36-9 Cardiac Conditions that Necessitate Antibiotic Endocarditis Prophylaxis

Prosthetic valves (bioprosthetic and homograft)
Previous bacterial endocarditis
Complex cyanotic heart disease
Systemic pulmonary shunts (e.g., Blalock-Taussig shunt)
Unrepaired cyanotic heart disease
Completely repaired congenital heart defects with prosthetic material or device, whether by surgery or by catheter intervention, during the first 6 months after procedure
Cardiac transplant recipients who develop cardiac valvulopathy

Data from Wilson W, et al: Prevention of infective endocarditis: guidelines from the American Heart Association, *Circulation* 116:1736, 2007.

consumption that causes an increase in mixed venous oxygen saturation and subsequently higher arterial oxygen saturation when some of this blood is shunted right to left.

Minimization of right-to-left shunting at the atrial level is addressed primarily by increasing intravascular volume. Minimization of shunting at the ventricular and great vessel levels is primarily modulated by changes in pulmonary vascular resistance (PVR) and systemic vascular resistance. Increasing systemic resistance or decreasing PVR increases left-to-right shunting (or decreases right-to-left shunting) and vice versa. Although α-adrenergic receptors are found in the pulmonary circulation (stimulation of which can increase PVR), they are denser in the systemic circulation, and α-agonists increase systemic vascular resistance significantly more than they increase PVR, with a decrease in right-to-left shunting.

Nitrous oxide is a mild myocardial depressant. In adult patients, it can increase PVR, particularly in patients in whom PVR is already elevated. However, in children, no significant increase in PVR has been observed with 50% nitrous oxide, regardless of the preexisting PVR (Hickey et al., 1986).

Patients who are cyanotic, and in particular patients with elevated central venous pressure, are at risk for increased perioperative blood loss and require adequate IV access. Not only do all patients with cyanotic disease need IV catheters to be kept clear of air bubbles to avoid systemic air emboli, but small amounts of transient right-to-left shunting can occur during the cardiac cycle, even with lesions thought of as left-to-right shunting lesions. Therefore, IV catheters must be cleared of air for all patients with shunt lesions, regardless of predominant direction of shunt flow. Stopcocks are common sites where air can be introduced inadvertently.

End-tidal Pco_2 correlates with arterial Pco_2 in acyanotic patients. However, in children and adults with cyanotic congenital heart disease, end-tidal Pco_2 tends to underestimate arterial Pco_2 (Burrows, 1989).

Postoperative Period

The specific length of observation in a postanesthesia care unit is dependent on the patient and the surgical procedure and cannot be generalized. Patients with good hemodynamic function may undergo relatively minor noncardiac surgery on an ambulatory basis and are not automatically excluded because of their cardiac disease.

When not under anesthesia, patients with cyanotic disease have relatively little increase in systemic oxygen saturation in response to supplemental oxygen. Similarly, oxygen saturation is not markedly decreased by removing supplemental oxygen (other causes for postoperative hypoxemia being absent). Knowledge of the patient's normal preoperative range of oxygen saturation helps avoid unnecessary prolongation of the PACU stay for fear of removing supplemental oxygen.

Hypovolemia from continued surgical blood or fluid loss postoperatively can worsen right-to-left shunting in patients with cyanosis and should be rapidly corrected. The onset of hypovolemia can be insidious if it is as a result of gradual oozing from surgical drains. Patients with cyanotic disease should have repeated measurement of Hb after surgery, especially after significant blood loss. They may require a higher than normal hematocrit level to ensure adequate oxygen delivery. In general, a level similar to the preoperative hematocrit should be maintained.

Patients with labile pulmonary arterial hypertension particularly benefit from good postoperative analgesia, because pain increases pulmonary vascular tone. Even patients with cyanosis have a normal ventilatory response to hypercarbia and respond in a normal fashion to appropriate doses of parenteral, intrathecal, or epidural opiates; therefore, age- and weight-appropriate doses of analgesic drugs should be given. Patients who have had a Glenn or Fontan procedure are dependent on low PVR for maintenance of adequate pulmonary blood flow. If these patients should require postoperative ventilation, PVR should be minimized by limiting positive inspiratory pressure and using low levels of positive end-expiratory pressure to optimize functional residual capacity, which in turn, minimizes PVR.

The Child with a Murmur and Possible Heart Disease

Cardiac murmurs are exceedingly common in healthy children, with an overall lifetime incidence of at least 50%. Most of these are the somewhat inappropriately named *functional* murmurs (also called *innocent*). The incidence of functional murmurs is highest at 3 to 4 years of age. Functional murmurs represent the sound of blood flowing through a structurally normal heart (Fig. 36-7). No anesthetic concern is associated with these murmurs, and the family should be reassured. Several functional murmurs are commonly recognized, almost all of which are short and soft but become louder when the patient lies supine.

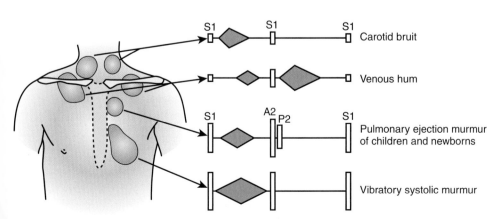

Carotid bruit

Venous hum

Pulmonary ejection murmur of children and newborns

Vibratory systolic murmur

■ **FIGURE 36-7.** Innocent murmurs. Not shown is the mammary souffle over the breast of a pregnant or lactating woman. The pulmonary ejection murmur is similar to the murmur of peripheral pulmonic stenosis in neonates. Vibratory systolic murmur is also called *Still murmur. (From Park MK: Pediatric cardiology for practitioners, ed 5, Philadelphia, 2008, Mosby.)*

Most functional murmurs become louder with increased cardiac output, as would occur with anemia, fever, exercise, or anxiety.

The most common functional murmur is the Still murmur, which has a typical musical or vibratory quality and is a midsystolic murmur heard between the midleft sternal border and the apex. Soft pulmonary flow murmurs at the upper left sternal border are commonly heard in thin-chested older children and adolescents. The murmur is softer than true pulmonic stenosis and is unaccompanied by a systolic ejection click. Peripheral pulmonic stenosis generates an ejection murmur from the left upper sternal border to the axillae and back and is common in neonates. It is generated by turbulent flow when blood passes from the main to the branch pulmonary arteries. In the neonate, the branch pulmonary arteries, unaccustomed to accommodating large amounts of pulmonary blood flow in utero, form an acute angle with the main pulmonary artery. By approximately 6 months of age the vessels remodel and the murmur disappears. Less common innocent murmurs are the *venous hum* and the *mammary souffle,* both of which are continuous murmurs and are thus exceptions to the rule that diastolic murmurs are always pathologic. The venous hum represents blood draining down the jugular into the subclavian veins. It is heard over the left or right upper chest with the patient upright and disappears when the patient lies down, with gentle compression of the jugular vein, or with a Valsalva maneuver. The mammary souffle can be heard over the breasts of pregnant or lactating women. Unlike functional murmurs, pathologic murmurs are generated by a normal amount of blood across an abnormal valve or opening or by an abnormal amount of blood passing through normal valves.

Occasionally, a murmur is appreciated for the first time when children arrive for a preanesthetic evaluation. The exact method of evaluation remains somewhat controversial (Yu et al., 2002). Isolated chest radiographs and electrocardiograms are generally a poor investment (Yu et al., 2002). In addition, electrocardiograms that are interpreted by computer or an adult cardiologist may need to be reinterpreted using age-appropriate normal values. Location of the murmur can also aid in the diagnosis (see Chapter 9, Preoperative Preparation, Fig. 9-3).

In general, children who are acyanotic and growing well, with a soft systolic murmur and good exercise tolerance, tolerate anesthesia well. Signs of heart disease in infants differ somewhat from those in adults and older children. Perioral cyanosis can be a normal finding in neonates, especially with crying, and must be differentiated from central cyanosis (confirmed by pulse oximetry). Heart failure is often manifested in young infants by tachypnea, diaphoresis with eating (in excess of the normal sweating of the head that many infants have), and hepatomegaly. Increased pulmonary blood flow can impinge upon small bronchioles, causing airway obstruction and expiratory wheezing ("cardiac asthma"). Peripheral edema as a result of congestive failure is distinctly uncommon in children. Blood pressure measurements in both arms and a leg help detect or exclude coarctation of the aorta.

When caring for children with known heart disease or a history of cardiac surgery, the child's pediatrician or cardiologist should be contacted, and a copy of the most recent evaluation should be obtained.

Noncardiac Manifestations of Congenital Heart Disease

Longstanding cyanotic and acyanotic congenital disease can have effects on the function of a variety of other organ systems. Some of these effects may not become clinically apparent until years after surgical correction of the underlying cardiac defect (Table 36-16).

TABLE 36-16. Potential Noncardiac Manifestations of Congenital Heart Disease

System	Causes/Implications for Anesthetic Management
Pulmonary/Thoracic	
Decreased lung compliance	Occurs in lesions with increased pulmonary blood flow (i.e., left-to-right shunting) or pulmonary venous obstruction; can require higher airway pressure for ventilation; can impinge on small airways, resulting in air trapping, wheezing
Scoliosis	More common with cyanotic lesions; can manifest in adolescence, years after corrective cardiac surgery
Hemoptysis	Can occur in end-stage Eisenmenger syndrome (pulmonary hypertension caused by prolonged excessive pulmonary blood flow)
Phrenic nerve injury	From prior surgery; more common after surgery at the apices of the thorax (e.g., patent ductus arteriosus ligation, coarctation, pulmonary artery banding, or Blalock-Taussig shunt)
Recurrent laryngeal nerve injury	From prior surgery or from an enlarged hypertensive pulmonary artery; see phrenic nerve injury (above)
Blunted ventilatory response to hypoxemia	In cyanotic patients; normalizes after surgical repair; normal ventilatory response to hypercarbia
Hematologic	
Symptomatic hyperviscosity	Due to chronic hypoxemia; occurs with hematocrit above approximately 65% (or lower if iron deficient); may cause neurologic symptoms
Bleeding diathesis	Abnormalities of a variety of factors have been described in patients who have cyanosis with no consistent pattern; elevated central venous pressure can cause increased operative bleeding, as can increased tissue vascularity with cyanotic disease (collateral blood vessel formation); increased risk of bleeding with prior thoracic surgery during subsequent thoracic procedures
Gallstones	Calcium bilirubinate stones from increased heme turnover in cyanotic disease; may not become symptomatic until years after corrective cardiac surgery

TABLE 36-16. Potential Noncardiac Manifestations of Congenital Heart Disease—cont'd

System	Causes/Implications for Anesthetic Management
Neurologic	
Paradoxical emboli to central nervous system	Can manifest even with a predominantly left-to-right shunt lesion
Brain abscess in patients with right-to-left shunts	Can manifest with seizure focus years later
Cerebral thrombosis	In children with erythrocytosis but not in adults
Compression of nerve by vascular structure	Recurrent laryngeal nerve by enlarged, hypertensive pulmonary artery
Nerve injury during prior surgery	Recurrent laryngeal, phrenic, or sympathetic chain; see phrenic nerve injury (above) for high-risk surgeries
Vascular	
Femoral vein complications	Thrombosis or ligation from prior cardiac catheterization
Anatomic discontinuity of inferior vena cava and right atrium	Congenital, associated with polysplenia syndrome
Anatomic discontinuity of right internal jugular and innominate vein with right atrium	As a result of Glenn shunt
Reduced lower extremity blood pressure	Coarctation of the aorta; left arm involvement is variable
Discontinuity of subclavian artery	With classic Blalock-Taussig anastomosis; stenosis of the subclavian artery after the modified Blalock-Taussig anastomosis; currently, classic Blalock-Taussig shunt is rarely performed
Artifactually elevated right arm blood pressure	Supravalvar aortic stenosis (the Coanda effect)

Kawasaki Disease

Originally named *mucocutaneous lymph node syndrome* after its major manifestations, Kawasaki disease is the most common cause of acquired heart disease in children in the United States. The etiology for this disease, with characteristics of an infectious disease without an identifiable agent and a vasculitis that is not easily treated with steroids, has yet to be determined. In the United States, the peak incidence occurs between 13 and 24 months of age. Diagnosis and therapy have been reviewed in detail, and a general overview has been presented by Burns (2007) (Newburger et al., 2004). No diagnostic test has been developed. The acute illness is associated with fever; intense conjunctival injection; red, cracked lips and oral mucosa; erythema of the palms and soles; and less commonly, cervical lymphadenitis of the neck followed weeks later by desquamation of the skin of the fingers and toes. Arthritis and arthralgia can also develop. Other uncommon systemic manifestations include transient high-frequency hearing loss, gastrointestinal complaints, hepatomegaly, and hydrops of the gallbladder. Erythema and induration at the site of a previous bacillus Calmette-Guérin (BCG) vaccination can also occur. The most concerning feature of the disease is that it causes an infantile periarteritis nodosa-like vasculitis of medium and large arteries in 10% to 15% of children. Of particular concern is involvement of coronary arteries, with the risk of subsequent thrombosis or, less commonly, rupture (Fig. 36-8). The risk of coronary artery aneurysms is higher in infants. In addition, the acute phase of the illness can be associated with myocarditis—usually mild but sometimes associated with heart failure. Myocarditis is usually transient, lasting several weeks. Laboratory findings during the acute phase reveal an intense acute-phase response that includes neutrophilia, elevated sedimentation rate and C-reactive protein, and thrombocytosis to over 800,000/mcL^3.

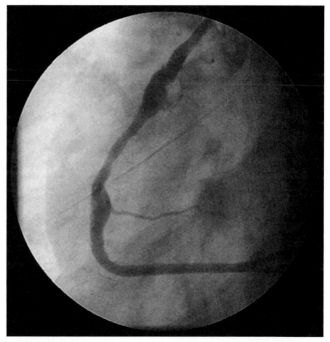

■ **FIGURE 36-8.** Angiogram of the left main coronary artery in a young child with Kawasaki disease showing multiple fusiform aneurysms of both the right and left coronary arteries. *(Courtesy Jonathan Rome, MD.)*

Coronary artery aneurysms become apparent within the first 2 weeks of disease in 3% to 5% of children who have been treated with IV gamma globulin (IVIG) and in 20% to 25% of children who have not. Early aneurysms can resolve spontaneously or progress.

Treatment in the acute phase includes IVIG and aspirin. Aspirin is begun at a high dosage (80 to 100 mg/kg per day) and continued either until the child is afebrile or until day 14 of illness, after which the high antiinflammatory dose is decreased to antiplatelet levels (3 to 5 mg/kg per day). The lower dose is continued until the child shows no evidence of aneurysm formation (6 to 8 weeks after onset) or is continued indefinitely if coronary aneurysms develop. Although the mechanism is undetermined, IVIG (2 g/kg) is an effective acute therapy that is successful in approximately 80% of cases. If IVIG therapy fails, children are at high risk for the development of coronary artery complications, which may be treatable with steroids, although a recent study suggests this may not be effective (Newburger et al., 2007).

If coronary artery aneurysms do develop, approximately one half to two thirds regress within 2 years, and approximately one fifth develop coronary stenoses. Smaller aneurysms (less than 8 mm in diameter) and fusiform aneurysms are more likely to regress than larger or saccular aneurysms. Larger aneurysms can develop thromboses or stenoses with subsequent ischemia, or they can rupture. Rupture is rare and usually occurs within the first month or two of disease. Ischemia can develop years after the acute illness. Even if aneurysms regress, intimal proliferation can result in endothelial dysfunction (Furuyama et al., 2003). Warfarin has been used at some centers to treat children with giant aneurysms. Angioplasty has been attempted at several centers with mixed results, and surgical bypass grafting has been performed on occasion for high-grade obstruction of the left main coronary artery or at least two of the major coronary arteries. Because of the young age of the patients, grafting is completed with arterial rather than venous grafts (Kitamura et al., 1994).

Takayasu Arteritis

Takayasu arteritis, a vasculitis of the aorta and its major branches that is sometimes known by its catchy synonym "pulseless disease," is an uncommon disease in children. However, 75% of patients will have begun to develop symptoms during adolescence. An important cause of hypertension in teenagers in Asia, where it is more common, it occurs 8 times more often in females. Narrowing of major arteries results in limb claudication or end-organ disease. Blood pressure in limbs can be artifactually low or unobtainable. Early vessel inflammation is followed by fibrosis. Headaches are a common symptom. The subclavian artery is involved in 90% of cases, and two thirds of all cases involve the aorta, both supradiaphragmatic and infradiaphragmatic. The carotid artery, almost always the left, is involved in half of cases. Stenoses are more common than occlusion, and occlusion is more common than aneurysm formation. Mural inflammation and thickening occur, and coronary and pulmonary arteries are uncommonly affected. Aortic root dilation can result in aortic valve insufficiency. Initial treatment is with corticosteroids. Long-term therapy is often required, and cytotoxic drugs are sometimes added. Once fibrosis has occurred, treatment is by stenting or surgery (Rigby et al., 2002; Kalangos et al., 2006). Unfortunately, there is often recurrence with tapering of steroid therapy or with time after surgical treatment (Maksimowicz-McKinnon et al., 2007).

HEMATOLOGY AND ONCOLOGY ISSUES: HEREDITARY AND CONGENITAL DISORDERS

Hemoglobinopathies

Hemoglobin Structure, Development, and Function

A Hb molecule is composed of two pairs of subunits comprised of protoheme and globin. The globin imparts the spatial structure responsible for characteristics of Hb, including oxygen affinity. Globin chains differ in the number and sequence of amino acids and are designated by α, β, γ, δ, ϵ, ζ, and θ. Human adult red blood cells (RBCs) contain three types of Hb: 95% HbA (α_2, β_2), 2% to 3% HbA$_2$ (α_2, δ_2), and less than 2% HbF (α_2, γ_2). The physical properties and spatial relationships of the four chains determine oxygen affinity and Hb solubility.

At birth, erythrocytes contain 70% to 90% HbF, and HbF predominates until 2 to 4 months of age in normal patients. β-chain production begins and γ-chain production decreases before birth, resulting in a normal adult Hb profile by the age of 4 months. Therefore, disorders of β-chain production do not manifest clinically, nor can they be reliably detected by Hb precipitation tests, before 4 months of age. However, neonatal Hb electrophoresis screening is included as part of testing for inborn errors of metabolism and detects most newborn patients with sickle cell disease (SCD) in the nursery. Persistence of HbF may occur naturally; it also results from hydroxyurea administration. An elevated HbF concentration is protective against complications of SCD.

Hemoglobinopathies result from either production of abnormal Hb or decreased production of a chain. The most relevant example of the former mechanism is amino acid substitution. Decreased chain production results in thalassemia. Hb profiles for clinically relevant hemoglobinopathies are detailed in Table 36-17 (Lane, 1996).

Genetics and Pathophysiology of Sickle Cell Disease

SCD refers to a clinical phenotype marked by erythrocyte deformation, hemolysis, anemia, microvascular occlusion, and recurrent ischemic injury in all organ systems. In the United States, 8% of the African American population carries one of the recessive genes that result in the sickle cell trait (HbAS, SCT), and one in 625 African Americans is homozygous for mutant alleles that result in sickle cell anemia (HbSS, SCA). SCD is a leading cause of morbidity and mortality among African Americans and is associated with important considerations for perioperative management.

The expression of the SCD phenotype is not limited to patients with SCA. Its expression is caused by the inclusion of a mutant β-globin chain in the Hb tetramer, resulting in clinical courses of variable severity. SCD phenotypes of clinical relevance include the following genotypes: sickle cell anemia (HbSS, SCA), HbSCD (HbSC), sickle-β^0 thalassemia (S-β^0), sickle-β^+ thalassemia (S-β^+), and HbS-O$_{Arab}$ (HbS-O$_{Arab}$).

By definition, patients with the sickle cell trait (HbAS) have at least 50% HbA. Under physiologic conditions, clinical problems are rare. Hb polymerization begins below oxygen saturations of 85% in patients with HbSS, but this does not occur in patients with HbAS until saturations are less than 40%. Thus, it is accepted that patients with HbAS do not require preoperative

TABLE 36-17. Clinical Severity and Diagnostic Testing for the Common Sickle Cell Syndromes

		Relative Clinical Severity			Hemoglobin Electrophoresis in Older Children					
Syndrome	Genotype	Hemolysis	Vasoocclusion	Neonatal Screening*	HbA (%)	HbS (%)	HbF (%)	HbA$_2$ (%)	HbC (%)	Solubility Test†
Sickle cell anemia (HbSS)	S-S	++++	++++	FS	0	80-95	2-20	<3.5	0	Pos
Sickle β⁰ thalassemia‡	S-β⁰	+++	+++	FS	0	80-92	2-15	3.5-7	0	Pos
Sickle HbC disease (HbSC)	S-C	+	++	FSC	0	45-50	1-5	NA§	45-50	Pos
Sickle β⁺ thalassemia‡	S-beta⁺	+	+	FSA or FS¶	5-30	65-90	2-10	35-6	0	Pos
Sickle cell trait	A-S	0	0	FAS	50-60	35-45	<2	<3.5	0	Pos
Normal	A-A	0	0	FA	95-98	0	<2	<3.5	0	Neg

From Lane PA: Sickle cell disease, *Pediatr Clin North Am* 43:639, 1996.
*Hemoglobin reported in order of quantity (e.g., FSA = F > S > A).
†False-negative results occur during infancy in all sickle syndromes.
‡β⁰ indicates thalassemia mutation with absent production of β-globin; β⁺ indicates thalassemia mutation with reduced (but not absent) production of β-globin.
§Quantity of HbA$_2$ cannot be measured in presence of HbC.
¶Quantity of HbA at birth sometimes insufficient for detection.
F, Fetal Hb; *S*, sickle Hb; *C*, HbC: *A*, HbA.

transfusion and are managed with standard attention to hydration, oxygenation, and temperature control.

The fundamental defect in SCD genotypes is amino acid substitution of valine for glutamine at position 6 of the β chain. The resulting HbS is prone to polymerization under conditions of oxygen desaturation caused by formation of bonds between the β-6 valine and the β chains of adjacent tetramers, resulting in the formation of erythrocyte-deforming Hb polymers, erythrocyte cell membrane dysfunction, intracellular oxidant injury, cellular dehydration, and irreversible erythrocyte membrane deformity (Eaton and Hofrichter, 1987; Hebbel et al., 1988; Repka and Hebbel, 1991; Aslan et al., 2000). Deformed erythrocytes obstruct the microvasculature, resulting in tissue ischemia and organ injury. Polymerization is not initially irreversible, however, and prompt return of damaged erythrocytes to the oxygenated state can result in restoration of Hb and cell membrane properties.

Survival of sickle cells in vivo is 5 to 15 days, compared with 120 days for RBCs that contain HbA. The oxygen-dissociation curve in SCA is shifted to the right (i.e., the Hb molecules' affinity for oxygen is less), and theoretically the cells are predisposed to sickling. The cause of this rightward shift is not known, but it is probably related to increased 2,3-diphosphoglycerate levels and to increased mean corpuscular Hb concentration. Of interest is the heterogeneous nature of the P$_{50}$ (Pao$_2$ at 50% Hb saturation) values among the erythrocyte population of individuals with sickle cell disease (Fig. 36-9) (Seakins et al., 1973).

Although it is apparent that erythrocyte and Hb factors are critical in the pathogenesis of the complications of SCD, recent investigations have identified other important contributors that include the coagulation cascade, platelets, leukocytes, endothelial cells, systemic inflammation, oxidant-mediated injury, and abnormalities of NO metabolism (Hammerman et al., 1999; Belcher et al., 2000; Morris et al., 2000a; Aslan et al., 2001; Pawloski et al., 2001; Cosby et al., 2003; Assis et al., 2005; Morris et al., 2005). The endothelium interacts with sickle erythrocytes, platelets, leukocytes, and the coagulation cascade through the expression of vascular cell adhesion molecule-1 (VCAM-1) and elaboration of potent vasoconstrictor compounds responsible for exacerbation

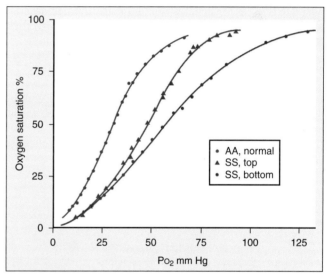

FIGURE 36-9. Oxygen-Hb dissociation curves from top and bottom layers of HbS RBCs. Notice the heterogeneous nature of the P$_{50}$ values. *(From Seakins M, et al: Erythrocyte HbS concentration: an important factor in the low oxygen affinity of blood in sickle cell anemia, J Clin Invest 52:422, 1973.)*

of tissue ischemia and pulmonary artery hypertension (PAH) (Mehta and Mehta, 1980; Brittain et al., 1993; Kurantsin-Mills et al., 1994; Peters et al., 1994; Gee and Platt, 1995; Hagger et al., 1995; Hammerman et al., 1997, 1999; Hebbel, 1997; Graido-Gonzalez et al., 1998; Liesner et al., 1998; Belcher et al., 2000; Assis et al., 2005). Systemic inflammation and oxidant-mediated injury also appear to propagate endothelial injury and tissue ischemia (Hebbel et al., 1982; Schacter et al., 1988; Dias-Da-Motta et al., 1996; Xia et al., 1996; Solovey et al., 1997; Demiryurek et al., 1998; Belcher et al., 2000; Aslan et al., 2001; Assis et al., 2005). SCD is a systemic vasculopathy adversely affecting every organ system in the body.

Abnormalities in the arginine-NO pathway are well described in SCD. Arginine, the precursor for the production of NO, is deficient in SCD and is depleted further during acute chest syndrome (ACS) and vasoocclusive crisis (VOC) (Enwonwu et al., 1990; McDonald et al., 1997; Morris et al., 2000a, 2000b, 2005). The pathophysiology of vasoocclusion and its biochemical contributors are detailed in Figure 36-10 (Gladwin and Vichinsky, 2008). NO is bound by Hb and is exported to the peripheral vasculature in the forms of nitrite and S-nitrosohemoglobin (Pawloski et al., 2001; Cosby et al., 2003). Deficient NO bioactivity occurs secondary to excessive NO and arginine consumption, arginase-mediated destruction of arginine, and abnormal conversion of arginine and NO to injurious oxidative metabolites (Boucher et al., 1999; Hammerman et al., 1999; Mori and Gotoh, 2000; Morris et al., 2000a). Deficient NO bioactivity contributes to the pathogenesis of SCD through diminished inhibitory effects of NO on VCAM-1 expression, leukocyte adhesion, coagulation cascade, and platelet activation, and through diminished NO-mediated vasodilation, which promotes vasoconstriction, ischemia, and resultant erythrocyte sickling. The interactions of deoxygenated sickle Hb, deformed erythrocyte cell membranes, and activated endothelial cells can be summarized by the "four S's"; unstable Hb that precipitates and becomes insoluble, leading to sickling deformation of erythrocyte membranes, which stick to activated endothelial cells.

Acute Complications of Sickle Cell Disease Relevant to Pediatric Anesthesia

Pediatric anesthesiologists encounter patients with SCD when the patients are experiencing acute complications of their disease. Acute splenic sequestration usually occurs in children between the ages of 5 months and 2 years and may appear as late as teenage years in patients with sickle-thalassemia (S-β⁺). This condition results from the pooling of large quantities of blood in the spleen and leads to shock with profound anemia. Aplastic crisis results when the normal brisk reticulocytosis associated with SCD is suppressed, usually as a result of an intercurrent viral infection with parvovirus B19. Hemolytic crisis occurs when a patient with SCD is exposed to a precipitant that causes an abrupt increase in hemolytic stress (infection or medication). Many patients with hemolytic crisis are also deficient in the enzyme glucose-6-phosphate dehydrogenase (G6PD). These disorders are treated with intravascular volume expansion and transfusion of packed RBCs. Treatment of infection and discontinuation of offending medications are also required for hemolytic crisis. Sepsis and septic shock are serious complications that occur in patients with SCD, who generally experience autoinfarction of the spleen in early childhood, rendering them susceptible to infection with encapsulated organisms. The importance of aseptic techniques and wound infection prophylaxis cannot be overstated.

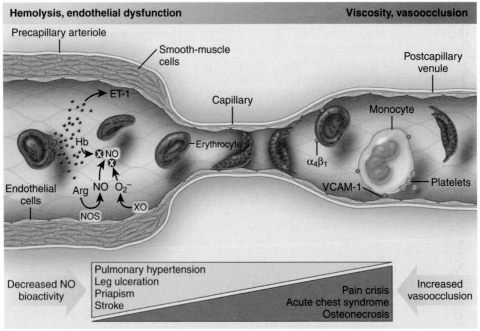

■ **FIGURE 36-10.** Hypothetical mechanisms of clinical subphenotypes of SCD. It is hypothesized that many of the complications of SCD can be divided into two overlapping subtypes, each driven by distinct mechanisms. Cutaneous leg ulceration, priapism, pulmonary hypertension, sudden death, and stroke are associated with low steady-state Hb levels and an increased rate of intravascular hemolysis, shown on the left side of the figure. These vasculopathic complications probably result from endothelial dysfunction, mediated by inactivation of NO by plasma-free Hb and vascular reactive oxygen species, and by arginine catabolism by plasma arginase. The process of hemolysis-associated endothelial dysfunction may also cause hemostatic activation and intimal and smooth muscle proliferation. Such clinical complications (e.g., VOC, ACS, avascular necrosis of bones, and retinal vasculopathy) are associated with high steady-state leukocyte counts and high Hb levels and are likely to result from obstruction of capillaries and postcapillary venules by erythrocytes that contain polymerized HbS and by leukocytes (a monocyte is shown), as shown on the right side of the figure. *ET-1,* Endothelin 1; *NOS,* nitric oxide synthase; *O₂⁻,* superoxide, *VCAM-1,* vascular cell adhesion molecule 1; *XO,* xanthine oxidase. *(From Gladwin MT, Vichinsky E: Pulmonary complications of sickle cell disease,* N Engl J Med *359:2254, 2008.)*

VOC manifests as episodes of painful ischemia and tissue infarction that result from small-vessel occlusion by sickle cells. The most common types of VOC include dactylitis (hand-foot crisis) in infancy, painful crisis in children and adolescents, and priapism in male patients. Stroke and ACS are the most serious forms of VOC that warrant further discussion.

ACS is a common and potentially lethal complication of SCD with complex pathophysiology that can occur in the perioperative period (Fig. 36-11). ACS is the second most common cause of hospital admission and is a leading cause of premature death (mortality rates of 2% to 12%) (Castro et al., 1994; Vichinsky et al., 1997). The etiology of ACS is multifactorial and includes regional hypoxemia secondary to atelectasis or pneumonia, pulmonary vasoocclusion, abnormal NO metabolism, fat emboli, and systemic liberation of inflammatory mediators (Garza, 1990; Vichinsky et al., 1994; Castro, 1996; Styles et al., 1996). ACS occurs in the setting of pulmonary infection or painful crisis, and the symptoms of pneumonia (i.e., fever, pleuritic chest pain, cough, dyspnea, hypoxemia, and progressive infiltrates on chest radiograph) may be difficult to distinguish

from ACS. Respiratory failure may develop quickly, and patients with ACS are treated with hydration, oxygen, antibiotics, simple transfusion, and in severe cases, exchange transfusion. Case reports have described treatment with inhaled NO and extracorporeal membrane oxygenation (Atz and Wessel, 1997; Pelidis et al., 1997; Sullivan et al., 1999). The best treatment for ACS is prevention.

Stroke is the other serious complication of SCD that may occur in the perioperative period. Stroke in children with SCD is most commonly ischemic, but one third of strokes in adult patients with SCD are hemorrhagic (Pavlakis et al., 1989). Many more patients with SCD suffer silent ischemic infarcts that are evident only on neuroimaging, and their presence predicts future ischemic neurologic injury. Indeed, 20% of asymptomatic adolescents have evidence of silent cerebral infarction on neuroimaging studies. Because of the prevalence of silent infarcts in the SCD population, hematologists monitor middle cerebral artery flow velocity with transcranial Doppler (TCD) ultrasonography. Patients who suffer stroke, as well as those with abnormally elevated TCD flow rates, are treated with chronic HbS erythrocyte

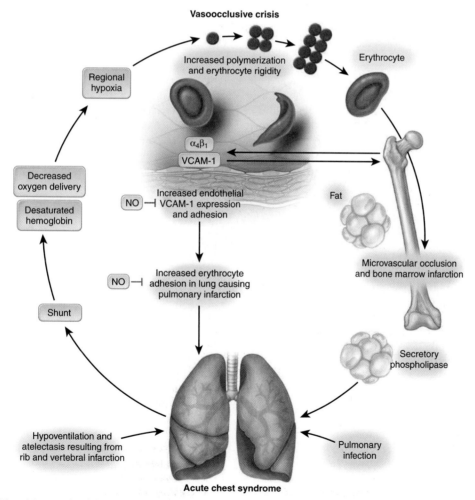

■ **FIGURE 36-11.** The vicious cycle of the ACS. ACS is a lung-injury syndrome initiated by three major triggers, all related to vasoocclusion by sickle cells: infection, embolization of bone marrow fat, and intravascular sequestration of red cells. All of these cause lung injury and infarction. Lung injury results in ventilation-perfusion mismatch and hypoxemia, which leads to increased deoxygenation of HbS, followed by Hb polymerization and erythrocyte vasoocclusion, which in turn promotes bone marrow infarction and pulmonary vasoocclusion. *NO*, Nitric oxide; *VCAM-1*, vascular cell adhesion molecule 1. *(From Gladwin MT, Vichinsky E: Pulmonary complications of sickle cell disease,* N Engl J Med *359:2254, 2008.)*

transfusion to keep HbA at less than 30%. Patients are treated with chronic transfusion for 10 years or longer, because cessation of therapy is associated with increased risk of stroke and recurrence of abnormal TCD flow rates (Adams and Brambilla, 2005). Alloimmunization to erythrocyte antigens is associated with chronic transfusion. Iron overload may also result and may require parenteral deferoxamine or oral deferasirox chelation therapy. Extended phenotypical matching of patient and donor red-cell antigens may result in decreased alloimmunization.

Angiographic and pathologic studies of patients with SCD who have experienced stroke have demonstrated proximal intracranial arterial stenosis of the internal carotid artery, which can be associated with segmental thickening of the arterial wall, and intimal hyperplasia, which tends to occur at sites of arterial bifurcation. A subset of patients with SCD may also demonstrate predominantly small-vessel disease of the CNS vasculature. The potential for presence of flow-limiting lesions in the CNS should be considered when modulating mean arterial blood pressure in the anesthetic management of patients with SCD.

Chronic Complications of Sickle Cell Disease Relevant to Pediatric Anesthesia

Chronic complications of SCD reflect the accumulation of a lifetime of ischemic insults and subsequent decrements in function in all organ systems. Complications include decreased growth and maturation, increased nutritional requirements, retinopathy, stroke, cognitive dysfunction, cardiac dysfunction, elevated PVR, chronic lung injury, diminished renal tubular function, icterus, bone and joint destruction, leg ulceration, and splenic infarction with consequent susceptibility to infectious risk. Of particular importance to the perioperative physician is an appreciation for chronic changes that occur with time in the cardiovascular, respiratory, and renal systems.

The effects of SCD on the cardiovascular system may not be clinically evident to the anesthesiologist. Patients with chronic anemia maintain systemic oxygen delivery through increases in stroke volume and, to a lesser degree, heart rate (in older children and adolescents). Stroke volume increases secondary to increased end-diastolic volume with minimal change in ejection fraction. This condition manifests clinically as cardiomegaly with ventricular dilation.

More ominous than the common changes evident in the left heart is the development of PAH and right ventricular dysfunction. Children with SCD may demonstrate elevated pulmonary vascular resistance during adolescence and early adulthood, and the development of PAH is a robust predictor of premature death (Castro et al., 2003). Most concerning is that in several series of echocardiographic evaluations of patients with SCD, the incidence of PAH was found to be between 20% and 32%, and many of the patients were asymptomatic (Sutton et al., 1994; Gladwin et al., 2004). The mechanisms for the development of PAH in patients who have SCD have been postulated to include diffuse arteriolar thrombosis, scavenging of NO by free Hb in the circulation, arginase-mediated destruction of arginine (limiting NO bioavailability), systemic oxidant-mediated vascular injury, and increased expression of cellular adhesion molecules. SCD patients with or without acute lung injury may have significant PAH and right ventricular dysfunction.

Older patients with SCD may also have significant chronic deterioration of pulmonary function. Sickle cell chronic lung disease is marked by recurrent episodes of chest pain associated with progressive pulmonary fibrosis and dyspnea (Powars et al., 1988). The etiology of this disease is not known but is associated with chronic hemolysis and increased plasma arginase activity. Anesthesiologists should be aware that restrictive lung disease, obstructive lung disease, airway smooth muscle hyperreactivity, and significant derangements of ventilation-perfusion matching have all been described in SCD.

Repeated ischemic insults to the kidneys may result in significant deterioration in glomerular and tubular function in patients who have SCD. Although this condition is rare in children, older patients may suffer impairment severe enough to require dialysis or transplantation. Patients with SCD demonstrate isosthenuria—an inability to concentrate urine—making the patient prone to dehydration. The potential for presence of renal dysfunction should be considered in the management of perioperative fluids, acid-base balance, electrolyte levels, and medications.

Anesthetic Management of Patients with Sickle Cell Disease

Patients with SCD are surviving later into adulthood as a consequence of availability of more effective immunization, antimicrobial prophylaxis and treatment of sepsis, surveillance measures to detect PAH and impending stroke, and disease-altering therapies such as hydroxyurea, chronic transfusion, and stem cell transplantation. Optimal perioperative management of this population requires an understanding of the pathophysiology of the serious complications of SCD and emphasizes basic strategies to minimize their occurrence. Perioperative care of these patients can be considered in terms of preoperative care (including the role for prophylactic preoperative RBC transfusion), intraoperative care, and postoperative care.

Preoperative Preparation of Patients with Sickle Cell Disease

The goal of preoperative preparation of the patient with SCD is to optimize medical conditions that impact the patient's surgery. Identification of patients with SCD is accomplished through newborn Hb electrophoresis screening. Most patients with a SCD phenotype will have been referred to a pediatric hematology practice for longitudinal follow-up care. Rarely, a child may elude detection, with potentially catastrophic results caused by lack of daily antibiotic prophylaxis. Patients older than 6 months can be screened for sickle hemoglobinopathies with "sickle prep" tests in which Hb polymerization is provoked in vitro. In the presence of significant HbF concentrations, these sickle prep examinations lack sensitivity, and Hb electrophoresis is required. Children younger than 6 months and older children with positive sickle prep results require Hb electrophoresis to delineate their hemoglobinopathy. By their tenth birthday, 90% of patients with SCD have clinical manifestations of their disease. Cardiovascular, respiratory, and renal systems, as well as the CNS should be screened for dysfunction that may impact perioperative management. Patients should be treated for infection when appropriate, because infection and systemic inflammation contribute to development of VOC and ACS.

In that dehydration may predispose to VOC and ACS, patients with SCD should be well hydrated before surgery. Administration of IV hydration at 1.5 times the maintenance rate overnight before surgery has been recommended in the past; however, this is not a practice supported by randomized trials. A recent small retrospective study demonstrated the safety and effectiveness of outpatient preoperative management (transfusion and liberal oral hydration) and goal-directed postoperative management, which obviated the need for preoperative admission and extended postoperative observation in this cohort of patients with SCD who were undergoing adenotonsillectomy (Duke et al., 2006). In short, patients with SCD should not be permitted to become dehydrated or volume overloaded during any phase of perioperative management.

Role of Routine Preoperative Blood Transfusion for Patients with Sickle Cell Disease

The most debated topic relevant to the perioperative management of patients with SCD concerns the role of prophylactic preoperative blood transfusion. It has long been appreciated that surgical morbidity and mortality are increased in this population. Early reviews reported mortality rates as high as 10% and complication rates of 50% (Holzmann et al., 1969). Data reflective of more recent advances in anesthetic monitoring and pharmacology demonstrate a 1.1% perioperative mortality rate among adult and pediatric patients with SCD—a level still clearly greater than that of the general population (Koshy et al., 1995). No perioperative deaths were reported in children younger than 14 years of age, nor were perioperative deaths noted in 54 children who underwent 66 elective surgical procedures without preoperative transfusion (Griffin and Buchanan, 1993; Koshy et al., 1995). Although perioperative mortality among patients with SCD is recognized to be more common in older children and adults, serious complications and mortality are well described in all age groups and warrant meticulous attention to perioperative management.

Beginning in the late 1980s, anesthesiologists, hematologists, and surgeons became interested in preoperative transfusion as a means of decreasing the perceived risk associated with surgery and anesthesia for patients with SCD. *Simple transfusion* strategies refer to the transfusion of small aliquots of blood with the goal of increasing the Hb level to 10 g/dL without regard to the final HbS percentage. *Aggressive transfusion* strategies refer to either repetitive, simple transfusions over time or acute exchange transfusion with the goals of Hb concentration of 10 g/dL and HbS less than 30%. The rationale for preoperative transfusion in both cases is to increase the oxygen-carrying capacity of the blood and in the case of aggressive transfusion to decrease the percentage of HbS in the circulation to prevent red cell sickling.

Potential detrimental effects of preoperative prophylactic transfusion include increased risk for acquisition of blood-borne infection, hemolytic transfusion reactions, febrile reactions to leukocyte antigens, transfusion-associated acute lung injury, iron overload, and immunosuppression. Alloimmunization to foreign RBC antigens may develop, which results in difficulty in cross-matching RBCs for transfusion.

The past two decades have witnessed the publication of numerous trials of variable quality and size that have attempted to define the utility of routine preoperative transfusion in the population with SCD. A succinct answer to whether preoperative transfusion is beneficial remains elusive because of confounding variables that include the following:

- Different surgical procedures appear to be associated with different degrees of risk for morbidity and mortality;
- Perioperative morbidity and mortality risk from the same surgical procedures may not be equivalent in infants, children, adolescents, and young adults;
- Changes in surgical and anesthetic techniques, as well as advances in disease-altering medical therapies for SCD, may result in changes in perioperative morbidity and mortality;
- Differing thresholds among studies for exclusion and inclusion of perioperative complications to be considered as clinically relevant endpoints to warrant transfusion in an effort to minimize its occurrence; and
- Lack of randomized prospective data that compare outcomes in patients with SCD who are managed with simple transfusion or exchange transfusion with those who are managed without preoperative transfusion.

Despite the difficulties discussed above, approximately 14 studies published during the past 20 years addressed, in some fashion, the utility of preoperative transfusion (Bischoff et al., 1988; Griffin and Buchanan, 1993; Koshy et al., 1995; Vichinsky et al., 1995, 1999; Haberkern et al., 1997; Neumayr et al., 1998; Waldron et al., 1999; Hirst and Williamson, 2001; Wali et al., 2003; Buck et al., 2005; Fu et al., 2005; Leff et al., 2007; Al-Samak et al., 2008). Considering these studies together, the practitioner can glean the following conclusions:

- Patients with SCD are at much higher risk for perioperative morbidity and mortality, and meticulous attention to preoperative, intraoperative, and postoperative care is warranted.
- Different surgical procedures are associated with different degrees of perioperative risk, and it may not be reasonable to require the same preoperative therapy and preparation for all surgical procedures.
- Among surgical procedures, adenotonsillectomy, laparotomy, and thoracotomy are common procedures associated with the greatest perioperative risk.
- Preoperative transfusion may be associated with improved perioperative outcomes (but not as low as in the population without SCD).
- When transfusion is used for preoperative management, simple transfusion is as effective as exchange transfusion in decreasing SCD-related morbidity for most patients.
- Simple transfusion is more effective than exchange transfusion in reducing transfusion related morbidity (Table 36-18) (Vichinsky et al., 1995).

Data from large, randomized, prospective studies that stratify patients according to age, hemoglobinopathy, surgical procedure, and prior morbidity have not been published. Therefore, the approach to preoperative transfusion should be appropriately individualized after considering the patient's comorbidities, history of SCD-related complications, proposed surgical procedure, and the opinions of the surgeon, anesthesiologist, and hematologist involved in the patient's care. Typically, patients with SCD who are undergoing procedures associated with moderate and increased risk (i.e., laparotomy, thoracotomy, and adenotonsillectomy) are managed with simple transfusion to correct anemia. High-risk patients, such as those with stroke and recurrent ACS, and patients who

TABLE 36-18. Aggressive vs. Simple Transfusion Protocols for Sickle Cell Patients

Characteristic	Aggressive Arm	Simple Arm
Hemoglobin S (HbS)	31%	59%
Hemoglobin (Hb)	11.1 g/dL	10.6 g/dL
Units transfused	5	2.5
Hospital days (for transfusion)	4	2.5
Complications	31%	35%
Transfusion-related	14%	7%
Acute chest syndrome	10%	10%
Death	1%	0

Data from Vichinsky EP, et al: A comparison of conservative and aggressive transfusion regimens in the perioperative management of sickle cell disease: the preoperative transfusion in sickle cell disease study group, *N Engl J Med* 333:206, 1995.

are undergoing very high-risk procedures (i.e., cardiovascular and cerebrovascular surgery) may require an aggressive exchange-transfusion approach that targets a particular HbS percentage (less than 30%).

Many patients with a history of stroke are treated with a chronic-transfusion protocol designed to maintain the Hb concentration at 10 to 11 g/dL and the HbS percentage at less than 30% to 40%. For such patients, further preoperative transfusion therapy is probably not necessary provided the patients have been compliant with the chronic-transfusion regimen. Verification of appropriate Hb concentration and HbS percentage through consultation with the referring hematology staff is appropriate in these circumstances.

In summary, in most patients undergoing most procedures, some form of simple transfusion to correct anemia is usually provided. Close consultation with the hematology service should be sought to help to determine which low-risk patients and low-risk procedures may be managed without transfusion. To maximize the benefit of transfusion therapy while preventing acute increase in viscosity and risk of stroke, the targeted Hb concentration after transfusion should be 10 to 11 g/dL.

Operative Anesthetic Management of Patients with Sickle Cell Disease

Monitoring and maintenance of arterial oxygenation are recommended in the anesthetic management of all patients. Although it is intuitive that maintenance of oxygenation is particularly critical in patients who have SCD, the medical literature contains many descriptions of patients with SCD who were exposed to hypoxemia (i.e., cyanotic congenital heart disease, occlusive tourniquet use, experimental inhalation of hypoxic gas mixtures, and chronic lung disease) and did not suffer immediate SCD-related complications. Similarly, postoperative SCD-related complications continue to occur despite administration of supplemental oxygen and avoidance of intraoperative hypoxemia. Nevertheless, close monitoring of arterial oxygenation and administration of supplemental oxygen are recommended to maintain arterial oxygen saturations in the normal range.

The consequences of Hb desaturation may be mitigated if Hb is promptly reoxygenated after short transit time through the circulation. It is imperative to avoid physiologic perturbations that result in both Hb desaturation and vascular stasis. Preservation of cardiac output, oxygen-carrying capacity, and oxygen saturation, and avoidance of dehydration, hypotension, and vasoconstriction are recommended to minimize conditions conducive to Hb desaturation and prolonged vascular transit time.

Maintenance of normal body temperature is also probably advisable during the anesthetic management of patients with SCD. Whereas hypothermia inhibits oxygen unloading at the tissue level and in this sense might be protective against Hb polymerization, it also results in vasoconstriction in vascular beds and prolongs vascular transit time, thus promoting Hb polymerization. Hyperthermia promotes oxygen unloading at the tissue level and may be associated with vasoconstriction or vasodilation. Close monitoring and maintenance of normal body thermal homeostasis are the basic tenets of critical care and anesthetic management.

At the tissue level, systemic acidosis promotes—and alkalosis inhibits—oxygen unloading. Clinical evidence linking acidosis to precipitation of SCD events is lacking, and sodium bicarbonate administration has not been shown to prevent SCD complications. Further, it is usually difficult to separate the clinical effects of acidosis from its underlying cause. It is recommended to keep systemic acid-base balance close to the normal range.

No particular anesthetic management technique has proven to be more or less effective than others. Arguments can be made for and against regional techniques for patients with SCD. In The Cooperative Study of Sickle Cell Disease, non–SCD-related complications of fever and infection were noted more often in the patients who received regional anesthesia than in those who received general anesthesia (Koshy et al., 1995). However, the group that received regional anesthesia contained more obstetric patients, a subpopulation known to have higher complication rates than other surgical groups. The theoretical rationale for the development of more complications in the regional group includes the presence of compensatory vasoconstriction in areas above the block, lack of controlled ventilation, and the potential for vascular stasis during regional anesthesia (Scott-Conner and Brunson, 1994). Other authors feel that regional techniques do not increase SCD complication risk and, in fact, have used them to treat complications of SCD, including painful crisis and priapism (Yaster et al., 1994). The anesthetic technique chosen is probably not as important as proper preoperative preparation and meticulous intraoperative attention to control of precipitating physiologic factors.

The safety of tourniquet use in orthopedic surgery for patients with SCD has been debated. Although prospective studies that examine the safety of tourniquet use in this population are lacking, retrospective studies supporting its safety have been published (Adu-Gyamfi et al., 1993). If a tourniquet is to be used, it is recommended that the extremity be meticulously exsanguinated before inflating the tourniquet.

Otolaryngology procedures are among the most common surgical procedures performed on children. In a 1999 study that compared patients who underwent adenotonsillectomy and myringotomy after simple and aggressive transfusion, 118 patients were enrolled and randomized to one of the two preoperative transfusion regimens, and an additional 47 patients were enrolled and not randomized; 20 of the 47 nonrandomized patients were not transfused (Waldron et al., 1999). No differences between transfusion strategies were reported with respect to complications. History of pulmonary disease predicted perioperative SCD-related complications in adenotonsillectomy patients. The authors speculated that because myringotomy is associated with short duration of surgery, minimal blood loss, and surgery remote from the airway, preoperative transfusion might not improve the safety of myringotomy. However, this hypothesis was not specifically studied, and the importance of attention to all other aspects of perioperative care (hydration, oxygenation, and temperature control) was emphasized. Patients with SCD who have sleep-disordered breathing require meticulous perioperative observation, because they have particularly severe nocturnal oxygen desaturation and hypercarbia when compared with age- and gender-matched patients in a control group (who do not have SCD) with sleep-disordered breathing (Kaleyias et al., 2008).

Cholecystectomy is another common procedure performed in patients with SCD (Haberkern et al., 1997). Increased use of laparoscopic techniques for gall bladder removal results in less postoperative pain, splinting, and atelectasis. Wales and colleagues (2001) examined the effect of laparoscopic vs. open cholecystectomy in this patient population. Increased risk for ACS in all types of abdominal surgery was noted, irrespective of technique (20% overall, 22% in laparoscopic cases, 15% in open cases), but most of these patients were not transfused. The authors concluded that the postoperative benefits of laparoscopic surgery do not result in decreased SCD complications, but they questioned whether more liberal preoperative transfusion would have resulted in improved outcomes.

Postoperative Management of the Patient with Sickle Cell Disease

Most serious SCD-related complications occur in the postoperative period, and therefore the advisability of outpatient surgery for patients with SCD is questionable. VOC is the most common postoperative SCD-related complication. For this reason, it is prudent to comply with the paradigm used by the Preoperative Transfusion in Sickle Cell Disease Study Group, which included postoperative hospitalization, oxygen supplementation, hydration, and pulse-oximeter monitoring. The importance of adequate postoperative analgesia (e.g., oral or IV opioids, NSAIDs, and regional anesthesia techniques) cannot be overstated, because inadequate pain management results in pulmonary splinting, hypoventilation, and ACS. On the other hand, excessive administration of pain medication may result in hypoventilation, atelectasis, and ACS. Postoperative length of stay in the hospital is dictated to a large degree by the type of surgery performed, but patients can be considered for discharge when they are able to sustain oral hydration, are free from fever, can demonstrate good oxygen saturations and pulmonary toilet, and when pain is well controlled on oral analgesics.

Other groups have advocated an individualized approach to the perioperative management of surgical patients with SCD. For children undergoing adenotonsillectomy, Duke and colleagues (2006) recommended preoperative outpatient transfusion, liberal oral clear liquid hydration at home, postoperative monitoring with pulse oximeter, and oxygen administration only to those patients with saturations of less than 94%. With this paradigm, which mandated controlled responses to hypoxemia and fever in the postoperative period, complications were noted

that included 20% with hypoxemia, 10% with fever, and 8% with ACS. Most of their patients were discharged from the hospital after fewer than 24 hours without adverse sequelae.

Thalassemia

Thalassemia refers to any of several genetic defects in the production of globin chains of Hb. Patients may have deficient production of the α-globin chain (α thalassemia) or the β-globin chain (β thalassemia). The clinical thalassemic syndromes can be understood in terms of the corresponding genotypes.

The α-thalassemia syndromes, which contain four allele loci, have more genotypical possibilities than the β thalassemias. The severity of the syndrome is dependent on how many of the four α-globin genes are absent. The absence of functional α-globin genes (–/–) is not compatible with life and leads to death in utero (hydrops fetalis). One functional α-globin gene (–/α-) leads to a severe microcytic, hemolytic anemia called *HbH disease*. Two nonfunctional genes (αα/–) gives rise to a mild anemia (α thalassemia minor syndrome). A single nonfunctional α-globin gene is clinically silent.

For the β thalassemias (with two β-globin gene loci), mutations on both of the β-globin gene loci result in homozygous disease; however, each locus has more than 60 possible mutations that result in heterogeneous clinical syndromes for homozygous patients, depending on which mutant alleles are present at the two loci. For some patients with very dysfunctional mutant genes present at the two loci, severe anemia results with a lifelong transfusion requirement—referred to as β-*thalassemia major*. Other patients with more functional mutant alleles at these loci also have severe anemia but do not require lifelong transfusions—this condition is referred to as β-*thalassemia intermedia*. Patients who are heterozygous (one normal β-globin gene and one mutant β-globin) have more moderate anemia and produce enough β-globin chains to obviate the need for ongoing transfusions—referred to as β-*thalassemia trait*, or β-*thalassemia minor*.

In patients with thalassemia, the issues encountered by the anesthesiologist are anemia, the problems associated with chronic anemia, and numerous transfusions. These patients do not recover from surgical blood loss with RBC production, as is expected in other patients. It should be remembered that thalassemia patients can be heterozygous for two different disorders of β-globin production. The most clinically relevant examples are patients who have both a sickle gene and a mutant β-thalassemia gene at the β-globin chain loci. The modifiers $β^+$ and $β^0$ are included as descriptive terminology for these patients. $β^0$ indicates that the patient cannot produce any normal β-globin chains; therefore, patients with S-$β^0$ thalassemia have no HbA. Their clinical course is similar to those of patients with HbSS disease. $β^+$ does not refer to a specific genotype but indicates that the patients can produce variable quantities of normal β-globin chains (depending upon the mutant gene present). Patients with S-$β^+$ thalassemia produce variable amounts of HbA and generally have a more benign clinical course than patients with HbSS. Both groups of heterozygotes warrant the same meticulous perioperative management that is provided to patients with sickle cell anemia.

Oncology Issues

Relationship to the Pediatric Anesthesiologist

As anesthesiologists play greater roles in the management of pediatric patients with cancer, their interactions with these patients and their families have become increasingly important. From the time children are diagnosed with malignancy until the end of a successful treatment, the anesthesiologist has assumed an increasingly important role in their care. Historically, repetitive painful procedures such as lumbar puncture, bone marrow aspiration, and others were performed with physical restraint under local anesthesia and without sedation. This protocol was minimally effective in relieving pain and anxiety, and families were confronted not only with the anxiety and uncertainty of the diagnosis and prognosis of their children, but also with the dread of repetitive painful procedures.

In many pediatric hospitals, an anesthesiologist is present when diagnostic procedures are performed, tumors are removed, central venous access devices are implanted and removed, and radiation treatments are administered. Increasingly, anesthesiologists are also being asked to assist with pain management during end-of-life care, in response to painful complications of chemotherapy, and during recovery from hematopoietic stem cell transplantation (HSCT).

Childhood cancer remains one of the leading causes of disease-related mortality among pediatric patients, but progressive advances in its management have led to increased numbers of long-term survivors. Indeed, 79% of children diagnosed with cancer before the age of 15 survive for at least 5 years (Jemal et al., 2006). Acute lymphoblastic leukemia and CNS tumors are the two most common malignancies in children, and advances in their management have exposed the anesthesiologist to increased numbers of surviving children with delayed organ toxicity related to treatment. The following section is a review of the anesthetic implications of chemotherapy, radiation therapy, and HSCT.

Myelosuppression

Acute and delayed toxicities result from the administration of chemotherapy. Acute toxicities common to most chemotherapy agents include myelosuppression, alopecia, nausea, vomiting, mucositis, and liver dysfunction. Myelosuppression results in profound pancytopenia and is of concern in perioperative management. Neutropenia renders patients susceptible to bacterial and viral infections. Recommended precautions to prevent introduction of bacterial infections include protective and reverse isolation, avoidance of rectal temperature measurement and medication administration, strict hand washing, and aseptic technique during procedures, including before and during medication administration through central venous catheters.

Thrombocytopenia is common in oncology patients, and the need for perioperative platelet transfusion is dependent on the type of procedure to be performed, the potential for bleeding, and the function of the existing platelets. Neuraxial anesthesia may be contraindicated in these situations. These decisions should be made in consultation with the patient, the family, and the hematologist directing the patient's care. The decision as to when to transfuse packed RBCs should also be discussed with the hematologist. In the absence of significant cardiac or pulmonary disease or the need for increased oxygen-carrying capacity, hematocrit values in the low to mid 20s are common and well tolerated. RBCs may require radiation to prevent graft-versus-host disease (GVHD) in the immunocompromised oncology patient, as well as leukocyte depletion to prevent transmission of cytomegalovirus.

Individual chemotherapeutic drugs and radiation produce unique toxicities that are of concern in the anesthetic management of oncology patients (Table 36-19) (Bleyer, 2007). Particularly important among them are medications that, alone or in combination with anesthetic drugs, result in cardiac and pulmonary toxicity, and these are discussed in detail.

Cardiac Toxicity

Anthracycline Antibiotics

Several chemotherapeutic agents cause cardiac toxicity that may be acute or chronic. The agents most commonly associated with cardiac toxicity are the anthracycline antibiotics doxorubicin, daunorubicin, epirubicin, and idarubicin (Giantris et al., 1998; Singal and Iliskovic, 1998; Balis et al., 2002). Acute cardiac changes associated with anthracycline administration include decreased QRS amplitude, nonspecific ST-T wave changes, supraventricular and ventricular rhythm disturbances, and reduction in ventricular ejection fraction, reaching a nadir at 24 hours after administration. A severe form of this constellation of effects, called *myocarditis-pericarditis syndrome*, results in congestive heart failure with cardiogenic shock.

Chronic toxicity may also occur weeks, months (early form), and years (late form) after anthracycline administration. The early form is associated with cytoplasmic vacuolization, myofibrillary lysis, and degeneration of nuclei and mitochondria. Oxidative damage that results from anthracycline metabolism is believed to be responsible for these changes. Myocardial dysfunction with congestive heart failure that is poorly responsive to cardiotonic medications occurs with a cumulative dose-dependent risk. Acute myocardial injury occurs in fewer than 1% of pediatric patients; the incidence of congestive heart failure increases with doxorubicin doses higher than 450 mg/m^2 but has been observed with doses as low as 220 mg/m^2 (Giantris et al., 1998). The toxic threshold for idarubicin is not known, but doses up to 150 mg/m^2 appear to be tolerated (Allen, 1992; Swafford and Gibbs, 1998). Mediastinal irradiation increases the risk of anthracycline-induced myocardial dysfunction.

Late-form cardiotoxicity, which occurs 7 to 14 years after therapy, is more common in children and may be related to the inability of the heart to grow with the child. Late toxicity is associated with cumulative doses of doxorubicin more than 300 mg/m^2 but has been described to occur in children after lower doses. Children treated with these medications receive follow-up care with baseline and serial echocardiograms for many years after treatment. Risk for death from cardiac-related events is eight times higher among survivors of pediatric malignancies than it is in the general population (Green et al., 2001; Mertens et al., 2001). Risk factors for anthracycline-mediated cardiac toxicity are listed in Table 36-20 (Swafford and Gibbs, 1998).

Methods to prevent or minimize anthracycline-induced cardiac disease have been and continue to be investigated. These include limiting cumulative dose and altering administration methods of anthracycline, coupling anthracyclines with liposomal carriers and polyethylene glycol, using anthracycline analogues, and adding cardioprotective medications

TABLE 36-19. Common Chemotherapeutic Agents Used In Children

Drug	Mechanism of Action or Classification	Indication(s)	Adverse Reactions	Monitory Drug Level	Comments
Methotrexate	Folic acid antagonist; inhibits dihydrofolate reductase	ALL non-Hodgkin lymphoma, osteosarcoma, Hodgkin lymphoma, medulloblastoma	Myelosuppression, mucositis, stomatitis, dermatitis, hepatitis; With long-term administration, osteopenia and bone fractures; With high-dose administration, renal and CNS toxicity; With intrathecal administration, arachnoiditis, leukoencephalopathy, leukomyelopathy	Plasma levels must be monitored with high-dose therapy and when low doses are administered to patients with renal dysfunction and leucovorin rescue applied accordingly	Systemic administration may be PO, IM, or IV; also may be administered intrathecally
6-Mercaptopurine (Purinethol)	Purine analogue; inhibits purine synthesis	ALL	Myelosuppression, hepatic necrosis, mucositis; allopurinol increases toxicity	Therapeutic drug monitoring not available or indicated	Allopurinol inhibits metabolism
Cytarabine (Ara-C)	Pyrimidine analogue; inhibits DNA polymerase	ALL, AML, non-Hodgkin lymphoma, Hodgkin lymphoma	Nausea, vomiting, myelosuppression, conjunctivitis, mucositis, CNS dysfunction; With intrathecal administration, arachnoiditis, leukoencephalopathy, leukomyelopathy	Therapeutic drug monitoring not available or indicated	Systemic administration may be PO, IM, or IV; may also be administered intrathecally
Cyclophosphamide (Cytoxan)	Alkylates guanine; inhibits DNA synthesis	ALL, non-Hodgkin lymphoma, Hodgkin lymphoma, soft tissue sarcoma, Ewing sarcoma	Nausea, vomiting, myelosuppression, hemorrhagic cystitis, pulmonary fibrosis, inappropriate ADH secretion, bladder cancer, anaphylaxis	Therapeutic drug monitoring not available or indicated	Requires hepatic activation and is thus less effective in presence of liver dysfunction
Ifosfamide (Ifex)	Alkylates guanine; inhibits DNA synthesis	Non-Hodgkin lymphoma, Wilms tumor, sarcoma, germ cell and testicular tumors	Nausea, vomiting myelosuppression, hemorrhagic cystitis, pulmonary fibrosis, inappropriate ADH secretion, bladder cancer, CNS dysfunction, cardiac toxicity, anaphylaxis	Therapeutic drug monitoring not available or indicated	
Doxorubicin (Adriamycin) and daunorubicin (Cerubidine)	Binds to DNA, intercalation	ALL, AML, osteosarcoma, Ewing sarcoma, Hodgkin lymphoma, non-Hodgkin lymphoma, neuroblastoma	Nausea, vomiting, cardiomyopathy, red urine, tissue necrosis on extravasation, myelosuppression, conjunctivitis, radiation dermatitis, arrhythmia	Therapeutic drug monitoring not available or indicated	
Dactinomycin	Binds to DNA, inhibits transcription	Wilms tumor, rhabdomyosarcoma, Ewing sarcoma	Nausea, vomiting, tissue necrosis on extravasation, myelosuppression, radiosensitizer, mucosal ulceration	Therapeutic drug monitoring not available or indicated	
Bleomycin (Blenoxane)	Binds to DNA cleaves DNA strands	Hodgkin disease, non-Hodgkin lymphoma, germ cell tumors	Nausea, vomiting, pneumonitis, stomatitis, Raynaud phenomenon, pulmonary fibrosis, dermatitis	Therapeutic drug monitoring not available or indicated	

Continued

TABLE 36-19. Common Chemotherapeutic Agents Used In Children—cont'd

Drug	Mechanism of Action or Classification	Indication(s)	Adverse Reactions	Monitory Drug Level	Comments
Vincristine (Oncovin)	Inhibits microtubule formation	ALL, non-Hodgkin lymphoma, Hodgkin disease, Wilms tumor, Ewing sarcoma, neuroblastoma rhabdomyosarcoma	Local cellulitis, peripheral neuropathy, constipation, ileus, jaw pain, inappropriate ADH secretion, seizures, ptosis, minimal myelosuppression	Therapeutic drug monitoring not available or indicated	IV administration only; must not be allowed to extravasate
Vinblastine (Velban)	Inhibits microtubule formation	Hodgkin disease; Langerhans cell histiocytosis	Local cellulitis, leukopenia	Therapeutic drug monitoring not available or indicated	IV administration only; must not be allowed to extravasate
L-Asparaginase	Depletion of L-asparagine	ALL; AML, when used in combination with asparaginase	Allergic reaction pancreatitis, hyperglycemia, platelet dysfunction and coagulopathy, encephalopathy	Therapeutic drug monitoring not available or indicated	PEG-asparaginase now preferred to L-asparaginase
Pegaspargase (Pegaspar)	Polyethylene glycol conjugate of L-asparaginase	ALL	Indicated for prolonged asparagine depletion and for patients with allergy to L-asparaginase	Therapeutic drug monitoring not available or indicated	
Prednisone and dexamethasone (Decadron)	Lymphatic cell lysis	ALL; Hodgkin disease, non-Hodgkin lymphoma	Cushing's is syndrome, cataracts, diabetes, hypertension, myopathy, osteoporosis, infection, peptic ulceration, psychosis	Therapeutic drug monitoring not available or indicated	
Carmustine (nitrosourea)	Carbamylation of DNA; inhibits DNA synthesis	CNS tumors, non-Hodgkin lymphoma, Hodgkin disease	Nausea, vomiting, delayed myelosuppression (4-6 wk); pulmonary fibrosis, carcinogenic stomatitis	Therapeutic drug monitoring not available or indicated	Phenobarbital increases metabolism, decreases activity
Carboplatin and cisplatin (Platinol)	Inhibits DNA synthesis	Gonadal tumors; osteosarcoma, neuroblastoma, CNS, tumors, germ cell tumors	Nausea, vomiting, renal dysfunction, myelosuppression, ototoxicity, tetany, neurotoxicity, hemolytic-uremic syndrome, anaphylaxis	Therapeutic drug monitoring not available or indicated	Aminoglycosides may increase nephrotoxicity
Etoposide (VePesid)	Topoisomerase inhibitor	ALL, non-Hodgkin lymphoma, germ cell tumor	Nausea, vomiting, myelosuppression, secondary eukemia	Therapeutic drug monitoring not available or indicated	
Etretinate (Tegison) (vitamin A analogue) and tretinoin	Enhances normal differentiation	Acute progranulocytic leukemia, neuroblastoma	Dry mouth, hair loss, pseudotumor cerebri, premature epiphyseal closure	Therapeutic drug monitoring not available or indicated	

From Bleyer A: Principles of treatment. In Kliegman RM, et al., editors: *Nelson textbook of Pediatrics*, ed 18, Philadelphia, 2007, Saunders.
IM, Intramuscularly; *IV*, intravenously; *PO*, orally.

TABLE 36-20. Risk Factors for Anthracycline Cardiac Toxicity

Risk Factor	Description
Cumulative dose	Risk <1% for doses <300 mg/m² 5%-10% for doses 350-450 mg/m² 30% for doses >550 mg/m²
Schedule of administration	Risk greatest with bolus administration Less risk with continuous infusion Less risk with dexrazoxane
Mediastinal irradiation	Strong association with increasing risk
Cardiac disease	Preexisting coronary artery disease, valvular heart disease, hypertension
Age	Young children Adults aged >70 years

From Swafford J, Gibbs HR: Cardiac complications of cancer treatment, *Anesth Clin N Am* 16:598, 1998.

such as dexrazoxane (that chelate iron molecules and prevent anthracycline-induced oxidative injury) into the chemotherapy regimen (Legha et al., 1982; Shapira et al., 1990; Dorr et al., 1991; Herman et al., 1997; Cottin et al., 1998; Creutzig et al., 2001; Lipshultz et al., 2002a; O'Byrne et al., 2002; Safra, 2003; Levitt and Dorup, 2004; O'Brien et al., 2004; Barry et al., 2007).

Patients who suffer from anthracycline-induced cardiotoxicity are treated with afterload-reducing medications to minimize ventricular wall stress. The most common medications used for this purpose are the angiotensin-converting enzyme (ACE) inhibitors. ACE inhibitors administered to survivors of pediatric cancers have been beneficial in improving left-ventricle dimensions, fractional shortening, left-ventricle mass, and decreasing afterload (Lipshultz et al., 2002b). However, this benefit appears to be transient, because many patients regress to baseline and deteriorate further after 6 to 10 years of treatment (Lipshultz et al., 2002b, 2004). Other medications used for cardiac dysfunction and congestive heart failure include β-blockers such as carvedilol. The beneficial effects of β-blockers in the setting of idiopathic dilated cardiomyopathy and ischemic heart disease with congestive heart failure in adult patients include reduction in mortality, increase in left-ventricular ejection fraction, and prevention of adrenergically mediated intrinsic myocardial dysfunction and remodeling (Bristow, 1997; Lechat et al., 1998).

Cyclophosphamide

Cyclophosphamide, especially in high doses (exceeding 100 to 200 mg/kg), can cause severe congestive heart failure and hemorrhagic myocarditis. Pericardial tamponade has also been described with cyclophosphamide and has resulted in cardiac tamponade. Toxicity occurs with lower doses in children who have also received anthracyclines.

Radiation

Radiation, when used for the treatment of thoracic tumors, has also resulted in cardiac toxicity, with early toxicity associated with pericarditis, pericardial effusions, and tamponade.

Radiation dose is expressed in terms of joules deposited per kilogram of body weight (J/kg), which is denoted as Gray (Gy) units. One Gy is equal to 100 rads in the old system; thus, 1 rad is equivalent to 1 cGy. Most long-term effects occur with cumulative doses that exceed 40 Gy and may not become manifest for up to 10 years after treatment (Applefield et al., 1982).

The anesthetic management of patients with known or suspected cardiomyopathy necessarily includes cardiology consultation and echocardiographic assessment of myocardial and valvular function. Oncology patients may have clinically silent deterioration in cardiovascular function for many years after completion of therapy. Selection of induction agents, maintenance agents, and invasive hemodynamic monitors is made on the basis of cardiovascular status. Intraoperative fatalities have occurred in children with chemotherapy-induced cardiomyopathy.

Pulmonary Toxicity

Many chemotherapeutic agents have some element of pulmonary toxicity. The etiology of pulmonary dysfunction in the immunosuppressed, and especially in stem cell-transplant recipients, may include infectious etiologies, nonspecific lung injury related to dysregulated inflammation and immune function, and toxic injury from medications and radiation. Because of the multifactorial causes for lung injury in oncology patients, it is often difficult to pinpoint the offending agent responsible for the injury.

Alkylating agents

Drugs such as carmustine, lomustine, busulfan, melphalan, chlorambucil, and cyclophosphamide are all associated with cytotoxic lung injury. Busulfan may cause lung injury when given as a single agent, whereas the other medications usually do so only in high doses or when part of multidrug therapy. Busulfan lung injury occurs 6 weeks to 10 years after therapy, with an average time interval from treatment to symptoms of 3 years. Dyspnea, fatigue, nonproductive cough, weight loss, unexplained fever, and bi-basilar pulmonary infiltrates are hallmarks of this complication, and it carries a poor prognosis.

Bleomycin (a cytotoxic antibiotic) and mitomycin (an alkylating agent) have pulmonary toxicities. Bleomycin lung injury is the prototype for interstitial pneumonitis and pulmonary fibrosis. It has been clearly recognized that a toxic synergistic relationship exists between high inspired-oxygen concentration and bleomycin. Although the exact mechanism is unclear, oxygen concentrations above 30% can rapidly precipitate acute lung injury and acute respiratory distress syndrome in patients who have previously received bleomycin (Maher and Daley, 1993; Mathes, 1995). Mortality from this injury ranges between 13% and 83% in various studies. High-dose corticosteroids have had a beneficial effect in the treatment of this injury (Maher and Daley, 1993). Antimetabolites such as cytosine arabinoside, fludarabine, methotrexate, and 6-mercaptopurine also cause varying degrees of lung injury in dose-related fashion but generally carry better long-term prognoses than does bleomycin-mediated pulmonary toxicity.

Radiation

Thoracic radiation causes clinically significant lung injury in 5% to 15% of patients. Several phases of lung injury are described.

The latent or early phase occurs within 1 to 2 months of exposure; the exudative phase occurs 4 to 6 months afterward, and symptoms of pneumonitis develop. The late phase is heralded by the development of pulmonary fibrosis from 6 to 12 months after exposure. Factors that influence the development of pulmonary toxicity include the total dose of irradiation, volume of lung treated, fraction size (radiation given per treatment), and patient age at the time of treatment (younger patients are more prone to toxicity). Pulmonary toxicity has decreased significantly over the past decade because of refined techniques of radiotherapy (Hassink et al., 1993). Toxicity usually does not occur until more than 30 Gy are delivered to more than 50% of the lung when radiation is used alone in adults. The mechanism of injury appears to be different in children younger than 3 years of age, in whom interference with lung and chest wall growth may occur (Miller et al., 1986). In these children, restrictive lung disease has developed with radiation doses as low as 11 to 14 Gy.

Anesthetic management of patients who have—or who are at risk for the development of—radiation or chemotherapy-induced pulmonary toxicity requires careful preoperative assessment and intraoperative management. Preoperative assessment may include chest x-ray or CT, spirometric assessment, oxygen saturation or arterial blood gas measurement, and pulmonology consultation. Children at risk for pulmonary toxicity should be treated with the lowest inspired oxygen concentration that provides acceptable oxygen saturation values, and the lowest airway pressures (peak inspiratory pressure and positive end-expiratory pressure) that provide adequate ventilation and preservation of functional residual capacity should be selected.

Hematopoietic Stem Cell Transplantation

HSCT has become an accepted therapy for many pediatric disorders, including hematologic malignancies, aplastic anemia, immunodeficiency disorders, congenital hematologic defects, inborn errors of metabolism, and some solid tumors. Pediatric patients who have received HSCT present several unique considerations for anesthetic management, including pretransplant conditioning, acute and chronic GVHD, adverse organ system effects of GVHD, non–GVHD-related morbidity, and unique pharmacologic considerations.

Pretransplant Conditioning

All patients who have undergone HSCT first undergo pretransplant conditioning to ablate or impair the native bone marrow. Chemotherapeutic agents commonly employed for this conditioning include cyclophosphamide, busulfan, and fludarabine with or without total body irradiation. In addition to the adverse effects of the chemotherapy agents already discussed, adverse effects of cyclophosphamide include hemorrhagic cystitis and pulmonary fibrosis, and busulfan causes hepatic venoocclusive disease and seizures (Stein et al., 1990; Culshaw et al., 2003). Patients with hemorrhagic cystitis may require blood transfusion or may need anesthesia for cystoscopy and possible suprapubic tube placement. Total body irradiation is associated with restrictive cardiomyopathy, interstitial pneumonitis, and hypothyroidism. Appropriate preoperative evaluation, induction and maintenance drug selection, placement of invasive hemodynamic monitors, and

provision for postoperative analgesia and monitoring are dictated by cardiovascular status and pulmonary reserve.

Graft-versus-Host Disease

Acute GVHD is a clinical syndrome that usually develops in 40% to 60% of patients receiving HSCT by 60 to 100 days after allogeneic HSCT. It is characterized by the development of erythematous skin rash; hepatic involvement with cholestatic jaundice; GI disease marked by the presence of abdominal pain, excessive vomiting, ileus, bleeding, and diarrhea; fever, thrombocytopenia, and anemia; and occasional pulmonary involvement with vascular leak. Chronic GVHD occurs in 20% to 40% of patients who have undergone HSCT and may occur as an extension of acute GVHD, or it may occur in the absence of preceding GVHD (Table 36-21) (Venkatesan and Jacob, 2007). The diagnosis is occasionally made after day 100 of HSCT and is rarely made after more than 500 days after HSCT (Arai and Vogelsang, 2000). Chronic GVHD is a distinctive syndrome that resembles autoimmune collagen vascular disease, with manifestations evident in every organ in the body.

Organ System Considerations in Patients with HSCT

The respiratory system is a major source of morbidity among patients receiving HSCT. Diffuse lung injury is a major

TABLE 36-21. Clinicopathologic Features of Chronic Graft-Versus-Host Disease

System	Features
Systemic	Recurrent infections with immunodeficiency, weight loss, sicca syndrome, debility
Skin	Lichen planus, scleroderma, hyperpigmentation or hypopigmentation, dry scale, ulcerated, freckling, flexion contractures
Hair	Alopecia
Mouth	Sicca syndrome, depapillation of tongue with variegations scalloping of lateral margins, lichen planus and ulcer, angular tightness, salivary gland inflammation, fibrosis
Joints	Decreased range of motion, diffuse myositis/ tendonitis
Eyes	Decreased tearing, injected sclerae, conjunctivae
Liver	Cholestasis, cirrhosis
Gastrointestinal	Failure to thrive, esophageal strictures, malabsorption, chronic diarrhea
Lung	Bronchiolitis obliterans can manifest as dyspnea, cough, wheezing with normal CT scan and marked obstructive ventilatory defects, pneumothorax, chronic sinopulmonary symptoms and/or infections
Heart	Bradycardia, chest pain
Hematopoietic	Refractory thrombocytopenia, eosinophilia
Immune system	Profound immunodeficiency, functional asplenia, risk of pneumococcal sepsis

From Venkatesan T, Jacob R: Anesthesia and graft-versus-host disease after hematopoietic stem cell transplantation, *Pediatr Anesth* 17:7, 2007.

complication of HSCT that accounts for 50% of transplant-related mortality and may be classified as either infectious or noninfectious. Acute noninfectious lung injury is called *idiopathic pneumonia syndrome* and refers to widespread alveolar injury that occurs in the absence of left-ventricular dysfunction or respiratory tract infection. Current treatment strategies for idiopathic pneumonia syndrome include oxygen administration, mechanical ventilation with small tidal volumes and low peak-inspiratory pressures, broad-spectrum antibiotic administration, and increased immune suppression.

Chronic GVHD may involve the respiratory system, resulting in recurrent sinopulmonary infections and restrictive or obstructive lung disease. A severe form of obstructive lung disease associated with chronic GVHD is bronchiolitis obliterans, which is characterized by progressive dyspnea, cough, wheezing, reduced FEV_1, reduced expiratory flow rates, and increased residual lung volume. Small-airway plugging with inflammatory cells, emphysematous distal airways, hyperinflation, interstitial pneumatosis, and pneumothorax may be noted. Patients with bronchiolitis obliterans have a very poor prognosis, and no therapies have been demonstrated to favorably influence the outcome of this disease.

Therapy for pulmonary disease with expiratory obstruction associated with chronic GVHD includes administration of supplemental oxygen, bronchodilators, enhanced immune suppression, antimicrobial prophylaxis, and IV immune globulin (Arai and Vogelsang, 2000; Yanik and Cooke, 2006). Patients with pulmonary involvement may need anesthesia for bronchoscopy with bronchoalveolar lavage or biopsy to discern the etiology of pulmonary disease (e.g., infectious vs. bronchiolitis obliterans). Pulmonary function may temporarily worsen after bronchoscopy, especially if bronchoalveolar lavage is performed. The parent/guardian should be informed of this possibility during the consent process. Preoperative evaluation of patients with advanced respiratory disease may include chest radiographs, spirometry, arterial blood gas measurement, and pulse oximetry. Intraoperative management emphasizes monitoring of airway pressure, humidification and warming of airway gases, and continuation of perioperative antibiotics. Patients with severe lung disease may require postoperative mechanical ventilation or placement of an arterial catheter for blood gas analysis.

The skin and its appendages are targets in chronic GVHD, resulting in dermal sclerosis with loss of hair and sweat glands. Patients with sclerotic disease have fragile skin prone to tissue trauma and have impaired ability to sweat, resulting in predisposition to the development of hyperthermia. The oral manifestations of acute and chronic GVHD can result in severe mucositis, restricted mouth opening, and difficult orotracheal intubation (Schubert et al., 1984; Arai and Vogelsang, 2000). Ocular manifestations of chronic GVHD include decreased lacrimation, which predisposes patients to corneal ulceration (Grover et al., 1998). The musculoskeletal system may be adversely affected by HSCT, resulting in polymyositis, polyserositis, and myopathy (Reyes et al., 1983; Beredjiklian et al., 1998). Joint involvement in the form of flexion contractures and ulcerations may be present. Decreased range of motion between cervical vertebrae and diminished mouth opening should be sought in sclerodermoid chronic GVHD, as these may complicate airway management. Polyserositis may be associated with ascites as well as pericardial and pleural effusions. Careful attention to assessment of potential for oral airway difficulties, positioning,

padding, monitoring of temperature, application of warming devices, eye lubrication, and eye protection is required.

The immune system can be assumed to be significantly impaired in recipients of HSCT (Atkinson et al., 1982; Lapp et al., 1985). Continuation of antibacterial, antiviral, and antifungal therapies during the perioperative period is imperative, and many clinicians insert bacterial and viral filters into the breathing circuit. Strict aseptic technique is required during invasive procedures. The rectal route of medication administration and temperature monitoring is discouraged.

The GI tract is a major source of morbidity in recipients of HSCT. Acute GVHD manifests with diarrhea, abdominal pain, GI bleeding, ileus, and loss of electrolytes, fluid, and blood. GI tract signs seen in chronic GVHD include esophageal, gastric, and duodenal ulcerations, esophageal web, diarrhea, vomiting, chronic malabsorption, and gastroesophageal reflux (Arai and Vogelsang, 2000). Because of mucosal abnormalities, it is prudent to avoid the use of esophageal stethoscopes and rectal temperature probes. Rapid-sequence induction and intubation should be considered if GI dysfunction appears to put the patient at risk for aspiration pneumonia. Mucositis and swelling of oral structures may impede visualization of airway structures.

Hepatic dysfunction is common in GVHD. Acute GVHD results in cholestatic jaundice, and chronic GVHD is associated with elevation of alkaline phosphatase, bilirubin, and transaminases. Many patients with GVHD are also dependent on parenteral nutrition, which may exacerbate hepatic injury. Selection of anesthetic agents with minimal hepatic metabolism and toxicity and minimal effects on hepatic blood flow may be indicated. Close attention to glucose homeostasis is necessary to prevent hypoglycemia under anesthesia. Monitoring and correction of coagulation parameters are essential for operative procedures associated with significant bleeding and when regional anesthesia is contemplated.

Hematologic dysfunction after HSCT may manifest as refractory thrombocytopenia, isolated neutropenia or anemia, or pancytopenia. Adequate blood and blood products should be available for cases in which blood loss is expected to be high and when hemostasis is critically important at the surgical site (CNS and ocular cases).

Non–Graft-versus-Host Disease HSCT Complications

Complications of HSCT not related to GVHD include renal dysfunction, hepatic venoocclusive disease, and impaired thyroid and adrenal function. Renal dysfunction occurs commonly as a result of nephrotoxic medications and immunosuppressive therapy. Preoperative assessment of renal function, careful attention to intravascular volume status, preservation of cardiac output, and avoidance of nephrotoxic medications (when possible) are the cornerstones of preservation of renal function. Hepatic venoocclusive disease is a nonspecific hepatic injury that occurs after the administration of some drugs used for pretransplant conditioning (e.g., busulfan or actinomycin D). The mechanism is unclear, but pathology involves vasculitis of the sinusoids of the hepatic venules. Hepatic venoocclusive disease initially presents as jaundice, right upper-quadrant pain, and ascites, but it may progress to include coagulopathy and encephalopathy. Thyroid and adrenal function are critical for cardiovascular stability and drug clearance. Endocrinology consultation and appropriate hormone replacement are recommended.

Pharmacologic Considerations

Immune-modulating medications used in HSCT include cyclosporine A, azathioprine, tacrolimus, mycophenolate mofetil, and corticosteroids. Relevant side effects of azathioprine include pancytopenia, and those of steroids include hypertension, diabetes, and neurotoxicity. Hypertension, seizures, diabetes, and renal insufficiency are toxicities associated with cyclosporine and tacrolimus (Kostopanagiotou et al., 2003). Adverse effects of immunosuppressive medications particularly relevant to children include growth retardation, hirsutism, obesity, and osteoporosis (Ellis et al., 2000).

In the presence of adequate renal and hepatic function, no contraindications exist to the use of anesthetic agents. Sevoflurane can be used for the induction of anesthesia, and sevoflurane, desflurane, and isoflurane, can be used for the maintenance of anesthesia. IV agents and local anesthetics can also be used. Cyclosporine increases the effects of nondepolarizing muscle relaxants, resulting in decreased dosage requirement. Neuromuscular blockade should be monitored closely to prevent inadvertent overdose. The use of cisatracurium is preferred with renal or hepatic impairment.

Nitrous oxide inhibits bone marrow function after prolonged exposure (longer than 6 hours) at high concentrations (Weimann, 2003). Methotrexate inhibits folate metabolism as well as marrow function. Nitrous oxide may amplify the side effects of methotrexate therapy and therefore should probably be avoided for long procedures in patients who are treated with methotrexate and in patients with marginal marrow function. NSAIDs may potentiate nephrotoxicity of cyclosporine and tacrolimus.

Potent anesthetic opioids (e.g., fentanyl, sufentanil, and alfentanil) and some of the benzodiazepines (e.g., midazolam and diazepam) are metabolized by the cytochrome P_{450} enzymes (Leather, 2004). Serum concentrations of these drugs are elevated if drugs that inhibit the cytochrome P_{450} system (e.g., azole antifungals, calcium-channel blockers, and macrolide antibiotics) are coadministered. Calcium-channel blockers, azole antifungals, and macrolide antibiotics increase levels of tacrolimus and cyclosporine through enzyme inhibition.

Children with extensive systemic involvement after HSCT as well as patients undergoing extensive surgical procedures may require postoperative admission to an intensive care unit as a result of limited physiologic reserve. Neuraxial blocks, local anesthesia infiltration, and parenteral opioids are appropriate methods for the provision of postoperative analgesia under close monitoring.

COAGULATION: DEVELOPMENTAL ASPECTS, DISORDERS OF COAGULATION, AND PERIOPERATIVE MANAGEMENT OF HEMOSTASIS

Coagulation abnormalities provide many challenges for the pediatric anesthesiologist. Children with known coagulation disorders require disease-specific perioperative management and must often be treated for complications of their bleeding diathesis. More challenging is the intraoperative investigation and management of children who develop a coagulopathy in the OR, either from preexisting, albeit undiagnosed, diseases or from acquired disorders. The following sections focus on endogenous control of hemostasis, developmental changes in coagulation, and commonly inherited coagulopathies and their management.

Overview of Hemostasis

The hemostatic system is designed to maintain blood in a fluid state until vessel injury occurs, at which point an explosive cascade of events terminates blood loss by sealing off the vascular defect. Hemorrhage occurs if the response is inadequate; thrombosis occurs if the response is dysregulated. The vascular endothelial cell is at the fulcrum of this delicate balance. The normal endothelial cell maintains blood in its fluid state by inhibiting platelet aggregation and blood coagulation through the production of prostacyclin, NO, and the ectonucleotidase CD39, as well as by promoting fibrinolysis through the antithrombin III-mediated conversion of plasminogen to plasmin (Ignarro et al., 1987; Marcus et al., 2005).

Physically, the endothelial cell is a barrier between the platelets and procoagulant proteins derived from reactive components present in the deeper layers of the vessel wall. These components include collagen, fibronectin, von Willebrand factor (vWF), and tissue factor (TF), all of which stimulate platelet adhesion and aggregation and trigger the coagulation cascade (Fig. 36-12).

Primary Phase of Hemostasis

The platelet is central to the primary phase of hemostasis (Fig. 36-13). The normal circulating platelet count ranges from 150,000 to 400,000/mL. An additional 33% of all platelets are

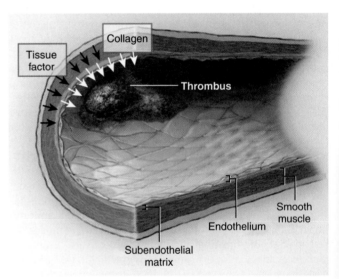

■ **FIGURE 36-12.** Response to vascular injury. Collagen and tissue factor (TF) associated with the vessel wall provide a hemostatic barrier to maintain the high-pressure circulatory system. Collagen *(white arrows),* located in the subendothelial matrix beneath the endothelium, is not exposed to flowing blood under normal conditions. TF *(black arrows),* located in the medial (smooth muscle) and adventitial layers of the vessel wall, comes in contact with flowing blood when the vessel is disrupted or punctured. Both collagen and thrombin initiate thrombus formation. Collagen is a first line of defense, and TF is a second line of defense. *(From Furie B, Furie BC: Mechanisms of thrombus formation, N Engl J Med 359:938, 2008.)*

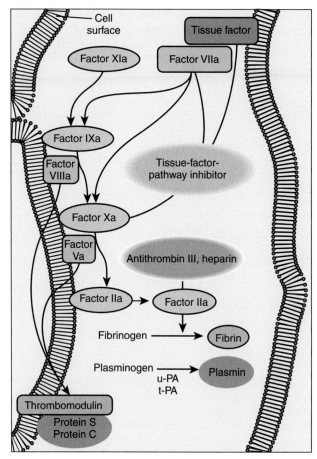

■ FIGURE 36-13. The clotting cascade. Coagulation is initiated by the exposure of blood to TF bound to cell membranes. TF interacts with factor VIIa to convert factor IX to factor IXa and factor X to factor Xa (only the activated forms are shown). Factor IXa converts factor X to factor Xa. Factor Xa generates factor IIa (thrombin) from factor II (prothrombin). Each of these reactions takes place on an activated cell surface. Once factor IIa is generated, it cleaves plasma fibrinogen to generate fibrin. The TF-pathway inhibitor forms a quaternary structure with TF, factor VIIa, and factor Xa *(shown in blue)*. The thrombomodulin-protein C-protein S pathway *(shown in yellow)* inactivates factors Va and VIIIa. Antithrombin III inactivates factors XIa, IXa, Xa, and IIa *(shown in orange)* in a reaction that is accelerated by the presence of heparin sulfate. In the fibrinolytic pathway, tissue-type plasminogen activator (t-PA) and urokinase-type plasminogen activator (u-PA) convert plasminogen to plasmin. Once generated, plasmin proteolytically degrades fibrin *(shown in purple)*. *(From Rosenberg RD, Aird WC: Vascular-bed-specific hemostasis and hypercoagulable states, N Engl J Med 340:1555, 1999.)*

sequestered within the spleen. After vascular injury, the affected vessel constricts proximally, diverting blood flow away from the site of endothelial disruption. Extravasated blood is exposed to subendothelial structures, and the platelets are stimulated by their contact with collagen. The platelets become adherent to the subendothelial infrastructure, anchored by the binding of vWF to the platelet surface glycoprotein Ib, as well as by the interaction of platelet glycoprotein VI with collagen (Ruggeri, 2000). Once platelet adhesion occurs, platelet activation results in the glycoprotein VI-mediated release of platelet agonists such as epinephrine and serotonin from the dense granules (Furie

and Furie, 2008). The synthesis of thromboxane-A$_2$ (TXA$_2$) from arachidonic acid by COX and thromboxane is then released from the platelet lipid membrane, and there is a 50% increase in the number of platelets and a conformational change in the platelet surface glycoprotein receptor IIb-IIIa (GPIIb-IIIa), which binds to fibrinogen, vWF, and fibronectin (Shattil et al., 1998). GPIIb-IIIa is now referred to as $\alpha_{IIb}\beta_3$ (Bennett, 2005).

TF can also trigger platelet activation independent of endothelial disruption, vWF contact, or glycoprotein VI (Dubois et al., 2006). The TF VIIa (factor VIIa) complex activates factor IX, which ultimately generates thrombin. Thrombin then cleaves the platelet surface receptor Par1, activating the platelet (Dubois et al., 2007).

A developing thrombus recruits unstimulated platelets. Platelet activation increases integrin $\alpha_{IIb}\beta_3$'s affinity for fibrinogen and vWF, clustering this receptor on the platelet surface (Bennett, 2005). Platelet aggregation, through the linkage of $\alpha_{IIb}\beta_3$ to the $\alpha_{IIb}\beta_3$ on other platelets bridged by fibrinogen or vWF, increases the size of the initial platelet plug, creating a mass of aggregated platelets at the injury site. At low shear rates, fibrinogen is the principle ligand, whereas at higher shear rates vWF plays a predominant role (Goto et al., 1998). Synthesized TXA$_2$ induces aggregation of other platelets and promotes vascular smooth muscle constriction, producing local vasoconstriction, which limits blood loss and increases the effectiveness of the platelet plug by decreasing the effective surface area that the platelet plug needs to cover. TXA$_2$ amplifies the platelet's responses to weak agonists such as ADP and epinephrine (Funk, 2001). Not all of the recruited platelets undergo activation. Many remain loosely associated but inactive and ultimately fall away from the initial platelet plug (Dubois et al., 2007).

TXA$_2$ binds to a G protein-coupled receptor on the platelet surface, leading to an increase in intracellular calcium and activation of protein kinase C. The initial platelet plug is friable. It is stabilized by the increase in platelet cytosolic calcium, which initiates actin filament turnover that in turn modulates the cytoskeletal changes. These changes enable integrin $a_{IIb}\beta_3$ clustering and the binding of both fibrinogen and vWF. The conformational change of $a_{IIb}\beta_3$, induced through ligand binding, exposes new ligand binding sites and further merging of platelet surface receptors, resulting in clot retraction (Warltier et al., 2002).

Secondary Phase of Hemostasis

The exposure of subendothelial structures to circulating blood simultaneously activates the coagulation cascade (the secondary phase of hemostasis) to produce a cross-linked fibrin clot. Of the coagulation proteins, prothrombin (II), protein C, protein S, and factors VII, IX, and X are synthesized as prozymogens and activated to serine proteases through a vitamin K-dependent hepatic enzyme (Furie and Furie, 1990). This modification is required for calcium binding, serving as a bridge for binding the factors to the phospholipid surface.

New Model of Cell-Based Coagulation

In earlier schemes, the coagulation cascade had been divided into intrinsic (e.g., factors XII, XI, IX, and VIII) and extrinsic (e.g., TF and factor VII) pathways (Fig. 36-14). This model is primarily useful for the interpretation of the in vitro laboratory

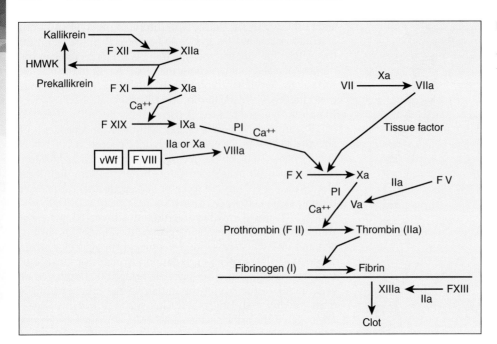

■ **FIGURE 36-14.** Mechanism of hemostasis. *HMWK,* High-molecular-weight kininogen; *vWF,* von Willebrand factor.

tests, the activated partial thromboplastin time (aPTT) and the prothrombin time (PT). The common pathway of the clotting cascade is the production of factor Xa, which in concert with factor Va, cleaves prothrombin to thrombin, resulting in fibrin production. It became apparent that deficiencies in the intrinsic pathway did not produce bleeding conditions and that the model was not clinically relevant.

In vivo, the critical component in coagulation initiation is TF, a membrane protein receptor for factor VII. TF is expressed constitutively on cells that are not in direct contact with blood, such as vascular smooth muscle, fibroblasts, and macrophages, forming a hemostatic envelope around the vascular endothelium (Mann et al., 1998). The endothelium acts as a barrier that separates the cellular sources of TF from factor VIIa in flowing blood, preventing inadvertent coagulation initiation. Once endothelial injury occurs, activated endothelial cells and platelets activate TF through the release of protein disulfide isomerases (Cho et al., 2008; Reinhardt et al., 2008). Activated TF forms a complex with factor VII, producing factor VIIa. The TF/factor VIIa complex then activates factors X and IX (Orfeo et al., 2005). Factor IXa binds to factor VIII, forming the "tenase complex" (factor IXa/VIII). This complex inefficiently activates factor X. The TF/factor VIIa complex also converts factor X to factor Xa directly. Factor Xa combines with its cofactor (factor Va) on the TF-bearing cell and generates small amounts of thrombin. Although this limited amount of thrombin is sufficient to activate platelets in the local area and to activate factors V, VIII, and IX, it is insufficient to cleave fibrinogen. Factor VIII is cleaved off vWF and is then activated to factor VIIIa, which complexes with factor IXa to form the "activated tenase complex" (factor VIIIa/IXa).

The activated tenase complex binds to the negatively charged phospholipids that coat the surface of activated platelets and produce factor Xa. This platelet-localized factor Xa binds to factor Va, also bound to the platelet surface, and catalyzes the conversion of prothrombin to thrombin at the rapid rate necessary for adequate hemostasis. Thrombin formation is accelerated, fibrinogen is cleaved, and the coagulation complex is

further activated, augmenting thrombin production. The fibrin monomers undergo spontaneous polymerization to form the fibrin clot, which is then stabilized by crosslinking, mediated by factor XIIIa. A firm platelet-fibrin clot results, which over the course of time, mediated by platelets, decreases in size. The graphic representation of this new model of cell-based coagulation, which replaces the former intrinsic pathway, is shown in Figure 36-15 (Gailani and Broze, 1991).

Although factor XII is not involved in physiologic hemostasis, accruing evidence suggests that it plays a key role in abnormal thrombosis (Renne and Gailani, 2007). Extracellular ribonucleic acid (RNA) released from damaged cells induces arterial thrombosis through factor XII activation (Kannemeier et al., 2007). Inorganic polyphosphates released from activated platelets trigger factor XII activation and provide an additional pathway for fibrin formation by stimulated platelets (Johne et al., 2006).

Modulators of Coagulation

Coagulation is modulated by a number of plasma proteins, the most important of which are antithrombin III, thrombomodulin, TF pathway inhibitor, protein C, protein S, and factor V. Antithrombin III is a potent inhibitor of thrombin and factors IXa, Xa, and XIIIa. Heparin potentiates the inhibition of thrombin by antithrombin III. Thrombomodulin, expressed on the endothelial cell surface, binds and neutralizes thrombin. TF pathway inhibitor limits factor Xa production by the activated tenase complex (factor IXa/VIIIa). Activated protein C (APC), activated by the presence of thrombin and accelerated by thrombin-thrombomodulin, proteolytically inactivates factor VIII/ VIIIa and factor V/Va, thereby down-regulating the production of factor Xa and thrombin. Protein S has two anticoagulant roles; it acts as a cofactor for APC in the inactivation of factors Va and VIIIa and as a cofactor for TF pathway inhibitor in the inactivation of factors Xa and VIIa (Castoldi and Hackeng, 2008). Factor V uniquely has procoagulant and anticoagulant

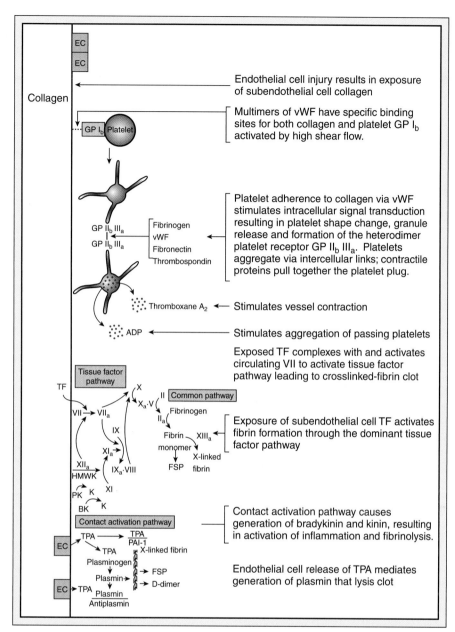

FIGURE 36-15. Hemostatic mechanism: cell-based coagulation model. *BK,* Bradykinin; *EC,* endothelial cell; *FSP,* fibrin split products; *GP,* glycoprotein; *K,* kallikrein; *PAI,* plasminogen activator inhibitor; *PK,* prekallikrein; *TF,* tissue factor; *TPA,* tissue plasminogen activator; *vWF,* von Willebrand factor. (*Redrawn from Manco-Johnson M, Nuss R: Hemostasis in the neonate,* Neoreviews 1:191, 2000.)

activities. Genetic alterations in factor V (i.e., factor V Leiden) or deficiencies of protein C may result in excessive procoagulant activity, which may lead to venous thromboembolism (Tormene et al., 2002). When factor V is cleaved by thrombin, a number of intermediates are formed in addition to factor Va, the essential cofactor to factor Xa. These intermediates are cofactors for APC and act as anticoagulants. APC can cleave factor V directly, producing an anticoagulant and precluding factor V's transformation to factor Va (Thorelli, 1999).

Fibrinolysis

Fibrinolysis occurs simultaneously with the initiation of clot formation, limits thrombosis to the local area of injury, and begins the processes of clot revision, vascular damage repair, and ultimately, vessel recanalization. During the initial phase of hemostasis, endothelial cells and platelets release plasminogen activator inhibitors (PAIs), which facilitate fibrin formation. In response to thrombin, endothelial cells begin to release tissue plasminogen activator (TPA) that along with prourokinase, converts plasminogen to plasmin. The plasminogen, which is bound to fibrin in the hemostatic plug, is much more reactive to TPA than circulating plasminogen. After plasmin is produced locally at the site of the hemostatic plug, fibrinolysis or fibrin degradation can occur. Fibrinolysis at the hemostatic plug is opposed by ongoing coagulation and by antifibrinolysis, mediated by α_2-plasmin inhibitor, which is also bound to fibrin.

The spectrum of endothelial cell and platelet interactions in the setting of clotting factors, adhesive proteins, fibrinolytic proteins, and the myriad inhibitors promotes an equilibrium that promotes fluidity of circulating blood, and localization of hemostasis and injury repair. Derangements in any portion of this precariously balanced mechanism can lead to a hemorrhagic or thrombotic complication. A defect in clot formation in the setting of physiologic fibrinolysis leads to bleeding, as does normal clot formation in the setting of premature fibrinolysis. Thrombosis can occur in the setting of endothelial cells expression of TF, reduction in antithrombin function, and when platelet aggregation and activation are excessive.

Antiplatelet and Anticoagulant Drugs

The increased understanding of physiologic hemostasis has led to the development of new antithrombotic agents to modulate the consequences of thrombosis in critical illness and many systemic diseases. Antiplatelet drugs target key steps in platelet secretion, adhesion, and activation. COX-1 inhibitors such as acetylsalicylic acid (ASA) inactivate platelet COX-1, a pivotal enzyme in TXA_2 and prostacyclin synthesis, important for platelet secretion and aggregation. Some COX-1 drugs inhibit the enzyme transiently, whereas others (e.g., ASA) permanently inhibit TXA_2 production for the lifespan of the platelet. ADP antagonists such as ticlopidine irreversibly block platelet receptor P2Y12, inhibiting platelet aggregation by the platelet agonists, thrombin, epinephrine, ADP, and collagen (Savi and Herbert, 2005). $\alpha_{IIb}\beta_3$-receptor antagonists block platelet integrin $\alpha_{IIb}\beta_3$ from binding to fibrinogen and vWF on activated platelets, thus reducing platelet aggregation by 80% (Warltier et al., 2002; Patrono et al., 2004).

Anticoagulant drugs are designed to perturb the precariously balanced factor-based physiologic coagulation system and its modulators. Vitamin K antagonists, exemplified by warfarin, inhibit the vitamin K-dependent γ-carboxylation of factors II, VII, IX, and X, and proteins C and S (Levy et al., 2008). The antithrombin (AT) III agonist unfractionated heparin binds to AT, resulting in a 1000-fold increase in both thrombin and factor Xa inactivation. Factor Xa inhibitors such as low-molecular-weight heparin (LMWH) and fondaparinux also bind to AT, augmenting factor Xa inhibition; however, these drugs are too small to simultaneously bind both AT and thrombin, which is necessary for thrombin inactivation. Increasingly, LMWH is replacing unfractionated heparin in the treatment of pediatric thrombotic disease (Dix et al., 2000; Merkel et al., 2006). Direct thrombin inhibitors lepirudin, bivalirudin, and argatroban, bind to thrombin's active site, preventing the conversion of fibrinogen to fibrin, both in the circulation as well as on the evolving thrombus. Argatroban has been successfully used as an anticoagulant for cardiopulmonary bypass in an infant with heparin-induced thrombocytopenia (Malherbe et al., 2004).

Laboratory Evaluation of Coagulation

The panel of tests routinely used to evaluate coagulation includes the platelet count, PT, aPTT, and bleeding time. The normal platelet count is between 150,000 and 500,000/mcL, but increased bleeding as a result of thrombocytopenia rarely occurs at counts above 50,000/mcL. Bleeding may also occur when platelets are relatively normal in number but dysfunctional with regard to their role in coagulation.

The normal PT, which ranges from 11.5 to 14 seconds, reflects normal amounts of factors II, V, VII, and X, which are the vitamin K–dependent factors. Defects in vitamin K–dependent clotting factors may be caused by a deficiency of the vitamin, poor responsiveness to the vitamin because of liver disease, or exposure to warfarin agents that impair vitamin K's transition to the reduced form. The International Normalized Ratio (INR) can be used to estimate the degree of factor deficiency. An INR in the range of 2 to 3 correlates with factor concentrations of 10%; between 3 and 4 correlates with concentrations of 5%; and an INR higher than 4 correlates with concentrations of 1% (Boulis et al., 1999).

The normal aPTT is between 25 and 40 seconds and requires normal levels of vWF and factors XII, XI, IX, and VIII.

The bleeding time test assesses the integrity of the vascular and platelet aspects of coagulation and is prolonged in patients with reduced numbers of platelets (fewer than 100,000/mcL), in patients with defective platelet function (e.g., after aspirin, NSAID, or valproic acid administration), and in patients with vWD. The test is performed using a standardized template device to guide the incision with a tourniquet placed on the arm at 40 mm Hg for children, 30 mm Hg for newborns at term, and 20 mm Hg for premature infants. The bleeding-time evaluation has suffered from a reputation of being difficult to perform and poorly reproducible, especially in newborns and infants. Results may be affected by skin thickness and the device used to puncture the skin (e.g., surgical blade or manufactured bleeding time device), location of incision, and body temperature. Recently, a bleeding-time device (Surgicutt; ITC, Edison, New Jersey) has been developed that comes in three sizes for adults, children (5 months to 15 years), and newborns (up to 5 months). The blades are different lengths (and depths for newborns) and afford a standardized incision rather than a puncture. This standardization should decrease the variability in bleeding times that result from varying incision techniques and skin thicknesses related to age, but this hypothesis has not yet been studied in a controlled fashion. The blood is blotted with filter paper every 30 seconds. Normal bleeding time is between 4 and 8 minutes in adults and may be as low as 2 minutes in newborns. The bleeding time is prolonged in very–low-birth-weight infants with hematocrit of less than 28%; bleeding time may be reduced in these infants after transfusion to hematocrit of more than 28% (Sola et al., 2001). It is unknown whether the longer bleeding times at lower hematocrits are associated with an increased risk of clinical bleeding.

Developmental Hemostasis

The hemostatic system of the newborn and young child is significantly different than that of the adult. Although considered immature, the hemostatic system is functional; the young child is successfully protected from hemorrhagic and thrombotic complications. These differences are most exaggerated in the hemostatic mechanism of the newborn. As the coagulation and fibrinolytic factors do not cross the placenta, the proposed causes for the differences in the newborn's hemostatic system include decreased factor synthesis, enhanced clearance, general activation of the coagulation system with resulting factor consumption, and the synthesis of less active fetal forms of some proteins.

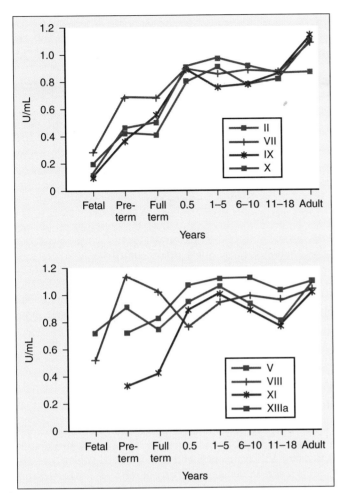

■ FIGURE 36-16. Developmental hemostasis: changes in plasma concentration of coagulation proteins over the course of development. *(Redrawn from Andrew M: Developmental hemostasis: relevance to thromboembolic complications in pediatric patients,* Thromb Haemost *74[Suppl]:415, 1995.)*

TABLE 36-22. Concentration of Coagulation Factors in the Term and Preterm Newborn Relative to Adult Values

Factor	Level at Term (% of Adult Value)	Level at Preterm (% of Adult Value)
Thrombin	50	40
Factor VII	66	66
Factor IX	50	35
Factor X	40	40
Fibrinogen	100	100
Factor V	75	88
Factor VIII	100	110
Factor X	40	40
Factor XI	40	40
Factor XII	50	30
Factor XIII	75	80
Heparin cofactor II	25	33
Antithrombin	50	40
α_2-Macroglobulin	150-200	150-200
Protein C	25	10
Protein S	40	25
Plasminogen	50	55
α_2-Antiplasmin	100	130
Tissue plasminogen activator	200	200
Plasminogen activator inhibitor	180	180

One of the most notable features of the coagulation system of the infant is that plasma clotting factors are inconsistently different from adult levels (Fig. 36-16). The most well-known ontogenetic differences in the hemostatic system involve the vitamin K–dependent factors. These proteins are present in low levels at birth, and coagulation is severely impaired in the absence of vitamin K supplementation; this is called hemorrhagic disease of the newborn (discussed more fully in the next section). The levels of the four vitamin K–dependent coagulation factors (factors II, VII, IX, and X) and the contact factors (factors XI and XII, prekallikrein, and kininogen) are all less than 50% of adult values and slowly rise to within 20% of adult levels by 6 months of age (Andrew et al., 1990a). Factor VII levels increase rapidly after birth in premature and full-term infants. Factors II and VII remain less than adult values for most of childhood (Andrew et al., 1992). Factor IX activity can be as low as 15% of adult levels and reach adult levels at 9 months of age. On the other hand, the levels of fibrinogen and factors V, VIII, and XIII are normal at birth; fibrinogen and factor VIII levels are at the high end of the normal range (Andrew, 1997). vWF levels are increased during the first weeks of life and return to adult levels between 2 and 6 months of life (Thomas et al., 1995). The net effect of these differences in the newborn's hemostatic system is delayed thrombin generation, similar to that seen in adults on receiving anticoagulant medications such as warfarin or subcutaneous heparin (Andrew et al., 1990b).

The concentration of coagulation factors in term and preterm infants relative to adult values is summarized in Table 36-22.

Laboratory Evaluation of Coagulation in the Newborn

Newborns with suspected coagulopathies are evaluated with PT, aPTT, platelet count, and levels of fibrinogen and fibrin degradation products. In newborns, as a result of the developmental differences in the coagulation protein levels, both PT and aPTT are prolonged compared with adult values. Because of the low plasma concentrations of many of the clotting factors in the newborn, the aPTT is markedly elevated. The developmental progression of the PT and aPTT in term and preterm infants is summarized in Table 36-23. Infants with vitamin-K deficiency have a prolonged PT when compared with age-appropriate norms. Fibrinogen concentrations less than 100 mg/dL and platelet counts of less than 100,000/mcL are indicative of a pathologic process (Manco-Johnson, 2008).

TABLE 36-23. Developmental Changes in the Prothrombin Time and Activated Partial Thromboplastin Time

Age of Infant	Day 1	Day 5	Day 30	Day 90	Adult
Term					
PT	13 ± 1.4	12.4 ± 2.5	11.8 ± 1.3	11.9 ± 1.2	12.4 ± 0.8
aPTT	42.9 ± 5.8	42.6 ± 8.6	40.4 ± 7.4	37.1 ± 6.5	33.5 ± 3.4
Preterm (30-36 weeks)					
PT	13 ± 1.5	12.5 ± 1.3	11.8 ± 0.9	12.3 ± 1.2	12.4 ± 0.8
aPTT	53.6 ± 13	50.5 ± 12	44.7 ± 9	50.5 ± 12	33.5 ± 3.4

Developmental Changes Beyond the Neonatal Period

Many of the proteins that regulate coagulation and thrombin generation are also decreased in early infancy. Antithrombin III and heparin cofactor II are markedly decreased to levels that might predispose to spontaneous thromboembolic events. The α_2 macroglobulin levels at birth are greater than those of adults and remain so until the third decade of life. By 6 months of life, AT III levels exceed levels seen in adults. Protein C and protein S concentrations at birth are also substantially less than those seen in adults and remain low throughout childhood (Andrew et al., 1992). Fibrinolysis is suppressed throughout childhood. During childhood, plasminogen levels increase to adult levels, but the TPA/PAI-1 ratio is significantly lower than that in adults, which explains the decrease in fibrinolysis in children (Siegbahn and Ruusuvaara, 1988).

Developmental Aspects of Platelet Number and Function

Although normal in number, neonatal platelets are hyporeactive. Neonatal platelet aggregation is diminished in response to certain physiologic agonists such as ADP, thromboxane, and epinephrine (Levy-Shraga et al., 2006). Intracellular calcium transport is decreased as well, resulting in diminished granule release and slowed conformational change (Kuhne and Imbach, 1998). Increased vWF levels in the newborn period contribute to decreased bleeding times (Andrew, 1997). Platelet function in the neonate is aided by a relatively high hematocrit, causing an increased concentration of platelets directed to the wall by the dynamics of laminar flow. Platelet function improves over the first 2 weeks of life (Israels, 2009).

The most serious manifestation of thrombocytopenia in the newborn period is intraparenchymal brain hemorrhage. Of neonates with spontaneous intraparenchymal hemorrhage, one third have an associated coagulopathy such as vitamin-K deficiency, hemophilia, or thrombocytopenia. Neonates with a platelet count of less than 50,000/mcL are at significant risk for intraparenchymal hemorrhage (Sandberg et al., 2001; Jhawar et al., 2003).

Inherited Coagulopathies

Hemostasis usually requires activity levels of coagulation factors at least 30% of normal. The aPTT may be normal with a factor level as low as 15% to 18% of normal. Past medical history and family history are invaluable tools in the evaluation of a bleeding patient. Substantial hemorrhage after oral cavity manipulation (whether by dentist or toothbrush) is often a sign of an underlying bleeding disorder, reflecting an imbalance between abnormal clot formation and normal salivary fibrinolysis. Patients with mild bleeding disorders who have never had trauma or surgery may experience symptoms rather late in life and may have normal screening tests. Prenatal diagnosis of most congenital factor deficiencies can now be made from fetal DNA.

Hemophilia

Of the inherited deficiencies of coagulation factors, the most common are the X-linked recessive hemophilias; hemophilia A is factor VIII deficiency, and hemophilia B (Christmas disease) is factor IX deficiency. Thirty percent of cases arise from spontaneous mutation. Approximately 50% of mutations of factor VIII result from inversions of the DNA sequence within intron 22. The incidence of hemophilia A is 1 in 5000 male live births, and that of hemophilia B is 1 in 30,000. Hemophilia B can result from spontaneous mutations, which cause decreased rates of activation of factor IX, altered binding of factor IX to phospholipid membranes, or reduced circulation times. Patients with hemophilia B, Leyden, a single nucleotide substitution in the transcriptional promoter, have severe hemophilia until puberty, at which point, factor IX spontaneously increases to 50%, suggesting that transcription of the factor IX gene is in part hormonally mediated. Factor IX is a smaller molecule than factor VIII and has a greater volume of distribution.

The clinical severity of hemophilia is usually dictated by the degree of clotting factor deficiency. Patients with severe hemophilia, less than 1% of normal plasma levels, have an annual average of 20 to 30 bleeds; these are bleeding events that may be spontaneous or marked by excessive bleeding after minor trauma, characteristically into joints or muscle. These patients are usually diagnosed within the first 2 years of life. Bleeding is less common in the newborn period than in later months, but when it occurs, it is most common after circumcision. In a study of newborns with hemophilia, 30% bled from circumcision sites, 27% had intracranial hemorrhage, 16% had persistent bleeding from puncture sites, and 1% had subgaleal hematomas or cephalohematomas (Kulkarni and Lusher, 2001). Infants with severe hemophilia A or B have a 2% to 8% risk of spontaneous intracranial hemorrhage (Rodriguez et al., 2005).

Hemophilia A and hemophilia B are characterized by a prolonged aPTT with a normal PT. Because the neonate's aPTT is physiologically prolonged, a factor VIII level must be directly measured to establish the diagnosis. Factor IX levels are physiologically low at birth and do not reach adult levels until 6 months of age, making confirmation of the diagnosis of hemophilia B uncertain until later infancy, except in severe cases. The treatment of hemophilia has changed dramatically over the past three decades from the availability of plasma-derived replacement factors in the 1970s to the engineering of recombinant factors in the 1990s to the recently begun trials of gene replacement therapy (Mannucci and Tuddenham, 2001).

Patients with mild and moderate disease, corresponding to 6% to 30% and 1% to 5% of normal factor levels, respectively, usually bleed excessively only after trauma or surgery and are managed with on-demand factor replacement. These patients are often diagnosed later in life.

Preoperative Preparation of the Child with Hemophilia

Preparation of the child with hemophilia for surgery depends on the severity of the patient's disease and the proposed procedure. Patients with mild hemophilia A who have demonstrated an adequate response to DDAVP in the past can undergo minor procedures after IV DDAVP administration (0.3 mcg/kg) 30 minutes before surgery (Mannucci, 1997; Rodriguez and Hoots, 2008).

Factor Replacement

Hemophilia A. The type, timing, and dose of factor to be administered should be decided in advance in consultation with the patient's hematologist. In general, children with hemophilia A who require major procedures should have their factor VIII level maintained close to 100% of normal from 30 minutes before surgery through the first 2 to 7 days of the postoperative period. Factor VIII levels can then be reduced to 30% to 50% of normal for the next 3 to 7 days. Children who undergo minor procedures can be adequately covered with factor VIII levels of 50% after the second postoperative day (Martlew, 2000). In determining factor replacement, it should be remembered that the plasma volume is 45 to 50 mL/kg. Because 1 mL of plasma contains 1 unit of factor VIII, 50 units/kg of factor VIII will increase the patient's level to 100% (rise of 2% per unit of factor VIII/kg). In the absence of inhibitors, the half-life of factor VIII in vivo is 8 to 12 hours; subsequent doses are timed to maintain the desired level of activity. The first dose has a somewhat shorter half-life than subsequent doses. Therefore, the second dose should be given after a somewhat shorter interval (6 hours). Factor VIII may be administered as cryoprecipitate (0.2 bags/kg should raise factor VIII level to 50%), but the factor VIII level in cryoprecipitate is variable, and plasma levels should be followed if bleeding is not well controlled. The use of heat- or detergent-treated factor concentrates (e.g., Monoclate-P and Hemofil-M) has been replaced with recombinant factor VIII (rFVIII) preparations (e.g., Humate-P). Although the treated factor concentrates had a lower risk of transmission of viruses (e.g., human immunodeficiency virus [HIV] and hepatitis A, B, or C) compared with cryoprecipitate, rFVIII carries no risk of viral transmission; however, it is unknown whether the albumin in the recombinant preparation may have a risk of prion

transmission. Albumin-free rFVIII concentrate has become available, which may eliminate concerns about infection (Josephson and Abshire, 2004).

Hemophilia B. As in the case of hemophilia A, rFIX has started to replace plasma-derived factor IX concentrate for prophylaxis and treatment of bleeding in children with hemophilia B (Shapiro et al., 2005). In adults, 1 IU/kg of rFIX increased circulating factor IX activity by 0.8 IU/dL. Children have been found to have a smaller increase—0.68 IU/dL per 1 IU/kg infused in children 1 month to 12 years, 0.46 IU/dL in neonates, and 0.93 IU/dL in adolescents, but sample sizes were small. A mean dose of 90 IU/kg (range 29 to 260 IU/kg) was given to 23 patients before surgery (Shapiro et al., 2005). Because of the low yield of circulating factor IX in neonates after rFIX administration, as noted, higher doses are required in this population with regular measurement of serum factor IX levels. A recent report described the administration of rFIX by continuous infusion at a rate of 30 to 35 IU/kg per hour for successful treatment of intracranial and extracranial hemorrhages in the neonate (Guilcher et al., 2005). Because the half-life of factor IX is 12 to 24 hours, it requires less frequent dosing than does factor VIII to maintain adequate levels. As with factor VIII, the second dose should be given at a somewhat shorter interval than subsequent doses (6 to 8 hours). If rFIX is unavailable, the factor IX level is raised 1% for each unit of factor IX concentrate/kg.

Hemophilia C. Hemophilia C is factor XI deficiency (Rosenthal syndrome), an autosomally recessive disease that is most commonly reported in Askhenazic Jews. The incidence in the Ashkenazic population is 3 in 1000, compared with a rate of 1 in 1,000,000 in the general population (Gomez and Bolton-Maggs, 2008). Incidence of hemophilia C is increased among people with Noonan syndrome (Bertola et al., 2003). Factor IX deficiency presents with a prolongation of the aPTT, with a normal PT. There is an incomplete correlation between the severity of factor deficiency and hemorrhagic symptoms, in that some patients with very low factor levels have no history of bleeding. Bleeding typically occurs after trauma or surgery and is commonly seen in sites that have a high fibrinolytic rate, such as the genitourinary tract, and after circumcision (Andrew, 1997). Because factor XI levels are physiologically low in the neonatal period, the diagnosis is confirmed through levels obtained in later infancy. The perioperative management of these patients is dictated by their bleeding risk. Patients with factor XI levels of more than 15% without a previous history of bleeding, or patients with levels of 5% to 14% who have had previous surgery without significant bleeding in the absence of fresh frozen plasma (FFP) administration can be considered to be at low risk. Patients with factor levels of less than 15%, a history of spontaneous bleeding, bleeding during previous surgeries, or those with a family history of such bleeding complications can be considered to be at high risk. Depending on the surgical procedure, patients who are considered to be at low risk for bleeding can be managed with FFP immediately available. High-risk patients should receive FFP 2 hours before surgery.

Factor Inhibitors in Patients with Hemophilia A and B

Factor replacement results in the development of neutralizing antibodies called *inhibitors*, which complicates the treatment of affected hemophiliacs. The incidence of inhibitors in hemophilia

A is 30%; in hemophilia B, it is 5% (Astermark, 2006). These antibodies are classified as low- or high-titer inhibitors. Patients with low-titer inhibitors may be treated with high doses of factor replacement. Patients with high titers of these inhibitors often develop severe bleeding complications that are recalcitrant to standard factor replacement algorithms and require bypassing agents such as rFVIIa or activated prothrombin complex concentrates (Matthew, 2006; Young, 2006; Rodriguez and Hoots, 2008). For patients with inhibitory antibodies, immunomodulation therapy should be instituted concomitantly with hemostatic therapy. No consensus has been reached on the optimal regimen. IV immune globulin, corticosteroids, and alkylating agents all have been shown to reduce inhibitor levels.

Adjuvant Treatment Options for Hemophilia Patients

Antifibrinolytics. These agents (ε-aminocaproic acid [EACA] and tranexamic acid) are very useful adjuvants for patients with mild to severe hemophilia who are experiencing mucosal bleeding, primarily of oral, nasal, and menstrual origins. They are discussed in greater detail below.

Recombinant Factor VIIa (rFVIIa). rFVIIa was initially licensed for use in hemophilia patients with inhibitors (Roberts, 2001). rFVIIa binds to TF and to the surface of activated platelets, both of which result in factor X activation and thrombin production. The standard dose is 90 to 120 mcg/kg every 2 to 3 hours until hemostasis is achieved. More than 90% of patients with hemophilia who have a low risk for thrombosis have an effective response to rFVIIa (O'Connell et al., 2002). Anecdotally, a child with hemophilia A and inhibitors was successfully managed intraoperatively with rFVIIa in combination with EACA (Simic and Milojevic, 2007).

von Willebrand Disease

Characteristics

vWD, the most common congenital bleeding disorder, is a deficiency or dysfunction of the adhesive glycoprotein, which is produced in endothelial cells and megakaryocytes and is stored in Weibel-Palade bodies in endothelial cells and platelets. vWF is fundamental in the binding of platelets to damaged endothelial surfaces, promotes the secretion of factor VIII, and binds, carries, and protects factor VIII in plasma. vWD affects 1 in 100 individuals and is inherited in an autosomal fashion (usually dominant), with males and females affected equally. It is characterized by impaired platelet adhesion to exposed subendothelium in high shear vessels (Federici, 2006). Because of the reduced or defective vWF, factor VIII is reduced to a mild and variable degree because of decreased secretion and enhanced clearance. Because vWD is a disorder of the protein responsible for the adherence of platelets to damaged endothelial surfaces, the clinical manifestations in affected individuals resemble those seen in patients with platelet disorders (i.e., mucocutaneous bleeding [e.g., nose or gingiva], menorrhagia, and increased bleeding with trauma or surgery).

vWD has three variants. Patients with the type 1 variant, the most common (80%), have a heterozygous quantitative deficiency of vWF (20% to 40% of normal) associated with diminished factor VIII levels. Patients with type 1 vWD often have menorrhagia or mild to moderate bleeding from mucocutaneous sites. Medications that affect platelet function (e.g., NSAIDS)

can cause hemorrhage in a previously asymptomatic patient with type 1 vWD. Type 2 vWD (17% of patients with vWD) is characterized by the production of qualitatively abnormal vWF. Some of these patients have an associated thrombocytopenia, whereas others have a factor VIII deficiency that is out of proportion to the level of vWF. Type 3 vWD (3%) is marked by profound deficiencies of vWF and factor VIII. Homozygous patients may experience severe bleeding and spontaneous hemarthrosis. Because vWF levels are higher at birth and the proportion of the most functional high-molecular-weight multimeric units is increased, the incidence of bleeding in newborns is very low. When newborns with vWD bleed, it is the result of concomitantly low factor VIII levels. Acquired vWD has been associated with Wilms tumor, systemic lupus erythematosus (SLE), congenital heart defects, and HbE thalassemia.

The laboratory diagnosis of vWD is based on a prolonged bleeding time and on decreased levels of vWF antigen and factor VIII in the face of normal PT, fibrinogen, and platelet count. The aPTT may be normal or mildly prolonged. Ristocetin cofactor assay, which measures vWF-induced platelet agglutination, is used to identify type 2 vWD. It is recommended that screening be performed on three separate occasions before ruling out vWD, because functional and antigenic vWF levels may overlap those of normal patients and vWF levels can fluctuate in unpredictable ways. The vWF levels rise during pregnancy. There is a significant linkage between ABO locus and the vWF antigen, such that patients with A and B blood types have markedly higher levels (100% to 115%) of factor than those with type O (75%) (Souto et al., 2000).

Preoperative Preparation

Most patients with type 1 disease respond to the IV administration of 0.3 mcg/kg of DDAVP 30 minutes before surgery. DDAVP induces the release of vWF from endothelial storage granules (Weibel-Palade bodies) into the circulation and results in a 2- to 3-fold increase in plasma von Willebrand antigen levels within 30 to 60 minutes, with the effect lasting more than 6 hours (Mannucci, 1997; Robertson et al., 2008). DDAVP may be administered two to three times a day, although tachyphylaxis may develop (Federici, 2008). Because 10% of patients with type 1 vWD fail to respond to DDAVP, the response (increased factor VIII levels and normalization of bleeding time) should be documented before surgery to make sure it is adequate to prevent excessive perioperative bleeding (Nolan et al., 2000). If it is effective, it may be used as the sole agent for the treatment of minor bleeding (e.g., epistaxis) or perioperatively for minor surgery, such as dental extraction.

Patients with type 2 or type 3 diseases usually require replacement factor VIII and vWF to control bleeding. DDAVP is contraindicated in type 2b disease, because it may exacerbate thrombocytopenia. Those who do respond to DDAVP may also need factor replacement before major surgical procedures or for major trauma. Plasma-derived human factor VIII concentrate, which has a high concentration of vWF (e.g., Humate-P), is effective and is approved for replacement therapy in vWD (Federici et al., 2002).

If the patient's response to DDAVP is adequate and bleeding is not a problem, liberal DDAVP administration may be substituted for factor concentrate in the postoperative period. Close monitoring of bleeding and communication with the hematologist should guide postoperative management of these patients.

Factor XIII Deficiency

The role of factor XIII in hemostasis is to stabilize newly formed clots by crosslinking fibrin monomers. Plasma levels as low as 1% to 2% are usually adequate for hemostasis. Patients with factor XIII deficiency have bleeding despite a normal PT, aPTT, and platelet count. Factor XIII deficiency is a rare bleeding disorder that is inherited in an autosomal-recessive manner and has an estimated incidence of 1 in 2 million. Typical symptoms are delayed hemorrhages after mild trauma. The most common manifestation is prolonged bleeding from the newborn's umbilical stump, which is virtually pathognomonic for this deficiency, or after circumcision. The major morbidity in children with factor XIII deficiency is a marked propensity for intracranial hemorrhages (Gordon et al., 2008). Seriously affected patients are treated with cryoprecipitate or purified factor concentrate. All traumatic brain or closed-head injuries are treated prophylactically.

Factor VII Deficiency

Factor VII has the shortest half-life of all of the clotting factors, estimated to be 6 hours. Factor VII deficiency is a rare autosomal-recessive disorder. The severity of the hemorrhagic diathesis does not correlate with factor VII levels. Many individuals have mutations of factor VII but are asymptomatic, and they come to medical attention as a result of an isolated PT prolongation. Much more common than an inherited factor VII deficiency is an acquired factor VII deficiency. Because of the exquisitely short half-life of factor VII, liver failure, vitamin-K deprivation, or oral anticoagulant toxicity first manifests as factor VII deficiency with an isolated increased PT value.

Platelet Abnormalities

Congenital Coagulopathies as a Result of Platelet Abnormalities

Inherited coagulopathies also include diseases associated with quantitative and qualitative platelet dysfunction. Wiskott-Aldrich syndrome is an X-linked syndrome characterized by thrombocytopenia, immunodeficiency, and eczema. Newborns typically have thrombocytopenia caused by underproduction. These platelets are abnormally small. The disease results from the mutation of the Wiskott-Aldrich syndrome protein (WASP), a cytoskeletal regulatory protein found in megakaryocytes and lymphocytes (Caron, 2002). Symptomatic bleeding is treated with platelet transfusions. Congenital bone-marrow–failure syndromes that result in congenital thrombocytopenia include Diamond-Blackfan syndrome anemia, Schwachman-Diamond syndrome, and Fanconi anemia. These infants have severe mucocutaneous bleeding or intracranial hemorrhage as a result of profound thrombocytopenia, and they depend on platelet transfusions. Thrombocytopenia with absent radii is another cause of neonatal thrombocytopenia that is associated with skeletal anomalies. The thrombocytopenia is most pronounced in the first year of life, when mucocutaneous bleeding commonly occurs, and platelet transfusions are required.

Thrombocytopenia of Critical Illness

Thrombocytopenia is a common problem in the neonatal and pediatric intensive care units, with a prevalence of 25%. A manifestation of endothelial activation in critically ill children, thrombocytopenia is an independent predictor of mortality and prolonged length of hospital stay (Krishnan et al., 2008).

Thrombocytopenia of Immune Origin

Immune-mediated thrombocytopenias occur in the setting of isoimmunization, with transplacental transfer of maternal alloantibodies directed against paternally inherited antigens present on fetal platelets or with transfer of maternal autoimmune diseases such as idiopathic thrombocytopenic purpura (ITP) and SLE. Isoimmune thrombocytopenia occurs in 1 of 1000 deliveries. The distinguishing characteristic is the maternal platelet count, which is normal in isoimmune disease and decreased in autoimmune disease. Infants are usually asymptomatic unless the platelet count is less than 10,000. Mucocutaneous, spinal cord, and intracranial hemorrhages are seen prenatally and postnatally in isoimmune disease (Abel et al., 2003). The bleeding in autoimmune thrombocytopenia is usually not as severe, but the risk of intracranial hemorrhage increases when the platelet count is less than 40,000 in the newborn. Both diseases are treated with platelet transfusions, IVIG, and corticosteroids. The established treatment of alloimmune thrombocytopenia is the administration of washed, irradiated maternal platelets (10 mL/kg), but donor platelets screened for the absence of human platelet antigen 1a (HPA-1a) have been shown to be effective (Rothenberger, 2002; Rayment et al., 2003).

Thrombocytopathies

Inherited qualitative platelet defects are uncommon conditions that also present with bleeding in the newborn period. Glanzmann thrombasthenia is an autosomal-recessive deficiency of $\alpha_{IIb}\beta_3$ that impairs fibrinogen binding to platelets. Patients experience mucocutaneous bleeding in the neonatal period and have a lifelong risk of bleeding. Platelet count and morphology are normal; however, bleeding time, clot retraction, and platelet aggregation tests are all abnormal, and flow cytometry is required to confirm the $\alpha_{IIb}\beta_3$ deficiency. Bleeding is managed with platelet transfusions. Bernard-Soulier syndrome is an autosomal-recessive deficiency of the platelet vWF receptor. These patients have mild to moderate bleeding and have unusually large platelets. The diagnosis is confirmed by failure of agglutination in the presence of ristocetin.

Bleeding Diathesis Associated with Blood Vessel Abnormalities

Hereditary blood vessel disorders associated with bleeding diathesis include uncommon connective tissue diseases such as Ehlers-Danlos and Marfan syndromes. Osteogenesis imperfecta, a heterogeneous group of disorders of collagen synthesis, may have increased perioperative bleeding as a result of increased capillary fragility and abnormalities in collagen-induced platelet aggregation (Edge et al., 1997).

Acquired Coagulopathies

Vitamin K Deficiency

Hemorrhagic disease of the newborn is a bleeding disorder that is caused by a deficiency of vitamin K. Clinical bleeding occurs in 1 in 1000 to 1 in 10,000 babies who do not receive vitamin K supplementation. Vitamin K is poorly transferred across the placenta and is present only in low concentration in breast milk. Hemorrhagic disease of the newborn can be temporally divided into three types: early, classic, and late onset. Bleeding within the first 24 hours of life is defined as *early disease* and is generally seen in infants born to mothers who receive oral anticoagulants or antiepileptic drugs. These infants often have serious bleeding, including intracranial hemorrhage. Bleeding within the first week of life is *classic disease* and usually involves cutaneous, GI, or circumcision bleeding in infants who did not receive vitamin K supplementation at birth and who are usually breastfed. Bleeding in the first 3 months of life is referred to as *late-onset disease*, and it is seen in exclusively infants who were breastfed and in those with disorders of fat absorption such as CF, biliary atresia, and celiac disease. The diagnosis is confirmed with a prolonged PT, increased levels of proteins produced in the absence of vitamin K, and a low vitamin K level. Administration of vitamin K subcutaneously or intravenously increases coagulation factors within 2 hours, with complete correction within 24 hours. Serious bleeding may be treated with FFP (10 to 20 mL/kg) or with purified factor IX product.

Hepatic Dysfunction-Related Coagulopathy

Liver disease that results in synthetic dysfunction has a major impact on hemostasis because many of the coagulation factors are synthesized in the liver. Levels of these proteins are the first to decline with worsening liver disease, especially the very short-lived factor VII. Measurement of factor V, a hepatically synthesized, non–vitamin K-dependent protein, which is present in similar amounts in the newborn and the adult, is useful in differentiating vitamin K deficiency from hepatic dysfunction. Fibrin-degradation products are increased as a result of their decreased clearance in the setting of hepatic dysfunction. The development of ascites results in further loss of coagulation proteins.

Perioperative management of these patients includes determination of their exact deficiencies and correcting them with targeted management. Prolongation of the PT, resulting from depletion of vitamin K-dependent factors, can be treated with vitamin K or FFP. Vitamin K should normalize the PT in as little as 6 to 8 hours. Hypofibrinogenemia should be treated with cryoprecipitate. rFVIIa has been used successfully to correct the coagulopathy associated with liver failure (Atkison et al., 2005). Factor VIIa has been used in small numbers of patients to decrease transfusion requirements during liver transplantation, despite the fact that bleeding in that setting is multifactorial in nature (Busani et al., 2008).

Anticoagulant-Related Coagulopathy

Pediatric thrombotic complications are being recognized, diagnosed, and treated in great numbers; neonates are at higher risk for thromboembolic complications than are older children

(Kenet and Nowak-Gottl, 2006). Patients who receive therapeutic anticoagulation are at risk for devastating hemorrhagic complications. They have a 0.25% to 1% annual risk of intracranial hemorrhage, either intracerebral or subdural, both associated with high morbidity and mortality rates (Leissinger et al., 2008). If surgery is contemplated or when procedural heparinization must be reversed, protamine can be administered IV over 10 minutes. The dosage of protamine is based on the time since the last dose of heparin and can be calculated using the formula shown in Table 36-24 (Monagle, et al., 2008).

LMWH anticoagulation is also reversed with protamine, in a dose of 1 mg of protamine per 1 mg (100 units) of LMWH (Monagle et al., 2001). Protamine is given slowly, because rapid administration may cause profound hypotension. It only partially (60%) reverses the anti-Xa effects of LMWH administered within the previous 3 to 4 hours (Monagle et al., 2001). Although fondaparinux and the direct thrombin inhibitors have no specific reversal agents, some experience with using rFVIIa has been reported (Bijsterveld et al., 2002).

Children receiving oral anticoagulation may be difficult to maintain in a therapeutic range because of variations in diet, concurrent medications, and underlying disease processes. Breastfed infants are very sensitive to oral anticoagulants because of low concentrations of vitamin K in breast milk. Many of the common medications that are prescribed for children, including prednisone, amoxicillin, trimethoprim-sulfamethoxazole, and ranitidine, increase the INR of children taking oral anticoagulants. In preparation for elective surgery, vitamin K antagonists can be discontinued 4 days before the procedure, with the goal to restore the patient's INR to the range of 0.8 to 1.2 (Ansell et al., 2008). In this setting, vitamin K supplementation normalizes the INR within 18 to 24 hours after IV administration (Douketis et al., 2008). In situations of acute bleeding or when more rapid reversal is necessary, both IV vitamin K and either FFP or prothrombin complex concentrate should be used. In adults, the INR is corrected at a rate of 0.18 INR/hour after FFP and IV vitamin K administration (Boulis et al., 1999). Prothrombin complex concentrate rapidly normalizes the INR more effectively than does FFP, at a much smaller volume, with a low risk of thrombotic events (Leissinger et al., 2008; Levy et al., 2008). rFVIIa has been used as an alternative agent; it quickly corrects elevated INR in the setting of intracranial hemorrhage, which has been reported to allow for rapid neurosurgical intervention or, in some cases, to actually successfully halt the progression of hemorrhage, obviating the need for a craniotomy (Bartal et al., 2007).

TABLE 36-24. Protamine Reversal of Heparin Therapy

Time Since Last Heparin Dose (minutes)	Protamine Dose* (mg/100 units Heparin)
<30	1
30-60	0.5-0.75
60-120	0.375-0.5
>120	0.25-0.375

Data from Monagle P, et al.: Antithrombotic therapy in neonates and children. In American College of Chest Physicians evidence-based clinical practice guidelines, ed 8, *Chest* 133:887S, 2008.
*Maximum protamine dose = 50 mg; Infusion rate should not exceed 5 mg/min.

Acquired Thrombocytopathy

Aspirin and NSAIDs are the most commonly used medications that affect the coagulation system. These medications inhibit platelet COX, blocking thromboxane synthesis and leading to a partial impairment of platelet function. Two COX isoenzymes have been characterized: COX-1, which is always present on platelets and the gastric mucosa, and COX-2, which is up-regulated during inflammation. Nonspecific COX inhibitors have been shown to increase perioperative bleeding complications after adenoidectomy. Aspirin ingestion prolongs the bleeding time by 2 to 3 minutes. Perioperative administration of NSAIDs (e.g., ketorolac) increased the number of children with bleeding after tonsillectomy (Marret et al., 2003; Dsida and Cote, 2004).

Many anesthetic agents have been implicated in platelet dysfunction, as measured by platelet aggregometry; among them are inhaled anesthetics such as sevoflurane and the IV anesthetics propofol and ketamine (Nakagawa et al., 2002). However, no data demonstrate that these agents increase perioperative bleeding or transfusion requirements in the clinical setting.

Another class of drugs that may interfere with platelet function is the anticonvulsants such as sodium valproate. Valproate has caused mild thrombocytopenia, neutropenia, and even red cell aplasia, and patients taking valproate should be evaluated before surgery with a complete blood count with platelet count. Bone marrow suppression usually occurs with levels higher than 100 mcg/mL and usually responds to a decrease in dose (Acharya and Bussel, 2000). Bleeding time may be prolonged in patients taking valproic acid but usually not to a clinically significant extent. In a small series of patients taking valproic acid, 20% were shown to have acquired vWD, with low ristocetin cofactor activity, although only 2 of 6 affected children were symptomatic (epistaxis) (Serdaroglu et al., 2002; Koenig et al., 2008). One case report documented profound factor XIII deficiency that resulted in severe intracranial bleeding after craniotomy for epilepsy surgery (Pohlmann-Eden et al., 2003). This deficiency was resolved after discontinuation of valproic acid therapy. In a small study of children with cerebral palsy who underwent femoral osteotomy, those children who took valproic acid had greater blood loss and need for transfusion than did those with cerebral palsy who were either taking no anticonvulsants or anticonvulsants other than valproic acid (Carney and Minter, 2005). Therefore, the anesthesiologist should have a heightened awareness of the possibility of excessive surgical bleeding, especially during and after craniotomy, in patients taking valproic acid. Some hematologists recommend a bleeding time for children who are taking valproic acid and who are scheduled for craniotomy, with further investigation including vWF and ristocetin cofactor, as well as possible preoperative administration of DDAVP if indicated (Acharya and Bussel, 2000; Koenig et al., 2008)

Disseminated Intravascular Coagulation

Disseminated intravascular coagulation (DIC) is the unregulated activation of the hemostatic system characterized by the generation of activated clotting factors, fibrin, and accelerated fibrinolysis. Conditions associated with DIC are listed in Box 36-10. Patients can have bleeding or thrombosis or may have only laboratory evidence of DIC. DIC is the result of significant

---

Box 36-10 Conditions Associated with Disseminated Intravascular Coagulation

Sepsis
Shock
Heat stroke
Acidosis
Hypoxia*
Trauma
Head injury
Fat embolism
Crush injury
Burn injury
Toxin exposure[†]
Severe allergic reaction
Intravascular hemolysis
Liver disease
Cancer
   Myeloproliferative disease
Vascular anomalies
   Kasabach-Merritt syndrome
Extracorporeal circulation
Obstetric complications
   Amniotic fluid embolism
   Placental abruption
   Preeclampsia

*Antenatal hypoxia, from Hannam S et al: Neonatal coagulopathy in preterm, small-for-gestational-age infants, *Biol Neonate* 83:177, 2003.
[†]Snake bite, from Gold BS et al.: Bites of venomous snakes, *N Engl J Med* 83:177, 2003.

---

exposure of circulating blood to TF, commonly from endothelial disruption or from hypoxia, acidosis, and sepsis.

No single laboratory test can establish or exclude the diagnosis of DIC. The most common laboratory abnormalities include thrombocytopenia or a rapidly falling platelet count and elevated D-dimer levels. Less commonly, microangiopathic hemolytic anemia, hypofibrinogenemia, and PT and aPTT prolongation are seen. D-dimers may be present in premature infants without DIC. Antithrombin III levels can be markedly depressed as well. The treatment of DIC is principally focused on eradicating the precipitating process; treatment of the consequences without treating the underlying cause is certain to fail. No evidence exists that prophylactic administration of platelets or plasma improves the outcome of a patient who is not bleeding. FFP, cryoprecipitate, and platelet transfusions are used only to treat active bleeding in the older child. However, in the neonatal period, because of the risk of intracerebral hemorrhage, many aim to correct platelet counts of less than 50,000, fibrinogen levels of less than 100 mg/dL, and INR of higher than 1.5. Sequential thromboelastograms (TEGs) are useful in monitoring the correction of DIC in the perioperative period (see "Thromboelastograph").

Nutritional Coagulopathies

In addition to vitamin K deficiency, vitamin C deficiency (i.e., scurvy) can result in a bleeding diathesis. Because vitamin C plays a fundamental role in collagen formation, patients with vitamin C deficiency have impaired collagen synthesis and capillary fragility, which leads to gingival bleeding and petechiae. Children with scurvy are at risk for significant oropharyngeal bleeding during airway manipulation (Disma et al., 2008).

Acquired Hemophilia

Antibodies to coagulation factors develop in patients with hemophilia who are treated with factor replacement and in patients who do not have hemophilia who have no prior exposure to hemostatic therapy. These acquired inhibitors to coagulation factors occur most commonly against factor VIII. Although many patients with acquired hemophilia are elderly, children can be affected in a devastating manner. Patients who develop inhibitors commonly have coexisting diseases such as lupus or rheumatoid arthritis, or they have been recently treated for rheumatic fever or nephrotic syndrome (Sakai et al., 2005). Transplacental transfer of acquired inhibitors has been reported, resulting in hemorrhagic complications in the newborn period. Patients with acquired inhibitors most commonly have bleeding into fascial planes and mucous membranes, rather than into joints. The diagnosis is elusive because of inconsistent test results. No correlation exists between inhibitor titers and the severity or pattern of bleeding (Huth-Kuhne et al., 2009).

In patients with inhibitors, even large amounts of cryoprecipitate or FFP may not promote satisfactory hemostasis. FFP administration leads to an anamnestic response, increasing inhibitor levels. Factor VIII autoantibodies in acquired hemophilia are usually incompletely inhibitory, so that factor VIII levels are usually detectable and may be as high as 10% to 20% of normal values. First-line therapy for inhibitor-associated hemorrhage is either rFVIIa or one of the commercially available activated prothrombin complexes. If one of these agents is not immediately available, DDAVP can be employed (Huth-Kuhne et al., 2009).

Recombinant Factor VIIa (rFVIIa)

The success of rFVIIa, a synthetic clotting factor, originally developed for use in patients with hemophilia and inhibitors to factors VIII or IX, dramatizes the new paradigm of cell-based hemostasis presented earlier and offers an additional therapeutic option for other bleeding situations in the perioperative period (Roberts et al., 2004). Because of deficiencies in either factors VIII or IX, patients with hemophilia are unable to generate the platelet-localized factor Xa that is necessary for explosive thrombin production. rFVIIa forms a complex with TF exposed at areas of vascular injury, acting as a local catalyst for coagulation. The resultant rFVIIa-TF-Xa complex can overcome a deficiency of factor VIII or IX, the foundation for rFVIIa's primary indication. rFVIIa also binds to activated platelets and enhances thrombin generation. rFVIIa's mechanism of action is illustrated in Figure 36-17 (Mannucci and Levi, 2007).

Intraoperative Coagulopathies

Patients with no preoperative disorders of coagulation who have surgery may develop coagulopathy because of a combination of blood loss, fluid replacement, and other intraoperative circumstances. Conditions associated with the development of intraoperative coagulopathy are listed in Box 36-11.

Colloid-Induced von Willebrand Syndrome

The administration of some synthetic colloids as volume expanders may be associated with the development of acquired vWD (Chappell et al., 2008; Bailey et al., 2010). Large amounts of dextran decrease vWF and factor VIII levels and enhance fibrinolysis. The increase in bleeding times after dextran infusion can be completely normalized by the administration of DDAVP.

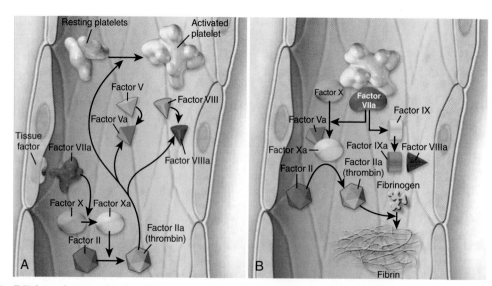

■ **FIGURE 36-17.** rFVIIa's mechanism of action. When the vessel wall is disrupted, subendothelial TF becomes exposed to circulating blood and may bind factor VIIa **(A).** This binding activates factor X, and activated factor X (factor Xa) generates small amounts of thrombin. The thrombin (factor IIa) in turn activates platelets and factors V and VIII. Activated platelets bind circulating factor VIIa **(B),** resulting in further factor Xa generation, as well as activation of factor IX. Activated factor IX (factor IXa) (with its cofactor VIIIa) yields additional factor Xa. The complex of factor Xa and its cofactor Va then converts prothrombin (factor II) into thrombin (factor IIa) in amounts that are sufficient to induce the conversion of fibrinogen to fibrin. *(From Mannucci PM, Levi M: Prevention and treatment of major blood loss, N Engl J Med 356:2301, 2007.)*

Box 36-11 Conditions Associated with the Development of Intraoperative Coagulopathy

NEUROLOGIC CONDITIONS
Intracranial surgery
Traumatic brain injury

CARDIOVASCULAR CONDITIONS
Congenital heart disease
Shock
Kasabach-Merritt syndrome

TRAUMA
ORTHOPEDIC CONDITIONS
Fat embolism
Scoliosis surgery
Osteogenesis imperfecta
Intramedullary nailing of long-bone fractures

MISCELLANEOUS CONDITIONS
Citrate-induced hypocalcemia
Factor V inhibition from exposure to bovine topical thrombin

Data from Iberti TJ, Miller M, Abalos A, et al: Abnormal coagulation profile in brain tumor patients during surgery, *Neurosurgery* 34:389–394, 1994; Vavilala MS, Dunbar PJ, Rivara FP, et al: Coagulopathy predicts poor outcome following head injury in children less than 16 years of age, *J Neurosurg Anesthesiol* 13:13–18, 2001; Murshid WR, Gader AG. The coagulopathy in acute head injury: comparison of cerebral versus peripheral measurements of haemostatic activation markers, *Br J Neurosurg* 16:362–369, 2002; Hymel KP, Absire TC, Luckey DW, et al: Coagulopathy in pediatric abusive head trauma, *Pediatrics* 99:371–375, 1997; Robinson CM, Ludlam CA, Ray DC, et al: The coagulative and cardiorespiratory responses to reamed intramedullary nailing of isolated fractures, *J Bone Joint Surg Br* 83:963–973, 2001; Keegan MT, Whatcott BD, Harrison BA: Osteogenesis imperfecta, perioperative bleeding, and desmopressin, *Anesthesiology* 97:1011–1013, 2002; Neschis DG, Heyman MR, Cheanvechai V, et al: Coagulopathy as a result of factory V inhibitor after exposure to bovine topical thrombin, *J Vasc Surg* 35:400–402, 2002.

Of the available colloids, children commonly receive human serum albumin and only rarely receive hydroxyethyl starch. Human serum albumin has minimal effects on coagulation (Schramko et al., 2009). However, albumin does prolong the bleeding time based on impairment of platelet aggregation. In adult studies, when albumin is compared with dextran and high-molecular-weight hydroxyethyl starch, albumin is associated with less postoperative blood loss. Preliminary studies comparing middle-molecular-weight hydroxyethyl starch and albumin suggest that a minimal difference exists between them in postoperative blood loss. In patients with even mild forms of vWD, the administration of artificial colloid in patients can be associated with significant hemorrhagic complications; albumin or crystalloid should be used preferentially (De Jonge and Levi, 2001).

Hypothermia

Substantial data suggest that hypothermia is an independent and dramatic contributor to coagulopathy. Mild hypothermia of 35° C significantly prolongs the PT, aPTT, and bleeding time. At a core temperature of 34° C, coagulation and platelet function are severely altered, despite normal fibrinolytic function (Wolberg et al., 2004). The coagulopathy of hypothermia is exacerbated by acidosis (Dirkman et al., 2008). Transfusion of platelets and clotting factors does not correct the hypothermic coagulopathy completely in the absence of rewarming.

Both components of the hemostatic mechanism appear to be deleteriously affected by hypothermia. Platelet function is seriously impaired by mild hypothermia as a result of a reduction in TXA_2 release. The clotting cascade involves a series of enzymatic reactions, all of which are slowed by hypothermia (Hoffman and Monroe, 2007). The laboratory detection of hypothermic coagulopathy is often missed because most laboratories perform clotting tests at 37° C (Rossaint and Spahn, 2006). The results of the PT and aPTT performed at the patient's actual core temperature are prolonged. TEG data suggest that hypothermia impairs clot formation rather than enhancing fibrinolysis (Dirkman et al., 2008). Thromboelastography can be adjusted to a patient's core body temperature to adequately evaluate the role played by hypothermia in hypothermic coagulopathy (Ramaker et al., 2009).

Hemodilution

Acute normovolemic hemodilution to minimize red cell transfusion requirements often results in alterations of hemostasis, especially when colloid is used as the diluent. Quantitative modeling of acute normovolemic hemodilution demonstrates that patients often develop inadequate fibrinogen levels (less than 100 mg/dL) before they reach the hematocrit threshold for red cell transfusion or the threshold for platelet transfusions (Singbartl et al., 2003). Fibrinogen administration has been shown to reverse the hemostatic consequences of colloid hemodilution (Mittermayr et al., 2007).

Massive Transfusion

Massive blood loss is defined as the loss of more than 1 blood volume in a 24-hour period, the normal blood volume being 7% of ideal body weight in an adult and 8% to 9% in an infant. In the operating room, early recognition of major blood loss can be appreciated using the definitions of massive blood loss as occurring at the rate of 2 to 3 mL/kg per minute or 50% of blood volume in over 3 hours.

The progression from dilutional coagulopathy to dilutional thrombocytopenia is seen in massive transfusion and in extreme hemodilution. During the era of whole-blood administration, thrombocytopenia was the initial coagulopathic event. Currently, blood loss is most often replaced with plasma-poor RBC products that are devoid of most coagulation factors. Under these conditions, the initial coagulopathic event is the dilution of coagulation factors (marked by prolongation of the PT); hypofibrinogenemia is the first factor deficiency that occurs, at a time when the platelet count remains more than 150,000/mcL (Perkins et al., 2008). The PT becomes prolonged when less than 1 blood volume is lost, but a clinical coagulopathy does not occur until the PT and PTT exceed 1.5 to 1.8 times the control values (Hirshberg et al., 2003). In the clinical setting, fibrinogen concentrations fall below the hemostatically critical level of 100 mg/dL when blood loss is in excess of 150% of the patient's blood volume, and the remaining coagulation factors fall below 25% after 200% blood loss. A platelet count of less than 50,000 should be anticipated when more than 2 blood volumes have been lost (Stainsby et al., 2000).

FFP is the first choice in treating a coagulopathy that results from massive transfusion (Gonzalez et al., 2007). Although the optimal FFP/RBC ratio is unknown, aggressive adherence to a ratio of 1:1 to 1:2 helps prevent the onset of a dilutional coagulopathy and minimize the need for cryoprecipitate (Hirshberg et al., 2003; Ho et al., 2005). These authors have also suggested an ideal platelet-to-RBC ratio of 0.8:1 for the massively transfused patient (Hirshberg et al., 2003). Survival in both civilian and combat victims requiring massive transfusions was dependent on the FFP/RBC ratio that they received; mortality was lowest when this ratio was approximately 1:1.5 (Borgman et al., 2007; Sperry et al., 2008). In this setting, if rapid laboratory corroboration is possible, a complete coagulation profile should be obtained to determine the patient's specific replacement needs. In the absence of timely data, or with continuing hemorrhage, empirical therapy with FFP is justified. FFP at a dose of 20 mL/kg increases fibrinogen by approximately 60 mg/dL and increases clotting factors by 20%.

Traumatic Coagulopathy Independent of Blood Loss or Replacement

Laboratory manifestations of trauma-related coagulopathy include abnormal PT and aPTT, decreased protein C levels, and an increase in plasma thrombomodulin. These patients have increased transfusion requirements. Abnormal aPTT and low protein C are independent predictors of mortality (Macleod et al., 2003; Brohi et al., 2007a).

Traumatic coagulopathy manifests as a hypocoagulable state associated with hypothermia, acidosis, clotting factor dilution, and tissue destruction, all of which are directly proportional to the severity of the traumatic injury (Hess et al., 2008). Nearly 25% of trauma patients arrive at the emergency department with an established clinically significant coagulopathy, and these patients are four times more likely to die than are trauma victims without a coagulopathy (Brohi et al., 2007b). The variables responsible for this coagulopathy include tissue trauma, shock, dilution, hypothermia, acidemia, and inflammation (Armand and Hess, 2003). Mild to moderate hypothermia affects coagulation and platelet function and is associated with clinical bleeding (Martini et al., 2005). Animal investigation confirms that acidemia slows the kinetics of coagulation reactions and enhances fibrinolysis (Martini et al., 2007).

Shock and the hemodilution that result from fluid resuscitation are the early instigators of the traumatic coagulopathy process. The aggressive fluid management required by these trauma patients produces a concomitant dilutional coagulopathy as well. Vigorous fluid resuscitation can result in a confluence of circumstances that in and of itself contributes to the traumatic coagulopathy. By increasing intravascular volume, blood pressure, and vasodilation, hemorrhage is further potentiated. These hemodynamic and rheologic perturbations increase the likelihood that hemostatic plug formation will not occur.

Specific injuries modulate the course of the coagulopathy. Extensive tissue destruction releases tissue thromboplastins, which activate the clotting process and result in a consumptive coagulopathy. tPA and PAI-1 are released from the extensively damaged tissue bed. In the first few hours after traumatic injury, tPA increases out of proportion to PAI-1 and produces a systemic activation of fibrinolysis (Brohi et al., 2008). This coagulopathy resembles that of DIC, but the diffuse microthrombi that are classically seen in DIC are not seen in traumatic coagulopathy.

Traumatic brain injury produces a consumptive coagulopathy as the result of the release of TF and other tissue thromboplastins into the circulation and fibrinolysis activation, which is associated with a dramatic increase in mortality (Stein and Smith, 2004; Talving et al., 2009). Long-bone fractures are also associated with coagulopathy, perhaps through the mechanism of subclincial fat embolism.

Intraoperative Evaluation of the Bleeding Patient

Activated clotting time (ACT) is a modification of a whole-blood clotting test that uses kaolin or Celite to accelerate coagulation by activating the contact pathway (Box 36-12). A fixed volume of blood is placed into a tube with activator at 37° C for 60 seconds, after which the contents are stirred until a clot is formed. The normal ACT range is 80 to 120 seconds. This test can be performed easily at the bedside using commercially available equipment. ACT levels correlate well with antifactor Xa heparin levels in the precardiopulmonary bypass period and are commonly used to monitor the adequacy of heparin anticoagulation

---

Box 36-12 Evaluation of the Bleeding Child

PLATELET ASSESSMENTS
Abnormal number: thrombocytopenias, hemangiomas
Abnormal morphology: inherited platelet defects
Abnormal function: inherited or acquired

PT AND APTT ASSESSMENTS
Abnormal PT, normal aPTT
   Factor VII deficiency
   Vitamin K deficiency, liver disease
   Factor deficiencies: II, V, VII, and X
   Drug related: Coumadin
Normal PT, abnormal aPTT
   Factor deficiencies: VIII, IX, XI, XII, kallikrein, prekallikrein, high-molecular-weight kininogen, and vWF
   Drug related: heparin
Abnormal PT, abnormal aPTT
   Vitamin K deficiency, liver disease
   Factor deficiencies: II, V, and X
   Dysfibrinogenemia
   Drug related: heparin and coumadin
Abnormal PT, abnormal aPTT, thrombocytopenia
   • DIC
   • Liver disease
   • Dysfibrinogenemia
Normal PT, normal aPTT, normal platelets
   Factor XIII deficiency
   α_2-antiplasmin deficiency

THROMBIN TIME*
Normal
   Liver disease, vitamin K deficiency
   Factor deficiencies: II, V, X
   Drug related: Coumadin
Abnormal
   Liver disease
   DIC
   Dysfibrinogenemia
   Drug related: heparin

*Useful in cases of abnormal PT and abnormal aPTT.

levels during extracorporeal circulation. The relationship of ACT with heparin dosing is linear in the setting of normal antithrombin III concentrations and factor XII activity, normothermia, a platelet count of more than 50,000, intact platelet function, and a fibrinogen level of more than 100 mg/mL. However, in the absence of extracorporeal circulation, ACT has a much poorer correlation with plasma heparin concentrations than does the aPTT. ACT is insensitive to many coagulation abnormalities; clotting deficiencies and platelet abnormalities can be present with a normal ACT (Girardi et al., 2000). Nevertheless, in the setting of major trauma, intraoperative ACT measurements were able to discriminate between patients who became coagulopathic and those who did not. However, because the ACT test is performed at 37° C, the contribution of hypothermia to the development of this coagulopathy is underappreciated (Aucar et al., 2003). ACT levels do not correlate well with LMWH anti-Xa levels.

Thromboelastograph

The TEG is a point-of-care evaluation of a patient's hemostatic balance, from initial clot formation to clot retraction or dissolution. Coagulation of blood has been compared with the building of a house: TEG profiling does not end when the foundation stone is laid, as do the other clinically employed clotting studies. The TEG also reflects the speed of the building process, whether the building will be sturdy, and whether it is likely to be damaged soon after it is built. The TEG examines the viscoelastic properties of blood as it clots. Placed into a rotating cup with an immersed pin, liquid blood begins to clot by forming fibers between the cup and the pin, transmitting motion to the pin. The TEG measures the elastic shear modulus of the clot, providing information about the rate of clot formation, clot strength, platelet function, and fibrinolytic activity, reflected in the characteristics of the tracing produced (Venkatesh et al., 2001). The maximal elastic sheer modulus depends on platelet count and function and the amount of fibrin deposited on the pin.

A typical TEG tracing and the parameters of the TEG are illustrated in Figure 36-18 and described in the following list:

R (reaction time): Latency to initial clot formation; from onset of tracing until a 2-mm amplitude on tracing. This

is similar to whole-blood clotting time; it depends on an intact intrinsic pathway and an adequate generation of thrombin. Prolonged R is associated with clotting deficiencies, heparin administration, and thrombocytopenia. The coagulation test that correlates with R is aPTT.

K (coagulation rate): Rate of fibrin buildup and crosslinking, occurring from 2 to 20 mm. Prolonged K is associated with clotting deficiencies, platelet dysfunction, thrombocytopenia, and hypofibrinogenemia.

a angle (rate of increase in elastic shear modulus): The rate of fibrin buildup and crosslinking; slope of divergence of tracing from R.

MA (maximal elastic shear modulus): Measured at maximal divergence of the graph, after the clot is entirely formed, this is the maximal clot strength. A typical clot has an MA of 50 mm, which is equivalent to 5000 dynes/cm^2. MA is the best description of the competency of the clot. It depends on platelet count and function and on the fibrinogen level (Chandler, 1995):

Decreased MA is associated with thrombocytopenia, platelet dysfunction hypofibrinogenemia, and deficiencies of factors VIII and XIII. Increased MA is associated with a prothrombotic state.

The tracings seen on the TEG for common disorders of hemostasis are shown in Figure 36-19. The TEG is a global measure of hemostasis, useful when multiple hemostatic defects are present. The weakness of TEG is its inability to identify specific clotting abnormalities. The TEG is a sensitive indicator of hypocoagulable and hypercoagulable perturbations. The typical hypercoagulable TEG profile has the appearance of a cognac glass (Traverso et al., 1995).

The R of patients receiving coumadin increases with increased INR, but it may remain within a normal range. Patients with decreased clotting factors have decreased R and K values and prolonged PT, or they have decreased angle and prolonged aPTT. Hypofibrinogenemia is associated with decreased R and K times, decreased angle, and decreased MA. Hyperfibrinolysis is characterized by reduced amplitude at 30 and 60 minutes (decreased A_{30}, A_{60}).

In addition to its point-of-care availability, the conditions under which a TEG is performed can be optimized to best define the clinical scenario. TEG offers a number of other advantages

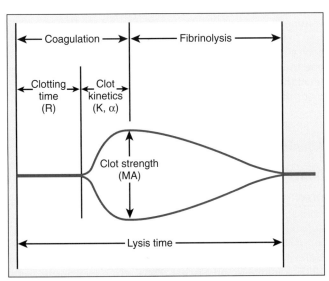

■ FIGURE 36-18. Parameters of the thromboelastograph.

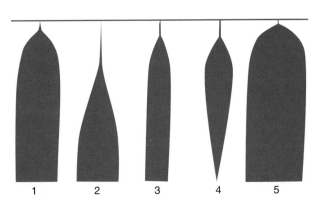

■ FIGURE 36-19. Thromboelastographic tracings of common hemostatic abnormalities. *1,* Normal; *2,* hemophilia; *3,* thrombocytopenia; *4,* fibrinolysis; *5,* hypercoagulation.

in the assessment of hemostasis that conventional coagulation tests do not. It is performed at the patient's temperature to reflect its effects on hemostasis; conventional parameters are measured at 37° C. The anticoagulation effects of LMWH can be rapidly assessed with TEG tests, whereas factor Xa measurements are not readily available (Coppell et al., 2006). Hypercoagulability can be diagnosed by TEG but usually cannot be determined through conventional means (Ganter and Hofer, 2008). The patient's state of coagulability can be quantified with the coagulation index (CI) (Chan et al., 2007):

$$CI = (-0.6516)R - (0.3772)K + (0.1224)MA + (0.0759)\alpha - 7.7922$$

CI > 3, hypercoagulable stage

CI < 3, hypocoagulable stage

TEG has been employed in the pediatric population. The parameters of children younger than 1 year of age undergoing noncardiac surgery were different from those of an adult control group. The rates of clot initiation and clot buildup, as well as clot strength were all greater in the infant groups. Despite their observations of developmental differences in clotting factor concentrations, the authors concluded that the hemostatic mechanism of the infant is balanced (Chan et al., 2007). TEG has been used in a variety of clinical pediatric perioperative settings, including cardiac surgery, extracorporeal membrane oxygenation, liver transplantation, and neurosurgery (Miller et al., 2000; Goobie et al., 2001; Davis et al., 2006;).

Because TEG has been a registered trademark since 1996 and because of the availability of other similar devices (rotation thromboelastometry [ROTEM] and Sonoclot), it has been suggested that the term *viscoelastic point-of-care coagulation analysis* should replace TEG as the generic term for this methodology. As of this writing, these newer devices have not been extensively used in children.

TREATMENT OF THE BLEEDING PATIENT

Safety of Transfusion and Factor Replacement

Complications of life-threatening bloodborne virus transmission have been markedly reduced by the institution of multiple screening steps in the procurement of donor-derived plasma products. However, the risks of transfusion-associated transmission of thermostable viruses such as hepatitis A and parvovirus B19 remain. Reports of transfusion-associated transmission of West Nile virus highlight the continued risks of using the blood supply as the principal source for hemostatic agents. Nucleic acid amplification testing for West Nile virus has now been shown to be effective in detecting virus in asymptomatic donors (Busch et al., 2005). The list of potential bloodborne pathogens is long and continues to grow, although not all bloodborne viruses have been demonstrated to be pathogenic to humans. Unfortunately, these concerns are not completely alleviated by the use of recombinant factor concentrates. With the outbreak of variant Creutzfeldt-Jakob disease in the United Kingdom, concern has been raised that the human albumin used in the manufacture and formulation of some recombinant factors may contain and transmit prion proteins. In countries where bovine spongiform encephalopathy has occurred, strategies to minimize the risk of transmission of Creutzfeldt-Jakob disease have

been developed, including screening potential blood, plasma, and platelet donors and leukoreducing whole-blood and red cell products (Ludlam and Turner, 2006).

Safety of Hemostatic Agents

Recently, the medications that have been most extensively evaluated as alternative or adjunctive hemostatic agents include the antifibrinolytic lysine analogues, EACA and tranexamic acid (a bovine-derived protease inhibitor), DDAVP, and rFVIIa. Designed to assess therapeutic efficacy, most trials were not optimally designed to assess potential adverse effects; therefore, definitive safety data are lacking for all agents. Although these drugs are often associated with dramatic success—"the liquid intracranial hemorrhage became a clot pancake before my eyes"—they are not panaceas. Adverse events should be anticipated when tightly regulated systems such as the hemostatic and fibrinolytic systems are pharmacologically perturbed. Of particular concern are the thrombotic adverse events associated with these hemostatic agents (Mannucci and Levi, 2007).

Most safety data regarding the complications of these hemostatic agents are based on results of studies in adult patients. Is it reasonable for pediatric providers to extrapolate safety concerns from the adult experience? Until sufficiently large pediatric studies are conducted to evaluate the safety of these agents, they must certainly pay close attention to the concerns raised by the adult studies. Given that these drugs have life-saving potential, the dilemma, as Twite and Hammer (2008) point out, is that in the absence of data, providers must balance "do what is best" with "do no harm." Informed consent, when deemed necessary, and heightened vigilance for the occurrence of adverse events must accompany the use of such agents in children.

Anticoagulant-Induced Coagulopathy

Patients who are experiencing severe bleeding should receive FFP in a dose of 20 mL/kg until vitamin K administration increases endogenous synthesis. Infusion of factor IX complex concentrate, which contains high concentrations of the activated vitamin K–dependent factors (II, VII, IX, and X) can correct the effects of anticoagulants rapidly without the excessive volume exposure of FFP. Factor IX complex (40 IU/kg) in addition to FFP infusion (as compared with FFP alone) successfully corrected the INR in patients with intracranial hemorrhage in one third of the time with 9% of total fluid volume administered (Boulis et al., 1999). rFVIIa can also correct oral anticoagulant-induced coagulopathy.

Agents Used to Control Bleeding

DDAVP

DDAVP is an analogue of vasopressin that recruits factor VIII from storage sites within endothelial cells via activation of the endothelial vasopressin V2 receptor and cAMP-mediated signaling; it may raise baseline factor VIII levels by 2- to 20-fold in normal patients and in patients with mild hemophilia (Mannucci, 1997; Kaufmann and Vischer, 2003). This increase in factor level is often sufficient to prevent or limit minor bleeding.

DDAVP also increases the release of ultra large vWF multimers from the endothelium. DDAVP is the treatment of choice for children with type 1 vWD, mild hemophilia, or platelet dysfunction, including uremia and drug-induced bleeding diatheses. DDAVP is also effective in treating hemorrhage in patients with acquired inhibitors to factors VIII or IX. Anecdotally, DDAVP has controlled perioperative bleeding in patients with Ehlers-Danlos syndrome, Marfan syndrome, and osteogenesis imperfecta, in which bleeding is thought to be the result of dysfunctional platelet aggregation caused by abnormal collagen (Keegan et al., 2002; Franchini, 2007).

DDAVP has been employed in a variety of pediatric procedures associated with risk of large blood loss in an attempt to decrease perioperative blood loss and transfusion requirements. Despite early studies to suggest that DDAVP reduced blood loss in cardiac surgery patients, most studies suggest that DDAVP is not efficacious in uncomplicated cardiac surgery. Children undergoing complex congenital heart repair did not have any reduction in bleeding or transfusion requirements with the prophylactic use of DDAVP (Oliver et al., 2000). Similarly, DDAVP does not appear to reduce blood loss in spinal fusion in patients with idiopathic scoliosis or in those with cerebral palsy-associated neuromuscular scoliosis (Theroux et al., 1997; Alanay et al., 1999).

A dose of 0.3 mcg/kg administered IV over 20 to 30 minutes or intranasally (150 mcg for children weighing less than 50 kg, and 300 mcg for those weighing more than 50 kg) increases factor VIII levels by 62%, and this dose may be repeated every 8 to 12 hours to control bleeding. Peak effects occur within 30 to 60 minutes after IV infusion and 60 to 90 minutes after intranasal administration. Tachyphylaxis may occur after three or four doses. Because severe hyponatremia-associated seizures have been reported with the use of DDAVP, close observation of fluid status and electrolyte balance is mandated. Although thrombotic complications have been reported, in two meta-analyses of DDAVP use in the adult perioperative period, no significant difference in the incidence of these complications between DDAVP and placebo was reported (Mannucci, 1997; Crescenzi et al., 2008).

Antifibrinolytics

Two classes of antifibrinolytics have been employed to optimize hemostasis in the setting of a bleeding diathesis and to reduce blood loss and transfusion requirements during major procedures: the synthetic lysine analogues EACA and tranexamic acid, and the serine protease inhibitor aprotinin. Their mechanism of action is illustrated in Figure 36-20. Antifibrinolytic drugs are commonly employed when bleeding occurs in sites that are rich in plasminogen activator and other fibrinolytic enzymes, such as the endometrium, the GI tract, and the urinary tract (Mannucci, 1998). These drugs are contraindicated in the setting of hematuria, DIC, or thromboembolic disease. EACA has been successfully used in managing bleeding crises in patients with hemophilia and inhibitors (Ghosh et al., 2004). EACA binds to the lysine site on plasminogen and plasmin, preventing plasmin from binding to fibrin; fibrinolysis is inhibited and clot stabilization continues. EACA has been shown to be

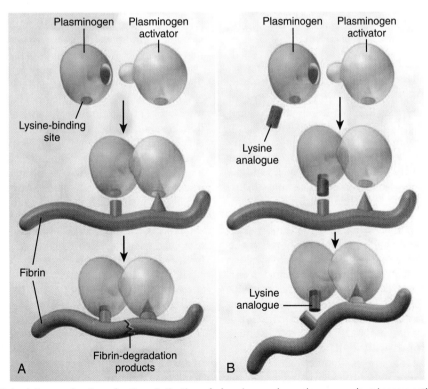

■ **FIGURE 36-20.** Antifibrinolytics mechanism of action. Activation of plasminogen by endogenous plasminogen activators results in plasmin, which causes degradation of fibrin. Binding of plasminogen to fibrin makes this process more efficient and occurs through lysine residues in fibrin that bind to lysine-binding sites on plasminogen **(A).** In the presence of lysine analogues, these lysine-binding sites are occupied, resulting in an inhibition of fibrin binding to plasminogen and impairment of endogenous fibrinolysis **(B).** *(From Mannucci PM, Levi M: Prevention and treatment of major blood loss, N Engl J Med 356:2301, 2007.)*

effective in decreasing blood loss in children undergoing cardiac surgery (Eaton, 2008). Children undergoing posterior lumbar fusion who received 100 mg/kg of EACA followed by an infusion of 10 mg/kg per hour had less blood loss and required less RBC transfusions than did a randomized control group (Florentino-Pineda et al., 2001).

Aprotinin is a naturally occurring serine protease inhibitor that affects hemostasis through several mechanisms; it is an antifibrinolytic and inhibits kallikrein, plasmin, trypsin, and APC. Aprotinin inhibits the initiation of fibrinolysis and the contact phase of coagulation, but it has no effects on platelet function. It is inactive when given orally. Aprotinin was first shown to be effective in reducing blood loss in coronary-artery–bypass graft operations and subsequently was shown to be effective in reducing perioperative bleeding and transfusion requirements in pediatric cardiac surgery, liver transplantation, hip replacements, and posterior spine fusion (Lemmer et al., 1996; Urban et al., 2001; Samama et al., 2002; Eaton, 2008).

Mouth bleeding is common in hemophilia patients, resulting in part from the potent fibrinolytic activity of saliva. For oral or GI bleeding in patients with hemophilia, EACA is often very effective and may dramatically reduce the need for additional coagulation factor infusions when given at a dose of 100 mg/kg orally every 6 hours for 5 to 10 days after a hemorrhagic episode. Antifibrinolytic mouthwashes allow for the performance of dental extractions on patients receiving long-term oral anticoagulant treatment without lowering the degree of anticoagulation (Patatanian and Fugate, 2006).

Safety of Antifibrinolytic Agents

Clinical trials demonstrate that all three drugs (EACA, aprotinin, and tranexamic acid) are effective at reducing transfusion requirements as compared with placebo (Henry et al., 2007). Recent studies of aprotinin's use in adult patients have documented an increased incidence of renal failure and cardiovascular complications; a study called *Blood Conservation Using Antifibrinolytics in a Randomized Trial (BART)* reported an increase in perioperative mortality (Mangano et al., 2006; Fergusson et al., 2008). Safety data on pediatric aprotinin use are limited. The largest pediatric review of aprotinin usage (865 children) was designed to evaluate the incidence and impact of aprotinin hypersensitivity reactions; this study was not designed to identify thrombotic events or renal impairment, and none was reported (Jaquiss et al., 2002). In a retrospective review of aprotinin's use in pediatric cardiac surgery, using historical controls, no differences in the complication rates were reported; however, thrombotic events were not one of the primary end points (Backer et al., 2007). Recent retrospective studies found no increase in renal dysfunction in neonates who received aprotinin during cardiopulmonary bypass (Guzzetta et al., 2009a; Manrique et al., 2009). At the current time, the issue of whether aprotinin is safe and effective in children is moot, as the manufacturer has removed the drug from the market because of concerns raised by the BART trial.

Recombinant Activated Factor VIIa (rFVIIa)

rFVIIa is a synthetic clotting factor that was originally developed for use in patients with hemophilia who developed inhibitors to factors VIII or IX. The rationale behind the development and clinical success of rFVIIa underscores the new paradigm of cell-based hemostasis presented earlier. Those with hemophilia are unable to generate the platelet-localized factor Xa necessary for explosive thrombin production because of deficiencies in factors VIII or IX. Administered factor VIIa is effective in improving hemostasis in patients who have hemophilia by complexing with TF exposed at areas of vascular injury and by binding to activated platelets and restoring platelet surface-thrombin generation. This augmented thrombin production further increases platelet activation and thrombin-activatable fibrinolysis inhibitor (TAFI), which decreases fibrinolysis. In this way, the resultant factor VIIa-TF-Xa complex thus overcomes a deficiency of factor VIII or IX. For patients with hemophilia who have high inhibitor titers, randomized, controlled trials in adults and children have shown that rFVIIa minimizes spontaneous bleeding and decreases intraoperative blood loss (O'Connell et al., 2002).

After rFVIIa's dramatic use in an exsanguinating 19-year-old soldier with a vascular injury, an increasing number of anecdotal and small case series have described rFVIIa's successful use in mitigating uncontrollable bleeding in patients without hemophilia in a variety of clinical situations—hepatic dysfunction, thrombocytopenia, platelet dysfunction, dilutional coagulopathies, DIC, and after cardiopulmonary bypass (Kenet et al., 1999; Poon et al., 1999; Martinowitz et al., 2001; Blajchman, 2003; Goodnough, 2003; Tobias et al., 2003a, 2003b; Guzzetta et al., 2009b). Because factor VII is the first of the clotting factors to become deficient in liver failure, rFVIIa has been used in the setting of hepatic dysfunction and vitamin K antagonism. The enhanced platelet activation that results from increased thrombin production has led to the use of rFVIIa in treating quantitative and qualitative platelet dysfunction (Patel et al., 2001). rFVIIa resulted in a reduction in bleeding time in 50% of patients with thrombocytopenia. The clot formed with rFVIIa use has a denser mesh of fibrin fibers that is more resistant to plasmin degradation (Hedner, 1998). rFVIIa has been used in the patient receiving massive transfusions whose coagulopathy has been unresponsive to conventional plasma-component therapy.

The recommended dose of rFVIIa is 90 mcg/kg administered over 2 to 5 minutes. Because of its short half-life, additional doses must be given every 2 to 4 hours until hemostasis is achieved. The dose for patients with factor VII-deficiency is 25 mcg/kg.

rFVIIa has many advantages. It is completely synthetic, decreasing the risks of infectious complications; it can be quickly reconstituted from powder, eliminating the time needed for thawing and procurement of products from the blood bank; and it is dissolved in a small volume, minimizing excessive volume load, electrolyte perturbations, and the latency between institution of treatment and correction of the hemostatic defect. rFVIIa has limitations as well. Its efficacy depends on the presence of the other clotting factors. In the setting of a massive transfusion, factor VIIa is not the only clotting factor that is deficient. Most anecdotal reports concerning the use of rFVIIa in massive transfusion-associated bleeding are in the context of earlier administration of FFP. rFVIIa has a short half-life, necessitating frequent dosing. In the context of liver failure or dilutional coagulopathy, dosing is required every 12 hours. In the presence of inhibitors to factors VIII or IX, doses must be given every 2 to 4 hours until hemostasis is maintained.

The risk of rFVIIa's thrombotic complications in hemophiliacs appears to be low. In contrast, most of the rFVIIa's thrombotic complications are in the context of its "off-label usage" and are associated with serious morbidity and mortality (O'Connell et al., 2006; Abshire, 2008; Abshire and Kenet, 2008).

Although potentially promising, at the present time the role of rFVIIa in the treatment of perioperative bleeding should be restricted to that of rescue therapy for the intractably bleeding patient unresponsive to conventional transfusion treatment. Specifically, rFVIIa should be used cautiously in patients at risk for catastrophic thrombotic complications (e.g., as children with small-vessel anastomoses or palliative cardiac shunts) until further experience is garnered. After randomized, controlled trials have been completed to better define the thrombotic and pulmonary risks, rFVIIa could become a first-line agent for many of the coagulopathies that plague patients in the perioperative period (Alten et al., 2009).

Hemostatic Formulary

The blood-based components available for treatment of the bleeding patient, their constituents, and indications for their use are summarized in Table 36-25.

The American Society of Anesthesiologists Task Force on Blood Component Therapy (2006) recommended that the triggers for treatment of the patient who is at risk for bleeding be multiple and not depend on a single factor. Often, the critically ill child may require an emergent invasive procedure before a complete hemostatic profile has been determined. In these circumstances, bleeding from puncture sites or general oozing in the surgical field may necessitate empirical treatment with FFP. Generally accepted treatment triggers for component therapy are listed in Box 36-13.

Platelets

Each unit of platelets contains 5.5 to 7.5×10^{10} platelets diluted in 50 mL of plasma. An apheresis platelet unit contains more than 3×10^{11} platelets in 250 to 300 mL of plasma. Normally, one third of all transfused platelets undergo splenic sequestration.

Box 36-13 Recommendations for Blood-Component Therapy

PLATELETS
Less than 50 k for acute bleeding
Less than 100 k for intracranial, subarachnoid, or extracorporeal circulation procedures

FFP
aPTT more than 1.5 times normal
PT more than 1.5 times normal

FIBRINOGEN
Less than 100 mg/dL

In nonsurgical patients with platelet counts of more than 20,000/mcL, spontaneous bleeding is uncommon. ASA guidelines suggest that patients receive transfusions for platelet counts less than 50,000/mcL and that platelet transfusions be considered for platelet counts between 50,000 and 100,000/mcL, taking into consideration the risks and consequences of postoperative bleeding from the surgical site. A platelet count of 50,000/mcL is considered sufficient for spinal anesthesia, 80,000/mcL for epidural anesthesia, and 100,000/mcL is recommended for neurosurgical or posterior ophthalmologic procedures (Rochon and Shore-Lesserson, 2006). Because of the risk of intracranial hemorrhage, sick premature infants are transfused when their platelet counts fall below 50,000/mcL (Roseff et al., 2006). If concurrent platelet dysfunction exists, the threshold for platelet transfusion should be lowered. The ideal platelet dose is between 0.07 and 0.15×10^{11} platelets/kg, which is approximately 10 mL/kg. A dose of 5 to 10 mL/kg or 1 unit/10 kg increases the platelet count by 50,000/mcL.

Platelets are much more likely than RBCs to cause bacterial sepsis, because they are stored at room temperature for up to 5 days and potentially have a higher bacterial load. The reported incidence of bacterial contamination of platelet products is 1 case per 2000 units (Blajchman et al., 2005). Storing the

TABLE 36-25. Hemostatic Formulary

Component	Contents	Indications	Dose	Outcome
Whole blood	Hematocrit: 30%-40% Most clotting factors ↓ FV, FVIII No platelets	Neonatal surgery Massive transfusion		
Fresh frozen plasma, 225 mL	All clotting factors 2 mg/mL fibrinogen	Hemodilution Liver failure DIC Warfarin toxicity FXI deficiency	10-15 mL/kg (max, 2 units) 5-8 mL/kg	↑15% in factors ↑40 mg/dL fibrinogen
Platelets, 50 mL	>5.5 × 10¹⁰ 50 mL plasma	Thrombocytopenia Platelet dysfunction	1 unit/10 kg (max, 10 units)	↑50,000
Cryoprecipitate, 25 mL*	Fibrinogen >150 mg Factor VIII >80 units von Willebrand factor >80 units FXIII >80 units	↓ fibrinogen Hemophilia A vWD	1-2 units/10 kg (max, 10 units)	↑ 60-100 mg/dL fibrinogen

*Cryo units = [(desired fibrinogen - initial fibrinogen) × plasma volume (dL)]/150 mg fibrinogen/unit.
DIC, Disseminated intravascular coagulation; *vWD*, von Willebrand disease.

platelets in galactose-containing solution has been found to preserve platelet function despite chilling, and this approach may reduce the risk of bacterial contamination (Jhang and Spitalnik, 2005; Hornsey et al., 2008).

Platelet transfusions can also be associated with the development of pulmonary microvascular injury, called *transfusion-related acute lung injury (TRALI)*. TRALI is clinically similar to acute respiratory distress syndrome (discussed in a later section). Within 6 hours of receiving a plasma-containing product, fever, tachypnea, dyspnea, progressive hypoxemia, radiographic evidence of pulmonary edema, and hypotension occur. The prevalence of TRALI in patients who have received platelet transfusions is estimated to be 3 per 1000 units of concentrate (Silliman, 1999).

Fresh Frozen Plasma

FFP contains 250 mL of plasma and 500 mg of fibrinogen in a citrate anticoagulant. One unit of FFP has a concentration of coagulation factors similar to that of 4 to 5 units of platelet concentrates, 1 apheresis unit of platelets, and 1 unit of fresh whole blood. FFP, 1 mL/kg, raises most factor levels by approximately 1%. After a dose of 10 to 15 mL/kg of FFP, plasma clotting factors rise approximately 15%, and the fibrinogen rises by 40 mg/dL. However, FFP contains only 0.6% of factor VIII.

FFP use is indicated for treatment of microvascular bleeding in patients who have had massive transfusions, for documented coagulopathy (PT more than 1.5 times normal) in patients who have had massive transfusions, for urgent reversal of anticoagulant therapy, and for active bleeding in patients with history or course suggestive of an inherited or acquired coagulopathy for which specific factor concentrates are not available.

Cryoprecipitate

Cryoprecipitate is the most practical source for fibrinogen replacement. Each unit contains approximately 200 mg of fibrinogen, as well as more than 80 units of factor VIII, vWF, fibronectin, and factor XIII. Achieving fibrinogen plasma levels of 80 to 100 mg/dL and maintaining this level above 50 to 60 mg/dL usually controls hemorrhagic symptoms. To raise the fibrinogen level 100 mg/dL, 0.17 unit of cryoprecipitate per 1 kg of body weight should be infused. Fibrinogen has a long half-life; therefore, replacement therapy can be given at intervals of 3 to 4 days.

Cryoprecipitate is indicated for several uses:

- For prophylactic use in patients with congenital fibrinogen deficiencies, vWD unresponsive to DDAVP, and factor VIII deficiency when factor VIII concentrate is not available;
- In bleeding patients with vWD or factor VIII deficiency when factor VIII concentrate is not available;
- For consumptive coagulopathies when the fibrinogen level is less than 80 to 100 mg/dL; and
- For microvascular bleeding in the patient who has had massive transfusion when hypofibrinogenemia cannot be immediately documented.

Factors V, X, XI, and XIII

The only current source of factor V is FFP. Normal hemostasis is achieved with levels higher than 25 units/dL. These levels can be achieved with a loading dose of 20 mL/kg of FFP followed by infusions of 6 mL/kg every 12 hours. Factor V is very labile in FFP, and recently donated FFP should be used. FFP (1 mL/kg) increases the plasma level of factor X by 1 unit/dL. FFP (1 mL/kg) increases circulating factor XI by 1.5 unit/dL. Hemostatic levels of factor XIII are 2 to 3 units/dL. FFP (5 to 10 mL/kg) is adequate to achieve therapeutic levels. Cryoprecipitate may also be used. One bag of cryoprecipitate contains 75 units of factor XIII.

Complications of Blood Product Administration

Citrate Intoxication

Citrate, when infused rapidly as the storage solution of blood products, can cause a temporary reduction in ionized calcium levels. FFP has considerably more citrate than do RBCs in citrate-phosphate-dextrose-adenine (CPDA-1). The signs of citrate intoxication include hypotension, narrow pulse pressure, flattening of the instantaneous slope of the arterial catheter tracing, elevated end-diastolic pressures, prolongation of the QT interval, widening of the QRS complexes, and flattening of the T waves. Hypocalcemia is directly related to the rate of citrate administration and is unlikely to occur unless transfusions exceed 1 mL/kg per minute. Impaired perfusion or liver dysfunction lowers this threshold for potential hypocalcemia. Slow calcium administration during rapid or large-volume blood product administration can avert this induced hypocalcemia.

Transfusion-Related Acute Lung Injury (TRALI)

TRALI usually manifests as bilateral pulmonary infiltrates within 4 hours of transfusion. The clinical picture consists of acute respiratory distress syndrome, with hypoxia, hypotension, and bilateral pulmonary edema, leading to radiographic opacification and fever within 2 to 6 hours of transfusion (Roseff et al., 2006). Although in most patients, TRALI symptoms usually resolve within 48 to 72 hours, a 5% to 10% mortality rate is associated. TRALI has two proposed mechanisms. In the first mechanism, leukocytes from transfused blood products interact with antibodies in the pulmonary microvasculature, leading to endothelial injury and alveolar exudation. Antileukocyte antibodies are found in this group of patients (Roseff et al., 2006). The other proposed mechanism involves clinical settings such as trauma, sepsis, or massive transfusion, in which cytokine production partially activates endogenous neutrophils. These neutrophils become adherent to the pulmonary microvascular endothelium. On exposure to the lipids contained in transfused blood products, neutrophil activation becomes complete and endothelial damage results in the clinical picture of TRALI (Silliman, 1999). The care of the patient with TRALI is supportive; the role of diuretics and steroids is unproven.

Transfusion-Associated Graft-Versus-Host Disease

Transfusion-associated GHVD (TA-GVHD) results when immunocompetent donor lymphocytes are transfused into an immunodeficient host patient who is unable to destroy them. These transfused lymphocytes react with host antigens, producing fever, skin rash, pancytopenia, diarrhea, and abnormal liver function test results. TA-GVHD can occur 4 to 30 days after transfusion (Alter and Klein, 2008). The pancytopenia is profound, and mortality approaches 100% (Slichter, 2007). Median survival is only 21 days after transfusion. Patients who are at high risk for developing TA-GVHD include neonates; patients with congenital immunodeficiency, leukemia, or lymphoma; and those who have received intensive chemotherapy and bone marrow or solid-organ transplants. Infants and children with severe combined immunodeficiency syndrome (SCIDS) are of most concern, in part because SCIDS is often unrecognized at birth or in early infancy. Although many children with SCIDS are diagnosed by 6 months of age, children have been diagnosed with SCIDS up until 2 years of age. Children with the DiGeorge syndrome (22q11 deletion) and those with conotruncal defects or tetralogy of Fallot in whom immunodeficiency has not been excluded should be considered at risk for TA-GVHD as well. Patients with HIV do not appear to be at increased risk for TA-GVHD. The absence of TA-GVHD in HIV patients may underscore the key role of the recipient's CD4 cells (depleted early in the course of HIV infection) in the pathogenesis of TA-GVHD (Alter and Klein, 2008).

TA-GVHD can occur in patients who do not have an immunodeficiency. Patients who receive products from a donor who is homozygous for a shared haplotype are also at risk for TA-GVHD. The chance of receiving haplotype-homozygous blood from an unrelated donor varies among countries, ranging from 1 in 874 in Japan to 1 in 7147 whites in the United States, and 1 in 16,835 in France. Trauma patients with no known risk factors for TA-GVHD had evidence of microchimerism for as long as 1.5 years after transfusion (Lee et al., 1999). The spectrum of patients who are at potential risk for TA-GVHD is likely to increase with the use of immunosuppressive regimens in the treatment of autoimmune and inflammatory bowel diseases.

The prevention of TA-GVHD lies in attenuation of donor lymphocyte reactivity. The only method approved by the FDA is irradiation (Alter and Klein, 2008). Irradiation damages the DNA in donated T cells, which precludes their proliferation and prevents the development of TA-GVHD (Shlomchik et al., 1999). Most blood centers rely on a nominal dose of 25 Gy. Patients at risk for TA-GVHD should receive only irradiated RBCs, platelets, and granulocytes. A summary of situations in which irradiated blood products should be administered is presented in Box 36-14.

Box 36-14 Indications for Irradiated Blood Products

Intrauterine transfusions
Patients younger than 2 years old
Transplantation
　Bone marrow transplantation
　Organ transplantation
Oncologic conditions
　Lymphoma
　Neuroblastoma
　Glioblastoma
　Rhabdomyosarcoma
Immunodeficiency
　Congenital immunodeficiency
　● Wiskott-Aldrich syndrome
　● Conotruncal abnormalities
　Acquired immunodeficiency
　● HIV infection
　● Patients receiving immunosuppressive drugs
Recipients of blood products from first-degree relatives

To avoid the risk of TA-GVHD in patients with late-presenting SCIDS, many blood banks routinely irradiate all cellular blood products given to young children. At present, no consensus exists as to the cut-off age for this practice (Roseff et al., 2006). The Children's Hospital of Philadelphia irradiates products for children who are younger than 3 months of age, whereas Johns Hopkins Hospital irradiates all products for recipients younger than 6 years of age. Blood components donated from first- or second-degree relatives should be irradiated because of the possibility of HLA haplotype homozygosity. FFP and cryoprecipitate need not be irradiated, because most authorities feel that the freezing and thawing process destroys any donor T cells (Luban, 2002).

Hyperkalemia

Acute hemodynamic decompensation after red cell transfusions should be considered hyperkalemia, until proved otherwise. Large volumes (more than 25 mL/kg) of stored red cells given rapidly to infants have been associated with hyperkalemic cardiac arrest (Smith et al., 2008). The combination of perturbations of calcium and potassium concentrations in the context of central venous blood administration may be sufficient to produce hyperkalemic dysrhythmia (Eder, 2002).

MISCELLANEOUS PROBLEMS

Acquired Immunodeficiency Syndrome

Epidemiology

The epidemic of HIV and acquired immunodeficiency syndrome (AIDS) has had an enormous deleterious impact on worldwide health, and children have not been spared. In 2007, the World Health Organization (WHO) estimated that 33 million people worldwide were infected with HIV. Of this number, 2 million were younger than 15 years of age (WHO, 2007). Most of those infected with HIV live outside of the United States. The Centers for Disease Control and Prevention (CDC) estimated that 1 to 1.2 million people in the United States were infected with HIV in 2003; during 2006, the most recent year with complete statistics, approximately 50,000 new HIV infections were reported (Glynn, 2005; CDC, 2007a; Hall et al., 2008). The incidence of HIV infection varies by both ethnicity and geography. In the United States, AIDS is seen more often in Hispanic and African American children than in Caucasians. In 2008, the HIV/AIDS surveillance system of the CDC reported that 49% of children with AIDS were African American, 18% were Hispanic, and 30% were Caucasian. Most cases in the United States have been reported in the Northeast (23%) and South (25%), primarily in the large metropolitan areas (CDC, 2007a).

Transmission of HIV can occur through parenteral exposure to blood, sexual contact, or through vertical transmission from mother to child. In the United States, nearly all HIV infections in children younger than 13 years are the result of vertical transmission. Approximately 6000 to 7000 children are born to HIV-positive mothers annually in the United States. Women of childbearing age comprise one of the fastest growing groups with HIV infection in the United States, accounting for more than 27% of adult HIV cases reported (CDC, 2007b). Although transmission of HIV from mother to child can occur before, during, or after delivery, the highest percentage of HIV-infected children acquire the virus during delivery, most likely through exposure to infected blood and secretions during delivery. Chance of transmission is increased with preterm birth, low birth weight, low maternal CD4 counts, and IV drug use during pregnancy. With cesarean section and prenatal, intrapartum, and neonatal antiretroviral treatment, vertical transmission in the United States has been decreased dramatically (AAP Committee on Pediatric AIDS, 2000; CDC, 2007b). In the United States, postpartum transmission via breastfeeding is the least common mode of perinatal transmission; however, it is quite common in developing countries. The number of perinatally acquired HIV cases in the United States peaked in 1992 at nearly 1000 and decreased to fewer than 100 in 2006 (Mofenson et al., 2006). This decline is thought to be related to more widespread use of the Public Health Service guidelines for universal counseling and voluntary HIV testing of pregnant women and more effective use of retroviral therapy in these patients (AAP Committee on Pediatric AIDS, 2000).

Although adolescents account for a small percentage of AIDS cases, the number of adolescents with AIDS is growing rapidly. In 2007, nearly 2000 young people in the United States were diagnosed with HIV infection or AIDS (CDC, 2007a). Transmission of HIV through contaminated blood or blood products accounts for approximately 3% of cases of HIV infection in the United States. Screening of blood products for HIV began in the United States in 1985, and since then the risk of transmission has decreased dramatically. Sexual transmission of HIV, although relatively rare in pediatrics, is a growing problem (Romero et al., 2007). The age at which HIV infection is diagnosed in children varies with the mode of transmission. Children who were infected by transfusion of contaminated blood or blood products, primarily between the years of 1978 and 1985, are now adults (Grubman et al., 1995). Children who

acquired the disease during birth can be diagnosed as infants, with detection of the virus as early as 1 week of age. The viral load increases with time, and the virus is detectable in the peripheral blood of almost all infected infants by the age of 4 months. HIV has three patterns of progression. Newborns who were infected during gestation develop symptoms within the first few months of life and have detectable virus early in life. Without treatment, they often die before their first birthday. Most newborns with HIV have acquired the infection during birth, and these infants have a much slower progression of disease. The viral load increases in the first few months of life and then declines over the subsequent 2 years. A small percentage of infants with perinatal infection survive for an extended time with minimal progression of the disease.

Children infected with HIV have generally the same immunologic manifestations as adults. Because infants and children have a lymphocytosis at baseline, true lymphopenia is relatively rare. However, relentless depletion of CD4 lymphocytes occurs, resulting in the development of opportunistic infections. Infants and children with HIV/AIDS have many opportunistic infections. The most common serious infections are pneumonia, bacteremia, and sepsis, and nearly every organ system may be affected. The CDC has classified HIV in young children based on the presence of signs and symptoms, the state of immunodeficiency, and the immunologic category of the disease (Caldwell et al., 1994). The current recommendations for initiation of antiretroviral therapy in infants, children, and adolescents were summarized in 2008 by the Working Group on Antiretroviral Therapy and Medical Management of HIV Infected Children, and these guidelines can be found on the CDC website and in Box 36-15 (Guidelines for Use of Antiretroviral Agents, 2009).

Box 36-15 Guidelines for the Use of Antiretroviral Agents in Pediatric HIV Infection

Preferred Regimen
Children 3 years and older: two NRTIs plus efavirenz*
Children younger than 3 years old or who cannot swallow capsules: two NRTIs plus nevirapine

Alternative
Two NRTIs plus nevirapine[1] (children 3 years and older)

PROTEASE INHIBITOR-BASED REGIMENS
Preferred Regimen
Two NRTIs plus lopinavir/ritonavir

Alternative
Two NRTIs plus atazanavir plus low-dose ritonavir (children older than 6 years)
Two NRTIs plus fosamprenavir plus low-dose ritonavir (children older than 6 years)
Two NRTIs plus nelfinavir (children older than 2 years)

USE IN SPECIAL CIRCUMSTANCES
Two NRTIs plus atazanavir unboosted (for treatment-naïve adolescents older than 13 years and weighing more than 39 kg)

Two NRTIs plus fosamprenavir unboosted (children older than 2 years)
Two NRTIs plus saquinavir plus low-dose ritonavir only in post-pubertal adolescents who weigh enough to receive adult doses
Zidovudine plus lamivudine plus abacavir

TWO NRTI BACKBONE OPTIONS
Preferred
Abacavir plus (lamivudine or emtricitabine)
Didanosine plus emtricitabine
Tenofovir plus (lamivudine or emtricitabine) (for Tanner stage 4 or postpubertal adolescents only)
Zidovudine plus (lamivudine or emtricitabine)

Alternative
Abacavir plus zidovudine
Zidovudine plus didanosine

Use In Special Circumstances
Stavudine plus (lamivudine or emtricitabine)

From Working Group on Antiretroviral Therapy and Medical Management of HIV-Infected Children, 2009: *Guidelines for the use of antiretroviral agents in pediatric HIV infection*. Available at http://aidsinfo.nih.gov/ContentFiles/PediatricGuidelines.pdf; accessed May 8, 2009.
*Efavirenz (a nonnucleoside reverse transcriptase inhibitor [NNRTI]) is currently available only in capsule form and should only be used in children aged 3 years and older who weigh 10 kg or more; nevirapine would be the preferred NNRTI for children aged younger than 3 years or who require a liquid formulation. Unless adequate contraception can be assured, efavirenz-based therapy is not recommended for adolescent females who are sexually active and may become pregnant.
PI, Protease inhibitor; *NRTI:* nucleoside/nucleotide reverse transcriptase inhibitors.

Clinical Presentation

In the perioperative environment, caring for children with HIV/AIDS is focused on two major considerations: effects of this systemic infection and its treatment on a child's readiness for anesthesia and surgery, and protection of health care workers from acquiring infection as a result of exposure to the blood or secretions of these children.

As many as 80% of children with HIV develop lung disease (McSherry, 1996). Pulmonary function is compromised by bacterial and viral infections, but in addition many children with AIDS also develop lipoid interstitial pneumonia (LIP) (Rubinstein et al., 1986). The incidence of LIP in children infected by HIV is 20% to 30%. Clinical characteristics of this condition include tachypnea, wheezing and cough, hypoxemia, and even clubbing. This condition presents with bilateral infiltrates. Severely affected children may have bronchiectasis and lung cysts. The most common opportunistic infection responsible for pneumonia in children with HIV infection is *Pneumocystis carinii* pneumonia. Most people are infected with this common organism in childhood, but disease is caused only in immunocompromised individuals. The peak incidence of this infection occurs in children who are younger than 1 year of age. *P. carinii* is often characterized by the acute onset of fever, hypoxemia, and respiratory distress, but a disease with a more desultory onset is also seen (Simonds et al., 1998). Infection with respiratory viruses in children with HIV is common and often more severe in these patients. In children with AIDS, infections with RSV, parainfluenza, and influenza viruses are more likely to be symptomatic, and infections with adenovirus or measles may lead to serious morbidity (Englund et al., 1998).

Children with LIP or infectious pneumonia may come to the operating room for bronchoscopy and bronchoalveolar lavage for diagnosis (Birriel et al., 1991). They are often hypoxemic and in respiratory distress before the procedure. These cases are often quite challenging, because the diagnosis must be established to prescribe the correct therapy; the procedure cannot be delayed until the child's condition improves. Children who are infected in the perinatal period with HIV often have involvement of the CNS, although opportunistic infections of the CNS are uncommon. In children infected during birth, encephalopathy is seen in 10% of those infected with HIV and in 23% of those diagnosed with AIDS (Navarro and Hanson, 1996). In toddlers, the presentation is that of a progressive encephalopathy with loss of developmental milestones or arrest of development. CNS pathology includes low brain weight, acquired microcephaly, inflammatory infiltrates, and calcific vasculopathy of the basal ganglia vessels. As the encephalopathy progresses, loss of fine and gross motor skills and language skills may occur and behavioral problems may develop. In older children, the clinical picture often becomes one of a static encephalopathy (Bowers et al., 1998). Seizures and focal neurologic signs are unusual and their presence should prompt a search for other causes, such as infection, stroke, or a tumor. It is important to document signs and symptoms of encephalopathy or other CNS involvement in the preoperative evaluation.

Approximately 10% to 20% of children with HIV infections have clinically significant cardiovascular involvement. Careful echocardiographic and electrocardiographic evaluations of children with HIV infections may uncover subtle abnormalities in a much higher percentage of patients (Lipshultz et al., 1989). Common abnormalities include resting sinus tachycardia, sinus dysrhythmias, and ventricular hypertrophy. Echocardiography studies of children with HIV infection have demonstrated both left ventricular diastolic and systolic dysfunction. One center reported that 10% of children with HIV required temporary treatment for congestive heart failure, generally during an intercurrent illness (Luginbuhl et al., 1993; Keesler et al., 2001). Hepatosplenomegaly and a gallop are indications of congestive heart failure in these patients, and medical therapy has been generally effective in reversing the symptoms. In children with advanced AIDS, hemodynamic instability may occur (Evenhouse et al., 1987; Stewart et al., 1989).

Children with AIDS often have lowered counts of all the formed elements of the blood. Poor bone marrow function in these patients may be caused by the disease itself, by poor nutrition, or as a side effect of the medications used to treat the disease. As with many chronic conditions, the anemia seen in AIDS patients is often normochromic and normocytic, with low reticulocyte counts. In the preoperative evaluation of these children, other causes for anemia, such as occult bleeding, should be ruled out (Russell and Nedeljkovic, 2001). Treatment of anemia in HIV-infected children should address the cause and should include administration of erythropoietin (rh-EPO). Perioperative transfusion of RBCs should be undertaken only to provide a minimum level of oxygen delivery and after careful consideration of the possible deleterious effects in patients with HIV/AIDS (Hillyer et al., 1999). Only cytomegalovirus-negative, leukocyte-depleted RBCs should be used. Patients with HIV have a high prevalence of thrombocytopenia. The cause is sometimes difficult to determine, but both impaired production and increased destruction have been found in patients with AIDS. In addition, a lupus-type anticoagulant was found in 20% of AIDS patients undergoing routine coagulation testing (Cohen et al., 1986).

GI and nutritional problems can be common and difficult to treat in children with AIDS. Infections of the GI tract cause major morbidity and can be quite severe (Doyle and Pickering, 1990). Oral infections with *Candida* or ulcerative gingivitis are seen in children infected with HIV. Bacterial, viral, or fungal infections may cause diarrhea. With recurrent or chronic diarrhea, children develop malnutrition and failure to thrive. Growth failure in these children can result from malabsorption, poor nutrient intake, and possibly altered energy use. Hepatosplenomegaly is seen in up to 80% to 90% of children infected with HIV and is associated elevated serum aminotransferases. Coinfection with hepatitis B or C virus is more prevalent in children with HIV than in the general population. Pancreatitis can occur, usually as a complication of the drug therapy used to treat HIV or one of the opportunistic infections. Other clinical signs of HIV infection include various skin rashes such as eczema or seborrhea and manifestations of renal dysfunction such as proteinuria, hematuria, hypoalbuminemia, and edema.

Anesthesia and Procedures

Children with HIV/AIDS often undergo diagnostic bronchoscopies with bronchoalveolar lavage or biopsy, diagnostic upper and lower endoscopies, placement of gastrostomy tubes for nutritional support, and placement of central venous catheters (Birriel et al., 1991). In addition to procedures specific to their underlying systemic viral infection, these children can require anesthesia for any other routine or emergent surgical or diagnostic procedure such as myringotomy or herniorraphy. In the evaluation of these children before anesthesia, the effects of the infection on organ systems as outlined above should be evaluated. The anesthesiologist should be aware of medications taken, their effects, and their side effects. In addition to medications specific for the treatment of AIDS, these children are often being treated with antibiotics and corticosteroids. Pulmonary insufficiency is often seen in patients with AIDS and despite meticulous management during the procedure, clinical deterioration commonly occurs after the procedure. During the preanesthetic visit, the anesthesiologist should, when indicated, discuss the possibility of postoperative intubation and ventilation. In an advanced case in which a do not resuscitate (DNR) order or other advance directive is in place, the anesthesiologist should discuss these thoroughly with the child and family (Truog et al., 1999). It may be that the person caring for the child is not a biological parent, necessitating additional administrative steps in the informed consent process.

Although the specific agents and techniques chosen for a case depend on the particular child and situation, the physician should consider several points when making those choices. CNS involvement is relatively common; therefore, CNS depressants such as barbiturates, benzodiazepines, and opioids should be carefully titrated. If liver or renal dysfunction is present, drug metabolism and elimination are impaired. Attention to sterile technique, often not a priority among anesthesiologists, is paramount in these children who are severely immunocompromised.

Pain Management

Children with HIV/AIDS may have many causes for pain and suffering independent of postoperative pain (Box 36-16) (Nedeljkovic, 2001). The anesthesiologist or pediatric pain specialist should be prepared to participate in the management of both the acute and chronic pain that afflicts these children. In one report, 59% of children with HIV described pain as having an important impact on their lives (Hirschfeld et al., 1996; Yaster and Schecter, 1996). The clinical presentations of pain and suffering in children with AIDS are varied, and the pharmacologic and nonpharmacologic treatments that may be employed are broad (Box 36-16) (Gaughan et al., 2002). Assessment is often difficult because of the nature of the discomfort and the difficulty in communicating with children who are afflicted with encephalopathy.

Box 36-16 Common Pain Syndromes in HIV/AIDS Patients

GASTROINTESTINAL TRACT
Visceral pain
Esophagitis
Pancreatitis
Sclerosing cholangitis

NERVOUS SYSTEM
Headache
Peripheral neuropathies

MUSCULOSKELETAL SYSTEM
Arthralgia
Myositis

HIV/AIDS and Health Care Providers

Individuals who care for HIV-infected children must take prudent steps to prevent transmission (CDC, 2002). Although HIV has been isolated from saliva, the titer is generally low. Studies of hundreds of household contacts have confirmed that the risk of transmission from casual contact is nearly zero. It is therefore unlikely that operating-room personnel would contract HIV from passive contact with an child who is HIV positive. Exposures that place these health care personnel at risk for contracting HIV include needlesticks, cuts with sharp objects, and contact of mucous membranes or nonintact skin with blood, tissue, or other body fluids. The greatest risk of contracting HIV for health care workers is via needlestick with a contaminated needle. Hollow-bore needles (those used to administer medications) give a much larger inoculum of blood and infectious agent than do solid needles. Estimates of the average risk for various types of exposure are 0.3% to 0.4% after percutaneous exposure (needlestick or laceration), 0.09% after mucous membrane exposure, and less than 0.09% after exposure to nonintact skin.

After parenteral exposure to HIV, specific steps should be taken; within existing state and local laws, evaluation of the HIV status of the source of the exposure, postexposure prophylaxis, postexposure treatment, and follow-up care should occur. A health care worker who has a parenteral exposure to blood or body fluids from a child known or suspected to be infected with HIV should have the wound thoroughly washed and then irrigated with saline. Exposed mucous membranes should be thoroughly irrigated with saline. The exposure should be immediately reported to the institutional employee health service or to the "stick" team if one exists. In addition, the patient should be tested for hepatitis, which may coexist with HIV. If the source is known to be HIV positive, details of the infection (such as CD4+ count, viral-load tests, and the source's current treatment) should be gathered quickly, so that the medications for postexposure prophylaxis can be chosen. Postexposure prophylaxis should be undertaken as close to immediately after parenteral exposure to the blood or body fluid from a child suspected of having or known to have HIV (Panlilio et al., 2005). In situations in which the HIV status is not known, prophylaxis should be given on a case-by-case basis. In most cases, administration of two antiretroviral drugs is indicated. The addition of a third medication should be considered in cases with increased risk for transmission. Before prophylaxis is begun, the employee should be tested to document HIV status, with subsequent testing at 6 and 12 weeks.

A retrospective study undertaken by the CDC to determine the rate of seroconversion of health care workers in England, France, and the United States reported three conclusions: exposure to a large quantity of blood was associated with a higher rate of seroconversion; seroconversion was more likely when the exposure was from a patient in the terminal stages of AIDS; and a 79% decrease in seroconversion occurred when zidovudine was begun after exposure. Anesthesiologists should be familiar with the needlestick policies of their institutions and be prepared to follow them and advise others of the policies in the event of an exposure. Universal precautions, as recommended by the CDC, should be followed by all health care workers who have direct patient contact or exposure to a patient's body fluids (CDC, 2009).

Latex Allergy

The first published report in an American medical journal about an allergy to rubber gloves appeared in 1933 (Downing, 1933). Sporadic reports followed until the late 1980s and early 1990s, when reporting of allergic reactions to latex rose sharply. This increase is thought to have been the result of increased exposure of health care workers and patients after the publication of the Universal Precautions Guidelines by the CDC in 1987 (CDC, 1987). After 1987 the use of surgical gloves in the United States increased by a factor of 25, from 800 million to 20 billion annually. Allergic reactions to latex were first reported by pediatric anesthesiologists in 1991, before circulation of the Medical Alert (in 1991) by the FDA that warned health care workers of this emerging problem (Holzman, 1993). Latex allergy is a significant problem in health care. As of 1997, through its mandatory reporting mechanism, the FDA had received more than 2300 reports of allergic reactions involving medical products that contain latex, with 225 cases of anaphylaxis, 53 cardiac arrests, and 17 deaths. Individuals at high risk for latex allergy have certain common characteristics, which are listed in Box 36-17 (Hochleitner et al., 2001; Randolph, 2001; Hourihane et al., 2002).

Many children who have had latex reactions in the operating room have had spina bifida or urinary tract anomalies (Cremer et al., 2007). These two groups, not surprisingly, undergo multiple surgical procedures, making it difficult to ascertain whether the high prevalence of latex allergy is simply the result of repeated exposure or to an immunologic response associated with specific conditions. Reactions to latex have been divided into three types: irritant contact dermatitis, type IV hypersensitivity (skin reactions similar to poison ivy), and type I, or IgE-mediated, hypersensitivity. Type I hypersensitivity is by far the more severe reaction. All 17 of the above-mentioned deaths reported to the FDA were the result of type I hypersensitivity. This type of response to latex has been reported in many clinical settings, including intraabdominal surgery, genitourinary surgery, and dental procedures. Some have reported reactions associated with airborne exposure as a result of being in the vicinity of someone donning latex-containing gloves. Manifestations of type I hypersensitivity are listed in Box 36-18.

Box 36-17 Individuals at High Risk for Latex Allergy

Patients who have undergone multiple surgical procedures
Patients with spina bifida (meningomyelocele)
Health care personnel
Individuals with a history of atopy
Individuals with a history of allergy to tropical fruits

Box 36-18 Manifestations of Type I (IgE-Mediated) Hypersensitivity

Hives, urticaria, red eyes, angioedema of the eyelids
Nasal congestion
GI cramping, nausea, diarrhea
Headache, anxiety
Shortness of breath, bronchospasm, tachycardia, hypotension, anaphylaxis

Generally, intraoperative type I hypersensitivity does not occur immediately at the beginning of a surgical procedure, but rather after exposure of the peritoneum or other mucous membranes to latex. The presentation includes bronchospasm, hypoxemia, hypotension, and tachycardia. Skin manifestations, such as urticaria or flushing, may also occur. In a series of patients reported by Holzman, the mean SpO_2 fell from 100% to 92% (Holzman, 1993). Bronchospasm and hypotension are difficult to treat, even with IV epinephrine, and the manifestations may persist until the exposure is stopped.

Treatment of Intraoperative Anaphylaxis

As increasingly more latex-free medical equipment is manufactured, it is important to remain vigilant for the possibility of inadvertent latex exposure with an at-risk patient. Delay in diagnosis of an episode of latex anaphylaxis only makes treatment more difficult and likely continues exposure to the offending allergen. The mainstays of treatment are stopping the latex exposure and resuscitation. All latex must be removed from the surgical field, as well as those materials for which the latex content is unknown, and the procedure must be ended as rapidly as possible. If blood or antibiotics are being administered, this administration should be stopped. Consideration should be given to evaluating the patient for a transfusion reaction if the symptoms and signs of anaphylaxis began during blood administration. Resuscitation efforts are directed toward stabilization of vital signs and reversal of the pathophysiology of anaphylaxis. Because these reactions often occur during intraabdominal surgery, patients are often already intubated when the reaction occurs. If the patient is not intubated, strong consideration should be given to intubation. If possible, based on the progress of the surgery and the patient's vital signs, administration of anesthetic agents should be stopped. IV fluid and epinephrine doses (starting at 0.001 mg/kg) should be given to maintain blood pressure in the normal range for the patient, a Foley catheter should be placed, invasive hemodynamic monitoring should be instituted, and if bronchospasm is present, inhaled bronchodilators should be given through the ETT. If repeated doses of epinephrine are needed, as often occurs, an infusion of 0.05 to 0.1 mcg/kg per minute should be started. The patient may require treatment as outlined above for several hours, and admission to the intensive care should be arranged. A *Latex Alert* sign should be placed outside of the patient's operating room and in the intensive care unit, and the condition should be noted prominently in and on the medical record. Once the vital signs are stable, secondary treatments can be instituted, including administration of diphenhydramine, ranitidine, and hydrocortisone. Further therapy depends on the patient's condition as the resuscitation progresses.

Diagnosis of Latex Anaphylaxis

After the patient is stabilized, tests to document the diagnosis of latex allergy can be performed. Although many tests are available to confirm diagnosis, a universally accepted serum test for the diagnosis of a type I hypersensitivity reaction is not available. An elevated level of serum tryptase occurs within the first 4 hours in patients who have experienced anaphylaxis with mast-cell degranulation, regardless of the cause. The radioallergosorbent (RAST) or enzymeallergosorbent (EAST) tests are available for specific proteins. Blood should be sent for testing, with the realization that a specific individual may or may not react to that particular protein. To determine type I hypersensitivity to latex, current practice is to use a skin prick test that employs antigen extracted from latex similar to that in medical products. Testing materials and methods have been standardized for some time (Hamilton et al., 2002). The patient should be referred to a specialist in allergy and immunology for complete evaluation. Skin testing should be delayed for 4 to 6 weeks after the episode of anaphylaxis to allow time for cellular inflammatory mediators released during the reaction to be reconstituted (Dakin and Yentis, 1998). Testing before allowing time for these proteins to be reconstituted increases the risk for false-negative results. This testing must be performed carefully and in the proper setting; severe reactions have been seen in sensitive individuals even with the minimal exposure that occurs with this test (Kelly et al., 1993). Once the diagnosis is confirmed, patients should be encouraged to wear a medical alert bracelet.

Recommendations

Avoidance of latex exposure is by far the best safeguard against the risks associated with latex sensitivity (Holzman, 1997). Although operating rooms nationwide are working toward becoming completely free of latex, 100% compliance has not yet been achieved. Avoidance, therefore, depends on recognizing those at risk for latex sensitivity (Box 36-17). Most pediatric anesthesiologists in the United States avoid latex exposure from birth in patients with meningomyelocele because of the high prevalence of sensitivity. In some hospitals, children with bladder exstrophy are treated similarly. The preanesthetic assessment should include questions about atopy and allergies to foods, especially tropical fruits. Children thought to be at risk based on history simply should not be exposed to latex. If a child who is thought to be at risk for latex sensitivity by virtue of a medical or surgical condition denies (or the parents deny) facial redness after touching balloons or after dental care and has not undergone latex-sensitivity testing, it still seems prudent to avoid latex-containing products, especially as more and more products are manufactured to be free of latex. All equipment used by anesthesiologists can be obtained in forms that are free of latex, including IV sets and tubing, breathing circuits and breathing bags, and sterile and nonsterile gloves. Most multidose vials are made with latex-free stoppers. *Latex Alert* warning signs should be placed outside the operating room door to avoid inadvertent latex exposure in these patients. Clinicians must keep themselves informed about the progress in this area. It is important to note that not all medical equipment and products are free of latex; therefore, each new product should be checked for possible latex content. It is true that products that were formerly unsafe become safe with a change in manufacturing. However, given the high morbidity of an anaphylactic reaction, it is essential that caregivers be certain of the safety of medical products used in children at risk for latex sensitivity.

The FDA approved the marketing of a patient-examination glove that is produced from a new form of natural rubber latex made from the guayule bush, a desert plant found in the American Southwest. Available data on this glove show that individuals who are allergic to latex made from the sap of the rubber tree *(heva braziliensis)* do not, on first exposure, react to the guayule latex (FDA, 2008).

Prophylaxis and Desensitization

Although it is difficult to create a completely latex-free environment, the current consensus seems to be that prophylaxis of patients with known or suspected latex sensitivity need not be undertaken. Those who endorse prophylaxis propose administration of diphenhydramine, ranitidine, and corticosteroids from the preoperative through the postoperative period. The literature contains case reports of patients who developed anaphylaxis after exposure to latex despite preoperative administration of the recommended prophylactic medication (Kwittken et al., 1992; Setlock et al., 1993). Desensitization has been successful in a limited number of reported cases (Patriarca et al., 2002a, 2002b). Many of the participants in these efforts were actually health care workers with documented IgE-mediated latex allergy, but none of them had previously suffered anaphylaxis after exposure to latex. The clinical manifestations of latex allergy included asthma, angioedema, and urticaria. Although most patients were adults, one report included subjects as young as 8 years of age. Techniques used were cutaneous exposure over a 12-month period and 4-day desensitization via sublingual exposure. At this point, however, desensitization does not appear to be an option for children with type I hypersensitivity to latex. As more details of the immunologic basis for latex reactions become known, new and safer desensitization programs may be developed (Rolland and O'Hehir, 2008).

Occupational Latex Allergy

In 1998, a report of latex sensitivity among the staff of the Department of Anesthesiology at the Johns Hopkins University School of Medicine documented a 24% incidence of irritant or contact dermatitis and nearly 13% incidence of latex-specific IgE positivity, although pediatric anesthesiologists may have a somewhat lower incidence (Brown et al., 1998; Greenberg et al., 1999). A large meta-analysis of studies in health care workers showed a 0% to 30% prevalence of type I latex allergy in that group. The authors did not have data that elucidated the reasons for the large variation in prevalence (Garabrant and Schweitzer, 2002). Other reports suggest that avoidance of latex reverses the sensitivity, at least in health care workers (Zeldin et al., 1996). The creation of a latex-free operating room environment will benefit both the patients and those who care for them.

Epidermolysis Bullosa

Epidermolysis bullosa (EB) encompasses a heterogeneous group of congenital, hereditary, blistering disorders and is subdivided into three major subtypes: EB simplex, junctional EB, and dystrophic EB. These types differ in histology, clinical severity, and mode of inheritance, but all are characterized by the easy development of blisters after minor trauma or friction. The literature contains several reviews of the perioperative and anesthetic care of children with one of the variants of EB (Tetzlaff and Fleisher, 2005; Lin and Golianu, 2006; Lindemeyer et al., 2009). Junctional EB is often clinically apparent early in life and heals with scarring. A discriminating feature of this variant is the relative sparing of the hands and feet. However, involvement of the mucous membranes may be severe, and ulceration of the respiratory epithelium has been documented. The recessive variant of dystrophic EB may be the most severe form of the condition, in which mucous membrane lesions are common. Treatment of children with this condition is supportive. Infections are common and should be promptly treated. Adequate nutrition is paramount but often difficult to provide in cases with esophageal blisters with subsequent stricture formation. Children with the more severe forms may come to the operating room for a variety of procedures such as scar revisions, corrections of digital fusions, placement of gastrostomy tubes, or even colonic interpositions.

Anesthetic Management

The preanesthetic evaluation of a child with EB should involve the patient's dermatologist and pediatrician, who can advise the anesthesiologist of the child's general course with regard to blistering, skin infections, nutritional status, and the possible usefulness of additional steroid administration. In addition to assessing the child's general condition and health, the physical examination should focus on the airway (that may be compromised by scarring around the mouth), IV access sites, and the location and condition of existing and recent blisters.

Friction and, secondarily, pressure must be avoided in caring for children with this condition in the perioperative period. Monitoring must adhere to the ASA standards, but the application of the monitors should be modified. Pulse oximetry may be accomplished with an adult clip-on probe (that may be impossible if the patient has complete pseudosyndactyly of the fingers and toes), or the adhesive strip oximeter probe may be placed over a clear plastic bag covering the hand or foot that is then wrapped with Webril or Coban (3M; Saint Paul, Minnesota) (Fig. 36-21). The precordial stethoscopes should simply be placed (without adhesive) onto the chest; temperature should be monitored with an axillary probe; soft padding should be placed between the skin and noninvasive blood pressure cuffs; electrocardiograph leads should be nonadhesive (e.g., needle electrodes); and IV and arterial catheters should be sutured and lightly covered with a gauze bandage (e.g., Webril or Coban). A nonadhesive, silicone-based dressing (Mepilex; Mölnlycke Health Care AB, Göteborg, Sweden) that is used for protecting blistered areas in these patients has recently become available. It has been found to be useful for securing venous and arterial catheters, holding precordial stethoscopes in place, and facilitating contact of electrocardiograph gel pads in which the adhesive has been removed (Figs. 36-22, 36-23, and 36-24). It can also be used to cover the contact surfaces of the anesthesia mask to substitute for the previous practice of coating the mask surface with steroid ointment, which creates a slippery environment for subsequent handling of the patient. The eyes should be lubricated but not taped closed with adhesive tape. (Mepilex may be used.)

A variety of techniques for anesthetic induction and maintenance have been reported for procedures performed on these challenging patients (Holzman et al., 1987; Farber et al., 1995; Herod et al., 2002; Lindemeyer et al., 2009). An oral premedication may be useful in children with EB who are taken to the operating room, because a struggling child who is restrained may develop blisters where held by the operating team. Alternatively, intramuscular ketamine has been used to both induce and maintain anesthesia in these patients (Ames et al., 1999). The

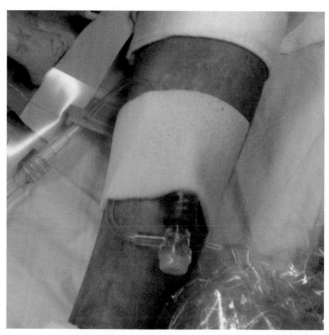

■ **FIGURE 36-22.** The IV cannula and tubing are held in place with a strip of Mepilex transfer.

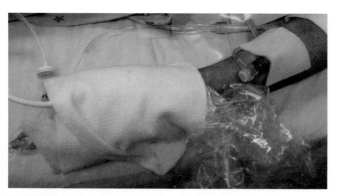

■ **FIGURE 36-21.** A thin plastic bag is placed over the digit; the adhesive pulse oximeter probe is then placed over the plastic bag. The extremity is then wrapped with Webril to keep the pulse oximeter bag assembly in place.

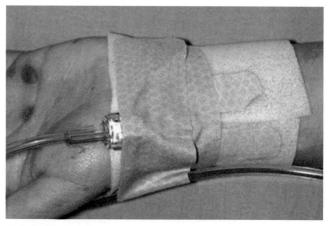

■ **FIGURE 36-23.** An arterial cannula and tubing are held in place with Mepilex transfer strips on the skin and adhesive tape applied to the Mepilex transfer.

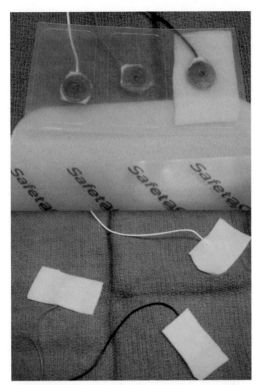

■ **FIGURE 36-24.** Adhesive is trimmed from the contact area of infant electrocardiograph pads. Contacts consisting only of gel and wire are secured to patient with strips of Mepilex transfer.

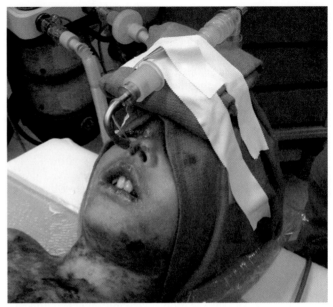

■ **FIGURE 36-25.** A nasal ETT is secured to a head wrap. No adhesive is applied to the face.

induction technique chosen depends on the preoperative assessment and the planned procedure. The induction of general anesthesia can be via an inhalational technique, but contact with the child's face must be gentle. Oropharyngeal airways should be avoided. Laryngoscopy with a straight blade without contact with the epiglottis is preferred, and intubation with a smaller-than-predicted, softened (in warm, sterile saline), lubricated ETT after administration of muscle relaxant will minimize trauma to the oral, supraglottic, and tracheal mucosa. Most physicians recommend securing the tube with umbilical tape tied around the back of the head. If there are no contraindications, a deep extubation decreases tracheal trauma caused by coughing. Cases of postoperative bullae in the pharynx, some of which caused airway obstruction, have been reported, but predisposing factors are difficult to identify (James and Wark, 1982). Most series report no airway complications despite the formation of new oral bullae.

Limited mouth opening in many patients with EB necessitates fiberoptic nasotracheal intubation. This route is a good choice for all patients with EB—even those with adequate mouth opening—because oral intubation causes more trauma and bulla formation to the tongue and oral mucosa because of pressure of the laryngoscope on the supraglottic area (Baum and O'Flaherty, 2006). The nasal mucosa is composed of pseudostratified cylindrical ciliated epithelium with goblet cells (i.e., respiratory epithelium), stratified cuboidal epithelium, and stratified squamous nonkeratinized epithelium. The first two types of epithelium are less vulnerable to bulla formation than the latter two, which comprise the epithelium of the oral mucosa. In addition, the nasotracheal tube may be secured more easily without tape than an oral tube (Fig. 36-25). Care should be taken to use a tube small enough to avoid pressure on the skin surface at the entrance to the naris. As is customary for

nasal intubation, the nare should be prepared with lubrication and vasoconstriction (e.g., oxymetazoline 0.05% or phenylephrine 0.25%), and the tube should be softened as described.

Oral rehabilitation procedures, commonly required by EB patients because of the inability to brush their teeth, are more easily accomplished with a nasotracheal tube (Griffin and Mayou, 1993). Some clinicians have recommended nasal intubation (with fiberoptic guidance) to eliminate the trauma and friction of direct laryngoscopy. It is also thought that the passage of the tube is not as traumatic and the nasopharyngeal mucosa is not as vulnerable to bulla formation as is the oral, gingival, and supraglottic mucosa, especially with the pressure of a laryngoscope blade. In addition, a nasal tube can be secured to a head-wrap dressing, eliminating the need for any ties that may abrade the face. The decision to admit these children after the procedure must be made on an individual basis. However, they warrant careful observation in a well-monitored environment after surgery and anesthesia. Even though general anesthesia is used often in these patients, reports of successful regional techniques have been published (Kaplan and Strauch, 1987; Cakmakkaya et al., 2008; Nasr et al., 2008).

Down Syndrome

The incidence of Trisomy 21 is 1 in 600 to 800 live births. More than half of Trisomy conceptions spontaneously abort early in pregnancy. The syndrome has many clinical manifestations, some of which are of particular note to the anesthesiologist.

Approximately 40% of children with Trisomy 21 have anomalies of the cardiovascular system. The three most common anomalies seen in these children are complete atrioventricular canal (CAVC) (comprising approximately 40% of the total), ventricular septal defect (25%), and atrial septal defect (10% to 15%). Children with Down syndrome who undergo repair of CAVC have significantly higher perioperative mortality than those without Trisomy 21. However, the outcome after surgery is not different for other cardiac anomalies. These defects have in common the propensity for increased pulmonary blood flow, which the anesthetic management should plan to minimize. Repair or palliation of a cardiac defect does not eliminate the need for particular attention to the cardiovascular system in the evaluation of these patients preoperatively.

Children with Down syndrome have varying degrees of mental retardation, and it is important to be aware of the degree of intellectual impairment when meeting and talking with them. Hypotonia is one of the most common clinical features seen in these children, and it may affect the patency of their upper airways. The relatively large tongue, short neck, and crowded midface and laryngomalacia contribute to upper airway obstruction (Kanamori et al., 2000; Mitchell et al., 2003). Partial airway obstruction, while awake and during sleep, is often seen in children with Trisomy 21. This situation is exacerbated by the administration of sedatives and during inhalation induction (Luscri and Tobias, 2006; Ng et al., 2006). Children with Trisomy 21 have an increased incidence of subglottic stenosis, and often the proper size of ETT for a given child is smaller than would have been predicted. The incidence of tracheal stenosis is also significant because of complete tracheal rings. An orthopedic anomaly of great concern in these children is ligamentous laxity of the atlantoaxial joint, which may predispose affected individuals to C_1-C_2 subluxation and possible spinal cord damage. The incidence of this anomaly is 12% to 32%, depending on the ages of the children studied and the exact definition of laxity used (Hata and Todd, 2005; Pizzutillo and Herman, 2005). The incidence of hearing loss and of hypothyroidism is increased in these children (Tuysuz and Beker, 2001). Other associated findings in patients with Down syndrome are included in Box 36-19.

Perioperative Management

The preoperative evaluation of a child with Down syndrome should give particular attention to the organ systems commonly affected by this condition (Mitchell et al., 1995). The history of prior surgeries should be reviewed. These children may have undergone cardiac procedures, removal of the tonsils and adenoids, myringotomy tube placement, and other common pediatric procedures. Records from other doctors may contain helpful information about associated conditions such as obstructive sleep apnea syndrome, atlantoaxial laxity, or subluxation. Management of these children regarding possible C_1-C_2 subluxation is a difficult matter. The American Academy of Pediatrics (AAP) has published statements by the AAP Committee on Genetics and AAP Committee on Sports Medicine and Fitness that include a discussion of this clinical problem. The Committee on Genetics policy statement on health care supervision of children with Down syndrome recommends that radiographs looking for evidence of atlantoaxial instability or subluxation be obtained at between 3 and 5 years of age (AAP Committee on Genetics, 2001). The Committee on Sports Medicine and Fitness reviewed the topic of atlantoaxial instability in Down syndrome in a 1995 publication and tentatively concluded that lateral plain films are of potential but unproved value in detecting patients at risk for developing spinal cord injury during participation in sports (AAP Committee on Sports Medicine and Fitness, 1995). The Special Olympics does not plan to remove its requirement that all athletes with Down syndrome receive lateral spine radiographs (Special Olympics,

Box 36-19 Associated Findings in Patients with Down Syndrome

GENERAL FINDINGS
Low birth weight
Short stature

CARDIOVASCULAR FINDINGS
Congenital heart disease
Increased susceptibility to pulmonary hypertension
Atropine sensitivity

RESPIRATORY FINDINGS
High-arched narrow palate
Macroglossia
Micrognathia
Increased susceptibility to respiratory infections
Subglottic stenosis
Postextubation stridor
Upper airway obstruction, sleep apnea

GI FINDINGS
Dental abnormalities
Duodenal obstruction
Gastroesophageal reflux
Hirschprung disease

CNS FINDINGS
Mental retardation
Epilepsy
Strabismus

MUSCULOSKELETAL FINDINGS
Hypotonia
Hyperextensibility or flexibility
Dysplastic pelvis
Atlantoaxial subluxation

IMMUNE SYSTEM FINDINGS
Immunosuppression
Leukemia (acute lymphoblastic, acute myeloid forms)

HEMATOLOGIC FINDINGS
Neonatal polycythemia

ENDOCRINE FINDINGS
Low circulating level of catecholamine
Hypothyroidism

1983). Some conclusions can be drawn from the published case reports summarized in the AAP Committee on Sports Medicine Subject Review and the recommendations cited above.

The preoperative history and physical examination should include a careful search for evidence of cervical instability. Of course, the parent should be questioned about past cervical x-rays, if they were taken. The family and patient should be questioned about the occurrence of any type of neck pain, limitation of neck mobility, tortocollis, head tilt, abnormalities of gait, or other signs of upper motor neuron dysfunction. The examination should also look for spasticity, hyperreflexia, extensor-plantar reflex, or clonus. If the history and physical examination reveal problems or the cervical radiographs show an atlan-todens interval of greater than 5 mm, the child's elective surgery should be delayed and neurosurgical consultation sought (Hata and Todd, 2005). If the child had previous negative radiographs and the history and physical do not suggest a problem, it is not clear whether the films should be repeated (Pueschel, 1998).

Although the incidence of worsening of the atlantodens interval over time is low, some patients do show progression. Even in asymptomatic patients, the possibility exists that a postoperative neurologic disability may occur (Williams et al., 1987; Litman and Perkins, 1994). Whatever the result of the evaluations, if surgery and anesthesia are undertaken, the general consensus is that the heads and necks of these patients should be kept in the neutral position throughout the perioperative period. A reassuring study of children with Down syndrome with normal cervical radiographs who underwent tonsillectomy and adenoidectomy in the usual position showed no changes in the latency or amplitude of the somatosensory potentials (Abramson et al., 1995). Atlantoaxial instability occurs in conditions other than Down syndrome and at a higher rate (Box 36-20).

GENETIC MUSCLE DISORDERS

The last decade has seen a tremendous increase in genetic and genomics research, which has allowed researchers to reach a clearer picture of the molecular causes of genetic-based muscle diseases. In most cases, identification of the proteins altered in the disease states has added to the understanding of the development of muscle and the neuromuscular junction, and the anesthetic management suggested for these diseases and syndromes is beginning to be modified as a result of this knowledge. This section contains a review of what is presently known concerning the molecular nature of diseases of the neuromuscular system and their clinical presentations. A general overview of the generation of muscle contraction in a normal cell (Fig. 36-26) is followed by a discussion of recent molecular and genetic studies that involve the major muscle diseases, because knowledge of their results may be of use to the clinician in the near future.

General Overview

The genetic muscle diseases can be divided into 4 broad categories—muscular dystrophies, myotonic syndromes, mitochondrial myopathies, and myasthenic syndromes. To these,

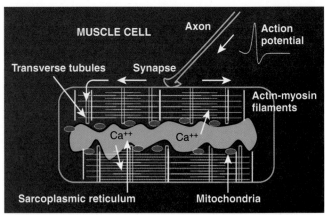

■ **FIGURE 36-26.** Schematic diagram of the muscle cell and motor neuron. An action potential (AP), generated in the membrane of the muscle by sodium influx through voltage-gated sodium channels, travels down the motor neuron, causing the release of acetylcholine at the synapse. It travels along the membrane and down the transverse tubules. There it causes the influx of calcium at the base of the tubules (through the dihydropyridine receptor). The small calcium currents trigger release of larger amounts of calcium (through the ryanodine receptor) from the sarcoplasmic reticulum into the matrix of the muscle cell, activating the actin-myosin filaments to contract. The filaments attach (not shown) to the surface of the cell and the extracellular matrix to cause effective mechanical contraction (see Fig. 36-27, *D*).

malignant hyperthermia (MH) must be added as a separate category, though some overlap between MH and the other diseases does exist (see Chapter 37, Malignant Hyperthermia). Of course, a few muscle diseases do not easily fit into these groupings. Each of these categories is discussed separately and related to the MH syndrome where possible. The general locations in the muscle cell of the molecular changes that lead to these classes of disease are shown in Figure 36-27. The syndromes are caused by changes listed below:

- The myasthenic syndromes affect transmission of the action potential (AP) from the motor neuron to the muscle cell; this involves a disruption of the signal carried by the neurotransmitter, acetylcholine, at the synapse (see Fig. 36-27, *A*).
- Myotonic syndromes affect transmission of the AP along the muscle membrane and are caused by abnormalities in sodium, chloride, potassium, or calcium channels (see Fig. 36-27, *B*). These changes cause a prolonged depolarization of the muscle membrane, which leads to prolonged contraction of the muscle.
- Mitochondrial myopathies are (as their name implies) caused by abnormalities in mitochondrial function. Because mitochondria are important for supplying ATP in most tissues (most importantly nerve and muscle), the symptoms often involve the nervous system and muscle (see Fig. 36-27, *C*). The lack of ATP in muscle leads primarily to weakness and wasting of muscle. Mitochondria are also important in triggering cell death, or apoptosis; therefore, mitochondrial diseases may also lead to muscle wasting via this mechanism.

Box 36-20 Conditions Associated with Atlantoaxial Dislocation

Congenital abnormalities
   Trisomy 21
   Klippel-Feil syndrome
   Larsen syndrome
   Mucopolysaccharidoses
   Spondyloepiphyseal dysplasia
   Metatropic dwarfism
   Kniest syndrome
   Chondodysplasia punctata
   22q syndrome
Infection
   Pharyngeal
Tumors
Trauma
Postoperative complications (especially after airway surgery)
Arthritis
   Rheumatoid
   Ankylosing spondylitis

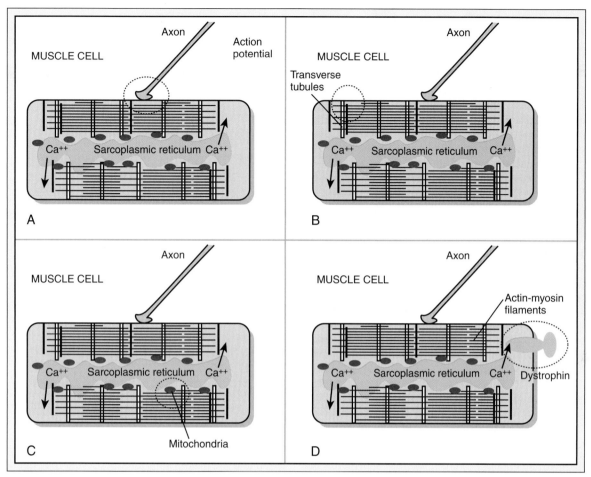

■ **FIGURE 36-27.** Detail of Figure 36-26 that shows the main areas of defects that lead to muscle disease. **A,** Disruption of the signal across the synapse leads to myasthenic syndromes. **B,** Defects in the calcium, potassium, and sodium channels in the muscle cell membrane give rise to myotonias. The membranes remain depolarized too long, causing the inability to relax. **C,** Mitochondrial dysfunction leads to decreased intracellular levels of ATP and to cell death. The decreased ATP concentration is responsible for the inability of the muscles to contract strongly and for insufficient reuptake of calcium into the sarcoplasmic reticulum. The latter effect may lead to inability to relax under certain circumstances. **D,** Defects in the attachment of the actin-myosin filaments to the cell surface and extracellular matrix produce muscular dystrophies. These attachments are important for mechanical force and for organizing and stabilizing the membrane.

● Muscular dystrophies result from the dissociation of contractile force from the muscle to the surrounding connective tissue. The actin-myosin filaments contract, but they are no longer connected well to the cell membrane or the surrounding tissue. As a result, the equivalent of electromechanical dissociation occurs; i.e., the electrical signal is not translated into effective mechanical force (see Fig. 36-27, *D*). In addition, the membrane defects cause instability in the cell membrane integrity that may result in deleterious responses to anesthetic agents.

The dotted circles in each panel of Figure 36-27 indicate the locations of the molecular changes. It is important to note that this figure is an oversimplification, but it gives the general pattern of the molecular causes of the syndromes.

Skeletal muscle contraction is accomplished by the generation of a neuronal AP that terminates at the neuromuscular synapse (see Fig. 36-26). The neuronal AP stimulates sodium channels in the neuronal axon that propagate the signal along the axon. As the AP reaches the end of the axon, voltage-gated calcium channels are activated that allow the influx of calcium into the neuron. This influx of calcium, in turn, stimulates the release of a neurotransmitter, acetylcholine, from the nerve terminal into the synapse. The acetylcholine binds to receptors on the cell surface of the postsynaptic cell—the muscle, in this case. Binding of the acetylcholine to its receptors allows influx of sodium into the muscle and generates a new AP, which propagates a transmembrane signal that spreads along the membrane of the cell.

The AP is carried from the cell surface into the interior of the cell by a series of invaginations of the cell membrane known as *T tubules*. These structures allow for transmembrane electrical depolarizations to be carried deeply within the cell, where they would otherwise not be generated. At the ends of the T tubules, the sodium currents are again replaced by calcium currents, resulting from the activation of a voltage-gated calcium channel known as the *dihydropyridine receptor* (Fig. 36-28). These calcium currents, in their turn, stimulate larger calcium release from the sarcoplasmic reticulum through a calcium-sensitive calcium channel called the *ryanodine receptor*. These larger fluxes of calcium stimulate movement of the

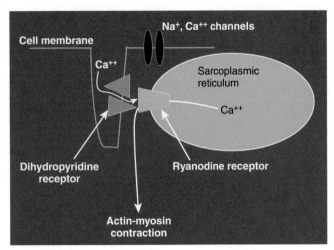

■ **FIGURE 36-28.** Further detail of the region of the T tubules. Sodium, potassium, and calcium channels on the cell surface are responsible for propagation of the AP along the cell membrane and into the T tubules. When the AP reaches the terminus of the T tubule, the sodium currents are replaced by calcium currents through the voltage-gated dihydropyridine receptor. These calcium currents trigger release of calcium through the ryanodine receptor from the large calcium stores in the sarcoplasmic reticulum.

actin-myosin filaments, an ATP-requiring step (and therefore dependent on functioning mitochondria). The filaments are attached to the surface of the muscle and the surrounding matrix through a variety of proteins, most notably, *dystrophin*. Movement of the filaments is transduced into shortening of the cell (muscle contraction) by the connection to the cell surface and surrounding matrix. Relaxation is accomplished by reuptake of the intracellular calcium primarily back into the sarcoplasmic reticulum. This reuptake is energy requiring and dependent on mitochondrial function, ATP generation, and ATP-dependent calcium pumps. Loss of this energy source is the cause of rigor mortis.

The normal flow of electrical signal transduced to mechanical force can be disrupted at many places. Anesthesiologists often inhibit the transmission of the signal across the neuromuscular junction with the use of neuromuscular blockers (NMBs) such as vecuronium. Such an effect is conceptually similar to a myasthenic syndrome. Local anesthetics applied to the motor neuron inhibit the propagation of an AP along the neuron, resulting in decreased release of neurotransmitters. In this manner, they also mimic the effect of myasthenia. The use of local anesthetics directly on muscle blocks voltage-gated sodium channels in the muscle membrane, with the resulting inhibition of AP propagation, acting in the opposite manner to the changes seen in myotonic syndromes. Volatile anesthetics are also inhibitors of the voltage-gated membrane channels (e.g., sodium, potassium, and calcium) and thus also act in a manner opposite to that seen in myotonia. However, these drugs also inhibit mitochondria and are capable of causing a relaxation effect in a manner similar to a mitochondrial myopathy. These examples are given only to further acquaint the anesthetist with the underlying causes of the myopathies; drugs certainly do not cause these diseases. However, these similar effects help explain the interaction of the drugs with the disease states.

Myasthenic Syndromes

Myasthenic syndromes are the result of the failure of transmission of the signal from the terminal of a motor neuron to the muscle innervated by the neuron. Most myasthenic syndromes are the result of immune responses against components of the neuromuscular junction (primarily the postsynaptic acetylcholine receptors) and are not classic genetic diseases. The symptoms result from decreased neurotransmission across the neuromuscular junction, and task-specific fatigue is the hallmark of these diseases (see Fig. 36-27, *A*). The well-known disease *myasthenia gravis (MG)* is an example of such a disorder, although it is primarily a disease of adulthood. MG can occur in the neonatal period because of placental transfer of maternal antibodies. In addition, juvenile-onset MG is seen in association with thymoma (Kiran et al., 2000).

Congenital myasthenic syndromes (CMSs) are genetic in origin, and analyses have identified more than ten different genes that are important in development of the neuromuscular synapse (Palace and Beeson, 2008). Rarely, inherited disorders of neuromuscular transmission (CMSs), can result from acetylcholine receptor mutations or other mutations that involve the release of acetylcholine. Included in this group are familial infantile myasthenia, familial limb-girdle myasthenia, endplate acetylcholinesterase deficiency, and syndromes with altered or deficient acetylcholine receptors (Menold et al., 1998; Maselli et al., 2001). In addition, CMS may result from defects in development of the synapse. One such form of congenital myasthenia is caused by a defect in the gene DOK7, which is important in the formation or maintenance of synaptic structure (Müller et al., 2007). These genetic diseases mimic MG in their presentation and implications for anesthesia, and they manifest during infancy or childhood (Dalal et al., 1972).

Anesthetic Considerations for Myasthenic Syndromes

The primary concern during the perioperative period for patients with myasthenic syndromes is to avoid respiratory compromise from weakened respiratory muscles or upper airway muscles (Brown et al., 1990; Abel and Eisenkraft, 2002). For this reason, nondepolarizing muscle relaxants are used sparingly, if at all, in these patients. As a result of the blockade and destruction of acetylcholine receptors, patients with MG or myasthenic syndromes are often resistant to succinylcholine (Baraka, 2001). It is important to remember that patients can appear strong on awakening only to become fatigued later in the recovery period. Itoh and others (2002) showed that seronegativity for the antiacetylcholine receptor antibody did not predict a normal response to muscle relaxants. In particular, patients with MG who were successfully treated with thymectomy may also retain a high sensitivity to muscle relaxants. The conclusion of these reports is that the anesthesiologist must presume a high sensitivity to muscle relaxants in all patients with myasthenic syndromes, even if they are functioning well after medical or surgical treatment.

Techniques that employ a variety of short-acting anesthetics without the addition of muscle relaxants have been very successful (Della Rocca et al., 2003; Bouaggad et al., 2005). Others have reported encouraging results after use of regional anesthesia in these patients (Caliskan et al., 2008). However, one report cautions that even with a stable anesthetic, tourniquet release may trigger an exacerbation of symptoms (Brodsky and Smith, 2007).

Myotonias

Myotonia is a temporary involuntary contraction of muscle fibers caused by transient hyperexcitability of the surface membrane (Miller, 1989; Bernard and Shevell, 2008). The persistent contracture of the skeletal muscle generally occurs after muscle stimulation but may be triggered by other stimuli such as cold, pain, or stress. A classic finding in patients with myotonia is the inability to easily relax after a firm handshake. Myotonias can be subdivided into 2 general groups — dystrophic and nondystrophic. The dystrophic group (represented by myotonic dystrophy [DM]) shows a progressive wasting of muscle mass and strength; the nondystrophic group does not show such progressive changes.

In general, the myotonias may be thought of as a family of channelopathies that mostly affect muscle (Jurkat-Rott et al., 2002; Rosenbaum and Miller, 2002; Bernard and Shevell, 2008). The abnormalities in the channels lead to prolonged depolarization in the membrane once an AP is generated (Fig. 36-28). This in turn leads to prolonged or increased release of calcium into the cell, resulting in prolonged contraction. Two forms of myotonia (myotonia congenita and Becker disease) result from defects in the same skeletal muscle chloride channel (termed *CLC1*) (Jurkat-Rott et al., 2002; Pusch, 2002; Renner and Ptacek, 2002). Myotonia congenita (Thomsen disease) is an autosomal-dominant disease that manifests in childhood and is associated with a normal life expectancy and minimal symptoms (Grunnet et al., 2003). Becker disease, not to be confused with Becker muscular dystrophy (BMD), is an autosomal recessive form of this channelopathy that also appears in childhood (Pusch, 2002). In addition, some mutations in this chloride channel cause a variant of dominant myotonia with a milder phenotype, myotonia levior (Ryan et al., 2002; Farbu et al., 2003). These myotonic diseases are nonprogressive and do not have a dystrophic component (i.e., the muscle does not deteriorate over time). Other less severe myotonias result from abnormalities in sodium or potassium channels on the muscle cell membrane. These include paramytonia congenita (sodium channel), hyperkalemic periodic paralysis (sodium channel), and hypokalemic periodic paralysis (calcium, sodium, or potassium channel) (Jurkat-Rott et al., 2002).

As noted above, myotonic contractions may be precipitated by stress, cold, and pain. Thus, these triggering factors must be aggressively avoided in this population during the perioperative period. Regional anesthesia and NMBs do not reverse the contractions, because they act upstream from the molecular causes of the syndrome (compare Fig. 36-27, *A* and *B*). However, succinylcholine has been noted to precipitate contractions, as have anticholinesterases when used for NMB reversal. These contractions have been most notable in the occurrence of masseter spasm after the use of succinylcholine but can also involve other muscles and lead to extreme difficulty with positive pressure ventilation and intubation (Farbu et al., 2003). For these reasons, the use of succinylcholine is discouraged in patients with myotonia. If an episode of myotonia occurs during anesthesia, volatile anesthetics, quinine, or procainamide can be used for relaxation. If a myotonic episode occurs in patients with periodic paralysis, use of the carbonic anhydrase inhibitor dichlorphenamide has been shown to be useful (Cleland and Griggs, 2008). In that the myotonias occur as the result of abnormal ion channels, great care must be taken to keep electrolytes normal at all times. Whereas myotonic syndromes may have symptoms in common with MH, they are not associated with true MH (see Chapter 37, Malignant Hyperthermia).

Steinert muscular dystrophy (DM) is the most common form of myotonia (Anderson and Brown, 1989). This disease is a form of muscular dystrophy and includes congenital DM. It is discussed here rather than with other muscular dystrophies, because its presentation is different—it more closely resembles the myotonias.

DM was shown to actually include two different molecular diseases (Ranum and Day, 2002). DM type 1 (DM1) results from alterations in the human dystrophia myotonica-protein kinase gene (DMPK), leading to an increase in unstable CTG repeats in the 3′ untranslated region of the DMPK gene (Amack and Mahadevan, 2004; Botta et al., 2008; Orengo et al., 2008). DMPK codes for a serine-threonine protein kinase. The changes in DMPK lead to abnormal splicing of the message for the calcium channel protein CLCN1, with resulting defects in function of the channel (Lueck et al., 2007). The myotonia may then result from defects in calcium channels, resulting in altered transmembrane potentials in muscle (Kaliman and Llagostera, 2008). However, others have suggested that the myotonia is probably the result of abnormal phosphorylation of sodium channels, resulting in delayed inactivation after channel opening (Lee et al., 2003). The precise mechanisms by which this mutation causes the changes in muscle function are not yet clear, but they appear to involve several pathways (Dansithong et al., 2008). As noted above, the changes in the protein kinase gene are in the promoter or starting region of the gene and are the result of duplications in short repetitive sequences (CTG triplets). The number of repetitive sequences is often increased in the offspring compared with an affected parent. As a result, each successive generation tends to exhibit a more severe form of the disease.

DM type 2, or DM2, has a clinically diverse presentation, including myotonia, proximal muscle wasting, and endocrine, cardiac, and cerebral abnormalities. It results from expansion of a similar sequence in an intron of a gene; however, the gene is separate from the one that causes DM1 and codes for a probable transcription factor, ZFN9 (Liquori et al., 2001; Finsterer, 2002; Liquori et al., 2003). The precise physiologic changes that lead to myotonic or dystrophic changes are not known. In both disease states, the abnormalities result from abnormal RNA species that disrupt normal development of the cells (Mankodi and Thornton, 2002).

Anesthetic Considerations for Myotonias

Attainment of muscle relaxation can be difficult in these patients. As with the other forms of myotonia discussed previously, cold, stress, pain, and succinylcholine can precipitate myotonia. Additionally, because this is a dystrophy with muscle wasting, succinylcholine can elicit a hyperkalemic response and should be avoided. Unlike the other myotonias, DM leads to deterioration of the muscle fibers and is associated with weakness and hypotonia in the infant and child. Paradoxically, however, these patients can still experience a myotonic episode as well. They can have profound respiratory depression, severe cardiac conduction abnormalities, cardiomyopathy, developmental delay, dysphagia, and decreased gastric motility. Muscle relaxants must be used with great care, if at all, in these patients. Smaller doses are probably indicated, and an NMB monitor is advised. As with nondystrophic myotonias, reversal agents may induce myotonic episodes.

Because respiratory muscle weakness is notable in these patients, the respiratory status is potentially fragile when any narcotic or general anesthetic is used. Thus, their care presents challenges involving several physiologic systems. White and Bass (2003) presented a thoughtful review of the anesthetic care of patients with DM. DM is also commonly thought to be associated with MH. However, as with the myotonias discussed above, although this syndrome shares features with MH, it is not associated with true MH (see Chapter 37, Malignant Hyperthermia).

Mitochondrial Myopathies

Mitochondrial dysfunction is being recognized as the cause of an increasingly large list of disease syndromes. The more commonly seen mitochondrial syndromes are Leigh disease, Kearns-Sayre syndrome, and Leber hereditary optic neuropathy. However, mitochondrial dysfunction is also associated with unnamed myopathies and encephalopathies and with symptoms of failure to thrive. Mitochondrial abnormalities have been shown to be involved with some forms of autism and Parkinson's disease (Shoffner et al., 1991; Schaefer et al., 2004). It is clear that the presentation of mitochondrial disease may be quite varied.

Mitochondria are the principal source of energy metabolism within cells, especially those of nerve and muscle (see Fig. 36-27, *C*). Within mitochondria reside the enzymes responsible for the Krebs cycle, fatty acid β oxidation, and most importantly, oxidative phosphorylation (Fig. 36-29). Mitochondria contain the enzymes that metabolize glucose, fatty acids, and amino acids to generate NADH and succinate, which in turn, are used as electron donors for the electron transport chain (ETC). By passing electrons down the ETC (complexes I to IV), a proton gradient is generated across the

mitochondrial inner membrane and electrons are donated to oxygen to generate water. The proton gradient is then used to drive an ATP synthase (complex V). The coupling of electron transfer to phosphorylation is known as *oxidative phosphorylation* and is overwhelmingly the major source of ATP and other high-energy phosphate bonds that supply energy to the cell.

Mitochondrial complexes are composed of groups of proteins, ranging from just a few (complex II) to over 40 (complex I). In addition, the dehydrogenases, membrane transporters, and structural proteins raise the number of functional proteins in the mitochondria into the hundreds. Genes in the cell's chromosomes encode for most of the proteins of the ETC, whereas mitochondrial DNA encodes a minority of the ETC proteins. The other enzymes in the mitochondria are entirely encoded by the nuclear genome. The genetics of mitochondrial disease are complicated by the fact that mitochondria are inherited from the mother. However, different populations of the maternal mitochondria may be passed to different offspring, so the inheritance pattern can be quite varied. Finally, mitochondrial dysfunction has effects other than energy depletion. Increased free radical damage to other cellular components and alterations in protein phosphorylation may be seen with mitochondrial disease. Each of these effects can give rise to mixed but wide-ranging functional changes in affected individuals.

It is a common mistake to group all mitochondrial diseases together as similar entities; however, mutations in any of the mitochondrial proteins may result in dramatically different functional changes. In addition, mitochondria in different tissues can be quite varied in their activity. The differences between tissues in sensitivity to abnormalities of mitochondrial function (and the varied inheritance pattern discussed previously) give rise to different symptoms even within members of a family who carry the identical mutation. Because of this variability, it is dangerous to imply that because an anesthetic

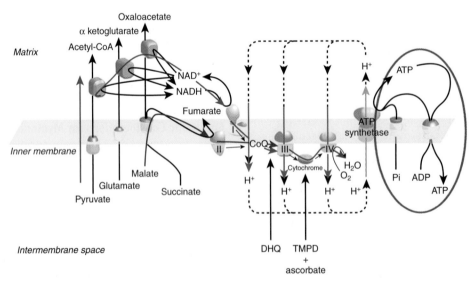

■ **FIGURE 36-29.** ETC of mitochondria. Substrates for the ETC are transported into the mitochondria *(light blue arrow)* and NADH, or succinate, is generated via the Krebs cycle. NADH donates electrons to the ETC at complex I; they then follow the path indicated by the *dark blue arrows.* Succinate donates electrons to complex II; they follow the path indicated by the *red arrows.* Once the electrons reach complex III, their paths are functionally the same *(gray arrow).* Protons are pumped into the intermembrane space *(green arrows)* to generate a transmembrane gradient. The protons then leak back into the matrix through complex V to generate the energy to drive the ATPase *(red oval).* DHQ and TMPD/ascorbate are indicated and are artificial electron donors that can be used experimentally to drive complexes III and IV, respectively. *DHQ,* Dihydroquinidine; *TMPD,* tetramethyl-p phenylenediamine.

technique was successful in a few patients with mitochondrial disease, the technique is safe for all patients with mitochondrial dysfunction.

Muscle and nerve cells are uniquely dependent on the energy delivered by the mitochondria. Mutations in mitochondrial proteins are responsible for striking clinical features in those two tissues, including myopathy, cardiomyopathy, encephalopathy, seizures, and cerebellar ataxia. Of course, cardiac muscle and the CNS are also the two main targets of general anesthetics. Thus, particular care must be taken when exposing such a patient to these agents. As motor neurons may be affected, a hyperkalemic response to succinylcholine may be seen. Lastly, MH is thought to be associated with some forms of mitochondrial myopathies, but the nature of this relationship is unclear (Keyes et al., 1996; Fricker et al., 2002).

Anesthetic Considerations for Mitochondrial Myopathies

The perioperative period is a time during which a patient may be exposed to periods of stress. Under conditions of stress, ATP levels may be inadequate to meet demand. Shivering caused by hypothermia probably represents the greatest threat to these patients. However, hyperthermia and stress from untreated pain also represent serious risks. The failure of ATP production to meet metabolic demands inevitably leads to lactic acidosis, often of profound significance. To avoid such problems, great care must be taken to keep patients normothermic during surgical cases and to provide adequate treatment for postoperative pain. Postoperative pain represents a particularly troublesome problem, because narcotics can further compromise respiratory status.

Mitochondrial patients may become acidotic, caused by high levels of lactate as a result of hypovolemia. Prolonged preoperative fasting should be avoided in these patients. If fasting is necessary, IV fluids should be started with glucose added to avoid anaerobic metabolism. As cyanide inhibits the respiratory chain, sodium nitroprusside should probably be avoided. For similar reasons, tourniquets should be avoided if possible. It is not clear what hematocrit value is adequate in these patients, but it is probably wise to maintain hematocrit at closer to normal levels than at the reduced levels allowed in other patients. Lastly, whereas mild levels of hypotension are commonly used in many patients to avoid blood loss, such an approach is less desirable in patients with mitochondrial disease. These patients are probably less able to compensate for decreased oxygen delivery.

Essentially, every general anesthetic studied has been shown to depress mitochondrial function. The most notable of these are the volatile anesthetics and propofol. It is often said that these agents only depress mitochondria at doses higher than their clinical concentrations. However, Miro and colleagues (1999) showed that even at doses commonly used in the operating room, anesthetics cause a significant depression of mitochondria in normal patients. Studies in model organisms have shown that when complex I is abnormal, sensitivity to volatile anesthetics is markedly increased (Kayser et al., 1999). Case reports have also indicated that some children exhibit an increased sensitivity to sevoflurane (Morgan et al., 2002). In addition, a strong clinical impression exists that children with mitochondrial myopathies have an increased risk during surgery (Morgan et al., 2002; Bolton et al., 2003; Farag et al., 2005). Because metabolism is altered in patients with mitochondrial

disease, the abilities of the cell to generate ATP and to effectively use oxygen are diminished, and exposure to anesthetics may represent an increased risk compared with other patients (Bolton et al., 2003). In contrast, others have found in retrospective studies that patients with mitochondrial defects did not appear to have an increased rate of perioperative complications (Driessen et al., 2007). Clearly, a prospective study is warranted to resolve these concerns. The use of regional anesthetics should be considered if appropriate for the case. However, it has also been noted that mitochondria are the probable target for the cardiac complications of bupivacaine; thus, patients with mitochondrial myopathies may be at increased risk with this drug as well (Weinberg et al., 2000).

From an anesthesiologist's point of view, the primary complications of mitochondrial myopathies include respiratory failure, impairment of myocardial function, conduction defects, and dysphagia. Each of the volatile anesthetics depresses respiration, though to varying degrees. Isoflurane and desflurane depress the ventilatory response to CO_2 more than does sevoflurane. In addition, isoflurane and desflurane cause more direct muscle relaxation. Thus, from this standpoint, sevoflurane would seem to be advantageous. However, isoflurane and desflurane are noted for their ability to maintain cardiac output to a greater degree than does sevoflurane (Weiskopf, 1995; Lowe et al., 1996). In short, each of the volatile anesthetics presently in use is capable of interacting negatively with a mitochondrial myopathy. Fortunately, patients may be supported during the perioperative period to avoid the theoretic or real side effects of these drugs. The volatile anesthetics do not require metabolism for excretion; rather, they are removed by ventilation, thus representing an advantage over IV anesthetics, which are dependent on energy-requiring metabolism. Lastly, the respiratory status of these patients (as with all patients with myopathies) must not be stressed, even when not exposed to anesthetics. Great care must be exercised while weaning them from ventilatory support to ensure adequate spontaneous ventilation.

During the past decade, the IV anesthetic propofol has become increasingly popular as a maintenance anesthetic. However, it has many of the same side effects as volatile anesthetics and is a profound inhibitor of several aspects of mitochondrial function. One notable exception is that it is not known to cause much muscle relaxation. However, it is quite capable of decreasing ventilatory drive as well as cardiac output and contractility. Although it is viewed as a short-acting drug, its ultimate elimination is metabolism dependent. Theoretic concern exists that patients with mitochondrial myopathy may have an increased risk of developing propofol-infusion syndrome during prolonged exposure. However, propofol has been used successfully both as an induction agent and as an infusion and seems to have little effect in this setting (Driessen, 2008). All of the general anesthetic agents are known to directly inhibit mitochondrial function and may add to preoperative problems. However, each of the anesthetics already discussed has been used successfully when caring for patients with mitochondrial disease. It may be that, as the various types of mitochondrial disease are better defined, anesthetic preferences in certain cases may become clear. However, such a recommendation cannot be made at the present time. What is clear is that these patients must be monitored more closely than other patients when a general anesthetic is used and that great care must be exercised to document that the effects of the anesthetics are largely gone before assuming that the patient can ventilate adequately.

Patients with mitochondrial myopathies respond well to the nondepolarizing relaxants, although they probably have an increased sensitivity. These drugs should be titrated to the desired effect and monitored closely by nerve stimulation. As noted for general anesthetics, great care must be exercised to ensure that these patients are fully reversed before removing them from ventilatory support. As motor neurons may be affected, a hyperkalemic response to succinylcholine may be seen. This drug should only be used when absolutely necessary in these patients. Succinylcholine and volatile anesthetics are also known as triggers for MH. MH is thought to be associated with some forms of mitochondrial myopathies, but the nature of this relationship is unclear. It may be that a group of mitochondrial myopathies mimics MH by having inadequate ATP for reuptake of calcium from the cytoplasm of muscle cells into the sarcoplasmic reticulum. Such a failure could cause prolonged muscle contraction and lead to increased metabolism. Clearly, this represents a complicated problem in these patients. Whether they increase their temperature or become acidemic depends on the nature and severity of their disease.

In general, regional anesthesia is well tolerated by patients with mitochondrial myopathies. This tolerance is in spite of data that indicate that local anesthetics, especially bupivacaine, are capable of potently depressing mitochondrial function. Although most neural blockade uses doses of anesthetic that are well below the doses necessary for mitochondrial effects, it is important to be aware that these drugs are also capable of such effects, especially on the heart. Despite this risk, however, because of the low doses commonly used, regional anesthesia represents a valuable mode of treatment. Ideally, such blocks avoid exposure of the CNS and cardiac muscle to potentially toxic side effects. Not all cases can be completed solely with regional anesthesia, especially in children. However, consideration should be given to this approach when possible, owing to the benefits of effective postoperative analgesia without sedation or respiratory compromise. It is important to remember that mitochondria are inhibited by local anesthetics. If a muscle biopsy is being performed for the diagnosis of mitochondrial disease, the muscle itself must not be exposed to the local anesthetic. Such exposure would likely lead to a false defect in mitochondrial function. A similar concern can be raised for the use of propofol in muscle biopsy cases, although it would be expected that the concentration of propofol in the muscle should be quite low.

At the present time, there is no perfect anesthetic for these patients. When possible, consideration should be given to the use of local anesthetics in small amounts for a regional anesthetic. When a general anesthetic is necessary, probably each of the general anesthetics in use has its place. At present it is not possible to entirely eliminate one group as less safe than others. What is clear is that these patients must be monitored more closely than other patients. The use CNS monitors to gauge their depth of anesthesia more closely may allow anesthesiologists to expose these patients only to the minimum amount of drug necessary to carry out the surgical procedure.

Muscular Dystrophy

At least five forms of muscular dystrophy are clinically relevant for anesthesiologists: Becker, Duchenne, facioscapulohumeral, Emery-Dreifuss, and limb-girdle muscular dystrophies (Farrell, 1994). These entities vary greatly in severity of presentation;

however, many of their implications for anesthesiologists are similar (Kerr et al., 2001; Schmidt et al., 2003). Duchenne's muscular dystrophy (DMD) is an X-linked disorder that results from deletion mutations in the dystrophin gene and leads to a complete lack of dystrophin in skeletal muscles (see Fig. 36-27, D). The defect is present in approximately 1 in 3500 live births, with the onset of disease often before school age and progressing to wheelchair dependence by the second decade of life. Dystrophin is a large protein that helps to anchor the contractile components (the actin myosin filaments) to the cell membrane and indirectly to the surrounding extracellular matrix (Fig. 36-30). Loss of this protein leads to profound muscle weakness and then respiratory failure, cardiomyopathy, cardiac conduction defects, and occasionally, mild mental retardation (Finsterer and Stollberger, 2003; Muntoni et al., 2003). Other, less global changes in this same gene cause Becker Muscular Dystrophy (BMD) and the related disease, X-linked dilated cardiomyopathy. Cardiomyopathy is occasionally seen in female carriers of the mutation. The clinical presentation of patients with various forms of muscular dystrophy are known to most anesthesiologists and are not reviewed in detail here other than as affects their anesthetic implications.

Anesthetic Considerations for Muscular Dystrophy

The approach to patients with DMD or BMD has changed in recent years. The main anesthetic implications of DMD and BMD are related to the severity of these profound myopathies. As would be expected in patients with muscle weakness, significant respiratory insufficiency can occur postoperatively with either disease. Cardiac muscle and conduction are also involved, and drugs that further depress cardiac function or that increase the likelihood of dysrhythmias should be avoided. All patients with DMD or BMD should receive a full cardiology evaluation with echocardiography within 3 months of surgery and pulmonary function testing before any surgery. Lastly, dysphagia is common, and gastric motility may be decreased, requiring expeditious control of the airway. The specific history of each patient

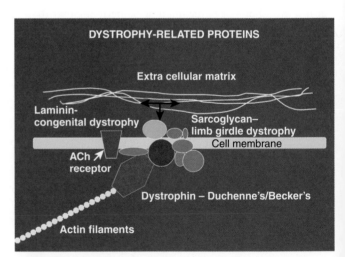

■ **FIGURE 36-30.** Dystrophy-related proteins; attachments of the actin filaments to the cell membrane and extracellular matrix. Disruption of these attachments alters protein distribution in the membrane and membrane stability. Some of the specific proteins (e.g., laminin, sarcoglycan, and dystrophin) that cause dystrophies are shown. *ACh,* Acetylcholine.

with DMD or BMD must be evaluated closely to determine the best technique to secure the airway.

In addition to playing a key role in anchoring contractile components to the cell membrane and the surrounding extracellular matrix, dystrophin is also important in organizing the postsynaptic acetylcholine receptors (Muntoni et al., 2003). In its absence, abnormalities occur both in the types of receptors and in their number and location, which may lead to abnormal responses to depolarizing muscle relaxants. Patients with BMD or DMD can have rhabdomyolysis and hyperkalemia in response to succinylcholine; thus, succinylcholine is contraindicated for them. It should also be noted that congenital forms of muscular dystrophy exist that probably involve other proteins necessary for attaching the contractile machinery to the extracellular matrix (see Fig. 36-30). Although this is a heterogeneous group of mutations, it is probably best to treat these patients as if they had DMD.

In the past few years, appreciation has increased concerning the risk of rhabdomyolysis and hyperkalemia in patients with DMD (and BMD) from exposure to volatile anesthetics alone. Hayes and colleagues (2008) present an important review of patients who had apparent hyperkalemic arrest after exposure to volatile anesthetics. These patients were felt to not have MH but to be still at risk for an untoward response to a volatile anesthetic. Although these events may be confused with MH, the association of DMD and BMD with true MH appears to be only coincidental. As a result, the authors strongly suggest using a "trigger-free" anesthetic in patients with known muscular dystrophy. This opinion is reinforced in a Consensus Statement from the American College of Chest Physicians (Birnkrant et al., 2007). However, at present no such recommendation has come from the ASA. The Association of Unusual Enzymopathies, Channelopathies, and Muscular Disorders with MH has been reviewed in a series of articles (Benca and Hogan, 2009; Davis and Brandom, 2009; Gurnaney et al., 2009; Hogan and Vladutiu, 2009; Klingler et al., 2009; Litman and Rosenberg, 2009; Parness et al., 2009).

Other Dystrophies

The remaining dystrophies—facioscapulohumeral (FSH), Emery-Dreifuss, and limb-girdle muscular dystrophy (LG)—are much milder in their presentations (Emery, 2002). FSH is one of the most common dystrophies; it is the most benign and usually is associated with little respiratory involvement (Fitzsimons, 1999). However, the neck, face, and scapular stabilizing muscles are often weak, and the ability to raise the head may be of little use in determining respiratory muscle strength (Dresner and Ali, 1989). Defects in the gene FRG1 are associated with FSH and with disrupted muscle growth in vertebrates; however, the function of FRG1 is unknown at present (Hanel et al., 2009).

Emery-Dreifuss muscular dystrophy usually has its onset in the teenage years and results from mutations in lamin (part of the nuclear matrix) or in emerin, an inner nuclear membrane protein that interacts with lamin and transcription regulators (Bione et al., 1994; Méjat et al., 2009). These patients have cardiac conduction defects, dilated cardiomyopathy, contractures (positioning problems), and often, fusion of C_3 to C_5, resulting in a less mobile neck (associated with difficult intubation) (Aldwinckle and Carr, 2002; Shende and Agarwal, 2002).

LG results from mutations in several proteins (at least 11 known), such as α-sarcoglycan, which associate with dystrophin. Some of these mutations are in proteins that overlap with those causing congenital muscular dystrophy. As in Emery-Dreifuss muscular dystrophy, LG is associated with some respiratory muscle weakness and cardiac conduction abnormalities, and at least some cases result from a defect in a protein that interacts with muscle cell membrane and is implicated in membrane repair (Capanni et al., 2003). The literature contains little regarding experience with the interaction of anesthetics with LG dystrophy (Pash et al., 1996).

In all three forms of muscular dystrophy, succinylcholine should be avoided, because hyperkalemia can result. MH is not reported in these three milder forms of muscular dystrophy. Thus, although not universal, the recurring themes with muscular dystrophy are to avoid succinylcholine, to watch for respiratory depression, and to avoid cardiac depressants and arrhythmogenic drugs. Volatile agents must be used with extreme caution because they are associated with rhabdomyolysis.

It is important to note that anesthetic complications have been reported in most of these types of muscular dystrophy (Farrell, 1994). These events most commonly involve a hyperkalemic episode, and sudden cardiac arrest may occur. Such events can occur in patients who are still in a subclinical stage of their disease and in whom the crisis may be the first manifestation. For this reason, many clinicians reserve their use of succinylcholine in children to only those cases in which there exists a specific indication for its use.

Metabolic Diseases

Several other genetic diseases of muscle exist that are of interest to anesthesiologists, including primary diseases of metabolism that lead to chronically weak muscles or muscles that are prone to damage when exposed to high metabolic stress. McArdle disease, an inherited disorder of muscle phosphorylase activity that down-regulates a Na^+K^+ membrane pump, is a prototypical disorder of this type (Clausen, 2003). Muscle from patients with McArdle disease can function normally until stressed by exercise or ischemia, at which time severely painful, electrically silent contracture develops, which can be followed by rhabdomyolysis, myoglobinuria, renal failure, and death. This sequence shares many elements with anesthesia-induced MH. Several MH-susceptible patients exhibited altered energy balance in response to caffeine, raising the possibility that disorders of intracellular energy production may contribute to the MH phenotype (Textor et al., 2003).

Patients with other less common diseases, such as Schwartz-Jampel syndrome, King-Denborough syndrome, and Brody disease, are also prone to anesthetic complications. In each case, MH-like responses have been reported, but their exact relationship to MH is not clear. King-Denborough syndrome is a progressive myopathy in which patients have short stature, severe scoliosis, pectus deformities, ptosis, low-set ears, and cryptorchism (Heiman-Patterson et al., 1986). Anesthesia-related deaths, fulminant episodes of MH, and positive in vitro contracture test results have been commonly associated with this disorder (Isaacs and Badenhorst, 1992). Because this disease is so rare, information about its genetic etiology is still lacking.

Patients with Brody disease (also known as Lambert-Brody disease) elicit a decreased ability to relax on repeated activation of their muscle, which results from an identified defect of the sarcoplasmic reticulum Ca^{2+}-ATPase (Odermatt et al., 2000). An in vitro contracture test performed on muscle from such a patient was abnormal, which may indicate that such patients may be at risk for MH-like syndrome (Froemming and Ohlendieck, 2001). Severe myotonia or neuromyotonia is a common feature of Schwartz-Jampel syndrome, in which hyperexcitability can be exacerbated by anesthetic agents and muscle relaxants are considered to be triggering agents for MH (Seay and Ziter, 1978; Ray and Rubin, 1994). It is unclear whether true MH is associated with this syndrome. In addition, difficult intubation because of neck and laryngeal anatomic abnormalities has been reported (Stephen and Beighton, 2002).

Clearly, these studies present as many questions as they do answers. Precise recommendations for the anesthetic care of these patients are not available. However, in general, the anesthesiologist probably should avoid the use of succinylcholine and volatile anesthetics while otherwise delivering normal meticulous anesthetic care. At present, the use of nontriggering anesthetics seems safe for this population, although any muscle relaxant must be used with the utmost caution. These patients should have prolonged observation for prolonged or recurrent weakness in the postoperative period.

The Undiagnosed Myopathy

In reviewing the above suggestions, an unpleasant scenario becomes apparent. What is the best anesthetic approach in the child with an undiagnosed myopathy? Depending on the molecular basis for the myopathy, the patient may turn out to have a diagnosis of mitochondrial defect or muscular dystrophy and may possibly be at risk for MH. The first possibility carries the recommendation to avoid propofol, and the second and third scenarios carry the recommendation to avoid volatile anesthetics (absolutely, if MH, and if possible, if muscular dystrophy). An insightful discussion of this conundrum was presented by Ross (2007) and Davis and Brandom (2009).

It is clear that volatile agents should be avoided if MH is a serious possibility. In those cases in which MH is not a concern, the choice of anesthetics depends on the likelihood of a mitochondrial defect vs. muscular dystrophy. Two reports of anesthetic management of children with muscle weakness who underwent muscle biopsy found that the likelihood of untoward effects using either class of drugs was low, in the range of 1% or lower (Driessen et al., 2007; Flick et al., 2007). To improve this number, it is incumbent on the anesthesiologist consult, the referring neurologist, and the geneticist/metabolism specialist to be aware of all aspects of the patient's history to determine which disease group is more likely. Until further information is available to guide the anesthesiologist, it remains crucial to closely monitor these patients during any anesthetic exposure and to maintain the close observation for several hours postoperatively.

SUMMARY

The anesthetic care of the pediatric patient with a systemic disorder provides myriad challenges for the anesthesiologist. A thorough understanding of the patient's disease and the effect that the anesthetic will have on the disease process are the two most important issues the anesthesiologist must address. For some of these patients, appropriate consultation with the surgeon, pediatrician, and pediatric subspecialist is essential to the proper management of these potentially difficult and challenging anesthetics.

For questions and answers on topics in this chapter, go to "Chapter Questions" at www.expertconsult.com.

REFERENCES

Complete references used in this text can be found online at www.expertconsult.com.

Malignant Hyperthermia

CHAPTER

37

Barbara W. Brandom

Deaths during anesthesia associated with high fever and tachycardia were described repeatedly in the first half of the 20th century (Moschcowitz, 1916; Burford, 1940). These deaths were sometimes ascribed to heat stroke and dehydration, because at that time intravenous hydration and air conditioning were not available. In 1915 and 1919, two deaths in one family occurred during chloroform anesthesia; in these cases, severe muscle spasm was observed before cardiac arrest. In 1987 a young child from this same family died during anesthesia for dental surgery. Subsequent in vitro contracture testing demonstrated susceptibility to malignant hyperthermia (MH) in several relatives in the family (Harrison and Isaacs, 1992). Even though MH is often suspected in cases such as these, in the 21st century it can still take years to complete MH diagnostic testing for a family.

Denborough was the first to investigate MH as a clinical entity (Denborough and Lovell, 1960; Denborough et al., 1962). Dr. James Villiers anesthetized a young Australian man for repair of a broken leg; the man was afraid to undergo general anesthesia because many of his relatives had died during ether anesthesia. Although during halothane anesthesia the patient became febrile, tachycardic, cyanotic, and hypotensive, he was aggressively cooled in the recovery room and he survived. Villiers asked his medical colleagues to investigate this patient and family. They found a pattern of anesthetic deaths consistent with an autosomal dominant trait. In 2009, despite many investigations, the genetic change associated with abnormal muscle calcium homeostasis in this family was still not identified (Ball, 2007).

An episode of MH is recognized by documentation of an increasing metabolic rate after exposure to a triggering agent such as a potent inhalation anesthetic. Rhabdomyolysis may also be observed. Susceptibility to MH is rarely associated with clinically evident hypermetabolism in the absence of drugs used during anesthesia (Gronert et al., 1980; Tobin et al., 2001). Halothane and succinylcholine, two drugs formerly used often in pediatric anesthesia, are two of the most potent triggers of MH. A review of 25 years of halothane anesthetics in one pediatric hospital found the incidence of acute MH episodes to range from 1:20,000 to 1:40,000 anesthesia procedures (Warner et al., 1984). Because choices of anesthetic and neuromuscular blocker influence the development of this potentially lethal syndrome, MH is a disease of particular concern to the pediatric anesthesiologist who chooses to administer inhalation anesthetics or succinylcholine. Indeed, in 2008 administration of succinylcholine during potent inhalation anesthesia precipitated cardiac arrest and death from MH (North American Malignant Hyperthermia Registry, 2008). The purpose of this chapter is to review the clinical manifestations, management, and underlying pathophysiology of MH.

MUSCLE PHYSIOLOGY

Normal Muscle Physiology

The propagation of an action potential down a motor nerve fiber produces depolarization of that fiber and release of acetylcholine (ACh) at the neuromuscular junction. When two molecules of ACh interact with the ACh receptor, the channel opens, allowing sodium to enter the cell and potassium to flow out. This initiates a wave of depolarization along the muscle cell membrane or sarcolemma. The propagated depolarization wave spreads internally via transverse tubules that abut onto the sarcoplasmic reticulum (SR) (Fig. 37-1). The SR is an internal cellular structure and a major storage site for calcium ions. The wall of the transverse tubule contains the dihydropyridine receptor, a voltage-dependent calcium channel that interacts with the calcium-sensitive ryanodine receptor (RYR), the footplate between the transverse tubule and the SR. Within a voltage window, calcium is released from the SR (Melzer and Dietze, 2001) into the sarcoplasm through RYR type 1 (RYR1). Increased calcium in the sarcoplasm also induces further calcium release from the SR.

Furthermore, when calcium has been depleted from the SR, a process known as store-operated calcium entry (SOCE) allows calcium entry into the sarcoplasm from the extracellular milieu (Fig. 37-2) (Zhao et al., 2006). Excitation-coupled calcium entry (ECCE) refers to the process by which extracellular calcium enters the sarcoplasm through the plasma membrane after depolarization (Cherednichenko et al., 2004; Lyfenko and Dirksen, 2008). The RYR has influence on both SOCE and ECCE.

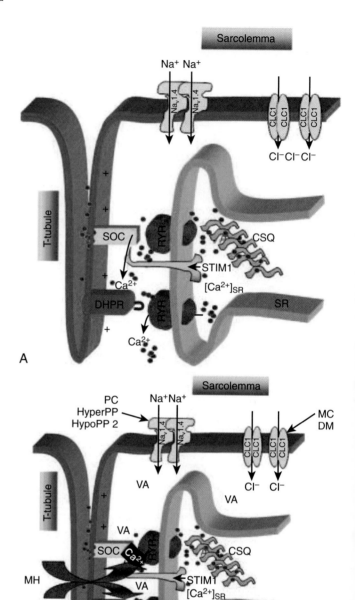

A

B

FIGURE 37-2. This diagram illustrates movement of calcium through the muscle cell after depolarization of the sarcolemma. Note several processes that contribute to elevation of calcium in the sarcoplasm during excitation-contraction coupling. *(Modified from Parness J et al.: The myotonias and susceptibility to malignant hyperthermia, Anesth Analg 109:1054, 2009.)*

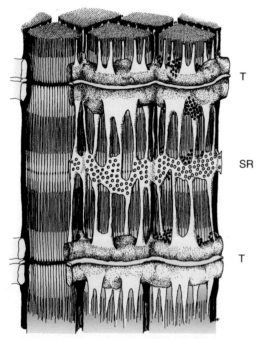

FIGURE 37-1. This three-dimensional reconstruction of the sarcoplasmic reticulum *(SR)* illustrates the continuity of the transverse tubules *(T)* surrounding the myofibrils and the fenestrations of the collar of the sarcoplasmic reticulum overlying the center of the A band of the myofibril. *(From Engel AG, Banker BQ, editors:* Myology basic and clinical, *New York, 1986, McGraw-Hill; modified from Peachey LD: The sarcoplasmic reticulum and transverse tubules of the frog's sartorius,* J Cell Biol *25:209, 1965.)*

Type 1 RYRs are found in all skeletal muscle, smooth muscle, neurons, and B lymphocytes. Type 2 RYRs are found in cardiac muscle, brain, and some hematopoietic cells. Type 3 RYRs are found in skeletal and smooth muscle and to a lesser extent in the brain. The function of RYR1 is modified by other proteins and by the redox state of the cell (Fig. 37-3) (Aracena-Parks et al., 2006; Goonasekera et al., 2007; Durham et al., 2008; Cornea et al., 2009; Protasi et al., 2009).

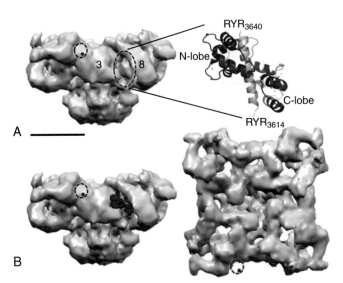

■ FIGURE 37-3. This cryoelectron microscopic model illustrates the shape of the ryanodine receptor (RYR1) and indicates areas where two other proteins interact with RYRY1. On the left is a side view of RYR1. The red dashed circle is the FK506 protein-binding site. The dashed blue oval is the approximate binding site of Ca^{2+} calmodulin *(CaM)* binding, between RYR1 cytoplasmic domains 3 and 8. On the top right is an atomic model of Ca^{2+} CaM in complex with RYR1 amino acids 3614-3640. The lower row is a space filling representation of CaM-RYR1 interaction from the side and from the cytoplasmic face of RYR1. *(From Cornea RL et al: FRET-based mapping of calmodulin bound to the RyR1 Ca^{2+} release channel,* Proc Natl Acad Sci USA *106:6128, 2009.)*

Calcium released from the SR combines with troponin, allowing cross-bridges to form between actin and myosin filaments and muscle to contract. When the wave of depolarization ceases, calcium ions dissociate from troponin and are removed from the sarcoplasm by adenosine triphosphate (ATP), requiring calcium pumps in the SR and other organelles. Thus, coupling of the excitation of the muscle membrane and contraction of the muscle cell entails changes in intracellular calcium concentration. Calcium increase in the sarcoplasm also initiates the breakdown of ATP and metabolic processes that support the energy needed for muscle contraction (e.g., glycolysis).

Pathophysiology of Malignant Hyperthermia

In classic MH, mutation of the *RYR1* gene produces enhanced activation of RYR1 by intraluminal calcium and reduced threshold for spontaneous calcium release during store calcium overload (store-overload–induced calcium release) (Jiang et al., 2008). In pigs, a specific single-point mutation in the RYR1 exists in all major breeds that are susceptible to malignant hyperthermia (Fuji et al., 1991). This point mutation is seen in a minority of human families who are susceptible to MH; however *RYR1* on chromosome 19q13.1 has been linked to MH susceptibility in the majority of families studied. Of the four other loci proposed as linked to MH susceptibility, only the *CACNA1S* on chromosome 1q13.1, coding for the α$_1$ subunit of the dihydropyridine receptor, has been linked to MH in more than two human families (Carpenter et al., 2009). The heterogeneous nature of human MH may be the result of a number of different mutations in *RYR1* or to abnormalities in other proteins such as the dihydropyridine receptor (Gallant and Lentz, 1992). In humans who have MH susceptibility, *RYR1* compound heterozygotes have been observed in several countries. This supports the claim that the incidence of a MH-causative genotype could be as great as 1 in 3000 people (Monnier et al., 2002; Ibarra et al., 2006).

The metabolic dysfunction of MH is caused by increased intracellular ionized calcium (Mickelson and Louis, 1996). A direct result of increased intracellular calcium is an increased need for intracellular ATP to drive pumps that transfer calcium into the SR, across the sarcolemma into the extracellular fluid, or into mitochondria. Increased demands for ATP lead to the clinically detectable manifestations of MH (e.g., an increase in metabolism). The elevation of intracellular calcium observed in MH muscle is decreased by dantrolene (Lopez et al., 1985; Mickelson and Louis, 1996; Cherednichenko et al., 2008).

Motor nerve activity and neuromuscular transmission are normal in patients who have MH susceptibility (Gronert, 1980). However, susceptible porcine muscle has a lower mechanical threshold than does normal muscle, and compared with normal muscle, less depolarization is required to initiate contraction (Moulds and Denborough, 1974; Okumura et al., 1979; Gronert, 1980). Calcium release from the SR occurs at more negative potentials in the presence of *RYR1* MH mutations, and calcium-induced calcium release from the SR is abnormal in subjects susceptible to MH. The abnormal RYR1 is resistant to the inhibitory effects of both calcium and magnesium (Mickelson and Louis, 1996).

During an episode of MH in pigs, lactate release from muscle increases before mixed venous oxygen tension decreases (Gronert and Theye, 1976a). This sequence is consistent with intracellular ATP depletion. Magnetic resonance imaging (MRI) techniques showed an increased ratio of inorganic phosphate to phosphocreatine in vivo in human muscle susceptible to MH. This ratio is an indicator of the energy state of the muscle (Chance et al., 1985a, 1985b). An increased ratio suggests either impaired synthesis of ATP or increased breakdown of ATP.

Mechanism of Action of Dantrolene

Since dantrolene was introduced in the 1970s, its use has remarkably improved the treatment and survival of patients with MH. It has been claimed that dantrolene inhibits the release of calcium from the SR by limiting the activation of the calcium-dependent RYR1, but more recently it was shown that dantrolene blocks ECCE across the plasma membrane (Fruen et al., 1997; Cherednichenko et al., 2008). Dantrolene does not act at the neuromuscular junction and has no effect on the passive or active electrical properties of the surface and tubular membranes of skeletal muscle fibers. Patients who have been given dantrolene have normal neuromuscular transmission and depressed force of muscle contraction. The protective effects of dantrolene against MH require significant depression of the force of contraction (Flewellen et al., 1983). Dantrolene can produce clinically significant weakness and decreased metabolism in normal muscle as well as in MH-susceptible muscle (Flewellen et al., 1983). It can reduce elevated creatine kinase (CK) in diseased muscle, independent of the presence of *RYR1* mutations (Bertorini et al., 1991; Kamper and Rodemann, 1992).

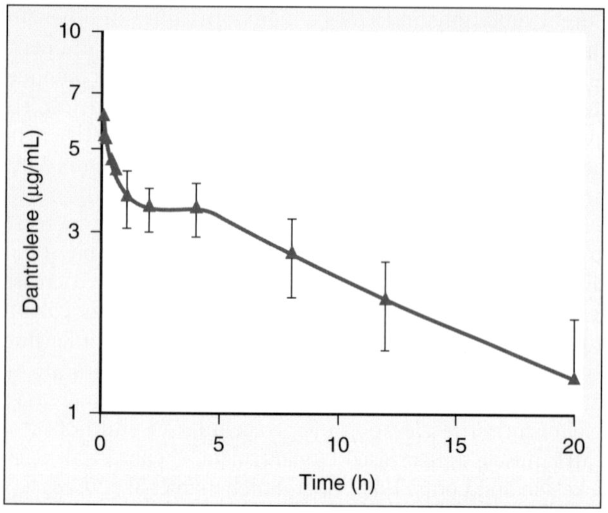

FIGURE 37-4. Plasma decay of dantrolene in children. *(From Lerman J et al: Pharmacokinetics of intravenous dantrolene in children, Anesthesiology 70:625, 1989.)*

The dose-response relationship of dantrolene in children has not been reported. Available data suggest that the half-life of dantrolene in children is somewhat shorter than that in adults: 7.3 to 9.8 hours and 12.1 hours, respectively (Fig. 37-4) (Lietman et al., 1974; Flewellen et al., 1983; Lerman et al., 1989). In adults, a cumulative dose of 2.2 to 2.5 mg/kg of dantrolene administered intravenously over 125 minutes produced a steady plasma concentration of dantrolene for longer than 5 hours (Flewellen et al., 1983). Orally administered dantrolene, a total of 5 mg/kg in 3 or 4 divided doses administered every 6 hours to adults with MH susceptibility, has also been shown to produce protective plasma concentrations of dantrolene for at least 6 hours after induction of anesthesia (Allen et al., 1988). In children, intravenous administration of 2.4 mg/kg of dantrolene infused over 10 minutes produced stable blood levels of about 3.5 mcg/mL for 4 hours, after which a slow decline in plasma concentration occurred (Lerman et al., 1989). Hence, it may be reasonable to repeat 1 mg/kg of dantrolene every 5 to 7 hours for prophylaxis. Alternatively, pharmacokinetic modeling with parameters derived in adults recommends a continuous infusion of dantrolene (Podranski et al., 2005). It is likely that when plasma concentrations of dantrolene are sufficient to inhibit an episode of MH, the patient experiences weakness and possibly disequilibrium.

A dynamometer could be used to assess grip strength objectively, but this requires the patient's cooperation. In a study of adults, the dose of dantrolene that produced maximal depression of grip strength and evoked force of thumb contraction had no significant effect on vital capacity (Flewellen et al., 1983). Similar studies have not been performed in children. Clinical experience suggests that less than 2 mg/kg of dantrolene administered intravenously to a child preoperatively can be associated with significant hypotonia in the postoperative period (Brandom and Carroll, unpublished observations). Weakness induced by dantrolene could compromise the ability to swallow and even necessitate artificial protection of the airway and mechanical ventilation, although this has never been reported in the literature (Flewellen et al., 1983). Intravenous dantrolene should be administered in settings where support of airway and ventilation can be easily provided.

CLINICAL PRESENTATION

The initial clinical signs of an impending episode of MH are nonspecific. The most commonly reported initial signs are hypercarbia, sinus tachycardia, and masseter spasm or jaw rigidity (Larach et al., 2010). Arrhythmias and tachypnea may be present (Box 37-1). Increased or rapidly increasing temperature is often an early sign of MH, and metabolic acidosis is often not observed before treatment of MH (Larach et al., 2010).

Rigidity of the extremities and the entire body are signs of fulminant MH. When MH is fulminant, there is severe metabolic acidosis (base deficit often greater than 8 mEq/L), respiratory acidosis (arterial carbon dioxide tension [Paco$_2$] of greater than 60 mm Hg), tachycardia with arrhythmias, a rapid increase in body temperature to 39.5° C or greater, hyperkalemia, myoglobinuria, and often, but not always, a marked increase in serum CK (Gronert, 1980; Newmark et al., 2007). However, because of modern comprehensive monitoring and increased awareness of MH, fulminant MH is rarely observed. The clinical diagnosis of MH is often considered before metabolism and temperature reach these extremes (Karan et al., 1994). The

---

Box 37-1 Steps in Identifying and Treating Malignant Hyperthermia

CLINICAL EVENTS DURING MH

Increased oxygen consumption
Increased minute ventilation with respiratory acidosis
Petco$_2$ > 55 mm Hg with appropriately controlled ventilation
Total body rigidity
Masseter spasm
Inappropriate sinus tachycardia
Ventricular tachycardia or ventricular fibrillation
Inappropriate increase in temperature; rapidly rising temperature (>1.5° C over 5 min) or temperature >38.8° C
Profuse sweating
Mottled, cyanotic skin
Cola-colored urine

- If any two or more of these events occur, determine venous blood Pco$_2$, Po$_2$, base excess, lactate, potassium ion, creatine phosphokinase, and myoglobin and consider discontinuing trigger agents. If temperature is >40° C, check clotting function and serum creatinine.
- If total body rigidity is present, without a neurologic explanation, send blood for laboratory evaluation as above, discontinue trigger agents, and begin treatment for acute MH episode.

LABORATORY EVALUATION: POSITIVE FINDINGS CONSISTENT WITH MH

Venous Pco$_2$ > 65 mm Hg with increased minute ventilation
Arterial Pco$_2$ > 60 mm Hg or 65 mm Hg with spontaneous ventilation > normal
Arterial base excess more negative than −8 mEq/L
Arterial pH < 7.25
Potassium ion > 6 mEq/L
Creatine kinase >10,000 IU/L after anesthetic without succinylcholine
Myoglobin in serum > 170 mcg/L
Myoglobin in urine > 60 mcg/L

Petco$_2$, End-tidal carbon dioxide tension; *Pco$_2$,* partial pressure of carbon dioxide; *Po$_2$,* partial pressure of oxygen.

patient's medical history and clinical course usually, but not always, help to differentiate fulminant MH from other metabolic crises such as porphyria, thyroid storm, untreated pheochromocytoma, and Ecstasy exposure (Allen and Rosenberg, 1990). Some other conditions that produce signs similar to MH are sepsis, allergic drug reactions, intracranial trauma, and hypoxic encephalitis.

Ideally, MH should be recognized and treated before it becomes fulminant. Treatment is more likely to be successful the earlier it is started, but because the signs of MH are not highly specific it is difficult for anesthesia practitioners to distinguish between early MH and many other complications. If there are only mild symptoms or signs suggestive of MH (e.g., moderate increases in heart rate, blood pressure, and temperature along with a slight metabolic or respiratory acidosis), yet evidence is later obtained that the patient is indeed susceptible to MH, this constellation of clinical findings could be called *abortive MH*. In such cases, masseter spasm may or may not occur (Ellis et al., 1990). There may be a moderate increase in CK and serum myoglobin. When considering the implications of these tests, note that myoglobin appears in the plasma within minutes of muscle injury by succinylcholine. However, CK continues to increase for 8 to 20 hours after a transient injury, even in patients who are not susceptible to MH (Florence et al., 1985). The incidence of abortive MH is as high as 1:4200 anesthesias when succinylcholine is used in combination with potent inhalation anesthetics (Ording, 1985). However, in the first decade of the 21st century, the incidence of MH cases identified by hospital discharge diagnosis codes was estimated to be about 1:100,000 anesthesias (Brady et al., 2009).

The diagnosis of MH may be mistakenly applied to patients suffering hyperkalemic cardiac arrest or sudden exacerbation of chronic rhabdomyolysis, which has occurred in pediatric patients after the administration of succinylcholine (Kovarik and Morray, 1995; Larach et al., 1997; Piotrowski and Fendler, 2007). In this condition, the sudden severe increase in plasma potassium can be fatal, but metabolic abnormalities are secondary to cardiac failure and not increased metabolism in skeletal muscle, as in MH (Delphin et al., 1987; Rosenberg and Gronert, 1992; Tang et al., 1992; Larach et al., 2001).

In a group of 48 children, 17 of whom later proved to be susceptible to MH by muscle biopsy, two or more adverse signs or abnormal laboratory findings were present in all patients with positive in vitro contracture tests (Larach et al., 1987). However, similar adverse events occurred in 83% of the children who had negative muscle-biopsy findings. Generalized muscle rigidity was the single factor significantly associated with positive biopsy findings for MH. However, generalized muscle rigidity is not an absolute predictor of MH susceptibility. Three of 24 patients, who were referred for muscle-contracture testing to evaluate MH susceptibility and had negative contracture test results, had experienced generalized muscle rigidity during induction of anesthesia. Signs consistent with abortive MH, such as tachycardia, premature ventricular contractions, elevated end-tidal carbon dioxide, and increase in tension of the masseter muscle may be observed in the normal pediatric patient who is given halothane or sevoflurane and succinylcholine (Van der Spek et al., 1987; 1988; Lanier et al., 1990). Larach and others (1987) could not identify the patient with MH susceptibility on the basis of these signs (Hackl et al., 1990). Therefore, when MH is suspected clinically, after treating the patient arrangements should be made for confirmatory testing (see related sections in this chapter).

If events during the induction of anesthesia require explanation beyond light anesthesia, transient rigidity and tachycardia during inhalation of sevoflurane, or hypoventilation, further investigation to rule out the diagnosis of MH must be undertaken immediately, before surgery begins. The anesthesiologist must document the presence of increased metabolic rate, rather than the decreased metabolic rate that usually follows induction of anesthesia. Venous or arterial blood should be obtained for measurement of partial pressure of carbon dioxide [Pco_2], lactate, potassium, and CK. Mixed venous blood is most likely to show significant alterations in Pco_2, but it may not be readily available (Gronert and Theye, 1976a, 1976b). During anesthesia there is increased arterial-to-venous shunting through the skin. Despite this fact, blood from a large peripheral vein, femoral or antecubital, may demonstrate increasing Pco_2 and worsening base deficit before these changes are found in arterial blood. Increasing end-tidal carbon dioxide concentrations, particularly with increased minute ventilation, supports the presumptive diagnosis of MH. Evidence of muscle injury, such as the presence of myoglobin in the serum and urine and elevated CK and other enzymes in the blood, may not be observed if MH is treated very quickly. With anesthesia techniques common in the 21st century, MH may not be recognized until the second or third hour of anesthesia. MH may first be recognized in the postoperative recovery room. Fatal MH can occur without exposure to anesthetics (Brown et al., 2000). Once a hypermetabolic state is recognized, appropriate actions must be taken without delay, as described later.

MASSETER SPASM

Masseter spasm (also termed *masseter muscle rigidity* or *trismus*) is a marked increase in tension of the masseter that prevents opening of the mouth when succinylcholine has produced neuromuscular blockade. Masseter spasm may be an early sign of MH. However, succinylcholine can produce increased tension in normal muscle at the same time that it produces block of neuromuscular transmission (van der Spek et al., 1987, 1988). Many anesthesiologists believe that only if the jaw cannot be forced open should this phenomenon be called masseter spasm.

Hannallah and Kaplan (1994) distinguish between masseter muscle rigidity and trismus. In masseter muscle rigidity, the mouth cannot be fully opened even with firm pressure on the incisors, but the mouth can be opened far enough to permit intubation of the trachea. In trismus, the mouth cannot be opened enough to permit intubation of the trachea. Using these definitions, Hannallah and Kaplan (1994) noted rigidity in 0.2% of 500 children anesthetized with halothane and administered succinylcholine, but none of these 500 patients experienced trismus. It may be that the several-fold greater incidence of masseter spasm noted in the 1980s included cases of incomplete jaw relaxation (i.e., the mouth opens fully with firm manual separation of the teeth), which was observed in 4.4% of these 500 pediatric patients. The 22 patients with incomplete jaw relaxation in this study continued to receive halothane anesthesia with no apparent complications. Masseter spasm has been touted as a specific early warning sign of MH. Undoubtedly, deaths from MH have occurred during anesthetic procedures in which masseter spasm was observed and in cases in which it was not observed. It may be that when masseter spasm is accompanied by rigidity of the entire body, MH is likely to occur. However, transient increase in jaw stiffness, or resting tension of jaw muscles, is a normal response to succinylcholine (van der Spek et al., 1987, 1988; Plumley et al., 1990). Increase in masseter muscle tension occurs in normal mammals after the administration of succinylcholine with prior administration of epinephrine (Pryn and van der Spek, 1990). There is a greater increase in jaw tension after administration of succinylcholine during halothane anesthesia than in the presence of barbiturates. Jaw tension is also increased in animals that are febrile as opposed to those that are normothermic (Storella et al., 1993). Temporomandibular joint abnormalities may confuse the diagnosis of masseter spasm by interfering with jaw opening.

Although masseter spasm usually occurs after anesthesia induction with halothane and the administration of succinylcholine, it may occur with other anesthetic agents (Larach et al., 1987; Marohn and Nagia, 1992; Takamatsu et al., 1996). Masseter spasm occurs despite abolition of evoked muscle function in the extremities. Tachycardia or other nonspecific arrhythmias may accompany masseter spasm. MH may follow masseter spasm immediately; in the continued presence of anesthetic trigger agents, however, a period of 10 or more minutes often intervenes between masseter spasm and the clinical presentation of MH when the clinical presentation of MH is defined as arterial Pco_2 greater than or equal to 50 mm Hg, pH less than 7.25, and base deficit more negative than 8 mEq/L (O'Flynn et al., 1994).

Anesthesia with halothane has been continued after isolated masseter spasm with no increased metabolism or cardiovascular instability. Littleford and others (1991) reported on 57 such children, of whom 33% experienced transient arrhythmias intraoperatively. Most of these children also had some degree of hypercarbia or metabolic acidosis. CK levels measured 18 to 24 hours postoperatively were elevated in all but one of these children, and CK levels greater than 20,000 units/L were observed in many. However, there were 11 children who experienced generalized rigidity in combination with masseter muscle spasm. Anesthesia was aborted for four of these children and continued without inhalation agents in three of the children. None of these children developed fulminant MH in the perioperative period. The remaining four patients who developed generalized rigidity received dantrolene. Kaplan and Rushing (1992) documented a case of masseter spasm in which clinical abnormalities prompted administration of dantrolene, and postoperative CK was 40,000 IU. Nine years later, this healthy adolescent had completed extensive evaluation for neuromuscular disorders, including in vitro testing for MH with the caffeine-halothane contracture test (CHCT). The patient and family remained without signs, symptoms, or diagnosis of any myopathy. If this patient had been labeled as susceptible to MH, it would have been a misdiagnosis. Total body rigidity accompanying masseter muscle rigidity does not absolutely guarantee that the patient has MH (Larach et al., 1987). Anesthetic depth may have been misjudged; however, if rigidity does not abate when deep neuromuscular block was produced with nondepolarizing blockers, muscle must be abnormal. Either fulminant MH is occurring or the patient may have occult myotonia (Neuman and Kopman, 1993).

Inhalation anesthesia without succinylcholine was associated with fewer episodes of both fulminant (2 vs. 8) and abortive (17 vs. 110) MH than was succinylcholine with potent inhalation anesthetics in a Danish population (Ording, 1985). Thus, avoiding succinylcholine administration to pediatric patients anesthetized with inhalation anesthetics not only avoids the diagnostic uncertainties associated with masseter spasm but also produces fewer episodes of MH and other adverse events (Delphin et al., 1987; Rosenberg and Gronert, 1992). Pediatric anesthesiologists may choose to administer succinylcholine only when definite, strong indications for this drug have been identified.

Management of Masseter Spasm

There is no agreement among experienced clinicians concerning the preferred management of patients with incomplete relaxation of the masseter after the administration of succinylcholine (Kaplan et al., 1993). If jaw stiffness is mild, so that the mouth can be opened with increased effort, there is no rigidity in the rest of the body, and cardiovascular function is stable, anesthesia may be continued with careful documentation of capnography and core temperature. Fluid deficits should be replaced completely so that urine output is greater than 3 mL/kg per hour. Urine should be obtained in the early postoperative period to check for the presence of myoglobin. Blood should be obtained for measurement of electrolytes and CK. It is not necessary to terminate anesthetic administration unless signs of increasing metabolic rate occur. If jaw stiffness is so great that the mouth cannot be opened, there are several reasons to terminate elective anesthetic administration, not the least of which may be the need to clear the upper airway. If trismus and extensor rigidity are present, biochemical signs of MH should be sought and treatment of MH initiated. Venous blood should be obtained for gas analysis and measurement of electrolytes, myoglobin, and CK. If rigidity persists in the presence of neuromuscular blockade either the patient has MH or a form of myotonia.

After an episode of masseter spasm, myalgia and occasionally weakness may be present for several days or longer. In patients who were not susceptible to MH and undergoing ophthalmic surgery with halothane anesthesia who received succinylcholine intraoperatively, an increase in CK level was noted 24 hours after surgery. The highest postanesthetic CK level in these otherwise healthy patients was 40 times that of normal (Inness and Stromme, 1973). Myoglobin appears quickly in the plasma after halothane anesthesia and succinylcholine administration, even in children who had no masseter spasm (Plotz and Braun, 1982). If radioimmunoassay is used to measure serum myoglobin concentrations, increases in myoglobin can be measured within the first hour after succinylcholine administration in normal children anesthetized with isoflurane or halothane.

If surgery must continue, inhalation anesthesia can be stopped and intravenous anesthetics given. Intraarterial, central venous, and bladder catheters are useful if evidence of increased metabolism is found and dantrolene is administered. Muscle tension of the rest of the body should be noted.

Postoperative renal failure has occurred in patients who had myoglobinuria after administration of succinylcholine during anesthesia. In any situation in which injury to muscle may occur, it is important to document that myoglobinuria is not present. If increased muscle stiffness is noted after administration of succinylcholine or the if child complains of muscle pain postoperatively, urine should be obtained. If there is no blood in the urine as assessed by orthotolidine (Hematest), then there is no myoglobin present (Bosch et al., 2009). If the response to blood is positive on the dipstick, urine should be examined for the presence of red blood cells, and free hemoglobin and myoglobin should be measured. If myoglobin is present, the patient should remain in the hospital. The patient should be observed for signs of MH, evaluated for the presence of occult muscle disease, and well hydrated. Alkaline urine may reduce the risk of renal tubular injury from myoglobin (Elsayed and Reilly, 2010).

TREATMENT OF AN ACUTE EPISODE OF MALIGNANT HYPERTHERMIA

When the diagnosis of MH is strongly suspected, the most important step to take is to administer dantrolene. The other steps in management are to discontinue the triggering anesthetic agents immediately, increase minute ventilation several-fold with 100% oxygen at the highest possible flow rate, check core temperature, and alert the surgeon that the procedure must be concluded promptly. Other anesthesiologists, paramedical personnel, or both should be called in at once for assistance. If core temperature is higher than 39° C, cooling measures should be applied until temperature is below 38° C (see *www.mhaus.org*).

Dantrolene must be diluted with sterile, preservative-free, distilled water that should be stored in large quantities with the drug (Table 37-1). It is important to store sterile water in clearly labeled containers of a different size from those used for routine intravenous solutions and to keep a mixing system nearby. New formulations of dantrolene may go into solution faster than did dantrolene manufactured before 2008. The initial intravenous dantrolene dose should be 2.5 mg/kg, although more than 10 mg/kg may be needed to control the episode (Larach et al., 2010). Repeated dosing should be guided by clinical and laboratory signs. A flow sheet including minute ventilation, end-tidal carbon dioxide concentration, heart rate and rhythm, arterial

blood pressure, central venous pressure, core temperature, and urine output, along with arterial and venous blood gas tensions, serum electrolytes, and glucose and total fluid intake, provides a useful guide for continued therapeutic interventions. Dantrolene must be administered until respiratory and metabolic acidosis, tachycardia and stiffness have resolved. The usual upper limit of 10 mg/kg may be exceeded as necessary. The most common side effects of this drug are muscle weakness and phlebitis.

The anesthesia machine need not always be switched to a standby unit that has been kept free of inhalation anesthetics. However, because of both the increased internal gas volume of and the increased anesthetic solubility in modern anesthesia work stations, more time may be required to eliminate traces of anesthetic. For example, over 100 minutes of 10 L/min fresh gas flow (10 L/min FGF) was needed to reduce residual inhalation anesthetic to 5 ppm in the Drager Fabius anesthesia machine, whereas after 20 minutes residual sevoflurane was less than 5 ppm in the Drager Narcomed GS machine (Gunter et al., 2008; Whitty et al., 2009). Isoflurane washout can require more than 45 minutes of 10 L/min FGF in the Drager Primus machine, more than 50 minutes in the Datex-Ohmeda machine, and more than 75 minutes in the Aestiva machine (Crawford et al., 2007; Birgenheier et al., 2009). If the carbon dioxide absorber and circuit tubing are not changed, 30 minutes of 10 L/min FGF is needed to reach 2 ppm isoflurane in the Datex-Ohmeda work station (Schonell et al., 2003). In summary, replacement of all exposed elements, including the ventilator diaphragm and breathing system with autoclaved or new parts, provides the fastest preparation of the anesthetic work station without the addition of charcoal filters. Continuation of 10 L/min FGF for the duration of the anesthesia has been recommended to avoid increasing concentrations of agent (Crawford et al., 2007; Whitty et al., 2009). If MH occurs after the first hour of exposure to an inhalation anesthetic, there is a substantial volume of the anesthetic trigger agent in the patient's body. It is likely that placement of a charcoal filter on the inspiratory limb of the anesthesia circuit and administration of 10 L/min FGF could greatly speed elimination of potent anesthetic from the breathing circuit (Gunter et al., 2008; Birgenheier et al., 2009.)

Procedures to cool the body should be instituted quickly. The goal is to reduce muscle metabolism and avoid exposure to a critical core temperature of greater than 40° C (Bouchama and Knochel, 2002). Furthermore, a temperature that is higher than normal may accelerate an MH episode in humans, as has been observed in animals (Chelu et al., 2006; Dainese et al., 2009). Drapes should be removed, heated humidifiers and hot air blowers should be turned off, and water mattresses should be turned to cooling temperatures. Room temperature normal saline solution should be given intravenously to maintain normal central venous pressure. The stomach can be irrigated with iced saline solution through an orogastric tube. Open body cavities can also be lavaged with iced saline solution, and ice packs can be placed in the groin and axillae where large vessels come close to the skin surface.

An arterial catheter should be inserted to observe the patient's hemodynamic status and acid-base balance. A central venous catheter is useful for obtaining cardiac filling pressures and blood gas tensions, as well as for administering intravenous fluids. A pulmonary artery catheter allows measurement of mixed venous blood gases and lactate and adjustment of cardiac filling pressures in the patient with pulmonary edema. Mixed

TABLE 37-1. Drugs and Dosages Used to Treat an Acute Episode of Malignant Hyperthermia

Dantrolene*	2.5-10 mg/kg or more (Sterile water must be available to dilute dantrolene.)
Sodium bicarbonate	2 mmol/kg as needed
Iced normal saline solution	As needed (10-12 L for 50-kg patient)
Mannitol	300 mg/kg (Note that there is 150 mg of mannitol per milligram of dantrolene in the vial.)
Furosemide	0.5-1 mg/kg
Insulin (regular)	10 units regular insulin in 50 mL of 50% dextrose titrated to produce normokalemia
Lidocaine	1 mg/kg

*Dantrolene administration should be repeated until physical and chemical signs have returned to normal. When this degree of physiologic stability has been obtained, dantrolene (1 mg/kg or more) should be repeated approximately every 6 hours until all signs of MH, including muscle stiffness, have abated and creatine kinase has decreased consistently. If the patient is metabolically stable, vital signs are normal, and muscle weakness is present, the interval between dantrolene doses can be increased to 8 hours.

venous blood is a more sensitive indicator of the patient's acid-base status than arterial blood. A blood sample should be taken to determine the blood gases and pH, potassium, glucose, CK, myoglobin, creatinine, and clotting profile as soon as feasible.

Hyperkalemia results when cell membranes are disrupted and when acidosis is severe. This is recognized on the electrocardiogram as increased T-wave amplitude in the early stages and later by widening QRS complexes, intraventricular conduction delays and blocks, and finally no organized rhythm at all. Intravenous calcium is appropriate emergency treatment of the hyperkalemia associated with MH (Gronert et al., 1986). Glucose and insulin (10 units of regular insulin in 50 mL of 50% glucose titrated to effect) can be administered to lower serum potassium temporarily. β-agonists can also be useful to move potassium intracellularly.

Large losses of intravascular volume should be anticipated; evaporative loss of fluid may be great, and edema formation may occur in muscles and in other tissues during fulminant MH. Intravenous fluids should be given to maintain normal cardiac filling pressures, as evidenced by adequate perfusion pressure, urine output, and capillary refill. Alkaline osmotic diuresis is induced by mannitol in the current formulation of dantrolene (150 mg of mannitol/mg of dantrolene in Dantrium). This protects renal tubule function in the presence of myoglobinuria and promotes acute intravascular volume loss. The management of the acute MH episode is summarized in Box 37-2.

Because calcium channel blockers might interfere with excitation-contraction coupling and conserve energy reserves, it is reasonable to ask what effects such drugs might have on MH-susceptible muscle (Lynch et al., 1986). Not all calcium channel-blocking drugs have the same effects in subjects with

MH susceptibility. Diltiazem inhibits halothane-induced contracture in MH-susceptible pig muscle, thus confirming a single similar observation in human muscle (Illias et al., 1985). Verapamil, however, is not a therapeutic agent in porcine MH (Gallant et al., 1985). Furthermore, verapamil and dantrolene can interact to produce severe hyperkalemia and myocardial depression (Lynch et al., 1986; Rubin and Zablocki, 1987). Nifedipine administration has been associated with the development of MH in a child with underlying neuromuscular disease (Cook and Henderson-Tilton, 1985). At this time, it seems prudent to administer calcium channel-blocking drugs to patients with a history of MH or neuromuscular disease only with caution. Calcium channel blockers are not recommended in the management of acute MH. If dantrolene must be administered to a patient who is also receiving calcium channel-blocking drugs, invasive hemodynamic monitoring and frequent measurement of serum potassium levels have been recommended (Lynch et al., 1986; Rubin and Zablocki, 1987).

Postanesthesia Considerations

A patient who has been successfully treated for MH in the operating room requires intensive care to continue treatment and to monitor for late manifestations of the disorder. Continuation of treatment is necessary, because recrudescence of MH can occur after an episode that has apparently been successfully treated. This usually happens in the first few hours after the initial event. Patients with a muscular body type, temperature increase, or longer interval between induction of anesthesia and beginning of the MH reaction had increased risk of recrudescence (Burkman et al., 2007). As much as 12 mg/kg of dantrolene has been required to treat recurrences over 12 hours (Pollock et al., 1992). Continuous monitoring of vital signs and minute ventilation, and frequent measurement of venous lactate, blood gases, and electrolytes should detect metabolic changes. Dantrolene should be administered intravenously as necessary, not only until no evidence of metabolic acidosis remains, but also until serum myoglobin levels decrease toward normal or there is no myoglobinuria. The half-life of myoglobin in the blood is normally 1 to 3 hours. In contrast, CK peaks 24 to 36 hours after injury and usually decreases about 40% per day thereafter (Salluzzo, 1992).

After an acute episode, the patient with MH may die of a recrudescence, disseminated intravascular coagulopathy, or other nonspecific systemic injury. Disseminated intravascular coagulopathy is a common finding in fatal MH (Larach et al., 2008). The administration of dantrolene should be continued to stop the disruption of muscle, the presumed underlying cause of disseminated intravascular coagulopathy. Supportive intensive care should be given as indicated, and coagulation function must be carefully monitored during and after an episode of MH.

Late manifestations of an episode of MH range from mild muscle pain to multiorgan system failure. Cerebral edema may occur. Fulminant cases of MH may have permanent neurologic sequelae (e.g., coma or paralysis) for no apparent reason. Even satisfactory care during anesthesia may not prevent these neurologic complications (Gronert, 1980). Rehabilitation can take months after an episode of fulminant MH.

Pulmonary edema may occur because of marked shifts in intravascular volume, myocardial dysfunction, and the effects

---

Box 37-2 Management of the Acute Malignant Hyperthermia Episode

Follow treatment guidelines prepared by MHAUS (see *www.mhaus.org*).

- Stop inhalation anesthetics immediately.
- Cancel or conclude surgery as soon as possible.
- Hyperventilate with >10 L/min of 100% oxygen.
- Administer dantrolene (2.5 mg/kg) intravenously over 5 minutes and repeat as needed. Give more dantrolene if signs of MH reappear.
- Initiate cooling with intravenous cold saline solution (15 mL/kg over 10 minutes), ice packs in the axillae and groin, and lavage of body cavities with cold saline solution if the core temperature is greater than 39° C. Stop cooling when the core temperature falls to 38° C.
- Correct metabolic acidosis with 1 to 2 mEq/kg of sodium bicarbonate as an initial dose.
- Administer calcium (10 mg/kg of calcium chloride) or insulin (0.2 mcg/kg) in 50% dextrose in water (1 mL/kg) to treat the effects of hyperkalemia.
- Follow Advanced Cardiac Life Support algorithm to treat dysrhythmias. Lidocaine may be given during an MH crisis.
- Maintain urine output of 2 mL/kg per hour with additional mannitol and furosemide (1 mg/kg) if needed.
- Insert arterial and central venous catheters.
- Repeat venous blood gas and electrolyte analyses every 15 minutes until these and vital signs normalize.

of heat shock. The presence of pulmonary edema requires more careful assessment of the circulatory status to improve cardiac filling pressures and inotropic state. Areas of myocardium may have abnormal conduction, decreased contractility, or both. It is important to maintain adequate renal perfusion, because massive myoglobinuria produced by fulminant MH can cause acute renal failure. Sufficient muscle damage to produce myoglobinuria and acute renal failure can occur in the absence of pigmenturia or dramatic elevation of CK (Grossman et al., 1974). If myoglobin (or hemoglobin) is present, urine gives a positive reaction with orthotolidine (Hematest). In the presence of myoglobinuria, normal saline solution should be given to force a diuresis of at least 3 mL/kg per hour; if urine output is less than this, then mannitol (1 mL of 25% solution) and bicarbonate (1 mEq) in 5% dextrose in water (D$_5$W; 8 mL) should be given at twice the maintenance fluid rate. Rapidly increasing serum creatinine signals the onset of renal failure.

All cases of MH, anesthetic-related episodes of increased metabolism or rhabdomyolysis, isolated masseter spasm, and anesthetics administered to patients who have undergone a CHCT should be reported to the Malignant Hyperthermia Registry, so that the epidemiologic study of MH may have as broad a scope and as complete a collection of data as possible. Report forms may be obtained by telephone (888-274-7899) or printed from *www.mhreg.org*.

PROPHYLACTIC MANAGEMENT

Indications for Muscle Biopsy and Genetic Evaluation of Type 1 Ryanodine Receptor

Indications may vary depending on the particular goals being addressed. Individuals, both patients and physicians, concerned with improving the diagnostic tests for MH may urge all patients with any symptoms consistent with MH and those with a clear history of fulminant MH to undergo muscle biopsy and CHCT. Others prefer to advise that this invasive test be performed only when the predictive value of the test is likely to be helpful for patient management. The CHCT is currently the only method that can rule out MH susceptibility. The Clinical Grading Scale (CGS) was developed using the Delphi process to provide clinical definition of a case that is almost certain to be MH for the purpose of defining the diagnostic criteria of the CHCT (Larach et al., 1994). Box 37-1 contains many of the elements of the CGS. The five processes evaluated by the CGS (rigidity, muscle breakdown, respiratory acidosis, temperature increase, and cardiac involvement) each contribute a limited number of points to the score. Scores are further divided into categories of likelihood of the patient having MH. Category 6 is almost certain MH; category 5 indicates that MH is very likely; category 4 means that MH is somewhat greater than likely; category 3 indicates that MH is somewhat less than likely; category 2 implies that MH is unlikely; and in category 1, the chance of a patient having MH is almost none. If the total score of the CGS is 50 or more, the case is category 6, almost certain to be MH. If the score is between 35 and 49 the case is category 5, very likely to be MH. The CGS must be applied with medical judgment to estimate the probability that a given anesthesia event was MH. It is important to document the adequacy of minute ventilation when interpreting carbon

dioxide tensions. Increased minute ventilation may be the only sign of MH. This produces a category 3 score on the CGS, indicating that MH is somewhat less than likely and might suggest that further testing is not warranted. However, if the anesthesiologist feels that carbon dioxide production was increased and this was reversed by elimination of potent anesthetic, the patient should be referred for testing of MH susceptibility. On the other hand, a child who has sepsis with cerebral palsy, or one of many other medical conditions, may have a high score on the CGS. Referral of a patient whose illness is explained by other processes for evaluation of MH susceptibility would be a costly waste of effort.

A new benefit of undergoing CHCT is that patients with contracture tests indicating MH susceptibility are candidates for genetic study. Initial studies of the *RYR1* gene in these subjects with MH susceptibility were limited to the three hot spots in *RYR1*. However, as a larger proportion of the *RYR1* gene is studied, the percentage of patients who have MH susceptibility with *RYR1* mutations or variants of unknown significance (VUS) has increased to 50% or more (Robinson et al., 2003; Sambuughin et al., 2005; Ibarra et al., 2006; Levano et al., 2009). The process of evaluating MH susceptibility in relatives can begin with genetic evaluation in search of the familial mutation (Urwyler et al., 2001; Girard et al., 2004) after an *RYR1* mutation has been identified in the proband. Because fewer than 50% of all people who undergo contracture testing may be diagnosed as susceptible to MH by this test, if evaluation of MH status begins with screen of *RYR1,* the yield of positive diagnoses will be low (Girard et al., 2004).

A panel of 17 *RYR1* exons, encompassing all the acknowledged MH mutations, is available as a clinically useful genetic test of MH susceptibility (Sei et al., 2004) (see *www.mhaus.org* for the addresses of the diagnostic laboratories). It may detect a *RYR1* abnormality in about 30% of North American patients who would be diagnosed as susceptible to MH by CHCT. With this test, genetic counseling is available at the University of Pittsburgh, Center for Medial Genetics (800-54-8155). It is expected that genetic testing of MH susceptibility will be less sensitive but also less invasive and less costly than muscle biopsy and CHCT, because the genetics of MH susceptibility is not completely known (Nelson et al., 2004). Therefore, clinical genetic testing is of most value for determining affected family members in a family in which an *RYR1* mutation has been found in an individual who experienced severe MH or had a positive CHCT. The incidence of compound heterozygotes is relatively high when the entire *RYR1* gene is examined. Therefore, if an individual does not have the familial *RYR1* variant, contracture testing must be performed to prove that the patient is not susceptible to MH.

Individuals who have had positive muscle contracture tests after experiencing MH episodes should undergo genetic screening and document the result in the MH Registry (*www.mhreg.org*; 888-74-7899). If no abnormality is found in the *RYR1* gene in such patients, these are important subjects for experimental study of MH genetics.

The sensitivity and specificity of the CHCT have been determined; therefore, general statements about the predictive value of this test can be made (Larach et al., 1992; Larach, 1993; Ording et al., 1997; Allen et al., 1998). The clinician needs to know the predictive value of the test because the clinician can obtain the results of the diagnostic test. Before applying the test, the clinician cannot be sure whether or not the patient really has the disease.

The positive predictive value (PPV) of a test is the probability that an individual whose test result indicates that the disease is present does indeed have the disease of interest. The negative predictive value (NPV) of a test is the probability that an individual whose test result indicates that disease is absent does not have the disease in question. By definition, the predictive value depends on the probability that the individual has the disease in question before the test results are obtained, as well as the sensitivity and specificity of the test (Rosner, 1990). The sensitivity of a diagnostic test is the probability that a test result will indicate the disease is present, when in fact the individual tested has the disease in question. Specificity is the probability that a test result will indicate disease is not present, when in fact the individual tested does not have the disease in question. The definition of a positive result of the CHCT was set to make this test sensitive, so that fewer than 1% of the people who would be at risk of MH events would fail to be identified by the CHCT. Therefore, the CHCT could not also be highly specific. To apply Bayes Theorem and estimate the PPV or NPV, given the sensitivity and specificity of the CHCT, a clinician also has to make a decision about the probability that the patient is MH susceptible before the diagnostic results are known (Rosner, 1990). This probability may be thought of as the prior probability of the individual having the disease of interest or, if a population rather than an individual is considered, the incidence of the disease in the population (Box 37-3).

Rather than speculate on what a group of clinical findings suggests about the probability of MH susceptibility in an individual, it is possible to use the test characteristics (sensitivity and specificity) to calculate the predictive value of the CHCT over a wide range of prior probabilities (Fig. 37-5, *A* and *B*). For example, if a patient with a history of isolated masseter spasm is thought to have less than a 25% chance of having MH, then if the sensitivity of the CHCT is 99% and the specificity

is 85%, the positive predictive value of the CHCT in that individual is less than 69% and the negative predictive value is greater than 99%. In other words, the chance of that individual having a false-positive result of CHCT is at least 30%, and the chance of a false-negative result is less than 1%. In contrast, if a patient with a strong family history of MH has many of the clinical signs of MH, it might be judged that the probability of that individual having MH, before obtaining the result of the CHCT, would be 80%. The positive and negative predictive values of the CHCT would be 96% and 99%, respectively, for such a patient. These statements are oversimplifications in that these calculations assume that the disease being tested for has similar manifestations in all affected individuals. Certainly this is not the case for MH. Nevertheless, appreciation of the concept of

---

Box 37-3 Interpretation of a Test

Sensitivity = Pr (T^+/D^+): The sensitivity of a test is the probability (Pr) that the test result is positive (T^+) given that the disease is present (D^+).

Specificity = Pr (T^-/D^-): The specificity of a test is the probability (Pr) that the test result is not positive (T^-) given that the disease is not present (D^-)

Predictive value of a positive test = Pr (D^+/T^+): The predictive value of a positive test, also known as the *positive predictive value (PPV)*, is the probability that the disease is present given that the test result was positive.

Predictive value of a negative test = Pr (D^-/T^-): The predictive value of a negative test, also known as the *negative predictive value (NPV)*, is the probability that the disease is present given that the test result was positive.

Prior probability and prevalence may be used interchangeably in these equations.

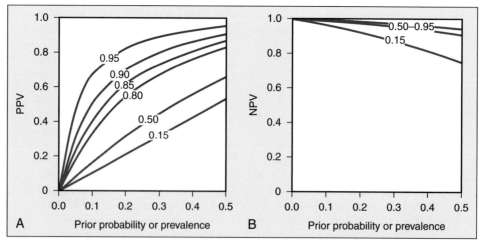

FIGURE 37-5. A, The y-axis is the PPV of the CHCT. This figure illustrates the fact that when the sensitivity is 95% and the specificity is 85%, the positive predictive value is less than 50% when the prior probability is less than 15%. **B,** The y-axis is the NPV of the CHCT. NPV is less altered by specificity than PPV when prior probability is less than 50%. Thus, the NPVs coincide for specificities from 85% to 95%. These two images illustrate the relationship between the sensitivity and specificity of a test, the prior probability of the disease, and the predictive value of that test (see definitions in Box 37-3). The probabilities on the graphs are shown as decimals between 0 and 1. In both figures, the x-axis is prior probability of MH susceptibility in the individual under consideration. This may be thought of as the probability that the individual under examination is susceptible to MH before the results of the CHCT are considered. This probability ranges from 0 to 0.5, or 50%, in these figures. In both figures, the sensitivity of the test is 0.95, or 95%. In both figures, the specificity of the CHCT varies between 0.95 (95%) and 0.15 (15%), as labeled on the dotted lines. The heavy line is the predictive value of the CHCT when sensitivity is 95% and specificity is 85%.

the predictive value of a test is important when questions arise regarding the meaning of clinical events and test results. These concepts have been used to argue that the index case should be the first person to undergo contracture testing, followed by first-degree relatives (Loke and MacLennan, 1998a; Larach and MacLennan, 1999). The same order of testing is appropriate for genetic analysis.

Currently, muscle biopsy and contracture testing of viable muscle is the only method that can confirm the diagnosis of not MH susceptible. The procedure can be viewed at *www.mhaus.org*. For satisfactory in vitro testing, 1 g of muscle must be removed from the thigh. A child weighing less than 20 kg may be too small to undergo muscle biopsy for CHCT. In general, children younger than 10 years of age are too young to undergo CHCT. Diagnostic standards were developed in adults.

Parents of an affected child may wish to have a muscle biopsy and contracture test performed (Figs. 37-6 and 37-7 and *www.mhaus.org*). The relatives of the parent whose findings are negative (assuming autosomal dominant inheritance) can then be reassured, without further testing, that they have no increased risk of MH. Ideally, siblings and first cousins on the affected side should be informed and offered diagnostic testing. Financial and geographic considerations often discourage families in these endeavors. However, the costs are less for genetic testing than for muscle contracture testing. Clinical genetic testing does not require travel to the location of the testing lab, as is necessary for CHCT. At the very

least, relatives of an patient with MH susceptibility should be informed about the presence of MH susceptibility in their family and its implications.

A valuable self-help resource is the Malignant Hyperthermia Association of the United States (MHAUS; PO Box 1069, 11 East State St., Sherburne, NY 13460; fax 1-607-674-7910). This organization offers information, expert consultation and referral, and many useful resources for families and health care providers. The MHAUS newsletter contains up-to-date information and reviews of the recent professional literature on topics related to MH. MHAUS maintains a 24-hour, professionally staffed telephone line to provide information on diagnosis, treatment, and referral of patients with MH (1-800-644-9737). See *www.mhaus.org* for addresses of the clinical laboratories at which genetic testing and muscle contracture testing are performed.

Care of Patients with a History of Malignant Hyperthermia

When a patient is referred preoperatively because of "possible MH," the anesthesiologist should determine what led to this diagnosis. At times, patients are erroneously told that they "must have had an episode of MH" because a slight increase in temperature or transient ventricular arrhythmias occurred and no diligent effort was made to clarify the causes or to obtain

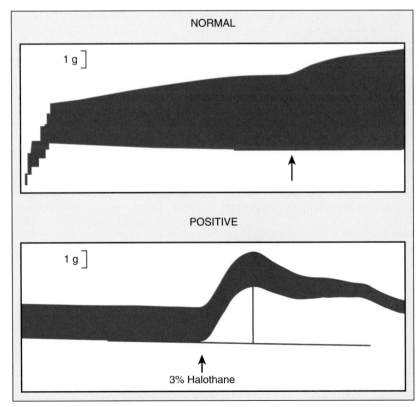

■ **FIGURE 37-6.** The muscle fiber contraction in response to an electrical stimulus and subsequent relaxation produces a black mark on the polygraph. Time is increasing from left to right. At the arrow, 3% halothane is added to the bath surrounding the fiber. The strength of normal muscle contraction *(top)* increases, but the muscle still relaxes to baseline. The MH susceptible muscle *(bottom)* does not relax back to baseline after exposure to halothane. In this case the contracture, the increase in baseline tension is over 2.5 g. *(Courtesy of Dr. Muldoon and the MH Diagnostic Laboratory at the Uniformed Services of the Health Sciences.)*

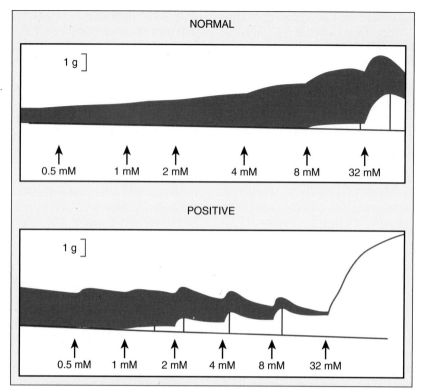

FIGURE 37-7. The muscle fiber contraction in response to an electrical stimulus and subsequent relaxation produces a black mark on the polygraph. Time is increasing from left to right. At the arrows increments of caffeine are added to the bath surrounding the fiber. The strength of normal muscle contraction *(top)* increases, but the muscle still relaxes to baseline until exposed to 8 mmol caffeine. The MH-susceptible muscle *(bottom)* does not relax back to baseline after exposure to low concentrations of caffeine. In this case the contracture, the increase in baseline tension is over 0.6 g in the presence of 2 mmol caffeine. *(Courtesy of Dr. Muldoon and the MH Diagnostic Laboratory at the Uniformed Services of the Health Sciences.)*

biochemical evidence of hypermetabolism or rhabdomyolysis. Many cases of increased jaw tension, arrhythmia, or mild elevation of myoglobin or CK after the administration of succinylcholine occur in the absence of MH susceptibility. When the issue of MH susceptibility has been raised, the personal and family history should be examined for adverse sequelae to anesthetics, sudden cardiovascular collapse suggestive of arrhythmias or heatstroke, and any evidence of musculoskeletal disorders, including cramping with exercise. A positive finding suggests that consultation with a neurologist and further testing (possibly including a muscle biopsy with in vitro contracture testing) may be warranted.

CK levels, at rest, are of no predictive value in the general population (Britt et al., 1976; Paasuke and Brownell, 1986). If a relative of a patient known to be susceptible to MH has an elevated CK level, that individual has an increased likelihood of susceptibility; however, this will not hold true for patients with other problems producing CK elevations (e.g., Duchenne's muscular dystrophy [DMD]). In some populations, more than 25% of the patients with elevated CK levels were not susceptible to MH on in vitro testing (Ellis et al., 1975).

Preoperative Care of Patients Who Are Susceptible to Malignant Hyperthermia

When it is clear that the suspected episode was MH, and especially when contracture testing has already been done and shows a typical MH pattern, several decisions must be made. If it is

at all possible, regional or local anesthesia should be chosen. Although some theoretic objections to amide-type local anesthetics exist, data in animals and humans have not shown any local anesthetic to trigger MH. Review of anesthetics during muscle biopsy suggests that nerve blocks with small volumes of amide local anesthetics do not provoke an episode of MH (Berkowitz and Rosenberg, 1985). Regional anesthesia with lidocaine, bupivacaine, ropivacaine, or another local anesthetic is an acceptable choice for the patient who is susceptible to MH.

Preoperative prophylactic dantrolene is not indicated. Because many muscle biopsies and other operations without preoperative administration of dantrolene or postoperative complications have been performed in patients with positive CHCT, it is considered acceptable to withhold preoperative dantrolene (Ording et al., 1991). These patients must be closely monitored during anesthesia with nontriggering agents (Table 37-2). If there are no signs of increased metabolism or rhabdomyolysis, and if no dantrolene was administered, then patients with MH susceptibility may be safely discharged on the day of surgery, even as soon as 2.5 hours after leaving the operating room (Yentis et al., 1992; Pollock et al., 2004, 2006).

Perioperative Care of Patients Who Are Suspected of Being Susceptible to Malignant Hyperthermia

An anesthesiologist may encounter patients who have had an anesthetic course or who have a family history that suggests susceptibility to MH but who have not had that possibility

TABLE 37-2. Malignant Hyperthermia and Drugs Used During Anesthesia

Drugs Likely to Trigger MH	Drugs that Do Not Trigger MH
Potent inhalation anesthetics:	Narcotics:
Sevoflurane	Benzodiazepines
Desflurane	Barbiturates
Isoflurane	Propofol
Halothane	Ketamine
Enflurane	Nondepolarizing (competitive) blockers
Ether	Anticholinesterases and anticholinergics
Depolarizing neuromuscular blocker succinylcholine	Local anesthetics
	Nonsteroidal antiinflammatory drugs
	Calcium

evaluated by means of muscle biopsy and in vitro contracture testing. A reasonable approach to providing anesthesia for such patients is to administer a nontriggering anesthetic and monitor the patient carefully for signs of MH (when this is consistent with safe anesthesia in that patient). It may not be possible to diagnose the underlying muscle disorder, but it is practical to watch for the processes that may hurt the patient postoperatively if an occult myopathy is present; these processes are hyperkalemic cardiac arrest, MH in the postanesthesia care unit (PACU), hyperthermia later resulting in multiorgan system failure, and myoglobinuric renal failure. Electrocardiogram can be monitored in the PACU in children. If there are no signs of MH in the first hour postoperatively, MH is unlikely to occur later (Litman et al., 2008). Rectal acetaminophen could block the increase in thermoregulatory setpoint that may produce postoperative temperature elevation and appropriate fluid replacement can promote dissipation of heat during recovery from anesthesia. Urine should be examined before discharge if a diagnosis of MH or other occult muscle disease is suspected. Dipstick of the urine with no blood demonstrates that there is no myoglobin in the urine; if there is no myoglobin in the urine, the patient has no increased risk of renal injury.

ANESTHESIA TECHNIQUES

Physiologic responses to stress may play a part in the initiation of an episode of MH in humans, as well as in pigs (Gronert and Theye, 1976a, 1976b; Gronert et al., 1980). Anesthesia for the patient who is susceptible to MH should be designed to be as stress free as possible, so that any tachycardia and arrhythmias that may occur are more likely to be associated with impending MH than with the stress of anesthetic, induction, or surgery.

There are many nontriggering techniques for general anesthesia (see Table 37-2). Local anesthetic cream can produce topical analgesia of the skin, which may facilitate intravenous catheter placement. Preoperative medication with midazolam, 0.3 to 0.7 mg/kg orally or 0.2 to 0.3 mg/kg nasally, often produces sedation adequate to facilitate the placement of an

intravenous catheter in a child. In the opinion of some anesthesiologists, preoperative sedation is an important part of the anesthetic management for patients who are susceptible to MH. After placement of an intravenous catheter, anesthesia may be induced with barbiturates or propofol. narcotics, and α_2-agonists (e.g., dexmedetomidine), as indicated by the planned surgery and other characteristics of the patient (Raff and Harrison, 1989; Harrison, 1991). Intramuscular administration of general anesthetics may be an alternative. Prior administration of benzodiazepine can reduce chest and truncal rigidity commonly observed after the administration of a synthetic narcotic. A nondepolarizing neuromuscular blocking agent may be administered if necessary. It is helpful to use a peripheral nerve stimulator when a neuromuscular blocker is administered so that the dose of drug can be titrated to the desired effect. Similarly, an anticholinesterase should be administered as indicated by the results of peripheral nerve stimulation.

There are rare reports of changes compatible with MH occurring after the use of such "safe" general anesthetic drugs (Fitzgibbons, 1980; Pollock et al., 1992; Shukry et al., 2006). For susceptible patients, there is no absolutely safe general anesthetic technique—merely drugs that are less likely to trigger MH. It is advisable to avoid drugs that may affect temperature regulation and sympathetic tone to such an extent that it might be difficult to detect early signs of insidious MH. Furthermore, serotonergic agonists and some psychotropic drugs (e.g., Ecstasy) have produced MH episodes in susceptible pigs (Wappler et al., 1997; Fiege et al., 2003). Large doses of phenothiazines and anticholinergics are not drugs of choice for the patient who is susceptible to MH. Atropine is administered only when there is significant risk of bradycardia. However, some anesthesiologists have found ketamine to be a useful anesthetic in patients who are susceptible to MH.

Monitoring and preparedness to treat acute MH are of the utmost importance. In addition to precordial heart tones, electrocardiogram, blood pressure, minute ventilation, and oxygen saturation, end-tidal oxygen and carbon dioxide concentrations should be monitored. Core temperature should be measured. Arterial and urinary bladder catheters are not needed for all surgery in patients with susceptibility to MH, but they are convenient for repeated blood sampling and close monitoring of hemodynamic stability and urine myoglobin.

It is helpful to keep drugs and supplies to treat MH in a portable container, such as a carry-all or rolling cart that is immediately accessible in the operating room and recovery room and can easily be transported to other areas of the hospital (see Table 37-1). The necessary supplies include at least 5 to 10 mg/kg of dantrolene and liter quantities of sterile, preservative-free, distilled water in which to dissolve the dantrolene. Ice or cold packs should be available, and large volumes of normal saline solution should be available in a nearby refrigerator.

Anesthetic Management for Muscle Biopsy for Contracture Testing

The preceding recommendations for the anesthetic care of patients with MH susceptibility apply to the patient undergoing diagnostic muscle biopsy. Biopsy for CHCT can be done only in one of the four specialized centers in the United States that support the performance of this in vitro test. The list of currently active centers may be obtained from *www.mhaus.org*.

The child scheduled for a biopsy usually weighs more than 20 kg, and some biopsy center directors will test only children who are at least 10 years old. The patient may be mature enough to have regional anesthesia before biopsy; in a cooperative child the use of lateral femoral-cutaneous nerve block and intravenous sedation is often successful (Berkowitz and Rosenberg, 1985). If the child cannot cooperate, general anesthesia may be induced and maintained with various agents, including benzodiazepines, narcotics, propofol or barbiturates, dexmedetomidine, nondepolarizing relaxants, or nitrous oxide.

Postoperative Care of Patients Who Are Susceptible to Malignant Hyperthermia

If anesthesia has proceeded uneventfully and prophylactic dantrolene has not been administered, the patient should be transported to the recovery room for the usual monitoring of vital signs, electrocardiogram, mental status, and urine output and color. A dipstick should be used to check urine for blood. The reaction of heme with orthotolidine occurs if myoglobin, free hemoglobin, or red blood cells are present (Bosch et al., 2009). If no sign of MH appears, the patient may be transferred to the floor after an ordinary length of stay in the recovery room. After observing such a patient for 2.5 hours after the end of anesthesia without any sign of MH, the patient may be discharged from the hospital. In this way, it is possible for a child who is susceptible to MH to be treated successfully as an outpatient (Yentis et al., 1992; Pollock et al., 2004, 2006).

If there is any evidence of hypermetabolism, or if continued treatment with intravenous dantrolene is contemplated, the patient should be cared for in an intensive care area. In a patient who has MH postoperatively, the anesthesiologist should be called to evaluate fever or tachycardia; the causes are usually related to pain, dehydration, or bacteremia. Nevertheless, MH has rarely been reported to occur several hours postoperatively. The patient must be examined carefully for signs of MH or altered mental status, venous blood gas tension and lactate should be measured, and urine should be tested for myoglobin. If signs of hypermetabolism or rhabdomyolysis are present, the patient should be treated with intravenous dantrolene and transferred to an intensive care unit.

DISORDERS ASSOCIATED WITH MALIGNANT HYPERTHERMIA

A number of disorders have been thought to be related to the MH syndrome because their presence appears to increase the risk of MH during anesthesia, but solid evidence is often lacking (Table 37-3) (Davis and Brandom, 2009). A complete understanding of these syndromes could contribute to understanding the pathophysiology of MH. Although not all myopathic patients are susceptible to MH, the presence of a known or suspected myopathy should alert the anesthesiologist that there may be increased potential for MH susceptibility or anesthesia complications that may mimic MH (Heytens et al., 1992).

Many patients with DMD have received potent inhalation anesthetics without occurrence of MH, but dystrophic muscle

TABLE 37-3. Association of Various Diseases with Malignant Hyperthermia

Disease	Observed Anesthetic Complications
Duchenne's muscular dystrophy (DMD)	Rarely, chronic rhabdomyolysis increases and may result in hyperkalemic cardiac arrest.
Becker muscular dystrophy	As in DMD, and growth of new muscle increases likelihood of hyperkalemia after succinylcholine.
Noonan syndrome	Not related to MH
Osteogenesis imperfecta	Increase in temperature is common but not related to MH.
King-Denborough syndrome	Susceptible to MH
Carnitine palmitoyltransferase II deficiency	MH susceptibility plausible but unproven
Myophosphorylase B deficiency (McArdle disease)	Rhabdomyolysis is common with any stress; CHCT may be diagnostic of susceptibility to MH, but few anesthesia experiences have been recorded.
Myoadenylate deaminase deficiency	As in McArdle disease
Brodie disease	Not susceptible to MH
Asymptomatic hyperkalemia	Causes of this syndrome may be many. Patients are likely to have hyperkalemia after succinylcholine and may have normal CHCT. Alternatively, an individual with increased CK may be a patient with central core disease (CCD) who is asymptomatic. MH is likely in CCD.
Myotonia congenita	No increased risk of MH over that in the general population
Paramyotonia congenita	No increased risk of MH over that in the general population
Potassium-aggravated myotonia	No increased risk of MH over that in the general population
Myotonia fluctuans	No increased risk of MH over that in the general population
Myotonia permanens	No increased risk of MH over that in the general population
Acetazolamide-responsive myotonia	No increased risk of MH over that in the general population
Hyperkalemic periodic paralysis ± myotonia	No increased risk of MH over that in the general population
Myotonic dystrophy type I (Steinert disease)	No increased risk of MH over that in the general population

TABLE 37-3. Association of Various Diseases with Malignant Hyperthermia—cont'd

Disease	Observed Anesthetic Complications
Myotonic dystrophy type II	No increased risk of MH over that in the general population, but there is greatly increased risk of adverse respiratory events postoperatively, as well as heart block. See detailed texts on this disease.
Hypokalemic periodic paralysis	Unclear, but there may be greater risk of MH than in the general population. There is potential for dangerous stiffness after succinylcholine, but metabolism may not increase as it does in MH.
Central core myopathy (CCD)	Susceptible to MH
Multiminicore disease with *RYR1* mutation	Susceptible to MH
Multiminicore disease without *RYR1* mutation	Maybe susceptible to MH
Nemaline rod myopathy without *RYR1* mutation	Maybe susceptible to MH
Nemaline rod myopathy with *RYR1* mutation	Susceptible to MH

From Davis PJ, Brandom BW: The association of malignant hyperthermia and unusual disease: when you are hot you are hot or maybe not, *Anesth Analg* 109:1001, 2009.

is fragile and can have RYR1 dysfunction (Peluso and Bianchini, 1992; Bellinger et al., 2009). Even mild exercise in patients with DMD results in a marked egress of sarcoplasmic components into the plasma, most notably myoglobin, CK, and potassium (Florence et al., 1985). These patients can have rhabdomyolysis during anesthesia with potent inhalation anesthetics even without the administration of succinylcholine (Rubiano et al., 1987). It is not surprising that anesthetic complications with many of the qualities of MH occur in patients with abnormal dystrophin (Kleopa et al., 2000) (see Chapter 32, Systemic Disorders). Nevertheless, there has been at least one patient who had dystrophinopathy and a negative contracture test, which ruled out MH susceptibility in that patient (Gronert et al., 1992).

Less common than dystrophinopathy, enzyme deficiencies and mitochondrial disease in muscle may also produce rhabdomyolysis, which can be easily exacerbated. Nonspecific signs of MH may occur during anesthesia (Hogan and Vladutiu, 2009). If the patient has a history of recurrent rhabdomyolysis, blood-based genetic testing of carnitine palmitoyltransferase II (CTP2), myophosphorylase (PYGM; deficiency of PYGM is McArdle disease), and myoadenylate deaminase (AMPD1) may determine the cause. When these blood tests are not diagnostic, muscle biopsy may be useful for diagnosis of these enzyme deficiencies as well as deficiencies in the glycolytic pathway and mitochondrial diseases.

Several extensive family studies of central core disease (CCD) have documented morphologically abnormal muscle—i.e., central cores of oddly aligned fibers—in some patients with MH (Shy and Magee, 1956; Byrne et al., 1982; Jeong et al., 2008). CCD is the first myopathy for which a definite link to MH was shown. Multiminicore disease is a different histologic diagnosis that has also been associated with susceptibility to MH and may be related to CCD (Ferreiro et al., 2002; Jeong et al., 2008). Several mutations in *RYR1* cause both CCD and MH susceptibility; therefore, it is advisable to treat a patient with CCD as susceptible to MH (Loke and MacLennan, 1998b; Tilgen et al., 2001; Robinson et al., 2006). The risk of MH in CCD, multiminicore disease, and nemaline rod myopathy was recently reviewed by Klinger and colleagues (2009).

Another familial myopathy, the King-Denborough syndrome, is associated with MH susceptibility (King and Denborough, 1973). Affected individuals have proximal muscle weakness, postural imbalances, cryptorchidism, webbed neck, pectus deformities, delayed development, and elevated levels of CK (Jurkat-Rott et al., 2000). Variants in the *RYR1* gene have been found in some patients with King-Denborough syndrome.

In the past, other disorders in which patients appeared to have MH susceptibility included myotonia congenita, osteogenesis imperfecta, Schwartz-Jampel syndrome (dwarfism, craniofacial and skeletal abnormalities, blepharophimosis, and muscle stiffness), and possibly arthrogryposis (Fowler et al., 1974; Rampton et al., 1984; Baines et al., 1986). These syndromes may be associated with many of the symptoms of MH, but these symptoms are not specific for MH. Many patients with these and other muscular disorders have received inhalation anesthetics without complications. For example, a pyloromyotomy was performed in an infant with paramyotonia congenita during sevoflurane anesthesia (Ay et al., 2004). Sometimes evaluation of suspect cases has found CHCT to be negative (Hopkins et al., 1991). A recent review of myotonias concluded that with the exception of hypokalemic periodic paralysis (hypoKPP), the risk of MH in myotonic patients is not increased (Parness et al., 2009). For theoretic reasons, although there are no published case reports of MH-like adverse events in patients with hypoKPP, risk of MH may be increased in this condition. Definitive diagnosis of myotonias and other channelopathies (including MH) should be pursued, because specific treatment may be available (Lehmann-Horn et al., 2008).

The neuroleptic malignant syndrome (NMS) is a potentially fatal disorder recognized by psychiatrists that may clinically resemble MH (Cohen et al., 1985; Guzé and Baxter, 1985; Mann et al., 2003). It occurs in 1:200 patients taking neuroleptic drugs that produce dopaminergic blockade. A 24-hour consultant service is available through the Neuroleptic Malignant Syndrome Information Service (NMSIS; *www.nmsis.org;* 888-667-8367). Most patients with NMS are young men with schizophrenia or mania treated with the potent piperazine phenothiazines or haloperidol, but more than 25 drugs have been implicated (Heiman-Patterson, 1993). NMS may also occur when the administration of antiparkinsonian drugs is stopped. The manifestations of NMS are altered mental status, hypermetabolism with fever, tachycardia, muscle rigidity, and myoglobinuria. NMS has all of the clinical features of MH, including acute renal failure and multiorgan failure, but it progresses over hours to days rather than minutes.

The inciting events of NMS differ from those of MH. Blockade of dopamine receptors can produce hyperthermia and rigidity, and bromoscriptine, (dopamine agonist) as well as dantrolene and benzodiazepines have been used to successfully treat this syndrome (Caroff, 1980; Granati et al., 1983; Heiman-Patterson, 1993). The results of CHCT in patients with a history of NMS have been inconsistent (Caroff et al., 1987; Adnet et al., 1989). Drugs that are known triggers of MH have been well tolerated in patients who have had NMS. Repeated exposure of pigs with MH susceptibility to a serotonin-2 receptor agonist can also induce typical MH symptoms without causing the same syndrome in normal animals (Gerbershagen et al., 2003). Mann et al. (2003) demonstrated that in humans the serotonin syndrome (tremor, diaphoresis, shivering, and myoclonus in the presence of serotonergic medication) could be elicited easily in individuals susceptible to MH. Dantrolene can delay serotonin-induced contractures (Wappler et al., 1997).

CONTRACTURE TEST

The CHCT is the best laboratory test available to investigate susceptibility to MH. The methods for performance of the test have been standardized in North America and slightly differently in Europe (Larach et al., 1989; Ording and Bendixen, 1992). Both tests provide consistent normal population values for comparison with diagnostic biopsies. In both North America and Europe, the CHCT is a concentration-response curve to caffeine alone and halothane alone. Unlike usual concentration-response phenomena, differences between persons susceptible to MH and those who are not do not appear as altered (median effective dose) ED_{50} or as a change in slope, but as a change in threshold. Patients must travel to the MH diagnostic center where this bioassay can be performed. The muscle strips to be tested must respond with active twitch to electrical stimulation (i.e., they must be viable). The test should be completed within 5 hours of the excision of muscle from the patient's thigh.

The North American protocol includes exposure of muscle strips to 0.5, 1, 2, 4, 8, and 32 mmol/L caffeine. A positive CHCT is often defined as an increase in tension of 0.2 g in the presence of 2 mmol/L caffeine or less. However, a cutoff of 0.3 g or 0.4 g may be preferred to increase the specificity of the test (Larach, 1989). A positive halothane contracture test is the development of more than 0.2 g to 0.7 g tension (depending on the controls in that laboratory) in the presence of 3% halothane (Larach et al., 1989). In the United States, if one muscle strip produces a positive reaction in either caffeine or halothane, the patient is said to be susceptible to MH.

Other laboratory tests have been evaluated for their diagnostic usefulness in MH; these include calcium uptake into frozen muscle, skinned fiber testing, platelet nucleotide depletion measurement, and the measurement of abnormal proteins in MH muscle. None of these is generally accepted, because none has been shown to reproduce the results of the in vitro muscle contracture tests (Lee et al., 1985; Britt and Scott, 1986; Whistler et al., 1986; Nagarjan et al., 1987). Several of the proposed tests produced inconsistent results (Ording et al., 1990; Quinlan et al., 1990).

MH is a disorder of muscle that is usually subclinical until the muscle is stressed. Tests discern MH susceptibility only if they impose a stress on the intact tissue or organism or detect a genetic difference that has been demonstrated to be causative

(Urwyler et al., 2003). MH muscle testing is generally designed to avoid false-negative diagnoses; hence, there may be false-positive results of the CHCT. Findings suggest that as with all tests, there are some rare false-negative contracture test results (Larach, 1993). However, overall MH contracture testing appears accurate, and patients with negative findings on CHCT can receive safe anesthetics with drugs that could trigger MH (Ording et al., 1991).

Failure to detect an *RYR1* mutation does not imply that the patient is not susceptible to MH. If a patient undergoes genetic evaluation before contracture testing and no MH-causative mutation is found, the patient must undergo contracture testing in order to support the diagnosis of not susceptible to MH. All patients should be monitored for signs of MH during anesthesia. Furthermore, MH can occur without the use of triggering drugs such as succinylcholine and potent inhalation anesthetics (Fitzgibbons, 1980; Pollock et al., 1992; Shukry et al., 2006).

ANESTHESIOLOGISTS' RESPONSIBILITY TO OTHER PHYSICIANS

MH has been known for more than 40 years, yet many primary care physicians, dentists, and surgeons are still unaware of its life-and-death significance. In 1986 the Malignant Hyperthermia Association of the United States published a letter from a parent:

> *Your information will be most helpful for my married, out-of-state, pregnant daughter who tried to explain that MH existed in our family... . They told her nobody could be allergic to anesthetics, which was the same thing I was told 22 years ago when my son's tonsils were removed. We had lost many relatives to ether for minor surgery over the years. Trying to explain MH in places that don't have large amounts of it is difficult. Some won't listen... .*

Anonymous, 1986

Physicians who are aware of the potential seriousness of MH may ask what the implications of the diagnosis of MH susceptibility are for the patient's daily life. MH susceptibility has been associated with fourfold increases in plasma catecholamines with graded exercise and rapid exhaustion after intense exercise; however, individuals susceptible to MS have performed farm labor in the hot sun without precipitating an MH attack (Wappler et al., 2000; Rueffert et al., 2004). Early studies of metabolic responses during noncompetitive, low-intensity, steady-state exercise found no difference between control and patients with MH susceptibility (Green et al., 1987). Slower recovery of muscle pH and phosphocreatine/inorganic phosphate ratios have been observed in patients with MH susceptibility (Allsop et al., 1991; Olgin et al., 1991). Patients who are susceptible to MH should be encouraged to refrain from strenuous exercise if they experience cramps or fever under such circumstances (Davis et al., 2002). Some people with MH susceptibility are unable to sustain exercise in the heat as well as they do in cool environments, and some patients with exertional heat stroke are actually susceptible to MH (Bendahan et al., 2001; Tobin et al., 2001; Wappler et al., 2001). Dantrolene may be therapeutic when these symptoms occur (Gronert, 1980).

Sudden death from undetermined cause may be common in the history of families with MH susceptibility. In adults these sudden deaths may be the result of arrhythmias. As of yet there are no published data regarding possible changes in muscle function with age in patients susceptible to MH, but it is noteworthy that in some families with MH susceptibility the young adults are muscular and strong, whereas the older adults may fatigue easily. CCD may be found in some individuals who are susceptible to MH.

The North American Malignant Hyperthermia Registry, now at the University of Pittsburgh Medical Center in Pittsburgh, Pennsylvania (Dr. Barbara W. Brandom, Director), collects data from health care providers, affected families, and testing centers in Canada and the United States. This registry provides a database through which to define clinical MH and to study aspects of its presentation, treatment, and diagnostic methods. Because MH is a rare event, it is necessary to collect clinical reports from a large geographic area over an extended period of time to improve understanding of the clinical problem. Because MH is rare, all health care providers have a responsibility to report such cases or suspected cases to the Registry.

SUMMARY

MH is a potentially lethal pharmacogenetic syndrome. It has been of particular concern to pediatric anesthesiologists because succinylcholine and inhalation anesthetics are potent triggers of MH and may be administered often in the practice of pediatric anesthesia. With the advent of improved monitoring techniques and universal availability of intravenous dantrolene, mortality from MH has plummeted. However, the definitive diagnosis of MH is still not simple or easy. It falls to anesthesiologists to choose anesthetic agents and adjuvants that maximize the safety of the patient, to identify as potentially susceptible to MH those individuals who experience adverse reactions consistent with MH, and to counsel and refer those individuals and families to appropriate diagnostic centers. Anesthesiologists must also make fellow physicians and other health care providers aware of the existence and the seriousness of MH and its effective treatment and prevention. When capnography, blood gas analysis, temperature monitoring, and dantrolene are available, patients with a history of MH susceptibility may safely receive routine anesthetic care with nontriggering anesthetics.

For questions and answers on topics in this chapter, go to "Chapter Questions" at www.expertconsult.com.

ACKNOWLEDGMENTS

We would like to acknowledge the extensive contributions of Joan Carroll, Henry Rosenberg, and Gerald Gronert to previous editions of this chapter.

REFERENCES

Complete references used in this text can be found online at www.expertconsult.com.

CHAPTER

38

Cardiopulmonary Resuscitation

**Jamie McElrath Schwartz, Eugenie S. Heitmiller,
Elizabeth A. Hunt, and Donald H. Shaffner**

CONTENTS

I n the late 1950s, children suffering cardiac arrest during anesthesia received 1.5 minutes of knee-to-chest "artificial respiration" followed by a thoracotomy for internal cardiac massage (Rainer, 1957). In 1958, closed-chest compressions were successfully performed on a 2-year-old child (Sladen, 1984). The resuscitation of that child, along with several successful resuscitations of subsequent patients (many undergoing anesthesia) led to reporting of closed-chest compressions for cardiac resuscitation (Kouwenhoven et al., 1960). Currently, 50% to 60% of

children who have perioperative cardiac arrest are successfully resuscitated (Bhananker et al., 2007). Despite the success rate of resuscitation during anesthesia, the potential for disaster and the increased likelihood of cardiac arrests in younger children and infants require that pediatric anesthesiologists have a complete understanding of the physiology and pharmacology of cardiopulmonary resuscitation (CPR). "No more depressing shadow can darken an operating room than that occasioned by the death of a child" (Leigh and Belton, 1949).

CARDIAC ARREST DURING ANESTHESIA

Incidence of Cardiac Arrest During Anesthesia

Perioperative cardiac arrest generally refers to an event that requires chest compressions while a patient is under an anesthesiologist's care during either the intraoperative or immediate postoperative period. Cardiac arrest may be the result of factors related to anesthesia, surgical procedure, or patient comorbidities. When comparing reports of anesthesia-related cardiac arrest, definitions and timeframes vary, with some including only the intraoperative period and others including the time from premedication through 24 hours postoperatively or longer. Some studies are based on electronic databases, and others depend on voluntary reporting to registries. The inclusion of events occurring during cardiac surgery by some studies and not others further complicates this comparison.

Results of studies that examined the incidence of pediatric perioperative cardiac arrest for all types of procedures, including cardiac surgery, are listed in Table 38-1. The overall incidence for pediatric perioperative cardiac arrest for all age groups undergoing all types of surgeries ranged from 7.2 to 22.9 per 10,000 procedures (Cohen et al., 1990a; Braz et al., 2006; Flick et al., 2007). Studies that excluded cardiac surgery reported a lower overall incidence, ranging from 2.9 to 7.4 per 10,000 (Murat et al., 2004; Flick et al., 2007; Bharti et al., 2009). When only anesthesia-related cardiac arrest was included, the incidence for all types of surgery (including cardiac) ranged from 0.8 to 4.58 per 10,000. The highest incidence of cardiac arrest was seen in patients undergoing cardiac surgery, ranging from 79 to 127 per 10,000 (Flick et al., 2007; Odegard et al., 2007). This information is helpful when estimating risk, but whatever the risk of pediatric perioperative cardiac arrest, the anesthesiologist must be ready and able to treat the cause and resuscitate the child.

As shown in Table 38-1, risk factors for pediatric perioperative cardiac arrest were consistently found in all studies to be associated with younger patient age. The highest risk was seen in infants younger than 1 month of age, followed by those younger than 1 year old. The Perioperative Cardiac Arrest (POCA) registry compared age groups in anesthesia-related cardiac arrests and found that between 1994 and 1997, 56% of cases were infants younger than 1 year old, whereas between 1998 and 2004, only 38% of the cases were infants younger than 1 year old. This significant decrease in the percentage of cardiac arrest in infants is attributed to the declining use of halothane and increasing use of sevoflurane, which is associated with less bradycardia and myocardial depression (Bhananker et al., 2007). Anesthesia-related cardiac arrest is reported to be higher overall for children (1.4 to 4.6 per 10,000) than adults (0.5 to 1 per 10,000), although the incidence in some studies is similar, presumably because both groups have high-risk patients at the extremes of age (Zuercher and Ummenhofer, 2008).

The patient's physical condition impacts cardiac arrest risk. Risk significantly increases when American Society of Anesthesiology (ASA) physical status (PS) is 3 or higher (Morray et al., 2000; Murat et al., 2004; Braz et al., 2006; Bhananker et al., 2007; Flick et al., 2007). Patients at ASA PS 5 are often not included in reports of anesthesia-related events, because by definition they have a low likelihood of survival, making it difficult to determine whether events are a result of their condition or related to anesthesia. Patients with ASA PS 4 and 5 have a 30 to 300 times greater risk of cardiac arrest than patients with ASA PS 1 or 2 (Rackow et al., 1961; Newland et al., 2002). Prematurity, congenital heart disease, and congenital defects are common pediatric comorbidities that increase the risk for children (Morray et al., 2000; Bhananker et al., 2007; Odegard et al., 2007).

The designation of emergency status to a patient's procedure was a risk factor for both cardiac arrest and mortality in some studies but not in others. Emergency surgery was associated with a significantly increased incidence of perioperative cardiac arrest, with 123 per 10,000 anesthesia procedures vs. 15 to 16 per 10,000 for nonemergent cases (p < 0.05) (Braz et al., 2006). In addition to a higher incidence of arrests during an emergency procedure, a poorer outcome was also reported (Vacanti et al., 1970; Marx et al., 1973; Olsson and Hallen, 1988; Morray et al., 2000; Biboulet et al., 2001; Newland et al., 2002;

TABLE 38-1. Incidence of Pediatric Perioperative Cardiac Arrest by Age Group for All Types of Surgery

Author, Year	Years of Study	Age Range	Number of Patients per Age Group	Cases of Cardiac Arrest per Age Group	Incidence of Cardiac Arrest per 10,000
Cohen et al., 1990a	1982-1987	<1 mo	361	3	83.1
		1 mo-1 yr	2,544	4	15.7
		1-5 yr	13,484	7	5.2
		6-10 yr	7,184	4	5.6
		>11 yr	5,647	3	5.3
		Total	29,220	21	7.2
Braz et al., 2006	1996-2004	<1 mo	697	14	200.9
		31 d-1 yr	2,368	10	42.2
		1-12 yr	8,856	8	9.0
		13-17 yr	3,332	3	9.0
		Total	15,253	35	22.9
Flick et al., 2007	1988-2005	<1 mo	1,451	23	158
		1 mo-1 yr	7,807	18	23
		1-3 yr	19,205	15	7.8
		4-9 yr	25,650	11	4.3
		10-18 yr	38,768	13	3.4
		Total	92,881	80	8.6

Sprung et al., 2003; Bharti et al., 2009). In contrast, several studies did not find a statistically significant trend to decreased survival as a result of emergency status (Biboulet et al., 2001; Flick et al., 2007; Zuercher and Ummenhofer, 2008). It is not clear whether emergency procedures have increased perioperative risk because of the patient's condition, the lack of optimal personnel, or both.

Etiology of Cardiac Arrest During Anesthesia

Causes of cardiac arrest during anesthesia are typically grouped either by organ systems involved or interventions applied. A summary of the etiologies and timing of cardiac arrest during anesthesia as reported in the literature is listed in Table 38-2. The pediatric POCA registry uses a classification system that involved both interventions and organ systems, thus grouping cardiac arrests as being related to medication, cardiovascular factors, respiratory factors, or equipment (Morray et al., 2000; Odegard et al., 2007). Some etiologies may be difficult to classify because they fit into several grouping schemes. For example, succinylcholine-induced dysrhythmia may be classified as either a medication-related or a cardiovascular cause of cardiac arrest. A set of guidelines for reporting cardiac arrest data in children, known as the pediatric Utstein guidelines, suggested a classification based on organ systems for etiologies (Zaritsky et al., 1995). The Utstein guidelines used three groups consisting of cardiac, pulmonary, and cardiopulmonary factors for comparison of etiologies of cardiac arrest in children. The Utstein guidelines have not yet been widely incorporated into anesthesia-related cardiac arrest literature. The anesthesia literature generally groups the etiology of cardiac arrest into those related to medication, cardiovascular, or respiratory categories, as shown in Box 38-1.

Previously, medication-related etiologies were the most common reasons for cardiac arrest related to anesthesia in children, representing approximately 35% of cardiac arrests (range of 4% to 54%) (Rackow et al., 1961; Salem et al., 1975; Keenan and Boyan, 1985; Olsson and Hallen, 1988; Morgan et al., 1993; Morray et al., 2000, Biboulet et al., 2001; Newland et al., 2002; Kawashima et al., 2003; Sprung et al., 2003). There has been a decrease in reports of medication-related etiologies to between 18% and 28%, and cardiac and respiratory causes are now the most commonly reported (Fig. 38-1) (Braz et al., 2006; Bhananker et al., 2007). This may be the result of a decrease in incidence of inhalation-agent overdose when use of sevoflurane replaced halothane for anesthetic induction. It is not clear whether sevoflurane is less cardiotoxic than halothane or the delivered dose of sevoflurane is lower because of vaporizer limits relative to a higher minimum alveolar concentration (MAC) for sevoflurane. Similarly, a decrease in succinylcholine-induced dysrhythmias was reported after a warning was issued related to use of succinylcholine in children. Other medication-related causes of cardiac arrest include those associated with regional anesthesia: intravenous (IV) administration of local anesthetic intended for caudal space, high spinal anesthesia, and local anesthesia toxicity. Inadequate reversal of a paralytic agent and opioid-induced respiratory depression are medication-related causes of cardiac arrest that more often present in the postoperative period.

Cardiovascular-related causes of cardiac arrest now represent approximately over 40% of cardiac arrests related to anesthesia in children (Braz et al., 2006; Bhananker et al., 2007).

Cardiac arrests caused by decreased intravascular volume are most commonly reported in this group, and causes include inadequate volume administration, excessive hemorrhage, and inappropriate volume or transfusion administration (Braz et al., 2006; Bhananker et al., 2007; Flick et al., 2007). Dysrhythmias caused by hyperkalemia are seen with succinylcholine administration, transfusion, reperfusion, myopathy, or renal insufficiency (Larach et al., 1997). Dysrhythmia or cardiovascular collapse (asystole) may have a vagal etiology as a result of traction, pressures, or insufflations of the abdomen, eyes, neck, or heart. Cardiovascular collapse can occur with anaphylaxis from exposure to latex, contrast, drugs, or dextran. Venous air embolism is another important cause of cardiovascular collapse and cardiac arrest in patients who are under anesthesia. Malignant hyperthermia is a seldom-reported cause of cardiac arrest in this group.

Respiratory-related causes are responsible for approximately 31% (range of 15% to 71%) of cardiac arrest related to anesthesia in children and adults (Rackow et al., 1961; Salem et al., 1975; Keenan and Boyan, 1985; Olsson and Hallen, 1988; Morgan et al., 1993; Morray et al., 2000; Biboulet et al., 2001; Newland et al., 2002; Kawashima et al., 2003; Sprung et al., 2003; Braz et al., 2006; Bhananker et al., 2007; Flick et al., 2007). Respiratory-related events as the primary cause of cardiac arrest have declined over the years as a source of malpractice claims, from 51% in the 1970s to 41% in the 1980s and 23% from 1990 through 2000 (Jimenez et al., 2007). Inadequate ventilation and oxygenation are broad categories often listed in this group as causes of cardiac arrest. "Loss of the airway" may involve laryngospasm or bronchospasm; an anatomy that is difficult to manage; or a misplaced, kinked, plugged, or inadvertently removed endotracheal tube (ETT). Aspiration remains a cause of respiratory-related cardiac arrest but is not often mentioned in the recent literature.

Equipment-related causes involve approximately 4% (range of 0% to 20%) of cardiac arrest related to anesthesia in children and adults (Rackow et al., 1961; Salem et al., 1975; Keenan and Boyan, 1985; Olsson and Hallen, 1988; Morgan et al., 1993; Morray et al., 2000; Biboulet et al., 2001; Newland et al., 2002; Kawashima et al., 2003; Sprung et al., 2003). Categories of equipment-related cardiac arrest most commonly described include central-venous-catheter–induced bleeding, dysrhythmias, and breathing circuit disconnection. Other etiology groups of cardiac arrest reported in some studies include multiple events (3%), inadequate vigilance (6%), or an unclear etiology (9%, range of 1% to 18%) (Olsson and Hallen, 1988; Morray et al., 2000; Biboulet et al., 2001; Kawashima et al., 2003).

Determination that a cardiac arrest is anesthesia related is subjective, as is the extent that a cardiac arrest is related to anesthesia care. Patient-related factors, procedure-related factors, and anesthesia care-related factors are the three most important determinants of etiology of operating-room cardiac arrests. Attempts to determine extent of contribution of anesthesia care in cardiac arrest has produced terms such as *anesthesia-associated* and *anesthesia-attributable* cardiac arrest. Determination of an anesthesia-related contribution is complicated by the contribution of patient- and procedure-related factors. To what extent does anesthesia care contribute to a cardiac arrest related to surgical bleeding in a patient with a coagulopathic condition? Is failing to keep up with major hemorrhage or to correct a coagulopathy related to the procedure, to the patient, or to the

TABLE 38-2. Etiology and Timing of Pediatric Perioperative Cardiac Arrest

Author, Year	Types of Surgery	No. of Cardiac Arrests		Etiology of Cardiac Arrest						Timing of Cardiac Arrest (%)		
		All	Anesthesia-Related	Cardiac	Respiratory	Medication	Embolic	Hemorrhage	Other	Induction	Maintenance	Emergence or Later
Morray et al., 2000	All	289	150*	38	30	55	2	8	17	37%	45%	18%
Murat et al., 2004	Non cardiac	8*	2	3	3	1	—	1	—	—	—	—
Braz et al., 2006	All	35*	7	18	5	2	—	10	—	71%	29%	—
Flick et al., 2007	Non cardiac†	26*	6	8	5	—	3	10	—	7 (27%)	19 (73%)	—
Bhananker et al., 2007	All	397	193*	79	53	35	4	23	26	46 (24%)	111 (58%)	36 (19%)
Bharti et al., 2009	Non cardiac	27*	9	3	5	1	—	6	12	33%	67%	—

*Denotes group with results for cardiac arrest etiology.
†Flick et al. (2007) reported the results of cardiac arrest separately for cardiac and noncardiac cases. None of the cardiac arrests during cardiac procedures were considered to be anesthetic related.

Box 38-1 Causes of Cardiac Arrest During Anesthesia

MEDICATION-RELATED CAUSES

Anesthetic overdose, or relative overdose, of inhalation or intravenous agent
Succinylcholine-induced dysrhythmia
Neostigmine-induced dysrhythmia
Medication "swaps"
Drug reactions
Unintended intravascular injection of local anesthetic
High spinal anesthesia
Local anesthesia toxicity
Inadequate reversal of a paralytic agent
Opioid-induced respiratory depression

CARDIOVASCULAR-RELATED CAUSES

Hypovolemia
Hemorrhage
Inadequate or inappropriate volume administration
Hyperkalemia as a result of succinylcholine, rapid or large-volume transfusion, reperfusion, myopathy, potassium administration, or renal insufficiency
Hypocalcemia from citrate intoxication during rapid blood product administration
Hypoglycemia

Vagal episodes as a result of traction, pressure, or insufflation involving the abdomen, eyes, neck, or heart
Central venous catheter related dysrhythmia, hemorrhage or tamponade
Anaphylaxis after exposure to latex, contrast agents, drugs, or dextran
Embolism of air, clot, or fat
Malignant hyperthermia
Hypothermia
Myocardial ischemia
Sepsis
Adrenal insufficiency

RESPIRATORY-RELATED CAUSES

Inadequate ventilation and oxygenation
Inability to ventilate as a result of laryngospasm, bronchospasm, airway mass, endotracheal tube misplacement, kink, plug, or inadvertent removal
Difficult-to-manage airway anatomy
Residual neuromuscular weakness
Aspiration
Pneumothorax

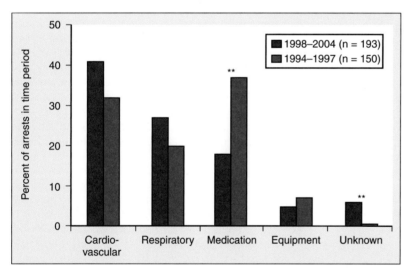

■ **FIGURE 38-1.** Causes of anesthesia-related cardiac arrest in 1998 through 2004 compared with 1994 through 1997. Multiple and miscellaneous other causes (3% from 1998 to 2004 vs. 4% from 1994 to 1997) not shown.** P < 0.01, 1998 to 2004 vs. 1994 to 1997 by Z test. *(Data for 1994 to 1997 from Morray et al: Anesthesia-related cardiac arrest in children: initial findings of the Pediatric Perioperative Cardiac Arrest [POCA] Registry, Anesthesiology 93:6, 2000.)*

anesthesia care? Many studies simply use the term *anesthesia-related* to describe a cardiac arrest after an anesthesiologist has been involved in care of the patient.

Anesthesia-related cardiac arrest may be preventable 53% of the time, and anesthesia-related mortality is preventable 22% of the time (Kawashima et al., 2003). Human error may be the most important factor in deaths attributable to anesthesia and usually manifests not as a fundamental ignorance but as a failure in application of existing knowledge (Olsson and Hallen, 1988). Poor preoperative preparation and inadequate vigilance are often reported as avoidable errors. Examples of poor preoperative preparation relevant to the pediatric anesthesiologist include failure to identify patients with symptoms of an undiagnosed skeletal myopathy, coronary involvement from Williams syndrome, prolonged QT syndrome, or a cardiomyopathy. Another category of preventable causes is inadequate

vigilance, such as failure to recognize progressive bradycardia and failure to respond to persistent hypotension. In addition to improving preparation and vigilance, the use of "test doses" or divided dosing when administering medications (especially drugs that may cause hypotension in unstable patients) is suggested to minimize medication errors. Other important and preventable causes of anesthesia-related cardiac arrest include transfusion-related hyperkalemia, local anesthetic toxicity, and inhalation-anesthetic overdose (Morray et al., 2000).

Cardiac arrest that is not related to anesthesia is most often the result of the patient's underlying condition or the procedure being performed. Trauma, exsanguination, and failure to wean from cardiopulmonary bypass (CPB) are three of the most commonly reported causes of cardiac arrest that are not anesthesia related. Myocardial infarction, pulmonary embolus, sepsis, and ruptured aneurysm are other, less often observed, patient-related causes of cardiac arrest. Procedure-related causes include technical problems, caval compression, vagal asystole related to traction or insufflation, and complications related to transplantation.

Outcomes of Cardiac Arrest During Anesthesia

What is the risk of a child dying during the perioperative period? Studies that have investigated this question have reported varied results, depending on whether they include only anesthesia-related causes or all causes of cardiac arrest. Although survival is the outcome most commonly viewed as a measure of successful resuscitation after cardiac arrest, mortality is the rate most commonly reported. Anesthesia-related mortality is currently reported to be 0.1 to 1.6 per 10,000 cases, which is down from 2.9 per 10,000 cases between 1947 and 1958 (Rackow et al., 1961; Morita et al., 2001; Morray et al., 2000; Flick et al., 2007). Some studies have even reported no anesthesia-related deaths (Tay et al., 2001; Murat et al., 2004; Braz et al., 2006). When all causes of perioperative cardiac arrest are included (i.e., anesthesia-related, surgical, and patient disease), risk of mortality is higher, ranging from 3.8 to 9.8 per 10,000 cases (Cohen et al., 1990a; Morita et al., 2001; Braz et al., 2006; Flick et al., 2007). Compared with neonates and infants, older children had a lower incidence of both cardiac arrest and mortality.

Although survival is used to describe a positive outcome for a patient who suffers a cardiac arrest, it is imprecise as to duration or quality of patient outcome. A patient may survive initial resuscitation attempts but subsequently die in the intensive care unit (ICU) from persistent hemodynamic instability or devastating neurologic injury. Initial survival from cardiac arrest after successful resuscitation efforts is defined as return of spontaneous circulation (ROSC), meaning that native heartbeat and blood pressure are adequate for at least 20 minutes. Although ROSC indicates a successful reversal of cardiac arrest, it may not be a meaningful indicator if many patients subsequently die in the ICU. The number of patients with ROSC after cardiac arrest is usually much greater than the number that has a longer, more meaningful, period of survival, such as survival to discharge from the hospital. Although survival to discharge indicates a longer survival than ROSC, surviving for a longer time does not address the quality of that outcome. An assessment of the quality of survival should acknowledge either the presence of a new neurologic deficit or a return to the patient's neurologic baseline. These terms are found in some descriptions in the anesthesia-related literature on outcomes of children who suffer cardiac arrest. Full recovery after intraoperative cardiac arrest in children is reported to range from 48% to 61% (Bharti et al., 2009; Bhananker et al., 2007; Flick et al., 2007).

It is often presumed that the duration and quality of survival from a cardiac arrest that occurred in the operating room should be good, because personnel who witness the cardiac arrest and provide resuscitation are trained and prepared. A review of the anesthesia literature reveals that cardiac arrest can be reversed in over 80% of anesthesia-related episodes (Sprung et al., 2003; Bhananker et al., 2007; Bharti et al., 2009). The likelihood of ROSC decreases to 50% or 60% if the cause of arrest includes those causes not related to anesthesia. Survival to hospital discharge after an anesthesia-related cardiac arrest appears to be approximately 65% to 68% (the range for pediatric studies of this variable is large). Survival to discharge is 30% if causes of

cardiac arrest unrelated to anesthesia are included. Comparing these data with data in literature not related to anesthesia reveals that studies of in-hospital cardiac arrest (IHCA) in children show a 23% rate of survival to discharge (range of 8% to 42%) (Gillis et al., 1986; Von Seggern et al., 1986; Davies et al., 1987; Carpenter and Stenmark, 1997; Parra et al., 2000; Suominen et al., 2000; Reis et al., 2002; Nadkarni et al., 2006, Tibballs and Kinney, 2006). This 23% survival-to-discharge rate is comparable with the 30% rate for all causes and much lower than the 65% rate for anesthesia-related causes of cardiac arrest in the operating room. The presence of anesthesiologists may account, in part, for the better survival outcomes in anesthesia-related cardiac arrests.

Outcome studies for cardiac arrest should include a determination of the presence of new neurologic injuries. Pediatric studies of IHCA show a 71% favorable neurologic outcome for the survivors (range of 45% to 90%) (Gillis et al., 1986; Davies et al., 1987; Carpenter and Stenmark, 1997; Parra et al., 2000; Suominen et al., 2000; Reis et al., 2002). Compilation of the available anesthesia-related literature indicates that 57% of children who suffer perioperative cardiac arrest survive and return to their baseline neurologic status, whereas 5% survive with a new neurologic deficit. Thus, for anesthetic-related cardiac arrest, a child has a 62% chance of surviving, and survivors have a 92% chance of having a favorable neurologic outcome. This percentage for pediatric survivors falls to 22% for those who return to neurologic baseline out of a rate of 36% for total survivors, or a 61% favorable neurologic outcome when all causes of cardiac arrest are included. The 71% favorable neurologic outcome for IHCA is comparable with the 61% rate for all causes and lower than the 92% rate for anesthesia-related causes of cardiac arrest in the operating room. It is noteworthy to mention that the number of studies and patients for these estimates are small and the ranges are large. These data indicate that both the duration and quality of survival are favorable for children who experience cardiac arrest from anesthesia-related causes.

There are many potential explanations for a higher resuscitation rate from anesthesia-related cardiac arrest. Factors such as the resuscitation skills of the anesthesiologist, preparation for emergencies by the anesthesiologist, reversible causes of cardiac arrest in the operating room, and increased monitoring during anesthesia to provide early recognition of problems may contribute to improved resuscitation rates during anesthesia care. The survival rate after cardiac arrest is affected by many factors, some of which are the same that predispose a patient to cardiac arrest: age of patient, ASA PS, and emergency procedures.

The etiology of cardiac arrest also impacts likelihood of successful resuscitation and survival. Mortality is increased if the cause of cardiac arrest is hemorrhage or is associated with protracted hypotension (both have a $P < 0.001$) (Girardi and Barie, 1995; Newland et al., 2002; Sprung et al., 2003). Resuscitation-related factors have an effect on outcome. These factors include cardiac rhythm during resuscitation, duration of resuscitation, and duration of no-flow and low-flow states during cardiac arrest and resuscitation. A no-flow state occurs when a patient is in cardiac arrest before receiving resuscitation efforts. A low-flow state occurs when a patient is in cardiac arrest and receiving resuscitation that is unable to provide adequate circulation. The longer the patient is in a no-flow or low-flow state, the worse the outcome is likely to be.

Asystole is a rhythm that, if present during resuscitation, has been associated with a decreased rate of both ROSC and survival to discharge for children with cardiac arrest outside of the operating room. Usually asystole is caused by prolonged hypoxia or myocardial ischemia and represents a terminal rhythm. Prolonged hypoxia causes the myocardium to be more resistant to resuscitation efforts and is more likely to result in neurologic injury. Thus, if the heart can be resuscitated, there is still the possibility of a poor outcome. In the operating room, continuous patient monitoring decreases the risk of prolonged periods of hypoxia or ischemia. Instead of asystole being a terminal rhythm, asystole in the operating room is often an initial rhythm that results from a vagal stimulation. As an initial rhythm, asystole is more likely to be reversed. Usually discontinuation of the vagal stimulus and chemical support of the heart rate are effective resuscitation measures. Unlike with cardiac arrests that occur outside the operating room, asystole is a commonly reported rhythm with anesthesia-related cardiac arrest and is associated with a good prognosis (Sprung et al., 2003).

The duration of the resuscitative efforts has an effect on patient outcome. Prolonged duration of CPR increases the possibility of low-flow intervals, thereby resulting in myocardial and cerebral injury. The need for CPR for more than 15 minutes has been determined to be a predictor of mortality in anesthesia-related cardiac arrests (P < 0.001) (Girardi and Barie, 1995). The interpretation of these data is complicated by reports of successful outcomes even after prolonged periods of resuscitation efforts. Up to 3 hours of CPR has been reported in anesthetic-related cardiac arrests, with eventual resuscitation and a good outcome (Cleveland, 1971; Lee et al., 1994). In summary, the cause of the cardiac arrest, the rhythm disturbance, and the duration of CPR can impact outcome from cardiac arrest that takes place in the operating room.

CARDIOPULMONARY RESUSCITATION

Recognition of the Need for Cardiopulmonary Resuscitation

Early recognition that a child's vital signs are inadequate and a response with rapid initiation of CPR reduces potential for injury from low-flow or no-flow intervals. It is difficult to give guidelines for the limit of each vital sign at which vital organ blood perfusion becomes inadequate for each child under anesthesia (Table 38-3). These limits depend on many factors, including the patient's general health, the patient's age, the type and depth of anesthesia, and the intensity and duration of deterioration of the vital signs. Pediatric training and experience are valuable in these uncommon but critical situations to help with the decision about when to initiate CPR.

In general, CPR including chest compressions should be initiated when it is felt that perfusion is inadequate to deliver oxygen, substrates, or resuscitative medications to the heart or brain. Extensive monitoring and continuous presence of anesthesia personnel should be optimal for early detection of inadequate perfusion or ventilation in the operating room. In the absence of adequate monitoring, health care personnel should palpate the umbilical artery in the newborn, the brachial artery in the infant, and the carotid artery in the

TABLE 38-3. Adequate Vital Signs for Children

| Age | Heart Rate (bpm)* | | | Blood Pressure (mm Hg) |
	Bradycardia	Normal PALS/HLH	Tachycardia	Hypotension
Term neonate	<60	80 to 205 95 to 180	>220	SBP <60
Infant	<60	75 to 190 110 to 180	>190	SBP <70
Child	<60	60 to 140 60 to 150	>180	SBP <70 + (2× age in years)
>10 years	<60	50 to 100 60 to 100	>150	SBP <90

Modified from Ralston M et al., editors: *Pediatric advanced life support provider manual*, American Heart Association, 2006; AHA /ILCOR Guidelines, part 12: pediatric advanced life support, *Circulation* 112(IV):167, 2005; Robertson J, Shilkofski N, editors: *Harriet Lane handbook: a manual for pediatric house officers*, ed 7, Philadelphia, 2005, Mosby, p 174.
*Bradycardia is the rate at which chest compressions should be considered; note that normal for >10 years may be below the level recommended and signs of inadequate perfusion should be assessed. Tachycardia listings are estimated rates at which symptoms usually occur.
PALS, Heart rate range from the 2006 PALS provider manual; *HLH*, heart rate range from 2005 *Harriet Lane Handbook*; *SBP*, systolic blood pressure.

child to detect an abnormal heart rate (Cavallaro and Melker, 1983; Lee and Bullock, 1991; AHA, 2006a). The analysis of a pulse in anesthetized and slightly hypotensive (systolic pressure lower than 70 mm Hg) infants revealed that detection of a pulse within 10 seconds was best with auscultation; brachial palpation was less successful than auscultation but better than carotid or femoral palpation by operating room nurses (Inagawa et al., 2003). Femoral palpation of pulse was more successful than carotid or brachial in anesthetized and hypotensive (systolic pressure lower than 70 mm Hg) infants in a subsequent study with personnel who had more pediatric resuscitation training (Sarti et al., 2006). Both authors agree that successful counting of heart rate over a brief time was better with auscultation.

In the operating room, monitoring is usually available to help determine vital signs of an anesthetized child. When the monitoring is unavailable or the readings are in question, having one rescuer auscultate and another palpate may increase reliability and decrease time needed to count a heart rate and determine the palpability of a pulse. Whereas either unresponsiveness or apnea is an indication to resuscitate in most situations, the administration of anesthesia masks these signs, and bradycardia by auscultation or lack of pulse by palpation may be valid indicators to start CPR.

Physiology of Cardiopulmonary Resuscitation: Reestablishment of Ventilation

The fraction of inspired oxygen (Fio_2) that should be administered during CPR is important, because either too much or too little may be detrimental. A report by Elam et al. (1954) showed that exhaled air from the rescuer (16% oxygen) provided adequate oxygenation of the victim (arterial oxygen level

[Sao$_2$] of 90% or greater) and became the basis for ventilation during CPR when supplemental oxygen is not available. In the operating room, the anesthesiologist has the ability to administer 100% oxygen via tracheal intubation during CPR. The anesthesiologist is faced with the theoretic concern that delivery of high oxygen levels during reperfusion may increase formation of oxygen free radicals and increase cellular injury. This concern is weighed against the knowledge that CPR is less effective in restoring oxygen delivery to the brain and heart than is native circulation and that during CPR the administration of low levels of oxygen may increase the delay in restoration of oxygen delivery. Adequacy of oxygen delivery during CPR depends on many variables, including the cause of cardiac arrest, the length of decreased perfusion, the effectiveness of CPR, and the patient's metabolic demands. The complexity of the determination makes it unlikely that oxygen delivery during CPR can be measured or predicted. A review of newborn resuscitation using 21% or 100% Fio$_2$ found that newborns with depressed (but not arrested) cardiac function can be effectively resuscitated with either 21% or 100% oxygen and that 21% oxygen administration is associated with less markers of oxidative stress. This review also found that for cardiac arrest in newborns there is no evidence that 21% is as effective as 100% oxygen in resuscitation of circulation, and that animal studies suggest 100% oxygen administration is more effective (Ten and Matsiukevich, 2009). A model of brain-tissue oxygen monitoring in piglets during CPR for cardiac arrest showed that despite administration of 100% Fio$_2$, the brain-tissue oxygen levels remained either at or below the levels before cardiac arrest until after ROSC, when they became dramatically elevated (Cavus et al., 2006). This finding implies that maximal oxygen administration is needed during CPR, but that it can create hyperoxic conditions after ROSC. Without adequate data to resolve this question, it seems reasonable to continue to use 100% Fio$_2$ during CPR for intraoperative cardiac arrest to help maximize the oxygen delivery during this low flow-state but to reduce oxygen levels once reliable oxygen monitoring shows adequate oxygenation during the hyperdynamic phase that occurs after ROSC (see Postresuscitation Care). The exception to the use of 100% O$_2$ for resuscitation may be the child with a circulatory condition such as a hypoplastic left heart, whose poor systemic perfusion is the result of pulmonary overcirculation. In such a case, the anesthesiologist needs to decide whether high levels of oxygen administration would contribute to the poor systemic circulation.

The contribution of chest compressions to ventilation during CPR impacts the decision of how much ventilation to provide to victims of cardiac arrest. Early in the study of external compressions, researchers did not add ventilation during CPR because they believed that closed-chest compression alone provided adequate ventilation (Kouwenhoven et al., 1960). The findings, that chest compressions alone provide some ventilation for adult victims and that minimal ventilation is necessary shortly after a sudden fibrillatory arrest, have resulted in over-the-phone instruction for CPR with compressions alone to untrained bystanders or those unwilling to provide mouth-to-mouth ventilation. It is difficult to determine how much chest compressions contribute to ventilation; their adequacy may vary with the cause of cardiac arrest, duration of cardiac arrest, the child's age, an underlying medical condition, the efficacy of resuscitation, and the child's metabolic needs. Requirements to administer oxygen and remove carbon dioxide (CO$_2$) differ by type of cardiac arrest; a sudden fibrillatory arrest has little loss of oxygen reserve or accumulation of CO$_2$, and a gradual asphyxial cardiac arrest has greatly depleted oxygen reserve and large accumulation of CO$_2$. Asphyxial cardiac arrest derives a greater benefit from ventilation efforts. A model of asphyxial arrest in piglets shows greatest benefit with delivery of both compressions and ventilations compared with compression or ventilation alone (Berg et al., 2000). Provision of ventilation early in resuscitation from cardiac arrest may be less necessary and has the potential to cause a respiratory alkalosis, resulting in unwanted effects on brain circulation and oxygen delivery. As the duration of cardiac arrest continues, despite CPR efforts, metabolic acidosis predominates and respiratory compensation may be difficult. Lack of data usually leads the pediatric anesthesiologist to choose a rate based on recommendations for age (10 ventilations per minute in children and 30 ventilations per minute for newborns) and to adjust the rate if blood-gas analysis becomes available during resuscitation (Table 38-4).

Intubation of the trachea by the anesthesiologist is recommended for the management of ventilation during intraoperative cardiac arrest. Without intubation and positive pressure ventilation, soft-tissue obstruction may prevent adequate ventilation in some victims (Safar et al., 1961). An unprotected airway puts patients at greater risk for aspiration during CPR because of loss of the airway's protective reflexes and increased likelihood of stomach distention with positive pressure ventilation. At onset of cardiac arrest, the lower esophageal sphincter

TABLE 38-4. Intraoperative Basic Life Support Procedures

	Newborn	Infant (<1 yr)	Child (1-8 yr)	Adult (>8 yr)
Breaths, intubated	30/min	8-10/min	8-10/min	8-10/min
Pulse check	Umbilical/brachial	Brachial/femoral	Carotid/femoral	Carotid/femoral
Compression landmark	Lower ⅓ sternum	Just below nipples	Between nipples	Between nipples
Compress using	2 thumbs encircling	2 thumbs encircling	1 or 2 hands	2 hands
Compression depth	⅓ chest AP diameter	⅓ to ½ chest AP diameter	⅓ to ½ chest AP diameter	1.5-2 inches
Compression rate (intubated patient)	90/min*	100/min	100/min	100/min

Modified from AHA /ILCOR Guidelines, part 12: pediatric advanced life support, *Circulation* 112(IV):167, 2005.
*In the newborn there are 120 events per minute. These events include 90 compressions and 30 breaths.

competency falls from approximately 20 cm H_2O to 5 cm H_2O (Gabrielli et al., 2005). The laryngeal mask airway (LMA) compares favorably with mouth-to mouth ventilation, mask ventilation, and other airway adjuncts during CPR, but there are limited data for a comparison with tracheal intubation during CPR and non-intubation technique may be less protective of gastric distention or aspiration (Samarkandi et al., 1994; Rumball and MacDonald, 1997; Stone et al., 1998). Airway adjuncts are not recommended as a replacement for tracheal intubation during CPR in children, especially when an anesthesiologist is available (Grayling et al., 2002). Tracheal intubation is optimal to assure ventilation during CPR for pediatric anesthesiologists, because they maintain training to use this procedure.

The appropriate placement of the ETT during cardiac arrest can be verified in most instances by the presence of end-tidal CO_2 (E_{TCO_2}). The incidence of accidentally placing an ETT in the esophagus of a child is greater during cardiac arrest (19% to 26%) than during an intubation that is not involved with cardiac arrest (3%) (Bhende and Thomson, 1992; Bhende and Thomson, 1995). Demonstration of persistent E_{TCO_2} wave forms after intubation is extremely reliable to confirm correct placement of the ETT in children with spontaneous circulation (Bhende et al., 1992). The lack of a measurable E_{TCO_2} level in the ETT usually indicates esophageal intubation. In resuscitation from a cardiac arrest, the pulmonary blood flow is decreased during CPR and the E_{TCO_2} level may be falsely low or absent despite a correctly placed ETT. This finding of no E_{TCO_2} detected during CPR in children experiencing cardiac arrest was seen in 14% to 15% of correctly placed ETTs (Bhende et al., 1992; Bhende and Thomson, 1995). Continually detectable E_{TCO_2} is proof of tracheal intubation even during cardiac arrest. The absence of E_{TCO_2} on placement of the ETT indicates that the larynx should be visually inspected to discriminate esophageal intubation. Loss of E_{TCO_2} during resuscitation efforts may indicate the ETT is dislodged and should be reinspected or replaced, that the ETT is plugged or kinked and a suction catheter should be passed, or that pulmonary blood flow is diminished and resuscitation efforts need to be increased. Tracheal intubation for resuscitation also offers the option of access (although limited) to the circulation for drug administration.

Interruption of chest compressions for delivery of ventilation increases the percentage of time that there is an absence of perfusion to vital organs; this percentage of CPR without perfusion is referred to as the *no-flow fraction (NFF)*. In addition to producing times with no perfusion, interruptions in the delivery of compressions result in a pooling of blood in the vasculature that causes the need for several compressions to be delivered before perfusion is back to the preinterruption level (Berg et al., 2001). Thus, there are both no-flow and low-flow problems caused by pausing compressions for ventilation or any other reason. The presence of an ETT during CPR eliminates concern for ventilation attempts contributing to the NFF. During CPR performed by bystanders compressions are held, ventilations are delivered, and then compressions are resumed. These pauses in chest compressions make it easier for ventilation provided by mouth-to-mouth or bag-mask ventilation to be delivered to the lungs, thereby improving the patient's ventilation and reducing the probability of gastric inflation. The need to interpose ventilations, thus interrupting compressions, during CPR is eliminated by placement of an ETT. A significant amount of research compares the effects of chest compression with ventilation ratios of 15:2, 30:2, and longer (continuous compressions) with varying results for fibrillatory and asphyxial cardiac arrest in prehospital settings. These ratios become irrelevant to the anesthesiologist when an ETT is placed, and compressions can be performed without interruptions for ventilation in a 10:1 ratio, generating 100 compressions and 10 ventilations per minute. The goal for the anesthesiologist is to maintain continuous delivery of compressions with interruption only at the 2-minute intervals necessary for switching of compression providers to prevent fatigue, pulse checks to determine ROSC, and when needed, the delivery of shocks. Intubation, central line placement, and placement of adhesive pads for defibrillation are other commonly reported interruptions to chest compressions and should be minimized and compressions should be continued when possible. It is important to remember the negative impact of holding compressions during intubation attempts and to absolutely minimize the duration of procedures that require these interruptions.

It is important to understand the effect of positive-pressure ventilation on perfusion produced by chest compression. In the previous section, the importance of minimizing NFF by maintaining compressions and not interrupting for ventilations was discussed. There are other physiologic interactions that cause ventilation to influence the effectiveness of chest compressions. Factors affected by these interactions include increased intrathoracic pressure, affecting the ability of chest compressions to move blood out of the thorax; intracranial pressure (ICP), reducing perfusion of the brain; myocardial perfusion pressure (MPP), and venous return to the thorax.

A comparison of different methods of delivery of ventilation during chest compressions revealed differences in oxygenation, ventilation, and hemodynamics (Wilder et al., 1963). Delivery of ventilations independent of compressions, interposed between compressions, and synchronized with compressions allows both adequate oxygenation and ventilation, but their effects on hemodynamic pressures vary. Delivery of positive pressure ventilation has an impact on the hemodynamic variables caused by changes in intrathoracic pressure. CPR with simultaneous compression and ventilation increases intrathoracic pressure at the time of compression and yields improvement in blood flow and survival in a canine model, but it has not shown the same benefit in humans. The simultaneous increase in intrathoracic pressure may lead to increased ejection of blood from the thorax, but elevation of intrathoracic pressure also leads to increases in intracardiac and ICP. Increasing intracardiac pressure at the time of compression may result in no change in the MPP and no overall benefit to the heart. Increases in ICP occur with increases in intrathoracic pressure and may result in no change in the cerebral perfusion pressure (CPP) and no overall benefit to the brain (see section that follows, Physiology of Cardiopulmonary Resuscitation: Reestablishment of Circulation, for mechanism). Increasing intrathoracic pressure during the relaxation phase of chest compressions has the potential to decrease venous return and may have significant impact on the effectiveness of subsequent compressions, depending on the duration of ventilation pressure. Attention to rate, duration, and pressure used during delivery of ventilations can prevent excessive ventilation that is common during these high-stress events and the impact overventilation has on venous return. Use of the impedance threshold device, the intrathoracic pressure regulator (ITPR), and decompression during CPR are techniques used to increase venous return by lowering intrathoracic pressure and are discussed in later sections.

Overventilation or underventilation can be detrimental during CPR. As discussed previously, overventilation can have hemodynamic effects or result in hypocarbia; either of these could result in decreased perfusion of the brain. Underventilation could result in a decrease in perfusion either from reduced pulmonic blood flow during CPR secondary to the increased vascular resistance that results from atelectasis or from the systemic effects of hypercarbia in addition to metabolic acidosis. The determination of a ventilation rate during CPR depends on the age of the child, whether the airway is secured, the number of rescuers, the type of cardiac arrest, and duration of the cardiac arrest. The young child has an increased baseline metabolic activity and a greater need for an increase in the number of ventilations during CPR. Recommendations for newborns include rates of about 30 breaths per minute, whether there are 1 or 2 rescuers and whether or not the child is intubated. The infant, the child between 1 and 8 years old, the child older than 8 years, and the adult share recommendations for 8 to 10 breaths per minute with intubation (Table 38-4). The newborn has both the highest metabolic activity and baseline CO_2 production and a greater chance of having a cardiac arrest with a prolonged ischemic period, resulting in a greater need to eliminate CO_2. There may be an ideal range for ventilation during CPR; overventilation may increase intrathoracic pressure (causing reduced venous return and increased ICP) and lower arterial carbon dioxide tension ($Paco_2$). Causing cerebral vasoconstriction while under ventilation may allow lung collapse and atelectasis, reducing pulmonary blood flow, MPP, and CPP. The decrease in pulmonary blood flow during CPR for cardiac arrest produces higher levels of venous CO_2 and lower levels of arterial and $ETco_2$. Determining the adequacy of ventilation efforts during CPR is difficult, because low pulmonary blood flow impacts the CO_2 levels of both $ETco_2$ and blood-gas monitoring. These techniques regain their usefulness in monitoring ventilation efforts as pulmonary blood is improved with resuscitation or ROSC.

The anesthesiologist will encounter the decision of whether to use mechanical or manual ventilation during CPR for intraoperative cardiac arrest. There are no data available to use to recommend one technique or the other.

Physiology of Cardiopulmonary Resuscitation: Reestablishment of Circulation

Mechanisms of Blood Flow During Cardiopulmonary Resuscitation

Kouwenhoven et al. (1960) proposed that external chest compressions squeeze the heart between the sternum and the vertebral column, forcing blood to be ejected. This assumption about direct cardiac compression during external CPR became known as the *cardiac-pump mechanism* of blood flow. The cardiac pump mechanism proposes that the atrioventricular (AV) valves close during ventricular compression and that ventricular volume decreases during ejection of blood. During chest relaxation, ventricular pressures fall below atrial pressures, enabling the AV valves to open and the ventricles to fill. This sequence of events resembles the normal cardiac cycle and occurs with use of direct cardiac compression during open-chest CPR.

Several observations of hemodynamics during external CPR are inconsistent with the cardiac pump mechanism for blood

TABLE 38-5. Comparison of Mechanisms of Blood Flow During Closed-Chest Compressions

Proposed Mechanism	Cardiac Pump	Thoracic Pump
	Sternum and spine compress heart	General increase in intrathoracic pressure
Findings During Compression		
Atrioventricular valves	Close	Stay open
Aortic diameter	Increases	Decreases
Blood movement	Left ventricle to aorta	Pulmonary veins to aorta
Ventricular volume	Decreases	Little change
Compression rate	Dependent	Little effect
Duty cycle	Little effect	Dependent
Compression force	Increases role	Decreases role
Patient Physiology		
	Small chest	Large chest
	High compliance	Low compliance

flow (Table 38-5). First, similar elevations in arterial and venous intrathoracic pressures during closed-chest CPR suggest a generalized increase in intrathoracic pressure (Weale and Rothwell-Jackson, 1962). Second, reconstructing thoracic integrity in patients with flail sternums improves blood pressure during CPR (unexpected, because a flail sternum should allow direct cardiac compression during closed-chest CPR) (Rudikoff et al., 1980). Third, patients who develop ventricular fibrillation (VF) produce enough blood flow by repetitive coughing or deep breathing to maintain consciousness; there are examples in which no compression of the heart occurs, only an increase in intrathoracic pressure (MacKenzie et al., 1964; Criley et al., 1976; Niemann et al., 1980; Harada et al., 1991). These observations suggest a generalized increase in intrathoracic pressure may contribute to the production of blood flow during CPR. The finding that changes in intrathoracic pressure without direct cardiac compression (i.e., a cough) produce blood flow epitomizes the *thoracic-pump mechanism* of blood flow during CPR. Familiarity with the thoracic pump and cardiac pump mechanisms of blood flow during CPR help with understanding of how alternative methods of CPR might be advantageous.

Thoracic-Pump Mechanism

Chest compression during CPR generates almost equal pressures in the left ventricle, aorta, right atrium, pulmonary artery, airway, and esophagus. Because all intrathoracic vascular pressures are equal, the suprathoracic arterial pressures must be greater than the suprathoracic venous pressures for a cerebral perfusion gradient to exist. Venous valves, either functional or anatomic, prevent direct transmission of the rise in intrathoracic pressure to the suprathoracic veins (Niemann et al., 1981; Swenson et al., 1988; Paradis et al., 1989; Chandra et al., 1990; Goetting and Paradis, 1991; Goetting et al., 1991). This unequal transmission of intrathoracic pressure to the suprathoracic vasculature establishes the gradient necessary for cerebral blood flow during closed chest CPR.

During normal cardiac activity, the lowest pressure measurement occurs on the atrial side of the AV valves, providing a downstream effect that allows venous return to the pump. The extrathoracic shift of this low-pressure area to the cephalic side of jugular venous valves during the thoracic pump mechanism implies that the heart is merely serving as part of a conduit for blood flow. Angiographic studies show that during a single chest compression, blood passes from the vena cavae through the right heart to the pulmonary artery and from the pulmonary veins through the left heart to the aorta (Niemann et al., 1981; Cohen et al., 1982). Unlike during normal cardiac activity and open-chest CPR, echocardiographic studies during closed-chest CPR have shown that AV valves remain open during blood ejection (Rich et al., 1981; Werner et al., 1981; Clements et al., 1986). In addition, unlike during native cardiac activity and open-chest CPR, aortic diameter decreases instead of increasing during blood ejection (Niemann et al., 1981; Werner et al., 1981). These findings about closed-chest CPR support the thoracic-pump theory that the chest becomes the "bellows," producing blood flow during CPR, and that the heart is a passive conduit.

Cardiac-Pump Mechanism

Despite evidence for the importance of the thoracic-pump mechanism of blood flow during external chest compressions, there are specific situations in which the cardiac pump mechanism predominates during closed-chest CPR. First, applying more force during chest compressions (as in high-impulse CPR, see related section) increases the likelihood of direct cardiac compression and closure of AV valves (Feneley et al., 1987; Hackl et al., 1990). Second, a small chest size allows for more direct cardiac compression, causing better hemodynamics during closed-chest CPR in a canine model (Babbs et al., 1982a). Third, the compliant infant chest should permit more direct cardiac compression, as shown in a closed-chest CPR model in piglets, in which excellent blood flows are produced as compared with most adult models (Schleien et al., 1986). Transesophageal echocardiography studies have demonstrated the closing of AV valves during the compression phase of CPR in humans (Higano et al., 1990; Kuhn et al., 1991). These findings support the occurrence of cardiac compression during conventional CPR, suggesting that both mechanisms of blood flow may occur during CPR. As will be seen in a later section, varying the method of CPR may alter the contribution of each mechanism.

Efficacy of Blood Flow During Cardiopulmonary Resuscitation

The level of blood flow to vital organs produced by conventional closed-chest CPR without pharmacologic support (basic life-support models) is disappointingly low. The range of cerebral blood flow in dogs during CPR is 3% to 14% of levels before cardiac arrest (Bircher and Satar, 1981; Koehler et al., 1983; Koehler and Michael, 1985; Luce et al., 1984; Jackson et al., 1984). CPPs are also low, at 4% to 24% of levels before cardiac arrest in animals and only 21 mm Hg in humans (Bircher et al., 1981; Koehler et al., 1983; Luce et al., 1984; Goetting et al., 1991). Myocardial blood flows in this basic CPR mode are also discouragingly low at 1% to 15% of pre–cardiac arrest levels in dogs (Chandra et al.,

1981a; Voorhees et al., 1983; Koehler et al., 1985; Halperin et al., 1986a; Shaffner et al., 1990). MPPs correlate with myocardial blood flow in a one-to-one relationship between myocardial blood flow (when measured in mL/min per 100 g) and MPP (mm Hg) (Voorhees et al., 1983; Ralston et al., 1984). Several factors affect cerebral and myocardial blood flow during CPR, and these disappointing results in basic life support models can be improved with addition of pharmacologic support.

Physiologic thresholds for minimal vital organ blood flow during CPR have been described. The inability to maintain blood flow above these thresholds during CPR results in organ malfunction. A myocardial blood flow of 20 mL/min per 100 g or greater is necessary for successful defibrillation in dogs (Guerci et al., 1985; Sanders et al., 1985a). A cerebral blood flow of greater than 15 to 20 mL/min per 100 g is necessary to maintain normal electrical activity during CPR (Michael et al., 1984). Models of basic life support often do not achieve these thresholds; the addition of advanced life support measures, such as epinephrine administration, is associated with blood flow levels above these thresholds.

Maintenance of Circulation During Cardiopulmonary Resuscitation

The goal of CPR is to improve a no-flow or low-flow state by restoring and maintaining the best flow possible to the brain and heart until an adequate spontaneous circulation can be recovered. Factors related to the patient, the ventilation technique, and the compression technique contribute to restoration and maintenance of blood flow during CPR. The pediatric anesthesiologist should understand how these factors affect restoration and maintenance of blood flow during an intraoperative arrest.

Patient-Related Factors

Patient-related factors that influence the effectiveness of CPR to maintain circulation include the victim's age, the duration of CPR, the duration of preresuscitation ischemia, ICP, and volume status.

Based on limited data, young age appears related to higher cerebral blood flow during closed-chest CPR. A piglet model has substantially higher cerebral blood flow (50% of those before cardiac arrest) and slightly higher myocardial flows (17% of that before cardiac arrest) than those reported for adult models (Schleien et al., 1986). Studies on slightly older pigs yielded opposing results (Brown et al., 1987b; Sharff et al., 1984). The cerebral blood flow in the first of these two studies was markedly higher than that in adult models during closed-chest CPR, and neither of the myocardial flows was different from adult models. No human data exist with blood flows at different ages during CPR.

Age-related physical factors that affect the blood flow produced during CPR include chest wall compliance and chest wall deformability. Chest wall compliance impacts both the ability to produce anteroposterior displacement and to directly compress the heart. Young children have increased chest wall compliance that facilitates the achievement of adequate compression depth and increases the chance of direct cardiac compression, either of which can result in better blood-flow production by chest compressions. These benefits of the more compliant infant chest may account for high flows that resemble those produced by open-chest cardiac massage in a piglet model (Schleien et al., 1986). Chest wall deformability is another factor that relates to the ability to maintain flows during prolonged periods of chest compressions. Chest deformation occurs as CPR becomes prolonged. The chest assumes a flatter shape as compressions continue, producing larger decreases in cross-sectional area at the same displacement. Progressive deformation may be beneficial if it leads to more direct cardiac compression. Unfortunately, too much deformation may result in loss of recoil of the chest wall during release of compression. Decreased chest recoil with progressive deformation limits displacement and produces less effective compression and less venous return during release of compression.

A model of conventional CPR in piglets shows a progressive decrease in the effectiveness of prolonged chest compressions to produce blood flow (Schleien et al., 1986; Dean et al., 1991). The permanent deformation of the chest in this model approaches 30% of original anteroposterior diameter. An attempt to limit deformation by increasing intrathoracic pressure during compression with simultaneous-ventilation CPR resulted in no improvement in either amount of deformation or time to deterioration of flow (Berkowitz et al., 1989). Investigators used a third mode of infant-animal CPR by using a vest to deliver compressions in an attempt to limit production of deformation. The vest distributes compression force diffusely around the thorax and greatly decreases permanent deformation (3% vs. 30%) (Schleien et al., 1986; Shaffner et al., 1990). Unfortunately, the deterioration of blood flow with time still occurs and appears to be unrelated to the amount of deformation in this model and is more likely related to the duration of prolonged CPR. There has not been a direct comparison of adult and pediatric CPR in humans. The increased compliance and deformability of the infant's chest make it likely that CPR would be more effective in children than in adults (as seen in animal models).

An increased duration of CPR has a negative effect on cerebral blood flow and seems to be most detrimental in the infant preparation (Schleien et al., 1986; Sharff et al., 1984). The length of the no-flow period before CPR begins also has a negative effect on cerebral blood flow that is produced with CPR (Shaffner et al., 1999; Lee et al., 1984). The supratentorial brain blood flow during CPR is reduced more than brain-stem flow, because the preceding ischemic interval is increased (Shaffner et al., 1998, 1999). The cause of these detrimental effects on cerebral blood flow is unclear. Tissue hypoxia resulting in loss of vascular tone that eventually becomes unresponsive to vasoconstrictors, pulmonary edema, capillary leak, and (with prolonged duration of CPR) chest wall deformity are factors that are likely to contribute. It remains obvious that a short ischemic period and quick resuscitation improve the eventual outcome.

ICP is another patient-related factor with effect on the circulation produced during CPR. ICP can represent the downstream pressure for cerebral blood flow, and if elevated it can inhibit cerebral perfusion. Increases in intrathoracic pressure with closed-chest CPR cause ICP increases (Rogers et al., 1979). This relationship is linear, and one third of the increase in intrathoracic pressure generated by chest compression is transmitted to ICP (Guerci et al., 1985). The carotid arteries and jugular veins do not appear to be involved in the transmission of intrathoracic pressure to the intracranial contents. The transmission can be partially blocked by occluding cerebrospinal fluid or vertebral vein flow (Guerci et al., 1985). The rise in ICP with chest compressions becomes more significant in

the setting of baseline increased ICP (an increase to two thirds of intrathoracic pressure is transmitted to ICP). The efficacy of CPR to perfuse the brain deteriorates markedly in the face of elevated ICP. When increased ICP is suspected (i.e., a child with hydrocephalus or head trauma) the ICP should be lowered early in the resuscitation (i.e., shunt tapped, or hematoma drained) to increase effectiveness of chest compressions to perfuse the brain.

Volume status, more specifically, hypovolemia, is another patient-related factor that can have an impact on effectiveness of chest compressions. There are little data to address the impact of volume status on blood flow during chest compression. Animal models include the administration of fluid (30 mL/kg or to a right atrial pressure of 6 to 8 mm Hg) before inducing cardiac arrest in fasted animals to improve the effectiveness of CPR (Sanders et al., 1990; Eleff et al., 1995).

Ventilation-Related Factors

Ventilation-related factors that affect compression-related blood flow during CPR have been discussed in the earlier section on the reestablishment of ventilation during CPR. These factors include the need for intubation of the trachea, avoiding interruptions of compressions to deliver ventilations, the effect of ventilation rate, the effect of ventilation pressure, and the decision to mechanically or manually ventilate, and they are discussed in detail in that section.

Compression-Related Factors

Factors related to chest compression that affect blood flow during CPR include compression rate (including NFF and number of compressions delivered), compression duty cycle, compression force, compression depth, and opportunity for full recoil (avoiding pressure during relaxation and leaning).

Compression Rate and Duty Cycle

Compression rate is the number of cycles per minute. Duty cycle is the ratio of the duration of compression phase to the entire compression-relaxation cycle, expressed as a percentage. For example, at the recommended rate of 100 compressions per minute, the total cycle for compression and relaxation is 0.6 seconds (100 compressions × 0.6 seconds/compressions = 1 minute). A 0.36-second compression time produces a 60% duty cycle (0.36 sec/0.6 sec = 60%). The impact of duty cycle differs between the two mechanisms of blood flow (Table 38-5). In 1986 the American Heart Association Guidelines for CPR and Emergency Cardiac Care recommended increasing the rate of chest compressions from 60 to 100 per minute. This change represented a compromise between advocates of the thoracic-pump mechanism and those of the cardiac-pump mechanism (Feneley et al., 1988). The mechanics of these two theories of blood flow differ, but a faster compression rate could augment both.

In the cardiac-pump mechanism of blood flow during CPR, direct cardiac compression generates blood flow, and the force of compression determines the stroke volume per compression. Prolonging the compression (increasing the duty cycle) beyond the time necessary for full ventricular ejection fails to produce any additional increase in stroke volume in this model. Also, increasing rate of compressions increases cardiac output, because a fixed ventricular blood volume ejects with each cardiac compression.

Therefore, in the cardiac-pump mechanism, blood flow is rate sensitive and duty-cycle insensitive. In the thoracic-pump mechanism, the reservoir of blood to be ejected is the large capacitance of the intrathoracic vasculature. With the thoracic pump mechanism, increasing either force of compression or duty cycle enhances flow by emptying more of the large intrathoracic capacity. Changes in compression rate have less effect on flow over a wide range of rates (Halperin et al., 1986a). Blood flow in the thoracic pump mechanism is generally duty-cycle sensitive but rate insensitive. With an increase in duty cycle, the percentage of time in compression is prolonged, but time for relaxation becomes decreased and venous return may become inhibited. At slow compression rates, the ability to hold a compression to prolong the duty cycle becomes physically demanding. The increased ability of a rescuer to produce a 50% duty cycle at a rate of 100 (compared with 60) compressions per minute is the reason behind the compression rate change recommendation in the 1986 American Heart Association guidelines for CPR.

The no-flow fraction and measurement of compressions delivered are important factors in the continued recommendation of a rate of 100 compressions per minute. The NFF is the percentage of time that compressions are interrupted. The interruption of compressions not only produces a no-flow time but also reduces effectiveness of the initial compressions on the resumption of chest compressions. The NFF in CPR performed by bystanders during out-of-hospital cardiac arrest (OHCA) has been reported to be 48% (Wik et al., 2005). For IHCA, a NFF of 24% has been reported with a sensing monitor and defibrillator (Abella et al., 2005). Reducing the pauses for ventilations from a compression/ventilation ratio of 15:2 to 30:2 in a bystander model of CPR on a manikin reduced NFF from 33% to 22% (Betz et al., 2008). Tracheal intubation in OHCA resulted in a reduction of NFF from 61% to 41% (p = 0.001) (Kramer-Johansen et al., 2006). Preshock pause also contributes to the NFF. Automatic external defibrillators (AEDs) create a variable preshock pause of 5 to 28 seconds. A 5-second increase in preshock pause was associated with a decrease in shock success (p = 0.02), and shock success fell from 94% if the pause was for fewer than 10 seconds to only 38% if it was longer than 30 seconds (Edelson et al., 2006). Interruptions of compressions for delivery of ventilation by tracheal intubation and for AED analysis can be eliminated by using a manual defibrillator. The goal is to have only a 10-second interruption every 2 minutes (120 seconds) for compressor change and rhythm analysis, resulting in an 8% NFF.

The number of compressions delivered per minute may differ from the compression rate. The compressor (see later section on teamwork for roles assumed during intraoperative CPR) may be delivering compressions at a rate of 0.6 seconds per cycle (100 compressions per minute), but if each minute there are 10 seconds of held compressions, then the number of compressions delivered at this rate falls to 83 compressions per minute. In the analysis of a 1-minute segment in which there were 15 seconds of held compressions, this same compression rate (0.6 seconds per cycle) resulted in a decrease to 75 compressions delivered to the patient. In an OHCA study of adults, the use of a compression rate of 121 resulted in the number of compressions being delivered at 64 per minute (Wik et al., 2005). The accomplishment of 80 chest compressions per minute has been correlated with successful resuscitation in an animal model (Yu et al., 2002). Resuscitation team members in the roles of compressor and leader need to be aware of how many actual compressions

per minute are occurring and minimize interruptions to keep the rate of compressions delivered above 80 per minute. In an intubated patient, compressing at a rate of 100 per minute and only stopping for 10 seconds every 2 minutes to change compressors and perform pulse checks and rhythm analysis results in 92 compressions delivered per minute.

Compression force is the pressure and the acceleration applied to the chest. There are accelerometers available to monitor and provide feedback about the compression force applied with each compression, but they are not typically available in intraoperative resuscitation. The compression depth is the amount of anterior-posterior displacement provided by a compression and is related to the compression force applied and the compliance of the chest wall. Compression depth for adult patients is recommended as 38 to 50 mm (1.5 to 2 in) and as one third to one half of the anterior-posterior chest diameter for children and infants. Literature on adults indicates that a depth of 38 mm is not often achieved during resuscitation. Compression depths less than 38 mm occurred for 37% of compressions during IHCA on adults (mean depth 43 mm for all compressions) and for 62% of compressions during OHCA (mean depth 34 mm) (Abella et al., 2005; Wik et al., 2005). When studying the importance of adequate compression depth on the success of shocks delivered during IHCA, it was found to be that a 5-mm increase in compression depth improved first shock success (p = 0.028) (Edelson et al., 2006). Compression depth in a pediatric manikin model was 14 mm with the two-thumbs techniques vs. 9 mm with the two-finger technique (p < 0.001), indicating that the two-thumb technique is more effective for depth of compression (Udassi et al., 2009). In the operating room, the leader and recorder can assess the depth of compressions provided by the compressor and remind the compressor to achieve the suggested depth. The improvement in E_{TCO_2} production should be noted when increasing compression depth with a goal of maximizing E_{TCO_2} levels, which should correlate with blood flow through the lungs and vital organs.

Full recoil of the chest and avoiding any pressure during the release of compression (avoiding leaning on chest) is a key concept in the performance of chest compressions. The native chest recoil leads to increased negative intrathoracic pressure that augments venous blood return and blood ejection with subsequent compression. An animal model of incomplete recoil during active compression-decompression CPR resulted in increased intrathoracic pressure and reduced systemic arterial pressure, MPP, and CPP. The decrease in cerebral perfusion was related to the decrease in systemic arterial pressure rather than an increase in ICP (Yannopoulos et al., 2005b). In humans the effect of incomplete recoil on intrathoracic pressure can be similar to the use of excessive rates or durations of ventilation and is likely to result in less effective CPR because of poor venous return (Aufderheide and Lurie, 2004). In a study of pediatric IHCA, a feedback device alerted the compressor to leaning. Leaning was present in 97% of nonfeedback compressions and 89% of feedback compressions when defined as force applied to the chest of more than 0.5 kg and present in 83% of the nonfeedback compressions and 71% of the feedback compressions when defined as depth applied to the chest of more than 2 mm (Niles et al., 2009). It is interesting that a feedback device during CPR was effective in causing a lower rate of leaning, but the majority of compressions still resulted in this complication in their patients despite feedback. The importance of this concept, that venous return and blood flow are related to chest recoil, has led to the development of alternative methods of providing compressions or ventilations to improve chest recoil during release of compression (active decompression CPR and some other techniques are discussed in a later section). Prevention of leaning on the chest during release of compression is difficult and may require the use of both visual and audio feedback devices and alternative methods of CPR. A team approach can be tried during an intraoperative cardiac arrest with the recorder and leader assessing the compressor and advising if full recoil appears to be inhibited by leaning on the chest between compressions.

Distribution of Blood Flow During Cardiopulmonary Resuscitation

Overall blood flow to tissues is decreased during CPR as compared with the normal physiologic state. A redistribution of blood flow during CPR favors perfusion to the heart and brain. This redistribution toward vital organs should enhance outcome. Maintenance of myocardial blood flow during CPR is necessary for ROSC, and maintenance of cerebral blood flow determines quality of neurologic outcome.

Distribution of blood flow to both the heart and brain during CPR is influenced by the development of regional gradients. Distribution of blood flow to the brain depends on development of three regional gradients: the intrathoracic-suprathoracic gradient, the intracranial-extracranial gradient, and the caudal-rostral gradient. The intrathoracic-suprathoracic gradient provides flow of oxygenated blood from the chest to the upper extremities and head. Either venous collapse secondary to elevated intrathoracic pressure or closure of anatomic valves in the jugular system prevents the transmission of intrathoracic pressure to the suprathoracic venous system (Rudikoff et al., 1980; Niemann et al., 1981; Fisher et al., 1982). When CPR is effective, arterial collapse does not occur and elevated intrathoracic pressure results in a gradient that promotes suprathoracic blood flow. The intracranial-extracranial gradient directs blood to the brain away from extracranial suprathoracic vessels and toward intracranial vessels. α-Adrenergic agonists constrict extracranial vessels but have little effect on intracranial vessels, resulting in increased intracranial blood flow. Use of the vasoconstrictor epinephrine increases intracranial blood flow while decreasing flow in the extracranial structures of skin, muscle, and tongue (Schleien et al., 1986). The caudal-rostral gradient occurs within intracranial vessels. The relatively low-flow state of CPR seems to increase the distribution of flow to caudal areas of the brain. Ischemia preceding CPR significantly increases the distribution of flow to these areas (Michael et al., 1984; Shaffner et al., 1998, 1999). This pattern of caudal redistribution of flow also occurs in other models of global ischemia and provides preferential perfusion of the brain stem (Jackson et al., 1981). Although brain-stem resuscitation is necessary for survival, this propensity for sparing of caudal circulation after either prolonged ischemia or prolonged CPR raises the concern for producing a victim who survives with only brain-stem function.

Myocardial blood flow does not have the advantage of a large extrathoracic pressure gradient that augments cerebral flow. The thoracic pump generates equal increases in all intrathoracic structures. This lack of a gradient can result in poor myocardial blood flow during external chest compressions. Several studies have shown much lower blood flow to the myocardium compared with the cerebrum during closed-chest CPR (Ditchey

et al., 1982; Michael et al., 1984; Schleien et al., 1986). The type of CPR influences the production of myocardial blood flow. Methods that are more likely to cause direct cardiac compression, such as high-impulse CPR, result in increased myocardial blood flow (Ditchey et al., 1982; Maier et al., 1984). Myocardial blood flow may be present only during relaxation of chest compression, correlating with a diastolic pressure, or in other methods seen during compressions correlating with a systolic pressure (Cohen et al., 1982; Maier et al., 1984; Michael et al., 1984; Schleien et al., 1986). Regional flow within the heart also changes during CPR, with a shift in the ratio of subendocardial/subepicardial blood flow from the normal 1.5:1 to 0.8:1 (Schleien et al., 1986). This ratio reverts to normal with epinephrine administration.

Conventional Cardiopulmonary Resuscitation

Conventional CPR includes closed-chest compressions delivered manually with ventilations interposed after every fifth, fifteenth, or thirtieth compression (see Table 38-4 for basic life support procedures). This method of CPR can be delivered in any setting without additional equipment and with a minimum of training. No large randomized study exists to demonstrate the superiority of any alternative method of CPR over conventional CPR.

Rescuer fatigue is a major problem with manual CPR in the field. Individual variation among rescuers performing manual CPR is another problem both in the field and in the laboratory. Mechanical devices are available to deliver chest compressions to prevent fatigue and to standardize compression delivery. Mechanical devices are presently limited to adult CPR and are not recommended for children (AHA, 2006a). The overall low efficacy of conventional CPR has led to investigations of multiple CPR modalities. The methods usually reflect attempts to enhance the contribution of the thoracic pump or cardiac pump to blood flow during CPR (Table 38-5). For example, the use of both hands to encircle the chest of an infant while using the thumbs to apply sternal compression attempts to both raise intrathoracic pressure and compress the heart (Todres and Rogers, 1975; David, 1988). This two-thumb encircling technique of CPR generates higher blood pressures and is recommended over the two-finger technique for infants (Dorfsman et al., 2000).

Blood flow to other organs during CPR is usually reduced compared with flow to the brain and heart. The lack of valves in infrathoracic veins causes retrograde transmission of venous pressure and decreases the gradient for blood flow below the diaphragm in animals (Brown et al., 1987b). Regional blood flows for infrathoracic organs (e.g., small intestine, pancreas, liver, kidneys, and spleen) during CPR are usually less than 20% of arrest rates before cardiac arrest and often close to zero (Koehler et al., 1983; Voorhees et al., 1983; Michael et al., 1984; Sharff et al., 1984). The addition of abdominal compressions does not alter the infrathoracic organ blood flow (Koehler et al., 1983; Voorhees et al., 1983). Administration of epinephrine during closed-chest CPR almost eliminates flow to the subdiaphragmatic organs, with the exception of the adrenal glands (Ralston et al., 1984). There are little data available regarding blood flow to the lungs during CPR. Pulmonary blood flow occurs primarily at times of low intrathoracic pressure during closed-chest CPR (Cohen et al., 1982). High extrathoracic venous pressure builds up during compression and results in pulmonary filling during relaxation as intrathoracic pressure falls. Resuscitation methods that lower intrathoracic pressure may augment pulmonary vascular filling. Leaning on the chest during relaxation of compression and maintenance of increased ventilation pressures may prevent the fall in intrathoracic pressure between chest compressions and decrease pulmonary venous return and blood flow.

Alternative Methods of Cardiopulmonary Resuscitation

Simultaneous Compression-Ventilation Cardiopulmonary Resuscitation

Simultaneous compression-ventilation CPR (SCV-CPR) represents a technique designed to augment conventional CPR by increasing the contribution of the thoracic pump mechanism to blood flow. Delivering ventilation simultaneously with every compression (instead of interposed after every fifth compression) adds to intrathoracic pressure and potentially augments blood flow produced by conventional chest compressions. This method is felt to increase the perfusion gradient to the brain but has little effect on the myocardial perfusion gradient perfusion to the heart. Animal models suggested that SCV-CPR increases carotid blood flow compared with conventional CPR and show an advantage of SCV-CPR in large canine models (Koehler et al., 1983; Luce et al., 1983). No advantage is seen over conventional CPR in infant pigs and small dogs, perhaps because in small animals the compliance of the chest allows more direct cardiac compression and higher intravascular pressure than with conventional CPR (Babbs et al., 1982a, 1982b; Sanders et al., 1982; Schleien et al., 1986; Dean et al., 1987, 1990; Berkowitz et al., 1989). Human studies comparing SCV-CPR with conventional CPR show minimal improvement or detrimental effect on the coronary perfusion pressure (Harris et al., 1967; Martin et al., 1986). Survival is worse in both animals and humans when SCV-CPR is compared with conventional CPR (Sanders et al., 1982; Krischer et al., 1989). No study has shown an increased survival with this CPR technique despite the potential for increased brain perfusion.

Intraoperative arrest should be managed with endotracheal intubation, and compressions should be delivered at a 10:1 ratio with ventilations. Compressions do not have to be held for ventilations once the patient is intubated. The delivery of a ventilation breath that occurs simultaneously with a chest compression mimics SCV-CPR and may have some benefit on cerebral perfusion but is unlikely to help myocardial perfusion. The team members in the roles of airway, monitor, and leader should be careful that the rate and duration of ventilations do not significantly increase the percentage of time with increased intrathoracic pressure and inhibit venous return.

High-Impulse Cardiopulmonary Resuscitation

High-impulse CPR involves the application of force that is greater than usual during chest compression. This increase in force can be in the form of greater mass, greater velocity, or both. It is hypothesized that the larger impulses result in greater chest deflection, causing more contact with the heart (Kernstine et al., 1982). Direct cardiac compression is more likely with this form of closed-chest CPR. High-impulse CPR can generate myocardial blood flows as high as 60% to 75%

of values before cardiac arrest (Maier et al., 1984). In humans, high-impulse CPR generates increased aortic pressures (Swenson et al., 1988). An outcome study in dogs compared high-impulse CPR with conventional closed-chest CPR and found no significant improvement in resuscitation, survival, or neurologic outcome (Kern et al., 1986). The application of this benefit of greater force is the same for an intraoperative cardiac arrest, resulting in an increased likelihood of cardiac compression, which then results in higher myocardial and cerebral blood flow; however, the risk is that there is potential for increasing chest deformation and trauma.

Negative Intrathoracic Pressure Methods

Active compression-decompression CPR (ACD-CPR) requires a device that attaches to the chest and allows the rescuer to pull up on the sternum and decompress the thorax between compressions. The theoretical advantages of decompressing the chest between compressions include restoring chest wall shape and creating a negative intrathoracic pressure that pulls gas into the lungs and pulls blood into intrathoracic vessels. These characteristics allow for more effect from the subsequent compression, because more intrathoracic pressure can be generated and more blood is available to be ejected. Preliminary studies in humans have shown that after advanced cardiac life support failed, ACD-CPR was more effective than standard CPR at improving hemodynamic variables (Cohen et al., 1992). After IHCA, more patients had ROSC, survival at 24 hours, and a better Glasgow coma score when they received ACD-CPR then when standard CPR was given (Cohen et al., 1993). A larger study of IHCA victims failed to show any difference in resuscitation or outcomes between patients receiving ACD-CPR or standard CPR (Stiell et al., 1996). Several large studies of patients who suffered an OHCA did not find a difference in effectiveness of ACD-CPR or standard CPR for improving ROSC incidence, hospital admission, hospital discharge, or short-term neurologic outcome (Lurie et al., 1994; Schwab et al., 1995; Mauer et al., 1996; Stiell et al., 1996; Nolan et al., 1998).

Complication rates were not different after ACD-CPR or standard CPR in most studies (Lurie et al., 1994; Schwab et al., 1995; Mauer et al., 1996). It is interesting that the same study that showed that ACD-CPR had more complications than standard CPR (hemoptysis and sternal dislodgment) was also one of the few large studies that found ACD-CPR more effective than standard CPR for OHCA (Plaisance et al., 1997). ACD-CPR has been combined with an airway device to increase negative intrathoracic pressure—the impedance threshold device (ITD; see the next paragraph)—and has been mechanized to allow continuous application without the need to change rescuers and ease use during transport (see the section on mechanical methods). ACD-CPR is considered an optional technique for adults, and there are no data on which to base a recommendation for children.

The ITD is a device on the ETT or face mask that impedes inflow of inspiratory gas during chest reexpansion between CPR compressions when rescuers are not actively ventilating the patient. Impedance of gas inflow promotes negative intrathoracic pressure development during chest reexpansion. This increase in the negative intrathoracic pressure facilitates, by chest recoil, blood return to the thorax before the next chest compression (Lurie et al., 2002). The use of an ITD has been shown to improve coronary perfusion pressure and vital organ blood flow with both standard and ACD-CPR in adult and pediatric animal models (Langhelle et al., 2002; Voelckel et al., 2002). Improved levels of E_{TCO_2}, diastolic pressure, and coronary perfusion pressure occurred in a prospective, randomized controlled trial in adults undergoing ACD-CPR with ITD compared with ACD-CPR without ITD. A decrease in time to achieve a ROSC was also seen with ACD-CPR with ITD (Plaisance et al., 2000). A prospective controlled trial comparing standard CPR without an ITD and ACD-CPR with an ITD found significantly improved short-term survival (24 hours) in adult patients in the group that had ACD-CPR and an ITD (Wolcke et al., 2003). The use of an ITD with standard CPR in an OHCA trial adult of adults failed to show significant improvements in outcome for ITD vs. a sham ITD except in a subgroup with pulseless electrical activity (PEA) (Aufderheide et al., 2005). A separate study showed an improvement in short-term survival for standard CPR with an ITD vs. historical controls (Thayne et al., 2005). A no-ventilation study showed hypoxemia developing in animals that received either standard CPR with ITD or ACD-CPR with ITD but not in the animals that received standard CPR alone (Herff et al., 2007). Standard CPR with and without ITD in a ventricular-fibrillation cardiac arrest (VFCA) model in pigs showed no effect on MPP and no effect on survival in one study and worse survival with ITD in another study (Menegazzi et al., 2007; Mader et al., 2008). Further studies are needed to determine the effectiveness of the use of an ITD for pediatric resuscitation.

The ITPR combines an ITD with a vacuum to maintain a negative intratracheal gradient (-10 cm H_2O) during CPR while allowing positive pressure ventilation. An ITD relies on chest elastic properties such as outward recoil of thorax and proper CPR technique (no leaning during relaxation) to allow full recoil and generation of a negative intrathoracic pressure, whereas ITPR overcomes these limitations. An ITPR in a porcine model of VFCA was able to maintain negative intrathoracic pressure with ACD-CPR; the result was improved hemodynamic measurements and survival with no effect on ventilation (Yannopoulos et al., 2005a, 2006). ITPR has not been evaluated on asphyxial cardiac arrest or a pediatric model.

Abdominal Methods

Abdominal binding and military antishock trousers (MASTs) have been used to augment closed-chest CPR. Both methods apply continuous compression circumferentially below the diaphragm. Abdominal binding theoretically augments CPR by decreasing the compliance of the diaphragm that results in increased intrathoracic pressure, forcing blood out of the subthoracic structures to increase the circulating blood volume (an autotransfusion effect), and increasing the resistance in subdiaphragmatic vasculature, which increases suprathoracic blood flow. The increases in intrathoracic pressure and blood volume lead to increases in aortic pressure and carotid blood flow in both animals and humans (Chandra et al., 1981b; Lilja et al., 1981; Lee et al., 1981; Koehler et al., 1983; Niemann et al., 1984). Unfortunately, as the aortic pressure increases, the right atrial diastolic pressure increases to a greater extent, resulting in a decrease in the coronary perfusion pressure (Sanders et al., 1982; Niemann et al., 1984). This deterioration of coronary perfusion pressure is coincidental with a decreased myocardial blood flow (Niemann et al., 1984). This technique also decreases CPP because transmission of the intrathoracic pressure to the

intracranial vault raises the ICP (Guerci et al., 1985). Use of abdominal binders or MASTs to augment CPR does not increase survival in clinical studies (Sanders et al., 1982; Mahoney and Mirick, 1983; Niemann et al., 1990). Liver laceration from CPR performed with an abdominal binder has been reported but is no more common than with conventional CPR (Harris et al., 1967; Redding, 1971; Rudikoff et al., 1980; Mahoney and Mirick, 1983; Niemann et al., 1984). A recent study using a contoured abdominal cuff in a VFCA model in pigs found that at pressures over 200 mm Hg, abdominal binding increased MPP over standard CPR and urges a reconsideration of this technique (Lottes et al., 2007). The potential benefits over vasoconstrictor medications are that there is no need for access to the circulation, and a brisk withdrawal is possible when spontaneous circulation returns, avoiding the postresuscitation issues typical of vasoconstrictor administration. There is a lack of data in children to support the use of these techniques clinically during CPR, and potential for complications would discourage their application.

Only abdominal compression CPR (OAC-CPR) is a new method that uses only rhythmic compressions of the abdomen during resuscitation efforts to avoid the rib fractures that occur with standard chest compressions. A VFCA model in pigs comparing OAC-CPR to standard CPR showed 60% greater myocardial perfusion than did standard CPR (Geddes et al., 2007). Further evaluation is needed of the potential benefits of this technique in situations in which chest compressions need to be held, such as in the postsurgical cardiac patient when the chest is reopened during resuscitative efforts. This technique could potentially provide some brain and heart perfusion during the no-flow state while initial or subsequent sternotomy takes place (Adam et al., 2009).

Combined Abdominal and Chest Compression Methods

Interposed abdominal compression CPR (IAC-CPR) is the delivery of an abdominal compression during the relaxation phase of chest compression. IAC-CPR may augment conventional CPR by increasing venous return to the chest during the abdominal compression-chest relaxation phase and "priming the pump"; increasing intrathoracic pressure during abdominal compression, adding to the duty cycle of the chest compression; and sending blood retrograde to the carotids or coronaries because of abdominal compression on the aorta (Ralston et al., 1982; Voorhees et al., 1983; Einagle et al., 1988). Several studies have shown hemodynamic improvements secondary to IAC-CPR. In animals, cardiac output and cerebral and coronary blood flow improved when IAC-CPR was compared with conventional CPR in adult models but not in an infant swine model (Ralston et al., 1982; Voorhees et al., 1983; Walker et al., 1984; Einagle et al., 1988; Eberle et al., 1990). Studies in humans have also shown an increase in aortic pressure and coronary perfusion pressure during IAC-CPR compared with conventional CPR (Berryman and Phillips, 1984; Howard et al., 1984, 1987; Ward et al., 1989; Barranco et al., 1990; Chandra et al., 1990). Although one study reports a 10% aspiration rate, most report no aspiration or liver lacerations (Voorhees et al., 1983; Berryman and Phillips, 1984; Walker et al., 1984; Mateer et al., 1985; Einagle et al., 1988; Ward et al., 1989; Barranco et al., 1990; Sack et al., 1992). Clinically, IAC-CPR requires extra manpower or equipment and remains experimental. Outcome studies have mixed results, showing no increase in survival with OHCAs but increased survival with

IHCAs (Mateer et al., 1985; Sack et al., 1992). Whereas IAC-CPR may serve as an alternative technique for in-hospital CPR in adults, a lack of data prevents a recommendation for the use of IAC-CPR in children.

Phased chest abdominal compression-decompression CPR (PCACD-CPR) is another manual method that combines chest and abdominal compressions (Tang et al., 1997). PCACD-CPR resembles a combination of ACD-CPR and IAC-CPR. It requires a device (Lifestick) that attaches to both the abdomen and chest and alternately compresses and reexpands both structures. It offers the theoretic advantages of both methods, because the chest shape is restored and blood and gas are pulled into the thorax during active chest decompression and blood flow is augmented because of compression and active decompression of the abdomen. MPP, ROSC, short-term survival, and neurologic outcome were improved in a porcine model of VFCA with resuscitation using PCACD-CPR (Tang et al., 1997). The use of the Lifestick proved safe and feasible in adults with cardiac arrest in the emergency room (Havel et al., 2008). Further information is required before these methods can be recommended for pediatric patients.

Mechanical Methods

Mechanical methods of producing chest compressions have continued interest, with the focus on minimizing interruption of compressions (to change compressors who fatigue) and reducing the NFF. Mechanical devices that provide compressions would not have pauses every 2 minutes to replace the compressor team member, would provide consistent quality of compressions, and improve the quality of compressions during patient transport. Compressions during radiation exposure for interventional procedures would be less hazardous. Several mechanical devices are currently being used for CPR.

Vest CPR uses an inflatable bladder that is wrapped circumferentially around the chest and is cyclically inflated. This method of delivering chest compressions by diffuse application of pressure has two unique characteristics. First, the increase in intrathoracic pressure occurs with only minimal change in chest dimensions, making direct cardiac compression unlikely (an almost pure thoracic-pump technique). Second, the diffuse distribution of pressure decreases the likelihood of trauma. Vest CPR in dogs improves cerebral and myocardial blood flows as well as survival when compared with conventional CPR (Luce et al., 1983; Criley et al., 1986; Halperin et al., 1986a, 1986b). In a pediatric model of vest CPR, only 3% permanent chest deformation occurred after 50 minutes of vest CPR compared with almost 30% deformation produced by an equivalent period of conventional CPR (Schleien et al., 1986; Shaffner et al., 1990). In humans, vest CPR increases aortic systolic pressure but does not significantly increase diastolic pressure compared with conventional CPR (Swenson et al., 1988). In a preliminary study of vest CPR in victims of OHCA, increased aortic and coronary perfusion pressure were demonstrated, and there was a trend toward a greater ROSC compared with standard CPR (Halperin et al., 1993). Clinically, use of vest CPR depends on sophisticated equipment, and the technique remains experimental at this time.

Load-distributing band CPR (LDB-CPR) is a modification of vest CPR that uses an automated device to provide compressions with a self-adjusting band across the anterior chest. Less equipment is required than with the use of the vest, making this technique better for OHCA. Both the vest and LDB-CPR provide compressions over a broader area of the chest than standard CPR,

reducing potential for inducing trauma during compressions. An initial study with LDB-CPR for adult OHCA showed an increase of ROSC vs. historical controls receiving standard CPR (Casner et al., 2005). LDB-CPR showed improved survival to discharge vs. standard CPR with historical controls for adult OHCA (Ong et al., 2006). A randomized study of LDB-CPR vs. standard CPR was halted for worse neurologic outcome and a trend toward worse survival than manual CPR (Hallstrom et al., 2006).

The Lund University Cardiopulmonary Assist System (LUCAS) is a mechanical device developed in Sweden to provide active compression-decompression CPR. In adult OHCA with LUCAS for CPR, the 30-day survival was 25% when it was applied within 15 minutes for witnessed cardiac arrests and 0% when applied after 15 minutes of cardiac arrest (Steen et al., 2005). The incidence and patterns of injury with the LUCAS are similar to those with manual CPR (Smekal et al., 2009). A report of five patients with IHCA showed that LUCAS ensured effective uninterrupted compressions during transport and during procedures in the cardiac catheterization laboratory (Bonnemeier et al., 2009).

Periodic acceleration CPR (pGz-CPR) is a method that produces rapid motion of the supine body in a headward-footward pattern that produces both circulation and ventilation with a decreased risk of rib fractures compared with standard CPR. In a VFCA model in pigs, pGz-CPR produced superior neurologic outcome compared with standard CPR (Adams et al., 2003). In an asphyxial cardiac arrest model in pigs, pGz-CPR produced equivalent outcomes with no broken ribs compared with standard CPR, during which 25% of animals received rib fractures (Adams et al., 2008).

In summary, multiple models of mechanical CPR are available and have the potential to provide continuous high quality compressions in many situations that would make compressions difficult (transport) or risky (fluoroscopy). None is sufficiently studied to deserve recommendation for intraoperative use in children.

Monitoring the Effectiveness of Resuscitative Efforts

The brain and heart are the organs most likely to suffer irreversible damage if resuscitation efforts do not provide adequate blood flow and oxygen delivery. The table below lists several methods that can be used during resuscitation to determine whether efforts are effective in the restoration of adequate perfusion to these vital organs (Table 38-6). It is important to determine whether restoration of perfusion by these efforts is adequate to prevent neurologic injury and to allow ROSC. The determination that resuscitation efforts are ineffective can prompt attempts to improve resuscitation or, if improvement attempts fail, to decide that resuscitation is futile and terminate efforts. If resuscitation efforts are determined to be inadequate, then interventions can be made to improve effectiveness and eventual patient outcome. These interventions include improving performance of compressions (i.e., increasing depth or replacing the fatigued compressor), administering fluid to improve intravascular volume, or administering vasoconstrictors to improve vascular tone. When the resuscitation efforts are determined to be ineffective and unable to be improved (as in prolonged cardiac arrest before CPR) this information aids in the decision that continued resuscitation is futile and efforts should be stopped.

TABLE 38-6. Techniques for Monitoring Cardiopulmonary Resuscitation Effectiveness

Technique	Monitoring Device	Goal
Level of consciousness	Examination	Consciousness
Return of spontaneous circulation	Examination, arterial catheter, E_{TCO_2}	Spontaneous circulation
Pulse during compressions	Examination	Arterial pulsation
E_{TCO_2}	Quantitative E_{TCO_2}	>10 mm Hg
Arterial diastolic (relaxation) pressure	Arterial catheter	>15 mm Hg
Mixed venous saturation	Central venous catheter	>30%
Venous-arterial CO_2 difference	Arterial and central catheter	Decreased difference
Amplitude of VF	Electrocardiogram	Increased amplitude
Frequency of VF	Electrocardiogram	Decreased frequency
AMSA	ECG and software for analysis	>13 mV Hz
Transthoracic impedance	AED and software for analysis	Decreased by compression

E_{TCO_2}, End-tidal carbon dioxide; CO_2, carbon dioxide; *VF*, ventricular fibrillation; *AMSA*, amplitude spectrum area; *ECG*, electrocardiogram; *AED*, automated external defibrillator; *mm Hg*, millimeters of mercury, *mV*, millivolts; *Hz*, hertz.

The level of consciousness can improve if resuscitation efforts are effective. Occasionally, a patient with a nonperfusing rhythm regains consciousness during chest compressions only to become unresponsive when compressions are held and perfusion falls. This may recur repeatedly until a perfusing rhythm is restored. Return of consciousness is evidence of highly effective resuscitative efforts, but it is rare that the level of perfusion required for this to occur can be accomplished. Additionally, in the operating room the victim of cardiac arrest may have the evaluation of their level of consciousness masked by the use of anesthetic agents. This technique is unlikely to be helpful in most intraoperative arrests.

The restoration of spontaneous circulation is another indicator of adequate resuscitative efforts. This is usually a sign that perfusion to the heart muscle is adequate to allow effective contractions. The temptation is often to hold resuscitation efforts when spontaneous ejection occurs, but spontaneous circulation may not be adequate or sustained, and continued resuscitation efforts may be required. Compressions must be continued if spontaneous circulation does not adequately perfuse vital organs.

The palpation of a pulse during chest or cardiac compressions may be a sign that significant arterial pressure is being generated. Unfortunately, the palpable pulse may represent only peak arterial pressure during compression and be accompanied by a lack of significant relaxation (diastolic equivalent) pressure necessary for coronary perfusion. Because significant coronary perfusion occurs during relaxation, a palpable peak pulse may not represent effective CPR. Additional concerns about the reliance on palpation to determine the effectiveness of resuscitation are

that the palpated artery is usually next to a large vein and that retrograde venous pulsations may occur in the absence of significant arterial blood flow. There are no data on when, or if, palpation of pulsations during chest compressions correlates with ROSC or outcome.

One of the most useful ways to measure the effectiveness of chest or cardiac compressions to generate blood flow is the use of quantitative E_{TCO_2} monitoring. These monitoring devices are readily available in areas where anesthesia is administered. The detection of E_{TCO_2} during compressions demonstrates that venous blood is being moved through the lungs in sufficient quantity that CO_2 is available for measurement with ventilation. The level of E_{TCO_2} increases as compressions are more effective in increasing the pulmonary blood flow and the delivery of carbon dioxide in the venous blood to the lungs.

Low levels of E_{TCO_2} generated during compressions correlate with decreased levels of blood flow and decreased likelihood of ROSC. E_{TCO_2} levels measured during CPR that are less than 10 mm Hg predict an inability to restore spontaneous circulation in adults (Callaham and Barton, 1990; Wayne et al., 1995; Levine et al., 1997). Levels of E_{TCO_2} during CPR that are greater than 15 mm Hg predict ROSC in adults and children (Sanders et al., 1989; Bhende and Thomson, 1995; Barton and Callaham, 1991). E_{TCO_2} levels lower than 10 to 15 mm Hg during CPR indicate a decreased likelihood of success and should prompt institution of methods to improve resuscitation (i.e., better compressions and fluid or vasoconstrictor administration).

The measurement of E_{TCO_2} during CPR has also been used to detect low levels of cardiac output during PEA, ROSC during compressions, and the presence of spontaneous circulation during CPB (Garnett et al., 1987; Barton and Callaham, 1991; Gazmuri et al., 1991).

The technique of using E_{TCO_2} measurement during CPR does not require an ETT. E_{TCO_2} levels measured during CPR with bag mask or laryngeal mask ventilations also correlate with the likelihood of achieving ROSC (Nakatani et al., 1999). Another important consideration when using this technique is that the administration of bicarbonate to the victim causes a transient elevation in E_{TCO_2} without an elevation in blood flow that may be misinterpreted as improving CPR. Epinephrine administration has been associated with a transient drop in E_{TCO_2} despite an increase in MPP and may be misinterpreted as a worsening of CPR (Martin et al., 1990b). The cause of cardiac arrest may influence the initial E_{TCO_2} levels during resuscitation; higher levels of E_{TCO_2} are found with asphyxial arrest than with fibrillatory arrest (Grmec et al., 2003).

Invasive monitoring may be in use at the time of a cardiac arrest and may be helpful to determine the effectiveness of resuscitative efforts. An arterial catheter is necessary to determine aortic diastolic pressure during the relaxation phase of compressions. If an arterial catheter is present, arterial diastolic pressure (relaxation pressure) represents the MPP, and levels greater than 15 mm Hg are necessary for, but do not guarantee, ROSC in adult patients (Paradis et al., 1990). A central venous catheter is another invasive monitor that, if present, may be used to determine the central venous oxygen saturation during resuscitative efforts. The level of venous blood oxygen saturation correlates with effectiveness of resuscitation to produce blood flow and correlates with likelihood of ROSC (Snyder et al., 1991; Rivers et al., 1992). Patients with a mixed-venous oxygen saturation of less than 30% were unlikely to have ROSC (Rivers et al., 1992). The presence of both arterial and venous catheters allow sampling of simultaneous gases. The venous-arterial CO_2 difference is approximately 5 mm Hg during native circulation, and this difference increases significantly as perfusion falls. During hypoperfusion tissue CO_2 increases, venous CO_2 increases, pulmonary blood flow falls, and ventilation removes a greater percentage of CO_2 resulting in lower arterial CO_2. As CPR is made more effective, this venous-arterial gradient decreases again.

The amplitude and frequency of VF can be determined from the electrocardiogram (ECG) or specific software built into AEDs and used to determine effectiveness of resuscitation. Typically, the VF waveform is initially coarse (high amplitude, low frequency) and deteriorates over time during ineffective CPR or prolonged cardiac arrest to fine (low amplitude, high frequency) VF. As blood flow perfusing the heart during CPR improves, VF reverts back to a coarse pattern that indicates that the heart is more readily converted by shock to allow ROSC. An index of amplitude and frequency-amplitude spectral area (AMSA) has been correlated with the use of the MPP, E_{TCO_2} and likelihood of ROSC in a porcine model of VF arrest (Li et al., 2008). This index is calculated by software built into the AED, and a value of at least 13 mV Hz has been regarded as a critical threshold for defibrillation success.

The transthoracic impedance (TTI) is measured between the gel-coated pads applied to the chest during CPR by the use of an AED. The TTI can be continuously measured by these devices, and impedance decreases during compression in relation to the amount of blood movement through the chest. The potential exists to use this technique to monitor the amount of blood flow generated by compressions and determine whether there is continued effectiveness or if deterioration of compressions occurs with rescuer fatigue.

Analysis of the TTI waveform using an investigational monitor or defibrillator has been used to detect ROSC in adults. Like a sudden spike in E_{TCO_2} during CPR, changes in the TTI waveforms can signify ROSC. These methods can lead to earlier detection of ROSC, potentially eliminate the need to pause compressions to check pulse to determine ROSC, and eliminate the simultaneous no-flow state if ROSC has not yet occurred (Losert et al., 2007). Similar impedance measurements have been shown to detect the difference between pulsatile and pulseless rhythms during pulse checks that occur with in-hospital resuscitation (Risdal et al., 2008). The rapid determination of a pulseless rhythm would prompt resumption of compressions and reduce the no-flow interval during pulse checks. A brisk fall in E_{TCO_2} during pulse check would be another indication that a no-flow state is occurring and compressions should be restarted.

An additional monitoring benefit of TTI during CPR is the detection of ventilation or the loss of ventilation. Entry of gas into the lungs with ventilation causes an increase in TTI. The sudden loss of the cyclic decreases in TTI with ventilation may indicate displacement of the ETT during CPR (Pytte et al., 2007). Although loss of E_{TCO_2} is also used to indicate displacement of the ETT, E_{TCO_2} levels may be markedly diminished by low pulmonary blood flow during CPR. There is potential that the disappearance of impedance changes related to the failure of air entry with ETT displacement may be more reliable in situations of very low E_{TCO_2}. The use of TTI to indicate loss of ventilation or ETT displacement might also eliminate the need to stop compressions to perform auscultation when ETT displacement is suspected. TTI also can be used as a training technique to review the number of compressions and

ventilations delivered over the course of resuscitation at post-resuscitation feedback sessions.

The anesthesiologist may have many methods to choose from to determine the effectiveness of intraoperative resuscitation efforts. The equipment for quantitative determination of E_{TCO_2} is the most likely to be available in the majority of perioperative situations. In fibrillatory arrest, the restoration of a coarse pattern demonstrates effective CPR and when defibrillation attempts are most likely to be successful (Hayes et al., 2003). In the near future, TTI measurements by the defibrillator or AED may be available to monitor the amount of blood flow produced by resuscitative efforts, recognize ETT displacement, recognize ROSC or pulseless rhythms, and serve as training tools for feedback during debriefing sessions.

Vascular Access for Drug and Fluid Administration

Peripheral and Central Vascular Access

Vascular access is crucial to the effective administration of drugs and fluids for resuscitation, but it may be difficult to achieve in pediatric patients. During cardiac arrest, attempts to obtain peripheral venous access in infants and children should be limited, and if they are unsuccessful an intraosseous (IO) needle should be placed and or the administration of drugs may be started in the ETT. The American Heart Association (AHA) and the International Liaison Committee on Resuscitation (ILCOR) recommendations prioritize IO drug administration over endotracheal administration because of variable blood concentrations if a drug is given endotracheally (AHA, 2006b; ILCOR, 2006). Central venous access may be attempted during cardiac arrest by skilled providers, but attempts should not delay administration of life-saving medications via the peripheral IV or IO route.

The ideal placement of an intravascular catheter during CPR provides ready access to the anesthesiologist and minimizes interruption of resuscitation efforts. Peripheral venous access, IO access, and femoral venous access can usually be accomplished without interruption of airway management or chest compressions. The use of a saline flush for medications administered in peripheral IV access, IO access, and central lines with the catheter tip below the diaphragm improves medication delivery to the heart in the low-flow state of CPR. A flush with 5 to 20 mL of normal saline should drive the medication into the central circulation (0.25 mL/kg was effective in an animal model) (Orlowski et al., 1990). For most instances of CPR, peripheral IV access should be adequate for administration of resuscitation medications (Table 38-7).

Intraosseous Access

IO cannulation provides a rapid and safe route to vascular access via the bone marrow; this space is a noncompressible venous plexus and therefore reliably available when peripheral venous access is limited as a result of dehydration or peripheral vasoconstriction. Trained providers can obtain IO access within 30 to 60 seconds with a first-attempt success rate of approximately 80% (Brunette and Fischer, 1988; Guy et al., 1993; Fiorito et al., 2005). All drugs, crystalloids, colloids, and blood can be administered via this route. The onset and duration of action of emergency medications are the same when given by IO, central, or peripheral access during native circulation in dogs (Orlowski et al., 1990).

TABLE 38-7. Vascular Access During CPR

Route	Characteristics
Peripheral venous access (IV)	Route of first choice if vascular access not present
	Rapidly and easily placed
	Any drug or fluid may be administered
	Flush each drug with 0.25 mL/kg normal saline (20 mL in adults)
Intraosseous access (IO)	Easier to obtain in <6-year-old, can use for any age
	Any drug or fluid may be administered
	Flush with 0.25 mL/kg normal saline (20 mL in adult)
Endotracheal route (ETT)	Use only if no IV or IO access
	Only administer naloxone, atropine, vasopressin, epinephrine, and lidocaine (NAVEL) drugs by ETT
	Note: ETT drug delivery requires 2-10 times IV dose
	Use 5 mL of normal saline in ETT to increase distribution into distal bronchial tree (10 mL in adults)
Central venous catheter	Central access is first choice if already in place
	Place if no IV or IO is obtained
	Requires flush if catheter tip is below diaphragm
Cut-down saphenous	Use when other options have failed
	Requires special skill, high complication rate

CPR, Cardiopulmonary resuscitation; *IV*, intravenous; *IO*, intraosseous; *ETT*, endotracheal tube.

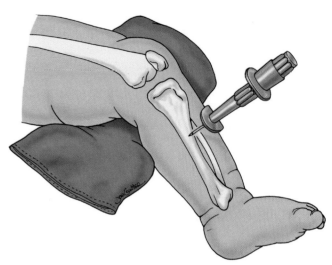

■ **FIGURE 38-2.** IO needle in proximal tibia.

The preferred site for an IO needle in a child is the anterior tibia. Alternative sites include the distal femur, medial malleolus, and iliac crest. In older children and adults, the distal radius, distal ulna, proximal humerus, and the sternum (risk of cardiac laceration) are also considered appropriate sites (Fig. 38-2) (Glaeser et al., 1993; Guy et al., 1993; Waisman and Waisman, 1997; Calkins et al., 2000). Specially designed IO needles should be readily available to the pediatric anesthesiologist for such emergencies. Rapid deployment devices for IO needles have been developed and may increase ease of IO placement (Horton et al., 2008; Schwartz et al., 2008). The most common complication from IO access is displacement of the needle and extravasation of fluid and medication (12%) (Fiorito et al., 2005). Other rare complications include bone fracture, compartment syndrome, osteomyelitis, and fat embolism (Orlowski et al., 1989).

Intratracheal Medication Administration

The intratracheal route may be used for administration of lipid-soluble resuscitation medications. Because most anesthetized children have this route available, it should be considered early, particularly if vascular access is a problem or access to

extremities is limited. Concerns related to variable delivery of medication and duration of effect make IO administration preferable to endotracheal administration in situations where IV access is not available.

Medications that can be administered via the ETT include the "NAVEL" drugs (naloxone, atropine, vasopressin, epinephrine, and lidocaine) (Wenzel et al., 1997; Efrati et al., 2003a). Studies suggest that similar doses given via the trachea achieve lower serum concentrations than when given by IV route (McDonald, 1985; Quniton et al., 1987; Jørgensen and Ostergaard, 1997; Kleinman et al., 1999). Lower serum concentrations of epinephrine may produce predominately β_2-adrenergic effects, causing vasodilation and decreased coronary perfusion pressures (Vaknin et al., 2001; Efrati et al., 2003b). Because of this concern, the recommended intratracheal dose of epinephrine is 10 times the intravascular dose, with a maximum dose of 2 to 2.5 mg (Manisterski et al., 2002). Recommended intratracheal doses of atropine and lidocaine are two times the intravascular dose; there is no optimal dose recommendation for naloxone or vasopressin. Drugs administered via the endotracheal route may have prolonged effect because of the reservoir of drug in the pulmonary tree (Hornchen et al., 1989). Prolonged effects of resuscitative medications can be detrimental in the patient after cardiac arrest because of sustained afterload and myocardial oxygen demand.

The technique for tracheal administration is to flush the medication with 2 to 5 mL (2 mL in children, 5 mL in adolescents) of normal saline into the ETT and provide five manual ventilation breaths to deliver medication into distal airways and alveoli. This technique is favored over delivery via catheter or feeding tube because of ease and practicality (Jasani et al., 1994).

DRUGS FOR RESUSCITATION

Vasoactive Drugs

Adrenergic Agonists

Epinephrine has been the drug of choice during CPR since the 1960s. Redding and Pearson (1963) first described the use of adrenergic agonists during CPR and demonstrated that early administration of epinephrine during cardiac arrest improved the resuscitation success rate. The increase in diastolic pressure from increased systemic vascular resistance was shown to be responsible for the success of resuscitation when using adrenergic agents (Pearson and Redding, 1965).

In order to investigate the relative importance of α-adrenergic and β-adrenergic agonist actions during resuscitation, Yakaitis et al. (1979) used a canine model of cardiac arrest and found they could resuscitate only one in four animals that received both the pure β-adrenergic agonist, isoproterenol, and an α-adrenergic antagonist. In contrast, all the dogs treated with both an α-adrenergic agonist drug and a β-adrenergic antagonist were successfully resuscitated (Yakaitis et al., 1979). These data suggest that the α-adrenergic agonist action of epinephrine is responsible for successful resuscitation after cardiac arrest. Support for this theory was reported by Michael et al. (1984) who demonstrated that the effects of epinephrine during CPR are mediated by selective vasoconstriction of peripheral vessels, excluding those supplying the brain and heart. Epinephrine infusions maintain a higher aortic pressure and result in a higher perfusion pressure to both the heart and brain (Michael et al., 1984). Even with increases in both mean and diastolic aortic pressure, the flow to other, nonvital organs, such as the kidneys and small intestine, becomes compromised with intense vasoconstriction of their blood supply (Schleien et al., 1986; Michael et al., 1984; Koehler et al., 1985).

Effects on Coronary Blood Flow

The increase and maintenance of aortic diastolic pressure associated with administration of α-adrenergic agonists during CPR are critical for coronary blood flow and ultimately successful resuscitation. In the beating heart, the contractile state of the myocardium is increased by β-adrenergic receptor agonist action. During CPR, β-adrenergic drugs may stimulate spontaneous myocardial contractions and increase intensity of VF, but this ionotropic effect can result in increasing intramyocardial wall pressure, decreased coronary perfusion pressure, and diminished myocardial blood flow (Livesay et al., 1978). In addition, β-adrenergic stimulation increases myocardial oxygen demand by increasing cellular metabolism and oxygen consumption. The superimposition of an increased oxygen demand on the low myocardial blood flow available during CPR probably contributes to ischemia.

The increase in and maintenance of aortic diastolic pressure associated with administration of α-adrenergic agonists during CPR are critical for coronary blood flow and ultimately successful resuscitation. Drugs that are pure α-adrenergic agonist drugs (such as methoxamine and phenylephrine) have been used successfully during CPR. The absence of direct β-adrenergic stimulation avoids an increase in myocardial oxygen uptake, resulting in a more favorable oxygen demand-to-supply ratio in the ischemic heart. These nonepinephrine, α-adrenergic agonists have been reported to be used in successful resuscitation and to maintain myocardial blood flow during CPR as effectively as epinephrine (Redding and Pearson, 1963; Pearson and Redding, 1965, Yakaitis et al., 1979; Schleien et al., 1989). Schleien et al. (1989) found that high aortic pressures can be sustained in a canine model of CPR with phenylephrine, a pure α-adrenergic agonist. The long-standing debate continues about the merits of pure α-adrenergic agonist drugs for resuscitation because of

confusion regarding benefit vs. detriment of the β-adrenergic effects of epinephrine (Holmes et al., 1980; Brown et al., 1987a, 1987c).

Effects on Cerebral Blood Flow

During CPR, the generation of cerebral blood flow, similar to coronary blood flow, depends on the vasoconstriction of peripheral vessels, and this vasoconstriction is enhanced by administration of α-adrenergic agonists. Epinephrine and other α-agonist drugs produce selective vasoconstriction of noncerebral peripheral vessels, supplying areas of the head and scalp (i.e., tongue, facial muscle, and skin) without causing cerebral vasoconstriction models of CPR in adults and infants (Koehler et al., 1983; Schleien et al., 1986; Beattie et al., 1991). Infusion of either epinephrine or phenylephrine maintained cerebral blood flow and oxygen uptake at prearrest levels for 20 minutes in a canine model of CPR. There were no differences in neurologic outcome 24 hours after resuscitation when either epinephrine or phenylephrine was administered 9 minutes after VF (Brillman et al., 1985). Other investigators found epinephrine to be more beneficial medication in generating vital organ blood flow (Brown et al., 1986b, 1987a, 1987c). This may have been because of the use of drug dosages that were not equipotent in generating vascular pressure and subsequent blood flow. In addition, epinephrine may have either a vasoconstriction or vasodilation effect on cerebral vessels, depending on the balance between α- and β-adrenergic actions (Winquist et al., 1982).

Cerebral oxygen uptake may be increased by a central β-adrenergic receptor effect if sufficient amounts of epinephrine cross the blood-brain barrier (BBB) during or after resuscitation (Carlsson et al., 1977; MacKenzie et al., 1976). When cerebral ischemia is brief and the BBB remains intact, epinephrine and phenylephrine have similar effects on cerebral blood flow and metabolism (Schleien et al., 1989). Catecholamines may cross the BBB when mechanical disruption occurs or when enzymatic barriers to vasopressors (i.e., monoamine oxidase inhibitors) are overwhelmed during tissue hypoxia (Edvinsson et al., 1978; Lasbennes et al., 1983). During CPR, the BBB may be disrupted by the generation of large fluctuations in cerebral venous and arterial pressures during chest compressions. In addition, permeability of the BBB may increase because of arterial pressure surge that occurs in a maximally dilated vascular bed after resuscitation (Arai et al., 1981). An increase in cerebral oxygen demand when cerebral blood flow is limited could affect cerebral recovery adversely. In an infant model of 8 minutes of cardiac arrest with CPR, disruption of the BBB was present 4 hours after defibrillation (Schleien et al., 1991). In similar protocols involving 8 minutes of cardiac arrest, endothelial vacuolization has been shown, with extravasation of protein through the BBB (Schleien et al., 1992a). These theoretic effects of catecholamines on cerebral circulation need to be further clarified and do not represent a contraindication to administration of epinephrine during cardiac arrest.

Dosage

High-dose epinephrine (0.1 mg/kg) is not recommended for resuscitation because of lack of evidence for benefit over standard dosing (0.01 mg/kg) and concern for harm (AHA, 2006b). Although early animal models of cardiac arrest and clinical studies indicated that high-dose epinephrine may be beneficial through increased cerebral and coronary blood flow (Brillman et al., 1985; Berkowitz et al., 1991; Brown et al., 1986a), other studies in animal models suggested that high-dose epinephrine is associated with a disproportionate rise in myocardial oxygen consumption (Maier et al., 1984; Jackson et al., 1984; Brown et al., 1988a, 1988b; Ditchey and Lindenfeld, 1988). Initial case series in adults reported increased diastolic blood pressure and successful ROSC when high-dose epinephrine was administered (Gonzalez et al., 1988, 1989; Paradis et al., 1990; Martin et al., 1990a; Cipolotti et al., 1991). In a nonrandomized, unblinded study, Goetting and Paradis (1989) reported on seven pediatric patients treated successfully with 0.2 mg/kg of epinephrine; three survived. Several large randomized controlled studies of high-dose and standard-dose epinephrine showed no benefit of high dose on survival or neurologic outcome (Brown et al., 1992; Callaham et al., 1992; Stiell et al., 1992). A prospective, randomized, double-blinded trial in children comparing high-dose epinephrine (0.1 mg/kg) with standard-dose epinephrine (0.01 mg/kg) for inpatient cardiac arrest after failure of initial standard epinephrine dose found that whereas the high-dose and standard-dose arms had equal ROSC (21 out of 34 vs. 20 out of 34), there was significantly better survival at 24 hours (7 out of 34 vs. 1 out of 34, p = 0.05) and discharge (4 out of 34 vs. 0 out of 34) in the standard dose patients (Perondi et al., 2004). Finally, a meta-analysis of these and other randomized, double-blinded studies found that whereas high-dose epinephrine may have benefit for the endpoint of ROSC, there was no improvement in survival to discharge; in fact, there was a trend toward negative impact on this endpoint (Vandycke and Martens, 2000). High-dose epinephrine may account for some of the adverse effects that occur after resuscitation by worsening myocardial ischemia that results in arrhythmias, hypertensive crisis, pulmonary edema, digitalis toxicity, hypoxemia, and cardiac arrest (Brown et al., 1992; Schleien et al., 1992b).

The 2005 AHA guidelines recommend epinephrine at 0.01 mg/kg IV or IO as the first and subsequent doses for pulseless cardiac arrest: asystole, PEA, ventricular tachycardia (VT), and VF. A dosing interval of 3 to 5 minutes is usually recommended; more frequent dosing may result in increased side effects similar to those with the use of high doses. Dosing every 4 minutes is within the recommendations and can be timed with every other 2-minute break for change in compressor and rhythm analysis. When IV or IO access is unavailable, epinephrine may be administered via the ETT at 0.1 mg/kg, although the 2005 guidelines emphasize IV and IO dosing over ETT dosing because of more reliable drug absorption and effect. The high dosage of epinephrine (0.1 mg/kg) may be considered in clinical situations refractory to standard dosing, such as β-blocker or calcium channel overdose, severe anaphylaxis, or septic shock (AHA, 2006b) (Table 38-8).

Other Adrenergic Agents

Dopamine and dobutamine are additional agents used for vasopressor support after cardiac arrest in infants and children. Guidelines for postresuscitation support advocate their use, because they cause less tachycardia, myocardial ectopy, and hypertension than epinephrine in the patient who has experienced cardiac arrest. Dopamine hydrochloride is administered as an infusion of 2 to 20 mcg/kg per minute. At higher doses (more than 10 mcg/kg per minute), α-adrenergic activity

TABLE 38-8. Epinephrine Administration During CPR

Actions	Decreases perfusion to nonvital organs (α-adrenergic effect)
	Improves coronary perfusion (aortic diastolic pressure) (α-adrenergic effect)
	Increases intensity of ventricular fibrillation (β-adrenergic effect)
	Stimulates cardiac contractions (β-adrenergic effect)
	Intensifies cardiac contractions (β-adrenergic effect)
Indications	Bradyarrhythmia with hemodynamic compromise
	Asystole or pulseless arrest
Dosage	Bradycardia: 0.0l mg/kg intravenous or intraosseous or 0.1 mg/kg ETT
	Repeat every 3 5 min at the same dosage
	Pulseless
	First dose: 0.01 mg/kg intravenous or intraosseous or 0.1 mg/kg ETT
	Repeat every 3-5 min

Data from AHA: 2005 American Heart Association (AHA) guidelines for cardiopulmonary resuscitation (CPR) and emergency cardiovascular care (ECC) of pediatric and neonatal patients: pediatric advanced life support. American Heart Association, *Pediatrics* 117:e1005, 2006b.
CPR, Cardiopulmonary resuscitation; *ETT,* endotracheal tube.

TABLE 38-9. Vasopressor Infusions in the Post-Arrest Period

Agent	Dosage	Comments
Epinephrine	0.05-1.0 mcg/kg/min	Inotrope, chronotrope
Dopamine	2-20 mcg/kg/min	Inotrope, chronotrope; dilates the splanchnic vasculature at lower doses, pressor effect at higher doses
Dobutamine	2-20 mcg/kg/min	Inotrope, decreased SVR
Milrinone	Load: 50-75 mcg/kg Infusion: 0.5-1 mcg/kg/min	Inotrope, improve diastolic relaxation, decreased SVR

SVR, Systemic vascular resistance.

is dominant. Dobutamine hydrochloride is another adrenergic agent used for inotropic support. Infusions rates range from 2 to 20 mcg/kg per minute. Decreases in systemic vascular resistance can be seen as a result of β-adrenergic effects (Table 38-9).

Phosphodiesterase Inhibitors

Milrinone is commonly used as an inotrope to support myocardial function during the perioperative period in children undergoing congenital heart surgery and may be useful in the postresuscitation period. The benefits of this agent are: increased inotropy (force of left ventricular contraction), increased dromotropy (speed and efficiency of myocardial conductive pathways) and increased lusitropy (left ventricular diastolic relaxation). There is no effect on chronotropy (rate of contraction); thus, minimal impact on myocardial oxygen consumption and the risk of arrhythmias is low. The side effects of milrinone are predominately thrombocytopenia and a decrease in systemic vascular resistance. Milrinone is usually loaded with a dose of 50 mcg/kg over 30 minutes followed by an infusion of

0.5 to 1 mcg/kg per minute. In an animal model of CPR during VFCA, a loading dose and maintenance infusion of milrinone improved stroke volume and sustained rhythm after arrest (Niemann et al., 2003).

Vasopressin

Vasopressin is a pituitary hormone that binds to specific receptors located throughout the vasculature (V1 receptors) that are responsible for vasoconstriction and in renal tubules (V2 receptors) that facilitate water reabsorption. L-arginine vasopressin is the exogenously administered compound traditionally used to treat diabetes insipidus and gastric hemorrhage. More recent indications for vasopressin include vasoplegic shock and cardiac arrest. Both endogenous and administered vasopressin are cleared and inactivated from plasma during passage through the liver and kidneys. This results in an elimination half-life of about 10 to 20 minutes.

In cardiac arrest, vasopressin has a theoretic advantage compared with epinephrine, because it causes vasoconstriction without adrenergic activity; it does not increase myocardial oxygen demand at a time when oxygen delivery is limited. In addition, vasopressin may result in less ventricular ectopy and tachycardia in the postresuscitation period. These advantages may be offset by intense vasoconstriction after ROSC, potentially worsening myocardial ischemia (Prengel et al., 1996, 1998; Wenzel and Lindner, 2002).

A meta-analysis of animal studies of vasopressin in cardiac arrest found that vasopressin increases ROSC compared with placebo (93% vs. 19%, p < 0.001) or adrenaline (84% vs. 52%, p < 0.001) (Biondi-Zoccai et al., 2003). However, data in humans are not as strong. Wenzel et al. (2004) performed a large randomized trial of vasopressin and epinephrine for the treatment of OHCA and found no difference between the two drugs in hospital admission for patients with VF or PEA but did show improved hospital admission rate and survival discharge in patients with asystole treated with vasopressin. Additionally, there was improved hospital admission (25.7% vs. 16.4%, p = 0.002) and survival to discharge rate (6.2% vs. 1.7%, p = 0.002) among patients treated with vasopressin and then epinephrine vs. epinephrine alone (Wenzel et al., 2004). However, other large, randomized controlled trials have failed to demonstrate the beneficial effect of vasopressin alone or in combination with epinephrine vs. epinephrine alone for survival to discharge (Lindner et al., 1997; Stiell et al., 2001; Callaway et al., 2006; Gueugniaud et al., 2008).

The pediatric literature concerning the use of vasopressin during CPR is limited. A pediatric animal model of asphyxia cardiac arrest found that ROSC was significantly more likely in animals treated with epinephrine than with vasopressin (Voelckel et al., 2000). In a retrospective review, Mann showed that four of six children experiencing cardiac arrest had ROSC after administration of vasopressin (0.4 units/kg). Two patients survived to 24 hours, and one patient survived to discharge (Mann et al., 2002). An additional case series reported the use of terlipressin, a vasopressin analogue in seven children with asystole. ROSC was achieved in five children, and four children survived to discharge (Matok et al., 2007). A retrospective review of the National Registry of CPR (NRCPR) database of vasopressin use during pediatric IHCA from 1999 to 2004 showed only 5% of children received vasopressin during the management of cardiac arrest. Children who received vasopressin had a lon-

ger duration of cardiac arrest than those who did not (median 37 vs. 24 minutes, p = 0.004) and were more commonly in an intensive care setting (77%). After multivariate analysis, vasopressin was associated with worse ROSC and no difference in 24-hour or discharge survival (Duncan et al., 2009). Thus, the role of vasopressin in pediatric cardiac arrest is indeterminate and requires further study.

Indication and Dosage

AHA guidelines do not recommend for or against the use of vasopressin for pediatric cardiac arrest, but they do recommend the administration of two doses of 40 units of vasopressin intravenously for refractory VF in adults. Vasopressin may have an advantage over epinephrine in the resuscitation of a child with prolonged QTc syndrome, because epinephrine may potentiate ventricular dysrhythmias in this disease. The few reports of vasopressin use in pediatric cardiac arrest, or pediatric models of cardiac arrest use a 0.4 to 0.5 units/kg dose, with an adult dose of 40 units (Mann et al., 2002). There are insufficient data on which to base suggestions for repeating the dose for pediatric cardiac arrest.

Adverse Effects

The most common side effects seen with vasopressin treatment in children receiving treatment for diabetes insipidus and gastric hemorrhage are nausea, vomiting, and abdominal pain. These may be related to vasoconstriction of the splanchnic vasculature. Rare adult reports of bowel ischemia, skin necrosis, and myocardial ischemia have been made that may be related to the vasoconstrictive effects of vasopressin. Anaphylactic and other allergic reactions have also been reported but also are rare (Wenzel and Lindner, 2002).

Antiarrhythmic Drugs

Atropine

Atropine is a parasympatholytic agent that reduces vagal tone to the heart, resulting in an increased discharge rate of the sinus node, enhanced atrioventricular conduction, and activated latent ectopic pacemakers (Gillette and Garson, 1981). Atropine has minimal effects on systemic vascular resistance, myocardial perfusion, and myocardial contractility (Gilman et al., 1990).

Indications

Atropine is indicated for treatment of bradycardia associated with hypotension, second- and third-degree heart block, and slow idioventricular rhythms (Goldberg, 1974; Scheinman et al., 1975). Atropine is a useful drug for clinical states associated with excessive parasympathetic tone. Pediatric patients who experience cardiac arrest commonly have bradycardia or asystole as initial rhythms, making atropine a first-line drug for such patients. During the perioperative period, laryngoscopy or manipulation of viscera may result in severe bradycardia or even asystole secondary to enhanced parasympathetic tone, particularly in infants. Bradycardia as a result of the oculocardiac reflex during ophthalmologic surgery can occur in a child of any age. Although the first line of treatment is cessation of the precipitating stimuli, atropine has been shown to be helpful when given intravenously or intraglossally (Arnold et al., 2002)

Dosage

The pediatric dose for atropine is 0.02 mg/kg, with a minimal dose of 0.1 mg and a maximal total dose of 1 mg. The minimal dose is recommended because of the potential for paradoxical bradycardia caused by a primarily central stimulating effect on the medullary vagal nuclei with low doses (Kottmeier et al., 1968). Atropine may be given via many routes: IV, endotracheal, IO, intraglossal, intramuscular, or subcutaneous. However, the intramuscular and subcutaneous routes may not have adequate perfusion and absorption during cardiac arrest or CPR. Onset of action occurs within 30 seconds, and peak effect occurs 1 to 2 minutes after an IV dose. The adult dose of atropine is 0.5 mg IV given every 5 minutes until a desired heart rate is obtained or to a maximal dose of 2 mg. Full vagal blockade occurs in adults who receive a dose of 2 mg. Dosages larger than recommended may be required in special circumstances, such as organophosphate poisoning or nerve gas exposure.

Adverse Effects

Atropine should not be used in patients in whom tachycardia is undesirable. After myocardial infarction or ischemia with persistent bradycardia, atropine should be administered in the lowest dose possible that increases heart rate. Tachycardia, which increases myocardial oxygen consumption and can lead to VF, can occur after large doses of atropine in patients with myocardial ischemia. Caution should also be used when administering atropine to patients with pulmonary or systemic outflow tract obstruction or idiopathic hypertrophic subaortic stenosis, because tachycardia can decrease ventricular filling and lower cardiac output (Table 38-10). Electrical pacing may be a safer means of maintaining a desired heart rate in these patients.

Adenosine

Adenosine is a purine nucleoside that is a first line treatment for supraventricular tachycardia (SVT) for children and adults. Adenosine acts by binding directly to adenosine receptors in the myocardium and peripheral vasculature. Receptor binding initiates intracellular signaling via G proteins and results in prolonged AV-node refractory period and slowed conduction. This action of adenosine breaks the reentrant circuit responsible for most SVT (Crosson et al., 1994).

Indications

Treatment of narrow complex QRS tachyarrhythmia (fewer than 0.08 seconds) with adenosine results in conversion to sinus rhythm in 72% to 77% of patients with few side effects (Till et al., 1989; Losek et al., 1999). Adenosine can be used diagnostically to differentiate between VT and SVT, because the temporary AV block allows observation of isolated atrial node electric activity. The half-life is less than 10 seconds because of rapid uptake by red blood cells and endothelial cells and metabolism by adenosine deaminase on the red-cell surface. Adenosine is completely cleared from the plasma in less than 30 seconds, giving it rapid onset and short duration of action (Losek et al., 1999).

TABLE 38-10. First Line Antiarrhythmic Administration During CPR

Atropine	
Indications	Symptomatic bradycardia with AV node block Vagal bradycardia during intubation attempts After epinephrine for bradycardia with poor perfusion
Dosage	0.02 mg/kg IV or intraosseous after ensuring oxygenation (2.5 times dose if given ETT) Repeat every 3-5 min at the same dose Maximum single dose 0.5 mg in a child and 1.0 mg in an adolescent Maximum total dose 1.0 mg in a child and 2.0 mg in an adolescent
Adenosine	
Indications	First line after vagal maneuvers fail for supraventricular tachycardia
Dosage	First dose, 0.1 mg/kg rapid IV bolus; second dose, increase to 0.2 mg/kg rapid IV bolus (maximum single dose: 12 mg) Note: must be followed with 0.5-1 mL/kg normal saline flush over 1-2 seconds to have effect.
Amiodarone	
Indication	Supra-ventricular and ventricular tachyarrhythmias
Dosage	5 mg/kg IV over 30 minutes (push if pulseless).

Data from American Heart Association.
CPR, Cardiopulmonary resuscitation; *AV,* atrioventricular; *ETT,* endotracheal tube; *IV,* intravenous.

Dosage

A rapid bolus of 100 mcg/kg (to a maximum of 6 mg) is given. If SVT resumes or no electrical response is seen, another higher bolus of 200 mcg/kg (to a maximum of 12 mg) is given and may be repeated if no response is seen or there is a limited duration of effect. The technique of administration of adenosine is critical for success of therapy. Each dose should be followed by rapid injection of 10 mL of saline flush to allow the drug to reach the heart before plasma clearance. This can be achieved with a two-stopcock technique connecting both the adenosine and flush to the patient in series. Central administration is preferable when available. Effectiveness is improved when adenosine is given by central venous access. When administering adenosine, the ECG may be helpful in determining the source of the arrhythmia.

Adverse Effects

Reported complications are rare and include hypotension, bradycardia, and brief AV block. Less likely complications are bronchospasm, facial flushing, headache, dyspnea, chest pain, nausea, lightheadedness, complete AV block, and ventricular standstill. If complications do occur they are often short in duration secondary to the short duration of action of adenosine. Dosages may need to be increased for patients receiving methylxanthines (i.e., theophylline), because these agents are adenosine antagonists (Table 38-10).

Amiodarone

Amiodarone hydrochloride is a diiodinated benzofuran derivative containing a diethylated tertiary amine chain. It is strongly lipophilic and has extensive tissue distribution. The drug is metabolized by the liver with mainly bile elimination; there is little renal elimination. Amiodarone has a long elimination half-life that ranges from 20 to 47 days (Chow, 1996). Amiodarone has pharmacologic effects of all four antiarrhythmic classes (Singh et al., 1989). It blocks potassium channels, blocks inward sodium current, is a noncompetitive β-blocker, and has calcium-channel blocking properties. Interestingly, its major electrophysiologic effect is dependent on the route (and duration) of administration (Bauman, 1997). With long-term oral treatment, amiodarone's predominant activity is to increase the duration of the action potential in most cardiac tissue, a class III effect. When used intravenously, amiodarone increases AV node refractoriness and intranodal conduction interval time, a class II antiadrenergic effect, or a calcium-channel blocker effect (Nattel, 1993). Additionally, amiodarone causes both coronary and systemic vasodilation (Coté et al., 1979). It does have phosphodiesterase inhibition and is a selective inhibitor of thyroid hormone metabolism (Singh et al., 1989; Harris et al., 1993).

Indications

Amiodarone has been studied as both a prophylactic long-term medication for patients with high arrhythmogenic potential caused by organic heart disease and for use in acute life-threatening arrhythmias. Amiodarone has been shown to be most effective for VT or VF when compared with lidocaine and bretylium in over 15 adult studies (Bauman et al., 1987; Helmy et al., 1988; Roberts et al., 1994; Podrid, 1995; Chow, 1996). When IV amiodarone was compared with placebo in a randomized trial (ARREST trial), there was significant improvement in the number of patients surviving to the emergency department after OHCA (Gonzalez et al., 1998). Amiodarone was shown to improve survival to admission when given to adults with OHCA and shock-resistant VF (Kudenchuk et al., 1999). A study comparing the efficacy of lidocaine to amiodarone for shock-resistant VF in OHCA demonstrated a 15% vs. 27% survival of adult patients to admission (Dorian et al., 2002). These adult studies support the superior performance of amiodarone for ventricular arrhythmias.

Amiodarone has been studied in children with generally favorable outcome. Perry et al. (1993) showed arrhythmia resolution in six of 10 children (mean age of 6.8 years) who had not responded to multiple other antiarrhythmic drugs. Figa et al. (1994) studied 30 infants and children with life-threatening arrhythmias, including SVT and VT and showed amiodarone eliminated arrhythmias in 71% of patients; an additional 23% experienced a significant improvement in clinical status and rhythm. Burri et al. (2003) treated 23 infants with hemodynamically unstable tachycardias with amiodarone; dosages ranged from 5 to 26 mcg/kg per minute (mean dosage of 15 mcg/kg per minute). He found only one infant to be unresponsive and adverse effects in four infants. A review of amiodarone use entered in the NRCPR database from 2000 to 2005 revealed that approximately 20% of children with VF while hospitalized and pulseless VT received amiodarone (October et al., 2008). The 2005 AHA guidelines recommend amiodarone for treatment of VF or VT without a pulse. It may also be considered in the treatment of stable SVT and VT.

Dosage

There are limited data of amiodarone pharmacokinetics in children. IV administration for active arrhythmias is common practice, and it is often followed by a continuous infusion or transition to oral medication if ongoing treatment is indicated. An initial IV dose of 5 mg/kg may be followed by additional doses or a continuous infusion of 5 mcg/kg per minute. Increases in the infusion can occur up to maximum of 10 mcg/kg per minute or 20 mg/kg per 24 hours (Perry et al., 1996). Caution should be taken in the rate of administration of amiodarone, because cardiovascular collapse can occur with rapid administration, particularly in the patient with arrhythmias who may already have hemodynamic instability. For patients in a state of cardiac arrest, amiodarone is administered via bolus. For patients not in a state of cardiac arrest, administration should be over 30 to 60 minutes to avoid further hemodynamic instability. Pretreatment with calcium may help prevent hypotension during administration, especially if the patient is hypocalcemic.

Adverse Effects

All of the adverse effects of amiodarone appear to be less common at lower dosages (Singh, 1996). Cardiovascular effects appear to be the most common and include hypotension caused by acute vasodilation and negative inotropic effects. Bradyarrhythmias, congestive heart failure, cardiac arrest, and VT have all been reported. Proarrhythmias, although possible, are seen less often than with other class III antiarrhythmics. The incidence is thought to be approximately 2%. Torsades de pointes occurs in one third of these cases (Perry et al., 1993). The most common noncardiovascular toxicities are pulmonary complications. Interstitial pneumonitis is the most common, usually associated with long-term oral treatment. A hypersensitivity pneumonitis can occur early in the course of treatment. Symptoms include cough, low-grade fever, dyspnea, weight loss, respiratory associated chest pain, and bilateral interstitial infiltrates. These symptoms are usually reversible on cessation of the drug (Jessurun et al., 1998). Hepatotoxicity can occur and is more common with oral use. Thyroid dysfunction may occur in as many as 10% of patients, resulting in either hypothyroidism or hyperthyroidism. Optic neuritis or neuropathy resulting in decreased acuity or blurred vision can progress to permanent blindness. Neurologic symptoms include ataxia, tremor, peripheral neuropathy, malaise or fatigue, sleep disturbance, dizziness, and headache. Dermatologic reactions include allergic rash, photosensitivity, and blue-gray skin discoloration (Hilleman et al., 1998) (Table 38-10).

Lidocaine

Lidocaine, a class IB antiarrhythmic, depresses the fast inward sodium channel, which results in an increased refractory period and shortening of the total action potential. The drug is metabolized primarily in the liver by the microsomal enzyme system (Collingsworth et al., 1974). Up to 10% of lidocaine is excreted unchanged in the urine. The amount excreted unchanged increases in acidic urine. There is no biliary excretion or intestinal absorption in humans.

During CPR, lidocaine clearance is decreased because of inherent decrease in cardiac output and low hepatic blood flow. During conventional CPR in dogs who had a blood pressure of 20% of control values, an IV lidocaine bolus of 2 mg/kg resulted in elevated blood and tissue concentrations. Lidocaine distribution, which is usually complete in 20 minutes, was still not complete after 1 hour. Lidocaine clearance and distribution may also be altered as a result of changes in protein binding and metabolism during CPR (Chow et al., 1983). In humans, high peak blood and tissue concentrations of lidocaine occur during CPR, with a delay in time to peak concentration. Comparison of peripheral, central, and IO routes of administration of lidocaine during open-chest CPR in dogs showed no difference in time to peak serum concentration (Chow et al., 1981).

Electrophysiology

Lidocaine causes a decrease in automaticity and in spontaneous phase 4 depolarization of pacemaker tissue. The drug increases VF threshold, whereas it has essentially no effect on ventricular diastolic threshold for depolarization. It decreases action potential duration of Purkinje fibers and ventricular muscle and increases the effective refractory period of these fibers. Lidocaine does not affect conduction time through the AV node or intraventricular conduction time. By decreasing automaticity, lidocaine prevents or terminates ventricular arrhythmias caused by accelerated ectopic foci. Lidocaine abolishes reentrant ventricular arrhythmias by decreasing action potential duration and conduction time of Purkinje fibers, thus reducing the nonuniformity of action. The effect on ischemic tissues in which lidocaine delivery may be limited is unknown (Collingsworth et al., 1974).

Hemodynamic Effects

In animal models, rapid IV delivery of lidocaine causes a decrease in stroke work, blood pressure, systemic vascular resistance, left ventricular contractility, and a slight increase in heart rate (Austen and Moran, 1965; Constantino et al., 1967). In healthy adults, the drug does not appear to cause any change in heart rate or blood pressure, but patients with cardiac disease have a slight decrease in ventricular function (Jewitt et al., 1968; Schumacher et al., 1969). In most patients, even in those who have sustained a recent myocardial infarction, a 1- to 2-mg/kg bolus of lidocaine does not alter cardiac output, heart rate, or blood pressure (Jewitt et al., 1968). Excessive doses of lidocaine given by rapid infusion may decrease cardiac function in patients with cardiac disease, especially in those suffering an acute myocardial infarction. Therefore, slow IV administration, no faster than 50 to 100 mg/min in adults, is recommended (Collingsworth et al., 1974).

Antiarrhythmic Effects

Lidocaine is effective in terminating ventricular premature beats and VT in humans during the perioperative period of general or cardiac surgery, after an acute myocardial infarction, and in patients with digitalis intoxication. Lidocaine is also effective in preventing and treating ventricular arrhythmias during cardiac catheterization. The drug is a secondary line of therapy for VF, especially when VF or tachycardia recurs. Lidocaine is not effective in the treatment of atrial or AV junctional arrhythmias.

Dosage

To achieve and maintain therapeutic levels of lidocaine, a bolus dose should be given at the initiation of a constant infusion. In patients with normal cardiac and hepatic function, an initial IV bolus of 1 mg/kg lidocaine is given, followed by a constant infusion at a rate of 20 to 50 mcg/kg per minute. If the arrhythmia recurs, a second bolus of the same dose can be given (Greenblatt et al., 1976). When a bolus administration is used without an infusion, the ventricular arrhythmias often return within 15 to 20 minutes because of its rapid clearance (Bartlett et al., 1984). If an infusion is begun without an initial bolus, approximately five half-lives are required to approach a plateau serum concentration (half-life of 108 minutes) (Collingsworth et al., 1974).

Patients with severe diminution of cardiac output should receive a bolus no greater than 0.75 mg/kg followed by an infusion at a rate of 10 to 20 mcg/kg per minute. In patients with hepatic disease, dosages should be decreased to 50% of normal. Patients with chronic renal disease who are receiving treatment through hemodialysis have normal lidocaine pharmacokinetics.

Drug interactions with lidocaine are common. Phenobarbital increases lidocaine metabolism, requiring increased doses. Isoniazid and chloramphenicol decrease lidocaine metabolism, so a decreased dosage should be used. Any drug that decreases cardiac output increases the serum concentration of lidocaine, and drugs that increase cardiac output and hepatic blood flow cause the serum concentration to be lower than predicted.

Adverse Effects

Lidocaine toxicity with a serum concentration of greater than 7 to 8 mcg/mL occurs most commonly in patients with severe hepatic disease or severe congestive heart failure. Decreased cardiac output results in decreased hepatic blood flow, which leads to decreased lidocaine clearance.

The toxic effects of lidocaine generally involve the central nervous system and include seizures, psychosis, drowsiness, paresthesias, disorientation, muscle twitching, agitation, and respiratory arrest. Treatment for seizures and psychosis includes benzodiazepines or barbiturates. True allergic reactions to lidocaine are rare. Cardiovascular side effects (discussed previously) are usually observed in patients whose myocardial function is already decreased. Conversion of second-degree to complete heart block has been described (Lichstein et al., 1973). Further slowing of sinus bradycardia has also been observed. These effects are uncommon and occur with large-dose administration. These potential side effects do not prohibit the use of lidocaine in these patients (Table 38-11).

Magnesium

Only two clinical scenarios are indications for emergent magnesium therapy in children: hypomagnesemia and polymorphic VT (torsades de pointes VT). Magnesium is an intracellular cation with less than 1% of the body's store available in the serum. The ionized fraction is physiologically active, much like calcium, and serves as a cofactor in enzymatic reactions. Low serum magnesium levels often develop in critically ill patients and patients who have had CPB surgery.

TABLE 38-11. Second-Line Antiarrhythmic Administration During CPR

Lidocaine

Indications	Ventricular arrhythmias (not ventricular escape rhythm)
	Suppress ventricular ectopy
	Raise threshold for fibrillation
Dose	1 mg/kg intravenous or intraosseous bolus (2.5 times dose if ETT)
	30-50 mcg/kg/min intravenous or intraosseous infusion
	Reduce infusion rate if low cardiac output or liver failure

Magnesium

Indications	Torsades de pointes
	Hypomagnesemia
Dose	25-50 mg/kg intravenous or intraosseous (maximum: 2 g/dose)

Data from AHA: 2005 American Heart Association (AHA) guidelines for cardiopulmonary resuscitation (CPR) and emergency cardiovascular care (ECC) of pediatric and neonatal patients: pediatric advanced life support. American Heart Association, *Pediatrics* 117:e1005, 2006b.
CPR, Cardiopulmonary resuscitation, *ETT,* endotracheal tube.

Magnesium has been shown to be effective in children with torsade de pointes VT that is associated with acquired or congenital long QT interval (Tzivoni et al., 1988; Hoshino et al., 2006). Other situations such as myocardial ischemia, premature ventricular contractions, and atrial arrhythmias have been studied; however, the benefits of magnesium administration are controversial. Treatment with magnesium (whether by bolus or infusion) prevented falls in magnesium levels and resulted in a lower incidence of hemodynamically unstable arrhythmias than was found in a placebo group in children after surgery for congenital heart disease (Dorman et al., 2000; Dittrich et al., 2003). However, amiodarone may be more effective in dealing with these same postoperative arrhythmias, and other studies have not found an association between hypomagnesemia and postoperative arrhythmias (Hoffman et al., 2002; Batra et al., 2006a). The exact mechanism of magnesium on the conduction pathways of the heart is not known. Studies have demonstrated antagonism of calcium channels. Such antagonism of calcium has been shown to block the rise of intracellular calcium during periods of hypoxia.

Dosage

Treatment with magnesium sulfate is 25 to 50 mg/kg per dose (with a maximum of 2 g/dose) given intravenously over 20 to 30 minutes in nonurgent situations; it may be bolused if a patient has polymorphic VT. Serum levels should be monitored, with some controversy regarding the utility of monitoring ionized levels. Of note, 1 g of magnesium sulfate is equivalent to 4 mmol, 8 mEq, or 98 mg of elemental magnesium. Magnesium sulfate can be administered by the IV, IO, and oral routes.

Adverse Effects

A rapid rate of administration can cause a fall in systemic vascular resistance by as much as 30%. This hypotension can be treated by either slowing or stopping the dose. Apnea and weakness are possible complications but are not routinely seen until toxic levels that have reached more than 4 mmol/L. Potentiation of neuromuscular blockade and neuromuscular weakness has been reported at lower serum levels (Table 38-11).

Other Drugs

Sodium Bicarbonate

Sodium bicarbonate causes an acid-base reaction in which bicarbonate combines with hydrogen ion to form water and carbon dioxide, resulting in an elevated blood pH:

$$HCO_3^- + H^+ \rightarrow H_2CO_3 \rightarrow H_2O + CO_2$$

Because sodium bicarbonate generates CO_2, adequate alveolar ventilation must be present before its administration. As respiratory failure is the leading cause of cardiac arrest in children, caution should be taken before sodium bicarbonate administration in the face of preexisting respiratory acidosis. Sodium bicarbonate use during CPR is one of the most controversial issues in the literature related to cardiac arrest. This stems from lack of evidence of benefit during CPR in animals and humans, as well as the potential adverse effects associated with sodium bicarbonate administration.

Literature on sodium bicarbonate use in CPR dates back to the 1960s, but there are little data demonstrating a beneficial impact on human survival (Levy, 1998). In animal models of resuscitation from cardiac arrest, sodium bicarbonate has been associated with increased survival in few studies and with no difference in survival in many studies (Andersen et al., 1967; Redding and Pearson, 1968; Kirimli et al., 1969; Lathers et al., 1989; Bleske et al., 1992; Neumar et al., 1995; Vukmir et al., 1995). Administration of sodium bicarbonate to humans experiencing cardiopulmonary arrest has been associated with increased mortality in retrospective reviews and nonblinded prospective studies (Suljaga-Pechtel et al., 1984; Skovron et al., 1985; Delooz and Lewi, 1989).

Several studies in both humans and animals document deleterious effects on physiologic endpoints such as myocardial performance, arterial blood pressure, and partial pressure of venous CO_2 (Pco_2) after sodium bicarbonate administration during CPR (Wang and Katz, 1965; Bishop and Weisfeldt, 1976; Weil et al., 1985; Adrogue et al., 1989; Kette et al., 1991; Eleff et al., 1995). This literature is difficult to interpret because of large variations in dosage, timing, blood sampling, and testing conditions. Animal data and a retrospective review of OHCA in adults indicate improved outcomes in cardiac arrest when sodium bicarbonate is administered early in cardiac arrest (Vukmir et al., 1995; Bar-Joseph et al., 1998; 2005; Leong et al., 2001). Dybvik et al. (1995) conducted the only randomized control trial of sodium bicarbonate administration in humans during CPR. Researchers found no survival benefit, but the study may have been underpowered because survival from OHCA is low and a large cohort would be required to detect a difference. Overall, there are insufficient data to assess the impact of sodium bicarbonate administration on survival during CPR.

Indications

The AHA's 2005 guidelines for CPR recommend that sodium bicarbonate be considered in cases of prolonged cardiac arrest only after effective ventilations and chest compressions are established and after epinephrine administration. Sodium bicarbonate is used for correction of significant metabolic acidosis. Acidosis depresses myocardial function by decreasing spontaneous cardiac activity, electrical threshold for VF, myocardial inotropic state, and cardiac responsiveness to catecholamines, and by prolonging diastolic depolarization (Pannier and Leusen, 1968; Cingolani et al., 1970; Orlowski, 1980; Steinhart et al., 1983). Acidosis also decreases systemic vascular resistance and blunts the vasoconstrictive effects of catecholamines (Wood et al., 1963). In addition, pulmonary vascular resistance increases with acidosis in patients with a reactive pulmonary vasculature (Rudolph and Yuan, 1966). Therefore, correction of acidosis may be of help in resuscitating patients who have potential for right-to-left shunting.

Sodium bicarbonate is also indicated in hyperkalemic arrest, because the increase in pH drives potassium intracellularly, resulting in a lowered serum potassium concentration. Hypermagnesemia, tricyclic antidepressant overdose, and overdose from sodium-channel blocking medications including cocaine, β-blockers, and diphenhydramine are other indications for sodium bicarbonate (Kilecki et al., 1997; Donovan et al., 1999; Mullins et al., 1999; AHA, 2006b).

Dosage

When the partial pressure of arterial CO_2 ($Paco_2$) and pH are known, the dose of sodium bicarbonate needed to correct the pH to 7.40 can be calculated from the following formula:

$$(0.3 \times \text{Weight [kg]} \times \text{Base Deficit}) = \text{mEq Bicarbonate}$$

Because of the possible side effects of sodium bicarbonate and the large arterial-to-venous carbon dioxide gradient that develops during CPR, giving half the dose based on a volume of distribution of 0.6 is recommended. If blood gases are not available, an initial dose of 1 mEq/kg, followed by 0.5 mEq/kg every 10 minutes of ongoing arrest has been proposed (Martinez et al., 1979). Adequate alveolar ventilation is important to eliminate the CO_2 produced during bicarbonate administration (Table 38-12).

Adverse Effects

Multiple adverse effects occur with administration of sodium bicarbonate, including metabolic alkalosis, hypernatremia, hypercapnia, and hyperosmolarity; all are associated with an increased mortality rate (Mattar et al., 1974; Worthley, 1976). Metabolic alkalosis causes a leftward shift of the oxyhemoglobin dissociation curve that impairs release of oxygen from hemoglobin to tissues at a time of low cardiac output and low oxygen delivery (Bishop and Weisfeldt, 1976). Hypernatremia and hyperosmolarity may decrease organ perfusion by increasing interstitial edema in microvascular beds.

Various theoretic adverse effects are also created by administration of sodium bicarbonate. The marked hypercapnic acidosis in both systemic venous and coronary sinus blood that develops during cardiac arrest may be worsened by administration of sodium bicarbonate (Grundler et al., 1986; Weil et al., 1986). Hypercapnic acidosis in the coronary sinus may cause decreased myocardial contractility (Pannier and Leusen, 1968; Cingolani et al., 1970; Deshmukh et al., 1986). Falk et al. (1988) measured the mean venoarterial difference of $Paco_2$ as 23.8 + 15.1 mm Hg in five patients during CPR. In one patient,

TABLE 38-12. Sodium Bicarbonate Administration During CPR	
Indications	Hyperkalemia
	Preexisting metabolic acidosis
	Long CPR time without blood-gas availability
	Pulmonary hypertensive crisis
Dosage	1 mEq/kg intravenous or intraosseous empirically, or calculated from base deficit
	Ensure adequate ventilation when administering bicarbonate
Complications	Metabolic alkalosis
	Impairs O_2 delivery by shift of oxyhemoglobin dissociation
	Decreases cardiac contractility
	Increases possibility for fibrillation
	Decreases plasma K^+ and Ca^{2+} by intracellular shift
	Hypernatremia
	Hyperosmolarity
	Hypercapnia
	Paradoxical intracellular acidosis

CPR, Cardiopulmonary resuscitation; O_2, oxygen; K^+, potassium; Ca^{2+}, calcium.

the difference increased from 16 mm Hg to 69 mm Hg after administration of sodium bicarbonate.

An additional theoretic concern is intracellular acidosis from CO_2 diffusion across cell membranes despite increased serum pH with sodium bicarbonate administration. In the central nervous system, intracellular acidosis probably does not occur unless overcorrection of the pH occurs. After administration of two doses of bicarbonate of 5 mEq/kg to neonatal rabbits recovering from hypoxic acidosis, the arterial pH increased to 7.41 and the intracellular brain pH increased to prehypoxic levels (Sessler et al., 1987). A paradoxical intracellular acidosis did not develop. In a study in rats the intracellular brain adenosine triphosphate (ATP) concentration did not change during 70 minutes of extreme hypercarbia, despite a decrease in the intracellular brain pH to 6.5 (Cohen et al., 1990b). After hypercarbia, these animals could not be distinguished from normal controls, and their brains were not morphologically different from those of control animals. Eleff et al. (1995) used magnetic resonance spectroscopy to measure cerebral pH during cardiac arrest and CPR in a dog model where CPP was maintained and Pco_2 was normalized with controlled ventilation. In that model, cerebral pH paralleled blood pH; administration of sodium bicarbonate did not cause a paradoxical intracerebral acidosis and instead prevented cerebral acidosis that occurred in the control group.

Calcium

The calcium ion is essential in myocardial excitation-contraction coupling and myocardial contractility, and it enhances ventricular automaticity during asystole (Greenblatt et al., 1976). Ionized hypocalcemia leads to decreased ventricular performance, peripheral vasodilation, and blunting of the hemodynamic response to catecholamines (Bristow et al., 1977; Scheidegger et al., 1977; Drop and Scheidegger, 1980; Marquez et al., 1986; Urban et al., 1986).

Based on its role in myocardial function, calcium should be of benefit in cardiac arrest, particularly PEA and asystole. However, limited retrospective and prospective adult studies have failed to demonstrate a benefit of calcium in these conditions (Harrison and Amey, 1983; Stueven et al., 1983, 1985a, 1985b). As a result of this data and others like it, the AHA's 2000 guidelines limited recommendations for calcium administration to cardiac arrest associated with electrolyte abnormalities and toxic ingestions (Guidelines 2000 for Cardiopulmonary Resuscitation and Emergency Cardiovascular Care, 2000).

Calcium administration during CPR has been associated with poor survival and neurologic outcomes in pediatric patients. In a single center trial, de Mos et al. (2006) reviewed 91 cardiac arrests in critically ill children over 5.5 years. In a multivariate analysis, patients who received one or more calcium boluses during cardiac arrest were 5.4 times more likely to suffer hospital mortality. In a large review of pediatric IHCA in the NRCPR database, Srinivasan et al. (2008) found that calcium was used in 45% of CPR events, despite guidelines limiting calcium use in CPR. After controlling for confounding variables, calcium administration was independently associated with decreased survival to discharge and poor neurologic outcome. However, for children with electrolyte- or toxin-associated cardiac arrest, calcium administration was not associated with worse event-survival or survival to discharge.

Neonates have low intracellular calcium stores and are more dependent on serum calcium levels. Calcium administration to this population, particularly after cardiac surgery, theoretically seems indicated and has been postulated to be beneficial (Peddy et al., 2007). Srinivasan et al. (2008) analyzed calcium administration during cardiac arrest in infants after cardiac surgery as part of a large review of NRCPR (spanning 2000 to 2004); after adjusting for confounding variables, calcium administration was associated with worse event-survival but not reduced rates of survival to discharge or unfavorable neurologic outcome. However, adjusted odds ratios were low (0.4 to 0.6), and this was a subgroup analysis only.

Calcium's association with poor outcomes may be related to its role in cellular apoptosis. In the setting of ischemia-reperfusion injury, calcium administration may worsen postischemic hypoperfusion and hasten development of intracellular events that lead to cell death. Intracellular calcium overload occurs in many pathologic conditions, including ischemia, and may be a part of the common pathway of cell death (Katz and Reuter, 1979; White et al., 1983).

Indications

The few firm indications for calcium use during CPR include cardiac arrest secondary to total or ionized hypocalcemia, hyperkalemia, hypermagnesemia, or an overdose of a calcium channel blocker (AHA, 2006b). Hypocalcemia occurs with a number of conditions that predispose to low total-body calcium stores, including the long-term use of loop diuretics. Ionized hypocalcemia may coexist with a normal total plasma calcium concentration. This occurs in the presence of severe alkalosis, which may be seen in the operating room secondary to iatrogenic hyperventilation. Ionized hypocalcemia also follows massive or rapid transfusion of citrated blood products into patients during surgery. The degree of hypocalcemia caused by citrated products depends on the rate of administration, the total dose, and the hepatic and renal function of the patient.

Administration of 2 mL/kg per minute of citrated whole blood causes a significant but transient decrease in the ionized calcium in patients who have been anesthetized (Denlinger et al., 1976).

Intraoperative cardiac arrests are more likely to be caused by electrolyte abnormalities than pediatric cardiac arrests in other situations. Electrolyte imbalance, particularly hyperkalemia, caused 5% of pediatric perioperative cardiac arrests in the 2007 review of the POCA registry (Bhananker et al., 2007). Despite the limited recommendations for calcium during CPR, intraoperative cardiac arrest is more likely to have a cause for which calcium administration is beneficial.

Dosage

The dosage of calcium chloride solution is 20 mg/kg. Calcium gluconate is as effective as calcium chloride in raising ionized calcium concentration during CPR (Heining et al., 1984). However, calcium chloride is more effective than calcium gluconate in supporting blood pressure in the hypotensive child (Broner et al., 1990). Calcium gluconate can be given as a dose of 30 to 100 mg/kg, with a maximum dosage of 2 g in pediatric patients (Table 38-13). Equally rapid increases in ionized calcium levels seen in patients with anhepatic jaundice after administration of calcium chloride and gluconate suggest that hepatic function is not necessary for either drug to be effective (Martin et al., 1990a).

Adverse Effects

Calcium should be given slowly through a large-bore, free-flowing IV line, preferably a central venous catheter. Severe tissue necrosis can occur when calcium infiltrates into subcutaneous tissue. When administered too rapidly, calcium may cause severe bradycardia, heart block, or ventricular standstill.

Glucose

Glucose administration during and after CPR should be restricted to documented hypoglycemia because of the detrimental effects of hyperglycemia during brain ischemia. Myers (1979) first hypothesized that hyperglycemia worsens the neurologic outcome after cardiac arrest. Siemkowicz and Hansen (1978) confirmed this finding when they found that after 10 minutes of global brain ischemia, neurologic recovery of hyperglycemic rats was worse than in normoglycemic control animals. Hyperglycemia exaggerates ischemic neurologic injury by increasing lactic acid production in the brain by anaerobic metabolism. During ischemia under normoglycemic conditions, brain lactate concentration plateaus. However,

TABLE 38-13. Calcium Chloride Administration During CPR

Indications	Hyperkalemia
	Hypocalcemia
	Hypermagnesemia
	Calcium channel blocker overdose
Dosage	20 mg/kg intravenously or intraosseously

CPR, Cardiopulmonary resuscitation.

when hyperglycemia is present, lactate concentration in the brain continues to rise for the duration of the ischemic period (Siesjo, 1984). The severity of intracellular acidosis during brain ischemia is directly proportional to the preischemic plasma glucose concentration.

Clinical studies have shown a direct correlation between the initial glucose concentration after cardiac arrest and a poor neurologic outcome (Pulsinelli et al., 1983; Longstreth and Inui, 1984; Woo et al., 1988; Ashwal et al., 1990). Longstreth et al. (1986) suggested that a higher plasma glucose concentration at admission may be an endogenous response to severe stress and not the cause of more severe brain injury. Losert et al. (2008) retrospectively examined blood glucose levels in adults 12 hours after ROSC and found that after controlling for confounding variables, normoglycemia and even mild hyperglycemia were associated with survival 6 months after arrest and good neurologic outcome. They concluded that glucose control goals after cardiac arrest need not be strict normoglycemia. Despite a lack of evidence in children, given the likelihood of additional ischemic events during the postresuscitation period, it seems warranted to maintain serum glucose in the normal range.

Voll and Auer (1988) showed that administration of insulin to hyperglycemic rats after global brain ischemia improved the neurologic outcome. Similarly, Katz et al. (1998) found that insulin and glucose administration after asphyxial cardiac arrest in rats improved neurologic outcome and histologic findings; the combination of insulin and glucose had superior outcomes as compared with either drug individually or saline placebo. The effect of insulin may be independent of its glucose-lowering properties, because an additional study by Voll and Auer (1991) found that normoglycemic-treated rats had a better outcome than placebo-treated controls. Infants, patients with hepatic disease, and debilitated patients with low endogenous glycogen stores are prone to hypoglycemia when energy requirements rise. In these patients, bedside monitoring of serum glucose level is critical during the perioperative period and cardiac arrest episodes.

Dosage

To treat hypoglycemia, an IV dose of 1 mL/kg of 50% dextrose for adults, 2 mL/kg of 25% dextrose in children, or 3 to 5 mL/kg of 10% dextrose for infants can be administered.

ELECTRICAL INTERVENTIONS IN CARDIOPULMONARY RESUSCITATION

Defibrillation

Defibrillation is the delivery of an untimed electrical shock for pulseless VT or VF. It is a life-saving intervention for children and adults, and AHA guidelines for 2005 place emphasis on the skill and timeliness of defibrillation (AHA, 2006b). This skill is particularly important to the anesthesiologist. As team leader of perioperative arrest, the anesthesiologist is expected to have a mastery of skills associated with resuscitation, including defibrillation.

VF is not an uncommon rhythm during cardiac arrest; it occurs in 27% of pediatric cardiac arrests at some point during resuscitation (Nadkarni et al., 2006). Intraoperative cardiac arrests seem more likely to have arrhythmias as part of the

presentation, because arrest causes are most commonly caused by cardiovascular problems, such as hypovolemia, blood loss, and electrolyte disorders (Bhananker et al., 2007). Timeliness of defibrillation is crucial, because likelihood of successful defibrillation from ventricular defibrillation degrades by 5% to 10% with each minute of delay, and a graded association is seen between increasing time to defibrillation and lower survival to discharge for each minute of delay during in-hospital ventricular arrhythmias (Larsen et al., 1993; Chan et al., 2008). In adult studies, survival rates higher than 50% can be achieved if VF is defibrillated in fewer than 3 minutes (Valenzuela et al., 2000). Despite these facts, in a survey of anesthesiologists' knowledge of CPR guidelines, only 49% of anesthesiologists who care for children routinely knew the correct sequence of defibrillation for VT (Heitmiller et al., 2008). Similarly, only 51% of senior pediatric residents were able to provide a successful defibrillation on the first attempt in a simulation model of pulseless VT (Hunt et al., 2009). The only variable independently associated with time to defibrillation in Hunt's study was previous experience discharging a defibrillator, highlighting the importance of hands-on training and simulation in learning and practicing psychomotor skills such as defibrillation.

Monophasic vs. Biphasic Current

Monophasic waveforms deliver current of one polarity (direction), whereas biphasic waveforms deliver current in two directions (Fig. 38-3). Neither monophasic nor biphasic waveforms have been associated with higher ROSC or survival to discharge; however, the biphasic waveform variant appears to be more effective at producing defibrillation and cardio version at lower dosages, as well as potentially less tissue damage (White et al., 1999; Clark et al., 2001; Tang et al., 2002). The advantages of lower dose and potentially less risk of injury have made biphasic defibrillators appealing. Monophasic waveform defibrillators are no longer manufactured, although many are in use.

Energy Dosage

The optimum dosage of electrical energy to defibrillate the heart of an infant or child is not conclusively established for either monophasic or biphasic current. The recommended dose of 2 to 4 J/kg for external defibrillation was derived from an animal model and a retrospective review of 57 children with in-hospital VF using monophasic current (Geddes et al., 1974; Gutgesell et al., 1976). In a swine model of pediatric fibrillation, biphasic current was superior to monophasic current at terminating VF at lower dosages; the biphasic dosage

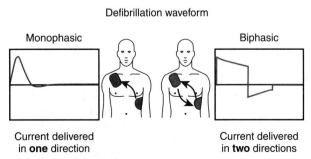

■ **FIGURE 38-3.** Monophasic and biphasic defibrillator waveforms. *(From Philips Healthcare, Andover, Mass.)*

that was required for 50% defibrillation success with first shock was 3 J/kg (Clark et al., 2001). Other data in both swine and children suggest that 2 J/kg is often ineffective at terminating fibrillation, particularly if the fibrillation is of longer duration (Berg et al., 2005a, 2005b). In a review of pediatric OHCA that received shocks for VF, a wide dosage range was documented, and 75% of children received more than the recommended dose; 45% of children received more than 6 J/kg energy doses (Rossano et al., 2006). The AHA guidelines for defibrillation dose in children are 2 J/kg initial dose and 4 J/kg subsequent doses with monophasic or biphasic current, but there is a lack of evidence to support that dosing regimen, and there is some evidence that required doses may be higher than what is recommended (AHA, 2006b). The biphasic dosage recommendations for adults are 150 to 200 J for the initial dose and equal or higher energy levels for subsequent doses (AHA, 2006b).

Paddle or Pad Type and Position

Correct paddle or self-adhesive pad size and position are important to the success of defibrillation. Two paddle sizes are available for external defibrillation: 8 to 13 cm in diameter for adults and children who weigh more than 10 kg, and 4.5 cm for infants and children who weigh less than 10 kg. Self-adhesive pads come in adult and pediatric sizes and are preferred to paddle defibrillation, because they have the correct gel interface prepackaged and are "hands-free," allowing for rapid return to chest compressions after defibrillation (Estes, 2005). The largest paddle or pad size that can be used without causing the paddles to touch should be used; large surface area reduces the density of current flow, TTI, and myocardial damage (Atkins and Kerber, 1994). Care should be taken that the entire paddle rests firmly on the chest wall; otherwise, a high-density current will be delivered to a small contact point on the skin. The paddles should be positioned on the chest wall with most of the myocardium included between them. If two paddles cannot be placed on the anterior chest, an alternate approach is to place one paddle anteriorly over the left precordium and the other paddle posteriorly between the scapulae; this technique works well in small infants (Garcia et al., 1998).

When providing defibrillation to patients with permanent pacemakers or automatic internal cardiac defibrillators (AICDs), care should be taken not to position paddles or pads over the device generators. The defibrillator current may cause device malfunction, and the device may block some current from reaching the myocardium. Pacemakers and AICDs should be checked for proper function after defibrillation.

The interface between the paddle and chest wall can be gel pads, electrode cream, paste, soap, or self-adhesive, monitoring defibrillation pads. The cream produces lower impedance than paste. Care should be taken not to allow the substance from one paddle to touch that from the other paddle, because electrical current follows the path of least resistance. This is especially important in infants, in whom the distance between electrodes is short.

Defibrillation Sequence and Technique

When the onset of VF or pulseless VT is observed, defibrillation should be attempted as soon as possible. AHA guidelines have changed to reflect the emphasis on reducing the time spent with the patient in a no-flow state; algorithms for ventricular arrhythmias no longer call for three rapidly administered shocks and multiple rhythm and pulse checks. Instead, with the onset of ventricular arrhythmia, CPR should be administered immediately while preparing for defibrillation. As soon as possible, defibrillation at 2 J/kg should be attempted with immediate return to CPR without a pulse or rhythm check. Epinephrine is administered during CPR, and a rhythm check can be performed after 2 minutes of CPR. If ventricular arrhythmia persists, additional defibrillation with 4 J/kg energy and return to CPR should be performed. Additional shocks at 4 J/kg are interspersed between CPR and antiarrhythmic medications (Fig. 38-4). The resuscitation should be seen as a continuous period of CPR with as brief as possible interruptions for defibrillation and rhythm checks (Fig. 38-5).

Although no studies compare the previously recommended three stacked shocks to the one-shock protocol, it has theoretic basis in multiple studies. Biphasic defibrillation has an initial-shock success rate of 90% in adults, and further shocks may not provide added benefit (Martens et al., 2001). Increased interruption of CPR for rhythm checks and defibrillation attempts (increasing no-flow time) is associated with lower coronary perfusion pressures and lower defibrillation success (Berg et al., 2001; Edelson et al., 2006).

Open-chest or internal defibrillation should be performed when the sternum is already open during surgery or is reopened after surgery. Paddles made specifically for this purpose are applied directly to the heart. Internal paddles have diameters of 6 cm for adults, 4 cm for children, and 2 cm for infants. The handles should be insulated. One electrode is placed behind the left ventricle, and the other is positioned over the right ventricle on the anterior surface of the heart, with saline soaked pads as conducting material. A dose 1 J/kg to a maximum of 10 J of delivered energy should be used, beginning with the lowest energy level available on the defibrillator.

Risk of Defibrillation

Skin erythema or first-degree burns have been documented after defibrillation; use of biphasic waveforms may decrease this complication (Ambler and Deakin, 2006). Reports exist of fire associated with defibrillation, particularly in an oxygen-rich environment (Miller, 1972; Theodorou et al., 2003). Care should be taken to remove disconnected oxygen tubing from the patient's immediate area during defibrillation. A review of the literature found no reports of life-threatening injury or long-term disability to rescuers and caregivers who were inadvertently shocked with a defibrillator, but defibrillation to the chest wall of a healthy individual can be life-threatening (Hoke et al., 2009).

Automated External Defibrillation

AEDs are preprogrammed defibrillators that analyze the ECG signal to distinguish shockable and nonshockable rhythms and direct providers to deliver shock when indicated. The devices are common in public settings where large numbers of people congregate and have been shown to increase the rate of survival from sudden cardiac arrest (MacDonald et al., 2002; Hallstrom et al., 2004). In a large, prospective randomized trial in public settings, lay-rescuer CPR combined with AED programs doubled survival

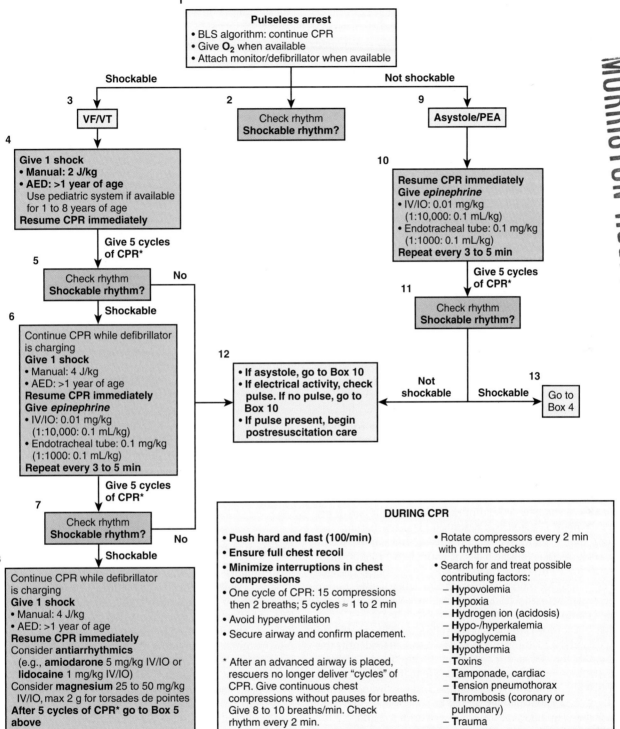

1

Pulseless arrest
- BLS algorithm: continue CPR
- Give **O₂** when available
- Attach monitor/defibrillator when available

Shockable   Not shockable

3   **2**   **9**

VF/VT   Check rhythm   **Asystole/PEA**
                 Shockable rhythm?

4   **10**

Give 1 shock
- **Manual: 2 J/kg**
- **AED: >1 year of age**
  Use pediatric system if available
  for 1 to 8 years of age
Resume CPR immediately

                                    Resume CPR immediately
                                    Give *epinephrine*
                                    - IV/IO: 0.01 mg/kg
                                      (1:10,000: 0.1 mL/kg)
                                    - Endotracheal tube: 0.1 mg/kg
                                      (1:1000: 0.1 mL/kg)
                                    Repeat every 3 to 5 min

Give 5 cycles
of CPR*   Give 5 cycles
                                                 of CPR*

5   **11**

Check rhythm   No   Check rhythm
Shockable rhythm?   **Shockable rhythm?**

Shockable   Not   13
6   **12**   shockable   Shockable
                                                                        Go to
Continue CPR while defibrillator   - **If asystole, go to Box 10**   Box 4
is charging   - **If electrical activity, check**
Give 1 shock   **pulse. If no pulse, go to**
- **Manual: 4 J/kg**   **Box 10**
- **AED: >1 year of age**   - **If pulse present, begin**
Resume CPR immediately   **postresuscitation care**
Give *epinephrine*
- IV/IO: 0.01 mg/kg
  (1:10,000: 0.1 mL/kg)
- Endotracheal tube: 0.1 mg/kg
  (1:1000: 0.1 mL/kg)
Repeat every 3 to 5 min

Give 5 cycles
of CPR*

7

Check rhythm
Shockable rhythm?   No

Shockable
8

Continue CPR while defibrillator
is charging
Give 1 shock
- **Manual: 4 J/kg**
- **AED: >1 year of age**
Resume CPR immediately
Consider **antiarrhythmics**
  (e.g., **amiodarone** 5 mg/kg IV/IO or
  lidocaine 1 mg/kg IV/IO)
Consider **magnesium** 25 to 50 mg/kg
IV/IO, max 2 g for torsades de pointes
After 5 cycles of CPR* go to Box 5
above

DURING CPR

- **Push hard and fast (100/min)**
- **Ensure full chest recoil**
- **Minimize interruptions in chest**
  compressions
- One cycle of CPR: 15 compressions
  then 2 breaths; 5 cycles ≈ 1 to 2 min
- Avoid hyperventilation
- Secure airway and confirm placement.

* After an advanced airway is placed,
rescuers no longer deliver "cycles" of
CPR. Give continuous chest
compressions without pauses for breaths.
Give 8 to 10 breaths/min. Check
rhythm every 2 min.

- Rotate compressors every 2 min
  with rhythm checks
- Search for and treat possible
  contributing factors:
  – **H**ypovolemia
  – **H**ypoxia
  – **H**ydrogen ion (acidosis)
  – **H**ypo-/hyperkalemia
  – **H**ypoglycemia
  – **H**ypothermia
  – **T**oxins
  – **T**amponade, cardiac
  – **T**ension pneumothorax
  – **T**hrombosis (coronary or
    pulmonary)
  – **T**rauma

■ **FIGURE 38-4.** PALS pulseless arrest algorithm, 2005. *(From Ralston M et al., editors:* Pediatric advanced life support provider manual, *Dallas, 2006, American Heart Association, p 168.)*

from out-of-hospital VF when compared with programs that provided early emergency medical services and CPR (Hallstrom et al., 2004).

Recommendations support the use of AEDs for early rhythm identification in children as young as 1 year of age. The algorithms are highly sensitive and specific for pediatric rhythms (Atkinson et al., 2003; Atkins et al., 2008). The energy dosage for AED use in adults is standardly set at 150 to 360 J and

often can be attenuated with a pediatric cable and pads for children younger than 8 years old (Berg, 2004). Attenuated pediatric energy doses range from 35 to 50 J for the initial dose and 80 to 90 J for subsequent doses. No adjustments are made for patient size or weight. Recommendations are to use pediatric attenuation cables and pads if they are available; if not, a standard AED should be used. AHA guidelines do not recommend for or against use of AED in infants younger than 1 year

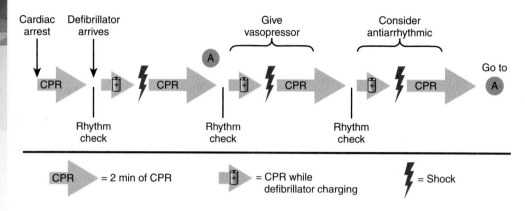

■ **FIGURE 38-5.** Continuum of CPR, 2005. *(From Ralston M et al., editors: Pediatric advanced life support provider manual, Dallas, 2006, American Heart Association, p 175.)*

of age, although termination of VF has been reported in infants with attenuated pediatric pads (Atkins and Jørgenson, 2005). A drawback of AED use in the operating room is that the time for rhythm recognition and delivery of shock needed by the AED may delay resuming chest compressions. This delay may be less with manual defibrillation by a trained provider.

Synchronized Cardioversion

Synchronized cardioversion involves timing the delivery of a shock with the cardiac cycle to treat organized arrhythmias such as atrial fibrillation and flutter or SVT. Delivery of low-dose, unsynchronized shocks in these rhythms may result in VF. Synchronized cardioversion is indicated for patients who have tachyarrhythmias but are hemodynamically stable; patients who are unstable should be defibrillated as described above.

The defibrillator or cardioversion device should be set in the synchronous mode ("sensing" on) to permit coordination of the countershock with electrical activity of the heart. Once a patient is adequately sedated (if necessary), paddles are positioned for optimal contact as described for defibrillation. The monitor should indicate adequate sensing and charge set to deliver 0.5 to 1 J/kg. Repeated dosing with up to 2 J/kg is sometimes required with the same technique. These energy dosages were developed for monophasic waveform defibrillators. Lower energies may be used with biphasic defibrillators (Batra et al., 2006b; Liberman et al., 2006).

After successful cardioversion, a follow-up ECG should be obtained and the rhythm strip should be reviewed to identify the resulting rhythm. Other antiarrhythmic therapy can be initiated if the rhythm is only transiently responsive to the cardioversion. For resistant tachycardias, hypoxemia, acidosis, hypoglycemia and electrolyte abnormalities should be sought and corrected, because they can interfere with success of cardioversion.

Transcutaneous Pacing

Most modern defibrillator and cardioversion units have capability for cardiac pacing. For transcutaneous pacing, external pacing electrodes should be positioned anteriorly on the left-sternal border and posteriorly between the scapulae. For most resuscitative efforts, asynchronous pacing should be selected. Initial settings should be set at the desired age-appropriate rate, and the output should be set at zero. Output should then be increased rapidly until capture and pacing occurs. Note that required output is

usually relative and not in a defined milliamperage (mA), as with epicardial or transvenous pacer units. Once electrical capture is seen on the monitor, mechanical association should be assessed by palpation of a pulse (Beland et al., 1988).

Transvenous Pacing

When transcutaneous pacing fails to provide results, transvenous pacing may be attempted. Experience with transvenous-pacing techniques in children has primarily occurred in the catheterization lab. Limited data are available using this technique in children during CPR. One study retrospectively reviewed experience with five children who had various causes for cardiac arrest. Four of the patients had restoration of cardiac output and stability for 10 to 60 minutes with subsequent cardiac arrest and death (Greissman et al., 1995). The pacing wire can be placed via a vascular introducer into the right atrium or right ventricle. The technique for setting output and sensitivity are the same as for epicardial pacing leads.

Epicardial Pacing

Many infants and children undergoing cardiac surgery have atrial and ventricular epicardial pacing wires placed during the procedure for postoperative management. During resuscitation, if both atrial and ventricular leads are available, ventricular leads should be used to maintain cardiac output. Note that most pacemaker generators can sense as well as pace, depending on the mode. It may be necessary to adjust the sensitivity and output to produce ventricular depolarization with every paced beat. Pacing in an asynchronous, ventricular, fixed-rate, or ventricular-inhibited pacing mode assures the most consistent cardiac output. Electrical activity should be monitored for electrical association, and pulses or arterial waveform should be monitored to evaluate mechanical capture and cardiac output.

ARRHYTHMIAS IN CARDIOPULMONARY RESUSCITATION

Bradycardia

Bradyarrhythmias are common complications in children during the perioperative period. Bradycardia is the rhythm seen most often before cardiac arrest in pediatric patients. Most bradycardic events are precipitated by hypoxemia, vagal stimuli, or side effects of medication. A sufficiently slow heart rate in an infant or child that results in hemodynamic instability should prompt CPR, diagnosis, and treatment. If resolution does not occur with ventilation, oxygenation, atropine, epinephrine, and chest compressions, then electrical pacing is indicated. The probability of successfully pacing after cardiac arrest decreases with increasing duration of CPR (Quan et al., 1992; Beland et al., 1988). If a bradyarrhythmia persists despite resuscitative and electrical support, other forms of cardiovascular support should be sought (e.g., extracorporeal membrane oxygenation). This therapy, although not curative, can provide time needed for diagnosis, treatment, and recovery.

Sinus Bradycardia

Great variability exists in infant and pediatric heart rates (Table 38-3). Lower limits of heart rates serve as guidelines but may not be indicative of pathology. Sinus bradycardia results from slowed or suppressed sinoatrial node depolarization. However, other pathologic causes can occur and should be considered in the settings of trauma, cardiac surgery, and structural heart disease. Diagnosis of sinus bradycardia implies that a normal P wave is visible on evaluation of a 12-lead ECG. Hemodynamic instability may or may not be present and is not essential for the diagnosis. Underlying causes, such as increased vagal tone, elevated ICP, hypoxia, metabolic abnormalities (hypokalemia or hypercalcemia), hypothermia, and drug effects, should be sought.

Sinus and Atrioventricular Block

Sinus block or sinus node arrest is characterized by absence of P waves from the ECG and is usually related to toxic ingestion or underlying cardiac disease. This can also present as asystole. In the absence of sinus node activity, the heart generates "escape" beats that originate from the atria, AV node, or ventricle. Atrial escape beats are characterized by P waves of varying morphology and timing associated with narrow QRS complexes. Junctional escape beats originate from the AV node and are narrow and complex; P waves from retrograde conduction may or may not be present. Ventricular escape rhythm is a wide, complex slow rate of approximately 30 to 40 beats per minute. Recognition and prompt initiation of transcutaneous pacing is crucial and can be lifesaving (Beland et al., 1988).

Varying degrees of heart block appear as a bradyarrhythmia (Fig. 38-6, A). Often a 12-lead ECG is needed to diagnose changes in the PR interval and potential conduction delays. First-degree heart block is the prolongation of the PR interval beyond normal for age. PR intervals vary but are usually less than 0.16 seconds. Such prolongation can be normal or a sign of underlying disease or medication effects. Most patients with first-degree heart block are hemodynamically stable and require monitoring for progression to other forms of heart blockage. No emergency intervention is required.

Second-degree AV block is characterized by the occurrence of a P wave without a QRS complex, where some but not all atrial impulses are conducted to the ventricle. Progressive lengthening of the PR interval until a P wave occurs alone and the QRS complex is "dropped" is called a *Wenckebach (Mobitz type I)* rhythm (Fig. 38-6, B). If the QRS complex is repeatedly absent without a change in the PR interval, it is termed a *Mobitz type*

II rhythm (Fig. 38-6, *C*). Both are forms of second-degree heart block caused by delayed or absent conduction through the AV node. Some medications, hypoxia, and myocarditis can create this problem. If the ventricular rate maintains adequate perfusion, no immediate treatment is necessary and determining and eliminating the causative factor is curative. However, if hemodynamic instability exists, attempts to increase conduction by increasing the heart rate with atropine or epinephrine may be useful, and a pediatric cardiologist should be consulted.

Third-degree AV block, or complete heart block, is characterized by consistent electrical and mechanical dissociation between the atrial and ventricular rates (Fig. 38-6, *D*). ECG analysis shows P waves at one rate and wide QRS complexes at a separate rate. As with other forms of heart block, finding and eliminating the causative agent are curative. If hemodynamically stable, observation is often suitable. However, if the rhythm deteriorates or the patient's condition becomes unstable, some form of supportive pacing is required. If the third-degree heart block is congenital in origin or is persistent from surgical correction of a congenital heart lesion, a permanent pacemaker is often required.

Treatment of Bradycardia

Therapy for all causes of bradycardia should focus on hemodynamic support and treatment of underlying causes. If the patient's condition is unstable, airway support and CPR should be initiated and immediate measures should be taken to improve the heart rate. In the operating room, potentially deleterious medications and exposures, including surgical stimulus, should be discontinued as therapy for bradycardia is initiated. The first line of therapy is administration of a vagolytic agent. The POCA registry has demonstrated that epinephrine with or without atropine is most successful in returning a stable heart rate and circulation (Morray, 2002). Potentially reversible causes of bradycardia that should prompt acute therapy can be recalled using the "H's and T's" mnemonic device (Box 38-2). If a patient is hypoxic, improved oxygenation and oxygen delivery often result in improvement in heart rate. Bradycardia secondary to vagal stimulus can be treated by the removal of the stimulus and the administration of a vagolytic agent. Further treatment with adrenergic agents, such as epinephrine, is reasonable and effective. Epinephrine may be the first choice treatment for bradycardia if it is associated with severe hypotension and causing inadequate cerebral or myocardial perfusion. Earlier recommendations have included the use of isoproterenol, a potent β-selective adrenergic agent, to provide chemical pacing. However, because of its tendency to vasodilate, resulting in inadequate coronary and cerebral perfusion, it is no longer recommended and the next line of therapy is electrical pacing (Fig. 38-7). Figure 38-8 shows additional algorithms that include pediatric advanced life support (PALS) guidelines as well as an emphasis on intraoperative factors and interventions, including evidence-based endpoints for quality care during cardiac arrest.

Tachycardia

Tachycardias include a variety of rhythms that occur at a rate greater than normal for age (Table 38-3). Analysis of a tachyarrhythmia must discriminate between sinus, supraventricular,

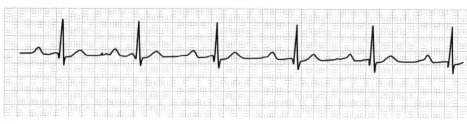

A First-degree heart block

■ **FIGURE 38-6. A,** ECG of first-degree heart block. **B,** ECG of second-degree heart block: Mobitz type I. **C,** ECG of second-degree heart block: Mobitz type II. **D,** ECG of third-degree heart block.

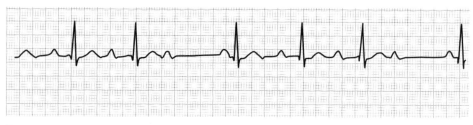

B Second-degree heart block, type 1: Wenckebach/Mobitz type I

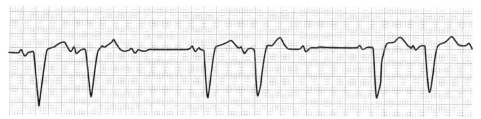

C Second-degree heart block, type 2: Mobitz type II

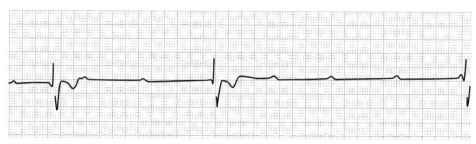

D Third degree—complete heart block

Box 38-2 Potentially Reversible Causes of Arrhythmias During Cardiopulmonary Arrest: The H's and T's

Hypovolemia
Hypoxia
Hydrogen ion (acidosis)
Hypokalemia/**H**yperkalemia
Hypoglycemia
Hypothermia
Hypervagal
Malignant **H**yperthermia
Toxins (consider medications)
Tamponade, cardiac
Tension pneumothorax
Thrombosis (coronary or pulmonary)
Trauma (hypovolemia)
Q**T** Prolongation
Pulmonary **H**yper**T**ension

junctional, or ventricular origins. The source of tachycardia, whether it is the sinus node, excitable focus, or reentrant pathway, creates variations of wide or narrow QRS complexes. Those tachycardias with narrow complexes (less than 0.08 seconds) are often atrial or high-junctional (between the atria) in origin. SVT, atrial fibrillation, atrial flutter, and junctional ectopic tachycardia (JET) present with narrow QRS complex. Wide-complex tachycardias originate from the ventricle or are SVTs with aberrant ventricular conduction. VT, often surprisingly well tolerated by pediatric patients, is the most common wide-complex tachycardia.

A patient with tachycardia may vary from showing no symptoms to being hemodynamically unstable, depending on underlying cause, other coexistent conditions, and duration and type of tachycardia. Increased myocardial oxygen consumption combined with reduced coronary perfusion caused by shortened diastolic time in rapid heart rates may cause myocardial failure when tachycardia persists or presents in an already diseased myocardium, such as cardiomyopathy.

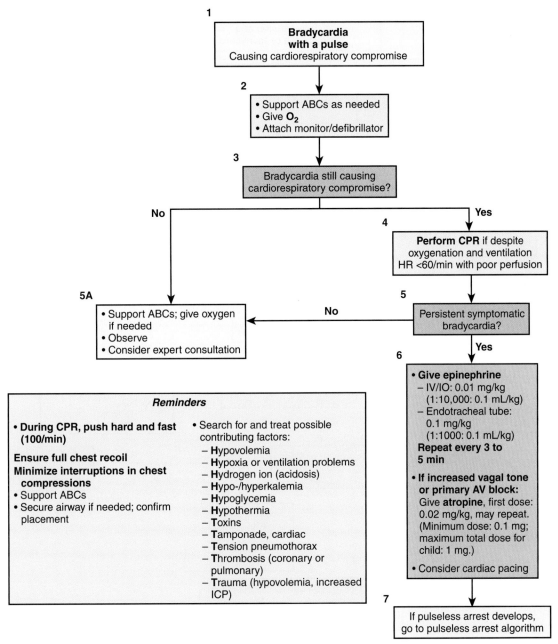

■ FIGURE 38-7. PALS bradycardia with a pulse, 2005. *(From Ralston M et al., editors:* Pediatric advanced life support provider manual, *Dallas, 2006, American Heart Association, p 123.)*

Evaluation should include assessment of hemodynamic stability and end-organ perfusion. A 12-lead ECG is often required to evaluate tachycardia. Treatment is directed at support of hemodynamics and diagnosis and treatment of tachycardia.

Sinus Tachycardia

Sinus tachycardia is the most common tachycardia seen in the pediatric patient who is under anesthesia. Common causes are pain, hyperthermia, light anesthesia, hypovolemia, anemia, hypercarbia, hypoxia, and hypoglycemia. Generally, these conditions are easily diagnosed and treated (Fig. 38-8). It is not uncommon to have a child with a heart rate that is 20% to 30% above baseline in the postoperative period because of

these factors. Sinus tachycardia has a heart rate that is not fixed; it varies with activity and intervention.

Supraventricular Tachycardia

SVT is the most common tachyarrhythmia in all ages. It is the most common nonarrest arrhythmia in children and the most common arrest arrhythmia in infancy (Fig. 38-9). The cause is often a reentrant mechanism that produces a rapid and narrow QRS complex (less than 0.08 seconds) on ECG. Rates are more than 220 beats per minute in infants and more than 180 beats per minute in children. The ability of a pediatric patient to tolerate SVT depends on coexistent pathology, possible initiating factors, and duration of arrhythmia.

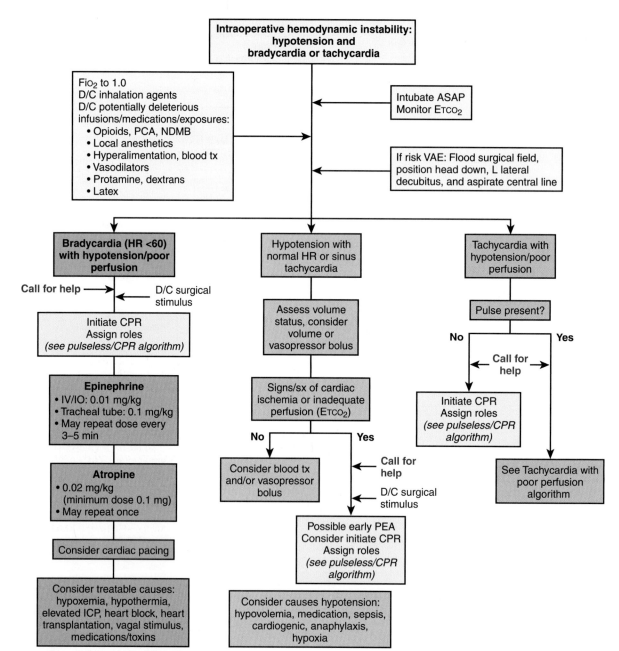

■ **FIGURE 38-8.** Intraoperative hemodynamic instability: hypotension and bradycardia or tachycardia. *ASAP,* As soon as possible; *Etco₂,* end-tidal carbon dioxide; *Fio₂,* fraction of inspired oxygen; *D/C,* discontinue; *PCA,* patient-controlled analgesia; *NDMB,* nondepolarizing muscle blockade; *tx,* transfusion; *VAE,* venous air embolus; *L,* left; *HR,* heart rate; *CPR,* cardiopulmonary resuscitation; *Sx,* symptom; *IV,* intravenous; *IO,* intraosseous; *PEA,* pulseless electrical activity; *ICP,* intracranial pressure. *(Modified from Ralston M et al., editors:* Pediatric advanced life support provider manual, *Dallas, 2006, American Heart Association.)*

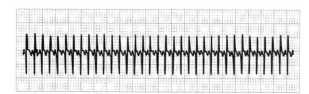

■ **FIGURE 38-9.** ECG of supraventricular tachycardia.

In infants, signs of SVT may be irritability and poor feeding. Older children often complain of lightheadedness, fatigue, and sometimes chest discomfort. Uncommonly, SVT can originate from an atrial focus that depolarizes faster than the intrinsic sinoatrial node rate. This tachycardia is termed *ectopic atrial tachycardia (EAT),* or *automatic tachycardia,* and is typically associated with cardiac surgery or congenitally acquired.

In patients who are under anesthesia, differentiating SVT from sinus tachycardia can be challenging. Lack of variability in the SVT rate compared with sinus tachycardia can be a clue. Additionally, most SVT has abrupt onset and offset, whereas sinus tachycardia tends to gradually increase and decrease. P waves in sinus tachycardia are normal and may be absent or abnormal in SVT. Ruling out possible causes of sinus tachycardia, such as fever, pain, hypovolemia, hypoxia, hypercarbia, and myocardial failure is helpful (Fig. 38-10).

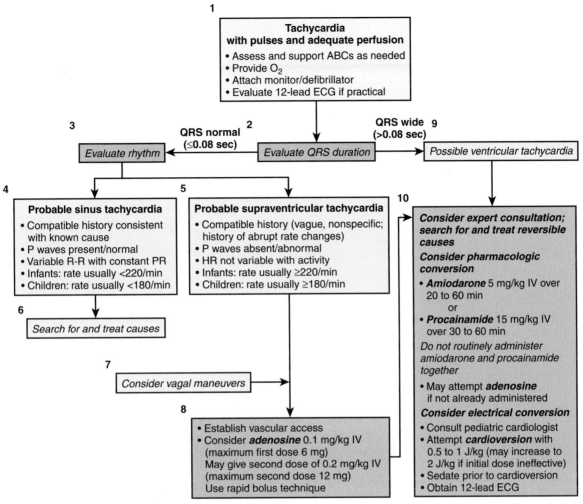

■ FIGURE 38-10. PALS tachycardia with adequate perfusion algorithm, 2005. *(From Ralston M et al., editors:* Pediatric advanced life support provider manual, *Dallas, 2006, American Heart Association, p 141.)*

SVT generally has a narrow, complex QRS appearance, but when ventricular aberrant conduction is present, the widened QRS complex and rapid rate can mimic VT. An ECG to evaluate P waves and the QRS complex can be helpful. SVT with aberrant conduction is quite rare, and in a patient whose condition is unstable, a wide-complex tachycardia should be assumed to be ventricular in origin.

If the patient is hemodynamically unstable, synchronized cardioversion is the treatment of choice at an initial dose of 0.5 to 1 J/kg. If SVT persists or recurs after countershock, additional synchronized cardioversion can occur with the dose increased to 2 J/kg. If both vascular access and adenosine are readily available, adenosine (see the related section on adenosine) can be attempted for hemodynamically unstable SVT; no delays for vascular access should occur (Figs. 38-11 and 38-12).

In a child with SVT whose state is hemodynamically stable, vagal maneuvers such as the gag and diving reflexes can be attempted as the first line of therapy. Ocular rubs are no longer recommended because of the risk for ocular trauma. Intraoperatively, some of these maneuvers will be unavailable. Ice to the face, Valsalva maneuvers, and carotid sinus massage have potential benefit and may be attempted until adenosine dosing is prepared. Failure of the above methods may indicate

a more complex arrhythmia and necessitate consultation with a pediatric cardiologist. Overdrive pacing with an esophageal or epicardial lead is an additional possible therapy in consultation with a pediatric cardiologist (Fig. 38-10).

Atrial Fibrillation and Atrial Flutter

Atrial flutter and fibrillation are extremely rare in children (Figs. 38-13 and 38-14). Atrial flutter is a rapid and regular rhythm, and in children it is often associated with structural heart disease. The underlying physiology is a macroreentry phenomenon creating a rapid, regular tachycardia. Atrial rates of 200 to 500 beats per minute are usually present and a "saw-toothed" wave or flutter waves are present on the ECG.

Atrial fibrillation is a rapid, irregular, tachycardia. Atrial rates can be as high as 600 beats per minute. The rhythm occurs because of multiple microreentrant circuits in the atria that create a variable ventricular response and irregular atrial rate. Treatment options are variable and depend on the underlying structural cause. If the rhythm is sustained and stable, consultation with a pediatric cardiologist should be sought. If it is unstable, synchronized cardioversion with 0.5 to 2 J/kg is the treatment of choice.

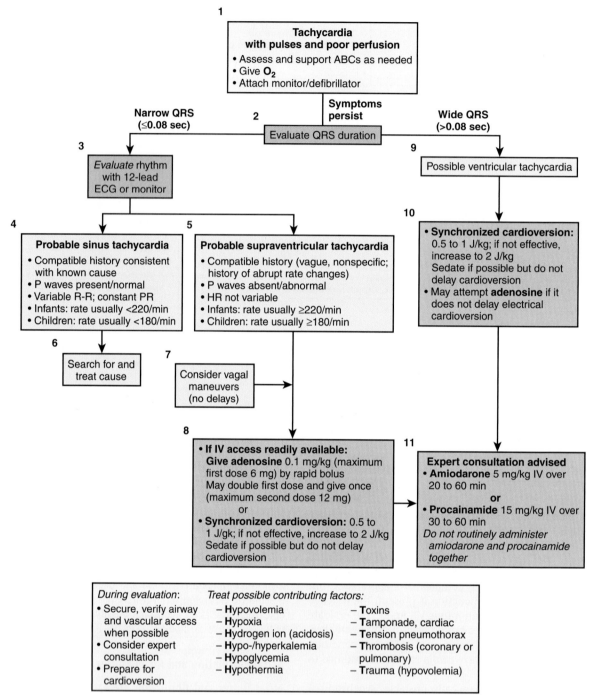

■ FIGURE 38-11. PALS tachycardia with pulses and poor perfusion algorithm, 2005. *(From Ralston M et al., editors:* Pediatric advanced life support provider manual, *Dallas, 2006, American Heart Association, p 145.)*

Junctional Ectopic Tachycardia

JET is most commonly seen after cardiac surgery for congenital heart disease. It is a narrow, complex, rapid rhythm with complete AV dissociation resulting in a ventricular rate that is more rapid than the atrial rate. Many describe the arrhythmia as a narrow complex SVT brought on by increased automaticity of the AV node or bundle of His. Occasional atrial beats are conducted through to the ventricles, depending on timing of the electrical pulse. Hemodynamic instability depends on heart rate

and degree of AV dissociation. If there is no instability, treatment is not needed. However, as cardiac output diminishes, more aggressive treatment is warranted. Therapy involves elimination of painful stimuli, metabolic acidosis, electrolyte abnormalities, endogenous and exogenous catecholamines, and fever. Further interventions involve cooling the child, IV amiodarone, and pacing the atria at a rate higher than the JET rate to provide improved AV synchrony. These efforts are supportive until the JET rhythm resolves over 2 to 4 days (Hoffman et al., 2002).

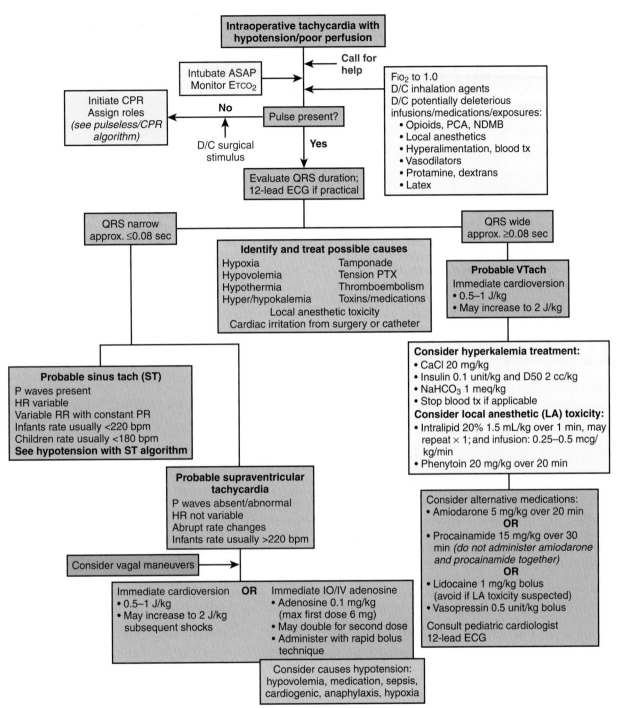

■ FIGURE 38-12. Intraoperative tachycardia with hypotension/poor perfusion. *ASAP,* As soon as possible; *E*τco$_2$, end-tidal carbon dioxide; *Fio$_2$,* fraction of inspired oxygen; *D/C,* discontinue; *PCA,* patient-controlled analgesia; *NDMB,* nondepolarizing muscle blockade; *tx,* transfusion; *CPR,* cardiopulmonary resuscitation; *ECG,* electrocardiogram; *PTX,* pneumothorax; *VT,* ventricular tachycardia; *CaCl,* calcium chloride; *D50,* 50% dextrose; *NaHCO$_3$,* sodium bicarbonate; *HR,* heart rate; *ST,* sinus tachycardia; *LA,* local anesthetic; *IO,* intraosseous, *IV,* intravenous. (*Modified from Ralston M et al., editors:* Pediatric advanced life support provider manual, *Dallas, 2006, American Heart Association.*)

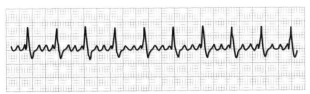

■ FIGURE 38-13. ECG of atrial flutter.

Ventricular Tachycardia

VT is defined as a rapid, wide complex QRS tachycardia (Fig. 38-15). The origin of the tachycardia is below the bifurcation of the bundle of His. This can result from either a reentrant phenomenon or from increased automaticity. At minimum, there are three wide QRS complexes with no evident P wave. When wide complex beats persist in runs of 30 seconds or more, sustained VT is present.

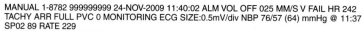
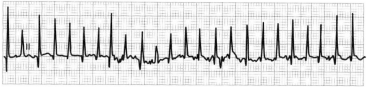
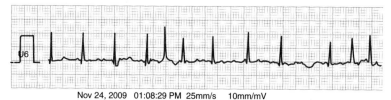

■ **FIGURE 38-14.** ECG of atrial fibrillation. Two examples of atrial fibrillation from the same patient after general anesthesia for MRI. The first shows irregular rhythm with a rate of 229; the second rhythm strip shows irregular rhythm with a rate of 130.

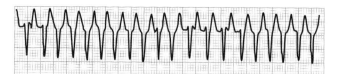

■ **FIGURE 38-15.** ECG of ventricular tachycardia.

If the patient has no pulse, defibrillation should be administered immediately at 2 J/kg followed by chest compressions. Changes in the 2005 AHA recommendations for the pulseless VT algorithm reflect the emphasis on sustained chest compressions and decreasing time when no cardiac output occurs (i.e., a no-flow state). Three stacked shocks are no longer recommended for pulseless VT; instead, recommendations are for a single defibrillation attempt followed by 2 minutes of chest compressions without pulse check (see Fig. 38-4; Fig. 38-16). Pharmacologic therapy in the algorithm includes epinephrine and in cases refractory to defibrillation and epinephrine, amiodarone or lidocaine.

VT with a pulse but poor perfusion should be treated as an emergency with synchronized cardioversion. Countershock should start with 0.5 to 1 J/kg and increase to 2 J/kg with subsequent countershocks (see Figs. 38-11 and 38-12). If the patient's condition is stable, then pharmacologic cardioversion can be attempted with the slow administration of IV amiodarone (see Fig. 38-10). The cause of VT should always be considered, and therapy should be instituted in parallel with the AHA PALS algorithms. The use of the H's and T's mnemonic device provides a method to recall likely causes (see Box 38-2). During anesthesia, electrolyte abnormalities, particularly hyperkalemia associated with rapid blood transfusion or succinylcholine, as well as other medication causes such as toxicity to local anesthetic should be considered. Surgical stimulus or venous air embolism can also cause ventricular arrhythmias (see Fig. 38-12).

After initial stabilization, electrolytes should be measured, medications should be reviewed for possible toxic or adverse effects, and potential structural or conductive abnormalities should be explored. Myocarditis and myocardial ischemia, although rare in pediatrics, should always be in the differential diagnosis.

Although most VT is monomorphic, VT can be polymorphic in nature when the QRS complexes vary in appearance. Torsades de pointes VT is a distinctive form of polymorphic VT in which the complexes increase and decrease in amplitude, seemingly undulating around the ECG isoelectric line (Fig. 38-17). Causes of torsades de pointes VT include long QT syndrome, hypomagnesemia, and drug toxicities. Torsades de pointes VT is an unstable, pulseless, preterminal rhythm, and treatment follows the pulseless algorithm with the addition of IV magnesium to treat presumed hypomagnesemia (Fig. 38-16).

Ventricular Fibrillation

VF is a sustained burst of multiple, uncoordinated, regional ventricular depolarizations and contractions that result in an ineffective cardiac output and cessation of myocardial blood flow. (Fig. 38-18). Reentrant impulses, generated within the ventricles with multiple shifting circuits, maintain VF. Several physiologic conditions lower the threshold for fibrillation, including hypoxia, hypercapnia, myocardial ischemia, hypothermia, metabolic acidosis, and electrolyte disturbances (such as imbalances of potassium, calcium, sodium, and magnesium). In addition to these causes of VF, surgical stimulus can trigger VF in the operative environment.

A review of outcomes of in-hospital VF arrests in children found that VF or pulseless VT was the presenting rhythm in 10% to 14% of patients and occurred at some point during the cardiac arrest in an additional 15% of patients. When VF or pulseless VT is the presenting rhythm in cardiac arrest, survival to hospital discharge is approximately 30% to 35%. Survival is significantly better in patients whose cardiac arrest presented with VF or VT than for those who developed it subsequently (35% vs. 11%, odds ratio = 2.6; 95% confidence interval 1.2 to 5.8). Additionally, survival to hospital discharge for patients with either VF or VT that developed subsequently during cardiac arrest was worse than for those patients with asystole or PEA. Presumably, VT or VF that develops later in cardiac arrest occurs as a result of other triggers, such as myocardial reperfusion injury (Samson et al., 2006; Nadkarni et al., 2006).

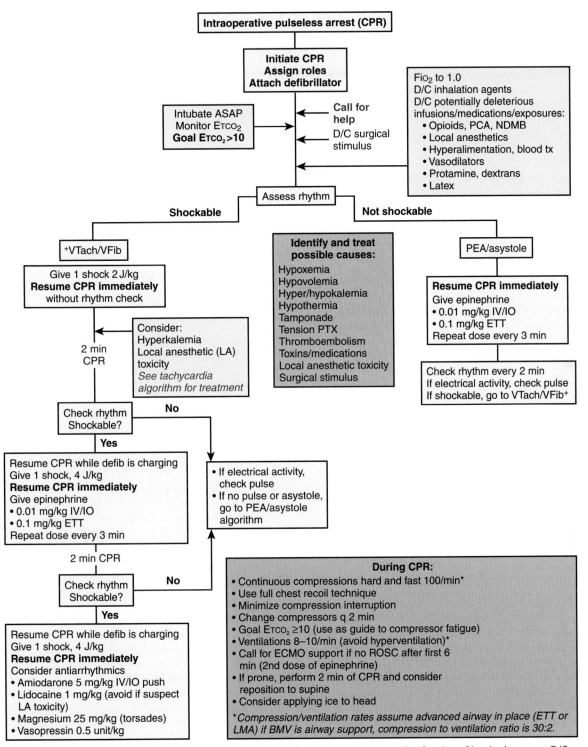

Intraoperative pulseless arrest (CPR)

Initiate CPR
Assign roles
Attach defibrillator

Intubate ASAP
Monitor ETco₂
Goal ETco₂ >10

Call for help
D/C surgical stimulus

Fio₂ to 1.0
D/C inhalation agents
D/C potentially deleterious infusions/medications/exposures:
• Opioids, PCA, NDMB
• Local anesthetics
• Hyperalimentation, blood tx
• Vasodilators
• Protamine, dextrans
• Latex

Assess rhythm

Shockable / **Not shockable**

⁺VTach/VFib

Give 1 shock 2 J/kg
Resume CPR immediately
without rhythm check

2 min CPR

Consider:
Hyperkalemia
Local anesthetic (LA) toxicity
See tachycardia algorithm for treatment

Identify and treat possible causes:
Hypoxemia
Hypovolemia
Hyper/hypokalemia
Hypothermia
Tamponade
Tension PTX
Thromboembolism
Toxins/medications
Local anesthetic toxicity
Surgical stimulus

PEA/asystole

Resume CPR immediately
Give epinephrine
• 0.01 mg/kg IV/IO
• 0.1 mg/kg ETT
Repeat dose every 3 min

Check rhythm every 2 min
If electrical activity, check pulse
If shockable, go to VTach/VFib⁺

Check rhythm
Shockable?   **No**   **Yes**

Resume CPR while defib is charging
Give 1 shock, 4 J/kg
Resume CPR immediately
Give epinephrine
• 0.01 mg/kg IV/IO
• 0.1 mg/kg ETT
Repeat dose every 3 min

• If electrical activity, check pulse
• If no pulse or asystole, go to PEA/asystole algorithm

2 min CPR

Check rhythm
Shockable?   **No**   **Yes**

Resume CPR while defib is charging
Give 1 shock, 4 J/kg
Resume CPR immediately
Consider antiarrhythmics
• Amiodarone 5 mg/kg IV/IO push
• Lidocaine 1 mg/kg (avoid if suspect LA toxicity)
• Magnesium 25 mg/kg (torsades)
• Vasopressin 0.5 unit/kg

During CPR:
• Continuous compressions hard and fast 100/min*
• Use full chest recoil technique
• Minimize compression interruption
• Change compressors q 2 min
• Goal ETco₂ ≥10 (use as guide to compressor fatigue)
• Ventilations 8–10/min (avoid hyperventilation)*
• Call for ECMO support if no ROSC after first 6 min (2nd dose of epinephrine)
• If prone, perform 2 min of CPR and consider reposition to supine
• Consider applying ice to head
Compression/ventilation rates assume advanced airway in place (ETT or LMA) if BMV is airway support, compression to ventilation ratio is 30:2.

■ **FIGURE 38-16.** CPR for intraoperative pulseless arrest. *CPR,* Cardiopulmonary resuscitation; *Fio₂,* fraction of inspired oxygen; *D/C,* discontinue; *PCA,* patient-controlled analgesia; *NDMB,* nondepolarizing muscle blockade; *tx,* transfusion; *ASAP,* as soon as possible; *ETco₂,* end-tidal carbon dioxide; *VT,* ventricular tachycardia; *VF,* ventricular fibrillation; *PTX,* pneumothorax; *PEA,* pulseless electrical activity; *IV,* intravenous; *IO,* intraosseous; *ETT,* endotracheal tube; *LA,* local anesthetic; *defib,* defibrillator. *(Modified from Ralston M et al., editors: Pediatric advanced life support provider manual, Dallas, 2006, American Heart Association.)*

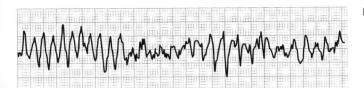

■ **FIGURE 38-17.** ECG of torsades de pointes.

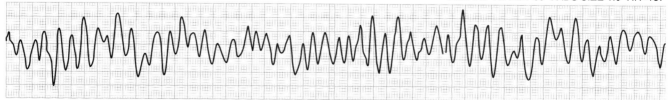

10:27:20 25-NOV-09 PADS SIZE 1.0 HR=137

■ **FIGURE 38-18.** ECG of ventricular fibrillation.

Treatment and causes of VF is the same as it is for pulseless VT—rapid single defibrillation and chest compressions (see Figs. 38-4 and 38-16).

Pulseless Electrical Activity

PEA is a clinical state characterized by the presence of electrical activity in the absence of detectable cardiac output. This is a preterminal condition that often leads to asystole. Typically, it is characterized by a slow, wide-complex rhythm in a child without a pulse who has experienced a prolonged period of hypoxia, ischemia, or hypercarbia. If the condition occurs rapidly, then it may result from a reversible cause. PEA was previously described as electromechanical dissociation (EMD). A review of the NRCPR data found that PEA is the presenting rhythm in 24% of pediatric cardiac arrests and has a rate of 27% for survival to hospital discharge. Over half of those cases of survival had good neurologic outcome (Nadkarni et al., 2006).

PEA should be managed according to the pulseless cardiac arrest algorithm (see Figs. 38-4 and 38-16).

During CPR for PEA, treatable causes of PEA should be considered; the H's and T's mnemonic device can be used to recall causes (see Box 38-2). In the setting of the operating room, many episodes of PEA in children are related to reversible causes that if promptly recognized and treated, result in survival.

Asystole

Asystole occurs when no electrical activity or mechanical contractions are present in the heart. Asystole is a presenting rhythm in 40% of IHCAs, and survival to hospital discharge from in-hospital asystolic cardiac arrest is 18% to 22% (Nadkarni et al., 2006). However, this rate includes patients who came to the emergency department in cardiac arrest and who were unmonitored on hospital medical or surgical floors. Although data are unavailable, perioperative cardiac arrest would be presumed to have a lower percentage of an asystolic presentation, because asystole more commonly occurs as other rhythms deteriorate, treatments fail, and patients are closely monitored in this setting. Asystole is treated according to the pulseless arrest algorithm (see Figs. 38-4 and 38-16).

In all arrhythmias that cause pulseless cardiac arrest, care should be taken to perform high-quality CPR while diagnosing and treating the rhythm and cause (see the inset boxes of Fig. 38-16). Compressions should be hard and fast, at 100 beats per minute, using full-chest–recoil technique, and minimizing compression interruption. E_{TCO_2} should be monitored with a goal of pressure higher than 15 mm Hg; hyperventilation should be avoided to improve venous return and cerebral

blood flow. Mechanical support, such as extracorporeal membrane oxygenation (ECMO), should be considered if ROSC is not achieved within the first 5 minutes.

ANESTHESIA-ASSOCIATED CONSIDERATIONS DURING CARDIOPULMONARY RESUSCITATION

Open-Chest Cardiopulmonary Resuscitation

Open-chest CPR involves a thoracotomy and application of direct compression of the heart to generate blood flow. The use of this technique requires a high level of preparation and training, as well as special equipment and facilities. These requirements limit open-chest CPR to certain hospital settings.

Open-chest CPR represents a model of the cardiac pump mechanism for generation of blood flow. In theory, this model eliminates production of intrathoracic pressure which, if transmitted, could reduce gradients for blood flow. This enhanced gradient combined with directly applied compression can result in near-normal blood flows. In experimental models, open-chest CPR produces cardiac outputs of 25% to 61% of values before cardiac arrest (Weiser et al., 1962; Bircher et al., 1981; Bartlett et al., 1984). These studies and others demonstrate cardiac outputs two to three times larger than with conventional closed-chest CPR (Weiser et al., 1962; Del Guercio et al., 1965; Bircher et al., 1980, 1981; Bartlett et al., 1984). Increases in CPP have been significant in some studies but not in others (Bircher et al., 1980, 1981; Del Guercio et al., 1965). MPPs are significantly increased compared with closed-chest CPR (Bircher et al., 1980; Sanders et al., 1984b). In dogs, cerebral blood flow of 150% of values before cardiac arrest can be produced with open-chest CPR (Jackson et al., 1984). Cross-clamping the descending aorta during open-chest CPR further increases carotid blood flow.

Survival in dogs can be improved by using of open-chest CPR after inadequate closed-chest CPR (Sanders et al., 1984a). Dogs with MPP of less than 30 mm Hg after 15 minutes of closed-chest CPR received 2 to 4 minutes of either open-chest or closed-chest external CPR before defibrillation was attempted. Dogs that received open-chest CPR had significantly greater MPPs and survival rates.

The length of time of preceding closed-chest CPR affects the success of subsequent open-chest CPR (Sanders et al., 1985b). After 20 and 25 minutes of closed-chest CPR, the success rate of open-chest CPR drops to 38% and 0%, respectively. This implies that the benefits from open-chest CPR are limited by time and that early application is crucial. There are no data to recommend routine use of open-chest CPR in the pediatric patient. Postoperative cardiac patients with a recent sternotomy may benefit from open-chest CPR. They have easier access, can be inspected for tamponade, and suture lines can be inspected and avoided.

Conventional Cardiopulmonary Resuscitation in the Prone Position

Conventional CPR is usually performed with sternal compressions applied to a supine patient. Prone positioning for surgical procedures provides an extra complication when cardiopulmonary arrest occurs. Patients who are prone and undergoing posterior cranial or spine surgery and suffer a cardiac arrest may not be able to be quickly repositioned to the supine position. An unstable spine, protruding stabilizers, and ongoing blood loss are factors that may delay turning the patient and necessitate starting CPR in the prone position. Additionally, repositioning the prone patient into a supine position requires multiple people, taking drapes down, and caution against dislodging tubes or lines. The time it takes to reposition delays life-saving CPR and defibrillation; therefore, resuscitation may be attempted before repositioning. Two methods for delivering posterior chest compressions to a patient in the prone position have been suggested. The first uses two hands with one hand spread over each scapula, and the second uses the heel of one hand on the spine with the second hand on top of the first, similar to the method for sternal compressions (Sun et al., 1992; Tobias et al., 1994; Dequin et al., 1996). Counter pressure under the sternum with another rescuer's hand or fist or a sand bag has also been suggested (Sun et al., 1992; Dequin et al., 1996; Mazer et al., 2003). In a high-fidelity simulation model of CPR with the patient in the prone position and using midline compressions with a counter pressure pad, effective or partially effective compression depth was able to be achieved 75% of the time (Atkinson, 2000). Prone CPR using a spine compression technique compared favorably with supine CPR in six intensive-care patients (Mazer et al., 2003). When possible, patients should be turned supine for CPR, but effective CPR may be able to be performed when a patient is in the prone position.

In addition to chest compressions, defibrillation may be necessary in a prone patient. Prone defibrillation may be attempted if the patient cannot be turned immediately. Placement of self-adhesive defibrillation pads is advised, because intraoperative placement of paddles may be difficult and require time. Gel pads placed on the back on either side of the surgical incision in the left midaxillary line and inferior to right scapula have been successful for defibrillation in a prone patient (Miranda and Newton, 2001).

Consideration of Etiology of Cardiopulmonary Arrest During Cardiopulmonary Resuscitation

Cardiopulmonary arrest in the perioperative period is likely to be caused by either surgical intervention or anesthesia in isolation or in combination with patient comorbidity. Therefore, the anesthesiologist is faced with the unique situation in which causes of cardiac arrest are diagnosed and treated in parallel with the delivery of standard resuscitation care. When possible, other skilled providers should be called to assist with CPR and the rapid processing of multiple algorithms and data that is required (see the section about roles in the operating room).

The most recent review of the POCA Registry found 193 perioperative cardiac arrests over 6 years. The most common causes of arrest include hypovolemia (15%), electrolyte imbalance including hyperkalemia (5%), and laryngospasm (6%). Other causes of cardiac arrest that require consideration perioperatively include venous air embolus, medication overdose, intravascular local anesthetic injection, anaphylaxis, and surgical stimulus (Bhananker et al., 2007). In addition to CPR, resuscitation for the patient in the perioperative period should include interventions targeted at likely causes for the cardiac arrest. There are algorithms that are based on the AHA guidelines for PALS but are focused on intraoperative management (see Figs. 38-8, 38-12, and 38-16).

Patients with Congenital Heart Disease and Cardiopulmonary Resuscitation

Pediatric anesthesiologists care for children with atypical cardiac anatomy and physiology that can have an effect on the cause of cardiac arrest, effectiveness of CPR, and the interventions required for resuscitation. Patients with congenital heart disease who are in or near cardiac arrest require thorough knowledge of patient-specific anatomy, physiology, and ECG. Patients with congenital heart disease have a higher likelihood of arrhythmia rather than respiratory insufficiency or failure as the primary cause of arrest (Peddy et al., 2007).

For patients with shunt-dependent pulmonary blood flow, occlusion of shunt flow is an emergency that may require urgent surgical intervention or mechanical support in addition to CPR. E_{TCO_2}, typically a marker for CPR effectiveness, should be evaluated in context of the patient's anatomy and potential for altered pulmonary blood flow. For example, the patient with shunt-dependent physiology and occluded shunt flow could have low E_{TCO_2} even when adequate CPR is being performed. E_{TCO_2} during CPR may not have the same prognostic value in patients with altered cardiac anatomy and pulmonary blood flow.

EXTRACORPOREAL SUPPORT AS ADJUNCTIVE THERAPY DURING CARDIOPULMONARY RESUSCITATION

The primary goal of CPR is to provide cerebral and coronary perfusion that is adequate to preserve organ function in anticipation of resumed circulation. Intuitively, extracorporeal support could aid in that goal by increasing oxygenation and blood flow in the low-flow and no-flow states of cardiopulmonary arrest. Additionally, extracorporeal support could prolong reliable organ perfusion while reversible causes of cardiac failure are treated.

CPB was the original model for extracorporeal support; its utility was documented in animal studies (Safar et al., 1990). In dogs, CPB increases 72-hour survival, recovery of consciousness, and preserves myocardium better than conventional CPR (Levine et al., 1987; Pretto et al., 1987). Additionally, CPB results in better neurologic outcome than continued conventional CPR after a 4-minute ischemic period in a canine model (Levine et al., 1987; Pretto et al., 1987). Survival for 24 hours is possible for at least 90% of dogs after 15 or 20 minutes of cardiac arrest but for only 10% of dogs after 30 minutes of cardiac arrest with CPB stabilization during defibrillation (Reich et al., 1990). In a model involving coronary artery occlusion, it was found that CPB decreases myocardial infarct size compared with conventional CPR (Angelos et al., 1990). Clinical use of CPB for CPR in humans is limited by equipment and technical constraints.

Improvements in gas-exchange apparatus permitted extracorporeal support to go beyond a few hours and allowed CPB techniques to move from the operating room into the intensive care unit. Because the gas-exchange portion of the circuit was very different than CPB, prolonged extracorporeal life support became known as extracorporeal membrane oxygenation (ECMO). Bartlett et al. (1976) first used of ECMO for neonatal cardiac failure after a mustard operation in 1972 and later published his case series about neonates with respiratory failure who were supported with ECMO.

Similar to CPB, ECMO removes deoxygenated blood from the venous system and returns oxygenated blood to the aorta using a mechanical pump and gas-exchange apparatus. In contrast to CPB, ECMO is designed for longer usage (days or weeks vs. hours). ECMO provides a gas-exchange apparatus— a membrane between the oxygen and blood interface—that causes less hemolysis than CPB. CPB is used intraoperatively to facilitate cardiac surgery by emptying the heart and supporting organ function during cardiac surgery; cannulae are typically placed directly in the heart or great vessels through sternotomy incision. ECMO can provide longer support to failing respiratory or cardiac systems when recovery is anticipated; arterial and venous cannulae can be placed percutaneously in large vessels more distal to the heart. Lower heparin dosages may be used in ECMO than in CPB, decreasing hemorrhagic risk over time.

The first use of ECMO for rescue in a pediatric patient receiving extracorporeal CPR (ECPR) was reported by Dalton in 1993. She reported the use of ECMO for cardiac failure in 29 patients with acquired or congenital heart disease after repair or transplantation; 11 of those were receiving CPR during cannulation. Survival to discharge in this group was six cases out of 11 (55%) despite CPR duration of 42 to 110 minutes (Dalton et al., 1993).

Since that time, multiple case series and reviews of ECMO data have replicated Dalton's findings. The majority of the reported cases concern patients with congenital or acquired heart disease and are inpatients that are younger than 1 year of age (Morris et al., 2004; Shah et al., 2005; Thourani et al., 2006; Alsoufi et al., 2007; Huang et al., 2008). Survival to hospital discharge in the series with larger numbers of patient is generally 33% to 41% (Morris et al., 2004; Shah et al., 2005; Alsoufi et al., 2007; Huang et al., 2008).

Few studies report neurologic outcomes or long-term follow-up issues; those that do have mixed results. Using the Pediatric Cerebral Performance Category Scale, Huang et al. (2008) reported normal or only mild disability in 10 of 11 survivors of ECPR in a population of pediatric patients 1 to 4 years after hospitalization. Morris et al. (2004) reported that 24% (five out of 21) of survivors of ECPR had significant neurologic impairment that was noted at the time of discharge.

Increased duration of CPR before ECMO cannulation has been found to increase the risk of mortality in two studies and to have no impact on survival in others (Dalton et al., 1993; Morris et al., 2004; Alsoufi et al., 2007; Huang et al., 2008; Tajik and Cardarelli, 2008). Notably, there are also reports of patients surviving nearly 2 hours of CPR before ECMO initiation without neurologic injury (Morris et al., 2004; Thourani et al., 2006; Alsoufi et al., 2007).

In the few studies that look at survival for noncardiac patients separately, outcomes may be much lower than for patients with cardiac disease. Alsoufi et al. (2007) reported nine patients without cardiac disease in his cohort of 80 patients; only one of those nine (11%) survived to discharge. Similarly, Morris et al. (2004) reported on 64 patients from a single institution who had received ECPR from 1995 to 2002. Only two of 21 (9.5%) noncardiac patients survived to discharge. The largest series of ECPR in noncardiac patients was reported by MacLaren in 2007. He reported on the use of ECMO in 45 pediatric patients with sepsis; 18 patients had CPR at the time of cannulation. In contrast to the findings of Morris and Alsoufi, 11 out of 18 (55%) survived to discharge (MacLaren et al., 2007).

Two large reviews of the Extracorporeal Life Support Organization (ELSO) database have demonstrated increased use of ECMO during CPR with stable survival outcomes. Cengiz et al. (2005) reviewed the ELSO database from 1981 to 2002 and found 161 reports of ECPR in children with and without cardiac disease, with survival to discharge in 64 of 161 (40%) patients. In a more recent review of the same database with overlapping dates with the Cengiz review, Thiagarajan et al. (2007) found 682 reports of ECPR in the ELSO database from 1992 to 2005; 499 were patients with heart disease. The median age was 0.25 years, and survival to discharge was 261 of 682 (38%). Patient age, weight, gender, or site of cannulation (thoracic vs. peripheral) did not impact survival. The duration of CPR before ECMO was not reported (Thiagarajan et al., 2007). Neither study reported neurologic outcomes.

Given that survival of prolonged IHCA (longer than 15 to 30 minutes) has been reported as low and that survival after ECPR may be as high as 33% to 41%, ECPR could provide an incremental increase in survival compared with refractory cardiac arrest that is treated with CPR alone (Suominen et al., 2000; Morris et al., 2004). Considering that this population would likely be deceased otherwise, ECMO is a potent and life-saving therapy.

ECPR perhaps has the greatest potential application for the intraoperative patient. Because patients are closely monitored by providers who are skilled in resuscitation at the time of cardiac arrest, the no-flow interval is minimal. Additionally, surgical staff is present at the time of cardiac arrest to assist with cannulation. There are multiple causes of reversible cardiac dysfunction in the operating room, including but not limited to hyperkalemia, local or general anesthetic overdose, and airway emergency. Dialysis to treat hyperkalemia and other drug or toxin overdose can be readily performed during ECMO; dialysis cannot be performed while CPR is in progress.

Survival from pediatric anesthesia-related cardiac arrest is reported to be 72%, but this number only represents survival from acute cardiopulmonary arrest; survival to discharge is not reported (Bhananker et al., 2007). A review of 91 cardiac arrests in the pediatric ICU (PICU) over 5 years similarly found an 82% survival rate for an acute cardiopulmonary arrest event but only 25% survival to discharge. Notably, use of ECMO in the first 24 hours after cardiac arrest in this population was associated with reduced hospital mortality (mortality reduced from 78% to 63%) in multivariate logistical regression analysis (odds ratio of 0.18; 95% confidence interval of 0.04 to 0.76) (de Mos et al., 2006). Data from the PICU patient population have mixed application to perioperative patients. Although the patients in the PICU are similar to those in the operating room in that the cardiac arrest is witnessed and acted on immediately by skilled providers, the PICU patients likely have significant comorbidities and may be an overall sicker population than operative patients. However, ECMO usage in the operating room would likely reduce mortality from perioperative cardiac arrest in select patients, similar to results seen in the PICU data.

There are issues and contraindications to ECMO that must be considered, however. ECMO is expensive, requires considerable technical support and experience, and is not universally available. ECMO provides support while reversible causes of CPA are treated and is not a therapy for CPA in itself. Contraindications to ECMO include nonreversible pathology or disability that precludes quality of life after ECMO. Heparinization is required, and bleeding can be a significant, but not insurmountable, problem after surgery. The anesthesiologist and surgeon should assess the cause of cardiac arrest, the potential reversibility of the etiology, and patient comorbidities before ECMO initiation.

The 2005 AHA recommendation regarding ECPR states: "Consider ECPR for IHCA refractory to initial resuscitation attempts if the condition leading to the arrest is reversible or amenable to heart transplantation, if excellent conventional CPR has been performed after no more than several minutes of no-flow cardiac arrest, and if the institution is able to rapidly perform ECMO" (AHA, 2006b). Because surgical and resuscitative staff members are present at the time of cardiac arrest, the no-flow period of cardiac arrest is virtually eliminated. If support for ECMO exits and can be rapidly mobilized, intraoperative cardiac arrests appear to be an ideal application for ECPR in children without contraindication to ECMO.

TEAMWORK DURING INTRAOPERATIVE CARDIAC ARREST

Complex, high-stake events that occur rarely, such as an intraoperative cardiac arrest in a child, often require multiple simultaneous interventions performed as rapidly as possible during a time of high stress. The response can be more effective and efficient, and the stress can be divided and reduced by using a well-organized team with the appropriate skills. Teamwork principles that can be applied to these situations are derived from airline industry's response to aviation disasters and referred to as *crew resource management (CRM)*. Application of these same principles to anesthesia-related emergencies led to the development of crisis-resource management (also CRM). The low incidence of intraoperative cardiac arrests makes it difficult to evaluate the application of CRM training on outcome. Simulation can be used to determine the effect that CRM training has on the improvement of attitudes or behaviors of the team (Cooper, 2004). Multiple reviews describe CRM in the fields of anesthesia and pediatrics (Sundar et al., 2007; Eppich et al., 2008; Weinstock and Halamek, 2008; Manser, 2009). Many of the principles and concepts of CRM are applicable to teams involved in responding to a cardiac arrest involving a child undergoing anesthesia for a procedure (Box 38-3).

A shared mental model is the concept that, without need for overt communication, all team members understand the organization and purpose of the team. It is difficult to develop this concept on an *ad hoc* basis. Even if they have not previously worked together, the individuals that will become the team in the event of an intraoperative arrest should have the same mental model for the team. Discussion and exploration of this

Box 38-3 Principles of Crew Resource Management that Apply to Teams Involved in Intraoperative Cardiac Arrests

SHARED MENTAL MODEL
Team composition
Individual roles
Team goal

TEAM-ORIENTED BEHAVIOR
Mutual respect
Mutual trust
Mutual performance monitoring
Back-up behavior
Conflict avoidance and resolution

CLARITY OF ROLES AND RESPONSIBILITIES
Effective leadership
Effective followership

RESOURCE MANAGEMENT
Access to equipment or staff needed
How to get it
Who will get it
When to get it

EFFECTIVE COMMUNICATION
Assertive
Directed
Closed-loop

SUPPORT MANAGEMENT
When to call for help
Who to call for help

REGULAR FEEDBACK AND DEBRIEFINGS
Team evaluation as opposed to evaluation of individuals

concept among individuals likely to be involved should occur before the event that will require the team formation.

Team-oriented behavior describes the willingness of individuals to work as members of a team and to accept the other members of that team. In the event of an intraoperative cardiac arrest, team members should treat the other members with respect due individuals who are willing to work hard under pressure to save the life of a child. A lack of respect that leads to the impression that offering suggestions will receive a condescending response could prevent the transfer of vital information. Team members should be observant of how the other team members are performing. If it is perceived that another team member is overwhelmed, other team members should be willing to offer assistance if they are able. If they have a conflict with another team member, they should postpone comments or actions that do not contribute to team performance until after the child is stabilized and the tension is decreased.

Having clarity of roles and responsibilities is a critical concept in the event of an intraoperative cardiac arrest. In the cardiac operating room, it is clear that the surgeon will compress the heart and deliver shocks for defibrillation, while the anesthesiologist will provide medications and fluids and manage ventilation. In this situation, in which the cardiac arrest is usually related to the surgical efforts, the surgeon initiates and leads the resuscitation. In contrast, when the cardiac arrest is related to problems with patient's response to anesthetics or difficulty with ventilation, the anesthesiologist becomes the leader.

The combination of a small number of pediatric cardiac surgeons and anesthesiologists at an institution and the common occurrence of cardiac arrests in their patients result in more opportunity to clarify their roles and responsibilities. In a surgery center during a hyperkalemic response (e.g., to the administration of succinylcholine for laryngospasm in a child with undiagnosed muscular dystrophy), it may not be clear who is best qualified to perform compressions, who should go for the defibrillator, who should perform IO access, who should administer defibrillation shocks, and who should record therapeutic interventions and responses while the anesthesiologist continues involvement in maintaining a secure airway, providing ventilation, and administering medications. Calling for help in these situations can complicate the situation by having the distraction of unnecessary staff who are unfamiliar with team roles during resuscitation and by causing roles or responsibilities to be missed or duplicated.

Clarity of roles and responsibilities is one of the team training concepts emphasized by the AHA in the PALS course. Six roles are recommended in the PALS course for pediatric arrests, the titles *Leader, Airway, Compressor, Access, Monitor,* and *Recorder*. These roles can be applied to the pediatric operating room environment, depending on the setting and available resources (Table 38-14). In the cardiac operating room the necessary resources (e.g., defibrillator, vasoactive medications, blood products, and CPB equipment) are available, and in this setting multiple roles are assumed by a few individuals. For example, the anesthesiologist performs the Airway, Access (medication), and Recorder roles while the surgeon performs Compressor and Monitor (defibrillator) roles, and either could be the Leader. In a general or ambulatory operating room, the necessary resources (e.g., code cart and defibrillator) often need to be brought to the room, and multiple roles may need to be assigned. It is a good idea to predetermine who will assume the Leader role in this setting; the anesthesiologist may have more

information about the cause of arrest, making it easier for him or her to solve problems in the Leader role. If enough staff is available, an additional anesthesiologist can assume the Airway role and maintain ventilation, allowing the primary anesthesiologist to focus on leadership. An otolaryngology surgeon may need to be in the Airway role during airway surgery. The Compressor role might need to be part of the surgical staff if the chest needs to be in the sterile field. The Access role is usually assumed by an anesthesiologist, ideally not the Leader or Airway designee, although combinations of roles may need to occur if an insufficient number of staff are available to provide all for all six roles. The Monitor role may require the participation of a surgeon if sterility is required, or it may be filled by an anesthesiologist if adhesive gel pads are to be applied under the surgical drapes. The Recorder role often falls to the anesthesiologist, who is already recording intraoperative events, but a circulating nurse performing this role could free the anesthesiologist for leadership or other roles. The Recorder role can also be expanded to include a list of desired goals, and the Recorder can use it to remind the Leader what has been accomplished and what needs to completed and when (See the section on documentation). Predetermining which roles are likely to be empty and which could be combined may save time and confusion during an actual event. In the event of insufficient staff, the primary anesthesiologist may be able to assume the Leader and Airway roles and delegate the Access and Monitor roles to additional responding anesthesiologists.

The principles of leadership and followership are very important in high-stress situations involving complex responses. It is important to have a clearly defined Leader who remains separate from resuscitative efforts, is able to assess the whole picture, determines the goals of resuscitation efforts, keeps focus on goals, monitors team effectiveness, redistributes work load for members who are overwhelmed or underused, frequently reassesses the situation, and makes clear decisions about the needs for resources and support. Followers need to be willing to assume their roles and responsibilities, act under the Leader's direction, offer feedback and ideas in a supportive manner, and own (and stick with) their assigned roles. The principles of leadership during resuscitation may not have received the proper focus in medical training. Residents in the field of internal medicine report not feeling qualified to lead a resuscitation team, and residents in pediatrics inadequately demonstrated leadership skills during mock pediatric arrests (Hayes et al., 2007; Hunt et al., 2008). Understanding and practicing the principles of leadership and followership should be incorporated into the goals of training for the management of intraoperative cardiac arrests.

Resource management may be one of the most important principles to apply to the situation of an intraoperative cardiac arrest. It is crucial to know what equipment, supplies, or information is needed and whether they are available when an intraoperative cardiac arrest is likely or occurring (Table 38-15). To have the code cart brought early requires that the team know where it is kept, whose responsibility it is to bring it, and what it contains. Pediatric anesthesiologists seldom use a defibrillator or AED, and issues often occur with paddle-size selection, switching to pediatric paddles, charging and discharging efficiently, understanding biphasic and monophasic dosing, and understanding defibrillator and AED differences (especially AED analysis and response time) (Heitmiller et al., 2008). Instruction in defibrillator use has a greater impact when the

---

TABLE 38-14. Roles and Responsibilities During Intraoperative Arrest

Role	Responsibility
Leader	Assigns roles Directs resuscitative efforts Monitors the performance of tasks
Airway	Equipment and oxygen preparation Airway and gastric intubation Ventilation
Compressor	Delivers chest compressions
Access (medication)	Obtains intravascular or intraosseous access Fluid and medication preparation and administration
Monitor (defibrillator)	Establishes and operates monitors and defibrillator Performs pulse checks
Recorder	Records resuscitative efforts Compares recorded efforts to goals of resuscitation list Reviews record as needed by the Leader/team

Modified from Ralston M et al., editors: *Pediatric advanced life support course guide,* Dallas, 2006, American Heart Association, p 31.

TABLE 38-15. Resources that May Be Needed During a Pediatric Intraoperative Cardiac Arrest

Resource	Indication
Backboard	Patient on stretcher or mattress
Stool	Improve compressor performance and endurance
Stretcher	Patient in prone position or on equipment that decreases CPR effectiveness
Code cart	Arrest is likely or in process
IO needles	Difficult access
Defibrillator	Shockable rhythm
Pacemaker	Dysrhythmia
Cognitive aids	Help with resuscitation algorithms
Blood products	Blood loss or coagulopathy
Ice, cooled IV fluids	Malignant hyperthermia or therapeutic hypothermia
Dantrolene	Malignant hyperthermia
Lipid emulsion	Local anesthetic toxicity
Emergency airway tools	Difficult airway

CPR, Cardiopulmonary resuscitation; *IO,* intraosseous; *IV,* intravenous.

trainees are required to demonstrate their use by having gone through the steps themselves rather than watching an instructor (Hunt et al., 2009). Cognitive aids may be attached to the code cart, so the Leader can review resuscitation algorithms if needed. Ice, cooled IV fluids, and dantrolene may be needed if malignant hyperthermia is encountered, as well as a small inflatable pool that may be placed under the patient to contain large quantities of ice. Keeping instructions with lipid emulsion can be helpful in the rare event of a toxic response to a local anesthetic. These and other issues of resource management during a resuscitation event can have a big effect on the response time and thus on outcome. It should be a goal of team training to have multiple (or all) members familiar with the resources needed and how they will be deployed in the event of intraoperative arrest.

Effective communication is another skill that is emphasized by the AHA in PALS training. Several CRM communication principles can be applied to team management during intraoperative resuscitation (Box 38-4). Assertive communication is important to ensure that all necessary information is communicated to the Leader and other team members. Failing to

Box 38-4 Important Principles of Effective Communication that Apply to Resuscitation

Be assertive.
Use direct communication to the appropriate team member using names and eye contact.
Deliver clear messages.
Use a closed-loop style of communication to show message has been received and understood as intended.

report necessary information because of concern about a condescending response may cost a child's life. Direct communication helps prevent information from being ignored because of not having the intended member's attention. Ideas should not be delivered in a general manner but instead directed to appropriate members after obtaining their attention. Team members should introduce themselves if they are not familiar with each other's names. The establishment of eye contact helps determine that the speaker has the attention of the appropriate members. Names of the appropriate members and eye contact should be used before information is delivered. The information should be delivered as clearly as possible. In the use of closed-loop style of communication, recipients should acknowledge and repeat the message to demonstrate that the information was received and understood as intended.

Support management is another team-training concept that is important to apply to pediatric intraoperative resuscitation. Support management involves knowing what help is available, how to access that help, and when to activate that help. The concept of activating "incremental help" means requesting only the necessary help rather than a broad request for all help, which may result in the chaos that can accompany too large of a response. In the setting of an intraoperative cardiac arrest, the concept of support management applies to many situations (Table 38-16).

Debriefing is the final team-management concept that should be applied to teams that respond to intraoperative arrests. Regular feedback and debriefing can be used to improve team performance for subsequent responses. It is recommended that feedback sessions be used to evaluate the team's performance and not that of an individual. Nontechnical skills improve with debriefing, and oral feedback alone may be sufficient and not enhanced by the use of accompanying video (Savoldelli et al., 2006).

One of the major differences between floor or operating-room resuscitations is that in the operating room there is rarely a team that responds with preconceived roles and responsibilities. In a code on a hospital ward, a senior resident responds as Leader, an anesthesiologist and respiratory therapist respond as Airway, a pharmacist and ICU nurse administer medications, a junior resident is responsible for the defibrillator (Monitor role),

TABLE 38-16. Support that May Be Needed During a Pediatric Intraoperative Cardiac Arrest

Support Needed	Situation
Additional resuscitation help	Unfilled team roles (any anesthesiologist call)
Otolaryngologist	Difficult airway management
General or thoracic surgeon	Vascular access or chest tube placement
PICU staff	Need for additional resuscitation support
Cardiologist	Arrhythmia management
ECMO or CPB	Failure to achieve return of circulation

PICU, Pediatric intensive care unit; *ECMO,* extracorporeal membrane oxygenation; *CPB,* cardiopulmonary bypass.

a ward nurse serves as Recorder. In noncardiac pediatric operating rooms there are individuals who have little experience with each other during resuscitation efforts who are suddenly put together in a critical high-stress situation. Discussing and practicing the concepts of CRM help teams perform better in simulated events and can be applied to the management of pediatric intraoperative cardiac arrest.

Documentation During a Pediatric Intraoperative Cardiac Arrest

The Recorder mentioned in the preceding section is tasked with documentation of resuscitative efforts performed during an intraoperative cardiac arrest. In addition to providing documentation for the patient's medical record, the information can be used by the Recorder to review for the Leader and team what has been accomplished and what has not been done that may still be of benefit to the patient. This documentation can also be used after the cardiac arrest for feedback and debriefing, and the documentation tool used by the Recorder should be designed with consideration of this potential use.

A potential additional use of the documentation tool that the Recorder uses may be as a cognitive aid to list resuscitation goals. A cognitive aid is a tool that can be used by the resuscitation team during a cardiac arrest to review the sequence of interventions described in a resuscitation algorithm. The design of the documentation used by the Recorder could be such that it incorporates a cognitive aid that allows the Recorder to review the resuscitative efforts against the suggested algorithms. The design of the documentation in this way would allow the Recorder to provide the Leader and team with time lines for interventions during resuscitation. For example, documentation could be designed in 2-minute intervals so that it reminds the Recorder when it is recommended to switch Compressors to prevent fatigue and to check for ROSC. A space for recording the initials of the Compressor and another for noting the state of the circulation every 2 minutes would serve to remind the Recorder of the need for these interventions. Every other 2-minute interval (every fourth-minute interval) could be designated to record the administration of epinephrine that is normally given every 3 to 5 minutes during resuscitation, again prompting the Recorder to note when epinephrine is due or overdue. A check-box at the 6-minute interval could be added to the documentation, asking whether resuscitation continues and if so whether ECMO has been activated. It takes time to assemble the necessary resources for ECMO; however, it is most effective when applied early. If it is forgotten until late in resuscitation, the benefit may be diminished. Six minutes into resuscitation is an appropriate time to consider the activation of ECMO, because it is long enough to show that initial resuscitation and the first dose of epinephrine have failed to have resuscitated the victim, but early enough to allow ECMO to be applied within the first hour of cardiac arrest. Additional check-boxes can be added for reminders of other significant tasks, such as bringing the code cart into the room or notifying the PICU. The design of the documentation tool should include a checklist of important tasks to accomplish that prompt the Recorder to make sure they are done on time. The Recorder can discuss these prompts with the Leader as necessary. Although this discussion with the Leader may be redundant in some cases, redundancy might help prevent important tasks from being missed during the stress of an intraoperative resuscitation.

POSTRESUSCITATION CARE

Close monitoring of vital-organ perfusion remains a priority in the postresuscitation period. Care should be taken that celebration of the team's success in resuscitation of the child does not interfere with patient care in the postresuscitation period. It is important to ensure that the patient is closely monitored during this postresuscitation period for several reasons.

First, the primary cause of the cardiac arrest may recur. For example, pulseless VT secondary to hyperkalemia from blood products is treated with medications that drive the potassium intracellularly. However, most of these acutely administered therapies do not actually remove potassium from the body (i.e., as opposed to furosemide, sodium polystyrene, and hemodialysis) and thus a rebound phenomenon, recurrence of VT, is not uncommon. It is essential that the team focus on how to fully reverse the primary cause of the event in order to decrease the chance of recurrence. Another example would be if a patient suffered a tension pneumothorax and a PEA cardiac arrest that was successfully treated with needle decompression. In this case, it is essential that the patient then have a chest tube placed to prevent recurrence of the event.

Second, invasive tubes and lines may have been disrupted during the cardiac arrest. In addition, lines placed during a cardiac arrest may not have been placed with the best technique (i.e., not truly sterile or placement not confirmed) because of the complexity of the event. It is essential that the anesthesiologist assess each of these tubes and lines to make sure they are in the location of choice (i.e., the central venous line is venous, not arterial, and in a safe location). Whereas it may not be appropriate to replace a line that was placed without fully using sterile technique in the immediate postresuscitation period, the details of the line placement should be shared with the intensivist who will manage the child later so a risk-benefit analysis about replacing the line and when it is safe to do so can be made.

Third, during reperfusion the patient is likely to be in a state that is more unstable than before the cardiac arrest, especially if it was a prolonged cardiac arrest. If the patient received multiple doses of vasoconstrictors or has elevated levels of endogenous catecholamines, the patient may be hypertensive and have increased cardiac ectopy. On the other hand, such a patient may be hypotensive, have a profound metabolic acidosis, or have developed disseminated intravascular coagulation (DIC) with bleeding. The patient may need interventions to maintain adequate metabolic supply, requiring attention to blood pressure, ventilation, and glucose levels. Avoiding increased metabolic demand involves prevention of hyperthermia and seizures. In the postresuscitation period, blood pressure should be maintained adequate for vital organ perfusion and may require the administration of fluids, vasoactive medication, or pacing. Ventilation should be normocapnic, avoiding hyperventilation and hypoventilation. Blood-glucose levels should also be normalized, avoiding hyperglycemia and hypoglycemia. Whereas it may not be feasible or necessary for the anesthesiologist to start an insulin infusion, particularly if the child is going to be rapidly transferred to the ICU, it is important to check a dextrose stick and remove any glucose-containing fluids that would exacerbate the situation if the child has developed hyperglycemia.

Postresuscitation hyperthermia is common, because patients are often excessively rewarmed. This overwarming can increase metabolic demands, thus worsening outcome, and overwarming should be avoided. In fact, hypothermia may be neuroprotective and has recently been recommended for adult victims of cardiac arrest. The International Liaison Committee on Resuscitation recommends that unconscious adult patients with spontaneous circulation after OHCA be cooled to 32° to 34° C for 12 to 24 hours when the initial rhythm was VF (Nolan et al., 2003). Consideration to cooling should also be given for other rhythms or IHCA. These recommendations are based on the results from two prospective randomized clinical studies that compared hypothermia with normothermia in comatose survivors of cardiac arrest (Hypothermia Study Group, 2002; Bernard et al., 2002). These European and Australian studies excluded children and patients who had cardiac arrests of noncardiac origin. Animal models of asphyxial arrest are reporting protective effects of hypothermia in rats and piglets (Xiao et al., 1998; Hicks et al., 2000; Hickey et al., 2000; Hachimi-Idrissi et al., 2001; Agnew et al., 2003). A recent multicenter, retrospective cohort study of 79 children who suffered cardiac arrests revealed that hypothermia was disproportionately applied to children at greater risk of a poor outcome, but adjusted analysis found no differences in outcomes based on the use of hypothermia (Doherty et al., 2009). There is currently insufficient evidence to make a recommendation on the use of therapeutic cooling for children resuscitated from cardiac arrest, and randomized controlled trials are ongoing. Thus, at this point, a primary goal of the anesthesiologist should be to avoid hyperthermia.

Finally, a very important issue to address is the role of the anesthesiologist in reporting information about the cardiac arrest to the surgeon, the family, and intensivist who will be caring for the child in the postresuscitation period. Each of these parties will be trying to determine the prognosis for the child. With regard to the intensivist, he or she will want a clear history of the child's baseline neurologic status and how the child was doing medically before the cardiac arrest. They will need details about all of the items on the following list:

1. How the event started
2. The proposed etiology of the event
3. The quality of basic life support and PALS delivered
4. The length of the cardiac arrest
5. The neurologic examination (i.e., pupils, breathing, movement, and drugs that may affect the examination, such as atropine or scopolamine),
6. Procedures that were performed during the event and whether any lines or tubes need to be checked or changed
7. Issues related to postresuscitation care
8. Information that was communicated to the family members (or patient) about the event

It is important to recall that little can be said about a patient's prognosis based on the neurologic examination that takes place immediately after the event. A patient can be fixed and dilated and in status epilepticus but make a full recovery. A patient may receive 90 minutes of compressions, receive ECMO during the event, make a full neurologic recovery; yet there are occasionally patients who have cardiac arrests of short duration who never wake up. Thus, it is important that the anesthesiologist avoid making comments about prognosis when talking to family about the likelihood of recovery.

CPR is not a definitive treatment for cardiac arrest but rather a means of maintaining respiration and circulation until the underlying pathology can be corrected. Because of the limited efficacy of CPR, it is important to identify the underlying pathology as early as possible and correct it so that spontaneous circulation can be restored.

Preparation for cardiopulmonary arrest during anesthetic management begins with an understanding of the surgical and patient-related risk factors and knowledge of the most current CPR recommendations. The anesthesiologist must also have at his or her disposal the appropriate medications and devices, as well as the skills to lead the operating room team in resuscitation. Because pediatric intraoperative cardiac arrest is a rare event, regular education and hands on practice will increase a team's confidence and effectiveness. A patient's chance for survival from intraoperative cardiac arrest will be maximized with thorough education, preparation, and practice.

For questions and answers on topics in this chapter, go to "Chapter Questions" at www.expertconsult.com.

REFERENCES

Complete references used in this text can be found online at www.expertconsult.com.

Critical Care Medicine

Kathryn Felmet

CONTENTS

In the 1960s and 1970s, pediatric anesthesiologists played a major role in the development of the pediatric intensive care unit (PICU), in part because the applied cardiopulmonary physiology in the operating room experience is similar to the initial resuscitation of patients with rapidly evolving illness such as multiple trauma and septic shock. With modern critical care, the job of the intensivist continues for days and weeks beyond the initial resuscitation.

Critical illness occurs in stages. The acute illness is followed by a plateau phase, which may be prolonged and is poorly understood. The biphasic response to stress exhibited by the hypothalamic pituitary adrenal axis is also poorly understood. In critically ill patients, an initial surge in adrenocorticotropic hormone (ACTH) and cortisol is followed by a prolonged state of decreased ACTH levels and persistently elevated cortisol (Beishuizen and Thijs, 2004). Persistent hypercortisolism may benefit the patient by promoting the availability of fuel substrates and minimizing inflammation, or it may be harmful, causing hyperglycemia, delayed wound healing, immune suppression, and myopathy. The immune or inflammatory response to injury follows a similar pattern (Hotchkiss and Karl, 2003).

An increasing number of studies have focused on long-term functional outcomes, and these are likely to change critical care practice in coming years. For example, although tolerance of relative hypoxia has become the norm for treating patients with acute respiratory distress syndrome (ARDS), outcome studies show that duration of saturation less than 90%, less than 85%, and less than 80% correlated with impairment in memory, attention, and processing speed, respectively (Hopkins et al., 1999). Pediatric patients undergoing arterial switch, a procedure that should leave them with normal long-term heart function, had a higher than expected incidence of neurodevelopmental disabilities at school age (Mehta and Arnold, 2004). As more information about how to promote good long-term functional outcomes becomes available, our practice will evolve.

The therapies we deliver in the ICU can be inherently dangerous, and the unintended consequences of the care constitute a large part of critical illness. The side effects of critical illness may be short term, merely prolonging ICU stay, or may last a lifetime. An important part of the discipline of critical care is anticipating these consequences. Prompt discontinuation of unnecessary therapies and the timely institution of prophylactic therapies can make a significant difference in the long-term outcomes of critically ill patients.

This chapter is organized by organ systems. In each section, the relevant pathophysiologic processes and support modalities are discussed, with a focus on recent discoveries and current controversies. The goal is to describe practices unique to intensive care, review some well-established protocols, and discuss the scientific foundation for some emerging therapies, as well as to provide a framework for the anesthesiologist who ventures into the ICU for extended periods.

RESPIRATORY SYSTEM

Actual or impending respiratory failure is a common reason for admission to the PICU, and one in six patients admitted requires mechanical ventilation (Epstein, 2009). Although some patients with healthy lungs require mechanical ventilation for nonrespiratory reasons, the majority have acute respiratory failure due to lung parenchymal disease. The treatment of acute respiratory failure remains primarily supportive. The goal of treatment is to avoid further damage to the lungs and other organ systems during the period required for the lungs to heal.

Modes of Mechanical Ventilation in the PICU

Ventilators commonly used in the PICU are capable of sophisticated measurements and analysis of airway pressure, gas flow, and carbon dioxide. All ventilator modes may be understood by identifying the variables that are controlled. In almost all cases, a preset rate is provided. The size of the breath delivered may be controlled either by setting a tidal volume to be delivered or by setting an airway pressure to be achieved.

Volume Control

In volume-control modes, the size of the breath is controlled by targeting a volume to be delivered. The ventilator senses air flow and calculates the volume as a product of flow and time. Most sophisticated volume ventilators measure and adjust the gas delivery on the basis of exhaled tidal volumes. When air leaks from the chest by routes other than the gas delivery circuit (e.g., a bronchopleural fistula or a leak around the endotracheal tube), volume delivery may be inaccurate. When compliance of the respiratory system is poor, a percentage of the tidal volume is lost in the circuit because of expansion of the ventilator tubing. The loss of tidal volume may be estimated using a compliance factor that is specific to the diameter of the ventilator tubing. The most sophisticated ventilators (the Servo 300i, Siemens Medical Solutions, Stockholm, Sweden) can adjust for this inaccuracy if that setting is selected. The most accurate measures of tidal volumes are obtained at the endotracheal tube using an in-line respiratory profile monitor (CO_2SMO Mainstream, Respironics). When the size of the breath is controlled by volume delivered, decreasing compliance in the lung will result in higher pressures achieved. An inspiratory pause gives the pressure in the circuit time to equilibrate between the proximal airway and the alveoli, and will help to determine if the alveoli are being distended by high pressures. In the setting of noncompliant, diseased lung, the duration of inhalation or inspiratory time will affect the pressures achieved in volume control modes.

Pressure Control

In pressure-control modes, the size of the breath delivered is determined by the target pressure and the inspiratory time. Pressure-control modes were developed for use in small infants before sophisticated methods existed to control delivery of very small tidal volumes. The volume delivered at a given airway pressure will depend on the compliance of the lungs. As the patient's disease process resolves and compliance improves, tidal volumes may become large, placing the patient at risk for

ventilator-induced lung injury (VILI). The very high initial flow rates necessary to achieve a given pressure for the duration of the inspiratory time can result in turbulence in a constricted airway, which results in decreased dynamic compliance and smaller tidal volumes delivered.

Pressure-Regulated Volume Control

Pressure-regulated volume control (PRVC) is a volume-controlled mode with a flow pattern similar to a pressure-controlled breath. A target tidal volume is set, and the ventilator applies constant pressure throughout inspiration to achieve that target volume. Volume delivered is measured on exhalation, and the pressure is adjusted in subsequent breaths to deliver the target tidal volume. Because exhalation volume is used to calculate the pressure needed for the next breath, PRVC may not be used when there is significant air leak outside the ventilatory circuit.

PRVC shares with pressure control the advantages of a larger area under the pressure-time curve, leading to higher mean airway pressure (MAP) and improvement in oxygenation. PRVC shares with volume control the safety of a controlled tidal volume that cannot increase as compliance improves or decrease as compliance worsens. This mode is particularly useful when dramatic improvement in compliance is expected, such as after the administration of surfactant. When PRVC is not available as a synchronized mode, significant inspiratory effort may result in breath stacking or extreme variability in tidal volumes delivered. For this reason, PRVC is usually used with very heavy sedation or neuromuscular blockade (or both), except with the Servo 300i, which can provide synchronized intermittent mandatory ventilation with PRVC.

Support Modes

Effort above a preset rate may or may not be supported. The most common form of support is pressure support. Pressure support has been shown to facilitate weaning, and it may also improve patient comfort. Pressure support is frequently used to recondition weakened respiratory muscles while still providing mandatory breaths to prevent atelectasis; however, data to support this approach do not exist (Turner and Arnold, 2007).

Positive End-Expiratory Pressure

All ventilation modes generate inhalation pressures above a set positive end-expiratory pressure (PEEP). The application of PEEP improves functional residual capacity and minimizes shearing forces that result from repeated opening and closing of lung units. Increasing PEEP also increases MAP, which improves ventilation/perfusion (V/Q) matching and oxygenation. High levels of PEEP may impair venous return to the thorax and thus cardiac preload. When there is significant resistance to exhalation, as in status asthmaticus, the patients may have an increase in intrinsic PEEP, which increases the resting lung volume and decreases inspiratory capacity. Intrinsic PEEP can be measured with an expiratory pause pressure.

Noninvasive Positive Pressure Ventilation

Over the past few years, there has been an increase in the use of noninvasive ventilation to prevent or delay endotracheal intubation. Noninvasive positive pressure ventilation (NPPV) includes continuous positive airway pressure (CPAP), which is used to increase functional residual capacity (FRC) and to overcome inspiratory airway collapse, and biphasic positive airway pressure, which also supports respiratory effort with positive inspiratory pressure. Studies in adults have shown clear benefit to NPPV, especially when endotracheal intubation can be avoided, with no decrement when endotracheal intubation is merely delayed (Pagano and Barazzone-Argiroffo, 2007). NPPV has been demonstrated successfully in pediatric patients with neuromuscular disease, upper airway obstruction, status asthmaticus, and cystic fibrosis (Deis, 2008).

There are many delivery devices for noninvasive ventilation, but most are poorly adapted to infants and toddlers. Skin breakdown under the mask or nasal delivery device is common, so strict attention to skin care is necessary when noninvasive ventilation goes on for more than a few hours. It is ideal to have more than one delivery device (e.g., nasal prongs and a mask) when NPPV is used for more than a few days, as rotation between devices can avoid skin breakdown. These devices are commonly used in the long term at home for children with neuromuscular disease.

Successful use of NPPV requires careful patient selection and close monitoring for signs of response or failure. NPPV should be used in patients with normal mental status and normal airway protective reflexes. Patient cooperation is necessary, and NPPV for a severely anxious patient is unlikely to succeed. It is also not very likely to succeed for patients with poor mask fit, copious secretions, or significant acid-base disturbances. NPPV should not be used in patients with upper gastrointestinal (GI) bleeding, recent upper airway or GI tract surgery, or hemodynamic instability.

Patients on NPPV should be carefully monitored for synchrony between patient and ventilator. A decrease in respiratory rate is a fairly reliable sign of effective response and is usually seen within 1 hour of initiation of therapy. In a patient with severe hypoxemic respiratory failure, converting to endotracheal intubation from a high level of support with NPPV can result in severe desaturations. The decision to intubate should be considered when the patient's fraction of inspired oxygen (Fio$_2$) requirement rises above 60%.

Ventilator-Induced Lung Injury

Ventilator-induced lung injury is caused by prolonged exposure to high Fio$_2$, by alveolar stretch from excessive tidal volumes (volutrauma), and by opening and closing of alveoli (shear stress trauma). Although hyperoxic inspired gas is essential for patients with lung injury, exposure to Fio$_2$ greater than 95% for 24 to 48 hours causes lung injury similar to ARDS and causes death within 48 to 72 hours due to oxygen toxicity (Adams et al., 2003).

Mechanical trauma from ventilation causes injury both through physical disruption of the architecture of the lung and through release of inflammatory mediators. Atelectatrauma, which is thought to occur when PEEP is set below the lower inflection point of the lung hysteresis curve, is particularly problematic in lung disease states associated with surfactant dysfunction, such as ARDS. Patients with heterogeneous lung disease are at increased risk for volutrauma. Transpulmonary pressure is not uniformly distributed to alveoli, and collapsed alveoli adjacent to inflated alveoli may be subject to extreme shearing forces. Mechanical trauma leads to release of inflammatory mediators, which may spill over to systemic circulation and play a role in the development of multiorgan failure (Plötz et al., 2004; Harris, 2005; Tremblay and Slutsky, 2006).

Use of Lung Hysteresis Curves

More sophisticated ventilators can calculate pressure-volume loops showing the difference in the pressure-volume relationship between the inspiratory and expiratory limbs of the respiratory cycle (Fig. 39-1). The sigmoidal shape of the hysteresis curve reflects differing compliance at different lung volumes. The lower inflection point represents the point during inspiration at which compliance improves. Below this point, the majority of alveoli are closed. The upper inflection point represents another change in compliance. Above a certain volume, more pressure is required to further distend alveoli, and the upper inflection point is thought to represent the beginning of a zone in which further pressure causes significant alveolar strain. The curve is steepest and nearly linear between these points, reflecting maximal compliance. Lung injury is thought to be minimized by keeping PEEP above the lower inflection point to maintain recruitment, and keeping tidal volumes below the upper inflection point by minimizing peak inspiratory pressure (Tremblay and Slutsky, 2006).

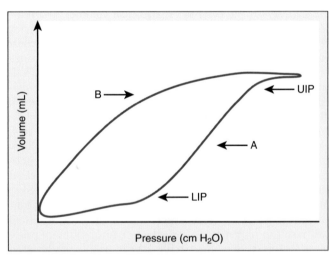

■ **FIGURE 39-1.** Pressure-versus-volume curve of the respiratory system. **A,** The inflation limb of the curve. **B,** The deflation limb of the curve. The point at which the curve touches the y-axis (zero pressure) is the functional residual capacity (FRC). The lower inflection point (LIP) represents the point during inspiration at which compliance improves. The upper inflection point (UIP) represents the point at which alveolar overdistention leads to worsening compliance. The curve is steepest between these points, reflecting the zone of best compliance. Lung injury is thought to be minimized by keeping positive end-expiratory pressure (PEEP) above the lower inflection point to maintain recruitment, and by keeping tidal volumes below the upper inflection point by minimizing peak inspiratory pressure. *(Reprinted with permission from Stawicki SP, Goyal M, Sarani B: High-frequency oscillatory ventilation [HFOV] and airway pressure release ventilation [APRV]: a practical guide, J Intensive Care Med 24:215, 2009.)*

Alternative Modes of Ventilation

High-Frequency Oscillatory Ventilation

Despite conventional ventilation strategies to reduce VILI, about one third of patients with ARDS die, and many of the survivors experience a significant decrement in function. The object of high-frequency oscillatory ventilation (HFOV) is to accomplish oxygenation and ventilation with less injury to the lung. HFOV uses laminar flow at high MAPs to maintain the lung open, and it uses an oscillating piston to create pressure displacement above and below the MAP to deliver very small tidal volumes in the range of the volume of the patient's anatomic dead space (Stawicki et al., 2009) (Fig. 39-2). The result, ideally, is ventilation only on the steep and linear part of the hysteresis curve. Compliant alveoli, which might receive an excessively large share of the delivered tidal volume in conventional ventilation, are protected from volutrauma. With this strategy, noncompliant alveoli—those with time constants long enough to preclude opening with conventional ventilation—may be recruited. Recruitment of new lung units may improve V/Q matching. A crossover trial comparing HFOV with conventional ventilation in children with severe lung disease showed that HFOV was associated with improved oxygenation and, despite higher MAPs, a reduced need for supplemental oxygen at 30 days (Arnold et al., 1994).

In HFOV, the variables controlled on the ventilator are frequency of respiration, (measured in cycles per second, or Hertz), amplitude of ventilation (power), and MAP. Frequency is measured in cycles per second. A frequency of 10 is 600 "breaths" per second, and a frequency of 3 is 180 breaths per second. A lower frequency functionally creates a longer inspiratory time and therefore a larger breath. The frequency is initially set at 10 for infants, and somewhat lower for older children. Amplitude, also referred to as *power,* is measured in centimeters of water. There is no standard starting pressure. The amplitude is initially set to produce a visible wiggling motion of the patient's

body to the level of the lower abdomen or groin. MAP is initially set to 5 cm H_2O greater than the last MAP on conventional ventilation (Stawicki et al., 2009). A chest radiograph performed within an hour or two after initiating HFOV should confirm an appropriate MAP setting by showing approximately nine visible ribs from the top of the thorax to the diaphragm.

Oxygenation can be improved by increasing Fio_2, MAP, or bias flow. Bias flow is an auxiliary flow of gas that crosses the oscillating gas flow to provide fresh gases and clear CO_2. Increasing MAP to the point where alveolar distention causes collapse of perialveolar vessels may result in hypotension or hypoxemia that may be responsive to administration of intravascular volume. Lung recruitment often allows a decrease in MAP within the first 24 hours. When the MAP can be weaned to near the last MAP recorded from conventional ventilation, conversion back to conventional ventilation should be considered.

Ventilation can be improved by increasing the amplitude and decreasing the frequency. As the frequency of breaths decreases, a higher percentage of the set amplitude will be delivered. This is like increasing the tidal volume in a conventional ventilator; decreasing frequency is a way to increase ventilation, thereby decreasing $Paco_2$. Frequencies less than 3 (180 cycles per minute) may increase the risk for volutrauma (Stawicki et al., 2009).

Patients on HFOV are usually treated with sedation and neuromuscular blockade. Because they are subject to a constant distending pressure, which may impede venous return, it is important to be attentive to maintaining a good intravascular volume and right ventricular filling pressure. Many patients require intravascular volume loading at the initiation of HFOV. Although nursing staff may be reluctant to suction patients on HFOV, secretions in the endotracheal tube can dramatically attenuate amplitude and should be removed. Finally, the appearance of a patient on HFOV, with the loud noise of the machine's diaphragm and the absence of tidal movement of the chest, can be disconcerting to patient's families. It is best to inform them of what to expect.

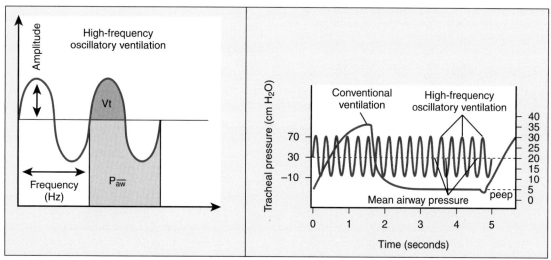

■ **FIGURE 39-2.** High-frequency oscillatory ventilation (HFOV). Both graphs depict pressure versus time in HFOV. The graph on the *left* depicts the ventilator cycle over only a fraction of a second, to illustrate the key variables that are controlled in HFOV. The graph on the *right* shows the pressure-versus-time curve of HFOV, with conventional ventilation superimposed for comparison. The y-axes are different, reflecting airway pressures in HFOV on the left and pressures in conventional ventilation on the right. The exhalation pressure in HFOV is actually negative, making expiration an active process. *(Reprinted with permission from Stawicki SP, Goyal M, Sarani B: High-frequency oscillatory ventilation [HFOV] and airway pressure release ventilation [APRV]: a practical guide,* J Intensive Care Med 24:215, 2009.)

For a more complete treatment of the mechanics of HFOV, see Stawicki and colleagues (2009).

Airway Pressure-Release Ventilation

Airway pressure-release ventilation (APRV) cycles between a high- (P_{high}) and a low-pressure level (P_{low}) in a high-flow CPAP circuit (Fig. 39-3). The continuous high flow allows spontaneous breathing throughout the ventilatory cycle, and it may reduce the need for heavy sedation and neuromuscular blockade. Spontaneous breathing is necessary to realize the benefits of this mode of ventilation (Stawicki et al., 2009).

Most of the respiratory cycle is spent at P_{high}, and pressure is briefly released to P_{low} several times per minute. Ideally, time spent at P_{high} will maximize recruitment and, by placing the lung on the steep part of the hysteresis curve, make spontaneous breathing easier. The time spent at P_{low} allows ventilation, but it is believed to be brief enough to prevent atelectasis of alveoli with long time constants (Stawicki et al., 2009).

Initially, P_{high} is set at the plateau pressure measured from an inspiratory pause on conventional ventilation and adjusted to allow weaning of Fio_2. P_{low} is set at zero to maximize the velocity of exhalation. The time (T) of T_{high} is initially set between 4 to 6 seconds and adjusted to maintain adequate oxygenation and ventilation. T_{low} is set at 0.4 to 0.5 seconds and adjusted to maintain a tidal volume of about 5 mL/kg, or such that expiration ends when the flow reaches 50% to 75% of the measured maximal expiratory flow. T_{low} is the critical variable that affects bulk air flow and thus ventilation. Oxygenation is increased by increasing Fio_2 or by increasing P_{high} or T_{high}, both of which will increase MAP. Ventilation is increased by encouraging spontaneous respiration or increasing T_{low} (Stawicki et al., 2009).

Although it was described in 1987, APRV is relatively new in pediatrics and has not been thoroughly studied. Case reports of APRV in pediatric patients have shown improvement in oxygenation with the ventilation strategy (Krishnan and Morrison, 2007; Kuruma et al., 2008). With a crossover design, the one randomized controlled trial of APRV in children demonstrated comparable ventilation at lower peak inspiratory and plateau pressures (Schultz et al., 2001). The potential advantages of decreasing mechanical ventilatory pressures and allowing spontaneous breathing and a reduced need for sedation and neuromuscular blockade in patients with severe lung disease make it worth considering despite the paucity of data. APRV may be contraindicated in patients with severe obstruction to exhalation, such as status asthmaticus.

Adjuncts to Mechanical Ventilation for Patients with Severe Lung Disease

Helium-Oxygen Mixtures (Heliox)

Helium is a low-density, biologically inert gas that can be safely mixed with oxygen. When air flow through a tube is turbulent, the flow rate depends on the density of the gas. With high helium concentrations, heliox can flow more rapidly through narrowed airways than nitrogen-oxygen mixtures. Additionally, carbon dioxide diffuses through helium faster than through air. The Fio_2 required by the patient may limit the use of heliox, as minimal benefit is believed to occur from heliox concentrations of less than 60%. When used with a spontaneously breathing patient, efforts should be made to prevent entrainment of room air with a well-fitting nonrebreather mask. Heliox can be delivered through the ventilator but may interfere with tidal volume measurements. This difficulty can be overcome with in-line monitors of respiratory mechanics (Myers, 2006).

Heliox may improve the delivery of nebulized medications. It improves dyspnea and peak expiratory flow in spontaneously breathing asthmatics, and it may limit peak inspiratory pressure in ventilated patients with status asthmaticus (Gupta and Cheifetz, 2005; Kissoon et al., 2008). Heliox improves respiratory distress associated with upper airway obstruction and improves the work of breathing in patients with bronchiolitis (Gupta and Cheifetz, 2005). No adverse effects of heliox have been reported. Despite a widespread belief that early application of heliox can prevent the need for intubation in select patients, there are no studies of heliox directed at patient outcomes.

Prone Positioning

In a supine patient, the dependent lung is underventilated and at risk for collapse, and the antidependent lung is aerated and at risk for overdistention. The mechanism by which prone

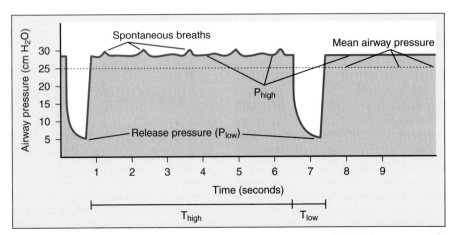

■ **FIGURE 39-3.** Airway pressure-release ventilation (APRV). In the pressure-versus-time curve for APRV, spontaneous breaths are present throughout the respiratory cycle. *(Reprinted with permission from Stawicki SP, Goyal M, Sarani B: High-frequency oscillatory ventilation [HFOV] and airway pressure release ventilation [APRV]: a practical guide,* J Intensive Care Med *24:215, 2009.)*

positioning can improve oxygenation is not completely clear, but it may improve V/Q matching by improving the aeration of the dependent lung (Ryu et al., 2008). Prone positioning can also improve lung mechanics by decreasing thoracoabdominal compliance. In adult patients, a protocol of prone positioning for 7 hr/day improved oxygenation but did not alter ventilator-free days or mortality (Gattinoni et al., 2001). In pediatric patients, a protocol of prone positioning for 20 hr/day improved efficiency of oxygenation but did not improve ventilator-free days or organ failure–free days (Curley et al., 2005).

Nitric Oxide

Inhaled nitric oxide (iNO) has been a mainstay of treatment for both primary and secondary pulmonary hypertension of the newborn since its introduction. In these patients, it causes a rapid and sustained improvement in efficiency of oxygenation by preferentially vasodilating ventilated lung units (Konduri and Kim, 2009). Because it is rapidly inactivated by hemoglobin, the effect of iNO is limited to the pulmonary vasculature (Adhikari et al., 2007).

Because the pathophysiology of ARDS and acute lung injury (ALI) involves V/Q mismatching, there has been interest in using iNO for patients outside the neonatal age range. In adult studies, iNO improved oxygenation (i.e., the ratio of pulmonary arterial oxygen pressure [Pao_2] to Fio_2, and the oxygenation index) but did not improve mortality. There has been some concern in adult patients that iNO may be associated with an increase in the need for new renal replacement therapy (Adhikari et al., 2007). In a randomized trial in children, iNO improved oxygenation without harmful side effects from methemoglobinemia at dosages up to 20 parts per million. The study was not powered to detect a difference in mortality (Tang et al., 1998).

Nitric oxide is commonly used at a level of 20 ppm. Very high concentrations of NO may paradoxically worsen V/Q matching by diffusing into nonventilated areas and improving the perfusion there. High concentrations also carry a significantly increased risk for methemoglobinemia. Methemoglobin should be monitored daily while therapy with iNO is used. If methemoglobin becomes elevated, it is usually sufficient to decrease the concentration of iNO. For very high methemoglobin levels, a scavenger, such as methylene blue, may be used. Exposure to NO for even a brief period can sensitize the pulmonary vasculature to its effects. Rapid weaning to low levels (5 ppm) is usually well tolerated, but thereafter, iNO should be weaned slowly to prevent rebound vasoconstriction (Adhikari et al., 2007).

Surfactant

Surfactant deficiency has been described in ARDS and ALI, particularly in the acute phase of the illness. The best-studied application of surfactant is in meconium aspiration syndrome, where significant clinical improvement is reported after surfactant installation (Willson et al., 2008). Surfactant instillation in infants mechanically ventilated for respiratory syncytial virus disease leads to improvement in oxygenation and decrease in duration of mechanical ventilation (Tibby et al., 2000; Luchetti et al., 2002).

Trials of endotracheal instillation or aerosolization of surfactant in adults have shown little or no benefit. In children, treatment with calfactant, a natural preparation relatively rich in surfactant specific protein B, has been associated with

improved oxygenation and mortality, with particular benefit seen in patients younger than 12 months (Willson et al., 2005). Although this trial generated significant interest in the use of calfactant for pediatric ARDS and ALI, an independent analysis of the data noted that the placebo arm of the trial had more immunocompromised patients, and that statistical significance was lost when controlling for immune status (Czaja, 2007). Surfactant therapy for ARDS/ALI in patients outside the neonatal age range remains controversial.

Surfactant is administered by direct endotracheal instillation through an endotracheal tube or bronchoscope at a dosage of 100 mg/kg body weight. The total volume of the drug preparation is significant. Complications of surfactant instillation include volume-responsive hypotension and transient hypoxia. Most authors cite pulmonary hemorrhage as a relative contraindication (Willson et al., 2008). Surfactant is probably best used early in the course of mechanical ventilation. Administration of surfactant in patients with severe hypoxia can provoke severe desaturation. In patients with severe hypoxia, surfactant may be safely given while the patient is supported with extracorporeal therapies.

Weaning and Extubation

Mechanical ventilation causes VILI, frequently necessitates invasive monitoring and heavy sedation, and predisposes patients to complications such as ventilator-associated pneumonia and gastric ulcer, so it should be discontinued as soon as the patient is capable of spontaneous breathing. The most common approach to weaning is gradual reduction of mechanical ventilatory support, often using pressure-support modes combined with mandatory breaths. Optimal sedation is crucial to weaning success. Oversedation may decrease respiratory drive, whereas undersedation may increase thrashing and the risk for airway injury, particularly in young children.

Not all patients require gradual weaning. An alternative approach is to perform a daily test of extubation readiness, such as a spontaneous breathing trial, and give higher amounts of support to provide periods of rest for the respiratory muscles between these tests. A third approach is to provide periods of rest interspersed with periods of lower support designed to exercise or train the muscles of respiration. Several adult studies have shown that protocolized weaning results in earlier extubation without an increase in complications (Newth et al., 2009). Studies of weaning protocols in children are ongoing. Pediatric studies have corroborated adult data showing that spontaneous breathing trials with a T-piece (i.e., a tracheotomy tube collar) or pressure support can predict successful extubation (Newth et al., 2009). A negative inspiratory force of –30 correlates with extubation success in adults but has not been validated in children.

Despite weaning and careful testing, 8% to 20% of patients fail extubation. Extubation failure is independently associated with a fivefold increased risk for mortality in children, and upper airway obstruction accounts for or contributes to 25% to 40% of extubation failures (Newth et al., 2009). Testing for a leak around the endotracheal tube may predict post-extubation stridor, particularly in patients with uncuffed endotracheal tubes and those whose intubation has been prolonged. The absence of a leak at 30 cm H_2O does not accurately predict extubation failure, but it is commonly a trigger for the use of steroids.

Dexamethasone given 24 hours in advance of extubation may reduce the inflammation associated with airway injury from the endotracheal tube (Randolph, 2009).

Specific Disease Processes Requiring Mechanical Ventilation

Asthma

Children who are ventilated for status asthmaticus are among the most difficult ventilated patients to manage. Resistance to exhalation may cause intrinsic PEEP, which can profoundly decrease the available inspiratory volume. In severe asthmatics, exhalation is an active process; under neuromuscular blockade, the loss of patient participation in exhalation almost always results in significant worsening of hypercarbia. The most important strategy for mechanical ventilation of the patient with status asthmaticus is to prevent the need for positive pressure ventilation with aggressive bronchodilator and steroid therapy. Helium-oxygen mixtures and intravenous magnesium can be useful adjuncts to these therapies.

NPPV, if applied early in patients with status asthmaticus, can take advantage of patient's respiratory efforts and prevent the muscle fatigue that leads to the need for intubation (Stather and Stewart, 2005). There is evidence that NPPV prevents hospitalization in patients presenting to the emergency department with status asthmaticus. Mental status changes, anxiety, exhaustion, or refractory hypoxemia preclude the use of NPPV, and it is these clinical changes rather than arterial blood gas analysis results that should guide the decision to intubate.

Once the patient is intubated, the primary strategy is to limit gas trapping, which causes intrinsic PEEP and forces the lung to operate on the less compliant portion of the hysteresis curve. Gas trapping is evident in flow-versus-time graphs, where inspiration is seen to start before flow returns to zero, or in graphs of end-tidal CO_2 versus time, where CO_2 fails to reach a plateau before the next inspiration begins (Stather and Stewart, 2005).

Significant controversy exists as to the best method for ventilating asthmatics. There are advocates for both pressure- and volume-control ventilation. Because of the high air-flow rates required to achieve targeted pressure in pressure-control ventilation, this mode may cause more turbulence in the airways of ventilated asthmatics. Volume-control modes may require higher set pressures to deliver adequate tidal volumes; however, because much of the pressure is lost in overcoming proximal airway resistance, alveolar hyperinflation may not occur. Alveolar pressure can be measured with an inspiratory pause pressure; complications are rare when this pressure does not exceed 30 cm H_2O (Stather and Stewart, 2005).

Intrinsic PEEP can be measured with an expiratory pause pressure in a muscle-relaxed patient. Because complete exhalation is the goal, some authors recommend minimizing PEEP with an initial setting from 0 to 5 cm H_2O. Others, acting on the theory that PEEP will stent airways open and ameliorate gas trapping, recommend setting PEEP at or slightly higher than the measured intrinsic PEEP. If a higher-PEEP strategy is used, intrinsic PEEP should be measured frequently, and the ventilator settings should be adjusted accordingly (Stather and Stewart, 2005).

There is general agreement that exhalation time should be as long as possible. Low respiratory rates and short inspiratory times give maximum exhalation time, but often at the expense of minute ventilation. Permissive hypercapnia (see Acute Respiratory Distress Syndrome and Acute Lung Injury, next) has been successfully used in the ventilation of asthmatics (Stather and Stewart, 2005). With permissive hypercapnia, patient ventilatory dyssynchrony is common. Neuromuscular blockade with adequate sedation is often necessary until severe bronchospasm resolves, usually within 24 hours. Weaning and extubation should be prompt, because spontaneous respiration is favorable for asthmatics. There are no generally agreed on criteria for extubating asthmatics, except that it should be performed as soon as possible. Negative inspiratory pressure with active exhalation is more effective than positive pressure in obstructive lung disease. Blood gas and ventilatory parameters that suggest the patient with asthma is improving include a normalizing partial pressure of CO_2 and pH, and a peak inspiratory pressure that begins to approach the inspiratory pause pressure. The difference between peak inspiratory pressure and inspiratory pause pressure correlates with airway resistance.

Acute Respiratory Distress Syndrome and Acute Lung Injury

The clinicopathologic picture of ARDS and ALI is diffuse alveolar damage, and four clinical parameters are involved: acute onset, severe arterial hypoxemia resistant to supplemental oxygen, bilateral infiltrates, and absence of left atrial hypertension. A Pao_2/Fio_2 ratio of less than 200 mm Hg defines ARDS, and a ratio of less than 300 mm Hg defines ALI (Randolph et al., 2003).

The most common cause of ARDS and ALI is lower respiratory tract infection, but it can be precipitated by a variety of systemic inflammatory conditions, including infection outside the respiratory tract, pancreatitis, and tissue necrosis. Overall mortality for children ranges between 8% and 15%, which is lower than that for adults (Randolph et al., 2003). Patients with bone marrow transplantation may have a significantly higher mortality. Because of the low mortality in children, duration of mechanical ventilation or number of ventilator-free days are both considered acceptable endpoints for studies of ARDS and ALI.

Although not a predictor of mortality in adults with ARDS, multiple single-center and multicenter studies of the epidemiology of ARDS and ALI in pediatric patients confirm that the ratio of the alveolar oxygen pressure (Pao_2) to Fio_2 at the onset of ARDS or ALI is an independent predictor of mortality (Flori et al., 2005; Erickson et al., 2007). Mortality rates for children with ARDS or ALI from studies in the past 10 years range from 8% to 35% (Willson et al., 2008; Randolph et al., 2003). A recent prospective multicenter observational study of 320 children with ARDS or ALI found that mortality in patients with a Pao_2/Fio_2 ratio of less than 200 is nearly twice the mortality in those with a ratio between 200 to 300 (26% versus 13%) (Erickson, 2007). The Pao_2/Fio_2 ratio also predicted the number of ventilator-free days (Flori et al., 2005). The severity of hypoxia is also sometimes measured by the oxygenation index, defined as $(MAP \times Fio_2)/Pao_2$ (Randolph, 2009).

Treatment of ARDS and ALI

Control of a persistent trigger of the inflammatory cascade is critical to eliminating the stimulus for ongoing lung injury. Because inflammation with capillary leak is part of the pathophysiology of ARDS, patients may benefit from a restrictive fluid strategy (Wiedemann et al., 2006). Fluid restriction should be initiated only after a patient with shock has been adequately resuscitated. Treatment of hypoproteinemia with albumin and furosemide may also be beneficial (Randolph, 2009).

Intensive care unit (ICU) stays for patients with ARDS or ALI may be prolonged, so is important to be attentive to other organ systems and to the prevention of iatrogenic injury. Strategies to avoid ICU-related pneumonia, critical care myopathy, central line infection, deep venous thrombosis, and gastritis, will be discussed later (see Prophylaxis).

Mechanical ventilation strategies for ARDS and ALI are designed to minimize VILI while protecting the patient from profound hypoxia. A Pao_2 target of 55 to 80 mm Hg (i.e., an arterial oxygen saturation as measured by pulse oximetry [SpO_2] of 88% to 95%) is commonly recommended for adult patients but may be too low for children, as the effect of prolonged marginal oxygenation on the developing brain is unknown. Most authors recommend an SpO_2 target of greater than 90% for children (Randolph, 2009).

In patients with ARDS and ALI, parenchymal lung damage occurs heterogeneously. The relatively normal aerated lung, which may be a relatively small proportion of the total lung volume, is at risk for overdistention. In 2000, the Acute Respiratory Distress Syndrome Network (ARDSNet) trial, in adults, a strategy aimed at reducing overdistention decreased mortality. The authors recommended reducing plateau pressure to 30 cm H_2O or less by targeting tidal volumes to 6 mL/kg or less. These data have not been replicated in children. Adoption of the target values from the adult study is controversial, particularly for younger children, as their more compliant chest wall and smaller airways may predispose them to atelectasis.

Alveolar collapse is possible with a low tidal volume strategy. Recruitment maneuvers with such a strategy include application of a sustained increase in airway pressure (i.e., a pressure of 40 mm Hg for 40 seconds) with a goal of opening the collapsed lung. After recruitment, PEEP is optimized to maintain the open lung (Randolph, 2009).

Permissive Hypercapnia

If the mode of ventilation that maintains ideal oxygenation and minimizes VILI is not capable of adequate CO_2 exchange, a lower pH and a higher Pco_2 may be tolerated. Patients in whom hypercapnia is being tolerated to minimize lung stretch will exhibit increased air hunger and anxiety and will require increased sedation. Hypercapnia is accompanied by acidosis in the acute phase, until renal compensation can buffer the pH. Hypercapnic acidosis (HCA) may benefit patients with ARDS or ALI apart from its association with ventilator strategies designed to decrease lung stretch. HCA increases cardiac output and organ blood flow (Rogovik and Goldman, 2008). It has antiinflammatory effects and attenuates free radical production. It may thus function to attenuate further lung injury from mechanical ventilation and from evolving infection.

HCA may have deleterious effects in select populations. Decreases in neutrophil chemotaxis and in the bactericidal activity of neutrophils and macrophages seen with HCA may be harmful, particularly in patients with sepsis (Curley et al., 2010). HCA increases pulmonary vascular resistance, and therefore it may not be appropriate for patients who are anticipated to

have reactive pulmonary vasculature, particularly those in the neonatal age range (Curley et al., 2010). The increase in organ blood flow with HCA can cause increased intracranial pressure (ICP) in at-risk patients. Higher levels of CO_2 are not believed to damage the brain, but rigorous long-term outcome studies in children have not been done (Curley et al., 2010).

Extracorporeal Membrane Oxygenation

Despite all the innovative therapies, deterioration of lung function in patients with acute respiratory failure may lead to a requirement for 100% oxygen and high ventilatory pressures. In some of these patients, extracorporeal membrane oxygenation (ECMO) can ensure adequate oxygenation and ventilation without high Fio_2 and without potentially injurious airway pressures, allowing time for the lungs to heal. ECMO has been a particularly effective treatment for neonates with persistent pulmonary hypertension of the newborn: the use of ECMO reduced mortality in this group from between 80% and 85% to about 20% (Roy et al., 2000). Although older trials had suggested that ECMO for acute respiratory failure in adults was futile, the Extracorporeal Life Support Organization registry reports a survival rate of 53% for the small number of adult patients treated with ECMO for respiratory failure (Zapol et al., 1979; Conrad et al., 2005). A recent randomized trial of ECMO for adults with acute respiratory failure found the therapy effective in terms of improving survival without disability, and in terms of cost effectiveness (Peek et al., 2009). The use of ECMO was associated with an improved survival in pediatric patients with respiratory failure (Green et al., 1996). In pediatric patients, the mortality reported by the Extracorporeal Life Support Organization registry was 56% (Conrad et al., 2005). A randomized controlled trial of ECMO in pediatric patients was attempted but failed because of an overall decrease in mortality, probably resulting from lung-protective ventilation strategies.

The general indication for ECMO is reversible lung disease that prevents adequate oxygenation with conventional therapy, or shock refractory to medical treatment in a patient who is believed to have reversible disease (see ECMO for Circulatory Support of the Patient with Shock, later).

It is difficult to precisely identify the indications for ECMO for the patient with respiratory failure. The issue is clearer in neonates, who may be expected to have a relatively rapid resolution of pulmonary hypertension and a good outcome with extracorporeal therapy. Before the advent of high-frequency oscillating ventilation and nitric oxide, an oxygenation index of 40 was the criterion for considering ECMO. A recent review of 174 newborns with respiratory failure suggested that using a lower oxygenation index (the authors suggested 33.2) as the criterion for ECMO resulted in a lower mortality rate and a lower rate of chronic lung disease (Bayrakci et al., 2007). As mechanical ventilation becomes more sophisticated, it becomes more difficult to identify its moment of failure. With continuous innovation, it is also difficult to collect historical data for criteria that would identify patients in whom mortality with conventional ventilation exceeds the expected mortality with ECMO.

ECMO should be considered in a patient with high airway pressures and high Fio_2 who may be expected to require a long course of mechanical ventilation, or when the clinician believes that the probability of chronic lung disease induced by mechanical ventilation outweighs the risk of ECMO. The best outcomes are seen in patients with single-organ dysfunction and viral pneumonia. Mortality is highest in patients with trauma, immune suppression, or multiple-organ dysfunction syndrome (MODS) at the time of ECMO initiation. Most authors consider prolonged ventilatory course (>10 to 14 days) with high pressures and high Fio_2 to contraindicate ECMO, because significant VILI has already occurred (Frenckner and Radell, 2008). Survival to hospital discharge is less likely in patients who have been ventilated longer than 10 days (Nehra et al., 2009). Absolute contraindications to ECMO include conditions that make cannulation impossible, including severe prematurity or small size (e.g., infants <34 weeks old and weighing <2 kg), any condition that would preclude systemic heparinization (e.g., major coagulopathy, active hemorrhage, or recent intracranial hemorrhage), or conditions amenable to surgical repair (e.g., total anomalous pulmonary venous return and lethal anomalies).

Once the need for ECMO is identified, the route of cannulation must be determined. Venoarterial ECMO, usually performed through the jugular vein and carotid artery, is used to provide both respiratory and cardiac support. In patients with respiratory failure who lack a significant component of cardiac insufficiency, venovenous ECMO may be preferable. Venovenous ECMO eliminates the risk for arterial embolic events and preserves the carotid artery, but, because of the inevitable recirculation, it may not allow complete oxygenation.

When ECMO is initiated, the ventilator is adjusted to settings that allow the lung to rest. Generally, this means reducing the Fio_2 to 21% and the airway pressures to the minimal settings that allow some lung inflation. In patients older than neonates, it can be very difficult to reopen lungs that have completely collapsed on ECMO.

The pulmonary hypertension that leads to neonates requiring ECMO resolves in a few days, but the lung damage that leads to pediatric patients requiring ECMO is much slower to heal. For pediatric patients, the mean time on ECMO is almost 2 weeks (Frenckner and Radell, 2008; Nehra et al., 2009). A recently published 8-year experience with ECMO from Massachusetts General Hospital described an average duration of ECMO for respiratory failure of 274 hours (11.4 days), with a range of 1 to 1154 hours (48 days) (Nehra et al., 2009). The duration of a course of ECMO should be considered on a case-by-case basis. In general, it is reasonable to continue ECMO support for a pediatric patient with respiratory failure until there is clear evidence that pulmonary disease is irreversible, or until complications preclude survival.

Every day on ECMO increases the risk for complications. Bleeding occurs in up to 16% of pediatric patients on ECMO, and it is most commonly seen at surgical sites, at cannula sites, and in the GI tract. Complications related to the ECMO circuit (e.g., oxygenator failure, cannula dysfunction, tubing rupture, pump malfunction) occur for 14% of pediatric patients (Frenckner and Radell, 2008). During prolonged ECMO runs, attention to the support and preservation of extrapulmonary organ systems becomes paramount. Patients who may require ECMO should be sent to a center with expertise in the procedure before the severity of lung disease prevents safe transport.

For a thorough review of management of the patient on ECMO, see Frenckner and Radell (2008). For the most complete resource on ECMO management, see Van Meurs and colleagues (2005).

CARDIOVASCULAR SYSTEM

Treatment of shock is the mainstay of emergent support of the cardiovascular system in the pediatric ICU. It is difficult to determine what percentage of shock seen in pediatric patients presenting to the PICU is septic shock, because nearly three fourths of children admitted to the PICU meet the criteria for systemic inflammatory response syndrome (SIRS) (Carvalho et al., 2005; Wessel and Laussen, 2006). Therefore, recommendations for treatment of shock are skewed toward SIRS, probably the most common cause of shock in the PICU. Despite their disparate causes, the various types of shock share a common pathophysiology and treatment, and classifying shock by etiology is not particularly useful in children. Pediatric patients with septic shock present with elements of hypovolemic, cardiogenic, and distributive shock (Zanotti-Cavazzoni and Dellinger, 2006).

Rapid resuscitation and management of shock are critical to the treatment of children with shock, and diagnosing the type of shock is secondary to initiating resuscitation (Brierley et al., 2009). Aggressive fluid resuscitation and initiation of inotropes and antibiotics should be accomplished within the first hour after presentation. In adults, an early and aggressive protocol for septic shock has proved vastly more effective than any pharmacologic intervention (Rivers et al., 2001). Pediatric shock resuscitation protocols call for symptomatic treatment of shock using clinical signs as endpoints. The guidelines are divided into specific tasks to be accomplished in the first 5 minutes, the first 15 minutes, and the first hour (Fig. 39-4). The guidelines from the American College of Critical Care Medicine (ACCM) have resulted in improved outcomes for children with septic shock (Han et al., 2003; de Oliveira et al., 2008).

Recognition of Shock and Initial Resuscitation

Outcomes are improved if shock is recognized by its early signs, before the onset of arterial hypotension (Han et al., 2003). Because of children's capacity to increase systemic vascular resistance, they may be normotensive in shock. Tachycardia is a sensitive but nonspecific indicator. Prolonged capillary refill in a central location, particularly when combined with tachycardia, is a more specific indicator of shock. Once the diagnosis of shock has been made, resolution of tachycardia is a useful indicator of successful treatment. Severe tachycardia (>180 beats/min in a child younger than 1 year, or >140 bpm in a younger child) in a severely ill child may be rapidly followed by a precipitous decline in blood pressure (Dabrowski et al., 2000). Treating shock in a timely manner, before hypotension develops, may prevent circulatory collapse.

The two distinct clinical presentations of shock are warm shock (characterized by full, bounding pulses, warm skin, and hypotension) and cold shock (characterized by hypotension and delayed capillary refill). Warm shock is more common in adults, but it is present in only 20% of children who present with septic shock (Zanotti-Cavazzoni and Hollenberg, 2009). Particularly in patients with cold shock, tissue hypoperfusion begins to occur long before compensatory mechanisms fail and hypotension develops (Dabrowski et al., 2000).

Shock resuscitation should begin with assessment of the airway, breathing, and circulation. All children with suspected shock should receive supplemental oxygen. Pulse oximetry is

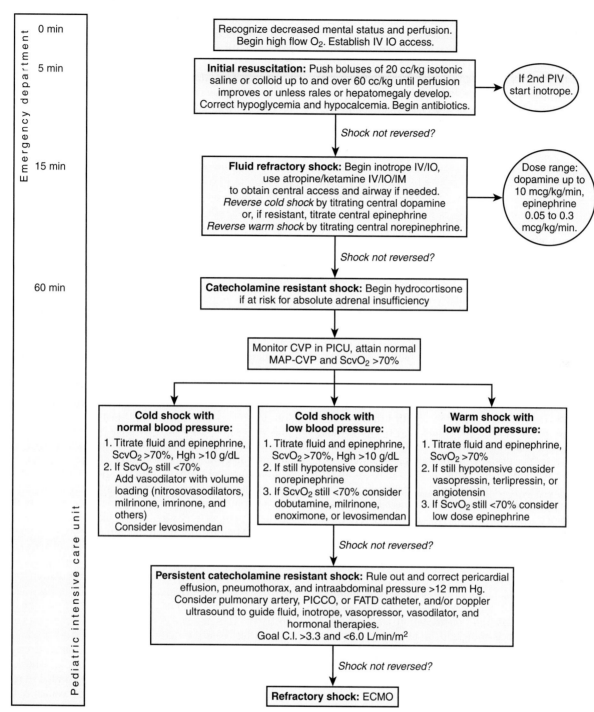

FIGURE 39-4. American College of Critical Care Medicine guidelines for resuscitation of pediatric patients with septic shock. *(From Brierley J, Carcillo JA, Choong K, et al: Clinical practice parameters for hemodynamic support of pediatric and neonatal septic shock: 2007 update from the American College of Critical Care Medicine,* Crit Care Med *37:666, 2009.)*

useful, not only to monitor adequacy of oxygenation but also because a poor signal indicative of poor perfusion may prompt a more aggressive resuscitation. Children with shock and severely increased work of breathing, or a Glasgow Coma Scale of less than 8, are at high risk for respiratory arrest, and the airway should be secured. Although etomidate as an induction agent favors hemodynamic stability, it impairs steroidogenesis and has been associated with increased mortality in patients with septic shock (Hildreth et al., 2008; Cuthbertson et al., 2009).

Ketamine, because of its favorable effects on hemodynamics and its antiinflammatory properties, may be the drug of choice for intubating patients in shock (Lois and De Kock, 2008).

Vascular access should be established as quickly as possible. Clinicians should have a low threshold for using the intraosseous route. Central venous access is recommended for fluid refractory shock, but resuscitation should begin via intravenous or intraosseous access (Brierley et al., 2009). Anything that can be given through an intravenous line can be given via the intraosseous route. For a child with impaired perfusion, the time to central circulation for drugs administered via the intraosseous route may be shorter than for drugs given though a peripheral intravenous line. A bedside glucose test is appropriate for any acutely ill child, as high metabolic rates and limited glycogen stores predispose infants and small children with sepsis to hypoglycemia. Hypocalcemia is an easily reversible contributor to myocardial dysfunction. An ionized calcium level should be obtained, and hypocalcemia should be treated in the initial phase of resuscitation (Brierley et al., 2009).

Fluid resuscitation should be accomplished as quickly as possible. No consensus exists with regard to the use of crystalloid versus colloid (Brierley et al., 2009). The most common initial resuscitation fluid is normal saline. Crystalloid resuscitation should be delivered in 20 mL/kg aliquots to most patients in 15 minutes or less (Brierley et al., 2009). Because it is impossible to administer large volumes rapidly via a standard intravenous pump, resuscitation fluids need to be pushed by hand in children larger than 10 to 15 kg. Children with shock may require large volumes of fluid resuscitation, often in excess of 100 mL/kg, and increased fluid requirements may persist for several days (Carcillo and Fields, 2002). Children can develop severe hypovolemia before presenting with obvious shock. They may also have significant ongoing losses from the intravascular space as a result of capillary leak. Outcomes are improved when at least 60 mL/kg are given within in the first hour of resuscitation (Carcillo et al., 1991). Large volumes of fluid given to pediatric patients with shock have not been shown to increase the rate of ARDS (Carcillo et al., 1991). Fluid resuscitation should continue until there is clinical improvement, with normalization of heart rate, perfusion, and mental status, or evidence of a hypervolemic state. Smaller fluid boluses (5 to 10 mL/kg) should be considered in some patients, particularly neonates and patients with suspected heart disease. The relatively thick right ventricle of the newborn may be less compliant and therefore less able to tolerate larger fluid boluses.

Fluid Refractory Shock

Vasoactive agents are an important adjunct to the stabilization of children in shock, but they should not be considered a replacement for adequate fluid resuscitation. Current ACCM guidelines recommend beginning with an inotrope (dopamine, up to 10 mcg/kg per minute, or lower-dosage epinephrine, beginning at 0.05 mcg/kg per minute). Mortality increases with delay in initiation of inotropes. Inotropes may be given through peripheral venous access (with close monitoring of the access site) or through an intraosseous line (Carcillo et al., 1991). In patients who require vasoactive medications, central venous access should be established. Warm shock should be treated with norepinephrine delivered via a central line (Carcillo et al., 1991).

Catecholamine-Resistant Shock

When shock is not reversed by the addition of centrally delivered inotropes or vasopressors, adrenal insufficiency should be considered (Carcillo et al., 1991). The diagnosis of relative adrenal insufficiency in patients with septic shock is controversial. Hypothalamic pituitary adrenal axis suppression can occur in patients with sepsis by a variety of mechanisms, as a result of dysfunction at any point along the hypothalamic pitu-

itary adrenal axis. A landmark study by Annane and colleagues (2002) found an improvement in mortality rates when septic patients with relative adrenal insufficiency were treated with steroid replacement. This study found a high incidence of relative adrenal insufficiency, which was probably related to a high rate of etomidate exposure in these patients, leading the author to recommend abandoning the use of etomidate (Annane, 2005). A subsequent multicenter randomized controlled trial failed to find a mortality benefit, although corticosteroid replacement did *hasten* reversal of shock in patients when shock could be reversed (Sprung et al., 2008). Exogenous corticosteroids have been shown to improve the vascular response to exogenous catecholamines in patients with shock (Oppert et al., 2005). The definition of an adequate circulating cortisol level is a subject of debate and probably depends on the severity of the illness. The most widely accepted definition in adults is a serum cortisol level of less than 15 mcg/dL, or an increase of less than 9 mcg/dL after ACTH stimulation (Annane et al., 2000). Because the dosage used in the ACTH stimulation test is supraphysiologic, some question its usefulness in identifying patients who could benefit from steroid replacement. Current recommendations for adult sepsis recommend use of low-dosage steroids (<300 mg/day of hydrocortisone) for shock that is resistant to fluid resuscitation and catecholamines without use of ACTH stimulation test (Dellinger et al., 2008; Marik et al., 2008). Because the P450 cytochrome system, which is responsible for steroidogenesis, matures to an adult level of functioning by about 1 year of age, infants and young children are at higher risk for adrenal insufficiency (Bartelink et al., 2006; Masumoto et al., 2008; Fernandez and Watterberg, 2009).

Adrenal insufficiency should be suspected in patients with fluid- and catecholamine-resistant shock who have risk factors for adrenal insufficiency, including a history of systemic steroid use, with a rapidly evolving purpuric rash, a history of panhypopituitarism, or exposure to etomidate (Brierley et al., 2009). The ACCM guidelines recommend hydrocortisone replacement for children with risk factors for adrenal insufficiency and catecholamine-resistant shock and for those with shock and inadequate response to the corticotropin stimulation test (peak cortisol, <18 mcg/dL after stimulation) (Brierley et al., 2009). A cortisol level should be drawn before the first dose of hydrocortisone. It is not always possible to wait for results of a stimulation test before initiating steroid replacement therapy. The recommended dosage for hydrocortisone ranges from 2 mg/kg per day (stress dosage) to 50 mg/kg per day (shock dosage) (Brierley et al., 2009). The dosage may be titrated to resolution of shock. Results of serum cortisol, when available, may lead to discontinuation of replacement hydrocortisone. The patient should be weaned from steroid therapy as soon as hemodynamics allow, because the impact of exogenous stress-dosage steroids on sensitive elements of the immune system is not fully understood. Prospective randomized controlled trials in children have not been done.

Increasing Oxygen Delivery and Normalizing Perfusion

The 2007 clinical practice parameters for hemodynamic support of pediatric and neonatal septic shock from the ACCM recommend use of clinical goals to direct shock resuscitation in the first hour. Shock resuscitation should be continued until therapeutic endpoints are reached (Box 39-1). Adult studies have shown improved outcomes when therapies for shock are titrated

Box 39-1 Therapeutic Endpoints for the Resuscitation of Shock

FIRST HOUR

- Maintain airway, oxygenation and ventilation
- Maintain hemodynamic variables
  - Heart rate below the 98th percentile of normal
  - Blood pressure above the 5th percentile of normal
- Maintain clinical indices of perfusion
- Capillary refill < 2 seconds
- Normal pulses, with no differential between central and peripheral pulses
- Warm extremities
- Urine output > 1 mL/kg per hour
- Normal mental status

BEYOND THE FIRST HOUR

- All of the above, plus the following:
- Perfusion pressure (mean arterial pressure and central venous pressure appropriate for age)
- Venous oxyhemoglobin saturation (Svo2) > 70%
- Cardiac index > 3.3 L/min per square meter; < 6 L/min per meter-squared

Adapted from Brierley J, Carcillo JA, Choong K, et al: Clinical practice parameters for hemodynamic support of pediatric and neonatal septic shock: 2007 update from the American College of Critical Care Medicine, *Crit Care Med* 37:666, 2009.

to maximize oxygen delivery, using venous oxyhemoglobin saturation (Svo_2) as a surrogate (Rivers et al., 2001). After the first hour of resuscitation in children, shock management should be directed to generating an Svo_2 of greater than 70% and, when pulmonary artery (PA) catheters are used, a cardiac index of 3.3 to 6.0 L/min per square meter (Brierley et al., 2009). A low Svo_2 may be treated with increasing inotropes or with blood transfusion, aiming for a hemoglobin level of about 10 mg/dL.

In adults, the use of PA catheters has not been shown to improve mortality, but comparable studies have not been done in children. PA catheters have been shown to identify incorrect assessment of hemodynamic status made on the basis of clinical parameters in children (Ceneviva et al., 1998). PA catheters may be useful in children when therapy directed by central venous pressure and Svo_2 is inadequate to reverse shock (Carcillo and Fields, 2002).

Children with cold shock and with poor perfusion often benefit from a reduction in cardiac afterload. Phosphodiesterase inhibitors such as milrinone are useful adjuncts to adrenergic agonists in these patients. Many of these children already have maximal adrenergic stimulation of the myocardium (whether exogenous or endogenous) and can benefit from the alternative pathway to increased inotropy provided by milrinone. As phosphodiesterase inhibitors are initiated, many patients will require further volume expansion. Loading dosages of phosphodiesterase inhibitors (e.g., milrinone) should not be used in pediatric patients with shock. Continuous intravascular monitoring is necessary when afterload reducers are used for patients with shock.

Vasopressin has been used in catecholamine refractory shock, particularly in the setting of decreased vascular tone. Children with severe shock often have high levels of endogenous catecholamines and some degree of catecholamine resistance.

This, coupled with the fact that catecholamines have some unfavorable effects on immune function and catabolism, have led investigators to consider other biochemical pathways to reverse shock. Vasopressin is a powerful vasoconstrictor, but at low dosages it has organ-specific vasodilatory effects (Holmes et al., 2003). Vasopressin deficiency has been described in vasodilatory shock states in both adults and children (Landry et al., 1997; Lodha et al., 2006). Studies in adults have shown that vasopressin improves blood pressure and urine output and allows lowering of the dosage of norepinephrine; however, a recent large randomized controlled trial of low-dosage vasopressin infusion found a good safety profile but no impact on mortality when compared with norepinephrine alone (Russell et al., 2008).

Vasopressin and its synthetic analogue, terlipressin, have been used in children in two ways: as a rescue therapy for severe shock, and as a catecholamine-sparing hormone replacement. Case series of the use of vasopressin in patients with refractory shock have described the use of dosages in the range of 0.00001 to 0.08 units/kg per minute (Matok et al., 2005; Choong and Kissoon, 2008; Yildizdas et al., 2008). When vasopressin is used as a hormone replacement, it is not titrated to clinical effect but used as a low-dosage continuous infusion. The only pediatric randomized controlled trial so far used a dosage of 0.0005 units/kg per minute, as in adult trials, and found an increase in MAP but no differences in time to hemodynamic stability or other clinical outcomes (Choong et al., 2009).

Reassessment of Fluid Balance and Hemodynamic Profile

Serial reassessments of patients admitted with shock are critical to good outcomes, and require continuous and meticulous attention to the maintenance of optimal preload, contractility, and afterload. Shock in neonates and children is more variable than in adults. Children who present in warm shock with an increased cardiac output and low systemic vascular resistance often progress to cold shock with myocardial dysfunction within 24 hours. Shock that is refractory to fluid resuscitation and vasoactive agents should prompt review of volume status. A high percentage of patients who have persistent shock after volume resuscitation have an underfilled ventricle, seen by echocardiography (Jardin et al., 1999). It should also raise the possibility of alternative diagnoses, including acquired cardiac disease, obstructive etiologies, toxins, occult blood loss, and inborn errors of metabolism.

Other Causes of Shock

Once shock resuscitation is initiated, the clinician should begin to consider the causes. Septic shock is the most common etiology of shock in the PICU. In patients with persistent shock, mechanical obstruction to flow in the form of pericardial effusion or elevated intraabdominal pressure should be considered. Other causes of shock, including occult hemorrhage, toxicologic causes, and acquired heart disease, should be addressed.

Causes of shock in the neonatal age range include congenital heart disease, particularly ductal-dependent lesions. An infusion of prostaglandin E_2 should be started immediately in neonates with shock until a ductal-dependent congenital heart lesion can be ruled out. Prostaglandin may cause apnea at higher dosages. Very young infants still transitioning from fetal to neonatal circulation are also at high risk for pulmonary hypertension and right-sided heart failure. Acidosis from shock and hypoxia can trigger this pathophysiology. Therapies that reduce pulmonary arterial pressure, including supplemental oxygen, sedation, maintenance of an alkalotic pH, and nitric oxide, are commonly needed for neonates with fluid-refractory shock and may be started empirically if necessary (Carcillo and Fields, 2002). Particular attention should be paid to maintenance of adequate temperature and glucose level in neonates with shock.

Early antibiotic administration is a high priority in patients presenting with septic shock. In adults with septic shock, a delay in antibiotic therapy is associated with worse survival, with mortality rates increasing by 7% for every 30 minutes that passes without delivery of appropriate antibiotic therapy (Kumar et al., 2006). Cultures are extremely important, but antibiotics should not be delayed if it is difficult to secure appropriate samples. In particular, lumbar puncture should be deferred until the patient is more stable and an evaluation of the coagulation system can be performed.

ECMO for Circulatory Support of the Patient with Shock

Shock that is refractory to medical interventions may be treated with extracorporeal support. ECMO for pediatric circulatory support was used in 29% of all cases in 2004, but most of these were cardiac patients requiring perioperative support (Conrad et al., 2005). Shock related to acute fulminant myocarditis has been successfully treated with extracorporeal support, with survival rates approaching 80% for patients on ECMO (Duncan et al., 2001). ECMO may be a bridge to myocardial recovery or to heart transplantation in these patients. It may be more effective in the support of shock characterized by inadequate cardiac output than of shock with a prominent component of vasoplegia or failure of oxygen extraction.

The use of ECMO for other causes of shock is uncommon and poorly studied. Historically, sepsis was considered a contraindication to ECMO because of concerns that the circuit would become irreversibly contaminated, but today, sepsis causing pulmonary hypertension is a standard indication for ECMO in neonates. Randomized controlled trials of ECMO for refractory septic shock are not possible, because the condition is rare and the options for treatment are few. A recent single-center report of 45 pediatric patients treated with ECMO for refractory circulatory failure due to sepsis, collected over 18 years, is the largest study published to date. These authors reported a 47% survival to hospital discharge despite the fact that 91% of the patients had three or more organ failures (Maclaren et al., 2007). Estimates of mortality without ECMO in case series of patients in which ECMO was used for this indication support the idea that ECMO as a treatment for septic shock significantly improves mortality rates (Bartlett, 2007). The reported average durations of ECMO for sepsis-related circulatory failure are 137 hours and 76 hours in case series of 9 and 12 patients, respectively (Beca and Butt, 1994; Goldman et al., 1997).

ECMO should be used for refractory shock when the clinician believes that other options are exhausted and the patient is unlikely to survive without it. In the treatment of septic shock, ECMO provides the treating team time to identify and treat the infectious agent, and it eliminates the problems of high dosages of vasoactive drugs and the toxicities associated with treatment of patients with ALI related to systemic inflammation.

Cardiac Arrest in Children

Management of the Patient after Cardiac Arrest

Protocols for the management of pediatric cardiac arrest have been developed by the American Heart Association and are covered in Chapter 38, Cardiopulmonary Resuscitation. The focus here is on the care of children after the return of spontaneous circulation.

The most important treatment for pediatric cardiac arrest is prevention. Because pediatric cardiac arrest is not usually sudden in onset, a window of opportunity exists in the period before it occurs. Medical emergency teams designed to respond to patients in danger of decompensation have been shown to decrease hospital mortality rates and the frequency of more serious codes (Topjian et al., 2009). In addition to early recognition of impending cardiac arrest, extracorporeal cardiopulmonary resuscitation (ECPR) has been used in an attempt to improve these outcomes. Intact survival from isolated respiratory arrest is the rule, but outcomes from in-hospital pediatric cardiac arrest remain poor. Return of spontaneous circulation is established in one half to two thirds of cases of in-hospital arrest, but less than 18% of patients survive with good neurologic outcome (Nadkarni et al., 2006). Survival rates and neurologic outcomes for out-of-hospital cardiac arrest are much poorer (Young et al., 2004). Cold-water submersion for cardiac arrest, even for relatively long duration, may be associated with a much higher rate of intact survival.

Extracorporeal Cardiopulmonary Resuscitation

Multiple physicians have examined the application of extracorporeal therapy as a rescue therapy during cardiac arrest before the return of spontaneous circulation. Survival to hospital discharge in these case series is surprisingly high—35%—despite a relatively long median duration of cardiopulmonary resuscitation (CPR) before the establishment of flow on ECMO (mean duration of 50 minutes) (Morris et al., 2004). With ECPR, survival to hospital discharge does not correlate with duration of CPR before ECMO. Neurologic outcomes have been encouraging: good neurologic outcomes are reported in greater than 75% of patients (Huang et al., 2008; Prodhan et al., 2009). It is important to select patients who have a reversible disease process for use of ECPR.

Management of Hypoxic-Ischemic Brain Injury after Resuscitation

Strategies aimed at preservation of brain function after cardiac arrest have been reported in adults and are under investigation in children. There is no single measure to decrease the impact of cardiopulmonary arrest on the brain.

Postischemic cytotoxicity occurs in animal models, so eliminating pathologic states known to increase active cerebral metabolism, such as seizure or hyperthermia, may be beneficial. The majority of cell injury may occur during the initial hypoxic ischemic event. However, cell death from apoptosis and as a result of reperfusion continues after the initial insult. After the event, an initial period of hyperemia is followed by a period of delayed postischemic hypoperfusion. Therapeutic strategies aimed at controlling this delayed cell death include maintenance of normoglycemia; avoidance of oxygen toxicity;

control of states characterized by increased cerebral metabolic rate, such as seizures and hyperthermia; and the application of therapeutic hypothermia.

Controlled hypothermia is associated with improved mortality rates and improved functional outcome after cardiac arrest in adults and in neonates with birth asphyxia (Bernard et al., 2002; Hypothermia after Cardiac Arrest Study Group, 2002; Gluckman et al., 2005; Shankaran et al., 2005). It is difficult to extrapolate these findings directly to children, because the circumstances surrounding cardiac arrest in children are different from those in adults. Ventricular fibrillation is the most common cause of cardiac arrest in adults, but cardiac arrest in children is predominately caused by asphyxia. Asphyxial arrest occurs after a period of hypoxia, and the total duration of cerebral insult (hypoxia plus anoxia) may be very long. Ischemic injury may be seen in brain cells after relatively short periods of interrupted circulation if they are preceded by a period of hypoxia (Vaagenes et al., 1997).

Clinical trials of therapeutic hypothermia after cardiac arrest in children are ongoing. Although there are not yet randomized controlled data supporting controlled hypothermia for pediatric patients after cardiac arrest, it is being used in the United States "consistently" by 9% of the pediatric intensivists surveyed and "sometimes" by 38% (Haque et al., 2006). Target temperatures vary widely, with most using temperatures of 32° to 35° for 12 to 24 hours (Haque et al., 2006). It is relatively labor intensive to rapidly achieve and maintain hypothermia. Neuromuscular blockade may be necessary to control shivering. Slow and controlled rewarming (0.5° C every 2 hours) is an important part of this therapy. Vigilance during the rewarming phase is necessary to avoid hyperthermia, which is known to exacerbate ischemic brain injury, but also to allow careful monitoring of the blood pressure and electrolyte disturbances that are common with rewarming (Wang et al., 2009; Fink et al., 2010a, 2010b). In a retrospective analysis of children after cardiac arrest, there was no increase in the number of hypothermia-associated adverse events in patients who received this therapy (Doherty et al., 2009).

Hypoglycemia has a synergistic, deleterious effect when coupled with neonatal asphyxia (Lubchenco and Bard, 1971). Hyperglycemia has been shown to be detrimental after near-drowning and traumatic brain injury, and, in general, glucose-containing solutions are not used in the first 48 hours after brain injury in older children (Ashwal et al., 1990; Chiaretti et al., 2002). Both hypotension and hypertension during reperfusion have been shown to have deleterious effects in animal models (Miller and Myers, 1972; Bleyaert et al., 1980).

Oxygen toxicity is posited to play a role in postischemic reperfusion injury. The brain is susceptible to oxygen free-radical damage (Siesjö et al., 1989). On the basis of this, there has been some interest in using room air to resuscitate newborns, particularly those with preserved circulation (Ten and Matsiukevich, 2009). In older patients, avoidance of hyperoxia may be beneficial.

Seizure activity increases cerebral metabolic rate and may worsen ischemic injury. Subclinical seizure activity is common after cardiac arrest, particularly in patients treated with therapeutic hypothermia, because of the requirement for neuromuscular blockade. Prophylactic use of antiepileptic drugs in patients who require paralysis is reasonable (Abend et al., 2009).

Prediction of Outcome after Cardiac Arrest

Attempts to use variables such as duration of cardiac arrest, initial pH, or early neurologic examination to predict neurologic outcome after cardiac arrest in children have been misleading. Electroencephalography can provide some prognostic information. The burst suppression pattern seen on the electroencephalogram after cardiac arrest is sensitive and specific for poor outcome (Wijdicks et al., 2006). No single test has been validated to predict outcome with a high sensitivity and specificity. High-quality CPR, and well-established ventilation and oxygenation in the period before the return of spontaneous circulation or the establishment of ECMO flow, may be the best predictors of outcome (Topjian et al., 2009).

RENAL SYSTEM

Fluid Balance and Renal Replacement

Fluid overload and renal insufficiency are common in critically ill patients because of requirements for fluid resuscitation, medications, and blood products. Fluid overload is associated with increased incidence of multiorgan failure in critically ill adults and children (Schuller et al., 1991; Rosenberg, 2003; Goldstein et al., 2005). Decreased fluid overload is associated with improved outcomes in neonates on ECMO, adults with ARDS, and children requiring continuous hemofiltration (Kelly et al., 1991; Foland et al., 2004; National Heart, Lung and Blood Institute, 2006). Diuretics and fluid restriction are routinely used to ameliorate the fluid overload accumulated with initial resuscitation. Fluid restriction may be necessary when fluid excretion is limited by kidney injury, but over time it may impair caloric intake.

Acute Kidney Injury

Acute kidney injury is fairly common in pediatric ICU patients and is independently associated with mortality (Plötz et al., 2008). The definition of acute renal failure is not mutually agreed on: it is described as a change from baseline in serum creatinine, or an elevation in blood urea nitrogen level, or urine output inadequate to match required intake (Plötz et al., 2008). A uniform definition of renal injury is important for research, but it does not yet inform clinical decision making. The RIFLE criteria (risk, injury, failure, loss, end-stage renal disease) have been proposed to classify renal injury in adult patients (Kellum et al., 2002). A pediatric modification of the adult RIFLE criteria has been proposed and independently evaluated (Table 39-1) (Akcan-Arikan et al., 2007). Among children requiring mechanical ventilation for less than 4 days, 58% met pediatric RIFLE criteria for acute kidney injury, most on the first day of admission. Patients with acute kidney injury according to the pediatric RIFLE scoring system had a mortality rate that was five times higher than patients without acute kidney injury (Akcan-Arikan et al., 2007; Plötz et al., 2008).

The primary treatment of acute kidney injury and failure is to remove the causative agent, if possible. The use of nephrotoxic medications should be reassessed; when they are deemed necessary, dosages should be based on drug levels and or creatinine

TABLE 39-1. Pediatric Modified RIFLE Criteria

	Estimated Creatinine Clearance Index	Urine Output
Risk	eCCI decreased by 25%	<0.5 mL/kg per hr for 8 hr
Injury	eCCI decreased by 50%	<0.5 mL/kg per hr for 16 hr
Failure	eCCI decreased by 75% or eCCI <35 mL/min per 1.73 square meter	<0.3 mL/kg per hr for 24 hr, or anuric for 12 hr
Loss	Persistent failure > 4 wk	—
End-stage renal disease	End-stage renal disease (persistent failure > 3 mo)	—

From Akcan-Arikan A, Zappitelli M, Loftis LL, et al: Modified RIFLE criteria in critically ill children with acute kidney injury, *Kidney Int* 71:1028, 2007.
eCCI, Estimated creatinine clearance index; *RIFLE*, risk, injury, failure, loss, and end-stage renal disease.

Box 39-2 Indications for Continuous Renal Replacement Therapy

- Fluid overload (defined as >10% weight gain from base-line) *and* acute renal dysfunction (defined as urine output <1 mL/kg per hour, unresponsive to diuretics infusion within 24 hours) *and* at least one of the following:
  - A change from baseline of >50% of serum creatinine, *or*
  - Elevated serum creatinine greater than 1.5 times the age-based normal value, *or*
  - A blood urea nitrogen level >40 mg/dL.
- Oliguric or anuric renal failure in patients who require administration of additional intravascular volume or whose nutritional status could be improved by increased fluid administration.
- Oliguric or anuric renal failure in patients with hepatic failure (continuous venovenous hemofiltration may remove hepatically cleared toxins).
- Electrolyte abnormalities requiring renal replacement (especially potassium and phosphorus).
- Metabolic derangements in which the production of noxious metabolic products is continuous, such as hyperammonemia
- Acute respiratory distress syndrome, defined as Fio_2/Pao_2 < 200, or oxygenation index > 10 in bone marrow transplantation patients. In this patient population, a high rate of clearance may be beneficial.

clearance. Consultation with a pharmacist, when one is available, can be invaluable for making these adjustments. Although acute kidney injury is associated with mortality, renal function usually returns in survivors, provided the offending agent is removed and attention is paid to preventing new medication and perfusion-related injury. While the kidney is healing, maintenance of appropriate fluid balance may require renal replacement therapy (RRT).

Renal Replacement Therapy

Criteria for Initiating Renal Replacement Therapy

There are no nationally published guidelines for the initiation of RRT, and there is wide variation among practitioners as to its timing of initiation and discontinuation. Absolute indications for renal replacement therapies include life-threatening electrolyte abnormalities and anuria. However, RRT is more commonly used for the relative indication of fluid overload with inadequate urine output (Gibney et al., 2008). The guidelines used at the Children's Hospital of Pittsburgh (University of Pittsburgh Medical Center) are shown in Box 39-2. There is increasing evidence that fluid overload contributes to mortality, particularly in children. Observational studies suggest that increasing severity of fluid overload before or at initiation of RRT is an independent predictor of mortality after controlling for severity of illness. RRT should be considered when accumulated fluid overload reaches 10% (Ricci and Ronco, 2008; Sutherland et al., 2010).

Practical Aspects of Renal Replacement Therapy

Continuous renal replacement therapy (CRRT) is the preferred mode of renal replacement therapy in ICU patients with hemodynamic instability. The advantages of CRRT over intermittent hemodialysis are that it allows correction of metabolic acidosis, provides temperature control, and provides constant fluid

hemostasis with better avoidance of intracerebral fluid shifts. Its main drawback is the need for anticoagulation. Although CRRT shows no survival benefit over intermittent therapy, it may predict renal recovery in survivors (Uchino et al., 2007).

CRRT can be accomplished with ultrafiltration alone (i.e., continuous venovenous hemofiltration [CVVH]) or with dialysis. With CVVH, both water and high-molecular-weight substances pass across the membrane because of a pressure gradient that creates convective flow. Convection, or passive movement of solute across a membrane along with water, allows phosphates and molecules such as urea and creatinine to clear at similar rates. Profound hypophosphatemia can easily develop, and patients on CVVH require phosphate replacement. Larger molecules such as heparin, insulin, and vancomycin, cleared in only negligible amounts during dialysis, are cleared more efficiently by CVVH.

With dialysis, blood flows along one side of a semipermeable membrane as a crystalloid solution is pumped along the other side of the membrane, countercurrent to the blood flow. Through the process of *diffusion*, molecules cross the membrane. The larger the molecule, the more slowly it moves across the membrane. Urea, a small molecule, is cleared efficiently, whereas creatinine, a larger molecule, is cleared less well. Phosphate ions have very low rates of clearance across the membrane.

Clinical Changes When Initiating CRRT

Clinicians should be alert to the risk for hypotension when CRRT is initiated. Hypotension may occur as a result of inadequate intravascular volume, hypocalcemia, or bradykinin release syndrome, particularly when patients are acidotic at the time of CRRT initiation. Once CRRT is begun, therapies aimed at preventing fluid overload should be discontinued. Diuretics should be decreased or stopped. Nutrition should be increased if it had been limited by fluid restriction. The amount of protein in parenteral nutrition should be increased to 1.5 to 4 mg/kg per day, because hemofiltration results in significant amino acid loss across the membrane (Maxvold et al., 2000). A low blood urea nitrogen level in a patient on RRT reflects inadequate nitrogen balance. A patient on CRRT requires additional potassium and phosphorus to replace that lost to the circuit. When CRRT is discontinued or interrupted, diuretics, fluid rate, TPN prescription, and electrolyte infusions should be returned to normal. The removal of medications across the CRRT membrane is difficult to predict. Consultation with a pharmacist is recommended with initiation of CRRT.

High-Clearance CRRT for Treatment of Sepsis

It is conventional to speak of the *dosage* of CRRT, meaning the quantity of blood purified per unit time. Higher-clearance CRRT (at least 35 mL/kg per hour versus 20 mL/kg per hour) is associated with improved survival in adults, with the greatest improvement seen in septic patients (Ronco et al., 2000). There has been some interest in using extremely high clearance CRRT to remove cytokines and modulate inflammation. This approach has shown some promise in patients with ARDS after bone marrow transplantation (DiCarlo et al., 2003). The pore size in most filters used for hemofiltration and dialysis admit passage of proteins whose size is in the range of 30 to 40 kDa, which is more than adequate for removal of interleukins 1, 6, 8, and 10, and tumor necrosis factor. Studies of high-clearance CRRT in septic patients have not shown significant and sustained decreases in cytokine levels, and high-clearance CRRT has not been conclusively shown to improve outcome (Joannidis, 2009).

Contraindications to CRRT

There are no absolute contraindications for the use of CRRT. Patients at risk for life-threatening bleeding with systemic heparinization may be put on CRRT with a citrate anticoagulation protocol. Citrate is added to the CRRT circuit, generating a level of hypocalcemia in the circuit sufficient to prevent clotting. Calcium must be infused centrally to replace the calcium lost in the circuit. Most of the citrate is removed in the circuit, and the liver metabolizes what remains. When citrate is used for anticoagulation, patients with liver failure who are unable to metabolize citrate are at risk for citrate lock, manifested by an increased ratio of total to ionized calcium (Morgera et al., 2004). Risks and benefits should be weighed carefully when considering the use of citrate CRRT in patients with liver failure.

Nutritional Support

Premorbid, protein-energy malnutrition is associated with poor immune function and wound healing, multiorgan failure, longer hospital stays, and poor outcomes, and the nutritional status of children deteriorates while they are in the PICU (Pollack et al., 1982; Pollack et al., 1985; Hulst et al., 2004). It can be difficult to assess the nutritional needs of PICU patients. Adults have a hypermetabolic response to critical illness. Calculations of resting energy expenditures and correction factors for a variety of critical illness states in children have been proposed, but, with the exception of burn injury,

for which the hypermetabolic state is well documented, these have not been validated. There are factors that both increase and decrease metabolic needs during critical illness. Resting energy expenditure may be higher than normal, but the energy used by muscle activity is much lower for healthy children. Metabolic calculations in critically ill children demonstrated that energy expenditure was lower than predicted by common formulas and was lowest in patients with multiple-organ dysfunction syndrome (Turi et al., 2001). Both overfeeding and underfeeding have deleterious consequences in critically ill children (Skillman and Wischmeyer, 2008). Optimal energy intake during the acute phase and the recovery phase of critical illness remains uncertain.

The recommended daily calorie requirements for healthy children are a reasonable starting target for critically ill children. A general estimate of calorie requirements by age is presented in Table 39-2 (Agus and Jaksic, 2002).

Enteral Feeding

Enteral feeding is usually withheld until cardiovascular stability is established, because generalized hypoperfusion and vasoactive agents limit intestinal blood flow. However, early enteral feeding may preserve gut mucosal integrity, may decrease septic episodes, and may decrease the incidence of ventilator-associated pneumonia (Jeejeebhoy, 2001; Kompan et al., 2004). Aspiration is thought to be a risk factor for ventilator-associated pneumonia (VAP), but enteral nutrition decreased the risk for VAP in adults. Similar studies have not been done in children. The frequent interruptions to enteral feeding (for many reasons, including perceived intolerance, procedures, diagnostic tests, medication administration) may result in inadequate nutrition delivery (de Neef et al., 2008). Attention should be given to calories *delivered,* not just calories *prescribed.* Feeding protocols may limit the impact of these factors on the delivery of adequate nutrition (Meyer et al., 2009). When complete enteral nutrition is impossible, low-dosage enteral nutrition in combination with parenteral nutrition is probably preferable to parenteral nutrition alone (Heidegger et al., 2008).

Transpyloric feeding may help to avoid unnecessary feeding interruptions, particularly in patients with gastroparesis or those who are at increased risk for aspiration, but it does not prevent aspiration of gastric contents (Meert et al., 2004). Because infants and children are at higher risk for malplacement of enteral feeding tubes, tube placement should be confirmed radiographically before use. Enteral formulas exist for special situations such as renal failure, general malabsorption, fat malabsorption, and pancreatitis. Although it is generally accepted that enteral nutrition is superior to parenteral nutrition, studies in pediatric patients are lacking.

TABLE 39-2. Estimated Calorie and Protein Requirements of Children During Critical Illness

Age	Calories	Protein (g/kg per day)
Premature infant	120	3.5
Term infant	100	2.5-3
Child, 1 to 12 years	70	1.5-2
Child, >12 years	70	1.5

Parenteral Nutrition

Total parenteral nutrition (TPN) is indicated for patients with contraindications to enteral feeding. TPN is associated with a number of complications, including intestinal mucosal atrophy with increased bacterial translocation, metabolic abnormalities including hyperglycema and hypertriglyceridemia, and immune dysfunction and infection. With long-term therapy, hepatic steatosis, cholestasis, and irreversible liver failure can occur. When there is risk for liver injury, TPN is often cycled to mimic the postabsorptive state (Kelly, 2006). Timing of initiation of parenteral nutrition is controversial. A recent review suggested starting it when enteral nutrition could not be used for 3 to 5 days (Skillman and Wischmeyer, 2008). In patients at high risk for malnutrition, it may be appropriate to initiate parenteral nutrition sooner.

In TPN, carbohydrates provide 60% to 75% of nonprotein calories. Carbohydrate concentrations are increased gradually to avoid hyperglycemia. The glucose infusion rate is calculated according as follows:

$$\text{Glucose infusion rate (mg/kg per minute)} =$$
$$\text{Volume (mL/kg per day)} \times$$
$$\text{Glucose concentration (as a decimal)} \div 1.44$$

The glucose infusion is typically started at 5 to 6 mg/kg per minute and increased by 0.5 to 1 mg/kg per minute per day for preterm infants, or 2 to 4 mg/kg per minute per day for older children. For patients with sepsis, the ACCM guidelines recommend at least 8 mg/kg per minute for neonates, 5 mg/kg per minute in children, and 2 mg/kg per minute in adolescents (Brierley et al., 2009). Glucose control may be important in critically ill patients (see later). Some of the negative effects of parenteral nutrition seen in studies done in the past two decades may be related to carbohydrate overfeeding and poor glycemic control.

Provision of adequate protein intake prevents negative nitrogen balance and skeletal muscle wasting and supports growth and wound healing. To prevent protein from being used as a calorie source and to preserve its availability for growth and repair, adequate nonprotein calories must be provided (see Table 39-2). In renal failure, it may be necessary to decrease the amount of protein delivered. When CRRT is initiated, protein delivery should increase to compensate for protein lost across the membrane.

Fats serve as an energy source and a source of essential fatty acids. About 30% to 40% of TPN calories are delivered as fat, providing both an energy source and a source of essential fatty acids. At least 3% to 4% of calories should be given as fat to prevent free fatty acid deficiency. If too much fat is given, the lipoprotein lipase system is overloaded and lipemia occurs. TPN fats are delivered as a 20% emulsion, which is low in osmolarity and thus safe for peripheral veins.

It is routine to provide a pediatric multivitamin in TPN. Other minerals, such as selenium, iodide zinc, and iron, may not be provided by standard TPN solutions but are available as additives.

Intensive Insulin Therapy in Critically Ill Patients

Hyperglycemia is common in critically ill patients. In children, hyperglycemia is associated with organ dysfunction and poor outcomes (Kyle et al., 2010). Maintenance of normal fasting blood glucose values (80 to 100 mg/dL) conferred a survival advantage over maintenance blood glucose values (180 to 200

mg/dL) in critically ill adult surgical patients and was associated with a shorter ICU and hospital stay, a shorter period of mechanical ventilation, and less renal injury in adult medical patients (van den Berghe et al., 2001, 2006). In a recently published trial of tight glucose control using age-stratified glucose targets in critically ill children, tight control was associated with improvement in morbidity and mortality over a glucose target of 180 to 214 mg/dL, despite episodes of hypoglycemia occurring in 25% of the treatment group. More than two thirds of the children in this study were postoperative cardiac surgery patients; this may hamper the study's generalizability to medical patients (Rouette et al., 2010).

The appropriate target for glycemic control in critically ill pediatric patients remains to be determined. Adoption of a tight glucose control strategy requires frequent monitoring and familiarity with glycemic control protocols at all levels of care. The long-term impact of hypoglycemia in the PICU is not known. These issues have prevented the widespread adoption of tight glycemic control in critically ill children.

NEUROLOGIC SYSTEMS

The special sensitivity of the brain to inflammation and the catastrophic effects of herniation generally lead physicians to prefer ICU monitoring for new neurologic impairment. Neurologic problems that are common in the ICU include status epilepticus and prolonged seizures leading to respiratory failure; meningitis and other intracranial infections; spontaneous vascular accidents including stroke and hemorrhage; and traumatic brain injury. Sensitivity to the possibility of adding to existing brain injury and to the possibility of herniation should guide ICU treatment of the patient with suspected intracranial pathology. General strategies to limit brain injury are similar to the treatments to limit worsening of hypoxic injury in cardiac arrest patients (see earlier) and include maintaining adequate blood pressure and oxygenation, avoidance of states that increase cerebral metabolic rate (e.g., fever and seizure), preservation of blood oncotic pressure with normal to high sodium levels, avoidance of hyperglycemia and hypoglycemia, and avoidance of preventable causes of increased ICP, such as hypercarbia and unsedated laryngoscopy.

Traumatic Brain Injury

See Adelson and colleagues (2003) for a thorough review of traumatic brain injury in infants, children, and adolescents. See Chapter 22, Anesthesia for Neurosurgery, for perioperative treatment of the pediatric trauma patient. Here, the focus is on the critical care management of traumatic brain injury (TBI).

Physiology of Traumatic Brain Injury

In the injured brain, there is an area of primary injury that cannot be ameliorated, a penumbra of brain tissue that is at risk for further injury, and normal brain distant from the site of initial injury. The goal of critical care after TBI is to keep that penumbra as small as possible and to protect the normal brain from further injury. Only part of the injury sustained in TBI occurs with the initial injury. The most important causes of secondary injury include hypoxia, hypotension, hyperglycemia and hyperthermia, seizures, and intracranial hypertension. The mechanisms for secondary brain injury, including excitotoxicity, have been reviewed by Kochanek and coworkers (2008).

Initial Management of the Brain-Injured Patient

Early management of airway, breathing, and circulation should take into account the devastating effect of even transient hypoxia and the impact of hypercarbia on ICP. Prevention of hypoxia by intubation is strongly associated with improved outcomes (Franschman et al., 2009; Zebrack et al., 2009). The initial management of TBI is presented in Box 39-3. The examiner should always be sensitive to signs of intracranial hypertension or impending herniation, including pupillary dilation, Cushing's triad, and extensor posturing. The Glasgow Coma Scale has been adapted for use in children and should be calculated for all patients with TBI on arrival and in subsequent examinations (Table 39-3). Brain injuries evolve over time, and the initial computed tomography scan might not reflect the current state of brain edema or intracranial hemorrhage. A sustained change in ICP or in the neurologic examination should prompt repeat imaging.

Minimizing Secondary Injury

Once the initial assessment and resuscitation are complete, further management is aimed at preventing and treating causes of secondary brain injury. The goals are to preserve delivery of fuel substrates, to prevent increases in cerebral metabolic needs, and to minimize ICP. The management for minimizing secondary injury is presented in Box 39-4 (Chiaretti et al., 2002; Adelson et al., 2003; Davis, 2008). Therapeutic hypothermia is under investigation for children with TBI, and although there are no data to support broad application of this therapy, it might be considered for severe refractory intracranial hypertension.

TABLE 39-3. Glasgow Coma Scale for Children and Adults

	Infants and Young Children	Older Children and Adults
Eye Opening		
4	Spontaneous	Spontaneous
3	To voice	To voice
2	To pain	To pain
1	None	None
Verbal		
5	Coos, babbles	Oriented
4	Irritable	Confused
3	Cries to pain	Inappropriate words
2	Moans to pain	Incomprehensible sounds
1	None	None
Motor		
6	Normal spontaneous movements	Obeys commands
5	Withdraws to touch	Localizes pain
4	Withdraws to pain	Withdraws to pain
3	Abnormal flexion	Abnormal flexion
2	Abnormal extension	Abnormal extension
1	Flaccid	None

Box 39-4 Minimizing Secondary Injury

- Treat hypotension with isotonic intravenous fluids.
- Do not treat hypertension in the presence of increased intracranial pressure.
- Maintain Pao_2 > 60 mm Hg.
- Maintain $Paco_2$ at 35 to 40 mm Hg.
- Maintain normal plasma glucose. Hyper/hypoglycemia worsen outcome.
- Hyponatremia may contribute to cerebral edema. Use isonatremic intravenous fluids.
- Treat fever aggressively with antipyretics.
- Early (1–7 days) prophylactic anticonvulsant medication is recommended.

Modified from Chiaretti A, Piastra M, Pulitanò S, et al: Prognostic factors and outcome of children with severe head injury: an 8-year experience, *Childs Nerv Syst* 18(3–4):129, 2002; Adelson PD, Bratton SL, Carney NA, et al; American Association for Surgery of Trauma; Child Neurology Society; International Society for Pediatric Neurosurgery; International Trauma Anesthesia and Critical Care Society; Society of Critical Care Medicine; World Federation of Pediatric Intensive and Critical Care Societies: Guidelines for the acute medical management of severe traumatic brain injury in infants, children, and adolescents. Chapter 5. Indications for intracranial pressure monitoring in pediatric patients with severe traumatic brain injury, *Pediatr Crit Care Med* 4(3 Suppl):S1, 2003; Davis DP: Early ventilation in traumatic brain injury, *Resuscitation* 76(3):333, 2008.

Box 39-3 Initial Management of Traumatic Brain Injury

AIRWAY (INDICATIONS FOR INTUBATION)
- Absence of protective reflexes
- Glasgow Coma Scale (GCS) < 8

BREATHING
- Maintain normal $Paco_2$ (35 to 40 mm Hg)

CIRCULATION
- Blunt sympathetic response to intubation with medication (lidocaine, 1 mg/kg)
- Maintain normal blood pressure
- Avoid nasogastric tube placement until cribriform plate injury is ruled out

INTRACRANIAL PRESSURE (ICP) MANAGEMENT
- Calculate pediatric GCS on arrival
- Head computed tomography scan
- Place ICP monitor for GCS < 8

Modified from Franschman G, Peerdeman SM, Greuters S, et al: ALARM-TBI investigators: Prehospital endotracheal intubation in patients with severe traumatic brain injury: guidelines versus reality, *Resuscitation* 80(10):147, 2009; Zebrack M, Dandoy C, Hansen K, et al: Early resuscitation of children with moderate to severe traumatic brain injury, *Pediatrics* 124(1):56, 2009.

Management of Intracranial Hypertension

Intracranial hypertension may impair cerebral blood flow and is associated with poor outcome. It results from osmolar shifts, cellular edema, vasogenic edema (blood-brain barrier breakdown),

Box 39-5 Management of Intracranial Hypertension

- Cerebral perfusion pressure should be maintained at 40 mm Hg or greater.
- Intracranial pressure (ICP) should be treated if greater than 20 mm Hg.
  - Consider ICP monitor for GCS < 8.
  - Head in midline position, and head of bed at 30 degrees.
  - Provide sedation and analgesia.
  - Use neuromuscular blockade to decrease metabolic demands.
  - Hyperosmolar therapy (3% normal saline, mannitol)
  - Hyperventilation for impending herniation
  - CSF drainage
  - Surgical evacuation of intracranial blood
  - Decompressive craniectomy

Adapted from Davis DP: Early ventilation in traumatic brain injury, *Resuscitation* 76(3):333, 2008; Adelson PD, Bratton SL, Carney NA, et al; American Association for Surgery of Trauma; Child Neurology Society International Society for Pediatric Neurosurgery; International Trauma Anesthesia and Critical Care Society; Society of Critical Care Medicine; World Federation of Pediatric Intensive and Critical Care Societies: Guidelines for the acute medical management of severe traumatic brain injury in infants, children, and adolescents. Chapter 5. Indications for intracranial pressure monitoring in pediatric patients with severe traumatic brain injury, *Pediatr Crit Care Med* 4(Suppl 3):S1, 2003.

mass lesions, and intracranial hemorrhage. Protocols exist for the management of intracranial hypertension, but they should not be seen as a surrogate for cooperative management with a neurosurgical team (Adelson et al., 2003). Therapies aimed at controlling intracranial pressure are applied in a stepwise fashion, beginning with the least invasive measures (Box 39-5).

HEMATOLOGY AND IMMUNOLOGY

Red Blood Cell Transfusion in the PICU

Critically ill patients are prone to anemia as a result of hemodilution, phlebotomy, and suppression of hematopoiesis by, for example, inflammation and malnutrition. Red blood cell transfusions are associated with significant risks related to immune suppression, transfusion reactions, transfusion associated lung injury, infection. Changes in the red blood cell that occur during storage may decrease oxygen delivery, negating the benefit expected from transfusion (Tinmouth et al., 2006). Adult studies have shown that setting a conservative threshold for transfusion (i.e., a hemoglobin level of 7 mg/dL) is safer than a threshold of 10 mg/dL. A conservative threshold reduced the number of transfusions and decreased the incidence of organ failure, cardiac complications, and mortality (Hébert et al., 1999).

Pediatric studies support that it is safer to use a conservative (7 mg/dL) than a liberal (9.5 mg/dL) threshold for stable critically ill children and postsurgical pediatric patients. This restrictive strategy reduces the number of transfusions per patient and dramatically reduces the number of patients who receive transfusions without worsening organ dysfunction (Lacroix et al., 2007; Rouette et al., 2010). The optimal transfusion threshold for unstable patients is unknown. It is probably appropriate to

target the normal range in children with profound hypoxemia and shock (Carcillo and Fields, 2002; Randolph, 2009).

Sepsis and Multiple Organ Dysfunction Syndrome

No treatment improves outcomes in pediatric patients with sepsis besides providing appropriate antibiotic therapy and rapidly and aggressively treating shock (for discussions on the latter, see Cardiovascular System, p. 1258). Administration of appropriate antimicrobial therapy should be considered urgent, as a delay of even 30 minutes has been shown to increase mortality in adults. It is appropriate to start with broad coverage, using local antimicrobial resistance patterns to guide antibiotic choice. The most common bacterial causes of sepsis vary by age and immunization status, with group B *Streptococcus* and *Escherichia coli* predominating in newborns, and *Streptococcus pneumonia, Staphylococcus aureus,* and *Neisseria meningitides* predominating in older children. Viruses and fungi can also cause sepsis, particularly in immunocompromised hosts. The pathophysiology of sepsis is complex and incompletely understood (but see Hotchkiss and Karl, 2003).

Activated protein C, which held some promise in adult patients with sepsis, is not recommended in children. In a randomized controlled trial of activated protein C in pediatric patients with sepsis, no difference in organ failure or mortality was found between groups, but there was an increase in central nervous system bleeding in the treatment group (Nadel et al., 2007).

Multiple organ dysfunction syndrome represents a continuum of physiologic abnormalities rather than a dichotomous state of organ function or failure. MODS develops quickly in children, with a maximum number of organ failures seen at 72 hours in most children (Proulx et al., 1994). Diagnostic criteria for organ failures are useful for comparing patients in research studies and evaluating outcome in clinical trials (Wilkinson et al., 1987; Leteurtre et al., 2003). Because overall mortality is lower in critically ill children than in adults, organ failure scores and time to resolution of organ failure are considered appropriate endpoints for clinical trials in pediatric intensive care. Children with MODS have a better chance of a good outcome than adults. Six months after discharge from the PICU, 60% of survivors of MODS have a normal quality of life, and 32% have ongoing health, emotional, or cognitive problems (Ambuehl et al., 2002). The number and severity of organ failures are associated with mortality, but it is rarely the case that failure of a specific organ can be implicated as a cause of death. Children with severe MODS usually die when the decision to withdraw support is made in response to an increasingly grim prognosis.

MODS is associated with shock states, including cardiogenic shock, sepsis, SIRS states not associated with infection, ARDS without systemic infection, and solid organ or bone marrow transplantations. The etiology of MODS is not completely understood, but it is almost certainly multifactorial and probably differs for different patients. The pathophysiology that is thought to contribute to MODS is worth reviewing, as it underscores the importance of many of the therapies already discussed here.

Shock states may cause relative hypoperfusion to abdominal organs, as sympathetic stimulation preferentially diverts blood flow from the periphery and the splanchnic circulation and toward the myocardium and the brain. This is particularly true in children, for whom the most common hemodynamic profile is cold shock. Elevated levels of both proinflammatory and antiinflammatory cytokines are associated with severity of MODS (Doughty et al., 1998; Whalen et al., 2000). Breakdown of the barrier function of intestinal mucosa has been postulated to contribute to MODS by initiating or exacerbating the inflammatory cascade (Proulx et al., 2009). Increased prothrombotic and antifibrinolytic activity in plasma is associated with severity of MODS. Dysregulation of normal clotting and fibrinolytic mechanisms may lead to microvascular thrombosis, impairing organ perfusion locally and perpetuating the inflammatory state (Proulx et al., 2009). Nitric oxide, which is present in increased amounts in the blood during shock states, may combine with superoxides to produce peroxynitrites. Peroxynitrites can damage lipid membranes and DNA and alter mitochondrial function (Wong et al., 1995; Burney et al., 1999).

Mechanical ventilation causing excessive stretch of poorly compliant lungs leads to the release of inflammatory mediators and has been implicated in the development of multiorgan failure in ARDS patients (Tremblay and Slutsky, 2006). The abnormalities of metabolism and neuroendocrine response noted in patients with multiorgan failure may represent other organ failures or may contribute to the syndrome (Proulx et al., 2009). Impairments in the immune response have also been noted in these patients. Failure of antigen presentation (i.e., immunoparalysis) and depletion of lymphoid elements predispose patients with MODS to secondary infection and may contribute to mortality (Peters et al., 1999; Felmet et al., 2005). Finally, mitochondrial dysfunction has been posited to be a part of the final common pathway of MODS and may some day be treatable (Singer, 2007).

The treatment of MODS is supportive. Treatments discussed earlier and later in this chapter are intended to minimize the development and severity of organ dysfunction. Treatments that have been associated with a decrease in the incidence or severity of MODS in adults include use of ventilator strategies that avoid of excessive stretch or atelectrauma, aggressive shock resuscitation, control of source of infection or inflammation, early enteric feeding to prevent intestinal mucosal atrophy, tight glycemic control, and a conservative transfusion threshold (Proulx et al., 2009).

PROPHYLAXIS

Gastritis

The association between severe stress and GI ulceration is well established. The incidence of clinically important GI bleeding in both adult and pediatric patients with critical illness is low (Quenot et al., 2009; Reveiz et al., 2010). The mechanism of stress ulcer formation is incompletely understood, but it includes impairment of blood flow to the intestinal mucosa and circulation of proinflammatory cytokines (Quenot et al., 2009). Direct damage to the epithelium by hydrogen ions is preventable to some degree, but this is only one of many factors. Options for prophylaxis include antacids, sucralfate, histamine type 2 (H_2) receptor antagonists (H_2RAs), and proton pump inhibitors (PPIs).

Sucralfate works by improving the neutralization capacity of the mucous layer of the gastric lining. It may decrease the absorption of concomitantly administered medications. Because it is not systemically absorbed, it may not be administered via duodenal or jejunostomy tubes. H_2RAs decrease gastric acid secretion through competitive inhibition of histamine-stimulated

acid secretion. PPIs irreversibly inhibit the final step in acid production (the transport of hydrogen), providing long-lasting acid suppression. PPIs inhibit both vagally mediated and histamine-induced acid secretion. Both PPIs and H_2RAs are superior to placebo in suppressing clinically significant stress-ulcer–related bleeding (Reveiz et al., 2010).

Stress-ulcer prophylaxis is not routinely indicated for ICU patients but should be reserved for patients at risk for stress ulcer–related bleeding. These include patients with sepsis, coagulopathy, or a history of ulcer or GI bleeding within the past year, and patients requiring mechanical ventilation for longer than 48 hours, a prolonged ICU stay, or high-dosage corticosteroids (Reveiz et al., 2010). A recent meta-analysis failed to find convincing evidence that PPIs are superior to H_2RAs in terms of preventing stress ulcer–related bleeding (Lin et al., 2010). Many clinicians discontinue stress ulcer prophylaxis when the patient begins an oral diet, begins a complete enteral diet, or discontinues steroid therapy.

Deep Venous Thrombosis

Among adult trauma patients, the risk for deep venous thrombosis (DVT) is greater than 50% without venous thromboembolism (VTE) prophylaxis. Prophylaxis reduces the incidence of new DVT in the adult medical and surgical ICU to between 10% and 33% (Cook et al., 2005). The incidence in pediatrics is much lower, but comprehensive screening studies have not been done. The reported incidence of DVT among pediatric trauma patients is 0.2 to 3.3 per 1000 trauma discharges. Older adolescents and young adults may be at higher risk than younger pediatric patients (O'Brien et al., 2008). For children who are critically ill after trauma, the incidence of symptomatic DVT is reported to be much higher (6.2%). The presence of central venous lines, poor perfusion and immobility, and a family history of thrombosis are risk factors. Studies screening for asymptomatic VTE found central venous line–associated VTE rates in critically ill children ranging from 8% to 35% (Hanson et al., 2010).

An algorithm for the use of VTE prophylaxis in pediatric trauma patients has been proposed (Fig. 39-5) (O'Brien et al., 2008). In critically ill pediatric patients without trauma, mechanical prophylaxis and vigilance for signs of DVT may be appropriate. Pulmonary embolus is rare in children, with about 40 per year occurring in the United States. The nonspecific symptoms of pulmonary embolus may be responsible for its underrecognition in critically ill patients. Massive pulmonary embolus in children is most often described at autopsy (Baird et al., 2010).

Ventilator-Associated Pneumonia

The frequency of VAP in pediatric patients is 2.9 episodes per 1000 ventilator days (Principi and Esposito, 2007). The presence of an endotracheal tube is the most important risk factor, and shortening the duration of ventilation is the most important preventative. Organisms responsible are typically *S. aureus* and gram-negative bacteria (Grohskopf et al., 2002). Early VAP may involve organisms commonly associated with community-acquired pneumonia. Specific measures for VAP prevention recommended in adult patients include raising the head of the bed by 30 to 45 degrees, instituting a daily sedation holiday with an extubation readiness trial, stress-ulcer prophylaxis, and DVT

Venous thromboembolism
prophylaxis in trauma patients

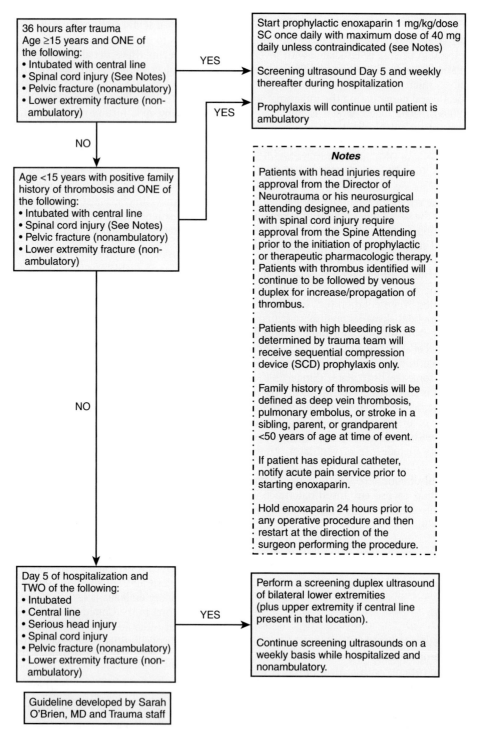

■ **FIGURE 39–5.** Deep venous thrombosis (DVT) prophylaxis for pediatric trauma patients. *(From O'Brien SH, Haley K, Kelleher KJ, et al: Variation in DVT prophylaxis for adolescent trauma patients: a survey of the Society of Trauma Nurses,* J Trauma Nurs *15:53, 2008.)*

prophylaxis (Grohskopf et al., 2002). It is essential to identify the causative agent. Because of antimicrobial resistance in hospital-acquired organisms, initial therapy should be broad and should be tailored once sensitivities are known. Compared with placebo, sucralfate and H_2 blockers do not alter the incidence of VAP or upper airway colonization in children (Lopriore et al., 2002).

Heparin-Induced Thrombocytopenia

Heparin-induced thrombocytopenia (HIT) is an immune response to platelet factor–heparin complexes that results in platelet activation and thrombocytopenia. These signs appear 4 to 5 days after initial heparin exposure, or more abruptly after reexposure. The primary complications are mostly thrombotic, although bleeding may occur, often as a postthrombotic complication. The diagnosis of HIT depends on demonstration of antibodies to platelet factor 4 (PF4)-heparin complexes, and on the appearance of the syndrome's clinical features, including a 50% fall in platelet count with appropriate timing and absence of a more likely cause of thrombocytopenia. Demonstration of PF4 heparin antibodies is necessary but not sufficient for diagnosis, as only a small fraction of patients with the antibody have the syndrome (Hassell, 2008).

Treatment consists of removal of all forms of heparin and using of alternative anticoagulants. Low-molecular-weight heparin has been used when platelet aggregation is not demonstrated. Warfarin and aspirin have been used in pediatric patients. Direct thrombin inhibitors such as argatroban, and anti-Xa agents such as fondaparanux have been used in adult patients. These drugs have been used in pediatric patients, but the efficacy and safety have not been well established (Rayapudi et al., 2008; Dhillon, 2009). Simple discontinuation of heparin without alternative anticoagulation is associated with severe complications (Hassell, 2008).

Trials in adults have reported an incidence of HIT that varies between 1% and 30%. The diagnosis can be challenging in severely ill patients, because heparin use is a ubiquitous part of intravenous and central line flushes in the pediatric ICU, and because most of these patients have a variety of potential reasons for thrombocytopenia. Venous clots around indwelling catheters may be more common in children because the diameter of central lines is larger than the size of the vessel (DeAngelis et al., 1996).

Critical Care Myopathy

Survivors of critical illness are at risk for polyneuropathy and myopathy syndromes causing weakness ranging in severity from brief and reversible skeletal muscle weakness to inability to wean from mechanical ventilation. There is an enormous deficit in knowledge about the incidence, causes, treatment, and prognosis of these syndromes, particularly in children (Williams et al., 2007). Pediatric patients with sepsis and SIRS are at particular risk, and in adult patients with sepsis and multiorgan failure the incidence of these syndromes approaches 100% (Berek et al., 1996; Latronico et al., 1996). Although data linking the combination of neuromuscular blockade and systemic steroids with ICU-acquired polyneuropathy and myopathy are limited, most clinicians agree that the combination should be avoided whenever possible. Hyperglycemia is a modifiable independent risk factor for critical care myopathy (Herridge et al., 2008). Tight glucose control may decrease its incidence in adults, but this preventive strategy not been investigated in children (van den Berghe et al., 2001).

A high index of suspicion is required for diagnosis. Identification of critical illness myopathy and polyneuropathy helps to predict respiratory failure after extubation and can help in planning rehabilitation. Neuropathy and myopathies are frequently lumped together because they are indistinguishable without relatively invasive tests, and because treatment for both syndromes is supportive. In both syndromes, weakness is usually symmetrical, and sensory symptoms are less common. Laboratory tests are usually normal and are of limited use. Nerve conduction studies and electromyography can help to differentiate between axonal neuropathy and muscle atrophy

or necrosis. Slow recovery over weeks to months is the norm, although many adults show diminished exercise capacity and quality of life years after critical illness (Herridge, 2009).

ICU-Acquired Infections

The National Nosocomial Infections Surveillance system found that nosocomial infections occur in ICUs at a rate of 13 per 1000 patient days. About 23% of nosocomial infections are urinary tract infections, and 97% of these are associated with urinary catheters. Central line–associated bloodstream infection (CLABSI) occurs in 1.0 to 5.6 per 1000 catheter days. Bloodstream infections associated with catheters are the most commonly reported nosocomial infection in pediatric intensive care. Duration of catheter use, TPN, and immunosuppression are correlated with CLABSI (Barsanti and Woeltje, 2009). The majority of pathogens causing CLABSI are found on the skin. A multidisciplinary strategy, involving, for example, maximum barrier precautions for catheter placement, antibiotic-coated catheters, handwashing campaigns, and use of chlorhexidine for dressing changes, significantly decreased rates of infection (Bhutta et al., 2007). The most important preventative for CLABSI is early removal of central venous catheters.

Clostridium difficile is increasingly recognized as a preventable cause of significant morbidity in the ICU. More virulent strains are emerging and have been implicated in ICU mortality. *C. difficile* spores can remain in the environment for a prolonged period of time and are spread by health care workers (Barsanti and Woeltje, 2009). Affected patients should be isolated, and general infection prevention measures should be in place for all patients. Use of broad-spectrum antibiotics increases the risk for *C. difficile* infection and should be carefully considered.

SUMMARY: THE ROLE OF THE INTENSIVIST

Pediatric critical care medicine is rapidly evolving. The initial resuscitation of the acutely ill patient is no longer a mystery. The difficulty lies in accomplishing what is needed during the first precious hours after their presentation. The most important area of growth in critical care is our understanding of the state of prolonged critical illness. We are only beginning to understand how ventilation practices, metabolic management, and hormone states affect the development of MODS and delayed mortality. In the next decade, we are likely to learn more about the impact of therapeutic strategies during the protracted phase of critical illness on long-term functional outcomes. Nowhere is this more important than in pediatric critical care, where most patients survive the acute illness but the disabilities in the survivors of ICU medicine may persist for many years. Incremental improvements are made in critical care. There are no miracle drugs; rather, attention to the small details improves the incidence of organ failure, the length of stay, and, we hope, the outcome.

As our support of individual organ systems becomes more complex, it is ever more tempting to refer to the organ-specific subspecialist to manage that aspect of care, but there is evidence that the continuous presence of a fellowship-trained intensivist improves outcomes and lowers cost (Pollack et al., 1988; Pronovost et al., 2002). Consultation with the specialist is invaluable, but each consultant focuses on the specialty's organ system. It is the job of the intensivist to consider the specialist's recommendations, and then negotiate the barriers of ego, control, and reimbursement to do what best serves the patient's long-term interests.

In addition to coordinating interaction of therapeutic approaches to various organ systems, the intensivist must coordinate the approach to patients' families. Parents are integral to good pediatric critical care. Because they often remain continuously at the bedside, they see a parade of doctors, who all have an opinion about the appropriate treatment for their child. Particularly when patients have a prolonged course in the ICU or when the end of life is near, the intensivist must ensure that the family receives one unambiguous message from the health care team.

Finally, no one person can provide perfect critical care. The intensivist needs a variety of specialists, surgeons, anesthesiologists, and primary care physicians to generate an ideal treatment plan. The intensivist relies on technicians to run the machines, and on respiratory therapists, perfusionists, and renal replacement staff. Nonphysician support staff, including nutritionists, pharmacists, social workers, psychologists, and physical and occupational therapists, are an important part of the patient's care and of the family's experience in the hospital. The care a patient receives ultimately depends on the nurses. The nurses, with their dedication, education, and support of critical care, are the intensivist's most important ally.

REFERENCES

Complete references used in this text can be found online at www.expertconsult.com.

Safety and Outcome in Pediatric Anesthesia

Brian P. Struyk, Donald C. Tyler, and Etsuro K. Motoyama

CHAPTER

40

CONTENTS

Anesthesiology has served as a model for patient safety and was the first medical specialty to recognize patient safety as an independent problem (Gaba, 2000). The safety of infants and children undergoing general anesthesia has improved considerably since the 1970s, as evidenced by significant decreases in anesthesia mortality despite the fact that more complicated surgical procedures have been performed on sicker children and more premature infants.

Since the 1980s, anesthesiologists' awareness of and interest in the subject of patient safety has reached a new peak, and a number of new steps have been taken to ensure perioperative patient safety (Keats and Siker, 1985; Smith and Norman, 1987; Runciman, 1988a; Runciman, 1988b). In addition to advanced technology for patient monitoring, standards for basic patient monitoring have been implemented (American Society of Anesthesiologists [ASA], 1986; Eichhorn et al., 1986). Documentation of the quality assurance (QA) process has been emphasized as an integral and essential component for hospital accreditation by the Joint Commission on Accreditation of Healthcare Organizations (JCAHO) in the United States. To further improve the quality of patient care, a number of national and international organizations have been created, including the International Committee on Prevention of Anesthesia Mortality and Morbidity, the Anesthesia Patient Safety Foundation, the Australian Patient Safety Foundation, and the ASA Committee on Patient Safety and Risk Management (Cooper and Pierce,

1986; Cooper, 1988; Pierce, 1984, 1988; Runciman, 1988b). The Institute of Medicine of the National Academies is an independent, nonprofit organization that seeks to ask and answer the nation's questions about health and health care. Their reports, such as the *Preventing Medication Errors* series, have analyzed complex problems in the modern health care industry and provided solutions that have been widely adopted. Sessions on patient safety topics have also been incorporated into the programs of the American Society of Anesthesiologists and Society for Pediatric Anesthesia annual meetings.

Nevertheless, anesthesia-related morbidity and mortality still do occur during the administration of anesthesia and can happen with any anesthesiologist under various situations. An analysis of anesthesia mishaps from closed anesthesia malpractice claims in the United States, before the new patient monitoring standards with pulse oximetry and capnography were instituted, indicated that at least 80% of the claims consisted of preventable hypoxic damage caused by human errors rather than mechanical failures (Davis, 1984).

Allnutt (1987), a member of the British Army Personnel Research Establishment, examined human factors in anesthesia-related mishaps in comparison with those in military aviation accidents. He stresses that "both pilots and doctors make many errors" (i.e., performance that deviates from the ideal). "Usually there is sufficient slack in the system for the error to be … noticed and corrected, but some apparently innocuous errors are not noticed and some systems are not so forgiving as others" (such as a high performance aircraft in flight). "Thus recovery from a control error when flying at high speed, low level may not be possible, whereas the same error in the cruise [at high altitude] might barely occasion comment." A basic tenet of Allnutt's theory is that "all human beings, without any exception whatsoever, make errors and that such errors are a completely normal and necessary part of human cognitive function." He goes on to state that "to claim exemption on the grounds of being a senior professor [or a] test pilot ... or of having 30 years' experience or 3000 accident-free hours, is the first step on the road to disaster." The first step toward the prevention of catastrophe is for the pilot or the anesthetist to accept that he or she is as likely as anyone else to make an error (Pierce, 1988).

In this chapter, some of the important aspects of patient safety, the incidence and causes of mortality and morbidity, and measures for the prevention of anesthesia-related mishaps are discussed.

ANESTHESIA-RELATED MORTALITY

Overall Anesthesia-Related Mortality

The number of deaths associated with general anesthesia has declined steadily over the past several decades as the standard of anesthesia practice has improved and as advances have been made in instrumentation, anesthetic and adjuvant drugs, and safety monitors and standards. An extensive survey of 10 university hospitals by Beecher and Todd (1954) involving nearly 600,000 anesthetic cases between 1948 and 1952 suggested that mortality primarily attributable to anesthesia occurred in 1:2680 anesthesia cases (3.7:10,000), whereas the overall anesthesia-associated mortality was 1:1580 (6.3:10,000) anesthesia procedures (Graff et al., 1964). A survey by Dornette and Orth (1956) showed similar mortality rates. Data from the Baltimore Anesthesia Study Committee (1953 to 1963) showed an anesthesia-related death rate of 2.7:10,000 cases. During the 1970s and 1980s, statistics on anesthesia-related mortality in the United States were scarce, apparently because of medicolegal concerns. Anesthesia-related mortality from Canadian, British, and European sources during this time ranged from 0.7 to 2.2:10,000 anesthetic procedures (Bodlander, 1975; Harrison, 1978; Hovi-Viander, 1980; Turnbull et al., 1980; Lunn and Mushin, 1982; Hatton et al., 1983; Vickers and Lunn, 1983).

In the 1980s, European and Australian studies showed much lower rates of operative mortality directly attributed to anesthesia. A report from the British Confidential Enquiry into Perioperative Deaths (CEPOD), a survey that was jointly organized by the Associations of Anaesthetists and Surgeons of Great Britain and Ireland during 1985 and 1986 and included more than 480,000 general anesthetic procedures, indicated that mortality attributable to anesthesia alone was 1:185,000 (0.054:10,000) procedures (Buck et al., 1987). However, anesthesia, along with other causes, was thought to be a contributory factor in the death of between 1.4 (surgeons' estimate) and 9.8 (anesthetists' estimate) per 10,000 cases. A prospective survey of anesthesia outcome by the French Health Ministry during the time from 1978 to 1982, in which nearly 200,000 general anesthetic cases were documented, revealed an intraoperative and early postoperative death rate solely attributable

TABLE 40-1. Historical Changes in Anesthesia-Related Mortality (All Ages)*

Authors (Country)	Years Included in Study	Incidence per 10,000
Beecher and Todd (United States)	1948 to 1952	3.7
Graff et al. (United States)	1953 to 1963	2.7
Hovi-Viander (Finland)	1975	2
Lunn and Mushin (United Kingdom)	1978 to 1979	1
Tikkanen (Finland)	1986	0.6
Tiret et al. (France)	1978 to 1982	0.76[†]
Buck et al., CEPOD (United Kingdom)	1985 to 1986	0.05[†]
Eichhorn (United States)	1976 to 1988 (ASA PS 1 or 2)	0.05[†]
Kawashima (Japan)	1994 to 1998	0.13[†]
Lagasse (United States)	1995 to 1999	0.75
Fasting and Gisvold (Canada)	1996 to 2000	0.12
Irita (Japan)	1999 to 2002	0.1[†]
Lienhart (France)	2006	0.12[†]

*For complete citations of studies, consult chapter reference list online at www.expertconsult.com.
[†]Anesthesia primarily responsible only; other factors may be involved.
ASA PS, American Society of Anesthesiologists physical status; *CEPOD,* Confidential Enquiry into Perioperative Death.

to anesthesia to be 0.76:10,000 procedures, and an intraoperative death rate of 0.44:10,000 cases (Table 40-1) (Tiret et al., 1986, 1988).

Clearly, it is difficult to compare the incidence of anesthesia-related death among reports from different parts of the world, because the definition and inclusion criteria (e.g., all inclusive vs. ASA physical status [PS] 1 and 2), perioperative duration (48 hours vs. 30 days), and the definition of anesthesia contributions (anesthesia contributory vs. primary cause) to mortality may differ markedly.

A longitudinal comprehensive anesthesia-related mortality study from New South Wales, Australia, which was continued by the same author using the same criteria since 1960 (interrupted between 1980 and 1983 because of the temporary loss of legal confidentiality), has indeed shown a steady decline in anesthetic mortality from 1.8:10,000 cases in 1960 to 0.38:10,000 cases by 1984 (Holland, 1984, 1987). Similarly, a longitudinal study from South Africa has also shown a decreasing trend in anesthesia-related mortality from 3.3:10,000 between 1956 and 1965 to 0.7:10,000 between 1983 and 1987 (Table 40-2) (Harrison, 1978, 1990).

In the United States, Eichhorn (1989) analyzed data from nine Harvard University–affiliated hospitals between 1976 and 1988. He reported 11 major anesthesia-related intraoperative accidents, including five deaths based on more than 1 million anesthetic procedures in relatively healthy patients (ASA PS 1 and 2); the anesthetic mortality was 0.05:10,000 cases;

TABLE 40-2. Anesthesia-Related Mortality: Longitudinal Studies at the Same Institution

Authors (Country)	Years Included in Study	Incidence per 10,000
Holland (Australia)	1960 to 1969	1.8
	1970 to 1980	0.97
	1983 to 1985	0.38
Harrison (South Africa)	1956 to 1965	3.3
	1967 to 1976	2.2
	1983 to 1985	0.7

From Holland R: Anaesthetic mortality in New South Wales, *Br J Anaesth* 59:834, 1987; Harrison GG: Death due to anesthesia at Groote Schuur Hospital, Cape Town: 1956-1987. Part II. Causes and changes in aetiological pattern of anesthetic-contributory death, *S Afr Med J* 77:416, 1990.

postoperative mortality, including two deaths from halothane hepatitis, was excluded from these statistics. After implementation of patient monitoring standards in 1985, there was only one serious accident (no mortality) in 319,000 general anesthesia procedures (Eichhorn et al., 1986). Of the 11 major accidents, eight cases were considered preventable with proper monitoring, especially with capnography. Unrecognized hypoventilation (seven cases) was the most common cause of major mishaps. Inadequate supervision of residents and nurse anesthetists was also contributory. Although Eichhorn's statistics were based on a malpractice insurance database and are likely different and considerably lower than the data based on a peer-review process, anesthesia-related safety appears to have improved significantly.

Irita and others (2004) analyzed morbidity and mortality statistics in Japan from 1999 to 2002 from the Japanese Society of Anesthesiologists annual survey. They reviewed 3,855,384 cases completed during that time. The incidence of cardiac arrest and mortality totally attributable to anesthesia management was 0.47 and 0.1 per 10,000 anesthesia procedures. Half of the anesthesia-related deaths were caused by airway or ventilatory problems; the other causes were medication-related and infusion/transfusion accidents.

Practitioners of anesthesiology have institutionalized patient safety in their scientific and governing bodies (such as the ASA Anesthesia Patient Safety Foundation and similar organizations in other countries) (Cooper and Gaba, 2002). In 1999, the Committee on Quality of Health Care in America for the Institute of Medicine published a report entitled *To Err Is Human: Building a Safer Health Care System* (Kohn et al., 1999). The report stated, "Anesthesia is an area in which very impressive improvements in safety have been made." This statement was based on the statistics that anesthesia-related mortality rates had decreased from two deaths per 10,000 anesthetic procedures in the 1980s to about 1 death per 200,000 to 300,000 anesthetic procedures administered at the time the report was published (probably quoting the report by Eichhorn [1989]). Such dramatic decreases in anesthetic mortality can be attributed to a variety of mechanisms, including wide acceptance of new monitoring guidelines, improvement in monitoring techniques, safer anesthetic drugs, and adoption of QA mechanisms and other systematic approaches for reducing human and systemic errors (Gaba, 2000; Stoelting, 2000; Lagasse, 2002).

Mortality in Infants and Children

Among the pediatric age group, the anesthesia-related mortality has been reported to be disproportionately high in the literature. In the 1950s, Beecher and Todd (1954) and Stevenson and others (1953) found that accidental deaths resulting from anesthesia were disproportionately high during the first decade of life. Between 1947 and 1956 at the Babies Hospital/Columbia-Presbyterian Medical Center, Rackow et al. (1961) found that the rate of cardiac arrest associated with anesthesia in infants younger than 1 year of age (1 in 617 cases, or 16.2:10,000) was higher than in children aged 1 to 12 years (1 in 1678, or 6.0:10,000) and in adults (1 in 2580, or 3.9:10,000) (Beecher and Todd, 1954). Hypoventilation and hypoxia from ether overdose were among the common causes of death. Smith (1956) emphasized the importance of certain factors contributing to the high anesthetic mortality in pediatric anesthesia. These factors included: lack of proper equipment, improper preoperative rehydration and stabilization, inadequate intraoperative monitoring, error in fluid replacement, and aspiration of vomitus. Today, half a century later, some of these factors are still applicable.

In a report by the Baltimore Anesthesia Study Committee, anesthesia-related mortality for children younger than 15 years of age was found to be 3.3:10,000 cases (vs. 0.6:10,000 for those aged 15 to 24 years) (Phillips and Frazier, 1957; Graff et al., 1964). These authors also found that the ratio of anesthesia deaths to total surgical deaths was higher in the neonatal period than in any other age group. Furthermore, 57% of the deaths related to anesthesia occurred in healthy children (ASA PS 1 and 2). Respiratory problems were implicated in 83% of the anesthesia-related deaths (Graff et al., 1964) (Table 40-3).

In contrast, in a review of 73 anesthesia-related cardiac arrests in children between 1960 and 1972 (33% resulted in death), Salem and others (1975) found that both respiratory (airway obstruction) and cardiovascular causes (blood loss,

TABLE 40-3. Anesthesia-Related Mortality in Children (n > 10,000)*

Authors (City)	Years Included in Study	Age (in years)	Incidence per 10,000
Rackow (New York City)	1947 to 1956	<1.0	16.2
		1 to 12	6
Graff et al. (Baltimore)	1957 to 1964	<15	3.3
		15 to 24	0.6
Smith (Boston)	1957 to 1966	<10	1.9
	1969 to 1978	<10	0.64
Elwyn (Salt Lake City)	1970 to 1975	<11	0.34
Morray et al. (POCA Registry)	1994 to 1997	<18	0.34[†]
Tay et al. (Singapore)	1997 to 1999	<18	0
Murat et al. (Paris)	2000 to 2002	<16	0

*For complete citations of studies, consult chapter reference list online at www.expertconsult.com.
[†]Estimated.
POCA, Perioperative cardiac arrest.

preoperative anemia, inappropriate injection of succinylcholine and potassium) were equally responsible. In retrospect, most of these accidents were preventable.

In an attempt to improve patient safety during anesthesia in infants and children, a number of important innovations and improvements in perioperative management and monitoring were made by the pioneering pediatric anesthesiologists in the 1950s and 1960s. These innovations include homemade pediatric blood pressure cuffs and precordial stethoscopes (by Robert Smith in Boston) and endotracheal intubation (by Margo Demming in Philadelphia). Fellowship training in pediatric anesthesia also began in several cities in North America and in the United Kingdom in the 1950s and spread across the continent by the early 1970s (see Chapter 41, History of Pediatric Anesthesia).

By the mid-1970s, anesthesia-related morbidity and mortality decreased considerably. Management of known hazards, such as the full stomach, preoperative fever, and hypovolemia, was greatly improved by increased experience and knowledge (Smith, 1975). Smith (1980) reported the anesthesia-related mortality rate of 2:10,000 general anesthesia cases in children (0 to 10 years old) during the decade ending in 1966 at the Children's Hospital in Boston; the mortality rate decreased to 0.6:10,000 anesthesia cases in the decade ending in 1978. Furthermore, there was a series of 35,710 consecutive tonsillectomies and adenoidectomies, mostly in children, without a single death at the Eye and Ear Hospital of Pittsburgh (Petruscak et al., 1974). There were 7500 consecutive anesthesia procedures for cleft lip and cleft palate repairs without a death at the Children's Hospital in Boston (Smith, 1975). Elwyn, in his 5-year study between 1970 and 1975 at the Primary Children's Hospital in Salt Lake City, reported one anesthetic death in 29,101 anesthetic procedures (0.34:10,000) in children under 11 years of age (Smith, 1980). Downes and Raphaely (1979) reported an anesthetic mortality of 0.2:10,000 cases (from a total of 50,000 patients) at Children's Hospital of Philadelphia. Most fatalities occur during the first year of life, beyond which the risk of mortality is no higher than that in teenagers and young adults (Table 40-3) (Smith, 1975).

Despite advances in pediatric anesthesia, statistics from the 1980s still showed anesthesia-related mortality rates in children that were three to four times higher than in the general patient population, although the mortality rates in children had decreased considerably and appeared to have reached a plateau (Keenan and Boyan, 1985; Gibbs, 1986; Olsson and Hallen, 1988).

As part of a study of closed malpractice claims by the Committee on Professional Liability of the ASA, Morray and others (1993) compared pediatric and adult closed claims and found a different distribution of serious outcomes in children compared with those in adults. Of 2400 closed malpractice claims, 238 (10%) were in the pediatric age group (15 years old or younger). A majority of cases involved children younger than 3 years of age, and 28% of all pediatric cases involved infants younger than 1 year of age. Respiratory events (mostly inadequate ventilation) were more common than among adult claims (43% vs. 30%), and mortality was higher (50% vs. 35%), mostly attributable to inadequate ventilation. Anesthesia care was judged inadequate more often. The authors concluded that 89% of the pediatric claims that were related to inadequate ventilation could have been prevented with proper monitoring through the use of pulse oximetry and capnography (Morray

et al., 1993). Jimenez and others (2007) reviewed 532 pediatric claims from 1973 to 2000. They concluded that claims for death (41%) and brain damage (21%) remained the dominant injuries in pediatric anesthesia claims in the 1990s. Half of the claims in 1990 to 2000 involved patients 3 years old or younger, and one fifth of the patients had ASA PS scores of 3 to 5. Cardiovascular (26%) and respiratory (23%) events were the most common damaging events. The proportion of claims reported as preventable by better monitoring decreased to 16% in the 1990s.

Analysis of anesthesia-related incidents reported to the Australian Incident Monitoring Study (AIMS) showed almost identical characteristics among pediatric age groups (van der Walt et al., 1993). Of the first 2000 cases reported, 10% involved infants and children. Incidents involving respiratory and breathing circuit systems accounted for nearly half of the adverse incidents. As with the ASA Closed Claims Project, the Australian reviewers estimated that 89% of all applicable problems in AIMS could have been detected and potentially prevented by the combination of pulse oximetry and capnography (van der Walt et al., 1993).

A study from Singapore, based on a QA database, reports no fatalities among 10,000 consecutive general pediatric anesthetic procedures from 1997 to 1999 (Tay et al., 2001). A 2004 QA database study from Hôpital d'Enfants Armand Trousseau in Paris also reports zero mortality among 24,165 general anesthesia procedures in children between 2000 and 2002 (Murat et al., 2004). On the other hand, from the Pediatric Perioperative Cardiac Arrest (POCA) Registry in the United States between 1994 and 1997, the anesthesia-related mortality rate was estimated to be 0.36:10,000 (Morray et al., 2000) (see related section). Obviously, a large-scale prospective and longitudinal study is needed to determine the overall pediatric anesthesia-related mortality in the early 21st century.

ANESTHESIA-RELATED MORBIDITY IN INFANTS AND CHILDREN

Perioperative Cardiac Arrests

Incidences of POCA have been reported from North America, Europe, and Australia. Estimated incidence of cardiac arrests ranged 17 to 24:10,000, and as with the mortality rates, the rates are three to 10 times higher in infants than in older children (Olsson and Hallen, 1988; Tiret et al., 1988; Cohen et al., 1990). Studies by Keenan and Boyan (1985) and by Morgan and others (1993) also showed higher incidences of cardiac arrest in younger children (younger than 10 to 12 years) than in older children. Most common causes leading to cardiac arrest involved respiratory and cardiovascular systems and included relative drug overdose, vagal stimulation, hypoventilation, and succinylcholine-induced asystole.

Keenan and others (1991) reported the effect of specialty training in pediatric anesthesia on the safety of children, especially in infants. In a single university hospital setting, the incidence of POCA in infants younger than 1 year of age was 19:10,000 with mortality when residents were supervised by nonpediatric attending anesthesiologists, whereas no cardiac arrest occurred when pediatric anesthesiologists were in charge.

Braz and others (2006) looked at the causes of POCA in children at a teaching hospital in Brazil. They reviewed 15,253 anesthesia procedures that took place between 1996 and 2004. There were 35 cardiac arrests (22.9:10,000) and 15 deaths (9.8:10,000). They identified seven anesthesia-related cardiac arrests but no deaths. The main causes of anesthesia-related cardiac arrest were respiratory events (71.5%) and medication-related events (28.5%). Major risk factors for cardiac arrest were neonates and children under 1 year of age with an ASA PS of 3 or poorer, emergency surgery, and general anesthesia.

Flick and others (2007) reviewed pediatric cardiac arrest data from 1998 to 2005 at the Mayo Clinic. A total of 92,881 anesthetics were administered to children under the age of 18 for noncardiac and cardiac procedures during the study period. The incidence of POCA and mortality during noncardiac procedures was 2.9:10,000 and 1.6:10,000, and the incidence of cardiac arrest during cardiac procedures was 127:10,000. The incidence of POCA attributable to anesthesia was 0.65:10,000, representing 7.5% of the 80 POCA. Both cardiac arrests and mortality were highest among neonates undergoing cardiac procedures. Regardless of procedure type, most patients who experienced POCA (88%) had congenital heart disease. Factors found to be associated with mortality included higher ASA PS, age, the need for mechanical ventilation before surgery, and the cause of the POCA.

Pediatric Perioperative Cardiac Arrest Registry

In order to accurately estimate the incidence of cardiac arrests and adverse outcomes, the Pediatric POCA Registry was formed in 1994 under the combined auspices of the ASA Committee on Professional Liability, the Quality Assurance Committee of the Section on Anesthesiology of the American Academy of Pediatrics (AAP) (Morray, 2004). The registry included 63 institutions, of which 75% were university hospitals and 40% were children's hospitals. All cardiac arrests requiring cardiopulmonary resuscitation during the immediate perioperative period are eligible for inclusion. During the first 4 years of the registry (1994 to 1997), participating institutions administered an estimated total of 1,089,200 anesthetics to children younger than 18 years old (Morray et al., 2000). A total of 289 cardiac arrests were registered, of which 150 cases were considered as anesthesia-related. The mean overall incidence of anesthesia-related cardiac arrest was 1.4:10,000 with a mortality rate of 26% (0.36:10,000). Of the total anesthesia-related cardiac arrests, 55% occurred in infants younger than 11 months of age (Morray et al., 2000).

Of the major causes of anesthesia-related cardiac arrests, medication-related (37%) and cardiovascular causes (32%) were most common, together accounting for 69% (Table 40-4). In contrast, the respiratory causes represented only 20%, a marked reduction from the incidence of 43% reported by the ASA Closed Claim Project (Morray et al., 2000). Equipment-related causes comprised 7% of the total (Morray et al., 2000). With regard to the patients' physical status, 33% were those with ASA PS 1 and 2, a significant decrease from earlier studies of pediatric mortality (57% of deaths), a significant improvement and a move in the right direction, although the percentage is still too high (Graff et al., 1964). Of medication-related cardiac arrests, cardiovascular depression with halothane alone or in combination with other drugs (mostly opioids) accounted for 66% of all medication-related arrests. In healthy children

with ASA PS 1 and 2, 64% of cardiac arrests were medication-related in comparison with 23% in those with ASA PS 3 to 5 (Fig. 40-1) (Morray et al., 2000; Mason, 2004). Among the patients who sustained anesthesia-related cardiac arrest in the POCA Registry, death was associated most strongly with an ASA

TABLE 40-4. Mechanisms of Cardiac Arrest

Mechanism	Number of Cardiac Arrests
Medication-related inhalation agents	55 (37%)
Halothane alone	26 (46%)
Halothane plus an intravenous medication	11 (20%)
Sevoflurane alone	2 (4%)
Intravenous medications	
Single	5 (9%)
Combination	5 (9%)
Intravenous injection of local anesthetic	5 (9%)
Succinylcholine-induced hyperkalemia	1 (2%)
Cardiovascular	48 (32%)
Presumed cardiovascular, unclear etiology	18 (38%)
Hemorrhage, transfusion related	8 (17%)
Inadequate/inappropriate fluid therapy	6 (13%)
Arrhythmia	5 (10%)
Hyperkalemia	4 (8%)
Air embolism	2 (4%)
Pacemaker related	2 (4%)
Vagal response	1 (2%)
Pulmonary hypertension	1 (2%)
Tetralogy hypercyanotic spell	1 (2%)
Respiratory	30 (20%)
Laryngospasm	9 (30%)
Airway obstruction	8 (27%)
Difficult intubation	4 (13%)
Inadequate oxygenation	3 (10%)
Inadvertent extubation	2 (7%)
Presumed respiratory, unclear etiology	2 (7%)
Inadequate ventilation	1 (3%)
Bronchospasm	1 (3%)
Equipment related	10 (7%)
Central line	4 (40%)
Breathing circuit	2 (20%)
Peripheral intravenous catheter	1 (10%)
Other	3 (30%)
Multiple events	5 (3%)
Hypothermia	1 (<1%)
Unclear etiology	1 (<1%)

Modified from Morray JP et al.: Anesthesia-related cardiac arrest in children: initial findings of the Pediatric Perioperative Cardiac Arrest (POCA) Registry, *Anesthesiology* 93:614, 2000.

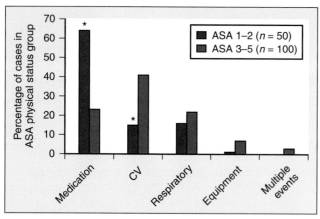

■ FIGURE 40-1. Primary cause of anesthesia-related cardiac arrest in patients of ASA PS 1 to 2 compared with patients of ASA PS 3 to 5; *p < 0.01. *(From Morray JP et al.: Anesthesia-related cardiac arrest in children: initial findings of the Pediatric Perioperative Cardiac Arrest [POCA] Registry, Anesthesiology 93:6, 2000.)*

PS 3 to 4 and emergency surgery (Morray et al., 2000). Similar correlations between cardiac arrest or death and ASA PS 3 to 4 were found in the earlier study by Keenan and Boyan (1985).

Since the last publication of the POCA Registry that was based on data between 1994 and 1997, more than 200 POCA cases have been added to the registry (from 2000 to 2003), and about one half of these cardiac arrests were found to be anesthesia-related (Morray, 2004). In a preliminary report on this new series of cardiac arrests, the cause profile has changed considerably from that of 1994 through 1997 (Fig. 40-2) (Morray, 2004). Medication-related cardiac arrests decreased markedly, from 37% to 12% of the total causes, primarily because of the near disappearance of cardiovascular depression by inhaled anesthetics causing cardiac arrest (Morray, 2004). These welcome changes appear to coincide with the replacement of halothane with sevoflurane (with its lower incidence

of causing myocardial depression and bradycardia) as an anesthetic of choice for induction,. As the consequence of reductions in cardiac arrests with medication (primarily from halothane), cardiovascular causes of cardiac arrest increased relatively, from 32% to 52%. Hypovolemia from hemorrhage and a metabolic consequence of massive transfusion and resultant hyperkalemia were the common causes of cardiac arrest under this category (Morray, 2004). Also, with a reduction in medication-related cardiac arrest in healthy infants, the incidence of cardiac arrest in patients with ASA PS 1 to 2 declined considerably from 33% to 19%, one of the most remarkable differences between the first and second databases (Table 40-5).

Bhananker and others (2007) subsequently published a study related to cases submitted to the POCA registry between 1998 and 2004. During that time, the registry received 397 reports of POCA in children. Of these cardiac arrests, 193 were judged as anesthesia related. Three quarters of the anesthesia-related arrests occurred in patients of ASA PS 3 to 5. Between 1998 and 2004, cardiovascular causes of cardiac arrest accounted for the highest proportion of anesthesia-related cardiac arrests (41%), in part because of a dramatic decrease in medication-related cardiac arrest. Among these, the most common identifiable cause was hypovolemia related to blood loss. The majority of these cardiac arrests resulted from blood loss that occurred during either spinal fusion or craniotomy and craniectomy. The most common anesthesia-related factors were underestimation of blood loss (48%) and inadequate venous access (22%). As reported in the preliminary communication by Morray (2004) on cases from the POCA Registry between 2000 and 2003, medication-related cardiac arrests decreased dramatically to 18% of all cardiac arrests (12% for 2000 to 2004, see above) from the 37% reported from

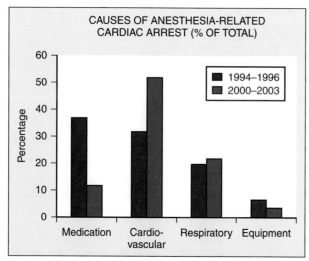

■ FIGURE 40-2. Causes of anesthesia-related cardiac arrest in children between 1994 and 1996 vs. between 2000 and 2003. *(From Morray JP: Unexpected cardiac arrest in the anesthetized child. Presented at the Society of Pediatric Anesthesia Spring Meeting, March 4-7, 2004.)*

TABLE 40-5. Demographic Data from Pediatric POCA Registry Cases, 1994 to 1997 vs. 2000 to 2003

	1994 to 1997	2000 to 2003
ASA PS		
1	15%	4%
2	18%	15%
3	37%	46%
4	27%	22%
5	2%	13%
Age		
<1 mo	15%	13%
1 to 5 mo	28%	25%
6 to 11 mo	13%	10%
12 mo to 5 yr	31%	25%
6 to 18 yr	13%	27%
Emergency surgery	21%	30%
Mortality	26%	27%

Modified from Morray JP: Unexpected cardiac arrest in the anesthetized child. Presented at the Society of Pediatric Anesthesia Spring Meeting, March 4-7, 2004.
POCA, Perioperative cardiac arrest; *ASA PS,* American Society of Anesthesiologists physical status.

1994 to 1997, apparently because of the decrease in the use of halothane for induction of anesthesia. However, it is important to remember that sevoflurane is also a cardiac depressant, and cardiac arrests related to its effects have been identified in the registry. Most cardiac arrests occurred during anesthesia maintenance (58%). Nearly one quarter (24%) occurred in the induction or preinduction phase, and 19% occurred during emergence, transport, or recovery (Fig. 40-3). Eight of 10 cardiac arrests caused by electrolyte imbalance were caused by hyperkalemia from the transfusion of stored blood. The use of fresh blood cells and saline washing of irradiated blood may help in reducing the incidence of transfusion-associated hyperkalemia. Equipment-related cardiac arrests accounted for 5% of the anesthesia-related incidents, and half of these were secondary to central venous catheter complications. Six percent of the causes of cardiac arrest were unknown. Mortality after anesthesia-related cardiac arrest was 28%. The only factors predictive of mortality after cardiac arrest were ASA PS and emergency surgery.

Information about POCA in children (younger than 18 years) between 1988 and 2005 was reported from the Mayo Clinic (Flick et al., 2007). Out of a total of 92,881 anesthesia procedures, of which about 5% were for the repair of congenital heart disease, the incidence of POCA for noncardiac procedures were 2.9:10,000 and the incidence during the cardiac surgery was 127:10,000. The incidence of cardiac arrest attributable to anesthesia, however, was 0.65:10,000 procedures, representing 7.5% of all POCA, much lower than in some of the published reports. Both the incidence of arrest as well as mortality rates were highest among neonates (younger than 30 days' postnatal life) undergoing cardiac procedures (POCA: 435:10,000; mortality: 389:10,000) (Flick et al., 2007).

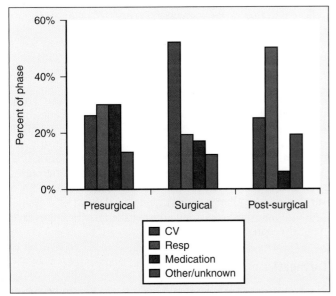

■ **FIGURE 40-3.** Cause of cardiac arrest by phase of care. Three cases of cardiac arrest during the "other" phase are excluded. p < 0.001; Fisher's exact test (Monte Carlo method of resembling). *Presurgical:* Preinduction and induction; *Surgical:* maintenance of anesthesia; *Postsurgical:* emergence, transport, and recovery. *(From Bhananker SM et al.: Anesthesia-related cardiac arrest in children,* Anesth Analg *105:347, 2007.)*

Other Perioperative Adverse Events

Computerized data acquisition on nonfatal adverse outcome has become commonplace in most hospitals for QA or quality improvement (QI); such information in pediatric anesthesia has started to appear in the literature. Excellent reviews on this subject have been published (Holzman, 1994; Duncan, 1995).

Cohen and others (1990) reviewed perioperative adverse events in over 29,000 children between 1982 and 1987 at Winnipeg Children's Hospital. Unlike the adult surgical population, a majority of children (70%) were healthy and had no preoperative medical problems. Infants younger than 1 year of age, particularly those younger than 1 month of age (61% of whom underwent intraabdominal, intrathoracic, or major cardiovascular surgery), had a significantly higher intraoperative incidence of airway obstruction and other adverse respiratory events (9.4%) and hypotension (3.9%) than did older children. Among children 1 to 10 years of age, the most common problem was arrhythmias (3.9% to 9.3%). In the recovery room, infants younger than 1 month of age had hypotension (13.9%), respiratory events (11.6%), and abnormal temperature (4.7%). In older children, the most common adverse event in the recovery period was vomiting (5.9%), followed by airway obstruction (3.2%). This study was performed during the pre-sevoflurane era, when essentially all inhalation inductions were performed with halothane, with potent myocardial depression and bradycardia (Table 40-6).

A report from Hôpital d'Enfants Armand Trousseau in Paris was based on a QA database involving over 24,000 pediatric anesthesia cases for a 30 months between 2000 and 2002, when halothane had been completely eliminated from clinical use (Murat et al., 2004). Although this database did not include open-heart and neurosurgical cases, the nature of adverse events and their incidence have changed considerably. As a whole, respiratory events were most common, representing 53% of all intraoperative events (Table 40-7). As with other reports, respiratory events were more common among infants (3.6:10,000 vs. fewer than 1.5:10,000 in older children); in ear, nose, and throat (ENT) surgery than in other surgery; in children who were intubated vs. those who were not intubated, and in those with ASA PS 3 to 5 vs. PS 1 or 2 (Murat et al., 2004). Cardiac events represented 12.5% of all intraoperative events and were mostly observed in sick children (ASA PS 3 to 5).

In contrast to earlier reports, the incidence of bradycardia was greatly decreased (13:10,000) and arrhythmias essentially disappeared. There were eight cardiac arrests (3.3:10,000), of which five children were in the ASA PS 3 to 5 category and four were infants 6 months old or younger (Table 40-7). There were no anesthesia-related deaths (Murat et al., 2004). Vomiting was the most common adverse event postoperatively, with an overall incidence of 6%. As with previous studies, vomiting was more common in older children than in infants and occurred more often after ENT surgery compared with other surgery and in children who were intubated vs. those who were not (Murat et al., 2004). Similarly, based on QA data of 10,000 surgical cases, Tay and others (2001) in Singapore found critical perioperative incidents four times higher in infants younger than 1 year of age than in older children (8.6% vs. 2.1%). Respiratory events were most common (77.4%) with laryngospasm accounting for 35.7%. There were no anesthesia-related deaths (Tay et al., 2001).

TABLE 40-6. Perioperative Events by Age of Child, 1982 to 1987 (Rate per 10,000 Anesthesia Cases)

	Age					
	<1 mo (n = 361)	1 to 12 mo (n = 2544)	1 to 5 yr (n = 12,484)	6 to 10 yr (n = 7184)	≥11 yr (n = 5647)	Total (n = 29,220)
Intraoperative						
Vomiting	28	47	56*	99	136*	81
Cardiac arrest	28	12	3	4	5	5
Arrhythmia	166	86	391	933	561	528[†]
Blood pressure	388*	55	22*	19	46	34
Temperature	83	24	13	8	16	14
Airway obstruction	222	200*	99	86	90	105
Other respiratory problems	720*	318*	118	82*	99	130
Drug incident		20	20	28	35	25
Surgical problems	28	31	39	43	39	39
Death	83*	8	3	1	2	4
Recovery Room						
Laryngospasm	28	43	187	177	165	166[†]
Vomiting		83	410	855	935	587[†]
Cardiac arrest	55*	4	2	1		2
Arrhythmia		12	8	15	9	10
Blood pressure	1385*	12	10*	15*	32	17
Temperature	471*	138	57*	86	159*	96
Airway obstruction	28	161	444	260	184	319[†]
Other respiratory problems	1163*	248*	105	78*	103	124
Drug incident		20	19	19	30	21
Surgical problems	28	63	131	167	76	122

Modified from Cohen MM et al.: Pediatric anesthesia morbidity and mortality in the perioperative period, *Anesth Analg* 70:160, 1990.
*p < 0.01, Exact tail probability calculation based on Poisson distribution.
[†]p < 0.01 χ^2 test for association.

Down syndrome is the most common autosomal chromosomal disorder in humans. Children with Down syndrome have a number of characteristics that place them at high risk for anesthesia complications, including craniofacial and cardiac anomalies. A study of 488 patients undergoing 930 procedures revealed several anesthesia-related complications. The most common complications were severe bradycardia (3.7%), natural airway obstruction (1.8%), difficult intubation (0.5%), postintubation croup (1.8%), and bronchospasm (0.4%) (Borland et al., 2004). The rates of bradycardia, obstruction, and postintubation croup were statistically significant and more than twice the rate of patients without Down syndrome, suggesting the need for increased vigilance in these patients.

Bradycardia

An outcome study from the Medical College of Virginia examined the incidence of bradycardia in nearly 8000 children younger than 4 years of age (Keenan et al., 1994). Bradycardia (fewer than 100 beats per minute) was more common in infants (1.27%) and decreased with age. The incidence in the group of children who were 4 years old was only 0.16%. Causes of bradycardia included disease or surgery (35%), inhalation anesthesia (35%), and hypoxemia (22%). Of these children, hypotension occurred in 30%, asystole or ventricular fibrillation in 10%, and death in 8%. Significant associated factors predisposing children to bradycardic events, based on multiple logistic regression analysis, were ASA PS, emergency surgery, duration of surgery (longer than 4 hours), and the absence of a trained pediatric anesthesiologist supervising the anesthetic management (Keenan et al., 1994).

Laryngospasm and Bronchospasm

The incidences of laryngospasm and bronchospasm have been studied in a series of large population studies in Stockholm by Olsson and Hallen (1984, 1988). The incidence of laryngospasm in children younger than 9 years of age was 1.7%. The presence of respiratory infection raises the incidence to 9.6%. The incidence of laryngospasm was also increased in patients with obstructive lung disease (6.4%) and in those with a history of previous anesthetic complications (5.5%). The incidence of

TABLE 40-7. Respiratory and Cardiac Adverse Events Observed During Anesthesia and in PACU by Age Group

	Age					
	0 to 1 yr	1 to 7 yr	8 to 16 yr	0 to 1 yr	1 to 7 yr	8 to 16 yr
Respiratory Event						
Number of cases	3681	12,495	6867	3681	12,495	6867
Bronchospasm	19	25	4	4	11	5
Hypercarbia	8	10	1	5	5	8
Hypoxemia	56	90	24	21	34	15
Aspiration	2	4	4	1	5	3
Unanticipated difficult intubation	9	7	6			
Esophageal intubation	3	2	1			
Endobronchial intubation	6	3	1	3	5	7
Laryngospasm	17	31	9	1	6	4
Pulmonary edema	0	0	2	1	9	7
Pneumothorax	0	2	0	1	7	6
Reintubation	13	17	7	5	11	9
Dental trauma				0	3	1
Respiratory depression				12	17	10
Total	133	191	59	54	113	75
Rate per 1000 anesthetics	36.1	15.3	8.6	14.7	9.0	10.9
Cardiac Event						
Number of cases	3681	12,495	6867	3681	12,495	6867
Cardiac arrest	4	2	2	0	0	0
Bradycardia	12	9	10	0	1	0
Hypertension	0	0	0	1	0	0
Hypotension	4	6	11	0	0	0
Hypovolemia	8	6	3	0	0	1
Circulatory insufficiency	3	2	1	1	0	0
Tachycardia	0	0	1	0	0	0
Arrhythmia	0	2	5	0	0	0
Total	31	27	33	2	1	1
Rate per 1000 anesthesia cases	8.4	2.2	4.8	0.5	0.1	0.2

Modified from Murat I et al.: Perioperative anaesthetic morbidity in children: a database of 24,165 anaesthetics over a 30-month period, *Pediatr Anesth* 14:161, 2004.

bronchospasm in the same age group increased from 0.4% to 4.1% in those with respiratory infection. The incidence of bronchospasm was also elevated (2.4%) in patients at high risk (ASA PS 3 or higher) (Olsson, 1987).

Up to 40% of children preparing for anesthesia have an upper respiratory tract infection (URI). Possible effects of recent or current URIs and the incidence of respiratory events have been studied by a number of investigators using parental interviews or written questionnaires. Of more than 1500 children, Schreiner and others (1996) found that patients who developed laryngospasm were more than twice as likely to have an active URI than were patients in the control group without URIs. A survey of more than 2000 children by Parnis and others (2001) did not find statistically significant differences in the long-term outcome of children with a recent history of URI. They did,

however, find that orotracheal intubation was associated with an increased probability of respiratory complications compared with the use of a face mask or laryngeal mask airway (LMA). Similarly, in more than 1000 children, Tait and others (2001) found no difference between children with active or recent URIs vs. asymptomatic children, with respect to the incidence of laryngospasm, bronchospasm, or long-term respiratory sequelae. However, children with current or recent URIs had significantly more overall adverse respiratory events, including breath-holding and major desaturation (arterial oxygen saturation [SpO_2] of less than 90%). Independent risk factors for adverse respiratory outcome in children with active URIs included tracheal intubation (younger than 5 years of age), history of prematurity, reactive airways disease, parental smoking, surgery involving the airway, and the presence of copious secretions and nasal congestion (Tait et al., 2001). A logistic regression analysis was created to look at the relationship between preoperative URI symptoms and adverse events during emergence from anesthesia. No association was found between particular URI symptoms and the rate of adverse events, but adverse events were increased if peak URI symptoms had occurred within the preceding 4 weeks (Homer et al., 2007).

The LMA has been advocated as an alternative to tracheal intubation for airway management in children with URIs. Von Ungern-Sternberg and others (2007) studied over 800 children having elective surgery with an LMA. A medical history of recent URI within the 2 weeks before anesthesia approximately doubled the risk of laryngospasm, oxygen desaturation, and coughing both intraoperatively and in the recovery room. This risk was further increased in younger children and in children undergoing ENT surgery (Tait et al., 2001). Flick and others (2008) reviewed 130 cases of laryngospasm in children at the Mayo Clinic and found that the use of an LMA was associated with laryngospasm even when adjusted for the presence of upper respiratory tract infections and airway anomaly.

Passive smoke exposure was studied in 405 children undergoing mask anesthesia procedures. The incidence of airway complications during anesthesia or postanesthesia recovery was significantly higher in children with passive smoke exposure. Intraoperative laryngospasm and airway obstruction were 4.9 and 2.8 times, respectively, more likely in children with passive smoke exposure (Jones and Bhattacharyya, 2006). Perioperative assessment of children undergoing surgery should include screening for passive smoke exposure to alert anesthesia providers to potential complications.

Aspiration

Studies before the 1970s reported high morbidity and mortality from pulmonary aspiration of gastric contents (Mendelson, 1946). The Baltimore Anesthesia Study Committee reported a mortality rate of 39% in children associated with pulmonary aspiration (Graff et al., 1964) (see Chapter 13, Induction, Maintenance, and Recovery). Studies reported since the 1980s, however, indicate marked improvements in outcome.

From a computer database covering the years between 1967 and 1985, Olsson and others (1986) reviewed more than 185,000 anesthesia cases in all ages and identified 83 cases of pulmonary aspiration of gastric contents (4.7:10,000 cases). The rate of gastric aspiration in children younger than 9 years of age (8.6:10,000) was nearly three times higher than that in young adults (20 to 49 years old). In 47% of patients with aspiration, pneumonia or atelectasis developed, as confirmed by chest radiograph. The mortality rate in children was relatively low (0.2:10,000) (Olsson et al., 1986). Risk factors associated with aspiration included the skill and experience of anesthetists, a number of coexisting diseases, ASA PS 3 to 5, emergency surgery, nighttime operation, history indicating an increased risk of regurgitation (e.g., esophageal disease, pregnancy), and difficult intubation. Other high-risk categories included children with intestinal obstruction, increased intracranial pressure, increased abdominal pressure, and obesity. Incidence of gastric aspiration was even lower in studies from the French-speaking countries (1.0:10,000) and from Norway (2.9:10,000) in the 1980s (Tiret et al., 1988; Mellin-Olsen et al., 1996). No fatalities were reported.

Borland and others (1998) studied the incidence and outcome of perioperative aspiration during the 5 years between 1988 and 1993 involving over 50,000 general anesthetic cases at Children's Hospital of Pittsburgh. They identified 52 cases of aspiration (10.2:10,000 cases), of which 25 patients aspirated gastric contents (4.9:10,000) (the rest were blood or pharyngeal secretions). Approximately 80% of aspirations occurred during induction. Most patients were treated aggressively with fiberoptic bronchoscopy through the endotracheal tube (ETT), removal of solid particles, and continuous positive pressure ventilation. Most patients had radiographic evidence of aspiration (e.g. infiltration, pneumonia, atelectasis, or pulmonary edema), but fulminant chemical pneumonitis secondary to aspiration, as reported in early publications, was absent (Mendelson, 1946). No death was attributable to aspiration. Among the different pediatric age groups, the incidence of aspiration was highest among children 6 to 11 years of age (0.22%). Several risk factors for intraoperative aspiration were identified: ASA PS 3 or higher, a history of previous esophageal surgery, and patients with previous chemotherapy undergoing central venous catheter (Broviac catheter) placement. Twenty-nine percent of these children were kept intubated in the postanesthesia care unit (PACU) for several hours or longer, but only 23% of these patients stayed overnight. None of these children developed clinically significant pneumonia, and there were no deaths (Borland et al., 1998).

Similarly, a study from the Mayo Clinic reported a low incidence of aspiration (3.8:10,000). In this report, however, the incidence of aspiration was similar to that of adults (3.1:10,000). There was no serious respiratory morbidity and no associated deaths (Warner et al., 1999). These epidemiologic studies suggest that the incidence of gastric aspiration and associated morbidity and mortality, especially in children, has declined considerably. The risk of aspiration in general, with the exception of the Mayo Clinic report, remained higher in infants and children than in adults (Olsson et al., 1986; Tiret et al., 1988; Warner et al., 1999; Flick et al., 2002).

Postoperative Complications

Postoperative Hypoxemia

During general anesthesia, static tension of the thoracic inspiratory muscle is abolished and the balance between the outward recoil of the thorax and the inward recoil of the lungs is altered. This change in balance results in the reduction of resting lung volume (functional residual capacity [FRC]), airway closure, collapse of alveoli (microatelectasis), and increased venous admixture, particularly in infants and young children (see Chapter 3, Respiratory Physiology in Infants and Children). By means of pulse oximetry, Motoyama and Glazener (1986) were the first to demonstrate that a large proportion of healthy infants and children undergoing simple elective surgical procedures (42%) become hypoxemic in the PACU. Patients sleeping in the PACU tend to be more hypoxemic and for a longer duration than those who are awake and sitting up, but the presence of hypoxemia is not clinically obvious and does not correlate with the recovery score (Motoyama and Glazener, 1986; Soliman et al., 1988). In a study involving a 1152 healthy infants, children, and adults (ASA PS 1) undergoing plastic surgical procedures, postoperative SpO_2 was monitored regularly for 2 hours. The incidences

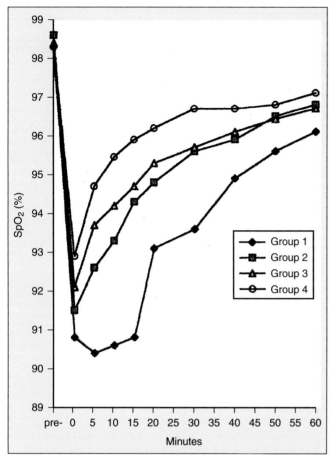

■ **FIGURE 40-4.** The recovery tendencies of arterial oxygen saturation (SpO$_2$) within the first hour after operation in four age groups. Group 1: infants younger than 1 year old; group 2: toddlers aged 1 to 3 years; group 3: children aged 3 to 14 years; group 4: teenagers and adults aged 14 to 58 years. *(From Xue FS et al.: A comparative study of early postoperative hypoxemia in infants, children, and adults undergoing elective plastic surgery,* Anesth Analg *83:709, 1996.)*

of both moderate (SpO$_2$, 86% to 90%) and severe (SpO$_2$, less than 86%) hypoxemia were the highest among infants (36.6% and 16.7%, respectively), followed by toddlers (20% and 10% in children 1 to 3 years old), children (14% and 3.3%), and adults (8% and 0.6%). The duration of hypoxemia was also significantly longer in infants than in older age groups (Fig. 40-4) (Xue et al., 1996).

Patients also become hypoxemic as often during the short transport from the operating room to the PACU, because the benefit of oxygen breathing to maintain oxygenation lasts only a few minutes (Pullerits et al., 1987). Children with upper respiratory infection and infants younger than 6 months of age are at increasing risk of developing hypoxemia (DeSoto et al., 1988; Kataria et al., 1988; Xue et al., 1996). Most pediatric anesthesiologists, therefore, recommend routine oxygen administration during the transport of children to and in the PACU (Duncan, 1995).

Postoperative Apnea

Postoperative apnea in prematurely born infants has become a major clinical concern since the early 1980s, when the number of premature infants surviving neonatal intensive care started

to increase. Apnea is usually defined as the cessation of breathing lasting longer than 15 to 20 seconds or lasting for a shorter duration when associated with bradycardia, cyanosis, or pallor (Thach, 1985). Apneic spells in these infants after simple surgical procedures are mostly central in origin (cessation of respiratory effort), although some infants have mixed (central and obstructive) apneas (Kurth and LeBard, 1991). Postoperative apnea occurs more commonly in infants with a previous history of apnea and those younger than 42 to 44 weeks' postconception (Liu et al., 1983). Apnea is uncommon after 44 weeks' postconception, although apnea in older expremature infants (up to 55 weeks' postconception) has been reported after more extensive surgical procedures (Kurth et al., 1987; Malviya et al., 1993). Malviya and others (1993) recommend that all former premature infants younger than 44 weeks' postconception be monitored for at least 12 hours postoperatively. Another important risk factor for postoperative apnea appears to be the presence of anemia (Welborn et al., 1991).

In 1995, Coté and others published the results of a meta-analysis of data from eight published reports of postoperative apnea between 1987 and 1993 involving 384 expremature infants after inguinal hernia repair. They concluded that apnea was strongly and inversely correlated both with gestational age and postconceptual age; an associated risk factor was continuing episodes of apnea at home; small-for-gestational-age infants seemed to be somewhat protected from apnea compared with those with normal or large-for-gestational-age infants; anemia (hematocrit less than 30) was a significant risk factor even beyond 43 weeks' postconceptual age; and relationships of postoperative apnea with history of necrotizing enterocolitis, neonatal apnea, respiratory distress syndrome, bronchopulmonary dysplasia, or operative use of opioids and muscle relaxants could not be determined (Coté et al., 1995). The probability of apnea in infants without anemia who are free of apnea in the recovery room decreases with postconceptual and postnatal ages but is not less than 5% (with 95% confidence limits) until the postconceptual age of 48 weeks (35 weeks' gestational age) and no less than 1% until postconceptual age of 56 weeks (with a gestational age of 32 weeks) or postconceptual age of 54 weeks (with a gestational age of 35 weeks) (Fig. 40-5) (Coté et al., 1995). In 2008, Murphy and others looked at the incidence of apneas in premature infants after inguinal hernia repair in 126 infants

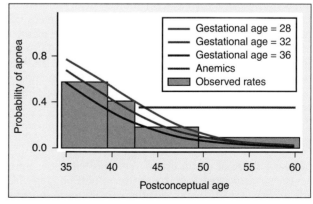

■ **FIGURE 40-5.** Probability of postoperative apnea vs. postconceptual and gestational ages of former preterm infants. *(From Coté CJ et al.: Postoperative apnea in former preterm infants after inguinal herniorrhaphy: a combined analysis,* Anesthesiology *82:809, 1995.)*

over a 5 years. Their data confirmed both the incidence and the risk factors for postoperative apnea of Coté's meta-analysis (Murphy et al., 2008).

Based on these findings, it is generally recommended in the United States that expremature infants younger than 44 to 46 weeks' postconception be admitted overnight for monitoring after general anesthesia. Whether the infant with postconceptual age between 46 and 48 weeks or even 52 weeks is admitted overnight depends on the decision made case by case between the anesthesiologist and the surgeon, based on a number of factors. These factors include the general health of the infant and his or her home environment (e.g., parents, passive smoking, and distance from the hospital). However, the decision often depends on the general policies of the hospital administration and insurance providers, and these policies do not necessarily represent the best interest of the patient or the health care providers. In countries like France and Japan, where economic pressure on health care resources is less stringent than in the United States, most infants younger than 60 weeks' postconception are admitted overnight for monitoring (Murat, 2002).

The incidence of postoperative apnea was reported to be lower after spinal anesthesia alone than after general (halothane or sevoflurane) anesthesia, but spinal anesthesia combined with ketamine increases the incidence of apnea more than that with general anesthesia (Welborn et al., 1990). Caffeine or methylxanthine may be helpful in preventing postoperative apnea and bradycardia in preterm infants (Welborn et al., 1988). Caffeine is usually preferred, because it has been proposed to have fewer hemodynamic consequences, a greater therapeutic index, and a longer half-life. A dose of 10 mg/kg of caffeine appears to be a safe and effective dose for prophylaxis of postoperative apnea. The infants treated with caffeine had a relative risk of 0.09 for postoperative apnea and bradycardia (McNamara et al., 2004). A long-term study on the effects of caffeine for apnea of prematurity (called the *CAP Study*) has been conducted (Schmidt, 2005).

Upper airway obstruction is an increasingly common indication for adenotonsillectomy in children. Adenotonsillectomy has established effectiveness for the treatment of obstructive sleep apnea (OSA). However, more than 20% of children with OSA have respiratory compromise requiring medical intervention in the postoperative period (Rosen et al., 1994). Nixon and others (2005) studied the postoperative course of children with OSA undergoing adenotonsillectomy surgery. They found that obstructive events occurred postoperatively in all children, but were more common and profound in those with severe OSA preoperatively. They recommend continuous pulse oximetry and overnight admission for children with severe OSA in a unit skilled in pediatric airway management. Schwengel and others (2009) reviewed the current literature on OSA in children and determined several clinical features that predict respiratory compromise after adenotonsillectomy (Box 40-1).

Postintubation Croup

The major cause of postintubation croup is subglottic injury and edema associated with traumatic intubation, especially with an oversized ETT. Koka and others (1977) made an important observation that the incidence of postintubation croup increases markedly when there is no air leak around the ETT with the airway pressure exceeding 40 cm H_2O. Consequently, it has become a standard practice in pediatric anesthesia to choose

Box 40-1 Predictors of Respiratory Compromise and Persistent Obstructive Sleep Apnea after Adenotonsillectomy

Severe obstructive sleep apnea on polysomnography
History of prematurity, especially with respiratory disease
Age less than 3 years
Morbid obesity
Nasal problems (e.g., deviated septum or enlarged turbinates)
Mallampati score 3 or 4
Neuromuscular disorders or disordered pharyngeal tone
Genetic or chromosomal disorders
Craniofacial disorders
Enlarged lingual tonsils
Upper respiratory infection within 4 weeks of surgery
Cor pulmonale
Systemic hypertension
Marked obstruction on inhalational induction
Disordered breathing in the PACU
Difficulty breathing during sleep
Growth impairment resulting from chronic obstructed breathing

Modified from Blum RH, McGowan FX: Chronic upper airway obstruction and cardiac dysfunction: anatomy, pathology, and anesthetic implications, *Paediatr Anaesth* 14(1):75–83, 2004; Guilleminault C, Huang YS, Glamman C, et al: Adenotonsillectomy and obstructive sleep apnea in children: a prospective survey, *Otolaryngol Head Neck Surg* 136(2):169–175, 2007; Gerber ME, O'Connor DM, Adler E, Myer CM 3rd: Selected risk factors in pediatric adenotonsillectomy, *Arch Otolaryngol Head Neck Surg* 122(8):811–814, 1996; McGowan FX, Kenna MA, Flemming JA, O'Connor T: Adenotonsillectomy for upper airway obstruction carries increased risk in children with a history of prematurity, *Pediatr Pulmonol* 13(4):222–226, 1992; Fricke BL, Donnelly LF, Shott SR, et al: Comparison of lingual tonsil size as depicted on MR imaging between children with obstructive sleep apnea despite previous tonsillectomy and adenoidectomy and normal controls, *Pediatr Radiol* 36(6):518–523, 2006.

an ETT that produces air leak around the tube with a pressure lower than 30 cm H_2O. With this preventive measure in clinical practice, the incidence of postintubation croup has decreased dramatically from 1% to less than 0.1%, along with reductions in the severity of croup (Litman and Keon, 1991). With the presence of a URI, however, the incidence of airway complications and the tendency for oxygen desaturation increase (Cohen and Cameron, 1991; Rolf and Coté, 1992).

Until the late 1980s and early 1990s, the use of cuffed ETTs was not generally recommended in most pediatric anesthesia textbooks for children younger than 5 to 8 years of age, depending on the authors (Fisher, 1989; Uejima, 1989). The primary reason for it had been that the inner diameter (ID) of a cuffed ETT had to be 1 to 2 sizes (0.5 to 1.0 mm) smaller than the uncuffed tube to accommodate the passage through the larynx of a bulky cuff, and consequently flow resistance would be drastically increased in those children most commonly breathing spontaneously under general anesthesia (with ether) before mechanical ventilation became a common practice (Gronert and Motoyama, 1996). More recently, cuffed ETTs have been used increasingly in young children and even in infants, and such practice has shown to be associated with decreased, rather than increased, incidence of postintubation croup (Motoyama, 2009). This decrease is in part a consequence of choosing a cuffed ETT that is 1 to 2 sizes smaller than a "properly" fitting uncuffed tube, thereby markedly reducing the need for reintubation attempts. (Keine, 1997; James, 2001; Fine and Borland,

2004; Cohen and Motoyama, 2006). Indeed, Murat (2001) reported that after a complete elimination of uncuffed ETTs at the Children's Hospital in Paris, there was not a single incidence of postintubation croup over 3 years. A new microcuff pediatric ETT has been developed that seals with a high-volume, low-pressure cuff (Dullenkopf et al., 2005). This tube uses an ultrathin, walled polyurethane cuff that is shorter and more distally placed. It can stay away from the cricoid mucosa while the airway is sealed at the upper to midtrachea, and away from the carina even in the neonate, where the posterior membranous wall can stretch and accommodate a complete seal with a low cuff pressure of less than 15 cm H_2O without increases in airway complications (Dullenkopf et al., 2005). In a study of 500 children, the microcuffed tube exchange rate was 1.6%, with only 0.4% having postintubation croup requiring therapy (Dullenkopf et al., 2005; Weiss and Gerber, 2006).

Postoperative Nausea and Vomiting

Although rarely life-threatening, postoperative nausea and vomiting (PONV) remains the single most common complication resulting in unscheduled overnight admissions in same-day surgery settings (Cohen et al., 1990; Patel and Rice, 1991). PONV occurs twice as often in children as in adults, increasing until puberty and then decreasing to adult incidence rates. The average incidence of PONV in children over 3 years of age is reported to be over 40%. The incidence of PONV has decreased considerably with newer anesthetics and techniques as well as with more effective medications (Murat et al., 2004). The incidence of PONV is higher after certain types of surgery, including adenotonsillectomy, eye-muscle surgery for strabismus, and orchiopexy. Other factors affecting the incidence of PONV include the gender and age of the child (uncommon in infants), PONV after previous surgery or history of motion sickness, anesthesia techniques (inhaled anesthetics and nitrous oxide vs. intravenous anesthesia with propofol), tracheal intubation, intraoperative opioids, inadequate pain control, gastric distention, and the skill of the anesthesiologist (Patel and Rice, 1991; Martin et al., 1993; Weir et al., 1993; Weinstein et al., 1994; Duncan, 1995; Villeret et al., 2002). A mandatory requirement for oral fluid intake and early ambulation before discharge from the short stay unit has also been associated with increased incidence of vomiting (Schreiner et al., 1992; Weinstein et al., 1994). Serotonin (5-HT$_3$) receptor antagonists (such as ondansetron and granisetron) have shown to be highly effective in preventing or treating PONV and are the preferred first-line agents for children, especially because ondansetron has become available as a less expensive generic drug (Fujii et al., 1996; Patel et al., 1996; Gan et al., 2007; Glass and White, 2007). Prophylactic use of dexamethasone and transdermal scopolomine were also found to be effective (Aouad et al., 2001) (see Chapter 11, Intraoperative and Postoperative Management). Gan and others (2003) developed consensus guidelines for the management of PONV. Strategies to reduce baseline PONV risk factors include the use of regional anesthesia, use of propofol for induction and maintenance of anesthesia, use of intraoperative supplemental oxygen, use of hydration, avoidance of nitrous oxide, avoidance of volatile anesthetics, minimization of intraoperative and postoperative opioids, and minimization of neostigmine (Gan et al., 2007). Droperidol has been effectively used for many years for PONV prophylaxis. However, because of the increased risk of extrapyramidal symptoms, high levels of sedation, and the United States Food and Drug Administration's (FDA's) "black box" warning about QT prolongation, droperidol was recommended to be reserved for patients in whom all other therapies have failed and who are being admitted to the hospital (Gan et al., 2003). Children at moderate to high risk for PONV should be given antiemetic prophylaxis with combination therapy with 2 or 3 prophylactic antiemetics from different antiemetic drug classes.

In comparison with PONV, the studies on postdischarge nausea and vomiting (PDNV) have been lacking. Oral opioid analgesics for postoperative pain management are a major factor contributing to PDNV in the ambulatory surgery facilities or after discharge from a hospital (Glass and White, 2007). Long-acting antiemetics (e.g., transdermal scopolamine or palonosetron) may offer an advantage over the commonly used antiemetics (Glass and White, 2007).

Complications of Regional Anesthesia

The potential benefits of peripheral nerve blocks for surgical procedures, when compared with general anesthesia, include improved postoperative analgesia, with an associated decrease in postoperative pain medication use, decreased nausea and vomiting, and quicker recovery and discharge times from the hospital (Hadzic et al., 2004). Regional anesthesia techniques in children have become more popular in the past decade. A survey by the ASA Closed Claims Project on the complication of regional anesthesia revealed that of 2400 closed anesthesia malpractice claims cases, 29 adult patients and 1 pediatric patient who developed cardiac arrest during regional anesthesia, resulting in death or severe brain damage, were identified (Morray et al., 1993). From the analysis of these data, mostly from the time before the ASA monitoring guidelines, including the mandatory use of pulse oximetry and capnography, had been adopted, it can be concluded that cardiac arrest resulting in death or other major outcomes can occur during apparently well-managed spinal or epidural anesthesia in young, healthy patients undergoing relatively minor procedures because respiratory insufficiency from sedation was not recognized; and that pulse oximetry would have given an early warning of respiratory insufficiency (Caplan et al., 1988; Cheney, 1988; Keats, 1988). An examination of the closed claims database from 1980 to 2000 by Lee and others showed that the most common complication associated with peripheral nerve block claims was nerve damage (31%) followed by pneumothorax (25%) and eye damage (18%). Block-needle trauma was the cause of 38% of these nerve injury claims. (Lee et al., 2008). The increasing use of ultrasound for the placement of peripheral nerve blocks has the promise of decreasing the incidence of nerve damage caused by block needle trauma (Marhoffer et al., 2005). Unintentional intravascular injection or signs of local anesthetic toxicity were associated with one third of the 19 claims with death or brain damage. Outcomes from this potentially lethal complication may be improved with the recent introduction of 20% intralipid as a rescue agent for local anesthetic toxicity (Lee et al., 2008).

The Japanese Society of Anesthesiology has conducted annual surveys concerning critical incidents in the operating room since 1994. Irita and others (2005) investigated critical incidents associated with regional anesthesia between 1999 and 2002. In patients receiving regional anesthesia, 628 critical incidents, including 108 cardiac arrests and 45 subsequent deaths were reported. The incidences of cardiac arrest and mortality resulting from anesthetic management were 0.54 and 0.02:10,000 with spinal anesthesia, 0.55 and 0:10,000 with combined spinal-epidural anesthesia, and 0.72 and 0.14:10,000 with epidural anesthesia, respectively (Irita et al., 2005).

Valley and Bailey (1991), in a retrospective survey involving 138 pediatric patients who received caudal morphine, reported 11 patients (8%) with postoperative respiratory depression. All but one incident occurred in infants younger than 12 months of age and within 12 hours of caudal morphine administration (70 mcg/kg). Krane (1988) reported a life-threatening delayed respiratory depression in a 2.5-year-old boy that occurred 3.5 hours after the administration of caudal morphine (100 mcg/kg, a much higher dose than today's standards of 30 to 50 mcg/kg) for postoperative analgesia. Intravenous naloxone was continued until 16.5 hours after caudal morphine to maintain adequate breathing. Jones and others (1984) used intrathecal morphine in 56 children undergoing open-heart surgery. Respiratory depression occurred (most commonly, 3.5 to 4.5 hours after morphine administration) in six of 27 patients (22%) who received 30 mcg/kg of morphine and in three of 29 children (10%) who received 20 mcg/kg. Patients receiving epidural or intrathecal morphine should therefore be admitted overnight and their respiration continuously monitored.

Giaufré et al. (1996) reported on a 1-year prospective study (1993 to 1994) of morbidity and mortality associated with regional anesthesia by the French Language Society of Pediatric Anesthesia. The study involved over 24,000 regional-block procedures out of about 85,000 pediatric anesthesia cases of which central blocks (approximately 15,000 cases [62%]) were the most common, followed by peripheral nerve blocks (17%) and others (22%). Of the central blocks, caudal block was most common (12,000, or 80% of central block or 50% of the total), followed by lumbar epidural (1700) and spinal anesthesia (500). A total of only 23 incidents was reported, with a morbidity rate of zero for peripheral blocks, 11 (0.7:1000) for caudal blocks, nine (3.7:1000) for lumbar epidural blocks, two (6.8:1000) for sacral epidural blocks, and one (2:1000) for spinal anesthesia (Giaufré et al., 1996). Complications included eight dural punctures (resulting in total spinal block in four cases), six intravascular injections (resulting in seizures or arrhythmias), two overdoses with arrhythmias, and one case of opioid-related apnea. No fatalities were reported. Thus, this study appears to establish the safety of regional anesthesia in children, although there had been some concerns and controversies about the safety of performing regional blocks in children under general anesthesia, because this is widely accepted as an unsafe practice in adults (Giaufré et al., 1996).

More recently, an analysis of a prospective audit of children receiving epidural infusion analgesia (EIA) in the United Kingdom and Ireland has been published; the audit included 10,633 EIA cases over 5 years (2001 to 2005) (Llewellyn and Moriarty, 2007). Of 96 incidents reported, 56 (1:198) were associated with the insertion and maintenance of EIA (mostly of low severity); five incidents were graded as 1 (serious) (1:2000); nine incidents were graded as 2 (moderate) (1:1100). Only one child had residual effects after 12 months after surgery (1:10,000). There were no reported deaths with EIA. There were four cases of compartment syndrome (1:1400), but none of them appeared to be masked by the presence of working epidural analgesia (Llewellyn and Moriarty, 2007).

Complications Arising from Sedation

According to the data compiled by the United States Department of Health and Human Services, more than 80 deaths attributable to midazolam occurred within 3 years after its introduction for clinical use in 1986. Midazolam was used, often in combination with fentanyl, for the sedation of patients undergoing various procedures without the supervision of anesthesiologists (Bailey et al., 1990). Of these deaths associated with midazolam, 78% were respiratory events, with opioids being used in 57% of these cases (Bailey et al., 1990).

A collaborative study by the American Society of Gastrointestinal Endoscopy and the United States Food and Drug Administration, involving over 21,000 endoscopic procedures with sedation, revealed the incidence of serious cardiorespiratory outcome to be 54:10,000 cases with a mortality rate of 3:10,000; that is 10 to 50 times higher than the reported deaths associated with general anesthesia (Tiret et al., 1986, 1988; Buck et al., 1987; Holland, 1987; Eichhorn, 1989; Arrowsmith et al., 1991). These extremely high morbidity and mortality rates of conscious and deep sedations (apparently including inadvertent general anesthesia and deaths) performed by clinicians who were not anesthesiologists and without adequate skills, proper monitoring, or supervision have led the way to the establishment and modifications of the new sedation guidelines by the AAP Section of Anesthesiology (Committee on Drugs, Section on Anesthesiology, American Academy of Pediatrics, 1985, 1992). Although the terms adopted (conscious sedation in particular) were misnomers (if not oxymorons), in hindsight the guidelines included the approach similar to that commonly practiced by anesthesiologists; that is, proper fasting, preprocedural history and physical examinations with a special attention to the airways, informed consent, monitoring including pulse oximetry, documentation of drugs used and vital signs during and after the procedure, and discharge criteria (Coté, 2004).

The JCAHO (1992) in the United States modified its regulations and published rules to develop new guidelines in each health care institution it accredits (available at *www.jcaho. org*). To further improve patient safety for sedation in accordance with the new JCAHO regulations, a task force by the ASA developed new guidelines for sedation by nonanesthesiologists (Gross et al., 2002). The sedation guidelines were again updated in 2002 (American Society of Anesthesiologists Task Force on Sedation and Analgesia by Non-Anesthesiologists, 2002) with the new terminology (available at *www.asahq.org/standards*) and were later incorporated by JCAHO and by the AAP (Committee on Drugs, Section on Anesthesiology, American Academy of Pediatrics, 2002). The term *conscious sedation* has been eliminated, and instead, three stages of procedural sedation are described: minimal, moderate, and deep stages (plus general anesthesia) (Coté, 2004).

Under the new JCAHO regulations, the director of anesthesia service in each institution has a responsibility for developing new "within-institution" sedation guidelines by nonanesthesiology services to further improve patient safety. General guidelines include onsite availability of oxygen and positive pressure oxygen delivery system (that can provide the minimum of 90% oxygen for 60 minutes), a resuscitation kit (including drugs, laryngoscope, and ETTs), a suction apparatus, and monitors (pulse oximeter, electrocardiography, and blood pressure apparatus). Documentation for sedation should include evaluation of health status before sedation, informed consent, record of drugs given (the time and doses), and vital signs (oxygen saturation, heart and respiratory rates). For deep sedation, there must be a dedicated person (e.g., registered nurse or respiratory therapist) in addition to the practitioner, whose only responsibility is monitoring and who is trained to perform resuscitation.

Using a QA database created specifically for procedural sedation, Malviya and others (1997) identified 239 adverse outcomes (20% of 1140 children), mostly after receiving recommended doses of chloral hydrate. Oxygen desaturation (5.5%) was the most common adverse outcome, and laryngospasm and apnea occurred in five children. Inadequate sedation occurred in 150 (13.2%) children. These findings appear to indicate that the establishment and enforcement of safety guidelines for procedural sedation have considerably reduced the incidence of adverse outcomes.

Analysis of adverse sedation events reported to the United States Food and Drug Administration (FDA) between 1969 and 1996 by Coté and others (2000) revealed that of 95 incidents reported, 60 ended in death (51) or permanent neurologic injury (9). Although the incidence of respiratory events (about 80% of all events; mostly hypoxia, laryngospasm, and apnea) was similar between hospital and nonhospital settings, inadequate resuscitation (57.1% vs. 2.3%) and death or permanent neurologic injury (92.8% vs. 37.2%) occurred more often in nonhospital vs. in hospital environments. Death or severe adverse outcome occurred disproportionately more often (32 of 95 cases) involving sedation for dental procedures (mostly at nonhospital settings). Ten children sustained death or permanent neurologic injury in the car or at home after being discharged from medical supervision despite deep levels of residual sedation. Unsupervised sedative medication by a parent at home (or by a technician at a facility) caused an additional two cardiac arrests in the car on the way to the hospital or clinic (Coté et al., 2000). The results of this report imply the inadequacy of existing (or the nonexistence of) discharge criteria and their practice. Two reports have further addressed these issues.

Motas and others (2004) studied the efficacy and safety of procedural (light or deep grade) sedation in 86 children under 12 years of age undergoing sedation by nonanesthesia services (for computed tomography scans, cardiac catheterizations, gastrointestinal endoscopy, and dental procedures). A variety of medications were used by different services, including intravenous pentobarbital, intravenous midazolam with fentanyl or meperidine, oral chloral hydrate with meperidine and hydroxyzine, and intramuscular or intravenous ketamine (Motas et al., 2004). An independent observer applied the Bispectral Index (BIS) monitor (40 to 60, general anesthesia; 61 to 70, deep sedation; 71 to 90, minimum, and over 90, awake) and the University of Michigan Sedation Scale (UMSS) (0 to 4 observational scale: 0, awake; 1, minimal sedation [tired, sleepy]; 2, moderately sedated [easily arousable]; 3, deeply sedated [deep sleep, arousable only with strong stimulus]; and 4, unarousable or general anesthesia) at 10-minute intervals for 1 hour. The goal of either light or deep sedation was attained in 53% (BIS) and 72% (UMSS) of cases. Depth consistent with general anesthesia was observed in 35% (BIS) and 0% (UMSS) of patients, and depth consistent with awake state (failure) was observed in 12% (BIS) and 28% (UMSS) of cases. About 8% of patients experienced desaturation and airway events. The patients were often sedated either too deeply or not enough, and the goal of either light or deep procedural sedation was not achieved in large numbers of children.

Malviya and others (2004) assessed the readiness for discharge in 29 children after procedural sedation for echocardiographic examinations with either chloral hydrate (93%) or midazolam with diphenhydramine (7%). A trained observer used a BIS monitor, UMSS scores every 10 to 15 minutes, a Modified Maintenance of Wakefulness Test (MMWT), and the visual observation of the time until the child was able to stay awake for 20 minutes, until revised discharge criteria were met (BIS greater than 90, UMSS of 0 or 1, MMWT greater than 20 minutes). There were moderate correlations among BIS, UMSS, and MMWT (p < 0.01). Revised criteria correctly identified wakefulness (BIS value greater than 90) in 88% of patients. However, when discharged by the nurse, only 55% of patients returned to the baseline BIS value (greater than 90); it took longer to meet the revised criteria (more appropriate and safer) compared with standard criteria (nursing judgment) (75 minutes vs. 13 minutes, p = 0.001).

Thus, Malviya and others (2004) clearly demonstrated that sedation with chloral hydrate can result in prolonged sedation even after the children reached currently used (but unsatisfactory) discharge criteria by nurses, with a potential for airway obstruction and adverse outcome (Coté et al., 2000). The results of this study have several important implications. First, the currently practiced guidelines are inadequate and need changes that make use of more reliable criteria, such as UMSS, MMWT, BIS monitor, or their combinations, to further improve patient safety associated with procedural sedations. Second, the duration of postsedation monitoring should be increased beyond what is currently practiced, and the hospital must respond to increase staffing needs for nurses in the recovery area and to provide additional space for adequate patient observation (quiet space for MMWT) and recovery, changes that have associated cost increases. Third, the anesthesia service should provide additional guidelines to nonanesthesiologists for the proper selection of sedative and hypnotic drugs, with shorter elimination half-life to shorten the recovery time (Coté, 2004). In addition, office-based procedures that are performed with the patient under sedation should either be performed under the care of anesthesiologists within the office setting or moved to hospital-based facilities to further decrease untoward events (see Chapter 35, Anesthesia for Office-Based Pediatric Anesthesia).

Cravero and others (2006) looked at data collected by the Pediatric Sedation Research Consortium (PSRC), a collaborative group of 35 institutions. A total of 26 institutions submitted data on 30,037 sedation and anesthesia procedures outside of the operating room from 2004 to 2005. Serious adverse events were rare in the institutions involved in the study; there were no deaths. Cardiopulmonary resuscitation (CPR) was required once. Less serious events were more common with oxygen desaturations below 90% for more than 30 seconds, occurring 157 times per 10,000 sedations. Unexpected apnea, excessive secretions, and vomiting had rates of 24, 41.6, and 47 per 10,000 encounters, respectively (Cravero et al., 2006). They concluded that pediatric sedation and analgesia for procedures outside of the operating room are unlikely to yield serious adverse outcomes in a collection of institutions with highly motivated and organized sedation services. However, the safety of this practice depends on the system's ability to manage less serious events (Cravero et al., 2006).

In 2008, Cravero and others looked at the safety of pediatric sedation and anesthesia with propofol for procedures outside of the operating room. Thirty-seven members of the PSRC submitted data on 49,836 propofol sedation and anesthesia cases from 2004 to 2007. There were no deaths, CPR was required twice, and aspiration during sedation or anesthesia occurred four times. Less serious events were more common with O_2 desaturation below 90% for more than 30 seconds, occurring 154 times per 10,000 sedation and anesthesia administrations. Central apnea or airway obstruction occurred 575 times per 10,000 sedations. Stridor, laryngospasm, excessive secretions, and vomiting had rates of 50, 96, 341, and 49 per 10,000 encounters, respectively. They concluded that, in the hospital setting of those institutions participating in the PSRC, the reported incidence of serious events in pediatric propofol sedation and anesthesia is low. However, the reported incidence of events that have the potential to harm and that require timely rescue interventions is significant, occurring once per 89 propofol administrations (Cravero et al., 2009).

Bhananker and others (2006) reviewed closed malpractice claims from the ASA database since 1990 to assess the patterns of injury and liability associated with monitored anesthesia care (MAC) compared with general and regional anesthesia. More than 40% of claims associated with MAC involved death or permanent brain damage, similar to general anesthesia claims. Respiratory depression (25%) was the most common damaging mechanism in MAC claims. Nearly half of these claims were judged as preventable by better monitoring.

COMMON CAUSES OF ANESTHESIA-RELATED MISHAPS

Judgment Errors

If one accepts the theory that "to err is human" and recognizes that "all human beings, without any exception whatsoever, make errors and [errors] are a completely normal and necessary part of human cognitive function," then it is not surprising to realize that most anesthetic mishaps involve human errors and are preventable (Salem et al., 1975; Cooper et al., 1978; Allnutt, 1987; Holland, 1987; Kohn et al., 1999). Cooper and others (1978), with the use of a carefully structured interview technique with a group of anesthesiologists, collected accounts of incidents in which human error or equipment failure occurred. These investigators found that 82% of incidents were caused by preventable human error; the remaining incidents were mostly caused by equipment failure. Analysis of 238 closed anesthesia malpractice claims involving pediatric patients revealed that 43% of these claims were related to inadequate ventilation and resulted in death or severe permanent neurologic damage (Morray et al., 1993). Morray and others concluded that 89% of these cases could have been prevented if they were monitored with pulse oximetry or capnography.

Holland (1987) compared incidences of various categories of mishaps during his three decades of investigation involving anesthesia-related mortality in patients of all ages (Table 40-8). In the 1960s, anesthetic overdose, wrong choice of anesthetics, inadequate preoperative preparation, and inadequate crisis management dominated as common causes of adverse outcomes, indicating inadequacy (according to today's standard) of equipment and the physicians' experience with administering anesthesia. The total incidence of management errors involving fatality was 2.7:10,000 anesthesia procedures. There has been a dramatic decrease in the incidence of management errors with time, as well as changes in the dominant categories of error in management over the decades. In the 1980s, inadequate preparation and inadequate postoperative management ranked high among the categories of errors causing anesthesia-related fatalities. Incidence of management errors decreased to 0.55:10,000 anesthetics, about one fifth that in the 1960s. Factors commonly associated with preventable adverse outcomes (both fatal and nonfatal) include a failure to perform proper review

TABLE 40-8. Errors of Management: Numbers and Ranked Order of Incidence

Error	1960 to 1969 No.	1960 to 1969 Rank	1970 to 1980 No.	1970 to 1980 Rank	1983 to 1985 No.	1983 to 1985 Rank	Whole Series No.	Whole Series Rank
Inadequate preparation	102	3	93	1	23	1	218	1
Wrong choice	120	2	65	3	13	4	198	4
Overdose	127	1	34	7	14	3	175	4
Aspiration	41	9	18	11	1	9	60	10
Inadequate resuscitation	63	7	49	4	6	5	118	6
Hypoxic mixture	14	12	0		0		14	12
Inadequate ventilation	68	5	21	9	1	9	90	7
Inadequate monitoring	22	11	19	10	6	5	47	11
Technical mishap	25	10	40	6	1	9	66	9
Inadequate crisis management	102	3	80	2	4	8	186	3
Inadequate reversal	52	8	22	8	5	7	79	8
Inadequate postoperative management	68	5	43	5	16	2	127	5
Total errors	804		484		90		1378	
Errors per patient	2.4		2.0		1.8		2.2	

Modified from Holland R: Anaesthetic mortality in New South Wales, *Br J Anaesth* 59:834, 1987.

of patients and anesthesia apparatus, distraction (e.g., inattention, haste, fatigue, and boredom), lack of experience, and lack of a skilled assistant (Craig and Wilson, 1981; Derrington and Smith, 1987).

Emergency or Urgent Cases

Inadequate preanesthetic preparation occurs most often with emergency or urgent cases and most commonly represents failure to appreciate the patient's degree of dehydration and electrolyte imbalance (Holland, 1987). In the CEPOD study cited previously, more than 20% of anesthesia-related deaths occurred after surgery performed as emergencies, and an additional 40% occurred in operations classified as urgent (Buck et al., 1987). In the New South Wales study, the risk of anesthesia-attributable death in patients undergoing emergency anesthesia is 10 times that of the overall incidence (Holland, 1987). In the British CEPOD study, anesthetists were dissatisfied with preoperative preparations in 14% of cases that ended with anesthesia-related deaths, but they presumably were pressured or persuaded by surgeons into administering anesthesia. On the basis of these findings, Lunn and Devlin (1987) emphasize the importance of proper preanesthetic preparation as an important deterrent of tragic outcome. In children, the incidence of bradycardic episodes, both fatal and nonfatal, during anesthesia was reported to be significantly higher among emergency surgical procedures (2.7%) than in elective procedures (1.1%) (Keenan et al., 1994).

Timing of Occurrence

Keenan and Boyan (1985) in a 15-year study of cardiac arrest resulting from anesthesia in a university hospital setting, found 18 of 27 cases that occurred during the induction of anesthesia, whereas the remaining nine occurred intraoperatively. However, in five of six patients in the pediatric age group who sustained cardiac arrest (aged 1 day to 6 years), the cardiac arrest occurred during the maintenance of anesthesia. In most other reports, critical incidents or mishaps, including the cardiac arrests reported from the POCA Registry as discussed earlier in this chapter, have occurred most often during the maintenance period of anesthesia (Cooper et al., 1978; Craig and Wilson, 1981; Gibbs, 1986; Bhananker et al., 2007). The maintenance period is not the quiet interlude between often stormy induction and emergence that many anesthesiologists had for a long time supposed (Epstein, 1978). In a survey involving 112,000 general anesthetic cases in a teaching hospital between 1975 and 1983, the incidence of intraoperative adverse events among adults was lower than events in the PACU (Cohen et al., 1988). In contrast, the incidence of adverse events in children tended to be higher during surgery than in the PACU (Tiret et al., 1988). Machine-patient disconnection was a common occurrence in the 1970s before the disconnect alarm became a standard feature of anesthesia machines, as mandated by the American National Standard Institute Z79 Committee on Anesthesia Equipment (Cooper et al., 1978).

Anesthetic Overdose

Drug overdose as the cause of anesthetic death occurs, although the incidence has decreased since the 1980s and it accounted for only 5.4% of anesthetic deaths reported to the Medical Defense Union of the United Kingdom between 1970 and 1979 (Utting et al., 1979; Holland, 1984, 1987). In a 15-year study between 1969 and 1983 by Keenan and Boyan (1985) an "absolute overdose" (a dose well in excess of the usual clinical range) caused one third of all cardiac arrests resulting from anesthesia. Of six incidents of cardiac arrest in children in this series, absolute overdose with halothane was responsible in five cases; the other resulted from airway obstruction during nitrous oxide-curare anesthesia.

As described earlier, the POCA Registry database revealed that from 1994 to 1997, cardiovascular depression with halothane accounted for 66% of all medication-related cardiac arrests. In healthy children with ASA PS 1 or 2, 64% of all cardiac arrests were medication-related, in comparison with 23% in those with ASA PS 3 to 5 (Morray et al., 2000). The database from 2000 to 2003, when halothane had been replaced by sevoflurane as the primary inhalation induction agent, showed a dramatic decrease in medication-related cardiac arrest, from 37% to 12% of the total arrests, indicating the importance of safer anesthetic drugs for reducing medication-related complications (Fig. 40-2) (Morray, 2004).

Risk Factors in Pediatric Anesthesia

A number of perioperative risk factors specific to infants and children have been identified.

Age

Infants younger than 1 year of age are at higher risk of developing complications (Tiret et al., 1988; Cohen et al., 1990). A prospective survey in France between 1978 and 1982 involving 440 institutions and a total of 40,240 anesthetic procedures found 27 major complications, of which nine occurred in infants (0.43:10,000 cases), an incidence significantly higher than that in children (0.05:10,000) (Tiret et al., 1988). Infants younger than 1 year of age also showed a significantly higher incidence of airway obstruction and other respiratory problems than did older children (Cohen et al., 1990). Cohen and others (1990) reported that the intraoperative incidence of complications in children was about the same as that in adults, but postoperative complications (35%) were twice as common as in adults (17%). The POCA Registry database from 1994 to 1997 revealed that 83 of 150 cases, or 55%, of anesthesia-related cardiac arrests occurred in infants younger than 12 months of age (Table 40-5) (Morray et al., 2000).

Physical Status

Correlation between POCA and ASA PS has been reported in adults (Keenan and Boyan, 1985). In a large-scale prospective survey in France involving infants and children, Tiret and others (1988) showed a highly significant correlation between the ASA PS classification and the incidence of major perianesthetic complications in children (Table 40-9). They also found a highly significant correlation between the perioperative adverse outcomes and the number of coexisting diseases. The POCA Registry database between 1994 and 1997 showed 100 of 150 (66.7%) of all anesthesia-related cardiac arrests occurred among children with ASA PS 3 to 5 (Morray et al., 2000) (Table 40-5).

Emergency Surgery

The French study by Tiret et al. (1988) showed a threefold increase in perioperative complications in pediatric emergency cases compared with the scheduled cases (Table 40-9). Similarly, Keenan and others (1994) found a highly significant increase of bradycardic episodes in children during emergency surgery compared with those with elective procedures (2.7% vs. 1.1%).

Training

Proper training or experience is particularly important for minimizing the incidence of adverse outcome in the field of pediatric anesthesia. In a retrospective study in a large university hospital over a span of 7 years, Keenan and others (1991) reviewed the incidence of cardiac arrests occurring in infants younger than 1 year of age. No anesthesia-related cardiac arrests occurred when trained pediatric anesthesiologists were in charge of pediatric cases. In contrast, when nonpediatric anesthesiologists were supervising, cardiac arrests (including deaths) occurred at a rate of 19.7:10,000 pediatric anesthesia procedures. In a subsequent prospective study from the same institution for the period of 9 years ending in 1992, the incidence of bradycardic episodes was significantly higher when

TABLE 40-9. Risks of Pediatric Anesthesia

	No. of Anesthetics	Rate of Complications (per 1000)	Significance
ASA PS			
1	36,903	0.4	p < 0.001
2	1461	3.4	
3	518	11.6	
4 and 5	122	16.4	
Number of Coexisting Diseases			
0	36,544	0.5	p < 0.001
1	3064	1.3	
2	490	4.1	
≥3	142	21.1	
Previous Anesthesia			
No	25,517	0.5	p < 0.05
Yes	11,343	1.1	
Duration of Preoperative Fasting (hours)			
<8	5189	1.5	p < 0.05
>8	34,067	0.6	
Emergency			
No	33,391	0.5	p < 0.05
Yes	5918	1.5	

Modified from Tiret L et al: Complications related to anaesthesia in infants and children: a prospective survey of 40,240 anaesthetics, *Br J Anaesth* 61:263, 1988. *ASA PS*, American Society of Anesthesiologists physical status.

pediatric anesthesiologists were not supervising the trainees administering anesthetics to infants (2.1%) compared with when pediatric anesthesiologists supervised the trainees (0.8%) (Keenan et al., 1994).

PREVENTION OF ANESTHESIA-RELATED MISHAPS

The first important step toward patient safety is prevention of critical events. As is clear from the foregoing discussion, a number of steps should be taken to achieve this goal.

Preanesthetic Preparation

Preoperatively, the patient's past medical history, especially the anesthetic history if there is any, should be reviewed thoroughly, and the patient should be examined carefully. The anesthesia machine, accessories, and drugs should also be checked carefully, because failure to perform these steps properly has been identified as a major cause of anesthesia-related mishaps, including death (Holland, 1984, 1987; Derrington and Smith, 1987). In an emergency or urgent situation (perhaps with the exception of exsanguination, cardiac tamponade, or acute upper airway obstruction), clinicians should try to take at least minimal necessary steps (e.g., fluid resuscitation, transfusion, correction of electrolytes, acid-base imbalance, and fever) to stabilize the patient for anesthesia and surgery in a coordinated effort with the surgeon. The anesthesiologist should not yield to unreasonable pressures to start the case before the patient is best prepared under these circumstances. Indeed, hypovolemia and anemia are reported to be the major causes of anesthesia-related cardiac arrest in infants and children (Salem et al., 1975).

If the anesthesiologist is unfamiliar or uncomfortable with uncommon pathophysiology (e.g., an infant with a cyanotic heart disease coming for noncardiac surgery or a child with craniopharyngioma and diabetes insipidus), the anesthesiologist should not hesitate to ask for consultation with a senior anesthesiologist or other specialists. In addition, especially in an emergency situation (such as posttonsillectomy bleeding or acute epiglottitis), an experienced assistant, preferably an attending pediatric anesthesiologist, should be standing by for the induction. Keenan and others (1994) found a significantly lower incidence of bradycardic events with the presence of a pediatric anesthesiologist during induction. In teaching institutions, resident trainees should always be supervised by a pediatric attending anesthesiologist for a pediatric patient. Lack of an experienced assistant has been associated with anesthesia-related mortality and a high rate of morbidity (Craig and Wilson, 1981; Derrington and Smith, 1987; Eichhorn, 1989; Keenan et al., 1994). A reluctance to ask for help, whether out of insecurity, pride, or ill-conceived heroism (or machismo), has no place in a pediatric anesthesia emergency and is the first step toward disaster.

Vigilance

A timely recovery from impending failure is the key to patient safety. It is therefore extremely important to recognize without delay that something is going wrong. Sustained attention or vigilance is essential for patient safety during the maintenance of anesthesia, because critical events most commonly occur at the time of presumably reduced mental and physical workload (Cooper et al., 1978; Craig and Wilson, 1981; Gibbs, 1986; Gaba et al., 1987). One should develop the habit of scanning all of the monitors regularly in an orderly fashion, as a pilot in flight scans the instrument panel at regular intervals, to keep up with minute deviations in the patient's cardiorespiratory stability. A survey by Cooper and others (1984), however, suggested that at least 33% of critical incidents occurring during the maintenance of anesthesia resulted from errors in judgment rather than from inattentiveness. Vigilance is an important deterrent but by itself is not sufficient for prevention of critical incidents. However, the notion that all human beings, including all anesthesiologists, make mistakes should not be used as an excuse to discount the importance of vigilance, especially in pediatric anesthesia (Allnutt, 1987). The anesthesiologist should aim for near perfection by minimizing factors that adversely affect vigilance, such as fatigue, distraction, and boredom. An audible tone for the pulse and oxygen saturation, as well as an audible tone for capnographic alarm limits and loss of pressure is advocated by the Anesthesia Patient Safety Foundation (APSF) as a method to enhance patient safety and improve vigilance. A better understanding and application of ergonomic principles may improve vigilance and help reduce anesthesia-related mishaps in the future (Gravenstein and Weinger, 1986).

Monitors and Monitoring Standards

The fact that most anesthesia-related fatalities involve human error clearly supports the concept that monitoring devices are essential for patient safety even for the experienced, conscientious, and vigilant anesthesiologist. The ASA Closed Claims Project indicated that in 28% of these cases, proper monitoring already available commercially could have averted the mishaps (Cheney, 1988). Of particular interest to anesthesiologists is that the median cost of legal settlement in cases in which improved monitoring would probably have prevented the complication or death was more than 10 times higher than in cases in which better monitoring would have had no effect on occurrence or outcome (Cheney, 1988). In a similar review involving 238 (10% of 2400 total claims) closed anesthesia malpractice claims concerning children, a vast majority (approximately 89%) of pediatric claims that were related to inadequate ventilation (43% of total) could have been prevented with pulse oximetry, capnography, or both (Morray et al., 1993). The proportion of claims assessed as preventable by better monitoring decreased from an average of 63% in the 1970s to 16% in the 1990s (Jimenez et al., 2007).

In 1985, minimum standards for patient monitoring during anesthesia at Harvard University teaching hospitals were adopted and later published (Eichhorn et al., 1986). Similar but slightly more specific standards for basic intraoperative monitoring, proposed by the ASA, were approved by the House of Delegates in 1986. Both sets of standards specifically mandate that oxygenation, ventilation, circulation, and body temperature be evaluated continually (at regular intervals) or continuously (without interruption). For each of the components, the clear objective to ensure adequacy, followed by specific methods, is stated (see Chapter 10, Equipment; Chapter 11, Monitoring; and Chapter 13, Induction, Maintenance, and Recovery). There

is a strong emphasis on combining clinical evaluation and technological methods. Although no specific methodology or instrumentation is mandated for monitoring cardiopulmonary and other indices, the ASA standards strongly encourage quantitative methods, such as pulse oximetry and capnography, over qualitative clinical assessment, with inspection and auscultation for cardiopulmonary monitoring. In addition, the New York State Hospital Code (1988) dictates that pulse oximetry and capnography be used to monitor all patients undergoing general anesthesia to reduce anesthesia-related morbidity and mortality. Eventually, most other states followed with similar laws mandating intraoperative monitoring with pulse oximetry and capnography. Accordingly, most malpractice liability insurers in the United States have required that anesthesiologists follow these standards whenever possible (Orkin, 1989). The APSF endorses the use of audible alarms on physiologic monitors.

Similar standards for basic patient monitoring have also been proposed in the United Kingdom, Australia, and other industrialized countries (Sykes, 1987; Cass et al., 1988; Runciman, 1988b). They are similar to the ASA standards in terms of machine monitoring (i.e., oxygen analyzer, low-flow alarm, and ventilator disconnect alarm). The standards for minimum patient monitoring, however, differ considerably, depending in part on the patient's physical status and the degree of surgical involvement (i.e., minor, standard, or major operation) (Sykes, 1987).

With the advent of pulse oximetry in the late 1980s, the anesthesiologist's ability to detect hypoxemia has improved markedly (see Chapters 10, Equipment, and 11, Monitoring). Coté and others (1988, 1991) have demonstrated that major hypoxemic events (arterial saturation of oxygen [Sao_2] equal to 80% lasting more than 30 seconds) can occur without visible cyanosis or obvious changes in the cardiorespiratory patterns in children and that pulse oximetry detects such events more quickly than other means of monitoring. Cooper and others (1987), as part of perianesthetic QA activity, found a significant reduction in undesirable anesthesia-related incidents that require intervention after the introduction of pulse oximetry in the operating room.

Technological Improvements

Another technological patient safety strategy is the use of engineered safety devices that physically prevent errors from occurring (Gaba, 2000). An example of this human factor design is the pin index safety system in pneumatic connections, which uses geometric features on the yoke to prevent a gas hose or cylinder from being connected to the wrong gas yoke. This system is not infallible, however, and misconnections can still occur without proper vigilance (Ellett et al., 2009). New technologies have also been developed to improve management of the patient's airway, including the video laryngoscope, improved fiberoptic laryngoscopes, and LMAs. These devices improve the management of the pediatric (upper) airway in both routine and emergency situations.

According to the APSF, the use of automated information management systems could improve the future ability to link intraoperative events to both short-term and long-term outcomes (Gravenstein, 2001). Collection of real-time data obtained from the millions of anesthetics administered annually worldwide could lead to a better understanding of best anesthesia practices and improved patient safety. Such data collection studies are increasingly common. In pediatric critical care, a collaborative project of over 70 pediatric intensive care units and Virtual Pediatric Systems has accumulated data on over 250,000 critically ill children and is providing benchmarking and quality data to guide critical care practice (Wetzel, 2009). The Society for Pediatric Anesthesia is sponsoring a similar prospective data collection methodology to collect detailed incident data across the field of pediatric anesthesia to provide benchmarking data.

Selection of Safer Anesthetics and Adjuvant Drugs

The POCA Registry data analyses have clearly demonstrated the safety of sevoflurane over halothane as the agent of choice for inhalation induction of anesthesia (Morray, 2004). Between 1994 and 1997, cardiac arrest associated with medication accounted for 37% of all cardiac arrests, from which halothane with or without other drugs accounted for 66% (Morray et al., 2000). From 2000 to 2003, when sevoflurane had replaced halothane as the inhalation induction agent of choice, medication-related causes of cardiac arrests decreased drastically, from 37% to 12%. Concomitantly, the incidence of cardiac arrests among healthy children (ASA PS 1 or 2) decreased from 33% to 19% of all cardiac arrests (Morray, 2004).

The developing nervous system is highly susceptible to neurotoxic insults during rapid synaptogenesis, during the brain growth spurts, and before neurons have migrated to their final destination and fully differentiated (Rabinowicz et al., 1996). In 2003, data were released that clearly showed that modern anesthetics cause widespread neurodegeneration in the developing rat brain (Jevtovic-Todorovic et al., 2003). Since that time, several more studies have confirmed that data by showing anesthesia-related increases in brain cell death and reductions in functional performance in rats. Although the exact mechanism of anesthesia-induced neurodegeneration in animals remains unclear, the evidence points toward the involvement of γ-aminobutyric acid (GABA) and N-methyl-D-aspartic acid (NMDA) receptors. All commonly used anesthetics are thought to exploit their effects on GABA or NMDA receptors to produce unconsciousness and immobility during painful stimulation. Moreover, all commonly used anesthetics that were investigated for their neurodegenerative properties, such as benzodiazepines, ketamine, propofol, nitrous oxide and isoflurane, have been shown to exacerbate neuronal cell death.(Loepke et al., 2008). Although the documented neurotoxic effects of anesthetics in the developing animal model are noteworthy and alarming, the implications of these findings for clinical practice remains uncertain. The complexity of the mammalian nervous-system development complicates the extrapolation of data derived from animal models to humans. The FDA convened an Advisory Committee Meeting in April of 2007 to review all of the available evidence regarding the potential neurodegenerative effects of anesthetics in infant and juvenile animals. The panel determined that, based on the current knowledge and lack of appropriate alternatives, there was no scientific basis to recommend changes in clinical practice. Future research in this area with animals and nonhuman primates is needed to further understand the exact mechanisms behind anesthesia-related neurodegeneration and the long-term effects of modern anesthetic agents on the development of the human brain. Increased research on the mechanisms of anesthetic action are needed to discover drugs with greater specificity or mechanisms of action

that do not involve the GABA and NMDA receptors, as well as adjuvant drugs and techniques that may limit their deleterious effects. Until the risk of neurocognitive injury is understood, pediatric surgical specialists, in conjunction with anesthesiologists and pediatricians, should identify surgical procedures that can be delayed until older ages without incurring additional risk (McGowan and Davis, 2008).

Improved Education and Training

The steady decline in anesthesia-related mortality and morbidity over the past several decades has been attributed to increases in better-trained and better-qualified physicians administering anesthesia (Holland, 1987). In a survey of potentially harmful anesthesia-related events, Cooper and others (1978) found that 25% of these events were associated with inadequate training or unfamiliarity with equipment or devices; further training of these anesthetists (presumably trainees) would have prevented some of these events. In addition, an anesthesia-related mortality study from Harvard University has shown that in 8 of 11 cases of fatalities attributed primarily to anesthesia, inadequate supervision of residents, medical students, and nurse anesthetists was considered contributory (Eichhorn, 1989).

As mentioned previously, Keenan and others (1991) reported the importance of specialty training in pediatric anesthesia for the reduction of cardiac arrests in infants. No anesthesia-related cardiac arrests occurred when trained pediatric anesthesiologists were in charge of pediatric cases, whereas cardiac arrests occurred at a rate of 19.7:10,000 when non–pediatric anesthesiologists were supervising trainees. The same investigators also reported in a subsequent prospective study that the incidence of bradycardic episodes was significantly higher when pediatric anesthesiologists were not supervising the trainees anesthetizing infants (2.1%) than when trained pediatric anesthesiologists were in charge (0.8%) (Keenan et al., 1994). These results emphasize the importance of training and experience for a better anesthetic outcome.

There has been an explosion of interest in patient safety over the last four decades, and sessions on patient safety are now common in the scientific programs of the ASA and SPA annual meetings. There is also an increasing amount of patient-safety research being done each year, with the APSF awarding grants for research funds since its inception in 1985. The results of this research are reported in anesthesiology journals, scientific and educational meetings, and textbooks. The availability of these data have raised physician awareness of patient safety. Realistic patient and infant simulators were introduced in the 1980s. Since that time there have been great advances in simulator technology and science, and these simulators are available at many anesthesia training programs and as a component of many scientific meetings. Anesthesia has become the leader in the application and adoption of simulators that provide strong patient safety implications through education, training, and research (Stoelting and Khuri, 2006).

Quality Assurance

Documentation of the QA or QI process, especially that of fatal and morbid events, has been mandated in an effort to reduce the risk to and improve the outcome of patients undergoing anesthesia. In a pilot prospective study, Currie and others (1988) found the QA survey helpful in identifying nonfatal, non-morbid, often transient events for peer review soon after such events took place. The survey demonstrated disproportionately high incidences of nonfatal events occurring with pediatric and emergency or out-of-hours cases. Induction and maintenance periods seem to be equally hazardous, up to four times more so than the emergence and recovery periods. As noted in other studies, airway events were most common (53%) (Cooper et al., 1978, 1984; Craig and Wilson, 1981). The authors concluded that the advantage of their method lies for the most part in its inherent lack of inertia: rapid evaluation, response, and feedback in a confidential and nonjudgmental atmosphere, resulting in the improvement of patient care in a unique manner (Cooper et al., 1978; Currie et al., 1988). QA or QI programs should be continued to prevent adverse events caused by human factors or errors (active failure) by learning from events and "near misses" as a group. Equally important, the QA program is the process of continually evaluating the environment in which anesthesia is practiced, and identifying systemic problems (environmental factors or latent failures) responsible for or potentially causing adverse events, which have not been obvious, so as to implement strategies or new guidelines to improve the structure or environment and prevent future occurrence of adverse events.

Environmental factors (latent failures) may play a major role and may be responsible for adverse outcomes impeding the safety and quality of patient care. These factors may include inadequate safety mechanisms (e.g., poor organization, unclear drug labeling), inadequate or nonfunctional monitoring systems, and poor communication among the surgeons, anesthesiologists, and operating room personnel. Indeed, in an analysis of 110 adverse events from more than 13,000 anesthetic procedures, Lagasse and others (1995) identified only 8% caused by human errors, whereas 92% of adverse events were attributable to system errors.

The impact of anesthetic management characteristics on severe morbidity and mortality in patients (between 62 and 65 years of age) was analyzed by the Dutch Association of Anesthesiology (Arbous et al., 2005). In a case-controlled study in the cohort of nearly 870,000 cases between 1995 and 1997, 807 patients who remained comatose or died within 24 hours of undergoing general anesthesia were identified and compared with 883 control cases without severe outcome. The incidence of postoperative death was 8.8:10,000 in this age group. Anesthetic management factors that were statistically significantly associated with a decreased risk included: equipment check with a protocol and checklist (odds ratio: 0.64), documentation of the equipment check (odds ratio: 0.61), a directly available anesthesiologist (odds ratio: 0.46), no change of anesthesia provider during the case (odds ratio: 0.44), two rather than one person present at emergence (odds ratio: 0.69), reversal of muscle relaxant or of the combination of relaxant and opioid (odds ratio: 0.1 and 0.29, respectively), and postoperative pain medication vs. no pain medication (Arbous et al., 2005).

Critical events related to anesthesia occur commonly during the practice of anesthesia. A well-trained, motivated, vigilant anesthesiologist normally detects these events in time and takes proper measures to prevent disaster. Anesthesia-related accidents causing catastrophic injury or death, therefore, are rare, especially in relation to the rate of such potentially harmful events. Because humans are imperfect and make mistakes as part of normal human cognitive behavior, catastrophic accidents can occur almost at random to any anesthesiologist (Allnutt, 1987). The availability of both machine and patient monitors and adherence to monitoring standards are indispensable.

From the preceding presentation, it is apparent that young children, especially infants, are more vulnerable to anesthesia-related mishaps, whereas such a risk in older, healthy children is relatively low. Because of the small size and physiologic differences in the cardiopulmonary and other organ systems in young infants, as outlined earlier in this book, safety in pediatric anesthesia demands additional clinical training and vigilance. Anesthetic complications in infants and children and their management, when applicable, have been discussed in appropriate chapters elsewhere in this book.

For the safety of infants and young children, a high-risk group in terms of anesthesia-related morbidity and mortality, more clinical training, adequate preoperative preparation, vigilance, and adherence to monitoring standards (especially the use of a pulse oximeter and precordial stethoscope continuously) are all important and indispensable. When in doubt, the clinician should not hesitate to transfer the young and unstable patient to a specialized center for pediatric anesthesia and surgery to provide them with a better opportunity for survival.

SUMMARY

Anesthesia-related mortality has declined steadily over the past several decades as the percentage of general anesthetics administered by trained anesthesiologists has increased and as newer and safer anesthetics and adjuvant drugs, anesthetic equipment, and monitoring and safety standards in the industrialized nations have improved. Yet, anesthesia-related adverse events remain relatively higher in infants younger than 1 year of age than in older children and adults. As in adults, anesthesia-related catastrophe is still caused predominantly by judgment errors and environmental factors that are potentially preventable (Lagasse, 2002). Critical incidents occur more often during the induction and maintenance of anesthesia than during emergence and recovery. Emergency and urgent surgeries are associated with a disproportionately high incidence of anesthesia-related adverse events, in part because of inadequate preanesthesia patient preparation.

Analyses of closed malpractice insurance claims as well as the POCA Registry sponsored by the ASA have been informative in developing a future strategy for preventing anesthesia-related mishaps. Emphasis on strict monitoring standards and QA surveillance, developed and sustained since the late 1980s, seem valuable both in preventing near misses and in heightening anesthesiologists' awareness of such events. For patient safety in pediatric anesthesia, better clinical training, adequate preanesthetic preparations, vigilance, and adherence to monitoring standards are essential. Anesthesiologists must remain motivated and continue to pursue harmless anesthesia, yet at the same time be proud leaders of patient safety (Cooper and Gaba, 2002).

REFERENCES

Complete references used in this text can be found online at www.expertconsult.com.

History of Pediatric Anesthesia

Robert M. Smith and Mark A. Rockoff

CONTENTS

T he pediatric anesthesiologist does not generally diagnose or cure patients but rather guides and supports each young patient through the operative experience with the least possible mental and physical stress. The history of pediatric anesthesia is best told by tracing the steps others have taken; steps toward increased precision in regulation and control of neurologic, respiratory, cardiovascular, and other body systems to serve both the surgeon and child (Smith, 1991).

The goals of pediatric anesthesiology as a specialty include the reduction of perioperative morbidity and mortality and the promotion of ancillary resuscitative and supportive fields through teaching, research, and organizational activity throughout the world.

PHASE I: PEDIATRIC ANESTHESIA BEFORE 1940

Primitive Period

Before the introduction of ether in 1846, circumcisions, amputations, tumor excisions, and correction of gross deformities were performed on infants and children without any relief of pain. Struggling was controlled by use of force, but pain was accepted as an unavoidable part of life. Crude attempts were occasionally made with alcoholic "spirits," nerve compression, or even brief strangling, coupled with headlong surgical

speed; however, these attempts resulted in predictably poor outcomes for both operation and patient. Harelip repair had been attempted without pain relief measures in many parts of the world for hundreds of years. In Japan, general anesthesia with the herb mixture *tsu san sen* was used successfully for breast cancer operations in 1804 by Seishu Hanaoka. In 1837, Gancho Homma reported a series of general anesthesia procedures with the use of the same herb mixture for children over 5 years of age for harelip repair, but it was withheld from use in younger patients because of its toxicity (Iwai and Satoyoshi, 1992). The conviction that small infants did not need anesthesia was not effectively suppressed until recently (Anand and Hickey, 1987). For many years, the "whiskey nipple" had been used widely as a sedative supplement to local anesthesia in infants undergoing abdominal procedures, and wine has been given for ritual circumcisions for millennia.

Early Control of Pain: Ether and Chloroform

The introduction of ether was the first giant step in the history of anesthesia. Although Crawford Long used ether in his rural practice in Georgia beginning in 1842, and his third ether-anesthesia procedure was for a toe amputation in a 7-year-old boy (Long, 1849), it was not until the famous public demonstration of ether anesthesia at the Massachusetts General Hospital in Boston in 1846 that ether was widely accepted for use during surgery (Morton, 1847). The discovery that sensation, or pain, and along with it consciousness and motion, could be abolished temporarily by ether was widely acclaimed; however, little was known about ether's actions, how to use it, or what its dangers might be. Ether was accepted only gradually over several years, with many surgeons retaining the belief that ordinary men (the wealthy excluded) should be able to tolerate surgery without anesthesia! However, for children and ladies, who were considered to be "more sensitive," anesthesia was considered appropriate, although Morton himself was reluctant to administer it to young subjects because of the high incidence of nausea and vomiting in this population (Bigelow, 1846; Warren, 1847; Pernick, 1975).

It was soon found that pouring ether onto a handkerchief or small cloth was a practical method of administration with small children. One simply pressed the cloth to the patient's face until the child was quiet and limp. The cloth was then withdrawn, and the surgeon was granted 3 or 4 minutes to operate as the child regained consciousness. The use of continuous administration of ether caught on slowly with gradual familiarization with the new agent. The early impression that ether was easy to administer, effective, and safe led to the belief that it was a trivial service that any inexperienced person, often an orderly or a parent, could perform. The unfortunate result was that throughout the rest of the century, the administration of anesthesia continued to be held in poor repute as a medical activity, rarely attracting physicians with special interest or ability in the field. Nurses eventually began to assume increasing responsibilities for providing anesthesia care. As late as 1940, a physician, in the lead article published in the first edition of the new journal *Anesthesiology*, noted, "During my internship I was trained by a nurse. I was given a cone, a can of ether, and a few empirical tricks" (Haggard, 1940).

In England, chloroform was accepted more readily because of its smoother and more rapid action. Soon, however, the incidence of deaths became so alarming that the British established a dictum that only physicians should be allowed to administer anesthesia (Eckenhoff, 1966). The fortunate result was that throughout the British Empire, anesthesia flourished as a medical specialty and its workers gained equal status with other physicians and became early leaders in the field.

Another great advantage for the British in the early development of anesthesia was the presence of the astounding John Snow (1813 to 1858), who made epidemiologic advances of national importance, ran an active medical practice, and kept notes on hundreds of anesthesia experiences and research experiments, mostly in the last 10 years of his life (1846 to 1856) (Griffith, 1934). Snow first described signs by which a practitioner could monitor and control the depth of anesthesia in patients of all ages (Snow, 1847). His five stages of anesthesia (excitement, loss of consciousness, relaxation, eye movement, and depth of respiration) served as a guideline throughout the remainder of the century and formed the basis of Guedel's important guide, *Inhalation Anesthesia,* published in 1937. Snow explored both ether and chloroform, preferring the latter, which he found well suited to infants and children. However, he warned of chloroform's danger with excessive depth (Snow, 1858). His record of successfully anesthetizing 147 infants for harelip repair is hardly conceivable in view of the mortality that this operation continued to bear well into the next century.

After the remarkable advances made by Snow, anesthesia in England progressed at a slower pace. For nearly 20 years,

chloroform and ether remained the only anesthetic agents available, and progress consisted mainly of developing methods of administration, comparing advantages and dangers, and simply studying how to keep children asleep and still for longer periods of time. Despite its recognized danger, chloroform remained the principal agent in England and throughout Europe. Efforts to reduce the complications associated with chloroform included many warnings, as well as attempts to increase its safety, such as diluting it with ether (CE) and with alcohol and ether (ACE). The introduction of nitrous oxide into general use by 1870 and ethyl chloride shortly after 1900 were important advances because they reduced or replaced the use of chloroform in many operations. Both of these agents were non-irritating and relatively acceptable, making them particularly adaptable for induction. Because induction had been seen as a troublesome stage of anesthesia, the use of these agents generated much interest.

British physician anesthetists began to publish articles and texts in increasing numbers. Buxton alone produced five editions of his *Anaesthetics: Their Uses and Administration* between 1888 and 1912. Many texts related to adult care contained advice on pediatric problems, of which harelip continued to attract the most attention. Numerous references to pediatric anesthesia could be found in *The Lancet*, Britain's premier medical journal, and in 1923, C. Langton Hewer wrote *Anaesthesia for Children*, the first text on pediatric anesthesia to be written in English.

In the United States, the special needs of children were given slight consideration for many years. The child was treated as "a little adult"; surgeons operated with large instruments, and all equipment was adult sized. Ether remained the principal agent. Although criticism of chloroform became more vehement, its use was advocated in the United States as recently as 1957 (Kopetsky, 1903; Schwartz, 1957). Progress was made by trial and error, with little communication among those using anesthesia. Most literature in the United States concerning anesthesia for children was written by surgeons before 1900.

Interest grew slowly around the turn of the century, and nurses and surgeons began to develop skills sufficient to carry children through longer and more difficult procedures. Thousands of tonsillectomies were being practiced by 1900, and appendectomy was an accepted, although often dangerous, procedure. Orthopedic surgery was the most active type of pediatric surgery during this time, and most procedures were easily managed by simple ether techniques. One of the first signs of concern for the child's anxiety when undergoing anesthesia was voiced by James Gwathmey in 1907. He recommended that one should "add a few drops of the mother's cologne to the ether mask and induce the child in the mother's arms." Another step toward easing induction came in 1928 with the introduction of tribromoethanol, the German Avertin, which was used widely as a rectal agent. It provided almost certain sleep in 7 to 8 minutes and was of special value before ether induction, because unlike the barbiturates used later, it had a bronchodilating effect that facilitated rather than retarded induction. However, the drug required preparation immediately before use. That, in addition to the repeated occurrence of fecal incontinence, led to its abandonment.

Between 1925 and 1940, activity in both pediatric surgery and anesthesia began to accelerate. William Ladd, whose interest stemmed from his experience in caring for children injured in a massive explosion in Halifax, Nova Scotia in 1917, led the

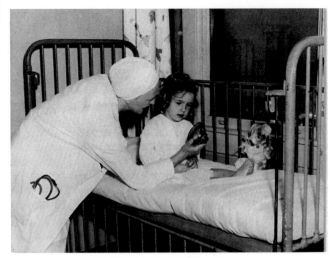

■ **FIGURE 41-1.** Ms. Betty Lank served as chief nurse anesthetist at Children's Hospital Boston from 1935 to 1969.

development of pediatric surgery in North America (Goldbloom, 1917; Steward, 1983; Smith, 1959). His work at Children's Hospital Boston was devoted to the correction of neonatal defects, including harelip. Ladd performed harelip repair seated, with the infant held facing him in the lap of a nurse. The anesthetist stood behind the nurse, directing ether from a vaporizing bottle into the infant's mouth via a metal mouth hook.*

The introduction of cyclopropane in 1930 proved particularly helpful for pediatric anesthetists in the management of infants, although it required assembly of a closed-system apparatus. Lamont and Harmel developed a miniaturization of the to-and-fro canisters Waters described in Wisconsin, and they used this technique for Blalock's "blue baby" (tetralogy of Fallot) operations at Johns Hopkins Hospital. In Boston, Betty Lank,[†] an enterprising nurse anesthetist, further redesigned the miniature to-and-fro apparatus with less dead space and shrank adult celluloid masks to infant size, enabling her to provide anesthesia, relaxation, and controlled respiration for Ladd's infants as well as for Robert Gross' widely heralded division of a patent ductus arteriosus in 1938—without endotracheal intubation (Fig. 41-1).

By 1940, considerable progress had been made in the ability of minimally trained anesthetists to provide satisfactory operating conditions for the surgeons of that time (Smith, 1959). Ladd strenuously corrected the previous concept by establishing the dictum "The child is not a little man." Supportive warming, preoperative correction of electrolyte balance, and intraoperative charting became standardized. Clinical signs of anesthetic depth, described by Guedel in 1937, served well. This might be termed the height of the art of pediatric anesthesia in the United States, where simple expedients still prevailed.

In England, there had been more progress in airway control. After World War I, Magill and Rowbotham popularized tracheal

intubation for adult procedures, and in 1937, Philip Ayre of Newcastle-Upon-Tyne reported his classic method of endotracheal intubation with a T-tube device for harelip repair in neonates (Ayre, 1937). Although Robson of Toronto had described intubation of children using digital guidance rather than a laryngoscope, it had received little attention (Robson, 1936).

PHASE II: EMERGENCE OF PEDIATRIC ANESTHESIA, 1940 TO 1960

Factors in the Rapid Development of Interest

Before and during this period, activity accelerated in related fields, and much information became available defining normal and abnormal infants in such texts as Clement Smith's *The Physiology of the Newborn Infant* (1945), Taussig's *Congenital Malformations of the Heart* (1947), and Nelson's *Textbook of Pediatrics* (1950). The practice of adult anesthesia had become established, providing fresh information on new agents and techniques easily adaptable to children. As yet, the only established pediatric anesthesiologist in North America was Charles Robson in Toronto; in England, it was Robert Cope at London's Hospital for Sick Children. Among those interested in pediatric anesthesia, M. Digby Leigh made himself well known (Fig. 41-2). Trained by Waters in Wisconsin, Leigh was appointed head of anesthesia at Montreal Children's Hospital, where he taught and (with his invaluable associate Kathleen Belton) authored *Paediatric Anaesthesia* (1948) the first North American text on this subject. Leigh and Belton described the use of spinal anesthesia for intrathoracic procedures, an original pediatric circle absorption apparatus, and a nonrebreathing valve. Leigh moved to Vancouver, British Columbia in 1947 and then to Los Angeles in 1954, where he started the first annual pediatric anesthesia teaching conference in America. He was a brilliant technician and a stern teacher, and he delighted his audiences with his

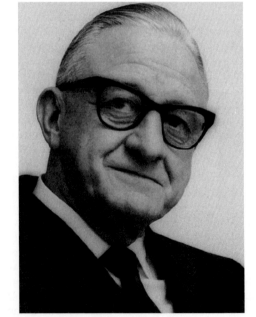

■ **FIGURE 41-2.** Dr. M. Digby Leigh.

---

*An accurate description of the first anesthetic agents given by one of the writers (RMS) for Dr. Ladd at Children's Hospital Boston in 1946.

[†]Ms. Lank, who served as chief nurse anesthetist at Children's Hospital Boston from 1935 to 1969, was one of several remarkable nurses who provided much of the anesthesia care for children at major pediatric centers in the United States until physician anesthesiologists trained and experienced during World War II returned home and began developing interest and expertise in pediatric care.

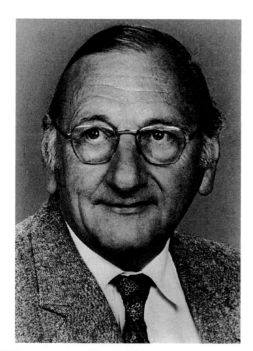

FIGURE 41-3. Dr. G. Jackson Rees.

stinging repartee. His foresighted attempts to monitor exhaled carbon dioxide in 1952, however, were rebuffed by incredulous scoffers (Conn, 1992).

In the meantime, in Liverpool, G. Jackson Rees (Fig. 41-3) had been named anesthetist at the Alder Hey Children's Hospital by his mentor and teacher, Cecil Grey. Together they conceived the idea that practically all surgery could be performed under the simple and nonexplosive combination of nitrous oxide and curare. Rees, adapting the Ayre T-tube system by adding an expiratory limb and breathing bag (the well-known Jackson-Rees system), proceeded to carry out this concept with astounding success. With minor alterations this technique was to survive through years of short-lived, complicated types of apparati. Rees' conviction that respiration should be controlled in infants with reduced tidal volumes and rates of 60 to 80 breaths per minute also met with criticism, but it proved to be rational when increased tidal volumes were found to cause barotrauma (volutrauma) and surfactant inactivation.

The new field of pediatric surgery, spearheaded by Gross, was calling for more skilled anesthetists, and at the end of World War II, large numbers of young physicians were released from military service, many of whom chose the uncharted field of pediatric anesthesia. McQuiston and Smith found posts at children's hospitals in Chicago and Boston, respectively, and Rackow worked at Columbia Presbyterian Hospital in New York, each to participate in early advances. In 1946, C. Everett Koop recruited Margo Deming to head the Department of Anesthesia at the Children's Hospital of Philadelphia as a teacher and investigator. Dr. Koop is currently a Professor at Dartmouth Medical School.

Little had happened in the field of anesthesia on the home front during World War II. After the war, numerous problems, many not even envisioned at the outset, were resolved by the exceptionally harmonious cooperation between pediatric surgeons and anesthesiologists. Whereas the success of individual operations is the natural goal of the surgeon, and improved

supportive measures are the steps noted by anesthesiologists, all are interdependent and are considered together.

Foundations of Clinical Control and Support

Neonatal Surgery and Anesthesia

Among the surgical challenges in the beginning of the 1940s, three congenital defects were dominant: tracheoesophageal fistula (TEF), omphalocele, and congenital diaphragmatic hernia (CDH). Both Leven and Ladd performed secondary multiprocedure repair of TEF in 1939 (Smith, 1959). Primary repair, first accomplished by Haight in 1941, then became the most important challenge in pediatric surgery, each case demanding all-day and all-night efforts of all participants. In Boston, the operation was carried out with the patient under the influence of cyclopropane via mask with a to-and-fro apparatus and the endotracheal intubation being reserved for emergency use during operation. Control of the exposed pleura during esophageal anastomosis required complete immobility, and the operation, in the words of Ladd, was "like stitching the wing of a butterfly" (Smith, 1959). Supportive management played a large part in the survival of these infants, both during and after the operation. Warmth was maintained by heating and humidifying the operating room, wrapping limbs in sheet-wadding, and using a semiclosed to-and-fro absorption technique. Blood pressure was measured by a locally introduced cuff with a latex bladder encircling the arm (Fig. 41-4). Fluids and blood were administered via a open-top burette with rubber tubing and "cut down" metal cannula in the saphenous vein. Postoperative survival depended largely on the remarkably able services of one or two very special nurses.

Repair of omphalocele posed different problems. Here the forceful closure of the abdomen over the extruded viscera often caused severe compression of the lungs and abdominal blood vessels. The challenge to the anesthetist was that of providing

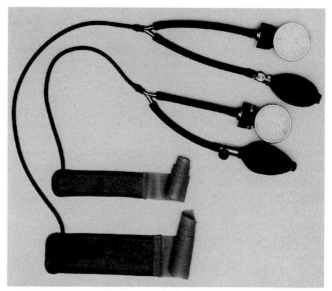

FIGURE 41-4. Smith's latex blood pressure cuffs: newborn and infant sizes.

adequate relaxation while preserving ventilation and circulation. Skin closure was possible only rarely, leaving the alternative of delayed closure, which often failed. The use of muscle relaxants facilitated closure but increased the risk of postoperative hypoventilation. Mortality was appreciable.

Of the three defects, CDH at first appeared to be the easiest to correct, and anesthesia often was managed with open-drop ether without mortality. By 1950, however, postoperative deaths became an obvious and unsolved problem. It later became evident that the CDH-related deaths occurred in the sickest of infants, who in an earlier time would have died before repair could be attempted. The management of CDH subsequently became, and still is, one of the most engrossing problems of neonatal surgery.

Herniorrhaphy and Pyloromyotomy

During this time period, herniorrhaphy and pyloromyotomy could be performed with a patient under local anesthesia by the average surgeon, but open-drop divinyl ether (Vinethene) was definitely preferable. The problem most often encountered in infants with inguinal hernia was whether to cancel the operation when the infant's hemoglobin was 9.8 g/dL instead of the "required" 10 g/dL, or to transfuse. Transfusion commonly was chosen. Before 1912, attempts to correct pyloric stenosis by gastroenterostomy had resulted in a 50% mortality rate. The Ramstedt pyloromyotomy effected one of the great achievements of pediatric surgery in creating a simple procedure for this common lesion, thereby saving the life of an otherwise normal child. Anesthetic management after early diagnosis was centered on the prevention of aspiration of the accumulated stomach contents and was best accomplished by drainage via a large-bore urethral catheter immediately before operation. In Boston, trachea intubation was not considered necessary unless contrast medium had been used for diagnosis, whereas intubation was routinely used in other centers. In cases of delayed diagnosis, the operation was postponed for rehydration and correction of electrolyte disorders or anemia.

Early Attempts to Control Fear

It soon became evident that for the small child, the fear of needles and the horrors of anesthetic induction were deeply upsetting and of long duration. Concern about this most unfortunate anesthetic by-product was voiced by psychologists, pediatricians, anesthesiologists, and others, as well as numerous mothers reporting prolonged night terrors, bed-wetting, and dependence (Levy, 1945; Jackson, 1951; Eckenhoff, 1953).

Some attention had been paid to premedication shortly before this time. French Armand-Delille (1932) recommended morphine, and Waters (1938) promoted the combination of morphine and scopolamine, but the response to the outburst of concern came in a flood of reports on a variety of ineffective agents. The basic error in most studies was, and still is, the use of age or weight for estimation of drug dosage, when neither reflects the child's state of mind. General use of intramuscular barbiturates plus morphine mixed with either atropine or scopolamine resulted in severe horror of needles, an uncomfortably dry mouth, and an unpredictable degree of sedation, seldom better than 65% successful. Attempts to improve this record continued to play a large part in the activities and literature of pediatric anesthesiologists with only slight improvement

with regard to the effectiveness of sedative drugs. However, the concentration of attention of numerous investigators on this problem did result in the development of close personal interest in each child studied, possibly responsible for much of the benefit credited to the drug being promoted.

Methods of induction showed somewhat more success than those of sedation. Thiopental replaced rectal tribromoethanol, providing greater ease of administration via either the intravenous or the rectal route, whereas induction with nitrous oxide, cyclopropane, or divinyl ether eliminated much use of the dreaded ether (Weinstein, 1939). With the repeated failure of sedative agents, greater skills were developed by caring anesthetists to gain the confidence of children in preoperative visits and then to divert their attention at induction by telling them stories or by simply lulling them to sleep. Hypnosis was used for induction by Betcher (1958), Marmer (1959), and a few others for the total operation in short procedures. It was particularly valuable for the repair of facial lacerations in small children who had recently eaten. Unfortunately, this potentially useful and harmless method gained only limited acceptance.

Control of the Airway

The importance of airway management became evident with the first anesthesia procedures, and after years of progress it still presents formidable difficulties. For patients of all ages, hypoxia resulting from laryngospasm, oral secretions or blood, abscesses or tumors, aspiration of vomitus, or simply blockage by the tongue has been an ever-present danger. Many deaths from early harelip procedures resulted primarily from hemorrhage, as did later deaths from tonsillectomy.

By 1940, two simple but extremely fundamental aids had been introduced. To prevent obstruction by the tongue, metal and rubber oral airways had been used successfully for a decade and were often fitted with a metal nipple for insufflation of vaporized ether. Suction apparatus was first available in the form of bulb syringes used alone or fitted with rubber catheters and then later as portable motorized pumps situated at the head of the operating table (ether and cyclopropane notwithstanding) or by means of a centrally operated pipeline.

Endotracheal Intubation

The greatest advance in pediatric anesthesia between 1940 and 1960 was in control of the airway by tracheal intubation. Early use in England and Canada met with little resistance. In the United States, however, opposition by surgeons raised the first major obstacle to progress in the new specialty. (It must be admitted that reasonable concern had been aroused in those who had witnessed the traumatic attempts of inexperienced individuals to perform unnecessary intubations.) It was the efforts of Rees in England; Leigh, then in Canada; the British-American Gillespie (1939); Americans Deming (1952), Pender (1954), and others; and their supportive younger surgeons that brought forth grudging acceptance of tracheal intubation of infants and children in the United States in the 1940s and 1950s.

The ongoing development of this technique led to an increased understanding of laryngeal anatomy; replacement of the "classic" hyperextension of the head by use of the "sniffing" position for intubation; a succession of different types of tracheal tubes, including the tapered tube of Cole (1945) that enjoyed more than a decade of popularity; a variety of tube materials progressing from coarse rubber to nonreactive plastic; and laryngoscopes of several types and sizes (Eckenhoff, 1951).

As with ether and other major advances, the advent of tracheal intubation brought a host of disadvantages and a few real dangers that in turn led to a glut of literature concerning complications, including subglottic stenosis, laryngeal irritation from large tubes, and tracheitis caused by contamination (Baron and Kohlmoos, 1951; Flagg, 1951; Smith, 1953a; Colgan and Keats, 1957). This proved to be just the beginning.

"Total Control" of Respiration: The Muscle Relaxants

After the first clinical use of d-tubocurarine by Griffith and Mitchell in Canada in 1942, Canadians and British accepted it readily and began extensive use in both children and adults, to be followed by much investigation in later years (Anderson, 1951; Stead, 1955; Leigh et al., 1957; Rees, 1958). Again, in the United States there was much opposition, this time by anesthesiologists as well as surgeons, to whom the concept of total "takeover" of an essential body function, termed *controlled respiration,* appeared to be a dangerous and unacceptable "physiologic trespass" (Gross, 1953; Beecher and Todd, 1954). Beecher threatened one of the authors of this chapter that "heads would roll" if he and others persisted in support of its use. In the meantime, Cullen (1943) had found it quite safe for adults and children, using it as a sole agent for infant surgery. This practice was abandoned after Scott Smith of Utah was tested under total curarization and suffered acutely on painful stimulation (Smith, 1947; Smith et al., 1947). As with tracheal intubation, the total acceptance of neuromuscular blocking agents in the United States required many years. By 1960, however, the terms *controlled respiration* and *assisted respiration* had gained widespread use.

Pediatric Breathing Systems: Assisted and Controlled Respiration

With the stimulating effect of ether on respiration in light surgical planes, assisted respiration was seldom needed. Open chest surgery, cyclopropane, and particularly muscle relaxants definitely changed this picture and led to a succession of considerably diverse devices (Dorsch and Dorsch, 1975). The to-and-fro absorption method, using soda-lime canisters of graduated sizes, was particularly adaptable to infants but caused heat retention and the aspiration of lime dust. For larger children, the canisters were bulky and heat retention was even more troublesome.

Special interest was taken in infant circle absorption systems. The Leigh, Ohio, and Bloomquist models were not only difficult to handle but also introduced the problems of valve resistance and dead space (Leigh and Belton, 1948).

To eliminate problems of carbon dioxide accumulation, several nonrebreathing valves were designed by Leigh and Belton (1948), Stephen and Slater (1948), and others. Although compact in design, they were not easy to manage and were definitely ill-suited for use with explosive agents.

The saga of apparatus variously called *rebreathing* (British), *nonrebreathing* (United States), and *partial rebreathing* (general) is complicated and involved numerous studies and modifications of the basic Ayre T system over 30 years (Fig. 41-5) (Ayre, 1937). After the Rees elongation of the expiratory limb

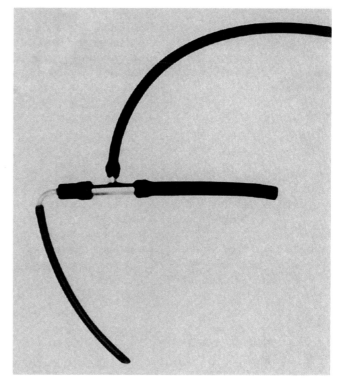

■ **FIGURE 41-5.** Original Ayre T-tube nonrebreathing system.

with an attached breathing bag, the addition of exhaust valves placed either proximal (Mapleson A) or distal (Mapleson D) to the face brought intensive examination, as did the estimation of proper flow rates of incoming gases. Evaluation by Mapleson (1954) and Inkster (1956) did much to clarify these issues at the time, but more problems lay ahead.

Cardiovascular and Thermal Control

Between 1940 and 1960, revolutionary advances were made in several areas involving the combined efforts of anesthesiologists and surgeons. The intentional reduction of arterial blood pressure, extensively explored by Enderby (1950) and others in England, was cautiously extended to pediatric use by Anderson (1955) with trimethaphan camphorsulfonate (Arfonad). This served as a reasonably safe agent. It was the initial step in induced hypotension to reduce surgical blood loss in major pediatric surgery and to prevent excessive blood pressure elevation during correction of coarctation of the aorta. However, the agent was unpredictable and soon was replaced by more controllable agents and techniques.

Controlled Reduction of Body Temperature and Cardiopulmonary Arrest

After Gross' ligation of a patent ductus arteriosus in 1938, correction of coarctation of the aorta, repair of vascular rings, and shunt procedures for tetralogy of Fallot were successfully performed under closed or semiclosed inhalation anesthesia, usually with cyclopropane (Harmel and Lamont, 1948; Harris, 1950; Smith, 1952). McQuiston, endeavoring to reduce the oxygen requirements of Dr. Potts' cyanotic infants, cooled them 3° to 4°C on a simple ice-water mattress, thereby introducing the practice of hypothermic control of body metabolism into pediatric anesthesia (McQuiston, 1949). Efforts to reduce oxygen demand by further lowering temperatures to 30° C with immersion in ice water provided surgeons time for simple intracardiac aortic or pulmonary valvotomy (Lewis and Taufic, 1953; Virtue, 1955).

The drive to bypass both the heart and lungs initiated by Gibbon in 1937 became exciting in the early 1950s, with competing surgeons Lillihei, Kirklin, and Kay and their respective anesthesiologists Matthews et al. (1957), Patrick et al. (1957), and Mendelsohn et al. (1957) all contributing toward the first practical use of the pump oxygenator in 1955, 2 years before publication of the articles cited.

The supplementation to bypass perfusion by moderate hypothermia (30° C) and different methods of induced cardiac arrest produced the greatest "takeover" of body function to date and the means of performing intracardiac surgery on all but small infants.

Mild and moderate hypothermia techniques were also used in this period for neurosurgery, orthopedic surgery, and harelip repair (Kilduff et al., 1956).

Control During Maintenance of Anesthesia

As more extensive procedures were developed and surgeons began to prefer accuracy to speed, 4-hour operations became more common and the methods of maintenance and support grew more demanding. Experience, skill, and constant observation were still primary factors that were assisted by a few simple devices (Fig. 41-6). During this time the precordial stethoscope became essential for use with every infant or child throughout the field of anesthesia (Smith, 1953b).

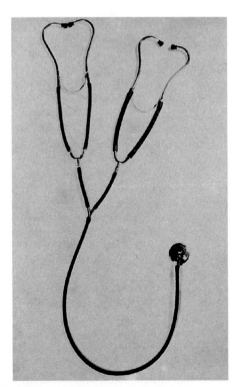

■ **FIGURE 41-6.** Smith's teaching precordial stethoscope with a single chest piece and two headpieces.

A precordial or esophageal stethoscope served first to keep the anesthetist in direct contact with the child at all times, providing unaltered information as to the clarity and strength of breath sounds and the rate, rhythm, and strength of heart sounds (Smith, 1991). Strength of heart sounds was an important guide to the degree of blood loss at that time. Arterial blood pressure could be obtainable with standard apparatus for larger children and with a specially constructed latex cuff with an inflatable bladder for infants (the Smith cuff). During this phase, the electrocardiograph was occasionally brought into operating rooms, encased in antiexplosive shielding (shaped like a torpedo) and serving relatively little purpose. Body temperature was measured intermittently at oral, nasal, or rectal sites, the standard glass thermometer giving way to the safer but less accurate thermostat devices. The anesthesia chart was considered a necessary item, gaining in importance as procedures grew increasingly complex and legal suits more common.

Control of Blood Loss

Methods of estimating blood loss at the time consisted of assessing blanching of conjunctivae, evaluating the strength of heart sounds, measuring arterial blood pressure, and weighing bloodied sponges, purposely used without moistening. Whereas speed was still considered essential in pediatric surgery during the excision of Wilms' and other large tumors, massive hemorrhage might exsanguinate small infants before replacement was possible. Attempts to restore the loss with cold, acidified blood brought failing hearts to irreversible cardiac arrest. A major advance to controlling these situations occurred when surgeons were persuaded to time their work by the advice of the anesthesiologist rather than by the clock. Although the cautery soon reduced blood loss drastically when used, it was not adopted immediately by all.

Progress in Local Anesthesia

Ladd had used local infiltration for abdominal procedures in premature infants in the late 1930s, and Leigh wrote of spinal anesthesia for open chest work in the 1940s, but improved inhalation methods outmoded both. Except for brachial plexus block, little attention was paid to these methods in the United States (Small, 1951; Eather, 1958; Smith, 1959). In many other countries, however, where inhalation anesthesia was less advanced, there was considerable dependence on regional and spinal anesthesia for both infants and children.

Halothane Opens a New Era

Although anesthesia with relaxants and nitrous oxide permitted the use of electrical instruments in the operating room, explosive gases were still popular until the introduction of halothane. After its first use in England by Johnstone in 1956 (in 10% concentration), this nonflammable, nonirritating, and potent agent was promptly introduced in Canada by Junkin et al. (1957) and in the United States by Stephen and colleagues (1958). Subsequently, flammable anesthetic agents were totally abolished in the United States, thus opening the way to revolutionary changes, first in the control of blood loss by cautery and then in the development of electronic devices for monitoring and physiologic control.

Supportive Care and Oxygen Therapy

Related fields brought important aid to pediatric anesthesiologists during this period. The time-honored rule developed by Holliday and Segar (1957) for pediatric fluid administration based on metabolic requirements serves to this day. Also of great importance, particularly in reducing the morbidity and mortality of small infants undergoing surgery, was the control of infection by the use of antibiotic agents.

The interest of pediatricians caring for neonates led to the development of enclosed incubators with regulated oxygen, warmth, and humidification for infants with respiratory distress syndrome. Improved oxygen tents were developed for older children, including those with cystic fibrosis. The poliomyelitis epidemics of the 1950s in Europe and North America initiated a succession of ventilating devices to replace the enclosed "iron lung" in use since 1929. Pediatric anesthesiologists and pediatricians shared responsibility for this work, which opened a new field for anesthesiologists.

In related areas, Virginia Apgar introduced her scoring system for neonatal assessment, Peter Safar launched his crusade for mouth-to-mouth ventilation and further work in cardiopulmonary resuscitation, and the first multidisciplinary adult intensive care unit in North America was developed (Apgar, 1953; Safar, 1958).

The first pediatric intensive care unit was established in Goteburg, Sweden, in 1955.* Similar units were established in Stockholm (Feychtung), Liverpool (Rees), and Melbourne (MacDonald and Stocks) between 1960 and 1964. In North America, the first pediatric intensive care unit was established by Downes at the Children's Hospital of Philadelphia in 1967, followed by Children's Hospital of Pittsburgh (Kampschulte), Yale-New Haven Hospital (Gilman), Massachusetts General Hospital (Todres and Shannon), and the Hospital for Sick Children in Toronto (Conn) within the next 4 years (Downes, 1992).

Teaching and Research

Throughout Europe and North America, communication among anesthesiologists began to accelerate. The Great Ormand Street Hospital for Sick Children in London and the Alder Hey Hospital in Liverpool became teaching centers in England; the Hospital for Sick Children in Toronto in Canada and the Children's Hospitals of Boston and Los Angeles in the United States became centers to which various novice and experienced anesthetists came from all parts of the world for clinical training. Residents on affiliation from teaching hospitals were rotated through brief training periods for instruction in basic, safe, and practical methods of anesthetic control of children undergoing standard operations and in special methods for those at higher risk.

On the heels of Leigh and Belton's *Pediatric Anesthesia* (1948), Stephen's *Elements of Pediatric Anesthesia* (1954) and Smith's *Anesthesia for Infants and Children* (1959) were published, with details of advances to date. Articles on new agents and techniques steadily increased in the anesthesia-related

literature. Whereas some reported personal early experiences based on limited numbers, many were of lasting value, including those involving tracheal abnormalities by Eckenhoff (1951) and Colgan and Keats (1957), tracheoesophageal repair by Zindler and Deming (1953), and the important warning of Leigh et al. (1957) concerning bradycardia after the intravenous administration of succinylcholine.

Research, on the other hand, was still in its infancy, there being little space, time, or funds for sophisticated investigation. As previously mentioned, many clinical studies offered practical current value concerning new agents and techniques. Whereas those concerning preoperative sedation outnumbered others, many reports covered airway resistance, valves, and dead space (Macon and Bruner, 1950; Mapleson, 1954; Orkin et al., 1954; Hunt, 1955; Inkster, 1956). The introduction of muscle relaxants initiated other studies, including those of Hodges (1955), Stead (1955), Telford and Keats (1957), and Bush and Stead (1962). The addition of halothane led to a more critical analysis of this agent than had been done for previous anesthetics.

This period established such fundamental techniques and basic concepts that Rees subsequently (1991) stated, "Paediatric anaesthesia in Great Britain and Ireland shows that by 1950 it had reached a point at which current practice is recognizable.... Future pediatric anaesthetists are therefore unlikely to experience the great excitement their predecessors enjoyed between 1930 and 1950, but will derive satisfaction from changes less dramatic as the curve of improvement approaches perfection."

PHASE III: ERA OF NONFLAMMABLE ANESTHETICS, 1960 TO 1980

With sound fundamental approaches defined and restrictions resulting from flammable agents eliminated, the way was cleared for rapid and extensive advances in all areas of pediatric anesthesia. Clinical control would drive ahead and research would become more productive, but this phase saw the greatest progress in the development of organized teaching and communication.

Unfortunately, progress was not marked in the control of fear. Despite continued efforts to address this problem by many skilled workers, sedatives were still unpredictable and intramuscular needles were still in general use (Poe and Karp, 1946; Rackow and Salanitre, 1962; Root, 1962). The introduction of ketamine (Ketalar) by Domino et al. (1965) created mixed feelings based on its early postoperative psychological reactions, but the agent found a place in pediatric use for uncontrollable patients and to accomplish minor but painful procedures.

A major change in the methods for controlling fear was in giving permission to parents to be at the child's bedside at all times, including "sleep-in" privileges, and later, to preinduction and induction areas. Whereas many parents were assuaged by these moves, statistics failed to show great help for the children (Schulman et al., 1967).

Increasing Clinical Precision

Modification of the partial rebreathing systems by Bain and Spoerel (1972), by which the exhalation tube passes inside the inhalation arm, provided a means of scavenging expired gases,

---

*The excellent first-hand report of Downes (1992) on the development of pediatric critical care is recommended.

thereby greatly enhancing the use of this popular pediatric method. This marked a major evolution of airway systems for pediatric anesthesia.

Steps toward greater precision in monitoring were taken in the measurement of infant blood pressure by Doppler sonography and by oscillotonometry (Dinamap) (Marcy and Cook, 1988). In the determination of arterial oxygen saturation, the transcutaneous electrode (ear oximetry) was used with limited success (Saunders et al., 1976). It was during this period that "control by the numbers" gained predominance over the unreliable art of anesthesia. Led by Downes of Philadelphia and others, arterial blood gas determinations, blood sugar, hemoglobin, electrolytes, and other measurements were serially evaluated intraoperatively in adjacent laboratories (Smith, 1990). Insertion of arterial and central venous catheters became commonplace, and urinary catheterization became an important guide to fluid and electrolyte replacement.

Progress in controlling fluid balance included the recognition of the importance of electrolytes in all intravenous solutions (Bennett et al., 1970; Herbert et al., 1971). New concepts concerning blood replacement included Davenport's practical recommendation to give blood when loss reached 10% of blood volume, followed later by Furman's more precise suggestion to maintain the hematocrit level above 28% to 30% in children and 40% in the newborn (Davenport and Barr, 1963; Furman et al., 1975). At this time, the concept of replacement of preoperative fluid deficit was widely adopted.

Airway problems presented ongoing challenges, and their management continued to register improved methods of control. Great emphasis was placed on the prevention of food aspiration and the damaging effects of hypoxia. The Sellick maneuver (1961) and many warnings from Salem (1970) about "the full stomach" were forever fixed in the mind of each new resident.

The treatment of acute epiglottitis by nasotracheal intubation instead of the former mandatory use of tracheostomy was a major change and clear advance, speeding recovery and significantly reducing serious complications (Oh and Motoyama, 1977).

Management of "the difficult airway" began to assume a larger role in both adult and pediatric anesthesia as more complicated procedures were undertaken on more deformed patients. By this time, some 120 different types of laryngoscope blades had been invented, each with some minor modifications to suit the designer, usually with no major advantage. It was the introduction of the fiberoptic laryngoscope that enabled anesthesiologists to intubate infants and children for whom this had been virtually impossible (Taylor and Towley, 1972; Stiles, 1974).

The startling appearance of what became known as malignant hyperthermia caused great concern, but widespread warnings about "triggering agents" and the discovery of a specific counteragent, dantrolene, usually brought it under reasonable control, at least when it was recognized early (Denborough et al., 1960; Britt, 1979; Gronert, 1980).

Surgical Progress

Interesting progress occurred in the evolution of infant surgery. TEF repair became a standardized procedure, and mortality was generally limited to infants with serious cardiac defects. Problems related to omphalocele repair were largely overcome by the introduction of Schuster's staged mesh sac closure (1967). CDH, however, brought about increasing difficulties as smaller

and more premature infants were encountered. Acidosis, shunting, and pulmonary hypertension posed problems yet to be solved (Raphaely and Downes, 1973; Dibbins, 1976). Attempts to use extracorporeal membrane oxygenation (ECMO) predicted later value for this procedure (Bartlett et al., 1979).

After the breakthrough in cardiac surgery accomplished by the establishment of extracorporeal circulation in larger children, the next step was to find a means of operating within the hearts of neonates without obstruction by intracardiac catheters. In 1965, the use of hyperbaric oxygenation served as a temporary answer, providing surgeons 3 to 5 minutes of inflow occlusion for the performance of aortic valvotomy and other brief procedures (Bernhard et al., 1966). The use of oxygen at 3 to 4 atmospheres of pressure substantially increased plasma oxygen-carrying capacity, while presenting increased potency of nitrous oxide and increased flammability (Smith et al., 1964).

The final hurdle in the approach to infant cardiac surgery was passed by the successful combination of deep hypothermia and extracorporeal circulation, providing time for the most complicated reconstruction of neonatal cardiac defects (Horiuchi et al., 1963; Hikasa et al., 1967). Rendering an infant virtually dead by complete cessation of respiration and circulation at a body temperature of 15° C appeared to be the ultimate in physiologic control. Agents and techniques have undergone several changes in subsequent years but remain fundamentally similar.

Somewhat less dramatic, but also of great importance, was the initiation of renal transplantation in 1954, which subsequently saved the lives of thousands of children and adults with end-stage renal disease.

Among many well-known tenets established, two of particular interest to anesthesiologists were the danger of succinylcholine in patients with elevated serum potassium levels and the evident tolerance to anesthesia in patients with hemoglobin levels as low as 6 g/dL (Powell and Miller, 1975).

The craniofacial repair devised by Tessier and others (1967) for correction of the disfiguring deformities of Apert syndrome and Crouzon disease was a bold undertaking. It was equally challenging for the anesthesiologists involved with difficult airway management, prolonged maintenance, marked fluid and blood loss, and a particularly precarious period of recovery while the child's head was so completely swathed in tight bandages that only the endotracheal tube was visible.

Anesthetic management to separate conjoined twins at birth was of such unique interest that any report of a single case was welcomed for publication. A separate team of surgeons and anesthesiologists was assigned to each twin, and multiple problems of shared organ systems, hemorrhage, and airway obstruction were noted (Furman et al., 1971; Winston et al., 1987).

Postoperative Patient Management: Ventilation, Resuscitation, and Intensive Care

For many years, much attention had been directed toward controlling the responses of children during the introductory phases of anesthesia. Postoperative care, however, often consisted of little more than a prompt return to the child's room with orders for checks every 4 hours, and nothing by mouth. The advent of various new and extensive operations made it evident that the survival of patients depended to a large extent on their supportive control during recovery—a third dimension of anesthesia.

One of the first needs to be met was the ability to provide prolonged tracheal intubation, fostered by Brandstater (1962), MacDonald and Stocks (1965), and Hatch (1968). The continuation of earlier efforts to devise ventilation machines for infants and children with cardiopulmonary pathology brought a succession of models, some as adaptations of those made for adults and others designed specifically for younger patients.

Recovery rooms or postanesthesia care units (PACUs) for routine postoperative care had been established in many hospitals over previous decades, but areas staffed by highly trained personnel and fully equipped for high-risk patient care became mandatory. The earliest units of this type, termed *critical care* or *intensive care units*, appeared in Goteburg, Sweden, in 1955; others were established in France in 1962, England in 1964, and Australia in 1963. In America they appeared in Philadelphia in 1967, Pittsburgh and Boston in 1969, and Toronto in 1971, where Conn established a prototype of the modern multidisciplinary unit for infants and children, including near-drowning survivors (Downes and Raphaely, 1975; Conn et al., 1980; Downes, 1992).

Important new approaches to resuscitation replaced such outmoded maneuvers as anal dilation, drugs promoted as respiratory stimulants, and the prone pressure method. During the trial-and-error development of pediatric cardiac surgery and the poliomyelitis epidemics, apparent death became an indication for immediate slashing into the chest and manual cardiac compression. When it became evident that the patients occasionally survived both the original insult and the therapeutic assault, the term "cardiac arrest" was coined (Singer, 1977). Because the exact cause of these mishaps commonly was uncertain, each was considered "an act of God," and successful resuscitation was considered a feather in the cap of any anesthesiologist who had been associated with one. Intelligent procedures of ventilation and closed-chest cardiac compression, combined with electric and pharmacologic stimulation, brought far greater reason, order, and success.

Organized Teaching

This period marked the definite establishment of teaching facilities for the specialized training of pediatric anesthesiologists. With markedly enlarged departmental staffs, didactic and clinical instruction became available in numerous institutions. Residents became capable of managing most types of cases and also received instruction in ancillary services. Accreditation for residency training in pediatric centers was established in Boston in 1970, to be followed by several others by 1980.

Teaching clinics were established for residents and others throughout the United States, Canada, and England. Edward Eger stood out as teacher par excellence over 3 decades. Annual symposia on pediatric anesthesia initiated by Leigh in 1962 were followed by those organized by Conn in Toronto, Downes in Philadelphia, Salem in Chicago, Ryan in Boston, and others. Literature became increasingly available in periodicals, including both new editions of previously published texts and added texts such as those by Davenport (1967) of Canada and an excellent Australian text by Brown and Fisk (1979). Early exponents of the specialty became popular at local and national meetings, and an international exchange of speakers grew rapidly, stimulating interest and exchanging information on the rapidly developing scene.

International Progress

At this time, it became evident that considerable progress was being made in many parts of the world. In France, Delegue pioneered the modern stage, her text *Memento a l'Usage de l'Anesthesiologiste-Reanimateur Pediatrique* passing through several editions. Rapid advances were taking place in France in many aspects of pediatric anesthesia. A marked difference in their approach appeared with the use of combinations of intravenous phenothiazines, antihistamines, and barbiturates in place of inhalation agents and had remarkable success (G. Durand-Gurry, personal communication, 1993). Their work in regional anesthesia and pharmacology was also outstanding (Saint Maurice et al., 1986; Murat et al., 1988). Early leaders in Europe included Suuterinen of Finland; Swensson, Feyting, and Ekstrom-Jodal of Sweden; and Rondio and Wezyk of Poland. South African and Australian workers, adopting British methods, also kept abreast or ahead of other areas. Douglas Wilson has been called the real pioneer of pediatric anesthesia in Western Australia, and Margaret McLellan, John Stocks, Ian McDonald, M.A. Denborough, and others contributed on local and international levels. Japanese interest in pediatric anesthesia began later, but proceeded vigorously beginning in 1958; the publication of *Pediatric Anesthesia* in 1958 by Onchi and Fujita served as a valuable guide (Iwai and Satoyoshi, 1992). Throughout Latin America, Brazilian physicians and others followed North American methods to some extent, but in these countries, especially in Mexico, local and regional anesthetic techniques were depended on and consequently more highly developed than inhalation anesthesia (Fortuna, 1967; Melman et al., 1975). The great number of students who studied in North America and Europe from India, the Philippine Islands, and other Asiatic areas resulted in the growth of this organized activity and clinical excellence in their respective nations.

Research Stimulated by Clinical Advances

The introduction of various breathing devices, new muscle relaxants, and halogenated agents provided material for extensive investigation. The demonstration of the more rapid uptake of anesthetic gases by infants than by adults became a classic study, as did Motoyama's measurements of pulmonary mechanics, with some of his contributions illuminating the pulmonary physiology of infants and children (Salanitre and Rackow, 1969; Motoyama, 1977; Motoyama and Cook, 1980). Bush and Stead (1962), Cook (1974), Goudsouzian et al. (1975), and other researchers did much to establish the comparable actions of successive neuromuscular blocking agents in the search for safer, shorter-acting, and reversible types (hence, greater control). The advent of new halogenated agents aroused the pharmacologic investigation of metabolism, toxicity, cardiovascular depression, and seizures, and the increased potency demanded vaporizers of greater accuracy (Brennan, 1957; Fabian et al., 1958; Lomaz, 1965). Other notable achievements included the establishment of minimum effective doses (ED_{50}) of halothane by Nicodemus and others (1969) and the minimum alveolar concentration (MAC) as a standard measure of potency, followed by the application of MAC to demonstrate the higher halothane requirement for infants than for adults (Eger et al., 1965; Gregory et al., 1969).

PHASE IV: PROGRESS AND SOPHISTICATION, 1980 TO PRESENT

This latest phase consists of many events now in progress that are described in this book. The entire scenario in the operating room has evolved enormously, with anesthesiologists setting multicomputerized monitors and infusion pumps, with numerous syringes loaded and coded, and with a large cabinet within reach that holds drugs and other equipment for all possible occasions. Children often receive an oral sedative, and anesthesia is induced with minimal resistance, often with a parent present. Variable time is then consumed while surgeons await the fixation of additional monitors, endotracheal tubes, and numerous catheters. Multiple medications are delivered by the intravenous route, generally measured by micrograms per kilogram. The ventilator is set at a prescribed rate and tidal volume or inspiratory pressure, and surgeons are allowed to approach and drape the patient, erecting a high sterile shield between themselves and the anesthesiologist. Charting is often automated. Communication occurs with other anesthesiologists and the surgeons and nurses. In long but simple cases, boredom can be a hazard, as is a tendency to watch the many monitors rather than the patient.

Fortunately, this is only one part of the picture. In the next room, a premature infant may be receiving spinal anesthesia for herniorrhaphy, and in another, a liver transplantation may have been in progress for the past 8 hours. In the many additional operating rooms, various procedures go on, more than half of which are outpatient cases.

Recognition of Risk

During this phase, there has been a widespread appreciation that infants and small children are at increased risk for complications from anesthesia and surgery. Previous reports had shown that these were often related to cardiovascular factors (including hypovolemia and anemia), respiratory difficulties (e.g., airway obstruction, hypoxia, and inadequate ventilation), or electrolyte imbalance (e.g., hyperkalemia, hyponatremia, and hypoglycemia) (Salem et al., 1975). Additional reports from the United States described some of the problems in greater detail, as did others from France, Scandinavia, Canada, and England (Olsson and Hallen, 1988; Tiret et al., 1988; Cohen et al., 1990; Lunn, 1992; Morray et al., 1993; Keenan et al., 1994; Holzman, 1994). In particular, postoperative apnea, especially in very premature infants, was noted by several investigators, and overnight hospitalization in these situations was widely adopted (Steward, 1982; Gregory and Steward, 1983; Liu et al., 1983). In addition, other groups of patients were noted to be at increased risk of postoperative respiratory complications, such as children with obstructive sleep apnea who appear more sensitive to the respiratory depressant effects of narcotics (Brown et al., 2004, 2006; Sanders et al., 2006). Furthermore, there were indications that risk in small children could be decreased if individuals specially trained and experienced in pediatric anesthesia provided the anesthesia care (Keenan et al., 1991; Morray, 1994; Berry, 1995; Downes, 1995). Although this concept remains controversial, surgeons, pediatricians, and parents increasingly have begun to appreciate the important role of pediatric anesthesiologists.

Growth in Pediatric Facilities

In part because the post-World War II "baby boomers" were now having their own children, pediatric facilities exhibited enormous growth during this period. Freestanding children's hospitals, which had existed for more than a century, expanded, and new pediatric hospitals were established. Some of these evolved as pediatric "hospitals within a hospital," whereby large general hospitals developed specific buildings, wings, or floors to provide specialized care for children. Currently, several large children's hospitals in the United States are performing more than 20,000 surgical procedures per year. Some children's hospitals perform more operations and have more operating rooms and staff than major hospitals caring for adult patients. Reports have been published indicating that the outcome (at least for some conditions in small children) is better when surgery is performed by pediatric specialists in large pediatric centers (Bratton et al., 2001; Kososka et al., 2001). The American Academy of Pediatrics (2002, 2003) has disseminated several policy statements emphasizing the need to have proper personnel and facilities available whenever children require surgery or anesthesia.

Changing Patterns of Care

There has also been a great impetus to perform surgical procedures in younger and younger patients. Whereas this was not possible or was fraught with danger in earlier eras, better equipment and surgeons well trained in pediatric subspecialties have made this not only feasible but also desirable for children. Outcome studies in several areas have shown that corrective procedures performed in infancy, rather than palliative procedures done initially and followed by full repair later in life, lead to improved long-term results. For example, in 1975 the American Academy of Pediatrics advocated surgical repair of elective urologic defects in children after the age of 4 years but by 1996 was recommending these repairs occur in infancy. Likewise, repair of congenital cardiac anomalies shifted from early palliative procedures (largely shunts) to corrective repairs in the neonatal period (Jenkins et al., 1995). This tendency to perform more complex surgical procedures in younger patients undoubtedly contributed to the growth of major pediatric centers.

At the opposite end of the age spectrum, pediatric institutions were also seeing an increasing population of older patients who had survived diseases generally considered pediatric in nature. For example, patients treated for cystic fibrosis, meningomyelocele and hydrocephalus, congenital heart disease, leukemias, and many "syndromes" were now routinely surviving into adulthood and arriving well past childhood for surgical procedures. Hospitals and their physicians catering to adults often exhibited a reluctance to manage these patients. This led to the interesting paradox of pediatric subspecialists and pediatric hospitals being involved in the ongoing management of patients who clearly are no longer children. Compounding this issue has been the growth of surgical specialties in which the care of children and adults is often undertaken simultaneously, such as fetal surgery or transplantation from living related donors. Thus, pediatric hospitals are now caring for patients well into their 20s, 30s, and beyond.

It is not simply the age of patients requiring surgery that has changed but also the setting of much of the surgery itself.

The vast majority of pediatric surgical procedures currently occurs in ambulatory patients who never remain overnight in the hospital. Patients often arrive for their procedure in the morning and go home later the same day. This creates additional challenges to anesthesiologists who must rely on surgeons to screen patients for significant coexisting medical problems, because patients are often not seen in advance of the procedure by their anesthesiologist. Even when postsurgical hospitalization is required, patients undergoing elective surgery are rarely admitted before the day of the procedure. This is the case even when the surgical procedure is quite complex, such as scoliosis repair, craniofacial reconstruction, or repair of congenital cardiac lesions. For these situations, patients can be evaluated in preoperative clinics by an anesthesiologist along with any necessary consultants. Laboratory and radiologic studies can also be obtained and blood cross-matched when necessary. This preoperative assessment also provides an opportunity to answer questions about anesthesia and the perioperative experience and to attempt to manage patient and parental anxiety.

Finally, pediatric anesthesiologists have become increasingly involved in caring for children outside the operating rooms when immobility or analgesia is required for nonsurgical procedures. This has largely occurred in the radiology departments, where increasingly sophisticated equipment and techniques have led to major advances in diagnosis (e.g., computed tomography, magnetic resonance imaging, and positron emission tomography) and new, less-invasive treatment options (e.g., in the catheterization laboratory or radiation therapy suite). Anesthesiologists are being requested to provide care for patients in several other areas of the hospital as well, including the gastrointestinal suite for endoscopy, the oncology unit for lumbar punctures and bone marrow aspirations, and so on. Whereas children clearly benefit from relief of pain and anxiety in these situations, this has greatly increased the demands for anesthesia services.

When anesthesiologists are unable or unwilling to assist in these areas, physicians from other specialties (including pediatricians, intensivists, and hospitalists) or nurses have stepped in (Malviya et al., 1997; Lowrie et al., 1998; Lightdale et al., 2008). Whether this affords a comparable degree of safety to administration of anesthesia by anesthesiologists in these situations remains to be seen. In any case, the large number of children requiring sedation or immobilization for nonoperative procedures has led to the development of sedation guidelines by several organizations representing anesthesiologists, pediatricians, emergency physicians, dentists, and others, with some variability among them (American Academy of Pediatrics, 1992; American Society of Anesthesiologists, 1996; American College of Emergency Physicians, 1997; American Academy of Pediatric Dentistry, 1997). A group of pediatric anesthesiologists at Dartmouth Hitchcock Medical Center convened in 2000 to develop a consensus among physicians from varied disciplines in this regard, and they continue to disseminate a bulletin via email to individuals interested in this ongoing issue (Dartmouth Sedation Project, 2000).

New Developments in Anesthesia

Although the scope of new developments in anesthesia is the subject of much of the remainder of this book, there are several major changes worth noting. The age-old, commonly used, restriction of preoperative intake ultimately underwent scrutiny, which resulted in changes in concept and reduction of fasting time (Coté, 1990; Ferrari et al., 1999). New, potent, inhalational anesthetic agents have been developed, virtually replacing halothane as the "standard" for the previous generation. To induce anesthesia via mask, sevoflurane is used almost exclusively, because it acts faster and results in less bradycardia and hypotension (Sarner et al., 1995; Holzman et al., 1996). This has been especially important in infants. Isoflurane is often used for maintenance of anesthesia, in part because it is currently cost effective. Desflurane may be used when particularly rapid awaking is desired, although the need for special, temperature-regulated vaporizers has limited its popularity. None of these newer agents, however, has the smooth induction properties of sevoflurane. Concerns have been raised about breakdown products that may develop when sevoflurane interacts with some carbon dioxide absorbents, especially when desiccated, leading to overheating of the absorbent system, carbon monoxide production, or both (Holak et al., 2003). The clinical significance of this remains unclear.

A new, major feature in airway management has been the promotion of the laryngeal mask airway to eliminate tracheal intubation for many simple procedures, as well as provide airway access in emergency situations when intubation is difficult (Brain, 1983; Mason and Bingham, 1990; Pennant and White, 1993). Endoscopes have also been developed that permit fiberoptic intubation even in small children.

Several "descendents" of fentanyl have been developed, with remifentanil capable of providing potent and transient analgesia when administered via constant intravenous infusion (Davis et al., 2001; Galinkin et al., 2001; Ross et al., 2001). Fentanyl transcutaneous "patches" have also been developed, largely to provide analgesia for chronic pain, and fentanyl is sometimes administered transnasally or transorally (Friesen et al., 1995; Viscusi et al., 2004). Potent opioids have been particularly useful for cardiac procedures when inhaled anesthetic agents are not well tolerated (Hickey and Hansen, 1984). Perhaps more significant, the prolonged debate over the need for anesthesia at all during surgery on small infants was finally terminated when Anand and Hickey (1987) produced evidence of physiologic stress in infants under light anesthesia. This brought general agreement that all infants should receive anesthesia during surgery, although the best method for doing this, especially when the patient is a fetus, remains to be fully elucidated.

However, concern has been expressed in recent years about potential adverse effects of many anesthetic agents on brain development. Studies in young animals receiving ketamine, midazolam, nitrous oxide, isoflurane, and other commonly used anesthetic agents have indicated increased apoptosis and cell death, at least in some experimental models, raising fears that similar findings could possibly occur when these drugs are administered to young children (Jevtovic-Todorovic and Olney, 2008). In view of the apparent increase in the incidence of autism and related disorders, much investigation is ongoing in this regard (Sun et al., 2008; Davidson et al., 2008). However, current consensus is that the benefits of a well-conducted anesthesia of the relatively brief duration necessary to perform most surgical procedures far outweigh the theoretical risk of anesthetic neurotoxicity (Soriano et al., 2005; Mellon et al., 2007; Loepke et al., 2008).

Propofol has become the most common intravenous induction agent for adults, but has not completely replaced thiopental in children because propofol causes some discomfort when injected into small peripheral veins. Midazolam has replaced diazepam as the intravenous benzodiazepine of choice for sedation in children; it is also the most popular oral sedative in the preoperative setting (Kain et al., 2000). Midazolam can be administered via several other routes (including intranasal) and is sometimes used rectally because production of methohexital, which is often used for this purpose, has ceased for economic reasons. The use of topical agents including lidocaine-prilocaine (EMLA; Freeman et al., 1993) or lidocaine-tetracaine (Synera; Sethna et al., 2005) for skin desensitization eases the discomfort of venipuncture for intravenous induction but requires adequate time to become effective. Intramuscular injections are now rarely necessary in pediatric anesthesia practice.

Several new, nondepolarizing muscle relaxants have replaced curare. Although pancuronium is commonly used for lengthy procedures, several shorter-acting agents (especially cisatracurium and vecuronium) are often administered for brief procedures and have fewer side effects. Rocuronium is often used to facilitate emergency endotracheal intubation, and succinylcholine is no longer administered without good cause because masseter spasm, malignant hyperthermia, or both occasionally develop after its administration, especially in the presence of potent inhaled anesthetic agents (Schwartz et al., 1984). In addition, the Food and Drug Administration (1997) issued a "black box" warning because of serious complications (including cardiac arrest resulting from acute hyperkalemia) associated with its use, particularly in young boys with unrecognized muscular dystrophy.

Although there was some use of local and regional anesthesia for children before 1940, the development of improved inhalation methods soon largely displaced other forms of anesthesia. Regional anesthesia became more commonplace in children, beginning in Europe with "single-shot" techniques (e.g., spinal, caudal, or peripheral nerve block) reducing the requirements for general anesthesia and providing postoperative analgesia (Abajian et al., 1984; Yaster and Maxwell, 1989; Dalens, 1989; Bosenberg and Ivani, 1998; Williams et al., 2006). Small, portable ultrasound machines have been introduced, which add great precision to the ability to deliver local anesthetic solutions to the desired location (Willschke et al., 2005, 2006; Marhofer et al., 2005; Marhofer and Chan, 2007; Tran et al., 2008). In addition, continuous infusions of local anesthetics with or without fentanyl are often delivered intraoperatively and postoperatively via catheters placed during surgery, especially via the epidural route. This reflects the much greater emphasis on the needs of the pediatric patient in the postoperative period. Pain control after surgery has been a major focus of pediatric anesthesiologists with patient-, parent-, or nurse-controlled analgesia available via computer-controlled infusion pumps for delivery of medications by the intravenous, epidural, or perineural route (Ganesh et al., 2007). Pain treatment services have become more important aspects of the mission of most departments of pediatric anesthesia to provide care for children with medical and surgical pain (Zeltzer et al., 1989; Berde and Sethna, 2002; Schecter et al., 2002).

In addition, outpatient pain treatment clinics evaluate and treat many chronic pain conditions in childhood; although largely directed by anesthesiologists, these are multidisciplinary (using nerve blocks, oral medications, acupuncture, hypnosis, and behavioral modification) and involve the participation of neurologists, neurosurgeons, physiatrists, physical therapists, psychologists, and many other ancillary medical and nursing

personnel. Greater attention has been directed toward assessing and allaying preoperative fears and anxiety of patients and their families. Preoperative clinics are used to evaluate many patients in advance of their procedures, and significant attention has been devoted to methods of easing induction of anesthesia, especially the use of oral premedicants and parental presence during mask induction (Kain et al., 1998a, 1998b, 2000, 2003). In all instances, kindness remains the essential feature in preoperative management.

Progress in Monitoring

Technical advances have also greatly enhanced patient monitoring. Smaller equipment is now readily available so that young patients can be monitored as carefully as critically ill adults. Percutaneous catheters can be inserted directly into virtually any peripheral vein or artery; the Seldinger technique (if necessary with ultrasound guidance) can be used to insert central catheters (Ganesh and Jobes, 2008). Echocardiography can be performed transthoracically or transesophageally in small children as well as in adults. Its use has greatly facilitated the ability of cardiac surgeons to assess the repair of congenital heart lesions intraoperatively (Ungerleider et al., 1990). "Standard" monitoring is now quite extensive and sophisticated as promulgated by the American Society of Anesthesiologists (1986) and includes continuous pulse oximetry and capnography. It appears that the average anesthesiologist is often able to manage a procedure with little or no direct observation of the patient, although a precordial or an esophageal stethoscope is still considered valuable by many pediatric anesthesiologists.

Advances in the intensive care unit also have been significant during this time and extend into the operating rooms. Patients with severe lung injury are now managed with several new forms of respiratory support, including advanced mechanical ventilators, inhaled nitric oxide, and extracorporeal membrane oxygenation or ECMO (Neonatal Inhaled Nitric Oxide Study Group, 1997; Bartlett et al., 2000; Aharon et al., 2001; Campbell et al., 2003). This latter technique can be used for weeks at a time and as an emergency method of resuscitation from cardiac arrest when a reversible condition is suspected (Laussen, 2002).

Advances in Surgery

Numerous developments have occurred in surgical techniques that have greatly influenced anesthesia practice and are discussed elsewhere in this text. However, it is worthwhile noting that laparoscopic techniques, robotics, and intraoperative imaging have progressed so extensively and rapidly into pediatric practice that anesthesiologists have had to accommodate the special problems and challenges presented by these situations. Perhaps nowhere is this more apparent than the field of fetal surgery where surgeons, obstetricians, anesthesiologists, and neonatologists must collaborate to care for two patients simultaneously, as techniques for surgical repair of prenatal anomalies are developed and assessed (Harrison et al., 1982, 1993; Rosen, 1992; Cauldwell, 2002). Controversy remains, however, about the best way to provide analgesia during fetal procedures (Benatar and Benatar, 2001; Myers et al., 2002; Schwartz and Galinken, 2003; Lee et al., 2005).

Organ transplantation has extended beyond kidneys, and transplantation of the liver has become a major challenge for pediatric surgeons and anesthesiologists (Starzl et al., 1963). To support a young patient with hepatic failure through a repeat liver transplant potentially requiring replacement of multiple blood volumes while monitoring and maintaining cardiac function, temperature, and many components of blood chemistry during an 8- to 12-hour operation is one of the most demanding anesthesia-related tasks known. The record of 1000 liver transplantations performed at the Children's Hospital of Pittsburgh between 1980 and 1990 with a nearly 70% survival rate stands as a remarkable accomplishment of both surgeons and anesthesiologists (Robertson and Borland, 1990). Transplantation of the heart, lungs, or both appears similarly impressive, although it is not associated with the same degree of blood loss (Jamieson et al., 1984). Intestinal transplants more recently have emerged as a potential method for treating children with short bowel syndrome (Mazariegos et al., 2008). In any case, a shortage of available organs, especially those of a small size, greatly limits pediatric transplantation, and attempts to grow organs in cell culture has evolved into the new and fascinating field of tissue engineering (Langer and Vacanti, 1993; Lanza et al., 2000; Dunn, 2008).

Research Efforts

Activity in research is reaching a new level of excellence and productivity, whereas demands for clinical service and limitations of funding make this an ongoing challenge, and old problems persist. As noted by Berry (1993), failure in the endless search for better preoperative sedation lies in controversies regarding basic ground rules for investigation, especially in children. In many fields, understanding of the problems has been gradually extended, with resultant improvement in the practical management of patients. Physiologic studies of cerebral circulation in the neonate by Rogers and colleagues (1980), gas exchange in cardiac patients, pharmacologic biotransformation of sedatives, the infant and the myoneural junction, and hypoxia in children who have undergone anesthesia are but a few of the important initial studies (Goudsouzian and Standaert, 1986; Motoyama and Glazener, 1986; Saint-Maurice et al., 1986; Lindahl, 1989; Fletcher, 1993). The report by Lerman and others (1986) concerning postanesthetic vomiting after strabismus surgery is another illustration of one of the problems of the conscious child that remains particularly difficult to control. Advances in molecular biology, mapping the human genome, and genomic pharmacology offer great hope that it will be possible to "customize" care for individual patients in a continuing attempt to drive the curve of improvement mentioned by Rees (1991) "closer to perfection" (Holtzman and Marteau, 2000).

Development of the Subspecialty

Pediatric anesthesia organizations have advanced greatly over the recent generation. Although a small group of anesthesiologists from the United States and Canada have had a section within the American Academy of Pediatrics since 1966 (now called the Section on Anesthesiology and Pain Medicine), it was not until 1973 that pediatric activities formally became a part of the American Society of Anesthesiologists. At this same time, a separate organization devoted to pediatric anesthesiology was established in the United Kingdom, but it was not until 1986 that the Society for Pediatric Anesthesia (SPA) was created in the United States. This is now the largest organization in the world devoted to pediatric anesthesiology with more than 4000 members largely from the United States. The SPA has held annual meetings since 1987 in association with the annual meeting of the American Society of Anesthesiologists. For several years, it has also organized an additional winter educational meeting. The goals of the SPA are listed in Box 41-1; the SPA's presidents are listed in Table 41-1.

The SPA collaborated with other pediatric anesthesiology groups in developing a proposal to have fellowship training formally accredited by the Accreditation Council for Graduate Medical Education (Rockoff and Hall, 1997). This was successful in 1997, and there are currently 45 programs in the United States that offer 1 year of training in pediatric anesthesiology to individuals who have completed a basic residency in anesthesiology (Accreditation Council for Graduate Medical Education, 2008). Furthermore, subspecialization within pediatric anesthesiology continues to advance informally with individuals developing additional experience in areas such as pediatric pain medicine, pediatric intensive care, pediatric cardiac anesthesiology, and others.

Box 41-1 Goals of the Society for Pediatric Anesthesia

1. To advance the practice of pediatric anesthesia through new knowledge
2. To provide educational programs on clinical, scientific, and political issues that are important to pediatric anesthesia practice
3. To promote scientific research in pediatric anesthesia and related disciplines
4. To provide a forum for exchange of ideas and knowledge among practitioners of pediatric anesthesia
5. To support the goals of the American Society of Anesthesiologists and the American Academy of Pediatrics

TABLE 41-1. Presidents of the Society for Pediatric Anesthesia

Year	President	Location
1986 to 1988	Myron Yaster, MD	Baltimore, Md.
1988 to 1990	Robert Crone, MD	Seattle, Wash.
1990 to 1992	Aubrey Maze, MD	Phoenix, Ariz.
1992 to 1994	Charles Lockhart, MD	Denver, Colo.
1994 to 1996	William Greeley, MD	Durham, N.C.
1996 to 1998	Mark Rockoff, MD	Boston, Mass.
1998 to 2000	Steven Hall, MD	Chicago, Ill.
2000 to 2002	Peter Davis, MD	Pittsburgh, Pa.
2002 to 2004	Anne Lynn, MD	Seattle, Wash.
2004 to 2006	Francis McGowan, MD	Boston, Mass.
2006 to 2008	Jayant Deshpande, MD	Nashville, Tenn.
2008 to 2010	Joseph Tobin, MD	Winston-Salem, N.C.

Finally, many additional textbooks directed to pediatric anesthesia have been published, and several have been updated into multiple editions; these include texts by Gregory (2002), Coté et al. (2009), Motoyama and Davis (2006), Berry (1990), Brown and Fisk (1992), Sumner and Hatch (1999), Steward and Lerman (2001), Bisonnette and Dalens (2002), and others. The further development of pediatric anesthesiology into subspecialties became evident in texts on topics such as uncommon diseases, neonatal anesthesia, pediatric pain regional anesthesia, cardiac anesthesia, and intensive care (Dalens et al., 1990; Saint-Maurice and Steinberg, 1990; Bush and Harkins, 1991; Katz and Steward, 1993; Hatch et al., 1995; Rogers, 1996; Tobias and Deshpande, 1996; Todres and Fugate, 1996; Schechter et al., 2002; Lake and Booker, 2004). The journal *Paediatric Anaesthesia*, originally edited by Bush in Liverpool and Saint-Maurice in Paris, became the first independent monthly publication devoted to this field. With its international editorial board members, it has led to enhanced worldwide relationships among pediatric anesthesiologists. *Anesthesia & Analgesia*, one of the largest anesthesia journals in the world, has also developed a separate section devoted to pediatric anesthesia. Furthermore, pediatric anesthesiologists are members of the editorial boards of *Anesthesiology* and several other well-respected international anesthesia journals.

SUMMARY

Pediatric anesthesia has advanced enormously from the days when anesthesiologists and surgeons adapted adult techniques and equipment to small children. It is clear that pediatric anesthesiology is a well-established and well-recognized subspecialty in its own right. It is one of the most popular fields to pursue for further training after the basic anesthesia residency, and its practitioners are desired by surgeons, pediatricians, and parents alike.

Challenges are ongoing as more complex surgical and diagnostic techniques are performed on younger and younger patients. Society will always have limited resources, and ensuring adequate allocation of funding, personnel, and research priorities is an increasing problem as the baby-boomer population ages, adults live longer with more complicated medical conditions, and geriatric problems demand society's greater attention.

Nevertheless, history has shown that talented and dedicated individuals can and will meet the challenges ahead, and there are few who doubt that things are better now for pediatric anesthesiologists—and their patients—than ever before.

REFERENCES

Complete references used in this text can be found online at www.expertconsult.com.

Medicolegal and Ethical Aspects

CHAPTER

42

Jessica Davis

Physicians are confronted with a variety of unique legal issues on a daily basis. It would be nearly impossible to cover all of them—even in broad strokes—in a single chapter. Accordingly, this chapter focuses on two issues that may be of specific importance to pediatric physicians: informed consent and related medical malpractice actions. It is important to note at the outset that this chapter is intended to provide only a broad overview of these issues; in most cases, the nuances of these issues are dictated by state laws. As such, the relevant state's laws should be consulted for more specific legal authority on these issues. This chapter attempts, however, to lay out the variety of considerations at play when determining whether both an adult and a minor patient have provided their informed consent to accept or decline the relevant medical treatment. It also provides an outline of two specific types of medical malpractice actions: one based on informed consent and one based on a negligence theory, which comprises the majority of malpractice actions in this country.

INFORMED CONSENT

Patient consent is one of the most prominent issues facing medical providers today. Consent becomes even more complicated when a patient is a minor. Recall the recent case of 12-year-old Parker Jensen, who was diagnosed with an extremely rare and aggressive cancer, Ewing's sarcoma, after physicians removed a tumor from the soft tissue of his mouth (Foy, 2003b; Watts, 2005). Parker's parents were undecided about the right course of treatment for their son and wanted to seek a second opinion (Foy, 2003a). Parker's physicians, however, sought a court order to remove Parker from his home in order for him to begin 49 weeks of chemotherapy that they—not necessarily Parker—believed was the appropriate course of treatment (Foy, 2003a). A battle ensued between Parker's parents and the state of Utah; the end result was that kidnapping and child neglect charges were filed against Parker's parents (Foy, 2003a). Parker's opinion was not nearly—if at all—as highly publicized.

The specific issues facing physicians are whose consent actually is required when the patient is a minor and what informed consent means for the practitioner.

Background

The notion of consent itself can be traced back to the laws of battery and trespass. In 1914 Judge Benjamin Cardozo likened assault to trespass of the body. He wrote, "Every human being of adult years and sound mind has a right to determine what shall be done with his own body; and a surgeon who performs an operation without his patient's consent commits an assault, for which he is liable in damages" (*Schloendorff v. Society of NY Hosp,* 1914). Thus, began the legal analysis of the notion of consent.

The issue of consent—and the circumstances under which a patient may be said to have consented to certain medical treatment—is an important one for physicians. Without patient consent to treatment, physicians may be sued for battery—the violation of a person's right to be free from unwanted touching (*McNeil v. Brewer,* 1999*; Syoboda et al., 2000). Subject to certain exceptions, such as emergencies that pose threats to a patient's life, any willful touching of another is unlawful without valid consent from the individual or another authorized to consent on that person's behalf (Syoboda et al., 2000). The requirement of consent primarily protects the patient's bodily integrity (Syoboda et al., 2000).

Informed Consent

Consent, however, gives the physician a privilege that protects him or her against liability for this tort as long as the patient is informed of the nature and consequences of treatment and

---

*For example, finding that an inmate's inclusion in a medical study did not constitute offensive conduct, an element of battery, when no blood was drawn without the inmate's consent.

gives knowing and intelligent consent to the proposed treatment the physician intends to provide (Schlam and Wood, 2000). "Informed consent" is designed to protect the individual's autonomy in medical decision making; in other words, it is a real-world application of the adage that "every person has the right to determine what is done to his own body" (Schlam and Wood, 2000).

In turn, physicians are obligated to provide the patient with a "reasonable amount of information" for the patient to be able to make an informed decision (Schlam and Wood, 2000). It is worth noting here that some jurisdictions reject this approach for one that shifts the focus to what a "reasonable patient would need to know," a standard that does not require expert testimony and thereby eases a patient's burden of proof (Altman et al., 1992; Schlam and Wood, 2000). In other words, the patient must know for what he or she is giving consent (Syoboda et al., 2000). Informed consent is the "autonomous authorization of medical intervention … by individual patients" (Beauchamp and Faden, 1995; Syoboda et al., 2000). It can really only follow after a discussion regarding the "nature of the proposed treatment procedures, possible alternative treatments, and the nature and the degree of the risk and benefits involved in accepting or rejecting treatment." Consent is then considered "informed" when it is given "knowingly, competently, and voluntarily" (Schlam and Wood, 2000). It is worth noting, however, that if a physician doesn't provide enough information to make an informed treatment and the patient consents, the physician may still be liable for negligence (Schlam and Wood, 2000).

Knowingly means that the physician has a duty of disclosure to provide adequate information to the patient in a manner that the patient can comprehend (Syoboda et al., 2000). "Adequate" means "the amount and kind of information that the average person in the patient's position would want to have in reaching an informed decision" (Syoboda et al., 2000). This usually means that the clinician must fully explain the proposed procedure, the expected short-term risks and long-term consequences, the available alternatives and their risks and benefits, and the consequences of declining or delaying treatment (Syoboda et al., 2000). In short, physicians must disclose all material information; i.e., all "information which the physician knows or should know would be regarded as significant by a reasonable person in the patient's position when deciding to accept or reject a recommended medical procedure" (*Arato v. Avedon,* 1993; Syoboda et al., 2000).

Competently means that the patient has the capacity, or ability, to understand "information relating to treatment decisions and to appreciate the consequences of a decision" (Syoboda et al., 2000). That a decision be made competently requires physicians to assess whether a patient can both understand the relevant medical information and make a rational decision based on that information (Syoboda et al., 2000).

The voluntariness requirement simply protects the patient's right to make health care decisions free from manipulation or undue influence (Syoboda et al., 2000). Because of the power imbalance between a physician and the patient and the sometimes vulnerable state of the patient, there is a great danger of undue influence; as such, the manner in which physicians present information can significantly influence the relative importance the patient may attach to certain information and could persuade the patient to favor the option emphasized by the physician. Accordingly, physicians have a duty to distance themselves from their personal preferences and allow their presentation of information to reflect an objective assessment of the various interests at stake for the patient (Syoboda et al., 2000).

Background: Consent by Minor

As outlined above, competent adults are entitled to make decisions regarding their medical care themselves. But the framework of consent changes if the patient is a minor (Syoboda et al., 2000). The legal framework of consent highlights the courts' recognition that the family must be protected by a broad right of privacy, limiting government interference in the intimate family workings (Watts, 2005). That right of privacy, however, is balanced by the fact that the state is permitted, in certain circumstances, to make determinations about the best interests of the child (Watts, 2005). When such a conflict arises—perhaps relating to the type, length, and necessity of medical treatments for a child, the question is about who possesses the ultimate right to make a child's medical decisions (Watts, 2005). When does a minor have the right to have a voice in medical decisions regarding his or her own well being? Even if the minor has a voice, when is that voice determinative?

An analysis of a minor's right to participate in his or her health care decisions reflects a huge variation from state to state over the amount, if any, of deference given to a minor to consent or refuse medical treatment (Watts, 2005). Traditionally, the view was that parents had total autonomy over a child's medical care. That idea can be traced back to a time when children were considered the property of their parents (Schlam and Wood, 2000). Before that time, children had no rights, and parents reared their children without government restraint (Schlam and Wood, 2000). The Supreme Court has articulated several justifications for total parental autonomy (*Parham v. JR,* 1979; Watts, 2005). Primarily, they rest in the presumptions that children lack the maturity, experience, and capacity to make appropriate decisions and that the "natural bonds of affection" between parents and children will lead parents to act in the best interest of their children (*Parham v. JR,* 1979; Watts, 2005). Since that time, however, the Supreme Court has modified the notion of absolute parental autonomy in order to account for the interest of minors, particularly in the arena of health care decisions (Watts, 2005). The idea is that there are better means for protecting parental autonomy than disregarding the desires of the children (Hawkins, 1996; Schlam and Wood, 2000). Jurisdictions vary in the deference given to parental autonomy over a child's health care (Watts, 2005).

Typically, the current view is that for most treatment provided to children, informed consent is provided by parents or guardians (*Health L Prac Guide,* 2008). Stated another way, parental permission for medical procedures on children, when appropriate and properly secured, constitutes an exception to the general requirement of personal consent to medical treatment (*Secretary, Dept Health and Comm Ser v. JWB and SMB,* 1992; Syoboda et al., 2000). In turn, parents are required to make decisions that are in the best interest of their children; they may not make decisions for their children that are likely to cause them physical harm or otherwise impair their healthy development (Syoboda et al., 2000). Parents, therefore, should be viewed as agents for their children, required to make decisions regarding medical interventions for their children in a manner consistent with the child's best interest. Medical professionals, in turn, owe a duty to their minor patients to assist parents in making decisions that conform to that standard (Syoboda et al., 2000). To assist "parents in making decisions that comport with their child's best interest, medical professionals must satisfy the same requirements of informed consent that apply to decision-making by adults as outlined above (Syoboda et al., 2000). In short, a minor has the right to consent to medical treatment without third-party involvement in two key situations. First, an unemancipated minor may consent to treatment of specific types of conditions for which either the state legislature or the courts have granted such authority (Vukadinovich, 2004). Such authority applies to any minor who is capable of giving meaningful informed consent and who has one of the specified medical conditions; in other words, if the minor can be said to be a "mature minor" (Vukadinovich, 2004). Secondly, a minor who qualifies as emancipated, either by court order or on other grounds, may consent to medical treatment as if he or she were an adult (Vukadinovich, 2004).

The Mature Minor

Most state laws provide that when minors reach a specified age, they are empowered to provide informed consent for the diagnosis and treatment for specific conditions (usually involving mental health, substance abuse, pregnancy, and sexually transmitted diseases) without the knowledge or consent of their parents (*Health L Prac Guide*, 2008). Then when they reach yet another, older age, they are given sole decision-making power over their own health care; at this point, they are no longer considered minors.

The law does recognize the "mature minor doctrine," which was developed to ensure treatment of minors when parental consent may cause intrafamily conflict or be difficult to obtain and to protect physicians who treat "mature minors" (Schlam and Wood, 2000). As a result of the mature minor doctrine, physicians may treat children even in the absence of parental consent or a court order, because it has become reasonable to assume that mature children are capable of providing informed consent pertaining to their own medical treatment in certain situations (Kreichman, 1989*; Schlam and Wood, 2000). Even if parents ultimately disagree with the treatment given, the physician should still be protected against liability by the doctrine, subject to any specific state law limitations that may apply.

Still, it is essential that physicians have a clear understanding of how to adequately determine and record indications of the maturity and decision-making competence of minor patients, as well as how to be assured that they have properly communicated with and obtained knowing and intelligent medical decisions from competent minor patients (Kreichman, 1989; Schlam and Wood, 2000). The Supreme Court has not been particularly helpful in offering guidance to physicians attempting to determine the maturity of a minor (Schlam and Wood, 2000). It did, however, hold in *Planned Parenthood of Central Missouri v. Danforth*, 428 US at 52-53, that a minor does not need parental consent if he or she "is sufficiently mature to understand the procedure and to make an intelligent assessment of" his or her circumstances. Jurisprudence has generally concluded that minors may be recognized as competent based on a vari-

ety of factors, including age (although it does not appear that any court has granted a patient younger than 14 years of age the right to consent), maturity, intelligence, and the nature and risks of the proposed treatment (Schlam and Wood, 2000). Accordingly, legal privileges are extended to these minors by allowing minors "who can understand the nature and consequences of the medical treatment offered" the right to consent to or refuse treatment (Schlam and Wood, 2000; O'Connor, 1994). That said, courts generally find children competent to consent or refuse treatment when the treatment has little risk, such as vaccinations, back pain, and cosmetic surgery (*Bishop v. Shurly*, 1926; *Gulf and SIR Co v. Sullivan*, 1928; *Younts v. St. Francis Hosp and Sch of Nursing*, 1970; *Cardwell v. Bechtol*, 1987; Schlam and Wood, 2000). However, ethicists agree that the ordinary indicia of competence should be balanced against the risks of treatment (Schlam and Wood, 2000). The mature minor doctrine has been consistently applied in cases in which the minor is nearing the age of majority, usually 15 years or older, the minor displays the capacity to understand the nature and risks of the treatment, and the nature of the treatment is not serious (Schlam and Wood, 2000). Courts will, however, generally protect physicians in their "non-negligent treatment of ... mature minor(s) who consent ... to a procedure after discussion with the physician" (Schlam and Wood, 2000). In addition, all states have statutes that give physicians the authority to treat minors, regardless of parental consent, in a variety of situations to "prevent certain negative consequences resulting from lack of medical care," including but not necessarily limited to the provision of care for emergency medical situations, to an emancipated minor, and if the minor seeks treatment for certain specific medical conditions, such as mental illness and sexually transmitted diseases (Schlam and Wood, 2000).

Notwithstanding any of the above, children's hospitals recognize an ethical obligation to involve children in the informed consent process to the maximum extent appropriate to their level of maturity (*Health L Prac Guide*, 2008). Where a minor expresses a reasonable desire to refuse offered care, an attempt is often made by the treatment team to reconcile the views of the child and the parents and to avoid invocations of any legal authority the parents may technically possess (*Health L Prac Guide*, 2008).

The Emancipated Minor

Notwithstanding the application of the mature minor doctrine, all states have statutes that give physicians the authority to treat minors, regardless of parental consent, to "prevent negative consequences resulting from lack of medical care," such as in emergency situations or if the patient suffers from certain medical conditions (Schlam and Wood, 2000). One such situation arises if the minor is considered an "emancipated minor." Emancipation for purposes of consenting to medical treatment may take various forms. It may be accomplished by court order when a child reaches a certain age. In such a case, often the State Department or Division of Motor Vehicles issues the minor an identification card reflecting the emancipated status, which the health care provider may request to see. It may also be accomplished by marriage. When a minor marries, that minor is deemed emancipated for purposes of consenting to or refusing medical treatment. Finally, a minor who is on active military duty has the authority to consent to medical treatment (Vukadinovich, 2004). The emancipated minor doctrine broadly

---

*Discussing mature minor doctrine and the capacity to understand the treatment as the primary concern with minor's consent to the proposed treatment.

conveys to the minor the right to consent to or refuse medical treatment without the involvement of the minor's parent, guardian, or other third party, obviously without regard to whether the minor has reached the age of majority (Vukadinovich, 2004). The contours of each state's emancipated minor doctrine varies, but generally it is intended to protect minors who are no longer dependent on their parents—those parents who have "relinquished control over their child's behavior and personal affairs" (Schlam and Wood, 2000).

Generally, an emancipated minor may consent to any type of medical treatment and is afforded the same confidentiality rights as an adult, regardless of the manner in which the minor is emancipated (Vukadinovich, 2004). Accordingly, with few exceptions, when treating an emancipated minor, the health care provider must deal with the minor as if that patient were an adult (Vukadinovich, 2004).

Informed Consent and HIPAA

The ability to authorize disclosure of health information usually goes hand in hand with the right to give informed consent, as discussed above (*Health L Prac Guide,* 2008). Accordingly, where the law recognizes the parent as the appropriate individual to give informed consent on behalf of a child, the parent may also exercise the child's rights to disclose health care related information (*Health L Prac Guide,* 2008). Likewise, where the minor is authorized to consent to medical care independently, only the minor has the authority to consent to the disclosure of such information (*Health L Prac Guide,* 2008).

The Health Insurance Portability and Accountability Act (HIPAA) of 1996 and its implementing regulations, as a general statement, defer to state laws addressing the ability of a parent or guardian to obtain or otherwise disclose protected health information concerning a minor (*Health L Prac Guide,* 2008). HIPAA does, however, specify the following three situations in which a parent does not function as the personal representative of the minor for the purpose of disclosing protected health information:

1. When state or other law does not require the consent of the parent or other person before a minor can obtain a particular health care service, and the minor consents to such service,
2. When a court determines or other law authorizes someone other than the parent to make treatment decisions for the minor, and
3. When a parent agrees to a confidential relationship between the minor and physician (Code of Federal Regulations, 2008; *Health L Prac Guide,* 2008).

MEDICAL MALPRACTICE LITIGATION

A health care professional is not liable to a patient merely because the care rendered produced a bad result, because a bad result was brought about by an error in judgment, when there is a reasonable doubt or difference of opinion as to the patient's condition or proper course of treatment, and when the physician acts with reasonable care in exercising judgment (*Roach v. Hockey,* 1981; McClellan, 2005). There are four theories of medical malpractice under which a plaintiff may be able to

recover: breach of contract, negligence, lack of informed consent, and respondeat superior (McClellan, 2005). Negligence cases compose most of the medical malpractice actions against individual health care providers (Mastroianni, 2006). Informed consent cases are particularly relevant to pediatric physicians and pose a set of unique issues, as discussed previously. Accordingly, this chapter focuses on those types of actions. As stated, however, it is important to note that this chapter is intended to provide only an overview of malpractice actions; in reality, such litigation is incredibly complex, and the burdens of proof and type of evidence required to meet that burden are governed more specifically by each individual state's law.

Negligence

Most medical malpractice actions are based on a negligence theory. In negligence-based malpractice actions, the plaintiff is essentially taking the position that the conduct in question "falls below the standard established by law for the protection of others against unreasonable risk of harm" (Mastroianni, 2006). Stated another way, the plaintiff is arguing that the professional did not possess or employ the degree of skill or knowledge required of a professional rendering such care under the circumstances (*Incollingo v. Ewing,* 1971; *Shilkret v. Annapolis Emergency Hosp Assoc,* 1975; McClellan, 2005). In such cases, the plaintiff, who is typically either the patient or the patient's family (in the event the patient is incompetent or has died) must prove four elements of malpractice: duty, breach of standard of care, injury, and causation.

Duty

First, the plaintiff must establish that the defendant—typically the physician or the institution with which the physician is affiliated—had a legal duty to the plaintiff (Mastroianni, 2006). In the context of medical malpractice actions, the "duty" can include any number of obligations that health care professionals incur on entering into a physician–patient relationship, including duties mandated by state or federal statute, either implicitly or explicitly (Mastroianni, 2006). Generally during the physician–patient relationship, the physician has a duty to exercise the degree of care, diligence, and skill that physicians of reasonable and ordinary prudence would exercise under the same or similar circumstances (Shandell et al., 1981).

Courts have held that this duty may include any of the following actions:

- Fully informing the patient of the condition
- Giving the patient the care and attention required by the known exigencies of the patient's case
- Continuing to provide medical care and giving proper instructions to a patient as to the patient's future conduct
- Obtaining the patient's informed consent to the treatment proposed
- Exercising reasonable care in prescribing treatment
- Referring the patient to a specialist or procuring another physician if necessary
- Exercising reasonable care in supervising resident physicians who are actually treating the patient
- Keeping the patient's condition confidential

- Keeping reasonably abreast of current advances in the field
- Otherwise exercising the utmost good faith in dealing with the patient (Shandell et al., 1981).

Breach of Standard of Care

The very existence of the physician's duty imposes on certain responsibilities to exercise due care, and the plaintiff must establish that the defendant breached that standard of care (Mastroianni, 2006). Stated differently, the plaintiff must establish that the physician undertook a form of treatment that a reasonable, prudent member of the medical profession would not have taken under the same or similar circumstances (Shandell et al., 1981). The standard of care, then, is what is reasonable under the circumstances (Shandell et al., 1981).

The first step for any plaintiff, after proving the existence of a duty, is to establish the appropriate medical standard of care (Shandell et al., 1981). Generally, a plaintiff must show that the defendant deviated from a standard of care and skill possessed by reasonably prudent physicians practicing in the same field of medicine. If the physician who renders the medical care to a patient in question specializes in a particular branch of medicine, that physician is required to use the care and judgment of a reasonably prudent person engaged in that specialty (McClellan, 2005). To be clear, a health care provider is not required to provide the highest degree of care possible—only the ordinary degree of skill and care exercised by his or her peers (Shandell et al., 1981). In order to establish the standard of care, the plaintiff must identify the person with whom the professional is being compared. There are jurisdictional differences as to the requirements of a geographic similarity and specialty training (McClellan, 2005). It appears that the current trend is to apply a national, rather than a local, standard to determine the standard of care required of a physician (*Naccarato v. Grob,* 1970; *Shildret v. Annapolis Emergency Hosp Assoc,* 1975; *Bruni v. Tatsumi,* 1976; *Zeller v. Greater Baltimore Med Cntr,* 1986; McClellan, 2005).

Injury

The plaintiff must also establish that he or she suffered a "compensable" injury—or one for which it is possible to be compensated for the actual harm suffered, including pain and suffering, with a monetary award. In most negligence cases, only compensatory damages are awarded. However, in cases where the defendant's actions is deemed to have been "reckless" or an "extreme departure from the standard of care" (gross negligence), some states do allow a plaintiff to recover punitive damages as well (Mastroianni, 2006). A bad result alone, however, cannot be equated with malpractice and typically does not create a presumption of negligence (Shandell et al., 1981).

Causation

Finally, the plaintiff must establish that the defendant's actions were the cause of the injury (Mastroianni, 2006). The fact that a physician erred does not necessarily warrant the conclusion that the error was the cause of the plaintiff's injury. In other words, the physician may have erred, and the patient may have suffered, but unless the error caused the injury, the physician may not be liable (PLI, *Med Malpractice).* The plaintiff is required to establish that the physician's departure from the standard of care was more likely than not to have been the proximate cause of the plaintiff's injury (PLI, *Med Malpractice).* It need not, however, be the sole cause—only a substantial factor in bringing about the injury (PLI, *Med Malpractice).* Typically, the plaintiff will establish the causation element through expert testimony, primarily because a jury must struggle to understand scientific processes that are unfamiliar and involve inherent uncertainty (Practicing Law Institute, 2009; Shandell et al., 1981).

Malpractice Resulting from Lack of Informed Consent

If certain requirements are met, a plaintiff may bring a cause of action against a physician for lack of informed consent. As previously stated, an action for lack of informed consent is an action for medical malpractice in which the practitioner failed to inform the patient of the alternatives to the proposed treatment or diagnosis and the reasonably foreseeable risks and benefits involved, such that the patient can make a knowledgeable evaluation (Practicing Law Institute, 2009). Generally, even when the physician adheres to the requisite standard of care in performing a procedure or conducting an examination, the patient may recover for injuries suffered as a result of the procedure or examination if the physician failed to obtain informed consent (*Armstrong v. Brookdale Univ Hosp and Med Cntr,* 2005).

An action for informed consent has the same four elements as any other action for medical malpractice: duty, breach, injury, and causation. The difference in an informed consent action is in the nature of the breach; that is, the physician was negligent in explaining the procedure rather than performing it. More specifically, in order to establish medical malpractice based on lack of informed consent, a plaintiff typically must establish that the medical procedure carried a specific risk that was not disclosed, the physician violated the applicable standard of disclosure, the undisclosed risk materialized, and the failure to disclose the information caused the patient's injury (Mastroianni, 2006).

Beyond those basic elements, each state has its own specific requirements for making a claim for informed consent, and more specifically, for how the plaintiff must go about establishing each of the requisite elements. By way of example, New York Public Health Law §2805-d(1) defines lack of informed consent as the "failure of the person providing the professional treatment or diagnosis to disclosure to the patient such alternatives thereto and the reasonably foreseeable risks and benefits involved as a reasonable medical ... practitioner under similar circumstances would have disclosed, in a manner permitting the patient to make a knowledgeable evaluation." Under New York's statute, one may only recover for lack of informed consent in cases involving either nonemergency treatment or a diagnostic procedure that involved invasion or disruption of bodily integrity (NY Pub Health Law §2805-d[2]). In order to recover, a plaintiff in New York must establish that "a reasonably prudent person in the patient's position would not have undergone the treatment or diagnosis if he had been fully informed and that the lack of informed consent is a proximate cause of the injury or condition for which recovery is sought" (NY Pub Health Law §2805-d[3]).

It is important to note that the court distinguishes a lack of informed consent case from a case of battery, which lies against one who "intentionally touches another person, without that person's consent, and causes an offensive bodily contact.... The intent required for battery is intent to cause a bodily contact that a reasonable person would find offensive" (*Jeffreys v. Griffin*, 2003; *Armstrong v. Brookdale Univ Hosp and Med Cntr*, 2005). In other words, in New York, a completely unpermitted touching by a medical practitioner is a battery, as distinct from a Section 2805-d claim (*Jeffreys v. Griffin*, 2003; *Armstrong v. Brookdale Univ Hosp and Med Cntr*, 2005). New Jersey also distinguishes a lack of informed consent case from a battery cause of action, reasoning that because physicians ordinarily lacked the intent to harm normally associated with the tort of battery, courts examining the nuances of the physician–patient relationship realized that conceptually a cause of action based on lack of patient consent fits better into the framework of a negligence cause of action. Accordingly, the framework for New Jersey's lack of informed consent cause of action can be characterized as a negligence type of action rather than an intentional tort (*Robinson v. Cutchin*, 2001; *Howard v. Univ of Medicine and Dentistry of New Jersey*, 2002).

New York has also provided, by statute, that five other classes of people may consent to medical care:

1. Anyone who is either 18 years old, married, or a parent, may give consent for his or her own care (because any such person is deemed to be emancipated).
2. Anyone who has been married or has given birth may consent to the child's care.
3. Anyone who is pregnant may consent to prenatal care.
4. A physician may consent to medical care for a minor in an emergency situation when delay would increase the risk for the patient's life or health.
5. A person with a parental relationship to a child may consent to the child's immunization (Practicing Law Institute, 2009; NY Pub Health Law §2804).

In New Jersey, a patient seeking to recover for lack of informed consent must prove that the physician withheld pertinent medical information concerning the risks of the procedure or treatment, the alternatives, or the potential results if the procedure or treatment were not undertaken (*Perna v. Pirozzi*, 1983; *Howard v. Univ of Medicine and Dentistry of New Jersey*, 2002). The information a physician must disclose depends on what a reasonably prudent patient would deem significant in determining whether to proceed with the proposed procedure (*Largey v. Rothman*, 1988; *Howard v. Univ of Medicine and Dentistry of New Jersey*, 2002). The plaintiff must also prove that a reasonably prudent patient in the plaintiff's position would have declined to undergo the treatment if informed of the risk that defendant failed to disclose (*Largey v. Rothman*, 1988; *Howard v. Univ of Medicine and Dentistry of New Jersey*, 2002).

REFERENCES

Complete references used in this text can be found online at www.expertconsult.com.

Note: Page numbers followed by *b* indicate boxes, *f* indicate figures, and *t* indicate tables.

G

  for catecholamine refractory shock, 1261
  deficiency of, 1102*b*
  for donor organ, 896*t*, 897, 898, 899*t*
  insensitivity to, 1102*b*
Vasopressin-resistant diabetes insipidus, 1102, 1102*b*
VATER association, 841, 843*t*
Vecuronium, 253–255
  classification by chemical structure and duration of
      action, 250*t*
  continuous infusion dose range for, 244*t*
  for fetal surgery, 598–599, 599*t*
  in heart transplantation, 662
  intubation and maintenance doses for, 244*t*
  in liver transplantation, 919
  for maintenance of anesthesia, 379
  metabolism and elimination of, 250*t*
  in open midgestation surgery, 600
  pharmacodynamics of, 244*t*
  pharmacokinetics of, 244*t*
  potency of, 242*t*
  recovery characteristics of, 247*f*
  time to onset of maximum block and recovery of, 242*t*
Velar repairs, 831, 832*f*
Velban. *See* Vinblastine
Velocity of circumferential fiber shortening, 108
Venous air embolism
  cardiac catheterization–related, 709
  in craniofacial surgery, 828–829
  in neurosurgery, 729–730, 729*f*
Venous cannula for cardiopulmonary bypass, 639, 639*t*
Venous drainage in cardiopulmonary bypass, 640–641
Venous hum, 1128
Venous malformation, 837
Venous thromboembolism, 1269
Venovenous bypass, 918
Ventilation, 54–57, 54*f*
  airway pressure-release ventilation, 1254, 1254*f*
  in burn injury, 1008
  clinical implications of, 56
  conjoined twins and, 962
  dead space and alveolar ventilation in, 54–55
  distribution of, 55–56, 55*f*, 56*f*
  high-frequency oscillatory ventilation, 1253–1254, 1253*f*
  maintenance of anesthesia and, 384
  mechanical, 1251–1252
      in acute respiratory distress syndrome, 1269
      after bariatric surgery, 785
      bronchopulmonary dysplasia and, 549
      in burn injury, 1020
      before neonatal surgery, 523
      potential organ donor and, 897–898
      pressure control, 1251
      pressure-regulated volume control, 1251
      support modes in, 1251–1252
      use of lung hysteresis curves in, 1252, 1252*f*
      ventilator-associated pneumonia and, 1265, 1269
      ventilator-induced lung injury and, 1252
      volume control, 1251
      weaning and extubation in, 1255–1256
  monitoring in neonatal surgery, 560–561
  reestablishment in cardiopulmonary resuscitation,
      1206–1209, 1207*t*
  in thoracic surgery, 764
  trauma patient and, 980
Ventilation/perfusion relationships, 59–60, 59*f*, 60*f*, 61*f*
Ventilator, 299–300
Ventilator-associated pneumonia, 1265, 1269
Ventilator-induced lung injury, 1252
Ventolin. *See* Albuterol
Ventral respiratory group of neurons, 28–29, 28*f*
Ventricular arrhythmias, 678
Ventricular dysfunction
  after Fontan procedure, 692*t*
  noncardiac surgery in child with, 676–677
Ventricular fibrillation, 1240–1242, 1242*f*
Ventricular outflow obstruction, 677
Ventricular pressure overload, 676
Ventricular septal defect, 612–614, 613*f*
  anesthesia management in, 614
      after cardiopulmonary bypass, 613*b*
      before cardiopulmonary bypass, 613*b*
  in atrioventricular canal defect, 614
  blood flows in, 609*f*
  noncardiac surgery in child with, 693–694

Ventricular septal defect *(Continued)*
  in tetralogy of Fallot, 615, 615*f*
  in transposition of great arteries, 623
  in tricuspid atresia, 619
  in truncus arteriosus, 627–628, 628*f*
Ventricular tachycardia, 1239–1240, 1240*f*, 1241*f*
Ventricular volume overload, 676
Ventriculoperitoneal shunt, 737
Venturi effect, 354
Venturi jet ventilation, 354
Venturi ventilation apparatus, 804, 804*f*
VePesid. *See* Etoposide
Verapamil, 447
Very low-birth weight infant, 516
  retinopathy of prematurity in, 560
Vesicoamniotic shunt, 599–600
Vesicoureteral reflux, 779–780, 780*f*
Vest cardiopulmonary resuscitation, 1216
Vicodin. *See* Hydrocodone
Video endoscopy, 745–746, 746*b*
Video laryngoscope, 317, 318*f*
  for difficult airway, 358
Video-assisted thoracoscopic surgery, 848
Vinblastine, 1139*t*
Vincristine, 1139*t*
Viral infection
  contraindication to heart transplantation, 657
  human immunodeficiency virus, 1165–1168
      antiretroviral agents for, 1166*b*
      clinical presentation of, 1167
      contraindication to heart transplantation, 657
      epidemiology of, 1165–1166
      healthcare providers and, 1168
      pain management in, 1168, 1168*b*
      post-transplant, 947
      transfusion-transmitted, 411*t*
  post-transplant, 947
  transfusion-associated, 411, 411*t*
  upper respiratory tract, 1112–1114
      after tracheoesophageal fistula repair, 579
      anesthetic decision making and, 1112–1113, 1113*f*,
          1114*f*
      induction of anesthesia and, 366
      outpatient procedures and, 1063–1064
      pathophysiology of, 1112
      perioperative risk and, 1112, 1281–1282
      preoperative evaluation of, 283
      signs and symptoms of, 1113*b*
Viscerocranium, 344–351
Viscoelastic point-of-care coagulation analysis, 1160
Visual analog pain scale, 392, 419
Visual evoked potentials, 338*t*, 342, 342*f*
Visual loss, postoperative, 855–856
Vital signs
  in cardiovascular assessment, 101, 101*f*, 101*t*, 102*f*
  recognition of need for cardiopulmonary
      resuscitation and, 1206, 1206*t*
Vitamin C deficiency, 1155
Vitamin K deficiency, 538, 1154
Vitamin-K dependent coagulation factors, 1149
Vitrectomy, 886
Vitreoretinal disorders, 887, 887*f*
Vitreous humor, 871
Vocal cord paralysis, 808, 809*f*
Volatile anesthetics
  asthma and, 1065
  for burn injury, 1016
  characteristics of, 373*t*
  intraocular pressure and, 878
  in office-based procedures, 1089
  in thoracic surgery, 767
Volume control mode of mechanical ventilation, 1251
Volume loading, response of newborn heart to, 90, 90*f*
Volume of distribution, 180–182, 183*f*
  of neuromuscular blocking agents, 244, 244*t*, 245*t*
  of vecuronium, 254
Volume resuscitation in burn injury, 1017–1018, 1018*b*, 1018*t*
Volume-controlled ventilation, 300, 302
Volvulus, 587–588, 587*f*
Vomiting
  anticholinesterase-related, 256
  opioid-induced, 435
  postoperative, 390–391, 390*f*
      antiemetics during maintenance of anesthesia and,
          378–379

Vomiting *(Continued)*
  in dental surgery, 1037–1038
  in office-based procedures, 1091–1092
  in ophthalmic surgery, 881–882, 881*b*
  in outpatient procedures, 1074–1075, 1074*t*
  in tympanomastoidectomy, 788
  in pyloric stenosis, 750
von Hippel–Lindau syndrome, 873*t*, 1110
von Recklinghausen's disease, 873*t*
von Willebrand disease, 1152, 1156–1157

W

W score in trauma, 976–977
Wake-up test, 851
Walking, development of, 13
Wall stress, 90
Warm receptor, 159–160, 160*f*
Warming device, 302–303
Warming mattress, 177
Warming of intravenous fluids, 177
Wash-in of inhaled anesthetic agents, 225–228, 225*f*,
      226*f*, 227*f*, 228*f*
Wash-out of inhaled anesthetic agents, 228
Waterston shunt, 699
Wave-speed theory of expiratory flow limitation, 52
Weaning
  from mechanical ventilation, 1255–1256
  from opioids, 436–438, 437*t*, 438*t*
Weight
  as measurement of well-being, 11
  relation to body surface area, 7*t*, 8*t*
  typical patterns of physical growth and, 8*b*
Weight loss
  neonatal, 541–542, 542*f*
  in terminal illness, 450
Wellbutrin. *See* Bupropion
Wenckebach rhythm, 1233, 1234*f*
Werdnig-Hoffmann disease, 843*t*
Werner syndrome, 1110*t*
Wheezing, intraoperative, 1119–1120, 1119*b*
White blood cell count, 545, 545*t*
Whole blood transfusion, 407–408, 408*b*, 1163*t*
Wide dynamic range neuron, 423
Williams' syndrome, 149–150
Wilms tumor, 751–754, 753*f*, 753*t*
Wilson's disease, 912
Wire-reinforced anode tube, 305, 305*f*
Wisdom teeth, 1025
Wis-Hipple blade, 316*t*, 317, 317*f*, 318*f*, 357
Wiskott-Aldrich syndrome, 413, 1153
Withdrawal from opioids, 436–438, 437*t*, 438*t*
Wong-Baker FACES Pain Rating Scale, 392
Wood units, 107
Word combination stage of language development, 17
Wound assessment in burn injury, 1003–1006, 1004*t*,
      1005*f*, 1006*f*, 1006*t*
Wound closure in craniopagus twins, 963
Wrapping and draping with plastic sheet, 302–303

X

Xenon
  hemodynamic effects of, 115
  pharmacology and solubility of, 224*t*
  thermoregulation and, 173*f*
Xerostomia, 1039
Xiphopagus conjunction, 954*t*
Xopenex. *See* Levalbuterol

Y

Yersinia enterocolitica, 412

Z

Z disc, 527
Z score in trauma, 976–977
Zaroxolyn. *See* Metolazone
Zellweger syndrome, 873*t*
Zones of thermal injury, 1007*f*

A1AT	α_1-antitrypsin
A-a o₂ gradient	alveolar-arterial oxygen gradient
AAP	American Academy of Pediatrics
ABCs	basics of resuscitation; i.e., airway, breathing, and circulation
ACD-CPR	active compression-decompression CPR
ACE	angiotensin-converting enzyme
ACP	antegrade cerebral perfusion
ACR	acute cellular rejection
ACS	acute chest syndrome
ACT	activated clotting (coagulation) time
ACTH	adrenocorticotropic hormone
ADARPEF	translated to French-Language Society of Pediatric Anesthesiologists
ADH	antidiuretic hormone
AED	automatic external defibrillator
AGA	appropriate for gestational age, >5th percentile, <90th percentile for gestational age
AHA	American Heart Association
AICD	automatic internal cardiac defibrillator
ALG	antilymphocyte globulin
ALTE	apparent life-threatening events ("near-miss SIDS")
AMC	arthrogryposis multiplex congenita
AMSA	amplitude spectral area
ANA	antinuclear antibody
ANH	acute normovolemic hemodilution
Ao	aorta
AP	action potential
APC	activated protein C
aPTT	activated partial thromboplastin time
APV	absent pulmonary valve
ARDS	acute (adult) respiratory distress syndrome
ASA	acetylsalicylic acid
ASA	American Society of Anesthesiology
ASD	atrial septal defect
ASIS	anterior-superior iliac spine
ALD	arginosuccinate lyase deficiency
ASO	arterial switch operation
ASS	argininosuccinate synthetase deficiency (citrulinnemia)
ASTM	American Society for Testing and Materials
AT III	antithrombin type III
AT	antithrombin
ATG	antithymocyte globulin
ATLS	advanced trauma life support
ATN	acute tubular necrosis
ATP	adenosine triphosphate
AV	aortic valve
AV	atrioventricular
AVM	arteriovenous malformation
BAS	balloon atrial septostomy
BBB	blood-brain barrier
BCKD	branched-chain α-ketoacid dehydrogenase
BD	base deficit
BDG	bidirectional Glenn (shunt/operation)
BiPAP	bilevel positive airway pressure
BIS	Bispectral Index
BMD	Becker muscular dystrophy
BMP	bone morphogenetic protein
BPD	bronchopulmonary dysplasia
bpm	beats per minute
BTX-A	botulinum toxin A
cAMP	cyclic adenosine monophosphate
CAVC	complete atrioventricular canal
CBF	cerebral blood flow
CBFV	cerebral blood flow velocity
CD	cadaveric donor
CDC	Centers for Disease Control and Prevention
CDH	congenital diaphragmatic hernia
CF	cystic fibrosis
CFTR	cystic fibrosis transmembrane conductance regulator
cGMP	cyclic guanosine monophosphate

CHD	congenital heart disease
CHF	congestive heart failure
CIBMTR	Center for International Blood and Marrow Transplant Research
C_L	compliance of lungs
CLD	chronic lung disease
cm	centimeter
CMR	cerebral metabolic rate
CMRGlc	cerebral metabolic rate for glucose
CMRo₂	cerebral metabolic rate of oxygen
CMS	congenital myasthenic syndrome
CMV	cytomegalovirus
CNS	central nervous system
CO₂	carbon dioxide
CO₂R	reactivity to carbon dioxide
COX	cyclooxygenase
COX-2	cyclooxygenase-2
CP	cerebral palsy
CPAP	continuous positive airway pressure
CPB	cardiopulmonary bypass
CPM	central pontine myelinolysis
CPP	cerebral perfusion pressure
CPR	cardiopulmonary resuscitation
CPS I deficiency	carbamoyl phosphatase I deficiency
CRM	crew resource management
Crs	compliance of respiratory system
CS	cold storage
CS	coronary sinus
CS	cortical stimulation
CSF	cerebrospinal fluid
CSW	cerebral salt wasting
CT	computed tomography
CTP	Child-Turcotte-Pugh (score)
CVA	cerebrovascular accident
CVP	central venous pressure
CVR	cerebrovascular resistance
Cw	compliance of chest wall
CyA	cyclosporine A
D10W	10% dextrose in water
DCD	donation after cardiac death
DD	deceased donor
DDAVP	1-desamino-8-D-arginine vasopressin (desmopressin)
DGF	delayed graft function
DHCA	deep hypothermic circulatory arrest
DI	diabetes insipidus
DIC	disseminated intravascular coagulation
DILV	double-inlet left ventricle
DKS	Damus-Kaye-Stansel (procedure)
DM	myotonic dystrophy
DMD	Duchenne's muscular dystrophy
DMPK	dystrophia myotonica-protein kinase (gene)
DORV	double-outlet right ventricle
DPG	diphosphoglycerate
DRG	dorsal respiratory group neurons (vs. VRG)
EACA	ε-aminocaproic acid
EAST	enzyme allergosorbent test
EAT	ectopic atrial tachycardia
EB	epidermolysis bullosa
EBD	epidermolysis bullosa dystrophica
EBV	Epstein-Barr virus
EBV	estimated blood volume
ECG	electrocardiogram/electrocardiograph/electrocardiography
ECMO	extracorporeal membrane oxygenation
ECoG	electrocorticography
ED₅₀	dose or concentration at which effectiveness occurs at a rate of 50%
ED₉₅	dose or concentration at which effectiveness occurs at a rate of 95%
EEG	electroencephalogram/electroencephalograph/electroencephalography
EGF	epidermal growth factor
ELBW	extremely low birth weight, <1000 g

ELSO	Extracorporeal Life Support Organization
EMD	electromechanical dissociation
EMG	electromyogram/electromyograph/electromyography
EMLA	eutectic mixture of local anesthetic
ERA	enthesitis-related arthritis
ERV	expiratory reserve volume
ESLD	end-stage liver disease
ESRD	end-stage renal disease
ET	endotracheal
ET-1	endothelin-1
ETC	electron transport chain
ET_{CO_2}	end-tidal CO_2
ETT	endotracheal tube
f	respiratory frequency
FEF	forced expiratory flow
FEF_{25-75}	see MMEFR
FENa	fractional excretion of sodium
FES	fat embolism syndrome
FEV_1	Forced expiratory volume at 1 second
FFP	fresh frozen plasma
FIO_2	fraction of inspired oxygen
FRC	functional residual capacity
FSH	facioscapulohumeral dystrophy
FVC	forced vital capacity
G	gauge
G6PD	glucose-6-phosphate dehydrogenase
GABA	γ-aminobutyric acid
Gaw	airway conductance (reciprocal of Raw)
GCS	Glasgow Coma Scale
GFR	glomerular filtration rate
GI	gastrointestinal
$GPII_b/III_a$	Platelet surface glycoprotein receptor $α_{IIb}β_3$
GVHD	graft-versus-host disease
HAT	hepatic artery thrombosis
$Hb\ A_2$	hemoglobin A_2
Hb AS	sickle cell trait
Hb E	hemoglobin E
Hb F	hemoglobin F
Hb S	hemoglobin S
Hb SS	sickle cell disease
Hb	hemoglobin
HBV	hepatitis B virus
HCV	hepatitis C virus
HDV	hepatitis D (delta) virus
HIV	human immunodeficiency virus
HLA	human lymphocyte antigen
HLHS	hypoplastic left heart syndrome
HMD	hyaline membrane disease (IRDS)
HME	heat and moisture exchanger
HMP	hypothermic machine perfusion
HPA	hypothalamic-pituitary-adrenal
HPA-1a	human platelet antigen 1a
HPN	home parenteral nutrition
HPS	hepatopulmonary syndrome
HPV	hypoxic pulmonary vasoconstriction
HR	Hoffman reflex
HSCT	hematopoietic stem cell transplantation
HT	hepatocyte transplantation
HTK	histidine- tryptophan-ketoglutarate
Hz	hertz
IAA	interrupted aortic arch
IAC-CPR	interposed abdominal compression CPR
IC	inspiratory capacity
ICP	intracranial pressure
ICPM	intracranial pressure monitoring
ICS	inhaled corticosteroids
ICT	islet cell transplantation
ICU	intensive care unit
ID	internal diameter
IHAST	Intraoperative Hypothermia in Aneurysm Surgery Trial
IHCA	in-hospital cardiac arrest
ILCOR	International Liaison Committee on Resuscitation
ILIH	ilioinguinal/iliohypogastric
IM	intramuscular/intramuscularly
INR	International Normalized Ratio
IO	intraosseous
IRDS	idiopathic (infantile) respiratory distress syndrome (HMD)
IRV	inspiratory reserve volume
ISC	irreversibly sickled cell
ITD	impedance threshold device
ITP	idiopathic thrombocytopenic purpura
ITPR	intrathoracic pressure regulator
IV	intravenous/intravenously
IVC	inferior vena cava
IVIG	IV gamma globulin
IVRA	intravenous regional anesthesia
IVS	intact ventricular septum
JET	junctional ectopic tachycardia
JIA	juvenile idiopathic arthritis
kg	kilogram
L	liter
L	levo-
LA	left atrium
LABA	long-acting $β_2$-agonist

LAP	left atrial pressure
LBW	Low birth weight, <2500 g
LD_{50}	dose or concentration at which lethality occurs at a ra
LDB-CPR	load distributing band CPR
LDLT	living donor liver transplantation
LFC	lateral femoral cutaneous (nerve)
LG	limb-girdle (muscular dystrophy)
LGA	Large for gestational age, >90th percentile for gestat
LIP	lipoid interstitial pneumonia
LLA	lower limit of autoregulation
LMA	Laryngeal Mask Airway
LMAU	Laryngeal Mask Airway Unique
LMWH	low–molecular-weight heparin
LOP	limb occlusion pressure
LT	laryngeal tube
LT	leukotriene
LT-D	laryngeal tube disposable
LTS	laryngeal tube suction
LUCAS	Lund University Cardiopulmonary Assist System
LV	left ventricle
LVIBP	lateral vertical infraclavicular brachial plexus
LVOTO	left ventricular outflow tract obstruction
M	meter
mA	milliAmperes
MABL	maximum allowable blood loss
MAC	minimum alveoloar concentration
MAP	mean arterial pressure
MAPCA	major aortopulmonary collateral artery
MAST	military anti-shock trousers
MBTS	modified Blalock-Taussig shunt
mcg	microgram
MCHC	mean corpuscular hemoglobin content
MCV	mean corpuscular volume
MEFV	maximum expiratory flow-volume (curve)
MELD	model for end-stage liver disease (in patients older than 12 years)
MEN	multiple endocrine neoplasia (syndrome)
MEP	motor evoked potential
MFS	Marfan syndrome
mg	milligram
MG	myasthenia gravis
MH	malignant hyperthermia
MHC	major histocompatibility (antigens)
MHz	megahertz
min	minute
mL	milliliter
mm Hg	millimeters of mercury
mm	millimeter
MMEFR	maximum mid-expiratory flow rate (same as FEF_{25-75})
MMF	mycophenolate mofetil
MPP	myocardial perfusion pressure
MPS	mucopolysaccharidosis
MRA	magnetic resonance angiography
MRI	magnetic resonance imaging
MSUD	maple syrup urine disease
MUF	modified ultrafiltration
MV	mitral valve
MVT	multivisceral transplantation
NAFLD	nonalcoholic fatty liver disease
NAGSD	N-acetylglutamate synthetase deficiency
NAPRTCS	North American Pediatric Renal Transplant Cooperative Study
NASH	nonalcoholic steatohepatitis
NATCO	North American Transplant Coordinators Organization
NEC	necrotizing enterocolitis
NFF	no-flow fraction
NICU	neonatal intensive care unit
NIDDK	National Institute of Diabetes and Digestive and Kidney Diseases Liver Transplantation Database
NIH	National Institutes of Health
NIRS	near-infrared spectroscopy
NMB	neuromuscular block(er)
NMDR	nondepolarizing muscle relaxant
NO	nitric oxide
NOS	nitric oxide synthase
NPH	neutral protamine Hagedorn
NPO	nothing by mouth
NRCPR	National Registry of CPR
NRGA	normally related great arteries
NS	nerve stimulation
NSAIDs	nonsteroidal antiinflammatory drugs
O_2	oxygen
OAC-CPR	only abdominal compression CPR
OD	outer diameter
OHCA	out-of-hospital cardiac arrest
OI	osteogenesis imperfecta
OLT, OLTx	orthotopic liver transplantation
OMIM	Online Mendelian Inheritance in Man
OPO	Organ Procurement Organization
OPTN	Organ Procurement and Transplantation Network
OR	operating room
OSHA	Occupational Safety and Health Administration
OTCD	ornithine transcarbamylase deficiency
P_{50}	Arterial oxygen tension (Pa_{O_2}) at 50% hemoglobin saturation
Pa	Pulmonary arterial pressure
P_A	Alveolar pressure